# Textbook of

# GASTROINTESTINAL

# RADIOLOGY

VOLUME ONE

# *Textbook of*

# GASTROINTESTINAL

# RADIOLOGY

## VOLUME ONE

**Richard M. Gore, M.D.**

Professor of Radiology
Northwestern University Medical School
Chief of Gastrointestinal Radiology
Evanston Hospital–McGaw Medical Center of
Northwestern University
Evanston, Illinois

**Marc S. Levine, M.D.**

Professor of Radiology
University of Pennsylvania School of Medicine
Gastrointestinal Radiology Section
Hospital of the University of Pennsylvania
Philadelphia, Pennsylvania

**Igor Laufer, M.D.**

Professor of Radiology
University of Pennsylvania School of Medicine
Chief of Gastrointestinal Radiology
Hospital of the University of Pennsylvania
Philadelphia, Pennsylvania

**W.B. SAUNDERS COMPANY**
*A Division of Harcourt Brace & Company*
Philadelphia    London    Toronto    Montreal    Sydney    Tokyo

**W.B. SAUNDERS COMPANY**
*A Division of*
*Harcourt Brace & Company*

The Curtis Center
Independence Square West
Philadelphia, Pennsylvania 19106

**Library of Congress Cataloging-in-Publication Data**

Textbook of gastrointestinal radiology / [edited by] Richard M. Gore,
    Marc S. Levine, Igor Laufer.—1st ed.
        p. cm.

ISBN 0–7216–3977–1 (2 v. set).—ISBN 0–7216–3978–X (v. 1).—
    ISBN 0–7216–3979–8 (v. 2)

1. Gastrointestinal System—radiography.     I. Gore, Richard M.
    II. Levine, Marc S.     III. Laufer, Igor.

[DNLM: 1. Gastrointestinal System—radiography.
2. Gastrointestinal System—pathology.     3. Radiography—
    methods.     4. Gastrointestinal Diseases—diagnosis.
    WI 141 T355 1994]

RC804.R6T46 1994

616.3′407572—dc20

DNLM/DLC

for Library of Congress                                    93–20475

Textbook of Gastrointestinal Radiology          Volume One   ISBN 0–7216–3978–X
                                                Volume Two   ISBN 0–7216–3979 –8
                                                2 Volume Set   ISBN 0–7216–3977 –1

Printed in the United States of America

Last digit is the print number:     9    8    7    6    5    4    3    2    1

*To Margaret,*

    *and my children,*

        *Diana, Elizabeth, and George*

            RICHARD M. GORE

---

*To Deborah,*

    *For everything*

            MARC S. LEVINE

---

*To Bernice,*

*. . . that indefinable beauty that comes from happiness, enthusiasm, success—a beauty that is nothing more or less than a harmony of temperament and circumstances.*

    Gustave Flaubert

           IGOR LAUFER

# Contributors

## Section Editors

**James S. Donaldson, M.D.**
*Section XVI* **Pediatric Diseases of the Solid Organs**
Associate Professor of Radiology, Northwestern University Medical School; Head, Section of Body Imaging, Children's Memorial Hospital, Chicago, Illinois

**Sandra K. Fernbach, M.D.**
*Section IX* **Pediatric Diseases**
Associate Professor of Radiology, Northwestern University Medical School; Head, Section of Gastrointestinal and Genitourinary Radiology, Children's Memorial Hospital, Chicago, Illinois

**Hans Herlinger, M.D.**
*Section VII* **Small Bowel**
Professor of Radiology (Emeritus), University of Pennsylvania School of Medicine; Gastrointestinal Radiology Section, Hospital of the University of Pennsylvania, Philadelphia, Pennsylvania

**Stephen E. Rubesin, M.D.**
*Section III* **Pharynx**
Associate Professor of Radiology, University of Pennsylvania School of Medicine; Gastrointestinal Radiology Section, Hospital of the University of Pennsylvania, Philadelphia, Pennsylvania

---

**Abass Alavi, M.D.**
Professor of Radiology, University of Pennsylvania School of Medicine; Chief, Division of Nuclear Medicine, Department of Radiology, Hospital of the University of Pennsylvania, Philadelphia, Pennsylvania

**M. Mazen Anbari, M.D.**
Research Assistant, Department of Radiology, and Medical Intern, Hospital of the University of Pennsylvania, Philadelphia, Pennsylvania

**Stephen R. Baker, M.D.**
Professor and Chairman, Department of Radiology, New Jersey Medical School; Director of Radiology, University Hospital, University of Medicine and Dentistry, Newark, New Jersey

**Dennis M. Balfe, M.D.**
Professor of Radiology, Washington University School of Medicine; Radiologist, Barnes Hospital and Children's Hospital, St. Louis, Missouri

**Emil J. Balthazar, M.D.**
Professor of Radiology, New York University–Tisch–Bellevue Medical Center; Attending Radiologist, New York University–Tisch Hospital and Bellevue Hospital, New York, New York

**Raul Barreda, M.D.**
Research Fellow, Department of Radiology, University of Florida College of Medicine, Gainesville, Florida

**Bernard A. Birnbaum, M.D.**
Assistant Professor of Radiology, New York University Medical Center, New York, New York

**Jeffrey C. Brandon, M.D.**
Assistant Professor, Department of Radiology, University of California, Irvine, Orange, California

**Hazel B. Breitz, M.B., B.Ch.**
Clinical Assistant Professor, University of Washington; Nuclear Medicine Consultant,

Virginia Mason Medical Center, Seattle, Washington

**Frank P. Brooks, M.D., Sc.D.**
Late Professor of Medicine and Physiology, University of Pennsylvania; Chief of Gastroenterology Section, Hospital of the University of Pennsylvania, Philadelphia, Pennsylvania

**James L. Buck, M.D.**
Chairman and Registrar, Department of Radiologic Pathology, Armed Forces Institute of Pathology, Washington, D.C.; Associate Professor of Radiology, Uniformed Services University of the Health Sciences; Clinical Consultant in Radiology, National Naval Medical Center, Bethesda, Maryland

**Dina F. Caroline, M.D.**
Professor of Radiology, Temple University School of Medicine; Chief, Gastrointestinal Radiology Section, Temple University Hospital, Philadelphia, Pennsylvania

**Cirrelda Cooper, M.D.**
Assistant Professor of Radiology, Georgetown University Medical School and Hospital, Washington, D.C.

**Constantin Cope, M.D.**
Professor of Radiology, University of Pennsylvania; Staff Radiologist, Hospital of the University of Pennsylvania, Philadelphia, Pennsylvania

**Abraham H. Dachman, M.D.**
Professor, Uniformed Services University of the Health Sciences, Bethesda, Maryland; Chief, Abdominal Radiology, Walter Reed Army Medical Center, Washington, D.C.

**Antonio De Franco, M.D.**
Assistant Professor of Radiology, Istituto di Radiologia, Università Cattolica del Sacro Cuore; Policlinico Universitario Agostino Gemelli, Rome, Italy

**Martin W. Donner, M.D., F.A.C.R.**
Late Professor of Radiology, The Johns Hopkins School of Medicine; Director Emeritus, The Russell H. Morgan Department of Radiology and Radiological Science; Founder, The Johns Hopkins Swallowing Center, Baltimore, Maryland

**Brian Eisenberg, M.D.**
Clinical Assistant Professor, Department of Radiology, University of Washington School of Medicine; Staff Radiologist, Virginia Mason Clinic, Seattle, Washington

**Ronald L. Eisenberg, M.D., F.A.C.R.**
Clinical Professor of Radiology, University of California, San Francisco, and University of California, Davis; Chairman of Radiology, Highland General Hospital, Oakland, California

**Olle Ekberg, M.D.**
Docent, University of Lund; Head of Gastrointestinal Radiology, Malmö General Hospital, Malmö, Sweden

**Michael P. Federle, M.D.**
Professor of Radiology, University of Pittsburgh; Staff, Presbyterian-University Hospital, Pittsburgh, Pennsylvania

**Kate A. Feinstein, M.D.**
Assistant Professor of Radiology, Northwestern University Medical School; Staff Radiologist, Children's Memorial Hospital, Chicago, Illinois

**Elliot K. Fishman, M.D.**
Professor of Radiology, Department of Radiology, The Johns Hopkins Medical School and Hospital, Baltimore, Maryland

**Steven W. Fitzgerald, M.D.**
Assistant Professor of Radiology, Northwestern University Medical School; Director, Magnetic Resonance Imaging, Northwestern Memorial Hospital, Chicago, Illinois

**Arnold C. Friedman, M.D.**
Professor and Acting Chairman, Department of Radiology, Medical College of Pennsylvania, Philadelphia, Pennsylvania

**Emma E. Furth, M.D.**
Assistant Professor, University of Pennsylvania School of Medicine; Staff, Department of Anatomic Pathology and Laboratory Medicine, Hospital of the University of Pennsylvania, Philadelphia, Pennsylvania

**R. Kristina Gedgaudas-McClees, M.D.**
Clinical Professor of Radiology, Emory University School of Medicine and Hospital; Staff, St. Joseph's Hospital, Atlanta, Georgia

**David W. Gelfand, M.D.**
Professor of Radiology and Chief of Abdominal Radiology, Bowman Gray School of Medicine; Attending Radiologist, North Carolina

Baptist Hospital, Winston-Salem, North Carolina

**Stephen G. Gerzof, M.D., F.A.C.R.**
Professor of Radiology, Tufts University School of Medicine; Chief, Sectional Imaging, Boston Veterans Administration Medical Center, Boston, Massachusetts

**Gary G. Ghahremani, M.D.**
Professor and Chairman, Department of Diagnostic Radiology, Evanston Hospital–McGaw Medical Center of Northwestern University, Evanston, Illinois

**Seth N. Glick, M.D.**
Professor of Radiology, Hahnemann University Hospital; Acting Chairman, Director of Gastrointestinal Radiology, and Co-Director, Body Computed Tomography, Hahnemann University Hospital, Philadelphia, Pennsylvania

**Margaret D. Gore, M.D.**
Assistant Professor, Department of Radiology and Nuclear Medicine, Rush Medical College; Attending Pediatric Radiologist, Rush–Presbyterian–St. Luke's Medical Center, Chicago, Illinois

**Richard M. Gore, M.D., F.A.C.R., F.A.C.G.**
Professor of Radiology, Northwestern University Medical School; Chief of Gastrointestinal Radiology, Evanston Hospital–McGaw Medical Center of Northwestern University, Evanston, Illinois

**Herbert F. Gramm, M.D.**
Assistant Professor of Radiology, Harvard Medical School; Vice Chairman, Department of Radiology, New England Deaconess Hospital, Boston, Massachusetts

**Deborah A. Hall, M.D.**
Assistant Professor, Harvard Medical School; Radiologist, Massachusetts General Hospital and Harvard Medical School, Boston, Massachusetts

**Robert A. Halvorsen, Jr., M.D.**
Professor and Vice Chairman, Department of Radiology, University of California, San Francisco; Chief of Radiology, San Francisco General Hospital, San Francisco, California

**Roger K. Harned, M.D.**
Professor of Radiology, University of Nebraska College of Medicine and Medical Center; Visiting Professor, Department of Radiologic Pathology, Armed Forces Institute of Pathology, Washington, D.C.; Consultant Physician, Omaha Veterans Administration Hospital, Omaha, Nebraska

**David L. Harshfield, M.D.**
Chief of Radiology, McClellan Veterans Administration Hospital; Assistant Professor of Radiology, University Hospital, University of Arkansas for Medical Sciences, and Arkansas Children's Hospital, Little Rock, Arkansas

**Jay P. Heiken, M.D.**
Professor of Radiology and Codirector, Body Computed Tomography, Mallinckrodt Institute of Radiology, Washington University School of Medicine, St. Louis, Missouri

**Charles Hyde, M.D.**
Assistant Professor of Radiology, Tufts University School of Medicine; Chief, Ultrasound, Boston Veterans Administration Medical Center, Boston, Massachusetts

**Bernadette V. Jakomin, M.D.**
Instructor in Diagnostic Radiology, Tufts University School of Medicine; Assistant in Diagnostic Radiology, New England Medical Center, Boston, Massachusetts

**Bruce R. Javors, M.D.**
Associate Professor of Clinical Radiology, University of Medicine and Dentistry–New Jersey Medical School, Newark; Chief of Radiology, Department of Veterans Affairs Medical Center, East Orange, New Jersey

**R. Brooke Jeffrey, M.D.**
Professor of Radiology and Chief of Abdominal Imaging, Stanford University School of Medicine and Hospital, Stanford, California

**Bronwyn Jones, M.D., M.B., B.S., F.R.A.C.P., F.R.C.R.**
Professor of Radiology, The Johns Hopkins School of Medicine; Director, The Johns Hopkins Swallowing Center; Associate Director, Abdominal Imaging; Section Head, Gastrointestinal Radiology, The Johns Hopkins Hospital, Baltimore, Maryland

**Peter J. Kahrilas, M.D.**
Associate Professor of Medicine, Northwestern University Medical School; Medical Director, GI Laboratory, Northwestern Memorial Hospital, Chicago, Illinois

**Akira Kawashima, M.D.**
Instructor of Radiology, Department of Radiology, The Johns Hopkins Medical School; Instructor of Radiology, The Johns Hopkins Hospital, Baltimore, Maryland

**Herbert Y. Kressel, M.D.**
Professor of Radiology, University of Pennsylvania Medical School; Chief, Magnetic Resonance Imaging, Hospital of the University of Pennsylvania, Philadelphia, Pennsylvania

**Gerbail T. Krishnamurthy, M.D., F.A.C.P.**
Professor of Radiology, Adjunct Professor of Medicine and Pathology, and Director, Nuclear Medicine Residency Program, Oregon Health Sciences University; Chief, Nuclear Medicine Service, Veterans Affairs Medical Center, Portland, Oregon

**Shakuntala Krishnamurthy, M.D.**
Clinical Assistant Professor of Radiology, Oregon Health Sciences University, Portland; Director, Nuclear Medicine Department, Tuality Community Hospital, Hillsboro, Oregon

**John C. Lappas, M.D.**
Professor of Radiology, Indiana University School of Medicine; Diagnostic Radiologist, Indiana University Medical Center, Indianapolis, Indiana

**Igor Laufer, M.D., F.A.C.R., F.A.C.P.(C)**
Professor of Radiology, University of Pennsylvania School of Medicine; Chief of Gastrointestinal Radiology, Hospital of the University of Pennsylvania, Philadelphia, Pennsylvania

**Marie E. Lee, M.D.**
Assistant Clinical Professor, University of Washington; Radiologist, Virginia Mason Hospital, Seattle, Washington

**Richard F. Lee, B.S., R.T.N.M.**
Supervisor of Nuclear Medicine and Clinical Supervisor—Nuclear Medicine Technology Program, Virginia Mason Medical Center, Seattle, Washington

**Janis Gissel Letourneau, M.D.**
Professor of Radiology, University of Minnesota, Minneapolis, Minnesota

**Marc S. Levine, M.D.**
Professor of Radiology, University of Pennsylvania School of Medicine; Gastrointestinal Radiology Section, Hospital of the University of Pennsylvania, Philadelphia, Pennsylvania

**Joel E. Lichtenstein, M.D.**
Professor of Radiology, University of Cincinnati and University Hospital, Cincinnati, Ohio

**Deborah G. Longley, M.D.**
Assistant Professor of Radiology, University of Minnesota, Minneapolis, Minnesota

**Robert L. MacCarty, M.D.**
Professor of Diagnostic Radiology, Mayo Medical School; Consultant in Diagnostic Radiology, Mayo Clinic and Mayo Foundation, Rochester, Minnesota

**Dean D. T. Maglinte, M.D.**
Clinical Professor of Radiology, Indiana University School of Medicine; Chief, Gastrointestinal Radiology Section, Department of Radiology, Methodist Hospital of Indiana, Indianapolis, Indiana

**Giulia Maresca, M.D.**
Associate Professor of Radiology, Istituto di Radiologia, Università Cattolica del Sacro Cuore; Policlinico Universitario Agostino Gemelli, Rome, Italy

**Charles S. Marn, M.D.**
Assistant Professor, Department of Radiology, University of Michigan Medical School and University of Michigan Hospitals, Ann Arbor, Michigan

**Terence A. S. Matalon, M.D.**
Associate Professor of Radiology, Rush Medical College; Associate Attending, Department of Radiology and Nuclear Medicine, Rush–Presbyterian–St. Luke's Medical Center, Chicago, Illinois

**Alan H. Maurer, M.D.**
Professor, Diagnostic Imaging, and Director, Nuclear Medicine, Temple University School of Medicine and Hospital, Philadelphia, Pennsylvania

**John P. McGahan, M.D.**
Professor of Radiology, University of California, Davis, School of Medicine; Professor and Head of Abdominal Imaging and Ultrasound, University of California, Davis, Medical Center, Sacramento, California

**Alec J. Megibow, M.D.**
Professor of Radiology, New York University School of Medicine and Medical Center; Chief, Computed Tomography and Gastrointestinal Radiology, Tisch Hospital, New York, New York

**James M. Messmer, M.D.**
Associate Professor of Radiology and Associate Dean for Academic Affairs, Medical College of Virginia/Virginia Commonwealth University Hospital, Richmond, Virginia

**Jonathan I. Meyer, M.D.**
Instructor of Radiology, University of Illinois; Radiologist, University of Illinois Hospital, Chicago, Illinois

**Morton A. Meyers, M.D.**
Professor of Radiology, School of Medicine, Health Sciences Center, State University of New York at Stony Brook, Stony Brook, New York

**David L. Nahrwold, M.D.**
Loyal and Edith Davis Professor and Chairman, Department of Surgery, Northwestern University Medical School; Surgeon-in-Chief, Northwestern Memorial Hospital, Chicago, Illinois

**Albert A. Nemcek, Jr., M.D.**
Assistant Professor of Clinical Radiology, Northwestern University Medical School; Chief, Section of Ultrasonography, and Associate Chief, Section of Cardiovascular and Interventional Radiology, Northwestern Memorial Hospital, Chicago, Illinois

**Daniel J. Nolan, M.D.**
Chief of Gastrointestinal Radiology, Consultant Radiologist, John Radcliffe Hospital, Oxford, England

**William W. Olmsted, M.D.**
Professor of Radiology, The George Washington University School of Medicine and Medical Center, Washington, D.C.

**David J. Ott, M.D.**
Professor of Radiology, Bowman Gray School of Medicine, Wake Forest University, Winston-Salem, North Carolina

**Robert V. Rege, M.D.**
Associate Professor of Surgery, Northwestern University Medical School; Chief, Surgical Services, Northwestern Memorial Hospital; Director, Surgical Intensive Care Unit, Veterans Administration Lakeside Medical Center, Chicago, Illinois

**Charles A. Rohrmann, Jr., M.D.**
Professor of Radiology, University of Washington and University of Washington Medical Center, Seattle, Washington

**Pablo R. Ros, M.D., F.A.C.R.**
Professor of Radiology, University of Florida College of Medicine; Director, Division of Abdominal Imaging and MRI, Shands Hospital, Gainesville, Florida

**Ernest F. Rosato, M.D.**
Professor of Surgery, University of Pennsylvania School of Medicine, Philadelphia, Pennsylvania

**Mitchell D. Schnall, M.D., Ph.D.**
Assistant Professor of Radiology, University of Pennsylvania School of Medicine; Magnetic Resonance Imaging Section, Hospital of the University of Pennsylvania, Philadelphia, Pennsylvania

**Francis J. Scholz, M.D.**
Radiologist, Lahey Clinic Medical Center, Burlington, Massachusetts

**Jane Chrestman Share, M.D.**
Assistant Professor of Radiology, Harvard Medical School; Radiologist and Director, Section of Ultrasound, Children's Hospital, Boston, Massachusetts

**Richard M. Shore, M.D.**
Assistant Professor of Clinical Radiology, Northwestern University Medical School; Staff Radiologist, Children's Memorial Hospital, Chicago, Illinois

**Alan Siegel, M.D.**
Director of Nuclear Medicine, Department of Radiology, Dartmouth–Hitchcock Medical Center, Lebanon, New Hampshire

**Bruce Silver, M.D.**
Associate Professor of Radiology, Rush Medical College; Senior Attending, Department of Radiology and Nuclear Medicine, Rush–Presbyterian–St. Luke's Medical Center, Chicago, Illinois

**Paul M. Silverman, M.D.**
Professor of Radiology and Director of Computed Tomography, Co-Director, Abdominal Imaging, Georgetown University Medical School and Hospital, Washington, D.C.

**Keith C. Simpkins, M.D.**
Senior Clinical Lecturer, University of Leeds; Consultant Radiologist, The General Infirmary at Leeds, Leeds, England

**Jovitas Skucas, M.D.**
Professor of Radiology, Department of Radiology, University of Rochester School of Med-

icine and Dentistry; Attending Radiologist; Co-Director, Diagnostic Division; Head, Gastrointestinal and Genitourinary Radiology, Strong Memorial Hospital, Rochester, New York

**James H. Sloves, M.D.**
Department of Radiology, North Shore University Hospital–Cornell University Medical College, Manhasset, New York

**Claire Smith, M.D., F.A.C.R.**
Professor of Radiology and Assistant Professor of Anatomy, Rush Medical College; Senior Attending Physician and Section Chief, Gastrointestinal Radiology, Department of Diagnostic Radiology and Nuclear Medicine, Rush–Presbyterian–St. Luke's Medical Center, Chicago, Illinois

**Sat Somers, M.D., F.R.C.P.(C)**
Professor of Radiology, Department of Radiology, McMaster University; Head of Gastrointestinal Radiology, McMaster University Medical Centre, Hamilton, Ontario, Canada

**Marshall S. Sparberg, M.D.**
Professor of Clinical Medicine, Northwestern University Medical School; Attending Physician, Northwestern Memorial Hospital, Chicago, Illinois

**Stewart M. Spies, M.D.**
Professor of Clinical Radiology, Northwestern University Medical School; Director of Nuclear Medicine, Northwestern Memorial Hospital, Chicago, Illinois

**William G. Spies, M.D.**
Associate Professor of Radiology, Northwestern University Medical School; Associate Director of Nuclear Medicine, Northwestern Memorial Hospital; Attending Radiologist, Veterans Administration Lakeside Hospital, Chicago, Illinois

**David H. Stephens, M.D.**
Professor of Diagnostic Radiology, Mayo Medical School; Consultant in Diagnostic Radiology, Mayo Clinic and Mayo Foundation, Rochester, Minnesota

**Giles W. Stevenson, M.D., F.R.C.R.,
F.R.C.P., F.R.C.P.(C), F.R.C.S.(I)**
Professor and Chairman of Radiology, McMaster University; Head of Radiology Section, Chedoke-McMaster Hospitals, Hamilton, Ontario, Canada

**Rita Littlewood Teele, M.D.**
Senior Lecturer in the Department of Radiology, Christchurch School of Medicine, University of Otago; Radiologist, Department of Radiology, Christchurch Hospital and Christchurch Women's Hospital, Christchurch; Consultant in Radiology, Auckland Children's Hospital, Auckland, New Zealand

**Steven K. Teplick, M.D.**
Professor/Vice Chairman, University of Arkansas for Medical Sciences; Professor of Radiology, University Hospital, McClellan Veterans Administration Hospital, and Arkansas Children's Hospital, Little Rock, Arkansas

**Ruedi F. Thoeni, M.D.**
Associate Professor of Radiology and Chief, Section of Computed Tomography/Gastrointestinal Radiology—Magnetic Resonance, Department of Radiology, University of California, San Francisco, Medical School and Hospital, San Francisco, California

**Gladys M. Torres, M.D.**
Assistant Professor, University of Florida; Radiologist, Shands Hospital, Gainesville, Florida

**William E. Torres, M.D.**
Associate Professor of Radiology, Emory University School of Medicine; Director, Outpatient Radiology, Emory Clinic; Staff Radiologist, Grady Memorial Hospital, Crawford Long Hospital, and Emory Hospital, Atlanta, Georgia

**Mary Ann Turner, M.D.**
Professor of Radiology, Department of Radiology, Medical College of Virginia; Director, Gastrointestinal Radiology, Medical College of Virginia Hospital, Richmond, Virginia

**Amorino Vecchioli, M.D.**
Associate Professor of Radiology, Istituto di Radiologia, Università Cattolica del Sacro Cuore; Policlinico Universitario Agostino Gemelli, Rome, Italy

**Robert L. Vogelzang, M.D.**
Associate Professor of Clinical Radiology, Northwestern University Medical School; Chief, Section of Angiography and Interventional Radiology, Northwestern Memorial Hospital, Chicago, Illinois

**Susan D. Wall, M.D.**
Associate Professor of Radiology, University of California, San Francisco; Assistant Chief

of Radiology, San Francisco Veterans Administration Medical Center, San Francisco, California

**Ellen M. Ward, M.D.**
Assistant Professor, Mayo Medical School; Consultant, Diagnostic Radiology, Mayo Clinic, Rochester, Minnesota

**Evelyn Maureen White, M.D.**
Associate Professor of Clinical Radiology, Northwestern University Medical School; Director, Abdominal Imaging Section, Evanston Hospital, Evanston, Illinois

**Susan M. Williams, M.D.**
Clinical Associate Professor of Radiology, University of Nebraska Medical Center, Omaha, Nebraska

**Stephanie R. Wilson, M.D.**
Professor, Department of Radiology, University of Toronto; Head, Division of Ultrasound, The Toronto Hospital, Toronto, Ontario, Canada

**Franz J. Wippold II, M.D.**
Assistant Professor (Neuroradiology), Washington University School of Medicine; Radiologist, Barnes Hospital and Children's Hospital, St. Louis, Missouri

**Ellen L. Wolf, M.D.**
Associate Professor of Radiology, Albert Einstein College of Medicine, Montefiore Medical Center; Associate Attending Physician, Montefiore Medical Center, Bronx, New York

**David M. Yousem, M.D.**
Associate Professor of Radiology, University of Pennsylvania School of Medicine; Neuroradiology Section, Hospital of the University of Pennsylvania, Philadelphia, Pennsylvania

**Robert K. Zeman, M.D.**
Professor of Radiology, Georgetown University School of Medicine; Clinical Director of Diagnostic Radiology, Georgetown University Medical Center, Washington, D.C.

# Preface

The practice of gastrointestinal radiology today bears little resemblance to its predecessor of just 20 years ago. Advances in conventional radiologic and scintigraphic techniques and the advent of cross-sectional imaging have revolutionized the field. We can now diagnose certain common lesions at much earlier stages and detect entire classes of lesions not seen before. These profound changes in diagnostic gastrointestinal radiology have been paralleled by equally dramatic developments in interventional procedures. Advanced technology and the acquisition of high-quality images are only starting points, however, because our ultimate objective is to apply our knowledge of pathology to the interpretation of morphologic findings so that we can more accurately diagnose and treat gastrointestinal disease.

The goal of this book is to provide complete and up-to-date coverage of the state of knowledge in gastrointestinal radiology in a practical and usable way. We have used two organizing principles in structuring this work to cover this enormous, ever-changing field. First is the integration of expanding information and proliferating technologies into an orderly, commonsense approach to radiologic diagnosis and treatment. To this end, the text contains sections on general radiologic principles for evaluating the hollow viscera and solid organs, as well as for performing and applying specific imaging and therapeutic techniques. Other sections present the clinical, radiologic, and pathologic aspects of disease in the various gastrointestinal organs. These chapters are designed to illustrate and integrate the spectrum of abnormalities seen on all diagnostic modalities available to the radiologist: plain films, barium studies, cholangiography, computed tomography, ultrasonography, magnetic resonance imaging, scintigraphy, and angiography.

An emphasis on image quality represents the second organizing principle of this textbook. In assembling our outstanding group of contributors, we chose authors whose work illustrates the highest respect for the quality of the radiologic image. This principle stresses the importance of excellent imaging technique for demonstrating the radiologic findings. For only when the abnormal findings are clearly shown can we fully use our knowlege of pathology to arrive at a correct diagnosis.

Three special features of this textbook deserve mention because we believe they greatly increase its utility for the practicing physician. Because patients present with signs and symptoms, rather than diagnoses, Section XVII was designed to present the most efficacious diagnostic approach to common gastrointestinal problems such as jaundice, dyspepsia, and hemorrhage. Similarly, radiographs, scintiscans, and cross-sectional images offer radiologic signs rather than specific diagnoses, so we have included selectively placed chapters presenting capsule reviews of the differential diagnosis of well-defined radiologic signs. Finally, because many disorders affecting the gastrointestinal tract, such as acquired immunodeficiency syndrome and Crohn's disease, involve multiple organs, Section XVIII presents the clinical and radiologic manifestations of these diseases in a unified fashion, with the complete spectrum of disease involvement discussed in an individual chapter.

As editors, we have tried to strike a balance between uniformity of style and individuality of authors, so that each contributor is allowed to speak with his or her unique voice. For some diseases, we include the views of several authors as discussions of a complex subject. We believe this overlap allows completeness of coverage within each chapter and emphasizes the complementary or equivalent roles of the various imaging technologies in certain disorders.

We hope that the readers will find this an efficient and effective way of approaching this diverse and fascinating topic. We invite the reader to communicate to us any gaps of coverage and to suggest any improvements for future editions.

RICHARD M. GORE, M.D.
MARC S. LEVINE, M.D.
IGOR LAUFER, M.D.

# Contents

# SECTION | VI

## Stomach and Duodenum

# SECTION | VII

## Small Bowel
### Section Editor, Hans Herlinger, M.D.

**SECTION ▮ *VIII*▮**

# Colon

## SECTION    IX

# Pediatric Diseases
### Section Editor, Sandra K. Fernbach, M.D.

### VOLUME TWO
## SECTION    X

# General Radiologic Principles

### SECTION ■ XI

# Gallbladder and Biliary Tract

## SECTION | XII

# Liver

---

**SECTION    XIII**

# Pancreas

**SECTION    XIV**

# Spleen

**SECTION    XV**

# Peritoneal Cavity, Omentum, and Abdominal Wall

## SECTION     XVI

# Pediatric Diseases of the Solid Organs
### Section Editor, James S. Donaldson, M.D.

## SECTION | XVII

# Common Clinical Problems

## SECTION | XVIII

# Generalized Clinical Problems: Multiorgan Involvement

# General Radiologic Principles

# Development of Gastrointestinal Radiology

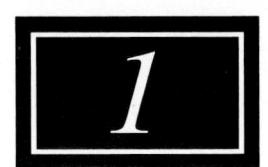

**M. Mazen Anbari, M.D.**

**Igor Laufer, M.D.**

## INTRODUCTION

The field of gastrointestinal radiology had its beginnings just a few months after Röntgen's discovery of x-rays in 1895. It has since progressed with incredible speed and now encompasses a variety of diagnostic modalities that make possible precise diagnoses, as well as therapeutic interventions that complement and often replace more invasive surgical procedures. What follows is a selective account of milestones in the development of gastrointestinal radiology (Table 1–1).

## UPPER GASTROINTESTINAL TRACT

### Early Days

The early clinical applications of the new x-rays did not involve the gastrointestinal tract; rather, they centered on the limbs and the localization of foreign bodies, because natural differences in opacity made examinations possible.[1-4] The first gastrointestinal applications went no further than the occasional visualization of an air-filled stomach[5] or the detection of foreign bodies in the gastrointestinal tract. One such early detection in the esophagus was reported by J. William White of the University of Pennsylvania.[6]

## Contrast Agents

The birth of gastrointestinal radiology awaited the fundamental idea of artificial contrast. The first idea about contrast that occurred to some who were experimenting with x-rays at that time was the use of a metallic wire. Carl Wegele suggested, without reporting any actual cases, that a thin metal wire, opaque to x-rays, could be passed through a gastric tube to track the greater curvature of the stomach down to the pylorus.[7] Radiographic images illustrating this technique were subsequently published.[8] Variations on this theme included the use of a bag swallowed into the stomach and then filled through an esophageal tube with lead acetate until the bag filled the stomach entirely.[3, 9] Another variation was the use of gelatin capsules containing opaque material. These were swallowed and observed with a fluoroscope as they outlined the greater curvature of the stomach.[9]

The idea of a liquid contrast medium slowly emerged, eventually leading to more comfortable examinations for the patient. Wolf Becher in Germany was probably the first person to perform a gastrointestinal study with liquid contrast medium—in mice and guinea pigs. He used mixtures of lead salts and was able to opacify the stomach and portions of the intestine.[10] Human applications followed soon thereafter.

## TABLE 1–1. SELECTED MILESTONES IN THE DEVELOPMENT OF GASTROINTESTINAL RADIOLOGY

| YEAR | EVENT |
| --- | --- |
| 1895 | W. C. Röntgen discovers x-rays |
| 1896 | Foreign body is detected in the esophagus |
| 1896 | Gastrointestinal study on a guinea pig is reported by Becher |
| 1897 | Rumpel reports bismuth study of the stomach |
| 1898 | Cannon reports radiologic observations on peristalsis |
| 1900 | American radiographs of gallstones in vivo |
| 1904 | Rieder meal method |
| 1904 | Single contrast examination of colon is reported by Schüle |
| 1910 | Barium is popularized by Bachem and Günther |
| 1911 | Lewis Gregory Cole reports first use of duodenal tube |
| 1914 | George and Gerber describe the radiologic appearance of duodenal ulcer |
| 1914 | Coolidge's tube |
| 1917 | Carman and Miller publish first comprehensive gastrointestinal radiology book |
| 1921 | Carman's meniscus sign |
| 1921 | Direct gallbladder puncture |
| 1923 | Double contrast study of the colon |
| 1924 | Cholecystography is developed by Graham and Cole |
| 1929 | Thorium is discovered |
| 1929 | Enteroclysis |
| 1932 | Crohn's disease is described |
| 1937 | Hampton reports double contrast study of stomach |
| 1937 | Percutaneous transhepatic cholangiography |
| 1945 | The beginnings of nuclear magnetic resonance spectroscopy |
| 1947 | Thorium-related neoplasm is first reported |
| 1951 | Iopanoic acid (Telepaque) is introduced |
| 1953 | Seldinger introduces percutaneous catheterization technique |
| 1950s | Early gastric cancer detection studies in Japan |
| 1960s | Welin's double contrast technique for study of the colon is reported |
| 1962 | Retained gallstones are extracted through a T tube |
| 1963 | Holmes and Howry report on ultrasound abdominal scanning |
| 1964 | Cormack publishes mathematic basis of computed tomography |
| 1971 | Damadian uses nuclear magnetic resonance to distinguish normal from malignant tissue |
| 1971 | Society of Gastrointestinal Radiologists is founded |
| 1973 | Retained gallstones are extracted by remote-controlled catheter |
| 1973 | Hounsfield publishes description of first computed tomographic apparatus |
| 1973 | Lauterbur reports magnetic resonance images of various rat tissues |
| 1974 | Skinny needle for invasive diagnostic procedures |
| 1975 | Appearance of gastric erosions on double contrast examination |
| 1975 | Technetium-labeled dimethyliminodiacetic acid is introduced for gallbladder imaging |
| 1975 | Earliest computed tomographic images of liver and pancreas |
| 1976 | A new journal, *Gastrointestinal Radiology,* is published |
| 1977 | First in vivo magnetic resonance human images |
| 1978 | Herlinger introduces a methylcellulose enteroclysis technique |
| 1981 | First magnetic resonance images of liver and pancreas |
| 1991 | Human immunodeficiency virus–related ulcers of esophagus are described |

Bismuth was the first practical gastrointestinal contrast medium. During the latter part of the 19th century, bismuth was often used as medication to treat gastric ulcer, "in doses so large that 60 grams of bismuth might well have been found in the stomach at one time. An x-ray taken at such a time would have astonished the

radiologist."[1] There are several reports of physicians who had noticed bismuth in the stomach but failed to appreciate the diagnostic potential of their observations.[1, 9] Two outstanding examples are Charles Lester Leonard of the University of Pennsylvania, who reported his observation in the *Journal of the American Medical Association* in 1897 while describing a case of gastroptosis, and George Edward Pfahler, who made his observations while an intern at Philadelphia General Hospital.[11]

Finally, reports of purposeful and successful examinations of the upper gastrointestinal tract using bismuth as a contrast medium came from Rumpel in Germany and were reported in the German literature in 1897.[12] Two months later, the first American observations were made by Walter B. Cannon, one of the most important figures in early 20th century gastrointestinal radiology and physiology (Fig. 1–1). His early research is worthy of somewhat detailed treatment.

## Walter B. Cannon

Walter B. Cannon is distinguished not only for his practical use of bismuth subnitrate as a contrast medium but also for his elucidation of valuable physiologic information about the workings of the gastrointestinal tract from what he saw with the fluoroscope. In addition to observations on esophageal peristalsis,[13] he reported his findings on the peristaltic movements in the stomach

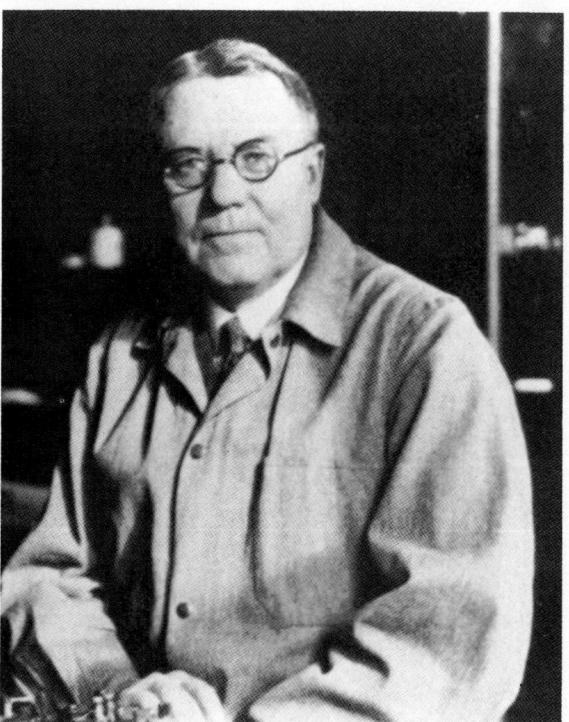

**Figure 1–1. Walter B. Cannon (1871–1945).** A pioneer in the use of radiology for the study of gastrointestinal physiology. (Courtesy of Countway Library, Boston, MA. Reprinted in Eisenberg RL: Radiology: An Illustrated History. St. Louis: Mosby–Year Book, 1992, p 259.)

and the functioning of the pyloric valve.[14] To make illustrations for his paper, "Cannon placed toilet paper over the fluoroscopic screen and traced an outline of the stomach at various times after the bismuth meal"[9] (Fig. 1–2). One of his most important insights occurred to him while studying gastric contractions in a cat:

> [The cat] suddenly changed from her peaceful sleepiness, began to breathe quickly, and struggled to get loose. As soon as the change took place, the movements in the stomach entirely disappeared; the pyloric portion relaxed and presented a smooth rounded outline. I continued observing, and stroked the cat reassuringly. In a moment she became quiet and began to purr. As soon as this happened, movements commenced again in the stomach; first a few constrictions were visible near the end of the antrum, then a few near the sharp bend in the lesser curvature, and finally the waves were running normally from their habitual starting place.

> By holding the cat's mouth closed between the thumb and last three fingers and covering her nostrils with the index finger, she could be kept from breathing. At the first sign of discomfort the fingers were removed. The experiment was repeated a great many times on different cats, and invariably the evidence of distress was accompanied by a total suspension of the motor activities of the stomach.[14]

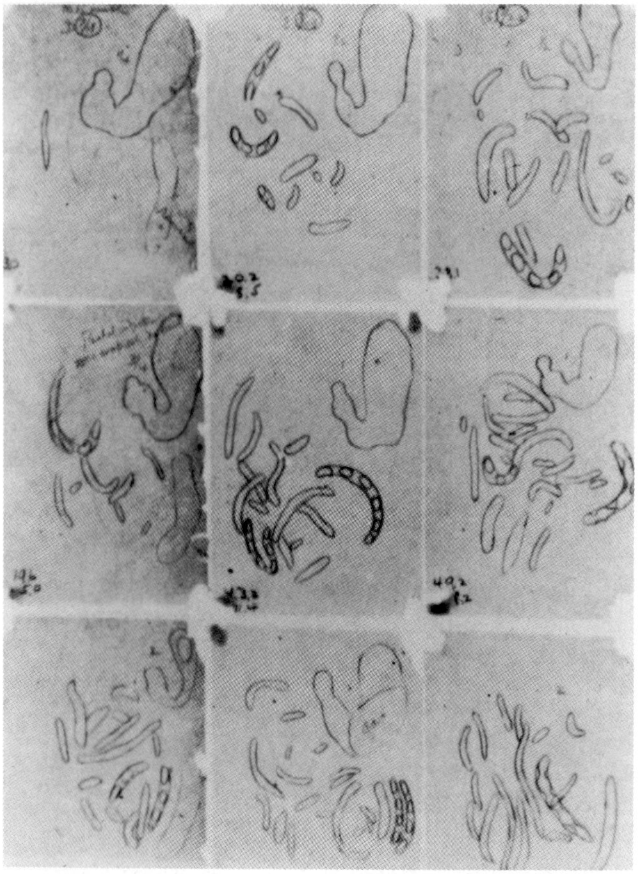

These words not only heralded Cannon's subsequent distinction between functional and mechanical disorders of the gastrointestinal tract but also provided impetus for much additional research on the autonomic nervous system.

The use of bismuth subnitrate in radiologic examinations was standardized and popularized by Hermann Rieder of Germany.[15] He stressed the use of large amounts of bismuth either with food or water, or alone as a thick paste. This became known as the Rieder meal and his method as the Rieder method. He favored the production of a large number of radiographs over fluoroscopy (Fig. 1–3).

The use of bismuth became widespread, but case reports of poisoning caused by the reduction of the nitrate to the highly toxic nitrite started appearing, and there was a need for a safer contrast medium. Cannon had used barium as well as bismuth in his experiments as early as 1896. He reported specifically on the advantages of barium sulfate in 1904.[16] The use of barium did not become standard, however, until it was popularized in Europe after a 1910 report by Bachem and Günther.[17]

## Technologic Advances

Meanwhile, a number of technologic advances had a profound impact on all of radiology including gastrointestinal radiology. These advances made it easier and safer for radiologists to do their work and made possible the orderly and methodical description of the radiologic appearance of various disorders.

Until 1914, x-rays were produced by the use of so-called Crookes tubes or other "gas tubes."[18] They were inadequately evacuated tubes with two metal electrodes sealed in the glass wall of the tube, usually at opposite ends. When a high voltage was applied between the two electrodes, electrons were accelerated, struck the anode, and produced x-rays. The tubes behaved unpredictably and inconsistently. The variance from tube to tube was high, rendering each tube essentially one of a kind and making control of beam intensity and penetration extremely difficult.[18] Thus, scientific advancement was hampered by technologic difficulty. In December 1913, W. D. Coolidge described his new tube in the physics literature; a report in the *American Journal of Roentgenology* soon followed.[19] The Coolidge tube was meticulously evacuated and permitted a large measure of control. Large scale radiologic adoption of the tube was not far behind.[20] Another important advance was the development of the universal radiographic-fluoroscopic table. Horizontal versions of the table were in existence as early as 1902; hand tilt models became available around 1907 and 1908, and the first motor-driven model was introduced in 1916.[2, 21]

## Radiography Versus Fluoroscopy

These technologic advances served to inflame a conflict among radiologists about the respective merits of

**Figure 1–2. Tracings by Walter B. Cannon.** Photograph of Cannon's toilet paper tracings made during gastrointestinal motility studies. (Courtesy of Countway Library, Boston, MA. Reprinted in AC Barger, New technology for a new century: Walter B. Cannon and the invisible rays, AJR, 136, 1, 187–193, 1981, © by American Roentgen Ray Society.)

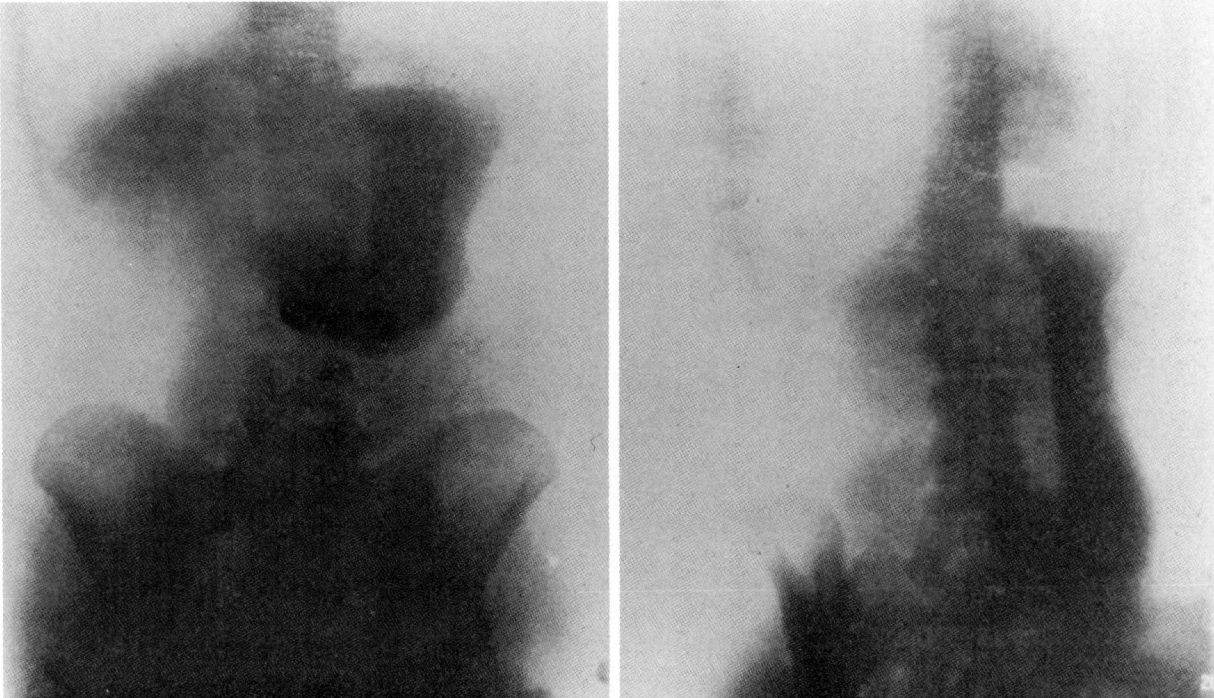

**Figure 1–3. Rieder meal.** Two illustrations of radiographs taken after a Rieder bismuth meal. (From Rieder H: Beitrage zur Topographie des Magendarm Kanales beim lebenden Menschen nebst Untersuchungen uber den zeitlichen Ablauf der Verdauung. Fortschr Geb Roentgenstr 8:141–172, 1905. Reprinted in Bruwer AJ: Classic Descriptions in Diagnostic Roentgenology, 1964, p 1857. Courtesy of Charles C Thomas, Publisher, Springfield, Illinois.)

fluoroscopy and radiography. Behind this conflict was a disagreement of a more medical than technical nature, about whether diagnosis should be made by visualizing the abnormality on a radiograph (the "direct method") or by observing fluoroscopically a certain pattern supposedly associated with specific entities (the "indirect method")[1, 9] (Fig. 1–4). Both of these methods had their proponents. Russell D. Carman, author of a major early work on gastrointestinal radiology,[22] was a proponent of fluoroscopy and the use of "symptom-complexes" to reach diagnoses (Fig. 1–5). Lewis Gregory Cole, a leader in radiologic-pathologic correlation (which he called "retrospectoscopy") preferred the use of a vast number of plates[1] (Fig. 1–6).

To this day, the descendants of these two schools can still be identified. The Mayo school[23] relies almost entirely on fluoroscopic observation, whereas the double contrast school relies on high-quality radiographs.[24] The two schools may be reaching a common ground with the development of high-resolution fluoroscopy and digital spot filming.

## Radiologic Pathology

The earliest radiologic descriptions of the gastrointestinal tract included the findings in the normal stomach and in those with gastric and duodenal ulcers.[25–27] Russell Carman of the Mayo Clinic published extensively on the diagnosis of gastric carcinoma. In 1921 he described the

meniscus sign that bears his name, which indicates an ulcerating gastric cancer[28] (Fig. 1–7). Ironically, Carman ended up diagnosing gastric cancer on his own radiographs in October 1925, and he died of the disease 8 months later.[1, 9] It was a usual practice at that time to illustrate radiologic reports with drawings showing the particular findings described (Fig. 1–8; see Fig. 1–2).

By the beginning of the second decade of this century, gastrointestinal radiologic studies had been performed on large series of patients. For example, in 1919, Carman and his staff at the Mayo Clinic performed more than 50,000 examinations.[1, 9] Numbers like these made it possible for Lewis Gregory Cole to establish the fundamental principle of the negative diagnosis. He followed a series of patients who had exploratory surgery for suspected ulcer even though they had no lesion on the radiograph and found that virtually none of them had ulcers. Thus, patients were assured they did not have ulcers when Cole did not see any on the radiographs. This showed that the radiologic method of diagnosis was both highly sensitive and highly specific. This basic principle reinforced the usefulness of radiology for medicine and surgery and led to the avoidance of much exploratory surgery, with its associated mortality and morbidity.

## Double Contrast

It is interesting that the idea of distending the stomach with gas to facilitate diagnosis may date back to 1901.

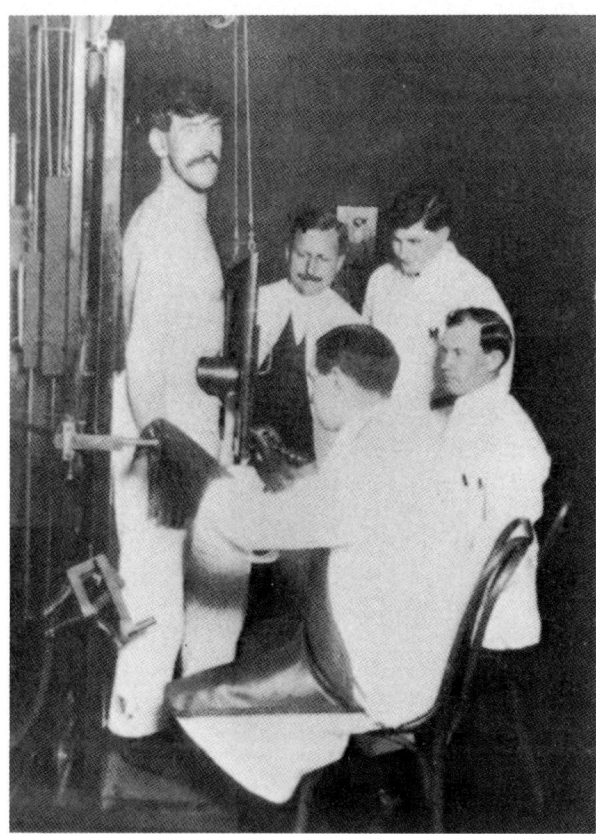

Figure 1–4. Fluoroscopic diagnosis. Direct fluoroscopy performed by a group in 1915. (From CW Lippman, Cylinder with bucky effect, AJR, 3, 452–453, 1915, © by American Roentgen Ray Society.)

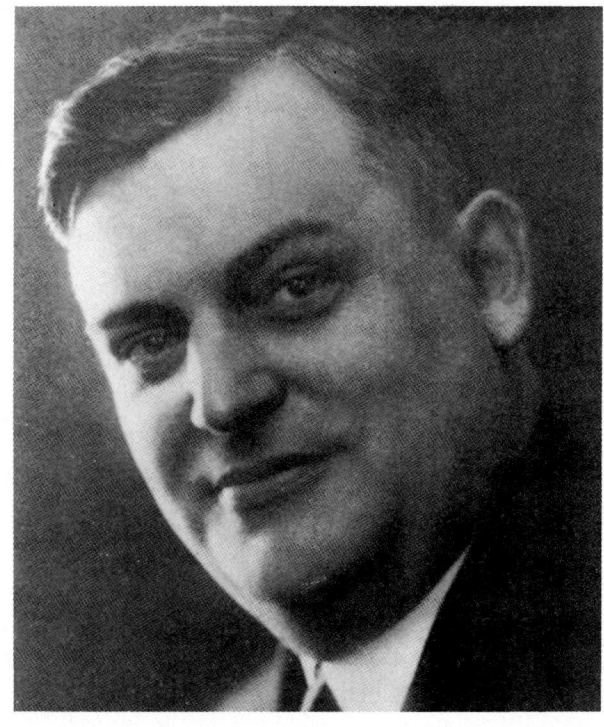

Figure 1–5. Russell D. Carman (1875–1926). Major proponent of fluoroscopic diagnosis and author of an early textbook on gastrointestinal radiology. (From the Mayo Clinic, Rochester, MN. Reprinted in Bruwer AJ: Classic Descriptions in Diagnostic Roentgenology, 1964, p 1983. Courtesy of Charles C Thomas, Publisher, Springfield, Illinois.)

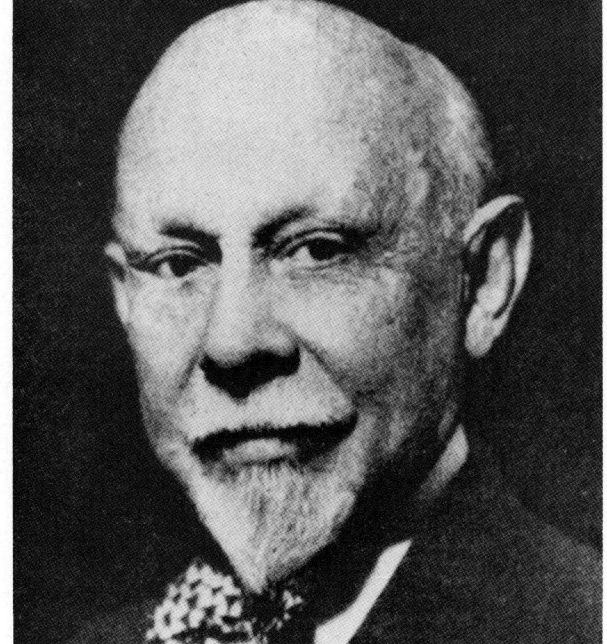

**Figure 1–6. Lewis Gregory Cole (1874–1954).** Major proponent of radiographic diagnosis and radiologic-pathologic correlation. (From AC Christie, Lewis Gregory Cole, 1874–1954, AJR, 73, 127–128, 1955, © by American Roentgen Ray Society.)

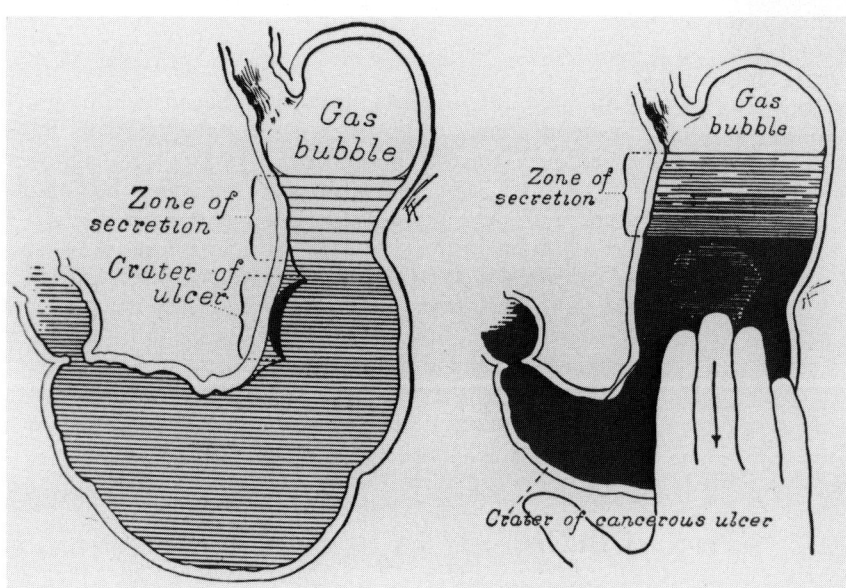

**Figure 1–7. Carman's drawings of the meniscus sign. Left.** Meniscus-like crater near the lesser curvature. **Right.** Visualization of an ulcer crater by manual compression of the stomach. (From Carman RD: A new roentgenray sign of ulcerating gastric cancer. JAMA 77:990–992, 1921. Copyright 1921, American Medical Association.)

**Figure 1–8. Gastric fold patterns as drawn by Eisler and Lenk. Left.** Normal appearance. **Middle.** Radiating folds and ulcer niche. **Right.** Radiating folds without evidence of an ulcer niche. (From Eisler F, Lenk R: The importance of the pattern of stomach folds in the diagnosis of gastric ulcer. Dtsch Med Wochenschr 1: 1449–1461, 1921. Reprinted in Bruwer AJ: Classic Descriptions in Diagnostic Roentgenology, 1964, pp 1896–1897. Courtesy of Charles C Thomas, Publisher, Springfield, Illinois.)

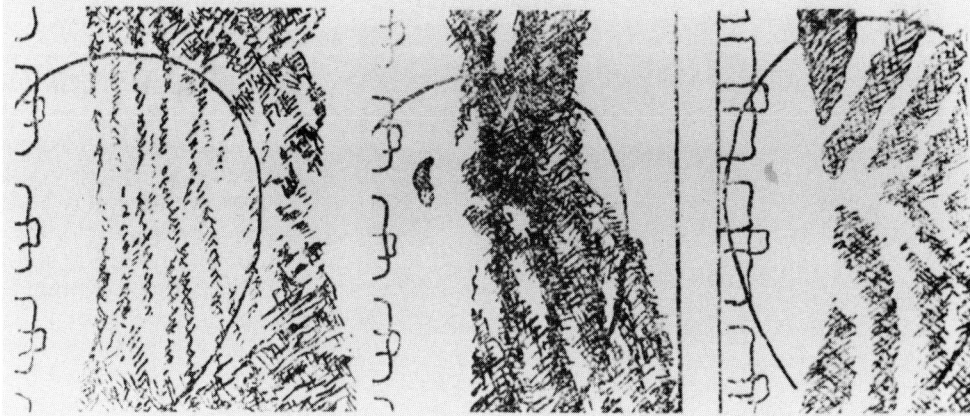

During that year, Francis Henry Williams published the 658-page book *The Roentgen Rays in Medicine and Surgery*.[29] He alluded to the idea of ingesting "seidlitz powder" to produce gas in the stomach. Guido Holzknecht of Vienna used a combination of bismuth and gas in 1906.[9] In 1913, Charles Lester Leonard of the University of Pennsylvania wrote, "if a method of coating the mucosa uniformly with an opaque salt can be combined with [gas distention of the stomach], the lesser lesions of the mucosa might be revealed."[30]

But it was not until 1937 that a report by Hampton showed examples of duodenal ulcers and a prepyloric carcinoma through the use of swallowed air and a barium suspension.[31] Several major papers elaborated on this theme in the following years. For example, Wasch and Epstein showed the special value of double contrast radiography in demonstrating tumors of the cardia.[32] In 1951, Ruzicka and Rigler described a method for double contrast examination of the stomach.[33] In 1958, Schatzki and Gary demonstrated the importance of en face views of the stomach for the diagnosis of ulcers[34] (Fig. 1–9).

In the 1950s, a group of Japanese gastroenterologists under the leadership of Professor Hikoo Shirakabe developed a double contrast technique for the examination of the stomach[35] (Fig. 1–10). Their initial interest was the diagnosis of gastric ulcers, but they soon directed their attention to the diagnosis of and screening for early gastric cancer, which is particularly prevalent in Japan. Their techniques became standard and the result was a marked improvement in outcome for patients with early gastric cancer, for whom the 5-year survival rate now approaches 90% or better.[36] Initially, these results

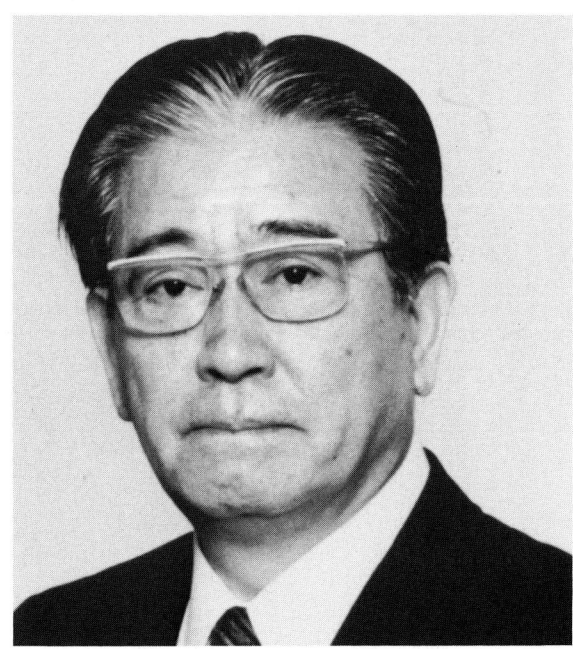

**Figure 1–10. Professor Hikoo Shirakabe.** Headed the team that developed double contrast study of the stomach for diagnosis of early gastric cancer. (Courtesy of H. Shirakabe, M.D., Tokyo, Japan.)

generated little interest in the West because of the much lower incidence of gastric cancer, but eventually these techniques were adopted for a variety of diagnoses. Important modifications of the Japanese techniques were published in the late 1960s and early 1970s.[37–39] New barium suspensions were developed and were specifically designed to produce high-quality radiographs of the stomach.[40] Soon thereafter, double contrast examination techniques were used by Laufer[41, 42] and Poplack[43, 44] and their associates to make diagnoses of entities more prevalent in the West, such as gastric erosions, linear ulcers, and ulcer scars—lesions that were rarely diagnosed with older techniques.

## COLON

### Early Days

Attempts to image the colon lagged no more than a few years behind imaging of the stomach. Still, as early as 1901, Francis Henry Williams discussed the use of air as a contrast medium and stated that "air may be pumped into the large bowel, and the outline of the sigmoid flexure and the descending colon may be easily followed."[29] He also commented on the idea that the "large intestine may be injected with fluid containing an opaque substance like subnitrate of bismuth, and its outline and position studied."[29] On the whole, however, he disapproved of this, fearing that the "heavy" opaque liquid might threaten the integrity of the bowel.[29]

The first reported single contrast examination of the colon was performed by Schüle in 1904[45] (Fig. 1–11A). As a contrast medium he used an oily suspension of

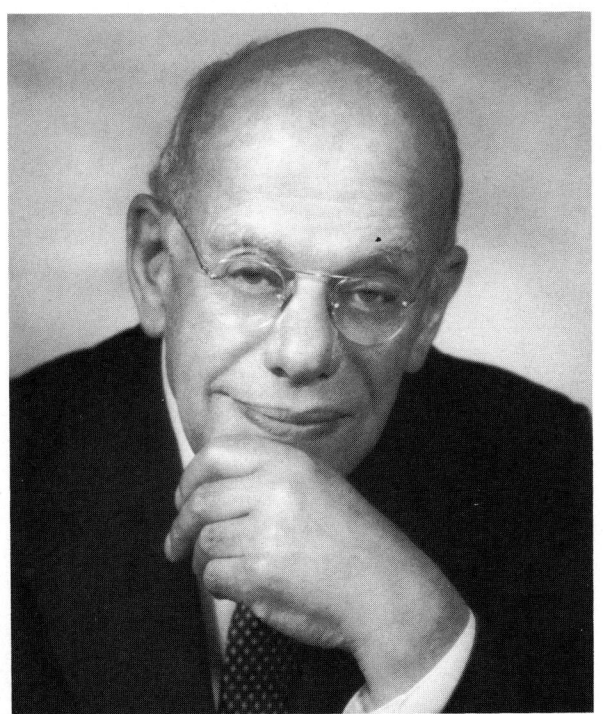

**Figure 1–9. Richard Schatzki (1901–1992).** Pioneer in gastrointestinal radiology with many original observations including the Schatzki ring. (Courtesy of Stefan C. Schatzki, M.D., Cambridge, MA.)

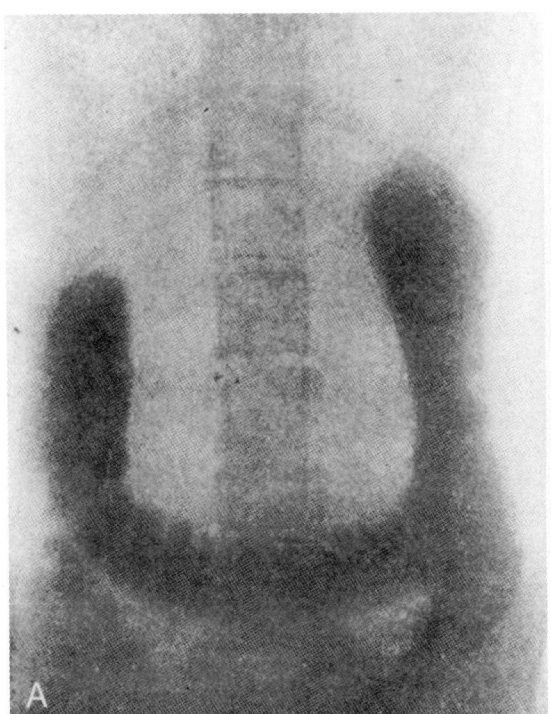
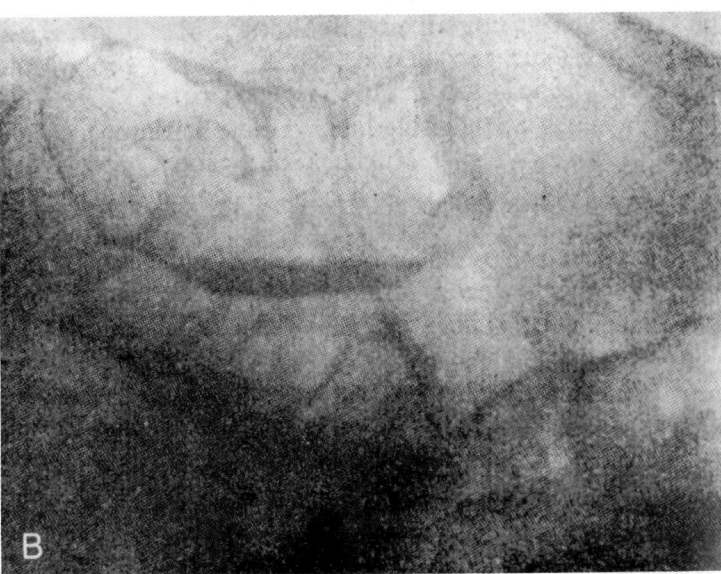

**Figure 1–11. Early contrast studies of the colon. A.** Bismuth enema by Schüle (1904). (From Schüle A: Intubation and radiography of the large intestine. Arch Verdau Kr 10:111–118, 1904. Reprinted in Bruwer AJ: Classic Descriptions in Diagnostic Roentgenology, 1964, p 1948. Courtesy of Charles C Thomas, Publisher, Springfield, Illinois.) **B.** Double contrast enema by Fischer in 1923, showing a cecal filling defect caused by tuberculosis. (From Fischer AW: A new roentgenologic method for examination of the large intestine: a combination of the contrast material enema and insufflation of air. Klin Wochenschr 2:1595–1598, 1923. Reprinted in Bruwer AJ: Classic Descriptions in Diagnostic Roentgenology, 1964, p 1976. Courtesy of Charles C Thomas, Publisher, Springfield, Illinois.)

bismuth subnitrate, already well established as a contrast medium for the upper gastrointestinal tract, given to the patient in enema form. He did not do so under fluoroscopic control; rather, he performed the x-ray examination after the enema was administered. In 1910, Georg Fedor Haenisch used a horizontal table equipped with facilities for fluoroscopy to follow the progress of the bismuth-based contrast medium in the body.[46] He argued that any obstruction to flow might indicate a narrowing caused by a tumor. Even at that time, he emphasized the value of cleansing the colon with cathartics and enemas and the necessity of examination after evacuation of the contrast medium.

As in the case of upper tract examination, once a reasonably reliable technique was established for the colon, descriptions of various pathologic entities followed. Thus by 1917, when Russell Carman and Albert Miller wrote the first definitive gastrointestinal radiology textbook, topics such as carcinoma, tuberculosis, diverticulosis, megacolon, and polyps were included.[22] Carman also stated that "lack of haustration, shortening of length, absence of flexures, stenoses and granularity of the mucosa" pointed to the diagnosis of ulcerative colitis.[47]

## Double Contrast

Double contrast was first used systematically in the colon. Fischer in Germany in 1923 combined the contrast medium enema with insufflation of air (see Fig. 1–11B).[48] This technique soon made its way to the United States, to be improved on by Weber and Kirklin at the Mayo Clinic during the 1930s.[9] They concentrated their efforts on developing criteria for identifying malignancy in the colon.[47] Much attention was also directed to the characterization and description of the radiologic appearance of colitis. In 1932, Crohn, Ginzburg, and Oppenheimer reported the radiologic appearance and clinical characteristics of an inflammatory process in the terminal ileum without a recognizable causative organism.[49] This entity, then called terminal ileitis, eventually was found to occur throughout the gastrointestinal tract and became known as regional enteritis or Crohn's disease. The differences between it and ulcerative colitis were subsequently clearly defined.[50–52]

Since the 1950s, intensive efforts have been directed at demonstrating small polypoid lesions of the colon.[47] Major progress in this area was made by Welin in Malmö, Sweden, where more than 70,000 double contrast examinations had been performed by 1967.[53] Welin and associates' 1963 report on the rates and patterns of growth of colonic and rectal tumors followed by double contrast imaging[54] continues to be heavily cited in the literature.[55] The Welin technique slowly became widespread in the United States, largely through the efforts of Roscoe E. Miller, who made the examination more practicable through the development of new apparatus, barium suspensions, and accessories (Fig. 1–12).

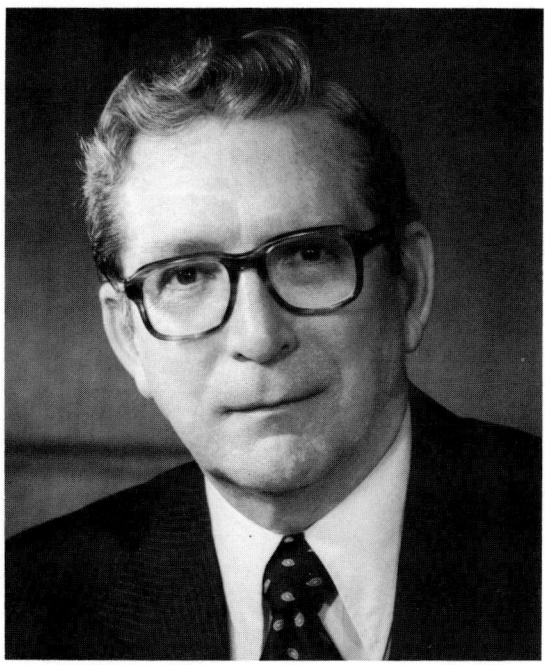

**Figure 1–12. Roscoe E. Miller (1918–1984).** Resurrected interest in the double contrast approach to gastrointestinal radiology.

## SMALL BOWEL

### Follow-through Studies

Follow-through studies of the small bowel evolved naturally from contrast studies of the stomach. The improved resolution and clarity of radiographs made it possible for radiologists to characterize the radiologic appearance of a variety of small bowel disorders, ranging from carcinoma and colitis to malabsorption and collagen-vascular diseases. The late Richard Marshak was a recognized leader in this regard[56] (Fig. 1–13).

### Enteroclysis

Small bowel enteroclysis had its origins in attempts to better visualize the duodenum. In 1911, Lewis Gregory Cole used a tube to obstruct the distal duodenum by balloon inflation to ensure complete filling of the duodenum with the bismuth-buttermilk mixture he was using.[57] Cole suggested that a modification of the tube may permit direct introduction of the contrast material into the duodenum. Building on earlier efforts,[58, 59] Gilberto S. Pesquera in New York recommended in 1929 the use of a duodenal tube for continuous and controlled filling of the small intestine.[60] The term barium enteroclysis was coined 10 years later by Gershon-Cohen and Shay of Philadelphia.[61] The next major improvement in this procedure was the introduction of new types of tubes, including the use of a guidewire, to make intubations more manageable and easier.[62–64]

The next hurdle was the choice of appropriate contrast solutions, and hydroxymethylcellulose was found to be better than water because it does not mix readily with barium.[65] The use of large volumes of barium combined with a 0.5% solution of methylcellulose in water was introduced by Herlinger in 1978.[66] Since then, this method has been used for the characterization of various small bowel diseases, and its superiority to follow-through studies has been shown.[59]

## CURRENT STATE OF CONTRAST RADIOLOGY

Although it originated almost a century ago, contrast examination of the gastrointestinal tract retains its vitality and continues to provide descriptions of new entities and improve our understanding of pathologic processes. For example, the last decade has seen reports of drug-induced esophagitis[67, 68] and carpet lesions of the colon and rectum.[69] The gastrointestinal manifestations of acquired immunodeficiency syndrome presented new diagnostic challenges, and the response of gastrointestinal radiology has been swift. Descriptions of herpes esophagitis,[70] *Candida* esophagitis,[71] cytomegalovirus esophagitis,[72] and esophagitis caused by the human immunodeficiency virus itself,[73] as well as gastrointestinal Kaposi's sarcoma,[74] quickly appeared.

Challenges by endoscopy and by newer imaging modalities made it necessary for contrast radiology of the gastrointestinal tract to maximize accuracy, sensitivity, and specificity. Radiologists therefore have directed their attention to the investigation of these issues, and the results have confirmed the clinical value of these techniques.[75–83]

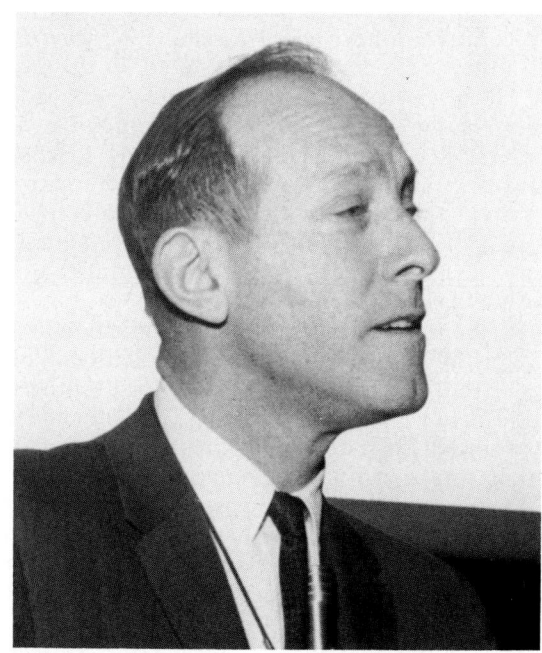

**Figure 1–13. Richard H. Marshak (1912–1982).** Pre-eminent proponent of radiologic-pathologic diagnosis, with particularly important contributions to the radiology of the small bowel and inflammatory bowel disease.

# GALLBLADDER AND BILIARY TRACT

## Stages of Development

Feld and colleagues have divided the history of gallbladder imaging into four periods, the plain film era (1895 to 1924); the contrast media era (1924 to 1960); the era of expanding technology, including the advent of percutaneous transhepatic cholangiography, scintigraphy, and sonography (1961 to 1979); and the interventional therapeutic era (since 1980).[84]

As with imaging of the hollow viscera, gallbladder-related imaging started soon after the discovery of x-rays. No more than 3 months after that discovery, reports of visualization of surgically removed gallstones appeared.[85, 86] A report in Europe[2] describing gallstones in vivo appeared in 1898 and a report in the United States by Carl Beck in 1900.[87] During the next two decades, the technique was streamlined and improved, but radiologists realized that only a minority of gallstones were radiopaque.[2, 9]

## Contrast Studies

Oral cholecystography began through the work of Evarts Graham and Warren H. Cole in 1923.[88] When they set out to inject dogs with an iodine or bromine derivative of phenolphthalein, they theorized that it would make the gallbladder visible because it would be excreted almost entirely through the bile. More than 200 futile attempts had been made before a gallbladder was finally visualized. The reason for this success turned out to be that the animal caretaker had forgotten to feed the particular dog that morning.[9]

Human applications soon followed but were hampered by the severe adverse reactions some patients had to the intravenous contrast agent. This problem led to a search for an effective oral contrast agent, supported by the knowledge of the workings of the enterohepatic circulation. In early 1925, two groups working independently reported successful oral cholecystography images.[89, 90] These were followed by various reports of efforts to develop better-tolerated and safer oral compounds for the procedure. In 1951, Hoppe and Archer described iopanoic acid (Telepaque),[91] which was both a safer compound and one that produced increased gallbladder opacification. Thus, oral cholecystography achieved the standards known today.[84]

## Isotopes and Ultrasound

The next two decades saw the application to gallbladder studies of two rapidly advancing modalities, nuclear medicine and ultrasound. The early developments of nuclear medicine in general have been reviewed in detail.[9, 92, 93] The major breakthrough[9] in radionuclide imaging of the gallbladder was the successful labeling of a molecule of iminodiacetic acid with technetium. In 1975, Harvey and co-workers showed that technetium-labeled dimethyliminodiacetic acid could be used to visualize the liver, bile ducts, and gallbladder with serial gamma camera images.[94] Subsequently, several other iminodiacetic acid molecules were produced to provide better visualization, including such compounds as technetium-labeled diisopropyl-iminodiacetic acid (DISIDA), permitting visualization even in the presence of significant jaundice.[84] Persistent nonvisualization of the gallbladder in a fasting individual with normal hepatic uptake and excretion is considered reliable evidence of acute cholecystitis.[95]

Like nuclear medicine techniques, ultrasound had been developing gradually for some time before it was finally applied to gallbladder imaging. The early development of ultrasound has been reviewed.[9, 96] Application of A-mode ultrasound to the abdomen was first reported in the mid-1960s. A landmark article in 1963 by Joseph Holmes and Douglass Howry, both ultrasound pioneers, reported on their experience with B-mode scanning of intra-abdominal structures.[97] Progress was quickly made and gallbladder-specific applications were described in the early 1970s.[98–100] Ultrasound has now virtually replaced oral cholecystography.

## Interventional Radiology

The major advances of recent years related to the gallbladder are various interventional techniques, both diagnostic and therapeutic. The advances have been in the making for decades. In 1921, Burckhardt and Mueller inserted a needle into the gallbladder cavity by direct transhepatic puncture.[101] Their purpose was to inject contrast medium to visualize gallstones, but even at that time the authors wondered whether it would one day be possible "by injection of a narcotic agent into the gallbladder to abort temporarily an acute attack of gallstone colic . . . to influence cholecystitis by direct injections into the gallbladder . . . by the injection of certain fluids into the gallbladder to dissolve gallstones or to reduce their size."[9] A few years later, postoperative cholangiography was performed in 1925 by Cotte of Lyon, France, and intraoperative cholangiography was performed by Mirrizzi and Losada of Argentina.[9] Nonsurgical percutaneous transhepatic cholangiography originated in Indochina in 1937[102] (Fig. 1–14). The first American report of this procedure, as well as a percutaneous method for drainage of an obstructed biliary tract, appeared in 1951.[103] The procedure did not become standard, however, because of two common side effects, internal bleeding and bile peritonitis. The introduction in 1974 of a flexible, skinny needle for use in transhepatic puncture changed that dramatically.[104]

A central insight in the area of interventional radiology of the gallbladder was that the techniques used to *diagnose* an entity, such as a retained gallstone after surgery, might be useful, when properly modified, to *treat* that entity. Drainage of an obstructed biliary tract may be seen as the beginning of this approach. Removal

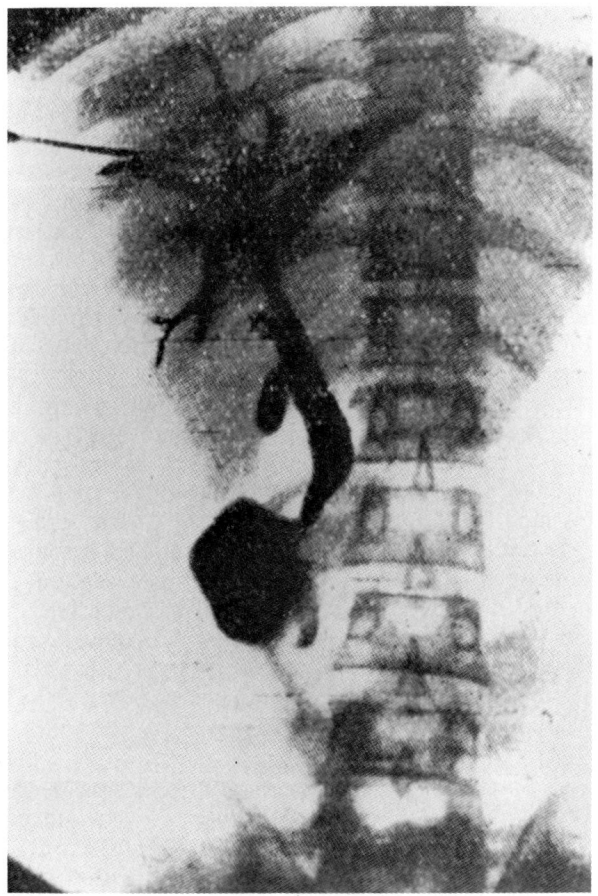

**Figure 1–14. Percutaneous transhepatic cholangiography (1937).** (From the National Library of Medicine. Reprinted in Bruwer AJ: Classic Descriptions in Diagnostic Roentgenology, 1964, p 1224. Courtesy of Charles C Thomas, Publisher, Springfield, Illinois.)

of retained stones, avoiding the risk associated with reoperation, was the end sought by these therapeutic interventions. Important early contributions were made by Mondet in Argentina and by Mazzariello and Mahorner in the United States.[105–107] These beginnings, ushered into existence by surgeons, were streamlined into a standard procedure by Burhenne. A series of papers by him starting in 1973[108] established the techniques not only for stone extraction but also for dilatation of benign biliary strictures.[105, 109]

## SOLID ORGANS

### Early Efforts

Early attempts at visualization consisted of the creation of artificial pneumomediastinum or pneumoperitoneum.[2] In 1929, opacification of the spleen with thorium was accidentally discovered, and thorium became useful in the localization of tumors, cysts, and abscesses.[9] In 1947, however, this came to an end, as a report of a human neoplasm attributable to thorium was published.[110] Useful imaging of these organs became possible

and widespread only after the application of modalities that developed independently, such as ultrasound, angiography, computed tomography (CT), and magnetic resonance (MR) imaging, and these have become the mainstay of solid organ imaging.

## Angiography

The idea of opacifying vessels to obtain diagnostic information dates back to 1896, when a contrast mixture composed of lime, cinnabar, and petroleum was injected into the brachial artery of a cadaver.[111] The search for contrast media safe for human injection centered on the halogens, which were known to be opaque to x-rays. Bromide and iodide salts were used based on the initial experience with these agents in the imaging of the urinary tract.[2, 9]

The first angiograms were obtained by direct injection of contrast medium into peripheral vessels through a needle placed by a surgical cutdown. Reaching such vessels as the aorta or portal vein proved problematic. Thus, angiographers relied on direct injection at laparotomy, or used a translumbar approach, or waited for the peripherally injected contrast medium to reach the desired area in retrograde fashion.[112, 113]

After initial efforts by Farinas and by Peirce to use femoral arterial catheterization to reach the aorta,[114, 115] Sven Ivar Seldinger of Sweden introduced his percutaneous catheter technique in 1953.[116] It involved the introduction of a catheter over a guidewire and soon became internationally known. Seldinger's 1953 report describing the technique became the most frequently cited radiologic paper of all time.[117] More recent advances in angiography have included the advent of digital subtraction angiography and low-osmolality contrast media.

## Computed Tomography

Excellent and detailed reviews of the development of CT[11, 118, 119] and MR[11, 118–120] have been published. The mathematic basis of CT was developed as early as 1917 by Radon, an Austrian mathematician, who was working with equations that described gravitational forces.[118] The principles he established were used in the 1950s and 1960s to solve imaging problems in solar astronomy and electron microscopy. In 1955, Allan MacLeod Cormack, a South African physicist, started working part-time in the radiation therapy department of a Cape Town hospital. He noted the problem of tissue inhomogeneity, which created difficulty in radiation therapy planning. His 1964 paper[121] developing a mathematic approach to this problem generated virtually no response, and his ideas were not acknowledged until several years later. Unaware of Cormack's work, Godfrey Hounsfield, an engineer with Electronic Musical Instruments in Britain, suggested in 1968 that an image might be constructed by computer from multiple x-ray images taken from multiple angles. He presented his early clinical results in April 1972 to the annual congress of the British Institute of Radiology.[119] Hounsfield's report[122] in the *British Journal of Radiology* in 1973 describing the CT system became the second most frequently cited radiology paper of all time.[55] Hounsfield and Cormack shared a Nobel Prize in 1979. The news soon reached the United States and preliminary reports of clinical applications followed.

## Magnetic Resonance Imaging

The development of MR imaging trailed that of CT by a few years. In 1945, Felix Bloch and Edward Purcell independently measured the magnetic moment of the proton to an accuracy of 1 per million. They received the Nobel Prize in physics in 1952 for their discovery, which led to the development of nuclear magnetic resonance (NMR) spectroscopy.[118, 120] Early use centered on chemical and biochemical applications, but NMR research on biologic systems soon followed. Two investigators, Thomas Shaw and Erik Odeblad, led the way, with the latter producing articles on the NMR properties of a variety of human tissues, fluids, and secretions.[120] In 1971, Raymond Damadian reported that NMR could distinguish malignant tumors from normal tissue.[123] Then, in 1973, Paul Lauterbur published a seminal paper in *Nature* on the NMR spectra of different rat tissues.[124] The first human in vivo image was published in 1977.[125]

## LIVER AND SPLEEN

Before the advent of ultrasound and CT, three angiographic techniques played an important part in the study of the liver and spleen. In the mid-1940s, direct injection of the portal vein at laparotomy was introduced, but the diagnostic value of the images obtained was limited.[112, 126] Another technique was splenoportography, which was introduced in the 1950s. It involved the injection of

contrast material directly into the spleen, and the material soon flowed into the splenic and portal veins.[127] As might be expected, the procedure was fraught with complications. The third technique was arterial portography, which is based on the observation that the portal system was occasionally visualized after aortography. The images obtained in this manner became useful only after the introduction of selective catheterization of the celiac, superior mesenteric, and splenic arteries.[128, 129]

The application of CT imaging to the abdomen initially presented a technical problem. Bodily movements made thorax and abdomen imaging difficult, because scanning time then was measured in minutes. Rapid technical advances decreased the scanning time and greatly improved resolution. Applications to abdominal imaging quickly proliferated.[130–132] The application of MR to liver imaging was also dependent on technologic progress in improving resolution and decreasing imaging time. Clinical reports on the use of MR imaging in diagnosis started appearing with frequency in the 1980s[133] (Fig. 1–15). Abdominal applications are gradually becoming standardized and widely used.[134]

## PANCREAS

For much of radiologic history, the pancreas was an imagined organ surrounded by the stomach and duodenum. Abnormalities of the pancreas could only be inferred from their effect on adjacent organs. Radiology of the pancreas came of age only in the past two decades or so, when invasive as well as cross-sectional techniques such as ultrasound, CT, and MR imaging were applied and could demonstrate the pancreas directly. Ultrasound was the first cross-sectional technique used to image the pancreas.[135] Improvement in resolution and image quality made it possible to visualize the pancreatic ducts. As with the liver and other abdominal organs, CT use for pancreatic imaging awaited improved resolution and decreased scanning time. Early reports on pancreatic

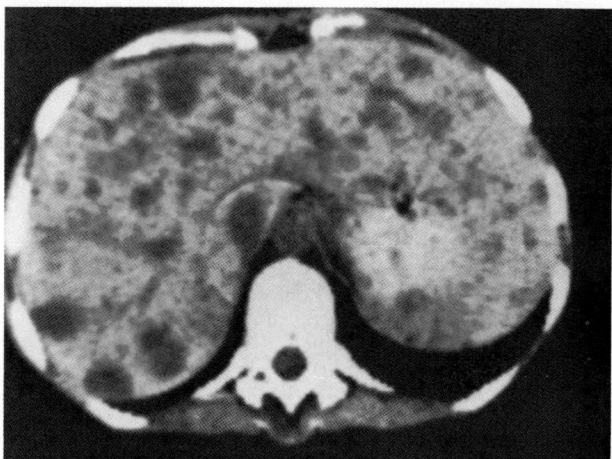 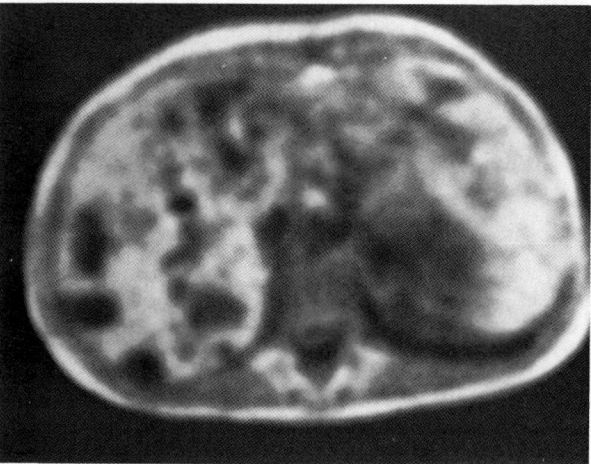

**Figure 1–15. Early abdominal MR imaging.** Carcinoma metastatic to the liver as shown by CT **(left)** and MR **(right)** (1982). (From FH Doyle, JM Pennock, LM Banks, et al, Nuclear magnetic resonance imaging of the liver: initial experience, AJR, 138, 2, 193–200, 1982, © by American Roentgen Ray Society.)

CT were published in the mid-1970s.[136, 137] MR imaging of the pancreas has not yet been widely used and its role remains to be defined.[135]

Pancreatic imaging benefited greatly from the introduction of the skinny needle for percutaneous transhepatic cholangiography. This needle was eventually used for aspiration biopsy and direct opacification of the pancreatic duct under sonographic guidance.[138] Superselective vessel catheterization resulted in significant improvement in the diagnosis of pancreatic neoplasms.[139] Currently, a combination of these techniques permits the precise diagnosis of pancreatitis and of a variety of pancreatic cancers.

## ORGANIZATION

Until the early 1970s, gastrointestinal radiology was generally considered a major component of the field of general diagnostic radiology. In 1971, the Society of Gastrointestinal Radiologists was founded under the leadership of Alexander Margulis and Joachim Burhenne. This was followed in 1990 by the organization of the European Society of Gastrointestinal Radiology. In 1976, the first edition of a new journal, *Gastrointestinal Radiology*, was published with Morton Meyers and Gary Gharemani as editors. These organizations and publications have helped define the subspecialty of gastrointestinal radiology and have provided a rich forum for the presentation of new work.

## CONCLUSION

The century-old contrast imaging of the gastrointestinal tract continues to develop in response to new diseases and new needs. Newer imaging modalities such as CT and MR imaging still have great potential for development and improvement. As gastrointestinal radiology enters its second century, new modalities such as positron emission tomography and others still unimaginable will probably find gastrointestinal applications. Also in the next few years, gastrointestinal radiology, like other subspecialties of radiology, will adopt some form of computer storage and digital imaging systems that will significantly alter the day-to-day practice of the specialty.

## References

1. Brecher R, Brecher E: The Rays: A History of Radiology in the United States and Canada. Baltimore: Williams & Wilkins, 1969.
2. Goodman P: History. *In* Margulis AR, Burhenne HJ (eds): Alimentary Tract Roentgenology (4th ed). St. Louis: CV Mosby, 1989, pp 1–30.
3. Kirsner, JB: The Development of American Gastroenterology. New York: Raven Press, 1990.
4. Bordley J, Harvey AM: Two Centuries of American Medicine, 1776–1976. Philadelphia: WB Saunders, 1976.
5. Morton, WJ, Hammer EW: The X-ray. New York: American Technical Book, 1896.
6. White JW: A foreign body in the esophagus detected and located by Rontgen rays. Univ Med Mag 8:710–715, 1896.
7. Wegele C: A proposal for the use of Roentgen procedures in medicine. Dtsch Med Wochenschr 22:287, 1896.
8. Lindemann E: Demonstration of Roentgen pictures of the normal and distended stomach. Dtsch Med Wochenschr 23:266–267, 1897.
9. Eisenberg RL: Radiology: An Illustrated History. St. Louis: Mosby–Year Book, 1992.
10. Becher W: The use of the Roentgen procedure in medicine. Dtsch Med Wochenschr 22:202–203, 1896.
11. Skinner EH: American Roentgen Ray Society 1900–1950. Springfield, IL: Charles C Thomas, 1950.
12. Rumpel T: Visualization of esophagus of patient with dysphagia with bismuth. Muench Med Wochenschr 44:420–421, 1897.
13. Cannon WB, Moser A: The movements of food in the oesophagus. Am J Physiol 1:435–444, 1898.
14. Cannon WB: The movements of the stomach studied by means of the Roentgen rays. Am J Physiol 1:359–382, 1898.
15. Rieder H: Radiologic examination of the stomach and intestines in the living man. Muench Med Wochenschr 51:1548–1551, 1904.
16. Cannon WB: The passage of different food-stuffs from the stomach and through the small intestine. Am J Physiol 12:387–418, 1904.
17. Bachem C, Günther H: Barium sulfate as a shadow-forming contrast agent in roentgenologic examinations. Röentgenkd 12:369–376, 1910.
18. Feldman A: A sketch of the technical history of radiology from 1896 to 1920. Radiographics 9:1113–1128, 1989.
19. Coolidge WD: A powerful Röntgen ray tube with a pure electron discharge. AJR 1:115–124, 1914.
20. Cole LG: A preliminary report on the diagnostic and therapeutic application of the Coolidge tube. AJR 1:125–131, 1914.
21. Angus WM: A commentary on the development of diagnostic imaging technology. Radiographics 9:1225–1244, 1989.
22. Carman RD, Miller A: The Roentgen Diagnosis of Diseases of the Alimentary Tract. Philadelphia: WB Saunders, 1917.
23. Teefey SA, Carlson HC: The fluoroscopic barium enema in colonic polyp detection. AJR 141:1279–1281, 1983.
24. Laufer I, Levine MS (eds): Double Contrast Gastrointestinal Radiology (2nd ed). Philadelphia: WB Saunders, 1992.
25. Rigler LG, Weiner M: History of radiology of the gastrointestinal tube. In Margulis AR, Burhenne HJ (eds): Alimentary Tract Roentgenology (3rd ed). St. Louis: CV Mosby, 1983, pp 3–17.
26. George AW, Gerber I: The direct method of diagnosis of duodenal ulcer by means of the Roentgen ray. AJR 1:277–293, 1914.
27. Eisler F, Lenk R: The importance of the pattern of stomach folds in the diagnosis of gastric ulcer. Dtsch Med Wochenschr 1:1459–1461, 1921.
28. Carman RD: A new roentgen-ray sign of ulcerating gastric cancer. JAMA 77:990–992, 1921.
29. Williams FH: The Roentgen Rays in Medicine and Surgery. New York: Macmillan, 1901.
30. Leonard CL: The radiography of the stomach and intestines. AJR 1:1–42, 1913.
31. Hampton AO: A safe method for the Roentgen demonstration of bleeding duodenal ulcers. AJR 38:565–570, 1937.
32. Wasch MG, Epstein BS: The Roentgen visualization of tumors of cardia. AJR 51:564–571, 1944.
33. Ruzicka FF, Rigler LG: Inflation of the stomach with double contrast: a roentgen study. JAMA 145:696–702, 1951.
34. Schatzki R, Gary JE: Face-on demonstration of ulcers in the upper stomach in a dependent position. AJR 79:722–780, 1958.
35. Shirakabe H: Double Contrast Studies of the Stomach. Stuttgart: Georg Thieme Verlag, 1972.
36. Yamada E, Nakazato H, Koite A, et al: Surgical results of early gastric cancer. Int Surg 59:7–14, 1974.
37. Obata WG: A double contrast technique for examination of the stomach using barium sulfate with simethicone. AJR 115:275–280, 1972.
38. Gelfand DW: The Japanese-style double contrast examination of the stomach. Gastrointest Radiol 1:7–12, 1976.

39. Scott-Harden WG: Radiological investigation of peptic ulcer. Br J Hosp Med 10:149–153, 1973.
40. Gelfand DW: High-density, low-viscosity barium for fine mucosal detail on double-contrast upper gastrointestinal examinations. AJR 130:831–833, 1978.
41. Laufer I, Hamilton J, Mullens JE: Demonstration of superficial gastric erosions by double contrast radiology. Gastroenterology 68:387–391, 1975.
42. Laufer I: Assessment of the accuracy of double contrast gastro-duodenal radiology. Gastroenterology 71:874–878, 1976.
43. Poplack W, Paul RE, Goldsmith M, et al: Demonstration of erosive gastritis by the double contrast technique. Radiology 117:519–521, 1975.
44. Poplack W, Paul RE, Goldsmith M, et al: Linear and rod-shaped peptic ulcers. Radiology 122:317–319, 1977.
45. Schüle A: Intubation and radiography of the large intestine. Arch Verdau Kr 10:111–118, 1904.
46. Haenisch GF: Roentgenologic examination in narrowing of the large intestine: the early roentgenologic diagnosis of carcinoma of the large intestine. Muench Med Wochenschr 45:2331–2375, 1911.
47. Stevenson CA: The development of gastrointestinal roentgenology. AJR 75:230–237, 1956.
48. Fischer AW: A new roentgenologic method for examination of the large intestine: a combination of the contrast material enema and insufflation of air. Klin Wochenschr 2:1595–1598, 1923.
49. Crohn B, Ginzburg L, Oppenheimer GD: Regional ileitis. JAMA 99:1323–1329, 1932.
50. Marshak RH, Wolf BS: Roentgen findings in regional enteritis. AJR 74:1000–1014, 1955.
51. Marshak RH, Wolf BS, Eliasoph J: Segmental colitis. Radiology 73:707–716, 1959.
52. Lockhart-Mummery HE, Morson BC: Crohn's disease (regional enteritis) of the large intestine and its distinction from ulcerative colitis. Gut 1:87–105, 1960.
53. Welin S: Results of the Malmö technique of colon examination. JAMA 199:369–372, 1967.
54. Welin S, Youker J, Spratt JS Jr, et al: The rates and patterns of growth of 375 tumors of the large intestine and rectum observed serially by double contrast enema study (Malmö technique). AJR 90:673–687, 1963.
55. Chew FS: AJR: the 50 most frequently cited papers in the past fifty years. AJR 150:227–233, 1988.
56. Marshak RH, Lindner AE: Radiology of the Small Intestine (2nd ed). Philadelphia: WB Saunders, 1976.
57. Cole LG: Artificial dilatation of the duodenum for radiographic examination. Am Q Roentgenol 3:204–205, 1911.
58. Einhorn, M, The Duodenal Tube and Its Possibilities (2nd ed). Philadelphia: FA Davis, 1926.
59. Herlinger H: Small bowel. In Laufer I, Levine MS (eds): Double Contrast Gastrointestinal Radiology (2nd ed). Philadelphia: WB Saunders, 1992, pp 363–422.
60. Pesquera GS: A method for the direct visualization of lesions in the small intestine. AJR 22:254–257, 1929.
61. Gershon-Cohen J, Shay H: Barium enteroclysis. AJR 42:456–458, 1939.
62. McLaren JW (ed): Modern Trends in Diagnostic Radiology (3rd series). London: Butterworth, 1960.
63. Bilbao MK, Frische LH, Dotter CT, et al: Hypotonic duoden-ography. Radiology 89:438–443, 1967.
64. Gianturco C: Rapid fluoroscopic duodenal intubation. Radiology 88:1165–1166, 1967.
65. Trickey SE, Halls J, Hobson CJ: A further development of the small bowel enema. Proc Soc Med 56:1070–1073, 1963.
66. Herlinger H: A modified technique for the double contrast small bowel enema. Gastrointest Radiol 3:201–207, 1978.
67. Creteur V, Laufer I, Kressel HY, et al: Drug-induced esophagitis detected by double-contrast radiography. Radiology 147:365–368, 1983.
68. Bova JG, Dutton NE, Goldstein HM, et al: Medication-induced esophagitis: diagnosis by double contrast esophagography. AJR 148:731–732, 1987.
69. Rubesin SE, Saul SH, Laufer I, et al: Carpet lesions of the colon. Radiographics 5:537–552, 1985.
70. Levine MS, Loevner LA, Saul SH, et al: Herpes esophagitis: sensitivity of double contrast esophagography. AJR 151:57–62, 1988.
71. Levine MS, Macones AJ, Laufer I: Candida esophagitis: accuracy of radiologic diagnosis. Radiology 154:581–587, 1985.
72. Balthazar EJ, Megibow AJ, Hulnick D, et al: Cytomegalovirus esophagitis in AIDS: radiographic features in 16 patients. AJR 149:919–923, 1987.
73. Levine MS, Loercher G, Katzka DA, et al: Giant HIV-related ulcers in the esophagus. Radiology 180:323–326, 1991.
74. Wall SD, Friedman SL, Margulis AR: Gastrointestinal Kaposi's sarcoma in AIDS: radiographic manifestations. J Clin Gastro-enterol 6:165–171, 1984.
75. Gelfand DW, Ott DJ: Single- vs. double-contrast gastrointestinal studies: critical analysis of reported statistics. AJR 137:523–528, 1981.
76. Gelfand DW, Dale WJ, Ott DJ, et al: The radiologic detection of duodenal ulcers: effects of examiner variability, ulcer size and location, and technique. AJR 145:551–553, 1985.
77. Ott DJ, Chen YM, Gelfand DW, et al: Peroral small bowel examination vs. enteroclysis. II. Radiologic accuracy. Radiology 155:31–34, 1985.
78. Simpkins KC, Stevenson GW: The modified Malmö double-contrast barium enema in colitis: an assessment of its accuracy in reflecting sigmoidoscopic findings. Br J Radiol 45:486–492, 1972.
79. Williams HJ Jr, Stephens DH, Carlson HC: Double contrast radiography: colonic inflammatory disease. AJR 137:315–322, 1981.
80. Laufer I, Mullens JE, Hamilton J: Correlation of endoscopy and double-contrast radiography in the early stages of ulcerative and granulomatous colitis. Radiology 118:1–5, 1976.
81. Eddy DM: Benefits and costs of screening for colorectal cancer. In Gelfand DW, Laufer I (eds): Colon Cancer: Diagnosis in an Era of Cost Containment. Reston, VA: American College of Radiology, 1989, pp 37–40.
82. Levine MS, Creteur V, Kressel HY, et al: Benign gastric ulcers: diagnosis and follow-up with double contrast radiology. Radiology 164:9–13, 1987.
83. Thompson G, Somers S, Stevenson GW: Benign gastric ulcer: a reliable radiologic diagnosis? AJR 141:331–333, 1983.
84. Feld R, Kurtz AB, Zeman RK: Imaging the gallbladder: a historical perspective. AJR 156:737–740, 1991.
85. Wakely TH: The new photographic discovery. Lancet 1:310, 1896.
86. Cattel HW: Roentgen's discovery: its application in medicine. Med News 68:169–171, 1896.
87. Beck C: On the detection of calculi in the liver and gallbladder. N Y Med J 71:73–77, 1900.
88. Graham EA, Cole WH: Roentgenologic examination of the gallbladder: new method utilizing intravenous injection of tetra-bromphenolphthalein. JAMA 82:613–614, 1924.
89. Whitaker LR, Milliken G, Vogt EC: The oral administration of sodium tetraiodophenolphthalein for cholecystography. Surg Gynecol Obstet 40:847–851, 1925.
90. Menees TO, Robinson HC: Oral administration of tetraiodo-phenolphthalein: preliminary report. AJR 13:368–369, 1925.
91. Hoppe JO, Archer S: Triiodoalkanoic acid derivatives as chole-cystographic media. Fed Proc 10:975–977, 1951.
92. Grigg ERN: The beginnings of nuclear medicine. In Gottschalk A, Hoffer PB, Potchen EJ (eds): Diagnostic Nuclear Medicine. Baltimore: Williams & Wilkins, 1988, pp 1–3.
93. Lindeman JF, Quinn JL: The history of nuclear medicine instru-mentation and clinical procedures. In Gottschalk A, Hoffer PB, Potchen EJ (eds): Diagnostic Nuclear Medicine. Baltimore: Williams & Wilkins, 1988, pp 4–10.
94. Harvey J, Loberg M, Cooper M: 99m Tc-HIDA: a new radio-pharmaceutical for hepatobiliary imaging. J Nucl Med 16:533, 1975.
95. Weissmann HS, Frank M, Bernstein LH, et al: Rapid and accurate diagnosis of acute cholecystitis with 99m Tc-HIDA cholescintigraphy. AJR 132:523–528, 1979.
96. Holm HH, Kristensen JK, Rasmussen SN, et al: Abdominal

Ultrasound: Static and Dynamic Scanning. Baltimore: University Park Press, 1980.

97. Holmes JH, Howry DH: Ultrasonic diagnosis of abdominal disease. Am J Dig Dis 8:12–32, 1963.
98. Doust BD, Malakad NF: Ultrasonic B-mode examination of the gallbladder. Radiology 110:643–647, 1974.
99. Hublitz VF, Kahn PC, Sell LA: Cholecystosonography: an approach to the non-visualized bladder. Radiology 103:645–649, 1972.
100. Leopold GR, Sokoloff J: Ultrasonic scanning in the diagnosis of biliary tract diseases. Surg Clin North Am 53:1043–1052, 1973.
101. Burckhardt H, Mueller W: Experiments on puncture of the gallbladder and its visualization with roentgen rays. Dtsch Z Chir 162:168–197, 1921.
102. Huard P, Do-Xuan-Hop: Transhepatic puncture of the bile ducts. Bull Soc Med Chir Indochine 15:1090–1100, 1937.
103. Carter R, Saypol GM: Transabdominal cholangiography. JAMA 148:253–255, 1952.
104. Okuda K, Tanikawa K, Emuro T, et al: Non-surgical percutaneous transhepatic cholangiography: diagnostic significance in medical problems of the liver. Am J Dig Dis 19:21–36, 1974.
105. Burhenne HJ: The history of interventional radiology of the biliary tract. Radiol Clin North Am 28:1139–1144, 1990.
106. Mazzariello RM: Removal of residual biliary tract calculi without reoperation. Surgery 67:566–573, 1970.
107. Mahorner H, Bean WJ: Removal of residual stone from common bile duct without surgery. Ann Surg 173:857–863, 1971.
108. Burhenne HJ: Nonoperative retained biliary tract stone extraction: a new roentgenologic technique. AJR 117:388–399, 1973.
109. Burhenne HJ: Percutaneous extraction of retained biliary tract stone: 661 patients. AJR 134:888–898, 1980.
110. MacMahon HE, Murphy AS, Bates MI: Endothelial cell sarcoma of the liver following thorotrast injections. Am J Pathol 23:585–611, 1947.
111. Haschek E, Lindenthal OT: A contribution to the practical use of photography according to Roentgen. Wien Klin Wochenschr 9:63–64, 1896.
112. Whipple AO: The problem of portal hypertension in relation to the hepatosplenopathies. Ann Surg 122:449–475, 1945.
113. Castellanos A, Pereiras R: Countercurrent aortography. Rev Cuba Cardiol 2:187–201, 1939.
114. Farinas PL: A new technique for the arteriographic examination of the abdominal aorta and its branches. AJR 46:641–645, 1941.
115. Peirce EC: Percutaneous femoral artery catheterization in man with special reference to aortography. Surg Gynecol Obstet 93:56–74, 1951.
116. Seldinger SI: Catheter replacement of the needle in percutaneous arteriography: a new technique. Acta Radiol 39:368–376, 1953.
117. Siegelman SS: The cat's meow: the most frequently cited papers in radiology 1955–1986. Radiology 168:414–420, 1988.
118. Hendee WR: Cross sectional medical imaging: a history. Radiographics 9:1115–1180, 1989.
119. Evens RG: The history, economics and politics of CT and MRI. *In* Lee JKT, Sagel SS, Stanley RJ (eds): Computed Body Tomography with MRI Correlation (2nd ed). New York: Raven Press, 1989, pp 1113–1124.
120. Mourino MR: From Thales to Lauterbur, or from the lodestone to MR imaging: magnetism and medicine. Radiology 180:593–612, 1991.
121. Cormack AM: Representation of a function by its line integrals with some radiological applications (I). J Appl Phys 35:2722–2727, 1964.
122. Hounsfield GN: Computerized transverse axial scanning (tomography). I. Description of system. Br J Radiol 46:1016–1022, 1973.
123. Damadian R: Tumor detection by nuclear magnetic resonance. Science 171:1151–1153, 1971.
124. Lauterbur PC: Image formation by induced local interactions: examples employing nuclear magnetic resonance. Nature 242:190–191, 1973.
125. Damadian R, Goldsmith M, Minkoff L: NMR in cancer: XVI. FONAR image of the live human body. Physiol Chem Phys 9:97–100, 1977.
126. Blakemore AH, Lord JW: Technique of using Vitallium tubes in establishing portacaval shunts for portal hypertension. Ann Surg 122:476–489, 1945.
127. Abeatici S, Campi L: On the possibilities of hepatic angiography—visualization of the portal system (experimental studies). Acta Radiol 36:383–392, 1951.
128. Boijsen E, Eckman CA, Olin T: Coeliac and superior mesenteric angiography in portal hypertension. Acta Chir Scand 126:315–325, 1963.
129. Pollard JJ, Nebesar RA: Catheterization of the splenic artery for portal venography. N Engl J Med 271:234–237, 1964.
130. Alfidi RJ, Haaga JR, Meaney TF, et al: Computed tomography of the thorax and abdomen: a preliminary report. Radiology 117:257–264, 1975.
131. Haaga JR, Alfidi RJ, Havrilla TR, et al: CT detection and aspiration of abdominal abscesses. AJR 128:465–474, 1977.
132. Stephens DH, Sheedy PF, Hattery RR, et al: Computed tomography of the liver. AJR 128:579–590, 1977.
133. Doyle FH, Pennock JM, Banks LM, et al: Nuclear magnetic resonance imaging of the liver: initial experience. AJR 138:193–200, 1982.
134. Lee JKT, Sagel SS, Stanley RJ (eds): Computed Body Tomography with MRI Correlation (2nd ed). New York: Raven Press, 1989.
135. Freeny PC: Radiology of the pancreas: two decades of progress in imaging and intervention. AJR 150:975–981, 1988.
136. Haaga JR, Alfidi RJ, Zelch MG, et al: Computed tomography of the pancreas. Radiology 120:589–595, 1976.
137. Stanley RJ, Sagel SS, Levitt RG: Computed tomographic evaluation of the pancreas. Radiology 124:715–722, 1977.
138. Ohto M, Karasawa E, Tsuchiya Y, et al: Ultrasonically guided percutaneous contrast medium injection and aspiration biopsy: a real time puncture transducer. Radiology 136:171–176, 1980.
139. Rösch J, Holman DC: Superselective arteriography of the pancreas. *In* Anacker H (ed): Efficiency and Limits of Radiologic Examination of the Pancreas. Acton, MA: Publishing Sciences, 1975, pp 159–167.

# Contrast Media

| 2 |

**Jovitas Skucas, M.D.**

**ORAL CONTRAST AGENTS**
Barium Sulfate
Water-Soluble Agents
Negative Contrast Agents

**INTRAVASCULAR CONTRAST AGENTS FOR COMPUTED TOMOGRAPHY**
Basic Properties

**Contrast Agent Distribution**
**Adverse Reactions**

## ORAL CONTRAST AGENTS

### Barium Sulfate

#### Physical Characteristics

Barium sulfate is common in numerous deposits throughout the earth's crust. Some of these deposits are mined, and the barium sulfate is used in a number of manufacturing and petrochemical applications. Because of the toxic impurities in many mined barium deposits, their application is limited in medicine. Eliminating these impurities tends to be economically not feasible; it is easier to obtain barium sulfate for medical use by precipitation from other compounds, a process in which impurities can be controlled more readily.

#### Particle Size

Depending on the precipitation process, the barium sulfate particles can be made in a variety of sizes. Extremely small particles are generally used as additives in other formulations. Larger particles, from 5 to 12 μm in diameter, are commonly used in commercial "high-density" products. In fact, some of the barium formulations specifically designed for double contrast gastric studies contain a significant number of particles 18 μm or larger in diameter. Generally, products designed for gastric coating have extreme heterogeneity in particle sizes, whereas products designed for single contrast studies tend to be more homogeneous.

#### Sedimentation

Any barium sulfate formulation eventually settles out. Larger particles settle faster and form a "denser" cake than smaller particles. Thus, products that contain the larger particles tend to form a relatively hard cake at the bottom of a storage jug; considerable shaking is required to force the particles back into suspension. Some of the tall storage jugs are best stored on their side.

Sedimentation also occurs when a suspension is poured into individual cups for patients; therefore, these should be filled just before use. The barium manufacturers try to decrease the sedimentation rate through use of a number of additives, with varying degrees of success. The sedimentation rate can also be decreased by using smaller barium particles, although a decrease in particle size results in an increase in viscosity. Depending on the intended application, a product can be formulated so that the physical characteristics reflect a compromise best suited for such use.

The large particle, high-density barium suspensions designed for double contrast examinations should not be simply diluted and used for single contrast studies. When such a diluted suspension is ingested there is rapid sedimentation of the barium particles in the gastrointestinal tract. As a result, the nondependent lumen may contain little barium and lesions here may be missed. The products designed primarily for single contrast examinations can be diluted considerably before any settling occurs, mainly because of the relatively small size of the barium particles.

#### Flocculation

Flocculation is not the same as sedimentation. It is a chemical process that results in a coarse precipitate of barium particles. Manufacturers attempt to decrease flocculation by adding a number of protective agents.

Over the years, commercial barium sulfate product preparation has evolved to the point at which flocculation is now only a minor problem with commercially available products. Even in the presence of diseases such as sprue, flocculation is now rarely encountered.

#### Viscosity

Most barium sulfate products exhibit non-newtonian flow; the viscosity thus varies with flow rate. Viscosity of the various commercial products varies considerably, with different flow characteristics needed for different clinical applications. The viscosity not only determines the flow rate through tubing but also influences the subsequent mucosal coating. Ideally, a relatively thick mucosal coat is desired throughout the gastrointestinal tract; unfortunately, viscosity can be increased only to a certain point before the barium suspension starts to form a paste and coating properties are then degraded.

The terms *thick* and *thin* should be used only when referring to the actual viscosity of a suspension or solution. They should not be misused to refer to radiodensity, which is the result of many other factors.

### Additives

Numerous known and proprietary additives are present in the commercial formulations. These include stabilizing, flavoring, coating, and viscosity-varying agents. They range from natural flavors and gums, such as lemon, pectin, and guar, to synthetic products, such as the various methylcelluloses.

The flavoring agents currently employed have been adapted empirically over the years for "best" acceptance by patients. The chalk-like taste common in the past is rarely encountered today. It is surprising that some of the barium formulations designed primarily for barium enema studies also contain flavoring agents, perhaps reflecting the manufacturers' hope for more generalized use.

Although barium sulfate itself is inert and does not support bacterial growth, some of the additives are organic products. When a container is opened or reconstituted with tap water, the suspension should be refrigerated if it is to be kept overnight. Although many commercial formulations contain preservatives, bacterial growth can occur.

### Measuring Systems

Three standardized systems are used in measuring the amount of barium sulfate present in a liquid suspension. These are based on specific gravity, weight to volume, and weight to weight.

The specific gravity is the ratio of the mass of a substance to the mass of an equal volume of water.

With the weight-to-volume system, a certain weight of barium sulfate is added to sufficient water to obtain a predetermined total volume. For example, a 40% weight-to-volume (w/v) suspension is prepared by adding 40 g of barium sulfate to enough water to obtain a total volume of 100 mL.

With the weight-to-weight system, a certain weight of barium sulfate is added to enough water to obtain a predetermined final total weight. Thus, a 40% weight-to-weight (w/w) suspension is prepared by adding 40 g of barium sulfate to 60 g (60 mL) of water; the total weight is 100 g. A 100% w/w suspension represents the dry powder.

In the United States, the weight-to-volume and weight-to-weight systems are generally used. In Asia and Europe, the specific gravity method is more common. Although the three systems are interrelated, they are not easily interchangeable. Conversion tables exist to convert from one system to another[1] (Fig. 2–1). Because of differences in the amount of additives in various commercial products, some error can be introduced in the conversion of one system to another, especially at the higher densities.

### Cost

Because the commercial barium preparations are used as liquid suspensions, cost should be estimated on a per examination basis or on a volume basis. The cost of dry

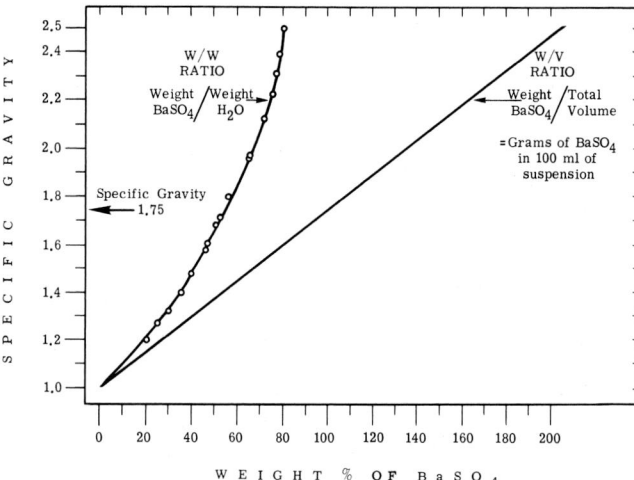

ALL PURPOSE COMPARISON CHART FOR BARIUM SULFATE SUSPENSIONS

**Figure 2–1. Conversion chart for one barium sulfate formulation.** Because there are different amounts of additives in the various commercial formulations, this chart should be used only as an approximation. The error can be significant at the higher specific gravities. (Reprinted from Radiographic Contrast Agents, 2nd ed., by J. Skucas, p 14, with permission of Aspen Publishers, Inc., © 1989.)

powder can be misleading. The cost of associated supplies, such as tubing, cups, and straws, should also be included in the total cost. Although prepackaged liquid products generally cost more per unit volume than the corresponding dry powder, when the cost of pharmacy use, mixing, and accessories is included, the liquid formulation is often comparable in cost. Yet, in spite of cost comparisons, the major factor in product selection should be the resultant examination quality.

### Ideal Suspension

Some commercial formulations are advertised as being applicable throughout the gastrointestinal tract. Invariably these represent a compromise. The gastrointestinal tract varies in pH, composition of mucus, type of mucosa, and so forth, and optimal coating in one part does not mean that a similar coating can be expected in another. Even in the same bowel segment, coating the mucosa with barium or simply opacifying the bowel lumen requires completely different barium formulations.

The ideal barium suspension that would be equally applicable throughout the gastrointestinal tract is not available. For each clinical application the suspension should not be too fluid; it should coat the mucosa sufficiently to be adequately visualized on radiographs. Once coated, the barium film should adhere to the mucosa without flocculation for a sufficiently long period to allow completion of the study.

## Clinical Application

### Pharynx

Radiographic examination of the pharynx was already established in the 1960s, when cineradiography was used to evaluate dysphagia. Although conventional "spot" radiography in the frontal and lateral projections produces the highest anatomic resolution, dynamic swallowing is best evaluated with either videofluorography or cineradiography.[2]

The indications for a pharyngogram vary considerably. In some patients the detection of aspiration may provide the etiology of chronic pneumonia. In others, differentiation between aspiration and a tracheoesophageal fistula is desired. After a stroke, the best way to feed a patient without inducing aspiration can be determined by using barium suspensions of different viscosities and barium-coated solid food.[3] In general, pharyngeal and laryngeal neoplasms are initially detected by indirect laryngoscopy; subsequent pharyngography is requested to evaluate tumor extension and is best performed by double contrast study.

Anatomic detail is studied with high-density products, such as the 250% w/v suspensions designed for gastric double contrast examinations. Fistulas are also probably best studied with such a contrast agent. A barium paste can also be used to study anatomy; the higher viscosity of the paste limits its application in fistula detection.

Pharyngeal function should be studied with both a low-viscosity and a high-viscosity barium suspension. The low-viscosity suspension should have a viscosity close to that of water, and the high-viscosity suspension should have a viscosity like that of a thick milkshake or honey. It should be emphasized that some of the high-density double contrast barium products are relatively fluid and are not applicable as high-viscosity preparations. Complicating this issue further is the observation that high-density and low-density barium suspensions, even with similar viscosities, are handled differently by the oropharynx.[4]

The volume of barium used should be individualized. Thus, in patients suspected of aspiration a several-milliliter bolus is swallowed initially; if no aspiration is detected, the bolus is gradually increased in volume. Both aspiration and a tracheoesophageal fistula are easier to detect fluoroscopically with the patient in the lateral position. If the patient is in the frontal position, when barium outlines the trachea it may not be possible to determine whether the barium was aspirated or a fistula is present (Fig. 2–2).

The choice of a low-viscosity barium formulation is least critical. Many such products are available on the market; as an alternative, a high-viscosity product can be diluted. Mucosal coating and sedimentation are not relevant for this part of the pharyngogram. The radiologist should, however, choose a product that has at least a modicum of palatable taste.

## Esophagus

In general, a study of the esophagus should include single contrast, double contrast, and mucosal relief views, together with a fluoroscopic evaluation of motility.[5] Normal esophageal tonicity leads to collapse of esophageal lumen when the primary bolus has passed.

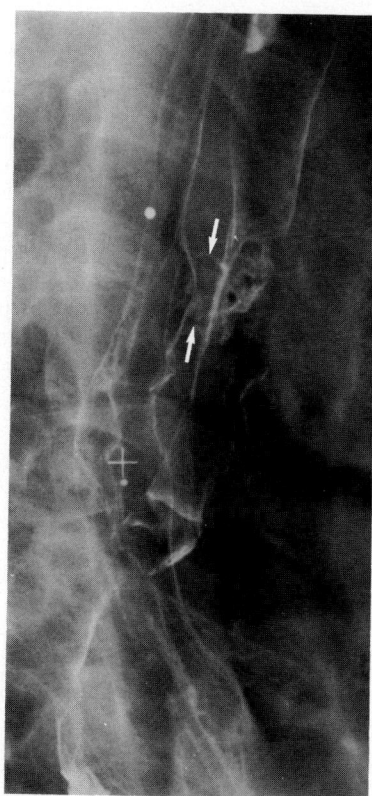

**Figure 2–2. Tracheoesophageal fistula.** The fistula *(arrows)* was best seen in the lateral position. (From Skucas J, Spataro RF: Radiology of the Acute Abdomen. Churchill Livingstone, New York, 1986, p 87.)

Therefore, regardless of which method is used, the study must be performed with reasonable dispatch.

Previous reports have suggested that some patients' symptoms could be reproduced by using a cold contrast medium or an acidic medium. Although some find acidified media useful,[6] they are not commonly employed.

In some patients with poor esophageal motility or with gastroesophageal reflux, sufficient air is introduced into the esophagus to obtain a double contrast study. In most patients, however, both a barium suspension and a negative contrast agent are necessary for a double contrast examination. The high-density, low-viscosity barium products used for the stomach and duodenum also coat the esophagus well. One useful method is to have the patient drink, in quick succession, first one and then another liquid effervescent solution, followed immediately by 60 to 120 mL of a barium suspension. The two effervescent agents distend the esophagus by releasing carbon dioxide, and the barium suspension then coats the esophageal mucosa.

Visualization of the esophagus is impaired if the barium is given before the effervescent agents. On the other hand, the quality of the gastric mucosal coating may be improved if the barium suspension is given first. Thus, optimal mucosal coating in both the esophagus and the stomach may be achieved by changing the sequence of ingestion of barium and effervescent agents.

With most patients, the sequence of ingestion can be tailored to the patient's primary symptoms: if disease involving the esophagus is suspected, the effervescent agents are given first; if gastroduodenal disease is suggested, the barium suspension is given first.

Esophageal varices tend to be more prominent with the esophagus collapsed. Thus, the yield of variceal detection increases if the esophagus is maintained in a collapsed state for some time. Although the high-density, low-viscosity barium products detect the more prominent esophageal varices, commercially available barium pastes are the product of choice. Some of these pastes are too viscous and tend to flow in a bolus. These should be diluted with water. The paste viscosity should be similar to that of honey.

In a patient with acute dysphagia, an esophagram can be therapeutic. With the patient in an upright position, the weight of a barium column can dislodge a foreign body into the stomach. In some patients, the addition of liquid effervescent agents increases the intraluminal pressure and aids esophageal distention, allowing a foreign body to pass into the stomach.[7] Glucagon has been proposed to help relieve spasm.[8] It is not known whether it has a significant role in acute dysphagia.

Commercial barium sulfate tablets with a diameter of 12.5 mm are available and can be used to evaluate the caliber of esophageal strictures. These tablets contain 650 mg of barium sulfate plus a number of additives. The tablets dissolve with time in either the esophagus or the stomach (Fig. 2–3). Relatively fresh tablets should be used because older tablets may take longer to dissolve.[9]

In patients with suspected esophageal perforation, it is not unusual to study the esophagus with a water-soluble agent and not see any abnormality; changing to barium sulfate may allow detection of subtle extravasation.

### Stomach and Duodenum

Occasionally, small lesions can be missed by either a single contrast or a double contrast study.[10] A combined study that also includes mucosal relief and compression views, called a biphasic examination, is commonly performed.[11] Some studies suggest that the quality of the examination is decreased in elderly patients.[12]

High-density, low-viscosity barium preparations specifically designed for the upper gastrointestinal tract produce the best double contrast results. Suspensions up to 250% w/v are available. A volume of 60 to 120 mL is generally sufficient. A good barium formulation should result in routine identification of the areae gastricae. Small cancers, ulcers, gastritis, and duodenitis should be readily detectable with a high-quality examination.

When the appropriate double contrast views have been obtained, a lower-density barium suspension can be ingested for a subsequent single contrast study. For this part of the examination, barium suspensions varying from 35 to 80% w/v are used. Various external compression paddles are available and are helpful in obtaining mucosal relief views.

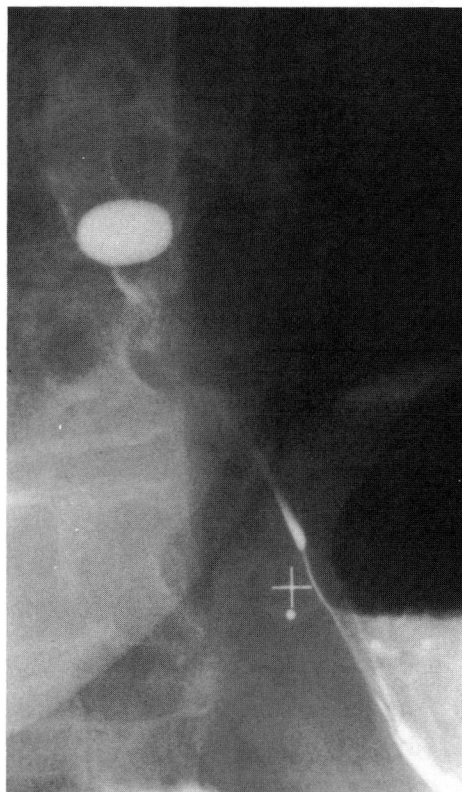

**Figure 2–3. Barium sulfate tablet proximal to a stricture.** A previous esophagram suggested narrowing at this site and the tablet confirmed this finding. (From Schabel SI, Skucas J: Esophageal obstruction following administration of "aged" barium sulfate tablets—a warning. Radiology 122:835–836, 1977.)

### Small Bowel

Four radiographic techniques are used in studying the small bowel: conventional antegrade examination, enteroclysis, retrograde ileography, and peroral pneumocolon. The type of examination performed varies with the clinical indication. Each examination requires modification of the type of barium suspension used and possible inclusion of a second contrast agent (see also Chapter 43).

#### ANTEGRADE SMALL BOWEL EXAMINATION

The antegrade examination (small bowel series) is the simplest and traditional way of studying the small bowel. Serial radiographs of the small bowel are obtained after the patient ingests a barium suspension. The primary requirement of the contrast agent is that it does not flocculate or precipitate during small bowel transit. The barium does not have to coat the mucosa well; visualization is obtained primarily by filling the bowel lumen with the radiopaque barium suspension. A 40 to 60% w/v suspension is typical. The volume required is controversial; many radiologists prefer 500 to 800 mL.

The contraindications to an antegrade barium study

are suspected colonic obstruction or bowel perforation. Small bowel obstruction is not a contraindication. Barium proximal to a small bowel obstruction continues to stay in suspension and therefore barium inspissation does not occur. In the setting of a small bowel obstruction, a study with a large volume of barium suspension is safe and can not only detect the site of obstruction but at times also suggest the etiology.

### ENTEROCLYSIS (SMALL BOWEL ENEMA)

Steerable guidewires and catheters are commercially available. These are maneuvered through the pylorus into the duodenum or proximal jejunum. The contrast agent is then injected through the catheter directly into the small bowel. The rate of injection can be controlled and the natural flow-limiting function of the pylorus thus bypassed.

The barium suspension can be infused by gravity, hand-held syringes, or a variety of infusion pumps.[13] The rate of infusion can be varied precisely with a pump. In most practices, however, such a system is not needed and injection by syringes at an appropriate rate should be adequate. Typical infusion rates are 75 to 100 mL/min, although the flow rate should be individualized. If the rate is too low, excessive peristalsis is present and the study is similar to a conventional antegrade small bowel examination. If the flow rate is too high, overdistention leads to small bowel atonia and lack of progression through the small bowel.

It is debatable whether a single contrast or double contrast enteroclysis study yields better results.[14] Water can be used as the second contrast agent, although water tends to wash off any barium sulfate particles adhering to the mucosa. For the double contrast portion of the examination, most American investigators use a 0.5% or greater solution of methylcellulose in water. The liquid methylcellulose solution helps propel a barium suspension ahead of it. The total volume of the two contrast agents is tailored for each examination. In some patients, up to 2 L may be required. The contrast agents are instilled until either a lesion is detected or the agents reach the right colon. If needed, glucagon can be administered to produce hypotonia.

Air as a second contrast agent is used more commonly by Japanese and some European investigators. It results in considerably more radiographic contrast than is obtainable with methylcellulose. Air does not propel the barium ahead of it as much as the methylcellulose solution; it tends to percolate through the barium-filled loops of small bowel.

Some investigators believe that small fistulas and polyps are not as well seen if air is used.[15] Air bubbles can result in confusing shadows. Others believe that better diagnostic results are achieved with air even in patients with inflammatory bowel disease.[16] With overlapping loops of bowel, as are commonly encountered in the pelvis, infusion of air can be helpful.

Barium sulfate formulations specifically designed for enteroclysis are commercially available. For a single contrast study, a barium sulfate suspension having a specific gravity of 1.27 (equivalent to approximately 34% w/v) is preferred. For a double contrast study, a barium suspension of a higher specific gravity is used. A range of 50 to 95% w/v is typical.[17, 18]

### RETROGRADE ILEOGRAPHY

In this examination, initially a single contrast barium enema is performed, but the infusion of barium is then continued retrogradely into the ileum. Because flow can be controlled by the examiner, the ileum can be readily studied without overlapping loops from more proximal small bowel. Premedication with glucagon increases the patient's comfort and also relaxes the ileocecal valve. In one double-blind barium study, approximately half the patients received glucagon and half did not.[19] Of 52 patients not given glucagon, 15 achieved barium reflux into the ileum. Of 50 patients who did receive glucagon, 37 had reflux into the ileum. The barium suspension is instilled until the area in question is reached. If a redundant sigmoid colon obscures part of the small bowel, the barium enema can be followed by a saline solution; such a solution pushes the barium ahead of it and leads to a see-through effect. A 20% w/v or somewhat greater concentration of barium is typical in retrograde ileography.

It is not unusual to achieve a double contrast study of the terminal ileum whenever a double contrast barium enema is performed, especially if glucagon is used.[19] Such a study is useful for suspected distal ileal Crohn's disease or gynecologic malignancies involving the ileum.[20]

### PERORAL PNEUMOCOLON

This study consists of both antegrade and retrograde components. Either the distal ileum or the right side of the colon can be studied. Initially a conventional antegrade small bowel examination is performed. When barium outlines the terminal ileum, air is instilled through the rectum to obtain a double contrast examination of the distal small bowel or proximal colon.[21] This study can also be combined with enteroclysis.

## Colon

Both single contrast and double contrast techniques are well established. Some radiologists prefer a single contrast study in elderly or debilitated patients.[22] Most double contrast examinations require that the patient lie prone for at least part of the time; in patients who cannot lie prone a single contrast examination is thus performed. A double contrast study can, however, be readily performed in elderly patients.[23] Unfortunately, inadequate bowel preparation continues to plague this examination[24] and direct supervision of the preparation process by the radiologist is mandatory.

Numerous studies have compared the relative accuracy of a single contrast versus a double contrast barium enema, generally evaluating specific findings. A summary of many of the earlier studies has been published.[25]

Quite often the technique of examination is different between the two studies. In many comparison studies it is not mentioned whether any pharmacologic agent has been used.

Disposable, barium-prefilled enema bags are available from several vendors. Some bags contain the barium in powder form and one simply adds the correct amount of water. These bags must be shaken vigorously and for a prolonged time to achieve adequate wetting of the barium particles. After such shaking, the bags should be kept on their sides; even then, considerable settling can occur if the bags are kept for some time before use.

Both dry and liquid commercial barium formulations are available. If the dry barium formulation is used, the amount of water added and degree of subsequent shaking to achieve wettability should be standardized. In particular, the level marking generally inscribed on the enema bag should not be used to gauge the amount of water needed; the resultant dilutions tend to be erratic. Rather, the amount of water needed to achieve the desired specific gravity should be measured with a graduated container.

The same commercial barium preparation should not be used for both the single contrast and the double contrast studies. The primary aim in a double contrast study is to achieve good mucosal coating. For the single contrast study, on the other hand, the aim is to achieve a homogeneous barium particle suspension throughout the bowel lumen. The low concentration of barium used for the single contrast examination is insufficient to produce good mucosal coating.

### SINGLE CONTRAST BARIUM ENEMA

A 12 to 25% w/v barium suspension is commonly used for a single contrast barium enema. The main requirement of the barium suspension is that it not flocculate or settle while the examination is in progress.

Most commercial formulations designed for single contrast examinations consist of small barium sulfate particles. Because the sedimentation rate also depends, in part, on the amount and type of additives present, some products that are well suspended at higher concentrations settle readily when diluted. If there is any doubt about a commercial product's sedimentation rate, a radiograph obtained with a horizontal x-ray beam will reveal any tendency toward settling.

### DOUBLE CONTRAST BARIUM ENEMA

Barium suspensions designed for double contrast barium enemas should have relatively high concentrations of barium but still be sufficiently fluid to flow readily through enema tubing. The mucosal coating should be uniform without significant artifacts. The suspension should not dry out during the time the examination is performed. These barium formulations are generally 60 to 120% w/v. Of necessity, their viscosity is greater than that of the lower-concentration barium formulations designed for single contrast studies.

Even when all conditions for use are standardized, the subsequent mucosal coating can vary from one radiology practice to another. Variations in local water hardness and the type of water used (distilled water or cold or hot tap water) influence the suspension's physical characteristics and subsequent mucosal coating. To avoid such variations, the manufacturers sell premixed liquid formulations. The barium suspension is simply poured into an enema bag without further dilution. Because of a tendency of the barium particles to settle out, vigorous shaking of the barium jugs before dispensing is required. With some of the tall jugs currently available, faster resuspension can be achieved if the jugs are routinely stored on their side rather than upright.

The relatively high viscosity of these products can lead to slow flow through the enema tubing, especially if narrow diameter tubing is used. As a result, the examination time can be prolonged. Large bore tubing, such as 12.5 mm diameter, is commercially available. Some manufacturers have introduced so-called low-viscosity barium preparations. The lower viscosity is achieved simply by using less barium sulfate and by other changes in the additives. Unfortunately, some of these products result in a rather thin and suboptimal mucosal coating by barium.

Some radiologists perform colonic lavage before a barium enema. Such lavage invariably results in water retention and subsequent dilution of the barium suspension. Some of the barium manufacturers recognize this difference and market two slightly different preparations; the one designed to be used after colonic lavage has a barium suspension of slightly greater specific gravity.

## Use in Computed Tomography

A full-strength barium sulfate preparation should not be diluted to the low concentrations needed for computed tomography (CT). The barium sulfate particles tend to settle out after ingestion of such a diluted preparation, leading to inhomogeneous opacification of the bowel lumen; the uppermost portion of a loop of bowel may not contain enough barium for visualization, while excess barium in the dependent portion can result in streak artifacts.

Barium manufacturers have recognized the need for a stable but rather low concentration barium formulation in CT and have developed appropriate contrast agents. Most oral CT products contain rather small barium sulfate particles that resist settling. The additives used also prevent barium sedimentation. Generally a 1 to 3% w/v barium sulfate suspension is used and several such products are commercially available.

Patients accept barium contrast agents better than the corresponding iodinated products. Both result in similar bowel opacification. At the low concentrations used, the barium particles do not coat the mucosa but simply opacify the lumen. Because of the better acceptance by patients, many investigators prefer the barium sulfate suspensions except when bowel perforation is suspected.

In CT evaluation of the thorax it is useful to outline the esophagus with contrast agent. The low-concentration, low-viscosity agents used in the rest of the gastrointestinal tract do not coat the esophageal mucosa long enough. As a result, a high-viscosity, low-concentration barium paste has been developed for coating the esophagus.[26] High viscosity is achieved by use of various nonopaque additives; mucosal adherence of the mixture is sufficiently long that a typical examination can be completed. Another option is to have the patient drink small sips of a conventional CT contrast agent before each scan.

One way to opacify the stomach and small bowel is to have the patient drink approximately 500 mL of the dilute CT contrast agent several hours before the examination. A similar amount is ingested immediately before the scan. In most patients, the stomach, small bowel, and varying amounts of colon are opacified enough that the bowel can be differentiated from surrounding structures.

If colonic distention is needed, a dilute contrast enema can be administered before the scan. Generally, 150 to 250 mL is sufficient to outline the rectosigmoid. Larger amounts are required if the proximal colon is to be opacified or if colonic distention is needed.

## Toxicity and Complications

Barium sulfate is a white crystalline powder having a molecular weight of 233. Because of its specific gravity of 4.5, patients often observe that a cup of barium suspension is "heavy." It is poorly soluble in water. It is not surprising, however, that a portion of any soluble barium is absorbed from the gastrointestinal tract. Atomic absorption spectrometry reveals that after oral ingestion of a commercial barium sulfate preparation, approximately $0.2 \times 10^{-6}$ of the ingested dose is subsequently excreted via the urinary tract.[27] Such minuscule absorption should be viewed as an example of equipment sophistication rather than an indication of any toxicity.

The constipating tendency of barium sulfate is well known to most radiologists. Through the judicious use of various additives, this possible complication can be minimized with most present-day formulations.

### Barium Aspiration

Aspiration of small amounts of commercial barium formulations should be of little clinical significance. Although initially readily identifiable on radiographs, such barium clears the major bronchi and trachea within hours. Aspiration of any fluid, including a barium suspension, can obviously result in pneumonia or compromise of pulmonary function.

After barium aspiration, most of the barium is cleared, although some is retained in the interstitium and in macrophages. This residue is generally not visualized on radiographs. Alveolarization of barium, however, can result in prolonged retention.[28]

In any patient, if aspiration is suspected clinically, barium sulfate rather than one of the ionic contrast agents is preferred. The place of the nonionic agents in a setting of aspiration is still not clear.

### Hypersensitivity

Hypersensitivity reactions during gastrointestinal examinations have been rare, although lately the reported incidence has increased. Most reactions are mild and consist of urticaria or pruritus. Erythema multiforme, respiratory complications, anaphylaxis, and death[29] have been reported. Patients with a history of asthma may be at increased risk for these reactions.[30] Gastrointestinal angioedema has been reported during an apparent allergic reaction to a barium suspension.[31]

Previously, the incidence of reactions was about equal in upper gastrointestinal examinations and barium enemas,[32] but currently reactions to the latter have increased. The incidence of reactions appears to be more commonly associated with a double contrast than a single contrast study. Any possible role of the effervescent agents in these reactions is speculative.

Theoretically, barium sulfate should be inert. The commercial barium preparations, however, contain numerous additives. These consist of naturally occurring substances and also synthetic materials, such as the celluloses. Older radiologists are familiar with chocolate-flavored barium products; these are not longer used because of the relatively common allergy to chocolate.

For many years methylparaben (methyl-*p*-hydroxybenzoate) and similar compounds were used as preservatives. Methylparaben-induced hypersensitivity reactions occur,[33] but currently the commercial barium manufacturers have replaced it by other, more innocuous preservatives. In spite of this, hypersensitivity reactions have continued.[34]

Some reactions have occurred even before barium sulfate was instilled. Such agents as the natural latex used in some enema balloons have been implicated in these reactions.[35, 36] In 1990 the major manufacturer of barium sulfate products in the United States recalled all enema tips containing natural latex balloons.

There is an extensive literature on allergy to latex. The offending antigen in latex is believed to be a water-soluble protein that is heat stable. It is found on the surface of the cured latex and probably is a contaminant of the natural latex when it is obtained from the *Hevea brasiliensis* tree. Latex gloves are commonly used and can result in sensitization. Contact with skin has been associated with urticaria, and subsequent contact with mucous membranes can lead to more severe anaphylactic reactions.[37] It is thought that the offending protein can be removed by prolonged washing. Currently, nonlatex and synthetic latex balloons are available on the market.

Occasional hypersensitivity reactions have also been reported after intravenous injection of glucagon.

The etiology of many hypersensitivity reactions during a barium study is not known. In general, the incriminating agent has not been sought and no further testing has been performed in most patients who do have a reaction.

### Extraperitoneal Perforation

Esophageal perforation and spill of barium into the mediastinum result in an immediate inflammatory reaction, followed by eventual fibrosis. Barium can persist in the mediastinum for prolonged periods. Such prior extravasation into the mediastinal soft tissues can be recognized radiographically as dense linear radiopacities. In spite of such obvious radiographic visualization, there is no solid evidence that the pathologic sequelae are significantly more severe than with the water-soluble agents.

Most extraperitoneal perforations associated with a barium enema occur in the rectum and are not immediately detected by fluoroscopy. Most such perforations have been associated with injudicious insufflation of the enema balloon. Two decades ago, a survey in Australia and New Zealand found one extraperitoneal perforation for every 40,000 barium enemas performed.[38]

Barium in the perirectal tissues incites an inflammatory reaction that eventually results in fibrosis. Such progressive fibrosis can narrow the rectosigmoid lumen and mimic a carcinoma. There is, however, no convincing evidence that such barium in the soft tissues is a carcinogen (Fig. 2–4).

Barium intravasation can occur into either the systemic veins or the portal venous system. Some of these patients have no predisposing factors to account for the intravasation. The mortality rate is greater than 50%.[39]

With a chronic or loculated perforation, the higher radiographic visibility of barium sulfate can yield more information than is obtained with the water-soluble contrast agents. Thus, a chronic abscess or other cavity that is in continuity with the bowel lumen can be safely studied with barium sulfate. If there is a possible communication with the peritoneal cavity, however, the water-soluble agents are preferred and barium sulfate is generally contraindicated.

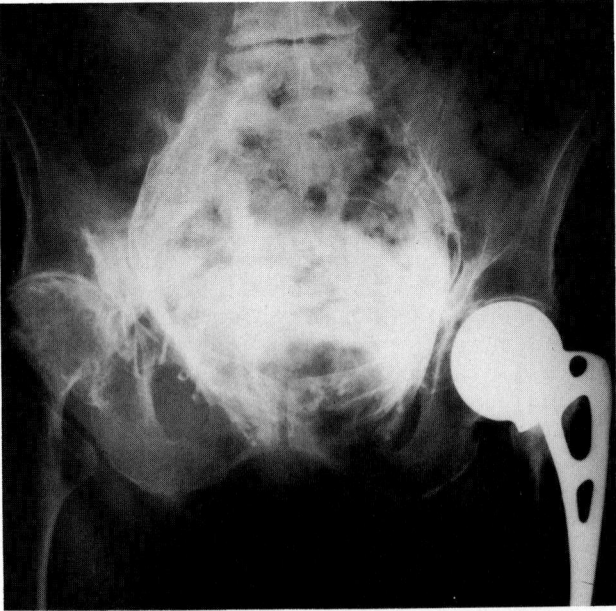

**Figure 2–4. Prior colon perforation during a barium enema.** The barium should now be encased by dense adhesions that also involve bowel. (Reprinted from Radiographic Contrast Agents by R. E. Miller and J. Skucas, p 137, with permission of Aspen Publishers, Inc., © 1977.)

### Barium Peritonitis

The incidence of acute barium peritonitis after a barium radiographic study is not known. The resultant mortality is significant and in some reviews has approached 50%. Even sterile barium sulfate introduced into the peritoneal cavity results in peritonitis. Spill of barium into the peritoneal cavity can be secondary to a preprocedure perforation, such as an ulcer. Some perforations, however, occur during the barium study and have been reported to occur during an upper gastrointestinal examination, during a barium enema, and even during enteroclysis.[40]

Initially, there is a concentration of leukocytes in the peritoneal cavity, together with a marked inpouring of fluid, and eventually the barium crystals become coated by a fibrin membrane. The additional introduction of bacterial contamination during the perforation can result in overwhelming sepsis and shock within hours. If the massive inpouring of fluid into the peritoneal cavity is untreated, the patient can develop profound hypovolemia.

The immediate management of barium peritonitis includes infusion of a relatively large volume of intravenous fluid. Antibiotics are commonly administered because of possible associated bacterial contamination. Most of these patients undergo surgery, in which the site of perforation is closed and an attempt is made to evacuate barium from the peritoneal cavity. Invariably, there is considerable residual barium that cannot be removed. The barium crystals are embedded on the peritoneal surface and resist dislodgement. Attempts to remove the barium particles with a wet sponge result in diffuse bleeding from the peritoneum. The residual barium can be subsequently well defined by either conventional radiography or CT.

Extensive fibrosis and granulomatous formation develop if the patient survives the acute episode. As with an extraperitoneal perforation, the dense fibrosis can involve adjacent structures; depending on the location of the contrast agent, subsequent ureteral obstruction or bowel deformity and stenosis may develop.

## Water-Soluble Agents

### Indications

The water-soluble organic iodine compounds designed for use in the gastrointestinal tract were introduced in the 1950s. Since then, there has been considerable controversy about the relative merit of these agents and their role in the gastrointestinal tract. These agents do not coat the gastrointestinal mucosa; rather, they allow bowel visualization by passive filling of the intestinal lumen.

For most examinations, experienced radiologists generally find the choice between barium and the water-soluble agents straightforward. Some surgeons, however, were taught by their seniors about the purported dangers of barium sulfate in the small or large bowel and insist on the use of water-soluble agents. In general, the water-soluble agents are preferred more often by surgeons than by radiologists, although exceptions exist. The stimulation of peristalsis in postoperative patients and the lack of radiographically visible sequelae of spill from the gastrointestinal tract are additional reasons why some surgeons prefer water-soluble agents.

Water-soluble agents are indicated if an acute perforation is suspected. The examination generally either confirms or excludes a perforation. Small perforations can, however, be missed. Likewise, walled-off perforations or a perforation in an area of spasm can be difficult to detect. Occasionally, visualization of an abnormality with a water-soluble medium is insufficient and in some patients it may be necessary to complete the examination with barium.

## Contraindications

In young children and in adults with hypovolemia, the introduction of large volumes of a hypertonic agent into the gastrointestinal tract can result in further hypovolemia, shock, and possibly death. In such a clinical setting, adequate intravascular fluid replacement and, where appropriate, use of a nonionic contrast agent should be considered.

If aspiration or an esophagotracheal fistula is suspected, use of the hyperosmolar ionic contrast agents is contraindicated because they can cause pneumonia, pulmonary edema, or death. The nonionic agents may be reasonable substitutes in some patients. In most adults, however, barium sulfate is the preferred contrast agent.

## Ionic Agents

In general, to achieve adequate radiographic opacification of most structures at least a 60% solution of the ionic contrast agents is needed. The resultant iodine concentration is 282 to 292 mg/mL for the more commonly used commercial products.[41] The resultant osmolality ranges from 1400 to 1540 mOsm/kg, or approximately five times that of serum. Because of this hyperosmolarity, fluid is drawn into the bowel lumen. Diarrhea is common after their use. All patients, but especially infants, should be well hydrated when these agents are used.

Because the ionic contrast agents stimulate intestinal peristalsis, faster visualization of the distal small bowel can be achieved than with barium sulfate. The need for such a faster examination should be balanced against the decreased radiographic contrast and resolution obtained with these agents. In general, best results are obtained in the stomach and proximal small bowel; intraluminal dilution leads to poor visualization of the ileum. When these agents are used to study the small bowel, radiographs should be obtained more frequently than when a similar study is performed with barium; invariably the transit time is shorter.

## Nonionic Agents

The available nonionic contrast agents with an iodine concentration of approximately 300 mg/mL have an os-

molality of 600 to 710 mOsm/kg, which is less than half that of the ionic agents. At this concentration, however, they are still hyperosmolar compared to serum.

The nonionic contrast agents are preferred because of their lower osmolarity. Ideally, one of the nonionic agents should be used whenever a water-soluble agent is indicated. Their high cost, however, precludes use in most adults. If a perforation into the pleural or peritoneal cavity is suspected in an adult, the nonionic agents probably do not offer any significant advantage over their ionic counterparts. In neonates or young children, on the other hand, the nonionic agents are generally preferred if there is a question of perforation. In routine studies of the gastrointestinal tract in infants and children in which perforation was not at issue, a study comparing iohexol and barium concluded that barium is the preferred contrast agent.[42]

In a neonate with suspected necrotizing enterocolitis, radiologists still use barium for the contrast enema. The nonionic agents are the contrast agents of choice, however, if there is a risk of perforation.

## Use in Computed Tomography

Dilute solutions of the ionic water-soluble contrast agents have been extensively used in CT. Ideally, such an agent should readily differentiate bowel from surrounding structures without any significant artifacts. The major limitation of the water-soluble agents is their poor taste and hence poor acceptance by patients, especially children and cancer patients. When instilled through a nasogastric tube or used in an enema, however, they produce adequate bowel opacification.

Some of the commercial contrast agents, such as the diatrizoate meglumine preparations Gastrografin and oral Hypaque, contain flavoring agents. These are preferred to their counterpart nonflavored products designed primarily for intravenous use. Some radiologists add fruit juice or other flavoring to improve their taste further.

Most radiologists use a 2 to 5% solution of Gastrografin or similar agent. At such dilution, the solution is hyposmolar, yet some patients still develop diarrhea after the examination.

If the indication for a CT examination is suspected pelvic disease, the patient can drink a contrast agent the evening before the examination. In such a situation, even 20 to 30 mL of full-strength Gastrografin can be ingested; overnight dilution within the bowel should be sufficient to eliminate most streak artifacts. There is better opacification of the rectosigmoid with ingestion of such a full-strength water-soluble contrast agent than with dilute barium, probably because of the hyperperistalsis induced by the full-strength ionic contrast agent.

At the dilutions used in CT, the nonionic contrast agents do not have any real advantage over the ionic agents. In addition, no flavored nonionic contrast agent specifically designed for oral use is currently available in the United States.

## Negative Contrast Agents

### *Conventional Radiography*

When performing double contrast gastrointestinal studies, by far the cheapest second contrast agent is air. In fact, in such applications as double contrast barium enemas and upper gastrointestinal studies using nasogastric tubes, air is the preferred agent. Excellent double contrast esophageal views can be obtained if the patient swallows air together with the barium preparation. Such a study can be performed by having the patient drink a barium suspension through a large bore straw containing side holes that draw in air.[43] With the patient in a prone position, small swallows of barium tend to produce gastroesophageal reflux of air.[44]

In one commercial preparation, an attempt was made to incorporate carbon dioxide directly in the barium suspension; when the can was opened, the patient drank the "bubbly barium," thus releasing carbon dioxide into the esophagus and stomach. The effect was similar to that of drinking a bottle of club soda. The amount of gas produced with the product was less than with conventional effervescent agents, and this product did not achieve ready acceptance.[45]

Effervescent tablets, granules, and powders are commercially available. They produce carbon dioxide on contact with water and most are satisfactory in achieving adequate gastric and duodenal distention. There is, however, considerable variation in the dissolution time of the various products; whenever evaluating a new product, it is best to experiment with the amount to be used until a satisfactory result is achieved.

Most of the commercial effervescent powders and granules come in single-dose packages. In clinical use, the patient places the effervescent agent in the mouth and uses small amounts of water to wash it down. This is immediately followed by the barium suspension. Double contrast views of the esophagus are then obtained. The swallowed gas can subsequently be used to obtain double contrast radiographs of the stomach and duodenum.

Liquid effervescent agents are available commercially or can be prepared locally by a hospital pharmacy. One manufacturer provides a built-in measuring cup for accurate volume dispensing of the separate acid and base solutions. In general, the acid consists of citric or tartaric acid and the base portion is sodium bicarbonate. A dose of 12 to 15 mL is satisfactory for most patients.

Carbon dioxide can be used in place of air in double contrast barium enemas. Carbon dioxide is absorbed faster than air from the gut lumen and is thought to result in greater comfort of the patient. Of 151 patients who were randomly assigned to either a carbon dioxide or an air category, 11% of the carbon dioxide–insufflated patients had pain and 30% of the air-insufflated patients had similar pain.[46] Patients in both groups received 1 mg of glucagon intravenously. The type of gas or air used probably does not influence the quality of the examination.

Some double contrast preparations result in excessive gas bubbles that can interfere with diagnosis. If excessive bubbles occur on a regular basis, an antifoam agent should be added empirically. Although many commercial barium preparations already include such an agent, in some localities the amount is not sufficient. A commonly such used antifoam agent is dimethyl polysiloxane (simethicone); addition of 1.5 mL of simethicone (equivalent to 100 mg) is often sufficient.

### *Computed Tomography*

Residual gas in the bowel often serves as a marker, especially in the colon. If a nasogastric tube is in place, air can be injected into the stomach and small bowel. With some of the earlier scanners, excessive air in the stomach resulted in streak artifacts; these have been essentially eliminated with most of the current fast scanners. If significant amounts of gas are present, filming with window settings slightly wider than usual can be helpful.

In the past, a number of products containing fat, such as mineral oil, have been proposed.[47] These have limited current application.

For a discussion of contrast agents used for magnetic resonance studies of the gastrointestinal tract, see Chapter 9.

## INTRAVASCULAR CONTRAST AGENTS FOR COMPUTED TOMOGRAPHY

### Basic Properties

In CT, a number of structures can be outlined in the abdomen without the introduction of any contrast agent. Yet, as with the use of oral contrast agents to define the bowel, opacification of blood vessels is advantageous in a number of clinical settings. For instance, opacification of the liver vasculature with a contrast agent allows identification of metastases that have a different vascularity compared with surrounding normal liver parenchyma. Differentiation of the major intrahepatic vessels from bile ducts can be achieved with greater certainty if intravascular contrast agents are employed. In the extraperitoneal para-aortic regions, an intravascular contrast agent is helpful in differentiating between blood vessels and lymph nodes.

The relative attenuation of an x-ray beam passing through soft tissue depends primarily on two factors: the Compton effect, which predominates with the body soft tissues, and the photoelectric effect, which predominates when x-rays interact with iodine. As with conventional radiography, at the energies used in CT the mass attenuation coefficient for iodine is considerably greater than that for the surrounding soft tissues or blood. Thus, after intravascular injection of an iodinated contrast agent, CT images initially reveal enhancement of the aorta and associated arterial structures, followed by a capillary or parenchymal "blush" and eventually opacification of the venous structures, including the vena cava. Thus, the rate of injection of contrast agent and timing of the subsequent CT scans determine the structures that are enhanced on any one image. A number of strategies of contrast agent administration for CT have been developed. Rapid bolus injection, slow infusion during part or all of the scanning time, or various combinations of the two can be used effectively, with the specific strategy adopted depending on the clinical questions to be answered by the examination. These various techniques of intravascular contrast agent administration are not covered here but are discussed elsewhere in the book (see Chapters 8 and 80).

From a simplistic viewpoint, the various intravascular contrast agents currently available in clinical practice can be viewed merely as vehicles that deliver a certain concentration of iodine to the blood vessel or structure in question. The complex delivery molecules that have evolved over the years simply represent an attempt to deliver the greatest concentration of iodine with the least possible toxicity.

The initially developed intravascular contrast agents had only one iodine atom per molecule. The next major advance was introduction of the acetrizoates, which are triiodobenzoate derivatives; these contrast agents have been in general angiographic and urographic use for years.

## Ionic Contrast Agents

Ionic contrast agents are formulated as salts and consist of a cation and an anion. The two commonly used cations are sodium and meglumine. The anion portion of the molecule consists of a benzene ring containing iodine substituted at positions 2, 4, and 6 plus a number of other side chains. These side chains determine the overall water solubility and indirectly affect the resultant toxicity of the compound. The benzene ring can be viewed as a scaffold for the iodine and other associated side chains. These compounds are highly hypertonic at concentrations useful for vascular opacification, and considerable effort has been spent in an attempt to decrease their osmolality.

In general, the sodium salt tends to be more toxic than the corresponding meglumine salt. On the other hand, the viscosity of the sodium salt is less than that of the corresponding meglumine salt. As a result, for various selective angiographic applications either one or a mixture of the cations has been preferred by angiographers to achieve the low toxicity and low viscosity needed. The toxicity and viscosity limitations encountered in direct intra-arterial injections are not as relevant with the intravenous injections used with CT, in which much lower intravascular and parenchymal concentrations of iodine can be readily quantified than in conventional radiography.

All currently available ionic monomer contrast agents have a carboxyl attachment at position 1. The cation, as mentioned, can be either sodium or a meglumine salt. Thus, when the molecule dissociates, three iodine atoms are available for every two particles in solution, or a ratio of 1.5.

Further refinements of ionic contrast media include the attachment of two monomer triiodinated benzene rings at one of their side groups. Such a dimer, containing two benzene rings with each having three iodine atoms and only one cation particle, thus has six iodine atoms per two particles, or a ratio of 3 (Fig. 2–5).

## Nonionic Contrast Agents

If the carboxyl group in position 1 on the benzene ring is replaced with a stable side group, the molecule no longer dissociates when in solution. As a result, there are three iodine atoms per particle in solution for these monomer-type nonionic contrast agents. They have a ratio of 3. A dimer structure can also be achieved by eliminating the single carboxyl group from the paired benzene ring, thus achieving six iodine atoms per particle, or a ratio of 6.

Various manufacturers have taken different approaches to the type of side chains used with both the ionic and nonionic contrast agents. As a result, there are differences in viscosities among these compounds. Within limits, however, for each group of contrast media the viscosity varies directly with the iodine concentration. The interaction with other molecules also differs between the ionic and nonionic agents and is affected by the type of side branches present.

## Contrast Agent Distribution

After intravascular injection, both ionic and nonionic contrast agents are eventually distributed throughout the extracellular space. They are then excreted by glomerular filtration by the kidneys. There have been

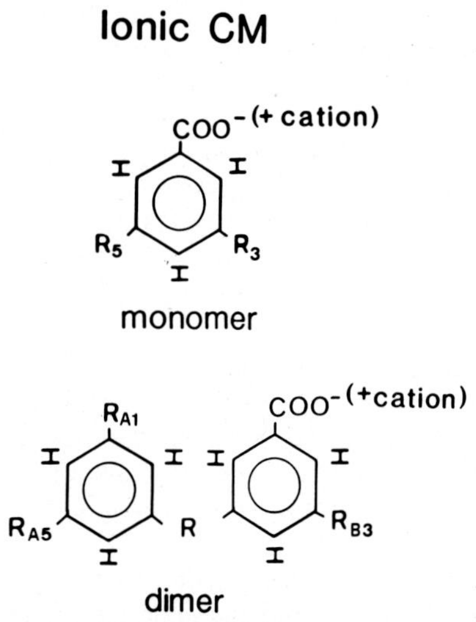

**Figure 2–5. Molecular structure of the monomeric and dimeric forms of contrast media in use today.** Changes in the R groups of the molecules greatly affect solubility, viscosity, and toxicity. (Reprinted from Radiographic Contrast Agents, 2nd ed., by J. Skucas (ed), p 123, with permission of Aspen Publishers, Inc., © 1989.)

numerous studies of the relative time-dependent blood iodine concentrations and renal excretion of the various contrast agents. Spataro has summarized this topic.[48]

Dynamic CT scanning after a single bolus injection relies on enhancement of the vascular structures above baseline. Depending on the clinical indication, it is desirable to have a sufficient iodine concentration in the vascular structures of interest to elevate them above baseline by up to 100 Hounsfield units. With such a degree of enhancement, major vessel thrombosis can be detected and vascular fistulas and related conditions evaluated. A relatively large caliber venous catheter and a power injector allow reproducible intravascular injection rates. Power injection through a central venous catheter at a rate of 1 mL/s has been proposed as a safe procedure.[49] Patency of the catheter can be checked by manual saline injection.

A typical sequence is a scan before contrast agent injection, followed by scanning after the initial bolus has arrived in the structure of interest. Contrast agent arrives in the renal veins considerably sooner than in the infrarenal inferior vena cava. The prediction of bolus arrival in a structure is somewhat empirical because, among other factors, decreased cardiac output can result in prolonged vascular flow times.

Whether early dynamic scanning is superior to delayed scanning after contrast agent equilibration depends on the clinical information desired.

## Adverse Reactions

### Types of Reactions

The risk of serious adverse reactions is quite low with both ionic and nonionic contrast agents.[50] These reactions can vary from minor effects that require no therapy to life-threatening, severe reactions. In general, reactions such as nausea, vomiting, a flushing sensation, or otherwise asymptomatic hives do not require any therapy. Moderate reactions, such as mild changes in blood pressure or mild wheezing, may be self-limited or may progress to more severe reactions. Unless such a reaction is self-limited, an intravenous line should be established early. The catheter used for contrast agent injection can be kept in place, ensuring intravascular access, until the possibility of a reaction has passed. With progressive hypotension it becomes increasingly difficult to find a peripheral vein.

Severe reactions, such as severe bronchospasm, convulsions, or significant cardiopulmonary reactions, require prompt therapy. Any physician injecting a contrast agent intravascularly can expect to encounter the broad spectrum from mild to severe reactions and must be prepared to deal with them.

Serious reactions, including death, have occurred with both ionic and nonionic agents. The overall rate of adverse reactions with the nonionic agents, however, appears to be less than that encountered with ionic agents. Because of this, some radiologists have adopted a policy of administering nonionic agents to patients in certain high-risk groups. Other radiologists have chosen empirically to administer the nonionic agents to all patients, in spite of the considerably higher cost. The American College of Radiology has established guidelines for situations in which it believes that the nonionic agents are preferred[51] (Table 2–1).

## Premedication

Premedication should be considered for patients who have had a previous reaction to a contrast agent. Regimens that have been proposed in the literature range from 3 days before the examination to immediately before the scan. At the University of Rochester, we currently recommend that patients who have had a significant prior reaction to intravenous contrast agents be pretreated as follows:

1. 50 mg prednisone orally every 12 hours for a total of three doses; the last dose should be given approximately 1 hour before the procedure.
2. 25 to 50 mg diphenhydramine hydrochloride (Benadryl) orally, 2 hours before the procedure.

In a multi-institutional study involving ionic contrast agents, Lasser and colleagues pretreated patients with corticosteroids before intravenous contrast studies.[52] They found that pretreatment with methylprednisolone, 32 mg, 12 hours and 2 hours before administration of an intravenous contrast agent, significantly reduced the incidence of reactions. In fact, they found that with the two-dose regimen the incidence of contrast reactions in patients receiving ionic contrast agents approximated that seen with the nonionic agents and no pretreatment.

Although seizures after intravenous contrast agent injection are rare, the incidence increases in patients with brain metastases. The capillaries in brain metastases do not exhibit normal blood-brain barrier integrity and are permeable to the contrast agent. It has been suggested that these patients be premedicated with diazepam, 5 mg intravenously, before contrast agent administration to decrease the risk of seizure.[53]

---

**TABLE 2–1. SUMMARY OF AMERICAN COLLEGE OF RADIOLOGY GUIDELINES FOR THE USE OF LOWER-OSMOLALITY CONTRAST AGENTS**

1. History of a previous adverse reaction to contrast material, with the exception of a sensation of heat, flushing, or a single episode of nausea or vomiting
2. History of asthma or allergy
3. Known cardiac dysfunction, including cardiac decompensation, severe arrhythmias, unstable angina, recent myocardial infarction, and pulmonary hypertension
4. Generalized debilitation
5. Any other circumstance in which the radiologist believes there is an indication to use lower-osmolality contrast agents

From American College of Radiology Committee on Drugs and Contrast Media: Appendix A—report of the current criteria for the use of water soluble contrast agents for intravenous injections. *In* Manual on Iodinated Contrast Media. Reston, VA: American College of Radiology, 1991, pp 27–29.

## *Therapy*

In general, mild reactions such as flushing or mild urticaria require no treatment and most reactions resolve spontaneously. Likewise, nausea and vomiting require general support and observation only. In some patients, however, these mild symptoms can progress to more severe reactions, so the patient should be monitored closely. If these symptoms occur before all of the contrast agent has been administered, either the rate of injection should be slowed or the injection postponed until the symptoms clear.

Moderate urticaria developing in the absence of any other significant symptoms should be treated with diphenhydramine 25 to 50 mg, given orally or injected intramuscularly or intravenously. With a moderate or severe urticarial reaction, one should also consider an $H_2$ blocking agent such as cimetidine (Tagamet), 300 mg injected slowly (diluted) intravenously. For severe urticaria, epinephrine, 0.1 to 0.3 mL (1:1000) should be given subcutaneously unless contraindicated. If needed, the dose can be repeated in 15 minutes. Epinephrine, however, should be used with caution in elderly patients, who may have significant cardiovascular disease. Electrocardiographic monitoring should be considered early for these patients.

Bronchospasm and laryngeal edema generally respond to subcutaneous epinephrine. If needed, the epinephrine dose can be repeated. Diphenhydramine and corticosteroids, such as hydrocortisone, 100 to 300 mg intravenously, are also often employed. Oxygen should be administered by mask or nasal cannula. Beta-agonist inhalers alone may be successful in mild bronchospasm or can be used in conjunction with aminophylline therapy. With refractory bronchospasm, aminophylline, 250 to 400 mg diluted in dextrose and water, can be administered intravenously over a 10- to 20-minute period. Aminophylline should be used with caution because it may exacerbate coexisting hypotension. Tracheal intubation should be considered early in the course of these symptoms; later, severe laryngeal edema may make intubation difficult if not impossible.

The initial therapy for moderately severe hypotension should be oxygen and rapid infusion of isotonic intravenous fluids. Epinephrine should be considered. Although subcutaneous injections are adequate for a mild to moderate reaction, intravenous administration is needed for moderate to severe hypotension. For intravenous administration, epinephrine should be diluted to 1:10,000; 1.0 to 3.0 mL should be administered slowly. If needed, the dose can be repeated in 15 minutes. The rate of injection can be titrated to achieve the desired result. For unresponsive hypotension, other agents are available for treatment of the underlying shock.

An $H_2$ blocker such as cimetidine can be added (300 mg in dextrose and water infused slowly). Likewise, diphenhydramine in a dose of 25 to 50 mg can be injected intravenously. Corticosteroids are also often employed. A typical dose of hydrocortisone is 500 mg intravenously. It should be realized that steroids probably have no immediate effect on the reaction. Their main use is to decrease the possibility of delayed reactions.

It has been suggested that severe hypotension in these patients may be corrected with vigorous hydration alone.[54] Such therapy avoids the complications and dangers encountered with epinephrine. One the other hand, overhydration of patients with underlying cardiovascular and renal disease also carries a risk. Thus, initiation of therapy by adequate hydration sounds reasonable, but appropriate pharmacologic therapy should be instituted without undue delay.[55]

Because hypotension in a setting of tachycardia or bradycardia requires different therapy, the pulse rate should be monitored during the reaction. A pulse may not be palpable in a hypotensive patient; cardiac auscultation or even electrocardiographic evaluation may be needed to determine the pulse rate.

Isolated hypotension in the absence of other significant signs of an anaphylactic reaction should initially be treated with oxygen and rapid administration of intravenous fluids. If needed, subcutaneous or intravenous epinephrine may be added. Likewise, a vasopressor agent such as dopamine, 2 to 5 µg/kg/min, can be added to sustain blood pressure.

Hypotension in the presence of bradycardia should signify a vasovagal reaction. Some patients respond to being placed in a Trendelenburg position. The hypotension should be treated with rapid intravenous infusion of isotonic saline. Oxygen should be administered. The bradycardia should be treated with atropine (0.5 to 1.0 mg intravenously), with the dose repeated every 5 minutes to a maximal total dose of 3.0 mg.

Some patients are receiving long-term therapy with beta-blocking agents, such as propranolol. A contrast reaction in a patient in this subgroup can be confusing because even in a setting of anaphylactic shock the beta-blocker–induced bradycardia can persist. Glucagon therapy for the bradycardia in these patients may be useful.[56, 57] An intravenous dose of 1.0 mg or more may be needed. Dopamine is also effective in such a clinical setting. The usual doses of epinephrine may not be effective in reversing hypotension.

With cardiovascular collapse, emergency cardiopulmonary resuscitation should be initiated. Refractory seizures can be treated with intravenous diazepam (Valium) and/or phenobarbital.

The foregoing outline is meant to be a guide only. All reactions should be individualized. The suggested doses are those for an average adult.

## References

1. Skucas J: Barium sulfate: clinical application. *In* Skucas J (ed): Radiographic Contrast Agents (2nd ed). Rockville, MD: Aspen Publishers, 1989, pp 14–17.
2. Dodds WJ, Stewart ET, Logemann JA: Physiology and radiology of the normal oral and pharyngeal phases of swallowing. AJR 154:953–963, 1990.
3. Chen MY, Ott DJ, Peele VN, et al: Oropharynx in patients with cerebrovascular disease: evaluation with videofluoroscopy. Radiology 176:641–643, 1990.

4. Dantas RO, Dodds WJ, Massey BT, et al: The effect of high- vs low-density barium preparations on the quantitative features of swallowing. AJR 153:1191–1195, 1989.

5. Maglinte DDT, Schultheis TE, Krol KL, et al: Survey of the esophagus during the upper gastrointestinal examination in 500 patients. Radiology 147:65–70, 1983.

6. Jones B, Donner MW: Examination of the patient with dysphagia. Radiology 167:319–326, 1988.

7. Rice BT, Spiegel PK, Dombrowski PJ: Acute esophageal food impaction treated by gas-forming agents. Radiology 146:299–301, 1983.

8. Kaszar-Seibert DJ, Korn WT, Bindman DJ, et al: Treatment of acute esophageal food impaction with a combination of glucagon, effervescent agent, and water. AJR 154:533–534, 1990.

9. Schabel SI, Skucas J: Esophageal obstruction following administration of "aged" barium sulfate tablets—a warning. Radiology 122:835–836, 1977.

10. Montagne J-P, Moss AA, Margulis AR: Double-blind study of single and double contrast upper gastrointestinal examinations using endoscopy as a control. AJR 130:1041–1045, 1978.

11. Op den Orth JO: The Standard Biphasic-Contrast Examination of the Stomach and Duodenum. The Hague: Martinus Nijhoff, 1979.

12. Hawkins SP, Rowlands PC, Shorvon PJ: Barium meals in the elderly—a quality reassurance. Br J Radiol 64:113–115, 1991.

13. Maglinte DDT, Miller RE: A comparison of pumps used for enteroclysis. Radiology 152:815, 1984.

14. Taverne PP, van der Jagt EJ: Small-bowel radiography. A prospective comparative study of three techniques in 200 patients. ROFO 143:293–297, 1985.

15. Ekberg O: Crohn's disease of the small bowel examined by double contrast technique: a comparison with oral technique. Gastrointest Radiol 1:355–359, 1977.

16. Geyer L, Reisinger W: Air or methylcellulose as a double contrast medium in x-ray studies of the small intestine? Radiol Diagn (Berl) 31:359–363, 1990.

17. Thoeni RF: Radiography of the small bowel and enteroclysis. A perspective. Invest Radiol 22:930–936, 1987.

18. Herlinger H: Double contrast enteroclysis. _In_ Margulis AR, Burhenne HJ (eds): Alimentary Tract Radiology (3rd ed). St. Louis: CV Mosby, 1983, p 892.

19. Violon D, Steppe R, Potvliege R: Improved retrograde ileography with glucagon. AJR 136:833–839, 1981.

20. Mandell GA, Teplick SK: Glucagon—its application to childhood gastrointestinal radiology. Gastrointest Radiol 7:7–13, 1982.

21. Fitzgerald EJ, Thompson GT, Sommers SS, et al: Pneumocolon as an aid to small-bowel studies. Clin Radiol 36:633–637, 1985.

22. Ott DJ, Chen YM, Gelfand DW, et al: Single-contrast vs double-contrast barium enema in the detection of colonic polyps. AJR 146:993–996, 1986.

23. Wolf EL, Frager D, Beneventano TC: Feasibility of double-contrast barium enema in the elderly. AJR 145:47–48, 1985.

24. Tinetti ME, Stone L, Cooney L, et al: Inadequate barium enemas in hospitalized elderly patients. Incidence and risk factors. Arch Intern Med 149:2014–2016, 1989.

25. Miller RE, Skucas J: The Radiological Examination of the Colon. The Hague: Martinus Nijhoff, 1983.

26. Cayea PD, Seltzer SE: A new barium paste for computed tomography of the esophagus. J Comput Assist Tomogr 9:214–216, 1985.

27. Clavel JP, Lorillot ML, Buthiau D, et al: Absorption intestinale du baryum lors d'explorations radiologiques. Therapie 42:239–243, 1987.

28. Buschman DL: Barium sulfate bronchography. Report of a complication. Chest 99:747–749, 1991.

29. Feczko PJ, Simms SM, Bakirci N: Fatal hypersensitivity reaction during a barium enema. AJR 153:275–276, 1989.

30. Feczko PJ: Increased frequency of reactions to contrast materials during gastrointestinal studies. Radiology 174:367–368, 1990.

31. Shaffer HA Jr, Eckard DA, de Lange EE, et al: Allergy to barium sulfate suspension with angioedema of the stomach and small bowel. Gastrointest Radiol 13:221–223, 1988.

32. Janower ML: Hypersensitivity reactions after barium studies of the upper and lower gastrointestinal tract. Radiology 161:139–140, 1986.

33. Nagel JE, Fuscaldo JT, Fireman P: Paraben allergy. JAMA 237:1594–1595, 1977.

34. Gelfand DW, Sowers JC, DePonte KA, et al: Anaphylactic and allergic reactions during double-contrast studies: is glucagon or barium suspension the allergen? AJR 144:405–406, 1985.

35. Morales C, Basomba A, Carreira J, et al: Anaphylaxis produced by rubber glove contact. Clin Exp Allergy 19:425–430, 1989.

36. Ownby DR, Tomlanovich M, Sammons N, et al: Anaphylaxis associated with latex allergy during barium enema examinations. AJR 156:903–908, 1991.

37. Sondheimer JM, Pearlman DS, Bailey WC: Systemic anaphylaxis during rectal manometry with a latex balloon. Am J Gastroenterol 84:975–977, 1989.

38. Masel H, Masel JP, Casey KV: A survey of colon examination techniques in Australia and New Zealand, with a review of complications. Australas Radiol 15:140–147, 1971.

39. Chan F-L, Tso W-K, Wong L-C, et al: Barium intravasation: radiographic and CT findings in a nonfatal case. Radiology 163:311–312, 1987.

40. Ginaldi S: Small bowel perforation during enteroclysis. Gastrointest Radiol 16:29–31, 1991.

41. Fischer HW: Catalog of intravascular contrast media. Radiology 159:561–563, 1986.

42. Cohen MD, Towbin R, Baker S, et al: Comparison of iohexol with barium in gastrointestinal studies of infants and children. AJR 156:345–350, 1991.

43. Koehler RE, Moss AA, Margulis AR: Early radiographic manifestations of carcinoma of the esophagus. Radiology 119:1–5, 1976.

44. Cassel DM, Anderson MF, Zboralske FF: Double-contrast esophagram. The prone technique. Radiology 139:737–739, 1981.

45. Bagnall RD, Galloway RW, Annis JAD: Double contrast preparations: an in vitro study of some antifoaming agents. Br J Radiol 50:546–550, 1977.

46. Coblentz CL, Frost RA, Molinaro V, et al: Pain after barium enema: effect of $CO_2$ and air on double-contrast study. Radiology 157:35–36, 1985.

47. Raptopoulos V, Davis MA, Davidoff A, et al: Fat-density oral contrast agent for abdominal CT. Radiology 164:653–656, 1987.

48. Spataro RE: Urography. _In_ Skucas J (ed): Radiographic Contrast Agents (2nd ed). Rockville, MD: Aspen Publishers, 1989, pp 245–269.

49. Carlson JE, Hedlund LJ, Trenkner SW, et al: Safety considerations in the power injection of contrast media via central venous catheters during computed tomographic examinations. Invest Radiol 27:337–340, 1992.

50. Lawrence V, Matthai W, Hartmaier S: Comparative safety of high-osmolality and low-osmolality radiographic contrast agents. Report of a multidisciplinary working group. Invest Radiol 27:2–28, 1992.

51. American College of Radiology Committee on Drugs and Contrast Media: Appendix A—report of the current criteria for the use of water soluble contrast agents for intravenous injections. _In_ Manual on Iodinated Contrast Media. Reston, VA: American College of Radiology, 1991, pp 27–29.

52. Lasser EC, Berry CC, Talner LB, et al: Pretreatment with corticosteroids to alleviate reactions to intravenous contrast material. N Engl J Med 317:845–849, 1987.

53. Pagani JJ, Hayman LA, Bigelow RH, et al: Diazepam prophylaxis of contrast media–induced seizures during computed tomography of patients with brain metastases. AJNR 4:67–72, 1983.

54. vanSonnenberg E, Neff CC, Pfister RC: Life-threatening hypotensive reactions to contrast media administration: comparison of pharmacologic and fluid therapy. Radiology 162:15–19, 1987.

55. Addlestone RB, Roach AC: Pharmacologic treatment of contrast media reactions. Radiology 165:876, 1987 (letter).

56. Zaloga GP, Delacey W, Holmboe E, et al: Glucagon reversal of hypotension in a case of anaphylactoid shock. Ann Intern Med 105:65–66, 1986.

57. Lee ML: Glucagon in anaphylaxis. J Allergy Clin Immunol 69:331–332, 1982.

# Pharmacoradiology

Jovitas Skucas, M.D.

---

INTRODUCTION

HYPOTONIC AGENTS
Glucagon
Anticholinergic Agents

HYPERTONIC AGENTS
Metoclopramide
Domperidone
Cisapride
Neostigmine

MIXED ACTION AGENTS
Cholecystokinin
Ceruletide

---

## INTRODUCTION

Discussed here are some of the pharmacologic agents of actual or potential use in radiographic examinations of the gastrointestinal tract. Agents useful during angiography are not included. Likewise, experimental agents and those considered to have little potential are excluded.

From a radiologist's viewpoint, the pharmacologic agents of interest can be divided into those that increase gastrointestinal tonicity and motility and those that decrease these functions. Some agents have different effects on different parts of the gastrointestinal tract. They are discussed separately in the section on mixed action agents.

Bowel tonicity is not the same as peristalsis. In general, however, the pharmacologic agents used in radiology that increase bowel tonicity also result in increased peristalsis. For instance, agents that induce gastric hypertonia tend to result in faster gastric emptying, hypertonic small bowel agents result in faster small bowel transit, and so on. The hypotonic agents have the opposite effect.

## HYPOTONIC AGENTS

Bowel hypotonia is helpful in a number of radiographic examinations. For instance, a segment of spastic colon can mimic a benign stricture or a malignancy. Likewise, polyps and diverticula in the small bowel can be detected more readily if the bowel is atonic.

A number of spasmolytic pharmacologic agents are available. These can be divided into anticholinergic agents, such as atropine, and hormonal agents, of which glucagon is a classic example.

### Glucagon

#### Introduction

Human glucagon is a single chain polypeptide containing 29 amino acid residues. It has a molecular weight of 3485. In animals, the glucagon amino acid sequence ranges from one similar to that in humans to completely different sequences. The amino acid sequence is identical in humans, pigs, and cattle.

Glucagon is generated by the alpha cells in the islets of Langerhans. In some species, glucagon is also produced in the stomach; whether any gastric glucagon is produced in humans is controversial.

Glucagon is a hormone having significant metabolic influence on a number of organ systems. It binds at specific receptor cell membranes in the target organs. In the liver, it stimulates glucose output and hepatic ketogenesis. It also lyses adipose tissue and leads to a reduction of circulating cholesterol and triglyceride levels. It stimulates insulin release and appears to be involved in liver regeneration, in which its full role is not known. Glucagon increases blood flow to the kidneys. Specific effects are also present in the adrenal glands and the heart.

In smooth muscle, glucagon is a relatively potent spasmolytic agent. This spasmolytic action accounts for the extensive use of glucagon in radiology, in which pharmacologic doses are employed. The smooth muscle in different segments of the gastrointestinal tract has varying sensitivity to glucagon. For example, 0.1 mg given intravenously is sufficient to induce gastroduodenal and small bowel hypotonia in most adults.[1] Such a dose is inadequate for colonic hypotonia, for which a dose up to 10 times greater may be needed.

#### Upper Gastrointestinal Tract

Among the hypotonic agents that have been evaluated for use in the upper gastrointestinal tract are morphine,[2] propantheline bromide (Pro-Banthine),[3–5] atropine, and related compounds. With some, after initial enthusiasm, the recognition of toxicity and undesirable side effects led to their abandonment.

In the early 1970s, in a study of the effect of glucagon on the gallbladder, the radiologist member of the research team noticed that after glucagon injection duodenal hypotonia was routinely detected on the test subject's radiographs.[6] A subsequent study of glucagon in hypotonic duodenography confirmed this finding.[7] A double-blind crossover study found that this hypotonic effect on the upper gastrointestinal tract was greater with glucagon than with either propantheline or atropine.[8] Glucagon decreases both intragastric and intraduodenal mean pressures.[9]

Hypotonicity of the upper gastrointestinal tract can be achieved both with glucagon and with some of the anticholinergic agents. The main advantage of glucagon over the anticholinergic agents is its lack of side effects.[10] In the United States, glucagon is generally used for this purpose. In some countries, however, the anticholinergic agent scopolamine butylbromide (Buscopan) is often employed. Presumably, one reason for using an anticholinergic agent is the higher cost of glucagon. The price ratio of glucagon to Buscopan fluctuates considerably throughout the world.

One author considered the quality of the barium mucosal coating in the stomach and duodenum to be better with the anticholinergic agents.[11] The rationale was that the anticholinergics decrease gastric secretions, whereas glucagon has no such effect. Another study found that Buscopan and glucagon produced equal distention and coating of both the stomach and duodenum.[12]

A more basic question is whether induced hypotonia of the stomach and duodenum improves one's ability to detect a lesion. The answer is controversial, and many radiologists in the United States do not induce hypotonia. At least one study found that the diagnostic quality with and that without glucagon did not differ significantly.[13]

## Small Bowel

### Enteroclysis

In enteroclysis, barium is instilled until either a lesion or an obstruction is reached or the terminal ileum is filled. When a suspicious area is seen or if for some other reason it is deemed desirable to slow down the barium progression through the bowel, glucagon can be administered. In general, 0.25 mg given intravenously is sufficient to induce enough hypotonia that a leisurely study of the area in question can be performed.

### Retrograde Ileography

While studying the effects of several drugs on the colon, it was discovered that with glucagon it was easier to reflux barium into the distal small bowel.[14] Another study using a double contrast barium enema, in which approximately half of the patients received glucagon and half did not, found that ileal reflux was achieved in more than twice as many patients in the glucagon group.[15] This tendency of glucagon to relax the ileocecal valve and allow barium reflux has been confirmed.[16, 17] Thus, if retrograde ileography is being performed for suspected disease in the distal ileum, it appears reasonable to administer glucagon almost routinely.

Some investigators believe that in the radiologic therapy of meconium ileus and the ileal plug syndrome glucagon also has a role.[18]

### Peroral Pneumocolon

The peroral pneumocolon examination is useful in achieving a double contrast study of the terminal ileum and right side of the colon. Barium is generally introduced via a conventional small bowel examination, although an enteroclysis approach can also be used. Because glucagon relaxes the ileocecal valve, it may increase the success rate of the double contrast portion of this examination.[19]

## Large Bowel

### Diagnostic Barium Enema

Colon hypotonia can be achieved by injecting 2 mg of glucagon intramuscularly.[10] The hypotonia begins several minutes after injection and generally lasts about 15 minutes. Hypotonia can also be achieved by injecting 0.25 to 0.5 mg of glucagon intravenously, although in some patients up to 1.0 mg may be necessary; the onset of hypotonia with an intravenous injection is almost immediate and lasts approximately 10 to 15 minutes. In general, the smaller intravenous dose is used because of cost considerations. In infants and children, an intravenous dose of 0.8 to 1.25 $\mu$g/kg has been recommended.[20]

Whether glucagon is administered before a barium enema varies considerably among radiologists. In general, it is more commonly used in hospitalized, elderly, and ill patients, for whom some investigators use it routinely. In some practices it is used routinely when double contrast barium enemas are performed but individualized with single contrast studies. In an outpatient setting, many radiologists use glucagon when the patient has painful spasm, has visualized spasm that interferes with diagnosis, or is unable to retain the enema.

Glucagon decreases both the extent and the severity of colonic spasm during a barium enema.[14, 21, 22] Thus, patients premedicated with glucagon before a barium enema should be more comfortable.[23] As a result, the radiologist should be under less pressure to speed up the examination and may obtain a better examination that clarifies the diagnosis.

Few studies have evaluated whether use of glucagon indeed results in a more accurate diagnosis. One prospective double-blind crossover study comparing glucagon with a placebo found that although both sensitivity and specificity were improved after glucagon, the results were not statistically significant.[24] It was recommended that glucagon be used only for patients who have considerable discomfort during the examination, colon spasm, difficulty retaining the enema, or suspected colitis or diverticulitis. This study was questioned on methodologic grounds,[25] yet further extension of the study to 120 patients in each category did not change the conclusions.[26] Another study concluded that glucagon degrades the examination because it promotes small bowel reflux,[17] a conclusion that has been questioned by others.[27]

Colonic spasm that persists in spite of glucagon is occasionally encountered. It has been my empirical observation that patients with long-standing diabetes have more glucagon-resistant colonic spasm than non-diabetic patients. The reason for such a possible decreased response in diabetics is not known. Many diabetics have high blood glucagon levels, although the levels are in the physiologic rather than the pharmacologic range. The presence of autonomic neuropathy in some of the diabetics may also be a factor. At times, refilling the colon several minutes later can result in marked decrease of spasm.[28, 29]

### Reduction of Intussusception

It was thought that, because of its spasmolytic effect and tendency to relax the ileocecal valve, glucagon should be useful in the hydrostatic reduction of an ileocolic intussusception. A number of case reports described intussusception reduction after administration of glucagon.[30–32] In one series, a success rate of 84% was achieved when glucagon was part of the intussusception reduction regimen.[33] Several controlled studies, however, found similar success rates for intussusception reduction with and without glucagon.[34–36] In one study, the children in the control group who had three unsuccessful attempts at hydrostatic reduction then received glucagon; during this fourth attempt a success rate of 59% was achieved. The authors recommended that if two attempts at hydrostatic reduction are not successful, glucagon should be administered before the next attempt.[35]

The current use of glucagon in the reduction of childhood intussusception is ambiguous. One approach is to attempt hydrostatic reduction of the intussusception without glucagon first; if such an attempt fails, glucagon can then be administered. Such empirical use does not imply that any eventual reduction can be attributed to glucagon, because even a second or third attempt at simple hydrostatic reduction improves the overall success rate.

## Biliary Tract

The gallbladder relaxes after an injection of glucagon.[6] The mean systolic and diastolic pressures decrease in the papilla of Vater.[9] Currently, little clinical use is made of these findings.

There is little current application of glucagon in percutaneous transhepatic cholangiography or in the various biliary drainage procedures. In an occasional patient who has persistent narrowing of the distal common bile duct, glucagon is helpful in differentiating among tumor, an impacted stone, and spasm. In most patients, however, judicious use of fluoroscopy is sufficient.

Most operative cholangiography is performed without fluoroscopic monitoring. Although some surgeons believe that glucagon improves the quality of the examination,[37] a double-blind prospective study found no improvement after glucagon injection.[38] Some have found that if persistent narrowing of the distal common bile duct is seen on the initial radiographs, glucagon may help relieve spasm.[39]

Hypotonic agents are commonly used during endoscopic retrograde cholangiography to induce duodenal hypotonia and aid in cannulation of the ampulla.[40] In the United States, glucagon is used almost exclusively for this purpose; in a number of other countries one of the anticholinergic drugs is more commonly employed.[41]

## Glucagon in Computed Tomography

Both glucagon[42] and somatostatin[43] have been used to decrease motion artifacts when using older scanners with prolonged examination times. A syringe pump can be used to infuse the glucagon.[44] There is less need for induced bowel hypotonia with most currently used fast scanners.

One study found that administration of glucagon (1.0 mg intravenously) and intravenous contrast medium was helpful in evaluating the full extent of a colorectal cancer.[45] Bowel lumen distention by a contrast enema and the lack of spasm aid in better defining the full extent of bowel wall infiltration.

## Glucagon in Ultrasonography

In abdominal ultrasonography there is occasionally a need to induce bowel atonia. At times a sonic window to the biliary tract can be obtained by filling the stomach with fluid and producing hypotonia of the surrounding gastrointestinal tract.[46]

## Contraindications

The contraindications to the use of glucagon include prior sensitivity to glucagon, a suspected pheochromocytoma, or an insulinoma.

Severe life-threatening reactions have been reported in patients with a pheochromocytoma.[47] Release of catecholamines from the tumor can result in sudden onset of hypertension. Such sudden hypertension can be countered with the alpha-adrenergic blocking agent phentolamine mesylate (Regitine Mesylate). In adults, a dose of 5 mg intravenously appears useful, although there is considerable variability in treatment requirements.

Glucagon can stimulate an insulinoma to release insulin, resulting in a sudden drop in blood glucose level; severe hypoglycemia obviously would be treated with glucose.

## Side Effects

The incidence of nausea or vomiting after injection of glucagon is dose dependent.[48] When glucagon is used intravenously, injecting it slowly tends to decrease the incidence of nausea.

Studies of several pharmacologic agents during various barium examinations revealed that the side effects with glucagon were less than those with atropine or propantheline.[8, 14] In fact, in one study the side effects with glucagon were similar to those seen with a placebo.[49]

Anaphylactic reactions have been associated with glucagon.[50] Glucagon is a naturally occurring polypeptide and in pure form should not result in hypersensitivity reaction. Commercially available glucagon may also contain as contaminants bovine and porcine insulins, protoinsulins, and other nonglucagon proteins. Any of these may be associated with a hypersensitivity reaction. A rash, periorbital edema, erythema multiforme, respiratory distress, and hypotension have been reported after glucagon injection.[51]

## Anticholinergic Agents

The anticholinergic agents as a group are effective in tissues having receptors supplied by cholinergic postganglionic autonomic nerves. They block the effect of acetylcholine liberated from nerve endings. Their main effect on the alimentary tract is to reduce tonicity, motility, and the amount of secretions.

Some of these agents are used in the therapy of peptic ulcer disease in conjunction with antacids and $H_2$ receptor antagonists. Such application has led to inconclusive results and is controversial. These agents also play a role in the therapy of irritable bowel syndrome. Some physicians have also used them as supplemental therapy in treating biliary and ureteral colic to help relax smooth muscle spasm. Here also the results have been inconsistent.

### Useful Agents

Several anticholinergic pharmacologic agents are commercially available. Perhaps the most widely used is atropine sulfate. It is available in tablet form and as a parenteral injectable liquid. Among senior radiologists in North America the best-known anticholinergic agent is propantheline bromide. Propantheline was in vogue in the United States in the 1960s and early 1970s as a gastrointestinal hypotonic agent. The delayed gastric emptying prolonged the examination, and to overcome this problem some radiologists then gave metoclopramide to induce gastric contractions.[52] Currently, propantheline bromide has been almost universally supplanted by other agents.

In other countries, however, the anticholinergic agents continue to be used for a number of reasons. The short-acting anticholinergic scopolamine butylbromide has been and still is the agent used most extensively. A common dose of scopolamine butylbromide is 20 mg before an upper gastrointestinal examination. Its hypotonic effect generally lasts for 15 to 20 minutes. For radiographic studies it is generally administered intravenously. Although other anticholinergic agents are available, generally their side effects and longer action than that of scopolamine butylbromide limit their application in radiology. Scopolamine butylbromide is not available in the United States. Although scopolamine hydrobromide is available, it is not used in radiologic examinations because of untoward side effects.

Chemically, atropine and scopolamine are natural tertiary amines. Propantheline is a quaternary ammonium compound.

In general, the anticholinergic agents reduce motility and secretions in the gastrointestinal tract, decrease tonicity in the urinary tract, and may also have a hypotonic effect on the bile ducts. Scopolamine butylbromide inhibits contractions of the sphincter of Oddi and is thought to aid in duodenal intubation during endoscopic cholangiopancreatography.[53] It is thought that scopolamine butylbromide does not induce gastroesophageal reflux, nor does it have any significant effect on the visualization of a hiatal hernia.[54]

In addition to effects on the gastrointestinal tract, these agents decrease salivary and bronchial secretions, dilate the pupils, and increase heart rate. The duration of action and specific effect on the various target organs depend on the specific compound and its dose.

## Complications

Several relative contraindications and complications are associated with use of anticholinergic drugs. In general, a history of glaucoma is a contraindication to use of these agents. In patients predisposed to glaucoma, the increased intraocular pressure may precipitate an acute attack. Unfortunately, most patients with a history of glaucoma have chronic glaucoma. A patient may have acute angle-closure glaucoma and not be aware of it.[55] Acute glaucoma should be suspected if there is any eye pain or loss of vision after administration of one of the anticholinergic agents.

The effect on the autonomic nervous system can result in urine retention. This complication is exacerbated in patients with prostatic hypertrophy or other predisposition to urine retention. Allergic reactions to anticholinergic agents are not common but have been recorded.[56, 57]

## HYPERTONIC AGENTS

Some patients have faster gastric emptying if the volume of the contrast agent is increased. A cold suspension not only is better tolerated but also leads to faster gastric emptying. Faster small bowel transit can be achieved by adding a hyperosmolar product to the barium suspension; in the past a small amount of diatrizoate meglumine preparation (Gastrografin) was often added to the oral barium suspension, although this is rarely done today. High-osmolality sorbitol has been added to oral CT contrast medium to speed up bowel opacification.[58] Sorbitol is also present in some conventional barium sulfate products.

## Metoclopramide

Metoclopramide (Maxolon) has been investigated extensively for use as an antiemetic agent and for various gastrointestinal disorders.[59] Its primary effects in the gastrointestinal tract are increased gastric peristalsis, relaxation of the pylorus, and increased small bowel peristalsis. It has no major effect on the colon.

A number of studies suggested that administration of metoclopramide before an upper gastrointestinal study would decrease gastric secretions and thus improve barium coating of the gastroduodenal mucosa. Prospective studies, however, have not shown that metoclopramide improves the quality of these studies.[60]

Metoclopramide has been used to accelerate small bowel transit.[61] In a study involving abdominal computed tomography, 10 mg of metoclopramide was administered orally 45 to 60 minutes before the scan (together with 500 mL of a 2% solution of sodium diatrizoate). Compared with a corresponding control population, the metoclopramide group had significantly better opacification of the ileum, right colon, and transverse colon.[62] The degree of opacification of the stomach, duodenum, and jejunum was similar for both groups. The authors recommended routine oral administration of metoclopramide before abdominal and pelvic computed tomographic examinations.

Metoclopramide has also been found useful in visualizing the pancreas in abdominal sonography.[63] Its primary benefit was in decreasing gastric and duodenal gas artifacts.

A typical dose of metoclopramide is 10 to 20 mg either parenterally or orally. It is a relatively safe drug; however, extrapyramidal side effects, such as dystonic reactions, have been reported.

Several authors have commented that the combination of ceruletide and metoclopramide aids ileal visualization.[64, 65] Longitudinal contractions and foreshortening of ileal loops tended to elevate the ileum out of the pelvis. A small bowel examination could be performed faster when both drugs were administered.[64]

## Domperidone

Domperidone, a potent dopamine antagonist, increases the rate of gastric emptying and accelerates small bowel transit. The effect on the small bowel appears to be less than that with metoclopramide. A study comparing intravenous domperidone (8 mg) and intravenous metoclopramide (10 mg) found that metoclopramide resulted in significantly faster small bowel transit.[66] No significant difference was seen in the quality of the examinations with the two agents.

## Cisapride

Cisapride is a gastrointestinal prokinetic substance that induces gastric and small bowel peristalsis.[67] It also enhances lower esophageal sphincter tone and is a relatively potent esophageal motor stimulator.[68, 69] It has been proposed for therapy in diabetic patients with gastroparesis[70] and as an antigastroesophageal reflux agent.

## Neostigmine

Neostigmine methyl sulfate (Prostigmin) is a synthetic preparation with cholinergic action. It increases gastric and small bowel peristalsis, leading to faster gastric emptying and shorter transit time through the small bowel. This pharmacologic agent is rarely employed because of extensive side effects and associated contraindications.

## MIXED ACTION AGENTS

### Cholecystokinin

Cholecystokinin induces gallbladder contraction and increases bowel peristalsis. Thus, its use results in faster small bowel transit.[71] Generally, the COOH-terminal octapeptide of cholecystokinin is used; this fragment is more potent than the entire molecule.

The effect on the gallbladder has been used to help increase radiographic contrast during oral cholecystography. It has also been used to evaluate gallbladder function.[72] Cholecystokinin also relaxes the sphincter of Oddi and, in the appropriate clinical setting, has been used to assist passage of bile duct stones.

### Ceruletide

Ceruletide is a synthetic compound similar to cholecystokinin in pharmacologic effects, namely delayed gastric emptying, hypoperistalsis of the duodenum, and hyperperistalsis of the jejunum, ileum, and colon. Ceruletide has an effect on the gallbladder similar to that of cholecystokinin or a fatty meal.[73]

The primary radiographic use of ceruletide has been to induce increased small bowel peristalsis and thus shorten the duration of a small bowel examination.[74–77] When given intravenously, ceruletide can induce nausea, vomiting, and abdominal cramps. These side effects are decreased if the drug is given intramuscularly. For acceleration of small bowel transit, a dose of 0.25 to 0.3 µg/kg is typical.

Whether the shorter small bowel transit time and pronounced contractions result in a better small bowel study is controversial; some investigators have reported a decrease in anatomic detail, particularly in the distal ileum.[74, 75]

Because ceruletide induces gastric hypotonia, it should not be administered before significant amounts of barium reach the jejunum. Some investigators overcome such gastric stasis by administering metoclopramide before the start of the examination.[64, 65]

# References

1. Miller RE, Chernish SM, Greenman GF, et al: Gastrointestinal response to minute doses of glucagon. Radiology 143:317–320, 1982.
2. Porcher P: La stase duodénale provoquée. Procédé simple, rapide et fidéle, d'améliorer la visibilité radiologique et les détails de l'image du bulbe ulcéreux. Arch Mal Appar Dig 33:24–26, 1944.
3. Baum M, Howe CT: Hypotonic duodenography in the diagnosis of carcinoma of the pancreas and its further use when combined with percutaneous cholangiography and pancreatic scintiscanning. Am J Surg 115:519–525, 1968.
4. Bilbao MR, Rösch J, Frische LH, et al: Hypotonic duodenography in the diagnosis of pancreatic disease. Semin Roentgenol 3:280–287, 1968.
5. Merlo RB, Stone M, Baugus P, et al: The use of Pro-Banthine to induce gastrointestinal hypotonia. Radiology 127:61–62, 1978.
6. Chernish SM, Miller RE, Rosenak BD, et al: Effect of glucagon on size of visualized human gallbladder before and after a fat meal. Gastroenterology 62:1218–1226, 1972.
7. Chernish SM, Miller RE, Rosenak BD, et al: Hypotonic duodenography with the use of glucagon. Gastroenterology 63:392–398, 1972.
8. Miller RE, Chernish SM, Skucas J, et al: Hypotonic roentgenography with glucagon. AJR 121:264–274, 1974.
9. Takemoto T, Okia K, Tada M, et al: Glucagon in digestive endoscopy—its usefulness for premedication. *In* Picazo J (ed): Glucagon in 1987. Lancaster, England: MTP Press, 1987, pp 55–66.
10. Miller RE, Chernish SM, Brunelle RL: Gastrointestinal radiography with glucagon. Gastrointest Radiol 4:1–10, 1979.
11. Maruyama M: Glucagon in upper gastrointestinal radiology. *In* Picazo J (ed): Glucagon in 1987. Lancaster, England: MTP Press, 1987, p 30.
12. Heron CW, Lynn AH, Marshall JH, et al: A comparison of paralysing agents in double-contrast barium meal examinations. Clin Radiol 36:391–393, 1985.
13. Rothe AJ, Young JWR, Keramati B: The value of glucagon in routine barium investigations of the gastrointestinal tract. Invest Radiol 22:786–791, 1987.
14. Miller RE, Chernish SM, Skucas J, et al: Hypotonic colon examination with glucagon. Radiology 113:555–562, 1974.
15. Violon D, Steppe R, Potvliege R: Improved retrograde ileography with glucagon. AJR 136:833–834, 1981.
16. Monsein LH, Halpert RD, Harris ED, et al: Retrograde ileography: value of glucagon. Radiology 161:558–559, 1986.
17. Stone EE, Conte FA: Glucagon-induced small bowel air reflux: degrading effects on double-contrast colon examinations. Gastrointest Radiol 13:212–214, 1988.
18. Mandell GA, Teplick SK: Glucagon—its application to childhood gastrointestinal radiology. Gastrointest Radiol 7:7–13, 1982.
19. Kelvin FM, Gedgaudas RK, Thompson WM, et al: The peroral pneumocolon: its role in evaluating the terminal ileum. AJR 139:115–121, 1982.
20. Ratcliffe JF: Glucagon in barium examinations in infants and children: special reference to dosage. Br J Radiol 53:860–862, 1980.
21. Gohel VK, Dalinka MK, Coren GS: Hypotonic examination of the colon with glucagon. Radiology 115:1–4, 1975.
22. Meeroff JC, Jorgens J, Isenberg JI: The effect of glucagon on barium-enema examination. Radiology 115:5–7, 1975.
23. Harned RK, Stelling CB, Williams S, et al: Glucagon and barium enema examinations: a controlled clinical trial. AJR 126:981–984, 1976.
24. Thoeni RF, Vandeman F, Wall SD: Effect of glucagon on the diagnostic accuracy of double-contrast barium enema examinations. AJR 142:111–114, 1984.
25. Marinelli D, Levine MS, Young M: Importance of sample size for statistical significance. AJR 143:923–924, 1984 (letter).
26. Thoeni RFL: Importance of sample size for statistical significance. AJR 143:924, 1984 (letter).
27. Maglinte DDT, Chernish SM: Glucagon-induced small bowel air reflux: degrading effects on double-contrast colon examination. Gastrointest Radiol 14:85–87, 1989 (letter).
28. Levine MS, Gasparaitis AE: Barium filling for glucagon-resistant spasm on double-contrast barium enema examinations. Radiology 160:264–265, 1986.
29. Demas BE, Margulis AR: Combined use of double- and single-contrast barium enema in the evaluation of suspected colonic disease. Gastrointest Radiol 9:241–245, 1984.
30. Fisher JK, Germann DR: Glucagon-aided reduction of intussusception. Radiology 122:197–198, 1977.
31. Lanocita M, Castiglioni G: Impiego del glucagone nella riduzione dell'invaginazione intestinale; presentazione di un caso. Radiol Med (Torino) 66:513–516, 1980.
32. Coppola V, Verrengia D, Esposito F, et al: L'ausilio del glucagone nella riduzione idrostatica dell'invaginazione in corso di clisma opaco. Minerva Pediatr 35:881–884, 1983.
33. Hoy GR, Dunbar D, Boles ET Jr: The use of glucagon in the diagnosis and management of ileocolic intussusception. J Pediatr Surg 12:939–944, 1977.
34. Franken EA Jr, Smith WL, Chernish SM, et al: The use of glucagon in hydrostatic reduction of intussusception: a double-blind study of 30 patients. Radiology 146:687–689, 1983.
35. Mortensson W, Eklöf O, Laurin S: Hydrostatic reduction of childhood intussusception. Acta Radiol Diagn 25:261–264, 1984.
36. Hsiao J-Y, Kao H-A, Shih S-L: Intravenous glucagon in hydrostatic reduction of intussusception: a controlled study of 63 patients. Acta Paediatr Sin 29:242–247, 1988.
37. Tabak CA, Tuxen PL, Bruce DL, et al: Glucagon enhancement of cholangiography. A preliminary report. Arch Surg 118:84–85, 1983.
38. Cofer JB, Barnett RM, Major GR, et al: Effect of intravenous glucagon on intraoperative cholangiography. South Med J 81:455–456, 1988.
39. McCammon RL, Stoelting R, Madura JA: Reversal of fentanyl induced spasm of the sphincter of Oddi. Surg Gynecol Obstet 156:329–334, 1983.
40. Silvis SE, Vennes JA: The role of glucagon in endoscopic cholangiopancreatography. Gastrointest Endosc 21:162–163, 1975.
41. Hannigan BF, Axon ATR, Avery S, et al: Buscopan or glucagon for endoscopic cannulation of ampulla of Vater. J R Soc Med 75:21–22, 1982.
42. Marks WM, Goldberg HI, Moss AA, et al: Intestinal pseudotumors: a problem in abdominal computed tomography solved by directed techniques. Gastrointest Radiol 5:155–160, 1980.
43. Efendic S, Mattson O, Luft R: Somatostatin in computer tomography of the abdomen. Acta Radiol Diagn 20:369–371, 1979.
44. Kreel L, Bydder G: Use of a portable syringe pump for glucagon administration in abdominal computed tomography. Radiology 136:507–508, 1980.
45. Hamlin DJ, Burgener FA, Sischy B: New techniques to stage early rectal carcinoma by computed tomography. Radiology 141:539–540, 1981.
46. Op den Orth JO: Sonography of the pancreatic head aided by water and glucagon. Radiographics 7:85–100, 1987.
47. McLoughlin MJ, Langer B, Wilson DR: Life-threatening reaction to glucagon in a patient with pheochromocytoma. Radiology 140:841–842, 1981.
48. Chernish SM, Maglinte DDT: Glucagon: common untoward reactions—review and recommendations. Radiology 177:145–146, 1990.
49. Chernish SM, Davidson JA, Brunelle RL, et al: Response of normal subjects to a single 2-milligram dose of glucagon administered intramuscularly. Arch Int Pharmacodyn Ther 218:312–327, 1975.
50. Zavras GM, Papadaki PJ, Kounis NG, et al: Glucagon-induced severe anaphylactic reaction. ROFO 152:110, 1990.
51. Edell SL: Erythema multiforme secondary to intravenous glucagon. AJR 134:385–386, 1980.
52. Margieson GR, Williams HBL: Radiopharmacology of the stomach, with special reference to the effects of metoclopramide. Australas Radiol 12:239–244, 1968.
53. Allescher HD, Neuhaus H, Hagenmüller F, et al: Effect of *N*-butylscopolamine on sphincter of Oddi motility in patients during routine ERCP—a manometric study. Endoscopy 22:160–163, 1990.

54. Rajah RR: Effects of Buscopan on gastro-oesophageal reflux and hiatus hernia. Clin Radiol 41:250–252, 1990.

55. Doran KML, Gray R, Virjee JP: Buscopan and glaucoma. Br J Radiol 60:417, 1987.

56. Thomas AMK, Kubie AM, Britt RP: Acute angioneurotic oedema following a barium meal. Br J Radiol 59:1055–1056, 1986.

57. Treweeke P, Barrett NK: Allergic reaction to Buscopan. Br J Radiol 60:417–418, 1987.

58. Lunderquist A, Ivancev K, Stridbeck H: Gastrografin-sorbitol solution for CT opacification of bowel. AJR 150:949, 1988.

59. Pinder RM, Brogden RN, Sawyer PR, et al: Metoclopramide: review of its pharmacological properties and clinical use. Drugs 12:81–131, 1976.

60. Gopichandran TD, Ring NJ, Beckly DE: Metoclopramide in double contrast barium meals. Clin Radiol 31:485–488, 1980.

61. Maglinte DDT, Lappas JC, Kelvin FM, et al: Small bowel radiography: how, when, and why? Radiology 163:297–305, 1987.

62. Thoeni RF, Filson RG: Abdominal and pelvic CT: use of oral metoclopramide to enhance bowel opacification. Radiology 169:391–393, 1988.

63. duCret RP, Jackson VP, Rees C, et al: Pancreatic sonography: enhancement by metoclopramide. AJR 146:341–343, 1986.

64. Grumbach K, Herlinger H, Laufer I, et al: Metoclopramide-ceruletide assisted small bowel examination. ROFO 149:47–51, 1988.

65. Weidenmaier W, Friedrich JM, Schif A, et al: Medikamentöse Beeinflussung der fraktionierten Dünndarmdoppelkontrastdarstellung. ROFO 152:137–141, 1990.

66. Morewood DJW, Whitehouse GH: A comparison of three methods for performing barium follow-through studies of the small intestine. Br J Radiol 59:971–973, 1986.

67. Schuurkes JAJ, Van Neuten JM: Gastrointestinal motor stimulating properties of cisapride in conscious dogs. Digestion 34:137, 1986.

68. Wienbeck M, Cuder-Wiesinger E, Berges W: Comparative study of cisepride's versus metoclopramide's effect on esophageal motility. Digestion 34:141–142, 1986.

69. Corazziari E, Bontempo I, Anzini F: Effects of cisapride on distal esophageal motility in humans. Dig Dis Sci 34:1600–1605, 1989.

70. Vogelberg KH, Dalügge A: Sonographische Untersuchungen bei der medikamentösen Behandlung der diabetischen Gastroparese. Dtsch Med Wochenschr 113:967–971, 1988.

71. Efsing HO, Lindroth B: Small bowel examination after injection of cholecystokinin. Clin Radiol 31:225–226, 1980.

72. Masclee AAM, Hopman WPM, Corstens FHM, et al: Simultaneous measurement of gallbladder emptying with cholescintigraphy and US during infusion of physiologic doses of cholecystokinin: a comparison. Radiology 173:407–410, 1989.

73. Wetzner SM, Vincent ME, Robbins AH: Ceruletide-assisted cholecystography: a clinical assessment. Radiology 131:23–26, 1979.

74. Sargent EN, Halls JM, Colletti P, et al: Efficacy and tolerance of ceruletide in radiography of the small intestine. Radiology 136:57–60, 1980.

75. Robbins AH, Wetzner SM, Landy MD: Ceruletide-assisted examination of the small bowel. AJR 134:343–347, 1980.

76. Novak D: Acceleration of small intestine contrast study by ceruletide. Gastrointest Radiol 5:61–65, 1980.

77. Thompson WM, Halvorsen RA, Shaw M, et al: Evaluation of intramuscular ceruletide for shortening small bowel transit time. Gastrointest Radiol 7:141–147, 1982.

# Barium Studies: Principles of Double Contrast Diagnosis

### Igor Laufer, M.D.

## INTRODUCTION

Although barium studies once reigned supreme in the arena of morphologic diagnosis in the gastrointestinal tract, these responsibilities are now shared with endoscopy and, to a lesser extent, cross-sectional imaging techniques.[1] As would be expected, the development of competition in the field has led to improvements in barium studies—in particular, the emergence of double contrast techniques as a competitive choice for the diagnosis of mucosal lesions in the gastrointestinal tract.[2]

In general terms, barium contrast studies can demonstrate the mucosal surface in three different ways. Mucosal relief views are obtained with a small amount of barium, just sufficient to demonstrate the mucosal folds (Fig. 4–1A). These views are particularly valuable

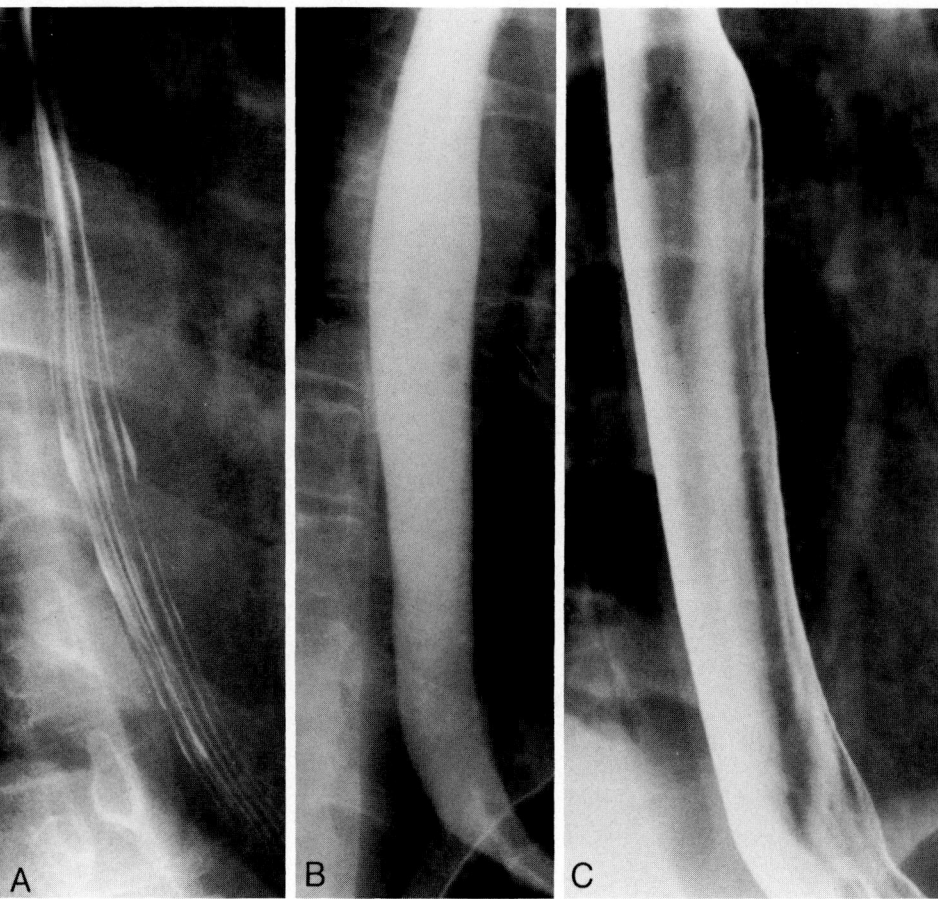

Figure 4–1. Approaches to the gastrointestinal tract as illustrated in the esophagus. A. Mucosal relief. With the esophagus collapsed and coated, the normal longitudinal folds are seen. B. Barium filling. With the patient in the prone position and with continuous drinking, the barium-filled esophagus is demonstrated. C. Double contrast. With the patient in the upright position, the smooth featureless surface of the esophagus is seen.

for demonstrating abnormalities affecting the mucosal folds, such as esophageal varices or some of the mucosal abnormalities in patients with inflammatory bowel disease. Barium filling is achieved with a larger volume of low-density barium (Fig. 4–1B). These views are particularly valuable for the demonstration of contour abnormalities, strictures, and large polypoid filling defects. Double contrast views are obtained after the mucosal surface has been coated with a thin layer of high-density barium and the viscus has been distended with air (Fig. 4–1C). These views are particularly valuable for the demonstration of subtle mucosal lesions such as the early changes of various inflammatory and neoplastic diseases.

Although these three types of views are incorporated to varying degrees in both single and double contrast examinations,[3] single contrast studies tend to rely more heavily on diagnostic fluoroscopy, mucosal relief, and barium filling. On the other hand, double contrast techniques emphasize the interpretation of double contrast radiographs but not to the exclusion of barium filling or mucosal relief.

There is still considerable controversy regarding the relative virtues of single and double contrast techniques.[4, 5] However, most authors believe, as I do, that double contrast techniques provide superior mucosal detail and allow earlier detection of subtle lesions. In the past decade, the proportion of barium studies performed using double contrast techniques has increased from 20% to more than 40%.

This chapter deals with the principles that must be understood for the proper performance and interpretation of double contrast studies.[6] These principles are illustrated with examples drawn from the entire gastrointestinal tract. The principles applicable to single contrast examinations are discussed in Chapter 6.

# PERFORMANCE

The yield of diagnostic information from double contrast studies can be maximized only with meticulous attention to the technical aspects of the examination. The major principles of performance include mucosal coating, distention, and projection.

## Mucosal Coating

The diagnostic quality of a double contrast study depends on the quality of mucosal coating. In the absence of good coating, lesions can be missed or patchy coating can be mistaken for a lesion. Good mucosal coating requires the optimal interaction between the barium suspension and the mucosal surface. A proper barium suspension must be chosen; it must be prepared properly[7] and the mucosal surface must be adequately prepared to receive the barium coating. Even when mucosal coating is only slightly impaired, extensive abnormalities can be missed (Fig. 4–2).

## Distention

Normal mucosal folds are soft and pliable and are therefore effaced with moderate distention. Thus, the optimal degree of distention is that which just effaces the normal mucosal folds. It is easy to understand that inadequate distention may hide lesions, but it must also be appreciated that overdistention can obscure lesions such as shallow ulcers. For the demonstration of complex or subtle lesions, the principle of varying degrees of distention should be used. Overdistention accentuates areas of rigidity, and partial collapse may accentuate

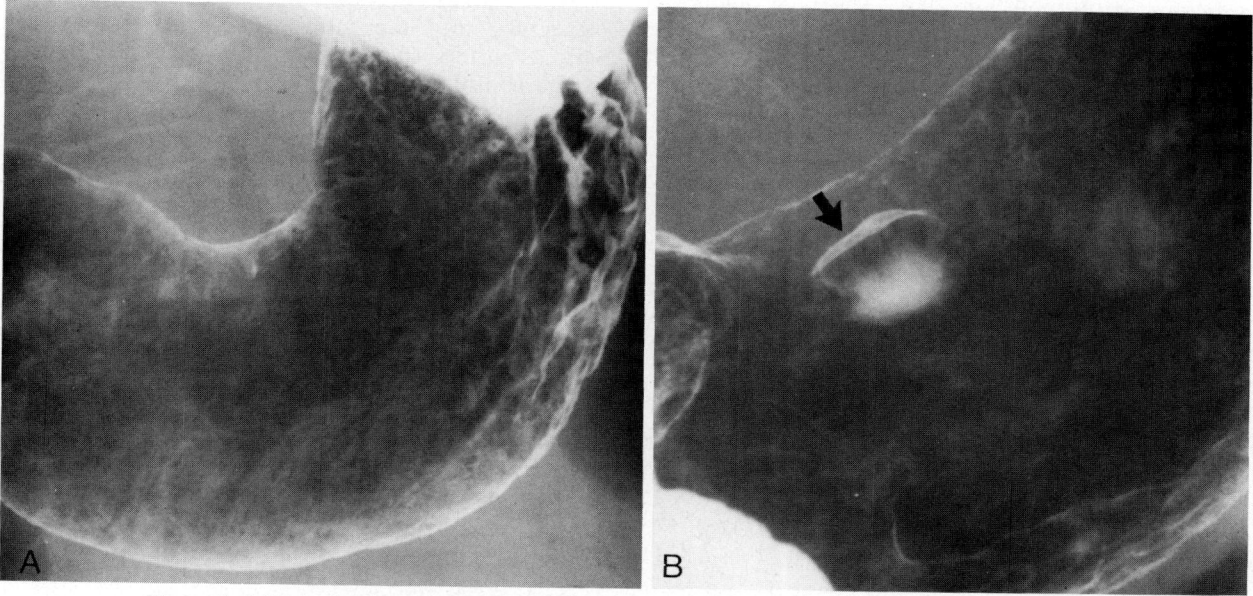

**Figure 4–2. Risk of suboptimal coating. A.** On the initial film, an ulcer crater is barely recognizable along the lesser curvature. **B.** With additional rotation and improved coating, the large ulcer crater *(arrow)* is clearly recognized.

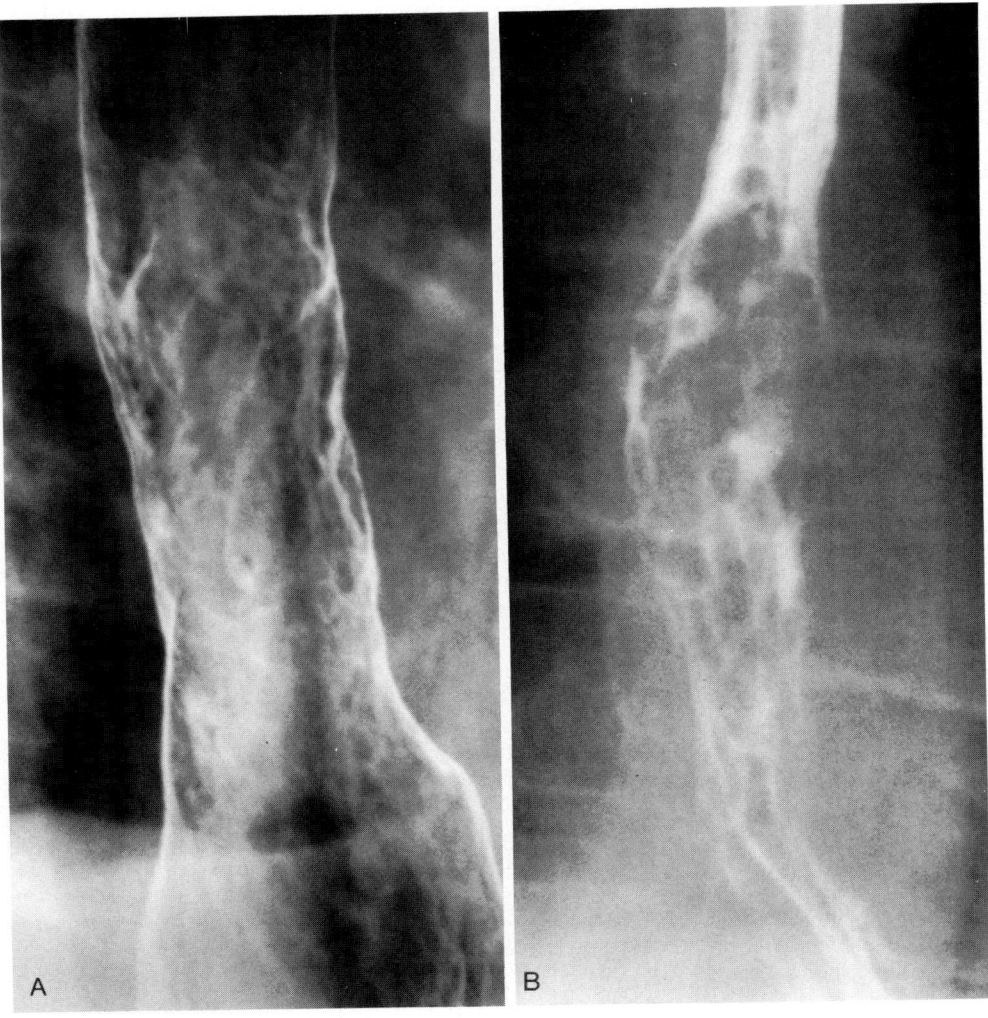

Figure 4–3. Adenocarcinoma in Barrett's esophagus. **A**. The double contrast view shows ulceration and slight rigidity of the contour. **B**. The mucosal relief film shows the polypoid nature of the lesion.

abnormalities of the mucosal folds. The final diagnosis represents a synthesis of the information obtained with the various views (Fig. 4–3).

## Projection

An adequate number of views should be obtained so that each loop of bowel is projected free of overlapping loops. Furthermore, each segment of the bowel should be demonstrated in profile. Nevertheless, these goals cannot always be accomplished, and it is important to get in the habit of looking through loops of bowel and recognizing abnormalities of the lumen when seen en face as well as in profile. This is particularly important for the recognition of short, annular lesions in the colon, where it may be difficult to demonstrate every bend in profile (Fig. 4–4).

## INTERPRETATION

After the effort is made to obtain excellent films, it is important to extract all the diagnostic information that is on the films. To accomplish this, it is important to recognize that the interpretation of double contrast studies differs substantially from the interpretation of single contrast studies.

## Dependent and Nondependent Surfaces

The distinction between the dependent and nondependent surfaces must be clearly understood. The nondependent surface has a thin coating of barium because all the free barium falls onto the dependent surface. The dependent surface, therefore, has a thicker coating of barium and in any depression or concavity a barium pool or puddle accumulates. The usual double contrast film made with a vertical beam results in a superimposition of the dependent and nondependent surfaces and any barium pool that might be present. The distinction between these surfaces is more clearly demonstrated on a horizontal beam radiograph (Fig. 4–5).

Lesions in the gastrointestinal tract can generally be classified as protruded or depressed, and their appearance depends on whether they are situated on the

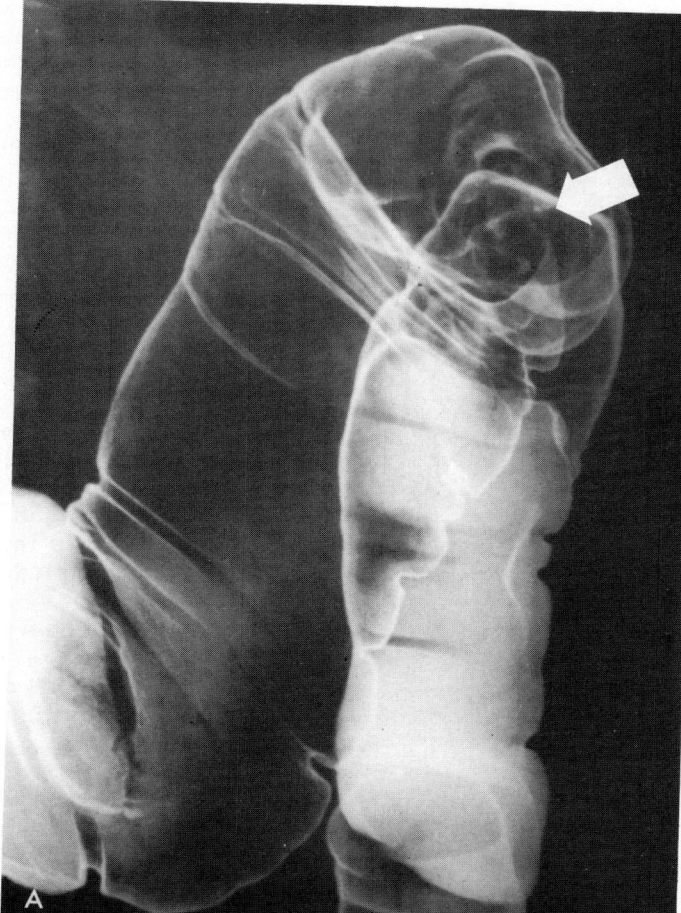

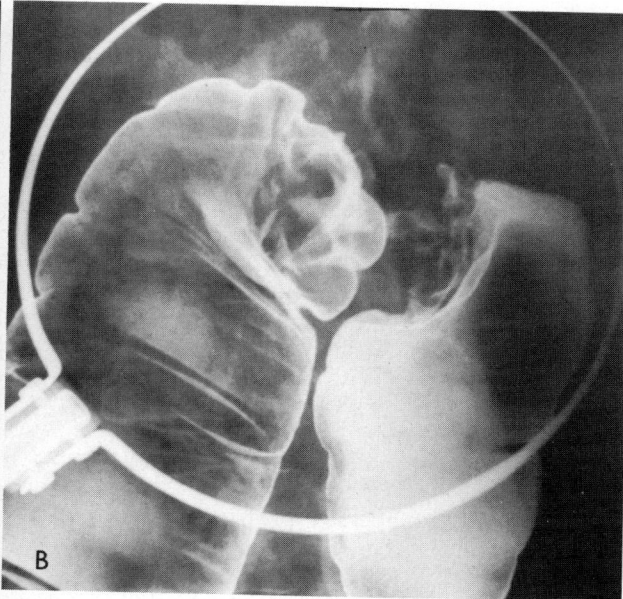

**Figure 4–4. Annular carcinoma seen en face and in profile.**
**A**. The irregularity of the lumen seen end on *(arrow)* is the result of an annular carcinoma. **B**. Carcinoma is confirmed on the appropriate oblique projection.

**Figure 4–5. Dependent and nondependent surfaces.** The distinction between the dependent and nondependent surfaces is clearly shown on this horizontal beam radiograph of the colon. The nondependent surface has a thin coating of barium, while the dependent surface contains barium pools.

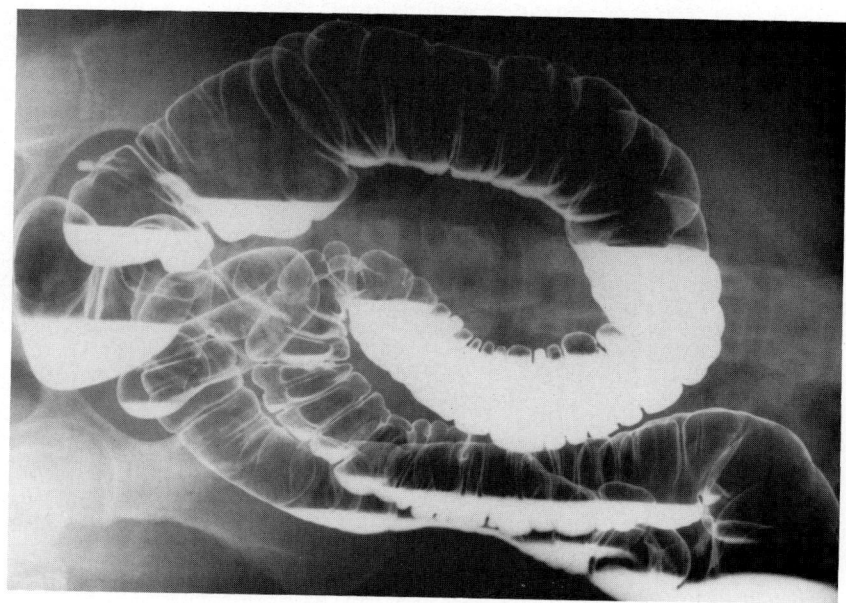

dependent or nondependent surface. Their appearance can also be modified or masked by the presence of a barium pool.

## Protrusions

Protrusions into the lumen of a hollow viscus can be either normal structures such as mucosal folds or pathologic lesions such as polypoid tumors. The radiographic principles underlying the appearance of protrusions are illustrated in Figure 4–6, which represents a cross section through the stomach with rugal folds on the anterior and posterior walls. With the patient in the supine position, the posterior wall is dependent and the anterior wall is nondependent.

A protrusion on the dependent surface displaces barium from the barium pool and is therefore seen as a radiolucent filling defect. A protrusion on the nondependent surface is coated with barium and the x-ray

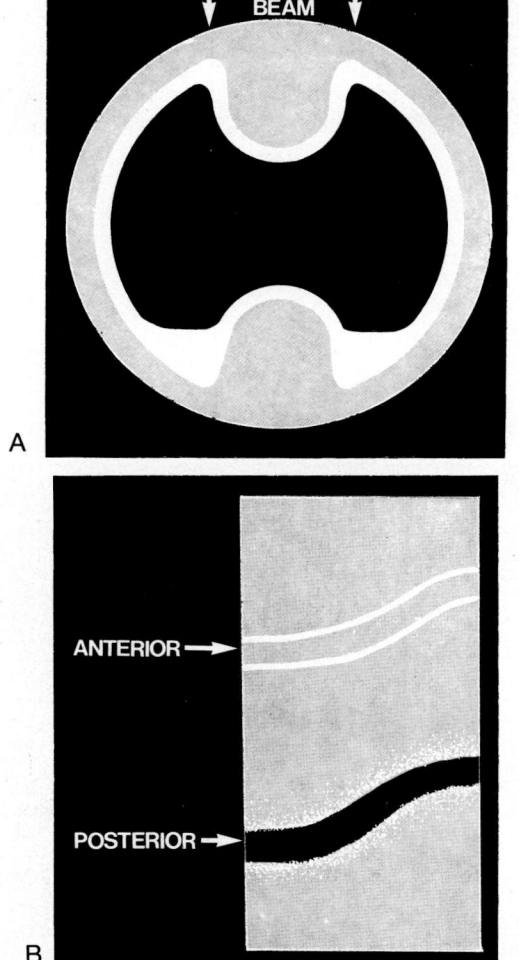

**Figure 4–6. Principles underlying the appearance of protrusions.** **A** and **B**. Diagrammatic representation of the appearances of a rugal fold on the anterior and posterior walls of the stomach.

beam catches the edges of the protrusions, which are then "etched in white." Figure 4–7 illustrates the different appearances of a lesion when it is located on the dependent surface and then on the nondependent surface.

In general, the density of the etching depends on the thickness of the lesion, and the etching of a slightly protruded or plaque-like lesion may be extremely faint indeed. Such lesions are best demonstrated on the dependent surface with a shallow barium pool. The flow technique[8] is particularly valuable for such lesions (see later).

Several other appearances are associated with protruded lesions. The stalactite phenomenon[9] (Fig. 4–8) represents a barium droplet hanging from a protrusion on the nondependent surface. These should not be mistaken for ulcers because they are always associated with protrusions on the nondependent surface and disappear as the droplet falls away. Nevertheless, it is important to recognize these stalactites because they may be the only clue to the presence of a protruded lesion on the nondependent surface.[10]

The "bowler hat" sign (Fig. 4–9) may be seen with either a polypoid lesion or a diverticulum. However, in the case of a polyp the dome of the hat points in toward the long axis of the bowel, whereas with a diverticulum the dome of the hat points outward.[11]

The "Mexican hat" sign (Fig. 4–10) represents a pedunculated polyp hanging from the nondependent surface. The outer ring represents the head of the polyp and the inner ring represents the stalk seen end on.

## Depressed Lesions

Depressed lesions are lesions that extend beyond the normal contour of the bowel, such as ulcers or diverticula. When located on the dependent surface, they trap the barium and therefore are seen as a focal barium collection (Fig. 4–11A). When located on the nondependent surface, they empty of barium. However, if there is adequate coating of the sides of the depressed lesion, it is seen as a ring shadow (Fig. 4–11B and C). For this reason, in patients with colonic diverticulosis, some of the diverticula are barium filled whereas others are recognized as ring shadows (Fig. 4–12).

This concept is particularly important for the recognition of anterior wall doudenal ulcers. With the patient in the supine or left posterior oblique position, the ulcer may be recognizable only as a ring or a crescent (see Fig. 4–11B). However, if the patient is put into the prone position, the ulcer fills with barium (see Fig. 4–11C).

## Barium Pool

The barium pool is the paint of the radiologic artist. The double contrast examination, in essence, represents a manipulation of the barium pool to coat the entire mucosal surface. However, the barium pool can also act

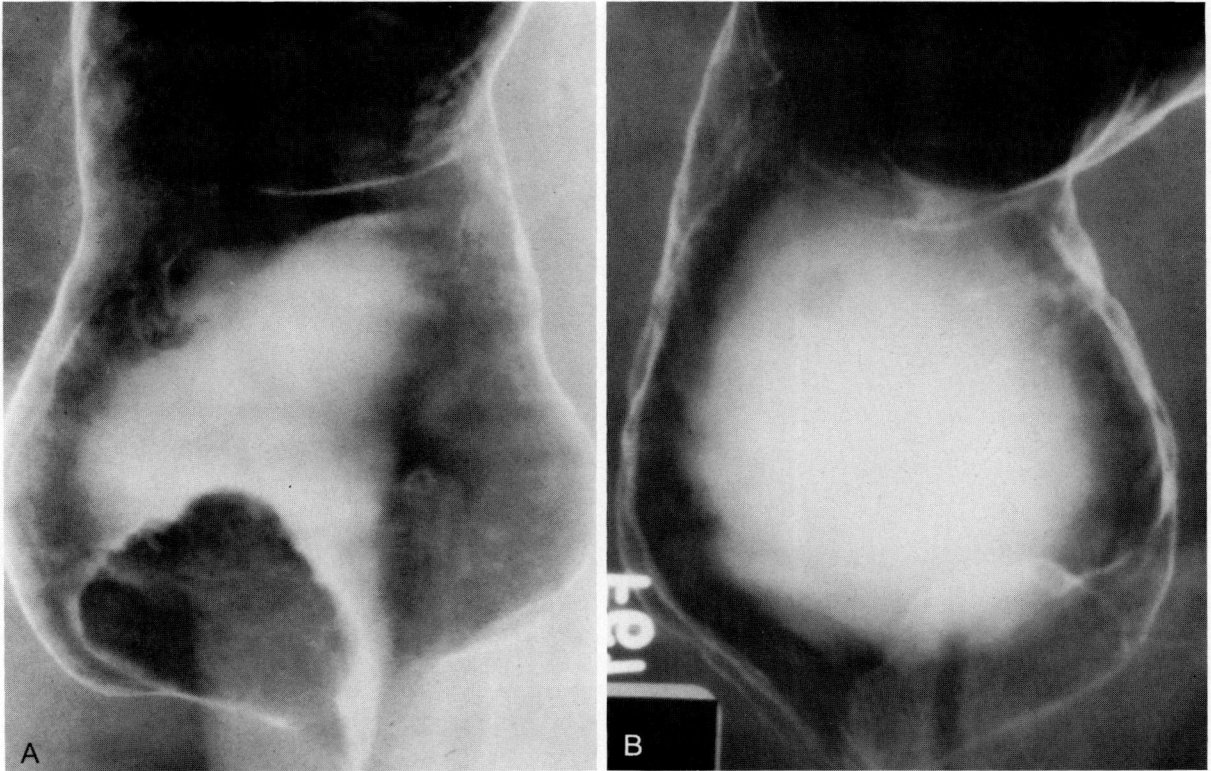

**Figure 4–7. Effect of position on the appearance of a rectal carcinoma. A**. With the patient in the supine position, there is a lobulated filling defect in the distal rectum. The plaque-like carcinoma is therefore on the posterior wall. **B**. With the patient turned into the prone position, the carcinoma is now etched in white because it is on the nondependent surface.

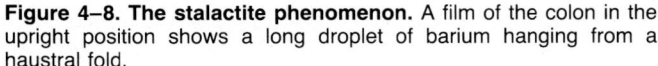

**Figure 4–8. The stalactite phenomenon.** A film of the colon in the upright position shows a long droplet of barium hanging from a haustral fold.

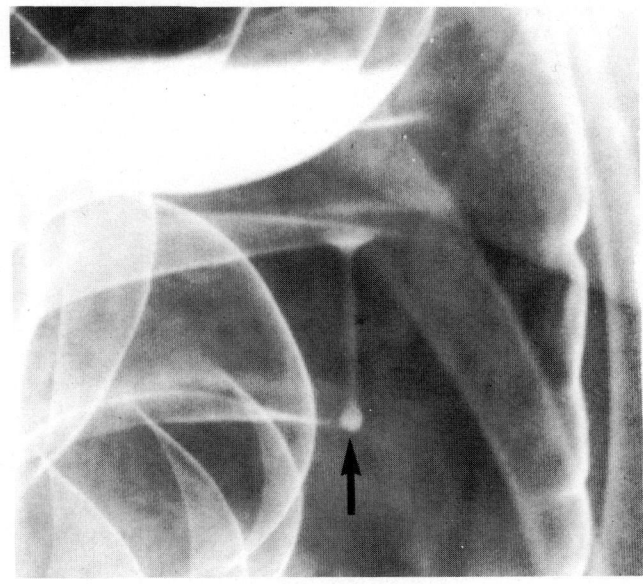

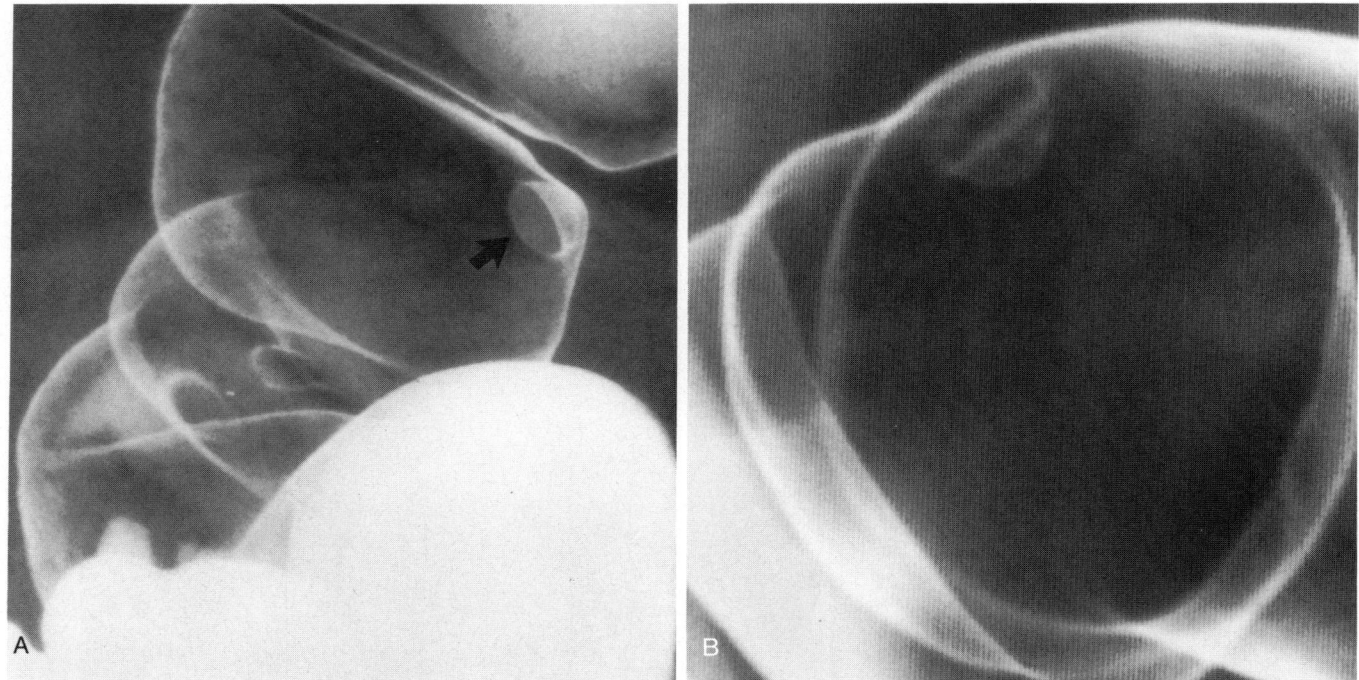

**Figure 4–9. Bowler hat: diverticulum or polyp? A**. When the dome of the hat points away from the axis of the bowel, it is a diverticulum. **B**. When the dome of the hat points toward the lumen of the bowel, it is a polyp.

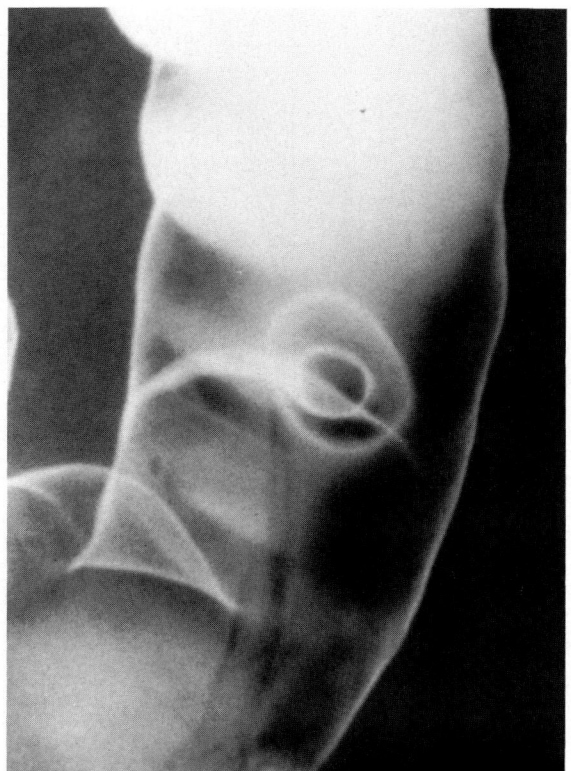

**Figure 4–10. The Mexican hat sign.** Typical appearance of pedunculated polyp seen end on. The outer ring represents the head of the polyp and the inner ring represents the stalk.

**Figure 4–11. Depressed lesions. A**. Dependent wall ulcer. Film of the stomach in the right posterior oblique projection shows a typical high lesser curve ulcer en face. **B**. Anterior wall ulcer. A film in the left posterior oblique projection shows a ring shadow representing the ulcer crater on the anterior wall in a deformed duodenal cap. **C**. With the patient in the prone position, the ring shadow fills with barium *(arrow)*, indicating an anterior wall duodenal ulcer.

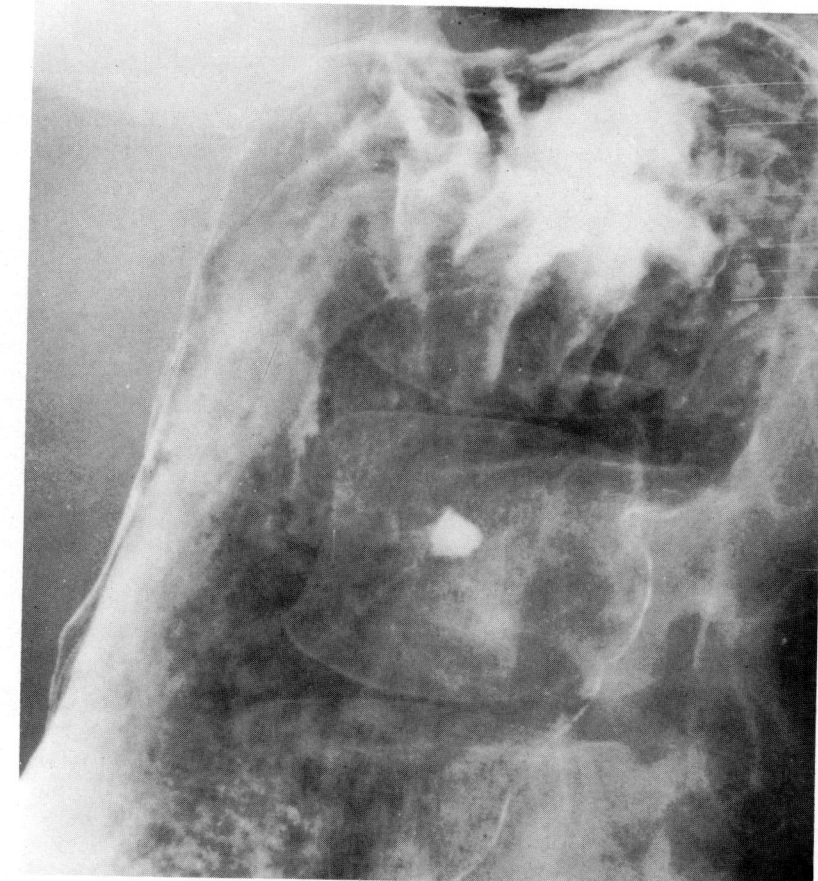

A

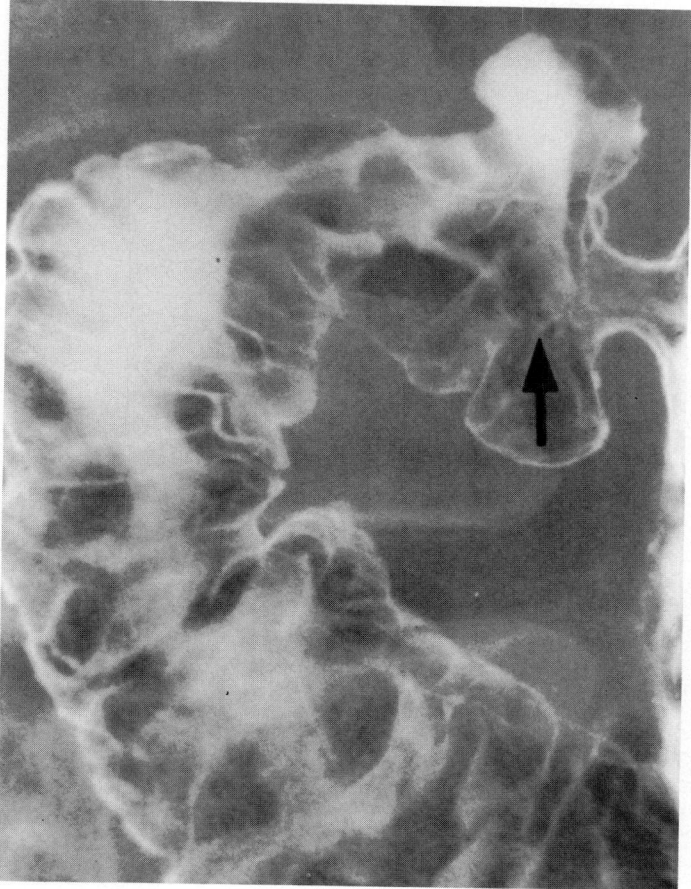

B

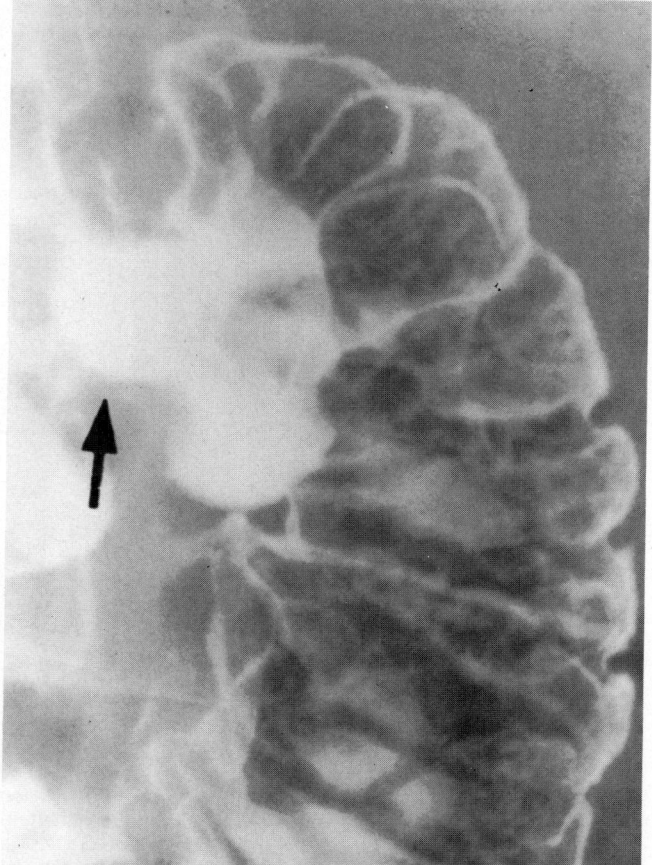

C

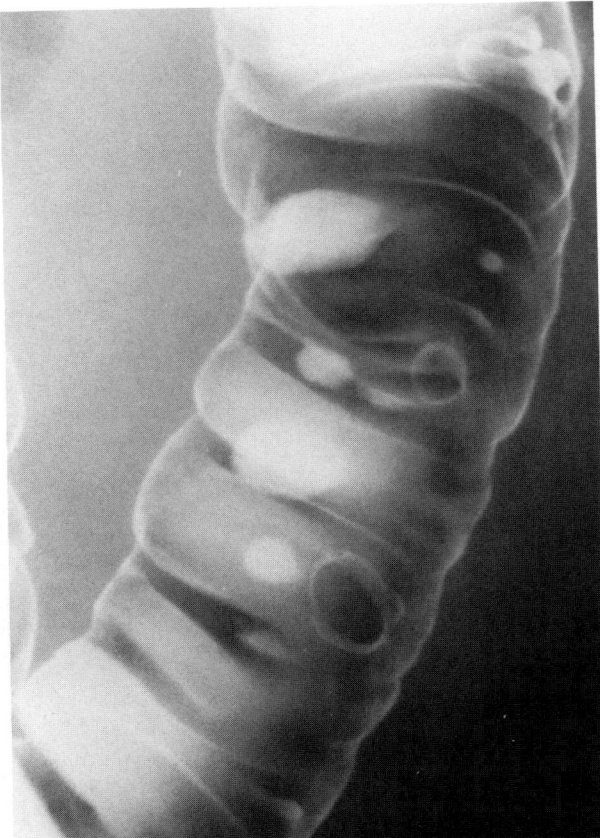

**Figure 4–12. Depressed lesions on the dependent and nondependent surfaces.** In a segment of colonic diverticulosis, there are barium-filled diverticula on the dependent surface, and the diverticula on the nondependent surface are seen as ring shadows.

as a hindrance in many ways (Fig. 4–13). It can cover over and submerge a lesion on the dependent surface. Even a small barium pool on the dependent surface can obscure the etching of a lesion on the nondependent surface (Fig. 4–14). Furthermore, a barium pool in an overlapping loop of bowel can also obscure lesions.

In general terms, lesions on the dependent surface are best demonstrated with an extremely shallow barium pool. Recognition of lesions on the nondependent surface requires that the barium pool on the dependent surface be entirely eliminated. These varying requirements can be met by using the flow technique (Fig. 4–15). As the patient is turned under fluoroscopic control, the flow of the barium pool is observed across the dependent surface. Thus, shallow lesions can be demonstrated on the dependent surface, and when the barium pool flows away, the nondependent surface lesions are seen. The concept of flow technique is important for demonstrating subtle lesions and avoiding diagnostic error.

## ARTIFACTS

Many of the artifactual appearances associated with double contrast studies are obvious to the radiologist.[12] These include findings caused by barium precipitation (Fig. 4–16A), patchy mucosal coating, and extraneous debris. However, a few artifacts may be confusing because they closely resemble pathologic states.

In the colon, some barium suspensions may crack or flake, producing an appearance suggestive of inflammatory bowel disease (Fig. 4–16B). In some patients,

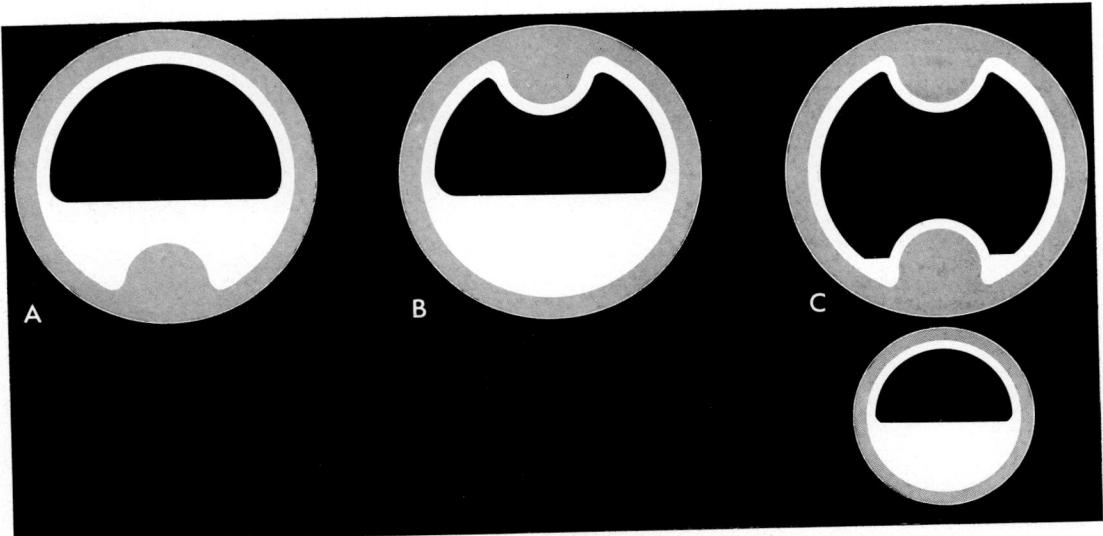

**Figure 4–13. Diagrammatic representation of the hazards of the barium pool. A.** Barium pool obscures the lesion on the dependent surface. **B.** The barium pool obscures the fine white etching of the lesion on the nondependent surface. **C.** The barium pool in the overlapping loop of bowel may obscure a lesion on either the dependent or the nondependent surface.

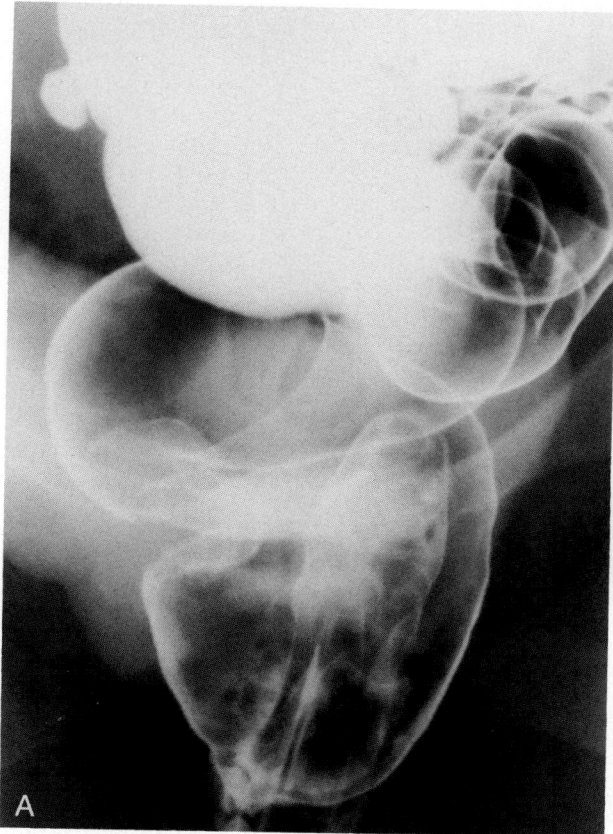

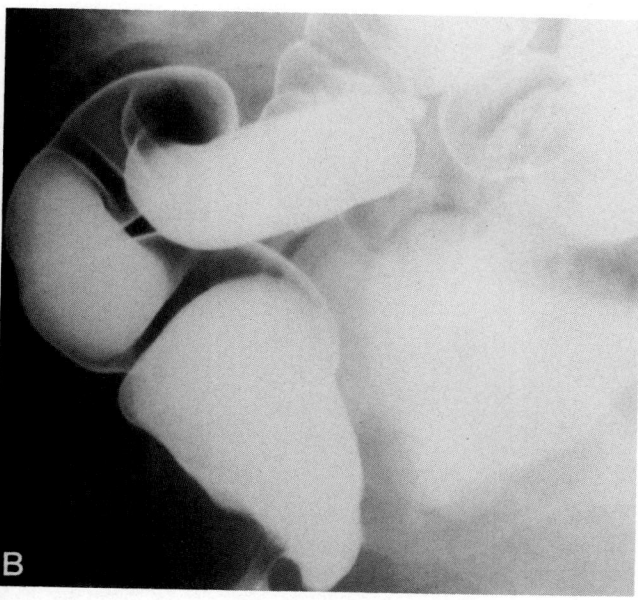

**Figure 4–14. Barium pool obscuring a lesion on the nondependent surface. A.** In the frontal projection, a polypoid carcinoma is seen along the right lateral wall of the rectum. **B.** In the left lateral projection, the rectal carcinoma is on the nondependent surface and its outline is obscured by the barium pool on the left lateral wall of the rectum.

**Figure 4–15. Flow technique.** There is a 1-cm sessile polyp in the cecum. Its appearance varies as barium flows across the dependent surface of the cecum.

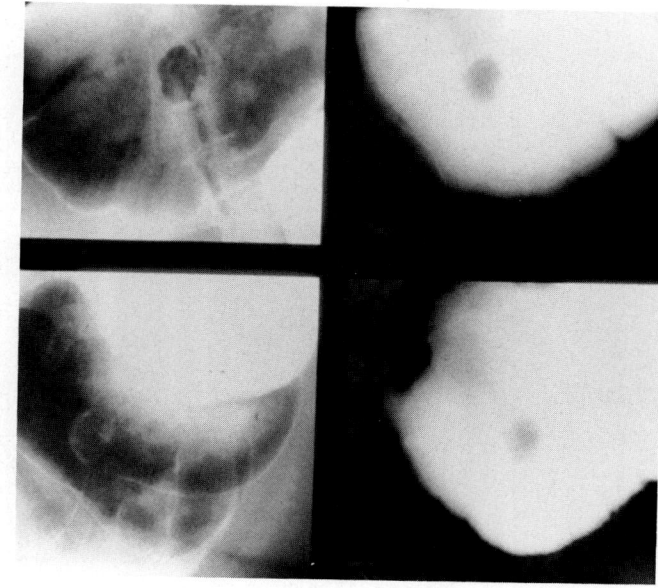

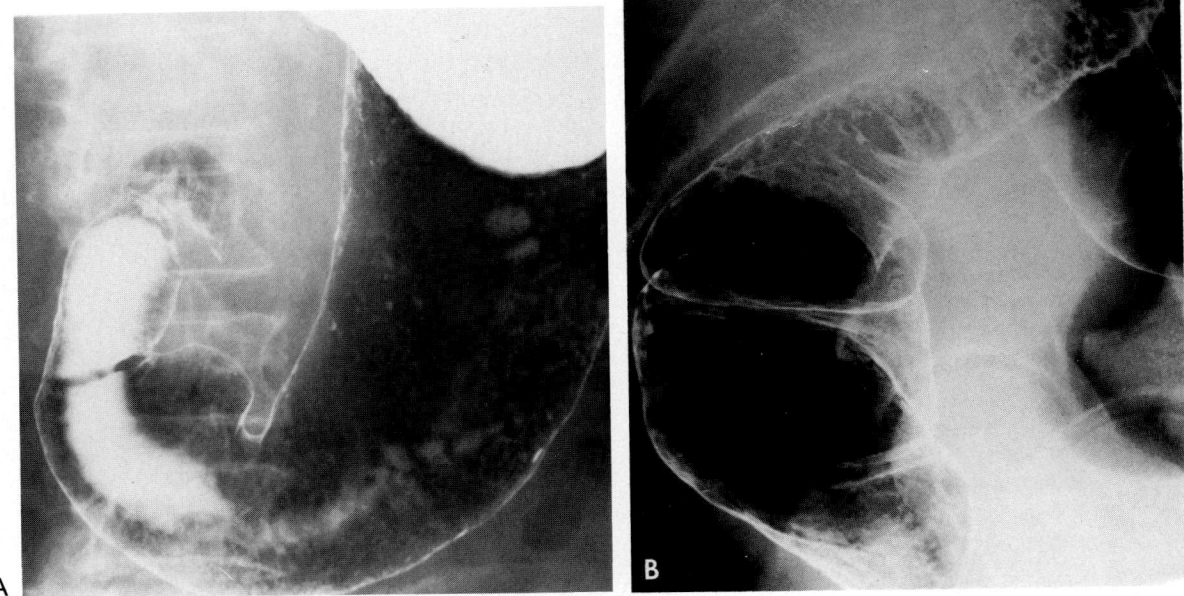

**Figure 4–16. Double contrast artifacts. A.** Barium precipitates. These are clearly recognized as sharp, dense barium collections on top of the mucosal surface. **B.** Flaking of the barium suspension simulating inflammatory bowel disease. (**B** from Laufer I: Air contrast studies of the colon in inflammatory bowel disease. Crit Rev Diagn Imaging 9:421–447, 1977. Copyright CRC Press, Inc., Boca Raton, FL.)

there may be inadequate distention to separate the anterior and posterior walls. The area of apposition is outlined and may resemble a mass lesion (Fig. 4–17A). This has been termed a "kissing" artifact. In other patients, this kissing artifact is produced by extrinsic compression (Fig. 4–17B) causing the anterior and posterior walls to appose. In such cases, the appropriate projection should be obtained to search for an extrinsic mass.

Because the air-filled bowel is transradiant, structures in front of or behind the bowel may be projected over the bowel and appear to represent lesions within the bowel. It is particularly important to recognize the true nature of barium-filled diverticula and calcified structures and not to mistake them for polypoid or ulcerated lesions in the bowel (Fig. 4–18).

Other double contrast artifacts are discussed in chapters dealing with specific organs.

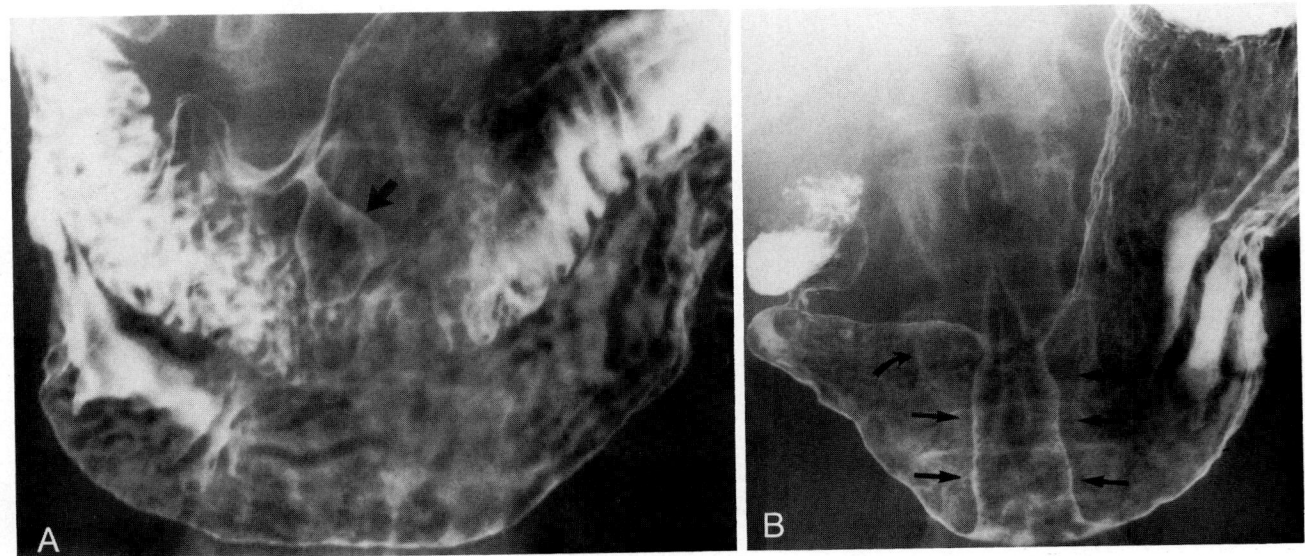

**Figure 4–17. Kissing artifact. A.** There is a kissing artifact along the lesser curve of the stomach, simulating a polypoid lesion *(arrow)*. **B.** A kissing artifact resulting from compression by the abdominal aorta *(arrows)*. The curved arrow indicates calcification in the wall of the aorta.

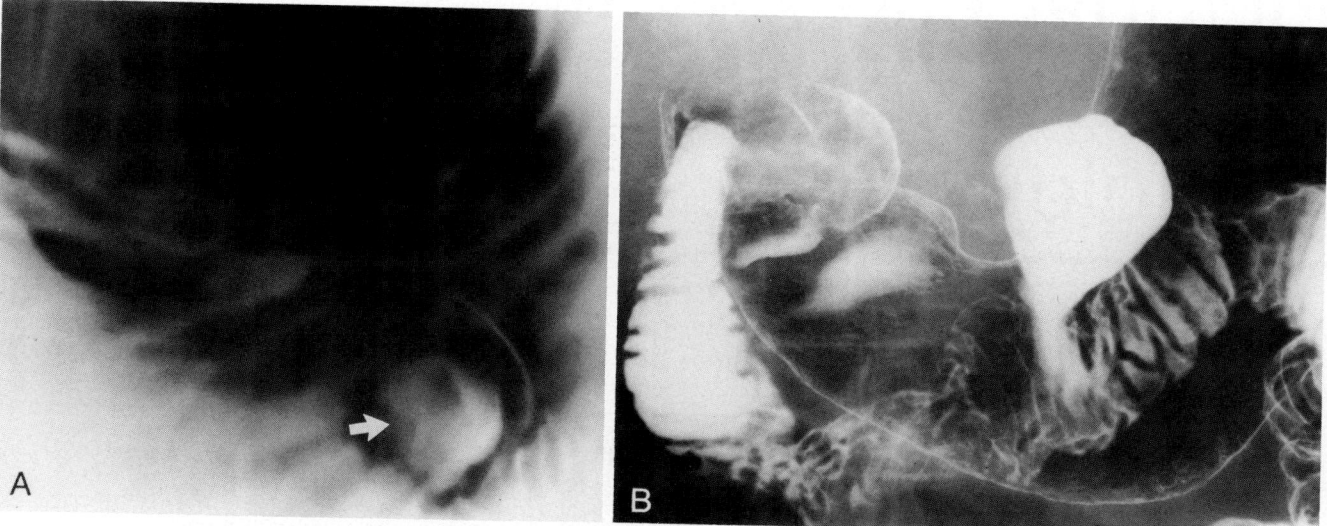

**Figure 4–18. Duodenal diverticulum simulating a gastric ulcer. A.** The compression film of the stomach shows a large barium collection suggestive of a gastric ulcer. **B.** Supine double contrast film shows that the barium-filled structure was a large diverticulum of the fourth portion of the duodenum.

### Acknowledgment

Figures 4–3A and B, 4–4A and B, 4–6A and B, 4–8, 4–9A and B, 4–11A to C, and 4–13A and B are reproduced from Laufer I, Levine MS (eds): Double Contrast Gastrointestinal Radiology (2nd ed). Philadelphia: WB Saunders, 1992.

# References

1. Gelfand DW, Ott DJ, Chen YM: Decreasing numbers of gastrointestinal studies: report of data from 69 radiologic practices. AJR 148:1133–1136, 1987.
2. Young JW, Ginthner TP, Keramati B: The competitive barium meal. Clin Radiol 36:43–46, 1985.
3. Dekker W, Op den Orth JO: Biphasic radiologic examination and endoscopy of the upper gastrointestinal tract. A comparative study. J Clin Gastroenterol 10:461–465, 1988.
4. Gelfand DW, Chen YM, Ott DJ: Multiphasic examinations of the stomach: efficacy of individual techniques and combinations of techniques in detecting 153 lesions. Radiology 162:829–834, 1987.
5. Gelfand DW, Ott DJ: Single vs. double-contrast gastrointestinal studies: critical analysis of reported statistics. AJR 137:523–528, 1981.
6. Laufer I, Kressel HY: Principles of double contrast diagnosis. *In* Laufer I, Levine MS (eds): Double Contrast Gastrointestinal Radiology (2nd ed). Philadelphia: WB Saunders, 1992, pp 9–54.
7. Miller RE: Recipes for gastrointestinal examinations. AJR 137:1285–1286, 1981.
8. Kikuchi Y, Levine MS, Laufer I, et al: Value of flow technique for double-contrast examination of the stomach. AJR 147:1183–1184, 1986.
9. Op den Orth JO, Ploem S: The stalactite phenomenon in double contrast studies of the stomach. Radiology 117:523–525, 1975.
10. Aronchick J, Laufer I, Glick S: Barium stalactites: observations on their nature and significance. Radiology 149:588–591, 1983.
11. Miller WT Jr, Levine MS, Rubesin SE, et al: Bowler-hat sign: a simple principle for differentiating polyps from diverticula. Radiology 173:615–617, 1989.
12. Gohel VK, Kressel HY, Laufer I: Double contrast artifacts. Gastrointest Radiol 3:139–146, 1978.

# Pictorial Glossary of Double Contrast Radiology

Stephen E. Rubesin, M.D.

Igor Laufer, M.D.

INTRODUCTION

DIFFUSE MUCOSAL LESIONS
Granularity
Nodularity
Shaggy
Villous Pattern
Reticular Pattern
Striae

FOCAL MASS LESIONS
Filling Defect
Polyp
Plaque
Carpet Lesion
Web
Contour Defect
Coil Spring Sign
Pliability

DEPRESSED LESIONS
Ulcer Niche (Crater)
Aphthoid Ulcer
Linear Ulcer
Varioliform Erosion
Collar Button Ulcer

MIXED LESIONS
Target Lesion

WALL LESIONS
Linitis Plastica
Submucosal Mass
Exoenteric Mass
Tracking

ABNORMAL FOLDS
Radiating Folds
Stack of Coins Appearance

Interspace Spikes
Thumbprinting
Cobblestoning
Polypoid Folds
Serpentine (Serpiginous) Folds

OTHER TERMS
String Sign
Annular Lesion
Sacculation

EXTRINSIC CHANGES
Extrinsic Mass Effect
Spiculation
Pleating
Tethering
Angulation

## INTRODUCTION

Careful use of descriptive terms aids in radiologic analysis of perceived abnormalities. By describing the radiographic characteristics of a lesion, a radiologist can localize the lesion to the mucosa, bowel wall, or tissue extrinsic to bowel. This radiographic description, in conjunction with the site and size of the lesion, the age of the patient, and the clinical history, enables the radiologist to make a specific diagnosis or formulate a graded differential diagnosis of the most likely possibilities. In addition, precise use of descriptive terms enhances communication between radiologist and clinician. A radiologist should be able to describe an abnormality so that the person reading or listening to the radiographic report can visualize the lesion without looking at the film.

This chapter is a pictorial glossary that visually defines common descriptive terms in gastrointestinal radiology. The terms are divided by whether they refer to mucosal, wall, or extrinsic lesions.

## DIFFUSE MUCOSAL LESIONS

### Granularity

*Granularity* implies subtle elevation of the mucosal surface seen en face as small radiolucencies in the shallow barium pool or as fine punctate dots of barium between lucencies (Fig. 5–1). The "granules" are barely perceptible elevations with indistinct borders, as if salt had been sprinkled on a plate. Granularity implies mucosa elevated by edema, inflammatory exudate, or

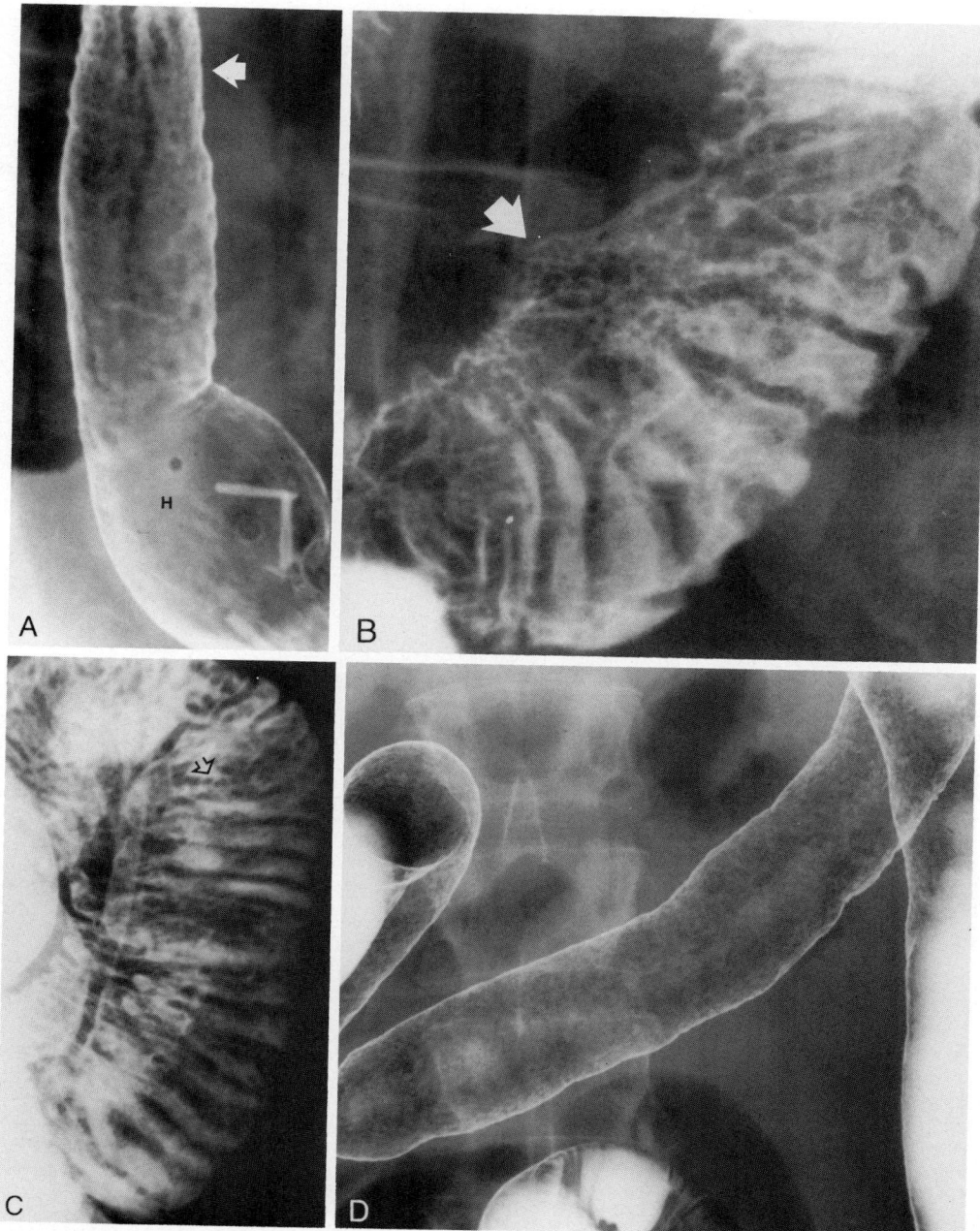

**Figure 5–1. Granularity. A.** Reflux esophagitis. Small, polygonal and round radiolucencies varying from less than 1 to 3 mm *(arrow)* diffusely involve the surface of the distal esophagus above a hiatal hernia (H). **B.** Crohn's disease. Along the mesenteric border of the ileum, mucosal granularity is seen *(arrow)*. The granular mucosa represents fusion and clubbing of villi and/or edema and inflammatory changes in the lamina propria that widen villi. (**B** from Rubesin SE, Bronner M: Radiologic-pathologic concepts in Crohn's disease. *In* Herlinger H, Megibow AJ [eds]: Advances in Gastrointestinal Radiology, Volume 1. Chicago: Mosby–Year Book, 1991, pp 27–55.) **C.** Whipple's disease. In the proximal jejunum, mildly thickened and undulating folds are seen. Subtle mucosal granularity *(arrow)* represents infiltration of the lamina propria by macrophages filled with Whipple's bacilli or fat. (**C** courtesy of E. Salomonwitz, M.D., Vienna, Austria.) **D.** Ulcerative colitis. In the transverse colon, granular mucosa is seen. The granular mucosa reflects mild edema and inflammatory changes. (**D** reprinted by permission of the publisher from Radiologic investigation of inflammatory bowel disease, by Rubesin SE, Laufer I, Dinsmore B, in Inflammatory Bowel Disease, pp 453–491. Copyright 1992 by Elsevier Science Publishing Co., Inc.)

tumor. Barium flocculated on the mucosal surface may mimic granular mucosa.

## Nodularity

Mucosal nodules are relatively well-circumscribed elevations seen en face as round to ovoid radiolucencies in the barium pool or as small rings etched in white

(Fig. 5–2). In profile, nodules are seen as small hemispheric elevations of the contour. Nodules may arise in the mucosa itself, the lamina propria, or the adjacent submucosa. If a mucosal nodule involves a bowel fold, especially the rugae of the stomach or the valvulae conniventes of the small bowel, the fold is eccentrically enlarged. Submucosal nodules involving a bowel fold, seen en face, symmetrically splay the parallel surfaces of the fold. Mucosal nodularity may be described as fine

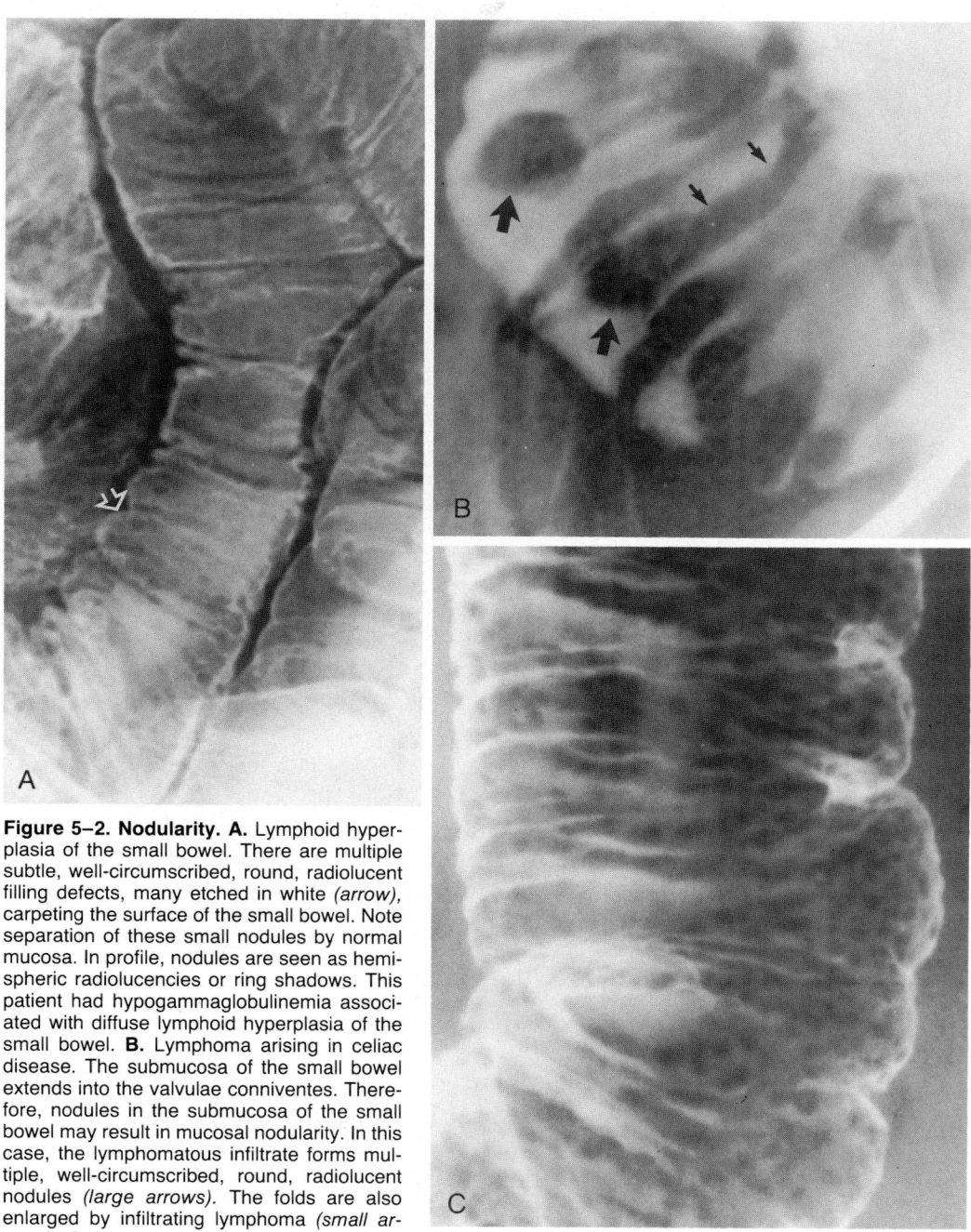

**Figure 5–2. Nodularity. A.** Lymphoid hyperplasia of the small bowel. There are multiple subtle, well-circumscribed, round, radiolucent filling defects, many etched in white *(arrow),* carpeting the surface of the small bowel. Note separation of these small nodules by normal mucosa. In profile, nodules are seen as hemispheric radiolucencies or ring shadows. This patient had hypogammaglobulinemia associated with diffuse lymphoid hyperplasia of the small bowel. **B.** Lymphoma arising in celiac disease. The submucosa of the small bowel extends into the valvulae conniventes. Therefore, nodules in the submucosa of the small bowel may result in mucosal nodularity. In this case, the lymphomatous infiltrate forms multiple, well-circumscribed, round, radiolucent nodules *(large arrows).* The folds are also enlarged by infiltrating lymphoma *(small arrows).* **C.** Lymphoid hyperplasia of colon in Crohn's disease. Numerous small, round, radiolucent nodules separated by normal mucosa are seen in this close-up view of the transverse colon.

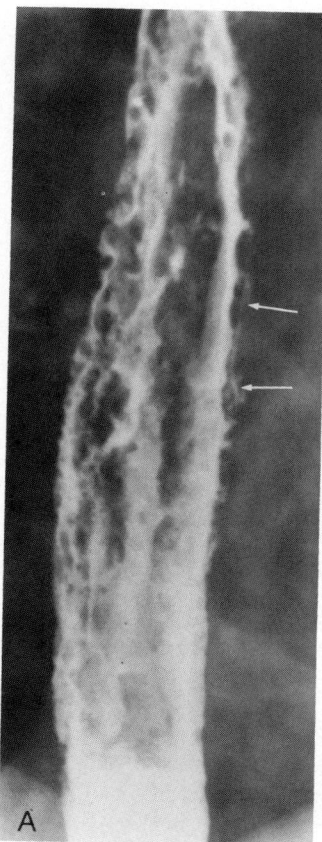

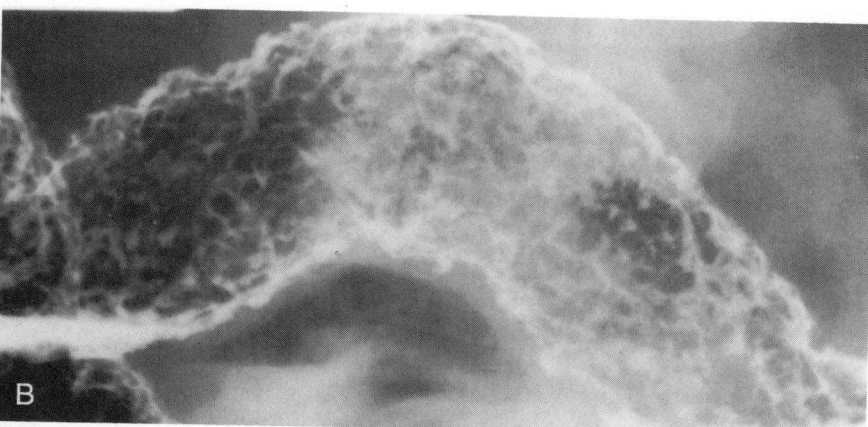

**Figure 5–3. Shaggy. A.** *Candida* esophagitis. The mucosal contour is markedly irregular. Barium appears to be beneath the mucosal surface *(arrows)*. In reality, this barium is trapped between sloughed epithelial debris and the ulcerated mucosa. En face, there are numerous and variable-sized plaques. (From Rubesin SE, Levine MS, Laufer I: Odynophagia. *In* Thompson WM [ed]: Common Problems in Gastrointestinal Radiology. Chicago: Year Book Medical, 1989, pp 108–117.) **B.** Ulcerative colitis. Irregular mucosal surface and contour in extensive ulcerative colitis.

or coarse. The distinction between fine nodularity and mucosal granularity is somewhat arbitrary, although in general, mucosal nodules are relatively larger and more discrete.

## Shaggy

*Shaggy* describes such severe mucosal abnormality that it is difficult to distinguish ulcerated mucosa from sloughed epithelium and inflammatory detritus (Fig. 5–3). In profile, the contour is jagged. En face, numerous barium lines fill the interstices between ulcerated mucosa and debris. Shaggy is frequently used to describe the radiographic findings in severe *Candida* esophagitis and ulcerative colitis (see Fig. 5–3).

## Villous Pattern

The villi of the small intestine are at the radiographic limits of resolution. Some villi may be seen if the mucosa is well coated and slightly magnified. This *villous pattern* is manifest as barely perceptible radiolucencies surrounded by barium in the interstices between villi (Fig. 5–4).

## Reticular Pattern

*Reticular* means net-like (Fig. 5–5). The net is formed by barium in the interstices of a mucosal lesion, such as a carpet lesion. The intervening radiolucent mucosa may be round, ovoid, or polygonal. There is no definite dividing line between a villous pattern and a reticular pattern on the mucosal surface. A reticular pattern typically occurs in abnormalities arising in columnar mucosa. For example, a reticular pattern is seen in the columnar metaplasia of Barrett's esophagus (see Fig. 5–5B) or in the colonic urticarial pattern (see Fig. 5–5C).

## Striae

Gastrointestinal mucosa must be distensible. This is accomplished by redundant folds and stretchable mucosa: the longitudinal folds of the esophagus, the rugal folds of the stomach, and the valvulae conniventes of the small bowel. When a viscus is less than fully distended, transverse striations appear. Examples are the "feline esophagus" (Fig. 5–6A), gastric striae (Fig. 5–6B), and innominate grooves of the colon (Fig. 5–6C).

## FOCAL MASS LESIONS

### Filling Defect

A *filling defect* is a radiolucency in the barium pool caused by displacement of the barium by a protruding lesion (Fig. 5–7).

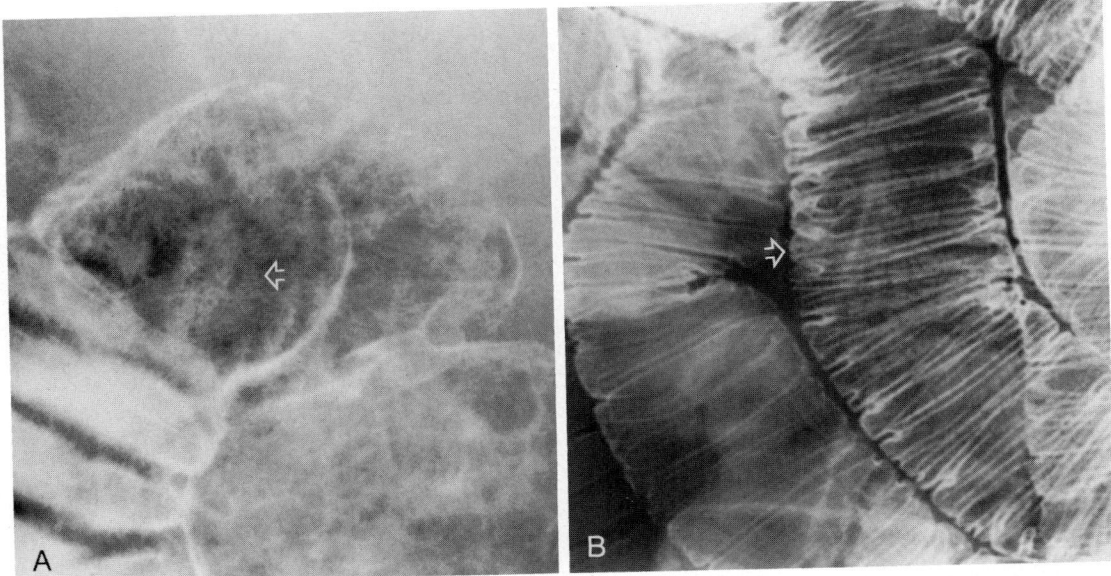

**Figure 5–4. Villous pattern. A.** Normal duodenal mucosa. Multiple, small, punctate radiolucencies are etched by barium. In some regions, a reticular pattern is seen *(arrow)*. **B.** Normal small bowel mucosa. Multiple punctate radiolucencies are seen in the small bowel mucosa *(arrow)*. In some loops of small intestine the villous pattern is not seen.

## Polyp

A *polyp* is a protrusion from a mucous membrane. In general, the height of a polyp is comparable to its width, but a polyp is relatively tall in comparison to a mucosal plaque. Polyps may be seen as radiolucent filling defects on the dependent surface or may be etched in white when on the nondependent surface (Fig. 5–8). They have many shapes and many radiographic appearances depending on whether they are small or large, sessile or pedunculated (see Fig. 5–8) (see Chapter 4). However, a polyp is a polyp is a polyp. Polyp is not a histologically definitive term and does not imply adenomatous (dysplastic) change.

## Plaque

A *plaque* is a shallow surface elevation much broader than it is high. Plaques are so distinct that their margins are etched in white by barium trapped between the edges of the plaque and the underlying mucosa (Fig. 5–9). Plaques may vary greatly in size, from the small plaques of *Candida* esophagitis to plaque-like tumors.

## Carpet Lesion

*Carpet lesions* are focal, flat, well-circumscribed surface elevations. En face, the margin of the lesion is etched in white by barium (Fig. 5–10). When barium fills the interstices of the lesion, multiple small, polygonal radiolucent filling defects are seen surrounded by barium. In profile, the contour may be finally spiculated or relatively normal. The most characteristic carpet lesions are flat colonic adenomas.

## Web

A *web* is a thin band of mucosa with or without submucosa that crosses a variable portion of the intestinal lumen. Webs vary from small shelf-like lesions to hemispheric bars to circumferential rings (Fig. 5–11). Webs may be normal variants or the sequelae of inflammatory disease.

## Contour Defect

A *contour defect* is a disruption of the expected luminal contour by a sessile lesion protruding into the gastrointestinal lumen (Fig. 5–12). A contour defect is not, in itself, a sign of malignancy. However, because the size of the contour defect is related to the size of the lesion, the larger the contour defect, the greater the likelihood of malignancy.

## Coil Spring Sign

If barium is forced between one loop of bowel intussuscepting into another loop, the barium may coat the mucosal folds of the outer loop. The result is concentric rings of barium coating the mucosa and resembling a coil spring (Fig. 5–13).

**Figure 5–5. Reticular pattern. A.** Areae gastricae. In general, columnar mucosa in the gastrointestinal tract is divided into islands of tissue surrounded by shallow grooves. This pattern is best exemplified in the areae gastricae of the stomach. The areae gastricae are seen as well-circumscribed, polygonal radiolucencies surrounded by barium-filled grooves, often in a reticular arrangement. **B.** Barrett's esophagus. The columnar mucosa of Barrett's esophagus may appear radiographically as a net-like collection of barium lines *(open arrows)*. It is difficult to differentiate fine nodularity from reticular mucosa or a villous pattern. The reticular pattern in Barrett's esophagus is often seen below a reflux-induced stricture *(white arrow)*. Note the mucosal ulceration *(black arrows)* related to reflux esophagitis proximal to the stricture. (**B** from Levine MS, Kressel HY, Caroline DF, et al: Barrett esophagus: reticular pattern of the mucosa. Radiology 147:663–667, 1983.) **C.** Urticarial pattern in colon. When colonic mucosa is slightly elevated by edema and/or mild inflammation, the colonic surface may assume a reticular pattern. Barium etches sharply polygonal epithelial islands. This has been termed the *urticarial pattern* because it was first described in colonic urticaria. However, any disease that causes mild edema, inflammation, or ischemia of the mucosa may cause the columnar mucosa of the colon to assume an urticarial pattern, including ischemia caused by obstruction, Crohn's disease, or viral infections. (**C** from Rubesin SE, Saul SH, Laufer I, et al: Carpet lesions of the colon. Radiographics 5:537–552, 1985.)

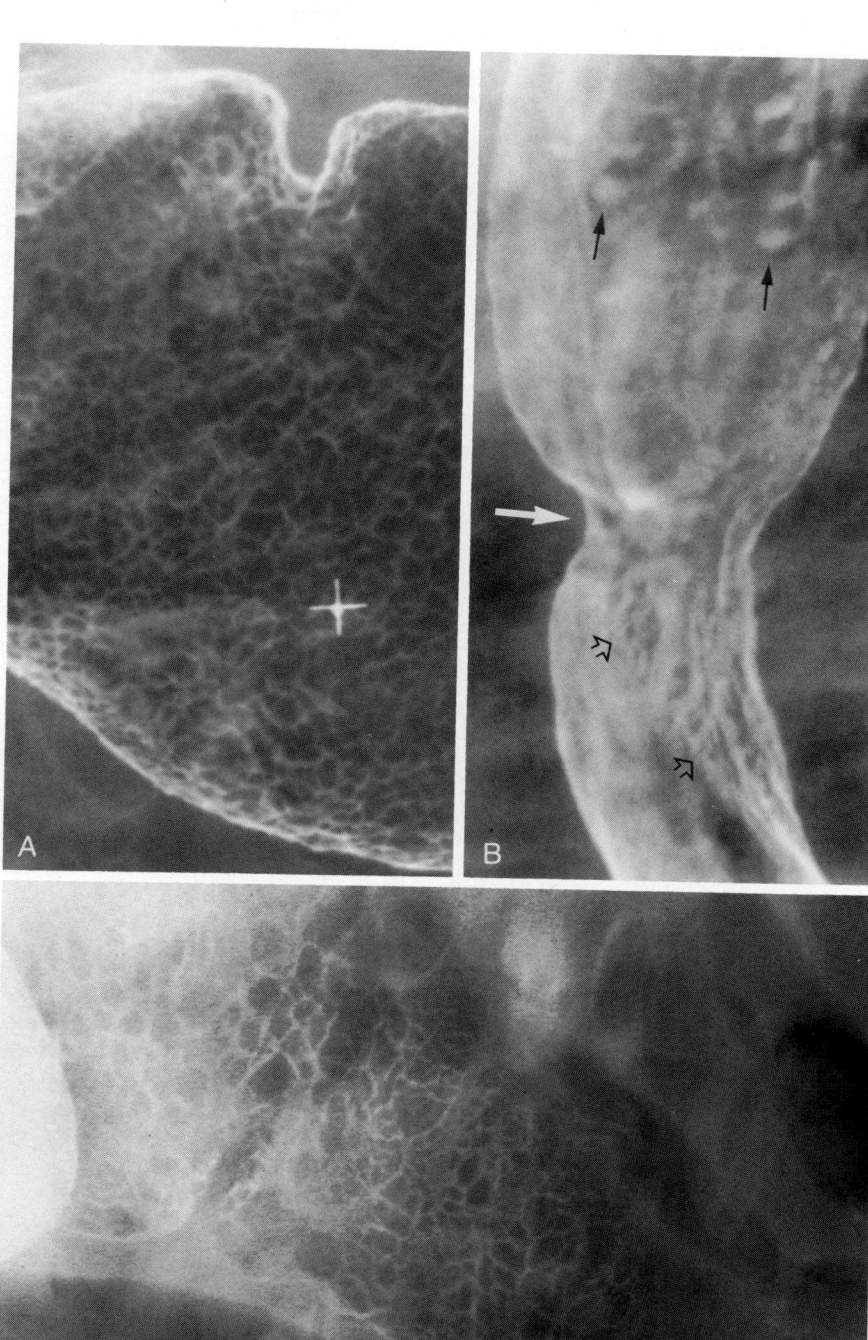

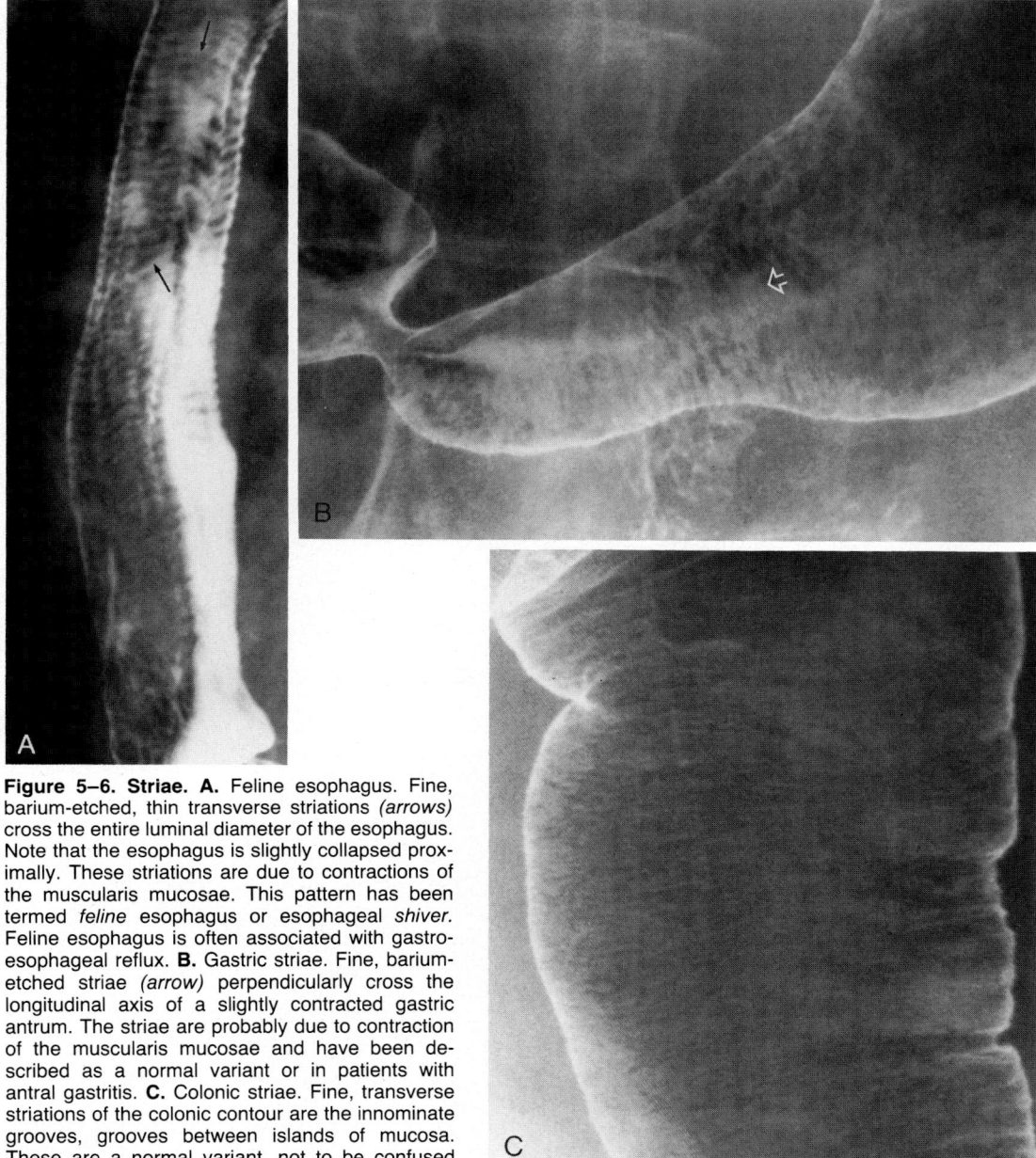

**Figure 5–6. Striae. A.** Feline esophagus. Fine, barium-etched, thin transverse striations *(arrows)* cross the entire luminal diameter of the esophagus. Note that the esophagus is slightly collapsed proximally. These striations are due to contractions of the muscularis mucosae. This pattern has been termed *feline* esophagus or esophageal *shiver.* Feline esophagus is often associated with gastro-esophageal reflux. **B.** Gastric striae. Fine, barium-etched striae *(arrow)* perpendicularly cross the longitudinal axis of a slightly contracted gastric antrum. The striae are probably due to contraction of the muscularis mucosae and have been described as a normal variant or in patients with antral gastritis. **C.** Colonic striae. Fine, transverse striations of the colonic contour are the innominate grooves, grooves between islands of mucosa. These are a normal variant, not to be confused with inflammation of the mucosa.

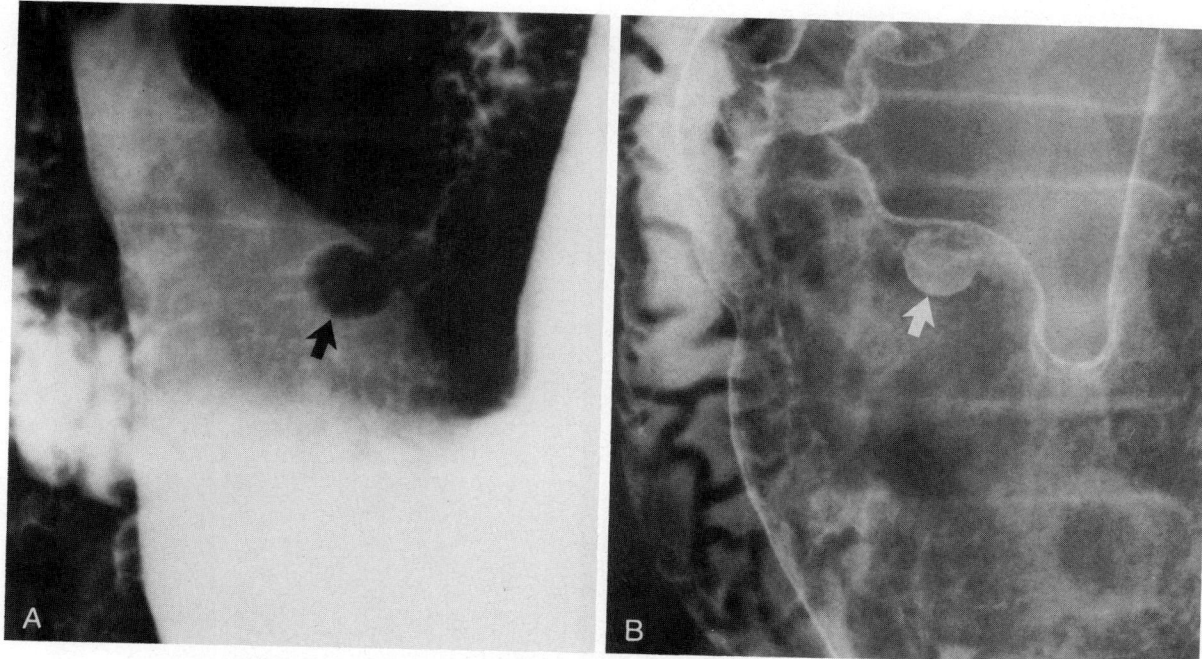

**Figure 5–7. Filling defect. A.** Hyperplastic polyp in the gastric antrum. A filling defect *(arrow)* is seen in the barium pool. **B.** The same polyp is seen in air contrast as a round, increased radiodensity etched in white *(arrow).*

## Pliability

Change or lack of change in the size and shape of a lesion is a clue to its composition (Fig. 5–14). Lesions that change in size or shape depending on the amount of luminal distention or manual compression are often composed of fat, fluid, or blood.

## DEPRESSED LESIONS

### Ulcer Niche (Crater)

The term *niche* or *crater* refers to the defect or the hole in the mucosal surface representing an ulcer. The niche may be visualized in profile as a projection of barium beyond the mucosal surface. Alternatively, the niche may be seen en face as a barium collection or the edges of the crater may be etched in white (Fig. 5–15).

### Aphthoid Ulcer

An aphthoid ulcer is a small ulcer occurring on a mucous membrane. This is a nonspecific pathologic term derived from the Greek root *aphthai*, which meant "to set on fire or to inflame" and referred to the oral lesions of thrush, which are raised white plaques. Later, the term was used by the Greeks to refer to small ulcers on the mucous membrane of the mouth. Aphth*oid* means "resembling aphthae." Aphth*ous* means "related to

aphthae." Radiologists use the terms aphthoid ulcer and aphthous ulcer interchangeably, but the preferred term is *aphthoid* ulcer. The most common causes of aphthoid ulcers are Crohn's disease, viral infections, varioliform erosions, and amebiasis (Fig. 5–16).

### Linear Ulcer

Ulcers of the gastrointestinal tract need not be round or ovoid. Linear ulcers are not infrequently seen and have a variety of etiologies, especially Crohn's disease (Fig. 5–17), trauma resulting from intubation or vomiting, or the toxic effects of drugs such as aspirin and other nonsteroidal anti-inflammatory agents.

### Varioliform Erosion

*Varioliform* means "resembling smallpox" (Fig. 5–18). This term refers to erosions characterized by a small central barium collection and a surrounding radiolucency associated with edema. These have also been referred to as "complete" erosions, and the radiographic appearance is identical to that of aphthoid ulcers seen throughout the gastrointestinal tract. In many cases, there is no known cause for varioliform gastritis, but in some patients the condition may be due to ingestion of aspirin or other nonsteroidal anti-inflammatory drugs, viral infection, or alcohol ingestion.

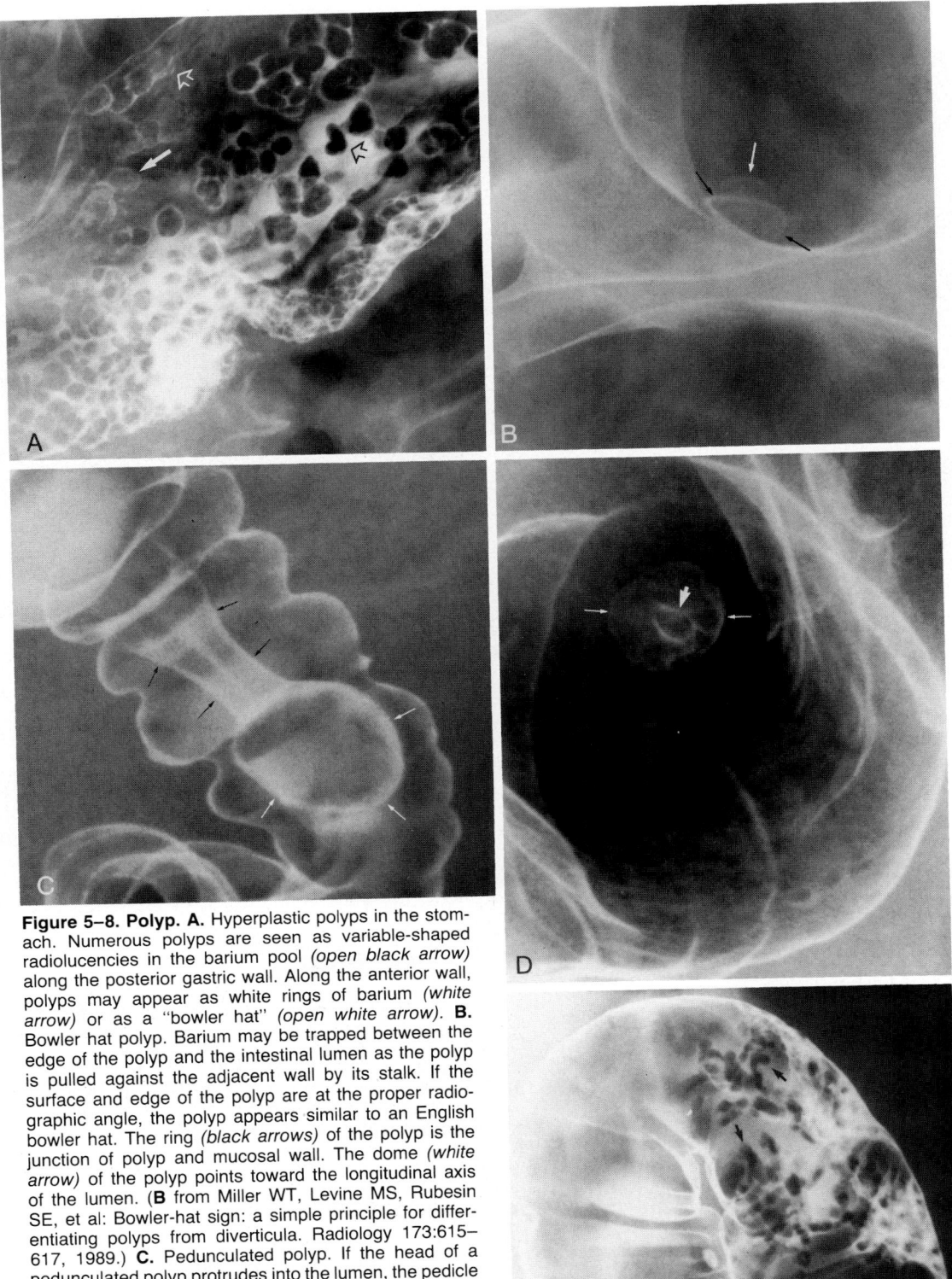

**Figure 5–8. Polyp. A.** Hyperplastic polyps in the stomach. Numerous polyps are seen as variable-shaped radiolucencies in the barium pool *(open black arrow)* along the posterior gastric wall. Along the anterior wall, polyps may appear as white rings of barium *(white arrow)* or as a "bowler hat" *(open white arrow).* **B.** Bowler hat polyp. Barium may be trapped between the edge of the polyp and the intestinal lumen as the polyp is pulled against the adjacent wall by its stalk. If the surface and edge of the polyp are at the proper radiographic angle, the polyp appears similar to an English bowler hat. The ring *(black arrows)* of the polyp is the junction of polyp and mucosal wall. The dome *(white arrow)* of the polyp points toward the longitudinal axis of the lumen. (**B** from Miller WT, Levine MS, Rubesin SE, et al: Bowler-hat sign: a simple principle for differentiating polyps from diverticula. Radiology 173:615–617, 1989.) **C.** Pedunculated polyp. If the head of a pedunculated polyp protrudes into the lumen, the pedicle of the polyp is seen in profile as parallel barium-etched lines *(black arrows)* or as a tubular radiolucency in the barium pool. The head of the polyp *(white arrows)* is seen as a round or ovoid filling defect in the barium pool or etched in white. **D.** Mexican hat polyp. If a pedunculated polyp is seen en face, the pedicle appears as a ring shadow *(thick arrow)* central to the larger ring shadow of the head of the polyp *(thin arrows).* These concentric ring shadows have been termed the *sombrero* or *Mexican hat* sign. **E.** Filiform polyp. A filiform polyp is a tubular or branched polyp, often with a clubbed head. Filiform polyps imply that there has been prior inflammatory disease involving the mucosal surface of the bowel. When residual inflamed and/or hyperplastic or reparative tissue protrudes into the lumen, the resulting projections appear in a filiform shape. In this patient with quiescent Crohn's disease, numerous filiform polyps *(arrows)* are seen in the splenic flexure.

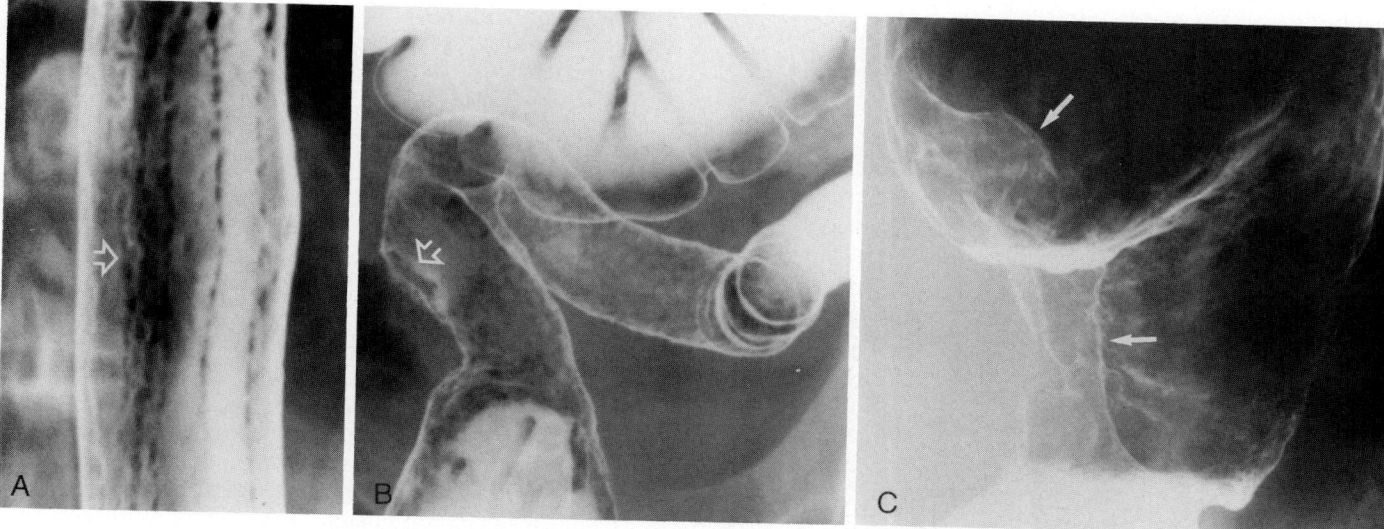

**Figure 5–9. Plaques. A.** *Candida* esophagitis. Small, well-circumscribed radiolucencies etched in white *(arrow)* are aligned longitudinally along the esophageal mucosa. Note normal intervening esophageal mucosa. (From Rubesin SE, Levine MS, Laufer I: Odynophagia. *In* Thompson WM [ed]: Common Problems in Gastrointestinal Radiology. Chicago: Year Book Medical, 1989, pp 108–117.) **B.** Dysplasia in ulcerative colitis. A 2-cm-long, slightly raised radiolucency is etched by barium *(arrow)*. This plaque is mass-like dysplasia associated with ulcerative colitis. Also note the tubular rectosigmoid colon with granular mucosa and the normal transverse colon. (Reprinted by permission of the publisher from Radiologic investigation of inflammatory bowel disease, by Rubesin SE, Laufer I, Dinsmore B, in Inflammatory Bowel Disease, pp 453–491. Copyright 1992 by Elsevier Science Publishing Co., Inc.) **C.** Adenocarcinoma of the stomach. The high lesser curvature of the stomach has a slightly abnormal contour. Several linear barium lines appear where they do not belong *(arrows)* and are associated with a slightly increased radiodensity of the lesser curvature.

**Figure 5–10. Carpet lesion. A.** Tubulovillous adenoma. A small carpet lesion of the colon is seen en face as a focal reticular pattern of intersecting barium lines *(large arrow)* disrupting the relatively smooth colonic mucosa. Note that the colonic contour *(small arrow)* is relatively normal. Also note the difference between the haustral fold carpeted by the tumor *(white arrowheads)* and the haustral fold covered by normal mucosa *(black arrowhead)*. (From Rubesin SE, Saul SH, Laufer I, et al: Carpet lesions of the colon. Radiographics 5:537–552, 1985.) **B.** Tubulovillous adenoma with carcinoma. A focal reticular network of barium lines courses across the circumference of the ascending colon *(thin arrows)*. The contour of the colon is relatively maintained in one region *(open arrow)*. In an area where carcinoma is present, the contour is indented and angulated *(thick arrows)*.

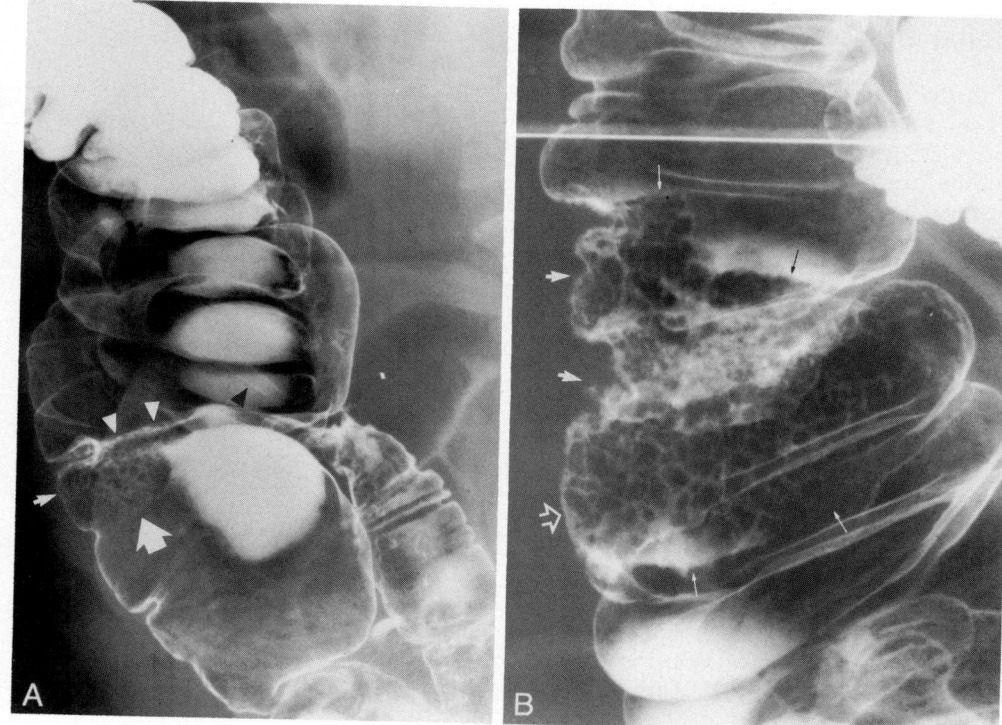

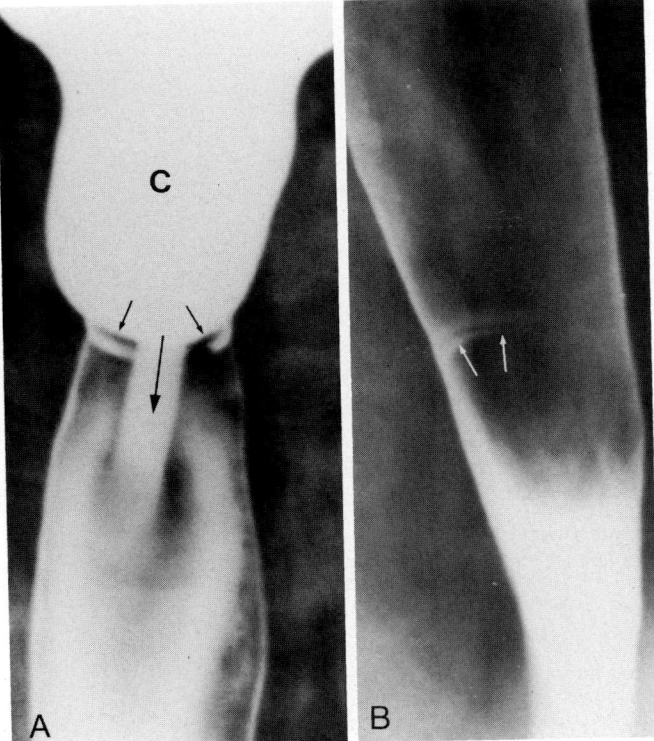

**Figure 5–11. Web. A.** Cervical esophageal web. A thin, radiolucent bar *(short arrows)* crosses the cervical esophagus. Obstruction is implied by dilatation of the proximal cervical esophagus (c) and spurt of barium through the web (the jet phenomenon) *(long arrow).* **B.** Web in distal esophagus. A thin, radiolucent bar *(arrows)* is etched in white and crosses part of the circumference of the distal esophagus. Distal esophageal webs are usually related to gastroesophageal reflux disease.

## Collar Button Ulcer

*Collar button ulcers* are ulcers with a narrow neck and a broad base (Fig. 5–19). These ulcers are formed when the ulcerative process spreads in the soft fat of the lamina propria and submucosa, parallel to the mucosal surface. This lateral extension gives the ulcer a relatively broad base in the submucosa and a narrow neck as it passes through the mucosa. In the colon, common causes of collar button ulcers are amebiasis, ulcerative colitis, and Crohn's disease.

## MIXED LESIONS

Lesions that have both a depressed and an elevated component are typically ulcerated masses of either mucosal or submucosal origin (Fig. 5–20).

## Target Lesion

A *target* or *bull's-eye lesion* is a mass with a central ulcer crater (Fig. 5–21). Target lesions are typically ulcerated *submucosal* masses caused by primary tumors

such as leiomyomas or by metastases, especially metastatic melanoma, Kaposi's sarcoma, or disseminated lymphoma.

## WALL LESIONS

### Linitis Plastica

*Linitis plastica* refers to diffuse narrowing and loss of pliability of a gastrointestinal organ. The linitis pattern is most commonly seen in scirrhous carcinoma of the stomach (Fig. 5–22). This type of cancer is also seen in the colon, especially in patients with chronic ulcerative colitis. Both inflammatory and neoplastic processes can result in a linitis appearance. For example, linitis plastica of the stomach may be due to lye ingestion or metastatic breast carcinoma. Because these infiltrative processes are primarily in a submucosal location, endoscopic biopsy may be negative.

### Submucosal Mass

The term *submucosal mass* refers to lesions arising in the submucosa and muscularis propria. These are typically benign or malignant tumors of smooth muscle, fat, or neural origin. The edge of a submucosal mass typically forms a right angle with the luminal contour (Fig. 5–23). The overlying mucosa is stretched and may be ulcerated.

Radiographically, in profile, a smooth-surfaced mass is seen forming right angles to the luminal contour (see

*Text continued on page 66*

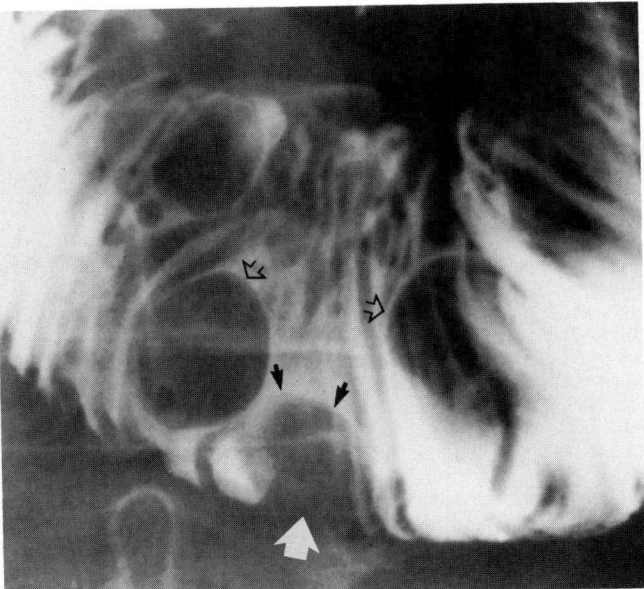

**Figure 5–12. Contour defect.** Metastatic melanoma in small intestine. A contour defect *(white arrow)* is seen as loss of the expected normal contour of bowel. The contour of the lumen is pushed toward the center of the bowel loop. In this case, a submucosal metastasis is seen in profile *(black arrows).* Other metastases are seen en face as smooth-surfaced, ovoid filling defects *(open arrows)* in the barium pool.

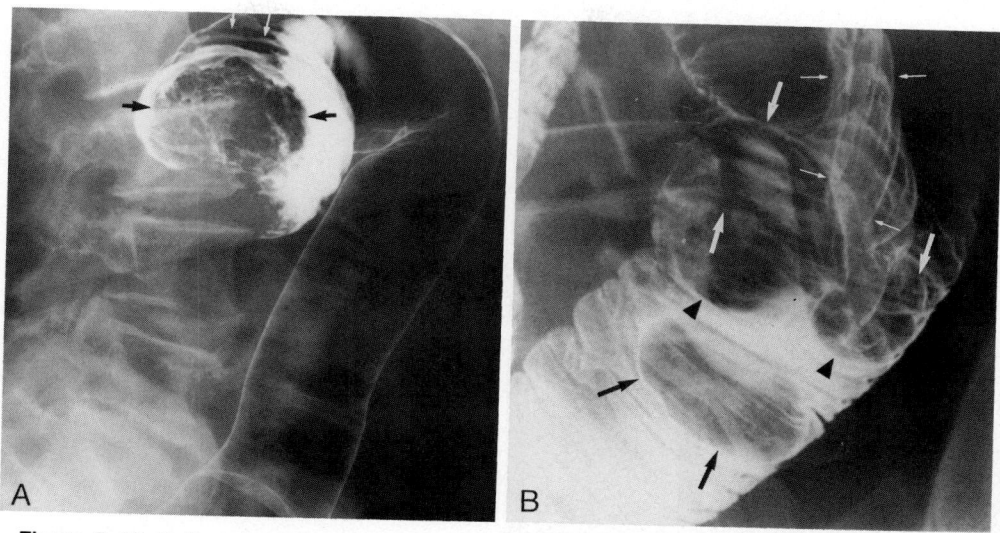

**Figure 5–13. Coil spring sign. A.** Colonic carcinoma causing intussusception. Parallel, barium-etched folds *(small white arrows)* are seen just distal to an intussuscepting mass in the splenic flexure. The mass *(black arrows)* has a reticular surface pattern and was a carcinoma arising in a villous adenoma. **B.** Metastatic melanoma causing intussusception of small bowel. Barium refluxes in a retrograde direction into the space between the prolapsing loop of the intussusception (intussusceptum) and the outer loop (intussuscipiens). The parallel folds of the coil spring are identified *(large white arrows)*. The intussusceptum is seen as a radiolucency *(arrowheads)* within the intussuscipiens. The lumen of the intussusceptum is narrow *(small white arrows)*. The lead point of the intussusceptum is a polypoid mass *(black arrows)*.

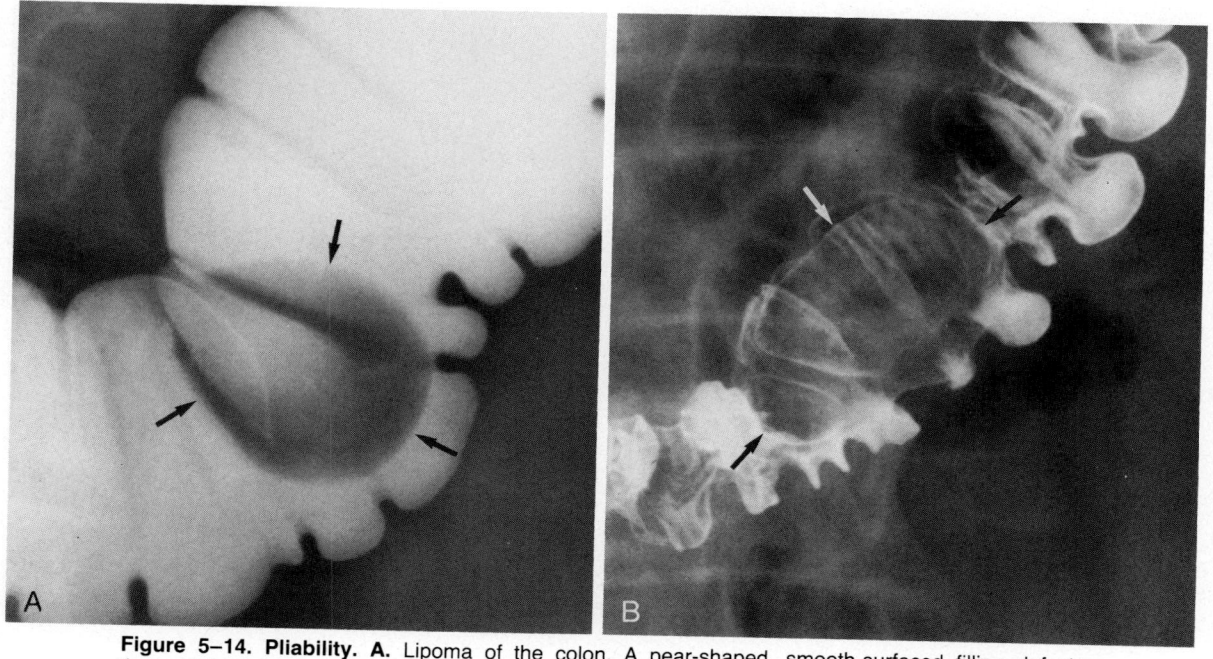

**Figure 5–14. Pliability. A.** Lipoma of the colon. A pear-shaped, smooth-surfaced filling defect *(arrows)* is seen in the barium column. **B.** A postevacuation film (same patient) shows that the polypoid mass has elongated *(arrows)* to conform to the collapsed lumen. These are the classic findings of a colonic lipoma.

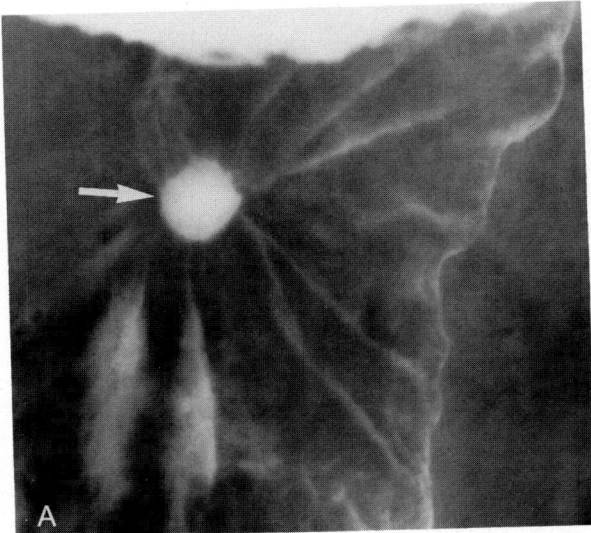

**Figure 5–15. Ulcer niche (crater). A.** Benign gastric ulcer. The ulcer niche (crater) is seen as a focal barium collection *(arrow).* The benign nature of the lesion is indicated by smooth folds that radiate to the ulcer's margin. **B.** Benign gastric ulcer. The ulcer crater is seen en face as a hemispheric ring shadow etched in white by barium *(arrows).* **C.** As this patient is turned, the ulcer is projected out of the expected contour of lesser curvature. The ulcer crater is now seen as a hemispheric line *(arrows)* protruding from the lesser curve of the stomach.

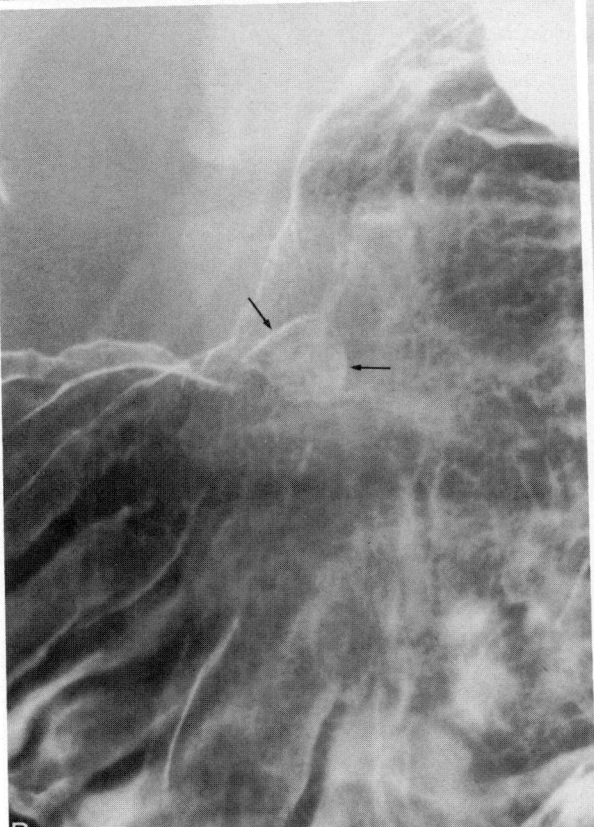

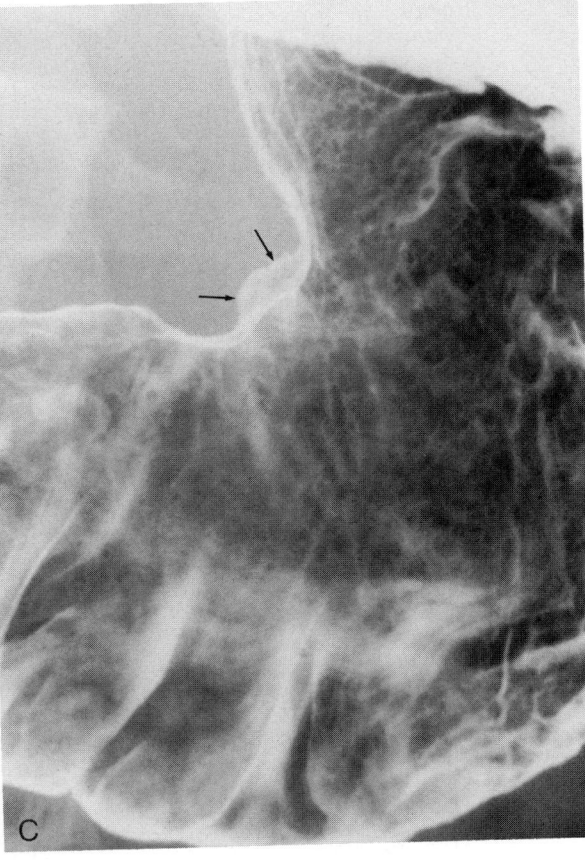

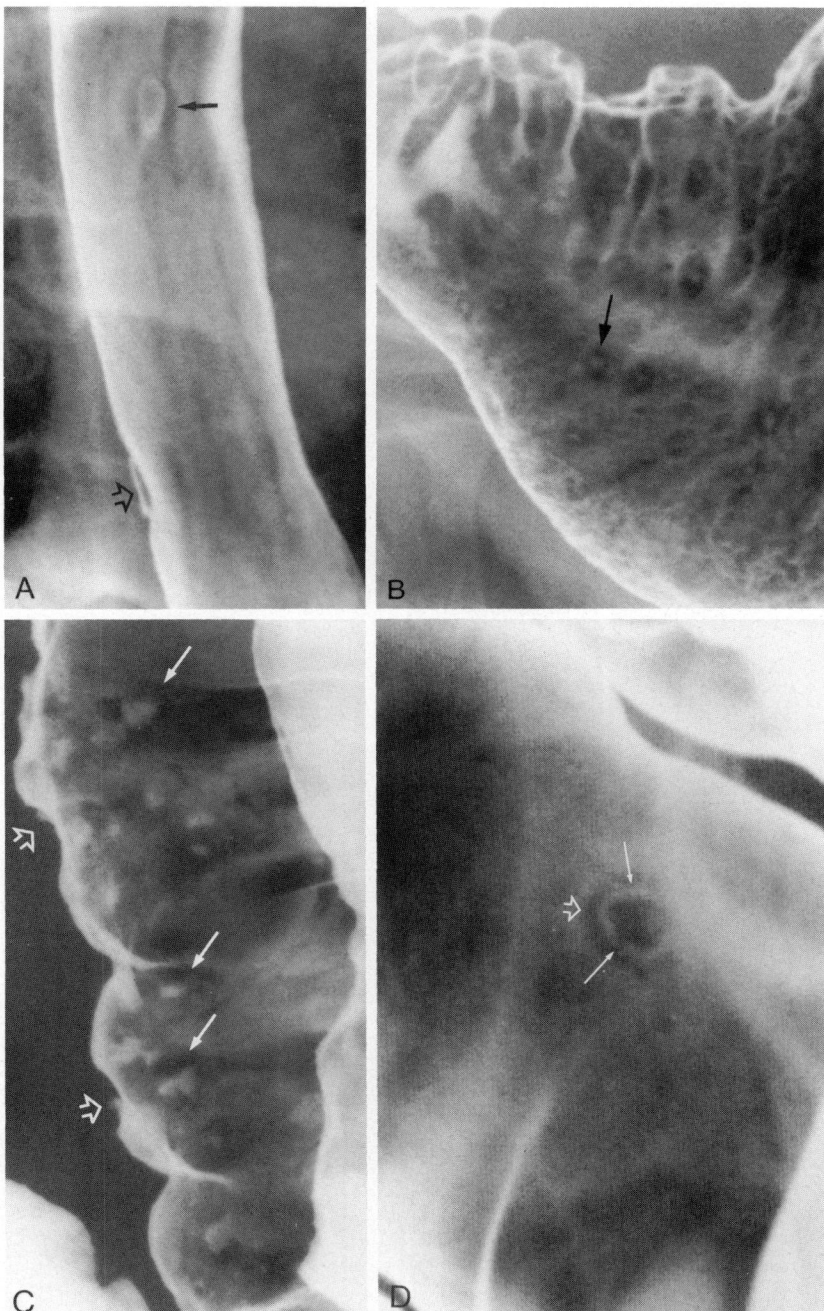

**Figure 5–16. Aphthoid ulcers. A.** Crohn's disease involving the esophagus. An aphthoid ulcer is seen en face as a focal barium collection surrounded by a radiolucent halo (of edema and inflammation) *(solid arrow)*. Another aphthoid ulcer is seen in profile as a shallow barium collection (ulcer) within a smooth-surfaced shallow protrusion of the contour (mound of edema) *(open arrow)*. (From V Gohel, WB Long, G Richter, Aphthous ulcers in the esophagus with Crohn disease, AJR, 137, 872–873, 1981, © by American Roentgen Ray Society.) **B.** Crohn's disease involving the gastric antrum. Numerous punctate barium collections *(arrow)* are surrounded by radiolucent halos of edema. (Reprinted by permission of the publisher from Radiologic investigation of inflammatory bowel disease, by Rubesin SE, Laufer I, Dinsmore B, in Inflammatory Bowel Disease, pp 453–491. Copyright 1992 by Elsevier Science Publishing Co., Inc.) **C.** Crohn's disease involving the splenic flexure of the colon. Numerous aphthoid ulcers are seen en face as punctate barium collections surrounded by radiolucent halos of edema *(solid arrows)*. In profile, small ulcers are seen within edematous mounds of mucosa *(open arrows)*. **D.** Crohn's disease involving colon. Barium has coated and spilled out of an aphthoid ulcer. Thus, a ring shadow *(solid arrows)* is seen peripheral to a radiolucency. The halo of edema is seen surrounding the edge of the ulcer *(open arrow)*.

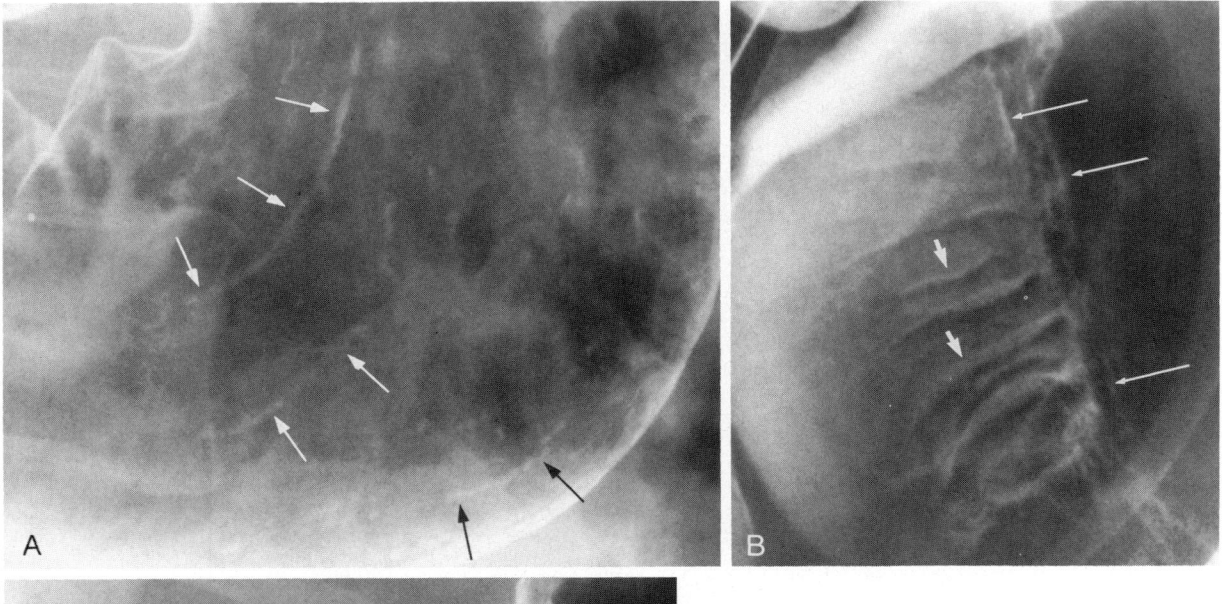

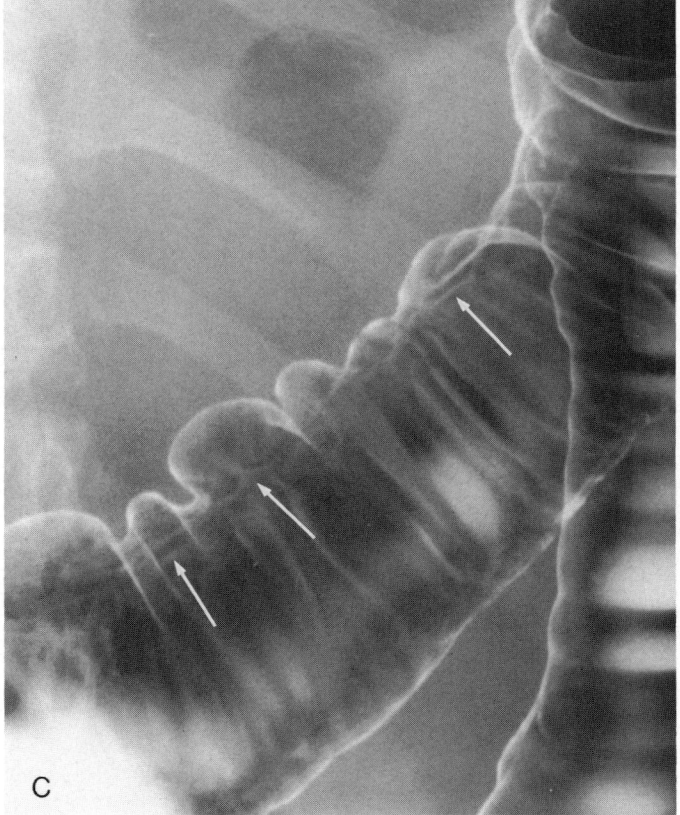

**Figure 5–17. Linear ulcers. A.** Ibuprofen-induced gastric ulceration. Long, linear collections of barium *(arrows)* are seen in the proximal gastric antrum. **B.** Crohn's disease involving the small bowel. Linear ulcers are seen as irregular barium collections *(long arrows)* along the mesenteric border of the ileum. Note the folds *(short arrows)* radiating toward the mesenteric border ulcer. **C.** Crohn's disease involving the colon. Linear ulcers are seen as barium-filled lines *(arrows)* along the upper border of the transverse colon. (**B** and **C** from Rubesin SE, Bronner M: Radiologic-pathologic concepts in Crohn's disease. *In* Herlinger H, Megibow AJ [eds]: Advances in Gastrointestinal Radiology, Volume 1. Chicago, Mosby–Year Book, 1991, pp 27–55.)

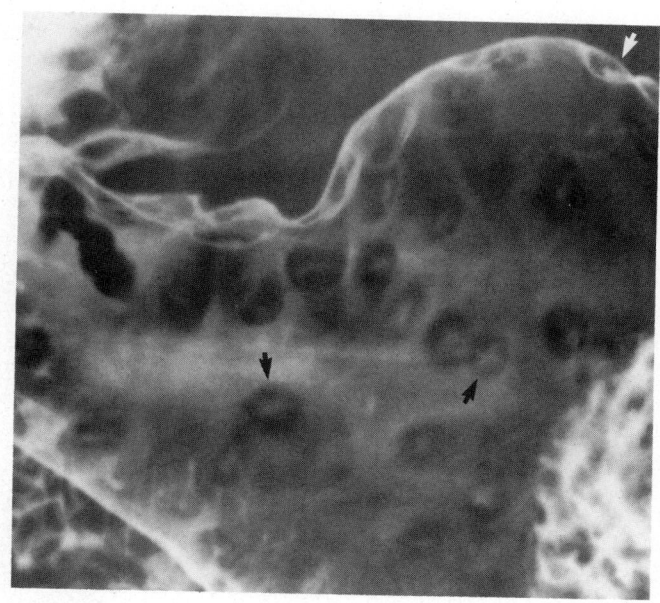

**Figure 5–18. Varioliform erosions.** Numerous linear and ovoid collections of barium *(arrows)* are surrounded by radiolucent halos (of edema). This erosive gastritis was due to aspirin use.

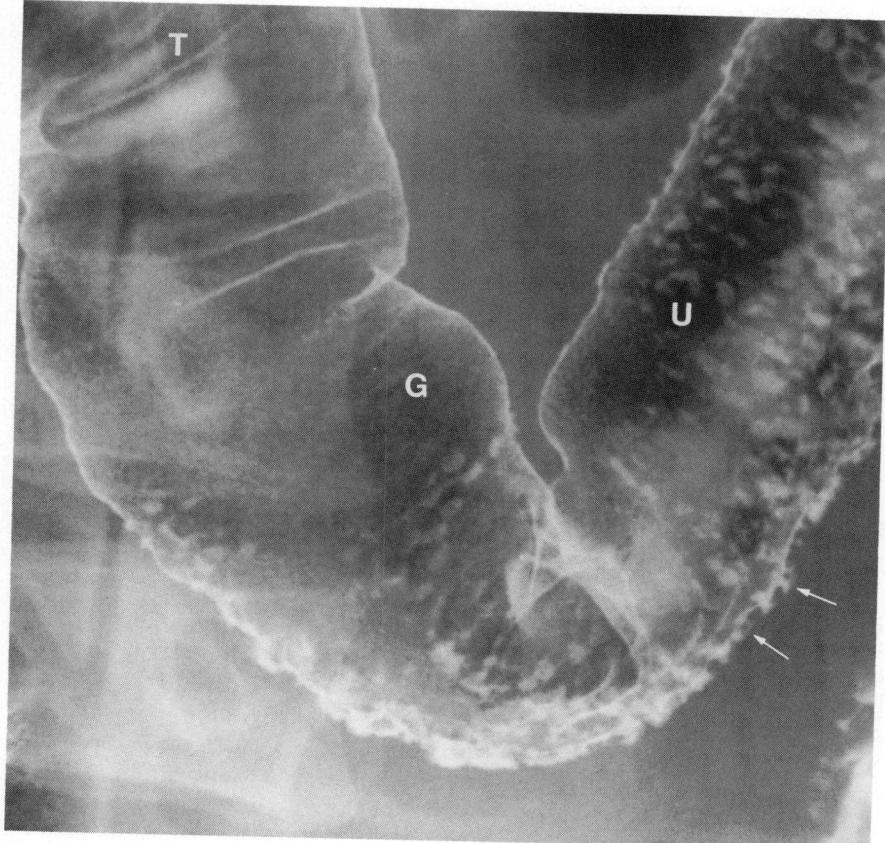

**Figure 5–19. Collar button ulcers.** The spectrum of inflammatory changes in ulcerative colitis is illustrated. In the proximal transverse colon (T) there is relatively smooth mucosa. This progresses to a granular pattern (G). Distally, there is superficial ulceration (U). When the superficial ulcers penetrate the mucosa, lateral spread of inflammation in the submucosa results in collar button ulcers *(arrows)*. (Reprinted by permission of the publisher from Radiologic investigation of inflammatory bowel disease, by Rubesin SE, Laufer I, Dinsmore B, in Inflammatory Bowel Disease, pp 453–491. Copyright 1992 by Elsevier Science Publishing Co., Inc.)

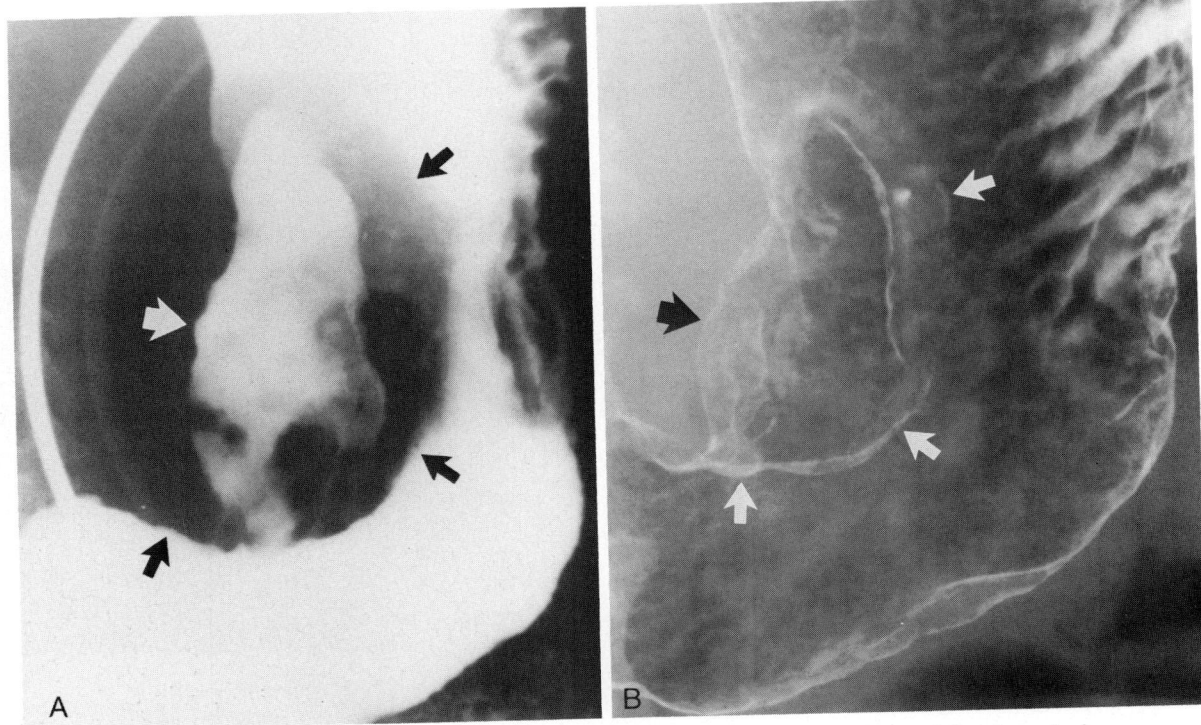

**Figure 5–20. Ulcerated mass. A.** Adenocarcinoma involving the lesser curvature of the stomach. A single contrast compression view of the lesser curvature shows an ulcerated mass seen as an irregular barium collection *(white arrow)* within a radiolucent mass *(black arrows)* that protrudes into the gastric lumen. **B.** With air contrast, barium has spilled from the ulcer crater and etched the mass (shown in **A**). The rim of the mass is seen en face as a curved increased radiodensity etched in white *(white arrows)*. The irregular contour of the lesser curvature represents the ulcer seen in profile *(black arrow)*.

Fig. 5–23A). En face, barium trapped in the abrupt margin results in a well-defined tumor (see Fig. 5–23B). Central ulcers are seen in about one half of submucosal masses. Small submucosal masses in a fold symmetrically splay the edges of the fold. Although the radiographic findings are distinctive for large lesions, small (0.5 to 2.0 cm) mucosal polyps are difficult to distinguish from small submucosal masses.

## Exoenteric Mass

*Exoenteric masses* are masses of gastrointestinal origin that extend predominantly outside the bowel rather than into the lumen of the bowel. They often extend into the mesentery or omentum. These lesions may cavitate, with the cavity extending outside the expected contour of the bowel (Fig. 5–24). The most common neoplastic exoenteric masses are lymphomas, metastatic melanoma, and stomal tumors (smooth muscle tumors).

## Tracking

Linear collections of contrast medium within the bowel wall are termed *intramural tracks*. Linear collections of contrast medium outside the expected confines

of the bowel are referred to as *extramural tracks*. Intramural tracks frequently course perpendicular to the longitudinal axis of the bowel (Fig. 5–25). Extramural tracks caused by diverticulitis often spread longitudinally in the pericolic fat (see Fig. 5–25). Tracks associated with radiation damage, trauma, Crohn's disease, or iatrogenic perforation spread in any direction.

## ABNORMAL FOLDS

Folds in the gastrointestinal tract are composed of mucosa (epithelium, lamina propria, and muscularis mucosae) and submucosa. Therefore, when a radiograph demonstrates abnormal folds, the process usually involves the mucosal and/or submucosal layers. Several radiographic terms are used to describe fold patterns.

## Radiating Folds

Folds radiating toward an area guide the radiologist's eye to the gastrointestinal lesion. Radiographic analysis of the radiating folds aids in differential diagnosis. Smooth radiating folds to a mucosal lesion indicate an active inflammatory process or scarring (Fig. 5–26). Lobulated, pointed, or clubbed radiating folds indicate

*Text continued on page 72*

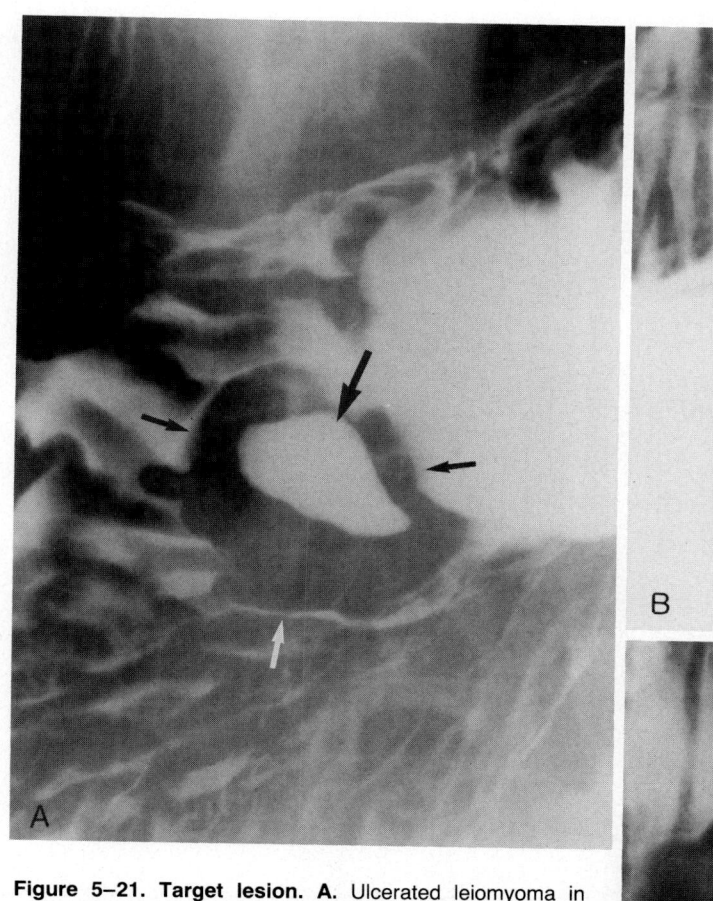

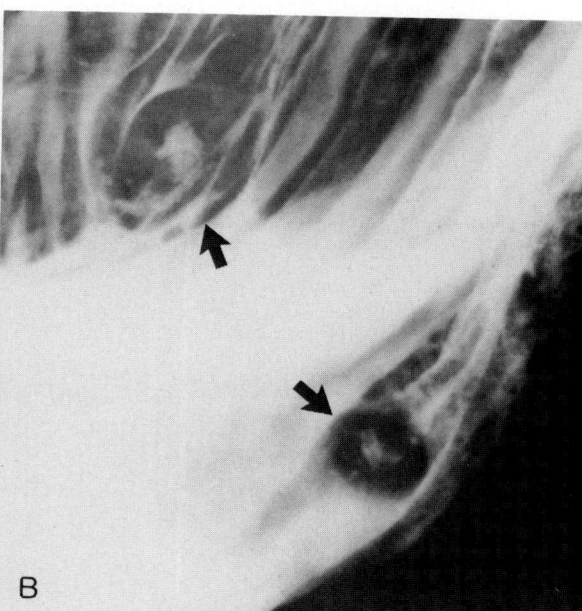

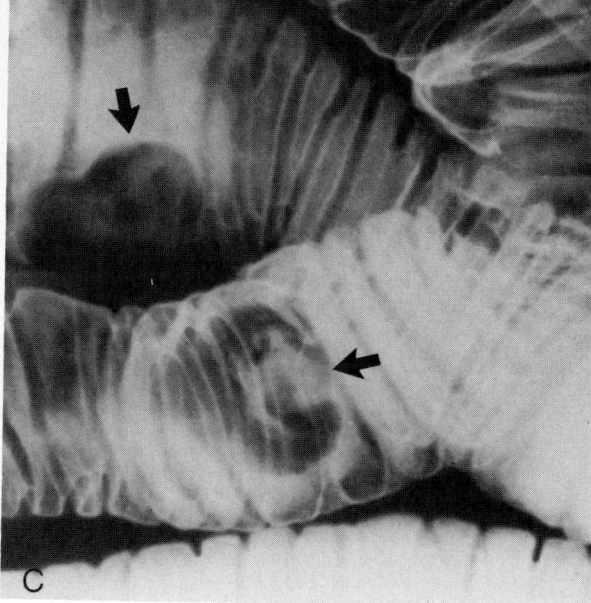

**Figure 5–21. Target lesion. A.** Ulcerated leiomyoma in gastric fundus. A relatively smooth-surfaced, sharply circumscribed mass *(short arrows)* is seen in the gastric fundus. A triangular-shaped barium collection *(long arrow)* fills the central ulcer crater. **B.** Disseminated lymphoma involving stomach. Ovoid, well-circumscribed, 2-cm-diameter masses *(arrows)* with small, central barium collections are seen along the greater curvature of the gastric body. (**B** from Rubesin SE, Gilchrist AM, Bronner M, et al: Non-Hodgkin lymphoma of the small intestine. Radiographics 10:985–998, 1990.) **C.** Metastatic melanoma involving small intestine. Several filling defects with bosselated margins and irregularly shaped, shallow, central barium collections *(arrows)* are seen in profile and en face.

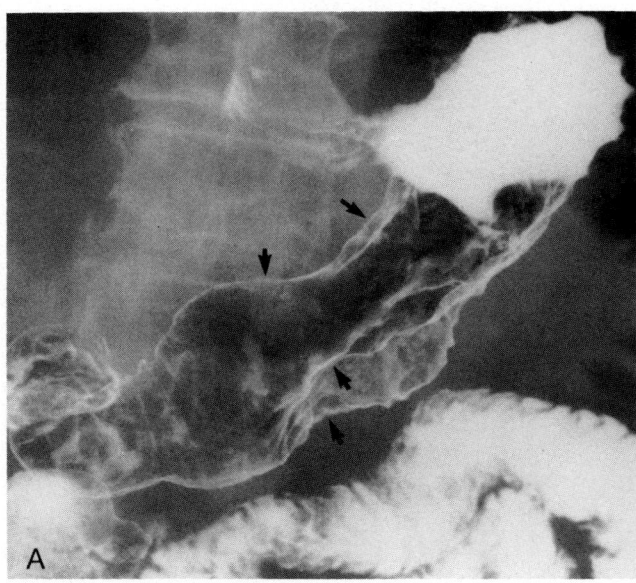

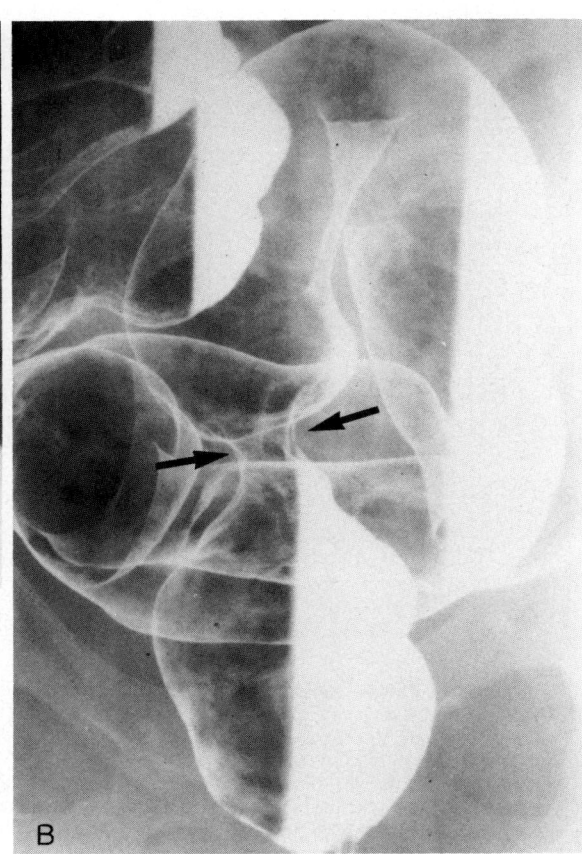

**Figure 5–22. Linitis plastica. A.** Adenocarcinoma of the stomach. The fundus and body of the stomach are diffusely narrowed. The luminal contour is altered by nodular, broad-based indentations *(arrows),* but the mucosa is relatively smooth. These findings indicate the submucosal location of the infiltrating tumor. **B.** Adenocarcinoma complicating ulcerative colitis. There is a short, circumferential narrowing *(arrow)* in the distal sigmoid colon with tapered margins and smooth mucosa. Despite the benign appearance, this was an adenocarcinoma arising in a patient with long-standing ulcerative colitis.

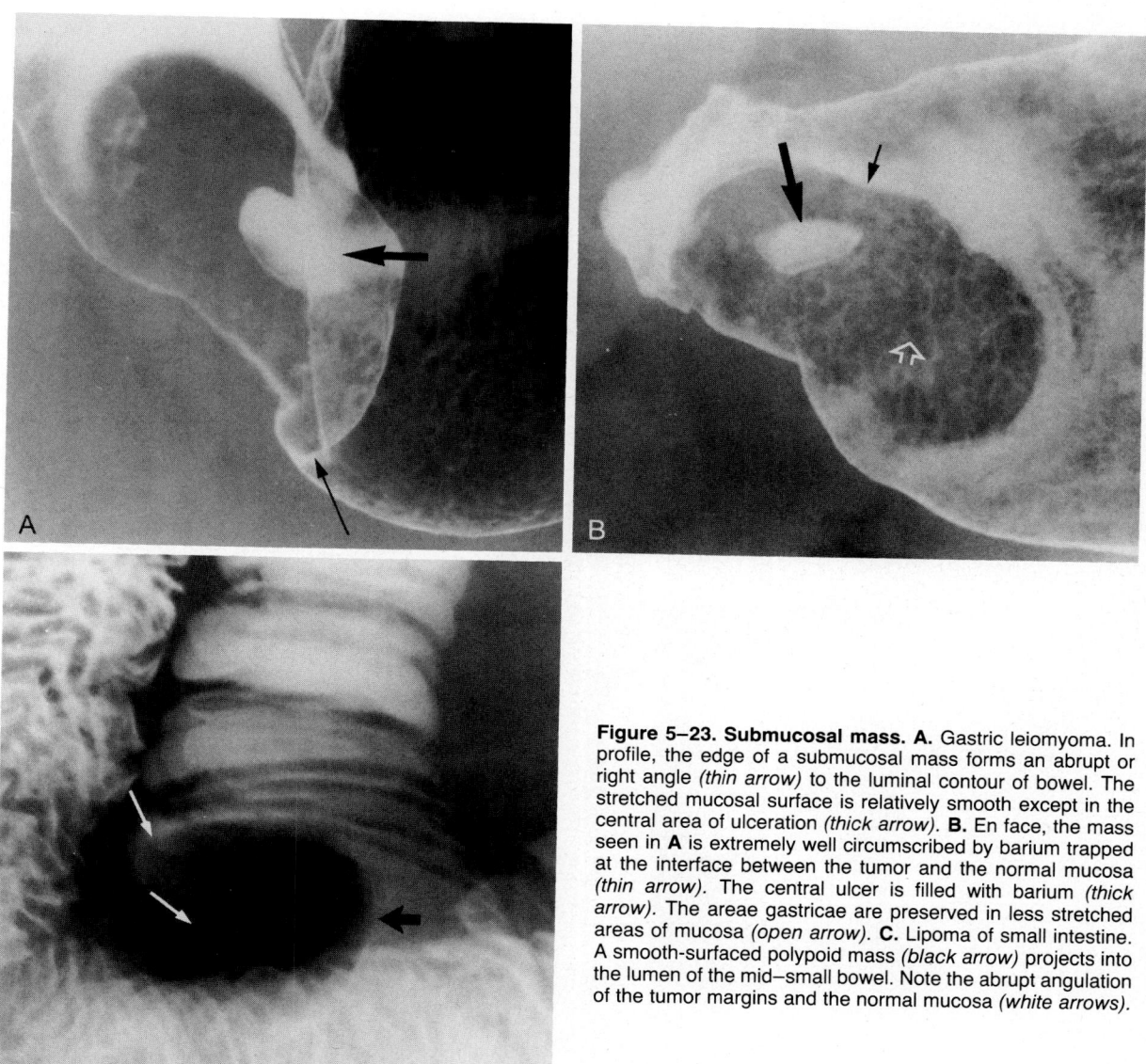

**Figure 5–23. Submucosal mass. A.** Gastric leiomyoma. In profile, the edge of a submucosal mass forms an abrupt or right angle *(thin arrow)* to the luminal contour of bowel. The stretched mucosal surface is relatively smooth except in the central area of ulceration *(thick arrow).* **B.** En face, the mass seen in **A** is extremely well circumscribed by barium trapped at the interface between the tumor and the normal mucosa *(thin arrow).* The central ulcer is filled with barium *(thick arrow).* The areae gastricae are preserved in less stretched areas of mucosa *(open arrow).* **C.** Lipoma of small intestine. A smooth-surfaced polypoid mass *(black arrow)* projects into the lumen of the mid–small bowel. Note the abrupt angulation of the tumor margins and the normal mucosa *(white arrows).*

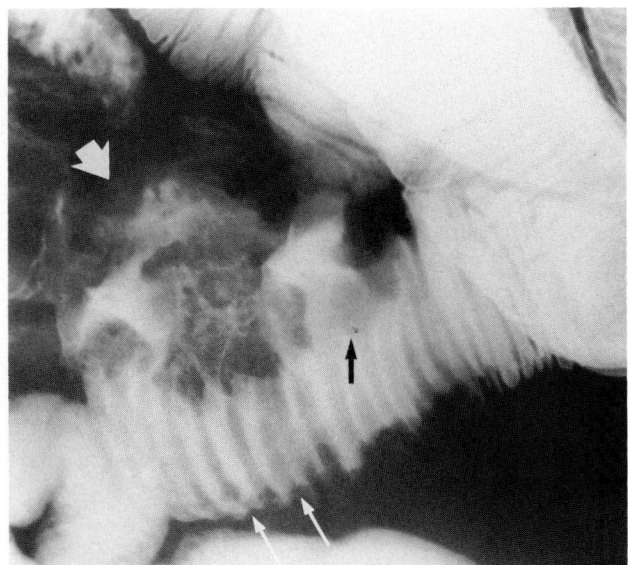

**Figure 5–24. Exoenteric mass.** Primary lymphoma of the small intestine. A large barium-filled excavation *(thick white arrow)* projects from the mesenteric border of the small bowel. Note other radiographic findings of primary small bowel lymphoma: thick, nodular folds *(thin white arrows)* and mucosal nodularity *(black arrow)*.

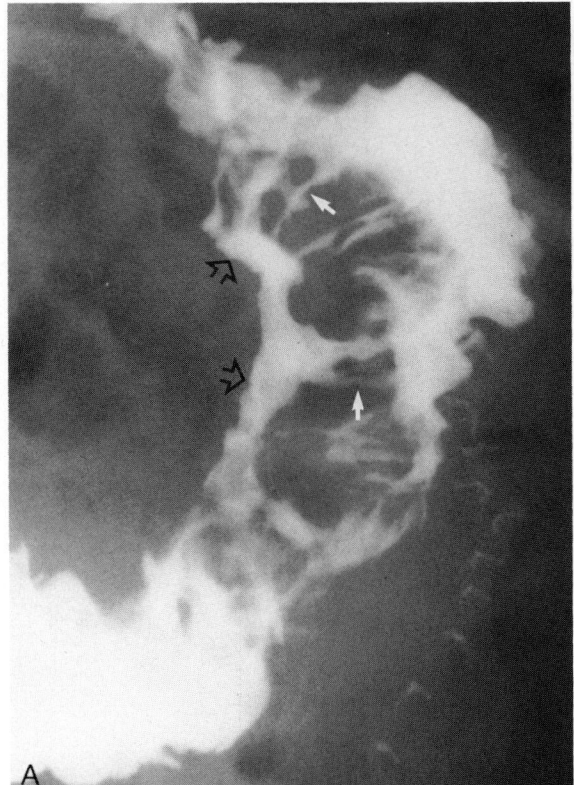

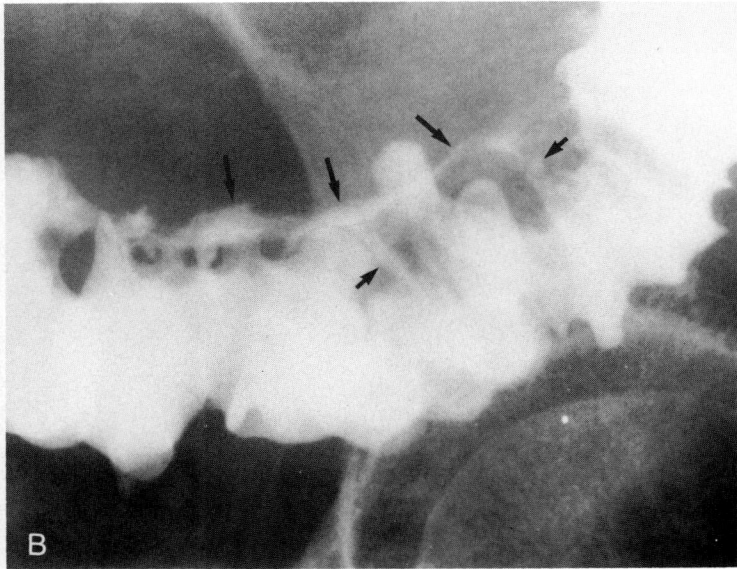

**Figure 5–25. Tracking. A.** Crohn's disease involving the descending colon. Numerous intramural tracks *(white arrows)* extend from the colonic lumen into the pericolic space. The intramural tracks course perpendicular to the lumen, through the muscularis propria. A large, linear, extramural barium collection *(open arrows)* (an extramural track) lies in the pericolic fat, parallel to the bowel lumen. **B.** Diverticulitis involving the sigmoid colon. A long extramural track *(long arrows)* lies in the mesenteric fat of the sigmoid colon. Note the intramural tracks *(short arrows)* extending into the extramural barium collection.

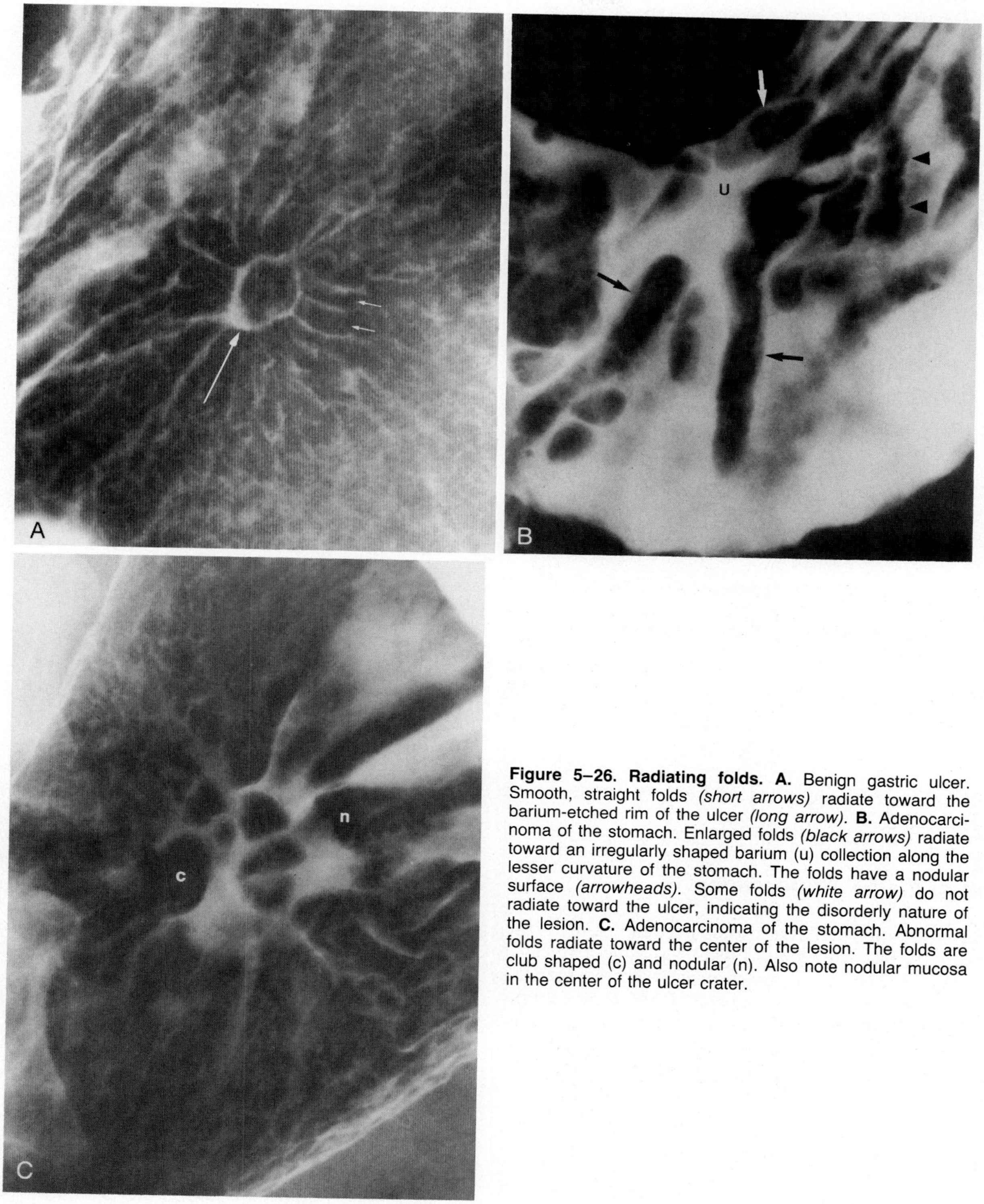

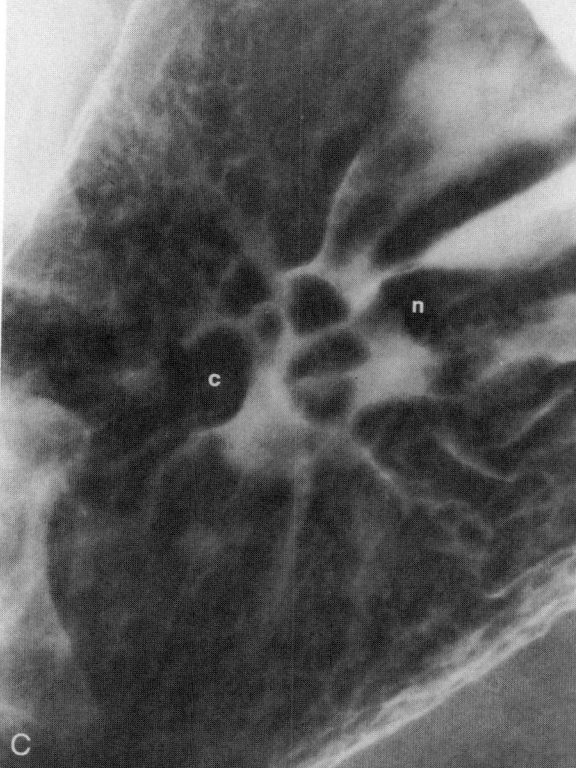

**Figure 5–26. Radiating folds. A.** Benign gastric ulcer. Smooth, straight folds *(short arrows)* radiate toward the barium-etched rim of the ulcer *(long arrow).* **B.** Adenocarcinoma of the stomach. Enlarged folds *(black arrows)* radiate toward an irregularly shaped barium (u) collection along the lesser curvature of the stomach. The folds have a nodular surface *(arrowheads).* Some folds *(white arrow)* do not radiate toward the ulcer, indicating the disorderly nature of the lesion. **C.** Adenocarcinoma of the stomach. Abnormal folds radiate toward the center of the lesion. The folds are club shaped (c) and nodular (n). Also note nodular mucosa in the center of the ulcer crater.

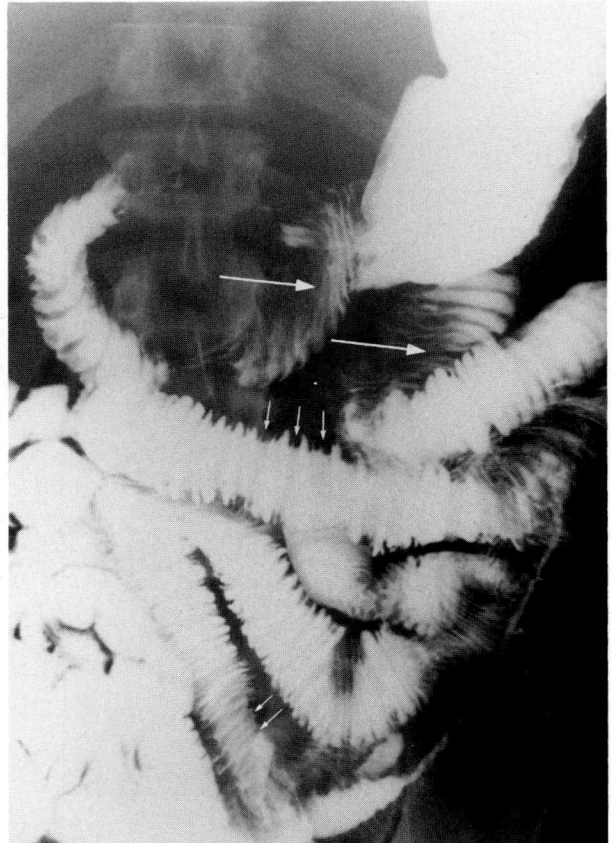

**Figure 5–27. Stack of coins appearance.** Small bowel ischemia caused by pancreatic carcinoma infiltrating mesenteric vessels. Enlarged, smooth, straight, parallel folds *(short arrows)* in the jejunum resemble a stack of coins or a picket fence. Also note extrinsic mass impression of the enlarged head and body of the pancreas on the duodenum and the first loop of the jejunum *(long arrows)*.

the presence of a malignant or severe inflammatory process (see Fig. 5–26).

## Stack of Coins Appearance

Smooth, straight, enlarged folds perpendicular to the longitudinal axis of the small bowel resemble a stack of coins (Fig. 5–27). This appearance indicates marked submucosal edema or hemorrhage. Causes of submucosal hemorrhage include trauma, ischemia, radiation damage, and bleeding diathesis resulting from anticoagulants, hemophilia, thrombocytopenic purpura, and so forth.

## Interspace Spikes

Barium trapped between moderately enlarged small bowel folds gives a spike-like appearance (Fig. 5–28). This radiographic finding indicates moderate to marked submucosal infiltration and is especially seen in radiation damage.

## Thumbprinting

Submucosal hemorrhage occurs to a greater degree along the mesenteric border of the small bowel and is radiographically manifested as *thumbprinting* (Fig. 5–29).

## Cobblestoning

Transverse and longitudinal fissuring of the mucosal surface with residual mucosa and inflammatory reaction in the submucosa results in a carpet of nodules on the luminal surface resembling cobblestones. This fissuring typically occurs in Crohn's disease, especially in the small intestine (Fig. 5–30).

## Polypoid Folds

Folds with a lobulated contour may appear polypoid (Fig. 5–31). Diseases that cause polypoid folds originate in the mucosa and submucosa and may also cause distinct polyps.

## Serpentine (Serpiginous) Folds

Serpentine (snake-like) and serpiginous (from the Latin, "to creep") folds are sinuous or wavy and are

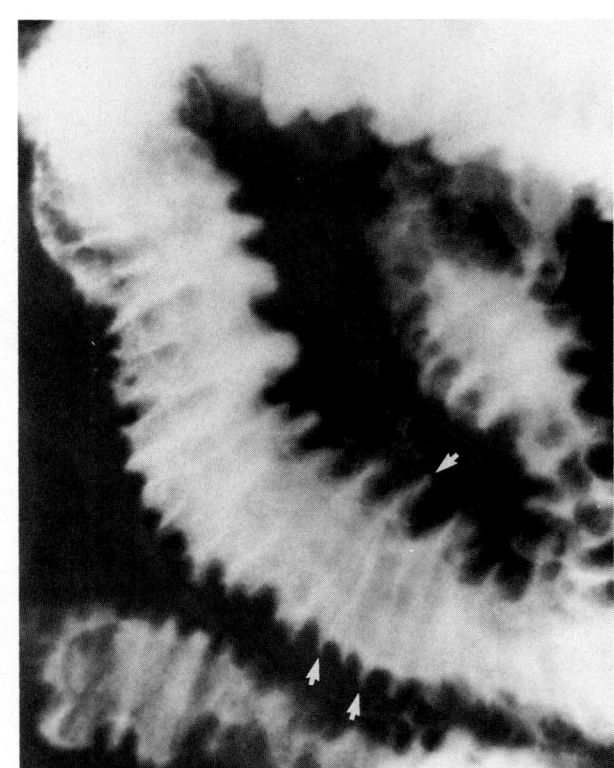

**Figure 5–28. Interspace spikes.** Radiation enteropathy. Barium trapped between enlarged, straight, parallel folds creates the appearance of interspace spikes *(arrows)*.

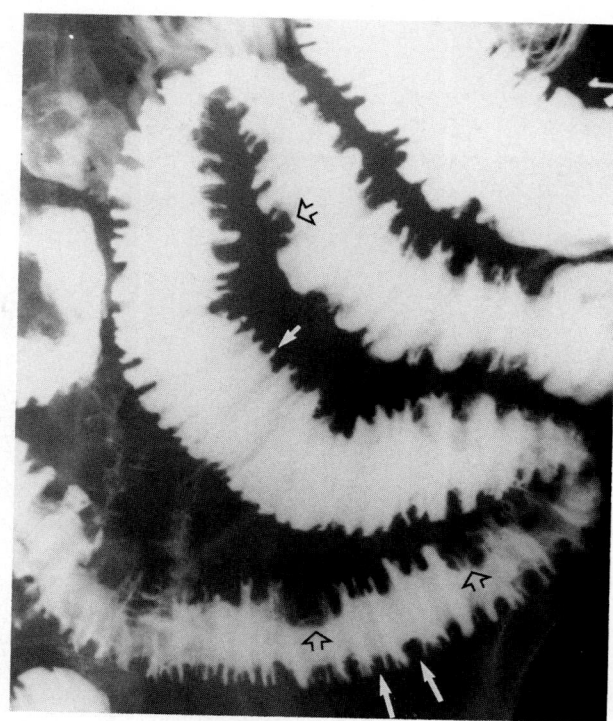

**Figure 5–29. Thumbprinting.** Small bowel vasculitis. Polypoid projections are seen along the mesenteric border *(open arrows)* of the ileum. Note abrupt angulation of the protrusions and smooth surfaces, radiographic findings typical of a submucosal lesion. The thumbprinting reflects the submucosal hemorrhage in vasculitis. Also note smooth, straight, parallel folds *(long white arrows)*—the stack of coins appearance—and interspace spikes *(short white arrow).*

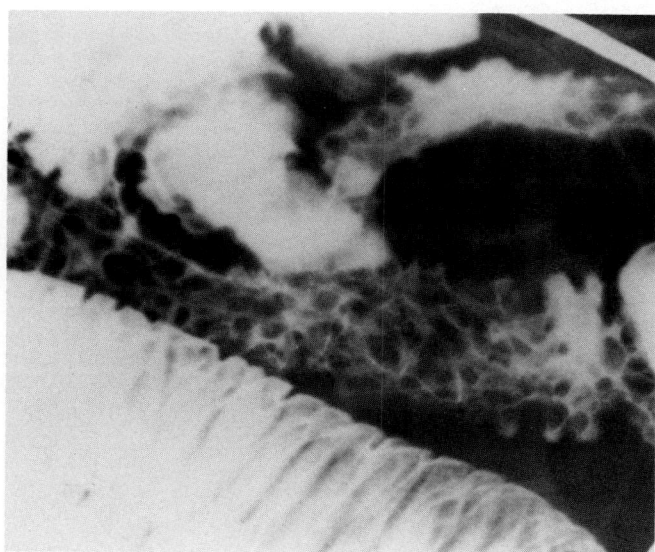

**Figure 5–30. Cobblestoning.** Crohn's disease involving the small intestine. Multiple round to ovoid radiolucencies are surrounded by barium-filled transverse and longitudinal fissures. This is also termed the *ulceronodular pattern*. Narrowing of the bowel lumen reflects the transmural inflammatory reaction and bowel wall thickening. (Reprinted by permission of the publisher from Radiologic investigation of inflammatory bowel disease, by Rubesin SE, Laufer I, Dinsmore B, in Inflammatory Bowel Disease, pp 453–491. Copyright 1992 by Elsevier Science Publishing Co., Inc.)

**Figure 5–31. Polypoid folds.** Hypertrophic gastropathy. Large lobulated folds *(arrows)* are present along the greater curvature of the stomach.

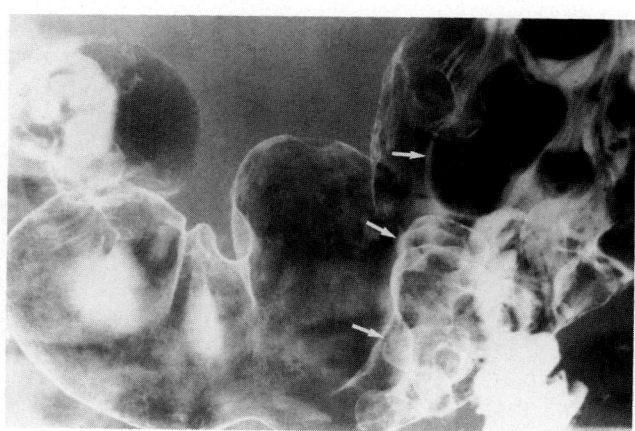

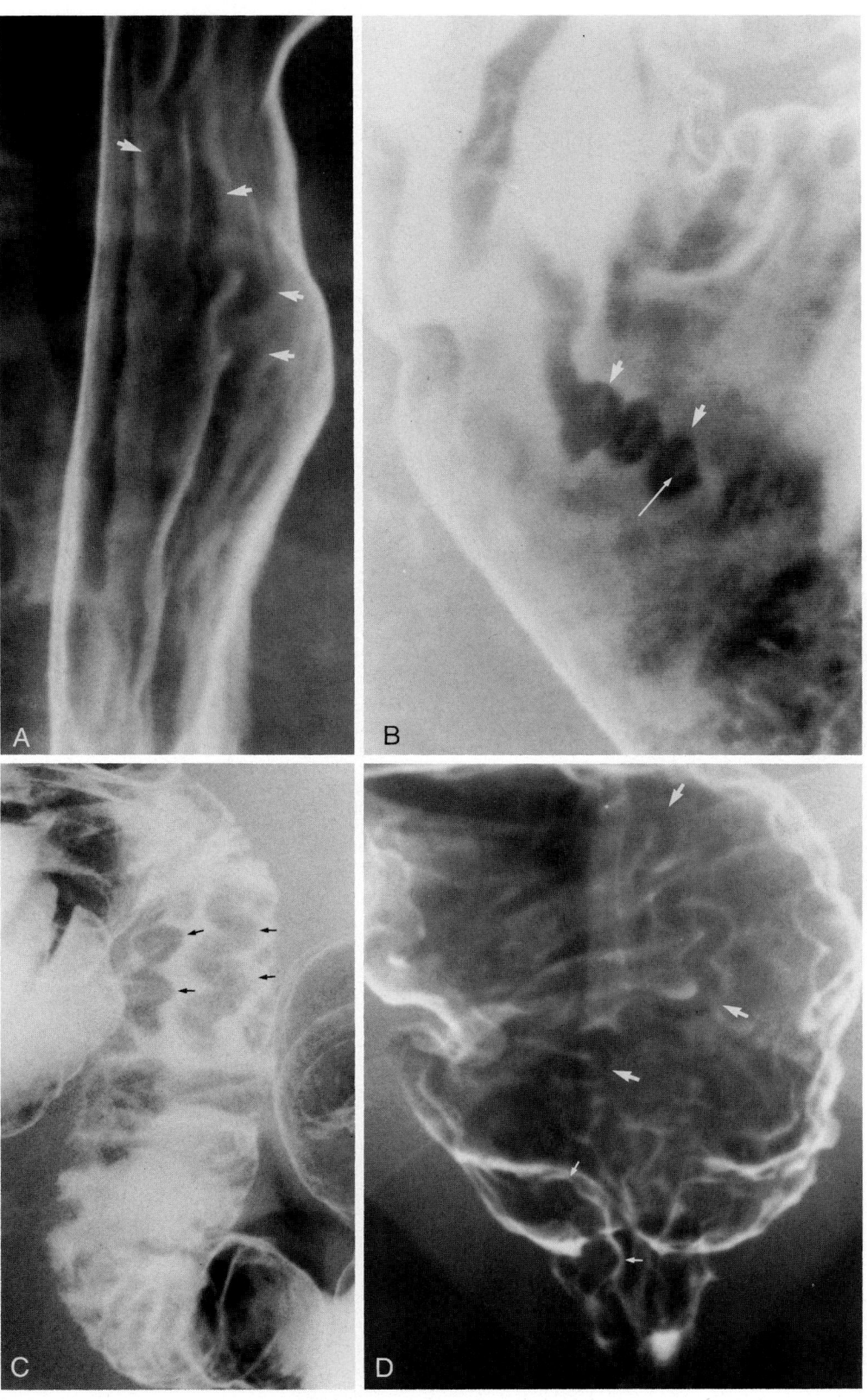

**Figure 5–32. Serpentine (serpiginous) folds. A.** Esophageal varices. Smooth-surfaced, sinuous folds *(arrows)* course longitudinally in the midesophagus. **B.** Antral erosions caused by aspirin use. The contour of an antral fold is scalloped *(short arrows)*, with a serpentine configuration. Note focal linear barium collections (erosions) *(long arrow)* on the surface of the fold. **C.** *Yersinia* enteritis involving the terminal ileum. Wavy, enlarged, radiolucent folds *(arrows)* course parallel to the longitudinal axis of the terminal ileum. **D.** Rectal varices. A sinuous radiolucent rectal fold *(large arrows)* is etched in white by barium. In the collapsed distal rectum, the contours of overlapped varices create undulating lines *(small arrows)* in an abnormal location.

often aligned parallel to the longitudinal axis of the bowel. Serpentine folds are seen in mucosal and submucosal inflammatory or vascular processes (Fig. 5–32), especially varices.

## OTHER TERMS

### String Sign

The term *string sign* is used when severe narrowing of a bowel loop results in a lumen resembling a string.

This term is especially applied in Crohn's disease when severe narrowing is caused by edema, spasm, and inflammation (Fig. 5–33). Narrowing may not reflect the true luminal diameter because of the component of spasm.

### Annular Lesion

Lesions that extend circumferentially around the bowel lumen are termed *annular* or *circumferential*.

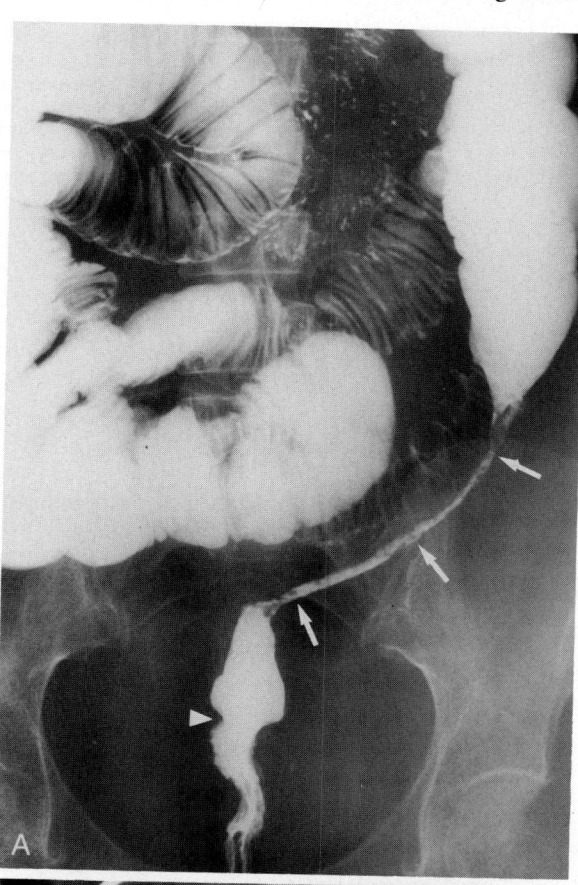

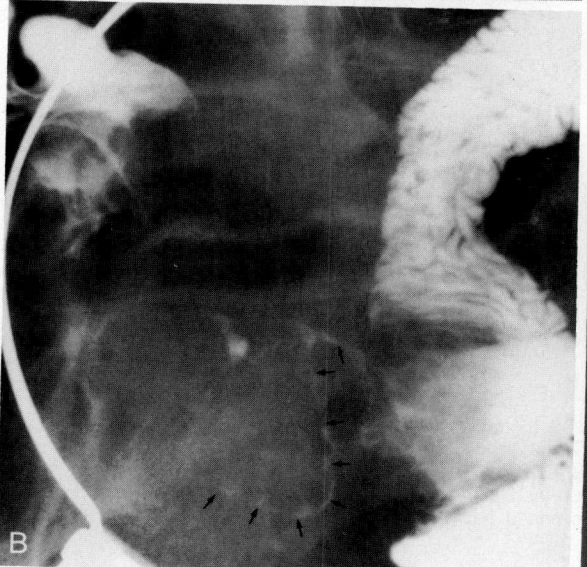

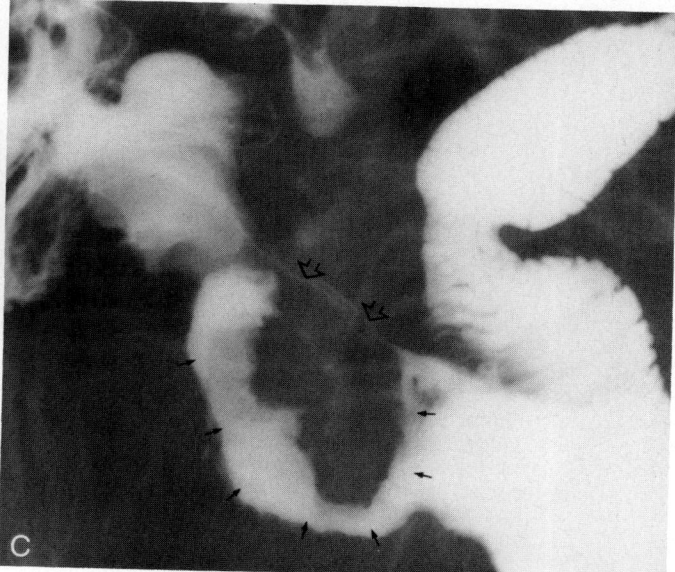

**Figure 5–33. String sign. A.** Recurrent Crohn's disease involving neoterminal ileum. Diffuse narrowing *(arrows)* of the neoterminal ileum is seen proximal to the ileorectal anastomosis *(arrowhead)*. **B.** Crohn's disease of the distal ileum. Barium fills a small track *(arrows)* resembling a string. It is difficult to distinguish bowel lumen from a fistula in this radiograph. **C.** After intravenous injection of metoclopramide, the barium-filled track (seen in **B**) becomes much wider *(small solid arrows)*, revealing an ulcerated bowel loop. Also note an ileo-ileal fistula *(open arrows)* and mesenteric mass effect.

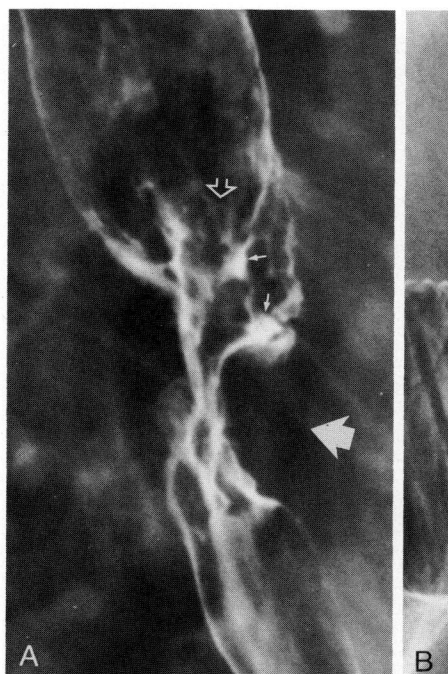

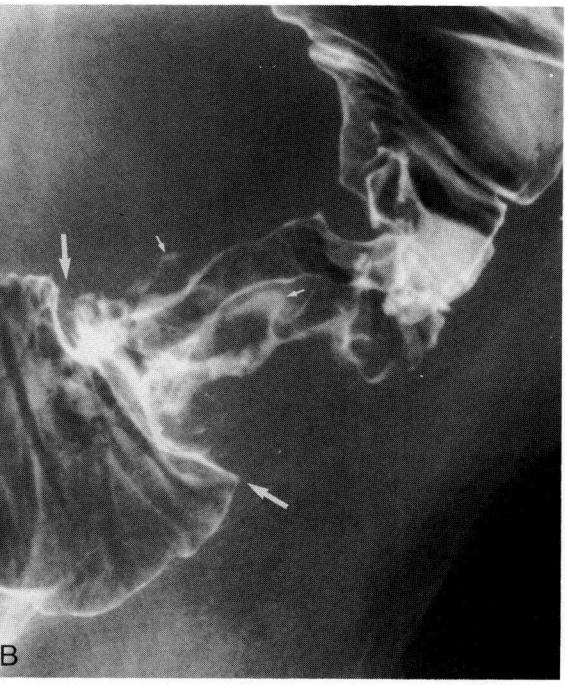

**Figure 5–34. Annular lesion. A.** Squamous cell carcinoma of the esophagus. An asymmetric circumferential narrowing *(large arrow)* of the esophagus is present. Note that the mucosa is nodular *(open arrow)*, with focal barium collections *(small arrows)* trapped in ulcerated areas. **B.** Adenocarcinoma of the sigmoid colon. An annular narrowing of the luminal contour is present. Note that the lesion has abrupt, shelving margins *(long arrows)* and mildly nodular and ulcerated mucosa *(short arrows)*.

Circumferential spread around the lumen implies that the neoplastic or inflammatory process has at least spread into the submucosa. Annular configurations are seen in benign strictures caused by ischemia, radiation therapy, or diverticulitis or in malignancies such as primary tumors or metastases (Fig. 5–34).

## Sacculation

*Sacculation* refers to broad-based outpouchings of bowel wall. Relatively normal bowel wall may appear sacculated between folds radiating toward a neoplastic or desmoplastic process. This form of sacculation occurs

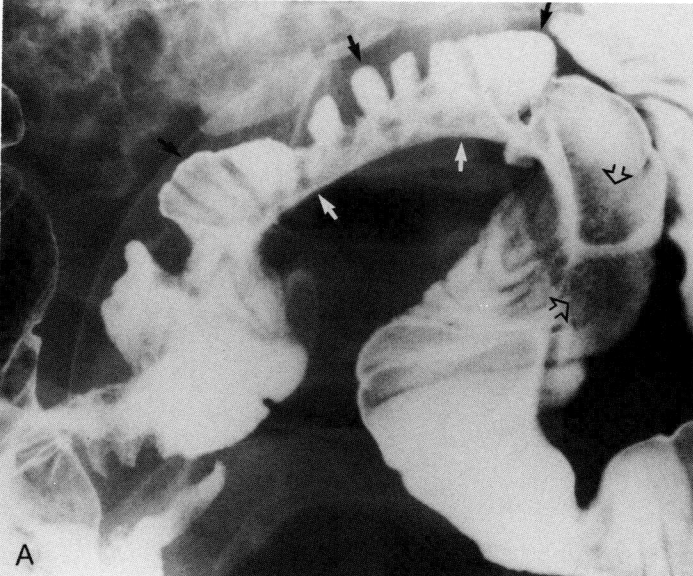

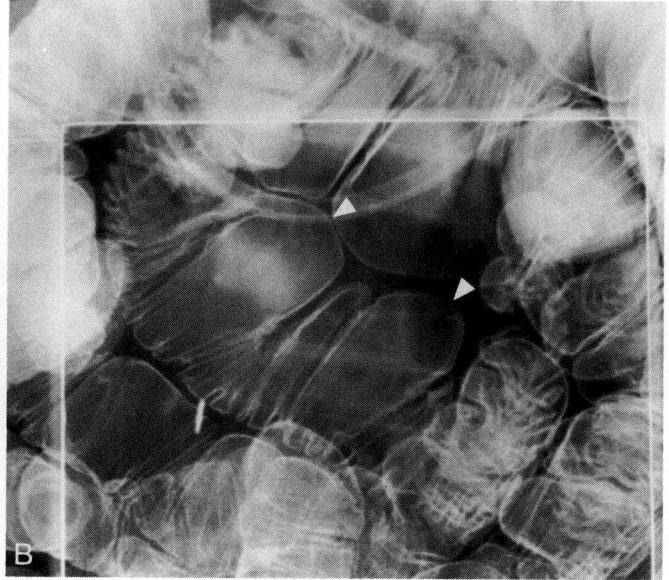

**Figure 5–35. Sacculation. A.** Crohn's disease involving the terminal ileum. The ileal contour is sacculated *(black arrows)* opposite a longitudinal ulcer *(white arrows)* on the mesenteric border. Note folds radiating toward the mesenteric border ulcer. Also note a reticular or granular mucosa *(open arrows)* reflecting mild mucosal changes. (Courtesy of Henrik DeGryse, M.D., Antwerp, Belgium.) **B.** Scleroderma involving the small intestine. Large broad-based sacculations *(arrowheads)* protrude from the expected contour of the mesenteric border.

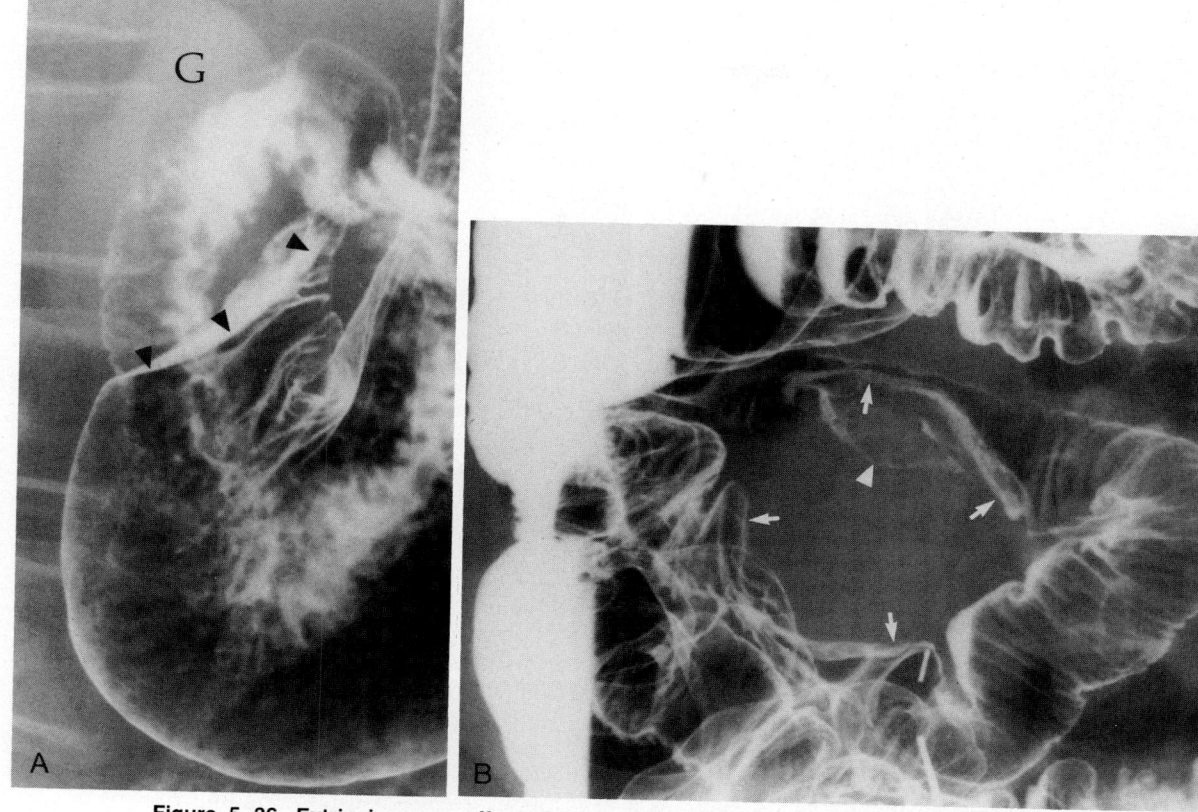

**Figure 5–36. Extrinsic mass effect. A.** Gallbladder impression on the stomach. The contrast medium–filled gallbladder (G) (by oral cholecystogram) makes a smooth, broad-based extrinsic mass impression *(arrowheads)* on the greater curvature of the distal gastric antrum. **B.** Peritoneal metastases from ovarian carcinoma. A loop of distal ileum is splayed by a mass on the mesenteric border. Note the broad-based indentation *(arrows)* at obtuse angles to the axis of the bowel. The indentation does not symmetrically impress the bowel *(arrowhead)*. The mucosal surface is not smooth, indicating mild involvement of the serosal surface by the extrinsic process.

across from the mesenteric changes of Crohn's disease (Fig. 5–35A), ischemia, or diverticulitis. These sacculations do not protrude from the expected contour of the bowel. Bowel wall weakened by atrophy or fibrosis of the muscularis propria may also appear sacculated, especially in scleroderma (Fig. 5–35B). Sacculation related to weakening protrudes from the expected contour of the bowel.

## EXTRINSIC CHANGES

### Extrinsic Mass Effect

Masses arising outside the gastrointestinal tract or gastrointestinal processes extending outside the luminal contour may indent the bowel wall. In profile, an extrinsic mass impression appears as a broad-based indentation with shallow angles to the contour (Fig. 5–36). En face, an extrinsic mass may appear as an ill-defined radiolucency. If imaged obliquely, an extrinsic mass effect may appear as a line.

### Spiculation

A desmoplastic process, resulting from either extrinsic inflammatory or neoplastic disease, may pull the luminal contour into spike-like points, termed *spiculation* (Fig. 5–37).

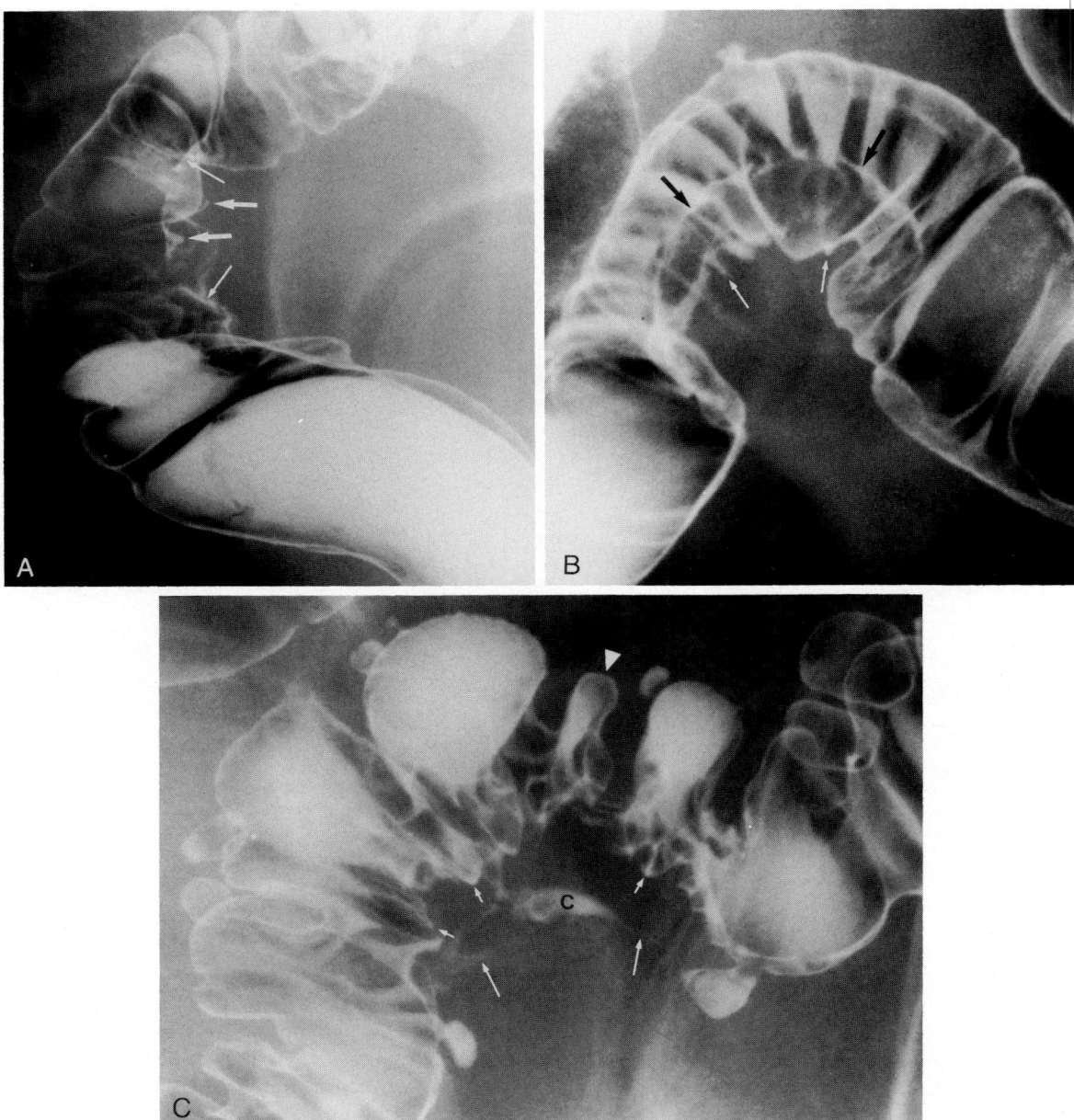

**Figure 5–37. Spiculation. A.** Pelvic abscess involving the rectosigmoid colon. The contour of the anterior wall of the rectosigmoid junction is spiculated *(thick arrows)*. A broad-based extrinsic mass impression *(thin arrows)* is seen, asymmetrically narrowing the luminal contour. **B.** Endometriosis involving the sigmoid colon. The contour of the inferior border of the sigmoid colon is spiculated *(white arrows)*. A smooth-surfaced "submucosal" mass *(black arrows)* is seen, reflecting deep extension of the endometrial tissue into the muscularis propria, with resultant muscular hyperplasia. **C.** Diverticulitis of the sigmoid colon. Even though diverticulitis is a primary disease of the colon, the pathologic changes are those of the extrinsic pericolic abscess. Diverticula that perforate lie in the pericolic fat. In this case, note multiple extramural tracks *(long arrows)* leading to an extracolic barium collection (C). The contour is spiculated *(short arrows)* adjacent to the pericolic abscess. There is a mild mass effect of the abscess on the adjacent sigmoid colon. The uninvolved colonic wall opposite the pericolic abscess is sacculated *(arrowhead)* as folds radiate toward the inflammatory process.

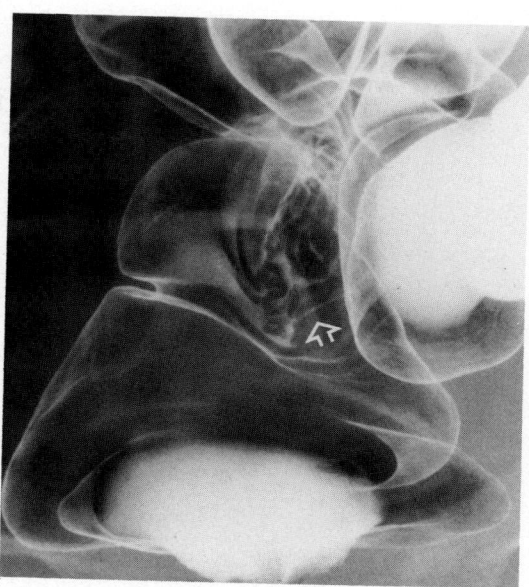

**Figure 5–38. Pleating of the mucosa.** Endometriosis involving the rectosigmoid junction. The colonic mucosa is thrown into sinuous folds *(arrow)* by a desmoplastic process in the serosa and muscular layers.

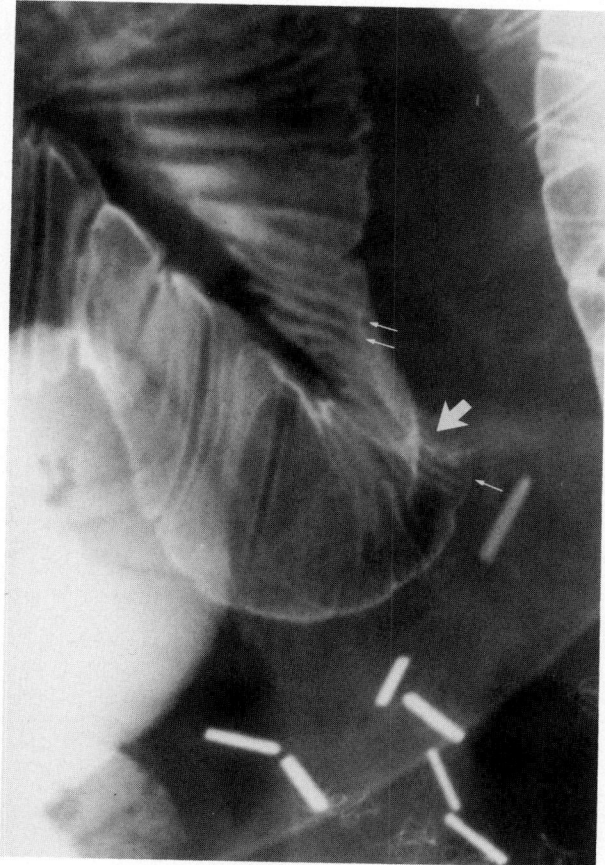

**Figure 5–39. Tethering of mucosal folds.** Postoperative adhesions involving the pelvic ileum. Smooth mucosal folds *(thin arrows)* are pulled toward an adhesive band. Note narrowing of the lumen and angulation of the bowel contour at the site of adhesion *(thick arrow).*

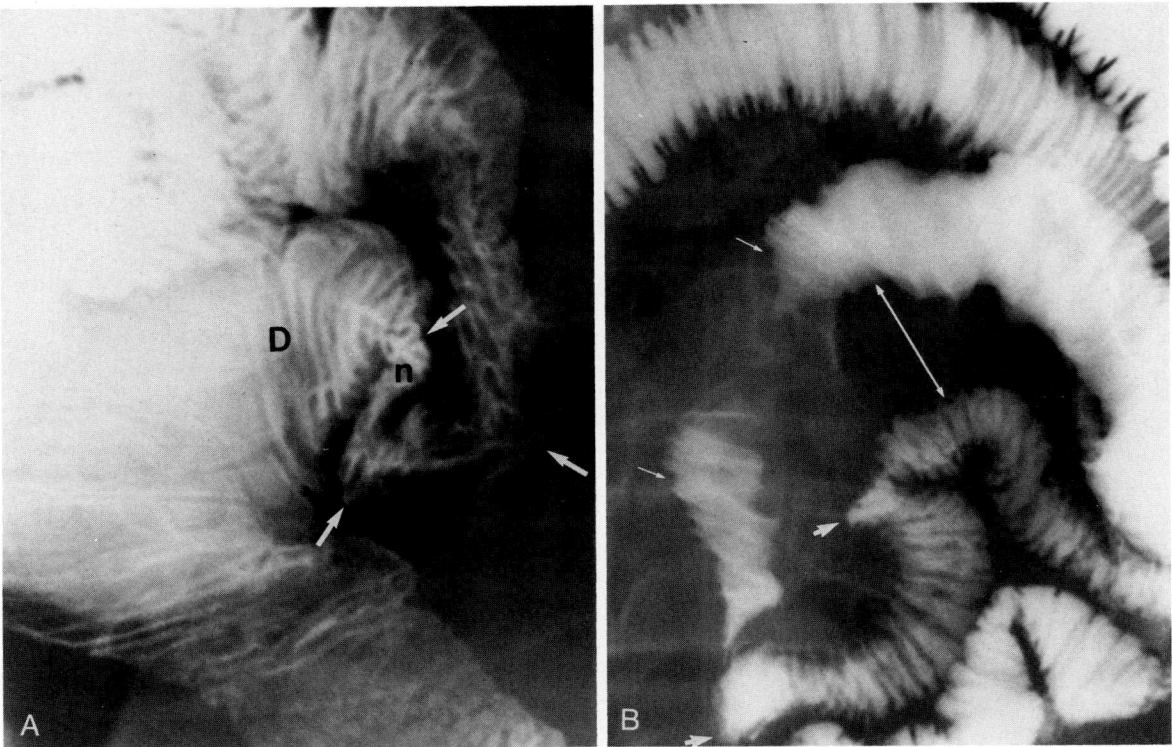

**Figure 5–40. Angulation of bowel loops. A.** Adhesions involving the pelvic ileum. The small bowel is abruptly angulated *(arrows)* in several locations. Note narrowing of the lumen distal to the obstruction (n) and dilatation of the lumen (D) proximal to the angulation. The mucosa is intact. **B.** Mesenteric lymphoma invading the small intestine. Two ileal loops are abruptly angulated *(thick arrows)* where mesenteric tumor invades the serosa. Also note separation of bowel loops *(double arrow)* and mass effect of the mesenteric tumor. In this case, thickened small bowel folds *(thin arrows)* were due to edema secondary to venous or lymphatic obstruction by mesenteric tumor. (**B** from Rubesin SE, Gilchrist AM, Bronner M, et al: Non-Hodgkin lymphoma of the small intestine. Radiographics 10:985–998, 1990.)

## Pleating

If the desmoplastic process extends deep into the bowel wall, the overlying mucosa may be thrown into thin folds, termed *pleating* (Fig. 5–38). For example, this finding suggests endometriosis or intraperitoneal metastases involving the colon.

## Tethering

Mucosal folds may be pulled toward the extrinsic process, resulting in tethering of the folds (Fig. 5–39).

## Angulation

Gross angulation of the bowel may occur (Fig. 5–40) as the desmoplastic process tethers the bowel wall.

### Acknowledgment

Figures 5–1C and 5–33B and C are reproduced from Herlinger H, Maglinte D (eds): Clinical Radiology of the Small Intestine. Philadelphia: WB Saunders, 1989.

Figures 5–11A and 5–32C are reproduced from Laufer I, Levine MS (eds): Double Contrast Gastrointestinal Radiology (2nd ed). Philadelphia: WB Saunders, 1992.

Figure 5–22B is reproduced from Laufer I: Double Contrast Gastrointestinal Radiology with Endoscopic Correlation. Philadelphia: WB Saunders, 1979.

# Barium Studies: Single Contrast

**6**

David W. Gelfand, M.D.

## INTRODUCTION

Major advances in gastrointestinal radiology in the past two decades have been made in the field of double contrast examinations. Nevertheless, single contrast studies continue to make up the majority of examinations performed in the United States. It has been estimated by the largest supplier of barium sulfate suspensions (personal communication, E-Z-EM Company, Westbury, NY), that approximately two thirds of fluoroscopic examinations employing barium sulfate suspension are performed as single contrast studies. Use of single contrast examinations is particularly appropriate when an extremely rapid or economic examination is required or for elderly or infirm patients who are unable to cooperate sufficiently for double contrast studies.[1]

## DIAGNOSTIC PRINCIPLES

Careful compression under fluoroscopic control should always be employed during single contrast examinations if acceptable accuracy is to be achieved. Compression pushes aside the mass of barium that may obscure small lesions. To be visible en face, a small neoplasm projecting into the lumen must displace most of the thickness of the barium column during compression (Fig. 6–1A). Similarly, the barium within the lumen of an organ must be thinned sufficiently to be radiolucent if the small collection of barium suspension in an ulcer is to be detected en face (Fig. 6–1B). In my opinion, the skill of a fluoroscopist in performing single contrast studies is directly exhibited in the skill and care used in the application of compression.

A more crude but still useful form of information is provided by the outline of the organ distended by barium suspension but without compression applied. Under this circumstance, ulcers and neoplasms are seen as projections and indentations, respectively, of the contour of the barium suspension (Fig. 6–2). Large ulcers and bulky circumferential tumors are easily detected by this means, particularly if multiple views of the barium-filled organ

are obtained. However, small ulcers and small polypoid lesions are likely to be detected only if they lie on the margin of the organ being cut tangentially by the x-ray beam. Many small lesions are therefore invisible on films of the barium-distended organ.

## EQUIPMENT

Single contrast examinations can be successfully performed with both conventional and remote control fluoroscopes. The major requirement for either type of machinery is that careful compression be easily performed. With the conventional fluoroscope, compression can be accomplished by manual palpation if the spot film device is not too bulky. Alternatively, the compression cone on the undersurface of the spot film device can be used to apply compression. In the latter case, the compression cone must project sufficiently from the base of the spot film device to allow truly effective compression to be applied. Also, the spot film device should be easily movable so that finely graded compression can be applied via the compression cone. It should be noted that the institution making greatest use of single contrast fluoroscopy, the Mayo Clinic, uses a spot film device containing only an image intensifier and 100-mm camera. This compact spot film device permits easy access for manual palpation.

With remote control fluoroscopes, compression is applied by a mechanical compression device incorporated in the machine. These compression devices vary considerably in effectiveness. I perform approximately half of gastrointestinal fluoroscopic examinations as single contrast studies and perform all studies with remote control fluoroscopes. The manufacturer of the machinery used (Seimens, Erlangen, Germany) provides an excellent compression device that easily accomplishes carefully graded compression and angled compression as well. The compression cone is a large, slightly rounded, pyramidal device of molded plastic that is useful for both upper and lower gastrointestinal studies. The compression cone is sufficiently large to encompass

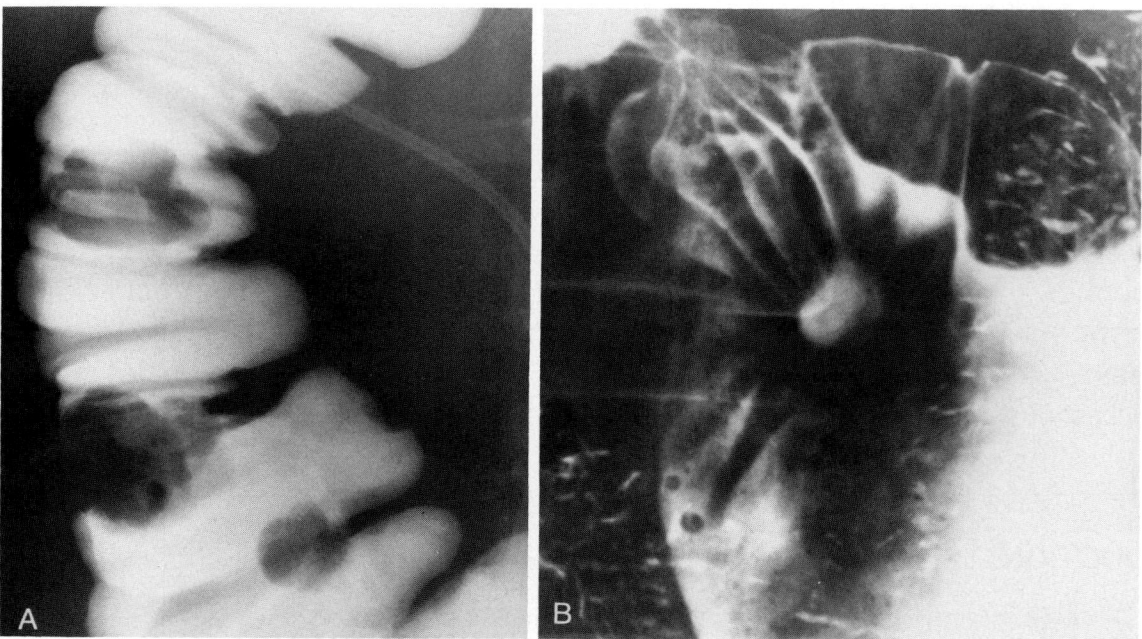

**Figure 6–1. Compression films demonstrating small lesions that become easily visible when the mass of barium is pushed aside by application of compression. A.** Five polypoid lesions of various sizes seen in the ascending colon during application of compression. **B.** Antral ulcer with converging folds as seen during compression filming of the stomach.

a 24 × 30 cm film, allowing broad areas of the stomach, small bowel, or colon to be compressed and filmed simultaneously. This large cone is specifically useful in applying compression during single contrast barium enemas.

## BARIUM SUSPENSIONS

The characteristic necessary for any barium suspension used during single contrast examinations is that it stay well suspended.[2] Good coating properties are also desirable, especially during mucosal relief filming of the upper gastrointestinal tract, postevacuation filming of the colon, and double contrast spot filming of the gastric antrum and duodenal bulb.

The densities of the barium suspensions suggested for single contrast examinations are as follows:

1. The esophagram requires a barium suspension of 50 to 100% w/v for barium-filled films and a barium suspension or paste of 250% w/v for mucosal relief films.
2. The upper gastrointestinal series employs a 50 to 100% w/v barium suspension that allows a combination of compression filming of the stomach and duodenum plus penetrative radiography of the barium-filled esophagus and duodenum.
3. The standard small bowel examination uses a 50 to 100% w/v barium suspension identical with that employed during the upper gastrointestinal series. This density allows effective compression filming of the individual loops of small bowel.

4. Single contrast enteroclysis uses a 15 to 20% w/v barium suspension that allows penetrative radiography of the distended small bowel loops.
5. The barium enema examination uses 15 to 20% w/v barium suspension, the low density permitting penetrative radiography of all portions of the filled colon.

## KILOVOLTAGE

The ideal kilovoltage for single contrast examinations is a balance between the requirement for adequate penetration of the barium column and the degradation of image contrast that occurs with high kilovoltages. In my opinion, the best range is 100 to 110 kV(p). Below 100 kV(p), radiographic penetration of barium-filled organs often cannot be accomplished. Above 110 kV(p), the image-degrading effects of scattered radiation increase dramatically. For example, Leininger, using a simulated model of the colon, established that a combination of 100 kV(p) and a 15% w/v barium suspension gave the most consistent visibility of small polyps during the single contrast barium enema.[3]

## QUALITY CONTROLS

The most important quality control for single contrast examinations requires that barium density, kilovoltage, and thickness of the barium column (with or without compression) be balanced to provide translucency of the

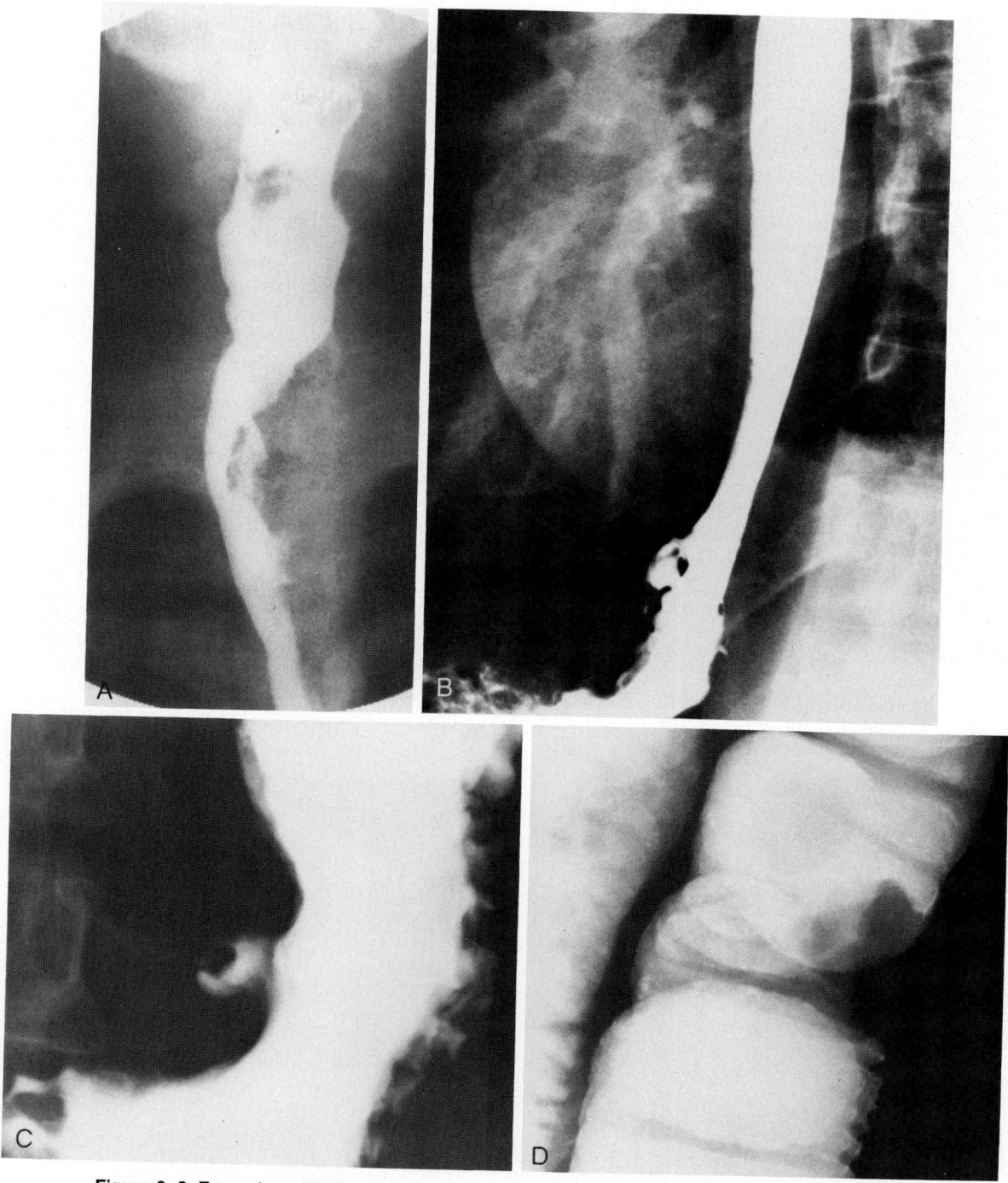

**Figure 6–2. Examples of lesions shown on films of the barium-filled organ as contour defects.**
**A.** Carcinoma of the cervical esophagus shown on an electronic spot film made from videotape. **B.** Ulcerating lesion of the distal esophagus in Crohn's disease. **C.** Lesser curvature gastric ulcer with a Hampton line crossing the neck of the ulcer. **D.** Partially circumferential carcinoma of the lateral aspect of the descending colon.

barium-filled viscus. Adequate radiographic penetration is required to ensure reliable en face visualization of lesions, because the outlines of the barium-filled organ provide limited information.

An easy way to determine that sufficient radiolucency of the barium column has been achieved is to note whether skeletal shadows are visible through the barium column (Fig. 6–3; see Fig. 6–1). This is important when obtaining compression films during any type of single contrast examination, and it is particularly important when obtaining the large films of the barium-filled colon, because penetration of the barium column is necessary for detection of small colonic polyps. Visibility of bone shadows through the barium column indicates that small filling defects displacing the barium suspension will also be visible.

A second quality control useful during both the barium enema examination and enteroclysis is the ability to see through two overlapping loops of bowel. During barium enema studies, loops of the sigmoid colon may be sufficiently tortuous that overlap of sigmoid loops cannot be completely avoided, even with multiple films taken at various angles. Also, it may be impossible to avoid overlap of small bowel loops within the pelvis during enteroclysis examinations. Use of a technique that provides radiographic penetration of overlapping loops minimizes the possibility of failing to detect lesions under this circumstance.

## ESOPHAGRAM

Two single contrast methods of examining the esophagus are available: the barium-filling technique and the mucosal relief technique. Also, in conjunction films of the barium-filled esophagus, motion recording may be used to record esophageal peristalsis on video tape or cine. Motion recording should be employed for any patient presenting with dysphagia, aspiration, or other swallowing difficulties.

The basic film obtained when examining the esophagus by single contrast technique is the full-length view of the esophagus distended with barium. The two most serious lesions of the esophagus, carcinoma and stricture, are reliably detected by this means (Fig. 6–4). Films of the barium-filled esophagus also allow reliable detection of the common structural abnormalities of the esophagogastric junction such as hiatal hernias and lower esophageal mucosal rings. Indeed, the lower esophageal mucosal ring is detected more reliably with a film of the barium-distended distal esophagus of the patient in the prone position than via any other radiographic or endoscopic means.[4]

Views of the full length of the barium-distended esophagus are usually obtained with the patient in the right anterior oblique position (with respect to the table). With the patient swallowing continuously, esophageal peristalsis is reflexly inhibited and the esophagus becomes fully distended. Full-length spot films of the entire esophagus should be obtained on a 30-cm or larger film. Errors may occur when filming is limited to the distal esophagus and esophagogastric junction with the use of smaller spot films, which decreases accuracy for detection of lesions in the proximal esophagus.

Maximal distention is required in the esophagogastric junction region and distal esophagus for accurate detection of hiatal hernia and lower esophageal rings.[4, 5] This is best achieved by asking the patient to perform a

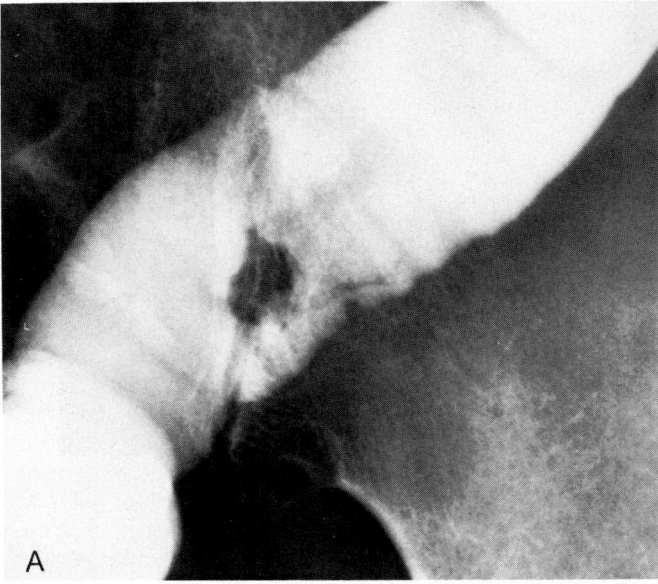
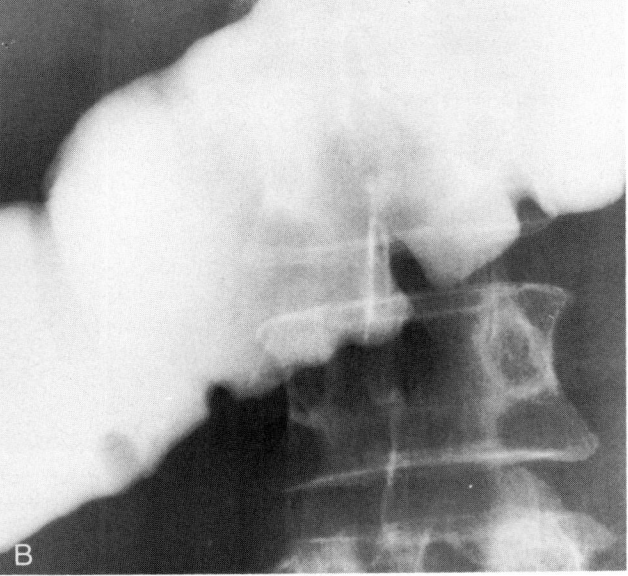

**Figure 6–3. Examples of visibility of bone shadows through the barium column as a means of quality control during barium enema examinations. A.** A 1-cm polyp in the descending colon shown on a compression spot film. **B.** A 5-mm polyp of the transverse colon shown on a film of the barium-filled colon with the patient in the prone position.

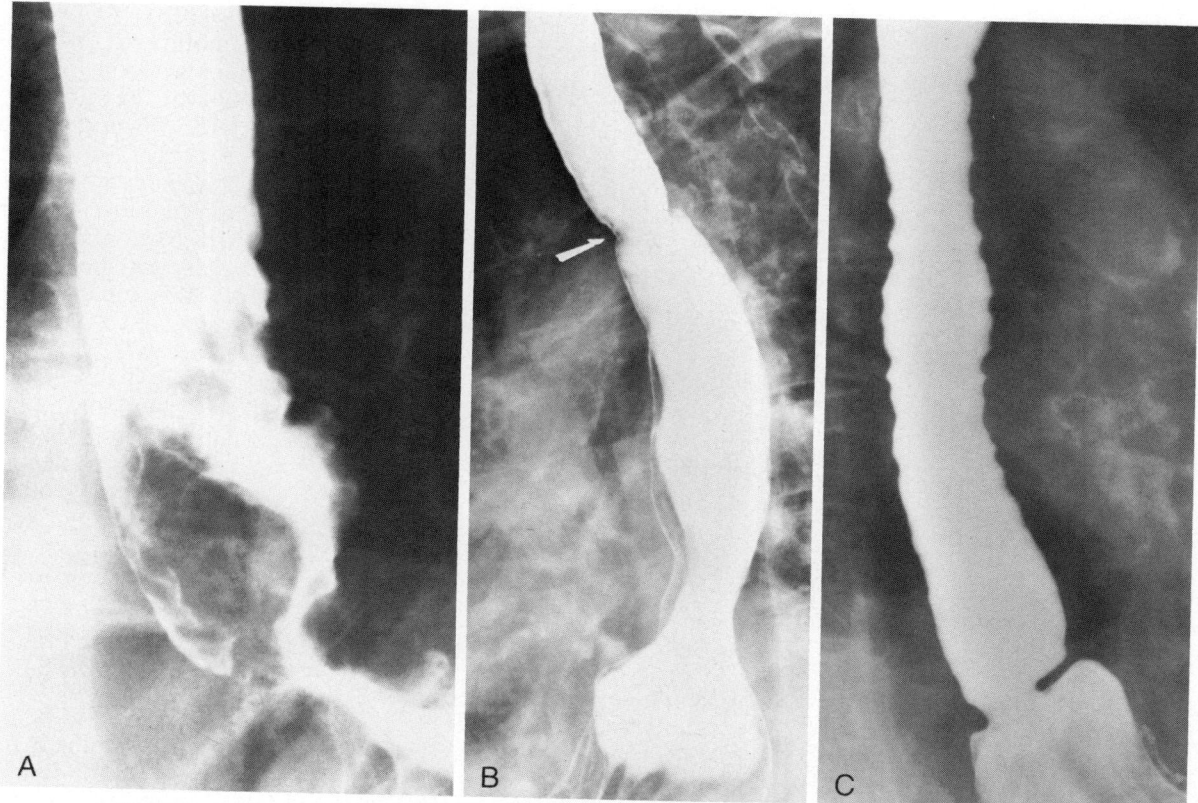

**Figure 6–4. Examples of common lesions shown on films of the barium-filled esophagus. A.** Carcinoma of the distal esophagus and fundus of the stomach. **B.** Stricture of the midesophagus *(arrow)* in a patient with Barrett's esophagus. **C.** Lower esophageal ring and hiatal hernia, demonstrated on films of the barium-filled esophagus with the patient in the prone position.

Valsalva maneuver when the esophagus has become maximally distended after five or six swallows of barium suspension. Films should be obtained under fluoroscopic control to ensure full distention of the esophagogastric junction and to increase detection of occasional lesions that may be visible only intermittently during swallowing or transmission of peristalsis.

Mucosal relief films are defined as films taken of the collapsed esophagus with the esophageal folds visible and coated with barium suspension. This technique is a second means of examining the esophagus during a single contrast examination and provides a reasonably detailed view of the esophageal mucosa. For mucosal relief filming, a barium paste or dense liquid barium suspension is used. The high-density barium suspension used for the double contrast upper gastrointestinal series[6] is ideal for this purpose and usually is readily available. The patient is asked to take a swallow or two of the dense barium suspension, and after peristalsis has stripped most of the barium into the stomach the coating remaining on the esophageal folds is radiographed.

Mucosal relief films are extremely useful in the diagnosis of reflux esophagitis, which is easily detected as irregularity and/or thickening of folds in the distal esophagus[7, 8] (Fig. 6–5A and B). Infectious esophagitis can similarly be demonstrated via the mucosal relief technique (Fig. 6–5C), but the differential diagnosis of the specific type of infectious esophagitis is more difficult and less accurate than with double contrast films. However, an advantage of single contrast examination of the esophagus in this situation is that patients in poor physical condition can be examined by this means.

Esophageal varices are most easily diagnosed using the single contrast mucosal relief technique.[9] Atropine, 0.4 mg intravenously, should be used to enhance variceal filling by inducing esophageal atony. The resulting decrease in intraluminal pressure promotes filling of the submucosally located varices (Fig. 6–6). Careful fluoroscopy is necessary to ensure optimal radiography of the varices, because they may appear only intermittently.

A motion-recording device, most commonly video tape (see Fig. 6–2A), should be employed in examinations of patients complaining of dysphasia or aspiration. For accurate evaluation of esophageal peristalsis, the barium suspension should be ingested as single swallows separated by approximately 10 seconds.[10, 11] Several of these single, separated swallows are required to determine the character and reliability of primary peristalsis. Multiple swallows at short intervals cannot be used to evaluate peristalsis, because they cause reflex inhibition of esophageal peristalsis.

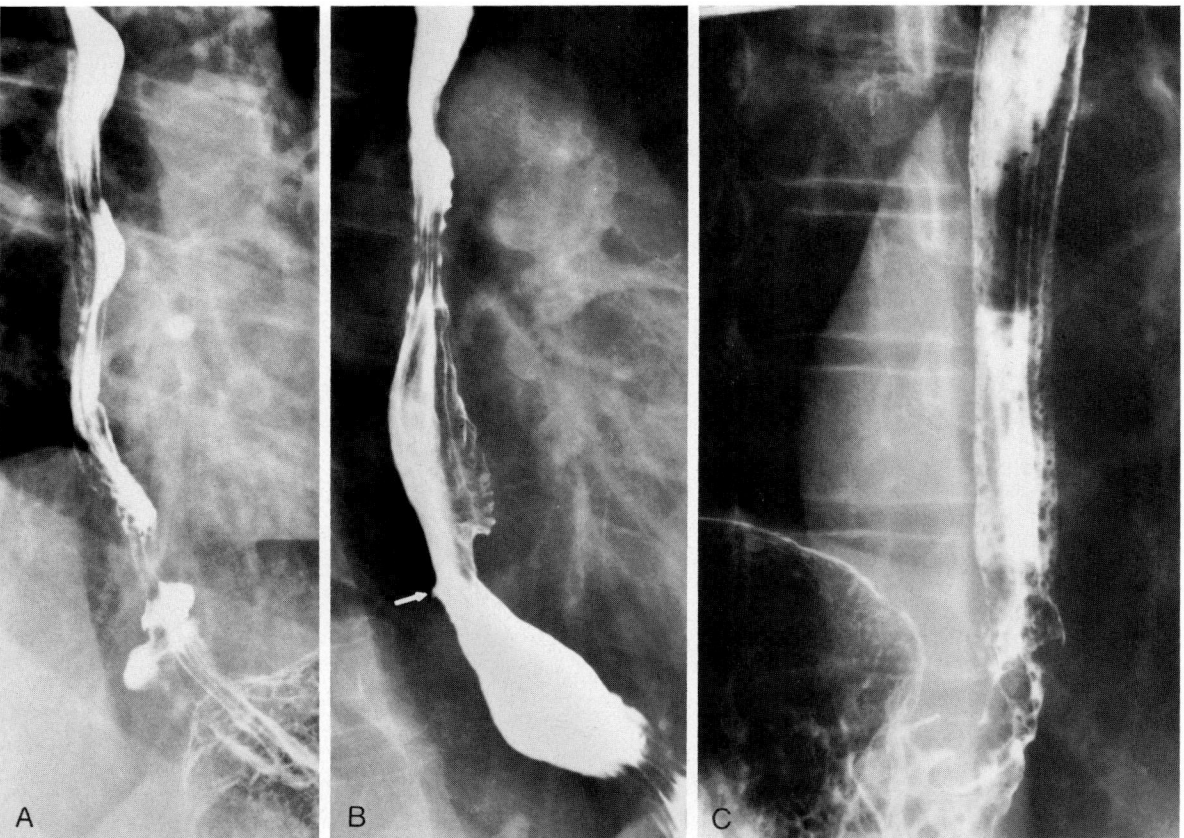

**Figure 6–5. Examples of esophagitis shown on mucosal relief films. A.** Hiatal hernia with reflux esophagitis shown as irregularity of the distal esophageal folds. **B.** Irregular thickening of folds in reflux esophagitis with associated stricture and ulcer *(arrow)*. **C.** *Candida* esophagitis and a distal esophageal carcinoma.

## UPPER GASTROINTESTINAL SERIES

A properly performed single contrast upper gastrointestinal series is a complex examination requiring careful application of compression, fluoroscopic observation, and regulation of filling of the various portions of the upper gastrointestinal tract.[12] Despite these requirements, the examination can be rapidly performed.

The examination begins with the table upright. The patient ingests four swallows of barium suspension and a visual search of the esophagus for stricture or cancer is made as barium suspension passes through the esophagus. The gloved hand or a compression device is used to compress carefully that portion of the stomach that lies below the margin of the ribs (see Fig. 6–1B). A quality control for this part of the examination is that the compression films should provide clear visualization of the gastric rugae. The distal three fourths of the stomach should be spot filmed while in optimal compression. Compression is also employed to determine the pliability of the gastric wall and thus detect any rigid area caused by tumor infiltration.

With the patient still upright, a similar compression examination of the duodenal bulb is performed (Fig. 6–

7). If the duodenal bulb fails to fill with barium suspension at this time, examination of the bulb with compression should be performed during a later phase of the examination.

Mucosal relief films of the stomach are employed to increase the accuracy of the examination. These are obtained while the stomach still contains a small amount of barium suspension, and images are obtained with the patient in the supine and prone positions. Mucosal relief films may serve as a partial substitute for compression filming (Fig. 6–8) when the latter cannot be easily performed because the patient is muscular or obese or the stomach is located beneath the ribs.

With the patient now recumbent and in the right anterior oblique position, the duodenal bulb fills with barium suspension. The contour of the distal stomach and duodenal bulb is observed, and spot films should be taken to include both regions (Fig. 6–9) because gastric ulcers most commonly occur in the antrum. Compression filming of both the distal stomach and duodenal bulb can be achieved at this time using an inflatable balloon paddle placed under the patient. This is specifically necessary if the upright compression examination of the stomach and duodenum has not been satisfactory.

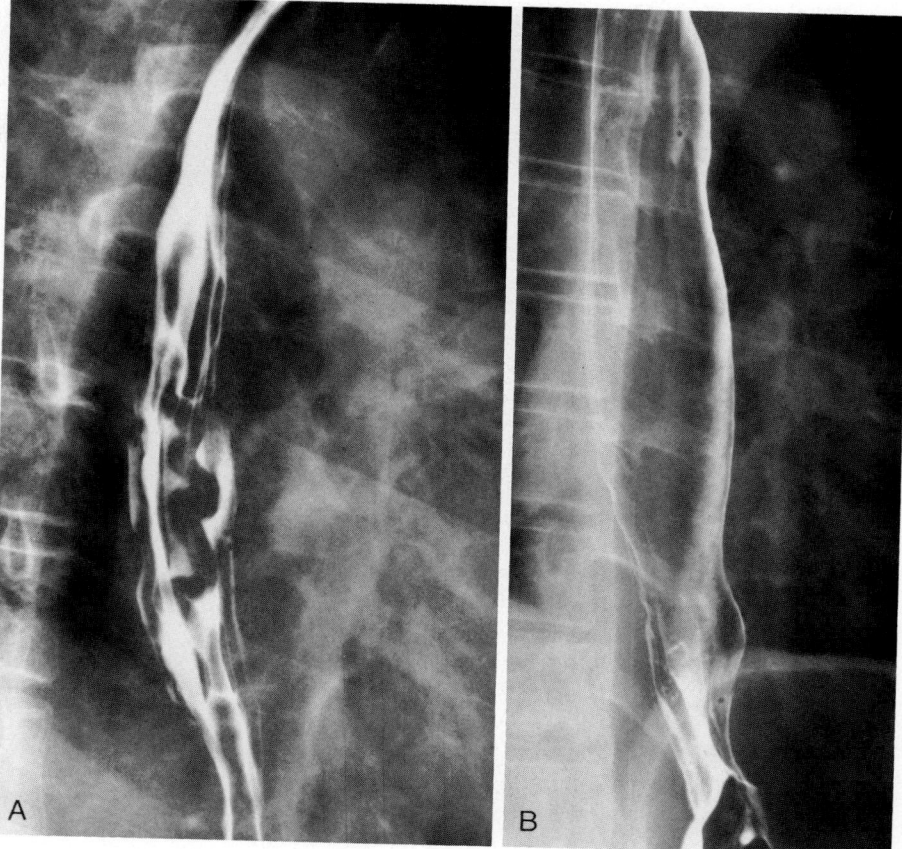

**Figure 6–6. Mucosal relief and double contrast films in a patient with esophageal varices. A.** Mucosal relief film clearly shows the varices. **B.** Distention and increased intraluminal pressure flatten the varices during double contrast filming.

While the patient remains in the right anterior oblique position, full-length films of the esophagus are obtained with the patient drinking barium suspension rapidly. A Valsalva maneuver is used to promote maximal disten-tion of the esophagogastric region for detection of lower esophageal rings, distal esophageal strictures, and hiatal hernias (see Figs. 6–2 and 6–4). After this, a small amount of dense barium suspension or paste is admin-istered and a mucosal relief film of the esophagus is obtained (see Fig. 6–5).

With the patient turned to the supine left posterior

**Figure 6–7. Compression film of the duodenal bulb showing extreme nodularity and thickening of folds in a patient with duodenitis.** At least one small erosion *(arrow)* is visible.

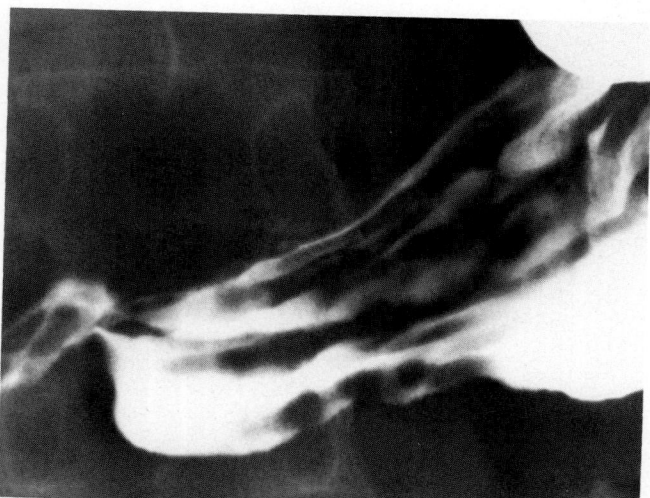

**Figure 6–8. Mucosal relief film of the distal stomach showing nodular thickening of folds in a supine patient found to have erosive gastritis at endoscopy.**

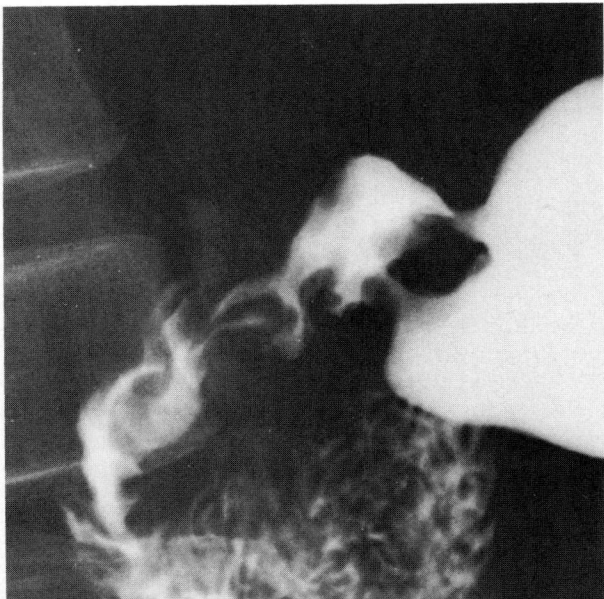

**Figure 6–9. Films of the barium-filled distal gastric antrum and duodenal bulb demonstrating a double pylorus resulting from peptic ulcer disease.**

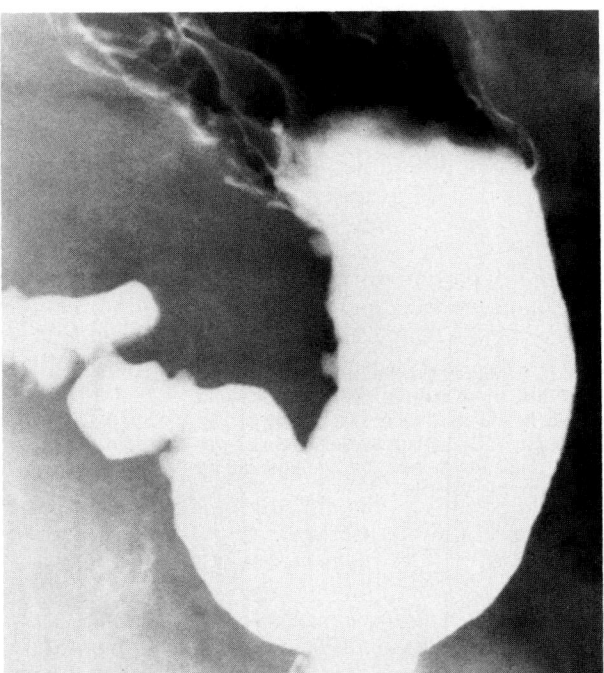

**Figure 6–11. Film of the barium-filled stomach showing at least three small ulcers in profile.**

oblique position, air in the stomach rises into the gastric antrum and duodenal bulb, and double contrast spot films of these regions should be obtained. The visibility of the barium suspension coating the gastric antrum and duodenum can be enhanced by temporarily lowering the kilovoltage to 80 to 90 kV(p) (Fig. 6–10).

After the fluoroscopic examination is completed, overhead films of the barium-filled stomach and duo-

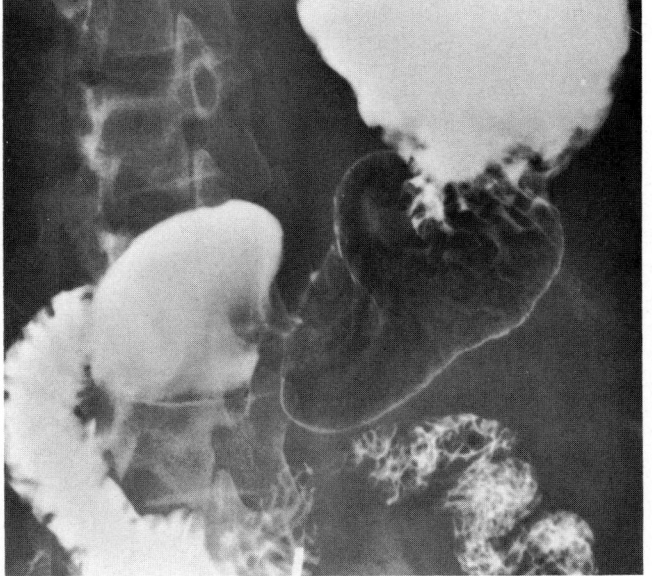

**Figure 6–10. Double contrast film of the distal stomach acquired during a single contrast examination using the normally ingested air in the stomach.** The coating of the 72% w/v barium suspension is enhanced by lowering the kilovoltage to 90 kV(p).

denum are obtained (Fig. 6–11). The technologist may briefly examine the stomach and duodenum fluoroscopically to achieve optimal positioning of each film. On remote control devices, these films are obtained during the fluoroscopic examination. A thorough set of overhead films is as follows:

1. Prone projection of the stomach and duodenum
2. Right anterior oblique projection of the stomach and duodenum
3. Right lateral projection of the stomach and duodenum
4. Supine projection of the stomach and duodenum
5. Left posterior oblique projection of the stomach and duodenum

## SMALL BOWEL

The peroral examination of the small bowel can be performed after a single contrast upper gastrointestinal series or as a separate examination. Properly performed, it is equally accurate when obtained as either a follow-on or a separate study. The accuracy of the peroral small bowel study is almost entirely dependent on the care taken during the fluoroscopic compression examination of the individual loops of the small intestine.

Most radiologists currently use at least 500 mL of barium suspension. This large volume of barium suspension accelerates the examination by distending the small bowel, thus stimulating intestinal peristalsis.[13] Also, opacification of the entire small intestine from duodenum to terminal ileum can be achieved if the patient continues to drink the barium suspension during the course of the examination. With the entire small intestine opacified, careful compression under fluoroscopic control is used to separate the individual loops of small intestine for fluoroscopic inspection and filming.

I use the following method for the peroral small bowel examination. The patient initially ingests a minimum of 500 mL of an isotonic, well-suspended barium suspension. I employ undiluted 72% w/v Liquid Solopake (E-Z-EM), which was formulated specifically for optimal performance during peroral small bowel studies. Any upper gastrointestinal series done before the small bowel examination is performed by single contrast methodology with the same barium suspension employed to examine the small bowel. Films of the small intestine with the patient prone are taken at 15 minutes, 30 minutes, 1 hour, 2 hours, 3 hours, and so on until the barium suspension fills the distal ileum. Because this barium suspension is isotonic, it reaches the cecum in 1 hour in most patients. The stomach is kept full of barium during the study so that barium suspension is constantly ejected from the stomach into the small bowel.

Compression filming (Fig. 6–12) should be performed at two points in the examination. When the proximal three fourths of the small bowel has been opacified, compression is used to separate the loops of proximal small intestine, and compression films should be obtained of every opacified loop at this time. When barium suspension has reached the cecum, compression filming

of the distal small bowel and terminal ileum is similarly performed. When examining the small intestine fluoroscopically, it should be noted that the small intestine lies in a curved plane that coincides with the contour of the anterior abdominal wall. For this reason, the lateral loops of the small intestine should be examined fluoroscopically and filmed with the patient in an oblique position to minimize overlap of loops. Also, the small intestinal loops are mobile and thus separation of the loops for fluoroscopic observation and radiography can be achieved by application of compression. This is by far the most important component of the small bowel examination. The terminal ileum is most easily filmed with the patient either supine or turned slightly to a left posterior oblique position. Loops of the small bowel obscuring the terminal ileum usually can be displaced by compression, providing a clear view of the terminal ileum.

Because the pelvic loops of the small intestine are often overlapped and may be difficult to displace or separate by compression, their clear visualization may not always be possible. However, several maneuvers are quite effective. First, the patient should be asked to avoid urination during the examination. This results in a full bladder that displaces the pelvic loops superiorly and out of the pelvis. Also, an air enema may be used to fill the rectum, which similarly displaces the pelvic loops upward. In addition, the lower abdominal region may be compressed while the patient forcibly exhales,

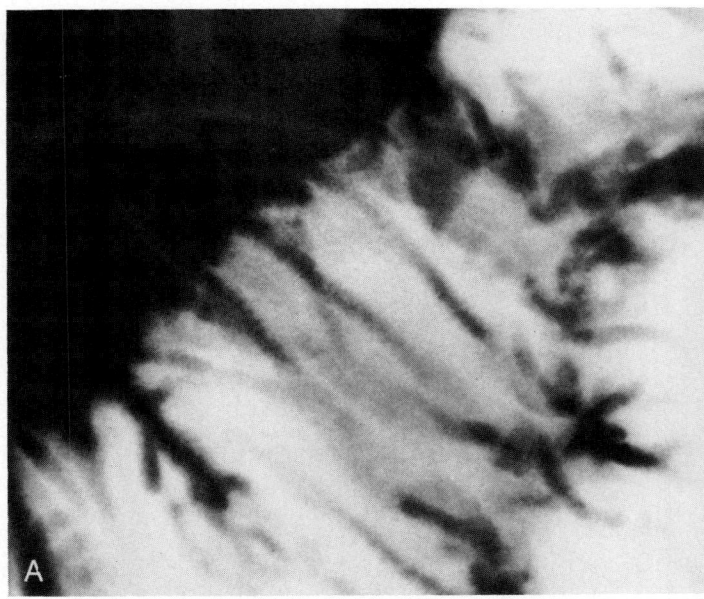
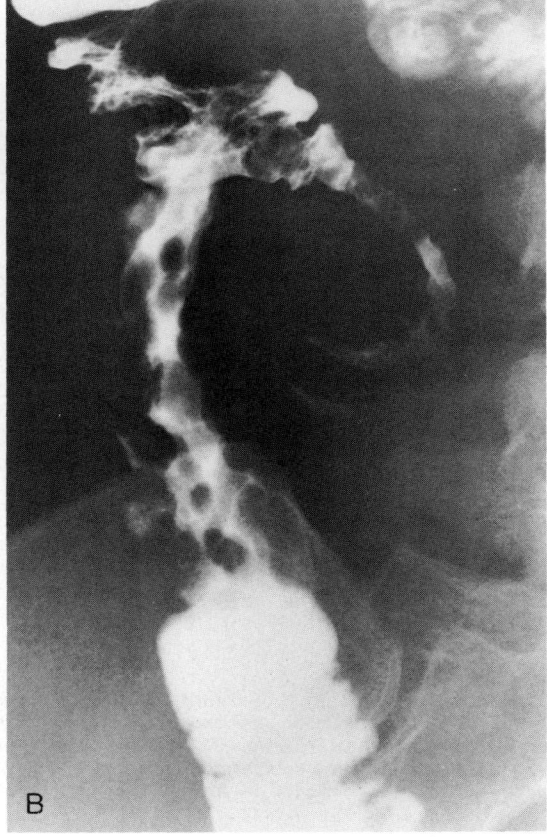

**Figure 6–12. Examples of compression films obtained during the peroral small bowel examination. A.** Villi visible as tiny nodular defects. **B.** Crohn's disease of the distal ileum with nodularity and transmural ulcers.

which encourages the small bowel loops to migrate superiorly and out of the pelvis. Finally, the patient can be placed in the prone Trendelenburg position with a bolster under the lower abdomen and pelvis. This causes the pelvic region to be the highest point within the abdominal cavity, and gravity then helps displace the loops of small intestine out of the pelvis.

## ENTEROCLYSIS

This examination was developed to perfection by Sellink and is accomplished via a tube placed in the proximal small intestine.[14] Several enteroclysis tubes are available and are well suited to the task, including the Bilbao-Dotter, Nolan, Herlinger, and Maglinte tubes. The Maglinte tube has a small balloon on its end to prevent reflux of contrast material into the stomach. The others are single lumen tubes without a balloon. In my opinion, the fastest and most direct method of intubation is via the mouth, which provides the greatest control and avoids any possibility of damage to the nasal turbinates. It also allows any of these tubes to reach the proximal jejunum.

After the tube has been swallowed, the guidewire is inserted and the tube is advanced along the greater curvature of the stomach. The guidewire is withdrawn slightly as the tube traverses the pylorus into the duodenum. The tube should be placed in the jejunum if

possible, because jejunal injection of the barium suspension prevents significant gastric reflux. When using the Maglinte tube, duodenogastric reflux is prevented by inflation of the balloon within the duodenum.

The barium suspension of 15 to 20% w/v is prepared to a volume of 800 mL. Diatrizoate meglumine (Gastrografin) (30 mL) is added to stimulate peristalsis and provide a more rapid examination. A well-suspended barium suspension diluted to the foregoing density is used (Liquid Solopake) and is allowed to flow through the tube by gravity without use of a pump. The flow rate of the barium suspension should be approximately 80 to 120 mL/min. If barium suspension is administered too slowly, adequate distention is not achieved. On the other hand, too rapid injection of barium suspension causes reflex paralysis of the small intestine and the barium column then progresses very slowly to the distal ileum. Initially, the bag of barium suspension is placed 2 ft above the table. By raising or lowering the bag, the flow rate can be adjusted so that it provides adequate distention yet avoids small bowel paralysis.

The examination should be performed under fluoroscopic control with the patient in the supine position. The most critical aspect of the examination is careful compression, separation, and spot filming of each loop of the small intestine as it fills (Fig. 6–13). When the entire small intestine has been opacified, the tube is removed and a large film of the entire small bowel is obtained with the patient in the prone position.

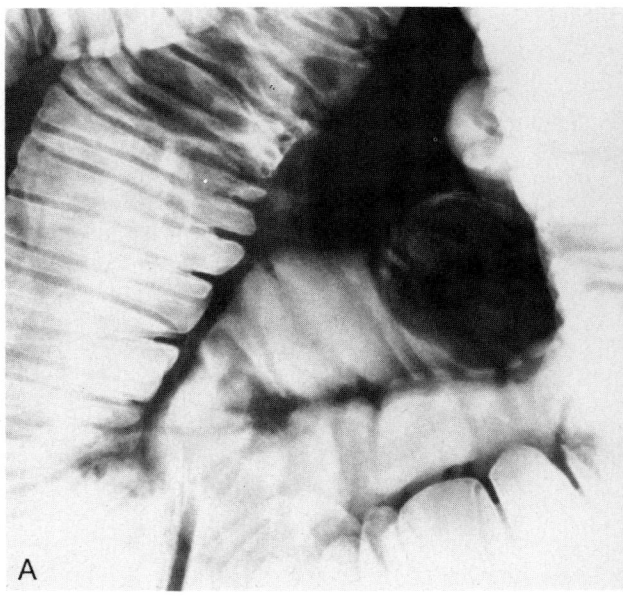
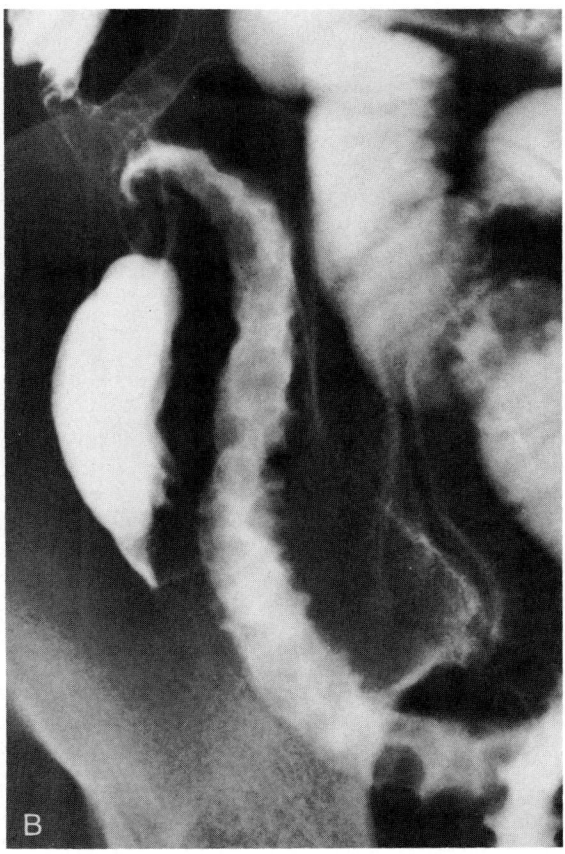

**Figure 6–13. Examples of compression films taken during single contrast enteroclysis examinations. A.** Large leiomyoma of the mid–small bowel. **B.** Extensive Crohn's disease of the distal ileum with a cobblestone appearance.

# BARIUM ENEMA

Accurate examination of the colon during a single contrast examination depends on careful use of fluoroscopically guided compression and an understanding of the technical factors that allow detection of small lesions in the barium-filled colon. Although slightly less accurate than the double contrast examination for the detection of small polypoid lesions[1, 15, 16] and for the evaluation of inflammatory bowel disease, the single contrast barium enema is ideal for examining patients who are immobile, elderly, or seriously ill.[1]

Apart from the examination itself, the most important aspect of a single contrast barium enema is the preparation of the patient. In the absence of fecal material, the diagnosis of neoplasms, including polyps smaller than 1 cm, is both easy and reliable. On the other hand, fecal material within the colon almost invariably decreases the detection of polyps and also decreases confidence that an apparently normal colon is in fact normal.

All effective preparations for the barium enema examination include the sequential use of dietary restriction, increased fluid intake, a saline cathartic, and a second irritant cathartic. Cleansing enemas can be employed to ensure complete cleansing of all patients. The following regimen is employed at Bowman Gray School of Medicine and was found to provide a totally clean colon in more than 97% of patients:[17]

1. A 24-hour clear liquid diet
2. A glass of clear liquid every hour the day before the examination
3. Magnesium citrate solution, 300 mL at 4:00 PM the day before the examination
4. Flavored castor oil, 60 mL at 8:00 PM the day before the examination
5. A tap water cleansing enema of 1500 mL the morning of the barium enema examination, which is repeated as necessary

After the cleansing enema, the patient should wait for 30 minutes before a single contrast enema (60 minutes before a double contrast enema) to allow the water to be expelled or absorbed. The waiting period prevents dilution of the barium suspension by retained fluid during the subsequent examination.

Certain principles must be adhered to for an accurate single contrast barium enema. First, the colon must be radiographed so that every segment is seen in profile and without overlapping on at least two films. This allows verification of any suspected lesion seen on a single film. During the examination, combined fluoroscopy, compression, and spot filming of the entire colon are performed. Subsequently, overhead films of the barium-filled colon are obtained in a manner that provides a clear view of all colonic segments.

As stated earlier, compression and spot filming under fluoroscopic control are the most important component of the single contrast barium enema examination. The large diameter of the barium-filled colon can otherwise prevent detection of small filling defects. Compression

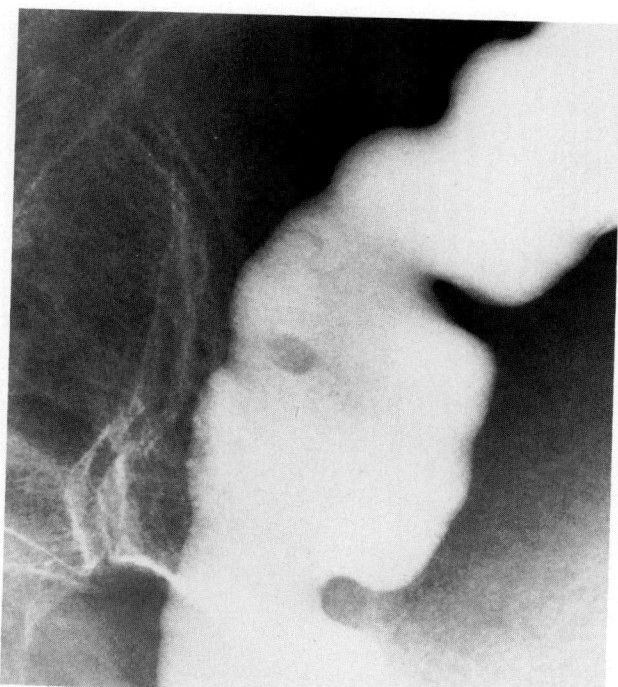

**Figure 6–14. Compression film of the descending colon showing a 5-mm polyp.** Compression filming of the entire colon must be performed for maximal detection of small polyps.

is applied under fluoroscopic control to thin down the barium column, ensuring that small lesions displace a large fraction of the barium suspension and can thus be seen easily (Fig. 6–14; see Figs. 6–1A, 6–2B, and 6–3).

The following describes a thorough single contrast barium enema examination. The patient is placed in the left posterior oblique position, the flow of barium suspension is started, and a spot film of the rectosigmoid region is taken while distention is still minimal. This allows small lesions in this noncompressible area to be more easily detected. The rectosigmoid region is then filmed again when fully distended. Sufficient films should be taken to demonstrate the entire sigmoid colon without overlapping of loops. After complete filling of the colon, spot films of the remaining segments of the colon are taken. Careful manual palpation or mechanical compression or both are employed over each segment of the colon. A thorough examination usually requires 8 to 10 spot films. After fluoroscopy, the following overhead films are obtained. When using a remote control fluoroscope, however, the following films are taken during the fluoroscopic examination.

1. Left lateral projection of the rectum
2. Prone projection of the colon
3. Right anterior oblique projection of the colon
4. Left anterior oblique projection of the colon
5. Prone angled projection of the rectum and sigmoid colon

Although there have been far fewer investigations of the accuracy of the single contrast barium enema than

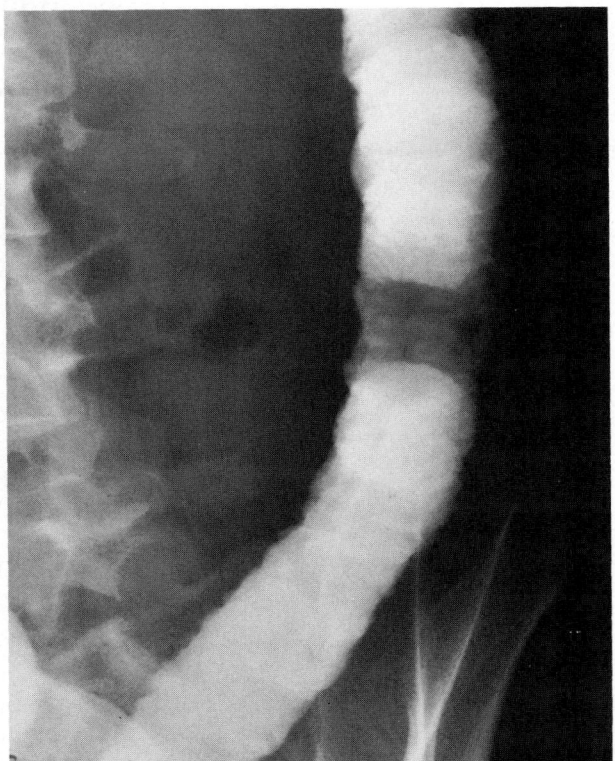

**Figure 6–15.** Extensive ulcerative colitis seen as marginal ulcerations on a single contrast barium enema examination.

ally useful for confirmation of an otherwise poorly seen neoplasm. However, the postevacuation film is mandatory for accurate evaluation of ulcerative colitis or Crohn's disease on a single contrast examination. In these patients, the postevacuation film provides the best assessment of the changes of early or minimal disease.

of the double contrast study, sufficient information is available to characterize the abilities of the single contrast examination. It has been found that the single contrast study has a sensitivity of 90 to 95% for lesions 1 cm or larger and also that a sensitivity of approximately 60 to 70% for detection of polyps under 1 cm can be achieved.[1, 15, 16] Detection of carcinomas of the colon and rectum approaches 100% if the examination is carefully performed.[18] Although the earliest manifestations of inflammatory bowel disease require a double contrast examination for accurate detection, more advanced cases of ulcerative colitis and Crohn's disease are easily and adequately assessed with a single contrast study (Fig. 6–15).

The postevacuation film has been stressed in the past, but it is my experience that the postevacuation film can be dispensed with in most single contrast examinations, greatly speeding the flow of patients through the fluoroscopy suite. The postevacuation film is only occasion-

## References

1. Gelfand DW, Chen YM, Ott DJ: Detection of colonic polyps on single-contrast barium enema study: emphasis on the elderly. Radiology 164:333–337, 1987.
2. Gelfand DW, Ott DJ: Barium sulfate suspensions: an evaluation of available products. AJR 138:935–941, 1982.
3. Leininger V: The concentration of enema materials. *In* Miller R (ed): Detection of Colon Lesions—First Standardization Conference—1969. Chicago, American College of Radiology, 1973.
4. Ott DJ, Chen YM, Wu WC, et al: Radiographic and endoscopic sensitivity in detecting lower esophageal mucosal ring. AJR 147:261–265, 1986.
5. Schatzki R, Gary JE: Dysphagia due to a diaphragm-like localized narrowing in the lower esophagus ("lower esophageal ring"). AJR 70:911–922, 1953.
6. Gelfand DW: High density, low viscosity barium for fine mucosal detail on double-contrast upper gastrointestinal examinations. AJR 130:831–833, 1978.
7. Gelfand DW, Ott DJ: Anatomy and technique in evaluating the esophagus. Semin Roentgenol 16:168–182, 1981.
8. Ott DJ, Gelfand DW, Wu WC: Sensitivity of single-contrast radiology in esophageal disease: a study of 240 patients with endoscopically verified abnormality. Gastrointest Radiol 8:105–110, 1983.
9. Cockerill EM, Miller RE, Chernish SM, et al: Optimal visualization of esophageal varices. AJR 126:512–523, 1976.
10. Ott DJ, Richter JE, Chen YM, et al: Esophageal radiography and manometry: correlation in 172 patients with dysphagia. AJR 149:307–311, 1987.
11. Ott DJ, Gelfand DW, Wu WC, et al: Radiological evaluation of dysphagia. JAMA 256:2718–2721, 1986.
12. Gelfand DW, Chen YM, Ott DJ: Multiphasic examinations of the stomach: efficacy of individual techniques and combinations of techniques in detecting 153 lesions. Radiology 162:829–834, 1987.
13. Caldwell WL, Floch MH: Evaluation of the small bowel barium motor meal with emphasis on the effect of volume of barium suspensions ingested. Radiology 80:383–391, 1963.
14. Sellink JL: Radiological Atlas of Common Diseases of the Small Bowel. Leiden: HE Stenfert Kroese, 1976.
15. Ott DJ, Chen YM, Gelfand DW, et al: Single-contrast vs double-contrast barium enema in the detection of colonic polyps. AJR 146:993–996, 1986.
16. Kaude JV, Harty RF: Sensitivity of single contrast barium enema with regard to colorectal disease as diagnosed by colonoscopy. Eur J Radiol 2:290–292, 1982.
17. Gelfand DW, Chen YM, Ott DJ: Preparing the colon for the barium enema examination. Radiology 178:609–613, 1991.
18. Gelfand DW, Chen YM, Ott DJ: Radiologic detection of colonic neoplasms: benefits of a systems analysis approach. AJR 156:303–306, 1991.

# Ultrasonography of the Hollow Viscera

Stephanie R. Wilson, M.D.

INTRODUCTION

SONOGRAPHIC TECHNIQUE

NORMAL GUT

ABNORMAL GUT
Mural Thickening
Mural Masses

PERITONEAL, MESENTERIC, AND
OMENTAL ABNORMALITIES

## INTRODUCTION

The significant artifact arising from gas in the lumen of the gastrointestinal tract has led many investigators to ignore the hollow viscera when performing routine abdominal sonography. This is regrettable because sonography is an excellent means of assessing a wide variety of gastrointestinal tract diseases, notably those that produce mural abnormality (either gut wall thickening or gut wall masses), and abnormality of the adjacent soft tissues including the peritoneum, mesentery, omentum, and solid organs. Although mucosal abnormalities and small mass lesions are beneath its spatial resolution, sonography, like computed tomography (CT), excels in demonstrating the nonmucosal aspects of gastrointestinal tract disease and in detecting extraintestinal complications.

In some patients, sonography is performed specifically to detect gastrointestinal tract disease and characterize its nature and extent. In other patients, a gastrointestinal abnormality may be detected on sonograms performed for nonspecific reasons, such as evaluation of a palpable abdominal mass or abdominal pain. Last, gut-related disease may be an occasional incidental observation on sonography. In all instances, recognition of the gastrointestinal origin of a sonographic finding should lead to appropriate further investigation.

## SONOGRAPHIC TECHNIQUE

Abdominal sonograms are ideally performed after an overnight fast to minimize luminal gas and fluid content. Oral or rectal fluid is not routinely administered, although filling the stomach with water may be helpful in patients with suspected mural or intraluminal gastric masses. Routine survey of the peritoneal cavity should be performed with a transducer that visualizes both deep (e.g., gastroesophageal junction) and more superficial (e.g., small bowel loops) structures. In large patients this may require survey with both a 3.5- and a 5-MHz transducer. The region of interest must be assessed within the focal zone of the transducer; transducers with short focal zones or variable focusing are best. Scans should be performed before and after bladder emptying. Suspicious gut loops should then receive detailed analysis using graded compression sonography (Fig. 7–1), a technique popularized by Julien Puylaert for patients with suspected appendicitis.[1] Although a 7.5-MHz linear array transducer was utilized initially, mechanical and convex linear probes work equally well; the critical transducer factor is a short focal zone. Gradually increasing pressure is applied to the region of interest. Normal loops of intestine are displaced or compressed, but abnormally thickened or obstructed loops are noncompressible and are trapped between the transducer anteriorly and the body wall musculature posteriorly. This optimizes visualization of the region of interest without annoying interference from luminal gas. In patients with peritoneal irritation or localized abdominal pain, it is important to use gentle graded compression; rapid or jerky movements of the transducer result in a nondiagnostic study and an unhappy patient.

## NORMAL GUT

The normal gut is a long hollow tube made of multiple concentric layers. On sonography, these layers are seen as five alternating echogenic and hypoechoic rings that correspond to the histologic layers from the lumen outward as follows (Fig. 7–2):

1. Echogenic: superficial mucosa and luminal content–mucous membrane interface
2. Hypoechoic: deep mucosa including muscularis mucosae
3. Echogenic: submucosa and submucosa–muscularis propria interface
4. Hypoechoic: muscularis propria
5. Echogenic: serosa or adventitia and muscularis propria–serosa interface[2]

The patient's habitus, the scan quality, and the transducer frequency all affect the delineation of the gut wall layers (Fig. 7–3).

Both the location and the morphology of the gut are

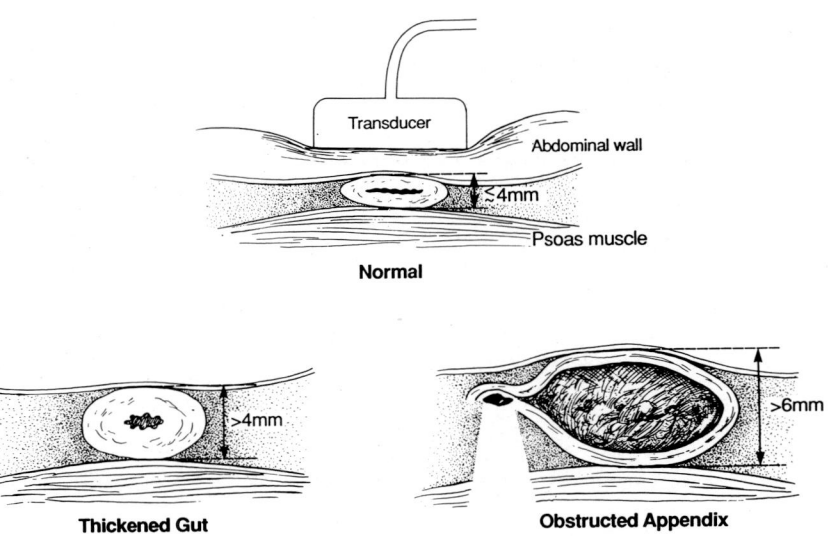

**Figure 7–1. Compression sonography, schematic depiction.** Normal gut is compressible. Abnormally thickened gut or an obstructed segment (e.g., acute appendicitis) is noncompressible. (Modified from Puylaert JBCM. From Wilson SR: Gastrointestinal tract sonography. *In* Rumack C, Wilson SR, Charboneau JW [eds]: Diagnostic Ultrasound. St. Louis: Mosby–Year Book, 1991, pp 181–207.)

helpful in determining the portion of the gut studied. The segments of the gastrointestinal tract that, by virtue of their peritoneal attachments, are relatively fixed in location are easiest to identify. Therefore, the gastroesophageal junction, antral-pyloric part of the stomach, duodenum, terminal ileum, ascending colon, descending colon, and rectum can usually be identified. The remainder of the gastrointestinal tract is localized by inference with somewhat less accuracy.

Identified morphologic features, such as gastric rugae, valvulae conniventes (Fig. 7–4), colonic haustra (Fig. 7–5), and appendices epiploicae, are all helpful localizers. However, these tend to be more frequently visualized in patients with an abnormally fluid-filled gastrointestinal tract or ascites than in the normal fasting patient.[3]

The normal thickness of the gut wall is 3 to 5 mm,

varying with luminal distention. The stomach wall in the fasting patient may normally appear somewhat thicker. In a fasting patient the gastrointestinal content is usually quite minimal, although variable amounts of fluid and particulate material may be seen throughout the bowel.

Peristaltic activity is frequently observed in the small bowel and the stomach and may be a useful sonographic observation. The presence of gut activity is particularly helpful in determining whether a sonographically identified "collection" represents a fluid-filled hollow viscus or a true collection such as an abscess, hematoma, or seroma. Furthermore, peristaltic activity is increased with infectious enteritides and mechanical bowel obstruction. Decreased peristaltic activity associated with paralytic ileus is much harder to appreciate sonographically, although a local ileus with associated focal fluid-filled loops may be readily seen.

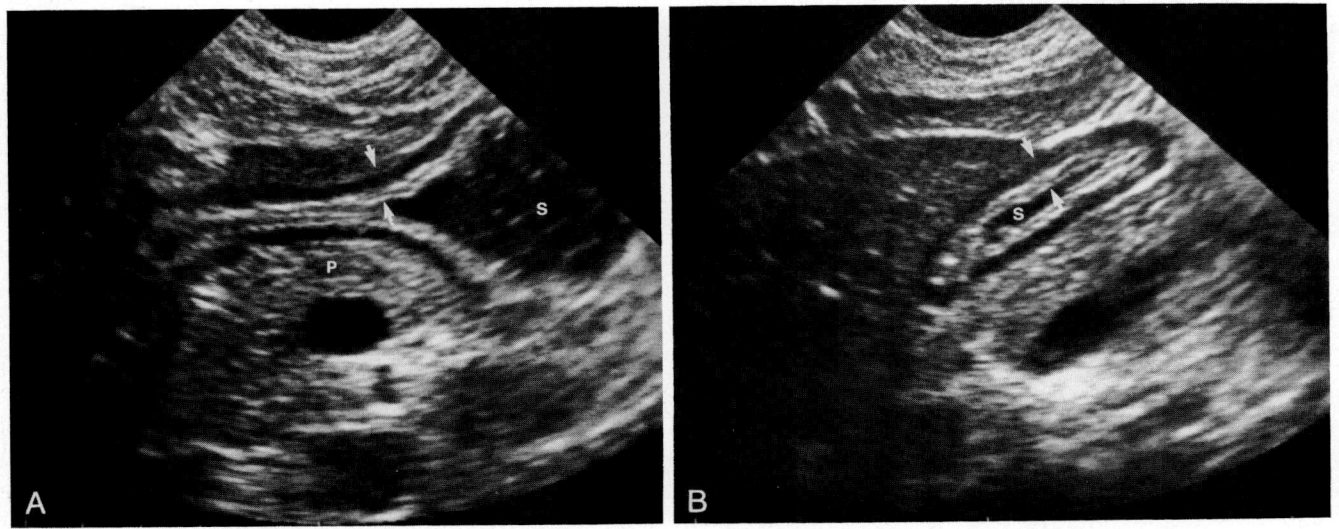

**Figure 7–2. Normal gut signature. A.** Long axis. **B.** Cross section. Images of the gastric antrum show the five normal layers of the gut wall *(arrows)*. The lumen (S) of the gastric body is filled with a moderate amount of fluid. P = pancreas.

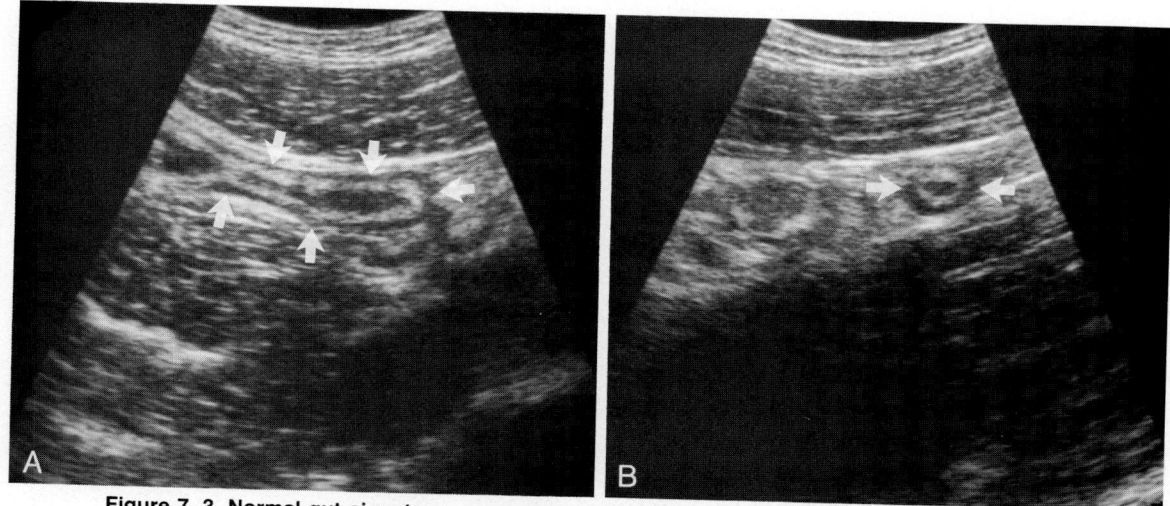

**Figure 7–3. Normal gut signature: appendix. A.** Long axis. **B.** Cross section. Images of a normal appendix *(arrows)* show only the two dominant layers of the gut wall: the echogenic submucosa and the hypoechoic muscularis propria.

## ABNORMAL GUT

The sonographic morphology of an abnormal segment of gut can occasionally suggest a specific diagnosis. Relevant features include gut wall thickening in either a symmetric or an asymmetric pattern; preservation or destruction of the normal gut wall layers; a gut wall mass with or without ulceration; the location, length, and number of involved segments; and the appearance of the external gut surface.[4] Adjacent soft tissue changes may suggest inflammatory complications such as perforation, phlegmon, or abscess. Similarly, neoplasm is suggested if metastases or tumor invasion is present.

## Mural Thickening

The "pseudokidney" or "target" sign is the familiar sonographic abnormality seen with gut wall thickening, the central echogenicity representing the lumen of the gut and the hypoechoic rim representing the thickening gut wall[5, 6] (Fig. 7–6). Ulcerations containing gas appear as bright echogenic foci within the wall with associated shadowing or "ring-down" artifact (Figs. 7–7 and 7–8). Benign thickening may be focal or diffuse, is usually symmetric, and maintains some preservation of the gut wall layers, whereas malignant thickening is more often focal, is frequently asymmetric, and is without preser-

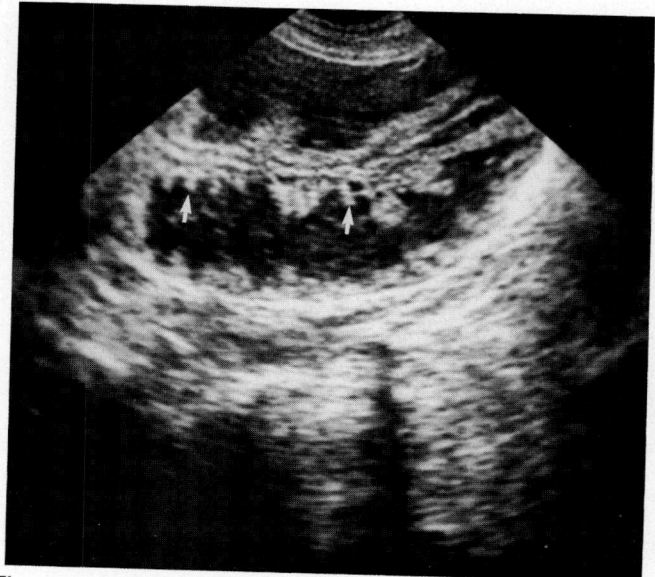

**Figure 7–4. Valvulae conniventes.** Visualization of the valvulae conniventes *(arrows)* indicates the small bowel origin of this dilated fluid-filled loop of gut in a patient with closed loop obstruction.

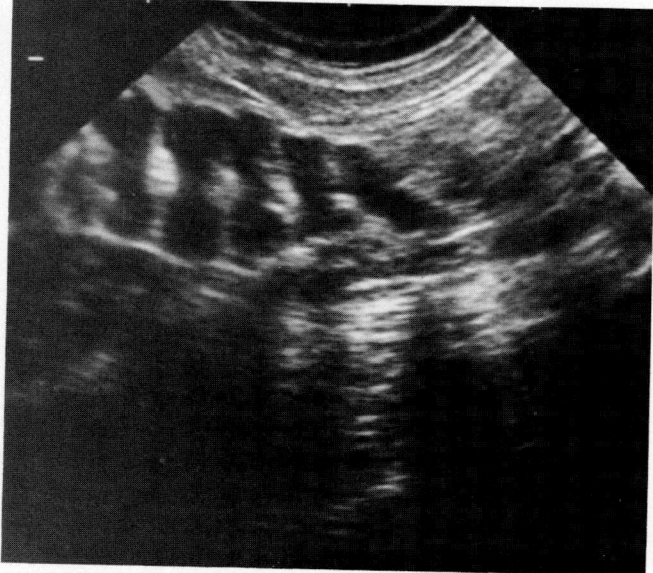

**Figure 7–5. Colonic haustra.** Long-axis sonogram of the ascending colon demonstrates the normal haustral pattern in this patient. A moderate amount of intraluminal fluid is present.

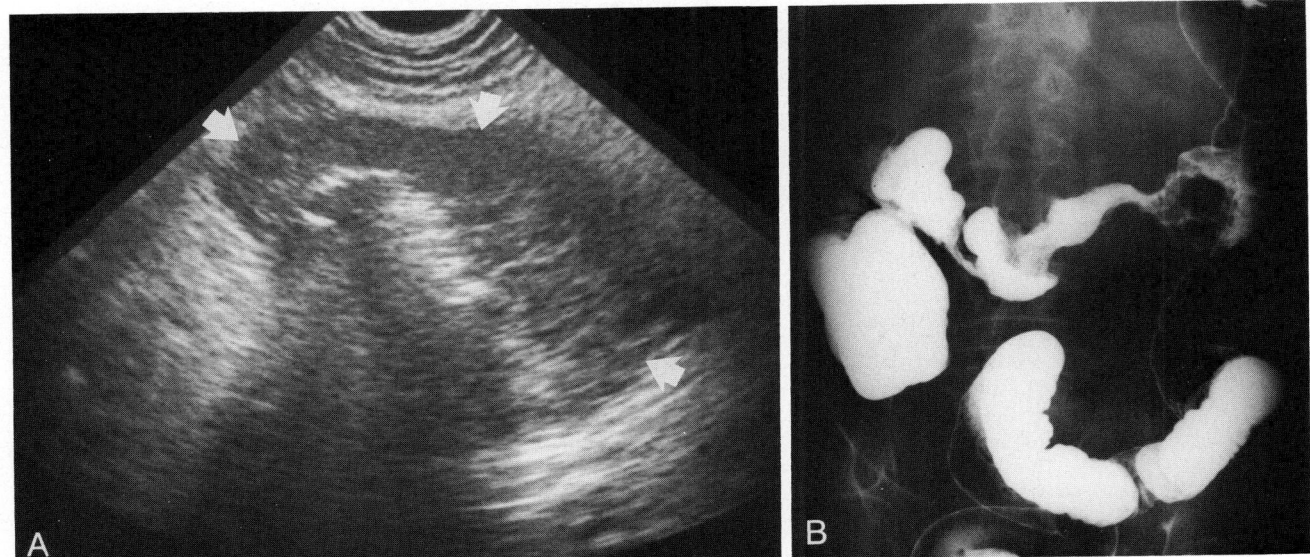

**Figure 7–6. Pseudokidney sign: carcinoma of the transverse colon. A**. Long-axis sonogram shows a large focal hypoechoic mass *(arrows)* with central echogenicity. The ring down and shadowing from the echogenic region confirm its gaseous origin. **B**. Confirmatory barium enema.

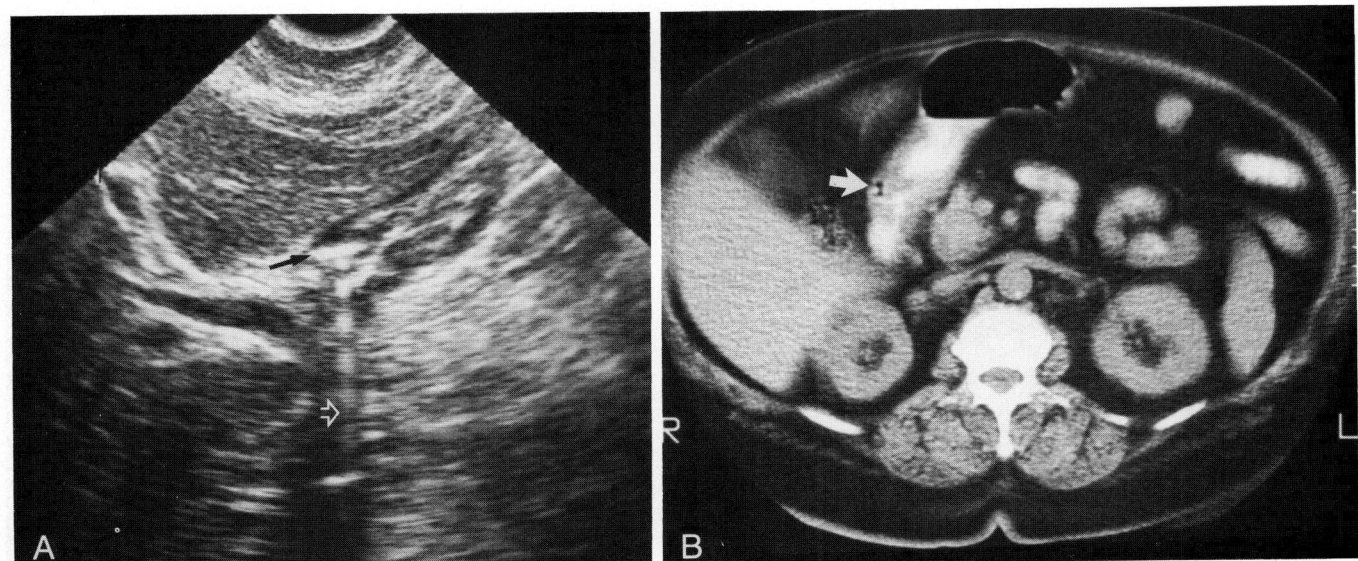

**Figure 7–7. Extraluminal gas: peptic ulcer disease. A**. Long-axis sonogram shows the irregular mural thickening of the antrum. An echogenic focus *(solid arrow)* within the thickened gut wall shows ring-down artifact *(open arrow)*. This is indicative of an ulcer crater with a gas bubble. **B**. Confirmatory CT scan. Arrow = ulcer.

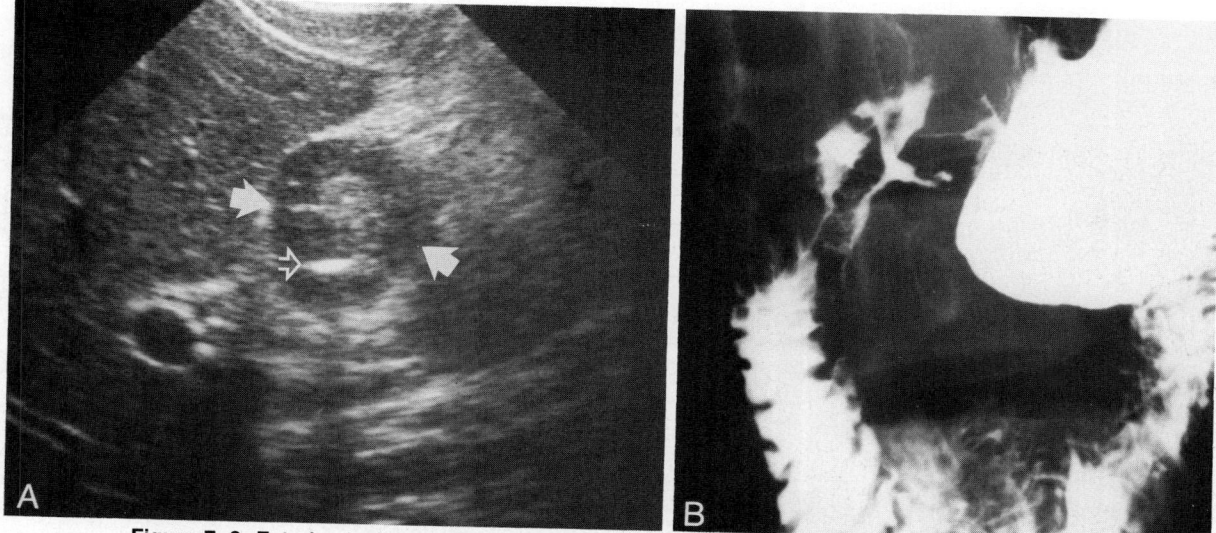

**Figure 7–8. Extraluminal gas: Crohn's disease of the duodenum. A.** Sagittal sonogram shows the duodenal bulb in cross section. The wall is uniformly thickened and appears hypoechoic *(solid arrows)*. The linear reflector *(open arrow)* with acoustic shadowing indicates air within the thickened duodenal wall. **B.** Upper gastrointestinal series confirms duodenal distortion, lumen narrowing, and ulceration.

vation of gut wall stratification. Sonographic features are not always specific, and the clinical picture should be considered in conjunction with the sonographic abnormalities (Fig. 7–9). Pathologic considerations include inflammatory (Fig. 7–10), neoplastic (Fig. 7–11), and edematous (Fig. 7–12) diseases of the gut wall.[7, 8]

## Mural Masses

Intramural masses affecting the gastrointestinal tract are frequently solid or complex. If these masses are large, their origin may not always be obvious. Accordingly, gastrointestinal tumors should be considered if intraperitoneal or appropriately positioned retroperitoneal masses are identified that do not arise from the abdominal solid organs. With ulceration, pockets of gas are often seen within the mass, and their typical ring down artifact is helpful in localizing the origin of the abnormality to the gastrointestinal tract (Fig. 7–13). Pathologic considerations for gut wall masses include mesenchymal tumors (Fig. 7–14), lymphoma (see Fig. 7–13), gut metastases, and adenocarcinoma with local tumor extension. Smooth muscle tumors and lymphomas

**Figure 7–9. Asymmetric gut wall thickening: intramural abscess from diverticulitis.** Longitudinal sonogram demonstrates asymmetric focal thickening of the superficial gut wall with multiple tiny echogenic foci indicative of gas bubbles within the abscess cavity *(arrows)*.

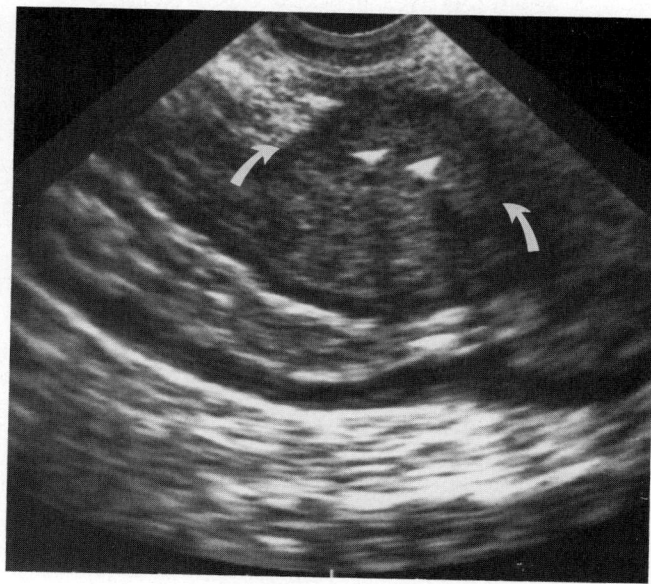

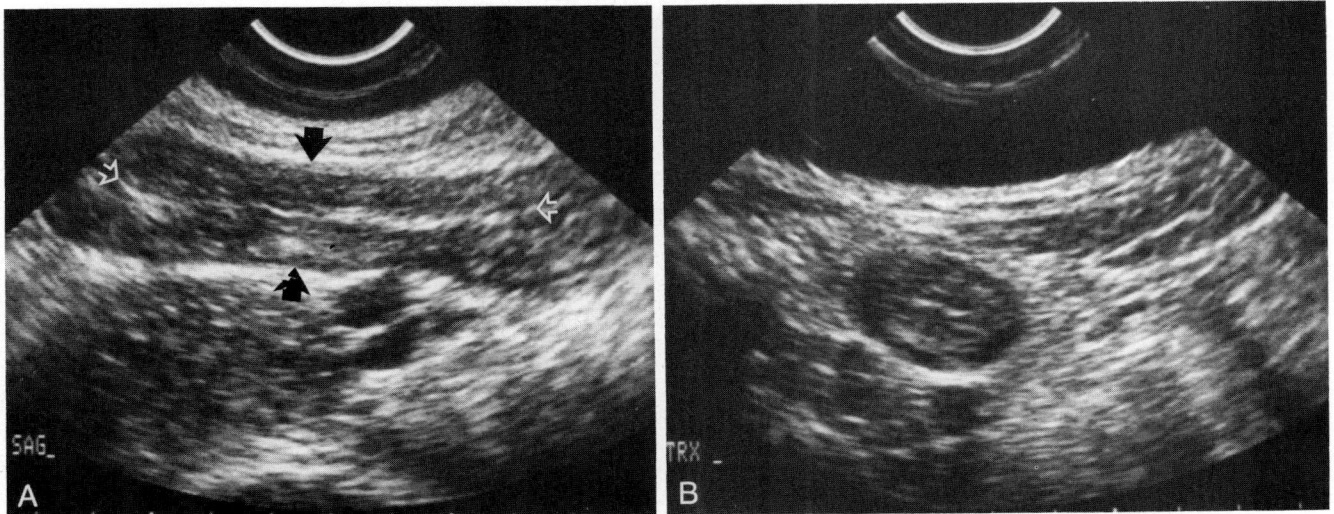

**Figure 7–10. Inflammatory thickening of the gut: Crohn's disease. A**. Long axis. **B**. Cross section. Sonograms show a uniformly thickened loop of terminal ileum *(solid arrows)*. The central echogenic line *(open arrows)* represents the stenotic lumen. Stratification of the normal gut wall layers is partially preserved.

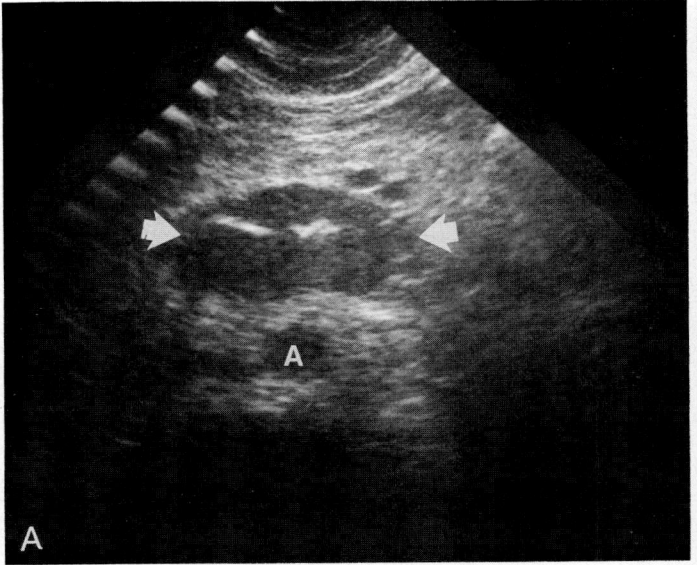

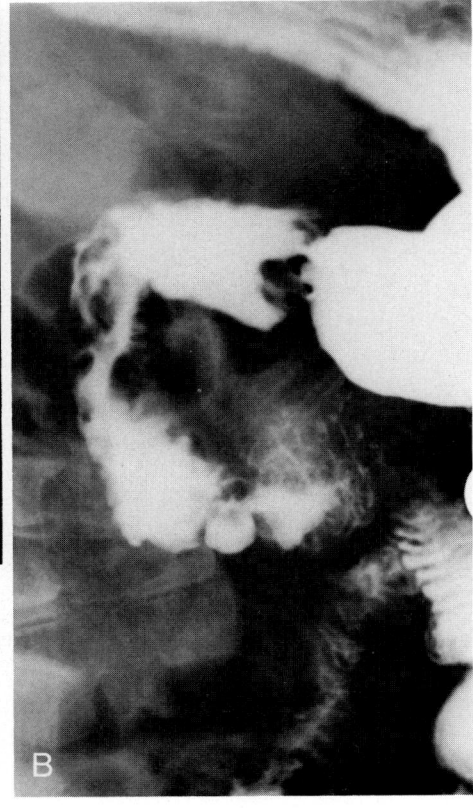

**Figure 7–11. Carcinoma of the duodenum. A**. Midline transverse sonogram shows a pseudokidney sign *(arrows)* between the aorta (A) posteriorly and the superior mesenteric vessels anteriorly. The eccentric echogenicity represents ulceration within the mass and suggests its gastrointestinal origin. **B**. Confirmatory upper gastrointestinal examination.

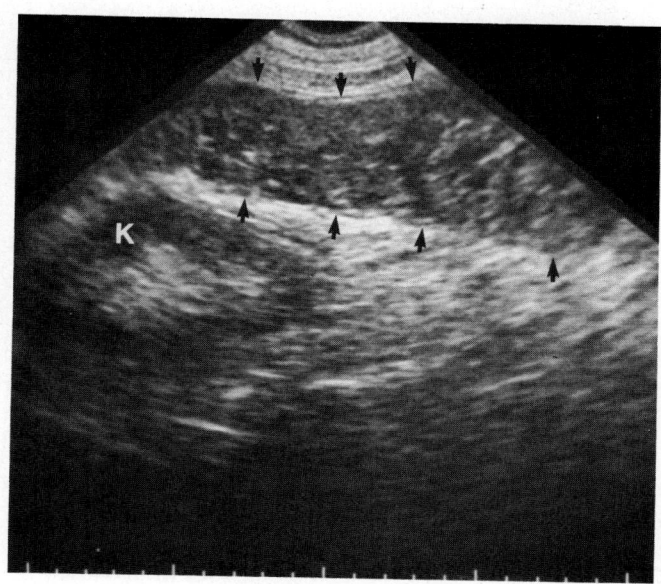

**Figure 7–12. Infectious-edematous thickening of the gut: pseudomembranous colitis.** Sagittal left flank sonogram shows a diffusely thickened gasless descending colon *(arrows)*. The mucosal surfaces are in virtual apposition. K = left kidney.

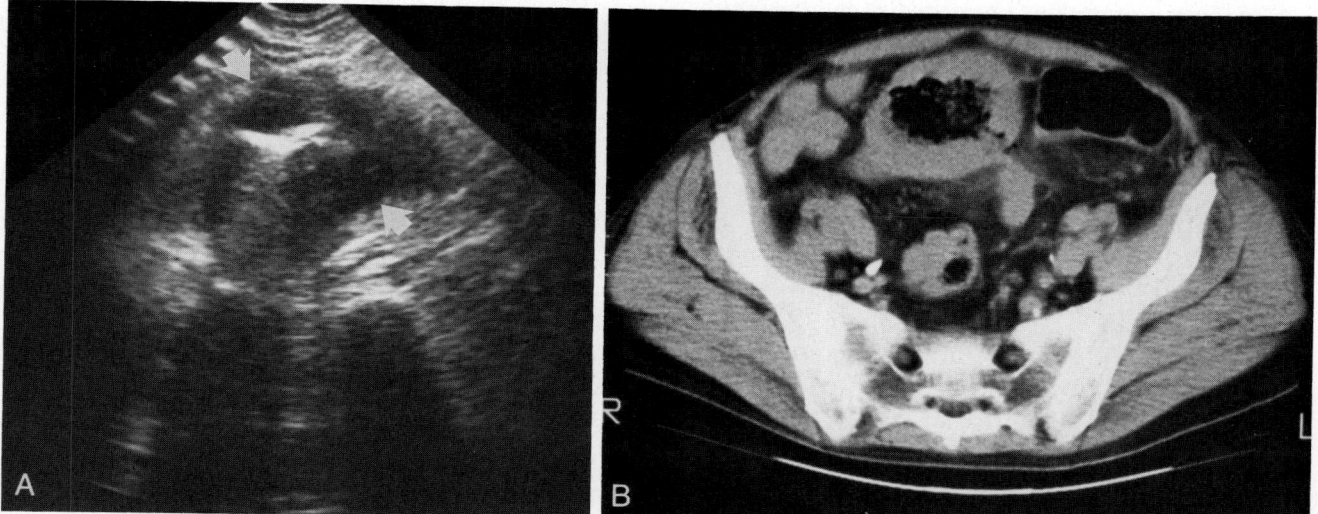

**Figure 7–13. Neoplastic mural thickening: small bowel lymphoma. A**. Midabdominal sonogram shows a focal hypoechoic mass *(arrows)* with an echogenic center. The ring-down artifact indicates the gas within the ulcerated lumen of the gut mass. **B**. Confirmatory CT scan.

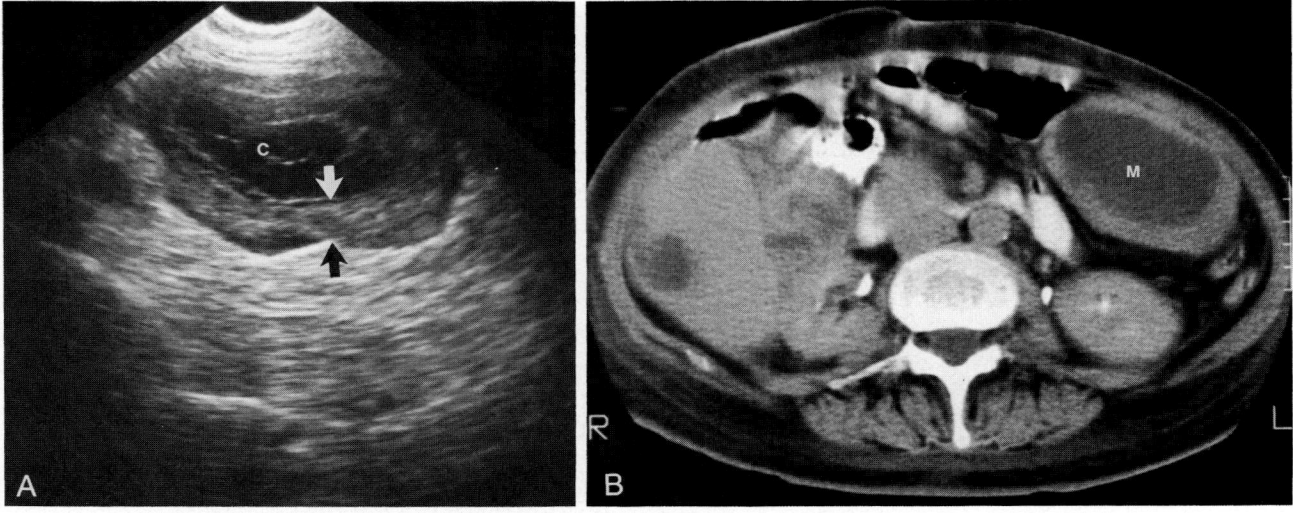

**Figure 7–14. Smooth muscle tumor: leiomyosarcoma of small bowel. A.** Transverse left flank sonogram reveals a complex mass lesion with a solid rim *(arrows)* and a irregular cystic center (C). Although the gut origin is not evident on this film, the morphology is highly suggestive of a smooth muscle tumor. **B.** Confirmatory CT scan shows the necrotic left flank mass (M) as well as a liver metastasis.

are the most commonly encountered causes of this sonographic morphology. Their sonographic detection is usually relatively easy because these tumors are often large at the time of presentation. In addition, both of these tumors have highly suggestive sonographic features. The tendency of smooth muscle tumors to undergo central necrosis frequently results in complex masses with both cystic and solid components (see Fig. 7–14). This morphology is virtually pathognomonic.[9] Lymphoma typically is strikingly hypoechoic and may suggest a cyst or fluid collection sonographically[10] (see Fig. 7–13).

## PERITONEAL, MESENTERIC, AND OMENTAL ABNORMALITIES

Although CT is often superior to sonography in its ability to determine the extent of extraintestinal disease, the experienced sonographer is frequently able to identify specific soft tissue changes (Fig. 7–15).

Inflammatory disorders, notably Crohn's disease, appendicitis, and diverticulitis, are often associated with fibrofatty proliferation of the mesentery (Fig. 7–16), edema, mesenteric adenopathy, or abscess (Fig. 7–17).

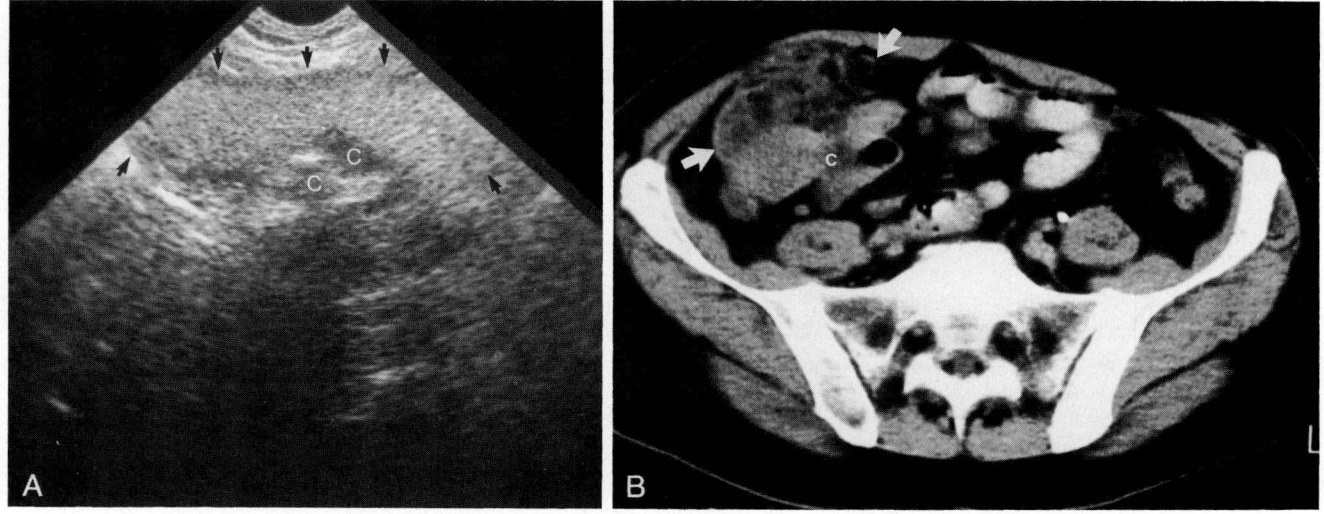

**Figure 7–15. Extraintestinal inflammatory change.** Thickened omentum secondary to perforated carcinoma of cecum. **A.** Sagittal sonogram shows thick echogenic mass, the inflamed omentum *(arrows)*, lying superficial to a colon carcinoma (C) that has a poorly defined pseudokidney appearance. **B.** Confirmatory CT scan. C = neoplasm; L = colon lumen; arrows = infiltrated omentum.

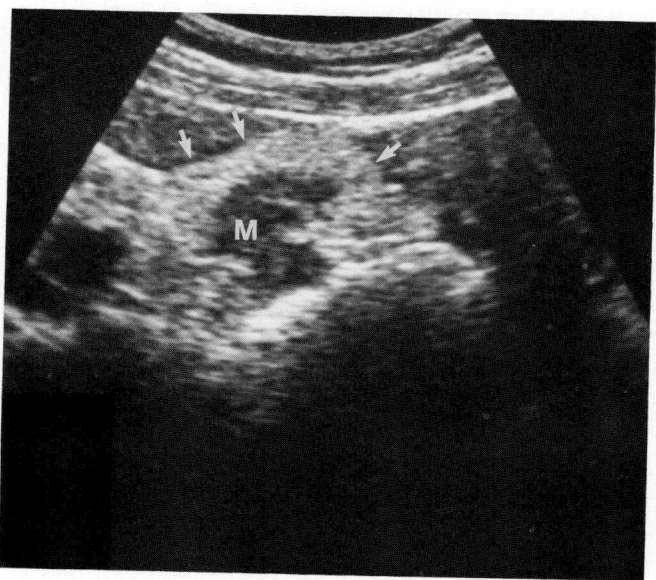

**Figure 7–16. Fibrofatty proliferation of the mesentery: perforated appendicitis.** Sagittal pelvic sonogram shows a uniform halo of increased echogenicity *(arrows)* surrounding a focal hypoechoic mass (M).

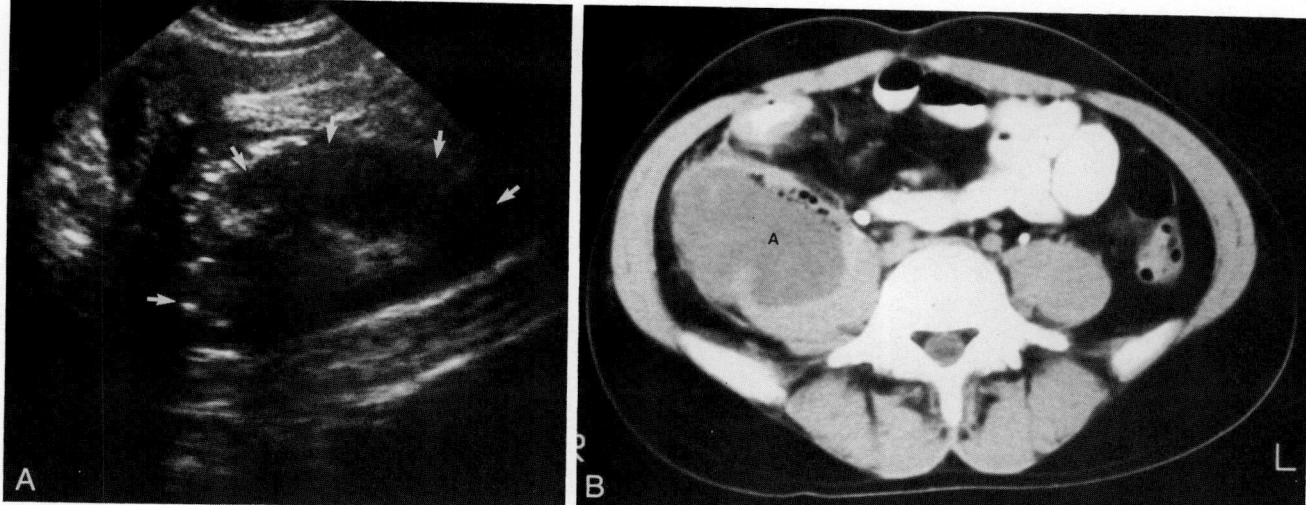

**Figure 7–17. Gas-containing abscess. A**. Sagittal sonogram shows a large focal hypoechoic mass *(arrows)* in the right psoas. Multiple bright echogenic foci indicative of gas bubbles are noted anteriorly. **B**. Confirmatory CT scan. A = abscess.

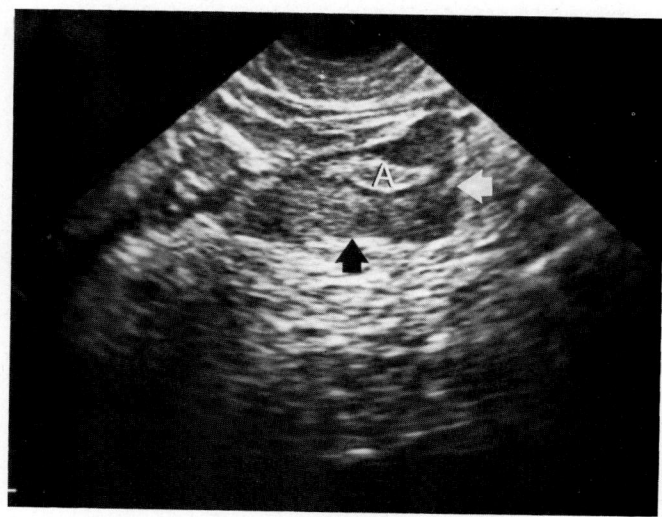

**Figure 7–18. Serosal implants from ovarian carcinoma.** Sagittal midline sonogram shows the gastric antrum (A) in cross section surrounded by a hypoechoic mass *(arrows)*.

Fistulous communications to the bladder, other loops of intestine, and skin usually produce hypoechoic tracts that are easily identified in the soft tissues adjacent to loops of diseased gut. Detection of neoplastic invasion and metastatic adenopathy is related to the size of the tumor deposits. Visualization of peritoneal implants (Fig. 7–18) and omental cakes is enhanced by the presence of intraperitoneal fluid.

## References

1. Puylaert JBCM: Acute appendicitis: US evaluation using graded compression. Radiology 158:355–360, 1986.
2. Heyder N, Kaarmann H, Giedi J: Experimental investigations into the possibility of differentiating early from invasive carcinoma of the stomach by means of ultrasound. Endoscopy 19:228–232, 1987.
3. Fleischer AC, Muhletaler CA, James AE Jr: Sonographic assessment of the bowel wall. AJR 136:887–891, 1981.
4. Wilson SR: Gastrointestinal tract sonography. In Rumack C, Wilson SR, Charboneau JW (eds): Diagnostic Ultrasound. St. Louis: Mosby–Year Book, 1991, pp 109–138.
5. Lutz H, Petzoldt R: Ultrasonic patterns of space occupying lesions of the stomach and intestine. Ultrasound Med Biol 2:129–131, 1976.
6. Bluth EL, Merritt CRB, Sullivan MA: Ultrasonic evaluation of the stomach, small bowel, and colon. Radiology 133:677–680, 1979.
7. Khaw KT, Yeoman LJ, Saverymuttu SH, et al: Ultrasonic patterns in inflammatory bowel disease. Clin Radiol 43:171–175, 1991.
8. Downey DB, Wilson SR: Pseudomembranous colitis: sonographic features. Radiology 180:61–64, 1991.
9. Kaftori JK, Aharon M, Kleinhaus U: Sonographic features of gastrointestinal leiomyosarcoma. JCU 9:11–15, 1981.
10. Derchi LE, Bandereali A, Bossi MC, et al: Sonographic appearance of gastric lymphoma. J Ultrasound Med 3:251–256, 1984.

# Computed Tomography of the Gastrointestinal Tract: Techniques and Principles of Interpretation

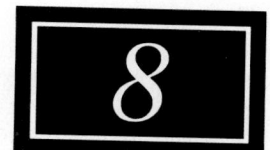

Alec J. Megibow, M.D.

## INTRODUCTION

Computed tomography (CT) has become a routine procedure for evaluation of alimentary tract disease because of its speed, accuracy, and cross-sectional imaging capabilities. Accurate interpretation of CT scans requires reliable bowel and vascular opacification. This chapter describes the techniques needed to optimize CT scans for the detection and diagnosis of luminal, mural, and mesenteric abnormalities of the gastrointestinal tract.

## LUMEN OPACIFICATION

### Positive Contrast Agents

Complete bowel opacification is essential for proper interpretation of all abdominal CT examinations.[1] Indeed, one of the most common sources of diagnostic error in interpreting abdominal CT scans is mistaking poorly opacified bowel loops for abdominal masses (Figs. 8–1 and 8–2). Consequently, rigorous attention to technique is vital.

The gut is usually opacified by giving oral positive contrast agents, either water-soluble iodinated or barium solutions. Both agents must be used in considerably lower concentrations than in plain film radiography. Barium preparations are administered as 1 to 2% suspensions, and water-soluble agents are prepared as 2 to 3% solutions. The low concentration of barium requires commercial preparations made specifically for CT, in which additives are used to ensure that the barium remains in suspension. Barium products are flavored, and water-soluble agents can be flavored with commercially available powdered agents.[1]

Sufficient time must be allotted for the contrast agent to distribute evenly throughout the alimentary canal. Most patients have contrast agent in the distal ileum within 45 minutes after initiation of drinking. Obviously, the clinical status of the patient must be considered. A gravely ill or recent postoperative patient may have significantly slower intestinal transit because of ileus. Prolonged transit time is also observed in patients with electrolyte disturbances, collagen-vascular diseases (e.g., scleroderma), and intestinal obstruction. Conversely, patients who are hyperthyroid, have syndromes with associated increased intestinal motility (e.g., carcinoid, islet cell tumor), or have a variety of infections (e.g., cryptosporidiosis, giardiasis) have a significantly accelerated intestinal transit time.

The choice between oral barium suspensions and water-soluble agents is dictated by the experience and preference of the radiologist. I prefer barium suspensions because the mucosal coating appears to be somewhat better, allowing more confident recognition of intestinal fold patterns (see later). Acceptance by patients is equivalent provided the water-soluble solutions are flavored with commercially available powdered agents (e.g., Tang). In my experience, there is no significant difference between the transit times of the barium and water-soluble agents. I routinely utilize

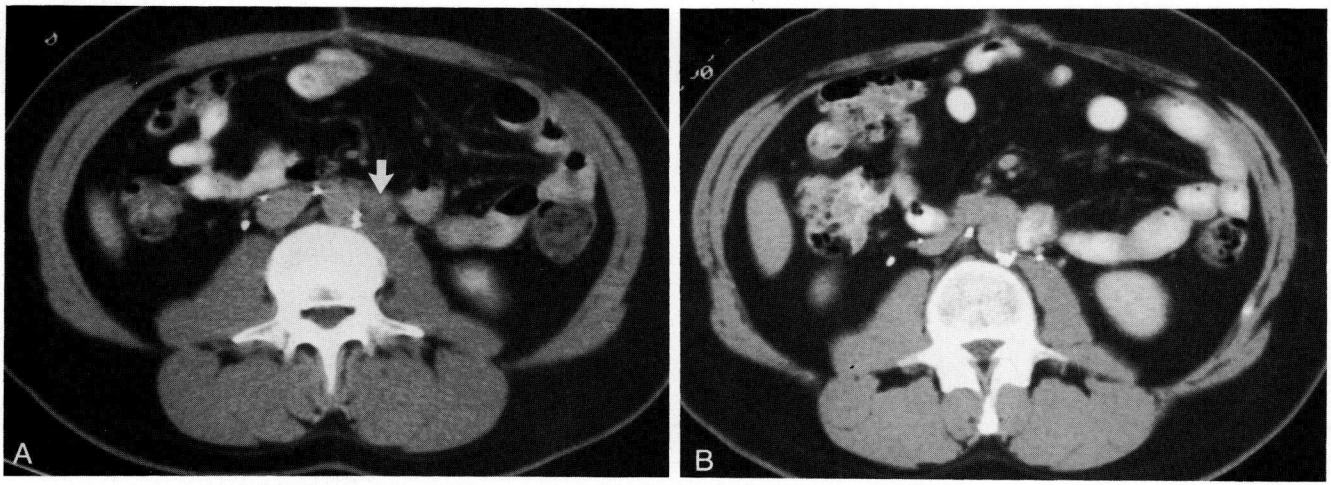

**Figure 8–1. Retroperitoneal pseudomass resulting from unopacified bowel. A.** Follow-up CT scan in patient with seminoma reveals apparent left para-aortic adenopathy. **B.** Another scan after flooding bowel with contrast agent clearly shows that the "node" is actually unopacified bowel.

water-soluble agents for patients with abdominal trauma or suspected perforated viscus, for patients who may go from CT to the operating room, or for percutaneous CT biopsy or other interventional procedures.

When a pelvic pathologic condition is suspected, opacification of the pelvic colon is critical. This is accomplished by giving a positive contrast enema at the time of the study. Approximately 50 to 100 mL of a dilute barium suspension or water-soluble solution is sufficient. An alternative method is to have the patient consume the contrast medium the night before the study to opacify the distal colon. Drawbacks of the latter method include logistic difficulties with the nursing station, outpatient compliance, and questionable incremental gain in information over and above recognizing the colon because of its normal content. Furthermore, as hospital stays are curtailed, patients are admitted the night before surgical procedures and may undergo preoperative colonic cleansing, which would obviously negate any effect of this regimen.

## Negative Contrast Agents

Negative contrast agents have several advantages over positive contrast agents for evaluating luminal gastrointestinal pathologic changes by CT.[2] They are related to the increase in subject contrast between the "dark" lumen and the "brighter" soft tissue density gut wall. Increasing the conspicuity of the bowel wall makes regions of mural thickening become apparent, increasing the confidence and scope of CT diagnosis. Negative contrast agents require some modification of routine scanning protocols. However, when these methods are adopted in a department, they can be implemented even in the presence of a busy schedule.

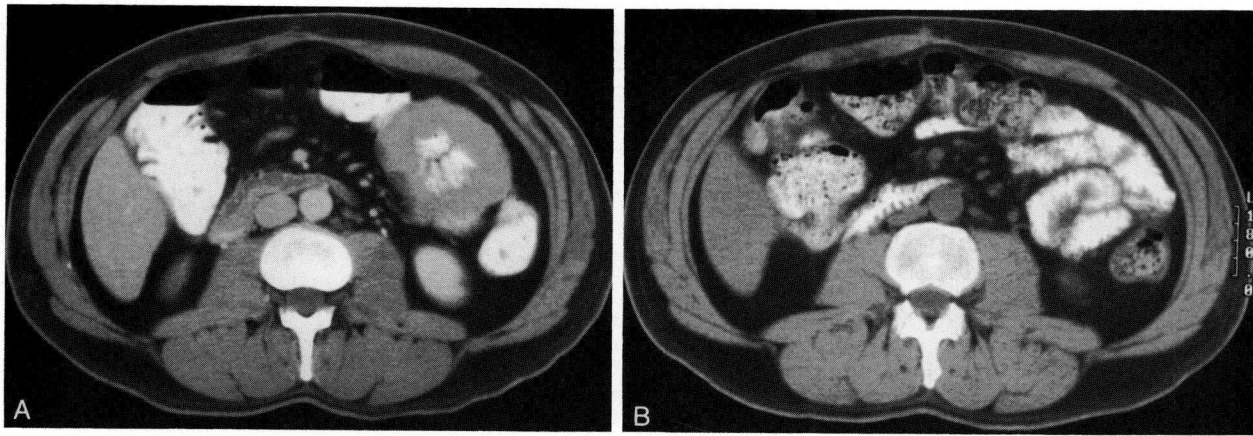

**Figure 8–2. Mesenteric pseudomass created by unopacified bowel. A.** CT scan of a patient with lymphoma shows an apparent mass related to jejunal loops. **B.** Another scan after flooding bowel with contrast agent reveals that the "mass" is only unopacified bowel surrounding opacified loops.

Three negative agents have been evaluated: air (or $CO_2$), water, and corn oil emulsion.[1-3] Water is simple to use and provides reliable bowel distention.[3a] Corn oil emulsion has been clinically evaluated but is no longer commercially manufactured.[4] I routinely utilize air in practice. Air is easily insufflated into the colon or can be administered orally by giving an effervescent agent to distend the stomach. Gas is safer than fluid: if it is expelled from the colon, the electrical integrity of expensive equipment is not threatened. If the patient vomits during dynamic bolus CT, a stomach filled with air is relatively safer than one filled with fluid. Modification of the patient's position may be needed to maximize air distention of targeted regions. Because of the relatively posterior orientation of the rectosigmoid, pelvic scanning with the patient in the prone position produces greater luminal distention. Accordingly, this position is used for staging rectal cancer and evaluating pelvic masses (Fig. 8–3). The prone position is also useful for distending and visualizing the gastric fundus and esophagogastric junction region (Fig. 8–4). If the duodenum or gastric antrum is being evaluated, scans taken with the patient in the left decubitus position should be obtained. Experience in double contrast barium radiography can help determine the most efficacious way to manipulate the air (Fig. 8–5).

Water and corn oil emulsion provide negative contrast and predictable luminal distention.[4] In theory, there should be greater contrast with corn oil emulsion because of its fat content, but in clinical practice only a minimal decrease in CT number is achieved. Furthermore, the high cost and poor palatability of corn oil emulsion compared with water have limited its acceptance. The remainder of this discussion, therefore, focuses on the use of water as a contrast agent.

Water provides reproducible luminal distention. In the stomach, water distends the fundus and gastroesophageal junction regions; the distal stomach is somewhat

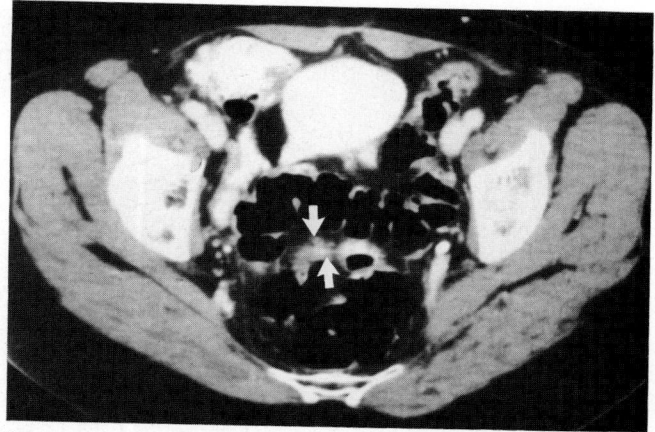

**Figure 8–3. Air-contrast CT scan in ovarian cancer follow-up.** The pelvic colon is distended with air, aiding identification of localized soft tissue thickening *(arrows)* that represents recurrent tumor.

less distended. Water given as an enema can distend the entire colon. Furthermore, in the range of clinically useful CT windows and levels, water maximizes appreciation of bowel wall thickness. With improving CT resolution, use of thin sections, and appropriate contrast enhancement techniques, actual layers of the bowel wall can be seen on the images obtained with water distention.[3] The gastric wall appears thicker, measuring approximately 0.4 cm (Fig. 8–6). Similarly, the colonic wall appears thicker than in a study with air insufflation, measuring approximately 0.2 cm in the rectum and 0.1 to 0.2 cm throughout the colon. This discrepancy, however, is simply the result of windowing.

There are advocates of both methods of negative contrast bowel opacification. The relative non–position-dependent distention and the ability to see the layered appearance of the bowel wall are the major advantages of the technique. Air minimizes visualization of the

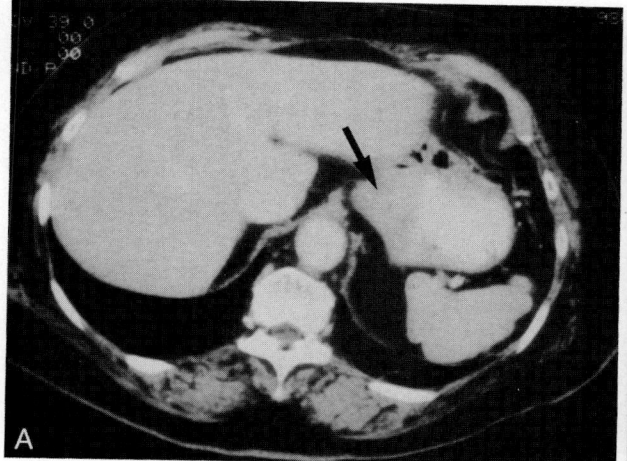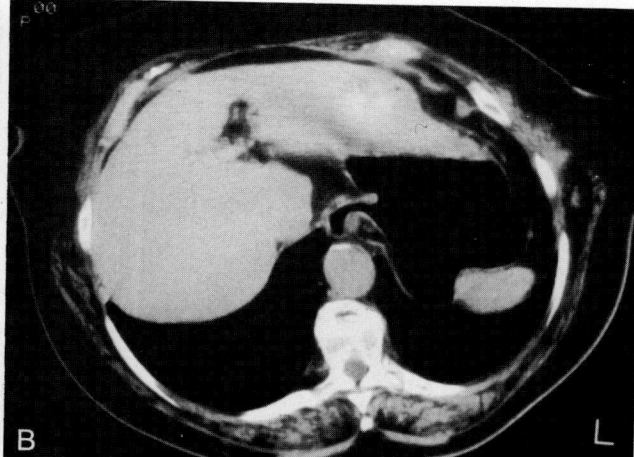

**Figure 8–4. Air-contrast CT scan: evaluation of gastric fundus. A.** Image with the patient supine suggests pathologic thickening at the esophagogastric junction *(arrow)*. **B.** After administration of an oral effervescent agent, repeated scanning with the patient in the prone position shows that the region is normal.

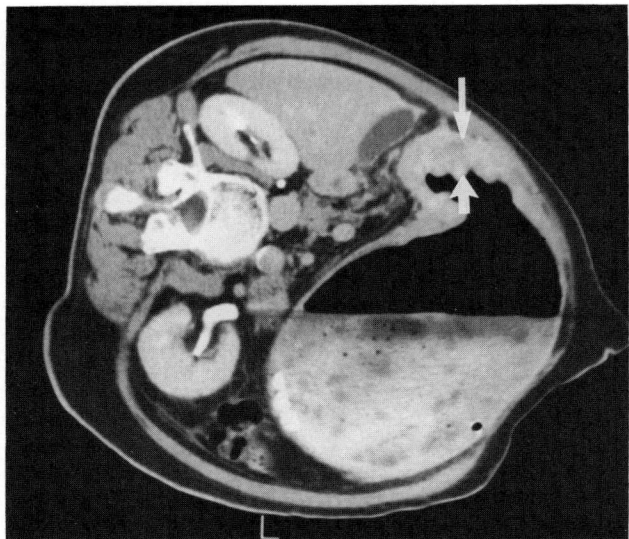

**Figure 8–5. Air-contrast CT scan showing the importance of positioning.** CT scan of a patient with gastric outlet obstruction performed with the patient in the left decubitus position promotes distention of the distal stomach, improving visualization of stenotic antral carcinoma *(arrows)*.

normal bowel wall, increasing the conspicuity of smaller lesions. Air is also easier to administer and is somewhat less risky for both the patient and the equipment (Fig. 8–7). Water as a contrast agent has several disadvantages: it can be degraded by the presence of residual opacification of the jejunum and ileum; barium or a water-soluble agent is necessary. As some of this material may admix with the water, the benefits of the negative contrast may be lessened. In either case, using negative contrast permits more thorough analysis of the intestinal wall, ultimately improving diagnostic ability.

## Indications for Negative Contrast

Negative contrast techniques are used to facilitate visualization of luminal diseases of the alimentary tube. They permit absolute identification of bowel loops and can serve as a method of bowel loop marking. In my practice, any patient referred for suspected colonic neoplasm or colonic inflammatory disease (who can clinically tolerate a contrast enema) is examined with air insufflation. All patients with suspected pelvic masses and all female patients with known pelvic neoplasms are similarly studied. Finally, all female patients with a history of treated gynecologic malignancy are scanned after colonic air insufflation.

Contraindications to prerectal colonic distention with any agent (air, water, barium, or water-soluble media) include any acute inflammatory condition of the colon, particularly when there are systemic signs of sepsis such as fever and leukocytosis. I do not like to perform nonfluoroscopic insufflation in patients with history of pelvic irradiation and symptomatic radiation proctitis.

## Schedule of Contrast Agent Administration

Uniform bowel opacification is achieved by drinking sufficient quantities of contrast agent to fill all of the loops and allowing enough time for the entire lumen to be filled. This is most reliably accomplished by having the patient drink at a steady, even rate during the period when contrast agent is administered. At my institution, the patient is asked to drink a 7-oz cup of contrast agent every 10 minutes over a 45- to 60-minute period before the scan begins. A total of 4 cups with a total volume of 800 to 900 mL is consumed. I routinely give 10 mg of oral metoclopramide with the first cup of contrast

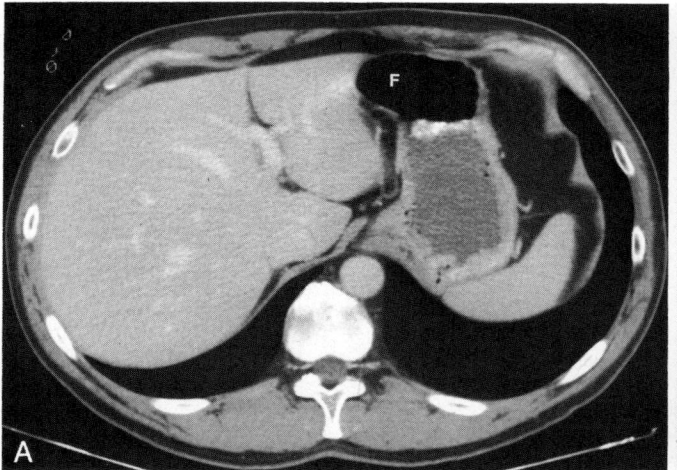
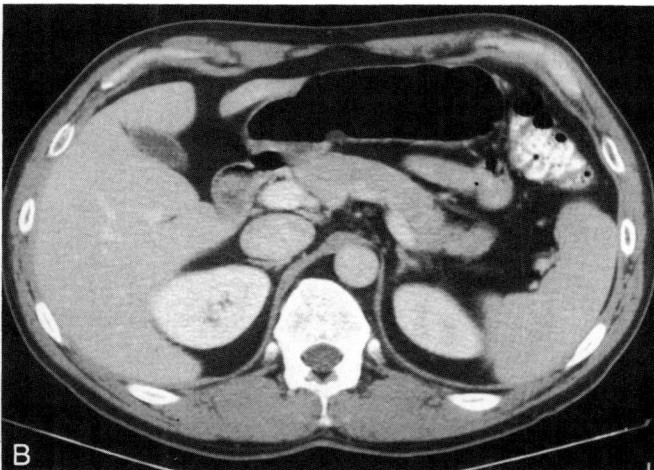

**Figure 8–6. Combined air-water contrast technique for gastric evaluation. A.** The fundus (F) has been distended with air. Note the layered appearance of the gastric wall. **B.** In the same patient, the distal stomach and antrum are distended with gas generated from an orally administered effervescent agent. The gastric wall appears considerably thinner. The disparate thicknesses are a function of windowing.

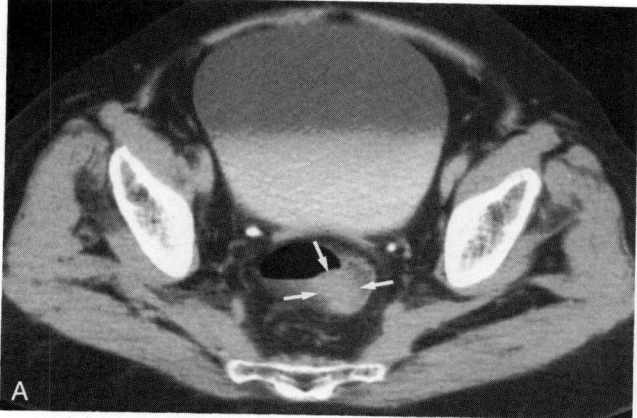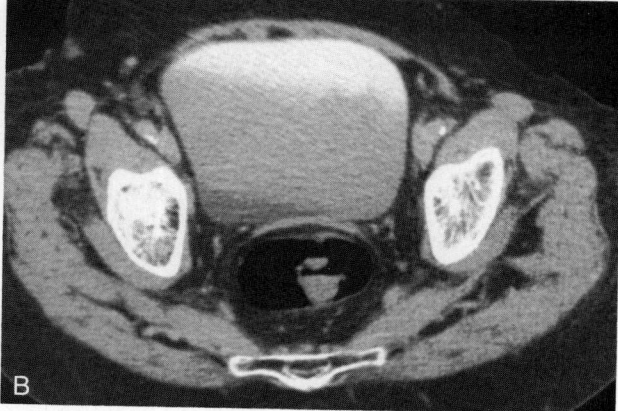

**Figure 8–7. Air versus water: rectal carcinoma. A.** Scan of a supine patient with a water-filled rectum shows a polypoid filling defect representing a known carcinoma *(arrows).* **B.** The lesion is more conspicuous when the patient is scanned in the prone position after air insufflation.

agent, which significantly improves distal ileal opacification. Metoclopramide is contraindicated in patients with mechanical intestinal obstruction and in patients with pheochromocytoma.[5]

It is often difficult to maintain good contrast in the proximal small intestine. This is related to physiologic secretion of fluid into the duodenum and relative increased transit through this area. Slow, steady oral intake minimizes these problems. I rely on orally administered positive contrast material to visualize the bowel from the duodenum to the ileocecal valve; negative contrast agents are too unreliable in these areas. I evaluate the stomach and colon with air. If one chooses to use positive contrast distention of the stomach, the patient should drink a fifth cup of contrast agent immediately before lying on the scanner. This fills and distends the stomach and proximal small intestine. Scan quality is improved with routine use of 0.1 mg of intravenous glucagon to diminish peristalsis artifact, even on scanners with scanning times less than 2 seconds. Glucagon is administered into the intravenous line just before iodinated contrast agent is given. If the colon is to be insufflated, 0.5 mg is administered.

When patients are referred from intensive care units, I ask the house staff or aides to administer the contrast material slowly via a nasogastric tube during a 1-hour period. These patients frequently have prolonged intestinal transit times, and an even more protracted period of bowel filling may be required. Contrast solutions are mixed in the department and brought to the patient's bedside for administration. With this protocol, the transported patient can be immediately placed on the scanner. The radiologist must permit sufficient "gut opacification" time before the scan is initiated. All too often, a rushed scan results in a delay and a rescan or, even worse, an erroneous diagnosis.

Negative contrast techniques for the stomach require little modification of standard protocols. Instead of giving a final cup of positive contrast medium, one can substitute a full cup of water or a mixture of water with

effervescent agent. This provides excellent gas $(CO_2)$ distention of the stomach. Diagnostic results obtained with colonic air insufflation are maximized by prior colonic cleansing.[6] I use an oral cathartic preparation (Fleet Kit 1, Fleet Co., Lynchburg, VA). If the patient is not prepared, a 2000-mL tap water enema can be given in the department; 20 mg of liquid bisacodyl added to the enema maximizes colonic contraction. The patient may be scanned immediately after the evacuation.

## COMPUTED TOMOGRAPHIC TECHNICAL PARAMETERS

Proper CT technique is necessary to optimize the information available for diagnosis. The radiologist has control of several aspects of the CT study, including intravenous contrast medium infusion rates, radiographic parameters of kV(p) and mAs, and collimation. Current scanners are capable of acquiring images in 2 seconds or less. Furthermore, most scans are performed with dynamic incremental protocols. Usually, images are acquired with 8- to 10-mm collimation and minimal slice gaps. Thinner collimation (4 to 5 mm) improves image "crispness" by minimizing z axis–related volume averaging effects. The penalty for using thinner slices is that an increase in dose (either milliamperes or exposure time) is necessary to offset the decreased photon flux resulting from a 50% reduction in collimator width. Although the patient's exposure is only slightly increased (effect of collimation), there is a significant increase in tube heating. Tube cooling may limit the number of scans. Therefore, I obtain thin, closely spaced scans only over the region of interest—right lower quadrant for suspected appendicitis, pelvis for acute diverticulitis, and so forth. "Coning down" only in the area of suspected pathology allows the entire abdomen and pelvis to be studied within the tube-heating capabilities of most modern third- and fourth-generation machines.

Intravenous contrast protocols and their rationale are

described in Chapters 80 and 101. Most sophisticated intravenous injection protocols are directed at optimizing the detection of liver lesions. Scanning during infusion of the contrast agent also enables subtle alterations in bowel wall enhancement to be appreciated, enhancing the conspicuity of lesions. I advise all patients being investigated for gastrointestinal pathology to undergo contrast-enhanced CT if there are no medical or allergic contraindications.

## PRINCIPLES OF INTERPRETATION

On CT, most gastrointestinal pathologic conditions are manifested as a region of thickening of the intestinal wall.[7, 8] When mural thickening is discovered, follow-up barium studies or endoscopy or both often provide a definitive diagnosis. Combining CT scanning and barium radiography can improve diagnostic confidence and help appreciate disease extent.[8] As experience with CT accumulates, it is becoming increasingly apparent that many primary alimentary tract disorders are associated with a constellation of findings that allows a precise diagnosis to be made, resulting in a diminishing role for follow-up examinations.[9] In the next section, the diagnostic parameters that are useful in narrowing the differential diagnosis of the thickened intestinal wall are discussed.

### Bowel Wall

Mural thickening on a CT scan is the hallmark of alimentary tract disease. The wall may be thickened in neoplastic diseases, in non-neoplastic disorders, or as a result of poor distention of the viscus. The last cause must be ruled out before considering a pathologic process. Accordingly, the radiologist must first examine the images to ensure that there is adequate bowel opacification, judge the extent and degree of filling of neighboring loops, and ensure that intravenous contrast agent has been appropriately administered. The patient's position must also be considered when assessing mural thickening. Several targeted scans after giving additional contrast material and repositioning the patient to distend the questionable region maximally often resolve the problem.

When a segment of bowel is determined to be truly thickened, several other diagnostic parameters must be evaluated: the contour of the contrast agent–filled lumen, preservation or obliteration of the normal fold pattern, presence and nature of contrast enhancement, perienteric changes, and associated local and distant findings.[10]

The most prevalent diseases of the alimentary canal often originate in the intestinal mucosa and variably involve the bowel wall and perienteric regions. The diseases with the greatest perienteric component are more efficaciously imaged with CT.[11]

### Fold Pattern

CT is inferior to barium studies in evaluating subtle changes in the intestinal folds or nodularity. Nevertheless, abnormalities (Fig. 8–8) of the intestinal folds suggested by CT should not be ignored, remembering that lack of visualization of abnormal folds does not exclude their presence.

### Wall Thickness

The normal intestinal wall is barely perceptible and should be no more than 3 mm thick. The normal stomach and rectum may appear somewhat thicker because these regions are invested by a third layer of oblique muscle fibers.

With proper utilization of intravenous contrast agent and dynamic scanning protocols, it is possible to display certain features of the intestinal wall that help distinguish neoplastic from non-neoplastic causes of mural thickening. A variably thick, lucent strip paralleling the intestinal lumen within the intramural portion of the bowel represents submucosal edema, and its identification almost always excludes a neoplasm. This may be seen in disorders involving the entire alimentary canal but is most frequently observed in the small intestine and colon. This phenomenon, originally described in Crohn's disease, is called the *target sign*.[12]

The differential diagnosis of the target sign includes Crohn's disease, ulcerative colitis, infections, vascular diseases, radiation, secondary effects of contiguous inflammatory processes (such as pancreatitis), and strangulated obstruction. The target sign is best observed with high levels of iodinated contrast agent, so there is a relatively short imaging window (approximately 5

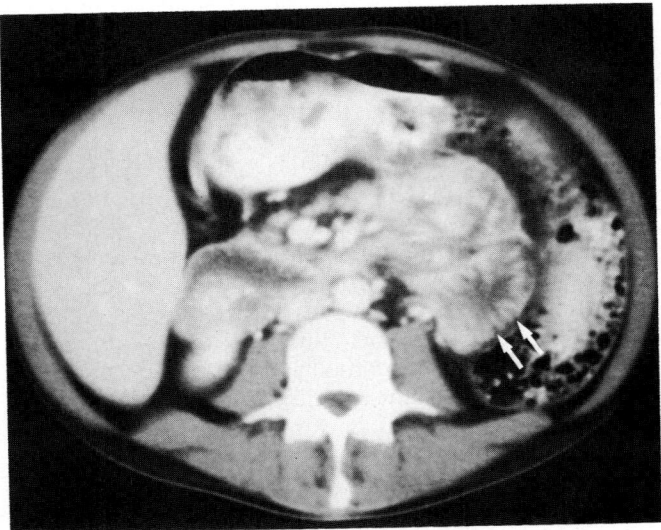

**Figure 8–8.** *Mycobacterium avium-intracellulare* **infection in a patient with acquired immunodeficiency syndrome.** Note the abnormal jejunal folds *(arrows)*.

minutes), which makes dynamic scanning essential (Fig. 8–9). The target sign may also be visible on unenhanced scans in patients with long-standing colitides in which there has been fatty metamorphosis within the intestinal wall. This finding therefore has major diagnostic implications and helps narrow the differential diagnosis for an individual patient. Not every benign disease process causes the target appearance; it is a sign that is helpful only when visualized.

Intramural hemorrhage and neoplasms typically thicken the intestinal wall but do not result in submucosal edema. With scirrhous, infiltrating neoplasms, the intestinal wall may appear brightly enhanced when studied by dynamic CT, which makes the lesion more conspicuous and allows more precise delineation of the tumor margins. Hemorrhage appears as a homogeneous, relatively high attenuation (50 to 60 Hounsfield units) region of mural thickening.

Adenocarcinomas throughout the gut result in thickening of the intestinal wall over a relatively focal region.

The thickened wall is usually of uniform soft tissue density and does not display low-attenuation regions paralleling the long axis of the bowel as seen in inflammatory disease.[12–14] When the luminal surface is visualized with negative contrast, the irregular, nodular, mass-like, or occasionally ulcerated luminal component can be seen. Associated findings, such as distant metastases and lymphadenopathy, favor a neoplastic cause for the thickened wall. Sarcomas grow exophytically from the affected bowel loop. Lymphomas tend to display homogeneous soft tissue attenuation regardless of their large size, whereas leiomyosarcomas characteristically undergo extensive cavitation and liquefaction. The point of attachment may be difficult to visualize, and cystic lesions in adjacent structures should be included in the differential diagnosis.

At times, CT alone cannot differentiate inflammatory from neoplastic diseases.[14] For example, in patients with sigmoid diverticulitis, the question of underlying neoplasm should be raised when the wall thickness is greater

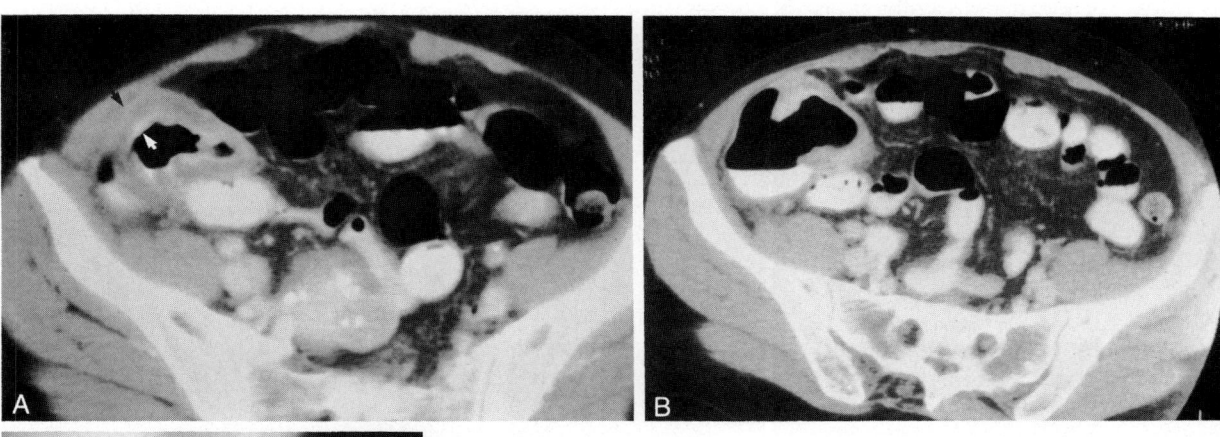

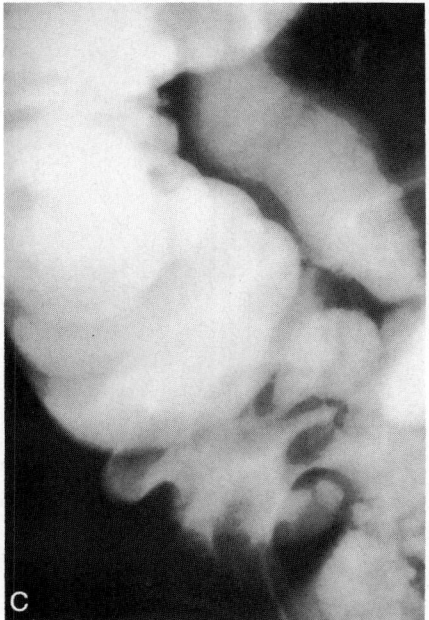

**Figure 8–9. Value of target sign. A.** Dynamic scan reveals lobulated appearance of cecum with a thickened wall *(arrows)*. The lucency within the wall, indicative of edema, is strongly suggestive of a non-neoplastic etiology. **B.** Scan performed approximately 5 minutes after that in **A**; the "target" appearance is no longer seen. Visualization requires dynamic scanning protocol. **C.** A barium enema on the following day confirms the inflammatory nature of the lesion.

than usually found with this entity (>5 mm). In these cases, barium enema or endoscopy may be necessary to differentiate these entities (see Chapter 61).

## Perienteric Changes

The ability of CT to image changes outside the intestinal lumen accounts for its unique contribution to the imaging of gastrointestinal disease. Several characteristic findings are indicative of extraluminal disease extension. The peritoneal ligaments and reflections define the course and appearance of these findings and guide the radiologist in a systemic assessment based on the location of the pathologic change.

There are several key observations to be made when attempting to interpret perienteric changes. First, the nature of the increased density must be assessed. There is a spectrum of variability that correlates with the severity of the process. Minimal disease is manifested by wispy linear strands of soft tissue density within the perienteric fat. In more severe cases, these strands may coalesce to form a cloud-like region of increased attenuation that may be termed a *phlegmon*. In the most severe cases, localized fluid collections (abscesses) are seen.[15] Fistulas and sinus tracts should be noted; they present as sharply defined, jagged, soft tissue attenuation lines within the mesentery or perienteric fat (Fig. 8–10). Recognition of fistulas is important because CT is inadequate to map their origin, course, or terminus. Barium studies are indicated in these instances.

The second observation to be made is the presence or absence of local fascial thickening (Fig. 8–11). Fascial thickening is classically found in pancreatitis (Gerota's fascia), sigmoid diverticulitis (sigmoid mesocolon), appendicitis (mesoappendix), and tuberculous peritonitis where the entire parietal peritoneal surface appears enhanced and retracted from the abdominal wall. The pathophysiology of this fascial thickening has not been elucidated; it seems to be a nonspecific response to a contiguous inflammatory process.

Neoplasms can incite or result in perienteric fat changes. Recognition of these changes is critical in attempting to accurately assess the presence and degree of transmural tumor extension. Although there is some overlap in the perienteric fat changes found in neoplastic and inflammatory diseases, in the presence of tumor the changes are qualitatively different from those in inflammation. Specifically, tumor extension into the pericolic fat is often more sharply defined and thicker than is found with inflammatory change (Fig. 8–12). Detection of these perienteric changes is helpful in localizing an abnormality and in narrowing the differential diagnosis.[16] Because of the relatively subtle nature of these changes, particularly in cases with minimal disease, I recommend using thin (≤5 mm) sections over the region of interest as determined from the patient's clinical history.

## Mesenteric Changes

These changes are distinguished from perienteric changes in that they are visualized over the entire portion of the mesentery subtending an affected bowel loop.[17] Diseases with these characteristic mesenteric abnormalities include Crohn's disease, retractile mesenteritis and lipodystrophies, carcinoid, local lymphadenopathy, peritonitis, and carcinomatosis.

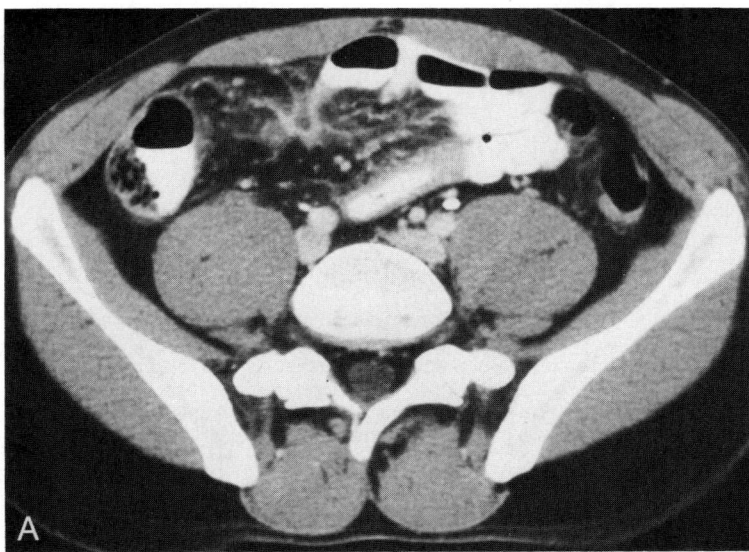
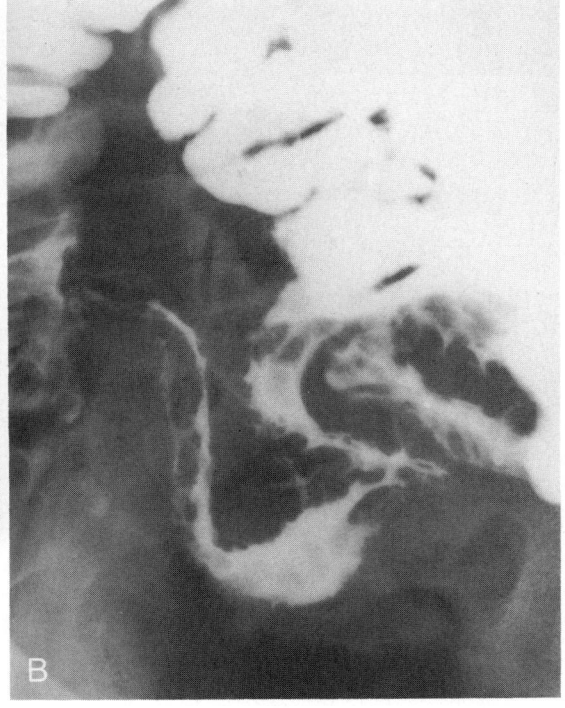

**Figure 8–10. Mesenteric fistulas: CT appearance. A.** CT scan of a patient with Crohn's disease reveals sharply defined, jagged lines in the mesenteric fat. These findings suggest fistulous disease. The patient should be investigated with barium studies to map their exact location. **B.** Barium study of same patient showing ileoileal fistulas.

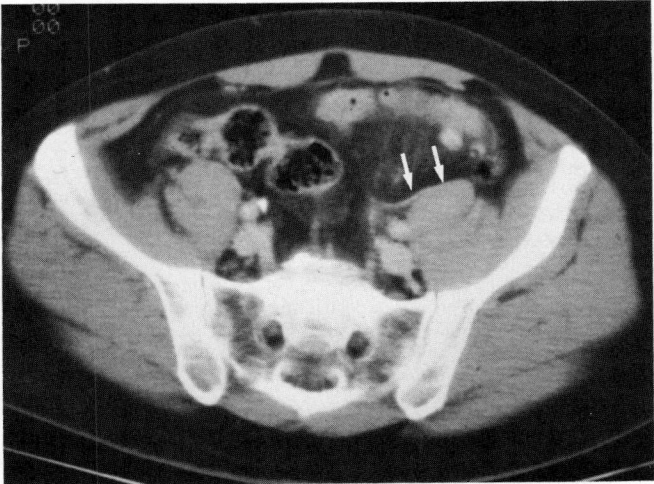

**Figure 8–11. Diverticulitis: associated mesenteric changes.** CT image reveals hazy clouding of sigmoid mesocolon and thickening of the mesocolic reflection along the left pelvic side wall *(arrows)*.

In all of these disorders there is increased density in the fat with variable-thickness, linear densities. In cases with associated adenopathy, multiple masses are present. Poor margination of mesenteric reflections progressing to frank loculated fluid collections is also seen. In patients with malignant ascites or complex infected ascites (as seen in tuberculosis), nodules can be identified along peritoneal reflections. If the neoplasm has a mucinous component, calcification may be present. A lacy, reticular, nodular, or cake-like mass may develop in the greater omentum in peritoneal carcinomatosis and in some cases of tuberculosis (see Chapters 131 to 133).

It is difficult to predict serosal involvement by peritoneal seeding, unless mural thickening in the immediate vicinity of a peritoneal nodule or fluid collection is identified.[16, 17]

Crohn's disease is unique in that these changes are

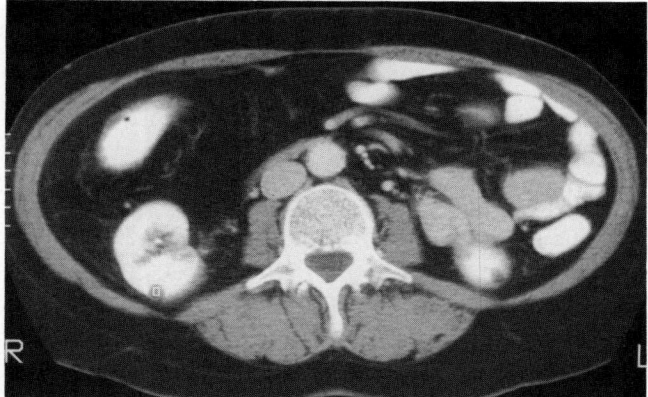

**Figure 8–13. Crohn's disease of colon with mesenteric fat hypertrophy.**

accompanied by hypertrophy of fat and associated regional inflammatory changes resulting in the separation of bowel loops so frequently observed on barium radiography (Fig. 8–13). Lipodystrophies also result in fat hypertrophy, but inflammatory stranding is not observed in these cases. Carcinoids induce an intense desmoplastic reaction, creating a retractile appearance.

Adenopathy is a nonspecific finding in that it can be seen in both benign and malignant disorders. Its presence, however, aids in differential diagnosis of right lower quadrant disease. Appendicitis almost never results in enlarged nodes, whereas Crohn's disease, tuberculosis, and other infections (e.g., *Salmonella*) are often associated with adenopathy. These nodes may overlap with the appearance of lymphoma, but generally they do not reach the large size of lymphomatous adenopathy. In carcinoid tumors, local adenopathy may calcify, and the diagnosis is suggested when these nodes are seen within the typical desmoplastic mesenteric reactions incited by the tumor.

# References

1. Megibow AJ, Balthazar EJ: Computed Tomography of the Gastrointestinal Tract. St. Louis: CV Mosby, 1986.
2. Megibow AJ, Zerhouni EA, Hulnick DH, et al: Air opacification of the colon as adjunct in CT evaluation of the pelvis. J Comput Assist Tomogr 8:797–800, 1983.
3. Baert AL, Roex L, Marchal G, et al: Computed tomography of the stomach with water as an oral contrast agent: technique and preliminary results. J Comput Assist Tomogr 13:633–636, 1989.
3a. Gossios KJ, Tsianos EV, Kontogiannis DS, et al: Water as contrast medium for computed tomography study of colonic wall lesions. Gastrointest Radiol 17:125–128, 1992.
4. Raptopoulis V, Davis MA, Davidoff A, et al: Fat density oral contrast agent for abdominal CT. Radiology 164:653–658, 1987.
5. Thoeni RF, Filson RG: Abdominal and pelvic CT: use of oral metoclopramide to enhance bowel opacification. Radiology 169:391–396, 1988.
6. Balthazar EJ, Megibow AJ, Hulnick DH, et al: Carcinoma of the colon: detection and preoperative staging by CT. AJR 150:301–306, 1988.
7. Desai RK, Tagliabue JR, Wegryn SA, et al: CT evaluation of wall thickening in the alimentary tract. Radiographics 11:771–783, 1991.

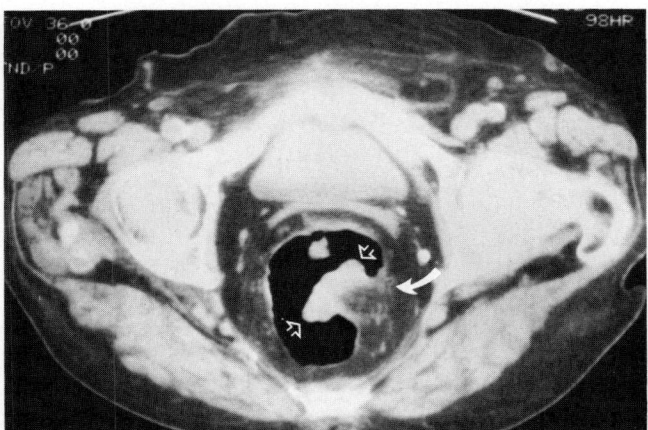

**Figure 8–12. Rectal carcinoma: local changes in perirectal fat.** Scanning with the patient in the prone position allows maximal distention of the rectum and optimal visualization of the rectal lesion *(open arrows)*. There are sharply defined soft tissue extensions of the tumor into the perirectal fat *(solid arrow)* indicative of local invasion.

8. Johnson CD: Invited commentary. Radiographics 11:784, 1991.
9. Coscina WF, Arger PH, Levine MS, et al: Gastrointestinal tract focal mass lesions: role of CT and barium evaluations. Radiology 158:581–587, 1986.
10. James S, Balfe DM, Lee JK, et al: Small-bowel disease: categorization by CT examination. AJR 148:863–886, 1987.
11. Balthazar EJ: CT of the gastrointestinal tract: principles and interpretation. AJR 156:23–32, 1991.
12. Karantanas AH, Tsianos EB, Kontogiannis DS, et al: CT demonstration of normal gastric wall thickness: the value of administering gas-producing and paralytic agents. Comput Med Imaging Graph 12:333–337, 1988.
12a. Hori S, Tsuda K, Muryama S, et al: CT of gastric carcinoma: preliminary results with a new scanning technique. Radiographics 12:257–268, 1992.
13. Megibow AJ: Imaging insights in gastrointestinal radiology. The target sign. RSNA Today 4:1, 1990.
14. Miyake H, Maeda H, Kurauchi S, et al: Thickened gastric walls showing diffuse low attenuation on CT. J Comput Assist Tomogr 13:253–255, 1989.
15. Balthazar EJ, Megibow AJ, Schinella RA, et al: Limitations in the CT diagnosis of acute diverticulitis: comparison of CT, contrast enema, and pathologic findings in 16 patients. AJR 154:281–287, 1990.
16. Megibow AJ: Imaging insights in gastrointestinal radiology. Perienteric changes—signs and significance in abdominal CT. RSNA Today 4:5, 1990.
17. Solomon A, Papo J, Pikielny S, et al: Computed tomographic investigation of serosal and intramural gastrointestinal pathology. Gastrointest Radiol 12:13–17, 1987.

# Magnetic Resonance of the Hollow Viscera

**Mitchell D. Schnall, M.D.**

INTRODUCTION

TECHNIQUE
Coils
Pulse Sequences
Preparation of the Patient and
Luminal Contrast

HIGH-RESOLUTION STUDIES OF
BOWEL WALL SPECIMENS

ESOPHAGUS

STOMACH AND DUODENUM

SMALL INTESTINE

COLORECTUM

## INTRODUCTION

Magnetic resonance (MR) imaging is potentially the most powerful cross-sectional imaging tool in the arsenal of the radiologist. This position is derived from its versatility in terms of imaging resolution, plane of section, and soft tissue contrast. These advantages have led to the application of MR as the primary imaging technique in the central nervous system and spine; however, its applications to the abdomen have proceeded more slowly. This is due to problems with motion artifacts and limited spatial resolution. Reports on the use of MR in the study of the hollow viscera are primarily limited to staging esophageal and rectal cancer and to case reports of other pathologic conditions. Advances in coil design that improve resolution and in software that reduce imaging time have provided more favorable abdominal MR results. Indeed, with proper technique, MR can be a useful means of studying a number of disorders of the hollow viscera of the gastrointestinal tract. This chapter presents an approach to evaluation of the gastrointestinal tract with MR. Basic MR physics is not discussed, however; the reader is referred to one of several sources for material related to MR physics and Chapter 82.[1-3]

## TECHNIQUE

### Coils

As in all applications of MR, the technique employed is dependent on the type of information that is sought. The anatomic region studied determines the coil system used. If the area to be studied is small, then a surface coil system can be used to enhance the signal/noise ratio (SNR) of the examination.[4] The increased SNR can be used to provide improved resolution, particularly in dealing with traditionally SNR-starved fast imaging techniques. It is possible to switch coils during an examination to study one area with particularly high resolution while the remainder of the abdomen is surveyed. For example, the local extent of a rectal carcinoma is best evaluated with use of a surface coil, whereas the remainder of the staging evaluation of the same patient (lymph nodes and liver) is best performed with a larger body coil.

The multicoil array represents a significant technical advance that has important implications for abdominal imaging.[5] This technology provides a means for using more than one surface coil at the same time. The commercially available versions of this system can use up to four coils simultaneously (General Electric, Milwaukee, WI). This allows creative coil design. In particular, arrays of coils that surround the entire pelvis or abdomen (Fig. 9–1) have been created.[6] These coils are particularly valuable for studying the abdominal and

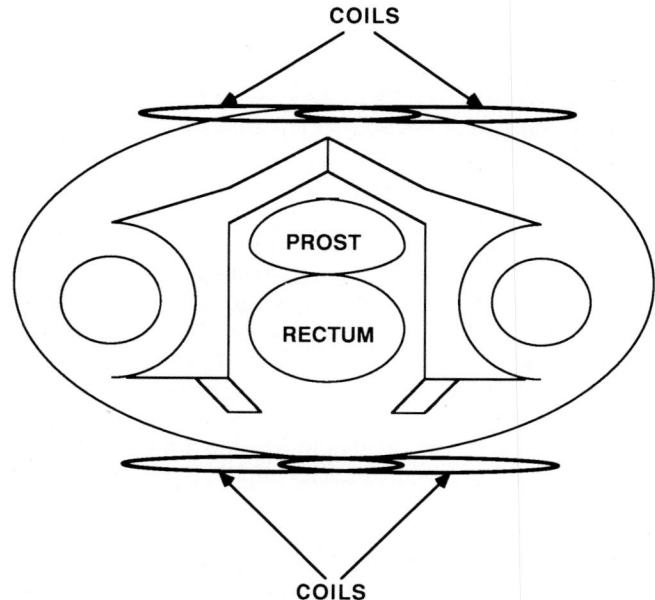

**Figure 9–1. Diagram depicting a volume multicoil for pelvic imaging.** The pelvis is surrounded by four coils, each of which is connected to a separate receiver.

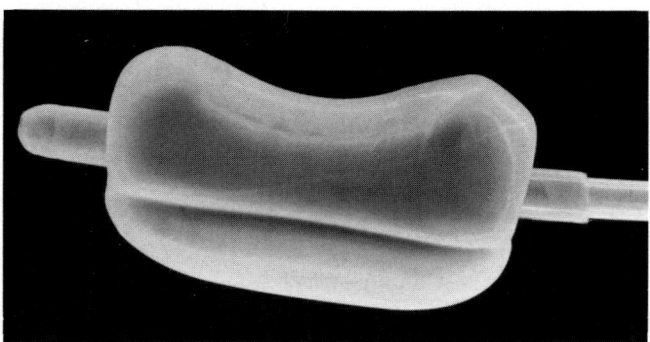

**Figure 9–2. Endorectal surface coil for high-resolution rectal and prostatic imaging.**

pelvic viscera. In the abdomen, the requirement for fast breath hold imaging necessitates the use of imaging techniques that have an intrinsically low SNR and thus benefit from the surface coils. In the pelvis, the use of a coil array provides a means for imaging the entire pelvis with high resolution.

For improving resolution yet further, endorectal coils have been applied to the pelvis.[7–9] These coils consist of a surface coil mounted on the inner surface of a balloon (Fig. 9–2). The balloon is in turn placed onto a flexible shaft. A commercial version of an endorectal coil is available for imaging the prostate (Med Rad, Pittsburgh, PA). Other balloon shapes for cervical and rectal imaging are under investigation. The use of the endorectal coils is exciting because it provides the capability of imaging with 300-μm resolution while the high contrast of MR is maintained. The combination of external coils with endorectal coils as part of an external-endorectal coil array adds improved spatial coverage to the ultra-high resolution available with the endorectal surface coils.[10] Endoluminal coils designed for imaging other parts of the gut are likely to be designed in the future.

## Pulse Sequences

Traditional spin-echo pulse sequences have been the mainstay of MR imaging. However, in imaging of the viscera, liberal use of faster sequences is important for obtaining a top-quality examination. Both fast gradient-echo and spin-echo techniques are valuable in this regard. Gradient-echo pulse sequences can be used to provide images with T1 contrast. In general, the spoiled gradient-echo techniques are preferred to those obtained without spoiling because improved soft tissue contrast results from spoiling the residual transverse magnetization after each excitation pulse. In the absence of spoiling, the steady-state magnetization that builds up during a short repetition time (less than 50 ms) sequence alters the expected T1-weighted contrast by increasing the amplitude of signal from species with a long T2 (which usually have a long T1). This tends to oppose the T1 contrast of partial saturation and thus results in a low-contrast image. Thus, spoiled gradient echos are important for providing traditional T1 contrast.[11]

These images can be obtained during a single breath hold, which makes them free of motion artifacts. Fat saturation is often useful for providing maximal soft tissue contrast, particularly when gadolinium is administered. Manufacturers of MR equipment now provide several different types of fast spoiled gradient-echo imaging sequences. The traditional spoiled gradient-echo sequence can be used to provide one image in each breath hold. Faster sequences that support repetition times of 8 to 10 ms and echo times of 2 to 3 ms have been developed. These sequences can provide three or four images in a single breath hold; however, the SNR and thus potential resolution are diminished. The speed of image acquisition of these single slice, ultrafast gradient-echo imaging sequences allows imaging after the preparation of the spin system with contrast by inversion recovery or spin-echo techniques. These add significant amounts of contrast to ultrafast gradient-echo images.

A slice interleaved gradient-echo sequence can be used to take advantage of the ultrashort echo times (2 to 3 ms) of the newer fast gradient-echo sequences with a longer repetition time (30 to 50 ms) in a slice inter-leaved fashion. This provides images with the SNR of the traditional spoiled gradient-echo images and allows three or four images to be obtained during each breath hold. The choice of technique depends on software availability and particular examination requirements.[12, 13]

Fast versions of spin-echo pulse sequences can provide T2-weighted images. These techniques are based on a multiecho spin-echo sequence. They differ from the traditional sequences in that each echo is obtained with a different amount of phase encoding, thus representing a different view of the image. If 16 views are obtained in a single echo train, then only 1/16 of the repetition time period is needed to obtain a fast spin-echo image, compared with the traditional technique.[14, 15] The decreased time of the examination reduces artifacts from motion of the patient.[16] In some cases, it is possible to obtain T2-weighted spin-echo images in a single breath hold. Another advantage of the fast spin-echo technique in imaging the hollow viscera is that the reduced examination time allows the use of an extremely long repetition time. This eliminates the residual T1 effects on traditional T2-weighted images, which improves image contrast. This is particularly helpful in the pelvis, in imaging the fluid-filled bowel, because the high signal intensity fluid becomes distinct.[17]

## Preparation of the Patient and Luminal Contrast

No specific bowel preparation is required to perform MR imaging of the viscera. For studying the upper gastrointestinal tract, it is helpful to have the patient fast for at least 8 hours before the examination. In all cases of gastrointestinal imaging, glucagon is essential for reducing artifacts from bowel peristalsis. The long duration of MR examinations dictates that the glucagon be administered subcutaneously or intramuscularly. In selected circumstances, an intravenous injection of glucagon before a particularly important imaging sequence may be helpful.

Many different intraluminal contrast agents for MR have been described, but none is clearly superior for all portions of the gut. There are two major classes of contrast agents: those that create positive contrast, and those that create negative contrast. In comparing various contrast agents, a major point of concern centers on the amplitude of motion artifacts that emanate from moving bowel filled with contrast material. The amplitude of these artifacts is dependent on the amount of motion and the contrast between the bowel lumen and the periluminal tissue. Although positive contrast agents are associated with larger artifact because of a larger signal gradient between luminal contents and periluminal tissues, negative contrast agents can suffer from the same effects. The best contrast agent results in a reproducible intraluminal signal that is only moderately different from the periluminal tissue.

The major negative contrast agents include suspensions of ferromagnetic particles, suspensions of barium sulfate, suspensions of clay compound such as attapulgite (found in the new formulation of Kaopectate), perfluorocytlbromide, and gas. Gas has the advantage of being inexpensive. It is most often used in the rectum and upper gastrointestinal tract. Air can be easily delivered to the rectum via a small catheter. Commercially available granules that create carbon dioxide provide gaseous distention of the upper gastrointestinal tract.[18] However, gas cannot be used to obtain acceptable contrast throughout the gastrointestinal tract.

Ferromagnetic particle suspensions provide excellent contrast in the stomach and small intestine but become diluted and provide only marginal contrast in the colon.[19] The ferromagnetic agents and gas share the common problem of creating a large susceptibility interface at the bowel wall. Although not a significant problem with spin-echo images, this can result in artifact in the bowel wall and periluminal tissue on fast gradient-echo sequences. It may also present a problem in trying to perform chemical shift–selective saturation.

Barium sulfate has been employed for endoluminal contrast by several groups.[20] It provides a negative contrast but is not associated with a large susceptibility interface at the lumen-wall interface. Although it provides adequate contrast on T1-weighted images, when diluted in the bowel, it does not provide good negative contrast on T2-weighted images. In fact, it often results in positive contrast on T2-weighted images. Suspensions of clay such as attapulgite have been shown to provide better negative contrast in T2-weighted images than does barium.[21] Barium has the advantages of availability and low cost.

Perfluorocytlbromide has many properties that make it a potentially useful endoluminal contrast agent. First, it contains no protons and thus has no signal on all MR pulse sequences. Second, it is immiscible with water, so it does not dilute in the bowel. Although this agent is experimental, it may prove to be an important endoluminal contrast agent.[22]

Several types of positive contrast agent have been described. Most contain paramagnetic species that provide contrast by shortening the T1 of the water in the bowel. The paramagnetic agents include preparations of ferric ammonium citrate (e.g., Geritol) and gadolinium mixed with mannitol, which permits dispersion through the entire bowel.[23–25] The major problem with these agents is the fact that endoluminal signal intensity depends on the concentration of these water-soluble species in bowel. The variability of their signal intensities makes it difficult to reliably label the entire gastrointestinal tract. These agents also promote peristalsis, which can create significant motion artifacts if they are not administered with glucagon.

It is clear that no ideal endoluminal MR contrast agent exists at this time. I use agents that are found routinely in most radiology departments, such as barium or gas, to provide contrast for the stomach and duodenum (from above) or the rectum and sigmoid colon (from below). Opacification of the small bowel has been less reliable.

## HIGH-RESOLUTION STUDIES OF BOWEL WALL SPECIMENS

For understanding the MR appearance of bowel wall, MR pathologic-correlative studies of resected specimens have been performed.[26] T1-weighted images demonstrate little contrast between the various layers; the bowel wall is homogeneously low to intermediate in signal intensity, contrasted with the high signal intensity of serosal fat and variable signal intensity of the luminal contents (Fig. 9–3A). Close inspection may reveal a layer of higher signal intensity on the surface of the bowel wall, correlating with the mucosa. This distinction is rarely identified on in vivo imaging and is most pronounced on fixed specimen images. T2-weighted images demonstrate the intramural anatomy of the bowel wall well (Fig. 9–3B). Six layers of signal intensity can be demonstrated on the resected specimen images. The high signal intensity on the luminal side of the specimen represents mucus and fluid. The thin, undulating, low signal intensity layer represents the combination of the mucosa and muscularis mucosae. The next higher signal intensity layer represents the submucosa. The thick low signal intensity layer represents the muscularis propria. Occasionally, a plane is demonstrated between the two layers of the muscularis propria. A thin layer of high signal intensity is just outside the muscularis propria that represents a subserosal layer. The serosal fat is lower in signal intensity.

For demonstration of this mural stratification, images with 0.5-mm resolution are required. Thus, with body coil technique, the normal bowel appears homogeneous on T2-weighted images with a low-intermediate signal intensity. The layers can be demonstrated in vivo under two conditions: with pathologic enlargement of the layers and with use of higher-resolution images. External surface coils can occasionally demonstrate the layers of

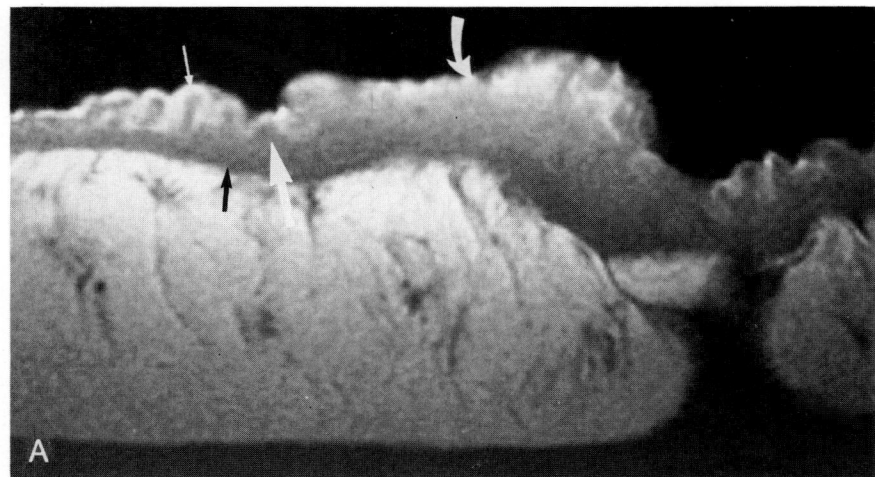

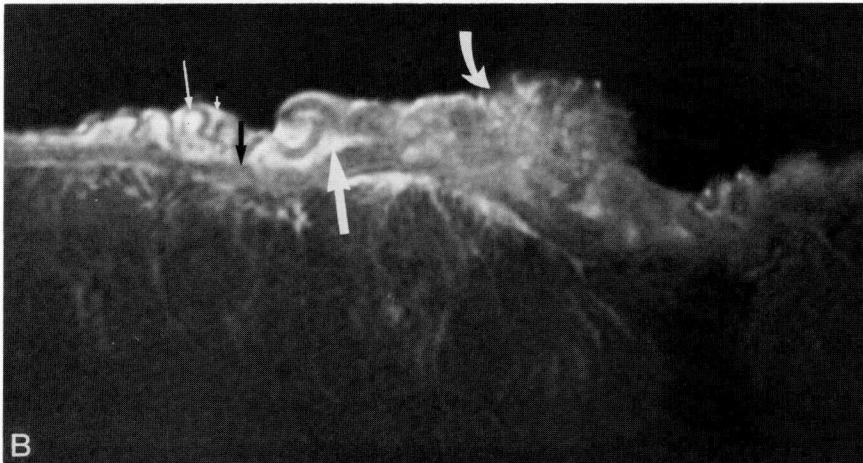

**Figure 9–3. Colon carcinoma.** T1-weighted **(A)** and T2-weighted **(B)** images of a fixed surgical colectomy specimen. Small white arrow = mucus; middle white arrow = mucosa; large white arrow = submucosa; black arrow = muscularis propria; curved arrow = colon carcinoma.

the gut wall. These layers are routinely demonstrated by the use of intraluminal (rectal) coils.[9]

## ESOPHAGUS

Esophageal MR imaging is compromised by respiratory and cardiac motion. The esophagus is most often imaged in the body coil because the respiratory artifacts produced by a surface coil positioned on the rib cage can be difficult to eliminate. Respiratory artifacts can be minimized by respiratory compensation of breath hold techniques. In addition, cardiac gating and gradient moment nulling help reduce artifacts from great vessel and cardiac pulsation. Spatially selective presaturation pulses on spin-echo sequences also minimize artifacts from flowing blood.

The esophagus appears as a low signal intensity structure contrasted by high signal intensity fat on T1-weighted images. On T2-weighted images, the muscular wall of the esophagus has low signal intensity, whereas intraluminal contents have high signal intensity (Fig. 9–4). The muscular wall of the esophagus enhances moderately after the injection of intravenous gadolinium diethylenetriaminepentaacetic acid (Gd-DTPA).

Although not a primary means for imaging the esophagus, MR can serve as an alternative technique to computed tomography (CT) and represents an important supplemental imaging method. Little has been written about MR of the esophagus; however, there have been several reports on its use to stage esophageal tumors. Tumors of the esophagus appear as focal thickening of the esophageal wall on MR. Leiomyomas are isointense to the esophageal wall on T2-weighted images; carcinoma tends to have a higher signal intensity than the normal esophagus on T2-weighted images (Fig. 9–5).

Criteria developed for determining the resectability of esophageal cancer on MR are identical to those used for CT.[27–29] Their accuracy in determining resectability is similar: 87% for CT and 84% for MR.[27–29] MR demonstrates osseous involvement and compression of the spinal cord better than CT does. MR can also image vascular structures without use of contrast agents. Thus, in patients with a contraindication to the use of intravenous contrast agents, MR can help differentiate lymph nodes from vascular structures.

On MR, esophageal cysts are characterized by high signal intensity on T2-weighted images and lack of enhancement after Gd-DTPA injection.[30, 31] Mediastinal

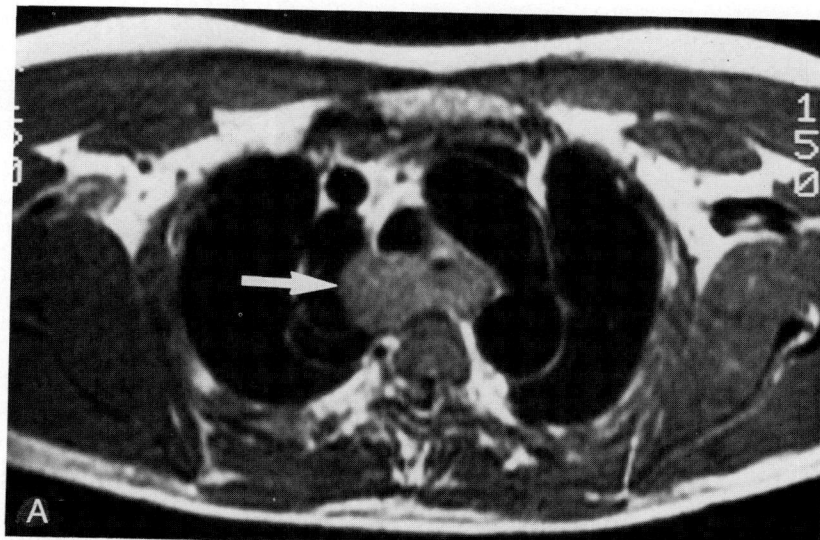

**Figure 9–4. Leiomyoma of the esophagus.** Axial T1 **(A)** and T2 **(B)** and coronal T1 **(C)** images of a patient with leiomyoma of the esophagus. On the T2-weighted image, the esophageal lumen has high signal intensity *(large black arrow)* contrasted by the low signal intensity esophageal wall *(small black arrows)*. The large right-sided esophageal mass *(large white arrow)* can be identified extending below the trachea. The coronal image **(C)** helps demonstrate the relationship of the mass *(large white arrow)* to other structures in the mediastinum.

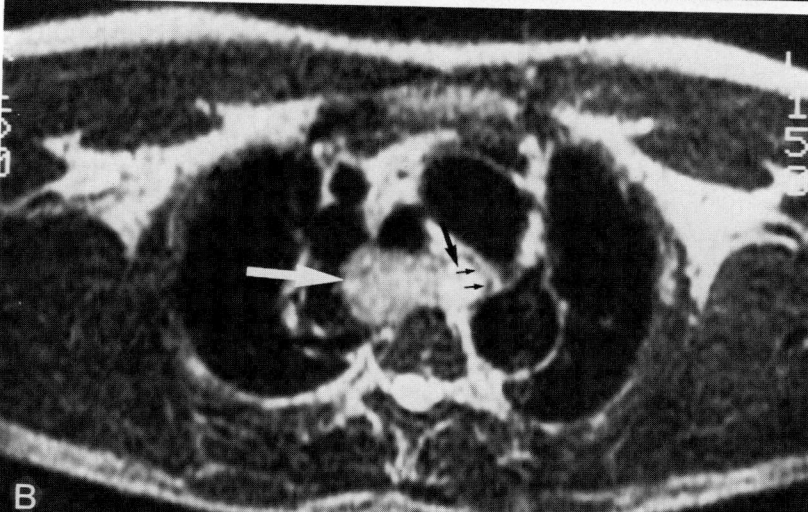

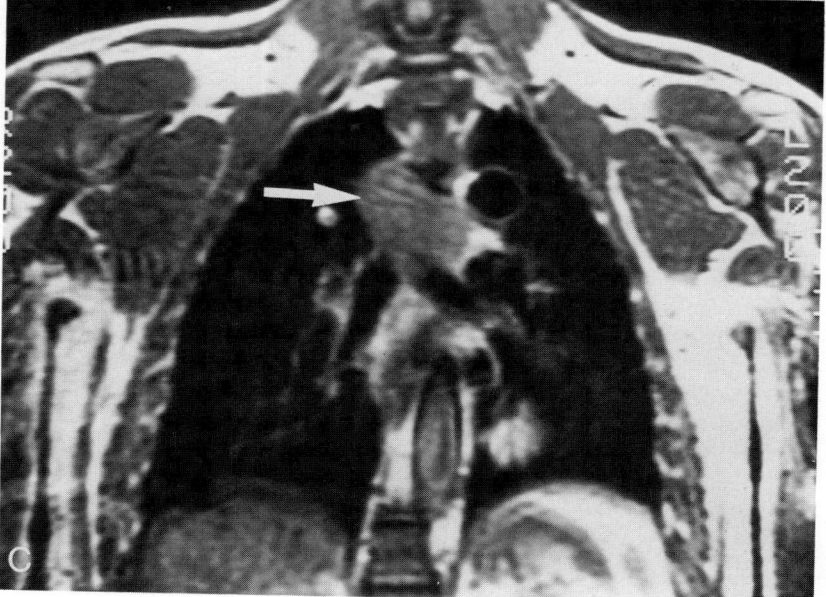

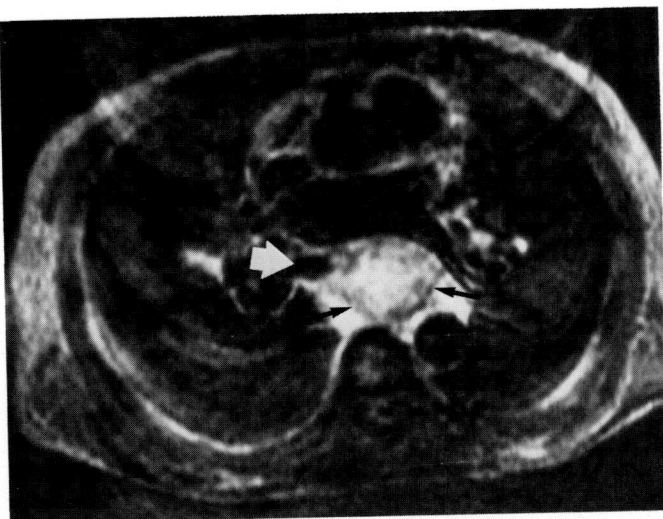

**Figure 9–5. Carcinoma of the esophagus.** Axial T2-weighted image demonstrates a medium to high signal intensity esophageal carcinoma *(black arrows)* adjacent to the bronchus intermedius *(white arrow)*.

cysts have variable signal intensity on T1-weighted images because of their varied contents. The multiplanar capability of MR is valuable for demonstrating the anatomic relationship of the lesion to other chest structures before resection.

## STOMACH AND DUODENUM

Little has been published concerning the use of MR in evaluating the stomach and duodenum. This is primarily due to technical problems associated with obtaining reliable high-quality images in the presence of respiration and peristaltic motion. These structures are best imaged after glucagon has been administered. Respiratory compensation techniques and breath hold fast imaging are essential. Breath hold T1-weighted spoiled gradient-echo images after the administration of Gd-DTPA are particularly helpful (Fig. 9–6). Barium and gas are used to opacify and distend the stomach and duodenum.

On T1-weighted images, the wall of the stomach and the duodenum have a low signal intensity. On most T2-weighted images, these structures also have a low signal intensity (Fig. 9–7). When motion artifacts are well suppressed, layers of the gastric wall can be identified on high-resolution surface coil T2-weighted images and images performed in the dynamic phase after injection of contrast agent.[32] As in the colon, the mucosa and muscularis propria are lower in signal intensity and enhance more after intravenous administration of Gd-DTPA than the submucosa does.

Gastric cancer appears as thickening of the gastric wall on T1-weighted images (Fig. 9–8). On T2-weighted images, the signal intensity of tumor is high relative to the surrounding gastric wall. No reports on the accuracy

of MR in demonstrating or staging gastric cancer have appeared in the literature.

High-resolution MR with surface coils can be helpful in imaging the complex anatomy of the duodenum. The clinical utility of MR in this region has yet to be demonstrated (Fig. 9–9).

## SMALL INTESTINE

MR of the small bowel is limited by the mobility of the bowel and by the lack of reliable intraluminal contrast agents. Although not a primary imaging method for the small bowel, MR represents a useful imaging adjunct. It is most helpful in the setting of extensive inflammatory disease or scarring that tends to immobilize the bowel. This is often the case in postoperative patients. In this setting, it may be difficult to image the intestinal wall with CT; however, the soft tissue contrast of MR allows better demonstration of small bowel anatomy (Fig. 9–10). MR can also provide valuable information concerning the architecture of thickened bowel wall. Submucosal thickening attributable to edema can be differentiated from other causes of bowel wall thickening, such as tumor invasion, on high-resolution T2-weighted images. The thickened high signal intensity submucosa surrounded by the low signal intensity muscularis propria and muscularis mucosae causes a "bull's-eye" pattern (Fig. 9–11) similar to that seen on dynamic-enhanced CT. MR evaluation of thickened small bowel is more reliable in the pelvis, where the respiratory artifacts are less pronounced.

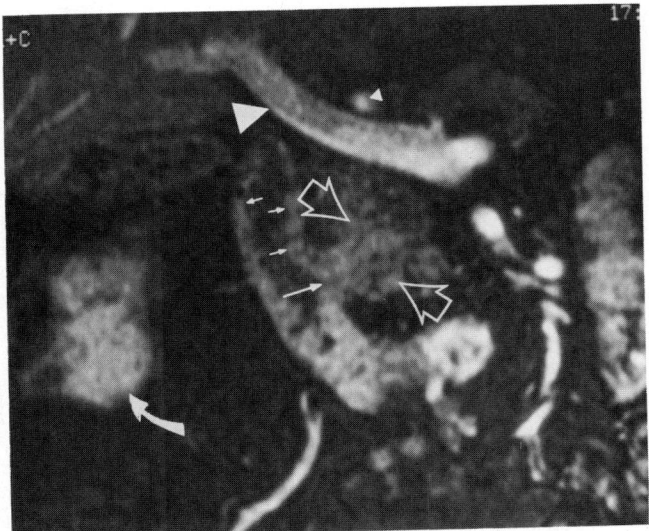

**Figure 9–6. Normal duodenal anatomy.** Breath hold T1-weighted spoiled gradient-echo image with fat saturation obtained after gadolinium injection. The wall of the second part of the duodenum *(small arrows)* and the ampulla of Vater *(large arrow)* are well seen. Large arrowhead = portal vein; small arrowhead = hepatic artery; open arrows = pancreas; curved arrow = right kidney.

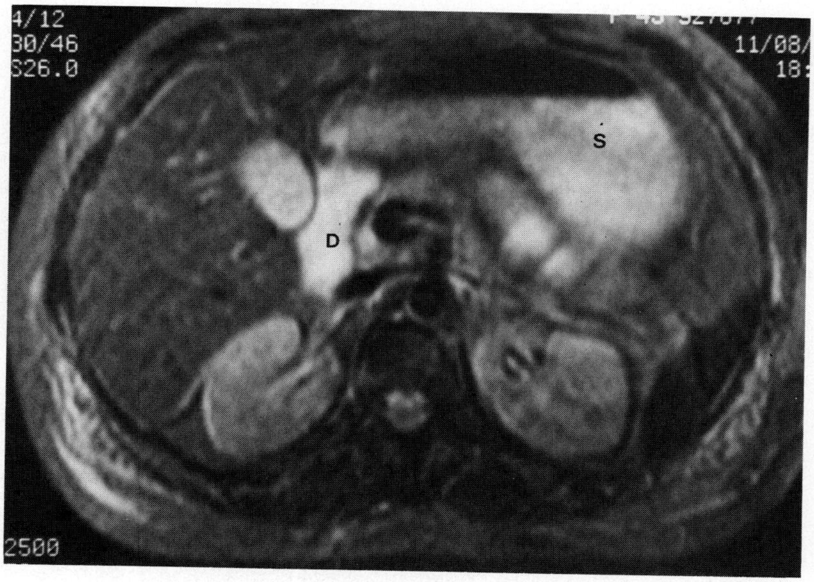

**Figure 9–7. Normal gastroduodenal anatomy.** Standard T2-weighted axial spin-echo image demonstrates the stomach (S) and proximal duodenum (D). The stomach was opacified with water for this T2-weighted image.

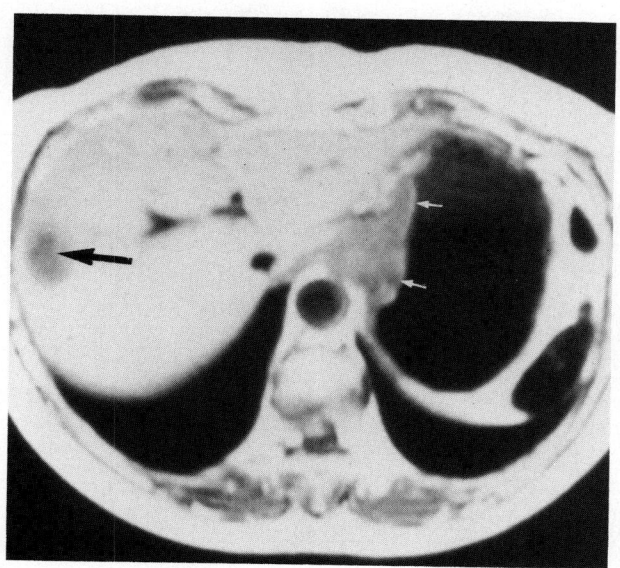

**Figure 9–8. Carcinoma of the stomach.** A T1-weighted spin-echo image demonstrates an area of low signal intensity gastric mural thickening in the region of the lesser curve *(white arrows)* that represents gastric carcinoma. Note the lesion of low signal intensity in the liver *(black arrow)* representing a hepatic metastasis.

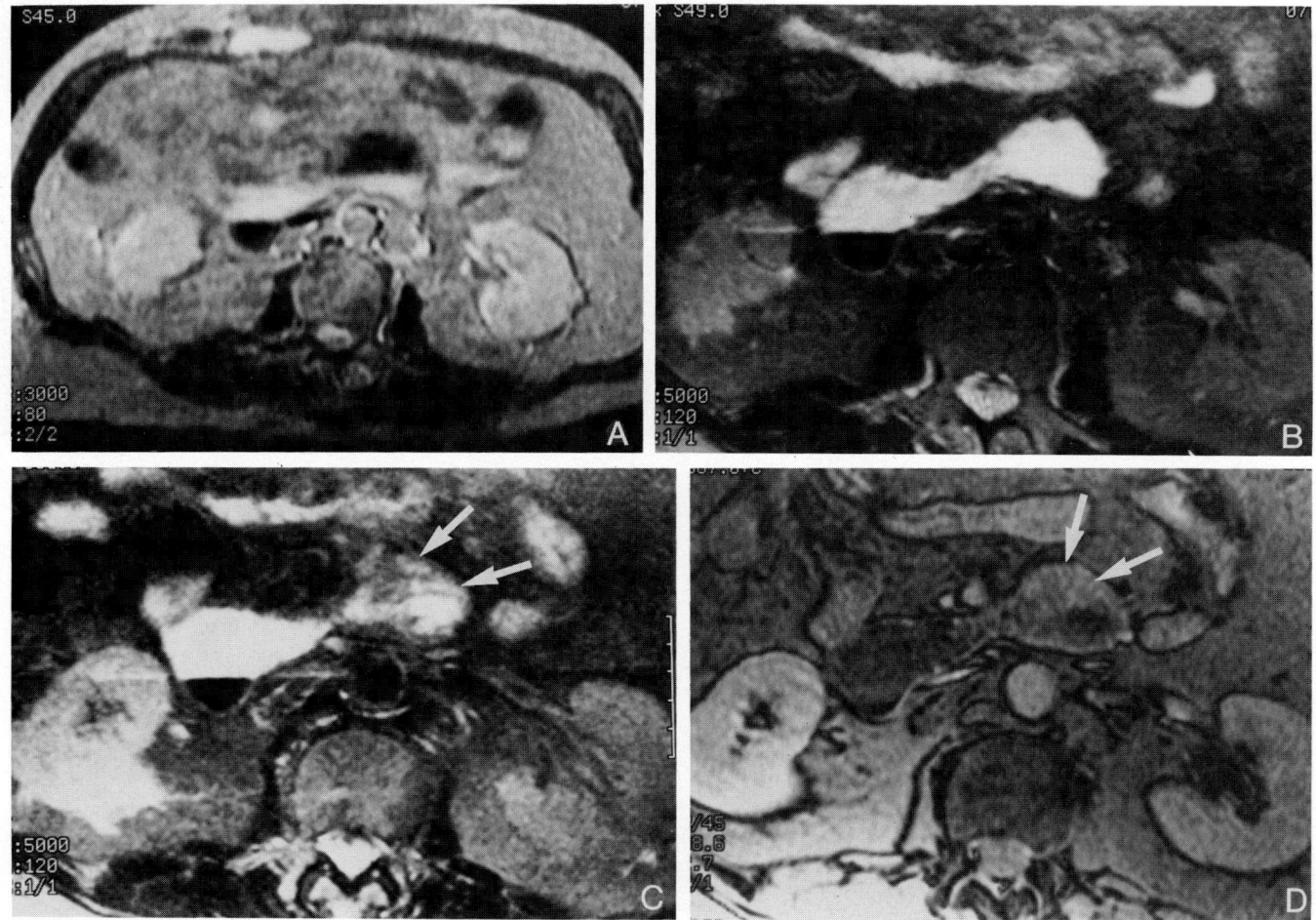

**Figure 9–9. Body coil versus external surface coil imaging.** Body coil **(A)** and external surface coil **(B)** images through a normal portion of the duodenum demonstrate the resolution advantages that may result from the use of an external surface coil. Image **B** was obtained with fat saturation; the duodenum was opacified with 70% barium initially (dependent low signal intensity layer); however, the patient refused further barium, and water was administered to further distend the duodenum. T2-weighted **(C)** and post–gadolinium breath hold spoiled gradient-echo **(D)** images at a different level demonstrate irregular thickening of the duodenal wall *(arrows)* attributable to a duodenal carcinoma.

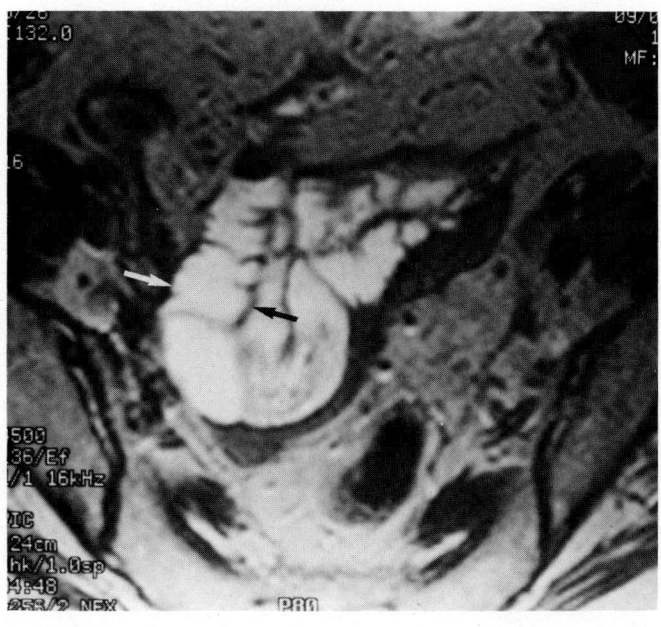

**Figure 9–10. Small bowel imaged with a surface coil.** T2-weighted fast spin-echo image through the pelvis obtained with an external multicoil array in a patient who has had several prior abdominal procedures demonstrates dilated, fluid-filled small bowel *(arrows)*. No intraluminal contrast agent was administered.

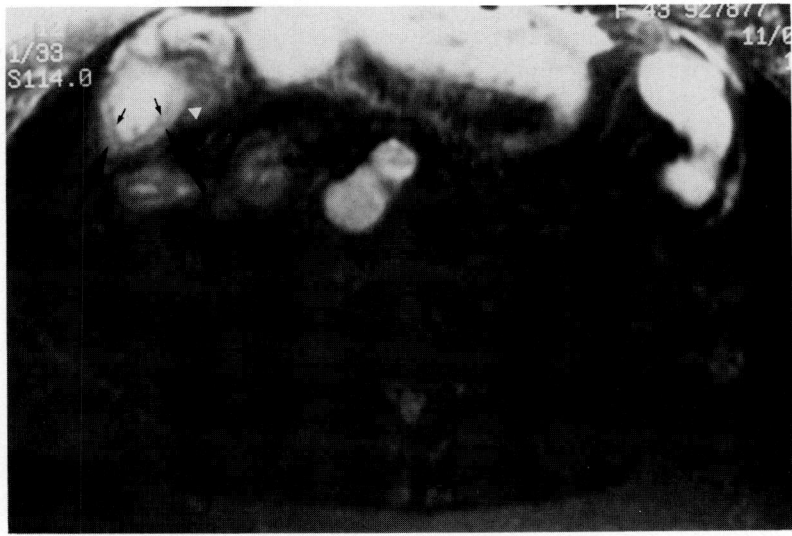

**Figure 9–11. Radiation enteritis: MR findings.** Fat-saturated T2-weighted fast spin-echo image through the pelvis in a patient with radiation enteritis demonstrates a thick high signal intensity layer that represents submucosal edema *(large arrows)*. Small arrows = low signal intensity mucosal layer; arrowhead = muscularis propria.

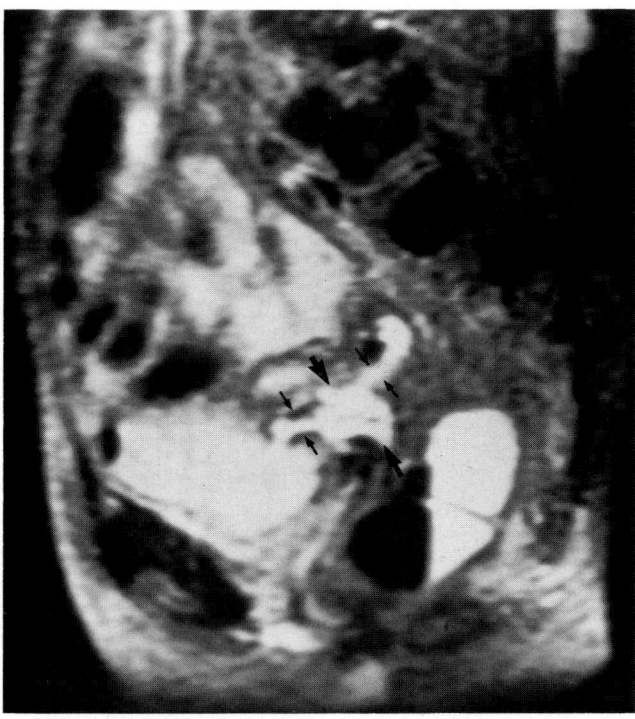

**Figure 9–12. Fistula: MR demonstration.** T2-weighted fat-saturated sagittal image obtained with the body coil demonstrates a fistula *(small arrows)* between the sigmoid colon and the bladder and an associated abscess cavity *(large arrows)*.

MR can demonstrate bowel fistulas in the setting of visceral inflammatory disease.[33, 34] Heavily T2-weighted images (best performed with fast spin-echo technique) have been shown to demonstrate the anatomy of fistulous tracts better than CT scanning (Fig. 9–12). The fluid in the tract appears as a high signal, well contrasted by soft tissue and fat on these images.

## COLORECTUM

MR is becoming an important imaging technique for the sigmoid colon and rectum. This is primarily due to the relatively fixed positions of these structures and the low amplitude of respiratory motion in the pelvis. The use of external surface coils to image the sigmoid colon and endorectal coils to image the rectum has also contributed to the success of MR in imaging these regions.

Inflammatory diseases are well demonstrated on MR because of the exquisite sensitivity of T2-weighted images to the presence of increased fluid content. It is particularly valuable in patients with suspected diverticulitis; MR dramatically demonstrates thickening of the bowel wall and high signal intensity in the pericolonic region associated with the inflammation[35] (Fig. 9–13). MR is also good at depicting the discrete fluid collections of pericolic abscesses. Other types of inflammatory disease, such as inflammatory bowel disease, infection, and radiation enteritis, are also well demonstrated.

MR is valuable in evaluating rectosigmoid tumors. Annular lesions or lesions of the sigmoid colon are best studied with the body coil or external surface coil, whereas lesions of the rectum are amenable to study with an endorectal surface coil (Fig. 9–14). MR is also useful in demonstrating invasion of the rectosigmoid colon by extrinsic masses such as gynecologic and prostatic malignant neoplasms (Fig. 9–15).

On high-resolution endorectal coil images, colorectal adenocarcinomas manifest as focal thickening of the mucosal layer[26] (Fig. 9–16). The epithelial component of the tumor has a signal intensity that is isointense to the mucosa on T2-weighted images. As the tumor grows, associated mucus-producing components or lakes of colloid have high signal intensity on T2-weighted images. Tumor-associated desmoplastic change has low signal intensity on all sequences. On images obtained with external surface coils or the body coil, the individual components of the bowel wall are often not demonstrated, so that the tumor cannot be recognized until it causes focal mural thickening.[36] It usually has intermediate signal intensity on T2-weighted images with low-resolution technique, which reflects the averaging of various signal intensity components.

MR has been used to stage colorectal malignant disease by several groups of investigators. The accuracy of MR in determining pericolonic involvement or local lymphadenopathy is similar to that demonstrated by CT.[36-38] A study comparing staging accuracy of MR with transrectal ultrasound demonstrated a slight advantage of ultrasound over MR (84% versus 76%).[39] The number of patients included in this study was small, and only low-resolution body coil imaging was employed in these studies. A single study on the use of an external surface

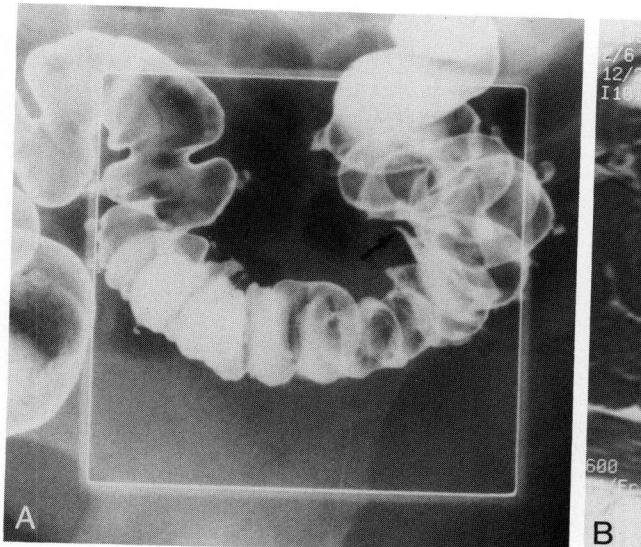

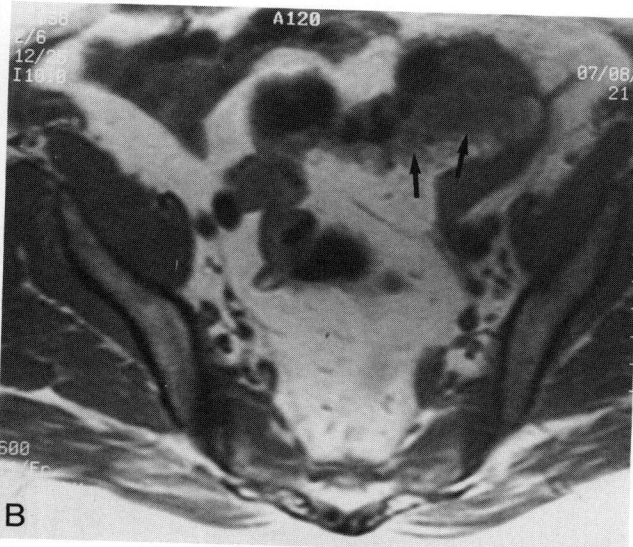

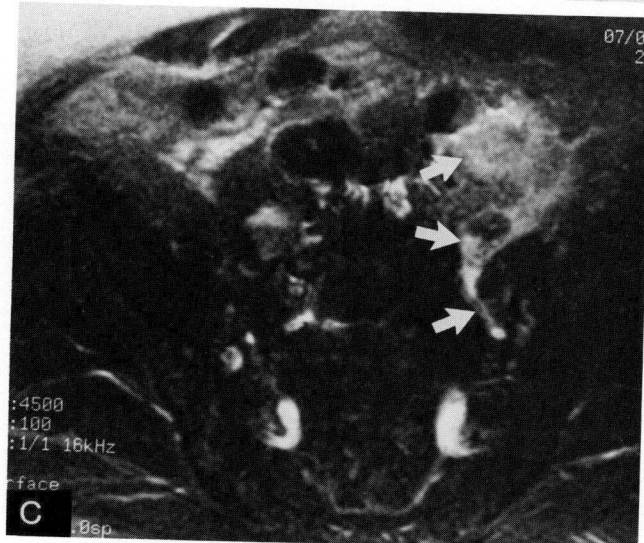

**Figure 9–13. Diverticulitis: barium enema and MR findings. A.** Double contrast barium enema study demonstrates diverticulosis and associated circular muscle hypertrophy. An irregular diverticulum *(arrow)* is suggestive of diverticulitis. **B.** T1-weighted axial image obtained with an external multicoil array demonstrates an area of focal thickening of the sigmoid colon with associated stranding in the pericolonic fat *(arrows)*. **C.** T2-weighted fast spin-echo image with fat saturation demonstrates high signal intensity in the area of bowel wall thickening and edema tracking along the mesentery *(arrows)* consistent with diverticulitis.

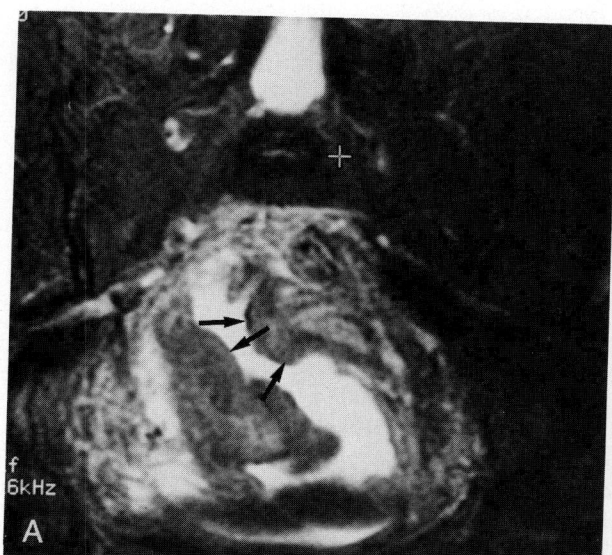

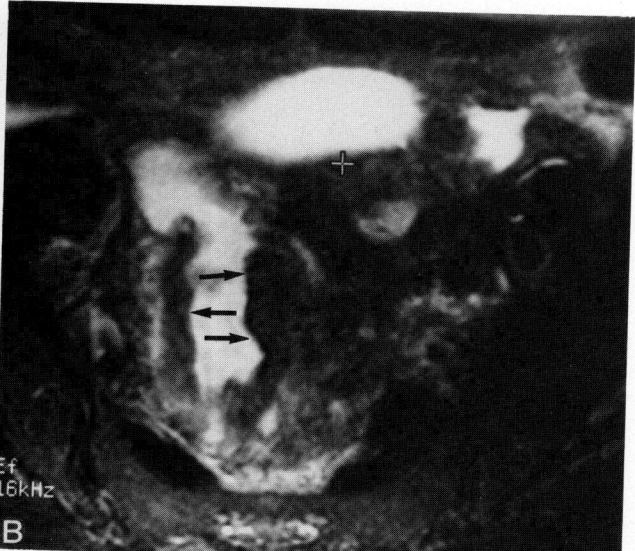

**Figure 9–14. Carcinoma of the colon: MR findings.** Fat-saturated coronal **(A)** and axial **(B)** T2-weighted fast spin-echo images through the pelvis with an external multicoil array demonstrate irregular thickening *(arrows)* of the rectosigmoid junction from an annular carcinoma.

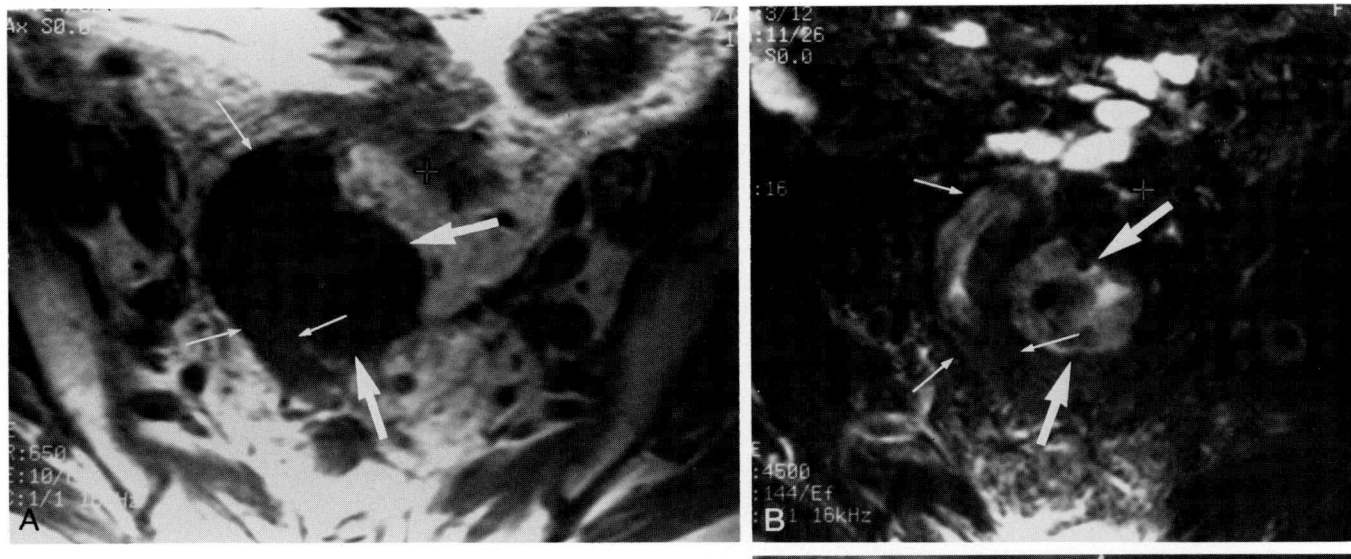

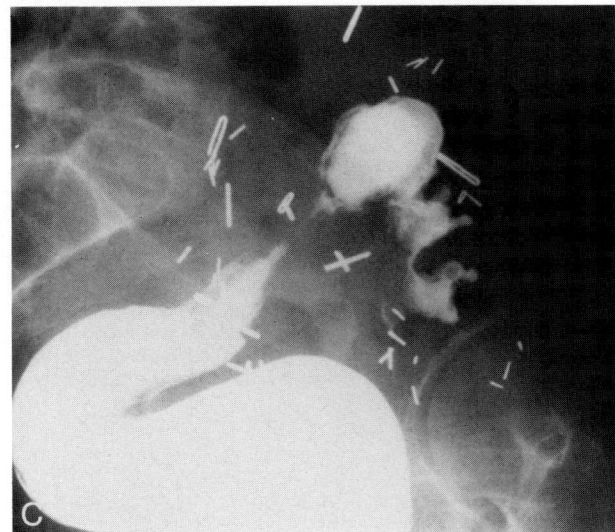

**Figure 9–15. Obstructive mesenteric mass: MR–barium enema correlation.** T1-weighted **(A)** and T2-weighted **(B)** fast spin-echo images of the pelvis obtained with an external multicoil array demonstrate a large mass in the mesentery *(large arrows)* invading and obstructing the distal sigmoid colon *(small arrows)*. **C.** Single contrast barium enema study demonstrates the high-grade obstruction.

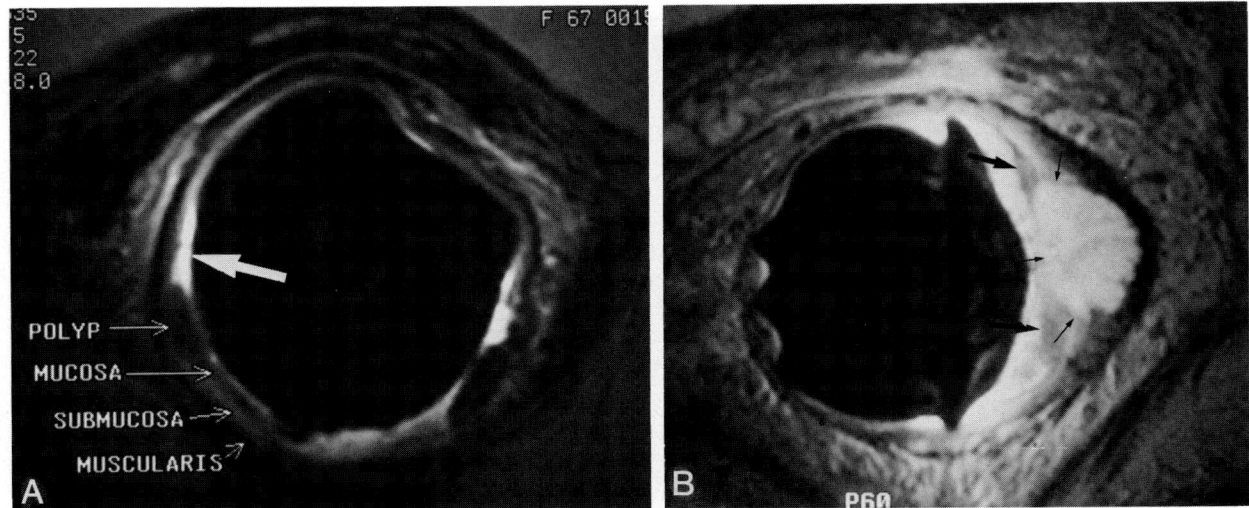

**Figure 9–16. Carcinoma of the colon: endorectal surface coil MR findings. A.** T2-weighted fast spin-echo image obtained with an endorectal surface coil demonstrates an area of focal thickening of the mucosa, which represents a small polyp that contained microscopic foci of carcinoma. The layers of the rectal wall are labeled. The unlabeled arrow points to high signal intensity luminal fluid. **B.** A similar image in a patient with a more advanced lesion demonstrates the lower signal intensity epithelial component *(large arrows)* and a high signal intensity colloid-producing component of disease *(small arrows)* invading the muscularis propria.

coil to stage the local extent of rectal carcinoma reported an accuracy of 89% in 29 cases. There was a tendency to overestimate tumor invasion.[39, 40] However, the results for detection of metastatic perirectal adenopathy were disappointing. There have been no reports on the accuracy of rectal cancer staging with an external multicoil.

A study of high-resolution imaging of resected specimens from patients with colorectal cancer has demonstrated a great potential for high-resolution MR to stage these lesions accurately. The exact level of involvement within the bowel wall was accurately determined in 14 of 15 cases. A preliminary report on the application of an endorectal surface coil for studying rectal cancers in vivo with resolution similar to that of the in vitro specimen studies revealed 92% accuracy of MR in assessing the level of invasion of these lesions. Although still early in its development, high-resolution endorectal surface coil MR holds great promise for studying rectal lesions.

Another important role of MR in the imaging of rectal cancer is the detection of recurrence. Locally recurrent tumor can be difficult to distinguish from postoperative fibrosis clinically and on CT examination. Although immature fibrosis (less than 1 year old) may have high signal intensity on T2-weighted images, it has been shown that mature fibrosis has low signal intensity on T2-weighted images. This fact has been used to detect recurrent cervical carcinoma as high signal intensity tissue within low signal intensity fibrosis.[41] Similar results have been shown for rectal carcinoma.[40, 42]

# References

1. Wherli FW: Principles of magnetic resonance. *In* Stark DD, Bradley WG (eds): Magnetic Resonance Imaging (2nd ed). St. Louis: Mosby–Year Book, 1992, pp 3–37.
2. Edelman RR, Kleefield J, Wentz KU, et al: Basic principles of magnetic resonance imaging. *In* Edelman RR, Hesselink JR (eds): Clinical Magnetic Resonance Imaging. Philadelphia: WB Saunders, 1990, pp 3–38.
3. Mansfield P, Morris PG: NMR Imaging in Biomedicine. New York: Academic Press, 1982, pp 29–56.
4. Axel L: Surface coil magnetic resonance imaging. J Comput Assist Tomogr 8:831–834, 1984.
5. Roemer PB, Edelstein WA, Hayes CE, et al: The NMR phased array. Magn Reson Med 16:192–225, 1990.
6. Hayes CE, Hattes N, Roemer PB: Volume imaging with phased arrays. Magn Reson Med 18:308–309, 1991.
7. Schnall MD: E-coil. *In* Book of Abstracts: Society of Magnetic Resonance in Medicine 1986. Berkeley, CA: Society of Magnetic Resonance in Medicine, 1986, p 57.
8. Schnall MD, Lenkinski RL, Pollack HM, et al: Prostate: MR imaging with an endorectal surface coil. Radiology 172:570–574, 1989.
9. Chan TW, Kressel HY, Milestone B, et al: Rectal carcinoma: staging at MR imaging with endorectal surface coil. Work in progress. Radiology 181:461–468, 1991.
10. Schnall MD, Connick T, Hayes CE, et al: MR imaging of the pelvis with an endorectal-external multicoil array. JMRI 2:229–232, 1992.
11. Frahm J, Hanicke W, Merboldt KD: Transverse coherence in rapid FLASH NMR imaging. J Magn Reson 72:304–307, 1987.
12. Hasse A: Snapshot FLASH MRI: application to T1, T2 and chemical shift imaging. Magn Reson Med 13:77–83, 1990.
13. Holsinger AE, Reiderer SJ: The importance of phase encoding order in ultrashort TR snapshot MR imaging. Magn Reson Med 16:481–488, 1990.
14. Hennig J, Nauerth A, Friedburg H: RARE imaging: a fast imaging method for clinical MR. Magn Reson Med 3:823–833, 1986.
15. Melki PS, Mulkern RV, Panych ZP, et al: Comparing the Faise method with the conventional dual-echo sequences. Magn Reson Med 1:319–326, 1991.
16. Smith RC, Reinhold C, McCauley T, et al: Multicoil high resolution fast spin-echo imaging of the female pelvis. Radiology 184:671–676, 1992.
17. Listerud J, Mulkern R: The J coupling hypothesis for bright fat observed on FSE. *In* Book of Abstracts: Society of Magnetic Resonance in Medicine 1992. Berkeley, CA: Society of Magnetic Resonance in Medicine, 1992, p 45.
18. Tart RP, Lik C, Storm BL, et al: Enteric MRI contrast agents: comparative study of five potential agents in humans. Magn Reson Imaging 9:559–568, 1991.
19. Hahn PF, Stark DD, Lewis JM, et al: First clinical trial of a new superparamagnetic iron oxide for use as an oral gastrointestinal contrast agent in MR imaging. Radiology 175:695–700, 1990.
20. Ros PR, Steinman RM, Torres GM, et al: The value of barium as a gastrointestinal contrast agent in MR imaging: a comparison study in normal volunteers. AJR 157:761–767, 1991.
21. Mitchell DG, Vinitski S, Mohamed FB, et al: Comparison of Kaopectate with barium for negative and positive enteric contrast at MR imaging. Radiology 181:475–480, 1991.
22. Brown JJ, Duncan JR, Heiken JP, et al: Perfluorocytlbromide as a gastrointestinal contrast for MR imaging: use with and without glucagon. Radiology 181:455–460, 1991.
23. Wesbey GE, Brasch RC, Goldberg HI, et al: Dilute oral iron solutions as gastrointestinal contrast agents for magnetic resonance imaging: initial clinical experience. Magn Reson Imaging 3:57–64, 1985.
24. Kaminski S, Laniado M, Gugall M, et al: Gadopentate dimeglumine as a bowel contrast agent: safety and efficacy. Radiology 178:50–58, 1991.
25. Li KC, Ang PG, Tart RP, et al: Paramagnetic oil emulsions as oral magnetic resonance imaging contrast agents. Magn Reson Imaging 8: 589–598, 1990.
26. Imai Y, Kressel HY, Saul SH, et al: Colorectal tumors: an in vitro study of high-resolution MR imaging. Radiology 177:695–701, 1990.
27. Takashima S, Takeuchi N, Shiozaki H, et al: Carcinoma of the esophagus: CT vs MR imaging in determining resectability. AJR 156:297–302, 1991.
28. Petrillo R, Balzarini L, Bidoli P, et al: Esophageal squamous cell carcinoma: MRI evaluation of mediastinum. Gastrointest Radiol 15:275–278, 1990.
29. Lenr L, Rupp N, Siewert JR: Assessment of resectability of esophageal cancer by computed tomography and magnetic resonance imaging. Surgery 103:344–350, 1988.
30. Bondestam S, Salo JA, Salonen OL, et al: Imaging of congenital esophageal cysts in adults. Gastrointest Radiol 15:279–281, 1990.
31. Lupetin AR, Dash N: MRI appearance of esophageal duplication cyst. Gastrointest Radiol 12:7–9, 1987.
32. Hamed MM, Hamm B, Ibrahim ME, et al: Dynamic MR imaging of the abdomen with gadopentetate dimeglumine: normal enhancement patterns of the liver, spleen, stomach, and pancreas. AJR 158:303–307, 1992.
33. Outwater E, Sheibler M, Schnall M, et al. Pelvic fistulas: findings on MR images. AJR (in press).
34. Koelbel G, Schmiedle V, Mayer MC, et al: Diagnosis of fistula and sinus tracts in patients with Crohn's disease: value of MR imaging. AJR 152:999–1003, 1989.
35. Hricak H: The rectum and sigmoid colon. *In* Hricak H, Carrington B (eds): MRI of the Pelvis. London: Martin Dunitz, 1991, pp 463–579.
36. Hodgman CG, MacCarthy RL, Wolff BG, et al: Preoperative staging of rectal carcinoma by computed tomography and 0.15T magnetic resonance imaging. Dis Colon Rectum 29:446–450, 1986.
37. Butch RJ, Stark DD, Wittenberg J, et al: Staging rectal cancer by MR and CT. AJR 146:1155–1160, 1986.

38. Guinet C, Buy JN, Sezeur A, et al: Preoperative assessment of the extension of rectal carcinoma: correlation of MR, surgical, and histopathologic findings. J Comput Assist Tomogr 12:209–214, 1988.

39. deLange EE, Fechner RE, Edge SB, et al: Preoperative staging of rectal carcinoma with MR imaging: surgical and histopathologic correlation. Radiology 176:623–627, 1990.

40. Waizer A, Powsner E, Russo I, et al: Prospective comparative study of magnetic resonance imaging versus transrectal ultrasound for preoperative staging and follow-up of rectal cancer. Preliminary report. Dis Colon Rectum 34:1068–1072, 1991.

41. Ebner F, Kressel HY, Mintz MC, et al: Tumor recurrence vs. fibrosis in the female pelvis: differentiation with MR imaging at 1.5T. Radiology 166:333–340, 1988.

42. Rafto SE, Amendola MA, Gefter WB: MR imaging of recurrent colorectal carcinoma versus fibrosis. J Comput Assist Tomogr 12:521–523, 1988.

# Endoscopic Ultrasonography

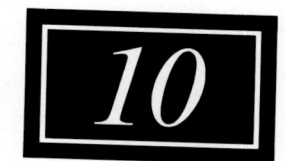

**Gladys M. Torres, M.D.**

INTRODUCTION

INSTRUMENTATION AND
TECHNIQUE
Upper Gastrointestinal
Endosonography
Colonic Endosonography
Limitations

NORMAL SONOGRAPHIC
ANATOMY
Esophagus
Stomach and Duodenum
Colorectum

PATHOLOGY
Esophagus
Stomach and Duodenum
Colorectum

CONCLUSIONS

## INTRODUCTION

Endoscopic ultrasonography (EUS) is an evolving imaging technique that combines fiberoptic endoscopy and high-frequency ultrasonography in the evaluation of the gastrointestinal tract and surrounding structures. It has the advantage of direct endoscopic visualization of the bowel wall and identification of the different wall layers with the use of a high-frequency transducer.[1-3] EUS is most efficacious in the evaluation of intramural extension of tumors and staging of gastrointestinal malignancies. Indeed, this technique has proved to be quite accurate in the preoperative staging of gastrointestinal tumors according to the tumor, node, metastasis (TNM) classification.[4-8] This chapter provides a general overview of this technique and its potential applications.

## INSTRUMENTATION AND TECHNIQUE

The initial version of the current echoendoscope was introduced about 10 years ago by Olympus (Tokyo, Japan). Since then, four echoendoscopic prototypes have been developed for clinical evaluation. The GF-UM3/EU-M3 (Olympus, Tokyo, Japan) is one of the most commonly employed units. It incorporates a radial scanning system (rotating piezoelectric tranducer) with a fiberoptic endoscope and an accompanying display unit[9] (Fig. 10–1). This system produces a 360-degree real-time ultrasound image, allowing circumferential visualization of the intestinal wall.

The GF-UM3/EU-M3 has the advantage of being able to image with either a 7.5- or 12-MHz transducer, offering a choice of imaging depth. With these high-frequency transducers, the depth of sound penetration is decreased but the resolution is better. This limits evaluation of surrounding deep structures to some extent. The equipment specifications are listed in Table 10–1.

## Upper Gastrointestinal Endosonography

The preparation and sedation of the patient for EUS are identical to those used for routine endoscopies. The patient is placed in the left lateral decubitus position and, after topical anesthetic is applied to the pharynx, the echoendoscope is advanced into the esophagus, stomach, and duodenum.[10, 11] The instrument is inserted in the lowest portion of the descending duodenum and slowly retracted into the esophagus.

Several techniques are used to improve contact between the gut wall and the transducer; the water-filled balloon and the water immersion method are most widely used. In the water immersion method, 300 to 600 mL of deaerated water is instilled through a Luer-Lok attachment in the echoendoscope. This serves as an excellent acoustic medium for conducting the sound wave and is used mainly for evaluating the stomach.[12-14]

**TABLE 10–1. TECHNICAL SPECIFICATIONS FOR A TYPICAL ECHOENDOSCOPE***

| PARAMETER | TYPE OR VALUE |
| --- | --- |
| Display mode | B-mode |
| Scanning method | Mechanical, radial |
| Frequency | 7.5 MHz, 12 MHz |
| Diameter of transducer | 7 mm |
| Focusing point | 25 mm (12 MHz), 30 mm (7.5 MHz) |
| Direction of view | Oblique 65 degrees |
| Field of view | 80 degrees |
| Depth of field | 5.4 mm |
| Biopsy channel size | 2 mm |
| Distal tip outer diameter | 13.0 mm |
| Insertion tube outer diameter | 11.2 mm |
| Working length | 130 cm |
| Angulation (up-down, right-left) | 90/90 |

*Olympus GF-UM3/EU-M3, Tokyo, Japan.

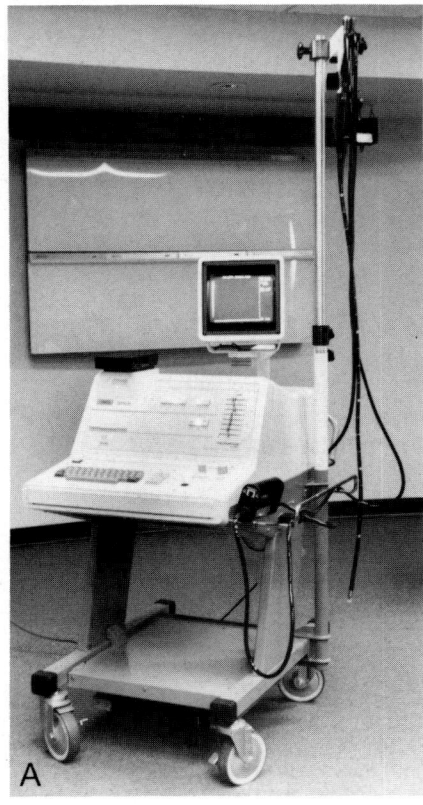
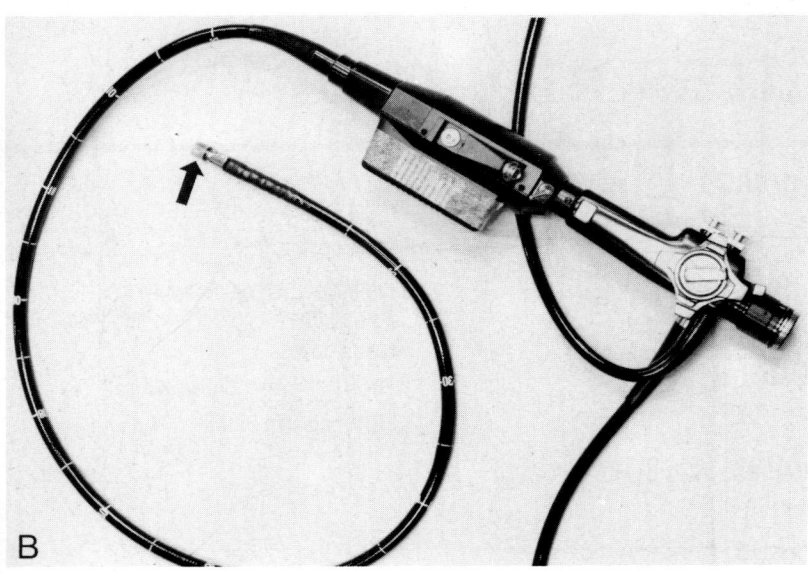

**Figure 10–1. The echoendoscope. A.** Olympus GF-UM3/EU-M3 unit with rotating piezoelectric transducer incorporated with a fiberoptic endoscope and an accompanying display unit. **B.** Close-up view of the echoendoscope demonstrating the transducer from the distal tip of the scope *(arrow).*

With the balloon contact method, water is also used as the acoustic coupling agent. The water-filled balloon enables the gut wall to be placed in the focal zone of the transducer, improving resolution of the different wall layers. The esophagus and duodenal wall are best evaluated with this technique.

The last method used is direct apposition of the transducer against the gut wall. This maximizes visualization of extraluminal structures adjacent to the wall: mediastinum, heart, aorta, spleen, and liver. This method requires aspirating all the intraluminal air, which degrades the image.

Routine fiberoptic endoscopy should be performed before EUS to determine the exact location of the lesion.

## Colonic Endosonography

Historically, studies of the rectum were performed with a rigid ultrasound probe that was devised for evaluating the prostate gland. Two types of transducers were available with this probe: linear and sector. The linear probe requires manual rotation through 360 degrees to evaluate the entire rectum and surrounding structures. For this reason, the sector scanner has gained wider acceptance.[15, 16] EUS using these probes is limited to the rectum.

A new echoendoscope has been developed for evaluating the entire colon. It is a forward-viewing instrument with a 7.5-MHz transducer and 320-degree field of view.

Preparation for this study includes a conventional water or phosphate enema. The patient is placed in the left lateral decubitus position. Scanning can be performed using the water-filled balloon technique and/or the water immersion technique. Preliminary studies have shown that in the majority of patients (95%) the entire colon can be evaluated to the cecum.[17, 18]

## Limitations

Technically, EUS is more difficult to perform than standard endoscopy because of the longer and more rigid tip used. Consequently, greater skill is required to traverse areas such as the proximal esophagus, pylorus, and areas of lumen narrowing. In about 15% of cases, the inexperienced echoendoscopist cannot negotiate the duodenum, resulting in an incomplete study.[19]

## NORMAL SONOGRAPHIC ANATOMY

### Esophagus

When performing EUS, it is vital to understand the normal sonographic anatomy of the gut and adjacent structures. Sonographically, the normal esophagus is divided in three parts: upper, middle and lower.[13, 14]

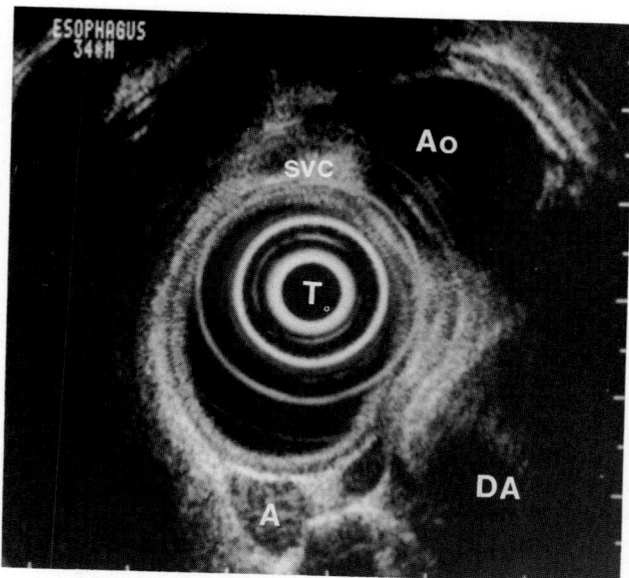

**Figure 10–2. EUS: midthoracic esophagus.** Hypoechoic vascular structures on the left of the esophagus represent the ascending (Ao) and descending (DA) thoracic aorta. The azygos vein (A) lies anterior to the spine. SVC = superior vena cava; T = transducer.

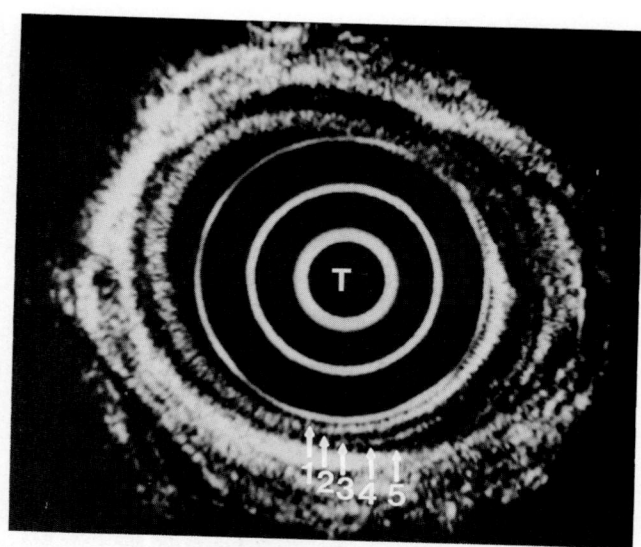

**Figure 10–4. Normal layers of the esophageal wall: EUS.** Layers 1, 3, and 5 are hyperechoic; layers 2 and 4 are hypoechoic. 1 = superficial mucosa; 2 = deep mucosa; 3 = interface between the submucosa and the muscularis; 4 = muscularis propria; 5 = adventitia and periesophageal fat; T = transducer.

The upper portion extends from the oropharynx to the superior region of the aortic arch. The great vessels can be imaged as they emerge from the aortic arch and extend to the neck. The middle portion extends from the aortic arch to the subcarinal region, where the aortic arch and descending aorta project posteriorly (Fig. 10–2). The distal portion extends from the subcarinal region to the level of the cardia. The left atrium projects anteriorly and the descending aorta posteriorly[13, 14] (Fig. 10–3).

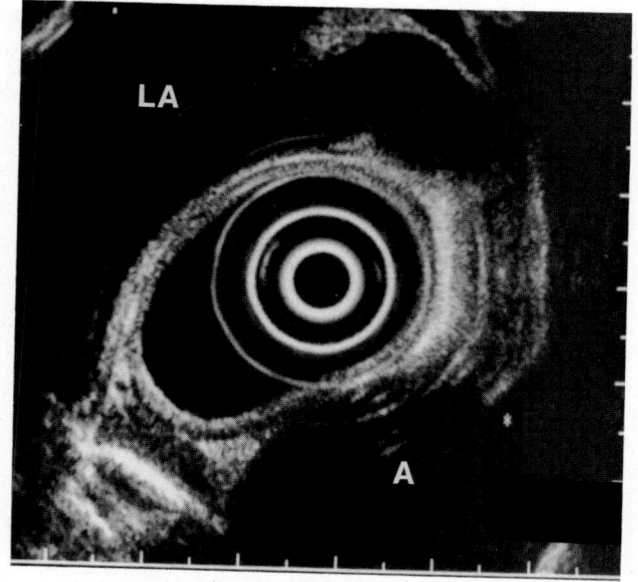

**Figure 10–3. EUS: lower esophagus.** Note the relationship between the left atrium (LA) anterior and toward the right and the descending aorta (A), which lies posterior to the esophagus.

The gut wall is stratified into five layers sonographically.[20-23] The first layer is hyperechoic and corresponds to the superficial mucosa. The second layer is hypoechoic and corresponds to the deep mucosa. The third layer is hyperechoic and corresponds to the submucosa and the interface between the submucosa and the muscularis propria. The fourth, hypoechoic, layer corresponds to the muscularis propria, and the fifth layer corresponds to the serosa, the subserosal fat, and, in the case of the esophagus, the adventitia (Fig. 10–4).

The esophagus is best evaluated with the balloon technique. Often only three layers are visualized because the wall is not entirely within the focal zone of the transducer or the inflated balloon pushes the wall away from the transducer. The hyperechoic first layer corresponds to the balloon-mucosa-submucosa and the interface between the submucosa and the muscularis. The hypoechoic second layer corresponds to the muscularis propria and the hyperechoic third layer to the interface between the muscularis propria and the periesophageal surrounding tissues[24] (Fig. 10–5).

## Stomach and Duodenum

With the water immersion technique, the five sonographic layers of the gastric and duodenal walls are usually delineated (Fig. 10–6). The hypoechoic fourth layer in the distal antrum and pylorus is slightly more prominent. A well-distended stomach has a wall thickness of approximately 3 mm.[13] The duodenum is evaluated with the water immersion and balloon techniques.

The stomach is used as an acoustic window to evaluate intra-abdominal and retroperitoneal structures echoendoscopically. The liver is viewed from the perspective of the lesser curvature of the stomach or the duodenum,

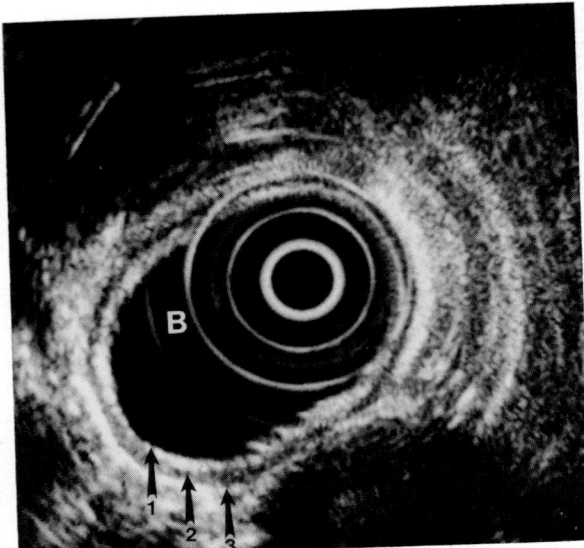

**Figure 10–5. Normal esophageal wall: balloon technique.** Three wall layers are identified. 1 = balloon (B)-mucosa-submucosa and the interface between the submucosa and the muscularis; 2 = muscularis propria; 3 = interface between muscularis propria and periesophageal tissues.

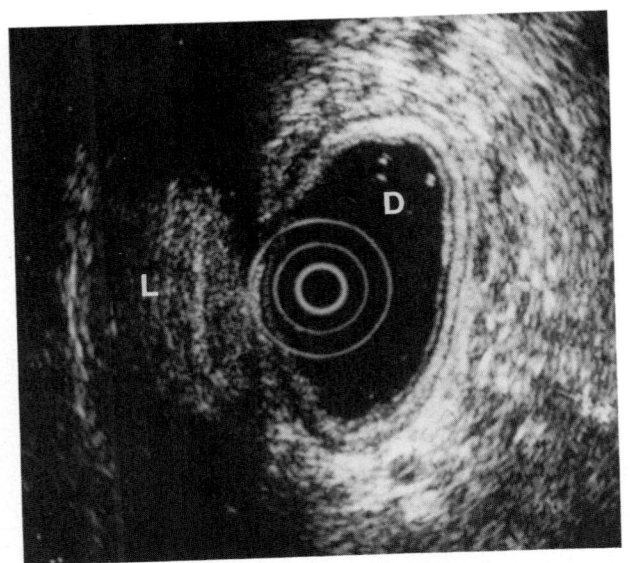

**Figure 10–7. Normal liver: EUS.** The right liver lobe (L) is seen from the duodenum (D). The lateral mural layers of the duodenum cannot be identified because the transducer abuts the wall, which is out of its focal zone.

the left lobe is seen from the fundus or body of the stomach, the midportion is seen from the antrum, and the right lobe is viewed from the distal stomach and duodenum (Fig. 10–7). The spleen is best seen from the superior portion of the lesser curvature of the stomach. Two gastric lumina can be seen as the ultrasound beam passes through the angularis, imaging the stomach, body, and antrum simultaneously (Fig. 10–8).

The pancreas is visualized from the posterior aspect of the midportion of the body of the stomach, anterior to the splenic vein (Fig. 10–9). The pancreatic body and

tail are visualized better from the region of the fundus of the stomach.

The evaluation of the head of the pancreas begins distally, at the level of the ampulla. The endoscope is slowly withdrawn and the head is best seen in the region of the duodenal bulb and proximal descending duodenum. The portal vein and its confluence with the splenic vein are sonographic landmarks for localizing the head of the pancreas, as in transabdominal ultrasonography. The pancreas has homogeneous echogenicity, and the normal pancreatic duct should not be more than 1 to 2 mm in diameter (Fig. 10–10).

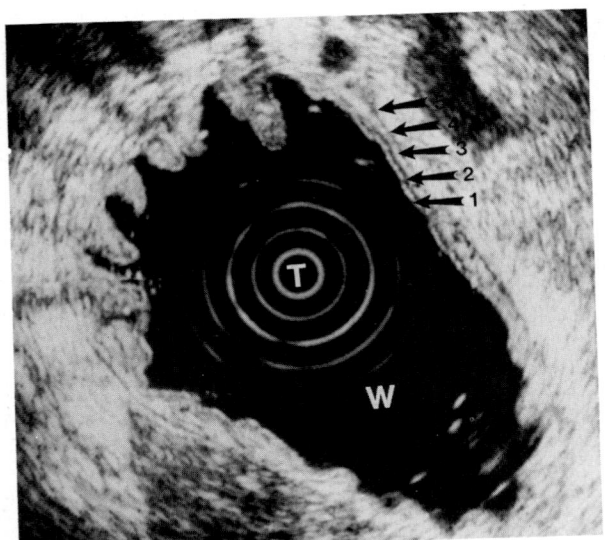

**Figure 10–6. Normal stomach: EUS with water immersion technique.** As in the rest of the gastrointestinal tract, five normal layers are identified *(arrows)*. W = water; T = transducer.

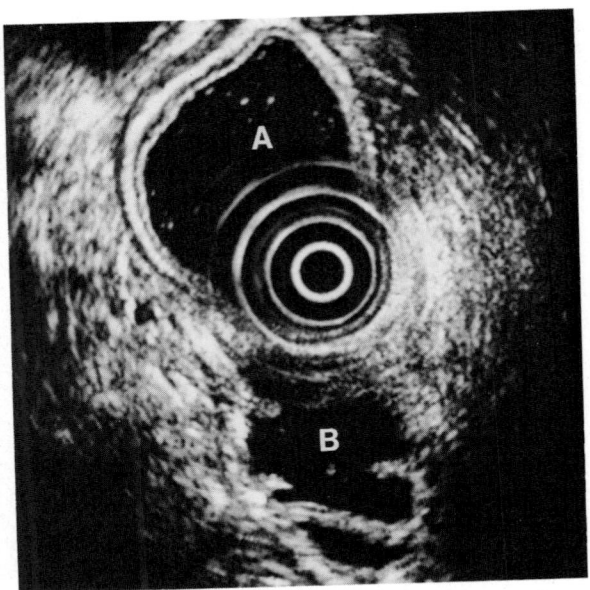

**Figure 10–8. Normal gastric angulis: EUS.** EUS through the region of the angulis shows two gastric lumina which represent the antrum (A) and body (B) of the stomach.

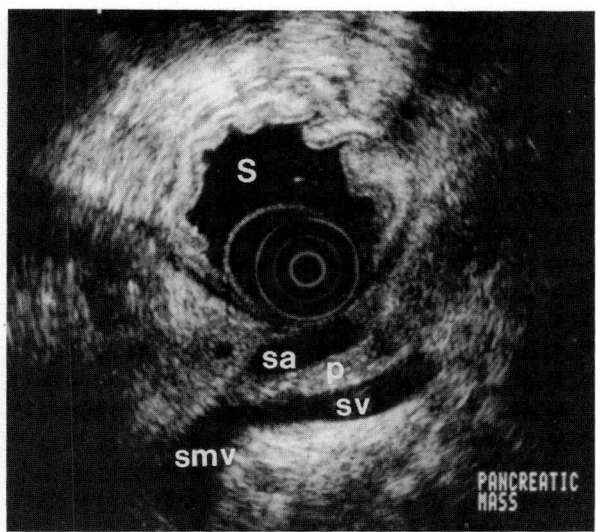

**Figure 10–9. Normal pancreas: EUS.** Splenic vein (sv) serves as landmark to localize the pancreas (p). View from the posterior wall of the stomach (S). sa = splenic artery; smv = superior mesenteric vein.

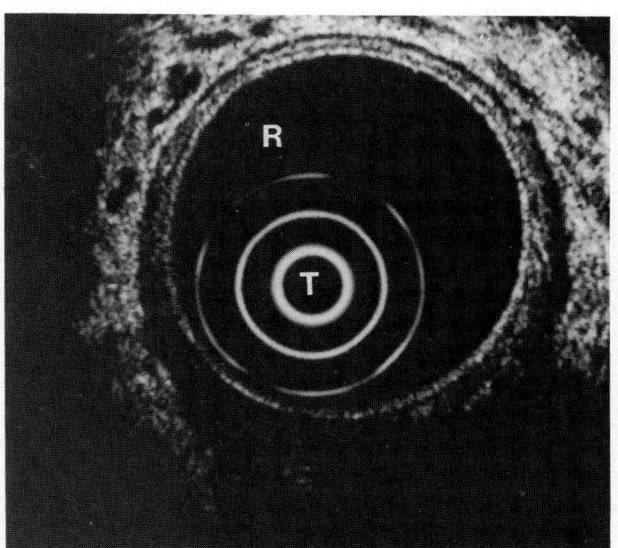

**Figure 10–11. Normal rectum: EUS.** The five sonographic layers are demonstrated on this circumferential view. R = rectum; T = transducer.

## Colorectum

As in other regions of the gut, five different echogenic layers have been described within the colon wall (Fig. 10–11). However, some in vitro studies using different transducer frequencies have shown up to seven to nine different sonographic layers. In the rectum, the fourth layer, representing the muscularis propria, is the thickest layer and can be subdivided into two sublayers, which represent the longitudinal and circular muscle coats.[24]

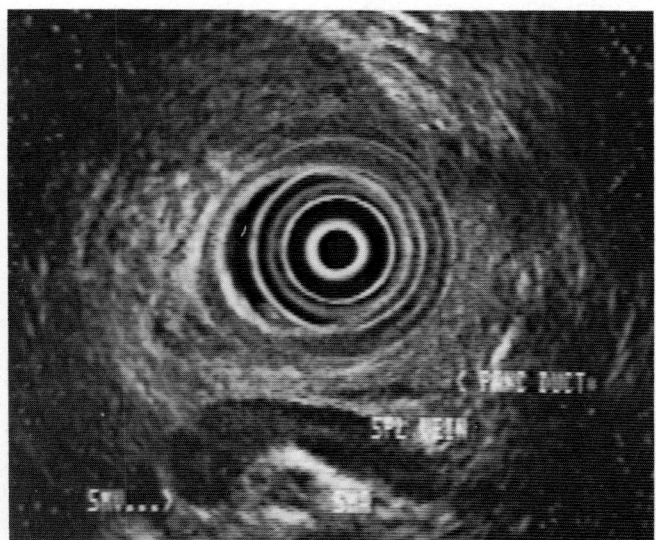

**Figure 10–10. Normal pancreatic duct: EUS.** Confluence of splenic vein and superior mesenteric vein. Pancreas shows homogeneous echogenicity and pancreatic duct serves as landmark. SMA = superior mesenteric artery. (Case courtesy of Maria Vilaró, M.D., Bayamón, Puerto Rico.)

## PATHOLOGY

### Esophagus

EUS provides a unique perspective for evaluating esophageal carcinoma that has profoundly influenced the new TNM classification (Table 10–2) for staging this tumor.[5–8] Several factors influence the therapeutic approach based on the clinical staging. These include tumor location, longitudinal extent (>5 cm has a worse prognosis), and depth of penetration.[25] The overall accuracy of assessing these factors ranges from 72 to 89%.[26]

Endosonographically, esophageal carcinoma is manifested as a hypoechoic lesion that disrupts the normal esophageal wall layer (Fig. 10–12). The relationship between tumor and aortic or tracheal wall must be carefully evaluated because of the risk of intraoperative bleeding if invasion is present[25] (Fig. 10–13).

The overall accuracy of EUS in diagnosing periesophageal lymph node metastasis ranges from 71 to 84%.[26] Sonographic findings suggesting lymph node metastases include well-defined nodes, round nodes, and nodes that are hypo- or isoechoic compared with the primary tu-

#### TABLE 10–2. TUMOR, NODE, METASTASIS STAGING OF ESOPHAGEAL CARCINOMA

| STAGE | DESCRIPTION |
| --- | --- |
| TX | Primary tumor cannot be assessed |
| T0 | No evidence of primary tumor |
| Tis | Carcinoma in situ |
| T1 | Tumor invades lamina propria or submucosa |
| T2 | Tumor invades muscularis propria |
| T3 | Tumor invades adventitia |
| T4 | Tumor invades adjacent structures |

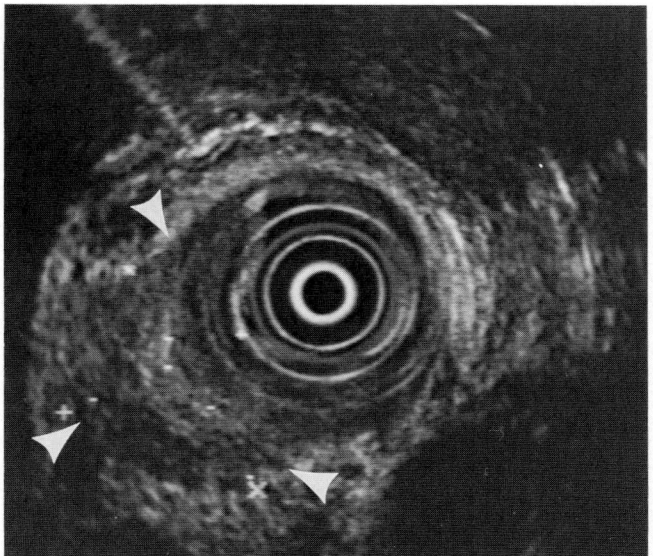

**Figure 10–12. Carcinoma of the esophagus.** EUS of the esophagus shows a hypoechoic mass disrupting the mural layers, extending through the adventitia *(arrowheads).* (Case courtesy of Maria Vilaró, M.D., Bayamón, Puerto Rico.)

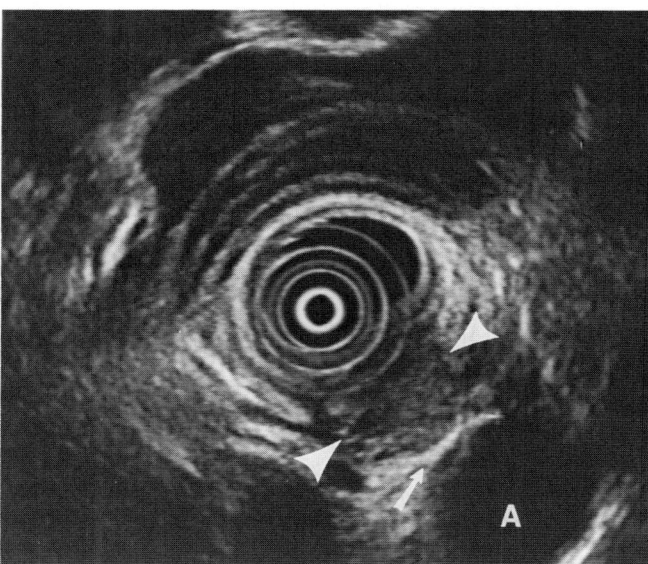

**Figure 10–13. T3 carcinoma of the esophagus.** EUS of an esophageal tumor that entends through the adventitia *(arrowheads).* Note that there is no tumor extension to the aorta (A) *(arrow).* (Case courtesy of Maria Vilaró, M.D., Bayamón, Puerto Rico.)

mor. Lymph node size cannot accurately predict tumor involvement because malignant lymph nodes measuring only 3 to 5 mm have been reported. For the purposes of staging, involvement of the mediastinal and perigastric lymph nodes is considered regional and involvement of the celiac axis nodes is considered distant metastasis (Fig. 10–14). With progression of tumor penetration, there is a higher incidence of lymph node metastasis. The accuracy of EUS for diagnosing nonmetastatic nodes is low (<56%) because of the difficulty in distinguishing between inflammation and microscopic metastasis.[13, 27]

Because of the limited depth of penetration of EUS, computed tomography (CT) should be performed to evaluate distant metastasis to the chest or abdomen.

## Stomach and Duodenum

Gastric carcinoma is the third most common malignancy of the gastrointestinal tract and the sixth leading cause of cancer death.[28] Efforts have been made to promote early diagnosis because the survival rate is

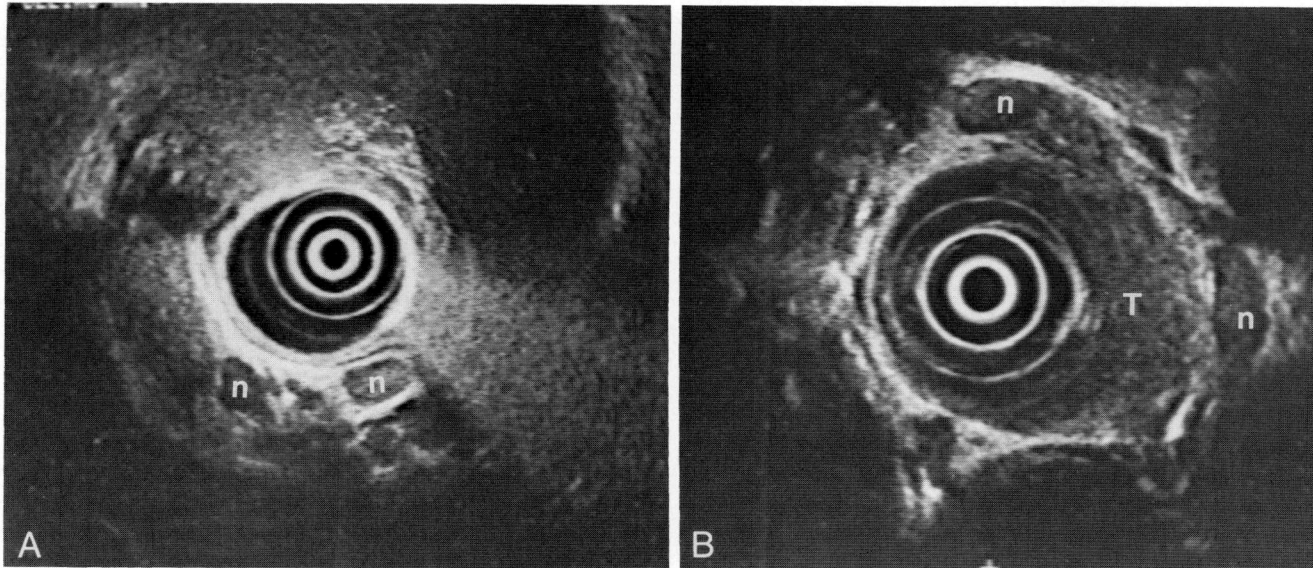

**Figure 10–14. Carcinoma of the esophagus: regional and distant metastases. A.** The primary esophageal tumor is associated with regional (mediastinal) adenopathy (n). **B.** Distant celiac adenopathy (n) is present as well. T = primary tumor. (Case courtesy of Maria Vilaró, M.D., Bayamón, Puerto Rico.)

higher for localized tumors. Indeed, the 5-year survival rate after gastrectomy is 90% for the early carcinomas.[29, 30] The EUS pattern seen in gastric carcinoma is a hypoechoic lesion with disruption of the five normal gastric wall layers[31] (Fig. 10–15). Tumor growth is predominately vertical with early invasion of the deeper layers of the wall (Fig. 10–16). The TNM staging of gastric cancer is listed in Table 10–3.

The overall accuracy of EUS in the diagnosis of lymph node metastasis ranges from 68 to 80% and that for nonmetastatic nodes is 56% or less. Endosonographically, malignant gastric nodes are round, sharply defined, and hypoechoic[7, 12, 31] (Fig. 10–17).

The major limitations of EUS in evaluating gastric carcinomas are limited depth of penetration and severe luminal stenosis that prevents passage of the echoendoscope.[32] Again, CT should be performed to detect distant metastasis. In general, EUS is accurate in the staging of local spread of gastric cancer but is not clinically useful in differentiating between benign and malignant gastric ulcers or in the primary diagnosis of gastric carcinoma.[33]

Several studies comparing EUS staging of gastric carcinoma with histopathology show an overall accuracy of 73 to 84%.[33] The differentiation between T2 and T3 carcinomas is problematic because of the difficulty in distinguishing gastric serosal from subserosal layers.[4] There is an overall overstaging rate of about 10% with EUS.

Locally recurrent gastric carcinoma is an important problem after gastric surgery. Routine endoscopy and CT have proved to be of limited value when the anastomotic tumor recurrence develops in the submucosa. Anastomotic recurrence is suggested by irregular, hy-

| TABLE 10–3. TUMOR, NODE, METASTASIS STAGING OF GASTRIC CANCER | |
| --- | --- |
| **STAGE** | **DESCRIPTION** |
| TX | Primary tumor cannot be assessed |
| T0 | No evidence of primary tumor |
| Tis | Carcinoma in situ |
| T1 | Tumor invades lamina propria or submucosa |
| T2 | Tumor invades the muscularis propria or the subserosa |
| T3 | Tumor penetrates the serosa without invasion of adjacent structures |
| T4 | Tumor invades adjacent structures |

poechoic thickening in the area of the anastomosis[34] (Fig. 10–18). EUS has difficulty in differentiating between inflammatory changes and tumor recurrence, however.

Gastric lymphoma represents about 2 to 5% of gastric tumors.[35] It is usually diagnosed in an advanced stage because early tumor involving the lamina propria and submucosa is not detected with conventional endoscopy.[36] Several sonographic features help distinguish lymphoma from epithelial neoplasms. Gastric wall infiltration by lymphoma occurs mainly by longitudinal growth, whereas the growth of carcinoma is primarily vertical. Extensive infiltration of the second and third layers associated with localized mucosal ulceration is considered pathognomonic of lymphoma. In early cases, there is thickening of the second and third layers with preserved mural stratification, whereas in advanced disease there is diffuse mural thickening with a hypoechoic pattern and loss of individual wall layers[36] (Fig. 10–19).

Three distinct patterns have been described in patients with thickened gastric folds: (1) diffuse hypertrophy of the layers of the gastric wall usually occurs in patients with benign processes such as gastritis, peptic ulcer disease, and Zollinger-Ellison syndrome; (2) diffuse fold enlargement with disruption of the gastric layers is found in lymphoma and linitis plastica; and (3) hypoechoic spaces within the gastric wall correspond to submucosal varices.[37]

Other indications for EUS include the evaluation of submucosal tumors (Fig. 10–20) and the differentiation of intrinsic wall lesions from extrinsic compression by adjacent structures. Although EUS cannot provide a pathologic diagnosis, the sonographic appearance of some lesions can be most instructive. Leiomyoma and leiomyosarcoma are hypoechoic lesions that arise from the muscularis propria. Lipomas are hyperechoic lesions within the submucosal layers. Ectopic pancreas presents as hypoechoic lesions with a central ductular structure. Gastric varices present as anechoic, submucosal, serpiginous lesions (Fig. 10–21). The ability to establish the last diagnosis can be lifesaving if a biopsy is contemplated.[38]

EUS has a reported overall accuracy of 92% for the diagnosis and staging of pancreatic carcinoma and 88% for ampullary neoplasms. Partial or total destruction of the normal wall of the papilla of Vater strongly suggests an ampullary tumor. Localized tumor in the papilla can

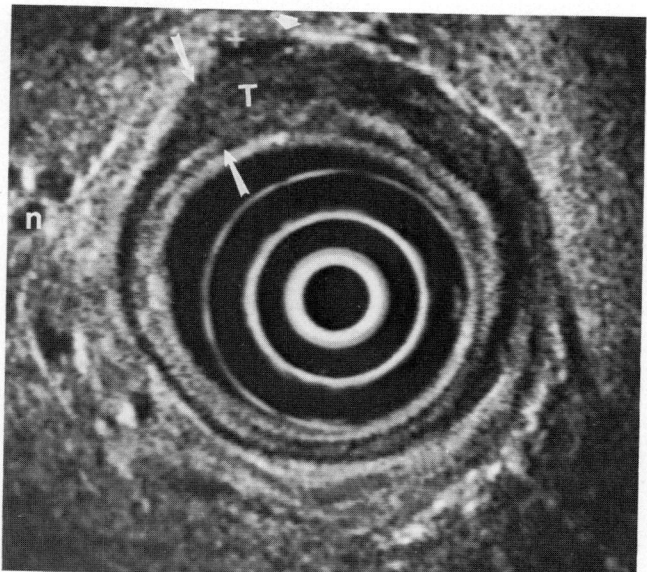

**Figure 10–15. Gastric carcinoma.** EUS of the stomach shows a hypoechoic submucosal lesion (T) *(large arrows)* that extends through the serosa *(small arrow).* Several small hypoechoic nodes (n) are seen adjacent to the stomach.

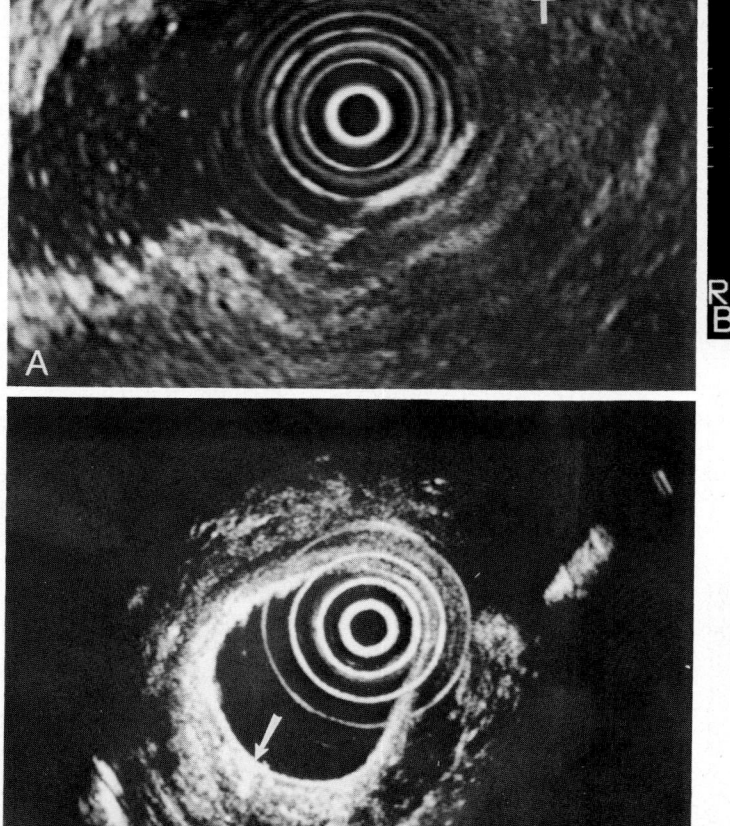

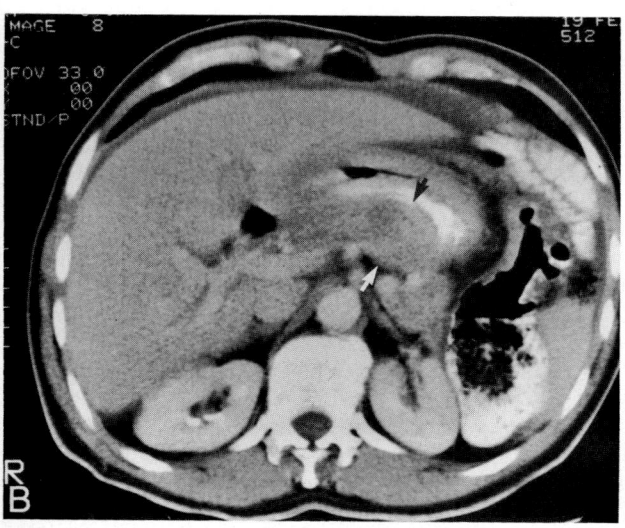

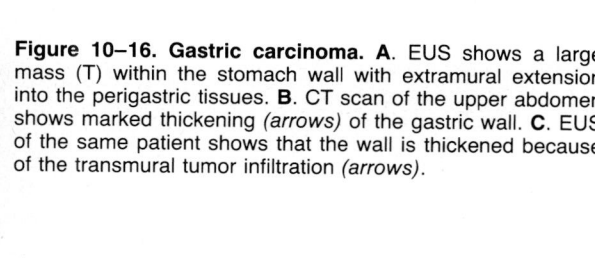

**Figure 10–16. Gastric carcinoma. A**. EUS shows a large mass (T) within the stomach wall with extramural extension into the perigastric tissues. **B**. CT scan of the upper abdomen shows marked thickening *(arrows)* of the gastric wall. **C**. EUS of the same patient shows that the wall is thickened because of the transmural tumor infiltration *(arrows)*.

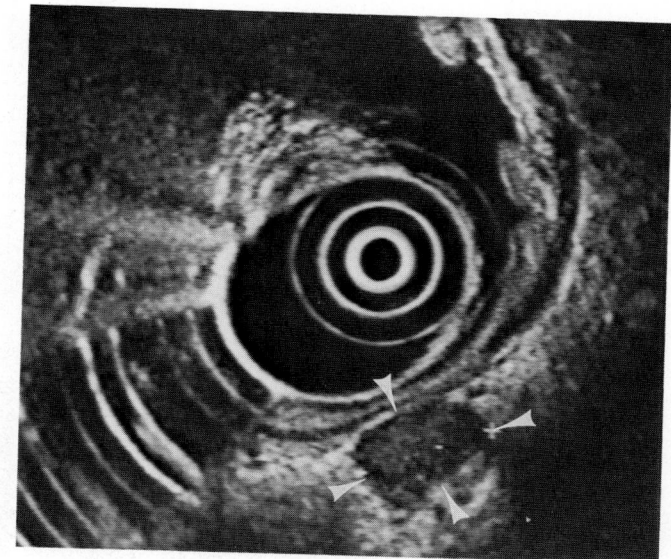

**Figure 10–17. Gastric carcinoma.** Malignant celiac lymph node in a patient with gastric carcinoma *(arrowheads).* Malignant nodes typically are well defined, rounded, and hypoechoic. (Case courtesy of Maria Vilaró, M.D., Bayamón, Puerto Rico.)

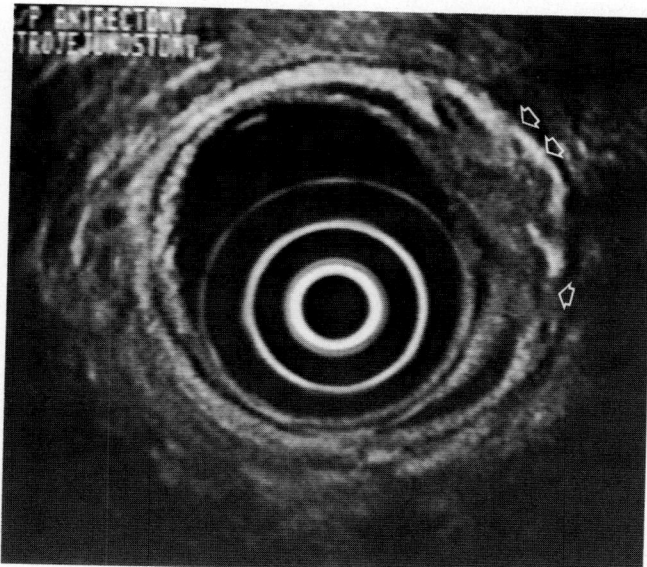

**Figure 10–18. EUS of gastric tumor recurrence.** Gastric recurrence *(arrows)* at anastomosis after antrectomy and gastrojejunostomy. (Case courtesy of Maria Vilaró, M.D., Bayamón, Puerto Rico.)

**Figure 10–19. Gastric lymphoma.** EUS of a gastric lymphoma shows circumscribed, hypoechoic thickening of the gastric wall *(arrowheads)* underlying an endoscopically visible ulceration. (From Bolondi L, Cassanova P, Caletti GC, et al: Primary gastric lymphoma versus gastric carcinoma: endoscopic US evaluation. Radiology 165:821–826, 1987.)

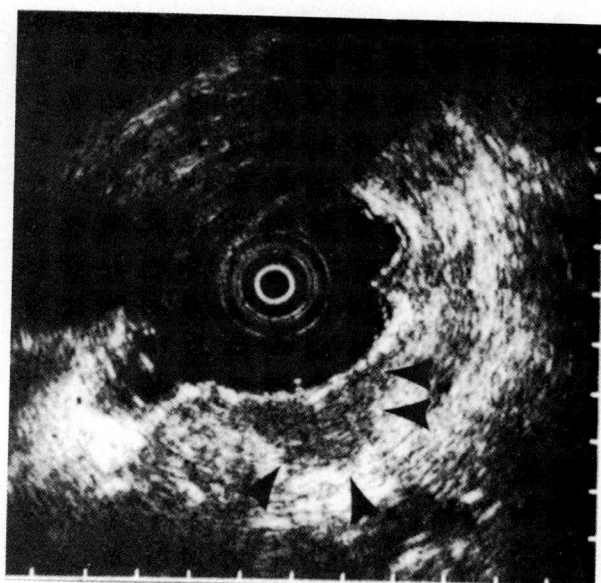

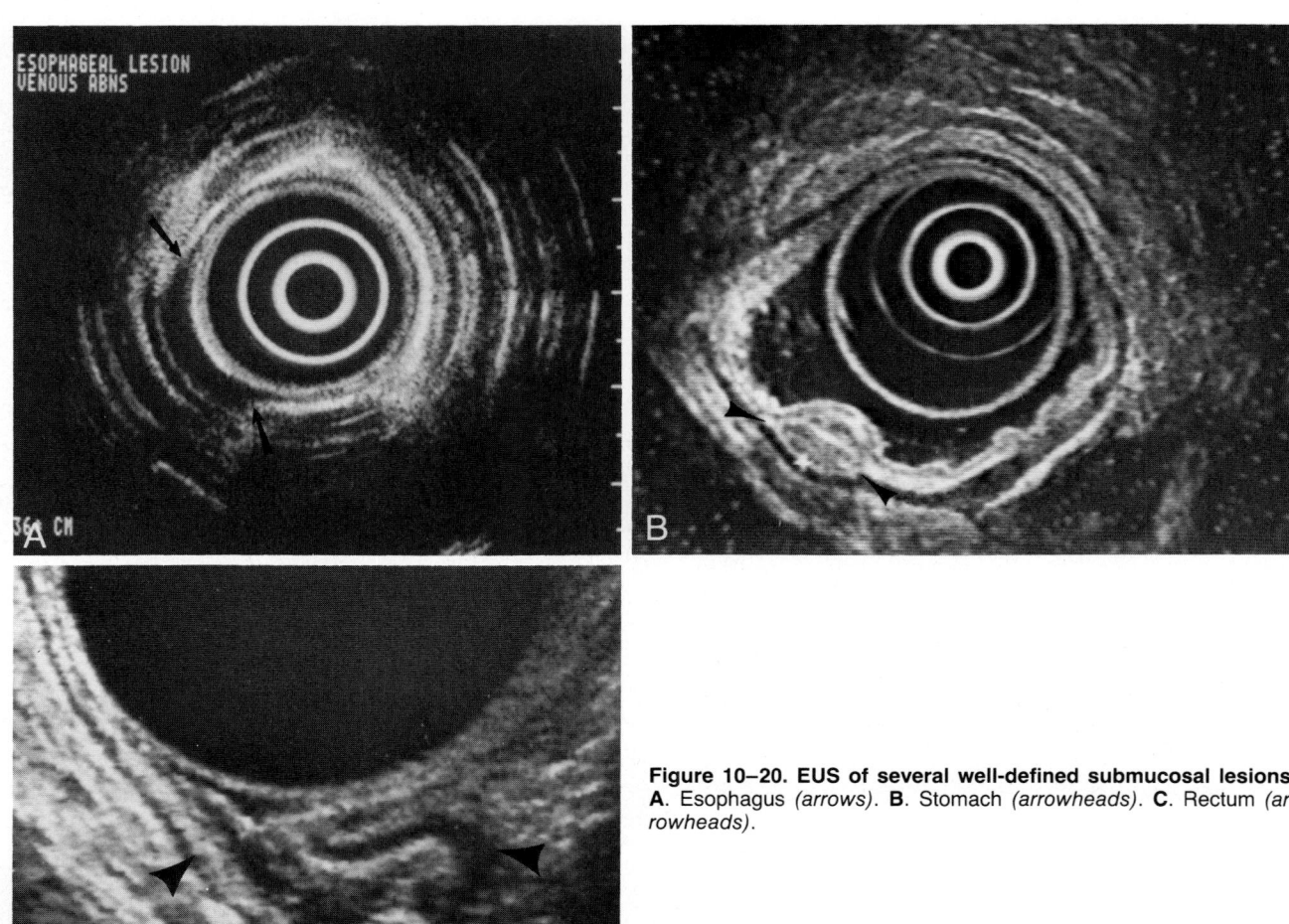

**Figure 10–20. EUS of several well-defined submucosal lesions.**
**A**. Esophagus *(arrows)*. **B**. Stomach *(arrowheads)*. **C**. Rectum *(arrowheads)*.

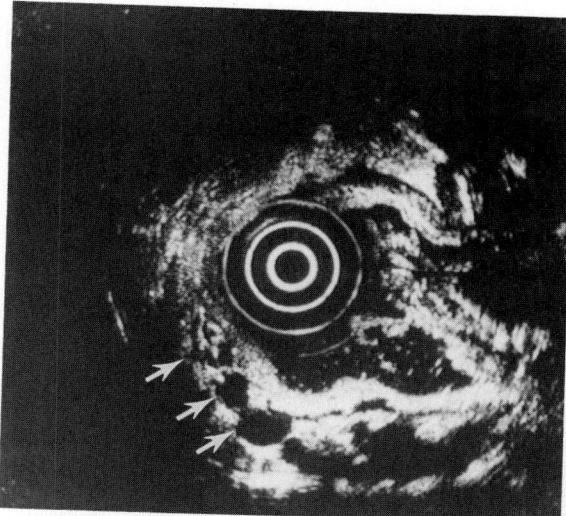

**Figure 10–21. Gastric varices.** EUS of the stomach shows anechoic serpinginous submucosal and extramural lesions *(arrows)*.

be differentiated from pancreatic neoplasms except when there is deep penetration into the adjacent pancreas.[39, 40]

## Colorectum

Colon cancer is one of the most prevalent malignant diseases in the United States, accounting for more than 69,000 deaths annually. Despite advances in diagnostic and surgical techniques, the 5-year survival rate remains at approximately 50%.[41, 42] It is hoped that increased use of cross-sectional imaging and endoscopy for screening and diagnosis of colorectal cancer will help lower the

### TABLE 10–4. TUMOR, NODE, METASTASIS STAGING OF COLORECTAL CANCER BASED ON ENDOSCOPIC ULTRASONOGRAPHY

| STAGE | DESCRIPTION |
| --- | --- |
| T1 | Tumor extends through first three layers of bowel wall |
| T2 | Tumor extends to fourth layer |
| T3 | Tumor extends through outer layer into perirectal fat |
| T4 | Tumor extends to adjacent organs |

mortality rate. Distant metastasis and nodal involvement can be accurately assessed by CT, but preoperative local wall extension is probably best assessed by rectal ultrasonography.[43–46] Anal sphincter preservation operations and multimodality therapy (surgery and radiation) require precise delineation of wall invasion. This information is nicely displayed by EUS.[47]

Colorectal carcinoma is seen as a hypoechoic or isoechoic mass that disrupts the bowel wall layers and spreads toward the perirectal and pericolic tissues. Internal echos may be present if there are areas of fibrosis or calcification (Fig. 10–22). Tumor penetration is staged by the TNM classification (Table 10–4) as well as by lymph node involvement (Figs. 10–23 and 10–24). EUS has an overall accuracy of 85 to 90% for staging this neoplasm.[48, 49]

As found elsewhere in the gut, EUS and CT are limited in the evaluation of lymphadenopathy. Reactive nodes cannot be differentiated from metastatic nodes. EUS is not accurate in evaluating depth of tumor extension because of its limited depth of sound penetration.[50, 51]

Local recurrence is a major concern after surgical resection of the primary colorectal neoplasm. EUS is sensitive in detecting local recurrence (100%) and is superior to endoscopy alone (50%) and CT (33%).[52]

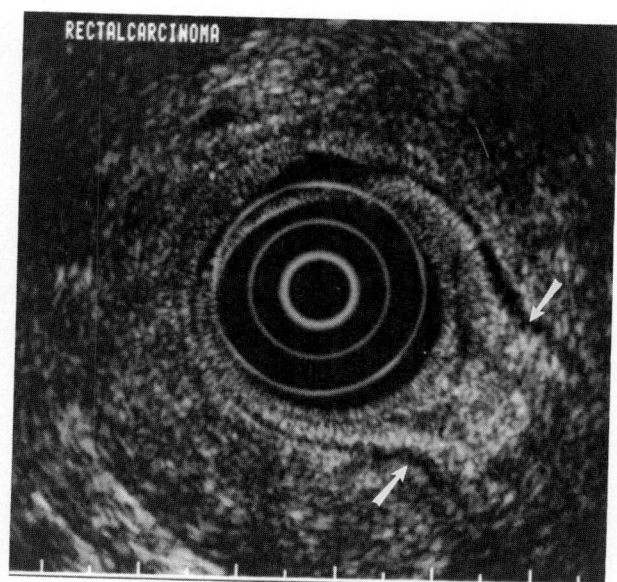

**Figure 10–22. Mural mass: radiation fibrosis.** EUS of patient with history of rectal cancer who received preoperative radiation therapy. There is a hyperechoic mass within the wall of the rectum *(arrows)*.

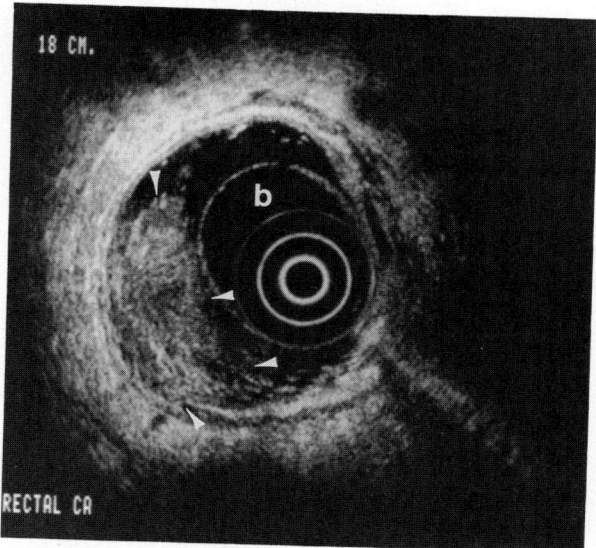

**Figure 10–23. Rectal cancer.** EUS of the rectum using the balloon (b) technique shows a superficial mucosal lesion *(arrowheads)* that extends into the rectal lumen.

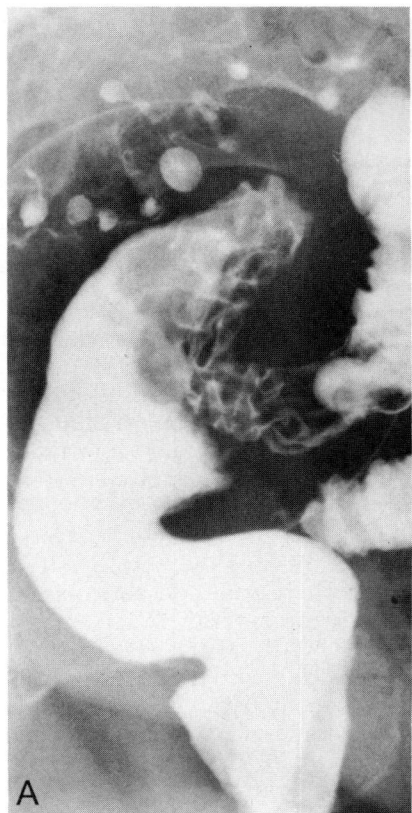

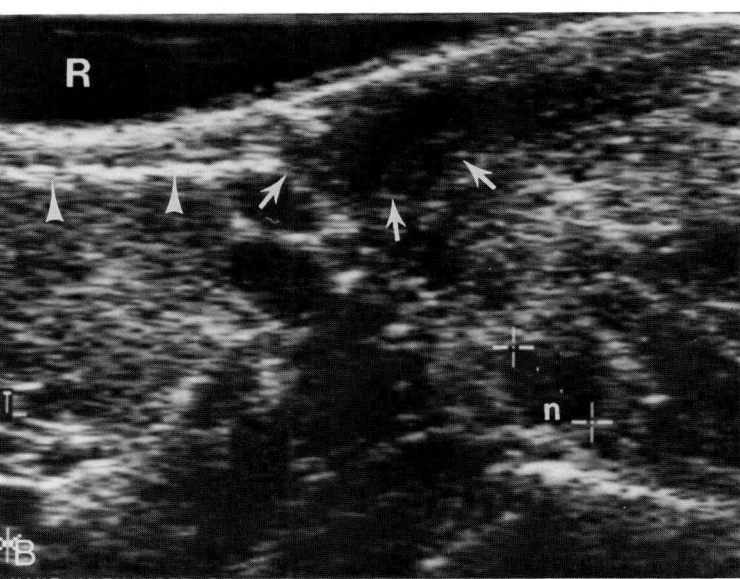

**Figure 10–24. Recurrent rectal cancer.** Patient with history of rectal carcinoma. **A.** Barium enema shows a polypoid mass in the rectum. **B.** Longitudinal view of the rectum (R) using a prostate transducer shows a hypoechoic mass extending to the perirectal soft tissues *(arrows)*. There is a hypoechoic lymph node (n). Note the normal rectal wall *(arrowheads)* and the abrupt transition with tumor.

False-positive findings occur in the presence of fibrosis or inflammation, and biopsy is needed for histologic confirmation. After abdominoperineal resection of rectal cancer, magnetic resonance or CT should be routinely used to detect tumor recurrence.

### TABLE 10–5. INDICATIONS FOR ENDOSCOPIC ULTRASONOGRAPHY

| REGION | INDICATION |
|---|---|
| Esophagus | Cancer staging |
| | Tumor recurrence |
| | Submucosal tumors |
| | Esophageal varices |
| |   Diagnosis |
| |   Treatment follow-up |
| Stomach | Adenocarcinoma |
| |   Staging |
| |   Local recurrence |
| |   Diagnosis |
| | Lymphoma |
| |   Staging |
| |   Diagnosis |
| | Submucosal tumors |
| | Gastric varices |
| |   Diagnosis |
| |   Treatment follow-up |
| Duodenum | Ampullary carcinoma |
| |   Staging |
| | Submucosal tumors |
| Colon-rectum | Carcinoma |
| |   Staging |
| |   Local recurrence |
| | Inflammatory disease |

EUS has also been used in evaluating inflammatory diseases of the colon. The findings are not specific and can be seen in both acute and chronic inflammatory processes. There is diffuse mural thickening of the bowel with preservation of the normal layers.[53, 54]

In general, higher-frequency transducers allow superior visualization of small tumors, adjacent lymph nodes, and local tumor invasion, and low-frequency transducers are better in assessing distant lymph nodes and perirectal disease.[48]

## CONCLUSIONS

The clinical applications of EUS are expanding (Table 10–5). The technique should become an increasingly important imaging procedure for clinical TNM staging and planning treatment strategy. There are still some limitations of the technique, but with technical improvements the clinical utility of EUS should increase.

## References

1. DiMagno EP, Regan PT, Clain JE, et al: Human endoscopic ultrasonography. Gastroenterology 83:824–829, 1982.
2. Tio TL, Tytgat GNJ: Endoscopic ultrasonography of normal and pathologic upper gastrointestinal wall structure. Comparison of studies in vivo and in vitro with histology. Scand J Gastroenterol 21(suppl 123):27–33, 1986.
3. Tio TL: Endosonography in Gastroenterology. Berlin: Springer-Verlag, 1988.
4. Tio TL, Schouwink MH, Cikot RJLM, et al: Preoperative TNM

classification of gastric carcinoma by endosonography in comparison with the pathological TNM system: a prospective study of 72 cases. Hepatogastroenterology 36:51–56, 1989.

5. Hermanek P, Sobin LH: International Union Against Cancer: TNM Classification of Malignant Tumors. Berlin: Springer-Verlag, 1987.

6. Sobin LH, Hermanek P, Hutter RVP: TNM classification of malignant tumors: a comparison between the new (1987) and the old editions. Cancer 61:2310–2314, 1988.

7. Tio TL, Coene PPLO, Schouwink MH, et al: Esophagogastric carcinoma: preoperative TNM classification with endosonography. Radiology 173:411–417, 1989.

8. Spiessl B, Beahrs OH, Hermanek P, et al: International Union Against Cancer (UICC): TNM Atlas (3rd ed). Berlin: Springer-Verlag, 1989, pp 118–133.

9. Caletti G, Bolondi L, Barbara L: Instrumentation and scanning techniques. *In* Kawai K (ed): Endoscopic Ultrasonography in Gastroenterology. Tokyo: Igaku-Shoin, 1988, pp 1–96.

10. Rifkin MD: Endoscopic ultrasonography of the gastrointestinal tract. *In* Rifkin MD (ed): Intraoperative and Endoscopic Ultrasonography. New York: Churchill-Livingstone, 1987, pp 167–189.

11. Fornage BD: Endosonography. *In* Rifkin MD (ed): Upper Abdominal Endoscopic Sonography. Boston: Kluwer Academic Publishers, 1989, pp 9–23.

12. Caletti GC, Bolondi L, Zani L, et al: Technique of endoscopic ultrasonography investigation: esophagus, stomach and duodenum. Scand J Gastroenterol 21(suppl 123):1–5, 1986.

12a. Rosch T, Lorenz R, Danoggier H, et al: Endoscopic diagnosis of submucosal upper gastrointestinal tract tumors. Scand J Gastroenterol 27:1–8, 1992.

13. Botet JF, Lightdale CJ: Endoscopic sonography of the upper gastrointestinal tract. AJR 156:63–68, 1991.

14. Lightdale CJ: Normal EUS anatomy: esophagus and stomach. *In* Endoscopic Ultrasonography: A Tutorial. Cleveland, OH: Cleveland Clinic Foundation, 1991, pp 43–56.

15. Hidelbrandt U, Feifel G, Ecker K: Rectal ultrasonography. Baillieres Clin Gastroenterol 3:531–541, 1989.

16. Van Dam J: Endoscopic ultrasonography (EUS): instrumentation. *In* Endoscopic Ultrasonography: A Tutorial. Cleveland, OH: Cleveland Clinic Foundation, 1991, pp 5–15.

17. Rosch T, Lorenz R, Suchy R, et al: Colonic endoscopic ultrasonography: first results of a new technique. Gastrointest Endosc 36:382–386, 1990.

18. Rosch T, Lorenz R, Classen M: Endoscopic rectal disease. Gastrointest Endosc 22:31–34, 1990.

19. Nickl NJ, Cotton PB: Clinical application of endoscopic ultrasonography. Am J Gastroenterol 85:675–682, 1990.

20. Kimmey MB, Martin RW, Hagitt RC, et al: Histologic correlates of gastrointestinal ultrasound images. Gastroenterology 96:433–441, 1989.

21. Bolondi L, Caletti GC, Casanova P, et al: Problems and variations in the interpretations of the ultrasound feature of the normal upper and lower GI tract wall. Scand J Gastroenterol 21(suppl 123):16–26, 1986.

22. Bolondi L, Casanova P, Santi V, et al: The sonographic appearance of the normal gastric wall: an in vitro study. Ultrasound Med Biol 12:991–998, 1986.

23. Torres GM, Ros PR, Kaude J, et al: High-frequency ultrasound—subgross pathologic correlation in colorectal and gastric adenocarcinoma. *In* 17th International Congress of Radiology, July 1–8, 1989, Paris, France, p 246.

24. Caletti G: Normal EUS anatomy: the gut wall. *In* Endoscopic Ultrasonography: A Tutorial. Cleveland, OH: Cleveland Clinic Foundation, 1991, pp 35–42.

25. Bolondi L, Caletti GC, Barbara L: Endoscopic sonography of the esophagus. *In* Fornage BD (ed): Endosonography. Boston: Kluwer Academic Publishers, 1989, pp 25–34.

26. Rosch T: Experience with staging of esophageal cancer. *In* Endoscopic Ultrasonography: A Tutorial. Cleveland, OH: Cleveland Clinic Foundation, 1991, pp 113–124.

27. Tio TL, Tytgat GNJ: Endoscopic ultrasonography in analysing peri-intestinal lymph node abnormality: preliminary results of studies in vitro and in vivo. Scand J Gastroenterol 21(suppl 123):158–163, 1986.

28. Dahnert W: Radiology Review Manual. Baltimore: Williams & Wilkins, 1991, pp 399–400.

29. Pointner R, Schwab G, Konigsrainer A, et al: Early cancer of the gastric remnant. Gut 29:298–301, 1988.

30. Abe S, Ogawa N, Nagasue N, et al: Early gastric cancer: results in a general hospital in Japan. World J Surg 8:308–314, 1984.

31. Lightdale C: EUS staging of gastric cancer. *In* Endoscopic Ultrasonography: A Tutorial. Cleveland, OH: Cleveland Clinic Foundation, 1991, pp 219–231.

32. Albe T, Fujimura H, Noguchi T, et al: Endosonographic detection of early gastric cancer. Z Gastroenterol (suppl):71–78, 1989.

33. Rosch T: Staging stomach cancer by EUS: clinical usefulness. *In* Endoscopic Ultrasonography: A Tutorial. Cleveland, OH: Cleveland Clinic Foundation, 1991, pp 205–214.

34. Lightdale CJ, Botet JF, Kelsen DP, et al: Diagnosis of recurrent upper gastrointestinal cancer at the surgical anastomosis by endoscopic ultrasound. Gastrointest Endosc 35:407–412, 1989.

35. Shimm DS, Dosoretz DE, Anderson T, et al: Primary gastric lymphoma: an analysis with emphasis on prognostic factors and radiation therapy. Cancer 52:2044–2048, 1983.

36. Bolondi L, Casanova P, Caletti GC, et al: Primary gastric lymphoma versus gastric carcinoma: endoscopic US evaluation. Radiology 165:821–826, 1987.

37. Botet JF: Endoscopic US in the evaluation of patients with large gastric folds. Radiology 177(P):115, 1990.

38. Boyce G: Subepithelial lesions. *In* Endoscopic Ultrasonography: A Tutorial. Cleveland, OH: Cleveland Clinic Foundation, 1991, pp 163–193.

39. Tio TL, Guido NJ, Tytgat GNJ, et al: Ampullopancreatic carcinoma: preoperative TNM classification with endosonography. Radiology 175:455–461, 1990.

40. Tio TL, Mulder CJJ, Egginx WF: Endosonography in staging early carcinoma of the ampulla of Vater. Gastroenterology 102:1392–1395, 1992.

41. Silverg E: Cancer statistics. Cancer 36:9–25, 1986.

42. Ackerman LV, Del Regato JA: Cancer Diagnosis, Treatment, and Prognosis (4th ed). St. Louis: CV Mosby, 1970, pp 426–464.

43. Rifkin MP, Marks GJ: Transrectal ultrasound as an adjunct in the diagnosis of rectal and extrarectal tumors. Radiology 157:499–502, 1985.

44. Katsura Y, Yamada K, Ishizawa T, et al: Endorectal ultrasonography for the assessment of wall invasion and lymph node metastasis in rectal cancer. Dis Colon Rectum 35:362–368, 1992.

45. Rifkin MP, Ehrlich SM, Marks G: Staging of rectal carcinoma: prospective comparison of endorectal ultrasound and computed tomography. Radiology 170:319–322, 1989.

46. Reading CC: Endorectal sonography. Crit Rev Diagn Imaging 33:1–28, 1992.

47. Mohiuddin M, Derdel J, Marks G, et al: Results of adjuvant radiation therapy in cancer of the rectum. Cancer 55:350–353, 1985.

48. Hawes RH: Staging colorectal cancer by ultrasonography. *In* Endoscopic Ultrasonography: A Tutorial. Cleveland, OH: Cleveland Clinic Foundation, 1991, pp 263–267.

49. Tschmlitsch J, Glaser K, Schwarz C, et al: Endosonography (ES) in the diagnosis of recurrent cancer of the rectum. J Ultrasound Med 11:149–153, 1992.

50. Tio TL: TNM classification of colorectal carcinoma by endosonography (ES): preoperative staging and follow-up. *In* Endoscopic Ultrasonography: A Tutorial. Cleveland, OH: Cleveland Clinic Foundation, 1991, pp 255–262.

51. Mortenson N: Rectal and anal sonography. Gut 33:148–149, 1992.

52. Rosch T: Colonic endosonography. *In* Endoscopic Ultrasonography: A Tutorial. Cleveland, OH: Cleveland Clinic Foundation, 1991, pp 277–289.

53. Candio GD, Mosca F, Fornage B: Endosonography of the rectum. *In* Fornage BD (ed): Endosonography. Boston: Kluwer Academic Publishers, 1989, pp 43–69.

54. Hill MC, Smith LE, Huntington DK, et al: Endorectal sonography in the evaluation of the rectum. Ultrasound Q 10:29–56, 1992.

# Introduction to Angiography of the Hollow Viscera

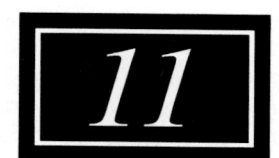

Albert A. Nemcek, Jr., M.D.

Robert L. Vogelzang, M.D.

## INTRODUCTION

The role of angiography in the diagnosis and treatment of gastrointestinal disease has significantly changed in the last two decades. This reflects, in part, newer and more effective methods of care of patients. The incidence of gastrointestinal bleeding, for example, has decreased because of improved medical therapy, particularly the use of $H_2$ blockers. In addition, more sophisticated endoscopic equipment and therapies and cross-sectional imaging have resulted in fewer indications for both diagnostic and therapeutic angiographic procedures. Nevertheless, certain disorders are still best evaluated and/or treated angiographically. This chapter provides general technical and procedural points about gastrointestinal angiography as well as a discussion of the vascular anatomy of the hollow viscera.

## PREPARATION OF PATIENTS

Certain preprocedural steps can enhance the ease and diagnostic quality of a visceral angiogram. When the study is ordered on an elective basis, a standard bowel cleansing should be considered to delineate vessels and pathologic findings more clearly. Intravenous administration of glucagon (1.0 mg) at the time of the procedure is helpful in reducing the effects of bowel motion, particularly in studies utilizing digital subtraction.[1]

A Foley catheter placed to drain the bladder is useful in studies of the inferior mesenteric artery (IMA) because a contrast agent filling the bladder can obscure vascular visualization. It also increases the patient's comfort and helps prevent unnecessary delays during long examinations.

Unless contraindicated, we routinely premedicate patients undergoing visceral angiography with fentanyl (Sublimaze) and midazolam (Versed) in an attempt to achieve the analgesic, anxiolytic, and amnestic effects of these combined agents while maintaining the patient's ability to cooperate. All patients have intraprocedural monitoring of pulse, electrocardiogram, arterial oxygenation (via a pulse oximeter), and blood pressure.

## TECHNICAL FACTORS

### Vascular Access

In general, the femoral arterial route of catheterization is used for abdominal aortography as well as selective visceral angiography; the safety and ease of this approach are well established. The brachial or axillary route may be necessary or helpful in cases of difficult femoral access or when there is a need to advance a catheter more deeply into a vessel that has a steep downgoing course.

### Catheter Selection

Our catheter of choice for celiac and superior mesenteric arteriography is a simple angled visceral hook with a single side hole; for inferior mesenteric arteriography we prefer a catheter with a short curved tip (Rösch inferior mesenteric). We also make frequent use of cobra-shaped catheters. For most indications, 5 French catheters are used to minimize puncture site complications. These sometimes fail to provide a stable catheter position, especially with high flow rates and volumes of injection. If multiple catheter exchanges are anticipated, we place an angiographic sheath with a check flow valve in the femoral artery to facilitate the exchanges.

Advances in guidewire and catheter technology have made subselective catheterization of visceral vessels easier. These advances include the development of flexible torque control guidewires such as the Terumo Glidewire (Medi-Tech, Watertown, MA) and the Wholey Hi-Torque wire (Advanced Cardiovascular Systems, Mountain View, CA) and of catheters such as the Tracker catheter (Target Therapeutics, San Jose, CA), which have low coefficients of friction that allow them more readily to follow wires around complex or tight curves.

## Equipment

Although advances in digital subtraction arteriography (DSA) have increased the utility of this technique for peripheral angiography, DSA is used less extensively for visceral angiography. This is largely due to the greater potential for misregistration artifacts secondary to breathing, motion of the patient, and bowel peristalsis, which impair the diagnostic quality of the study, as well as the inferior spatial resolution inherent in current DSA technology. Nevertheless, investigators have assessed the role of DSA for gastrointestinal hemorrhage and arterial portography and have found that this technique is diagnostically useful and has certain advantages over standard techniques: shorter time of examination, limitation of contrast agent dose, increased contrast resolution, and savings on cost of film.[2–5] For cooperative patients without significant bowel peristalsis, we consider DSA an excellent method for performing arterial portography (Fig. 11–1). We also prefer DSA for the initial portions of studies performed to evaluate mesenteric ischemia because it provides a rapid screen for patency of major mesenteric vessels. However, the search for small emboli in this setting generally requires the improved spatial resolution of standard filming. For gastrointestinal bleeding, DSA can sometimes provide extremely rapid localization of a bleeding site. Unfor-

tunately, many patients with acute bleeding are restless and uncooperative, making interpretation of digital subtraction studies difficult at best. Finally, if an abnormality requiring intervention has already been identified, DSA offers superior procedural guidance.[2–5]

## ANGIOGRAPHY OF THE MAJOR VISCERAL VESSELS

Visceral angiography begins with injection of contrast medium into the aorta or into one of the three major abdominal visceral vessels: the celiac artery, the superior mesenteric artery (SMA), or the IMA. Aortic injection is usually limited to situations in which there is a suspicion of severe narrowing or occlusion of one or more of the origins of the major visceral vessels: in patients with acute or chronic intestinal ischemia clinically or those with severe aortic atherosclerosis. In these cases, attempts at selective catheterization may cause damage to visceral arteries.

It is helpful at the beginning of any procedure to consider the questions that need to be answered by the angiogram and how best to answer them. The order of examination of the visceral vessels depends on the clinical situation. For example, in the search for a site of gastrointestinal bleeding, the patient's clinical history and the results of prior diagnostic studies should be carefully evaluated. Angiography should then begin with the vessel most likely to be bleeding. It is also critical not to perform too limited a study despite what might seem to be reasonable indications. Again, using the example of gastrointestinal bleeding, a patient who has clear clinical and endoscopic evidence for acute hemorrhage into the colon may nonetheless have a bleeding source in the celiac territory.[6]

Before pulling the catheter, the questions asked of the examination should be answered as well as possible given limitations imposed by contrast agent dose and the patient's safety.

Selective catheterization of the visceral arteries can be performed as an initial step or after aortography. The celiac artery generally arises from the aorta anteriorly, at level of middle T-12 to upper L-1. The SMA originates slightly caudal to the celiac trunk. Generally, 7 to 10 mL of contrast medium is injected into these arteries for a total of 35 to 60 mL; the rate is based on test injections. Certain clinical situations require an alteration in these rates and volumes. For example, when evaluation of the mesenteric and portal venous systems is important, particularly in patients with portal hypertension, high rates and volumes are needed (e.g., 8 to 10 mL/s for a total of 80 to 100 mL). For the IMA, which usually arises to the left of midline from the abdominal aorta at the lower aspect of the L-3 vertebral body, injection at a rate of 3 to 4 mL/s for a total of 12 to 16 mL is generally appropriate. Injection rates are proportionately decreased for mesenteric branches.

Filming rates are rapid during the early arterial phase, with progressive slowing as the venous phase is approached. Longer filming is necessary when the venous

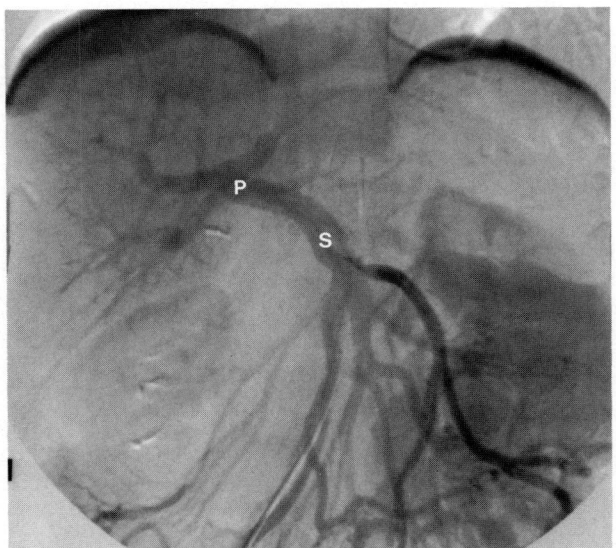

**Figure 11–1. Arterial portography obtained during digital subtraction angiography.** Excellent opacification of the mesenteric and portal venous system is achieved after superior mesenteric arterial injection. S = superior mesenteric vein; P = portal vein.

phase is of particular interest. Our standard filming rate includes an injection delay of 0.7 second after the first film (to obtain a scout), with initial filming at two films per second for 3 seconds, followed by one film per second for 3 seconds, followed by one film every 3 seconds for 6 to 30 seconds, depending on the indication for the study. When using digital subtraction, we generally record images at a fixed rate of two to three per second for an appropriate period.

## Arterial Anatomy of Specific Segments of the Gut

The vascular anatomy of the hollow abdominal viscera is quite complex. We have utilized a number of excellent general references in preparing this chapter; the reader is referred to these for more detailed discussions of angiographic and gross anatomy and of the embryologic basis for many of the observed anatomic variations.[7–12] Vascular anatomy of the solid abdominal organs is discussed in Chapters 101, 103, 113, 114, 122, and 123.

### *Esophagus*

From a practical standpoint, only the arterial supply of the distal esophagus is important for angiographers because the lower esophagus and gastroesophageal junction can be a site of arterial hemorrhage potentially

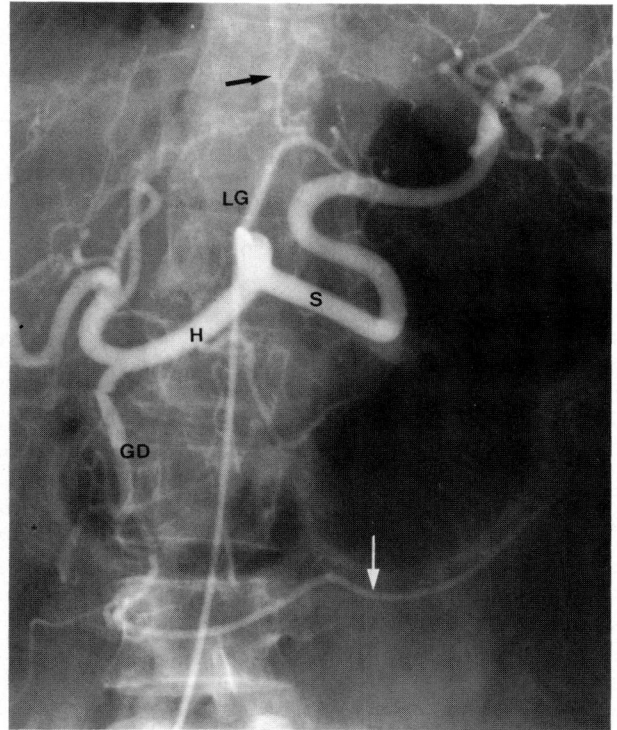

**Figure 11–2. Celiac arteriogram.** LG = left gastric artery; H = common hepatic artery; S = splenic artery; GD = gastroduodenal artery; black arrow = branches of left gastric artery supplying lower esophagus; white arrow = right gastro-omental artery.

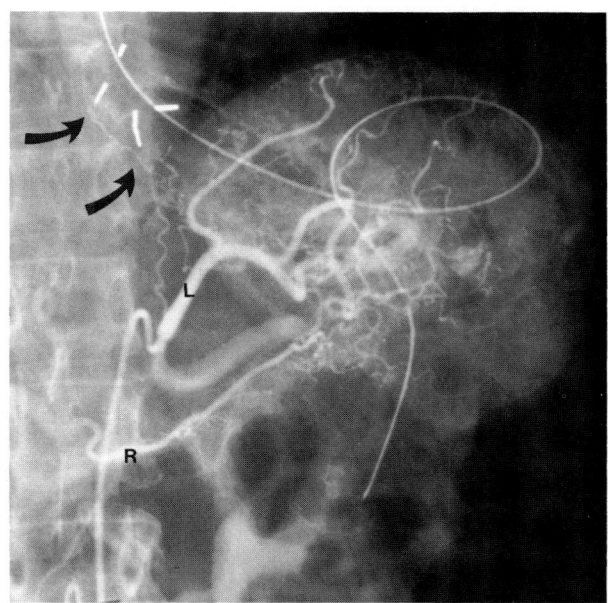

**Figure 11–3. Selective left gastric artery injection.** L = left gastric artery; R = right gastric artery (filling retrograde via left gastric branches); arrows = branches of left gastric artery supplying lower esophagus.

treatable by embolization or vasopressin infusion.[13, 14] This region is typically supplied by branches of the left gastric artery (discussed later) or the left inferior phrenic artery[8, 12, 15–17] (Figs. 11–2 and 11–3).

Catheterization of the upper and middle portions of the esophagus is difficult but fortunately rarely necessary. The cervical esophagus typically receives its arterial supply from the inferior thyroid arteries (branches of the subclavian arteries), with predominant supply from the right. Subclavian, common carotid, or aortic branches may also supply this segment. The thoracic esophageal arteries arise either directly from the aorta or as branches of the intercostal and/or bronchial arteries.[8, 15, 17] Esophageal arteries anastomose along the length of the esophagus.

### *Stomach*

The stomach has two major vascular arcades, one along the lesser curve formed by the right and left gastric arteries and the other along the greater curve consisting of what are commonly termed the right and left gastroepiploic arteries but now are preferably called the right and left gastro-omental arteries.[8, 12, 15, 16]

The left gastric artery (Figs. 11–4 to 11–6; see Figs. 11–2 and 11–3) usually arises as one of the three major branches of the celiac trunk, originating anywhere from the orifice of the trunk to the hepatic splenic bifurcation.[8, 9, 12, 15, 18] In 2 to 6% of patients this vessel arises separately from the aorta.[12, 18, 19]

A replaced or accessory left hepatic artery arises from the left gastric artery in about 20 to 30% of cases.[8, 12, 18, 20] This has important clinical implications in patients for whom embolization or infusion therapy of hepatic

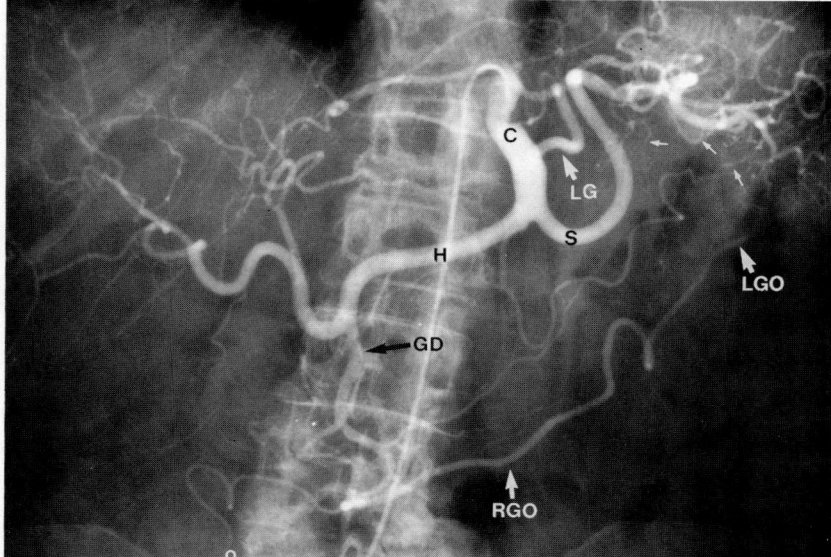

**Figure 11–4. Celiac arteriogram.** C = celiac artery; LG = left gastric artery; GD = gastroduodenal artery; RGO = right gastro-omental artery; LGO = left gastro-omental artery; S = splenic artery; H = common hepatic artery; o = omental branch of right gastro-omental artery; small white arrows = short gastric branches. A well-formed gastro-omental anastomosis is present.

or gastric arteries is anticipated; unintended damage to the stomach or liver could result. When this variant is present, the relative blood supply to the stomach and liver can vary so that minimal supply to either may be present.[18] In about 5% of cases, one or both inferior phrenic arteries arise from the left gastric trunk; this association is much higher when the left gastric artery arises as a separate aortic branch.[18, 20] The importance of this variant is emphasized by the reported association of hypertension and cardiac arrhythmias with vasopressin infusion into the phrenic artery.[21] Accessory left gastric arteries are common.[9, 15]

Because most gastric angiography is performed for diagnosis and treatment of gastrointestinal bleeding and

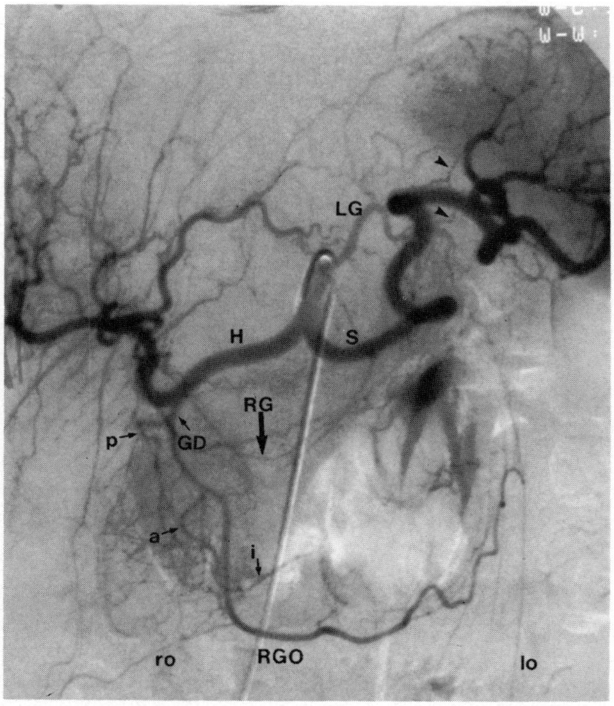

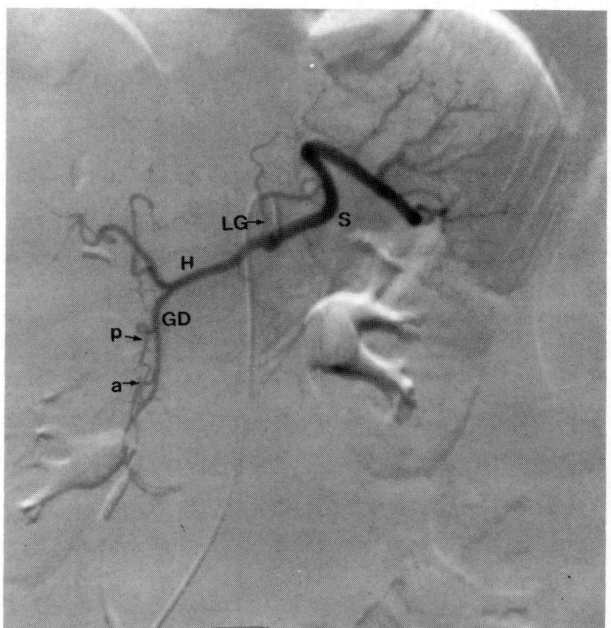

**Figure 11–5. Celiac arteriogram.** LG = left gastric artery; GD = gastroduodenal artery; S = splenic artery; H = common hepatic artery; RGO = right gastro-omental artery (the left gastro-omental is not well opacified); p = posterior superior pancreaticoduodenal branch; a = anterior superior pancreaticoduodenal branch; i = inferior pancreaticoduodenal branch (filling retrograde via pancreaticoduodenal arcades); ro = right omental branch; lo = left omental branch; arrowheads = short gastric branches.

**Figure 11–6. Early arterial phase, celiac arteriogram.** LG = left gastric artery; S = splenic artery; H = common hepatic artery; GD = gastroduodenal artery; p = posterior superior pancreaticoduodenal branch; a = anterior superior pancreaticoduodenal branch.

the left gastric arterial ramifications account for about 85% of gastric hemorrhage,[20] this is clearly an important vessel for subselective catheterization.

Unfortunately, the celiac artery is most readily catheterized with a caudally directed catheter, but the course of the left gastric artery is cephalad. This may make selective catheterization difficult. A number of articles and texts detail methods that facilitate catheterization of this sometimes elusive vessel.[10, 22-26] The basic principle of these methods is initial selection of the celiac artery with a catheter that has a downgoing tip, followed by intraceliac exchange for, conversion to, or coaxial insertion of the catheter with a tip that points upward. Failing direct catheterization of the left gastric artery with the initial selective catheter, we next place a guidewire deeply into the common hepatic or splenic artery and exchange it for a preformed Rösch left gastric catheter. As this catheter is slowly pulled back, small injections of contrast medium are made. The catheter frequently flips into the orifice of the left gastric artery when it is pulled back far enough. If left gastric embolization is needed for hemostasis, a Tracker 18 catheter (Target Therapeutics) and 0.018-inch steerable guidewire can often catheterize the left gastric artery by coaxial placement through a catheter that has engaged the celiac orifice. This catheter, however, is expensive and cannot accommodate sufficient flow and volume of contrast medium to provide studies of diagnostic quality.

The right gastric artery (see Figs. 11–3 and 11–5) is a small and generally unimportant vessel for arteriographers. In 98% of cases it arises at or distal to the common hepatic artery bifurcation, usually from the proper hepatic but occasionally from left or right hepatic branches, at the origin or proximal portion of the gastroduodenal artery.[12]

The right gastro-omental artery (see Figs. 11–2, 11–4, and 11–5) is typically the larger of the two gastro-omental vessels. It is the terminal branch of the gastroduodenal artery. The left gastro-omental artery (see Fig. 11–4) arises from either the main splenic artery or a splenic arterial branch, usually an inferior branch. These two vessels anastomose in a well-formed arcade along the greater curve of the stomach in 65 to 75% of cases; in most other instances an anastomosis is still present but not as well developed. In slightly fewer than half of individuals, a parallel anastomotic arcade called the arc of Barkow is present in the greater omentum, joining right and left omental arteries (see Figs. 11–4, and 11–5), which are branches (respectively) of the right and left gastro-omental arteries.[12, 15, 27]

The supply from the gastric and gastro-omental arcades is supplemented by a number of other branches. A variable number of short gastric arteries (see Figs. 11–4 and 11–5) supply the fundus and superior aspect of the greater curve of the stomach and originate most often from splenic hilar vessels. In 36 to 60% of individuals, a posterior gastric artery arises from the main splenic artery to supply the posterior wall of the stomach as well as parts of the fundus and gastroesophageal junction.[8, 12, 15, 28] The pyloric region typically receives part of its supply via branches of the gastroduodenal artery.

## Small Bowel

Much of the blood supply to the duodenum is via a series of freely anastomosing vessels: the anterior and posterior pancreaticoduodenal arcades provide a rich source of collaterals for the duodenum and head of the pancreas and between the celiac artery and the SMA.[8-12, 15] These arcades (usually dual but occasionally more numerous) form a continuous loop along the descending and transverse duodenum and the pancreatic head. The superior origin of this complex is usually dual, both branches of the gastroduodenal artery, with the posterior arcade typically arising more cephalad than the anterior (Fig. 11–7; see Figs. 11–5 and 11–6). The inferior origin is most often a single trunk (see Figs. 11–5 and 11–7), usually arising from the SMA or its first or second jejunal branch.

Other sources of duodenal blood supply are branches of the right gastro-omental artery, the supraduodenal artery (which has many possible origins including the hepatic artery, the gastroduodenal artery, the posterior pancreaticoduodenal arcade, or the right gastric artery), and smaller gastroduodenal branches.

In addition to the pancreaticoduodenal arcades, another potential collateral route between the celiac and superior mesenteric territories is the arc of Bühler, which represents persistence of an embryologic anastomosis between the celiac and superior mesenteric trunks.[10, 15, 27]

The jejunum and ileum are supplied primarily by multiple branches arising from the left side of the SMA (Figs. 11–8 and 11–9); the level of the ileocolic artery origin is a good general indicator of the division between jejunal and ileal territories. The distal ileum also re-

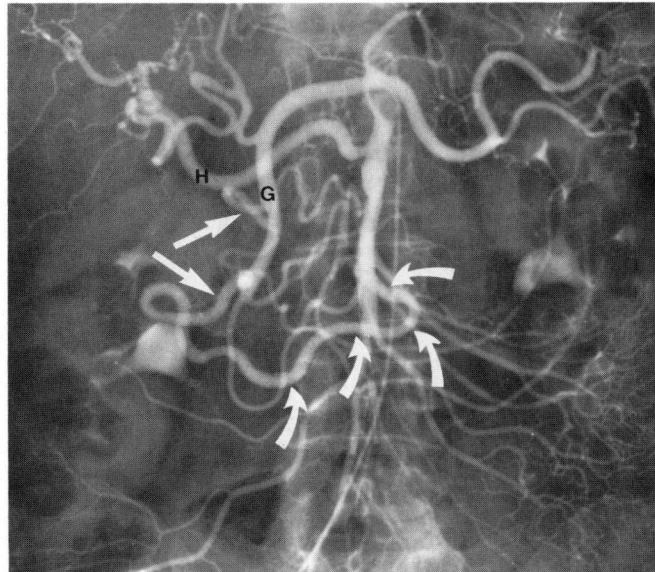

**Figure 11–7. Superior mesenteric arteriogram.** There are enlarged pancreaticoduodenal arcades that provide collaterals to the celiac territory in a patient with occlusion of the proximal celiac artery. Inferior pancreaticoduodenal branch *(curved arrows)* arises from the SMA and anastomoses with superior pancreaticoduodenal branches *(straight arrows)* to reconstitute the gastroduodenal artery (G). H = replaced right hepatic artery arising from the SMA.

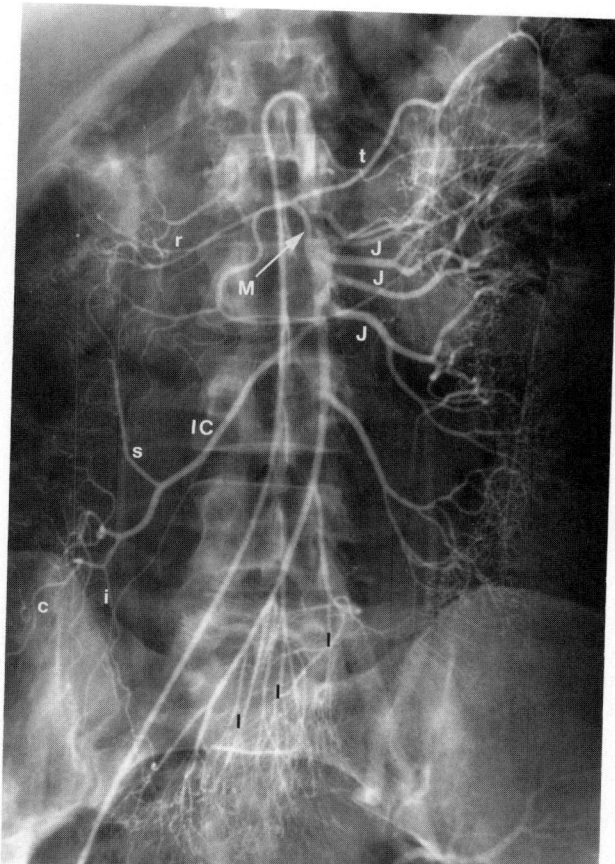

**Figure 11–8. Superior mesenteric arteriogram.** J = jejunal branches; I = ileal branches; IC = ileocolic artery; s = superior colic branch of the ileocolic artery, supplying the ascending colon and anastomosing with branches of the middle colic artery; c = cecal branches of ileocolic artery; i = ileal branch of ileocolic artery, anastomosing with terminal branches of the main superior mesenteric trunk; M = middle colic artery, with branches to the right colonic flexure (r) and the transverse colon (t).

ceives blood from the ileocolic artery (discussed later). There is an extensive network of vascular arcades connecting the jejunal and ileal branches; along the mesenteric border of the small bowel the distal arcades give rise to multiple straight vasa recta that enter the bowel wall. Palmaz and colleagues have noted that the number of arcades increases and the length of the vasa recta decreases more distally in the small bowel and that these anatomic factors must be considered when performing small bowel embolization.[29]

## Colon and Rectum

The right colon and transverse colon are usually supplied by the SMA. Most anatomic descriptions note three main branches: the ileocolic, the right colic, and the middle colic arteries.[8–11, 15] However, in their excellent treatises VanDamme and associates have noted that although the ileocolic is a constant vessel, a true right colic artery is uncommon and the middle colic "artery" frequently is variable in extent and branching pattern, consisting of one or more of five distinct vessels.[12, 30]

The ileocolic artery (see Figs. 11–8 and 11–9) supplies the transition between the small bowel and colon, with branches to the terminal ileum, the cecum, the ascending colon, and the appendix. It is the last branch arising from the right side of the superior mesenteric trunk and is constant enough to be an important angiographic landmark. Most often it consists of a main stem branching into two cecal branches distally, with anastomotic branches arising along the main stem.[12] A nearly constant branch of the ileocolic artery is the superior colic, which anastomoses with the next colic artery arising from the SMA, whether the right colic or part of the middle colic complex.

A true right colic artery, defined as one arising directly from the superior mesenteric trunk and supplying the middle portion of the ascending colon, has been found by VanDamme and Bonte in only 13% of individuals.[12, 30] This portion of the ascending colon is usually supplied via an arcade formed by the ileocolic artery and the middle colic system.[12, 30]

The middle colic artery has been classically described as the major proximal branch of the SMA that supplies the right colonic flexure and transverse colon.[8–11, 15] VanDamme and colleagues have observed a true middle colic artery in slightly fewer than half of their cases. In other instances, variant arteries or combinations of these arteries supply the vascular territory between the ileocolic or right colic artery and the left colic artery; a single vessel is present 75% of the time (see Figs. 11–8 and 11–9).

The middle colic artery or accessory arteries to the

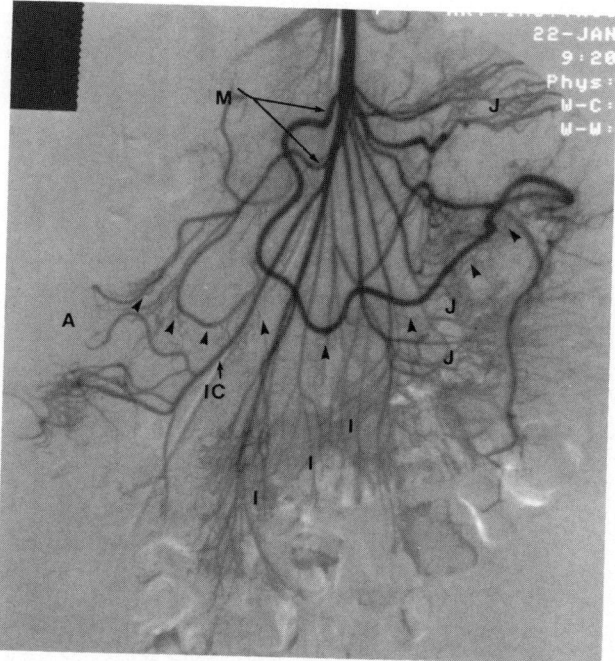

**Figure 11–9. Superior mesenteric arteriogram.** The middle colic territory *(arrowheads)* is supplied by two anastomosing superior mesenteric branches (M, *arrows*), one of which supplies the right colonic flexure and the other the mid- to distal transverse colon. No discrete right colic artery to the ascending colon is present. IC = ileocolic artery; J = jejunal branches; I = ileal branches; A = postion of ascending colon.

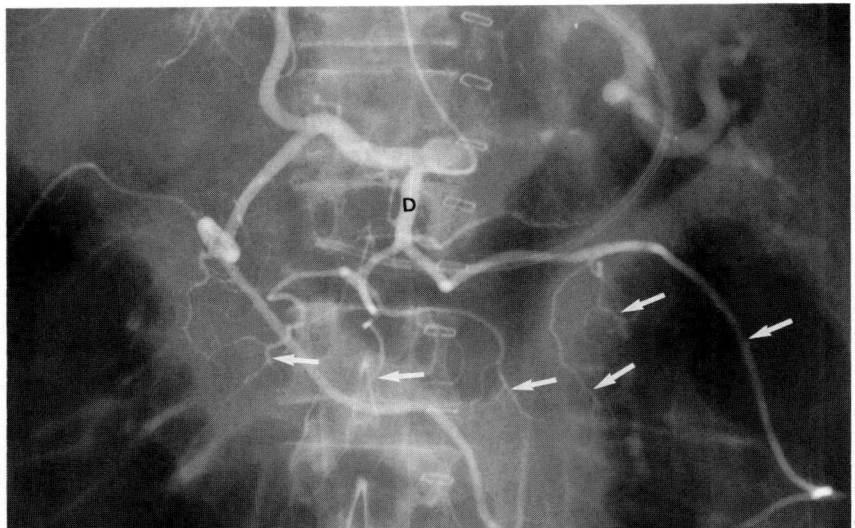

**Figure 11–10. Variant middle colic supply.** Celiac injection reveals an enlarged dorsal pancreatic artery (D), from which branches arise that course to the middle colic territory and the transverse mesocolon *(arrows)*.

middle colic territory can arise from the celiac, splenic, hepatic, or pancreatic arteries (especially the dorsal pancreatic artery)[10–12, 15, 30] (Fig. 11–10). Thus, angiographic assessment of the entire colon may require injection of the celiac artery or its branches.

In unusual situations, portions of the blood supply to the colon can arise directly from the aorta between the origins of the SMA and IMA.[31–33] In two radiologic publications, such a variant has been called the "middle mesenteric artery," although in one the artery supplied the distal transverse and proximal descending colon and in the other the artery supplied the entire proximal colon up to and including the splenic flexure.[31, 32]

The IMA (Figs. 11–11 to 11–14) most often supplies the left colonic flexure, the descending colon, the sigmoid colon, and the upper rectum.[8, 10–12, 15, 34] However,

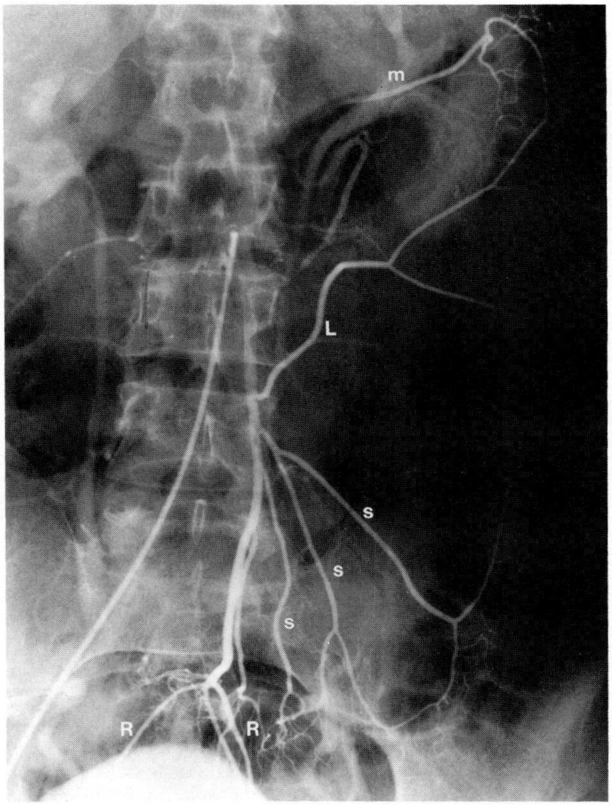

**Figure 11–11. Inferior mesenteric arteriogram.** L = left colic artery; s = sigmoid branches; R = superior rectal (hemorrhoidal) arteries; m = partial filling of middle colic territory via marginal artery.

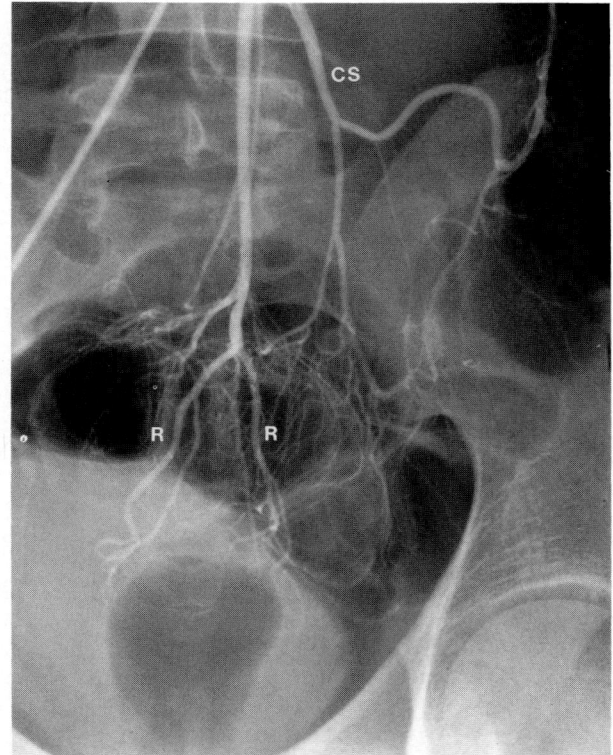

**Figure 11–12. Caudal branches of inferior mesenteric trunk.** CS = colosigmoid trunk; R = superior rectal (hemorrhoidal) arteries.

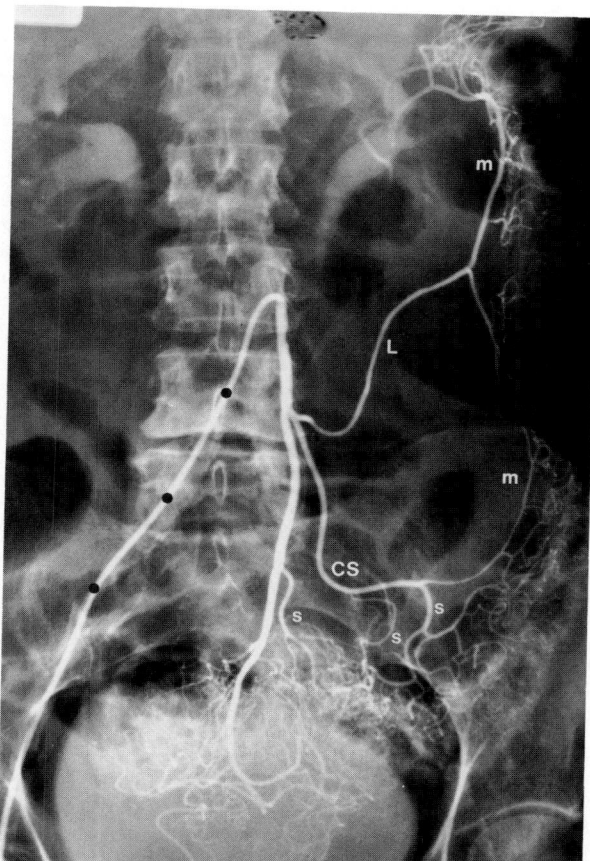

**Figure 11–13. Inferior mesenteric arteriogram.** L = left colic artery; CS = colosigmoid branch; s = sigmoid branches; m = marginal artery; black dots = selective catheter.

of the IMA origin in the elderly. The terminology can be confusing. The marginal artery of Drummond[10, 11, 15, 35, 36] (Figs. 11–15 and 11–16; see Figs. 11–11, 11–13, and 11–14) designates a vascular arcade that runs along the mesenteric border of the colon, where it gives off its nutrient vessels. Defined in this way, the major colic arteries can parallel the marginal artery or constitute part of it.[10, 11, 15, 35, 36] The paracolic arcade can be considered part of the generalized system of paraintestinal arcades present throughout the abdominal gastrointestinal tract.[12, 37] An enlarged marginal artery frequently provides a collateral pathway between the SMA and IMA territories (see Figs. 11–15 and 11–16). The marginal artery is not always reliably complete along its entire length. Griffith's point, for example, represents an area of a potentially poor anastomotic connection between the SMA territory and the marginal artery of the descending colon at the splenic flexure.[36] The arc of Riolan refers to a more central anastomotic pathway within the mesentery between the IMA and SMA.[10, 11, 15, 27, 35] The term "meandering mesenteric artery" has also been used.[38] According to VanDamme and Bonte, this actually represents an enlarged and tortuous left colic artery (see Figs. 11–15 and 11–16) acting as part of a collateral pathway.[12]

The more distal rectum is supplied by branches of the internal iliac artery.[8, 12, 34, 39] As is the case with the most proximal portion of the gut, angiography of this region is infrequently performed. Collateralization via the rectal arteries between the IMA and the internal iliac

the boundary between the parts of the colon supplied by the SMA and the IMA can be variable—proximal or distal to the splenic flexure. The IMA terminates in two superior rectal (hemorrhoidal) branches (see Figs. 11–11 and 11–12). It gives off branches from its left side. The first is the left colic artery (see Figs. 11–11, 11–13, and 11–14), which courses toward the splenic flexure. Its branches anastomose with branches of the middle colic territory (see Figs. 11–11 and 11–14). The left colic artery is frequently absent if there is an accessory left colic vessel arising as a portion of the middle colic supply.[12, 34] Other branches arise from the left colic artery or the IMA trunk proximal to the superior rectal arteries to supply the descending and sigmoid colon and the upper rectum. A colosigmoid artery or branch (see Figs. 11–12 and 11–13) can usually be identified as a large vessel supplying the transition between the descending colon and sigmoid.[12, 34]

Potential anastomotic pathways between the superior and inferior mesenteric supply to the colon are often discussed in the angiographic literature. They can occur in cases of proximal superior mesenteric or inferior mesenteric stenosis or occlusion or when there is stenosis of occlusion of the abdominal aorta between the SMA and IMA. On arteriograms, they are most commonly noted as a manifestation of atherosclerotic involvement

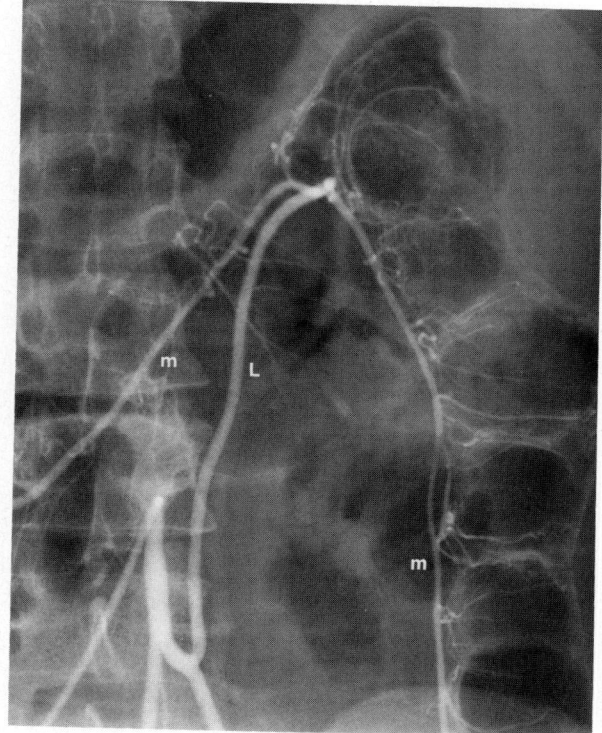

**Figure 11–14. Inferior mesenteric injection.** Left colic artery (L) ascends toward left colonic flexure, and the marginal artery (m) is opacified in a continuous fashion from the transverse colon to the descending colon.

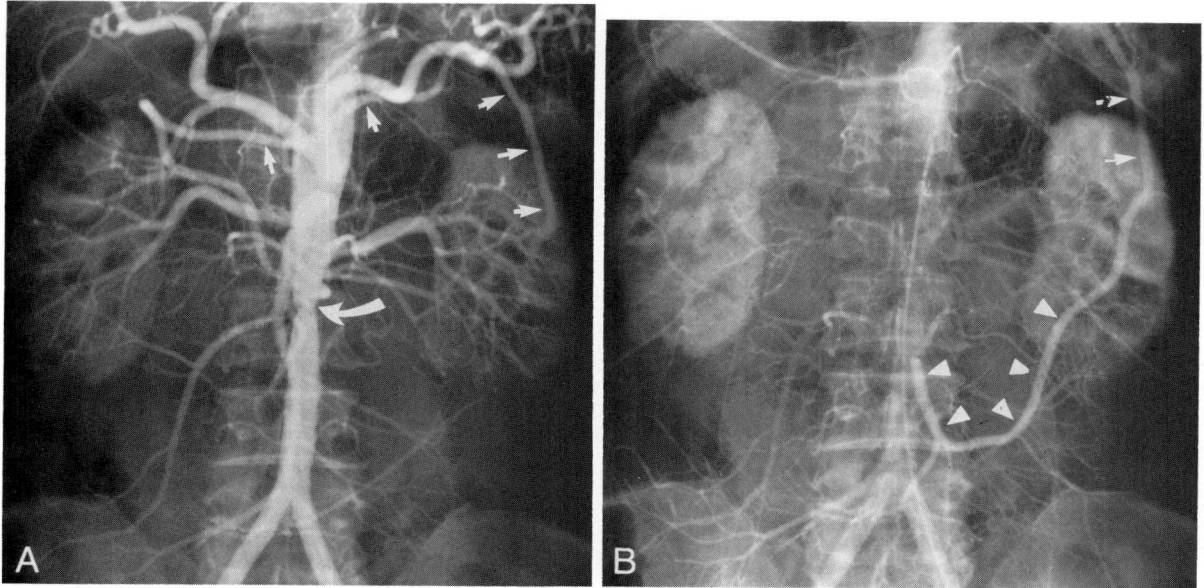

**Figure 11–15. Collateral blood supply of the colon.** Early **(A)** and delayed **(B)** films from an abdominal aortogram show a dilated marginal artery fed by the middle colic artery, which courses along the transverse and proximal descending colon *(straight arrows)* and reconstitutes the IMA via the left colic artery *(arrowheads)*. Stenosis of the abdominal aorta is present between the origins of the SMA and IMA *(curved arrow)* and may contribute to diminished flow at the origin of the IMA.

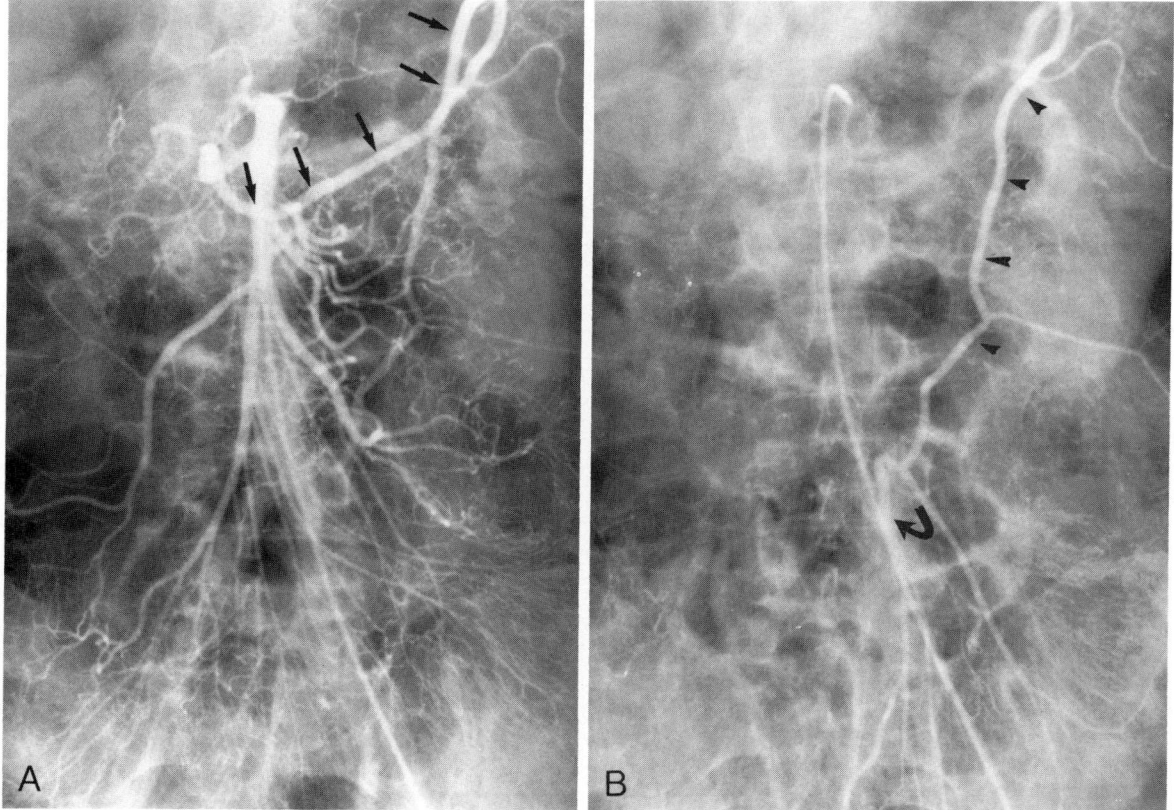

**Figure 11–16. Collateral blood supply of the colon.** Early **(A)** and delayed **(B)** films from a superior mesenteric arteriogram demonstrated an enlarged marginal artery arising from the middle colic in **A** *(arrows)*. In **B** the marginal artery fills the left colic artery *(arrowheads)* in a retrograde fashion, allowing reconstitution of the inferior mesenteric trunk *(curved arrow)*. The dilated, tortuous collateral pathway has been called a meandering mesenteric artery.

system can become important in occlusive disease of the aorta and common iliac arteries.[36]

## Venous Anatomy

The mesenteric venous system is studied for two main indications: 1) evaluation of the patency of the mesenteric veins in the setting of suspected mesenteric ischemia and 2) evaluation of the patency and direction of flow in the mesenteric, splenic, and portal veins and potential collateral pathways in portal hypertension. As noted earlier, in patients with portal hypertension, large flow rates and volumes of contrast medium are needed for optimal visualization of these vessels, and DSA may be useful in cooperative patients. Tolazoline (Priscoline), a vasodilator that acts directly on smooth muscle, injected into the SMA improves visualization of the mesenteric and portal veins. We dilute 25 mg in 10 mL of normal saline and inject it slowly for 2 minutes; contrast medium injection and filming commence immediately after drug administration.

The most important gastric vein is the left gastric, or coronary, vein, which courses along the lesser curve of the stomach and joins the splenic-portal venous system at variable sites. It is a frequent pathway for portal-systemic collateralization in portal hypertension and splenic-portal collateralization in splenic vein occlusion. Gastro-omental and short gastric veins parallel their respective arteries and can be important collateral pathways as well. The superior mesenteric and inferior mesenteric veins run to the right of and parallel to, and drain the respective territories of, the SMA and IMA. The superior mesenteric vein (see Fig. 11–1) joins the splenic vein behind the pancreatic neck to form the portal vein; the inferior mesenteric vein (Fig. 11–17) can join either the splenic or superior mesenteric vein or their confluence.[10, 40]

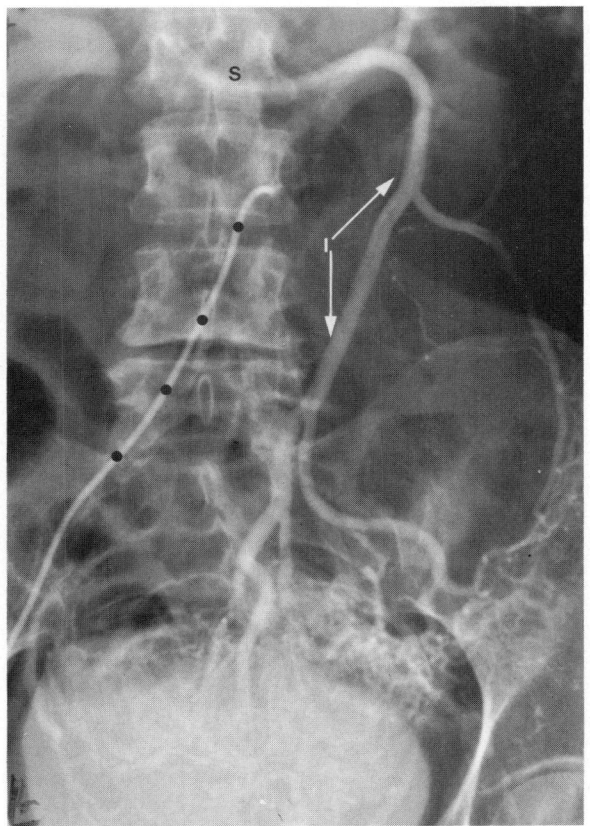

**Figure 11–17. Venous phase of inferior mesenteric artery injection.** The inferior mesenteric vein (I) joins the splenic vein (S). Black dots: catheter placed selectively into the IMA.

## References

1. Rabe FE, Yune HY, Klatte EC, et al: Efficacy of glucagon for abdominal digital angiography. AJR 139:618–619, 1982.
2. Rees CR, Palmaz JC, Alvarado R, et al: DSA in acute gastrointestinal hemorrhage: clinical and in vitro studies. Radiology 169:499–503, 1988.
3. Foley WD, Stewart ET, Milbrath JR, et al: Digital subtraction angiography of the portal venous system. AJR 140:497–499, 1983.
4. Sussman SK, Braun SD, Perlmutt GE, et al: Digital indirect portography. AJR 147:39–43, 1986.
5. Rossi P, Simonetti G, Passariello R, et al: Digital celiac arteriography. Radiology 154:229–231, 1985.
6. Walker TG, Geller SC, Waltman AC: Splenic artery pseudoaneurysms causing lower gastrointestinal hemorrhage. AJR 150:433–434, 1988.
7. Kadir S (ed): Atlas of Normal and Variant Angiographic Anatomy. Philadelphia: WB Saunders, 1991.
8. Lippert H, Pabst R: Arterial Variations in Man: Classification and Frequency. New York: Springer-Verlag, 1985.
9. Michels NA: Blood Supply and Anatomy of the Upper Abdominal Organs. Philadelphia: JB Lippincott, 1955.
10. Reuter SR, Redman HC, Cho KJ: Gastrointestinal Angiography (3rd ed). Philadelphia: WB Saunders, 1986.
11. Ruzika FF Jr, Rossi P: Normal vascular anatomy of the abdominal viscera. Radiol Clin North Am 8:3–29, 1970.
12. VanDamme J-P, Bonte J: Vascular Anatomy in Abdominal Surgery. New York: Thieme Medical Publishers, 1990.
13. Fischer RG, Schwartz JT, Graham DY: Angiotherapy with Mallory-Weiss tear. AJR 134:679–684, 1980.
14. Lang EV, Picus D, Marx VM, et al: Massive arterial hemorrhage from the stomach and lower esophagus: impact of embolotherapy on survival. Radiology 177:249–252, 1990.
15. Kadir S, Lundell C, Saeed M: Celiac, superior, and inferior mesenteric arteries. In Kadir S (ed): Atlas of Normal and Variant Angiographic Anatomy. Philadelphia: WB Saunders, 1991, pp 297–364.
16. El-Eishi HI, Ayoub SF, Abd-El-Khalek M: The arterial supply of the human stomach. Acta Anat 86:565–580, 1973.
17. Caix M, Descottes B, Rousseau DG, et al: The arterial vascularization of the middle thoracic and lower esophagus. Anat Clin 3:95–106, 1981.
18. Naidich JB, Naidich TP, Sprayregen S, et al: The origin of the left gastric artery. Radiology 126:623–626, 1978.
19. Sundgren R: Selective angiography of the left gastric artery. Acta Radiol Suppl (Stockh) 299:1–100, 1970.
20. Kelemouridis V, Athanasoulis CA, Waltman AC: Gastric bleeding sites: an angiographic study. Radiology 149:643–648, 1983.
21. Athanasoulis CA: Angiographic methods for the control of gastric hemorrhage. Am J Dig Dis 21:174–181, 1976.
22. Waltman AC, Courey WR, Athanasoulis C, et al: Technique for left gastric artery catheterization. Radiology 105:573–578, 1972.
23. Reuter SR, Atkin TW: High-dose left gastric angiography for demonstration of esophageal varices. Radiology 105:573–578, 1972.
24. Rösch J, Grollman JH Jr: Superselective arteriography in the diagnosis of abdominal pathology: technical considerations. Radiology 92:1008–1013, 1969.

25. Gerlock AJ Jr, Mirfakhraee M: Essentials of Diagnostic and Interventional Angiographic Techniques. Philadelphia: WB Saunders, 1985.
26. Kadir S: Diagnostic Angiography. Philadelphia: WB Saunders, 1986.
27. Michels NA, Siddharth P, Kornblith PL, et al: Routes of collateral circulation of the gastrointestinal tract as ascertained in a dissection of 500 bodies. Int Surg 49:8–28, 1968.
28. Didio LJA, Christoforidis AJ, Chandnani PC: Posterior gastric artery and its significance as seen in angiograms. Am J Surg 139:333–337, 1980.
29. Palmaz JC, Walter JF, Cho KJ: Therapeutic embolization of the small-bowel arteries. Radiology 152:377–382, 1984.
30. Vandamme JPJ, Van der Schuren G: Re-evaluation of the colic irrigation from the superior mesenteric artery. Acta Anat 95:578–588, 1976.
31. Lawdahl RB, Keller FS: The middle mesenteric artery. Radiology 165:371–372, 1987.
32. LeQuire MH, Sorge DG, Brantley SD: The middle mesenteric artery: an unusual source for colonic hemorrhage. J Vasc Interv Radiol 2:141–145, 1991.
33. Benton RS, Cotter WB: An unusual variation of the arterial supply of the transverse and descending colon. Anat Rec 142:215, 1962.
34. Vandamme JPJ, Bonte J, Van der Schueren G: Re-evaluation of the colic irrigation from the inferior mesenteric artery. Acta Anat 112:18–30, 1982.
35. Kahn P, Abrams HL: Inferior mesenteric arterial patterns: an angiographic study. Radiology 82:429–441, 1984.
36. Meyers MA: Griffith's point: critical anastomosis at the splenic flexure. Significance in ischemia of the colon. AJR 126:77–94, 1976.
37. Vandamme JPJ, Bonte J: Arcus paracolicus. Acta Anat 118:50–53, 1984.
38. Moskowitz M, Zimmerman H, Felson B: The meandering mesenteric artery of the colon. AJR 92:1088–1099, 1964.
39. Kadir S: Abdominal aorta and pelvis. _In_ Kadir S (ed): Atlas of Normal and Variant Angiographic Anatomy. Philadelphia: WB Saunders, 1991, pp 97–121.
40. Lundell C, Kadir S: The portal venous system and hepatic veins. _In_ Kadir S (ed): Atlas of Normal and Variant Angiographic Anatomy. Philadelphia: WB Saunders, 1991, pp 365–385.

# Abdominal Plain Film

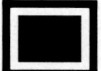

# Technique and Normal Anatomy

Susan M. Williams, M.D.

## INTRODUCTION

The development of cross-sectional imaging has altered traditional approaches for the diagnosis of abdominal disease. Although the abdominal plain film is usually less critical to diagnosis, it is still helpful in diagnosing a variety of pathologic conditions and in directing subsequent radiologic evaluation, when used judiciously. When it is ordered as a screening procedure, the yield of abnormal findings is low, and most abnormalities that are detected are nonspecific.[1-3] Eisenberg and associates reviewed 1780 abdominal plain film examinations and found abnormalities in only 10% of cases.[2] In this large series, no significant disease would have been missed if plain films had been obtained only for patients who had strong clinical indications of disease or moderate to severe abdominal symptoms. The plain film is most efficacious when obtained for patients who have significant abdominal tenderness or who are strongly suspected of having bowel obstruction or perforation, urinary calculi, or ischemia. The plain film examination is least effective as a screening study in patients with mild or nonspecific symptoms. The major value of normal findings from a plain film examination is that they exclude bowel obstruction or a large perforation.

The traditional practice of obtaining a preliminary plain film before performing an upper gastrointestinal examination or barium enema has been challenged by several authors.[4-6] These authors have suggested that the preliminary film is unlikely to reveal significant disease that would otherwise be overlooked. The preliminary film is most helpful in patients whose clinical condition suggests bowel obstruction, perforation, or fulminant inflammatory bowel disease, which could modify or even serve as a contraindication for a contrast study. Some authors also believe that the preliminary film is useful in assessing the adequacy of colonic preparation for a barium enema, but others have found that it is unreliable.[4, 5]

The plain film is invaluable in assessing the positions of intra-abdominal tubes and catheters and is commonly used for this purpose in the hospital setting.

## TECHNIQUE

### Standard Projections

The anteroposterior radiograph taken with the patient in a supine position is the basis of the plain film examination of the abdomen (Fig. 12–1). Careful attention to technical detail is important, so that the final radiograph has the greatest possible diagnostic information. The patient should be positioned comfortably on the back with no rotation of the pelvis. Maximal relaxation of the abdominal musculature is important in reducing film artifact caused by motion. Such relaxation is facilitated by supporting and slightly flexing the patient's knees. A 14 × 17 inch film should be positioned with its lower edge at the symphysis pubis and the x-ray beam centered at the iliac crest. The exposure is made during expiration and should begin 1 to 2 seconds after respiration is suspended.[7]

The delineation of intra-abdominal soft tissues on the plain film depends on inherent contrast provided by fat and intraluminal gas. Subject contrast seen on the radiograph is caused by differential attenuation of the x-ray beam in the patient. Photoelectric interactions, which

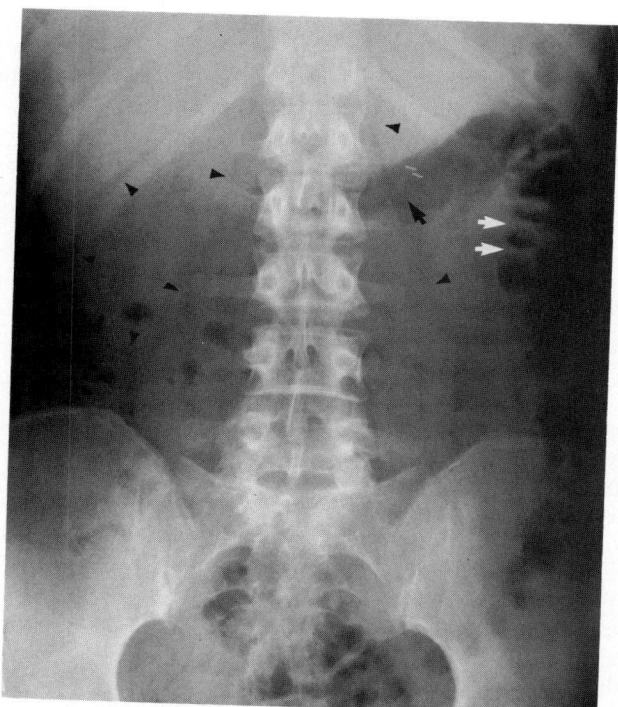

**Figure 12–1. Anteroposterior supine abdominal film.** This patient has a normal gas pattern for the adult bowel. Gas is present in nondilated stomach and colon. Note the typical appearance of the rugal folds *(black arrow)* of the stomach and haustral folds *(white arrows)* of the colon. The kidneys are a relatively constant landmark and are outlined by perirenal fat *(black arrowheads)*.

allow tissue differentiation based on atomic number, result in the best subject contrast.[8] Unfortunately, the proportion of photoelectric reactions decreases rapidly with incident energies greater than 30 kV(p), which is too low to penetrate a thick body part such as the abdomen. Most plain films of the abdomen are exposed at 60 to 75 kV(p), depending on the equipment and size of the patient.[7] At these levels of energy, Compton's scatter is the predominant mode of attenuation, and soft tissue discrimination depends entirely on density.[8] Short exposure times are desirable to avoid unsharpness caused by motion. However, an increase in peak kilovoltage also increases scattered radiation, which degrades the contrast. Optimal technique should therefore incorporate the lowest possible peak kilovoltage that can penetrate the patient and that has an acceptable exposure time. A reciprocating (Potter-Bucky) grid and careful collimation are employed to reduce scatter.[7] In males with reproductive potential, gonadal shielding should be used if the gonads lie within 5 cm of the primary beam and if such shielding does not compromise the clinical objectives of the examination.

Portable films are useful in extremely ill patients; however, the resultant radiographs are of lower technical quality than standard abdominal plain films. The patients are frequently too ill to cooperate in breath holding, and many portable units have fixed milliampere settings, which may necessitate techniques of higher peak kilovoltage, which reduce contrast. In addition, a stationary grid, rather than a Potter-Bucky grid, must be used to control scatter. Accurate positioning of the grid is often difficult. Abdominal films should therefore be obtained in the x-ray department whenever possible.

## Supplemental Projections

In addition to the anteroposterior supine view, supplemental projections may be helpful in specific clinical situations and are frequently obtained as part of a routine abdominal plain film series. In a patient with abdominal pain, a chest film taken with the patient in an upright position is useful for two reasons: it facilitates the detection of small amounts of free intraperitoneal air, and it may demonstrate unsuspected thoracic disease that is causing abdominal pain.

The abdominal film obtained with the patient in an erect position is often ordered on a routine basis but only rarely adds significant information. Mirvis and associates reviewed 252 emergency department examinations consisting of a series of radiographs, which included films of the abdomen obtained with the patient in supine and erect positions and a chest film taken with the patient in an upright position.[3] The film of the abdomen in the erect position did not contribute to the management of any patients with acute abdominal conditions. This film therefore could have been omitted to reduce the time and cost of the examination without sacrificing important diagnostic information. However, this film may be helpful in patients with suspected bowel obstruction, to assess the proportion of gas and fluid in the distended bowel. Alternatively, this information can be obtained on a film of the abdomen taken with the patient in the lateral decubitus position. For extremely ill patients who cannot stand, a lateral decubitus view is far more helpful than a slouched, sitting "erect" view.

Miller and Nelson have shown that when a perforated viscus is suspected clinically, a specific sequence of filming is most likely to demonstrate extra-alimentary gas.[9] Before films are obtained, the patient should be in the left-side-down position for at least 10 minutes. This position allows gas to rise out of the lesser sac of the peritoneal cavity (where it may be loculated) and accumulate beneath the iliac crest or over the right margin of the liver. If the patient is unable to stand, a film of the patient in the left lateral decubitus position should be obtained with a horizontal x-ray beam, using a short exposure technique. This method results in underpenetration of the abdominal viscera but good visualization of small amounts of extra-alimentary gas (Fig. 12–2). If the patient is able to stand, the table is tilted upright, and a posteroanterior chest film with the patient in an upright position is obtained. Films of the abdomen in erect and supine positions are also obtained to complete the "perforation series." Posteroanterior chest films taken with the patient upright are more sensitive for detecting pneumoperitoneum than are abdominal films taken with the patient in an erect position.[9] This difference in sensitivity occurs because the x-ray beam is centered at the iliac crest on abdominal films, so that it penetrates air beneath the diaphragm obliquely rather

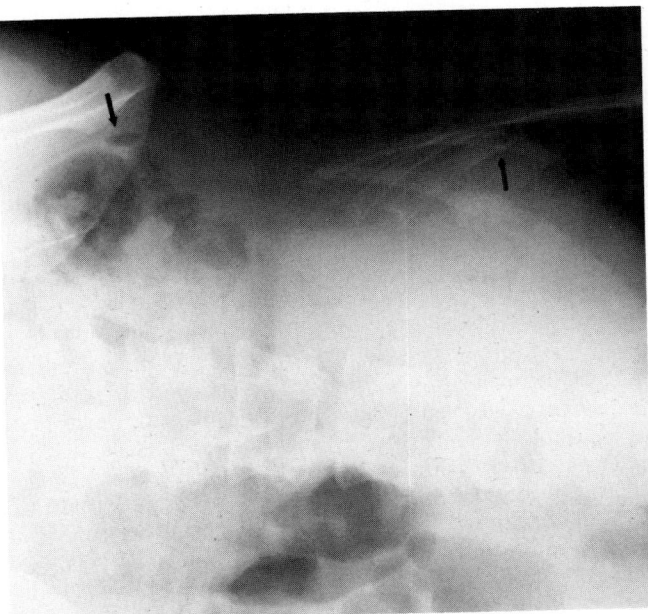

**Figure 12–2. Pneumoperitoneum on a left lateral decubitus film of the abdomen.** Small collections of intraperitoneal gas *(arrows)* appear adjacent to the right lateral border of the liver and right iliac crest.

than tangentially, making small gas collections undetectable. In addition, the exposure technique that is required to penetrate the abdomen results in excessive penetration at the lung interface, obscuring small collections of free intraperitoneal air. Nevertheless, the erect and supine abdominal films are a useful part of the perforation series for detecting other intra-abdominal disease in these patients.

Depending on the clinical setting, additional projections such as prone, oblique, lateral, or coned views may be helpful for better definition and location of mass lesions, calcifications, or herniations. Because colonic gas tends to occupy the more anterior transverse and sigmoid segments of the colon in the supine position, a distal colonic obstruction may be difficult to distinguish from adynamic neuromuscular dysfunction or pseudo-obstruction on supine and erect views.[10, 11] In this situation, a left lateral view of the rectum has been found to be useful, as this position allows air to fill the rectosigmoid if no mechanical obstruction is present.[12]

## RETROPERITONEUM AND ABDOMINAL WALL

Intra-abdominal tissue planes and visceral surfaces are visible on plain films because of the natural contrast created by surrounding fat. The best visualized interfaces are those that are smoothly marginated and oriented in a sagittal or transverse plane tangential to the incident x-ray beam. Familiarity with the most commonly visualized tissue planes is helpful in identifying normal anatomic structures and in recognizing and localizing pathologic processes.

The anatomy of the retroperitoneal space has been well described by Meyers.[13] Nevertheless, this anatomy is reviewed here, because it is helpful in understanding abdominal plain films. The retroperitoneal space lies posterior to the parietal peritoneum and anterior to the transversalis fascia. Anatomically, it is divided into three distinct compartments: the perirenal space, the posterior pararenal space, and the anterior pararenal space.

## Perirenal Space: Kidneys and Adrenal Glands

The right and left perirenal spaces are confined by the anterior and posterior layers of renal fascia (Gerota's fascia) and are not continuous across the midline. These spaces contain the adrenal glands, the kidneys, and abundant fat. The perirenal fat allows plain film visualization of the renal outlines in most patients (see Fig. 12–1). The adrenal glands are small and triangular and are not discernible on plain films unless they have become calcified as a result of previous hemorrhage or granulomatous disease (Fig. 12–3). The perirenal fat is also responsible for plain film visualization of the upper half of the psoas muscle and the medial aspects of the hepatic and splenic angles. Obliteration of the perirenal fat by inflammation, blood, or urine may prevent visualization of these structures. Medially, the perirenal space is in continuity with the aorta and often fills with blood in patients with ruptured abdominal aortic aneurysms.[14] Laterally, the anterior and posterior layers of perirenal fascia fuse to form the lateroconal fascia, which continues laterally and ventrally to fuse with the parietal peritoneum along the lateral abdominal wall. In patients with abundant fat, the lateroconal fascia may be visible on plain films as a thin line separating the posterior pararenal and anterior pararenal fat[15] (Fig. 12–4). (See

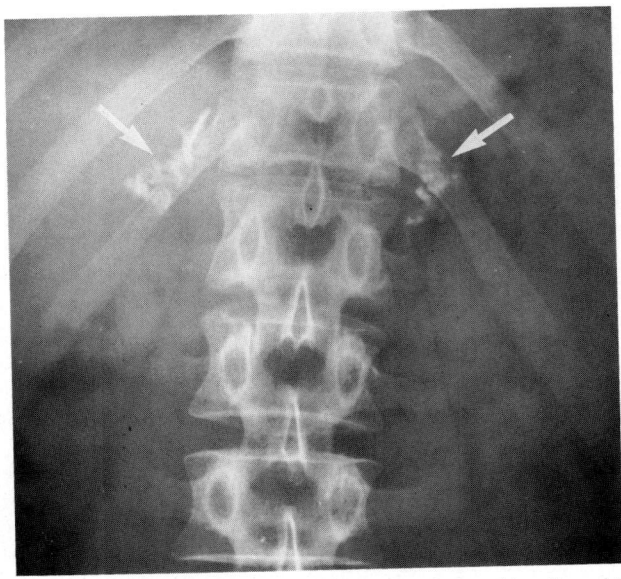

**Figure 12–3. Calcified adrenal glands.** The size and location of the adrenal glands *(arrows)* are apparent in this patient with bilateral calcification of the glands.

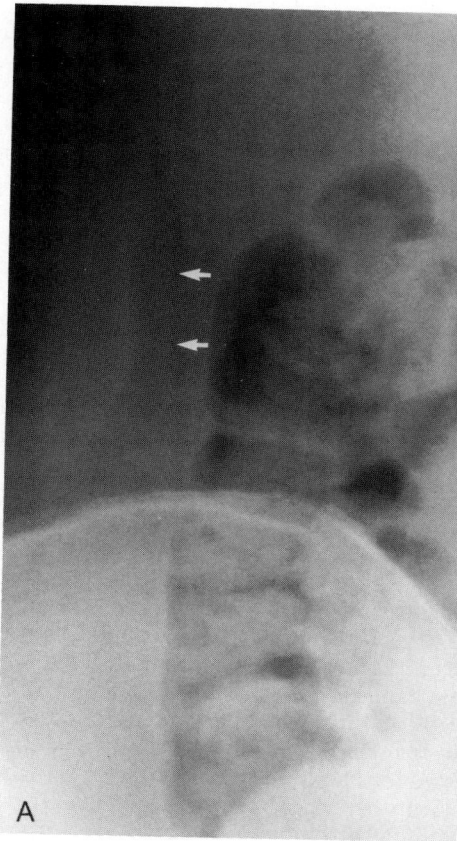

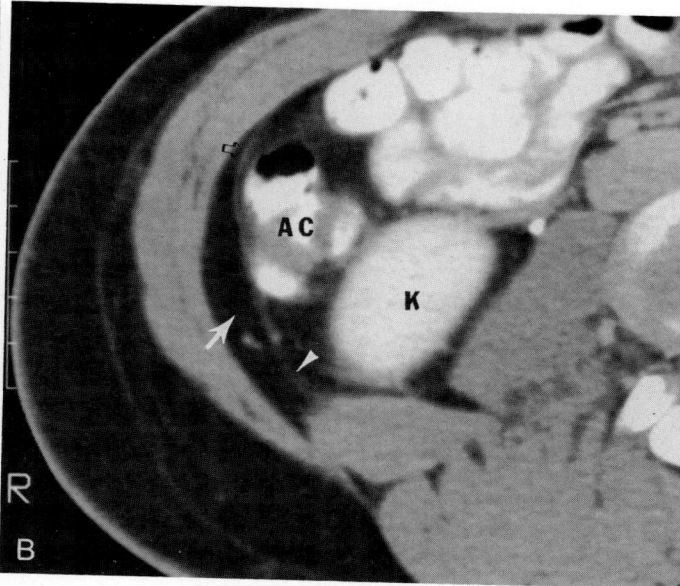

**Figure 12–4. Lateroconal and perirenal fasciae. A.** The lateroconal fascia *(arrows)* appears on an abdominal plain film as a thin, white line extending inferiorly from the hepatic angle. **B.** A computed tomographic (CT) scan shows how the anterior and posterior layers of perirenal fascia fuse laterally to form the lateroconal fascia *(open arrow)*, which courses along the lateral abdominal wall to fuse with the parietal peritoneum. The posterior pararenal fat *(solid arrow)* is posterior and lateral to the lateroconal fascia and posterior perirenal fascia *(arrowhead)*. The ascending colon (AC) is located in the anterior pararenal space. K = kidney.

later sections in this chapter for more detailed description of this anatomy.)

## Posterior Pararenal Space

The posterior pararenal space lies posterior to the posterior perirenal and lateroconal fascia and anterior to the transversalis fascia lining the abdominal wall[13] (see Fig. 12–4B). This space contains a variable amount of fat, but no organs. Medially, the posterior pararenal space originates at the lateral margin of the psoas muscle and is not continuous across the midline. Laterally, the posterior pararenal fat continues around the flank to become continuous with the properitoneal fat of the lateral abdominal wall, forming the "flank stripe" (Fig. 12–5). The width of the flank stripe is quite variable and depends on body habitus. The posterior pararenal fat is continuous inferiorly with extraperitoneal fat in the pelvis.

## Anterior Pararenal Space: Ascending and Descending Colon, Duodenum, and Pancreas

The anterior pararenal space lies anterior to the perirenal space and lateroconal fascia[13] (see Fig. 12–4B). It is potentially continuous across the midline and contains the ascending and descending colon, retroperitoneal duodenum, and pancreas. Like the posterior pararenal space, the anterior pararenal space communicates inferiorly with the pelvis. In most patients, the ascending and descending colon can be identified by intraluminal fecal material and gas medial to the flank stripes (see Fig. 12–5). Semisolid fecal material in the cecum and ascending colon often has a characteristic bubbly appearance. The retroperitoneal duodenum is usually not visible on plain films unless it is filled with gas as a result of ileus or adjacent inflammation. The pancreas is not visualized on plain films either, because it has undulating, lobulated borders. The head of the pancreas, which is its most caudal portion, lies just to the right of the midline within the duodenal loop. The body and tail extend posteriorly and superiorly toward the hilum of the spleen in the left upper quadrant. The normal location of the pancreas may be recognized on plain films in patients with chronic calcific pancreatitis (Fig. 12–6).

## Psoas Muscle

The psoas muscle forms one of the classic landmarks on abdominal plain films. This muscle arises from the T12-L5 vertebrae. It extends inferiorly to join the iliac muscle below the iliac crest and continues as the iliopsoas muscle to the lesser trochanter.[16] The lateral to its junction with the iliac muscle[17, 18] (Fig. 12–7). Blood or inflammatory exudate in the adjacent retroperitoneal fat may cause obliteration of the margin of the psoas muscle. For example, loss of one or both shadows of the psoas muscle is a common plain film finding in patients who have a ruptured abdominal aortic aneurysm with blood infiltrating the perirenal and posterior pararenal spaces.[14]

The psoas muscle is best visualized when its lateral margin is straight and nearly parallel to the incident x-ray beam. Absence of the psoas margin on plain films must be interpreted with caution. In some patients, lumbar scoliosis may result in nonvisualization of the psoas shadow.[18] In such patients, rotation of the spinal column causes the psoas muscle on the concave side to assume a more flattened, horizontal configuration. Its margin is then more nearly perpendicular to the incident x-ray, so that it may not be visible on plain films (Fig. 12–8). This phenomenon occurs not only in patients with structural scoliosis, but also in those with positional scoliosis, in whom muscle spasm causes contraction of the muscles of the flank. In some normal patients with a limited amount of retroperitoneal fat, the peritoneal cavity extends posteriorly, so that fluid-filled bowel loops may come to lie directly adjacent to the psoas muscle and obscure its margin. The kidney may also occasionally abut the psoas muscle, causing segmental nonvisualization. This abutment may occur in normal patients or in patients with splenomegaly, in whom the kidney is displaced medially by the enlarged spleen.[18] Thus, the psoas margin may not be visualized as a result of retroperitoneal or intraperitoneal disease, scoliosis, or normal variation.

## Quadratus Lumborum Muscle

Just lateral and roughly parallel to the psoas muscle is the lateral margin of the quadratus lumborum muscle, which is often seen to extend to its origin at the iliac crest (see Fig. 12–7). The quadratus lumborum muscle is part of the posterior abdominal wall and lies dorsal to the transversalis fascia, which passes between it and the psoas muscle.[16] However, visualization of the quadratus lumborum muscle depends on the integrity of the posterior pararenal fat, which outlines its lateral margin.

## Diaphragmatic Crura

Retroperitoneal fat that is continuous with the origin of the psoas muscle may outline the diaphragmatic crura (Fig. 12–9). The crura are best seen on plain films when the x-ray beam is centered near the level of the diaphragm. Posterior pararenal fat continues superiorly beneath the diaphragm, where it may occasionally simulate pneumoperitoneum. In such cases, a film of the patient in the left lateral decubitus position should differentiate pneumoperitoneum from pararenal fat, because the lucency associated with fat is not affected by changes in position.

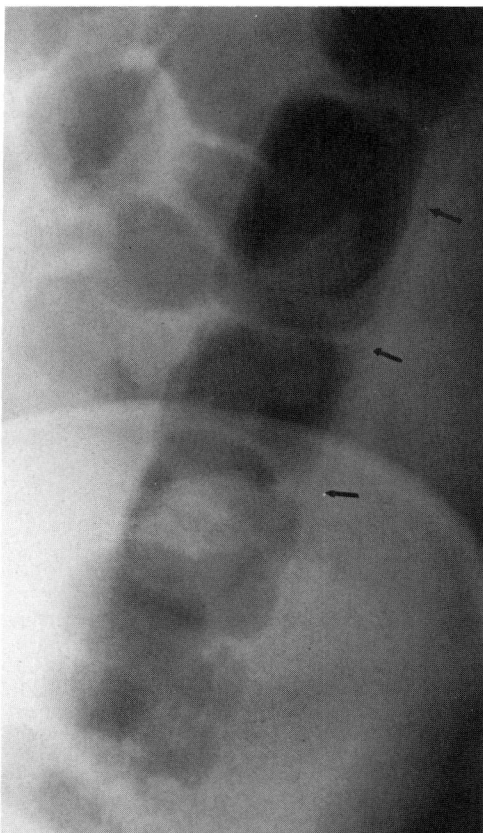

**Figure 12–5. Flank stripe.** A coned view of the left side of the abdomen shows the flank stripe *(arrows)* caused by properitoneal fat just lateral to the descending colon. This fat is contiguous with retroperitoneal fat in the posterior pararenal space. It is separated from the descending colon by parietal and visceral peritoneum, the potential space of the left paracolic gutter. This space is several millimeters or less when the paracolic gutter contains no intraperitoneal fluid.

margin of the psoas muscle is outlined by perirenal fat superiorly and posterior pararenal fat below the level of the kidneys. In about 75% of normal patients, the psoas muscle is seen to extend from the diaphragmatic crura

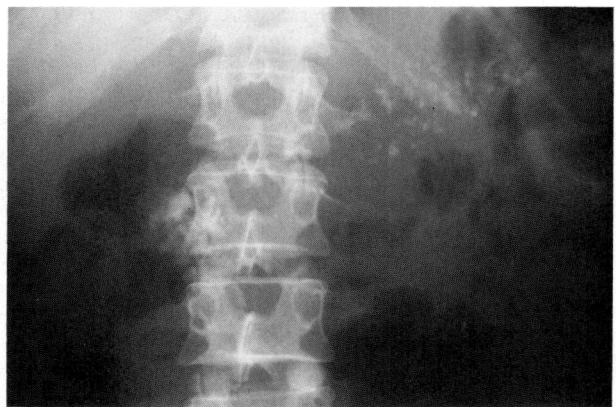

**Figure 12–6. Chronic calcific pancreatitis.** The location of the pancreas is apparent in this patient with diffuse pancreatic calcification. The normal pancreas is not visible on abdominal plain films.

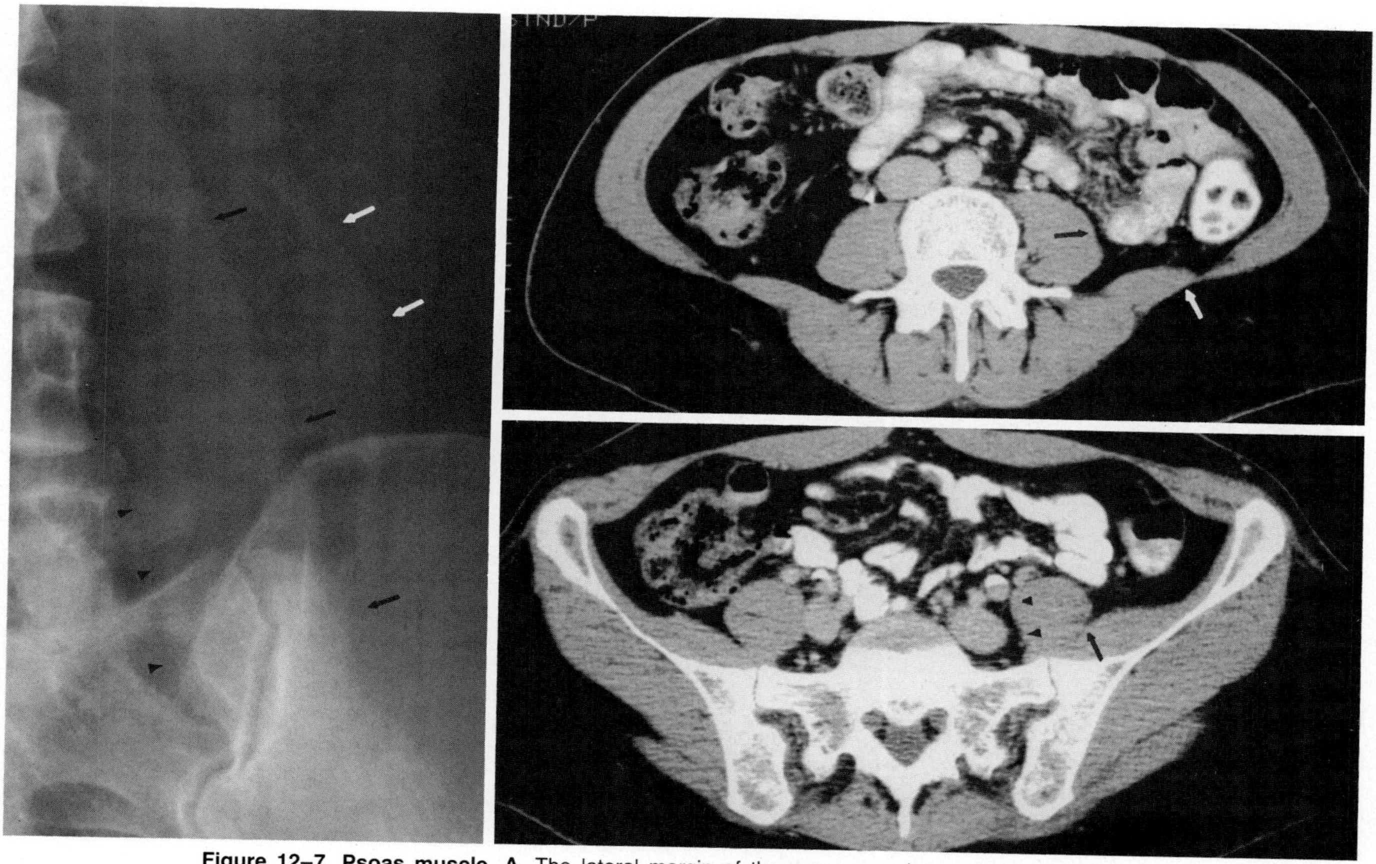

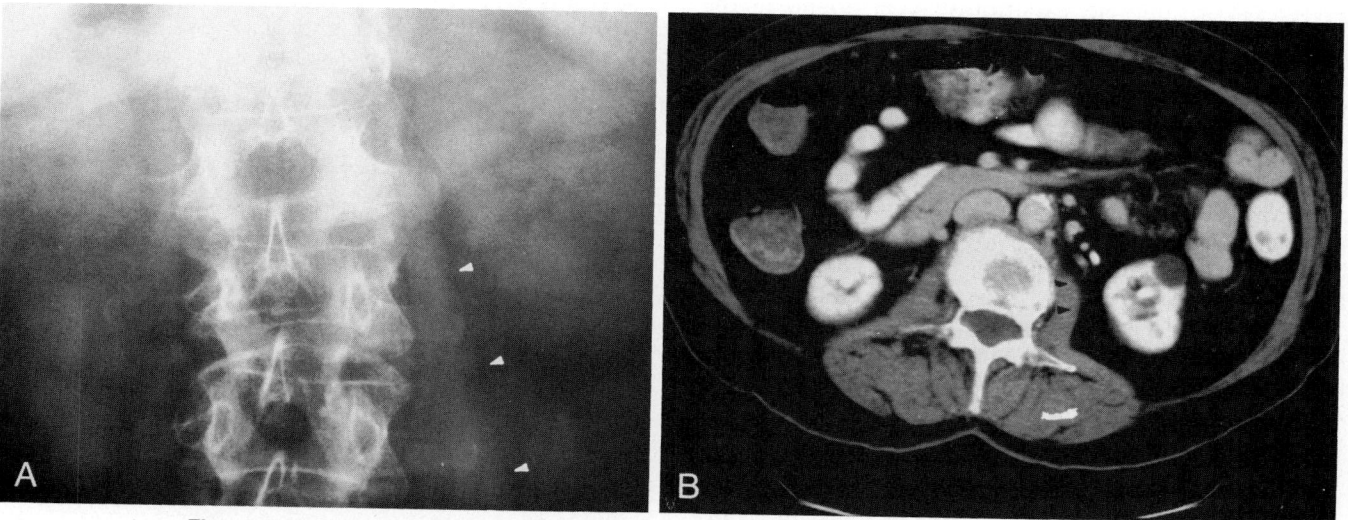

**Figure 12–7. Psoas muscle. A.** The lateral margin of the psoas muscle can be seen to extend inferiorly from the diaphragmatic crura to just below the left iliac crest *(black arrows)*. The medial margin of the psoas muscle is also located inferiorly *(arrowheads)*. The lateral border of the quadratus lumborum muscle *(white arrows)* is located lateral to the psoas muscle. **B.** A CT scan shows how the posterior pararenal fat outlines the lateral margin of the psoas muscle *(black arrow)* and quadratus lumborum muscle *(white arrow)*. **C.** A more caudal CT scan shows that the lateral margin of the psoas shadow visualized on plain films ends below the iliac crest at the junction of the psoas and iliac muscles *(arrow)*. The medial margin of the psoas muscle is outlined by retroperitoneal fat *(arrowheads)*, which accounts for its visualization on the plain film.

**Figure 12–8. Effect of scoliosis on visualization of the psoas muscle. A.** In this patient with lumbar scoliosis that is convex on the left side, the psoas margin is clearly visible *(arrowheads)*. On the right or concave side of the spinal curvature, however, the psoas margin is not well delineated. **B.** A CT scan shows why the psoas muscle is likely to be visualized on only one side in patients with scoliosis. The orientation of the psoas muscle *(arrowheads)* is more nearly vertical on the convex side of the scoliosis, and the muscle is tangential to the incident x-ray beam. It is therefore more clearly visible on anteroposterior radiographs.

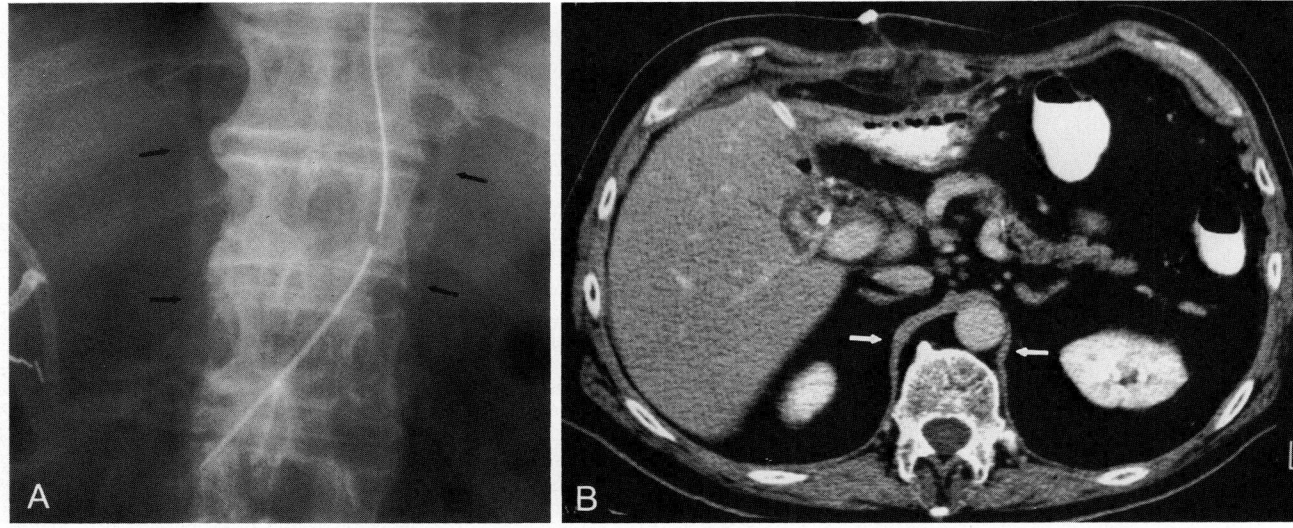

**Figure 12–9. Diaphragmatic crura. A.** The diaphragmatic crura *(arrows)* are well visualized on this film centered near the diaphragm. **B.** A CT scan from the same patient shows the crura *(arrows)* outlined by retroperitoneal fat.

# PERITONEAL CAVITY

## Liver

The liver is primarily an intraperitoneal structure that occupies the right upper quadrant of the abdomen. It is suspended from the posterior abdominal wall by a peritoneal fold, known as the *coronary ligament.* The surface of the liver between the superior and inferior reflections of the right coronary ligament is the liver's only nonperitonealized portion and is known as the *bare area of the liver.*[19] The adult liver measures about 20 to 22 cm in its greatest transverse dimension and 15 to 17 cm in its greatest vertical dimension, near its right lateral border.[16] Considerable variation may be found in the normal shape of the liver.[20] The superior aspect is commonly S shaped or concave, with its most cephalad portion lying just beneath the dome of the right hemidiaphragm. The inferior edge is most commonly triangular, with its apex directed caudally toward the right lower quadrant. About 4 to 14% of the population have a prominent inferior extension of the right lower lobe, known as *Riedel's lobe.* This lobe may extend caudally below the iliac crest and does not by itself indicate hepatomegaly.

No consistent intraperitoneal fat is present around the liver. However, the right inferior edge of the liver (hepatic angle) is often visible on plain films, because it indents the extraperitoneal fat pad that surrounds the parietal peritoneum[15] (Fig. 12–10). This fat pad consists of posterior pararenal fat laterally and perirenal fat medially. The perirenal fat may outline not only the medial aspect of the hepatic angle, but also the more cephalad portion of the posteromedial surface of the right lobe of the liver (Fig. 12–11). The hepatic angle may not be visualized because of effusions or blood that infiltrates the retroperitoneal fat, or because of ascites, which displaces the liver edge away from the adjacent

fat.[21] The posterior edge of the liver is directly visible on plain films, whereas the anterior and left lateral margins of the liver are not. Conversely, the anterior margin of an enlarged liver is usually palpated on

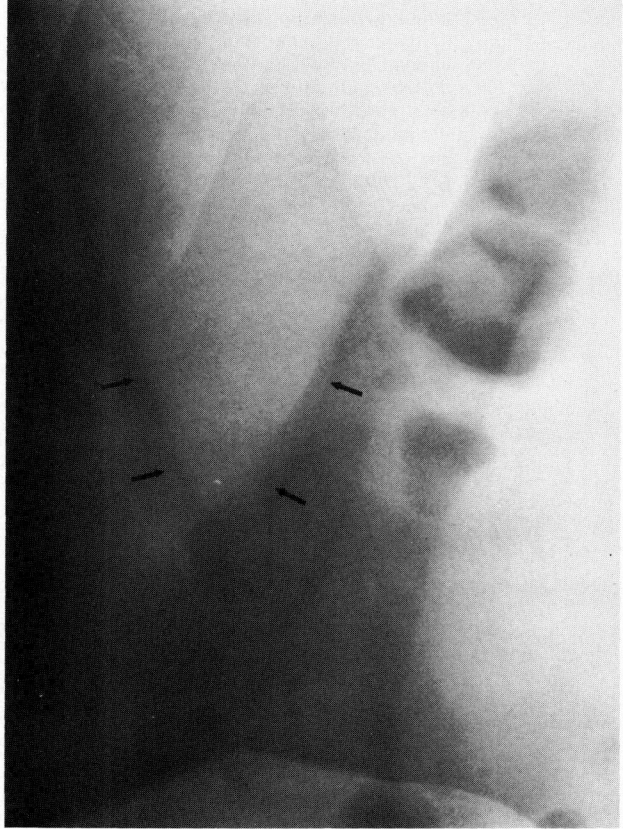

**Figure 12–10. Hepatic angle.** The hepatic angle *(arrows)* is outlined by surrounding extraperitoneal fat.

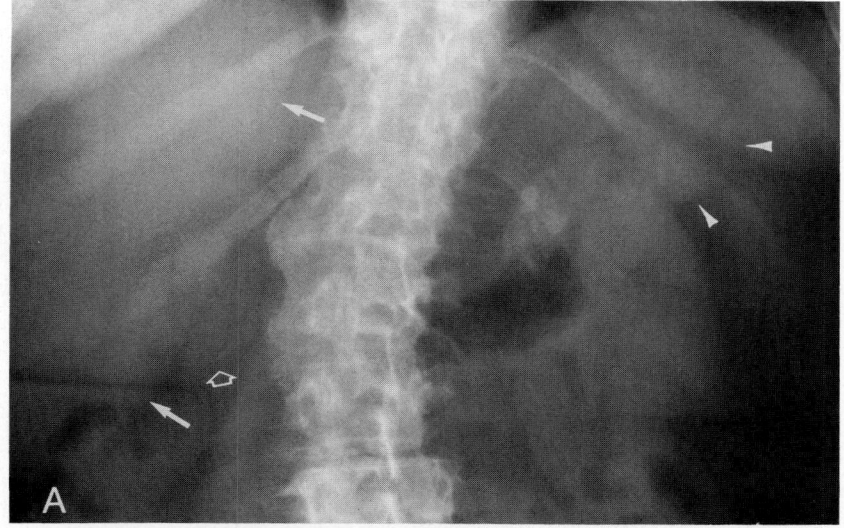

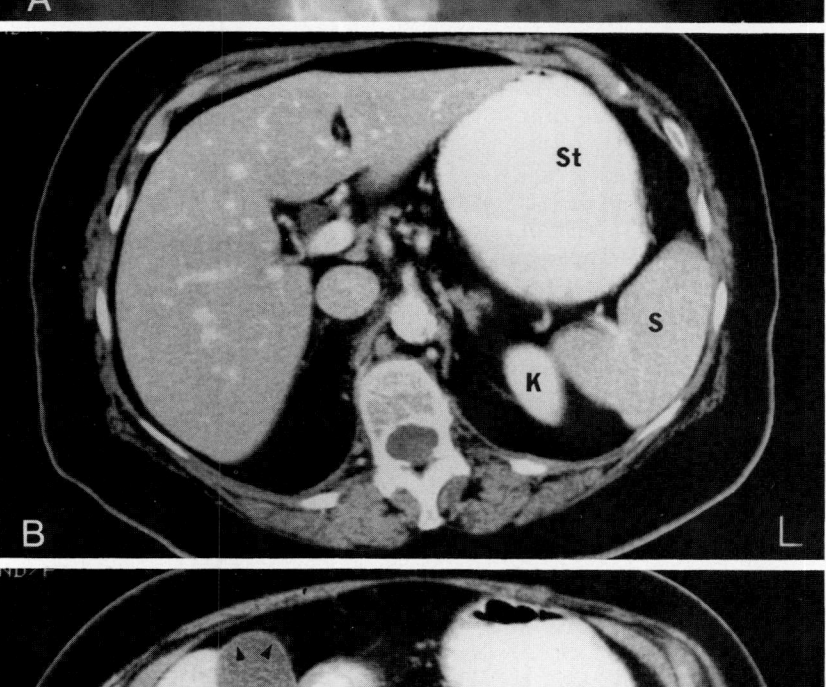

**Figure 12–11. Right lobe of the liver. A.** Perirenal fat outlines the posteromedial surface of the right lobe of the liver *(solid arrows)*. The anterior liver edge is not visible on this film. Note how the fundus of the gallbladder *(open arrow)* and fluid-filled gastric fundus *(arrowheads)* are visible on this film because of surrounding fat. **B.** A CT scan from the same patient shows the fluid-filled stomach (St) outlined by surrounding fat. The location of the spleen (S) is posterior and lateral to the gastric fundus and lateral to the left kidney (K). **C.** A more caudal CT scan shows the fundus of the gallbladder indenting fat in the lesser omentum *(arrowheads)*. Note that the gallbladder is just lateral to the gastric antrum (A). Posteriorly, the medial aspect of the right lobe of the liver is outlined by perirenal fat *(solid arrows)*. The tip of the spleen (S) is outlined by posterior pararenal fat laterally and perirenal fat medially *(open arrows)*.

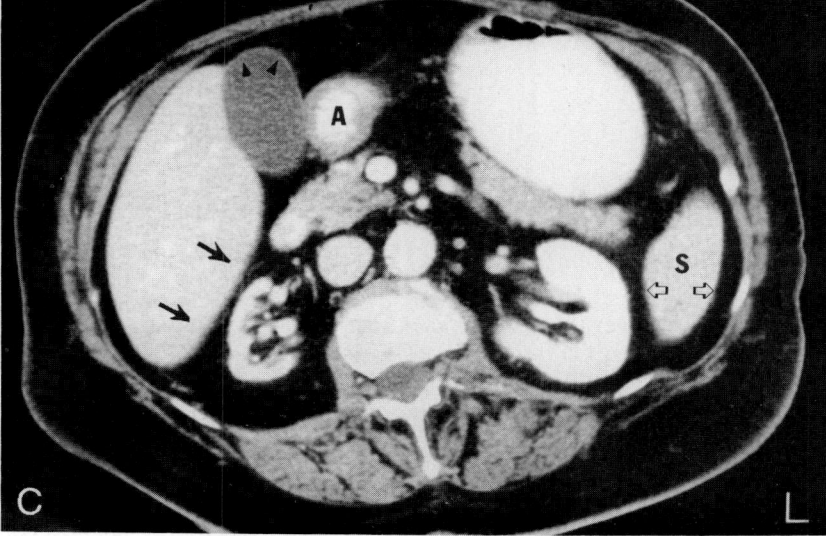

physical examination.[15] As a result, a discrepancy may arise between the clinical and radiographic findings. Enlargement of the liver on plain films may be inferred by elevation of the right hemidiaphragm, inferior displacement of the hepatic flexure of the colon, and lateral displacement of the lesser curvature of the stomach.[22]

## Gallbladder

The gallbladder occupies a shallow fossa on the inferior surface of the liver between the right and left lobes and is not often visualized on plain films. It lies just superior and lateral to the duodenal bulb and gastric antrum and just above the transverse colon. Occasionally, the fundus of the gallbladder may be visualized in normal patients if it indents the surrounding fat (see Fig. 12–11A). Only about 15% of gallstones are sufficiently calcified to be seen on plain films, so that the abdominal radiograph is a poor screening study for gallbladder disease.

## Spleen

The spleen is located in the left upper quadrant of the peritoneal cavity, beneath the left hemidiaphragm and posterolateral to the gastric fundus (see Fig. 12–11B and C).[23] The average adult spleen is 12 cm in length and 7 cm in width.[16] The lower edge of its inferolateral surface often indents extraperitoneal fat and is therefore visible on plain films[22] (Fig. 12–12).

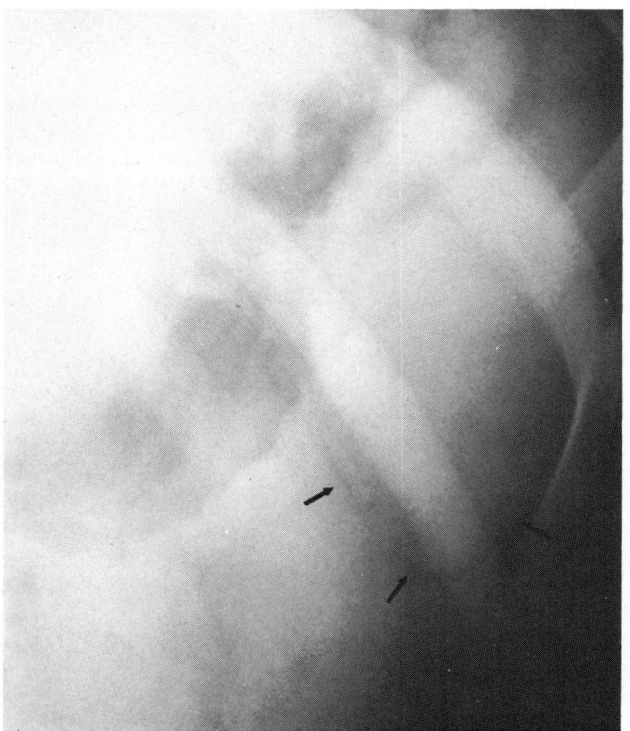

**Figure 12–12. Spleen.** The inferior tip of the spleen *(arrows)* is outlined by perirenal fat medially and posterior pararenal fat laterally.

The lower medial aspect of the spleen is adjacent to the left kidney and is occasionally outlined by perirenal fat. However, the bulk of the spleen extends medially behind the stomach, where it is not visible on plain films. Thus, splenomegaly cannot always be diagnosed on abdominal radiographs. Nevertheless, an enlarged spleen should be suspected when plain films show elevation of the left hemidiaphragm, medial displacement of the gastric air bubble and left kidney, or the splenic tip below the costal margin.[22]

The most inferior surface of the spleen abuts the phrenicocolic ligament, a thick peritoneal fold that marks the anatomic splenic flexure of the colon. The left lateral pleural recess may extend inferiorly along the lateral margin of the spleen to the splenic tip.[23]

## Stomach

The stomach almost always contains air and fluid, so that it can be recognized in the left upper quadrant by its characteristic shape and pattern of rugal folds (see Fig. 12–1). When the patient is in the supine position, gas in the stomach rises to the anteriorly located antrum while fluid gravitates to the fundus. When the fluid-filled fundus is visible on plain films, it may occasionally be mistaken for a soft tissue mass (see Fig. 12–11). However, confusion may be eliminated by the use of the upright films, which should allow gas to enter the fundus. The stomach is a valuable landmark for identifying space-occupying lesions in surrounding structures, such as the spleen laterally, the liver medially, and the lesser sac and pancreas posteriorly.

## Small Intestine

The small bowel and its associated mesentery occupy the central portion of the peritoneal cavity. In most normal adults, the transit time through the small bowel is sufficiently rapid to prevent swallowed air from accumulating in small bowel loops, so that these loops are usually not visible on plain films. Large amounts of air and fluid in dilated small bowel therefore indicate prolonged transit time due to mechanical obstruction or adynamic neuromuscular dysfunction. Scattered gas and fluid within normal to minimally dilated small bowel loops may occur in a variety of normal or pathologic conditions, including gastroenteritis, pancreatitis, inflammatory bowel disease, and aerophagia. Unfortunately, considerable interobserver variation occurs in interpretation of small bowel gas.[10] The term nonspecific gas pattern has been used to describe plain films showing more than the average amount of small bowel gas without a clear indication of bowel obstruction. However, this term is vague or even misleading and is not particularly helpful to the referring physician.[10] Radiologists should therefore avoid the use of this term, instead providing a clear description of the radiographic findings and the most reasonable diagnostic considerations. The gas-filled small bowel is distinguished from the colon by its smaller caliber and typical mucosal folds, the valvulae

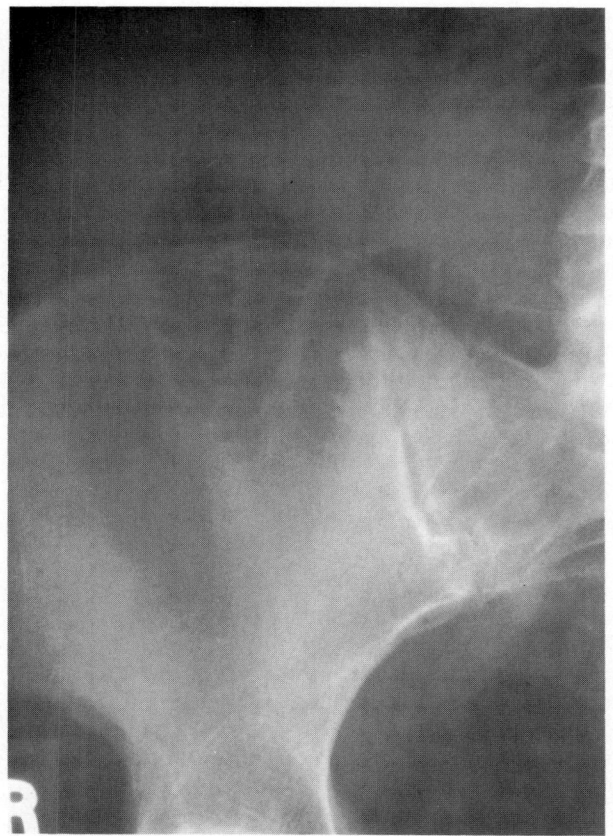

**Figure 12–13. Normal gas pattern of small bowel.** Note how the valvulae conniventes cross the entire circumference of the gas-filled lumen.

conniventes. When visualized, folds of the small bowel are usually thin and extend across the entire lumen of the bowel (Fig. 12–13).

## Colon

The adult colon almost always contains some gas and fecal material. The more anterior transverse and sigmoid segments often contain the greatest amount of gas when the patient is in the supine position. The typical configuration of the haustral folds is useful in identifying the colon (see Fig. 12–1). Haustra are infoldings of the colonic wall, formed by contraction of the taeniae coli, three longitudinal bands of muscle that run along the surface of the colon. Unlike the valvulae conniventes of the small bowel, these indentations are more widely spaced and usually do not cross the entire lumen. The caliber of the colon varies from 3 to 8 cm, with the largest diameter found in the cecum. Persistent cecal diameters of 10 cm or greater suggest mechanical obstruction or ileus and may indicate a risk of impending perforation.[24]

The sigmoid and transverse segments of the colon are intraperitoneal structures that are suspended by the sigmoid mesentery and transverse mesocolon, respectively. Conversely, the ascending and descending colon

and rectum are retroperitoneal structures that are fixed to the posterior abdominal wall. In about 20% of the population, the cecum and a variable portion of the ascending colon have a persistent mesentery.[25] In such cases, the gas-filled cecum is mobile, and its position may be more anterior and medial than usual. Although most such patients are asymptomatic, this anatomic variation predisposes them to cecal ileus or volvulus. The sigmoid colon is an intraperitoneal structure, but sigmoid diverticula are frequently oriented toward the sigmoid mesentery, so that rupture of a diverticulum may result in retroperitoneal gas.[13]

Air-fluid levels in the bowel are often interpreted as a sign of bowel obstruction on films of patients in an upright position. However, air-fluid levels may also accompany a variety of nonobstructive conditions and may occur in normal patients. Air-fluid levels are particularly common in the right side of the colon after cathartic preparation.[26]

## Potential Intraperitoneal Spaces

The reflections of the peritoneum from the posterior abdominal wall over the viscera give rise to potential spaces in which blood, fluid, or pus may localize in the peritoneal cavity.[13] In a normal abdomen, these compartments are not directly visible on plain films, but their location can be inferred from the location of adjacent organs. Familiarity with the anatomy facilitates interpretation of abdominal radiographs. The right subphrenic space is located between the right hemidiaphragm and the liver, above the superior reflection of the right coronary ligament. It is continuous around the lateral edge of the liver with the right subhepatic space. The anterior subhepatic space lies just above the transverse colon and mesocolon and anterior to the right kidney and duodenum. The posterior subhepatic space, also known as Morison's pouch, continues posteriorly and superiorly to the inferior reflection of the coronary ligament. On plain films, Morison's pouch overlies the superior pole of the right kidney.[13] This pouch is the most dependent portion of the peritoneal cavity when the patient is in the supine position, and it is a frequent site of abscess formation. The subhepatic space is continuous with the right paracolic gutter between the ascending colon and properitoneal fat. The right paracolic gutter is deeper and wider than the left paracolic gutter. Fluid and abscesses are often visible here and can be recognized on plain films by separation of the ascending colon and properitoneal fat (Fig. 12–14). The left subphrenic space is separated from the right subphrenic space by the falciform ligament. It surrounds the left lobe of the liver and spleen and is limited inferiorly by the phrenicocolic ligament. Below the phrenicocolic ligament, the shallow left paracolic gutter extends inferiorly into the portion of the pelvis lateral to the descending colon (see Fig. 12–5).

The lesser sac of the peritoneal cavity is a potential space in the midabdomen, extending into the left upper quadrant. It is bounded superiorly by the left lobe of

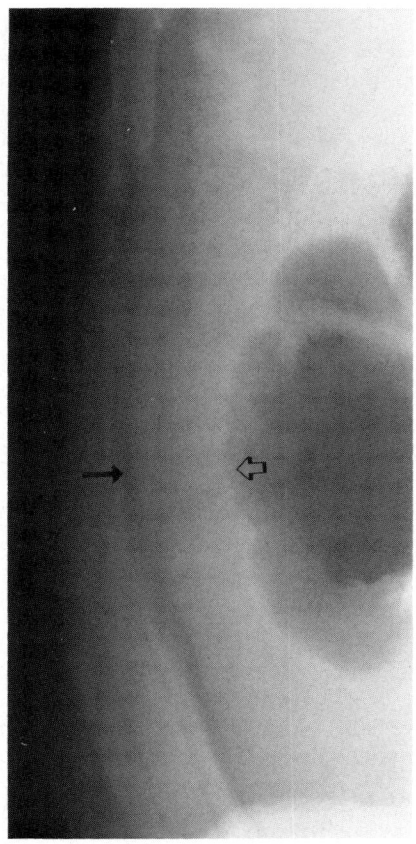

**Figure 12–14. Intraperitoneal fluid in the right paracolic gutter.** Note how fluid in this space separates the ascending colon *(open arrow)* from the properitoneal fat *(solid arrow)*. Ascitic fluid has also displaced the hepatic angle from the surrounding extraperitoneal fat, so that it is no longer visible in this patient.

the liver; posteriorly by the pancreas; anteriorly by the stomach, lesser omentum, and gastrocolic ligament; and inferiorly by the transverse colon and mesocolon[16] (Fig. 12–15A). Its left lateral borders are formed by the gastrosplenic and splenorenal ligaments. The sac opens into the right subhepatic space via the foramen of Winslow at a site just posterior and superior to the duodenal bulb, beneath the free margin of the hepato-duodenal ligament. Dodds and associates have described the lesser sac as an area defined by placing the right hand over the upper abdomen with the thumb extended over the midline and the fingers directed toward the hilum of the spleen[27] (Fig. 12–15B). Space-occupying lesions or fluid collections in the lesser sac may displace the transverse colon inferiorly and the stomach anteriorly, laterally, or medially.

## PELVIS

Extraperitoneal fat in the pelvis often allows plain film identification of various pelvic muscles and viscera. Delineation of these structures is highly variable and depends on the bowel content, degree of bladder distention, angulation of the x-ray beam, position of the patient, and body habitus. Absence of these pelvic interfaces on radiographs must therefore be interpreted with caution and is not necessarily a sign of disease.

## Piriformis Muscle

The piriformis muscle lies in the superolateral aspect of the pelvis along its posterior wall.[16] The inferior

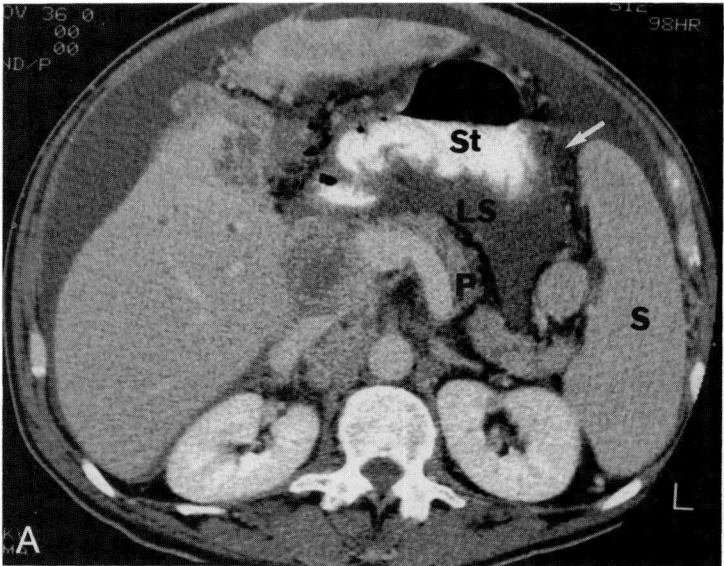
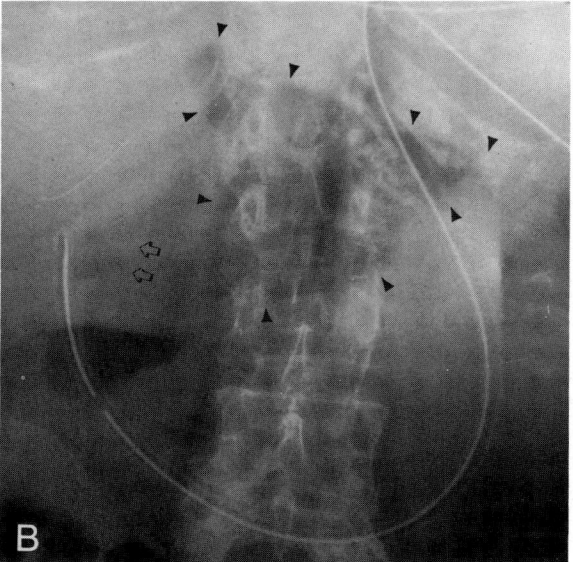

**Figure 12–15. Lesser peritoneal sac. A.** A CT scan in a patient with fluid in the lesser sac (LS) shows the anatomic boundaries of this space. Note posterior location of the pancreas (P), lateral locations of the spleen (S) and gastrosplenic ligament *(arrow),* and anterior location of the stomach (St). **B.** The boundaries of the lesser sac *(arrowheads)* are well delineated on a supine abdominal radiograph in another patient, who has gas in the lesser sac due to an abscess. The superior recess of the lesser sac extends toward the diaphragm just to the right of the spine. The foramen of Winslow is denoted by the open arrows. A nasogastric tube is present in the stomach.

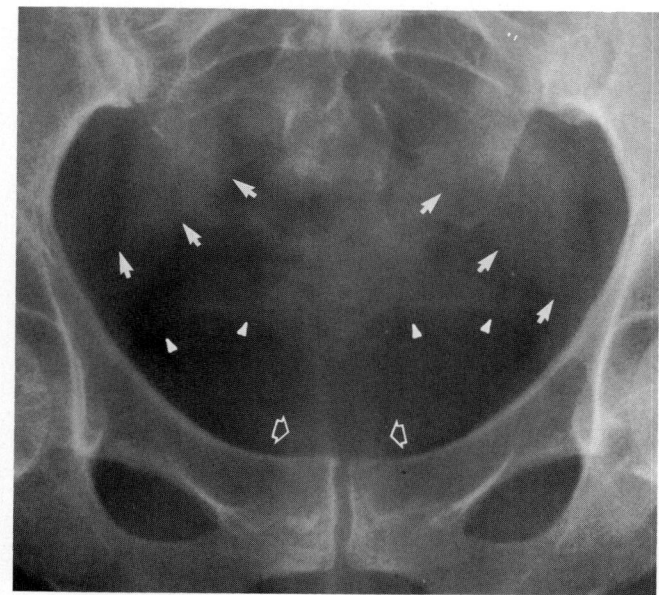

**Figure 12–16. Piriformis muscle.** The inferior margin of the piriformis muscle is seen bilaterally on this abdominal plain film as a smooth, convex line *(solid arrows)* in the superolateral aspect of the pelvis. Just inferior to the piriformis muscle, the edge of the sacrospinous ligament and the closely associated coccygeus muscle outline the roof of the ischiorectal fossa *(arrowheads)*. The perineum forms the medial boundary of the ischiorectal fossa *(open arrows)*.

border of the piriformis muscle may be visualized as a smooth, convex interface passing from the sacrum to the greater sciatic foramen (Figs. 12–16 and 12–17). The site at which the sciatic nerve passes out of the pelvis is just caudal to the piriformis muscle. Internal hernias containing bowel, bladder, or ureter may extend through the greater sciatic foramen into the buttocks.

## Obturator Internus Muscle

The obturator internus muscle lies along the lateral pelvic side wall and surrounds the greater portion of the obturator foramen.[16] The muscle arises from the ramus of the pubis, the ischium, and the pelvic wall, and its tendon exits the pelvis at the lesser sciatic foramen just below the sacrospinous ligament. The obturator internus muscle may be seen on plain films as a result of subperitoneal fat that surrounds it superiorly and ischiorectal

fat that surrounds it inferiorly, below the origin of the levator ani muscle (Fig. 12–18). The obturator canal is located on the superolateral aspect of the obturator foramen and transmits the obturator vessels and nerve.[16] It may be a site of herniation, particularly in elderly women. These hernias are often associated with characteristic neuralgia in the thigh attributable to nerve compression.[28, 29]

## Sacrospinous Ligament and Coccygeus Muscle

Just inferior to the piriformis muscle, a smooth band arching from the tip of the sacrum to the ischial spine is frequently observed (see Fig. 12–16). This band represents the edge of the sacrospinous ligament and closely associated coccygeus muscle outlined by underlying ischiorectal fat[16] (Fig. 12–19).

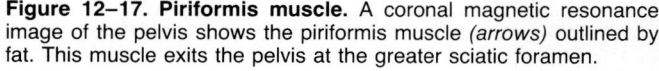

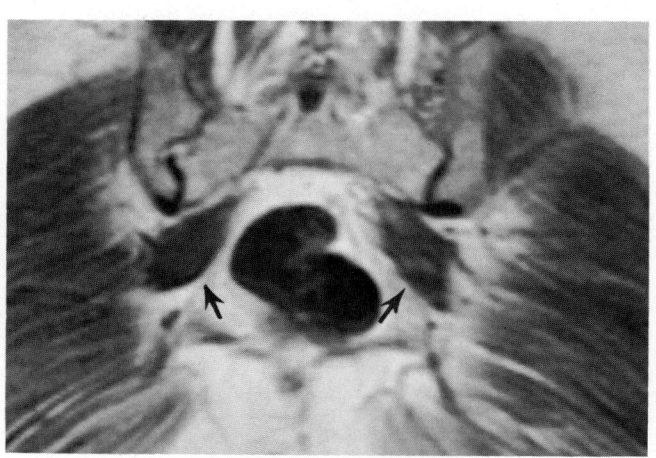

**Figure 12–17. Piriformis muscle.** A coronal magnetic resonance image of the pelvis shows the piriformis muscle *(arrows)* outlined by fat. This muscle exits the pelvis at the greater sciatic foramen.

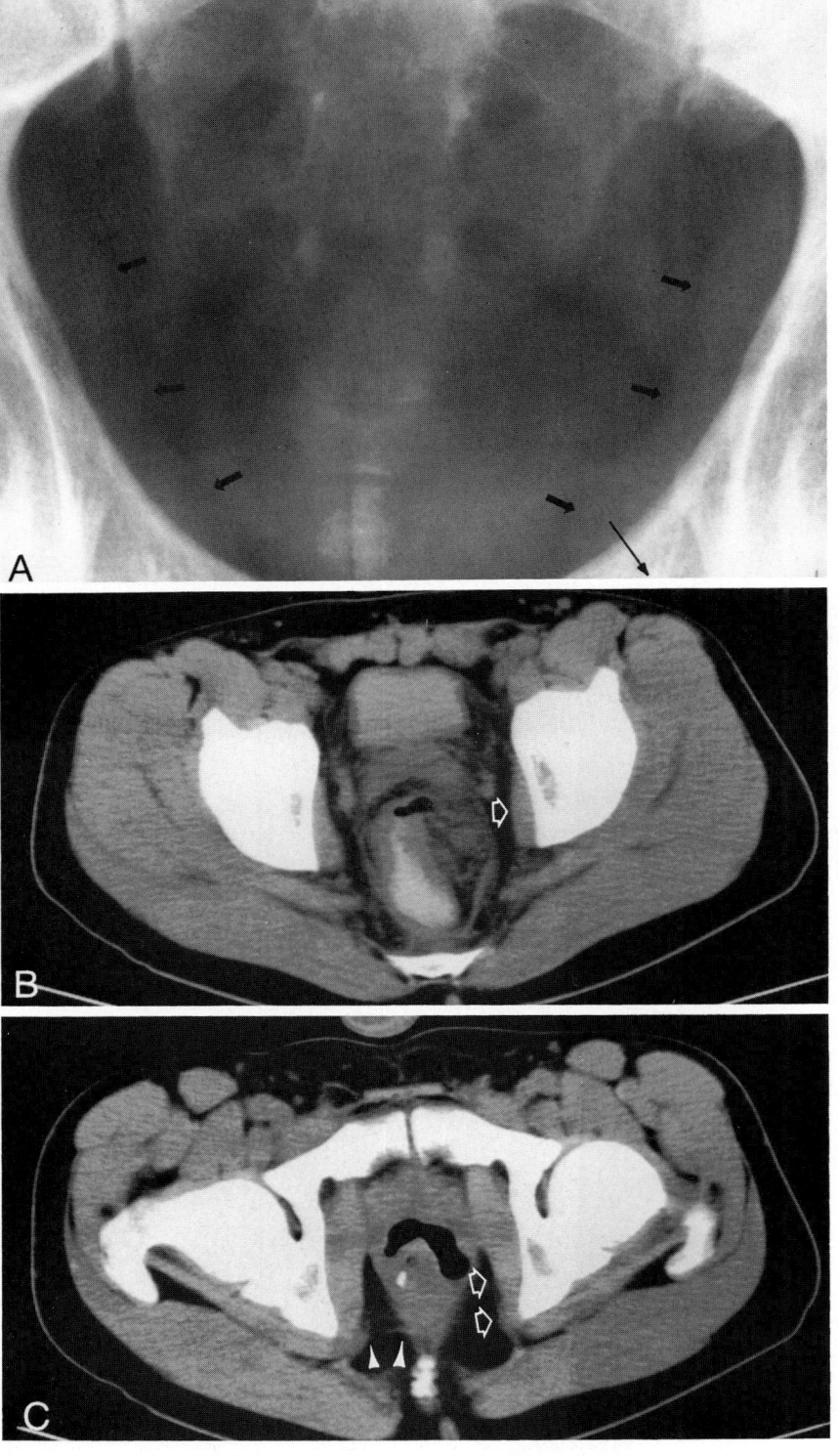

**Figure 12–18. Obturator internus muscle. A.**
The obturator internus muscle lines the pelvic side-wall *(short arrows)*. The obturator canal leaves the pelvis beneath the pubic ramus *(long arrow)*. **B.** A CT scan above the level of the ischial spines shows the most superior portion of the obturator internus muscle outlined by extraperitoneal fat *(arrow)*. **C.** Between the ischial spine and pubis, a thickened band of obturator fascia gives rise to the levator ani muscle, which stretches across the pelvic floor to the perineum *(arrowheads)*. Below the origin of the levator ani muscle, the inferior portion of the obturator internus muscle is outlined by ischiorectal fat *(arrows)*.

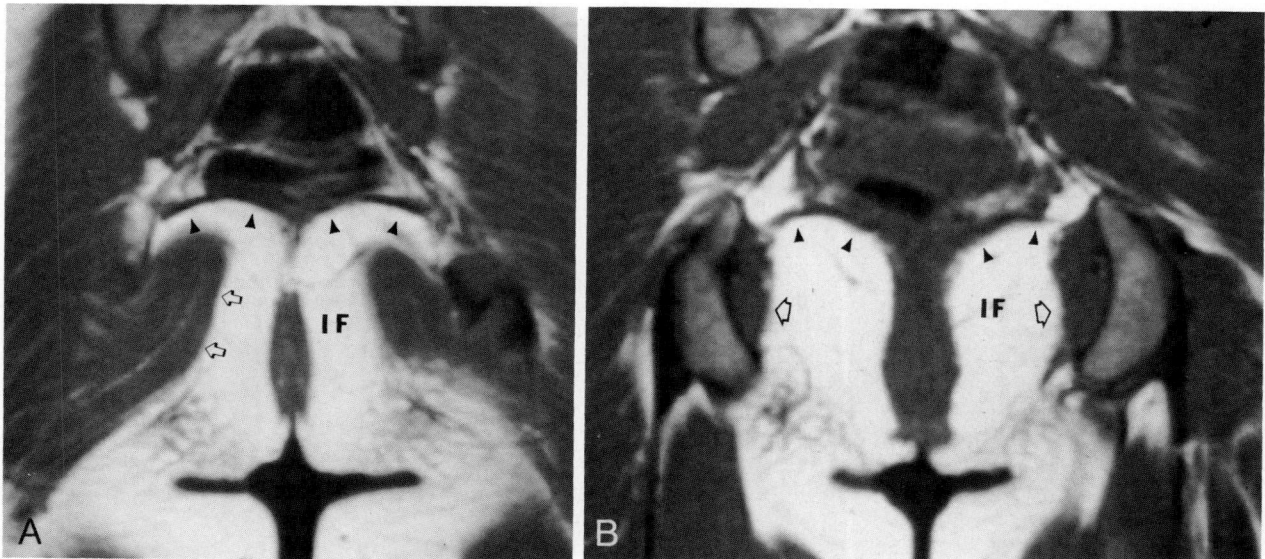

**Figure 12–19. Sacrospinous ligament and coccygeus muscle. A.** A coronal magnetic resonance image shows the inferior edge *(arrowheads)* of the sacrospinous ligament and the coccygeus muscle above the ischiorectal fossa (IF). Note that the gluteus maximus muscle *(arrows)* forms the posterolateral border of the ischiorectal fossa. **B.** A coronal magnetic resonance image more anteriorly shows the levator ani muscle *(arrowheads)* supporting the pelvic viscera and forming the anterior roof of the ischiorectal fossa (IF). The obturator internus muscles *(arrows)* form the lateral border of the ischiorectal fossa.

## Levator Ani Muscle

The floor of the pelvis is formed by the coccygeus muscle posteriorly and the levator ani muscle anteriorly.[16] These muscles stretch across the pelvis like a sling and support the pelvic viscera, closing the abdominal cavity caudally (Fig. 12–20). The levator ani muscle arises along the lateral aspect of the pelvis from the superior ramus of the pubis, the ischial spine, and a thickened band of fascia covering the inner surface of the obturator internus muscle.[16] It passes downward and

medially to the anal sphincter and central tendon of the perineum (see Figs. 12–18C and 12–19B). The thin fasciculi of the muscle are not often visualized on abdominal radiographs.

## Ischiorectal Fossa

The ischiorectal fossa is a wedge-shaped collection of subcutaneous fat, with its base at the perineum and its apex at the junction of the obturator internus and levator

**Figure 12–20. Levator ani muscle and ischiorectal fossa.** A sagittal magnetic resonance image through the pelvis and lateral to the midline shows the coccygeus muscle posteriorly *(open arrow)* and the levator ani muscle anteriorly *(solid arrows)*, stretching across the floor of the pelvis. These muscles form the roof of the ischiorectal fossa (IF). The gluteus maximus muscle (GM) forms the posterior border of the ischiorectal fossa. B = bladder.

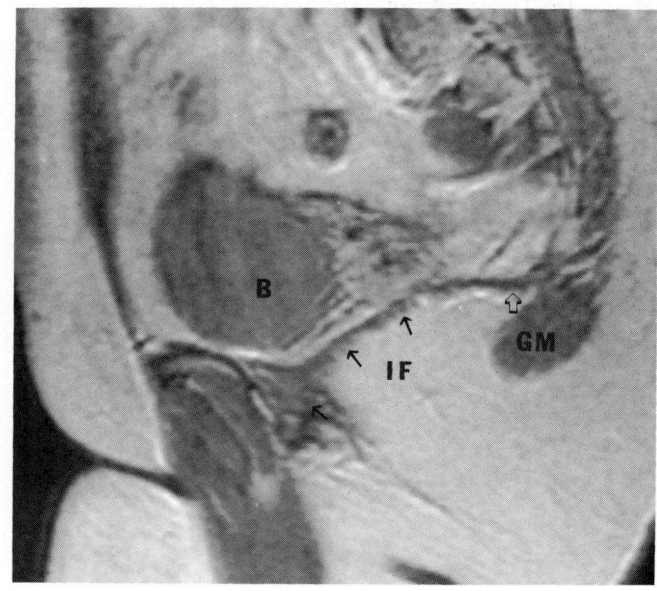

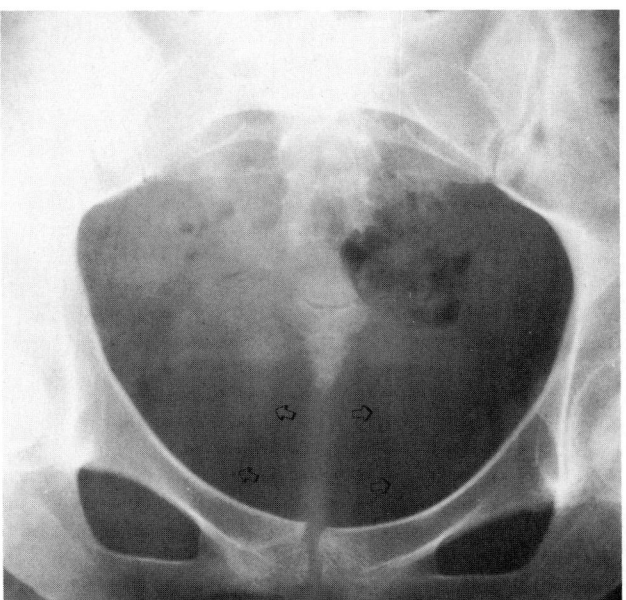

**Figure 12–21. Gluteus maximus muscle.** The medial edge of this muscle *(arrows)* is visualized on plain film because of adjacent ischiorectal fat.

ani muscles[16] (see Figs. 12–19 and 12–20). Its margins are often discernible on plain films (see Figs. 12–16 and 12–21).

## Gluteus Maximus Muscle

The posterior border of the ischiorectal fossa is formed by the gluteus maximus muscle[16] (see Figs. 12–19 and 12–20). Because the medial edge of this muscle is outlined by subcutaneous fat, it often appears on plain films as a smooth line extending inferiorly and laterally from the tip of the sacrum (Fig. 12–21).

## Pelvic Viscera

Subperitoneal fat in the pelvis may outline the superior and lateral aspects of the fluid-filled urinary bladder (Fig. 12–22). The uterus may also be visible in the pelvis, particularly if the fundus is anteverted and impresses adjacent fat (Fig. 12–23). The prostate gland is caudal to the urinary bladder and is not visible unless prostatic calculi are present (Fig. 12–24). Posterior to the bladder and uterus, the rectum can usually be recognized by the presence of intraluminal gas and stool (see Fig. 12–22).

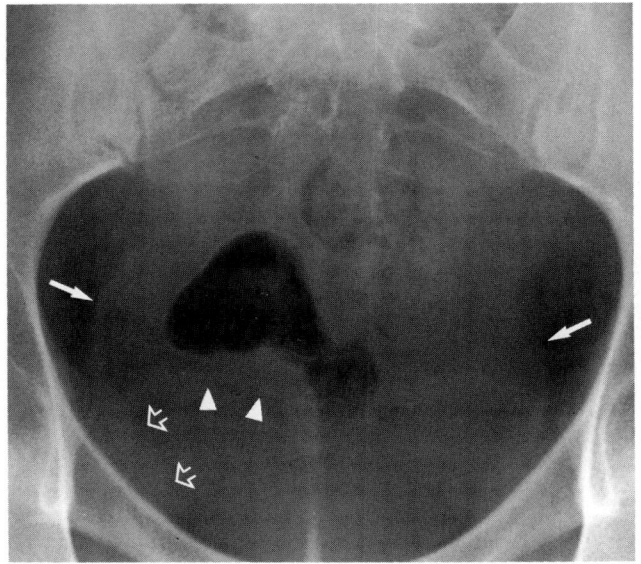

**Figure 12–22. Urinary bladder.** The lateral margins of the filled urinary bladder are outlined by subperitoneal fat *(solid arrows)*. Note the margins of the ischiorectal fossa, formed by the obturator internus muscle *(open arrows)* and the sacrospinous ligament and coccygeus muscles *(arrowheads)*. The rectum contains gas and formed stool.

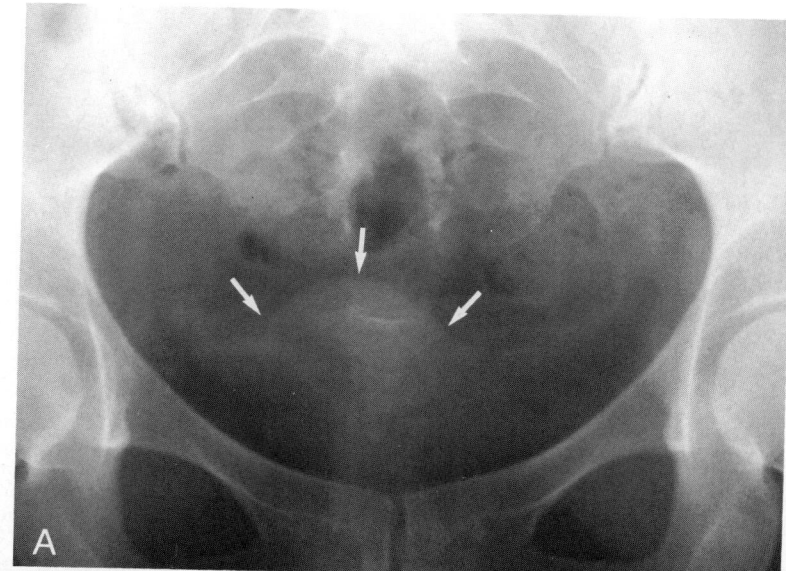

**Figure 12–23. Uterus. A.** This patient has an anteverted uterus *(arrows)* that is visible on abdominal plain film. **B.** A CT scan shows the uterine fundus (U) surrounded by fat. This scan, obtained at the apex of the ischiorectal fossa, shows the sacrospinous ligament and coccygeus muscle *(arrows)* extending from the sacrum (S) to the ischial spine. The subperitoneal fat around the uterus also outlines the upper aspect of the obturator internus muscle (O).

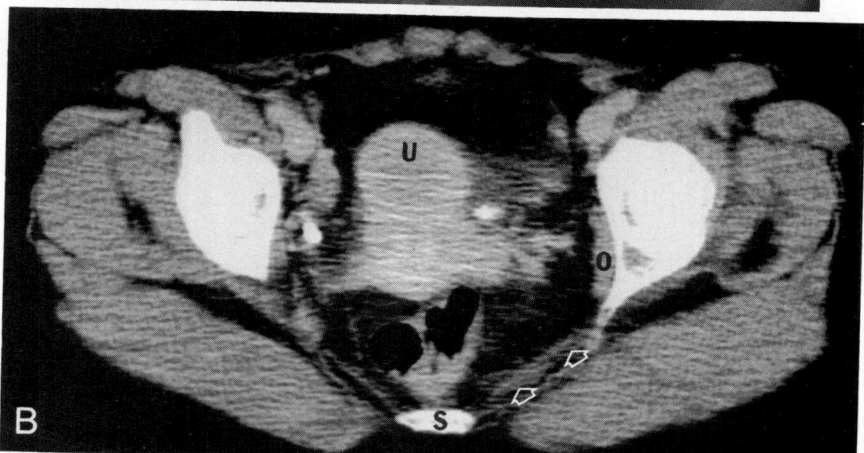

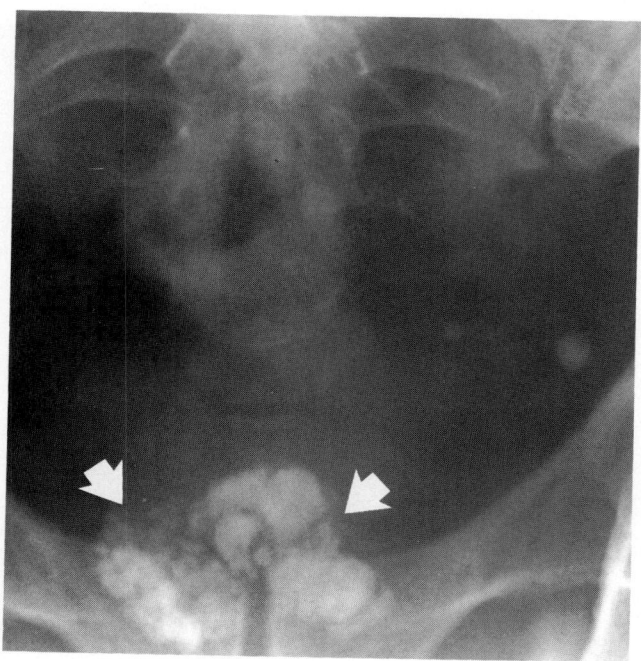

**Figure 12–24. Prostate gland.** An enlarged, calcified prostate *(arrows)* is visible in its normal location beneath the symphysis pubis.

# References

1. Brewer RJ, Golden GT, Hitch DC, et al: Abdominal pain: an analysis of 1000 consecutive cases in a university hospital emergency room. Am Surg 131:219–224, 1976.

2. Eisenberg RL, Heineken P, Hedgcock MW, et al: Evaluation of plain abdominal radiographs in the diagnosis of abdominal pain. Ann Surg 197:464–469, 1983.

3. Mirvis SE, Young JWR, Keramati B, et al: Plain film evaluation of patients with abdominal pain: are three radiographs necessary? AJR 147:501–503, 1986.

4. Eisenberg RL, Hedgcock MW: Preliminary radiograph for barium enema examination: is it necessary? AJR 136:115–116, 1981.

5. Harned RK, Wolf GL, Williams SM: Preliminary abdominal films for gastrointestinal examinations: how efficacious? Gastrointest Radiol 5:343–347, 1980.

6. Schwab FJ, Glick SN, Teplick SK, et al: The barium enema scout film: cost effectiveness and clinical efficacy. Radiology 160:619–622, 1986.

7. Ballinger PW: Merrill's Atlas of Radiographic Positions and Radiologic Procedures, Volume 2 (6th ed). St. Louis: CV Mosby, 1986, pp 32–38.

8. Curry TS, Dowdey JE, Murry RC: Christensen's Physics of Diagnostic Radiology (4th ed). Philadelphia: Lea & Febiger, 1990.

9. Miller RE, Nelson SW: The roentgenologic demonstration of tiny amounts of free intraperitoneal gas: experimental and clinical studies. AJR 112:574–585, 1971.

10. Markus JB, Somers S, Slobodan EF, et al: Interobserver variation in the interpretation of abdominal radiographs. Radiology 171:69–71, 1989.

11. Tibblin S: Diagnosis of intestinal obstruction with special regard to plain roentgen examination of the abdomen. Acta Chir Scand 135:249–252, 1969.

12. Laufer I: The left lateral view in the plain film assessment of abdominal distention. Radiology 119:265–269, 1976.

13. Meyers MA: Dynamic Radiology of the Abdomen. New York: Springer-Verlag, 1979, pp 113–194.

14. Loughran CF: A review of the plain abdominal radiograph in acute rupture of abdominal aortic aneurysms. Clin Radiol 37:383–387, 1986.

15. Whalen JP, Berne AS, Riemenschneider PA: The extraperitoneal perivisceral fat pad. Radiology 92:466–480, 1969.

16. Goss CM, Gray H (eds): Gray's Anatomy of the Human Body (28th ed). Philadelphia: Lea & Febiger, 1968.

17. Elkin M, Cohen G: Diagnostic value of the psoas shadow. Clin Radiol 13:210–217, 1962.

18. Williams SM, Harned RK, Hultman SA, et al: The psoas sign: a reevaluation. Radiographics 5:525–536, 1985.

19. Boyd DP: The anatomy and pathology of the subphrenic spaces. Surg Clin North Am 38:619–626, 1958.

20. Mould RF: An investigation of the variations in normal liver shape. Br J Radiol 45:586–590, 1972.

21. Bundrick TJ, Cho SR, Brewer WH: Ascites: comparison of plain film radiographs with ultrasonograms. Radiology 152:503–506, 1984.

22. Riemenschneider PA, Whalen JP: The relative accuracy of estimation of enlargement of the liver and spleen by radiologic and clinical methods. AJR 94:462–468, 1965.

23. Dodds WJ, Taylor AJ, Erickson SJ, et al: Radiologic imaging of splenic anomalies. AJR 155:805–810, 1990.

24. Johnson CD, Rice RP, Kelvin FM, et al: The radiologic evaluation of gross cecal distension: emphasis on cecal ileus. AJR 145:1211–1217, 1985.

25. Weinstein M: Volvulus of the cecum and ascending colon. Am Surg 107:248–259, 1938.

26. Gammill SL, Nice CM: Air fluid levels: their occurrence in normal patients and their role in the analysis of ileus. Surgery 71:771–780, 1972.

27. Dodds WJ, Foley WD, Lawson TL: Anatomy and imaging of the lesser peritoneal sac. AJR 144:567–575, 1985.

28. Wechsler RJ, Kurtz AB, Needleman L, et al: Cross-sectional imaging of abdominal wall hernias. AJR 153:517–521, 1989.

29. Glicklich M, Eliasoph J: Incarcerated obturator hernia: case diagnosed at barium enema fluoroscopy. Radiology 172:51–52, 1989.

# Gas and Soft Tissue Abnormalities

**James M. Messmer, M.D.**

## INTRODUCTION

The plain abdominal radiograph is one of the most commonly ordered films in radiologic practice. Although the advent of ultrasound and computed tomography (CT) has challenged its worth, plain film radiography has the advantages of relatively low cost, ease of acquisition, and low level of necessary cooperation of the patient, which make it extremely valuable as a simple diagnostic study to the trained and perceptive observer. The film has also been called a KUB, signifying kidneys, ureters (which are not visible), and bladder. The term flat plate of the abdomen is dated and refers to a time when glass plates were used to produce images. *Plain abdominal radiograph, plain film of the abdomen,* and *abdominal plain film* are the preferred terms.

A wealth of diagnostic information can be gained from correct interpretation of abdominal plain films, and several excellent texts are available on the subject.[1-3] This chapter reviews abnormalities of gas and soft tissues that can be detected on these films.

## NORMAL BOWEL GAS PATTERNS

The intestinal tract of adults usually contains less than 200 mL of gas. Intestinal gas has three sources: swallowing of air, bacterial production, and diffusion from the blood.[4, 5] The distribution of this gas appearing on radiographs taken with the patient in the supine position is determined by the patient's position and the quantity of intestinal gas present. Gas rises and accumulates in the anteriorly placed segments of intestine, including the body of the stomach, transverse colon, and sigmoid colon. Gas is also frequently found in the rest of the colon, particularly in the rectum. Gas tends to accumulate in the stomach and colon because of the slower exit of fluid and gas from these structures.

The radiographic evaluation of intestinal gas should include 1) identification of the bowel segment containing the gas; 2) assessment of the caliber of the segment; 3) assessment of the most distal point of passage of the gas; and 4) evaluation of the mucosa outlined by the gas.

The normal bowel gas pattern is readily visible on abdominal plain films taken with the patient in the supine position (Fig. 13–1). The first collection of gas encountered from the top of the film downward is usually in the middle and distal stomach. Gas may also be seen in the transverse colon at a site immediately inferior to the stomach. Gas in the ascending and descending portions of the colon tends to "frame" the abdomen, occupying the lateral margins of the peritoneal cavity. The sigmoid colon occupies the inferior aspect of the abdomen and may be recognized by its characteristic shape and haustra. Rectal gas occupies a midline position in the pelvis and generally extends to the level of the pubic symphysis. The gas-filled small intestine tends to occupy the central portion of the abdomen and has a smaller caliber than the colon.

Although the location of intestinal gas in the abdominal cavity is helpful in differentiating colon from small bowel, recognition of mucosal features is also important. Haustra of the colon tend to be 2 to 3 cm wide and

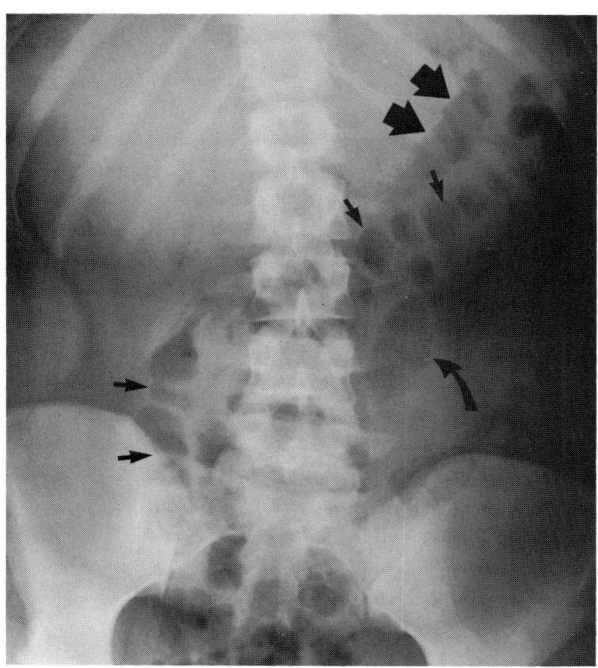

**Figure 13–1. Normal bowel gas pattern.** The most superior collection of intestinal gas is contained in the stomach *(large arrows)*. Gas and stool outline the ascending and transverse colon *(small arrows),* respectively. Gas can also be seen in a portion of the small intestine *(curved arrow).*

occur at intervals of 1 cm, whereas the plicae circulares, or circular folds of the small bowel, are 1 to 2 mm wide and occur at intervals of 1 mm (see Fig. 13–1). Extension of the folds across the entire width of the bowel lumen is not thought to be a helpful point of distinction. The width and spacing of the folds and the location of the bowel loop are believed to be more important distinguishing features. Occasionally, however, the differentiation of colon from small bowel is difficult without a positive contrast study. The small bowel is usually less than 3 cm in diameter, and the colon is less than 5 cm in diameter.

Intestinal gas should be considered a natural contrast agent in the interpretation of abdominal plain films. When the patient is in the supine position, the gastric antrum and body tend to distend with air. A long, narrowed segment of air-filled stomach may indicate a diffuse infiltrating process such as linitis plastica. Gastric ulcerations and malignant masses are also occasionally visible (Fig. 13–2A). In the colon, a narrowed lumen associated with lack of haustra or with a nodular mucosa may be seen in patients with granulomatous or ulcerative colitis (Fig. 13–2B and C). Annular colonic carcinomas may also be visible. Benign colonic polyps are usually small lesions that are indistinguishable from stool on abdominal radiographs, so that they cannot be diagnosed with confidence on the basis of these films.

## ABNORMAL BOWEL GAS PATTERNS

### Gastric Outlet Obstruction

Recognition of gastric outlet obstruction on abdominal plain films depends on the degree of distention of the stomach by air or fluid. The duration of obstruction, the position of the patient, and the frequency of emesis also affect the radiographic appearance. The dilated, air-filled stomach is usually recognized without difficulty because of its characteristic shape and location. Occasionally, however, a massively dilated, fluid-filled stomach can mimic the appearance of ascites or hepatomegaly (Fig. 13–3). Displacement of the transverse colon inferiorly and the characteristic contour of the soft tissue density should help establish that the stomach is dilated. Furthermore, a small amount of air is almost always present within the stomach, so that a film of the chest taken with the patient in an upright position or a film of the abdomen taken with the patient in the right lateral decubitus position should confirm that the soft tissue density represents fluid in the stomach.

The antrum or pyloric region is the usual site of gastric outlet obstruction. The most common causes of obstruction include edema and spasm resulting from an acute pyloric channel ulcer and antral scarring caused by previous ulcers. Other causes include scirrhous gastric carcinomas and scarring from previous ingestion of a caustic substance.

Not all patients with gastric distention have a mechanical obstruction. Metabolic or drug-induced alterations of gastric peristalsis may cause the stomach to become dilated. Gastric atony may also occur in patients with chronic diabetes (i.e., gastroparesis diabeticorum) and is almost always associated with evidence of peripheral neuropathy.[6, 7] The degree of gastric distention does not correlate with blood glucose levels but is an intestinal manifestation of the diabetic neuropathy. Other causes of gastric dilatation include morphine and other atropine-like drugs, uremia, hypokalemia, porphyria, lead poisoning, and previous truncal vagotomy. Pancreatitis

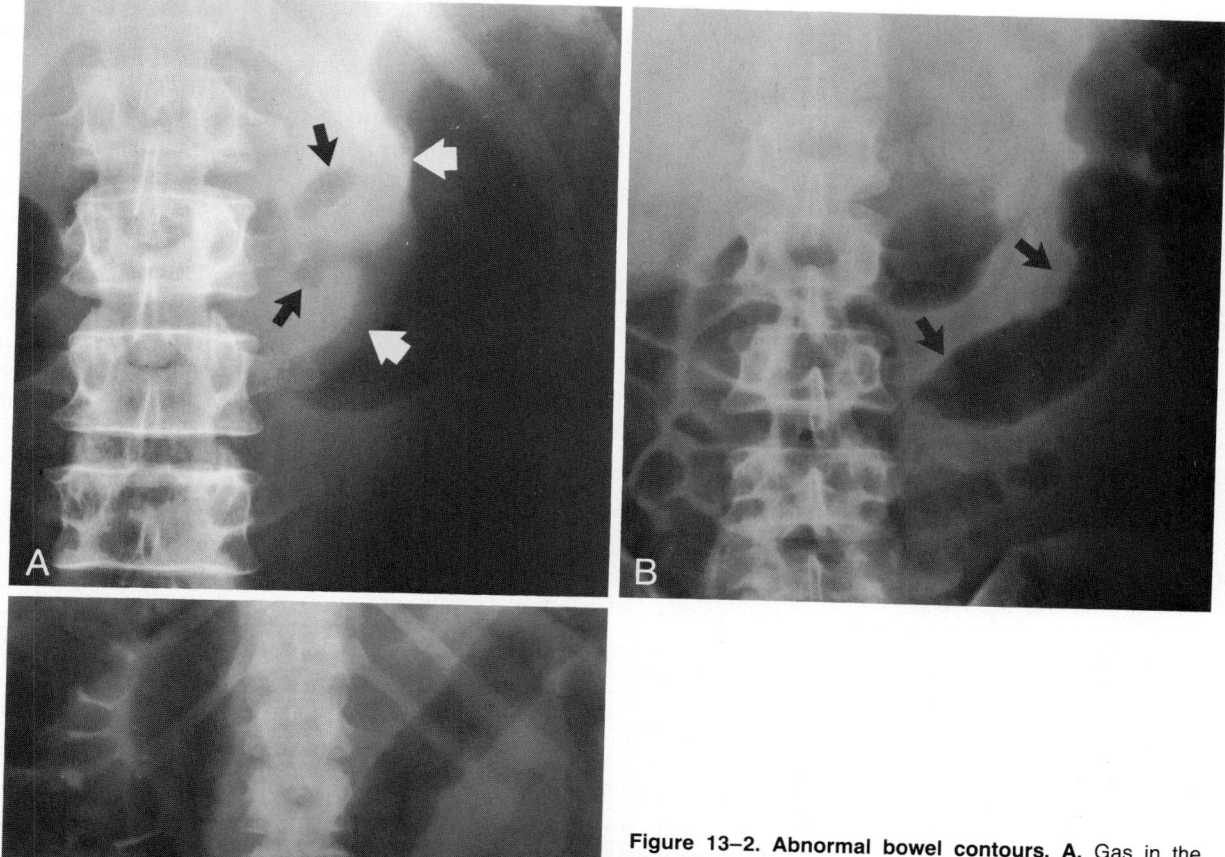

**Figure 13–2. Abnormal bowel contours. A.** Gas in the stomach outlines a mass on the lesser curvature *(white arrows)* with an irregular collection of central gas *(black arrows)*, representing a large benign ulcer with surrounding edema. **B.** Air in the transverse colon outlines a narrowed segment with a nodular contour *(arrows)* attributable to granulomatous colitis. **C.** Narrowing and loss of the haustral pattern are evident in the transverse and descending colon in another patient with ulcerative colitis. A nodular mucosal contour is best demonstrated in the distal descending colon *(arrows)*. (**A** to **C** courtesy of Timothy J. Cole, M.D., Richmond, VA.)

or gastritis may also result in reflex gastric atony, and general anesthesia may occasionally cause marked gastric dilatation.

Patients with obstructive lesions in the duodenum may have the same clinical presentation as patients with gastric outlet obstruction. However, the duodenum may be filled with fluid, so that it is not readily visible on radiographs taken with the patient in the supine position. A left lateral decubitus view of the abdomen may allow air to enter the dilated duodenum, indicating that the obstruction is distal to the pylorus. Contrast studies

are often performed to confirm the presence of gastric outlet obstruction, so that the duodenum must be examined if the stomach appears normal.

## Adynamic Ileus

The term *adynamic ileus* refers to dilated bowel, usually small intestine, in the absence of mechanical obstruction. It is used synonymously with the terms paralytic ileus and nonobstructive ileus. Other authors

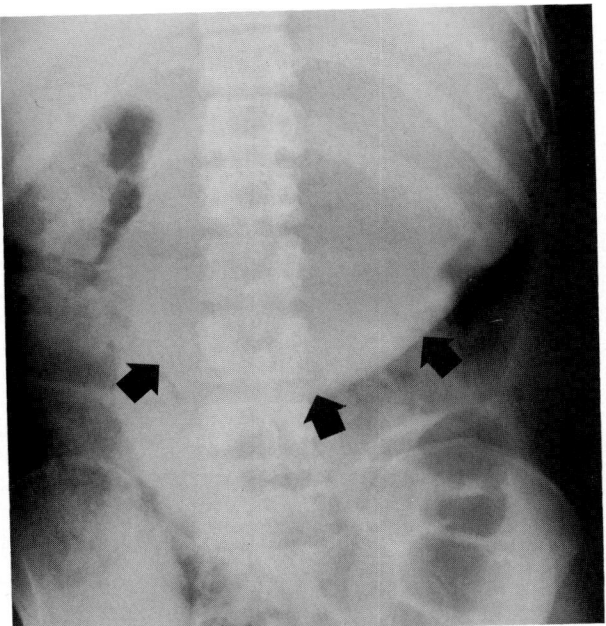

**Figure 13–3. Dilated, fluid-filled stomach.** The large soft tissue density in the left upper quadrant *(arrows)* is due to a dilated stomach filled with fluid in a severely burned patient with gastric atony.

prefer the term nonspecific bowel gas pattern. A more specific term, postoperative ileus, is limited to patients who have undergone recent surgical procedures (Fig. 13–4).

All of these terms refer to a state of absent or decreased intestinal peristalsis, which allows swallowed

air to accumulate in dilated small intestine.[8] The presence of colonic gas may be helpful in distinguishing this condition from a mechanical small bowel obstruction. An adynamic ileus may result from a variety of causes, including electrolyte imbalances, sepsis, generalized peritonitis, blunt abdominal trauma, and infiltration of the mesentery by tumor.[9]

## Small Bowel Obstruction

Small bowel obstruction is often difficult to diagnose on the basis of abdominal plain films. The duration of obstruction, the frequency of emesis, and the use of nasogastric suction may affect the radiographic appearance. False-positive and false-negative rates of 20% have been reported in the diagnosis of intestinal obstruction based solely on the radiographic findings.[10] The diagnostic sensitivity can be increased by correlating the films with the presence or absence of bowel sounds. Sequential films over 12 to 24 hours may be helpful in demonstrating an evolving obstructive pattern. Bryk suggested that films be obtained at 5-minute intervals to distinguish a mechanical obstruction with hyperperistalsis from an adynamic ileus.[11]

When the small intestine becomes completely obstructed, accumulation of swallowed air and intestinal secretions causes proximal dilatation of bowel. Normal peristalsis and colonic contractions eventually eliminate intestinal contents distal to the site of obstruction. This process takes approximately 12 to 24 hours. Abdominal plain films may reveal dilated small bowel loops, usually measuring greater than 3 cm in diameter (allowing for

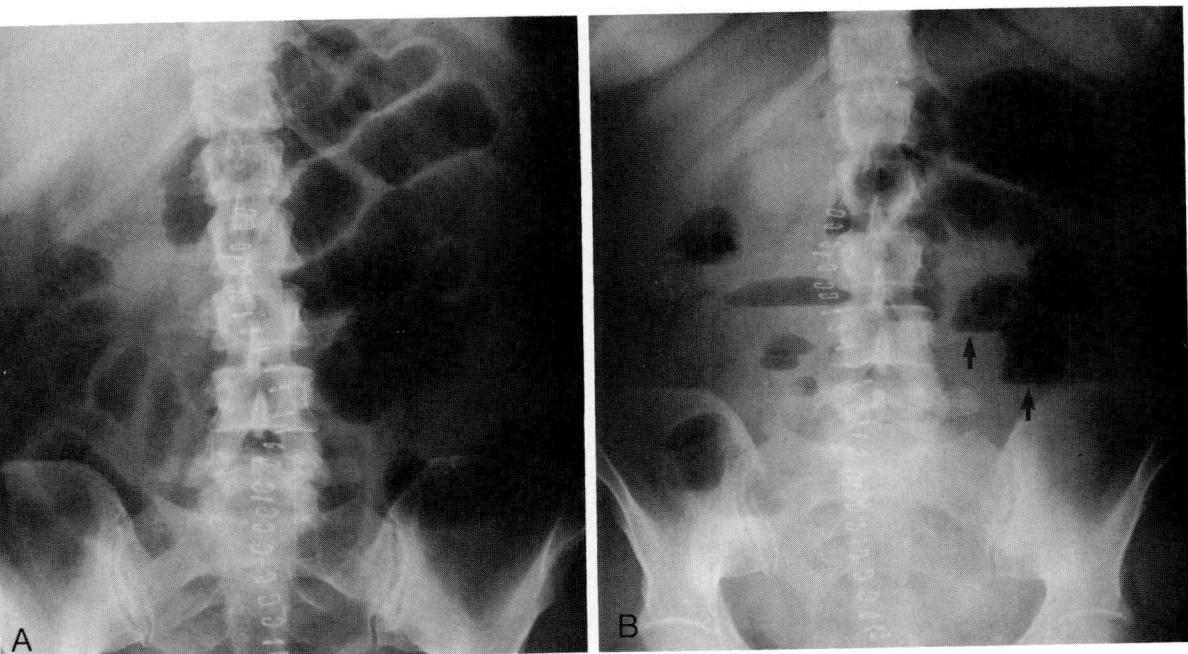

**Figure 13–4. Postoperative ileus. A.** This supine film in a postoperative patient with absent bowel sounds shows multiple loops of mildly dilated small bowel in the abdomen. **B.** The upright film shows differential air-fluid levels *(arrows)* in the same loop of small bowel. This finding may be caused by an ileus or obstruction. Normal intestinal function returned within 48 hours.

magnification), with little if any gas appearing distally in the colon (Fig. 13–5).

Air-fluid levels are often present on films taken in patients with small bowel obstruction who are in an upright or decubitus position. In his classic work on the acute abdomen, Frimann-Dahl stated that the presence of air-fluid levels at two different levels in the same segment of bowel indicated a hyperperistaltic small intestine and was therefore a sign of obstruction.[12] However, subsequent investigators have found that differential air-fluid levels may be present in any tubular structure filled with air and fluid that can be altered with changes in the patient's position.[13–15] Thus, air-fluid levels should be recognized as a nonspecific finding that can accompany an adynamic ileus or mechanical obstruction.

The degree of small bowel dilatation tends to be greater in patients with true mechanical obstruction than in those with an adynamic ileus. As the loops fill with air, they may assume a "stepladder" configuration in the abdomen. In other patients, air may be resorbed through the intestinal wall as fluid accumulates in the bowel lumen, occasionally producing a "gasless" abdomen. Small amounts of air trapped between the plicae circulares on films of patients in an upright position may also produce an appearance that has been likened to a string of beads or pearls (see Fig. 13–5B). This radiographic finding is seldom found in adynamic ileus and therefore suggests mechanical obstruction.

Distinguishing mechanical obstruction from adynamic ileus on the basis of a single set of abdominal films may not be possible. If immediate surgery is not contemplated, further radiographic work-up with contrast studies may be indicated. This topic is discussed in detail in Chapter 52. In general, however, barium studies are helpful in determining the presence, site, and cause of obstruction. Whether orally administered barium and a routine small bowel follow-through is sufficient, or whether enteroclysis is required to evaluate these patients, is controversial. As a rule, the diagnosis can be established more quickly when barium is introduced directly through an indwelling tube or catheter in the small bowel.

In general, water-soluble contrast agents should not be used to determine the presence or site of obstruction in the small bowel. The only exception may be for patients with extremely proximal obstructions. Although water-soluble contrast agents usually offer little or no diagnostic information, they may be used therapeutically to stimulate an adynamic intestine and may occasionally help relieve a partial small bowel obstruction. The mode of action is presumed to be a combination of a direct irritant effect and the drawing of more fluid into the bowel.

Most small bowel obstructions are caused by postoperative adhesions. Such adhesions may occur as early as 1 week after surgery, but more typically the surgery is remote. Although most patients are knowledgeable of their own surgical history, they may not recall having undergone laparoscopy or other surgical procedures during childhood. In the absence of a surgical history, an obstructive hernia should be suspected. Ninety-five percent of such hernias are external (i.e., inguinal, femoral, umbilical, or incisional). The presence of air-filled bowel below the pubic ramus should suggest the possibility of an obstructive inguinal hernia. Internal hernias such as paraduodenal or mesenteric hernias are an uncommon cause of intestinal obstruction and are

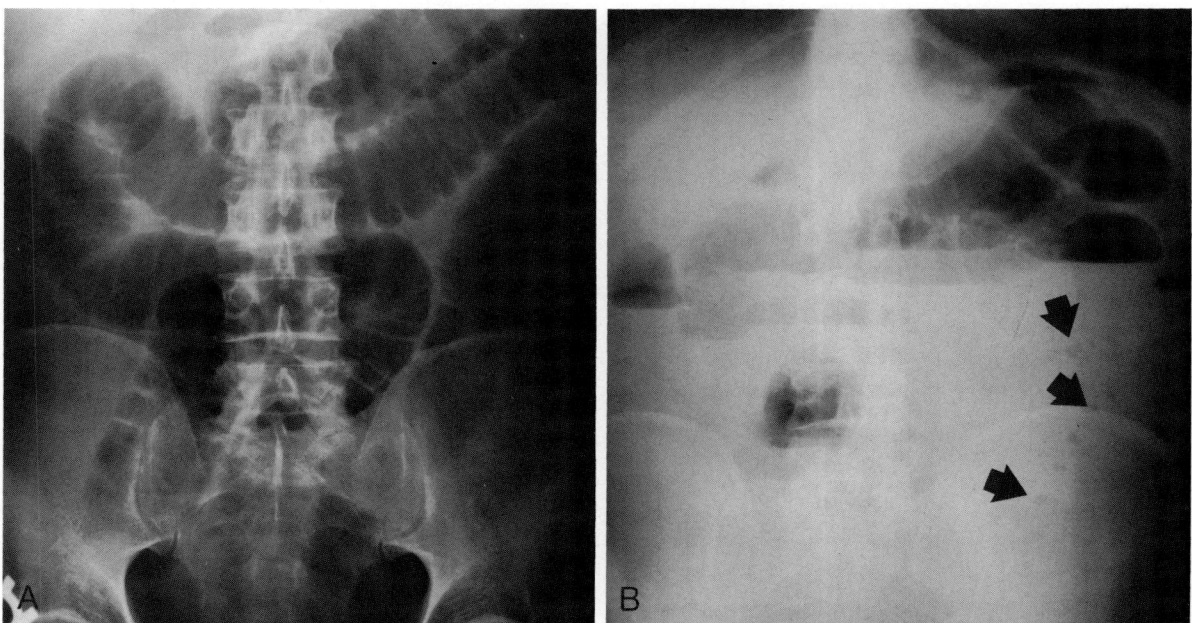

**Figure 13–5. Small bowel obstruction. A.** The supine film demonstrates long segments of dilated small bowel in the abdomen. **B.** The upright film demonstrates multiple air-fluid levels. Also note small amounts of gas trapped between the plicae circulares in the left lower quadrant *(arrows)*, producing the "string of pearls" sign.

rarely suspected in the evaluation of plain films. Other less common causes of small bowel obstruction include tumors of the small intestine, ectopic gallstones, acute appendicitis, and occasionally, intestinal parasites, food, and antiobesity gastric balloons.[16–27]

## Colonic Obstruction

More than 50% of colonic obstructions are caused by primary adenocarcinomas of the colon.[28–30] The obstruction usually occurs in the sigmoid colon, where the bowel tends to have a narrower caliber and the stool is more solid. Conversely, carcinomas of the cecum and ascending colon are less likely to cause obstruction because of the wider caliber of the bowel and more liquid content of the stool. During the past 40 years, the distribution of colonic carcinoma has been noted to shift proximally toward the right side of the colon, most likely because of increased surveillance and the development of flexible sigmoidoscopy.[31–34] In any case, this shift in the distribution of colonic carcinoma should lead to a lower incidence of obstruction from these lesions.

Colonic obstruction is typically manifested on abdominal plain films by dilated, gas-filled loops of colon proximal to the site of obstruction and a paucity or absence of gas in the distal colon and rectum (Fig. 13–6A). A single contrast barium enema may be performed to confirm the presence of obstruction and determine its cause (Fig. 13–6B). In patients with a competent ileocecal valve, the colon (particularly the cecum) may become markedly dilated, and little, if any, gas may be seen in the small bowel. As the cecal diameter increases, the risk of perforation also increases. In various series,

colonic perforations have been reported in as many as 7% of all large bowel obstructions and 2% of obstructing colonic carcinomas.[35–37] Perforations tend to occur at the site of obstruction but may also result from ischemic change that is located more proximally in the dilated colon or cecum.[37]

An incompetent ileocecal valve allows gas to reflux proximally into the small bowel, producing findings on plain film that can mimic those of small bowel obstruction. A close search for colonic gas is therefore required. A right lateral decubitus view may be used to facilitate passage of gas distally into the descending colon and rectosigmoid. The presence of occult blood in the stool in an elderly patient may also suggest the correct diagnosis. The distinction between colonic obstruction and small bowel obstruction has important diagnostic implications, because orally administered barium may inspissate above an unsuspected colonic obstruction. A single contrast barium enema or water-soluble contrast enema should therefore be considered in any patient with apparent obstruction of the distal small bowel on abdominal plain films to rule out an underlying colonic obstruction (see Fig. 13–6). If an obstructing carcinoma is encountered in the colon, the fluoroscopist should try to minimize reflux of barium above the level of the tumor (see Chapter 67).

## Colonic Ileus

Acute colonic pseudo-obstruction was first described in 1948 by Ogilvie, who postulated that progressive colonic dilatation was caused by interruption of sympathetic innervation with unopposed parasympathetic in-

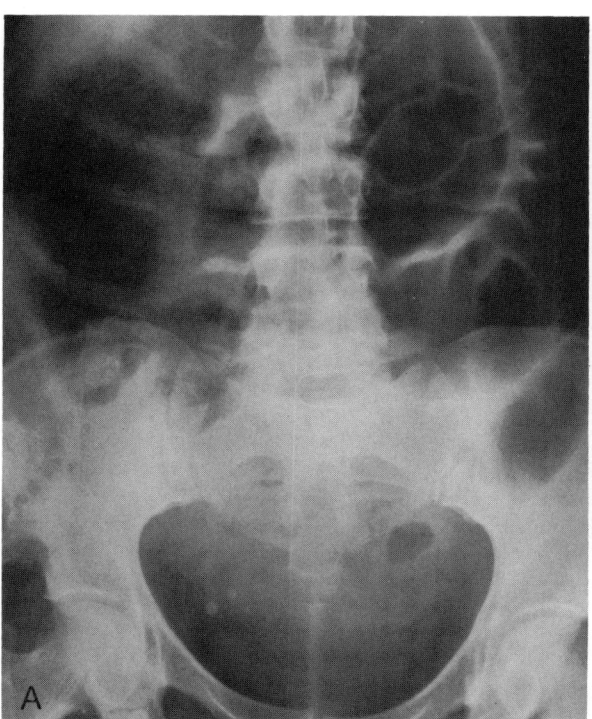

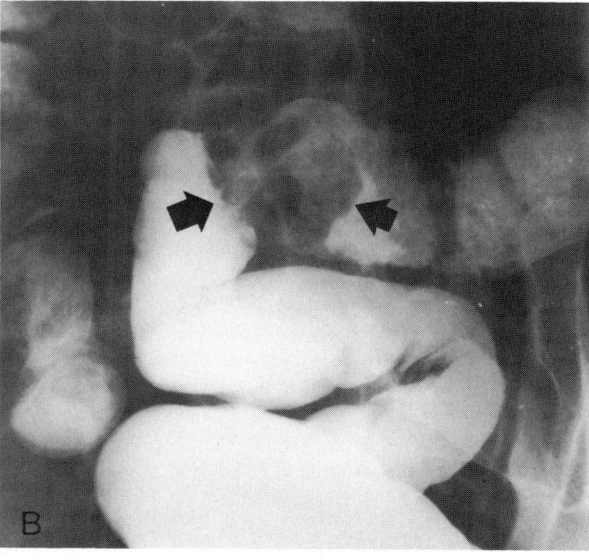

**Figure 13–6. Distal colonic obstruction attributable to colonic carcinoma. A.** The supine film shows dilated colon with little gas in the sigmoid colon or rectum. **B.** A limited single contrast barium enema reveals an annular carcinoma *(arrows)* in the proximal sigmoid colon.

nervation of the colon.[38] The most common clinical presentation is acute abdominal distention, occurring within 10 days of the onset of the precipitating pathologic process. Intra-abdominal inflammation, alcoholism, cardiac disease, burns, retroperitoneal disease, trauma, and normal pregnancy with spontaneous delivery or cesarean section have all been described as precipitating causes.[39–45]

Abdominal plain films may demonstrate marked colonic distention, which is usually confined to the cecum, ascending colon, and transverse colon. Occasionally, however, gas may extend to the level of the sigmoid colon. The underlying clinical condition and rapid onset of colonic distention usually suggest the diagnosis of colonic pseudo-obstruction, but a limited contrast enema may be performed to rule out obstructive lesions in the colon.

Prediction of impending perforation of the cecum, as judged by cecal diameter, is fraught with difficulty. Although some authors have indicated that a cecal diameter of 9 to 12 cm suggests impending perforation, cecal diameters of 15 to 20 cm are commonly observed in patients who recover spontaneously.[44, 46–49] When a portable technique is used to obtain radiographs in supine obese patients who have an anteriorly placed cecum, marked radiographic magnification may occur. A film taken with the patient in a prone or decubitus position should lessen the effect of magnification. Serial radiographs showing a change in cecal diameter at 12- to 24-hour intervals may be more helpful than a single film showing a dilated cecum. Prolonged cecal distention beyond 2 to 3 days should prompt surgical or colonoscopic decompression.[50] The presence of intramural gas in the region of the dilated cecum strongly suggests infarction and impending perforation.

## Closed Loop Obstruction

A closed loop obstruction refers to a segment of bowel that is obstructed at two points. These obstructions usually involve the small bowel and are caused by an adhesion, internal hernia, or volvulus. The plain film findings are often nonspecific in these patients. Occasionally, the dilated, air-filled segment of bowel may assume a "coffee bean" configuration. Persistence of such an air-filled loop on sequential films for several days suggests the possibility of a closed loop obstruction. Vascular compromise may lead to edema and thickening of the bowel wall. The normally thin plicae circulares may become thickened or effaced. If the obstructed segment becomes filled with fluid, a rounded soft tissue density outlined by intra-abdominal fat may appear as a pseudotumor.[16] The clinical presentation may contribute to the correct diagnosis in these patients. Intermittent, crampy abdominal pain that is replaced by steady, unrelenting pain suggests vascular compromise. However, a definitive diagnosis of a closed loop obstruction can be made only at surgery.

## Volvulus

Any segment of intestine that has a mesenteric attachment has the potential to undergo a volvulus. Some patients may have intermittent intestinal twists associated with recurrent episodes of abdominal pain or emesis. If the twist is greater than 360 degrees, it is unlikely to resolve spontaneously. In some cases, air and intestinal contents may enter the twisted segment of bowel, producing abdominal distention and pain. The risk of vascular compromise in the twisted segment is more important than the mechanical effects of the volvulus. Severe vascular compromise may result in necrosis and perforation of bowel, causing sepsis and even death. Gastric volvulus is discussed in Chapter 40.

### Sigmoid Colon

Approximately 60 to 75% of cases of colonic volvulus involve the sigmoid colon. Overall, sigmoid volvulus accounts for 1 to 2% of all cases of intestinal obstruction in the United States.[51, 52] In some areas of South America and Africa, the incidence of this type of volvulus is extraordinarily high, reportedly because of a high-fiber diet and the resultant large, bulky stools, which produce a chronically dilated, elongated sigmoid colon. The incidence of sigmoid volvulus also appears to be increased in people living at higher altitudes in South America and Africa.[53, 54] In the United States, sigmoid volvulus tends to occur in elderly males and residents of nursing homes and mental hospitals, in whom chronic constipation and obtundation from medication are predisposing factors for gaseous distention of the sigmoid colon.

Patients with sigmoid volvulus may present with abdominal pain and distention attributable to colonic obstruction. Obstipation and vomiting are also common findings. The symptoms are usually acute, but they may have a gradual onset in some patients.[55]

Findings on abdominal plain films are diagnostic of sigmoid volvulus in 75% of patients with this condition. The classic radiographic appearance consists of a dilated loop of sigmoid colon that has an inverted U configuration and absent haustra (Fig. 13–7A). The dilated bowel commonly extends into the upper abdomen above the transverse colon. The bowel may be located in the midline, or it may be directed toward the right or left upper quadrants, where it can elevate the hemidiaphragm. Because sigmoid volvulus represents a closed loop obstruction, there is usually a considerable amount of gas in the more proximal colon. Gas may also be present in the small intestine. The apposed inner walls of the sigmoid colon may occasionally form a dense white line that points toward the pelvis[56] (see Fig. 13–7A). Absence of rectal gas is also an important finding. Prone or decubitus views should facilitate passage of gas into the rectum and exclude the diagnosis of sigmoid volvulus.

Therapy usually consists of emergent sigmoidoscopic

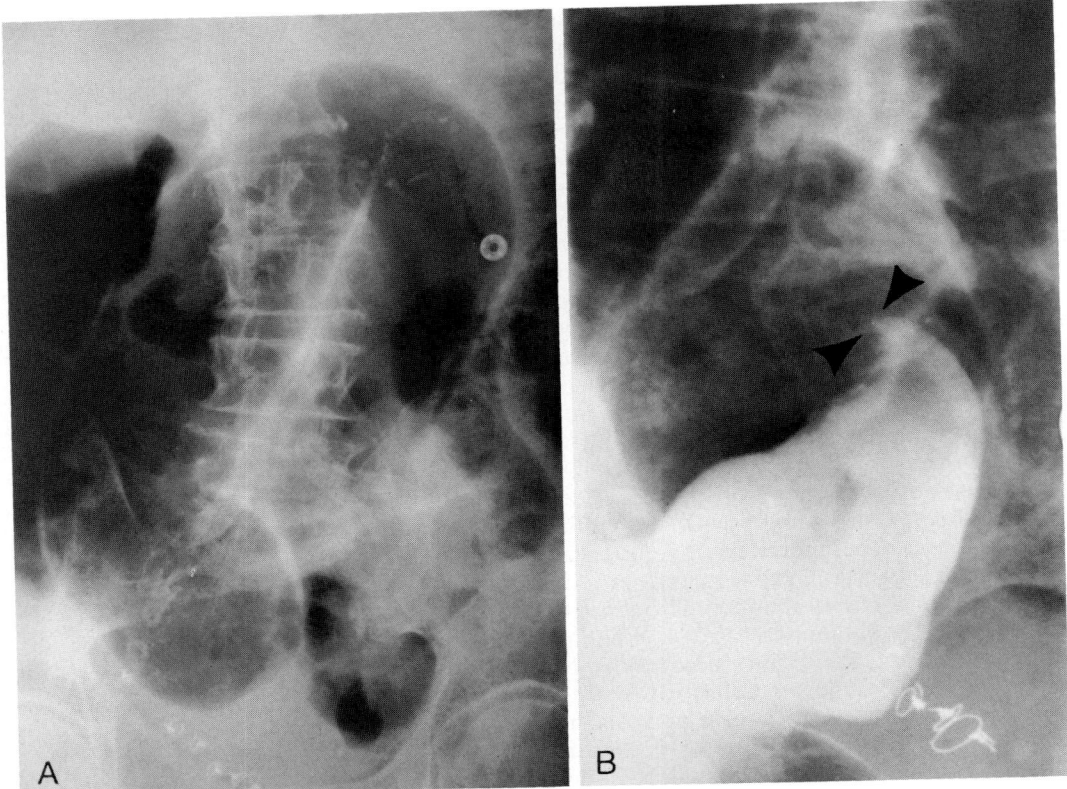

**Figure 13–7. Sigmoid volvulus. A.** A supine abdominal film in a patient with sigmoid volvulus shows the characteristic loop of dilated sigmoid colon with a vertically oriented soft tissue stripe, representing the two apposed walls of the obstructed sigmoid colon. No gas is seen in the rectum. **B.** A subsequent barium enema reveals smooth, tapered narrowing *(arrowheads),* or beaking, of the sigmoid colon at the site of the volvulus.

decompression and placement of a rectal tube. This approach has been successful in up to 90% of cases.[52, 57, 58] However, recurrence of the volvulus after detorsion is common, occurring in more than 50% of cases.[59] A contrast enema may occasionally be required in patients with suspected sigmoid volvulus. A low-pressure barium enema performed without inflation of a rectal balloon should demonstrate smooth, tapered narrowing, or "beaking," at the rectosigmoid junction (Fig. 13–7B). After decompression and stabilization of the patient, a follow-up barium enema may be performed to rule out underlying colonic neoplasms.

## Transverse Colon

Volvulus of the transverse colon is an uncommon condition, accounting for about 4% of all cases of colonic volvulus in the United States.[52] As with sigmoid volvulus, elongation of the transverse mesocolon and close approximation of the hepatic and splenic flexures may allow the transverse colon to rotate. Failure of normal fixation of the mesentery may lead to increased mobility of the ascending colon and hepatic flexure, predisposing the patient to volvulus of the transverse colon.[60, 61] Compression of the duodenojejunal junction at the root of the mesentery may cause severe vomiting. Mortality rates in these patients have been as high as 33%.[62]

Abdominal plain films are usually not helpful in patients with volvulus of the transverse colon and may erroneously suggest sigmoid volvulus. A barium enema can confirm the diagnosis if it demonstrates the typical beaking at the level of the transverse colon. The presence of two air-fluid levels can often be seen in the dilated transverse colon and is helpful in distinguishing volvulus of the transverse colon from cecal volvulus.

## Splenic Flexure of the Colon

The least common site for a colonic volvulus is the splenic flexure. Postoperative adhesions, chronic constipation, and congenital or postsurgical absence of the normal peritoneal attachments may predispose patients to this uncommon condition.[63–65] Abdominal plain films may suggest the diagnosis of volvulus of the splenic flexure, but as with volvulus of the transverse colon, a barium enema is often needed to confirm this diagnosis.[66] The only plain film finding may be a dilated, featureless, air-filled loop of bowel that is located in the left upper quadrant and is separate from the stomach.[67]

## Cecum

The term *cecal volvulus* refers to a condition characterized by a rotational twist of the right colon on its axis associated with folding of the right colon, so that the cecum is located in the midabdomen or left upper quadrant. Cecal volvulus can occur only when the right colon is incompletely fused to the posterior parietal peritoneum, an embryologic variant present in 10 to 37% of normal adults.[52, 68, 69] The term cecal volvulus is actually a misnomer, because the twist is distal to the ileocecal valve. Cecal volvulus is less common than sigmoid volvulus, accounting for 2 to 3% of all colonic obstructions and about one third of all cases of colonic volvulus.

Abdominal plain film findings are diagnostic of cecal volvulus in about 75% of patients with this condition. Plain films characteristically reveal a dilated, air-filled cecum in an ectopic location, usually with the cecal apex in the left upper quadrant (Fig. 13–8A). The medially placed ileocecal valve may produce a soft tissue indentation, so that the gas-filled cecum has the appearance of a coffee bean or kidney (Fig. 13–8B). Usually, little gas is seen distally in the colon. If the ileocecal valve is incompetent, refluxed gas in the small bowel may erroneously suggest a small bowel obstruction and obscure the diagnosis. A contrast enema shows typical beaking at the point of the volvulus in the mid–ascending colon.[69, 70]

Cecal volvulus is likely to occur in a variety of clinical settings, including colonoscopy, barium enema, obstructive lesions in the distal colon, and pregnancy.[52, 71–74]

In 1938, Weinstein described a condition known as *cecal bascule*, which involved folding of the right colon without twisting, so that the cecum occupied a position in the midabdomen.[75] The term bascule is derived from *bascula*, the Latin word for scale.[1] The point at which the ascending colon is folded represents the fulcrum of the scale. This entity also requires a loosely attached right colon.[76] The concept of a cecal bascule was challenged by Johnson and colleagues, who believed that these patients have a focal adynamic ileus of the cecum.[50] Twenty percent of their patients had cecal perforation. They emphasized that the duration of cecal distention was more important than cecal diameter in predicting impending perforation.

Whether cecal bascule represents an actual anatomic folding of the right colon or an adynamic ileus is not as important as the recognition of a dilated, ectopically located cecum as a source of symptoms and potential perforation.

## APPENDICITIS

The development of acute appendicitis requires obliteration of the appendiceal lumen, usually by a concretion that may be visible on abdominal plain films. The concretion has been called a fecalith or coprolith, but the preferred term is *appendicolith*. This concretion forms around a nidus such as a piece of vegetable matter. Inspissated feces and calcium salts may adhere to this nidus, so that it eventually reaches a size that occludes the appendiceal lumen. Accumulation of mucus proximal to the obstruction may distend the appendix, causing infection, ischemia, and subsequent perforation.

Acute appendicitis is a common cause of abdominal

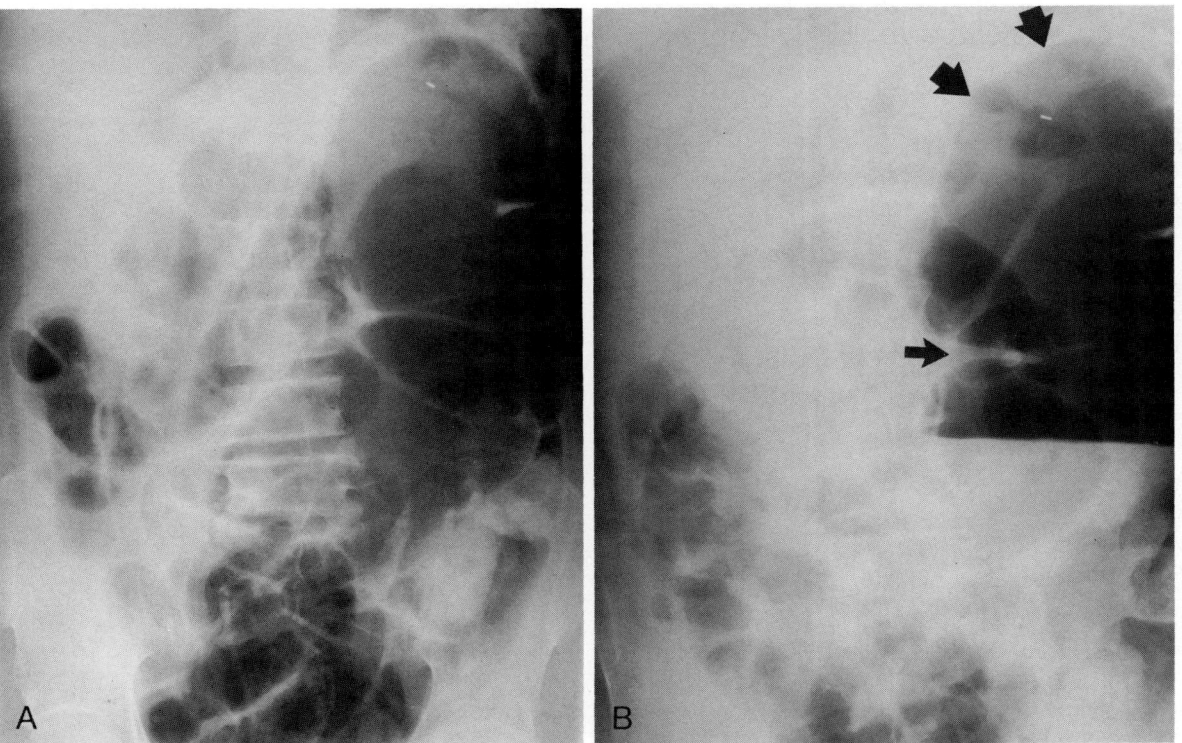

**Figure 13–8. Cecal volvulus. A.** A supine abdominal film shows a markedly dilated viscus in the left upper quadrant, representing the obstructed cecum. Note multiple loops of dilated small bowel. **B.** The upright film shows the caput of the cecum *(thick arrows)* and the ileocecal valve *(thin arrow)* with a single air-fluid level in the dilated cecum.

pain. Some investigators believe that abdominal plain films have little value in patients with suspected appendicitis.[77, 78] Nevertheless, such films are frequently obtained as the first imaging study in these patients. The plain film findings of appendicitis include the following:

1. *Appendicolith.* The appearance of an appendicolith is the most helpful plain film finding. Appendicoliths are found in about 10% of patients with acute appendicitis. They typically appear as round or oval calcified densities and are frequently laminated (Fig. 13–9A). Appendicoliths usually range from 1 to 2 cm in size but may be as large as 4 cm.[79–83] They are usually located in the right lower quadrant but can also be located in the pelvis, right upper quadrant, or even the left upper quadrant.[83] The presence of an appendicolith has important clinical implications, as it often indicates appendicitis complicated by perforation and abscess formation.

2. *Abnormal bowel gas pattern.* About 25% of patients with appendicitis have an abnormal bowel gas pattern—most commonly an adynamic ileus, but occasionally a partial or even complete small bowel obstruction (see Fig. 13–9).[84] An adynamic ileus occurs as a response to focal inflammation and may be localized to the right lower quadrant. Air-fluid levels in the jejunum have been described in up to 50% of cases.[85] A dilated transverse colon may also be seen as an early sign of appendiceal perforation.[86] A mechanical obstruction may occur if the terminal ileum is compressed by the appendix or is bound by adhesive bands. The small bowel may also herniate through a loop formed by the inflamed appendix.[24–27]

3. *Abnormal cecum and ascending colon.* Local inflammation and edema may cause thickening of the cecal wall and widening of the haustra. A cecal air-fluid level may also be present on films of the patient in an upright or decubitus position;[86, 87] this finding is transient and nonspecific.

4. *Extraluminal soft tissue mass.* A soft tissue mass can be found in up to one third of patients with perforation. It may be caused by a combination of edema, fluid, and fluid-filled loops of small bowel in the right lower quadrant. The presence of mottled gas within the soft tissue mass indicates an abscess.

5. *Gas in the appendix.* This sign has been described as one of acute appendicitis,[88, 89] but an air-filled appendix may be a normal finding and simply reflects the position of the appendix in relation to the cecum. An ascending retrocecal appendix is more likely to contain gas.

6. *Free intraperitoneal air.* A ruptured appendix may rarely lead to the development of a small amount of free intraperitoneal air. The obstructed appendiceal lumen prevents larger collections of gas from escaping into the peritoneal cavity, except in the case of a ruptured gas-containing abscess.[90–94]

7. *Obliteration of normal fat planes.* Inflammation and edema may alter the water content of surrounding fat and obscure the normal fat planes of the psoas muscle, obturator muscle, or properitoneal flank stripe (Fig. 13–10). This finding is nonspecific and usually associated with other plain film signs of appendicitis.

8. *Scoliosis of the lumbar spine.* Some patients with appendicitis may develop lumbar scoliosis as a result of splinting. However, this finding is non-

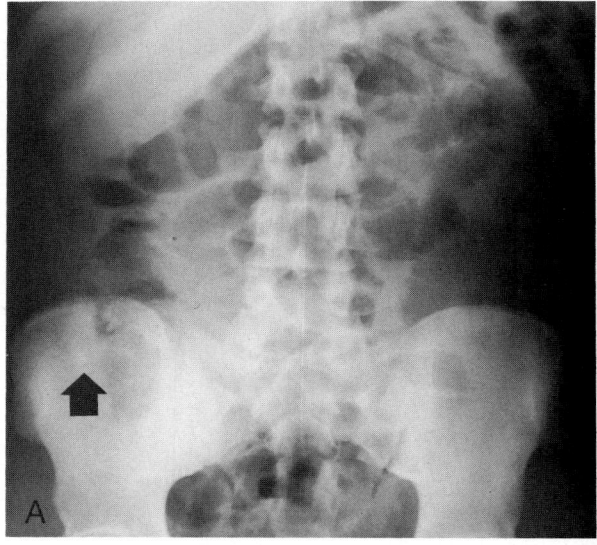
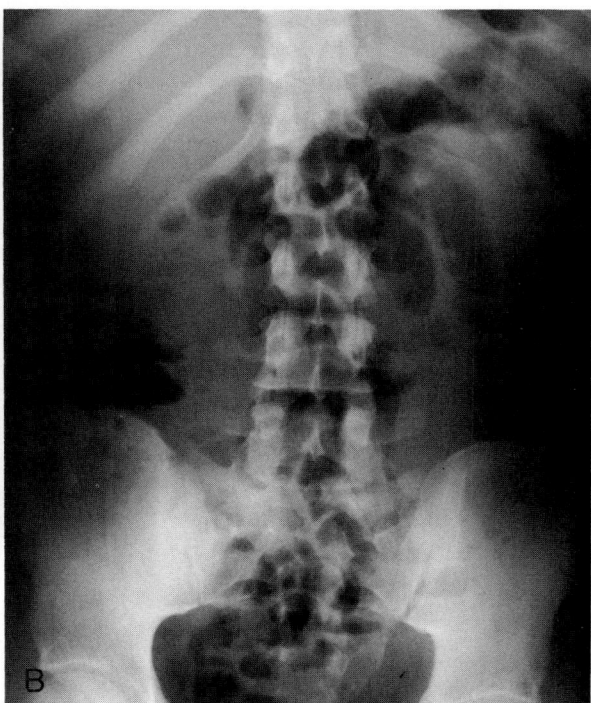

**Figure 13–9. Acute appendicitis with partial small bowel obstruction. A.** The supine film shows mildly dilated small bowel with a laminated appendicolith *(arrow)* in the right lower quadrant. **B.** An upright film shows air-fluid levels in the small bowel. Note the relative paucity of colonic gas.

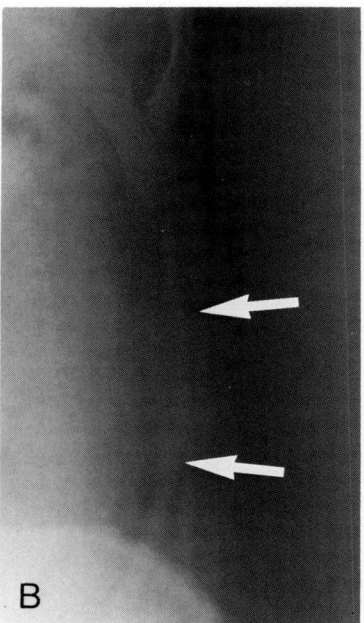

**Figure 13–10. Acute appendicitis with obliteration of the flank stripe. A.** The right flank stripe is not seen on this supine film obtained in a patient with inflammation and edema in the right lower quadrant attributable to appendicitis. **B.** Note preservation of the left flank stripe *(arrows)* in the same patient.

specific and can be related to positioning of the patient.

Surgeons have long believed that false-negative laparotomies are acceptable in some patients with right lower quadrant pain, because of the serious, potentially life-threatening complications of untreated acute appendicitis. The newer imaging techniques of ultrasound and CT have shown significant promise in improving the preoperative work-up of patients with suspected appendicitis (see Chapter 69).[95–104]

An emergent single contrast barium enema has also been advocated for the evaluation of patients with right lower quadrant pain in whom laboratory and clinical findings are equivocal. This study is performed on an unprepared colon for the primary purpose of refluxing barium into the appendix to demonstrate an unobstructed appendiceal lumen and to rule out acute appendicitis. However, the normal appendix is not always visualized with a barium enema, so that the absence of appendiceal filling does not necessarily indicate appendicitis. When the appendix is not visualized, mass effect on the cecum or terminal ileum is an ancillary finding that supports the diagnosis of appendicitis. Unless plain films reveal free intraperitoneal air, barium is the contrast agent of choice for evaluating these patients. Because of the pathophysiology of appendicitis, the risk of intraperitoneal spillage of barium is small; however, the study should always be performed with a minimal amount of hydrostatic pressure to prevent this complication. Performing gentle palpation of the right lower quadrant, exercising patience, and obtaining a postevacuation film may facilitate appendiceal visualization.[105–109]

## TOXIC MEGACOLON

Toxic megacolon, or toxic dilatation of the colon, may be diagnosed on the basis of a dilated colon on abdominal plain films in a patient with fever, tachycardia, and hypotension. Toxic megacolon is traditionally associated with ulcerative colitis, but it can occur in patients with granulomatous colitis, amebiasis, cholera, pseudomembranous colitis, and ischemic colitis.[110] Toxic megacolon may develop in 5 to 10% of patients with ulcerative colitis but in only 2 to 4% of patients with granulomatous colitis.[111–114] Surprisingly, the duration of disease has no relationship to the development of toxic megacolon. In fact, 70% of patients with toxic megacolon develop this complication during their first episode of colitis.[113]

When toxic megacolon is suspected on clinical grounds, assessment must be made not only of the degree of bowel dilatation, but also of the appearance of the colonic mucosa outlined by air and the presence or absence of free intraperitoneal air. In general, the transverse and ascending portions of the colon tend to dilate, but this tendency is a reflection more of their anterior position within the abdomen or their underlying capacity to dilate than of a predisposition to disease.[115] Although magnification may be a factor in obese patients, the upper normal limit for the transverse colonic diameter is about 6 cm. In toxic megacolon, the diameter of the transverse colon ranges from 6 to 15 cm.[116] A nodular, inflamed mucosa may be readily visible in the dilated transverse colon[117] (Fig. 13–11). Perforation may occur in 30 to 50% of cases and is associated with a high mortality rate.[113, 118] Thus, a delay in the diagnosis of toxic megacolon based on abdominal radiographs may have disastrous consequences for these patients.

The diagnosis of toxic megacolon is made by use of a combination of the plain film and clinical findings, so that a contrast enema does not need to be performed in these patients. Although some patients with toxic megacolon have undergone barium enema examinations without complications,[119] many authors believe that contrast enemas are contraindicated in patients suspected of having this condition.

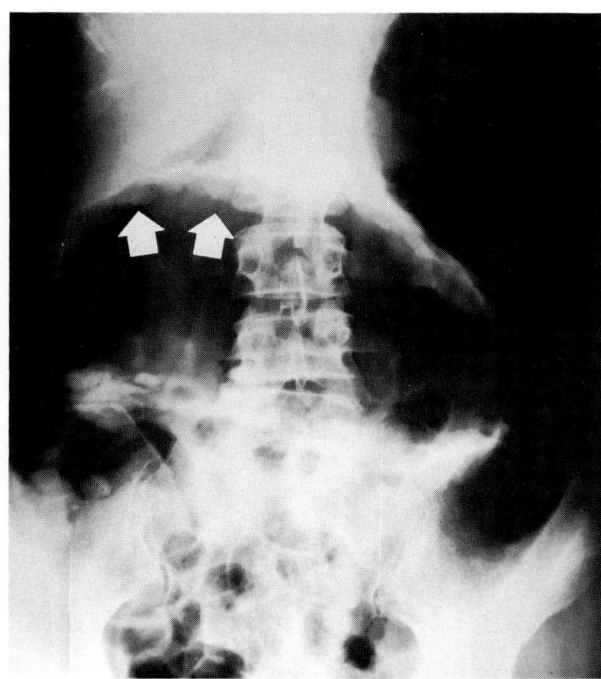

**Figure 13–11. Toxic megacolon.** This film demonstrates marked colonic distention in a patient with ulcerative colitis and toxic megacolon. Note the nodular mucosal contour *(arrows)* in the transverse colon.

## PNEUMOPERITONEUM

The presence of intraperitoneal air in acutely ill patients is an important radiographic observation that usually indicates bowel perforation. Classic experimental studies by Miller and Nelson showed that as little as 1 mL of air could be detected below the right hemidiaphragm on properly exposed chest films taken with the patient in an upright position.[120] These investigators emphasized the importance of placing the patient in the left lateral decubitus position for 15 to 20 minutes before obtaining a film with the patient in an upright position, to maximize the possibility of detecting small amounts of free air. Films obtained in midinspiration or midexpiration are even more likely to reveal tiny amounts of free air.[121] Chest films taken with the patient in an upright position are ideal for demonstrating free air, because the x-ray beam strikes the hemidiaphragms tangentially at their highest point. In contrast, the more inferior centering of the beam required for abdominal films taken with the patient in an upright position results in an oblique view of the hemidiaphragms that may obscure free air. Left lateral decubitus views of the abdomen are also sensitive for detecting small amounts of free air that become interposed between the free edge of the liver and the lateral wall of the peritoneal cavity. Care should be taken to include the upper abdomen, because air rises to the highest point in the abdomen, which frequently is beneath the lower ribs. Films taken with the patient in the right lateral decubitus position are also helpful, but gas in the stomach or colon

may obscure small amounts of free air. A cross-table lateral view of the abdomen with the patient in a supine position may demonstrate free air in individuals who are physically unable to roll onto their sides.

All of these horizontal beam views are based on the principle that air rises to the highest point in the peritoneal cavity. If for various reasons, however, horizontal beam views cannot be obtained, the radiologist must be able to recognize the presence of intraperitoneal air on abdominal films taken with the patient in a supine position. Although small amounts of air cannot usually be detected, larger amounts may result in the following radiographic signs:

1. *Serosal or Rigler's sign.* Normally, gas outlines only the luminal side of the bowel. However, gas on both sides of the bowel may outline the bowel wall as a thin, linear stripe (Fig. 13–12A and B). Since its original description by Rigler in 1941,[122] this sign has been recognized as an important indication of pneumoperitoneum on abdominal films taken with the patient in a supine position, although a moderate amount of free air must be present. Overlapping loops of dilated small bowel in the midabdomen can mimic this sign, so that it is helpful to evaluate the periphery of the film. Air trapped between loops of bowel may assume a triangular configuration (Fig. 13–12C).
2. *Increased lucency in the right upper quadrant.* Air accumulating superiorly in the free space between the anterior aspect of the liver and the abdominal wall may cause increased lucency in the right upper quadrant (Fig. 13–13A). This sign may be quite subtle. Depending on the habitus of the patient, the lateral border of the air collection may be linear.
3. *Visualization of the undersurface of the diaphragm.* Air may be trapped anteriorly in the cupula of the diaphragm, permitting visualization of the undersurface of the central portion of the diaphragm (Fig. 13–13B). This sign is affected by the amount of air present and the orientation of the diaphragm.[123]
4. *Air in Morison's pouch (posterior hepatorenal space).* Morison's pouch is an intraperitoneal recess that is bounded anteriorly by the liver and posteriorly by the right kidney. In the supine position, fluid may gravitate to this space. Air escaping from a perforated viscus may become loculated in this space because of surrounding inflammation. Air in Morison's pouch is characterized radiographically by a linear or triangular collection of gas in the right upper quadrant outside the expected location of the bowel[124–126] (Fig. 13–13C).
5. *Outline of the normal peritoneal ligaments.* With larger amounts of free air, the falciform ligament in the upper abdomen (Fig. 13–13D), the lateral umbilical ligaments (inverted V sign) in the lower abdomen, and the urachus may occasionally be visualized.[127, 128]
6. *"Football" sign.* Originally described by Miller in infants, this sign indicates a large amount of free

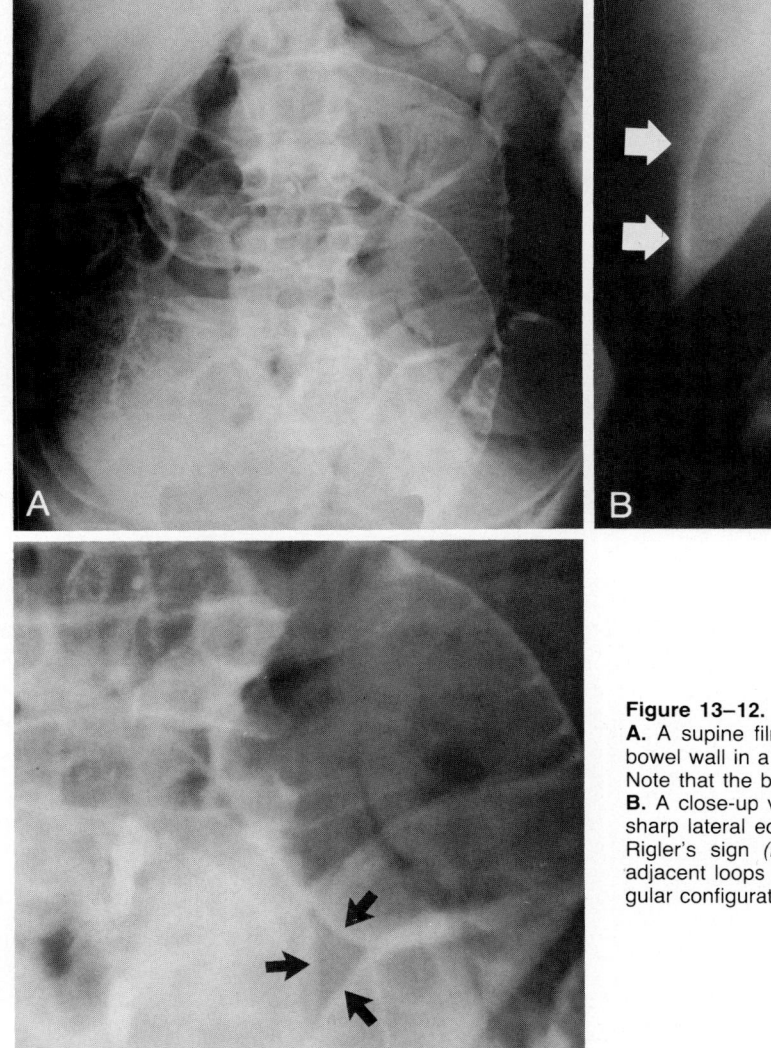

**Figure 13–12. Pneumoperitoneum with Rigler's sign.**
**A.** A supine film shows gas outlining both sides of the bowel wall in a patient with massive pneumoperitoneum. Note that the bowel wall appears as a thin, white stripe. **B.** A close-up view of the right upper quadrant shows a sharp lateral edge of the liver *(white arrows)* as well as Rigler's sign *(black arrows)*. **C.** Air trapped between adjacent loops of bowel may have a characteristic triangular configuration *(arrows)*.

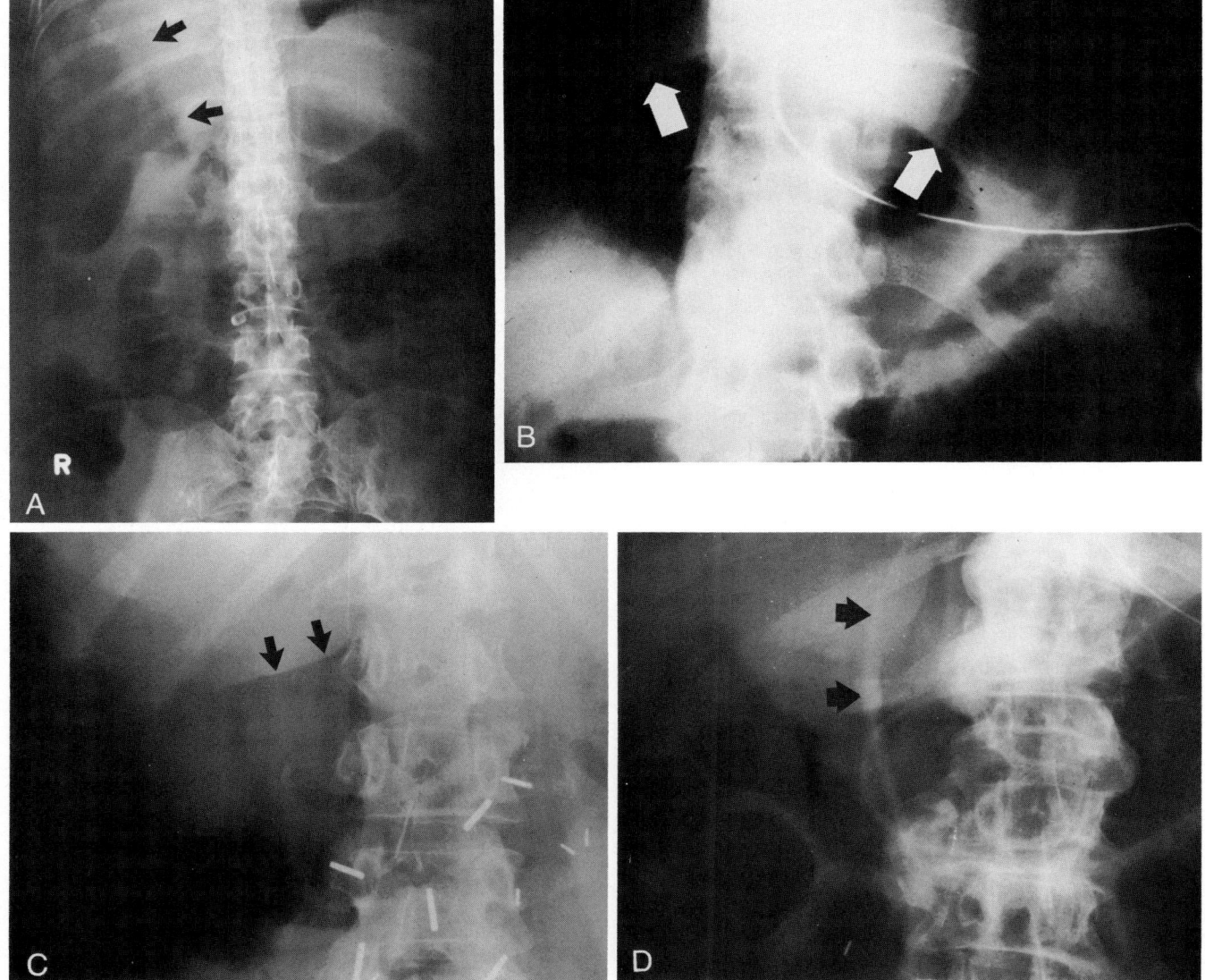

**Figure 13–13. Other signs of pneumoperitoneum on supine abdominal films. A.** Increased radiolucency can be seen in the right upper quadrant *(arrows)* and is due to air interposed between the anterior abdominal wall and the liver. **B.** A supine chest film shows air trapped anteriorly beneath the hemidiaphragms *(arrows)*, producing the "cupula" sign. **C.** Air collecting in Morison's pouch outlines the inferior border of the liver *(arrows)*. **D.** The falciform ligament *(arrows)* is outlined by air.

## TABLE 13–1. CAUSES OF PNEUMOPERITONEUM

**BOWEL**
Perforation of benign ulcer
Perforation of neoplasm
Perforation of appendix
Jejunal diverticulosis
Diverticulitis of sigmoid colon
Pneumatosis cystoides intestinalis
Foreign body perforation

**TRAUMA**
Abdominal surgery
Anastomotic leak
Peritoneal tap
Endoscopy or biopsy
Penetrating injury
Percutaneous endoscopic gastrostomy

**FEMALE GENITAL TRACT**
Rubin's test
Sexual intercourse or cunnilingus
Pelvic examination
Athletic activities such as water-skiing

air filling the oval-shaped peritoneal cavity, mimicking an American football.[129] This sign has limited value in adults.

7. *Air in the lesser sac of the peritoneal cavity.* Intraperitoneal air occasionally may enter the foramen of Winslow and become loculated in the lesser sac. This gas may be manifested by an ill-defined lucency above the lesser curvature of the stomach.[130]

The presence of pneumoperitoneum does not always indicate an acute abdominal emergency. Various causes of free air are listed in Table 13–1.

## PNEUMORETROPERITONEUM

Gas that enters the retroperitoneal spaces usually can be distinguished easily from intraperitoneal gas. Because retroperitoneal gas is bound by fascial planes, it collects in a linear fashion along the margins of the psoas muscle, the renal outlines, and the medial undersurface of the hemidiaphragms. Meyers has described the various pathways that retroperitoneal gas can travel.[131] The retroperitoneal portions of the intestines, such as the duodenum, ascending and descending colon, and rectum, can serve as sources. In patients with sigmoid diverticulitis, gas can extend laterally along the left margin of the psoas muscle, or if the perforation involves the root of the sigmoid mesocolon, along both margins of the psoas muscle (Fig. 13–14).

The location of the retroperitoneal gas may provide a clue to its site of origin. Gas escaping from duodenal perforations tends to be confined to the right anterior pararenal space. Gas may extend medially across the anterior aspect of the psoas muscle, sparing the lateral margin of the muscle. Less commonly, gas may enter the perirenal space and outline the right kidney. Duodenal ulcers, iatrogenic duodenal injuries, and blunt abdominal trauma can all result in perforation of the extraperitoneal portion of the duodenum.[132]

Peripancreatic abscesses may appear as gas collections in the anterior pararenal space. These collections tend to have a mottled rather than a linear appearance, and they can extend inferiorly in the abdomen. Similarly, renal infection by gas-forming organisms that spread through the renal capsule may be manifested by mottled gas collections that are confined to the perirenal space.

Gas from a rectal perforation may be limited to the perirectal space, or it may extend into both the anterior and the posterior retroperitoneal spaces (Fig. 13–15). Iatrogenic trauma is a common cause of rectal perforation. Radiologists must be aware of the potential danger of causing a rectal perforation when insufflating a balloon during barium enema examinations.[133] Rarely, gas from a rectal perforation may extend into the mediastinum.[134]

## PNEUMOBILIA

Gas in the bile ducts, or pneumobilia, is characterized radiographically by thin, branched, tubular areas of lucency in the central portion of the liver (Fig. 13–16). This central location can be explained by the flow of bile from the periphery of the liver toward the porta hepatis.

Pneumobilia almost always results from some type of communication between the bile duct and the intestine. One of its most common causes is surgical creation of a biliary-enteric fistula such as a choledochoduodenostomy, choledochojejunostomy, or cholecystoenterostomy. A choledochoduodenal fistula secondary to a penetrating duodenal ulcer represents the most common nonsurgical communication between the common bile duct and the duodenum.[135] In contrast, a cholecystoduodenal fistula secondary to a gallstone that erodes into

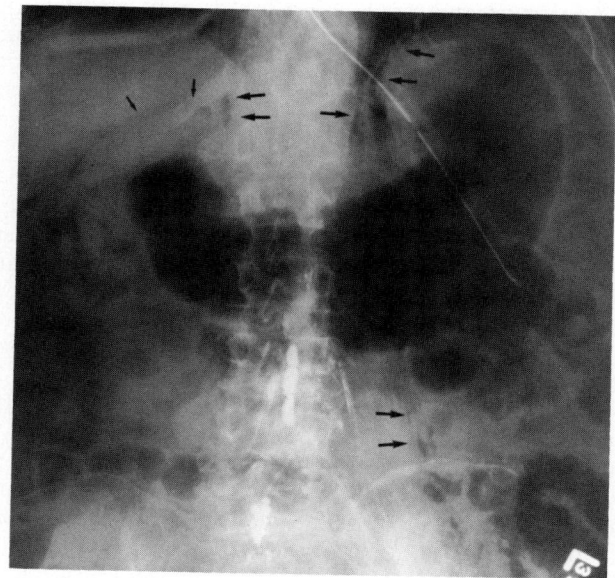

**Figure 13–14. Retroperitoneal air in a patient with diverticulitis of the sigmoid colon.** The retroperitoneal air is manifested by linear gas collections *(arrows)* dissecting along the left margin of the psoas muscle, upper retroperitoneum, and right kidney.

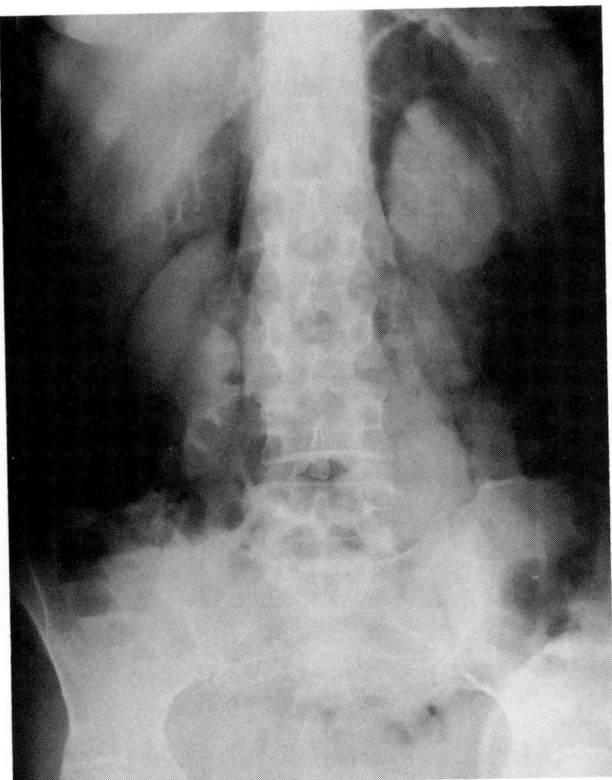

**Figure 13–15, Retroperitoneal air after a rectal biopsy.** Extensive air in the retroperitoneum outlines the margins of the psoas muscle and both kidneys.

the duodenum represents the most common nonsurgical communication between the gallbladder and the duodenum. In some patients with a cholecystoduodenal fistula, a patent cystic duct may allow air to enter the intrahepatic biliary ducts.[136, 137] If the ectopic gallstone is 2.5 cm or greater in diameter, it may obstruct the intestine, usually at or near the ileocecal valve, producing a "gallstone ileus." The classic triad of air in the biliary tree, small bowel obstruction, and an ectopic gallstone (i.e., Rigler's triad) is virtually diagnostic of gallstone ileus.[138]

Emphysematous cholecystitis, caused by gallbladder ischemia, may also be manifested by gas in the lumen and wall of the gallbladder. If the cystic duct remains patent, luminal gas may communicate with the biliary tree. Anomalous insertions of the biliary tree, recent passage of a common duct stone, and even infestation of the biliary tree by *Ascaris* organisms are other causes of pneumobilia.[139, 140]

The radiographic appearance of pneumobilia is sufficiently characteristic to permit a confident diagnosis on the basis of abdominal plain films. Occasionally, periportal fat or fat around the ligamentum teres hepatis may be manifested by faint lucency over the liver, but its appearance is different from that of pneumobilia.[141, 142] The most important consideration in the differential diagnosis of pneumobilia is the presence of gas in the portal venous system.

# PORTAL VENOUS GAS

The first report of portal venous gas in adults is attributed to Susman and Senturia in 1960.[143] This ominous radiographic finding is manifested by thin, branching, tubular areas of lucency that occupy the periphery of the liver and extend almost to the liver surface (Fig. 13–17). The peripheral location of the gas reflects the hepatopetal flow of blood in the portal venous system. In advanced cases, air can be seen outlining the more centrally located main portal vein, but this finding is less common. A film of the abdomen taken with the patient in the left lateral decubitus position may facilitate visualization of portal venous gas. Unless the gas has been introduced iatrogenically by vascular catheterization, the source of the gas is almost invariably the intestine. Intraluminal intestinal air can breach a damaged mucosa, enter the blood stream, and eventually reach the portal venous system of the liver.

The most important cause of portal venous gas is intestinal ischemia or infarction. In adults, death often occurs shortly after portal venous gas has been observed.[144, 145] The finding of portal venous gas should therefore lead to a careful search for gas in the wall of the bowel that is due to intestinal infarction.

Portal venous gas may occasionally have other benign causes. Dilatation of the stomach, and even of the small bowel, may allow some air to enter the intestinal mucosa, eventually reaching the liver.[146] Double contrast barium enemas and colonoscopy performed on patients with inflammatory bowel disease or sigmoid diverticulitis have also resulted in nonfatal cases of portal venous gas.[147–151] Doppler ultrasound has been used to detect gas in the portal vein in the immediate postoperative period after liver transplantation.[152]

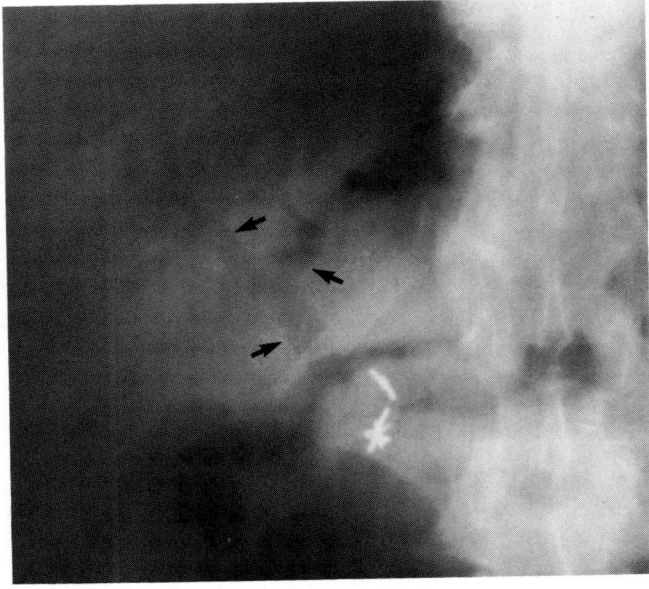

**Figure 13–16. Pneumobilia.** Air is seen in the biliary tree *(arrows)* in a patient who had undergone an earlier choledochojejunostomy.

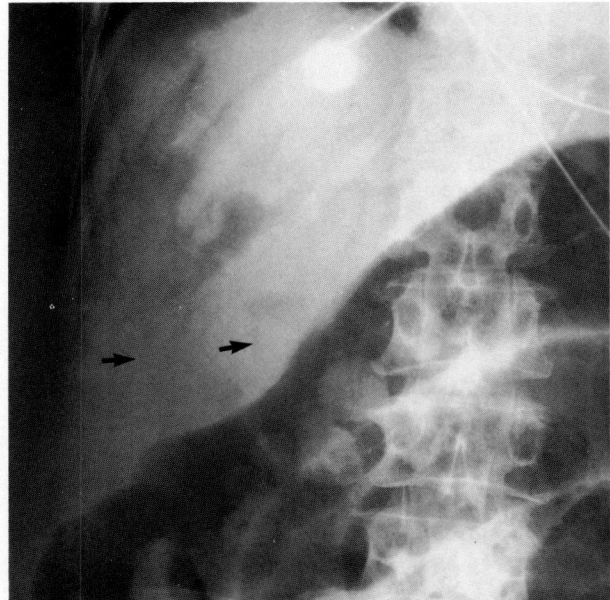

**Figure 13–17. Portal venous gas.** Tiny, branching gas collections *(arrows)* can be seen extending toward the periphery of the liver. This radiograph was taken in an elderly woman with necrosis of the small bowel.

## HEPATIC ARTERIAL GAS

Gas in the hepatic artery has been anecdotally reported in a patient in whom the hepatic artery was ligated for the treatment of an unresectable hepatic adenoma.[153] The smaller caliber of the hepatic artery and relative paucity of intrahepatic branches should differentiate this finding from portal venous gas. Hepatic arterial gas may be reported more frequently as the use of aggressive interventional radiographic techniques increases for the treatment of hepatic neoplasms.

## INTRAMURAL GAS (PNEUMATOSIS)

Gas in the wall of the intestine, or pneumatosis, may be characterized by two radiographic patterns: a bubbly appearance and thin, linear streaks. Unfortunately, the bubbly appearance of intramural gas is easily mimicked by fecal material within the colon. In patients with this form of pneumatosis, however, close inspection may reveal small bubbles of gas outside the confines of the bowel, leading to the correct diagnosis. In contrast, linear gas collections tend to be more readily apparent and should always be considered a significant plain film finding, regardless of their location (Fig. 13–18). In combination with portal venous gas (see earlier), linear gas collections in the intestinal wall are almost always a sign of bowel infarction in adult patients.[154] Other plain film findings of bowel ischemia or infarction include dilatation of bowel and nodular thickening or thumbprinting of the bowel wall. CT may also reveal characteristic findings in patients with bowel ischemia or infarction.[155] Pneumatosis and intravascular air are particularly well demonstrated by CT.[156]

Air in the wall of the stomach is a focal form of pneumatosis. *Emphysematous gastritis* is the term used to describe the rare fulminant variant of phlegmonous gastritis that results from infection of the gastric wall. Hemolytic streptococcus is the most commonly implicated organism.[157] Ingestion of caustic substances, gastroduodenal surgery, gastroenteritis, intubation injury, ulceration, and gastric outlet obstruction are other causes of air in the gastric wall.[158–160] The plain film findings must be correlated with the clinical history and presentation.

Pneumatosis cystoides coli is a rare, benign condition characterized by multiple gas-filled blebs or cysts in the wall of the colon. These cysts appear radiographically as grape-like clusters of gas, usually segmental in distribution (Fig. 13–19). The left colon tends to be more frequently involved than the right colon. The cystic collections may protrude into the bowel lumen, so that the colon may have a scalloped appearance on barium studies. The cysts tend to resolve spontaneously, but oxygen inhalation therapy has been used to facilitate resolution of these lesions.[161–163]

## ABSCESSES

Although CT is the most definitive radiologic test for diagnosing an abscess, abdominal radiographs may also be helpful in these patients.[157, 164, 165] An abscess may be manifested by an extraluminal soft tissue mass that displaces adjacent bowel or by an extraluminal collection

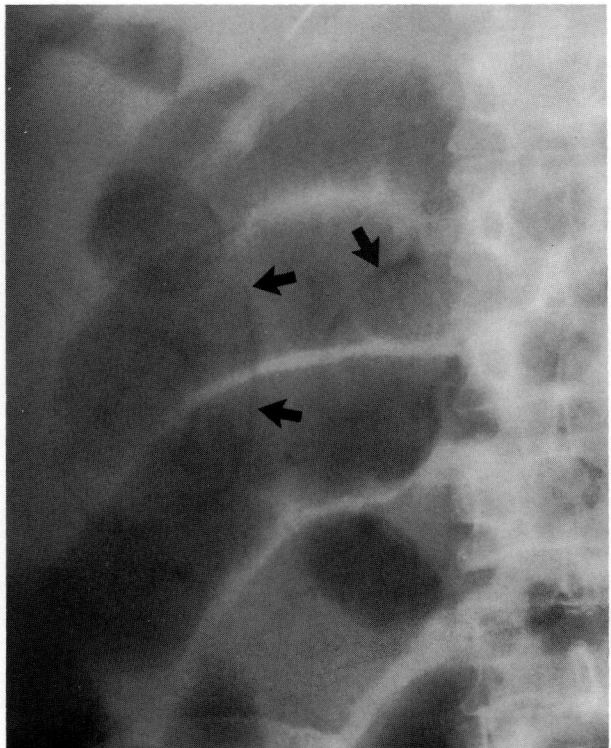

**Figure 13–18. Infarcted bowel with intramural gas.** Linear gas collections *(arrows)* are seen in the wall of several moderately dilated small bowel loops in a patient with bowel infarction.

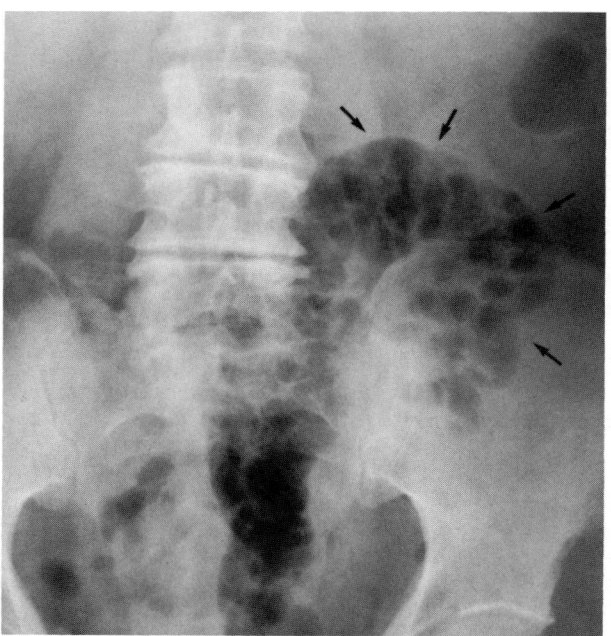

**Figure 13–19. Pneumatosis cystoides coli.** Multiple rounded, grape-like collections of gas *(arrows)* are seen in the wall of the sigmoid colon in a patient with benign pneumatosis cystoides coli.

of gas. The most characteristic plain film finding is a localized, mottled, or bubbly gas collection (Fig. 13–20). Other patients may have a single, rounded or oval collection of gas with an air-fluid level on horizontal beam views. Fecal material can mimic the appearance of a mottled collection of gas but usually is distinguished by its location within the colon. A gastric bezoar can also mimic an abscess (Fig. 13–21).

# NORMAL SOFT TISSUE STRUCTURES

The ability to discern the edge of intra-abdominal organs on abdominal radiographs taken with the patient in a supine position depends on the differences in x-ray attenuation between water density, fat density, and air. Intraperitoneal fat and retroperitoneal fat are present in varying degrees even in the thinnest patients. The liver, spleen, kidneys, psoas muscles, and urinary bladder can often be readily demonstrated because of surrounding fat (Fig. 13–22). In patients with sufficient fat, the serosal surface of the stomach may also appear as a faint edge. This subtle radiographic observation should not be confused with the much more distinct appearance of the serosa when it is outlined by air in patients with pneumoperitoneum. Fluid-filled loops of small and large bowel may also appear as tubular densities on a backdrop of abdominal fat.

Recognition of normal organs is important, because an abnormal contour or size of these organs on abdominal plain films may be the first indication of intraabdominal disease.

# SOFT TISSUE ABNORMALITIES

## Liver

Liver size was estimated on abdominal radiographs by Pfahler as early as 1926.[166] Usually, the inferior tip of the liver does not extend below the iliac crest, except in asthenic individuals. Generalized hepatic enlargement tends to displace the hepatic flexure and transverse colon inferiorly and the stomach to the left (Fig. 13–23). Other

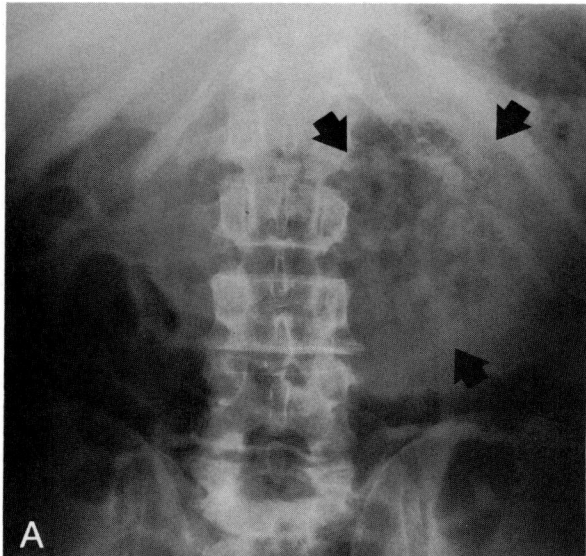
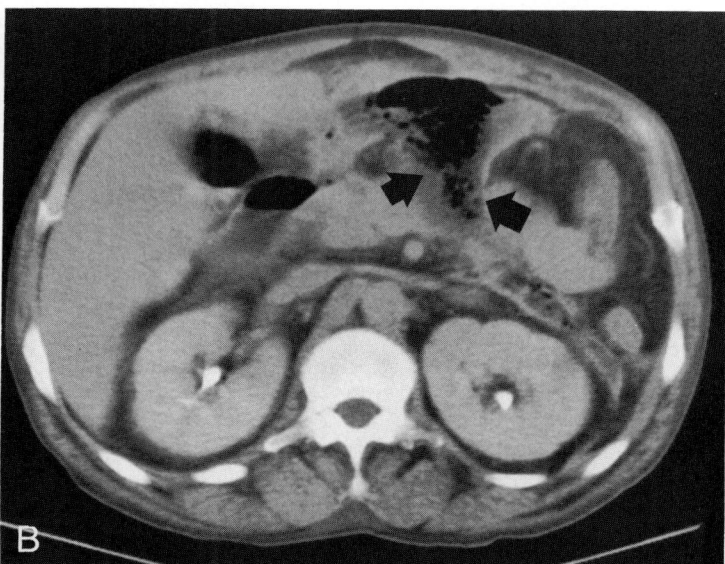

**Figure 13–20. Lesser sac abscess attributable to pancreatitis. A.** A mottled collection of gas *(arrows)* is present in the upper abdomen. **B.** A CT scan shows gas and fluid in the abscess cavity *(arrows)* in a patient with underlying pancreatitis.

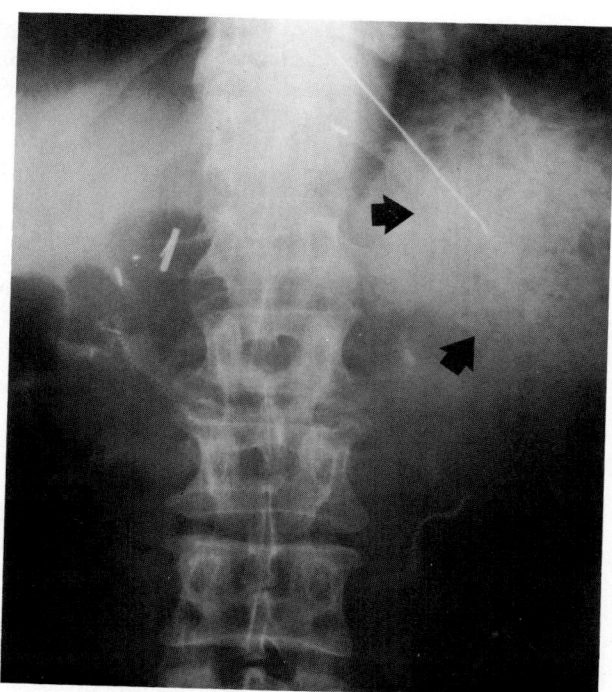

**Figure 13–21. Gastric bezoar after gastrojejunostomy.** Note the similarity between the mottled gas collection *(arrows)* in the left upper quadrant and the lesser sac abscess in Figure 13–20. (Courtesy of Gilbert E. Parker, M.D., Richmond, VA.)

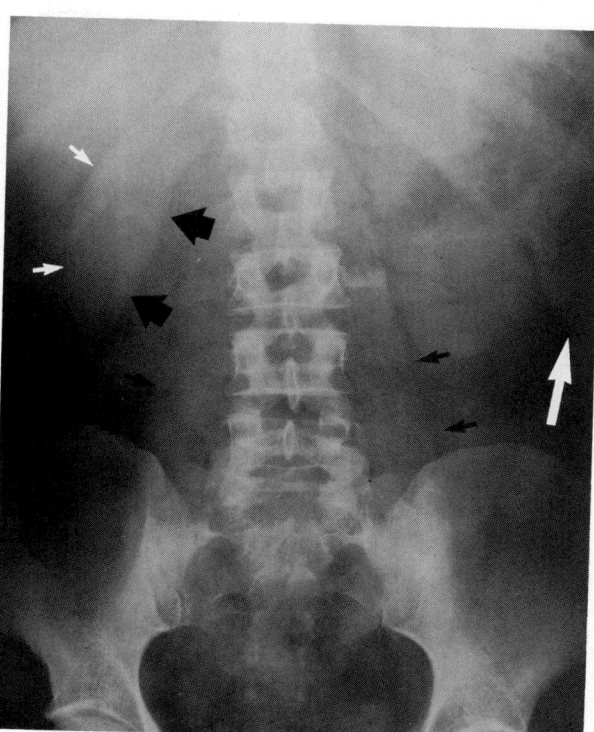

**Figure 13–22. Normal soft tissue planes outlined by fat.** The liver edge *(large black arrows),* right renal outline *(small white arrows),* margins of the psoas muscle *(small black arrows),* and splenic tip *(large white arrow)* can be identified.

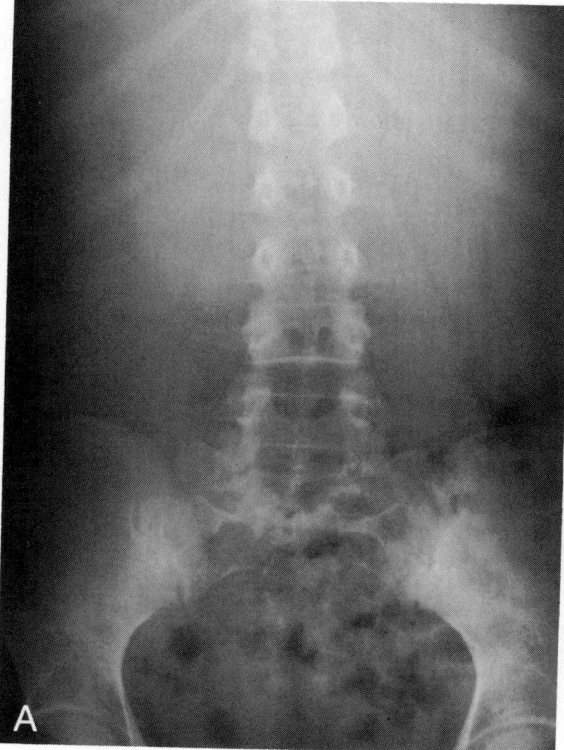

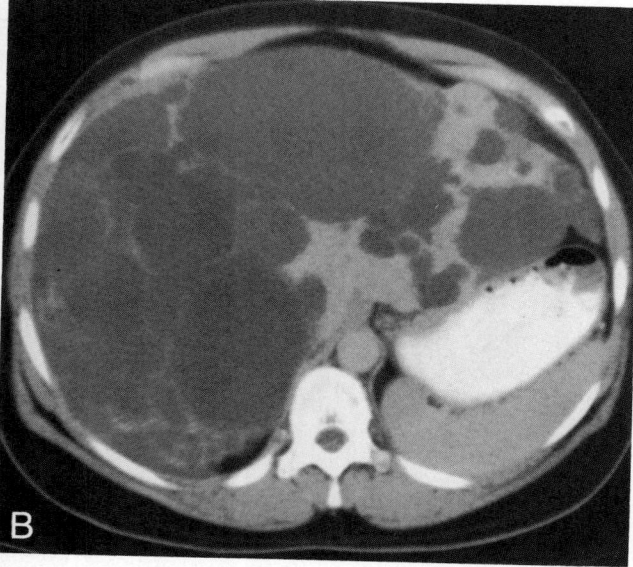

**Figure 13–23. Hepatomegaly. A.** Marked hepatic enlargement causes displacement of bowel gas into the left lower quadrant of the abdomen. **B.** A CT scan shows multiple large cysts in the liver to be the cause of the patient's hepatomegaly.

signs of hepatic enlargement include 1) displacement of the inferior edge of the liver beyond the right margin of the psoas muscle; 2) displacement of the duodenal bulb below the L-2 vertebral body or to the left of the midline; 3) inferior displacement of the right kidney; 4) enlargement or marked rounding of the hepatic angle; 5) elevation of the right hemidiaphragm with decreased motion on normal respiration; 6) inferior displacement of the gastric fundus away from the diaphragm with left lobe enlargement; and 7) anterior displacement of the duodenal bulb on lateral films with caudate lobe enlargement.[167–171]

A small liver may result in reversal of some of these findings, with the right kidney higher than the left, the stomach displaced upward and to the right, and the duodenal bulb displaced above the level of the right 12th rib.

## Spleen

Brogdon and Cros found that the inferior tip of the spleen could be seen on abdominal radiographs in 44% of patients who had no evidence of splenomegaly.[172] Normally, the superior margin of the spleen lies just beneath the left hemidiaphragm, and its lateral edge approximates the lateral abdominal wall. As the spleen increases in size, its tip extends inferiorly below the 12th rib (Fig. 13–24). The enlarged spleen also tends to become directed anteriorly, so that it may be readily palpated on physical examination. Displacement of the splenic flexure of the colon is an uncommon finding because the splenic flexure usually lies anterior to the spleen. Marked splenomegaly may also displace the stomach medially.

## Kidneys

Because of surrounding fat, the renal outlines are visible on the majority of abdominal films taken with the patient in a supine position. Moel studied 100 men and 100 women between 20 and 49 years of age and found that the average renal length on plain films was 13.0 cm for men and 12.5 cm for women.[173] Estimates of renal size must also take into account the foreshortening of the kidney that occurs because of angulation of this structure in normal individuals. Because of its retroperitoneal location, an enlarged kidney does not displace intra-abdominal organs, except in extreme cases. Renal cysts or tumors that produce contour abnormalities in the kidney may be readily apparent.

## Other Structures

Retroperitoneal fat and intraperitoneal fat that permit visualization of adjacent water-density organs are also helpful in evaluating contiguous pathologic processes in the abdomen. Surrounding inflammation may cause the fat to become edematous, so that it takes in more water. This process may lead to a change in tissue characteristics, so that the normal radiolucency of fat approximates soft tissue density, thus obliterating contiguous planes. These changes are exemplified in patients with appendicitis. The properitoneal fat planes that demarcate the internal oblique, external oblique, and transversalis muscles of the abdomen may become obliterated. Similarly, the fat surrounding the psoas muscle may become edematous, obscuring the normal margin of the psoas muscle. Although obliteration of these fat planes is an important sign of inflammation, it seldom occurs as an

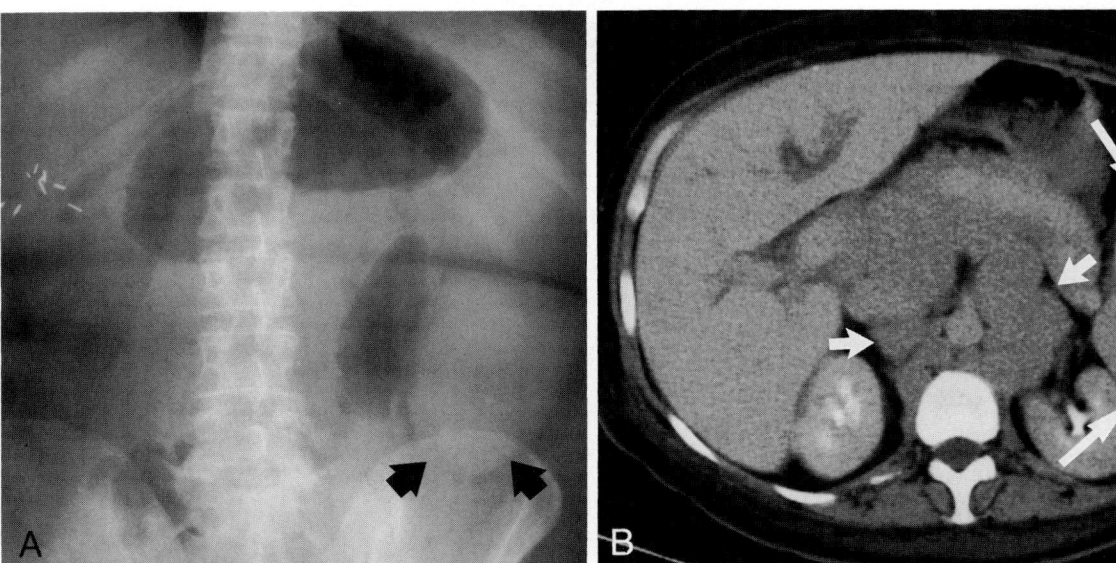

**Figure 13–24. Splenomegaly. A.** A supine abdominal film demonstrates marked splenic enlargement with the tip of the spleen *(arrows)* projecting over the left iliac wing. **B.** A CT scan shows the enlarged spleen *(long arrows)* and para-aortic adenopathy *(short arrows)* in a patient with lymphoma.

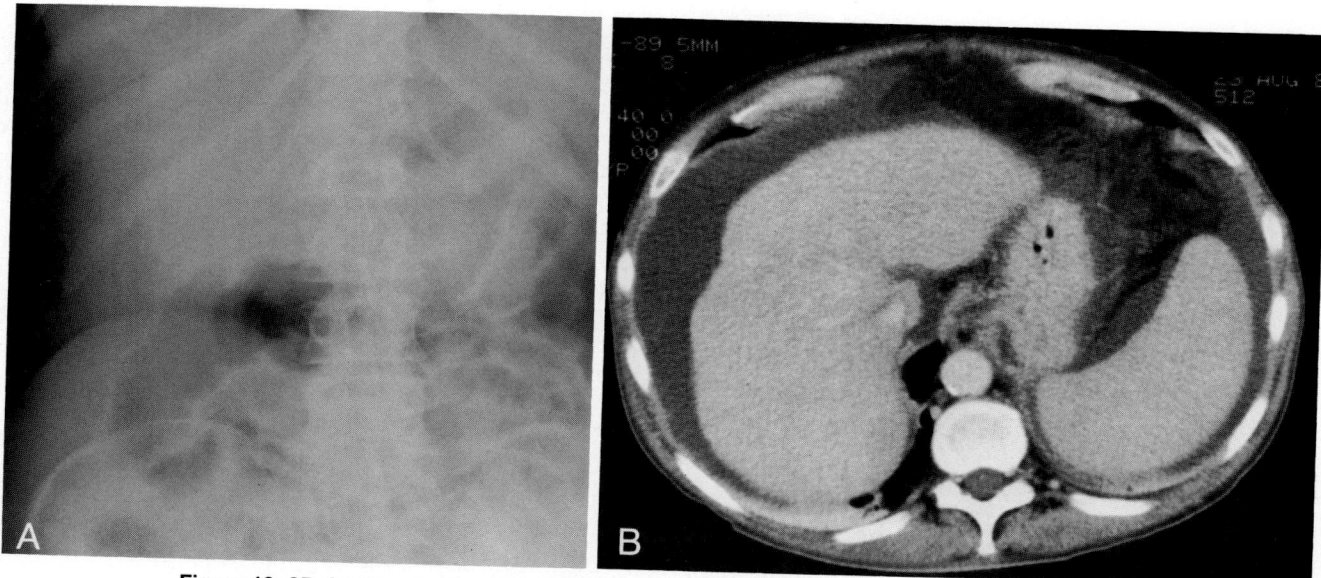

**Figure 13–25. Ascites. A.** The normal liver edge is obscured in a patient with ascites. **B.** A CT scan confirms the presence of perihepatic ascites.

isolated finding, so that it should be interpreted with caution and in conjunction with other signs of abdominal disease.

## ASCITES

The widespread use of ultrasound and CT has lessened the emphasis placed on the plain film findings of ascites. These signs are still important to recognize, however, because plain film radiography of the abdomen is frequently one of the first imaging studies performed in patients with abdominal distention. In general, only large amounts of ascites can be identified on abdominal radiographs. The following plain film findings for ascites have been described:

1. *Obliteration of the inferior edge of the liver* (Fig. 13–25). This sign can be extremely helpful. Proper technique in which low kilovoltage is used is essential. However, the liver edge may be preserved in patients with loculated ascites, and excessive feces in the hepatic flexure of the colon may falsely obliterate the liver edge.[174]
2. *Widening of the distance between the flank stripe and the ascending colon.* This distance is normally 2 to 3 mm, but it may increase as fluid fills the right paracolic gutter. This finding may be accentuated by placing the patient in a right lateral decubitus position for several minutes before obtaining a film with the patient in the supine position.
3. *Medial displacement of the lateral edge of the liver (Hellmer's sign).* This finding usually requires a large amount of ascites and is more common with malignant ascites than with cirrhosis, probably because the fat content of the cirrhotic liver approximates the density of ascites.[175]

4. *Fluid accumulation in the pelvis.* As the most inferior intraperitoneal recess, the pouch of Douglas, or cul de sac, readily accumulates intraperitoneal fluid. A distended bladder or rectum may impress centrally on this fluid, causing symmetric bulges that have been described as "dog ears."
5. *Separation of bowel loops.* This sign is seldom an isolated finding and requires a large amount of ascites. It can easily be mimicked by a disproportionately large amount of fluid and smaller amount of air in juxtaposed bowel loops.
6. *Centrally located bowel loops with bulging flanks.* With large amounts of ascites, the bowel loops may float to the highest central portion of the abdomen.
7. *Ground-glass appearance.* This radiographic finding also requires large amounts of fluid and may erroneously be suggested by improper radiographic technique or marked obesity.

## MISCELLANEOUS ABNORMALITIES

Whenever a soft tissue density that projects over the abdomen has a sharp margin, the possibility of a skin lesion should be considered. Umbilical hernias, stomas, and neurofibromas may all be sufficiently protuberant to be recognized on plain films. However, they seldom pose a diagnostic dilemma when correlated with the clinical findings.

## References

1. Baker SR: The Abdominal Plain Film. East Norwalk, CT: Appleton & Lange, 1990.
2. McCort JJ (ed): Abdominal Radiology. Baltimore: Williams & Wilkins, 1981.

3. Welch JP: Bowel Obstruction: Differential Diagnosis and Clinical Management. Philadelphia: WB Saunders, 1990.

4. Levitt MD, Bond JH Jr: Volume, composition and source of intestinal gas. Gastroenterology 59:921–929, 1970.

5. Anderson K, Ringsted A: Clinical and experimental investigation of ileus with particular reference to the genesis of intestinal gas. Acta Chir Scand 88:475–502, 1943.

6. Goyal RK, Spiro HM: Gastrointestinal manifestations of diabetes mellitus. Med Clin North Am 55:1031–1040, 1971.

7. Kassander P: Asymptomatic gastric retention in diabetes (gastroparesis diabeticorum). Ann Intern Med 48:797–812, 1958.

8. Seaman WB: Motor dysfunction of the gastrointestinal tract. AJR 116:235–248, 1972.

9. Cantor MO: Ileus. Am J Gastroenterol 47:461–484, 1967.

10. Tibblin S: Diagnosis of intestinal obstruction with special regard to plain roentgen examination of the abdomen. Acta Chir Scand 135:249–252, 1969.

11. Bryk D: Functional evaluation of small bowel obstruction by successive abdominal roentgenograms. AJR 116:262–275, 1972.

12. Frimann-Dahl J: Roentgen findings in intestinal knots. Acta Radiol 23:22–33, 1942.

13. Gammill SL, Nice CM Jr: Air-fluid levels: their occurrence in normal patients and their role in the analysis of ileus. Surgery 71:771–780, 1972.

14. Donahue JK, Hunter C, Balch HH: Significance of fluid levels in x-ray films of the abdomen. N Engl J Med 259:13–15, 1958.

15. Hodges P, Miller RE: Intestinal obstruction. AJR 74:1015–1025, 1955.

16. Mellins HZ, Rigler LG: The roentgen findings in strangulating obstructions of the small intestine. AJR 71:404–416, 1954.

17. Holder LE, Schneider HJ: Spigelian hernias: anatomy and roentgenographic manifestations. Radiology 112:309–313, 1974.

18. Spiers TC, Rosenbloom MB, Palayew MJ: Spigelian hernia: plain film diagnosis. J Can Assoc Radiol 31:147–148, 1980.

19. Strauss S, Rubinstein ZJ, Shapiro Z: Food as a cause of small intestinal obstruction. A report of five cases without previous gastric surgery. Gastrointest Radiol 2:17–20, 1977.

20. Weissberg DL, Berk RN: Ascariasis of the gastrointestinal tract. Gastrointest Radiol 3:415–418, 1978.

21. Ellman BA, Wynee JM, Freeman A: Intestinal ascariasis: new plain film features. AJR 135:37–42, 1980.

22. Conti PS, Warner CH, Fleisher AG, et al: Bowel obstruction caused by gastric balloons. AJR 151:313–314, 1988.

23. Kirby DF, Mills PR, Kellum J, et al: Incomplete small bowel obstruction by the Garrens-Edwards gastric bubble necessitating surgical intervention. Am J Gastroenterol 82:251–253, 1987.

24. Bose SM, Talwar BL: Appendicitis causing acute intestinal obstruction with strangulation. Aust N Z J Surg 43:56–57, 1973.

25. Buckwalter JA, Modlin M: Acute appendicitis with intestinal obstruction. JAMA 155:1577–1578, 1954.

26. Cohn S, Felmus RD: Volvulus with partial intestinal obstruction caused by an abnormally placed appendix. N Y State J Med 50:2965–2966, 1950.

27. Gupta S, Vaidya MP: Mechanical small bowel obstruction caused by acute appendicitis. Am Surg 35:670–674, 1969.

28. Welch CE, Ottinger LW, Welch JP: Manual of Lower Gastrointestinal Surgery. New York: Springer-Verlag, 1980.

29. Phillips RK, Hittinger R, Fry JS, et al: Malignant large bowel obstruction. Br J Surg 72:296–302, 1985.

30. Falterman KW, Hill CB, Markey JC, et al: Cancer of the colon, rectum, and anus: a review of 2313 cases. Cancer 34:951–959, 1974.

31. Abrams JS, Reines HD: Increasing incidence of right-sided lesions in colorectal cancer. Am J Surg 137:522–526, 1979.

32. Cady B, Persson AV, Monson DO, et al: Changing patterns of colorectal carcinoma. Cancer 33:422–426, 1984.

33. Maglinte DD, Keller KJ, Miller RE, et al: Colon and rectal carcinoma: spatial distribution and detection. Radiology 147:669–672, 1983.

34. Rhodes JB, Holmes FF, Clark GM: Changing distribution of primary cancers in the large bowel. JAMA 238:1641–1643, 1977.

35. Albers JH, Smith LL, Carter R: Perforation of the cecum. Ann Surg 143:251–255, 1956.

36. Crowder VH Jr, Cohn I Jr: Perforation in cancer of the colon and rectum. Dis Colon Rectum 10:415–420, 1967.

37. Glenn F, McSherry CK: Obstruction and perforation in colorectal cancer. Ann Surg 173:983–992, 1971.

38. Ogilvie H: Large intestine colic due to sympathetic deprivation. Br Med J 2:671–673, 1948.

39. Lescher TJ, Teegarden DK, Pruitt BA: Acute pseudo-obstruction of the colon in thermally injured patients. Dis Colon Rectum 21:618–622, 1978.

40. Wojtalik RS, Lindenauer SM, Kahn SS: Perforation of the colon associated with adynamic ileus. Am J Surg 125:601–606, 1973.

41. Nivatvongs S, Vermeulen FD, Fang DT: Colonoscopic decompression of acute pseudo-obstruction of the colon. Ann Surg 196:598–600, 1982.

42. Caccese WJ, Bronzo RL, Wadler G, et al: Ogilvie's syndrome associated with herpes zoster infection. J Clin Gastroenterol 7:309–313, 1985.

43. MacManus Q, Krippaehne WW: Diastatic perforation of the cecum without distal obstruction. Arch Surg 112:1227–1230, 1977.

44. Nanni C, Garbini A, Luchett P, et al: Ogilvie's syndrome (acute colonic pseudo-obstruction): review of the literature (October 1948 to March 1980) and report of four additional cases. Dis Colon Rectum 25:157–166, 1982.

45. Ravo B, Pollane M, Ger R: Pseudo-obstruction of the colon following caesarean section: a review. Dis Colon Rectum 26:440–444, 1983.

46. Nakhgevany KB: Colonoscopic decompression of the colon in patients with Ogilvie's syndrome. Am J Surg 148:317–320, 1984.

47. Davis L, Lowman EM: Roentgen criteria of impending perforation of the cecum. Radiology 68:542–547, 1957.

48. Shirazi KK, Agha FP, Strodel WE, et al: Nonobstructive colonic dilation: radiologic findings in 50 patients following colonoscopic treatment. J Can Assoc Radiol 35:116–119, 1984.

49. Strodel WE, Nostrant TT, Eckhauser FE, et al: Therapeutic and diagnostic colonoscopy in nonobstructive colonic dilatation. Ann Surg 197:416–421, 1983.

50. Johnson CD, Rice RP, Kelvin FM, et al: The radiological evaluation of gross cecal distensions: emphasis on cecal ileus. AJR 145:1211–1217, 1985.

51. Ballantyne GH: Review of sigmoid volvulus: clinical patterns and pathogenesis. Dis Colon Rectum 25:823–830, 1982.

52. Ballantyne GH, Brandner MD, Beart RW Jr, et al: Volvulus of the colon. Incidence and mortality. Ann Surg 202:83–92, 1985.

53. McAdam IWJ: Geographical pathology: East Africa. Clin Radiol 14:193–199, 1963.

54. Figiel LS, Figiel SJ: Lesions of the large intestine producing acute symptoms. Radiol Clin North Am 2:33–54, 1964.

55. Arnold GJ, Nance FC: Volvulus of the sigmoid colon. Ann Surg 177:527–537, 1973.

56. Essenson L, Ginzburg L: Volvulus of the sigmoid. Am J Surg 77:240–249, 1949.

57. Bruusgaard C: Volvulus of the sigmoid colon and its treatment. Surgery 22:466–478, 1947.

58. Shepherd JJ: Treatment of volvulus of the sigmoid colon: a review of 425 cases. Br Med J 1:280–283, 1968.

59. Wertkin MG, Aufses AH Jr: Management of volvulus of the colon. Dis Colon Rectum 21:40–45, 1978.

60. Newton NA, Reines HD: Transverse colon volvulus: case reports and review. AJR 128:69–72, 1977.

61. Zinken LD, Katz LD, Rosin JD: Volvulus of the transverse colon: report of a case and review of the literature. Dis Colon Rectum 22:492–496, 1979.

62. Kerry RL, Ransom HK: Volvulus of the colon. Etiology, diagnosis, and treatment. Arch Surg 99:215–222, 1963.

63. Ghahremani GG, Bowie JD: Volvulus of the splenic flexure. Dis Colon Rectum 17:100–102, 1974.

64. Ballantyne GH: Volvulus of the splenic flexure: report of a case and review of the literature. Dis Colon Rectum 24:630–632, 1981.

65. Lantieri R, Teplick SK, Labell MJ: Splenic flexure volvulus: two case reports and review. AJR 132:463–464, 1979.

66. Buenger RE: Volvulus of the splenic flexure of the colon. AJR 71:81–83, 1954.

67. Sachidananthan CK, Soehrer B: Volvulus of the splenic flexure of the colon: report of a case and review of the literature. Dis Colon Rectum 15:466–469, 1972.

68. Young WS: Further radiological observations in caecal volvulus. Clin Radiol 31:479–483, 1980.

69. Anderson JR, Mills JOM: Cecal volvulus: a frequently missed diagnosis? Clin Radiol 35:65–69, 1985.

70. Anderson JR, Lee D: Acute cecal volvulus. Br J Surg 67:39–41, 1980.

71. Anderson JR, Spence RA, Wilson BG, et al: Gangrenous cecal volvulus after colonoscopy. Br Med J 286:439–440, 1983.

72. Hemingway AP: Cecal volvulus—a new twist to the barium enema. Br J Radiol 53:806–807, 1980.

73. Howard RS, Catto J: Cecal volvulus. A case for non-resectional therapy. Arch Surg 115:273–277, 1980.

74. Ritvo M, Farrell GE Jr, Shauffer IA: The association of volvulus of the cecum and ascending colon with other obstructive colonic lesions. AJR 78:587–598, 1957.

75. Weinstein M: Volvulus of the cecum and ascending colon. Ann Surg 107:248–259, 1938.

76. Bobroff LM, Messinger NH, Subbarao K, et al: The cecal bascule. AJR 115:249–252, 1972.

77. Campbell JP, Gunn AA: Plain abdominal radiographs and acute abdominal pain. Br J Surg 75:554–556, 1988.

78. Olutola PS: Plain film radiographic diagnosis of acute appendicitis: an evaluation of the signs. Can Assoc Radiol J 39:254–256, 1988.

79. Nitecki S, Karmeli R, Sarr MG: Appendiceal calculi and fecaliths as indications for appendectomy. Surg Gynecol Obstet 171:185–188, 1990.

80. Faegenburg D: Fecaliths of the appendix: incidence and significance. AJR 89:752–759, 1963.

81. Thomas SF: Appendiceal coproliths: their surgical importance. Radiology 49:39–49, 1947.

82. Bunch GH, Adcock DF: Giant faceted calculus. Ann Surg 109:143–146, 1939.

83. Brady BM, Carroll DS: The significance of the calcified appendiceal enterolith. Radiology 68:648–653, 1957.

84. Lewis FR, Holcroft JW, Boey J, et al: Appendicitis: a critical review of diagnosis and treatment in 1000 cases. Arch Surg 110:677–684, 1975.

85. Mowji PJ, Jones MD, Cohen AJ: Localized ileus of the proximal jejunum: a new sign for acute appendicitis. Gastrointest Radiol 14:173–175, 1989.

86. Hayden CK, Swischuk LE: Appendicitis with perforation: the dilated transverse colon sign. AJR 135:687–689, 1980.

87. May LM, O'Neill FE, Allen SW: Cecal ileus—an undescribed and helpful sign in acute appendicitis. Tex Med 54:92–95, 1958.

88. Soteropoluos C, Gilmore JH: Roentgen diagnosis of acute appendicitis. Radiology 71:246–256, 1958.

89. Killen DA, Brooks DW Jr: Gas-filled appendix: a roentgen sign of acute appendicitis. Ann Surg 161:474–478, 1965.

90. Lim MS: Gas-filled appendix: lack of diagnostic specificity. AJR 128:209–210, 1977.

91. Chavez MC, Morgan BD: Acute appendicitis with pneumoperitoneum. Radiographic diagnosis and report of five cases. Am Surg 32:604–608, 1968.

92. Farman J, Kassner EG, Dallemand S, et al: Pneumoperitoneum and appendicitis. Gastrointest Radiol 1:277–279, 1976.

93. McCort JJ: Extra-alimentary gas in perforated appendicitis: report of six cases. AJR 77:647–651, 1977.

94. Rucker CR, Midler RE, Nay HR: Pneumoperitoneum secondary to perforated appendicitis. Am Surg 33:188–190, 1967.

95. Puylaert JBCM: Acute appendicitis: US evaluation using graded compression. Radiology 158:355–360, 1986.

96. Puylaert JBCM, Rutgers PH, Lalisang RI, et al: A prospective study for ultrasonography in the diagnosis of appendicitis. N Engl J Med 317:666–669, 1987.

97. Larson JM, Peirce JC, Ellinger DM, et al: The validity and utility of sonography on the diagnosis of acute appendicitis in the community setting. AJR 153:687–691, 1989.

98. Jeffrey RB, Laing FC, Townsend RR: Acute appendicitis: sonographic criteria based on 250 cases. Radiology 167:327–329, 1988.

99. Vignault F, Filiatrault D, Brandt ML, et al: Acute appendicitis in children: evaluation with US. Radiology 176:501, 1990.

100. Scatarige JC, DiSantis DJ, Allen HA, et al: CT demonstration of the appendix in asymptomatic adults. Gastrointest Radiol 14:271–273, 1989.

101. Balthazar EJ, Gordon RB: CT of appendicitis. Semin Ultrasound CT MR 10:326–340, 1989.

102. Balthazar EJ, Megibow AJ, Gordon RB, et al: Computed tomography of the abdominal appendix. J Comput Assist Tomogr 12:595–601, 1988.

103. Shapiro MP, Gale ME, Gerzot SG: CT of appendicitis: diagnosis and treatment. Radiol Clin North Am 27:753–762, 1989.

104. Balthazar EJ, Megibow AJ, Siegel SE, et al: Appendicitis: prospective evaluation with high resolution CT. Radiology 180:21–24, 1991.

105. Sakover RP, Del Fava RL: Frequency of visualization of the normal appendix with the barium enema examination. AJR 121:312–317, 1974.

106. Fedyshin P, Kelvin FM, Rice RP: Non-specificity of barium enema findings in acute appendicitis. AJR 143:99–102, 1984.

107. Kelvin FM, Rice RP: Radiologic evaluation of acute abdominal pain arising from the alimentary tract. Radiol Clin North Am 16:25–36, 1978.

108. Garcia CJ, Rosenfield NS: The barium enema in the diagnosis of acute appendicitis. Semin Ultrasound CT MR 10:314–320, 1989.

109. El Ferzli G, Ozuner G, Davidson PG, et al: Barium enema in the diagnosis of acute appendicitis. Surg Gynecol Obstet 171:40–42, 1990.

110. Wruble LD, Dachsworth JK, Duke DD, et al: Toxic dilatation of the colon in a case of amebiasis. N Engl J Med 275:926–928, 1966.

111. Greenstein AJ, Sachar DB, Gibas A, et al: Outcome of toxic dilatation in ulcerative colitis and Crohn's colitis. J Clin Gastroenterol 7:137–144, 1985.

112. Jalan KN, Sircus W, Card WI, et al: An experience of ulcerative colitis: I. Toxic dilatation in 55 cases. Gastroenterology 8:213–220, 1947.

113. Roys G, Kaplan MS, Juler GL: Surgical management of toxic megacolon. Am J Gastroenterol 68:161–166, 1977.

114. Katzka I, Katz S, Morris E: Management of toxic megacolon: the significance of early recognition in medical management. J Clin Gastroenterol 1:307–311, 1979.

115. Kramer P, Wittenberg J: Colonic gas distribution in toxic megacolon. Gastroenterology 80:433–437, 1981.

116. Norland CC, Kirsner JB: Toxic dilatation of the colon (toxic megacolon): etiology, treatment and prognosis in 42 patients. Medicine (Baltimore) 48:229–250, 1969.

117. Halpert RD: Toxic dilatation of the colon. Radiol Clin North Am 25:147–155, 1987.

118. Greenstein AJ, Aufses AH: Differences in pathogenesis, incidence and outcome of perforation in inflammatory bowel disease. Surg Gynecol Obstet 160:63–69, 1985.

119. Wolf BS, Marshak RH: Toxic segmental dilatation of the colon during the course of fulminating ulcerative colitis: roentgen findings. AJR 82:985–995, 1959.

120. Miller RE, Nelson SW: The roentgenological demonstration of tiny amounts of free intraperitoneal gas: experimental and clinical studies. AJR 112:574–585, 1971.

121. Miller RE, Becker GJ, Slabaugh RA: Detection of pneumoperitoneum: optimum body position and respiratory phase. AJR 135:487–490, 1980.

122. Rigler LG: Spontaneous pneumoperitoneum: a roentgenologic sign found in supine position. Radiology 37:604–607, 1941.

123. Mindelzun RE, McCort JJ: Cupola sign of pneumoperitoneum in the supine patient. Gastrointest Radiol 11:283–285, 1986.

124. Hajdu N, de Lacy G: The Rutherford Morison pouch: a characteristic appearance on abdominal radiographs. Br J Radiol 43:706–709, 1970.

125. Brill PW, Olson SR, Winchester P: Neonatal necrotizing enterocolitis: air in Morison pouch. Radiology 174:469–471, 1990.

126. Menuck L, Siemers PT: Pneumoperitoneum: importance of right upper quadrant features. AJR 127:753–756, 1976.

127. Jelaso DV, Schultz EH Jr: The urachus—an aid to the diagnosis of pneumoperitoneum. Radiology 92:295–296, 1969.

128. Weiner CI, Diaconis JN, Dennis JM: The "inverted V": a new sign of pneumoperitoneum. Radiology 107:47–48, 1973.

129. Miller RE: Perforated viscus in infants: a new roentgen sign. Radiology 74:65–67, 1960.

130. Walker LA, Weens HS: Radiological observations on the lesser peritoneal sac. Radiology 80:727–737, 1963.

131. Meyers MA: Radiological features of the spread and localization of extraperitoneal gas and their relationship to its source. An anatomical approach. Radiology 111:17–26, 1974.

132. Walker CW, Purnell GL, Diner WC: Complications from extravasated retroperitoneal barium: case report and review of the literature. Radiology 173:618–620, 1989.

133. Peterson N, Rohrmann CA Jr, Lennard ES: Diagnosis and treatment of retroperitoneal perforation complicating double-contrast barium enema examination. Radiology 144:249–252, 1982.

134. Beerman PJ, Gelfand DW, Ott DJ: Pneumomediastinum after double-contrast barium enema examination: a sign of colonic perforation. AJR 136:197–198, 1981.

135. Balthazar EJ, Gurkin S: Cholecystoenteric fistulas: significance and radiographic diagnosis. Am J Gastroenterol 65:168–173, 1976.

136. Balthazar EJ, Schecter LS: Air in gallbladder: a frequent finding in gallstone ileus. AJR 131:219–222, 1978.

137. Ulreich S, Massi J: Recurrent gallstone ileus. AJR 133:921–923, 1979.

138. Rigler LG, Borman DN, Noble JF: Gallstone obstruction. Pathogenesis and roentgen manifestations. JAMA 117:1753–1759, 1941.

139. Cremin BJ: Biliary parasites. Br J Radiol 42:506–508, 1969.

140. Mindelzun R, McCort JJ: Hepatic and perihepatic radiolucencies. Radiol Clin North Am 18:221–238, 1980.

141. Govoni AF, Meyers MD: Pseudopneumobilia. Radiology 118:526, 1976.

142. Halber MD, Daffner RH: Fat in the intrahepatic fissure. AJR 132:842–843, 1979.

143. Susman N, Senturia HR: Gas embolization of the portal venous system. AJR 83:847–850, 1960.

144. Sisk PB: Gas in the portal venous system. Radiology 77:103–107, 1981.

145. McClandless RL: Portal vein gas: a grave prognostic sign. AJR 92:1162–1165, 1964.

146. Benson MD: Adult survival with intrahepatic portal venous gas secondary to acute gastric dilatation, with a review of portal venous gas. Clin Radiol 36:441–443, 1985.

147. Graham GA, Bernstein RB, Gronner AT: Gas in the portal and inferior mesenteric veins caused by diverticulitis of the sigmoid colon. Report of a case with survival. Radiology 114:601–602, 1975.

148. Stein MG, Cruez JV III, Hamlin JA: Portal venous air associated with barium enema. AJR 140:1171–1172, 1983.

149. Birnberg FA, Gore RM, Shragg B, et al: Hepatic portal venous gas. A benign finding in a patient with ulcerative colitis. J Clin Gastroenterol 5:89–91, 1983.

150. Sadler VK, Brennan RE, Madan V: Portal vein gas following air-contrast barium enema in granulomatous colitis: report of a case. Gastrointest Radiol 4:163–164, 1979.

151. Haber I: Hepatic portal vein gas following colonoscopy in ulcerative colitis—report of a case. Acta Gastroenterol Belg 46:14–17, 1983.

152. Chezmar JL, Nelson RC, Bernardino ME: Portal venous gas after hepatic transplantation: sonographic detection and clinical significance. AJR 153:1203–1205, 1989.

153. Marks WM, Filly RA: Computed tomographic demonstration of intraarterial air following hepatic artery ligation. Radiology 132:665–666, 1979.

154. Tomchik FS, Wittenberg J, Ottinger LW. The roentgenographic spectrum of bowel infarction. Radiology 96:249–260, 1970.

155. Smerud MJ, Johnson CD, Stephens DH: Diagnosis of bowel infarction: a comparison of plain films and CT scans in 23 cases. AJR 154:99–103, 1990.

156. Lund EC, Han SY, Holley HC, et al: Intestinal ischemia: comparison of plain radiographic and computed tomographic findings. Radiographics 8:1083–1108, 1988.

157. Zweig GJ, Yuk-Pui L, Srinantaswamy S, et al: Gas forming infections of the abdomen: plain film findings. Appl Radiol 19:37–42, 1990.

158. Meyers HI, Parker JJ: Emphysematous gastritis. Radiology 89:426–434, 1967.

159. Berens SV, Moskowitz H, Mellins HZ: Air within the wall of the stomach: roentgen manifestations and a new roentgenographic sign. AJR 103:310–313, 1968.

160. Seaman WB, Fleming RJ: Intramural gastric emphysema. AJR 101:431–436, 1967.

161. Marshak RH, Lindner AE, Milano AM: Pneumatosis coli. Am J Gastroenterol 56:68–73, 1971.

162. Bloch C: The natural history of pneumatosis coli. Radiology 123:311–314, 1977.

163. Simons NM, Hyman KE, Divertie MB, et al: Pneumatosis cystoides intestinalis. Treatment with oxygen via close-fitting mask. JAMA 231:1354–1356, 1975.

164. Sands WW: Extraluminal localized gas vesicles: an aid in the diagnosis of abdominal abscesses from plain roentgenograms. AJR 74:195–203, 1955.

165. Rice RP, Masters SJ: Intraabdominal abscess. Semin Roentgenol 8:365–374, 1973.

166. Pfahler GE: Measurement of the liver by means of roentgen rays based upon a study of 502 subjects. AJR 16:558–564, 1926.

167. Gelfand DW: The liver. Plain film diagnosis. Semin Roentgenol 10:177–185, 1975.

168. Chon H, Arger PH, Miller WT: Displacement of duodenum by an enlarged liver. AJR 119:85–88, 1987.

169. Kattan KR, Moskowitz M: Position of the duodenal bulb and liver size. AJR 119:78–84, 1973.

170. Epstein BS: Diaphragmatic changes incident to hepatic neoplasms. AJR 82:114–119, 1959.

171. Whalen JP, Evans JA, Meyers MS: Vector principle in the differential diagnosis of abdominal masses. II. Right upper quadrant. AJR 115:318–333, 1972.

172. Brogdon BG, Cros NE: Observations on the "normal" spleen. Radiology 72:412–414, 1959.

173. Moel H: Size of the normal kidneys. Acta Radiol Diagn 46:640, 1956.

174. Proto AV, Lane EJ: Visualization of differences in soft tissue densities: the liver in ascites. Radiology 121:19–23, 1976.

175. Wixson D, Kazam E, Whalen JP: Displaced lateral surface of the liver (Hellmer's sign) secondary to an extraperitoneal fluid collection. AJR 127:679–682, 1976.

# Abdominal Calcifications

Stephen R. Baker, M.D.

## INTRODUCTION

The abdomen is a closely packed space containing numerous conduits and organs related to each other in a complex spatial arrangement. Each of these structures is subject to a unique range of diseases, all having specific causes and characteristic manifestations. However, the spectrum of plain film findings produced by various abdominal diseases is surprisingly limited. Important signs include displacement, enlargement, or atrophy of organs; distention of bowel; extraluminal gas; and calcification in parenchymal and supporting tissues. In many cases, the pattern of calcium deposition is the most informative and distinctive radiographic finding.

Calcification may occur in the wall of blood vessels or other conduits, the lumen of hollow structures, and the solid substance of viscera or neoplasms. Despite the variety of causes of abdominal calcification, a systematic evaluation of the morphologic features, location, and mobility of an abnormal opacity usually narrows the diagnostic considerations to just a few likely possibilities. In many cases, analysis of the plain film appearance of an abdominal calcification provides sufficient information for an unequivocal diagnosis without need for additional examinations. In other cases, careful assessment of the morphology, location, and mobility of an abdominal calcification helps focus the choice and sequence of subsequent imaging examinations.

## PHYSIOLOGY

The precipitation of calcareous substances requires an alkaline medium and high local concentrations of ionic calcium. The term *metastatic calcification* refers to the deposition of calcium salts in normal tissues as the result of hypercalcemia and an elevated pH. Although the stomach and kidneys are the most frequent sites of metastatic calcification in the abdomen, the degree of parenchymal opacification in these organs is usually too faint to be detected on abdominal plain films. The most common cause of radiographically detectable metastatic calcification is chronic renal failure with secondary hyperparathyroidism.[1] As a result of this pathologic process, diffuse opacification of the kidneys is often accompanied by osteomalacia or osteoporosis.

The term *dystrophic calcification* refers to a phenomenon, far more frequent than metastatic calcification, that occurs despite normal serum levels of calcium. Dystrophic calcification may be caused by trauma, ischemia, infarction, or other pathologic processes resulting in a predisposition to calcium deposition. In some tumors, the rapid breakdown of lipids releases fatty acids that bind calcium with particular avidity. Mucin-producing adenocarcinomas of the gastrointestinal tract possess a glycoprotein that is similar in chemical configuration to cartilage and shares with it an affinity for calcium aggregation.[2] Although some structures in the abdomen have a propensity for dystrophic calcification, the mechanisms and kinetics of calcium deposition have not been fully elucidated.

Some devitalized or degenerative tissues are also associated with new bone formation. However, ossification is less common than dystrophic calcification. Calcified osteoid may be found as an isolated finding, or it may coexist with adjacent areas of calcium deposition that lack the histologic structure of bone. In either case, local tissue damage appears to be the precipitating factor. Ossification may occur in ovarian or retroperitoneal teratomas (Fig. 14–1), abdominal scars, and, rarely, other colonic and retroperitoneal neoplasms.

Papillary serous cystadenocarcinomas of the ovary may contain a distinctive form of calcification that is characterized by a psammomatous or cloud-like opacity attributable to intracellular deposition of calcium salts in the lesion[3] (Fig. 14–2). In contrast, dystrophic calcification associated with other metastatic tumors is caused by extracellular precipitation of calcium salts. Both psammomatous and dystrophic calcification may be manifested by amorphous, poorly outlined areas of increased density. Nevertheless, the distribution of calcified metastases may suggest the correct diagnosis in these patients.

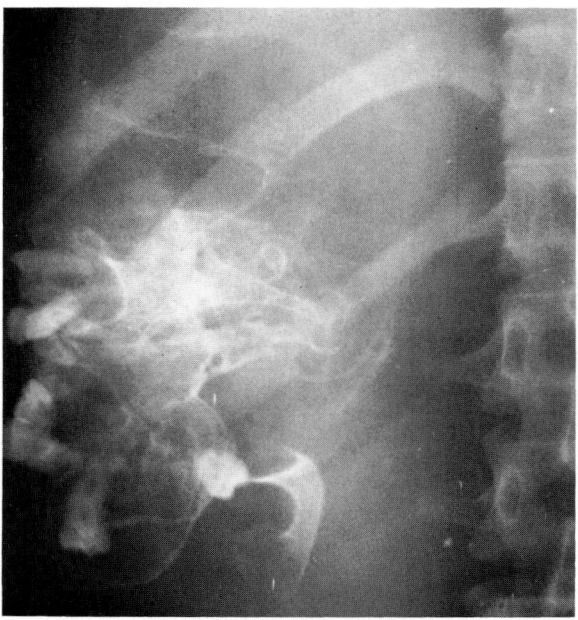

**Figure 14–1. Retroperitoneal teratoma.** Both teeth and bone are visualized. Note the cortex and trabecula in the disordered pattern of ossification.

## MORPHOLOGY

The recognition of specific abdominal calcifications has been aided by the attribution of vivid, descriptive names to particular radiopacities. For example, a "staghorn calculus" is a large, branching opacity in the renal pelvis. Such appellations are highly evocative and easily remembered; however, they do not help generate a differential diagnosis encompassing the many causes of abdominal calcification. Unfortunately, most surveys of abdominal calcification have relied primarily on these

descriptive designations and have failed to emphasize diagnostic features that might help to organize the various opacities into categories with shared characteristics.

This chapter describes a logical scheme for classifying almost all abdominal calcifications. These calcifications may be distinguished radiographically on the basis of various morphologic features, including contour, border, sharpness, marginal continuity, and internal architecture. Consideration of these features permits a grouping of calcifications into one of four classes: concretions, conduit wall calcification, cystic calcification, and solid mass calcification. In the following sections, the distinguishing features of each class are discussed in detail. Potential pitfalls and notable exceptions are also considered.

## Concretions

Concretions are precipitates removed from solution of the liquid medium inside a vessel or hollow viscus. They often contain a central nidus, composed of an insoluble substance such as an inorganic foreign body, ingested vegetable matter, thrombus, or focal collection of pus and cellular debris. In pelvic veins and in the gastrointestinal and genitourinary tracts, concretions are likely to calcify. They can be brightly or faintly opaque; the radiographic density depends on the size of the opacity and the amount of calcium per unit volume. Concretions do not have a common shape. Biliary calculi are usually oval or rounded, whereas gallstones are often faceted (Fig. 14–3). Ureteral and pancreatic stones

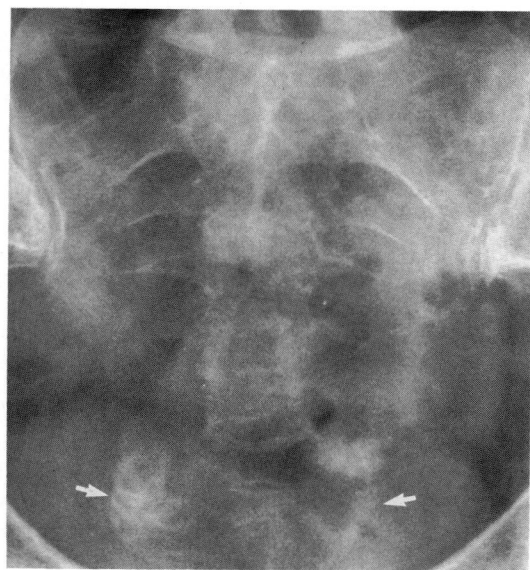

**Figure 14–2. Papillary serous cystadenocarcinoma.** Patches of psammomatous calcification are seen in the lower pelvis *(arrows)* and over the sacrum near the midline.

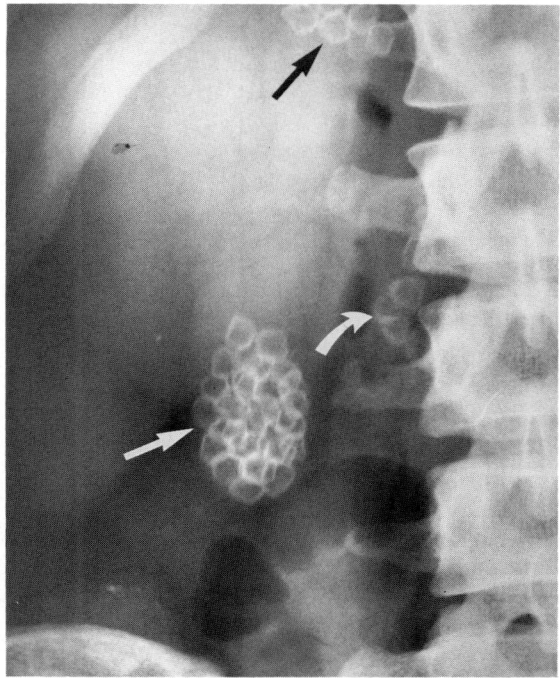

**Figure 14–3. Biliary stones.** Numerous stones are seen in the gallbladder *(straight white arrow)*, cystic duct *(black arrow)*, and common bile duct *(curved white arrow)*. Note how the stones have faceted margins.

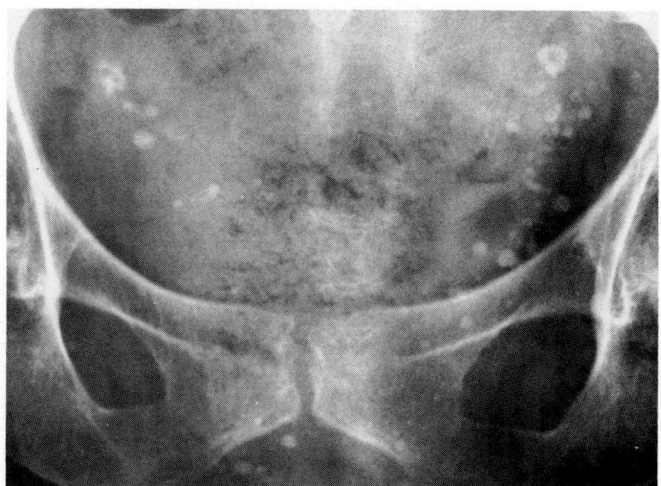

**Figure 14–4. Phleboliths scattered in the veins of the broad ligament.** Uterine prolapse has displaced the lower phleboliths below the pubic symphysis. Note the pronounced lucent centers of the uppermost stones on the left.

often have jagged edges, but in hollow viscera such as the urinary bladder and gallbladder, concretions usually have smooth margins.

A sharply defined external margin is a unifying feature of concretions. Stones are almost always characterized by a continuous edge of calcification throughout the entire perimeter, with no lucent gaps or discontinuities along the interface with the surrounding medium. This unique feature may permit differentiation of small stones with radiolucent centers from calcified vessels seen on end. The uninterrupted opacification of the perimeter of large stones also helps distinguish them from calcified cysts on abdominal plain films.

Concretions may vary greatly in their internal architecture. A stone may be homogeneously dense, a pattern often encountered in urinary calculi, or it may contain a slightly eccentric area of lucency, an appearance typical of phleboliths (Fig. 14–4). Concentric lamina-

tions are characteristically seen in gallstones, bladder concretions, and appendicoliths (Fig. 14–5). Each of these various internal configurations has a certain predictability and uniformity. A central lucency is often present. Stones seldom have a mottled, speckled, or patchy appearance. The deposition of calcium on only one surface of the stone is extremely rare.

Unlike calcified solid lesions or cysts, which are pathologic tumefactions that distort or displace normal organs and supporting structures, stones tend to be confined within pre-existing vessels or fluid-filled viscera. When multiple stones are present, they may outline the course of a hollow tube or the dimensions of a distensible reservoir. Concretions appearing outside expected anatomic locations are unusual; examples are multiple phleboliths in a hemangioma, ectopic gallstones in the distal small bowel, and appendicoliths from a ruptured appendix in the peritoneal cavity.

## Conduit Wall Calcification

Conduits are fluid-conducting hollow tubes. In the abdomen, they include the ureter, urethra, vas deferens, pancreatic ducts, bile ducts, and vascular structures. The vast majority of conduit wall calcifications are located in the aorta and its branches. The tubular configuration characteristic of conduits is readily appreciated if the calcification is circumferential. When the vessel is parallel to the radiographic beam, a ring-like density is often observed (Fig. 14–6). In contrast to calculi, conduit wall calcifications often have gaps in the opaque ring. Because calcification in conduit walls is not uniform, alternating radiopaque and radiolucent areas may be seen along the course of the vessel. Because internal radiopacities are not a feature of conduit wall calcifications, central radiopaque areas should suggest another class of abdominal calcifications. Even when there is extensive mural calcification, the lateral walls of the conduit provide a longer path for the x-ray beam to traverse than either the anterior or posterior walls, so that they appear more opaque. As a result, a conduit

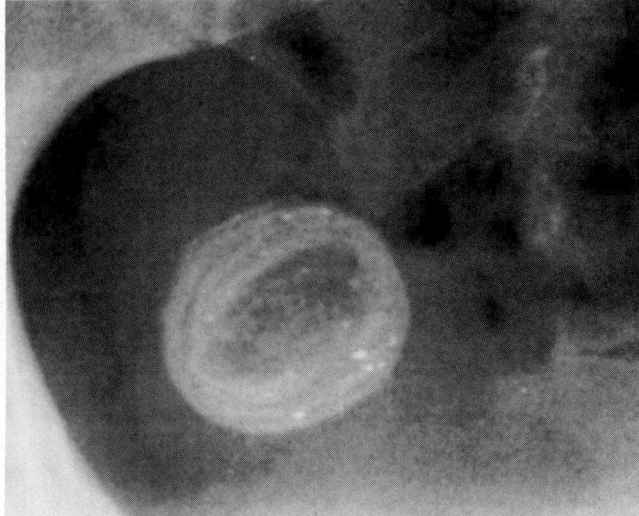

**Figure 14–5. Large calcified appendicolith.** Concentric laminations and flecks of barium are visualized within the growing stone.

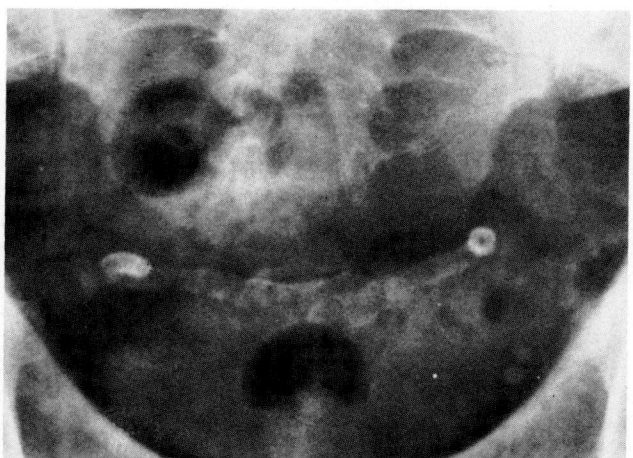

**Figure 14–6. Conduit wall calcification in the vas deferens.** Marginal opacities are seen en face and in profile.

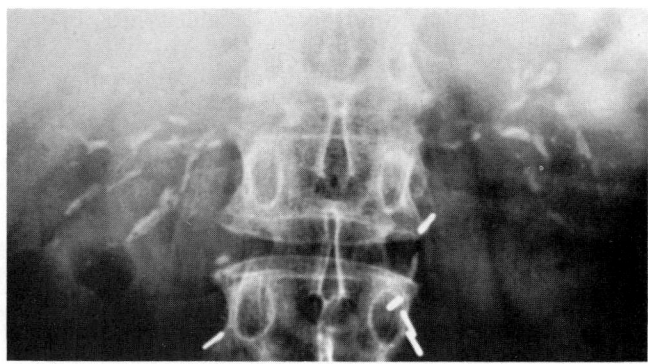

**Figure 14–7. Calcification of the renal arteries and their intrarenal branches.** These opacities have the typical configuration of conduit wall calcification.

wall calcification is usually manifested by parallel, linear opacities or, en face, by a circle of radiopacity. A marginal branching pattern may be observed at the bifurcation of the abdominal aorta or in the intrarenal arteries (Fig. 14–7). Calcification of narrow-caliber vessels occasionally produces a string-like appearance. In the female pelvis, calcification of the uterine artery may be evident by a horizontal or slightly undulating linear opacity.

Conduit wall calcification is clearly discernible only if deposition of calcium is extensive. A single fleck of calcification can simulate a small calculus or even a thin piece of cortical bone, particularly in the renal pelvis. Conversely, the lateral margin of the transverse process of a lumbar vertebra can mimic calcification in the renal artery. However, the lateral margin of the transverse process has a vertical orientation, whereas the renal artery is oriented horizontally (see Fig. 14–7).

Conduit wall calcification is usually found at the expected location of vessels; thus, it is not seen at the lateral margin of the spleen or in other peripheral locations. As arteries become tortuous and dilated, however, their walls may eventually be displaced several centimeters or more from their expected location. As a result, the wall of a dilated, calcified aorta may be seen to overlie the midline, or even to lie to the right of the spine, on abdominal plain films.

## Cystic Calcification

Cystic calcification is characterized by the deposition of calcium in the wall of abnormal fluid-filled masses, including true epithelial cysts, pseudocysts, and aneurysmally dilated arteries. Despite the diversity of cystic structures in the abdomen, cystic calcification exhibits remarkably uniform radiographic findings.

A cystic pattern of calcification is characterized by the presence of a smooth, curvilinear rim of radiopacity in the wall of the cyst (Fig. 14–8). Although arcuate opacities may be present in both cysts and conduits, the calcified rim of a cyst has a larger diameter than that of a conduit. Unlike stones, this calcified rim is often incomplete, and in many cases, only a small section of the wall contains visible calcium. Moreover, cysts have

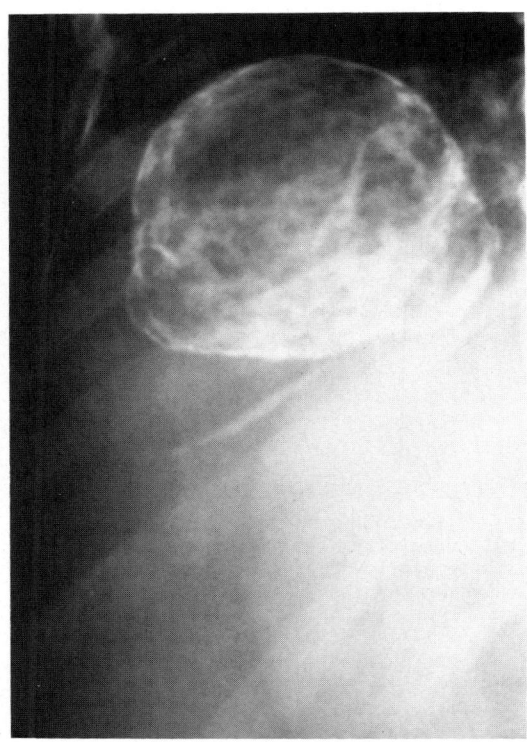

**Figure 14–8. Large echinococcus cyst in the liver.** Note how the calcified wall of the cyst is flattened inferiorly.

only a single encircling wall, so that when calcified, they do not have a laminated appearance. Cysts need not be perfectly round; some can be compressed on one side, producing an ovoid configuration (see Fig. 14–8).

The configuration of cysts depends on their location. They may displace and distort adjacent structures, or they themselves may be displaced by nearby solid organs or vessels. Usually, differentiation of cystic calcification from the diffuse opacification of solid masses is not difficult. Nevertheless, uterine leiomyomas may contain curvilinear calcifications at their margins, mimicking the appearance of cystic calcification.

Unlike concretions and conduit wall calcifications,

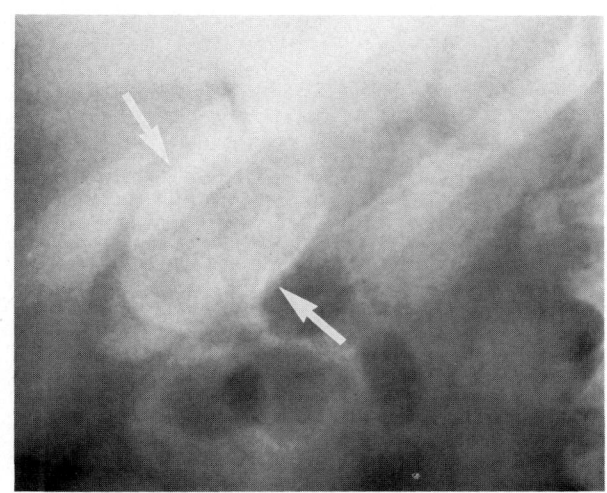

**Figure 14–9. Cystic calcification in the gallbladder wall** *(arrows)*.

which occur at expected locations, the cystic pattern of calcification may be found almost anywhere in the abdomen. Cystic calcification most commonly occurs in abdominal aortic aneurysms. It is usually associated with conduit wall calcification in contiguous sections of the aorta and in the common iliac arteries. Cystic calcification may also occur in aneurysms of the splenic artery in the left upper quadrant. Other patients may have cystic calcification in a variety of urinary tract lesions, including aneurysms of the renal artery, echinococcus cysts, perirenal hematomas, multicystic kidneys, adrenal cysts, and renal carcinomas. Echinococcus cysts are the most common cause of cystic calcification in the liver, but a calcified gallbladder (i.e., a "porcelain" gallbladder) may occasionally produce similar findings (Fig. 14–9). Other causes of cystic calcification in the lower abdomen include mesenteric cysts, calcified appendiceal mucoceles, and calcified benign tumors of the ovary.

## Solid Mass Calcification

Of all the classes of abdominal calcification, solid mass calcification includes the greatest variety of pathologic abnormalities. Solid masses may appear as mottled densities with scattered radiolucencies on a calcified background, an appearance typical of calcified mesenteric lymph nodes (Fig. 14–10). A whorled configuration with incomplete bands and arcs of calcification is a feature of uterine leiomyomas. Calcified leiomyomas may also be manifested by numerous flocculent densities superimposed on a radiolucent background. Solid calcifications share the unifying feature of a nongeometric inner architecture and an irregular, often incomplete margin.

Calcified solid masses can be located anywhere in the abdomen. Calcified mesenteric lymph nodes are usually found in middle-aged or elderly individuals. They tend

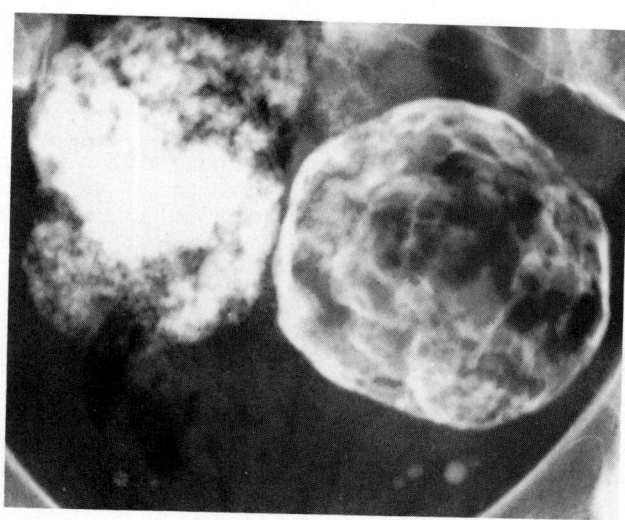

**Figure 14–11. Calcified uterine leiomyomas.** Dense areas of flocculent calcification on the right and cystic calcification on the left.

to be located in a broad arc along the course of the mesentery of the small bowel from the left upper quadrant to the right lower quadrant of the abdomen. Multiple calcified nodes are often present, and individual nodes may vary widely in diameter.

Uterine leiomyomas are the most common calcified solid masses in the female pelvis. Some patients have multiple leiomyomas that may become calcified as they grow to enormous sizes (Fig. 14–11). Although leiomyomas are usually located in the pelvis, they may occasionally be found almost anywhere in the abdomen (Fig. 14–12).

All other types of solid mass calcification are much less common than calcified mesenteric lymph nodes or

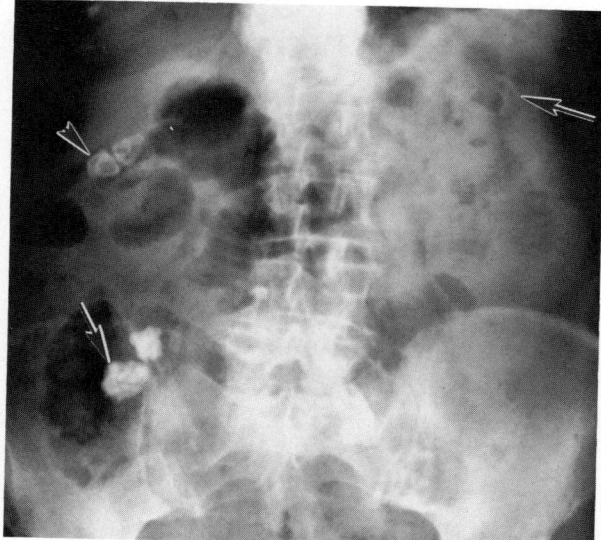

**Figure 14–10. Calcified mesenteric nodes.** The mottled interior of the nodes *(lower arrow)* contrasts with the geometric laminations of calcified gallstones *(arrowhead)* and the linear tracks of a section of the splenic artery *(upper arrow)*.

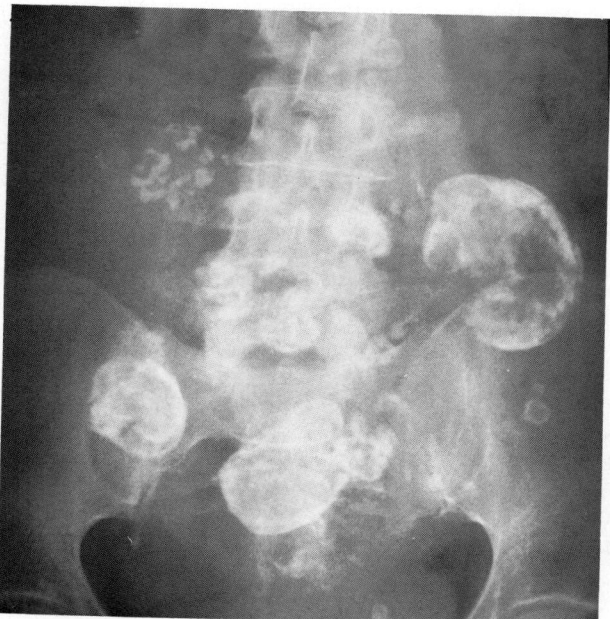

**Figure 14–12. Multiple calcified leiomyomas.** This patient has different patterns of calcification in leiomyomas extending from the pelvis to the midabdomen.

calcified uterine leiomyomas. A solid pattern of calcification may occasionally be found in adenomas, hamartomas, and carcinomas of the kidney as well as in tuberculous and chronic pyogenic abscesses of the kidney. Calcified pancreatic masses are quite rare. Small calcified densities in the liver and spleen usually represent granulomas. However, the presence of poorly defined radiopaque areas in the liver should be considered an indication of calcified metastases from colonic carcinoma until proved otherwise.

## Difficulty in Classification

This classification scheme can be applied broadly to most abdominal calcifications. However, some calcifications cannot be separated into one of the four classes. If the density is too faint to have a definite inner architecture or margin, morphologic analysis is not possible. In addition, if the calcification is extremely small, a concretion may be difficult to distinguish from a solid opacity. Other calcifications may have an appearance suggestive of more than one morphologic class. For example, numerous pancreatic stones clustered together may resemble a solid mass, although the area of radiopacity actually represents innumerable intraductal concretions with irregular margins (Fig. 14–13). Thus, one must be aware of potential pitfalls in the classification of abdominal calcifications. Nevertheless, a specific abdominal calcification can usually be classified into one of the four morphologic categories with a reasonable degree of confidence.

## LOCATION

The location of abdominal radiopacities also provides important clues about the origin of the calcifications. Most calcifications in the right upper quadrant are related to the gallbladder or right kidney. Gallstones are often multiple and are frequently laminated. Gallbladder wall calcification is much less common but can be clearly recognized by its marginal arcuate configuration. A transverse orientation and conduit morphologic features indicate calcification of the renal artery. Stones in the renal pelvis and ureters have characteristic appearances and are oriented along the course of the urinary tract.

In both upper quadrants, adrenal calcification may assume various forms, including the solid opacities of calcified granulomas and the eggshell calcification of cysts and pheochromocytomas. Multiple calcifications crossing the midline of the upper abdomen are characteristic of pancreatic lithiasis. Calcified mesenteric lymph nodes may also cross the midline but are usually located more inferiorly, along an oblique path extending from the left midabdomen to the right lower quadrant.

Appendicoliths typically appear as a single or a tight cluster of laminated calcifications in the right lower quadrant. However, the appendix may be located anywhere between the lower pelvis and the right upper quadrant, so that the diagnosis of an appendicolith should not be excluded simply because the concretion is found at a considerable distance from its expected location in the right iliac fossa.

In the lower abdomen and pelvis, calcifications that appear as concretions should arouse suspicion of ureteral calculi; however, a small ureteral stone is often difficult to distinguish from a phlebolith on a single film. Reference should therefore be made to previous or subsequent films. Calculi may move freely within the ureteral lumen, whereas pelvic phleboliths are fixed in position unless displaced by an enlarging extraperitoneal mass. Bladder stones are usually readily recognizable. Because of their protean manifestations, however, calcified uterine leiomyomas may be confused with other calcified lesions in the pelvis, such as ovarian tumors and mesenteric lymph nodes. Cystic teratomas of the ovary can

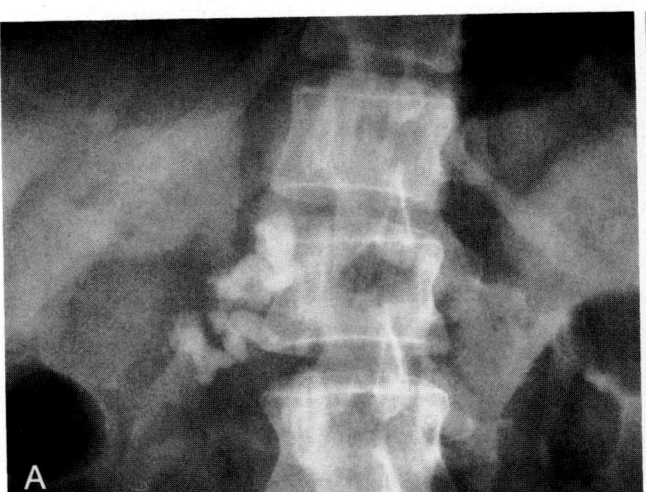
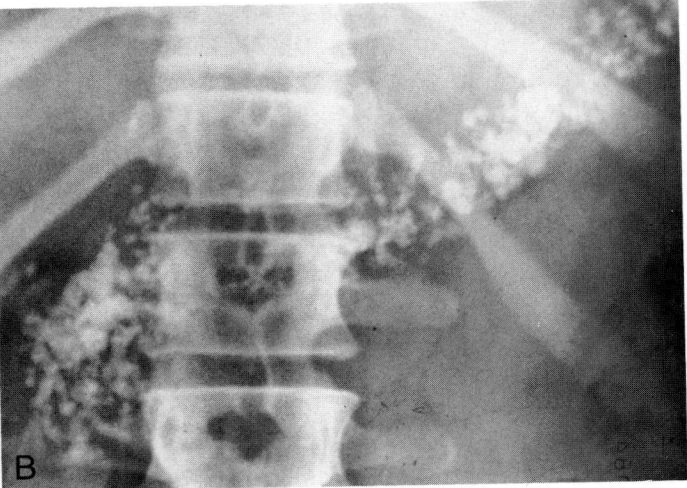

**Figure 14–13. Two calcification patterns in pancreatic lithiasis. A.** A conglomerate of stones filling larger ducts in the pancreatic head could be mistaken for calcification in conduits. **B.** Pancreatic stones can be seen throughout the pancreas. Each stone is located within a duct, but the cumulative appearance suggests diffuse acinar opacification.

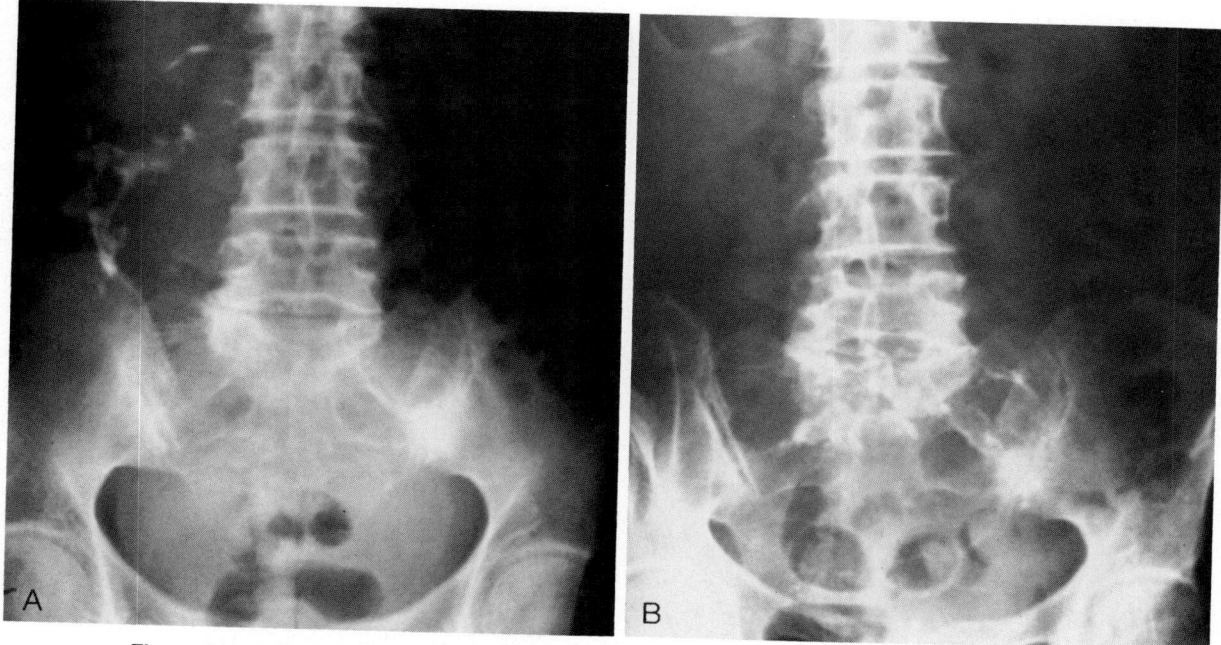

**Figure 14–14. Mobility of ovarian dermoid. A.** When the bladder is full, the tumor rises into the lower abdomen. **B.** After voiding of the bladder, the calcified mass overlies the sacrum.

be recognized by the presence of teeth and bone, which are often accompanied by a large homogenous lucency, indicating fat, within the tumor.

## MOBILITY

The movement of abdominal calcifications, either during a single examination or over a longer period,

provides additional information that may lead to a specific plain film diagnosis. Gravity, respiration, peristaltic activity, and growth of masses may all cause changes in location. Stones that are located in a fluid medium may undergo layering on films obtained using upright or decubitus projections. Such manipulation of position may be helpful in the diagnosis of gallstones or of calculi in hydronephrotic sacs. Epiploic appendices that have become amputated or appendicoliths that lie

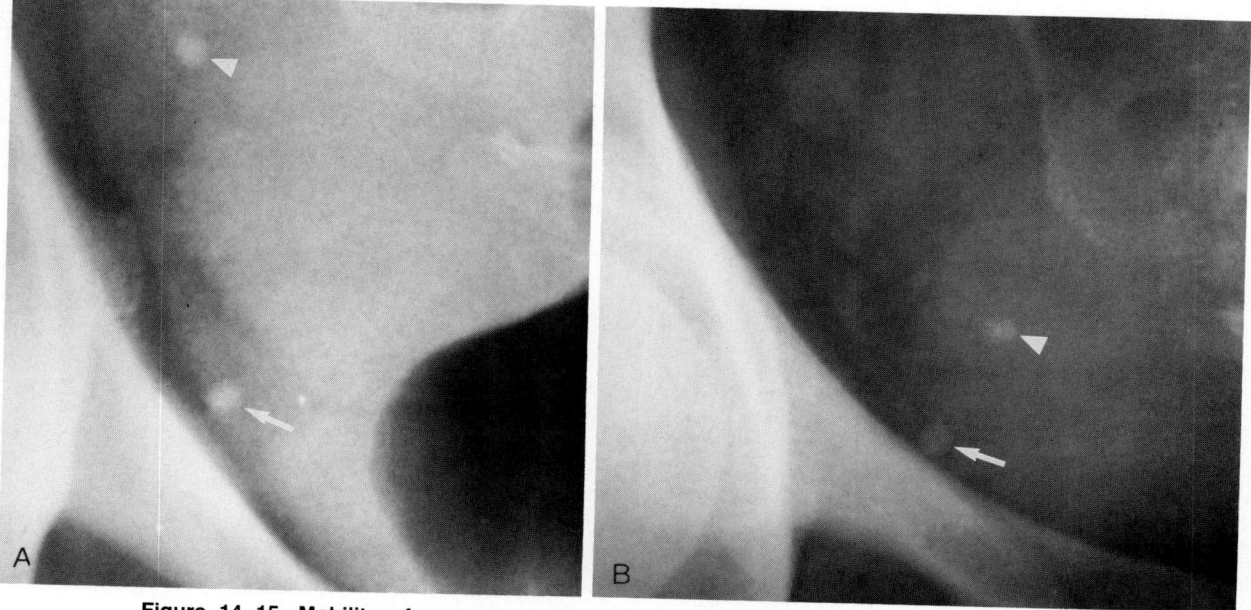

**Figure 14–15. Mobility of ureteral calculus. A.** A phlebolith *(arrow)* and a ureteral calculus *(arrowhead)* are morphologically identical on the initial plain film. **B.** However, the venous stone *(arrow)* maintains a fixed position, and the ureteral stone *(arrowhead)* has migrated distally on a subsequent film.

free in the peritoneal cavity may exhibit a great range of movement on sequential films. Whereas mesenteric nodes move slightly with positional changes, ovarian teratomas may move considerably as the bladder fills and empties (Fig. 14–14). Because of the effects of peristalsis, stones in the lumen of the gastrointestinal tract and pelvicaliceal system can migrate on successive films. Consideration of this migration is particularly important in diagnosing ectopic gallstones and in differentiating distal ureteral calculi from stones in pelvic veins (Fig. 14–15). When films are taken over a period of weeks or months, enlargement or shrinkage of abdominal masses may be recognized by the movement of calcifications that lie within or adjacent to these lesions.

Even pelvic phleboliths can be displaced by hematomas or other masses.[4]

## References

1. Hilbish TF, Bartter FC: Roentgen findings in abnormal deposition of calcium in tissues. AJR 87:1128–1129, 1962.
2. Kurturna P: A contribution to the problem of calcifications in malignant tumors: a case of late calcified retroperitoneal metastasis of an ovarian carcinoma. Neoplasma 11:633–642, 1964.
3. Widmann BF, Ostrum AW, Fried H: Practical aspects of calcification and ossification in the various body tissues. Radiology 30:598–609, 1938.
4. Steinbach HL: Identification of pelvic masses by phlebolith displacement. AJR 83:1063–1066, 1960.

# SECTION III

# Pharynx

*Section Editor*

Stephen E. Rubesin, M.D.

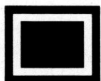

# Pharynx: Normal Anatomy and Techniques

**Stephen E. Rubesin, M.D.**

**David M. Yousem, M.D.**

## INTRODUCTION

The pharynx is the "crossroads" of speech, swallowing, and respiration. During swallowing, the pharynx directs the bolus into the esophagus and prevents the bolus from entering the tracheobronchial tree. During respiration, the pharynx is an active conduit from nasopharynx to laryngeal aditus. During speech, the pharynx functions as a resonating chamber, changing size and shape to alter sounds.

Disorders of the pharynx may be manifested by swallowing, respiratory, or speech dysfunction. Patients may complain of dysphagia, odynophagia, choking, or a feeling of a lump in the throat not associated with swallowing. Soft palate insufficiency may be suggested by nasal regurgitation or a nasal quality of voice. Recurrent pneumonia, asthma, chronic bronchitis, or coughing may indicate pharyngeal dysfunction. Routine barium studies may be useful in assessing pharyngeal function in patients with known cerebrovascular accident, neuromuscular disease, pharyngeal tumor, or prior head and neck surgery or radiation.

Chapters 15 through 18 focus on the main gastrointestinal function of the pharynx—swallowing. This chapter presents the anatomy of the pharynx as a basis for understanding both structural and motility disorders. Chapter 16 presents the neurologic anatomy necessary for understanding motility disorders.

## ANATOMY

### Location

The pharynx is a funnel-shaped tube of skeletal muscle extending from the cranial base to the lower margin of the cricoid cartilage (Figs. 15–1 and 15–2A). The pharynx lies anterior to the vertebral bodies of the cervical spine, prevertebral muscles, and loose connective tissue of the retropharyngeal space.[1] The pharynx is confined laterally by the muscles of the neck, the lateral portions of the hyoid bone and thyroid cartilage, and the carotid sheath[2] (Fig. 15–2B).

### Divisions

The pharynx is arbitrarily divided into three parts: the nasopharynx (epipharynx), the oropharynx (mesopharynx), and the laryngopharynx (hypopharynx).[3] The nasopharynx is primarily a respiratory tract structure continuous anteriorly with the nasal cavity. The superior and posterior walls of the nasopharynx abut the basisphenoid and basilar part of the occipital bone. Inferiorly, the nasopharynx is separated from the oropharynx by the soft palate.

The oropharynx (Fig. 15–3) lies posterior to the oral cavity, extending from the soft palate to its arbitrary division from the hypopharynx at the level of the hyoid bone. Some anatomists divide the oropharynx from the hypopharynx at the level of the pharyngoepiglottic fold (Fig. 15–4), a mucosal fold overlying the stylopharyngeal muscle.[1] The base of the tongue forms the lower anterior wall of the oropharynx.

The hypopharynx lies behind and lateral to the larynx, extending from the level of the hyoid bone to the lower border of the cricopharyngeal muscle at the level of the inferior margin of the cricoid cartilage. These divisions are arbitrary, as the soft palate and hyoid bone change position with phonation, swallowing, and respiration.

The oropharynx and hypopharynx are the divisions of the pharynx that participate in swallowing. The oro-

**Figure 15–1. Basic structures of the normal pharynx. A.** Double contrast film in the frontal view shows the contours of the superior surface of the tongue *(black arrow)*, the tonsillar fossa *(white arrow)*, the valleculae (v), and the lateral wall *(open arrow)* of the piriform sinus (p). The surface of the base of the tongue (t), seen en face, has a reticular appearance because of the underlying lingual tonsil. **B.** Double contrast radiograph in the lateral view shows the contours of the soft palate (s), the base of the tongue (t), the epiglottis (e), the valleculae (v), the posterior pharyngeal wall *(arrow)*, barium pooling in the lower piriform sinus (p), and collapsed region of the pharyngoesophageal segment *(arrowheads)*. **(B** from SE Rubesin, B Jones, MW Donner, Contrast pharyngography: the importance of phonation, AJR, 148, 2, 269–272, 1987, © by American Roentgen Ray Society.)

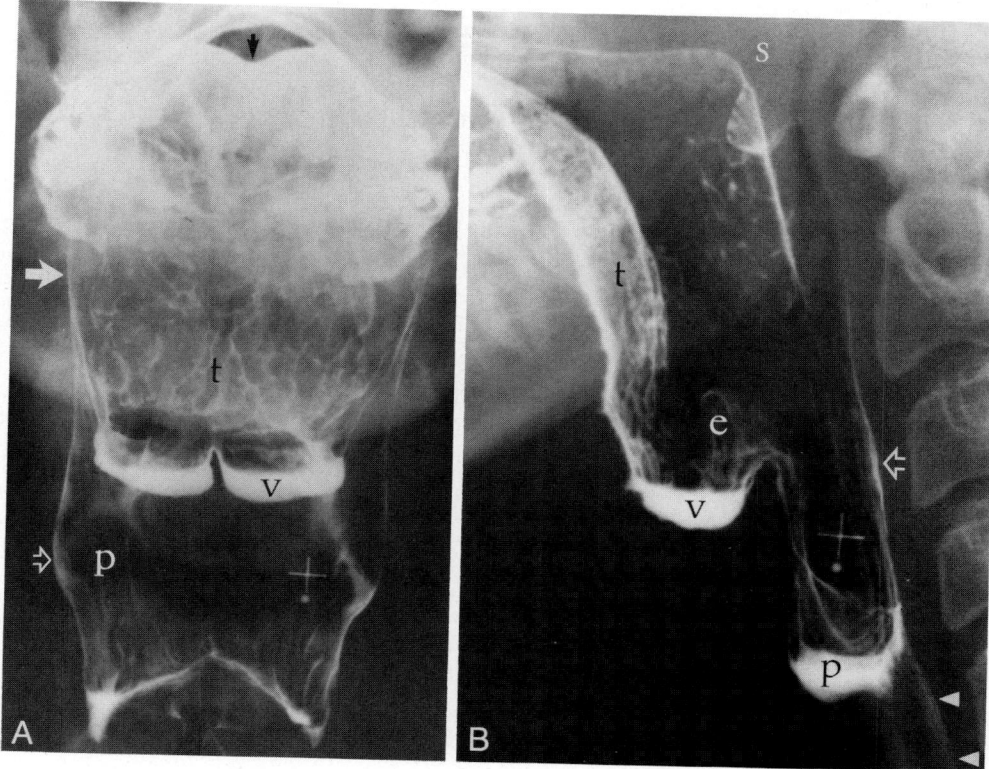

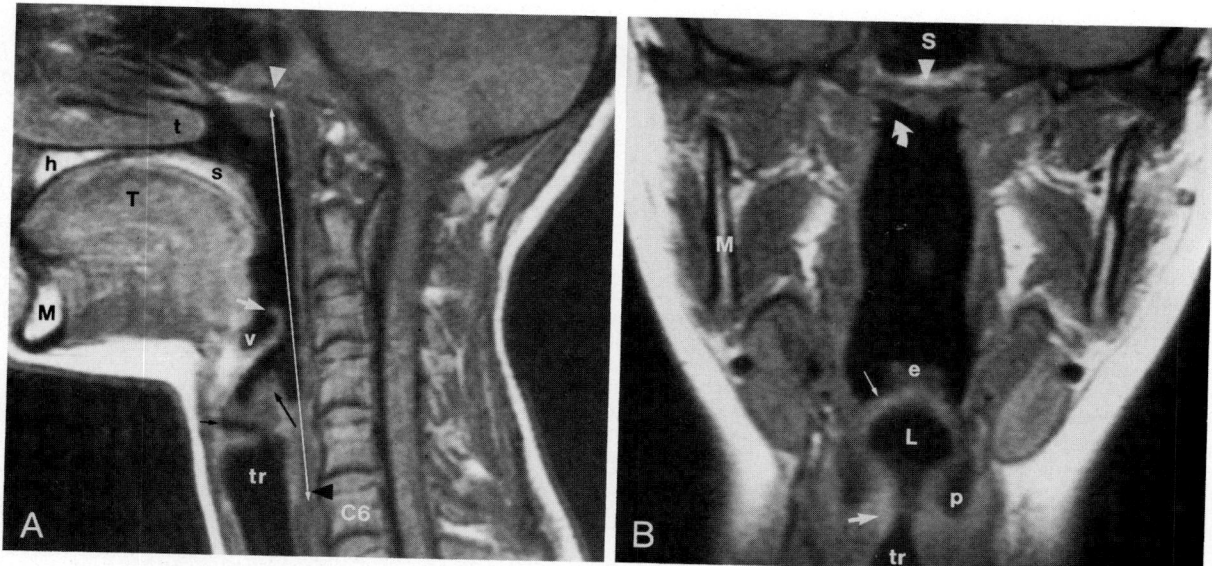

**Figure 15–2. Location of the pharynx. A.** Sagittal T1-weighted magnetic resonance (MR) image of the head and neck shows the pharynx *(double arrow)* extending from the basisphenoid *(white arrowhead)* to the C-6 vertebral body (C6) and pharyngoesophageal segment *(black arrowhead)*. The pharynx is confined posteriorly by the cervical spine. The tongue (T) is apposed to the hard palate (h) and soft palate (s). Also shown are the inferior turbinate (t), the mandible in cross section (M), the epiglottis *(white arrow)*, the vallecula (v), the laryngeal ventricle *(small black arrow)*, the bulge of the arytenoid glands *(large black arrow)*, and the trachea (tr). **B.** Coronal T1-weighted MR image of the neck shows the relationship of the pharynx to the basisphenoid *(arrowhead)* and to the sphenoidal sinus (S). The epiglottis (e), aryepiglottic folds *(thin white arrow)*, and piriform sinus (p) are well depicted. Also note fossa of Rosenmüller *(curved arrow)*, the laryngeal vestibule (L), the mandible (M), the true vocal cord *(thick white arrow)*, and the trachea (tr).

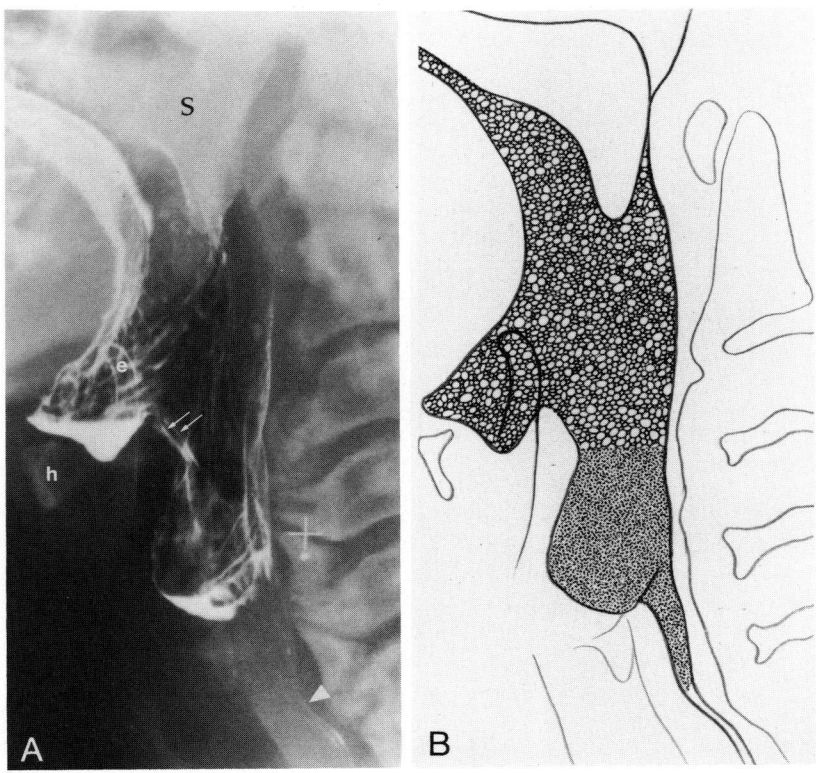

**Figure 15–3. Divisions of the pharynx.** A lateral double contrast image of the pharynx **(A)** with its corresponding drawing **(B)**. The divisions of the pharynx involved with swallowing are the oropharynx *(bubble pattern)* and the hypopharynx *(granular pattern)*. The oropharynx extends from the soft palate (S) to the level of the hyoid bone (h). The hypopharynx extends from the level of the hyoid bone to the inferior portion of the collapsed pharyngoesophageal segment *(arrowhead)*. Note the epiglottis (e) and the aryepiglottic folds *(arrows)* spanning the oropharynx and hypopharynx. (**A** and **B** from Rubesin SE, Jesserun J, Robertson D, et al: Lines of the pharynx. Radiographics 7:217–237, 1987.)

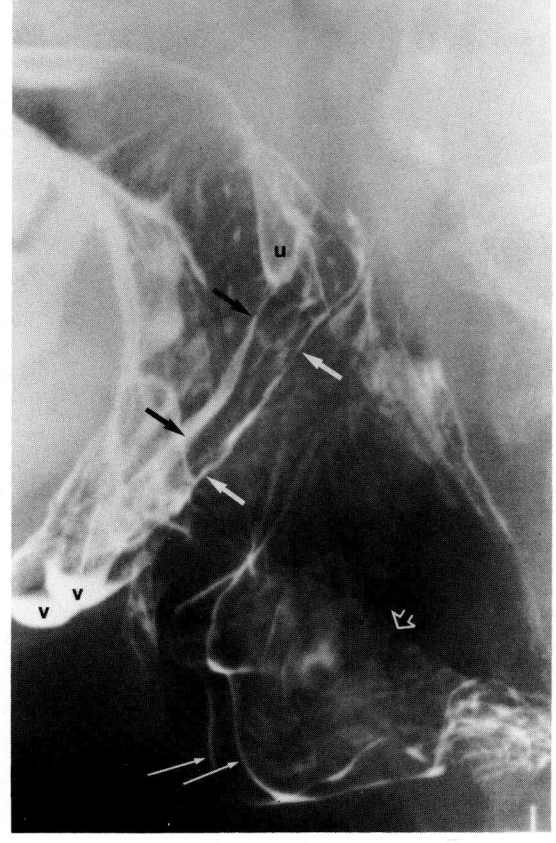

**Figure 15–4. The pharyngoepiglottic folds.** A spot film obtained in the lateral projection shows the paired pharyngoepiglottic folds *(short arrows)* coursing as oblique lines across the lateral wall of the pharynx. The pharyngoepiglottic fold overlies the stylopharyngeal muscle, which extends from the styloid process to the posterior wall of valleculae (v). The uvular tip (u) is seen. The anterior wall of the piriform sinuses *(long arrows)* is well visualized. The mucosa overlying the muscular processes of the arytenoid cartilages *(open arrow)* is demonstrated. (Reprinted with permission from Rubesin SE, Glick SN: The tailored double-contrast pharyngogram. Crit Rev Diagn Imaging 28:133–179, 1988. Copyright CRC Press, Inc. Boca Raton, FL.)

pharynx and hypopharynx have four openings: superiorly, the velopharyngeal portal between the nasopharynx and the oropharynx; anteriorly, the opening to the oral cavity; anteroinferiorly, the laryngeal aditus; and posteroinferiorly, the opening into the esophagus.

## Muscles

Oropharyngeal function depends on coordinated, sequential contraction of the extrinsic muscles of the pharynx, which arise from the skull base, neck, tongue, mandible, and hyoid bone, and the intrinsic skeletal muscles of the pharynx and larynx[3] (Fig. 15–5). The pharynx and larynx are suspended as a unit from the skull base, tongue, and hyoid bone. The suspensory muscles of the hyoid bone, or the suprahyoid muscles, include the following (with their cranial nerve innervation given in parentheses): from the tongue and/or mandible, the anterior belly of the digastric muscle (V), the geniohyoid muscle (XII), the hyoglossal muscle (XII), and the mylohyoid muscle (V); from the skull base, the posterior belly of the digastric muscle (VII), and the stylohyoid muscle (VII)[4–6] (see Fig. 15–5). The major activity of the suprahyoid muscle group that is related to pharyngeal function is to elevate and fix the hyoid bone, a motion that contributes to elevating and widening the pharynx and opening the cricopharyngeal muscle during the passage of a bolus.

The soft palate is formed by an interweaving of muscles from the skull base (tensor veli palatini and levator veli palatini), the tongue (palatoglossus muscle) and the pharynx (palatopharyngeal muscle)[1, 3, 7] (Figs. 15–6 and 15–7). The musculus uvulae is the only intrinsic muscle of the soft palate.

The tendon of the tensor veli palatini (V) forms the fibrous skeleton of the anterior portion of the soft palate. This muscle depresses the anterior soft palate during swallowing. The levator veli palatini (pharyngeal plexus [X]) suspends the midportion of the soft palate (see Figs. 15–6 and 15–7). During swallowing, the levator veli palatini pulls the mid–soft palate superiorly and posteriorly.[8] The palatopharyngeal muscle (pharyngeal plexus [X]) depresses the posterolateral part of the soft palate, elevates the pharynx, and constricts the faucial isthmus. The palatoglossus muscle (X) pulls the soft palate and tongue toward each other. The musculus uvulae (pharyngeal plexus [X]) shortens, thickens, and elevates the uvula.

The thyrohyoid muscle (C1-2) courses from the hyoid bone to the thyroid cartilage (see Fig. 15–5). Its main function is approximation of the hyoid bone and thyroid cartilage, an action that is partly responsible for closing the laryngeal orifice (see Chapter 16). The infrahyoid depressors include the sternohyoid (C1-3), sternothyroid (C1-3), and omohyoid (C1-3) muscles.

The muscular tube of the pharynx is surrounded by the buccopharyngeal fascia. The buccopharyngeal fascia is separated from the prevertebral muscles and fascia by the retropharyngeal space. The retropharyngeal space is an important site for the spread of malignant and inflammatory processes.

The muscular tube of the pharynx is formed by two layers: the inner longitudinal layer and the outer circular (constrictor) layer. The constrictor muscle layer (pharyngeal plexus [X]) forms a ring that is incomplete anteriorly. The relationship of these muscles to the double contrast appearance of the pharynx is illustrated in Figure 15–8. During swallowing, the constrictor muscles contract sequentially to propel the bolus into the esophagus.[9] Contraction of the superior constrictor muscle also apposes the lateral pharyngeal wall with the soft palate, closing the lateral portion of the velopharyngeal portal.[10–12]

During swallowing, the inner longitudinal muscle layer (see Figs. 15–5 to 15–7), which includes the stylopharyngeal muscle (IX), the salpingopharyngeal muscle (pharyngeal plexus [X]), and the palatopharyngeal muscle (pharyngeal plexus [X]), elevates the pharynx up and over the descending bolus of food.[13] The palatopharyngeal muscle also constricts the posterior portion of the pharynx, channeling the bolus into the hypopharynx and helping to prevent nasal regurgitation.

The double contrast appearances and landmarks of the pharynx depend to a large extent on the inner longitudinal muscle layer.[3] Folds of mucosa are elevated into the pharyngeal lumen by the inner longitudinal layer of muscles. These muscular elevations are seen as the palatoglossal fold (anterior tonsillar pillar), the palatopharyngeal fold (posterior tonsillar pillar) (Fig. 15–9), and the pharyngoepiglottic fold[1, 3] (see Fig. 15–4).

## Basic Structures and Mucosal Surface Patterns

The shape of the pharynx is determined by the underlying musculature, the laryngeal cartilages, the supporting skeleton, and the hyoid sling (Fig. 15–10). Although the nasopharynx is primarily a respiratory tract structure, certain nasopharyngeal structures participate in the act of swallowing. The eustachian tube connects the middle ear with the nasopharynx, allowing equilibration of air pressures on the internal and external aspects of the tympanic membrane during swallowing. During breathing, the eustachian tube is closed. The eustachian tube cartilage bulges into the lateral nasopharyngeal wall at the torus tubarius[14, 15] (Fig. 15–11). Radiographically, a C-shaped prominence appears near the torus tubarius[8] (Fig. 15–12). The salpingopharyngeal fold overlying the salpingopharyngeal muscle courses inferiorly from the torus along the lateral pharyngeal wall to the level of the soft palate.[16] The posterior nasopharyngeal wall has a variably nodular surface because of underlying adenoidal tissue.[17, 18]

The oropharynx communicates anteriorly with the oral cavity. The vertical (pharyngeal) surface of the tongue (base of the tongue) is variably nodular because of underlying lymphoid tissue of the lingual tonsil[19] (Fig. 15–13). The median glossoepiglottic fold overlies the glossoepiglottic ligament, which courses from the base of the tongue to the epiglottis. The glossoepiglottic fold divides the space between the tongue and the epiglottis into two sacs—the valleculae (Fig. 15–14). The lateral

*Text continued on page 210*

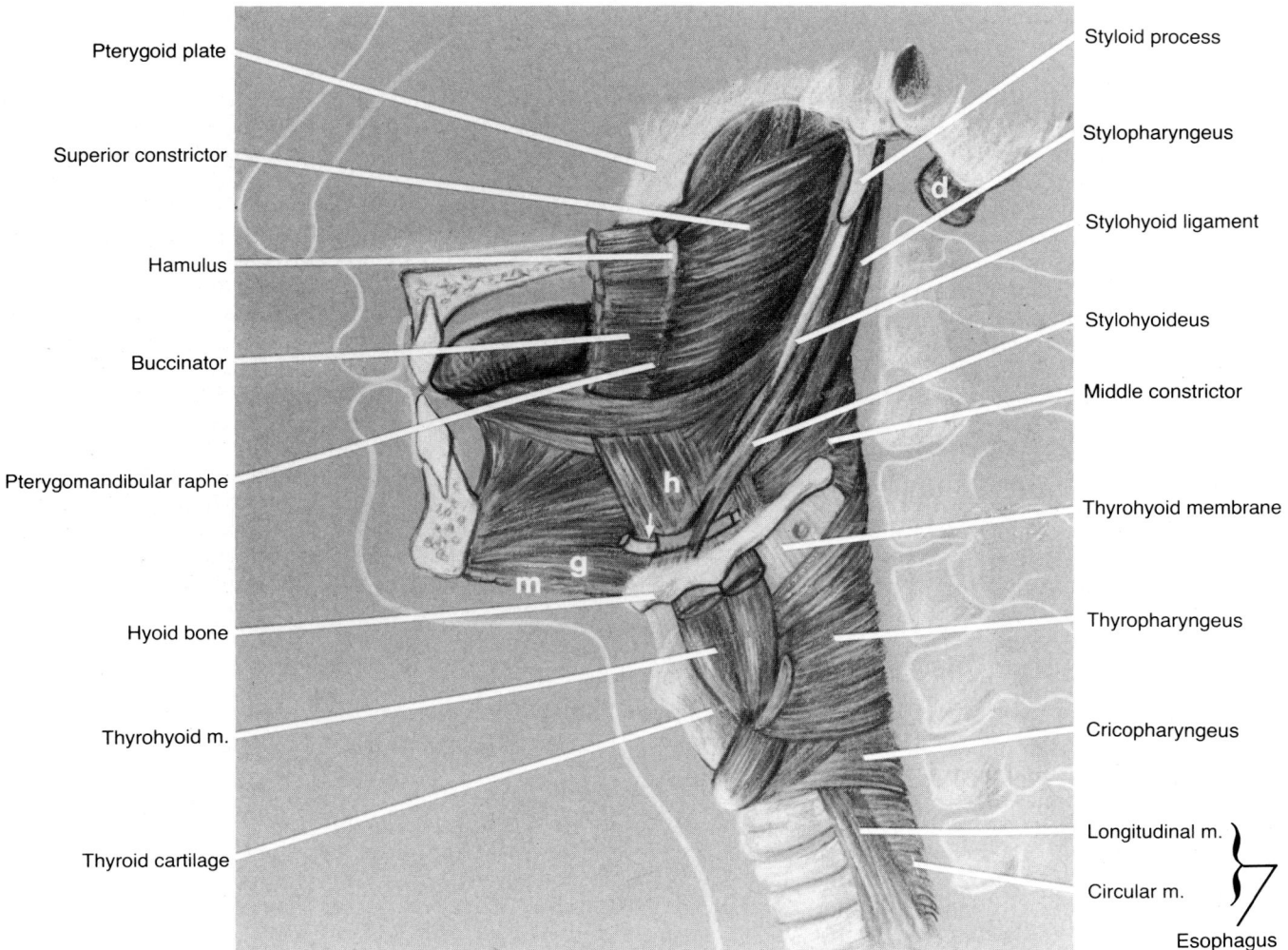

Pterygoid plate

Superior constrictor

Hamulus

Buccinator

Pterygomandibular raphe

Hyoid bone

Thyrohyoid m.

Thyroid cartilage

Styloid process

Stylopharyngeus

Stylohyoid ligament

Stylohyoideus

Middle constrictor

Thyrohyoid membrane

Thyropharyngeus

Cricopharyngeus

Longitudinal m.

Circular m.

Esophagus

**Figure 15–5. Lateral view of the muscles of the pharynx.** The superficial muscles, nerves, arteries, and veins have been removed. The suspensory and constrictor muscles of the normal pharynx are demonstrated. The hyoid bone is suspended anteriorly by the geniohyoid muscle (g), the mylohyoid muscle (m, cut in cross section), the hyoglossus muscle (h), and the anterior belly of the digastric muscle (resected). The tendon connecting the anterior and posterior belly of the digastric muscle is shown *(arrow)*. Posteriorly, the hyoid bone is suspended by the stylohyoid ligament, the stylohyoid muscle and the posterior belly of the digastric muscle (d) (resected). The thyrohyoid muscle and ligament suspend the thyroid cartilage from the hyoid bone. The overlying depressors of the hyoid bone, the omohyoid and sternohyoid muscles, have been resected. The constrictor muscles of the pharynx (superior, middle, and inferior) are incomplete anteriorly. The superior constrictor muscle originates at the pterygoid plate and hamulus, at the pterygomandibular raphe, and in the longitudinal muscles of the tongue; it inserts along the median raphe of the pharynx. The middle constrictor muscle originates on the greater and lesser horns of the hyoid bone and along the lower stylohyoid ligament; it inserts along the median raphe of the pharynx. The thyropharyngeal muscle (upper portion of the superior constrictor muscle) originates from the oblique line of the thyroid cartilage; it inserts into the median raphe of the pharynx. The lower portion of the inferior constrictor muscle, the cricopharyngeal muscle, arises from the lateral surface of the cricoid cartilages, encircles the pharynx, and inserts on the opposite side of the cricoid cartilage. (Photographed directly from Rubesin S, et al: Lines of the pharynx. Poster presented at the 71st Scientific Assembly and Annual Meeting, Radiological Society of North America, Chicago, IL, 1985.)

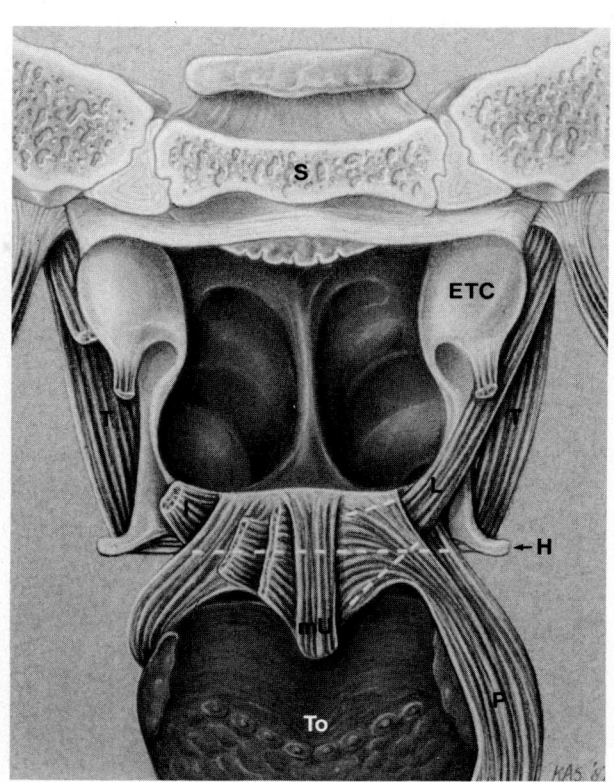

**Figure 15–6. Muscles of the soft palate.** The muscles forming the soft palate are viewed from behind, looking toward the tongue (To), nasal cavity, and sphenoid bone (S). The levator veli palatini (L) joins its partner (l) (partly resected in drawing) from the opposite side to form a sling, which supports the mid–soft palate. The tensor veli palatini (T) forms a tendon that hooks around the pterygoid hamulus (H) to joint its partner from the other side, forming the fibrous skeleton of the anterior soft palate. Also shown are the musculus uvulae (mU), palatopharyngeal muscle (P), and eustachian tube cartilage (ETC). (From Rubesin SE, Rabischong P, Bilaniuk LT, et al: Contrast examination of the soft palate with cross sectional correlation. Radiographics 8:641–665, 1988.)

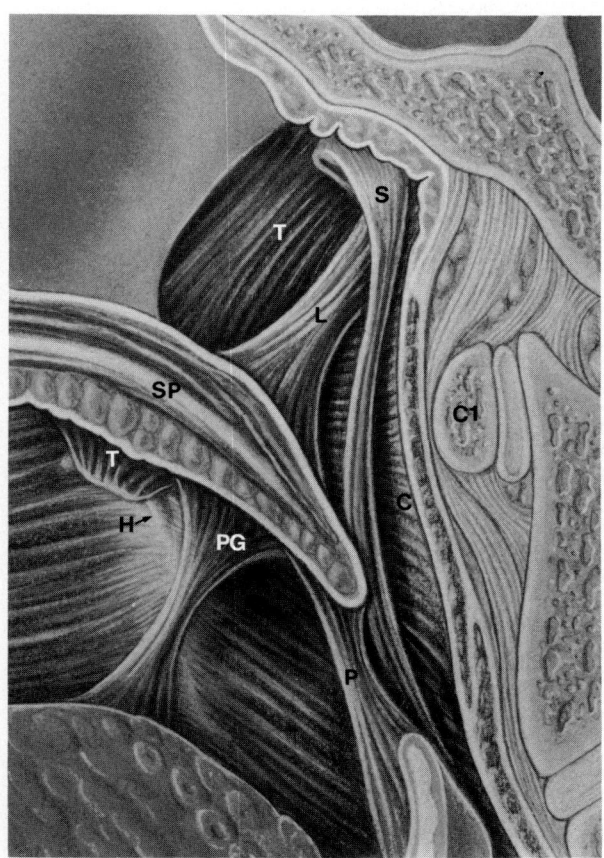

**Figure 15–7. Muscles of the soft palate and tonsilar fossa.** A drawing of the sagittal view of the nasopharynx and oropharynx after removal of the overlying mucosal layer. The levator veli palatini (L) pulls the midportion of the soft palate (SP) superiorly and posteriorly. The relationship between the tensor veli palatini (T) and the pterygoid hamulus (H) is shown. The palatoglossus muscle (PG) pulls the midtongue and mid–soft palate together. The salpingopharyngeal muscle (S) arises from the eustachian tube cartilage and forms the salpingopharyngeal fold. Also shown are the superior constrictor muscle (C) and the palatopharyngeal muscle (P). The anterior arch of C-1 (C1) is shown. (From Rubesin SE, Rabischong P, Bilaniuk LT, et al: Contrast examination of the soft palate with cross-sectional correlation. Radiographics 8:641–665, 1988.)

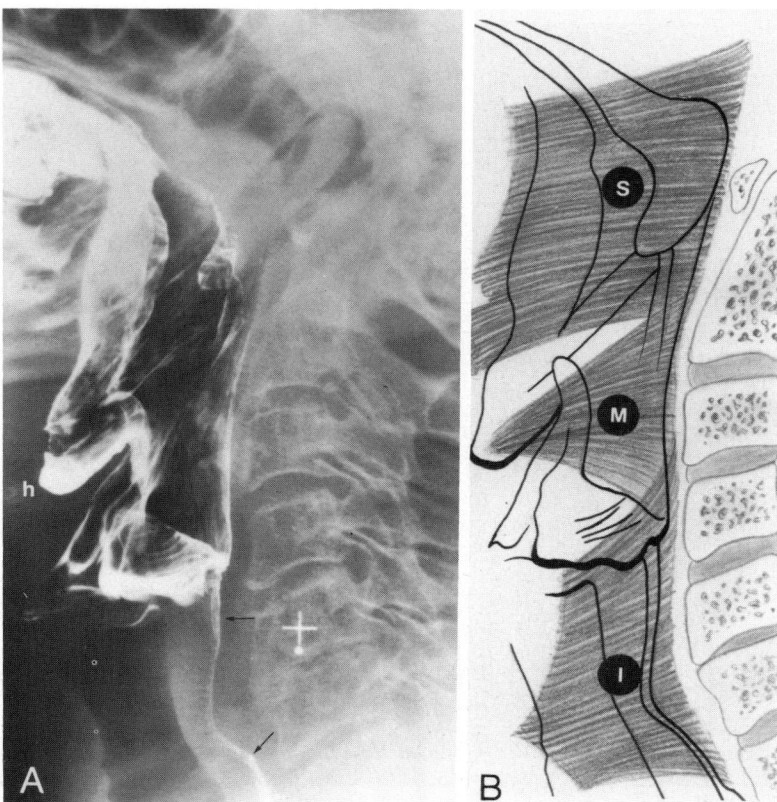

**Figure 15–8. Constrictor muscle layer.** A lateral radiograph taken during phonation **(A)** and its corresponding anatomic drawing **(B)** show the relationship of the superior (S), middle (M), and inferior (I) constrictor muscles to the lateral view of the pharynx. The inferior border of the middle constrictor is at the level of the hyoid bone (h). Note that a long segment of the lower hypopharynx *(arrows)* remains collapsed during phonation (and during suspended respiration). (**A** and **B** from Rubesin SE, Jesserun J, Robertson D, et al: Lines of the pharynx. Radiographics 7:217–237, 1987.)

**Figure 15–9. The palatopharyngeal folds.** A lateral view of the pharynx shows the paired palatopharyngeal folds (posterior tonsillar pillars) *(white arrow)* coursing from the mid–soft palate to the lateral wall of the pharynx. The paired palatoglossal folds *(black arrows)* form the anterior tonsillar pillars. U = uvula. (From Rubesin SE, Jesserun J, Robertson D, et al: Lines of the pharynx. Radiographics 7:217–237, 1987.)

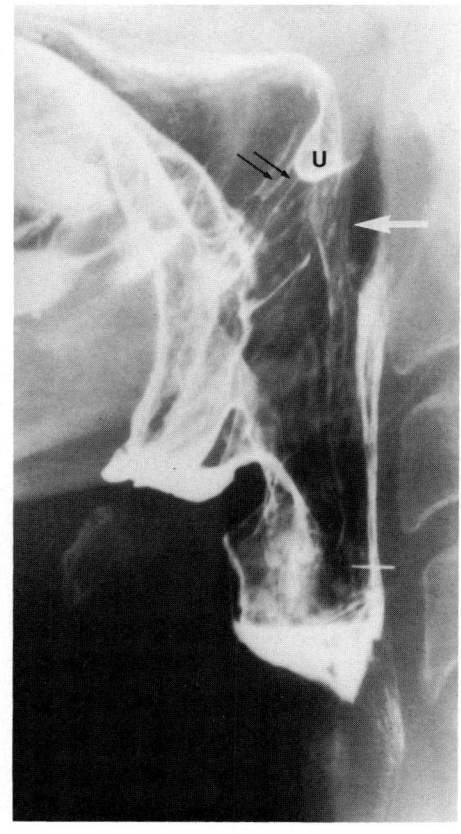

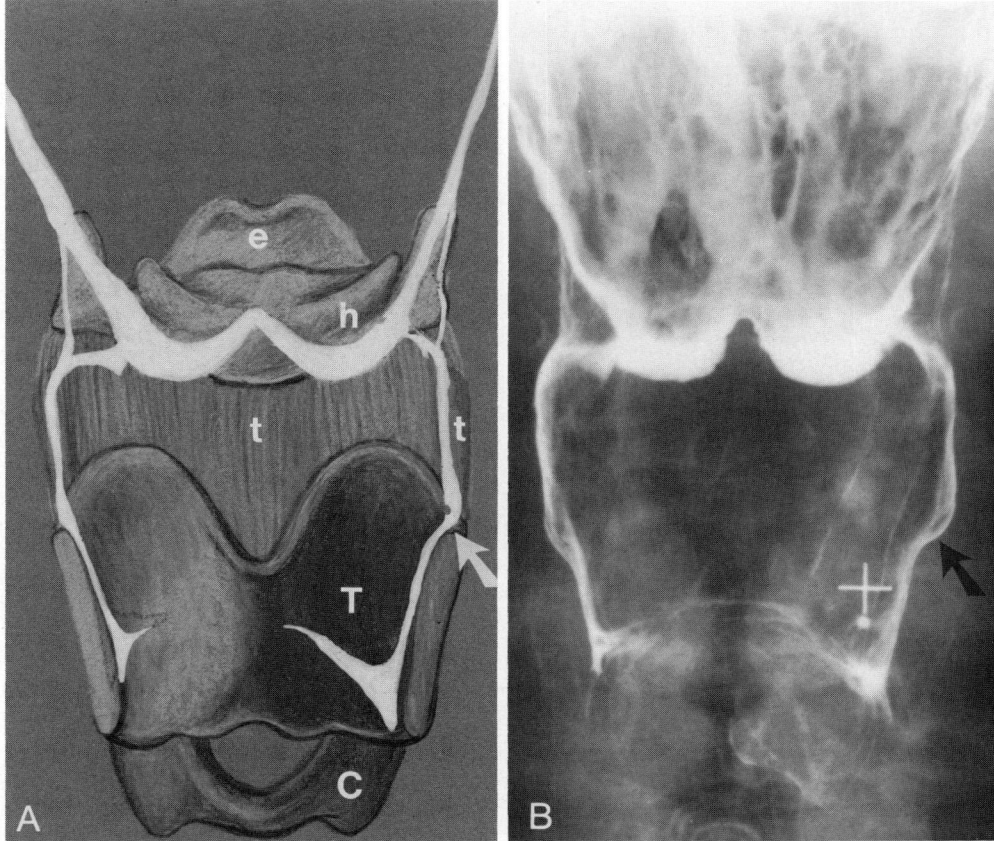

Figure 15–10. Relationship of the laryngeal cartilages to the double contrast view of the pharynx. The laryngeal cartilages, including the epiglottis (e), thyroid cartilage (T), and cricoid cartilage (C), and the hyoid bone (h), are shown in relationship to the barium-coated pharynx in **A** and **B**. The thyrohyoid membrane (t) connects the hyoid bone to the thyroid cartilage. The junction of the ala of the thyroid cartilage and the thyrohyoid membrane *(white arrow)* is seen as a notch in the lateral wall of the hypopharynx on the double contrast view *(black arrow)*. (**A** and **B** from Rubesin SE, Jesserun J, Robertson D, et al: Lines of the pharynx. Radiographics 7:217–237, 1987.)

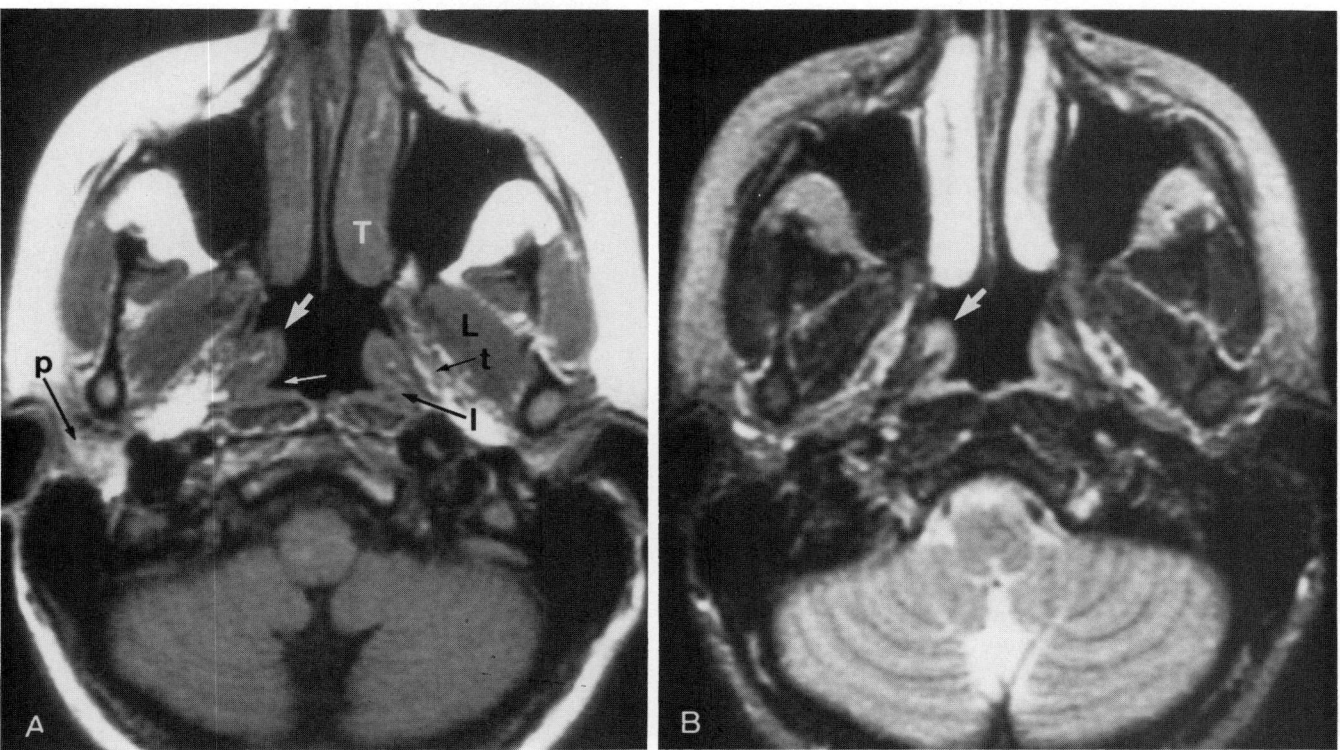

Figure 15–11. The nasopharynx. **A**. Image from an axial T1-weighted scan through the nasopharynx shows the torus tubarius protruding from the lateral nasopharyngeal wall *(thick arrow)*. The fossa of Rosenmüller *(thin arrow)* lies posterior to the torus tubarius. Also shown are the inferior turbinate (T), the tensor veli palatini (t), the levator veli palatini (l), the lateral pterygoid muscles (L), and deep lobe of the parotid gland (p). **B**. Image from an axial T2-weighted scan through the nasopharynx shows that the nasal turbinates are bright. The mucosa of the nasopharynx *(arrow)* is also bright, because of edema.

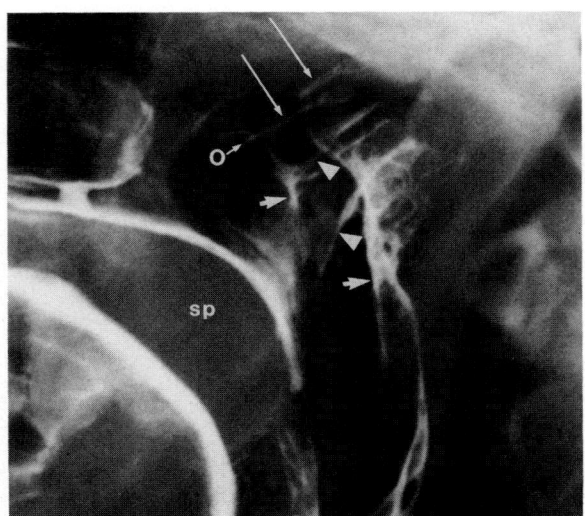

**Figure 15–12. Lines of the nasopharynx.** A lateral view of the nasopharynx after intranasal instillation of 1 mL of barium shows paired, barium-filled eustachian tubes *(long arrows)*. The orifice of one eustachian tube (O) is seen under the C-shaped slit of the torus tubarius. The paired salpingopharyngeal folds *(short arrows)* are seen. The levator veli palatini forms slight bulges in the lateral nasopharyngeal wall—the levator ridge. The inferior border of these bulges is marked with arrowheads. sp = soft palate. (From Rubesin SE, Rabischong P, Bilaniuk LT, et al: Contrast examination of the soft palate with cross sectional correlation. Radiographics 8:641–665, 1988.)

glossoepiglottic folds form the lateral wall of the valleculae. The pharyngoepiglottic folds course from the posterolateral valleculae into the lateral pharyngeal wall[1] (Fig. 15–15). These folds overlie the stylopharyngeal muscle.

The tonsillar fossa forms part of the lateral oropharyngeal wall. The tonsillar fossa is bounded anteriorly by the palatoglossal fold (anterior tonsillar or faucial pillar) (Figs. 15–16 and 15–17). Posteriorly, the tonsillar fossa is bounded by the palatopharyngeal fold overlying the palatopharyngeal muscle (see Figs. 15–16 and 15–17).

The rounded epiglottic tip rises above the level of the valleculae.[20] The aryepiglottic folds connect the epiglottis with the muscular processes of the arytenoid cartilages. Occasionally, round bulges are seen in the lower aryepiglottic folds, reflecting the small cuneiform and corniculate cartilages embedded in the lower aryepiglottic folds.

The shape of the hypopharynx is created mainly by its relationship to the posteriorly protruding larynx (Fig. 15–18). The protrusion of the larynx into the pharynx creates two grooves in the anterolateral hypopharynx—the piriform sinuses (recesses)—pear-shaped structures that open posteriorly into the hypopharynx (see Figs. 15–4 and 15–18). Each piriform sinus is bounded medially by the aryepiglottic fold and mucosa overlying the muscular process of the arytenoid cartilage, and laterally by the hyoid bone, thyrohyoid membrane, and thyroid cartilage[1, 3] (see Figs. 15–10 and 15–18).

The lower end of the hypopharynx is collapsed except during the passage of a bolus. The posterior portion of

the larynx (including the arytenoid cartilages, arytenoid muscles, and cricoid cartilages) protrudes deeply into the lower hypopharynx. The upper esophageal sphincter (formed predominantly by the cricopharyngeal muscle) is tonically contracted at rest, closing the pharyngoesophageal segment (see Fig. 15–10). Thus, the lower hypopharynx is markedly constricted in an anteroposterior direction and is often not appreciated on a frontal radiograph. The arcuate "lower border" of the hypopharynx seen on the frontal view reflects only the protrusion of the larynx into the hypopharynx[3] (see Fig. 15–18).

The squamous mucosa of the lateral and posterior pharyngeal walls is closely apposed to the longitudinally striated inner longitudinal muscle layer and its aponeurosis. Only a thin tunica propria separates the epithelium from the muscle or the elastic tissue of the aponeurosis. Thus, on double contrast views, longitudinally oriented lines are frequently seen in the lateral and posterior pharyngeal walls, reflecting apposition of epithelium to muscle[3] (Fig. 15–19A).

Transversely oriented lines are seen in the anterior hypopharyngeal wall, where redundant squamous mu-

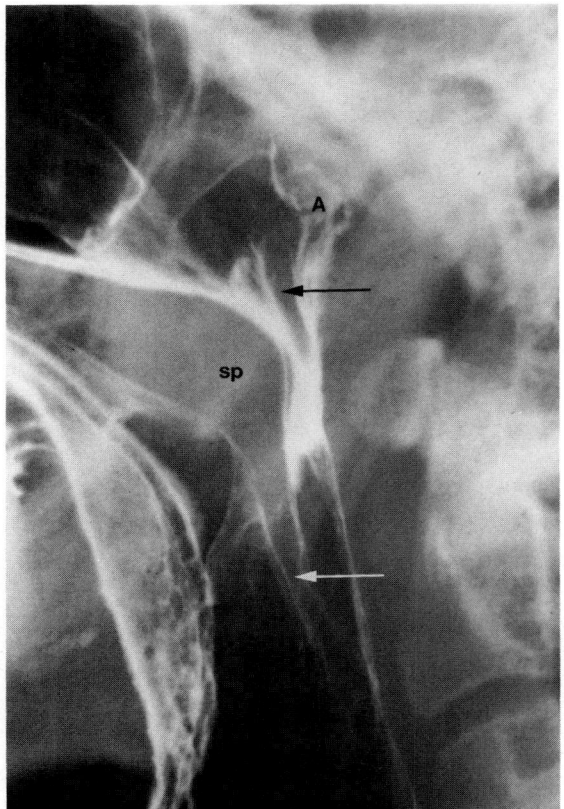

**Figure 15–13. The salpingopharyngeal fold and adenoids.** Lateral view of nasopharynx during phonation after intranasal instillation of 1 mL of barium shows the salpingopharyngeal folds *(black arrow)*. The posterior wall of the nasopharynx is slightly irregular because of the underlying adenoidal lymphoid tissue (A). The soft palate (sp) and palatopharyngeal fold *(white arrow)* are also demonstrated. (From Rubesin SE, Rabischong P, Bilaniuk LT, et al: Contrast examination of the soft palate with cross sectional correlation. Radiographics 8:641–665, 1988.)

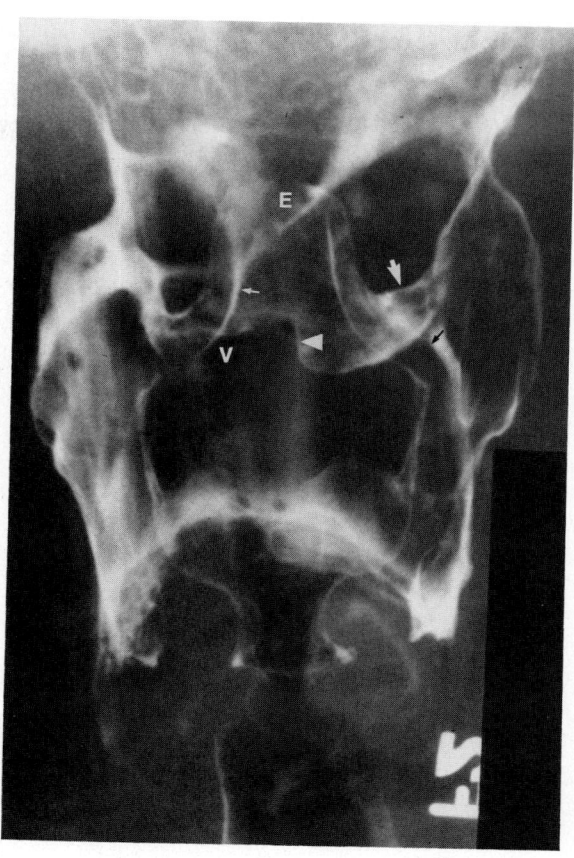

**Figure 15–14. Frontal (supine) view of pharynx demonstrates the folds of the valleculae.** The median glossoepiglottic fold *(arrowhead)* divides the retroglottic space into the two valleculae (V). The pharyngoepiglottic fold *(large white arrow)* overlies the stylopharyngeal muscle. Also shown are the epiglottic tip (E) and aryepiglottic fold *(black arrow)*. Barium coating the laryngeal surface of the epiglottis *(small white arrow)* is due to laryngeal penetration.

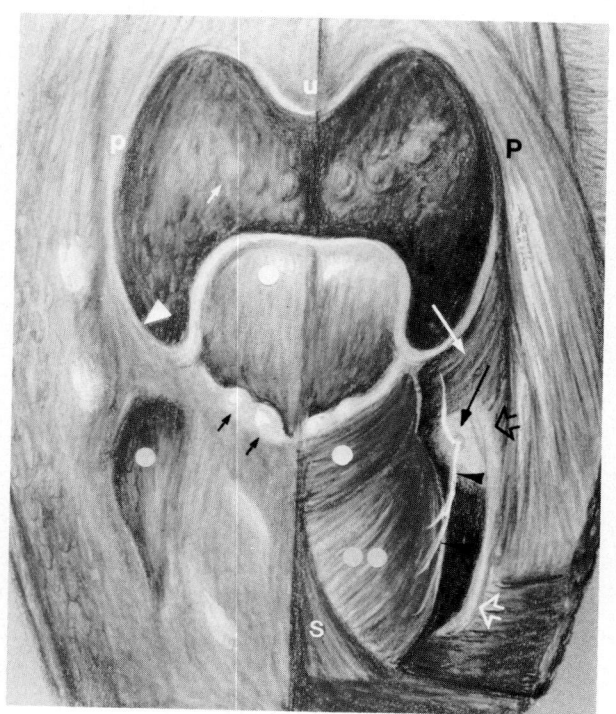

**Figure 15–15. Posterior view of pharynx opened from behind.** On the viewer's left, the mucosa has been left intact. The uvula (u), palatopharyngeal fold (p), piriform sinus *(left dot)*, and laryngeal surface of the epiglottis *(uppermost dot)* are seen en face. The pharyngoepiglottic fold *(white arrowhead)* separates the oropharynx from the hypopharynx. Bulges in the aryepiglottic fold overlie the cuneiform and corniculate cartilages *(short black arrows)*. The circumvallate papillae *(short white arrow)* form a V-shaped protruberance along the base of the tongue. On the right side, the mucosa has been removed. The palatopharyngeal muscle (P) forms the palatopharyngeal fold. This muscle has been retracted laterally. The stylopharyngeal muscle *(long white arrow)* underlies the pharyngoepiglottic fold. The thyroid cartilage forms the lateral boundary of the pharynx. Its superior horn *(open black arrow)* and posterior border of the right lamina *(open white arrow)* form the lateral boundary of the piriform sinus. The thyrohyoid membrane *(long black arrow)* and the internal branch of the superior laryngeal nerve *(black arrowhead)* are identified. The transverse arytenoid muscle *(single dot on right)*, posterior cricoarytenoid muscle *(two adjacent dots)*, and suspensory ligament of the esophagus (s) are identified. (Photographed directly from Rubesin S, et al: Lines of the pharynx. Poster presented at the 71st Scientific Assembly and Annual Meeting, Radiological Society of North America, Chicago, IL, 1985.)

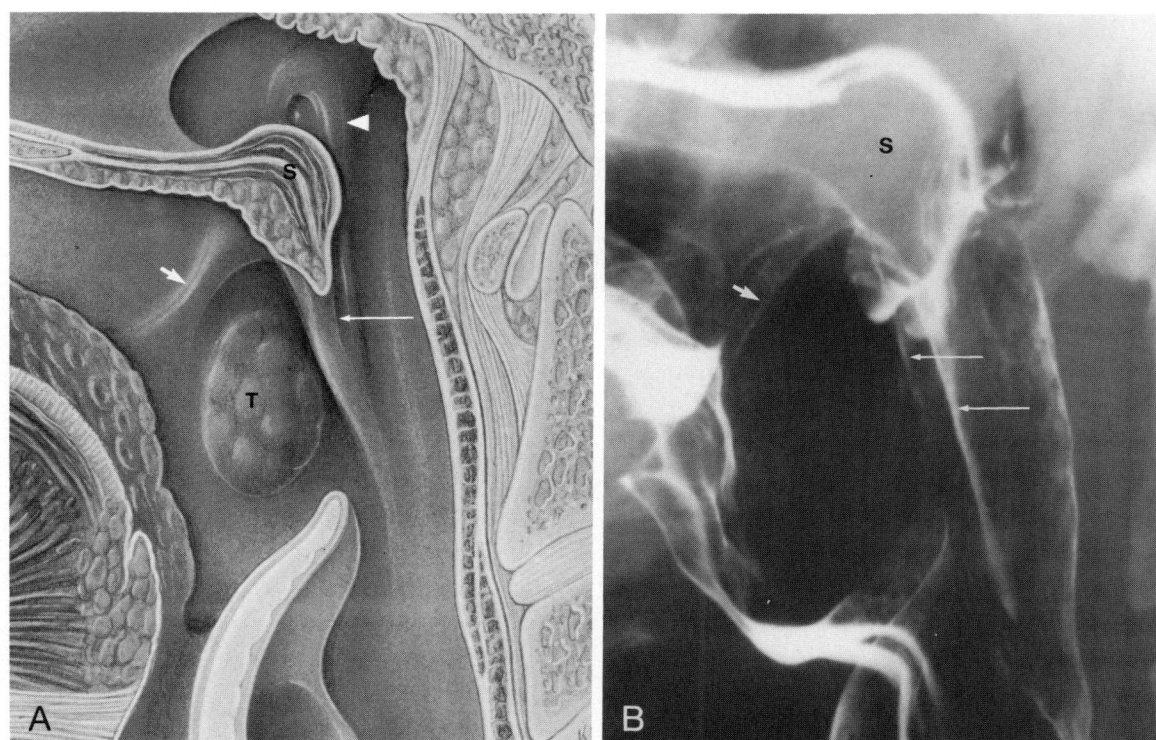

**Figure 15–16. The tonsillar fossa.** A lateral drawing **(A)** and its corresponding radiograph **(B)** demonstrate the tonsillar fossa during soft palate elevation by phonation. The palatine tonsil (T) is surrounded by the palatoglossal fold *(short arrow)* and palatopharyngeal fold *(long arrows)*. Also shown is the salpingopharyngeal fold *(arrowhead)*. S = soft palate. (**A** and **B** from Rubesin SE, Rabischong P, Bilaniuk LT, et al: Contrast examination of the soft palate with cross sectional correlation. Radiographics 8:641–665, 1988.)

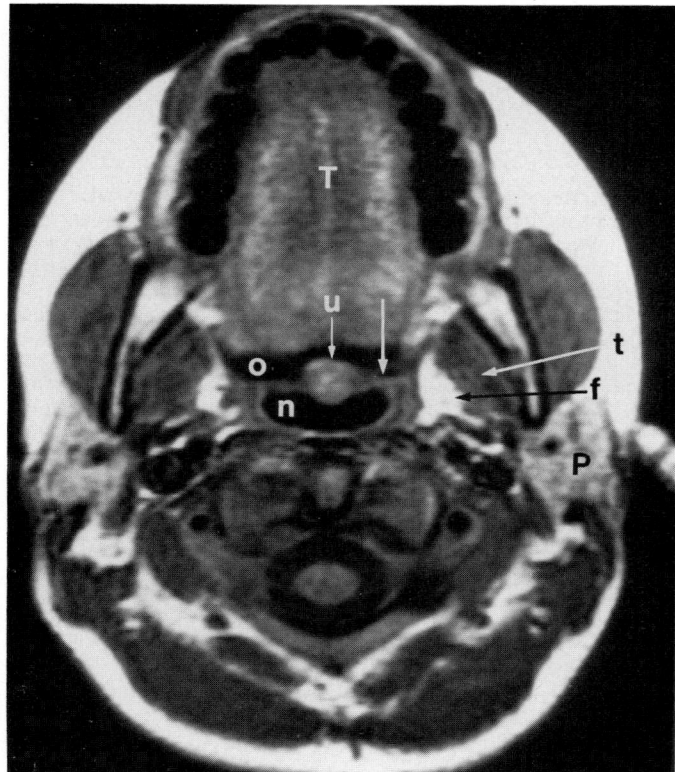

**Figure 15–17. Palatopharyngeal fold.** T1-weighted MR image of the pharynx shows the uvula *(white arrow,* u) and palatopharyngeal folds *(white arrow, alone)* separating the oropharynx (o) from the nasopharynx (n). Parapharyngeal fat *(black arrow,* f) separates the pharynx from the masticator space, pterygoid muscle *(white arrow,* t), and parotid gland (P) posterolaterally. The region of the retromolar trigone is anterolateral to the parapharyngeal fat. T = tongue.

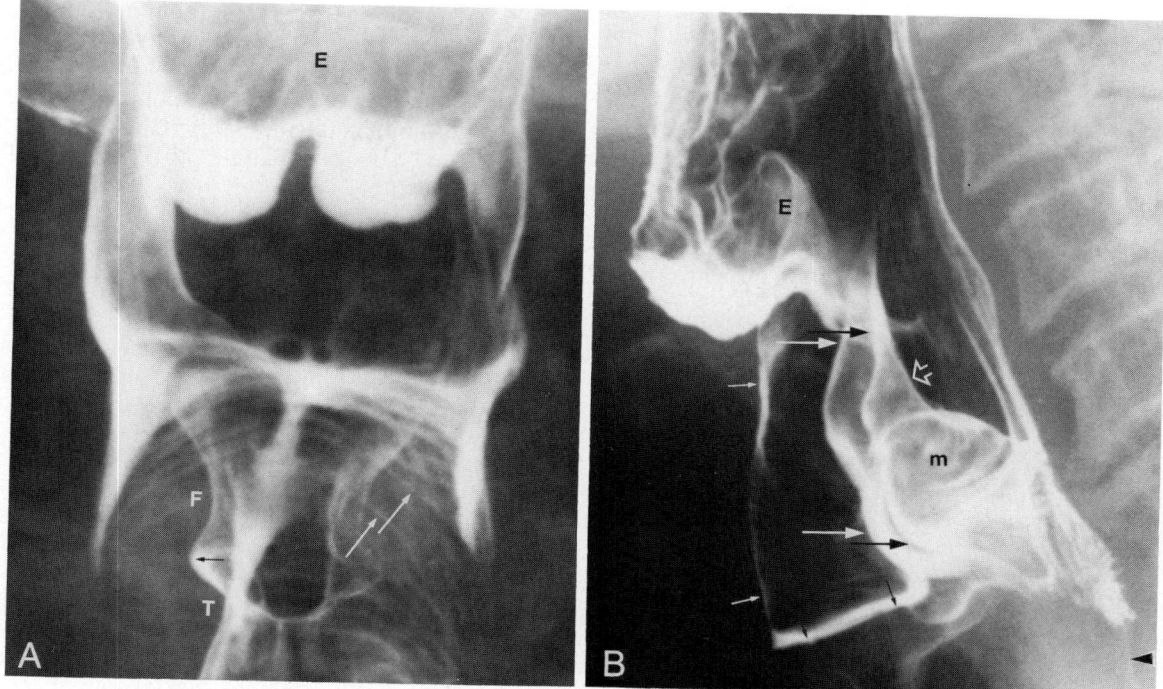

**Figure 15–18. Relationship of larynx to pharynx. A**. In a patient with larnygeal penetration, barium coats the false vocal cords (F), the true vocal cords (T), and the laryngeal ventricle *(black arrow)*. As the larynx protrudes into the mid-hypopharynx, arcuate lines *(white arrows)* are formed. E = epiglottis. **B**. The relationship of the barium-coated laryngeal vestibule *(small white arrows)* to the laryngeal ventricle *(small black arrows)* is shown. The anterior walls of the right piriform sinus *(large white arrows)* and of the left piriform sinus *(large black arrows)* are seen as anteriorly convex lines. The mucosa (M) overlying the muscular process of the arytenoid cartilages lies below the aryepiglottic fold *(open arrow)*. The lower hypopharynx *(arrowhead)* is closed at rest. E = epiglottis. (**B** reprinted with permission from Rubesin SE, Glick SN: The tailored double-contrast pharyngogram. Crit Rev Diagn Imaging 28:133–179, 1988. Copyright CRC Press, Inc. Boca Raton, FL.)

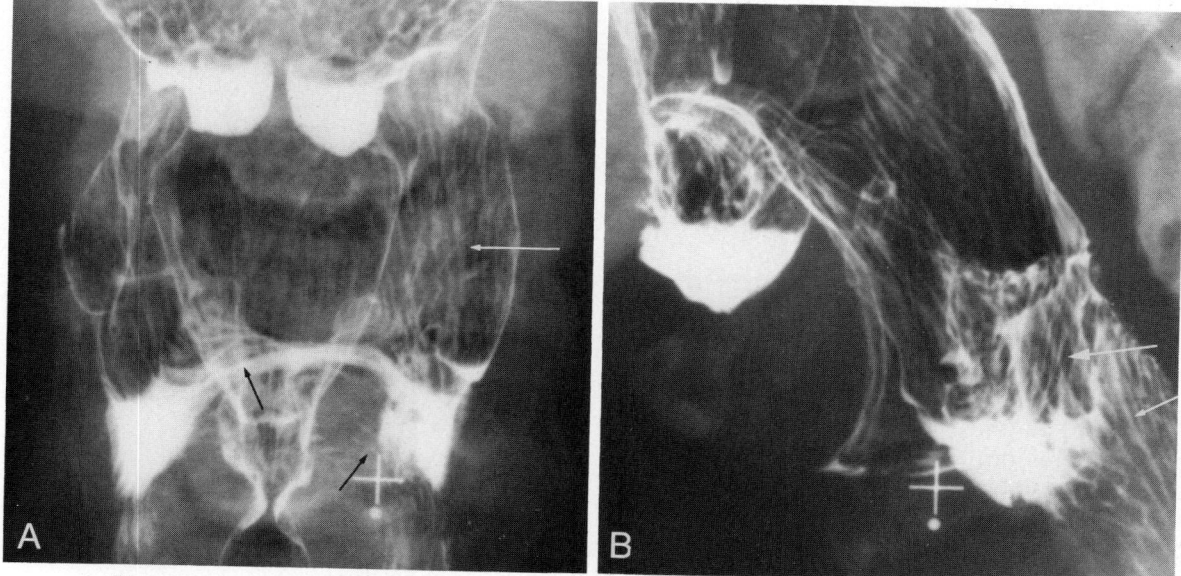

**Figure 15–19. Lines of the pharynx. A**. Longitudinally striated mucosa *(white arrow)* reflects close apposition of the squamous mucosa to the underlying longitudinal muscle layer of the pharynx. Arcuate lines of the anterior hypopharyngeal wall are identified *(black arrows)*. **B**. Arcuate lines and transversely oriented lines overlying the muscular processes of the arytenoid cartilage *(large arrow)* and the lower hypopharynx *(small arrow)* reflect redundant mucosa in this region. (**B** reprinted with permission from Rubesin SE, Glick SN: The tailored double-contrast pharyngogram. Crit Rev Diagn Imaging 28:133–179, 1988. Copyright CRC Press, Inc. Boca Raton, FL.)

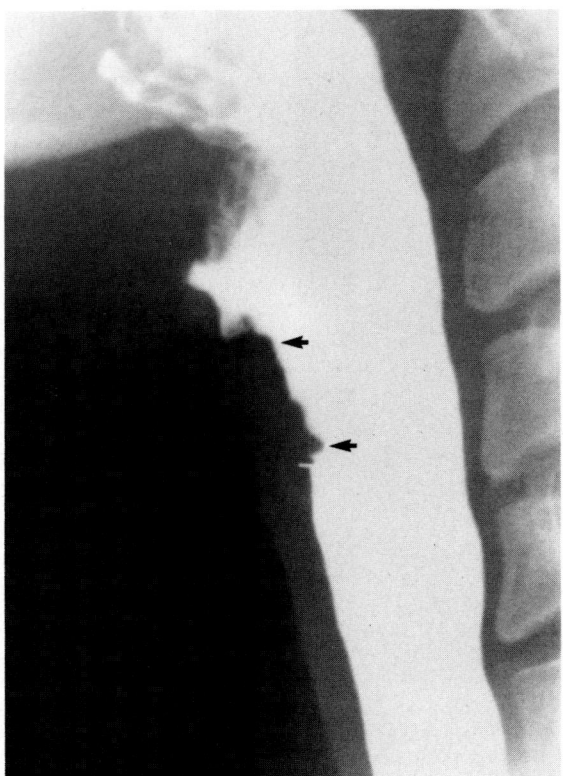

**Figure 15–20. Postcricoid defect.** During swallowing, redundant mucosa along the anterior wall of the distal hypopharynx may create an undulating or plaque-like contour *(arrows)*. To rule out a subtle stricture, web, or infiltrating lesion, the radiologist must be sure that this region changes size and shape.

cosa and submucosa overlie the muscular processes of the arytenoid cartilages and cricoid cartilage (Fig. 15–19B). Transverse lines and tissue bulging from the anterior hypopharyngeal wall have been previously described as a "venous plexus."[21] The radiographic findings described as the *postcricoid venous plexus*, however, are mainly due to redundant mucosa and submucosa in the anterior hypopharyngeal wall[3, 22] (Fig. 15–20).

## PRINCIPLES OF TECHNIQUE

### Preparation of Patients

High-density barium adheres to dry pharyngeal mucosa. Therefore, in the preparation of patients, the pharynx is made as dry as possible despite continuing salivary secretion. Patients are instructed not to eat or drink after midnight on the day of the examination. In the morning, regular oral medications may be taken with small amounts of water. Insulin-dependent diabetics should not take insulin on the morning of examination. Oral antacid medications impair barium coating and should be avoided. If possible, the patient should refrain from activities that stimulate salivary secretion, such as sucking throat lozenges, smoking, or chewing gum.

Contrast examination of the pharynx may be dangerous in patients with suspected airway obstruction, especially in those with acute epiglottitis.[23] Therefore, the initial examination should consist of plain film radiography of the neck if airway obstruction is suspected (Fig. 15–21). Plain film images are also obtained for suspected foreign body, fistula, abscess, perforation (Fig. 15–22), or palpable neck mass.

## Components of Routine Examination

Routine examination of the pharynx and esophagus includes 1) videofluoroscopy or cineradiography of the oral, pharyngeal, and esophageal phases of swallowing; 2) double contrast spot film examination of the pharynx, esophagus, and gastric cardia; and 3) single contrast and mucosal relief views of the esophagus[24–29] (Table 15–1). The examination is tailored to the patient's clinical history, symptoms, and initial fluoroscopic findings. The pharyngoesophagram is an interactive study: if a motility disorder is the major radiologic finding, dynamic techniques (videofluoroscopy or cineradiography) are emphasized.[29] If a structural abnormality is the major radiographic finding, a spot film examination predominates. Both static and dynamic images are obtained,

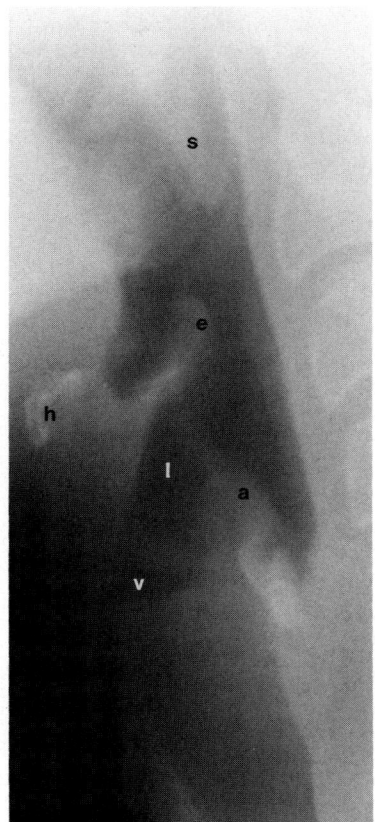

**Figure 15–21. Lateral plain film image of normal pharynx.** The soft palate (s), the epiglottis (e), the hyoid bone (h), the laryngeal vestibule (l), the laryngeal ventricle (v), and the mucosa overlying the muscular process of the arytenoid cartilage (a) are shown.

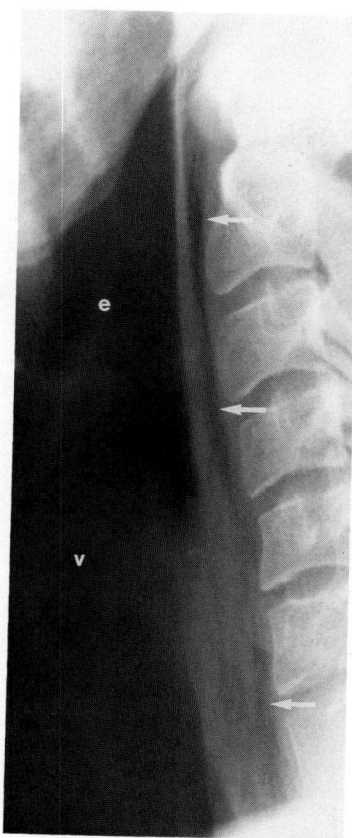

**Figure 15–22. Neck pain after ingestion of taco chips.** A lateral plain film image of the neck shows a large amount of retropharyngeal air *(arrows)*. e = epiglottis; v = laryngeal ventricle.

| TABLE 15–1. ROUTINE PHARYNGOESOPHAGRAM FOR RESPIRATORY OR PHARYNGEAL SYMPTOMS* | | |
|---|---|---|
| **VIEW** | **TECHNIQUE** | **ORGAN** |
| Erect, left lateral | Videofluoroscopy Double contrast (R,P) (two 2:1 films) | Mouth and pharynx |
| Erect, frontal | Videofluoroscopy Double contrast (R,V) (two 2:1 films) | Pharynx |
| Oblique | Double contrast (V) (one 2:1 film) | Pharynx |
| ***Effervescent Agent and Water*** | | |
| Erect, LPO | Double contrast (two 2:1 films) | Esophagus |
| Prone, RAO | Single contrast (one 2:1 film) | Esophagus |
| Right lateral | Double contrast | Gastric cardia |

*LPO = left posterior oblique with respect to table top; P = phonation; R = suspended respiration; RAO = right anterior oblique with respect to table top; V = modified Valsalva maneuver.

however, because 1) structural disorders often alter pharyngeal motility (Fig. 15–23); 2) structural features of motility disorders are often well demonstrated on static images (Fig. 15–24); and 3) structural lesions and motility disorders may coexist.

The oral and pharyngeal phases of swallowing should be evaluated first if symptoms suggest an oral or pharyngeal disorder (see Table 15–1). If clinical history and symptoms suggest thoracic esophageal disease, a double contrast examination of the esophagus should be performed first, followed by examination of the oral and pharyngeal phases of swallowing (Table 15–2). The radiologist must remember that symptoms poorly reflect the site of a lesion, especially esophageal symptoms referred to the neck or suprasternal region.[30] Furthermore, patients may have an esophageal disorder that secondarily affects pharyngeal function (Fig. 15–25), or a disease that involves both pharynx and esophagus intrinsically. Some patients have more than one abnormality in the pharynx or esophagus, or in both.

## Double Contrast Interpretation

The principles of double contrast interpretation in studying the pharynx are the same as in studying structures elsewhere in the gastrointestinal tract. The double contrast examination requires good mucosal coating, an adequate number of projections, and varying degrees of luminal distention.

## Mucosal Coating

Adequate mucosal coating depends primarily on two factors: dry pharyngeal mucosa and properly prepared high-density barium (250% w/v). If the barium is too thin, the barium is of insufficient radiodensity to outline the pharyngeal mucosa. If the barium is too thick, mucosal coating may be patchy or may obscure mucosal detail. Barium that is too viscous may be unable to wash and scrub the mucosa, resulting in artifactual strands of mucus. Several swallows of high-density barium may be needed in each projection to achieve uniform coating.

| TABLE 15–2. ROUTINE PHARYNGOESOPHAGRAM FOR ESOPHAGEAL SYMPTOMS* | | |
|---|---|---|
| **VIEW** | **TECHNIQUE** | **ORGAN** |
| ***Effervescent Agent and Water*** | | |
| Erect, LPO | Double contrast (two 2:1 films) | Esophagus |
| Right lateral | Double contrast | Gastric cardia |
| Prone, RAO | Videofluoroscopy (2–5 swallows) | Esophagus |
| | Single contrast (one or two 2:1 films) | Esophagus |
| | Mucosal relief (one film) | Esophagus |
| Erect, lateral | Videofluoroscopy Double contrast (R,P) (one film) | Pharynx |
| Erect, frontal | Videofluoroscopy Double contrast (R,P) (one film) | Pharynx |

*LPO = left posterior oblique with respect to table top; P = phonation; R = suspended respiration; RAO = right anterior oblique with respect to table top.

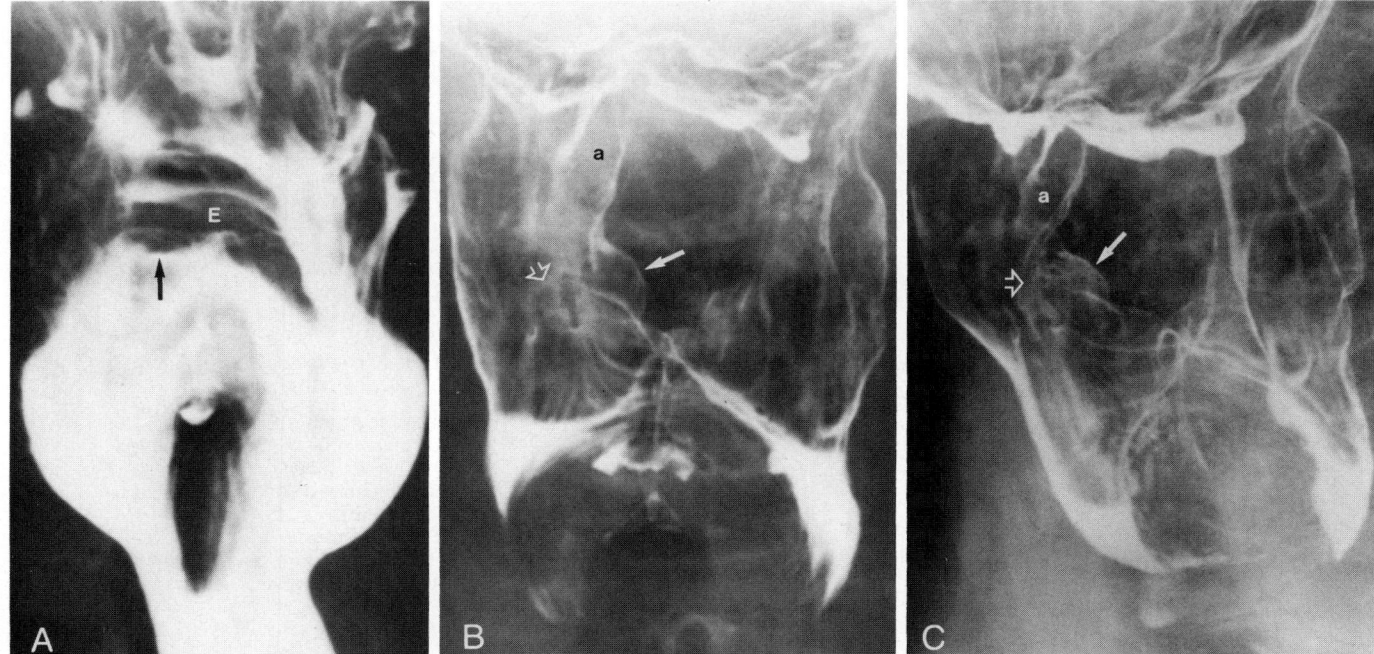

**Figure 15–23. Abnormal epiglottic tilt attributable to squamous cell carcinoma involving right aryepiglottic fold and mucosa overlying the arytenoid cartilage.** During swallowing, tilt of epiglottis (E) is diminished on the right, as indicated by the arrow **(A)**. Frontal **(B)** and slight right oblique **(C)** spot films show a small mass *(arrow)* and thickening of the aryepiglottic fold (a) and nodular mucosa *(open arrow)*. A small squamous cell carcinoma was found to involve the aryepiglottic fold and mucosa overlying the right arytenoid process. (**A** to **C** from Rubesin SE: Pharyngeal dysfunction. *In* Gore R [ed]: Syllabus for Categorical Course on Gastrointestinal Radiology. Reston, VA: American College of Radiology, 1991, pp 1–9.)

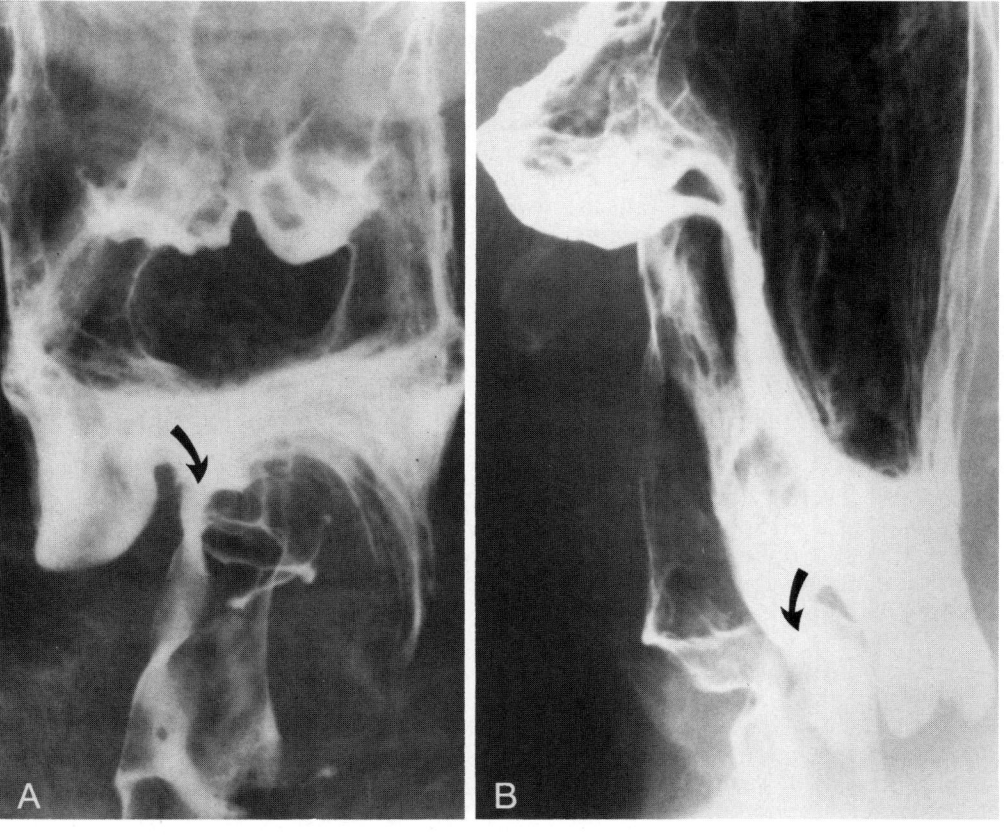

**Figure 15–24. Overflow aspiration in patient 1 month after high-speed vehicular head trauma.** Frontal **(A)** and lateral **(B)** films show moderate stasis of barium that is greater in the right piriform sinus than in the left piriform sinus and overflow of barium *(arrows)* through the vocal cords into the trachea. Note ballooning of the right piriform sinus and vocal cord asymmetry.

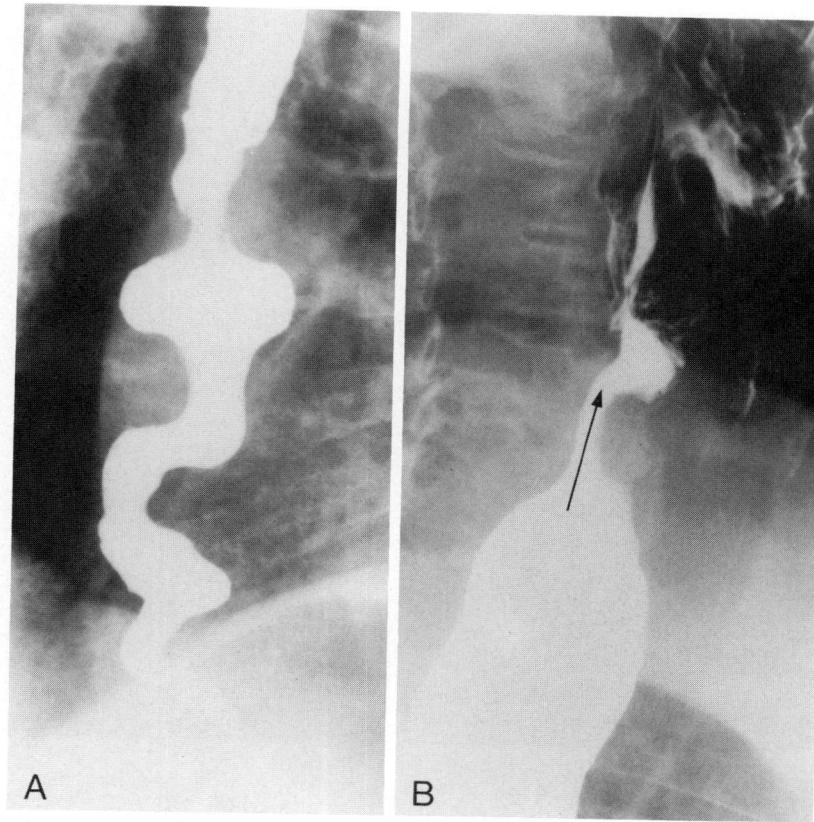

**Figure 15–25. Example of interrelationship of pharynx and esophagus. A.** Upright spot film image of esophagus shows diffuse esophageal spasm. **B.** Upright spot film image of neck shows barium refluxing into the pharynx *(arrow)*. During this episode of esophagopharyngeal reflux, the patient complained of neck discomfort.

## Projection

Films taken in the frontal and lateral projection suffice for most examinations. The frontal view shows the surface of the base of the tongue en face and the contours of the median and lateral glossoepiglottic folds, the tonsillar fossa, the valleculae, and the hypopharynx in profile (see Figs. 15–1, 15–14, and 15–18). The lateral view best demonstrates the tonsillar fossa en face and the contours of the soft palate, base of the tongue, posterior pharyngeal wall, epiglottis, aryepiglottic folds, anterior hypopharyngeal wall, and region of the cricopharyngeal muscle in profile (Fig. 15–26; see Figs. 15–1, 15–16, and 15–18). The lateral view is crucial for

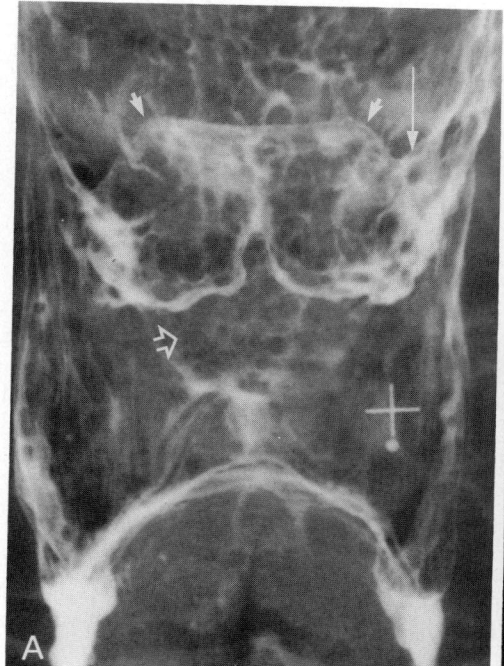
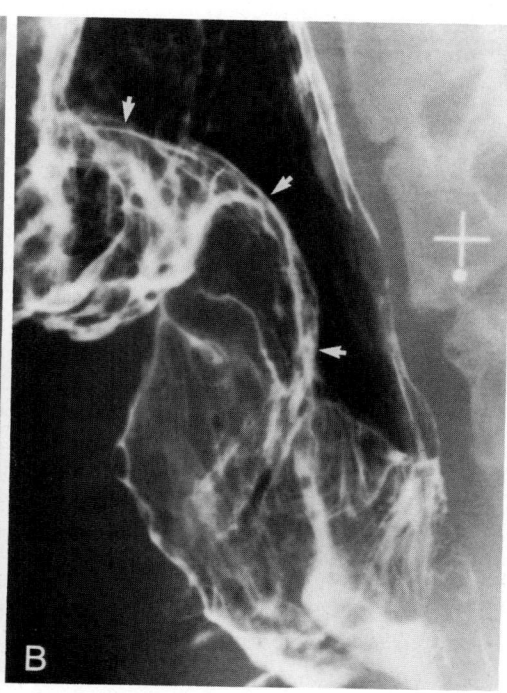

**Figure 15–26. Effect of projection. A.** Frontal view of pharynx shows subtle enlargement of the epiglottic tip *(small arrows)*, elevation of the left pharyngoepiglottic fold *(arrow)* and nodular mucosa overlying the region of the base of the tongue, extending below the valleculae into the region of the laryngeal vestibule *(open arrow)* and laryngeal surface of the epiglottis. **B.** Lateral view during phonation shows a markedly enlarged epiglottis and the aryepiglottic folds *(arrows)*. A supraglottic squamous cell carcinoma was confirmed at endoscopy and surgery. (**B** from SE Rubesin, B Jones, MW Donner, Contrast pharyngography: the importance of phonation, AJR, 148, 2, 269–272, 1987, © by American Roentgen Ray Society.)

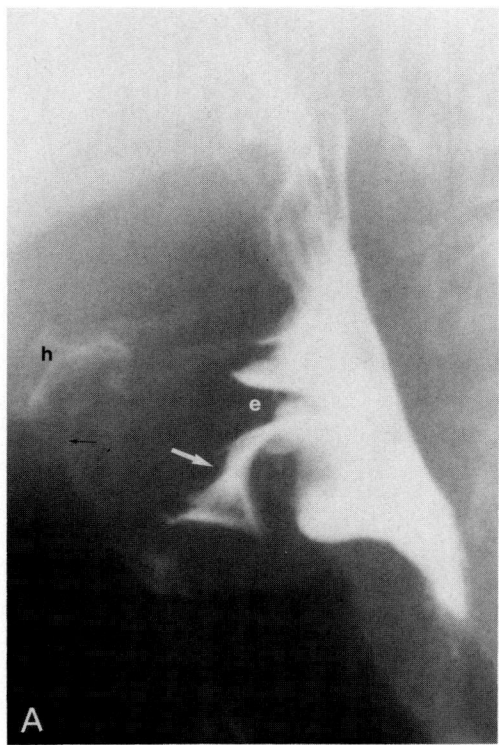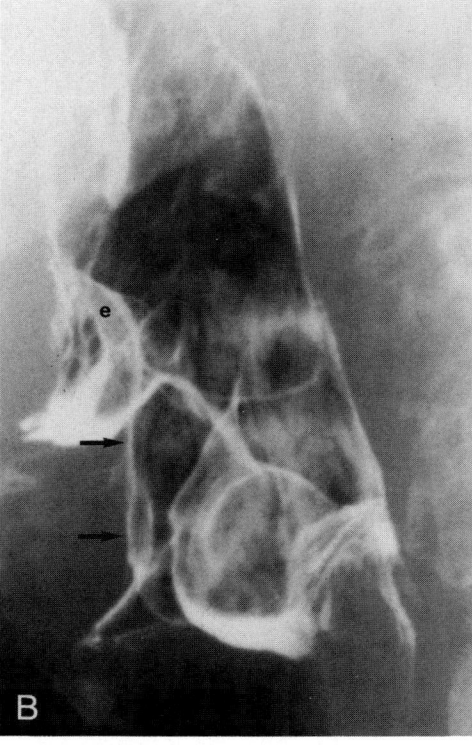

**Figure 15–27. Laryngeal penetration. A.** In an image obtained during swallowing, barium can be seen entering the laryngeal vestibule *(white arrow)*. Note apposition of the hyoid bone (h) to the calcified edge of the thyroid cartilage *(black arrow)*. e = epiglottis. **B.** Spot-film radiography performed during phonation documents coating of the laryngeal vestibule with barium *(arrows)*. e = epiglottis.

evaluating penetration of barium into the laryngeal vestibule (Fig. 15–27). Oblique films are valuable in some patients for demonstrating the obliquely oriented aryepiglottic folds, the anterior walls of the piriform sinuses, and the region of the pharyngoesophageal segment.[23, 31]

## Distention

Adequate distention is important for the demonstration of mucosal surface and contour. The pharynx cannot be distended by the use of effervescent agents or tube insufflation, as in other regions of the gastrointestinal tract. Instead, pharyngeal distention is achieved with either phonation (the long vowel sounds "eee . . ." or "ooo . . .") or some form of modified Valsalva maneuver (blowing against pursed or closed lips or whistling).[32, 33]

Phonation with "eee . . . " expands the pharynx, resulting in better visualization of the soft palate, tonsillar fossa, base of the tongue, valleculae, epiglottic tip, aryepiglottic folds, and mucosa overlying the muscular processes of the arytenoid cartilages in the lateral view (see Fig. 15–1). The distal 2 cm of hypopharynx, however, remains collapsed during phonation, because the pharyngoesophageal sphincter remains contracted and the larynx impresses on this region. The distal 2 cm of hypopharynx, the pharyngoesophageal segment, and the proximal cervical esophagus are most distended during

swallowing and best visualized during dynamic examination.

Pharyngeal distention in the frontal view is best performed with a modified Valsalva procedure (Fig. 15–28). Alternatively, the patient is asked to whistle or blow air out of the mouth as if blowing out a candle. To optimize visualization of pharyngeal structures, the patient is positioned so that the mandible and hard palate are superimposed over the occiput. Flexion or extension of the neck, or protrusion or retraction of the tongue, may improve visualization of various anatomic structures, such as the uvula, epiglottic tip, and lateral walls of the hypopharynx.

## Motility Examination

Cineradiography and videofluoroscopy are the best methods for studying pharyngeal motility.[22, 24, 25] Spot films or rapid-sequence 105-mm spot films are insufficient to detect all functional abnormalities. Rapid-sequence 105-mm spot films are easier than dynamic images to retrieve, however, and are easier to use when demonstrating abnormalities to clinicians. The dynamic portion of the pharyngoesophagram focuses on bolus holding; tongue motion; hyoid, laryngeal, and pharyngeal elevation; soft palate elevation; formation of Passavant's cushion; pharyngeal constrictor motion; epiglottic tilt; laryngeal penetration (see Fig. 15–27); and

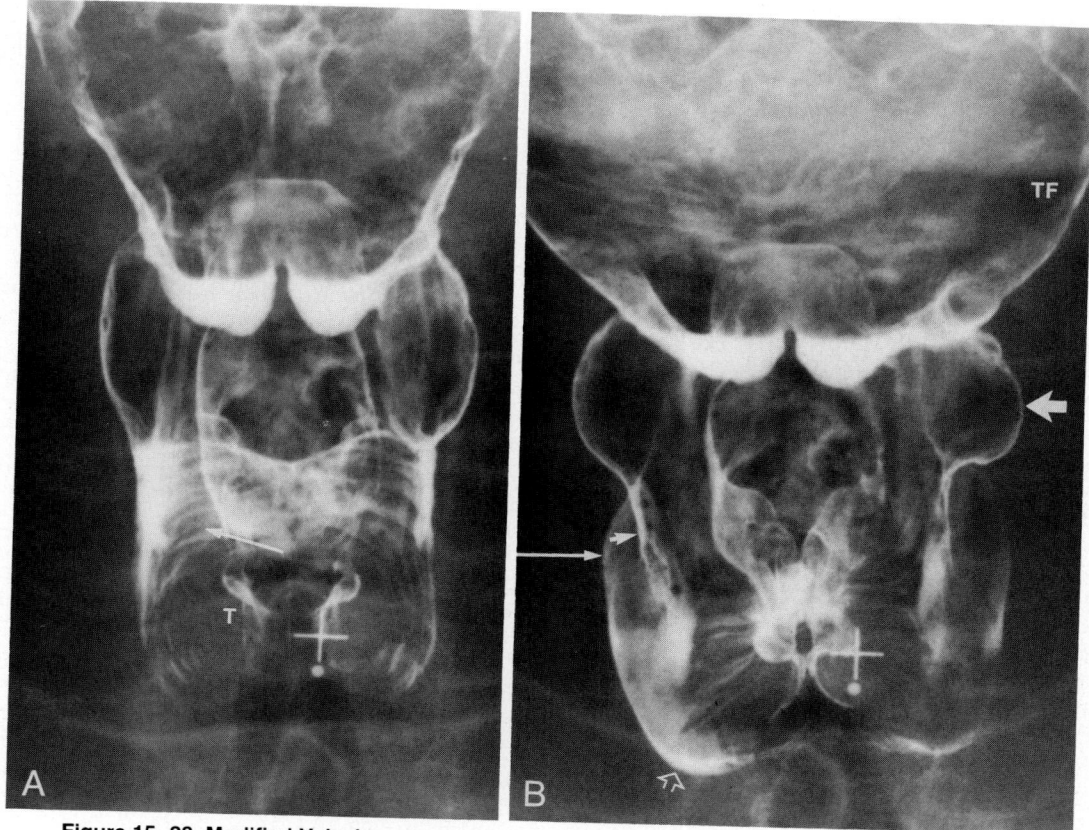

**Figure 15–28. Modified Valsalva procedure. A.** During quiet inspiration, the true (T) and false vocal cords are open. The pharynx is mildly distended. Note arcuate lines in collapsed mid-hypopharynx *(arrow)*. **B.** During the modified Valsalva maneuver, marked distention of the oral cavity and pharynx occurs. Note ballooning of the tonsillar fossae (TF). Lateral pharyngeal pouches *(short thick arrow)* protrude from the region of the thyrohyoid membrane. The lateral hypopharynx protrudes posterolaterally *(long thin arrow)* from the confines of the ala of the thyroid cartilage *(short thin arrow)*. The lower hypopharynx, which was not apparent during inspiration, is now visible *(open arrow)*. Demonstration of the lower hypopharynx is a sign of weakness of the pharyngeal muscle or the pharyngoesophageal segment or of both. (**A** and **B** reprinted with permission from Rubesin SE, Glick SN: The tailored double-contrast pharyngogram. Crit Rev Diagn Imaging 28:133–179, 1988. Copyright CRC Press, Inc. Boca Raton, FL.)

the cricopharyngeal muscle activity. Analysis of motility disorders is presented in Chapter 16.

## Choice of Contrast Agents

In general, the pharynx manipulates a cohesive bolus more readily than a liquid bolus.[34] Therefore, the pharyngeal phase of swallowing is usually safer with barium paste than with thick barium, and safer with thick barium than with thin barium. We usually begin an examination with thick, high-density barium, however, because this barium best demonstrates morphologic characteristics of the pharynx. Usually, we then proceed to barium paste. However, if a motility disorder is seen during fluoroscopy, swallows of thin barium are videotaped in the lateral and frontal projections after double contrast imaging of the pharynx and esophagus. Epiglottic motility is better assessed with thin barium, because thick barium often obscures the epiglottic tip.

Thin barium is also valuable because some patients show laryngeal penetration only with thin barium, not with thick barium or barium paste.

In general, the pharynx can manipulate small, nonphysiologic boluses (2 to 5 mL) more safely than larger physiologic boluses (8 to 10 mL).[35, 36] If any indication of abnormal pharyngeal function exists, the patient should be given small boluses first, and then larger boluses. However, we routinely ask usual outpatients to "take a normal-sized swallow of barium."

For the patient who is massively aspirating barium, the clinical status of the patient determines the number of barium swallows deemed safe. A radiologic finding that indicates that the examination should be discontinued is barium penetration to the carina. Usually, even in the patient with massive aspiration, views of one swallow in the lateral projection and one swallow in the frontal projection are obtained. A suction apparatus should be available for prompt removal of barium that enters the distal trachea.

## Position of the Patient

The patient is first examined in the erect lateral position—the best position for visualizing entry of barium into the laryngeal vestibule either during swallowing (penetration) or during normal breathing (aspiration). If unable to stand, the patient is strapped and seated in a chair or on the footboard of a fluoroscope in a lateral position. If unable to sit, the patient is placed on the fluoroscopic table in as lateral a position as possible. Dentures are left in place, as denture removal may alter swallowing dynamics. If a portable or fixed C-arm fluoroscope is available, patients may be studied while they are confined to a wheelchair or as they lie on a stretcher.[37]

## Soft Palate Examination

Barium may be instilled into the nares to coat the superior surface of the soft palate. Use of intranasal barium enhances visualization of the soft palate and is helpful in patients who have nasal speech; cleft palate or cleft palate repair; known or suspected oropharyngeal or nasopharyngeal tumor; cranial nerve deficits attributable to stroke, tumor, or poliomyelitis; prior cranial or neck surgery; or irradiation.[8, 17, 38, 39] Although not commonly performed, intranasal instillation of barium may demonstrate abnormalities that may not be appreciated otherwise (Fig. 15–29). One to 2 mL of high-density barium is injected into the nares through a small tube-syringe combination while the patient looks upward

and swallows.[27] The patient then swallows additional high-density barium, and videotape and spot film examinations of the pharynx are made in the lateral, frontal, and sphinx positions.[17]

## Therapeutic Examination

A "therapeutic" examination of the pharynx may be performed to 1) discover modifications of swallowing that prevent or diminish laryngeal penetration and 2) educate the patient in swallowing.[36] This examination is usually performed in conjunction with a swallowing therapist from the department of rehabilitation medicine or speech pathology. We prefer to perform diagnostic and therapeutic examinations at different times because of the demands and length of each examination. During the therapeutic examination, various types of boluses, head positions, and breathing techniques are used to determine which foods can be safely swallowed. The patient swallows a series of barium-impregnated foods such as gels, pastes, mashed potatoes, puddings, and hamburger. In general, the safest bolus is of homogeneous consistency and resistant to separation or deformity by the pharynx. Barium paste and barium-impregnated pudding are examples of boluses safe for swallowing in patients with pharyngeal dysmotility.[34] A thin, watery substance similar to thin barium is the most dangerous bolus. The effects of flexed, neutral, and extended positions of the head and neck are examined. Flexing the neck (tilting the chin against the chest) facilitates laryngeal elevation and usually diminishes

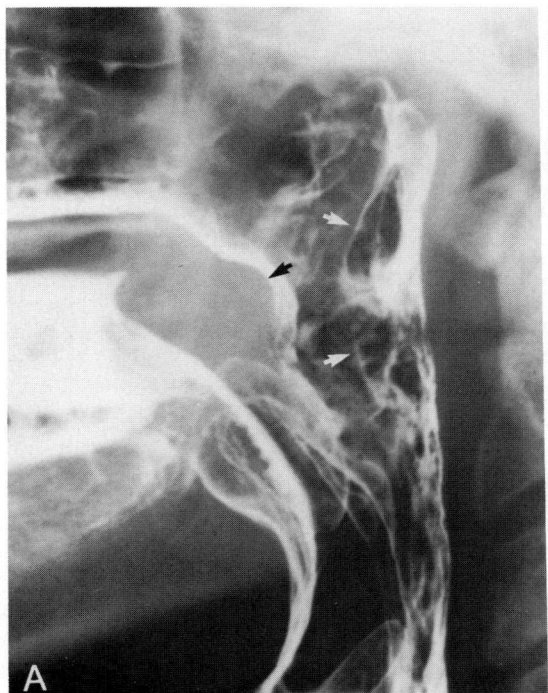

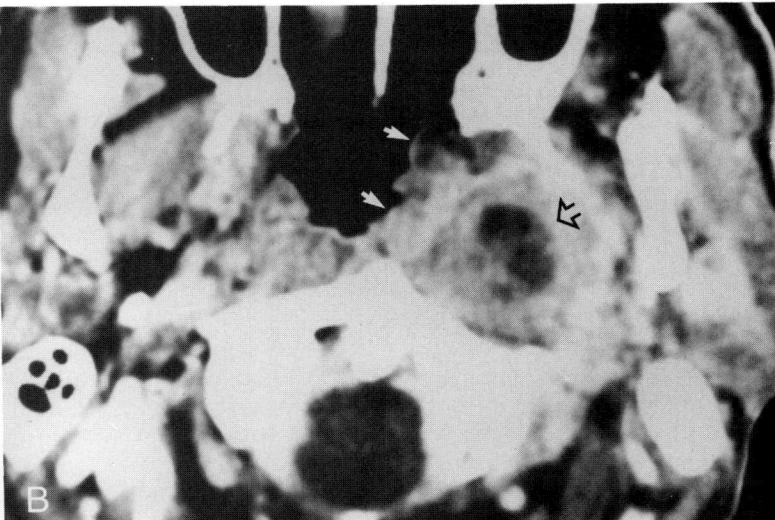

**Figure 15–29. Unsuspected squamous cell carcinoma of the soft palate. A.** Because mild nasal regurgitation and an abnormal contour of the soft palate were initially detected during pharyngography, 1 to 2 mL of barium was instilled into each naris. A large, broad-based, nodular mass protrudes from the posterior nasopharyngeal wall *(white arrows)*. The soft palate is deformed *(black arrow)*. (Reprinted with permission from Rubesin SE, Glick SN: The tailored double-contrast pharyngogram. Crit Rev Diagn Imaging 28:133–179, 1988. Copyright CRC Press, Inc. Boca Raton, FL.) **B.** CT scan through the nasopharynx shows a large mass with a low-density center *(open arrow)* causing asymmetry of the lateral and posterior nasopharyngeal wall *(solid arrows)*.

laryngeal penetration. Swallowing is made more difficult by extending the neck. Breathing techniques may diminish aspiration into the trachea and lungs. Aspirated material may be cleared from the larynx and proximal trachea by exhaling after swallowing. The patient is instructed to inhale, to swallow, and then to exhale to allow clearance of aspirated material from the trachea and larynx.

## Cross-sectional Imaging

Cross-sectional imaging techniques are used primarily 1) to stage neoplastic diseases, such as squamous cell carcinoma, lymphoma, rhabdomyosarcoma, and minor salivary gland tumors; 2) to search for an occult primary lesion in patients with squamous cell carcinoma metastases to neck nodes; 3) to identify a lesion in the peripheral or central nervous system that causes a swallowing disorder; and 4) to evaluate the acutely injured larynx. Whereas the most superficial aspect of a mucosal lesion is best evaluated with barium studies and endoscopy, submucosal tumor spread and spread outside of pharyngeal tissue are best evaluated with cross-sectional techniques.

Currently, computed tomography (CT) is the cross-sectional method of choice for imaging the oropharynx and hypopharynx; magnetic resonance (MR) is the method of choice for imaging the nasopharynx.[40-43] The rapid scanning times of CT prevent motion artifacts. Currently, MR requires a longer scanning time and thus may result in image degradation caused by swallowing, jaw motion, labored breathing, or a combination of these factors. CT is superior to MR in demonstration of 1) small cervical and retropharyngeal nodal metastases in patients with metastatic squamous cell carcinoma and 2) early extranodal spread of tumor. MR is superior to CT in demonstration of 1) perineural spread of tumor and 2) tumor infiltration of the intrinsic muscles of the base of the tongue, superior constrictor muscle, and structures of the carotid sheath. The superior contrast quality of MR allows excellent demonstration of lymphoid tissue. Whether CT or MR is superior to the other in the demonstration of early cartilage invasion by tumor is not clear.

CT scans through the pharynx are typically performed in the straight transaxial plane with 5-mm-thick sections. In a high-volume contrast technique, an initial bolus of 50 mL is followed by rapid infusion via an injector system or through a large gauge catheter. The rapid infusion technique is often combined with "dynamic" rapid scanning to ensure optimal opacification of blood vessels in the neck, allowing them to be easily distinguished from lymph nodes. Typical CT parameters are 140 kV and 120 mA with 2-second scanning. The patient is told to breathe shallowly and not to swallow or speak during the examination. Standard soft tissue windows are used for filming. Bone windows are required when there is clinical or radiographic suggestion of cartilaginous or bony invasion, or when degenerative arthritis or osteophytes could account for pharyngeal symptoms or neck pain. Coronal reconstructions can be obtained

with contiguous sectioning; however, these are improved with an overlap of 1 to 2 mm.

A standard MR evaluation of the pharynx includes both sagittal and axial short repetition time (TR) T1-weighted and axial long TR, long time to echo (TE) T2-weighted scans extending from the cavernous sinus to the thoracic inlet. Thus, the most superior extent of a lesion (into the intracranial space) and the most inferior extent of a lesion (lymphatic spread to the supraclavicular lymph nodes) are included in the examination. Coronal or sagittal images, or both, usually T1 weighted, should be included for direct visualization of the lesion. In cases in which perineural spread of tumor is suspected, postgadolinium T1-weighted images with or without fat suppression are a necessity. For definition of perineural spread, a fat-suppressed postgadolinium T1-weighted scan is helpful in identifying the nerve amid the fat in the skull base or parapharyngeal tissues. Without fat suppression, both fat and enhancing tissue or nerves are bright on T1-weighted scans. Fat-suppressed long-TR proton density and T2-weighted images may render masses in the head and neck more conspicuous.

For fine definition of pharyngeal lesions, spin-echo imaging with slice thicknesses in the range of 3 to 5 mm should be performed. When carotid invasion, perineural spread, or absolute boundaries of tumors must be demonstrated, an imaging matrix that is $256 \times 192$ or $256 \times 256$ should be used. Flow compensation techniques (gradient moment nulling) are helpful in reducing motion artifacts from pulsating blood vessels.

The signal intensity of the pharyngeal mucosa is usually similar to that of muscle on both T1- and T2-weighted images. However, the lingual tonsils, the adenoids, and the palatine tonsils have longer T2 relaxation times and are bright on T2-weighted images. The mucosa of the pharynx enhances with gadolinium. The salivary glands, adenoidal tissue, and slow-flowing venous structures are enhanced with gadolinium.

The muscular structures of the pharynx are well visualized by MR.[44, 45] Within the nasopharynx, tensor veli palatini, levator veli palatini, constrictor muscles, and muscles of the soft palate can be identified (Fig. 15–30). Inferior to these structures are the palatopharyngeal muscle (Fig. 15–31) and the palatoglossus muscle. The muscles of the base of the tongue, including the genioglossus, styloglossus, hyoglossus, mylohyoid, and digastric, can be seen (Figs. 15–32 to 15–35). The vascular structures of the carotid and jugular system can be differentiated from adjacent lymphadenopathy. Although difficulty may be encountered distinguishing lymph nodes from muscle on T1-weighted images, the lymph nodes on T2-weighted images are of intermediate to high intensity whereas the muscle is of low intensity. On T2-weighted images obtained with flow compensation techniques, lymph nodes may be difficult to distinguish from jugular venous structures. A phase-encoded direction flow artifact may be helpful if it is identified. Gradient-echo flow imaging is an alternative method of distinguishing the two types of structures, as flowing vessels appear bright and lymph nodes appear isointense to muscle.

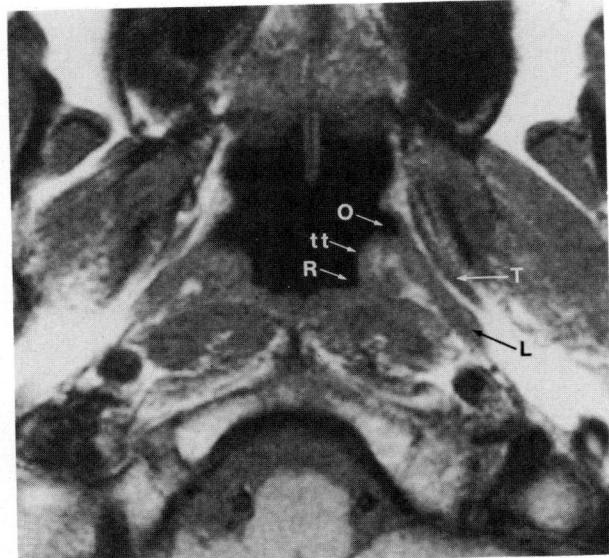

**Figure 15–30.** Axial T1-weighted MR image of nasopharynx shows the relationship of the torus tubarius (tt) to the tensor veli palatini (T) and the levator veli palatini (L). Also shown are the eustachian tube orifice (O), and fossa of Rosenmüller (R). (From Rubesin SE, Rabischong P, Bilaniuk LT, et al: Contrast examination of the soft palate with cross sectional correlation. Radiographics 8:641–665, 1988.)

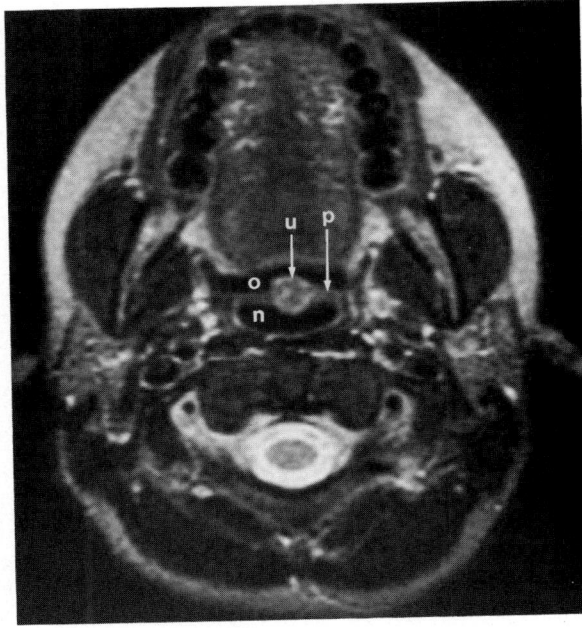

**Figure 15–31.** Axial T2-weighted MR image through the level of the uvula (u) demonstrates the palatopharyngeal fold and the underlying palatopharyngeal muscle (p). The soft palate and the palatopharyngeal fold separate the nasopharynx (n) from the oropharynx (o).

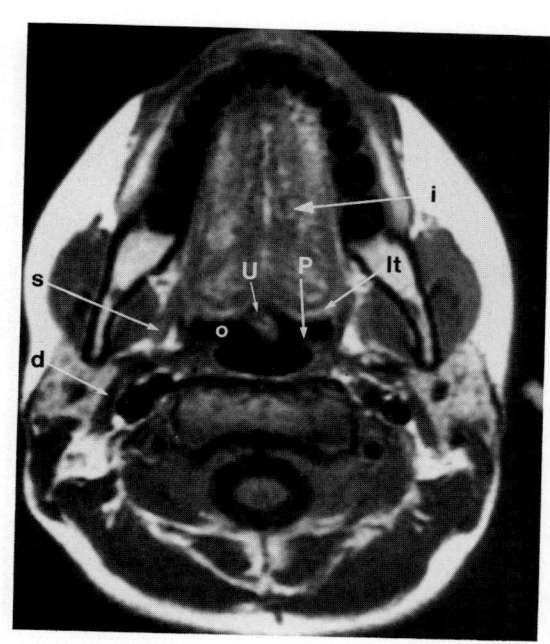

**Figure 15–32.** Axial T1-weighted MR image through the oropharynx (o) demonstrates the tip of the uvula (U) and the palatopharyngeal fold (P) overlying the palatopharyngeal muscle. The lingual tonsil (lt) appears as a bright signal along the surface of the base of the tongue. The intrinsic muscles of the tongue (i), the styloglossus muscle (s), and the posterior belly of the digastric muscle (d) are identified.

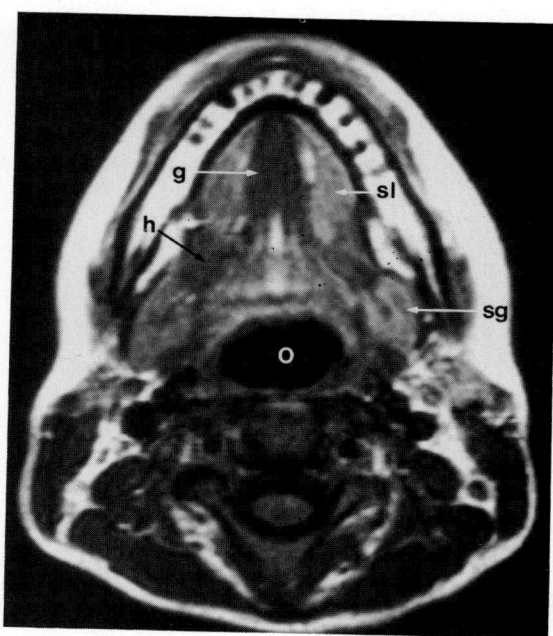

**Figure 15–33.** Axial T1-weighted MR image through the level of the oropharynx (o) demonstrates the genioglossus muscle (g), the hyoglossus muscle (h), and the submandibular gland (sg). The sublingual space (sl) has a relatively high signal intensity because of fat intermixed in this tissue.

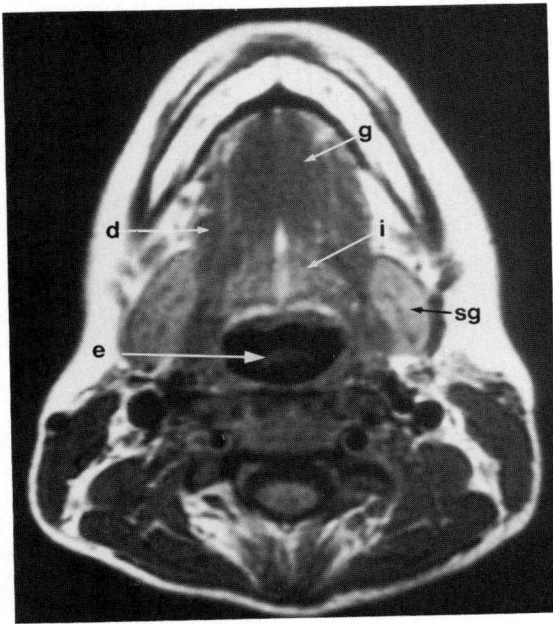

**Figure 15–34.** Axial T1-weighted MR image through the level of the epiglottic tip (e) demonstrates the intermingled genioglossus and geniohyoid muscles (g), the lower part of the intrinsic muscles of the tongue (i), the upper part of the anterior belly of the digastric muscle (d), and the submandibular gland (sg).

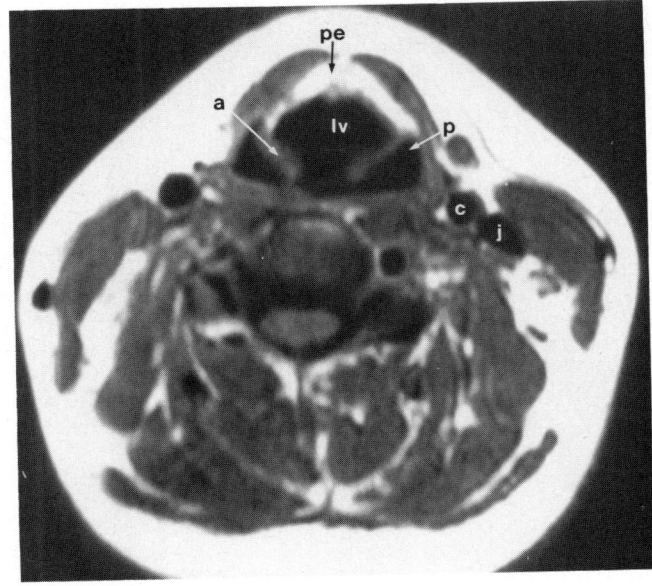

**Figure 15–35.** Axial T1-weighted MR image through the level of the hypopharynx demonstrates the left aryepiglottic fold (a) forming the medial wall of the piriform sinus (p). The laryngeal vestibule (lv) is bounded posteriorly by the left and right aryepiglottic folds. The pre-epiglottic space (pe) has a high signal intensity because it is filled with fat. The carotid artery (c) and jugular vein (j) are identified. p = right piriform sinus.

## Acknowledgment

Figure 15–27A and B is reproduced from Laufer I, Levine MS (eds): Double Contrast Gastrointestinal Radiology (2nd ed). Philadelphia: WB Saunders, 1992.

# References

1. DuBrul EL: Sicher's Oral Anatomy (7th ed). St. Louis: CV Mosby, 1980, pp 319–350.
2. Pernkopf E: Anatomy, Volume I, Head and Neck (3rd ed). Baltimore: Urban & Schwarzenberg, 1989.
3. Rubesin SE, Jesserun J, Robertson D, et al: Lines of the pharynx. Radiographics 7:217–237, 1987.
4. Bosma JF, Donner MW, Tanako E, et al: Anatomy of the pharynx, pertinent to swallowing. Dysphagia 1:23–33, 1986.
5. Dodds WJ: The physiology of swallowing. Dysphagia 3:171–178, 1989.
6. Dodds WJ, Stewart ET, Logemann JA: Physiology and radiology of the normal oral and pharyngeal phases of swallowing. AJR 154:953–963, 1990.
7. Dickson DR: Anatomy of the normal velopharyngeal mechanism. Clin Plast Surg 2:235–248, 1975.
8. Rubesin SE, Rabischong P, Bilaniuk LT, et al: Contrast examination of the soft palate with cross-sectional correlation. Radiographics 4:641–665, 1988.
9. Doty RW, Bosma JF: An electromyographic analysis of reflex deglutition. J Neurophysiol 19:44–60, 1956.
10. Shprintzen RJ, McCall GN, Skolnick ML, et al: Selective movement of the lateral aspects of the pharyngeal walls during velopharyngeal closure for speech, blowing, and whistling in normals. Cleft Palate J 12:51–58, 1975.
11. Skolnick ML, McCall GN, Barnes M: The sphincteric mechanism of velopharyngeal closure. Cleft Palate J 10:286–305, 1973.
12. Skolnick ML: Video fluoroscopic examination of the velopharyngeal portal during phonation in lateral and base projections—a new technique for studying the mechanism of closure. Cleft Palate J 7:803–816, 1970.
13. Donner MW, Bosma JF, Robertson DL: Anatomy and physiology of the pharynx. Gastrointest Radiol 10:196–212, 1985.
14. Silver AJ, Sane P, Hilal SK: CT of the nasopharyngeal region: normal and pathologic anatomy. Radiol Clin North Am 22:161–176, 1984.
15. Sobotta J, Figge FHJ: Atlas of Human Anatomy, Volume 2. Baltimore: Urban & Schwarzenberg, 1977.
16. McMyn JK: The anatomy of the salpingopharyngeus muscle. J Laryngol Otol 55:1–22, 1940.
17. Rubesin SE, Jones B, Donner MW: Radiology of the adult soft palate. Dysphagia 2:8–17, 1987.
18. Capitanio MA, Kirkpatrick JA: Nasopharyngeal lymphoid tissue. Roentgen observations in 257 children two years of age or less. Radiology 96:389–391, 1970.
19. Gromet M, Homer MJ, Carter BL: Lymphoid hyperplasia at the base of the tongue. Radiology 144:825–828, 1982.
20. Curtis DJ, Hudson T: Laryngotracheal aspiration: analysis of specific neuromuscular factors. Radiology 149:517–522, 1983.
21. Pitman RG, Fraser GM: The post-cricoid impression of the esophagus. Clin Radiol 16:34–39, 1965.
22. Dodds WJ, Logemann JA, Stewart ET: Radiologic assessment of abnormal oral and pharyngeal phases of swallowing. AJR 154:965–974, 1990.
23. Balfe DM, Heiken JP: Contrast evaluation of structural lesions of the pharynx. Curr Probl Diagn Radiol 15:73–160, 1986.
24. Jones B, Donner MW: Examination of the patient with dysphagia. Radiology 167:319–326, 1988.
25. Jones B, Kramer SS, Donner MW: Dynamic imaging of the pharynx. Gastrointest Radiol 10:213–224, 1985.
26. Levine MS, Rubesin SE: Radiologic investigation of dysphagia. AJR 154:1157–1163, 1990.
27. Rubesin SE, Glick SN: The tailored double-contrast pharyngogram. Crit Rev Diagn Imaging 28:133–179, 1988.
28. Ekberg O, Nylander G: Double contrast examination of the pharynx. Gastrointest Radiol 10:263–271, 1985.
29. Rubesin SE, Laufer I: Pictorial review: principles of double contrast pharyngography. Dysphagia 6:170–178, 1991.
30. Jones B, Ravich WJ, Donner MW, et al: Pharyngoesophageal interrelationships: observations and working concepts. Gastrointest Radiol 10:225–233, 1985.
31. Taylor AJ, Dodds WJ, Stewart ET: Pharynx: value of oblique projections for radiographic examination. Radiology 178:59–61, 1991.
32. Rubesin SE, Jones B, Donner MW: Contrast pharyngography: the importance of phonation. AJR 148:269–272, 1987.
33. Jing BS: The pharynx and larynx: roentgenographic technique. Semin Roentgenol 9:259–265, 1974.
34. Dantas RO, Dodds WJ, Massey BT, et al: The effect of high- vs. low-density barium preparations on the quantitative features of swallowing. AJR 153:1191–1195, 1989.
35. Dodds WJ, Man KM, Cook IJ, et al: Influence of bolus volume on swallow-induced hyoid movement in normal subjects. AJR 150:1307–1309, 1988.
36. Logemann J: Anatomy and physiology of normal deglutition. In Logemann J (ed): Evaluation and Treatment of Swallowing Disorders. San Diego: College Hill Press, 1983, pp 9–36.
37. Davis M, Palmer P, Kelsey C: Use of C-arm fluoroscope to examine patients with swallowing disorders. AJR 155:986–988, 1990.
38. Khoo FY, Chia KB, Nalpon J: A new technique of contrast examination of the nasopharynx with cinefluorography and roentgenography. Am J Roentgenol 99:238–248, 1967.
39. Khoo FY, Kanagasuntheram R, Chia KB, et al: The normal nasopharyngogram. AJR 147:145–148, 1986.
40. Teresi LM, Luftkin RB, Vinuela F, et al: MR imaging of the nasopharynx and floor of the middle cranial fossa. Part I: Normal anatomy. Radiology 164:811–816, 1987.
41. Christianson R, Lufkin R, Hanafee W: Normal magnetic resonance imaging anatomy of the tongue, oropharynx, hypopharynx, and larynx. Dysphagia 1:119–127, 1987.
42. Silver AJ, Mawad ME, Hilal SK, et al: Computed tomography of the nasopharynx and related space. I. Anatomy. Radiology 147:725–731, 1983.
43. Silver AJ, Mawad ME, Hilal SK, et al: Computed tomography of the nasopharynx and related spaces. Radiology 147:733–738, 1983.
44. Lufkin RB, Hanafee WN, Wortham D, et al: MRI of the larynx and hypopharynx using surface coils. Radiology 158:747–754, 1986.
45. Lufkin RB, Wortham DG, Dietrich RB, et al: Tongue and oropharynx findings on MRI. Radiology 161:69–75, 1986.
46. Rubesin SE: Pharyngeal dysfunction. In Gore R (ed): Syllabus for Categorical Course on Gastrointestinal Radiology. Reston, VA: American College of Radiology, 1991, pp 1–9.
47. Rubesin SE: Pharynx. In Laufer I, Levine MS (eds): Double Contrast Gastrointestinal Radiology (2nd ed). Philadelphia: WB Saunders, 1991, pp 73–105.

# Abnormalities of Pharyngeal Function

**Bronwyn Jones, M.D.**

**Martin W. Donner, M.D.**

## ANALYSIS OF THE FUNCTIONAL ASPECTS OF SWALLOWING

In reviewing examinations of the pharynx and esophagus, the slow-motion, reverse, and stop-frame capabilities of cineradiography or videofluoroscopy are essential. With these capabilities, the movement of individual structures can be analyzed, first in isolation and then in combination with other structures. The tongue, palate, pharyngeal stripping wave, epiglottis, hyoid bone, larynx, cricopharyngeus, and esophageal peristalsis should be evaluated (Table 16–1).

A familiarity with the anatomy, the radiographic anatomy, and the physiology of the pharynx and related structures is required for abnormalities to be appreciated. Any lack of movement, or abnormalities indicating compensation or decompensation, must be noted.

Two important principles must be considered when reviewing pharyngeal studies: 1) *Dynamic imaging is vital.* Pharyngeal events take place too rapidly for the eye to detect subtle (but clinically important) abnormalities. In addition, a lesion such as a web or a ring may appear on only 1 or 2 frames at 30 frames per second. 2) *The entire swallowing chain must be examined.* Such extensive examination is necessary because the level of symptoms is not a reliable indicator of the site of the abnormality.[1] Also, several lesions could be producing dysphagia, and esophageal disease may result in pharyngeal disease.[2]

## Neurophysiologic Control of Swallowing

Swallowing involves the close cooperation of many muscles, six cranial nerves (trigeminal, facial, glossopharyngeal, vagus, spinal branch of accessory, and hypoglossal), and the first, second, and third cervical nerves (through the ansa cervicalis). Afferent sensory information is integrated in the brain stem in the "swallowing center," and efferent signals originate in the motor ganglia of the cranial nerves; movements are then effected peripherally.[3–8]

The vagus nerve, or 10th cranial nerve (CN X), supplies motor efferent fibers to all the intrinsic pharyngeal muscles (constrictors, palatopharyngeus, and salpingopharyngeus) except the stylopharyngeus, which is supplied by the glossopharyngeal nerve (CN IX). The vagus nerve also supplies motor efferent fibers to all the palatal muscles except the tensor veli palatini, which is supplied by the trigeminal nerve (CN V). The trigeminal nerve also supplies the anterior digastricus and mylohyoideus. The facial nerve (CN VII) supplies the posterior digastricus and stylohyoideus. Although the vagus nerve carries the efferent fibers that innervate the striated pharyngeal musculature, most of these fibers probably emerge from the brain stem in the bulbar part of the accessory nerve (CN XI).

Pharyngeal branches of the glossopharyngeal and the vagus nerves and rami of the sympathetic trunk and the

## TABLE 16–1. CHECK LIST FOR REVIEWING SWALLOWING STUDIES

**HEAD AND NECK POSTURE**
Swan neck or flexion at rest
Flexion during swallowing

**MOUTH-TONGUE COORDINATION**
Bolus transfer
Drooling or dribbling

**TONGUE**
Atrophy, resection, or increased bulk
Bolus control
Abnormal movements

**HYOID BONE MOTION**
Original position
Elevation with swallowing

**TONGUE AND PALATE**
Premature leakage

**PALATE AND POSTERIOR PHARYNGEAL WALL**
Elevation with speech
Elevation and apposition to posterior pharyngeal wall with swallow
  (Passavant's cushion)

**PHARYNGEAL STRIPPING WAVE**
Wave normal, deeper than usual, absent, disordered
Cervical spine disease

**EPIGLOTTIS**
Tilt or asymmetry

**LARYNGEAL PENETRATION**
During, before, and after swallowing
Contrast medium squeezed out by larynx
Entry of contrast medium into trachea
Cough

**ASPIRATION**
Elevation of larynx
Closure of larynx
Cough

**CRICOPHARYNGEUS**
Opening complete and on time
Early closure

**ESOPHAGUS**
Normal motility
Emptying
Gastroesophageal reflux
Stricture or ring
Mucosal abnormality

Modified from Jones B, Gayler BW, Donner MW: Pharynx and cervical esophagus. *In* Levine MS (ed): Radiology of the Esophagus. Philadelphia: WB Saunders, 1989, pp 311–336.

## TABLE 16–2. INNERVATION OF MUSCLES USED IN SWALLOWING

| MUSCLES | NERVE* |
|---|---|
| All soft palate muscles (except tensor veli palatini) | CN X |
| All pharyngeal muscles (except stylopharyngeus) | CN X |
| | CN IX |
| All laryngeal muscles (except cricothyroideus) | RLN |
| | SLN |
| All tongue muscles (except palatoglossus) | CN XII |
| | CN X |
| Suprahyoid muscles | CN V |
| | CN VII |
| Infrahyoid muscles | Ansa cervicalis |

*CN = cranial nerve; RLN = recurrent laryngeal nerve; SLN = superior laryngeal nerve.

## Functional Components of Swallowing

### Oropharyngeal Phase

#### Tongue and Palate

Swallowing begins with the lips engulfing the bolus (Figs. 16–1 and 16–2). The bolus is then manipulated by the tongue and teeth until it is judged "swallowable." Two positions of the bolus preparatory to swallowing have been identified: the *dipper position* (in which the bolus is positioned anteriorly underneath the tongue in the floor of the mouth) and the *tipper position* (in which the bolus is held in a midline groove of the tongue against the alveolar ridge and hard palate).[9]

The back of the tongue blade and the soft palate form a seal that prevents premature leakage of bolus into the pharynx before swallowing (see Figs. 16–1A and 16–2A). Weakness, atrophy, or resection of the tongue or soft palate can lead to leakage of a bolus into the open, unprotected larynx before swallowing. Viewed in the frontal position, unilateral leakage indicates decompensation.

As the bolus is propelled into the oropharynx by an upward and backward movement of the tongue, the soft palate elevates to a right angle to appose the posterior pharyngeal wall. At the same time, a focally converging segment of the superior pharyngeal wall, Passavant's cushion, moves anteriorly to seal the palatopharyngeal isthmus. Passavant's cushion is formed by focal contraction of the upper fibers of the superior constrictor muscle of the pharynx (Fig. 16–3A; see Figs. 16–1B, 16–2B, 16–10A, and 16–11A and B). Tongue thrust (involving both blade and base of the tongue), combined with pharyngeal constriction and intrabolus pressure, contributes to bolus compression and propulsion.

#### Pharynx

The constrictor stripping wave can be observed in the lateral position as a progressive forward movement of the posterior pharyngeal wall at the tail of the bolus (see Figs. 16–1C to F and 16–2C to E). In the frontal view, the wave appears to squeeze the back of the bolus,

superior cervical ganglion form a plexus in the connective tissue outside the constrictor muscles (the pharyngeal plexus). In this plexus, autonomic (parasympathetic and sympathetic) and afferent and efferent branchial fibers intermingle and branch into the muscles and the mucosal lining. Damage to this plexus can produce dysphagia.

Pharyngeal sensation (including sensation of the tonsil and the postsulcal part of the tongue) appears to be mediated by the glossopharyngeal nerve. This nerve also supplies motor innervation to the stylopharyngeus and parasympathetic secretomotor fibers to the parotid gland. A summary of the innervation of the muscles involved in swallowing is presented in Table 16–2.

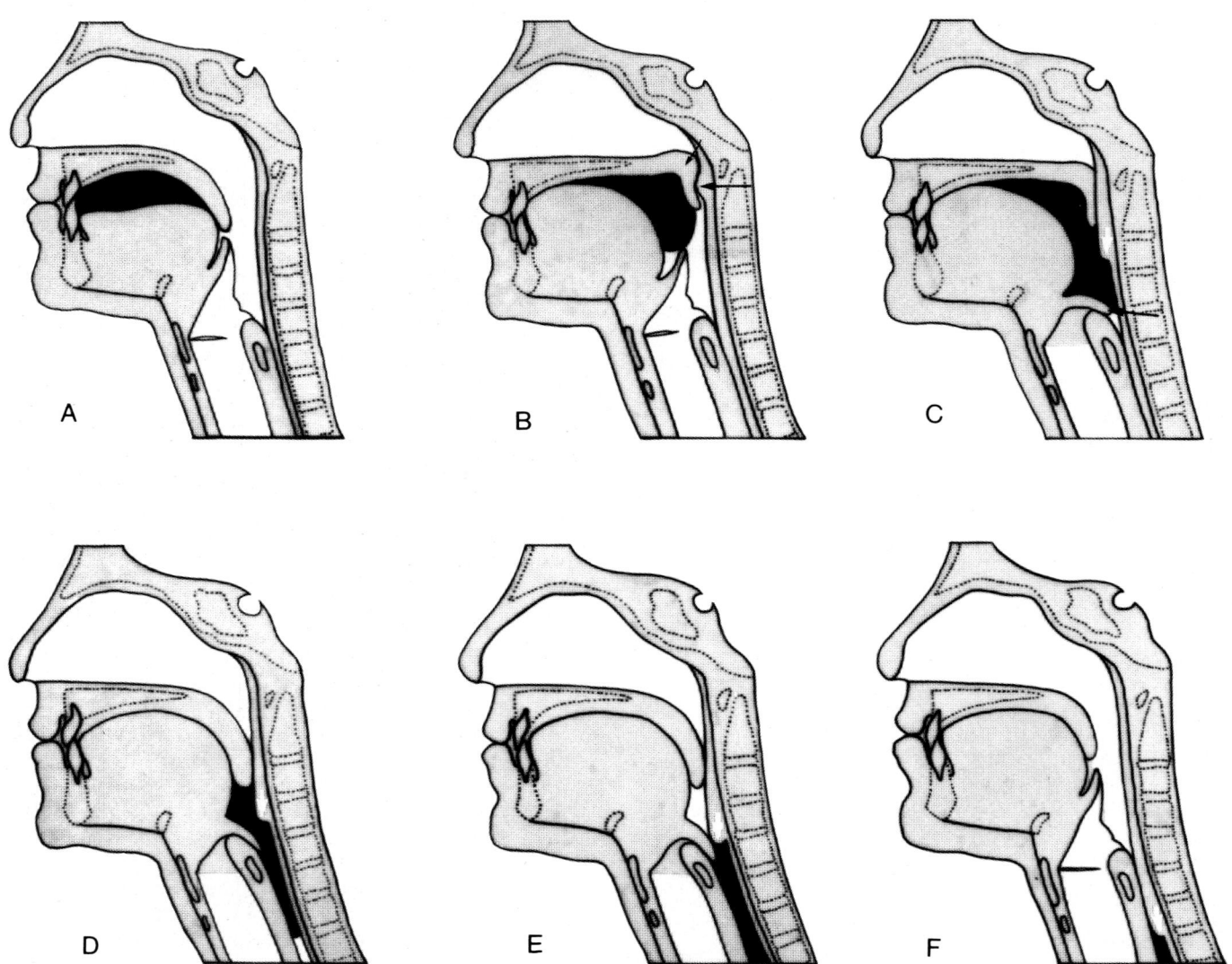

**Figure 16–1. Line drawing of normal swallowing (lateral view). A**. Bolus is held in the oral cavity by apposition of the soft palate and back of the tongue. **B**. As bolus is presented to the oropharnyx, the soft palate *(short arrow)* elevates to appose Passavant's cushion *(long arrow)* to prevent nasopharyngeal regurgitation. **C**. As the bolus passes through the pharynx, the beginning of the posterior pharyngeal stripping wave *(white arrow)* can be seen. The epiglottis *(black arrow)* is completely tilted to cover the laryngeal aperture, which is completely closed. **D**. As the bolus descends further, the back of tongue, the soft palate, and the pharyngeal stripping wave *(arrow)* continue to seal the nasopharyngeal inlet. The epiglottis remains tilted, and the larynx remains closed. The cricopharyngeus has opened completely to allow unimpeded bolus passage. **E**. As the bolus descends past the level of the cricopharyngeus, the tongue base begins to move forward and the soft palate begins to elevate. **F**. As the bolus passes into the thoracic esophagus, the tongue base moves forward, the epiglottis flips up, and the larynx returns to its resting, open position. (**A** to **F** from Donner MW, Bosma JF, Robertson DL: Anatomy and physiology of the pharynx. Gastrointest Radiol 10:196–212, 1985.)

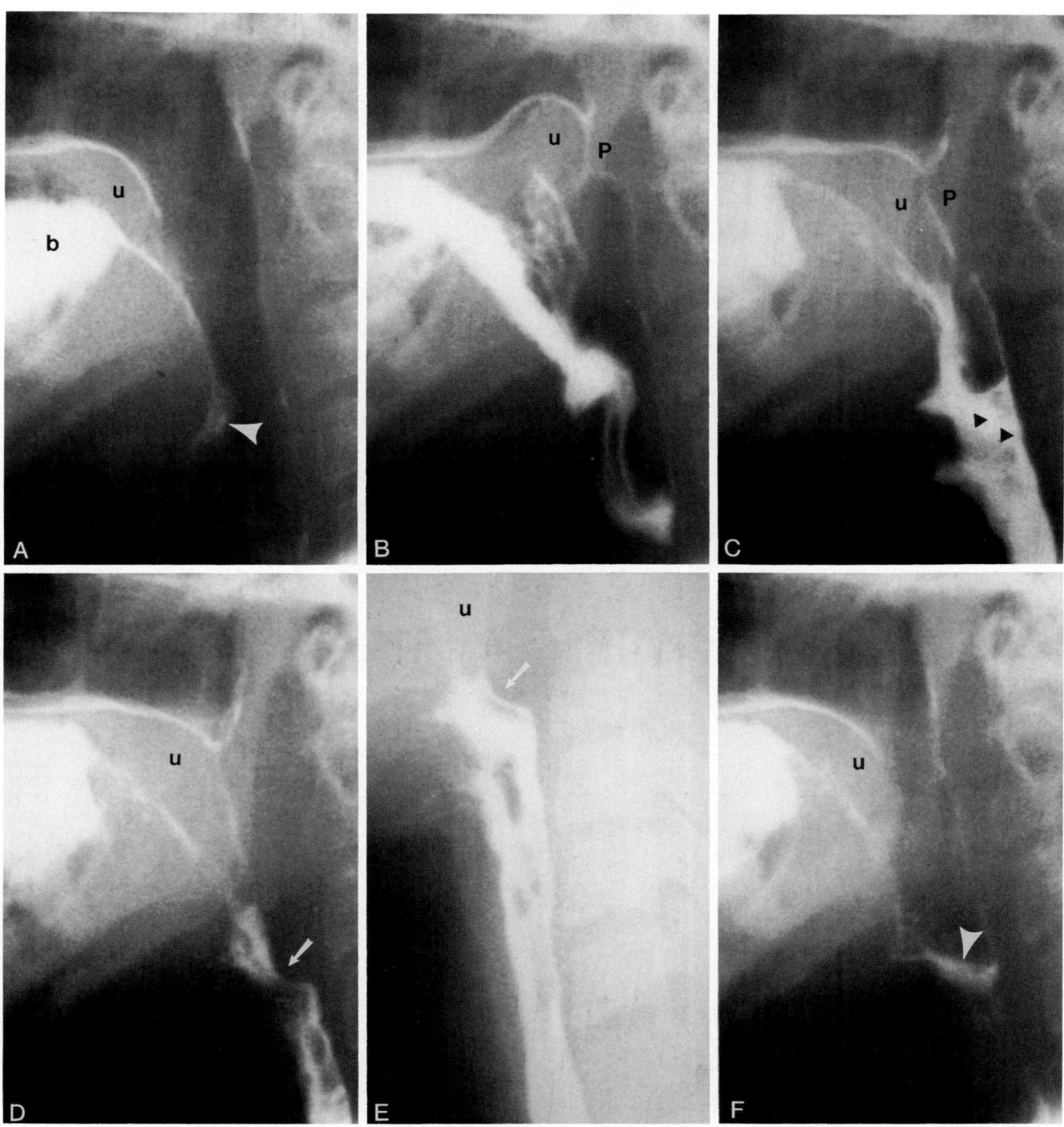

**Figure 16–2. Normal swallowing. A** to **F**. A series of stop-frame images from a cinepharyngoeso-phagram demonstrates normal swallowing as it appears on the dynamic imaging study in the lateral position. The epiglottis *(arrowheads)* and stripping wave *(arrow)* are identified. Note that the superior and posterior surfaces of the soft palate (u) have been coated by intranasal injection of barium. Also, note that in **F** the epiglottis is beginning to re-elevate and has not yet returned to its resting position. b = bolus; P = Passavant's cushion.

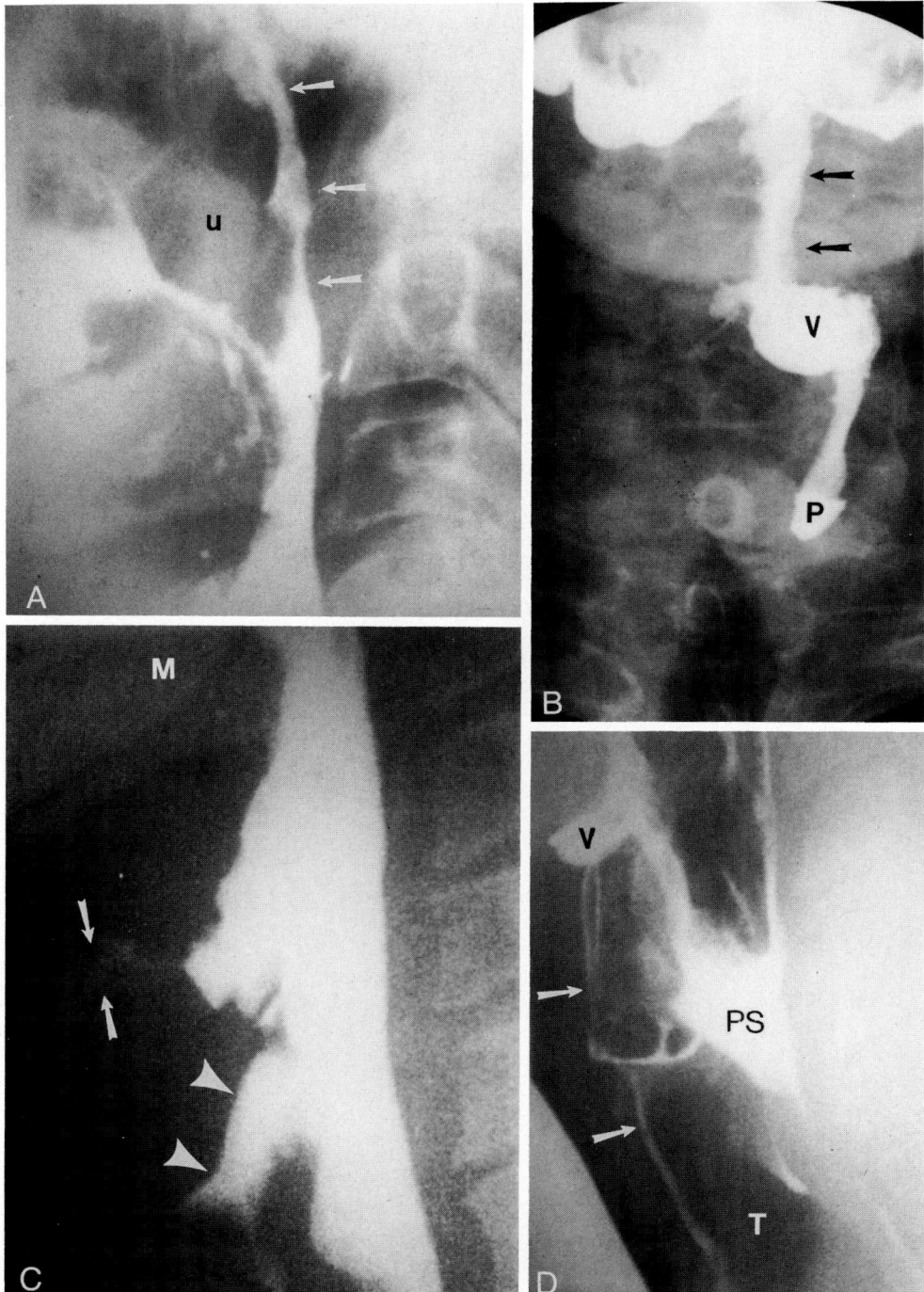

**Figure 16–3. Stop-frame images from four patients showing four different types of decompensation. A**. A somewhat magnified lateral view of the oropharynx and nasopharynx demonstrates incomplete elevation of the soft palate (u) and marked nasopharyngeal regurgitation *(arrows)*. **B**. An anteroposterior view shows unilateral leakage over the back of the tongue *(arrows)*, into the left vallecula (V), and then into the piriform sinus (P). (**B** from Jones B, Donner MW: Interpreting the study. *In* Jones B, Donner MW [eds]: Normal and Abnormal Swallowing: Imaging in Diagnosis and Therapy. New York: Springer-Verlag, 1991, p 60.) **C**. A lateral view shows marked laryngeal penetration into the wide-open laryngeal vestibule *(arrowheads)* and incomplete elevation of the hyoid bone *(arrows)*; normally the hyoid bone is elevated almost to the level of the angle of the mandible (M). **D**. Marked retention in the valleculae (V) and piriform sinuses (PS) is demonstrated after swallowing, and overflow aspiration *(arrows)* downward into the larynx and trachea (T) can be seen.

obliterating the lumen. Unilateral weakness results in asymmetry in the frontal view; the contracting normal side throws the bolus across to the atonic side, so that the bolus passes down the paralyzed side. The contracting normal side may be misinterpreted as a mass, whereas the abnormality is actually on the noncontracting bulging side.

Because pharyngeal contraction occurs much more rapidly than does esophageal contraction (12 to 25 cm/s versus 1 to 4 cm/s), dynamic imaging is essential in examination of the pharynx. Contraction of the constrictor muscles may be affected by intrinsic disease of the pharyngeal muscles (e.g., polymyositis), neuromuscular disorders (e.g., amyotrophic lateral sclerosis, multiple sclerosis, or cerebrovascular accident), or by local factors such as scarring, radiation, or cervical spine disease. Diseases that restrict laryngeal elevation compound the problem. Depending on their location, large osteophytes may hinder or prevent epiglottic tilt.[10]

### Laryngeal Dynamics

Respiration is suspended during swallowing and resumes after swallowing. As the bolus enters the oropharynx, the larynx begins to elevate, moving upward and forward, and the true vocal cords, false vocal cords, and laryngeal vestibule close inferiorly to superiorly, with the vestibule closing last. Laryngeal elevation begins simultaneously with elevation of the hyoid bone but continues for a short time after the hyoid bone has reached its peak elevation. Laryngeal movement can be appreciated by observing the hyoid bone rising to appose the angle of the mandible. An excellent review of laryngeal dynamics has been written by Curtis.[23] A direct correlation exists between hyoid bone excursion and bolus volume,[24] with larger volumes producing more elevation. Hyoid bone elevation may occur in one step (20%) or in two steps (80%), whereas descent occurs in one step,[25] simultaneously with return of the epiglottis to the upright position.

### Epiglottic Tilt

Epiglottic tilt deflects food and liquid into the lateral food channels away from the larynx, and when completely inverted, the epiglottis covers the laryngeal aperture. In many people, this movement occurs in two steps: the first movement (to a horizontal position) is probably a passive one caused by elevation of the hyoid bone; the second movement (to complete inversion) is probably due to contraction of the thyroepiglotticus.[26] In a minority of people, the epiglottis fails to invert, tilting only to the horizontal or oblique position. In the frontal view, the completely inverted epiglottis produces a "sea gull"–shaped filling defect. Flow of bolus into the lateral food channels may produce a flow defect.

### Cricopharyngeal Opening

Activity of the constrictor muscles must be coordinated with cricopharyngeal relaxation and opening. The cricopharyngeus must relax and open completely to allow unimpeded passage of the bolus.[11–22] Complete opening of the lumen at the pharyngoesophageal junction involves several actions: 1) cricopharyngeal relaxation; 2) superior and anterior movement of the larynx; 3) pharyngeal constriction, producing thrust; and 4) intrabolus pressure. Thus, cricopharyngeal prominence is often observed in patients with pharyngeal paresis or in patients with a frozen larynx. In such circumstances, the pharyngeal milieu, rather than the muscle itself, is abnormal.

*Cricopharyngeal achalasia* is a manometric term referring to complete failure of cricopharyngeal relaxation—an unusual entity. Radiographic examinations reveal luminal opening, not cricopharyngeal relaxation. Findings that are commonly associated with cricopharyngeal prominence include pharyngeal paresis; gastroesophageal reflux; an esophageal motility disturbance, such as spasm or achalasia[2, 19] (Fig. 16–4); aging, and Zenker's diverticulum (see section on Zenker's diverticulum). The resultant luminal compromise may be minimal or marked. In severe cases, a horizontal "bar" may be observed. The luminal narrowing usually responds to bougienage.

## Prevention of Aspiration

Many mechanisms protect the larynx against aspiration (Table 16–3; see Figs. 16–3 and 16–11). Laryngeal elevation and closure of the vocal cords, arytenoid cartilages, and laryngeal vestibule are as important as epiglottic tilt.[27] Thus, a frozen larynx can result in aspiration.

If aspiration is observed, all factors that prevent aspiration should be analyzed and the following questions asked. Does the epiglottis tilt and does the larynx (hyoid bone) elevate adequately? Do the vocal cords and laryngeal vestibule close? Also, swallowing should be analyzed for timing of oral and pharyngeal events. Laryngeal penetration or aspiration through the vocal cords into the trachea may occur *during* swallowing, *before* swallowing (premature leakage from the mouth), or *after* swallowing (overflow aspiration of retained bolus or regurgitated or refluxed material). The timing and

---

**TABLE 16–3. AIRWAY PROTECTION**

Momentary suspension of respiration
Adduction of the true and false vocal cords
Posterior tilt of the epiglottis
Constrictor contraction compressing the inverted epiglottis against the laryngeal aperture
Deflection of bolus away from the laryngeal vestibule into lateral food channels formed by the piriform sinuses
Elevation of the larynx
Closure of the laryngeal aperture (apposition of arytenoid masses)
Approximation of the thyroid cartilage to the hyoid bone
Coughing

Modified from Jones B, Gayler BW, Donner MW: Pharynx and cervical esophagus. *In* Levine MS (ed): Radiology of the Esophagus. Philadelphia: WB Saunders, 1989, pp 311–336.

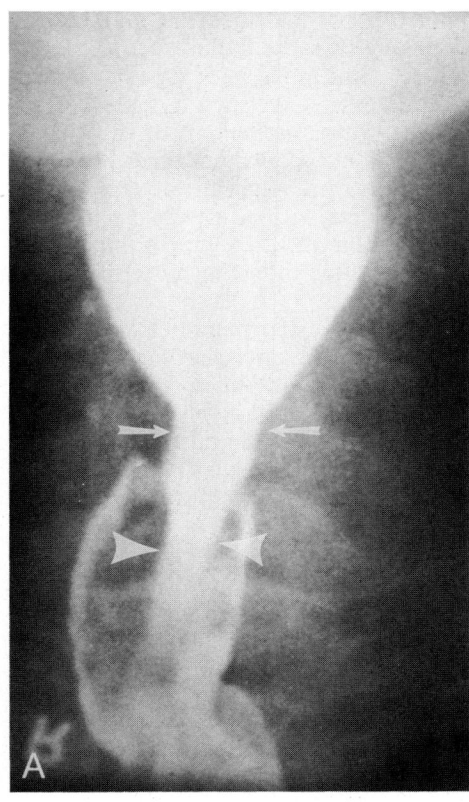 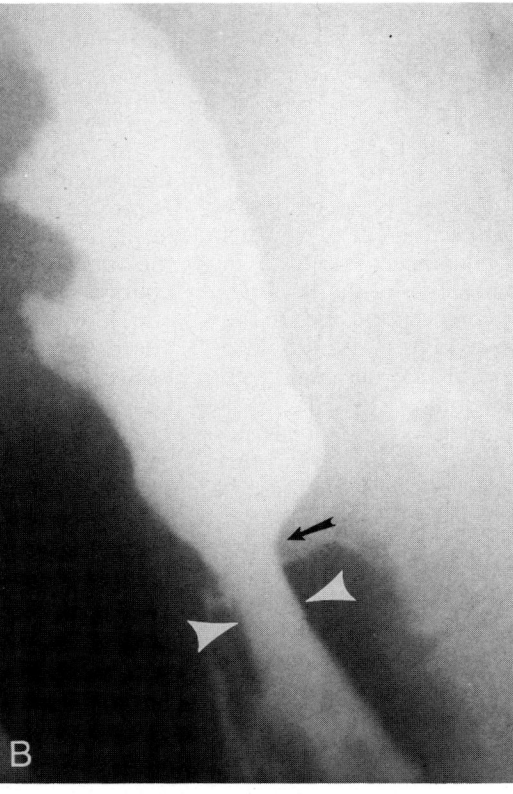

**Figure 16–4. Cricopharyngeal prominence.** Frontal **(A)** and lateral **(B)** views show prominence of the cricopharyngeus *(arrows)*. Note the jet effect *(arrowheads)* below the narrowing, simulating a stenotic lesion, especially in the lateral view. The lumen of the cervical esophagus is actually dilated, as the patient has achalasia. (**A** and **B** from Jones B, Donner MW, Rubesin SE, et al: Pharyngeal findings in 21 patients with achalasia of the esophagus. Dysphagia 2:87–92, 1987.)

causes of the patient's aspiration have therapeutic implications; varying the bolus volume or consistency, repositioning the head, and instituting breathing techniques are useful therapeutic strategies.[28]

The important role that oral decompensation can have in aspiration has been underestimated until recently. Feinberg and Ekberg studied a group of 50 patients with known aspiration and found that the aspiration was the result of oral decompensation in 23 patients, a combination of oral and pharyngeal decompensation in 17 patients, and pharyngeal decompensation in only 10 patients.[29]

Another important observation is whether the aspirated material precipitates a cough; this observation needs to be conveyed to the referring physician in the radiologic report. Some patients with chronic aspiration are silent aspirators (presumably because of loss of laryngeal sensation). Bedside evaluation of these patients does not reveal the severity of decompensation.

## ADAPTATION, COMPENSATION, AND DECOMPENSATION

The pharynx is an extremely flexible organ that must adapt to its various functions, namely respiration, speech, and swallowing. In addition, it adapts to different stimuli and compensates when one of its parts is defective (Tables 16–4 and 16–5). The process of adjustment of normal swallowing to different stimuli is called *adaptation*. The pharynx must adjust to the bolus, which may vary in volume, temperature, consistency, viscosity, and elasticity. The effect of different boluses can be seen on videofluoroscopy by watching the difference between a swallow of thin liquid barium and one of the same volume of barium paste.[30]

Signs of *compensation* (visible on dynamic studies) indicate that swallowing is already impaired.[31] Some types of compensation for impaired swallowing may be conscious and voluntary. For example, a patient may change the types of food eaten, perhaps omitting solid foods and substituting purées, or may even restrict the diet to liquids only. Certain postures, such as tilting or flexing the head and neck, may help a patient to swallow more effectively, reducing laryngeal penetration or clearing a retained bolus.

Swallowing can be considered to have five distinct stages (see Table 16–4), each of which has a characteristic pattern of compensation and decompensation.[31] The five stages are

1. Control of junction of mouth and pharynx (palatoglossal seal) (Fig. 16–5)
2. Closure of the palatopharyngeal isthmus (Fig. 16–6)
3. Compression of the bolus (Fig. 16–7)
4. Closure of the larynx (Fig. 16–8)
5. Opening of the pharyngoesophageal (PE) segment (Fig. 16–9)

At the first stage, for example, downward displacement of the soft palate may compensate for deficiency of the

## TABLE 16–4. PHARYNGEAL DEFICIENCY IN RELATION TO FIVE STAGES OF SWALLOWING

| STAGE OF SWALLOWING | SITE OF DEFICIENCY | SIGNS OF COMPENSATION | SIGNS OF DECOMPENSATION |
|---|---|---|---|
| 1. Control of junction of mouth and pharynx (tongue/palate competence) | Tongue | Palate kinks to appose tongue. (This is normal in the supine position.) | Leakage into pharynx before swallowing |
| | Palate | Posterior aspect of tongue displaced upward | As above |
| 2. Closure of palatopharyngeal isthmus (palate/constrictor muscle competence) | Palate | Greater convergence of pharyngeal wall by pharyngeal contraction (prominent Passavant's cushion) | Nasopharyngeal regurgitation |
| 3. Compression of bolus | Constrictor muscles | Tongue and larynx displaced posteriorly | Retention in valleculae and piriform sinuses after swallowing |
| | Tongue base | Greater convergence of pharyngeal wall of constrictor muscles (prominent stripping wave) | As above |
| 4. Closure of larynx | Intrinsic laryngeal muscles | Further displacement of larynx upward and forward | Laryngeal penetration |
| 5. Opening of pharyngoesophageal segment | Pharyngoesophageal segment opening | Head flexion | Overflow aspiration of retained bolus |

tongue (resulting from atrophy, weakness, or surgical resection); conversely, upward displacement of the tongue may compensate for weakness of the soft palate. (See Table 16–4 and Figs. 16–5 to 16–9 for compensation occurring in the other stages.)

Another compensatory phenomenon is the development of a deeper pharyngeal stripping wave, which is observed in the presence of a partially obstructing lesion in the cervical esophagus, such as a web or prominent cricopharyngeus.

Any radiographic findings of compensation must be communicated to the referring physician, so that the patient can be informed that swallowing is impaired and

## TABLE 16–5. COMMON ABNORMALITIES OF SWALLOWING

| FINDING | CAUSES |
|---|---|
| Leakage | Weakness, atrophy, resection of tongue |
| | Edentulous or missing teeth or ill-fitting dentures |
| | Paralysis of soft palate |
| Nasal regurgitation | Weakness of soft palate or superior constrictor |
| Penetration or aspiration, or both | Poor or absent epiglottic tilt |
| | Poor or absent elevation of larynx |
| | Poor or absent closure of larynx |
| Retention (in valleculae or piriform sinuses) | Poor push |
| | Weakness of stripping wave |
| | Relative obstruction such as prominent cricopharyngeus or web |

Modified from Jones B, Gayler BW, Donner MW: Pharynx and cervical esophagus. *In* Levine MS (ed): Radiology of the Esophagus. Philadelphia: WB Saunders, 1989, pp 311–336.

can be instructed to take additional care when eating or drinking quickly, for example, in a restaurant or in other social situations.

## FUNCTIONAL ASPECTS OF ZENKER'S DIVERTICULUM

Zenker's diverticulum is a pulsion diverticulum located at the level of the pharyngoesophageal junction, with the most common site being between the oblique and horizontal fibers of the cricopharyngeus through a triangular area known as *Killian's dehiscence* (Fig. 16–10). It is a posterior diverticulum, it may fill during or after swallowing, and if large, it may flop to one or the other side. Once swallowing is completed, the diverticulum may empty back into the pharynx, filling the piriform sinus. This occurrence often precipitates a second swallow, but it also places the patient at risk for overflow aspiration.

The pathogenesis of Zenker's diverticulum remains unclear, although incoordination between pharyngeal contraction and cricopharyngeal opening may be a contributing factor.[32, 33] Some manometric and cineradiographic studies have demonstrated premature sphincter closure in some patients with Zenker's diverticulum. Other studies performed in patients with fully developed diverticula showed that timing of pharyngeal contraction and cricopharyngeal relaxation appears to be normal.

Cook and colleagues demonstrated decreased compliance of the upper esophageal sphincter (UES) in a group of patients who had Zenker's diverticulum and in whom inadequate sphincter opening resulted in increased intrabolus pressure.[34, 35] Shaw and associates subsequently demonstrated that with cricopharyngeal myotomy and pouch ablation, the intrabolus pressure

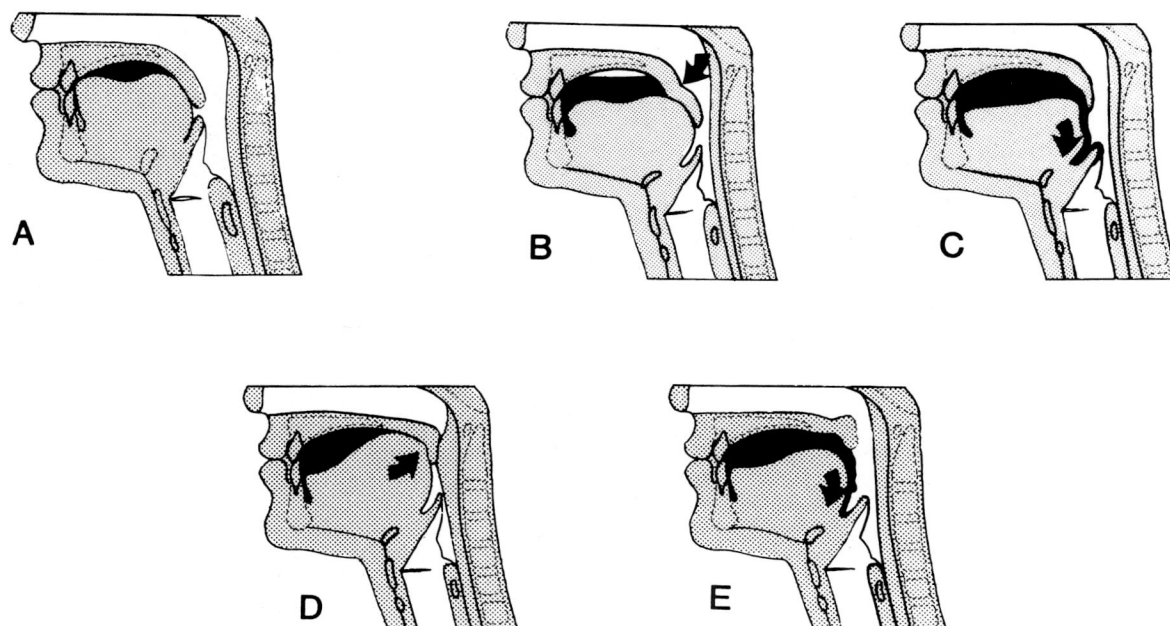

**Figure 16–5. Control of junction of mouth and pharynx (stage 1 of swallowing).** Leakage from the back of the mouth is prevented in the normal patient **(A)** when the soft palate abuts the posterior portion of the tongue. Deficiency of the tongue **(B)** caused by atrophy, weakness, incoordination, or postsurgical defect may be compensated by downward displacement of the palate *(arrow* in **B)**, with the palate "kinking" to appose the tongue. Conversely, palatal deficiency **(D)** is compensated by upward displacement of the tongue *(arrow* in **D)**. Note that the bolus is held farther forward in the mouth under these circumstances. Decompensation **(C** and **E)** in which the oral contents leak prematurely into the pharynx *(arrow* in **C** and **E)** creates the potential for overflow aspiration. **(A** to **E** from Buchholz DW, Bosma JF, Donner MW: Adaptation, compensation, and decompensation of the pharyngeal swallow. Gastrointest Radiol 10:235–239, 1985.)

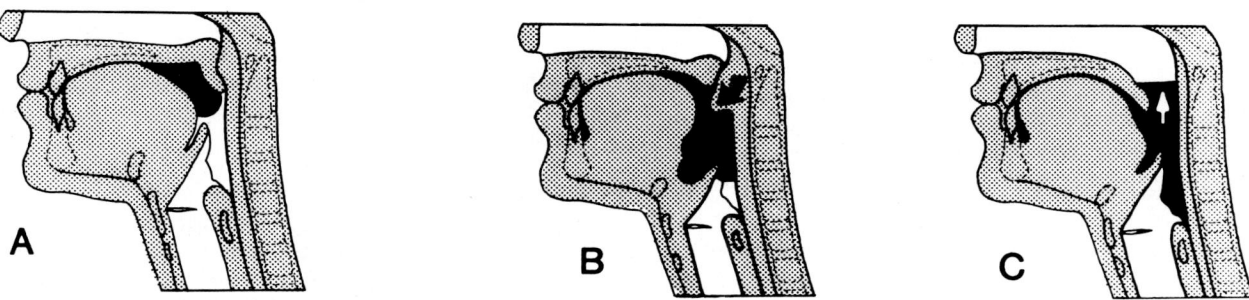

**Figure 16–6. Closure of palatopharyngeal isthmus during swallowing (stage 2 of swallowing).**
**A**. Normal closure, in which the soft palate has elevated to a right angle to abut Passavant's cushion.
**B**. Deficiency of the pharyngeal palate may be compensated by increasing convergence of the pharyngeal constrictor muscles *(arrow)*, resulting in a prominent Passavant's cushion. **C**. Decompensation results in nasopharyngeal regurgitation through the palatopharyngeal isthmus *(arrow)*. **(A** to **C** from Buchholz DW, Bosma JF, Donner MW: Adaptation, compensation, and decompensation of the pharyngeal swallow. Gastrointest Radiol 10:235–239, 1985.)

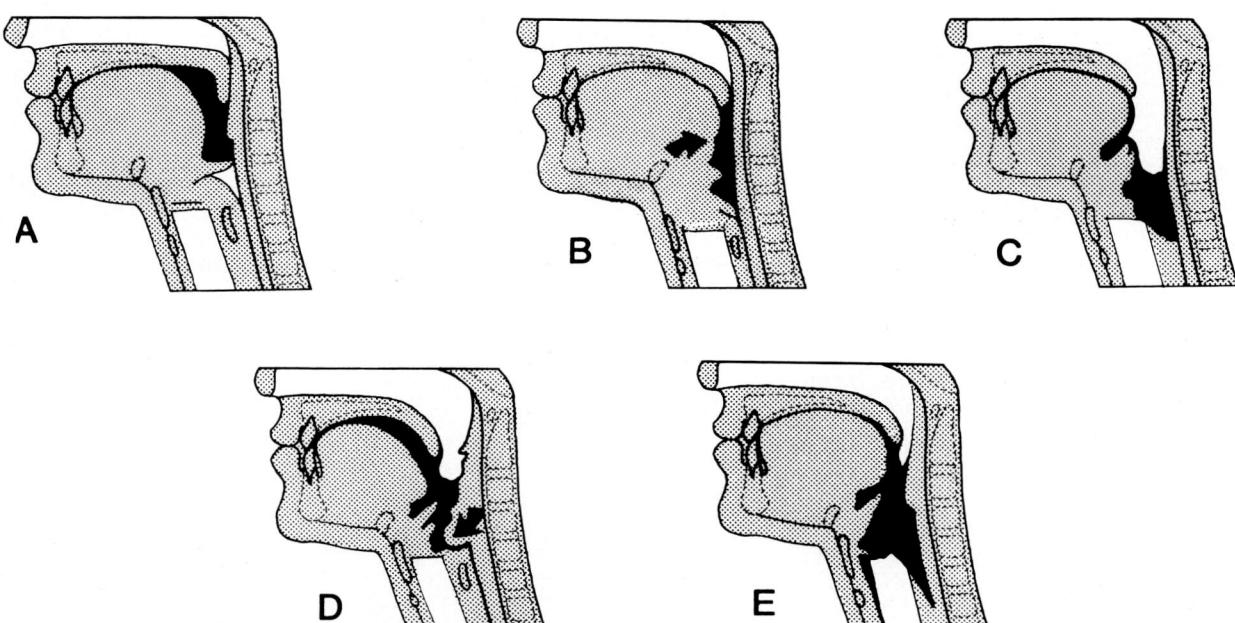

**Figure 16–7. Compression of the bolus (stage 3 of swallowing).** Normal compression is shown (**A**). Deficiency of the constrictor muscles (**B**) may be compensated by upward and posterior displacement of the tongue and larynx (*arrow* in **B**). Deficiency of the tongue in bolus compression (**D**) may be followed by anterior displacement of the constrictor muscle wall (*arrow* in **D**), resulting in a prominent pharyngeal stripping wave. Decompensation attributable to inadequate bolus compression (**C** and **E**) results in bolus retention in the valleculae and piriform sinuses after swallowing, with the potential for overflow aspiration. (**A** to **E** from Buchholz DW, Bosma JF, Donner MW: Adaptation, compensation, and decompensation of the pharyngeal swallow. Gastrointest Radiol 10:235–239, 1985.)

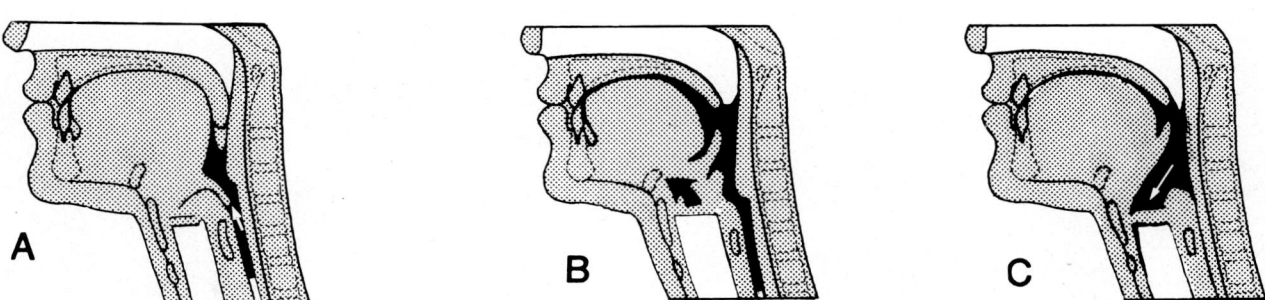

**Figure 16–8. Closure of the larynx (stage 4 of swallowing). A.** The normal condition, in which the larynx is elevated and closed and the epiglottis *(arrow)* is completely tilted downward to cover the entrance to the laryngeal aperture. **B.** With deficiency of epiglottic tilting or of glottic closure, upward and anterior displacement of the larynx *(arrow)* may occur. Occasionally under these circumstances, the arytenoid masses are enlarged as an additional sign of compensation (not illustrated). **C.** Failure of compensation results in penetration of the bolus *(arrow)* into the laryngeal vestibule, and even through the incompletely closed cords, causing aspiration. (**A** to **C** from Buchholz DW, Bosma JF, Donner MW: Adaptation, compensation, and decompensation of the pharyngeal swallow. Gastrointest Radiol 10:235–239, 1985.)

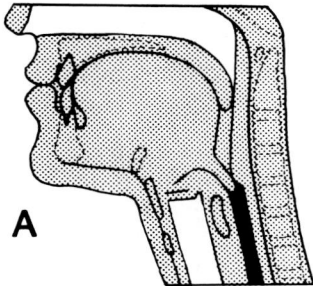 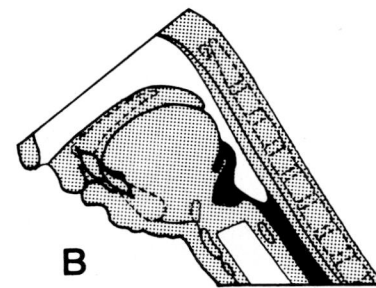 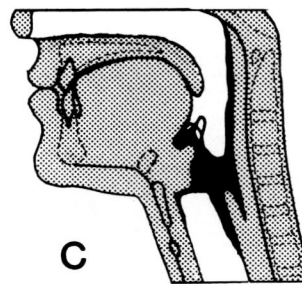

**Figure 16–9. Opening of the pharyngoesophageal (PE) segment (stage 5 of swallowing). A.** Normal opening of PE segment. **B.** Deficiency of upward laryngeal displacement (which contributes to opening of the PE segment) may result in flexion of the neck or in forward thrusting of the jaw or in both, during swallowing. **C.** Failure of compensation results in poor opening of the PE segment, causing retention in the piriform sinuses and the risk of overflow aspiration. (**A** to **C** from Buchholz DW, Bosma JF, Donner MW: Adaptation, compensation, and decompensation of the pharyngeal swallow. Gastrointest Radiol 10:235–239, 1985.)

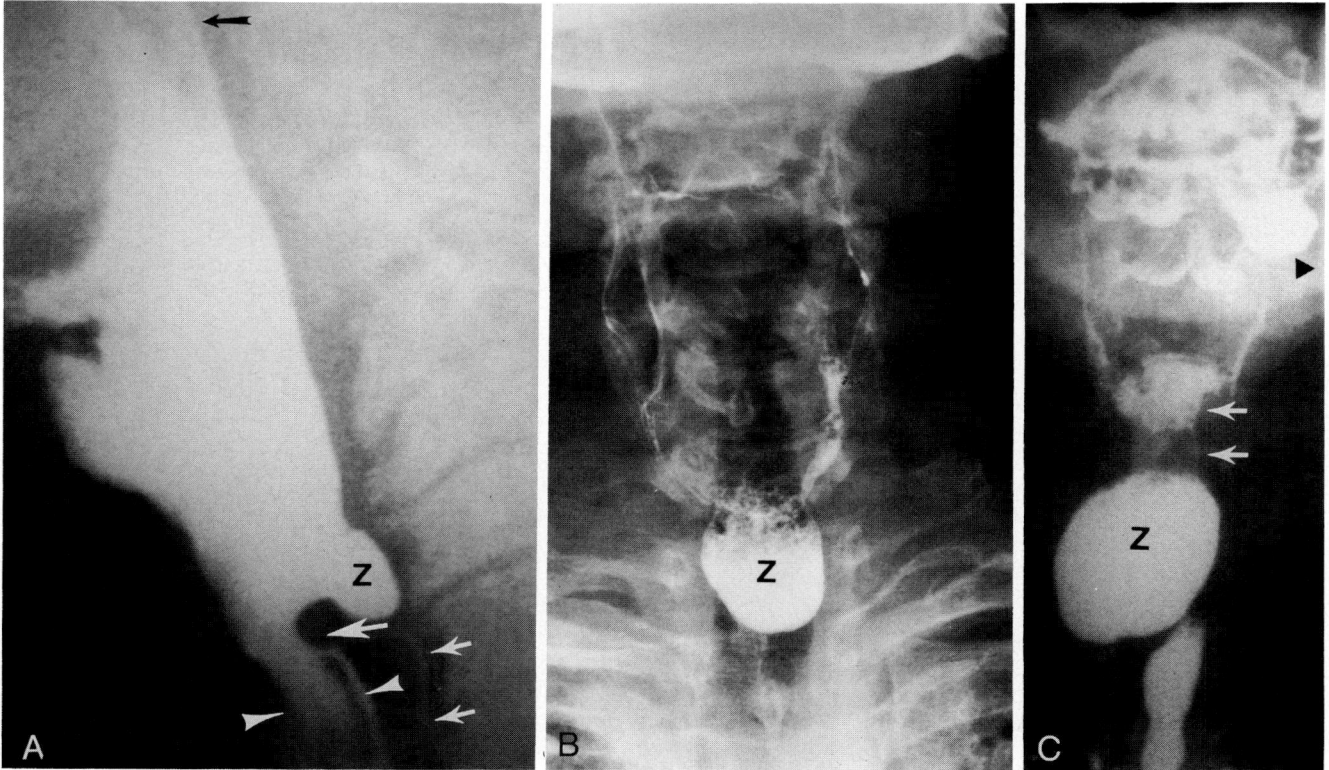

**Figure 16–10. Zenker's diverticulum demonstrated from three aspects. A.** Lateral view shows a small diverticulum (Z) lying above a prominent cricopharyngeus *(large white arrow)*, which causes luminal narrowing of at least 50%. A jet of barium *(arrowheads)* spurts through the prominent cricopharyngeus. Note that the cervical esophageal lumen is actually abutting the spine *(small white arrows)*. Also note nasopharyngeal regurgitation *(black arrow)* and marked degenerative change in the cervical spine. **B.** After swallowing, Zenker's diverticulum (Z) remains filled (anteroposterior view). **C.** Frontal view of another patient shows emptying of the diverticulum (Z) back into the pharynx *(arrows)* after swallowing, which causes this patient to be at risk for overflow aspiration. Note also the buccal pouch on the left side *(arrowhead)*. (**C** from Jones B, Donner MW: Common structural diseases. *In* Jones B, Donner MW [eds]: Normal and Abnormal Swallowing: Imaging in Diagnosis and Therapy. New York: Springer-Verlag, 1991, p 99.)

fell, and full UES opening was restored.[36] These studies suggest that decreased UES compliance may have a major role in the development of Zenker's diverticulum.

Gastroesophageal reflux may contribute to the development of Zenker's diverticulum.[37, 38] In our experience of 36 patients with Zenker's diverticulum, all but 1 had free gastroesophageal reflux, segmental spasm, acid-induced spasm, hiatal hernia, or Schatzki's ring (unpublished observation).

Radiologically, Zenker's diverticulum is almost always associated with prominence of the cricopharyngeus. Esophageal disease may produce prominence of the cricopharyngeus (perhaps with decreased compliance), which in turn may raise intrapharyngeal (and intrabolus) pressure, necessitating more forceful contraction.

Further studies are necessary, including those addressing the early developmental stages of Zenker's diverticulum, before the pathophysiology can be understood.

# GASTROESOPHAGEAL REFLUX

Heartburn and indigestion are not the only effects of gastroesophageal reflux. Direct contact may produce inflammation such as erosive esophagitis and peptic stricture, and remote reflexes may produce other effects[39–41] (Tables 16–6 and 16–7).

Prominence of the cricopharyngeus, observed radiographically, is common in the patient with gastroesophageal reflux. One manometric study, however, failed to demonstrate any response of the UES to spontaneous gastroesophageal reflux in normal volunteers.[42] Another study from the same laboratory showed no change during spontaneous reflux or under experimental conditions in either volunteers or patients with esophagitis.[43]

## TABLE 16–6. REMOTE EFFECTS OF GASTROESOPHAGEAL REFLUX

**PHARYNX**
Pain, or lump or foreign body sensation
  (globus hystericus), or both
Prominent cricopharyngeus
Asymmetry of contraction
Lateral pharyngeal pouches
Zenker's diverticulum

**LARYNX**
Chronic cough
Pain and hoarseness
Laryngitis
Contact granuloma
Laryngeal ulcer
Laryngospasm
Laryngeal cancer (possibly)

**LUNG**
Aspiration pneumonia
Chronic lung disease
Asthma
Sleep apnea

**HEART**
Tachycardia
Bradycardia
Syncope

## TABLE 16–7. REFLEXES ASSOCIATED WITH SWALLOWING

| NORMAL REFLEXES | ABNORMAL REFLEXES |
| --- | --- |
| *Pharynx* | *Cardiovascular System* |
| Gag | Bradycardia or hypotension, |
| Breathing | syncope or seizures |
| Swallow | Tachycardia |
| Laryngeal closure | Hypertension |
| Respiratory suppression | Dysrhythmia |
| | Myocardial insufficiency |
| *Larynx* | |
| Cough | *Respiratory System* |
| Forced inspiration | Laryngospasm |
| Laryngeal closure | Prolonged apnea |
| Respiratory suppression | Bronchospasm |
| Bronchoconstriction | |
| Secretion of mucus | |
| Arousal | |
| | |
| *Esophagus* | |
| Deglutitive inhibition of | |
| peristalsis | |

This study also demonstrated no difference in the basal UES pressure between normal volunteers and patients with esophagitis. Further studies are needed in this area.

# SWALLOWING-RELATED REFLEXES

Many cardiorespiratory reflexes are related to swallowing, resulting from laryngeal, pharyngeal, or esophageal stimulation. Examples include syncope, change in heart rate, apnea, and bronchoconstriction leading to asthma[44–48] (see Table 16–7).

# FUNCTIONAL CHANGES AFTER RADIATION

The acute effects of radiation on pharyngeal function have not, to our knowledge, been studied radiographically. Within days or weeks, mucosal edema occurs. It is most marked over the arytenoid cartilages, although the epiglottis and posterior pharynx are also edematous. The mucosa becomes inflamed and friable, and lymphangiectasia adds to the edema. Endothelial vasculitis produces localized ischemia, which in the long term may result in fibrosis.[49]

The long-term effect of radiation on swallowing has been studied by Ekberg and Nylander in a postoperative study of a group of 13 patients with head and neck cancer who had received radiotherapy before tumor resection.[50] Abnormalities were present in 12 of the 13 patients and consisted of paresis of the constrictor muscle with bolus retention, laryngeal penetration, and cricopharyngeal incoordination. Interestingly, static films produced significant underestimations of the decompensation; dynamic imaging revealed the true extent of the abnormalities. Further studies are needed, especially in patients who receive radiotherapy without resection.

# AGING AND SWALLOWING (PRESBYPHAGIA)

Swallowing in elderly persons is termed *presbyphagia*,[51] and it may be considered under two separate categories:

1. The effects of the normal aging process on swallowing *(primary presbyphagia)*
2. The effects on swallowing of other diseases that affect elderly persons, such as cerebrovascular accidents or Parkinson's disease *(secondary presbyphagia)*

Prevalence studies of the incidence of dysphagia as a symptom of patients in general hospitals and of residents in nursing homes have yielded surprisingly high numbers, namely 12 to 20% of patients in general hospitals and 50% of residents in nursing homes.[52]

Little loss of functioning motoneurons has been shown to occur before 60 years of age, but a striking and progressive depletion has been found to occur subsequently, with deterioration of connective tissue, loss of elasticity, and atrophy of fat.[53] In the oropharynx, the suspensory ligaments of all structures become lax, resulting in premature leakage, low hyoid bone, squaring of the valleculae, and expansion of the pharyngeal cavity.[54-57] Loss of pliability may result in incomplete inversion of the epiglottis and incomplete closure of the larynx.[58] In one study, defective closure of the laryngeal vestibule with laryngeal penetration was found in 70 of 101 patients older than 80 years.[59] Thus, the significance of laryngeal penetration in elderly persons is unknown.

The laryngeal epithelium appears to become less sensitive to aspirated material with increasing age, which may explain why silent aspiration can be a problem.[60] In addition, airway protection may be further compromised by medications for depression, anxiety, or Parkinson's disease.

One study in patients whose ages ranged from younger than 40 to older than 75 years revealed no significant change in speed of peristalsis with increasing age.[61] In older patients, however, the oral and pharyngeal phases may become "uncoupled," resulting in delayed initiation of pharyngeal contraction and early cricopharyngeal closure.[55] Aging also causes a decrease in the time in which the PE segment remains open to allow passage of a bolus.[55]

Borgstrom and Ekberg studied swallowing function in an asymptomatic group of 56 patients whose ages ranged from 72 to 93 years. Normal deglutition (as defined in younger persons) was found in only 16% of patients. Oral abnormalities were found in 63%, pharyngeal abnormalities in 25%, PE segment abnormalities in 39%, and esophageal abnormalities in 36%.[62]

Changes in esophageal motility that occur with increasing age are outside the scope of this discussion.

# NEUROLOGIC DISEASE AND THE PHARYNX

Neuromuscular disorders can cause dysphagia by affecting the afferent or efferent portions of the swallow-

## TABLE 16–8. COMMON NEUROMUSCULAR CAUSES OF DYSPHAGIA

**BRAIN AND BRAIN STEM**
Cerebrovascular accident
Multiple sclerosis
Amyotrophic lateral sclerosis (motor neuron disease)

**MOVEMENT DISORDERS AND NEURODEGENERATIVE DISEASES**
Parkinson's disease
Spinocerebellar degeneration
Olivopontocerebellar atrophy
Huntington's disease
Alzheimer's disease
Dystonia and dyskinesia

**INFECTIONS**
Poliomyelitis
Neurosyphilis
Encephalitis, meningitis

**MYONEURONAL JUNCTION**
Myasthenia gravis
Botulism
Eaton-Lambert syndrome

**MUSCLE DISEASE**
Dystrophy
Polymyositis, dermatomyositis
Ragged red fiber disease (mitochondrial myopathy)

Adapted from Buchholz D: Neurologic causes of dysphagia. Dysphagia 1:152–156, 1987.

ing reflex and by producing abnormalities at many levels: the cerebral cortex, the cranial nerve nuclei in the brain stem, the cranial nerves themselves, the pharyngeal plexus, the neuromuscular junction, the muscles, or sensory feedback[63-65] (Table 16–8).

Dysphagia may be a minor or major symptom; occasionally, it is the predominant or only complaint. For example, acute onset of dysphagia may signal a focal brain stem stroke, or chronic dysphagia may be the presenting symptom of an unrecognized neuromuscular disease such as amyotrophic lateral sclerosis. At the Johns Hopkins Swallowing Center, for example, approximately 30% of our patients have dysphagia in the setting of neuromuscular disease; dysphagia was the predominant or only symptom in 10% of these patients (personal observation, B. Jones).

## Bulbar and Pseudobulbar Palsy

The term *bulbar palsy* implies dysfunction of the motor unit (i.e., a lower motor neuron and the muscle innervated by that lower motor neuron) and may involve cranial nerve nuclei, cranial nerves, the neuromuscular junction, or muscle. This kind of abnormality primarily affects the pharyngeal stage of swallowing. Characteristic signs are atrophy, fasciculation, weakness, flaccidity, and decreased reflexes.

The term *pseudobulbar palsy* refers to a disorder affecting the corticobulbar tract, which is therefore an upper motor neuron abnormality causing weakness accompanied by spasticity, increased reflexes, and spastic dysarthria. Emotional lability is characteristic. Pseudobulbar palsy primarily affects the initiation of the oral phase of swallowing.

Formerly, unilateral abnormality of one corticobulbar tract was not thought to produce a significant swallowing deficit, as each corticobulbar tract supplies both sides of the brain stem with cortical data. Despite the supposed bilateral representation of swallowing, however, dysphagia occurs in 20 to 40% of patients with cerebrovascular accidents, including those with "unilateral" stroke.[66, 67] Robbins and Levine have challenged the theory of bilateral representation of swallowing.[68] These authors studied patients with unilateral cortical strokes (as diagnosed by computed tomography) and compared swallowing abnormalities in the group with infarcts in the right cerebral cortex with those in the group with infarcts in the left cerebral cortex. Initiation of pharyngeal swallowing was delayed in all patients. The left cortical stroke group, however, showed impaired oral stage function, difficulty initiating coordinated motor activity, and apraxia, whereas pharyngeal pooling, penetration, and aspiration were prominent in patients with right cortical stroke. Studies using more sensitive imaging methods, such as magnetic resonance imaging, are in progress to validate these observations.

## Amyotrophic Lateral Sclerosis

Amyotrophic lateral sclerosis, also called *motor neuron disease* and *Lou Gehrig's disease*, can result in bulbar palsy or pseudobulbar palsy, or a combination of both. The disease can produce a wide spectrum of abnormal findings, including muscle weakness and atrophy of lips, tongue, palate, and constrictor muscles with various degrees of retention of secretions.[65, 69] Weakness of intrinsic laryngeal muscles leads to airway penetration and aspiration. The tongue, suprahyoid muscles, and larynx are weak and ptotic in the upright position. Often, the patient compensates by holding the head and neck in a position of sustained extension ("swan neck") to help maintain the airway and swallowing.

## Multiple Sclerosis

Corresponding to the course of the disease itself, impairment of swallowing in multiple sclerosis is relapsing and remitting. The radiographic appearance of the dysphagic pattern depends on the extent and location of the demyelinization, that is, in the white matter of the cerebral cortex, the periventricular areas, the brain stem, the spinal cord, or the cerebellar peduncles. Abnormalities may vary from difficult initiation of swallowing to episodes of choking on liquids or sticking of solid particles. Sensory loss may not reveal the severity of disease, and symptoms may be minimal or absent even in the presence of severe decompensation.[70]

## NEURODEGENERATIVE DISORDERS

Parkinson's disease is associated with dysphagia in as many as 50% of patients. Delayed initiation of swallowing and problems with oral transfer predominate. The findings include lingual tremor or rocking, squeezing of the bolus between tongue and palate, "piecemeal" deglutition, and hesitancy to propel the bolus into the pharynx.[64, 71] Airway penetration, silent aspiration, and retention in valleculae and piriform sinuses after a delayed swallowing reflex are also common.

The esophagus may also be involved in Parkinson's disease, with loss of the primary stripping wave. Whether this loss is an intrinsic problem of esophageal motility or whether the peristaltic wave is absent because there is no pharyngeal contraction (i.e., no "message" to the esophagus) is not known. Qualman and co-workers reported that patients with Parkinson's disease and achalasia had degeneration of the dorsal vagal motor nucleus. The same study demonstrated that Lewy's bodies, typically found in the vagal nucleus and substantia nigra in Parkinson's disease, could be found in the esophageal myenteric plexus in achalasia.[72]

Huntington's disease,[73] progressive supranuclear palsy, and Alzheimer's disease may also produce dysphagia and feeding difficulties. The oropharyngeal findings are similar to those of Parkinson's disease. Dementia, other cognitive problems, and uncontrolled movements may complicate feeding and rehabilitation.

Similarly, dystonia and dyskinesia may result in dysphagia or feeding difficulties because of the involuntary localized muscle contractions. In dystonia, the tonically contracted tongue, positioned in a tight mass in the back of the oral cavity, appears characteristically as "fisted." To swallow, the patient tilts the head into extreme extension, by which movement the bolus is "decanted" into the pharynx.[74]

## INFECTIONS

Viral infections of the nervous system may cause dysphagia.[63, 64] For example, a patient with bulbar poliomyelitis may present with pharyngeal paralysis, aspiration, and disturbance of vasomotor control if motoneurons in the medullary reticular formation, especially those in or near the nucleus ambiguus, are involved. Acute bulbar poliomyelitis is now rare in geographic areas with mass vaccination, but it is still observed in countries in which vaccination is not widespread.

A phenomenon called *postpolio syndrome* causes symptoms of increasing weakness beginning 20 or more years after an acute attack of poliomyelitis; symptoms may include dysphagia.[75, 76] In the minority of patients, the symptoms are progressive, and this progressive disorder has been called *postpolio progressive muscular atrophy*. Buchholz and Jones reported 13 patients with dysphagia who had a remote history of acute poliomyelitis.[77] We recently reviewed the dynamic imaging studies of 20 patients with dysphagia and a remote history of poliomyelitis.[78] Multiple abnormalities were present, including atrophy of prevertebral soft tissues, pharyngeal paresis or paralysis with retention after swallowing, incomplete or absent epiglottic tilt, laryngeal penetration or aspiration, luminal narrowing caused by a prominent cricopharyngeus, palatal weakness, incomplete laryngeal closure, and poor or absent laryngeal elevation (Fig. 16–11).

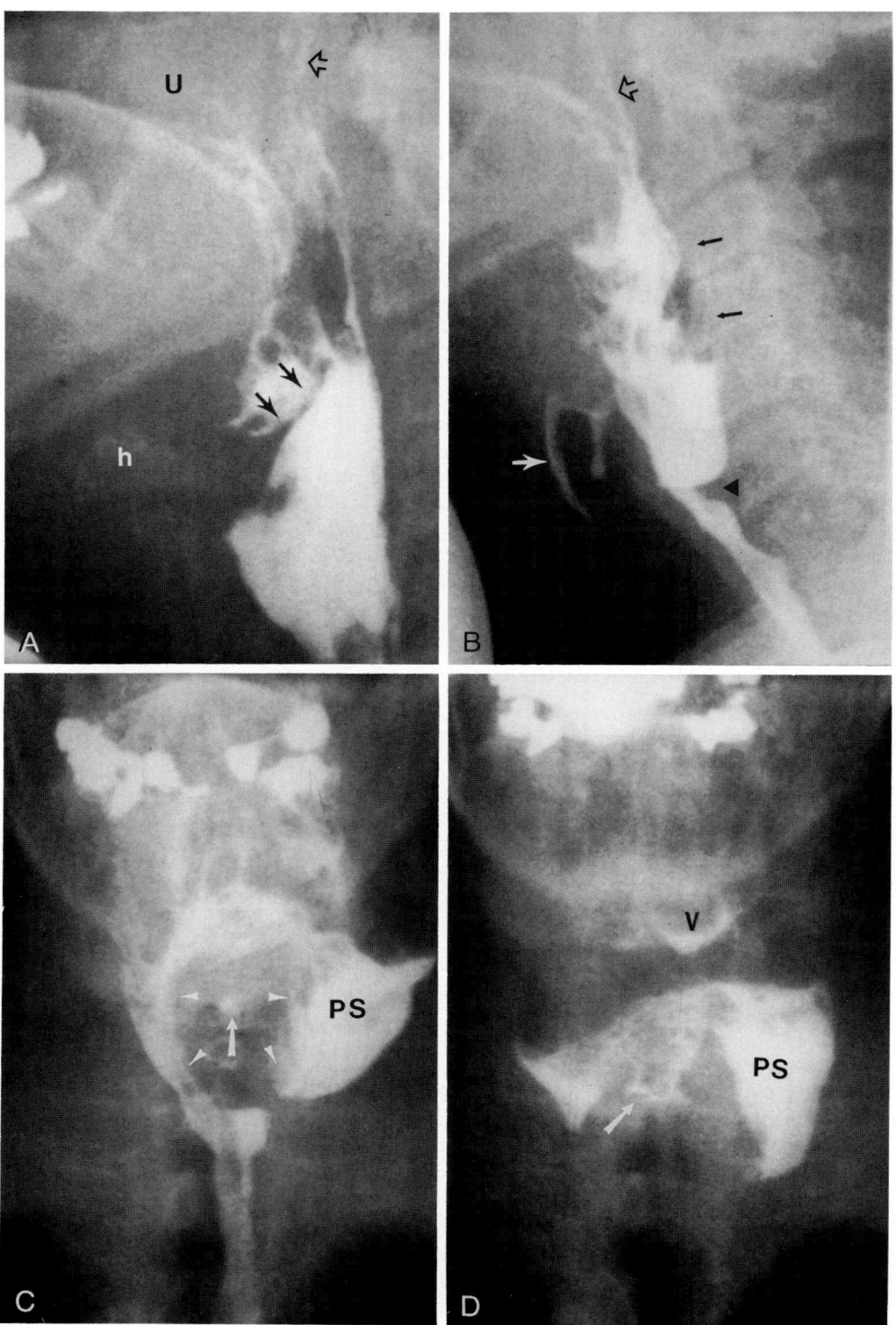

**Figure 16–11. Postpoliomyelitis dysphagia. A**. Lateral view shows incomplete elevation of the soft palate (U) and minimal nasopharyngeal regurgitation *(open arrow)*. Passavant's cushion is not evident. The bolus is past the epiglottis *(solid arrows)*, which has remained almost completely upright, and there is incomplete elevation of the hyoid bone (h), which has not moved anteriorly. **B**. Atrophy of the pharyngeal muscles is manifested as wrapping of the pharynx posteriorly around the cervical spine *(solid black arrows)*. Laryngeal penetration *(solid white arrow)* has occurred. Prominence of the cricopharyngeus *(arrowhead)* and poor distention of the cervical esophagus below the cricopharyngeus can be seen. Note nasopharyngeal regurgitation *(open arrow)*. **C**. Frontal view shows asymmetry of distention, with the left piriform sinus (PS) bulging much more than the right piriform sinus because of weakness of the constrictor muscles. A small amount of contrast medium is present in the laryngeal vestibule *(arrow)*, and a moderate flow defect *(arrowheads)* can be seen. **D**. After passage of the bolus, marked retention occurs in the left piriform sinus (PS), which is larger than the right piriform sinus, in which mild retention occurs. Also, the vallecula (V) shows asymmetric retention. Contrast medium also appears in the laryngeal vestibule and ventricle *(arrow)*.

Sonies and Dalakas evaluated 32 postpoliomyelitis patients with videofluoroscopy and ultrasound; 18 of the patients did not report dysphagia.[79] Despite the lack of symptoms in some, all but one of the patients had abnormalities of oropharyngeal function, which varied in severity.

## MYASTHENIA GRAVIS AND RELATED DISORDERS

Myasthenia gravis[80] and the Eaton-Lambert myasthenic-myopathic syndrome[81] are myoneural junction disorders involving diminished release or inadequate binding of acetylcholine. In addition to ocular and proximal limb weakness, dysphagia or choking may occur, characteristically appearing late in the day. Slowing of swallowing or decompensation after repetitive swallowing may suggest the diagnosis during dynamic studies.

Eaton-Lambert syndrome (carcinomatous neuropathy) is most often seen with oat cell carcinoma of the lung, but it has also been reported in association with carcinoma of the breast, prostate, stomach, and rectum.[81] Diplopia, dysarthria, and dysphagia may accompany weakness of muscles of the trunk, pelvis, and shoulder girdle, the most common sites affected.

Botulism also affects transmission at the myoneuronal junction and may result in dysphagia.[63, 64] Interestingly, botulin has been used to treat a variety of dystonias including torticollis; in a small number of patients, dysphagia may result as a side effect.[82]

## FAMILIAL DYSAUTONOMIA (RILEY-DAY SYNDROME)

Characteristic findings in this syndrome are delay in cricopharyngeal relaxation with airway penetration.[83]

## DISEASES OF MUSCLE

Diseases prominently affecting bulbar muscles may be due to inflammatory disease (polymyositis, dermatomyositis, sarcoidosis);[84] metabolic or endocrine disease (mitochondrial myopathy); dysthyroid myopathy (hypothyroidism or hyperthyroidism); a prolonged course of steroid medication; or muscular dystrophy. The last category includes myotonic dystrophy (pharyngeal and esophageal motility disturbances),[85] Duchenne's muscular dystrophy, and oculopharyngeal dystrophy.[86] Bilateral pharyngeal paresis occurs with bolus retention; the cricopharyngeus may be prominent but closes with normal timing. The cervical esophagus may also be abnormal with diminished or absent peristalsis. The use of chilled barium makes the abnormalities more prominent in myotonic dystrophy.[87]

## MEDICATIONS

Medications may induce or aggravate myasthenia gravis, dystonia,[74] myopathy, or neuropathy. More than 30 drugs in current clinical use may interfere with neuromuscular transmission, among them antibiotics such as neomycin, streptomycin, and certain tetracyclines,[88, 89] and immunosuppressant agents such as adrenocorticotropic hormone, prednisone, and azathioprine.[90, 91] Sedatives, antipsychotic drugs, and antidepressants may produce extrapyramidal symptoms and signs of muscle spasm or dystonia or may unmask a latent neuromuscular disease.[90] Ideally, such drugs are temporarily stopped for several days before a swallowing study. Use of tryptophan has been associated with the development of an eosinophilia-myalgia syndrome.[92–94] Studies suggest that the cause of this syndrome was related to a chemical constituent associated with the specific manufacturing conditions at one company rather than to tryptophan itself.[94]

## References

1. Edwards DAW: History and symptoms of esophageal disease of the esophagus. *In* Vantrappen G, Hellemans J (eds): Diseases of the Esophagus. New York: Springer-Verlag, 1972, pp 103–105.
2. Jones B, Ravich WJ, Donner MW, et al: Pharyngoesophageal interrelationships: observations and working concepts. Gastrointest Radiol 10:225–233, 1985.
3. Bosma JF: Deglutition: pharyngeal state. Physiol Rev 37:275–300, 1957.
4. Miller AJ: Deglutition. Physiol Rev 62:129–184, 1982.
5. Donner MW, Bosma JF, Robertson DL: Anatomy and physiology of the pharynx. Gastrointest Radiol 10:196–212, 1985.
6. Miller AJ: Neurophysiological basis of swallowing. Dysphagia 1:91–100, 1986.
7. Miller AJ: Swallowing: neurophysiologic control of the esophageal phase. Dysphagia 2:72–82, 1987.
8. Dodds WJ, Stewart ET, Logemann JA: Physiology and radiology of the normal oral and pharyngeal phases of swallowing. AJR 154:953–963, 1990.
9. Dodds WJ, Taylor AJ, Stewart ET, et al: Tipper and dipper types of oral swallows. AJR 153:1197–1199, 1989.
10. Zerhouni EA, Bosma JF, Donner MW: Relationship of cervical spine disorders to dysphagia. Dysphagia 1:129–144, 1987.
11. Torres WE, Clements JL, Austin GE, et al: Cricopharyngeal muscle hypertrophy: radiologic anatomic correlation. AJR 141:927–930, 1984.
12. Seaman WB: Functional disorders of the pharyngoesophageal junction: achalasia and chalasia. Radiol Clin North Am 7:113–119, 1969.
13. Sokol EM, Heitman P, Wolfe BS, et al: Simultaneous cineradiographic and manometric study of the pharynx, hypopharynx, and cervical esophagus. Gastroenterology 51:960–974, 1966.
14. Templeton RE, Kredel RA: Cricopharyngeal sphincter: roentgenologic study. Laryngoscope 53:1–12, 1943.
15. Crichlow TVL: Cricopharyngeus in radiography and cineradiography. Br J Radiol 29:546–556, 1956.
16. Seaman WB: Cineroentgenographic observations of the cricopharyngeus. AJR 96:922–931, 1966.
17. Palmer ED: Disorders of the cricopharyngeus muscle: a review. Gastroenterology 71:510–517, 1976.
18. Roed-Peterson K: The pharyngo-esophageal sphincter: a review of the literature. Dan Med Bull 26:275–281, 1979.
19. Ekberg O, Nylander B: Dysfunction of the cricopharyngeal muscle. Radiology 143:481–486, 1982.
20. Curtis DJ, Cruess DF, Berg T: The cricopharyngeal muscle: a videorecording review. AJR 142:497–500, 1984.

21. Kahrilas PJ, Dodds WJ, Dent J, et al: Upper esophageal sphincter function during deglutition. Gastroenterology 95:52–62, 1988.

22. Jacob P, Kahrilas PJ, Logemann JA, et al: Upper esophageal sphincter opening and modulation during swallowing. Gastroenterology 97:1469–1478, 1989.

23. Curtis DJ: Laryngeal dynamics. Crit Rev Diagn Imaging 19:29–80, 1982.

24. Dodds WJ, Man KM, Cook IJ, et al: Influence of bolus volume on swallow-induced hyoid movement in normal subjects. AJR 150:1307–1309, 1988.

25. Ekberg O: The normal movements of the hyoid bone during swallow. Invest Radiol 21:408–410, 1986.

26. Ekberg O, Sigurjonsson S: Movements of the epiglottis during deglutition: a cineradiographic study. Gastrointest Radiol 7:101–107, 1982.

27. Ekberg O, Hilderfors H: Defective closure of the laryngeal vestibule: frequency of pulmonary complications. AJR 145:1159–1164, 1985.

28. Palmer JB, DuChane AS, Donner MW: Role of radiology in rehabilitation of swallowing. *In* Jones B, Donner MW (eds): Normal and Abnormal Swallowing: Imaging in Diagnosis and Therapy. New York: Springer-Verlag, 1991, pp 215–225.

29. Feinberg MJ, Ekberg O: Deglutition after near-fatal choking episode: radiologic evaluation. Radiology 176:637–640, 1990.

30. Dantas RO, Dodds WJ, Massey BT, et al: The effect of high- vs. low-density barium preparations on the quantitative features of swallowing. AJR 153:1191–1195, 1989.

31. Buchholz DW, Bosma JF, Donner MW: Adaptation, compensation, and decompensation of the pharyngeal swallow. Gastrointest Radiol 10:235–240, 1985.

32. Dohlman G, Mattsson O: The role of the cricopharyngeal muscle in cases of hypopharyngeal diverticula. AJR 81:561–569, 1959.

33. Knuff TE, Benjamin SB, Castell DO: Pharyngoesophageal (Zenker's) diverticulum: a reappraisal. Gastroenterology 82:734–736, 1982.

34. Cook IJ, Gabb M, Panagopoulos V, et al: Zenker's diverticulum: a defect in upper esophageal sphincter compliance. Gastroenterology 96:A98, 1989 (abstract).

35. Cook IJ, Blumbergs P, Cash K, et al: Zenker's diverticulum: evidence for a restrictive cricopharyngeal myopathy. Gastroenterology 96:A98, 1989 (abstract).

36. Shaw DW, Cook IJ, Simula ME, et al: Restoration of normal upper esophageal sphincter compliance following cricopharyngeal myotomy in patients with Zenker's diverticulum. Gastroenterology 95:A122, 1990 (abstract).

37. Smiley TB, Caves PK, Porter DC: Relationship between posterior pharyngeal pouch and hiatus hernia. Thorax 25:725–731, 1970.

38. Delahunty JE, Margulies SE, Alonso UA, et al: The relationship of reflux esophagitis to pharyngeal pouch (Zenker's diverticulum). Laryngoscope 81:570–577, 1971.

39. Bain WM, Harriggton JW, Thomas LE, et al: Head and neck manifestations of gastroesophageal reflux. Laryngoscope 93:175–179, 1983.

40. Weiner GJ, Koufman JA, Wu WC, et al: Chronic hoarseness secondary to gastroesophageal reflux disease: documentation with 24-hour ambulatory pH monitoring. Am J Gastroenterol 84:1503–1508, 1989.

41. Deschner KW, Benjamin SB: Extraesophageal manifestations of reflux gastroesophageal reflux disease. Am J Gastroenterol 84:1–5, 1989.

42. Kahrilas PJ, Dodds WJ, Dent J, et al: Effect of sleep, spontaneous gastroesophageal reflux, and a meal on upper esophageal sphincter pressure in normal human volunteers. Gastroenterology 92:466–471, 1987.

43. Vakil NB, Kahrilas PJ, Dodds WJ, et al: Absence of an upper esophageal sphincter response to acid reflux. Am J Gastroenterol 84:606–610, 1989.

44. Thach BT, Davies AM, Koenig JS, et al: Reflex induced apneas. *In* Issa FG, Suratt PM, Remmers JE (eds): Sleep and Respiration. New York: Wiley-Liss, 1990, pp 77–87.

45. Loughlin GM: Respiratory consequences of dysfunctional swallowing and aspiration. Dysphagia 3:126–130, 1989.

46. Levin B, Posner JB: Swallow syncope: report of a case and review of the literature. Neurology 22:1086–1093, 1972.

47. Kalloo AN, Lewis JH, Maher K, et al: Swallowing: an unusual case of syncope. Dig Dis Sci 34:1117–1120, 1989.

48. Wright RA, Miller SA, Corsello BF: Acid-induced esophagobronchial-cardiac reflexes in humans. Gastroenterology 99:71–73, 1990.

49. Libshitz HI (ed): Diagnostic Roentgenology of Radiotherapy Change. Baltimore: Williams & Wilkins, 1979.

50. Ekberg O, Nylander G: Pharyngeal dysfunction after treatment for pharyngeal cancer with surgery and radiotherapy. Gastrointest Radiol 8:97–104, 1983.

51. Kashima HK: Presbyphagia: introduction. *In* Goldstein JC, Kashima HK, Koopmann CF (eds): Geriatric Otorhinolaryngology. Toronto: BC Decker, 1989, pp 122–123.

52. Groher ME, Bukatman R: The prevalence of swallowing disorders in two teaching hospitals. Dysphagia 1:3–6, 1986.

53. McComas AF, Lipton ARM, Sica REP: Motoneuron disease and aging. Lancet 2:1477–1480, 1973.

54. Baum BJ, Bodner L: Aging and oral motor function: evidence for altered performance among older persons. J Dent Res 62:2–6, 1983.

55. Tracy JF, Logemann JA, Kahrilas PJ, et al: Preliminary observations on the effects of age on oropharyngeal deglutition. Dysphagia 4:90–94, 1989.

56. Ekberg O, Feinberg MJ: Altered swallowing function in elderly patients without dysphagia: radiologic findings in 56 cases. AJR 156:1181–1184, 1991.

57. Shaker R, Dodds WJ, Hogan WJ, et al: Effect of aging on swallow induced lingual palatal closure pressure. Gastroenterology 96:A464, 1989 (abstract).

58. Sonies BC, Stone M, Shawker T: Speech and swallowing in the elderly. Gerodontology 3:115–123, 1984.

59. Kahane JC: Postnatal development and aging of the human larynx. Semin Speech Lang 4:189–203, 1983.

60. Borgstrom PS, Ekberg O: Pharyngeal dysfunction in the elderly. J Med Imaging 2:74–81, 1988.

61. Pontoppidan H, Beecher HK: Progressive loss of protective reflexes in the airway with the advance of age. JAMA 174:2209–2213, 1960.

62. Borgstrom PS, Ekberg O: Speed of peristalsis in pharyngeal constrictor musculature: correlations to age. Dysphagia 2:140–144, 1988.

63. Buchholz D: Neurologic causes of dysphagia. Dysphagia 1:152–156, 1987.

64. Kirshner S: Causes of neurogenic dysphagia. Dysphagia 3:184–188, 1989.

65. Silbiger ML, Pikheney R, Donner MW: Neuromuscular disorders affecting the pharynx: cineradiographic analysis. Invest Radiol 2:442–448, 1967.

66. Veis SL, Logemann JA: Swallowing disorders in persons with cerebrovascular accident. Arch Phys Med Rehabil 66:372–375, 1985.

67. Gordon C, Hewer RL, Wade DT: Dysphagia in acute stroke. Br Med J 295:411–414, 1987.

68. Robbins JA, Levine RL: Swallowing after unilateral stroke of the cerebral cortex: preliminary experience. Dysphagia 3:11–17, 1988.

69. Garfinkle TJ, Kimmelman CP: Neurologic disorders: amyotrophic lateral sclerosis, myasthenia gravis, multiple sclerosis and poliomyelitis. Am J Otolaryngol 3:204–212, 1982.

70. Daly DD, Code CF, Anderson HA: Disturbances of swallowing and esophageal motility in patients with multiple sclerosis. Neurology 59:250–256, 1962.

71. Lieberman AN, Horowitz L, Redmond P, et al: Dysphagia in Parkinson's disease. Am J Gastroenterol 74:157–160, 1980.

72. Qualman SJ, Haupt HM, Yang P, et al: Esophageal Lewy bodies associated with ganglion cell loss in achalasia. Gastroenterology 87:848–856, 1984.

73. Leopold NA, Kagel MC: Dysphagia in Huntington's disease. Neurology 42:57–60, 1985.

74. Bosma JF, Geoffrey VC, Thach BT, et al: A pattern of medication-induced persistent bulbar and cervical dystonia. Int J Orofacial Myology 8:5–18, 1982.

75. Dalakas MC, Elder G, Hallett M, et al: A long term follow-up study of patients with post-poliomyelitis neuromuscular symptoms. N Engl J Med 314:959–963, 1986.

76. Cashman NR, Maselli R, Wollmann RL, et al: Late denervation in patients with antecedent paralytic poliomyelitis. N Engl J Med 317:7–12, 1987.

77. Buchholz DW, Jones B: Dysphagia after polio. Dysphagia 6:165–169, 1991.

78. Jones B, Buchholz DW, Ravich WJ, et al: Swallowing dysfunction in the post-polio syndrome: a cinefluorographic study. AJR 158:283–286, 1992.

79. Sonies BC, Dalakas MC: Dysphagia in patients with the post-polio syndrome. N Engl J Med 324:1162–1167, 1991.

80. Murray JP: Deglutition in myasthenia gravis. Br J Radiol 35:43–52, 1962.

81. Eaton LM, Lambert EH: Electromyography and electric stimulation of nerves and diseases of motor unit: observations on myasthenia syndrome associated with malignant tumors. JAMA 163:1117–1124, 1957.

82. Jankovic J, Brin MF: Therapeutic uses of botulinum toxin. N Engl J Med 324:1186–1194, 1991.

83. Margulies SI, Bruint PW, Donner MW, et al: Familial dysautonomia: a cineradiographic study of the swallowing mechanism. Radiology 90:107–112, 1968.

84. Merieux P, Verity M, Clements P, et al: Esophageal abnormalities and dysphagia in polymyositis and dermatomyositis: clinical, radiographic, and pathologic features. Arthritis Rheum 26:961–968, 1983.

85. Siegel CI, Hendrix TR, Harvey JC: The swallowing disorder in myotonia dystrophica. Gastroenterology 50:541–550, 1966.

86. Duranceau A, Jamieson G, Clemont RJ: Oropharyngeal dysphagia in patients with oculopharyngeal muscular dystrophy. Can J Surg 21:326–329, 1978.

87. Bosma JF, Brodie DR: Cineradiographic demonstration of pharyngeal area myotonia in myotonic dystrophy patients. Radiology 92:104–109, 1969.

88. McQuillen MP, Cantor HE, O'Rourke JR Jr: Myasthenic syndrome associated with antibiotics. Arch Neurol 18:402–415, 1968.

89. Pittinger CB, Eryasa Y, Adamson R: Antibiotic-induced paralysis. Anesth Analg 49:487–501, 1970.

90. Swift TR: Disorders of neuromuscular transmission other than myasthenia gravis. Muscle Nerve 4:334–353, 1981.

91. Adams RD, Victor M: Principles of Neurology (4th ed). New York: McGraw-Hill, 1989.

92. Hertzman PA, Blevins WL, Mayer J, et al: Association of the eosinophilia-myalgia syndrome with the ingestion of tryptophan. N Engl J Med 322:869–873, 1990.

93. Dicker RM, James N, Cunha BA: The eosinophilia-myalgia syndrome with neuritis associated with L-tryptophan use. Ann Intern Med 112:957–958, 1990.

94. Belongia EA, Hederg CW, Gleich GJ, et al: An investigation of the cause of the eosinophilia-myalgia syndrome associated with tryptophan use. N Engl J Med 323:357–365, 1990.

# Structural Abnormalities

Stephen E. Rubesin, M.D.

David M. Yousem, M.D.

## INTRODUCTION

This chapter focuses on structural abnormalities of the pharynx. The background anatomy and techniques have been discussed in Chapter 15. The radiologist must remember that a dynamic examination (videofluoroscopy or cineradiography) of motility is integrated with a double contrast spot film examination of morphologic features. Furthermore, structural abnormalities may cause problems in motility, and motility disorders may be manifested by structural changes on spot films. Thus, the radiologist performs an interactive examination that tailors dynamic and morphologic studies to the clinical history, symptoms, and fluoroscopic findings.[1]

## PHARYNGEAL POUCHES AND DIVERTICULA

The terminology of pharyngeal pouches and diverticula is confusing. Knowledge of the muscular anatomy and embryology of the pharynx allows a classification of pharyngeal outpouchings into five main categories: 1) lateral pharyngeal pouches and diverticula; 2) laryngocele; 3) branchial cysts; 4) Zenker's diverticulum; and 5) Killian-Jamieson pouches and diverticula.

### Lateral Pharyngeal Pouches and Diverticula

The lateral pharyngeal wall may protrude out of the normal contour of the pharynx, especially in areas of weakness—namely, the regions of the tonsillar fossa and the thyrohyoid membrane. The tonsillar fossa is poorly supported laterally by the flat superior constrictor muscle and the palatopharyngeal muscle.[2] The tonsillar fossa wall is further weakened by tonsillectomy or by atrophy of the palatine tonsil with age. The upper lateral pharyngeal wall is poorly supported in the region of the posterior thyrohyoid membrane.[2] This region is bounded superiorly by the greater cornu of the hyoid bone, anteriorly by the thyrohyoid muscle, posteriorly by the superior cornu of the thyroid cartilage and the stylopharyngeal muscle, and inferiorly by the ala of the thyroid cartilage.[3] This unsupported part of the thyrohyoid membrane is perforated by the superior laryngeal artery and vein and the internal laryngeal branch of the superior laryngeal nerve.[2]

Patients with lateral pharyngeal pouches usually have no symptoms. Occasionally, patients may complain of dysphagia, choking, or regurgitation of undigested food.[4, 5] Lateral pharyngeal pouches are extremely common. The frequency of occurrence of lateral pharyngeal pouches increases with age.[2] Pouches are usually bilateral.

On frontal views during swallowing, pouches appear as transient, hemispheric, contrast-filled protrusions from the lateral hypopharyngeal wall, below the hyoid bone and above the calcified edge of the thyroid cartilage. The junction of the ala of the thyroid cartilage and the thyrohyoid membrane is seen on frontal views as a notch in the lateral pharyngeal wall.[3] During double contrast frontal views in which a modified Valsalva maneuver is used, pouches are seen as hemispheric, barium-coated protrusions above the "notch" in the

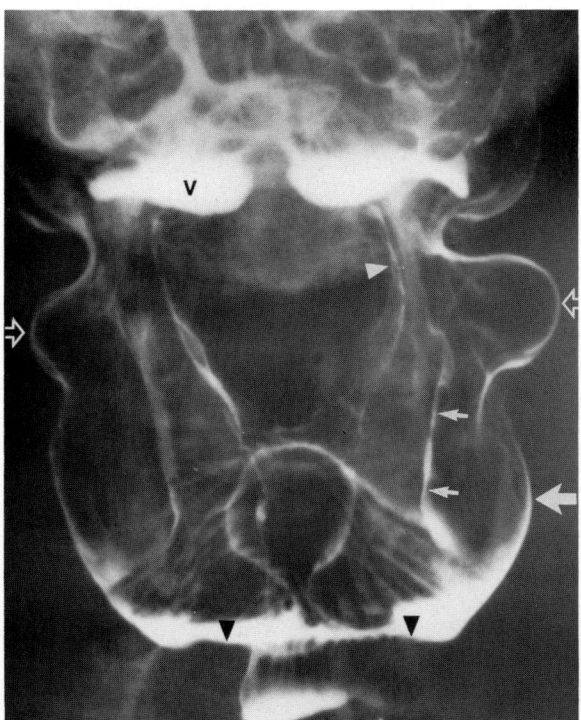

**Figure 17–1. Lateral pharyngeal pouches.** A frontal view of the pharynx during modified Valsalva maneuver shows right and left lateral pharyngeal pouches *(open arrows)* protruding through the region of the thyrohyoid membrane. The lower hypopharynx *(large arrow)* protrudes posteriorly and laterally beyond the confines of the ala of the thyroid cartilage *(small arrows)*. Laryngeal penetration is evidenced by barium coating of the laryngeal surface of the epiglottis and aryepiglottic folds *(white arrowhead)*. Pharyngeal muscle weakness is evidenced by ballooning of the lower hypopharynx *(black arrowheads)*, an area usually collapsed by tonicity of the pharyngoesophageal segment and protrusion of the larynx into the lower hypopharynx. V = vallecula. (From Rubesin SE: Pharyngeal dysfunction. *In* Gore R [ed]: Syllabus for Categorical Course on Gastrointestinal Radiology. Reston, VA: American College of Radiology, 1991, pp 1–9.)

lateral pharyngeal wall[3] (Fig. 17–1). On the lateral view, pouches are seen as oval ring shadows (occasionally filled with an air-contrast level) below the hyoid bone at the level of the valleculae, just behind the epiglottic plate, along the anterior hypopharyngeal wall.[2, 3] Barium that is retained in pouches during swallowing spills into the ipsilateral piriform sinus after the bolus passes. This spill may result in dysphagia or a choking sensation because of overflow aspiration.[5, 6]

Lateral pharyngeal diverticula are persistent protrusions of pharyngeal mucosa usually through the thyrohyoid membrane or, rarely, through the tonsillar fossa.[2, 4] The diverticula are lined by nonkeratinizing squamous epithelium that is surrounded by areolar connective tissue with many vascular spaces.[4] These protrusions are commonly associated with increased intrapharyngeal pressure (i.e., they are seen in wind instrument players, glass blowers, and patients with severe sneezing episodes). Clinical symptoms may include dysphagia, choking, cough, hoarseness, regurgitation of undigested

food, or a painless neck mass.[2, 4] Radiographically, the diverticula are persistent, barium-filled sacs of various sizes connected to a bulging lateral hypopharyngeal wall by a narrow neck (Fig. 17–2). They are usually unilateral.

## Laryngocele

Lateral pharyngeal diverticula should not be confused with laryngoceles. A laryngocele is an abnormal saccular dilatation of the appendix of the laryngeal ventricle. The laryngocele is a protrusion of ciliated pseudostratified columnar epithelium and loose areolar connective tissue arising in the larynx.[7] In contrast, a pharyngeal diverticulum is a protrusion of nonkeratinizing squamous mucosa originating in the pharynx.

The appendix (saccule) of the laryngeal ventricle arises from the anterior end of the lateral recess of the laryngeal ventricle.[8] The appendix courses superiorly in the paralaryngeal space and is lateral to the false vocal cord and aryepiglottic fold, medial to the thyroid cartilage, and anterior to the pharynx. If the saccular dilatation of the appendix is confined by the thyroid cartilage, it is termed *internal laryngocele*. If the dilatation extends above the thyroid cartilage and through the thyrohyoid membrane, the sac is termed *external laryngocele*. A combination of internal and external laryngocele is termed *mixed laryngocele*. Approximately 20% of these lesions are bilateral.[9] Approximately 15% of these lesions are associated with a laryngeal neoplasm.[8, 9]

Patients with laryngoceles and lateral pharyngeal diverticula have similar symptoms and physical findings. Most patients are asymptomatic and in the fifth to sixth decade of life.[7] Patients with external or mixed laryngoceles may have a compressible lateral neck mass. Patients with internal laryngoceles may complain of hoarseness, dysphagia, or choking. Laryngoceles are seen in patients with increased intralaryngeal pressure, such as glass blowers and wind instrument players.

Frontal plain films of patients with an external laryngocele show an air-filled sac above and lateral to the ala of the thyroid cartilage. The lateral plain film shows the air-filled sac anterior to the epiglottic plate, in contrast to a lateral pharyngeal diverticulum, which lies posterior to the epiglottic plate.[2] External and internal laryngoceles do not fill with barium on pharyngograms. However, barium studies may reveal enlargement of the aryepiglottic fold with a smooth overlying mucosa.

Cross-sectional imaging of internal laryngoceles may demonstrate a mass filled with air or fluid, or both, in the paralaryngeal space.[10] An external laryngocele appears as a mass that extends through the thyrohyoid membrane, is anterior to the jugular vein and carotid artery, and is medial to the sternocleidomastoid muscle[10] (Fig. 17–3). The density of the mass may be that of air, fluid, or soft tissue. Laryngoceles of soft tissue density are filled with either mucus or infected secretions (laryngopyocele).

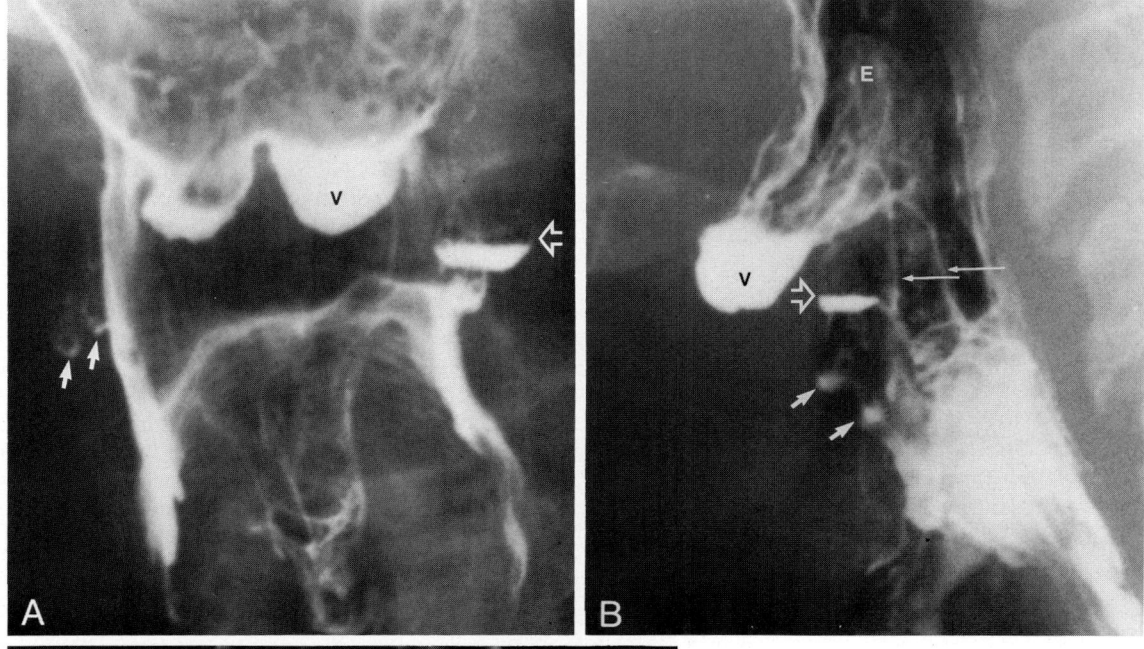

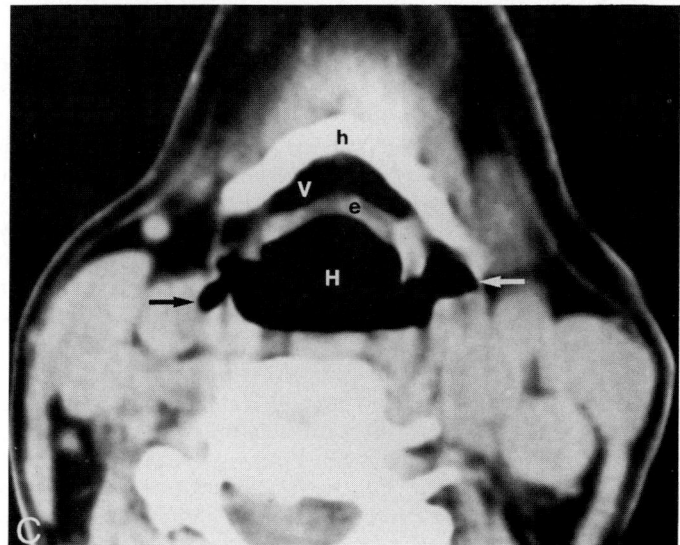

**Figure 17–2. Lateral pharyngeal diverticula. A.** A frontal view shows a round, sac-like structure protruding from the left lateral pharyngeal wall *(open arrow)*. The lateral pharyngeal diverticulum contains an air-contrast level. A right lateral diverticulum is faintly seen as a bilobate structure *(solid arrows)*. V = vallecula. **B.** A lateral view shows that the left lateral pharyngeal diverticulum *(open arrow)* is behind and at the level of the vallecula (V). In this slightly tilted view, the bilobate right lateral pharyngeal diverticulum is faintly seen *(short arrows)*. Long arrows indicate the aryepiglottic folds. E = epiglottic tip. (**A** and **B** modified from Rubesin SE, Glick SN: The tailored double-contrast pharyngogram. Crit Rev Diagn Imaging 28:133–179, 1988. Copyright CRC Press, Inc. Boca Raton, FL.) **C.** Computed tomography (CT) shows left and right lateral pharyngeal diverticula *(arrows)*. e = epiglottis; H = hypopharynx; h = hyoid; V = vallecula.

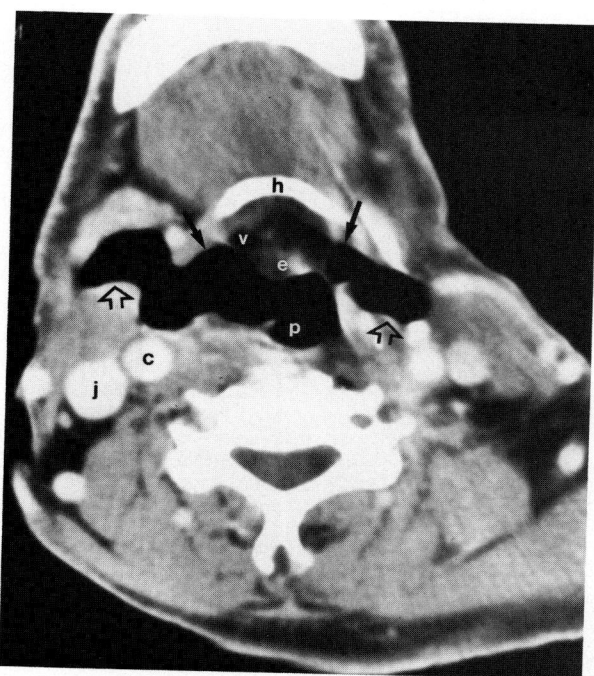

**Figure 17–3. Right and left mixed laryngoceles.** Axial CT scan through the level of the hyoid bone (h) shows air-filled sacs that extend through the thyrohyoid membrane and are anterior to the carotid artery (c) and jugular vein (j). The internal component of the mixed laryngocele is in the paralaryngeal space *(solid arrows).* The external component of the laryngoceles is indicated *(open arrows).* e = epiglottis; p = pharynx; v = vallecula.

## Branchial Cleft Cysts, Branchial Cleft Fistulas, and Branchial Pouch Sinuses

In the 4-week-old embryo, paired grooves appear on both sides of the neck region, leaving branchial ridges (arches) between them.[7, 11] The grooves are called *branchial clefts* and are of ectodermal origin. Four outpouchings from the pharynx meet the branchial clefts. These pharygeal outpouchings are of endodermal origin and are called *branchial pouches*. The first branchial cleft forms the external auditory meatus. The second branchial cleft forms the middle ear, the eustachian tube, and the floor of the tonsillar fossa. The third and fourth branchial pouches form the piriform sinus.[11] Persistence of either branchial pouches or clefts results in the formation of sinus tracts or cysts.

The most common branchial vestige is a cyst arising from the second branchial cleft. A second branchial cleft cyst is found at the level of the hyoid bone, deep to the sternocleidomastoid muscle.[7] Pathologically, a unilocular cyst is lined by keratinizing stratified squamous epithelium and is filled with desquamated keratinaceous debris. A zone of lymphoid tissue surrounds the epithelium.[7]

Patients with second branchial cleft cysts usually present between the ages of 10 and 40 years with a painless or fluctuant mass in the upper neck along the upper third of the anterior border of the sternocleidomastoid muscle.[12] When small, the cysts are anterior to the sternocleidomastoid muscle. When large, the cysts may extend posteriorly to the sternocleidomastoid muscle and displace the carotid sheath.

Cross-sectional imaging of noninfected cysts shows a smooth, thin-walled mass filled with a homogeneous water core.[13] If infected, the wall of the branchial cleft cyst becomes thick and may enhance with the use of intravenous contrast medium.[13] The second branchial cleft cyst may extend between the internal and external carotid arteries at a level superior to their bifurcation.[14] Rarely, branchial cleft cysts may communicate with the pharynx (branchial cleft fistulas) and may fill with barium during pharyngography.[2]

Branchial pouch sinuses or fistulas are tracts that extend from the pharynx and end blindly in the soft tissue of the neck (sinus) or extend to the skin (fistulas). These tracts are lined by ciliated columnar epithelium. Branchial pouch sinuses arise from the tonsillar fossa (second pouch), the upper anterolateral piriform fossa (third pouch), or the lower anterolateral piriform sinus (fourth pouch). Many of these fistulas are present at birth[12] and communicate with the skin. Sinus tracts that end blindly are occasionally seen in adults. Radiographically, second branchial pouch vestiges appear as sinus tracts that arise from the tonsillar fossa and extend along the sternocleidomastoid muscle in the deep cervical fascia (Fig. 17–4).

## Zenker's Diverticulum

Zenker's diverticulum (posterior hypopharyngeal diverticulum) is an acquired mucosal herniation through an area of anatomic weakness in the region of the cricopharyngeal muscle (Killian's dehiscence). The inferior constrictor muscle is composed of the thyropharyngeal and cricopharyngeal muscles. The thyropharyngeal muscle arises from the lateral ala of the thyroid cartilage, and it courses laterally and posteriorly to merge with its counterpart from the opposite side in a raphe in the posterior pharyngeal wall. The cricopharyngeal muscle constitutes the lower portion of the inferior constrictor muscle, arising from the lateral cricoid cartilage to encircle the lowermost hypopharynx. The cricopharyngeal muscle has no midline raphe. No overlap of fibers exists between the thyropharyngeal and cricopharyngeal muscles. Considerable variation is found in the arrangement of the muscle bundles of the thyropharyngeal and cricopharyngeal muscles. Killian's dehiscence has been variably described as arising between the thyropharyngeal and cricopharyngeal muscles or as arising between the oblique and horizontal fibers of the cricopharyngeal muscle.[15, 16] This area of weakness occurs in one third of patients.[17]

The pathogenesis of Zenker's diverticulum is as controversial as the muscular anatomy. Early radiographic and manometric studies suggested that either spasm (elevated pressure of the upper esophageal sphincter [UES]) or incoordination and abnormal relaxation of the UES (achalasia) occurred. However, manometric

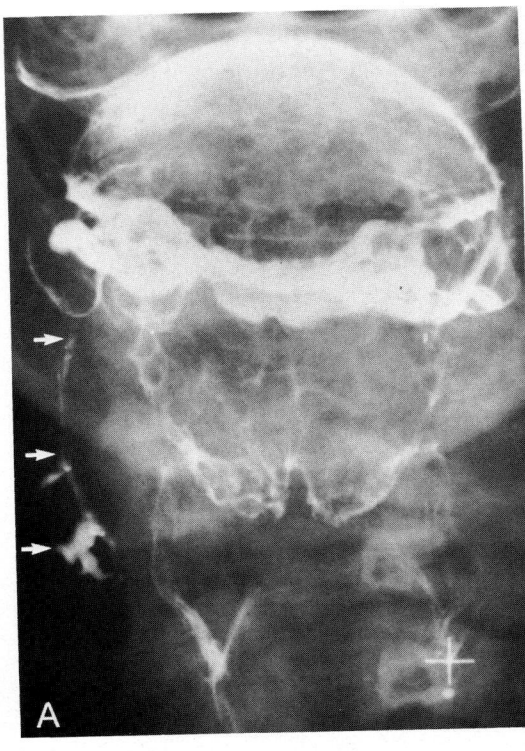
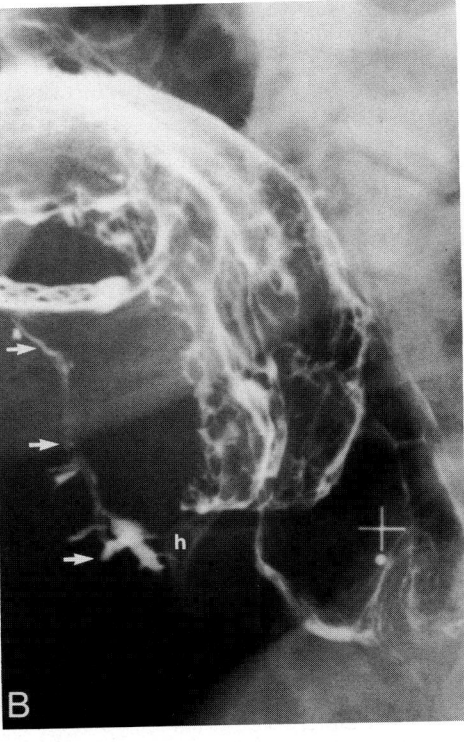

**Figure 17–4. Second branchial pouch sinus. A.** A frontal view shows a sinus tract *(arrows)* arising from the lateral side of the oral cavity. **B.** The lateral view shows the sinus tract *(arrows)* arising in the region of the retromolar trigone just anterior to the tonsillar fossa and extending inferiorly toward the hyoid bone (h). (**A** and **B** reprinted with permission from Rubesin SE, Glick SN: The tailored double-contrast pharyngogram. Crit Rev Diagn Imaging 28:133–179, 1988. Copyright CRC Press, Inc. Boca Raton, FL.)

studies have shown that 1) there is normal coordination between pharyngeal peristalsis and relaxation of the UES; 2) the UES relaxes completely during swallowing (i.e., there is no achalasia); and 3) the resting pressure of the UES is low (i.e., there is no spasm).[18, 19] The relationship between gastroesophageal reflux disease and Zenker's diverticulum is also controversial. Almost all patients with Zenker's diverticulum have an associated hiatal hernia,[20, 21] and many patients have radiographic evidence of gastroesophageal reflux or reflux esophagitis, or both. Whether gastroesophageal reflux predisposes patients with a large Killian's dehiscence to the formation of Zenker's diverticulum is unknown.

Zenker's diverticulum is found in elderly patients who have dysphagia, regurgitation of undigested food, halitosis, choking, hoarseness, or occasional neck mass.[22] Some patients with Zenker's diverticulum are asymptomatic.

During swallowing, Zenker's diverticulum appears as a posterior bulging of the distal pharyngeal wall above an anteriorly protruding pharyngoesophageal segment (cricopharyngeal muscle). At rest, the barium-filled diverticulum extends below the level of the cricopharyngeal muscle and is posterior to the proximal cervical esophagus (Figs. 17–5 to 17–7). A large diverticulum may protrude laterally to the left or compress the cervical esophagus. After swallowing, the patient regurgitates barium into the hypopharynx. In some patients, barium regurgitation may result in dysphagia or overflow aspiration.

True Zenker's diverticulum may be confused with barium trapped above a cricopharyngeal muscle that has closed before the pharyngeal peristaltic wave has passed.

This barium, trapped between downwardly progressing peristalsis and the cricopharyngeal muscle, is termed *pseudo–Zenker's diverticulum.*

The complications of Zenker's diverticulum include bronchitis, bronchiectasis, lung abscess, diverticulitis, ulceration, fistula formation, and carcinoma.[23] Any change in the character of dysphagia, or a bloody discharge in a patient known to have Zenker's diverticulum, suggests a complication.[24, 25] On barium studies, any irregularity of the contour of Zenker's diverticulum suggests either an inflammatory or a neoplastic complication. Carcinoma arises in only 0.3% of patients with Zenker's diverticulum,[25] but it is usually fatal.

## Killian-Jamieson Pouches and Diverticula

The Killian-Jamieson space is a triangular area of weakness in the cervical esophagus just below the cricopharyngeal muscle. This space is bounded 1) superiorly by the inferior margin of the cricopharyngeal muscle, 2) anteriorly by the inferior margin of the cricoid cartilage, and 3) inferomedially by the suspensory ligament of the esophagus originating from the posterior wall of the cricoid cartilage, just before the tendon forms the longitudinal muscle of the esophagus.[26]

Transient or persistent protrusions of the anterolateral cervical esophagus into the Killian-Jamieson space are termed *Killian-Jamieson pouches* or *Killian-Jamieson diverticula*, respectively. Most patients with Killian-Jamieson diverticula are asymptomatic, but some may complain of dysphagia or regurgitation.

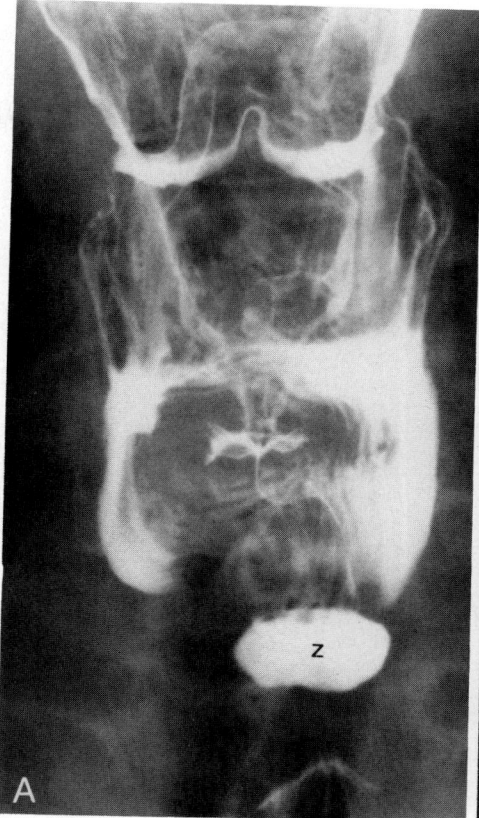
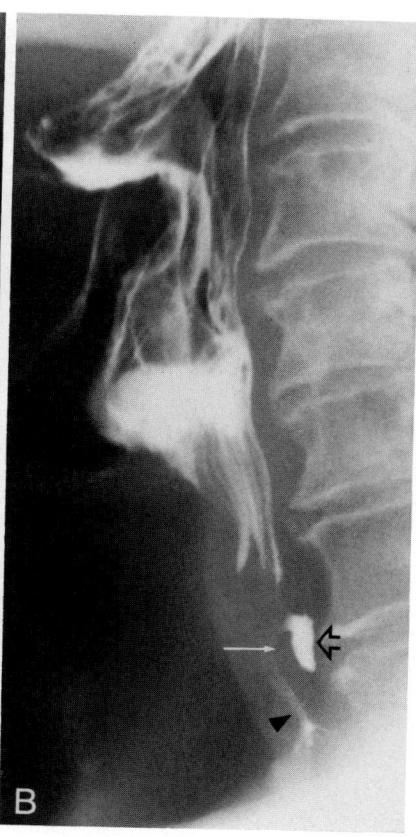

**Figure 17–5. Small Zenker's diverticulum. A.** A frontal view of the pharynx shows a barium-filled sac (Z) below the level of the hypopharynx. Neuromuscular weakness is indicated by barium stasis and ballooning of the lower hypopharynx. Barium also coats the vocal cords. **B.** In the lateral view, Zenker's diverticulum appears as a barium-filled sac *(open arrow)* posterior to the cervical esophagus *(arrowhead).* Note how flat the sac is in its anteroposterior dimension. Also note the prominent pharyngoesophageal segment *(solid arrow).*

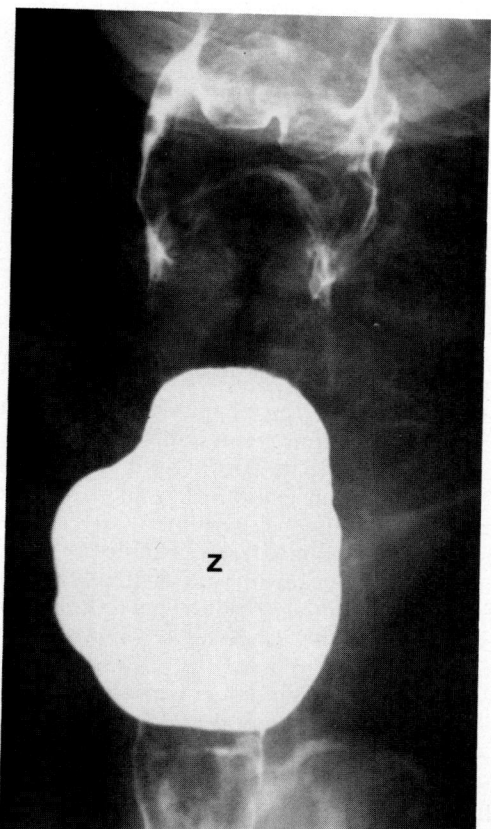

**Figure 17–6. Large Zenker's diverticulum.** A huge, barium-filled sac (Z) extends inferiorly into the mediastinum.

These pouches and diverticula are relatively common and may be confused radiographically with Zenker's diverticulum. Radiographically, a round to oval, smooth-surfaced outpouching that is 3 × 3 to 10 × 20 mm in diameter is seen just below the level of the cricopharyngeal muscle[26] (Figs. 17–8 and 17–9). On the frontal view, pouches appear as shallow, broad-based protrusions of the lateral upper esophageal wall that are effaced during swallowing and that empty after swallowing.[26] Diverticula appear as saccular protrusions that have narrow necks that do not empty as quickly after swallowing. On the lateral view, the sac is anterior to the cervical esophagus below the level of the cricopharyngeal muscle.[22] In contrast, the neck of Zenker's diverticulum is on the posterior hypopharyngeal wall, and the sac extends inferiorly behind the cervical esophagus.[22]

## PHARYNGEAL AND CERVICAL ESOPHAGEAL WEBS

Webs are thin mucosal folds most frequently located along the anterior wall of the lower hypopharynx and proximal cervical esophagus. They are usually composed of normal epithelium and lamina propria.[27] Some webs show inflammatory changes.

The etiology and clinical significance of webs are controversial. Most patients with cervical esophageal webs are asymptomatic. The webs are seen as isolated findings in 3 to 8% of patients undergoing upper gas-

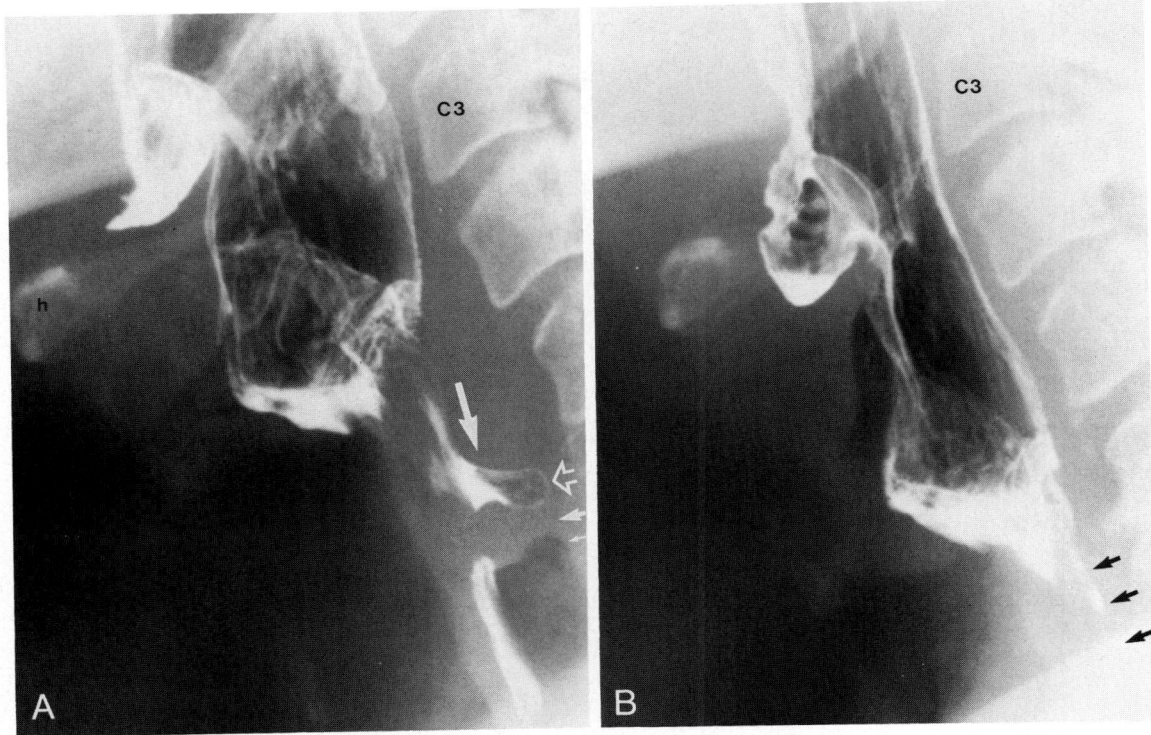

**Figure 17–7. Pseudo–Zenker's diverticulum.** A lateral view near the end of the swallow **(A)** is compared with a view taken in suspended respiration **(B)**. Note that near the end of the swallow, the pharynx and the hyoid bone (h) are still elevated. A sac-like collection of barium (pseudo–Zenker's diverticulum, *open arrow*) is trapped between the peristaltic wave *(large arrow* in **A)** and a prominent pharyngoesophageal segment ("cricopharyngeus") *(medium-sized arrow* in **A)**. Note, however, that the pseudo–Zenker's diverticulum does not extend posteriorly beyond the expected contour of the cervical esophagus *(small arrow* in **A)**. After the peristaltic wave has passed, during suspended respiration, the trapped barium has been cleared and the pseudo–Zenker's diverticulum is not evident *(black arrows* in **B)**. Note that the air-filled cervical esophagus is coated only on its anterior wall, because the prominent cricopharyngeus prevents barium from contacting with the posterior wall *(small arrow* in **A)**. C3 = third cervical vertebra.

trointestinal examination.[28–32] In one autopsy series, 16% of patients had incidental cervical esophageal webs.[27]

Some pharyngeal and cervical esophageal webs are associated with diseases that cause inflammation and scarring, such as epidermolysis bullosa or benign mucous membrane pemphigoid. A few older, northern European series showed an association of cervical esophageal webs, iron deficiency anemia, and pharyngeal or esophageal carcinoma.[33, 34] This association was termed *Plummer-Vinson syndrome* or *Paterson-Kelly syndrome*. In the United States, no association of cervical esophageal webs, iron deficiency anemia, and pharyngoesophageal carcinoma has been found. Webs in the distal esophagus have been associated with gastroesophageal reflux disease.[29] Perhaps, some cervical esophageal webs are associated with gastroesophageal reflux.

Some webs are present in the valleculae or lower piriform sinus. These vallecular and piriform sinus webs are composed of mucosa, lamina propria, and underlying blood vessels. These webs are thought to be normal variants in the valleculae and piriform sinuses.[35]

Radiographically, webs appear as 1- to 2-mm-wide, shelf-like filling defects along the anterior wall of the hypopharynx or cervical esophagus (Fig. 17–10). The webs protrude to various depths into the esophageal lumen. Webs may extend laterally, and a few extend circumferentially. Circumferential webs appear as ring-like shelves in the cervical esophagus. With severe luminal narrowing, dysphagia may result, especially in patients with circumferential cervical esophageal webs. Partial obstruction is suggested by a jet phenomenon,[36, 37] or by dilatation of the esophagus or pharynx proximal to the web. A dynamic examination reveals a higher percentage of webs than does a spot film examination alone.[31] Better demonstration of webs is achieved with the use of large boluses of barium.[31]

Webs may be confused radiographically with redundant mucosa in the anterior wall of the hypopharynx at the level of the cricoid cartilage. This redundant mucosa has been termed the *postcricoid defect,* and it was previously attributed to a venous plexus in this region.[38] However, the postcricoid defect is probably related only to redundancy of the mucosal and submucosal tissue in this area.[3]

Webs should also not be confused with a prominent cricopharyngeal muscle, which appears as a round, broad-based protrusion from the posterior pharyngeal wall at the level of the pharyngoesophageal segment.

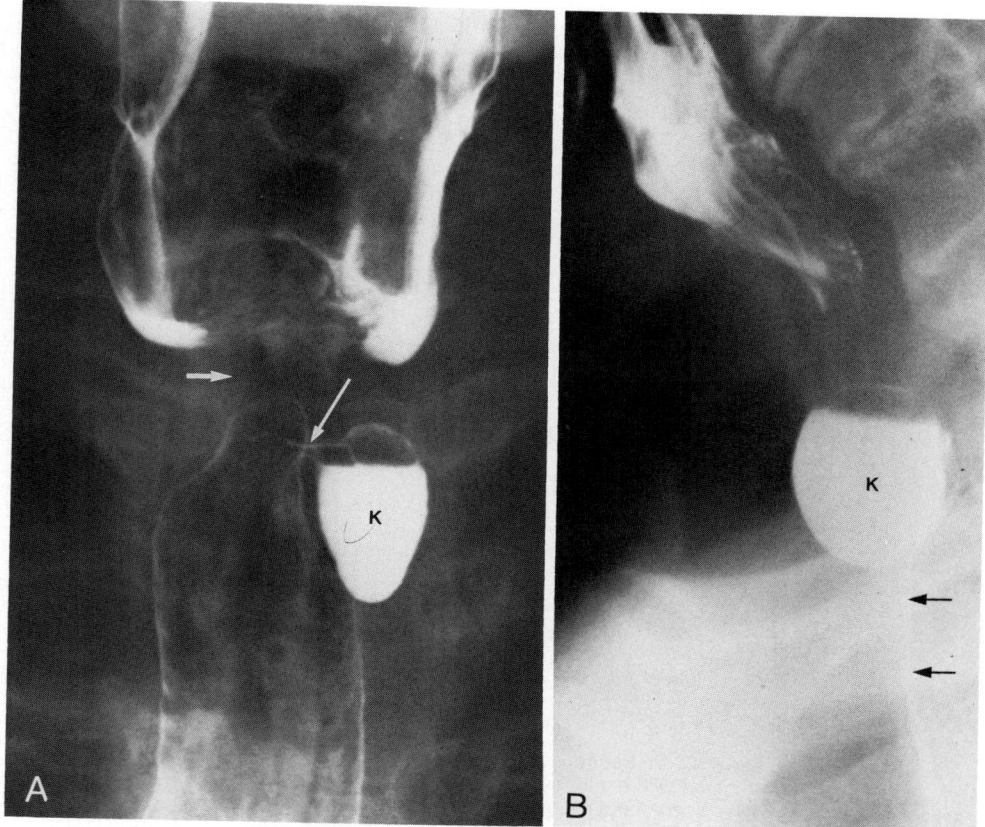

**Figure 17–8. Killian-Jamieson diverticulum. A.** A frontal view of the pharynx shows a barium-filled sac (K) to the left of the cervical esophagus. The neck of the diverticulum *(long arrow)* is below the level of the cricopharyngeal muscle *(short arrow)*. **B.** A lateral view shows the diverticulum (K) protruding anterior to the course of the cervical esophagus *(arrows)*.

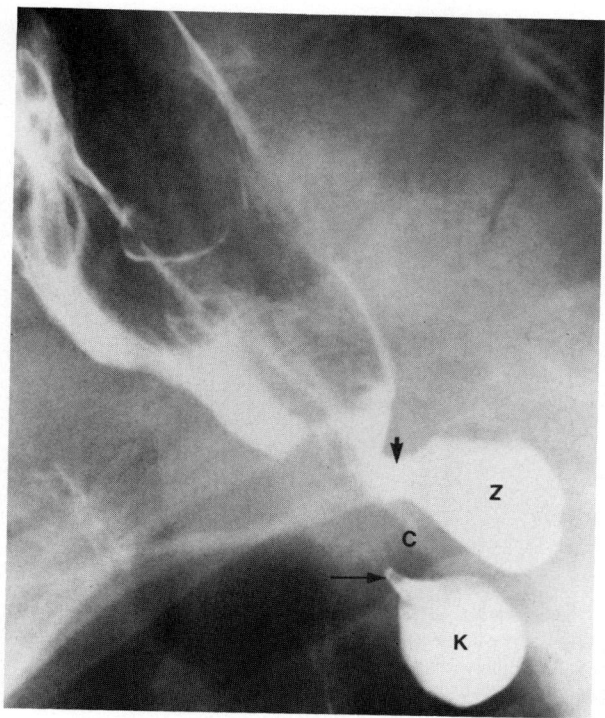

**Figure 17–9. Simultaneous Killian-Jamieson and Zenker's diverticula.** An oblique view of the pharynx shows Zenker's diverticulum (Z) with its opening *(short arrow)* above the prominent cricopharyngeus (C). The Killian-Jamieson diverticulum (K) has its opening *(long arrow)* below the prominent cricopharyngeus.

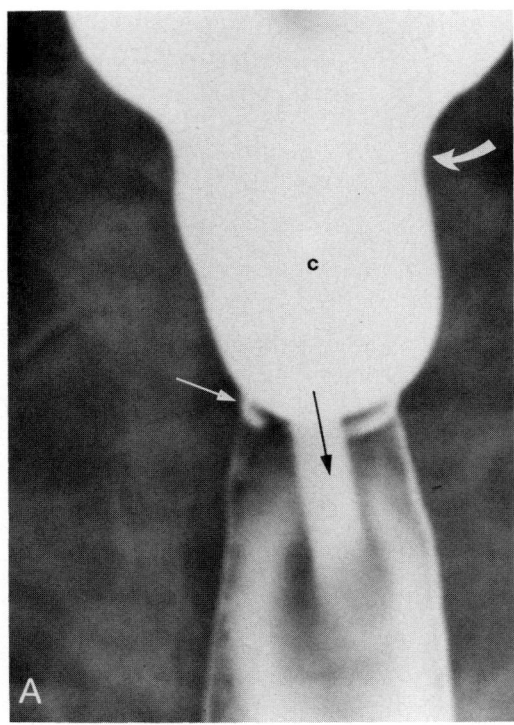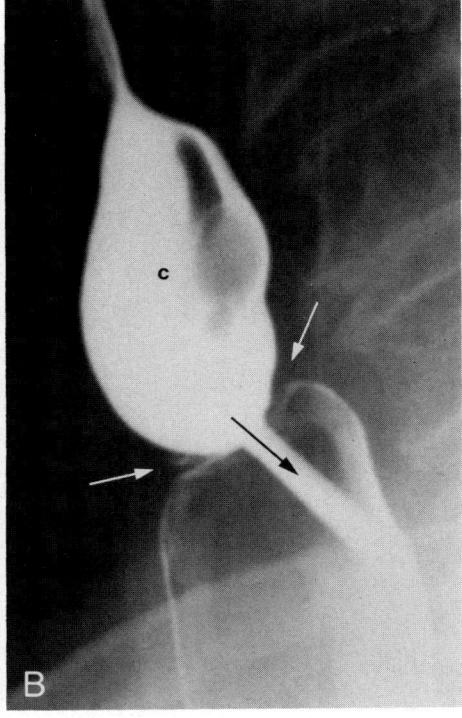

**Figure 17–10. Partially obstructive cervical esophageal web.** Frontal **(A)** and lateral **(B)** views show a circumferential, radiolucent ring *(straight white arrows)* in the proximal cervical esophagus. Partial obstruction is suggested by the jet phenomenon *(black arrows)*, with barium spurting through the ring, and by mild dilatation of the proximal cervical esophagus (c). The level of the cricopharyngeus is identified *(curved arrow in **A**)*.

## INFLAMMATORY LESIONS OF THE PHARYNX

Although acute epiglottitis usually affects children between 3 and 6 years of age, it occasionally causes severe stridor and sore throat in adults.[39] Plain film diagnosis of acute epiglottitis is important, even in adults, as manipulation of the tongue or pharynx may exacerbate edema and respiratory distress. Plain films show smooth enlargement of the epiglottis and aryepiglottic folds. Barium studies are contraindicated, as they may also exacerbate edema and trigger acute respiratory arrest.[40]

Barium studies of the pharynx are usually of limited value in patients with *acute* sore throat that is due to viral, bacterial, or fungal infection.[40] On pharyngograms, such patients usually demonstrate normal findings or evidence of nonspecific lymphoid hyperplasia of the palatine or lingual tonsils (Figs. 17–11 and 17–12).

In immunosuppressed patients with acute dysphagia, barium studies are directed toward the esophagus to demonstrate the presence, site, and type of esophagitis. A double contrast examination of the pharynx, however, may demonstrate the plaques of *Candida* pharyngitis or the ulcers of herpes pharyngitis, particularly in patients with acquired immunodeficiency syndrome[41] (Figs. 17–13 and 17–14).

In patients with *chronic* sore throat, barium studies may help to determine whether underlying gastroesophageal reflux and reflux esophagitis are present. Inflammatory disorders of the pharynx or gastroesophageal reflux can alter pharyngeal elevation, epiglottic tilt, or closure of the vocal cords and laryngeal vestibule. In-

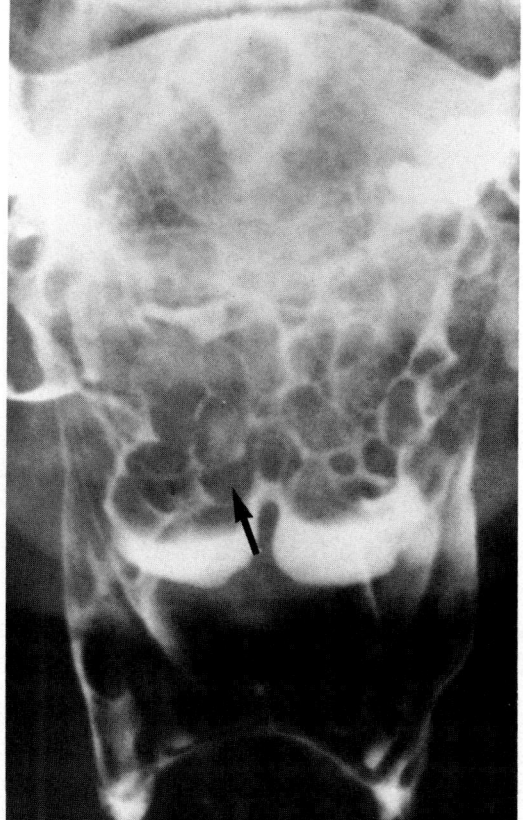

**Figure 17–11. Lymphoid hyperplasia of the base of the tongue.** A frontal view shows large, smooth-surfaced, round to ovoid nodules *(arrow)* symmetrically distributed over the surface of the base of the tongue.

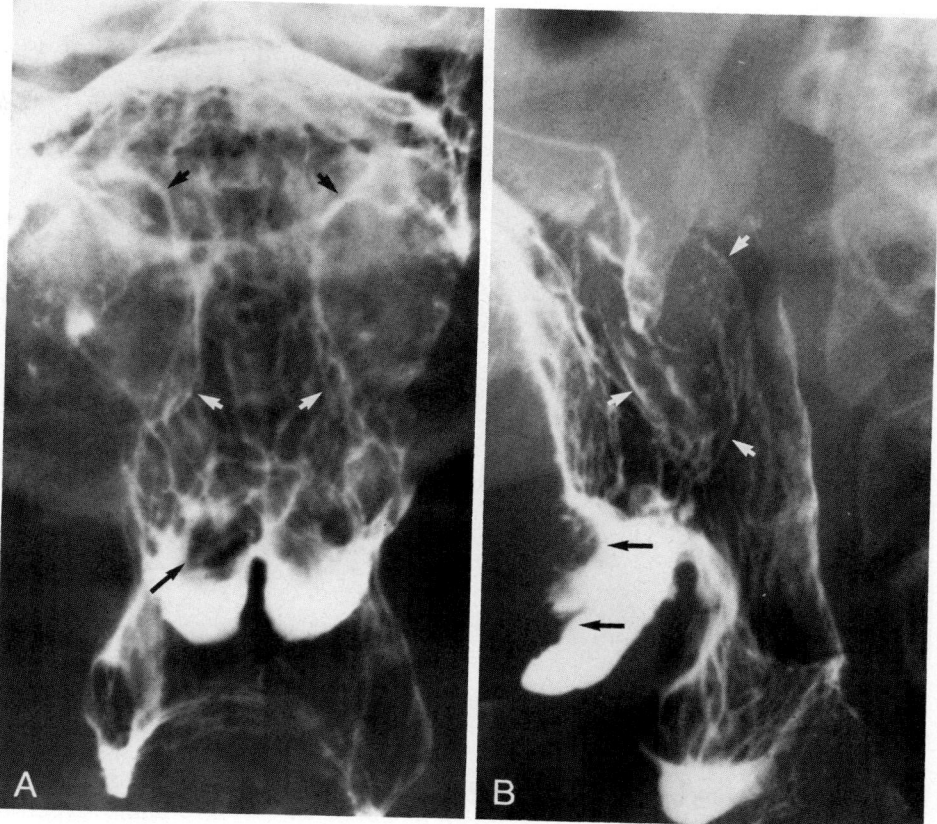

**Figure 17–12. Lymphoid hyperplasia of the palatine tonsils and base of the tongue in a young patient with a chronic sore throat.** Frontal **(A)** and lateral **(B)** views of the pharynx show moderate nodularity of the base of the tongue *(long arrows)* and bilateral, symmetric enlargement of the palatine tonsils *(short arrows)*.

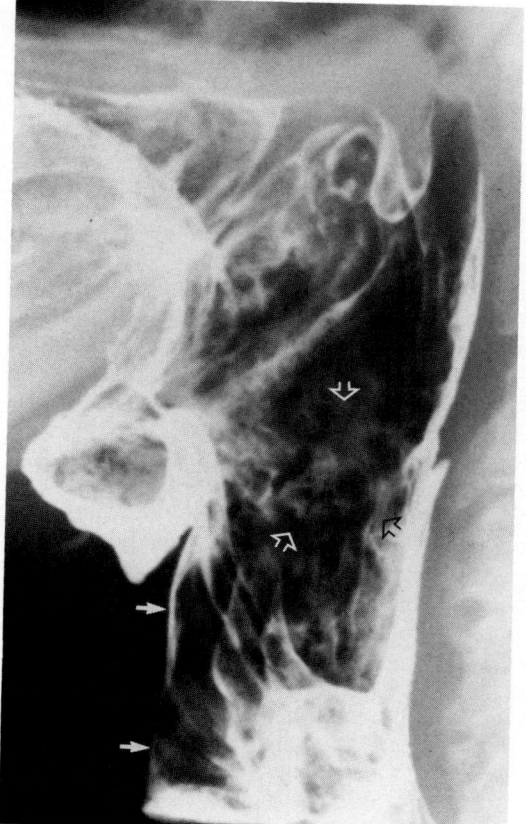

**Figure 17–13.** *Candida* **pharyngitis.** A lateral view of the pharynx shows well-circumscribed plaques *(open arrows)* at the level of the epiglottis. Note laryngeal vestibule penetration *(solid arrows)* due to abnormal pharyngeal motility associated with inflammatory pharyngitis.

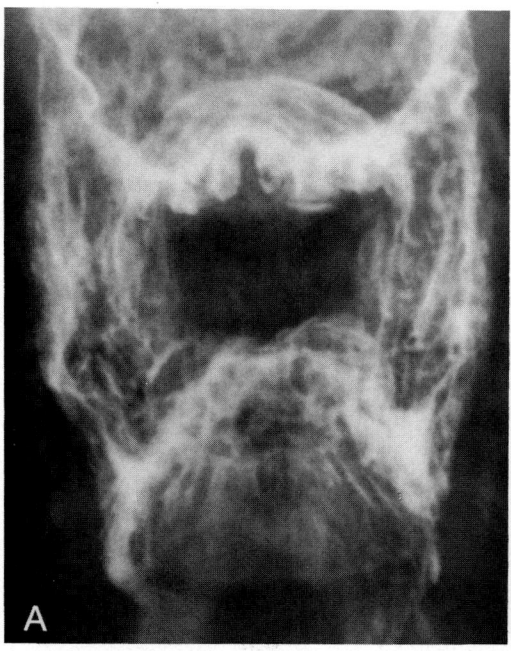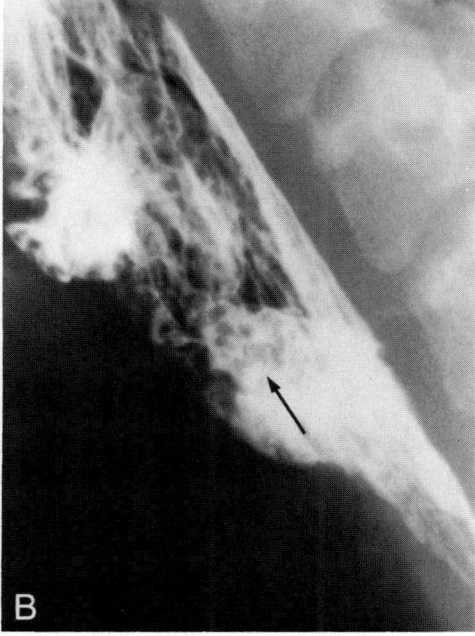

**Figure 17–14. Diffuse *Candida* pharyngitis.** Frontal **(A)** and lateral **(B)** views of the pharynx show innumerable plaques coating the entire mucosal surface of the pharynx. These well circumscribed plaques are seen as radiolucent filling defects in the barium pool *(arrow* in **B)** or as ring-like lines. This homosexual patient with acquired immunodeficiency syndrome and oral thrush complained of neck pain with swallowing. (**A** and **B** from Rubesin SE: Pharyngeal dysfunction. *In* Gore R [ed]: Syllabus for Categorical Course on Gastrointestinal Radiology. Reston, VA: American College of Radiology, 1991, pp 1–9.)

flammation-induced dysmotility may result in laryngeal penetration and stasis. Inflammatory dysmotility is discussed in Chapter 16.

Some diseases with diffuse mucous membrane ulceration affect the pharynx. Pharyngeal inflammation and ulceration may be seen in patients with Behçet's syndrome, Stevens-Johnson syndrome, Reiter's syndrome, epidermolysis bullosa,[42] and bullous pemphigoid.[43] Most of these patients have recurrent aphthous stomatitis and oropharyngeal ulceration. With severe ulceration, amputation of the uvula and tip of the epiglottis may be observed radiographically.[43] Scarring may cause distortion of the pharyngeal contours.

## Lymphoid Hyperplasia of the Lingual Tonsil

The lingual tonsil is an aggregate of 30 to 100 follicles along the pharyngeal surface of the tongue, extending from the circumvallate papillae to the root of the epiglottis.[44] This lymphoid tissue causes the normal surface of the base of the tongue to be divided into small nodules of varying size.

Hypertrophy of the lingual tonsil frequently occurs 1) after puberty, 2) as a compensatory response after tonsillectomy, or 3) as a nonspecific response to allergy or repeated infection.[44] Symptoms attributed to lymphoid hyperplasia of the lingual tonsil include throat discomfort and dysphagia. There are no criteria based on size for differentiating nodularity of the base of the tongue attributable to normal lingual tonsils from that attributable to reactive lymphoid hyperplasia. On frontal films obtained in patients with lymphoid hyperplasia, multiple smooth, round, or ovoid nodules are symmetrically distributed over the surface of the base of the tongue (see Fig. 17–11). On lateral films, the base of

the tongue may seem to protrude posteriorly. With severe lymphoid hyperplasia of the base of the tongue, nodules may extend into the valleculae, along the lingual surface of the epiglottis, or into the upper hypopharynx. Lymphoid hyperplasia can be coarsely nodular, asymmetrically distributed, or mass-like. However, any asymmetrically distributed coarse nodularity or mass must be viewed with suspicion. The use of endoscopy and magnetic resonance (MR) may help to rule out malignancy.

## BENIGN TUMORS OF THE PHARYNX

A wide variety of benign tumors occur in the pharynx.[7] Nonepithelial tumors arising from the supporting tissues of the pharynx are rare.[45, 46] However, tumor-like cysts of various histologic types are not uncommonly seen in the pharynx.[47] The most common benign lesions are retention cysts of the valleculae or aryepiglottic folds.

Symptoms are related primarily to location and to the polypoid or sessile nature of the lesion. Patients with benign tumors of the base of the tongue may be asymptomatic or may complain of throat irritation or dysphagia. Aryepiglottic fold nodules or mass lesions may cause dysphonia or respiratory symptoms such as stridor. Tumors of the epiglottis and aryepiglottic folds may also result in dysphagia, coughing, or choking because of laryngeal penetration. Pedunculated lesions (papilloma, lipoma,[48] fibrovascular polyp) may be coughed up into the mouth or may cause sudden death resulting from asphyxiation.

Tumors of various histologic types tend to occur at specific locations in the pharynx. Retention cysts and granular cell tumors are the most common benign tumors of the base of the tongue (Fig. 17–15). Ectopic thyroid tissue and thyroglossal duct cysts may occur in the base of the tongue but are rare. The tumor-like

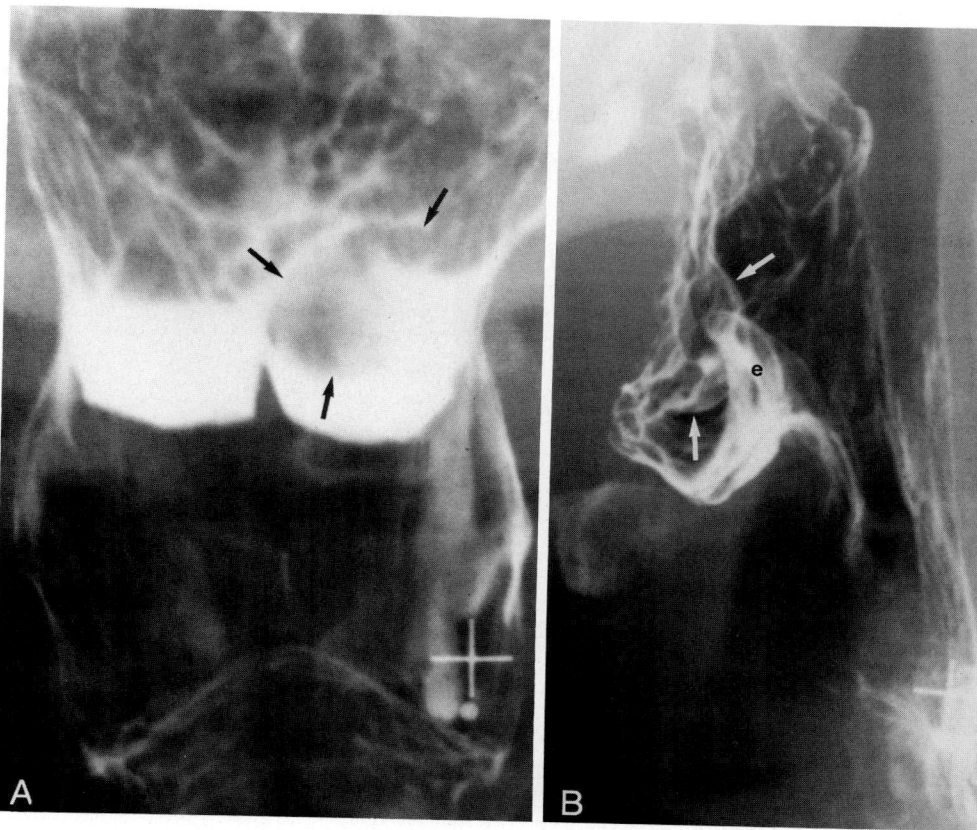

**Figure 17–15. Retention cyst in the base of the tongue. A.** A frontal view shows a faint, radiolucent filling defect in the barium pool *(arrows)* in the left vallecula. **B.** A lateral view shows a smooth-surfaced hemispheric mass *(arrows)* protruding posteriorly from the base of the tongue. The mass is partially obscured by the epiglottic tip (e). (**A** and **B** from Rubesin SE, Laufer I: Pictorial review: principles of double contrast pharyngography. Dysphagia 6:170–178, 1991.)

lesions that most commonly involve the aryepiglottic folds are saccular and retention cysts. Retention cysts of the aryepiglottic folds are lined by squamous epithelium and filled with desquamated squamous debris (Fig. 17–16). Saccular cysts of the aryepiglottic folds are filled with mucoid secretion, arising from the mucus-secreting glands of the appendix of the laryngeal ventricle. Sac-

cular cysts are the mucus-filled variant of an internal laryngocele. True soft tissue tumors of the aryepiglottic folds, such as lipoma, neurofibroma, hamartoma,[46] granular cell tumor, and oncocytoma, are rare.[7] Laryngeal involvement in neurofibromatosis (von Recklinghausen's disease) is rare, but it most frequently involves the region of the arytenoid cartilage and aryepiglottic folds[49]

**Figure 17–16. Retention cyst in mucosa overlying the muscular process of the right arytenoid cartilage.** A smooth-surfaced, well-circumscribed mass is seen in the region of the mucosa overlying the muscular process of the right arytenoid cartilage *(arrow)*. This 2.5-cm mass was not detected during fiberoptic examination. After another endoscopic examination confirmed the radiographically demonstrated mass, surgery was performed, and pathologic evaluation revealed a cyst lined by squamous epithelium. (Reprinted with permission from Rubesin SE, Glick SN: The tailored double-contrast pharyngogram. Crit Rev Diagn Imaging 28:133–179, 1988. Copyright CRC Press, Inc. Boca Raton, FL.)

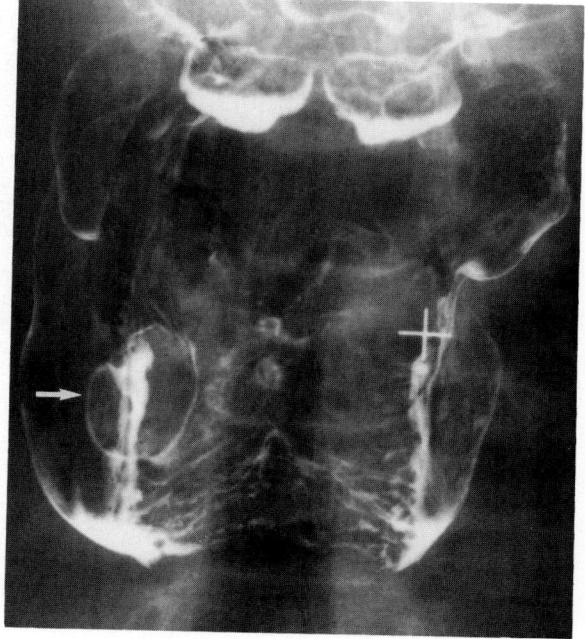

(Fig. 17–17). Benign tumors arising from the minor mucoserous salivary glands are most frequently seen in the oropharynx, in the region of the soft palate and the base of the tongue. Benign cartilaginous tumors involving the pharynx (chondromas) usually arise in the posterior lamina of the cricoid cartilage.[50]

Regardless of its underlying histologic characteristics, a benign pharyngeal tumor usually appears radiographically as a smooth, round, sharply circumscribed mass en face and as a hemispheric line with abrupt angulation in profile[40] (Fig. 17–18). Only rarely is a pedunculated, polypoid lesion (papilloma, fibrovascular polyp) seen.

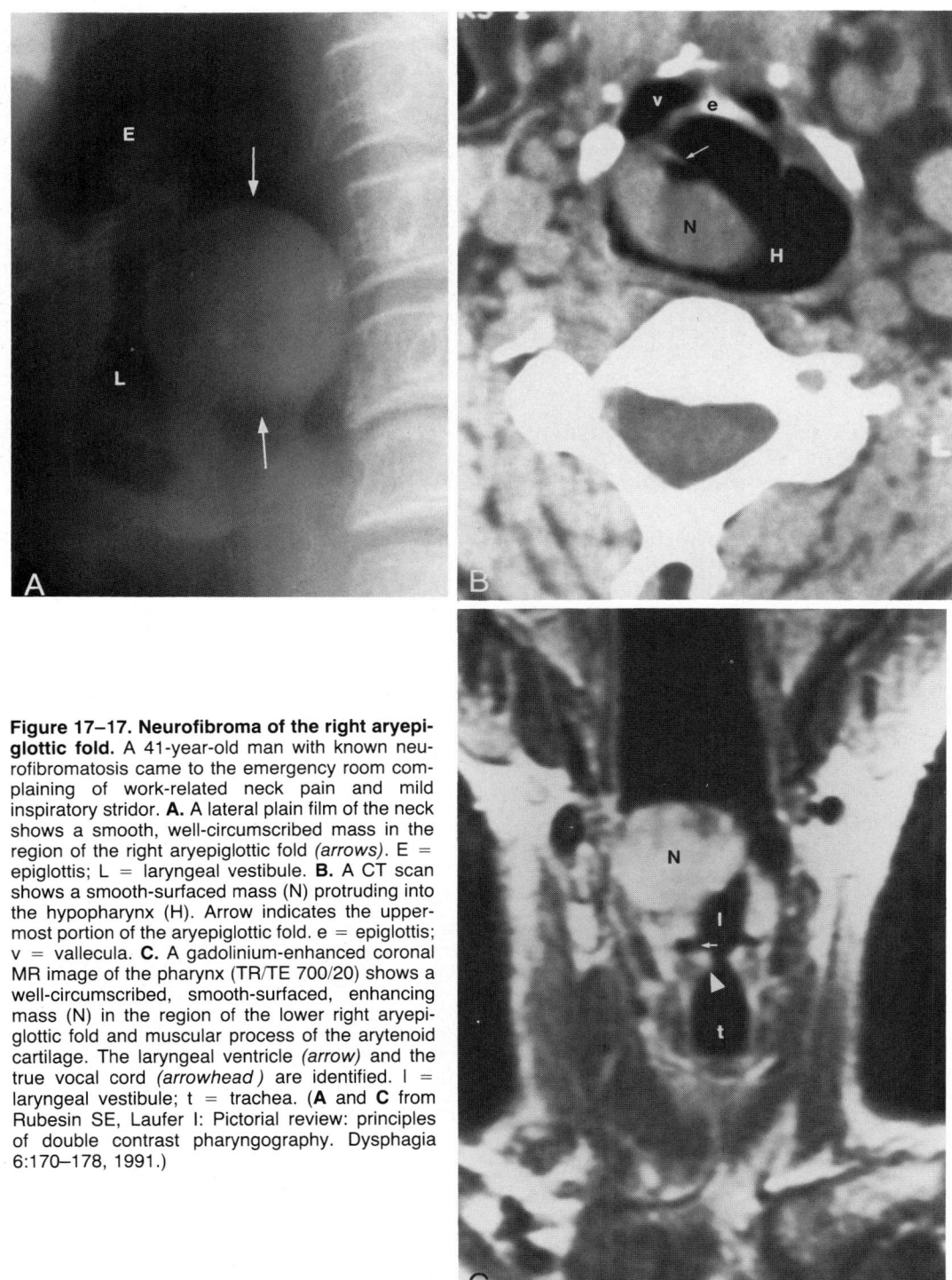

**Figure 17–17. Neurofibroma of the right aryepiglottic fold.** A 41-year-old man with known neurofibromatosis came to the emergency room complaining of work-related neck pain and mild inspiratory stridor. **A.** A lateral plain film of the neck shows a smooth, well-circumscribed mass in the region of the right aryepiglottic fold *(arrows)*. E = epiglottis; L = laryngeal vestibule. **B.** A CT scan shows a smooth-surfaced mass (N) protruding into the hypopharynx (H). Arrow indicates the uppermost portion of the aryepiglottic fold. e = epiglottis; v = vallecula. **C.** A gadolinium-enhanced coronal MR image of the pharynx (TR/TE 700/20) shows a well-circumscribed, smooth-surfaced, enhancing mass (N) in the region of the lower right aryepiglottic fold and muscular process of the arytenoid cartilage. The laryngeal ventricle *(arrow)* and the true vocal cord *(arrowhead)* are identified. l = laryngeal vestibule; t = trachea. (**A** and **C** from Rubesin SE, Laufer I: Pictorial review: principles of double contrast pharyngography. Dysphagia 6:170–178, 1991.)

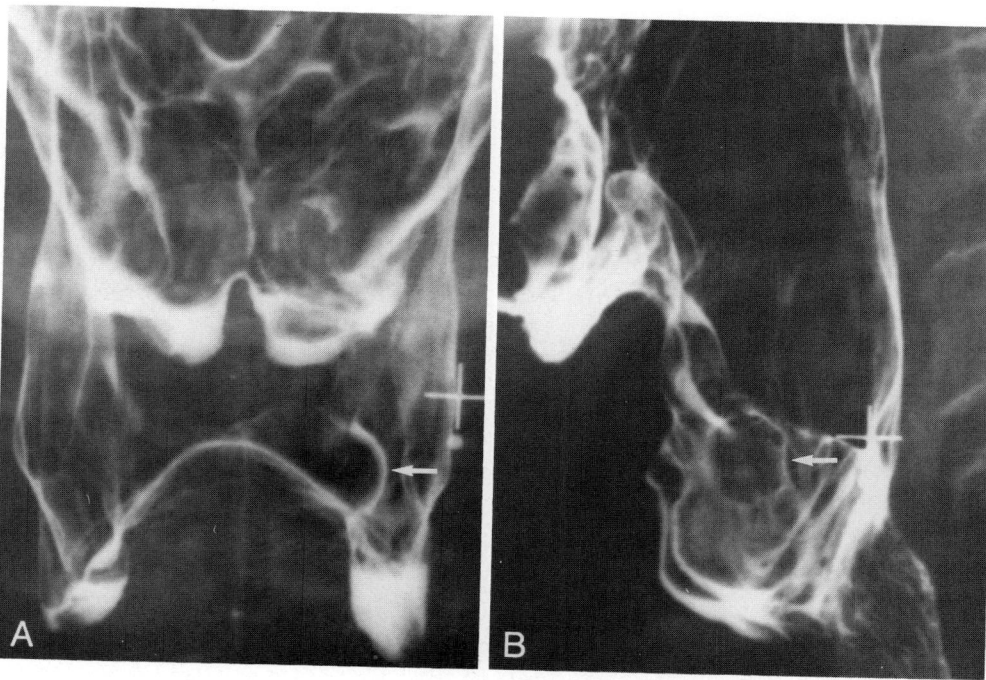

Figure 17-18. Submucosal mass of the left piriform sinus. A. A frontal view shows a smooth-surfaced mass arising from the medial wall of the left piriform sinus. The mass is 7 mm in diameter and demonstrates abrupt angulation (arrow) with the mucosal surface. B. A lateral view shows a sharply circumscribed, round, smooth-surfaced mass (arrow) overlying the muscular process of the arytenoid cartilage. (A and B reprinted with permission from Rubesin SE, Glick SN: The tailored double-contrast pharyngogram. Crit Rev Diagn Imaging 28:133–179, 1988. Copyright CRC Press, Inc. Boca Raton, FL.)

The benign nature of these lesions should be confirmed by endoscopic examination. Submucosal masses may not be visualized, however, by endoscopy.

## MALIGNANT TUMORS OF THE PHARYNX

Radiologists should be as thoroughly familiar with pharyngeal carcinoma as they are with esophageal carcinoma. Squamous cell carcinomas of the head and neck (e.g., of the tongue, pharynx, or larynx) constitute 5% of all cancers in the United States.[51] Esophageal carcinomas constitute 1% of all cancers in the United States. The prognosis of pharyngeal cancer is better than that of esophageal cancer. The 5-year survival rate for pharyngeal cancer is approximately 20 to 40%, whereas the 5-year survival rate for esophageal cancer is approximately 5 to 10%.

The radiologist is often the first physician to suggest a diagnosis of pharyngeal carcinoma (Fig. 17–19). Some tumors may be detected during barium studies performed for other reasons. Some patients with pharyngeal symptoms or a palpable neck mass undergo pharyngoesophagography as the initial diagnostic examination. In patients with known pharyngeal cancer, a contrast examination is of value to assist in planning proper workup and therapy. A barium examination can be used to rule out a second primary lesion in the esophagus. Furthermore, the examination can detect coexisting structural lesions (e.g., prominent cricopharyngeal muscle, Zenker's diverticulum, web, or stricture) that may be difficult to circumvent safely at endoscopy. Barium examination reveals the size, extent, and inferior limit of the tumor and the degree of functional impairment.

The barium examination also reveals areas behind bulky tumor that may be difficult to see even with fiberoptic examination.

Barium studies allow detection of more than 95% of structural lesions below the pharyngoesophageal fold.[52] These studies are especially valuable in the areas of the pharynx difficult to evaluate by endoscopy (i.e., the lower base of the tongue, the valleculae, the lower hypopharynx, and the pharyngoesophageal segment).

## Signs and Symptoms

The symptoms of pharyngeal carcinoma are nonspecific and usually of short duration (<4 months). They include sore throat, dysphagia, and odynophagia.[53] Choking or coughing may be due to laryngeal penetration during swallowing or aspiration of barium trapped in ulcerated tumor. Hoarseness occurs primarily in patients with laryngeal carcinoma, supraglottic carcinoma, or carcinoma of the medial piriform sinus infiltrating the arytenoid cartilage or cricoarytenoid joint. Referred earache may occur, especially when nasopharyngeal tumors block the eustachian tube.[53] Many patients are asymptomatic but present with a palpable neck mass. Most patients with squamous cell carcinoma are 50 to 70 years of age.[53, 54] Almost all patients (>95%) are moderate to heavy abusers of alcohol and tobacco.[51]

## Squamous Cell Carcinoma

### Pathology

Squamous cell carcinomas represent 90% of malignant lesions involving the oropharynx and hypopharynx.[7, 54, 55]

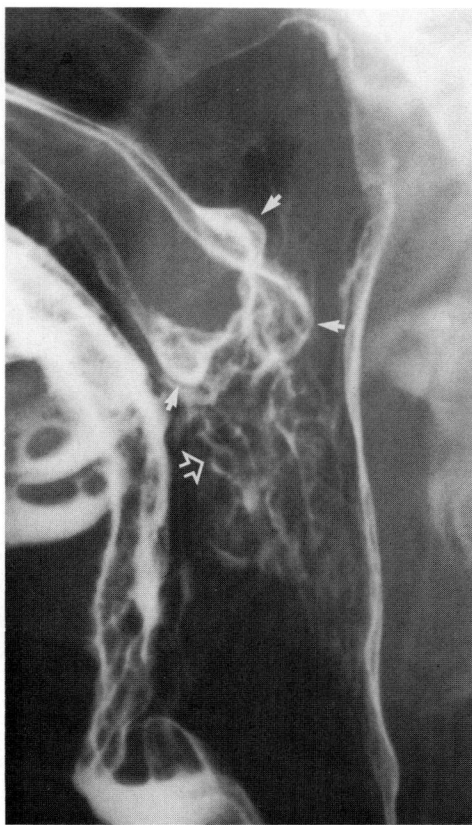

**Figure 17–19. Unsuspected soft palate carcinoma.** An 80-year-old patient with dementia was undergoing upper gastrointestinal tract examination for epigastric pain. Nasal regurgitation was observed during the initial double contrast swallow. A lateral spot film of the pharynx shows obliteration of the contour of the lower soft palate. The soft palate is replaced by a lobulated mass *(solid arrows)*. Nodular mucosa in the tonsillar fossa *(open arrow)* indicates spread of tumor into this region. (From Rubesin SE, Rabischong P, Bilaniuk LT, et al: Contrast examination of the soft palate with cross sectional correlation. Radiographics 8:641–665, 1988.)

Most of these tumors are keratinizing squamous cell carcinomas. In general, they occur in two macroscopic forms: 1) exophytic tumors that spread over the mucosa, and 2) infiltrative and ulcerative tumors that penetrate deeply into surrounding soft tissue, cartilage, and bone.[7] Multiple primary lesions of the oral cavity, pharynx, esophagus, and lung are seen in more than 20% of patients.[53] Because such a strong association exists between head and neck squamous cell carcinoma and esophageal carcinoma,[56, 57] a major goal of radiologic studies is to rule out a synchronous esophageal primary tumor. Between 1 and 15% of patients with head and neck squamous cell carcinoma later develop an esophageal squamous cell carcinoma.[56–58]

## Classification

Classification of tumors of the pharynx and larynx is confusing. Many authors discuss supraglottic, oropharyngeal, and hypopharyngeal tumors separately. Thus, interpretation of incidence and prognosis of tumors by specific region is slightly misleading. The major confu-

sion arises from the fact that the supraglottic laryngeal structures are derived from pharyngobuccal anlage and form part of the anterior pharyngeal wall, but supraglottic tumors are classified as laryngeal. Thus, tumors of the epiglottis, aryepiglottic folds, mucosa overlying the muscular processes of the arytenoid cartilages, false vocal cords, and laryngeal ventricle are defined as laryngeal (supraglottic) carcinomas.

The TNM classification of tumors is frequently used by clinicians. In this classification, T refers to the extent of tumor, N refers to the absence or the presence and extent of regional lymph node metastases, and M refers to the absence or presence of distant metastases. Although this classification is clinical or pathologic, it is presented as a guide to the radiologist[59] (Table 17–1).

## General Radiographic Findings

### Barium Studies

The radiographic findings of pharyngeal cancer are 1) intraluminal mass; 2) mucosal irregularity; and 3) impairment or loss of normal mobility or distensibility[40, 60–62] (Fig. 17–20). An intraluminal mass may be manifested radiographically as obliteration of the normal luminal contour, as extra barium-coated lines protruding into the expected pharyngeal air column, as a focal area of increased radiopacity, or as a filling defect in the barium pool.[40, 41, 60] Mucosal irregularity may be seen as abnormal barium collections resulting from surface ulceration or as a lobulated, finely nodular, or granular surface texture.[60] Asymmetric distensibility is seen as flattening of the pharyngeal contour that is due to fixation of structures by infiltrating tumor or to an extrinsic mass impinging on the pharynx.[41, 61, 62]

### Cross-sectional Imaging

Cross-sectional imaging studies are the examinations of choice for demonstrating spread of tumor into the submucosa, the intrinsic muscles, the tissue extrinsic to the pharynx, and the regional lymph nodes (see Chapter 15).[63, 64] Computed tomography (CT) and MR imaging may occasionally reveal lesions that are not visible even with modern endoscopes, typically submucosal masses.

On CT scans, squamous cell carcinoma appears as a soft tissue mass altering the contour of the pharynx (Fig. 17–21). On T1-weighted MR images, the signal intensity of squamous cell carcinoma is the same as that of muscle, and on T2-weighted MR images, it is the same or slightly higher than that of fat. Squamous cell carcinoma demonstrates minimal enhancement with the use of gadolinium. The tumor is frequently of inhomogeneous intensity. Areas of tumor necrosis demonstrate signal intensity similar to that of cerebrospinal fluid on long repetition time (TR), long echo time (TE) images.

Lymphomas of the pharynx are typically of homogeneous intensity. The signal intensity of lymphoma may be identical with that of squamous cell carcinoma on T1- and T2-weighted MR images. Signal intensity of lymphoma mimics that of normal lymphoid tissue. It may be brighter than fat on T2-weighted images.

## TABLE 17–1. TNM CLASSIFICATION OF PHARYNGEAL MALIGNANT TUMORS*

*T: Primary Tumor*
  TX: primary tumor cannot be assessed
  T0: no evidence of primary tumor
  Tis: carcinoma in situ

*Nasopharynx* (lateral wall and fossa of Rosenmüller, posterosuperior wall, superior surface of soft palate)
  T1: tumor is limited to one subsite
  T2: tumor invades more than one subsite
  T3: tumor invades nasal cavity and/or oropharynx
  T4: tumor invades skull base and/or cranial nerves

*Oropharynx* (tongue and valleculae, tonsillar fossa and faucial pillars, inferior surface of soft palate and uvula, posterior wall)
  T1: tumor ≤ 2 cm in greatest dimension
  T2: tumor > 2 cm but ≤ 4 cm in greatest dimension
  T3: tumor > 4 cm in greatest dimension
  T4: tumor invades adjacent structures: bone, soft tissue of neck, deep (extrinsic) muscle of tongue

*Hypopharynx* (piriform sinus, posterior pharyngeal wall, postcricoid area)
  T1: tumor is limited to one subsite
  T2: tumor invades more than one subsite in hypopharynx, or an adjacent site without fixation of hemilarynx
  T3: tumor invades more than one subsite, or an adjacent site with fixation of hemilarynx
  T4: tumor invades adjacent structures (cartilage, soft tissue of neck)

*Supraglottis* (epiglottis, including lingual and laryngeal surfaces; aryepiglottic folds; arytenoids; false vocal cords; laryngeal ventricles)
  T1: tumor is limited to one subsite, with normal vocal cord motility
  T2: tumor invades more than one subsite, with normal vocal cord motility
  T3: tumor limited to larynx with vocal cord fixation and/or tumor invades pre-epiglottic tissue, medial wall of piriform sinus, or postcricoid area
  T4: tumor invades through thyroid cartilage and/or extends to oropharynx or soft tissue of neck

*Regional Lymph Nodes*
  N0: no regional lymph node metastasis
  N1: metastasis in single, ipsilateral lymph node ≤ 3 cm in greatest dimension
  N2a: metastasis in single ipsilateral lymph node > 3 cm and < 6 cm
  N2b: metastasis in multiple ipsilateral lymph nodes, each ≤ 6 cm
  N2c: metastasis in bilateral or contralateral lymph nodes, each < 6 cm
  N3: metastasis in lymph node > 6 cm

*Subsites are listed in parentheses.
Modified from Spiessl B, Bearhs OH, Hermanek P, et al: TNM Atlas. Berlin: Springer-Verlag, 1990, p 143.

Squamous cell carcinoma metastases to lymph nodes (see Fig. 17–21)—especially small, necrotic cervical metastases—are better demonstrated on CT scans than on MR images. CT may identify necrosis as small as 5 mm in diameter in lymph nodes.

With the use of MR imaging, necrosis in small lymph nodes may be difficult to detect, and reactive inflammatory changes may be difficult to distinguish from necrosis. To date, postgadolinium fat-suppression techniques are the best methods for enhancing tissue differences between the periphery and the necrotic center of lymph nodes.

## Specific Sites

### Nasopharynx

Squamous cell carcinoma is the most common histologic type of nasopharyngeal malignant tumor. Its risk factors, age of presentation, and histologic type are more varied than those of the typical squamous cell carcinoma of the oropharynx and hypopharynx. In addition to alcohol and smoking abuse, poor ventilation, nasal balms, ingested carcinogens, and upper respiratory

viruses such as the Epstein-Barr virus have been implicated as causative factors.[7]

Nasopharyngeal squamous cell carcinoma appears clinically at a relatively younger age, with 20% of patients being younger than 30 years old.[7] Many squamous cell cancers are undifferentiated tumors, and many have a reactive lymphoid stroma. Approximately one half of patients complain of hearing loss attributable to eustachian tube involvement. One half of patients are asymptomatic and present with a neck mass caused by cervical nodal metastases. Other signs and symptoms include nasal obstruction, epistaxis, pain, headache, and damage to the fifth cranial nerve. The 5-year survival rate varies from 76% for patients with localized tumors to 10 to 20% for patients with cervical lymph node metastases.[65]

MR imaging is the method of choice for the nasopharynx.[66] The radiologist carefully searches for spread to the nasal cavity, sinuses, and cranial base, especially for cranial nerve involvement. Barium studies are used primarily to evaluate the symptoms of nasal regurgitation and voice changes that are due to soft palate insufficiency and to rule out a synchronous esophageal tumor (Fig. 17–22).

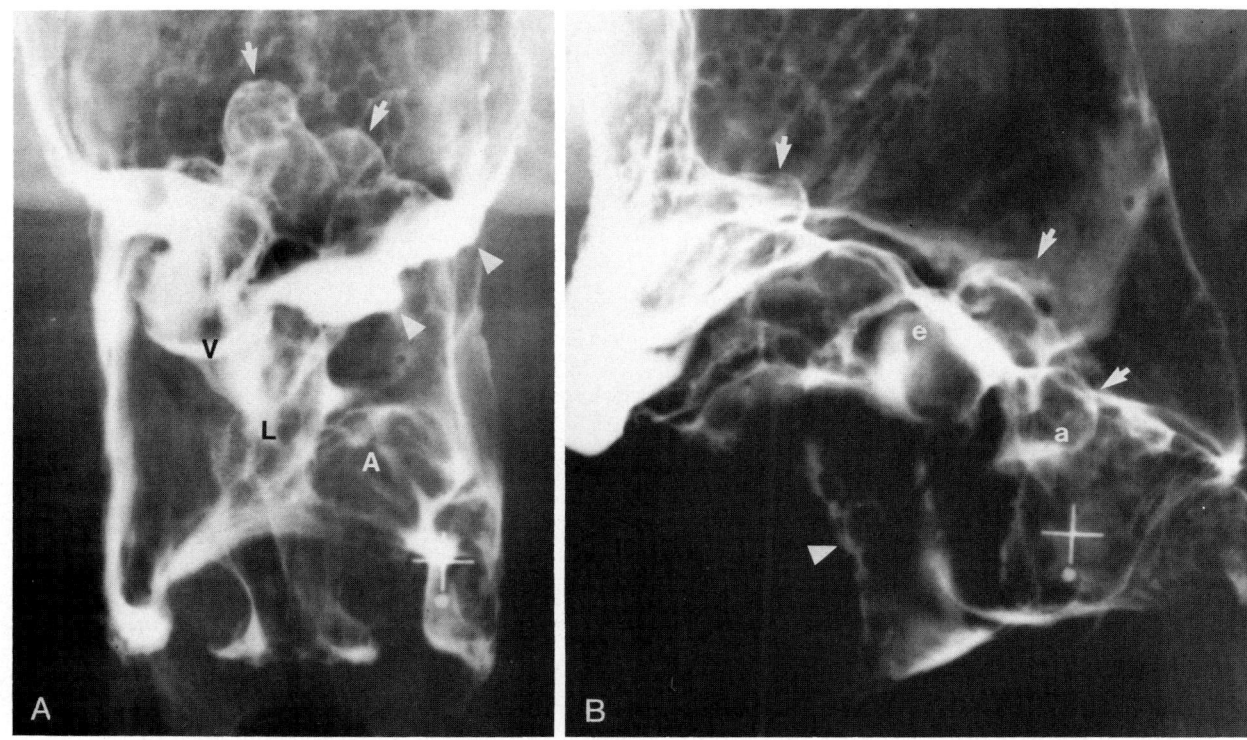

**Figure 17–20. Radiographic findings in pharyngeal carcinoma. A.** A large, supraglottic squamous cell carcinoma is shown. The normal contour of the epiglottis is obliterated and replaced by a lobulated contour *(white arrows)*. The left vallecula is flattened and nodular *(arrowheads)*. The right vallecula ( V ) is marked for comparison. Nodular mucosa is seen over the surface of the epiglottis, the laryngeal vestibule, which has been coated by barium (L), and the mucosa overlying the muscular process of the arytenoid cartilage (A). **B.** A lateral view shows loss of the normal contour of the epiglottis, with a huge lobulated mass *(arrows)* extending from the region of the epiglottis down the aryepiglottic folds (e) to the mucosa overlying the muscular process of the arytenoid cartilage (a). Barium coats the anterior wall of the laryngeal vestibule *(arrowhead)*. This wall appears irregular in its proximal portion, a finding compatible with tumor infiltration. (**A** and **B** reprinted with permission from Rubesin SE, Glick SN: The tailored double-contrast pharyngogram. Crit Rev Diagn Imaging 28:133–179, 1988. Copyright CRC Press, Inc. Boca Raton, FL.)

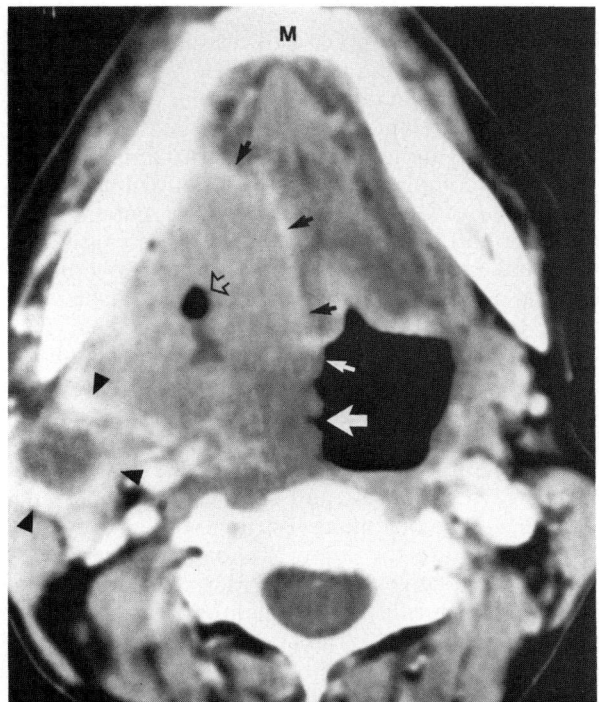

**Figure 17–21. Squamous cell carcinoma of the base of tongue and right tonsil.** An axial CT scan through the level of the oropharynx and mandible (M) shows obliteration of the space of the right oropharynx by a large mass involving the base of the tongue *(small white arrow)* and the right lateral pharyngeal wall *(large white arrow)*. The mass extends deep into the extrinsic and intrinsic muscles of the tongue *(small black arrows)*. It demonstrates mild enhancement with intravenous contrast medium. A central air-filled cavity is at a biopsy site *(open arrow)*. A metastatic lymph node has a low-density center that is due to necrosis and a peripherally enhancing rim *(arrowheads)* representing viable tissue with extranodal spread.

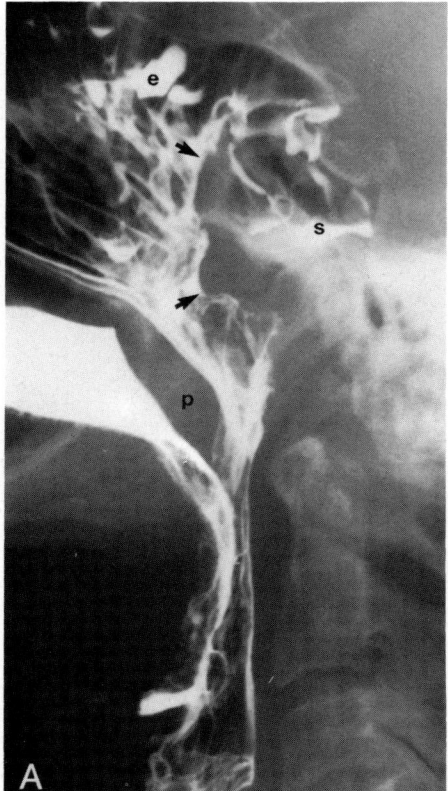

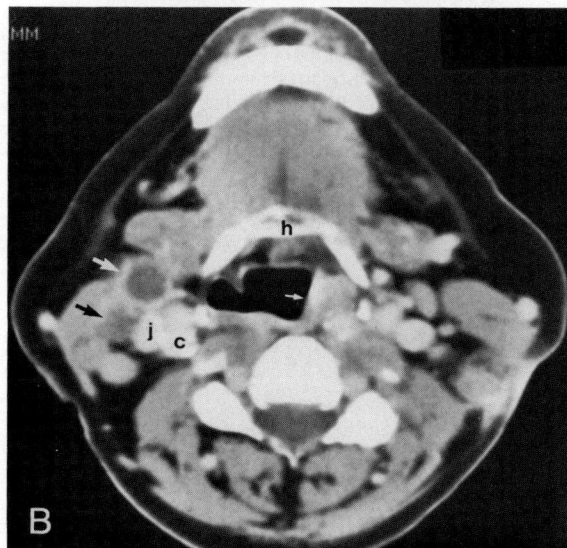

**Figure 17–22. Squamous cell carcinoma of the nasopharynx. A.** A large, lobulated tumor *(arrows)* of the posterior nasopharyngeal wall invades the region of the ostium of the sphenoidal sinus. The sphenoidal sinus (s) and ethmoidal air cells (e) are filled with a small amount of barium. The soft palate (p) is coated by barium. Note that 1 to 2 mL of barium was instilled into each naris before this radiograph was obtained. **B.** CT scan through the level of the hyoid bone (h) shows low-density necrotic cervical lymph node metastases *(large arrows)*. The left lateral wall of the pharynx is flattened *(small arrow)*. This flattening may have been caused by submucosal tumor infiltration. The calcified carotid artery (c) and the jugular vein (j) are identified.

## Palatine Tonsil

Squamous cell carcinoma of the palatine tonsil is the most common malignant tumor arising in the pharynx.[67] Well-differentiated tumors are usually exophytic and easily seen on barium studies[40] (Fig. 17–23). Poorly differentiated tumors are frequently of the ulcerative-infiltrative type and may be obscured on barium studies by the underlying nodular lymphoid tissue of the palatine tonsil.[41] Tonsillar tumors spread to the soft palate (Fig. 17–24), the base of the tongue, and the posterior pharyngeal wall. Approximately one half of patients develop cervical nodal metastases.[40]

## Base of the Tongue

Squamous cell carcinomas of the base of the tongue are poorly differentiated lesions that often present as advanced lesions with nodal metastases.[68–70] These tumors infiltrate deeply into the intrinsic and extrinsic muscles of the tongue. Patients with small lesions are often asymptomatic but present with enlarged cervical nodes. Initial results of diagnostic endoscopy may be negative.[71] Small or predominantly submucosal lesions may be hidden in the valleculae or the recess between the tongue and tonsil (glossotonsillar recess). Barium, MR, or CT studies may be extremely helpful in detecting clinically occult lesions with nodal metastases. Lymph node metastases are seen ipsilaterally or contralaterally in more than 70% of patients. The 5-year survival rate is approximately 20 to 40%.[54, 68, 72]

Radiographically, an exophytic lesion appears as a polypoid mass that projects into the oropharyngeal airspace[71, 72] (Fig. 17–25). An ulcerated lesion appears as an irregular barium collection disrupting the expected contour of the base of the tongue. Nodules of tumor may spread to the palatine tonsil, valleculae, or pharyngoepiglottic fold. Occasionally, a deeply infiltrating, primarily submucosal lesion is seen as a subtle, asymmetric enlargement of the base of the tongue (Fig. 17–26). A small plaque-like or ulcerative lesion may be easily missed on barium or endoscopic studies, but detected on MR or CT studies.

## Supraglottic Region

Squamous cell carcinomas that affect the epiglottis, aryepiglottic folds, mucosa overlying the arytenoid cartilages, false vocal cords, and laryngeal ventricles are defined as *supraglottic carcinomas*. These poorly differentiated or undifferentiated tumors spread rapidly to the entire supraglottic region and pre-epiglottic space.[40, 73] Exophytic lesions are more common[61, 74] (Fig. 17–27). Ulcerative lesions deeply penetrate the tongue and valleculae and invade the pre-epiglottic space[61] (Fig. 17–28). These tumors may spread laterally to the pharyngoepiglottic folds and lateral pharyngeal walls. Only rarely does this tumor extend through the laryngeal ventricles into the true vocal cords. Cervical nodal

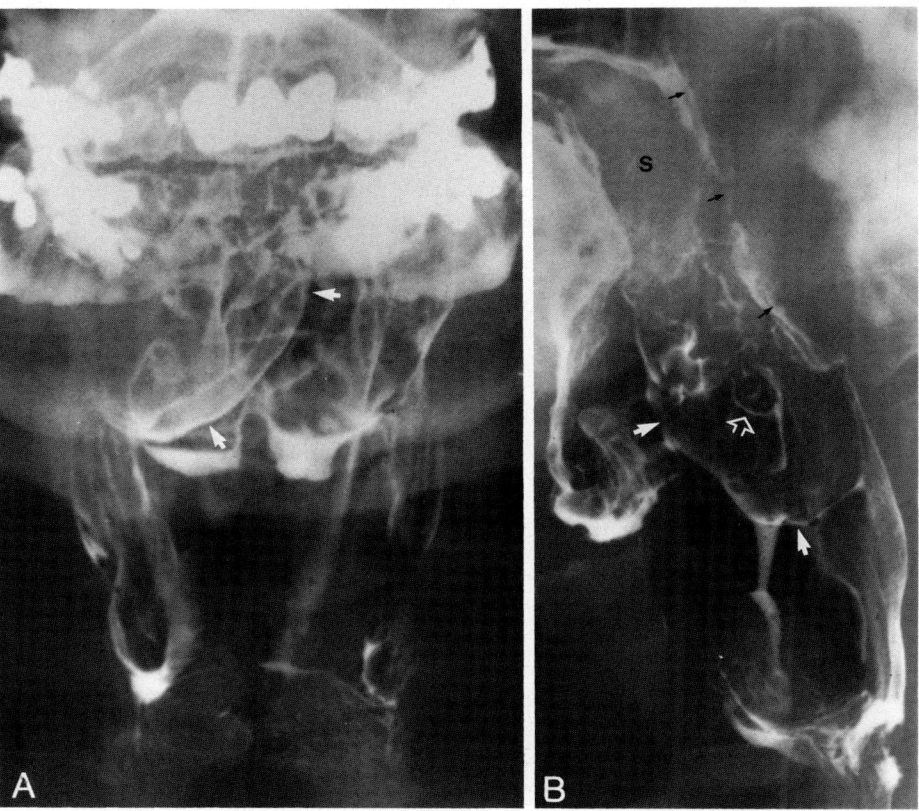

**Figure 17–23. Squamous cell carcinoma of the palatine tonsil. A.** A frontal view shows a large, polypoid mass *(arrows)* protruding into the oropharynx. The lateral wall of the tonsillar fossa has been obliterated. **B.** A lateral view shows a large, tonsillar fossa mass *(white arrows)* with a central ulcer *(open arrow)*. Tumor infiltration of the posterior pharyngeal wall is represented by enlargement of the soft tissue space in this region *(black arrows)*. The soft palate (S) is also widened and has an irregular contour. (**A** and **B** from MS Levine, SE Rubesin, Radiologic investigation of dysphagia, AJR, 154, 6, 1157–1163, 1990, © by American Roentgen Ray Society.)

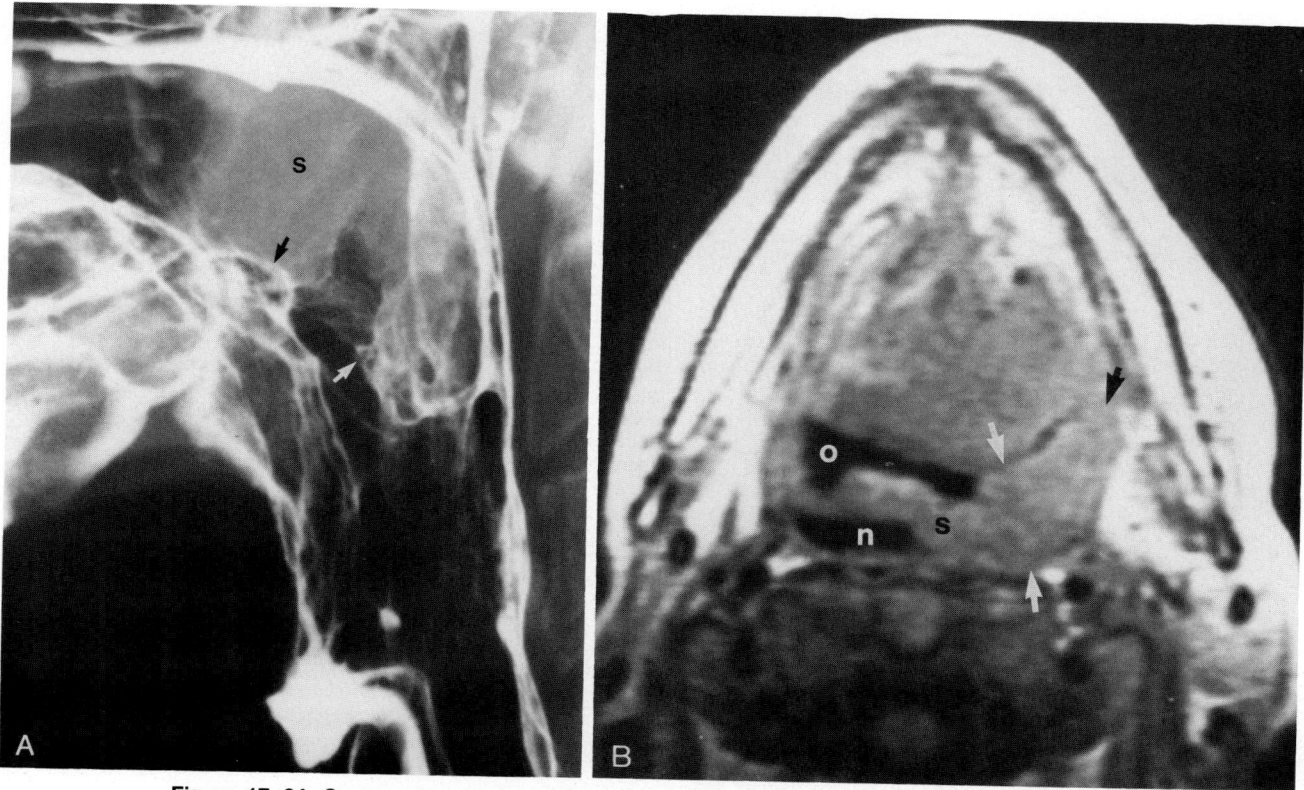

**Figure 17–24. Squamous cell carcinoma of the soft palate with spread to the base of the tongue and tonsillar fossa. A.** The soft palate (s) is markedly enlarged with a lobulated contour. Nodular mucosa is seen in the region of the tonsillar fossa *(white arrow)*. Spread of lobulated tumor to the base of the tongue *(black arrow)* is seen. **B.** A T1-weighted MR image obtained through the base of the tongue shows an enlarged soft palate (s) *(white arrows)*. Tumor extends to the lateral margin of the tongue *(black arrow)*. Note that the tumor is of the same signal intensity as that of the base of the tongue. n = nasopharynx; o = oropharynx.

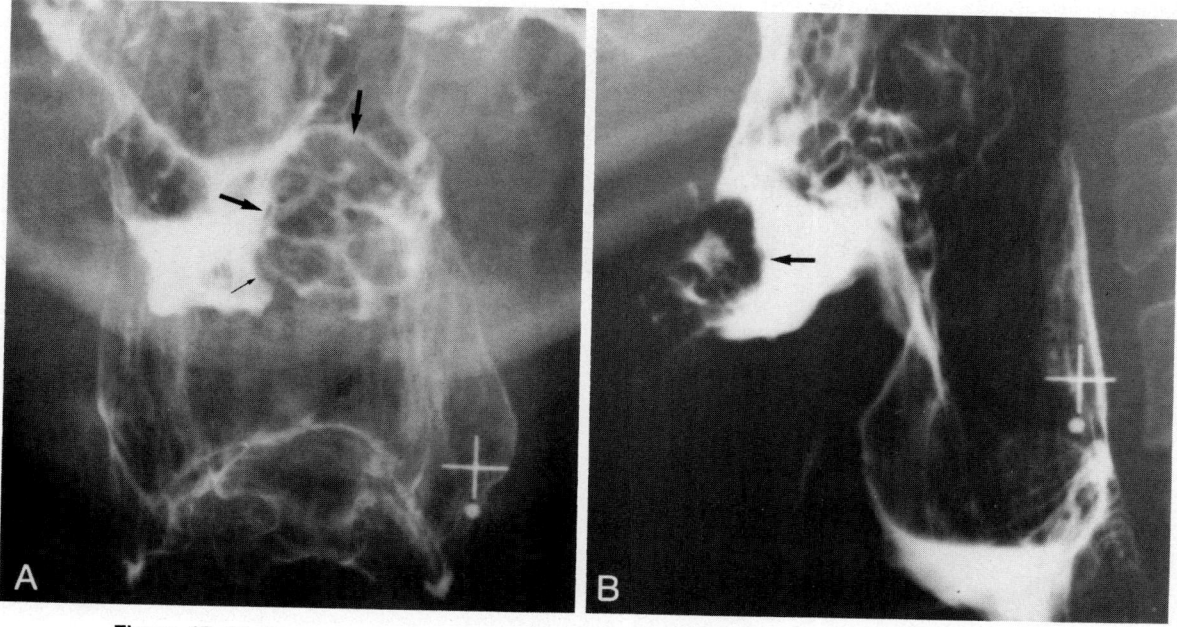

**Figure 17–25. Squamous cell carcinoma of the base of the tongue. A.** A frontal view shows obliteration of the contour of the left vallecula and a lobulated, soft tissue mass *(large arrows)* replacing the barium pool in the left vallecula. The median glossoepiglottic fold *(small arrow)* is deviated to the right. **B.** A lateral view shows a polypoid mass *(arrow)* protruding posteriorly into the vallecula. Deep ulcerations into the base of the tongue are filled with barium. (**A** and **B** reprinted with permission from Rubesin SE, Glick SN: The tailored double-contrast pharyngogram. Crit Rev Diagn Imaging 28:133–179, 1988. Copyright CRC Press, Inc. Boca Raton, FL.)

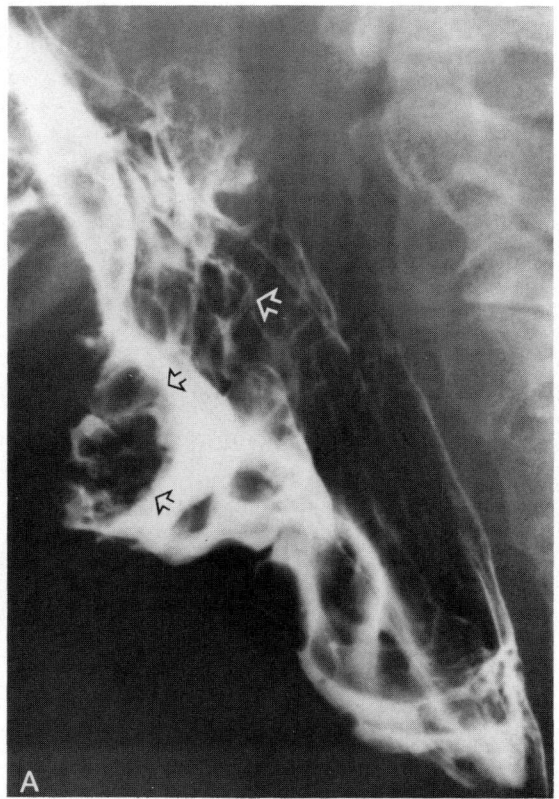

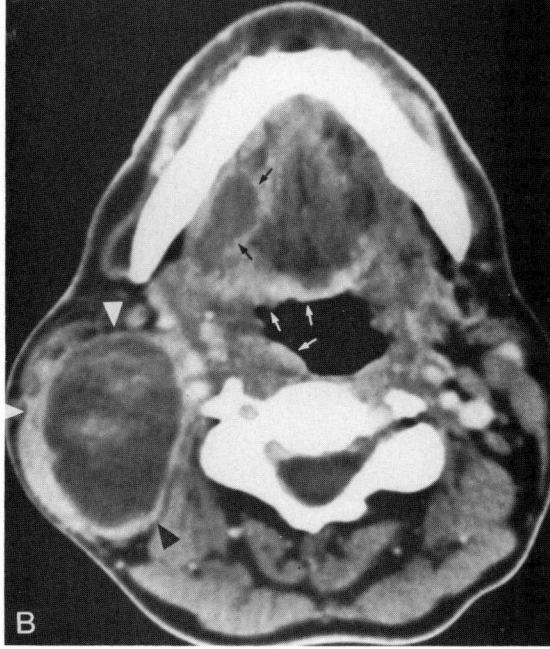

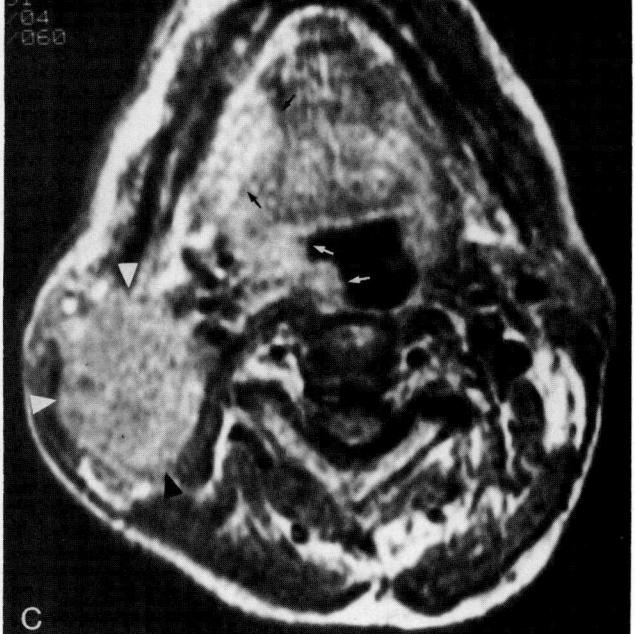

**Figure 17–26. Deeply infiltrating squamous cell carcinoma of the base of the tongue. A.** A lateral view of the pharynx shows a broad-based polypoid mass *(black arrows)*. Tumor nodules also extend into the tonsillar fossa *(white arrow)*. **B.** CT scan through the base of the tongue shows asymmetry of the base of the tongue and the lateral pharyngeal wall *(white arrows)*, with a peripherally enhanced mass also invading the sublingual space *(black arrows)*. A large, centrally necrotic cervical lymph node metastasis is identified *(arrowheads)*. **C.** Proton density MR image obtained through the same level as that in **B** shows asymmetry of the base of the tongue and lateral pharyngeal wall *(white arrows)*. The deeply infiltrating tumor *(black arrows)* has a signal intensity much higher than that of the muscles of the base of the tongue. The cervical lymph node metastasis *(arrowheads)*, which was identified as necrotic on the CT scan, has a higher signal intensity compared with muscle.

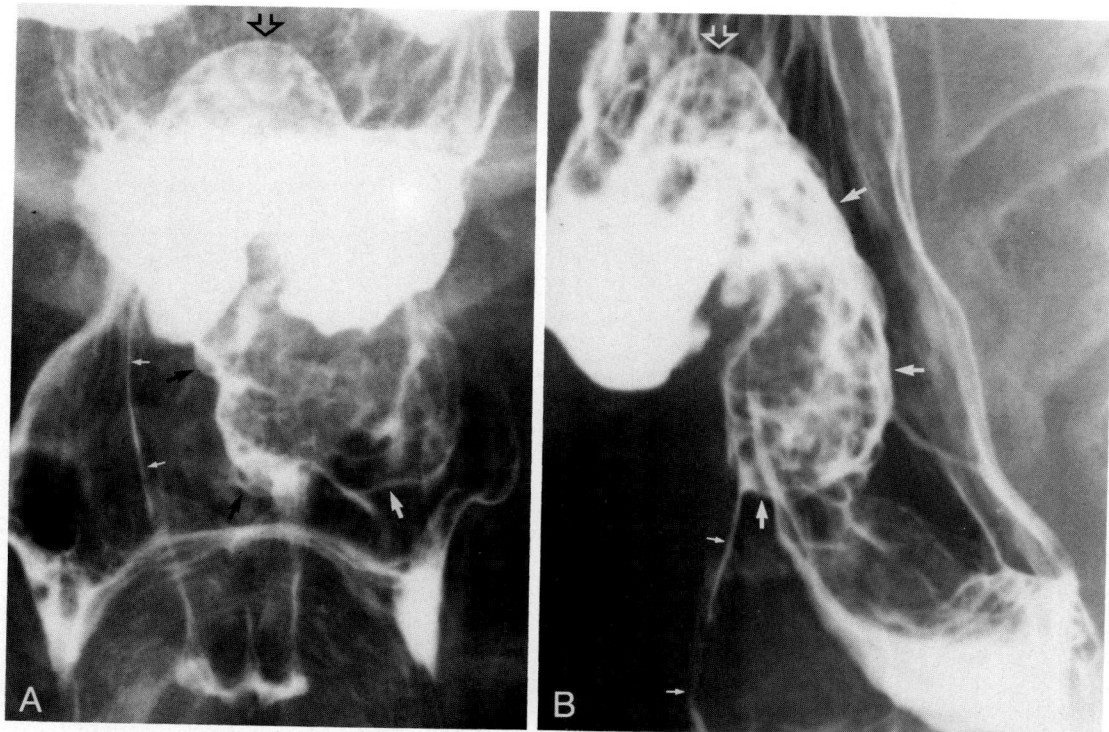

**Figure 17–27. Polypoid squamous cell carcinoma of the epiglottis. A.** A frontal view shows an enlarged, rounded epiglottic tip *(open arrow)* and an enlarged, nodular left aryepiglottic fold *(large solid arrows)*. Note excessive pooling of barium in the valleculae. Laryngeal penetration has occurred, coating the laryngeal vestibule. This barium coating shows that the tumor has not spread to the lower right side of the epiglottis and right aryepiglottic fold *(small solid arrows)*. **B.** The lateral view shows a bulbous, enlarged epiglottic tip *(open arrow)* and a large epiglottic mass *(large solid arrows)* extending down the aryepiglottic fold and along the anterior wall of the laryngeal vestibule. The lower portion of the laryngeal vestibule is spared from tumor *(small solid arrows)*.

metastases are seen in one third to one half of patients.[40, 74] The 5-year survival rate is approximately 40%.

### Piriform Sinus

Squamous cell carcinomas of the piriform sinuses are advanced lesions that spread quickly and metastasize widely.[60] Patients usually present with hoarseness or a neck mass.[60] Metastases to the lymph nodes are seen in 70 to 80% of patients.[40, 67] The 5-year survival rate is approximately 20 to 40%.[53, 74] Tumors involving the medial wall of the piriform sinus (Fig. 17–29) have a slightly better prognosis than do lateral wall tumors.[53] Medial wall tumors infiltrate the aryepiglottic fold, arytenoid and cricoid cartilages, and the paraglottic space, resulting in hoarseness.[60] Tumors involving the lateral wall infiltrate the thyrohyoid membrane, thyroid cartilage, and soft tissues of the neck, including the structures of the carotid sheath[40] (Fig. 17–30). Radiographically, an early lesion may appear as a subtle area of mucosal irregularity (Fig. 17–31). The more typical advanced lesions are bulky exophytic masses. Occasionally, infiltrative masses are seen.

### Posterior Pharyngeal Wall

Squamous cell carcinomas of the posterior pharyngeal wall are typically large but asymptomatic lesions whose first clinical manifestation is usually a neck mass that is due to cervical nodal metastasis.[40] These fungating lesions are usually longer than 5 cm (Fig. 17–32). They spread vertically into the nasopharynx or cervical esophagus. Approximately 50% of patients have either jugular or retropharyngeal lymphatic metastases, or both, at the time of initial diagnosis.[53] This form of pharyngeal cancer is the one most frequently associated with a synchronous or metachronous malignant lesion in the oral cavity, pharynx, or esophagus. The 5-year survival rate is approximately 21%.[53]

### Postcricoid Area

Postcricoid squamous cell carcinomas are rare except in Scandinavia.[60] In Scandinavia, primary postcricoid carcinomas may be associated with iron deficiency anemia and cervical esophageal webs—the Plummer-Vinson syndrome. In the United States, however, no association has been found between iron deficiency anemia and

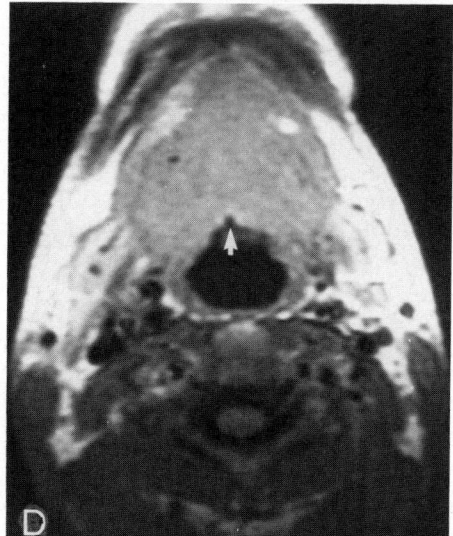

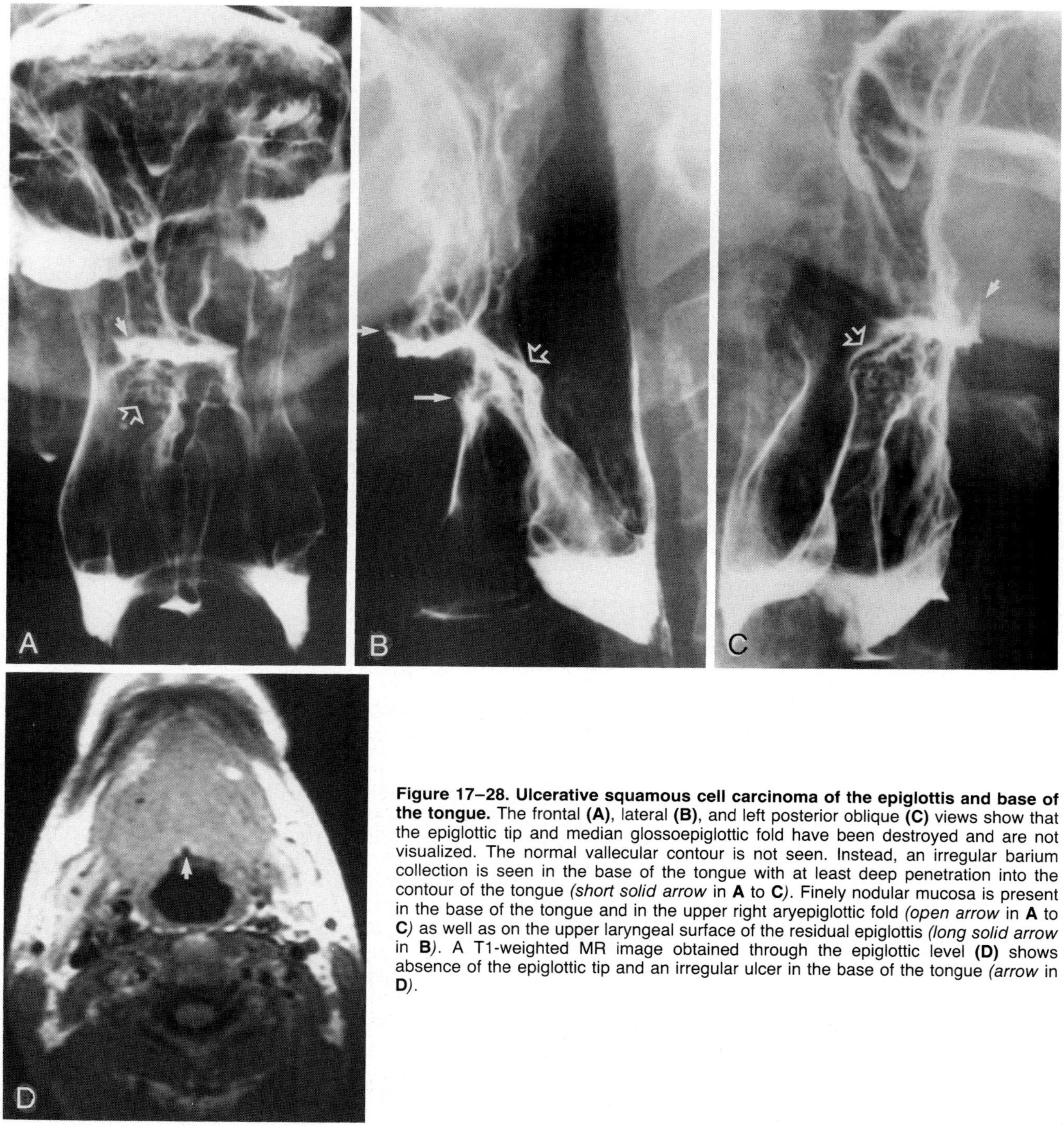

**Figure 17–28. Ulcerative squamous cell carcinoma of the epiglottis and base of the tongue.** The frontal **(A)**, lateral **(B)**, and left posterior oblique **(C)** views show that the epiglottic tip and median glossoepiglottic fold have been destroyed and are not visualized. The normal vallecular contour is not seen. Instead, an irregular barium collection is seen in the base of the tongue with at least deep penetration into the contour of the tongue *(short solid arrow* in **A** to **C)**. Finely nodular mucosa is present in the base of the tongue and in the upper right aryepiglottic fold *(open arrow* in **A** to **C)** as well as on the upper laryngeal surface of the residual epiglottis *(long solid arrow* in **B)**. A T1-weighted MR image obtained through the epiglottic level **(D)** shows absence of the epiglottic tip and an irregular ulcer in the base of the tongue *(arrow* in **D)**.

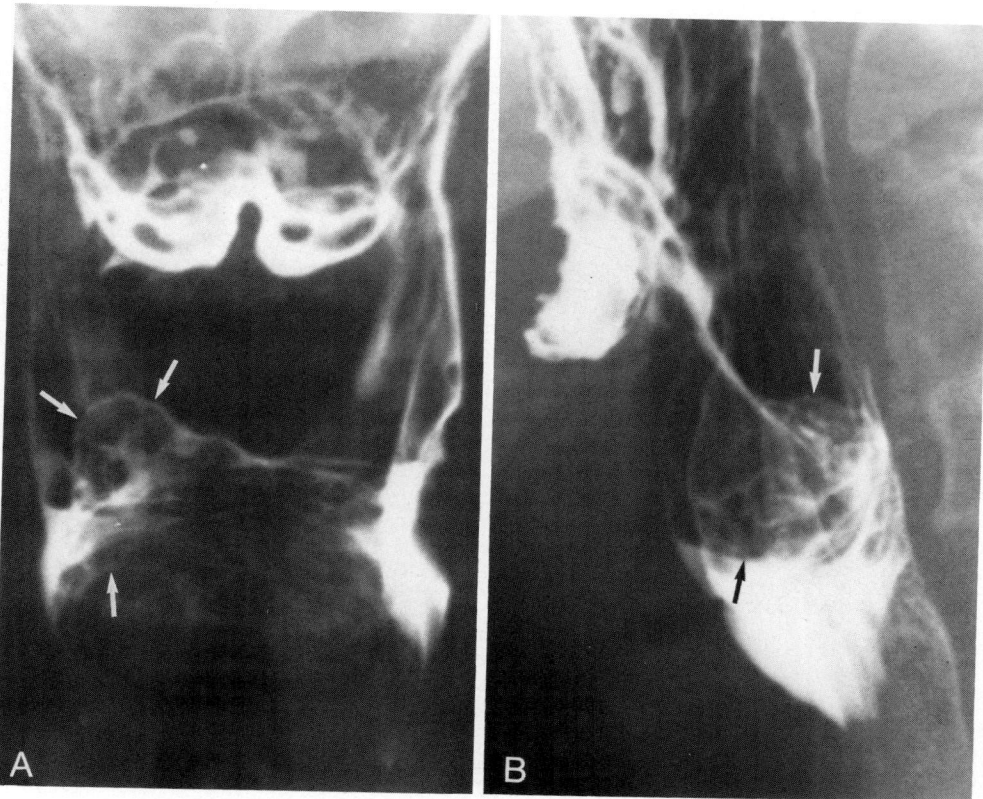

**Figure 17–29. Squamous cell carcinoma of the medial wall of the right piriform sinus. A.** A frontal view of the pharynx shows a polypoid mass involving the mucosa overlying the muscular process of the right arytenoid cartilage and medial wall of the right piriform sinus *(arrows)*. **B.** A lateral view of the pharynx shows elevation and nodularity of the mucosa overlying the muscular process of the arytenoid cartilage *(white arrow)* and nodular mucosa of the piriform sinus en face *(black arrow)*.

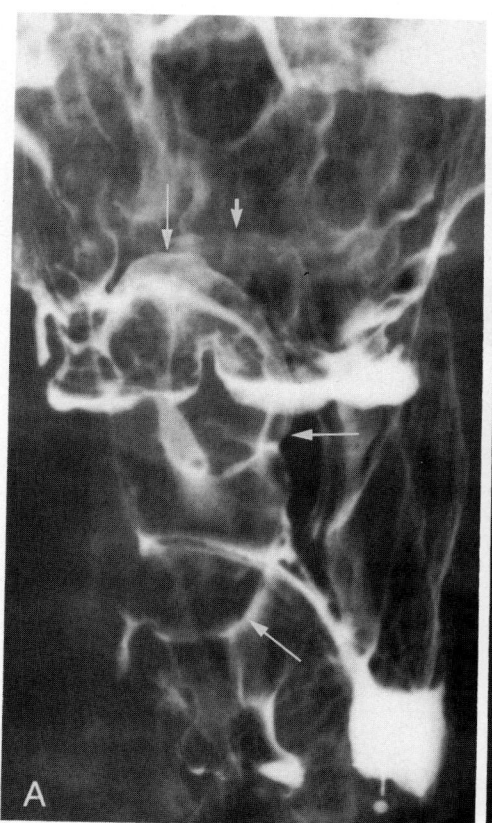

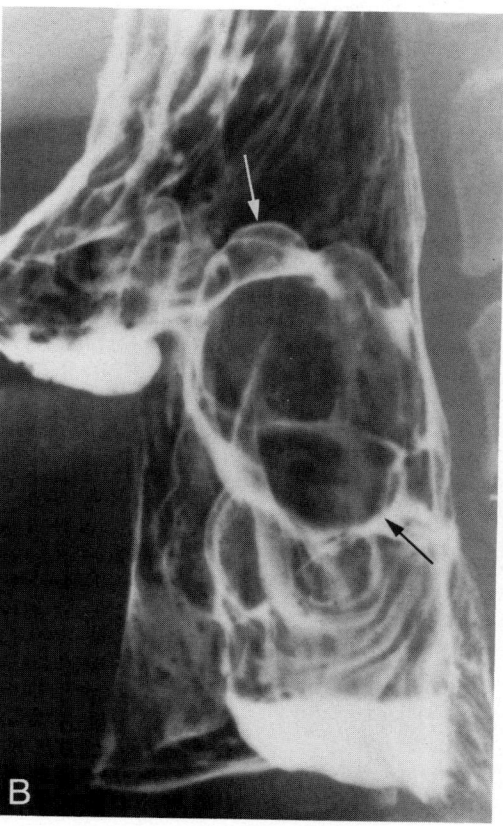

**Figure 17–30. Squamous cell carcinoma of the lateral wall of the right piriform sinus. A.** A frontal view shows obliteration of the right lateral wall of the piriform sinus. There is a large, polypoid mass *(long arrows)* protruding into the hypopharynx. The tip of the epiglottis *(short arrow)* is spared. **B.** A lateral view of the hypopharynx shows a large polypoid mass *(arrows)* en face. (**A** and **B** reprinted with permission from Rubesin SE, Glick SN: The tailored double-contrast pharyngogram. Crit Rev Diagn Imaging 28:133–179, 1988. Copyright CRC Press, Inc. Boca Raton, FL.)

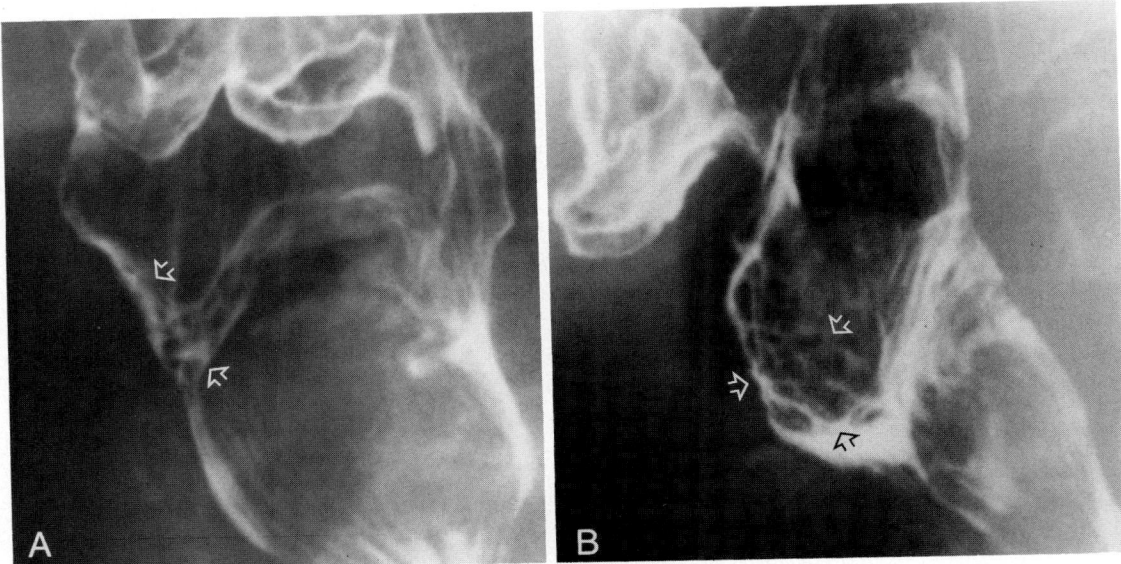

**Figure 17–31. Early squamous cell carcinoma of the right piriform sinus, extending into the submucosa.** Slight right posterior oblique **(A)** and lateral **(B)** views of the pharynx show a flat area of nodular mucosa along the lateral wall of the right piriform sinus *(arrows)*. (**A** and **B** from MS Levine, SE Rubesin, DJ Ott, Update on esophageal radiology, AJR 155, 5, 933–941, 1990, © by American Roentgen Ray Society.)

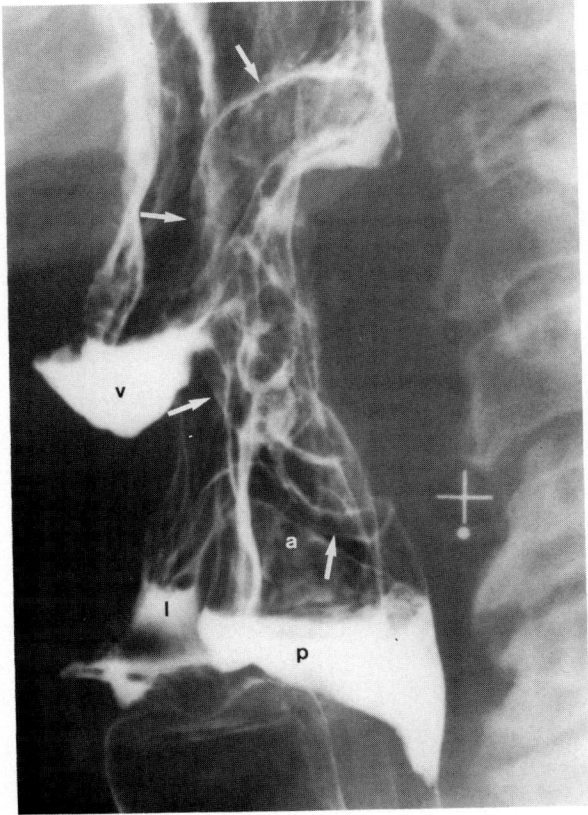

**Figure 17–32. Squamous cell carcinoma of the posterior pharyngeal wall.** A lateral spot film of the pharynx shows a large, fungating mass *(arrows)* extending from the level of the uvula to the level of the muscular processes of the arytenoid cartilages (a). Note evidence of significant pharyngeal dysfunction, with pooling in the valleculae (v), piriform sinus (p), and laryngeal vestibule (l). (Reprinted with permission from Rubesin SE, Glick SN: The tailored double-contrast pharyngogram. Crit Rev Diagn Imaging 28:133–179, 1988. Copyright CRC Press, Inc. Boca Raton, FL.)

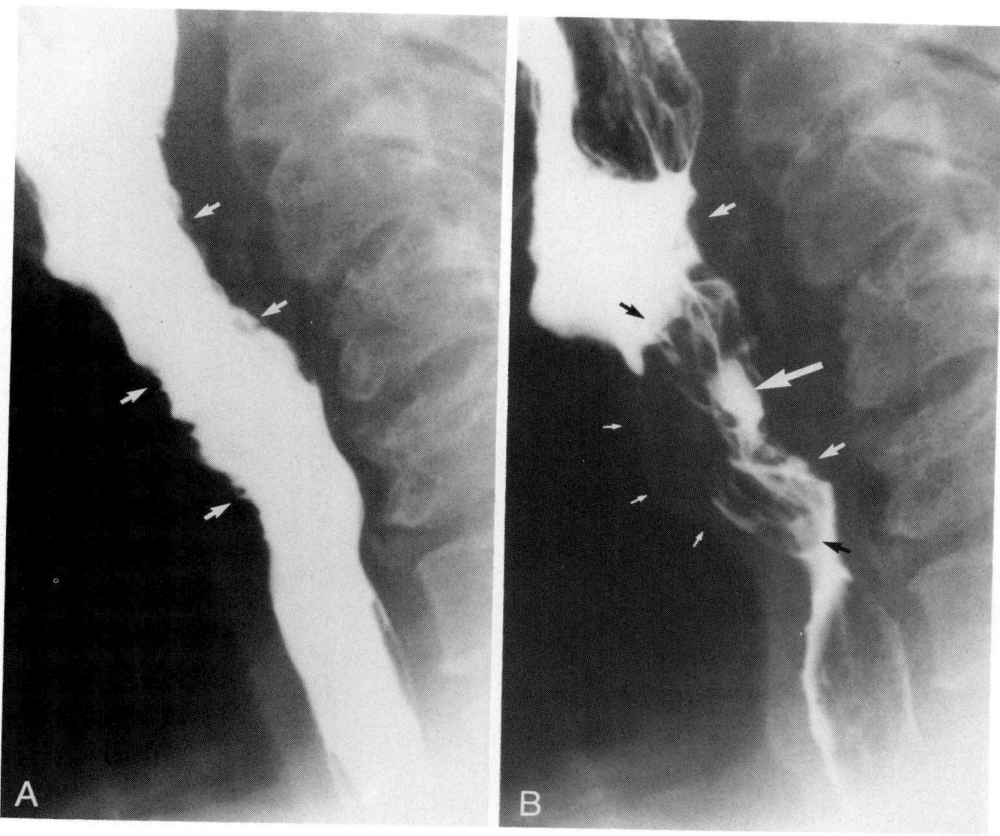

**Figure 17–33. Squamous cell carcinoma of the postcricoid region. A.** A spot film obtained during swallowing shows a finely lobulated contour of the anterior and posterior walls of the pharyngoesophageal segment *(arrows).* **B.** A spot film of the pharyngoesophageal segment during phonation shows an ulcerated mass. The central crater *(large white arrow)* is filled with barium. The mass is seen as a filling defect in the barium pool *(black arrows)* and as an irregular contour of the posterior pharyngeal wall *(medium-sized white arrows).* An impression of a smooth, extrinsic mass appears on the posterior wall of the trachea *(small white arrows).*

malignant pharyngeal tumors. The pharyngoesophageal segment is more frequently involved by direct extension of squamous cell cancer of the piriform sinus, posterior pharyngeal wall, or cervical esophagus.[60] Radiographically, postcricoid carcinomas appear as annular, infiltrating lesions that may extend into the lower hypopharynx or cervical esophagus[40] (Fig. 17–33). These annular lesions are best detected while the pharyngoesophageal segment is fully distended with barium—during dynamic examination and spot film examination obtained during swallowing.

## Lymphoma

Lymphomas of the pharynx represent approximately 10% of malignant pharyngeal tumors.[7, 75] Almost all pharyngeal lymphomas are of a non-Hodgkin type, arising in Waldeyer's ring: the adenoids, palatine tonsil, and lingual tonsil. Hodgkin's disease involving the pharynx is rare, despite the fact that Hodgkin's disease often begins in cervical lymph nodes.[76] Pharyngeal involvement occurs in only 1 to 2% of all patients with Hodgkin's disease, even those patients with disseminated tumor.

Most patients with pharyngeal lymphoma are in the fifth to sixth decade of life. Approximately one half of patients have cervical lymphadenopathy as the first clinical finding.[75] The cervical lymph nodes are involved in more than 60% of patients.[75] At the time of initial diagnosis, only 10% of patients have involvement of extranodal sites (lung and bones).[75] Approximately one half of patients have symptoms related to local pharyngeal involvement: nasal obstruction, earache, sore throat, or lump in the throat.

The most frequent pharyngeal locations of lymphoma are the palatine tonsil (in 40 to 60% of patients),[7, 75] the nasopharynx (in 18 to 28%),[75, 77] and the base of the tongue (in 10%). Approximately 25% of tumors involve multiple sites. Bilateral involvement of the palatine tonsils occurs in 15% of pharyngeal lymphomas.[75] Lymphomas only rarely arise in the hypopharynx.

Pharyngeal lymphomas are manifested radiographically as lobulated masses involving the nasopharynx, palatine tonsil (Fig. 17–34), base of the tongue, or a combination of these sites (Fig. 17–35). The mucosal surface landmarks are frequently obliterated by bulging submucosal masses[7, 22] (see Fig. 17–35). Thus, the normal lymphoid follicular pattern of the base of the tongue or palatine tonsil may be effaced by the submucosal mass.

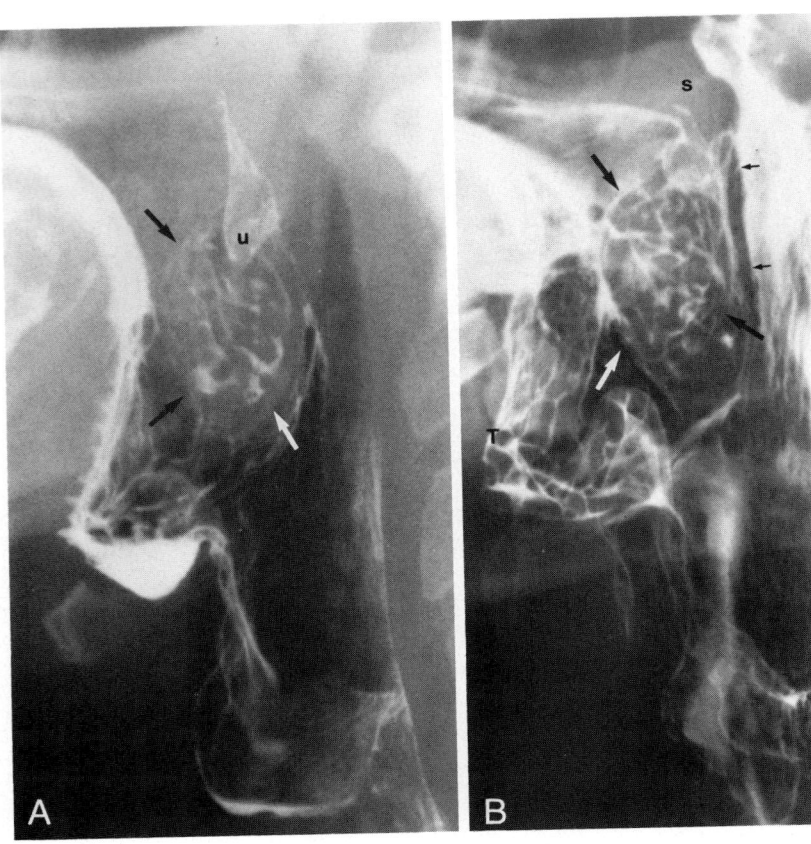

**Figure 17–34. Lymphoma of the palatine tonsil. A.** A large, lobulated palatine tonsil *(arrows)* is seen in this lateral view of the pharynx. In this elderly patient, the enlarged tonsil proved to be non-Hodgkin's lymphoma. u = uvula. **B.** A large, lobulated palatine tonsil *(long arrows)* is similar in appearance to the lymphoma in **A.** In this young patient with head trauma, the enlarged tonsil was due to lymphoid hyperplasia. Note the lymphoid hyperplasia of the base of the tongue ( T ) and lingual surface of the epiglottis. Nasopharyngeal reflux outlines the salpingopharyngeal fold *(short arrows)* and the posterior surface of the soft palate (s). Thus, tonsils that are enlarged and lobulated may be due to lymphoid hyperplasia of various causes or to infiltrating tumor, and they must be endoscopically evaluated.

**Figure 17–35. Lymphoma of the base of the tongue and the epiglottic tip. A.** A lateral view of the pharynx shows a large, lobulated mass involving the base of the tongue *(large arrows)* and tip of the epiglottis *(small arrow)*. Note that the normal contours of the valleculae have been obliterated. **B.** A frontal view of the pharynx shows complete effacement of the normal lymphoid surface pattern of the base of the tongue ( T ). Loss of contour of the valleculae is seen. Laryngeal penetration has occurred, with barium coating both surfaces of the epiglottis. The epiglottic tip *(arrow)* is smoothly enlarged. The relative lack of mucosal irregularity suggests that this huge base of the tongue mass is due to infiltrating tumor primarily in a submucosal location. (**A** and **B** from Rubesin SE, Laufer I: Pictorial review: principles of double contrast pharyngography. Dysphagia 6:170–178, 1991.)

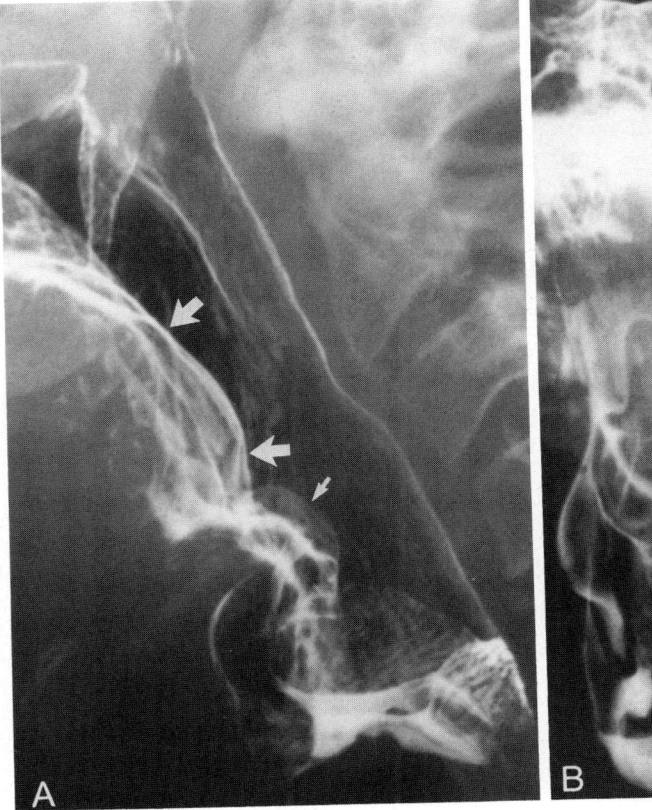

# Rare Malignant Tumors

## Carcinoma of the Minor Salivary Glands

Both benign and malignant tumors arise in the minor mucoserous salivary glands scattered deep to the epithelial layer of the pharynx. Minor salivary gland tumors constitute 20% of all salivary gland tumors and have diverse histologic features and a diverse clinical course (Fig. 17–36). Approximately 65 to 88% of minor salivary gland tumors are malignant.[78, 79] The most frequent malignant types are adenoid cystic carcinoma (35%), solid adenocarcinoma (22%) (Fig. 17–37), and muco-epidermoid carcinoma (16%).[78] By far, the most common pharyngeal location of minor salivary gland tumors is the soft palate. Palatal salivary gland tumors appear clinically as painless masses near the junction of the hard and soft palate (see Fig. 17–36). Palatal salivary gland tumors spread to the tongue, submandibular gland, lingual and hypoglossal nerves, and the mandible. In contrast to squamous cell carcinoma, cervical metastases are relatively infrequent, occurring in approximately 23% of malignant lesions.[78] Adenoid cystic carcinoma has a particular propensity for perineural tumor spread.

## Synovial Sarcoma

Synovial sarcomas of the pharynx are extremely rare. Most patients are 20 to 40 years old and complain of a painless neck mass.[80] At initial diagnosis, synovial sarcomas appear radiographically as large, bulky tumors involving the larynx, pharynx, and soft tissue of the neck.[81]

## Cartilaginous Tumors

Primary cartilaginous tumors of the pharynx are extremely rare. The pharynx may be invaded secondarily by cartilaginous tumors (chondroma, osteochondroma, and chondrosarcoma) arising in the larynx.[82] Cartilaginous tumors of the larynx are seen mainly in the fourth to sixth decade of life. Patients complain of hoarseness, poor voice, and dysphagia. Chondroid tumors usually arise in the cricoid cartilage.

Radiographically, a smooth-surfaced mass arises in the posterior lamina of the cricoid cartilage and presses and distorts the lower hypopharynx and pharyngoesophageal segment. Stippled calcification is seen in a central and/or peripheral location in more than 80% of patients.[7]

# PHARYNGEAL DAMAGE FROM RADIATION

Radiation therapy may be used as a primary or adjunctive form of treatment for pharyngeal tumors such as lymphoma or squamous cell carcinoma. The pharynx is included within the radiation portal during irradiation of tumors of the larynx and cervical lymph nodes. In the past, the pharynx was also included in the radiation portal during treatment for thyrotoxicosis or tuberculous lymphadenitis.[83]

Acute mucositis and edema occur early during the course of radiotherapy. Epithelial necrosis and ulceration result in a fibrinous exudate.[84, 85] Submucosal inflammation also occurs early. With time, the mucosa atrophies and submucosal fibrosis may occur. The majority of the chronic radiation damage results from vascular changes: thrombosis and fibrosis of capillaries and lymphatics, and subintimal fibrosis and hyalinization of veins and arteries.[86] Vascular damage leads to atrophy of the skin and to fibrosis of subcutaneous tissues, submucosal tissues, and muscle.[86] The most frequent localization of persistent edema is in the glottis and mucosa overlying the arytenoid cartilages. Severe complications such as life-threatening osteomyelitis and chondronecrosis may occur.

Five to 10 days after initial radiotherapy, the patient may complain of local discomfort, hoarseness, dryness, dysphagia, or a lump in the throat. The peak occurrence of symptoms occurs near the end of the typical 6-week course of radiation treatment. Most symptoms gradually subside 2 to 6 weeks after cessation of radiotherapy.[85] However, a substantial number of patients have persistent symptoms. For example, 15% of patients have persistent edema after radiotherapy for carcinoma of the vocal cord.[87] If parotid or other salivary glands have been damaged, xerostomia may cause persistent dysphagia. Persistent edema may suggest a serious underlying complication such as persistent carcinoma, osteomyelitis, or chondronecrosis.[87–91] Approximately one half of patients with persistent edema have recurrent or persistent tumor.[87]

The radiographic changes of radiation damage are seen in almost all patients after irradiation, with or without surgery.[92] The most frequent dynamic findings are those of epiglottic and laryngeal vestibular dysfunction and pharyngeal paresis.[92] Spot films show that the

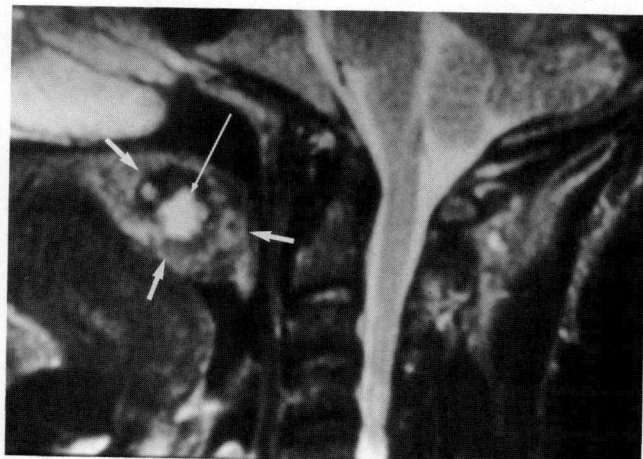

**Figure 17–36. Pleomorphic adenoma of the soft palate.** The midportion of the soft palate is markedly enlarged by a finely lobulated mass of mixed low and moderate signal intensity *(short arrows)*. On this T2-weighted image, the lobulated area of high signal intensity in the center of the mass *(long arrow)* is due to hemorrhage associated with a recent biopsy.

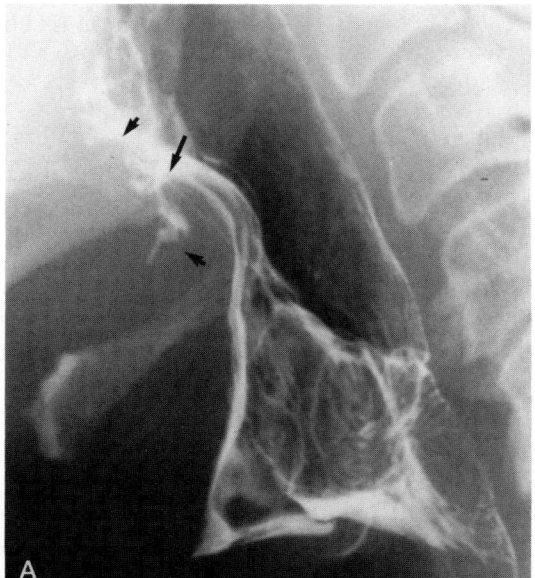

**Figure 17–37. Adenocarcinoma of the base of the tongue. A.** The epiglottic tip *(long arrow)* is apposed to the base of the tongue, and its vallecular surface is ulcerated. The valleculae are obliterated and filled by lobulated tumor *(short arrows)* arising in the base of the tongue. **B.** CT scan shows asymmetry *(arrow)* of the surface of the base of the tongue. Streak artifact from the spine and mandible makes it difficult to evaluate the depth of tumor invasion in this case. **C.** A proton density MR image obtained through the same area shows asymmetry of the tongue surface *(white arrow)* from a tumor of slightly increased signal intensity *(black arrows)* compared with that of muscle. This adenocarcinoma is macroscopically indistinguishable from the typical squamous cell carcinoma of the base of the tongue. This tumor presumably arose in minor salivary glands.

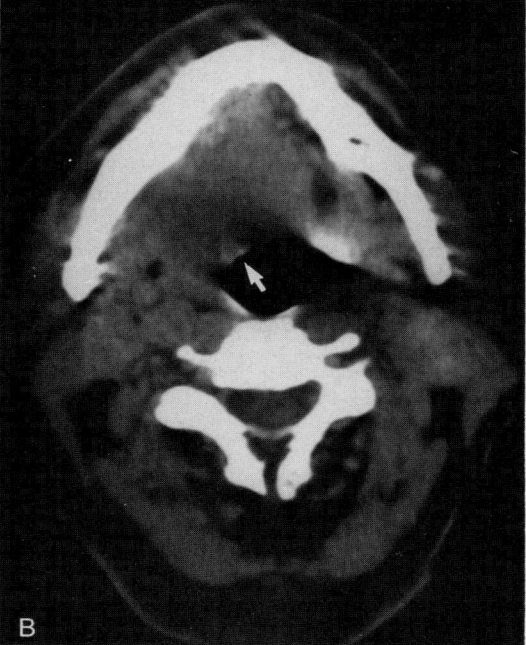

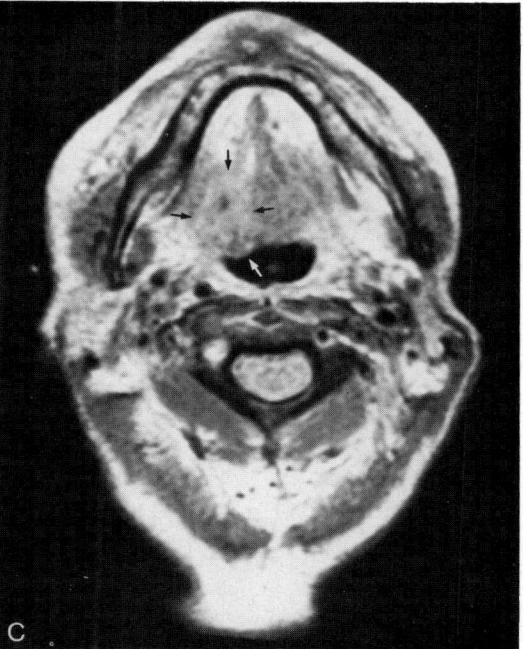

epiglottis and aryepiglottic folds are diffusely and smoothly enlarged (Fig. 17–38). The valleculae may be flattened. The mucosa overlying the muscular processes of the arytenoid cartilages is elevated. Edema from radiation may be asymmetric, especially in the region of the original tumor. Any surface irregularity on a postradiation pharyngogram suggests the possibility of persistent cancer, although radiation-induced ulceration may produce an identical radiographic finding (Fig. 17–39). Soft tissue atrophy is observed in patients with chronic radiation damage (Fig. 17–40).

Cross-sectional imaging in the patient who has undergone radiation treatment is used for detection of tumor recurrence in lymph nodes or soft tissue. Radiation changes detected by CT scanning include edema in subcutaneous tissue, or in the fat of the pre-epiglottic and the paralaryngeal spaces, and thickening of the mucosa overlying the arytenoid cartilages and aryepiglottic folds. Whether MR imaging will be able to distinguish radiation fibrosis from recurrent tumor, or from the severe inflammatory changes related to osteonecrosis or chondronecrosis, is unknown. Baseline stud-

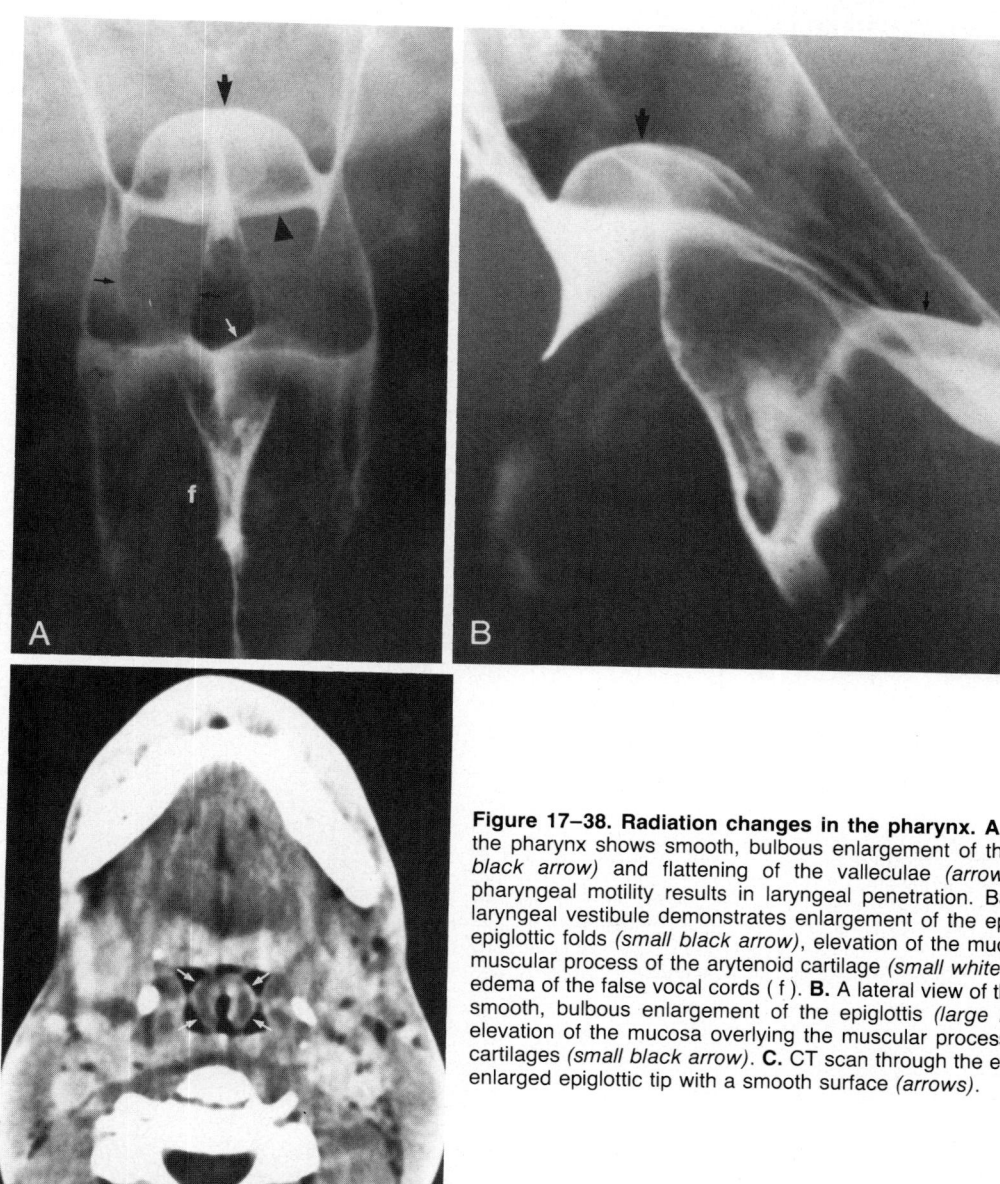

**Figure 17–38. Radiation changes in the pharynx. A.** A frontal view of the pharynx shows smooth, bulbous enlargement of the epiglottis *(large black arrow)* and flattening of the valleculae *(arrowhead)*. Abnormal pharyngeal motility results in laryngeal penetration. Barium coating the laryngeal vestibule demonstrates enlargement of the epiglottis, wide aryepiglottic folds *(small black arrow)*, elevation of the mucosa overlying the muscular process of the arytenoid cartilage *(small white arrow)*, and even edema of the false vocal cords ( f ). **B.** A lateral view of the pharynx shows smooth, bulbous enlargement of the epiglottis *(large black arrow)* and elevation of the mucosa overlying the muscular process of the arytenoid cartilages *(small black arrow)*. **C.** CT scan through the epiglottis shows an enlarged epiglottic tip with a smooth surface *(arrows)*.

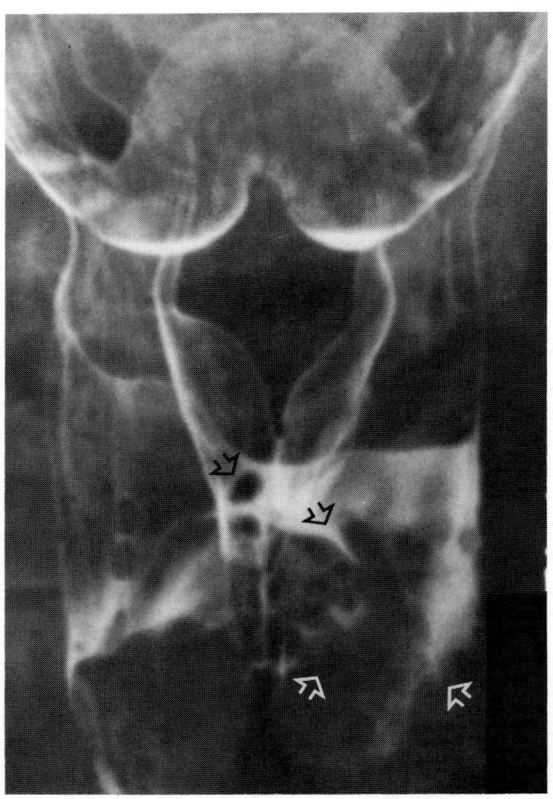

**Figure 17–39. Radiation damage to pharynx and recurrent squamous cell carcinoma in the piriform sinus.** A frontal view shows the typical findings of radiation damage, with smooth enlargement of the epiglottis, flattening of the valleculae, laryngeal penetration showing widening of the aryepiglottic folds, and elevation of the mucosa overlying the muscular process of the arytenoid cartilages. However, the lower contour of the left piriform sinus is irregular, and a nodular mucosa *(arrows)* carpets the left piriform sinus. A recurrent squamous cell carcinoma of the piriform sinus was diagnosed at endoscopy and biopsy.

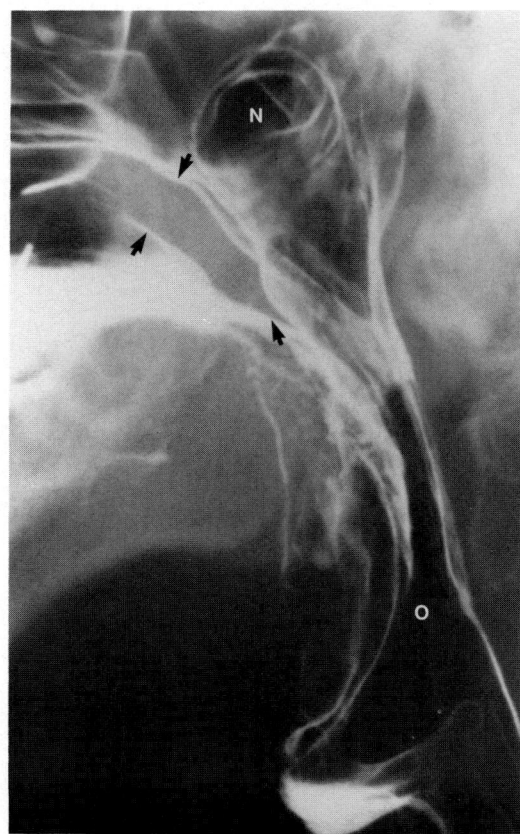

**Figure 17–40. Atrophy after radiotherapy.** This patient had two courses of radiotherapy for nasopharyngeal lymphoma, with recurrence 10 and 20 years before this examination was performed. A lateral view of the nasopharynx (N) and oropharynx (O) shows barium coating of the nasopharynx attributable to nasal regurgitation. The soft palate *(arrows)* is shortened and thinned, an indication of soft palate atrophy associated with radiotherapy. The nasal regurgitation is secondary to loss of soft palate function and volume.

ies after therapy are helpful when patients are evaluated for tumor recurrence at a later date.

### Acknowledgment

Figures 17–7, 17–8, 17–10, 17–13, and 17–27 are reproduced from Laufer I, Levine MS (eds): Double Contrast Gastrointestinal Radiology (2nd ed). Philadelphia: WB Saunders, 1992.

# References

1. Rubesin SE, Laufer I: Pictorial review: principles of double contrast pharyngography. Dysphagia 6:170–178, 1991.
2. Bachman AL, Seaman WB, Macken KL: Lateral pharyngeal diverticula. Radiology 91:774–782, 1968.
3. Rubesin SE, Jessurun J, Robertson D, et al: Lines of the pharynx. Radiographics 7:217–237, 1987.
4. Norris CW: Pharyngoceles of the hypopharynx. Laryngoscope 89:1788–1807, 1979.
5. Curtis DJ, Cruess DF, Crain M, et al: Lateral pharyngeal outpouchings: a comparison of dysphagic and asymptomatic patients. Dysphagia 2:156–161, 1988.
6. Jones B, Donner MW: Common structural lesions. In Jones B, Donner MW (eds): Normal and Abnormal Swallowing: Imaging in Diagnosis and Therapy. New York: Springer-Verlag, 1991, pp 93–107.
7. Hyams VJ, Batsakis JG, Michaels L: Tumors of the upper respiratory tract and ear. In Atlas of Tumor Pathology, Second Series, Fascicle 25. Bethesda: Armed Forces Institute of Pathology, 1988.
8. Lindell MM, Jing BS, Fischer EP, et al: Laryngocele. AJR 131:259–262, 1978.
9. Canalis RF, Maxwell DS, Hemenway WG: Laryngocele—an updated review. J Otolaryngol 6:191–199, 1977.
10. Glaser HS, Mauro MA, Aronberg DJ, et al: Computed tomography of laryngocele. AJR 140:549–552, 1983.
11. Maran AGD, Buchanan DR: Branchial cysts, sinuses and fistulae. Clin Otolaryngol 3:77–92, 1978.
12. Bhaskar SN, Bernier JL: Histogenesis of branchial cysts. Am J Pathol 35:407–414, 1959.
13. Som PM, Sacher M, Lanzieri CF, et al: Parenchymal cysts of the lower neck. Radiology 157:399–406, 1985.
14. Salazar JB, Duke RA, Ellis JV: Second branchial cleft cyst: unusual location and a new CT diagnostic sign. AJR 145:965–966, 1985.
15. Perrott JW: Anatomical aspects of hypopharyngeal diverticula. Aust N Z J Surg 31:307–317, 1962.
16. Zaino C, Jacobson HG, Lepow H, et al: The pharyngoesophageal sphincter. Radiology 89:639–645, 1967.
17. Zaino C, Jacobson HG, Lepow H, et al: The pharyngoesophageal sphincter. Springfield, IL: Charles C Thomas, 1970.
18. Knuff TE, Benjamin SB, Castell DO: Pharyngoesophageal (Zenker's) diverticulum: a reappraisal. Gastroenterology 82:734–736, 1982.
19. Frieling T, Berges W, Lubke HJ, et al: Upper esophageal sphincter function in patients with Zenker's diverticulum. Dysphagia 3:90–92, 1988.
20. Smiley TB, Caves PK, Porter DC: Relationship between posterior pharyngeal pouch and hiatus hernia. Thorax 25:725–731, 1970.
21. Delahunty JE, Margulies SE, Alonso UA, et al: The relationship of reflux esophagitis to pharyngeal pouch (Zenker's diverticulum). Laryngoscope 81:570–577, 1971.
22. Rubesin SE: Pharynx. In Laufer I, Levine MS (eds): Double Contrast Gastrointestinal Radiology (2nd ed). Philadelphia: WB Saunders, 1992, pp 73–105.
23. Shirazi KK, Daffner RH, Gaede JT: Ulcer occurring in Zenker's diverticulum. Gastrointest Radiol 2:117–118, 1977.
24. Nanson EM: Carcinoma in a long-standing pharyngeal diverticulum. Br J Surg 63:417–419, 1976.
25. Wychulis AR, Gunnulaugsson GH, Clagett OT: Carcinoma arising in pharyngoesophageal diverticulum. Surgery 66:976–979, 1969.
26. Ekberg O, Nylander G: Lateral diverticula from the pharyngoesophageal junction area. Radiology 146:117–122, 1983.
27. Clements JL, Cox GW, Torres WE, et al: Cervical esophageal webs—a roentgen-anatomic correlation. AJR 121:221–231, 1974.
28. Nosher JL, Campbell WL, Seaman WB: The clinical significance of cervical esophageal and hypopharyngeal webs. Radiology 117:45–47, 1975.
29. Weaver JW, Kaude JV, Hamlin DJ: Webs of the lower esophagus: a complication of gastroesophageal reflux? AJR 142:289–292, 1984.
30. Seaman WB: The significance of webs in the hypopharynx and upper esophagus. Radiology 89:32–38, 1967.
31. Ekberg O: Cervical oesophageal webs in patients with dysphagia. Clin Radiol 32:633–641, 1981.
32. Ekberg O, Nylander G: Webs and web-like formations in the pharynx and cervical esophagus. Diagn Imaging 52:10–18, 1983.
33. Waldenstrom J, Kjeulberg SR: The roentgenological diagnosis of sideropenic dysphagia (Plummer-Vinson's syndrome). Acta Radiol 20:618–638, 1939.
34. McNab Jones RF: The Paterson-Brown-Kelly syndrome: its relationship to iron deficiency and postcricoid carcinoma. J Laryngol Otol 71:529–561, 1961.
35. Ekberg O, Birch-lensen M, Lindstrom C: Mucosal folds in the valleculae. Dysphagia 1:68–72, 1986.
36. Shauffer IA, Phillips HE, Sequeira J: The jet phenomenon: a manifestation of esophageal web. AJR 129:747–748, 1977.
37. Taylor AJ, Stewart ET, Dodds WJ: The esophageal jet phenomenon revisited. AJR 155:289–290, 1990.
38. Pitman RG, Fraser GM: The post-cricoid impression on the oesophagus. Clin Radiol 16:34–39, 1965.
39. Harris RD, Berdon WE, Baker DH: Roentgen diagnosis of acute epiglottis in the adult. J Can Assoc Radiol 21:270–272, 1970.
40. Balfe DM, Heiken JP: Contrast evaluation of structural lesions of the pharynx. Curr Probl Diagn Radiol 15:73–160, 1986.
41. Rubesin SE, Glick SN: The tailored double-contrast pharyngogram. Crit Rev Diagn Imaging 28:133–179, 1988.
42. Kabakian HA, Dahmash MS: Pharyngoesophageal manifestations of epidermolysis bullosa. Clin Radiol 29:91–94, 1978.
43. Bosma JF, Gravkowski EA, Tryostad CW: Chronic ulcerative pharyngitis. Arch Otolaryngol 87:85–96, 1968.
44. Gromet M, Homer MJ, Carter BL: Lymphoid hyperplasia at the base of the tongue. Radiology 144:825–828, 1982.
45. Mansson T, Wilske J, Kindblom L-G: Lipoma of the hypopharynx: a case report and a review of the literature. J Laryngol Otol 92:1037–1043, 1978.
46. Patterson HC, Dickerson GR, Pilch BZ, et al: Hamartoma of the hypopharynx. Arch Otolaryngol 107:767–772, 1981.
47. Bachman AL: Benign, non-neoplastic conditions of the larynx and pharynx. Radiol Clin North Am 16:273–290, 1978.
48. DiBartolomeo JR, Olsen AR: Pedunculated lipoma of the epiglottis. Arch Otolaryngol 98:55–57, 1973.
49. Chang-Lo M: Laryngeal involvement in Von Recklinghausen's disease. Laryngoscope 87:435–442, 1977.
50. Hyams VJ, Rabuzzi DD: Cartilaginous tumors of the larynx. Laryngoscope 80:755–767, 1970.
51. Decker J, Goldstein JC: Current concepts in otolaryngology: risk factors in the head and neck cancer. N Engl J Med 306:1151–1155, 1982.
52. Semenkovich JW, Balfe DM, Weyman PJ, et al: Barium pharyngography: comparison of single and double contrast. AJR 144:715–720, 1985.
53. Carpenter RJ III, DeSanto LW, Devine KD, et al: Cancer of the hypopharynx. Arch Otolaryngol 102:716–721, 1976.
54. Cunningham MP, Catlin D: Cancer of the pharyngeal wall. Cancer 20:1859–1866, 1967.
55. Dockerty MD, Parkhill EM, Dahlin DC, et al: Tumors of the Oral Cavity and Pharynx. Washington, DC: Armed Forces Institute of Pathology, 1968.
56. Goldstein HM, Zornoza J: Association of squamous cell carcinoma of the head and neck with cancer of the esophagus. AJR 131:791–794, 1978.
57. Thompson WM, Oddson TA, Kelvin F, et al: Synchronous and metachronous squamous cell carcinoma of the head, neck, and esophagus. Gastrointest Radiol 3:123–127, 1978.

58. Wagonfeld DJH, Harwood AR, Bryce EP, et al: Second primary respiratory tract malignant neoplasms in supraglottic carcinoma. Arch Otolaryngol 107:135–137, 1981.

59. Spiessl B, Bearhs OH, Hermanek P, et al: TNM Atlas. Berlin: Springer-Verlag, 1990, p 143.

60. Jing BS: Roentgen examination of the larynx and hypopharynx. Radiol Clin North Am 8:361–386, 1970.

61. Seaman WB: Contrast radiography in neoplastic disease of the larynx and pharynx. Semin Roentgenol 9:301–309, 1974.

62. Levine MS, Rubesin SE, Ott DJ: Update on esophageal radiology. AJR 155:933–941, 1990.

63. Kassel E, Keller A, Kuchorczyk W: MRI of the floor of the mouth, tongue and orohypopharynx. Radiol Clin North Am 27:331–351, 1989.

64. Mancuso AA, Calcaterra TC, Hanafee WN: Computed tomography of the larynx. Radiol Clin North Am 16:195–208, 1978.

65. Hoppe RT, Goffinet DR, Bagshaw MA: Carcinoma of the nasopharynx. Cancer 37:2605–2612, 1976.

66. Vogl T, Dresel S, Bilaniuk LT, et al: Tumors of the nasopharynx and adjacent areas: MR imaging with Gd-DTPA. AJNR 11:187–194, 1990.

67. Silver CE: Surgical management of neoplasms of the larynx, hypopharynx and cervical esophagus. Curr Probl Surg 14:2–69, 1977.

68. Frazell EL, Lucas JC: Cancer of the tongue: report of the management of 1,554 patients. Cancer 15:1085–1099, 1962.

69. Barrs DM, DeSanto LW, O'Fallon WM: Squamous cell carcinoma of the tonsil and tongue-base region. Arch Otolaryngol 105:479–485, 1979.

70. Strong EW: Carcinoma of the tongue. Otolaryngol Clin North Am 12:107–114, 1979.

71. Jiminez JR: Roentgen examination of the oropharynx and oral cavity. Radiol Clin North Am 8:413–424, 1970.

72. Apter AJ, Levine MS, Glick SN: Carcinomas of the base of the tongue: diagnosis using double-contrast radiography of the pharynx. Radiology 151:123–126, 1984.

73. Chung CK, Stryker JA, Abt AB, et al: Histologic grading in the clinical evaluation of laryngeal carcinoma. Arch Otolaryngol 106:623–624, 1980.

74. Kirchner JA, Owen JR: Five hundred cancers of the larynx and pyriform sinus: results of treatment by radiation and surgery. Laryngoscope 87:1288–1303, 1977.

75. Banfi A, Bonadonna G, Carnevali G, et al: Lymphoreticular sarcomas with primary involvement of Waldeyer's ring. Cancer 26:341–351, 1970.

76. Todd GB, Michaels L: Hodgkin's disease involving Waldeyer's lymphoid ring. Cancer 34:1769–1778, 1974.

77. Al-Saleem T, Harwick R, Robbins R, et al: Malignant lymphomas of the pharynx. Cancer 26:1383–1387, 1970.

78. Spiro RH, Koss LG, Hajdu SI, et al: Tumors of minor salivary origin. Cancer 31:117–129, 1973.

79. Conley J, Dingman DL: Adenoid cystic carcinoma in the head and neck (cylindroma). Arch Otolaryngol 100:81–90, 1974.

80. Krugman ME, Rosin HD, Toker C: Synovial sarcoma of the head and neck. Arch Otolaryngol 98:53–54, 1973.

81. Gatti WM, Strom CG, Orfei E: Synovial sarcoma of the laryngopharynx. Arch Otolaryngol 101:633–636, 1975.

82. Huizenga C, Balogh K: Cartilaginous tumors of the larynx. Cancer 26:201–210, 1970.

83. Goolden AWG: Pharyngeal malignancy following irradiation of the neck. Br J Radiol 45:795, 1972 (abstract).

84. Fajardo LF: Radiation-induced pathology of the alimentary tract. *In* Whitehead R (ed): Gastrointestinal and Oesophageal Pathology. Edinburgh: Churchill Livingstone, 1984, pp 813–814.

85. Chandler JR: Radiation fibrosis and necrosis of the larynx. Ann Otol Rhinol Laryngol 88:509–514, 1979.

86. Keene M, Harwood AR, Bryce DP, et al: Histopathological study of radionecrosis in laryngeal carcinoma. Laryngoscope 92:173–180, 1982.

87. Fu KK, Woodhouse RJ, Quivey JM, et al: The significance of laryngeal edema following radiotherapy of carcinoma of the vocal cord. Cancer 49:655–658, 1982.

88. Kagan AR, Calcaterra T, Ward P, et al: Significance of edema of the endolarynx following curative irradiation for carcinoma. AJR 120:169–172, 1974.

89. Larson DL, Lindberg RD, Lane E, et al: Major complications of radiotherapy in cancer of the oral cavity and oropharynx. A 10 year retrospective study. Am J Surg 146:531–536, 1983.

90. Goffinet DR, Eltringham FR, Glatstein E, et al: Carcinoma of the larynx: results of radiation therapy in 213 patients. AJR 117:553–564, 1973.

91. Bedwinek JM, Shukovsky LJ, Fletcher GH, et al: Osteonecrosis in patients treated with definitive therapy for squamous cell carcinomas of the oral cavity and naso- and oropharynx. Radiology 119:665–667, 1976.

92. Ekberg O, Nylander G: Pharyngeal dysfunction after treatment for pharyngeal cancer with surgery and radiotherapy. Gastrointest Radiol 8:97–104, 1983.

# Imaging of the Postoperative Neck

Franz J. Wippold II, M.D.

Dennis M. Balfe, M.D.

## INTRODUCTION

Clinical management of patients who have undergone surgery for cancer of the larynx or pharynx is difficult. The contribution of a skilled clinical examination toward assessment of nodal recurrence is considerably reduced, because of the alterations of the normal anatomy resulting from surgery or radiation therapy. Although mucosal recurrence can be adequately detected by the use of direct laryngoscopy and biopsy, swelling of the residual laryngeal structures often obscures portions of the mucosal field. Moreover, random biopsies of an irradiated field are not without risk, because deep biopsy may induce chondronecrosis.[1, 2] For these reasons, radiologists asked to evaluate postoperative patients can provide uniquely valuable information for clinical management.

The most common indications for performing an imaging procedure in the patient who has undergone laryngectomy fall into two general categories: early surgical complications and late dysphagia. In the early recuperative phase, the most common clinical problems are fistula and abscess. The development of late dysphagia is usually caused by recurrent, persistent, or second primary cancer,[3–6] but benign processes such as fibrous stricture or recurrent aspiration are also frequently encountered.[7] Therefore, the radiologist must ask two questions: 1) What examination is most likely to be helpful in this clinical situation? 2) What is the expected appearance of the neck structures after a particular surgical procedure? These questions are the focus of this chapter.

The procedures available to the radiologist must first be determined. The simplest is pharyngography. Highly detailed images of the pharynx may be obtained by using standard air-contrast methods;[8, 9] these methods represent a well-established means of obtaining information about the mucosal surface. A water-soluble contrast medium or thin barium suspension can also identify fistulas. The most important contribution of videofluoroscopy, however, is its recording of dynamic functional information to assess a cause for dysphagia or aspiration.[10, 11] Videofluoroscopy is usually not useful in evaluating extra-alimentary regions, such as the submucosa and lymph nodes.

Computed tomography (CT) affords little information about the mucosa and cannot be used to assess dynamic function. Its major contribution is that it allows evaluation of lymph nodes and submucosal areas in the neck and upper thorax.[12] Proper technique is vital: collimation should be optimized for the structures of interest (5 mm is the most common choice), and the patient's neck should be extended as much as possible to profile the residual laryngeal structures in the optimal plane. In postoperative patients, evaluation should extend from the base of the skull to the thoracic inlet. Provided no contraindication exists, intravenous contrast medium should always be administered as a rapid bolus, and scans should be obtained as quickly as possible before intravascular contrast medium begins to equilibrate with the extracellular fluid space. CT is the preferred technique for evaluating patients for abscesses or possible tumor recurrence.

Magnetic resonance (MR) imaging is a method capable of displaying images in any plane of section. Its spatial resolution is poorer than that of CT, but its contrast sensitivity is considerably better. Unlike CT, MR imaging requires no iodinated contrast agents or ionizing radiation.[13–17] Artifacts from dental plates or shoulders are eliminated. However, MR imaging is slower than CT, and artifacts caused by motion can be introduced. This problem is particularly important in postoperative patients because of their inability to control secretions during long examinations and because of the high association of epidermoid cancer of the head and neck with chronic obstructive pulmonary disease. Furthermore, the strong magnetic field precludes the imaging of patients with clips for treatment of cerebral aneurysm or with cardiac pacemakers. Neither CT nor MR imaging has emerged as the definitively superior diagnostic technique for evaluating the postoperative patient. In our practice, MR imaging is used chiefly as a problem-solving technique to evaluate nonspecific CT findings.

Ultrasonography is available for some special indications. It is quite useful as a bedside method to evaluate the postoperative neck for the presence of an abscess. Color Doppler sonography may be of use in diagnosing vascular complications, such as arterial insufficiency of graft pedicles; this concept has not been tested on a clinical basis.

## EFFECTS OF ADJUNCTIVE PROCEDURES ON IMAGING

Before specific operations are considered, it is useful to define the radiologic effects of adjunctive procedures that are commonly performed. These procedures include radiation therapy, radical neck dissection, and flap grafts.

### Radiation Therapy

Radiation therapy may be administered either as a primary therapy (for inoperable patients or for patients with localized true vocal cord tumors) or as an adjunctive procedure (in surgical patients who have tumor at the margin of resection). For primary radiation therapy, the radiation oncologist attempts to deliver 7000 cGy to the primary tumor site and to the node-bearing regions of the neck. During the acute phase of radiation injury, mucosal edema occurs. Chronic radiation damage is characterized by fibrosis and vasculitis, which may persist for years.[1, 2, 18, 19]

Pharyngography performed after radiation therapy demonstrates thickening and reduced mobility of the epiglottis and arytenoid cartilages (Fig. 18–1). Some degree of vestibular penetration of barium is common and may result from the reduced mobility and associated sensory loss throughout the pharynx. Asymmetry in the degree of enlargement of the arytenoid cartilages or aryepiglottic folds is also common and does not suggest persistent cancer. Mucosal irregularity, discrete mass, and ulceration are not expected responses, however, and should be interpreted as highly suggestive of tumor recurrence (Fig. 18–2).

The most common reason to perform pharyngography in an irradiated patient is to determine a cause for dysphagia. Clinically occult aspiration may be demonstrated during pharyngography. For this reason, the optimal examination begins in the lateral projection, with the patient sipping small amounts of thin barium suspension. If florid aspiration occurs, the examination is terminated. Although the examination is limited, it should be possible to determine whether the aspiration is due to limited mobility or to mechanical obstruction.

CT scanning after radiation therapy shows thickening of the skin and platysma muscle. Linear soft tissue densities and subcutaneous fat thickening occur at doses of 6800 to 7000 cGy. Above 7000 cGy, the aryepiglottic folds and the pharyngeal walls become thickened. Also, the CT density of the paralaryngeal and pre-epiglottic spaces increases. Intralaryngeal edema may be symmetric or asymmetric and is therefore nonspecific for tumor

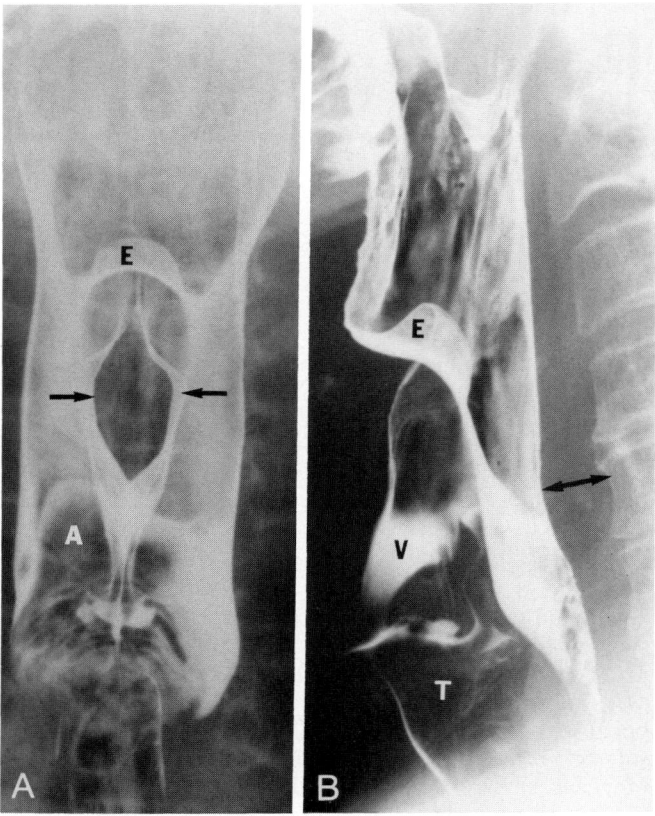

**Figure 18–1. The pharynx after radiation therapy: expected pharyngographic appearance.** This 71-year-old man was examined for mild dysphagia 7 months after undergoing full-course radiation therapy for right tonsillar epidermoid carcinoma. **A.** Anteroposterior view shows thickening of the epiglottis (E) and aryepiglottic folds *(arrows)*. There is asymmetric swelling of the mucosa overlying the arytenoid cartilages (A), so that the right side appears mass-like. No tumor was present; the patient has survived tumor free for 5 years. **B.** Lateral view of the same patient demonstrates the thickened epiglottis (E) and aryepiglottic folds. Note the increased prevertebral space *(double arrow)*. Silent aspiration has occurred, explaining the presence of barium in the laryngeal vestibule (V) and laryngeal ventricle and the coating of barium on the anterior surface of the trachea (T).

recurrence. Routine scanning should include bolus administration of contrast medium and rapid table incrementation. With the use of this technique, residual tumor is depicted as a low-attenuation mass, often with a more densely stained periphery (Fig. 18–3). It may, however, be quite difficult to distinguish an infiltrating tumor from an area of radiation-induced edema.

Some reports indicate that signal intensity of tumor on MR images tends to diminish with successful radiation therapy and with the development of fibrosis. Residual tumor usually maintains a high signal intensity. However, similar changes can also be seen in edema, hyperplastic lymphadenopathy, infection, and hemorrhage.

### Radical Neck Dissection

Radical neck dissection is occasionally performed as a primary procedure for primary cancer of unknown

**Figure 18–2. New primary tumor after full-course radiation therapy: pharyngographic appearance.** This 55-year-old woman was treated with full-course radiation therapy 18 months previously for epidermoid carcinoma of the left true vocal cord. **A.** Anteroposterior view shows a large mass (M) with ulceration on its inferior surface *(arrow)*, which has replaced the right aryepiglottic fold and extended into the right false vocal cord. **B.** Lateral view from the same examination shows the deep ulcer (U) that penetrated into the paralaryngeal space. Note the irregularity of the posterior surface of the swollen epiglottis *(arrows)*; this irregularity reflects tumor involvement of the laryngeal surface of the epiglottic mucosa.

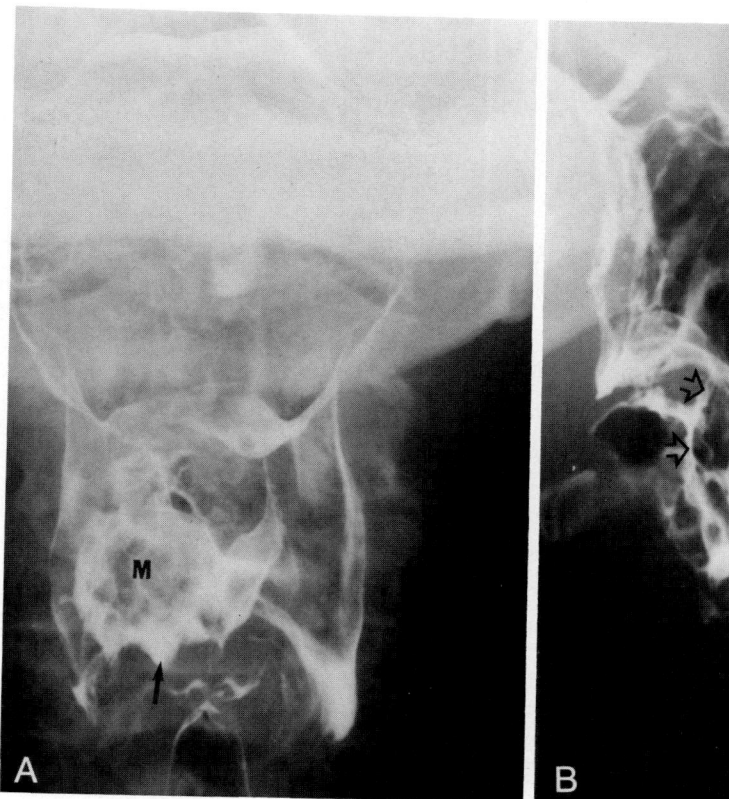

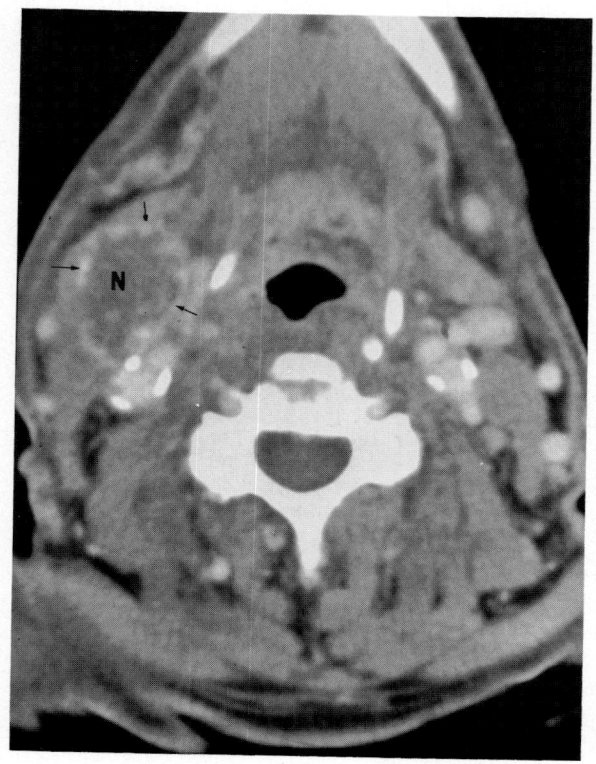

**Figure 18–3. Nodal metastasis after full-course radiation therapy: CT appearance.** This CT scan, which was obtained during rapid infusion of contrast medium, shows thickening of the skin and platysma muscle, and linear soft tissue strands within the subcutaneous fat. A low-attenuation nodal mass (N) is present within the jugular chain. The hypervascular rim *(arrows)* correctly predicted capsular invasion by the recurrent epidermoid tumor.

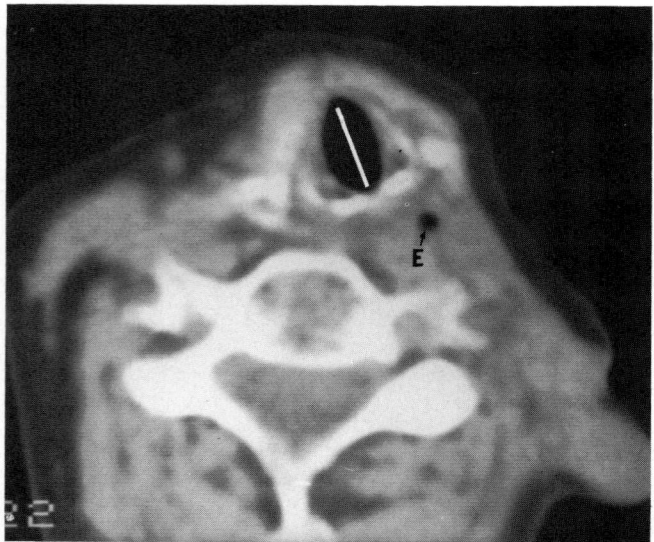

**Figure 18–4. Radical neck dissection: expected CT appearance.** This 70-year-old woman who had epidermoid cancer of unknown origin metastatic to left neck nodes was examined by CT 2 years after undergoing radical lymph node dissection. Note shift of the axis of the larynx *(white line),* and displacement of the esophagus (E), toward the dissected side.

origin detected in a cervical lymph node but is much more commonly performed in conjunction with laryngectomy. Because cancers of the supraglottis and piriform sinuses are so commonly associated with cervical adenopathy (which is often clinically occult), conservation surgery performed for these primary tumors is almost always accompanied by neck dissection.[20] The surgical procedure entails removal of the major cervical lymph nodes and their surrounding fat as well as of the sternocleidomastoid muscle. The observable effects of the procedure are due to the absence of these structures.

On pharyngograms, the lateral wall of the pharynx is straightened, and the piriform sinus on the resected side is usually narrower than that on the normal side. The cervical esophagus frequently shifts to the side of the resection but returns to the midline at the thoracic inlet.

Imaging with CT and MR likewise demonstrates deviation of the residual laryngeal cartilages and cervical esophagus toward the resected side (Fig. 18–4). Except for the absence of the sternocleidomastoid muscle, jugular vein, and perinodal fat, the neck anatomy is otherwise undisturbed (Fig. 18–5). Nodular masses in the surgical bed are unusual and suggest recurrent tumor (Figs. 18–6 to 18–8).

## Flap Grafts

One of the problems confronting a surgeon attempting to reconstruct the pharynx in a patient with extensive tumor is the absence of sufficient mucosa to form the neopharyngeal tube. Bakamjian's introduction of flap grafts in the 1960s markedly increased the number of successful reconstructions performed.[21] The major difficulty with the common myocutaneous grafts (taken from the region of the greater pectoral muscle or deltoid

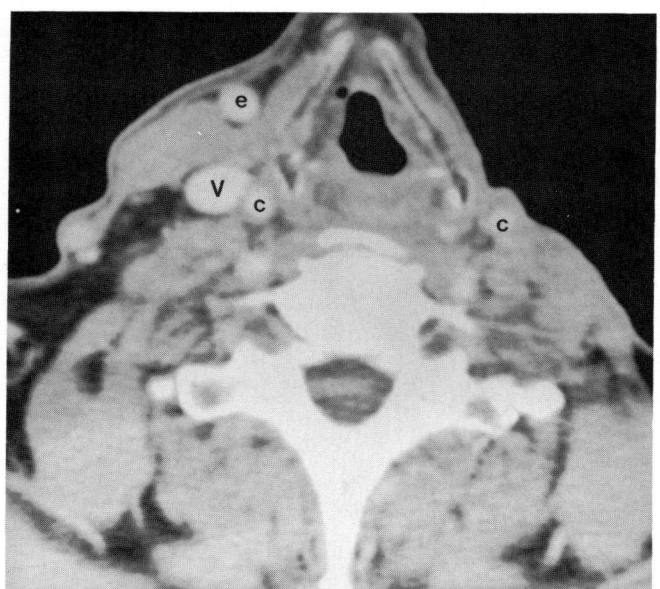

**Figure 18–5. Vascular alterations after radical neck dissection: CT appearance.** This 60-year-old man was examined by CT 15 months after undergoing left radical neck dissection for metastatic epidermoid carcinoma from an unknown primary site. Note opacification of the normal carotid artery (c), internal jugular vein (V), and external jugular vein (e) on the right side. The left carotid artery (c) lies just deep to the skin, and neither jugular vein is visualized on the operated side.

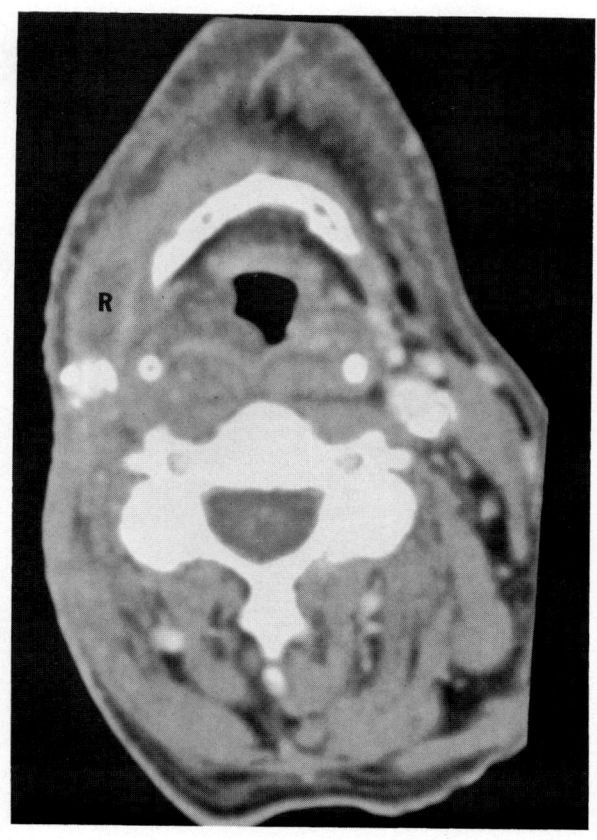

**Figure 18–6. Residual tumor after radical neck dissection: CT appearance.** This 72-year-old man developed right jugulodigastric recurrence of tumor 6 months after undergoing full-course radiation therapy for a left tonsillar primary cancer. The recurrent tumor was treated by right radical neck dissection 3 months before this CT scan was obtained. Physical examination revealed only nonspecific neck induration. CT scan performed during rapid bolus administration of intravenous contrast medium shows recurrence (R) of low attenuation within the bed of the radical neck dissection. Note the hypervascular periphery.

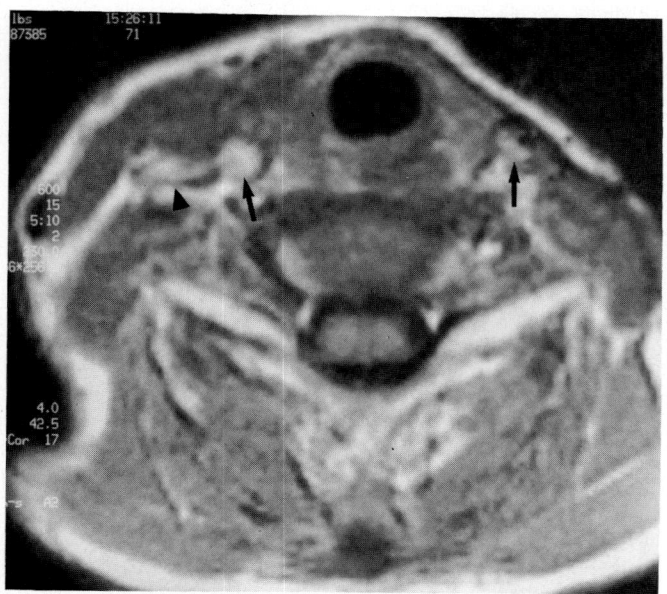

**Figure 18–7. Radical neck dissection: MR appearance.** This 53-year-old woman was examined by MR imaging 8 months after undergoing radical neck dissection. The T1-weighted MR image (600/15) displays the carotid arteries *(arrows)* and right internal jugular vein *(arrowhead)* with flow-related high signal intensity. On this sequence, fat is high in signal intensity and muscle low in signal intensity. The T1-weighted sequences are excellent for monitoring the appearance of metastatic lymph nodes, which tend to be isointense with muscle, within the bright fat.

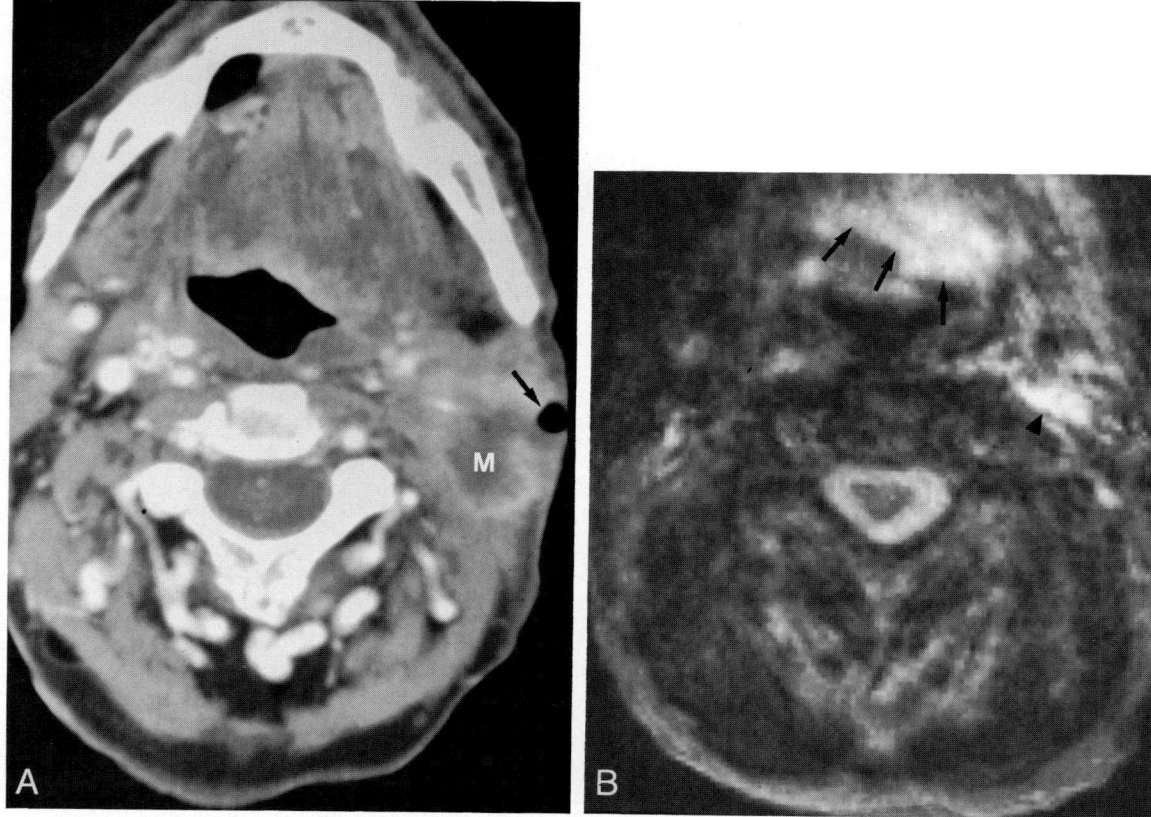

**Figure 18–8. Recurrent tumor after radical neck dissection: CT and MR appearances.** This 71-year-old man was examined by CT scanning and MR imaging 13 months after undergoing left radical neck dissection and radiation therapy for an epidermoid carcinoma. **A.** Contrast-enhanced CT scan demonstrates an irregular low-attenuation mass (M) with ring enhancement in the left side of the neck; the mass proved to be recurrent tumor. The thickened left base of the tongue did not contain cancer, and its appearance was attributed to surgical and radiation changes. The collection of air *(arrow)* is due to a biopsy. **B.** MR image (2500/90) enhanced by gadolinium diethylenetriaminepentaacetic acid (Gd-DTPA) obtained from the same patient. Corresponding regions of nonspecific high signal intensity, which are seen at the left base of the tongue *(arrows)*, were shown to be secondary to benign post-treatment changes. Similar high signal intensity is seen in the tumor recurrence in the left side of the neck *(arrowhead)*. Gd-DTPA enhancement for identification of lymph node necrosis is a promising technique.

muscle) is their bulk: they cannot be fashioned easily into tubular form. Advances in microvascular surgery have permitted the use of free flaps, obtained from more malleable donor sites such as the thigh. In all grafts, the muscle accompanying the skin and subcutaneous tissues atrophies quickly, and the graft has no intrinsic motility. The most important clinical problems associated with myocutaneous grafts are fistula formation and graft necrosis attributable to devascularization.

Pharyngography demonstrates the normal graft as a bulky, immobile smooth mass (Fig. 18–9). Pharyngograms may demonstrate postoperative fistulas, which occur along the margins of the graft, and which may extend into the tissues deep to the graft to form abscesses.

CT scanning and MR imaging show the striking fatty replacement of the muscular portion of the graft. These techniques are most useful in detecting abscesses unassociated with pharyngeal fistulas and in assessing the patient for extramucosal recurrence of tumor (Fig. 18–10).

# SPECIFIC PROCEDURES

## Total Laryngectomy

Total laryngectomy (TL) is conceptually the simplest of the surgical procedures for head and neck cancer. It is indicated for patients with stage T3 or T4 primary lesions and for patients with cancers of lower stages whose medical condition prohibits the extensive postoperative rehabilitation necessary for successful conservation therapy. In performing TL, the surgeon removes all of the laryngeal structures from the base of the tongue to the second tracheal cartilage, as well as all tumor-bearing mucosa in the pharynx. The trachea is then brought anteriorly to a stoma in the neck, and the pharyngeal defect is closed, using the inferior constrictor muscle of the pharynx and the cricopharyngeal muscle as part of the closure, if possible. The reconstructed tube that results from this closure is known as the *neopharynx*.

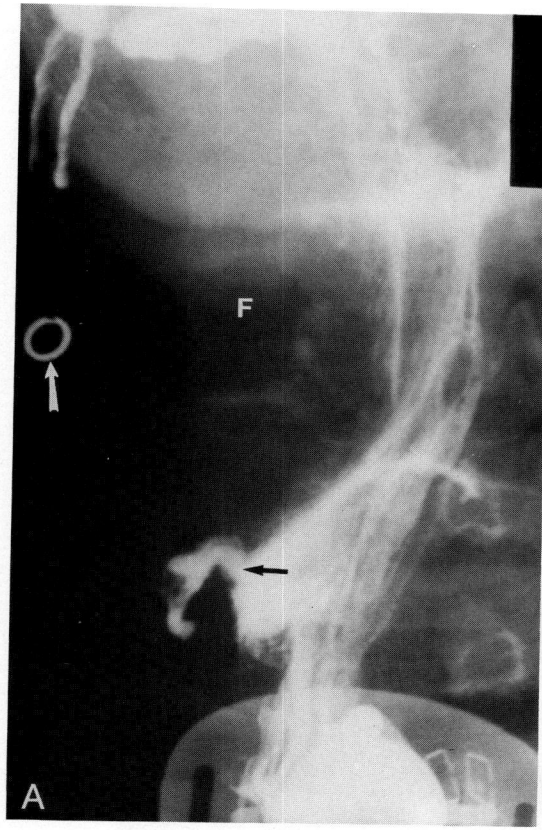 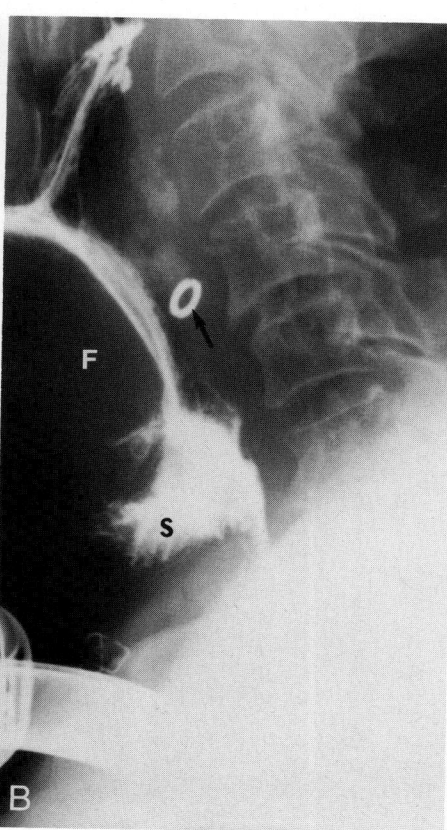

**Figure 18–9. Free flap graft: expected pharyngographic appearance.** This 78-year-old man underwent total laryngectomy (TL) 24 months previously for extensive epidermoid tumor of the right false vocal cord. A postoperative stricture necessitated revision of the neopharynx; the defect was repaired with a free flap graft harvested from the thigh. Pharyngography was requested because of clinical suspicion of a postoperative leak. **A.** Anteroposterior view from pharyngography performed with water-soluble contrast material shows the bulky, immobile flap (F) deforming the right side of the proximal neopharynx. At the inferior surface of the flap margin, a sinus tract *(black arrow)* extends into the subcutaneous tissues. Note ring *(white arrow)* marking graft of vascular pedicle from the thigh. **B.** On the lateral projection, the bulky flap (F) is noted on the anterior neopharyngeal surface. Contrast material has extended anteriorly through the sinus tract (S) at its inferior surface. The black arrow indicates the ring marking the vascular pedicle.

On pharyngograms, the appearance of the neopharynx is that of a simple cylinder extending from the oral cavity to the cervical esophagus[22] (Fig. 18–11). When the tumor resection is extensive, there may be narrowing of the cylinder at the site of the primary cancer. In the lateral projection, a posterior indentation attributable to the residual cricopharyngeal muscle is present and may be quite variable in size. An anterior outpouching at the top of the suture line (at the level of the tongue base) is also routinely observed. It may be large enough to trap food, which leads to dysphagia[23] (Fig. 18–12).

In the early postoperative period, pharyngography is used to assess clinically suspected fistula formation (Fig. 18–13). For this reason, water-soluble contrast agents are usually used first; if findings of the water-soluble examination are negative, however, thin barium suspension should be administered, because it is more sensitive in detecting leaks of small volume. The patient should be examined in the lateral projection, because a high percentage of the fistulas occurring in the early postoperative period arise from the top of the suture line and course anteriorly or anterolaterally. However, in patients who have had myocutaneous flap grafts, the most likely site of fistula formation is the margin of the graft.

In the late postoperative period, pharyngography is most useful in evaluating a mechanical cause for dysphagia. Direct visualization of the neopharynx is definitive in diagnosing mucosal recurrences of tumor when the entire neopharynx is visualized. However, pharyngeal strictures occur fairly commonly in patients who had locally extensive primary tumors (Fig. 18–14), and their presence may prevent endoscopic evaluation of the entire narrowed area. In the setting of neopharyngeal stricture, contrast evaluation reliably depicts mucosal detail and is of value in diagnosing mucosal recurrences of tumor. Of equal importance, pharyngography also demonstrates the anatomy of the esophagus (Fig. 18–15). Patients with a previous history of epidermoid cancer of the neck are at increased risk of developing a second primary tumor anywhere in the squamous mucosa, including the esophagus. Moreover, reflux esophagitis, with or without distal esophageal stricture formation, is a common entity for anyone in this age group and may result in dysphagia.

Pharyngography is also useful in evaluating neuromuscular causes of dysphagia in the laryngectomy patient. Extensive resection of the tongue base leads to diminished swallowing force, and the laryngectomy procedure itself leads to a reduction in normal esophageal peristaltic waves. Nasopharyngeal reflux may occur in individuals who required resection of the soft palate. It is important to administer solid bolus material as well as liquid contrast medium; apparently innocuous strictures that offer no impediment to the passage of barium may cause profound dysphagia when ingestion of solid or semisolid food is attempted.

The CT appearance of the neck after TL is also straightforward.[24] The neopharynx is readily identified as a midline tubular structure with a well-defined muscular wall approximately 1 cm thick, extending from the

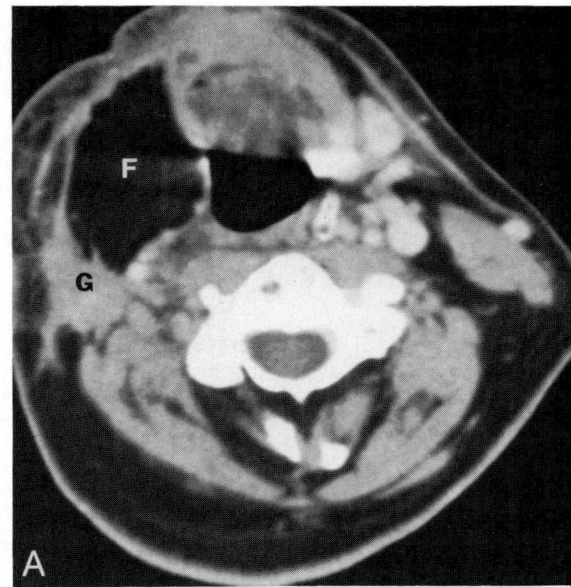

**Figure 18–10. Myocutaneous flap: expected CT and MR appearances.** This 39-year-old man underwent right hemi-mandibulectomy, tongue excision, and radical neck dissection for extensive carcinoma of the tongue. Imaging was performed 18 months after surgical creation of a myocutaneous dorsopectoral flap graft. **A.** CT image shows extensive fatty atrophy of the grafted muscle flap (F), which covers the extensive surgical defect. The ill-defined area of higher attenuation posterior to the fat (G) proved to be a combination of mature fibrosis and active granulation tissue. **B.** MR image (750/20) obtained at the same time shows the characteristic high-intensity fat within the flap (F). Note that the MR image differentiates between the fibrous tissue *(arrow)* and the area of granulation *(arrowhead).* **C.** MR image (2500/90) shows slightly higher intensity within the granulation tissue (G) than within the flap (F). Note that the fibrous tissue *(arrow)* remains low in intensity on the T2-weighted image.

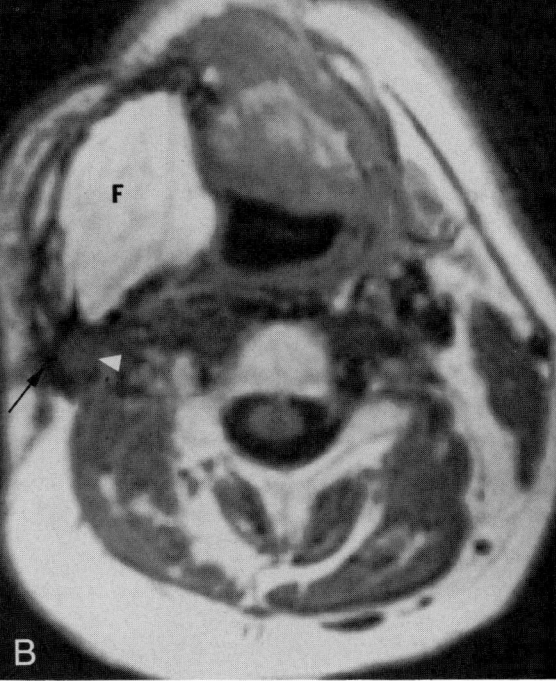

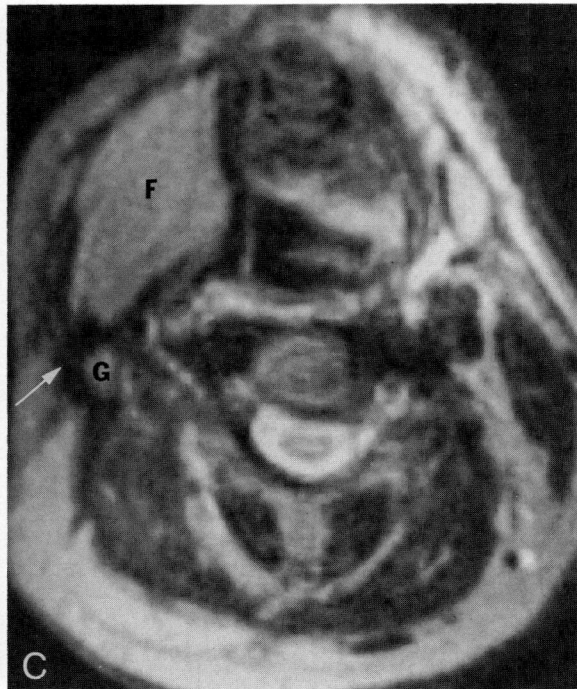

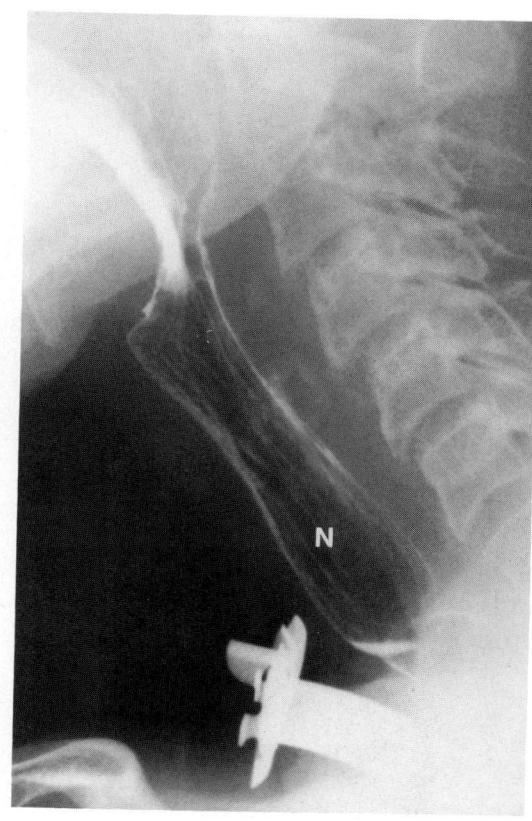

**Figure 18–11. The neopharynx after TL: expected pharyngographic appearance.** Lateral view of the neck in a 59-year-old woman who underwent TL 5 years previously is shown. The neopharynx (N) is a featureless cylindric tube extending from the tongue base to the cervical esophagus.

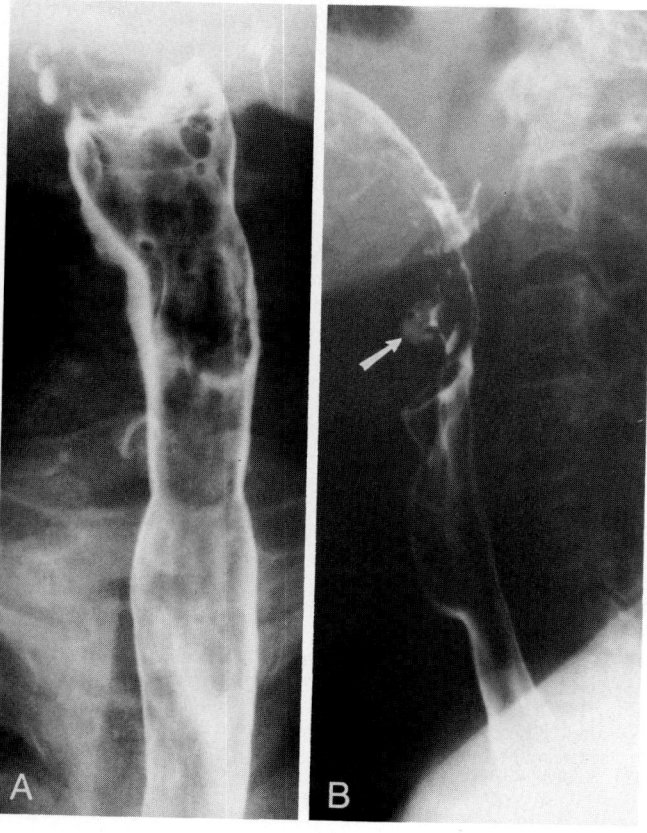

**Figure 18–12. The neopharynx after TL: expected pharyngographic appearance. A.** Anteroposterior view from barium pharyngography shows the neopharynx as a featureless tube with slight tapering at its junction with the proximal cervical esophagus. **B.** Lateral view from the same examination shows a small diverticulum *(arrow)* just inferior to the tongue base.

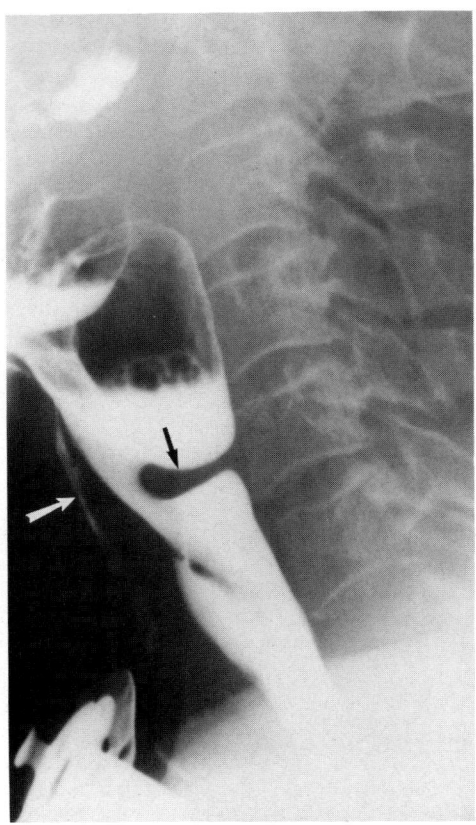

**Figure 18–13. Postoperative fistula after TL: pharyngographic appearance.** This 46-year-old man developed clinical evidence of a pharyngocutaneous fistula after TL. Lateral pharyngographic film shows a linear track *(white arrow)* extending from the junction of the tongue base with the anterior suture line, which is the most common site of postoperative fistulas. Note the prominent residual cricopharyngeal muscle *(black arrow)*.

tongue base to the cricopharyngeal muscle. The tracheal stoma is identified immediately above the sternal notch. Often, a radical lymph node dissection has been performed, so that the symmetry of the neck is disturbed by the absence of one sternocleidomastoid muscle. In such cases, the neopharynx often deviates from its midline position; usually, it courses to the side of the dissection.

CT is most useful in the immediate postoperative period for detecting abscesses, which are displayed as well-defined fluid attenuation masses in the soft tissues of the neck. Because postoperative hematomas may have a similar appearance, definitive diagnosis is obtained by needle aspiration. The presence of an abscess should prompt a search for an underlying fistula.

The major clinical application of CT in the long-term management of patients with head and neck cancer is in detecting submucosal tumor recurrence or nodal metastases. The entire neck and upper thorax should be examined from the skull base to the tracheal stoma. Intravenous contrast material should be administered as

a rapid bolus (1 to 2 mL/s), and images should be obtained as quickly as possible after a 30-second delay to allow optimal arterial opacification. With the use of this technique, epidermoid carcinoma, whether intranodal or extranodal, usually appears as a low-attenuation mass; a hypervascular rim in lymph nodes implies that tumor has invaded the capsule (Figs. 18–16 and 18–17). Solitary masses present little difficulty in diagnosis. However, many recurrent epidermoid cancers are infiltrative and may be difficult to distinguish from postoperative fibrosis (especially when radiation therapy has been administered). MR has been advocated as a means to solve this problem, because fibrous tissue has a low signal intensity, whereas active tumor has an intermediate signal intensity. Unfortunately, the edema and low-grade inflammation that accompany both surgery and radiation therapy produce variable amounts of edema within the treated field; the MR appearance in such cases is indistinguishable from that of metastasis. The potential contribution of positron emission tomography scanning, using metabolic tracers such as fludeoxyglucose F 18, has yet to be determined. At present, diagnosis depends on biopsy of the area combined with clinical judgment.

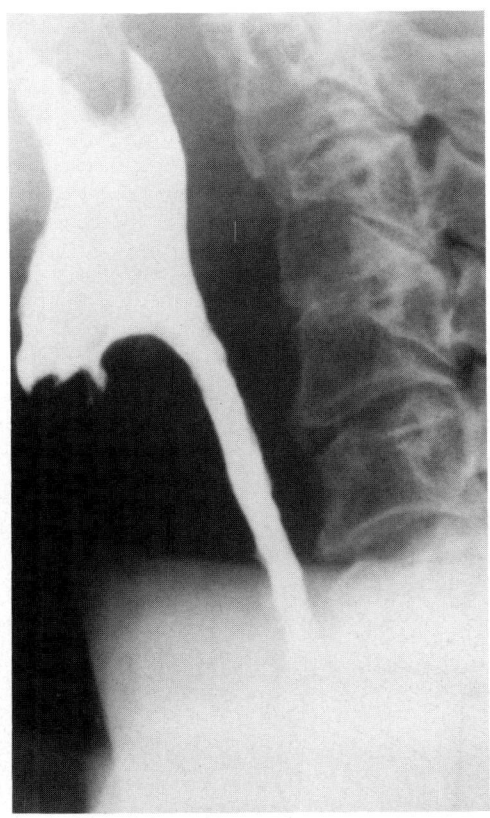

**Figure 18–14. Benign stricture after TL: pharyngographic appearance.** This 78-year-old man had progressive dysphagia 9 months after TL. He had been treated with full-course radiation therapy before his surgical procedure. Lateral pharyngogram shows marked narrowing of the entire neopharynx. Patient ultimately required reconstruction with a myocutaneous flap graft.

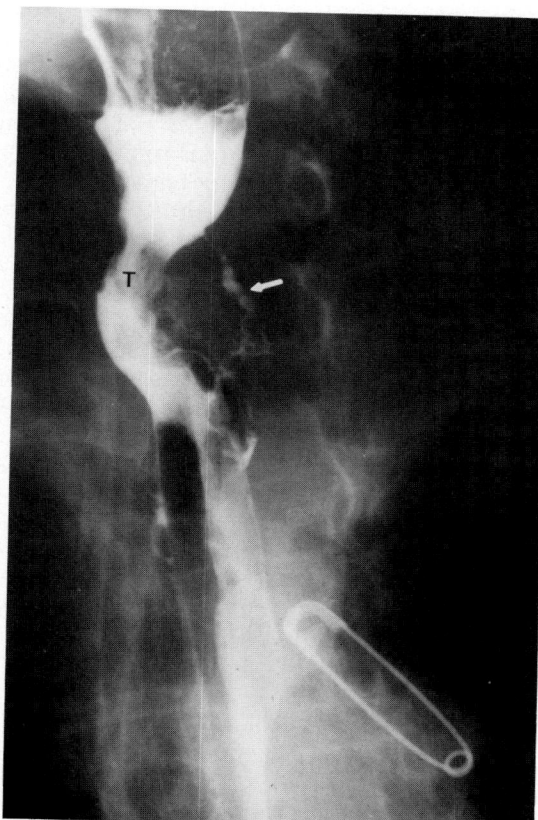

**Figure 18–15. Recurrence of tumor after TL: pharyngographic appearance.** This 70-year-old man who developed dysphagia after TL had a recent history of coughing with meals. Anteroposterior view of a barium swallow examination shows eccentric tumor (T) displacing esophageal lumen. A fistula *(arrow)* connecting the neopharynx to the trachea courses through a necrotic portion of the tumor.

## Subtotal Supraglottic Laryngectomy

Subtotal supraglottic laryngectomy (SSL) is a commonly performed procedure designed to preserve the voice in patients with relatively low-stage supraglottic carcinomas.[25] Patients with stage T1 or T2 lesions arising in the epiglottis, false vocal cords, or aryepiglottic folds are candidates for this procedure. The tumor may extend to only one arytenoid cartilage. The surgical procedure involves removal of the false vocal cords, epiglottis, superior half of the thyroid cartilage, and anterior portion of the hyoid bone. Continuity with the oral cavity is then re-established by suturing the remaining larynx and pharynx to the tongue base. Because two of the three normal laryngeal sphincters are surgically resected, only the true cords protect the trachea from a swallowed bolus. It is not surprising, then, that aspiration is a major postoperative complication; accordingly, debilitated patients or any patients who are unlikely to successfully cooperate in rehabilitation are best excluded from this surgical option.

On pharyngograms, the most striking feature is the absence of all supraglottic structures, so that the true vocal cords approximate the tongue base[26] (Fig. 18–18). The lateral pharyngeal wall is unaltered, but the piriform sinuses are less deep than usual. The impressions of the cricoid cartilage and the coated surfaces of the arytenoid cartilages are much more prominent than those in normal patients. A fold of tissue (resembling the aryepiglottic fold) extends from the lateral pharyngeal wall, over the arytenoid cartilages, and into the remaining anterior space just above the true vocal cords (see Fig. 18–18). The postoperative appearance of the pharynx is symmetric unless the surgeon also performs a radical neck dissection or extends the procedure to

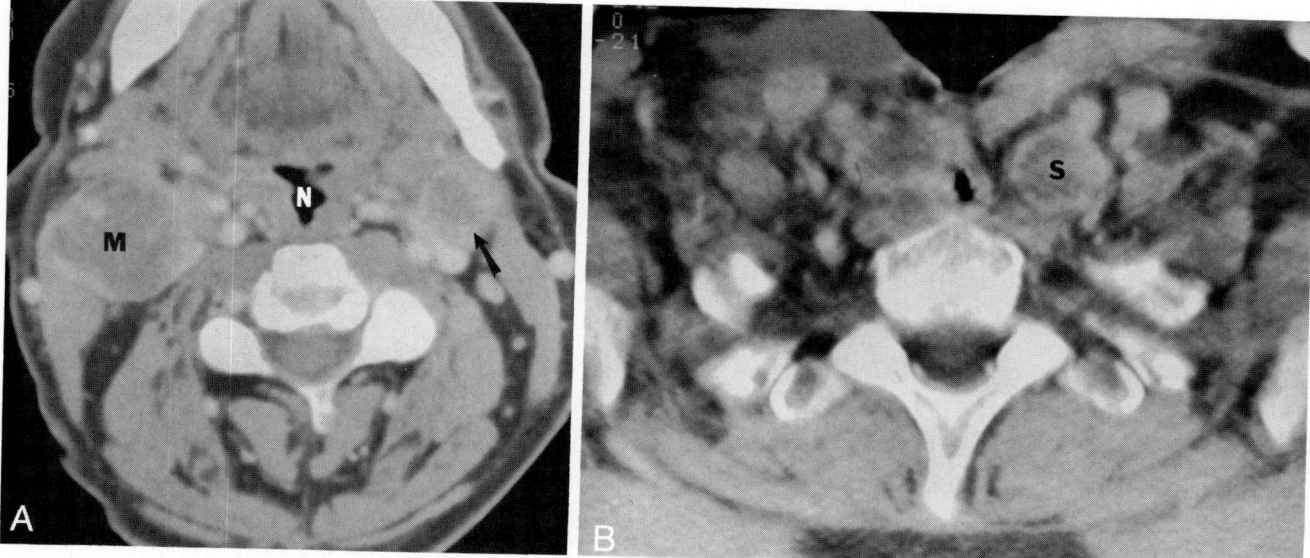

**Figure 18–16. Extensive tumor recurrence after TL: CT appearance. A.** Section through the tongue base shows the normal neopharynx (N). A large right nodal mass (M) and smaller left nodal mass *(arrow)* show characteristic peripheral enhancement. **B.** Section near the tracheal stoma shows the normal midline neopharynx immediately above its junction with the esophagus. A left peristomal node (S) is present at this level.

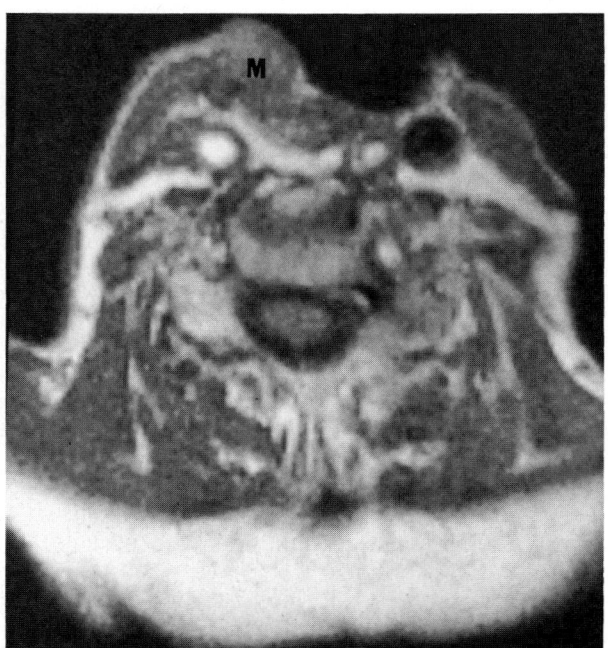

**Figure 18–17. Tumor recurrence after TL: MR appearance.** This 68-year-old man was examined 7 months after undergoing TL. MR image (600/15) shows mass (M) of intermediate signal intensity in the peristomal soft tissues. This location is a common one for postoperative recurrence of tumor and may represent an area of tumor seeding during the surgical procedure.

remove one arytenoid cartilage. All patients demonstrate barium coating of the superior margin of the true vocal cords, and most also have some degree of subglottic penetration of liquids.

Pharyngography is rarely used in the immediate postoperative period. When the clinical suspicion of a fistula arises, small volumes of dilute barium are preferred to ionic water-soluble contrast agents, because the risk of aspiration is high. Nonionic water-soluble agents are a reasonable alternative.

An important use of pharyngography in the long-term management of SSL patients is the evaluation of dysphagia. Recurrent or second primary esophageal cancer may cause mechanical obstruction leading to dysphagia (Fig. 18–19), but the most important clinical problem in SSL patients is aspiration. The majority of patients prevent aspiration by learning what is referred to as the supraglottic maneuver: the patient takes a deep breath, voluntarily closes the glottis, swallows forcefully, exhales briskly, and swallows again. This maneuver prevents that portion of the bolus that is retained in the pharynx from entering the unprotected airway at the end of the swallow. Swallowing abnormalities may result from a variety of mechanisms in this population. For example, sensory defects produce a delay in the swallowing reflex, permitting the bolus to enter the airway before the swallow. Misdirection of the bolus results from mechanical interference and may be due to recurrent tumor, stricture, or laryngeal edema. Reduced motor activity that is due to primary weakness of the tongue or pharynx or to distal obstruction produces retention of the bolus

within the pharynx and results in aspiration after the swallow. Assessment of these abnormalities is best performed with videofluoroscopy in the lateral projection. Because different consistencies are often tolerated differently, it is important to administer materials ranging from extremely thin to solid. We perform this evaluation with the assistance of a trained speech pathologist; this approach allows therapy to be directed toward the radiologically documented abnormalities and allows progress to be objectively recorded and followed.

The surgical changes in the soft tissues of the neck can easily be documented with CT[27] (Fig. 18–20). Below the level of the ventricle, the anatomy is undisturbed. Immediately above this level, sections demonstrate the prominent arytenoid cartilages and the folds of tissue that connect them with the lateral pharyngeal wall. Asymmetry of the upper neck is quite common, because a large percentage of patients undergo radical neck dissection on the side of greatest tumor involvement.

As is true after TL, the most important clinical use of CT after SSL is the diagnosis of extramucosal recurrence of cancer. The CT appearance of recurrent tumor in the submucosa and node-bearing regions in SSL patients is identical with that described for TL patients.

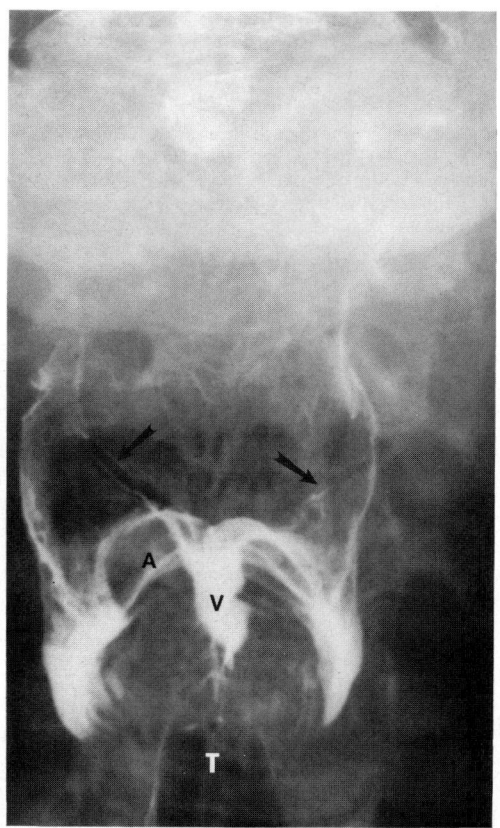

**Figure 18–18. SSL: expected pharyngographic appearance.** This 61-year-old man was asymptomatic 24 months after undergoing SSL without neck dissection. Anteroposterior view shows two folds of tissue *(arrows)* extending from the arytenoid cartilages posteriorly to the lateral pharyngeal wall. Note prominent arytenoid cartilages (A) bilaterally. Contrast medium has entered the fossa superior to the true vocal cords (pseudovestibule, V); some barium has penetrated into the trachea (T).

**Figure 18–19. Tumor recurrence after SSL: pharyngographic appearance.**
This 64-year-old man had dysphagia 2 years after undergoing SSL. Anteroposterior view demonstrates irregularity and a mass involving the residual aryepiglottic folds on the left *(arrows)* and extending to the left true vocal cord. Note the normal right true vocal cord (c).

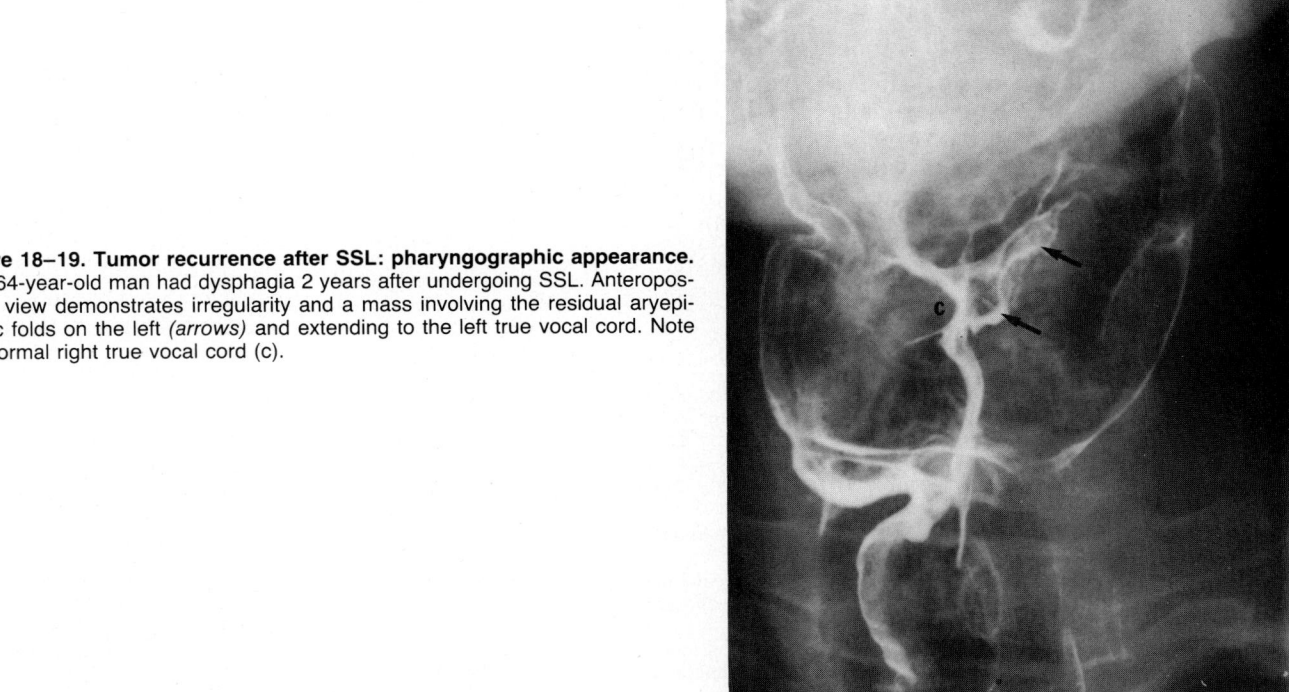

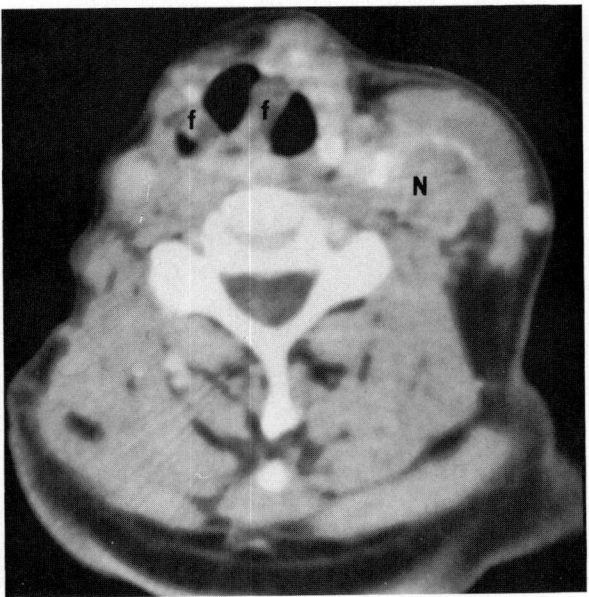

**Figure 18–20. Tumor recurrence after SSL: CT appearance.** This 49-year-old man underwent SSL combined with right radical neck dissection 7 months previously. Examination of the larynx shows two prominent folds (f) extending from the lateral pharyngeal wall to the arytenoid cartilages. These folds are remnants of the posterior part of the aryepiglottic folds. A large node (N) is present in the internal jugular chain. It proved to be recurrent epidermoid carcinoma.

Cancer can persist, or new primary cancers can arise, in the residual larynx; it is difficult to differentiate subtle neoplastic infiltration from surgically induced edema or radiation fibrosis. Distortion of paralaryngeal fat planes suggests a malignant process.

## SUMMARY

Radiologists have the opportunity to contribute greatly to the management of patients after head and neck surgery. Familiarity with the structural changes produced by specific procedures allows the interpreter to distinguish between the expected post-therapy appearance and the recurrence of cancer or other complications.

## References

1. Kagan AR, Calcaterra T, Ward P, et al: Significance of edema of the endolarynx following curative irradiation for carcinoma. AJR 120:169–172, 1974.
2. Fu KK, Woodhouse RJ, Quivey JM, et al: The significance of laryngeal edema following radiotherapy of carcinoma of the vocal cord. Cancer 49:655–658, 1982.
3. Jung TK, Adams GL: Dysphagia in laryngectomized patients. Otolaryngol Head Neck Surg 88:25–33, 1980.
4. Gluckman JL, Crissman JD, Donegan JO: Multicentric squamous-cell carcinoma of the upper aerodigestive tract. Head Neck Surg 3:90–96, 1980.
5. Wagenfeld DJH, Harwood AR, Bryce DP, et al: Second primary respiratory tract malignant neoplasms in supraglottic carcinoma. Arch Otolaryngol 107:135–137, 1981.
6. Ekberg O, Nylander G: Pharyngeal dysfunction after treatment for pharyngeal cancer with surgery and radiotherapy. Gastrointest Radiol 8:97–104, 1983.
7. Schobinger R: Spasm of the cricopharyngeal muscle as a cause of dysphagia with total laryngectomy. Arch Otolaryngol 67:271–274, 1958.
8. Semenkovich JW, Balfe DM, Weyman PJ, et al: Barium pharyngography: comparison of single and double contrast. AJR 144:717–718, 1985.
9. Ekberg O, Nylander G: Double-contrast examination of the pharynx. Gastrointest Radiol 10:263–271, 1985.
10. Donner MW, Siegel CI: The evaluation of pharyngeal neuromuscular disorders by cinefluorography. AJR 94:299–307, 1965.
11. Donner MW: Swallowing mechanisms and neuromuscular disorders. Semin Roentgenol 9:273–282, 1974.
12. van der Brekel MWM, Stel HV, Castelijns JA, et al: Cervical lymph node metastasis: assessment of radiologic criteria. Radiology 177:379–384, 1990.
13. Dooms GC, Hricak H, Crooks LE, et al: Magnetic resonance imaging of the lymph nodes: comparison with CT. Radiology 153:719–728, 1984.
14. Glazer HS, Niemeyer JH, Balfe DM, et al: Neck neoplasms: MR imaging. Part II. Posttreatment evaluation. Radiology 160:349–354, 1986.
15. Jabour BA, Lufkin RB, Layfield LJ, et al: Magnetic resonance imaging of metastatic cervical adenopathy. Top Magn Reson Imaging 2:69–75, 1990.
16. Jabour BA, Lufkin RB, Hanafee WN: Magnetic resonance imaging of the larynx. Top Magn Reson Imaging 2:60–68, 1990.
17. Lufkin RB, Hanafee WN: Applications of surface coils to MR anatomy of the larynx. AJNR 6:491–497, 1985.
18. Bronstein AD, Nyberg DA, Schwartz AN, et al: Soft-tissue changes after head and neck radiation: CT findings. AJNR 10:171–175, 1989.
19. Chandler JR: Radiation fibrosis and necrosis of the larynx. Ann Otol Rhinol Laryngol 88:509–514, 1979.
20. Thawley SE, Ogura JH: Conservation laryngeal surgery and radical neck dissection. *In* English GM (ed): Otolaryngology. Philadelphia: JB Lippincott, 1989, pp 41–50.
21. Johns ME: Myocutaneous flaps in head and neck surgery. *In* English GM (ed): Otolaryngology. Philadelphia: JB Lippincott, 1989, pp 1–21.
22. Balfe DM, Koehler RE, Setzen M, et al: Barium examination of the esophagus after total laryngectomy. Radiology 143:501–508, 1982.
23. Kirchner JA, Scatliff JH, Dey FL, et al: The pharynx after laryngectomy: changes in its structure and function. Laryngoscope 73:18–33, 1963.
24. DiSantis DJ, Balfe DM, Hayden RE, et al: The neck after total laryngectomy: CT study. Radiology 153:713–717, 1984.
25. De Santo LW: Surgical perspective. *In* Thawley SE, Pange WR, Batsakis JG, et al (eds): Comprehensive Management of Head and Neck Tumors. Philadelphia: WB Saunders, 1987, pp 1029–1039.
26. Ogura JH, Heeneman H: Conservation surgery of the larynx and hypopharynx—selection of patients and results. Can J Otolaryngol 2:11–16, 1973.
27. Niemeyer JH, Balfe DM, Hayden RE: Neck evaluation with barium-enhanced radiographs and CT scans after supraglottic subtotal laryngectomy. Radiology 162:493–498, 1987.

# Upper Gastrointestinal Tract: Technique and Normal Anatomy

# Barium Studies

Igor Laufer, M.D.

## INTRODUCTION

There are many ways to perform an upper gastrointestinal examination. Chapter 6 describes a technique relying primarily on barium filling and mucosal relief. The method described in this chapter relies primarily on double contrast, although, in truth, it is a biphasic technique that tries to combine the advantages of both single and double contrast. Individual practitioners undoubtedly develop their own particular routine techniques. Nevertheless, the techniques in this chapter and in Chapter 6 are presented as starting points that are representative of two approaches to the examination of the upper gastrointestinal tract.[1]

## GENERAL PRINCIPLES

The examination is designed to coat the mucosal surface with a thin layer of high-density barium while the lumen is distended with gas. The routine upper gastrointestinal examination should include at least the distal half of the esophagus, the stomach, and the duodenum to the duodenojejunal junction. The examination must be performed quickly to avoid overlap of duodenum and small bowel on the stomach. It is not critical that each segment be examined in its anatomic sequence. In some cases, it may be preferable to examine the antrum, pylorus, and duodenum before significant overlap has occurred. Likewise, in cases in which it is desirable to examine the pharynx, it may be preferable to perform this portion of the examination after the upper gastrointestinal examination has been completed. The specific details of the examination should always be tailored to the patient's presenting symptoms, anatomic configuration, or pathologic findings during fluoroscopy.

## MATERIALS

### Barium Suspensions

For our method of examination, we use a high-density barium of 250% w/v concentration (E-Z-EM Company, Westbury, NY). The preparation of these barium suspensions is critical because slight deviations in concentration can impair the quality of mucosal coating and cause artifacts.[2]

### Effervescent Agents

Various effervescent agents are available in powder, granular, or liquid form.[3] These agents release 300 to 400 mL of $CO_2$ on contact with fluid in the stomach.

### Hypotonia[4]

In our opinion, the use of a hypotonic agent to relax the stomach and duodenum provides a better examination and also allows the examiner additional time to achieve good mucosal coating. In the United States the only suitable agent is glucagon, and an injection of 0.1 mg intravenously generally produces a short-lived hypotonic state. In some patients, this may retard barium filling of the duodenum for a few minutes. In other parts of the world, butylscopolammonium bromide (Buscopan) is frequently used to achieve gastrointestinal hypotonia.

### Radiography

The choice of a radiographic system represents a tradeoff between resolution, contrast, and speed. In the past, we have preferred a 400-speed system with a preference for long scale contrast to achieve a relatively uniform density over the entire film. Spot films have been exposed at 105 kV(p). Digital spot filming has now become available[5] and it appears to present interesting opportunities for contrast resolution, although at the expense of spatial resolution. It also presents interesting opportunities for improving the communication and transmission of radiographic findings.[6]

## ROUTINE TECHNIQUE

Selected views from a normal upper gastrointestinal study are shown in Figure 19–1. We start with a short review of the patient's history and symptoms. In particular, we take special care to ask whether the patient has had any previous surgery and whether the patient is taking any ulcerogenic medication. The examination

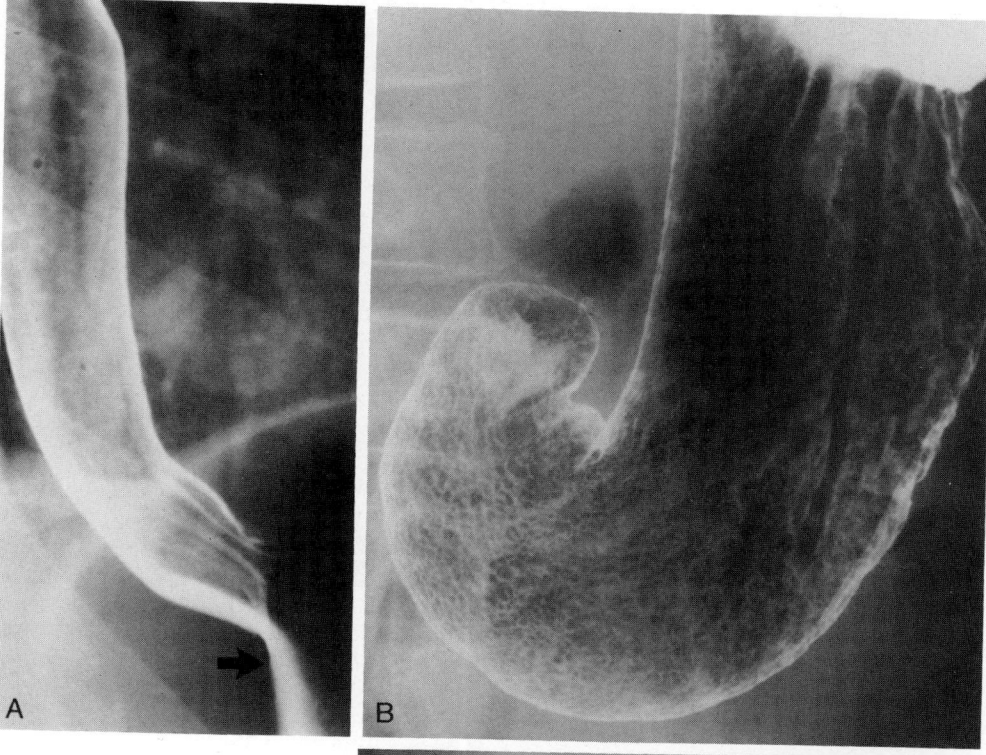

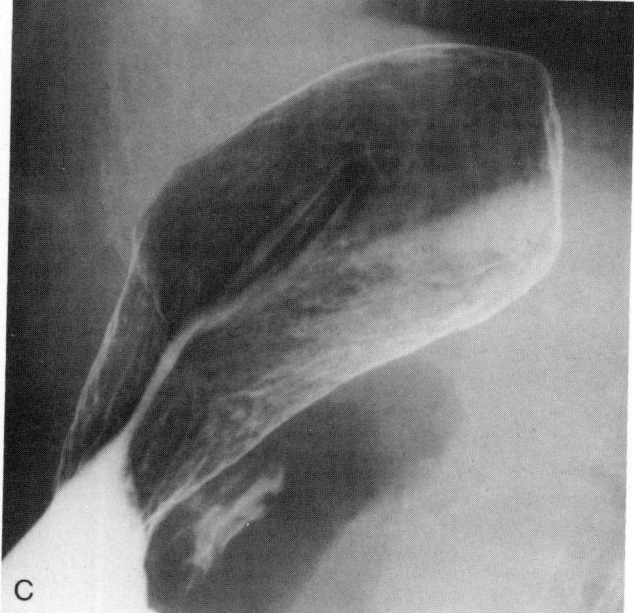

**Figure 19–1. Representative films from a normal study. A.** Double contrast view of the esophagus showing the distal esophagus with barium cascading like a waterfall *(arrow)* into the gas-distended stomach. **B.** Supine film of the stomach in the LPO projection showing rugal folds along the greater curvature of the body of the stomach and the areae gastricae pattern most clearly seen in the body and antrum. **C.** Right lateral view of the stomach with faint filling of the duodenum. This film is particularly good for the cardia and retrogastric region.

*Illustration continued on following page*

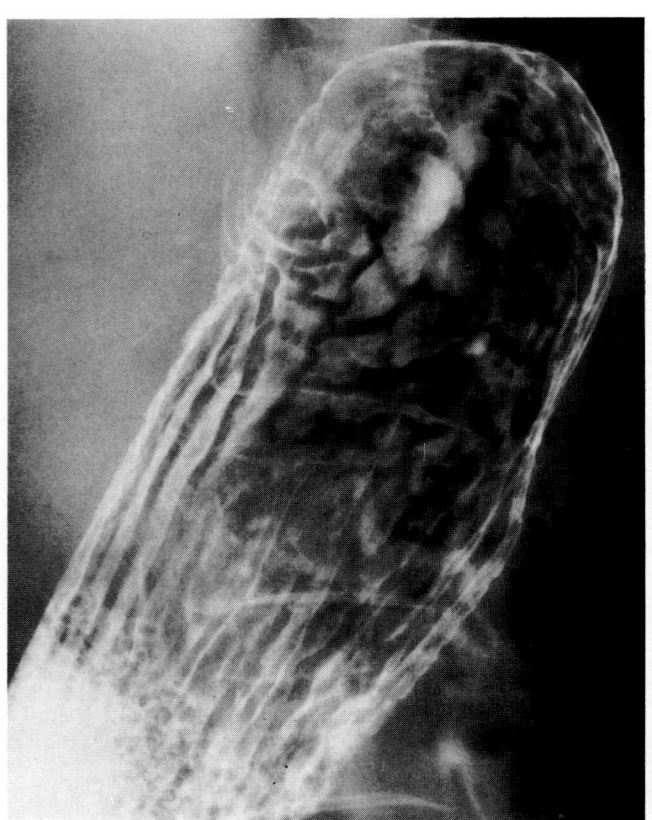

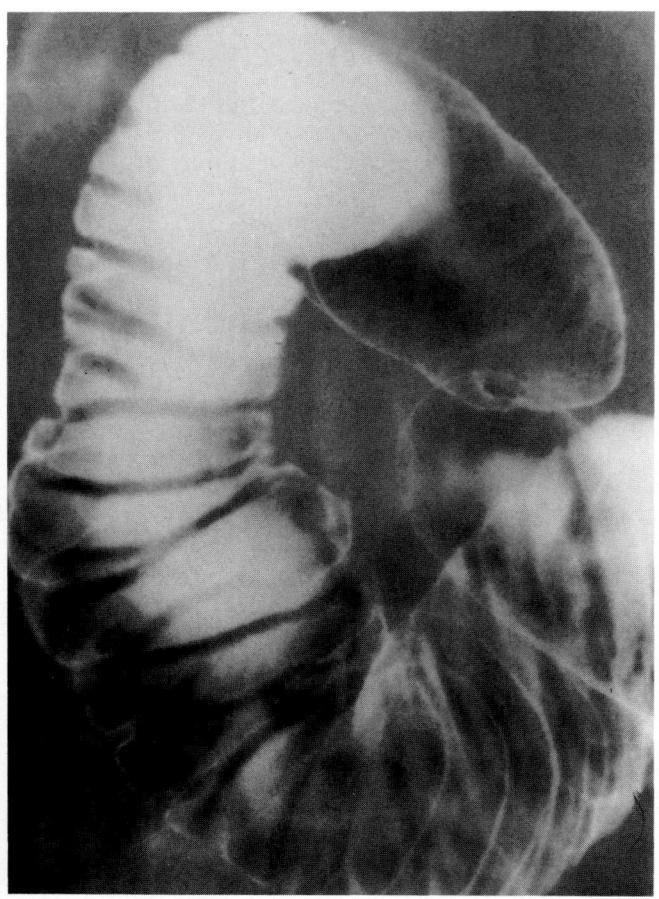

D

E

Figure 19–1 *Continued* **D.** Semiupright right posterior oblique view of high lesser curvature, upper body, and fundus. **E.** Ideal visualization of the duodenum in the left posterior oblique projection. Note the smooth, featureless appearance of the bulb.

usually starts with an intravenous injection of 0.1 mg of glucagon. The patient then ingests the effervescent agent, followed by 10 mL of water to facilitate the release of $CO_2$. The patient then stands upright in the left posterior oblique (LPO) position and is asked to gulp the contents of a cup containing 120 mL of high-density barium as rapidly as possible while two or three double contrast views of the esophagus are obtained in rapid succession. These views should include the distal esophagus and gastroesophageal junction. Barium is often seen cascading like a waterfall into the gas-dis-

tended stomach (see Fig. 19–1A). While the table is being lowered into the horizontal position, the patient turns to the left onto the stomach and onto the back again. With the table in the horizontal position, the first LPO view of the stomach is exposed (see Fig. 19–1B).

The remainder of the examination proceeds as outlined in Table 19–1 (see Fig. 19–1C to E). In cases in which barium filling of the duodenum is delayed, the examination of the esophagus can be completed and the duodenal films can be obtained at the end of the examination. It is important to keep in mind the value

### TABLE 19–1. ROUTINE UPPER GASTROINTESTINAL TECHNIQUE: DOUBLE CONTRAST

| POSITION | FILMS | PURPOSE |
|---|---|---|
| LPO, upright | 3 on 1 | Esophagus, double contrast |
| LPO | 1 on 1 | Stomach, body and antrum, double contrast |
| Right lateral | 1 on 1 | Fundus, double contrast, retrogastric area |
| LPO | 1 on 1 | Antrum, pylorus, and duodenum, double contrast |
| Right posterior oblique, semiupright | 1 on 1 | Cardia and fundus, double contrast |
| Prone | 4 on 1 | Antrum and duodenum, compression |
| Supine | 4 on 1 | Antrum and duodenum, flow technique |
| Right anterior oblique, prone | 2 on 1 | Esophagus, function and barium filling |
| Upright | 4 on 1 | Stomach and duodenum, compression |

of flow technique[7] for the demonstration of superficial lesions on the dependent surface (Fig. 19–2; see also Chapter 4, Fig. 4–15).

## ANATOMIC CONSIDERATIONS

Although the normal anatomy of the upper gastrointestinal tract is well known, a few of the features that are particularly well demonstrated by double contrast should be stressed.

### Esophagus

The normal mucosal surface of the esophagus is smooth and featureless (Fig. 19–3A). With partial collapse of the esophagus, the normal longitudinal folds are seen (Fig. 19–3B). In some patients, fine transverse folds may also be seen in the body of the esophagus[8] (Fig. 19–3C). We believe that these folds represent a transient contraction of the muscularis mucosae and may be seen in normal patients, although they are probably seen with increased frequency in patients with gastroesophageal reflux.[9] Occasionally, fine transverse folds may be seen as a normal variant in the proximal esophagus[10] (Fig. 19–3D). In older, asymptomatic patients, small nodules may be seen on the mucosal surface. These are due to glycogenic acanthosis,[11] a degenerative phenomenon of no clinical significance (Fig. 19–4). Normal extrinsic impressions are usually seen from the aorta, heart, and left main bronchus (Fig. 19–5A). Abnormal impressions may be caused by enlargement of normal structures such as the heart and aorta or by abnormal structures such as lymph nodes, mediastinal masses, or vertebral osteophytes (Fig. 19–5B).

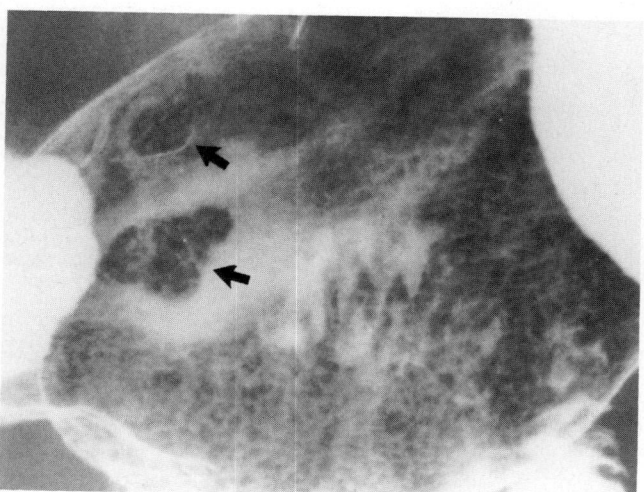

**Figure 19–2. Flow technique.** With barium flowing across the posterior wall of the stomach, at least two polypoid lesions *(arrows)* of Kaposi's sarcoma are identified.

### Stomach

The mucosal surface of the stomach can be studied at several different levels. The rugal fold pattern is clearly seen when the stomach is not fully distended and is most prominent along the greater curvature of the body of the stomach (Fig. 19–6A). As the normal rugal folds are effaced, the finer mucosal pattern, the areae gastricae,[12] are visualized. These can be seen by double contrast study (see Fig. 19–1B) or by single contrast study with high-density barium and compression (see Fig. 19–6A). This fine mucosal pattern can become distorted in patients with inflammatory or neoplastic lesions, and it also serves as a marker of the quality of mucosal coating. In some patients, fine transverse folds (striae) are seen as a normal variant in the gastric antrum[13] (Fig. 19–6B). In thin patients, the posterior wall of the stomach may be impressed by normal retrogastric structures, and these should not be mistaken for retrogastric masses (Fig. 19–6C).

The anatomy of the gastric cardia is particularly well seen on double contrast studies. A variety of appearances may be seen, including a filling defect, radiating folds representing the cardiac rosette, and a hooding fold[14] (Fig. 19–7). In patients with lax ligaments and a small hiatal hernia, the anatomic landmarks may not be seen. The landmarks are also obliterated or distorted in patients with tumors of the gastric cardia (see Chapters 32 and 38).

### Duodenum

The surface of the duodenal bulb is usually quite smooth. In some patients, a fine feathery or velvety surface is seen and probably represents the villous pattern of the duodenum[15] (Fig. 19–8A). In other patients, small angular filling defects are seen near the base of the bulb. These are characteristic of heterotopic gastric mucosa[16] (Fig. 19–8B). The clinical significance of this finding is uncertain. At the superior duodenal flexure, there is often a mass-like filling defect with a central barium collection on the inferior surface. This may resemble an ulcer but simply represents an infolding of mucosa. It has been termed the *duodenal pseudolesion* or *flexural fallacy*[17] (Fig. 19–8C). In some patients, the duodenal bulb is covered by small barium collections[18] (Fig. 19–8D). These appear to represent pits in the duodenal mucosa and should not be mistaken for duodenal erosions.

In the descending duodenum, the anatomy of the major papilla of Vater is particularly well demonstrated.[19] It is usually associated with a longitudinal fold as well as a hooding fold (Fig. 19–9A). The minor papilla is located on the anterior wall slightly proximal to the major papilla and is therefore usually seen only with the patient in the prone position (Fig. 19–9B).

*Text continued on page 302*

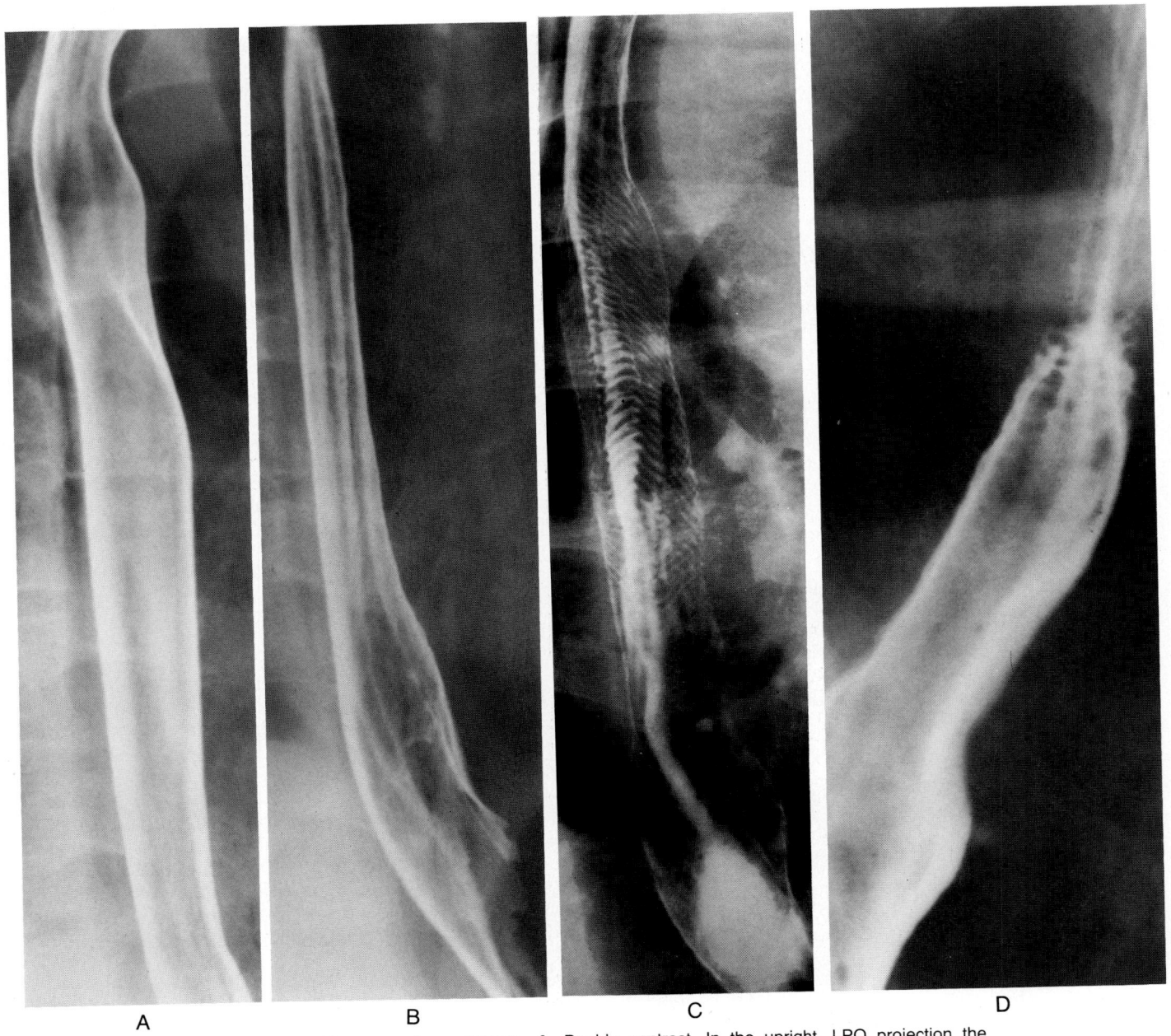

**Figure 19–3. The normal esophagus. A.** Double contrast. In the upright, LPO projection the esophagus is thrown off the spine. Note the smooth, featureless surface. **B.** Longitudinal folds. With the esophagus partially collapsed, the normal longitudinal folds are seen. **C.** Transverse folds. These transverse folds are thought to result from contraction of the longitudinally oriented muscularis mucosae. (**C** from Gohel VK, Edell SK, Laufer I, et al: Transverse folds in the human esophagus. Radiology 128:303–308, 1978.) **D.** Spiculation of the upper esophagus attributable to transverse folds.

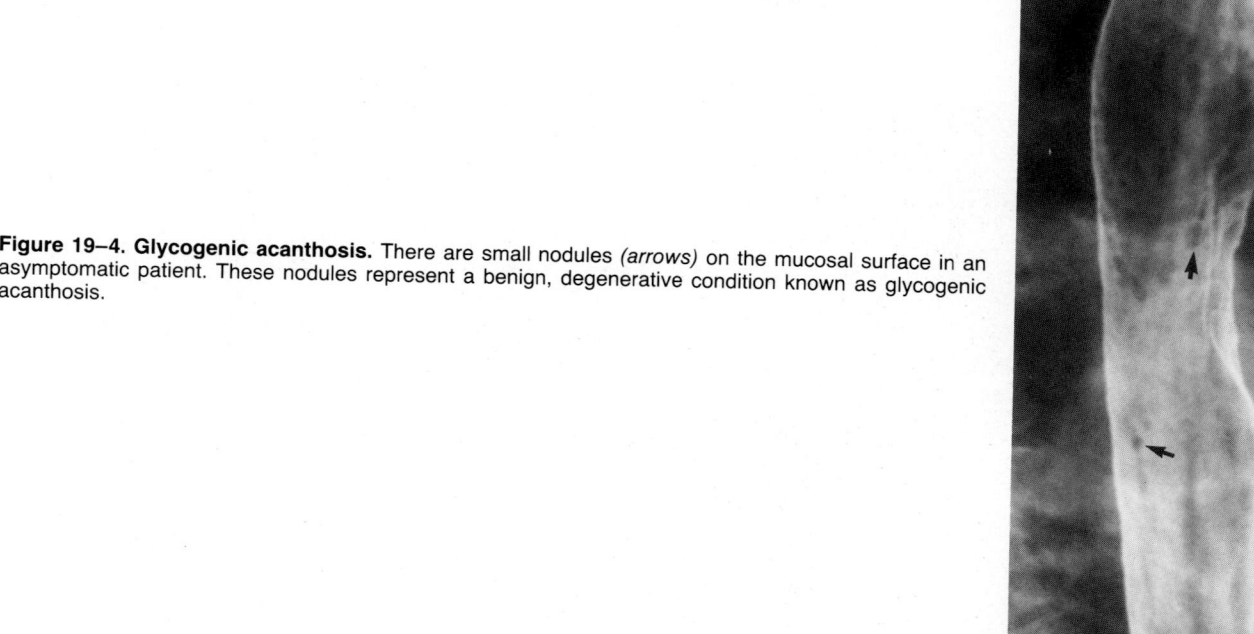

**Figure 19–4. Glycogenic acanthosis.** There are small nodules *(arrows)* on the mucosal surface in an asymptomatic patient. These nodules represent a benign, degenerative condition known as glycogenic acanthosis.

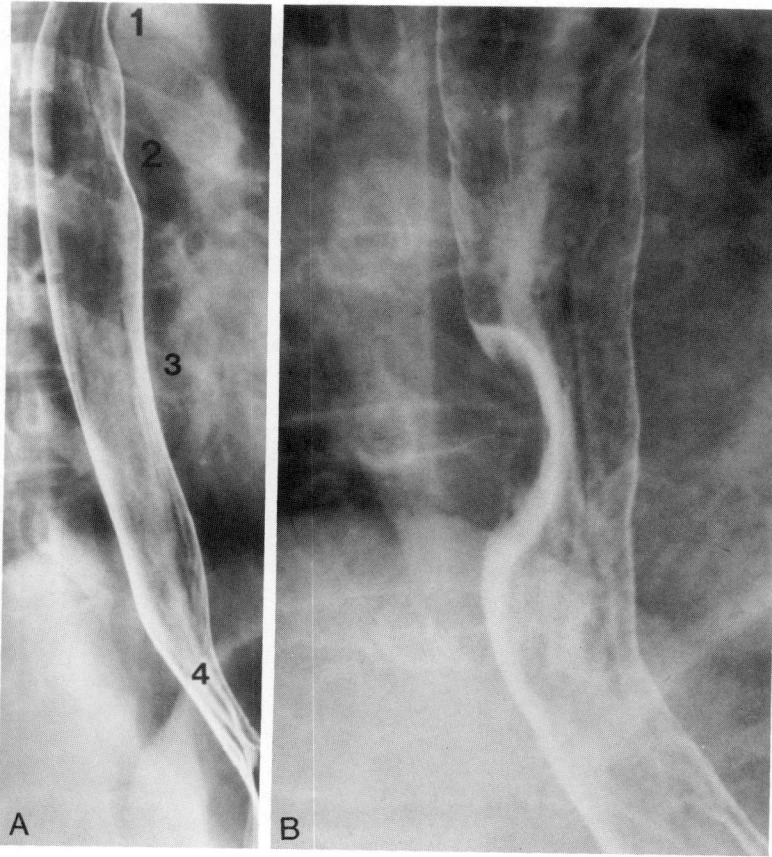

**Figure 19–5. Extrinsic impressions on the esophagus. A.** Normal impressions. 1 = aortic arch; 2 = left main bronchus; 3 = heart; 4 = esophageal hiatus. **B.** Abnormal extrinsic impression on the posterior wall of the esophagus resulting from a vertebral osteophyte.

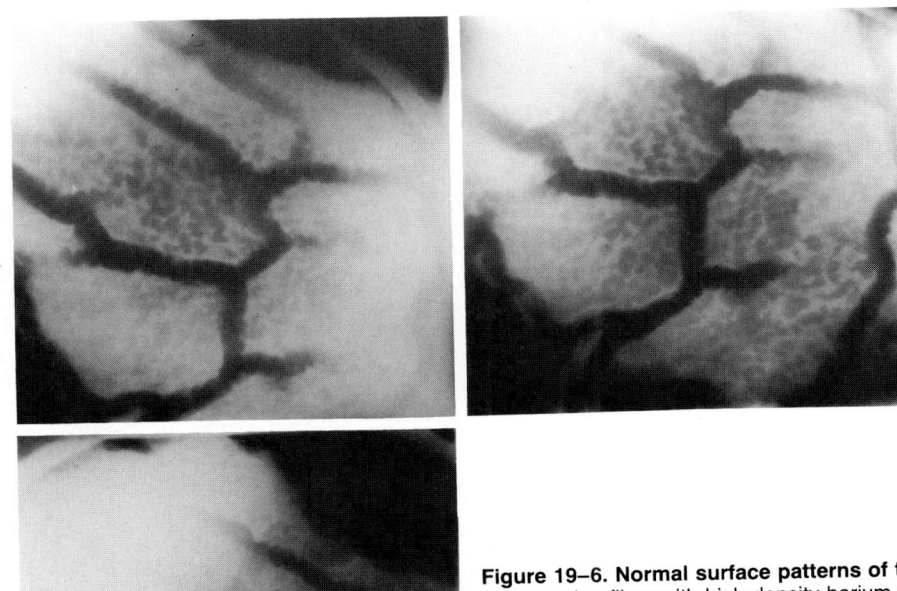

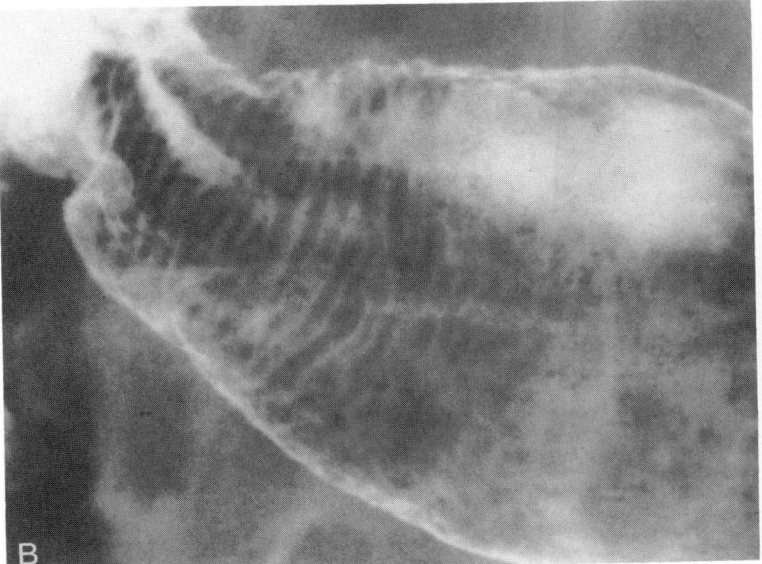

**Figure 19–6. Normal surface patterns of the stomach. A.** Prone compression films with high-density barium showing the rugal folds as branching linear filling defects. Superimposed is the fine reticular pattern of the areae gastricae. See also Figure 19–1B. **B.** Gastric striae in the distal antrum. The fine transverse folds represent the striae. **C.** Normal rectogastric impressions in a thin female.

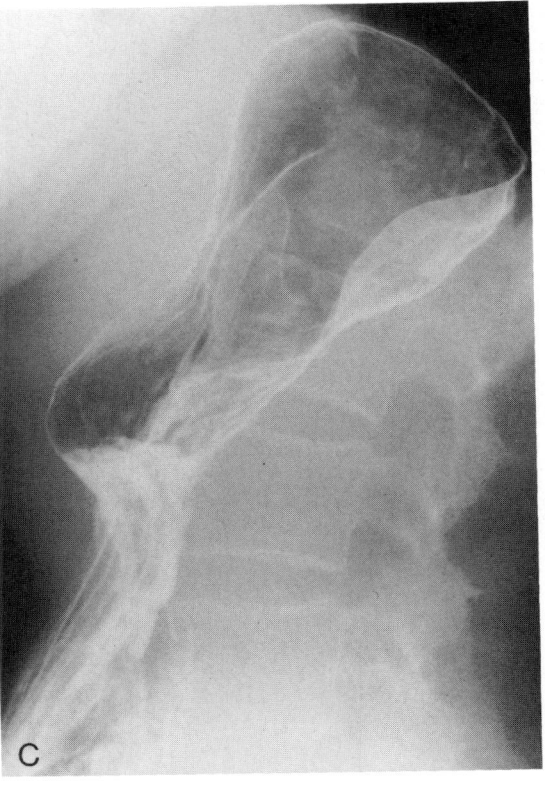

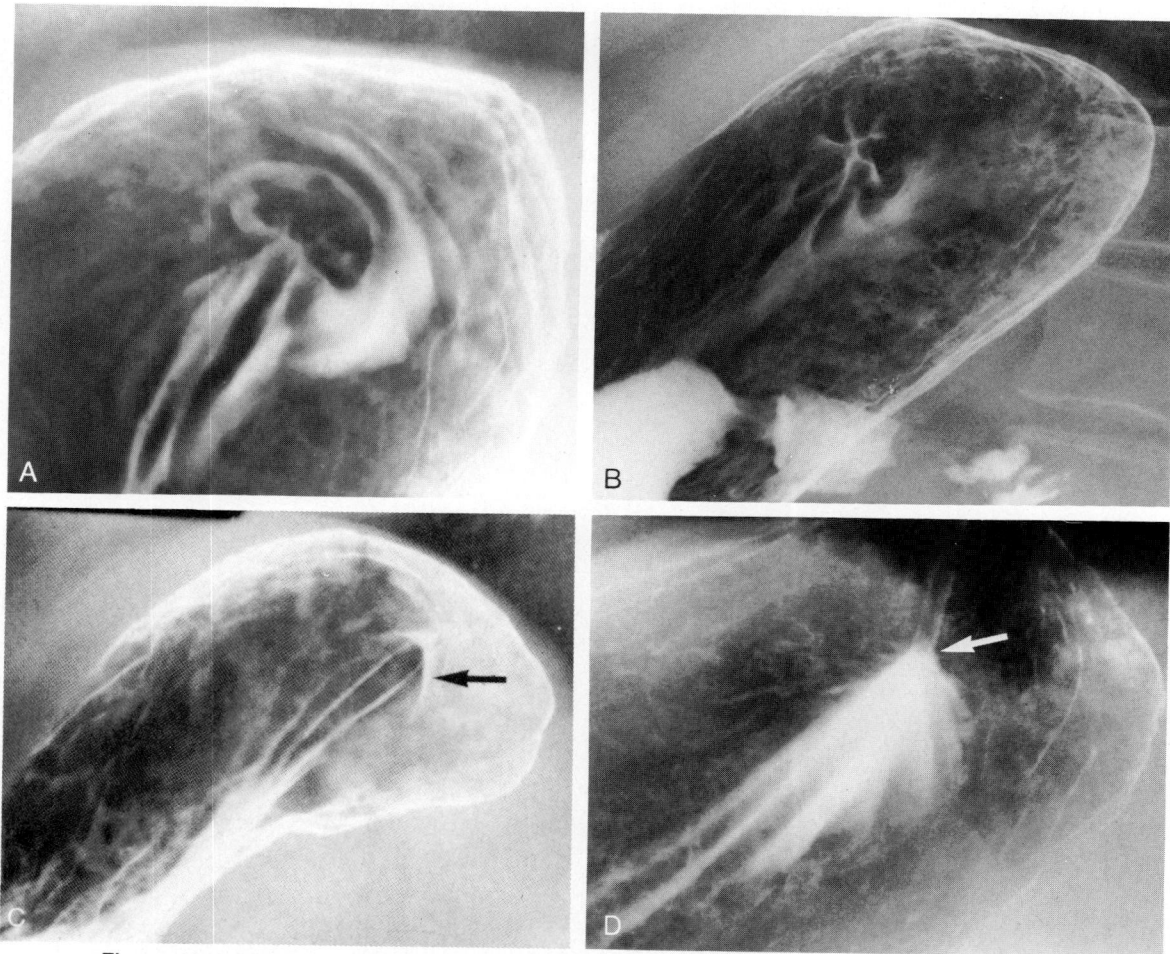

**Figure 19–7. Normal cardia and its variations. A.** Well-anchored cardia appearing as circular elevation with centrally radiating folds (the cardiac "rosette"). **B.** Stellate folds without surrounding elevation caused by laxity of ligamentous attachments. **C.** Further weakening of ligaments with obliteration of cardiac rosette. Note crescentic line *(arrow)* that crosses area of esophageal orifice. **D.** Severe ligamentous laxity with gastric folds in small hiatal hernia converging superiorly *(arrow)* above esophageal hiatus of diaphragm.

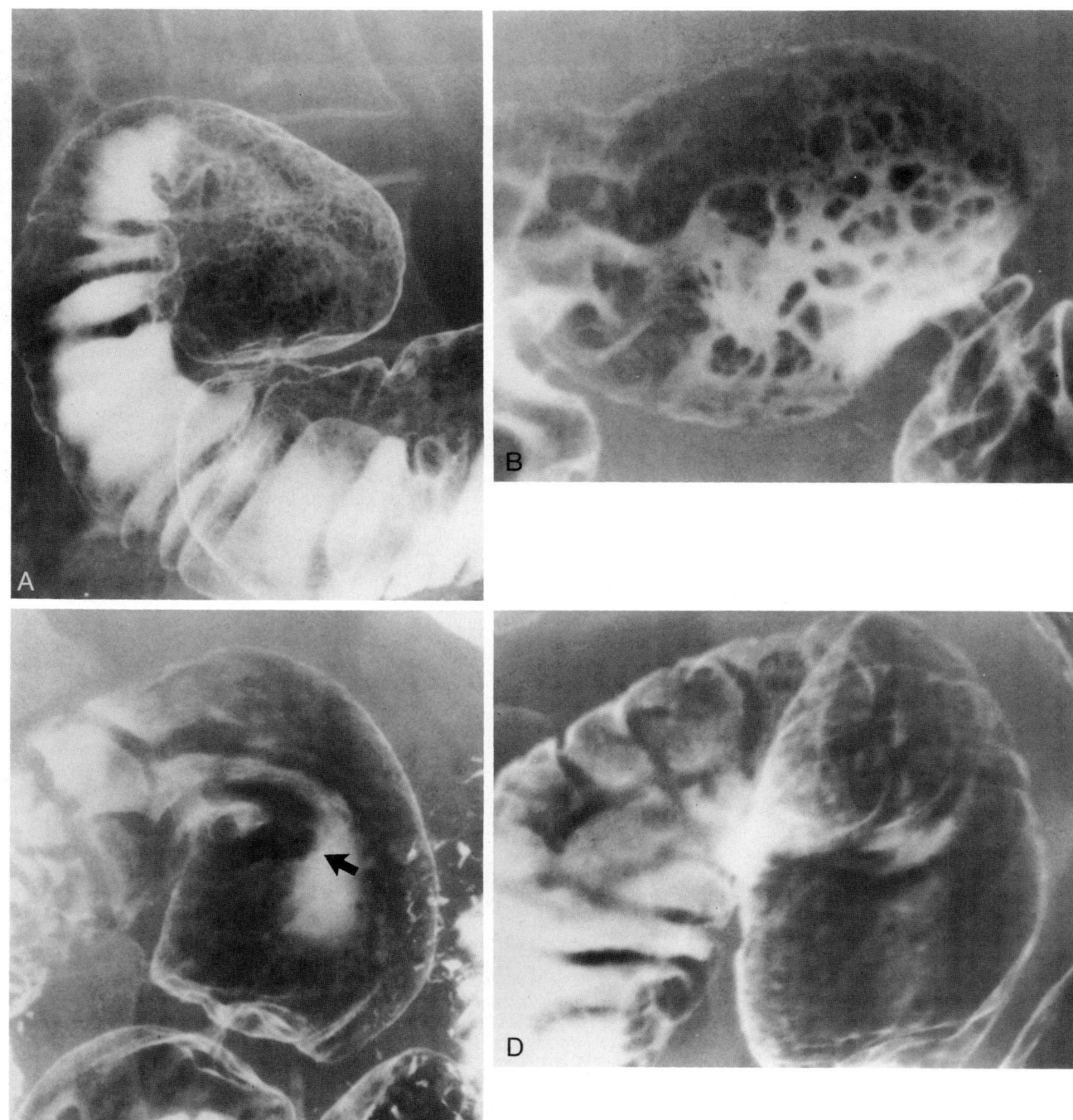

**Figure 19–8. Surface patterns in the duodenum. A.** A fine velvety pattern in the duodenal bulb. **B.** Angular filling defect caused by heterotopic gastric mucosa. **C.** The flexural pseudolesion *(arrow)* is due to infolding of the mucosa at the superior duodenal flexure. **D.** Multiple punctate collections in the duodenal bulb represent duodenal pits.

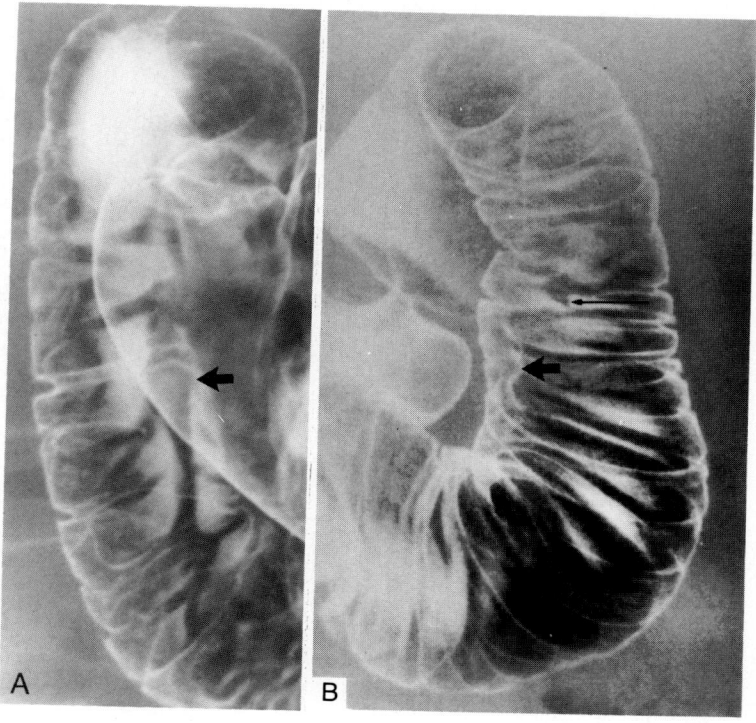

**Figure 19–9. The descending duodenum. A.** In the LPO projection, the descending duodenum is seen through the gas-filled antrum. Note the papilla *(arrow)* and its associated folds. **B.** Prone view shows major papilla *(short arrow)* on the medial wall of the descending duodenum with minor papilla *(long arrow)* seen anteriorly above this level.

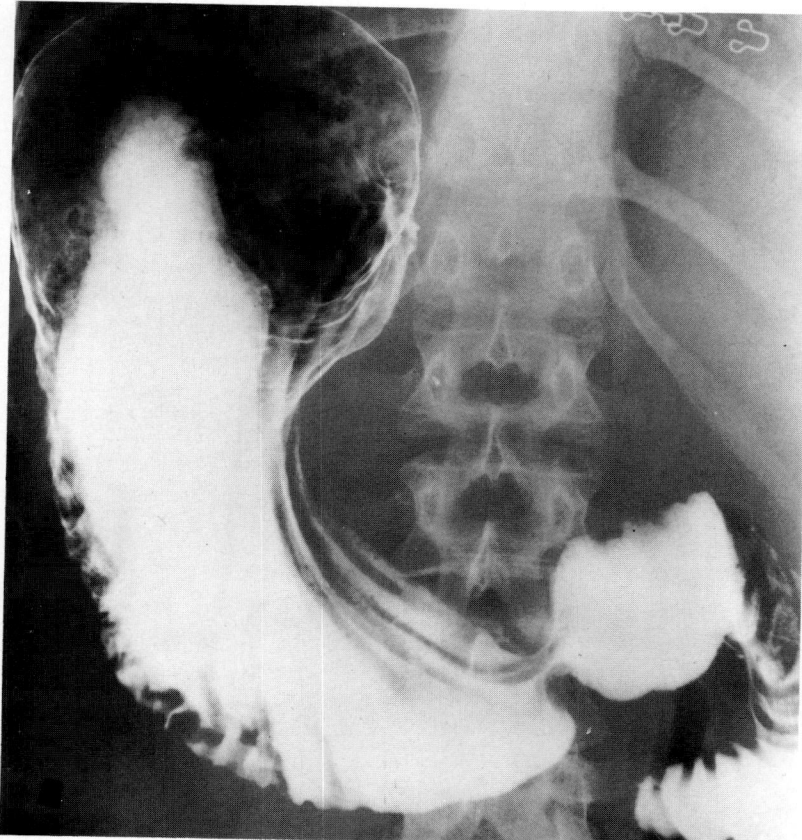

**Figure 19–10. Examination of the anterior wall of the stomach.** With the patient in the prone position, the rugal folds are seen on the anterior wall. The fundus is gas filled and coated.

# VARIATIONS IN TECHNIQUE

## Anterior Wall Lesions[20]

It is important to recognize that the routine technique as described is biased toward lesions on the posterior wall. Lesions on the anterior wall may be seen on films obtained with the patient supine as lesions etched in white. However, they are probably best seen on views obtained using compression with the patient in the prone position (Fig. 19–10). In addition, double contrast study of the anterior wall of the stomach can be performed with the patient in the prone position, turned slightly onto the left side with the head of the table lowered. Likewise, the anterior wall of the duodenum can be studied by double contrast with the patient in the prone position (see Fig. 19–9B).

## Possible Perforation

When a perforation of any portion of the gastrointestinal tract is suspected for reason of disease, iatrogenic cause, or surgery, a water-soluble contrast agent such as diatrizoate meglumine (Gastrografin) should be used.[21] If no extravasation is demonstrated, the examination should be completed with barium because the better definition achieved with barium may demonstrate a small leak that was undetected with the water-soluble contrast agent.

## After Gastric Resection[22]

After gastric resection for ulcer disease or tumor, the examination must be modified to compensate for the absence of the pylorus. The important modifications include an increase in the dose of glucagon to at least 0.5 mg and smaller amounts of effervescent agents. In addition, the examination should not be started with the patient in the upright position because that promotes rapid emptying of the gastric remnant. The details of the examination are discussed in Chapter 41 (Fig. 19–11).

## Gastric Outlet Obstruction

When gastric outlet obstruction is suspected, the examination should start with upright fluoroscopy to determine whether there is a fluid level in the stomach. If a fluid level is present, a single contrast barium examination is used to determine the site and nature of the obstruction.

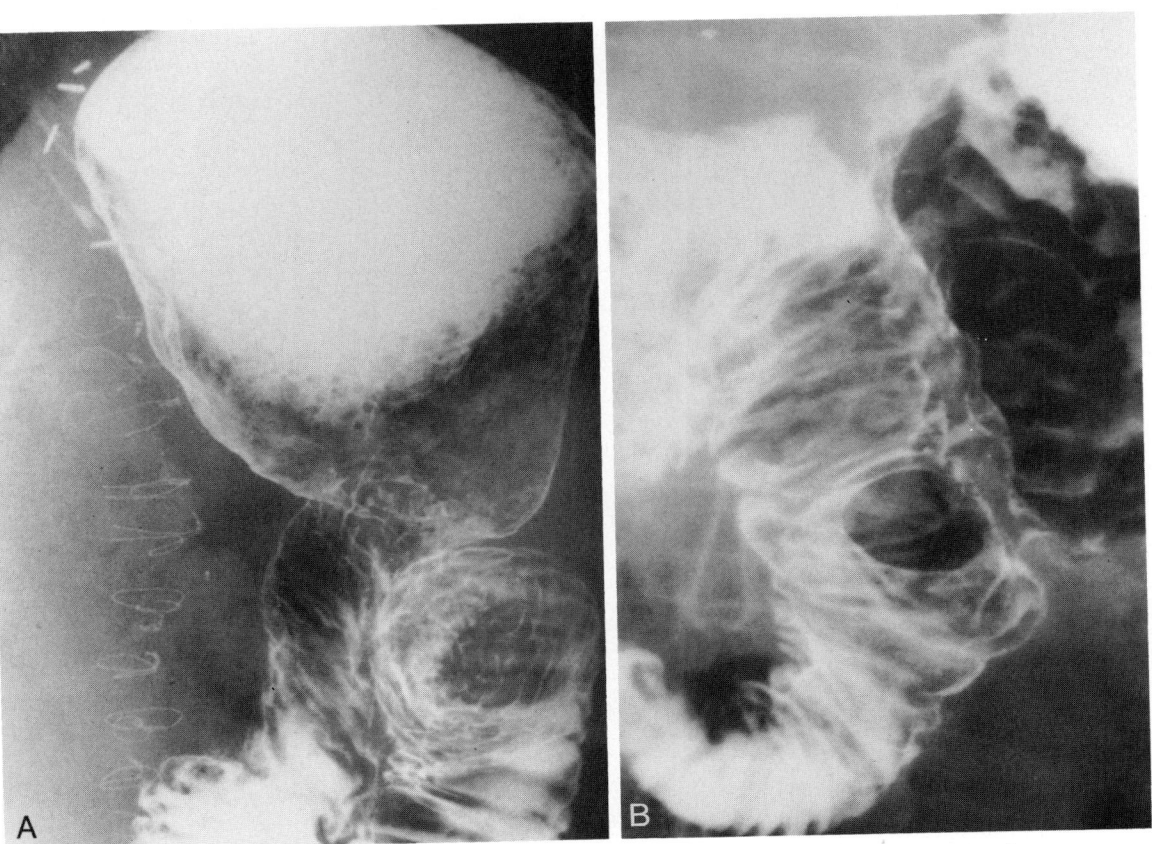

**Figure 19–11. Postoperative stomach. A.** Film showing a normal postoperative appearance after a Billroth II gastrectomy. **B.** Double contrast view of gastrojejunal anastomosis after partial gastrectomy.

## Esophageal Varices[23]

The subject of esophageal varices is discussed in Chapter 30. Esophageal varices are manifest as thickening and lobulation of the longitudinal esophageal folds and are best demonstrated with the patient in the recumbent position with the esophageal mucosa coated and the esophagus relaxed.

### Acknowledgment

Figures 19–1D and E, 19–7, 19–9B, and 19–10 are reproduced from Laufer I, Levine MS (eds): Double Contrast Gastrointestinal Radiology (2nd ed). Philadelphia: WB Saunders, 1992.

# References

1. Levine MS, Rubesin SE, Herlinger H, et al: Double-contrast upper gastrointestinal examination: technique and interpretation. Radiology 168:593–602, 1988.
2. Rubesin SE, Herlinger H: The effect of barium suspension viscosity on the delineation of areae gastricae. AJR 146:35–38, 1986.
3. Koehler RE, Weyman PJ, Stanley RJ, et al: Evaluation of three effervescent agents for double-contrast upper gastrointestinal radiography. Gastrointest Radiol 6:111–114, 1981.
4. Moeller G, Hughes JJ, Mangano FA, et al: Comparison of L-hyoscyamine, glucagon, and placebo for air-contrast upper gastrointestinal series. Gastrointest Radiol 17:195–198, 1992.
5. Kastan DJ, Ackerman LV, Feczko PJ: Digital gastrointestinal imaging: the effect of pixel size on detection of subtle mucosal abnormalities. Radiology 167:853–856, 1987.
6. Arenson RL, Chakraborty DP, Seshadri SB, et al: The digital imaging workstation. Radiology 176:303–315, 1990.
7. Kikuchi Y, Levine MS, Laufer I, et al: Value of flow technique for double-contrast examination of the stomach. AJR 174:1183–1184, 1986.
8. Gohel VK, Kressel HY, Laufer I: Double-contrast artifacts. Gastrointest Radiol 3:139–146, 1978.
9. Williams SM, Harned RK, Kaplan P, et al: Transverse striations of the esophagus: association with gastroesophageal reflux. Radiology 146:25–27, 1983.
10. Levine MS, Low V, Laufer I, et al: Focal spiculation of the upper thoracic esophagus: a normal variant on double-contrast esophagography. Radiology 183:807–810, 1992.
11. Glick SN, Teplick SK, Goldstein J, et al: Glycogenic acanthosis of the esophagus. AJR 139:683–688, 1982.
12. Mackintosh CE, Kreel L: Anatomy and radiology of the areae gastricae. Gut 18:855–864, 1977.
13. Cho KC, Gold BM, Printz DA: Multiple transverse folds in the gastric antrum. Radiology 164:339–341, 1987.
14. Herlinger H, Grossman R, Laufer I, et al: The gastric cardia in double-contrast study: its dynamic image. AJR 135:21–29, 1980.
15. Glick SN, Gohel VK, Laufer I: Mucosal surface patterns of the duodenal bulb. Radiology 150:317–322, 1984.
16. Langkemper R, Hoek AC, Dekker W, et al: Elevated lesions in the duodenal bulb caused by heterotopic gastric mucosa. Radiology 137:621–624, 1980.
17. Burrell M, Toffler R: Flexural pseudolesions of the duodenum. Radiology 120:313–315, 1976.
18. Bova JG, Kamath V, Tio FO, et al: The normal mucosal surface pattern of the duodenal bulb: radiologic-histologic correlation. AJR 145:735–738, 1985.
19. Levine MS, Laufer I, Stevenson G: Duodenum. In Laufer I, Levine MS (eds): Double Contrast Gastrointestinal Radiology (2nd ed). Philadelphia: WB Saunders, 1992, pp 321–361.
20. Goldsmith MR, Paul RE, Poplack WE, et al: evaluation of routine double-contrast views of the anterior wall of the stomach. AJR 126:1159–1163, 1976.
21. Dodds WJ, Stewart ET, Vlymen WJ: Appropriate contrast media for evaluation of esophageal disruption. Radiology 144:439–441, 1982.
22. Op den Orth JO: The postoperative stomach. In Laufer I, Levine MS (eds): Double Contrast Gastrointestinal Radiology (2nd ed). Philadelphia: WB Saunders, 1992, pp 287–320.
23. Cockerill EM, Miller RE, Chernish SM, et al: Optimal visualization of esophageal varices. AJR 126:512–523, 1976.

# Cross-sectional Imaging

**Richard M. Gore, M.D.**

## INTRODUCTION

Barium studies and endoscopy are the primary means of evaluating patients with suspected esophageal and gastroduodenal disease. These techniques provide exquisite delineation of mucosal pathologic features but cannot reliably detect, characterize, or differentiate the extramucosal component of many neoplastic, infectious, and traumatic disorders of the gastrointestinal tract. This chapter describes the applications of cross-sectional imaging in patients with known or suspected upper gastrointestinal tract disease.

## ULTRASOUND

Early in the development of ultrasound, the stomach and the duodenum were considered obstacles to the performance of upper abdominal sonography.[1-4] Technical advances in gray-scale ultrasound and high-resolution real-time sonography and the development of endoscopic ultrasound have dramatically expanded the applications of ultrasound in the evaluation of upper gastrointestinal tract disorders. Indeed, every complete sonographic examination of the upper abdomen should include assessment of the lumen, wall, and serosa of the stomach and duodenum. Because ultrasound is often the initial examination ordered for patients with abdominal complaints, the ultrasonographer is often in the position to make the initial diagnosis of upper gastrointestinal disease.[1-10] Transabdominal ultrasound has also become a primary means of assessing children with suspected hypertrophic pyloric stenosis.[11-17]

## Scanning Technique

Transabdominal real-time sonography should be performed with a transducer of the highest possible frequency, usually 3.5 or 5 MHz. Water can be given 1) to provide an acoustic "window" to the pancreas; 2) to assess distensibility of the stomach and peristalsis; and 3) to evaluate gastroesophageal reflux in children.[5]

The following elements must be carefully assessed when performing gastroduodenal sonography: 1) mural thickness; 2) mural symmetry; 3) mural homogeneity; 4) peristalsis; and 5) intraluminal contents.[1-10]

The technique of endoscopic ultrasound is described in Chapter 10.

## Normal Sonographic Anatomy

The gastrointestinal tract has a distinctive sonographic signature in which up to five layers are visualized within the wall[5-18] (Fig. 20–1). The normal gastric wall, when imaged axially, has a reniform, "target," or pseudokidney appearance (Fig. 20–2). Usually, only two layers, an echogenic center and a hypoechoic periphery, can be visualized on transabdominal scans. The gut wall measured from the lumen to the outer edge of the hypoechoic layer (wall) should be 3 mm or less when distended. If the bowel wall is thicker than 5 mm or appears asymmetrically thickened (Fig. 20–3), a pathologic process should be suspected.[5]

Peristalsis should be observed, and the stomach should be compressible.[19-21] If gastroduodenal disease is associated with an exophytic mass (Fig. 20–4), the pseudokidney appearance is deformed; ulcers within the gastroduodenal wall or within masses may produce shadowing and a "ring-down" artifact.[22, 23]

## Neoplasms

Intrinsic gastroduodenal neoplasms produce an abnormal appearance on abdominal ultrasound. Infiltrative lesions cause mural thickening, which can be localized or diffuse, smooth or irregular. The mean gastric wall thickness in patients with neoplasms is 15.9 mm.[24] Wall thickening may be quite pronounced and asymmetric, creating a globular mass that is nodular or irregular, that is poorly or irregularly echogenic, or that contains a necrotic cavity.[25] Peristalsis is often absent, and the involved gut cannot be compressed.[26-29]

**Figure 20–1. The sonographic signature of the normal gut. A.**
Diagram depicting the histologic layers of the gut wall. **B.** Corresponding axial and longitudinal representation of the five layers of gut wall.
(**A** and **B** from Wilson SR: The gastrointestinal tract. *In* Rumack CM, Wilson SR, Charboneau JW [eds]: Diagnostic Ultrasound. St. Louis: Mosby–Year Book, 1991, pp 181–207.)

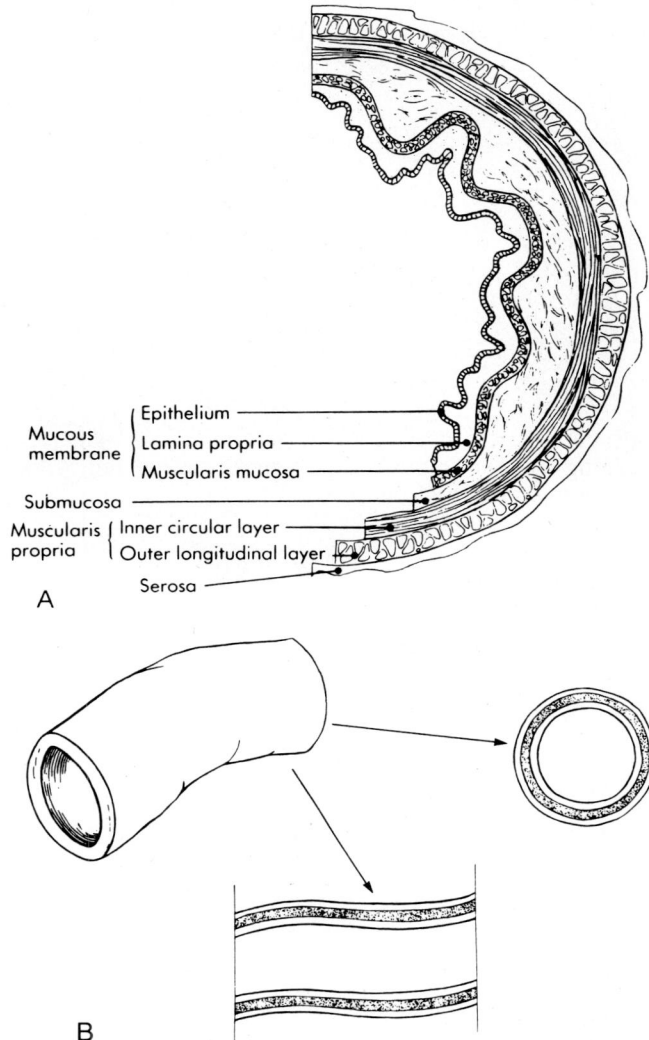

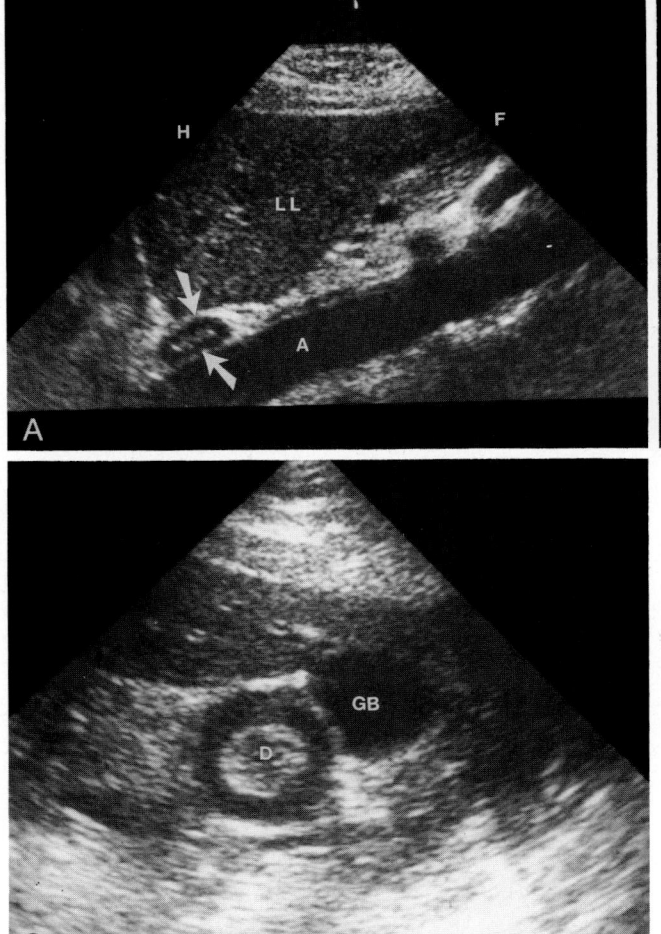

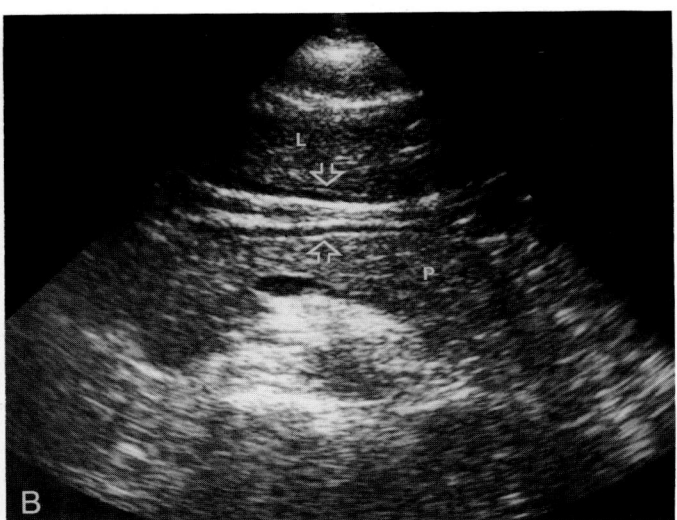

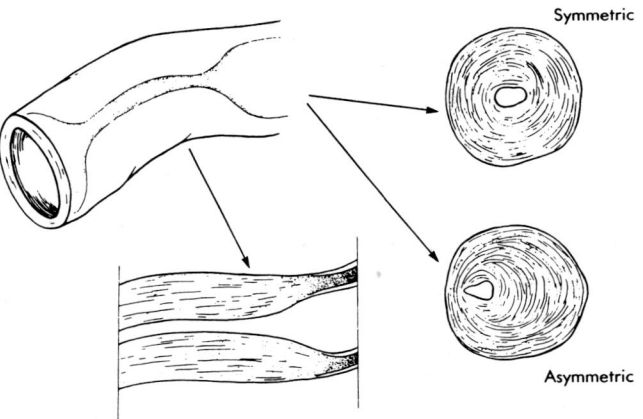

**Figure 20–2. Normal upper gastrointestinal tract: sonographic features. A.** Longitudinal scan of gastroesophageal junction. Note the reniform appearance *(arrows)* of the gut. A = aorta; F = caudal; H = cranial; LL = left lobe of liver. **B.** Axial scan of the stomach. The anterior and posterior walls of the stomach are opposed *(arrows)*. Mural stratification is present. L = liver; P = pancreas. **C.** Axially imaged duodenum (D) has a target appearance. It indents the gallbladder (GB) wall.

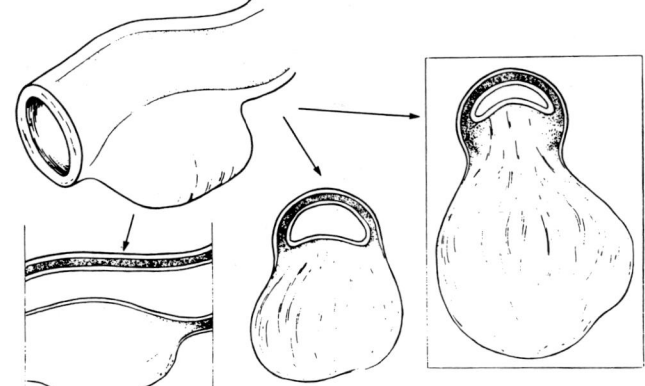

**Figure 20–3. Mural thickening of the gut.** Diagram depicts symmetric and asymmetric mural thickening with corresponding longitudinal and axial representations, showing an abnormal target or pseudokidney appearance. (From Wilson SR: The gastrointestinal tract. *In* Rumack CM, Wilson SR, Charboneau JW [eds]: Diagnostic Ultrasound. St. Louis: Mosby–Year Book, 1991, pp 181–207.)

**Figure 20–4. Exophytic gastric neoplasm.** Diagram depicting the longitudinal and axial sonographic appearance of such a mass. (From Wilson SR: The gastrointestinal tract. *In* Rumack CM, Wilson SR, Charboneau JW [eds]: Diagnostic Ultrasound. St. Louis: Mosby–Year Book, 1991, pp 181–207.)

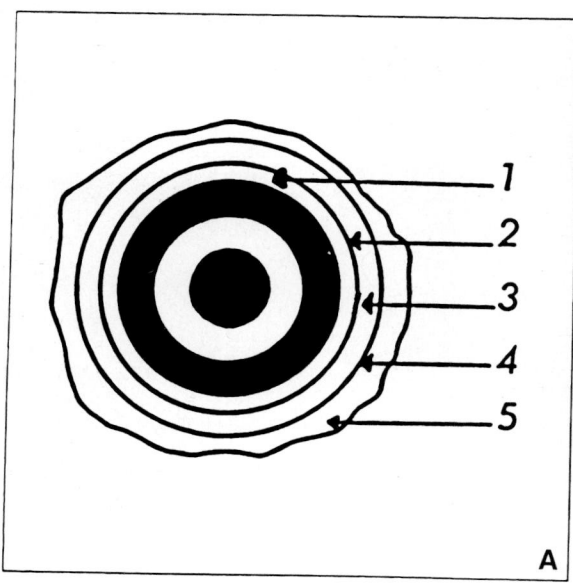

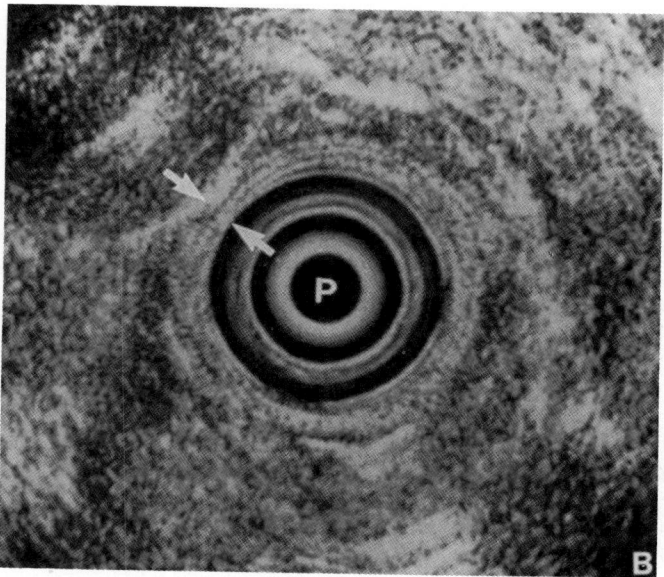

**Figure 20–5. Esophagus: normal anatomy and endoscopic ultrasound appearance. A.** Diagram showing the normal layers of the esophagus. 1 = interface between probe and balloon; 2 = muscularis mucosae; 3 = submucosa; 4 = muscularis propria; 5 = adventitia and periesophageal fat. **B.** Normal appearance of the esophagus on endoscopic ultrasound examination shows five layers. P (probe) = lumen of esophagus. (**A** and **B** from V Vilgrain, D Mompoint, L Palazzo, et al, Staging of esophageal carcinoma: comparison of results with endoscopic sonography and CT, AJR, 155, 277–281, 1990, © by American Roentgen Ray Society.)

In patients with gastric lymphoma, the stomach and adjacent lymph nodes often have a strikingly hypoechoic appearance. Mucosal folds outlined by strong intraluminal echoes arranged like the spokes of a wheel may also be seen.[30–33]

In several series, endoscopic ultrasound has proved statistically more accurate than dynamic computed to-mography (CT) in determining the extent of mural invasion in gastric and esophageal cancers[34–41] (Figs. 20–5 and 20–6). Endoscopic ultrasound also has the capacity to identify malignancy within normal-sized nodes on the basis of tissue texture and morphology. Diagnosis by CT and magnetic resonance (MR) is based on node size only, and these techniques cannot identify malignant

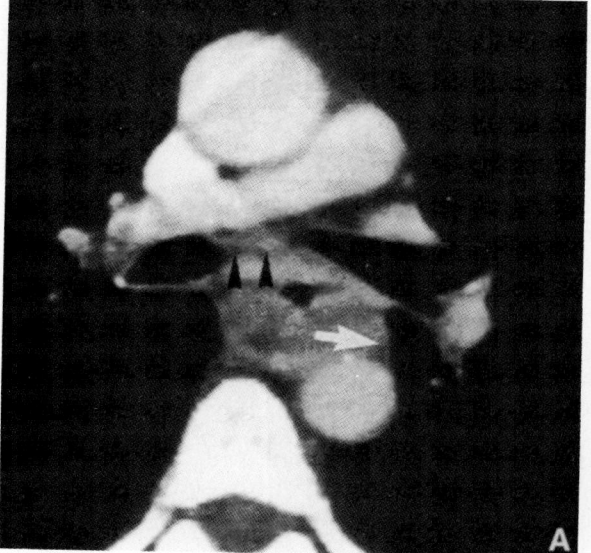

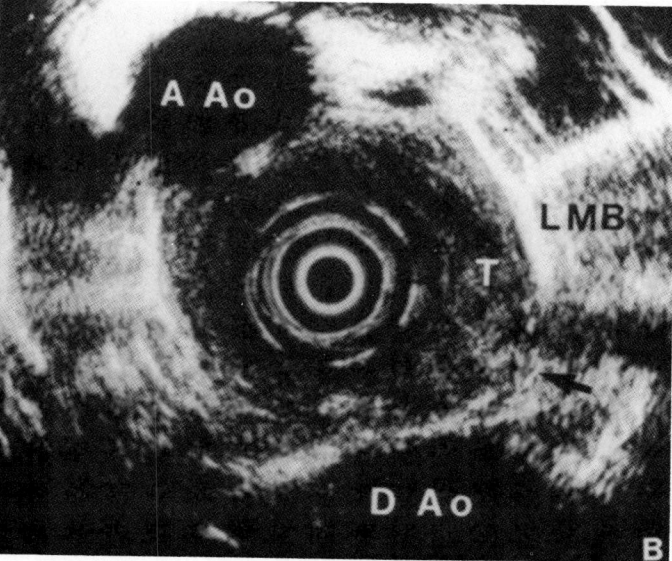

**Figure 20–6. Carcinoma of the esophagus: CT and endoscopic ultrasound findings.** This neoplasm extends between the descending aorta and left main bronchus. **A.** CT scan shows tumor displacing the left main stem bronchus and located between the aorta and the left main stem bronchus *(arrow)*, suggesting nonresectability. There is an enlarged subcarinal lymph node *(arrowheads)*. **B.** Endoscopic ultrasound scan shows mediastinal invasion *(arrow)* of tumor (T) between left main stem bronchus (LMB) and descending aorta (D Ao). A Ao = ascending aorta. (**A** and **B** from V Vilgrain, D Mompoint, L Palazzo, et al, Staging of esophageal carcinoma: comparison of results with endoscopic sonography and CT, AJR, 155, 277–281, 1990, © by American Roentgen Ray Society.)

disease with normal-sized nodes.[42] Endoscopic ultrasound is difficult to perform and requires the combined skills of an expert endoscopist and ultrasonographer. Also, most surgeons do not demand such detailed staging information. Distant disease is important to appreciate preoperatively, but preoperative recognition of mural invasion is less important.[43] Endoscopic ultrasound has also proved useful in the diagnosis of regional lymph node metastases in gastric cancer, with a positive predictive value of 87.5% and a negative predictive value of 82.1%.[44]

In patients with esophageal and gastric neoplasms, endoscopic ultrasound has proved useful for 1) diagnosing submucosal tumors; 2) establishing the layer of origin, direction of growth, and consistency of tumor; 3) differentiating extrinsic compression from submucosal tumors in difficult cases; 4) determining the depth of invasion; 5) detecting invasion of the wall by extrinsic tumors; 6) evaluating the effect of laser treatment of early carcinoma; 7) detecting lymph node metastasis; and 8) avoiding potentially dangerous biopsies.[45–46]

## Benign Disorders

Mural thickening of the stomach is the hallmark of benign gastric disease as well as of neoplasms.[24] In benign disease, the degree of thickening is usually less impressive, and mural stratification may be preserved. This finding has been reported in Ménétrier's disease, acute gastritis, Crohn's disease, lymphoid hyperplasia, eosinophilic gastritis, Zollinger-Ellison syndrome, varioliform gastritis, chronic granulomatous disease, and lymphangiectasia.[47]

The diagnosis of hypertrophic pyloric stenosis is being established sonographically in an increasing number of cases. The diameter, thickness, and length of the canal, as well as the correlation of diameter and thickness to age, must be considered.[48–50] Ultrasound can also be used to assess gastroesophageal reflux in children without using fluoroscopy or nuclear scintigraphy.[51]

## Peptic Ulcer Disease

Modest mural thickening in the region of ulceration is often found associated with spasm and deformity. Focal dense echoes with acoustic shadowing and ring-down artifact with air in the ulcer crater may be seen. The hyperechoic center may be surrounded by a hypoechoic halo, which represents duodenal wall edema and infiltration. With perforation, perigastric fluid and gas collections can develop.[24, 52–59]

## COMPUTED TOMOGRAPHY

## Esophagus

### Normal Anatomy

The esophagus is usually well delineated by CT (Fig. 20–7). The paraesophageal fat is visualized as an inter-

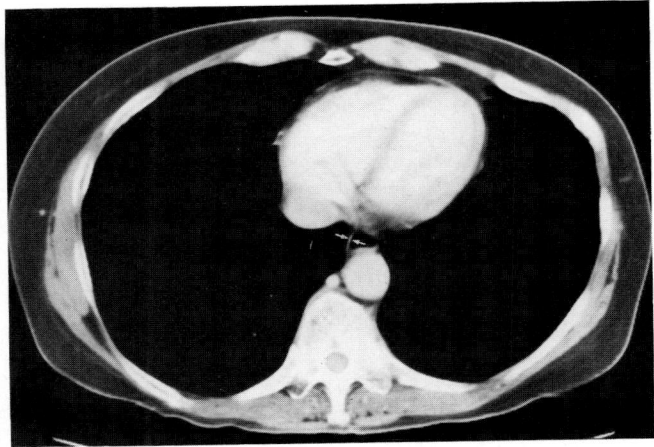

**Figure 20–7. Normal esophagus: CT appearance.** Air is seen in this normal esophagus. The wall (arrows) is barely perceptible.

face between the esophagus and adjacent vascular, cardiac, and connective tissue structures. The cervical esophagus lies near the midline, posterior to and occasionally indenting the trachea. It usually does not contain air. As the esophagus enters the thorax, it lies posterior and slightly to the left of the trachea, and the esophagotracheal fat pad is often thin. More inferiorly, the esophagus is situated close to the posterior surface of the left main stem bronchus, descending thoracic aorta, and thoracic spine. Tumors, adenopathy, and aneurysms can all displace and invade the esophagus.[60–65]

Small amounts of intraesophageal air are seen in approximately 65% of normal individuals. The presence of an air-fluid level, fluid-filled lumen, or lumen caliber greater than 10 mm usually indicates obstruction or severe esophageal dysmotility.[60–62, 64]

Although there are no normal standards for the cross-sectional diameter of the collapsed esophagus, the wall thickness of a distended esophagus should not exceed 3 mm.[60–65]

As the esophagus becomes intra-abdominal, it courses anteriorly and to the left to enter the stomach at the gastroesophageal junction. This region is often problematic, because in nearly one third of normal individuals, prominent soft tissue in this region projects into the gastric lumen. This soft tissue "mass" represents the combined thickness of the esophageal walls and medial gastric wall with its nondistended mucosal folds. A hiatal hernia can create a similar appearance. Rescanning the patient in the left lateral decubitus position with more contrast medium or air usually resolves the problem.[66, 67]

Hiatal hernias are manifested by widening of the esophageal hiatus associated with separation of the diaphragmatic crura and an increased distance between the crura and the esophageal wall.[68, 69]

### Esophageal Carcinoma

CT has been found useful in staging patients with advanced esophageal carcinoma (Fig. 20–8). Tumors that demonstrate evidence on CT scans of aortic or tracheobronchial invasion are considered unresectable.[70–80] In one series, CT had a sensitivity, specificity,

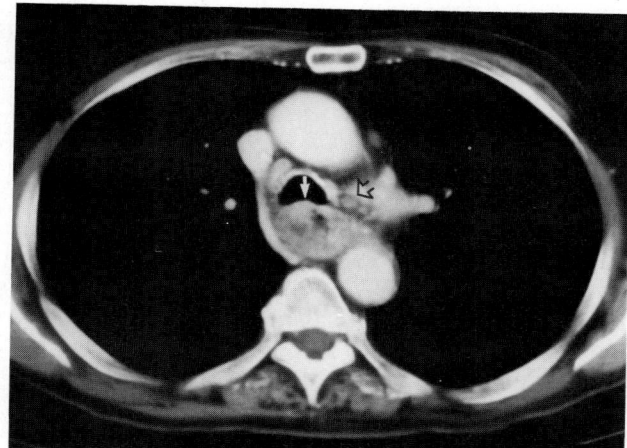

**Figure 20–8. Carcinoma of the esophagus: CT findings.** Scan at the level of the aortopulmonary window shows an esophageal mass that indents the trachea *(solid arrow)* and subtends a 90-degree arc with the aorta. Aortopulmonary adenopathy is also shown *(open arrow).*

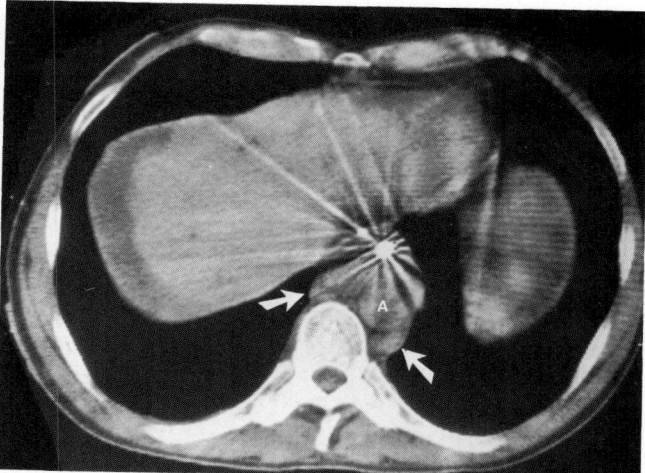

**Figure 20–9. Esophageal varices: CT findings.** Tubular enhanced structures *(arrows)* are adjacent to the aorta (A), azygos vein, and hemiazygos vein in this patient with ulcerative colitis, sclerosing cholangitis, and secondary biliary cirrhosis. Note the irregular hepatic contour and ascites.

and accuracy of 100, 84, and 87%, respectively, in staging esophageal cancers. CT can also provide information concerning the presence of metastatic disease in the liver, adrenal glands, and abdominal lymph nodes.

CT is also useful for detecting postoperative complications and extramucosal tumor recurrence.[81]

MR imaging has been shown to be as accurate as CT scanning in staging esophageal cancers, and it has the same limitations (see Chapter 28).[77, 80, 82]

## Benign Esophageal Lesions

**Perforation.** Although the definitive diagnosis of esophageal perforation is established by the contrast esophagram, CT can provide critical information concerning the extent of mediastinal, pleural, and parenchymal involvement.[83–86]

**Varices.** CT is useful in the detection of paraesophageal varices (Fig. 20–9) and of complications of esophageal sclerotherapy.[87–91]

**Infectious and Inflammatory Conditions.** CT has no role in the diagnosis of infectious esophagitis and intramural pseudodiverticulosis. These disorders, however, can cause focal or, more commonly, diffuse mural thickening of the esophagus.[92, 93]

**Extramural Lesions.** There are many causes of extrinsic compression of the esophagus, and CT is valuable in differentiating them: substernal goiter and vascular abnormalities involving the aorta and great vessels, including aneurysms, aberrant right and left subclavian arteries, double aortic arch anomalies, and pulmonary vascular sling (see Chapter 75).

## Stomach

### Normal Anatomy

Gastric CT requires meticulous attention to technique so that the stomach is distended with contrast medium or gas (see Chapter 9) (Fig. 20–10). The most common

diagnostic dilemma in gastric CT is the need to differentiate mural thickening that is truly pathologic from a focal area of incomplete distention. The stomach wall is usually less than 5 mm in thickness and homogeneous in attenuation. Perigastric fat is usually uniform in attenuation.[94–99]

For patients with previous gastric surgery, it is useful to administer oral contrast medium, an effervescent agent, and glucagon to slow motility. The patient is turned from the supine position to the right lateral decubitus position, to the prone position, to the left lateral decubitus position, and finally to the supine position. These maneuvers help fill the afferent loop resulting from a Billroth II procedure and the proximal limb resulting from Whipple's procedure.[60]

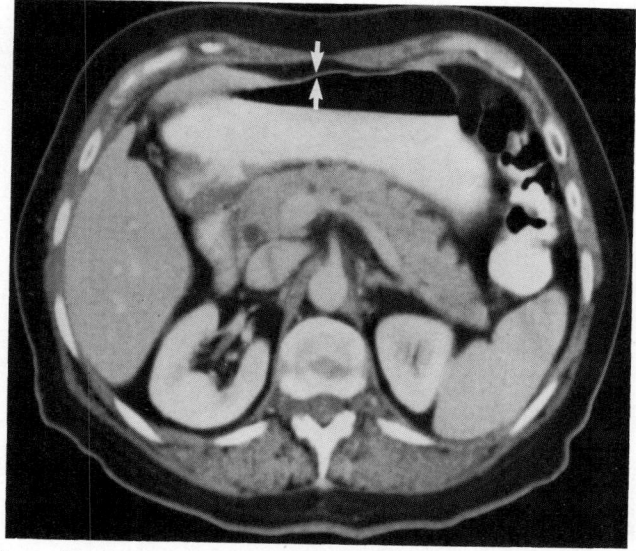

**Figure 20–10. Normal stomach: CT appearance.** Axial scan of the gastric antrum distended with contrast medium and air shows a thin, uniform gastric wall *(arrows).*

The gastric air-fluid level is helpful in differentiating apparent gastric wall thickening that is due to incomplete gastric distention from true pathologic wall thickening (Fig. 20–11). A transition in gastric wall thickness is often present at or slightly above the gastric air-fluid or air-contrast level. The apparently thickened gastric wall in the dependent portion of the stomach undergoes an abrupt change to normal thickness at or above the air-fluid level. This phenomenon has been observed in 22% of CT scans in patients without upper gastrointestinal symptoms. Although its occurrence does not obviate the need to perform additional diagnostic maneuvers or procedures in cases of suspected gastric disease, this phenomenon can allow a greater degree of confidence in dismissing apparent thickening when the stomach is included on scans performed for other indications.[100]

## Gastric Neoplasms

Double contrast barium studies and endoscopy are the primary means of establishing the diagnosis of gastric adenocarcinoma. CT, however, may uncover a gastric neoplasm incidentally, may help differentiate lymphoma from adenocarcinoma when biopsies are nonspecific, and may identify local and distant metastases. Gastric cancers usually cause focal or diffuse mural thickening of the stomach (Fig. 20–12). This finding is nonspecific, but it strongly suggests neoplasm when it is combined with one or more of the following findings: adjacent adenopathy, liver metastases, or disease in the adjacent omentum, gastrocolic ligament, or gastrohepatic ligament.[101–107]

Gastric lymphomas typically produce mural thickening of the stomach and distortion of the rugal fold pattern. Most patients have clearly defined lymphade-

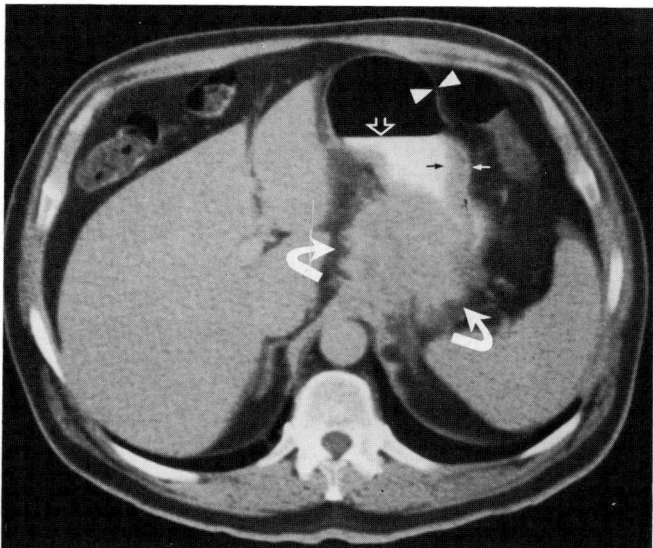

**Figure 20–11. True thickening and pseudothickening of the gastric wall.** A carcinoma of the gastric cardia *(curved arrows)* is invading adjacent fat, causing true mural thickening. Pseudothickening *(solid arrows)* is seen in the portion of stomach distended with contrast medium. Note the abrupt reduction of mural thickness *(arrowheads)* at the air-fluid interface *(open arrow).*

nopathy in the gastrohepatic ligament, gastrocolic ligament, or greater omentum. Adenopathy beneath the level of the renal hilum is unusual in carcinoma, and when present, it more likely indicates gastric lymphoma.[108]

## Gastritis and Peptic Ulcer Disease

Patients with severe gastritis caused by *Helicobacter pylori* have two major patterns of CT abnormalities: 1) circumferential antral wall thickening and 2) thickening of the posterior gastric wall along the greater curvature, with or without evidence of ulceration. The mural thickening can be impressive (1.5 to 2.0 cm), suggesting malignancy, but in gastritis, no associated adenopathy, obliteration of fat planes, or invasion of adjacent structures is observed.[109]

Although it has little application to the detection of uncomplicated peptic ulcer disease, CT is helpful in detecting acute free perforation and penetration. CT signs of complicated ulcer disease include bowel wall thickening and inflammatory changes in adjacent soft tissues, including the pancreas, liver, and lesser omentum.[110–113]

Other benign causes of mural thickening of the stomach include Zollinger-Ellison syndrome and Ménétrier's disease, Crohn's disease, cytomegalovirus infection, cryptosporidiosis, and graft-versus-host disease.[114]

## Duodenum

Because of its intimate relationship to the pancreas, hepatoduodenal ligament, duodenal-colic ligament, and transverse mesocolon, the duodenum may be involved by adjacent disease. Incomplete distention of the duodenum by air or contrast medium may simulate disease in these other structures.[115, 116]

The normal duodenal wall is usually thinner than the stomach wall, measuring approximately 1 mm in thickness. Duodenal diverticula may fill with air or contrast medium. In the latter case, the contrast medium–filled diverticulum may suggest a common bile duct stone. Accordingly, some authors suggest withholding oral contrast medium when using CT to diagnose choledocholithiasis (see Chapter 91).[117]

Intrinsic duodenitis and pancreatitis can lead to mural thickening of the duodenum. CT can also demonstrate perforating ulcers and sinus tracts from the duodenum.[118] Duodenal diverticulitis can also be diagnosed on CT (Fig. 20–13), which may clarify a confusing clinical picture.[119] CT is also useful in diagnosing subtle duodenal rupture that is due to trauma.[120]

Duodenal tumors are uncommon, and CT is useful in characterizing and staging these lesions.[121, 122]

## MAGNETIC RESONANCE IMAGING

Although it is used for routine imaging of the esophagus, stomach, and duodenum, MR has not been widely

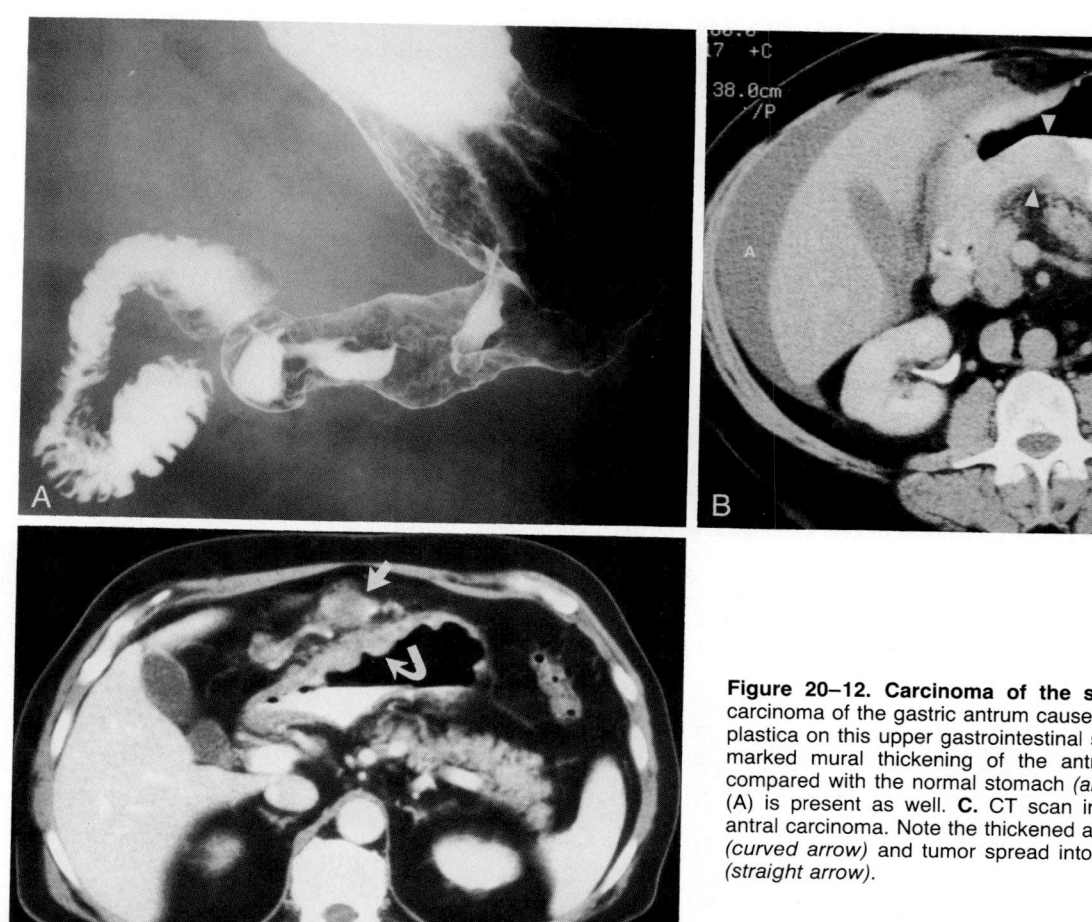

**Figure 20–12. Carcinoma of the stomach. A.** An annular carcinoma of the gastric antrum causes an appearance of linitis plastica on this upper gastrointestinal study. **B.** CT scan shows marked mural thickening of the antrum *(arrowheads)* when compared with the normal stomach *(arrows)*. Malignant ascites (A) is present as well. **C.** CT scan in a different patient with antral carcinoma. Note the thickened anterior wall of the antrum *(curved arrow)* and tumor spread into the gastrocolic ligament *(straight arrow)*.

**Figure 20–13. Duodenal diverticulitis: CT findings.** CT scan shows an abscess secondary to a perforated perivaterian duodenal diverticulum *(arrows)*.

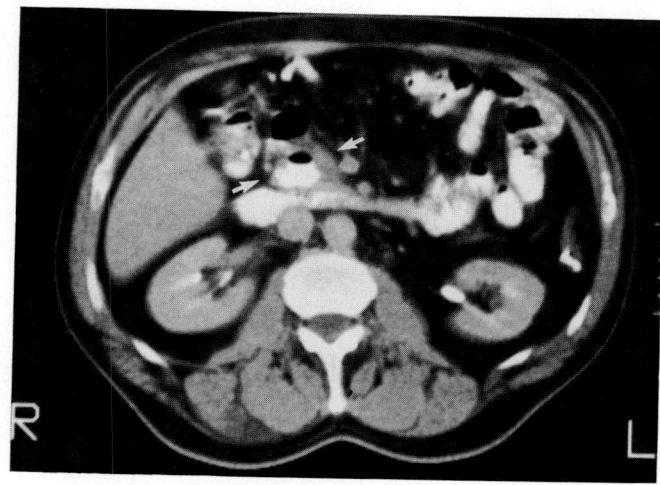

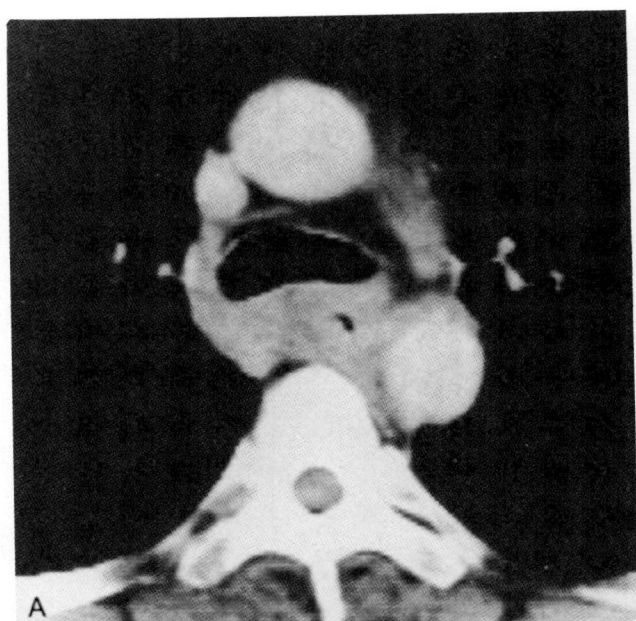
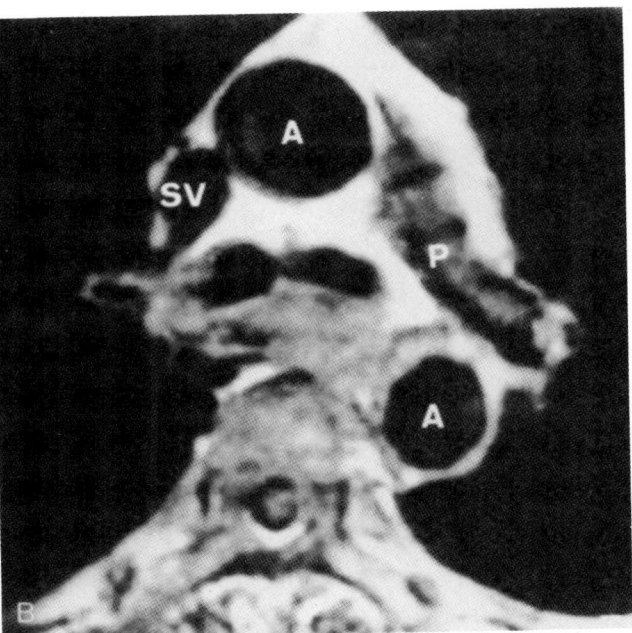

**Figure 20–14. Carcinoma of the esophagus: MR and CT correlation.** Carcinoma of the esophagus invades the aorta. **A.** CT scan shows obliteration of the triangular fat space between the esophagus, aorta, and spine, suggesting aortic invasion. **B.** Aortic invasion is also suggested on this T1-weighted (500/15) MR scan. A = aorta; p = left pulmonary artery; SV = superior vena cava. (**A** and **B** from S Takashima, N Takeuchi, H Shiozaki, et al, Carcinoma of the esophagus: CT vs MR imaging in determining resectability, AJR, 156, 297–302, 1991, © by American Roentgen Ray Society.)

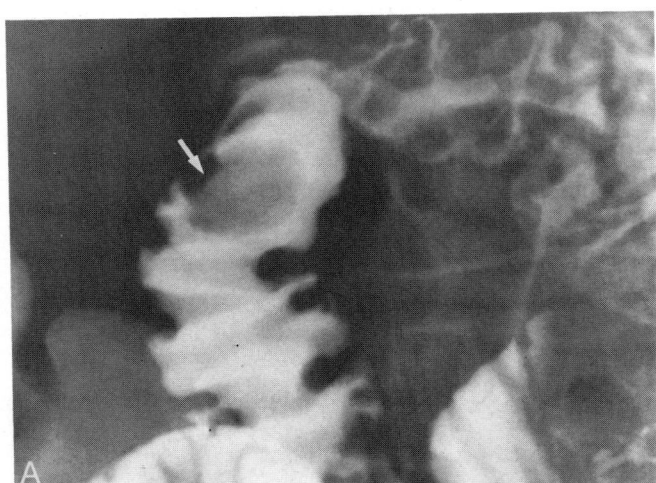
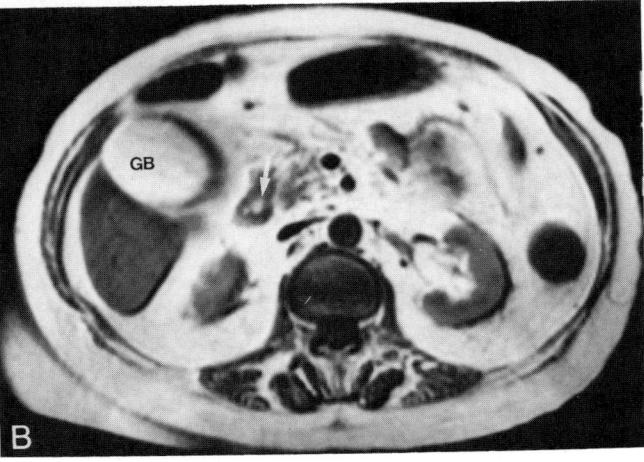

**Figure 20–15. Duodenal lipoma: MR findings. A.** A smooth filling defect *(arrow)* is present in the descending duodenum on this spot film from an upper gastrointestinal series. **B.** T1-weighted MR image shows high signal intensity in the region of this mass *(arrow)* indicating fat. Note the high signal intensity of the fasting gallbladder (GB). (**A** and **B** from Ros PR: Extrahepatic applications of magnetic resonance imaging. *In* Gore RM [ed]: Syllabus for Categorical Course on Gastrointestinal Radiology. Reston, VA: American College of Radiology, 1991, pp 121–128.)

used to evaluate these structures for a variety of reasons: artifact from motion caused by respiration, peristalsis, and cardiac pulsation; inferior spatial resolution; lack of optimal contrast agents; and most important, high cost and limited availability.[123-126]

Many medical centers have assessed the utility of MR in staging esophageal and gastric cancer (Figs. 20–14 and 20–15). At present, this imaging method appears to offer little advantage over CT and is limited by many of the same factors—for example, inability to determine the content of adjacent lymph nodes. With faster scanning times, better contrast agents, and better spatial resolution, the indications for MR of the upper gastrointestinal tract will no doubt expand (see Chapter 9).[127-131]

# References

1. Fleischer AC, Muhletaler CA, James AE: Detection of bowel lesions during abdominal and pelvic sonography. JAMA 244:2096–2099, 1980.
2. Fleischer AC, Dowling AD, Weinstein ML, et al: Sonographic patterns of distended, fluid-filled bowel. Radiology 133:681–685, 1979.
3. Fakhry JR, Berk RN: The "target" pattern: characteristic sonographic feature of stomach and bowel abnormalities. AJR 137:969–972, 1981.
4. Morgan CL, Trought WS, Oddson TA, et al: Ultrasound patterns of disorders affecting the gastrointestinal tract. Radiology 135:129–135, 1980.
5. Wilson SR: The gastrointestinal tract. *In* Rumack CM, Wilson SR, Charboneau JW (eds): Diagnostic Ultrasound. St. Louis: Mosby–Year Book, 1992, pp 181–207.
6. Wilson SR, Thurston WA: Gastrointestinal sonography. Curr Opin Radiol 4:69–77, 1992.
7. Rad BK, Fleischer AC: Sonography of the gastrointestinal tract. Curr Opin Radiol 2:207–212, 1990.
8. Carroll BA: US of the gastrointestinal tract. Radiology 172:605–608, 1989.
9. Wang KY, Kimmey MB: Intestinal ultrasound. Appl Radiol 15:59–66, July 1991.
10. Reading CC: Endorectal sonography. Crit Rev Diagn Imaging 33:1–28, 1992.
11. O'Keefe FN, Stansberry SD, Swischuk LE, et al: Antropyloric muscle thickness at US in infants: what is normal? Radiology 178:827–830, 1991.
12. Ball TI, Atkinson GO, Gay BB: Ultrasound diagnosis of hypertrophic pyloric stenosis: real-time application and the demonstration of a new sonographic sign. Radiology 147:499–502, 1983.
13. Miller JH, Kemberling CR: Ultrasound of the pediatric gastrointestinal tract. Semin Ultrasound CT MR 8:349–365, 1987.
14. Haller JO, Cohen HL: Hypertrophic pyloric stenosis: diagnosis using US. Radiology 161:335–339, 1986.
15. Lund Kofoed PE, Höcst A, Elle B, et al: Hypertrophic pyloric stenosis: determination of muscle dimensions by ultrasound. Br J Radiol 61:19–20, 1988.
16. Westra SJ, deGroot CJ, Smits NJ: Hypertrophic pyloric stenosis. Radiology 172:615–619, 1989.
17. Breaux CW, Georgeson KE, Royal SA, et al: Changing patterns in the diagnosis of hypertrophic pyloric stenosis. Pediatrics 81:213–217, 1988.
18. Kimmey MB, Martin RW, Haggitt RC, et al: Histologic correlates of gastrointestinal ultrasound images. Gastroenterology 96:433–441, 1989.
19. Smithius RHM, Opden Orth: Gastric fluid detected by sonography in fasting patients: relation to duodenal ulcer disease and gastric-outlet obstruction. AJR 153:731–733, 1989.
20. Hausken T, Odegaard S, Berstad A: Antroduodenal motility studied by real-time ultrasonography. Gastroenterology 100:59–63, 1991.
21. Worlicek H, Dunz D, Engelhard K: Ultrasonic examination of the wall of the fluid-filled stomach. JCU 17:5–14, 1989.
22. Martinez-Noguera A, Mata J, Matias-Guiu Y, et al: Echogenic focus in the gastrointestinal wall as a sign of ulceration. Gastrointest Radiol 14:295–299, 1989.
23. Lim LH, Lee DH, Ko YT: Sonographic detection of duodenal ulcer. J Ultrasound Med 11:91–94, 1992.
24. Rapaccini GL, Aliotta A, Pompili M, et al: Gastric wall thickness in normal and neoplastic subjects: a prospective study performed by abdominal ultrasound. Gastrointest Radiol 13:197–199, 1988.
25. Yeh HC, Rabinowitz JG: Ultrasonography and computed tomography of gastric wall lesions. Radiology 141:147–155, 1981.
26. Machi J, Takeda T, Sigel B, et al: Normal stomach wall and gastric cancer: evaluation with high resolution operative US. Radiology 159:85–87, 1986.
27. Miyamoto Y, Tsujimoto F, Tada S: Ultrasonographic diagnosis of submucosal tumors of the stomach: the "bridging layers" sign. JCU 16:251–258, 1988.
28. Derchi EE, Biggi E, Rolland GA, et al: Sonographic staging of gastric cancer. AJR 140:273–276, 1983.
29. Sandler MA, Ratanaprakarn S, Madrazo BL: Ultrasonic findings in intramural exogastric lesions. Radiology 128:189–192, 1978.
30. Derchi LE, Banderali A, Bossi MC, et al: The sonographic appearance of gastric lymphoma. J Ultrasound Med 3:251–256, 1984.
31. Francica G, Cozzolino G, Morange R, et al: Gastric lymphoma: diagnosis and follow-up of chemotherapy-induced changes using real-time ultrasonography: a report of three cases. Eur J Radiol 11:68–72, 1990.
32. Tio TL, den Hartog Jager FCA, Tytgat GNJ: Endoscopic ultrasonography of non-Hodgkins lymphoma. Gastroenterology 91:401–408, 1986.
33. Georg C, Schwerk WB, Georg K: Gastrointestinal lymphoma: sonographic findings in 54 patients. AJR 155:795–798, 1990.
34. Vilgrain V, Mompoint D, Palazzo L, et al: Staging of esophageal carcinoma: comparison of results with endoscopic sonography and CT. AJR 155:277–281, 1990.
35. Silva SA, Kovzo T, Ogino Y, et al: Endoscopic ultrasonography of esophageal tumors and compressions. JCU 16:149–158, 1988.
36. Dimagno EP, Regan PT, Clain JE, et al: Human endoscopic ultrasonography. Gastroenterology 83:824–829, 1982.
37. Tytgat GNJ, Tio TL: Esophageal ultrasonography. Gastroenterol Clin North Am 20:659–672, 1991.
38. Rosch T, Lorenz R, Dancygier H, et al: Endoscopic diagnosis of submucosal upper gastrointestinal tract tumors. Scand J Gastroenterol 27:1–8, 1992.
39. Bolondi L, Casanova P, Caletti GC, et al: Primary gastric lymphoma versus gastric carcinoma: endoscopic US evaluation. Radiology 165:821–826, 1987.
40. Green J, Katz S, Phillips G, et al: Percutaneous sonographic needle aspiration biopsy of endoscopically negative gastric carcinoma. Am J Gastroenterol 83:1150–1153, 1988.
41. Baker MK, Kopecky KK: Endoscopic US in the staging of esophageal and gastric cancer. Radiology 181:342–343, 1991.
42. Tio TL, Tytgat GNJ: Endoscopic ultrasonography in analysing peri-intestinal lymph node abnormality: preliminary results of studies in vitro and in vivo. Scand J Gastroenterol 21:158–163, 1986.
43. Tio TL, Den Hartog Jager FCA, Tytgat GNJ: The role of endoscopic ultrasonography in assessing local resectability of oesophagogastric malignancies: accuracy, pitfalls, and predictability. Scand J Gastroenterol 21:78–86, 1986.
44. Akahoshi K, Misawa T, Fujishima H, et al: Regional lymph node metastasis in gastric cancer: evaluation with endoscopic US. Radiology 182:559–564, 1992.
45. Fujishima H, Misawa T, Maruoka A, et al: Staging and follow-up of primary gastric lymphoma by endoscopic ultrasonography. Am J Gastroenterol 86:719–724, 1991.
46. George C, Schwerk WB, Neumann K, et al: Gastric lymphoma—ultrasound appearance due to isolated mucosal infiltration. J Clin Ultrasound 20:59–61, 1992.
47. Gassner I, Strasser K, Bart G, et al: Sonographic appearance of Ménétrier's disease in a child. J Ultrasound Med 9:537–539, 1990.

48. Blumhagen JD, Nobel HGS: Muscle thickness in hypertrophic pyloric stenosis: sonographic determination. AJR 140:221–223, 1983.

49. Strauss S, Itzchak Y, Manor A, et al: Sonography of hypertrophic pyloric stenosis. AJR 136:1057–1058, 1981.

50. Sauerbrei EE, Paloschi GGB: The ultrasonic features of hypertrophic pyloric stenosis, with emphasis on the postoperative appearance. Radiology 147:503–506, 1983.

51. Wright LL, Baker KR, Meny RG: Ultrasound demonstration of gastroesophageal reflux. J Ultrasound Med 7:471–476, 1988.

52. Joharjy IA, Mustafa MA, Zaidi AJ: Fluid-aided sonography of the stomach and duodenum in the diagnosis of peptic ulcer disease in adult patients. J Ultrasound Med 9:77–84, 1990.

53. Parulekar SG, Lubert M: Ultrasound demonstration of giant duodenal ulcer. Gastrointest Radiol 8:29–31, 1983.

54. Tomooka Y, Onitsuka H, Goya T, et al: Ultrasonography of benign gastric ulcers. J Ultrasound Med 8:513–517, 1989.

55. Madrazo BL, Hricak H, Sandler MA, et al: Sonographic findings in complicated peptic ulcer. Radiology 140:457–461, 1981.

56. Rosenberg ER, Morgan CL, Trought WS, et al: The ultrasonographic recognition of a gastric ulcer. Br J Radiol 53:1014–1016, 1980.

57. Derchi LE, Ierace T, DePra L, et al: The sonographic appearance of duodenal lesions. J Ultrasound Med 5:269–273, 1986.

58. Hayden CK, Swischuk LE, Rytting JE: Gastric ulcer disease in infants: US findings. Radiology 164:131–134, 1987.

59. Tuncel E: Ultrasonic features of duodenal ulcer. Gastrointest Radiol 15:207–210, 1990.

60. Koehler RE, Balfe DM, Stanley RJ: Gastrointestinal tract. *In* Lee JKT, Sagel SS, Stanley RJ (eds): Computed Body Tomography (2nd ed). St. Louis: CV Mosby, 1989, pp 477–521.

61. Naidich DP: Esophagus. *In* Megibow AJ, Balthazar EJ (eds): Computed Tomography of the Gastrointestinal Tract. St. Louis: CV Mosby, 1986, pp 33–98.

62. Marx MV, Balfe DM: Computed tomography of the esophagus. Semin Ultrasound CT MR 8:316–348, 1987.

63. Megibow AJ: The gastrointestinal tract. *In* Haaga JR, Alfidi RJ (eds): Computed Tomography of the Whole Body (2nd ed). St. Louis: CV Mosby, 1988, pp 1390–1428.

64. Halber MD, Daffner RH, Thompson WM: CT of the esophagus: I. Normal appearance. AJR 133:1047–1050, 1979.

65. Quint LE, Glazer GM, Orringer MB: Esophageal imaging by MR and CT: study of normal anatomy and neoplasms. Radiology 156:727–731, 1985.

66. Marks WM, Callen PW, Filly RA: Gastroesophageal region: source of confusion on CT. AJR 136:359–362, 1981.

67. Pillari G, Weinreb J, Vernace F, et al: CT of gastric masses: image patterns and a note on potential pitfalls. Gastrointest Radiol 8:11–17, 1983.

68. Pupols A, Ruzicka FF: Hiatal hernia causing a cardia pseudomass on computed tomography. J Comput Assist Tomogr 8:699–700, 1984.

69. Kaye MD, Young SW, Hayward R, et al: Gastric pseudotumor on CT scanning. AJR 135:190–193, 1980.

70. Halvorsen RA, Thompson WM: Computed tomographic staging of gastrointestinal tract malignancies. Part I. Esophagus and stomach. Invest Radiol 22:2–16, 1987.

71. Quint LE, Glazer GM, Orringer MB, et al: Esophageal carcinoma: CT findings. Radiology 155:171–175, 1985.

72. Moss AA, Schnyder P, Thoeni RF, et al: Esophageal carcinoma: pre-therapy staging by computed tomography. AJR 136:1051–1056, 1981.

73. Halvorsen RA, Magruder-Habib K, Foster WL, et al: Esophageal cancer staging by CT: long-term follow-up study. Radiology 161:147–151, 1986.

74. Becker CD, Barbier P, Porcellini B: CT evaluation of patients undergoing transhiatal esophagectomy for cancer. J Comput Assist Tomogr 10:607–611, 1986.

75. Legmann P, Marmuse JP, Rjob S, et al: Preoperative computed tomography for transhiatal esophagectomy. Invest Radiol 26:987–991, 1991.

76. vonMühling T, Kuklinski MC, Hübsch T, et al: Computed tomography of oesophageal carcinoma. Fortschr Geb Röntgenstr 143:189–193, 1985.

77. Glew D, Virjee J, Goddard P, et al: Staging of oesophageal cancer: comparison of CT with MRI. Clin MRI 1:135–137, 1992.

78. Halvorsen RA, Thompson WM: CT of esophageal neoplasms. Radiol Clin North Am 27:667–686, 1989.

79. Thompson WM: Computed tomographic staging of gastrointestinal malignancies. *In* Najarian JS, Delaney JP (eds): Progress in Gastrointestinal Malignancies. Chicago: Mosby–Year Book, 1989, pp 333–350.

80. Thompson WM, Trenkner S: Staging colon cancer and other gastrointestinal malignancies. *In* Gore RM (ed): Syllabus for Categorical Course on Gastrointestinal Radiology. Reston, VA: American College of Radiology, 1991, pp 55–64.

81. Heiken JP, Balfe DM, Roper CL: CT evaluation after esophagogastrectomy. AJR 143:555–560, 1984.

82. Takashima S, Takeuchi N, Shiozaki H, et al: Carcinoma of the esophagus: CT vs MR imaging in determining resectability. AJR 156:297–302, 1991.

83. Hans Y, McElvein RB, Aldrete JS, et al: Perforation of the esophagus: correlation of site and cause with plain film findings. AJR 145:537–540, 1985.

84. Brown BM: Case report: computed tomography of mediastinal abscess secondary to post-traumatic esophageal laceration. J Comput Assist Tomogr 8:765–767, 1984.

85. Pezzulli FA, Aronson D, Goldberg N: Computed tomography of mediastinal hematoma secondary to unusual esophageal laceration: A Boerhaave variant. J Comput Assist Tomogr 13:129–131, 1989.

86. Lee KS, Kim IY, Kim PN, et al: Dissecting intramural hematoma of the esophagus in Boerhaave syndrome: CT findings. AJR 157:197–198, 1991.

87. Herbetko J, Delany D, Ogilvie D, et al: Spontaneous intramural haematoma of the esophagus—appearance on computed tomography. Clin Radiol 44:327–328, 1991.

88. Balthazar EJ, Naidich DP, Megibow AJ, et al: CT evaluation of esophageal varices. AJR 148:131–135, 1987.

89. Ishiwaka T, Tsukune Y, Ohyama Y, et al: Venous abnormalities in portal hypertension demonstrated by CT. AJR 134:271–276, 1980.

90. Millward SF, Ramsewak W, Joseph G, et al: Pericardial varices demonstrated by computed tomography. J Comput Assist Tomogr 9:1106–1107, 1985.

91. Pearlberg JL, Sandler MA, Madrazo BL: Computer tomographic features of esophageal intramural pseudodiverticulosis. Radiology 147:189–190, 1983.

92. Williford ME, Thompson WM, Hamilton JD, et al: Esophageal tuberculosis: findings on barium swallow and computed tomography. Gastrointest Radiol 8:119–122, 1983.

93. Hori S, Tsuda K, Muryama S, et al: CT of gastric carcinoma: preliminary results with a new scanning technique. Radiographics 12:257–268, 1992.

94. Megibow AJ: Stomach. *In* Megibow AJ, Balthazar EJ (eds): Computed Tomography of the Gastrointestinal Tract. St. Louis: CV Mosby, 1986, pp 99–174.

95. Scatarige JC, Fishman EK, Jones B: CT of the stomach. *In* Fishman EK, Jones B (eds): Computed Tomography of the Gastrointestinal Tract. New York: Churchill Livingstone, 1988, pp 55–84.

96. Gossios KJ, Tsianos EV, Demou LL, et al: Use of water or air as oral contrast media for computed tomographic study of the gastric wall: comparison of the two techniques. Gastrointest Radiol 16:293–297, 1991.

97. Miyake H, Maeda H, Karauchi S, et al: Thickened gastric walls showing diffuse low attenuation on CT. J Comput Assist Tomogr 13:253–255, 1989.

98. Thompson WM, Halvorsen RA, Williford ME, et al: Computed tomography of the gastroesophageal junction. Radiographics 2:179–193, 1982.

99. Komaki S: Normal or benign gastric wall thickening demonstrated by computed tomography. J Comput Assist Tomogr 6:1103–1107, 1982.

100. Hammerman AM, Mirowitz SA, Susman N: The gastric air-fluid sign: aid in CT assessment of gastric wall thickening. Gastrointest Radiol 14:109–112, 1989.

101. Balfe DM, Koehler RE, Karstaedt N, et al: Computed tomography of gastric neoplasms. Radiology 140:431–436, 1981.
102. Moss AA, Schnyder P, Marks W, et al: Gastric adenocarcinoma: a comparison of the accuracy and economics of staging by computed tomography and surgery. Gastroenterology 80:45–50, 1991.
103. Sussman SK, Halvorsen RA, Illescas FF, et al: Gastric adenocarcinoma: CT versus surgical staging. Radiology 167:335–340, 1988.
104. Lee KR, Levine E, Moffat RE, et al: Computed tomographic staging of malignant gastric neoplasms. Radiology 133:151–155, 1979.
105. Moss AA, Schnyder P, Candardjis G, et al: Computed tomography of benign and malignant gastric abnormalities. J Clin Gastroenterol 2:401–409, 1980.
106. Balfe DM, Koehler RE, Karstaedt N, et al: Computed tomography of gastric neoplasms. Radiology 140:431–436, 1981.
107. Scatarige JC, DiSantis DJ: CT of the stomach and duodenum. Radiol Clin North Am 27:687–706, 1989.
108. Buy JN, Moss AA: Computed tomography of gastric lymphoma. AJR 138:859–865, 1982.
109. Urban BA, Fishman EK, Hruban RH: *Helicobacter pylori* gastritis mimicking gastric carcinoma at CT evaluation. Radiology 179:689–691, 1991.
110. Jacobs JM, Hill MC, Steinberg WM: Peptic ulcer disease: CT evaluation. Radiology 178:745–748, 1991.
111. Radin DR: Intramural and intraperitoneal hemorrhage due to duodenal ulcer. Radiology 157:45–46, 1991.
112. Glazer GM, Buy JN, Moss AA, et al: CT detection of duodenal perforation. AJR 137:333–336, 1981.
113. Glick SN, Levine MS, Teplick SK, et al: Splenic penetration by benign gastric ulcer: preoperative recognition with CT. Radiology 163:637–639, 1987.
114. Thoeni RF, Moss AA: The gastrointestinal tract. *In* Moss AA, Gamsu G, Genant HK (eds): Computed Tomography of the Body (2nd ed). Philadelphia: WB Saunders, 1992, pp 643–734.
115. Megibow AJ: Duodenum. *In* Megibow AJ, Balthazar EJ (eds): Computed Tomography of the Gastrointestinal Tract. St. Louis: CV Mosby, 1986, pp 175–216.
116. Scatarige J, diSantis DJ: CT of the stomach and duodenum. Radiol Clin North Am 27:687–706, 1989.
117. Baron RL: Computed tomography of the biliary tree. Radiol Clin North Am 29:1235–1250, 1991.
118. Glazer GM, Buy JN, Moss AA, et al: CT detection of duodenal perforation. AJR 137:333–336, 1981.
119. Gore RM, Ghahremani GG, Kirsch MD, et al: Diverticulitis of the duodenum: clinical and radiological manifestations of 7 cases. Am J Gastroenterol 86:981–985, 1991.
120. Karnaze GC, Sheedy PF, Stephens DH, et al: Computed tomography in duodenal rupture due to blunt abdominal trauma. J Comput Assist Tomogr 5:267–269, 1981.
121. Cwikiel W, Andrén-Sanberg A: Diagnostic difficulties with duodenal malignancies: a new strategy. Gastrointest Radiol 16:301–304, 1991.
122. Radin DR, Halls JM: Cavitating metastases of the stomach and duodenum. J Comput Assist Tomogr 11:283–287, 1987.
123. Weinreb JC: MR imaging of the abdomen: are we there yet? JMRI 1:393–397, 1991.
124. Hahn PF, Stark DD, Glastad K: Biliary system, pancreas, spleen, and alimentary tract. *In* Stark DD, Bradley WA (eds): Magnetic Resonance Imaging (2nd ed). St. Louis: CV Mosby, 1992, pp 1769–1853.
125. Werthmuller WC, Margulis AR: Magnetic resonance imaging of the alimentary tube. Invest Radiol 26:195–200, 1991.
126. Goldberg HI, Thoeni RF: MRI of the gastrointestinal tract. Radiol Clin North Am 27:805–812, 1989.
127. Winkler ML, Hricak H, Higgins CB: MR imaging of diffusely infiltrating gastric carcinoma. J Comput Assist Tomogr 11:337–339, 1987.
128. Semelka RC, Shoenut JP, Silverman R, et al: Bowel disease: prospective comparison of CT and 1.5-T pre- and postcontrast MR imaging with T1-weighted fat-suppressed and breath-hold FLASH sequences. JMRI 1:625–632, 1991.
129. Rubin DL, Muller HH, Nino-Murcia M, et al: Intraluminal contrast enhancement and MR visualization of the bowel wall: efficacy of PFOB. JMRI 1:371–380, 1991.
130. Patten RM, Moss AA, Fenton TA, et al: OMR, a positive bowel contrast agent for abdominal and pelvic imaging: safety and imaging characteristics. JMRI 2:25–34, 1992.
131. Hamed MM, Hamm B, Ibrahim ME, et al: Dynamic MR imaging of the abdomen with gadopentate dimeglumine: normal enhancement patterns of the liver, spleen, stomach and pancreas. AJR 158:303–307, 1992.

# Scintigraphic Evaluation

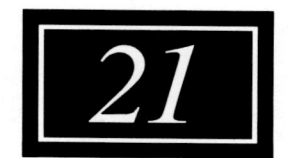

## Alan H. Maurer, M.D.

## INTRODUCTION

The advantages of radionuclide imaging for studying gastrointestinal tract function have remained the same since Griffith and colleagues first introduced the oral administration of sodium chromate to measure gastric emptying.[1] In contrast to invasive manometric methods, scintigraphy is simple to perform, does not disturb normal physiology, and permits accurate quantification of transit using physiologic markers. Compared with radiographic methods, scintigraphy results in low radiation exposure, is easily quantifiable, and uses commonly ingested liquids and solid foods rather than barium. By properly selecting radioisotopes that are specifically concentrated in certain tissues, radionuclide imaging can also be used to localize normal or abnormal tissue, such as gastric mucosa in Meckel's diverticulum or Barrett's esophagus.

Although scintigraphy has been used for studying transit and for imaging the entire gastrointestinal tract, this chapter is limited to applications involving the upper gastrointestinal tract.

## INSTRUMENTATION

Although any standard gamma camera can be used for gastrointestinal scintigraphy, a camera with a large field of view, which can image the distance from the mouth to the stomach, is preferable, especially for esophageal transit studies. For the performance of dual isotope imaging, in which solid and liquid tracers are measured simultaneously, the camera and collimators should be able to image both indium 111 ([111]In), with its higher energy (273 keV), and technetium 99m ([99m]Tc) (140 keV).

Because there is little need for high resolution or count rates, cameras that may not meet the latest standards for high-quality planar imaging or single photon emission computed tomography can be reserved for gastrointestinal scintigraphy. Thus, departments can use older cameras for gastrointestinal studies, which is particularly helpful because some studies such as gastric emptying may require use of the instrument for up to 2 hours. This broader range of suitable cameras makes functional gastrointestinal imaging widely available.

Because all gastrointestinal transit studies require quantification, the camera must be interfaced to a digital computer with region of interest analysis.

## RADIOPHARMACEUTICALS

The two most commonly used radioisotopes in upper gastrointestinal studies are [99m]Tc and [111]In. [99m]Tc is usually compounded to form the radiopharmaceutical technetium Tc 99m sulfur colloid ([99m]Tc-SC). [111]In is available as either indium In 111 oxine or indium In 111 chloride.

The ultimate form in which the radioisotope is delivered depends on the study to be performed. If [99m]Tc is given intravenously in its unbound form as pertechnetate, it is actively trapped by gastric mucosal cells. If given orally, the final radiopharmaceutical formulation (labeled compound) must be stable over a wide range of pH values and in the presence of digestive enzymes. The radiopharmaceutical must be nonabsorbable to reduce radiation exposure and to limit secretion into the gastrointestinal tract.

In the United States, the only radiopharmaceutical approved for oral administration by the Food and Drug Administration is [99m]Tc-SC. If given with liquid, it is nonabsorbable and can be used for esophageal transit and gastroesophageal reflux studies. When properly cooked with certain solid foods, [99m]Tc-SC does not dissociate from the solid. Historically, Meyer's approach to in vivo labeling of chicken liver was the first method described for radiolabeling of solid food.[2]

Such labeling is performed by injecting [99m]Tc-SC into the wing vein of a live chicken. The colloid is phagocytosed by the Kupffer cells of the liver, resulting in an intracellularly bound radiolabel. Chicken liver labeled

## TABLE 21–1. STABILITY OF RADIOLABELED SOLIDS TESTED IN VITRO

| FOOD | PERCENTAGE BOUND AFTER 3 h IN GASTRIC JUICE | PERCENTAGE BOUND AFTER 3 h IN 0.1 N HCl |
|---|---|---|
| [99m]Tc-SC egg | 81 | 97 |
| [99m]Tc aggregated albumin egg | 65 | 95 |
| [99m]Tc in vivo chicken liver | 98 | 94 |
| [99m]Tc surface-labeled chicken liver | 91 | |
| [99m]Tc Chelex resin | 98 (24 h) | |
| [131]I fiber | | 99 (48 h) |

Modified from Knight LC, Fisher RS, Malmud LS: Comparison of solid food markers in gastric emptying studies. *In* Raynaud C (ed): Nuclear Medicine and Biology. Copyright 1982, pp 2407–2410, with permission from Pergamon Press Ltd, Headington Hill Hall, Oxford OX3 0BW, UK.

in vivo has become the "gold standard" to which all other solid food labeling methods are compared.

Because of the inconvenience of maintaining and handling live chickens, numerous other radiolabeled solid meals have been proposed. Knight and associates found that of several meals tested, Meyer's in vivo chicken liver is the most stable in gastric juice.[3] Surface-labeled chicken liver, and Chelex resin also retain their radiolabels but to a lesser degree (Table 21–1).

Because of the ease of preparation and availability, most gastric emptying studies today are performed with eggs labeled with [99m]Tc-SC. Compared with in vivo labeled chicken liver, there is minimal breakdown at 2 hours (see Table 21–1).

For dual isotope, solid-liquid gastric emptying studies, the liquid phase is imaged with indium In 111 diethylenetriaminepentaacetic acid. It is readily available, is chemically inert, and is not absorbed by the gastric mucosa. Because the 243-keV photon emission of [111]In can be separated from the 140-keV photon emission of [99m]Tc, dual isotope imaging can be performed. Because oral [111]In is not approved for routine clinical use in the United States, a broad license is required for its use.

Table 21–2 summarizes typical doses and radiation exposures associated with several common gastrointestinal studies.

# RADIONUCLIDE ESOPHAGEAL TRANSIT STUDIES

The diagnostic approach to the evaluation of a patient with suspected esophageal dysmotility depends on the patient's symptoms. If dysphagia is present, a barium swallow or endoscopy is usually performed first to exclude an anatomic lesion. These studies demonstrate narrowing, obstruction, an endoluminal lesion, and extrinsic compression. Ulcerations and evidence of reflux can also be detected.

A negative result of a barium swallow or endoscopy does not exclude an esophageal cause for dysphagia. If anatomic studies are not diagnostic, manometric and motility studies are then indicated. It has been shown that as many as 50% of patients with dysphagia but with normal results of manometry and barium studies demonstrate objective evidence of esophageal dysmotility with a radiolabeled solid bolus.[4] Studies have suggested that manometry provides only an indirect measure of peristalsis, because the pressure waves recorded do not always correlate with the force applied aborally to a solid bolus at a given level of the esophagus.[5]

In 1972, Kazem first described the use of radionuclide esophageal transit (RET) scintigraphy and summarized the problems associated with cineradiography, endoscopy, and manometry: "none is a true physiologic test. Either investigation is performed under an unnatural condition of instrumentation, or a foreign material like barium is used as a test medium."[6]

In spite of its limitations, manometry has remained the gold standard for the diagnosis of esophageal motility disorders. Manometry does provide accurate definition of esophageal peristalsis, contraction amplitude, and pressures of the upper esophageal sphincter and of the lower esophageal sphincter (LES). Manometric studies are inconvenient, however, particularly when repetition of studies is desired to assess the response to a therapeutic intervention. It can be argued that the presence of the manometric tube itself can affect normal physiology and that the recordings reflect pressure changes and not the actual bulk transit of a solid or

## TABLE 21–2. RADIATION EXPOSURES FOR GASTROINTESTINAL SCINTIGRAPHY*

| TYPE OF STUDY | ORGAN DOSE (mrad) | | | | | | |
|---|---|---|---|---|---|---|---|
| | Stomach | Small Intestine | Upper Large Intestine | Lower Large Intestine | Ovaries | Testes | Total Body |
| Esophageal motility and GER with 300 µCi [99m]Tc-SC | 28 | 83 | 160 | 97 | 29 | 2 | 5 |
| Gastric emptying with | | | | | | | |
| 250 µCi [111]In-DTPA | 110 | 490 | 1100 | 2000 | 420 | 27 | 60 |
| 500 µCi [99m]Tc-SC or chicken liver | 120 | 120 | 230 | 230 | 42 | 2 | 9 |
| Imaging gastric mucosa with 10 mCi technetium Tc 99m pertechnetate (adult estimates) | 510 | | 1200 | 1100 | 300 | 90 | 110 |

*GER = gastroesophageal reflux; [111]In-DTPA = indium In-111 diethylenetriaminepentaacetic acid.
Modified from Siegel JA, Wu RK, Knight LC, et al: Radiation dose estimates for oral agents used in upper gastrointestinal disease. J Nucl Med 24:835–837, 1983.

liquid in the esophagus. Quantification of the volume of retained solids or liquids is difficult with either barium studies or manometry.

For many of the foregoing reasons, RET scintigraphy was developed as a simple, noninvasive, and quantitative method of assessing esophageal motility. Early studies reported a high sensitivity for detecting motility disorders. Later studies have indicated lower sensitivity, especially for detecting those disorders with intact peristalsis but high-amplitude contractions or with isolated elevation of LES pressures.[7, 8]

The simplest measure of esophageal transit is the mean transit time required for a liquid bolus to traverse the entire esophagus. This time has been determined with good reproducibility. Kazem first reported a normal total esophageal transit time of a single swallow of 10 to 20 mL of water as up to 8 seconds, with an observed delay in the distal esophagus of up to 5 seconds because of relaxation of the LES.[6] Russell and associates[9] and Blackwell and associates[10] reported similar values of 7.2 ± 1.7 and 7.3 ± 2.3 (SD) seconds, respectively. Holloway and co-workers reported a slightly longer normal mean transit time of 9.6 seconds (with a range of 6 to 15 seconds).[8]

Since Kazem's initial description, numerous methods for performing and analyzing results of RET scintigraphy have been proposed, using both solid and liquid boluses. Tolin and colleagues proposed recording total counts remaining in the esophagus after multiple swallows.[11] Russell and associates demonstrated that regional esophageal transit could be analyzed by a process similar to manometry, by dividing the esophagus into upper, middle, and distal thirds.[9]

With the method by Tolin and colleagues, the patient performs an initial single swallow of 15 mL of water containing 150 μCi of [99m]Tc-SC.[11] The patient is placed in a supine position to avoid the effects of gravity. A large-field-of-view gamma camera is used to image the distance from the mouth to the proximal stomach. After the initial swallow, the subject performs serial dry swallows at 15-second intervals for 10 minutes. An esophageal region of interest comprising the entire length of the esophagus is defined for computer analysis, and the total number of counts within the esophagus, $E_t$, is plotted as a percentage of the maximal number of counts, $E_{max}$, which is recorded during the initial swallow. The percentage of esophageal emptying at time t is given by the following equation:

$$\% \text{ esophageal emptying} = \frac{E_{max} - E_t}{E_{max}} \times 100\%$$

In normal individuals, total esophageal activity decreases rapidly. Within 5 to 10 seconds of the first swallow, no significant esophageal activity is visible. Quantitatively, up to 10% of peak activity may occur up to the time of the eighth swallow. By the 40th swallow (10 minutes), less than 5% of peak activity remains in the esophagus. With this method of analysis, Tolin and colleagues reported 100% sensitivity for detecting primary motor disorders, and there was good separation of patients based on the severity of impaired

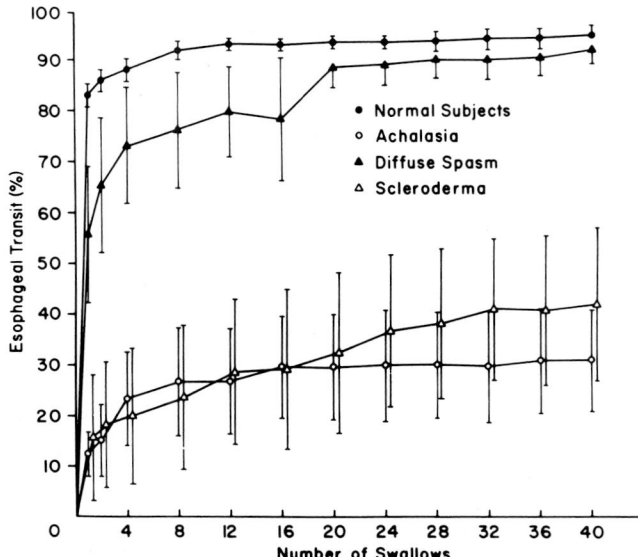

**Figure 21–1. Global esophageal transit curves after multiple swallows.** Each point represents the mean ± SEM for the percentage of esophageal clearance. (From Tolin RD, Malmud LS, Reillely J, et al: Esophageal scintigraphy to quantitate esophageal transit [quantitation of esophageal transit]. Gastroenterology 76:1402–1408, 1979.)

transit: achalasia involved greater impairment than scleroderma, which involved greater impairment than diffuse esophageal spasm (DES) (Fig. 21–1).

The method proposed by Russell and associates uses multiple esophageal regions of interest to characterize the progression of a liquid bolus after a single swallow of 250 μCi of [99m]Tc-SC in 10 mL of water, which the patient performs in the supine position.[9] Computer images are recorded at 0.25 to 0.40 second per frame for 60 seconds. Time-activity curves are generated for the upper, middle, and lower thirds of the esophagus. Activity in the mouth, pharynx, and stomach can also be monitored to help identify artifacts from delayed or multiple swallows and gastroesophageal reflux (GER).

The regional transit curves of Russell and associates appear similar to manometric tracings (Fig. 21–2), and the good correlation between the two methods localizes abnormal transit to the distal third of the esophagus in scleroderma and reflux esophagitis. Incoordinate peristalsis throughout the esophagus is seen in DES. Achalasia characteristically shows an adynamic esophagus with little activity seen to enter the stomach because of the hypertensive LES (Fig. 21–3).

Russell and colleagues found prolonged radionuclide transit times in 15 (100%) of 15 patients with dysphagia and abnormal manometric findings.[9] Of greater interest was the fact that 9 (64%) of 14 patients with dysphagia and normal manometric findings had abnormal esophageal transit detected with RET scintigraphy.

Because recording of the dynamics of a single swallow (the method of Russell and colleagues[9]) does not preclude analysis of global esophageal transit (the method of Tolin and colleagues[11]), both can easily be performed using an initial single swallow followed by multiple dry swallows. With this approach, Blackwell and associates

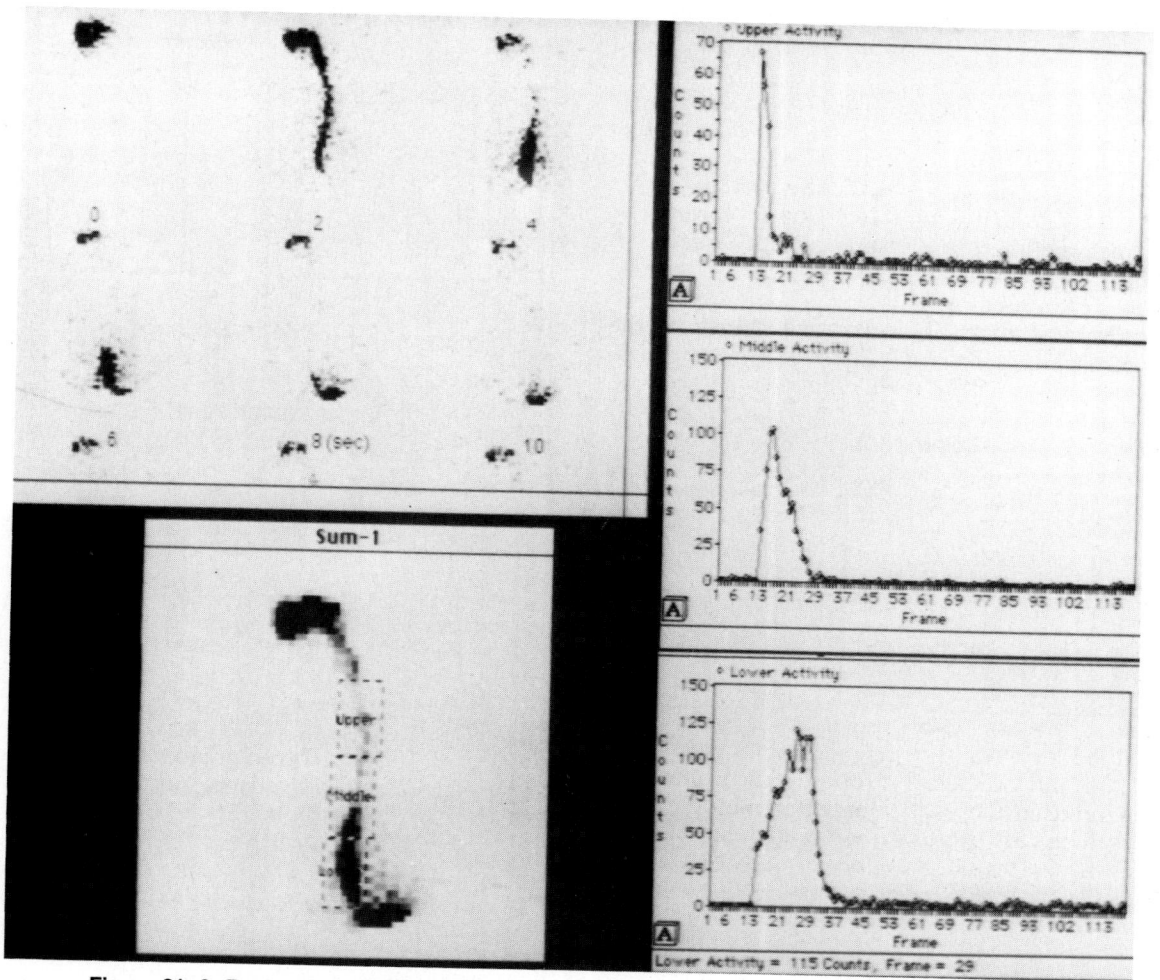

**Figure 21–2. Regional esophageal transit after a single swallow.** The time-activity curves *(right half)* for the upper, middle, and lower esophagus of a normal subject show smooth aboral progression of the bolus through the esophagus. Each frame lasts 0.25 second. The increased width of the distal esophageal curve *(lower right)* is due to the time required for relaxation of the LES. Serial images *(upper left)* are reformatted at 2 seconds each to demonstrate the appearance of the single swallow. A composite image *(lower left)* is formed by addition of all the images. The esophageal regions of interest are shown.

found agreement between scintigraphy and manometry in 42 (84%) of 50 patients.[10]

Based on these results, several authors proposed that RET scintigraphy could be used as a simple, sensitive screening test for esophageal dysmotility. Questions have been raised on the sensitivity of the test, particularly in patients with disorders characterized by high-amplitude contractions but normal peristalsis. Styles and co-workers reported good correlation between RET scintigraphy and manometry in only 22 (52%) of 42 patients with dysphagia and high-amplitude contractions. There was disagreement in 6 (14%) patients, and equivocal studies in 14 (33%) patients, from a total of 42 patients.[7] Only a measure of transit time was used in this study, however. Drane and colleagues evaluated esophageal transit time as well as the percentage of retained esophageal activity and found that the results of scintigraphy agreed with those of manometry in 13 (81%) of 16 patients with mean distal esophageal con-

tractile pressure amplitudes greater than 120 mm Hg, but in only 3 (20%) of 15 patients with pressures less than 120 mm Hg.[12]

The sensitivity of RET studies for the diagnosis of esophageal motility disorders therefore appears to depend on the disorder being evaluated. Sensitivity is highest for primary motor disorders with abnormal peristalsis, such as achalasia, DES, and scleroderma. Sensitivity is low in nutcracker esophagus or in those disorders in which peristalsis is preserved but manometry shows high-amplitude contractions.

Nonspecific esophageal motility disorders are characterized by one or more minor manometric abnormalities. Mughal and co-workers concluded that RET studies are not useful as a screening test for esophageal dysmotility because of the high prevalence of nonspecific esophageal motility disorders and low sensitivity (42%) for detecting this common disorder.[13]

Sensitivity for detecting abnormal esophageal motility

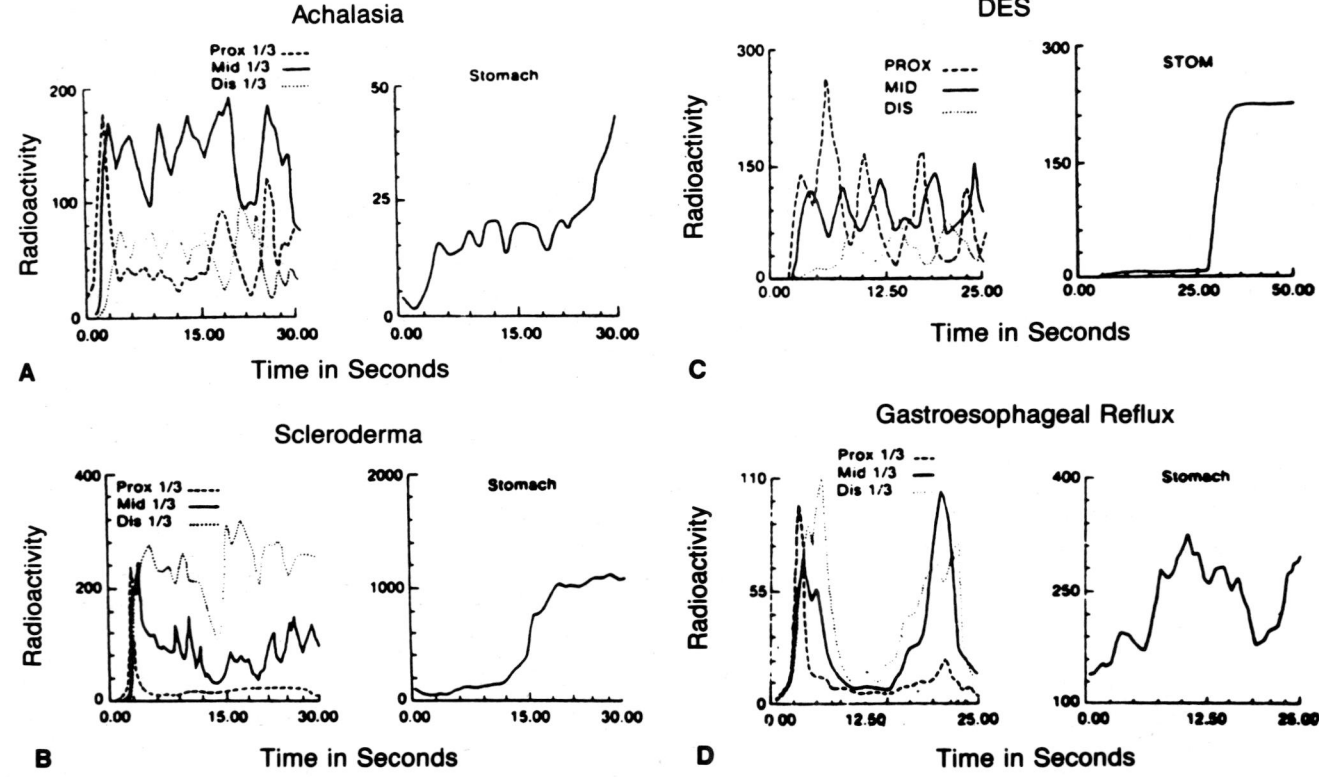

**Figure 21–3. Abnormal esophageal transit curves (single swallow). A.** Achalasia. **B.** Scleroderma. **C.** DES. **D.** GER. In achalasia, the upper esophagus empties, but there is aperistalsis of the middle and distal thirds of the esophagus. In DES, uncoordinated contractions occur throughout the entire esophagus. In scleroderma, abnormal motility is seen primarily in the distal third of the esophagus. With reflux, counts decrease in the stomach and reflux back into the middle and distal thirds of the esophagus. (**A** to **D** from Russell COH, Hill LD, Holmes ER 3rd, et al: Radionuclide transit: a sensitive screening test for esophageal dysfunction. Gastroenterology 80:887–892, 1981.)

can be improved if multiple criteria, including quantification of transit times, regional transit curves, and esophageal retention, are used. It is also important to play back and visually review as a cine loop the dynamic display of the swallow. Furthermore, most studies have relied on analysis of a single swallow. Experience with radiographic studies have shown that up to five swallows may be needed to achieve good correlation with the results of manometry.[14]

Although the exact role of RET scintigraphy in the diagnosis of esophageal dysmotility remains controversial, its unique ability to quantitate esophageal emptying has been shown to be valuable in assessing the response to therapeutic interventions, particularly in achalasia. Treatment of achalasia is usually directed at lowering pressures of the LES by mechanical dilatation or surgery. It has been shown that measurement of LES pressures is not sufficient to determine the response to treatment, because patients may report subjective improvement while their emptying abnormalities persist.[15, 16]

The effect of drugs such as nifedipine and isosorbide dinitrate has also been studied in achalasia and DES.[17, 18] This ability to assess the response to therapy quantitatively remains one of the most useful applications of RET scintigraphy.

## GASTROESOPHAGEAL REFLUX SCINTIGRAPHY

Symptoms of GER are common. An initial diagnosis of GER is usually based on clinical symptoms. A history of heartburn or retrosternal burning that is exacerbated by eating, bending, or lying down and is relieved by antacids is usually sufficient to make the diagnosis. Atypical chest pain, however, may be difficult to differentiate from cardiac chest pain and often leads to further diagnostic testing.

LES pressure was previously considered to be the most crucial factor controlling GER. Many factors, including diet, medications, and hormones, have been shown to affect this disorder.[19]

Numerous methods have been proposed for diagnosing GER. Indirect studies include examination of the distal esophagus with barium, endoscopic or histologic studies; evaluation of esophageal motility; or symptomatic evaluation of the response to intraesophageal acid (the Bernstein test).

Other studies are designed to document the presence of acid in the distal esophagus directly. Use of a pH probe in the distal esophagus was first proposed by Tuttle and Grossman in 1958.[20] They showed that symptoms of heartburn were correlated with a pH of less than 4 and that symptoms abated when the pH was greater than 4. A standardized acid reflux test was developed in which a pH probe was used to measure pH under basal conditions and after maneuvers to produce GER. Although this test has good sensitivity and specificity, it is invasive, is time-consuming, and is performed only over short periods.

The use of 24-hour pH probe monitoring was proposed to overcome some of these shortcomings. Early 24-hour studies demonstrated the importance of prolonged monitoring. They showed that factors such as bending, lifting, smoking, and diet contribute to the occurrence of reflux. Brief periods of postprandial reflux occur commonly in asymptomatic individuals, whereas patients with symptoms of reflux usually demonstrate the reflux at night and for longer periods. These results all emphasized the need for prolonged monitoring under the varying conditions of day-to-day activity.

GER scintigraphy was initially developed for use in adults to document and quantitate the presence of reflux. A method for performing GER scintigraphy was proposed by Fisher and colleagues in 1976.[21] The patient drinks 300 μCi of [99m]Tc-SC suspended in 150 mL of orange juice that has been mixed with an equal volume of 0.1 N HCl. The weak acidification decreases the LES pressure and delays gastric emptying, both of which actions increase the likelihood of detecting reflux. The patient is imaged in a supine position under a gamma camera, and an abdominal binder is used to increase abdominal pressures in 20-mm increments up to 100 mm Hg. At each level of binder pressure, computer images are recorded for 30 seconds.

In normal individuals, no reflux of gastric contents is seen (Fig. 21–4A). In studies of patients with GER, reflux can be seen in the distal esophagus (Fig. 21–4B). Esophageal activity present in the first image may be due to either reflux or abnormal esophageal transit. When such activity is present, the esophagus can be cleared by having the patient drink water. Before a GER study, it is helpful to perform an RET study to exclude abnormal transit. If activity is due to abnormal esophageal transit, the GER study can be repeated with direct placement of the labeled colloid into the stomach through a gastric tube.

Fisher and colleagues proposed quantification of GER for each level of pressure, using the following formula:

$$R = \frac{E_p - E_b}{G_o} \times 100\%$$

where R represents the GER index expressed as a percentage, $E_p$ represents the esophageal counts at abdominal pressure p, $E_b$ represents the background counts, and $G_o$ represents the gastric counts at the beginning of the study.[21]

In Fisher's initial study, the mean reflux index for patients with symptomatic GER was 11.7 ± 1.8% compared with 2.7 ± 0.3% for normal control subjects.[21] With an upper limit for reflux in the control subjects of 4%, reflux was detected in 90% of patients with confirmed reflux and in only 10% of control subjects, and then, only at the highest pressures.

Later studies have not confirmed the high sensitivity reported by Fisher and colleagues. Hoffman and Vansant reported a sensitivity of only 14% (4 of 29 reflux patients had positive test results). They also, however, reported the same sensitivity for the acid reflux test.[22]

Fung and associates reported a low sensitivity for GER scintigraphy with mean GER indices of 1.6 and 3.2% in symptomatic patients who had endoscopic evidence of severe and moderate esophagitis, respectively.[23] Similarly, Jenkins and associates reported only a 30% sensitivity for detecting reflux, designating a reflux index of greater than 4% as abnormal.[24] The authors of these later studies all concluded that an upper limit of normal for the GER index of 4% was of little value in the diagnosis of GER because almost all patients with documented esophagitis would have been within the normal range.

Many patients have visually obvious reflux, but they demonstrate reflux indices of less than 4% when calculated by the method of Fisher and colleagues. This discrepancy is due to failure to correct for attenuation of counts in the distal esophagus. Direct measurement of attenuation that is due to overlying tissues (the chest wall, the heart, and the cardiac blood pool) has shown that quantification of GER should employ correction for individual differences in soft tissue attenuation. When a point source is used in the esophagus to measure counts directly, errors of 10 to 35% have been shown to occur if no correction is made for attenuation.[25] Despite reports demonstrating the need for attenuation correction, no studies addressing GER scintigraphy with attenuation correction have been reported.

Experience with 24-hour pH probe monitoring has shown that patients should be studied under various conditions that may exacerbate reflux. If the result of GER scintigraphy is initially negative, and the clinical suspicion for GER is high, the study can be repeated under different dietary conditions or at different times of day. The study can easily be modified and performed under those clinical conditions that are likely to precipitate the patient's symptoms.

As with RET studies, GER scintigraphy is particularly useful for monitoring and quantifying changes in reflux that occur in response to medical or surgical treatment.[26, 27]

## GASTROESOPHAGEAL REFLUX AND PULMONARY ASPIRATION

Attempts have been made to image pulmonary aspiration to determine whether aspiration of gastric contents contributes to pulmonary symptoms in adults.[28] There are insufficient data reported, however, to evaluate the role of scintigraphy in detecting pulmonary aspiration in adults.

In children, GER has been implicated as a contributing factor to esophageal strictures, esophagitis, apnea, respiratory disease, and failure to thrive.[29] GER scintigraphy (the "milk scan") has been used to evaluate esophageal transit, GER, gastric emptying, and pulmo-

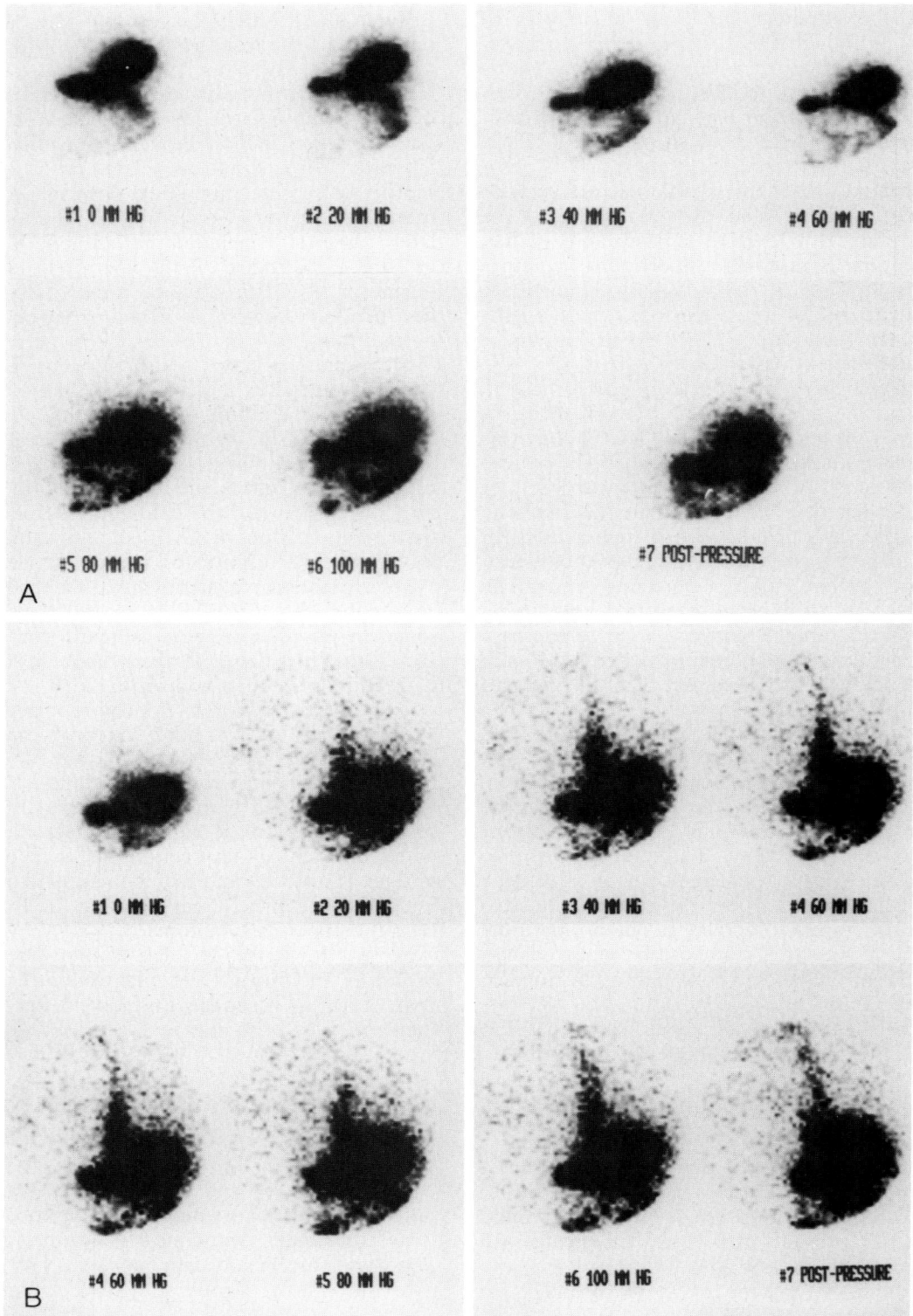

**Figure 21–4. GER study. A.** Negative findings. No reflux is visualized. **B.** Positive findings. The initial image before inflation of the abdominal binder (0 mm Hg) shows no activity in the distal esophagus. With increasing abdominal pressure, there is reflux into the distal esophagus.

nary aspiration.[30–32] As with adults, 24-hour pH probe monitoring is usually used to confirm the diagnosis of GER. Seibert and co-workers compared scintigraphy with simultaneous pH probe monitoring in children and reported a sensitivity and specificity of 79 and 93%, respectively.[33]

To perform GER scintigraphy in infants, 200 to 1000 μCi of $^{99m}$Tc-SC is mixed with the child's usual volume of milk, formula, apple juice, or glucose water and is given at the time of routine feeding. If a minimal dose of 200 μCi is given, 25 to 35 mrad is delivered to the whole body and 100 mrad is delivered to the bowel. The labeled colloid is mixed in about three quarters of the usual feeding volume, and the initial swallows are recorded from a posterior projection at 0.5 second per frame for 150 seconds with computer acquisition. Use of a high-sensitivity collimator increases counting efficiency. Swallowing curves can be generated to evaluate esophageal transit. After the labeled feeding is completed, the child is permitted to complete the unlabeled remainder of the meal to clear residual activity from the mouth and esophagus.

With the patient then lying supine on the camera, anterior or posterior images are obtained for at least 60 minutes at a framing rate of 3 seconds per frame. GER may be evident on analog film images, but computer-enhanced images are more sensitive and should always be obtained to demonstrate small reflux volumes. Time-activity curves are used to document the frequency of reflux and delayed esophageal clearance. Frequent imaging is important because transient reflux into the esophagus can be rapidly dissipated and missed. Delayed static images at 1, 2, and even 24 hours can be acquired to detect any pulmonary aspiration. Pulmonary aspiration is detected with this method in 35 to 55% of children with severe pulmonary disease.[33]

## GASTRIC EMPTYING

### Background

Symptoms of gastric stasis include nausea, vomiting, abdominal fullness or distention, early satiety, and weight loss. Functional studies of gastric emptying are indicated when an anatomic cause (ulcer, tumor, or foreign body) has been excluded by either endoscopy or barium examination. The introduction of drugs such as metoclopramide, domperidone, and cisapride, which can alleviate symptoms, increases the clinical importance of measuring gastric emptying to document gastroparesis and response to treatment.[34, 35]

Nonradionuclide methods have been used to quantitate gastric emptying. A simple method of quantifying emptying of liquids or a semisolid meal consists of gastric and gastroduodenal intubation and aspiration with a nonabsorbable marker. After the marker is added to the liquid or semisolid meal of known volume, the gastric contents are aspirated at different times. The amount remaining in the stomach can be calculated by sampling the volume and concentration of the marker in each aspirate. These studies require intubation, which itself may affect gastric function, and are limited to the use of liquid or semisolid meals. Radiologic measurements with barium are nonphysiologic, result in high radiation exposure, and are not amenable to accurate quantification.

All scintigraphic methods discussed so far have been compared with other invasive or physiologic studies, but as stated earlier, the use of a radiolabeled meal to measure gastric emptying has become the gold standard with which all other methods must be compared. Once the solid or liquid phase of a meal is radiolabeled and appropriate corrections are made for attenuation, the counts measured are directly proportional to the volume of solid or liquid remaining. These counts are easily monitored and quantified for all phases of gastric emptying.

## Physiology of Gastric Emptying

An understanding of the methods used to acquire and analyze data regarding gastric emptying requires knowledge of the physiology of this complex process. Cannon first observed that the fundus and antrum have separate roles in emptying liquids and solids.[36] He proposed that the fundus acts as a reservoir that undergoes receptive relaxation to receive food from the esophagus.[37] Normally, solid foods are temporarily stored in the fundus until slow sustained contractions transfer the solids to the antrum. This early segregation of solids in the fundus is apparent in the initial images of a radionuclide gastric emptying study (Fig. 21–5). Commonly, a persistent transverse band separating the fundus and antrum is observed (Fig. 21–6A), and it is believed to play a role in the regulation of emptying of solids.[38]

As solids move from the posteriorly located fundus to the more anteriorly located antrum, there is an apparent increase in measured counts, because the solids are moving closer to a camera positioned in front of the patient (Fig. 21–6B). This increasing count rate is due to the changing depth of the solids from the camera. A method of attenuation correction must therefore be applied to the analysis of data regarding gastric emptying of solids.

After the solids are in the antrum, peristaltic contractions work by a process called trituration, in which the solids are mixed with gastric digestive juices and are ground into particles of 1 to 2 mm, so that they are able to pass through the pylorus.[39, 40] The time required to complete trituration so that solid particles can then empty from the stomach is commonly referred to as the *lag phase.*

The contractile activity of the antrum is controlled by a pacemaker located high on the greater curvature, at the boundary between the fundus and the antrum. Normally, antral contractions occur at a rate of three per minute.[41]

The final rate of gastric emptying must be compatible with pancreatic digestion and intestinal absorption, which are determined by the composition of the meal.

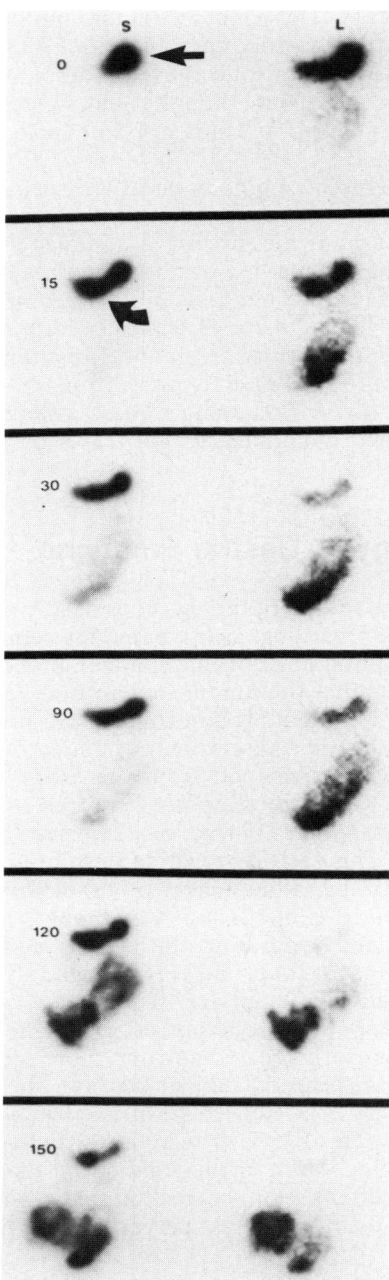

**Figure 21–5. Normal dual isotope solid (S) and liquid (L) gastric emptying study.** Anterior views only are shown to demonstrate the early uniform distribution of liquids throughout the stomach, with rapid emptying into the proximal duodenum (t = 0 minutes). This is in contrast to the initial localization of solids in the fundus *(straight arrow)*. With time, the solids redistribute distally into the antrum *(curved arrow)* and then begin to empty into the small bowel at 30 minutes.

Experimental studies in humans and animals have demonstrated that small intestinal receptors for acid, glucose, lipids, amino acids, and osmolality feed back to control the rate of gastric emptying.[42] Any test meal for measuring gastric emptying must then be standardized for volume, density, caloric content, and nutrients (amounts of protein, fat, and carbohydrate).

At present, no single standardized meal is universally used. Normal values for a variety of meals, including meats, porridge, pancakes, eggs, and chemical resins, have been reported (Table 21–3). For any test meal, the stability of the radiolabel to the solid phase must be established to ensure that the radioisotope does not dissociate in gastric juice.

In addition to establishing normal values for a given test meal, studies have shown that normal values depend on sex[43] and on the time of day the test is performed.[44]

Many early investigations emphasized the need for dual isotope studies of gastric emptying for both the solid and liquid phases. Emptying of liquids is controlled by a sustained pressure gradient generated by the fundus. Liquids require no trituration, are normally distributed throughout the stomach immediately after ingestion, and are rapidly emptied (see Fig. 21–5).

Studies have shown that the rate of liquid emptying from the stomach can be measured with less attenuation correction than the rate of solids emptying from the stomach[45, 46] (Fig. 21–7). Although some authors have attributed this difference to the higher energy of the $^{111}$In label (243 keV) used for liquids compared with that of the $^{99m}$Tc label (140 keV) used for solids, it is likely that the uniform distribution of liquids throughout the stomach results in a smaller percentage of changing counts from the posteriorly located fundus.

Liquids empty from the stomach monoexponentially (see Fig. 21–7), and in contrast to solids, they can be adequately described by a simple half-time ($T_{1/2}$) value, or the time to 50% emptying of initial gastric contents.[47] Technically, liquid studies are much simpler to acquire and analyze, because there is no need to perform radiolabeling of a solid meal or to make complicated attenuation corrections. These studies are of little clinical value, however, because liquid emptying does not become abnormal until gastroparesis is far advanced.[48]

Solid phase studies always reveal abnormal gastric emptying at an earlier stage than liquid phase studies. Occasionally, a liquid phase study is useful without a solid phase study in a patient unable to tolerate a solid meal because of severe nausea and vomiting. In these cases, if liquid emptying is abnormal, severe gastroparesis must be present.

The first step in performing a radionuclide gastric emptying study is preparation of the test meal. Although Meyer's in vivo labeling of chicken liver has become the gold standard, eggs labeled with $^{99m}$Tc-SC have become widely accepted because of their ease of preparation. A standardized meal in common use consists of two large scrambled eggs served between two pieces of white toasted bread and consumed with 300 mL of water. This meal has 270 calories, with 23% protein, 40% fat, and 37% carbohydrate. The eggs are labeled with 500 μCi of $^{99m}$Tc-SC. If a liquid study is also desired, 125 μCi of indium In 111 diethylenetriaminepentaacetic acid is added to the water. The patient is requested to consume the meal within 10 minutes.

Immediately after eating the meal, the patient is imaged either standing or in a supine position. The earliest studies of gastric emptying were often recorded from the front with the patient supine. The effect of

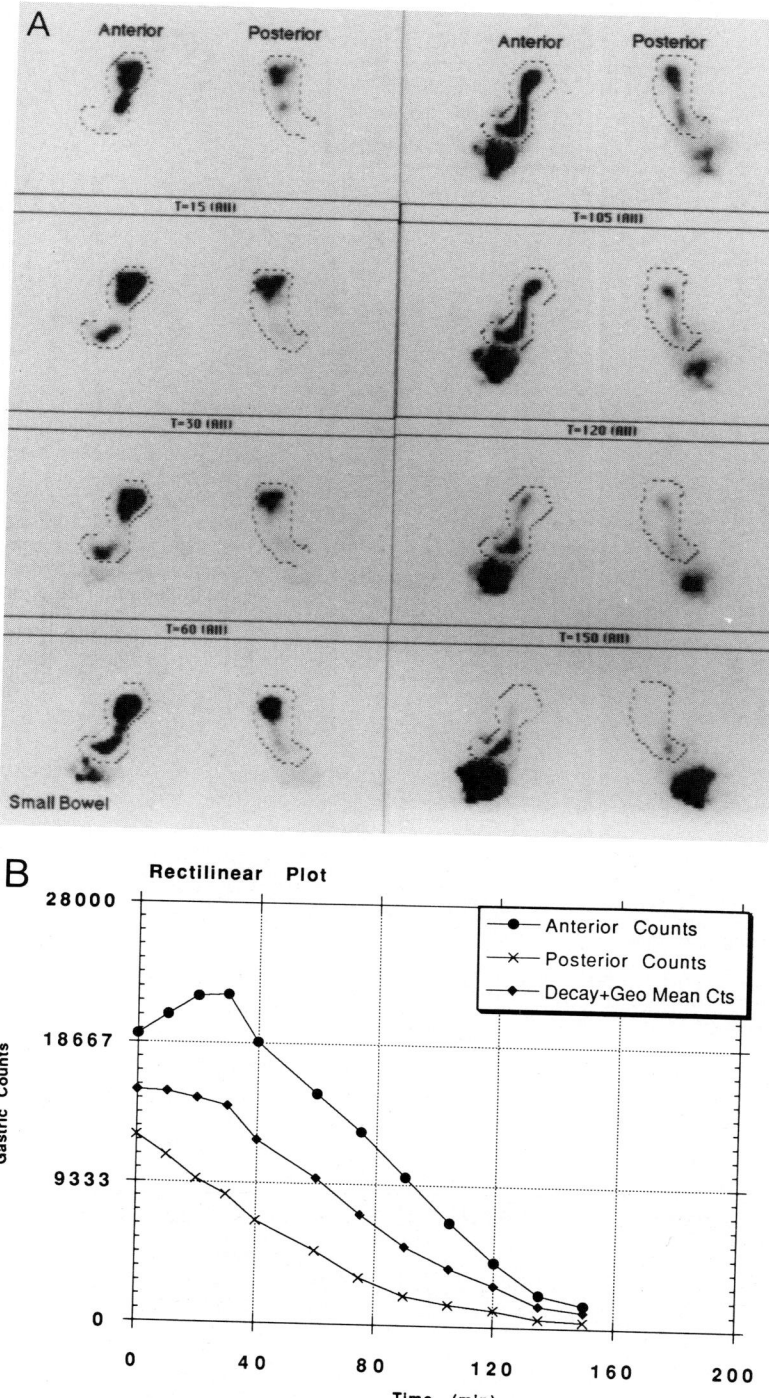

**Figure 21–6. Processing of solid phase gastric emptying studies. A.** Normal anterior and posterior images with gastric regions of interest are shown. In the early images, solids are preferentially stored in the fundus. By 15 to 30 minutes after ingestion, the solids begin to move into the distal stomach. At 30 to 60 minutes, solids can be seen in the small bowel. A transverse band of no activity separates the antrum and the fundus. **B.** Anterior, posterior, and decay-corrected geometric mean counts are plotted by using rectilinear coordinates. The increasing anterior gastric counts are shown as well as the posterior and geometric mean corrections.

*Illustration continued on following page*

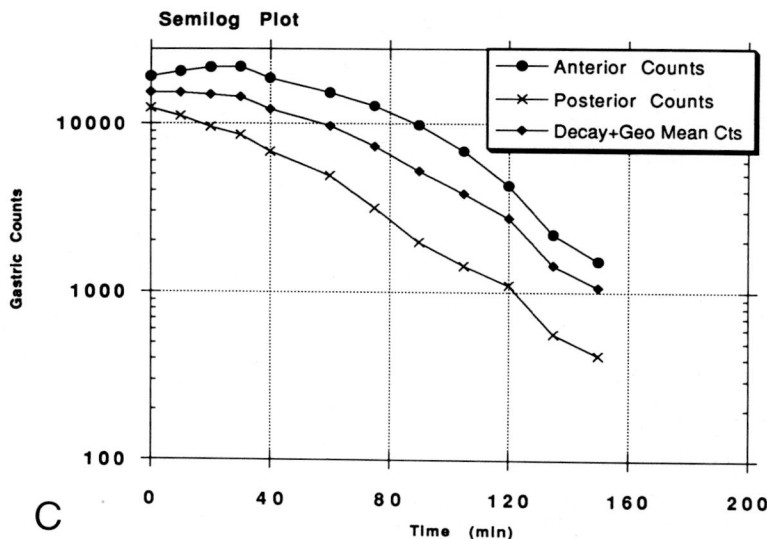

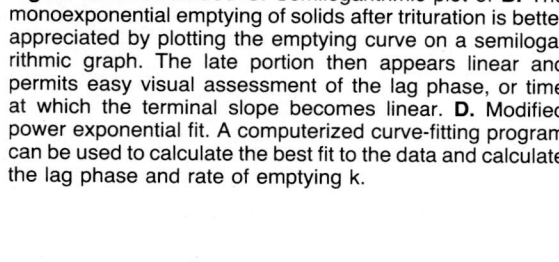

C

**Figure 21–6** *Continued* **C.** Semilogarithmic plot of **B.** The monoexponential emptying of solids after trituration is better appreciated by plotting the emptying curve on a semilogarithmic graph. The late portion then appears linear and permits easy visual assessment of the lag phase, or time at which the terminal slope becomes linear. **D.** Modified power exponential fit. A computerized curve-fitting program can be used to calculate the best fit to the data and calculate the lag phase and rate of emptying k.

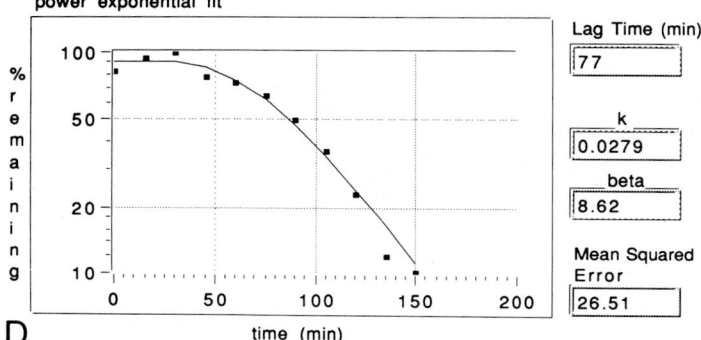

D

## TABLE 21–3. NORMAL GASTRIC EMPTYING HALF-TIME VALUES FOR VARIOUS MEALS*

| SOLID | LIQUID | $T_{1/2}$ SOLID (min) (±1 SEM) | $T_{1/2}$ LIQUID (min) (±1 SEM) | REFERENCE |
|---|---|---|---|---|
| Oatmeal and Chelex resin (15 g) | Milk (100 mL) | 44 ± 7.4 | | 83 |
| Chicken liver | Variable | | | |
|    300 g | | 77 ± 5 | | 53 |
|    900 g | | 146 ± 26 | | |
|    1692 g | | 277 ± 44 | | |
| Chicken liver with ground beef (100 g) | Water (150 mL) | 70 ± 7 | 15 ± 2 | 45 |
| | 25% dextrose (150 mL) | 105 ± 13 | 46 ± 7 | |
| Scrambled egg sandwich (142 g) | Water (300 mL) | 78 ± 11 | 28 ± 5 | 64 |

*$T_{1/2}$ = half-time.

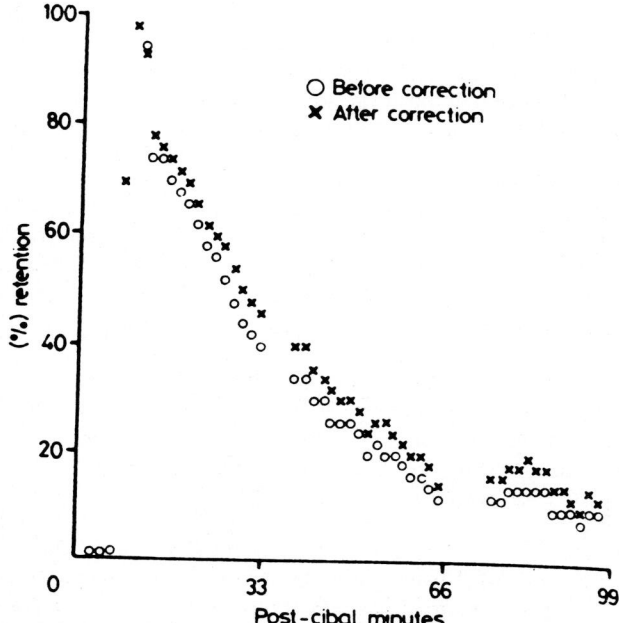

Figure 21–7. **Normal liquid gastric emptying curves with and without attenuation correction.** The shape of the emptying curve for liquids is monoexponential and is not significantly changed when depth correction is applied. (From Collins PJ, Horowitz M, Cook DJ, et al: Gastric emptying in normal subjects—a reproducible technique using a single scintillation camera and computer system. Gut 24:1117–1125, 1983.)

body posture on measurement of gastric emptying has been studied, and the results indicate that supine positioning can significantly slow gastric emptying of solids (20% emptying at 1 hour in a supine position versus 50% in an upright position).[49] Normal values must be established both for the meal and for the method used for image acquisition and processing.

Attenuation correction is needed for accurate measurement of the lag phase for solids.[50] Correction using a geometric mean—(anterior counts × posterior counts)$^{1/2}$—is most commonly used. Studies have shown that this correction results in only a 3 to 4% variation in counts for the depths typically encountered with gastric emptying studies.[51] Anterior and posterior 60-second images are acquired every 10 to 20 minutes for up to 2 hours. This imaging is easily accomplished with the patient standing, first facing the camera and then turning and placing his or her back against the camera. Because the process of gastric emptying of solids takes place slowly, no significant information is lost by acquiring images 60 seconds apart.[52, 53]

Computer regions of interest corresponding to the stomach are defined to obtain the gastric counts (see Fig. 21–6A). Because of the 6-hour half-life for the decay of $^{99m}$Tc, the counts must also be corrected for physical decay. After attenuation and decay correction, the percentage of activity remaining in the stomach is normalized to 100% for maximal gastric counts and then plotted for all times. Plotting the data on a semilogarithmic graph better demonstrates the linear nature of the late slope of the line (Fig. 21–6B and C). Programs available on small personal computer systems can be

used to perform curve fitting and automated analysis of the data[50] (Fig. 21–6D).

The major disadvantage associated with the use of geometric mean correction is the need to acquire and process two views. Other methods for performing attenuation correction have been proposed. These include use of a lateral view, a peak/scatter ratio, and a left anterior oblique image.[51, 54, 55]

The simplest approach to interpreting gastric emptying data has been to report the $T_{1/2}$ or to use a percentage of emptying measured at some fixed time after ingestion of the meal.[53, 56–58] Although these approaches have become common in clinical practice, they do not fully characterize the biphasic nature of gastric emptying.

There has been controversy over whether an initial lag phase for emptying of solid foods occurs. Moore and co-workers argued that the lag phase was an artifact created by failure to correct for attenuation.[46] Numerous studies, however, have confirmed the occurrence of a lag phase followed by emptying, during which the stomach expels solids at a characteristic rate.[39, 45, 51, 59–62]

To characterize all phases of gastric emptying completely, it is best to fit the data to a mathematic function such as the power exponential function, which was first proposed by Elashoff and associates.[63] A modified power exponential function was later introduced by Siegel and associates and has been used successfully to characterize lag phase differences that are due to food particle size and to the physical characteristics of different solids.[62, 64]

The modified power exponential function is given by the following equation:

$$y(t) = 1 - [1 - \exp(-kt)]^\beta$$

where y(t) is the percentage of gastric activity remaining at time t; k is the slope of the exponential fit to the terminal portion of the gastric emptying curve expressed in min$^{-1}$; and β is the extrapolated y intercept of a linear fit to the terminal portion of the emptying curve. In this equation, the lag phase is given by ln β/k. The lag phase corresponds to the inflection point of the gastric emptying curve where the second derivative of the function equals zero and to the time of peak activity in the distal stomach[62] (Fig. 21–8).

Use of the modified power exponential function for analyzing gastric emptying provides further insight into the function of both the proximal and the distal stomach. Physically, the lag phase corresponds to maximal filling of the distal stomach. It includes the time for redistribution of solids from the fundus to the antrum and for trituration. The end of the lag phase corresponds to the time taken for trituration to be completed so that the small suspended solids begin to empty at a uniform rate, k.

Normal values for the two-egg meal described earlier are as follows (mean ± 1 SD):[64]

$$k = 0.0142 \pm 0.0034 \text{ min}^{-1}$$
$$\text{lag phase (ln } \beta/k) = 31 \pm 7.5 \text{ min}$$
$$T_{1/2} = 77.6 \pm 11.2 \text{ min}$$

Definition of the lag phase remains controversial. Some authors have chosen to define the lag phase visually as "the part of the solid-emptying curve prior

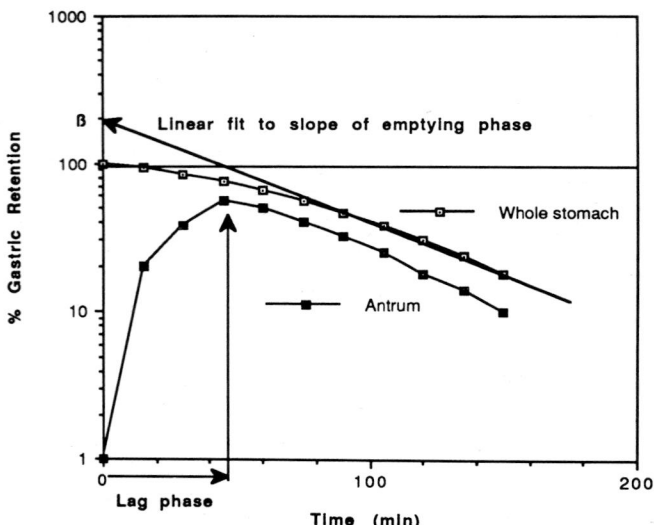

**Figure 21–8. Lag phase and antral emptying.** The physical significance of the lag phase as defined by the modified power exponential is best illustrated by separately plotting the antral and the whole stomach emptying curves. The lag phase corresponds to the peak in antral counts, which occurs just before the onset of emptying of solids from the antrum. (Modified from Urbain JL, Siegel JA, Charkes ND, et al: The two-component stomach: effects of meal particle size on fundal and antral emptying. Eur J Nucl Med 15:254–259, 1989.)

to the appearance of detectable amounts of radiolabel of the solid phase in the proximal small intestine".[60] Although there is no consensus on the best method of measuring the lag phase, there is no debate regarding its clinical significance. It is a sensitive indicator of the efficacy of drugs used to treat diabetic gastroparesis.[65] Analysis of the lag phase has also been used to study the effects of ulcer surgery on gastric emptying. Mayer and colleagues found obliteration of the lag phase without an effect on trituration after truncal vagotomy and pyloroplasty.[59] Siegel and co-workers showed that the lag phase increases with the density of the solid food. Once solids are triturated to a small size and are suspended with the liquid in the stomach, solids and liquids appear to empty at the same rate.[64]

Newer methods for analyzing radionuclide gastric emptying data that have been introduced permit analysis of the frequency of antral contractions.[66, 67] Because gastroparesis can result from a number of different mechanisms, including disease of the gastrointestinal smooth muscle and neurohormonal gastroduodenal motor control, these methods should enhance our ability to study normal and abnormal gastric motor function.

## IMAGING OF GASTRIC MUCOSA

### Meckel's Diverticulum

Meckel's diverticulum is a congenital remnant of the omphalomesenteric duct of the embryo. It is usually located in the terminal 100 cm of the ileum. It occurs in 1 to 3% of the population, and 25 to 40% of these

individuals develop symptoms.[68] Usually, complications such as bleeding occur early in life, with 50% of symptoms developing before the age of 2 years.[69] Of those Meckel's diverticula that are symptomatic, pathologic studies show that 57% contain ectopic gastric mucosa.

The anion technetium Tc 99m pertechnetate ($^{99m}TcO_4^-$) is actively accumulated and secreted by the mucoid surface cells of the gastric mucosa. A histologic diagnosis of ectopic gastric mucosa is usually based on the finding of parietal cells. These may be absent in Meckel's diverticulum, yet results of the pertechnetate imaging study may be positive if mucoid surface cells are present.[70]

False-positive studies can result from nonspecific pertechnetate accumulation in obstructed loops of bowel, intussusception, arteriovenous malformations, ulcers, inflammatory lesions, and some tumors of the bowel. Because of normal urinary excretion of pertechnetate, urinary tract structures may be confused with ectopic gastric mucosa. Ectopic gastric mucosa may also be found in duplication cysts, gastrogenic cysts, and enteric duplications. Care must be taken not to confuse ectopic gastric mucosa with normal duodenal and jejunal accumulation of pertechnetate that has been secreted into the stomach and has moved distally into the small bowel.

Both the location of the site of pertechnetate localization and the timing of its appearance must be evaluated. Lesions with increased blood pool or hyperemia appear early in the angiographic phase (the "flow study") or appear within 10 minutes and then fade. Gastric mucosa becomes more prominent with time, and the rate of uptake is similar to that of the normal stomach (Fig. 21–9).

Patients should have fasted for several hours before imaging, and barium studies should be avoided for 2 to 3 days before the scintigraphy. Certain drugs and hormones have been shown to improve detection rates. Cimetidine (300 mg three times per day) is given for 2 days before the study, because it does not block uptake but inhibits the intraluminal secretion and potential translocation of pertechnetate into the small bowel.[71] Glucagon may also be given to prevent peristaltic removal of pertechnetate from the lesion site and translocation of gastric secretions.[72] Pentagastrin (6 μg/kg) is administered subcutaneously just before imaging to enhance uptake in gastric mucosal cells.[73] Gastric suction is usually not necessary if imaging is limited to 60 minutes.

The patient is placed in a supine position under a gamma camera, and serial anterior images are obtained. After injection of 30 to 100 μCi/kg technetium 99m pertechnetate, a radionuclide angiogram is acquired at 1- to 5-second intervals for 30 to 60 seconds to record blood flow and vascular blood pool anatomy. Images are then recorded every 3 to 5 minutes for up to 60 minutes to document any site of pertechnetate localization.

With proper attention to technical details and with knowledge of potential pitfalls, there is an 85% detection rate for surgically proven cases.[74] When adults alone, however, are studied, the sensitivity (63%) and

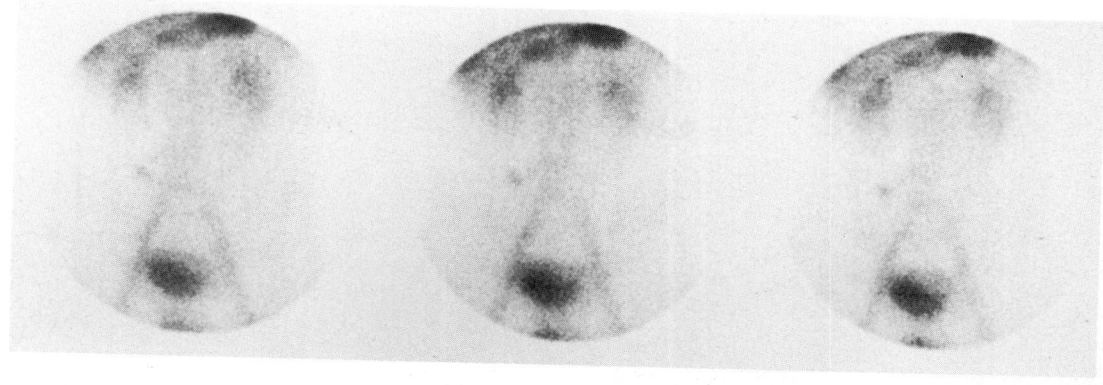

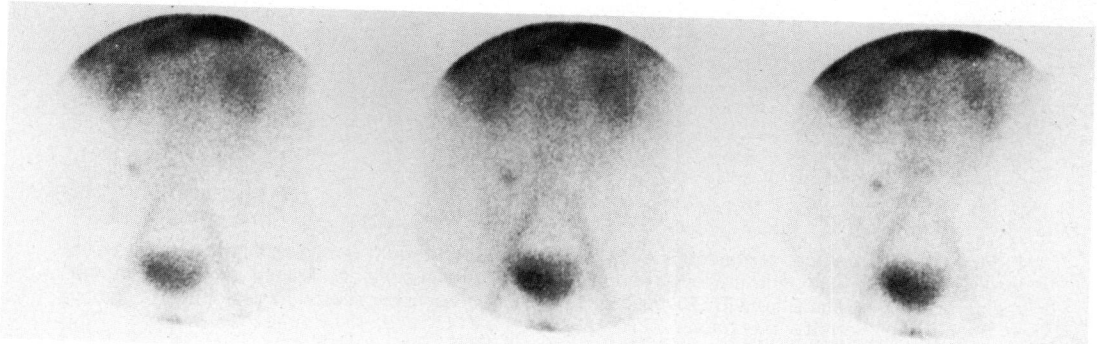

**Figure 21–9. Imaging of Meckel's diverticulum.** Serial anterior images of the abdomen every 5 minutes show localization of pertechnetate in the gastric mucosa as well as in an area in the distal ileum, the Meckel diverticulum.

specificity (9%) appear to be much lower. This finding is related to a .high number of false-positive studies associated with other surgically confirmed pathologic conditions[75] (Table 21–4).

## Barrett's Esophagus

The term *Barrett's esophagus* refers to the replacement of denuded squamous epithelial cells in the lower esophagus by columnar gastric epithelial cells. This phenomenon is most commonly due to chronic gastroesophageal reflux, although it has been associated with other factors such as bile reflux, lye ingestion, chemotherapy for malignancy, and *Campylobacter pylori*.[76–80]

Because patients with Barrett's esophagus are known to be at high risk for developing adenocarcinoma, methods for screening patients at high risk have been sought.

The gold standard for diagnosing Barrett's esophagus consists of multiple biopsies performed at the time of endoscopy. Because gastric mucus-secreting cells may be present, pertechnetate imaging can suggest the presence of Barrett's esophagus[70, 81] (Fig. 21–10).

Reflux of pertechnetate from the stomach into a hiatal hernia or the lower esophagus may reduce the specificity of the test. Best results are obtained when the patient is imaged in an upright position and with oral suction to remove swallowed pertechnetate from salivary secretions.

## Retained Gastric Antrum

The retained gastric antrum syndrome occurs in patients who have undergone a partial gastrectomy with a Billroth II anastomosis. The syndrome is caused by

**TABLE 21–4. PATHOLOGIC CONDITIONS ASSOCIATED WITH FALSE-POSITIVE RESULTS OF MECKEL'S DIVERTICULUM SCINTIGRAPHY**

Abnormalities characterized by hyperemia of the bowel
  Peptic ulcers
  Intussusception
  Obstruction
  Regional enteritis
Vascular masses
  Arteriovenous malformations
  Hemangioma
  Vascular tumors
  Uterine blush
Urinary tract abnormalities
  Hydronephrosis
  Ectopic or horseshoe kidney
  Vesicoureteral reflux
  Bladder diverticulum
Other lesions containing ectopic gastric mucosa
  Gastrogenic cyst
  Enteric duplication
  Duplication cysts
  Barrett's esophagus

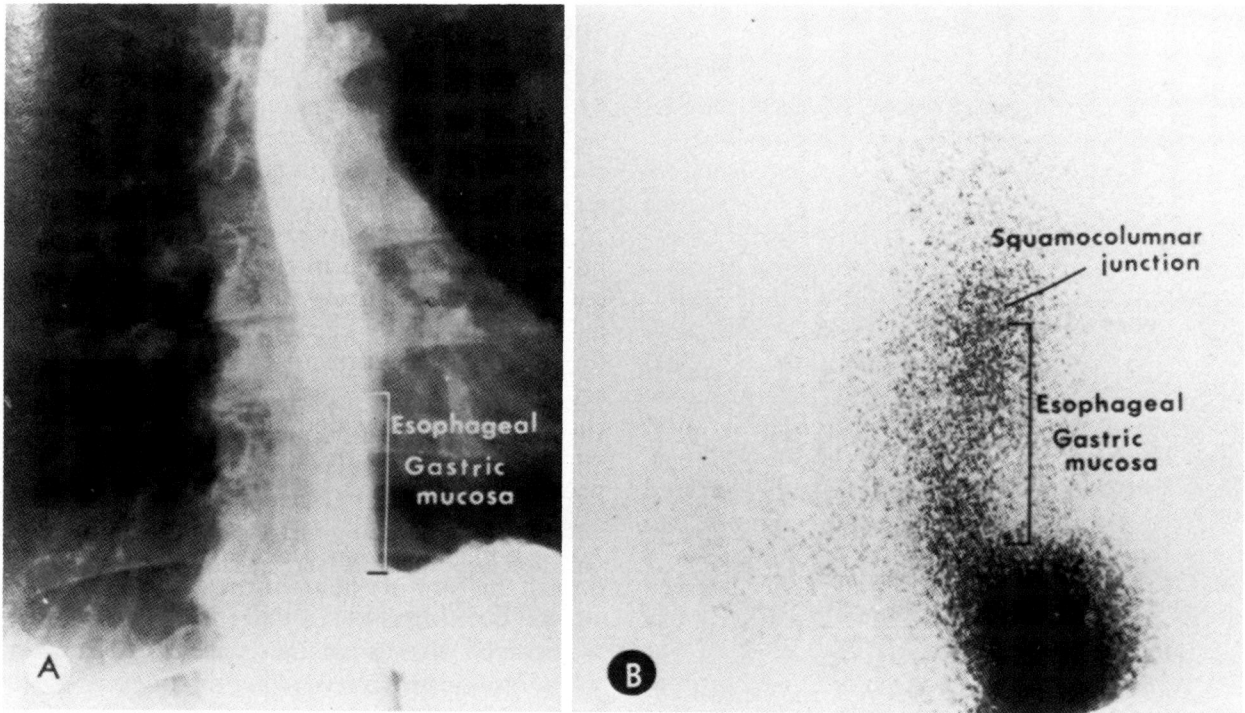

**Figure 21–10. Imaging of Barrett's esophagus with technetium 99m pertechnetate.** There is localization of the isotope in the lower esophagus (**B**), corresponding to the level of stricture on the radiograph (**A**). (**A** and **B** from TH Berquist, NG Nolan, DH Stephens, et al, Radioisotope scintigraphy in diagnosis of Barrett's esophagus, AJR, 123, 2, 401–411, 1975, © by American Roentgen Ray Society.)

gastrin-secreting cells from the antrum retained in the duodenal stump. Serum gastrin levels usually are elevated, because gastrin secretion by the remaining cells is not inhibited by gastric acidity. The increased acid output of the stomach leads to recurrent marginal ulceration, creating a clinical picture that may be confused with the Zollinger-Ellison syndrome.

Pertechnetate imaging can be used to identify retained gastric antrum. In the absence of retained gastric antrum, pertechnetate moves sequentially from the gastric pouch into the efferent loop of the jejunum and then into the ileum. Activity should not localize in the afferent loop near the duodenum or pylorus. Retrograde filling of the afferent loop can be best appreciated by using serial dynamic imaging and a cine mode for viewing. Pertechnetate imaging has a reported sensitivity of 73% and a reported specificity of 100% for identifying retained gastric antrum.[82]

# References

1. Griffith GH, Owen GM, Kirkman S: Measurement of rate of gastric emptying using chromium-51. Lancet 1:1244–1245, 1966.
2. Meyer JH: 99mTc–tagged chicken liver as a marker of solid food in the human stomach. Am J Dig Dis 21:296–304, 1976.
3. Knight LC, Fisher RS, Malmud LS: Comparison of solid food markers in gastric emptying studies. *In* Raynaud C (ed): Nuclear Medicine and Biology. Paris: Pergamon Press, 1982, pp 2407–2410.
4. Kjellen G, Svedberg JB, Tibbling L: Solid bolus transit by esophageal scintigraphy in patients with dysphagia and normal manometry and radiography. Dig Dis Sci 29:1–5, 1984.
5. Pope CE, Horton PF: Intraluminal force transducer measurements of human esophageal peristalsis. Gut 13:464–470, 1972.
6. Kazem I: A new scintigraphic technique for the study of the esophagus. AJR 115:681–688, 1972.
7. Styles CB, Holt S, Bowes KL, et al: Esophageal transit scintigraphy—a cautionary note. J Can Assoc Radiol 35:31–33, 1984.
8. Holloway RH, Lange RC, Plankey MW, et al: Detection of esophageal motor disorders by radionuclide transit studies. A reappraisal. Dig Dis Sci 34:905–912, 1989.
9. Russell COH, Hill LD, Holmes ER 3rd, et al: Radionuclide transit: a sensitive screening test for esophageal dysfunction. Gastroenterology 80:887–892, 1981.
10. Blackwell JN, Hannan WJ, Adam RD, et al: Radionuclide transit studies in the detection of oesophageal dysmotility. Gut 24:421–426, 1983.
11. Tolin RD, Malmud LS, Reilley J, et al: Esophageal scintigraphy to quantitate esophageal transit (quantitation of esophageal transit). Gastroenterology 76:1402–1408, 1979.
12. Drane WE, Johnson DA, Hagan DP, et al: "Nutcracker" esophagus: diagnosis with radionuclide esophageal scintigraphy versus manometry. Radiology 163:33–37, 1987.
13. Mughal MM, Marples M, Bancewicz J: Scintigraphic assessment of oesophageal motility: what does it show and how reliable is it? Gut 27:946–953, 1986.
14. Ott DJ, Chen YM, Hewson EG, et al: Esophageal motility: assessment with synchronous video tape fluoroscopy and manometry. Radiology 173:419–422, 1989.
15. Pope CE: Is LES enough? Gastroenterology 71:328–329, 1976.
16. VanTrappen G, Helleman J: Treatment of achalasia and related motor disorders. Gastroenterology 79:144–154, 1980.
17. McCallum RW: Radionuclide scanning in esophageal disease. J Clin Gastroenterol 4:67–70, 1982.
18. Rozen P, Gelfond M, Zaltzman S, et al: Dynamic, diagnostic, and pharmacological radionuclide studies of the esophagus in achalasia. Radiology 144:587–590, 1982.
19. Richter JE, Castell DO: Gastroesophageal reflux: pathogenesis, diagnosis, and therapy. Ann Intern Med 97:93–103, 1982.
20. Tuttle SG, Grossman MI: Detection of gastro-esophageal reflux

by simultaneous measurements of intraluminal pressure and pH. Proc Soc Exp Biol Med 98:225–227, 1958.

21. Fisher RS, Malmud LS, Roberts GS, et al: Gastroesophageal (GE) scintiscanning to detect and quantitate GE reflux. Gastroenterology 70:301–308, 1976.

22. Hoffman GC, Vansant JH: The gastroesophageal scintiscan: comparison of methods to demonstrate gastroesophageal reflux. Arch Surg 114:727–728, 1979.

23. Fung W, Schaaf AVD, Grieve JC: Gastroesophageal scintigraphy and endoscopy in the diagnosis of esophageal reflux and esophagitis. Am J Gastroenterology 80:245–247, 1985.

24. Jenkins AG, Cowan RJ, Richter JE: Gastroesophageal scintigraphy: is it a sensitive screening test for gastroesophageal reflux disease? J Clin Gastroenterol 7:127–131, 1985.

25. Maurer AH, Siegel JA, Denenberg BS, et al: Absolute left ventricular volume from gated blood pool imaging with use of esophageal transmission measurement. Am J Cardiol 51:853–858, 1983.

26. Fisher RS, Malmud LS, Lobis IF, et al: Antireflux surgery for symptomatic gastroesophageal reflux: mechanism of action. Am J Dig Dis 23:152–160, 1978.

27. Malmud LS, Fisher RS: The evaluation of gastroesophageal reflux before and after medical therapies. Semin Nucl Med 11:205–215, 1981.

28. Ghaed N, Stein MR: Assessment of a technique for scintigraphic monitoring of pulmonary aspiration of gastric contents in asthmatics with gastroesophageal reflux. Ann Allergy 42:306–308, 1979.

29. Sondheimer JM: Gastroesophageal reflux: update on pathogenesis and disagnosis. Pediatr Clin North Am 35:103–116, 1988.

30. Jona JZ, Sty JR, Glicklich M: Simplified radioisotope technique for assessing gastgroesophageal reflux in children. J Pediatr Surg 16:114–117, 1971.

31. Heyman S, Kirkpatrick JA, Winter HS, et al: An improved radionuclide method for the diagnosis of gastroesophageal reflux and aspiration in children (milk scan). Radiology 131:479–482, 1979.

32. Blumhagen JD, Rudd TG, Christie DL: Gastroesophageal reflux in children: Radionuclide gastroesophagography. AJR 135:1001–1004, 1980.

33. Seibert JJ, Byrne WJ, Euler AR, et al: Gastroesophageal reflux—the acid test: scintigraphy or pH probe? AJR 140:1087—1090, 1983.

34. Snape WJ, Brattle WM, Schwartz S, et al: Metoclopramide to treat gastroparesis due to diabetes mellitus. A double-blind controlled trial. Ann Intern Med 96:444–446, 1982.

35. Feldman M, Smith HJ: Effect of cisapride on gastric emptying of indigestible solids in patients with gastroparesis diabeticorum. Gastroenterology 92:171–174, 1987.

36. Cannon WB: The movements of the stomach studied by means of the Roentgen rays. Am J Physiol 1:359–382, 1898.

37. Cannon WB: The receptive relaxation of the stomach. Am J Physiol 29:267–273, 1911.

38. Moore JG, Dubois A, Christian PE, et al: Evidence for a midgastric transverse band in humans. Gastroenterology 91:540–545, 1986.

39. Meyer JH, Ohashi H, Jehn D, et al: Size of liver particles emptied from the human stomach. Gastroenterology 80:1489–1496, 1981.

40. Minami H, McCallum RW: The physiology and pathophysiology of gastric emptying in humans. Gastroenterology 86:1592–1610, 1984.

41. Kelly KA, Code CF, Elveback LR: Patterns of canine gastric electrical activity. Am J Physiol 217:461–470, 1969.

42. Hunt JN, Stubbs DE: The volume and energy content of meals as determinants of gastric emptying. Am J Physiol 245:209–225, 1975.

43. Datz FL, Christian PE, Moore J: Gender-related differences in gastric emptying. J Nucl Med 28:1204–1207, 1987.

44. Goo RH, Moore JG, Greenberg E, et al: Circadian variation in gastric emptying of meals in humans. Gastroenterology 93:515–518, 1987.

45. Collins PJ, Horowitz M, Cook DJ, et al: Gastric emptying in normal subjects—a reproducible technique using a single scintillation camera and computer system. Gut 24:1117–1125, 1983.

46. Moore JG, Christian PE, Taylor AT, et al: Gastric emptying

measurements: delayed and complex emptying patterns without appropriate correction. J Nucl Med 27:1206–1210, 1985.

47. Dugas MC, Schade RR, Lhotsky D, et al: Comparison of methods for analyzing gastric isotopic emptying. Am J Physiol 243:G237–G242, 1982.

48. Loo FD, Palmer DW, Soergel KH, et al: Gastric emptying in patients with diabetes mellitus. Gastroenterology 86:485–494, 1984.

49. Moore JG, Datz FL, Greenberg CE, et al: Effect of body posture on radionuclide measurements of gastric emptying. Dig Dis Sci 33:1592–1595, 1988.

50. Maurer AH, Knight LC, Vitti RA, et al: Geometric mean vs left anterior oblique attenuation correction: effect on half emptying time, lag phase, and rate of gastric emptying. J Nucl Med 32:2176–2180, 1991.

51. Collins PJ, Horowitz M, Shearman DJC, et al: Correction for tissue attenuation in radionuclide gastric emptying studies: a comparison of a lateral image method and a geometric mean method. Br J Radiol 57:689–695, 1984.

52. Tothill P, McLoughlin GP, Holt S, et al: The effect of posture on errors in gastric emptying measurements. Phys Med Biol 25:1071–1077, 1980.

53. Christian PE, Moore JG, Sorenson JA, et al: Effects of meal size and correction technique on gastric emptying time: studies with two tracers and opposed detectors. J Nucl Med 21:883–885, 1980.

54. Meyer JH, VanDeventer G, Graham LS, et al: Error and corrections with scintigraphic measurement of gastric emptying of solid foods. J Nucl Med 24:197–203, 1983.

55. Fahey FH, Ziessman HA, Collen MJ, et al: Left anterior oblique projection and peak-to-scatter ratio for attenuation compensation of gastric emptying studies. J Nucl Med 30:233–239, 1989.

56. Campbell IW, Heading RC, Tothill P, et al: Gastric emptying in diabetic autonomic neuropathy. Gut 18:462–467, 1977.

57. Hurwitz A, Robinson RG, Vats TS, et al: Effects of antacids on gastric emptying. Gastroenterology 71:268–273, 1976.

58. Fisher RS, Rock E, Malmud LS: Effects of meal composition on gallbladder and gastric emptying in man. Dig Dis Sci 32:1337–1344, 1987.

59. Mayer EA, Thomson JB, Jehn D, et al: Gastric emptying and sieving of solid food and pancreatic and biliary secretions after solid meals in patients with nonresective ulcer surgery. Gastroenterology 87:1264–71, 1984.

60. Camilleri M, Malagelada JR, Brown ML, et al: Relation between antral motility and gastric emptying of solids and liquids in humans. Am J Physiol 245:G580–G585, 1985.

61. Collins PJ, Horowitz M, Chatterton BE: Proximal, distal and total stomach emptying of a digestible solid meal in normal subjects. Br J Radiol 61:12–18, 1988.

62. Urbain JL, Siegel JA, Charkes ND, et al: The two-component stomach: effects of meal particle size on fundal and antral emptying. Eur J Nucl Med 15:254–259, 1989.

63. Elashoff JD, Reedy TJ, Meyer JH: Analysis of gastric emptying data. Gastroenterology 83:1306–1312, 1982.

64. Siegel JA, Urbain JL, Adler LP, et al: Biphasic nature of gastric emptying. Gut 29:85–89, 1988.

65. Horowitz M, Harding PE, Chatterton BE, et al: Acute and chronic effects of domperidone on gastric emptying in diabetic autonomic neuropathy. Dig Dis Sci 30:1–9, 1985.

66. Urbain JLC, VanCutsem E, Siegel JA, et al: Visualization and characterization of gastric contractions using a radionuclide technique. Am J Physiol 259:G1062–G1067, 1990.

67. Akkermans LM, Jacobs F, Hong-Yoe O, et al: A noninvasive method to quantify antral contractile activity in man and dog (a preliminary report). In Christensen J (ed): Gastrointestinal Motility. New York: Raven Press, 1980, pp 195–202.

68. Kilpatrick JM: Scanning in diagnosis of Meckel's diverticulum. Hosp Pract 9:131–138, 1974.

69. Rutherford RB, Akers DR: Meckel's diverticulum: a review of 148 pediatric patients, with special reference to the pattern of bleeding and to mesodiverticular vascular bands. Surgery 59:618–626, 1966.

70. Berquist TH, Nolan NG, Stephens DH, et al: Radioisotope scintigraphy in diagnosis of Barrett's esophagus. AJR 123:401–411, 1975.

71. Petrokubi RJ, Baum S, Rohrer GV: Cimetidine administration

resulting in improved pertechnetate imaging of Meckel's diverticulum. Clin Nucl Med 3:385–388, 1978.

72. Sfakianakis GN, Anderson GF, King DR, et al: The effect of intestinal hormones on the Tc-99m pertechnetate (TcO$_4$) imaging of ectopic gastric mucosa in experimental Meckel's diverticulum. J Nucl Med 22:678–683, 1981.

73. Treves S, Grand RJ, Eraklis AJ: Pentagastrin stimulation of technetium 99m uptake by ectopic gastric mucosa in a Meckel's diverticulum. Radiology 128:711–712, 1978.

74. Sfakianakis GN, Conway JJ: Detection of ectopic gastric mucosa in Meckel's diverticulum and in other aberrations by scintigraphy: II. Indications and methods—a 10-year experience. J Nucl Med 22:732–738, 1981.

75. Schwartz MJ, Lewis JH: Meckel's diverticulum: pitfalls in scintigraphic detection in the adult. Am J Gastroenterol 79:611–618, 1984.

76. Meyer W, Vollmar F, Bär W: Barrett-esophagus following total gastrectomy. A contribution to its pathogenesis. Endoscopy 11:121–126, 1979.

77. Fisher DR, Preston DF, Robinson RG, et al: Barrett's esophagus

78. Spechler SJ, Schimmel EM, Dalton JW, et al: Barrett's epithelium complicating lye ingestion with sparing of the distal esophagus. Gastroenterology 81:580–583, 1981.

79. Dahms BB, Greco MA, Strandjord SE: Barrett's esophagus in children after antileukemia chemotherapy. Cancer 60:2896–2900, 1987.

80. Paull G, Yardley JH: Gastric and esophageal *Campylobacter pylori* in patients with Barrett's esophagus. Gastroenterology 95:216–218, 1988.

81. Taillerfer R, Beauchamp G, Duranceau AC, et al: Nuclear medicine and esophageal surgery. Clin Nucl Med 11:445–460, 1986.

82. Lee C, P'eng FK, Yeh PH: Sodium pertechnetate Tc 99m antral scan in the diagnosis of retained gastric antrum. Arch Surg 119:309–311, 1984.

83. Wirth N, Swanson D, Shapiro B, et al: A conveniently prepared Tc-99m resin for semisolid gastric emptying studies. J Nucl Med 24:511–514, 1983.

complicating lye ingestion. Demonstration by pertechnetate scintigraphy. Clin Nucl Med 8:550–552, 1983.

# Angiography and Interventional Radiology

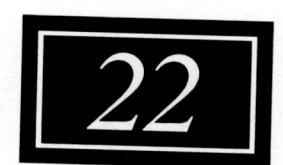

Albert A. Nemcek, Jr., M.D.

Robert L. Vogelzang, M.D.

**ANGIOGRAPHY OF THE UPPER GASTROINTESTINAL TRACT**
Vascular Lesions
Tumors

**NONVASCULAR INTERVENTIONAL RADIOLOGY OF THE UPPER GASTROINTESTINAL TRACT**
Gastrointestinal Intubations

Management of Enteric Strictures
Percutaneous Gastrostomy
Esophageal Fistulas
Foreign Bodies

## ANGIOGRAPHY OF THE UPPER GASTROINTESTINAL TRACT

### Vascular Lesions

Aneurysms can involve the main celiac trunk as well as its branches to the liver, spleen, and gut.[1] Causes of aneurysms include arteriosclerosis, medial degeneration, infection, inflammation, and trauma. Many of these lesions are discovered during the work-up for gastrointestinal and intraperitoneal hemorrhage.

Arteriovenous malformations, characterized by dilated, tortuous feeding arteries and prominent venous drainage, can occur throughout the gastrointestinal tract. They are thought to be developmental in origin, and they are frequently discovered during the angiographic work-up for gastrointestinal hemorrhage.[2, 3]

Vascular lesions may also occur in association with systemic disorders. Pseudoxanthoma elasticum is a hereditary, autosomal recessive disorder of connective tissue that involves systemic abnormalities of elastic fibers. Patients display characteristic ocular and cutaneous lesions. Cardiovascular manifestations occur because of fragmentation, degeneration, and calcification of the arterial elastic laminae and premature atherosclerosis.[4] A variety of splanchnic angiographic abnormalities have been described and include angiomatous malformations, vascular tortuosity, segments of vascular narrowing and occlusion, and small aneurysms.[5, 6] Upper gastrointestinal tract bleeding is common and probably results from submucosal vascular degeneration and inability of the abnormal vessels to constrict at sites adjacent to areas of erosion and hemorrhage. Embolization with absorbable gelatin sponge (Gelfoam) and coils has been used to treat hemorrhage in this disorder.[7]

Patients with hereditary hemorrhagic telangiectasia (Osler-Weber-Rendu disease) have multiple systemic vascular lesions involving the skin, mucous membranes, and gut. Abnormalities on abdominal visceral angiography include tangled masses of tortuous vessels with early venous filling, direct arteriovenous fistulas, arterial aneurysms, localized venous dilatations, and small focal accumulations of contrast medium representing angiomas and visualized during the arterial phase of injection of the contrast medium.[8] Thin, fragile walls are characteristic of these vascular lesions and help explain their propensity to bleed; recurrent gastrointestinal hemorrhage is common.[2, 8]

### Tumors

Upper gastrointestinal tract neoplasms may occasionally be detected on angiograms as incidental abnormalities or as the cause of gastrointestinal bleeding. Leiomyomas are typically hypervascular, are well defined, and have a tendency to bleed. Arteriovenous shunting, commonly found in small bowel leiomyomas, is not a typical feature of gastric leiomyomas.[9] Other primary and metastatic upper gastrointestinal tract tumors may demonstrate nonspecific signs of neoplasia, including neovascularity, vascular encasement, vascular displacement and stretching, and arteriovenous shunting.[10, 11]

## NONVASCULAR INTERVENTIONAL RADIOLOGY OF THE UPPER GASTROINTESTINAL TRACT

### Gastrointestinal Intubations

Gastrointestinal intubation refers to the passage of tubes, wires, and other devices into an intended location in the gastrointestinal tract. Techniques for intubation range from passive reliance on enteric peristalsis to carry a tube to a specific site to complex manipulations using endoscopic or interventional radiologic techniques. These techniques are used to optimize positioning of feeding or decompression tubes, catheterization of enteric strictures before balloon dilatation, or the performance of diagnostic studies like enteroclysis. Most often, transnasal or transoral access to the gastrointestinal tract is used. Manipulations can also be carried out transrectally, transhepatically, or via enterostomy sites.[12]

"Blind" passage of nasoenteric feeding or decompression tubes is common in clinical practice. In cooperative patients with adequate peristalsis and an intact swallowing mechanism, this method is usually reliable. Passage is more difficult and hazardous in patients with pathologic narrowing or other intrinsic disease of the gastrointestinal tract, surgical anastomoses, diminished peristalsis, enteric leaks, injuries to the gastrointestinal tract or surrounding structures, pharyngeal or esophageal neuromuscular dysfunction, or impaired mental status. Potential complications of enteric tube placement include malpositioning into or perforation of the lungs, pleural space, peritoneal cavity, mediastinum, neck, face, and even intracranial structures, resulting in such diverse clinical sequelae as pneumothorax, pneumonitis, empyema, mediastinitis, abdominal abscess, and cardiovascular or cerebral injury.[12-22] Plain films should routinely be obtained to confirm tube position and exclude potential complications.

Fluoroscopic guidance of enteric intubation has been advocated as a means of minimizing complications and achieving more rapid and optimal tube positioning.[12, 17, 18, 21-34] The techniques discussed later in this section are especially helpful in high-risk individuals, those in whom difficult intubation is anticipated, or those in whom reliance on blind methods has resulted in failure or unacceptable delay in spontaneous passage. Some authors have advocated fluoroscopically guided intubation in more routine situations, noting high rates of success and safety in placing tubes as well as a high rate of clinical acceptance.[23, 25] Indeed, nonguided tube placement has been virtually eliminated at their institutions.[25] Whether the reliability and safety of fluoroscopically guided placement outweigh the cost, the radiation exposure, and the time commitment in all patients remains to be determined.

Fluoroscopically aided intubation can be facilitated by several simple maneuvers. Preliminary steps include coating the tube with surgical lubricant and, when necessary, administering topical anesthesia to the pharynx. If the patient can swallow, fluoroscopy may be needed only to confirm passage into the stomach. If the patient cannot swallow, the tube can be gently and actively advanced with fluoroscopic monitoring. If placement into the jejunum is desired, the patient's position can be changed to take advantage of the effect of gravity on tube tips, many of which are weighted.[25, 35]

Collapse of the stomach or small intestine can hinder antegrade tube movement; this problem can be overcome with insufflation of moderate amounts of air.[12, 26, 35] Conversely, excessive dilation of the gut lumen may simply result in looping of the tube as attempts are made to direct its passage. Tube buckling or kinking also results from the distensibility and mobility of the gastrointestinal tract, problems compounded by the fact that most enteric tubes are relatively soft and flexible. In many cases, some type of stiffener or support for the tube is desirable. Many tubes come packaged with stiff wires or stylets to provide internal support.[12, 13, 26, 28, 31, 33, 34] These wires and stylets can often be preformed into gentle curves to facilitate directional guidance. Angiographic guidewires, which are less stiff, provide variable degrees of support and may be advanced ahead of the tube into a desired location. Standard enteric tubes can be modified to follow guidewires by cutting end or side holes into them. Tubes have also been designed specifically for this purpose with end holes already present.[27, 29] Many of the flexible tubes used for long-term alimentation or decompression can be difficult to manipulate over guidewires because of friction; liberal lubrication of wires or the use of hydrophilic wires may be necessary.

External support and guidance in tube placement can be provided by pressure from a lead-gloved hand. This method may be useful along the greater curvature of the stomach when passage beyond the pylorus proves difficult.[12, 13, 26] External support can also be accomplished by using stiff guiding catheters, peel-away sheaths, and other devices.[36-38] Endotracheal tubes have been placed through a gastrostomy site to help guide flexible tubes into the jejunum.[38] Another option is endoscopic stabilization, particularly when combined endoscopic-fluoroscopic intubation is indicated for other reasons.[12, 26]

An angiographic catheter with an appropriate shape can be used primarily or in exchange for a flexible tube.[12, 26, 30, 36, 37, 39] These catheters are used alone or in combination with guidewires. Angiographic catheters should be left in place for short-term purposes only; over longer periods, they become rigid and tend to erode into the bowel wall.[12, 32]

Areas of intestinal narrowing or anatomic distortion also make intubation challenging. These areas may result from normal anatomic structures, such as the pyloric channel; from intrinsic bowel disease; or from surgical anastomoses. Angiographic guidewires and catheters can be invaluable in traversing these regions.[12, 24, 26] Wires with atraumatic tips such as J-tipped wires or floppy-tipped torque control wires help prevent unintentional perforation in severely narrowed segments, especially if inflammation or tumor supervenes and makes the channel more irregular and friable. Torque control wires and appropriately shaped angiographic catheters can also allow the tube to be steered through tortuous paths when necessary.[12] Small amounts of contrast medium administered at the site of difficulty usually serves to define the anatomy; hypertonic water-soluble agents should be avoided in the upper esophagus, and in patients with severe reflux, to minimize the sequelae of aspiration.[12, 24, 26] Endoscopy can also be performed to define anatomy and is especially valuable in cases of chronic gastric outlet obstruction or poorly functioning gastroenterostomy when contrast studies are not diagnostic.[12, 26] Because endoscopic visualization past such sites of abnormality is impaired, fluoroscopy provides important information regarding the course and length of initial guidewire purchase and the final catheter position beyond the narrowed or distorted region.

Alternative routes of intubation can give rise to other difficulties.[12, 26, 37, 38] For example, loss of access and peritoneal leakage are concerns during attempts to catheterize the jejunum via a recently created gastrostomy tube. These concerns place limits on the size of the jejunal tube that can be used.[37] The use of enteric fixation devices (see section on percutaneous gastrostomy) may also provide a margin of safety in this setting.

## Management of Enteric Strictures

The majority of enteric strictures amenable to interventional radiologic methods involve the upper gastrointestinal tract and include narrowing attributable to previous inflammation, gastroesophageal reflux, achalasia, malignancy, surgical anastomoses, ingestion of caustic substances, and peptic disease of the gastric outlet.

Treatment options for enteric strictures fall into three major categories: surgical, endoscopic, and radiologic.[12] Surgical options include bypass or resection and reanastomosis of the involved area. Although long-term success rates are high, patients have higher rates of morbidity and mortality as well. Endoscopic methods include bougienage, in which blunt dilators of increasing size are passed through the area of narrowing, and balloon dilatation. Balloon dilatation is also the method used in radiologic stricture management.[12, 40–54]

Although bougienage has a long history of success and safety, balloon dilatation has become increasingly popular among endoscopists and interventional radiologists. The advantage of balloon dilatation is that the forces applied are radially directed except for the minor longitudinal shear induced by passage of the deflated balloon past the stricture (Fig. 22–1). With bougienage, there is significant generation of longitudinal shear forces during dilatation, which theoretically promotes tearing and perforation.[41, 55–57]

A prospective comparison of radiologic and endoscopic methods has not been performed, although both methods have definite clinical applications (Fig. 22–2). Endoscopy provides direct visualization of mucosa of the strictured area and allows biopsy. It should be performed even when radiologic management is chosen.[58, 59] Radiologic methods are particularly useful when endoscopic passage of balloon or bougie proves difficult. When the stricture is long, irregular, and tortuous, fluoroscopy aided by injection of small amounts of contrast medium can usually show the entire length of the stricture well and safely guide catheterization using the previously discussed techniques. In these cases, endoscopy may be limited in view, and attempts to pass devices under endoscopic guidance alone may be hazardous.

Strictures of the upper gastrointestinal tract are usually approached by transnasal or transoral intubation, although trans-stomal intubation can also be used in special circumstances. The initial goal is safe passage of a guidewire through the strictured area, followed by

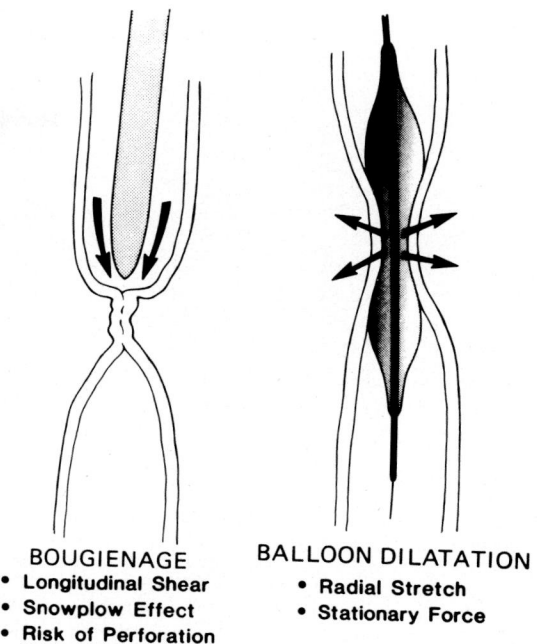

**BOUGIENAGE**
- Longitudinal Shear
- Snowplow Effect
- Risk of Perforation

**BALLOON DILATATION**
- Radial Stretch
- Stationary Force

**Figure 22–1. Bougienage versus balloon dilatation.** Diagram depicting the different dilating forces generated by bougienage technique versus balloon dilatation. Bougienage, which relies on longitudinal forces to dilate a stricture, can cause perforation. (From Dawson SL, Mueller PR, Ferrucci JT, et al: Severe esophageal strictures: indications for balloon catheter dilatation. Radiology 153:631–635, 1984.)

passage of a balloon dilatation catheter over the wire (Fig. 22–3). Once the balloon catheter is centered on the lesion, it is inflated to its maximal pressure tolerance, usually 4 to 6 atm.[12, 43] The length of time required for balloon inflation varies among investigators, from a range of 30 to 60 seconds up to 10 minutes.[12, 40, 42–45, 53] The number of inflations recommended also varies. The procedure should be terminated if the patient experiences severe pain, which may indicate perforation.[12, 42] After dilatation, contrast medium is injected to exclude perforation and to assess the dilated segment[12, 43] (Fig. 22–4). There is often poor correlation between the im-

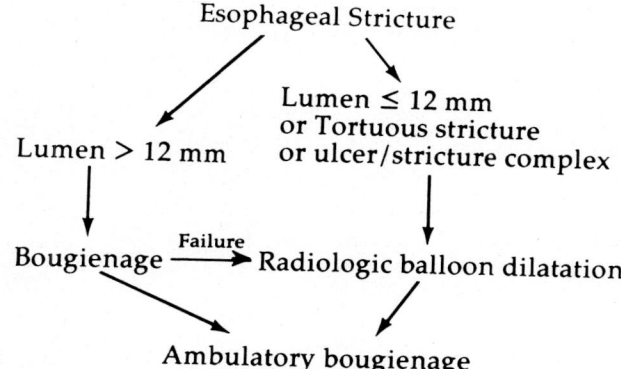

**Figure 22–2. Roles of bougienage and balloon dilatation in the management of esophageal strictures.** (From Dawson SL, Mueller PR, Ferrucci JT, et al: Severe esophageal strictures: indications for balloon catheter dilatation. Radiology 153:631–635, 1984.)

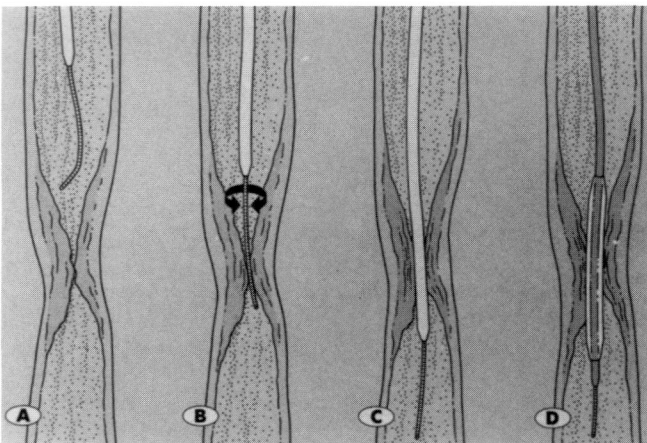

**Figure 22–3. Negotiation of an esophageal stricture. A.** A torque control guidewire has been introduced into the esophagus above the lesion, which has been demonstrated fluoroscopically. **B.** Careful manipulation directs the guidewire through the stricture. **C.** A straight catheter is then directed over the guidewire through the lesion, and an exchange-length guidewire is placed through the lesion. **D.** The balloon catheter is then inserted coaxially over the guidewire and centered across the stricture. (From Cope C, Burke DR, Meranze SG: Atlas of Interventional Radiology. New York: Gower Medical Publishing, 1990, p 12.10.)

mediate postprocedural radiologic appearance and the degree of symptom improvement.[53] The timing and need for repeated dilatation are determined by symptomatic response.

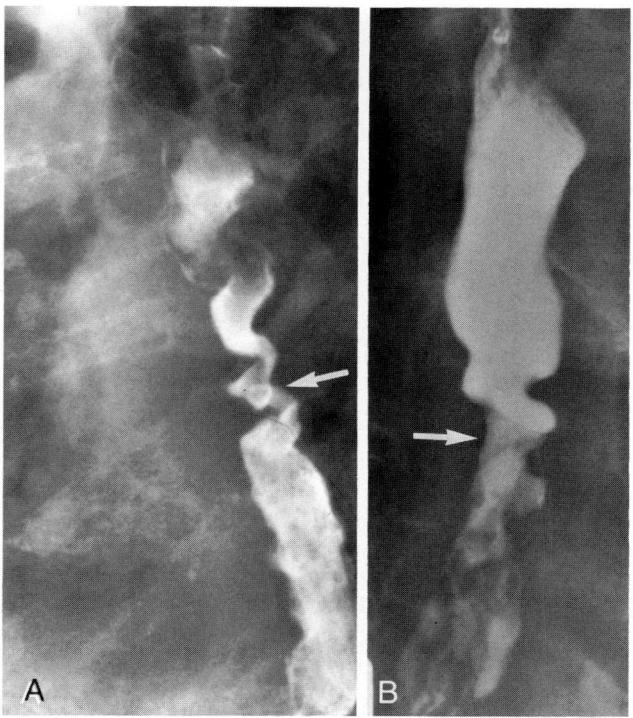

**Figure 22–4. Dilatation of a benign esophageal stricture.** Predilatation **(A)** and postdilatation **(B)** films. Endoscopic dilatation was first attempted but proved difficult in this elderly patient. A steerable wire was manipulated through the stenosis under fluoroscopic guidance. After dilatation of the stricture *(arrow)* to 15 mm, symptomatic improvement was noted.

Balloons used by radiologists for gastrointestinal stricture dilatation are usually 1 to 2 cm in diameter, although smaller balloons can be used for extremely tight strictures or for strictures in children. The use of balloons with diameters of up to 4 cm, or the simultaneous use of two or three balloons, is sometimes necessary for areas with a larger diameter.[12, 40, 43–45] Choice of a proper diameter is usually based on the severity of the stricture and on the size of the lumen measured proximally and distally to the stricture. Special circumstances, such as the dilatation of gastroplasty stomas in patients with morbid obesity, involve other factors, and the choice of an optimal balloon size requires close consultation with the referring physician.[12]

The major complication of balloon dilatation of gastrointestinal tract strictures is perforation. Various large series report perforation in 2% or less of cases.[42, 43, 46, 49] Malignant strictures are more prone to rupture than benign strictures.[12, 42, 43, 49, 60] Perforation, particularly if minor, is not necessarily an indication for urgent surgical repair. However, patients with documented perforation should be followed carefully.[12]

Successful dilatation is measured by improvement in symptoms such as dysphagia, nausea and vomiting, and aspiration. Overall success rates between 67 and 93% have been reported.[12, 40–43, 47, 49, 51] McLean and associates have reported that in those patients with initial success, 83% remained symptom free after 1 year, and 69% have remained so after 2 years.[46] Malignant strictures are less likely to respond than benign strictures, particularly over longer periods. Nevertheless, balloon dilatation represents a viable palliative option in patients with unresectable malignancies, because it is usually performed quickly and easily and can be repeated as often as needed.[12, 40, 42, 46]

Success of initial intubation depends on location: lesions distal to the esophagus are generally more difficult to intubate; proximal esophageal strictures tend to be more difficult to dilate than distal strictures.[47] However, once successful intubation and dilatation have been achieved, location does not have a major effect on long-term outcome.[46] Patients with anastomotic strictures are reportedly more difficult to intubate and a combined endoscopic-radiologic approach may be helpful.[12, 47]

## Percutaneous Gastrostomy

The major indications for gastrostomy tube placement are gastric decompression and nutritional support via enteral tube feedings. This procedure can also provide access for percutaneous transgastric drainage of pancreatic fluid collections and dilatation of upper gastrointestinal tract strictures.[61–66]

In the past, gastrostomy tubes were placed surgically. However, many patients who require gastrostomy tubes are poor operative risks because of malnutrition, debilitation, and coexistent illnesses. In the past decade, gastrostomy has been increasingly performed using two nonsurgical techniques: endoscopic and imaging-guided percutaneous methods.[12, 67–91] Both methods are safe and successful and have proved to be acceptable and cost-effective alternatives to operative placement.

The endoscopic method does not require exposure to ionizing radiation and can be performed easily and rapidly at the bedside. Although bedside placement using sonography or portable fluoroscopy is possible, it is rarely performed.[77] Endoscopic placement may be difficult or impossible when there is obstruction or high-grade narrowing of the esophagus or pharynx, leaving imaging-guided placement as the only feasible nonoperative alternative. Imaging guidance may also be critical in delineating and avoiding interposed structures (e.g., the colon) between the anterior abdominal wall and the stomach (Fig. 22–5). In patients prone to aspiration, imaging guidance is usually preferable, because endoscopy may require heavy sedation and be a lengthy procedure if tube placement into the jejunum is required.[90] Finally, tubes placed under imaging guidance are less likely to give rise to stomal wound infections than those inserted endoscopically; the endoscope must pass through the contaminated oral cavity rather than the scrubbed anterior abdominal wall.

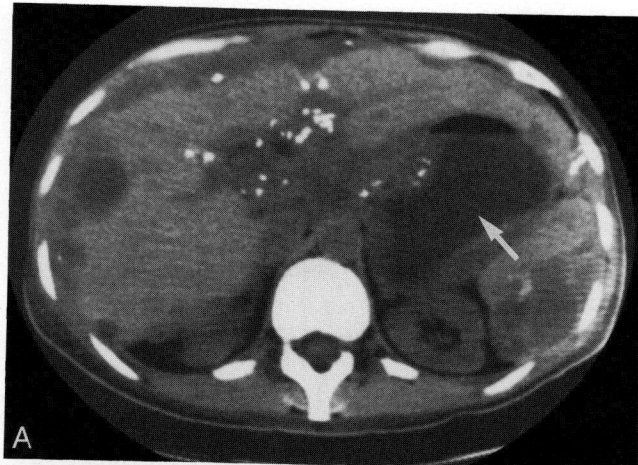

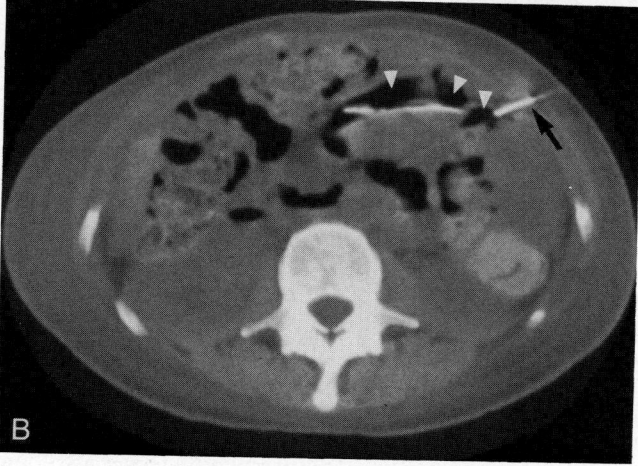

**Figure 22–5. CT-guided percutaneous gastrostomy. A.** CT scanning of the upper abdomen in a patient with pseudomyxoma peritonei attributable to ovarian carcinoma shows the stomach (arrow) surrounded by adjacent organs and peritoneal metastases. **B.** At a more caudal level, a safe window to the stomach is present. Percutaneous gastrostomy was successfully performed under CT guidance. Arrowheads = gastric lumen; arrow = initial puncture needle.

Complications of percutaneous gastrostomy include catheter dislodgment, pericatheter leakage, peritonitis, sepsis, pain, hemorrhage, inadvertent puncture of other organs, pulmonary aspiration, subcutaneous inflammation, and wound infection.[12, 78, 79, 79a, 83, 85–87, 89–95] Review of four of the larger series of percutaneous imaging-guided gastrostomies, reporting a total of 635 patients, indicates a procedure-related mortality of 0 to 9.8%, major complications in 0 to 6%, and minor complications in 4.4 to 12%.[85–87, 89] Thirty-day mortality in these series ranged from 11 to 26%, reflecting the poor overall condition of many patients requiring gastrostomy. These complication rates are comparable to those reported for surgical and endoscopic gastrostomy.[80, 81, 96–100] Unfortunately, basing conclusions on such comparisons is unreliable. Methods of reporting complications differ widely, and no direct prospective comparison with surgical or endoscopic methods has been undertaken. In a single retrospective comparison of percutaneous nonendoscopic gastrostomy and surgical gastrostomy, there were significantly fewer complications with the nonsurgical method.[95]

Percutaneous gastrostomy can be performed by a variety of methods. Before the procedure, the patient should be given nothing by mouth for at least 12 hours to minimize risks of aspiration and peritoneal leakage. Usually, prophylactic antibiotics are not necessary.[87, 90] Only mild sedation combined with local anesthesia at the puncture site is usually required.[12, 84, 85, 88]

An entry site is chosen in the anterior left upper quadrant, which allows direct puncture of the stomach with no transgression of bowel, liver, or vascular structures. Preprocedural ultrasonography or computed tomography (CT) provides delineation of these structures (see Fig. 22–5). Ultrasound is quickly and easily performed in the fluoroscopy suite and is often used routinely to demarcate a safe "window" on the skin surface.[12, 77, 90] If fluoroscopic puncture proves difficult because of interposed structures, cross-sectional imaging can be used to plan and follow a more precise puncture route[82, 84] (see Fig. 22–5). Another helpful adjunct in patients who have no obstruction or altered enteric motility is the administration of oral contrast medium the night before the examination, which provides good opacification of the colon at the time of the procedure.

One potential hazard of percutaneous gastrostomy is injury to the inferior epigastric artery, which lies at the junction of the medial two thirds and lateral third of the rectus abdominis. Therefore, skin puncture should be made at a site lateral to this muscle or close to the midline of the abdomen, depending on the position of the stomach.[77] A subcostal puncture site usually provides good access to the stomach, is more comfortable for the patient, and avoids pleural and pulmonary complications.

Gastric distention makes it easier to pierce the gastric wall, which tends to invaginate and move away from the puncture needle[77] (Fig. 22–6). Distention also helps bring the stomach closer to the anterior abdominal wall and displace any interposed bowel. Distention is provided by insufflation of the stomach with several hundred milliliters of room air administered via a pre-

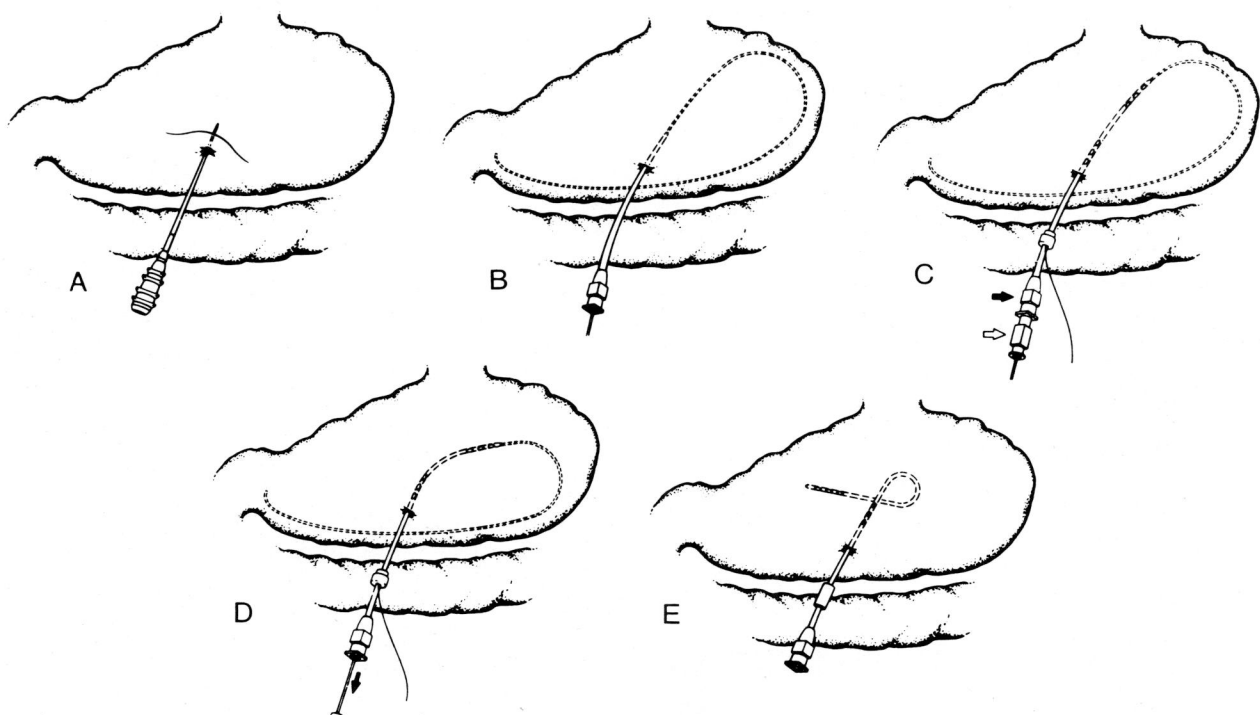

**Figure 22–6. Technique of percutaneous gastrostomy. A.** The sheathed needle is inserted into the midbody of the stomach; note the inward puckering of the gastric wall. **B.** After guidewire insertion, the tract is dilated to 12 French. The dilators closely follow the original path of the guidewire. **C.** The catheter introducer assembly is inserted over the guidewire into the gastric lumen. Gastric distention should be maintained. Solid arrow indicates catheter hub; open arrow indicates introducer hub. **D.** Once the appropriate length of catheter is inserted into the stomach, the metal introducer is removed *(arrow)*. **E.** The loop string is pulled to fix the loop. After satisfactory catheter position is confirmed, the string is knotted and covered by its sleeve. (**A** to **E** from Wills JS, Oglesby JT: Percutaneous gastrostomy. Radiology 167:41–43, 1988.)

viously placed nasogastric tube.[12, 77, 84, 88, 90] If a nasogastric tube cannot be placed, the stomach can be punctured with a Seldinger needle, and air can be injected through its lumen.[88] Another means of providing distention is the oral administration of effervescent granules that produce carbon dioxide.[88] Intravenous glucagon (1.0 mg in adults, 0.14 mg/kg in children) can be used to augment these measures by diminishing gastric peristalsis and decreasing passage of air through the pylorus.[12, 83, 84, 88]

One other option for providing distention is intragastric inflation of a latex balloon attached to the end of a nasogastric tube.[101] The balloon is inflated with diluted contrast medium or with air, providing an easily visualized and stable target for fluoroscopically or sonographically guided puncture. Bursting of the balloon confirms intragastric positioning of the needle tip. Although this device can be difficult for some patients to tolerate and is usually unnecessary, it may be helpful when simple insufflation is unsuccessful in providing gastric distention, as occurs in patients with a partial gastrectomy.[102]

The anterior wall of the stomach is usually punctured under fluoroscopy in its middle third toward the side of the greater curvature (Fig. 22–7). The greater and lesser curvatures should be avoided because the larger vascular arcades of the stomach are located in these regions.

Lateral fluoroscopy is used to access the proximity of the anterior gastric wall to the skin surface. If initial or delayed small bowel catheterization is anticipated, a "downhill" puncture angled toward the pyloric region makes manipulations of the guidewire and catheter easier.[78] Too great an angle, however, makes tract dilatation and catheter exchange difficult. If the tube is being placed for decompressive purposes only, it can be angled somewhat more vertically and toward the gastric fundus. Once the gastric wall is indented by the puncture needle, a short vigorous thrust is used to pierce its muscular layers.

Final catheter placement can be achieved by a variety of methods. One is the Seldinger technique and its variants, in which initial puncture is made with an 18- to 22-gauge Seldinger needle or a small sheathed needle. A wire is passed through the sheath or cannula, and successive guidewire and catheter exchange is used to place a final gastrostomy tube.[12, 78, 84, 88, 90] Techniques using a trocar, an instrument consisting of a catheter or sheath mounted on the puncture needle, have also been successfully used in placing gastrostomy tubes.[77, 78] The trocar technique allows larger and softer tubes to be inserted at the time of the initial procedure and requires fewer catheter and wire exchanges, each of which may

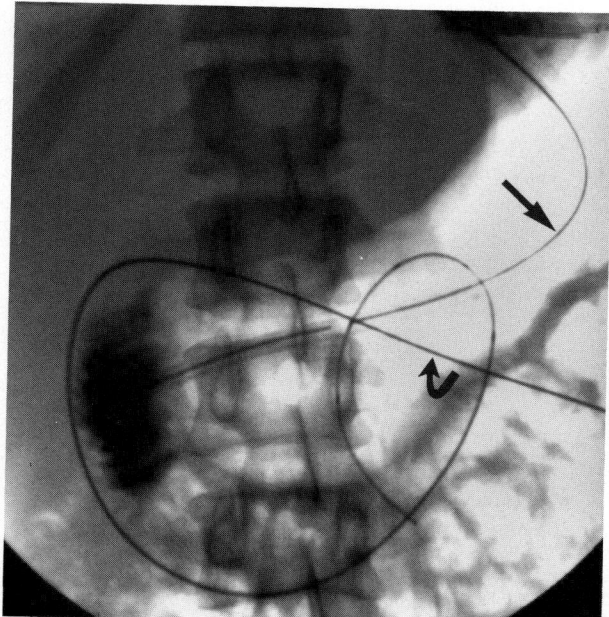

**Figure 22–7. Fluoroscopically guided percutaneous gastrostomy.** The midbody of the gas-filled stomach has been punctured at the site of the curved arrow with an 18-gauge Seldinger needle. It is angulated toward the pylorus, and a wire has been manipulated into the proximal jejunum. A gastrojejunostomy tube was subsequently placed. Straight arrow indicates the nasogastric tube used for insufflation of air.

result in loss of gastric access. Initial puncture, however, may be difficult and risky with trocars, which are usually larger devices.

When the Seldinger technique is used, a peel-away sheath may facilitate insertion if catheter exchange is difficult or if placement of a soft catheter or catheter without an end hole is desired. In addition, removal of the peel-away sheath may correct any gastric wall invagination that has occurred.[91] During passage of catheters or dilators, the stabilizing guidewire has a free end within the gastrointestinal tract and must not be displaced out of the gastric lumen. A method of preventing this problem in children has been described: the free end of the wire is secured and pulled from the stomach to the mouth by a wire basket or snare, allowing stable control of both ends of the wire in a manner analogous to that of endoscopic methods.[103, 104] In general, however, these maneuvers are unnecessary.

The use of fixation devices as an adjunct to percutaneous gastrostomy has generated some controversy. These devices are fasteners that can be placed through a small needle to affix the anterior gastric wall to the anterior abdominal wall at one or more sites (Fig. 22–8). Advocates of these devices cite a number of potential advantages, including reduced intraperitoneal leakage of gastric contents, facilitation of guidewire and catheter exchange and immediate placement of large catheters, easy reinsertion in cases of early catheter dislodgment (of greater concern in uncooperative patients), and possible tamponade of gastric hemorrhage induced at the gastrostomy site.[89, 105–108] In two published series

using two different fixation devices, no guidewire or tube dislodgments and no clinically apparent peritoneal leakage occurred in more than 200 percutaneous gastrostomies.[89, 107] Theoretic disadvantages of gastric fixation are interference with gastric peristalsis and excessive traction on the gastric wall resulting in pressure

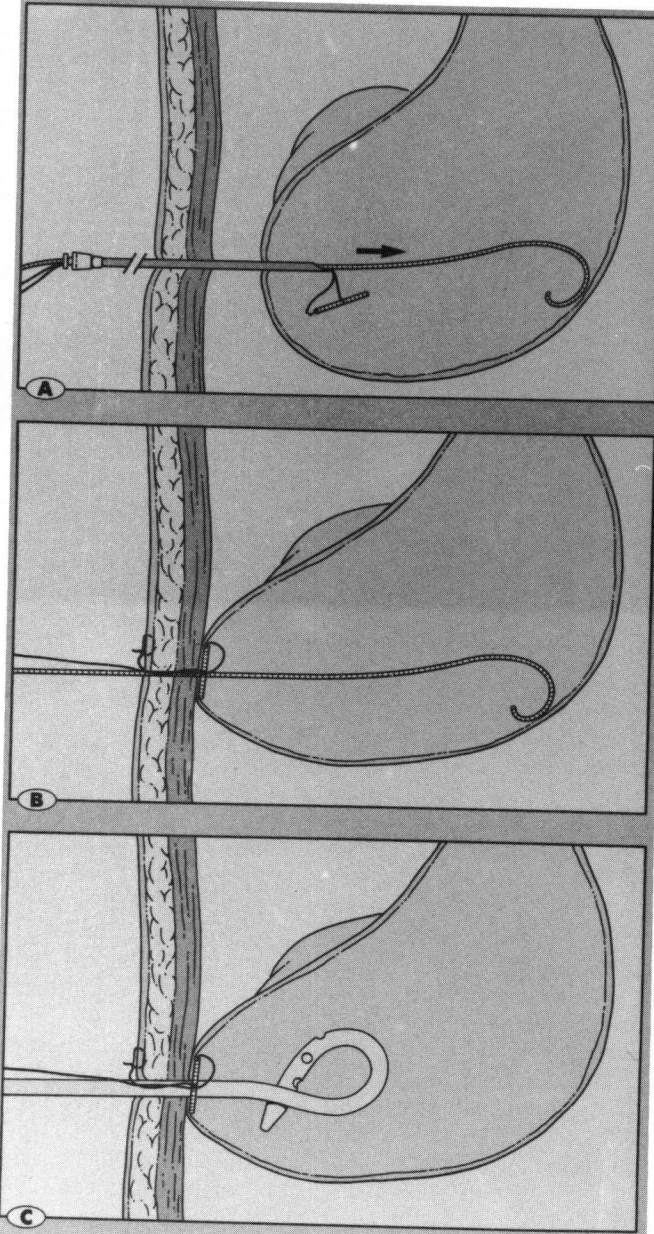

**Figure 22–8. Gastrostomy anchor. A.** A 17-gauge needle has been inserted into the stomach, and a guidewire has pushed the anchor, represented by the crossbar, into the stomach by applying traction to the middle suture. **B.** This procedure allows the stomach to be held closely against the abdominal wall. **C.** A catheter is inserted over the guidewire, which is then removed. The anchor is left in place for 7 to 10 days to prevent dehiscence of the stomach from the anterior abdominal wall. (From Cope C, Burke DR, Meranze SG: Atlas of Interventional Radiology. New York: Gower Medical Publishing, 1990, p 12.5.)

necrosis, bleeding, infection, or catheter dislodgment.[89, 109] Other potential disadvantages that can be obviated by careful technique include anchor misplacement into the peritoneal cavity and difficulty with tube passage immediately adjacent to the anchor.[107] Most of the controversy, however, has resulted from extensive clinical and laboratory experience with percutaneous gastrostomy accomplished without fixation devices, which suggests that the procedure can be performed easily, safely, and less expensively in most instances without their use.[109, 110] No large prospective comparisons have yet been made.

Another area of controversy is the final position of the tube. Some practitioners prefer that the tube be manipulated into the proximal jejunum at the time of the initial procedure. This method allows immediate catheter feeding, diminishes the risks of gastroesophageal reflux and aspiration of gastric contents, and provides additional insurance against catheter dislodgment.[79, 85, 90] Other practitioners have maintained that routine gastrojejunostomy is not indicated, and they have reserved jejunal placement for patients who are prone to reflux or aspiration, have impaired gastric motility, or have partial gastric obstruction.[84, 87] Even if the tube is left in the stomach initially, subsequent conversion to a gastrojejunostomy tube can usually be accomplished without difficulty.

A large variety of tubes have been used for percutaneous gastrostomy, including simple Cope loop catheters, Foley catheters, and catheters specially designed for percutaneous gastrostomy and gastrojejunostomy.[12, 78, 79, 84–87, 90, 91] Catheter sizes usually range from about 10 to 18 French. Because of its ease of insertion, the Cope loop is preferred by many investigators, except in patients who require gastrojejunostomy.

Although patients should be observed carefully after percutaneous gastrostomy for signs of complications, it should be noted that a number of postprocedural radiologic findings are common and should not by themselves cause alarm or prompt laparotomy. These radiologic findings include pneumoperitoneum and small abdominal wall and gastric hematomas. Subcutaneous emphysema, gastric pneumatosis, free or loculated intraperitoneal fluid (Fig. 22–9), and pneumoperitoneum that increases in volume are uncommon and should be viewed with more concern.[93, 93a, 94]

Long-term care of percutaneous gastrostomy catheters includes keeping the catheter entry site clean and maintaining tube patency after feeding with injection of saline.[84] A tract between the abdominal wall and the gastric lumen is usually well established in about 7 days, and exchange of an occluded tube or replacement of a recently dislodged tube after this time is generally easy.[77] If the tube is advertently removed at an earlier time, an attempt can be made to recatheterize the tract, but it is less likely to be successful. As noted earlier, one possible advantage to using gastric fixation devices is that it facilitates tube replacement or repeated puncture of the stomach in this early period. If pericatheter leakage is noted, the problem may respond to replacement of the tube with one slightly larger. Delayed pericatheter hemorrhage, presumably attributable to erosion into an adjacent vessel, has been described. Successful tampon-

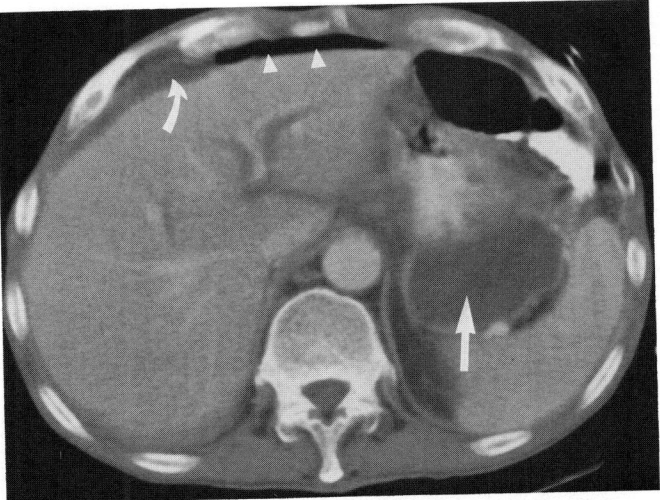

**Figure 22–9. Percutaneous gastrostomy: complication.** This CT scan was obtained 3 days after percutaneous gastrostomy. Although pneumoperitoneum *(arrowheads)* is often seen in the absence of clinically apparent complications, findings of loculated *(straight arrow)* and free *(curved arrow)* intraperitoneal fluid are atypical and are cause for concern. Peritoneal spillage in this case resulted from intraperitoneal positioning of a side hole of the gastrostomy tube. The patient required surgical treatment.

ade and long-term control of the bleeding can be achieved with gentle traction by a Foley catheter against the gastric wall.[92]

## Esophageal Fistulas

General aspects of management of enteric fistulas are discussed in Chapter 45. Esophageal leaks and fistulas have certain distinctive features. If an abscess results from an esophageal leak (Fig. 22–10), standard drainage methods can be used when combined with suction of esophageal secretions. There is a high rate of closure, when the leak is due to benign disease.[111, 112] When a percutaneous route is not available, an alternative approach of abscess drainage via the esophageal lumen, across the opening in the esophageal wall, can be used. This rather unique approach is made possible by fluoroscopy, which makes wires and catheters easy to manipulate in the esophagus. This technique has been performed transnasally as well as via a retrograde route, with access provided by percutaneous gastrostomy.[111, 113] Patients with leaks of this type typically require intravenous or enteric tube alimentation during the period of drainage. Another interesting approach is the use of balloon dilatation of esophageal anastomoses in patients with anastomotic leaks: narrowing at the anastomotic site may contribute to maintenance of the fistula; balloon dilatation should help promote its resolution.[48]

## Foreign Bodies

Radiologists play a role in removal of some foreign objects, either through conservative means or through

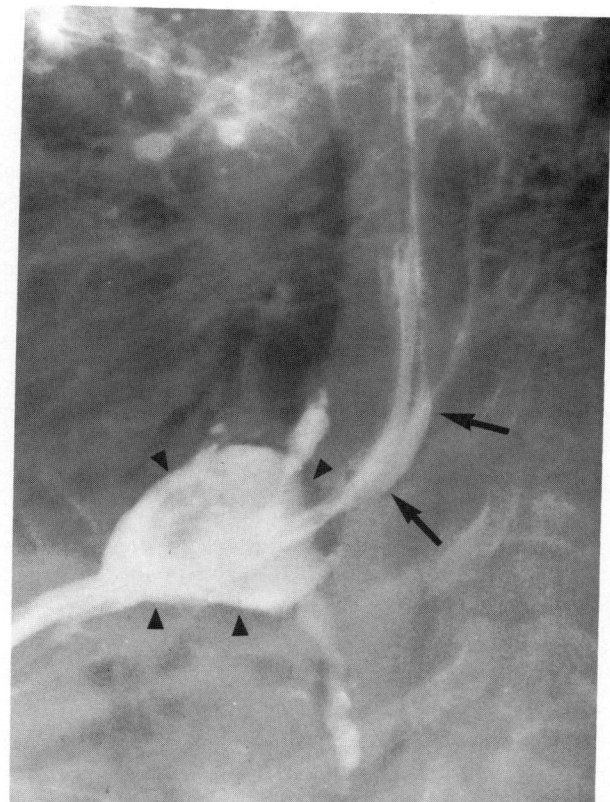

**Figure 22–10. Percutaneous drainage of esophageal leak.** Sinogram performed after CT-guided drainage of a juxtapleural fluid collection *(arrowheads)* shows communication with the esophagus *(arrows).*

more active manipulations. A foreign body that has caused or is likely to cause perforation indicates endoscopic or surgical removal rather than the radiologic methods described later.

Most foreign bodies become lodged above areas of esophageal narrowing. Gas-forming agents and glucagon have been successfully used in this setting.[114–119] The intended action of glucagon is relief of spasm associated with obstruction of the passage of the foreign body. It is ineffective on the skeletal muscle of the upper esophagus. Gas-forming agents act by transiently distending the esophageal lumen. Separately or in combination, gas-forming agents and glucagon allow some foreign bodies to pass into the stomach or to be vomited back up. It has been suggested that if either of these agents is to be used first, it should probably be the gas-forming agent, because a fixed esophageal lesion is more likely than esophageal spasm to be the cause of the impaction.[118] The idea of combining the agents is appealing, but a case report has raised the question of whether an esophageal perforation is induced by their simultaneous use.[115] A subsequent report describes a number of situations in which combined agents should not be used: a rigid and fixed esophageal obstruction, a prominent cricopharyngeus, an esophageal diverticulum, obstruction lasting longer than 24 hours, obstruction in the

proximal third of the stomach, and obstruction by an object with sharp edges.[114]

The inflated balloon of a Foley catheter can also be used to dislodge a blunt esophageal foreign body under fluoroscopic guidance.[120–124] This technique is quick, is readily performed with commonly available equipment, and typically requires little sedation of the patient. The uninflated balloon is passed transnasally to a level past the object. It is then inflated with saline, and the balloon is used to pull the object into the oropharynx, where it can be removed. Occasionally, the object can be pushed into the stomach. Because the balloon does not firmly grab the foreign body, it may slip away during the procedure, leading to the risk of tracheobronchial aspiration once the object is pulled into the oropharynx. Another theoretic problem is excessive distention of the esophagus leading to perforation. An alternative fluoroscopic method that overcomes these potential difficulties is the use of wire retrieval baskets similar to those used for percutaneous removal of gallstones.[125] These baskets are particularly useful for ovoid or spheric objects, less so for flat objects such as coins. A soft feeding tube is first advanced past the foreign body, and the basket is advanced through it to its tip. The basket is deployed at the level of the foreign body. The risk of esophageal perforation is small when this procedure is performed under fluoroscopic guidance, even when the esophageal lumen is severely narrowed.

Catheters have been designed with magnets at their tips for removal of magnetic, metallic foreign bodies, such as disk batteries.[126–129]

# References

1. Stanley JC, Thompson NW, Fry WJ: Splanchnic artery aneurysms. Arch Surg 107:689–697, 1970.
2. Moore JD, Thompson NW, Appelman HD, et al: Arteriovenous malformations of the gastrointestinal tract. Arch Surg 111:381–388, 1976.
3. Sheedy PF II, Fulton RE, Atwell DT: Angiographic evaluation of patients with chronic gastrointestinal bleeding. AJR 123:338–347, 1975.
4. Mendelsohn G, Bulkley BH, Hutchins GM: Cardiovascular manifestations of pseudoxanthoma elasticum. Arch Pathol Lab Med 102:298–302, 1987.
5. Bardsley JL, Koehler PR: Pseudoxanthoma elasticum: angiographic manifestations in abdominal vessels. Radiology 93:559–562, 1969.
6. Belli A, Cawthorne S: Visceral angiographic findings in pseudoxanthoma elasticum. Br J Radiol 61:368–371, 1988.
7. Cunningham JR, Lippman SM, Renie WA, et al: Pseudoxanthoma elasticum: treatment of gastrointestinal hemorrhage by arterial embolization and observations on autosomal dominant inheritance. Johns Hopkins Med J 147:168–173, 1980.
8. Halpern M, Turner AF, Citron BP, et al: Hereditary hemorrhagic telangiectasia. An angiographic study of abdominal visceral angiodysplasias associated with gastrointestinal hemorrhage. Radiology 90:1143–1149, 1968.
9. Kaude J, Silseth CH, Tylen U: Angiography in myomas of the gastrointestinal tract. Acta Radiol Diagn 12:691–704, 1972.
10. Kadir S: Diagnostic Angiography. Philadelphia: WB Saunders, 1986.
11. Reuter SR, Redman HC, Cho KJ: Gastrointestinal Angiography. Philadelphia: WB Saunders, 1986.
12. McLean GK: Interventional radiology of the gastrointestinal tract. Curr Probl Diagn Radiol 19:85–132, 1990.

13. Bilbao MK, Frische LH, Dotter CT, et al: Hypotonic duodenography. Radiology 89:438–443, 1967.
14. Wheeler PS: Complications due to inadvertent tracheobronchial placement of feeding tubes. Radiology 167:877, 1988 (letter).
15. Wheeler PS: Feeding tubes that pierce the lung: a case study in risk prevention and quality assurance. Radiology 165:861, 1987 (editorial).
16. Koch KJ, Becker GJ, Edwards MK: Intracranial placement of a nasogastric tube. AJNR 10:443–444, 1989.
17. McLean GK, Meranze SG, Burke DR: Inadvertent tracheobronchial placement of feeding tubes. Radiology 170:278, 1989 (letter).
18. Woodall BH, Winfield DF, Bisset GS 3rd: Inadvertent tracheobronchial placement of feeding tubes. Radiology 165:727–729, 1987.
19. Woodall BH, Winfield DF, Bisset GS 3rd: Complications due to inadvertent tracheobronchial placement of feeding tubes. Radiology 167:876, 1988 (letter).
20. Ghahremani GG, Turner MA, Prot RB: Iatrogenic intubation injuries of the upper gastrointestinal tract in adults. Gastrointest Radiol 5:1–10, 1980.
21. Ghahremani GG: Complications due to inadvertent tracheobronchial placement of feeding tubes. Radiology 167:875–876, 1988 (letter).
22. Gelfand DW, Ott DJ: Inadvertent pulmonary placement of feeding tubes. Radiology 167:283, 1988 (letter).
23. Grant JP, Curtas MS, Kelvin FM: Fluoroscopic placement of nasojejunal feeding tubes with immediate feeding using a nonelemental diet. JPEN 7:299–303, 1983.
24. Law RL: The value of fluoroscopy as an aid to problematic intubations of the fine bore feeding tubes. J Intervent Radiol 5:171–173, 1990.
25. Gutierrez ED, Balfe DM: Fluoroscopically guided nasoenteric feeding tube placement: results of a 1-year study. Radiology 178:759–762, 1991.
26. McLean GK, Ring EJ, Freiman DB: Applications and techniques of gastrointestinal intubation. Cardiovasc Intervent Radiol 5:108–116, 1982.
27. McLean GK, Meranze SG, Burke DR: Enteric alimentation: a radiologic approach. Radiology 160:555–556, 1986.
28. Gelfand DW: An easy method for passing an intestinal intubation tube under fluoroscopic guidance. Radiology 129:532, 1978.
29. McLean GK, Burke DR, Meranze SG: An enteric alimentation tube designed for rapid, guidewire-directed placement. J Intervent Radiol 2:43–44, 1987.
30. Rosenkrantz H, Healy JF: Rapid placement of small-bowel tubes using modified angiographic techniques and equipment. Radiology 143:564, 1982.
31. Hatfield DR, Beck JL: An improved technique for feeding tube placement. Radiology 141:823, 1981.
32. Frederick PR, Miller MH, Morrison WJ: Feeding tube for fluoroscopic placement. Radiology 145:847, 1982.
33. Sargent FN, Meyers H: Wire guide and technique for Cantor tube insertion. AJR 107:150–155, 1969.
34. Hanafee WN, Weiner M: External guided passage of an intestinal intubation tube. Radiology 89:1100–1102, 1967.
35. Kohn MI, Teplick SK, Glick SN. Useful techniques for passage of a Cantor tube into the small bowel. Appl Radiol 17:51–58, 1988.
36. Cardoza JD, Jeffrey RB Jr: Nasojejunal feeding tube placement in immobile patients. Radiology 166:893, 1988.
37. McLean GK, Rombeau JL, Caldwell MD, et al: Transgastrostomy jejunal intubation for enteric alimentation. AJR 139:1129–1133, 1982.
38. Strife JL, Dunbar JS, Rice S: Jejunal intubation via gastrostomy catheters in pediatric patients. Radiology 154:249, 1985.
39. Zornoza J, Chuang VP, Wallace S: Use of angiographic catheters for intestinal alimentation in patients with upper gastrointestinal obstruction. Radiology 134:240, 1980.
40. Grundy A, Mills P, Cawthorne SJ: Balloon dilatation of upper gastrointestinal anastomoses. J Intervent Radiol 5:7–12, 1990.
41. McLean GK, Meranze SG: Interventional radiologic management of enteric strictures. Radiology 170:1049–1053, 1989.
42. Nóbrega J: Esophageal balloon dilatation: a follow-up study in 74 patients. Cardiovasc Intervent Radiol 12:255–257, 1989.

43. Maynar M, Guerra C, Reyes R, et al: Esophageal strictures: balloon dilatation. Radiology 167:703–706, 1988.
44. Sato Y, Frey EE, Smith WL, et al: Balloon dilatation of esophageal stenosis in children. AJR 150:639–642, 1988.
45. de Lange EE, Shaffer HA Jr: Anastomotic strictures of the upper gastrointestinal tract: results of balloon dilatation. Radiology 167:45–50, 1988.
46. McLean GK, Cooper GS, Hartz WH, et al: Radiologically guided balloon dilatation of gastrointestinal strictures. Part II. Results of long-term follow-up. Radiology 165:41–43, 1987.
47. McLean GK, Cooper GS, Hartz WH, et al: Radiologically guided balloon dilatation of gastrointestinal strictures. Part I. Technique and factors influencing procedural success. Radiology 165:35–40, 1987.
48. de Lange EE, Shaffer HA Jr, Daniel TM, et al: Esophageal anastomotic leaks: preliminary results of treatment with balloon dilatation. Radiology 165:45–47, 1987.
49. Gotberg S, Hambraeus G, Hedenbro J, et al: Experience with balloon catheter dilatation of strictures in the upper digestive tract. Appl Radiol 15:124–130, 1986.
50. Hegedüs V, Raaschou HO: Radiologically guided dilatation of stenotic gastroduodenal anastomosis. Gastrointest Radiol 11:27–29, 1986.
51. Starck E, Paolucci V, Herzer M, et al: Esophageal stenosis: treatment with balloon catheters. Radiology 153:637–640, 1984.
52. Goldthorn JF, Ball WS Jr, Wilkinson LG, et al: Esophageal strictures in children: treatment by serial balloon catheter dilatations. Radiology 153:655–658, 1984.
53. Dawson SL, Mueller PR, Ferrucci JT Jr, et al: Severe esophageal strictures: indications for balloon catheter dilatation. Radiology 153:631–635, 1984.
53a. Song H-Y, Han Y-M, Kim H-N, et al: Corrosive esophageal stricture: safety and effectiveness of balloon dilation. Radiology 184:373–378, 1992.
54. Ball WS, Strife JL, Rosenkrantz J, et al: Esophageal strictures in children: treatment by balloon catheter dilatation. Radiology 150:263–264, 1984.
55. McLean GK, LeVeen RF. Shear stress in the performance of esophageal dilatation: comparison of balloon dilatation and bougienage. Radiology 172:983–986, 1989.
56. McLean GK, LeVeen RF. Shear stress in the performance of esophageal dilatation: comparison of balloon dilatation and bougienage. Radiology 172:983–986, 1989 (letter).
57. Lindahl H, Rintala R: Shear stress in the performance of esophageal dilatation: comparison of balloon dilatation and bougienage. Radiology 175:879, 1990 (letter).
58. Castañeda-Zuniga WR: Esophageal strictures: balloon dilatation. Radiology 171:285–286, 1989 (letter).
59. Cohen ME, Goldberg RI, Barkin JS: Esophageal strictures: balloon dilatation. Radiology 171:285–286, 1989 (letter).
60. LaBerge JM, Kerlan RK Jr, Pogany AC, et al: Esophageal rupture: complication of balloon dilatation. Radiology 157:56, 1985.
61. Bernardino ME, Amerson JR. Percutaneous gastrocystostomy: a new approach to pancreatic pseudocyst drainage. AJR 143:1096–1097, 1984.
62. Grosso M, Gandini G, Cassinis ME, et al: Percutaneous treatment (including pseudocystogastrostomy) of 74 pancreatic pseudocysts. Radiology 173:493–497, 1989.
63. Ho CS, Taylor B: Percutaneous transgastric drainage for pancreatic pseudocyst. AJR 143:623–625, 1984.
64. Kuligowska E, Olsen WL: Pancreatic pseudocysts drained through a percutaneous transgastric approach. Radiology 154:79–82, 1985.
65. Matzinger FRK, Ho C-S, Yee AC, et al: Pancreatic pseudocysts drained through a percutaneous transgastric approach: further experience. Radiology 167:431–434, 1988.
66. Wills JS: Percutaneous gastrostomy: applications in gastric carcinoma and gastroplasty stoma dilation. AJR 147:826–827, 1986.
67. Preshaw RM: A percutaneous method for inserting a feeding gastrostomy. Surg Gynecol Obstet 152:658–660, 1979.
68. Gauderer MWL, Ponsky JL, Izant RJ: Gastrostomy without laparotomy: a percutaneous endoscopic technique. J Pediatr Surg 15:872–875, 1980.
68a. Jarnagin WR, Duh Q-Y, Mulvihill SJ, et al: The efficacy and

limitations of percutaneous endoscopic gastrostomy. Arch Surg 127:261–264, 1992.

69. Ho C-S: Percutaneous gastrostomy for jejunal feeding. Radiology 149:595–596, 1983.

70. Wills JS, Oglesby JT: Percutaneous gastrostomy. Radiology 149:449–453, 1983.

71. Sacks BA, Vine HS, Palestrant AM, et al: A nonoperative technique for establishment of a gastrostomy in a dog. Invest Radiol 18:485–487, 1983.

72. Deutsch L-S, Kannegieter L, Vanson DT, et al: Simplified percutaneous gastrostomy. Radiology 184:181–183, 1992.

73. Tao HH, Gillies RR: Percutaneous feeding gastrostomy AJR 141:793–794, 1983.

74. Wills JS, Oglesby JT: Percutaneous gastrostomy: further experience. Radiology 154:71–74, 1985.

75. Ho C-S, Gray RR, Goldfinger M, et al: Percutaneous gastrostomy for enteral feeding. Radiology 156:349–351, 1985.

76. Malone JM, Koonce T, Larson DM, et al: Palliation of small bowel obstruction by percutaneous gastrostomy in patients with progressive ovarian carcinoma. Obstet Gynecol 68:431–433, 1986.

77. vanSonnenberg E, Wittich GR, Brown LK, et al: Percutaneous gastrostomy and gastroenterostomy: 1. Techniques derived from laboratory evaluation. AJR 146:577–580, 1986.

78. vanSonnenberg E, Wittich GR, Brown LK, et al: Percutaneous gastrostomy and gastroenterostomy: 2. Clinical experience. AJR 146:581–586, 1986.

79. Alzate GD, Coons HG, Elliott J, et al: Percutaneous gastrostomy for jejunal feeding: a new technique. AJR 147:822–825, 1986.

79a. Ho C-S, Yeung EY: Percutaneous gastrostomy and transgastric jejunostomy. AJR 185:251–257, 1992.

80. Foutch P: Percutaneous endoscopic gastrostomy (PEG): a new procedure comes of age. J Clin Gastroenterol 8:10–15, 1986.

81. Larson DE, Burton DD, Schroeder KW, et al: Percutaneous endoscopic gastrostomy: indications, success, complications, and mortality in 314 consecutive patients. Gastroenterology 93:48–52, 1987.

82. Picus D, Marx MV, Weyman PJ: Chronic intestinal obstruction: value of percutaneous gastrostomy tube placement. AJR 150:295–297, 1988.

82a. Yeung EY, MacPhadyen N, Ho C-S: Intractable gastroparesis: treatment with percutaneous fluoroscopically guided gastrostomies. Am J Gastroenterol 87:651–654, 1992.

83. Cory DA, Fitzgerald JF, Cohen MD: Percutaneous nonendoscopic gastrostomy in children. AJR 151:995–997, 1988.

84. Wills JS, Oglesby JT: Percutaneous gastrostomy. Radiology 167:41–43, 1988.

85. Halkier BK, Ho C-S, Yee ACN: Percutaneous feeding gastrostomy with the Seldinger technique: review of 252 patients. Radiology 171:359–362, 1989.

86. O'Keeffe F, Carrasco CH, Charnsangavej C, et al: Percutaneous drainage and feeding gastrostomies in 100 patients. Radiology 172:341–343, 1989.

87. Hicks ME, Surratt RS, Picus D, et al: Fluoroscopically guided percutaneous gastrostomy and gastroenterostomy: analysis of 158 consecutive cases. AJR 154:725–728, 1990.

88. Wittich G, vanSonnenberg E, Jantsch H: Percutaneous gastrostomy. *In* McGahan JP (ed): Interventional Ultrasound. Baltimore: Williams & Wilkins, 1990, pp 193–198.

89. Saini S, Mueller PR, Gaa J, et al: Percutaneous gastrostomy with gastropexy: experience in 125 patients. AJR 154:1003–1006, 1990.

90. Ho C-S: Percutaneous gastrostomy and transgastric jejunostomy. *In* Kadir S (ed): Current Practice of Interventional Radiology. Philadelphia: BC Decker, 1991, pp 444–449.

91. Gehman KE, Elliott JA, Inculet RI: Percutaneous gastrojejunostomy with a modified Cope loop catheter. AJR 155:79–80, 1990.

92. Rose DB, Wolman SL, Ho C-S: Gastric hemorrhage complicating percutaneous transgastric jejunostomy. Radiology 161:835–836, 1986.

93. Wojtowycz MM, Arata JA Jr, Micklos TJ, et al: CT findings after uncomplicated percutaneous gastrostomy. AJR 151:307–309, 1988.

93a. Sanches RB, van Sonnenberg E, D'Agostino HB, et al: CT guidance for percutaneous gastrostomy and gastroenterostomy. Radiology 184:201–205, 1992.

94. Wojtowycz MM, Arata JA Jr. Subcutaneous emphysema after percutaneous gastrostomy. AJR 151:311–312, 1988.

95. Ho C-S, Yee ACN, McPherson R: Complications of surgical and percutaneous nonendoscopic gastrostomy: review of 233 patients. Gastroenterology 95:1206–1210, 1988.

96. Kirby DF, Craig RM, Tsang T-K, et al: Percutaneous endoscopic gastrostomies: a prospective evaluation and review of the literature. JPEN 10:155–159, 1986.

97. Ponsky JL, Gauderer MWL, Stellato TA, et al: Percutaneous approaches to enteral alimentation. Am J Surg 149:102–105, 1985.

98. Ruge J, Vazquez RM: An analysis of the advantages of Stamm and percutaneous endoscopic gastrostomy. Surg Gynecol Obstet 162:13–16, 1986.

99. Shellito PC, Malt RA: Tube gastrostomy: techniques and complications. Ann Surg 201:180–184, 1985.

100. Wasilijew BK, Ujiki GT, Beal JM: Feeding gastrostomy: complication and mortality. Am J Surg 143:194–195, 1982.

101. vanSonnenberg E, Cubberley DA, Brown LK, et al: Percutaneous gastrostomy: use of intragastric balloon support. Radiology 152:531–532, 1984.

102. Varney RA, vanSonnenberg E, Casola G, et al: Balloon techniques for percutaneous gastrostomy in a patient with partial gastrectomy. Radiology 167:69–70, 1988.

103. Towbin RB, Ball WS Jr, Bissett GS III: Percutaneous gastrostomy and percutaneous gastrojejunostomy in children: antegrade approach. Radiology 168:473–476, 1988.

104. Keller MS, Lai S, Wagner DK. Percutaneous gastrostomy in a child. Radiology 160:261–262, 1986.

105. Brown AS, Mueller PR, Ferrucci JT Jr: Controlled percutaneous gastrostomy: nylon T-fastener for fixation of the anterior gastric wall. Radiology 158:543–545, 1986.

106. Brown AS, Mueller PR: Controlled percutaneous gastrostomy: nylon T-fastener for fixation of the anterior abdominal wall. Radiology 160:278, 1986 (letter).

107. Coleman CC, Coons HG, Cope C, et al: Percutaneous enterostomy with the Cope suture anchor. Radiology 174:889–891, 1990.

108. Cope C: Suture anchor for visceral drainage. AJR 146:160–161, 1986.

109. Moote DJ, Ho C-S, Felice V: Fluoroscopically guided percutaneous gastrostomy: is gastric fixation necessary? Can Assoc Radiol J 41:363–368, 1990.

110. Wills JS, Oglesby JT: Controlled percutaneous gastrostomy: nylon T-fastener for fixation of the anterior abdominal wall. Radiology 170:1055–1057, 1989 (letter).

111. Maroney TP, Ring EJ, Gordon RL, et al: Role of interventional radiology in the management of major esophageal leaks. Radiology 170:1055–1057, 1989.

112. Neff C, Lawson DW: Boerhaave syndrome: interventional radiologic management. AJR 145:819–820, 1985.

113. Meranze SG, LeVeen RF, Burke DR, et al: Transesophageal drainage of mediastinal abscesses. Radiology 165:395–398, 1987.

114. Kaszar-Seibert DJ, Korn WT, Bindman DJ, et al: Treatment of acute esophageal food impaction with a combination of glucagon, effervescent agent, and water. AJR 154:533–534, 1990.

115. Smith JC, Janower ML, Geiger AH: Use of glucagon and gas-forming agents in acute esophageal food impaction. Radiology 159:567–568, 1986 (letter).

116. Trenkner SW, Maglinte DDT, Lehman GA, et al: Esophageal food impaction: treatment with glucagon. Radiology 149:401–403, 1983.

117. Rice BT, Spiegel PK, Dombrowski PJ: Acute esophageal food impaction treated by gas-forming agents. Radiology 146:299–301, 1983.

118. Friedland GW: The treatment of acute esophageal food impaction. Radiology 149:601–602, 1983.

119. Ferrucci JT Jr, Long, JA Jr: Radiologic treatment of esophageal food impaction using intravenous glucagon. Radiology 125:25–28, 1977.

120. Alexander AA, Hayden CK Jr, Swischuk LE: Catheter removal of esophageal foreign bodies: push or pull? AJR 151:835, 1988 (letter).

121. Campbell JB, Quattromani FL, Foley LC: Foley catheter removal of blunt esophageal foreign bodies: experience with 100 consecutive children. Pediatr Radiol 13:116–119, 1983.
122. Nixon GW: Foley catheter method of esophageal foreign body removal: extension of applications. AJR 132:441–442, 1979.
123. Campbell JB, Davis WS: Catheter technique for extraction of blunt esophageal foreign bodies. Radiology 108:438–440, 1973.
124. Shackelford GD, McAlister WH, Robertson CL: The use of a Foley catheter for removal of blunt esophageal foreign bodies from children. Radiology 105:455–456, 1972.
125. Shaffer Jr HA, Alford BA, de Lange EE, et al: Basket extraction of esophageal foreign bodies. AJR 147:1010–1013, 1086.
126. Volle E, Hanel D, Beyer P: Ingested foreign bodies: removal by magnet. Radiology 160:407–409, 1986.
127. Volle E, Beyer P, Kaufmann HJ: Therapeutic approach to ingested button-type batteries. Pediatr Radiol 19:114–118, 1989.
128. Towbin RB, Dunbar JS, Rice S: Magnet catheter for removal of magnetic foreign bodies. AJR 154:149–150, 1990.
129. Jaffe RB, Corneli HM: Fluoroscopic removal of ingested alkaline batteries. Radiology 150:585–586, 1984.

# SECTION
# V

# Esophagus

# Motility Disorders

### David J. Ott, M.D.

## INTRODUCTION

Motility disorders of the esophagus are an important cause of esophageal complaints, especially when symptoms are not readily explained by a structural abnormality. An understanding of esophageal anatomy and physiology is required for proper radiographic evaluation of normal and abnormal esophageal function. This chapter first reviews normal anatomy and physiology of the esophagus and then discusses radiographic evaluation of esophageal function. The major portion of the chapter is devoted to the various esophageal motility disorders, particularly the primary motility disorders. Radiologic efficacy in evaluating esophageal function in relation to esophageal manometry and clinical symptoms is also considered.

## NORMAL ESOPHAGEAL ANATOMY

The esophagus is a muscular tube measuring 20 to 24 cm in length. It is composed of outer longitudinal and inner circular muscle fibers and is lined by stratified squamous epithelium.[1] Striated muscle predominates in the upper esophagus, and smooth muscle predominates in the lower half or lower two thirds of the esophagus. The transition from striated to smooth muscle varies in location but usually occurs at the level of the aortic arch.[1, 2] Although this transitional zone is not evident radiographically, certain motility disorders may selectively involve the smooth or striated muscle portions of the esophagus.

Opening and closing of the upper and lower ends of the esophagus are regulated by the upper esophageal sphincter (UES) and lower esophageal sphincter (LES), respectively. The UES is located at the pharyngoesophageal junction and is formed primarily by the cricopharyngeal muscle, which is the horizontal portion of the inferior pharyngeal constrictor. The LES is not a distinct muscular entity but is defined manometrically as a high-pressure zone measuring 2 to 4 cm in length in the esophagogastric region.[1, 3] This physiologic sphincter corresponds in location to the anatomic lower esophageal vestibule.[3, 4]

## NORMAL ESOPHAGEAL PHYSIOLOGY

In the resting state, the esophageal body is normally collapsed, and the UES and LES are closed to prevent retrograde flow of esophageal and gastric contents.[1, 5] The major function of the esophagus is the transport of solids and liquids from the oral cavity to the stomach. The chief mechanism of bolus transport is esophageal peristalsis, which is assisted by gravity in the upright position. However, radiographic and manometric evaluation of esophageal peristalsis usually is performed with the patient in a horizontal position to eliminate the effects of gravity.

Primary esophageal peristalsis is initiated by swallowing. A rapid wave of inhibition, not apparent radiographically, is followed by a slower wave of contraction, which traverses the entire length of the esophagus (Fig. 23–1). Relaxation of the UES occurs within 0.2 to 0.3 second of the initiation of swallowing, and relaxation of the LES occurs several seconds later.[1, 5, 6] The LES remains relaxed as the oncoming bolus approaches the distal esophagus. It then returns to its resting tone shortly after the bolus reaches the stomach. The primary peristaltic contraction wave propagates through the esophagus in about 6 to 8 seconds.

Secondary peristalsis and nonperistaltic contractions are other types of esophageal functional activity.[1, 6–9] Secondary peristalsis is similar to primary peristalsis, but it is initiated by local esophageal stimulation or distention. Once initiated, a secondary peristaltic contraction wave propagates aborally in the same way as primary peristalsis. In contrast, nonperistaltic or tertiary contractions are not propagated aborally. They typically involve the smooth muscle segment of the esophagus and may occur spontaneously or during swallowing. Nonperistaltic contractions may be single or multiple, simultaneous or repetitive, and feeble or strong. De-

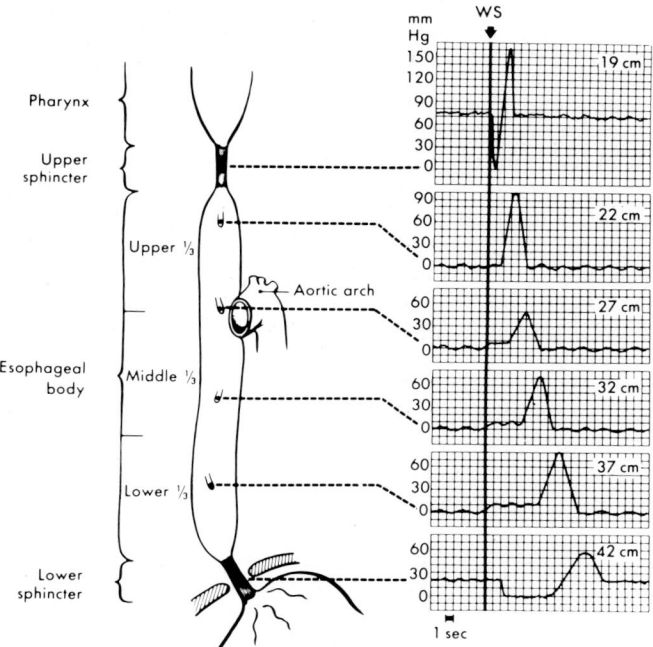

**Figure 23–1. Manometric representation of normal esophageal peristalsis.** Measurements are taken from multiple recording sites in the esophagus, including the UES and LES. After a wet swallow (WS), UES relaxation is followed almost immediately by prolonged LES relaxation. The primary peristaltic contraction wave is seen as an aborally progressing pressure peak. (From Dodds WJ: Normal motor physiology and motility disorders. *In* Margulis AR, Burhenne HJ [eds]: Alimentary Tract Radiology, Volume 1 [4th ed]. St. Louis: CV Mosby, 1989, p 430.)

pending on their severity, they may narrow or obliterate the esophageal lumen, producing a characteristic appearance on barium studies (Fig. 23–2). Nonperistaltic contractions may occur as a nonspecific finding, or they may be related to structural or motility disorders of the esophagus.

Variations in esophageal function that occur among individuals are primarily related to aging. In young adults, approximately 95% of "wet" swallows result in a complete peristaltic sequence, followed invariably by LES relaxation.[10] Nonperistaltic contractions are rare in this age group. However, older patients more often exhibit incomplete peristaltic sequences during swallowing, with occasional LES dysfunction and a higher prevalence and severity of nonperistaltic contractions.[11–13] The amplitude of peristalsis, as recorded manometrically, also decreases with age. Thus, mild functional disturbances of the esophagus that are observed in the elderly must be interpreted with caution and correlated with the clinical findings.

## RADIOGRAPHIC EVALUATION

Radiographic evaluation of esophageal motility includes an examination of the esophageal body and both sphincters.[1, 7–9, 14] During swallowing, the UES relaxes,

and the pharyngoesophageal segment opens widely in response to bolus distention. Abnormal relaxation or a persistent impression from the cricopharyngeal muscle may be observed in some patients. These abnormalities are often associated with other signs of pharyngeal dysmotility, such as aspiration or stasis of barium within the pharyngeal recesses. Motion recording techniques, using videotape or cineradiography, facilitate evaluation of the pharynx and UES.

The fluoroscopic examination is usually adequate to evaluate esophageal motility, but motion recording techniques may be used to document esophageal function. The patient is placed in the prone oblique position and is instructed to take single swallows of barium. At least five barium swallows are required for adequate evaluation of esophageal peristalsis and LES relaxation.[5, 15] Single swallows must be observed, because a second swallow taken before completion of a primary contraction wave would inhibit the propagating wave and be mistaken for a peristaltic abnormality. Rapid, repetitive swallowing does not allow assessment of primary esoph-

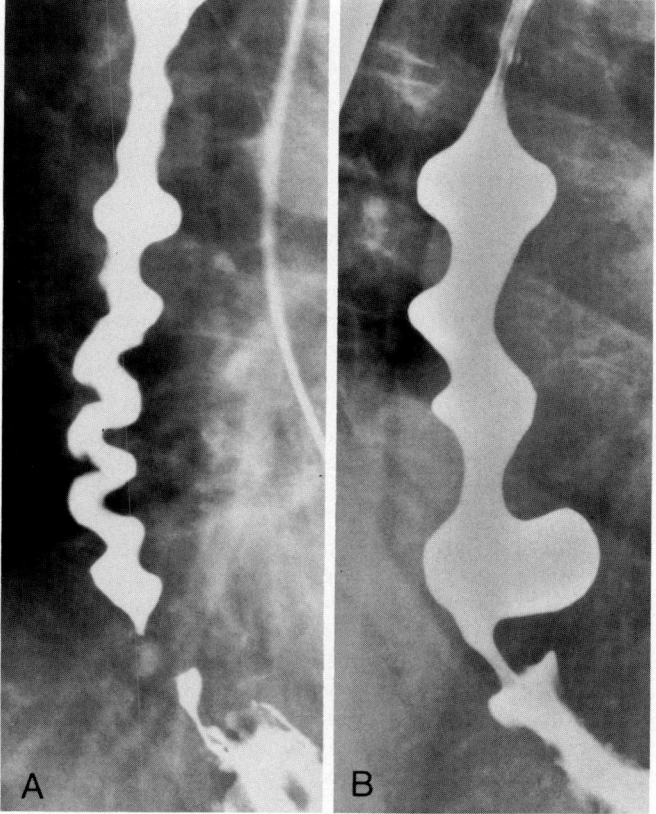

**Figure 23–2. Nonperistaltic contractions in the esophagus. A.** Barium study of an 89-year-old man with dysphagia but no chest pain. There is diffuse "curling" of the esophagus because of simultaneous nonperistaltic contractions. A nonspecific esophageal motility disorder (NEMD) was diagnosed on manometric examination. **B.** Another elderly man without esophageal symptoms has less severe simultaneous nonperistaltic contractions. (**A** and **B** from Ott DJ: Radiologic evaluation of esophageal dysphagia. Curr Probl Diagn Radiol 17:1–33, 1988.)

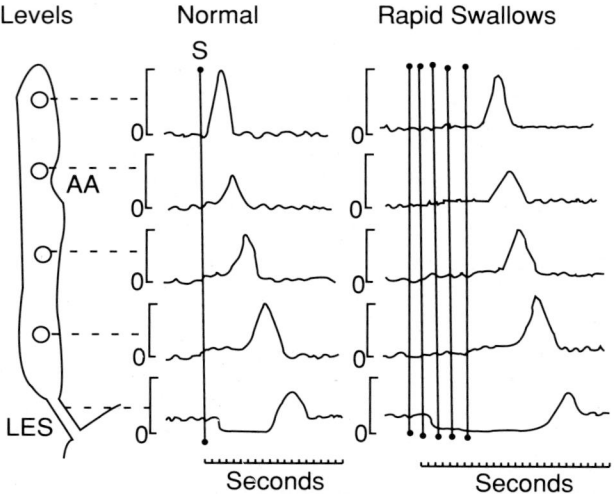

Levels        Normal        Rapid Swallows

**Figure 23–3. Manometric representation of normal esophageal peristalsis.** Measurements are taken from multiple recording levels in the esophagus. Rapid swallows cause prolonged LES relaxation but do not generate a primary peristaltic sequence until the final swallow. AA = aortic arch; S = swallow.

ageal peristalsis but distends the esophagus maximally for structural evaluation (Fig. 23–3).

As barium is propelled into the esophagus through the relaxed UES, a normal primary peristaltic sequence is seen as an aboral contraction wave that obliterates the esophageal lumen and progressively strips the barium bolus from the esophagus (Fig. 23–4). The lumen-obliterating wave imparts an inverted V configuration to the top of the barium column, which corresponds to the peristaltic pressure peak seen at manometry. In younger individuals, the peristaltic contraction wave normally strips all of the barium from the esophagus. Occasionally, however, some proximal escape of barium occurs at the level of the aortic arch (Fig. 23–5). This proximal escape is caused by a low-amplitude pressure trough at the junction of the striated and smooth muscle portions of the esophagus, which prevents complete obliteration of the esophageal lumen and allows retrograde flow of barium.[2, 5, 16] Proximal escape becomes more frequent with age and can be misinterpreted as a peristaltic abnormality. True esophageal motility disorders may be manifested by weakened or absent primary peristalsis, nonperistaltic contractions, or associated structural abnormalities in the esophagus.

Radiographic examination of the LES requires evaluation of functional and structural abnormalities. The LES relaxes shortly after swallowing, and the esophagogastric segment opens widely in response to bolus distention. In patients with achalasia, incomplete relaxation of the LES produces a smooth, tapered appearance at the lower end of the esophagus because of failure of the esophagogastric junction to distend normally. Mucosal irregularity or nodularity of the esophagogastric region should suggest an inflammatory or neoplastic process, which may cause a secondary motility disorder of the esophagus.

# ESOPHAGEAL MOTILITY DISORDERS

Esophageal motility disorders usually are classified as primary or secondary types[1, 7–9, 17–19] (Table 23–1). In primary motility disorders, the esophagus is the primary or only organ involved. Secondary esophageal motility disturbances result from a wide variety of systemic diseases or from physical or chemical injury of the esophagus. The classification of esophageal motility disorders, especially the primary types, is still evolving. New disorders have been described in recent years, and others have been reclassified or eliminated. As a result, there is overlap in the classification of these disorders, and some patients with esophageal dysmotility are not easily labeled.

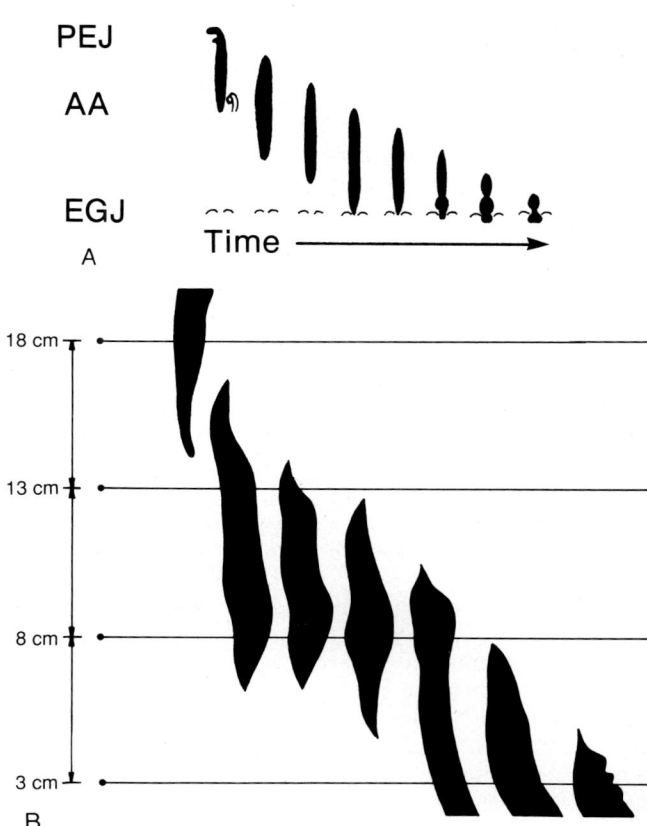

**Figure 23–4. Normal primary peristalsis. A.** Schematic representation of normal primary peristalsis with a lumen-obliterating contraction wave stripping all of the barium from the esophagus. AA = aortic arch; EGJ = esophagogastric junction; PEJ = pharyngoesophageal junction. (From Ott DJ: Radiologic evaluation of esophageal dysphagia. Curr Probl Diagn Radiol 17:1–33, 1988.) **B.** Videotaped temporal tracings of a 5-mL barium bolus at 1-second intervals show normal primary peristalsis. The tapered tops of the barium column correspond to the peristaltic contraction wave seen during synchronous manometry. The numbers on the vertical axis represent the positions of the manometric catheter ports above the LES. (From Ott DJ, Chen YM, Hewson EG, et al: Esophageal motility: assessment with synchronous video tape fluoroscopy and manometry. Radiology 173:419–422, 1989.)

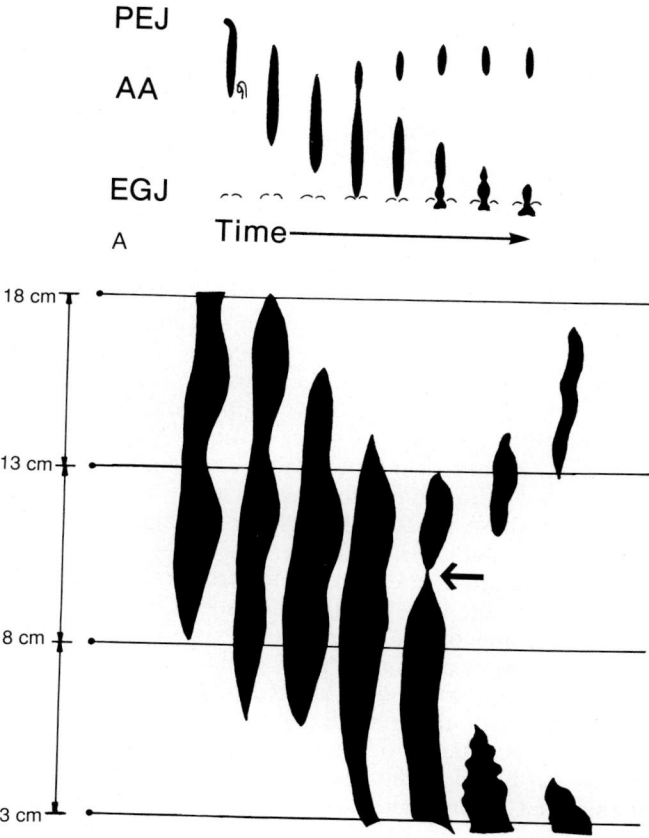

**Figure 23–5. Proximal excape. A.** A manometric representation showing normal primary peristalsis with proximal escape, as the contraction wave fails to obliterate the lumen completely at the level of the aortic arch (AA). Note that the peristaltic sequence continues aborally. EGJ = esophagogastric junction; PEJ = pharyngoesophageal junction. (From Ott DJ: Radiologic evaluation of esophageal dysphagia. Curr Probl Diagn Radiol 17:1–33, 1988.) **B.** Videotaped temporal tracing of a 5-mL barium bolus at 1-second intervals show normal primary peristalsis associated with proximal escape *(arrow).* The lower esophagus is normally stripped of barium below the area of escape. The numbers on the vertical axis represent the positions of the manometric catheter ports above the LES. (From Ott DJ, Chen YM, Hewson EG, et al: Esophageal motility: assessment with synchronous video tape fluoroscopy and manometry. Radiology 173:419–422, 1989.)

## Primary Motility Disorders

### *Achalasia*

Achalasia, the best known of the primary esophageal motility disorders, is characterized by aperistalsis and LES dysfunction.[7–9, 14, 17, 20] The cause of achalasia is unknown, but histologic lesions have been found in the dorsal vagal nucleus, vagal trunks, and myenteric ganglia of the esophagus.[20, 21] Ganglionic cells are decreased in number in achalasia, but a narrow aganglionic segment is not present, as in Hirschsprung's disease. Thus, achalasia appears to be a neurogenic disorder. This theory is supported by the hyper-responsiveness of the esoph-

ageal body to cholinergic stimulation (i.e., denervation hypersensitivity).

Achalasia is characterized pathologically by esophageal dilatation.[21] Some patients may have a massively dilated esophagus, or megaesophagus, but this finding is not specific for achalasia. Changes in smooth muscle are variable; both atrophy and hypertrophy have been described. Secondary stasis esophagitis is common and may be associated with ulceration. Achalasia may also be a precursor of esophageal carcinoma. The association with carcinoma varies but in a study of 1318 patients, the risk of carcinoma was found to be 2.7 to 14 times greater than that in the general population.[22]

Achalasia occurs equally among males and females and usually affects patients during the middle decades of life.[20, 21] The typical clinical presentation is slowly progressive dysphagia for both solids and liquids. Painful swallowing and chest pain are less common findings. Weight loss often occurs in more severe cases. Regurgitation is a common finding, and it can lead to pulmonary symptoms such as choking, coughing, aspiration, and pneumonia. If symptoms have a more rapid onset in older patients and are accompanied by chest pain or odynophagia, secondary achalasia attributable to malignancy is more likely.[23–25]

Achalasia is characterized manometrically by absence of primary peristalsis, elevated or normal resting LES pressures, and incomplete or absent LES relaxation[17, 20] (Fig. 23–6). Other patients may have variants of achalasia with atypical manometric findings. A variant called *vigorous achalasia* is characterized by high-amplitude, simultaneous, and repetitive contractions.[20, 26, 27] These patients may present with chest pain and have less

---

**TABLE 23–1. CLASSIFICATION OF ESOPHAGEAL MOTILITY DISORDERS**

**PRIMARY MOTILITY DISORDERS**
Achalasia and variants
Diffuse esophageal spasm
Nutcracker esophagus
Nonspecific esophageal motility disorder
Presbyesophagus?
Hypertensive LES

**SECONDARY MOTILITY DISORDERS**
Collagen-vascular disease
Chemical or physical agents
   Reflux esophagitis
   Caustic esophagitis
   Radiation therapy
Infectious causes
Diabetes mellitus
Alcoholism
Endocrine disease
Neuromuscular disorders
   Cerebrovascular disease
   Demyelinating disorders
   Chorea-related disorders
   Myasthenia gravis
   Muscular dystrophies
   Other rare causes
Idiopathic intestinal pseudo-obstruction

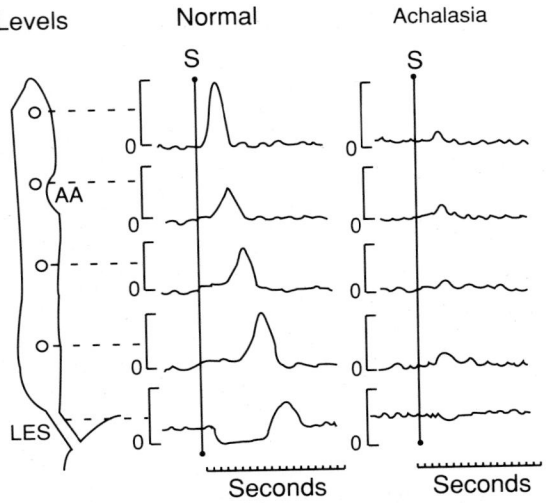

**Figure 23–6. Manometric representation of normal peristalsis and achalasia.** Measurements are taken from multiple recording levels in the esophagus. In this example of achalasia, peristalsis and LES relaxation are absent, and LES pressure is elevated. AA = aortic arch; LES = lower esophageal sphincter; S = swallow.

esophageal dilatation. Another variant, called *early achalasia*, is characterized by aperistalsis with normal LES relaxation.[20, 28, 29] Patients with this variant also have less esophageal dilatation and tend to be younger. Both of these variants may represent part of the spectrum of

achalasia or, alternatively, transitional motility disorders evolving toward classic achalasia.[30–34]

Radiographically, primary peristalsis is absent on all swallows observed.[1, 7–9, 14] Typically, the lower end of the esophagus has a smooth, tapered, beak-like appearance at the level of the esophageal hiatus (Fig. 23–7). This tapered appearance reflects LES dysfunction and failure of the barium bolus to distend the tonically contracted sphincter. Depending on the severity and duration of achalasia, the esophagus may become markedly dilated and tortuous, producing a sigmoid appearance. Some patients may have retained food, secretions, and barium in the dilated esophagus (Fig. 23–8A). Advanced achalasia can sometimes be recognized on chest radiographs when massive esophageal dilatation is present (Fig. 23–8B). In other patients with vigorous achalasia, repetitive nonperistaltic contractions may be observed. Radiographic findings in early achalasia are similar to those described in classic achalasia, but less esophageal dilatation is present.

Achalasia must be differentiated from other causes of narrowing at the lower end of the esophagus (Table 23–2). Carcinoma of the esophagogastric region must be excluded, especially in older patients who have abrupt onset of symptoms and associated odynophagia.[23–25] Although most of these malignancies are associated with mucosal irregularity or mass effect, carcinoma of the gastric cardia and other neoplasms may occasionally be manifested by smooth, tapered narrowing of the lower esophagus and aperistalsis, simulating achalasia (Fig. 23–9). Peptic strictures are usually associated with intact primary peristalsis, and these patients almost always have hiatal hernias, a rare finding in achalasia. Uncomplicated scleroderma can also be differentiated from achalasia, as it is characterized by a dilated esophagus with a patulous esophagogastric region. Occasionally, however, peptic strictures complicating scleroderma may produce an appearance that closely resembles achalasia.

Achalasia is treated by pneumatic dilatation or a Heller myotomy.[35–39] Radiographic evaluation of the esophagus immediately after pneumatic dilatation is helpful in detecting serious complications such as perforation.[40–44] After a Heller myotomy, an outpouching resembling a diverticulum is typically present at the lower end of the esophagus (Fig. 23–10A). The treatment of achalasia (especially after surgical myotomy) may also be complicated by reflux esophagitis and subsequent peptic strictures (Fig. 23–10B).

Radionuclide studies may be performed to facilitate the diagnosis and management of patients with achala-

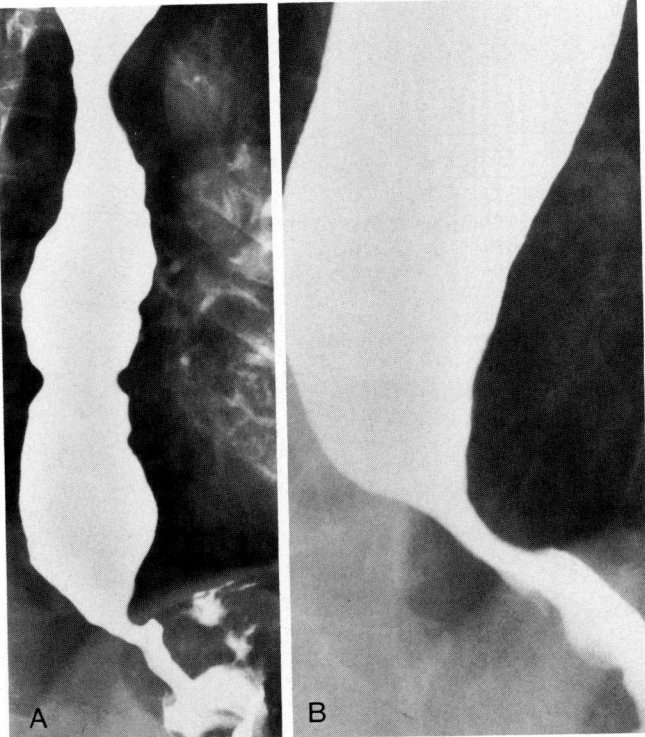

**Figure 23–7. Achalasia. A.** There is a dilated esophagus with smooth, tapered narrowing at the esophagogastric region. Esophageal aperistalsis was seen at fluoroscopy. **B.** A close-up view shows smooth, beak-like tapering at the lower end of the esophagus due to LES dysfunction.

---

**TABLE 23–2. DIFFERENTIAL DIAGNOSIS OF ACHALASIA**

Intrinsic neoplasms
Extrinsic neoplasms
Peptic stricture
Complicated scleroderma
Intestinal pseudo-obstruction
Chagas' disease
Hypertensive LES
Postvagotomy effect

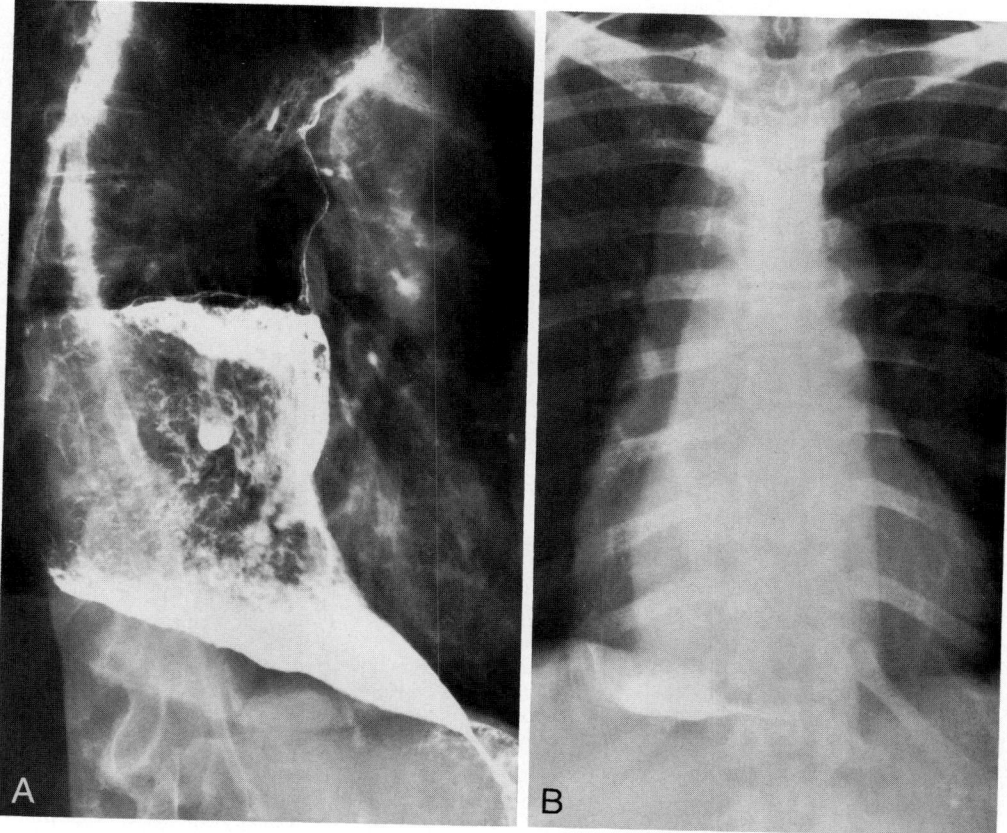

**Figure 23–8. Advanced achalasia. A.** There is a markedly dilated esophagus with retained secretions and food. **B.** A double contour of the right mediastinal border is seen in another patient with advanced achalasia. The outer border represents the dilated esophagus projecting beyond the shadows of the aorta and heart. A small amount of retained barium is present in the distal esophagus.

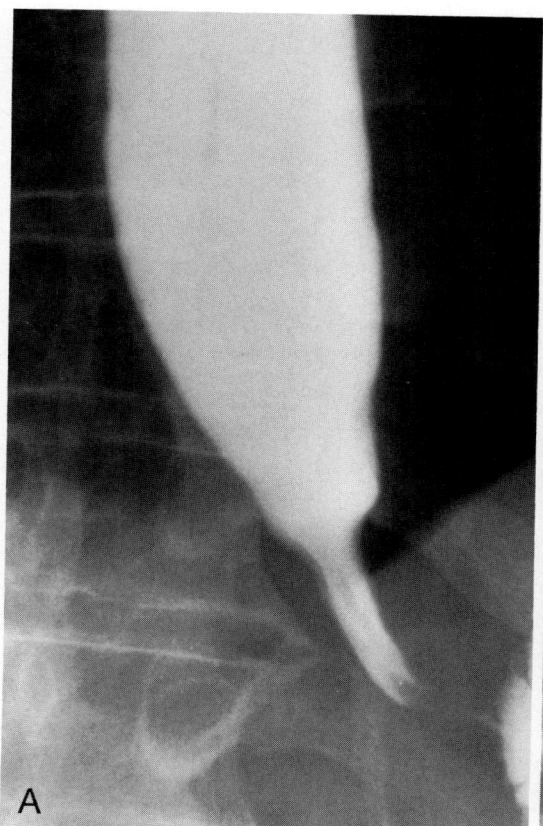
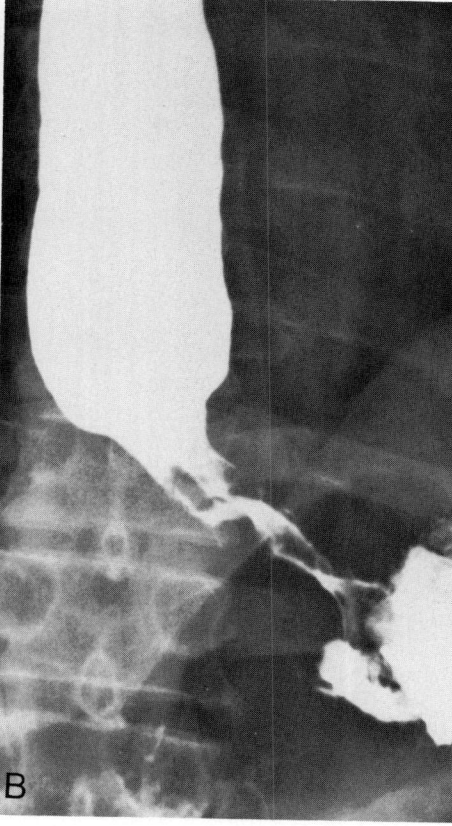

**Figure 23–9. Secondary achalasia, or pseudoachalasia. A.** Smooth narrowing of the esophagogastric junction simulates achalasia. This patient had a scirrhous carcinoma of the proximal stomach invading the distal esophagus. (From Ott DJ: Radiologic evaluation of esophageal dysphagia. Curr Probl Diagn Radiol 17:1–33, 1988.) **B.** Fluoroscopy in another patient revealed esophageal dilatation and aperistalsis. However, there is irregular tapering of the esophagogastric region due to gastric carcinoma.

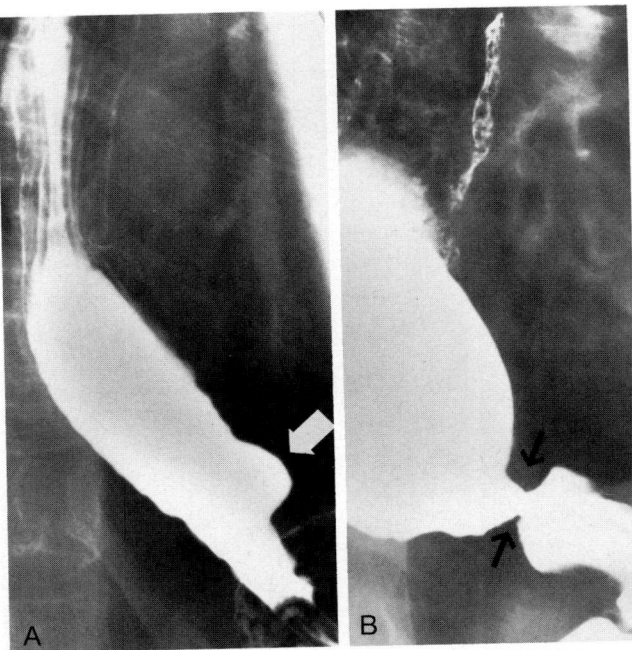

**Figure 23–10. Complications of a Heller myotomy. A.** A deformity *(arrow)* resembling a diverticulum is seen in this patient after a Heller myotomy for achalasia. **B.** A stricture *(arrows)* is present in the distal esophagus after a Heller myotomy in another patient with achalasia. The stricture was confirmed by endoscopy.

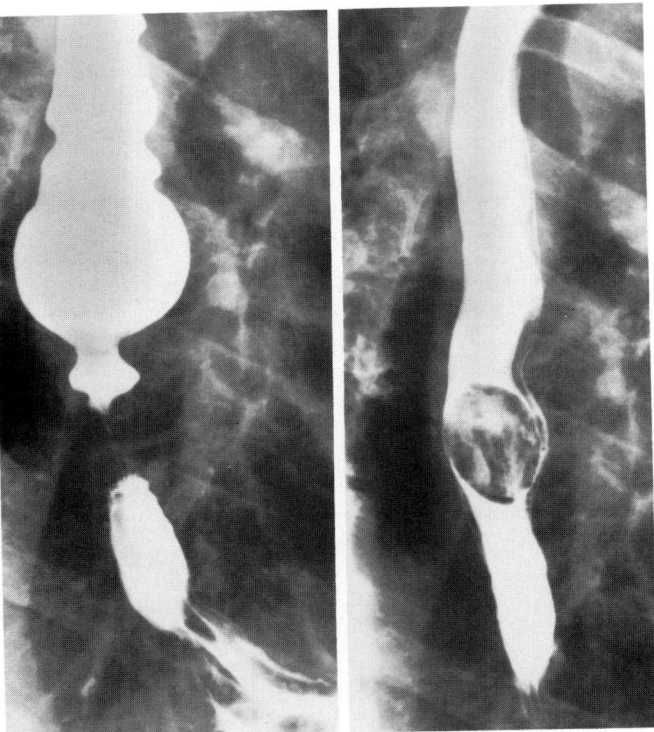

**Figure 23–11. Food impaction associated with DES.** This patient with DES complained of acute odynophagia after ingestion of a hot dog. On the left, an obliterative contraction of the lower esophagus obscures the food bolus. On the right, another film obtained moments later shows a piece of the hot dog. Endoscopic removal was required.

sia.[28, 29, 45–48] Radionuclide transit and emptying studies are particularly helpful in quantitating esophageal retention before and after therapy.

## Diffuse Esophageal Spasm

Diffuse esophageal spasm (DES) is an uncommon motility disorder characterized by chest pain, which is often accompanied by dysphagia, and intermittently abnormal esophageal motility.[35, 49] Although the cause of DES is unknown, a transition to other types of motility disorders has occasionally been described. DES, achalasia, and vigorous achalasia may be part of a spectrum of abnormal esophageal motility that is related to varying degrees of neurogenic damage and that accompanies changes in the esophageal wall.[30–34]

DES typically involves the smooth muscle portion of the esophagus. Pathologically, the esophageal musculature may be relatively normal or markedly thickened because of hypertrophy.[21, 50–52] If muscular hypertrophy is present, the circular layer of the muscularis propria is most often affected. However, some investigators have found that muscle thickening is a rare occurrence in DES.[53, 54] Unlike achalasia, DES usually does not involve the esophagogastric region, and the ganglionic cells are invariably preserved.

The most common clinical presentation of DES is chest pain, often accompanied by dysphagia.[35, 49] The chest pain is intermittent and can be mild or severe. Radiation of pain to the shoulder or back may simulate angina and may even be relieved by nitroglycerin. The pain is often spontaneous and not related to swallowing,

it can awake the patient from sleep, and it can worsen during emotional stress. Other patients with DES may have dysphagia for solids or liquids without associated chest pain. Food impaction is a dramatic but unusual feature of DES (Fig. 23–11).

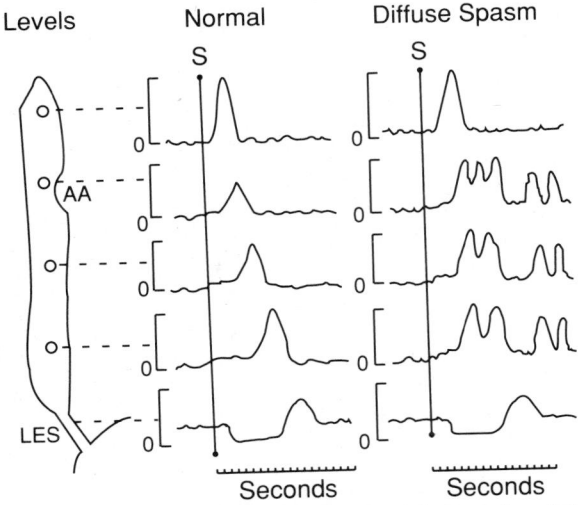

**Figure 23–12. Manometric representation of normal peristalsis and DES.** Measurements are taken from multiple recording levels in the esophagus. Normal peristalsis is present in the upper esophagus, but it is replaced by simultaneous, repetitive contractions below the aortic arch (AA). Normal LES relaxation is seen. S = swallow.

The major manometric criteria for DES are simultaneous contractions on more than 10% of wet swallows and intermittently normal primary peristalsis.[49] Associated findings include repetitive or prolonged-duration contractions, high-amplitude contractions, and frequent spontaneous contractions (Fig. 23–12). Most patients with DES have normal LES function with complete sphincter relaxation during swallowing. However, high resting sphincter pressures and incomplete LES relaxation are occasionally found.

The radiographic features of DES reflect the manometric findings.[1, 7–9, 14, 54] Primary peristalsis is present in the cervical esophagus but intermittently absent in the thoracic esophagus. Nonperistaltic contractions affect the smooth muscle portion of the esophagus, replacing the disrupted primary wave (Fig. 23–13). These contractions are often repetitive and simultaneous, and they may compartmentalize the esophageal lumen, producing the typical "corkscrew" or "rosary bead" appearance (see Fig. 23–13B). Coexisting pulsion diverticula may be present.

Muscular thickening of the esophagus is uncommon in DES, but a wall thickness of 2 cm or more is occasionally seen (normal wall thickness is less than 4 mm).[53, 54] Thickening of the esophageal wall is best estimated along the right border of the esophagus, where the wall is close to the pleural reflection line. Alternatively, wall thickness can be measured directly by endoscopic ultrasound.

The radiographic findings in DES can be minimal or nonspecific, so that correlation with clinical symptoms and esophageal manometry is required. As in achalasia, neoplastic lesions involving the esophagogastric region may cause a secondary motility disorder that mimics DES. Structural disorders of the esophagus, especially inflammatory diseases, may also cause esophageal dysmotility with nonperistaltic contractions. Similar radiographic findings are observed in other primary or secondary motility disorders and may sometimes occur in asymptomatic patients. Thus, the diagnosis of DES is made on the basis of clinical, radiographic, and manometric findings.

## Nutcracker Esophagus

Nutcracker esophagus is an esophageal motility disorder seen in some patients with chest pain or dysphagia.[18, 55–57] It is characterized on manometric examination by normal peristalsis with distal contractions of abnormally high amplitude and prolonged duration. Nutcracker esophagus has emerged as a potentially important motility disorder as a result of the increasing referral of patients with noncardiac chest pain for esophageal manometry. The cause of nutcracker esophagus is unknown, and debate has arisen over whether this entity is a true motility disorder, a result of improved manometric instrumentation, or part of the normal spectrum of esophageal function.[18, 55–61]

The specific manometric criteria for nutcracker esophagus include the presence of normal peristalsis with distal peristaltic pressure amplitudes greater than two standard deviations from normal and with prolonged duration of peristaltic contractions.[18] In our manometric laboratory, the normal mean distal esophageal amplitude is 100 ± 80 mm Hg (± 2 SD).[62] The diagnosis of nutcracker esophagus therefore requires peristaltic contractions with average amplitudes greater than 180 mm Hg (Fig. 23–14). The term *high-amplitude peristaltic esophageal contractions* has also been used to describe this entity.

Nutcracker esophagus is primarily a manometric diagnosis made in patients with appropriate symptoms. Usually, the radiographic examination is normal or reveals only nonspecific findings such as nonperistaltic contractions.[63, 64] This absence of specific findings is not surprising, because intact primary esophageal peristalsis is required for the diagnosis of nutcracker esophagus. In addition, esophageal transit is normal, despite some controversy regarding the results of radionuclide studies in patients with this disorder.[65–69] As currently understood, nutcracker esophagus is therefore not a radiologic diagnosis.

## Nonspecific Esophageal Motility Disorder

Nonspecific esophageal motility disorder (NEMD) is a "catchall" category used for symptomatic patients with

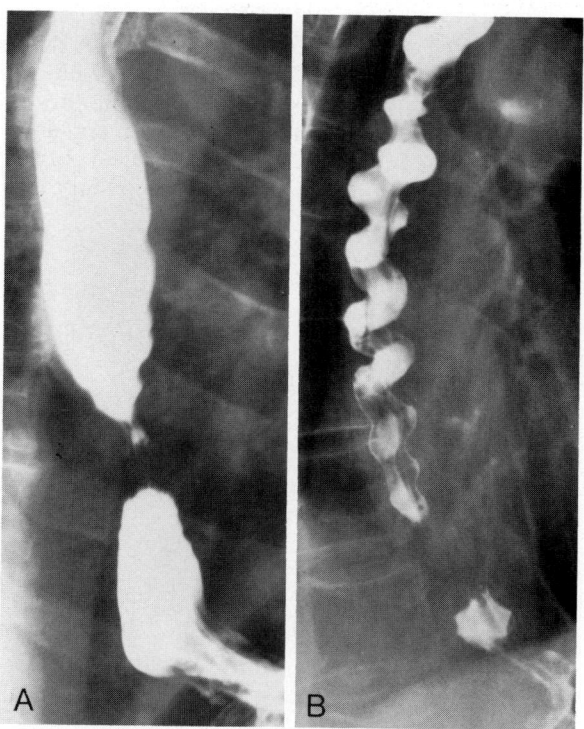

**Figure 23–13. DES. A.** This patient has DES with intermittent disruption of primary peristalsis associated with focally obliterative simultaneous contractions. **B.** Another patient has the typical "corkscrew" or "rosary bead" appearance of DES. Clinical and manometric correlations are required to confirm this diagnosis, because this appearance is nonspecific, especially in the elderly. (**A** and **B** from MS Levine, SE Rubesin, DJ Ott, Update on esophageal radiology, AJR, 155, 5, 933–941, 1990, © by American Roentgen Ray Society.)

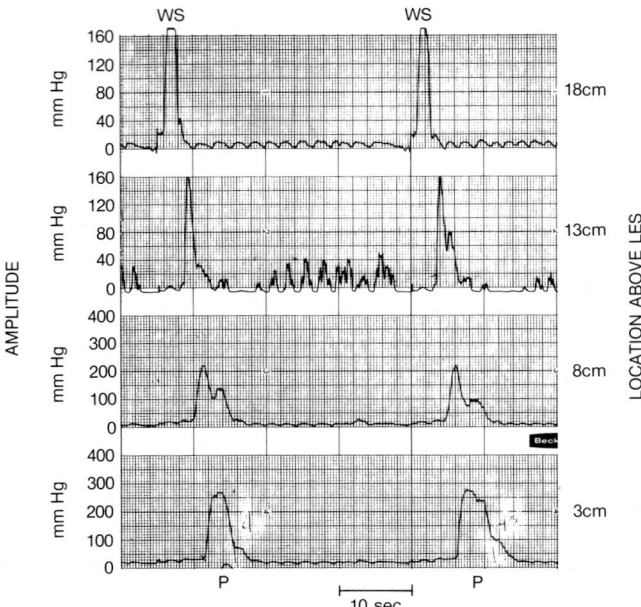

**Figure 23–14. Manometric representation of nutcracker esophagus.** This patient had a normal radiographic examination. There is normal peristalsis (P) manometrically with high-amplitude contractions (>200 mm Hg, *lower two leads*). Accentuated baseline activity in the 13-cm lead is cardiac artifact. LES = lower esophageal sphincter; WS = wet swallow. (From DJ Ott, JE Richter, YM Chen, et al, Esophageal radiography and manometry: correlation in 172 patients with dysphagia, AJR, 149, 2, 307–311, 1987, © by American Roentgen Ray Society.)

motility disturbances that defy specific classification.[14, 17, 18] Not infrequently, manometry reveals esophageal motility abnormalities that do not fit the criteria for specific motility disorders such as achalasia.[17, 18, 70, 71] Patients with NEMD often have dysphagia or chest pain, but symptoms may be minimal.

Manometric abnormalities include intermittent absence of peristalsis on 20% or more of wet swallows, low-amplitude peristalsis, prolonged duration of peristalsis, repetitive or triple-peaked contractions, or incomplete LES relaxation[17, 18, 70] (Fig. 23–15). Radiographic findings may reflect these manometric abnormalities.[14] Disruption of primary peristalsis and nonperistaltic contractions are typically seen (Fig. 23–16). However, the radiographic examination is often normal in patients with NEMD who have only minor manometric abnormalities.[14] The nonspecific abnormalities identified radiographically may also overlap the findings seen in other primary or secondary motility disorders, so that careful clinical correlation is required.

### Presbyesophagus

Presbyesophagus has become a controversial entity.[11, 12, 14] As originally described, the term *presbyesophagus* referred to esophageal motility dysfunction associated with aging.[72, 73] The major manometric criteria included decreased frequency of normal peristalsis, increased frequency of nonperistaltic contractions, and less commonly, incomplete LES relaxation. These manometric

changes are reflected by a wide spectrum of radiographic abnormalities. However, in early reports of presbyesophagus, many of the older patients had underlying neurologic disorders or diabetes, which could have accounted for their esophageal dysmotility. Later manometric studies in older patients have shown only minor changes in esophageal motility with aging.[11-13] Furthermore, many of the manometric criteria for presbyesophagus are similar to those for NEMD, which has become the preferred term to describe esophageal dysfunction in these patients.

### Hypertensive Lower Esophageal Sphincter

Hypertensive LES was first described in patients with esophageal symptoms who had unusually high resting LES pressures.[18, 74] The disorder is rare, and its cause is unknown. Nearly all patients have chest pain, and many also have dysphagia. The reported manometric criteria have usually included a resting LES pressure greater than 40 mm Hg with normal LES relaxation and esophageal peristalsis. Results of radiographic evaluation, including radionuclide emptying studies, are usually normal.[74] Like nutcracker esophagus, hypertensive LES is therefore a manometric diagnosis.

### Secondary Motility Disorders

The causes of secondary esophageal motility disorders are numerous and varied[1, 8, 9, 19, 75] (see Table 23–1). With some exceptions, the radiographic manifestations of these disorders are nonspecific and are similar to the findings described for NEMD. Thus, clinical correlation is critical for the proper diagnosis of secondary esophageal dysmotility.

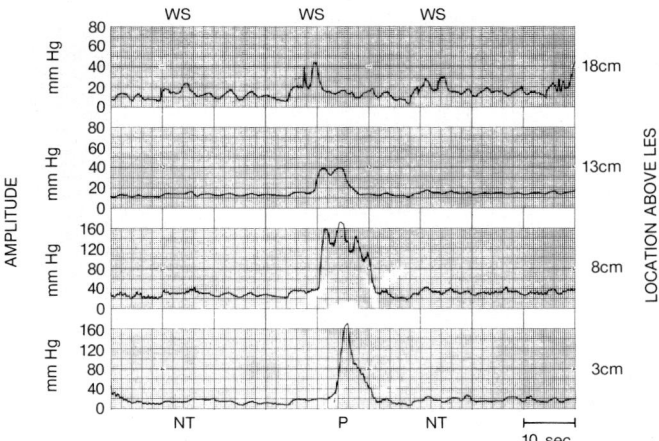

**Figure 23–15. Manometric representation of NEMD.** There is nontransmitted peristalsis (NT) in the lower leads and repetitive contractions during transmitted peristalsis (P). LES = lower esophageal sphincter; WS = wet swallow. (From DJ Ott, JE Richter, YM Chen, et al, Esophageal radiography and manometry: correlation in 172 patients with dysphagia, AJR, 149, 2, 307–311, 1987, © by American Roentgen Ray Society.)

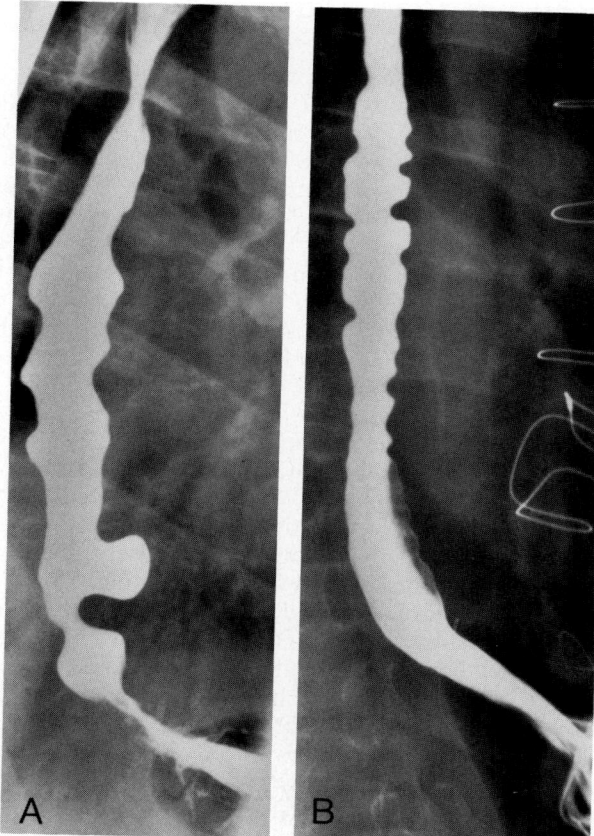

**Figure 23–16. NEMD. A**. This asymptomatic patient has simultaneous nonperistaltic contractions. Primary peristalsis was disrupted intermittently at fluoroscopy. NEMD was diagnosed by manometry. **B**. Multiple nonperistaltic contractions and disrupted primary peristalsis are seen in another patient with NEMD. Clinical and manometric correlations are needed to distinguish this appearance from DES. (**A** and **B** from MS Levine, SE Rubesin, DJ Ott, Update on esophageal radiology, AJR, 155, 5, 933–941, 1990, © by American Roentgen Ray Society.)

creased or absent resting LES pressure and weakened or absent peristalsis in the lower two thirds of the thoracic esophagus[19] (Fig. 23–17). These abnormalities are manifested radiographically by the absence of peristalsis in the smooth muscle portion of the esophagus, the presence of a hiatal hernia, and findings related to reflux esophagitis and peptic strictures (Fig. 23–18).

## Other Secondary Motility Disorders

A variety of conditions may be associated with motility disorders in the esophagus. Of the infectious causes, Chagas' disease has the most specific appearance.[19, 75] It occurs primarily in South America and is caused by the protozoan *Trypanosoma cruzi*. The disease affects multiple organs, including the myenteric plexus of the gastrointestinal tract, and it produces esophageal abnormalities that are identical with those in achalasia, both manometrically and radiographically.

A variety of metabolic and endocrine disorders may also affect esophageal motor function. In diabetic patients with peripheral neuropathy, manometric and radiographic abnormalities of the esophagus are common.[19, 75] These abnormalities are most likely caused by the degenerative effects of diabetes mellitus on the autonomic nervous system. The most common radiologic findings include decreased primary peristalsis, increased nonperistaltic contractions, mild esophageal dilatation, and hiatal hernia with gastroesophageal reflux (Fig. 23–19). Esophageal dysmotility is also common in alcoholic patients, even in the absence of esophagitis and neuropathy. The functional abnormalities seen in the esophagus may be reversed by withdrawal of alcohol.[79]

Esophageal motility may be affected by a number of neuromuscular disorders, so that clinical correlation is

## Collagen-Vascular Diseases

Collagen-vascular diseases compose a large group of acquired disorders of unknown origin that have multisystemic involvement with immunologic and inflammatory changes in connective tissue. The esophagus may be affected by nearly all of these collagen diseases, but it is most often involved by scleroderma, mixed connective tissue disease, dermatomyositis, and polymyositis.[19] Although these disorders produce similar manometric and radiologic abnormalities, diseases other than scleroderma may involve the striated muscle portion of the esophagus.

Scleroderma is characterized by fibrosis and degenerative changes in the skin, synovium, and parenchyma of multiple organs, including the esophagus. Esophageal involvement occurs in 75 to 87% of patients with scleroderma, with the smooth muscle segment, including the LES, being predominantly affected.[19, 76–78] Because of LES incompetence, symptoms of gastroesophageal reflux are common, and dysphagia may result from abnormal motility, reflux esophagitis, or peptic strictures. Manometric features of scleroderma include de-

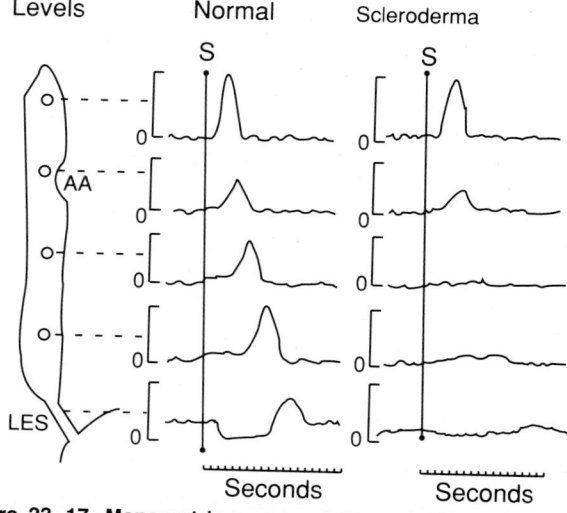

**Figure 23–17. Manometric representation of normal peristalsis and scleroderma.** Measurements are taken from multiple recording levels in the esophagus. Normal peristalsis is present in the upper esophagus with absence of peristalsis in the smooth muscle segment. The LES also shows low resting pressure. AA = aortic arch; S = swallow.

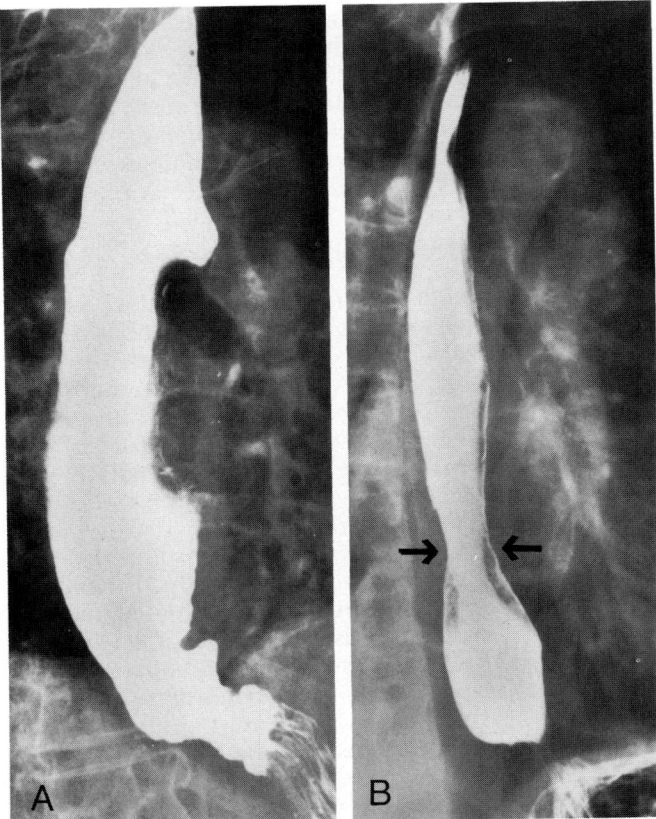

**Figure 23–18. Esophageal involvement by scleroderma. A**. This patient has a dilated esophagus and a patulous esophagogastric junction. There was aperistalsis at fluoroscopy. **B**. Another patient with scleroderma has developed a peptic stricture *(arrows)* as a complication of reflux disease.

mandatory. Most of these disorders also affect the pharynx and upper esophagus. Finally, idiopathic intestinal pseudo-obstruction is a poorly understood syndrome associated with intermittent signs and symptoms of intestinal obstruction.[19, 75] Various motility disorders throughout the bowel have been described in this syndrome. Most patients with intestinal pseudo-obstruction have abnormal esophageal motility with a radiographic appearance indistinguishable from that of achalasia (Fig. 23–20).

## RADIOLOGIC EFFICACY

The efficacy of radiologic evaluation of normal and abnormal esophageal motility depends on the quality of the examination performed and the types of motility disorders for which the patient is being evaluated.[14] Observation of multiple single swallows of barium is critical to the radiologic assessment of esophageal function if results are to correlate well with esophageal manometry.[1, 5, 15, 80, 81] This section reviews the radiologic efficacy in relation to manometry, the types of primary motility disorders being evaluated, and the clinical presentation of the patient.

## Manometric Correlation

In one study, normal esophageal motility and abnormal esophageal motility were assessed by using synchronous videofluoroscopy and manometry. A total of 98 swallows were correlated (58 normal and 40 abnormal), and 96% agreement was found in establishing the correct status of primary peristalsis.[15] Segregating swallows into groups of five showed a 92% concordance and led to the recommendation of using five barium swallows to evaluate esophageal motility by fluoroscopy. If two or more of the five barium swallows were abnormal, the patient was considered to have a motility disorder. Radiologic specificity in that study was 95%, similar to that in other reports.[5, 82]

Reported radiologic detection of esophageal motility disorders has been highly variable, depending primarily on the type of disorder for which the patient is being evaluated.[14, 82] In retrospective studies, the radiologic sensitivity for those primary motility disorders amenable to fluoroscopic diagnosis has varied from 46 to 95%.[54, 82] These studies have reported detection rates of about 95% for achalasia, 75% for DES, and 50% for NEMD. Nutcracker esophagus and hypertensive LES are not diagnosed radiographically, but their inclusion in correlative studies of esophageal motility obviously lowers the overall radiologic sensitivity. Synchronous manometric and fluoroscopic investigations have suggested

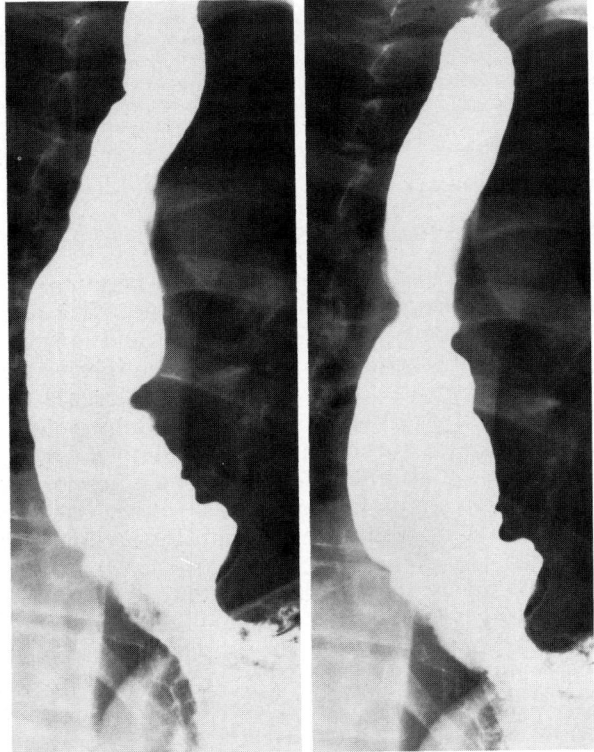

**Figure 23–19. Esophageal involvement by diabetes.** Two spot films, exposed seconds apart, reveal a secondary motility disorder in a patient with a hiatal hernia, esophageal dilatation, nonperistaltic contractions, and disrupted primary peristalsis at fluoroscopy.

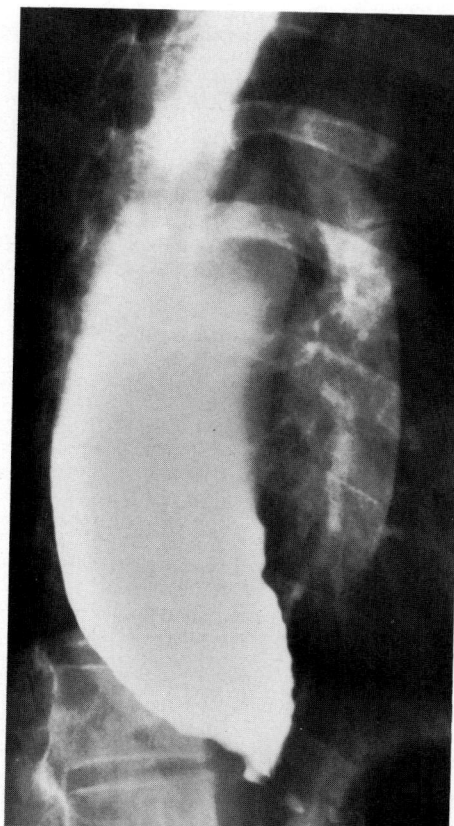

**Figure 23–20. Idiopathic intestinal pseudo-obstruction.** The appearance of the esophagus is indistinguishable from that in achalasia.

that observation of five barium swallows would improve radiologic detection of DES and NEMD.[15, 81]

## Clinical Considerations

Radiologic efficacy also depends on the clinical presentation of the patient.[83] Dysphagia and chest pain are the most common symptoms of esophageal motility disorders. However, the spectrum of motility disorders in patients with dysphagia is different from that in those with chest pain.[84] Dysphagia is a more specific esophageal complaint that often results from structural or functional disorders of the esophagus.[14] In a radiographic and manometric study of 172 patients with dysphagia, esophageal manometric findings were abnormal in 38% of the patients (66 of 172).[82] Achalasia was diagnosed in 29% (19 of 66) of those patients with abnormal manometric findings, and nutcracker esophagus was diagnosed in 18% (12 of 66) of the same group. Excluding the diagnosis of nutcracker esophagus, the overall radiographic sensitivity in this group of patients with dysphagia was 69%.

Recurrent chest pain is a less specific indicator of esophageal motility disorders, and cardiac disease must first be excluded.[84–86] Only 10 to 15% of patients with chest pain are found to have an esophageal cause, which is usually structural disease or gastroesophageal reflux

rather than a motility disorder. In a radiographic and manometric study of 170 patients with noncardiac chest pain, esophageal manometric findings were abnormal in 33% (56 of 170) of the patients.[87] Unlike patients with dysphagia, however, achalasia accounted for only 4% (2 of 56) of cases, and nutcracker esophagus for 29% (16 of 56) of cases. The overall radiographic sensitivity was only 36%. This lower figure presumably reflects a different spectrum of motility disorders occurring in patients with chest pain. In a more general population of individuals with chest pain, radiologic detection of abnormal motility would be detected radiologically in about only 1 to 2%.[88]

Before attributing dysphagia or chest pain to esophageal motility disorders, one should recognize that abnormal esophageal function does not prove an esophageal origin of the symptom.[84–88] Most patients with dysphagia or chest pain and abnormal esophageal motility do not have complaints during routine manometric or radiologic examinations. Provocative testing by esophageal acid perfusion or drugs usually produces negative results in these patients. Prolonged ambulatory monitoring of esophageal function has also shown changing motility patterns in the same patient, raising questions about the value of brief temporal sampling of esophageal pressures during a routine manometric study.[89–92] Finally, the occasional observation of transitional motility disorders emphasizes the difficulty of correlating symptoms with abnormal esophageal function.

## References

1. Dodds WJ: Normal motor physiology and motility disorders. *In* Margulis AR, Burhenne HJ (eds): Alimentary Tract Radiology, Volume 1 (3rd ed). St. Louis: CV Mosby, 1983, pp 530–553.
2. Meyer GW, Austin RM, Brady CE III, et al: Muscle anatomy of the human esophagus. J Clin Gastroenterol 8:131–134, 1986.
3. Ott DJ, Katz PO, Wu WC: Anti-reflux barrier. *In* Castell DO, Wu WC, Ott DJ (eds): Gastroesophageal Reflux Disease. Mt. Kisco, NY: Futura Publishing, 1985, pp 35–54.
4. Ott DJ, Gelfand DW, Wu WC, et al: Esophagogastric region and its rings. AJR 142:281–287, 1984.
5. Dodds WJ: Current concepts of esophageal motor function: clinical implications for radiology. AJR 128:549–561, 1977.
6. Castell DO: Anatomy and physiology of the esophagus and its sphincters. *In* Castell DO, Richter JE, Dalton CB (eds): Esophageal Motility Testing. New York: Elsevier, 1987, pp 13–27.
7. Margulis AR, Koehler RE: Radiologic diagnosis of disordered esophageal motility. Radiol Clin North Am 14:429–439, 1976.
8. Stewart ET: Radiographic evaluation of the esophagus and its motor disorders. Med Clin North Am 65:1173–1194, 1981.
9. Laufer I: Motor disorders of the esophagus. *In* Levine MS (ed): Radiology of the Esophagus. Philadelphia: WB Saunders, 1989, pp 229–246.
10. Dodds WJ, Hogan WJ, Reid DP, et al: A comparison between primary esophageal peristalsis following wet and dry swallows. J Appl Physiol 35:851–857, 1973.
11. Hollis JB, Castell DO: Esophageal function in elderly men—a new look at "presbyesophagus." Ann Intern Med 80:371–374, 1974.
12. Khan TA, Shragge BW, Crispin JS, et al: Esophageal motility in the elderly. Am J Dig Dis 22:1049–1054, 1977.
13. Eckardt VF, LeCompte PM: Esophageal ganglia and smooth muscle in the elderly. Dig Dis Sci 23:443–448, 1978.
14. Ott DJ: Radiologic evaluation of esophageal dysphagia. Curr Probl Diagn Radiol 17:1–33, 1988.

15. Ott DJ, Chen YM, Hewson EG, et al: Esophageal motility: assessment with synchronous video tape fluoroscopy and manometry. Radiology 173:419–422, 1989.

16. Dodds WJ: Instrumentation and method for intraluminal esophageal manometry. Arch Intern Med 136:515–523, 1976.

17. Katz PO, Castell DO: Review: esophageal motility disorders. Am J Med Sci 290:61–69, 1985.

18. Castell DO: The nutcracker esophagus and other primary esophageal motility disorders. In Castell DO, Richter JE, Dalton CB (eds): Esophageal Motility Testing. New York: Elsevier, 1987, pp 130–142.

19. Scobey MW: Secondary motility disorders. In Castell DO, Richter JE, Dalton CB (eds): Esophageal Motility Testing. New York: Elsevier, 1987, pp 163–182.

20. Katz PO: Achalasia. In Castell DO, Richter JE, Dalton CB (eds): Esophageal Motility Testing. New York: Elsevier, 1987, pp 107–117.

21. Enterline H, Thompson J: Pathology of the Esophagus. New York: Springer-Verlag, 1984, pp 55–71.

22. Wychulis AR, Woolam GL, Andersen HA, et al: Achalasia and carcinoma of the esophagus. JAMA 215:1638–1641, 1971.

23. Ott DJ, Gelfand DW, Wu WC, et al: Secondary achalasia in esophagogastric carcinoma: re-emphasis of a difficult differential problem. Rev Interam Radiol 4:135–138, 1979.

24. Dodds WJ, Stewart ET, Kishk SM, et al: Radiologic amyl nitrite test for distinguishing pseudoachalasia from idiopathic achalasia. AJR 146:21–23, 1986.

25. Kahrilas PJ, Kishk SM, Helm JF, et al: Comparison of pseudoachalasia and achalasia. Am J Med 82:439–446, 1987.

26. Sanderson DR, Ellis FH Jr, Schlegel JF, et al: Syndrome of vigorous achalasia: clinical and physiologic observations. Dis Chest 52:508–517, 1967.

27. Bondi JL, Godwin DH, Garrett JM: "Vigorous" achalasia. Am J Gastroenterol 58:145–155, 1972.

28. Katz PO, Richter JE, Cowan R, et al: Apparent complete lower esophageal sphincter relaxation in achalasia. Gastroenterology 90:978–983, 1986.

29. Ott DJ, Richter JE, Chen YM, et al: Radiographic and manometric correlation in achalasia with apparent relaxation of the lower esophageal sphincter. Gastrointest Radiol 14:1–5, 1989.

30. Hogan WJ, Caflisch CR, Winship DH: Unclassified oesophageal motor disorders simulating achalasia. Gut 10:234–240, 1969.

31. Millian MS, Bourdages R, Beck IT, et al: Transition from diffuse esophageal spasm to achalasia. J Clin Gastroenterol 1:107–117, 1979.

32. Vantrappen G, Janssens J, Hellemans J, et al: Achalasia, diffuse esophageal spasm, and related motility disorders. Gastroenterology 76:450–457, 1979.

33. Shiflett DW, Wu WC, Ott DJ: Transition from nonspecific motility disorder to achalasia. Am J Gastroenterol 73:325–328, 1980.

34. Rosenzweig S, Traube M: The diagnosis and misdiagnosis of achalasia. J Clin Gastroenterol 11:147–153, 1989.

35. Castell DO: Achalasia and diffuse esophageal spasm. Arch Intern Med 136:571–579, 1976.

36. Vantrappen G, Hellemans G: Treatment of achalasia and related motor disorders. Gastroenterology 79:144–154, 1980.

37. Csendes A, Velasco N, Braghetto I, et al: A prospective randomized study comparing forceful dilatation and esophagomyotomy in patients with achalasia of the esophagus. Gastroenterology 80:789–795, 1981.

38. Vantrappen G, Janssens J: To dilate or to operate? That is the question. Gut 24:1013–1019, 1983.

39. Donahue PE, Schlesinger PK, Bombeck CT, et al: Achalasia of the esophagus—treatment controversies and the method of choice. Ann Surg 203:505–510, 1986.

40. Stewart ET, Miller WN, Hogan WJ, et al: Desirability of roentgen esophageal examination immediately after pneumatic dilatation for achalasia. Radiology 130:589–591, 1979.

41. Ott DJ, Wu WC, Gelfand DW, et al: Radiographic evaluation of the achalasic esophagus immediately following pneumatic dilatation. Gastrointest Radiol 9:185–191, 1984.

42. Agha FP, Lee HH: The esophagus after endoscopic pneumatic balloon dilatation for achalasia. AJR 146:25–29, 1986.

43. Ott DJ, Richter JE, Wu WC, et al: Radiographic evaluation of the esophagus immediately after pneumatic dilatation for achalasia. Dig Dis Sci 32:962–967, 1987.

44. Stark GA, Castell DO, Richter JE, et al: Prospective randomized comparison of Brown-McHardy and Microvasive balloon dilators in treatment of achalasia. Am J Gastroenterol 85:1322–1326, 1990.

45. Gelfond M, Rozen P, Gilat T: Isosorbide dinitrate and nifedipine treatment of achalasia: a clinical, manometric and radionuclide evaluation. Gastroenterology 83:963–969, 1982.

46. Rozen P, Gelfond M, Zaltzman S, et al: Dynamic, diagnostic, and pharmacological radionuclide studies of the esophagus in achalasia. Radiology 144:587–590, 1982.

47. Holloway RH, Krosin G, Lange RC, et al: Radionuclide esophageal emptying of a solid meal to quantitate results of therapy in achalasia. Gastroenterology 84:771–776, 1983.

48. Cowan RJ: Gastroesophageal scintigraphy. In Castell DO, Wu WC, Ott DJ (eds): Gastroesophageal Reflux Disease. Mt. Kisco, NY: Futura Publishing, 1985, pp 185–207.

49. Richter JE: Diffuse esophageal spasm. In Castell DO, Richter JE, Dalton CB (eds): Esophageal Motility Testing. New York: Elsevier, 1987, pp 118–129.

50. Johnstone AS: Diffuse spasm and diffuse muscle hypertrophy of the lower oesophagus. Br J Radiol 33:723–735, 1960.

51. Craddock DR, Logan A, Walbaum PR: Diffuse oesophageal spasm. Thorax 21:511–517, 1966.

52. Gillies M, Nicks R, Skyring A: Clinical, manometric, and pathological studies in diffuse oesophageal spasm. Br Med J 2:527–530, 1967.

53. Loebenberg MJ, Lewis JH, Fleischer DE, et al: Endoscopic ultrasound (EUS) for evaluating esophageal wall thickness (EWT) in esophageal motility disorders (EMD). Gastroenterology 94:A267, 1989 (abstract).

54. Chen YM, Ott DJ, Hewson EG, et al: Diffuse esophageal spasm: radiographic and manometric correlation. Radiology 170:807–810, 1989.

55. Benjamin SB, Gerhardt DC, Castell DO: High amplitude, peristaltic esophageal contractions associated with chest pain and/or dysphagia. Gastroenterology 77:478–483, 1979.

56. Traube M, Albibi R, McCallum RW: High-amplitude peristaltic esophageal contractions associated with chest pain. JAMA 250:2655–2659, 1983.

57. Herrington JP, Burns TW, Balart LA: Chest pain and dysphagia in patients with prolonged peristaltic contractile duration of the esophagus. Dig Dis Sci 29:134–140, 1984.

58. Narducci F, Bassotti G, Gaburri M, et al: Transition from nutcracker esophagus to diffuse esophageal spasm. Am J Gastroenterol 80:242–244, 1985.

59. Richter JE, Obrecht WF, Bradley LA, et al: Psychological comparison of patients with nutcracker esophagus and irritable bowel syndrome. Dig Dis Sci 31:131–138, 1986.

60. Bassotti G, Bacci G, Biagini D, et al: Manometric investigation of the entire esophagus in healthy subjects and patients with high-amplitude peristaltic contractions. Dysphagia 3:93–96, 1988.

61. Valori RM: Nutcracker, neurosis, or sampling bias? Gut 31:736–737, 1990.

62. Richter JE, Wu WC, Johns DN, et al: Esophageal manometry in 95 healthy adult volunteers. Dig Dis Sci 32:583–592, 1987.

63. Chobanian SJ, Curtis DJ, Benjamin SB, et al: Radiology of the nutcracker esophagus. J Clin Gastroenterol 8:230–232, 1986.

64. Ott DJ, Richter JE, Wu WC, et al: Radiologic and manometric correlation in "nutcracker esophagus." AJR 147:692–695, 1986.

65. Benjamin SB, O'Donnell JK, Hancock J, et al: Prolonged radionuclide transit in "nutcracker esophagus." Dig Dis Sci 28:775–779, 1983.

66. De Caestecker JS, Blackwell JN, Adam RD, et al: Clinical value of radionuclide oesophageal transit measurement. Gut 27:659–666, 1986.

67. Holloway RH, Lange RC, Plankey MW, et al: Detection of esophageal motor disorders by radionuclide transit studies. Dig Dis Sci 34:905–912, 1989.

68. Drane WE, Johnson DA, Hagan DP, et al: "Nutcracker" esophagus: diagnosis with radionuclide esophageal scintigraphy versus manometry. Radiology 163:33–37, 1987.

69. Richter JE, Wu WC, Ott DJ, et al: "Nutcracker" esophagus: diagnosis with radionuclide esophageal scintigraphy versus manometry. Radiology 164:877–879, 1987 (letter).

70. Richter JE: Normal values for esophageal manometry. *In* Castell DO, Richter JE, Dalton CB (eds): Esophageal Motility Testing. New York: Elsevier, 1987, pp 79–90.

71. Clouse RE, Staiano A: Contraction abnormalities of the esophageal body in patients referred for manometry. Dig Dis Sci 28:784–791, 1983.

72. Soergel KH, Zboralske FF, Amberg JR: Presbyesophagus: esophageal motility in nonagenarians. J Clin Invest 43:1472–1479, 1964.

73. Zboralske FF, Amberg JR, Soergel KH. Presbyesophagus: cineradiographic manifestations. Radiology 82:463–467, 1964.

74. Waterman DC, Dalton CB, Ott DJ, et al: Hypertensive lower esophageal sphincter: what does it mean? J Clin Gastroenterol 11:139–146, 1989.

75. Chobanian SJ, Castell DO: Esophageal abnormalities in systemic disease. *In* Castell DO, Johnson LF (eds): Esophageal Function in Health and Disease. New York: Elsevier Biomedical, 1983, pp 273–294.

76. Turner R, Lipshutz W, Miller W, et al: Esophageal dysfunction in collagen disease. Am J Med Sci 265:191–199, 1973.

77. Clements PJ, Kadell B, Ippoliti A, et al: Esophageal motility in progressive systemic sclerosis (PSS)—comparison of cineradiographic and manometric evaluation. Dig Dis Sci 24:639–644, 1979.

78. Campbell WL, Schultz JC: Specificity and sensitivity of esophageal motor abnormality in systemic sclerosis (scleroderma) and related diseases: a cineradiographic study. Gastrointest Radiol 11:218–222, 1986.

79. Keshavarzian A, Iber FL, Ferguson Y: Esophageal manometry and radionuclide emptying in chronic alcoholics. Gastroenterology 92:651–657, 1987.

80. Kahrilas PJ, Dodds WJ, Hogan WJ: Effect of peristaltic dysfunction on esophageal volume clearance. Gastroenterology 94:73–80, 1988.

81. Hewson EG, Ott DJ, Dalton CB, et al: Manometry and radiology—complementary studies in the assessment of esophageal motility disorders. Gastroenterology 98:626–632, 1990.

82. Ott DJ, Richter JE, Chen YM, et al: Esophageal radiography and manometry: correlation in 172 patients with dysphagia. AJR 149:307–311, 1987.

83. DiPalma JA, Meyer GW: A rational clinical approach to esophageal motor disorders. Dysphagia 2:97–108, 1987.

84. Katz PO, Dalton CB, Richter JE, et al: Esophageal testing of patients with noncardiac chest pain or dysphagia. Ann Intern Med 106:593–597, 1987.

85. Richter JE, Bradley LA, Castell DO: Esophageal chest pain: current controversies in pathogenesis, diagnosis, and therapy. Ann Intern Med 110:66–78, 1989.

86. Richter JE: Noncardiac chest pain—use of esophageal manometry and provocative tests. *In* Castell DO, Richter JE, Dalton CB (eds): Esophageal Motility Testing. New York: Elsevier, 1987, pp 143–155.

87. Ott DJ, Abernethy WB, Chen MYM, et al: Radiologic evaluation of esophageal motility: results in 170 patients with chest pain. AJR 155:983–985, 1990.

88. Levine MS, Rubesin SE, Ott DJ: Update on esophageal radiology. AJR 155:933–941, 1990.

89. Peters L, Maas L, Petty D, et al: Spontaneous noncardiac chest pain—evaluation by 24-hour ambulatory esophageal motility and pH monitoring. Gastroenterology 94:878–886, 1988.

90. Vantrappen G, Janssens J: What is irritable esophagus? Gastroenterology 94:1092–1094, 1988.

91. Hewson EG, Dalton CB, Richter JE: Comparison of esophageal manometry, provocative testing, and ambulatory monitoring in patients with unexplained chest pain. Dig Dis Sci 35:302–309, 1990.

92. Ghillebert G, Janssens J, Vantrappen G, et al: Ambulatory 24 hour intraoesophageal pH and pressure recording vs provocation tests in the diagnosis of chest pain of oesophageal origin. Gut 31:738–744, 1990.

# Gastroesophageal Reflux Disease

### Marc S. Levine, M.D.

## INTRODUCTION

Gastroesophageal reflux disease is by far the most common inflammatory disease involving the esophagus. Barium studies have been advocated for patients with reflux symptoms primarily to show the presence of a hiatal hernia or gastroesophageal reflux, to detect complications such as deep ulcers or strictures, and to rule out other organic or motor abnormalities in the esophagus that can mimic reflux disease. By permitting a more detailed assessment of the esophageal mucosa, however, double contrast radiographic techniques have made it possible to detect superficial ulceration and other changes of mild or moderate esophagitis before the development of deep ulcers or strictures. Double contrast esophagography is also a useful screening examination for Barrett's esophagus to determine the need for endoscopy and biopsy in these patients. Thus, esophagography has become a valuable technique for evaluating patients with suspected gastroesophageal reflux disease.

## REFLUX ESOPHAGITIS

### Pathogenesis

Reflux esophagitis is thought to be a multifactorial process related to the frequency and duration of gastroesophageal reflux, the volume and potency of the refluxed material, and the intrinsic resistance of the esophageal mucosa.[1–4] Gastroesophageal reflux occurs when lower esophageal sphincter pressure is decreased or absent, so that the major barrier to reflux is lost.[1–3, 5] An incompetent lower esophageal sphincter may result either from a sustained decrease in resting sphincter pressure or from multiple transient sphincter relaxations occurring on a background of normal sphincter tone.[3, 4, 6] In any case, the severity of esophagitis depends not only on the frequency of reflux episodes but also on their duration. Because the duration of reflux is related to the efficacy of esophageal clearance by esophageal peristalsis, abnormal motility may exacerbate the pa-

tient's esophagitis by prolonging exposure to the refluxed material.[2, 3] Thus, esophageal involvement by scleroderma often leads to severe esophagitis due to absent peristalsis and extremely poor clearance of refluxed peptic acid from the esophagus. In one study, 60% of patients with scleroderma who underwent endoscopy had evidence of esophagitis.[7]

The severity of reflux esophagitis also depends on the potency or acidity of the refluxed material. The high prevalence of reflux esophagitis in patients with duodenal ulcers is presumably related to the damaging effect of hyperacidic gastric juices on the esophagus.[8, 9] Patients with Zollinger-Ellison syndrome may also develop severe esophagitis or strictures due to reflux of highly acidic peptic contents into the esophagus.[10–12] However, reflux esophagitis may occasionally occur in patients who have decreased secretion of acid or even achlorhydria.[13] This apparent paradox can probably be attributed to the damaging effects of refluxed biliary or pancreatic secretions on the esophagus.

Finally, the severity of reflux esophagitis depends on the intrinsic resistance of the esophageal mucosa.[2–4] Because mucosal resistance and esophageal motor function deteriorate with age, older patients are at greater risk for developing reflux esophagitis as a result of prolonged exposure of a susceptible mucosa to refluxed acid in the esophagus.

### Relationship Between Hiatal Hernia, Gastroesophageal Reflux, and Reflux Esophagitis

Sliding hiatal hernias occur more frequently in elderly patients as a result of a degenerative process in which there is progressive weakening and laxity of the ligaments that anchor the gastroesophageal junction to the surrounding esophageal hiatus of the diaphragm.[2, 14] However, there is considerable controversy about the relationship between a hiatal hernia and the subsequent development of gastroesophageal reflux or reflux esophagitis. Because most patients with clinically significant gastroesophageal reflux disease have evidence of a hiatal hernia, it has been postulated that a hernia predisposes to the development of gastroesophageal reflux and that it has a permissive role in the development of reflux esophagitis.[15, 16] However, many patients with a hiatal hernia have no evidence of gastroesophageal reflux, and many patients with gastroesophageal reflux have no evidence of a hernia.[17–19] Thus, intrinsic dysfunction of the lower esophageal sphincter (i.e., decreased sphincter tone or transient sphincter relaxations) is probably the major factor in the development of gastroesophageal reflux, independent of the anatomic location of the sphincter above or below the diaphragm.[1, 3, 17]

Although the presence of a sliding hiatal hernia is a poor predictor of gastroesophageal reflux disease, most patients with severe reflux esophagitis or peptic strictures have evidence of a hiatal hernia.[3, 20, 21] It has therefore been postulated that severe inflammation and scarring from reflux esophagitis cause longitudinal esophageal shortening that disrupts the ligaments surrounding the gastroesophageal junction and pulls the gastric fundus into the thorax.[20] Thus, the hiatal hernia may represent an effect rather than a cause of esophagitis in these patients.

Similarly, gastroesophageal reflux is a poor predictor of reflux esophagitis, as reflux may be demonstrated in some asymptomatic individuals but not in others with proven reflux esophagitis.[2, 3, 22] Thus, the diagnosis of reflux esophagitis should be based not on the presence or absence of a hiatal hernia or gastroesophageal reflux but on specific morphologic evidence of inflammatory changes in the esophagus.

## Clinical Findings

The classic history of episodic heartburn and regurgitation exacerbated by bending over or lying down should strongly suggest the diagnosis of reflux esophagitis.[1] However, many patients have symptoms that are nonspecific or misleading. The pain associated with reflux esophagitis may be difficult to distinguish from symptoms of ischemic heart disease. Other patients may have epigastric or right upper quadrant pain that erroneously is attributed to peptic ulcer disease or cholecystitis.[23] Still others may develop upper gastrointestinal bleeding with hematemesis, melena, or guaiac-positive stool.[1] However, major life-threatening hemorrhage from reflux esophagitis is extremely uncommon.

The severity of reflux symptoms correlates poorly with the severity of reflux esophagitis. Whereas some patients with marked reflux symptoms have normal endoscopic examinations, others with unequivocal endoscopic evidence of esophagitis are asymptomatic.[24] It has therefore been postulated that the development of reflux symptoms is related more to the "reactivity" or sensitivity of the esophageal mucosa to refluxed peptic acid than to the presence or degree of inflammation in the esophagus.[24, 25]

The development of a peptic stricture is usually manifested by slowly progressive dysphagia for solids superimposed on a history of long-standing reflux symptoms.[26] Subsequently, those reflux symptoms may subside or even disappear as the developing stricture forms a barrier against further episodes of gastroesophageal reflux. However, other patients with peptic strictures may develop dysphagia as the initial manifestation of their disease.[1] Occasionally, dysphagia may be caused by edema and spasm associated with severe esophagitis in the absence of fibrosis or scarring.[1] Thus, a peptic stricture cannot be diagnosed definitively on clinical grounds.

## Diagnosis

Patients with reflux symptoms may undergo a variety of clinical tests to determine if their symptoms are esophageal in origin and if there is objective evidence of gastroesophageal reflux or reflux esophagitis. Assessment of gastroesophageal reflux requires radiologic, scintigraphic, manometric, or pH-monitoring techniques. However, radiologic or endoscopic examinations are required for diagnosing reflux esophagitis.

### *Gastroesophageal Reflux*

Spontaneous gastroesophageal reflux can be demonstrated with barium studies in only about 20% of patients with reflux esophagitis.[3, 21, 27] Because gastroesophageal reflux may result from multiple transient relaxations of the lower esophageal sphincter that occur at random, intermittent episodes of reflux are often missed during the brief period of fluoroscopic observation. At the same time, spontaneous gastroesophageal reflux may be demonstrated with barium studies in 40% of asymptomatic volunteers.[22] Routine use of the water siphon test or other nonphysiologic maneuvers to induce reflux has been discouraged, as these techniques may allow gastroesophageal reflux to occur in normal individuals.[18, 28] Thus, fluoroscopy is neither a sensitive nor a specific technique for diagnosing gastroesophageal reflux. Nevertheless, free reflux of barium on the fluoroscopic examination is often associated with reflux esophagitis when it occurs spontaneously in patients with reflux symptoms.[21]

Gastroesophageal scintigraphy is an alternative technique that appears to be far more accurate than conventional barium studies for detecting and quantifying gastroesophageal reflux (see Chapter 21).[29, 30] Esophageal manometry can also be used to assess sphincter competence, but many patients with normal resting pressures have intermittent gastroesophageal reflux due to transient relaxation of the lower esophageal sphincter.[6] Thus, sphincter pressures alone should not be used to indicate the presence or absence of gastroesophageal reflux. Intraesophageal pH monitoring is now thought to be the most accurate diagnostic test for gastroesophageal reflux. However, it should be recognized that this test measures the acidity rather than the volume of refluxed material in the esophagus.

Because the severity of reflux esophagitis also depends on the duration of reflux, esophageal clearance may also be evaluated once reflux has occurred. Fluoroscopy, gastroesophageal scintigraphy, intraesophageal pH monitoring, and manometry can all be used to evaluate esophageal motility or clearance.[3, 21, 31, 32]

## Reflux Esophagitis

Conventional single contrast esophagography has been considered an unreliable technique for diagnosing reflux esophagitis, with an overall sensitivity of only 50 to 75%.[33–36] The use of double contrast esophagography has increased the radiographic sensitivity to almost 90%.[34, 36, 37] However, the greater sensitivity of the double contrast study has been compromised by the increased number of false-positive examinations with this technique.[34, 36] As a result, the overall accuracy of the barium study thus far has not significantly improved with the use of double contrast technique. Nevertheless, double contrast examinations permit a detailed assessment of the esophageal mucosa for superficial ulceration or other changes of mild or moderate esophagitis that cannot be detected with conventional barium studies. At the same time, single contrast esophagrams with the patient in the prone position are best for demonstrating contour abnormalities in the distal esophagus, such as lower esophageal rings and strictures.[38] A biphasic examination with upright double contrast and prone single contrast views of the esophagus therefore appears to be the best radiologic technique for evaluating patients with suspected reflux disease.

Endoscopy has become an increasingly popular technique for diagnosing reflux esophagitis. Various grading systems have been used to estimate the severity of esophagitis based on the endoscopic findings of erythema, friability, exudates, ulcers, and strictures.[39] A histologic diagnosis of reflux esophagitis can be made when endoscopic biopsies reveal acute inflammatory changes with accumulation of neutrophils and other round cells in the lamina propria. Basal cell hyperplasia of the squamous epithelium has also been recognized as an important sign of reflux disease on endoscopic biopsies.[40] This basal cell hyperplasia apparently results from accelerated epithelial turnover due to mucosal damage by refluxed peptic acid in the esophagus. Thus, endoscopy and biopsy should be considered the most definitive diagnostic test for reflux esophagitis.

## Radiographic Findings

### Abnormal Motility

Between 25 and 50% of patients with reflux esophagitis have abnormal esophageal motility, manifested by feeble or absent primary peristalsis associated with an increased frequency of nonperistaltic contractions.[2, 21, 41] Occasionally, esophageal aperistalsis may be the only radiographic finding in patients with reflux disease.[42] Abnormal motility may be secondary to neuronal damage in Auerbach's plexus caused by direct extension of the inflammatory process into the esophageal wall.[42] Conversely, pre-existing esophageal motor disorders may predispose to the development of reflux esophagitis by impairing clearance of refluxed peptic acid from the esophagus. In any case, the combination of abnormal motility and gastroesophageal reflux may lead to progressively severe esophagitis and stricture formation.[3]

In the past, acid barium was used to induce motor dysfunction in patients with reflux esophagitis who had normal motility with standard barium suspensions.[43] However, acid barium may also produce abnormal motility in asymptomatic patients who have no other objective evidence of esophagitis.[44] As a result, this test is no longer widely used to evaluate patients with suspected reflux disease.

Reflux esophagitis sometimes may be manifested radiographically by an abnormally wide cardiac segment of the esophagus, with a diameter greater than 2.5 cm.[37] The increased distensibility of the distal esophagus in these patients has been attributed to localized weakness of the esophageal wall because of inflammation in this region. In many cases, however, there is other radiographic evidence of reflux esophagitis. Thus, the practical value of a dilated distal esophagus as an isolated finding for diagnosing reflux esophagitis is uncertain.

## Mucosal Nodularity

In the early stages of reflux esophagitis, mucosal edema and inflammation may be manifested on double contrast radiographs by a granular or finely nodular appearance in the distal third or half of the thoracic esophagus[45–47] (Fig. 24–1). Although mucosal granularity

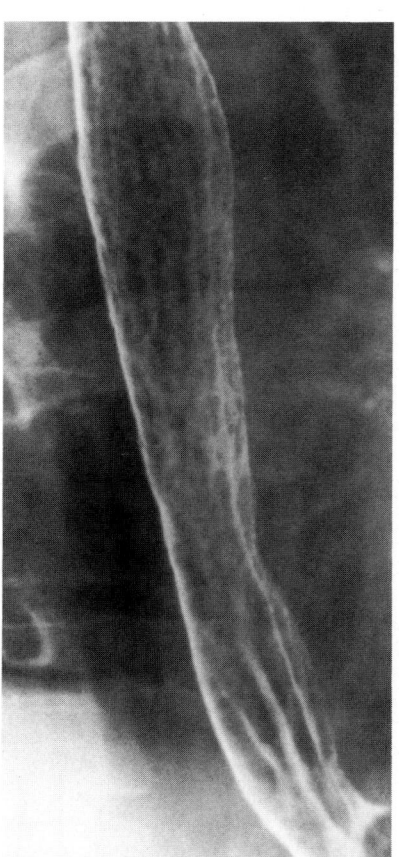

**Figure 24–1. Reflux esophagitis with a granular mucosa.** There is a finely nodular or granular appearance of the mucosa extending proximally from the gastroesophageal junction as a continuous area of disease.

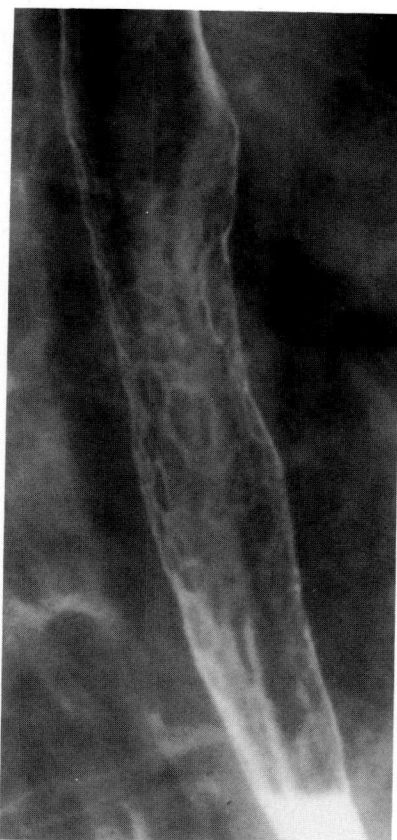

**Figure 24–2. Reflux esophagitis with pseudomembranes.** The pseudomembranes appear as discrete plaque-like defects that are indistinguishable from the plaques of candidiasis. (Courtesy of Howard Kessler, M.D., Philadelphia, PA.)

is best seen with maximal esophageal distention, it can also be recognized in the collapsed esophagus by lobulation or nodularity of the longitudinal folds.[45] Less frequently, these patients may have coarse nodularity of the mucosa. However, the nodules tend to have poorly defined borders that fade peripherally into the adjacent mucosa, so that discrete nodules are rarely detected in patients with reflux esophagitis.

Severe reflux esophagitis may occasionally be associated with inflammatory exudates or pseudomembranes that closely resemble the plaque-like lesions of *Candida* esophagitis[48] (Fig. 24–2). However, these patients usually present with reflux symptoms rather than odynophagia. A single, large pseudomembrane can also be mistaken for a plaque-like carcinoma, particularly an adenocarcinoma arising in Barrett's mucosa.[48] However, pseudomembrane formation may be suggested by the presence of other satellite lesions or by a change in the size or shape of the lesions at fluoroscopy. When the radiographic findings are equivocal, endoscopy and biopsy are required for a definitive diagnosis.

## Ulceration

Shallow ulcers and erosions associated with reflux esophagitis may appear on double contrast radiographs

as one or more tiny collections of barium in the distal esophagus near the gastroesophageal junction[45, 46, 49] (Fig. 24–3). Some ulcers may have an irregular appearance, and others may have a linear configuration with their long axis oriented perpendicular to the gastroesophageal junction[46] (Fig. 24–4). The ulcers are often associated with surrounding mounds of edematous mucosa, radiating folds, or puckering and sacculation of the adjacent esophageal wall[45, 46, 49] (see Fig. 24–4). Occasionally, longitudinally oriented ulcers may have a serpiginous, flowing appearance with multiple transverse folds straddling the ulcers[50] (Fig. 24–5).

When superficial ulceration is detected in patients with reflux esophagitis, the correct diagnosis is almost always suggested by the distal location of the ulcers, the presence of an associated hiatal hernia or gastroesophageal reflux, and the clinical presentation of the patient. Some individuals may have relatively diffuse ulceration in the distal half or even two thirds of the thoracic esophagus. However, ulceration in reflux esophagitis tends to occur as a continuous area of mucosal disease extending proximally from the gastroesophageal junction, so the presence of superficial ulcers in the mid-esophagus with distal esophageal sparing should suggest another cause of the esophagitis.

Reflux esophagitis may also be manifested by a soli-

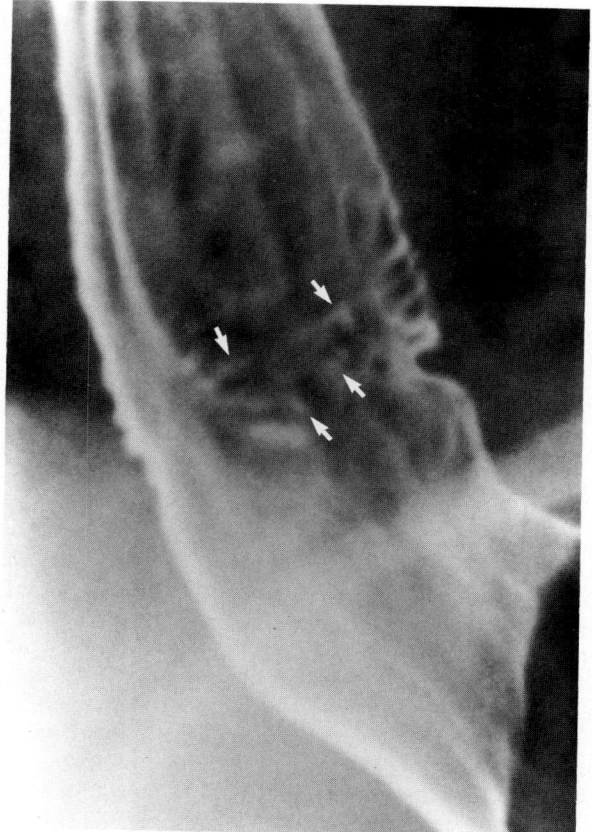

**Figure 24–3. Reflux esophagitis with superficial ulceration.** Multiple tiny ulcers *(arrows)* are seen en face in the distal esophagus near the gastroesophageal junction. Note radiating folds and puckering of the adjacent esophageal wall.

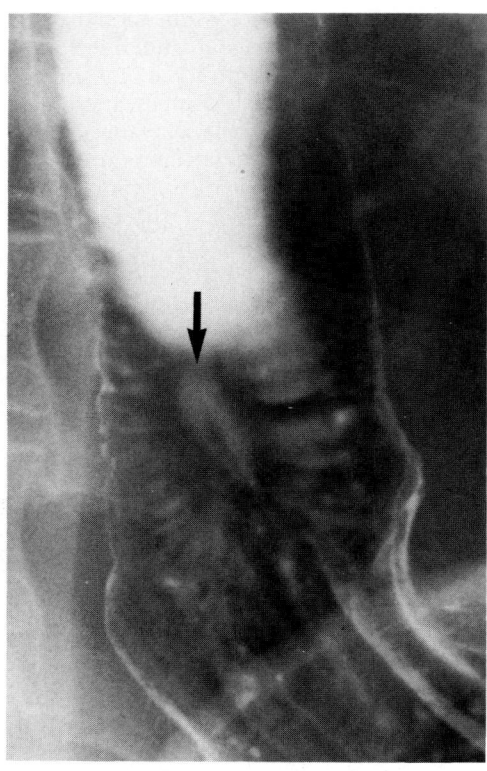

**Figure 24–4. Reflux esophagitis with a linear ulcer *(arrow)*.** Note the radiolucent halo of edematous mucosa and folds radiating toward the ulcer crater.

tary ulcer in the distal esophagus at or adjacent to the gastroesophageal junction.[51] These "marginal" ulcers may be recognized as discrete collections of barium en face (Fig. 24–6A) but are best visualized when the ulcers are projected tangentially beyond the normal contour of the esophagus (Fig. 24–6B). Associated spasm and edema of the distal esophagus erroneously may suggest a stricture. Occasionally, the narrowing, mass effect, and deformity associated with a deep ulcer crater can also mimic the appearance of a malignant lesion (Fig. 24–7). When the radiographic findings are equivocal, endoscopy and biopsy should be performed to rule out an ulcerated carcinoma.

In advanced reflux esophagitis, the esophagus may have a grossly irregular contour with serrated or spiculated margins, wall thickening, and decreased distensibility due to extensive ulceration, edema, and spasm[2, 21, 33, 35, 52] (Fig. 24–8). Without a clinical history, such cases may be difficult to distinguish from other types of severe esophagitis. However, predominant involvement of the distal esophagus and the presence of an associated hiatal hernia and gastroesophageal reflux should suggest the correct diagnosis.

## *Thickened Folds*

In some patients with reflux esophagitis, submucosal edema and inflammation may lead to the development of thickened longitudinal folds (Fig. 24–9). Thickened folds are best seen on mucosal relief views of the collapsed esophagus, where folds wider than 3 mm are thought to be abnormal.[35, 45] These thickened folds may have a smooth, nodular, or scalloped appearance. Oc-

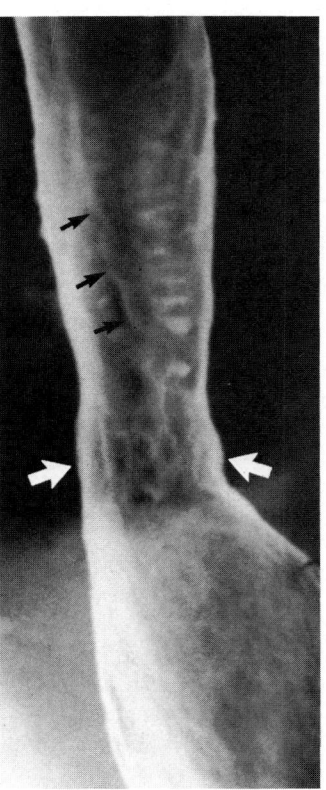

**Figure 24–5. Reflux esophagitis with serpiginous, flowing ulcers.** Multiple transverse folds straddle these longitudinally oriented ulcers *(black arrows)* in the distal esophagus. A mild peptic stricture *(white arrows)* is also present. (From MS Levine, HM Goldstein, Fixed transverse folds in the esophagus: a sign of reflux esophagitis, AJR, 143, 2, 275–278, © by American Roentgen Ray Society.)

**Figure 24–6. Reflux esophagitis with a discrete ulcer.** This small ulcer *(arrows)* is seen both en face **(A)** and in profile **(B)** in the distal esophagus above a hiatal hernia.

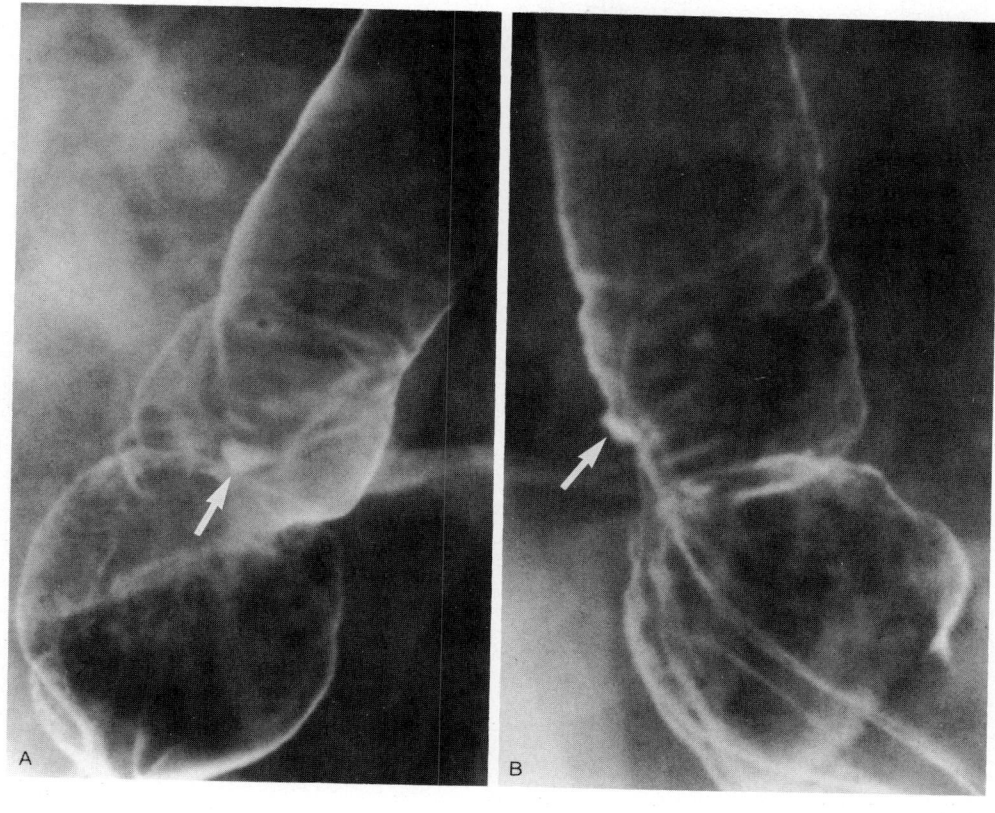

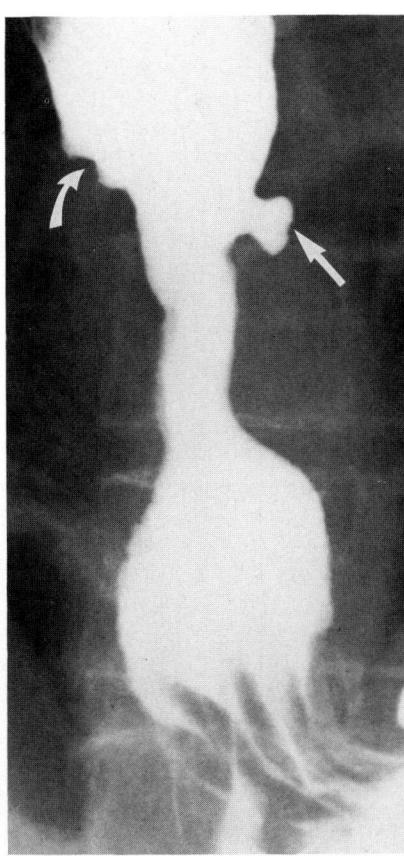

**Figure 24–7. Reflux esophagitis with a deep ulcer *(straight arrow)*.** There is also asymmetric narrowing of the distal esophagus with a relatively abrupt cutoff *(curved arrow)* at the proximal border of the narrowed segment. These findings were caused by edema and spasm, but the possibility of malignancy cannot be excluded on this film.

**Figure 24–8. Advanced reflux esophagitis.** There is decreased distensibility of the distal esophagus with an irregular, serrated esophageal contour due to extensive ulceration.

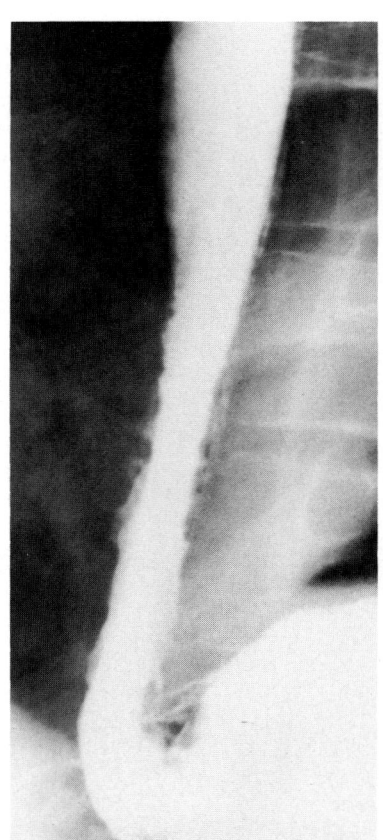

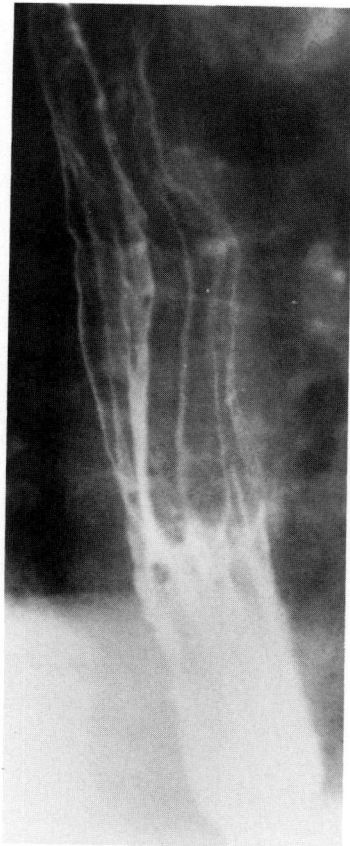

**Figure 24–9. Reflux esophagitis with thickened longitudinal folds.**

casionally, they may be quite tortuous or serpiginous, mimicking the appearance of esophageal varices.[53]

Multiple transverse folds may also be found in patients with gastroesophageal reflux disease[54, 55] (Figs. 24–10 and 24–11). These delicate transverse striations are only 1 to 2 mm wide and extend completely across the esophagus without interruption.[55] The folds occur as a transient phenomenon, so they may be seen on only one of a number of spot films obtained during the radiologic examination (see Fig. 24–11). Although transverse folds are often observed in patients with gastroesophageal reflux, this finding alone does not indicate the presence of esophagitis.[55] Occasionally, however, thickening of these transverse folds may occur as a nonspecific manifestation of esophagitis[45] (Fig. 24–12).

## Inflammatory Esophagogastric Polyps

Other patients with reflux esophagitis may have a single prominent fold that arises in the gastric fundus and extends above the gastroesophageal junction as a polypoid protuberance in the distal esophagus.[56–58] These "inflammatory" esophagogastric polyps are composed of inflammatory and granulation tissue and are thought to be a manifestation of chronic reflux esophagitis.[57, 58] The polyps have no malignant potential, so endoscopic resection is unwarranted.[57]

Inflammatory esophagogastric polyps are usually manifested radiographically by a smooth, ovoid, or club-shaped mass at the gastroesophageal junction atop a single, prominent mucosal fold that tapers distally in the gastric fundus[56, 57] (Fig. 24–13).Esophagogastric polyps frequently straddle a hiatal hernia and may be associated with other radiographic evidence of reflux esophagitis. When the characteristic findings of esophagogastric polyps are present on barium studies, endoscopic confirmation is unnecessary[57, 58] (see Fig. 24–13A). When these lesions are not associated with a mucosal fold or have a lobulated or irregular appearance (see Fig. 24–13B), however, endoscopy and biopsy should be performed to rule out a malignant lesion.

## Scarring and Strictures

Depending on the degree of scarring, reflux esophagitis eventually may lead to stricture formation. However, esophageal scarring may occur without the development of a circumferential stricture. It is often possible to detect slight flattening or puckering of the esophageal wall and/or radiating folds at the site of previous ulceration (Fig. 24–14). Scarring caused by reflux esophagitis may also lead to focal outpouching or sacculation of the distal esophagus with outward ballooning of the esoph-

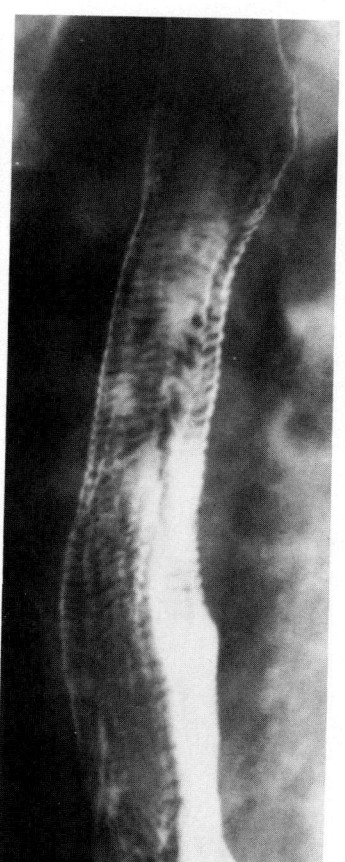

**Figure 24–10. "Feline" esophagus.** Multiple fine transverse folds are seen in the esophagus due to contraction of the longitudinally oriented muscularis mucosae.

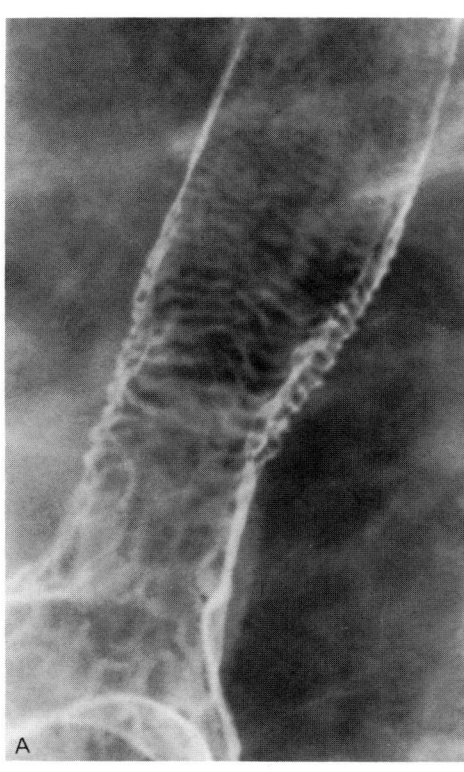
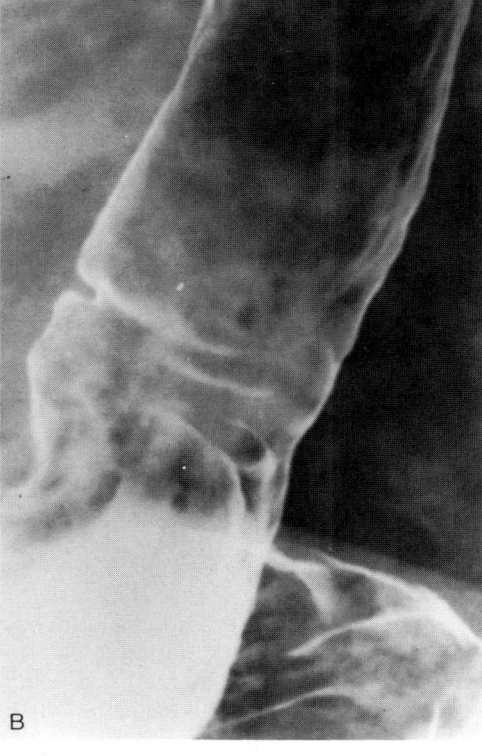

ageal wall between areas of fibrosis (Fig. 24–15). Sacculations are particularly common in patients with scleroderma as a result of the severe esophagitis that occurs in these individuals. Sacculations may resemble active

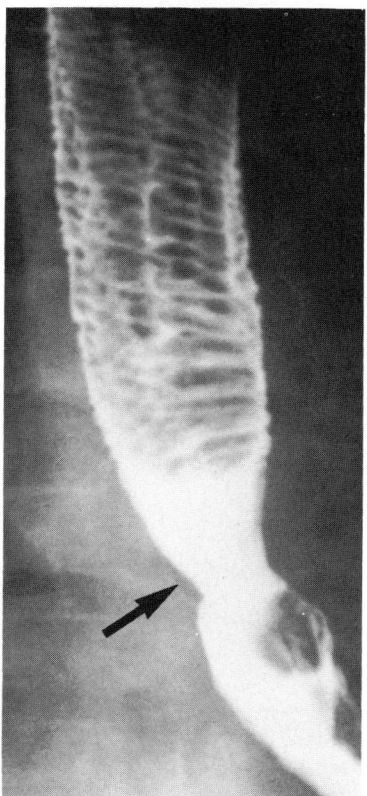

**Figure 24–12. Reflux esophagitis with thickened transverse folds.** There is also a peptic stricture *(arrow)* in the distal esophagus.

ulcer craters but usually can be differentiated from ulcers by their changing shape and appearance at fluoroscopy.

Scarring caused by reflux esophagitis may also be manifested by fixed transverse folds in the distal esophagus, producing a characteristic "stepladder" appearance due to pooling of barium between the folds[50] (Fig. 24–16). These transverse folds are usually 2 to 5 mm wide and do not extend more than halfway across the esophagus. The folds tend to be relatively few in number, and they cannot be obliterated with esophageal distention. In most cases, there is other evidence of scarring from reflux esophagitis, and these transverse folds extend proximally a variable distance from the site of a distal stricture or scar. The folds probably represent areas of heaped-up or crinkled mucosa caused by simultaneous longitudinal scarring from reflux esophagitis. These fixed transverse folds should be distinguished from the thin transverse striations that are sometimes a transient finding on double contrast studies[54, 55] (see Figs. 24–10 and 24–11).

Between 10 and 20% of patients with reflux esophagitis develop peptic strictures as a result of circumferential scarring of the distal esophagus.[36, 59] Accurate radiologic diagnosis of peptic strictures requires continuous drinking of low-density barium in the prone position for optimal esophageal distention to demonstrate mild or even moderate strictures that are not visible on the double contrast phase of the examination (Fig. 24–17). The routine esophagram should therefore be performed as a biphasic study that includes upright double contrast and prone single contrast views of the esophagus. With careful technique, esophagography has a sensitivity of almost 95% in diagnosing peptic strictures and occasionally may demonstrate strictures that are missed at endoscopy.[60, 61]

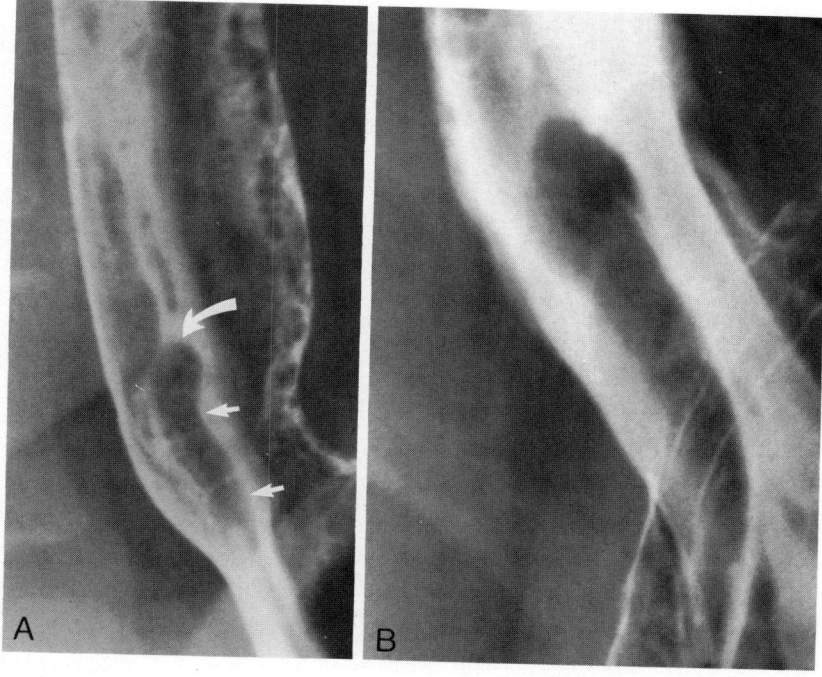

**Figure 24–13. Inflammatory esophagogastric polyps. A.** A prominent fold *(straight arrows)* is seen arising at the cardia and extending into the distal esophagus as a smooth, polypoid protuberance *(curved arrow).* This appearance is characteristic of inflammatory polyps. **B.** An inflammatory esophagogastric polyp is seen in the distal esophagus in another patient. This lesion is more lobulated than most inflammatory polyps, so it cannot be differentiated from an adenomatous polyp or even an adenocarcinoma.

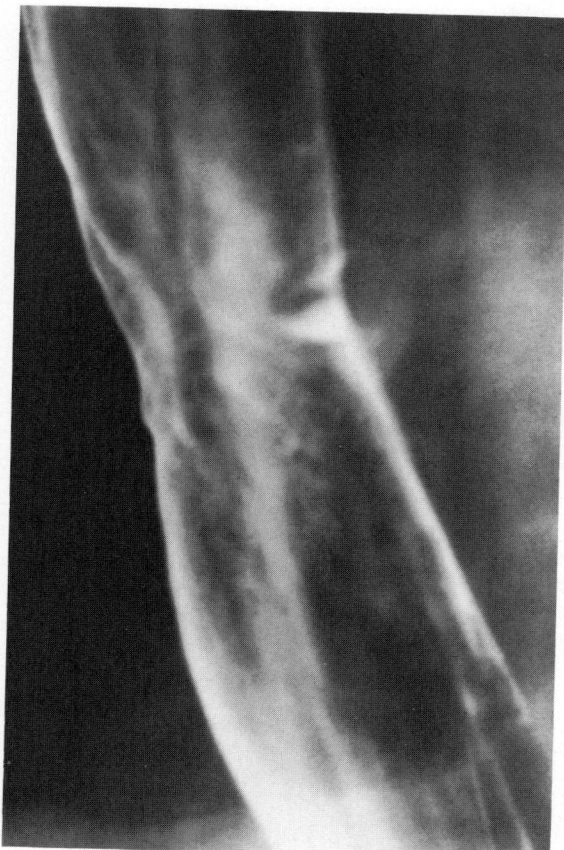

**Figure 24–14. Mild peptic scarring in the distal esophagus.** There is slight flattening and puckering of the distal esophagus with radiating folds in this region due to scarring from reflux esophagitis.

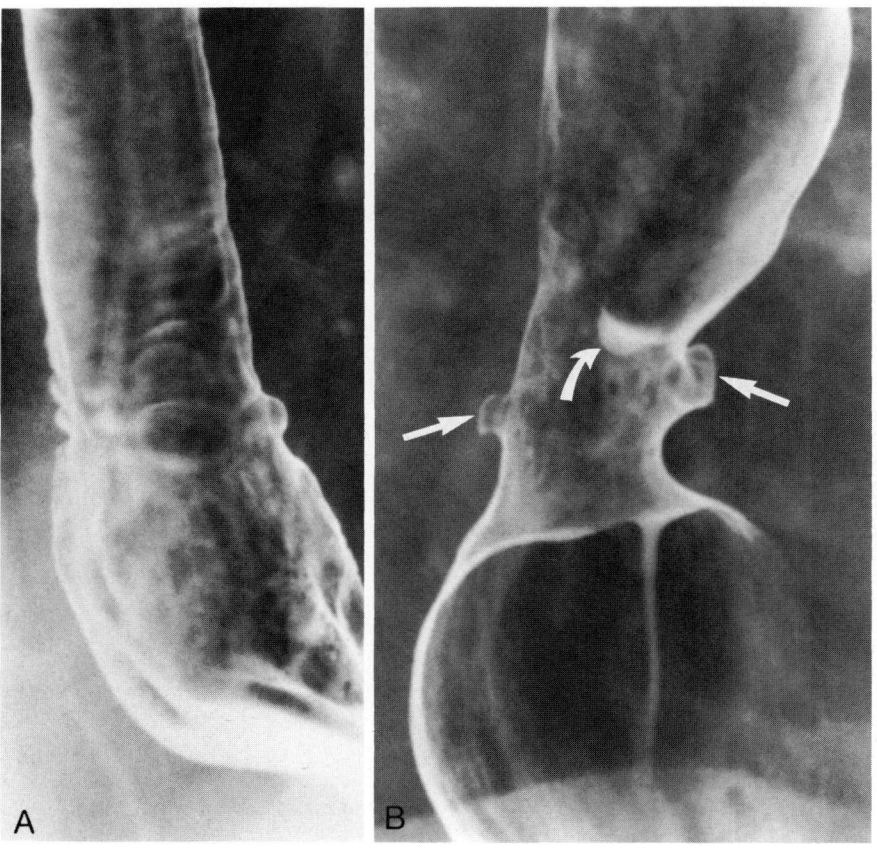

**Figure 24–15. Scarring from reflux esophagitis with sacculations. A.** There are sacculations and radiating folds in the distal esophagus without evidence of a stricture. (From MS Levine, HM Goldstein, Fixed transverse folds in the esophagus: a sign of reflux esophagitis, AJR, 143, 2, 275–278, 1984, © by American Roentgen Ray Society.) **B.** In another patient with greater scarring, there is a peptic stricture with several large sacculations seen en face *(curved arrow)* and in profile *(straight arrows)* in the distal esophagus.

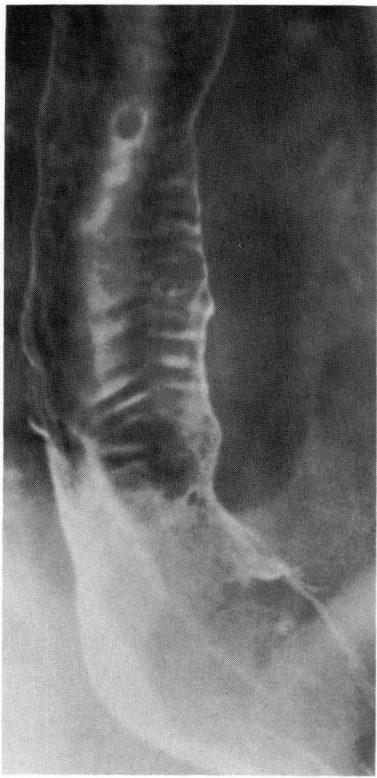

**Figure 24–16. Fixed transverse folds in the esophagus.** There are multiple transverse folds in the distal esophagus, producing a step-ladder appearance due to longitudinal scarring from reflux esophagitis. (From MS Levine, HM Goldstein, Fixed transverse folds in the esophagus: a sign of reflux esophagitis, AJR, 143, 2, 275–278, 1984, © by American Roentgen Ray Society.)

The vast majority of peptic strictures are located in the distal esophagus above a sliding hiatal hernia (Fig. 24–18). Because many patients with gastroesophageal reflux or mild reflux esophagitis do not have a concomitant hernia, it has been postulated that scarring from reflux esophagitis leads not only to circumferential narrowing of the esophagus but also to longitudinal shortening of the esophagus with subsequent hernia formation.[1, 20, 62] Whatever the explanation, a hiatal hernia is seen radiographically in more than 95% of patients with peptic strictures.[20] Thus, other causes of a distal esophageal stricture, particularly malignancy, should be considered when a hiatal hernia is not found.

The classic appearance of a smooth, tapered area of concentric narrowing in the distal esophagus above a sliding hiatal hernia should be virtually pathognomonic of a benign peptic stricture (see Fig. 24–18A). However, many peptic strictures have an asymmetric appearance with puckering, deformity, or sacculation of one wall of the stricture due to asymmetric scarring from reflux esophagitis (see Fig. 24–18B). Other strictures may involve a longer segment of the distal esophagus and may have irregular margins due to associated reflux esophagitis[60] (see Fig. 24–18C). As a result, a benign peptic stricture cannot always be distinguished from an infiltrating carcinoma, particularly an adenocarcinoma

arising in Barrett's esophagus (see Chapter 28). Endoscopy should therefore be performed to rule out a malignant lesion when the radiographic findings are equivocal.

Most peptic strictures range from 1 to 4 cm in length and from 0.2 to 2.0 cm in width.[60] Marked luminal narrowing may occur, but these strictures rarely cause esophageal obstruction. Occasionally, short peptic strictures may have an annular appearance and are difficult to distinguish from Schatzki rings (Fig. 24–19). However, Schatzki rings usually appear radiographically as symmetric, ring-like constrictions at the gastroesophageal junction with a vertical height of 2 to 4 mm[63, 64] (see Chapter 32). In contrast, annular peptic strictures tend to have a vertical height of more than 4 mm.[60]

Distal esophageal webs have also been recognized as a manifestation of scarring from reflux esophagitis.[65] The webs tend to occur at a discrete distance from the gastroesophageal junction, so they usually can be differentiated from Schatzki rings by their more proximal location (Fig. 24–20).

Longer peptic strictures involving the distal third or half of the thoracic esophagus are relatively unusual.

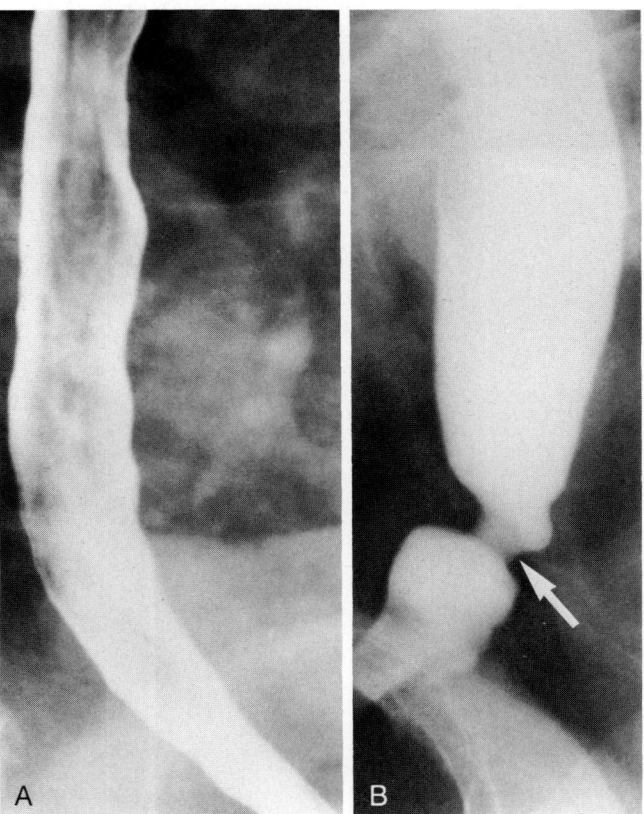

**Figure 24–17. Peptic stricture seen only on prone single contrast views of the esophagus. A.** A double contrast radiograph with the patient upright shows no evidence of narrowing in the distal esophagus. **B.** However, a single contrast radiograph from the same examination with the patient prone reveals an unequivocal peptic stricture *(arrow)* above a hiatal hernia. Even in retrospect, this stricture was not visible on double contrast radiographs because of inadequate distention of this region.

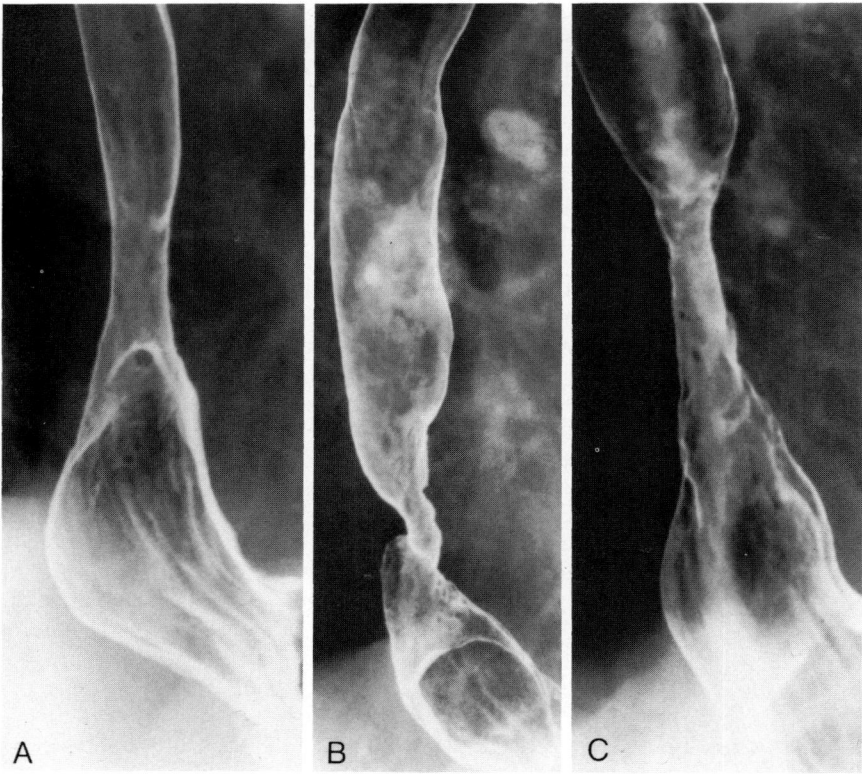

Figure 24–18. Peptic strictures. A. There is a concentric area of smooth, tapered narrowing in the distal esophagus above a hiatal hernia. This is the classic appearance of a peptic stricture. B. In another patient, there is an eccentric stricture with asymmetric narrowing and deformity of the distal esophagus. C. This peptic stricture involves a longer segment of the distal esophagus.

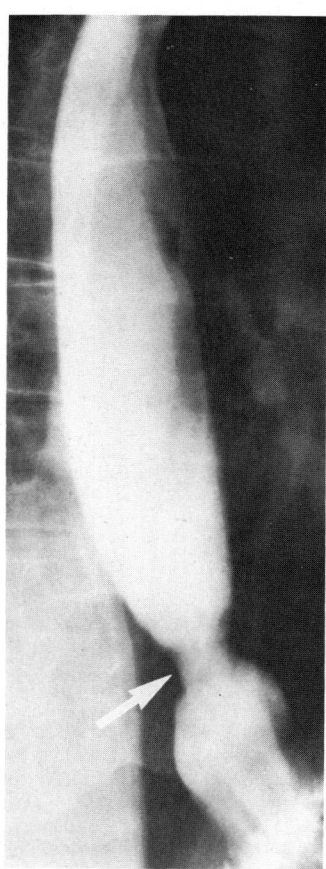

Figure 24–19. Annular peptic stricture. This stricture *(arrow)* could be mistaken for a Schatzki ring. However, it has a greater vertical height than expected for Schatzki rings.

They may occur as a result of nasogastric intubation, protracted vomiting, bile reflux after partial or total gastrectomy, and Zollinger-Ellison syndrome.[10–12, 26, 66–69] Although uncommon, severe esophagitis and rapidly progressive stricture formation may occur after nasogastric intubation[66, 67] (Fig. 24–21) (see Chapter 26). Patients with Zollinger-Ellison syndrome may also develop long strictures in the distal esophagus due to reflux of extremely acidic peptic contents[11] (Fig. 24–22). Occasionally, these individuals may present with an esophageal stricture as the initial manifestation of their disease.[11, 12]

Esophageal intramural pseudodiverticulosis may occasionally be detected radiographically in the region of a peptic stricture[70] (Fig. 24–23) (see Chapter 26). The pseudodiverticula probably occur as a sequela of chronic reflux esophagitis, but it is unclear why so few patients with esophagitis have this finding.

## Differential Diagnosis

### Artifacts

Shallow ulcers or nodules in the esophagus may be simulated by a variety of technical artifacts on the double contrast examination.[45, 71] When barium agents are improperly prepared, barium precipitates can be mistaken for numerous tiny ulcers (Fig. 24–24A). A similar appearance may also result from transient mucosal crinkling due to incomplete esophageal distention. Occasionally, an irregular Z line at the squamocolumnar junction may resemble a focal area of superficial ulceration. Even prominent interstitial lung markings or

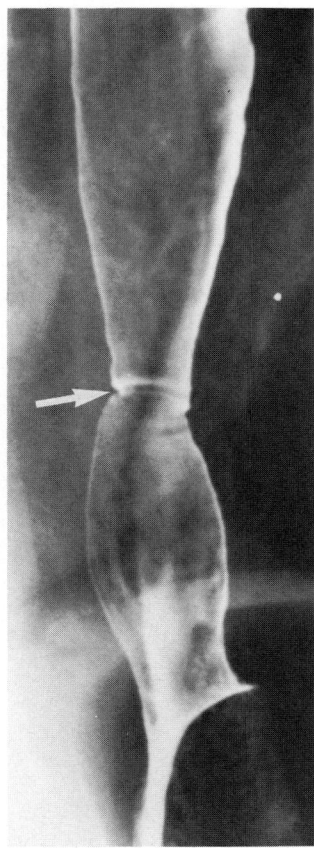

**Figure 24–20. Peptic stricture with an associated web *(arrow)*.** Note how the web is located a greater distance from the gastroesophageal junction than expected for lower esophageal rings.

vascular shadows seen through the esophagus may create the erroneous impression of ulceration.

Apparent nodularity may result from undissolved effervescent agents, gas bubbles, or debris in the esophagus (Fig. 24–24B). As a result, the increased sensitivity of the double contrast study has been compromised by the increased number of false-positive examinations with this technique.[34, 36] If an artifact is suspected, however, additional double contrast radiographs should be obtained to demonstrate the transient nature of these findings.

## Mucosal Nodularity

Glycogenic acanthosis should be the major consideration in the differential diagnosis of a nodular esophageal mucosa (see Chapter 27). This benign, degenerative condition is manifested radiographically by multiple small, rounded nodules or plaques in the middle or distal third of the esophagus, so it can resemble the nodular mucosa of reflux esophagitis[72, 73] (Fig. 24–25). However, the nodules of glycogenic acanthosis tend to be more well defined than those of reflux esophagitis and are usually more prominent in the midesophagus than in the distal esophagus. The clinical history is also helpful, as patients with glycogenic acanthosis are almost always asymptomatic.[72]

*Candida* esophagitis may occasionally produce finely nodular lesions in the middle or distal esophagus, mimicking the appearance of reflux esophagitis (Fig. 24–26). This form of *Candida* esophagitis has been observed more frequently in patients with acquired immunodeficiency syndrome.[74] Herpes esophagitis may also be manifested by an edematous, nodular mucosa in the distal esophagus, resembling that of reflux esophagitis. However, opportunistic esophagitis should be suggested by the typical history of odynophagia in an immunocompromised patient.

Rarely, superficial spreading carcinoma may produce a reticulonodular appearance of the mucosa, but the area of involvement is usually more localized and more well defined than that in reflux esophagitis.[75] Finally, leukoplakia, acanthosis nigricans, and squamous papillomatosis are rare causes of mucosal nodularity in the esophagus, and the diagnosis is usually made unexpectedly at endoscopy or autopsy in these patients (see Chapter 27).

## Ulceration

Although reflux esophagitis is the most common cause of superficial ulceration in the esophagus, shallow ulcers and erosions may be caused by other types of esophagitis, including herpes esophagitis, drug-induced esoph-

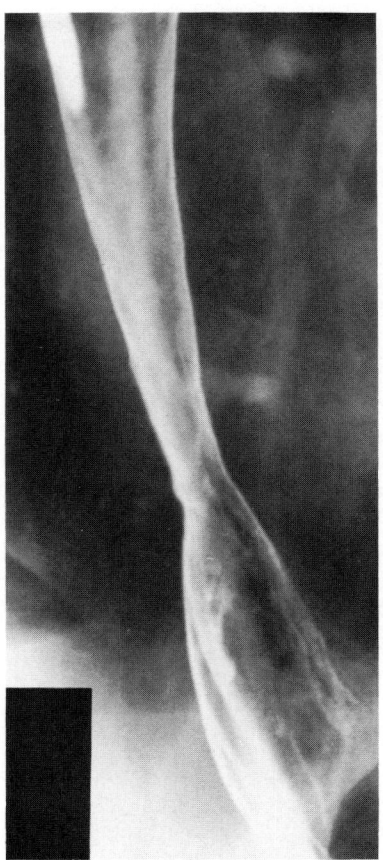

**Figure 24–21. Nasogastric intubation stricture.** The stricture is manifested by a long, tapered area of narrowing in the distal third of the esophagus.

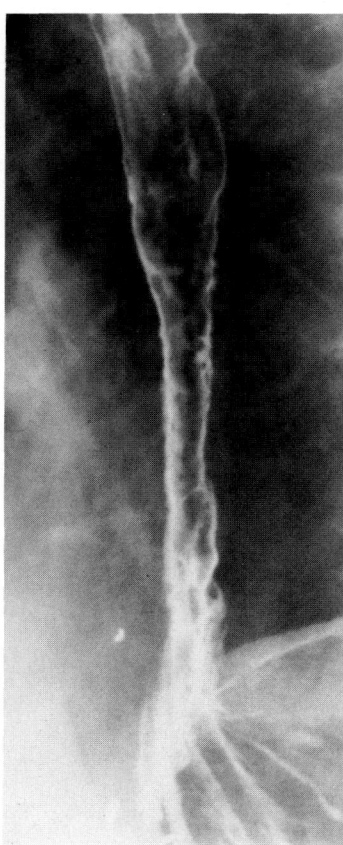

**Figure 24–22. Long peptic stricture caused by Zollinger-Ellison syndrome.** There is a long area of narrowing in the distal esophagus with extensive ulceration in the region of the stricture. The unusual length of the strictures in these patients is presumably related to the higher acidity of refluxed peptic contents in Zollinger-Ellison syndrome.

**Figure 24–23. Peptic strictures with esophageal intramural pseudodiverticulosis. A.** There is a mild peptic stricture in the distal esophagus with multiple intramural pseudodiverticula seen en face and in profile *(arrows)* in the region of the stricture. **B.** This patient has a more severe peptic stricture with several pseudodiverticula *(arrows)* adjacent to the stricture. Note how the pseudodiverticula seem to be floating outside the wall of the esophagus without apparent communication with the lumen. The latter feature is characteristic of these structures.

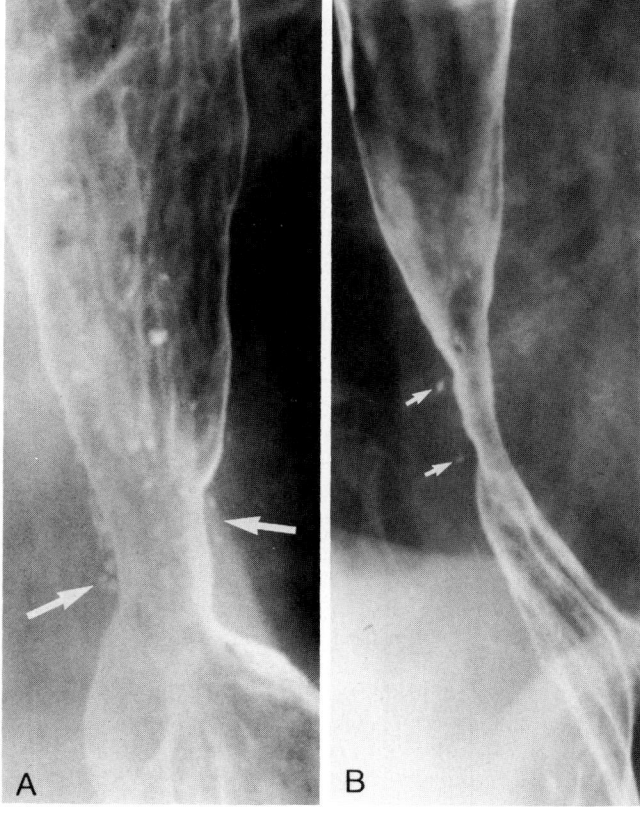

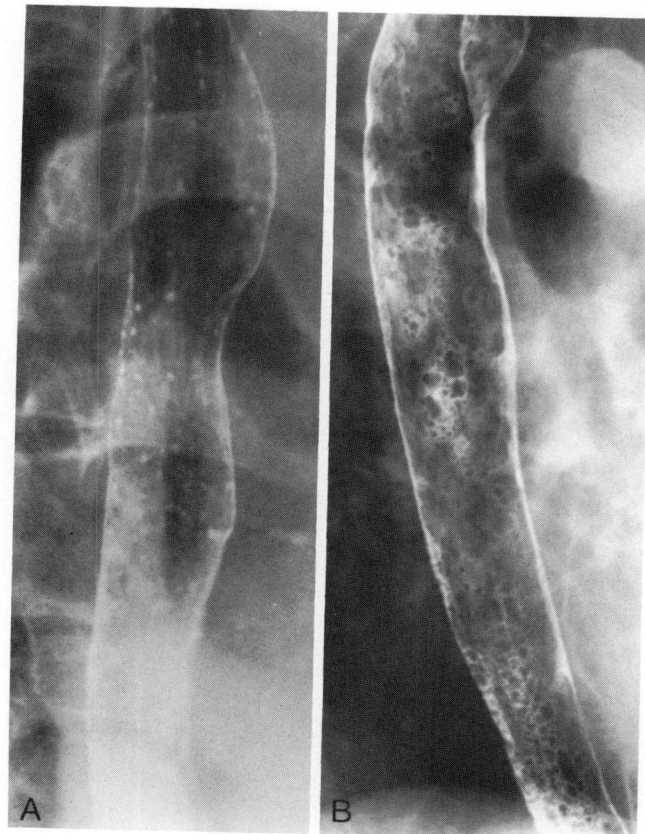

**Figure 24–24. Double contrast artifacts. A.** Barium precipitates are present in the esophagus. These punctate collections of barium could be mistaken for tiny ulcers. **B.** In another patient, undissolved effervescent agent and gas bubbles in the esophagus cause apparent nodularity of the mucosa. If an artifact is suspected, additional double contrast views should be obtained to demonstrate the transient nature of these findings.

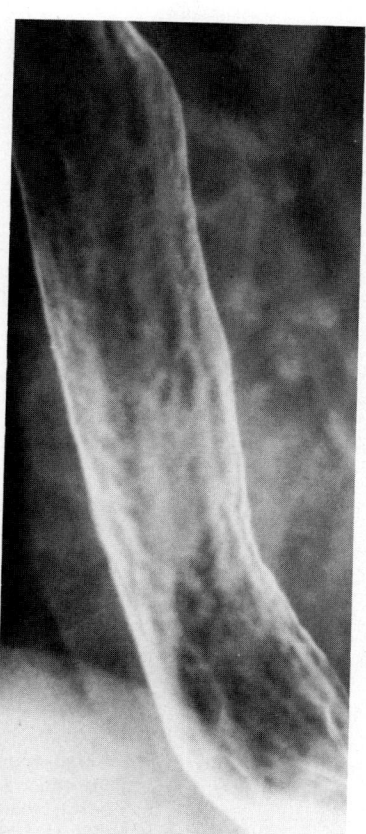

**Figure 24–25. Glycogenic acanthosis.** There are poorly defined nodules in the distal esophagus, mimicking the appearance of reflux esophagitis. However, this patient was asymptomatic.

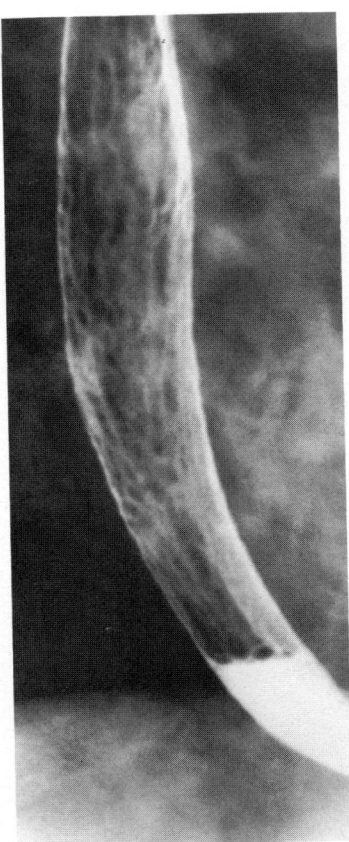

**Figure 24–26. Candida esophagitis.** There are finely nodular lesions in the distal half of the esophagus. Note the resemblance to the granular mucosa of reflux esophagitis. However, this was a patient who had acquired immunodeficiency syndrome with odynophagia.

neoplastic process that involves the submucosa. Although varices occasionally may resemble the thickened folds of esophagitis, they tend to be more tortuous or serpiginous and can usually be effaced to a greater degree or even obliterated by esophageal distention. Rarely, "varicoid" carcinomas may also be indistinguishable from varices or esophagitis on a single radiograph.[79] Because the folds are infiltrated by tumor, however, they are unaffected by esophageal peristalsis, respiration, and Valsalva maneuvers and cannot be significantly effaced by esophageal distention. Thus, these entities can usually be differentiated at fluoroscopy.

## Scarring and Strictures

Fixed transverse folds in the esophagus due to scarring from reflux esophagitis should be distinguished not only from delicate transverse striations in the esophagus but also from transverse bands associated with nonperistaltic contractions. However, the latter finding can easily be recognized as a transient phenomenon due to contraction of the muscularis propria.[54] The horizontal collections of barium pooling between these fixed transverse folds should also not be mistaken for areas of linear ulceration. However, the regularity and symmetry of

agitis, and esophageal involvement by Crohn's disease.[76–78] Unlike reflux esophagitis, however, herpes esophagitis and drug-induced esophagitis tend to involve the middle or upper third of the esophagus with distal esophageal sparing (Figs. 24–27 and 24–28), and they are usually not associated with evidence of a hiatal hernia or gastroesophageal reflux. The correct diagnosis should also be suggested by a clinical history of acute odynophagia in patients who are immunocompromised or who are taking oral medications such as tetracycline and doxycycline.

Occasionally, esophageal involvement by Crohn's disease may be manifested radiographically by one or more superficial ulcers, mimicking the appearance of reflux esophagitis. However, esophageal Crohn's disease is uncommon, and these patients almost always have evidence of advanced Crohn's disease in the small bowel or colon. More extensive ulceration may be caused by opportunistic infection, caustic ingestion, and mediastinal irradiation (see Chapters 25 and 26). In most cases, however, the correct diagnosis is suggested by the clinical history and presentation.

## Thickened Folds

Thickened longitudinal folds in the esophagus may be caused by esophageal varices or by any inflammatory or

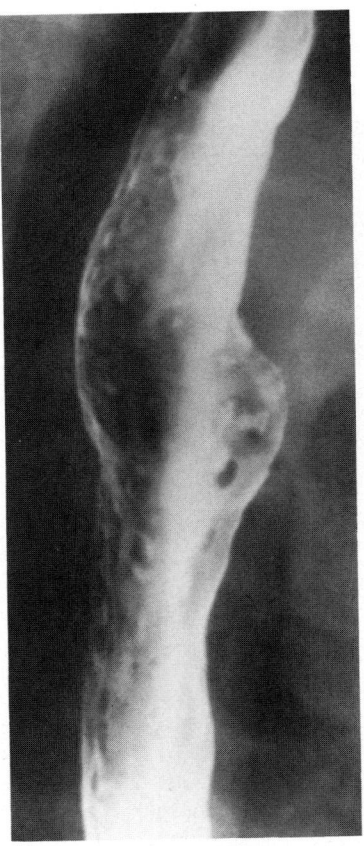

**Figure 24–27. Herpes esophagitis.** There are discrete, superficial ulcers in the midesophagus. In contrast, ulceration in reflux esophagitis predominantly involves the distal esophagus, extending proximally from the gastroesophageal junction as a continuous area of disease. (From Levine MS: Radiology of esophagitis: a pattern approach. Radiology 179:1–7, 1991.)

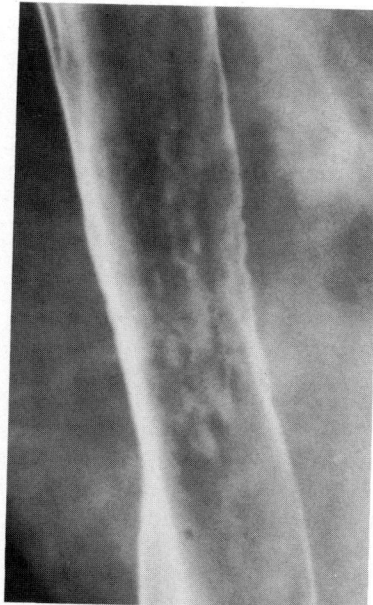

**Figure 24–28. Drug-induced esophagitis.** There are multiple tiny ulcers in the midesophagus with normal-appearing mucosa below this level. The absence of disease distally argues against a diagnosis of reflux esophagitis. This patient had a history of recent doxycycline ingestion.

is considerable evidence that it is a premalignant condition associated with a significantly increased risk of developing esophageal adenocarcinoma. It is widely believed that adenocarcinoma evolves through a sequence of progressively severe epithelial dysplasia, eventually leading to the development of invasive carcinoma. In various studies, the prevalence of adenocarcinoma in patients with Barrett's esophagus has ranged from 2.4 to 46.5%, with an overall prevalence of about 15%.[84, 86–90] Prevalence data may exaggerate the risk of cancer, as most patients with Barrett's esophagus do not seek medical attention until they develop complications such as ulcers, strictures, or malignancy. Nevertheless, prospective studies have found that the annual incidence of malignant transformation in Barrett's esophagus is 1 to 2%.[91, 92] Many investigators therefore advocate periodic endoscopic surveillance with biopsy and cytology at 6-month or yearly intervals for early detection of cancer in Barrett's esophagus (see Chapter 28).[84, 86–88, 93–96]

## Clinical Findings

Barrett's esophagus is most commonly found in older individuals but may also occur in young patients with

these collections should suggest the correct diagnosis.

A smooth, tapered area of concentric narrowing above a hiatal hernia poses little diagnostic dilemma, but not all peptic strictures have this classic appearance. If suspicious radiographic features such as asymmetry, abrupt margins, and mucosal nodularity or ulceration are identified on the barium study (Fig. 24–29), endoscopy and biopsy should be performed to rule out an infiltrating carcinoma. Alternatively, a tube esophagram may better delineate the radiographic features of the stricture to differentiate benign and malignant lesions.[80]

## BARRETT'S ESOPHAGUS

Barrett's esophagus is an acquired condition in which there is progressive columnar metaplasia of the distal esophagus due to long-standing gastroesophageal reflux and reflux esophagitis.[81–83] Current data suggest that Barrett's esophagus is a much more common condition than has previously been recognized. In various studies, the prevalence of Barrett's esophagus in patients with reflux esophagitis has ranged from 8 to 20%, with an overall prevalence of about 10%.[84–87] These figures may be skewed in favor of Barrett's esophagus, because patients with reflux symptoms who undergo endoscopy are more likely to have significant reflux disease. Nevertheless, Barrett's esophagus is being diagnosed with greater frequency as the number of patients who undergo endoscopy increases.

Despite its frequency, Barrett's esophagus would not be important if it were a benign entity. However, there

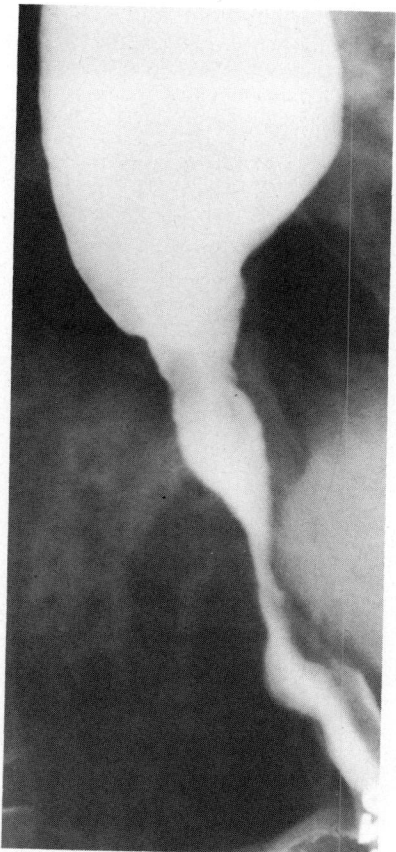

**Figure 24–29. Esophageal carcinoma.** There is a relatively long area of narrowing in the distal esophagus that could be mistaken for a benign peptic stricture. However, the asymmetric contour and relatively abrupt proximal borders of the narrowed segment should suggest the possibility of malignancy.

reflux esophagitis. There is no apparent sex predilection. Some patients have a long-standing history of reflux symptoms, whereas others may initially present with dysphagia due to the development of peptic strictures.[97] However, 20 to 40% of patients with Barrett's esophagus have no esophageal symptoms.[98, 99] Unfortunately, these patients may remain asymptomatic until the development of a superimposed esophageal adenocarcinoma. As a result, the tumors often are advanced, unresectable lesions at the time of clinical presentation. Barrett's carcinoma therefore has an extremely poor prognosis, with 5-year survival rates comparable to those of squamous cell carcinoma.[90, 96]

## Endoscopic and Histologic Findings

Barrett's esophagus may be recognized at endoscopy by the presence of velvety, pinkish red islands or tongues of columnar mucosa extending more than 2 cm above the gastroesophageal junction or an endoscopically identified hiatal hernia. Endoscopy has a sensitivity of greater than 90% in diagnosing Barrett's esophagus solely on the basis of the endoscopic appearance.[100, 101] However, a definitive diagnosis can be made only on histologic criteria. The columnar epithelium in Barrett's esophagus is not simply gastric mucosa but a mosaic of intimately admixed glandular and cell types from the stomach and small bowel, including a gastric-fundic–type epithelium with parietal and chief cells, a junctional-type epithelium with cardiac mucous glands, and a specialized columnar-type epithelium with a villiform surface, mucous glands, and intestinal-like goblet cells (i.e., intestinal metaplasia).[102, 103] One or more foci of low- or high-grade dysplasia, intramucosal carcinoma, or invasive carcinoma may be present in Barrett's mucosa. However, some investigators believe that the risk of malignant degeneration is greatest in pre-existing areas of intestinal metaplasia.[93]

## Radiographic Findings

The classic radiologic features of Barrett's esophagus consist of a high esophageal stricture or ulcer, often associated with a sliding hiatal hernia or gastroesophageal reflux[104–106] (Figs. 24–30 to 24–32). The unusual location of these strictures and ulcers can be attributed to the fact that they often occur in the proximal zone of columnar metaplasia near the squamocolumnar junction. The strictures may appear as ring-like constrictions or, less commonly, as smooth, tapered areas of narrowing in the midesophagus[104] (see Fig. 24–30). Barrett's ulcers typically appear as relatively deep ulcer craters within the columnar mucosa at a considerable distance from the gastroesophageal junction[107] (see Fig. 24–31). Other patients may have a high esophageal stricture associated with an ulcer (see Fig. 24–32). Because these

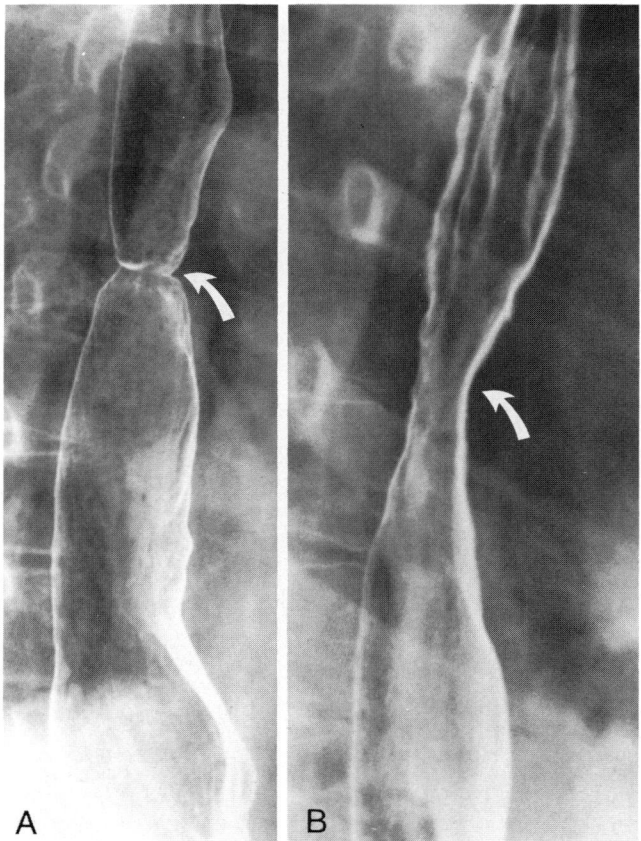

A   B

**Figure 24–30. Barrett's esophagus with high strictures. A.** There is a ring-like constriction *(arrow)* in the midesophagus. **B.** A smooth, tapered area of narrowing *(arrow)* is seen in the midesophagus. In the presence of a hiatal hernia and gastroesophageal reflux, a high esophageal stricture should be strongly suggestive of Barrett's esophagus.

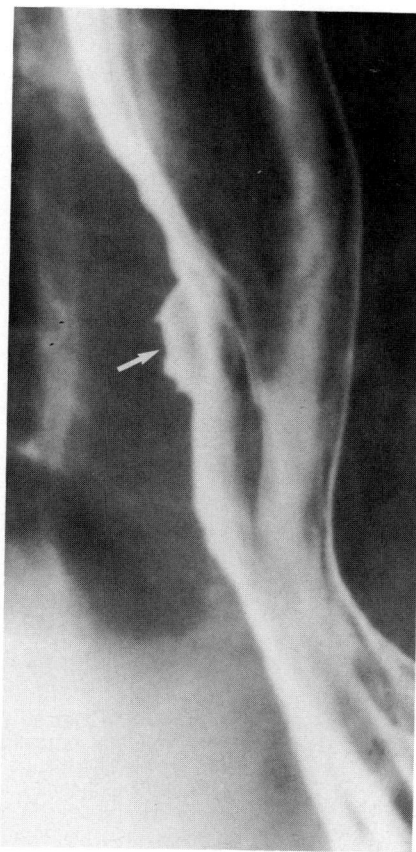

**Figure 24–31. Barrett's esophagus with a high ulcer.** There is a relatively deep ulcer crater *(arrow)* at a greater distance from the gastroesophageal junction than expected for uncomplicated reflux esophagitis. In the presence of a hiatal hernia and gastroesophageal reflux, a high ulcer should be strongly suggestive of Barrett's esophagus.

normality in Barrett's esophagus without evidence of strictures.[112] Whether or not a stricture is present, this distinctive reticular pattern should be highly suggestive of Barrett's esophagus, and endoscopy and biopsy should be performed for a definitive diagnosis. Nevertheless, this finding has been observed in only 5 to 30% of patients with Barrett's esophagus,[106, 109–111, 113] and its specificity has also been questioned.[114] Thus, most cases of Barrett's esophagus will be missed on double contrast esophagography if a reticular mucosal pattern is used as the primary radiologic criterion for diagnosing this condition.

Because Barrett's esophagus develops as the sequela of long-standing reflux esophagitis, it is not surprising that these patients often have radiologic evidence of hiatal hernias, gastroesophageal reflux, reflux esophagitis, and peptic strictures[105, 106, 108–111, 113] (Fig. 24–34). In one study, 97% of patients with Barrett's esophagus had esophagitis or strictures on double contrast studies.[106] However, these findings often occur in patients with uncomplicated reflux disease. As a result, inclusion of these findings as criteria for Barrett's esophagus increases the sensitivity of the radiologic examination but decreases its specificity, so that many patients would be referred unnecessarily for endoscopy and biopsy.[113] Thus, radiographic findings that are relatively specific for Barrett's esophagus are not sensitive, and those that

findings are unusual in uncomplicated reflux esophagitis, the presence of a high esophageal stricture or ulcer, particularly if associated with a hiatal hernia or gastroesophageal reflux, should be strongly suggestive of Barrett's esophagus. However, studies have found that strictures are actually more common in the distal esophagus and that most cases do not fit the classic stereotype of a high stricture or ulcer.[108–111] Thus, esophagography is an inadequate screening examination for Barrett's esophagus when the diagnosis is made only in patients who have the classic radiologic features of this condition.

A reticular mucosal pattern has also been described as a relatively specific sign of Barrett's esophagus, particularly if located adjacent to a stricture.[109] This delicate reticular pattern is characterized radiographically by innumerable tiny, barium-filled grooves or crevices on the esophageal mucosa, often resembling the areae gastricae pattern found on double contrast studies of the stomach (Fig. 24–33). In most cases, there is an adjacent stricture in the middle or, less commonly, distal esophagus, with the reticular pattern extending distally a short but variable distance from the stricture.[109] Occasionally, however, a reticular or villous pattern of the mucosa may be observed as the only morphologic ab-

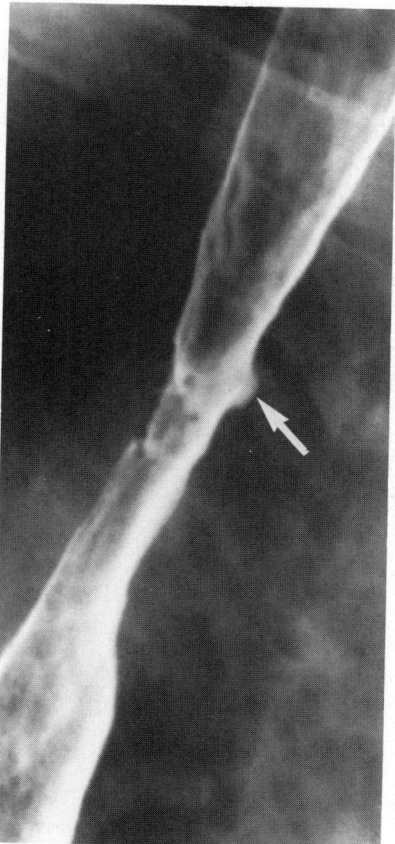

**Figure 24–32. Barrett's esophagus with a high stricture and ulcer.** There is a segmental stricture in the midesophagus with a discrete ulcer *(arrow)* in the region of the stricture.

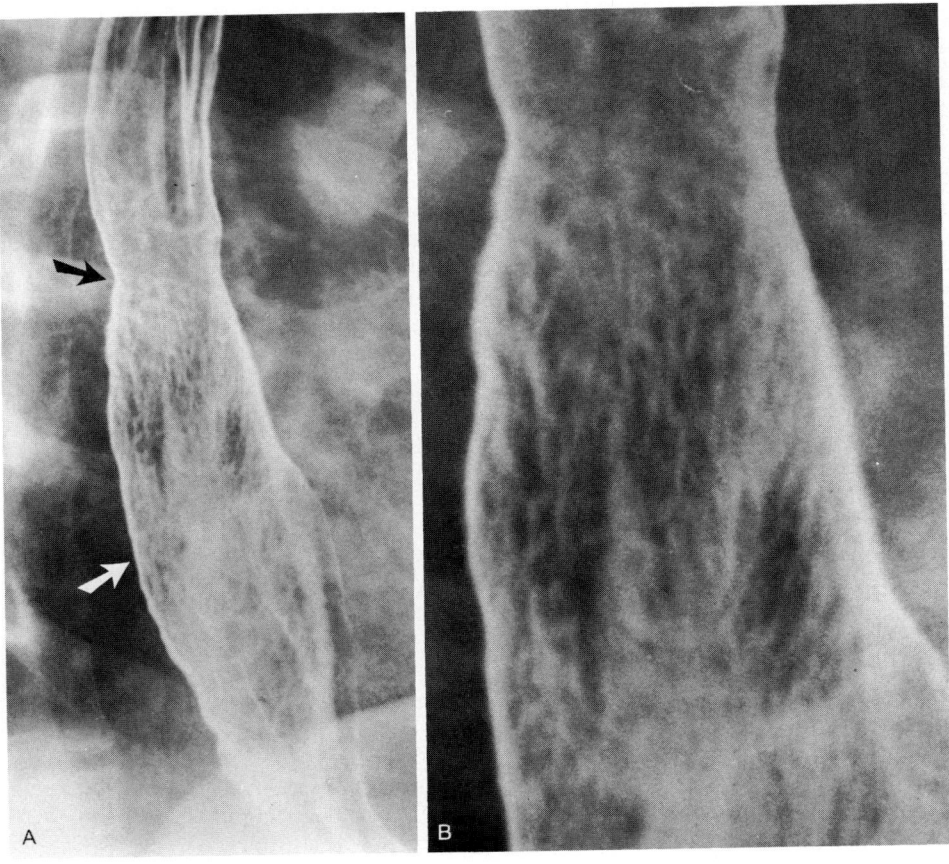

**Figure 24–33. Barrett's esophagus with a reticular mucosal pattern. A.** There is an early stricture *(black arrow)* in the midesophagus with a reticular pattern seen extending distally a considerable distance from the stricture (approximately to the level of the white arrow). **B.** A close-up view better delineates this delicate reticular pattern. (**A** and **B** from Levine MS, Kressel HY, Caroline DF, et al: Barrett esophagus: reticular pattern of the mucosa. Radiology 147:663–667, 1983.)

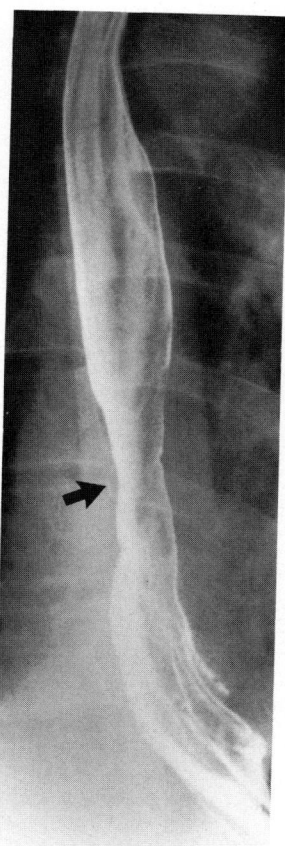

**Figure 24–34. Barrett's esophagus with a distal stricture.** There is a concentric area of narrowing *(arrow)* in the distal esophagus above a hiatal hernia. An ordinary peptic stricture without Barrett's esophagus could produce identical findings.

only 1 of 117 patients (<1%) at low risk for Barrett's esophagus. Although the overall sensitivity in diagnosing reflux esophagitis was only 53%, most cases of reflux esophagitis missed radiographically were mild and only one of those patients had Barrett's esophagus. The data suggest that esophagitis severe enough to cause Barrett's esophagus can almost always be detected on technically adequate double contrast examinations.

Based on their findings, Gilchrist and colleagues concluded that patients who are at high risk for Barrett's esophagus because of a high stricture or ulcer or a reticular mucosal pattern should undergo early endoscopy and biopsy for a definitive diagnosis.[115] A larger group of patients are at moderate risk for Barrett's esophagus because of reflux esophagitis or peptic strictures, so clinical judgment should be used regarding the decision for endoscopy in this group based on the severity of reflux symptoms, age, and overall health of the patient. However, the majority of patients have no radiologic evidence of esophagitis or strictures, and the risk of Barrett's esophagus is so low in this group that endoscopy does not appear to be warranted. Thus, the major value of double contrast esophagography is its ability to separate patients into high-, moderate-, and low-risk groups for Barrett's esophagus to determine the relative need for endoscopy and biopsy in these patients.

## Differential Diagnosis

Uncomplicated peptic strictures are almost always located in the distal esophagus, so the presence of a high esophageal stricture should strongly suggest the possibility of Barrett's esophagus, particularly if an associated hiatal hernia and gastroesophageal reflux are present. High esophageal strictures may also be caused by caustic ingestion (Fig. 24–35A), mediastinal irradiation (Fig. 24–35B), primary or metastatic tumors, and, rarely, esophageal involvement by dermatologic disorders such as epidermolysis bullosa dystrophica and benign mucous membrane pemphigoid. However, these conditions can usually be differentiated from Barrett's esophagus by the clinical history and presentation.

The presence of a reticular mucosal pattern appears to be a relatively specific radiologic criterion for Barrett's esophagus, particularly if located adjacent to the distal aspect of a high stricture.[109] Although a reticulonodular appearance may occasionally be seen in patients with superficial spreading carcinoma, it is a rare entity that is not classically associated with strictures.[75] Shallow ulceration or mucosal irregularity due to reflux esophagitis might also conceivably produce a similar appearance. However, reflux esophagitis usually occurs proximal to a peptic stricture, and it would be extremely unusual for an isolated area of esophagitis to occur at the distal aspect of a stricture. *Candida* esophagitis may also be manifested by mucosal nodularity, but the discrete plaque-like lesions of candidiasis can usually be differentiated from the reticular pattern of Barrett's mucosa.

are sensitive are not specific. Many investigators therefore believe that esophagography has limited value as a screening examination for Barrett's esophagus and that endoscopy and biopsy are required to diagnose this condition.

Gilchrist and colleagues performed a "blinded," retrospective study of 200 patients who had both double contrast esophagrams and endoscopy because of severe reflux symptoms.[115] The patients were classified into high-, moderate-, and low-risk groups for Barrett's esophagus on the basis of the radiographic findings. Patients were classified at high risk if the radiographs revealed the classic findings of a high stricture or ulcer or a reticular mucosal pattern, at moderate risk if the radiographs revealed a distal peptic stricture or reflux esophagitis (because previous studies have shown that about 45% of patients with peptic strictures and 10% with reflux esophagitis have Barrett's esophagus[84–87, 116]), and at low risk if none of these findings were present. When these radiologic criteria were used, 10 patients (5%) were thought to be at high risk, 73 (37%) at moderate risk, and 117 (58%) at low risk for Barrett's esophagus. Endoscopic correlation revealed biopsyproven Barrett's mucosa in 9 of 10 patients (90%) at high risk, 12 of 73 patients (16%) at moderate risk, and

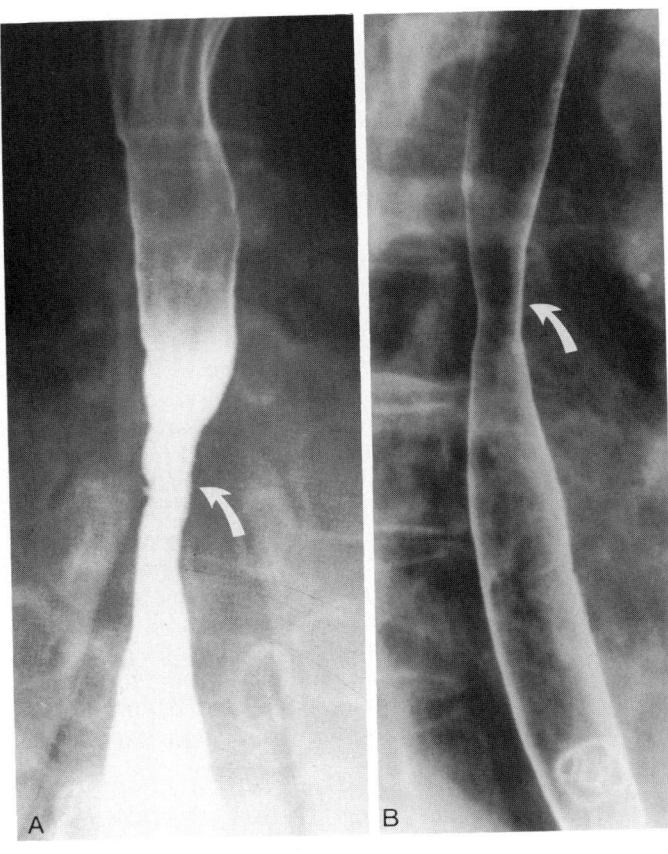

**Figure 24–35. Other causes of high esophageal strictures. A.** There is a segmental stricture *(arrow)* with shallow ulceration in the midesophagus due to prior lye ingestion. **B.** There is a smooth, tapered stricture *(arrow)* in the midesophagus due to mediastinal irradiation.

## Acknowledgment

Figures 24–1, 24–7 to 24–9, 24–11 to 24–13, 24–18A, 24–19 to 24–22, 24–23A, 24–24B, 24–25, 24–26, 24–28 to 24–31, 24–34, and 24–35 are reproduced from Levine MS: Radiology of the Esophagus. Philadelphia: WB Saunders, 1989.

Figures 24–4, 24–6A and B, 24–14, 24–15B, and 24–18B are reproduced from Laufer I, Levine MS (eds): Double Contrast Gastrointestinal Radiology (2nd ed). Philadelphia: WB Saunders, 1992.

# References

1. Behar J: Reflux esophagitis: pathogenesis, diagnosis, and management. Arch Intern Med 136:560–566, 1976.
2. Dodds WJ: Current concepts of esophageal motor function: clinical implications for radiology. AJR 128:549–561, 1977.
3. Dodds WJ, Hogan WJ, Helm JF, et al: Pathogenesis of reflux esophagitis. Gastroenterology 81:376–394, 1981.
4. Dodds WJ: The pathogenesis of gastroesophageal reflux disease. AJR 151:49–56, 1988.
5. Pope CE: Pathophysiology and diagnosis of reflux esophagitis. Gastroenterology 70:445–454, 1976.
6. Dodds WJ, Dent J, Hogan WJ, et al: Mechanisms of gastroesophageal reflux in patients with reflux esophagitis. N Engl J Med 307:1547–1552, 1982.
7. Zamost BJ, Hirschberg J, Ippoliti AF, et al: Esophagitis in scleroderma: prevalence and risk factors. Gastroenterology 92:421–428, 1987.
8. Goldman MS, Rasch JR, Wittsie DS, et al: Incidence of esophagitis in peptic ulcer disease. Am J Dig Dis 12:994–998, 1967.
9. Casten DF: Peptic esophagitis, hiatal hernia, and duodenal ulcer. Am J Surg 113:638–641, 1967.
10. Dodds WJ, Dehn TG, Hogan WJ, et al: Severe peptic esophagitis in a patient with Zollinger-Ellison syndrome. AJR 113:237–240, 1971.
11. Smith HJ, Chapa HJ, Kilman WJ, et al: Zollinger-Ellison syndrome presenting as esophageal stricture. Gastrointest Radiol 4:349–351, 1979.
12. Agha FP: Esophageal involvement in Zollinger-Ellison syndrome. AJR 144:721–725, 1985.
13. Orlando RC, Bozymski EM: Heartburn in pernicious anemia—a consequence of bile reflux. N Engl J Med 289:522–523, 1973.
14. Cohen S: The diagnosis and management of gastroesophageal reflux. Adv Intern Med 21:47–75, 1976.
15. Wright RA, Hurwitz AL: Relationship of hiatal hernia to endoscopically proved reflux esophagitis. Dig Dis Sci 24:311–313, 1979.
16. Ott DJ, Gelfand DW, Chen YM, et al: Predictive relationship of hiatal hernia to reflux esophagitis. Gastrointest Radiol 10:317–320, 1985.
17. Cohen S, Harris LD: Does hiatus hernia affect competence of the gastroesophageal sphincter? N Engl J Med 284:1053–1056, 1971.
18. Ellis FH: Current concepts: esophageal hiatal hernia. N Engl J Med 287:646–649, 1972.
19. Hiebert CA, Belsey R: Incompetency of the gastric cardia without radiologic evidence of hiatal hernia: the diagnosis and management of 71 cases. J Thorac Cardiovasc Surg 42:352–359, 1961.
20. Ho CS, Rodrigues PR: Lower esophageal strictures, benign or malignant? J Can Assoc Radiol 31:110–113, 1980.
21. Ott DJ, Dodds WJ, Wu WC, et al: Current status of radiology in evaluating for gastroesophageal reflux disease. J Clin Gastroenterol 4:365–375, 1982.
22. Skinner DB, Camp TF: Measurement of gastroesophageal reflux in the evaluation of hiatus hernia and chest pain in fliers. Aerosp Med 8:846–850, 1967.
23. Bernstein LM, Pacini R, Fruin RC, et al: Esophagitis as a cause of upper abdominal pain. JAMA 168:27–33, 1958.

24. Siegel CI, Hendrix TR: Esophageal motor abnormalities induced by acid perfusion in patients with heartburn. J Clin Invest 42:686–695, 1963.

25. Smith JL, Opekun AR, Larkai E, et al: Sensitivity of the esophageal mucosa to pH in gastroesophageal reflux disease. Gastroenterology 96:683–689, 1989.

26. Bennett JR: Oesophageal strictures. Clin Gastroenterol 7:555–569, 1978.

27. Kantrowitz PA, Corson JG, Fleischli DJ, et al: Measurement of gastroesophageal reflux. Gastroenterology 56:666–674, 1969.

28. Blumhagen JD, Christie DL: Gastroesophageal reflux in children: evaluation of the water siphon test. Radiology 131:345–349, 1979.

29. Blumhagen JD, Rudd TG, Christie DL: Gastroesophageal reflux in children: radionuclide gastroesophagography. AJR 135:1001–1004, 1980.

30. Malmud LS, Fisher RS: Gastroesophageal scintigraphy. Gastrointest Radiol 5:195–204, 1980.

31. Booth DJ, Kemmerer WT, Skinner DB: Acid clearing from the distal esophagus. Arch Surg 96:731–734, 1968.

32. Tolin RD, Malmud LS, Reilley J, et al: Esophageal scintigraphy to quantitate esophageal transit (quantitation of esophageal transit). Gastroenterology 76:1402–1408, 1979.

33. Ott DJ, Gelfand DW, Wu WC: Reflux esophagitis: radiographic and endoscopic correlation. Radiology 130:583–588, 1979.

34. Koehler RE, Weyman PJ, Oakley HF: Single- and double-contrast techniques in esophagitis. AJR 135:15–19, 1980.

35. Ott DJ, Wu WC, Gelfand DW: Reflux esophagitis revisited: prospective analysis of radiologic accuracy. Gastrointest Radiol 6:1–7, 1981.

36. Creteur V, Thoeni RF, Federle MP, et al: The role of single and double-contrast radiography in the diagnosis of reflux esophagitis. Radiology 147:71–75, 1983.

37. Graziani L, De Nigris E, Pesaresi A, et al: Reflux esophagitis: radiologic-endoscopic correlation in 39 symptomatic cases. Gastrointest Radiol 8:1–6, 1983.

38. Chen YM, Ott DJ, Gelfand DW, et al: Multiphasic examination of the esophagogastric region for strictures, rings, and hiatal hernia: evaluation of the individual techniques. Gastrointest Radiol 10:311–316, 1985.

39. Gibbs D: Endoscopy in the assessment of reflux oesophagitis. Clin Gastroenterol 5:135–142, 1976.

40. Ismail-Beigi F, Horton PF, Pope CE: Histological consequences of gastroesophageal reflux. Gastroenterology 58:163–174, 1970.

41. Kahrilas PJ, Dodds WJ, Hogan WJ, et al: Esophageal peristaltic dysfunction in peptic esophagitis. Gastroenterology 91:897–904, 1986.

42. Simeone JF, Burrell M, Toffler R, et al: Aperistalsis and esophagitis. Radiology 123:9–14, 1977.

43. Donner MW, Silbiger ML, Hookman P, et al: Acid-barium swallows in the radiographic evaluation of clinical esophagitis. Radiology 87:220–225, 1966.

44. Benz LJ, Hootkin LA, Margulies S, et al: A comparison of clinical measurements of gastroesophageal reflux. Gastroenterology 62:1–5, 1972.

45. Kressel HY, Glick SN, Laufer I, et al: Radiologic features of esophagitis. Gastrointest Radiol 6:103–108, 1981.

46. Laufer I: Radiology of esophagitis. Radiol Clin North Am 20:687–699, 1982.

47. Graziani L, Bearzi I, Romagnoli A, et al: Significance of diffuse granularity and nodularity of the esophageal mucosa at double-contrast radiography. Gastrointest Radiol 10:1–6, 1985.

48. Levine MS, Cajade AG, Herlinger H, et al: Pseudomembranes in reflux esophagitis. Radiology 159:43–45, 1986.

49. McDermott P, Wallers KJ, Holden R, et al: Double-contrast examination of the oesophagus: the radiological changes of peptic oesophagitis. Clin Radiol 33:259–264, 1982.

50. Levine MS, Goldstein HM: Fixed transverse folds in the esophagus: a sign of reflux esophagitis. AJR 143:275–278, 1984.

51. Wolf BS, Marshak RH, Som ML, et al: Peptic esophagitis, peptic ulcer of the esophagus, and marginal esophagogastric ulceration. Gastroenterology 29:744–766, 1955.

52. Wolf BS, Marshak RH, Som ML: Peptic esophagitis and peptic ulceration of the esophagus. AJR 79:741–759, 1958.

53. Rabin M, Schmaman IB: Reflux oesophagitis resembling varices. S Afr Med J 55:293–295, 1979.

54. Gohel VK, Edell SL, Laufer I, et al: Transverse folds in the human esophagus. Radiology 128:303–308, 1978.

55. Williams SM, Harned RK, Kaplan P, et al: Transverse striations of the esophagus: association with gastroesophageal reflux. Radiology 146:25–27, 1983.

56. Bleshman MH, Banner MP, Johnson RC, et al: The inflammatory esophagogastric polyp and fold. Radiology 128:589–593, 1978.

57. Ghahremani GG, Fisher MR, Rushovich AM: Prolapsing inflammatory pseudopolyp-fold complex of the oesophagogastric region. Eur J Radiol 4:47–51, 1984.

58. Styles RA, Gibb SP, Tarshis A, et al: Esophagogastric polyps: radiographic and endoscopic findings. Radiology 154:307–311, 1985.

59. Palmer ED: The hiatus hernia–esophagitis–esophageal stricture complex: twenty-year prospective study. Am J Med 44:566–579, 1968.

60. Ott DJ, Gelfand DW, Lane TG, et al: Radiologic detection and spectrum of appearances of esophageal strictures. J Clin Gastroenterol 4:11–15, 1982.

61. Ott DJ, Chen YM, Wu WC, et al: Endoscopic sensitivity in the detection of esophageal strictures. J Clin Gastroenterol 7:121–125, 1985.

62. Dodds WJ, Stewart ET, Stef JJ, et al: Longitudinal esophageal contractions: a possible factor in the genesis of hiatal hernia. Invest Radiol 11:375, 1976 (abstract).

63. Schatzki R, Gary JE: Dysphagia due to a diaphragm-like localized narrowing in the lower esophagus ("lower esophageal ring"). AJR 70:911–922, 1953.

64. Ingelfinger FJ, Kramer P: Dysphagia produced by a contractile ring in the lower esophagus. Gastroenterology 23:419–430, 1953.

65. Weaver JW, Kaude JV, Hamlin DJ: Webs of the lower esophagus: a complication of gastroesophageal reflux? AJR 142:289–292, 1984.

66. Douglas WK: Oesophageal strictures associated with gastroduodenal intubation. Br J Surg 43:404–409, 1956.

67. Graham J, Barnes N, Rubenstein AS: The nasogastric tube as a cause of esophagitis and stricture. Am J Surg 98:116–119, 1959.

68. McKeown KC: Oesophageal stenosis after partial gastrectomy. Br Med J 2:819–823, 1958.

69. Levine MS, Fisher AR, Rubesin SE, et al: Complications after total gastrectomy and esophagojejunostomy: radiologic evaluation. AJR 157:1189–1194, 1991.

70. Levine MS, Moolten DN, Herlinger H, et al: Esophageal intramural pseudodiverticulosis: a reevaluation. AJR 147:1165–1170, 1986.

71. Gohel VK, Kressel HY, Laufer I: Double contrast artifacts. Gastrointest Radiol 3:139–146, 1978.

72. Glick SN, Teplick SK, Goldstein J, et al: Glycogenic acanthosis of the esophagus. AJR 139:683–688, 1982.

73. Ghahremani GG, Rushovich AM: Glycogenic acanthosis of the esophagus: radiographic and pathologic features. Gastrointest Radiol 9:93–98, 1984.

74. Levine MS, Woldenberg R, Herlinger H, et al: Opportunistic esophagitis in AIDS: radiographic diagnosis. Radiology 165:815–820, 1987.

75. Itai Y, Kogure T, Okuyama Y, et al: Superficial esophageal carcinoma: radiological findings in double-contrast studies. Radiology 126:597–601, 1978.

76. Levine MS, Laufer I, Kressel HY, et al: Herpes esophagitis. AJR 136:863–866, 1981.

77. Bova JG, Dutton NE, Goldstein HM, et al: Medication-induced esophagitis: diagnosis by double-contrast esophagography. AJR 148:731–732, 1987.

78. DeGryse HR, De Schepper AM: Aphthoid esophageal ulcers in Crohn's disease of ileum and colon. Gastrointest Radiol 9:197–201, 1984.

79. Silver TM, Goldstein HM: Varicoid carcinoma of the esophagus. Am J Dig Dis 19:56–58, 1974.

80. Levine MS, Kressel HY, Laufer I, et al: The tube esophagram: a technique for obtaining a detailed double-contrast examination of the esophagus. AJR 142:293–298, 1984.

81. Bozymski EM, Herlihy KH, Orlando RC: Barrett's esophagus. Ann Intern Med 97:103–107, 1982.

82. Sjogren RW, Johnson LF: Barrett's esophagus: a review. Am J Med 74:313–321, 1983.

83. Spechler SJ, Goyal RK: Barrett's esophagus. N Engl J Med 315:362–371, 1986.

84. Naef AP, Savary M, Ozello L: Columnar-lined lower esophagus: an acquired lesion with malignant predisposition. J Thorac Cardiovasc Surg 70:826–835, 1975.

85. Burbige EJ, Radigan JJ: Characteristics of the columnar-cell lined (Barrett's) esophagus. Gastrointest Endosc 25:133–136, 1979.

86. Starnes VA, Adkins RB, Ballinger JF, et al: Barrett's esophagus: a surgical entity. Arch Surg 119:563–567, 1984.

87. Sarr MG, Hamilton SR, Marrone GC, et al: Barrett's esophagus: its prevalence and association with adenocarcinoma in patients with symptoms of gastroesophageal reflux. Am J Surg 149:187–192, 1985.

88. Hawe A, Payne WS, Weiland LH, et al: Adenocarcinoma in the columnar epithelial lined lower (Barrett) oesophagus. Thorax 28:511–514, 1973.

89. Levine MS, Caroline DF, Thompson JJ, et al: Adenocarcinoma of the esophagus: relationship to Barrett mucosa. Radiology 150:305–309, 1984.

90. Skinner DB, Walther BC, Riddell RH, et al: Barrett's esophagus: comparison of benign and malignant cases. Ann Surg 198:554–565, 1983.

91. Robertson CS, Mayberry JF, Nicholson DA, et al: Value of endoscopic surveillance in the detection of neoplastic change in Barrett's oesophagus. Br J Surg 75:760–763, 1988.

92. Hameeteman W, Tytgat GN, Houthoff HJ, et al: Barrett's esophagus: development of dysplasia and adenocarcinoma. Gastroenterology 96:1249–1256, 1989.

93. Berenson MM, Riddell RH, Skinner DB, et al: Malignant transformation of esophageal columnar epithelium. Cancer 41:554–561, 1978.

94. Haggitt RC, Tryzelaar J, Ellis FH, et al: Adenocarcinoma complicating columnar epithelium–lined (Barrett's) esophagus. Am J Clin Pathol 70:1–5, 1978.

95. Harle IA, Finley RJ, Belsheim M: Management of adenocarcinoma in a columnar-lined esophagus. Ann Thorac Surg 40:330–336, 1985.

96. Sanfey H, Hamilton SR, Smith RRL, et al: Carcinoma arising in Barrett's esophagus. Surg Gynecol Obstet 161:570–574, 1985.

97. Mangla JC: Barrett's esophagus: an old entity rediscovered. J Clin Gastroenterol 3:347–356, 1981.

98. Kerlin P, D'Mellow G, Van Deth A: Barrett's esophagus: clinical, endoscopic, and histologic spectrum in fifty patients. Aust N Z J Med 16:198–205, 1986.

99. Cooper BT, Barbezat GO: Barrett's oesophagus: a clinical study of 52 patients. Q J Med 62:97–108, 1987.

100. Katzka D, Plotkin A, Saul S, et al: A controlled study of toluidine blue staining in patients with Barrett's metaplasia of the esophagus. Gastroenterology 90:1485, 1986 (abstract).

101. Winters C, Spurling TJ, Chobanian SJ, et al: Barrett's esophagus: a prevalent, occult complication of gastroesophageal reflux disease. Gastroenterology 92:118–124, 1987.

102. Paull A, Trier JS, Dalton D, et al: The histologic spectrum of Barrett's esophagus. N Engl J Med 295:476–480, 1976.

103. Thompson JJ, Zinsser KR, Enterline HT: Barrett's metaplasia and adenocarcinoma of the esophagus and gastroesophageal junction. Hum Pathol 144:42–61, 1983.

104. Missakian MM, Carlson HC, Andersen HA: The roentgenologic features of the columnar epithelial-lined lower esophagus. AJR 99:212–217, 1967.

105. Robbins AH, Hermos JA, Schimmel EM, et al: The columnar-lined esophagus: analysis of 26 cases. Radiology 123:1–7, 1977.

106. Chen YM, Gelfand DW, Ott DJ, et al: Barrett esophagus as an extension of severe esophagitis: analysis of radiologic signs in 29 cases. AJR 145:275–281, 1985.

107. Adler RH: The lower esophagus lined by columnar epithelium: its association with hiatal hernia, ulcer, stricture, and tumor. J Thorac Cardiovasc Surg 45:13–34, 1963.

108. Robbins AH, Vincent ME, Saini M, et al: Revised radiologic concepts of the Barrett esophagus. Gastrointest Radiol 3:377–381, 1978.

109. Levine MS, Kressel HY, Caroline DF, et al: Barrett esophagus: reticular pattern of the mucosa. Radiology 147:663–667, 1983.

110. Shapir J, DuBrow R, Frank P: Barrett oesophagus: analysis of 19 cases. Br J Radiol 58:491–493, 1985.

111. Agha FP: Radiologic diagnosis of Barrett's esophagus: critical analysis of 65 cases. Gastrointest Radiol 11:123–130, 1986.

112. Glick SN, Teplick SK, Amenta PS, et al: The radiologic diagnosis of Barrett esophagus: importance of mucosal surface abnormalities on air-contrast barium studies. AJR 157:951–954, 1991.

113. Chernin MM, Amberg JR, Kogan FJ, et al: Efficacy of radiologic studies in the detection of Barrett's esophagus. AJR 147:257–260, 1986.

114. Vincent ME, Robbins AH, Spechler SJ, et al: The reticular pattern as a radiographic sign of the Barrett esophagus: an assessment. Radiology 153:333–335, 1984.

115. Gilchrist AM, Levine MS, Carr RF, et al: Barrett's esophagus: diagnosis by double-contrast esophagography. AJR 150:97–102, 1988.

116. Spechler SJ, Sperber H, Doos WG, et al: The prevalence of Barrett's esophagus in patients with chronic peptic esophageal strictures. Dig Dis Sci 28:769–774, 1983.

# Infectious Esophagitis

**Marc S. Levine, M.D.**

## INTRODUCTION

Because of the increased survival of immunocompromised patients with malignant neoplasms, organ transplants, and other debilitating diseases, infectious esophagitis has become an increasingly common problem in modern medical practice. *Candida albicans* is the usual offending organism, but herpes simplex virus and cytomegalovirus (CMV) have also been recognized with increased frequency as opportunistic invaders of the esophagus. The epidemic of acquired immunodeficiency syndrome (AIDS) has led to the development of more fulminant forms of fungal and viral esophagitis, accentuating the need for early diagnosis and treatment of these patients.

## *CANDIDA* ESOPHAGITIS

### Pathogenesis

Candidiasis is by far the most common cause of infectious esophagitis. Although *C. albicans* is almost always the offending organism, *C. tropicalis, C. pseudotropicalis,* and *C. kruzei* have been implicated in rare cases.[1] Because *C. albicans* is a normal commensal inhabitant of the pharynx, *Candida* esophagitis is presumably caused by downward spread of the fungus to the esophagus.[2] However, clinically significant esophagitis usually occurs when the host's immune system is impaired by underlying malignancy, debilitating illness, diabetes, or treatment with radiation, steroids, or other cytotoxic agents.[3–6] *Candida* esophagitis is particularly prevalent in patients with AIDS, a severe disorder of cellular immunity that has become one of the most feared medical illnesses in the world. At the time of clinical presentation, these patients often have a much more fulminant form of candidiasis than other immunocompromised patients.

Although *Candida* esophagitis typically occurs in patients who are immunocompromised, local esophageal stasis is another predisposing factor, accounting for nearly 25% of cases.[7] Esophageal stasis may be due to mechanical obstruction resulting from achalasia or strictures or to physiologic obstruction resulting from scleroderma or other causes of weakened or absent esophageal peristalsis.[7, 8] Delayed esophageal emptying in these individuals apparently permits the fungal organism to overgrow and colonize the esophagus, producing esophagitis.

Rarely, *Candida* esophagitis may occur in otherwise healthy, immunocompetent individuals who have no underlying systemic or esophageal diseases.[9, 10] The possibility of fungal infection should therefore not be excluded simply because the classic predisposing factors are not present in a particular patient.

### Clinical Findings

Most patients with *Candida* esophagitis have acute onset of odynophagia, characterized by intense substernal pain or burning during swallowing.[1–5] Others have more nonspecific findings such as dysphagia, chest pain, and, less commonly, upper gastrointestinal bleeding.[1, 4–6] There usually is rapid progression of symptoms, so untreated or inadequately treated patients may soon be unable to eat or even swallow their saliva. In some cases, the pain may be so severe that it simulates a myocardial infarction.[5] Occasionally, patients with chronic or recurrent *Candida* esophagitis may have persistent dysphagia due to the development of esophageal strictures.[11–14] Rarely, severe cases can also result in a potentially fatal, disseminated infection due to hematogenous spread of the fungal organism.[5] Other unusual but life-threatening complications include esophageal perforation, aortoesophageal fistulas, tracheoesophageal fistulas, and lung abscesses.[15–18]

*C. albicans* is by far the most common cause of opportunistic esophagitis, but the herpes simplex virus or, less commonly, CMV may produce identical clinical findings. The presence of oropharyngeal candidiasis (i.e., thrush) should suggest the correct diagnosis, but the majority of patients with *Candida* esophagitis do not have active infection of the oropharynx.[19] Other patients with thrush may have herpes or CMV esophagitis, so oropharyngeal candidiasis does not preclude the possibility of viral infection in the esophagus.[20] Thus, it may be difficult or impossible to differentiate fungal and viral esophagitis on clinical grounds.

The diagnosis of opportunistic esophagitis is further complicated by occasional cases in which the esophagus is simultaneously colonized by fungal and viral organisms. Cases of concomitant *Candida* and herpes esophagitis have been documented at endoscopy and at autopsy.[21, 22] In such cases, *Candida* esophagitis most likely results from fungal superinfection of herpetic ulcers.[22] As a result, there may be a small but significant incidence of coexisting fungal and viral esophagitis in patients treated for presumed candidiasis.

Oral nystatin is often used for the initial treatment of *Candida* esophagitis, particularly in unproven cases, as it is a relatively innocuous antifungal agent. However, ketoconazole and fluconazole are much more effective drugs for treating these patients. Marked clinical improvement usually occurs within several days of treatment. Some AIDS patients with *Candida* esophagitis may be more resistant to conventional antifungal therapy than other immunocompromised individuals.[23] These patients are also at risk for simultaneous or recurrent esophageal infections by other organisms.[20] Thus, infectious esophagitis is a particularly devastating problem in patients with AIDS.

## Endoscopic Findings

The characteristic endoscopic appearance of *Candida* esophagitis consists of patchy, white plaques covering a friable, erythematous mucosa.[1, 24] In more advanced disease, the mucosa becomes ulcerated and necrotic with extensive pseudomembrane formation. A definitive diagnosis of *Candida* esophagitis requires demonstration of fungal mycelia on cytologic specimens or evidence of tissue invasion on mucosal biopsy specimens from the esophagus.[1]

## Radiographic Findings

The radiographic diagnosis of *Candida* esophagitis has been limited by the fact that it tends to be a superficial disease with mucosal abnormalities that are difficult to detect on conventional single contrast barium studies. As a result, single contrast esophagography has been considered an unreliable technique for diagnosing *Candida* esophagitis, with an overall sensitivity of less than 50% reported in the medical literature.[1, 3, 4, 6, 10] However, studies have shown that double contrast esophagography has a sensitivity of about 90% in diagnosing *Candida* esophagitis.[7, 25] The major advantage of this technique is its ability to demonstrate mucosal plaques that cannot easily be seen on single contrast studies. As a result, only mild cases of *Candida* esophagitis are likely to be missed on the double contrast examination.

*Candida* esophagitis is usually manifested on double contrast radiographs by discrete plaque-like lesions corresponding to the characteristic white plaques seen at endoscopy. These plaques consist of heaped-up areas of necrotic epithelial debris or actual colonies of *C. albicans* on the esophageal mucosa. The plaque-like lesions tend to be longitudinally oriented, appearing en face as linear or irregular filling defects with normal intervening mucosa[7, 20, 26] (Fig. 25–1). The lesions often have discrete borders that are etched in white by a thin layer of barium trapped between the edge of the plaque and the adjacent mucosa. Whether they have a localized or diffuse distribution in the esophagus (Fig. 25–2), discrete

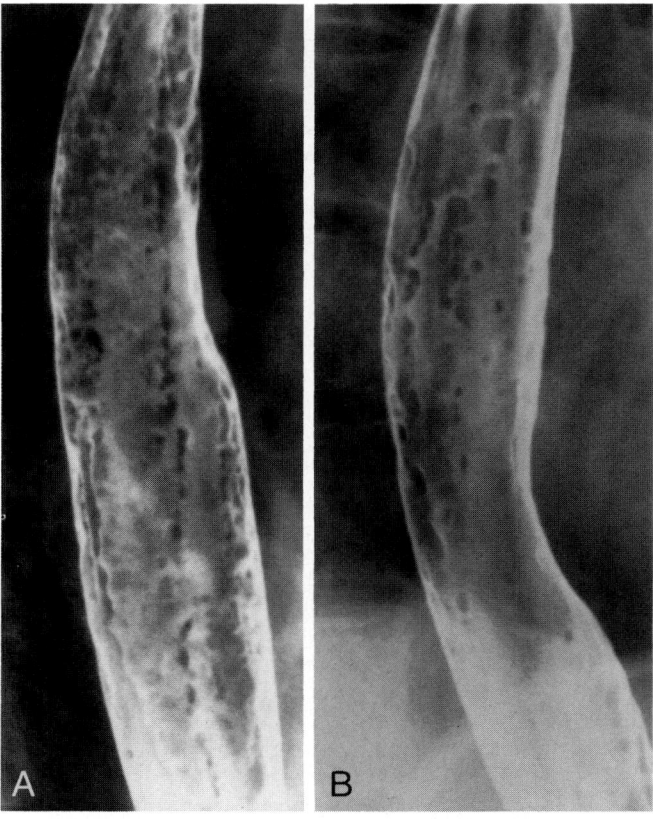

**Figure 25–1.** *Candida* **esophagitis with discrete plaques. A.** Multiple plaque-like lesions are present in the esophagus. Note how the plaques have a characteristic appearance with discrete borders and a predominantly longitudinal orientation. **B.** In another patient, the plaques have a more irregular configuration. However, they are still seen as discrete lesions separated by normal mucosa. (**A** and **B** from Levine MS, Macones AJ, Laufer I: *Candida* esophagitis: accuracy of radiographic diagnosis. Radiology 154:581–587, 1985.)

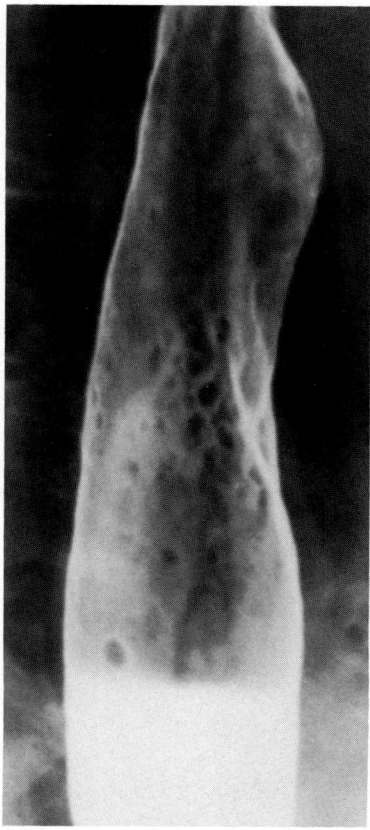

**Figure 25–2. Localized *Candida* esophagitis.** There are discrete plaque-like lesions clustered together in the midesophagus with normal-appearing mucosa above and below this level.

Because this degree of esophagitis rarely occurs in other immunocompromised patients, the possibility of AIDS should be suspected when a shaggy esophagus is detected on barium studies, particularly in high-risk patients.

*Candida* esophagitis occasionally may produce other unusual radiographic findings. In some patients, barium may dissect beneath plaques or pseudomembranes, producing an intramural track or "double-barreled" esophagus.[31] A coalescent mass of heaped-up necrotic debris and fungal mycelia (i.e., a fungus ball) may be indistinguishable from a polypoid esophageal carcinoma.[32, 33] Nodular masses of fungal organisms have also been reported in AIDS patients with severe *Candida* esophagitis.[34] Esophageal obstruction or perforation, aortoesophageal fistulas, and tracheoesophageal fistulas are other rare complications of this disease.[15–18, 35]

*Candida* esophagitis usually responds quickly to antifungal therapy. Dramatic regression of the lesions may be demonstrated on repeat esophagrams within several days of treatment. However, resolution of the radiographic findings sometimes lags behind the clinical recovery, so follow-up barium studies may still be abnormal in patients who are asymptomatic.[30] The immediate effects of antifungal therapy should therefore be assessed primarily on clinical grounds.

Although *Candida* esophagitis is usually self-limited

mucosal plaques should strongly suggest the diagnosis of *Candida* esophagitis.

In other patients, the esophagus may have a finely nodular or granular appearance due to mucosal edema and inflammation or tiny plaques on the mucosa[20, 27] (Fig. 25–3). When larger plaques are present, the lesions occasionally may coalesce, producing a distinctive "cobblestone" or "snakeskin" appearance due to confluent involvement of the mucosa by innumerable round, oval, or polygonal plaques[25, 28] (Fig. 25–4). In other patients, submucosal edema and inflammation may cause irregular thickening of the longitudinal esophageal folds, mimicking the appearance of varices.[2, 29, 30] Thus, the classic radiographic features of *Candida* esophagitis are not present in all patients.

In severe candidiasis, the esophagus eventually may have a grossly irregular or "shaggy" contour due to coalescent plaque and pseudomembrane formation with barium trapped between these plaques and pseudomembranes[2, 5, 7, 20, 30, 31] (Fig. 25–5). Ulceration may also be seen as a result of sloughing of necrotic pseudomembranes in advanced disease. This fulminant form of candidiasis has been recognized with increased frequency in patients with AIDS.[20] In fact, some AIDS patients may demonstrate the shaggy esophagus of candidiasis as the initial manifestation of their disease.[20]

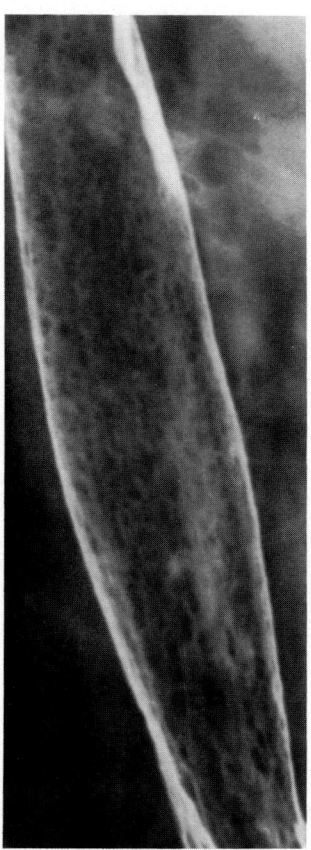

**Figure 25–3. *Candida* esophagitis with a granular mucosa.** This patient has innumerable tiny, nodular elevations in the esophagus rather than the typical plaque-like defects associated with candidiasis.

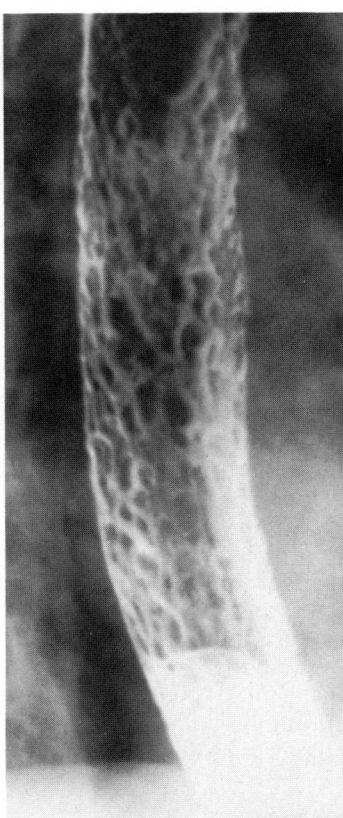

**Figure 25–4.** *Candida* **esophagitis with a cobblestone appearance.** There is confluent involvement of the mucosa by innumerable round, oval, and polygonal plaques.

**Figure 25–5.** *Candida* **esophagitis with a shaggy esophagus.** In both **A** and **B,** the esophagus has a grossly irregular contour due to multiple plaques and pseudomembranes with trapping of barium between these lesions. In **B,** a deep area of ulceration *(arrow)* is also seen. Both patients had AIDS. (**B** from Levine MS, Woldenberg R, Herlinger H, et al: Opportunistic esophagitis in AIDS: radiographic diagnosis. Radiology 165:815–820, 1987.)

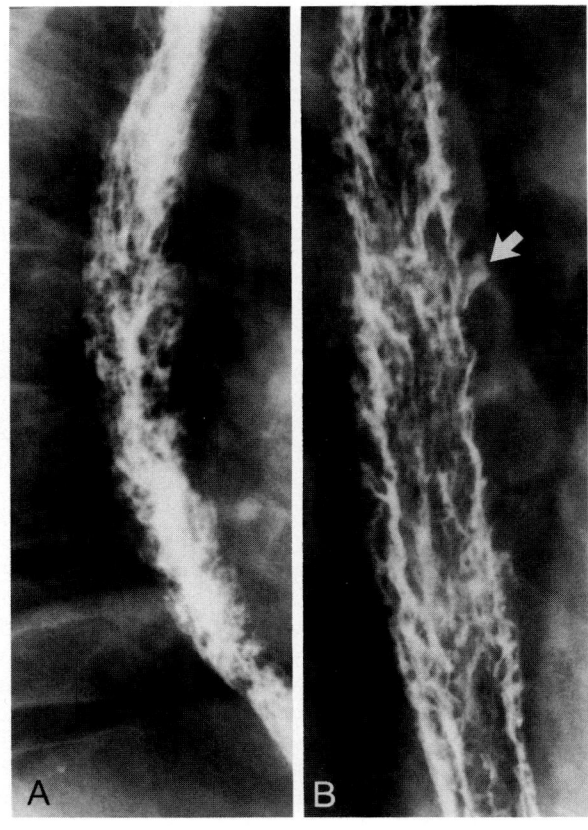

with proper treatment, occasional cases of stricture formation have been reported.[11-14] These strictures typically appear as long, tapered areas of narrowing in the esophagus[13, 14] (Fig. 25–6). *Candida*-induced strictures should be distinguished from pseudostrictures caused by esophageal spasm or the patient's inability to swallow an adequate bolus of barium.[24] For this reason, a second examination may be necessary after treatment to determine if a true stricture is present.

Because local esophageal stasis also predisposes to *Candida* esophagitis, patients with conditions such as achalasia and scleroderma are at increased risk for developing this disease.[7, 8] In such cases, *Candida* esophagitis may be manifested radiographically by tiny, nodular defects, polypoid folds, or a distinctive lacy appearance in the esophagus[8] (Fig. 25–7). These findings can be simulated by retained debris or undissolved effervescent agent in a dilated, obstructed esophagus, so esophageal lavage may be required to evacuate debris and secretions from the esophagus before performing the examination. Despite careful technique, double contrast esophagrams are often suboptimal in these patients due to pooling of barium in the distal esophagus, which obscures mucosal detail in this region. Thus, a false-negative radiologic examination is most likely to occur in patients with a mechanically or physiologically ob-

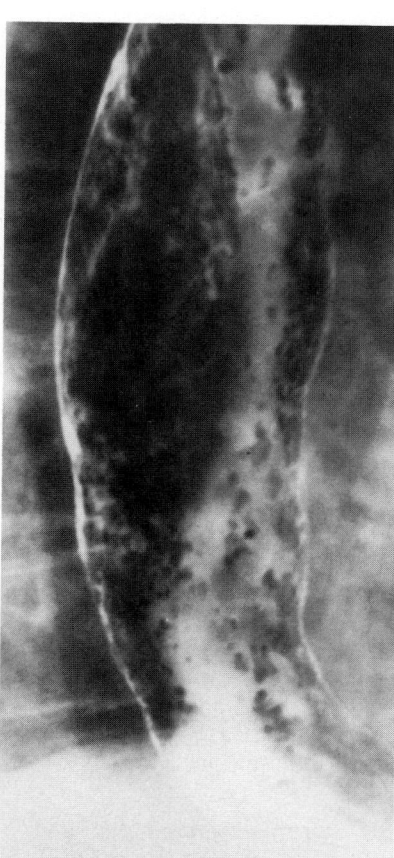

**Figure 25–7.** *Candida* **esophagitis in a patient with scleroderma.** There are tiny, nodular defects in the esophagus that could be mistaken for retained debris. Note how the esophagus is dilated because of underlying involvement by scleroderma.

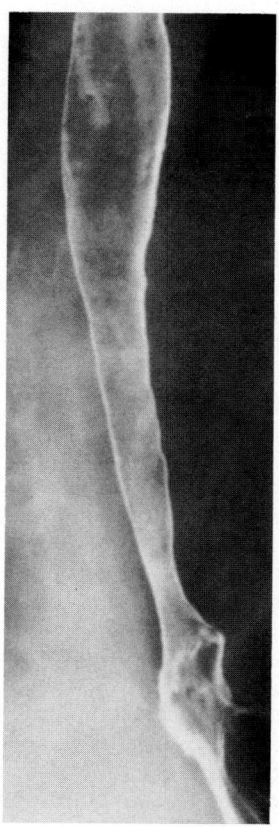

**Figure 25–6.** *Candida*-**induced esophageal stricture.** A long, tapered stricture in the distal esophagus is caused by scarring from severe *Candida* esophagitis.

structed esophagus because of the inherent limitations of the barium study in these patients.

*Candida* esophagitis is also known to be associated with esophageal intramural pseudodiverticulosis (see Chapter 26).[36-38] Esophageal cultures are positive for *C. albicans* in almost 50% of patients with this condition.[38] It therefore has been postulated that esophageal intramural pseudodiverticulosis develops as a complication of *Candida* esophagitis.[36] However, it is more widely believed that the fungal organism is a secondary invader due to local stasis in these intramural pseudodiverticula.[37, 38]

Patients with defects in their cell-mediated immune response to *C. albicans* may have an unusual disease known as chronic mucocutaneous candidiasis in which there is persistent fungal infection of the skin, mucous membranes, and nails.[12, 39] Although uncommon, esophageal involvement may lead to chronic esophageal candidiasis.[39] Unlike acute *Candida* esophagitis, this entity is characterized by chronic scarring and stricture formation in the esophagus with a relative absence of mucosal disease. The presence of a long esophageal stricture in patients with chronic mucocutaneous candidiasis should therefore suggest the possibility of esophageal involvement by this disease.

## Differential Diagnosis

Discrete mucosal plaques or nodules may also be caused by herpes esophagitis, reflux esophagitis, glycogenic acanthosis, and superficial spreading carcinoma.[27, 40–45] Although herpes esophagitis is typically manifested by discrete ulcers in the esophagus (see later section on herpes esophagitis), advanced herpetic infection may occasionally produce multiple plaque-like defects that are indistinguishable from the lesions in *Candida* esophagitis[40, 41] (Fig. 25–8).

Reflux esophagitis may also produce a nodular or granular appearance of the mucosa that can resemble candidiasis[27] (Fig. 25–9). However, the nodules of reflux esophagitis tend to have poorly defined borders that fade peripherally into the adjacent mucosa, whereas *Candida* esophagitis is usually manifested by discrete plaques. Furthermore, the nodular mucosa of reflux esophagitis almost always occurs as a continuous area of disease extending proximally from the gastroesophageal junction, whereas *Candida* esophagitis often spares the distal esophagus. Rarely, severe reflux esophagitis may produce inflammatory exudates or pseudomem-

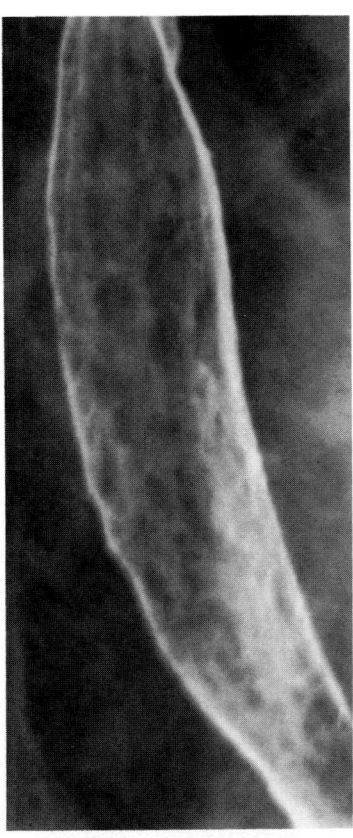

**Figure 25–9. Reflux esophagitis.** There is a nodular mucosa in the distal half of the esophagus, but the nodules are more poorly defined than the plaques of *Candida* esophagitis. (Courtesy of Harvey M. Goldstein, M.D., San Antonio, TX.)

branes that are indistinguishable on double contrast studies from the plaque-like lesions of candidiasis.[42]

Glycogenic acanthosis may also be manifested by discrete plaques or nodules in the middle or distal esophagus, mimicking the appearance of *Candida* esophagitis[43] (Fig. 25–10). However, the clinical history is extremely helpful in differentiating these conditions, as patients with glycogenic acanthosis are almost always asymptomatic.[43]

Superficial spreading carcinoma of the esophagus is also characterized by focal nodularity of the mucosa that could be mistaken for a localized area of *Candida* esophagitis[44, 45] (see Fig. 28–4). However, candidiasis usually produces discrete lesions, whereas the plaques or nodules of superficial spreading carcinoma tend to coalesce, producing a continuous area of disease.[44, 45] Rarely, advanced, infiltrating carcinomas extending longitudinally in the wall can mimic the shaggy esophagus of candidiasis (Fig. 25–11).

Finally, mucosal plaques may be simulated by technical artifacts on the double contrast examination, such as undissolved effervescent agent, air bubbles, and debris[27, 46] (Fig. 25–12). If an artifact is suspected, however, additional double contrast radiographs should be obtained to demonstrate the transient nature of these findings.

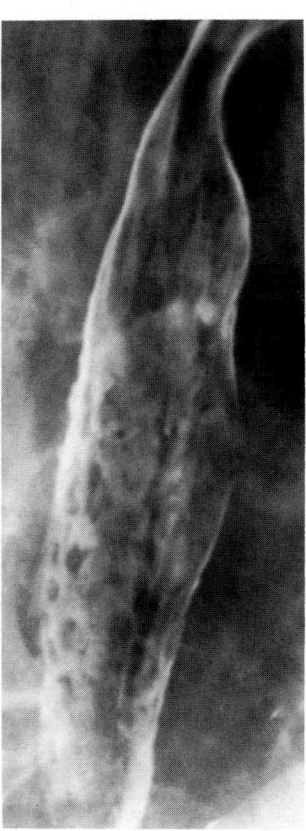

**Figure 25–8. Herpes esophagitis.** There are multiple plaque-like lesions in the midesophagus, mimicking the appearance of candidiasis. (From MS Levine, I Laufer, HY Kressel, et al, Herpes esophagitis, AJR, 136, 5, 863–866, 1981, © by American Roentgen Ray Society.)

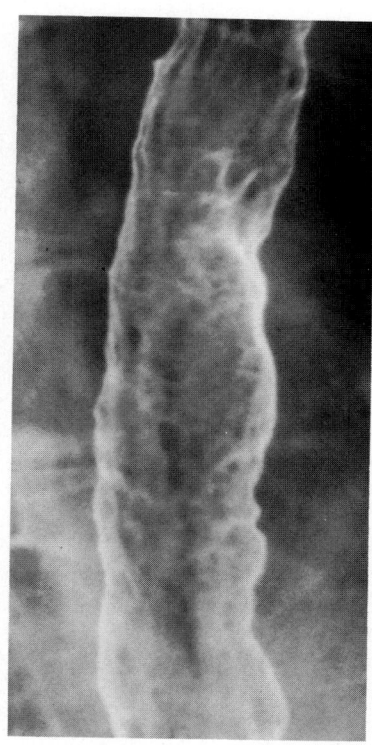

**Figure 25–10. Glycogenic acanthosis.** There are multiple plaques and nodules in the midesophagus, mimicking the appearance of *Candida* esophagitis. However, this patient was asymptomatic.

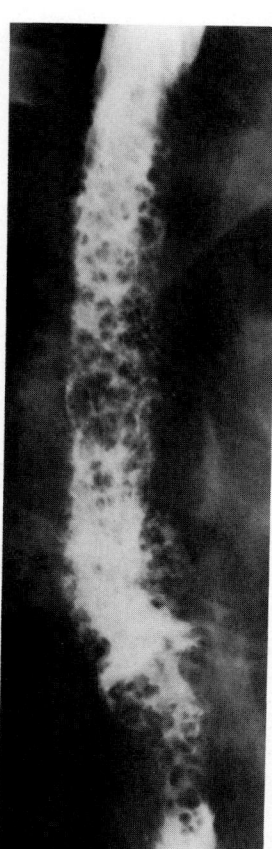

**Figure 25–11. Advanced esophageal carcinoma.** The esophagus has a grossly irregular or shaggy contour due to a highly invasive carcinoma extending longitudinally in the wall. (Courtesy of Hans Herlinger, M.D., Philadelphia, PA.)

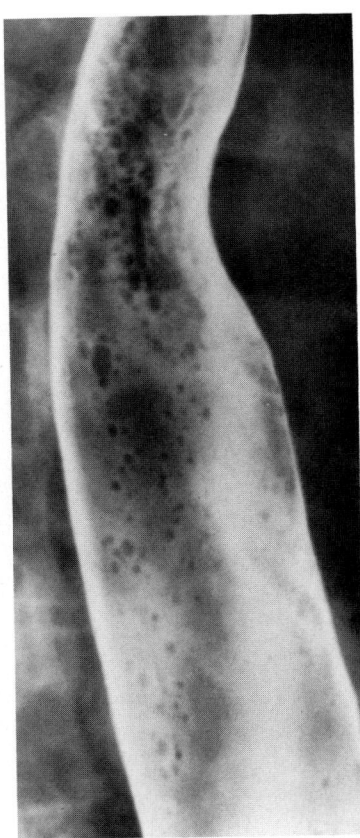

**Figure 25–12. Undissolved effervescent agent and bubbles in the esophagus.** Although this appearance could be mistaken for *Candida* esophagitis on a single radiograph, the transient nature of these artifacts can easily be confirmed by obtaining additional views.

## HERPES ESOPHAGITIS

### Pathogenesis

Herpes simplex virus type 1, a DNA core virus, has been recognized as the second most common cause of opportunistic esophagitis in patients who are clinically immunocompromised because of underlying malignancy; debilitating illness; treatment with radiation, steroids, or chemotherapy; or, most recently, AIDS.[20, 47–51] Herpes esophagitis should therefore be suspected in the same clinical setting as candidiasis. Occasionally, however, herpes esophagitis may occur as an acute, self-limited illness in otherwise healthy individuals who have no underlying immunologic problems.[52–56] Thus, the diagnosis of herpes esophagitis should not be excluded simply because the patient has a normal immunologic status.

### Clinical Findings

Patients with herpes esophagitis typically present with acute odynophagia, characterized by severe substernal chest pain during swallowing.[19, 57] Other patients may have dysphagia, chest pain, and, less commonly, upper gastrointestinal bleeding.[58, 59] The presence of herpetic lesions in the oropharynx should suggest the possibility of herpes esophagitis in immunocompromised patients with odynophagia. However, the majority of patients with herpes esophagitis do not have active infection of the oropharynx, so the absence of oropharyngeal lesions in no way precludes this diagnosis.[19, 57] Furthermore, some patients with herpetic lesions in the oropharynx may have *Candida* esophagitis. Thus, it is difficult to differentiate viral and fungal esophagitis on clinical grounds.

The natural history of herpes esophagitis is uncertain. Various autopsy series have shown that herpes esophagitis can be complicated by herpetic pneumonitis or even a disseminated herpetic infection in immunocompromised hosts.[48, 51, 60] However, most patients with herpes esophagitis have recovered spontaneously without sequelae.[57, 61, 62] These patients are usually managed with analgesia, sedation, and, if necessary, antiviral agents such as acyclovir. Although marked clinical improvement often occurs within several days of treatment, it is unclear whether antiviral therapy significantly affects the course of this disease.

Otherwise healthy patients with herpes esophagitis have a characteristic clinical presentation. They typically are young men who have a history of recent exposure to sexual partners with herpetic lesions on the lips or buccal mucosa.[53, 55] Before the development of esophageal symptoms, most of these patients have a 3- to 10-day influenza-like prodrome characterized by fever, sore throat, upper respiratory infection, or myalgias.[52, 53, 55, 56] This is followed by acute onset of odynophagia, which prompts the patient to seek medical attention. Although the odynophagia may be severe, herpes esophagitis in otherwise healthy subjects almost always occurs as an acute, self-limited illness with resolution of symptoms within 3 to 14 days after presentation.[52–55] As a result, these patients can be treated conservatively with topical anesthetics, analgesics, and antacids. Occasionally, however, patients with severe symptoms may require acyclovir to accelerate healing of the herpetic lesions.

### Endoscopic Findings

Herpes esophagitis is initially manifested on endoscopy by esophageal blisters or vesicles that subsequently rupture to form discrete, punched-out ulcers on the mucosa.[51, 61–63] With further progression, the ulcers may become covered by a fibrinous exudate or pseudomembranes.[51] Thus, early herpes esophagitis has a characteristic endoscopic appearance, whereas advanced herpes esophagitis may be indistinguishable from candidiasis at endoscopy. Whatever the stage of infection, the histologic or cytologic findings on brushings or biopsy specimens from the esophagus are relatively specific for the herpes virus group. The classic finding of Cowdry's type A intranuclear inclusions in intact epithelial cells adjacent to ulcers is virtually pathognomonic of herpes.[51, 64] The diagnosis of herpes esophagitis may also be confirmed by positive viral cultures from the esophagus or by direct immunofluorescent staining for the herpes simplex antigen.

## Radiographic Findings

Herpes esophagitis is usually manifested by discrete, superficial ulcers in the midesophagus without evidence of plaques.[20, 57, 65–67] These ulcers are visible on double contrast radiographs in more than 50% of patients with endoscopically proven disease.[67] The ulcers may have a punctate, linear, ring-like, or stellate configuration and are often surrounded by radiolucent halos of edematous mucosa[57] (Fig. 25–13). Ulceration may occasionally be present in patients with candidiasis, but it almost always occurs on a background of diffuse plaque formation.[7, 20] Thus, discrete ulcers on an otherwise normal mucosa should be highly suggestive of herpes esophagitis in immunocompromised patients with odynophagia.

More advanced herpes esophagitis may be associated with extensive ulceration, plaque formation, or a combination of ulcers and plaques in the esophagus[40, 41, 57, 65, 67] (see Fig. 25–8). Advanced herpes esophagitis may therefore be indistinguishable from *Candida* esophagitis. Rarely, herpes esophagitis may be manifested by a giant ulcer with a surrounding mound of edema, mimicking the appearance of an ulcerated carcinoma.[67]

The radiologist's ability to differentiate fungal and viral esophagitis is important for the treatment of all immunocompromised patients but particularly for the treatment of patients with AIDS, as many gastroenter-

ologists are reluctant to perform endoscopy on these individuals for fear of contaminating their endoscopic instruments or exposing themselves to the AIDS virus. However, there are data suggesting that *Candida* and herpes esophagitis can often be diagnosed in AIDS patients by their characteristic features on double contrast radiographs, eliminating the need for endoscopic intervention in many cases[20] (Fig. 25–14). Nevertheless, endoscopy may be required for a definitive diagnosis if the radiographic findings are equivocal or if appropriate treatment with antifungal or antiviral agents fails to produce an adequate clinical response in these patients.

Otherwise healthy patients with herpes esophagitis have remarkably similar findings on double contrast esophagography, with innumerable tiny ulcers, predominantly located in the midesophagus near the level of the left main bronchus[68, 69] (Fig. 25–15). The small size of the ulcers may be related to an intact immune system that contains the herpetic infection and prevents the ulcers from enlarging. In any case, this appearance should be highly suggestive of herpes esophagitis in otherwise healthy young men who have the characteristic influenza-like prodrome before the development of odynophagia.[69] Because it is a self-limited illness, these patients may undergo conservative treatment without need for endoscopy.

## Differential Diagnosis

In the appropriate clinical setting, discrete ulcers on an otherwise normal background mucosa should be

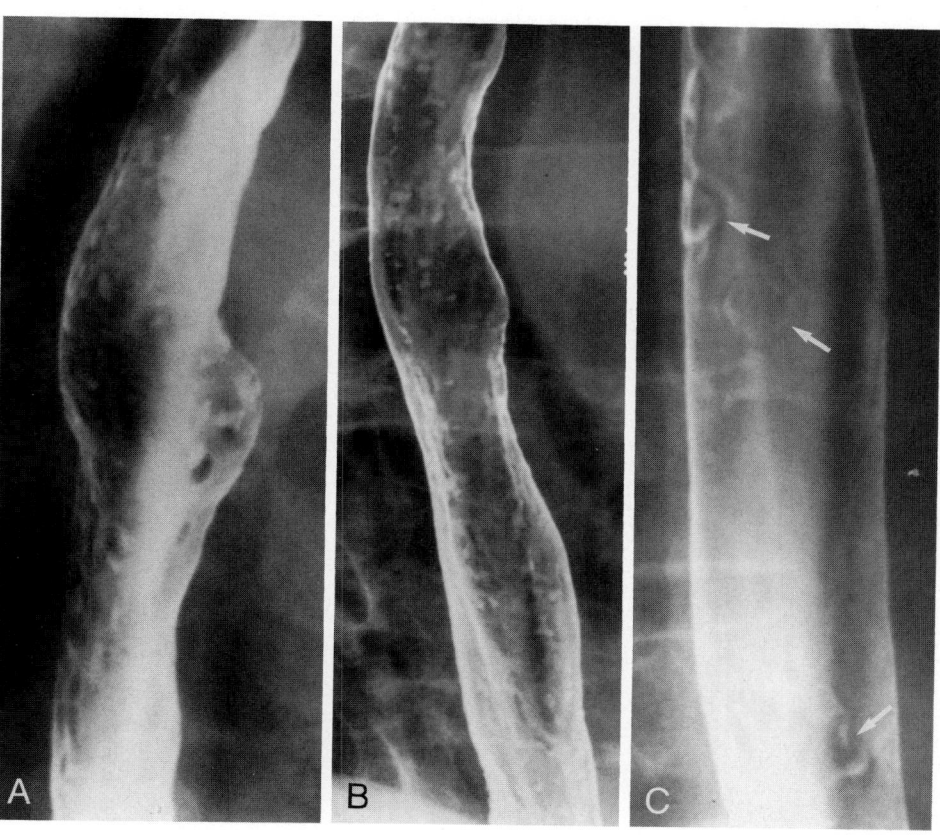

**Figure 25–13. Herpes esophagitis with discrete ulcers.** In **A** and **B**, there are multiple discrete, superficial ulcers in the midesophagus. Note how many of the ulcers are surrounded by radiolucent mounds of edema. In **C**, there are several widely separated ulcers *(arrows)* with a ring-like or stellate configuration. (**A** from Levine MS: Radiology of esophagitis: a pattern approach. Radiology 179:1–7, 1991. **B** courtesy of Harvey M. Goldstein, M.D., San Antonio, TX.)

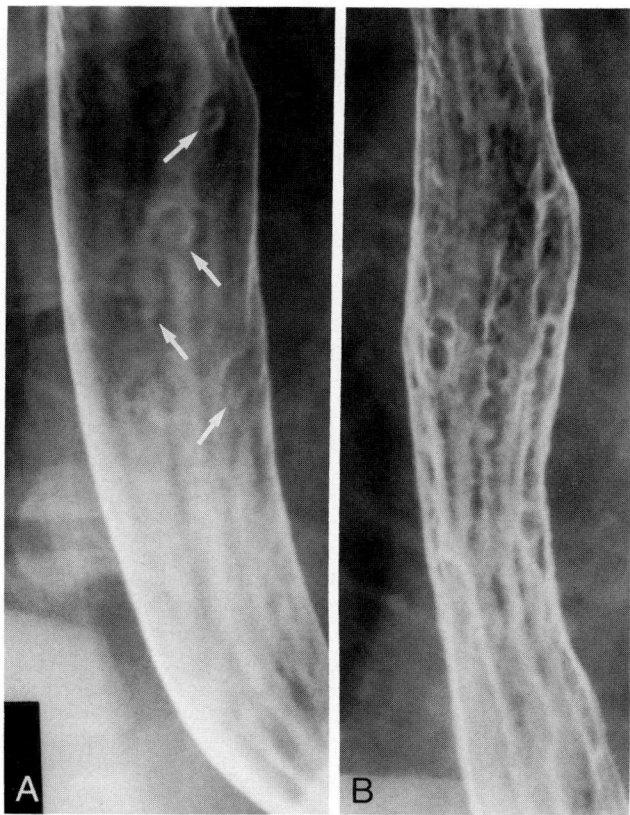

**Figure 25–14. Herpes and *Candida* esophagitis in a patient with AIDS. A.** The initial esophagram shows discrete, superficial ulcers *(arrows)* on an otherwise normal background mucosa without evidence of plaques. There are halos of edematous mucosa surrounding the ulcers. This patient was treated successfully for herpes esophagitis without undergoing endoscopy. **B.** Another esophagram 3 months later because of recurrent odynophagia shows linear plaque-like lesions compatible with *Candida* esophagitis. Antifungal treatment led to marked clinical improvement within several days. (**A** and **B** from Levine MS, Woldenberg R, Herlinger H, et al: Opportunistic esophagitis in AIDS: radiographic diagnosis. Radiology 165:815–820, 1987.)

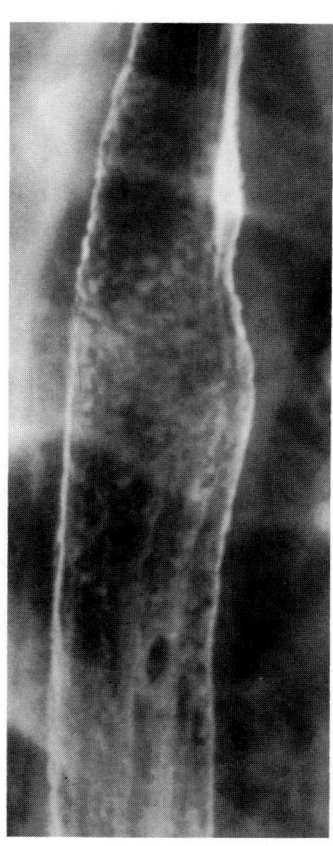

**Figure 25–15. Herpes esophagitis in an otherwise healthy patient.** There are multiple punctate and linear areas of ulceration in the midesophagus below the level of the left main bronchus. This appearance is characteristic of herpes esophagitis in immunocompetent patients. (From L DeGaeta, MS Levine, GE Guglielmi, et al, Herpes esophagitis in an otherwise healthy patient, AJR, 144, 6, 1205–1206, 1985, © by American Roentgen Ray Society.)

virtually pathognomonic of viral esophagitis. Although most cases are caused by the herpes simplex virus, CMV may occasionally produce similar findings. However, CMV esophagitis almost always occurs in patients with AIDS, and this condition is often manifested by the development of one or more giant, relatively flat ulcers in the esophagus (see the next section on cytomegalovirus esophagitis).

Other conditions may also be associated with superficial ulceration in the esophagus. Oral medications such as tetracycline and doxycycline may cause a focal contact esophagitis, manifested by multiple shallow ulcers that are indistinguishable from those of herpes esophagitis[70, 71] (Fig. 25–16). However, a temporal relationship between ingestion of the offending medication and the onset of esophagitis should suggest the correct diagnosis. Reflux esophagitis is a more common cause of ulceration, but it tends to involve the distal esophagus and is usually associated with a hiatal hernia or gastroesophageal reflux (Fig. 25–17). Radiation esophagitis, caustic esophagitis, and, rarely, esophageal involvement by Crohn's disease or Behçet's syndrome may be associated with superficial ulceration, but these entities usually can be differentiated from herpes esophagitis by the clinical history and presentation.

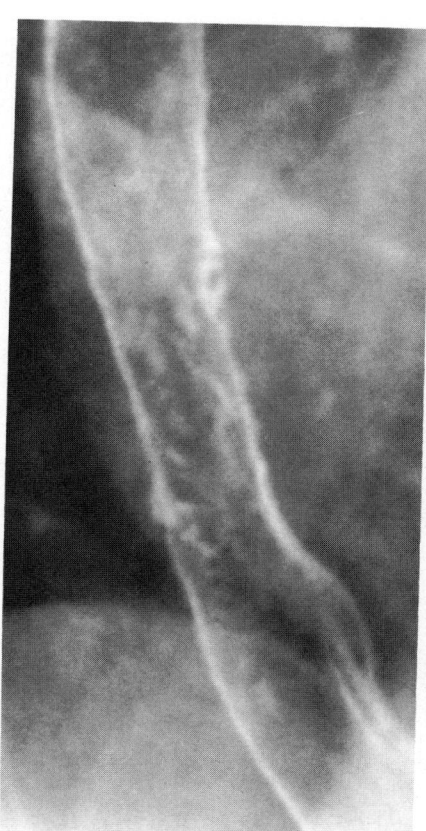

**Figure 25–17. Reflux esophagitis.** Superficial ulceration is present in the distal esophagus above a hiatal hernia. In contrast, herpes esophagitis tends to involve the upper or midesophagus with relative sparing of the distal esophagus.

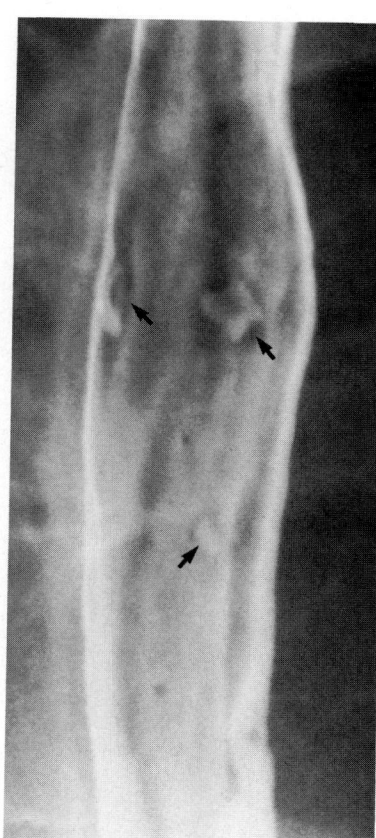

**Figure 25–16. Drug-induced esophagitis.** There are several widely separated ulcers *(arrows)* in the midesophagus. Although herpes esophagitis could produce identical findings, the correct diagnosis was suggested by a recent history of doxycycline ingestion.

## CYTOMEGALOVIRUS ESOPHAGITIS

CMV is another member of the herpesvirus group that has been recognized as a cause of opportunistic esophagitis in patients with AIDS.[72–74] Surprisingly, however, CMV esophagitis rarely occurs in other immunocompromised patients. Affected individuals usually present with severe odynophagia. Endoscopic examinations may demonstrate one or more shallow or deep ulcers in the esophagus. The diagnosis of CMV esophagitis may be confirmed on endoscopic brushings or biopsy specimens by characteristic intranuclear inclusions in endothelial cells or fibroblasts at or near the base of the ulcers.[72, 74] Because herpes esophagitis is characterized by intranuclear inclusions in squamous epithelial cells adjacent to ulcers, these infections usually can be differentiated on histologic criteria.

### Radiographic Findings

CMV esophagitis may be manifested radiographically by discrete, superficial ulcers that are indistinguishable from those of herpes esophagitis[72–74] (Fig. 25–18). Other patients may have localized ulceration, nodularity, or

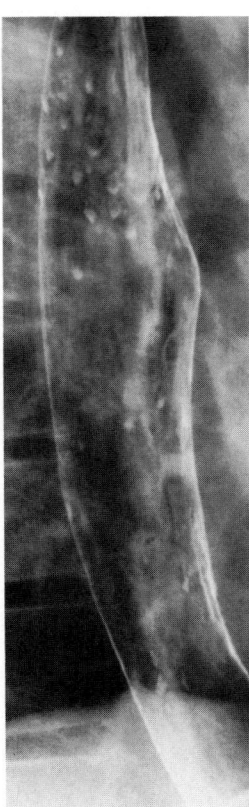

**Figure 25–18. CMV esophagitis.** There are multiple discrete, superficial ulcers, predominantly located in the midesophagus. Herpes esophagitis could produce identical radiographic findings.

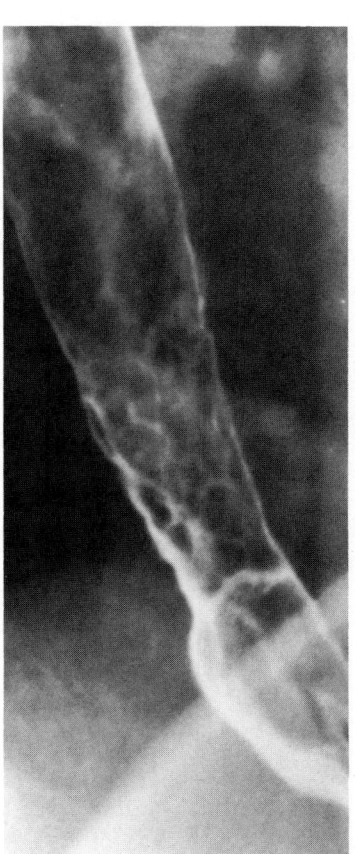

**Figure 25–19. CMV esophagitis.** Mucosal nodularity and shallow ulceration are seen in the distal esophagus, mimicking the appearance of reflux esophagitis. However, this patient had AIDS.

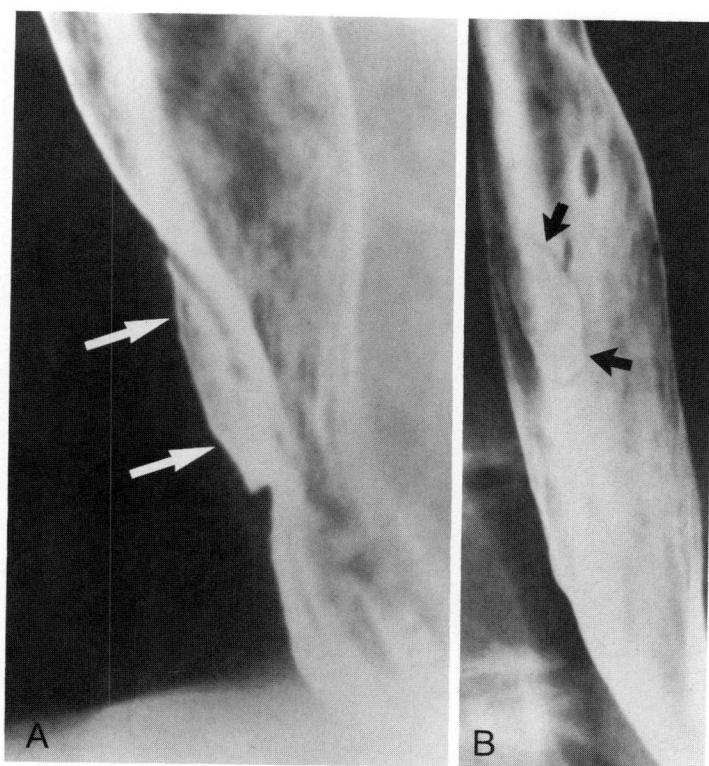

**Figure 25–20. CMV esophagitis. A.** A giant, relatively flat ulcer *(arrows)* is seen in profile in the distal esophagus. (Courtesy of Sidney W. Nelson, M.D., Seattle, WA.) **B.** A large, ovoid ulcer *(arrows)* in another patient is seen en face. Note the thin radiolucent rim of edema surrounding the ulcer. Because herpetic ulcers rarely become this large, the presence of one or more giant esophageal ulcers should raise the possibility of CMV esophagitis in patients with AIDS. (Courtesy of Kyunghee C. Cho, M.D., Newark, NJ.)

thickened folds in the distal esophagus, mimicking the appearance of reflux esophagitis[72] (Fig. 25–19). Still other patients may have one or more giant, relatively flat ulcers in the esophagus[20, 72, 73, 75] (Fig. 25–20). These ovoid or elongated ulcers may be surrounded by a radiolucent rim of edematous mucosa. Some of the ulcers may be several centimeters or more in length. Because herpetic ulcers rarely become this large, the presence of one or more giant esophageal ulcers should suggest the possibility of CMV esophagitis. However, human immunodeficiency virus (HIV) has also been implicated as a cause of giant esophageal ulcers in HIV-positive patients with odynophagia (see the next section on HIV esophagitis). Because HIV-related ulcers in the esophagus may produce the same radiographic findings as CMV ulcers, endoscopy is required to differentiate these conditions. If brushings or biopsy specimens reveal characteristic intranuclear inclusions or if viral cultures are positive for CMV, treatment can be initiated with potent antiviral agents such as ganciclovir.[76] However, ganciclovir may cause bone marrow suppression, with neutropenia, thrombocytopenia, or anemia.[77] This potentially toxic drug should therefore be used only if cytopathologic confirmation of CMV is obtained.

## HUMAN IMMUNODEFICIENCY VIRUS ESOPHAGITIS

A new clinical syndrome of odynophagia and giant esophageal ulcers has been recognized in patients with

HIV.[78–82] Brushings, biopsy specimens, and cultures from the esophagus have failed to reveal any signs of the usual fungal or viral organisms associated with opportunistic esophagitis in HIV-positive patients. Furthermore, electron microscopy of biopsy specimens from these ulcers has demonstrated viral particles with morphologic features of HIV infection, directly implicating HIV as the cause of the ulcers.[81] HIV-related esophageal ulcers may develop in patients who have recently become HIV-positive or in patients who have been HIV-positive for extended periods and have had other clinical signs of AIDS.[80–82] Thus, giant esophageal ulcers may occur as a manifestation of acute or chronic HIV infection.

## Clinical Findings

Patients with HIV-related esophageal ulcers typically present with acute onset of severe odynophagia.[79–82] The pain may be so intense that they are unable to swallow their saliva. Occasionally, these patients may develop hematemesis or other signs of upper gastrointestinal bleeding.[78] Others may have associated ulcers on the hard palate or a distinctive maculopapular rash involving the face, trunk, and upper extremities.[81] *Candida*, herpes, or CMV esophagitis more commonly causes odynophagia in HIV-positive patients, but the possibility of HIV-related ulcers should be suspected if these individuals have the characteristic maculopapular rash or develop symptoms at about the time of seroconversion.

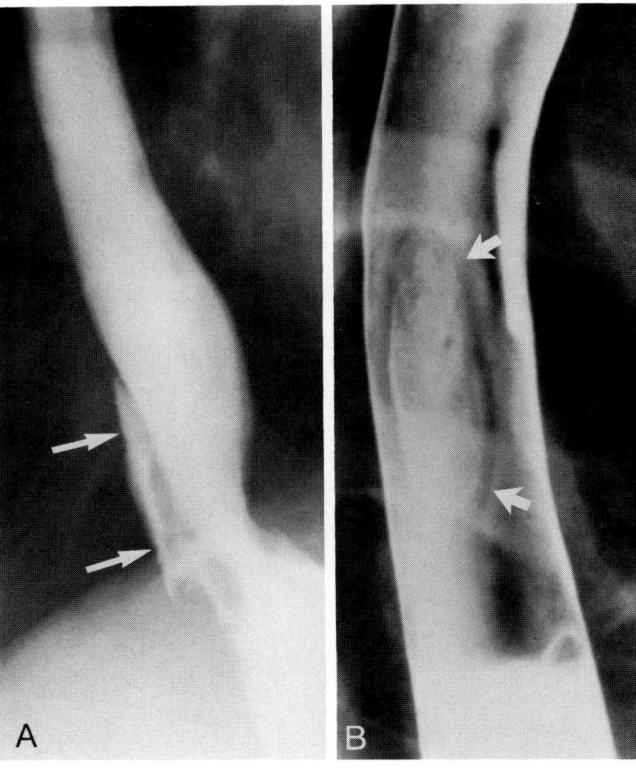

**Figure 25–21. Giant HIV-related ulcers in the esophagus. A.** A single contrast esophagram shows a giant, relatively flat ulcer *(arrows)* in profile in the distal esophagus. This patient was HIV-positive. **B.** A double contrast esophagram in another HIV-positive patient shows a giant ulcer *(arrows)* en face with a surrounding rim of edema. These ulcers are indistinguishable from the CMV ulcers illustrated in Figure 25–20. However, endoscopic brushings, biopsy specimens, and cultures were negative for CMV in both cases. (**B** from Levine MS, Loercher G, Katzka DA, et al: Giant, human immunodeficiency virus–related ulcers in the esophagus. Radiology 180:323–326, 1991.)

## Radiographic Findings

HIV-related ulcers in the esophagus usually appear on esophagrams as giant, relatively flat, ovoid or irregular collections of barium in the middle or, less commonly, the distal third of the esophagus[82] (Fig. 25–21). In some cases, small satellite ulcers may be located near the primary lesion. The ulcers may be demonstrated en face or in profile on double contrast radiographs. Because these patients are often incapable of swallowing multiple boluses of barium in different projections, double contrast technique is extremely helpful for detecting HIV-related ulcers that are seen en face during the initial examination[82] (Fig. 25–21B).

CMV esophagitis may also be manifested by the development of one or more giant, relatively flat ulcers that are indistinguishable from HIV-related ulcers in the esophagus[20, 72, 73, 75] (see Fig. 25–20). Endoscopy is therefore required to differentiate these conditions. Although it is not possible to diagnose HIV esophagitis definitively at endoscopy, HIV-related ulcers in the esophagus should be suspected if endoscopic brushings, biopsy specimens, and cultures are all negative for CMV or other opportunistic organisms. HIV-related esophageal ulcers may heal spontaneously or may respond to treatment with oral steroids, but they do not require treatment with potentially toxic antiviral agents such as ganciclovir.[79–81, 83] Thus, it is important to distinguish HIV-related ulcers from CMV ulcers so that appropriate treatment can be initiated in these patients.

Rarely, HIV-positive patients may develop giant ulcers due to mycobacterial esophagitis, but the ulcers tend to be deeper and may be associated with multiple sinus tracks or fistulas into the mediastinum (see the next section on tuberculous esophagitis).[84, 85] Other causes of giant ulcers include nasogastric intubation, endoscopic sclerotherapy, caustic ingestion, radiation, and oral medications such as quinidine, potassium chloride, and nonsteroidal anti-inflammatory agents. However, the correct diagnosis is usually suggested by the clinical history and presentation. Thus, for all practical purposes, giant esophageal ulcers in HIV-positive patients are most likely CMV- or HIV-related ulcers.

## TUBERCULOUS ESOPHAGITIS

Esophageal involvement by tuberculosis is extremely uncommon. When it occurs, the patients usually have advanced tuberculosis in the lungs or mediastinum.[86–88] However, occasional cases of primary tuberculous esophagitis have been reported in patients who had no evidence of tuberculosis elsewhere.[89] During the past decade, both *Mycobacterium tuberculosis* and *Mycobacterium avium* have also been implicated as causes of opportunistic esophagitis in patients with AIDS.[84, 85]

Esophageal involvement is most frequently caused by adjacent tuberculous nodes in the mediastinum that compress or erode into the esophagus, causing narrowing, ulceration, or fistula formation.[84–88] In patients with active pulmonary tuberculosis, esophageal infection may also be caused by swallowed sputum containing the tubercle bacilli, particularly if there is a pre-existing mucosal lesion or stricture in the esophagus.[86] Rarely,

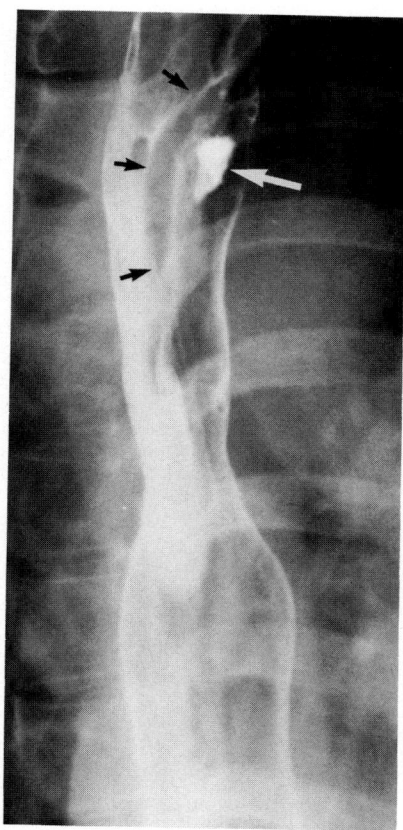

**Figure 25–22. Tuberculous esophagitis.** There is compression *(black arrows)* of the upper thoracic esophagus with associated ulceration *(white arrow)* due to caseating tuberculous nodes that have eroded into the esophagus. (Courtesy of Alan Grundy, M.D., London, England.)

hematogenous seeding of the esophagus may occur in patients with disseminated miliary tuberculosis.

Patients with tuberculous esophagitis may be asymptomatic or may present with dysphagia, odynophagia, or chest pain.[86, 88] Although the clinical findings are nonspecific, the possibility of esophageal tuberculosis should be considered in patients with persistent dysphagia who have active pulmonary tuberculosis. In such cases, the diagnosis may be confirmed at endoscopy by the presence of tubercle bacilli, or, rarely, caseating granulomas in esophageal brushings or biopsy specimens.[90]

## Radiographic Findings

Extrinsic esophageal involvement by tuberculous nodes in the mediastinum is usually manifested radiographically by compression, displacement, or narrowing of the esophagus by an adjacent mediastinal mass.[87, 90] These patients may also develop strictures or traction diverticula, most frequently at the level of the carina.[87, 88] Occasionally, caseating nodes in the mediastinum may erode into the esophagus, producing superficial or deep areas of ulceration, longitudinal or transverse sinus tracks, or fistulas into the mediastinum or tracheobronchial tree[87, 88] (Fig. 25–22). Sinus tracks and fistulas have been recognized as a prominent feature of tuberculous esophagitis in patients with AIDS[84, 85] (Fig. 25–23). Similar findings may be demonstrated in patients with Crohn's disease, trauma, radiation, and esophageal carcinoma, but the presence of pulmonary or mediastinal tuberculosis should suggest the correct diagnosis, particularly in patients with AIDS.

Intrinsic tuberculous esophagitis occurs much less frequently and is characterized on barium studies by mucosal irregularity, ulcers, plaques, fistulas, and, eventually, strictures[86, 87, 90] (Fig. 25–24). Tuberculous esophagitis may be indistinguishable from severe esophagitis due to caustic ingestion, radiation, or other causes. However, the possibility of tuberculous esophagitis should be considered in patients with active pulmonary tuberculosis.

## OTHER INFECTIONS

Although infectious esophagitis is usually caused by fungal or viral organisms, other rare causes include

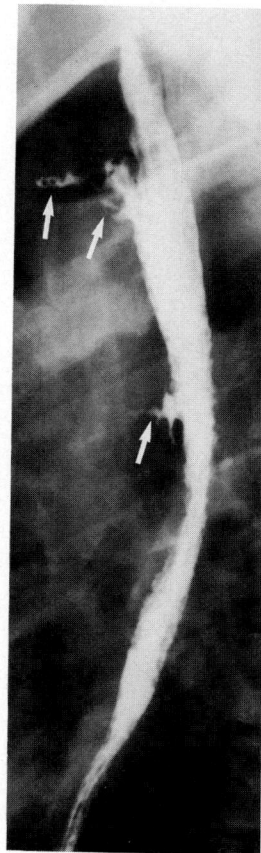

**Figure 25–23. Tuberculous esophagitis in a patient with AIDS.** There is diffuse esophagitis with several deep sinus tracks *(arrows)* extending anteriorly from the esophagus into the mediastinum. (From Goodman P, Pinero SS, Rance RM, et al: Mycobacterial esophagitis in AIDS. Gastrointest Radiol 14:103–105, 1989.)

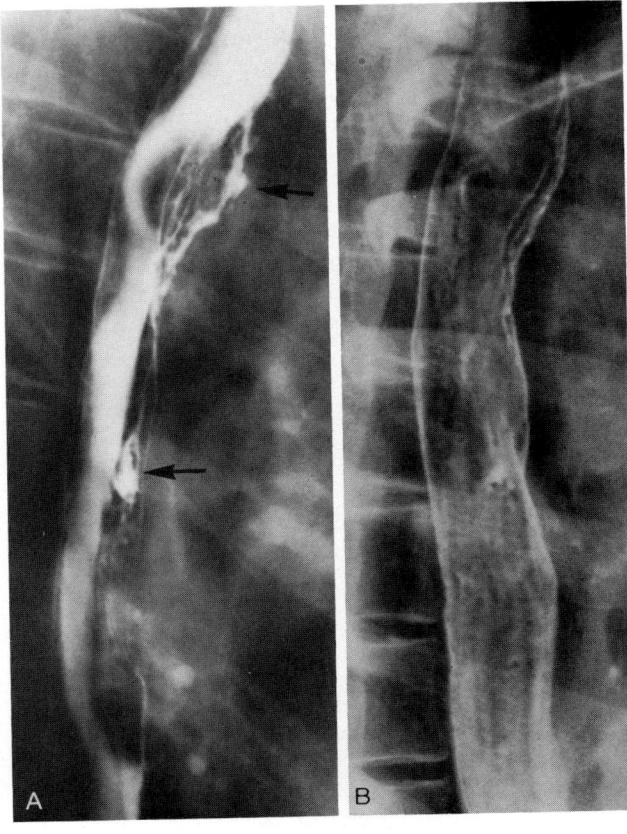

**Figure 25–24. Tuberculous esophagitis. A.** The initial esophagram shows two areas of irregular ulceration *(arrows)* in the midesophagus due to proven tuberculous esophagitis. **B.** Another esophagram after 6 months of antituberculous therapy shows healing of the ulcers. (From Savage PE, Grundy A: Oesophageal tuberculosis: an unusual cause of dysphagia. Br J Radiol 57:1153–1155, 1984.)

*Staphylococcus, Streptococcus, Klebsiella, Blastomyces, Cryptosporidium, Torulopsis glabrata,* and *Lactobacillus acidophilus.*[91–95]

## Acknowledgment

Figures 25–4, 25–5A, 25–6, 25–10 and 25–16 to 25–18 are reproduced from Levine MS: Radiology of the Esophagus. Philadelphia: WB Saunders, 1989.

## References

1. Mathieson R, Dutta SK: Candida esophagitis. Dig Dis Sci 28:365–370, 1983.
2. Lewicki AM, Moore JP: Esophageal moniliasis. AJR 125:218–225, 1975.
3. Jensen KB, Stenderup A, Thomsen JB, et al: Oesophageal moniliasis in malignant neoplastic disease. Acta Med Scand 175:455–459, 1964.
4. Holt JH: *Candida* infection of the esophagus. Gut 9:227–231, 1968.
5. Sheft DJ, Shrago G: Esophageal moniliasis: the spectrum of the disease. JAMA 213:1859–1862, 1970.
6. Eras P, Goldstein MJ, Sherlock P: *Candida* infection of the gastrointestinal tract. Medicine (Baltimore) 51:367–379, 1972.
7. Levine MS, Macones AJ, Laufer I: Candida esophagitis: accuracy of radiographic diagnosis. Radiology 154:581–587, 1985.
8. Gefter WB, Laufer I, Edell S, et al: Candidiasis in the obstructed esophagus. Radiology 138:25–28, 1981.
9. Brown JW, McKee WM: Acute monilial esophagitis occurring without underlying disease in a young male. Dig Dis Sci 17:85–88, 1972.
10. Kodsi BE, Wickremesinghe PC, Kozinn PJ, et al: Candida esophagitis. Gastroenterology 71:715–719, 1976.
11. Ott DJ, Gelfand DW: Esophageal stricture secondary to candidiasis. Gastrointest Radiol 2:323–325, 1978.
12. Kelvin FM, Clark WM, Thompson WM, et al: Chronic esophageal stricture due to moniliasis. Br J Radiol 51:826–828, 1978.
13. Orringer MB, Sloan H: Monilial esophagitis: an increasingly frequent cause of esophageal stenosis? Ann Thorac Surg 26:364–374, 1978.
14. Agha FP: Candidiasis-induced esophageal strictures. Gastrointest Radiol 9:283–286, 1984.
15. Gonzales-Crussi F, Iung DS: Esophageal moniliasis as a cause of death. Am J Surg 109:634–638, 1965.
16. Lefkowitz M, Louis EJ, Levine RS: Candidal infection complicating peptic esophageal ulcer. Arch Intern Med 113:672–675, 1964.
17. Obrecht WF, Richter JE, Olympio GA, et al: Tracheoesophageal fistula: a serious complication of infectious esophagitis. Gastroenterology 87:1174–1179, 1984.
18. Sehha S, Hazeghi K, Bajoghli M, et al: Oesophageal moniliasis causing fistula formation and lung abscess. Thorax 31:361–364, 1976.
19. Friedman HM, Gluckman SJ: Infections of the esophagus. *In* Cohen S, Soloway RD (eds): Diseases of the Esophagus. New York: Churchill Livingstone, 1982, pp 277–286.
20. Levine MS, Woldenberg R, Herlinger H, et al: Opportunistic esophagitis in AIDS: radiographic diagnosis. Radiology 165:815–820, 1987.
21. Brayko CM, Kozavek RA, Sanowski RA, et al: Type I herpes simplex esophagitis with concomitant esophageal moniliasis. J Clin Gastroenterol 4:351–355, 1982.
22. Mirra SS, Bryan JA, Butz WC, et al: Concomitant herpes-monilial esophagitis: case report with ultrastructural study. Hum Pathol 13:760–763, 1982.
23. Tavitian A, Raufman JP, Rosenthal LE, et al: Ketoconazole-

resistant Candida esophagitis in patients with acquired immuno-deficiency syndrome. Gastroenterology 90:443–445, 1986.

24. Hartong WA, Moeller DD, Laing RR: Esophageal moniliasis: radiographic, endoscopic, and pathologic criteria for diagnosis. J Kans Med Soc 73:470–474, 1972.

25. Vahey TN, Maglinte DDT, Chernish SM: State-of-the-art barium examination in opportunistic esophagitis. Dig Dis Sci 31:1192–1195, 1986.

26. Laufer I: Radiology of esophagitis. Radiol Clin North Am 20:687–699, 1982.

27. Kressel HY, Glick SN, Laufer I, et al: Radiologic features of esophagitis. Gastrointest Radiol 6:103–108, 1981.

28. Goldberg HI, Dodds WJ: Cobblestone esophagus due to monilial infection. AJR 104:608–612, 1968.

29. Kaufman SA, Scheff S, Levene G: Esophageal moniliasis. Radiology 75:726–731, 1960.

30. Athey PA, Goldstein HM, Dodd GD: Radiologic spectrum of opportunistic infections of the upper gastrointestinal tract. AJR 129:419–424, 1977.

31. Gonzalez G: Esophageal moniliasis. AJR 113:233–236, 1971.

32. Ho CS, Cullen JB, Gray RR: An unusual manifestation of esophageal moniliasis. Radiology 123:287–288, 1977.

33. Roberts L, Gibbons R, Gibbons G, et al: Adult esophageal candidiasis: a radiographic spectrum. Radiographics 7:289–307, 1987.

34. Farman J, Tivitian A, Rosenthal LE, et al: Focal esophageal candidiasis in acquired immunodeficiency syndrome (AIDS). Gastrointest Radiol 11:213–217, 1986.

35. Campero AA, Campbell GD: Complete oesophageal obstruction due to monilial infection. Aust N Z J Surg 43:244–246, 1973.

36. Troupin RH: Intramural esophageal diverticulosis and moniliasis: a possible association. AJR 104:613–616, 1968.

37. Beauchamp JM, Nice CM, Belanger MA, et al: Esophageal intramural pseudodiverticulosis. Radiology 113:273–276, 1974.

38. Castillo S, Abvrashed A, Kimmelman J, et al: Diffuse intramural esophageal pseudodiverticulosis. Gastroenterology 72:541–545, 1977.

39. Rohrmann CA, Kidd R: Chronic mucocutaneous candidiasis: radiologic abnormalities in the esophagus. AJR 130:473–476, 1978.

40. Meyers C, Durkin MG, Love L: Radiographic findings in herpetic esophagitis. Radiology 119:21–22, 1976.

41. Skucas J, Schrank WW, Meyer PC, et al: Herpes esophagitis: a case study by air-contrast esophagography. AJR 128:497–499, 1977.

42. Levine MS, Cajade AG, Herlinger H, et al: Pseudomembranes in reflux esophagitis. Radiology 159:43–45, 1986.

43. Glick SN, Teplick SK, Goldstein J, et al: Glycogenic acanthosis of the esophagus. AJR 139:683–688, 1982.

44. Itai Y, Kogure T, Okuyama Y, et al: Diffuse finely nodular lesions of the esophagus. AJR 128:563–566, 1977.

45. Itai Y, Kogure T, Okuyama Y, et al: Superficial esophageal carcinoma: radiological findings in double-contrast studies. Radiology 126:597–601, 1978.

46. Gohel VK, Kressel HY, Laufer I: Double-contrast artifacts. Gastrointest Radiol 3:139–146, 1978.

47. Montgomerie JZ, Becroft DMO, Croxson MC, et al: Herpes simplex virus infection after renal transplantation. Lancet 2:867–871, 1969.

48. Rosen P, Hajdu SI: Visceral herpes virus infections in patients with cancer. Am J Clin Pathol 56:459–465, 1971.

49. Muller SA, Herrmann EC, Winkelmann RK: Herpes simplex infections in hematologic malignancies. Am J Med 52:102–114, 1972.

50. Weiden PL, Schuffler MD: Herpes esophagitis complicating Hodgkin's disease. Cancer 33:1100–1102, 1974.

51. Nash G, Ross JS: Herpetic esophagitis: a common cause of esophageal ulceration. Hum Pathol 5:339–345, 1974.

52. Depew WT, Prentice RS, Beck IT, et al: Herpes simplex ulcerative esophagitis in a healthy subject. Am J Gastroenterol 68:381–385, 1977.

53. Owensby LC, Stammer JL: Esophagitis associated with herpes simplex infection in an immunocompetent host. Gastroenterology 74:1305–1306, 1978.

54. Springer DJ, Da Costa LR, Beck IT: A syndrome of acute self-limiting ulcerative esophagitis in young adults probably due to herpes simplex virus. Dig Dis Sci 24:535–539, 1979.

55. Deshmukh M, Shah R, McCallum RW: Experience with herpes esophagitis in otherwise healthy patients. Am J Gastroenterol 79:173–176, 1984.

56. Desigan G, Schneider RP: Herpes simplex esophagitis in healthy adults. South Med J 78:1135–1137, 1985.

57. Levine MS, Laufer I, Kressel HY, et al: Herpes esophagitis. AJR 136:863–866, 1981.

58. Fishbein PG, Tuthill R, Kressel HY, et al: Herpes simplex esophagitis: a cause of upper gastrointestinal bleeding. Am J Dig Dis 24:540–544, 1979.

59. Rattner HM, Cooper DJ, Zaman MB: Severe bleeding from herpes esophagitis. Am J Gastroenterol 80:523–525, 1985.

60. Nash G, Foley FD: Herpetic infection of the middle and lower respiratory tract. Am J Clin Pathol 54:857–863, 1970.

61. Lightdale CJ, Wolf DJ, Marcucci RA, et al: Herpetic esophagitis in patients with cancer: antemortem diagnosis by brush cytology. Cancer 39:223–226, 1977.

62. Lasser A: Herpes simplex virus esophagitis. Acta Cytol (Baltimore) 21:301–302, 1977.

63. Klotz DA, Silverman L: Herpes virus esophagitis, consistent with herpes simplex, visualized endoscopically. Gastrointest Endosc 21:71–73, 1974.

64. Pearce J, Dagradi A: Acute ulceration of the esophagus with associated intranuclear inclusion bodies. Arch Pathol 35:889–897, 1943.

65. Shortsleeve MJ, Gauvin GP, Gardner RC, et al: Herpetic esophagitis. Radiology 141:611–617, 1981.

66. Agha FP, Lee HH, Nostrant TT: Herpetic esophagitis: a diagnostic challenge in immunocompromised patients. Am J Gastroenterol 81:246–253, 1986.

67. Levine MS, Loevner LA, Saul SH, et al: Herpes esophagitis: sensitivity of double-contrast esophagography. AJR 151:57–62, 1988.

68. DeGaeta L, Levine MS, Guglielmi GE, et al: Herpes esophagitis in an otherwise healthy patient. AJR 144:1205–1206, 1985.

69. Shortsleeve MJ, Levine MS: Herpes esophagitis in otherwise healthy patients: clinical and radiographic findings. Radiology 182:859–861, 1992.

70. Creteur V, Laufer I, Kressel HY, et al: Drug-induced esophagitis detected by double-contrast radiography. Radiology 147:365–368, 1983.

71. Bova JG, Dutton NE, Goldstein HM, et al: Medication-induced esophagitis: diagnosis by double-contrast esophagography. AJR 148:731–732, 1987.

72. Balthazar EJ, Megibow AJ, Hulnick DH: Cytomegalovirus esophagitis and gastritis in AIDS. AJR 144:1201–1204, 1985.

73. Balthazar EJ, Megibow AJ, Hulnick D, et al: Cytomegalovirus esophagitis in AIDS: radiographic features in 16 patients. AJR 149:919–923, 1987.

74. Teixidor HS, Honig CL, Norsoph E, et al: Cytomegalovirus infection of the alimentary canal: radiologic findings with pathologic correlation. Radiology 163:317–323, 1987.

75. Frager DH, Frager JD, Brandt LJ, et al: Gastrointestinal complications of AIDS: radiologic features. Radiology 158:597–603, 1986.

76. Wilcox CM, Diehl DL, Cello JP, et al: Cytomegalovirus esophagitis in patients with AIDS: a clinical, endoscopic, and pathologic correlation. Ann Intern Med 113:589–593, 1990.

77. Buhles WC, Mastre BJ, Tinker AJ, et al: Ganciclovir treatment of life- or sight-threatening cytomegalovirus infection: experience in 314 immunocompromised patients. Rev Infect Dis 10(suppl 3):495–506, 1988.

78. Kumar A, Posner G, Colby S, et al: Giant esophageal ulcers in AIDS-related complex. Gastrointest Endosc 34:153–154, 1988.

79. Bach MC, Valenti AJ, Howell DA, et al: Odynophagia from aphthous ulcers of the pharynx and esophagus in the acquired immunodeficiency syndrome (AIDS). Ann Intern Med 109:338–339, 1988.

80. Bach MC, Howell DA, Valenti AJ, et al: Aphthous ulceration of the gastrointestinal tract in patients with the acquired immunodeficiency syndrome (AIDS). Ann Intern Med 112:465–466, 1990.

81. Rabeneck L, Popovic M, Gartner S, et al: Acute HIV infection presenting with painful swallowing and esophageal ulcers. JAMA 263:2318–2322, 1990.

82. Levine MS, Loercher G, Katzka DA, et al: Giant, human immunodeficiency virus–related ulcers in the esophagus. Radiology 180:323–326, 1991.

83. Dretler RH, Rausher DB: Giant esophageal ulcer healed with steroid therapy in an AIDS patient. Rev Infect Dis 11:768–769, 1989.

84. Goodman P, Pinero SS, Rance RM, et al: Mycobacterial esophagitis in AIDS. Gastrointest Radiol 14:103–105, 1989.

85. de Silva R, Stoopack PM, Raufman JP: Esophageal fistulas associated with mycobacterial infection in patients at risk for AIDS. Radiology 175:449–453, 1990.

86. Rubinstein BM, Patrana T, Jacobson HG: Tuberculosis of the esophagus. Radiology 70:401–403, 1958.

87. Schneider R: Tuberculosis of the mediastinum. Gastrointest Radiol 1:143–145, 1976.

88. Williford ME, Thompson WM, Hamilton JD, et al: Esophageal tuberculosis: findings on barium swallow and computed tomography. Gastrointest Radiol 8:119–122, 1983.

89. Fahmy AQ, Guindi R, Farid A: Tuberculosis of the oesophagus. Thorax 24:254–256, 1969.

90. Savage PE, Grundy A: Oesophageal tuberculosis: an unusual cause of dysphagia. Br J Radiol 57:1153–1155, 1984.

91. Walsh TJ, Belitsos NJ, Hamilton SR: Bacterial esophagitis in immunocompromised patients. Arch Intern Med 146:1345–1348, 1986.

92. McKenzie R, Khakoo R: Blastomycosis of the esophagus presenting with gastrointestinal bleeding. Gastroenterology 88:1271–1273, 1985.

93. Kazlow PG, Shah K, Benkov K, et al: Esophageal cryptosporidiosis in a child with acquired immune deficiency syndrome. Gastroenterology 91:1301–1303, 1986.

94. Bentlif PS, Widermann B: Esophagitis caused by *Torulopsis glabrata*. Am J Gastroenterol 71:395–397, 1979.

95. McManus JPA, Webb JN: A yeast-like infection of the esophagus caused by *Lactobacillus acidophilus*. Gastroenterology 68:583–586, 1975.

# Other Esophagitides

Marc S. Levine, M.D.

## DRUG-INDUCED ESOPHAGITIS

Although oral medications were not described as a cause of esophageal injury until 1970,[1] drug-induced esophagitis is recognized as a relatively common condition in today's pill-oriented society. The medications implicated most frequently are doxycycline and tetracycline.[2] These patients may have severe esophageal symptoms, but drug-induced esophagitis usually resolves rapidly after withdrawal of the offending agent. Conventional single contrast barium studies have been of limited value in detecting mucosal abnormalities associated with drug-induced esophagitis. However, double contrast esophagography appears to be a valuable technique for diagnosing this condition.

## Pathogenesis

The type and degree of injury that occurs in drug-induced esophagitis depend on the specific properties of the offending medication, which is usually given in the form of capsules or tablets. Prolonged retention of these capsules or tablets in the esophagus may cause ulceration of the adjacent mucosa through a focal contact esophagitis. However, the development of esophagitis is primarily related to the manner in which the medication is taken. In one study, orally ingested technetium 99m–labeled gelatin capsules remained in the esophagus considerably longer in subjects who were recumbent than in those who were upright, and, regardless of position, capsules were rapidly cleared only when taken with a 15-mL chaser of water.[3] In another study, esophageal retention of barium sulfate tablets was observed at fluoroscopy for intervals of 5 to 90 minutes in about 60% of patients who remained supine after taking the tablets.[4] Retention of pills is favored not only by recumbency but also by a marked decrease in salivation and swallowing that occurs during sleep.[5, 6] Thus, most patients with drug-induced esophagitis have a history of ingesting their medication with little or no water immediately before going to bed.[2, 4]

Drug-induced esophagitis usually occurs in the mid-esophagus, presumably because of delayed passage of the medication at this level due to extrinsic compression of the esophagus by the aortic arch or left main bronchus.[2] Less frequently, prolonged retention of the medication may result from esophageal compression by an enlarged heart.[7] Occasionally, drug-induced esophagitis may occur in patients who have abnormal motility or pre-existing strictures that delay transit of pills from the esophagus[8, 9] (see Fig. 26–4A).

## Etiologic Agents

### Doxycycline and Tetracycline

Doxycycline and tetracycline, two widely used antibiotics, account for about half the reported cases of drug-induced esophagitis.[2] About 90% of these cases are caused by doxycycline.[2] Both doxycycline and tetracycline are given in the form of capsules that are relatively acidic. As a result, prolonged retention of the capsules in the upper esophagus or midesophagus may cause superficial ulceration of the adjacent mucosa.[2, 10] Although tetracycline (pH 2.3) is slightly more acidic than doxycycline (pH 3.0), it dissolves rapidly, whereas doxycycline dissolves quite slowly and forms a thick gel.[11] Prolonged adherence of the slowly disintegrating doxycycline capsules to the adjacent mucosa may account for the higher frequency of esophagitis in patients taking this drug.

### Potassium Chloride

Potassium chloride tablets may produce a severe form of drug-induced esophagitis.[1, 2, 7, 12–14] These patients often have mitral valvular disease with an enlarged left atrium compressing the distal esophagus, so that passage of the potassium chloride tablets is impeded at this level. Subsequent release of potassium chloride over a localized area of esophageal mucosa may cause severe chemical injury with focal ulceration and stricture formation.[7, 13, 14] As a result, potassium supplements are sometimes given in liquid form to patients with known cardiomegaly to prevent this complication. However, even liquid potassium has been described as a cause of drug-induced esophagitis.[15]

### Quinidine

Because oral quinidine is often given for cardiac arrhythmias, these patients may have associated cardiomegaly, with compression of the distal esophagus by an enlarged left atrium or ventricle. Retained quinidine above this level may have a corrosive effect on the adjacent mucosa, causing ulceration and strictures.[2, 8, 15] Patients who are receiving long-term quinidine therapy are more likely to develop strictures.[15]

### Other Drugs

Other oral medications that have been implicated in the development of drug-induced esophagitis include aspirin and other nonsteroidal anti-inflammatory drugs, emepronium bromide, ferrous sulfate, alprenolol chloride, ascorbic acid, theophylline, cromolyn sodium, Clinitest tablets, and other antibiotics such as clindamycin and lincomycin.[2, 9, 16–25]

## Clinical Findings

Patients with drug-induced esophagitis typically present with odynophagia (painful swallowing) or unrelenting chest pain that is accentuated by swallowing.[2] Others may have dysphagia or a persistent foreign body sensation in the esophagus.[10] Symptoms usually develop rapidly within several hours to days after taking the medication.[2] The acute onset of odynophagia may suggest the possibility of esophageal infection by fungal or viral organisms. However, Candida or herpes esophagitis usually occurs in immunocompromised patients, whereas drug-induced esophagitis often develops in otherwise healthy individuals. Occasionally, chest pain may be so severe that it mimics angina pectoris or a myocardial infarction. However, the symptoms of drug-induced esophagitis tend to resolve rapidly after withdrawal of the offending agent, so that most patients are asymptomatic within 7 to 10 days after stopping the medication.[10] Rarely, drug-induced ulcers may be complicated by hemorrhage or perforation.[7, 12] Other patients may have persistent dysphagia due to the development of strictures.[7, 15, 25]

## Radiographic Findings

The radiographic findings in drug-induced esophagitis depend on the nature of the offending medication (Figs. 26–1 to 26–4). Doxycycline and tetracycline usually cause superficial ulceration in the esophagus without permanent sequelae. In contrast, potassium chloride and quinidine tend to produce a more severe esophagitis with deep ulcers and strictures. Although conventional single contrast barium studies may demonstrate deep ulcers and strictures, they are rarely able to detect superficial areas of ulceration. As a result, endoscopy has generally been advocated as the primary technique for diagnosing this condition.[2]

With double contrast technique, however, esophagography appears to be a more sensitive method for diagnosing drug-induced esophagitis than has been suggested in the earlier literature.[26–28] The major advantage of this technique is its ability to demonstrate shallow ulcers and other mucosal changes of drug-induced esophagitis that cannot easily be recognized on single contrast studies. Thus, experience suggests that double contrast esophagography is a valuable technique for diagnosing this condition.

Drug-induced esophagitis is typically manifested by a solitary ulcer (see Fig. 26–1A), several discrete ulcers (see Fig. 26–1B), or a localized cluster of tiny ulcers distributed circumferentially on a normal background mucosa[26–28] (see Fig. 26–1C). The ulcers are usually located in the midesophagus, near the level of the aortic arch or left main bronchus. The ulcers may be recog-

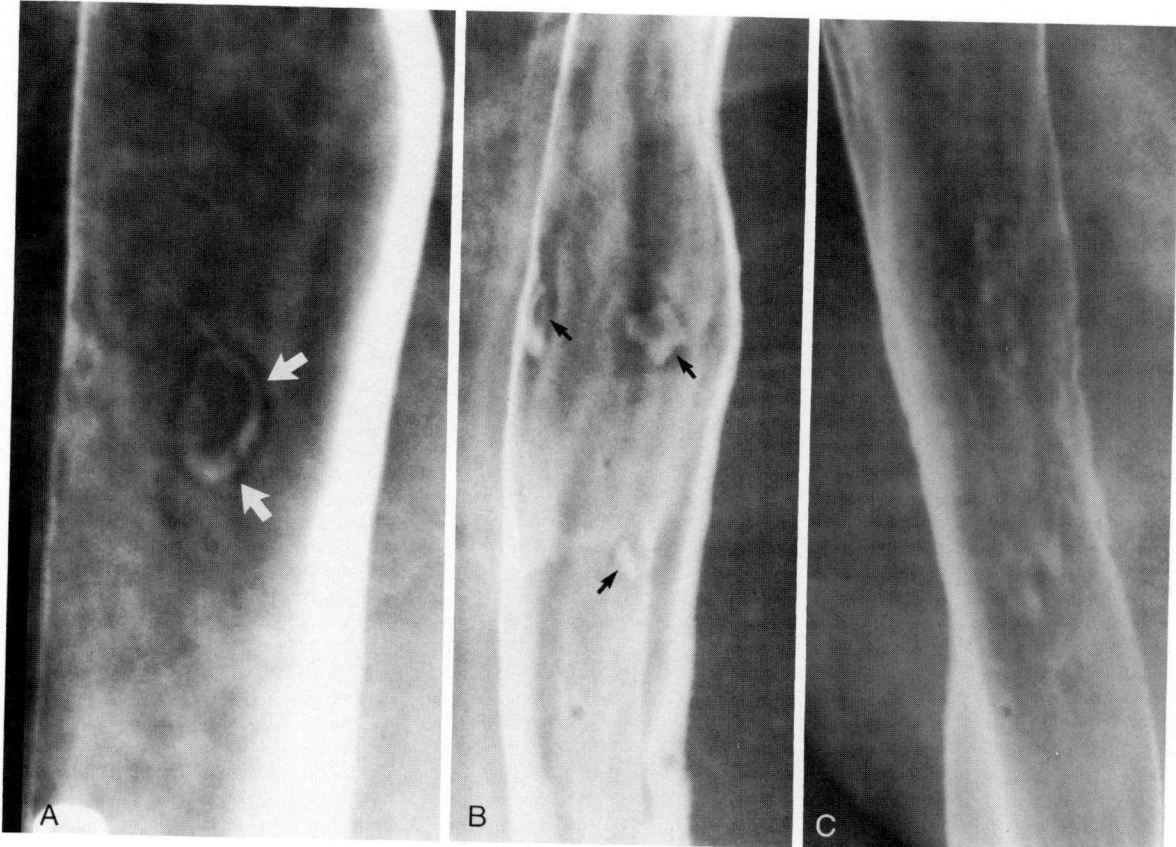

**Figure 26–1. Drug-induced esophagitis with superficial ulcers. A.** There is a solitary ring-like ulcer *(arrows)* in the midesophagus. Note the thin, radiolucent halo of edematous mucosa surrounding the ulcer. **B.** Several discrete ulcers *(arrows)* are seen in the midesophagus on a normal background mucosa. The largest ulcer has a stellate configuration. **C.** This patient has more extensive esophagitis with multiple tiny superficial ulcers clustered circumferentially in the midesophagus. The patients in **A** and **C** were taking doxycycline, and the patient in **B** was taking tetracycline.

**Figure 26–2. Drug-induced esophagitis with healing. A.** The initial double-contrast esophagram shows multiple serpiginous ulcers in the midesophagus with normal mucosa distally. **B.** Seven days after the patient stopped taking doxycycline, another esophagram shows complete healing of the ulcers. (Several air bubbles are present in the esophagus.)

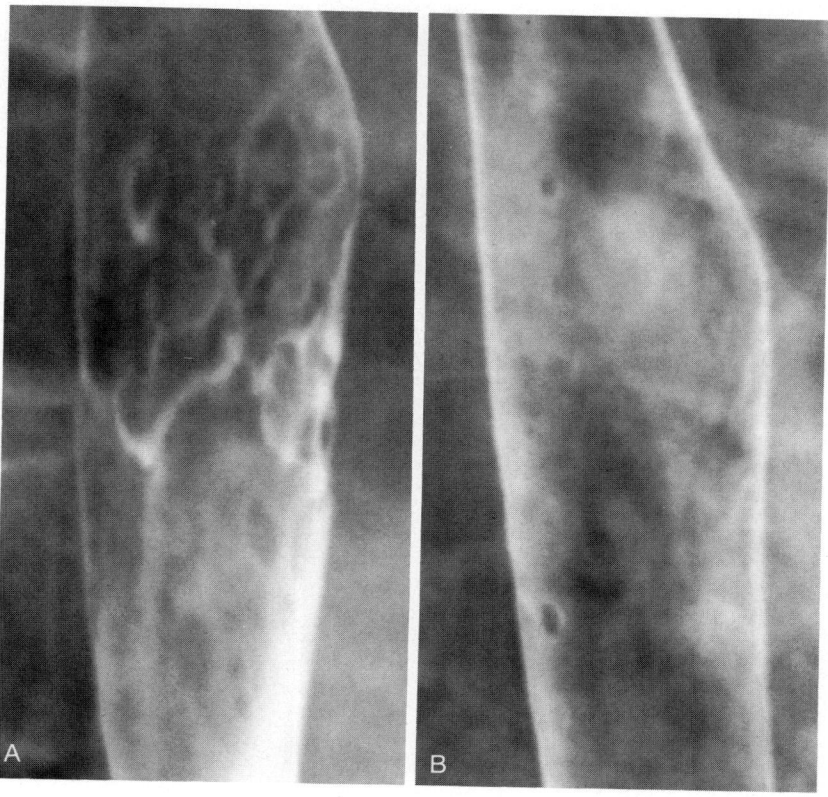

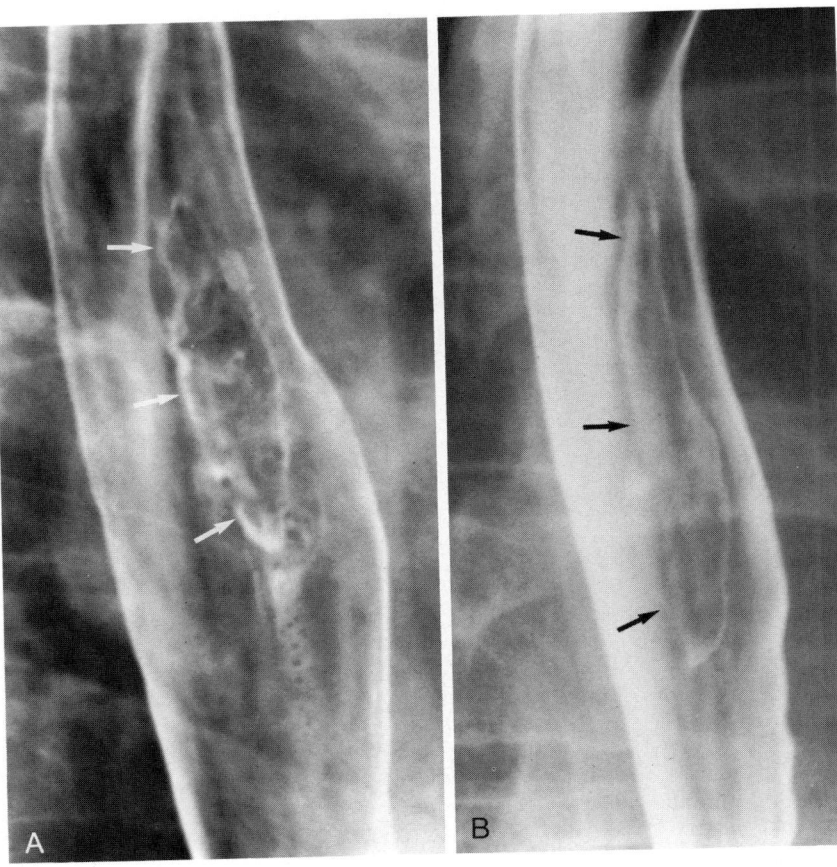

**Figure 26–3. Drug-induced esophagitis with a giant esophageal ulcer. A.** The initial double contrast esophagram shows a 7 × 2 cm ulcer *(arrows)* in the midesophagus below the level of the carina. Note how the ulcer crater has irregular margins. This patient was taking sulindac (Clinoril), a nonsteroidal anti-inflammatory agent. **B.** Another esophagram 6 months later shows a long, shallow depression with smooth borders *(arrows)* at the site of the previous ulcer. Endoscopy revealed that this was an ulcer scar with a re-epithelialized pit or depression. (**A** and **B** from MS Levine, RD Rothstein, I Laufer, Giant esophageal ulcer due to Clinoril, AJR, 156, 5, 955–956, 1991, © by American Roentgen Ray Society.)

**Figure 26–4. The spectrum of esophageal injury associated with potassium chloride ingestion. A.** A conglomerate of undissolved potassium chloride tablets is seen in the midesophagus. The tablets remained at this level during fluoroscopy because of abnormal motility with absent peristalsis in the esophagus. The patient subsequently developed severe drug-induced esophagitis. **B.** A giant ulcer *(white arrows)* is seen in the midesophagus with an associated area of mass effect *(black arrows)* due to a surrounding mound of edema. This lesion could be mistaken for an ulcerated carcinoma. **C.** A midesophageal stricture *(arrows)* is seen in a patient who had been taking slow-release potassium chloride tablets. The stricture has relatively tapered margins.

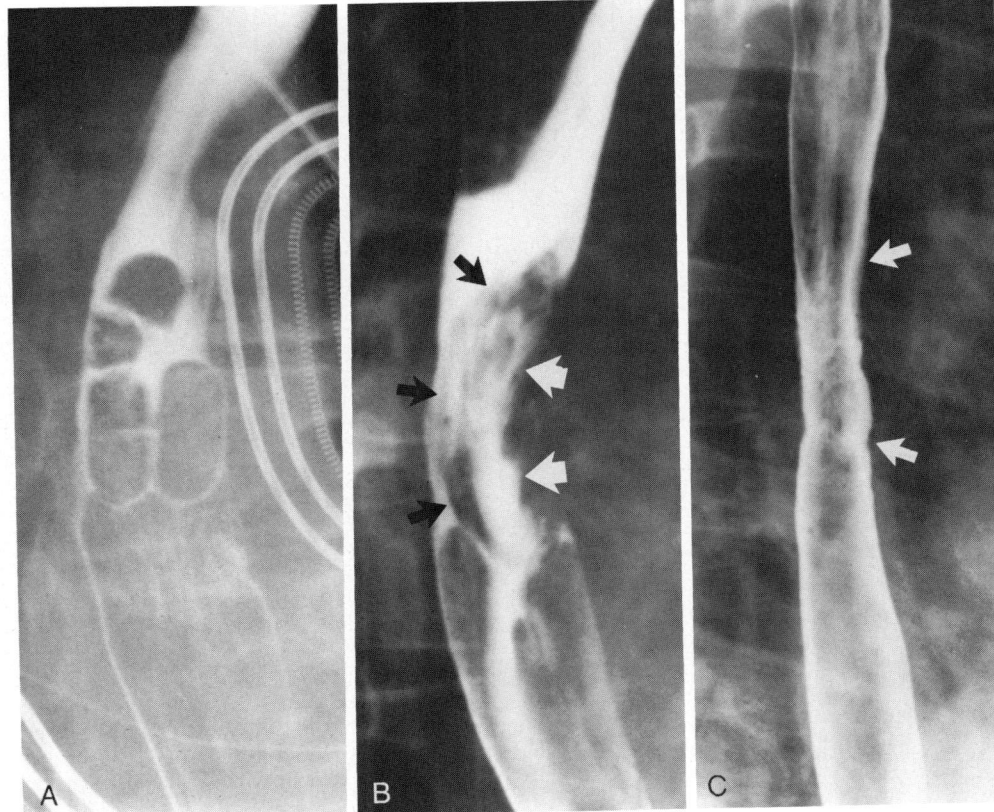

nized en face as punctate, linear, ovoid, stellate, or serpiginous collections of barium on the esophageal mucosa or in profile as shallow depressions[26-28] (see Figs. 26–1 and 26–2A). There may be slight nodularity of the adjacent mucosa or thickening and distortion of adjacent esophageal folds. When esophageal ulcers are drug induced, another esophagram 7 to 10 days after withdrawal of the offending agent may show dramatic healing of the lesions[26] (see Fig. 26–2B).

Drug-induced esophagitis may occasionally be manifested by giant, relatively flat ulcers that are several centimeters or more in length[17] (see Fig. 26–3A). Healing of these ulcers may lead to the development of smooth, re-epithelialized depressions that can be mistaken for active ulcer craters[17] (see Fig. 26–3B). Larger areas of ulceration are more likely to be caused by ingestion of potassium chloride or quinidine in patients with cardiomegaly. Because of associated edema and inflammation, there may be a considerable mass effect surrounding the ulcer, mimicking the appearance of an ulcerated carcinoma[15, 26, 29] (see Fig. 26–4B). However, the correct diagnosis should be suggested by the patient's drug history. Furthermore, a follow-up esophagram should show marked healing or disappearance of the ulcer after the offending agent has been withdrawn.

Because of the degree of ulceration associated with potassium chloride and quinidine, these drugs may also lead to the development of esophageal strictures.[7, 14, 15, 25] The strictures usually appear as segmental areas of concentric narrowing above the level of an enlarged left atrium[15] (see Fig. 26–4C). Occasionally, however, an apparent stricture may be caused by edema and spasm associated with severe esophagitis, so that a focal area of narrowing may resolve after stopping the medication.

## Differential Diagnosis

Herpes esophagitis is the major consideration in the differential diagnosis for discrete, superficial ulcers in the upper esophagus or midesophagus.[30] Although viral ulcers tend to have a more widespread distribution, they sometimes are indistinguishable from the ulcers of drug-induced esophagitis (Fig. 26–5). Because most patients with herpes esophagitis are immunocompromised, these entities can usually be differentiated on the basis of the clinical history. Occasionally, however, herpes esophagitis may occur in otherwise healthy patients who have no underlying immunologic problems (see Chapter 25).[31] Thus, the diagnosis of drug-induced esophagitis should be suggested only when there is a definite temporal relationship between ingestion of the offending medication and the onset of esophagitis.

Reflux esophagitis is a more common cause of superficial ulceration in the esophagus.[32] However, it would be unusual for patients with reflux esophagitis to have focal ulceration in the midesophagus with a normal-appearing mucosa below this level. Mediastinal irradiation and caustic ingestion are other causes of ulceration, but the correct diagnosis is usually suggested on clinical grounds. Crohn's disease may also be associated with

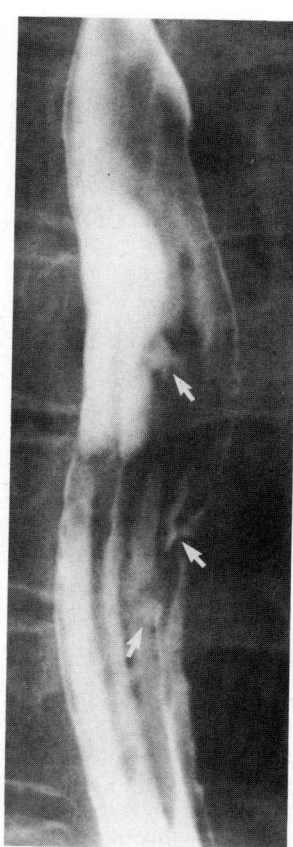

**Figure 26–5. Herpes esophagitis with discrete ulcers.** There are several widely separated ulcers *(arrows)* in the midesophagus on a normal background mucosa. Although the radiographic findings are indistinguishable from those of drug-induced esophagitis, the correct diagnosis is suggested by the clinical setting of odynophagia in an immunocompromised patient. (From MS Levine, I Laufer, HY Kressel, et al, Herpes esophagitis, AJR, 136, 5, 863–866, 1981, © by American Roentgen Ray Society.)

shallow ulcers in the esophagus, but these patients usually have advanced Crohn's disease in the small bowel or colon. Finally, giant drug-induced ulcers may be indistinguishable from cytomegalovirus or human immunodeficiency virus ulcers in patients with acquired immunodeficiency syndrome (see Chapter 25).[33] However, these conditions can usually be differentiated by the clinical history and presentation.

Because drug-induced strictures are usually located at a considerable distance from the gastroesophageal junction, they must be differentiated from other, more common causes of high esophageal strictures, such as Barrett's esophagus, mediastinal irradiation, caustic ingestion, and primary or metastatic tumors. However, the possibility of a drug-induced stricture should be suspected in patients with cardiomegaly who have a history of taking potassium chloride or quinidine.

## RADIATION ESOPHAGITIS

Malignant tumors involving the lungs, mediastinum, or thoracic spine are often treated by high-dose, external beam radiation to the chest. The major limiting factor with this form of treatment is esophageal damage by ionizing radiation. Total doses of 4500 to 6000 rad may lead to severe esophagitis with irreversible damage and stricture formation.[34] Smaller doses (2000 to 4500 rad) may cause a self-limited esophagitis without permanent sequelae. Most patients have clinical evidence of esophagitis shortly after the onset of radiotherapy.[35] However, barium studies are rarely performed during this period. Instead, esophagography has been used primarily to detect strictures or other signs of chronic radiation injury. Both the acute and the chronic forms of radiation esophagitis are considered in this chapter.

## Pathogenesis

Experiments on laboratory animals have shown that high-dose radiation to the esophagus may cause acute esophagitis with ulceration, necrosis, and sloughing of the irradiated mucosa within 1 to 2 weeks.[36–38] However, there is usually complete healing of the esophageal mucosa by 3 to 4 weeks.[36] These animal studies indicate that an acute, self-limited form of esophagitis almost always occurs after mediastinal irradiation within a relatively uniform time frame. Other investigators have shown that the early postirradiation changes in humans are comparable to those found in animal models.[35]

After the acute stage of radiation injury and subsequent epithelial repair, chronic radiation esophagitis is characterized by marked thickening of the submucosa due to edema and fibrosis.[34–36] In one laboratory study, the majority of irradiated animals had evidence of progressive submucosal fibrosis 3 to 4 months after radiotherapy.[36] The delayed appearance of strictures in humans can therefore be attributed to this gradual cicatrization process. The strictures usually develop 4 to 8 months after completion of radiotherapy at doses of 3000 to 5000 rad.[39] If the radiation dose is more than 6000 rad, however, esophageal strictures may develop within 3 to 4 months.[39] In various studies, stricture formation has been found to occur in 17 to 42% of patients who undergo mediastinal irradiation.[34, 35, 39]

Although most patients with radiation esophagitis receive doses of more than 3000 rad to the esophagus, a clinically distinct type of esophagitis may be caused by low-dose radiotherapy in patients who receive combined radiation and chemotherapy with adriamycin.[40–42] In such cases, severe esophagitis or stricture formation may occur after radiation doses to the mediastinum as low as 500 rad.[42] It has been postulated that adriamycin potentiates the effects of radiotherapy, possibly by inhibiting DNA repair and decreasing the chance of cellular recovery from sublethal radiation damage.[40, 41] The patients usually have received adriamycin within 1 week of radiotherapy, so synchronous treatment with radiation and chemotherapy appears to be critical to the development of esophagitis. These patients may have recurrent esophagitis after each subsequent course of adriamycin.[40, 42] This "recall" phenomenon may account for the increased frequency of strictures with this form of treatment.

## Clinical Findings

Most patients who receive mediastinal irradiation have varying degrees of esophagitis, manifested by acute onset of substernal burning, odynophagia, or dysphagia within 2 to 3 weeks after the initiation of radiotherapy.[35, 43] These symptoms may subside within 24 to 48 hours or may persist for several weeks after completion of radiotherapy.[35, 43] Because these patients are immunocompromised, the development of odynophagia may erroneously be attributed to opportunistic esophagitis. However, a temporal relationship between the onset of radiotherapy and the onset of symptoms should suggest the correct diagnosis. When acute radiation esophagitis is diagnosed on clinical grounds, these patients usually receive empirical treatment with viscous lidocaine (Xylocaine) and analgesics. As a result, radiologic or endoscopic examinations are not often performed during this period.

Chronic radiation injury to the esophagus may cause dysphagia within several months after completion of radiotherapy. Dysphagia may result from abnormal esophageal motility or, less commonly, from the development of strictures.[34, 39] Mild radiation strictures may be successfully dilated, but more severe strictures may necessitate feeding tube placement or other palliative measures.

Chronic radiation esophagitis occasionally may lead to life-threatening complications because of the development of deep ulcers, esophageal-airway fistulas, or esophageal perforations. However, these unusual complications of radiotherapy almost always occur in an area of esophagus involved by metastatic tumor or lymphadenopathy and rarely in normal irradiated tissue.[39, 44]

Both the acute and the chronic effects of radiation to the esophagus may be potentiated by adriamycin.[40–42] Even at low doses of radiotherapy, the possibility of esophagitis resulting from combined treatment with radiation and adriamycin should be considered when these patients develop dysphagia or other esophageal symptoms.[42] Because recurrent episodes of severe esophagitis may occur after subsequent courses of adriamycin, other chemotherapeutic agents should be substituted for adriamycin to prevent further radiation damage and stricture formation.

Although radiation injury to the esophagus often occurs in patients who are receiving mediastinal irradiation for bronchogenic carcinoma or other malignant tumors involving the mediastinum, patients who undergo radiotherapy for primary esophageal carcinoma rarely seem to develop clinical evidence of esophagitis. Because these patients usually have severe dysphagia before radiotherapy, it has been postulated that the adverse effects of radiation may be masked by the patient's underlying esophageal cancer.[35]

## Radiographic Findings

Most patients who are thought to have acute radiation esophagitis are treated empirically without undergoing

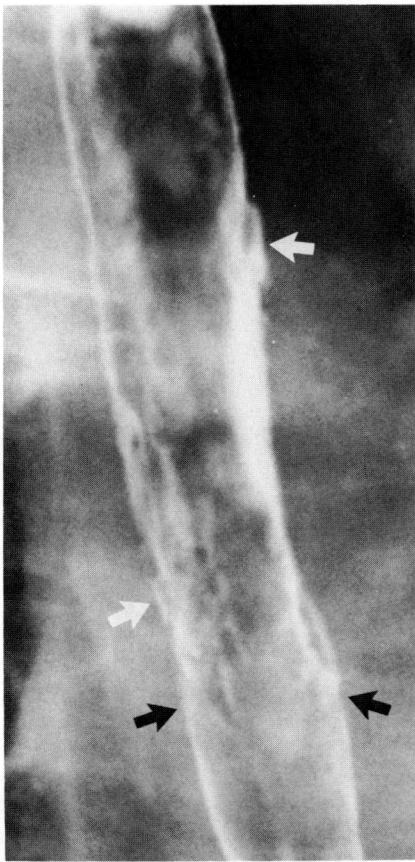

**Figure 26–6. Acute radiation esophagitis.** Multiple superficial ulcers are seen en face and in profile *(white arrows)* in the midesophagus. The area of ulceration has a relatively abrupt inferior demarcation *(black arrows),* which corresponds to the lower border of the radiation portal. This patient had undergone mediastinal irradiation for bronchogenic carcinoma several weeks earlier.

istaltic contractions occurring distal to the point of disruption of the primary wave.[34, 39] Less commonly, the irradiated segment may be totally aperistaltic.[39] Because these findings are nonspecific, documentation of normal motility before treatment may be helpful in implicating radiotherapy as the cause of the motor disorder.

Radiation strictures in the esophagus usually develop 4 to 8 months after completion of radiotherapy.[34, 39] Higher doses of radiation may shorten the interval for developing a stricture but have no effect on its length or caliber. The strictures typically appear as relatively smooth, tapered areas of narrowing in the upper esophagus or midesophagus within a pre-existing radiation portal[34, 39, 44] (Fig. 26–7B). Occasionally, there may be angulation or deformity of the stricture due to adherence of the narrowed segment to adjacent mediastinal structures.[34]

Chronic radiation esophagitis may also be manifested by the development of one or more ulcers, most frequently at the site of extrinsic compression of the esophagus by mediastinal lymphadenopathy or tumor.[39] These late-developing ulcers may be an ominous sign of impending fistula formation. Tracheoesophageal and esophagobronchial fistulas are potentially life-threaten-

radiologic tests to confirm the diagnosis. Nevertheless, double contrast esophagography can demonstrate superficial ulceration of the mucosa within 7 to 10 days of radiotherapy.[38] These superficial ulcers may be recognized as shallow, irregular collections of barium on the esophageal mucosa within a pre-existing radiation portal (Fig. 26–6). In other patients, acute radiation esophagitis may be manifested by a granular appearance of the mucosa with decreased distensibility of the irradiated segment due to punctate ulcers, edema, and spasm (Fig. 26–7A). With more severe disease, the esophagus may have a grossly irregular, serrated contour due to larger areas of ulceration and mucosal sloughing.[35]

After the acute phase of radiation injury, the most frequent finding on barium studies is abnormal esophageal motility.[34, 39] Disordered motility usually develops 4 to 8 weeks after completion of radiotherapy.[39] However, patients receiving combined treatment with radiotherapy and adriamycin may have abnormal motility as early as 1 week after completion of therapy.[39] The etiology is uncertain, but abnormal motility may be related to radiation-induced neuronal damage in Auerbach's plexus.[39] This motor dysfunction is usually characterized by interruption of primary peristalsis at the superior border of the radiation portal, with numerous nonper-

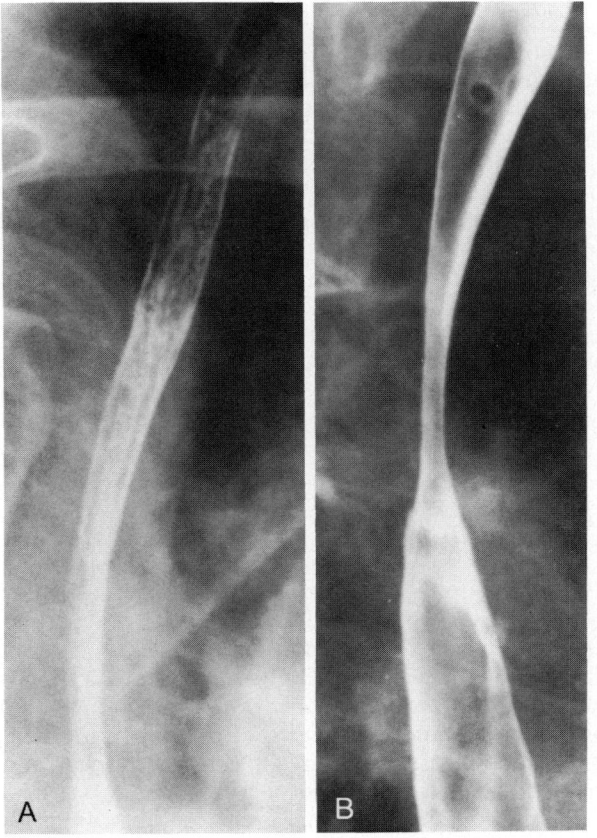

**Figure 26–7. Acute radiation esophagitis with subsequent stricture formation. A.** Mucosal granularity and decreased distensibility of the upper thoracic esophagus are seen. The patient presented with acute odynophagia 3 weeks after undergoing mediastinal irradiation for bronchogenic carcinoma. **B.** Another esophagram 6 months later because of recurrent dysphagia shows a smooth, tapered stricture within the radiation portal.

ing complications of mediastinal irradiation. The fistulas are usually caused by radiation necrosis, with erosion of tumor into the esophagus and adjacent airway.[44] The most frequent site of fistula formation is the left main bronchus, where it crosses the esophagus at the level of the fourth or fifth thoracic vertebra.[39] When an esophageal-airway fistula is suspected, the radiologic examination should be performed with barium sulfate, because water-soluble contrast material may cause severe pulmonary edema if it enters the lungs via a fistula.[45]

## Differential Diagnosis

When acute odynophagia or dysphagia develops several weeks after mediastinal irradiation, the major diagnostic considerations should be acute radiation esophagitis versus opportunistic esophagitis in an immunocompromised patient. If barium studies are performed, *Candida* esophagitis should be suggested by mucosal plaques, whereas herpes esophagitis should be suggested by discrete, superficial ulcers without plaque formation.[30] Radiation esophagitis may also be manifested by ulcers, but the location of the ulcers usually conforms to a known radiation portal with a sharp demarcation at the inferior border of the portal (see Fig. 26–6).

Although a variety of other conditions should be considered in the differential diagnosis for a high or midesophageal stricture, the major diagnostic consideration after mediastinal irradiation for bronchogenic or other intrathoracic neoplasms should be a benign radiation stricture versus esophageal involvement by recurrent mediastinal tumor (see Chapter 29). A concentric area of smooth, tapered narrowing should favor the diagnosis of a radiation stricture, whereas irregular, eccentric narrowing with extrinsic mass effect should suggest malignancy. When the radiographic findings are equivocal, endoscopy or computed tomography may be helpful for differentiating a radiation stricture from recurrent tumor in the mediastinum.

## CAUSTIC ESOPHAGITIS

Caustic esophagitis did not become a serious medical problem in the United States until 1967, when concentrated liquid lye solutions were made commercially available to the American public for use as drain cleaners.[46] Because they could be swallowed rapidly, liquid corrosives exposed all surfaces of the upper gastrointestinal tract to potentially life-threatening caustic injury. Thus, caustic esophagitis became an important clinical entity. Endoscopy has generally been advocated as the best means of assessing the extent and severity of esophageal injury, but radiologic studies may also provide valuable information during both the acute and chronic stages of the disease.

## Pathogenesis

Caustic injury to the esophagus may be caused by ingestion of alkali, acids, ammonium chloride, phenols, silver nitrate, and a variety of other common household products. Children usually ingest these corrosive substances accidentally, whereas adults take them intentionally to commit suicide. In either case, the degree of injury depends on the nature, concentration, and volume of the corrosive agent as well as the duration of tissue contact. In the United States, most patients with caustic esophagitis swallow some form of liquid lye (concentrated sodium hydroxide), which causes severe esophageal injury by liquefaction necrosis.[47, 48] In contrast, ingested acids cause tissue damage by coagulative necrosis, forming a protective eschar that tends to limit further tissue penetration.[47, 48] Because acidic agents may severely damage the stomach without damaging the esophagus, it has been postulated that the squamous epithelium in the esophagus is more resistant to acid than the columnar epithelium in the stomach. However, caustic esophagitis has become a relatively common condition in South America, where household cleaning products containing highly concentrated acids are readily available.[49] Thus, acidic agents may produce severe esophagitis and strictures comparable to those caused by lye.

Caustic esophagitis is characterized pathologically by three phases of injury: an acute necrotic phase, an ulceration-granulation phase, and a final phase of cicatrization and stricture formation.[50, 51] The initial phase of acute cellular necrosis begins immediately after caustic ingestion. This acute phase usually last 1 to 4 days and is accompanied by an intense inflammatory reaction in the surrounding tissues.[50, 51] The ulceration-granulation phase begins 3 to 5 days after caustic ingestion and is characterized by edema, ulceration, and sloughing of necrotic mucosa.[50, 51] During the next 7 to 14 days, subsequent healing leads to the production of granulation tissue in areas of mucosal sloughing. The esophagus is thought to be weakest and therefore most vulnerable to perforation during this period. The final phase of cicatrization begins 3 to 4 weeks after caustic ingestion.[50, 51] Depending on the degree of injury, this cicatrization process may lead to severe stricture formation in the esophagus.

## Clinical Findings

Acute caustic esophagitis may be manifested by the rapid onset of intense odynophagia, chest pain, drooling, vomiting, and/or hematemesis.[47, 48, 50] Severe substernal pain, fever, and shock usually indicate esophageal perforation and mediastinitis.[47, 48] Other complications of perforation include tracheoesophageal and aortoesophageal fistulas, lung abscess, empyema, and pericarditis.[52] Associated gastric injury or perforation may lead to the development of peritonitis.

If patients survive the acute illness, there may be a

latent period of several weeks during which they are no longer symptomatic.[47, 48, 50] Subsequently, however, these individuals often develop severe dysphagia due to progressive cicatrization and stricture formation 1 to 3 months after caustic ingestion.[47, 48]

## Diagnosis and Treatment

When caustic ingestion is suspected, examination of the mouth and oropharynx may reveal obvious tissue injury, with ulceration of the lingual, buccal, or pharyngeal mucosa. However, liquid corrosives may be swallowed rapidly, so caustic esophagitis often occurs without associated pharyngeal injury.[47, 48, 50] Thus, direct visualization of the esophagus is required to confirm the diagnosis of caustic esophagitis. A limited radiographic study may be performed with a water-soluble contrast agent such as diatrizoate meglumine (Gastrografin) to detect an esophageal or gastric perforation or other signs of caustic injury. However, most authors advocate endoscopy within 24 hours of caustic ingestion (assuming that there are no clinical or radiographic signs of perforation) to assess the extent and severity of esophageal injury.[47, 48, 50, 53]

Treatment of caustic esophagitis is generally aimed at preventing stricture formation. Some authors advocate early administration of steroids and antibiotics to inhibit collagen formation and decrease the risk of infection.[54, 55] Others believe that esophageal bougienage should be performed as early as 2 to 3 weeks after caustic ingestion. Despite these measures, between 10 and 40% of patients with caustic esophagitis develop strictures.[48, 56] Some may respond to periodic dilatations, but others require an esophageal bypass operation such as a jejunal or colonic interposition (see Chapter 33). When strictures develop after caustic ingestion, esophagography may be used to determine the site and extent of stricture formation as well as the response to treatment.

Patients with lye strictures are thought to have a significantly increased risk of developing esophageal carcinoma 20 to 40 years after the initial caustic injury.[57, 58] This subject is discussed in detail in Chapter 28.

## Radiographic Findings

Chest and abdominal radiographs should be obtained routinely for patients who have ingested caustic agents. With severe esophageal injury, posteroanterior and lateral films of the chest may demonstrate a dilated, gas-filled esophagus or, if esophageal perforation has occurred, mediastinal widening, pneumomediastinum, and/or pleural effusions.[59, 60] Similarly, abdominal plain films may demonstrate pneumoperitoneum or a localized gas-containing abscess due to gastric perforation.

When esophageal or gastric perforation is suspected in patients who have normal or equivocal plain films, a limited water-soluble contrast study should be performed to document the presence of a leak. Water-soluble contrast agents are used because barium in the mediastinum may cause mediastinal fibrosis and barium in the peritoneal cavity may cause severe peritonitis.[45] If there is no evidence of esophageal or gastric perforation, however, barium should then be given for a more detailed examination.

Acute caustic esophagitis may be manifested on esophagrams by abnormal esophageal motility with poor primary peristalsis, nonperistaltic contractions, diffuse esophageal spasm, or a dilated, atonic esophagus[59–61] (Fig. 26–8). Some authors believe that the latter finding indicates diffuse muscular necrosis and that it is an ominous sign of impending perforation.[59] In other patients, the motor disturbance can mimic achalasia, with markedly elevated lower esophageal sphincter pressures.[62] These various motor abnormalities have been attributed to edema, inflammation, or destruction of ganglion cells in Auerbach's plexus.[61, 62]

Single contrast esophagography has not generally been considered a sensitive technique for detecting morphologic changes of mild or moderate caustic esophagitis. With double contrast technique, however, shallow ulcers may appear as punctate, linear, or serpiginous collections of barium on the mucosa (Fig. 26–9). With more severe caustic injury, the esophagus may be diffusely narrowed and may have a grossly irregular con-

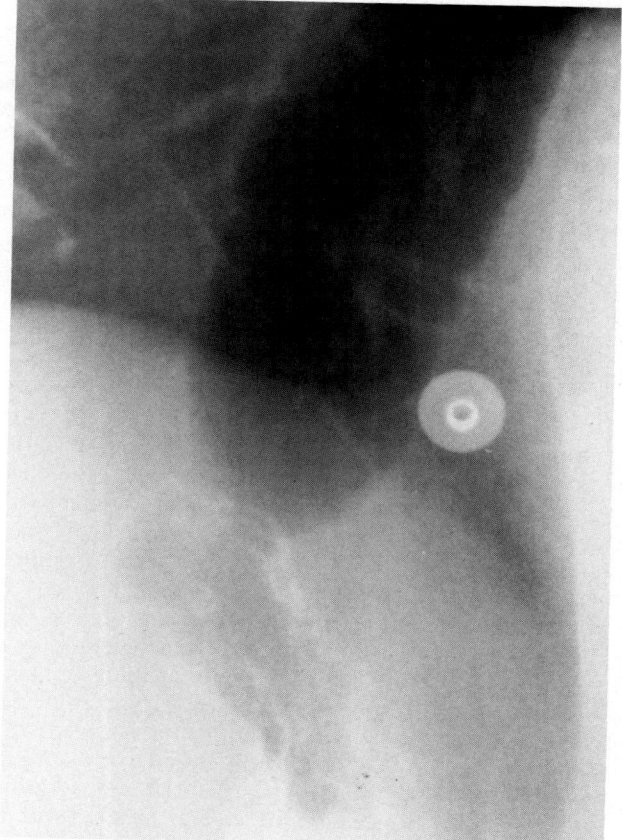

**Figure 26–8. Acute caustic esophagitis with a dilated, atonic esophagus.** There is a dilated, aperistaltic, gas-filled esophagus with a small amount of water-soluble contrast material in the stomach. This finding may indicate a high risk of perforation.

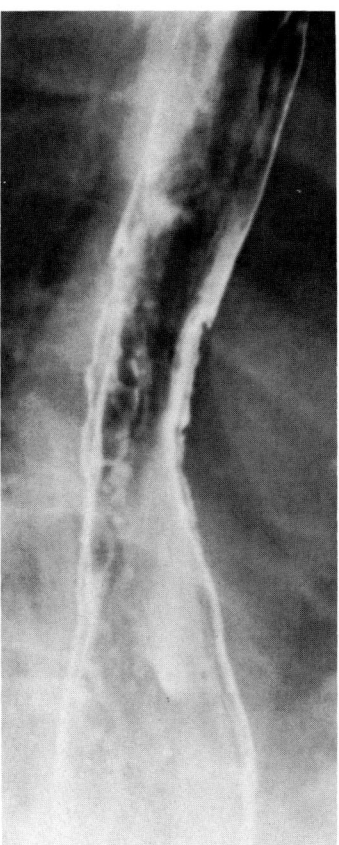

**Figure 26–9. Acute caustic esophagitis.** Multiple shallow, irregular ulcers are seen en face and in profile in the midesophagus. This patient had taken concentrated potassium hydroxide in a suicide attempt.

tour due to marked edema, spasm, and ulceration[49, 59, 60] (Fig. 26–10). Occasionally, contrast material may dissect beneath partially sloughed mucosal fragments, producing a double-barreled appearance, with linear or streaky collections in the esophageal wall.[59] Rarely, these intramural collections may remain visible on delayed radiographs after the lumen has emptied.[59]

Subsequent cicatrization and fibrosis may lead to the development of esophageal strictures 1 to 3 months after the acute injury. In the majority of patients, the strictures appear as relatively long areas of smooth, tapered narrowing in the cervical or upper thoracic esophagus[60, 63] (Fig. 26–11). However, some strictures may have an irregular contour or eccentric areas of sacculation because of asymmetric scarring (see Fig. 26–11). In other patients, one or more focal strictures may be present in random fashion throughout the esophagus because of unpredictable segmental injury that occurs when the caustic agent is ingested.[60] With severe scarring, the entire thoracic esophagus may have a thread-like, or filiform, appearance[60] (Fig. 26–12). This finding should be highly suggestive of a caustic stricture, as other conditions are rarely associated with such diffuse esophageal narrowing.

When the esophagus is examined radiographically after caustic ingestion, the stomach should also be evaluated to determine whether associated gastric injury has occurred. This subject is discussed in detail in Chapter 36.

## Differential Diagnosis

Acute caustic esophagitis may be difficult to differentiate from severe cases of reflux, infectious, drug-induced, or radiation esophagitis. However, reflux esophagitis tends to involve the distal esophagus, drug-induced esophagitis usually involves the midesophagus, and radiation esophagitis occurs within a previously determined radiation portal. In contrast, the site of caustic injury in the esophagus is unpredictable, as these patients may have diffuse or segmental esophagitis involving the cervical or thoracic esophagus. Whatever the radiographic findings, the diagnosis of caustic esophagitis is usually apparent from the clinical history.

The classic finding of a relatively long segment of smooth, tapered narrowing in the cervical or thoracic esophagus should suggest prior caustic ingestion. However, localized caustic strictures in the upper esophagus or midesophagus may be indistinguishable from other causes of high esophageal strictures, including Barrett's esophagus, mediastinal irradiation, oral medications,

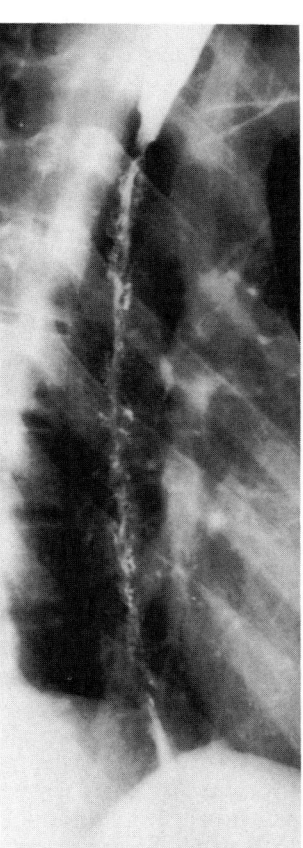

**Figure 26–10. Severe caustic esophagitis.** The thoracic esophagus is diffusely narrowed and has a grossly irregular contour with extensive ulceration due to ingestion of concentrated sodium hydroxide (liquid lye).

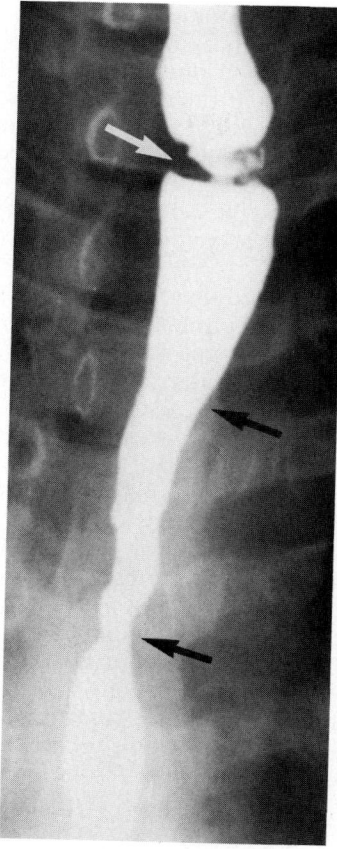

**Figure 26–11. Lye strictures.** There is a long, smooth, tapered stricture *(black arrows)* in the upper thoracic esophagus. A second area of irregular narrowing *(white arrow)* is seen more proximally at the thoracic inlet. The presence of one or more segmental strictures in the cervical or thoracic esophagus is characteristic of caustic injury.

metastatic tumor, or, rarely, dermatologic diseases such as epidermolysis bullosa dystrophica and benign mucous membrane pemphigoid. When a lye stricture has irregular margins or relatively abrupt borders, differentiation from an infiltrating carcinoma may also be difficult. The ability to distinguish benign from malignant lesions is particularly important because of the increased risk of developing esophageal carcinoma in long-standing lye strictures[57, 58] (Fig. 26–13). Thus, endoscopy and biopsy may be required for a definitive diagnosis.

## CROHN'S DISEASE

The esophagus is the rarest site of involvement by Crohn's disease in the gastrointestinal tract. When the esophagus is involved, the patients almost always have associated disease in the small bowel or colon. As a result, esophageal lesions are usually found after a clinical diagnosis of granulomatous ileocolitis has been established. Occasionally, however, the onset of esophageal Crohn's disease coincides with the onset of disease in the small bowel or colon, so that these patients do not necessarily have known Crohn's disease when they

seek medical attention. Rarely, isolated esophageal Crohn's disease may occur before the development of disease more distally in the bowel.[64]

A definitive diagnosis of esophageal Crohn's disease requires histologic confirmation. However, endoscopic biopsies often fail to reveal granulomas because of the superficial nature of the biopsies and the patchy distribution of the disease.[65] Thus, the absence of definitive histologic findings should not preclude a diagnosis of Crohn's disease if the clinical and radiographic findings suggest this condition.

## Clinical Findings

Most patients with esophageal Crohn's disease have advanced Crohn's disease in the lower gastrointestinal tract, so the clinical presentation is dominated by ileocolitis. Nevertheless, esophageal involvement may cause dysphagia or, less commonly, odynophagia, chest pain, or upper gastrointestinal bleeding.[66, 67] Because esophageal Crohn's disease is rarely an isolated finding, the diagnosis should be considered only in patients with known Crohn's disease elsewhere in the gastrointestinal

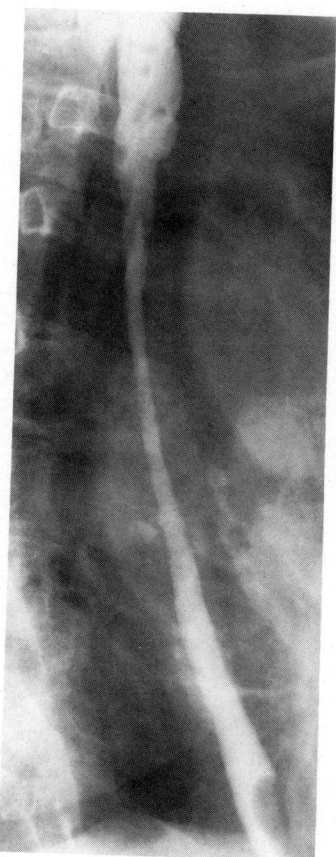

**Figure 26–12. Advanced lye stricture.** There is diffuse narrowing of the thoracic esophagus due to widespread fibrosis and scarring. This appearance should suggest caustic injury, as other conditions are rarely associated with such severe esophageal narrowing.

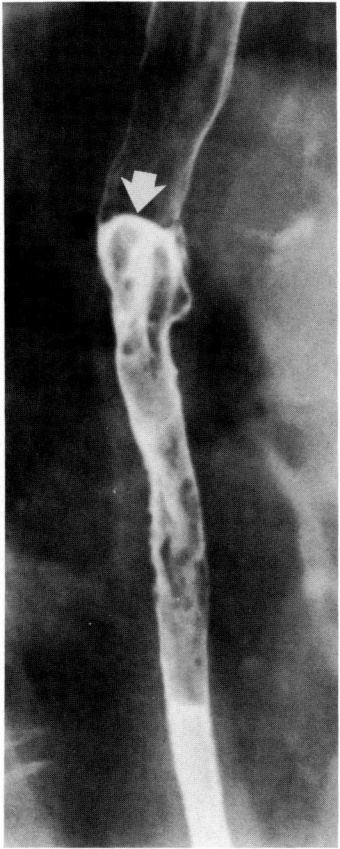

**Figure 26–13. Esophageal carcinoma arising in a lye stricture.**
There is a long stricture in the thoracic esophagus due to caustic
ingestion many years earlier. Note the irregular appearance and
abrupt proximal border *(arrow)* of the narrowed segment due to a
superimposed carcinoma.

tract who develop dysphagia or other esophageal symptoms. When esophageal disease is present, the clinical
course may parallel that of the patient's ileal or colonic
disease, with remission of both upper and lower gastrointestinal symptoms after medical treatment or ileo-
colectomy.[66]

## Radiographic Findings

Although Crohn's disease affects primarily the small
bowel and colon, esophageal involvement has been
recognized with increased frequency on double contrast
esophagography. The major advantage of double contrast technique is its ability to detect aphthous ulcers,
the earliest morphologic lesions of Crohn's disease.[68]
These aphthous ulcers are seen on double contrast
esophagrams in about 3% of patients with granulomatous ileocolitis.[67] As in the small bowel or colon,
aphthous ulcers may occur as isolated lesions in the
esophagus, or they may be associated with other, more
advanced changes of Crohn's disease. The aphthous
ulcers appear radiographically as punctate, slit-like, or

ring-like collections of barium surrounded by radiolucent halos of edematous mucosa[67, 69, 70] (Fig. 26–14).
They are usually few in number (two to five) and are
sporadically distributed throughout the esophagus with
long intervening segments of normal mucosa[70] (see Fig.
26–14A). As a result, these lesions may be quite subtle
and are recognized only with optimal double contrast
technique. Occasionally, however, numerous aphthous
ulcers may be present in the esophagus (see Fig. 26–
14B).

With more advanced disease, the size and number of
ulcers may increase, producing a localized or diffuse
esophagitis. The esophagus may also be involved by one
or more areas of deep ulceration.[71] Severe esophagitis
may also be manifested by thickened folds, pseudomembranes, and, rarely, a diffuse cobblestone appearance.[66, 71] Other patients may develop transverse or
longitudinal intramural tracks similar to those found in
the colon with granulomatous colitis[66, 71] (Fig. 26–15).
In advanced cases, esophageal perforation may lead to
esophagobronchial, esophagomediastinal, or esophagogastric fistulas.[66, 71]

Progressive scarring may eventually lead to the development of strictures, most commonly in the distal
third of the esophagus[64, 66, 72] (Fig. 26–16). The strictures
are almost always more than 1 cm in length and may
involve a considerable segment of the esophagus.
Rarely, advanced esophageal Crohn's disease may be
manifested by filiform polyposis of the esophagus, analogous to filiform polyposis of the colon in granulomatous
colitis.[73]

## Differential Diagnosis

Aphthous ulcers in the esophagus may be indistinguishable from discrete, superficial ulcers associated
with reflux, herpes, or drug-induced esophagitis. However, reflux esophagitis involves predominantly the distal
esophagus and usually occurs in patients who have a
history of reflux symptoms. Although herpetic ulcers in
the esophagus may closely resemble the aphthous ulcers
of Crohn's disease, a clinical history of odynophagia in
an immunocompromised patient should suggest the correct diagnosis.[30] Drug-induced esophagitis may also be
manifested by shallow ulcers, but they tend to be clustered in the region of the aortic arch or left main
bronchus, and there is usually a recent history of ingesting oral medications such as doxycycline or tetracycline.[26–28] Thus, the clinical history and presentation are
extremely helpful for differentiating these conditions.

More advanced esophageal Crohn's disease may be
indistinguishable from other types of severe esophagitis.
When intramural tracks or fistulas are present, the
differential diagnosis includes radiation, trauma, malignancy, and tuberculosis.[74, 75] Because esophageal Crohn's
disease is much less common than other types of esophagitis, this diagnosis should be considered only in patients who have clinical or radiographic findings of
Crohn's disease elsewhere in the gastrointestinal tract.

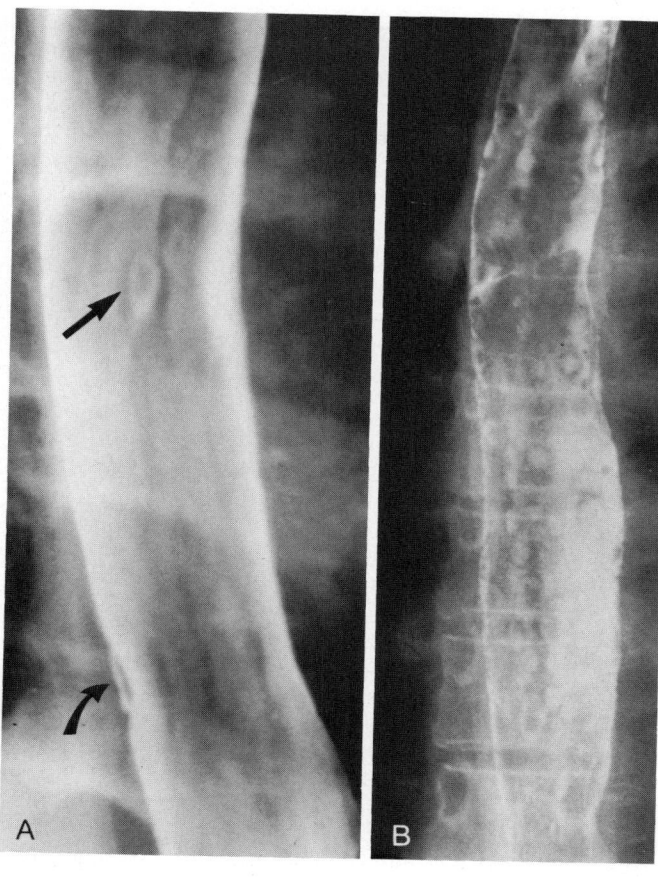

**Figure 26–14. Esophageal Crohn's disease with aphthous ulcers. A.** Discrete, widely separated aphthous ulcers are seen en face *(straight arrow)* and in profile *(curved arrow)* due to early esophageal involvement by Crohn's disease. (From V Gohel, BW Long, G Richter, Aphthous ulcers in the esophagus with Crohn colitis, AJR, 137, 4, 872–873, 1981, © by American Roentgen Ray Society.) **B.** This patient has more advanced Crohn's disease with multiple large aphthous ulcers in the mid- and distal esophagus. The ulcers are surrounded by radiolucent mounds of edema. (Courtesy of Peter J. Feczko, M.D., Royal Oak, MI.)

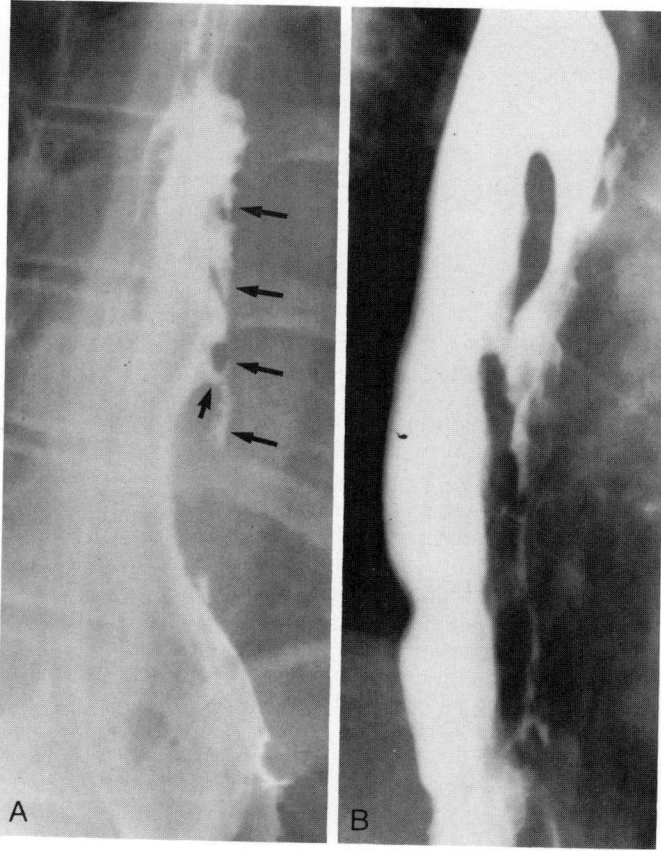

**Figure 26–15. Esophageal Crohn's disease with intramural tracks. A.** Longitudinal *(long arrows)* and transverse *(short arrow)* tracks are seen in the distal third of the esophagus due to transmural involvement by Crohn's disease. (Courtesy of Peter J. Feczko, M.D., Royal Oak, MI.) **B.** This patient has a "double-barreled" esophagus with a long intramural track due to advanced esophageal Crohn's disease. (Courtesy of Francis J. Scholz, M.D., Burlington, MA.)

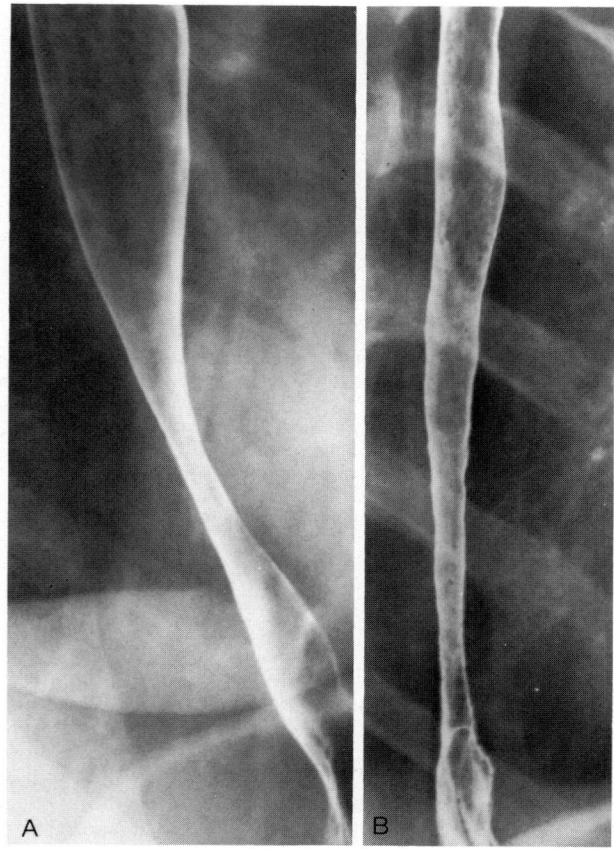

**Figure 26–16. Esophageal Crohn's disease with strictures.** Both patients (**A** and **B**) have long strictures in the distal esophagus due to severe scarring from Crohn's disease. (**B** reprinted from, by permission of the publisher, Tishler JMA, Hellman CA: Crohn's disease of the esophagus. Can Assoc Radiol J 35:28–30, 1984.)

# EPIDERMOLYSIS BULLOSA DYSTROPHICA

Epidermolysis bullosa is a rare hereditary skin disease in which minimal trauma causes separation of the epidermis and dermis with subsequent bullous formation. Two forms of the disease, epidermolysis bullosa simplex and epidermolysis bullosa dystrophica, have been described. In epidermolysis bullosa simplex, the bullae heal without scarring, and the disease usually subsides at puberty.[76] However, epidermolysis bullosa dystrophica is a mutilating, potentially lethal condition manifested by progressive scarring and deformity throughout the body.[76] Epidermolysis bullosa dystrophica may be transmitted by autosomal dominant and autosomal recessive forms of inheritance. The autosomal dominant form involves only the skin, whereas the autosomal recessive form also involves mucous membranes in other squamous epithelium–lined organs such as the oropharynx, esophagus, and anus.[76, 77]

## Pathogenesis

In patients with epidermolysis bullosa dystrophica, solid food in the esophagus repeatedly traumatizes an already fragile mucosa, causing extensive bulla formation.[76, 78] Some bullae rupture and heal without permanent sequelae, but others heal with severe scarring and stricture formation. Because these strictures further impede the passage of swallowed food, esophageal involvement may lead to a self-perpetuating cycle of blistering, scarring, and stenosis.[78]

## Clinical Findings

Skin involvement by epidermolysis bullosa dystrophica may be recognized at or shortly after birth. Other findings include flexion contractures of the hands and feet, webbed digits (syndactyly), dystrophic or absent nails, microstomia, retarded epiphyseal development, and overconstriction of the shafts of long bones.[79] These deformities can be disabling or even fatal.

Although the esophagus is usually affected during the first decade of life, clinical signs of esophageal involvement may not be seen until puberty.[80] Affected individuals may present with intermittent dysphagia or odynophagia due to recurrent bulla formation and healing.[77, 80, 81] Subsequently, they may develop severe dysphagia due to irreversible scarring and stricture formation.[78, 80, 81] Esophageal involvement should therefore be suspected in any patient with epidermolysis bullosa dystrophica who develops dysphagia or other esophageal symptoms. Occasionally, however, the skin disease may be less severe and may actually improve during early adulthood, so the diagnosis of epidermolysis bullosa is not necessarily known to the referring physician.

Endoscopy should be avoided in patients with known or suspected epidermolysis bullosa dystrophica involving the esophagus because of the risk of further traumatizing an already fragile mucosa and causing bleeding, perforation, or further scarring and stenosis. Once strictures have developed, however, balloon dilatation or bougienage of the esophagus may be required to alleviate symptoms.[76, 77, 79, 80] Occasionally, a major operation such as a colonic interposition may be performed as a last resort for patients with intractable strictures.[81]

## Radiographic Findings

Because of the risk of endoscopy, barium studies should be performed when esophageal involvement by epidermolysis bullosa dystrophica is suspected on clinical grounds. Early disease is manifested radiographically by abnormal motility, spasm, edema, bullae, or ulcers.[76, 80] Discrete bullae may be recognized as small, nodular filling defects in the esophagus, and extensive bulla formation may produce a diffusely serrated or spiculated esophageal contour.[80] Because of the reversible nature of the disease, these lesions may completely regress on follow-up examinations.

More advanced esophageal disease is characterized by scarring and stricture formation. These strictures tend to be located in the upper thoracic esophagus, possibly because of esophageal compression by the aortic arch, which exacerbates the traumatic effect of swallowed

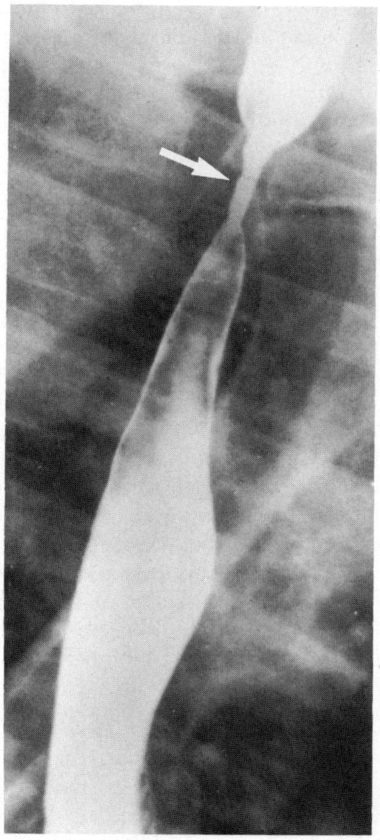

**Figure 26–17. Epidermolysis bullosa dystrophica with a high esophageal stricture *(arrow)*.** (From JM Tishler, SY Han, CA Hellman, Esophageal involvement in epidermolysis bullosa dystrophica, AJR, 141, 6, 1283–1286, 1983, © by American Roentgen Ray Society.)

food at this level.[76] The strictures usually appear as concentric areas of segmental narrowing, ranging from 2 to 6 cm in length[78, 80, 82] (Fig. 26–17). As a result, they may be indistinguishable from other, more common causes of high esophageal strictures, such as Barrett's esophagus, mediastinal irradiation, and caustic ingestion. Other patients with this condition may develop esophageal webs, most frequently in the cervical esophagus near the level of the cricopharyngeus.[80, 82] Esophageal involvement by epidermolysis bullosa dystrophica should be suspected when high esophageal strictures or webs are seen radiographically in children or young adults who have other clinical signs of this disease.

## PEMPHIGOID

Pemphigoid is a dermatologic disease characterized by chronic, recurrent bullous eruptions of the skin and mucous membranes. Two forms of pemphigoid, benign mucous membrane pemphigoid and bullous pemphigoid, have been described. However, benign mucous membrane pemphigoid is much more likely to involve mucous membranes, so esophageal abnormalities are primarily encountered in this form of the disease.

## Clinical Findings

Benign mucous membrane pemphigoid usually occurs in middle-aged patients and is twice as common in women.[83] About 75% of patients have involvement of the oral mucosa and conjunctiva, 50% have skin involvement, and 5 to 10% have esophageal involvement.[83–85] The most severe complications of this disease occur in the eye, where conjunctival scarring causes corneal destruction and blindness in 25% of patients.[84] Thus, despite its name, benign mucous membrane pemphigoid should not be considered a benign condition.

Esophageal involvement may be manifested by dysphagia resulting from edema, spasm, ulceration, or strictures.[83, 85] Severe esophageal involvement may occasionally result in massive sloughing of mucosa, with subsequent expulsion of a hollow membranous cast from the patient's mouth.[86] When these patients initially develop dysphagia, systemic administration of steroids may prevent further progression of esophageal disease and stricture formation. Once strictures have developed, however, one or more esophageal dilatation procedures may be required to alleviate symptoms.[87]

## Radiographic Findings

Although discrete bullae are rarely observed radiographically, barium studies may reveal edema, spasm, or superficial ulceration in the early stages of esophageal involvement by benign mucous membrane pemphigoid[83] (Fig. 26–18). Subsequent scarring may be manifested by the development of webs or strictures.[83, 85, 88] The webs usually appear as thin, shelf-like defects protruding a variable distance into the lumen of the cervical or upper thoracic esophagus. They cannot be distinguished from idiopathic webs or those associated with other diseases such as Plummer-Vinson syndrome and epidermolysis bullosa dystrophica. In other patients, scarring may produce one or more segmental strictures in the cervical or upper thoracic esophagus[83, 85, 88] (Fig. 26–19). The strictures may be of variable length and are difficult to distinguish from other, more common causes of high esophageal strictures, such as Barrett's esophagus, mediastinal irradiation, and caustic ingestion. However, the correct diagnosis may be suggested in patients who have a history of bullous eruptions on the skin.

## NASOGASTRIC INTUBATION ESOPHAGITIS

Nasogastric intubation has been recognized as an unusual cause of esophagitis and stricture formation.[89–91] Most patients develop strictures only after repeated or prolonged nasogastric intubation, but others with this complication have nasogastric tubes in place less than 48 hours.[89] The strictures may progress rapidly after removal of the tube, causing severe dysphagia. When all causes of esophageal strictures are considered, nasogastric intubation is probably second only to caustic

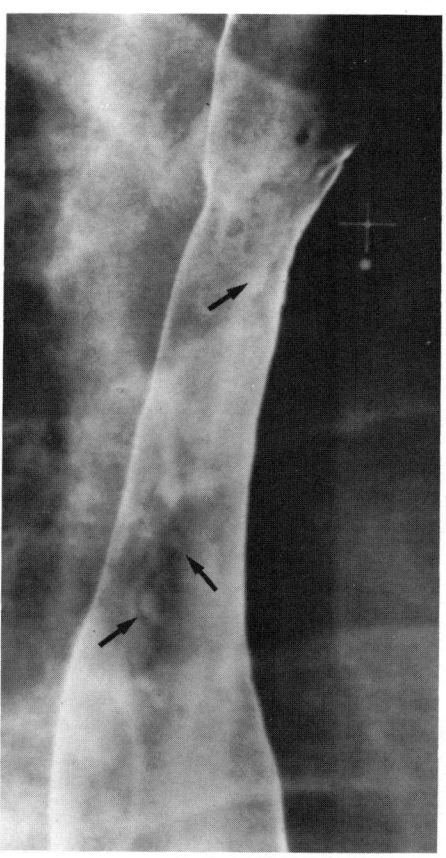

**Figure 26–18. Benign mucous membrane pemphigoid with superficial ulceration.** There are multiple shallow ulcers *(arrows)* in the midesophagus with decreased distensibility of this region. (Courtesy of Stephen E. Rubesin, M.D., Philadelphia, PA.)

ingestion in terms of the length and severity of stricture formation.

## Pathogenesis

The pathogenesis of esophageal injury is uncertain. Most patients who develop strictures have been intubated for a period of 3 to 15 days.[91] Some investigators believe that uncontrolled gastroesophageal reflux around the lower end of the nasogastric tube causes severe esophagitis and strictures, whereas others have found that the tube occludes the lower esophageal sphincter, preventing clearance of refluxed peptic acid from the esophagus when reflux has occurred.[89, 92] It has also been postulated that the trauma of intubation or the irritant effect of the tube itself may cause a direct contact type of esophagitis.[90, 93]

## Clinical Findings

Most patients with esophageal injury develop symptoms several weeks to months after removal of the tube.[90, 91] These patients may initially present with heartburn, substernal chest pain, or odynophagia due to esophagitis. Subsequently, they often develop severe dysphagia as a result of rapid stricture formation.[91] Despite the length and severity of the strictures, adequate relief from dysphagia may be obtained by periodic mechanical dilatations.

## Radiographic Findings

Nasogastric intubation esophagitis may be manifested by a long segment of extensive ulceration in the mid- and distal esophagus[93] (Fig. 26–20). Occasionally, large, flat ulcers in the distal esophagus are associated with a considerable mass effect due to an adjacent mound of edema, mimicking the appearance of an ulcerated esophageal carcinoma (Fig. 26–21). Subsequent stricture formation may be detected radiographically 1 to 4 months after removal of the tube.[89–91] Initially, the strictures may appear as smooth, tapered areas of concentric narrowing in the distal esophagus that are indistinguishable from ordinary peptic strictures.[89] However, they tend to progress rapidly, increasing in length and severity within a relatively short period (Fig. 26–22). Some strictures may have a corrugated appearance due to areas of sacculation within the narrowed segment. Because of the extent and severity of stricture formation,

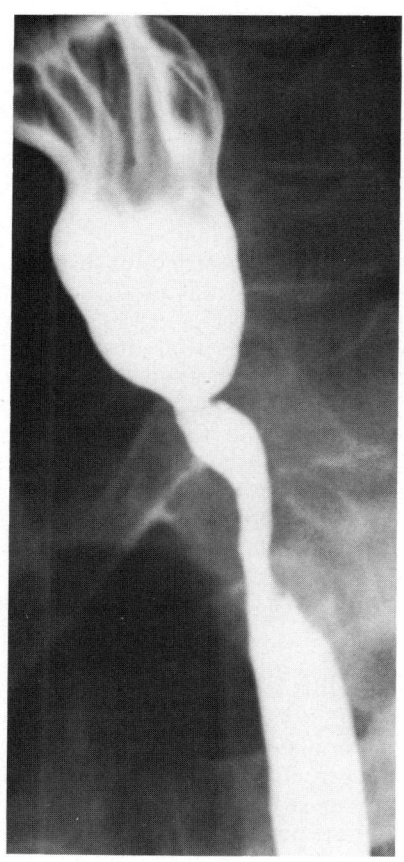

**Figure 26–19. Benign mucous membrane pemphigoid with a high esophageal stricture.** A long, asymmetric stricture is seen in the cervical and upper thoracic esophagus. (Courtesy of John A. Bonavita, M.D., Philadelphia, PA.)

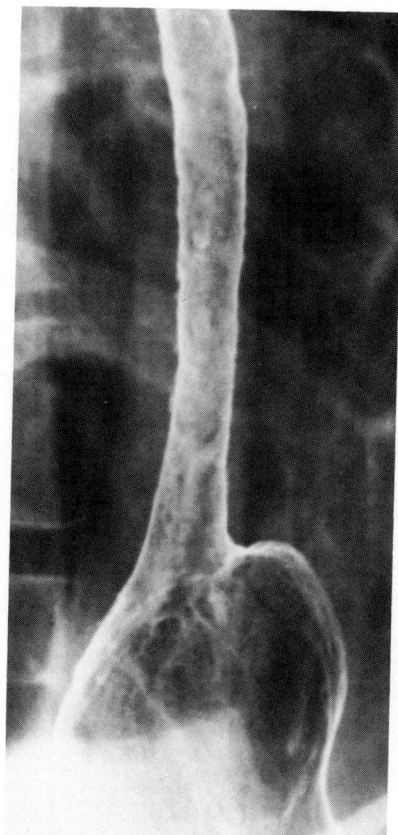

**Figure 26–20. Severe esophagitis caused by nasogastric intubation.** There are multiple areas of superficial ulceration and associated narrowing of the distal esophagus due to marked spasm and edema. A large hiatal hernia is also present.

these patients may be suspected of ingesting caustic agents. However, the presence of an unusually long or rapidly progressive stricture in the distal esophagus should suggest the possibility of prior nasogastric intubation.

## ALKALINE REFLUX ESOPHAGITIS

Alkaline reflux esophagitis is an unusual condition caused by reflux of bile and pancreatic secretions into the esophagus after total or, less commonly, partial gastrectomy.[94, 95] However, the development of esophagitis in these patients depends on the type of surgical reconstruction that is employed. Alkaline reflux esophagitis is a relatively common complication of total gastrectomy and simple loop esophagojejunostomy but rarely occurs after a Roux-en-Y esophagojejunostomy.[96–99] Thus, most surgeons now perform a Roux-en-Y reconstruction, placing the jejunojejunal anastomosis 40 cm or more distal to the esophagojejunal anastomosis to prevent reflux of bile and pancreatic secretions into the esophagus. Nevertheless, alkaline reflux esophagitis has occasionally been documented in these patients, so a Roux-en-Y reconstruction decreases the risk of esoph-

agitis or strictures but does not completely eliminate these complications.[100, 101] Some investigators have found that alkaline reflux esophagitis also predisposes to the development of Barrett's esophagus,[102, 103] but the significance of this observation is doubtful because of the limited life expectancy of most patients who undergo esophagojejunostomy.

## Clinical Findings

Alkaline reflux esophagitis may initially be manifested by retrosternal burning, chest pain, and regurgitation of bile.[96, 97] These patients may then develop rapidly progressive dysphagia within several months after surgery due to stricture formation.[96] In most cases, relief from dysphagia is obtained by mechanical dilatation of the stricture.

## Radiographic Findings

Alkaline reflux esophagitis is characterized by mucosal nodularity, thickened folds, and ulceration of the distal third or half of the esophagus above the esophagojejunal

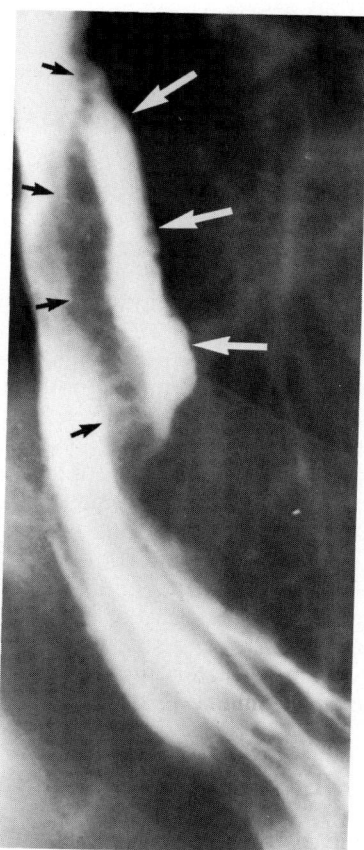

**Figure 26–21. Giant esophageal ulcer caused by nasogastric intubation.** There is a large, flat ulcer *(white arrows)* in the distal esophagus; an associated area of mass effect *(black arrows)* is due to an adjacent mound of edema. This appearance could be mistaken for that of an ulcerated esophageal carcinoma.

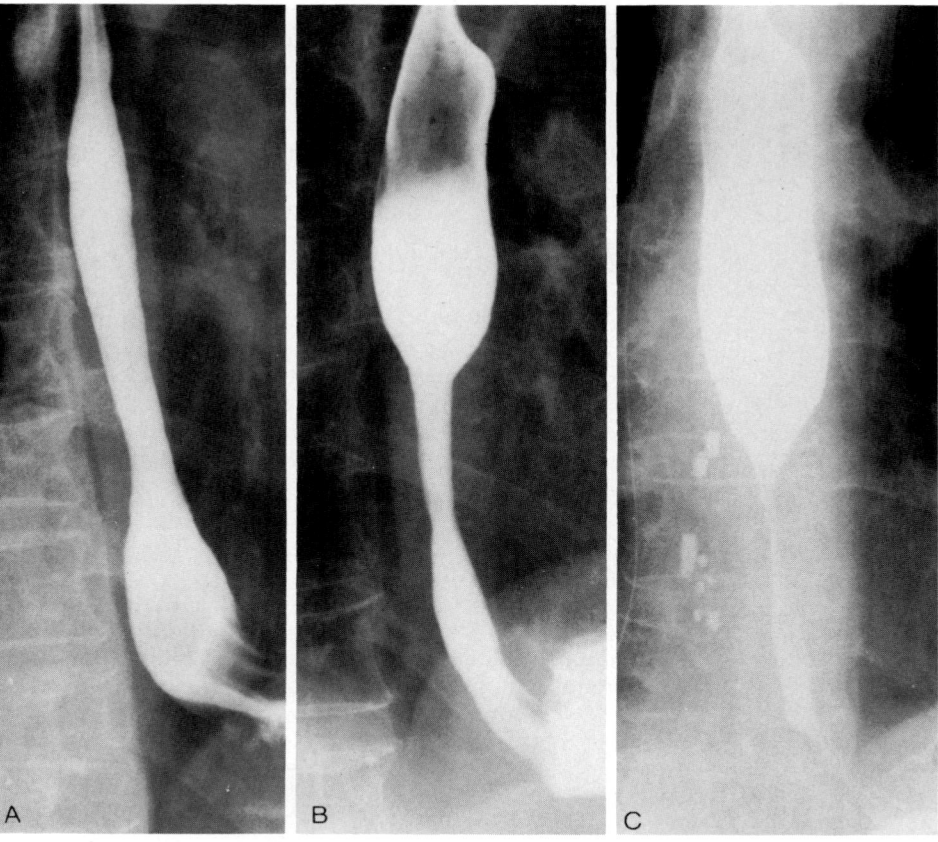

**Figure 26–22. Rapidly progressive stricture caused by nasogastric intubation. A.** The initial esophagram shows moderately decreased distensibility of the distal esophagus shortly after removal of a nasogastric tube. **B.** A second esophagram 3 weeks later shows rapid stricture formation with marked narrowing of the distal esophagus. **C.** A third esophagram 6 weeks later shows further progression of the stricture. There is now evidence of esophageal obstruction. (**A, B,** and **C** courtesy of Vijay Gohel, M.D., Philadelphia, PA.)

anastomosis[101] (Fig. 26–23). Subsequent stricture formation may be detected radiographically as early as 1 to 3 months after surgery.[96, 101] The strictures usually appear as smooth, tapered areas of narrowing in the distal esophagus, often extending a considerable distance above the esophagojejunal anastomosis.[96, 101] These strictures must be differentiated from benign anastomotic strictures or recurrent tumor involving the distal esophagus. However, anastomotic strictures usually appear as focal areas of symmetric narrowing at the esophagojejunal anastomosis, whereas recurrent tumor is manifested by more irregular esophageal narrowing, often associated with eccentric areas of mass effect.[101] Alkaline reflux strictures also tend to progress rapidly, increasing in length and severity within several months.[101] However, most patients are intubated at the time of surgery, and nasogastric intubation may also lead to rapidly progressive stricture formation. Thus, alkaline reflux and previous intubation may both contribute to the development of strictures in these patients.

## EOSINOPHILIC ESOPHAGITIS

Eosinophilic gastroenteritis is an uncommon condition characterized by eosinophilic infiltration of the stomach and small bowel. Almost all patients have a peripheral eosinophilia, ranging from 10 to 80%.[104] About half of the patients have a history of allergic diseases.[105] The

stomach and the small bowel are the major sites of involvement, but occasional cases of eosinophilic esophagitis have been described.[106–108] Eosinophilic esophagitis tends to involve the muscular layers of the esophageal wall, occasionally producing strictures in the upper thoracic esophagus.[107, 108] It has been postulated that a local allergic response may be triggered by a transient delay in the passage of food due to esophageal compression by the aortic arch.[107, 108] As with gastric or small bowel disease, eosinophilic esophagitis is almost always associated with a peripheral eosinophilia.

## Clinical Findings

Eosinophilic esophagitis may be manifested by intermittent or gradually worsening dysphagia, with a sensation of food sticking behind the upper sternum due to localized esophageal narrowing at this level.[107, 108] Occasionally, these patients may have acute episodes of dysphagia precipitated by specific food allergens.[108] When eosinophilic esophagitis is suspected, the diagnosis may be confirmed on endoscopic biopsy specimens by the presence of a dense, eosinophilic infiltrate in the esophageal wall.[107, 108] Treatment with steroids often produces a dramatic clinical response, but significant strictures may require mechanical dilatation for relief of symptoms.[107, 108]

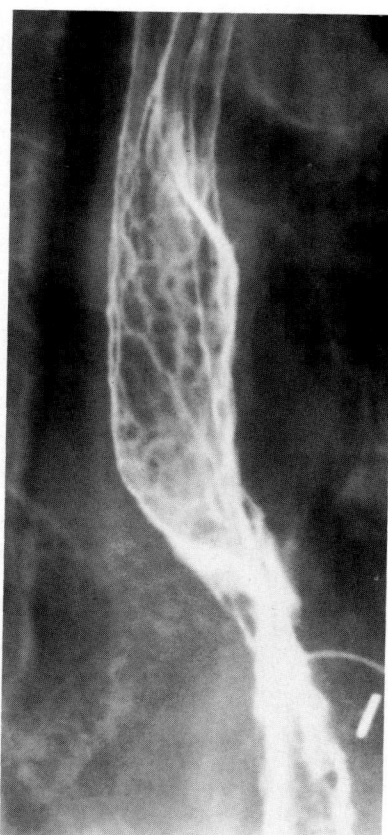

**Figure 26–23. Alkaline reflux esophagitis.** This patient had undergone a total gastrectomy and esophagojejunostomy. A nodular mucosa is seen in the distal esophagus above the anastomosis.

## Radiographic Findings

Eosinophilic esophagitis may be manifested by the development of one or more segmental strictures in the upper thoracic esophagus near the level of the aortic arch[107, 108] (Fig. 26–24A). Nodularity or ulceration may be found within the narrowed segment because of associated mucosal disease. However, these strictures cannot be differentiated from other, more common causes of high esophageal strictures, such as Barrett's esophagus, mediastinal irradiation, caustic ingestion, and metastatic tumor. Other patients may have abnormal motility, with an increased frequency of nonperistaltic contractions or even an achalasia-like syndrome.[106, 109] Rarely, small, sessile eosinophilic polyps may be found in the esophagus, analogous to those found in the stomach or duodenum[107, 108] (Fig. 26–24B).

Because of its rarity, eosinophilic esophagitis should be considered only in patients who have a known history of allergic diseases or a peripheral eosinophilia. When eosinophilic esophagitis is suspected radiographically, upper gastrointestinal and small bowel follow-through examinations should be performed to determine whether the stomach and small bowel are involved by this disease.

# ACUTE ALCOHOL-INDUCED ESOPHAGITIS

Alcohol abusers occasionally may develop an acute, transient esophagitis after an alcoholic binge.[110] The etiology is uncertain, but heavy alcohol consumption appears to have an effect on esophageal peristalsis and lower esophageal sphincter function. Several studies have shown that oral or intravenous ethanol in healthy volunteers produces a reversible esophageal motor disturbance with impaired primary peristalsis and decreased lower esophageal sphincter pressures.[111, 112] As a result, acute alcohol intoxication may cause increased gastroesophageal reflux with impaired clearance of refluxed peptic acid from the esophagus when reflux has occurred. Thus, alcohol-induced esophagitis may represent an acute, self-limited form of reflux esophagitis.

## Clinical Findings

Acute alcohol-induced esophagitis may be associated with abrupt onset of odynophagia, dysphagia, or hematemesis immediately after an alcoholic binge.[110]

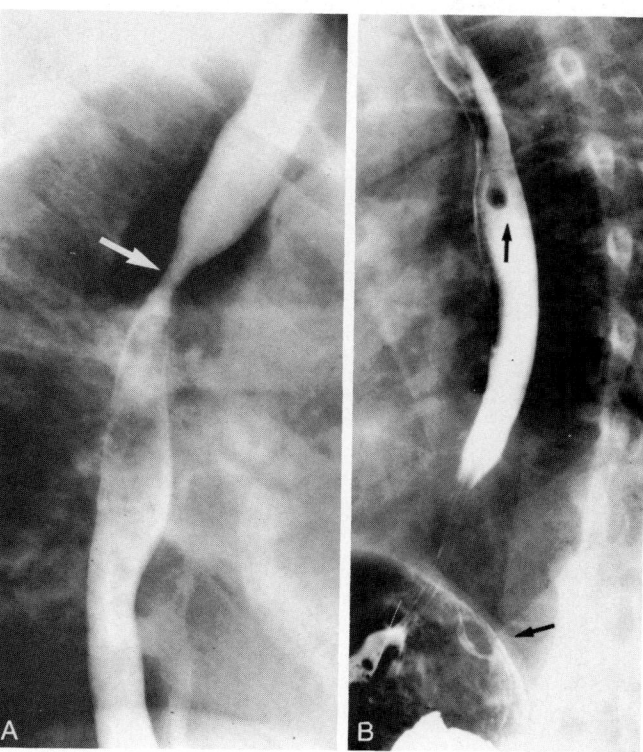

**Figure 26–24. Eosinophilic esophagitis. A.** There is a smooth, tapered stricture *(arrow)* in the midesophagus. Biopsies revealed localized eosinophilic infiltration of the esophageal wall. **B.** This patient has small, sessile polyps in the midesophagus *(upper arrow)* and gastric fundus *(lower arrow)*. These proved to be eosinophilic polyps. (**A** and **B** from Feczko PJ, Halpert RD, Zonca M: Radiographic abnormalities in eosinophilic esophagitis. Gastrointest Radiol 10:321–324, 1985.)

Marked clinical improvement occurs within 1 to 2 weeks after withdrawal of alcohol.[110] Although other conditions may have a similar presentation, the temporal relationship between an alcoholic binge and the development of esophagitis should suggest the correct diagnosis.

## Radiographic Findings

Acute alcohol-induced esophagitis is manifested radiographically by multiple areas of superficial ulceration in the distal third of the esophagus[110] (Fig. 26–25). Reflux esophagitis may produce identical radiographic findings. Nevertheless, the correct diagnosis may be suggested by the patient's recent drinking history.

## CHRONIC GRAFT-VERSUS-HOST DISEASE

Transplantation of bone marrow from matched sibling donors has become an accepted treatment for patients

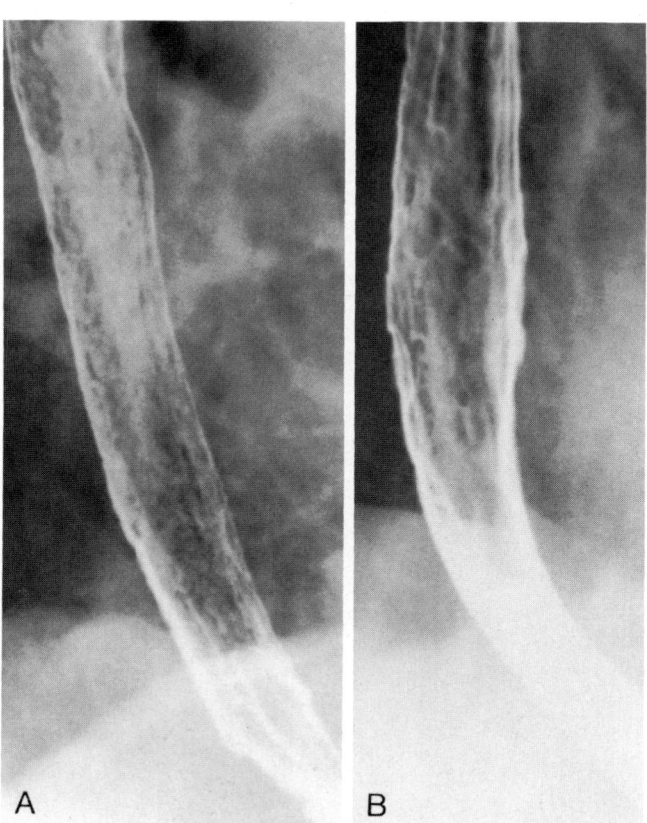

**Figure 26–25. Acute alcohol-induced esophagitis.** In both patients (**A** and **B**), multiple small, superficial ulcers are present in the mid- and distal esophagus. Reflux esophagitis could produce identical findings, but esophageal symptoms were precipitated by a recent alcoholic binge in both cases. (**A** and **B** reprinted from, by permission of the publisher, O'Riordan D, Levine MS, Laufer I: Acute alcoholic esophagitis. Can Assoc Radiol J 37:54–55, 1986.)

with aplastic anemia, acute leukemia, and other hematologic malignancies. Depending on the underlying disease, these patients have 5-year survival rates of 60 to 80% after marrow transplantation.[113] However, 30% of long-term survivors develop chronic graft-versus-host disease within 3 to 12 months after undergoing this procedure.[114] The disease is an immunologic disorder in which immunocompetent donor lymphocytes react against antigenic differences in host tissues, causing severe tissue damage. The most frequently involved target organs are the skin and liver, but the eyes, mucous membranes, and gastrointestinal tract may also be affected.[113–115]

Esophageal involvement occurs in about 15% of patients with chronic graft-versus-host disease.[116] The immunologic process causes desquamation and sloughing of esophageal mucosa. Subsequent scarring may lead to the development of webs or strictures.[116, 117] The pathologic findings appear to be similar to those of epidermolysis bullosa dystrophica, benign mucous membrane pemphigoid, and other diseases associated with severe scarring and stricture formation in the esophagus.

## Clinical Findings

Symptoms of esophageal involvement by chronic graft-versus-host disease include dysphagia, odynophagia, substernal chest pain, and weight loss.[114, 116] Esophageal symptoms usually develop 3 to 12 months after marrow transplantation.[116] Opportunistic esophagitis may produce similar findings in this clinical setting.[118] However, esophageal symptoms that occur within 1 to 8 weeks after transplantation are more likely to be caused by opportunistic infection, whereas symptoms that occur months to years after successful transplantation are more likely to be caused by chronic graft-versus-host disease.[116]

## Radiographic Findings

In early esophageal involvement by chronic graft-versus-host disease, the esophagus may have an irregular, serrated contour due to mucosal desquamation and sloughing.[116] With the development of scarring, barium studies may also demonstrate webs or strictures in the esophagus. Webs are usually found in the cervical esophagus near the level of the cricopharyngeus[116] (Fig. 26–26A). These lesions cannot be differentiated from idiopathic webs or those associated with other conditions such as epidermolysis bullosa dystrophica and benign mucous membrane pemphigoid. Other patients may develop ring-like or smoothly tapered strictures in the upper, middle, or, less commonly, distal esophagus[114, 116] (Fig. 26–26B). Although chronic graft-versus-host disease is a rare cause of esophageal webs and strictures, the correct diagnosis may be suggested in patients who are known to have undergone previous marrow transplantation.

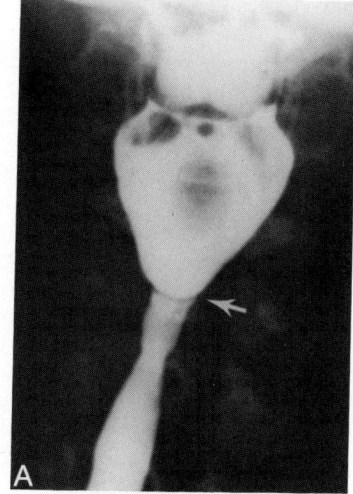

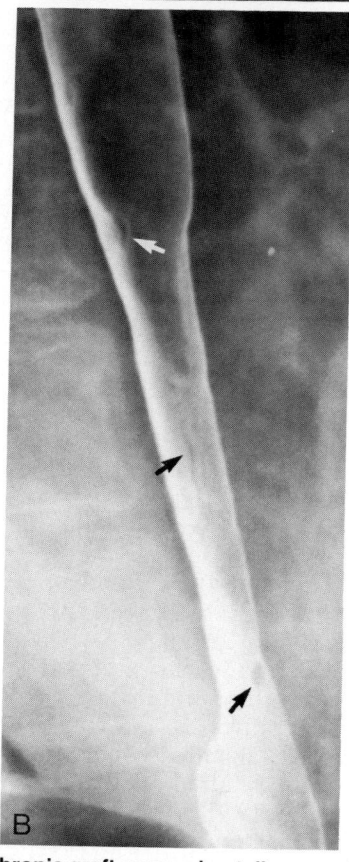

**Figure 26–26. Chronic graft-versus-host disease with esophageal involvement. A.** A web is seen en face *(arrow)* in the cervical esophagus. (From GB McDonald, KM Sullivan, TF Plumley, Radiographic features of esophageal involvement in chronic graft-vs.-host disease, AJR, 142, 3, 501–506, 1984, © by American Roentgen Ray Society.) **B.** A long, tapered stricture is present in the distal esophagus in another patient. Nodular and linear filling defects *(arrows)* are seen within the narrowed segment due to mucosal desquamation and sloughing. (Courtesy of Seth N. Glick, M.D., Philadelphia, PA.)

## BEHÇET'S DISEASE

Behçet's disease was first described by Behçet in 1937 as the clinical triad of oral and genital ulceration and ocular inflammation. However, it is now recognized as a multisystem disorder, also characterized by skin lesions, arthritis, colitis, thrombophlebitis, and, rarely, encephalitis.[119] In the gastrointestinal tract, Behçet's disease usually involves the colon and produces a localized or diffuse form of colitis in about 20% of patients.[119] However, esophageal involvement has occasionally been reported.[120–122] Affected individuals may present with odynophagia or upper gastrointestinal bleeding.[120, 121] Double contrast esophagography may reveal discrete, superficial ulcers in the mid- or distal esophagus (Fig. 26–27). Rarely, a single giant ulcer may be observed.[122] Because Behçet's disease is often treated with steroids or other immunosuppressive agents, herpes esophagitis should be suspected as a more likely cause of discrete esophageal ulcers in these patients. Endoscopic brushings, biopsies, and cultures are therefore required to differentiate this condition from viral esophagitis.

## ESOPHAGEAL INTRAMURAL PSEUDODIVERTICULOSIS

When esophageal intramural pseudodiverticulosis was first described in 1960, it was thought that mucosal herniation through defects in the esophageal wall produced true intramural diverticula, analogous to Rokitan-

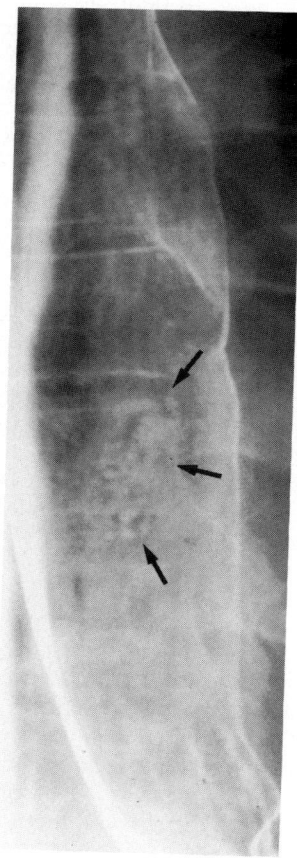

**Figure 26–27. Behçet's disease with superficial ulceration.** A cluster of tiny ulcers *(arrows)* is present in the midesophagus. Herpes esophagitis and drug-induced esophagitis are much more common causes of discrete ulcers in the midesophagus.

sky-Aschoff sinuses in the gallbladder.[123] Since that time, however, the pathologic basis for these structures has been well elucidated. Although esophageal intramural pseudodiverticulosis is a relatively uncommon condition, it has received considerable attention in the radiologic literature because of its often spectacular appearance on barium studies.

## Pathogenesis

The esophagus normally contains about 200 deep mucous glands that occur in longitudinal rows parallel to the long axis of the esophagus.[124] Within each gland, several short ducts converge to form a single main excretory duct that extends 2 to 5 mm through the esophageal wall, producing a small opening on the mucosa.[125] Pathologic studies have shown that esophageal intramural pseudodiverticula represent dilated excretory ducts of these deep mucous glands.[126-128]

Although the anatomic basis of these structures has been well delineated, the explanation for this ductal dilatation is unclear. One infectious organism, *Candida albicans,* has been cultured from the esophagus in 34 to 48% of patients.[124, 129, 130] As a result, it has been postulated that *Candida* esophagitis predisposes to the development of esophageal intramural pseudodiverticulosis.[131] However, most investigators believe that the fungal organisms are probably secondary esophageal invaders and are not important etiologic factors in the development of this condition.[127, 132-134]

Others have postulated that ductal dilatation results from plugging and obstruction of the ducts by thick, viscous mucus, inflammatory material, and desquamated epithelium.[125-127] Alternatively, the ducts may be extrinsically compressed by periductal inflammation and fibrosis due to chronic esophagitis.[128-130] In various series, 80 to 90% of patients with pseudodiverticulosis have had endoscopic or histologic evidence of inflammatory disease in the esophagus.[124, 130] In one study, the majority of patients with this condition had associated scarring or strictures in the distal esophagus due to reflux esophagitis.[135] Thus, esophageal intramural pseudodiverticulosis is probably a sequela of chronic esophagitis, particularly reflux esophagitis, but it is unclear why so few patients with esophagitis develop this condition.

About 90% of patients with esophageal intramural pseudodiverticulosis have associated strictures.[124, 129, 130] It has therefore been suggested that increased intraluminal pressure or stasis above the stricture may also cause ductal dilatation.[125] However, this theory is weakened by the observation that the pseudodiverticula are often found below the level of the stricture.[124, 136] Conversely, stricture formation could be caused by the development of microabscesses in the ducts, resulting in perforation, peridiverticulitis, and scarring.[134, 137] This hypothesis would explain why there often is no other apparent etiology for the development of high esophageal strictures in these patients.

## Clinical Findings

Esophageal intramural pseudodiverticulosis usually occurs in the elderly and is slightly more common in men.[124, 129, 130] About 20% of patients are diabetics, and 15% are alcoholics.[129, 130] Most patients present with intermittent or slowly progressive dysphagia due to the high prevalence of associated strictures.[124, 126, 129, 130, 133, 134] Treatment is usually directed toward the underlying stricture because the pseudodiverticula themselves rarely cause problems. Mechanical dilatation of strictures produces a dramatic clinical response in almost all patients.[134, 137] The intramural pseudodiverticula may persist or disappear after treatment, but the fate of these strictures has no relationship to the clinical course of the patient.

## Radiographic Findings

Esophageal intramural pseudodiverticulosis is diagnosed in fewer than 1% of all patients who undergo radiologic examinations of the esophagus.[135] Failure to visualize the pseudodiverticula may result from ductal obstruction by inflammatory material or debris that prevents barium from entering the ducts. Nevertheless, esophagography is more sensitive than endoscopy for detecting these lesions because the orifices of the dilated excretory ducts are extremely difficult to visualize at endoscopy.[129]

Esophageal intramural pseudodiverticulosis is classically manifested by innumerable, tiny (1 to 4 mm), flask-shaped outpouchings in longitudinal rows parallel to the long axis of the esophagus[124, 126, 129, 130, 132, 137] (Fig. 26–28). These barium-filled outpouchings tend to be oriented perpendicular to the esophagus or in a slightly oblique and caudad direction, with their tips aimed toward the stomach.[124] Because the necks of the pseudodiverticula are 1 mm or less in diameter, incomplete filling may erroneously suggest lack of communication with the esophageal lumen.[138] Occasionally, bridging may occur between adjacent pseudodiverticula, which produces discrete intramural tracks[129, 130, 132, 138] (Fig. 26–29). Rarely, pseudodiverticulosis may be associated with large, irregular extraluminal collections of barium due to massive ductal dilatation or sealed-off perforation of the ducts (Fig. 26–30). Because ductal perforation may lead to the development of a periesophageal inflammatory mass or abscess, this complication has been described as esophageal intramural pseudodiverticulitis.[139]

About half the reported patients with esophageal intramural pseudodiverticulosis have diffuse disease, and half have segmental disease.[124, 129, 130] Furthermore, 90% of patients have associated strictures, most frequently in the upper third of the esophagus[124, 129, 130] (see Fig. 26–28). In such cases, the pseudodiverticula often extend above and below the level of the stricture.[129] In contrast, one study found that the majority of patients had isolated involvement of the distal esophagus, with

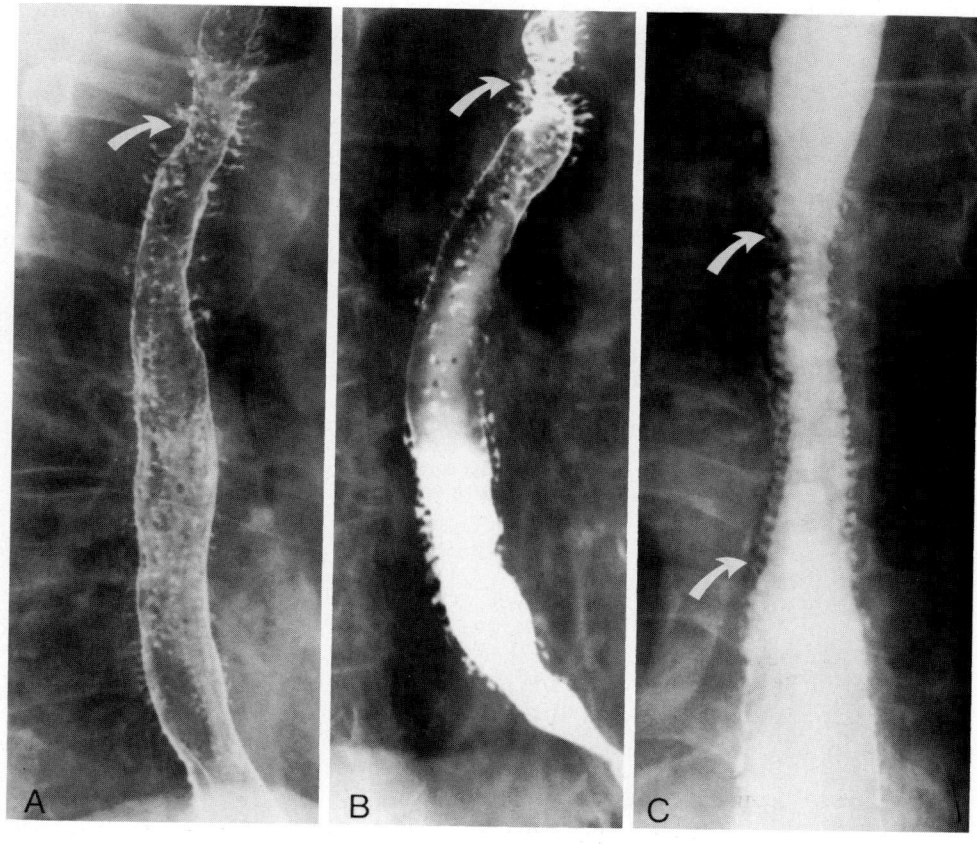

**Figure 26–28. Esophageal intramural pseudodiverticulosis associated with high strictures.** In all three patients **(A to C),** the pseudodiverticula appear as characteristic outpouchings in longitudinal rows parallel to the long axis of the esophagus. In all cases, associated strictures of varying length *(arrows)* are seen in the upper thoracic esophagus. The cause of the strictures was unknown. (**A** courtesy of Michael Davis, M.D., Albuquerque, NM. **C** from MS Levine, DN Moolten, H Herlinger, et al, Esophageal intramural pseudodiverticulosis: a reevaluation, AJR, 147, 6, 1165–1170, 1986, © by American Roentgen Ray Society.)

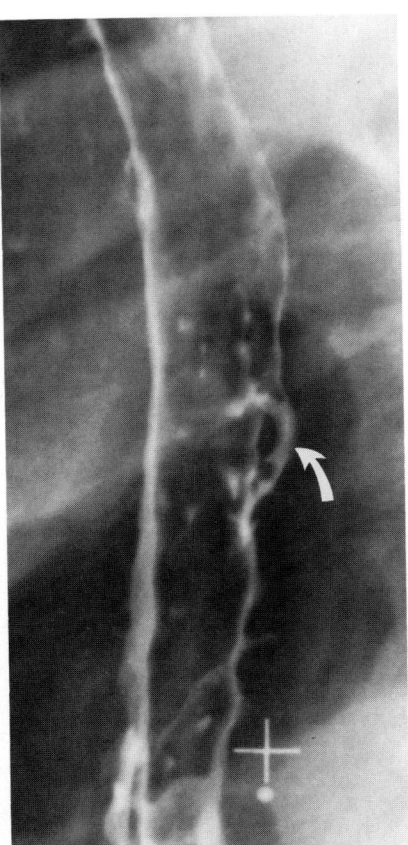

**Figure 26–29. Esophageal intramural pseudodiverticulosis with an intramural track.** This track *(arrow)* is caused by bridging of adjacent pseudodiverticula. Other pseudodiverticula seen en face could be mistaken for shallow ulcers. (Courtesy of Stephen E. Rubesin, M.D., Philadelphia, PA.)

a focal cluster of pseudodiverticula in the region of a peptic stricture.[135] The explanation for this discrepancy is unclear. However, most reports on the subject are anecdotal, and it seems likely that the more spectacular cases have been reported rather than the more subtle ones with fewer pseudodiverticula. In any case, it should be recognized that esophageal intramural pseudodiverticulosis often occurs as a localized phenomenon in the distal esophagus associated with scarring from reflux esophagitis (Fig. 26–31).

Although this condition is usually associated with chronic esophagitis or strictures, it may occasionally be observed in patients who have an otherwise normal-appearing esophagus[135] (Fig. 26–32). Rarely, pseudodiverticula may also be found in patients with infiltrating esophageal carcinomas.[135] Such cases could conceivably result from malignant degeneration of a previously benign stricture. Whatever the explanation, strictures associated with pseudodiverticulosis are not always benign, so cases should be evaluated individually for radiologic signs of malignancy.

Esophageal intramural pseudodiverticulosis may occasionally be recognized on computed tomography by marked thickening of the esophageal wall, diffuse irreg-

ularity of the lumen, and intramural gas collections corresponding to the pseudodiverticula.[140] When this condition is suspected on the basis of computed tomography, an esophagram should be obtained for a definitive diagnosis. Rarely, perforation of a pseudodiverticulum may result in peridiverticulitis and abscess formation, manifested on computed tomography by a periesophageal soft tissue mass with or without associated collections of gas.[139]

## Differential Diagnosis

The radiographic findings of esophageal intramural pseudodiverticulosis are virtually pathognomonic of this condition. Although pseudodiverticula may occasionally be confused with true diverticula, the latter structures are considerably larger and less numerous and should not pose a significant diagnostic dilemma. When viewed en face, intramural pseudodiverticula are sometimes mistaken for multiple discrete ulcers associated with various types of esophagitis. When viewed in profile, however, intramural pseudodiverticula have a typical flask-shaped configuration and often seem to be floating outside the esophageal wall without any apparent com-

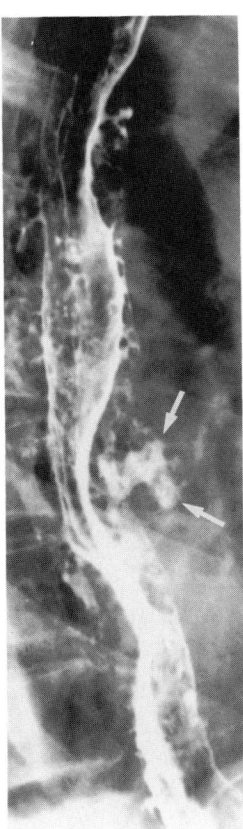

**Figure 26–30. Esophageal intramural pseudodiverticulosis with associated perforation.** There is a large, irregular, extraluminal barium collection *(arrows)*, presumably caused by a sealed-off perforation of a dilated duct. (Courtesy of Peter J. Feczko, M.D., Royal Oak, MI.)

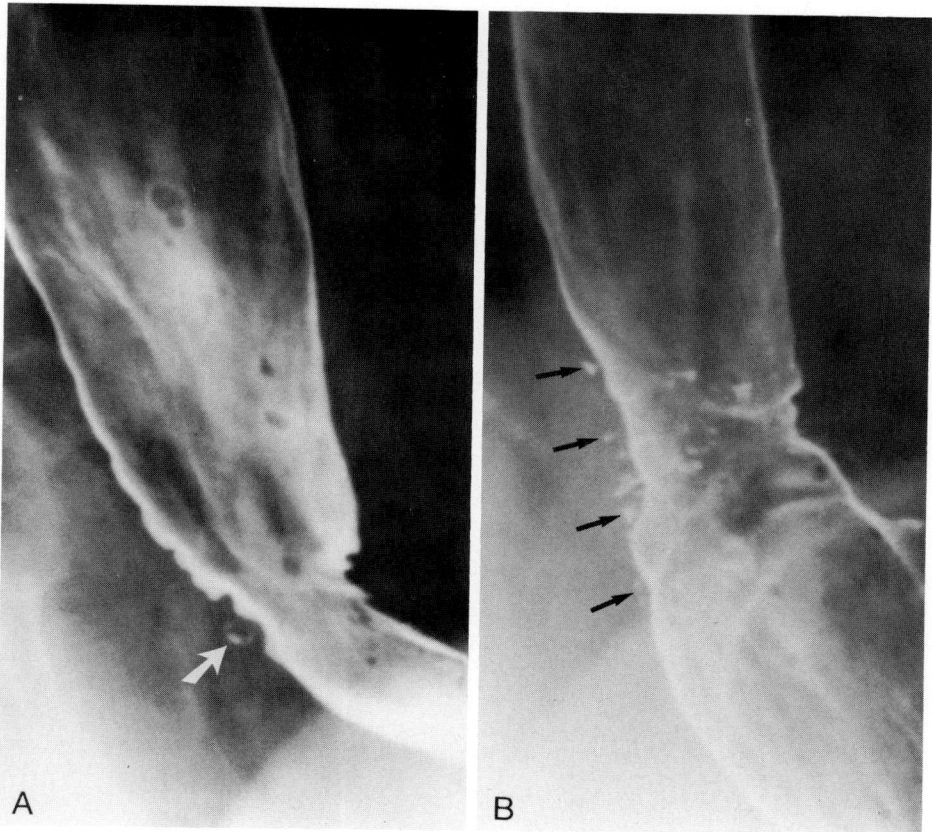

**Figure 26–31. Esophageal intramural pseudodiverticulosis with associated peptic strictures.** In both patients (**A** and **B**), the pseudodiverticula seen in profile *(arrows)* do not appear to communicate with the esophageal lumen. This is a characteristic feature that helps differentiate these structures from ulcers. (**A** from MS Levine, DN Moolten, H Herlinger, et al, Esophageal intramural diverticulosis: a reevaluation, AJR, 147, 6, 1165–1170, 1986, © by American Roentgen Ray Society.)

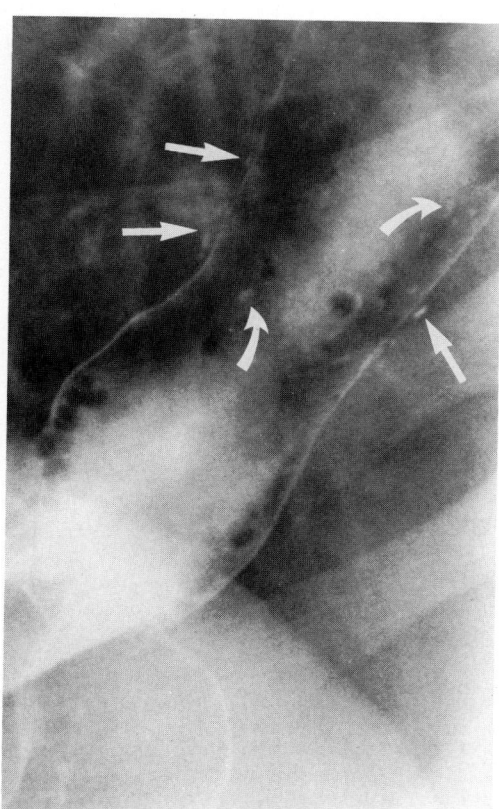

**Figure 26–32. Esophageal intramural pseudodiverticulosis in an otherwise normal-appearing esophagus.** The pseudodiverticula are visualized en face *(curved arrows)* and in profile *(straight arrows)* in this patient.

munication with the lumen, whereas true ulcers almost always communicate directly with the lumen. The characteristic tangenital appearance of the pseudodiverticula should therefore differentiate these structures from actual areas of ulceration.

## Acknowledgment

Figures 26–1, 26–2, 26–4C, 26–6, 26–9 to 26–12, 26–16A, 26–20, 26–21, 26–23, 26–27, 26–28B, and 26–32 are reproduced from Levine MS: Radiology of the Esophagus. Philadelphia: WB Saunders, 1989.

# References

 1. Pemberton J: Oesophageal obstruction and ulceration caused by oral potassium therapy. Br Heart J 32:267–268, 1970.
 2. Kikendall JW, Friedman AC, Oyewole MA, et al: Pill-induced esophageal injury: case reports and review of the medical literature. Dig Dis Sci 28:174–182, 1983.
 3. Fisher RS, Malmud LS, Applegate G, et al: Effect of bolus composition on esophageal transit: concise communication. J Nucl Med 23:878–882, 1982.
 4. Evans KT, Roberts GM: Where do all the tablets go? Lancet 2:1237–1239, 1976.
 5. Schneyer LH, Pigman W, Hanahan L, et al: Rate of flow of human parotid, sublingual and submaxillary secretions during sleep. J Dent Res 35:109–114, 1956.
 6. Dent J, Dodds WJ, Friedman RH, et al: Mechanisms of gastroesophageal reflux in recumbent asymptomatic human subjects. J Clin Invest 65:256–267, 1980.
 7. Whitney B, Croxon R: Dysphagia caused by cardiac enlargement. Clin Radiol 23:147–152, 1972.
 8. Mason SJ, O'Meara TF: Drug-induced esophagitis. J Clin Gastroenterol 3:115–120, 1981.
 9. Walta DC, Giddens JD, Johnson LF, et al: Localized proximal esophagitis secondary to ascorbic acid ingestion and esophageal motor disorder. Gastroenterology 70:766–769, 1976.
10. Bokey L, Hugh TB: Oesophageal ulceration associated with doxycycline therapy. Med J Aust 1:236–237, 1975.
11. Crowson TD, Head LH, Ferrante WA: Esophageal ulcers associated with tetracycline therapy. JAMA 235:2747–2748, 1976.
12. Rosenthal T, Adar R, Militianu J, et al: Esophageal ulceration and oral potassium chloride ingestion. Chest 65:463–465, 1974.
13. Lubbe WF, Cadogan ES, Kannemeyer AHR: Oesophageal ulceration due to slow-release potassium in the presence of left atrial enlargement. N Z Med J 90:377–379, 1979.
14. Peters JL: Benign oesophageal stricture following oral potassium chloride therapy. Br J Surg 63:698–699, 1976.
15. Teplick JG, Teplick SK, Ominsky SH, et al: Esophagitis caused by oral medication. Radiology 134:23–25, 1980.
16. Coates AG, Nostrand TT, Wilson JAP, et al: Esophagitis caused by nonsteroidal antiinflammatory medication. South Med J 79:1094–1097, 1986.
17. Levine MS, Rothstein RD, Laufer I: Giant esophageal ulcer due to Clinoril. AJR 156:955–956, 1991.
18. Kavin H: Oesophageal ulceration due to emepronium bromide. Lancet 1:424–425, 1977.
19. Abbarah TR, Fredell JE, Ellenz GB: Ulceration by oral ferrous sulfate. JAMA 236:2320, 1976.
20. Stiris MG, Oyen D: Oesophagitis caused by oral ingestion of Aptin (alprenolol chloride) durettes. Eur J Radiol 2:38–40, 1982.
21. Enzenauer RW, Bass JW, McDonnell JT: Esophageal ulceration associated with oral theophylline. N Engl J Med 310:261, 1984.
22. Israel RH, Wood J: Esophagitis related to cromolyn. JAMA 242:2758–2759, 1979.
23. Rabinowitz JG, Tchang S: Esophageal stricture following ingestion of Clinitest tablets. AJR 86:579–581, 1961.
24. Sutton DR, Gosnold JK: Oesophageal ulceration due to clindamycin. Br Med J 1:1598, 1977.
25. Bonavina L, DeMeester TR, McChesney L, et al: Drug-induced esophageal strictures. Ann Surg 206:173–183, 1987.
26. Creteur V, Laufer I, Kressel HY, et al: Drug-induced esophagitis detected by double contrast radiography. Radiology 147:365–368, 1983.
27. Agha FP, Wilson JAP, Nostrand TT: Medication-induced esophagitis. Gastrointest Radiol 11:7–11, 1986.
28. Bova JG, Dutton NE, Goldstein HM, et al: Medication-induced esophagitis: diagnosis by double-contrast esophagography. AJR 148:731–732, 1987.
29. Ravich WJ, Kashima H, Donner MW: Drug-induced esophagitis simulating esophageal carcinoma. Dysphagia 1:13–18, 1986.
30. Levine MS, Laufer I, Kressel HY, et al: Herpes esophagitis. AJR 136:863–866, 1981.
31. Shortsleeve MJ, Levine MS: Herpes esophagitis in otherwise healthy patients: clinical and radiographic findings. Radiology 182:859–861, 1992.
32. Kressel HY, Glick SN, Laufer I, et al: Radiologic features of esophagitis. Gastrointest Radiol 6:103–108, 1981.
33. Levine MS, Loercher G, Katzka DA, et al: Giant, human immunodeficiency virus-related ulcers in the esophagus. Radiology 180:323–326, 1991.
34. Goldstein HM, Rogers LF, Fletcher GH, et al: Radiological manifestations of radiation-induced injury to the normal upper gastrointestinal tract. Radiology 117:135–140, 1975.
35. Seaman WB, Ackerman LV: The effect of radiation on the esophagus: a clinical and histological study of the effects produced by the betatron. Radiology 68:534–540, 1957.
36. Jennings FL, Arden A: Acute radiation effects in the esophagus. Arch Pathol 69:407–412, 1960.
37. Phillips TL, Ross G: Time-dose relationships in the mouse esophagus. Radiology 113:435–440, 1974.
38. Northway MG, Libshitz HI, West JJ, et al: The opossum as an animal model for studying radiation esophagitis. Radiology 131:731–735, 1979.
39. Lepke RA, Libshitz HI: Radiation-induced injury of the esophagus. Radiology 148:375–378, 1983.
40. Greco FA, Brereton HD, Kent H, et al: Adriamycin and enhanced radiation reaction in normal esophagus and skin. Ann Intern Med 85:294–298, 1976.
41. McCormick B, Hopfan S, Wittes R: Esophageal complications in the treatment of oat cell carcinoma with combined irradiation and chemotherapy. Radiology 123:185–187, 1977.
42. Boal DKB, Newburger PE, Teele RL: Esophagitis induced by combined radiation and adriamycin. AJR 132:567–570, 1979.
43. Roswit B: Complications of radiation therapy: the alimentary tract. Semin Roentgenol 9:51–63, 1974.
44. Rubin P: The radiographic expression of radiotherapeutic injury: an overview. Semin Roentgenol 9:5–13, 1974.
45. Dodds WJ, Stewart ET, Vlymen WJ: Appropriate contrast media for evaluation of esophageal disruption. Radiology 144:439–441, 1982.
46. Leape LL, Ashcraft KW, Scarpelli DG, et al: Hazard to health: liquid lye. N Engl J Med 284:587–591, 1971.
47. Kirsh MM, Ritter F: Caustic ingestion and subsequent damage to the oropharyngeal and digestive passages. Ann Thorac Surg 21:74–82, 1976.
48. Goldman LP, Weigert JM: Corrosive substance ingestion: a review. Am J Gastroenterol 79:85–90, 1984.
49. Muhletaler CA, Gerlock AJ, de Soto L, et al: Acid corrosive esophagitis: radiographic findings. AJR 134:1137–1140, 1980.
50. Citron BP, Pincus IJ, Geokas MC, et al: Chemical trauma of the esophagus and stomach. Surg Clin North Am 48:1303–1311, 1968.
51. Dafoe CS, Ross CA: Acute corrosive oesophagitis. Thorax 24:291–294, 1969.
52. McCabe RE Jr, Scott JR, Knox WG: Fistulization between esophagus, aorta, and trachea as a complication of acute corrosive esophagitis: report of a case. Am Surg 35:450–454, 1969.
53. Holinger PH: Management of esophageal lesions caused by chemical burns. Ann Otol Rhinol Laryngol 77:819–829, 1968.
54. Webb WR, Koutras P, Ecker RR: An evaluation of steroids and antibiotics in caustic burns of the esophagus. Ann Thorac Surg 9:95–102, 1970.
55. Cardona JC, Daly JF: Current management of corrosive esophagitis: an evaluation of results in 239 cases. Ann Otol 80:521–527, 1971.

56. Neimark S, Rogers AI: Chemical injury of the esophagus. *In* Berk JA (ed): Bockus Gastroenterology (4th ed). Philadelphia: WB Saunders, 1985, pp 769–776.

57. Appelqvist P, Salmo M: Lye corrosion carcinoma of the esophagus: a review of 63 cases. Cancer 45:2655–2685, 1980.

58. Hopkins RA, Postlethwait RW: Caustic burns and carcinoma of the esophagus. Ann Surg 194:146–148, 1981.

59. Martel W: Radiologic features of esophagogastritis secondary to extremely caustic agents. Radiology 103:31–36, 1972.

60. Franken EA: Caustic damage of the gastrointestinal tract: roentgen features. AJR 118:77–85, 1973.

61. Guelrud M, Arocha M: Motor function abnormalities in acute caustic esophagitis. J Clin Gastroenterol 2:247–250, 1980.

62. Moody FG, Garrett JM: Esophageal achalasia following lye ingestion. Ann Surg 170:775–784, 1969.

63. Kinnman JEG, Lee BC, Lee CW, et al: Management of severe lye corrosions of the oesophagus. J Laryngol Otol 83:899–910, 1969.

64. LiVolsi VA, Jaretzki A: Granulomatous esophagitis: a case of Crohn's disease limited to the esophagus. Gastroenterology 64:313–319, 1973.

65. Danzi JT, Farmer RG, Sullivan BH, et al: Endoscopic features of gastroduodenal Crohn's disease. Gastroenterology 70:9–13, 1976.

66. Ghahremani GG, Gore RM, Breuer RI, et al: Esophageal manifestations of Crohn's disease. Gastrointest Radiol 7:199–203, 1982.

67. Tishler JMA, Helman CA: Crohn's disease of the esophagus. J Can Assoc Radiol 35:28–30, 1984.

68. Morson BC: The early histological lesion of Crohn's disease. Proc R Soc Med 65:71–72, 1972.

69. Gohel V, Long BW, Richter G: Aphthous ulcers in the esophagus with Crohn colitis. AJR 137:872–873, 1981.

70. Degryse HRM, De Schepper AM: Aphthoid esophageal ulcers in Crohn's disease of ileum and colon. Gastrointest Radiol 9:197–201, 1984.

71. Cynn WS, Chon H, Gureghian PA, et al: Crohn's disease of the esophagus. AJR 125:359–364, 1975.

72. Dyer NH, Cook PL, Harper RAK: Oesophageal stricture associated with Crohn's disease. Gut 10:549–554, 1969.

73. Cockey BM, Jones B, Bayless TM, et al: Filiform polyps of the esophagus with inflammatory bowel disease. AJR 144:1207–1208, 1985.

74. Schneider R: Tuberculous esophagitis. Gastrointest Radiol 1:143–145, 1976.

75. Spalding AR, Burney DP, Richie RE: Acquired benign bronchoesophageal fistulas in the adult. Ann Thorac Surg 28:378–383, 1979.

76. Katz J, Gryboski JD, Rosenbaum HM, et al: Dysphagia in children with epidermolysis bullosa. Gastroenterology 52:259–262, 1967.

77. Tishler JM, Han SY, Helman CA: Esophageal involvement in epidermolysis bullosa dystrophica. AJR 141:1283–1286, 1983.

78. Nix TE, Christianson HB: Epidermolysis bullosa of the esophagus: report of two cases and review of literature. South Med J 58:612–620, 1965.

79. Becker MH, Swinyard CA: Epidermolysis bullosa dystrophica in children: radiologic manifestations. Radiology 90:124–128, 1968.

80. Agha FP, Francis IR, Ellis CN: Esophageal involvement in epidermolysis bullosa dystrophica: clinical and roentgenographic manifestations. Gastrointest Radiol 8:111–117, 1983.

81. Schuman BM, Arciniegas E: The management of esophageal complications of epidermolysis bullosa. Am J Dig Dis 17:875–880, 1972.

82. Mauro MA, Parker LA, Hartley WS, et al: Epidermolysis bullosa: radiographic findings in 16 cases. AJR 149:925–927, 1987.

83. Agha FP, Raji MR: Esophageal involvement in pemphigoid: clinical and roentgen manifestations. Gastrointest Radiol 7:109–112, 1982.

84. Hardy KM, Perry HO, Pingree GC, et al: Benign mucous membrane pemphigoid. Arch Dermatol 104:467–475, 1971.

85. Al-kutoubi MA, Eliot C: Oesophageal involvement in benign mucous membrane pemphigoid. Clin Radiol 35:131–135, 1984.

86. Foroozan P, Enta T, Winship DH, et al: Loss and regeneration of esophageal mucosa in pemphigoid. Gastroenterology 52:548–558, 1967.

87. Soong C, Bynum TE: The endoscopic appearance of pemphigoid esophagitis. Gastrointest Endosc 19:17–18, 1972.

88. Karasick S, Mapp E, Karasick D: Esophageal involvement in benign mucous membrane pemphigoid. J Can Assoc Radiol 32:247–248, 1981.

89. Graham J, Barnes M, Rubenstein AS: The nasogastric tube as a cause of esophagitis and stricture. Am J Surg 98:116–119, 1959.

90. Waldman I, Berlin L: Stricture of the esophagus due to nasogastric intubation. AJR 94:321–324, 1965.

91. Banfield WJ, Hurwitz AL: Esophageal stricture associated with nasogastric intubation. Arch Intern Med 134:1083–1086, 1974.

92. Nagler R, Spiro HM: Persistent gastroesophageal reflux induced during prolonged gastric intubation. N Engl J Med 269:495–500, 1963.

93. Balkany TJ, Baker BB, Bloustein PA, et al: Cervical esophagostomy in dogs: endoscopic, radiographic, and histopathologic evaluation of esophagitis induced by feeding tubes. Ann Otol Rhinol Laryngol 86:1–6, 1977.

94. Helsingen N. Oesophagitis following total gastrectomy: a clinical and experimental study. Acta Chir Scand [Suppl] 273:1–21, 1961.

95. Salo JA, Kivilaakso E: Role of bile salts and trypsin in the pathogenesis of experimental alkaline esophagitis. Surgery 93:525–532, 1983.

96. Helsingen N: Oesophagitis following total gastrectomy: a follow-up study on 9 patients 5 years or more after operation. Acta Chir Scand 118:190–201, 1960.

97. Morrow D, Passaro ER: Alkaline reflux esophagitis after total gastrectomy. Am J Surg 132:287–290, 1976.

98. Sanchez RE, Gordon HE: Complications of total gastrectomy. Arch Surg 100:136–139, 1970.

99. Olbe L, Lundell L. Intestinal function after total gastrectomy and possible consequences of gastric replacement. World J Surg 11:713–719, 1987.

100. Salo J, Kivilaakso E. Failure of long limb Roux-en-Y reconstruction to prevent alkaline reflux esophagitis after total gastrectomy. Endoscopy 22:65–67, 1990.

101. Levine MS, Fisher AR, Rubesin SE, et al: Complications after total gastrectomy and esophagojejunostomy: radiologic evaluation. AJR 157:1189–1194, 1991.

102. Meyer W, Vollmar F, Bar W: Barrett-esophagus following total gastrectomy. Endoscopy 2:121–126, 1979.

103. Sandvik AK, Halvorsen TB: Barrett's esophagus after total gastrectomy. J Clin Gastroenterol 10:587–588, 1988.

104. Goldberg HI, O'Kieffe D, Jenis EH, et al: Diffuse eosinophilic gastroenteritis. AJR 119:342–351, 1973.

105. Edelman MJ, March TL: Eosinophilic gastroenteritis. AJR 91:773–778, 1964.

106. Dobbins JW, Sheahan DG, Behar J: Eosinophilic gastroenteritis with esophageal involvement. Gastroenterology 72:1312–1316, 1977.

107. Picus D, Frank PH: Eosinophilic esophagitis. AJR 136:1001–1003, 1981.

108. Feczko PJ, Halpert RD, Zonca M: Radiographic abnormalities in eosinophilic esophagitis. Gastrointest Radiol 10:321–324, 1985.

109. Landres RT, Kuster GGR, Strum WB: Eosinophilic esophagitis in a patient with vigorous achalasia. Gastroenterology 74:1298–1301, 1978.

110. O'Riordan D, Levine MS, Laufer I: Acute alcoholic esophagitis. J Can Assoc Radiol 37:54–55, 1986.

111. Hogan WJ, De Andrade SR, Winship DH: Ethanol-induced acute esophageal motor dysfunction. J Appl Physiol 32:755–760, 1972.

112. Kaufman SE, Kay MD: Induction of gastro-oesophageal reflux by alcohol. Gut 19:336–338, 1978.

113. McDonald GB, Shulman HM, Sullivan KM, et al: Intestinal and hepatic complications of human bone marrow transplantation. I. Gastroenterology 90:460–477, 1986.

114. McDonald GB, Shulman HM, Sullivan KM, et al: Intestinal and hepatic complications of human bone marrow transplantation. II. Gastroenterology 90:770–784, 1986.

115. Rosenberg HK, Serota FT, Hock P, et al: Radiographic features

of gastrointestinal graft-vs.-host disease. Radiology 138:371–374, 1981.

116. McDonald GB, Sullivan KM, Plumley TF: Radiographic features of esophageal involvement in chronic graft-vs.-host disease. AJR 142:501–506, 1984.

117. McDonald GB, Sullivan KM, Schuffler MD, et al: Esophageal abnormalities in chronic graft-vs.-host disease in humans. Gastroenterology 890:914–921, 1981.

118. McDonald GB, Sharma P, Hackman RC, et al: Esophageal infections in immunosuppressed patients after marrow transplantation. Gastroenterology 88:1111–1117, 1985.

119. O'Duffy JD: Suggested criteria for diagnosis of Behçet's disease. J Rheumatol 1:18, 1974 (abstract).

120. Lockhart JM, McIntyre W, Caperton EM: Esophageal ulceration in Behçet's syndrome. Ann Intern Med 84:572–573, 1976.

121. Kaplinsky N, Neumann G, Harzahav Y, et al: Esophageal ulceration in Behçet's syndrome. Gastrointest Endosc 23:160, 1977.

122. Lebwohl O, Forde KA, Berdon WE, et al: Ulcerative esophagitis and colitis in a pediatric patient with Behçet's syndrome. Am J Gastroenterol 68:550–555, 1977.

123. Mendl K, McKay JM, Tanner CH: Intramural diverticulosis of the oesophagus and Rokitansky-Aschoff sinuses in the gallbladder. Br J Radiol 33:496–501, 1960.

124. Cho SR, Sanders MM, Turner MA, et al: Esophageal intramural pseudodiverticulosis. Gastrointest Radiol 6:9–16, 1981.

125. Hammon JW, Rice RP, Postlethwait RW, et al: Esophageal intramural diverticulosis. Ann Thorac Surg 17:260–267, 1974.

126. Wightman AJA, Wright EA: Intramural esophageal diverticulosis: a correlation of radiological and pathological findings. Br J Radiol 47:496–498, 1974.

127. Umlas J, Sakhuja R: The pathology of esophageal intramural pseudodiverticulosis. Am J Clin Pathol 65:314–320, 1976.

128. Medeiros LJ, Doos WG, Balogh K: Esophageal intramural pseudodiverticulosis: a report of two cases with analysis of similar, less extensive changes in "normal" autopsy esophagi. Hum Pathol 19:928–931, 1988.

129. Bruhlmann WF, Zollikofer CL, Maranta E, et al: Intramural pseudodiverticulosis of the esophagus: report of seven cases and literature review. Gastrointest Radiol 6:199–208, 1981.

130. Sabanathan S, Salama FD, Morgan WE: Oesophageal intramural pseudodiverticulosis. Thorax 40:849–857, 1985.

131. Troupin RH: Intramural esophageal diverticulosis and moniliasis. AJR 104:613–616, 1968.

132. Boyd RM, Bogoch A, Greig JH, et al: Esophageal intramural pseudodiverticulosis. Radiology 113:267–270, 1974.

133. Beauchamp JM, Nice CM, Belanger MA, et al: Esophageal intramural pseudodiverticulosis. Radiology 113:273–276, 1974.

134. Castillo S, Aburashed A, Kimmelman J, et al: Diffuse intramural esophageal pseudodiverticulosis. Gastroenterology 72:541–545, 1977.

135. Levine MS, Moolten DN, Herlinger H, et al: Esophageal intramural pseudodiverticulosis: a reevaluation. AJR 147:1165–1170, 1986.

136. Culver GJ, Chaudhari KR: Intramural esophageal diverticulosis. AJR 99:210–211, 1967.

137. Graham DY, Goyal RK, Sparkman J, et al: Diffuse intramural esophageal diverticulosis. Gastroenterology 68:781–785, 1975.

138. Hodes PJ, Atkins JP, Hodes BL: Esophageal intramural diverticulosis. AJR 96:411–413, 1966.

139. Kim S, Choi C, Groskin SA: Esophageal intramural pseudodiverticulitis. Radiology 173:418–419, 1989.

140. Pearlberg JL, Sandler MA, Madrazo BL: Computed tomographic features of esophageal intramural pseudodiverticulosis. Radiology 147:189–190, 1983.

# Benign Tumors

### Marc S. Levine, M.D.

## INTRODUCTION

Benign tumors of the esophagus constitute only about 20% of all esophageal neoplasms.[1] The vast majority are small, asymptomatic lesions without malignant potential. As a result, they are usually discovered fortuitously on radiologic or endoscopic examinations. Occasionally, however, these lesions cause dysphagia, bleeding, or other symptoms. In such cases, endoscopic or surgical removal may be required. Depending on their site of origin, benign tumors may be classified as mucosal or submucosal lesions, which have typical radiographic and endoscopic features. Although most benign tumors are thought to be leiomyomas, small, asymptomatic papillomas have been recognized with increased frequency on double contrast studies.

## MUCOSAL LESIONS

### Papilloma

Squamous papillomas are benign neoplasms that appear grossly as coral-like excrescences on the mucosa. Histologically, they consist of a central fibrovascular core with multiple finger-like projections covered by hyperplastic squamous epithelium.[2] Papillomas are generally thought to be rare lesions in the esophagus, accounting for less than 5% of all benign esophageal tumors.[3] However, many of these lesions are never diagnosed because of their small size and lack of symptoms.[2] Some investigators have found that these small, asymptomatic papillomas are considerably more common than has previously been suspected.[4]

All squamous papillomas in the esophagus reported thus far have been benign lesions. However, malignant transformation has been documented in papillomas arising in other sites such as the oral cavity, larynx, and uterine cervix.[5–7] Malignant degeneration has also been observed in experimentally induced esophageal papillomas in rats.[8] The malignant potential of these lesions is therefore uncertain. Benign papillomas may also be confused histologically with verrucous carcinoma, an uncommon form of squamous cell carcinoma that is locally invasive but rarely metastasizes to distant structures.[9] Thus, some investigators believe that all esophageal papillomas should be resected because of the uncertain risk of malignant degeneration and potential confusion with verrucous carcinoma.[10]

Esophageal papillomas usually occur as solitary lesions, ranging from 0.5 to 1.5 cm in size. Most patients with papillomas are asymptomatic, but dysphagia is an occasional finding.[2, 10] Rarely, multiple papillomas may be present in the esophagus, a condition known as esophageal papillomatosis.[11, 12] Associated papillomas may also be found in the hypopharynx or larynx.[11] Despite the dramatic appearance of the lesions on radiologic or endoscopic examinations, most patients with esophageal papillomatosis are asymptomatic.

### Radiographic Findings

Squamous papillomas are difficult to detect on conventional single contrast esophagrams because of the small size of the lesions. However, Montesi and colleagues found that squamous papillomas accounted for about 65% of all benign tumors diagnosed on double contrast esophagography.[4] All of the papillomas detected were less than 1 cm in size. The high frequency of esophageal papillomas in this study presumably reflects the greater ability to detect small lesions by double contrast technique.

Esophageal papillomas usually appear on double contrast radiographs as small, sessile polyps with smooth or slightly lobulated contours[4] (Fig. 27–1). Some lesions may produce a ring shadow similar to that of colonic polyps on double contrast barium enema studies as a result of barium trapped between the edge of the papilloma and the adjacent esophageal wall.[4] Because early esophageal cancers may also appear radiographically as smooth or slightly lobulated polyps, endoscopy should be performed to exclude an early carcinoma. Occasionally, larger papillomas may appear as lobulated intraluminal masses. Such lesions may be difficult to distinguish

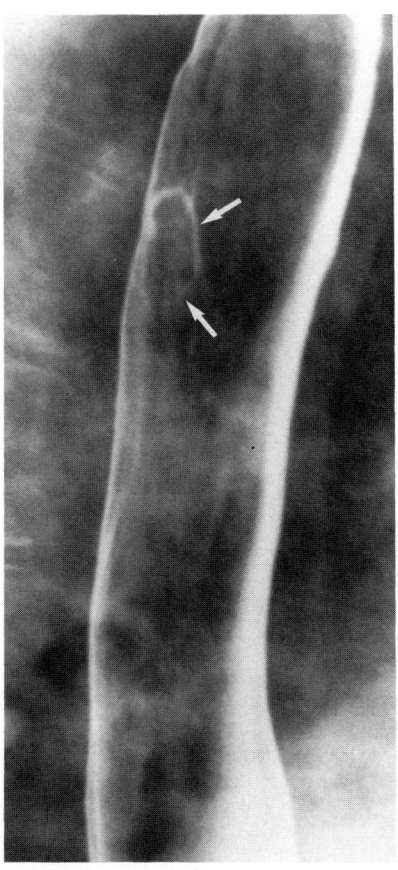

**Figure 27–1. Squamous papilloma.** The lesion appears as a sessile, slightly lobulated polyp *(arrows)* in the midesophagus. An early esophageal carcinoma could produce similar findings.

from polypoid esophageal carcinomas. Other papillomas may resemble submucosal tumors such as leiomyomas. Rarely, giant esophageal papillomas may have a bubbly appearance due to trapping of barium between the papillary fronds of the tumor[13] (Fig. 27–2).

Multiple papillomas may occasionally be seen radiographically in patients with esophageal papillomatosis.[11, 12] The diagnosis may be suggested on double contrast studies by the presence of multiple, discrete, wart-like excrescences on the esophageal mucosa (Fig. 27–3). Even when multiple papillomas are present, however, these lesions rarely cause esophageal obstruction.

## Adenoma

Adenomas account for less than 1% of all benign tumors in the esophagus.[14] These lesions originate in columnar rather than squamous epithelium, so they are traditionally thought to arise from ectopic gastric mucosa in the esophagus. However, it has been shown that most esophageal adenomas arise from Barrett's mucosa (see Chapter 28).[15, 16] These adenomas are important because of the risk of developing esophageal adenocarcinoma.[15, 16] Malignant degeneration apparently results from an adenoma-carcinoma sequence similar to

that found in the colon. Because esophageal adenomas are premalignant, they should be resected endoscopically or surgically whenever feasible.

### Radiographic Findings

Esophageal adenomas may appear radiographically as sessile or pedunculated polyps in the esophagus (Fig. 27–4). Larger, more lobulated lesions have a greater likelihood of harboring adenocarcinoma. Most adenomas are located in the distal esophagus at or adjacent to the gastroesophageal junction.[14–16] As a result, they can be mistaken for inflammatory esophagogastric polyps. However, nodularity, lobulation, or the large size of the lesion should favor an adenoma or adenocarcinoma. When an adenoma is suspected on barium studies, endoscopy and biopsy should be performed for a definitive diagnosis.

## Inflammatory Esophagogastric Polyp

Although the inflammatory esophagogastric polyp is not neoplastic, it is included in this chapter because it is characterized by the presence of a polypoid protuberance in the distal esophagus near the gastroesophageal junction. The inflammatory esophagogastric polyp represents the bulbous tip of a thickened gastric fold extending into the distal esophagus from the gastric fundus.[17–21] The lesion is composed of inflammatory and

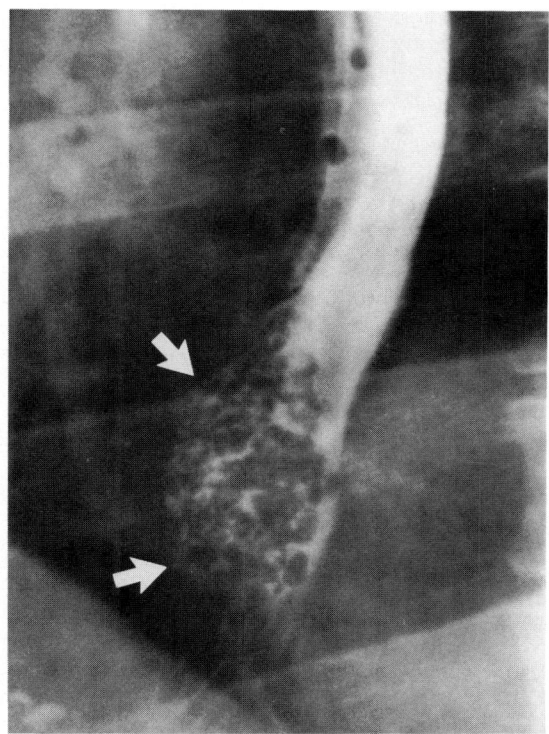

**Figure 27–2. Giant esophageal papilloma.** The lesion has a bubbly appearance *(arrows)* due to barium trapping between the papillary fronds of the tumor. (From JH Walker, Giant papilloma of the thoracic esophagus, AJR, 131, 3, 519–520, 1978, © by American Roentgen Ray Society.)

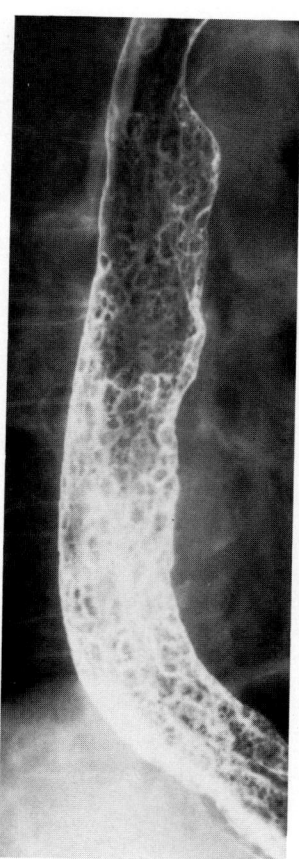

**Figure 27–3. Squamous papillomatosis.** There are innumerable wart-like excrescences on the esophageal mucosa. Despite the dramatic radiographic appearance, this patient had no esophageal symptoms. (Courtesy of Harvey M. Goldstein, M.D., San Antonio, TX.)

granulation tissue, and it is thought to be a sequela of chronic reflux esophagitis (see Chapter 24).[18, 19] As a result, these patients often have clinical signs of underlying reflux disease. However, the esophagogastric polyp has no malignant potential, so endoscopic resection is unwarranted.[21]

## Radiographic Findings

Inflammatory esophagogastric polyps are usually manifested radiographically by a single prominent mucosal fold arising in the gastric fundus and extending into the distal esophagus as a smooth, ovoid or club-shaped mass[17, 20, 21] (Fig. 27–5A and B). The lesion frequently straddles a hiatal hernia and may be associated with other findings of reflux esophagitis. When the characteristic features of inflammatory esophagogastric polyps are present on esophagrams, endoscopic confirmation is unnecessary. Occasionally, however, a prominent gastric fold can be mistaken for the stalk of a pedunculated polyp. Conversely, the gastric fold may not be recognized radiographically, and the bulbous tip of the polyp can be mistaken for a submucosal mass such as a leiomyoma. Occasionally, inflammatory esophagogastric polyps may have a more irregular, nodular, or lobulated appearance, so a malignant lesion cannot be excluded[20]

(Fig. 27–5C). When the radiographic findings are equivocal, endoscopy and biopsy are required for a definitive diagnosis.

## Glycogenic Acanthosis

Glycogenic acanthosis is a benign condition of unknown etiology in which there is accumulation of cytoplasmic glycogen within the squamous epithelium of the esophagus. Although glycogenic acanthosis is not considered to be a neoplastic condition, it is included in this chapter because it is characterized by mucosal nodules or plaques. Glycogenic acanthosis was not described until 1970, when two pathologists discovered this entity while examining the esophagus at autopsy.[22] Since that time, other investigators have found that it is a relatively common condition, with a prevalence of 3 to 15% reported at endoscopy.[23, 24]

Glycogenic acanthosis is characterized histologically by hyperplasia or swelling of squamous epithelial cells in the esophagus due to increased cytoplasmic glyco-

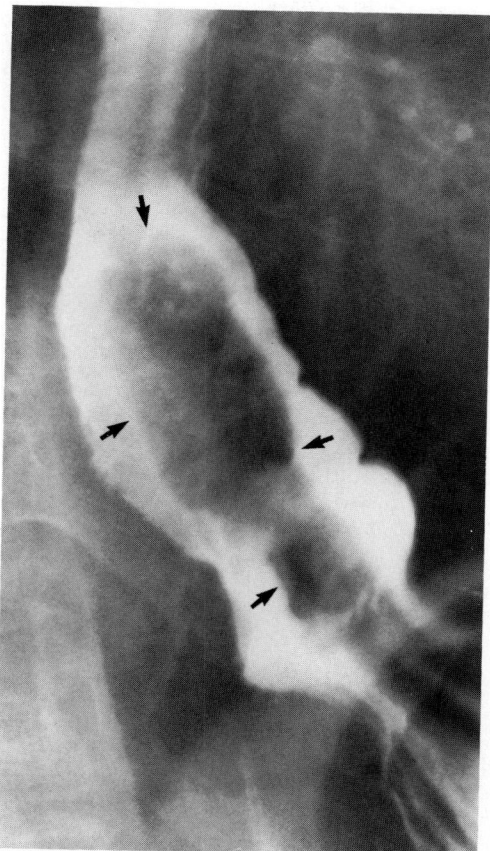

**Figure 27–4. Adenomatous polyp in Barrett's esophagus.** Note how the polyp (arrows) originates at the gastroesophageal junction and extends into the distal esophagus above a hiatal hernia. Although this lesion could be mistaken for an inflammatory esophagogastric polyp, it is larger and more lobulated than most inflammatory polyps. The resected specimen contained a solitary focus of adenocarcinoma. (From Levine MS, Caroline D, Thompson JJ, et al: Adenocarcinoma of the esophagus: relationship to Barrett mucosa. Radiology 150:305–309, 1984.)

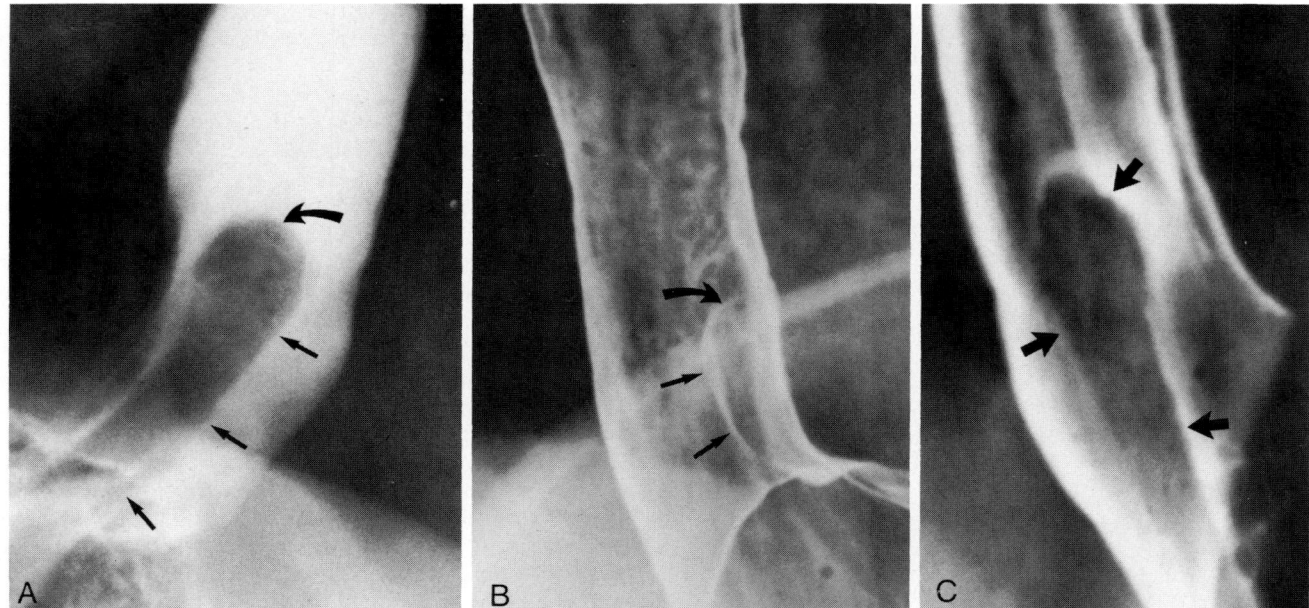

**Figure 27–5. An inflammatory esophagogastric polyps. A.** An inflammatory polyp is seen en face as a prominent fold *(straight arrows)* arising at the cardia and extending into the distal esophagus as a smooth, club-shaped mass *(curved arrow)*. **B.** An inflammatory polyp is seen in profile in another patient as a prominent fold *(straight arrows)* with a bulbous tip *(curved arrow)*. In both **A** and **B**, the radiographic findings are so characteristic that endoscopy is unwarranted. **C.** This inflammatory polyp has a more lobulated appearance *(arrows)*, so it cannot be differentiated from an adenomatous polyp or even an adenocarcinoma (see Fig. 27–4).

gen.[22] The resulting lesions appear grossly as white mucosal plaques or nodules, ranging from 2 to 15 mm in size.[23, 24] The diagnosis may be suggested on the basis of the gross findings at endoscopy, and a definitive diagnosis is made by demonstrating the characteristic glycogen-rich epithelial cells on biopsy specimens stained with periodic acid–Schiff material.[22]

Glycogenic acanthosis seems to be a degenerative, age-related phenomenon, with the lesions first appearing during the fifth and sixth decades of life and becoming larger and more numerous with increasing age.[25] It is a benign condition without any known risk of malignant degeneration.[26] Furthermore, it rarely causes esophageal symptoms. Thus, glycogenic acanthosis is usually an incidental finding in patients who undergo radiologic or endoscopic examinations for other reasons.

## Radiographic Findings

Glycogenic acanthosis was not described radiographically until 1981.[27] Nevertheless, it has been shown that glycogenic acanthosis is a relatively frequent finding on double contrast studies.[25, 26] In one series, this condition was detected in nearly 30% of patients who underwent double contrast esophagography.[26] In fact, glycogenic acanthosis may be easier to detect by double contrast studies than by endoscopy. In contrast, the small, often subtle lesions of glycogenic acanthosis may be difficult or impossible to detect with conventional single contrast barium studies.

Glycogenic acanthosis is usually manifested radio-graphically by multiple small, rounded nodules or plaques in the middle or, less commonly, distal third of the esophagus[26] (Fig. 27–6). The lesions are more obvious in the midesophagus because this segment is best seen on double contrast radiographs and the distal esophagus is often obscured by barium pooling in this region. The nodules usually range from 1 to 3 mm in size, but occasional plaques may be as large as several centimeters.[26, 27] Some lesions have well-defined borders, but others have hazy margins that fade peripherally into the adjacent mucosa without a discrete edge. When vertically contiguous, the nodules may cause slight thickening or scalloping of the longitudinal folds of the esophagus.[26]

## Differential Diagnosis

Although glycogenic acanthosis has little clinical significance, it should be distinguished radiographically from other causes of mucosal nodularity, such as superficial spreading carcinoma, squamous papillomatosis, acanthosis nigricans, leukoplakia, and esophagitis. Because of the rarity of most of these conditions, the major consideration in the differential diagnosis, for all practical purposes, is esophagitis. When glycogenic acanthosis involves the distal esophagus, the radiographic appearance can be mistaken for the nodular mucosa of reflux esophagitis. However, the nodules of glycogenic acanthosis tend to be more well defined than those of reflux esophagitis and are usually more prominent in the midesophagus than in the distal esophagus. Other

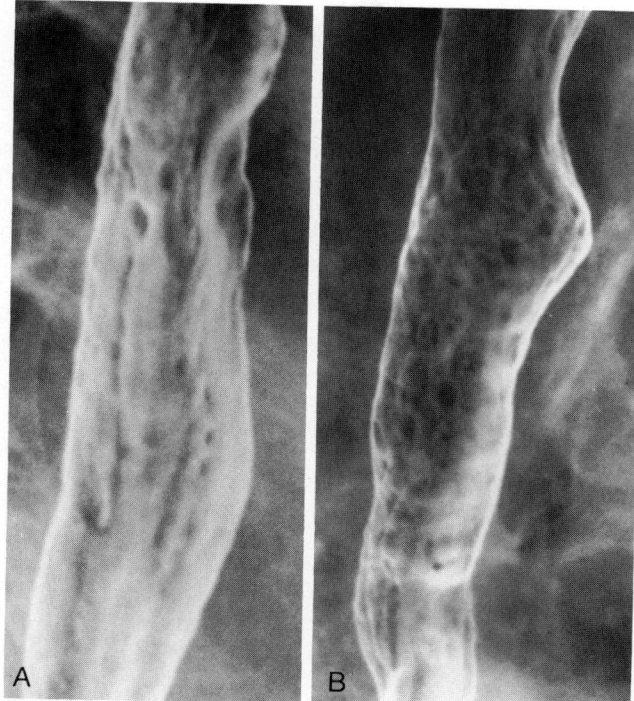

**Figure 27–6. Glycogenic acanthosis.** In both cases (**A** and **B**), this condition is manifested by multiple small plaques and nodules in the midesophagus. *Candida* esophagitis could produce similar findings, but patients with glycogenic acanthosis are almost always asymptomatic. (**A** from Levine MS, Macones AJ, Laufer I: *Candida* esophagitis: accuracy of radiographic diagnosis. Radiology 154:581–587, 1985.)

patients with glycogenic acanthosis may have discrete plaque-like defects indistinguishable from those of *Candida* esophagitis. However, the clinical history is extremely helpful, as patients with glycogenic acanthosis are almost always asymptomatic. Thus, it is usually possible to distinguish these entities on clinical and radiographic grounds.

## Leukoplakia

Oral leukoplakia is a relatively common condition characterized by white mucosal plaques that exhibit various combinations of hyperkeratosis, parakeratosis, epithelial dysplasia, and frank carcinoma on histologic examination. This condition often develops in the oral cavity but rarely occurs in the esophagus. Some investigators even doubt the existence of esophageal leukoplakia and suggest that, in retrospect, most reported cases probably represent glycogenic acanthosis.[26] However, there have been anecdotal cases of esophageal leukoplakia in which biopsies of the lesions clearly fulfilled the histologic criteria for this condition.[28, 29] Oral leukoplakia is a premalignant condition, but the malignant potential of esophageal leukoplakia is unknown.

Most reported patients with esophageal leukoplakia have been asymptomatic.[28] The lesions appear endoscopically as discrete, slightly raised, white mucosal plaques less than 1 cm in size.[28] These lesions may

occasionally be recognized on barium studies by the presence of tiny nodules or plaques.[29, 30] However, most asymptomatic patients with a nodular mucosa probably have glycogenic acanthosis.[26] Thus, esophageal leukoplakia should be considered a histologic diagnosis.

## Acanthosis Nigricans

Acanthosis nigricans is a dermatologic disorder characterized by the triad of papillomatosis, pigmentation, and hyperkeratosis. Some patients have a malignant type of acanthosis nigricans associated with adenocarcinomas of the gastrointestinal tract, ovary, lung, or breast. Esophageal involvement has occasionally been reported in patients with the malignant form of the disease.[30, 31] The esophageal lesions appear radiographically as numerous finely nodular elevations on the esophageal mucosa.[30, 31] Because this condition rarely involves the esophagus, the diagnosis should be suggested only for patients who have known acanthosis nigricans involving the skin.

## SUBMUCOSAL LESIONS

### Leiomyoma

More than 50% of all benign esophageal tumors are leiomyomas.[3, 32, 33] Histologically, these tumors consist of intersecting bands of smooth muscle and fibrous tissue in a well-defined capsule. About 60% of these lesions are located in the distal third of the esophagus, 30% in the middle third, and 10% in the proximal third.[34] Leiomyomas are less common above the level of the aortic arch because of the presence of striated rather than smooth muscle in this portion of the esophagus. These tumors appear grossly as discrete submucosal masses, usually ranging from 2 to 8 cm in size.[33] Occasionally, however, the lesions may have an exophytic, intraluminal, or circumferential growth pattern. Giant leiomyomas as large as 20 cm in size rarely have been described.[35, 36]

Most esophageal leiomyomas occur as solitary lesions, but multiple leiomyomas are present in 3 to 4% of patients.[33, 34] Rarely, these tumors may be associated with uterine or vulvar leiomyomas, apparently on a familial basis.[37, 38] Esophageal leiomyomas have also been documented in patients with hypertrophic osteoarthropathy, a condition characterized by clubbed fingers and toes, swollen joints, and subperiosteal new bone formation in the extremities.[39] An association between esophageal leiomyomas and Alport's syndrome has been recognized in children.[40]

### *Clinical Findings*

Most patients with esophageal leiomyomas are asymptomatic.[34] Even large masses significantly indenting the lumen may not produce symptoms. When these patients are symptomatic, they may present with intermittent, gradually worsening dysphagia or, less commonly, sub-

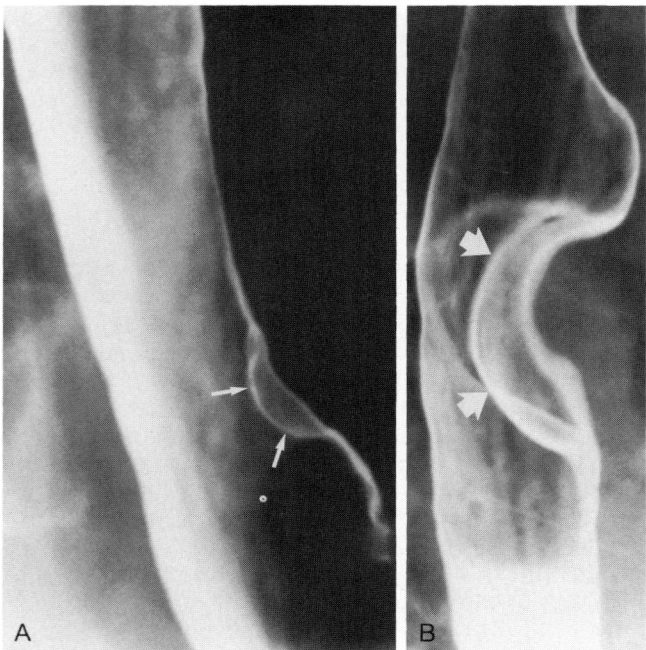

**Figure 27–7. Esophageal leiomyomas.** In both **A** and **B**, the lesions *(arrows)* have a smooth surface and slightly obtuse borders characteristic of submucosal masses.

sternal discomfort, vomiting, or weight loss.[34, 41] Unlike gastric leiomyomas, however, esophageal leiomyomas rarely undergo ulceration, so upper gastrointestinal bleeding is extremely uncommon.[41] Because of the slowly progressive nature of the lesion, symptoms may be present for several years before these patients seek medical attention.[34] The treatment of choice for symptomatic leiomyomas is surgical enucleation.[34] Occasionally, however, extensive lesions may necessitate more radical surgery.

Although leiomyomas are relatively common lesions in the esophagus, their malignant counterparts, leiomyosarcomas, are rare (see Chapter 29). Thus far, no case of malignant degeneration in an esophageal leiomyoma has been documented in the literature. In one series, patients with leiomyomas were followed for as long as 15 years without evidence of malignant transformation in the lesions.[42] Esophageal leiomyomas therefore have little if any tendency to undergo sarcomatous degeneration, so surgical removal of small, asymptomatic leiomyomas is probably unwarranted.

### Radiographic Findings

Esophageal leiomyomas may occasionally be recognized on chest radiographs by the presence of a soft tissue mass in the posterior mediastinum or by amorphous or punctate areas of calcification in the tumor.[43–45] In fact, the presence of a calcified esophageal mass should be virtually pathognomonic of a leiomyoma, as calcification almost never occurs in other benign or malignant esophageal tumors.[45] However, a case of a densely calcified esophageal leiomyosarcoma has been described.[46]

Esophageal leiomyomas are usually recognized on barium studies as discrete submucosal masses, ranging from 2 to 8 cm in size (Figs. 27–7 and 27–8). These tumors have the typical appearance of intramural lesions elsewhere in the gastrointestinal tract.[47] When viewed en face, the lesions appear as round or ovoid filling defects sharply outlined by barium on each side[33] (see Fig. 27–8A). As a result, splitting of barium around the tumor may produce a characteristic "forked stream" appearance.[48] When viewed in profile, the lesions have a smooth surface, and their upper and lower borders form abrupt right angles or slightly obtuse angles with the adjacent esophageal wall (see Figs. 27–7 and 27–8B). Occasionally, larger tumors may significantly com-

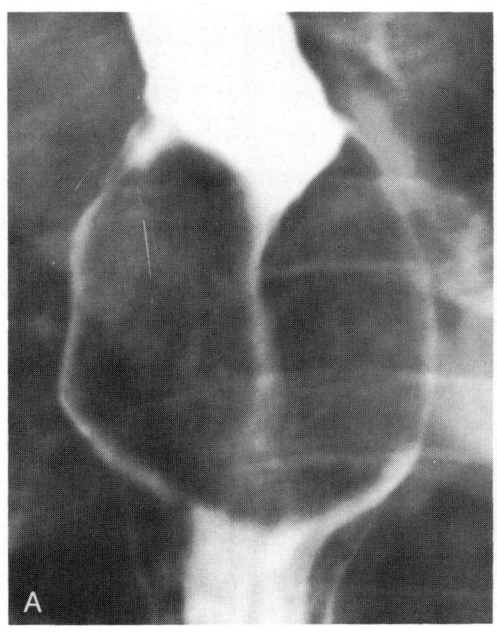
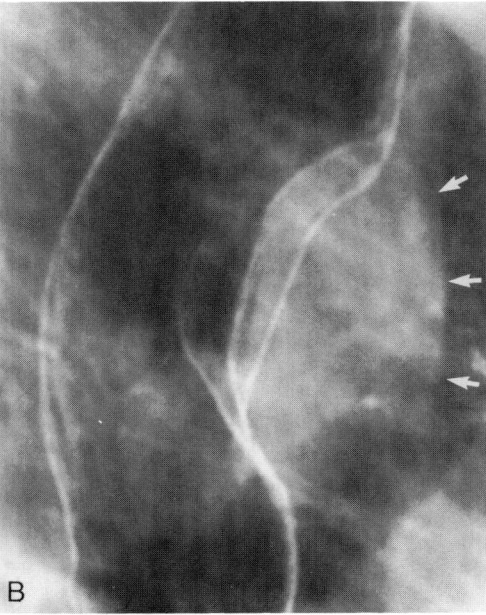

**Figure 27–8. Esophageal leiomyoma. A.** An en face view shows a smooth, rounded filling defect in the esophagus, with splitting of barium around the lesion. Also note how the esophagus appears widened at this level. **B.** A tangential view reveals the characteristic features of a submucosal lesion. Also note how the outer margin of the leiomyoma is seen as a soft tissue shadow *(arrows)* abutting the lung. (**A** and **B** courtesy of Marc P. Banner, M.D., Philadelphia, PA.)

press the lumen, causing the esophagus to appear narrowed in tangential projections but stretched and widened en face[47] (see Fig. 27–8). Although esophageal leiomyomas may gradually enlarge over a period of years, ulceration is rarely observed in these lesions. Occasionally, computed tomography (CT) may be helpful in demonstrating the intramural location of leiomyomas, which typically appear as homogeneous soft tissue densities.[49]

Most esophageal leiomyomas appear radiographically as discrete submucosal masses, but about 10% become annular lesions.[34] Even less commonly, leiomyomas may be manifested by giant intraluminal masses that are attached to the upper thoracic or cervical esophagus by a long, slender pedicle.[34, 50] However, most pedunculated, intraluminal tumors in the esophagus contain a variety of other mesenchymal elements and are classified together as fibrovascular polyps (see later section on fibrovascular polyps).

Occasionally, leiomyomas arising near the gastroesophageal junction may involve not only the distal esophagus but also the gastric cardia and fundus.[51] Leiomyomas in this location may cause severe dysphagia due to obstruction of the distal esophagus. These lesions may be difficult to distinguish radiographically from carcinoma of the cardia involving the distal esophagus.

About 3 to 4% of patients with esophageal leiomyomas have multiple lesions.[52, 53] These tumors may be recognized on barium studies by the presence of two or more discrete submucosal masses in the esophagus, but the size and number of lesions are variable. Other patients may have diffuse esophageal leiomyomatosis, a rare condition manifested by innumerable tiny submucosal nodules in the esophagus.[54] The lesions may be so confluent that it is impossible to delineate individual nodules in these patients.[40]

Another rare form of leiomyomatosis is idiopathic muscular hypertrophy of the esophagus, in which there is massive thickening of esophageal smooth muscle without discrete lesions.[40, 55, 56] This condition may be manifested on barium studies by marked narrowing of the distal esophagus and proximal dilatation (Fig. 27–9A), mimicking the appearance of an annular malignancy or achalasia.[40, 56] In such cases, however, CT scans may demonstrate massive esophageal wall thickening rather than a focal mass lesion[40] (Fig. 27–9B). Some patients with idiopathic muscular hypertrophy of the esophagus may have such severe dysphagia that an esophagectomy is required.

## Differential Diagnosis

Almost all submucosal masses in the esophagus are leiomyomas. However, other unusual submucosal tumors such as fibromas, neurofibromas, lipomas, hemangiomas, and granular cell tumors may produce identical radiographic findings (see later sections). Cystic lesions such as congenital duplication cysts and acquired retention cysts may also appear as submucosal masses (see

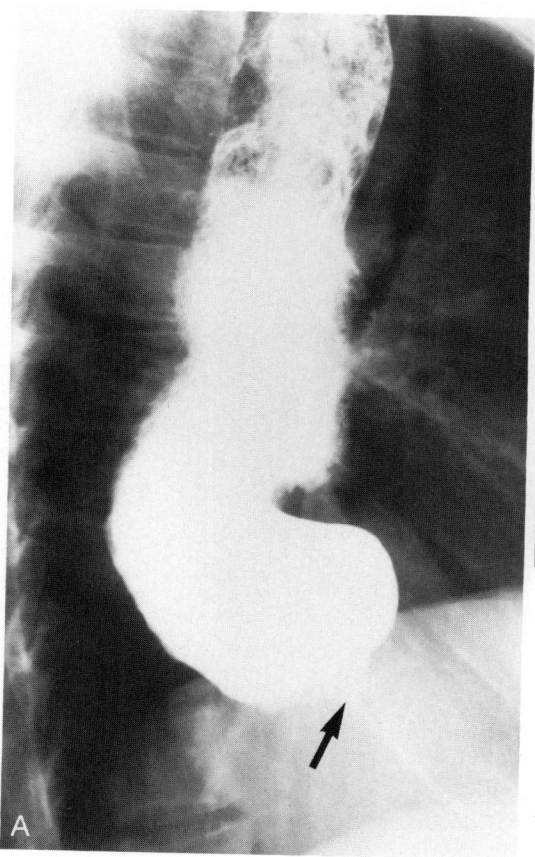

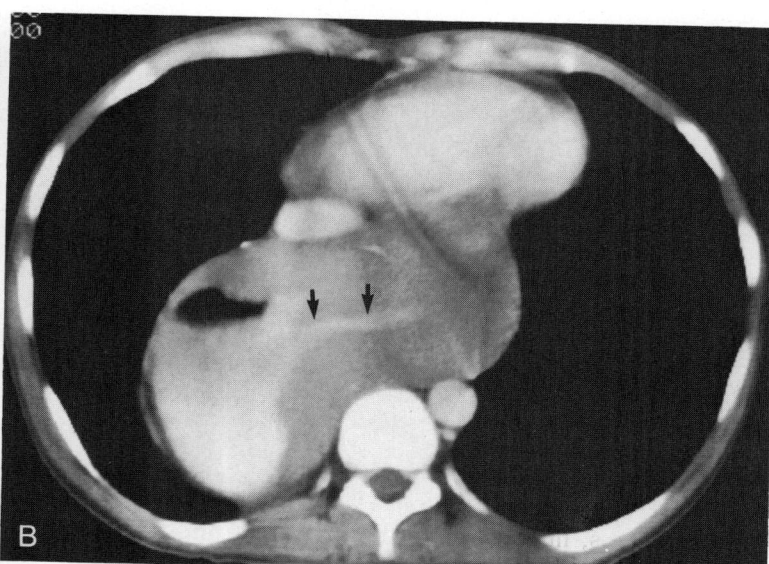

**Figure 27–9. Idiopathic muscular hypertrophy of the esophagus. A.** Esophagography reveals a markedly dilated esophagus with relatively abrupt narrowing *(arrow)* near the gastroesophageal junction. **B.** A CT scan near the level of the gastroesophageal junction shows massive thickening of the distal esophageal wall and narrowing of the lumen *(arrows)*. An air-contrast level is present in the dilated esophagus to the right. At surgery, there was a markedly thickened esophageal wall because of localized muscular hypertrophy without evidence of tumor. (**A** and **B** courtesy of Richard L. Baron, M.D., Pittsburgh, PA.)

later section on cysts). Rarely, an isolated esophageal varix may also resemble a submucosal tumor, but effacement or obliteration of the lesion by esophageal distention should suggest its vascular origin (see Chapter 30). When multiple submucosal masses are present in the esophagus, the differential diagnosis should include not only multiple leiomyomas but also esophageal retention cysts, hematogenous metastases, Kaposi's sarcoma, and lymphomatous or leukemic infiltrates in the esophagus (see Chapter 29).

Most leiomyomas are readily differentiated from mucosal lesions, which tend to have a more irregular or lobulated surface and are often associated with ulceration. However, some papillomas may be smooth, sessile lesions that are difficult to distinguish from leiomyomas or other submucosal masses in the esophagus.

Leiomyomas should also be distinguished from extramural lesions that are extrinsically compressing or indenting the esophagus. When viewed in profile, extrinsic lesions tend to have more obtuse, gently sloping margins than intramural lesions.[47] Another useful criterion for differentiating these lesions is the "spheroid" sign, which is based on the principle that the estimated center of the mass should lie outside the projected contour of the esophagus for extramural lesions but inside the projected contour for intramural lesions.[57] Finally, leiomyomas should move freely with the esophagus on breathing or deglutition, whereas the relationship of an extrinsic mediastinal mass to the esophagus may vary considerably with these maneuvers.[43] Despite these differentiating features, it may occasionally be difficult to distinguish an intramural lesion from an extrinsic mediastinal mass on barium studies. In such cases, a tube esophagram may help to differentiate these lesions, as extrinsic masses involving the esophagus can often be effaced with greater esophageal distention, whereas intramural lesions tend to maintain their typical submucosal appearance.[58] CT may also be helpful for differentiating a submucosal tumor from a mediastinal mass.[49]

## Fibrovascular Polyp

Fibrovascular polyps are uncommon neoplasms characterized by pedunculated, often gigantic intraluminal masses in the esophagus. These tumors consist histologically of varying amounts of fibrovascular and adipose tissue covered by normal squamous epithelium.[59–61] Depending on the predominant mesenchymal element, these lesions have variously been called hamartomas, fibromas, lipomas, fibrolipomas, fibromyxomas, and fibroepithelial polyps.[61, 62] Because of their similar clinical and pathologic features, however, many investigators have classified these tumors together as *fibrovascular polyps*.[59–62] Unlike leiomyomas, which tend to occur in the mid- or distal esophagus, fibrovascular polyps almost always arise in the cervical esophagus near the level of the cricopharyngeus.[60–62] Mesenchymal tumors in this location are particularly prone to enlarge and elongate, gradually forming a pedicle as a result of constant peristaltic activity in the esophagus and the traction of passing food.[63] Over a period of many years, continued peristalsis may "drag" the tumor downward in the esophagus until the intraluminal portion of the mass has attained gigantic proportions.

### Clinical Findings

Fibrovascular polyps are typically found in elderly men, who are often asymptomatic until the tumor has reached a massive size.[62] These patients eventually may develop dysphagia as a result of esophageal obstruction by the mass.[59–62] Others may have upper gastrointestinal bleeding, with hematemesis, melena, or iron deficiency anemia.[61] Occasionally, these pedunculated masses may be regurgitated into the oropharynx, so that affected individuals may transiently "vomit up" a fleshy, sausage-shaped mass into the mouth.[59, 61–63] Some distraught patients have even tried to bite off the tumor with their teeth or to remove it manually with their fingers.[63] Aside from the bizarre clinical features of this entity, regurgitated fibrovascular polyps in the pharynx are potentially dangerous, as they have occasionally been known to occlude the larynx, causing asphyxia and sudden death.[64]

Although fibrovascular polyps rarely if ever undergo malignant degeneration, endoscopic or surgical resection is warranted because of the risk of upper gastrointestinal bleeding or potentially life-threatening laryngeal obstruction. Small fibrovascular polyps may be resected endoscopically, but large tumors should be removed

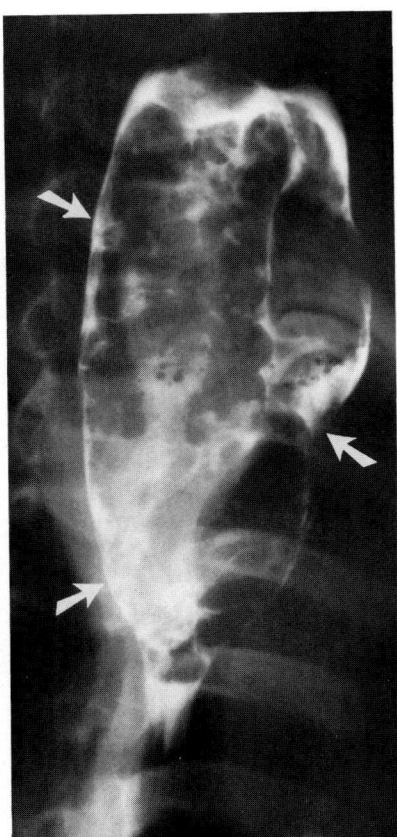

**Figure 27–10. Giant fibrovascular polyp.** The lesion appears as a smooth, sausage-shaped mass *(arrows)* that expands the lumen of the upper thoracic esophagus. (Courtesy of Duane G. Mezwa, M.D., Royal Oak, MI.)

surgically, as significant bleeding may occur when the stalk is transected.[60, 61]

## Radiographic Findings

Fibrovascular polyps appear on esophagrams as smooth or slightly lobulated intraluminal masses extending from the region of the cricopharyngeus into the middle or distal third of the esophagus[59, 61, 63] (Figs. 27–10 and 27–11A). These sausage-shaped masses should be completely surrounded by a thin layer of barium in all projections, because they are attached to the wall by a pedicle in the cervical esophagus. Although the bulbous tip of the polyp may be recognized radiographically, it is often difficult to demonstrate a pedicle, so the site of origin may be unclear. Because these lesions are pedunculated, they often move with deglutition and may dramatically change their position in the esophagus during the fluoroscopic examination.[59] Giant fibrovascular polyps may occupy the entire thoracic esophagus,

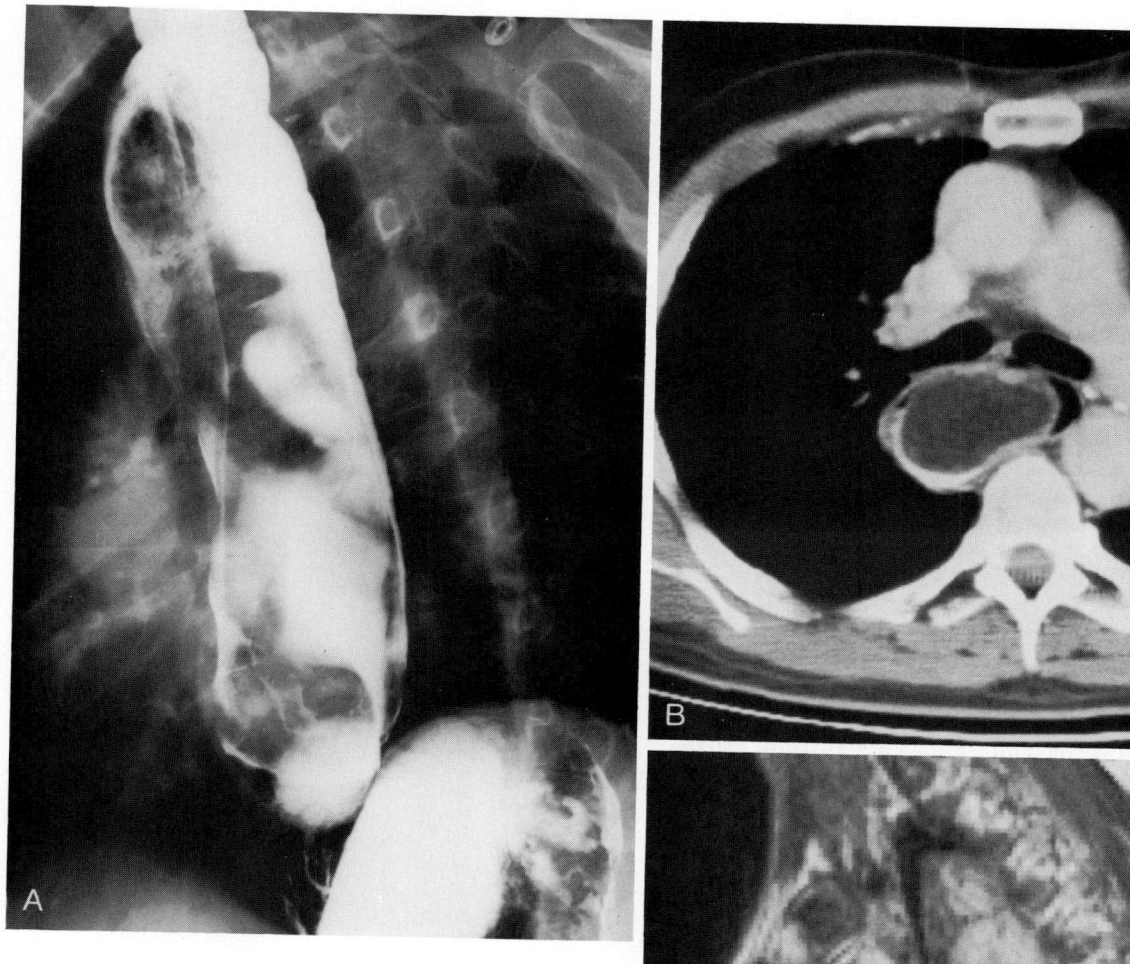

**Figure 27–11. Giant fibrovascular polyp. A.** An esophagram shows a giant, sausage-shaped mass extending into the distal esophagus. **B.** A contrast-enhanced CT scan at the level of the carina reveals a posterior mediastinal mass with lipid attenuation. Note how oral contrast material in the esophagus outlines the posterolateral aspect of the mass. **C.** A sagittal T1-weighted MR image shows a cylindric posterior mediastinal mass with high signal intensity. These features are characteristic of fibrovascular polyps on CT and MR scans. (**A, B,** and **C** from GJ Whitman, GP Borkowski, Giant fibrovascular polyp of the esophagus: CT and MR findings, AJR, 152, 3, 518–520, 1989, © by American Roentgen Ray Society.)

and some lesions may even prolapse through the cardia into the gastric fundus.[60–62, 65] Although fibrovascular polyps may expand or dilate the esophagus, they rarely cause evidence of obstruction. CT and magnetic resonance (MR) imaging may also be helpful for diagnosing these lesions. When a significant amount of adipose tissue is present, fibrovascular polyps may show lipid attenuation on CT scans (Fig. 27–11B) and high signal intensity on T1-weighted MR images[66] (Fig. 27–11C).

## Differential Diagnosis

Despite their size, fibrovascular polyps are sometimes difficult to diagnose on barium studies. The radiographic findings may erroneously suggest retained debris in a dilated esophagus due to achalasia. However, fibrovascular polyps are usually associated with a widely patent cardia rather than the distal beak-like narrowing associated with achalasia. These tumors can also be mistaken for giant, coalescent air bubbles in the esophagus. Even when a neoplastic process is suspected, the lesions may be confused with malignant tumors such as adenocarcinomas, spindle cell carcinomas, and leiomyosarcomas. However, these malignant tumors tend to have an irregular, lobulated contour, whereas fibrovascular polyps usually appear as smooth, sausage-shaped defects with discrete bulbous tips in the distal esophagus. The typical findings on CT or MR imaging should also suggest the correct diagnosis.

## Granular Cell Tumor

Since its original description by Abrikossoff in 1926, granular cell myoblastoma has been recognized as a rare benign tumor that predominantly involves the skin, tongue, breast, and subcutaneous tissues.[67, 68] Abrikossoff believed that these tumors had a myogenic origin, but pathologic data now suggest that they have a neural derivation, arising from Schwann cells.[69] Thus, the term granular cell myoblastoma is a misnomer, and these lesions have more aptly been described as granular cell tumors.[70–72] Histologically, these lesions consist of sheets of polygonal tumor cells containing an eosinophilic-staining granular cytoplasm.[70, 72] The tumors are covered by hyperplastic but otherwise normal squamous epithelium. About 7% of granular cell tumors are located in the gastrointestinal tract, and one third of these lesions are located in the esophagus.[68, 71]

Most granular cell tumors in the esophagus occur as solitary lesions, ranging from 0.5 to 2.0 cm in size.[70] Lesions less than 1 cm in size usually are incidental findings at autopsy, but larger lesions may cause dysphagia or other symptoms such as substernal chest pain, vomiting, and weight loss.[70, 72] The treatment of choice for symptomatic granular cell tumors is local excision, as these lesions virtually never recur after endoscopic or surgical removal.[68, 70–72] In contrast, asymptomatic granular cell tumors found by endoscopic biopsy can probably be left in the esophagus because of the negligible risk of malignant degeneration.[73] Occasionally, however, the findings on endoscopic biopsy can be mistaken for squamous cell carcinoma as a result of pseudoepitheliomatous hyperplasia of the overlying squamous mucosa.[70, 72, 73]

## Radiographic Findings

Granular cell tumors appear radiographically as round or oval submucosal masses in the distal or, less commonly, middle third of the esophagus[70, 72] (Fig. 27–12). They usually range from 0.5 to 2.0 cm in size.[70, 72] Because of their typical submucosal appearance, they are most often mistaken for esophageal leiomyomas.[70] Occasionally, granular cell tumors arising at the gastric cardia may be manifested by a polypoid or submucosal mass that distorts or obliterates the normal anatomic landmarks of this region.[72] Rarely, multiple granular cell tumors may be present in the esophagus or stomach[74] (Fig. 27–13).

## Other Mesenchymal Tumors

The vast majority of submucosal masses are leiomyomas. Other rare mesenchymal tumors in the esophagus

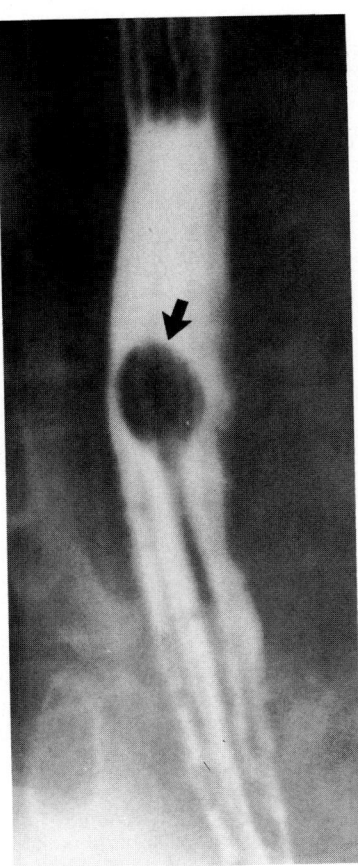

**Figure 27–12. Granular cell tumor.** There is a smooth submucosal mass *(arrow)* in the midesophagus. This lesion cannot be differentiated from other, more common submucosal lesions in the esophagus, such as leiomyomas.

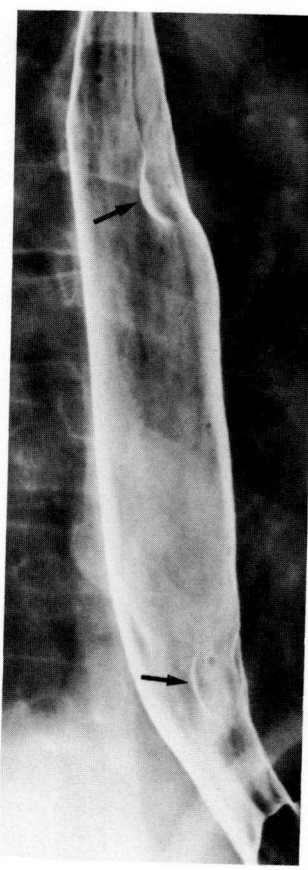

**Figure 27–13. Multiple granular cell tumors.** The lesions are seen as discrete submucosal masses *(arrows)* in the mid- and distal esophagus. This patient had additional granular cell tumors in the stomach.

## Hemangioma

The esophagus is the least common site of involvement by vascular tumors in the gastrointestinal tract. Rarely, multiple esophageal hemangiomas may be found in patients with Osler-Weber-Rendu disease, a hereditary disorder characterized by multiple telangiectasias of the face, lips, and mucous membranes.[83] However, most vascular tumors in the esophagus are solitary cavernous hemangiomas.[82] These highly vascular lesions may occasionally ulcerate, causing massive hematemesis and fatal exsanguination.[82] Esophageal hemangiomas usually appear radiographically as smooth or slightly lobulated submucosal masses that are indistinguishable from other, more common benign intramural tumors.[84] Because of the risk of significant bleeding, the treatment of choice is surgical enucleation.[82, 84]

## Hamartoma

Esophageal hamartomas are rare, benign tumors characterized histologically by metaplastic respiratory epithelium and islets of cartilage in a fibrous stroma.[85, 86] These tumors usually appear radiographically as pedunculated, intraluminal masses that are indistinguishable from fibrovascular polyps.[85] Rarely, multiple esophageal hamartomas may be found in patients with Cowden's

include fibromas, myxofibromas, neurofibromas, lipomas, hemangiomas, and hamartomas.[41, 75–86] These lesions usually appear as discrete submucosal masses that are indistinguishable from leiomyomas on clinical or radiographic criteria. When mesenchymal tumors contain a significant amount of fibrovascular or adipose tissue, they often elongate, forming pedunculated, intraluminal masses. Because the latter tumors have characteristic clinical and radiographic findings, they have been classified together as fibrovascular polyps (see earlier section on fibrovascular polyps).

## Lipoma

The esophagus is the rarest site of involvement by lipomas in the gastrointestinal tract. These tumors may appear radiographically as discrete submucosal masses (Fig. 27–14) or, more commonly, as pedunculated, intraluminal masses.[77–80] Like other pedunculated esophageal tumors, lipomas tend to arise in the cervical esophagus and occasionally may be regurgitated into the pharynx, causing asphyxia and sudden death.[79] Rarely, esophageal lipomas may be diagnosed preoperatively by their characteristic adipose density on CT scans.[81]

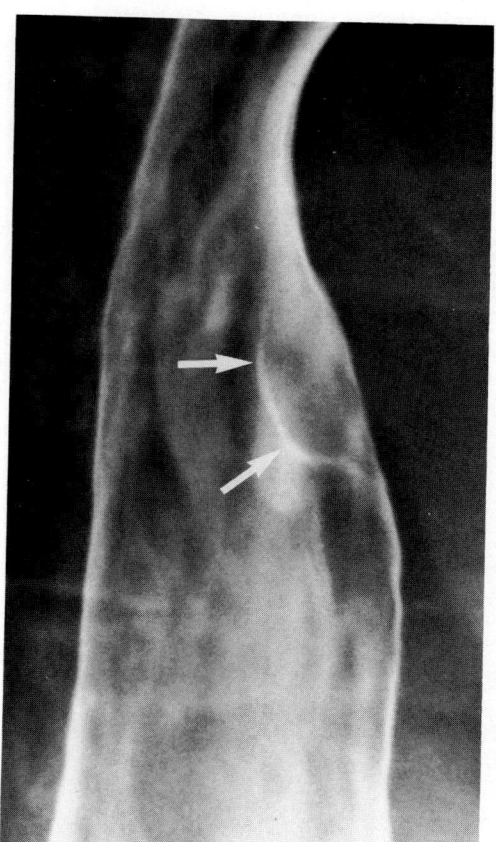

**Figure 27–14. Esophageal lipoma.** This patient has a discrete submucosal mass *(arrows)* that is indistinguishable from other, more common intramural tumors.

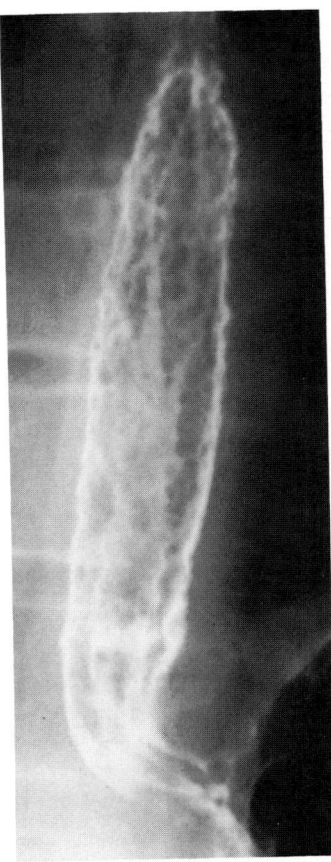

**Figure 27–15. Cowden's disease with multiple hamartomatous polyps in the esophagus.** The lesions appear as tiny, nodular elevations on the mucosa. (Courtesy of Wylie J. Dodds, M.D., Milwaukee, WI.)

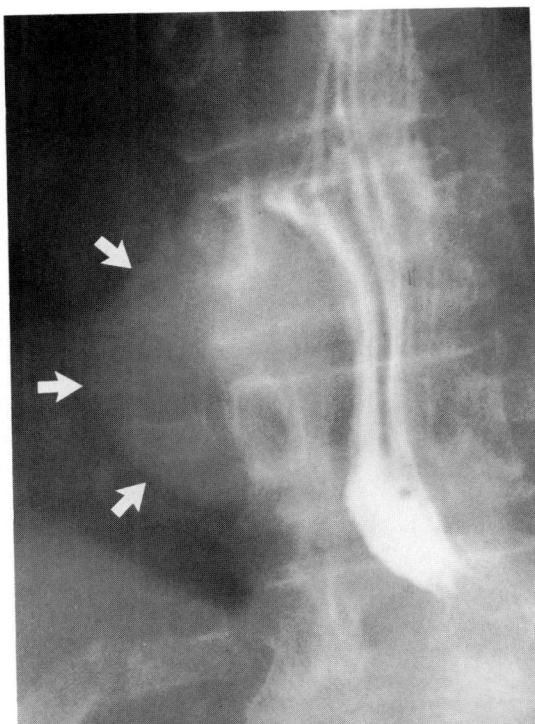

**Figure 27–16. Duplication cyst.** There is a large submucosal mass in the distal esophagus. The lateral border of the cyst *(arrows)* is readily visible where it abuts the right lung.

disease or multiple hamartoma syndrome, an autosomal dominant, hereditary disorder characterized by multiple hamartomatous malformations of ectodermal, mesodermal, and endodermal layers as well as by benign or malignant tumors of the skin, breast, gastrointestinal tract, and thyroid.[87, 88] Esophageal involvement may be manifested by innumerable tiny, hamartomatous polyps in the esophagus, producing a diffusely nodular mucosa on double contrast radiographs[87, 88] (Fig. 27–15). When the esophagus is involved by this disease, widespread polyposis of the gastrointestinal tract is usually present. However, Cowden's disease should be distinguished from other polyposis syndromes, which rarely involve the esophagus.

## Cysts

### Duplication Cyst

Most esophageal cysts are congenital duplication cysts caused by abnormal embryologic development in which nests of cells are sequestered from the primitive foregut.[89] Histologically, these cysts are lined by ciliated columnar or cuboidal epithelium.[89] Most patients with duplication cysts are asymptomatic, but symptoms may occasionally be caused by obstruction, bleeding, or infection of the cysts.[90, 91] Duplication cysts tend to be

located in the lower half of the posterior mediastinum, often projecting to the right of the esophagus. They usually appear on esophagrams as submucosal masses that are indistinguishable from solid mesenchymal tumors (Fig. 27–16). However, CT and MR imaging may be helpful for diagnosing these lesions. Because they are fluid-filled structures, the cysts typically have homogeneous low attenuation on CT scans and high signal intensity on T2-weighted MR images[92, 93] (Fig. 27–17).

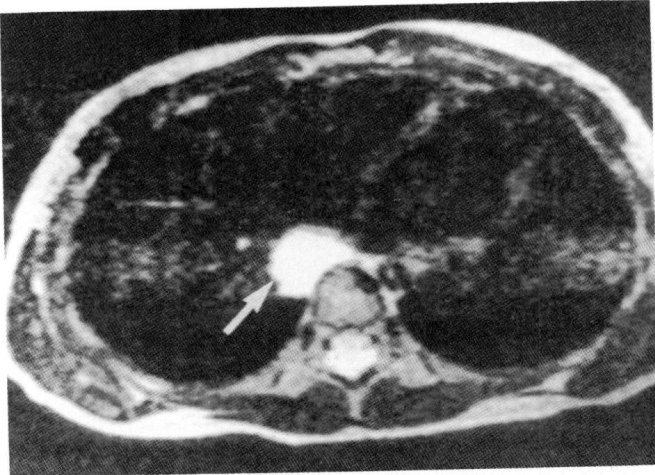

**Figure 27–17. Duplication cyst.** An axial T2-weighted MR image shows a fluid-filled, cystic mass *(arrow)* with high signal intensity in the right side of the mediastinum. (From Rafal RB, Markisz JA: Magnetic resonance imaging of an esophageal duplication cyst. Am J Gastroenterol 86:1809–1811, 1991. © 1991, the Williams & Wilkins Co., Baltimore.)

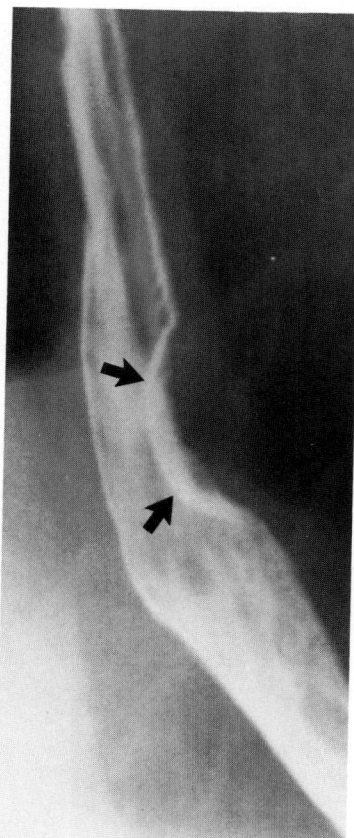

**Figure 27–18. Esophageal retention cyst.** The lesion is seen as a discrete submucosal mass *(arrows)* that is indistinguishable from other intramural lesions.

## *Retention Cyst*

Acquired esophageal cysts are much less common than congenital duplication cysts. They probably result from abnormal dilatation of columnar epithelium–lined mucous glands in the submucosa and are therefore called *esophageal retention cysts* or *mucoceles.*[94–97] Histologically, these cysts are lined by nonciliated, columnar, or cuboidal epithelium.[96] The pathogenesis of these lesions is uncertain, but it has been postulated that submucosal glands in the esophagus may become cystically dilated due to mechanical obstruction of the excretory ducts by mucous plugs or abnormally viscous mucus.[94, 95] This entity has sometimes been described as esophagitis cystica, but esophageal retention cyst is a more appropriate descriptive term, as only minimal inflammatory change may be present in these lesions.[94, 95]

Esophageal retention cysts may appear radiographically as solitary or, more commonly, multiple submucosal masses in the distal esophagus[94, 95, 97] (Fig. 27–18). As a result, the lesions cannot be distinguished from other submucosal tumors on barium studies. However, these patients usually are asymptomatic, so most esophageal retention cysts are incidental findings at autopsy.[94]

**Acknowledgment**

Figures 27–5B and C, 27–6B, 27–12 to 27–14, 27–16, and 27–18 are reproduced from Levine MS: Radiology of the Esophagus. Philadelphia: WB Saunders, 1989.

## References

1. Ming SC: Tumors of the esophagus and stomach. *In* Atlas of Tumor Pathology, Fascicle 7. Washington, DC: Armed Forces Institute of Pathology, 1973, pp 16–23.
2. Miller BJ, Murphy F, Lukie BE: Squamous cell papilloma of esophagus. Can J Surg 21:538–540, 1978.
3. Plachta A: Benign tumors of the esophagus: review of literature and report of 99 cases. Am J Gastroenterol 38:639–652, 1962.
4. Montesi A, Alessandro P, Graziani L, et al: Small benign tumors of the esophagus: radiological diagnosis with double-contrast examination. Gastrointest Radiol 8:207–212, 1983.
5. Samitz MH, Ackerman AB, Lantis LR: Squamous cell carcinoma arising at the site of oral florid papillomatosis. Arch Dermatol 96:286–290, 1967.
6. Toso G: Epithelial papillomas—benign or malignant? Laryngoscope 81:1524–1531, 1971.
7. Gilbert EF, Palladino A: Squamous papillomas of the uterine cervix: review of the literature and report of a giant papillary carcinoma. Am J Clin Pathol 46:115–121, 1966.
8. Napalkov NP, Pozharisski KM: Morphogenesis of experimental tumors of the esophagus. J Natl Cancer Inst 42:927–933, 1969.
9. Minielly JA, Harrison EG, Fontana RS, et al: Verrucous squamous cell carcinoma of the esophagus. Cancer 20:2078–2087, 1967.
10. Zeabart LE, Fabian J, Nord HJ: Squamous papilloma of the esophagus: a report of 3 cases. Gastrointest Endosc 25:18–20, 1979.
11. Nuwayhid NS, Ballard ET, Cotton R: Esophageal papillomatosis. Ann Otol Rhinol Laryngol 86:623–625, 1977.
12. Waterfall WE, Somers S, Desa DJ: Benign oesophageal papillomatosis. J Clin Pathol 31:111–115, 1978.
13. Walker JH: Giant papilloma of the thoracic esophagus. AJR 131:519–520, 1978.
14. Spin FP: Adenomas of the esophagus: a case report and review of the literature. Gastrointest Endosc 20:26–27, 1973.
15. McDonald GB, Brand DL, Thorning DR: Multiple adenomatous neoplasms arising in columnar-lined (Barrett's) esophagus. Gastroenterology 72:1317–1321, 1977.
16. Levine MS, Caroline D, Thompson JJ, et al: Adenocarcinoma of the esophagus: relationship to Barrett mucosa. Radiology 150:305–309, 1984.
17. Bleshman MH, Banner MP, Johnson RC, et al: The inflammatory esophagogastric polyp and fold. Radiology 128:589–593, 1978.
18. Staples DC, Knodell RG, Johnson LF: Inflammatory pseudotumor of the esophagus. Gastrointest Endosc 24:175–176, 1978.
19. Jones TB, Heller RM, Kirchner SG, et al: Inflammatory esophagogastric polyp in children. AJR 133:314–316, 1979.
20. Styles RA, Gibb SP, Tarshis A, et al: Esophagogastric polyps: radiographic and endoscopic findings. Radiology 154:307–311, 1985.
21. Ghahremani GG, Fisher MR, Rushovich AM: Prolapsing inflammatory pseudopolyp-fold complex of the oesophagogastric region. Eur J Radiol 4:47–51, 1984.
22. Rywlin AM, Ortega R: Glycogenic acanthosis of the esophagus. Arch Pathol 90:439–443, 1970.
23. Bender MD, Allison J, Cuartas F, et al: Glycogenic acanthosis of the esophagus: a form of benign epithelial hyperplasia. Gastroenterology 65:373–380, 1973.
24. Stern Z, Sharon P, Ligumsky M, et al: Glycogenic acanthosis of the esophagus: a benign but confusing endoscopic lesion. Am J Gastroenterol 74:261–263, 1980.

25. Ghahremani GG, Rushovich AM: Glycogenic acanthosis of the esophagus: radiographic and pathologic features. Gastrointest Radiol 9:93–98, 1984.

26. Glick SN, Teplick SK, Goldstein J, et al: Glycogenic acanthosis of the esophagus. AJR 139:683–688, 1982.

27. Berliner L, Redmond P, Horowitz L, et al: Glycogen plaques (glycogenic acanthosis) of the esophagus. Radiology 141:607–610, 1981.

28. Herschman BR, Uppaputhangkule V, Maas L, et al: Esophageal leukoplakia: a rare entity. JAMA 239:2021, 1978.

29. Graziani L, Bearzi I, Romagnoli A, et al: Significance of diffuse granularity and nodularity of the esophageal mucosa at double-contrast radiography. Gastrointest Radiol 10:1–6, 1985.

30. Itai Y, Kogure T, Okuyama Y, et al: Diffuse finely nodular lesions of the esophagus. AJR 128:563–566, 1977.

31. Itai Y, Kogure T, Okuyama Y, et al: Radiological manifestations of oesophageal involvement in acanthosis nigricans. Br J Radiol 49:592–593, 1976.

32. Attah EB, Hajdu SI: Benign and malignant tumors of the esophagus at autopsy. J Thorac Cardiovasc Surg 5:396–404, 1968.

33. Goldstein HM, Zornoza J, Hopens T: Intrinsic diseases of the adult esophagus: benign and malignant tumors. Semin Roentgenol 16:183–197, 1981.

34. Seremetis MG, Lyons WS, DeGuzman VC, et al: Leiomyomata of the esophagus: an analysis of 838 cases. Cancer 38:2166–2177, 1976.

35. Tsuzuki T, Kakegawa T, Arimori M, et al: Giant leiomyoma of the esophagus and cardia weighing more than 1,000 grams. Chest 60:396–399, 1971.

36. Barriero F, Seco JL, Molina J, et al: Giant esophageal leiomyoma with secondary megaesophagus. Surgery 7:436–439, 1976.

37. Wahlen T, Astedt B: Familial occurrence of coexisting leiomyomas of vulva and oesophagus. Acta Obstet Gynecol Scand 44:197–203, 1965.

38. Schapiro RL, Sandrock AR: Esophagogastric and vulvar leiomyomatosis: a new radiologic syndrome. J Can Assoc Radiol 24:184–187, 1973.

39. Ullal SR: Hypertrophic osteoarthropathy and leiomyoma of the esophagus. Am J Surg 123:356–358, 1972.

40. Rabushka LS, Fishman EK, Kuhlman JE, et al: Diffuse esophageal leiomyomatosis in a patient with Alport syndrome: CT demonstration. Radiology 179:176–178, 1991.

41. Totten RS, Stout AP, Humphreys GH, et al: Benign tumors and cysts of the esophagus. J Thorac Surg 25:606–622, 1953.

42. Glanz I, Grunebaum M: The radiological approach to leiomyoma of the oesophagus with a long-term follow-up. Clin Radiol 28:197–200, 1977.

43. Griff LC, Cooper J: Leiomyoma of the esophagus presenting as a mediastinal mass. AJR 101:472–481, 1967.

44. Gutman E: Posterior mediastinal calcification due to esophageal leiomyoma. Gastroenterology 63:665–666, 1972.

45. Ghahremani GG, Meyers MA, Port RB: Calcified primary tumors of the gastrointestinal tract. Gastrointest Radiol 2:331–339, 1978.

46. Itai Y, Shimazu H: Leiomyosarcoma of the oesophagus with dense calcification. Br J Radiol 51:469–471, 1978.

47. Schatzki R, Hawes LE: The roentgenological appearance of extramucosal tumors of the esophagus: analysis of intramural extramucosal lesions of the gastrointestinal tract in general. AJR 48:1–15, 1942.

48. Storey CF, Adams WC: Leiomyoma of the esophagus: a report of four cases and review of the surgical literature. Am J Surg 91:3–23, 1956.

49. Megibow AJ, Balthazar EJ, Hulnick DH, et al: CT evaluation of gastrointestinal leiomyomas and leiomyosarcomas. AJR 144:727–731, 1985.

50. Orchard JL, Peternel WW, Arena S: Remarkably large, benign esophageal tumor: difficulties in diagnosis. Dig Dis 22:266–269, 1977.

51. Schnug GE: Leiomyoma of the cardioesophageal junction. Arch Surg 65:342–346, 1952.

52. Godard JE, McCranie D: Multiple leiomyomas of the esophagus. AJR 117:259–262, 1973.

53. Shaffer HA: Multiple leiomyomas of the esophagus. Radiology 118:29–34, 1976.

54. Kabuto T, Taniguchi K, Iwanaga T, et al: Diffuse leiomyomatosis of the esophagus. Dig Dis Sci 25:388–391, 1980.

55. Fernandes JP, Mascarenhas MJ, daCosta JC, et al: Diffuse leiomyomatosis of the esophagus: a case report and review of the literature. Am J Dig Dis 20:684–690, 1975.

56. Zeller R, McLelland R, Meyers B, et al: Idiopathic muscular hypertrophy of the esophagus: a case report. Gastrointest Radiol 4:121–125, 1979.

57. Stein LA, Margulis AR: The spheroid sign: a new sign for accurate differentiation of intramural from extramural masses. AJR 123:420–426, 1975.

58. Levine MS, Kressel HY, Laufer I, et al: The tube esophagram: a technique for obtaining a detailed double-contrast examination of the esophagus. AJR 142:293–298, 1984.

59. Jang GC, Clouse ME, Fleischner FG: Fibrovascular polyp: a benign intraluminal tumor of the esophagus. Radiology 92:1196–1200, 1969.

60. Lolley D, Razzuk MA, Urschel HC: Giant fibrovascular polyp of the esophagus. Ann Thorac Surg 22:383–385, 1976.

61. Carter MM, Kulkarni MV: Giant fibrovascular polyp of the esophagus. Gastrointest Radiol 9:301–303, 1984.

62. Patel J, Kieffer RW, Martin M, et al: Giant fibrovascular polyp of the esophagus. Gastroenterology 87:953–956, 1984.

63. Beeler RC, Collins JN, Hall MF: Benign pedunculated tumors of the esophagus. AJR 60:466–470, 1948.

64. Cochet B, Hohl P, Sans M, et al: Asphyxia caused by laryngeal impaction of an esophageal polyp. Arch Otolaryngol 106:176–178, 1980.

65. Burrell M, Toffler R: Fibrovascular polyp of the esophagus. Am J Dig Dis 18:714–718, 1973.

66. Whitman GJ, Borkowski GP: Giant fibrovascular polyp of the esophagus: CT and MR findings. AJR 152:518–520, 1989.

67. Paskin DL, Hall JD, Cookson PJ: Granular cell myoblastoma: a comprehensive review of 15 years experience. Ann Surg 175:501–504, 1972.

68. Lack EE, Worsham GF, Callihan MD, et al: Granular cell tumor: a clinicopathologic study of 110 patients. J Surg Oncol 13:301–306, 1980.

69. Fisher ER, Wechsler H: Granular cell myoblastoma—a misnomer: electron microscopic and histochemical evidence concerning its Schwann cell derivation and nature (granular cell schwannoma). Cancer 15:936–954, 1962.

70. Gershwind ME, Chiat H, Addei KA, et al: Granular cell tumors of the esophagus. Gastrointest Radiol 2:327–330, 1978.

71. Johnston J, Helwig EB: Granular cell tumors of the gastrointestinal tract and perianal region: a study of 74 cases. Dig Dis Sci 26:807–816, 1981.

72. Rubesin S, Herlinger H, Sigal H: Granular cell tumors of the esophagus. Gastrointest Radiol 10:11–15, 1985.

73. Subramanyam K, Shannon CR, Patterson M, et al: Granular cell myoblastoma of the esophagus. J Clin Gastroenterol 6:113–118, 1984.

74. Radin DR, Zelner R, Ray MJ, et al: Multiple granular cell tumors of the skin and gastrointestinal tract. AJR 147:1305–1307, 1986.

75. Hyatt I, Kravitz SC: A benign tumor of the esophagus in an elderly female. Gastroenterology 37:774–778, 1959.

76. Engelking CF, Knight MD, Brauns WH, et al: Benign tumors of the esophagus: report of a case of neurofibroma. Arch Otolaryngol 52:150–156, 1950.

77. Kinnear JS: Report of case of intramural lipoma of the oesophagus. Br J Surg 42:439, 1955.

78. Nora PF: Lipoma of the esophagus. Am J Surg 108:353–356, 1964.

79. Allen MS, Talbot WH: Sudden death due to regurgitation of a pedunculated esophageal lipoma. J Thorac Cardiovasc Surg 54:756–758, 1967.

80. Liliequist B, Wiberg A: Pedunculated tumours of the oesophagus: two cases of lipoma. Acta Radiol Diagn (Stockh) 15:383–392, 1974.

81. Gandini G, Andreis M, Avataneo T, et al: A case of esophageal lipoma diagnosed by computed tomography. Diagn Radiol 10:55–60, 1985.

82. Grimes OF: Cavernous hemangioma of the esophagus. Dis Chest 48:384, 1965.

83. Loughry RW: Hemangiomas of the esophagus. Rocky Mt Med J 68:37–39, 1971.

84. Govoni AF: Hemangiomas of the esophagus. Gastrointest Radiol 7:113–117, 1982.

85. Dieter RA, Riker WL, Holinger P: Pedunculated esophageal hamartoma in a child. J Thorac Cardiovasc Surg 59:851–854, 1970.

86. Shah B, Unger L, Heimlich HJ: Hamartomatous polyp of the esophagus. Arch Surg 110:326–328, 1975.

87. Hauser H, Ody B, Plojoux O, et al: Radiological findings in multiple hamartoma syndrome (Cowden disease): a report of three cases. Radiology 137:317–323, 1980.

88. Chen YM, Ott DJ, Wu WC, et al: Cowden's disease: a case report and literature review. Gastrointest Radiol 12:325–329, 1987.

89. Vithespongse P, Blank S: Ciliated epithelial esophageal cyst. Am J Gastroenterol 56:436–440, 1971.

90. Gatzinsky P, Fasth S, Hansson G: Intramural oesophageal cyst with massive mediastinal bleeding. Scand J Thorac Cardiovasc Surg 12:143–145, 1978.

91. Whitaker JA, Deffenbaugh LD, Cooke AR: Esophageal duplication cyst. Am J Gastroenterol 73:329–332, 1980.

92. Bondestam S, Salo JA, Salonen OLM, et al: Imaging of congenital esophageal cysts in adults. Gastrointest Radiol 15:279–281, 1990.

93. Rafal RB, Markisz JA: Magnetic resonance imaging of an esophageal duplication cyst. Am J Gastroenterol 86:1809–1811, 1991.

94. Voirol MW, Welsh RA, Genet EF: Esophagitis cystica. Am J Gastroenterol 59:446–453, 1973.

95. Farman J, Rosen Y, Dallemand S, et al: Esophagitis cystica: lower esophageal retention cysts. AJR 128:495–496, 1977.

96. Edgin R, Mekhjian HS: Esophageal retention cyst: unusual cause for dysphagia. J Clin Gastroenterol 3:57–59, 1981.

97. Hover AR, Brady CE, Williams JR, et al: Multiple retention cysts of the lower esophagus. J Clin Gastroenterol 4:209–212, 1982.

# Esophageal Carcinoma

Marc S. Levine, M.D.
Robert A. Halvorsen, M.D.

## INTRODUCTION

Esophageal carcinoma constitutes only about 1% of all cancers and 7% of cancers in the gastrointestinal tract.[1] Nevertheless, esophageal carcinoma is a deadly disease with overall 5-year survival rates of less than 10%.[2] Most of these tumors are squamous cell carcinomas, but adenocarcinomas arising in Barrett's esophagus also account for a significant percentage of cases. Because these lesions have different clinical, radiographic, and pathophysiologic features, the chapter is divided into separate sections on squamous cell carcinoma and adenocarcinoma of the esophagus.

## SQUAMOUS CELL CARCINOMA

### Epidemiology

The development of squamous cell carcinoma of the esophagus is a multifactorial process associated with a variety of risk factors, including tobacco and alcohol consumption, other environmental carcinogens, nutritional deficiencies, and geographic location. The two major risk factors for esophageal cancer in the United States are tobacco and alcohol consumption.[3, 4] Furthermore, tobacco and alcohol have a synergistic effect, so those who smoke and drink have even higher rates of esophageal cancer.[5] Although tobacco smoke is known to contain a variety of carcinogens, the development of esophageal carcinoma in alcoholics may be related to other factors such as poor health and nutritional deficiencies. Some investigators believe that alcohol acts primarily by enhancing the carcinogenic effect of tobacco, so that heavy drinking increases the risk of developing esophageal cancer in smokers.

Esophageal cancer has striking geographic variations, with the highest incidences reported in China, Iran, South Africa, India, Sri Lanka, and France.[3] This high frequency of esophageal cancer in various parts of the world has been attributed primarily to environmental rather than hereditary factors. For example, nitrosamines and other nitroso compounds are potent carcinogens that occur in high concentration in the food and water supply of parts of northern China.[6] Epidemiologic studies in China and South Africa have shown that these areas also have unusually low levels of molybdenum in the soil.[6–8] Because molybdenum is required for the metabolism of nitrite to ammonia, low molybdenum levels in the soil could lead to accumulation of nitrites and potentially carcinogenic nitrosamines in plants consumed by humans. The high prevalence of esophageal cancer in parts of Saudi Arabia has been attributed to contamination of drinking water by impurities such as petroleum oils.[9] Other substances such as tannin, betel leaves, and asbestos fibers have also been implicated in the development of esophageal cancer.[10–12]

### Predisposing Conditions

Conditions that are thought to predispose patients to the development of squamous cell carcinoma of the esophagus include achalasia, lye strictures, head and neck tumors, celiac disease, Plummer-Vinson syndrome, radiation, and tylosis. Because of the increased risk of developing esophageal cancer, periodic surveillance has often been advocated for patients with these conditions.

#### Achalasia

Achalasia is thought to be a premalignant condition associated with a significantly increased risk of developing esophageal carcinoma. In various studies, the prevalence of esophageal cancer in patients with long-standing achalasia ranges from 2 to 8%.[13-16] Malignant degeneration may occur as a result of chronic stasis esophagitis caused by retained food and debris in a dilated, obstructed esophagus.[13, 15-17] Most patients have achalasia for at least 20 years before the development of cancer.[13, 16, 17] Unfortunately, a neoplastic lesion growing inside a massively dilated esophagus may not cause symptoms until it is an advanced, unresectable tumor.[16, 18] As a result, some authors believe that patients with long-standing achalasia should undergo annual radiologic or endoscopic screening examinations to detect developing cancers at the earliest possible stage.[13, 17, 18] However, other studies have failed to show an increased cancer risk in these patients.[19] Thus, not all investigators accept the need for surveillance.

## Lye Strictures

Patients with chronic lye strictures have a significantly increased risk of developing esophageal carcinoma. In various studies, the prevalence of cancer has ranged from 2 to 16%.[20, 21] Although the pathogenesis of these lesions is uncertain, it has been postulated that chronic inflammation and scarring from caustic esophagitis predispose patients to the development of esophageal carcinoma.[22] The average latent period between the ingestion of lye and the development of cancer is 40 to 45 years.[23, 24] These patients usually seek medical attention for recurrent or suddenly worsening dysphagia many years after lye ingestion.[25] Carcinomas arising in lye strictures have a better prognosis than most esophageal cancers, with 5-year survival rates of 8 to 33%.[23] This more favorable prognosis may be related to the presence of dense scar tissue surrounding the tumor, which prevents early invasion of adjacent mediastinal structures.[23-25] In any case, some investigators advocate periodic screening of patients with long-standing lye strictures to detect these cancers while they are still resectable. However, surveillance is not always feasible, as many patients who ingest lye are in socioeconomic groups least likely to be compliant.[24]

## Head and Neck Tumors

Patients with primary squamous cell carcinomas of the oral cavity, pharynx, and larynx have a significantly increased risk of developing separate primary esophageal carcinomas. In various studies, 2 to 8% of patients with head and neck tumors who underwent endoscopic surveillance have had synchronous esophageal cancers.[26-28] This association has been attributed to common predisposing factors, primarily smoking and drinking, as exposure to tobacco and alcohol considerably increases the risk of squamous cell carcinoma in both areas.[29] Radiologic or endoscopic evaluation of the esophagus has therefore been advocated in the initial work-up of all patients with head and neck tumors. Many of these synchronous esophageal cancers are small, asymptomatic lesions, so screening examinations may detect these tumors at an early stage, when they are potentially

curable.[28] Discovery of an advanced lesion in the esophagus is also important, as unnecessary radical head and neck surgery may be avoided in these patients. The risk of developing metachronous esophageal carcinomas is also significantly increased in patients with head and neck tumors. Thus, some form of ongoing surveillance is required to detect metachronous esophageal lesions.

## Celiac Disease

Celiac disease, or nontropical sprue, is thought to be associated with an increased risk of esophageal cancer.[30-32] The pathogenesis of cancer in these patients is uncertain, but it has been postulated that absorption of carcinogens occurs through an atrophic jejunal mucosa in patients with advanced celiac disease.[32] Most patients have long-standing disease, with malabsorption present for an average of 35 years before the development of cancer.[31] Some investigators therefore advocate radiologic or endoscopic surveillance of the esophagus in these patients.

## Plummer-Vinson Syndrome

Plummer-Vinson, or Paterson-Kelly, syndrome is characterized by iron deficiency anemia, glossitis, postcricoid webs, and dysphagia.[33] This syndrome has been described primarily in women of Scandinavian origin. In various studies, the prevalence of hypopharyngeal or esophageal carcinoma in patients with Plummer-Vinson syndrome has ranged from 4 to 16%.[33, 34] Almost all of these cancers are associated with postcricoid webs.[33, 34] Radiologic or endoscopic examinations are therefore required to differentiate webs from superimposed hypopharyngeal or esophageal carcinomas in these patients.

## Radiation

Esophageal cancer is a rare complication of chronic radiation injury to the esophagus. Most cases have occurred in the cervical or upper thoracic esophagus after radiation doses of 2000 to 5000 rad to the mediastinum or neck.[35, 36] However, the average latent period between radiation therapy and the development of cancer is about 30 years.[36] Thus, it is difficult to prove that these lesions are not coincidental cancers arising in a previously irradiated area.

## Tylosis

Tylosis (Howell-Evans syndrome) is a rare, hereditary, autosomal dominant disorder characterized by hyperkeratosis of the palms and soles, with thickening and fissuring of the skin. This disorder is associated with an extraordinarily high risk of developing esophageal cancer.[37-39] In one study, 95% of patients with tylosis had esophageal cancer by age 65.[38] Most of these patients are found to have advanced, unresectable tumors at the time of clinical presentation. However, asymptomatic individuals with tylosis may have hyperkeratotic esophageal plaques containing foci of dysplasia, intramucosal carcinoma, or invasive carcinoma.[39] Thus, periodic surveillance of asymptomatic family members has been advocated to detect these premalignant lesions before the development of overt carcinoma. Because of the inevitability of developing esophageal cancer, however, a prophylactic esophagectomy may be justified in these patients.

## Pathology

### Gross Features

Squamous cell carcinomas of the esophagus may appear grossly as infiltrating, polypoid, ulcerative, or superficial spreading lesions. Infiltrating lesions, the most common type, cause irregular narrowing and constriction of the lumen. Polypoid lesions are lobulated or fungating masses that protrude into the lumen. Primary ulcerative lesions are relatively flat masses in which the bulk of the tumor is replaced by ulceration. Less frequently, esophageal carcinoma may spread superficially without invading the deep muscle layers of the esophageal wall. The latter tumors tend to have a better prognosis than other, more invasive forms of esophageal cancer.

### Histologic Features

About 80 to 90% of malignant tumors in the esophagus are squamous cell carcinomas, and the remaining 10 to 20% are adenocarcinomas arising in Barrett's mucosa. Other rare esophageal malignancies are discussed in Chapter 29.

At the time of clinical presentation, most squamous cell carcinomas of the esophagus are advanced lesions that have already invaded regional lymph nodes or other local or distant structures. As a result, these tumors have a dismal prognosis, with overall 5-year survival rates of less than 10%. In contrast, early esophageal cancers are relatively curable lesions, with 5-year survival rates approaching 90%.[40, 41] According to the Japanese Society for Esophageal Diseases, *early esophageal cancer* is defined histologically as cancer limited to the mucosa or submucosa without lymph node involvement.[42] Most of these cases have been reported in the Chinese literature as a result of mass screening of the adult population because of the high incidence of esophageal cancer in that country.[6, 40, 41]

Considerable confusion exists in the literature regarding the terminology for "early" cancer. Early esophageal cancer, superficial esophageal cancer, and small esophageal cancer are terms that have been used interchangeably to describe malignant esophageal tumors diagnosed at an early stage. However, these lesions should not be considered synonymous, as they have different histopathologic features that may dramatically alter the prognosis of this disease. According to the Japanese Society for Esophageal Diseases, *superficial esophageal cancer* is also confined to the mucosa or submucosa, but unlike patients with early esophageal cancer, patients with superficial disease may have lymph node metastases.[42]

*Small esophageal cancer* is a term used to describe tumors less than 3.5 cm in size, regardless of the depth of invasion or the presence or absence of lymph node metastases.[43, 44] Previous studies have shown that the 5-year survival for esophageal cancer decreases dramatically when regional lymph nodes are involved by tumor.[45, 46] Thus, some superficial or small esophageal cancers may be early lesions histologically, whereas others may have invaded regional lymph nodes, with a prognosis comparable to that of advanced esophageal cancer.[44, 46]

### Distribution

Squamous cell carcinomas of the esophagus have a relatively even distribution in the upper, middle, and distal thirds of the esophagus.[45, 47] Unlike adenocarcinomas arising in Barrett's mucosa, squamous cell carcinomas of the distal esophagus rarely invade the stomach, and there is usually a discrete segment of normal esophagus between the tumor and the gastric cardia.

### Routes of Spread

Esophageal carcinoma may invade local, regional, or distant structures by various pathways, including direct extension, lymphatic spread, and hematogenous metastases.

### Direct Extension

Because the esophagus lacks a serosa and is attached to neighboring structures by only a loose adventitia, there is no anatomic barrier to prevent spread of tumor into the adjacent mediastinum. As a result, esophageal cancer has a marked tendency to invade contiguous structures in the neck or chest, such as the thyroid, larynx, trachea, bronchi (usually the left main bronchus), aorta, thoracic duct, lung, pericardium, and diaphragm.[45, 47] The tracheobronchial tree is a particularly common site of involvement, and tracheoesophageal or esophagobronchial fistulas develop in 5 to 10% of patients with esophageal cancer.[48, 49] Rarely, aortoesophageal fistulas may occur as a terminal complication of esophageal cancer due to aortic invasion by tumor.[50]

### Lymphatic Spread

Lymphatic metastases are found in 67 to 75% of patients with esophageal cancer.[51, 52] Because the esophagus contains a rich network of interconnecting lymphatic channels, lymphatic spread from esophageal cancer is unpredictable, with "jump" metastases to lymph nodes in the neck or mediastinum often occurring in the absence of segmental lymph node involvement.[52, 53] Submucosal esophageal lymphatics also communicate subdiaphragmatically with paracardial, lesser curvature, and celiac nodes in the upper abdomen, and these nodal groups may be involved by tumor in 25 to 50% of patients with esophageal cancer.[51-53] Although tumors in the distal esophagus are more likely to metastasize to the abdomen, lymphatic spread of cancers in the upper or midesophagus may also result in metastases to celiac or other abdominal lymph nodes.[51, 52]

Discrete lymphatic metastases or satellite nodules are found in the esophagus at autopsy in about 50% of patients with esophageal cancer.[52] These lesions should be distinguished pathologically from rare double primary carcinomas of the esophagus.[54, 55] However, it may be impossible to determine whether two discrete lesions represent synchronous primary tumors or a single cancer with lymphatic dissemination.

Between 2 and 15% of patients dying of esophageal cancer have gastric metastases at autopsy.[56] These lesions probably result from tumor emboli that seed the gastric fundus via submucosal esophageal lymphatics extending subdiaphragmatically to the stomach.[56, 57] In such cases, the primary esophageal cancer may be located a considerable distance from the gastroesophageal junction, with a normal esophageal segment below the lesion.

## Hematogenous Metastases

Hematogenous, or blood-borne, metastases are often found in patients with advanced esophageal carcinoma. The most common sites of metastases are the lungs, liver, adrenals, kidneys, pancreas, peritoneum, and bones.

## Clinical Aspects

Most patients with esophageal cancer develop dysphagia only when the lumen of the esophagus has been reduced by 50 to 75% of its normal circumference.[45, 47] By that time, malignant invasion of periesophageal lymph nodes or surrounding mediastinal structures has usually occurred.[45] Thus, most patients have advanced, unresectable tumors at the time of diagnosis.

Dysphagia is by far the most common complaint in patients with esophageal cancer.[45, 58] Dysphagia is usually present for a period of 2 to 4 months before these patients seek medical attention.[45] Some patients can accurately localize the level of obstruction, but others may have a sensation of blockage referred to the pharynx by a cancer in the middle or distal third of the esophagus.[47] The esophagus should therefore be carefully evaluated in all patients with unexplained pharyngeal dysphagia to rule out an esophageal cancer below the subjective site of obstruction.

Other common presenting findings include odynophagia, anorexia, weight loss, and persistent substernal chest pain unrelated to swallowing. The latter finding is a poor prognostic sign that suggests mediastinal invasion.[47] Patients with esophageal cancer occasionally may have guaiac-positive stool or iron deficiency anemia due to occult bleeding from the friable surface of the tumor.[45] However, frank hematemesis is uncommon.[59, 60] Rarely, fatal hemorrhage may result from an aortoesophageal fistula.[61, 62] The latter patients may have minimal hematemesis before the sudden development of massive hemorrhage, shock, and death.

Other patients with esophageal cancer may develop hoarseness as a result of direct extension of tumor into the larynx or involvement of the recurrent laryngeal nerve.[45] Recurrent aspiration may lead to a chronic cough. However, the presence of a paroxysmal cough on swallowing should suggest the development of a malignant tracheoesophageal or esophagobronchial fistula. Rarely, patients with esophageal cancer may have anorexia, weight loss, or other signs of widespread malignancy without experiencing dysphagia, so that localizing esophageal symptoms are not always present.[47]

## Endoscopic Findings

When adequate biopsy specimens and brushings are obtained, endoscopy has an overall sensitivity of 95 to 100% in diagnosing esophageal carcinoma.[63–65] Brush cytology is particularly helpful when the esophageal lumen is so compromised by tumor that adequate biopsy specimens cannot be obtained. Detection of suspicious lesions on barium studies should therefore lead to early endoscopy for a definitive histologic diagnosis. Occasionally, however, it is possible to detect small lesions by endoscopy that are missed radiographically.[64, 66] For this reason, a normal barium study should not preclude endoscopy when esophageal cancer is suspected on clinical grounds.

## Radiographic Findings

### Early Esophageal Cancer

Double contrast esophagography has been widely advocated as the best radiologic technique for diagnosing early esophageal cancer. Unfortunately, the increased sensitivity of this technique has resulted in lower specificity, as more subtle abnormalities are suspected of representing cancer.[43] Nevertheless, it is probably best to accept a certain percentage of false-positive findings to avoid missing early lesions. The diagnosis of esophageal cancer should therefore be considered for any lesion that does not have a classically benign appearance. Although the radiologic diagnosis of early esophageal cancer is generally limited by the late onset of symptoms, some patients do experience dysphagia, upper gastrointestinal bleeding, or other esophageal symptoms while the tumor is still at an early stage.[43, 67, 69–69] Thus, double contrast esophagrams may occasionally demonstrate early cancers in symptomatic patients. When a lesion is detected on barium studies, endoscopy and biopsy are required for a definitive diagnosis.

Early esophageal cancers classically appear radiographically as small, protruded lesions less than 3.5 cm in diameter.[43, 67, 69–71] They may be plaque-like lesions (often with central ulceration) (Fig. 28–1) or small, sessile polyps with a smooth or slightly lobulated contour (Fig. 28–2). Other early cancers may be superficial or

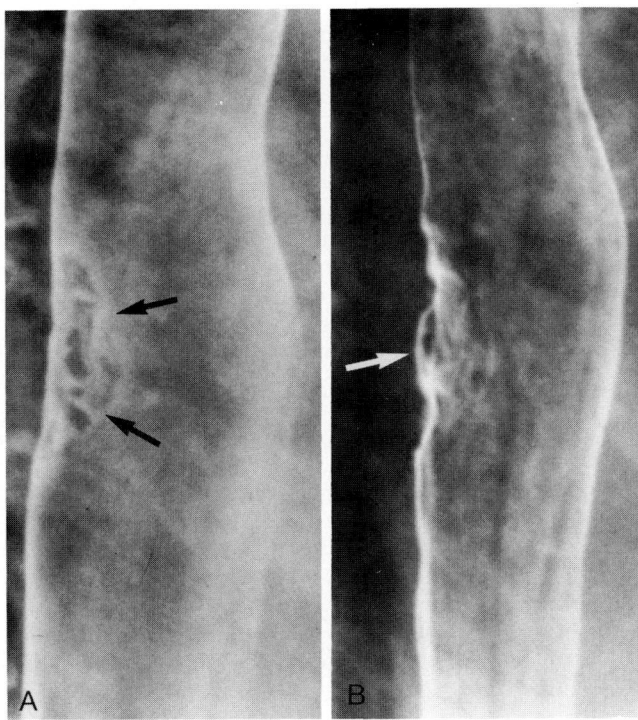

**Figure 28–1. Early esophageal cancer. A.** An en face view from a double contrast esophagram shows a poorly defined lesion *(arrows)* in the midesophagus. **B.** However, a tangential view reveals a characteristic plaque-like lesion containing a central area of ulceration *(arrow).*

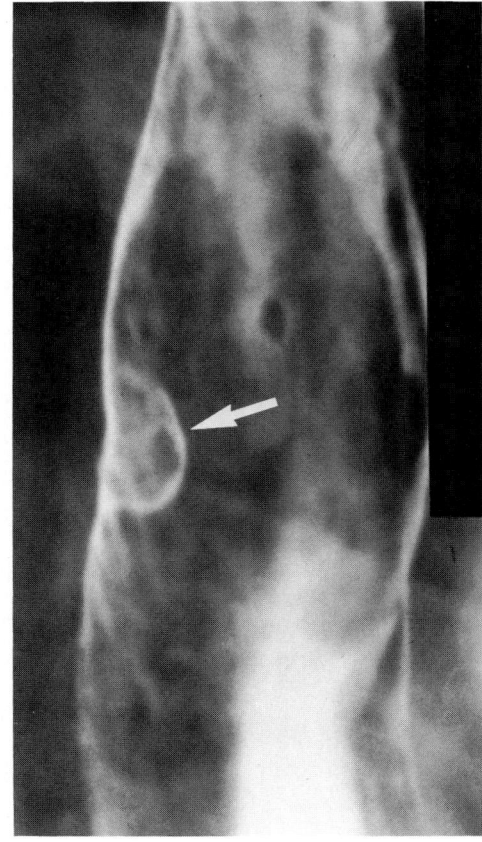

**Figure 28–2. Early esophageal cancer.** The lesion appears radiographically as a small, sessile polyp *(arrow)* in the midesophagus. (Courtesy of Seth N. Glick, M.D., Philadelphia, PA.)

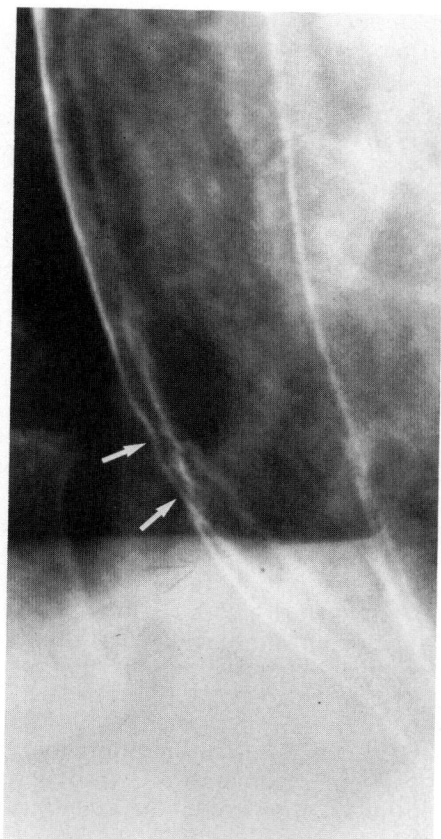

**Figure 28–3. Early esophageal cancer.** There is focal irregularity of the esophageal wall *(arrows)* without a discrete lesion. (Courtesy of Akiyoshi Yamada, M.D., Tokyo, Japan.)

depressed lesions, causing focal irregularity, nodularity, or ulceration of the mucosa[72–74] (Fig. 28–3). When a lesion is detected on double contrast studies, multiple projections should be obtained to determine its appearance both en face and in profile. Tangential views are particularly helpful for assessing the degree of intraluminal protrusion and the presence of associated ulceration (see Fig. 28–1B).

Although most early esophageal cancers appear radiographically as focal lesions, superficial spreading carcinoma is an unusual form of esophageal cancer that extends longitudinally in the wall without invading beyond the mucosa or submucosa. Superficial spreading carcinomas are manifested radiographically by tiny, coalescent nodules or plaques, causing nodularity or granularity of the mucosa[69, 72, 74, 75] (Fig. 28–4). These lesions may be relatively localized or may involve a considerable surface area of the esophagus.

Early esophageal cancers are generally thought to be small lesions, but some early cancers may appear radiographically as relatively large intraluminal masses more than 3.5 cm in size[69, 76] (Fig. 28–5). Such lesions may be indistinguishable from advanced carcinomas. Thus, early esophageal cancers are not necessarily small cancers, as they may undergo considerable intraluminal or intramural growth and still be classified histologically as early lesions.

## Advanced Carcinoma

### Plain Films

Nearly half of all patients with advanced esophageal cancers have abnormal chest radiographs.[77] The most common findings include mediastinal widening; a hilar, retrohilar, or retrocardiac mass; tracheal deviation; a widened retrotracheal stripe; and an air-fluid level in the esophagus[77–79] (Fig. 28–6). Anterior bowing of the posterior tracheal wall or thickening of the retrotracheal stripe beyond 3 mm in width may result from lymphatic infiltration or direct invasion of the retrotracheal area by tumor.[78, 79] Distally obstructing cancers may be recognized by an air-fluid level in the esophagus. However, esophageal obstruction by achalasia or benign strictures may also be manifested by anterior tracheal bowing or an esophageal air-fluid level.

### Barium Studies

Advanced esophageal carcinomas may appear on barium studies as infiltrating, polypoid, ulcerative, or varicoid lesions[80, 81] (Fig. 28–7). However, many esophageal cancers have mixed morphologic features, so there is considerable overlap in the classification of these tumors.

Infiltrating esophageal carcinomas are characterized by irregular narrowing and constriction of the lumen associated with a nodular or ulcerated mucosa and abrupt, well-defined proximal and distal borders (see Fig. 28–7A). Occasionally, these cancers have shelf-like,

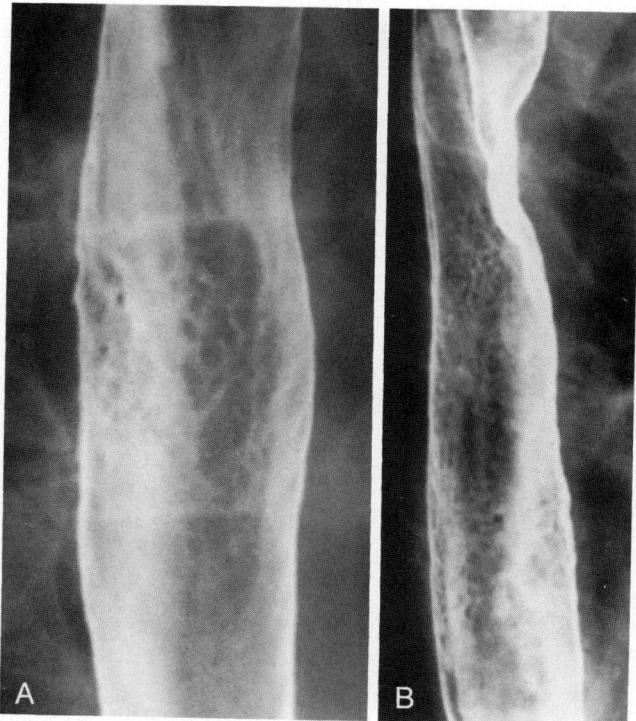

**Figure 28–4. Superficial spreading carcinoma. A.** There is focal nodularity in the midesophagus due to tiny, coalescent nodules and plaques. **B.** In another patient with a more extensive lesion, there is diffuse granularity of the mucosa.

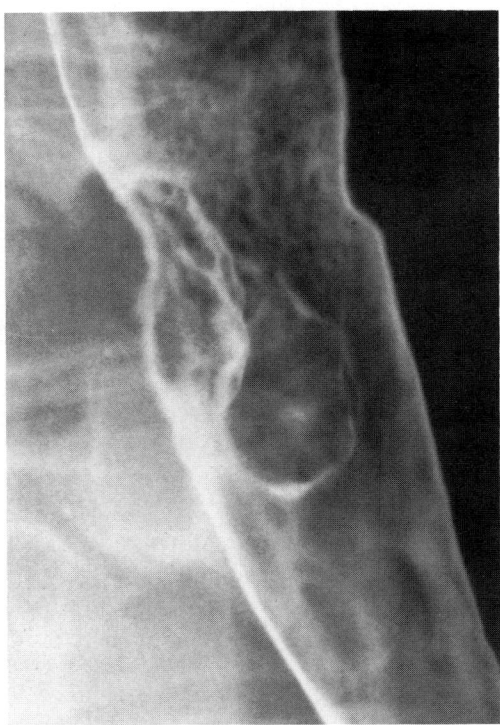

**Figure 28–5. Early esophageal cancer.** This lesion appears as a relatively large polypoid mass indistinguishable from an advanced carcinoma.

overhanging borders, producing true annular lesions analogous to annular carcinomas of the colon[80] (Fig. 28–8A). However, other infiltrating lesions may have more gradual, tapered borders, occasionally mimicking the appearance of benign strictures[81] (Fig. 28–8B). Infiltrating lesions may eventually cause partial or even complete esophageal obstruction, with proximal dilatation and minimal or no emptying of barium into the stomach.

Polypoid carcinomas appear as lobulated or fungating intraluminal masses, usually more than 3.5 cm in size[80, 81] (see Fig. 28–7B). They often contain areas of ulceration as a result of tumor necrosis. Bulky lesions may cause significant luminal encroachment and obstruction. However, squamous cell carcinomas are not generally polypoid, so other types of esophageal malignancy, such as adenocarcinoma and spindle cell carcinoma, should be suspected in these patients.

Primary ulcerative carcinomas are those in which the bulk of the tumor mass is replaced by ulceration. When viewed in profile, these lesions appear as well-defined meniscoid ulcers, with a radiolucent rim of tumor surrounding the ulcer[82] (see Fig. 28–7C). As in the stomach, this rim of tumor may be obscured when the lesions are detected en face. Multiple projections should therefore be obtained to demonstrate these lesions in profile.

Varicoid carcinomas are those in which submucosal spread of tumor results in thickened, tortuous or serpiginous longitudinal filling defects, mimicking the appearance of esophageal varices[83–85] (see Fig. 28–7D). However, these entities can usually be differentiated at fluoroscopy (see later section on differential diagnosis). Although varicoid carcinomas are uncommon, submucosal extension of tumor not infrequently produces a focal varicoid pattern adjacent to an obvious squamous cell carcinoma. In one study, a varicoid pattern was seen radiographically in 40% of patients with esophageal cancer.[86]

Mediastinal involvement by advanced esophageal car-

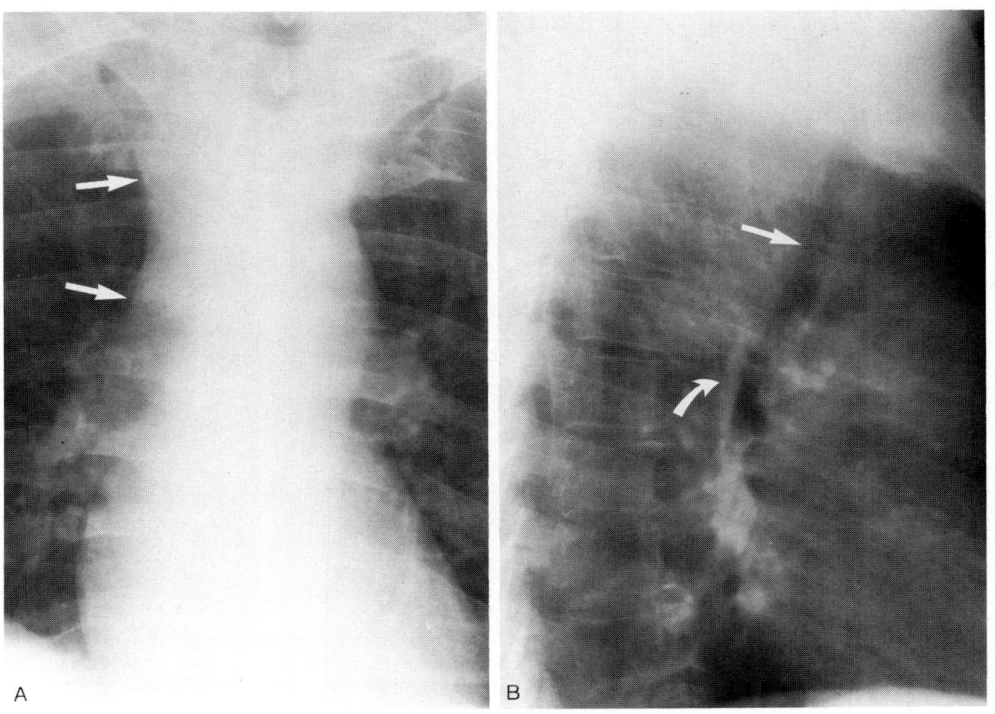

**Figure 28–6. Advanced esophageal carcinoma with abnormal chest radiographs. A.** A posteroanterior chest film shows widening of the superior mediastinum on the right *(arrows)*. **B.** A lateral film shows increased soft tissue density in the retrotracheal space with slight anterior bowing of the trachea *(straight arrow)* by an advanced esophageal cancer in this region. Also note thickening of the retrotracheal stripe inferiorly *(curved arrow)* due to direct invasion of this area by tumor. (**A** and **B** courtesy of Wallace T. Miller, M.D., Philadelphia, PA.)

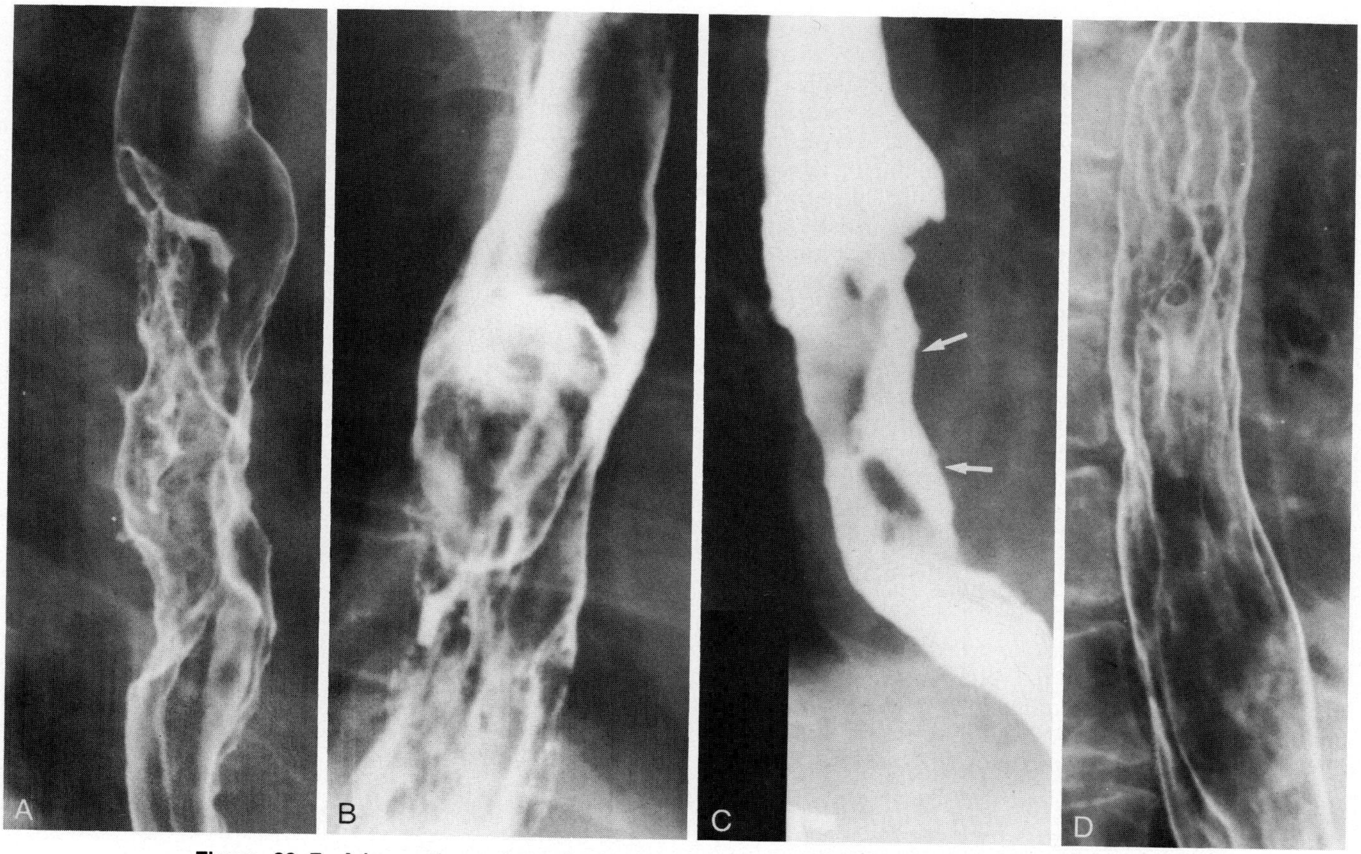

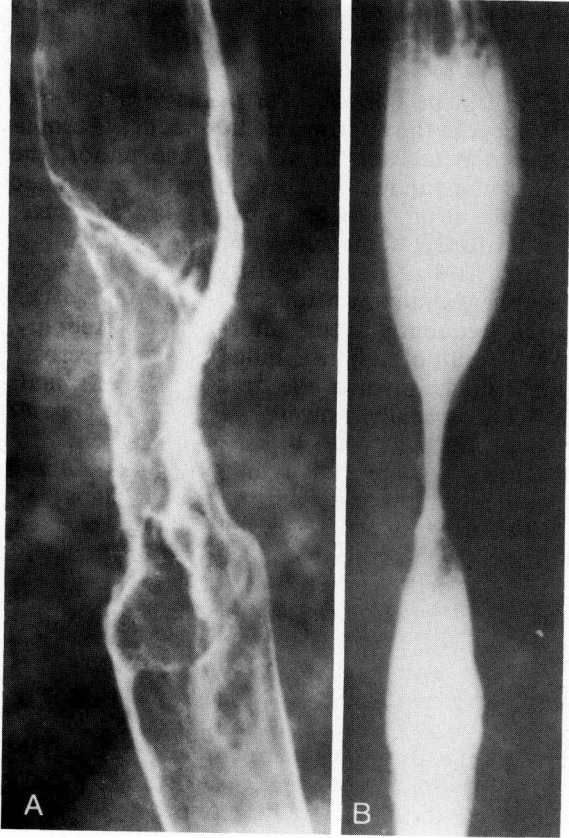

**Figure 28–7. Advanced esophageal carcinoma: patterns of tumor. A.** Infiltrating lesion. **B.** Polypoid lesion. **C.** Ulcerative lesion with a large, meniscoid ulcer *(arrows)* and a radiolucent rim of tumor. **D.** Varicoid lesion with thickened, tortuous folds in the midesophagus due to submucosal spread of tumor. (**D** courtesy of Akiyoshi Yamada, M.D., Tokyo, Japan.)

**Figure 28–8. Other forms of infiltrative esophageal carcinoma. A.** This lesion has an annular appearance with shelf-like proximal and distal borders. **B.** In another patient, the cancer is manifested by a relatively smooth, tapered area of narrowing that could be mistaken for a benign stricture.

cinoma can also be recognized on barium studies. Lymphatic spread of tumor to paratracheal, subcarinal, or paraesophageal lymph nodes may lead to extrinsic compression or displacement of the esophagus, often at a considerable distance from the primary lesion[51] (Fig. 28–9). Mediastinal lymphadenopathy is usually characterized by a smooth, extrinsic esophageal impression with gently sloping, obtuse borders. This finding almost always indicates an advanced, unresectable lesion.

Lymphatic metastases from esophageal cancer may be manifested by discrete implants adjacent to or remote from the primary lesion. These metastases may appear radiographically as small polypoid, plaque-like, or ulcerated lesions separated from the main tumor by normal intervening mucosa[87] (Fig. 28–10). Although most of these satellite lesions represent lymphatic metastases from the original cancer, the possibility of two primary carcinomas (double primaries) should be considered when the lesions are separated by an unusually long segment of normal mucosa.[54]

Squamous cell metastases to the stomach usually appear radiographically as solitary, large submucosal masses in the gastric fundus.[56, 57] These lesions often contain areas of ulceration and may resemble ulcerated leiomyomas or leiomyosarcomas (Fig. 28–11). Less fre-

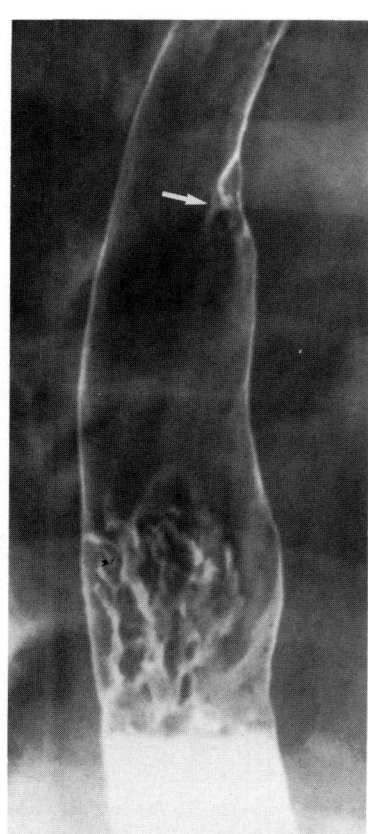

**Figure 28–10. Advanced esophageal carcinoma with a discrete lymphatic metastasis.** This patient has a large, ulcerated cancer in the midesophagus with a discrete metastatic implant *(arrow)* separated from the main lesion by normal intervening mucosa. The implant appears as a plaque-like lesion.

quently, they can be mistaken for primary gastric carcinomas.[88] Because the appropriate treatment for esophageal cancer depends on the stage of the tumor, the gastric cardia and fundus should be carefully examined radiographically in all patients with esophageal cancer to rule out unsuspected metastases to the stomach.

About 5 to 10% of patients with esophageal cancer develop esophageal-airway fistulas[48, 49] (Fig. 28–12). This complication frequently occurs after radiation therapy, probably as a result of radiation-induced tumor necrosis. Most such fistulas involve the trachea or left main bronchus.[49] Occasionally, however, a locally aggressive esophageal cancer may lead to the development of a necrotic, tumor-containing cavity in the mediastinum or lung that communicates directly with the esophagus (Fig. 28–13). When an esophageal-airway fistula is suspected, the radiologic examination should be performed with barium rather than meglumine diatrizoate (Gastrografin), as water-soluble contrast agents are hyperosmolar and may draw fluid into the lungs if a fistula is present, causing severe pulmonary edema.

Esophageal-airway fistulas are usually recognized on esophagrams by the presence of barium in the bronchi or distal trachea. In many cases, the origin of the fistulous track is identified within an obvious, infiltrating carcinoma (see Fig. 28–12B). Once barium has entered

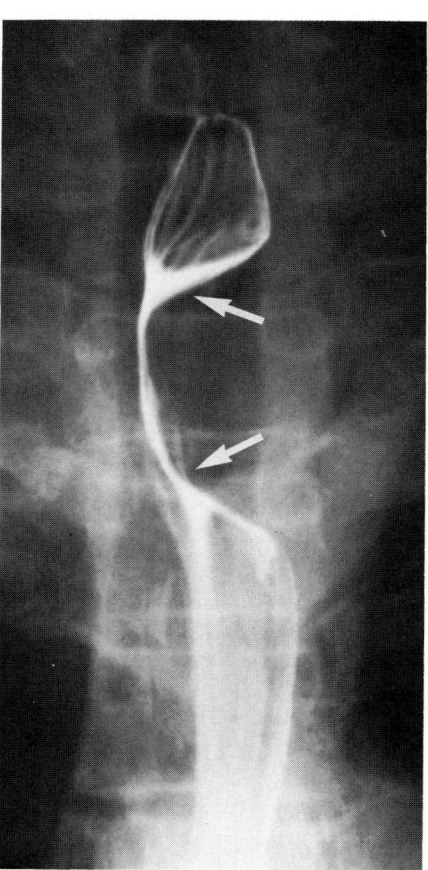

**Figure 28–9. Advanced esophageal carcinoma with mediastinal adenopathy.** There is a smooth, extrinsic area of mass effect on the left lateral wall of the upper thoracic esophagus *(arrows)* by mediastinal adenopathy from a distal esophageal cancer that is not shown on the film.

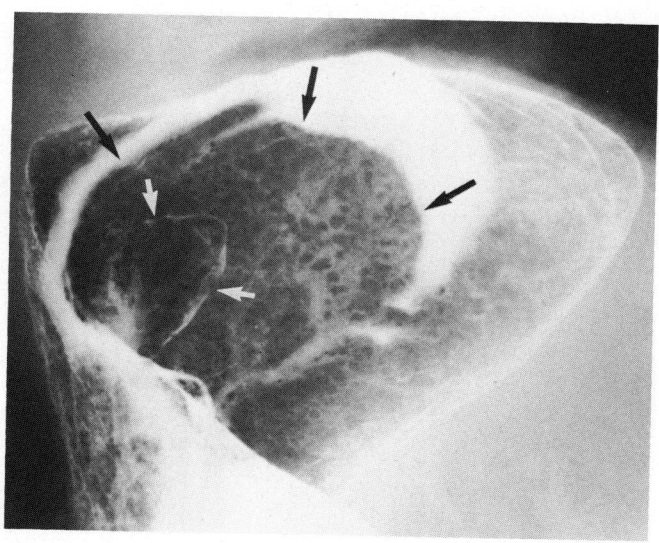

**Figure 28–11. Advanced esophageal carcinoma with a squamous cell metastasis to the stomach.** There is a giant submucosal mass *(black arrows)* in the gastric fundus, containing a triangular area of central ulceration *(white arrows).* An ulcerated leiomyosarcoma could produce similar findings. (From Glick SN, Teplick SK, Levine MS: Squamous cell metastases to the gastric cardia. Gastrointest Radiol 10:339–344, 1985.)

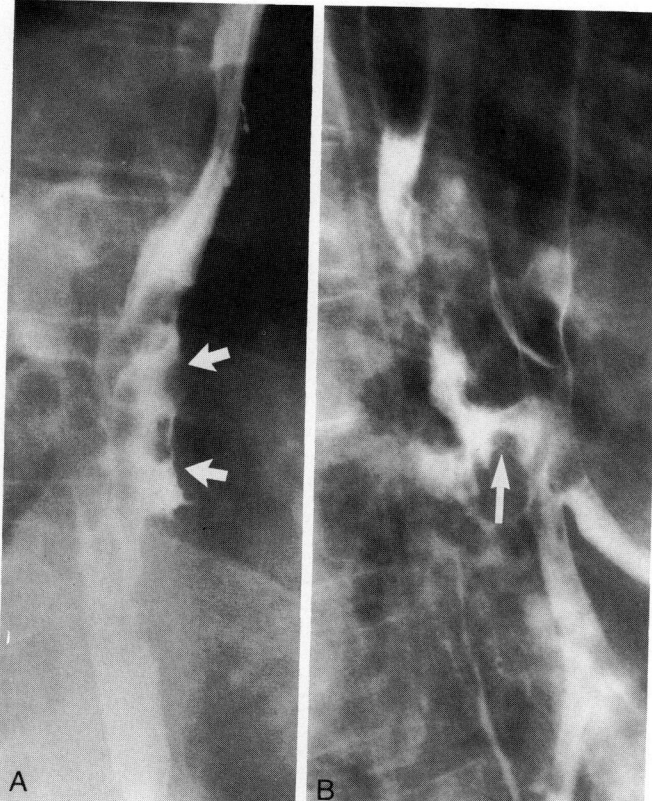

**Figure 28–12. Advanced esophageal carcinoma with a tracheoesophageal fistula. A.** An ulcerative esophageal carcinoma *(arrows)* is present in the midesophagus. **B.** A second esophagram 4 months after radiation therapy shows partial regression of the tumor with the development of a tracheoesophageal fistula *(arrow).*

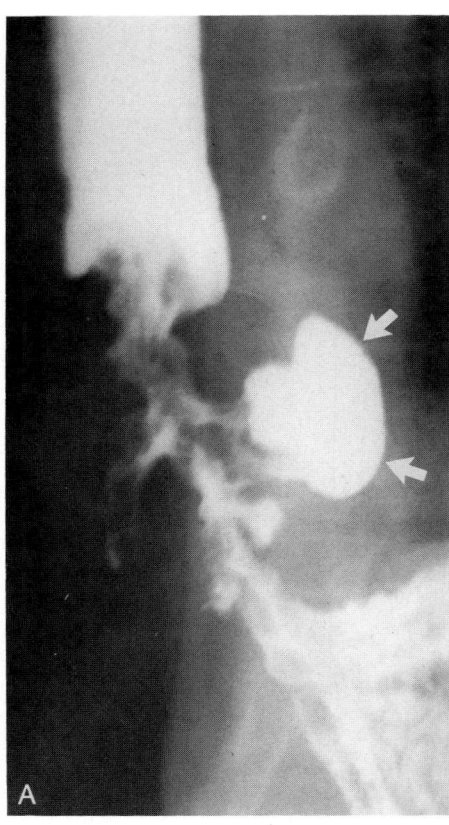

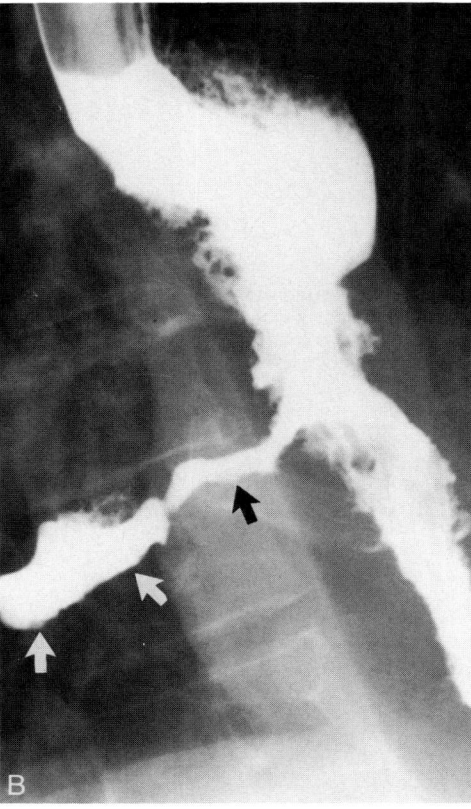

**Figure 28–13. Advanced esophageal carcinoma with fistulas to the mediastinum and lung.** In these two cases, there is direct communication between the cancer and necrotic, tumor-containing cavities *(arrows)* in the mediastinum **(A)** and the right lung **(B)**.

the trachea or left main bronchus, however, it can be coughed up into the proximal trachea or larynx, so that delayed overhead radiographs may erroneously suggest tracheobronchial aspiration. When an esophageal-airway fistula is suspected, the initial swallow should therefore be performed in a lateral projection with a video recording of the hypopharynx to differentiate a fistula from aspiration.

## Associated Conditions

### Achalasia

Esophageal carcinomas arising in patients with achalasia usually appear radiographically as polypoid masses in the middle or, less commonly, distal third of the esophagus[13, 14, 18] (Fig. 28–14). Because these lesions often develop in a massively dilated esophagus, they can reach enormous sizes, producing bulky intraluminal masses that have a fungating or "cauliflower" appearance.[18] Nevertheless, the lesions may be obscured by retained fluid and debris in a dilated, partially obstructed esophagus.[16–18] Careful esophageal lavage with a soft rubber catheter may therefore be required to cleanse the esophagus before performing the radiologic examination.

### Lye Strictures

The development of a lye cancer may be manifested radiographically by increasing stenosis, mass effect, nodularity, or ulceration within a pre-existing lye stricture[25] (Fig. 28–15). The underlying strictures are often located

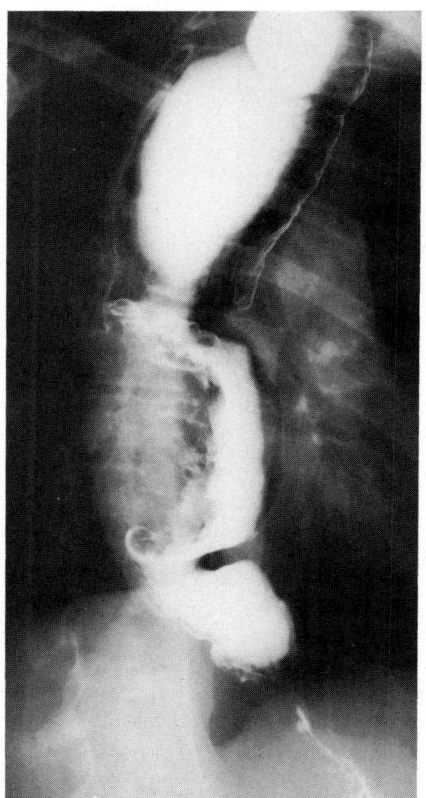

**Figure 28–14. Advanced esophageal carcinoma associated with achalasia.** There is a large, fungating mass in the midesophagus in a patient with long-standing achalasia. Note the beak-like narrowing of the distal esophagus caused by incomplete relaxation of the lower esophageal sphincter.

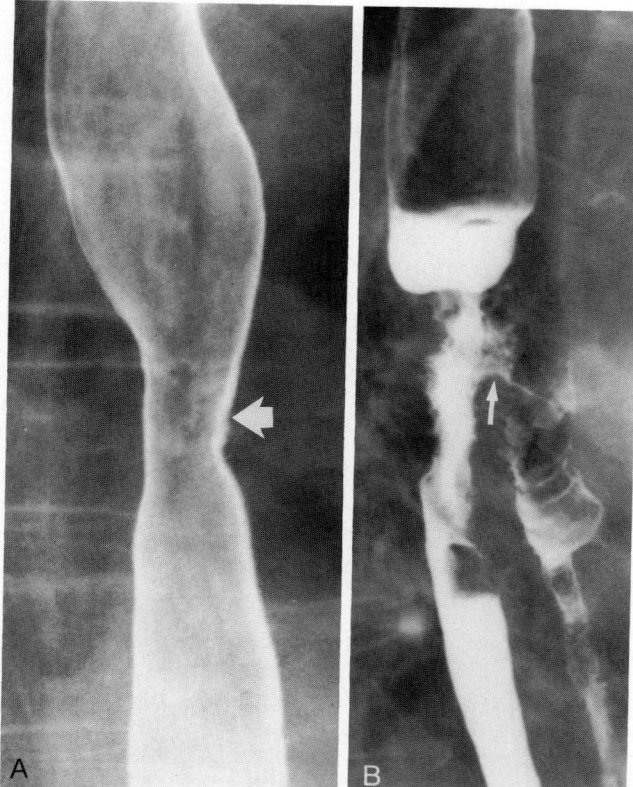

**Figure 28–15. Advanced esophageal carcinoma arising in a lye stricture. A.** The initial double contrast esophagram shows a focal stricture *(arrow)* in the midesophagus due to previous lye ingestion. Note the superficial ulceration and nodularity of the mucosa in the region of the stricture. The patient refused surgery at this time. **B.** Another study 2 years later shows an advanced, infiltrating carcinoma at the site of the previous stricture with an esophagobronchial fistula *(arrow).*

in the region of the tracheal bifurcation, so lye cancers may be complicated by the development of tracheo-esophageal or esophagobronchial fistulas.[23] Any change in the appearance of a chronic lye stricture should therefore be evaluated by endoscopy with multiple biopsy specimens and brushings to rule out a superimposed carcinoma.

### Tylosis

When patients with tylosis develop esophageal symptoms, they usually have advanced esophageal carcinomas, manifested radiographically by annular, infiltrating, or plaque-like lesions.[39] Occasionally, however, asymptomatic patients with tylosis may have discrete hyperkeratotic plaques containing one or more foci of dysplasia or intramucosal carcinoma.[39] These lesions may appear on esophagrams as large, well-defined plaques with normal intervening mucosa[39] (Fig. 28–16).

## ADENOCARCINOMA

Primary adenocarcinoma of the esophagus has traditionally been considered a rare lesion, accounting for

only 1 to 4% of all esophageal cancers.[89–92] Because most esophageal adenocarcinomas involve the gastro-esophageal junction or gastric fundus, they have generally been classified as primary gastric carcinomas secondarily invading the lower end of the esophagus.[89, 90] However, studies have shown that esophageal adenocarcinomas often spread distally to involve the gastric cardia or fundus.[93–96] Virtually all of these tumors are found to arise on a background of Barrett's mucosa in the esophagus. When these cases are included, adenocarcinoma accounts for 5 to 20% of all esophageal cancers.[95, 96] Nevertheless, many questions remain about the risk of malignant degeneration in Barrett's esophagus and the long-term management of patients with this condition.

## Epidemiology and Pathogenesis

Considerable attention has been focused on the relationship between esophageal adenocarcinoma and the columnar epithelium–lined or Barrett's esophagus. In various studies, 90 to 100% of all primary esophageal adenocarcinomas have been found to arise on a background of Barrett's mucosa.[95–97] Thus, not only is adenocarcinoma of the esophagus more common than has

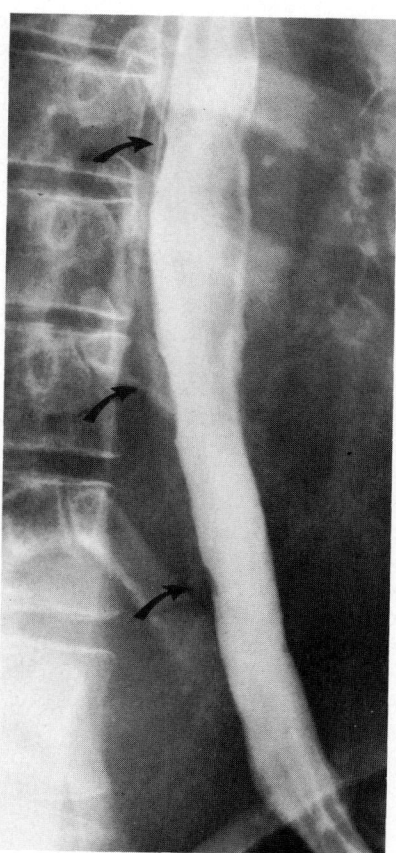

**Figure 28–16. Tylosis with hyperkeratotic plaques.** There are multiple discrete plaques *(arrows)* in the distal and midesophagus. These lesions were found to be hyperkeratotic plaques in a patient with long-standing tylosis. (From TP Munyer, AR Margulis, Tylosis, AJR, **136**, 5, 1026–1027, 1981. © by American Roentgen Ray Society.)

previously been recognized but also the vast majority of these tumors appear to result from malignant degeneration in Barrett's esophagus.

## Barrett's Esophagus

Barrett's esophagus is a well-recognized condition in which there is progressive columnar metaplasia of the distal esophagus due to long-standing gastroesophageal reflux and reflux esophagitis.[98–100] In various studies, the prevalence of Barrett's esophagus in patients with reflux esophagitis has ranged from 8 to 20%, with an overall prevalence of about 10%.[101–104] Histologically, the columnar epithelium in Barrett's esophagus is not simply gastric mucosa but a variety of intimately admixed epithelial patterns from the stomach and small bowel, including a gastric-fundic–type epithelium with parietal and chief cells, a junctional-type epithelium with cardiac mucous glands, and a specialized columnar-type epithelium with a villiform surface, mucous glands, and intestinal-like goblet cells.[105, 106] The clinical and radiographic aspects of Barrett's esophagus are presented in Chapter 24.

## Dysplasia-Carcinoma Sequence

Pathologic data strongly suggest that esophageal adenocarcinoma evolves through a sequence of progressively severe epithelial dysplasia in areas of pre-existing columnar metaplasia.[93, 97, 100, 107–111] These dysplastic or early carcinomatous changes can be recognized on endoscopic biopsy specimens or brushings. Many investigators therefore advocate periodic endoscopic surveillance with multiple biopsies and brushings at 6-month or yearly intervals for early detection of cancer in Barrett's esophagus.[97–101, 107–112] However, it is unclear what measures should be taken when endoscopy reveals dysplasia in these patients. Although the presence of high-grade dysplasia or intramucosal carcinoma may warrant an immediate esophagectomy in patients who are good surgical candidates, the frequency with which low-grade dysplasia progresses to invasive carcinoma is uncertain. Thus, many questions remain about the role of surveillance and its ultimate value in detecting early cancer in Barrett's esophagus.

Much less frequently, the development of cancer in Barrett's esophagus may result from an adenoma-carcinoma sequence similar to that found in the colon. Benign adenomatous polyps have occasionally been documented in Barrett's mucosa with or without focal areas of invasive adenocarcinoma.[95, 113, 114] Because malignant degeneration of these adenomas represents another potential pathway for the development of adenocarcinoma, endoscopic resection of adenomatous polyps in Barrett's esophagus may decrease the risk of cancer.

## Risk of Adenocarcinoma

Barrett's esophagus is thought to be a premalignant condition associated with a significantly increased risk of developing esophageal adenocarcinoma. In various series, the prevalence of adenocarcinoma in patients with Barrett's esophagus has ranged from 2.4 to 46.5%, with an overall prevalence of about 15%.[95, 101, 103, 104, 115, 116] However, prevalence data tend to exaggerate the risk of cancer, as most patients with Barrett's esophagus do not seek medical attention until the development of complications such as ulcers, strictures, or malignancy. Other studies of cancer-free patients with Barrett's esophagus who have been followed by endoscopy for a period of years provide lower estimates of the risk of developing cancer.[111, 117–119] Nevertheless, some of these prospective studies have found that the annual incidence of malignant transformation in Barrett's esophagus is 1 to 2% and that the overall risk of developing esophageal adenocarcinoma may be 125 times greater than that in the general population.[111, 119] Thus, most investigators accept the need for routine endoscopic surveillance.

## Relationship Between Scleroderma, Barrett's Esophagus, and Adenocarcinoma

Scleroderma, a connective tissue disease characterized by smooth muscle atrophy and fibrosis, affects the esophagus in about 75% of patients. Esophageal involvement is usually characterized by a patulous, incompetent lower esophageal sphincter and absent esophageal peristalsis with poor clearance of refluxed peptic acid from the esophagus once reflux has occurred. As a result, patients with scleroderma often have reflux esophagitis. Because of the severity of esophagitis, however, these individuals have an even greater risk of developing Barrett's esophagus than other patients with reflux disease. In one study, 37% of those with scleroderma who underwent endoscopy for reflux symptoms had biopsy-proven Barrett's esophagus.[120] Because Barrett's esophagus predisposes to esophageal adenocarcinoma, patients with scleroderma also appear to have an increased risk of developing esophageal cancer.[120, 121] Thus, scleroderma should indirectly be considered a premalignant condition in the esophagus.

## Pathology

### Gross Features

Adenocarcinomas arising in Barrett's mucosa appear grossly as infiltrating, polypoid, ulcerative, or varicoid lesions. These tumors tend to be located in the middle or, more commonly, distal third of the esophagus.[94–96] Unlike squamous cell carcinomas, adenocarcinomas of the distal esophagus frequently spread subdiaphragmatically to involve the gastric cardia or fundus.[93–96] In view of the traditional notion that adenocarcinomas at the gastroesophageal junction arise in the stomach,[89, 90] one might consider the possibility that these cases actually represent gastric carcinomas invading the distal esophagus and that the presence of Barrett's epithelium in the esophagus is a fortuitous, unrelated finding. In many cases, however, areas of dysplasia or intramucosal carcinoma have been identified within Barrett's mucosa adjacent to or remote from the proximal margin of the tumor.[94–96] Because dysplastic changes would not be expected to occur beyond the leading edge of a gastric carcinoma invading the esophagus, the pathologic data strongly suggest an esophageal origin of these lesions with subsequent spread into the stomach.

Studies have shown that adenocarcinomas arising in Barrett's esophagus constitute as many as 20 to 50% of all adenocarcinomas involving the gastroesophageal junction.[94–96] The remaining lesions are primary carcinomas of the gastric cardia or fundus with secondary esophageal involvement. Whether they arise in the esophagus or in the stomach, these tumors have similar morphologic features in terms of pattern of growth, degree of differentiation, and depth of invasion.[122] However, it is important to ascertain if the cancer has arisen in Barrett's esophagus, as it may be necessary to resect not only the primary tumor but all residual Barrett's mucosa. Detection of a malignancy at the cardia should therefore lead to a careful search for Barrett's epithelium in the esophagus.

### Histologic Features

At the time of diagnosis, most adenocarcinomas in Barrett's esophagus are advanced, unresectable tumors.[108, 112] Occasionally, however, early, potentially curable lesions may be detected by radiologic or endoscopic screening of patients with known Barrett's esophagus, or they may be fortuitous findings in patients undergoing barium studies or endoscopy because of their underlying reflux disease.[69, 108, 110, 123]

### Routes of Spread

Like squamous cell carcinoma, esophageal adenocarcinoma readily invades local, regional, or distant structures via direct extension, lymphatic spread, or hematogenous metastases. Unlike squamous cell carcinoma, however, adenocarcinoma in Barrett's esophagus has a marked tendency to spread distally into the stomach, with involvement of the gastric cardia or fundus in 35 to 60% of cases.[94–96]

### Clinical Aspects

Most patients with esophageal adenocarcinoma present clinically with dysphagia and weight loss.[99, 100, 108, 112, 116] Less common findings include upper gastrointestinal bleeding, odynophagia, and chest pain.[116] Because of their underlying reflux disease, some patients may have a history of long-standing reflux symptoms before the development of cancer.[99, 108, 112] By the time these tumors cause dysphagia, however, most patients have advanced, unresectable tumors. As a result, these individuals have an extremely poor prognosis, with 5-year survival rates comparable to those for squamous cell carcinoma.[112, 116]

Although most patients with early adenocarcinomas in Barrett's esophagus are asymptomatic, some patients may have melena, guaiac-positive stool, or iron deficiency anemia due to from low-grade bleeding from the friable surface of the tumor.[69] Other patients may seek medical attention because of their underlying gastroesophageal reflux disease, so these lesions may be detected fortuitously in patients with reflux symptoms.[69] Finally, early adenocarcinomas may be discovered during radiologic or endoscopic surveillance of asymptomatic patients with known Barrett's esophagus.

## Radiographic Findings

### Early Adenocarcinoma

Like squamous cell carcinomas, early adenocarcinomas in Barrett's esophagus may appear radiographically as plaque-like lesions or as flat, sessile polyps.[69] Sessile or pedunculated polyps in the distal esophagus may also represent adenomatous polyps in Barrett's mucosa with or without foci of invasive carcinoma[95, 114] (Fig. 28–17).

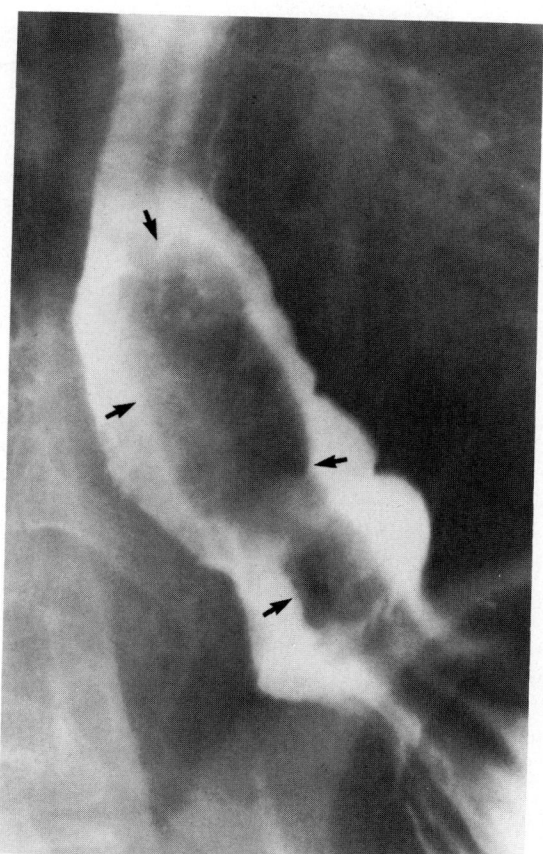

**Figure 28–17. Early adenocarcinoma in Barrett's esophagus.** There is a large, pedunculated polyp *(arrows)* in the distal esophagus. Pathologic examination of the resected specimen revealed an adenomatous polyp with a solitary focus of adenocarcinoma. (From Levine MS, Caroline D, Thompson JJ, et al: Adenocarcinoma of the esophagus: relationship to Barrett mucosa. Radiology 150:305–309, 1984.)

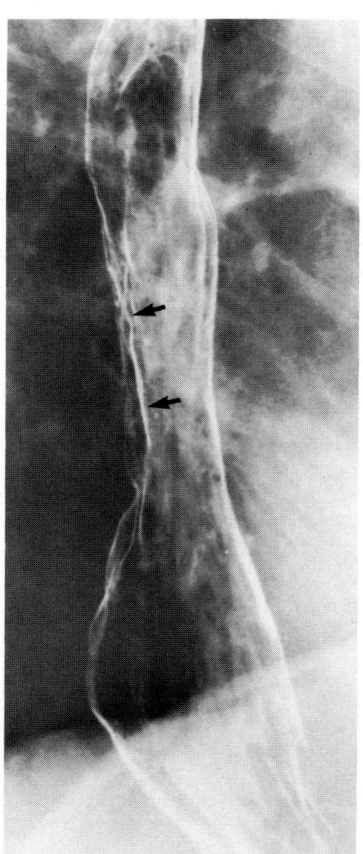

**Figure 28–18. Early adenocarcinoma in Barrett's esophagus.** There is a relatively long peptic stricture in the distal esophagus with slight flattening or stiffening of one wall of the stricture *(arrows).* Surgery revealed an intramucosal adenocarcinoma arising in Barrett's esophagus. (From Levine MS, Caroline D, Thompson JJ, et al: Adenocarcinoma of the esophagus: relationship to Barrett mucosa. Radiology 150:305–309, 1984.)

In patients with peptic strictures, the earliest manifestation of a developing adenocarcinoma may be a localized area of flattening or stiffening in one wall of the stricture[69, 95, 96] (Fig. 28–18). Other patients may have superficial spreading cancers with diffuse nodularity of the mucosa but no focal lesion.[69] Although early cancers are classically small lesions, some patients with early adenocarcinomas may have relatively large polypoid masses that are indistinguishable radiographically from advanced esophageal carcinomas.[69]

Most early adenocarcinomas in Barrett's esophagus reported in the radiologic literature have been discovered fortuitously during radiologic evaluation of patients with reflux symptoms.[69] However, asymptomatic lesions could also be detected by radiologic surveillance of patients with known Barrett's esophagus. In our opinion, an optimal screening program for these patients might therefore alternate double contrast esophagography and endoscopy at 6-month intervals in the hopes of detecting malignant change in Barrett's esophagus at the earliest possible stage.

## Advanced Adenocarcinoma

Advanced esophageal adenocarcinomas usually appear radiographically as infiltrating lesions with irregular luminal narrowing, nodularity or ulceration of the mucosa, and abrupt, asymmetric borders[94–96] (Fig. 28–19A). In general, these lesions cannot be distinguished radiographically from squamous cell carcinomas. In one study, however, esophageal adenocarcinomas were found to involve a longer vertical segment of the esophagus than is found in squamous cell carcinomas, so that the presence of an unusually long, infiltrating lesion should suggest the possibility of adenocarcinoma.[96]

Less frequently, these tumors may appear as polypoid intraluminal masses (Fig. 28–19B) or as primary ulcerative lesions with a meniscoid ulcer surrounded by a narrow ridge of tumor[95, 96] (Fig. 28–19C). Occasionally, these lesions may have a varicoid appearance due to submucosal spread of tumor[95, 96, 124] (Fig. 28–19D). Similar findings may be present in patients with squamous cell carcinoma. However, many patients with adenocarcinoma arising in Barrett's esophagus have associated hiatal hernias or gastroesophageal reflux.[95, 96] They may also have reflux esophagitis, a middle or distal esophageal stricture, or a reticular pattern of the mucosa.[96] Thus, the possibility of adenocarcinoma should be considered in any patient with esophageal cancer who has other clinical or radiologic signs of reflux disease.

When adenocarcinomas are located in the distal esophagus, they have a marked tendency to invade the gastric cardia or fundus.[93–96] Gastric involvement may be manifested radiographically by a polypoid or ulcerated mass in the fundus. In other patients, these tumors may cause obliteration of the normal anatomic landmarks at the cardia and irregular areas of ulceration without a discrete lesion[95] (Fig. 28–20). The findings may be quite subtle, so optimal double contrast views of the gastric cardia and fundus are required to demonstrate these lesions. In general, esophageal adenocarcinoma invading the gastric cardia or fundus cannot be distinguished radiographically from carcinoma of the cardia or fundus invading the distal esophagus. However, esophageal adenocarcinomas usually have a greater degree of esophageal involvement in relation to that of the stomach, whereas gastric cardiac carcinomas have a greater degree of fundal involvement. A significant history of reflux disease should also suggest the correct diagnosis.

## DIFFERENTIAL DIAGNOSIS

### Early Esophageal Cancer

Early squamous cell carcinomas and adenocarcinomas usually appear radiographically as plaque-like lesions or as flat, sessile polyps. However, other benign lesions may produce similar findings. Squamous papillomas often appear as small, sessile, slightly lobulated polyps indistinguishable from early esophageal cancers on dou-

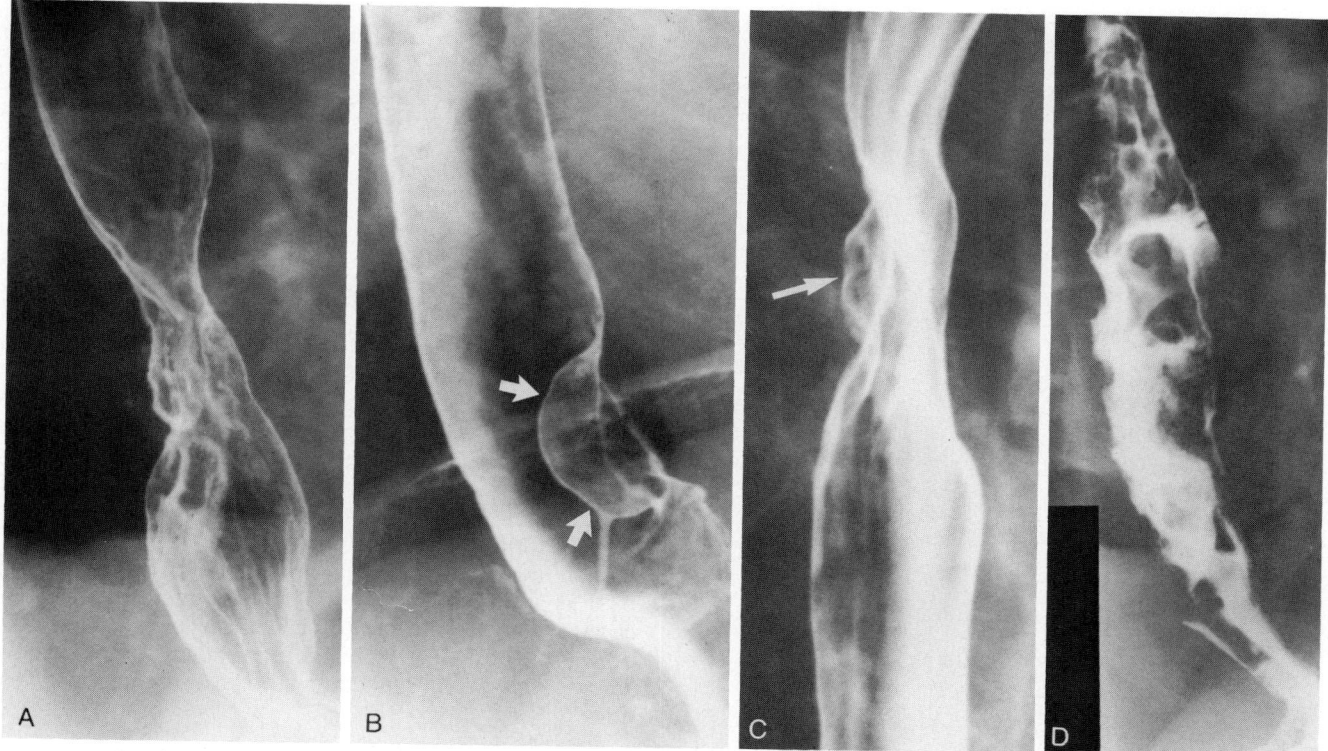

**Figure 28–19. Advanced adenocarcinoma in Barrett's esophagus: patterns of tumor. A.** Infiltrating lesion. **B.** Polypoid lesion *(arrows).* **C.** Ulcerative lesion *(arrow).* **D.** Varicoid lesion. (**C** and **D** from Levine MS, Caroline D, Thompson JJ, et al: Adenocarcinoma of the esophagus: relationship to Barrett mucosa. Radiology 150:305–309, 1984.)

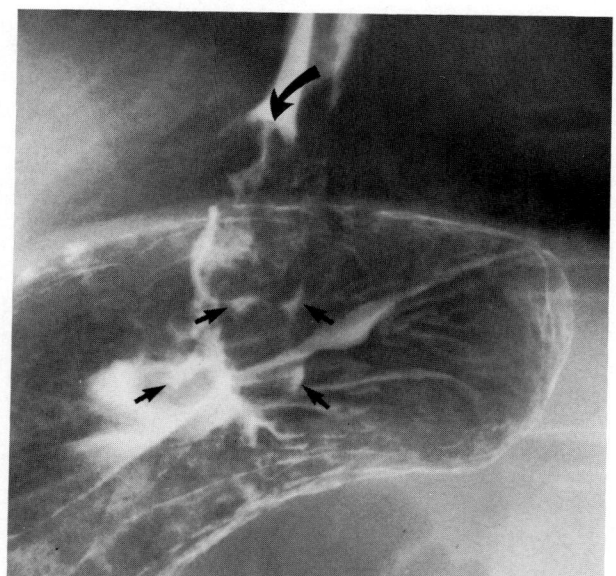

**Figure 28–20. Adenocarcinoma in Barrett's esophagus invading the stomach.** A double contrast view of the gastric fundus shows obliteration of the normal anatomic landmarks at the cardia with irregular areas of ulceration *(straight arrows).* Also note how the tumor involves the distal esophagus *(curved arrow).* At surgery, this patient had a primary adenocarcinoma arising in Barrett's mucosa with secondary gastric involvement. (From Levine MS, Caroline D, Thompson JJ, et al: Adenocarcinoma of the esophagus: relationship to Barrett mucosa. Radiology 150:305–309, 1984.)

ble contrast radiographs[125] (see Fig. 27–1). *Candida* esophagitis and glycogenic acanthosis usually produce multiple plaque-like defects in the esophagus, but a single large plaque can be mistaken for a plaque-like carcinoma. Occasionally, inflammatory exudates or pseudomembranes associated with severe reflux esophagitis may also appear radiographically as plaque-like defects indistinguishable from early adenocarcinomas arising in Barrett's esophagus[126] (Fig. 28–21). However, pseudomembrane formation may be suggested by the presence of other discrete satellite lesions or by a change in the size and appearance of the lesions during the radiologic examination. When the radiographic findings are equivocal, endoscopy and biopsy are required for a definitive diagnosis.

Because superficial spreading carcinomas are manifested radiographically by tiny nodules or plaques, a localized area of *Candida* esophagitis could conceivably produce a similar appearance[127] (Fig. 28–22). However, the plaque-like defects of candidiasis tend to be discrete lesions with well-defined borders and normal intervening mucosa, whereas the nodules or plaques of superficial spreading carcinoma tend to coalesce, producing a continuous area of disease. Superficial spreading carcinomas that are more extensive should be differentiated from other benign conditions causing a diffusely nodular mucosa, such as *Candida* esophagitis, glycogenic acanthosis, or, rarely, leukoplakia, acanthosis nigricans, and

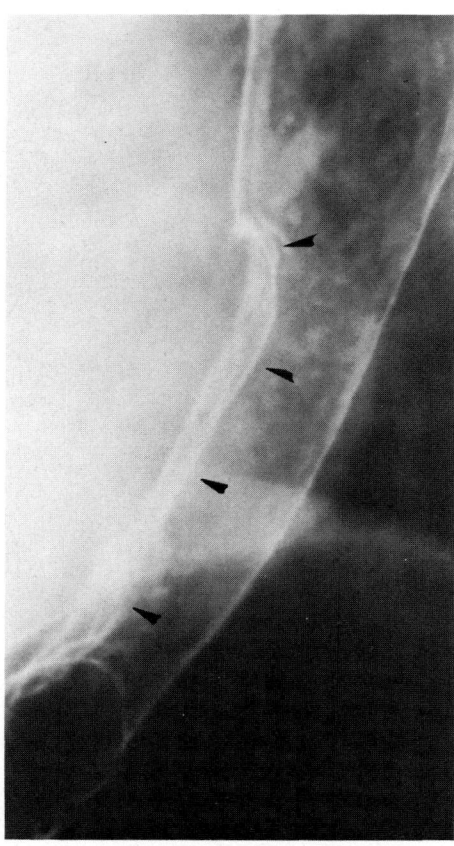

**Figure 28–21. Reflux esophagitis with a large pseudomembrane, mimicking a plaque-like adenocarcinoma.** There is a longitudinally oriented, plaque-like lesion *(arrowheads)* on the anterolateral wall of the distal esophagus. The radiographic findings raise suspicion of a plaque-like carcinoma, but endoscopy revealed pseudomembranes due to severe reflux esophagitis without evidence of tumor. (From Levine MS, Cajade AG, Herlinger H, et al: Pseudomembranes in reflux esophagitis. Radiology 159:43–45, 1986.)

squamous papillomatosis.[127–131] However, the latter conditions also tend to produce discrete lesions rather than a continuous area of disease. Finally, superficial spreading carcinoma may produce a reticulonodular appearance that closely resembles the reticular pattern of Barrett's mucosa.[132] However, the latter finding usually is associated with a mid- or distal esophageal stricture, with the reticular pattern extending distally from the stricture (see Fig. 24–33).

## Advanced Carcinoma

Infiltrating esophageal carcinomas usually have an obvious malignant appearance. Occasionally, however, these lesions may resemble benign strictures, with concentric narrowing and relatively smooth, tapered borders[81, 133] (see Fig. 28–8B). In such cases, the presence of focal irregularity, nodularity, or stiffening of one wall of the stricture should suggest the possibility of malignancy, particularly an adenocarcinoma in Barrett's esophagus.[95, 96] Fluoroscopic observation may also help differentiate benign and malignant strictures, as the

wall of the esophagus is immobile when infiltrated by tumor, whereas normal peristalsis is usually observed in a benign stricture.[134] Rarely, esophageal cancer may cause beak-like narrowing of the distal esophagus, mimicking the appearance of primary achalasia.[96] However, asymmetry, nodularity, or ulceration of the narrowed segment should suggest a malignant lesion.

When infiltrating cancers are detected in the esophagus, it may be difficult or impossible to differentiate a squamous cell carcinoma from an adenocarcinoma arising in Barrett's mucosa. However, adenocarcinomas tend to be located more distally in the esophagus and often invade the gastric cardia or fundus, whereas squamous cell carcinomas rarely extend subdiaphragmatically to involve the stomach.[94–96] Other clinical or radiographic signs of reflux esophagitis should also favor adenocarcinoma. As a result, it is often possible for the radiologist to suggest a histologic diagnosis in these patients. However, endoscopy and biopsy are required for a definitive diagnosis.

Esophageal adenocarcinomas are more likely to appear as polypoid intraluminal masses than squamous cell carcinomas, which tend to be infiltrating or mixed polypoid-infiltrating lesions. Other malignant tumors such as spindle cell carcinomas and leiomyosarcomas may also

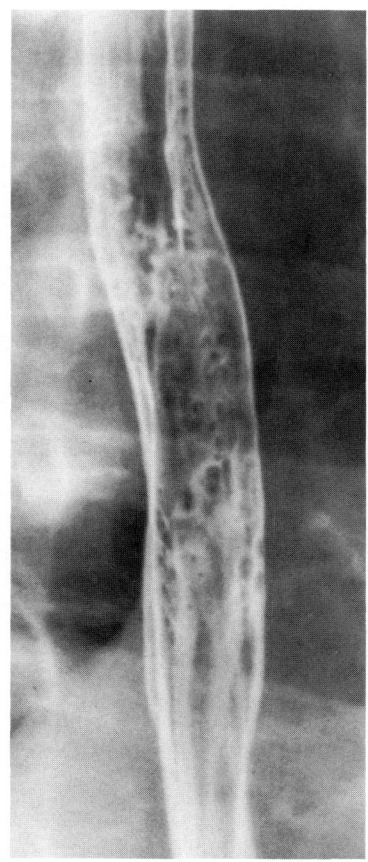

**Figure 28–22. Localized area of *Candida* esophagitis**. This appearance could be mistaken for a superficial spreading carcinoma. However, note how the plaques have discrete borders and are separated by short segments of normal mucosa.

appear as bulky intraluminal masses.[135, 136] Rarely, benign tumors such as giant fibrovascular polyps may be manifested by enormous sausage-shaped lesions that can be mistaken for cancer.[137] Finally, impacted food in the esophagus may be confused radiographically with polypoid carcinomas. However, the presence of a stricture directly below the polypoid defect should suggest the possibility of a food impaction. Impacted debris may also obstruct the esophagus, whereas polypoid carcinomas rarely produce high-grade esophageal obstruction. Obviously, a history of sudden onset of dysphagia while eating meat or other bulky food products should suggest this complication.

Primary ulcerative carcinomas usually appear as distinctive meniscoid ulcers surrounded by a thin rim of malignant tissue. However, the adjacent tumor mass may be relatively subtle, so these lesions can occasionally be mistaken for benign ulcers. Conversely, some patients with esophagitis may have large, flat ulcers with a surrounding mound of edema, erroneously suggesting an ulcerated carcinoma. Ulcers associated with potassium chloride or quinidine ingestion or nasogastric intubation may have a particularly ominous appearance. In such cases, endoscopy and biopsy are required to exclude a malignant lesion.

Although varicoid carcinoma can mimic the appearance of esophageal varices on a single radiograph, these entities can usually be differentiated at fluoroscopy.[83-85, 124] True varices tend to change in size and shape with peristalsis, respiration, and Valsalva maneuvers, whereas varicoid tumors have a rigid, fixed configuration, with an abrupt demarcation between the involved segment and the adjacent normal mucosa. Most varicoid carcinomas are squamous cell carcinomas or adenocarcinomas, but other malignant tumors such as lymphoma may occasionally produce similar findings.[138]

Rarely, localized submucosal extension of a squamous cell carcinoma or adenocarcinoma may produce a smooth submucosal mass, mimicking the appearance of a benign leiomyoma[139] (Fig. 28–23). However, a malignant lesion should be suspected if there is lobulation or eccentric ulceration of the mass.

## STAGING

Before the development of computed tomography (CT), there was no reliable preoperative means for detecting periesophageal invasion or regional lymph node involvement by esophageal carcinoma. However, the emergence of CT and other noninvasive imaging modalities has had a major impact on the preoperative evaluation of esophageal carcinoma, leading to the development of new tumor, node, metastases (TNM) staging criteria.[140] In the new system, the depth of primary tumor (T) invasion through the esophageal wall is carefully assessed, but the length of the tumor and percentage of wall involvement are not important. The new system also places greater emphasis on the presence of regional lymph node (N) involvement, which includes upper abdominal lymph nodes in patients with distal esophageal cancers. For the purposes of staging, the

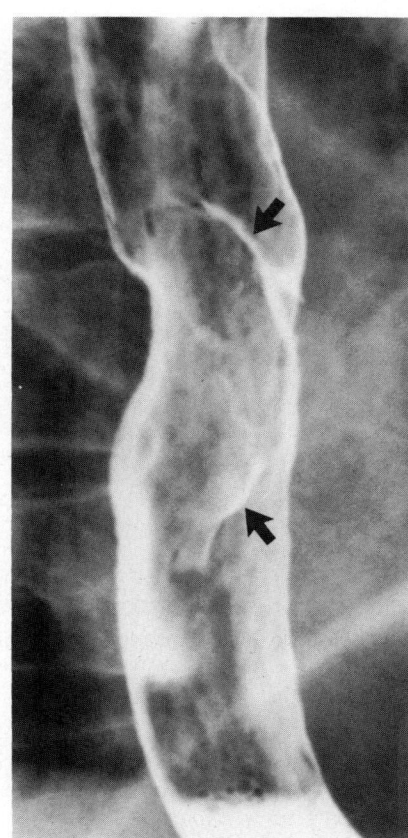

**Figure 28–23. Esophageal carcinoma resembling a benign submucosal mass (arrows).** However, this lesion is larger and has a more irregular contour than most leiomyomas.

esophagus consists of four segments. The cervical esophagus begins at the lower end of the cricoid cartilage and ends at the thoracic inlet. The thoracic esophagus is divided into thirds. The upper third extends from the thoracic inlet to the carina. The middle third extends from the carina halfway to the gastroesophageal junction. The lower third is the distal half of the esophagus between the carina and gastroesophageal junction.

## Routes of Spread

### Primary Site (T)

The new staging criteria for the primary tumor are listed in Table 28–1. Note that the length of the tumor and the presence of circumferential involvement are no

| TABLE 28–1. DEFINITION OF PRIMARY TUMOR | |
|---|---|
| TX | Primary tumor cannot be assessed |
| T0 | No evidence of primary tumor |
| Tis | Carcinoma in situ |
| T1 | Tumor invades lamina propria or submucosa |
| T2 | Tumor invades muscularis propria |
| T3 | Tumor invades adventitia |
| T4 | Tumor invades adjacent structures |

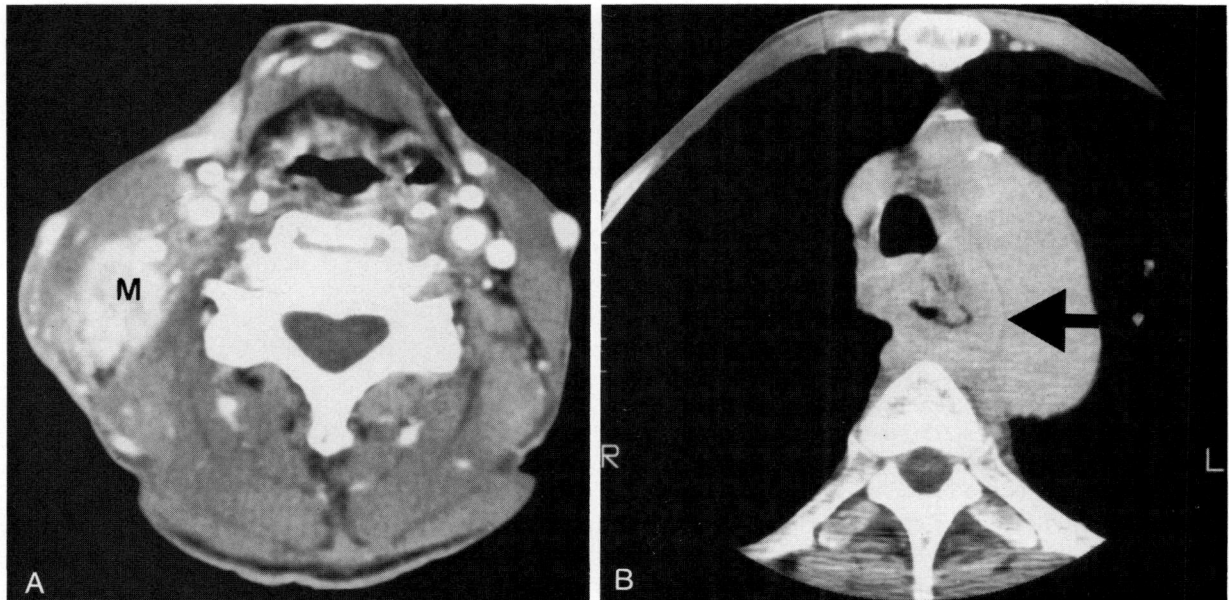

**Figure 28–24. Metastatic esophageal carcinoma. A.** There is a bulky, enhancing mass (M) in the right side of the neck due to biopsy-proven metastatic esophageal carcinoma. **B.** A CT scan at the level of the aortic arch shows the primary tumor *(arrow).*

longer used to define T. With these new criteria, the stage of the tumor is affected only by the depth of invasion and not by tumor size.

### Regional Lymph Nodes (N)

The classification of regional lymph nodes depends on the location of the primary tumor in patients with esophageal cancer. For cervical esophageal cancers, involved cervical and supraclavicular nodes are considered regional metastases. When lymph nodes in the mediastinum or upper abdomen are involved, they are classified as distant metastases. For upper or midthoracic esophageal cancers, involved cervical, supraclavicular, and abdominal lymph nodes are classified as distant metastases (Fig. 28–24). For lower esophageal cancers, involved mediastinal and upper abdominal lymph nodes (including perigastric nodes but excluding celiac nodes) are considered regional metastases. For staging purposes, regional lymph nodes are classified as follows: N0, no regional lymph node metastases; N1, regional lymph node metastases; and NX, regional lymph nodes cannot be assessed.

### Distant Metastases (M)

The most common sites of distant metastases from esophageal carcinoma are the liver, lungs, pleura, and kidneys. Distant metastases are classified as follows: M0, no distant metastases; M1, distant metastases; and MX, distant metastases cannot be assessed.

## Staging Criteria

Esophageal carcinoma may be classified by clinical and pathologic staging criteria. The clinical stage of the tumor can be determined preoperatively by endoscopy, CT, or other imaging tests; the pathologic stage depends on the surgical findings. The new TNM staging criteria for esophageal carcinoma are presented in Table 28–2. In the new system, stage II is subdivided into IIA and IIB.

CT and magnetic resonance (MR) imaging are both capable of detecting mediastinal invasion, mediastinal adenopathy, and distant metastases from esophageal carcinoma.[141] Although neither imaging modality can determine the depth of invasion in the wall of the esophagus, direct invasion of periesophageal structures can be accurately predicted by both CT and MR imaging. However, extension of tumor through the muscular wall and adventitia of the esophagus into the periesophageal fat does not necessarily preclude surgery, as an en bloc resection may still be performed. In contrast, invasion beyond the mediastinal fat into adjacent structures does preclude surgical resection. Obvious mediastinal invasion may be demonstrated by CT or MR imaging in patients with tracheoesophageal fistulas (Fig. 28–25). However, many patients have subtle evidence of mediastinal invasion, so specific signs are used to

### TABLE 28–2. DEFINITION OF TNM STAGES

| Stage 0 | Tis | N0 | M0 |
|---|---|---|---|
| Stage I | T1 | N0 | M0 |
| Stage IIA | T2 | N0 | M0 |
| | T3 | N0 | M0 |
| Stage IIB | T1 | N1 | M0 |
| | T2 | N1 | M0 |
| Stage III | T3 | N1 | M0 |
| | T4 | Any N | M0 |
| Stage IV | Any T | Any N | M1 |

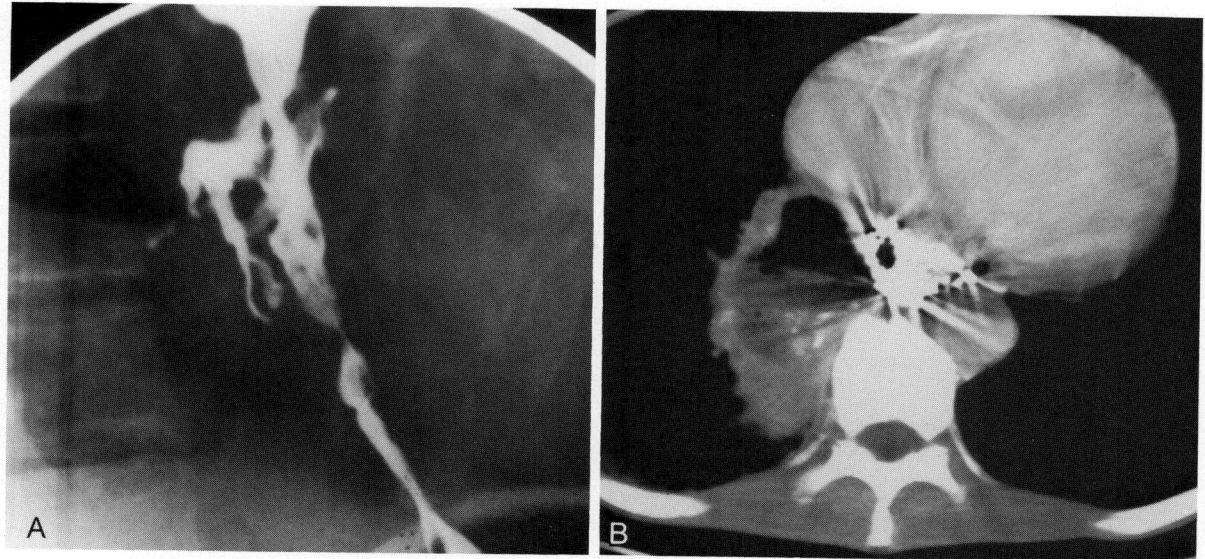

**Figure 28–25. Advanced esophageal carcinoma with a tracheoesophageal fistula and mediastinal abscess. A.** A barium study shows an advanced esophageal carcinoma with a fistula into the bronchial tree. **B.** A CT scan demonstrates an abscess in the right side of the mediastinum, containing air-fluid levels and barium.

detect this form of tumor spread, including mass effect and loss of fat planes (see later sections).

## Tracheobronchial Invasion

Carcinomas of the upper or midthoracic esophagus may directly invade the trachea or bronchus. However, the posterior wall of the trachea and left main bronchus directly abut the esophagus, so the absence of a fat plane between the trachea or bronchus and an esophageal mass cannot be used to predict invasion. Instead, demonstration of mass effect is required.[142] The presence of an esophageal mass that displaces the trachea or bronchus from the spine is diagnostic of invasion (Fig.

28–26). Tracheobronchial invasion by esophageal carcinoma may also be manifested by a discrete indentation on the posterior wall of the trachea or bronchus (Figs. 28–27 and 28–28). Posterior wall bowing and displacement of the trachea or bronchus have been reported to be the most accurate signs of mediastinal invasion on CT or MR images.

In evaluating these mass effect criteria for tracheobronchial invasion by esophageal carcinoma, however, the limitations of CT should be recognized. Because the posterior wall of the trachea lacks cartilaginous support, it often bows inward on expiration, whereas it is always flat or convex on inspiration.[143] Thus, inward bowing of the posterior wall of the trachea or bronchus is a valid

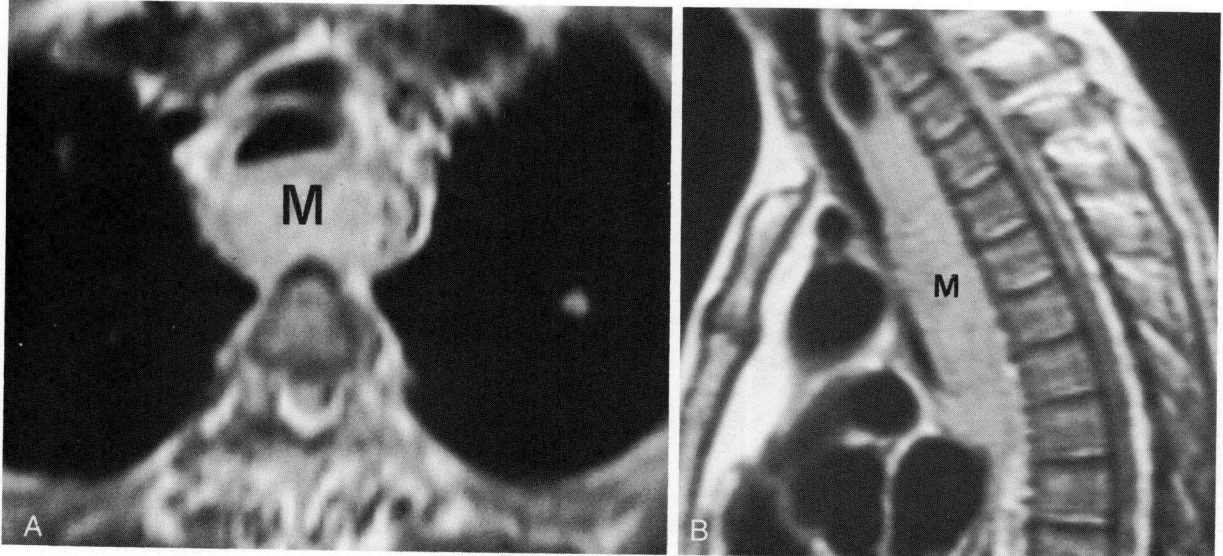

**Figure 28–26. Tracheal invasion by esophageal carcinoma. A.** An axial cardiac-gated MR scan shows a large esophageal mass (M) displacing the trachea anteriorly. **B.** A sagittal scan shows the elongated esophageal mass (M) compressing the posterior wall of the trachea.

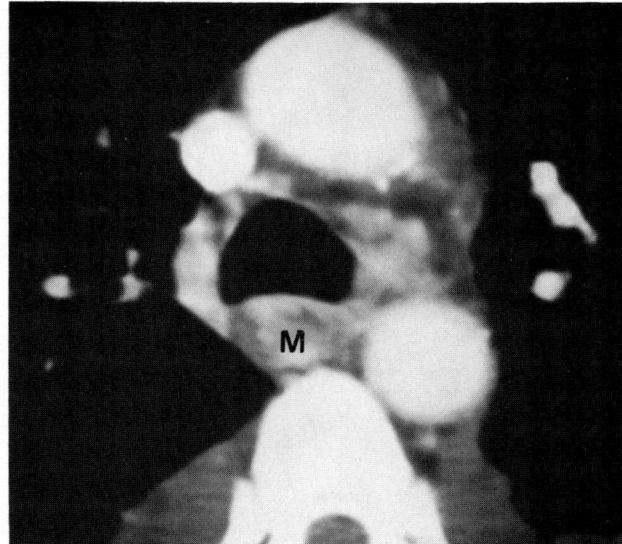

**Figure 28–27. Tracheal invasion by esophageal carcinoma.** An esophageal mass (M) indents the posterior wall of the trachea. This finding indicates tracheal invasion.

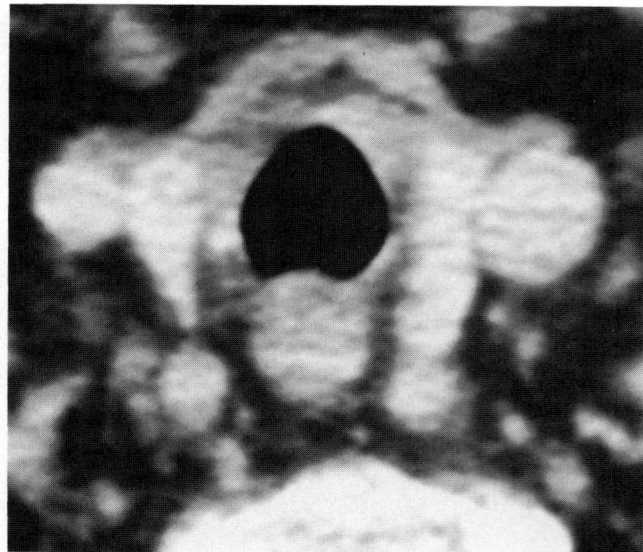

**Figure 28–29. Normal cervical CT scan.** Note how the cervical esophagus normally produces an indentation on the posterior wall of the trachea in the neck.

sign of invasion only if the CT scan is obtained during inspiration. Furthermore, these criteria for mass effect on the tracheobronchial tree should not be used to stage cervical esophageal carcinoma because indentation of the posterior wall of the cervical trachea by the cervical esophagus is a normal finding due to the narrow antero-posterior diameter of the neck (Fig. 28–29). Another pitfall occurs when a dilated, obstructed esophagus causes a posterior indentation on the mediastinal trachea, which mimics invasion (Fig. 28–30). Finally, these mass effect criteria should not be used for unusual tumors such as spindle cell carcinomas that appear as

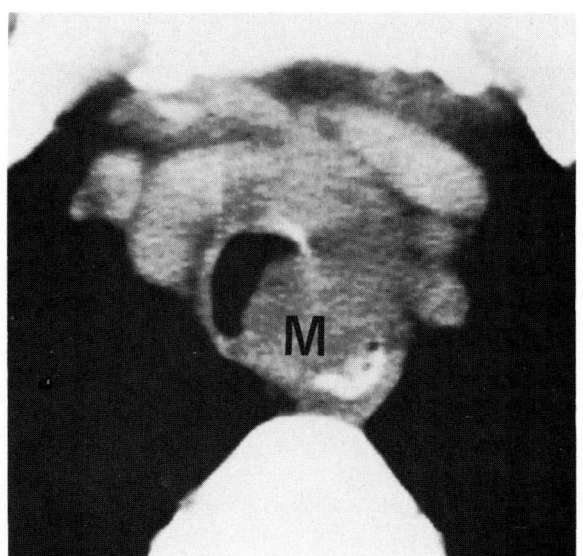

**Figure 28–28. Tracheal invasion by esophageal carcinoma.** A bulky esophageal mass (M) both displaces and indents the postero-lateral wall of the trachea.

bulky, intraluminal masses, because a displaced trachea or bronchus does not necessarily indicate invasion by these lesions[144] (Fig. 28–31).

### Aortic Invasion

Direct invasion of the aorta by esophageal carcinoma is an uncommon finding. In a review of 2400 autopsies, only 2% of patients dying of esophageal carcinoma had aortic invasion.[145] On CT evaluation, the esophagus abuts the descending thoracic aorta without an intervening fat plane, so absence of a fat plane between these structures is a normal finding. However, an esophageal carcinoma that directly invades the aorta may increase the area of contact between the aorta and esophagus. Picus and colleagues described a CT criterion for predicting aortic invasion based on the degree of contact between the tumor and aorta without intervening fat planes.[146] If the area of contact is less than 45 degrees (less than one eighth of the total aortic circumference), the aorta is not thought to be invaded by tumor. If the area of contact is greater than 90 degrees (more than one fourth of the aortic circumference), however, invasion is assumed to be present (Fig. 28–32). With this criterion, CT had an accuracy of 80% in detecting aortic invasion by esophageal carcinoma. Takashima and colleagues have described another criterion for predicting aortic invasion based on obliteration of the triangular fat space between the esophagus, aorta, and spine adjacent to the primary tumor.[147] In a study of 35 patients with esophageal carcinoma, they found that obliteration of this triangular fat space had a sensitivity of 100% and a specificity of 82% in detecting aortic invasion. Thus, CT is an excellent technique for assessing aortic invasion by these lesions.

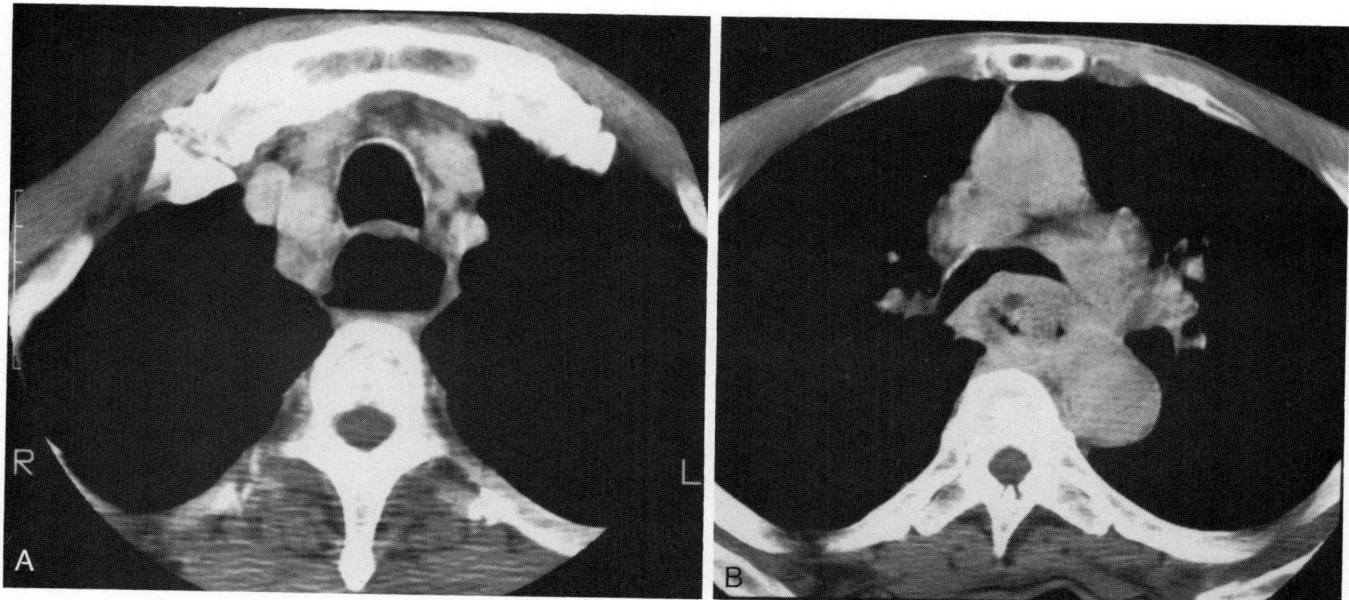

**Figure 28–30. Pseudotracheal invasion by a dilated esophagus. A.** A CT scan at the level of the trachea shows a dilated esophageal lumen displacing and indenting the posterior wall of the trachea. This is not tracheal invasion. **B.** Another scan at the level of the bronchus shows an esophageal mass indenting the posterior wall of the bronchus. Invasion of the bronchus but not the trachea was found at operation in this patient with an obstructing carcinoma of the distal esophagus.

## Pericardial Invasion

CT detection of pericardial invasion is based on either mass effect or obliteration of fat planes. Because a fat plane is often not present between the pericardium and esophagus, loss of fat planes between these structures does not necessarily indicate pericardial invasion by esophageal carcinoma. Multiple CT sections are therefore required to evaluate this criterion. If a fat plane separates the esophageal mass from the pericardium at all levels, the tumor is considered to be noninvasive. However, pericardial invasion by esophageal carcinoma is thought to be present if fat planes between the esophagus and pericardium are obliterated at the level of the mass but are present on other scans above and below this level (Fig. 28–33). Finally, CT is considered indeterminate for pericardial invasion if fat planes are not detected at any level. Another criterion for predicting pericardial invasion is the presence of mass effect with a concave deformity of the heart associated with loss of the normal fat planes in this region.[147]

## Mediastinal Adenopathy

CT has a number of limitations in detecting mediastinal lymph node metastases from esophageal carcinoma. Because the major criterion for adenopathy is size, CT cannot demonstrate lymph node metastases that have not caused significant enlargement of the nodes. In other patients, enlarged lymph nodes adjacent to an esophageal cancer may not be detected because they are inseparable from the primary lesion. Even when mediastinal adenopathy is detected, CT cannot differentiate benign causes of lymph node enlargement from metastatic tumor. In one study, benign enlargement of lymph nodes occurred more frequently when the primary esophageal cancer was large and necrotic.[148]

## Subdiaphragmatic Adenopathy

Abdominal lymphadenopathy is frequently encountered in patients with esophageal carcinoma. In one series of 205 patients with squamous cell carcinoma of the esophagus, the number of abdominal and mediastinal lymph nodes that contained tumor at surgery was virtually identical.[149] Involvement of abdominal lymph nodes was more common in patients with distal esophageal cancers. Abdominal adenopathy was present in more than two thirds of patients with cancers in the lower third of the esophagus, whereas subdiaphragmatic lymph node metastases were present in less than one third of patients with cancers in the upper third of the esophagus. As indicated earlier, upper abdominal lymph node metastases from carcinoma of the distal esophagus are classified as regional lymph node metastases rather than as distant metastases.

Because esophageal carcinoma often metastasizes to upper abdominal lymph nodes, CT staging of these tumors should include evaluation of the upper abdomen. Abdominal adenopathy is usually detected in lymph nodes at or above the celiac axis, frequently in the gastrohepatic ligament. The gastrohepatic ligament is a fat-containing structure extending from the lesser curvature of the stomach to the medial border of the liver. It normally contains the left gastric artery, coronary vein, and left gastric lymph node chain. Masses larger than 8 mm in diameter in the gastrohepatic ligament

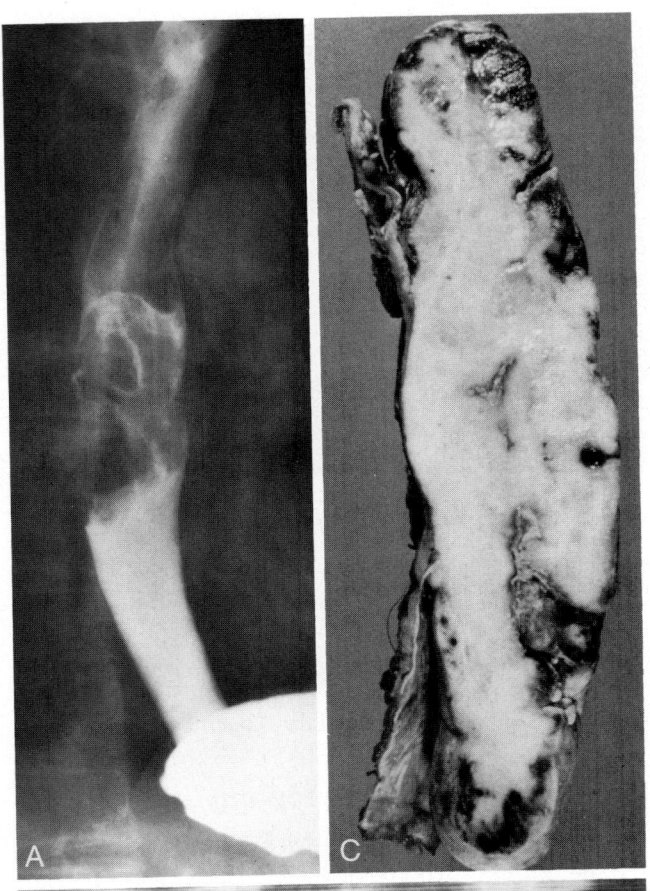

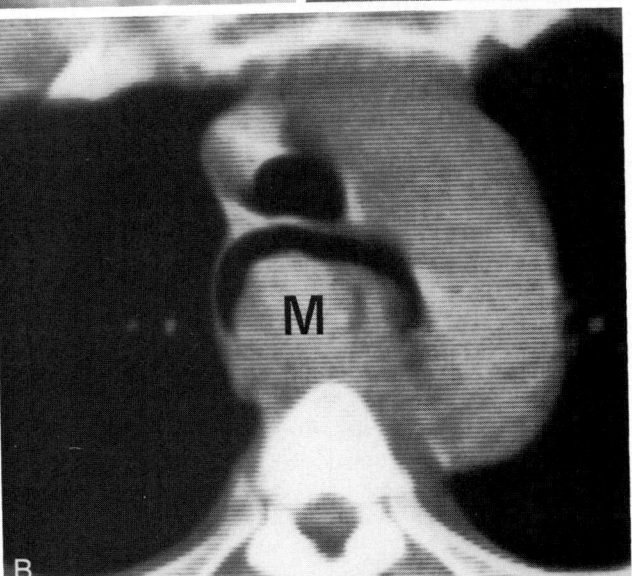

**Figure 28–31. Pseudotracheal invasion by spindle cell carcinoma of the esophagus. A.** A barium study reveals a bulky, intraluminal mass without evidence of esophageal narrowing. **B.** A CT scan shows this mass (M) indenting the posterior wall of the trachea. **C.** Gross specimen of tumor. There was no evidence of tracheal invasion at surgery.

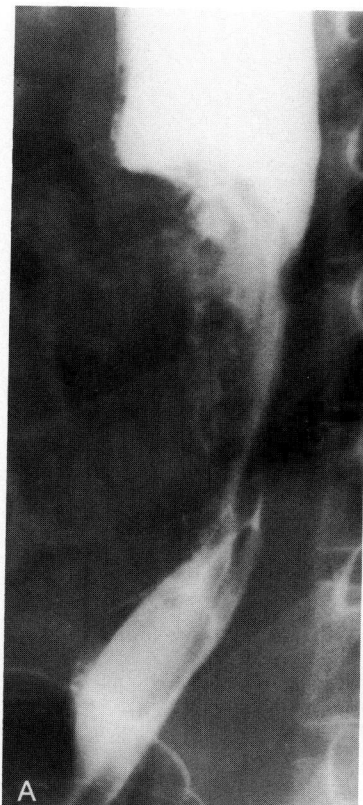
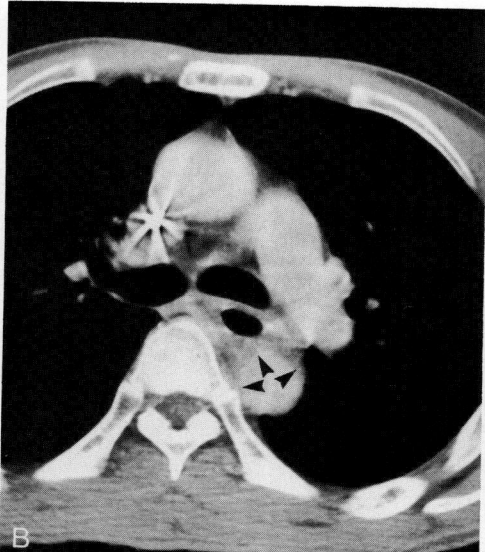
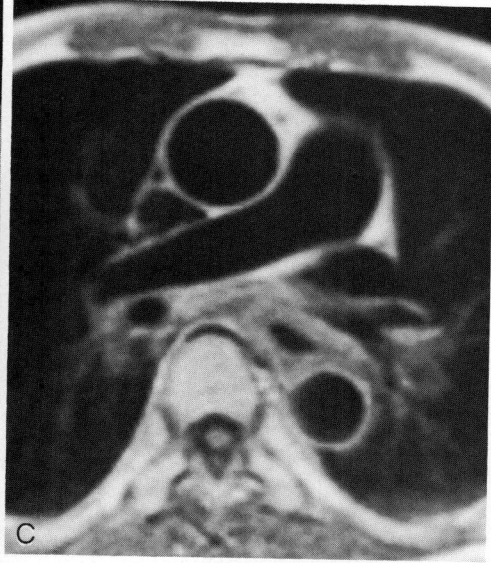

**Figure 28–32. Aortic invasion by esophageal carcinoma. A.** A barium study reveals an advanced carcinoma of the distal esophagus. **B.** A CT scan shows how the tumor encases the descending thoracic aorta, obliterating fat planes between these structures over 180 degrees of the aortic circumference (*arrowheads*). **C.** An MR scan at a different level shows obliteration of 120 degrees of the aortic circumference. Aortic invasion was found at operation.

usually represent enlarged lymph nodes[150] (Fig. 28–34). However, CT has several limitations in detecting adenopathy in the gastrohepatic ligament. Normal structures outside the gastrohepatic ligament may appear to lie within it because of a partial volume effect on CT. The upper portion of the body of the pancreas is the structure most commonly mistaken for enlarged lymph nodes in the gastrohepatic ligament (Fig. 28–35). Other abnormal structures in the gastrohepatic ligament, such as varices of the coronary vein, can also be mistaken for enlarged lymph nodes. However, varices can usually be distinguished from adenopathy by the marked degree of enhancement that occurs within these structures after intravenous infusion of contrast agent.

## Computed Tomography

CT currently is the best noninvasive test for staging patients with esophageal carcinoma. These patients can be placed in one of three groups on the basis of the CT findings. One group has no evidence of local invasion or distant metastases, so these patients have potentially curable lesions. A second group has obvious metastatic disease or local invasion, so these patients are candidates for only palliative treatment. A third group has inconclusive CT studies, so further preoperative or operative evaluation of the extent of disease is required. The last group of patients should not be denied an attempt at curative surgery solely on the basis of the CT findings.

Numerous articles have been published about the accuracy of CT for staging esophageal carcinoma. Early reports claiming high accuracy in detecting mediastinal invasion were limited by a lack of correlative data between the CT and surgical findings.[151] Subsequent studies found that CT had such a low sensitivity and specificity in detecting mediastinal invasion that many authors questioned whether CT had a legitimate role in staging esophageal carcinoma.[152–156] However, many of these studies were limited by a variety of flaws in study design and methodology, including questionable CT scanning techniques, inadequate "gold standards," poorly defined CT criteria for mediastinal invasion, and inappropriate inclusion of indeterminate CT scans as false-positives. Using more rigorous scientific methodology, other investigators have since found that CT is a relatively sensitive and specific imaging modality for predicting mediastinal invasion by esophageal carcinoma. The combined data from seven studies comparing CT with operative and histologic findings revealed that CT had an overall accuracy of 97% for detecting tracheobronchial invasion, 94% for aortic invasion, and 94% for pericardial invasion[141, 143, 146, 157–160] (Table 28–3). At the same time, CT was much less accurate in predicting mediastinal and subdiaphragmatic adenopathy. Although the sensitivity of CT was only 48 and 61% for detecting mediastinal and subdiaphragmatic adenopathy, respectively, the specificity of CT was about 90% in diagnosing lymph node metastases (see Table 28–3). The combination of low sensitivity and high

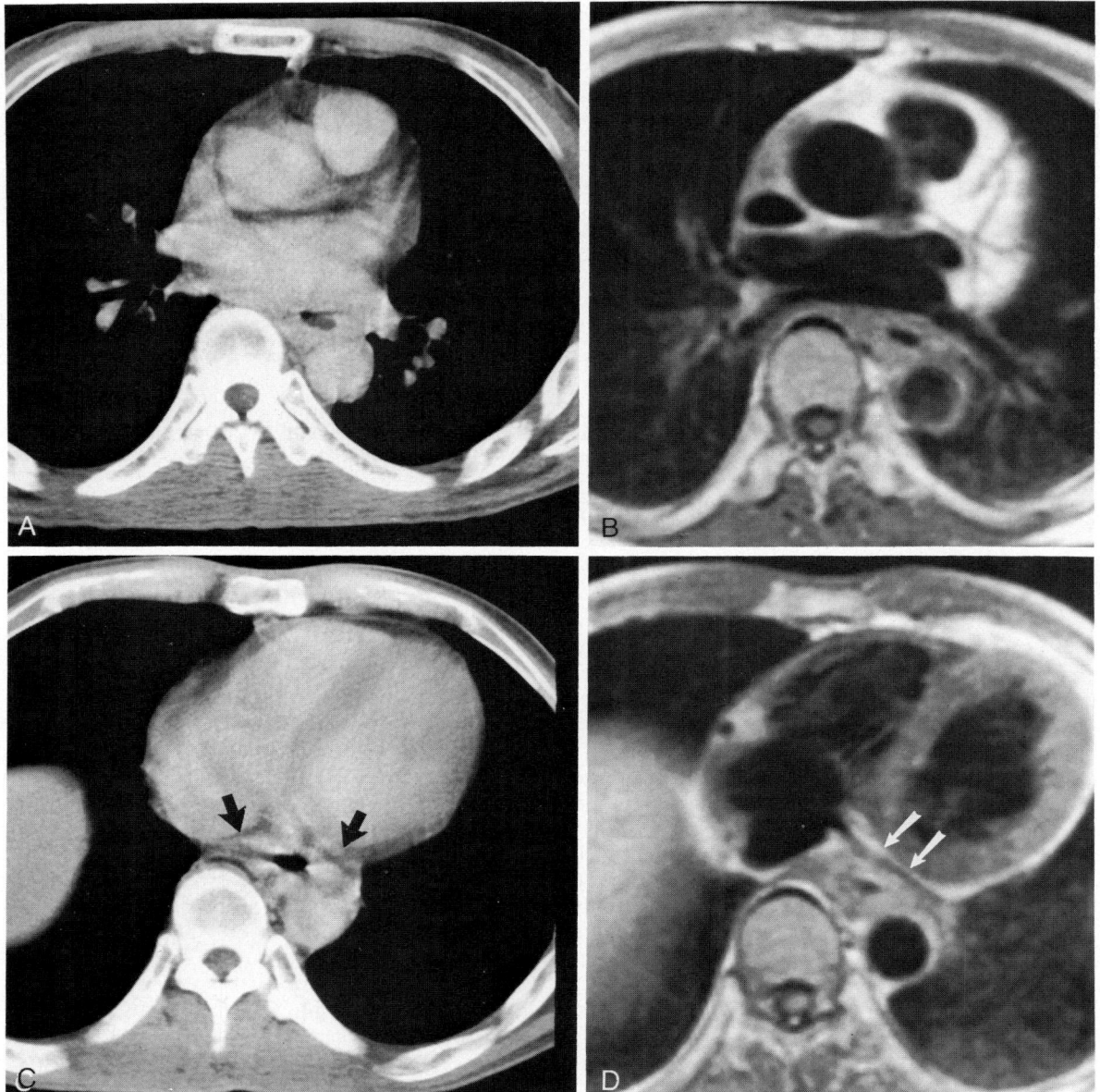

**Figure 28–33. Pericardial invasion by esophageal carcinoma. A.** A CT scan shows esophageal tumor obliterating the fat plane between the aorta and pericardium. **B.** An MR scan at the same level also shows an esophageal mass obliterating the fat plane between the aorta and pericardium. **C.** A CT scan at a lower level shows preservation of the fat plane (*arrows*) between the esophagus and pericardium. **D.** An MR scan at the same level also demonstrates a residual fat plane (*arrows*) between the esophageal tumor and heart. The preservation of fat at this level with obliteration of fat planes superiorly indicates pericardial invasion by tumor.

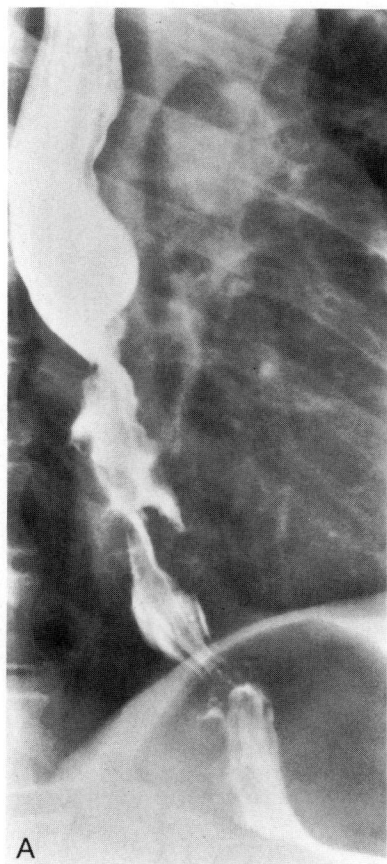

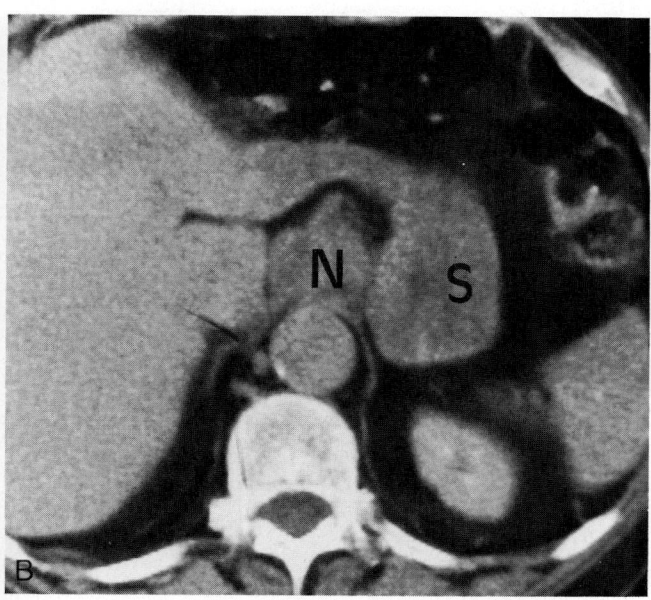

**Figure 28–34. Adenopathy in the gastrohepatic ligament. A.** A barium study reveals an advanced carcinoma of the distal esophagus. **B.** A CT scan of the upper abdomen shows enlarged nodes (N) in the gastrohepatic ligament between unopacified stomach (S) and liver.

**TABLE 28–3. COMPARISON OF COMPUTED TOMOGRAPHY WITH SURGICAL FINDINGS IN PATIENTS WITH ESOPHAGEAL CARCINOMA**

| FINDING | SENSITIVITY (%) | SPECIFICITY (%) | ACCURACY (%) |
|---|---|---|---|
| Tracheobronchial invasion | 93 | 98 | 97 |
| Aortic invasion | 88 | 96 | 94 |
| Pericardial invasion | 94 | 94 | 94 |
| Mediastinal adenopathy | 48 | 90 | 70 |
| Abdominal adenopathy | 61 | 94 | 82 |
| Liver metastases | 70 | 100 | 98 |

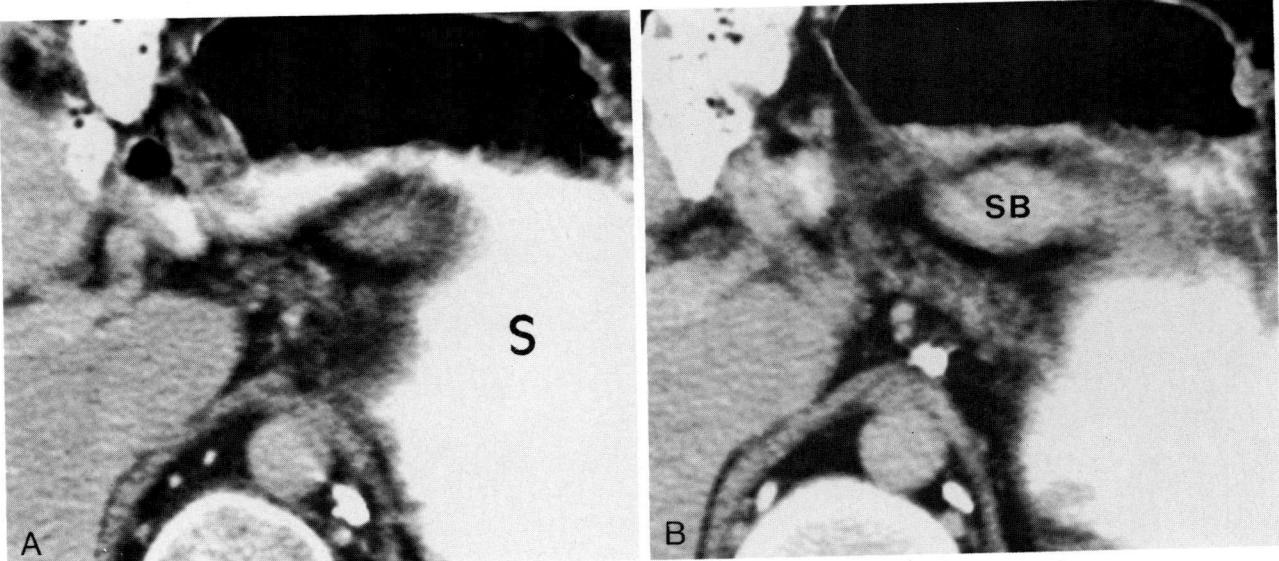

**Figure 28–35. Pseudoadenopathy in the gastrohepatic ligament. A.** A CT scan reveals one large soft tissue density and multiple smaller densities in the gastrohepatic ligament between the stomach (S) and liver. Are these enlarged lymph nodes? **B.** Another CT scan 1 cm below the level of the first scan explains the basis for these densities. The anterior structure represents a loop of small bowel (SB), whereas the more posterior densities actually represent the upper portion of the body of the pancreas.

specificity indicates that enlarged lymph nodes on CT scans are likely to be involved by metastatic tumor, whereas the absence of lymphadenopathy is an unreliable finding because normal-sized lymph nodes may also harbor metastases.

CT may have a role not only in the preoperative staging of esophageal carcinoma but also in predicting the patient's prognosis. In one study, patients with CT signs of mediastinal invasion or subdiaphragmatic adenopathy had a significantly shorter survival than patients who did not have these findings.[161] Specific CT criteria that indicated a poor prognosis included tracheal, aortic, or pericardial invasion. The mean survival of patients with evidence of mediastinal invasion and abdominal metastases was only 4 months. In contrast, patients who had no evidence of mediastinal invasion or abdominal metastases had a mean survival of more than 1 year. The presence of subdiaphragmatic adenopathy indicated a worse prognosis than any other individual criterion evaluated by CT, as these patients had a mean survival of only 90 days.

## Magnetic Resonance Imaging

In the preoperative staging of esophageal carcinoma, MR imaging is potentially superior to CT for detecting mediastinal invasion, as it permits easy differentiation of fat from soft tissue structures (see Figs. 28–26, 28–32, and 28–33). Nevertheless, MR imaging may be limited by motion artifacts due to long acquisition times. Early studies found that MR imaging was less accurate than CT in staging esophageal carcinoma.[162–164] However, more recent studies have found that MR imaging

and CT are comparable in predicting tumor resectability in patients with esophageal carcinoma.[147, 165] In one study, CT and MR imaging both had poor sensitivity in detecting mediastinal adenopathy but 100% sensitivity in detecting tracheobronchial invasion (see Fig. 28–26).[165] Overall, MR imaging appears to be slightly less accurate than CT for staging esophageal cancer with CT staging criteria.

## Endoscopic Ultrasound

The role of ultrasound in evaluating the esophagus is being reassessed due to the introduction of intracavitary technology[166] (Fig. 28–36). Endoscopic ultrasound has been found to be a useful technique for preoperative staging of upper gastrointestinal tract cancers.[167, 168] Other reports have suggested that endoscopic ultrasound may be more accurate than CT for staging esophageal carcinoma.[169, 170] Endoscopic ultrasound is particularly useful for evaluating the depth of tumor invasion (Fig. 28–37). This technique is also capable of differentiating benign and malignant lymph nodes in the mediastinum on the basis of the appearance of the nodes. Lymph nodes with a hypoechoic pattern and clearly defined borders are characteristic of metastatic tumor, whereas nodes with a hyperechoic pattern and indistinct borders are usually benign.[170] Endoscopic ultrasound is also an effective technique for visualizing mediastinal lymph nodes greater than 1 cm in diameter, but many of these enlarged nodes are not found to be involved by metastatic tumor.[171] Despite its advantages, endoscopic ultrasound is extremely operator dependent. Furthermore, in about 20% of patients with esophageal cancer, en-

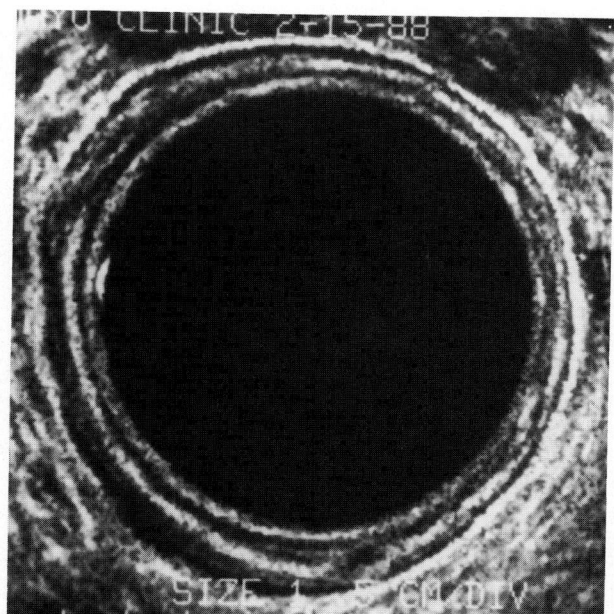

**Figure 28–36. Normal endoscopic ultrasound of the esophagus.** There are five distinct layers in the esophageal wall that have an alternating hyperechoic and hypoechoic appearance. The central hyperechoic layer represents submucosal fat.

doscopic ultrasound is limited by an inability to pass the esophageal ultrasound probe through a malignant stricture.[172, 173]

The eventual role of endoscopic ultrasound for staging esophageal carcinoma remains uncertain. Current data suggest that it is a useful technique for determining tumor invasion in about 80% of patients in whom the

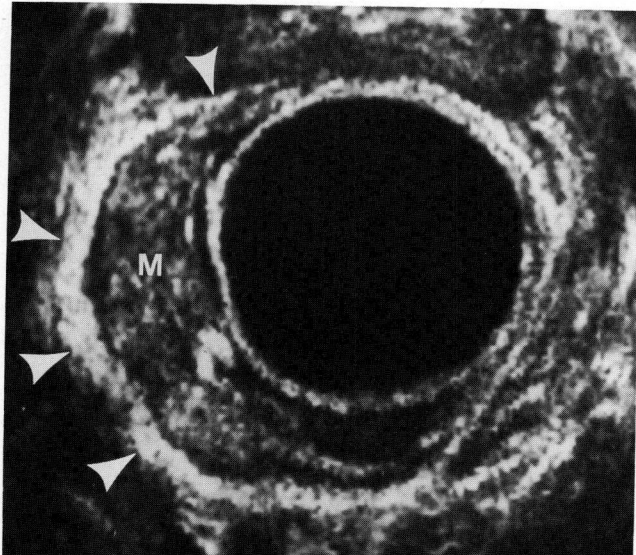

**Figure 28–37. Endoscopic ultrasound appearance of esophageal carcinoma.** There is an intact submucosal fat layer (*arrowheads*) surrounding the esophageal mass (M). (From Halvorsen RA, Thompson WM: Primary neoplasms of the hollow organs of the gastrointestinal tract: staging and follow-up. Cancer 67:1181–1188, 1991.)

probe can be passed through the tumor, permitting evaluation of adjacent mediastinal structures. However, inadequate depth of penetration with high-frequency transducers limits the ability of endoscopic ultrasound in detecting distant metastases. The role of endoscopic ultrasound in evaluating mediastinal lymph nodes is also controversial. Thus, other imaging modalities such as CT and MR imaging are still required for evaluating these patients.

## TREATMENT

Depending on the stage of the tumor at the time of diagnosis, esophageal cancer may be treated by curative or palliative measures. Curative therapy includes surgery, radiation, or surgery combined with preoperative or postoperative radiation or chemotherapy. Palliative therapy includes surgery, radiation, chemotherapy, placement of an indwelling esophageal prosthesis, or laser therapy. A detailed description of these treatment modalities or the rationale for selecting a particular modality as a palliative or curative form of therapy is beyond the scope of this chapter.

### Surgery

Curative resection of a carcinoma in the distal two thirds of the esophagus usually requires an esophagogastrectomy and gastric pull-through. Resection of a more proximal lesion may require a free jejunal graft for reconstruction of the pharyngoesophagus. Palliative surgery in patients with advanced esophageal cancer usually consists of an esophageal bypass procedure to control symptoms of obstruction or fistula formation. The most common bypass procedures include colonic interposition and creation of a gastric tube. Occasionally, palliation may be achieved by passage of a rigid tube or esophageal prosthesis (i.e., a Celestin tube) to bypass an obstruction or fistula. The normal and abnormal postoperative appearances after esophageal cancer surgery are presented in Chapter 33.

### Radiation Therapy

Radiation therapy may be used for either palliative or definitive treatment of esophageal cancer. Squamous cell carcinomas tend to be more radiosensitive than adenocarcinomas.[174] Tumors in the cervical or upper thoracic esophagus also tend to be more radiosensitive than those located in the middle or distal thoracic esophagus.[174] Partial or total regression of tumor occurs in most patients who undergo this form of treatment.[175–177] Although these patients may have significant relief from dysphagia in the initial months after therapy, the lesions subsequently recur locally in 30 to 85% of cases.[174, 177–179] Even when the tumor is eradicated from the esophagus, these patients often die as a result of widespread metastases to the liver, lungs, or mediastinum.[174, 177, 180] In-

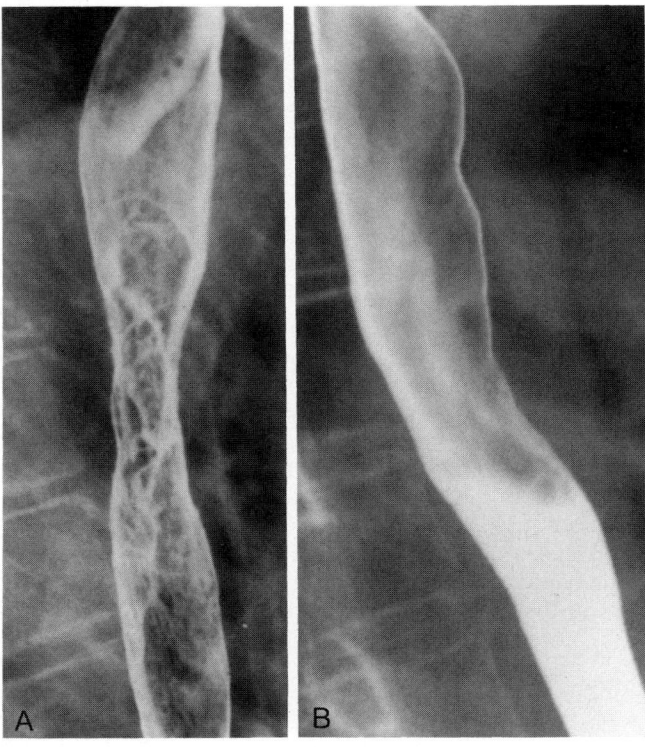

**Figure 28–38. Total regression of esophageal carcinoma after radiation therapy. A.** The initial esophagram reveals an infiltrating carcinoma of the midesophagus. **B.** A second study 1 year after radiation therapy shows a normal-appearing esophagus without evidence of a stricture or residual tumor in this region.

**Figure 28–39. Total regression of esophageal carcinoma after radiation therapy with a benign residual stricture. A.** The initial esophagram shows an advanced, infiltrating carcinoma in the midesophagus. **B.** A second study 4 months after radiation therapy shows partial regression of the tumor with residual areas of ulceration. **C.** A third study 2 months later shows total regression of the lesion with a smooth, tapered, benign-appearing radiation stricture in this region.

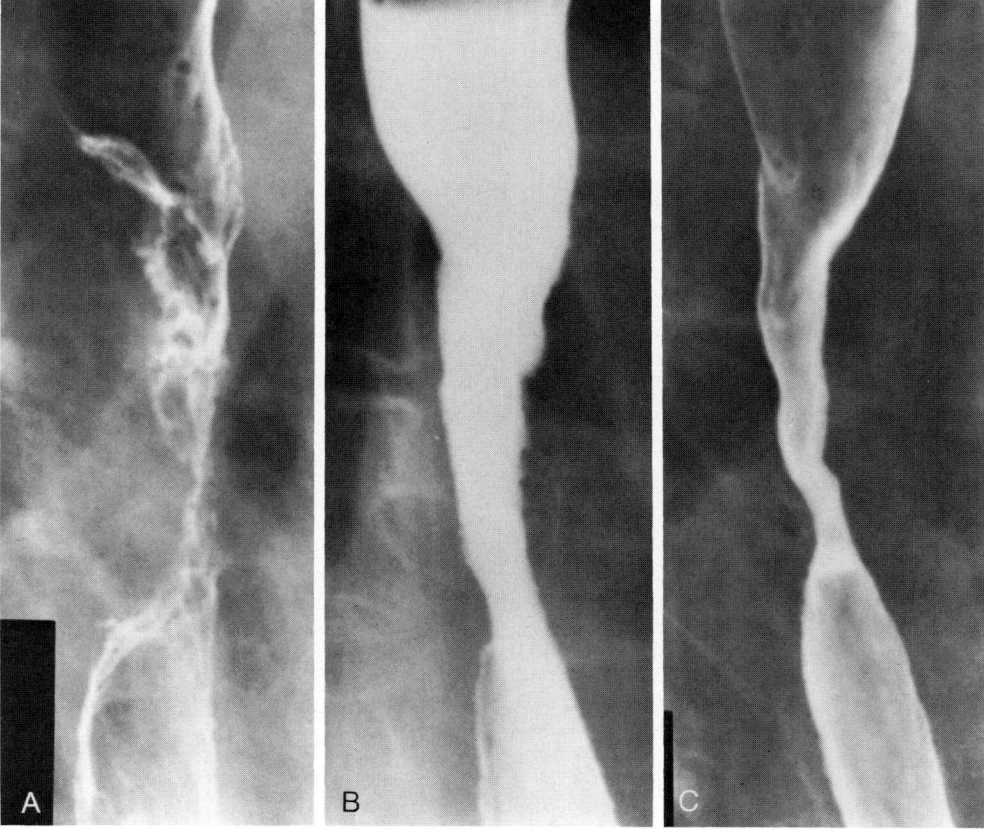

creased morbidity or mortality may also be attributed directly to complications of radiation therapy, such as esophageal ulceration, perforation, and fistula formation.[179, 181] As a result, the prognosis after radiation therapy is comparable to or slightly worse than that after surgery, with an average survival of only 9 to 10 months.

Partial regression of tumor after radiation therapy may be recognized on barium studies by a decrease in the size and bulk of the lesion compared with those before treatment. With total regression of tumor, esophagography may reveal a normal esophagus (Fig. 28–38) or a benign-appearing stricture at the site of the original lesion[177, 178, 182, 183] (Fig. 28–39). In most cases, these strictures appear as smooth, tapered areas of narrowing without evidence of nodularity, mass effect, or ulceration to suggest residual tumor. Even when there is total regression of tumor, these patients often die as a result of distant metastases, presumably because of unrecognized lymphatic involvement at the time of therapy.[177] Thus, disappearance of the cancer on radiologic or endoscopic studies does not necessarily indicate a cure.

Although most patients have an initial clinical response to radiation therapy, recurrent dysphagia often occurs within 3 to 9 months after treatment because of local recurrence of tumor.[174, 177, 178] Recurrent carcinoma may be recognized on barium studies by the development of a polypoid, ulcerative, or infiltrating lesion within or just beyond the margins of the original radiation portal.[177] However, exacerbation of symptoms in these patients may result not only from recurrent tumor but also from benign radiation strictures, fistula formation, perforation, or opportunistic esophageal infections such as *Candida* and herpes esophagitis.[177] Thus, radiologic studies may differentiate recurrent carcinoma from other esophageal complications in these patients.

## Acknowledgment

Figure 28–1A and B is reproduced from Laufer I, Levine MS (eds): Double Contrast Gastrointestinal Radiology (2nd ed). Philadelphia: WB Saunders, 1992.

Figures 28–4A, 28–5, 28–7A to C, 28–9, 28–12, 28–13, 28–14, 28–15A and B, 28–19B, 28–22, 28–23, and 28–39 are reproduced from Levine MS: Radiology of the Esophagus. Philadelphia: WB Saunders, 1989.

# References

1. Livstone EM, Skinner DB: Tumors of the esophagus. *In* Berk JE (ed): Gastroenterology. Philadelphia: WB Saunders, 1985, pp 818–850.
2. Cancer statistics, 1985. CA 35:19–35, 1985.
3. Wynder EL, Mabuchi K: Cancer of the esophagus: etiological and environmental factors. JAMA 226:1546–1548, 1973.
4. Pottern LM, Morris LE, Blot WJ, et al: Esophageal cancer among black men in Washington DC: alcohol, tobacco, and other risk factors. J Natl Cancer Inst 67:777–783, 1981.
5. Fielding JE: Smoking: health effects and control. N Engl J Med 313:491–498, 1985.
6. Yang CS: Research on esophageal cancer in China: a review. Cancer Res 40:2633–2644, 1980.
7. Warwick GP, Harington JS: Some aspects of the epidemiology and etiology of esophageal cancer with particular emphasis on the Transkei, South Africa. Adv Cancer Res 17:81–229, 1973.
8. Burrell RJW, Roach WA, Shadwell A: Esophageal cancer in the Bantu of the Transkei associated with mineral deficiency in garden plants. J Natl Cancer Inst 36:201–214, 1966.
9. Amer MH, El-Yazigi A, Hannan MA, et al: Water contamination and esophageal cancer at Gassim Region, Saudi Arabia. Gastroenterology 98:1141–1147, 1990.
10. Correa P: Precursors of gastric and esophageal cancer. Cancer 50:2554–2565, 1982.
11. Stephen SJ, Uragoda CG: Some observations on oesophageal carcinoma in Ceylon, including its relationship to betel chewing. Br J Cancer 24:11–15, 1970.
12. Craighead JE, Mossman BT: The pathogenesis of asbestos-associated diseases. N Engl J Med 306:1446–1455, 1982.
13. Just-Viera JO, Haight C: Achalasia and carcinoma of the esophagus. Surg Gynecol Obstet 128:1081–1093, 1969.
14. Lortat-Jacob JL, Richard CA, Fekete F, et al: Cardiospasm and esophageal carcinoma: report of 24 cases. Surgery 66:969–975, 1969.
15. Seliger G, Lee T, Schwartz S: Carcinoma of the proximal esophagus: a complication of long-standing achalasia. Am J Gastroenterol 57:20–25, 1972.
16. Carter R, Brewer LA: Achalasia and esophageal carcinoma. Am J Surg 130:114–118, 1975.
17. Wychulis AR, Woolam GL, Andersen HA, et al: Achalasia and carcinoma of the esophagus. JAMA 215:1638–1641, 1971.
18. Hankins JR, McLaughlin JS: The association of carcinoma of the esophagus with achalasia. J Thorac Cardiovasc Surg 69:355–360, 1975.
19. Chuong JJH, DuBovik S, McCallum RW: Achalasia as a risk factor for esophageal carcinoma: a reappraisal. Dig Dis Sci 29:1105–1108, 1984.
20. Bigger IA, Vinson PP: Carcinoma secondary to burn of the esophagus from ingestion of lye. Surgery 28:887–889, 1950.
21. Imre J, Kopp M: Arguments against long-term conservative treatment of oesophageal strictures due to corrosive burns. Thorax 27:594–598, 1972.
22. Bigelow NH: Carcinoma of the esophagus developing at the site of lye stricture. Cancer 6:1159–1164, 1953.
23. Appleqvist P, Salmo M: Lye corrosion carcinoma of the esophagus: a review of 63 cases. Cancer 45:2655–2658, 1980.
24. Hopkins RA, Postlethwait RW: Caustic burns and carcinoma of the esophagus. Ann Surg 194:146–148, 1981.
25. Lansing PB, Ferrante WA, Ochsner JL: Carcinoma of the esophagus at the site of lye stricture. Am J Surg 118:108–111, 1969.
26. Weaver A, Fleming SM, Knechtges TC, et al: Triple endoscopy: a neglected essential in head and neck cancer. Surgery 86:493–496, 1979.
27. Atkinson D, Fleming S, Weaver A: Triple endoscopy: a valuable procedure in head and neck surgery. Am J Surg 144:416–419, 1982.
28. McGuirt WF: Panendoscopy as a screening examination for simultaneous primary tumors in head and neck cancer: a prospective sequential study and review of the literature. Laryngoscope 92:569–576, 1982.
29. Wynder EL, Mushinski MH, Spivak JC: Tobacco and alcohol consumption in relation to the development of multiple primary cancers. Cancer 40:1872–1878, 1977.
30. Brechwa-Ajdukiewicz A, McCarthy CF, Austad WI, et al: Carcinoma, villous atrophy, and steatorrhea. Gut 7:572–577, 1966.
31. Harris OD, Cooke WT, Thompson H, et al: Malignancy in adult coeliac disease and idiopathic steatorrhea. Am J Med 42:899–912, 1967.
32. Collins SM, Hamilton JD, Lewis TD, et al: Small bowel malabsorption and gastrointestinal malignancy. Radiology 126:603–609, 1978.
33. Chisholm M: The association between webs, iron and postcricoid carcinoma. Postgrad Med J 50:215–219, 1974.
34. Wynder EL, Hultberg S, Jacobsson F, et al: Environmental factors in cancer of the upper alimentary tract: a Swedish study with special reference to Plummer-Vinson (Paterson-Kelly) syndrome. Cancer 10:470–487, 1957.
35. Chudecki B: Radiation cancer of the thoracic oesophagus. Br J Radiol 45:303–304, 1972.
36. O'Connell EW, Seaman WB, Ghahremani GG: Radiation-induced esophageal carcinoma. Gastrointest Radiol 9:287–291, 1984.

37. Shine I, Allison PR: Carcinoma of the oesophagus with tylosis. Lancet 1:951–953, 1966.
38. Harper PS, Harper RMJ, Howel-Evans AW: Carcinoma of the oesophagus with tylosis. Q J Med 39:317–333, 1970.
39. Munyer TP, Margulis AR: Tylosis. AJR 136:1026–1027, 1981.
40. Guojun H, Lingfang S, Dawei Z, et al: Diagnosis and surgical treatment of early esophageal carcinoma. Chin Med J [Engl] 94:229–232, 1981.
41. Shu YJ: Cytopathology of the esophagus: an overview of esophageal cytopathology in China. Acta Cytol (Baltimore) 27:7–16, 1983.
42. Japanese Society for Esophageal Diseases: Guidelines for the clinical and pathologic studies on carcinoma of the esophagus. Jpn J Surg 6:69–78, 1976.
43. Moss AA, Koehler RE, Margulis AR: Initial accuracy of esophagograms in detection of small esophageal carcinoma. AJR 127:909–913, 1976.
44. Zornoza J, Lindell MM: Radiologic evaluation of small esophageal carcinoma. Gastrointest Radiol 5:107–111, 1980.
45. Mannell A: Carcinoma of the esophagus. Curr Probl Surg 19:553–647, 1982.
46. Yamada A: Radiologic assessment of resectability and prognosis in esophageal carcinoma. Gastrointest Radiol 4:213–218, 1979.
47. Postlethwait RW: Carcinoma of the esophagus. Curr Probl Cancer 2:1–44, 1978.
48. Fitzgerald RH, Bartles DM, Parker EF: Tracheoesophageal fistulas secondary to carcinoma of the esophagus. J Thorac Cardiovasc Surg 82:194–197, 1981.
49. Little AG, Ferguson MK, DeMeester TR, et al: Esophageal carcinoma with respiratory tract fistula. Cancer 53:1322–1328, 1984.
50. Bottiglieri NG, Palmer ED, Briggs GW, et al: Aortoesophageal fistula complicating carcinoma of the esophagus. Am J Dig Dis 8:837–844, 1963.
51. McCort JJ: Radiographic identification of lymph node metastases from carcinoma of the esophagus. Radiology 59:694–711, 1952.
52. Mandard AM, Chasle J, Marnay J, et al: Autopsy findings in 111 cases of esophageal cancer. Cancer 48:329–335, 1981.
53. Sannohe Y, Hiratsuka R, Doki K: Lymph node metastases in cancer of the thoracic esophagus. Am J Surg 141:216–218, 1981.
54. Rosengren JE, Goldstein HM: Radiologic demonstration of multiple foci of malignancy in the esophagus. Gastrointest Radiol 3:11–13, 1978.
55. Davis M, Gogel H, McIntire C, et al: Esophageal carcinoma multiplex with gastric metastasis. Gastrointest Radiol 14:6–8, 1989.
56. Glick SN, Teplick SK, Levine MS, et al: Gastric cardia metastasis in esophageal carcinoma. Radiology 160:627–630, 1986.
57. Glick SN, Teplick SK, Levine MS: Squamous cell metastases to the gastric cardia. Gastrointest Radiol 10:339–344, 1985.
58. Postlethwait RW, Sealy WC, Emlet JKR, et al: Squamous cell carcinoma of the esophagus. Surg Gynecol Obstet 105:465–472, 1957.
59. Carey LC, Darin JC, Worman LW, et al: Upper gastrointestinal hemorrhage from carcinoma of esophagus. Arch Surg 90:460–464, 1965.
60. Barrie JR, Goodner JT: Hematemesis from cancer of the esophagus. J Thorac Cardiovasc Surg 56:289–292, 1968.
61. Ghosh BC, Choudhry KU, Beattie EJ: Massive bleeding from esophageal cancer. J Thorac Cardiovasc Surg 63:977–979, 1972.
62. Alrenga DP: Fatal hemorrhage complicating carcinoma of the esophagus: report of four cases. Am J Gastroenterol 65:422–426, 1976.
63. Sherlock P, Ehrlich AN, Winawer SJ: Diagnosis of gastrointestinal cancer: current status and recent progress. Gastroenterology 63:672–700, 1972.
64. Bruni HC, Nelson RS: Carcinoma of the esophagus and cardia. J Thorac Cardiovasc Surg 70:367–370, 1975.
65. Bemventui GA, Hattori K, Levin B, et al: Endoscopic sampling for tissue diagnosis in GI malignancy. Gastrointest Endosc 21:159–161, 1975.
66. Appleqvist P: Carcinoma of the oesophagus and gastric cardia. Acta Chir Scand [Suppl] 430:1–92, 1972.
67. Koehler RE, Moss AA, Margulis AR: Early radiographic man-

ifestations of carcinoma of the esophagus. Radiology 119:1–5, 1976.
68. Skinner DB: Surgical treatment for esophageal carcinoma. Semin Oncol 11:136–143, 1984.
69. Levine MS, Dillon EC, Saul SH, et al: Early esophageal cancer. AJR 146:507–512, 1986.
70. Suzuki H, Kobayashi S, Endo M, et al: Diagnosis of early esophageal cancer. Surgery 71:99–103, 1971.
71. Yamada A, Kobayashi S, Kawai B, et al: Study on x-ray findings of early oesophageal cancer. Australas Radiol 16:238–246, 1972.
72. Itai Y, Kogure T, Okuyama Y, et al: Superficial esophageal carcinoma: radiological findings in double-contrast studies. Radiology 126:597–601, 1978.
73. Zheng-Yan W: Radiological appearances in early oesophageal carcinoma. J R Soc Med 73:849–852, 1980.
74. Sato T, Sakai Y, Kajita A, et al: Radiographic microstructures of early esophageal carcinoma: correlation of specimen radiography with pathologic findings and clinical radiography. Gastrointest Radiol 11:12–19, 1986.
75. Itai Y, Kogure T, Okuyama Y, et al: Diffuse finely nodular lesions of the esophagus. AJR 128:563–566, 1977.
76. Schmidt LW, Dean PJ, Wilson RT: Superficially invasive squamous cell carcinoma of the esophagus. Gastroenterology 91:1456–1461, 1986.
77. Lindell MM, Hill CA, Libshitz HI: Esophageal cancer: radiographic chest findings and their prognostic significance. AJR 133:461–465, 1979.
78. Putman CE, Curtis A, Westfried M, et al: Thickening of the posterior tracheal stripe: a sign of squamous cell carcinoma of the esophagus. Radiology 121:533–536, 1976.
79. Daffner RH, Postlethwait RW, Putman CE: Retrotracheal abnormalities in esophageal carcinoma: prognostic implications. AJR 130:719–723, 1978.
80. Wiot JW, Felson B: Radiographic differential diagnosis of esophageal cancer. JAMA 226:1548–1552, 1973.
81. Goldstein HM, Zornoza J, Hopens T: Intrinsic diseases of the adult esophagus: benign and malignant tumors. Semin Roentgenol 16:183–197, 1981.
82. Gloyna RE, Zornoza J, Goldstein HM: Primary ulcerative carcinoma of the esophagus. AJR 129:599–600, 1977.
83. Lawson TL, Dodds WJ, Sheft DJ: Carcinoma of the esophagus simulating varices. AJR 107:83–85, 1969.
84. Silver TM, Goldstein HM: Varicoid carcinoma of the esophagus. Dig Dis 19:56–58, 1974.
85. Yates CW, LeVine MA, Jensen KM: Varicoid carcinoma of the esophagus. Radiology 122:605–608, 1977.
86. Cho SR, Schneider V, Beachley MC, et al: Carcinoma of the esophagus: assessment of submucosal extent. J Can Assoc Radiol 33:154–157, 1982.
87. Steiner H, Lammer J, Hackl A: Lymphatic metastases to the esophagus. Gastrointest Radiol 9:1–4, 1984.
88. Allen HA, Bush JE: Midesophageal carcinoma metastatic to the stomach: its unusual appearance on an upper gastrointestinal series. South Med J 76:1049–1051, 1983.
89. Raphael HA, Ellis FH, Dockerty MB: Primary adenocarcinoma of the esophagus: 18 year review and review of literature. Ann Surg 164:785–796, 1966.
90. Turnbull ADM, Goodner JT: Primary adenocarcinoma of the esophagus. Cancer 22:915–918, 1968.
91. Hankins JR, Cole FN, Attar S, et al: Adenocarcinoma involving the esophagus. J Thorac Cardiovasc Surg 68:148–158, 1974.
92. Bosch A, Frias Z, Caldwell WL: Adenocarcinoma of the esophagus. Cancer 43:1557–1561, 1979.
93. Thompson JJ, Zinsser KR, Enterline HT: Barrett's metaplasia and adenocarcinoma of the esophagus and gastroesophageal junction. Hum Pathol 14:42–61, 1983.
94. Keen SJ, Dodd GD, Smith JL: Adenocarcinoma arising in Barrett's esophagus: pathologic and radiologic features. Mt Sinai J Med 51:442–450, 1984.
95. Levine MS, Caroline D, Thompson JJ, et al: Adenocarcinoma of the esophagus: relationship to Barrett mucosa. Radiology 150:305–309, 1984.
96. Agha FP: Barrett carcinoma of the esophagus: clinical and radiographic analysis of 34 cases. AJR 145:41–46, 1985.

97. Haggitt RC, Tryzelaar J, Ellis FH, et al: Adenocarcinoma complicating columnar epithelium-lined (Barrett's) esophagus. Am J Clin Pathol 70:1–5, 1978.

98. Bozymski EM, Herlihy KJ, Orlando RC: Barrett's esophagus. Ann Intern Med 97:103–107, 1982.

99. Sjogren RW, Johnson LF: Barrett's esophagus: a review. Am J Med 74:313–321, 1983.

100. Spechler SJ, Goyal RK: Barrett's esophagus. N Engl J Med 315:362–371, 1986.

101. Naef AP, Savary M, Ozzello L: Columnar-lined lower esophagus: an acquired lesion with malignant predisposition. J Thorac Carciovasc Surg 70:826–835, 1975.

102. Burbige EJ, Radigan JJ: Characteristics of the columnar-cell lined (Barrett's) esophagus. Gastrointest Endosc 25:133–136, 1979.

103. Starnes VA, Adkins RB, Ballinger JF, et al: Barrett's esophagus: a surgical entity. Arch Surg 119:563–567, 1984.

104. Sarr MG, Hamilton SR, Marrone GC, et al: Barrett's esophagus: its prevalence and association with adenocarcinoma in patients with symptoms of gastroesophageal reflux. Am J Surg 149:187–192, 1985.

105. Trier JS: Morphology of the epithelium of the distal esophagus in patients with midesophageal peptic strictures. Gastroenterology 58:444–461, 1970.

106. Paull A, Trier JS, Dalton MD, et al: The histologic spectrum of Barrett's esophagus. N Engl J Med 295:476–480, 1976.

107. Berenson MM, Riddell RH, Skinner DB, et al: Malignant transformation of esophageal columnar epithelium. Cancer 41:554–561, 1978.

108. Harle IA, Finley RJ, Belsheim M: Management of adenocarcinoma in a columnar-lined esophagus. Ann Thorac Surg 40:330–336, 1985.

109. Hamilton SR, Smith RRL: The relationship between columnar epithelial dysplasia and invasive adenocarcinoma arising in Barrett's esophagus. Am J Clin Pathol 87:301–312, 1987.

110. Reid BJ, Weinstein WM, Lewin KJ, et al: Endoscopic biopsy can detect high-grade dysplasia or early adenocarcinoma in Barrett's esophagus without grossly recognizable neoplastic lesions. Gastroenterology 94:81–90, 1988.

111. Hameeteman W, Tytgat GNJ, Houthoff HJ, et al: Barrett's esophagus: development of dysplasia and adenocarcinoma. Gastroenterology 96:1249–1256, 1989.

112. Sanfey H, Hamilton SR, Smith RRL, et al: Carcinoma arising in Barrett's esophagus. Surg Gynecol Obstet 161:570–574, 1985.

113. McDonald GB, Brand DL, Thorning DR: Multiple adenomatous neoplasms arising in columnar-lined (Barrett's) esophagus. Gastroenterology 72:1317–1321, 1977.

114. Keeffe EB, Hiskin EC, Schubert F: Adenomatous polyp arising in Barrett's esophagus. J Clin Gastroenterol 8:271–274, 1986.

115. Radigan LR, Glover JL, Shipley FE, et al: Barrett esophagus. Arch Surg 112:486–491, 1977.

116. Skinner DB, Walther BC, Riddell RH, et al: Barrett's esophagus: comparison of benign and malignant cases. Ann Surg 198:554–565, 1983.

117. Spechler SJ, Robbins AH, Rubins HB, et al: Adenocarcinoma and Barrett's esophagus: an overrated risk? Gastroenterology 87:927–933, 1984.

118. Cameron AJ, Ott BJ, Payne WS: The incidence of adenocarcinoma in the columnar-lined (Barrett's) esophagus. N Engl J Med 313:857–859, 1985.

119. Robertson CS, Mayberry JF, Nicholson DA, et al: Value of endoscopic surveillance in the detection of neoplastic change in Barrett's oesophagus. Br J Surg 75:760–763, 1988.

120. Recht MP, Levine MS, Katzka DA, et al: Barrett's esophagus in scleroderma: increased prevalence and radiographic findings. Gastrointest Radiol 13:1–5, 1988.

121. Halpert RD, Laufer I, Thompson JJ, et al: Adenocarcinoma of the esophagus in patients with scleroderma. AJR 140:927–930, 1983.

122. Kalish RJ, Clancy PE, Orringer MB, et al: Clinical, epidemiologic, and morphologic comparison between adenocarcinomas arising in Barrett's esophageal mucosa and in the gastric cardia. Gastroenterology 86:461–467, 1984.

123. Dupas JL, Caproy JP, Lorriaux A: Endoscopic diagnosis of early primary adenocarcinoma in Barrett's columnar-lined esophagus. Endoscopy 7:98–101, 1975.

124. Odes HS, Maor E, Barki Y, et al: Varicoid carcinoma of the esophagus: report of a patient with adenocarcinoma and review of the literature. Am J Gastroenterol 73:141–145, 1980.

125. Montesi A, Alessandro P, Graziani L, et al: Small benign tumors of the esophagus: radiological diagnosis with double contrast examination. Gastrointest Radiol 8:207–212, 1983.

126. Levine MS, Cajade AG, Herlinger H, et al: Pseudomembranes in reflux esophagitis. Radiology 159:43–45, 1986.

127. Levine MS, Macones AJ, Laufer I: *Candida* esophagitis: accuracy of radiographic diagnosis. Radiology 154:581–587, 1985.

128. Glick SN, Teplick SK, Goldstein J, et al: Glycogenic acanthosis of the esophagus. AJR 139:683–688, 1982.

129. Itai Y, Kogure T, Okuyama Y, et al: Diffuse finely nodular lesions of the esophagus. AJR 128:563–566, 1977.

130. Itai Y, Kogure T, Okuyama Y, et al: Radiological manifestations of oesophageal involvement in acanthosis nigricans. Br J Radiol 49:592–593, 1976.

131. Nuwayhid NS, Ballard ET, Cotton R: Esophageal papillomatosis. Ann Otol Rhinol Laryngol 86:623–625, 1977.

132. Levine MS, Kressel HY, Caroline D, et al: Barrett esophagus: reticular pattern of the mucosa. Radiology 147:663–667, 1983.

133. Agha FP, Whitehouse WM: Carcinoma of the esophagus: its varied radiologic features. Mt Sinai J Med 51:430–441, 1984.

134. Berridge FR, Gregg D: The value of cinematography in the diagnosis of malignant strictures of the oesophagus. Br J Radiol 31:465–471, 1958.

135. Agha FP, Keren DF: Spindle-cell squamous carcinoma of the esophagus: a tumor with biphasic morphology. AJR 145:541–545, 1985.

136. Wolfel DA: Leiomyosarcoma of the esophagus. AJR 89:127–131, 1963.

137. Carter MM, Kulkarni MV: Giant fibrovascular polyp of the esophagus. Gastrointest Radiol 9:301–303, 1984.

138. Caruso RD, Berk RN: Lymphoma of the esophagus. Radiology 95:381–382, 1970.

139. Engelman RM, Scialla AV: Carcinoma of the esophagus presenting radiologically as a benign lesion. Dis Chest 53:652–655, 1968.

140. Beahrs OH, Henson DE, Hutter RVP, et al (eds): Manual for Staging of Cancer (3rd ed). Philadelphia: JB Lippincott, 1988, pp 63–67.

141. Halvorsen RA, Thompson WM: CT of esophageal neoplasms. Radiol Clin North Am 27:667–685, 1989.

142. Halvorsen RA, Thompson WM: Computed tomographic staging of gastrointestinal tract malignancies. Part I. Esophagus and stomach. Invest Radiol 22:2–16, 1987.

143. Thompson WM, Halvorsen RA, Fister WL, et al: Computed tomography for staging esophageal and gastroesophageal cancer: re-evaluation. AJR 141:951–958, 1983.

144. Halvorsen RA, Foster WL, Williford ME, et al: Pseudosarcoma of the esophagus: barium swallow and CT findings. J Can Assoc Radiol 34:278–281, 1983.

145. Postlethwait R: Squamous cell carcinoma of the esophagus. *In* Surgery of the Esophagus (2nd ed). East Norwalk, CT: Appleton-Century-Crofts, 1986, pp 369–442.

146. Picus D, Balfe DM, Koehler RE, et al: Computed tomography in the staging of esophageal carcinoma. Radiology 146:433–438, 1983.

147. Takashima S, Takeuchi N, Shiozaki H, et al: Carcinoma of the esophagus: CT vs. MR imaging in determining resectability. AJR 156:297–302, 1991.

148. Lackner K, Weiand G, Koster O, et al: Computed tomography for tumors of the esophagus and stomach. Fortschr Geb Rontgenstr Nuklearmed Erganzungsband 134:364–370, 1981.

149. Akiyama H, Tusurumaru M, Kawamura T, et al: Principles of surgical treatment for carcinoma of the esophagus. Analysis of lymph node involvement. Ann Surg 194:438–446, 1981.

150. Balfe DM, Mauro MA, Koehler RE, et al: Gastrohepatic ligament: normal and pathologic CT anatomy. Radiology 150:485–490, 1984.

151. Moss AA, Schnyder P, Thoeni RF: Esophageal carcinoma: pretherapy staging by computed tomography. AJR 136:1051–1056, 1981.

152. Schneekloth G, Terrier F, Fuchs WA: Computed tomography in carcinoma of the esophagus and cardia. Gastrointest Radiol 8:193–206, 1983.

153. Samuelson L, Hambraeus GM, Mercke E, et al: CT staging of esophageal carcinoma. Acta Radiol Diagn 25:7–11, 1984.

154. Lea JW, Prager RL, Bender HW: The questionable role of computed tomography in preoperative staging of esophageal cancer. Ann Thorac Surg 38:479–481, 1984.

155. Quint LE, Glazer GM, Orringer MB, et al: Esophageal carcinoma: CT findings. Radiology 155:171–175, 1985.

156. Mannell A, Epstein B, Patel V, et al: The spread of oesophageal cancer: an evaluation of clinical barium and computed tomography assessments. Aust N Z J Surg 54:119–126, 1984.

157. Coulomb M, Leas JF, Sarrazin R, et al: Computed tomography and esophageal carcinoma. J Radiol 62:475–487, 1981.

158. Grosser G, Wimmer B, Ruf G: Computed tomography for carcinoma of the esophagus. A prospective study. Fortschr Geb Rontgenstr Nuklearmed Erganzungsband 143:288–293, 1985.

159. Mühling T, Kuklinski ME, Hübsch T, et al: Computed tomography of oesophageal carcinoma. A correlation of computed tomographic and post-operative findings. ROFO 143:189–193, 1985.

160. Gayet B, Frija J, Cahuzac J, et al: The usefulness of computed tomography in esophageal carcinoma. A prospective and "blind" study. Gastroenterol Clin Biol 12:23–28, 1988.

161. Halvorsen RA, Magruder-Habib K, Foster W, et al: Esophageal cancer: long-term follow-up of staging by computed tomography. Radiology 161:147–151, 1986.

162. Quint LE, Glazer GM, Orringer MB: Esophageal imaging by MR and CT: study of normal anatomy and neoplasms. Radiology 156:727–731, 1985.

163. Kijima M, Kubo H, Nagao F, et al: MRI and CT findings of the paraesophageal organs and mediastinal lymph nodes with invasion or metastasis of esophageal carcinoma. In Siewert JR, Holscher AH (eds): Diseases of the Esophagus (1st ed). New York: Springer-Verlag, 1987, pp 149–151.

164. Lehr L, Rupp N, Siewert JR: Assessment of resectability of esophageal cancer by computed tomography and magnetic resonance imaging. Surgery 103:344–350, 1987.

165. Halvorsen RA, Herfkens RJ, Wolfe WG, et al: Comparison of magnetic resonance to computed tomography for staging esophageal carcinoma. Presented at American Roentgen Ray Society; May 1987; Miami Beach, FL.

166. Halvorsen RA, Thompson WM: Primary neoplasms of the hollow organs of the gastrointestinal tract: staging and follow-up. Cancer 67:1181–1188, 1991.

167. Murata Y, Muroi ML, Yoshida M, et al: Endoscopic ultrasonography in the diagnosis of esophageal carcinoma. Surg Endosc 1:11–16, 1987.

168. Hyder N: Endoscopic ultrasonography of tumors of the esophagus and the stomach. Surg Endosc 1:17–23, 1987.

169. Shorvon PJ, Lees WR, Frost RA, et al: Upper gastrointestinal endoscopic ultrasonography and gastroenterology. Br J Radiol 60:429–438, 1987.

170. Tio TL, Cohen P, Conne PP, et al: Endosonography and computed tomography of esophageal carcinoma: preoperative classification compared to the new (1987) TNM system. Gastroenterology 96:1478–1486, 1989.

171. Sugimachi K, Ohno S, Fujishima H, et al: Endoscopic ultrasonographic detection of carcinomatous invasion and of lymph nodes in the thoracic esophagus. Surgery 107:366–371, 1990.

172. Rice TW, Sivak MV, Loop FD: Esophageal ultrasound and the preoperative staging of carcinoma of the esophagus. J Thorac Cardiovasc Surg 101:536–544, 1991.

173. Ziegler K, Sanft C, Zeitz M, et al: Evaluation of endosonography in TN staging of esophageal cancer. Gut 32:16–20, 1991.

174. Beatty JD, DeBoer G, Rider WD: Carcinoma of the esophagus: pretreatment assessment, correlation of radiation treatment parameters with survival, and identification and management of radiation treatment failure. Cancer 43:2254–2267, 1979.

175. Parker EF, Gregorie HB: Carcinoma of the esophagus: long-term results. JAMA 235:1018–1020, 1976.

176. Rosenberg JS, Franklin B, Steiger Z: Esophageal cancer: an interdisciplinary approach. Curr Probl Cancer 11:1–52, 1981.

177. Levine MS, Langer J, Laufer I, et al: Radiation therapy of esophageal carcinoma: correlation of clinical and radiographic findings. Gastrointest Radiol 12:99–105, 1987.

178. Pearson JG: The value of radiotherapy in the management of esophageal cancer. AJR 105:500–513, 1969.

179. Drucker MH, Mansour KA, Hatcher CR, et al: Esophageal carcinoma: an aggressive approach. Ann Thorac Surg 28:133–137, 1979.

180. Fraser RW, Wara WM, Thomas AN, et al: Combined treatment methods for carcinoma of the esophagus. Radiology 128:461–465, 1978.

181. Elkon D, Lee MS, Hendrickson FR: Carcinoma of the esophagus: sites of recurrence and palliative benefits after definitive radiotherapy. Int J Radiat Oncol Biol Phys 4:615–620, 1978.

182. Leborgne R, Leborgne F, Barlocci L: Cancer of the oesophagus: results of radiotherapy. Br J Radiol 36:806–811, 1963.

183. Wara WM, Mauch PM, Thomas AN, et al: Palliation for carcinoma of the esophagus. Radiology 121:717–720, 1976.

# Other Malignant Tumors

**Marc S. Levine, M.D.**

## METASTASES

Esophageal metastases are found at autopsy in about 3% of patients dying of carcinoma.[1] Most cases result from direct invasion by primary malignant tumors of the stomach, lung, and neck or from contiguous involvement by tumor-containing lymph nodes in the mediastinum. These various forms of esophageal involvement by metastatic tumor produce characteristic radiographic findings that are discussed separately in later sections.

### Sites of Origin

Carcinoma of the stomach accounts for about 50% of all esophageal metastases.[1, 2] Tumors involving the gastric cardia or fundus may invade the distal esophagus by contiguous spread through the diaphragmatic hiatus. Carcinomas of the lung and breast are other less common causes of esophageal metastases.[3–6] Most cases result from direct extension of tumor to the esophagus or from contiguous esophageal involvement by lymphadenopathy in the posterior mediastinum. Patients with metastatic breast cancer involving the esophagus are almost always found to have widespread metastatic disease.[5] The esophagus may also be involved by contiguous spread of malignant tumors in the neck, such as laryngeal, pharyngeal, and thyroid carcinoma, or by transdiaphragmatic spread of pancreatic carcinoma.[7, 8] Rarely, the esophagus may be involved by hematogenous metastases from tumors arising in distant locations such as the kidney, liver, rectum, prostate, cervix, and skin.[9–14] Thus, most malignant tumors are capable of metastasizing to the esophagus.

### Clinical Findings

About 50% of patients with esophageal metastases present with dysphagia as a result of esophageal compression by enlarged mediastinal lymph nodes or actual invasion of the esophagus by tumor.[1] Although the presence of esophageal metastases usually indicates a poor prognosis, some patients (particularly those with breast or lung cancer) may present with dysphagia as the initial manifestation of their disease.[4, 15] Patients with breast cancer often develop esophageal symptoms many years after treatment of the original tumor, with a peak incidence of dysphagia 4 to 5 years after mastectomy.[6] The longest reported interval between removal of a breast cancer and the development of esophageal metastases is 19 years.[16] When dysphagia occurs, however, these patients usually have widespread metastatic disease.[5]

Other presenting findings in patients with esophageal metastases include vomiting, epigastric or chest pain, anorexia, and weight loss. Occasionally, esophageal metastases may cause odynophagia or upper gastrointestinal bleeding due to ulceration of the overlying mucosa.[17] Rarely, esophageal perforation may lead to the development of a mediastinal abscess or tracheoesophageal fistula.[6, 15]

## Radiographic Findings

### Direct Invasion

Direct invasion of the cervical or thoracic esophagus by carcinoma of the larynx, pharynx, thyroid, or lung produces characteristic findings on barium studies. Early invasion may be manifested by a smooth or slightly irregular contour defect in the esophagus with gently sloping, obtuse borders and a contiguous soft tissue mass in the adjacent neck or mediastinum (Fig. 29–1). The area of involvement may have a more serrated, scalloped, or nodular appearance as the esophageal wall is further infiltrated by tumor (Fig. 29–2). Eventually, there may be circumferential narrowing of the esophagus associated with fixed, irregular folds, mass effect, nodularity, ulceration, or obstruction (Fig. 29–3). Thus, the radiographic findings are similar to those caused by malignant spread elsewhere in the gastrointestinal tract.

Secondary esophageal involvement by carcinoma of the gastric cardia or fundus may be manifested radiographically by a polypoid mass extending from the fundus into the distal esophagus[18, 19] (Fig. 29–4). Other infiltrating tumors may cause irregular narrowing of the distal esophagus without a discrete mass.[18, 19] Esophageal involvement is usually confined to a short segment of the distal esophagus but may extend as far proximally as the aortic arch.[18] Occasionally, these tumors may cause smooth, tapered narrowing of the distal esophagus at or just above the gastroesophageal junction, mimick-ing the appearance of achalasia (see later section on secondary achalasia).

When the distal esophagus appears to be involved by tumor on barium studies, the gastric cardia and fundus should also be evaluated radiographically to determine if there is associated gastric involvement. In some cases, barium studies may demonstrate an obvious malignant tumor in the stomach (see Fig. 29–4). In others, however, the presence of tumor in the gastric fundus may be recognized only by distortion or obliteration of the normal anatomic landmarks at the cardia associated with relatively subtle areas of nodularity, mass effect, or ulceration[19, 20] (Fig. 29–5). Thus, a meticulous double contrast examination of the fundus is essential to rule out an underlying carcinoma of the cardia in these patients.

### Contiguous Involvement by Mediastinal Lymph Nodes

Although any neoplasm that metastasizes to mediastinal lymph nodes may secondarily involve the esophagus, carcinomas of the breast and lung are the most common underlying malignancies in these patients.[3] Because of the proximity of the midesophagus to subcarinal lymph nodes, esophageal involvement by mediastinal lymphadenopathy occurs most frequently at this level.[15, 21] Barium studies typically reveal a smooth or slightly lobulated indentation on the right anterolateral

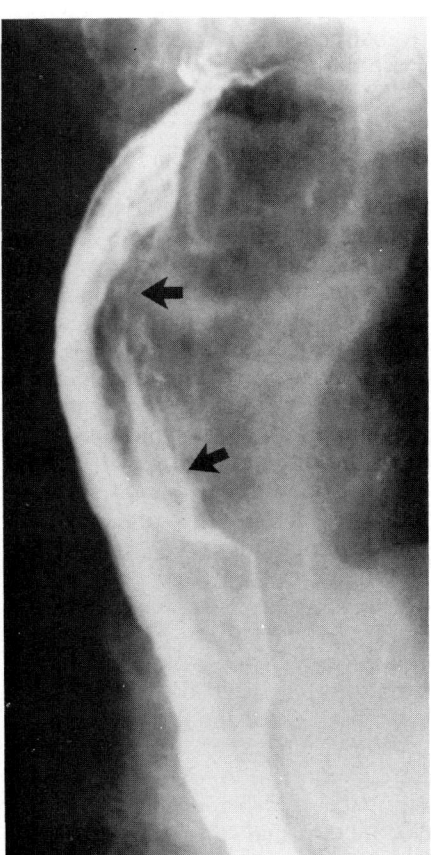

**Figure 29–1. Direct esophageal invasion by thyroid carcinoma.** The upper thoracic esophagus is compressed and displaced to the right *(arrows)* by a large thyroid mass. Note that the area of involvement has an irregular contour due to esophageal invasion by tumor.

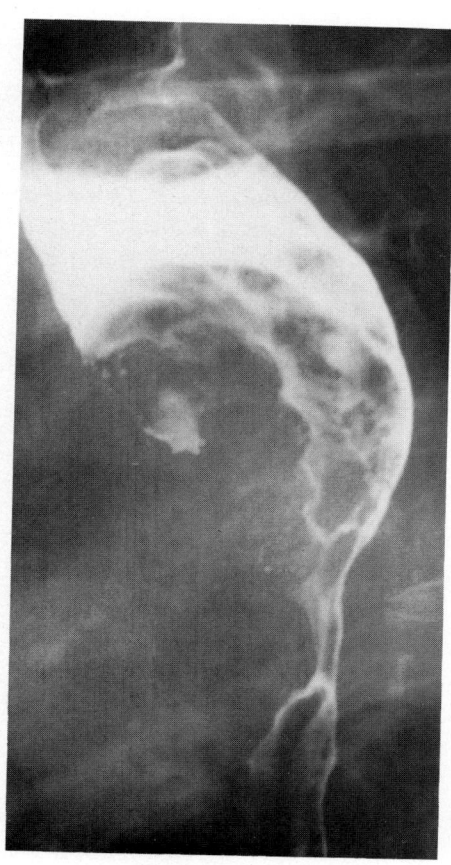

**Figure 29–2. Direct esophageal invasion by carcinoma of the lung.** There are eccentric mass effect and narrowing of the esophagus by tumor in the adjacent mediastinum. The scalloped contour of the esophagus in this region indicates direct invasion by tumor.

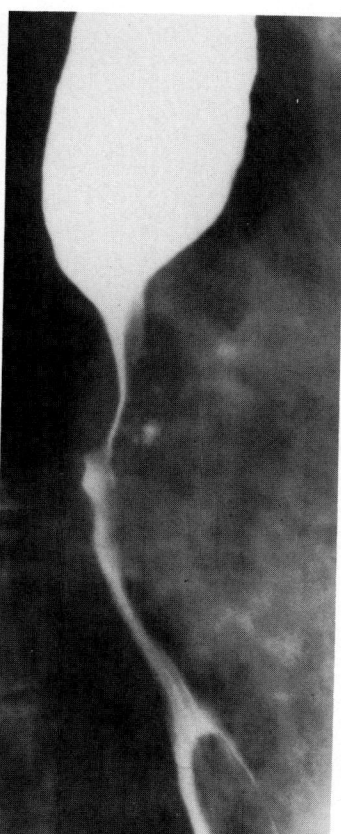

**Figure 29–3. Direct esophageal invasion by carcinoma of the lung.** This patient has a long segment of irregular narrowing in the upper thoracic esophagus due to circumferential involvement by metastatic tumor in the mediastinum. (Courtesy of Robert A. Goren, M.D., Philadelphia, PA.)

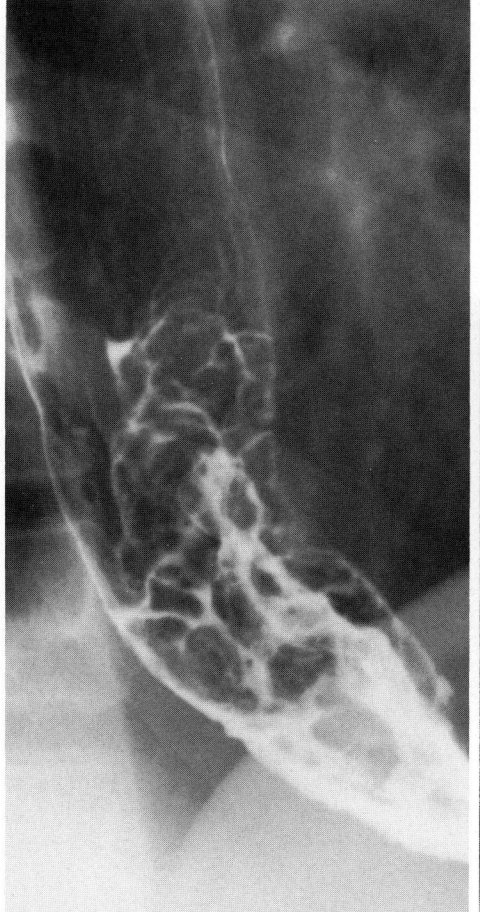

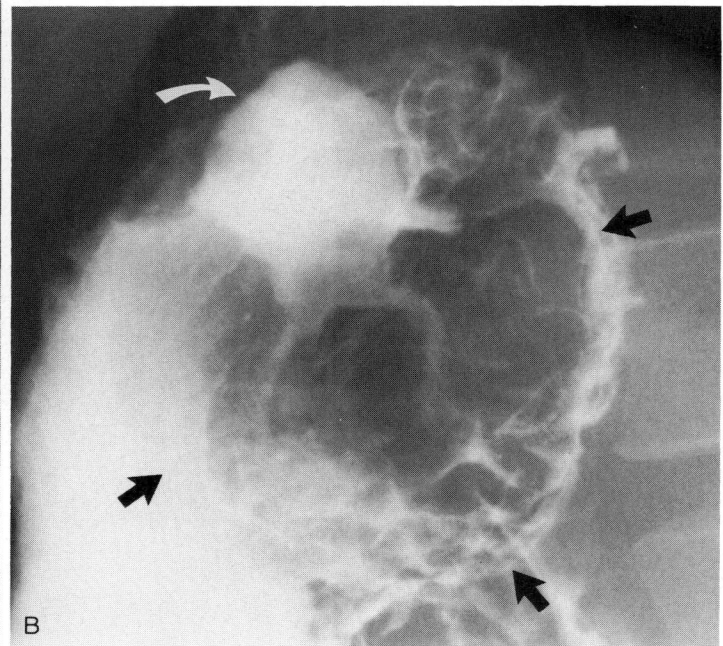

**Figure 29–4. Direct esophageal invasion by gastric carcinoma. A.** A double contrast esophagram shows a polypoid lesion in the distal esophagus, extending inferiorly to the gastroesophageal junction. **B.** A lateral view of the gastric fundus shows a large fundal mass *(black arrows)* containing an eccentric area of ulceration *(white arrow)*. This patient had a primary gastric carcinoma invading the distal esophagus.

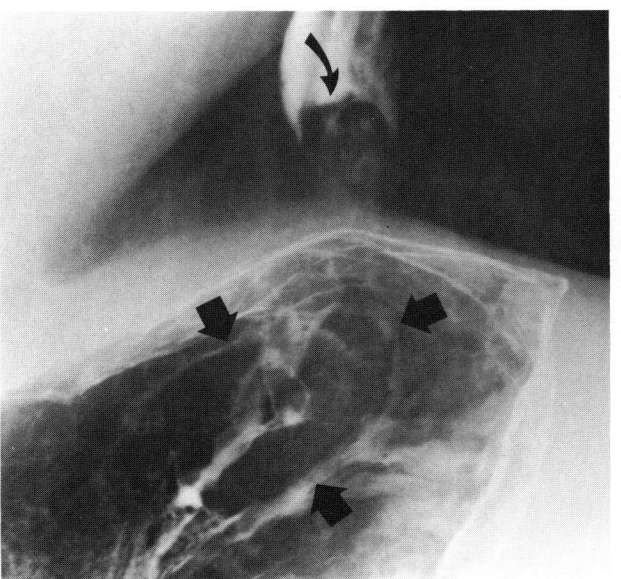

**Figure 29–5. Direct esophageal invasion by carcinoma of the gastric cardia.** A double contrast view of the fundus shows obliteration of the normal anatomic landmarks at the cardia with a centrally ulcerated polypoid lesion *(straight arrows)* extending into the distal esophagus *(curved arrow)*. (From MS Levine, I Laufer, JJ Thompson, Carcinoma of the gastric cardia in young people, AJR, 140, 1, 69–72, 1983, © by American Roentgen Ray Society.)

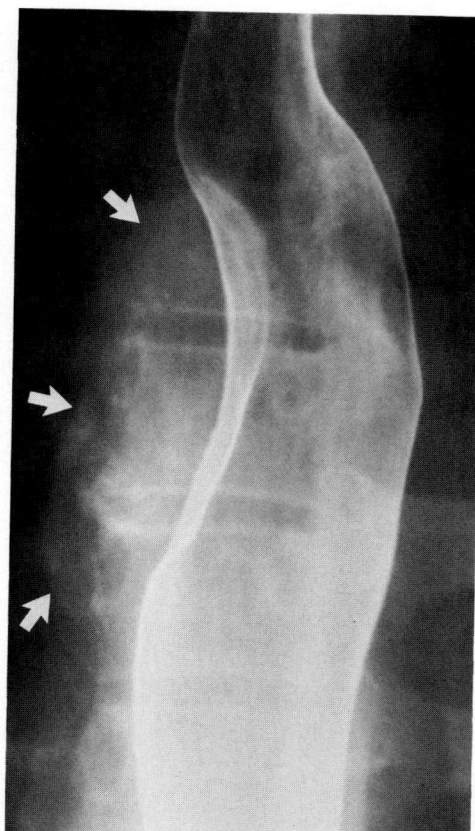

**Figure 29–6. Esophageal compression by mediastinal lymphadenopathy from carcinoma of the lung.** There is a smooth, gently sloping indentation on the right lateral wall of the midesophagus due to enlarged subcarinal lymph nodes *(arrows)* in the adjacent mediastinum.

wall of the esophagus at the level of the carina[15, 21] (Fig. 29–6). More extensive mediastinal lymphadenopathy may cause larger, more lobulated contour defects in the esophagus that are associated with ulceration or narrowing[2, 6, 12] (Fig. 29–7). Eventually, the wall of the esophagus may be circumferentially infiltrated by tumor, producing an area of concentric narrowing[4, 6, 12] (Fig. 29–8). In such patients, the presence of a soft tissue mass in the adjacent mediastinum should suggest esophageal involvement by tumor (see Fig. 29–8B). Computed tomography (CT) is often helpful for evaluating patients with suspected esophageal involvement by mediastinal lymphadenopathy.

## *Hematogenous Metastases*

True blood-borne or hematogenous metastases to the esophagus are extremely uncommon. Although most cases are caused by carcinoma of the breast, other distant tumors may also metastasize hematogenously to the esophagus. These lesions usually appear radiographically as short, eccentric strictures, most frequently in the middle third of the esophagus[2, 6, 12, 22] (Fig. 29–9). Rarely, hematogenous metastases, particularly those from malignant melanoma, may have a polypoid or

annular appearance indistinguishable from that of a primary esophageal carcinoma.[9, 11] Although blood-borne metastases to the esophagus tend to be manifested by infiltrating lesions, metastases from malignant melanoma may occasionally be manifested by one or more discrete submucosal masses[22] (Fig. 29–10). Rarely, hematogenous metastases may produce coalescent, nodular defects in the esophagus, mimicking the appearance of varices.

## Differential Diagnosis

A smooth or slightly lobulated indentation on the esophagus may be caused by a variety of extrinsic mass lesions, such as benign tumors and cysts in the mediastinum, aberrant vessels, and an ectatic aorta or aortic aneurysm compressing or displacing the esophagus. In contrast, esophageal invasion by metastatic tumor should be suspected when the area of mass effect has an irregular, serrated, or nodular contour associated with angulated, tethered folds or ulceration. As a result, malignant invasion of the esophagus usually can be distinguished radiographically from benign lesions in the

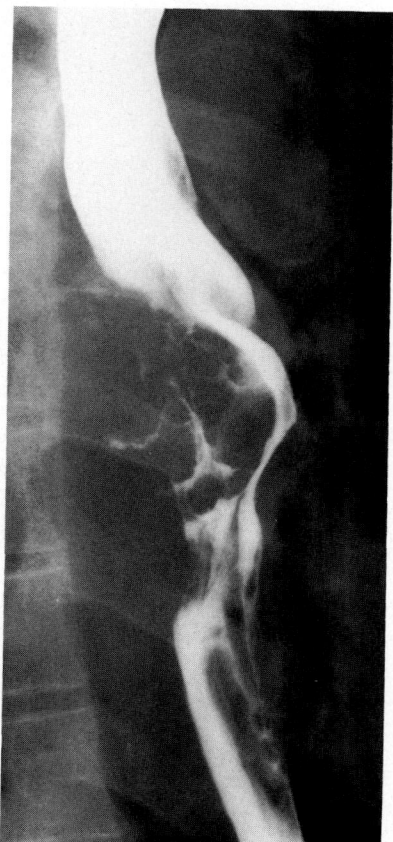

**Figure 29–7. Esophageal involvement by mediastinal lymphadenopathy from carcinoma of the cervix.** There is eccentric mass effect on the midesophagus with an irregular contour and ulceration due to esophageal invasion by tumor in adjacent subcarinal nodes.

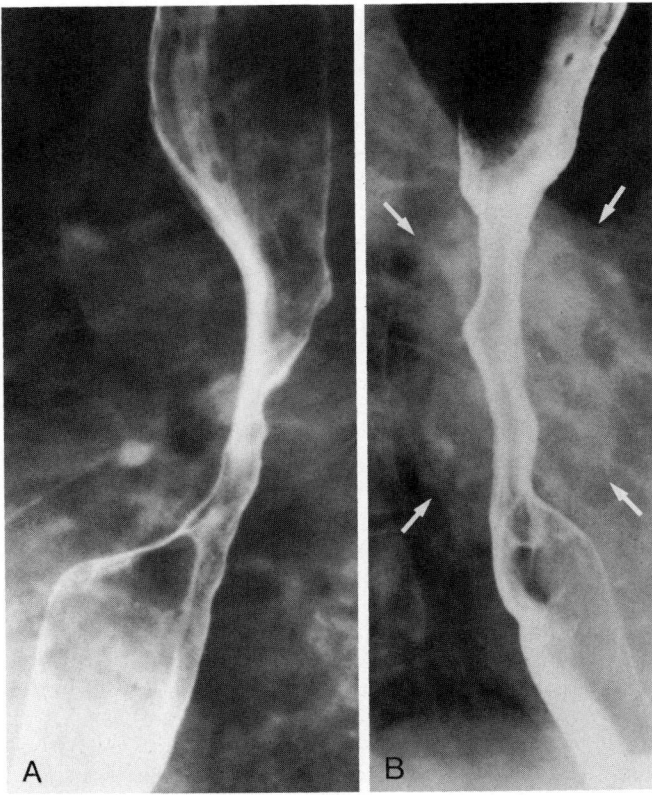

**Figure 29–8. Circumferential esophageal involvement by metastatic breast cancer in the mediastinum. A**. There are eccentric mass effect and narrowing of the midesophagus due to circumferential invasion by tumor in subcarinal nodes. **B**. In another patient, a relatively smooth, tapered area of narrowing is seen in the midesophagus. However, a surrounding soft tissue mass *(arrows)* in the mediastinum should suggest esophageal involvement by lymphadenopathy.

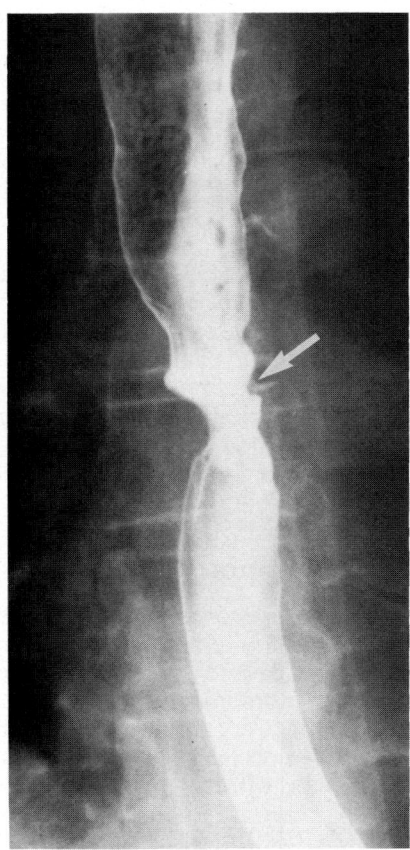

**Figure 29–9. Hematogenous metastasis to the esophagus from carcinoma of the breast.** The lesion is manifested by a short, benign-appearing stricture *(arrow)* in the midesophagus.

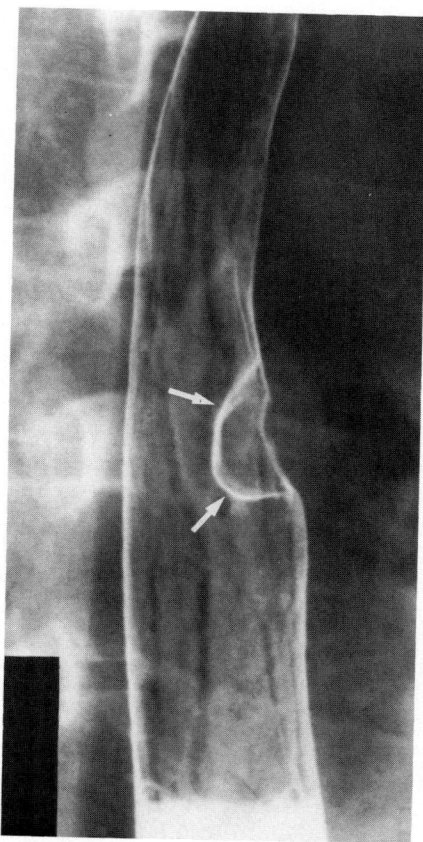

**Figure 29–10. Hematogenous metastasis to the esophagus from malignant melanoma.** A discrete submucosal mass *(arrows)* is seen in the midesophagus. This patient had additional metastatic lesions in the stomach.

mediastinum that are extrinsically compressing but not invading the esophagus.

In more advanced cases, circumferential narrowing of the esophagus by metastatic tumor can be mistaken for an infiltrating or annular esophageal carcinoma.[9] However, strictures caused by metastatic tumor often have a benign radiographic appearance, with intact overlying mucosa and smooth, tapered margins.[4, 6, 12, 22] When the strictures are located in the middle or upper third of the esophagus, the differential diagnosis includes Barrett's esophagus and scarring from mediastinal irradiation, caustic ingestion, *Candida* esophagitis, or oral medications such as potassium chloride and quinidine. When these patients are known to have a malignant, previously irradiated thoracic lesion, however, the major diagnostic consideration, for all practical purposes, is differentiation of recurrent tumor from a benign radiation stricture (see Chapter 26). In such cases, CT may confirm the presence of recurrent tumor by demonstrating a mediastinal mass or lymphadenopathy in the region of the stricture.

## SECONDARY ACHALASIA

The terms *secondary achalasia* and *pseudoachalasia* are used interchangeably to describe a condition in which the clinical, radiographic, endoscopic, and manometric features are indistinguishable from those of primary, or idiopathic, achalasia. Most cases of secondary achalasia are caused by carcinoma of the gastric cardia or fundus directly invading the gastroesophageal junction or distal esophagus.[23, 24] Less frequently, hematogenous metastases from breast, lung, pancreatic, or other malignant lesions may produce identical findings.[8, 14, 23] Occasionally, lymphoma or other benign conditions such as Chagas' disease and amyloidosis may also produce an achalasia-like syndrome.[25–27] It is important to differentiate primary and secondary achalasia, as primary achalasia may be treated by pneumatic dilatation, whereas secondary achalasia often necessitates exploratory laparotomy or other treatment for widespread metastatic disease.

## Pathogenesis

Both primary achalasia and secondary achalasia are characterized by absent esophageal peristalsis and a hypertensive lower esophageal sphincter that fails to relax normally in response to deglutition. In patients with primary achalasia, the motor disorder is thought to result in degeneration and loss of the ganglion cells of Auerbach's plexus in the esophagus. However, the precise mechanism by which metastases to the gastroesophageal junction produce this syndrome is uncertain. Some patients have tumor directly invading the distal esophagus with actual destruction of myenteric ganglia.[28] However, others have tumor confined to the gastroesophageal junction without involvement of the neural plexus in the esophagus.[29] It has therefore been suggested that this syndrome may also be caused by extraesophageal metastases to the vagus nerve or dorsal motor nucleus of the vagus nerve in the brain stem.[24, 29] Alternatively, secondary achalasia may be a paraneoplastic phenomenon caused by a circulating tumor product that alters esophageal motor function.[14] Finally, it has been postulated that high-grade obstruction of the esophagogastric region by metastatic tumor may cause esophageal decompensation with obliteration of normal peristalsis, mimicking the findings of primary achalasia.[14]

## Clinical Findings

Although dysphagia occurs in both primary achalasia and secondary achalasia, other clinical features are often helpful in distinguishing these entities. Most patients with primary achalasia are between 20 and 50 years of age, and they usually have dysphagia for 1 year or longer before seeking medical attention. In contrast, most patients with secondary achalasia are older than 50 years of age, and the duration of symptoms is usually less than 6 months.[23, 30] Also, secondary achalasia tends to be associated more frequently with weight loss and upper gastrointestinal bleeding.[23, 30] An underlying malignancy should therefore be suspected whenever achalasia is diagnosed radiographically or endoscopically in elderly patients who have recent onset of dysphagia,

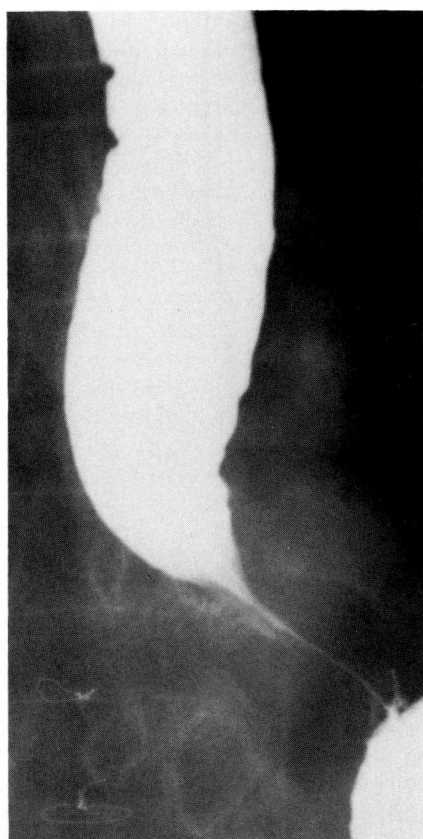

**Figure 29–11. Secondary achalasia.** There is smooth, tapered narrowing of the distal esophagus, producing an achalasia-like appearance due to a hematogenous metastasis to the gastroesophageal junction from colonic carcinoma.

weight loss, or upper gastrointestinal bleeding.[30] Nevertheless, some patients with primary achalasia may be older than 60 years of age, and some may have a relatively short duration of symptoms.[31] Thus, primary achalasia and secondary achalasia cannot always be differentiated by clinical criteria.

## Radiographic Findings

Secondary achalasia is classically manifested radiographically by absent peristalsis in the body of the esophagus associated with smooth, tapered narrowing of the distal esophagus, producing a "bird-beak" configuration at or just above the gastroesophageal junction[14, 23, 32] (Figs. 29–11 and 29–12). Although the radiographic appearance may closely resemble that of primary achalasia, certain morphologic features should suggest an underlying malignancy. Irregular, eccentric, or asymmetric involvement of the narrowed segment, abrupt transitions, rigidity, and mucosal nodularity or ulceration may be found in secondary achalasia due to infiltration of the distal esophagus by tumor[32] (Fig. 29–13). Another relatively subtle sign of malignancy is the length of the narrowed segment, which may extend several centimeters above the gastroesophageal junction in secondary achalasia but rarely extends as far proximally in the idiopathic form of the disease[32] (Fig. 29–14). Finally, abrupt angulation of the narrowed segment may result from elevation and encasement of the distal esophagus by tumor. Metastases from carcinoma of the tail of the pancreas have particularly been implicated as a cause of 90-degree or right-angled narrowing of the distal esophagus due to contiguous spread of tumor through the diaphragmatic hiatus.[8]

Because secondary achalasia usually is caused by carcinoma of the gastric cardia or fundus invading the distal esophagus, careful radiologic examination of the fundus is essential in these patients. Not infrequently, an obvious polypoid, ulcerated, or infiltrating malignancy may be demonstrated in the fundus (see Fig. 29–12). When significant esophageal obstruction prevents adequate filling of the fundus with barium, advanced

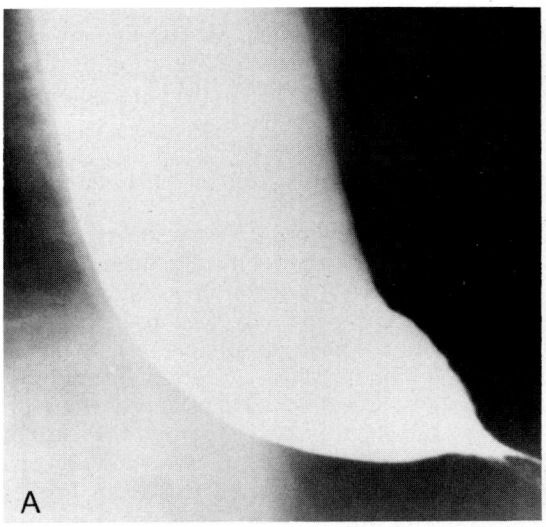
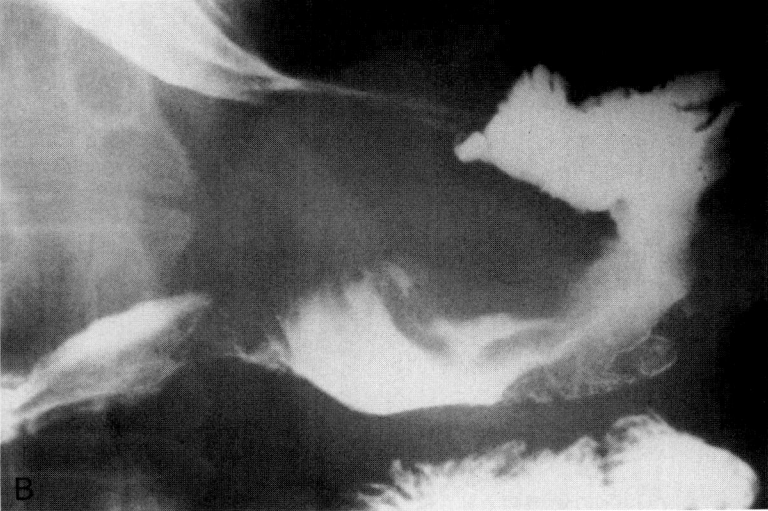

**Figure 29–12. Secondary achalasia caused by gastric carcinoma. A.** There is smooth, tapered narrowing of the distal esophagus, producing the characteristic bird-beak appearance of primary achalasia. **B.** However, a radiograph of the stomach reveals a diffusely infiltrating carcinoma of the gastric body and fundus that has invaded the distal esophagus.

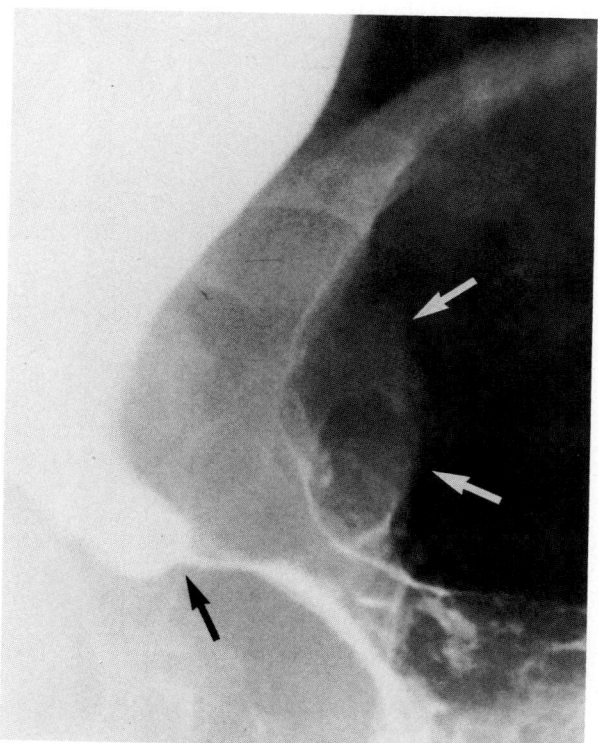

**Figure 29–13. Secondary achalasia caused by carcinoma of the gastric fundus.** In this patient, the relatively abrupt origin of the narrowed segment *(black arrow)* argues against a diagnosis of primary achalasia. Note the soft tissue defect *(white arrows)* in the fundus due to the patient's underlying fundal carcinoma.

tapered narrowing of the lower esophageal lumen, normal wall thickness, and no evidence of extrinsic compression.[35] The possibility of secondary achalasia should therefore be considered when there is mural thickening (particularly asymmetric mural thickening) or a soft tissue mass at the gastroesophageal junction.[35] CT is also helpful in identifying the site of the primary tumor (i.e., stomach, pancreas, or lung) in patients with secondary achalasia.

## LYMPHOMA

Esophageal lymphoma is a rare disease, accounting for only about 1 to 2% of all cases of lymphoma with gastrointestinal involvement.[36] Both non-Hodgkin's and, less commonly, Hodgkin's lymphoma may involve the esophagus. Whatever the cell type, these patients almost always have generalized lymphoma with direct invasion of the esophagus by lymphomatous nodes in the mediastinum, contiguous spread of lymphoma from the gastric fundus, or synchronous development of lymphoma in the wall of the esophagus.[37–41] Rarely, primary esophageal lymphoma may occur without extraesophageal disease.[42, 43]

Some investigators believe that esophageal involvement is an ominous finding in patients with lymphoma, usually leading to rapid deterioration and death within

lesions may still be recognized by the presence of a soft tissue defect in the fundal gas shadow or by an increased space between the fundus and diaphragm (see Fig. 29–13). With less advanced lesions, no gross abnormalities may be identified in the gastric fundus on conventional single contrast barium studies. However, double contrast studies of the fundus may demonstrate subtle evidence of tumor distorting or obliterating the normal anatomic landmarks at the cardia[19, 20] (see Fig. 29–14). In contrast, the esophageal "rosette" that demarcates the gastric cardia on double contrast studies should be normal in patients with primary achalasia.

Although secondary achalasia can often be diagnosed on barium studies, some cases may be difficult or impossible to distinguish from primary achalasia. A positive Mecholyl test is also nonspecific, as a response to the drug may be elicited in either condition.[33] However, it has been shown that inhalation of amyl nitrite, a smooth muscle relaxant, does not affect the narrowed esophageal segment in secondary achalasia but causes a measurable increase of 2 mm or more in the diameter of the segment in primary achalasia.[34] Thus, the use of amyl nitrite may be helpful in distinguishing these conditions.

CT may also have a role in evaluating patients with suspected achalasia when the findings on barium studies are equivocal. In primary achalasia, CT typically reveals moderate to marked esophageal dilatation, smooth,

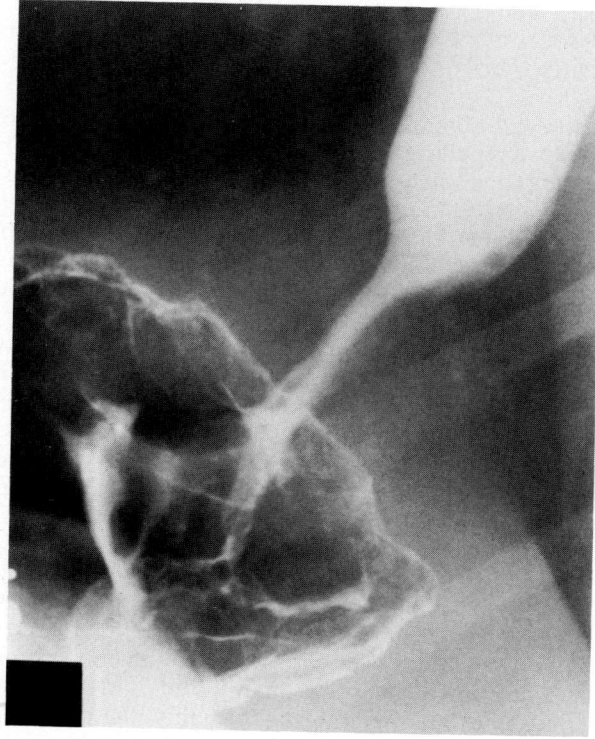

**Figure 29–14. Secondary achalasia caused by carcinoma of the gastric cardia.** Although smooth, tapered narrowing of the distal esophagus can occur in primary achalasia, the narrowed segment rarely extends as far proximally in primary achalasia as seen in this case. Note how the tumor is causing diffuse nodularity in the fundus with obliteration of the normal anatomic landmarks at the cardia.

6 to 12 months.[41] However, others have found that esophageal involvement does not significantly alter the overall prognosis of the disease and that long-term survival may still occur after radiation therapy or chemotherapy.[39, 44] When esophageal lymphoma is suspected, endoscopy should be performed with deep esophageal biopsies to confirm the diagnosis. However, false-negative biopsies have been reported in 25 to 35% of cases.[43, 45] Thus, some patients may require surgery for a definitive diagnosis.

## Clinical Findings

Most patients with esophageal lymphoma have no esophageal symptoms, so that the diagnosis usually is made at autopsy in patients with widespread disease.[36, 38] However, some patients may develop dysphagia as a result of esophageal narrowing or obstruction by tumor.[39–41, 44] Rarely, they may present with dysphagia as the initial manifestation of their disease.[46] Because many patients with lymphoma are treated with some form of immunosuppressive therapy, opportunistic esophagitis may be suspected as a more likely cause of dysphagia in these individuals. Occasionally, esophageal lymphoma may cause upper gastrointestinal bleeding, with hematemesis, melena, or guaiac-positive stool.[37] Rarely, esophageal perforation may lead to an esophagomediastinal, esophagobronchial, or tracheoesophageal fistula.[37, 47, 48]

## Radiographic Findings

Esophageal lymphoma may be manifested radiographically by irregular narrowing of the distal esophagus due to contiguous spread of tumor from the gastric fundus[39–41, 45] (Fig. 29–15). In such cases, careful radiologic examination of the gastric cardia and fundus may demonstrate a polypoid, ulcerated, or infiltrating lesion in the fundus due to associated gastric lymphoma. Transcardiac extension of gastric lymphoma is thought to occur in about 10% of patients.[45] However, these lesions cannot be distinguished radiographically from carcinoma of the gastric fundus invading the distal esophagus. Thus, the correct diagnosis can only be suggested in patients with a known history of gastric lymphoma. Rarely, lymphomatous involvement of the gastroesophageal junction may be manifested by smooth, tapered narrowing of the distal esophagus, mimicking the appearance of primary achalasia.[25]

Mediastinal lymphoma may cause extrinsic compression of the esophagus, resulting in a smooth indentation with obtuse, gently sloping borders.[38] Further esophageal involvement may be manifested by a more irregular or serrated contour abnormality due to invasion of the wall by tumor. Eventually, mediastinal lymphoma may cause diffuse esophageal narrowing (Fig. 29–16A). CT is particularly useful for determining the extent of disease in the mediastinum (Fig. 29–16B). Other patients may develop esophageal-airway fistulas, usually

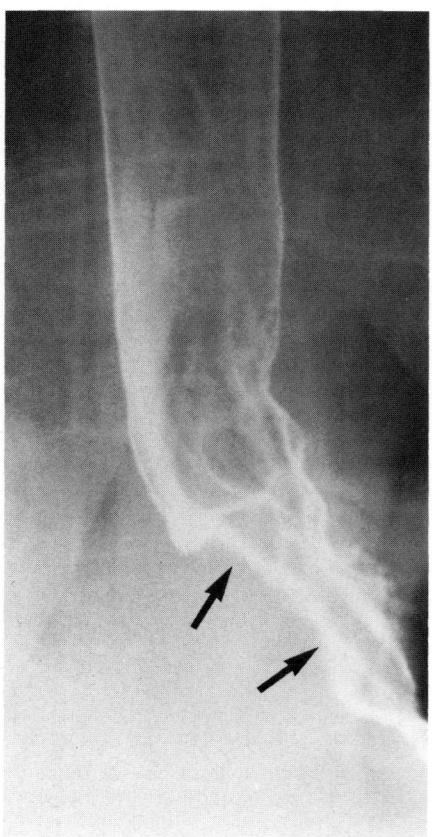

**Figure 29–15. Esophageal involvement by gastric lymphoma.** There is irregular narrowing *(arrows)* of the distal esophagus due to contiguous spread of lymphoma from the gastric fundus. Carcinoma of the gastric cardia invading the distal esophagus could produce identical findings.

as a complication of radiation therapy[37, 47, 48] (Fig. 29–17).

Depending on the pattern of growth, intrinsic esophageal lymphoma may be manifested by a spectrum of abnormalities, including submucosal nodules, enlarged folds, polypoid masses, or strictures. The most common finding is a polypoid or ulcerated mass or an infiltrating stricture indistinguishable from esophageal carcinoma[39–41, 44] (Fig. 29–18). Less frequently, lymphomatous infiltration of the submucosa may result in enlarged, tortuous longitudinal folds, mimicking the appearance of varices.[38–41] Occasionally, discrete submucosal masses may be found in the middle or distal third of the esophagus, suggesting multiple leiomyomas.[39, 40] In other patients, the esophagus may have a diffusely nodular appearance with innumerable tiny (3- to 10-mm) submucosal nodules extending from the thoracic inlet to the gastroesophageal junction[49, 50] (Fig. 29–19). Although these lesions can be mistaken for varices on conventional single contrast barium studies, the diffuse distribution and discrete margins of the lesions on double contrast studies allow them to be differentiated from varices.[49] *Candida* esophagitis may also produce a diffusely nodular appearance in the esophagus because of widespread plaque formation. However, the plaques of

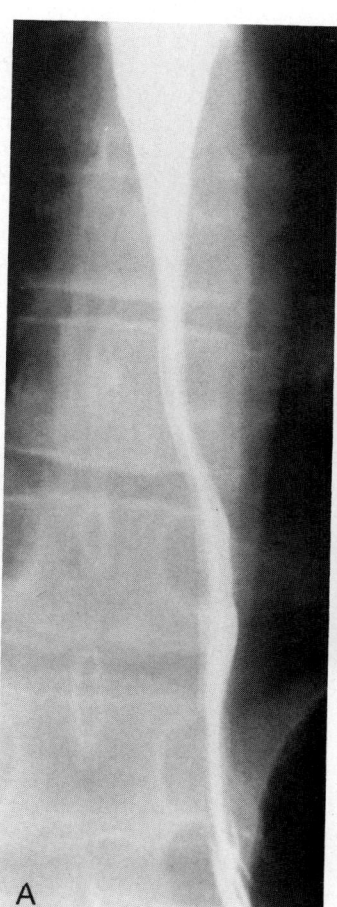

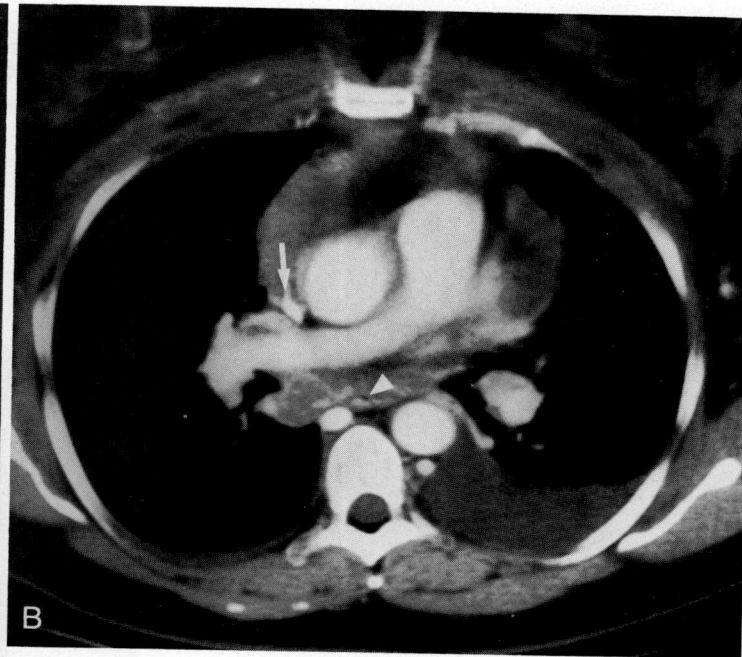

**Figure 29–16. Esophageal involvement by mediastinal lymphoma. A.** A barium study shows a long segment of smooth narrowing in the distal third of the esophagus due to circumferential involvement by mediastinal lymphoma. (Courtesy of Kyunghee C. Cho, M.D., Newark, NJ.) **B.** A CT scan in another patient with large cell lymphoma of the mediastinum shows extensive mediastinal adenopathy compressing the esophagus *(arrowhead)* and superior vena cava *(arrow)*. (Courtesy of Richard M. Gore, M.D., Evanston, IL.)

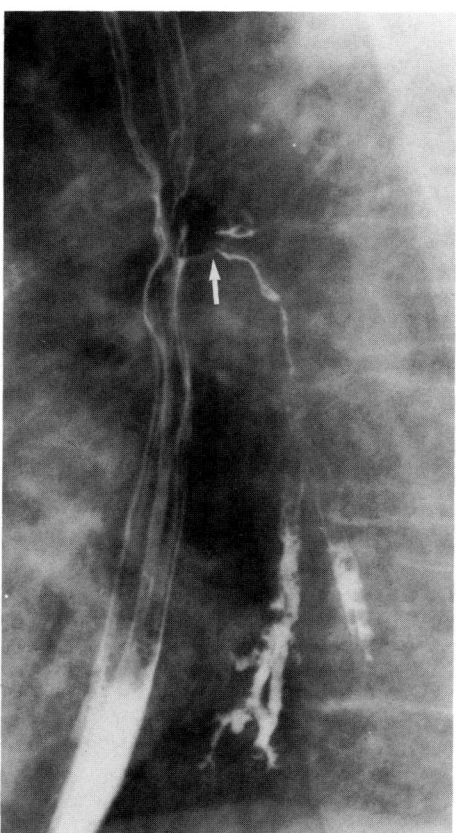

**Figure 29–17. Mediastinal lymphoma with an esophagobronchial fistula.** This patient developed an esophagobronchial fistula *(arrow)* several months after undergoing radiation therapy for mediastinal lymphoma.

candidiasis tend to have a more linear configuration and more discrete borders than the submucosal nodules of lymphoma. Leukemic infiltrates, hematogenous metastases, Kaposi's sarcoma, multiple leiomyomas, and esophageal retention cysts have also been described as rare causes of submucosal nodules, but the lesions tend to be larger and less numerous in these cases.

Follow-up barium studies after radiation therapy or chemotherapy may demonstrate partial or total regression of lymphomatous lesions in the esophagus[39, 49, 50] (see Fig. 29–19). However, recurrent esophageal involvement may be documented on subsequent studies, so that serial esophagrams can be extremely helpful in following these patients.

## SPINDLE CELL CARCINOMA

Polypoid epithelial malignant tumors of the esophagus containing both carcinomatous and sarcomatous elements are rare, accounting for only 0.5 to 1.5% of all esophageal neoplasms.[51] Terms used to describe these lesions include carcinosarcoma, pseudosarcoma, polypoid carcinoma, and spindle cell variant of squamous

cell carcinoma. However, many investigators have believed that these lesions represent various expressions of a single malignant tumor, which has been designated *spindle cell squamous carcinoma*, or simply *spindle cell carcinoma*.[52–54]

## Pathology

These polypoid epithelial malignant tumors, or spindle cell carcinomas, were originally classified as carcinosarcomas or pseudosarcomas, depending on the morphology and biologic behavior of the particular lesion. Classic carcinosarcomas contained a true mixture of carcinomatous and sarcomatous elements in which either element could metastasize to regional lymph nodes or distant structures.[55, 56] However, pseudosarcomas were composed primarily of sarcoma-like spindle cells with adjacent areas of early squamous cell carcinoma at the base of the lesions.[57–59] Because the sarcomatous portion of the tumor rarely seemed to metastasize to other structures, pseudosarcomas were thought to be less aggressive lesions and to have a better prognosis than carcinosarcomas.[56] Indeed, the term pseudosarcoma was

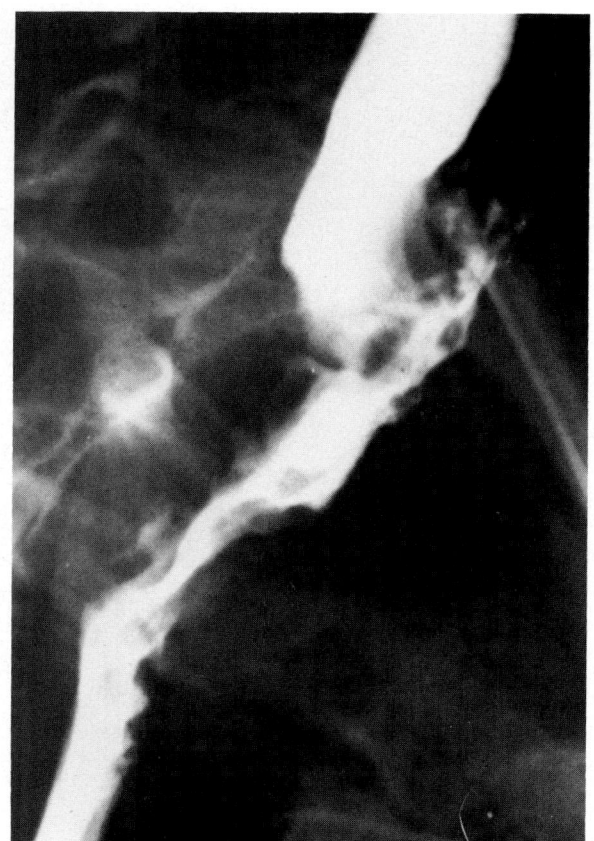

**Figure 29–18. Primary Hodgkin's disease of the esophagus.** There is an irregular, ulcerated area of narrowing in the upper thoracic esophagus. This lesion is indistinguishable from an esophageal carcinoma.

**Figure 29–19. Generalized non-Hodgkin's lymphoma involving the esophagus. A** and **B**. Double contrast radiographs of the middle **(A)** and distal **(B)** thoracic esophagus reveal innumerable 3- to 10-mm submucosal nodules extending from the thoracic inlet to the gastroesophageal junction. This appearance might initially be mistaken for that of varices, but the diffuse distribution and discrete margins of the lesions allow them to be differentiated from varices. **C**. An endoscopic photograph reveals multiple, discrete submucosal nodules that had a white or yellowish appearance on visual examination. **D**. A second esophagram obtained 2 months after chemotherapy reveals virtually complete healing of the submucosal nodules seen on the earlier study. (The rounded filling defects are air bubbles.) (**A** to **D** from MS Levine, AG Sunshine, JC Reynolds, et al, Diffuse nodularity in esophageal lymphoma, AJR, 145, 6, 1218–1220, 1985, © by American Roentgen Ray Society.)

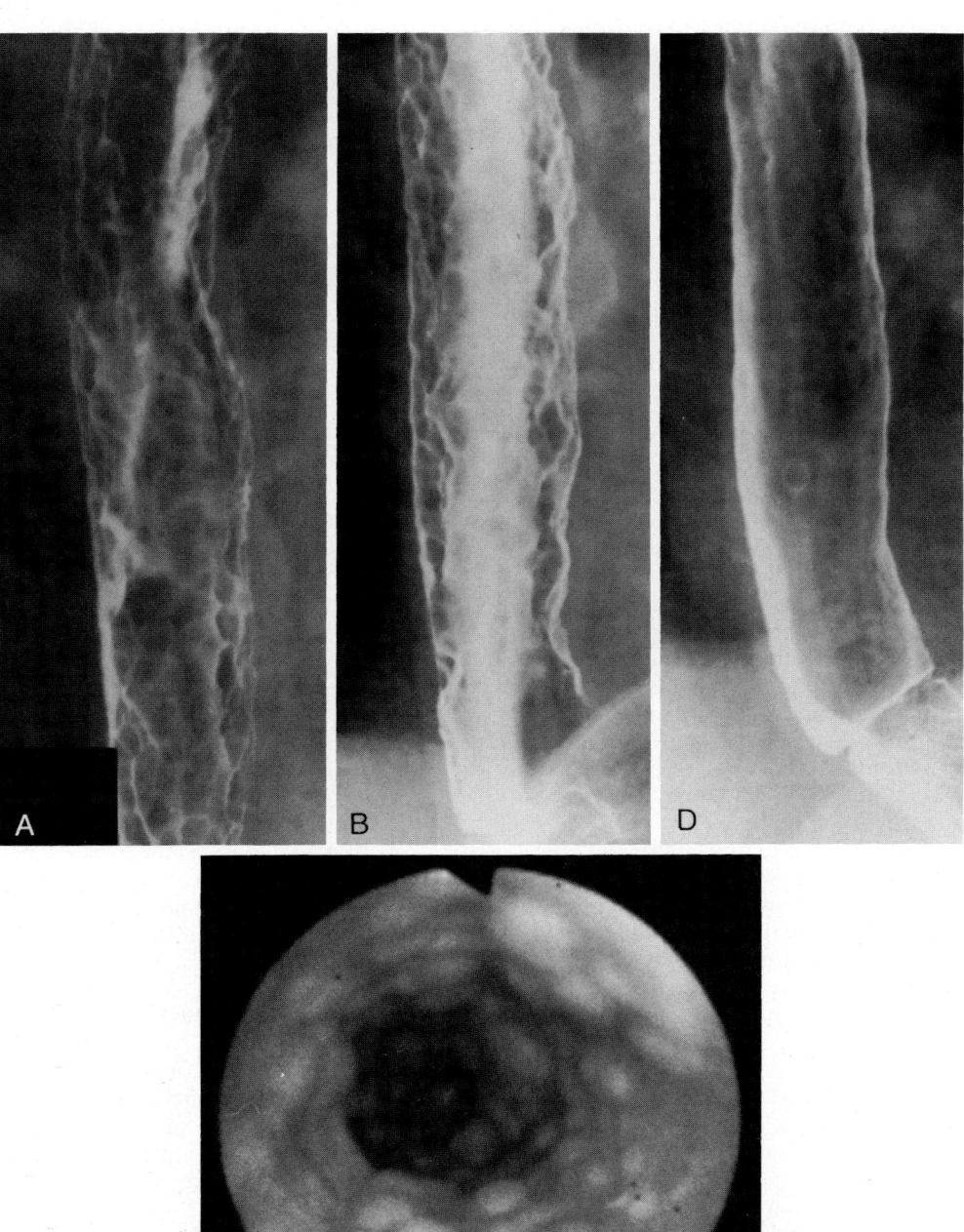

used to indicate the non-neoplastic nature of the spindle cell stroma, which could be mistaken histologically for a malignant sarcoma.[57]

Subsequently, however, the clinical and pathologic basis for differentiating these entities has been questioned. Several studies have shown that local or distant metastases may occur from the sarcomatous portion of so-called pseudosarcomas and that these lesions may behave as aggressively as carcinosarcomas.[52, 60] Furthermore, some reported pseudosarcomas have intimately admixed carcinomatous and spindle cell elements, so that the lesions are indistinguishable histologically from carcinosarcomas.[52] Instead, pseudosarcoma and carcinosarcoma appear to be the same pathologic entity with varying degrees of anaplastic spindle cell metaplasia of the carcinomatous portion of the tumor.[52, 54, 61] Thus, these lesions have been classified together as spindle cell carcinomas.

## Clinical Findings

Because spindle cell carcinomas are polypoid intraluminal tumors, affected individuals almost always present clinically with dysphagia and weight loss.[62] Other, less common findings include odynophagia, chest pain, and upper gastrointestinal bleeding.[51, 59, 63] Most patients are elderly men, who often have a significant history of smoking or drinking alcohol.[59, 62] The clinical presentation is therefore indistinguishable from that of squamous cell carcinoma.

It has previously been suggested that spindle cell carcinomas have a better prognosis than squamous cell carcinomas, as spindle cell carcinomas tend to remain superficial, with local invasion and regional or distant metastases occurring late in the course of the disease.[55, 63] However, other investigators have found that as many as 50% of patients with spindle cell carcinoma have metastatic disease at the time of diagnosis and that the overall 5-year survival rate is only 2 to 8%.[56, 62] Thus, the prognosis of this tumor is probably comparable to that of squamous cell carcinoma.

## Radiographic Findings

Spindle cell carcinomas almost always appear radiographically as polypoid intraluminal masses, ranging from 5 to 15 cm in size[53, 54, 56, 60, 63] (Fig. 29–20). They tend to occur in the middle or, less commonly, distal third of the esophagus.[54, 59, 62] These tumors usually have lobulated or scalloped borders.[53, 54] In some cases, barium may form a dome over the intraluminal portion of the tumor, producing a "cupula" effect.[53, 54, 56] Although these bulky tumors may locally expand and dilate the esophagus, they rarely cause radiographic evidence of obstruction.[54, 60] Occasionally, a broad-based or narrow pedicle may be observed radiographically.[53, 54, 59, 60] Rarely, torsion of the pedicle results in spontaneous sloughing of the tumor.[59] Most spindle cell carcinomas are polypoid lesions, but infiltrating or annular lesions

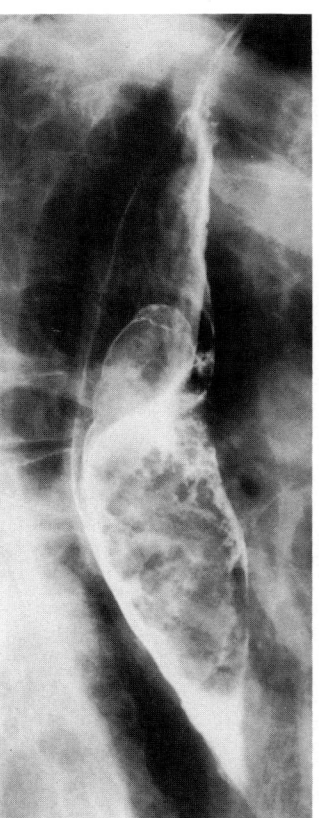

**Figure 29–20. Spindle cell carcinoma of the esophagus.** There is a polypoid intraluminal mass in the midesophagus that expands the lumen without causing obstruction. This appearance is typical of spindle cell carcinomas but can also be seen with other malignant lesions in the esophagus (see Figs. 29–21 and 29–22). (Courtesy of Robert A. Halvorsen, M.D., San Francisco, CA.)

have occasionally been reported.[56, 62, 64] Such lesions are indistinguishable radiographically from typical squamous cell carcinomas.

## Differential Diagnosis

The differential diagnosis for a bulky intraluminal mass includes other benign and malignant polypoid tumors in the esophagus. Benign lesions such as fibrovascular polyps and pedunculated lipomas or leiomyomas occasionally produce a similar appearance.[65] Although squamous cell carcinomas are not usually polypoid, adenocarcinomas arising in Barrett's mucosa may be bulky intraluminal tumors.[66, 67] Other sarcomatous lesions such as leiomyosarcomas, melanosarcomas, and lymphosarcomas may produce similar findings. Thus, a definitive diagnosis of spindle cell carcinoma can be made only on histologic grounds.

## LEIOMYOSARCOMA

Leiomyosarcomas are rare lesions, accounting for less than 1% of all malignant tumors in the esophagus.[68]

These lesions arise in smooth muscle, so that they rarely occur above the level of the aortic arch, because of the presence of striated rather than smooth muscle in this portion of the esophagus.[69] Nevertheless, leiomyosarcomas have occasionally been reported to occur in the cervical and upper thoracic esophagus.[70, 71] Although leiomyosarcomas might theoretically result from malignant degeneration of pre-existing leiomyomas, there is no evidence in the literature to support this contention (see Chapter 27).

Esophageal leiomyosarcomas tend to be indolent, low-grade sarcomas with relatively slow growth and infrequent metastases.[69] Both polypoid and infiltrating types have been described. The more common polypoid type occurs as a slowly growing intraluminal mass with little tendency to obstruct the lumen or produce metastases until late in the course of the disease.[69, 71] In contrast, the infiltrating type is a more invasive neoplasm that narrows and obstructs the esophagus and metastasizes to distant structures at an earlier stage.[71] Thus, polypoid leiomyosarcomas have a better overall prognosis than infiltrating lesions.[68, 72] However, both types of leiomyosarcoma have a better prognosis than esophageal carcinoma, with long-term survival reported in about 50% of patients.[70]

## Clinical Findings

Esophageal leiomyosarcomas usually are found in middle-aged or elderly patients.[71, 72] Unlike esophageal carcinoma, however, this tumor occurs more frequently in women.[71] Most patients present clinically with dysphagia.[69–71] Infiltrating lesions cause relatively rapid onset of dysphagia because of their tendency to narrow and obstruct the esophagus at an early stage. However, the more common polypoid type may reach enormous proportions before obstructive symptoms develop.[71] The absence of dysphagia in these patients is related to the tendency for this tumor to grow exophytically without significant encroachment of the esophageal lumen. When dysphagia does occur, it is slowly progressive, and the average duration of symptoms before the seeking of medical attention is about 9 months—an unusually long interval for esophageal carcinoma.[68] Although dysphagia is the most common symptom, these patients may also present with substernal chest pain, odynophagia, or upper gastrointestinal bleeding.[70] Rarely, they develop clinical signs of an abscess in the mediastinum or lung as the tumor spreads exophytically to invade these structures.[73]

Radical surgery is the treatment of choice for esophageal leiomyosarcoma.[68, 70] Because of its tendency to metastasize late, the polypoid type is particularly amenable to surgical resection. Even when metastases are present, resection of the primary tumor may still prolong survival of patients.[70] These tumors are relatively radiosensitive, so that bulky lesions can also be palliated by radiation therapy, with a dramatic clinical response.[69, 74]

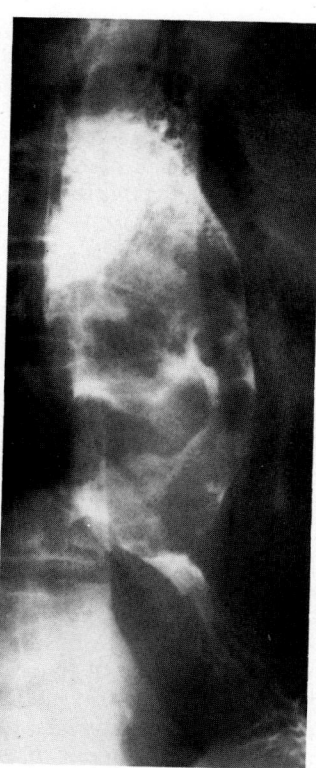

**Figure 29–21. Esophageal leiomyosarcoma.** There is a bulky intraluminal mass in the distal third of the esophagus. Note how the lesion expands the lumen without causing obstruction. (Courtesy of William M. Thompson, M.D., Minneapolis, MN.)

## Radiographic Findings

Because of their exophytic pattern of growth, polypoid leiomyosarcomas may be recognized on chest radiographs by the presence of a posterior mediastinal mass.[69, 71, 74] Rarely, these lesions may calcify.[75] Polypoid leiomyosarcomas usually appear on barium studies as bulky, expansile intraluminal masses in the middle or distal third of the esophagus[69, 71, 72, 74] (Fig. 29–21). Despite the size and extent of these lesions, they rarely cause radiographic evidence of obstruction.[69, 71] Thus, the presence of a bulky, nonobstructing intraluminal mass with a large exophytic component should raise the possibility of a leiomyosarcoma, despite its rarity, because this appearance would be extremely unusual for esophageal carcinoma. In contrast, infiltrating leiomyosarcomas cannot be distinguished radiographically from infiltrating esophageal cancers.

## Differential Diagnosis

Other, more common malignant tumors should be considered in the differential diagnosis of a polypoid leiomyosarcoma. Adenocarcinomas arising in Barrett's esophagus and spindle cell carcinomas may also appear as bulky intraluminal masses.[54, 60, 66, 67] Similarly, giant fibrovascular polyps may be expansile intraluminal lesions, but these benign tumors have a smooth contour and virtually never extend exophytically into the mediastinum.[65] Finally, an esophageal leiomyosarcoma can be mistaken for a large bolus of food impacted in the esophagus. However, patients with food impaction usually have acute onset of symptoms precipitated by the impaction.

## MALIGNANT MELANOMA

Malignant melanoma is a rare primary malignant tumor of the esophagus. For many years, the existence of primary melanoma of the esophagus was doubted because melanin-producing cells could not be demonstrated in the esophagus. Instead, these lesions were thought to represent metastases from occult melanomas of the eye, skin, or anus. However, esophageal metastases are rarely found in patients with documented melanomas elsewhere.[10, 11] Furthermore, it has been shown that melanoblasts are present in the esophageal mucosa at autopsy in 4 to 8% of patients.[76, 77] Because malignant melanoma results from malignant degeneration of these melanin-producing cells, most esophageal melanomas are now thought to be primary malignant tumors of the esophagus.

## Clinical Findings

Most patients with esophageal melanoma present clinically with dysphagia and weight loss.[78–80] However, these tumors tend to have a polypoid growth pattern and are usually advanced lesions with widespread metastases when obstructive symptoms develop.[78, 81] As a result, these patients have a poor prognosis, with an average survival of only 7 months from the time of diagnosis.[80]

## Radiographic Findings

Esophageal melanomas usually appear radiographically as bulky intraluminal masses in the middle or distal third of the esophagus[78–80, 82] (Fig. 29–22). These lesions are indistinguishable from other polypoid esophageal tumors. Occasionally, a discrete pedicle is observed.[78] Rarely, esophageal melanoma is manifested by a centrally ulcerated submucosal mass similar to the "bull's-eye" lesions associated with metastatic melanoma elsewhere in the gastrointestinal tract.[83]

## KAPOSI'S SARCOMA

Kaposi's sarcoma is a multifocal neoplasm of the reticuloendothelial system that is classically manifested

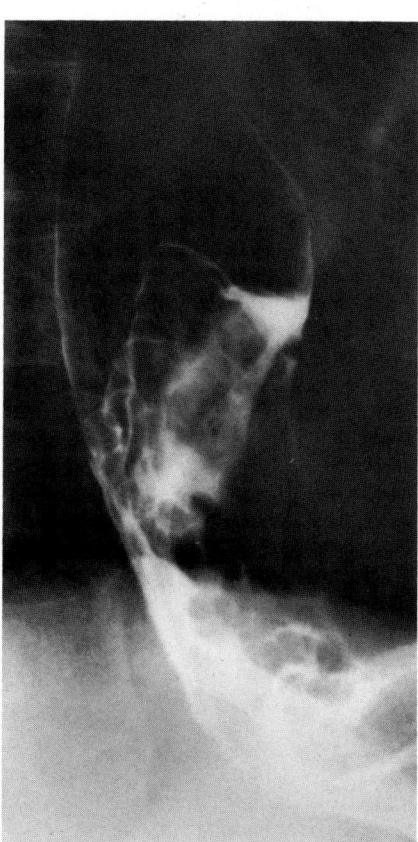

**Figure 29–22. Primary malignant melanoma of the esophagus.** There is a polypoid intraluminal mass in the distal esophagus. This lesion cannot be distinguished from other, more common polypoid tumors in the esophagus. (Courtesy of Akiyoshi Yamada, M.D., Tokyo, Japan.)

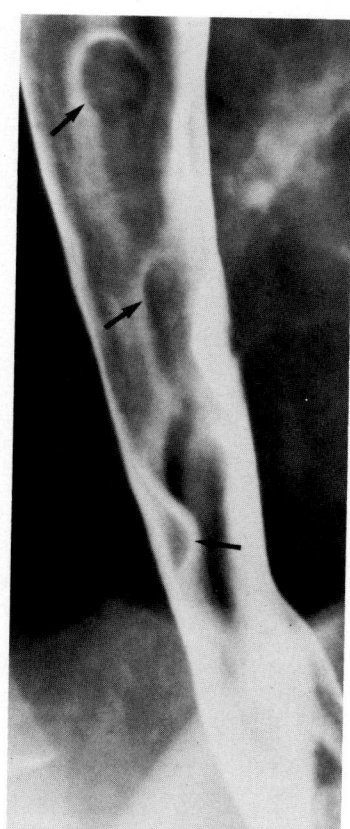

**Figure 29–23. Kaposi's sarcoma involving the esophagus.** There are multiple submucosal masses *(arrows)* in the esophagus. This patient had additional submucosal lesions elsewhere in the gastrointestinal tract. (Courtesy of Robert A. Goren, M.D., Philadelphia, PA.)

by slow-growing cutaneous lesions on the lower extremities. Formerly, this malignancy was rarely diagnosed in North America. Since 1979, however, an aggressive form of Kaposi's sarcoma has been recognized with increased frequency in patients with acquired immunodeficiency syndrome. More than 30% of patients with acquired immunodeficiency syndrome in the United States have Kaposi's sarcoma.[84] About 50% of patients with Kaposi's sarcoma have gastrointestinal involvement, manifested by submucosal nodules, polypoid lesions, or thickened folds in the stomach, duodenum, small bowel, or colon.[85, 86] Rarely, esophageal involvement has also been reported.[85, 87]

## Radiographic Findings

Esophageal involvement by Kaposi's sarcoma may be manifested radiographically by multiple submucosal lesions or by a single polypoid mass in the esophagus[85, 87] (Fig. 29–23). When multiple submucosal lesions are present, the differential diagnosis includes lymphoma, leukemia, metastases from malignant melanoma, retention cysts, and multiple leiomyomas. However, Kaposi's sarcoma should be suspected when one or more discrete esophageal lesions are found in patients with acquired immunodeficiency syndrome.

## LEUKEMIA

Although rarely diagnosed before death, esophageal involvement by leukemia has been reported at autopsy in 2 to 13% of patients.[88, 89] Most leukemic deposits in the esophagus are asymptomatic, but bulky lesions may obstruct the esophagus, causing dysphagia.[90, 91] These leukemic deposits may appear on barium studies as one or more discrete nodular elevations[88, 91] (Fig. 29–24). Coalescent intramural lesions may also be manifested by irregular areas of narrowing in the middle or distal third of the esophagus[91] (Fig. 29–25). Rarely, bulky leukemic deposits may appear as polypoid lesions in the esophagus.[90] These leukemic deposits may undergo marked regression after radiation therapy.[91] Thus, esophageal symptoms may be palliated by mediastinal irradiation, but the overall prognosis for this disease is unchanged.

## MISCELLANEOUS TUMORS

Other rare malignant tumors that have been reported in the esophagus include oat cell carcinomas, adenoid cystic carcinomas, rhabdomyosarcomas, fibrosarcomas, chondrosarcomas, synovial sarcomas, and malignant car-

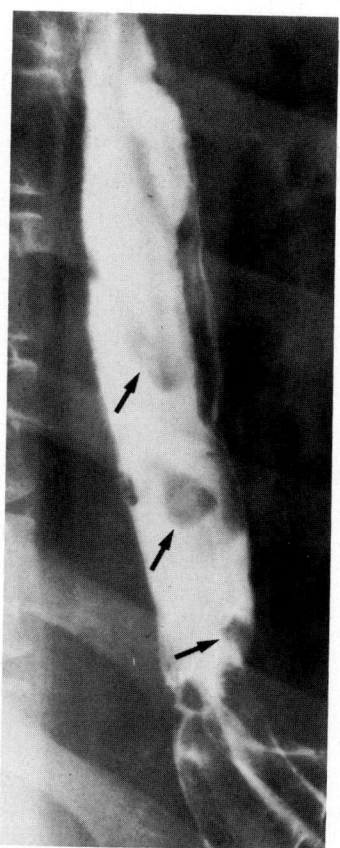

**Figure 29–24. Leukemic infiltration of the esophagus.** This patient has multiple submucosal masses *(arrows)* in the esophagus due to leukemic deposits. (Courtesy of Sadi R. Antonmattei, M.D., Arecibo, Puerto Rico.)

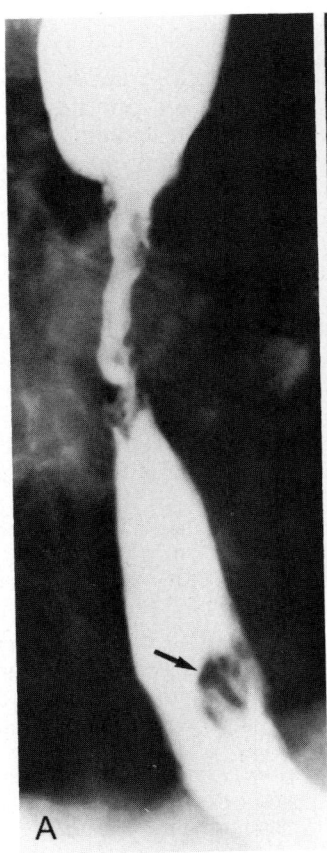

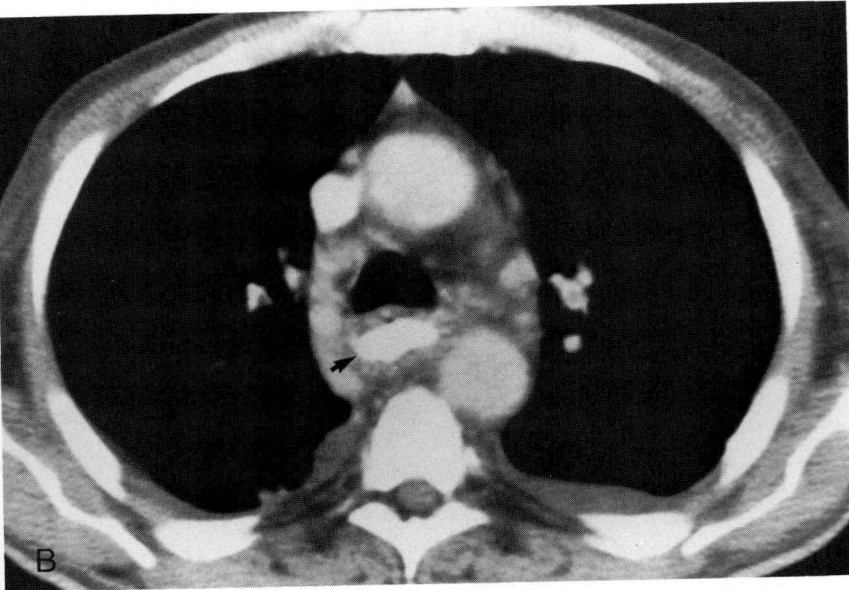

**Figure 29–25. Leukemic infiltration of the esophagus. A.** An esophagram shows irregular narrowing of the midesophagus due to leukemic infiltration of the wall. Note a discrete leukemic deposit *(arrow)* in the distal esophagus. **B.** A CT scan just above the level of the stricture shows contrast medium in a dilated lumen *(arrow)* with infiltration of the surrounding wall. (**A** and **B** courtesy of Duane G. Mezwa, M.D., Royal Oak, MI.)

cinoid tumors.[92–100] In general, sarcomas tend to be more polypoid and pedunculated than carcinomas, which are more infiltrating lesions. Nevertheless, a definitive diagnosis can be made only on histologic criteria.

### Acknowledgment

Figures 29–2, 29–4, 29–6, 29–7, 29–8B, 29–9 to 29–11, 29–13 to 29–15, and 29–18 are reproduced from Levine MS: Radiology of the Esophagus. Philadelphia: WB Saunders, 1989.

# References

1. Toreson WE: Secondary carcinoma of the esophagus as a cause of dysphagia. Arch Pathol 38:82–84, 1944.
2. Agha FP: Secondary neoplasms of the esophagus. Gastrointest Radiol 12:187–193, 1987.
3. Sanborn EB, Beattie EJ, Slaughter DP: Secondary neoplasms of the mediastinum. J Thorac Surg 35:678–682, 1958.
4. Polk HC, Camp FA, Walker AW: Dysphagia and esophageal stenosis: manifestation of metastatic mammary cancer. Cancer 20:2002–2007, 1967.
5. Holyoke ED, Nemoto T, Dao TL: Esophageal metastases and dysphagia in patients with carcinoma of the breast. J Surg Oncol 1:97–107, 1969.
6. Anderson MF, Harell GS: Secondary esophageal tumors. AJR 135:1243–1246, 1980.
7. Ward P: Pulmonary and oesophageal presentations of pancreatic carcinoma. Br J Radiol 37:27–33, 1964.
8. Joffe N: Right-angled narrowing of the distal oesophagus secon-

dary to carcinoma of the tail of the pancreas. Clin Radiol 30:33–37, 1979.
9. Sasson L: Metastatic neoplasms of esophagus simulating primary carcinoma. JAMA 174:2075–2076, 1960.
10. Das Gupta T, Brasfield R: Metastatic melanoma: a clinicopathological study. Cancer 17:1323–1339, 1964.
11. Wood CB, Wood RAB: Metastatic malignant melanoma of the esophagus. Am J Dig Dis 20:786–789, 1975.
12. Fisher MS: Metastasis to the esophagus. Gastrointest Radiol 1:249–251, 1976.
13. Gore RM, Sparberg M: Metastatic carcinoma of the prostate to the esophagus. Am J Gastroenterol 77:358–359, 1982.
14. Feczko PJ, Halpert RD: Achalasia secondary to nongastrointestinal malignancies. Gastrointest Radiol 10:273–276, 1985.
15. Stankey RM, Roshe J, Sogocio RM: Carcinoma of the lung and dysphagia. Dis Chest 55:13–17, 1969.
16. Stallone RJ, Benson BR: Breast carcinoma as a cause of dysphagia. Dis Chest 56:449–451, 1969.
17. Nussbaum M, Grossman M: Metastases to the esophagus causing gastrointestinal bleeding. Am J Gastroenterol 66:467–472, 1976.
18. Balthazar EJ, Goldfine S, Davidian NM: Carcinoma of the esophagogastric junction. Am J Gastroenterol 74:237–243, 1980.
19. Freeny PC, Marks WM: Adenocarcinoma of the gastroesophageal junction: barium and CT examination. AJR 138:1077–1084, 1982.
20. Levine MS, Laufer I, Thompson JJ: Carcinoma of the gastric cardia in young people. AJR 140:69–72, 1983.
21. Fleischner FG, Sachsse E: Retrotracheal lymphadenopathy in bronchial carcinoma, revealed by the barium-filled esophagus. AJR 90:792–798, 1963.
22. Libshitz HI, Lindell MM, Dodd GD: Metastases to the hollow viscera. Radiol Clin North Am 20:487–499, 1982.
23. Lawson TL, Dodds WJ: Infiltrating carcinoma simulating achalasia. Gastrointest Radiol 1:245–248, 1976.

24. McCallum RW: Esophageal achalasia secondary to gastric carcinoma: report of a case and review of the literature. Am J Gastroenterol 71:24–29, 1979.

25. Davis JA, Kantrowitz PA, Chandler HL, et al: Reversible achalasia due to reticulum-cell sarcoma. N Engl J Med 293:130–132, 1975.

26. Ferreira-Santos R: Aperistalsis of the esophagus and colon (megaesophagus and megacolon) etiologically related to Chagas' disease. Am J Dig Dis 6:700–726, 1961.

27. Costigan DJ, Clouse RE: Achalasia-like esophagus from amyloidosis. Dig Dis Sci 28:763–765, 1983.

28. Simeone J, Burrell M, Toffler R: Esophageal aperistalsis secondary to metastatic invasion of the myenteric plexus. AJR 127:862–864, 1976.

29. Shulze KS, Goresky CA, Jabbari M, et al: Esophageal achalasia associated with gastric carcinoma: lack of evidence for widespread plexus destruction. Can Med Assoc J 112:857–864, 1975.

30. Tucker HJ, Snape WJ, Cohen SC: Achalasia secondary to carcinoma: manometric and clinical features. Ann Intern Med 89:315–318, 1978.

31. Sandler RS, Bozymski EM, Orlando RC: Failure of clinical criteria to distinguish between primary achalasia and achalasia secondary to tumor. Dig Dis Sci 27:209–213, 1982.

32. Seaman WB, Wells J, Flood CA: Diagnostic problems of esophageal cancer: relationship to achalasia and hiatus hernia. AJR 90:778–791, 1963.

33. Ennis JT, Lewicki AM: Mecholyl esophagography. AJR 119:241–244, 1973.

34. Dodds WJ, Stewart ET, Kishk SM, et al: Radiologic amyl nitrite test for distinguishing pseudoachalasia from idiopathic achalasia. AJR 146:21–23, 1986.

35. Rabushka LS, Fishman EK, Kuhlman JE: CT evaluation of achalasia. J Comput Assist Tomogr 15:434–439, 1991.

36. Rosenberg SA, Diamond HD, Jaslowitz B, et al: Lymphosarcoma: a review of 1,269 cases. Medicine (Baltimore) 40:31–84, 1961.

37. Ehrlich AN, Stalder G, Geller W, et al: Gastrointestinal manifestations of malignant lymphoma. Gastroenterology 54:1115–1121, 1968.

38. Caruso RD, Berk RN: Lymphoma of the esophagus. Radiology 95:381–382, 1970.

39. Carnovale RL, Goldstein HM, Zornoza J, et al: Radiologic manifestations of esophageal lymphoma. AJR 128:751–754, 1977.

40. Zornoza J, Dodd GD: Lymphoma of the gastrointestinal tract. Semin Roentgenol 15:272–287, 1980.

41. Agha FP, Schnitzer B: Esophageal involvement in lymphoma. Am J Gastroenterol 80:412–416, 1985.

42. Stein HA, Murray D, Warner HA: Primary Hodgkin's disease of the esophagus. Dig Dis Sci 26:457–461, 1981.

43. Doki T, Hamada S, Murayama H, et al: Primary malignant lymphoma of the esophagus. Endoscopy 16:189–192, 1984.

44. Nissan S, Bar-Moar JA, Levy E: Lymphosarcoma of the esophagus. Cancer 34:1321–1323, 1974.

45. Hricak H, Thoeni RF, Margulis AR, et al: Extension of gastric lymphoma into the esophagus and duodenum. Radiology 135:309–312, 1980.

46. Traube M, Waldron JA, McCallum RW: Systemic lymphoma initially presenting as an esophageal mass. Am J Gastroenterol 77:835–837, 1982.

47. Lambert A: Malignant tracheoesophageal fistula secondary to Hodgkin's disease. J Thorac Cardiovasc Surg 69:820–826, 1975.

48. Kirsch HL, Cronin DW, Stein GN, et al: Esophageal perforation: an unusual presentation of esophageal lymphoma. Dig Dis Sci 28:371–374, 1983.

49. Levine MS, Sunshine AG, Reynolds JC, et al: Diffuse nodularity in esophageal lymphoma. AJR 145:1218–1220, 1985.

50. Gedgaudas-McClees RK, Maglinte DDT: Lymphomatous esophageal nodules: the difficulty in radiologic differential diagnosis. Am J Gastroenterol 80:529–530, 1985.

51. Xu L, Sun C, Wu L, et al: Clinical and pathological characteristics of carcinosarcoma of the esophagus: report of four cases. Ann Thorac Surg 37:197–203, 1984.

52. Martin MR, Kahn LB: So-called pseudosarcoma of the esophagus: nodal metastases of the spindle cell element. Arch Pathol Lab Med 101:604–609, 1977.

53. Olmsted WW, Lichtenstein JE, Hyams VJ: Polypoid epithelial malignancies of the esophagus. AJR 140:921–925, 1983.

54. Agha FP, Keren DF: Spindle-cell squamous carcinoma of the esophagus: a tumor with biphasic morphology. AJR 145:541–545, 1985.

55. Talbert JL, Cantrell JR: Clinical and pathological characteristics of carcinosarcoma of the esophagus. J Thorac Cardiovasc Surg 45:1–12, 1963.

56. McCort JJ: Esophageal carcinosarcoma and pseudosarcoma. Radiology 102:519–524, 1972.

57. Razzuk MA, Urschel HC, Race GJ, et al: Pseudosarcoma of the esophagus. J Thorac Cardiovasc Surg 61:650–653, 1971.

58. Postlethwait RW, Wechsler AS, Shelburne JD: Pseudosarcoma of the esophagus. Ann Thorac Surg 19:198–205, 1975.

59. Nichols T, Yokoo H, Craig RM, et al: Pseudosarcoma of the esophagus. Am J Gastroenterol 72:615–622, 1979.

60. Halvorsen RA, Foster WL, Williford ME, et al: Pseudosarcoma of the esophagus: barium swallow and CT findings. J Can Assoc Radiol 34:278–281, 1983.

61. Osamura RY, Shimamora K, Hata J: Polypoid carcinoma of the esophagus: a unifying term for carcinosarcoma and pseudosarcoma. Am J Surg Pathol 2:201–208, 1978.

62. Hinderleider CD, Aguam AS, Wilder JR: Carcinosarcoma of the esophagus: a case report and review of the literature. Int Surg 64:13–19, 1979.

63. Kenneweg DJ, Cimmino CV: Carcinosarcoma of the esophagus. AJR 101:482–484, 1967.

64. Ende N, Pizzolato P, Raider L, et al: An unusual case of carcinosarcoma of the esophagus. AJR 65:227–231, 1951.

65. Carter MM, Kulkarni MV: Giant fibrovascular polyp of the esophagus. Gastrointest Radiol 9:301–303, 1984.

66. Levine MS, Caroline D, Thompson JJ, et al: Adenocarcinoma of the esophagus: relationship to Barrett mucosa. Radiology 150:305–309, 1984.

67. Agha FP: Barrett carcinoma of the esophagus: clinical and radiographic analysis of 34 cases. AJR 145:41–46, 1985.

68. Goodner JT, Miller TR, Watson WL: Sarcoma of the esophagus. AJR 89:132–139, 1963.

69. Wolfel DA: Leiomyosarcoma of the esophagus. AJR 89:127–131, 1963.

70. Camishion RC, Gibbon JH, Templeton JY: Leiomyosarcoma of the esophagus: review of the literature and report of two cases. Ann Surg 153:951–956, 1961.

71. Berk RN, Scher GS, Bode DF: Unusual tumors of the gastrointestinal tract. AJR 113:159–169, 1971.

72. Rainer WG, Brus R: Leiomyosarcoma of the esophagus: review of the literature and report of 3 cases. Surgery 58:343–350, 1965.

73. Lipschultz BM, Fisher S: Leiomyosarcoma of the esophagus. Gastroenterology 27:661–666, 1954.

74. Athanasoulis CA, Aral IM: Leiomyosarcoma of the esophagus. Gastroenterology 54:271–274, 1968.

75. Itai Y, Shimazu H: Leiomyosarcoma of the oesophagus with dense calcification. Br J Radiol 51:469–471, 1978.

76. De la Pava S, Nigogosyan G, Pickren JW, et al: Melanosis of the esophagus. Cancer 16:48–50, 1963.

77. Tateishi R, Taniguchi H, Wada A, et al: Argyrophil cells and melanocytes in esophageal mucosa. Arch Pathol 98:87–89, 1974.

78. Suehs OW: Malignant melanoma of the esophagus. Ann Otol Rhinol Laryngol 70:1140–1147, 1961.

79. Moffat RC, Richard LB, Gnass JE: Primary malignant melanoma of the esophagus. Can J Surg 15:306–309, 1972.

80. Hendricks GL, Barnes WT, Suter HJ: Primary malignant melanoma of the esophagus. Am Surg 40:468–473, 1974.

81. Broderick PA, Allegra SR, Corvese N: Primary malignant melanoma of the esophagus. Acta Cytol (Baltimore) 16:159–164, 1972.

82. Raven RW, Dawson J: Malignant melanoma of the oesophagus. Br J Surg 51:551–555, 1964.

83. Musher DR, Linder AE: Primary melanoma of the esophagus. Am J Dig Dis 19:855–859, 1974.

84. Friedman SL, Wright TL, Altman DF: Gastrointestinal Kaposi's sarcoma in patients with acquired immunodeficiency syndrome: endoscopic and autopsy findings. Gastroenterology 89:102–108, 1985.

85. Rose HS, Balthazar EJ, Megibow AJ, et al: Alimentary tract involvement in Kaposi sarcoma: radiographic and endoscopic findings in 25 homosexual men. AJR 139:661–666, 1982.

86. Wall SD, Friedman SL, Margulis AR: Gastrointestinal Kaposi's sarcoma in AIDS: radiographic manifestations. J Clin Gastroenterol 6:165–171, 1984.

87. Umerah BC: Kaposi sarcoma of the oesophagus. Br J Radiol 53:807–808, 1980.

88. Prolla JC, Kirsner JB: The gastrointestinal lesions and complications of the leukemias. Ann Intern Med 61:1084–1103, 1964.

89. Givler RL: Esophageal lesions in leukemia and lymphoma. Am J Dig Dis 15:31–36, 1970.

90. Gildenhorn HL, Fahey JL, Solomon RD: Functional esophageal obstruction due to leukemic infiltration. AJR 88:736–740, 1962.

91. Thompson BC, Feczko PJ, Mezwa DG: Dysphagia caused by acute leukemic infiltration of the esophagus. AJR 155:654, 1990 (letter).

92. Reid HAS, Richardson WW, Corrin B: Oat cell carcinoma of the esophagus. Cancer 45:2342–2347, 1980.

93. Imai T, Sannohe Y, Okanu H: Oat cell carcinoma (apudoma) of the esophagus. Cancer 41:358–364, 1978.

94. O'Sullivan JP, Cockburn JS, Drew CE: Adenoid cystic carcinoma of the esophagus. Thorax 30:476–480, 1975.

95. Kabuto T, Taniguchi K, Iwanaga T, et al: Primary adenoid cystic carcinoma of the esophagus. Cancer 43:2452–2456, 1979.

96. Thorek P, Neiman BH: Rhabdomyosarcoma of the esophagus. J Thorac Surg 20:77–89, 1950.

97. Clark DE: Sarcoma of the esophagus: report of successful resection of a fibrosarcoma. Arch Surg 59:348–354, 1949.

98. Yaghmai I, Ghahremani GG: Chondrosarcoma of the esophagus. AJR 126:1175–1177, 1976.

99. Block MJ, Iozzo RV, Edmunds LH, et al: Polypoid synovial sarcoma of the esophagus. Gastroenterology 92:229–233, 1987.

100. Brenner S, Heimlich H, Widman M: Carcinoid of esophagus. N Y State J Med 69:1337–1339, 1969.

# Varices

Marc S. Levine, M.D.

## INTRODUCTION

Esophageal varices are usually caused by portal hypertension in patients with cirrhosis or other liver diseases. Because increased portal venous pressure leads to upward venous flow via dilated esophageal collaterals to the superior vena cava, these varices are called *uphill varices*. Less frequently, obstruction of the superior vena cava may lead to downward venous flow via esophageal collaterals to the portal vein and inferior vena cava. As a result, these varices are called *downhill varices*. Rarely, idiopathic varices may be found in patients who have no evidence of portal hypertension or superior vena caval obstruction. Although gastric varices often accompany esophageal varices in patients with portal hypertension, isolated gastric varices may occasionally be found in patients with portal hypertension or splenic vein obstruction. Whatever the underlying cause, esophageal and gastric varices are important because of the risk of variceal rupture and gastrointestinal bleeding.

## UPHILL VARICES

### Pathophysiology

The development of uphill varices results from changes in the venous drainage of the esophagus caused by altered flow dynamics in patients with portal hypertension. Normally, the cervical and upper thoracic esophagus is drained by the supreme intercostal vein, bronchial veins, inferior thyroid vein, and other mediastinal collaterals; the midthoracic esophagus is drained by the azygos and hemiazygos veins; and the distal thoracic esophagus is drained by a periesophageal plexus of veins that communicate distally with the coronary vein. In turn, the coronary vein drains into the splenic vein near its junction with the portal vein or directly into the portal vein. In portal hypertension, however, increased portal venous pressure leads to reversal of venous flow through the coronary vein into a plexus of dilated esophageal and periesophageal veins that anastomose superiorly with collaterals from the azygos and hemiazygos venous systems. Because the azygos vein drains directly into the superior vena cava, portal venous blood returns to the right side of the heart via the superior vena cava rather than the inferior vena cava, thus bypassing the obstructed portal system.

### Clinical Findings

Esophageal varices are important because of the potentially catastrophic consequences of variceal rupture and hemorrhage. In the past, bleeding varices have accounted for nearly one third of all deaths from cirrhosis.[1] Although major variceal bleeding may be manifested by one or more episodes of massive hematemesis, other patients may have intermittent, low-grade bleeding with melena, guaiac-positive stool, or iron deficiency anemia. Surprisingly, however, the size and extent of varices correlate poorly with the degree of bleeding.[2]

Esophageal varices are a common source of gastrointestinal bleeding, but they rarely cause dysphagia. The possibility of esophageal carcinoma or other, unrelated lesions should therefore be considered in patients with varices who develop dysphagia.

### Radiographic Findings

#### Plain Films

Esophageal varices may occasionally be manifested on chest radiographs by a retrocardiac posterior mediastinal mass. This finding is caused either by dilated esophageal or paraesophageal veins or, less commonly, by dilated azygos or hemiazygos veins.[3–5] The mass is usually more obvious on films taken with the patient in the recumbent position, as hydrostatic pressure tends to overcome portal pressure in the upright position, shifting blood flow to other, more dependent collateral vessels. Although there are many causes of a posterior mediastinal mass, the possibility of esophageal varices should be considered when this finding occurs in patients with portal hypertension.

## Barium Studies

Esophagography has traditionally been considered an unreliable technique for diagnosing esophageal varices. Some authors have advocated the use of anticholinergic agents such as propantheline bromide (Pro-Banthine) and hyoscine-N-butyl bromide (Buscopan) to improve visualization of varices.[6-8] Unlike glucagon, which has no effect on esophageal motor function, 20 to 30 mg of intravenous Pro-Banthine or Buscopan enhances variceal filling by significantly decreasing peristalsis and muscle tone in the esophagus. In various studies, 50 to 100% of patients with varices not seen on esophagography had definite radiologic evidence of varices after administration of these drugs.[6-8] However, anticholinergic agents such as Pro-Banthine may be contraindicated in patients with glaucoma, cardiac disease, or urinary retention. Although Buscopan has fewer side effects, it is not yet commercially available in the United States.

Whether or not pharmacologic agents are used, optimal demonstration of varices requires meticulous attention to radiographic technique, as varices can easily be obscured on overly distended or collapsed views of the esophagus (Fig. 30–1). The examination should be performed with the patient in a recumbent (usually prone, right anterior oblique) position and with use of a high-density barium suspension or paste to increase adherence of barium to the esophageal mucosa.[9, 10] Mucosal relief views of the collapsed esophagus are particularly helpful for demonstrating varices (see Fig. 30–1D). However, spot films should be taken between peristaltic waves, as peristalsis tends to squeeze blood from the thin-walled varices, rendering them invisible for as long as 15 to 30 seconds (see Fig. 30–1C). If necessary, patients should be asked to spit their saliva into a basin to avoid initiating a peristaltic sequence and collapsing the varices.

Because of the underlying venous anatomy, uphill varices tend to be most prominent in the distal third or half of the thoracic esophagus, fading gradually as they ascend to the level of entry of the azygos vein into the superior vena cava. Varices are usually best seen on mucosal relief views, appearing as tortuous or serpiginous longitudinal filling defects in the collapsed or partially collapsed esophagus (see Fig. 30–1D). Varices may also be seen on double contrast radiographs when they are etched in white as a result of barium trapped between the edge of the lesions and the adjacent esophageal wall (Fig. 30–2; see Fig. 30–1A). Because varices alternately distend and collapse with peristalsis, respiration, and varying degrees of esophageal distention, they may be observed as a transient finding, visible only on one or several spot films taken during the radiologic examination. In fact, the changeable nature of varices at fluoroscopy allows them to be differentiated from inflammatory or neoplastic conditions associated with thickened esophageal folds (see later section on differential diagnosis).

## Computed Tomography

Esophageal varices may be recognized on computed tomography (CT) scans by the presence of a thickened, lobulated esophageal wall that is markedly enhanced after a bolus injection of contrast medium[11, 12] (Fig. 30–3). Occasionally, dilated azygos, hemiazygos, or paraesophageal veins can be mistaken for a posterior mediastinal mass on unenhanced CT scans.[13] However, the marked degree of enhancement that occurs within these dilated vascular structures after infusion of contrast medium should establish the correct diagnosis.

## Angiography

Arteriograms of the celiac artery, selective arteriograms of the superior mesenteric or splenic artery, or, less frequently, portal venograms may be obtained to confirm the presence of uphill varices and to determine the nature and extent of underlying venous abnormalities. With portal hypertension, films taken during the venous phase of the examination usually fail to demonstrate the portal vein because of reversal of blood flow through numerous collateral vessels to bypass the obstructed venous system. In almost all cases, the coronary vein acts to shunt portal blood through a periesophageal plexus of veins, producing uphill varices, which subsequently communicate with the azygos venous system and superior vena cava (Fig. 30–4). Delineation of the angiographic anatomy is important when a surgical shunt to control variceal bleeding is contemplated.

## Differential Diagnosis

A confident diagnosis of esophageal varices can usually be made on the basis of radiologic criteria. Occasionally, however, submucosal edema and inflammation associated with esophagitis may be manifested by thickened, tortuous longitudinal folds, mimicking the appearance of varices.[14] Some esophageal carcinomas may also produce a varicoid appearance due to submucosal spread of tumor[15-17] (Fig. 30–5). However, varices can be differentiated from varicoid carcinomas at fluoroscopy, as varices tend to change dramatically in size and shape with respiration, peristalsis, and other maneuvers, whereas varicoid tumors have a more fixed, rigid appearance.[15-17] An abrupt demarcation between the involved segment and adjacent normal esophagus should also favor tumor, as uphill varices tend to fade superiorly without an obvious demarcation. Finally, varicoid carcinomas may cause dysphagia, whereas this symptom rarely occurs in patients with varices. Thus, it is usually possible to differentiate these entities on clinical and radiologic grounds.

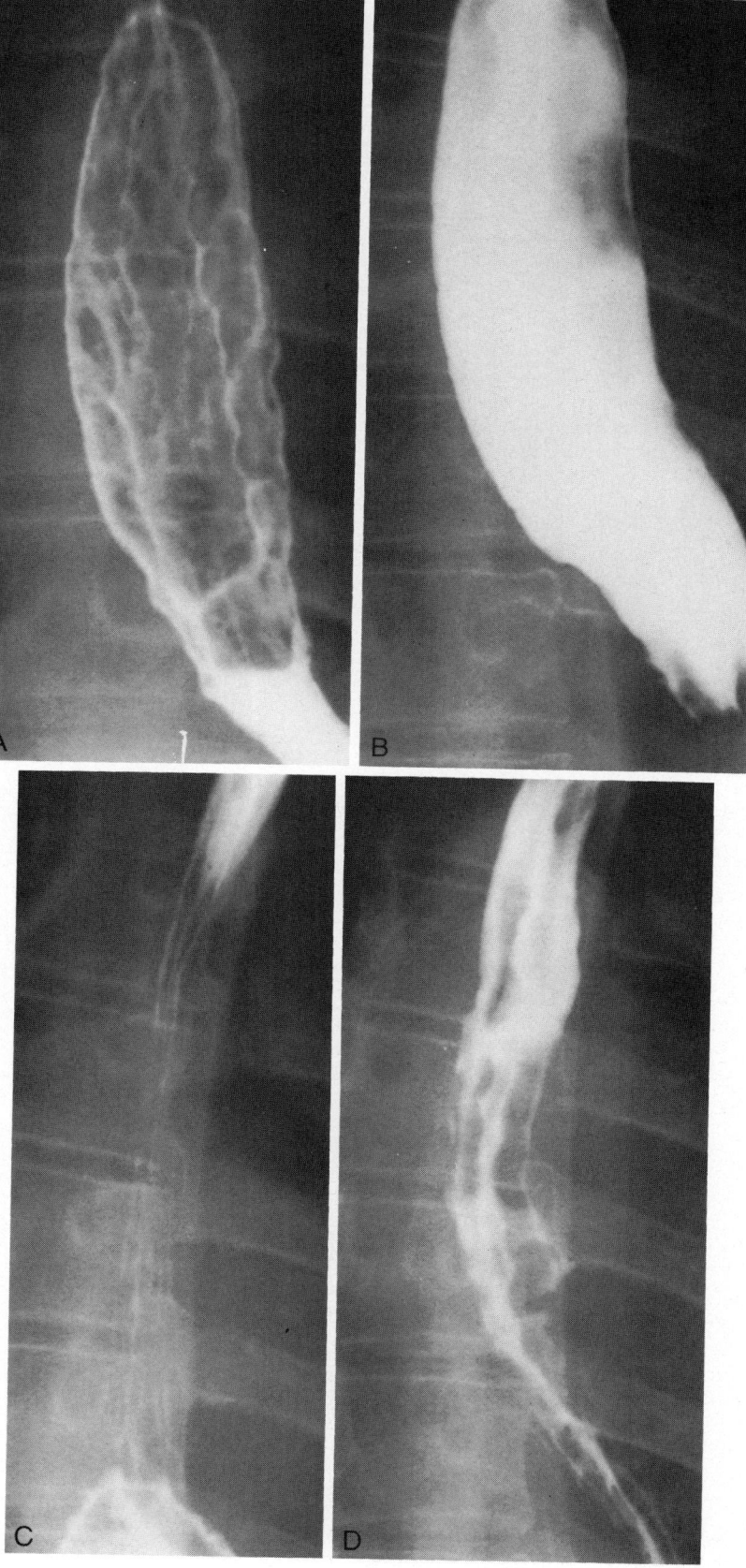

**Figure 30–1. Uphill esophageal varices. A.** Multiple varices are seen on a double contrast esophagram. Note how the varices are etched in white. **B.** The varices are obscured by intraluminal barium on a single contrast radiograph. **C.** The varices are also not visible on a mucosal relief view immediately after a peristaltic stripping wave that has squeezed blood from the dilated veins, causing them to collapse. **D.** However, the varices can be recognized as serpiginous filling defects on another view several seconds after passage of the peristaltic wave.

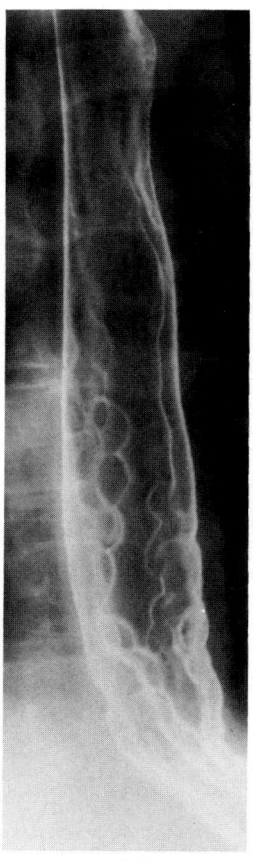

**Figure 30–2. Uphill esophageal varices.** Note how these large varices in the distal third of the esophagus are etched in white.

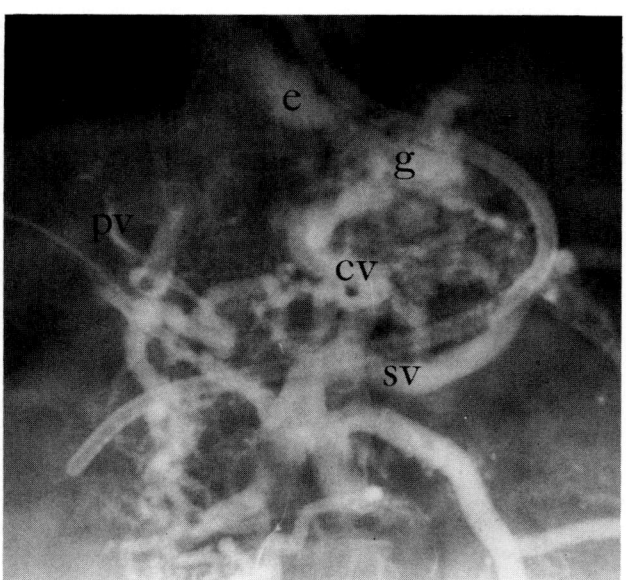

**Figure 30–4. Angiographic demonstration of esophageal and gastric varices due to portal hypertension.** This radiograph from a portal venogram shows cavernous transformation of the portal vein (pv) with reversal of blood flow through the coronary vein (cv) and splenic vein (sv), producing gastric (g) and esophageal (e) varices. (Courtesy of Dana R. Burke, M.D., Bethesda, MD.)

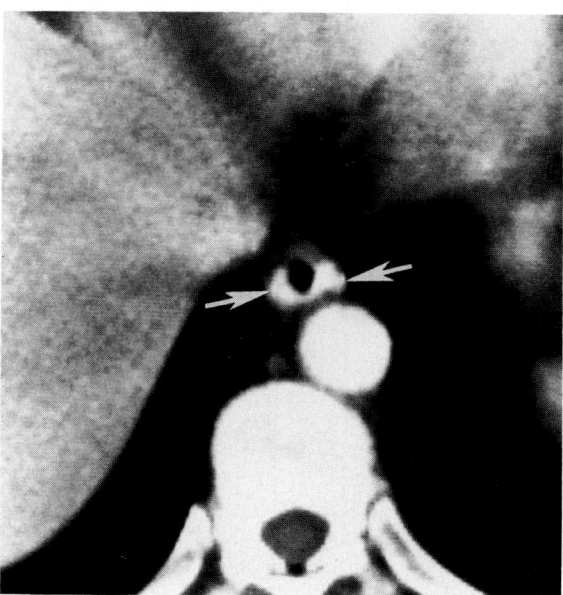

**Figure 30–3. Esophageal varices: CT findings.** A CT scan during rapid infusion of intravenous contrast medium shows dense enhancement of the varices *(arrows)*. (Courtesy of Robert A. Halvorsen, M.D., San Francisco, CA.)

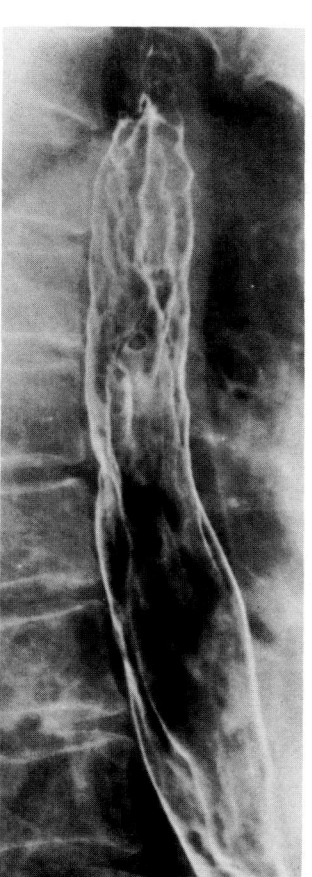

**Figure 30–5. Varicoid carcinoma.** Thickened, tortuous folds in the esophagus mimic the appearance of varices. This appearance is caused by submucosal spread of tumor. (Courtesy of Akiyoshi Yamada, M.D., Tokyo, Japan.)

# Treatment

The treatment for bleeding esophageal varices includes vasopressin infusion, esophageal balloon tamponade, portal-systemic shunt surgery, the Sugiura procedure, endoscopic sclerotherapy, and transjugular intrahepatic portal-systemic shunt—the TIPS procedure. The primary aims of therapy are to control active bleeding and to prevent rebleeding. Although portal-systemic shunts may control variceal bleeding, these procedures have a high operative mortality rate, and in controlled studies, they have not significantly prolonged survival of patients.[18, 19] Similarly, balloon tamponade of bleeding varices with a Sengstaken-Blakemore tube has a high mortality rate and produces only transient control of bleeding.[20] In another operation called the Sugiura procedure, the distal esophagus is transected and devascularized to control variceal bleeding (see Chapter 33).[21] However, this procedure has been performed primarily in Japan.

Endoscopic sclerotherapy has emerged as a viable alternative to surgery because of its ability to decrease the morbidity and mortality of bleeding varices with fewer complications than other forms of treatment.[22-24] Endoscopic sclerotherapy is performed by paravariceal injection or direct intraluminal injection of varices with a sclerosing solution via a fiberoptic endoscope. The sclerosing agent causes a severe inflammatory reaction and intramural fibrosis with mechanical obliteration of varices and shunting of blood from submucosal to muscular layers of the esophageal wall. Endoscopic sclerotherapy appears to be an effective technique for controlling variceal bleeding and decreasing the risk of recurrent bleeding. Nevertheless, complications occur in as many as 30% of patients who undergo this form of treatment.[25] Many patients have transient chest pain or dysphagia for several days after the procedure because of mild chemical esophagitis caused by the sclerosing agent.[26] With more severe damage, transmural inflammation and necrosis may lead to esophageal perforation with mediastinitis, mediastinal abscess, or empyema.[27] Other patients may have persistent dysphagia due to the development of strictures.[28]

Contrast studies performed immediately after sclerotherapy may reveal severe dysmotility, manifested by weakened or absent primary peristalsis, nonperistaltic contractions, and delayed emptying of contrast medium from the esophagus.[26, 29] Acute inflammation, edema, or hemorrhage in the wall may produce irregular luminal narrowing with multiple intramural defects or, less frequently, a large submucosal hematoma.[26, 29, 30] Occasionally, the narrowed segment may have abrupt, shelf-like borders, mimicking the appearance of esophageal carcinoma.[31] Mucosal sloughing at the injection sites may also be manifested by one or more areas of ulceration[26, 29] (Fig. 30–6A). In severe cases, transmural necrosis may lead to the development of transverse or longitudinal intramural tracks (Fig. 30–6B), esophago-esophageal or esophagopleural fistulas, or localized esophageal perforation[29, 32] (Fig. 30–6C). Other patients may develop esophageal strictures 30 days or more after sclerotherapy.[29] Most strictures appear as short, narrowed segments in the distal esophagus, but some patients with severe esophagitis may have extensive stricture formation with long, tapered areas of narrowing in the distal or midesophagus[29] (Fig. 30–6D).

Sclerosed varices are usually manifested on CT scans by a thickened esophageal wall with outer high-attenuation and inner low-attenuation regions on contrast-enhanced scans, producing a characteristic laminated appearance.[33, 34] This finding may result from a sclerosant-induced inflammatory reaction, edema, or hemorrhage within the esophageal wall, so that normal enhancement of varices no longer occurs. CT may also demonstrate a predominantly low-attenuation mediastinal effusion with obliteration of mediastinal fat planes due to an acute paraesophageal reaction after sclerotherapy.[34] In contrast, a mediastinal abscess due to esophageal perforation may be manifested on CT scans by a predominantly high-attenuation mediastinal effusion associated with mediastinal or pleural gas.[34] Thus, CT may be helpful in determining the nature and extent of postsclerotherapy complications in these patients.

# DOWNHILL VARICES

## Pathophysiology

Because the venous structures draining the cervical and upper thoracic esophagus communicate with the supreme intercostal vein, bronchial veins, inferior thyroid vein, and other mediastinal collaterals, obstruction of the superior vena cava may lead to reversal of flow through those vessels into esophageal and paraesophageal veins to bypass the obstruction. Because blood flows downward in them, the dilated esophageal veins are called *downhill varices*.[35]

The location and extent of downhill varices depend pathophysiologically on whether the superior vena cava is obstructed above or below the site of entry of the azygos vein into the vena cava.[35, 36] If the obstruction occurs above the entry of the azygos vein, downhill varices can return blood from the head and upper extremities via the azygos vein to the superior vena cava below the level of obstruction. As a result, downhill varices are always confined to the upper or midthoracic esophagus in these cases. If, however, the obstruction occurs at or below the site of entry of the azygos vein into the superior vena cava, the azygos venous system can no longer be used to bypass the obstruction. In such cases, venous flow continues via downhill varices to the distal esophagus, where the coronary vein diverts blood to the portal vein and inferior vena cava, bypassing the superior vena caval obstruction. Thus, downhill varices of this type may involve the entire thoracic esophagus.

Downhill varices are most commonly caused by mediastinal metastases from bronchogenic carcinoma obstructing the superior vena cava.[35-37] However, downhill varices may also result from other metastatic tumors or lymphoma in the mediastinum. When the superior vena

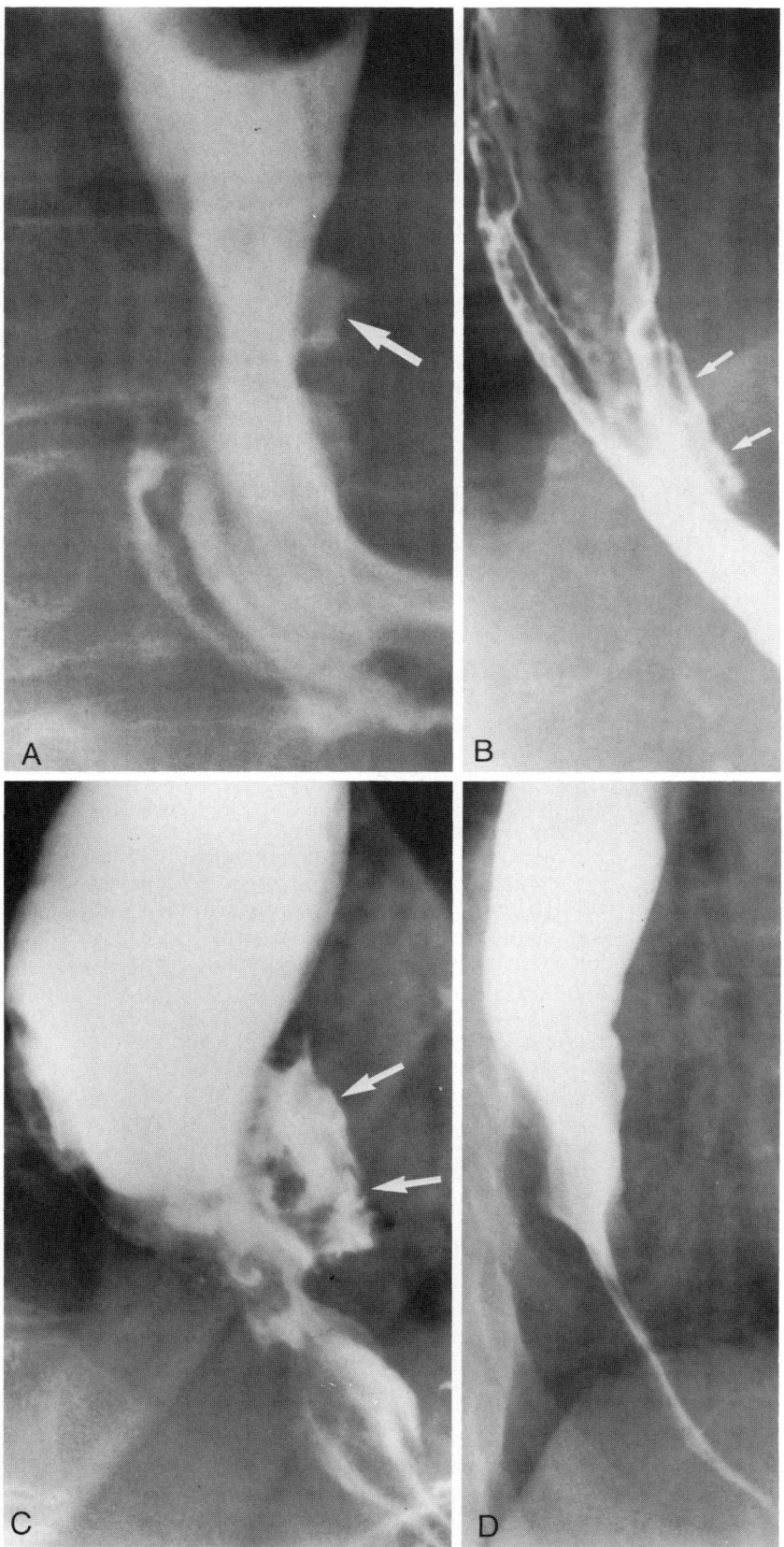

**Figure 30–6. Complications of endoscopic sclerotherapy of varices. A**. There is a relatively deep ulcer *(arrow)* with associated narrowing of the distal esophagus due to edema and spasm. **B**. This patient has a longitudinal intramural track *(arrows)* in the distal esophagus. **C**. Another patient has a focal, sealed-off perforation of the distal esophagus with contrast medium seen entering an extraluminal cavity *(arrows)*. **D**. This patient has a long, tapered stricture in the distal esophagus several months after endoscopic sclerotherapy.

cava is involved by a malignant process, the patient rarely survives long enough for the varices to extend distally, so that they are almost always confined to the upper thoracic esophagus, regardless of whether the obstruction occurs above or below the entry of the azygos vein into the vena cava.[35] Occasionally, however, obstruction of the superior vena cava may be caused by a substernal goiter or benign mediastinal fibrosis due to radiation or histoplasmosis (i.e., sclerosing mediastinitis).[38, 39] In such cases, gradually progressive, long-standing obstruction of the superior vena cava at or below the level of entry of the azygos vein may lead to the development of extensive downhill varices involving the entire thoracic esophagus.[35, 39]

## Clinical Findings

Whereas obstruction of the superior vena cava produces characteristic clinical findings (i.e., the superior vena cava syndrome), downhill varices are usually asymptomatic. Occasionally, however, they may cause hematemesis or low-grade gastrointestinal bleeding with melena, guaiac-positive stool, or iron deficiency anemia.[40] Downhill varices should therefore be suspected in any patient with superior vena caval obstruction who develops signs of upper gastrointestinal bleeding.

## Radiographic Findings

Like uphill varices, downhill varices appear on barium studies as serpiginous longitudinal filling defects in the esophagus[37] (Fig. 30–7). However, they can be differentiated from uphill varices by their location, as they are almost always confined to the upper or middle third of the thoracic esophagus, whereas uphill varices are predominantly located in the distal third. As expected, downhill varices are best visualized on mucosal relief views of the collapsed or partially collapsed esophagus with use of a high-density barium suspension.

When downhill varices are suspected on the basis of barium studies, the patient should be evaluated for other clinical or radiologic signs of superior vena caval obstruction. Chest radiographs or CT scans may reveal obvious widening of the superior mediastinum due to mediastinal lymphadenopathy (see Fig. 30–7A), tumor, substernal thyroid goiter, or, less commonly, mediastinal fibrosis. Venography may be required to confirm the diagnosis and to determine the level of obstruction and extent of collateral circulation, particularly if a surgical shunt is contemplated.

## Differential Diagnosis

Downhill varices may be confused radiographically with varicoid carcinomas that produce thickened, tortuous folds in the upper or midesophagus due to submucosal spread of tumor[15–17] (see Fig. 30–5). However, downhill varices tend to change in size and shape at fluoroscopy, whereas varicoid tumors have a more fixed appearance and more abrupt, well-defined borders. Although these conditions usually can be differentiated by esophagography, other studies such as endoscopy or venography may occasionally be required for a more definitive diagnosis.

## IDIOPATHIC VARICES

Rarely, esophageal varices may occur in patients who have no other signs of hepatic cirrhosis, portal hypertension, or superior vena caval obstruction.[41, 42] Because the mechanism of variceal formation is unknown, they have been called *idiopathic varices*. Occurrence of such varices in children, including monozygotic twins, has been described.[43] It has therefore been postulated that they develop as a result of a congenital weakness in the venous channels of the esophagus.[41–43] Idiopathic varices are extremely uncommon, but they are important because of the risk of variceal bleeding.[41]

## Radiographic Findings

Although uphill and downhill varices tend to occur as multiple lesions, a single idiopathic varix or several idiopathic varices may be manifested by one or more smooth submucosal masses in the esophagus[44] (Fig. 30–8A). As a result, the radiographic appearance may erroneously suggest a submucosal tumor such as a leiomyoma. However, an idiopathic varix usually can be effaced or even obliterated by esophageal distention (Fig. 30–8B), so that radiographs obtained in both upright and recumbent positions with variable esophageal distention should suggest the vascular origin of the lesion.[44] Endoscopists should be aware of this entity, so that a varix is not inadvertently biopsied without careful preliminary visual inspection.

## GASTRIC VARICES

## Pathophysiology

### Portal Hypertension

The gastric fundus contains a venous plexus that normally is drained by numerous short gastric veins that anastomose distally with the splenic vein and proximally with branches of the coronary vein as well as by venous channels surrounding the distal esophagus. Blood in the short gastric veins normally empties via the splenic vein into the portal venous system. In patients with portal hypertension, however, increased pressure in the portal and splenic veins leads to reversal of blood flow through the short gastric veins into the fundal venous plexus, producing fundal varices. Elevated portal pressure also causes reversal of flow through the coronary vein, producing uphill esophageal varices. Thus, portal hypertension is classically manifested by the combined presence

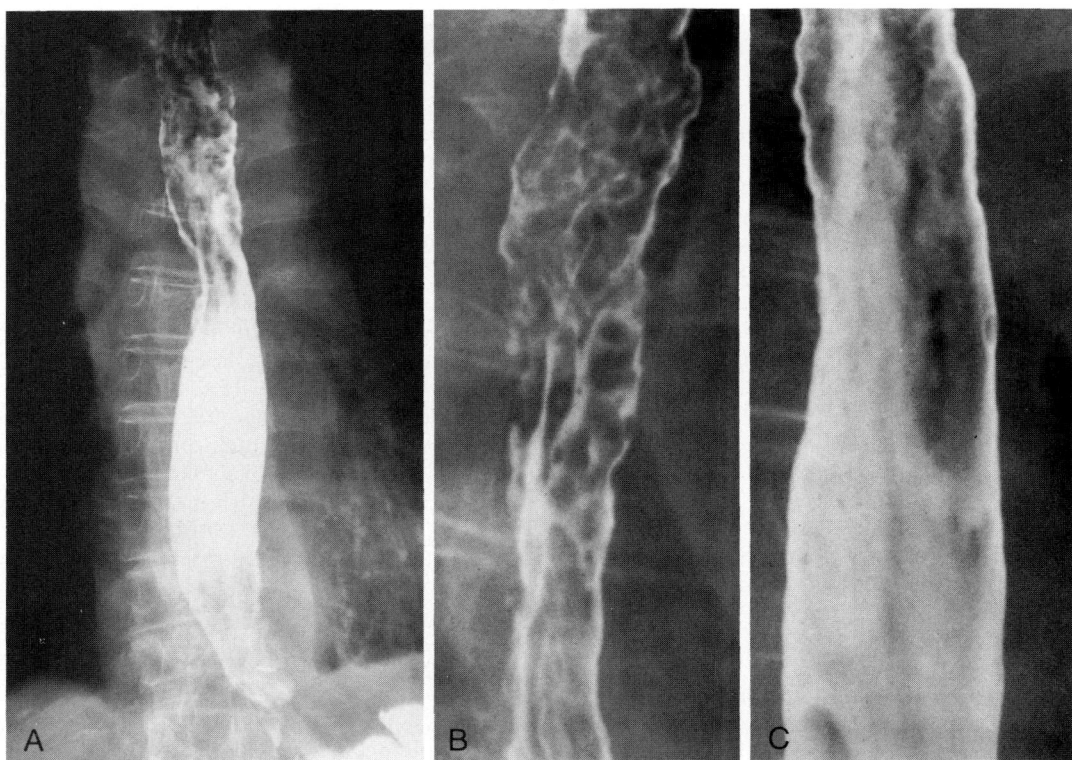

**Figure 30–7. Downhill esophageal varices due to superior vena caval obstruction by broncho-genic carcinoma. A**. A chest radiograph with barium in the esophagus shows thickened, nodular folds in the midesophagus with a normal-appearing esophagus below this level. Note how the superior mediastinum is widened because of adenopathy from metastatic lung cancer. **B**. A mucosal relief view of the esophagus shows prominent downhill varices. **C**. A second view moments later shows obliteration of the varices with greater esophageal distention.

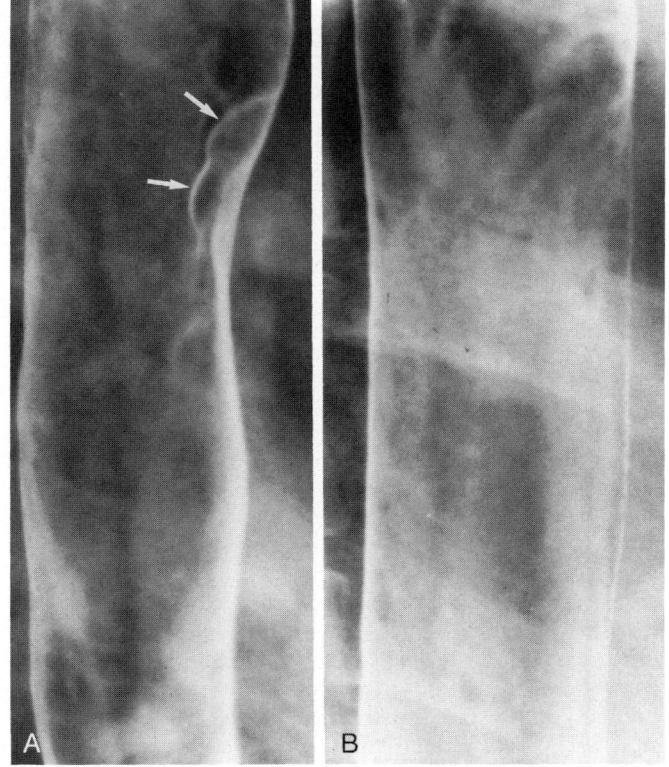

**Figure 30–8. Idiopathic varix. A**. There is a slightly lobulated, submucosal-appearing mass *(arrows)* that is indistinguishable from a leiomyoma or other submucosal tumor. **B**. A second view moments later shows obliteration of the varix with greater esophageal distention. (**A** and **B** courtesy of Seth N. Glick, M.D., Philadelphia, PA.)

of gastric and esophageal varices. However, some patients with portal hypertension have isolated gastric varices, and an even greater number have isolated esophageal varices. One explanation for the frequent failure to visualize gastric varices in patients with portal hypertension is that the venous channels in the gastric fundus have thicker, better connective tissue support than the thin-walled, loosely supported veins in the distal esophagus. As a result, varices may be more likely to form in the esophagus than in the stomach, despite comparable elevations in pressure.[9, 45] Even when gastric varices are present, they may be obscured on barium studies or endoscopy by overlying gastric rugae. As a result, gastric varices are seen radiographically in less than 50% of patients with uphill esophageal varices.[45]

### Splenic Vein Obstruction

In patients with splenic vein obstruction, increased pressure in the splenic vein beyond the obstruction leads to reversal of flow through the short gastric veins to the fundal plexus of veins, producing gastric varices. Because these patients have normal portal pressure, however, venous blood from the dilated fundal plexus can enter the portal venous system via the coronary vein without producing uphill esophageal varices. Unlike portal hypertension, splenic vein obstruction is therefore characterized by isolated varices in the gastric fundus without associated varices in the esophagus.

Splenic vein obstruction may result from intrinsic thrombosis or, more commonly, from extrinsic compression of the splenic vein by a variety of benign or malignant conditions. Because the splenic vein courses along the superior-posterior surface of the pancreas, it is particularly susceptible to entrapment or encasement by diseases in the body or tail of the pancreas. As a result, splenic vein obstruction is most commonly caused by chronic pancreatitis, pancreatic pseudocysts, or pancreatic carcinoma.[46, 47] Occasionally, splenic vein obstruction may result from peripancreatic lymphadenopathy due to metastatic disease or lymphoma or from retroperitoneal fibrosis or bleeding.[47–49] Intrinsic thrombosis of the splenic vein may be idiopathic or may result from polycythemia or other myeloproliferative disorders (see Chapter 109).[47]

### Clinical Findings

Regardless of whether they are associated with portal hypertension or splenic vein obstruction, gastric varices are important because of the risk of gastrointestinal bleeding. These individuals may have low-grade bleeding or massive hematemesis due to variceal rupture.[50, 51] However, gastric varices are less likely to bleed than esophageal varices, probably because of their subserosal location and the greater thickness of overlying gastric tissue.[52] In addition, because of their location, gastric varices may not have the typical bluish tint observed at endoscopy in patients with esophageal varices, so that inadvertent biopsy of a varix may lead to massive bleeding in these individuals.[52]

Most patients with gastric varices have associated esophageal varices with clinical signs and symptoms of portal hypertension. Patients with splenic vein obstruction do not have the stigmata of portal hypertension, but they may have abdominal pain, weight loss, or anemia because of underlying pancreatitis or pancreatic carcinoma.[47] Splenomegaly and hypersplenism are also frequent findings in splenic vein obstruction, but a normal-sized spleen does not exclude this condition.[53]

## Radiographic Findings

### Plain Films

Large gastric varices may occasionally be recognized on chest or abdominal radiographs as one or more lobulated soft tissue densities in the gas-filled fundus. Depending on the cause of the varices (portal hypertension or splenic vein obstruction), abdominal plain films may also demonstrate splenomegaly, ascites, or pancreatic calcification. When gastric varices are suspected on the basis of plain films, barium studies or endoscopy should be performed for a more definitive diagnosis.

### Barium Studies

Conventional single contrast barium studies are generally thought to be unreliable for diagnosing gastric varices. Double contrast technique has therefore been advocated to improve visualization of these structures.[49, 54] Gastric varices may be recognized by the presence of thickened, tortuous folds or lobulated filling defects in the gastric fundus, resembling a bunch of grapes[45, 47, 49] (Fig. 30–9). Less frequently, a conglomerate of varices may produce a single lobulated filling

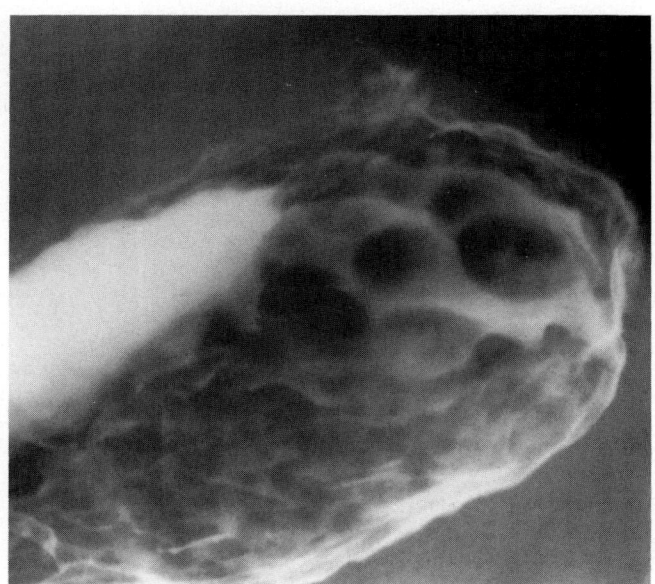

**Figure 30–9. Gastric varices.** Tortuous folds and lobulated filling defects seen in the gastric fundus resemble a bunch of grapes. (From Levine MS, Kieu K, Rubesin SE, et al: Isolated gastric varices: splenic vein obstruction or portal hypertension? Gastrointest Radiol 15:188–192, 1990.)

defect that may be mistaken for a polypoid fundal carcinoma[47, 54–56] (Figs. 30–10 and 30–11). Rarely, dilated gastroepiploic veins are manifested by varices in the antrum or body of the stomach[57] (Fig. 30–12).

When gastric varices are detected by barium studies, it is important to determine whether uphill esophageal varices are also present in these patients. The combined presence of esophageal and gastric varices almost always indicates portal hypertension as the underlying cause. In contrast, the presence of isolated gastric varices should raise the possibility of splenic vein obstruction with a patent portal vein[47, 49] (see Fig. 30–11). Nevertheless, portal hypertension is so much more common than splenic vein obstruction that most patients with gastric varices, even in the absence of esophageal varices, are found to have portal hypertension as the underlying cause[58] (see Fig. 30–10). If necessary, CT or angiography may be performed to document the presence of varices and elucidate the pathophysiology.

## Computed Tomography

Gastric varices are usually recognized on CT scans as enhancing, well-defined, round or tubular densities in the posterior or posteromedial wall of the gastric fundus[59] (Fig. 30–13). In fact, CT may be more sensitive than conventional radiologic examinations in diagnosing these lesions, as barium studies can demonstrate only varices that protrude into the lumen, whereas CT can delineate deeper intramural and perigastric varices.[59] CT may also reveal cirrhotic liver disease, splenomegaly, or ascites in patients with portal hypertension (see Fig. 30–13), and splenomegaly or pancreatic disease in patients with splenic vein obstruction.

## Angiography

Angiography may be performed to confirm the presence of gastric varices and to determine the nature of

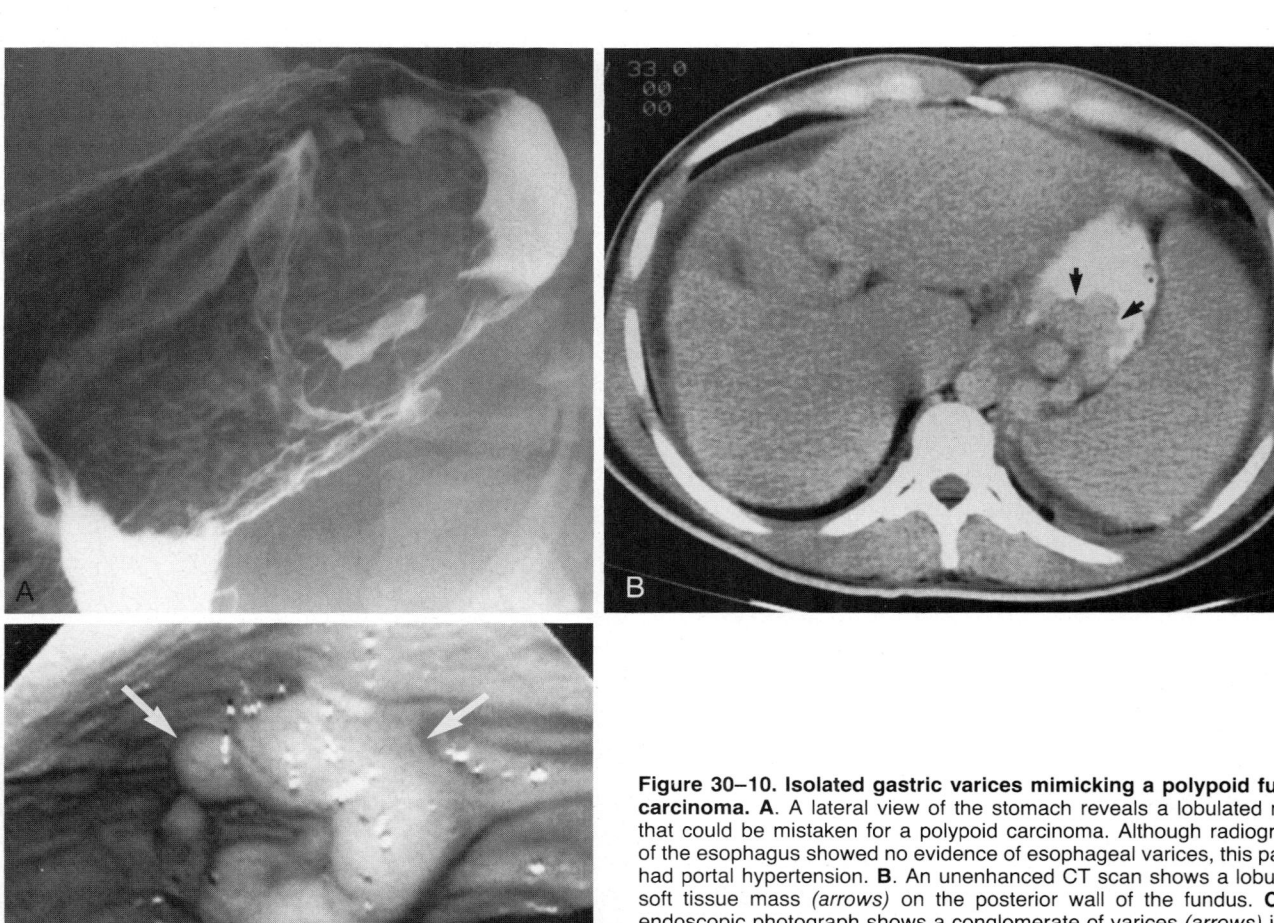

**Figure 30–10. Isolated gastric varices mimicking a polypoid fundal carcinoma. A.** A lateral view of the stomach reveals a lobulated mass that could be mistaken for a polypoid carcinoma. Although radiographs of the esophagus showed no evidence of esophageal varices, this patient had portal hypertension. **B.** An unenhanced CT scan shows a lobulated soft tissue mass *(arrows)* on the posterior wall of the fundus. **C.** An endoscopic photograph shows a conglomerate of varices *(arrows)* in the fundus, adjacent to the cardia. (From Levine MS, Kieu K, Rubesin SE, et al: Isolated gastric varices: splenic vein obstruction or portal hypertension? Gastrointest Radiol 15:188–192, 1990.)

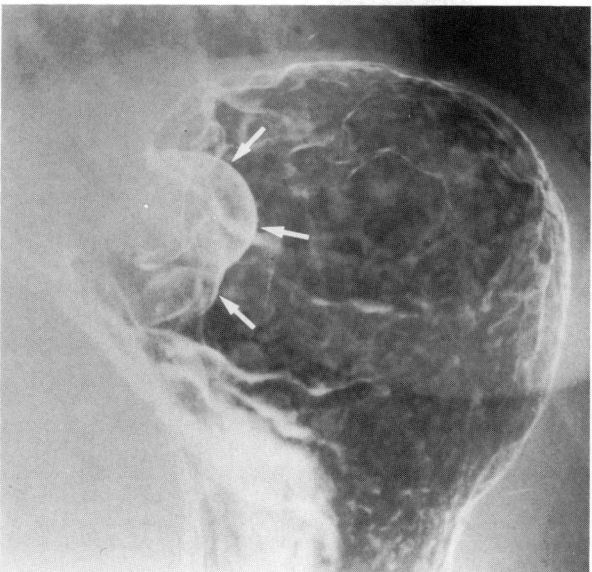

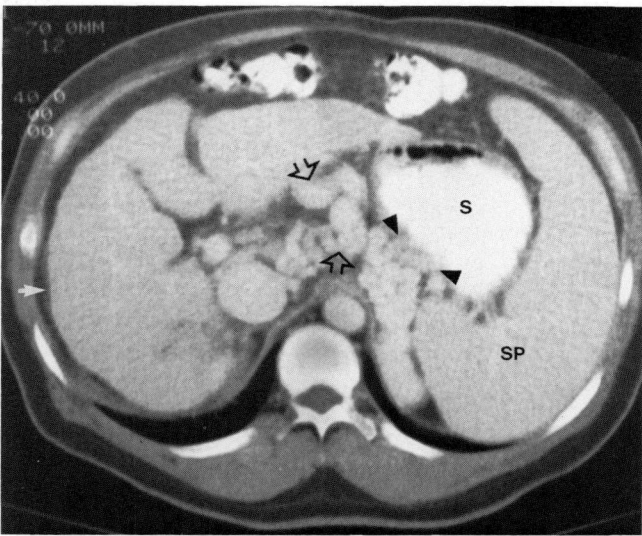

**Figure 30–13. Gastric varices: CT findings.** Enhanced collaterals are seen in the gastric wall *(arrowheads)*, gastrohepatic ligament *(open arrows)*, and left retroperitoneal space. This patient also has cirrhosis with splenomegaly and minimal ascites *(solid arrow)* due to portal hypertension. S = stomach; SP = spleen. (Courtesy of Richard M. Gore, M.D., Evanston, IL.)

**Figure 30–11. Isolated gastric varices *(arrows)* mimicking a polypoid fundal carcinoma.** This patient had underlying pancreatitis causing splenic vein obstruction. (Courtesy of William M. Thompson, M.D., Minneapolis, MN.)

the underlying venous abnormality. With portal hypertension, reversal of flow through the coronary and short gastric veins leads to the formation of esophageal and gastric varices, with absent visualization of the portal and splenic veins on angiograms. With splenic vein obstruction, however, delayed films reveal normal filling of a patent portal vein without evidence of esophageal varices, as blood is diverted from the fundal plexus of veins via the coronary vein to the portal venous system, bypassing the obstructed splenic vein (Fig. 30–14). Thus, portal hypertension can usually be differentiated from splenic vein obstruction by angiography, so that appropriate therapy can be instituted in these patients.

## Differential Diagnosis

When gastric varices appear as thickened, nodular folds in the fundus, the differential diagnosis for this finding includes hypertrophic gastritis, Ménétrier's disease, Zollinger-Ellison syndrome, pancreatitis, and lymphoma.[60] However, varices tend to be more tortuous or lobulated, often resembling a cluster of grapes. Less frequently, a conglomerate of varices in the fundus may produce a single lobulated lesion, mimicking the appearance of a polypoid fundal carcinoma[47, 54–56] (see Figs. 30–10 and 30–11). However, the presence of esophageal varices should suggest the possibility of associated fundal varices. In equivocal cases, angiography or CT may be required for a definitive diagnosis. It is particularly important to differentiate gastric varices from a fundal carcinoma before performing endoscopic biopsy or surgery, as inadvertent perforation of a varix may lead to catastrophic gastrointestinal bleeding.

## Treatment

Emergency treatment for bleeding gastric varices is rarely necessary. When significant bleeding does occur in patients with splenic vein obstruction, the patients

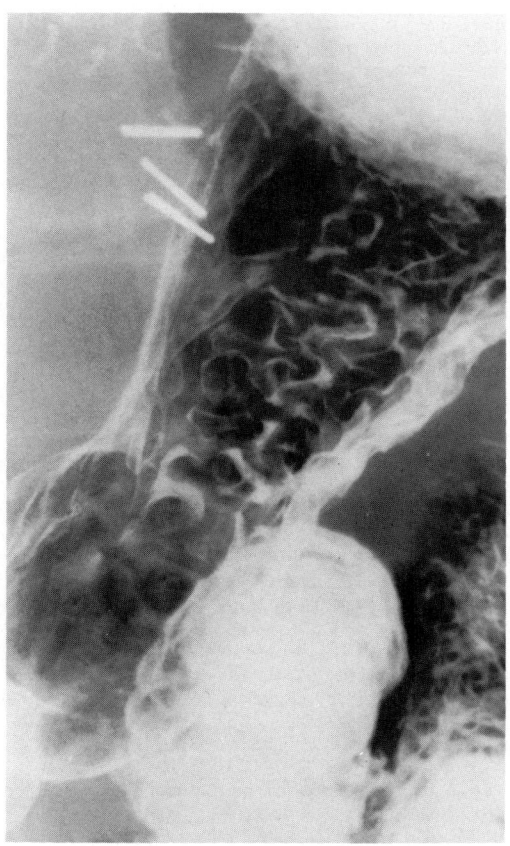

**Figure 30–12. Nonfundal gastric varices.** Thickened, tortuous folds are seen in the body of the stomach due to markedly dilated gastroepiploic veins. This patient had severe portal hypertension.

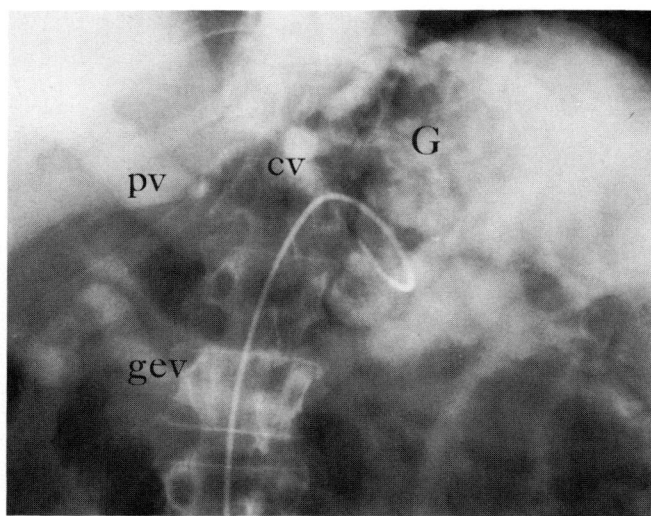

**Figure 30–14. Angiographic demonstration of gastric varices due to splenic vein obstruction.** A radiograph from the venous phase of a splenic arteriogram shows a densely opacified spleen with absent visualization of the splenic vein, extensive gastric varices (G), and a dilated coronary vein (cv) diverting blood from the fundal plexus of veins to the portal vein (pv). Note the presence of a dilated gastroepiploic vein (gev). (Courtesy of Dana R. Burke, M.D., Bethesda, MD.)

are almost always cured by simple splenectomy, as portal venous pressure is normal in these individuals.[61] In contrast, some form of portal-systemic shunt may be required for gastric varices caused by portal hypertension, as splenectomy alone has no effect on portal venous pressure in these patients. Thus, the choice of treatment for gastric varices depends on the underlying cause.

## Acknowledgment

Figures 30–1, 30–2, 30–6A, B, and D, 30–7A to C, 30–12, and 30–14 are reproduced from Levine MS: Radiology of the Esophagus. Philadelphia: WB Saunders, 1989.

# References

1. Kirsh IE, Blackwell CC, Bennett HD: Roentgen diagnosis of esophageal varices: comparison of roentgen and esophagoscopic findings in 502 cases. AJR 74:477–485, 1955.
2. Palmer ED, Brick IB: Correlation between the severity of esophageal varices in portal cirrhosis and their propensity toward hemorrhage. Gastroenterology 30:85–90, 1956.
3. Campbell HE, Baruch RJ: Aneurysm of hemiazygos vein associated with portal hypertension. AJR 83:1024–1026, 1960.
4. Jonsson K, Rian RL: Pseudotumoral esophageal varices associated with portal hypertension. Radiology 97:593–597, 1970.
5. Ishikawa T, Saeki M, Tsukune Y, et al: Detection of paraesophageal varices by plain films. AJR 144:701–704, 1985.
6. Dalinka MK, Smith EH, Wolfe RD, et al: Pharmacologically enhanced visualization of esophageal varices by Pro-Banthine. Radiology 102:281–282, 1972.
7. Ghahremani GG, Port RB, Winans CS, et al: Esophageal varices: enhanced radiologic visualization by anticholinergic drugs. Am J Dig Dis 17:703–712, 1972.
8. Liu CI: Enhanced visualization of esophageal varices by Buscopan. AJR 121:232–235, 1974.
9. Nelson SW: The roentgenologic diagnosis of esophageal varices. AJR 77:599–611, 1957.
10. Cockerill EM, Miller RE, Chernish SM, et al: Optimal visualization of esophageal varices. AJR 126:512–523, 1976.
11. Clark KE, Foley WD, Berland LL, et al: CT evaluation of esophageal and upper abdominal varices. J Comput Assist Tomogr 4:510–515, 1980.
12. Balthazar EJ, Naidich DP, Megibow AJ, et al: CT evaluation of esophageal varices. AJR 148:131–135, 1987.
13. Ishikawa T, Tsukune Y, Ohyama Y, et al: Venous abnormalities in portal hypertension demonstrated by CT. AJR 134:271–276, 1980.
14. Rabin M, Schmaman IB: Reflux esophagitis resembling varices. S Afr Med J 55:293–295, 1979.
15. Lawson TL, Dodds WJ, Sheft DJ: Carcinoma of the esophagus simulating varices. AJR 107:83–85, 1969.
16. Silver TM, Goldstein HM: Varicoid carcinoma of the esophagus. Dig Dis 19:56–58, 1974.
17. Yates CW, LeVine MA, Jensen KM: Varicoid carcinoma of the esophagus. Radiology 122:605–608, 1977.
18. Jackson FC, Perrin EB, Felix WR, et al: A clinical investigation of the portacaval shunt: survival analysis of the therapeutic operation. Ann Surg 174:672–698, 1971.
19. Rueff B, Prandi D, Degos F, et al: A controlled study of therapeutic portacaval shunt in alcoholic cirrhosis. Lancet 1:655–659, 1976.
20. Conn HO: Excessive mortality associated with balloon tamponade of bleeding varices: a critical reappraisal. JAMA 202:587–591, 1967.
21. Sugiura M, Futagawa S: A new technique for treating esophageal varices. J Thorac Cardiovasc Surg 66:677–685, 1973.
22. Macdougall BRD, Westaby D, Theodossi A, et al: Increased long-term survival in variceal haemorrhage using injection sclerotherapy: results of a controlled trial. Lancet 1:124–127, 1982.
23. Hootegem PV, Van Besien K, Broeckaert L, et al: Endoscopic sclerotherapy of esophageal varices: long-term follow-up, recurrence, and survival. J Clin Gastroenterol 10:368–372, 1988.
24. Infante-Rivard C, Esnaola S, Villeneuve JP: Role of endoscopic variceal sclerotherapy in the long-term management of variceal bleeding: a meta-analysis. Gastroenterology 96:1087–1092, 1989.
25. Barsoum MS, Abdel-Wahab MH, Bollous F, et al: The complications of injection sclerotherapy of bleeding oesophageal varices. Br J Surg 69:79–81, 1982.
26. Tihansky DP, Reilly JJ, Schade RR, et al: The esophagus after injection sclerotherapy of varices: immediate postoperative changes. Radiology 153:43–47, 1984.
27. Korula J, Pandya K, Yamada S: Perforation of esophagus after endoscopic variceal sclerotherapy. Dig Dis Sci 34:324–329, 1989.
28. Guynn TP, Eckhauser FE, Knol JA, et al: Injection sclerotherapy-induced esophageal strictures: risk factors and prognosis. Am Surg 57:567–571, 1991.
29. Agha FP: The esophagus after endoscopic injection sclerotherapy: acute and chronic changes. Radiology 153:37–42, 1984.
30. Steenbergen WV, Fevery J, Broeckaert L, et al: Intramural hematoma of the esophagus: unusual complication of variceal sclerotherapy. Gastrointest Radiol 9:293–295, 1984.
31. Bridges R, Runyon BA, Hamlin JA, et al: Sclerotherapy induced pseudo-carcinoma. J Can Assoc Radiol 35:199–201, 1984.
32. Wilbom SL, Rector WG, Schaefer JW: An esophagobronchial fistula after endoscopic variceal sclerotherapy. J Clin Gastroenterol 10:81–83, 1988.
33. Halden WJ, Harnsberger HR, Mancuso AA: Computed tomography of esophageal varices after sclerotherapy. AJR 140:1195–1196, 1983.
34. Mauro MA, Jaques PF, Swantkowski TM, et al: CT after uncomplicated esophageal sclerotherapy. AJR 147:57–60, 1986.
35. Felson B, Lessure AP: "Downhill" varices of the esophagus. Dis Chest 46:740–746, 1964.
36. Otto DL, Kurtzman RS: Esophageal varices in superior vena caval obstruction. AJR 92:1000–1012, 1964.
37. Mikkelsen WJ: Varices of the upper esophagus in superior vena caval obstruction. Radiology 81:945–948, 1963.
38. Salyer JM, Harrison HN, Winn DF, et al: Chronic fibrous medi-

astinitis and superior vena caval obstruction due to histoplasmosis. Dis Chest 35:364–377, 1959.

39. Sorokin JJ, Levine SM, Moss EG, et al: Downhill varices: report of a case 29 years after resection of a substernal thyroid gland. Gastroenterology 73:345–348, 1977.

40. Fleig WE, Stange EF, Ditschuneit H: Upper gastrointestinal hemorrhage from downhill esophageal varices. Dig Dis Sci 27:23–27, 1982.

41. Schaefer J, Bramschreiber J, Mistilis S, et al: Gastroesophageal variceal bleeding in the absence of hepatic cirrhosis or portal hypertension. Gastroenterology 46:583–588, 1964.

42. Kelsen K, Burbige J: Idiopathic esophageal varices. Am J Gastroenterol 77:539–540, 1982.

43. Harinck E, Fernandes J, Vervat D: Congenital esophageal varices in identical twins without portal hypertension. J Pediatr Surg 6:488, 1971.

44. Trenkner SW, Levine MS, Laufer I, et al: Idiopathic esophageal varix. AJR 141:43–44, 1983.

45. Evans JA, Delany F: Gastric varices. Radiology 60:46–51, 1953.

46. Sutton JP, Yarborough DY, Richards JT: Isolated splenic vein occlusion. Arch Surg 100:623–626, 1970.

47. Muhletaler C, Gerlock J, Goncharenko V, et al: Gastric varices secondary to splenic vein occlusion: radiographic diagnosis and clinical significance. Radiology 132:593–598, 1979.

48. Lavender S, Lloyd-Davies RW, Thomas ML: Retroperitoneal fibrosis causing localized portal hypertension. Br Med J 3:627–628, 1970.

49. Cho KJ, Martel W: Recognition of splenic vein occlusion. AJR 131:439–443, 1978.

50. Hershfield NB, Morrow I: Gastric bleeding due to splenic vein thrombosis. Can Med Assoc J 98:649–652, 1968.

51. Goldstein GB: Splenic vein thrombosis causing gastric varices and bleeding. Am J Gastroenterol 58:319–325, 1972.

52. Okuda K, Yasumoto M, Goto A, et al: Endoscopic observations of gastric varices. Am J Gastroenterol 60:357–365, 1973.

53. Itzchak Y, Glickman MG: Splenic vein thrombosis in patients with a normal size spleen. Invest Radiol 12:158–163, 1977.

54. Rice RP, Thompson WM, Kelvin FM, et al: Gastric varices without esophageal varices: an important preendoscopic diagnosis. JAMA 237:1976–1979, 1977.

55. Belgrad R, Carlson HC, Payne WS, et al: Pseudotumoral gastric varices. AJR 91:751–756, 1964.

56. Kaye JJ, Stassa G: Mimicry and deception in the diagnosis of tumors of the gastric cardia. AJR 110:295–303, 1970.

57. Sos T, Meyers MA, Baltaxe HA: Nonfundic gastric varices. Radiology 105:579–580, 1972.

58. Levine MS, Kieu K, Rubesin SE, et al: Isolated gastric varices: splenic vein obstruction or portal hypertension? Gastrointest Radiol 15:188–192, 1990.

59. Balthazar EJ, Megibow A, Naidich D, et al: Computed tomographic recognition of gastric varices. AJR 142:1121–1125, 1984.

60. Marshall JP, Smith PD, Hoyumpa AM: Gastric varices: problems in diagnosis. Am J Dig Dis 22:947–955, 1977.

61. Babb RR: Splenic vein obstruction: a curable cause of variceal bleeding. Am J Dig Dis 21:512–513, 1976.

# Miscellaneous Abnormalities

Marc S. Levine, M.D.

## MALLORY-WEISS TEAR

### Pathogenesis

Mallory-Weiss tears are recognized as a relatively common injury in which a sudden, dramatic increase in intraesophageal pressure produces a linear mucosal laceration at or near the gastric cardia. Although these tears are often caused by violent retching or vomiting after an alcoholic binge, severe vomiting for any reason may produce this injury.[1-3] Less commonly, Mallory-Weiss tears may be caused by prolonged hiccuping or coughing, seizures, straining at stool, childbirth, or blunt abdominal trauma.[4] Similar injuries may also result from direct laceration of the mucosa by an advancing endoscope or by a sharp foreign body in the esophagus, such as a piece of taco.[5, 6]

### Clinical Findings

Mallory-Weiss tears account for about 5 to 10% of all cases of acute upper gastrointestinal bleeding.[7, 8] The classic history of violent retching or vomiting after an alcoholic binge with abrupt onset of hematemesis should suggest the correct diagnosis.[9] However, a Mallory-Weiss tear should be suspected in any patient with hematemesis, even if a history of vomiting or a recent alcoholic binge cannot be documented. Some patients may have massive hematemesis, but most Mallory-Weiss tears heal spontaneously within 48 to 72 hours, so that bleeding is usually self-limited.[1, 4, 8] Patients with Mallory-Weiss tears therefore have an excellent prognosis, with an overall mortality rate of only about 3%.[2, 4] Although most patients can be managed conservatively, selective intra-arterial infusion of vasopressin, transcath-eter embolization, or surgical repair of the tear may occasionally be required to control bleeding.[10, 11]

### Radiographic Findings

About 95% of Mallory-Weiss tears are diagnosed by endoscopy.[3] Nevertheless, these lesions may occasionally be recognized on double contrast esophagrams as shallow, longitudinally oriented, linear 1- to 4-cm collections of barium in the distal esophagus at or slightly above the gastroesophageal junction (Fig. 31–1). The radiographic appearance may be indistinguishable from that of a linear ulcer in the distal esophagus caused by reflux esophagitis. However, a history of recent vomiting or hematemesis, particularly in an alcoholic, should suggest the correct diagnosis.

## ESOPHAGEAL HEMATOMA

### Pathogenesis

Most esophageal hematomas are caused by a mucosal laceration or tear in the distal esophagus. If the tear is partially or completely occluded by edema or blood clot, continued hemorrhage may lead to progressive submucosal dissection of blood, producing an intramural hematoma.[12, 13] As with Mallory-Weiss tears, the underlying laceration is usually caused by a sudden increase in intraesophageal pressure due to one or more episodes of violent retching or vomiting.[12-14] Esophageal hematomas may also be caused by esophageal instrumentation or, rarely, by blunt trauma to the chest or abdomen.[15-17] Although most hematomas are associated with underlying mucosal lacerations, spontaneous hematomas may occasionally develop in patients who have impaired

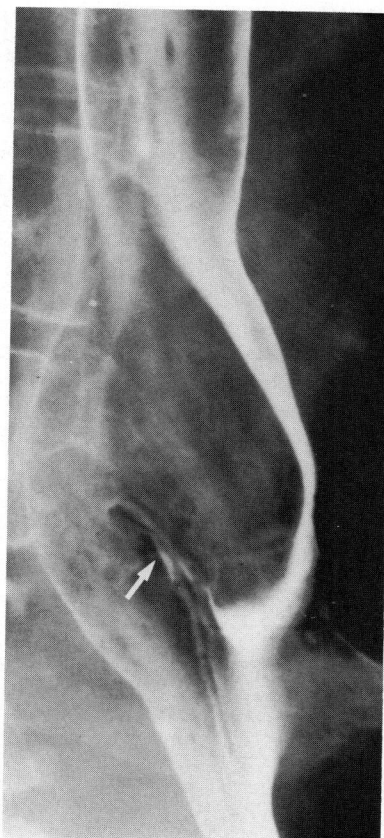

**Figure 31–1. Mallory-Weiss tear.** There is a linear collection of barium *(arrow)* in the distal esophagus just above the gastroesophageal junction. Although a linear ulcer from reflux esophagitis could produce a similar appearance, the correct diagnosis was suggested by the clinical history. (Courtesy of Harvey M. Goldstein, M.D., San Antonio, TX.)

hemostasis due to thrombocytopenia, hemophilia, other bleeding disorders, or anticoagulation.[18, 19] Unlike traumatic hematomas, which almost always occur as solitary lesions in the distal esophagus, spontaneous hematomas tend to spare the distal esophagus and occur at multiple sites.[14]

## Clinical Findings

Esophageal hematomas may be manifested clinically by the sudden onset of retrosternal chest pain, dysphagia, or hematemesis.[13, 19] Occasionally, chest pain may be so severe that it mimics a myocardial infarction or dissecting aortic aneurysm. However, an esophageal hematoma should be suspected if there is a recent history of vomiting, esophageal instrumentation, or abnormal hemostasis. In such cases, a study using a water-soluble contrast medium may be performed to determine if a hematoma or other esophageal injury is present.

Most esophageal hematomas resolve spontaneously on conservative treatment with nasogastric suction, antibiotics, and intravenous fluids.[13, 16, 19] These lesions should therefore be considered self-limited, as intramural hematomas almost never progress to complete

transmural perforation. An esophageal hematoma may be recognized at endoscopy as a large submucosal mass bulging into the lumen with dark blue discoloration of the overlying mucosa.[16] If an esophageal hematoma is demonstrated on barium studies, however, endoscopy is unnecessary because of the self-limited nature of the lesion.

## Radiographic Findings

Most esophageal hematomas appear radiographically as solitary, ovoid or elongated submucosal masses on the posterior or lateral wall of the distal esophagus[13, 16–18, 20] (Fig. 31–2). Like other submucosal lesions, hematomas tend to have smooth borders and, when viewed in profile, to form 90-degree or slightly obtuse angles with the adjacent esophageal wall. Rarely, circumferential hematomas may cause smooth, tapered narrowing of the esophagus with associated obstruction.

When a mucosal laceration is present, contrast medium may dissect beneath the mucosa into the hematoma. This intramural dissection may produce a characteristic "double-barreled" appearance due to parallel collections of contrast medium in both true and false

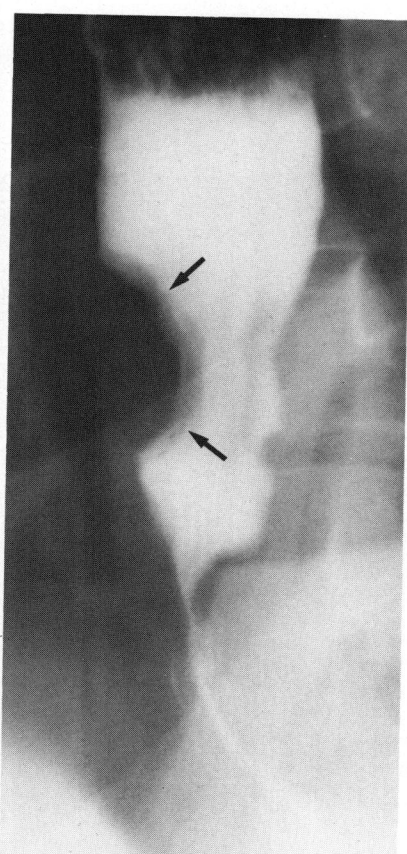

**Figure 31–2. Esophageal hematoma.** There is a smooth submucosal mass *(arrows)* in the distal esophagus. The hematoma was caused by a pneumatic dilatation procedure for achalasia. Note how the esophagus is markedly narrowed below the hematoma due to the patient's underlying achalasia.

lumens, separated by a thin, radiolucent stripe[12, 15, 20–23] (Fig. 31–3). This appearance has been compared with the angiographic findings in an aortic dissection.

Esophageal hematomas may be indistinguishable from leiomyomas or other benign submucosal tumors in the esophagus.[13] When intramural dissection of contrast medium produces a double-barreled esophagus, the radiographic findings may erroneously suggest a transmural perforation. However, extravasated contrast medium in the mediastinum has a more irregular appearance and is more persistent, whereas intramural contrast medium may empty rapidly into the lumen.[15, 22] Thus, it is usually possible to differentiate intramural dissection of contrast medium from a true perforation. A double-barreled esophagus may also result from intramural tracking due to Crohn's disease, *Candida* esophagitis, or tuberculous esophagitis.

## ESOPHAGEAL PERFORATION

Esophageal perforation is the most serious and rapidly fatal type of perforation in the gastrointestinal tract. Untreated thoracic esophageal perforations have a mortality rate of nearly 100% because of the fulminant mediastinitis that occurs after esophageal rupture.[24] Perforation of the cervical esophagus is a more common but less devastating injury. Early diagnosis of esophageal perforation is important, because of the need for prompt surgical intervention in most cases.

## Pathogenesis

### Instrumentation

Endoscopic procedures are responsible for 75 to 80% of all esophageal perforations.[25] This complication occurs in about 1 in 1000 patients who undergo endoscopic examinations with modern fiberoptic instruments.[25, 26] Most endoscopic perforations occur on the posterior wall of the cervical esophagus at or near the level of the cricopharyngeus.[25–27] This area is particularly susceptible to perforation when it is compressed against the cervical spine by the advancing endoscope. The presence of a pharyngeal diverticulum, cervical lordosis, or cervical osteophyte increases the risk of perforation.[27] The piriform sinus is another common site of high instrumental perforations.

Thoracic esophageal perforations usually occur at or near the gastroesophageal junction or, less commonly, at areas of normal anatomic narrowing due to extrinsic compression by the aortic arch or left main bronchus.[25] However, the thoracic esophagus may also be perforated at or above benign or malignant strictures, particularly when biopsies or dilatation procedures are performed.

Although endoscopy accounts for most iatrogenic perforations, the esophagus may occasionally be perforated by pneumatic dilatation balloons, nasogastric or endotracheal tubes, Celestin tubes, Sengstaken-Blakemore tubes, or esophageal obturator airways.[28] Perforation may also occur after esophageal surgery, most

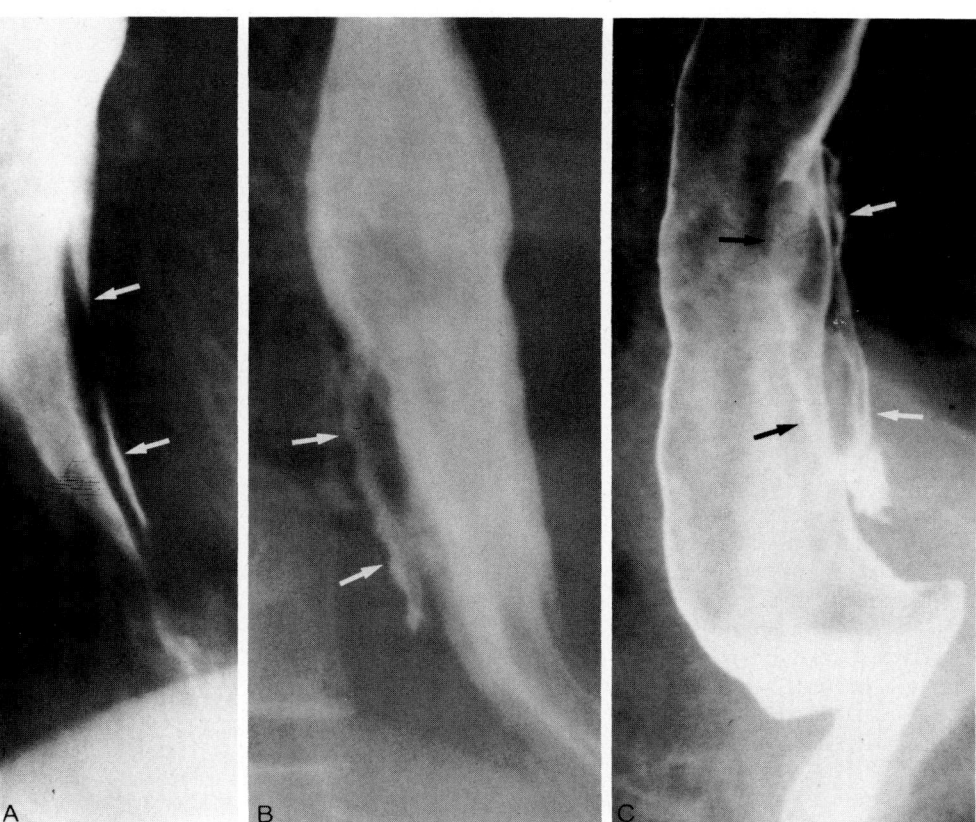

**Figure 31–3. Three examples of intramural dissections with a double-barreled esophagus.** In all cases (**A** to **C**) the longitudinal intramural tracks *(arrows)* are separated from the esophageal lumen by a radiolucent mucosal stripe (best seen in **A**). **A** and **B** show traumatic dissections that occurred during esophageal instrumentation, whereas **C** shows a spontaneous dissection detected as an incidental finding on a double contrast examination. (**A** courtesy of Sang Y. Han, M.D., Birmingham, AL. **C** courtesy of Seth N. Glick, M.D., Philadelphia, PA.)

A          B          C

frequently at the site of a ruptured anastomosis (see Chapter 33).

## Foreign Bodies

Most foreign body perforations in adults are caused by impacted animal or fish bones in the hypopharynx that erode through the piriform sinus or cervical esophagus at the level of the cricopharyngeus. Rarely, long-standing foreign body obstructions in the thoracic esophagus also lead to perforation as a result of transmural inflammation and pressure necrosis at the site of impaction (see later section on foreign bodies). Esophageal perforation may also be caused by accidental or intentional ingestion of caustic agents (see Chapter 26).

## Trauma

Penetrating injuries to the esophagus are almost always caused by knife or bullet wounds. Because the neck lacks the bony protection afforded by the thorax, these injuries usually involve the cervical esophagus.[25] Blunt trauma to the chest or abdomen may also lead to esophageal rupture or transection due to a sudden elevation in esophageal hydrostatic pressure (see next section).

## Spontaneous Esophageal Perforation (Boerhaave's Syndrome)

In spontaneous esophageal perforation, a sudden increase in intraluminal esophageal pressure causes a full-thickness perforation of normal underlying esophageal tissue, with ensuing mediastinitis, sepsis, and shock. Most cases result from violent retching or vomiting after an alcoholic binge.[29–31] Occasionally, however, spontaneous rupture of the esophagus may result from other causes of increased intraesophageal pressure, such as coughing, weightlifting, childbirth, defecation, seizures, status asthmaticus, and blunt trauma to the chest or abdomen.[30, 31]

Spontaneous esophageal perforations usually occur as 1- to 4-cm, vertically oriented, linear tears on the left posterolateral wall of the distal esophagus just above the gastroesophageal junction.[29–32] The distal esophagus is most vulnerable because of the lack of supporting mediastinal structures in this region. These perforations tend to be located on the left side of the distal esophagus, because the right side is protected by the descending thoracic aorta.[25, 31]

## Clinical Findings

### Cervical Esophageal Perforation

Most cervical esophageal perforations occur as direct complications of endoscopy, but the endoscopist may be unaware that a perforation has occurred at the time of the examination. Subsequently, patients may develop dysphagia, neck pain, and fever.[27] Physical examination often reveals subcutaneous emphysema in the neck due to gas escaping from the pharynx into the adjacent soft tissues. If untreated, these patients eventually may develop a retropharyngeal abscess associated with sepsis and shock.

Cervical esophageal perforations often heal after conservative treatment with antibiotics and intravenous hyperalimentation, so that small perforations can be treated nonoperatively. However, larger perforations usually require a cervical mediastinotomy and open drainage to prevent abscess formation.[33] With an overall mortality rate of less than 15%,[27] these injuries have a much better prognosis than do thoracic esophageal perforations.

### Thoracic Esophageal Perforation

Thoracic esophageal perforations are typically manifested by the sudden onset of excruciating substernal or lower thoracic chest pain.[29, 31] Swallowed food or saliva and refluxed peptic acid may enter the mediastinum, causing severe mediastinitis, fever, and shock.[29, 31, 32] As air escapes from the esophagus into the mediastinum and neck, these patients often develop subcutaneous emphysema with crepitus in the soft tissues of the anterior chest wall (i.e., mediastinal "crunch") or neck on physical examination.

The classic triad of vomiting, lower thoracic chest pain, and subcutaneous emphysema is virtually pathognomonic of spontaneous esophageal perforation.[29] However, some patients with thoracic esophageal perforations have atypical chest pain referred to the left shoulder or back.[29] Others have epigastric pain, particularly if the perforation involves the intra-abdominal segment of the esophagus below the diaphragmatic hiatus.[34] Furthermore, subcutaneous emphysema is not always present on physical examination. As a result, a thoracic esophageal perforation can be mistaken for a perforated peptic ulcer, myocardial infarction, spontaneous pneumothorax, pulmonary infarct, acute pancreatitis, dissecting aortic aneurysm, or mesenteric infarction.[29, 31] Because of this clinical confusion, spontaneous esophageal perforations are rarely diagnosed within 24 hours of their occurrence.[31] Unfortunately, the prognosis for these patients is directly related to the interval between the perforation and the initiation of therapy. After 24 hours, the mortality rate for thoracic perforations is about 70%.[29] Thus, early diagnosis and treatment are essential for improving survival of these patients.

Unlike cervical esophageal perforations, which can often be treated conservatively, thoracic esophageal perforations usually require immediate thoracotomy with surgical closure of the perforation and mediastinal drainage, to prevent the development of mediastinitis, sepsis, and death.[35] Rarely, thoracic esophageal perforations heal spontaneously without surgical intervention.[36] The overall mortality rate for all patients with thoracic esophageal perforations is about 25%.[27]

# Radiographic Findings

## Plain Films

### Cervical Esophageal Perforation

Subcutaneous emphysema may be visible on antero-posterior or lateral radiographs of the neck within 1 hour after a pharyngeal or cervical esophageal perforation[25] (Fig. 31–4A). Subsequently, air may dissect along fascial planes from the neck into the chest, producing pneumomediastinum.[25] Lateral films of the neck may also demonstrate widening of the prevertebral space, anterior deviation of the trachea, and, eventually, a retropharyngeal abscess containing mottled gas or a single air-fluid level. When a cervical esophageal perforation is suspected on the basis of plain films, a study using water-soluble contrast medium should be performed to determine the site and extent of perforation (Fig. 31–4B). Because subtle perforations are sometimes difficult to demonstrate with water-soluble contrast material, a barium study should be performed to decrease the chance of missing a perforation if the initial study using water-soluble contrast medium shows no evidence of a leak.

### Thoracic Esophageal Perforation

About 90% of patients with thoracic esophageal perforations have abnormal chest radiographs.[37, 38] The earliest plain film findings are mediastinal widening and pneumomediastinum.[25, 29–31, 38] Pneumomediastinum is usually recognized by the presence of radiolucent streaks of gas in the mediastinum along the left lateral border of the aortic arch and descending thoracic aorta, or along the right lateral border of the ascending aorta and heart (Fig. 31–5A). Subsequently, gas in the mediastinum may dissect along fascial planes superiorly to the supraclavicular area, producing subcutaneous emphysema in the neck within several hours of the perforation.[31]

Between 75 and 90% of thoracic esophageal perforations are associated with a pleural effusion or hydropneumothorax.[39] Distal esophageal perforations often result in a sympathetic left pleural effusion or atelectasis in the basilar segments of the left lung because of irritation of the adjacent mediastinal parietal pleura and pulmonary parenchyma (see Fig. 31–5A). Pleural effusions may be present within 12 hours of the perforation and are occasionally detected before the development of mediastinal or cervical emphysema. If the mediastinal pleura ruptures, gas and fluid may enter the pleural space directly from the mediastinum, producing a hydropneumothorax. Because the distal esophagus directly abuts the mediastinal parietal pleura on the left, 75% of hydropneumothoraces occur on the left side, whereas 5% occur on the right, and 20% are bilateral.[29, 32]

Pneumoperitoneum is rarely observed in patients with thoracic esophageal perforations. With perforation of

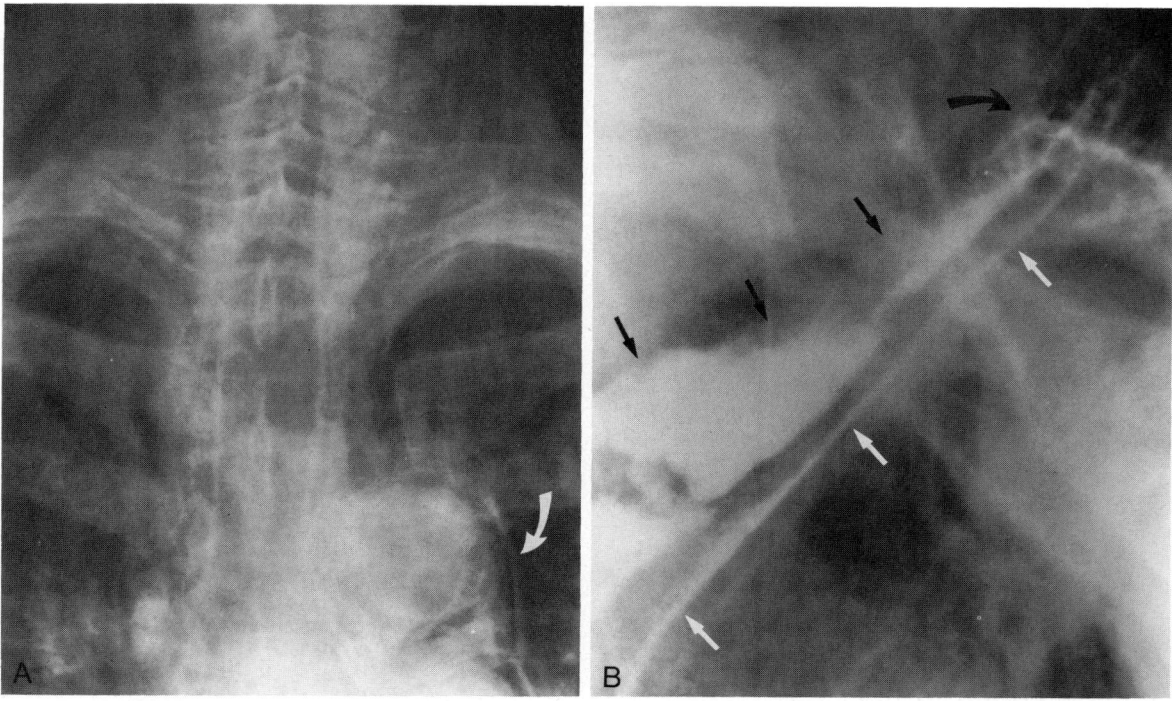

**Figure 31–4. Cervical esophageal perforation by traumatic endoscopy. A.** A close-up view from a posteroanterior (PA) chest radiograph obtained several hours after the procedure shows extensive subcutaneous emphysema in the neck and associated pneumomediastinum *(arrow)*. **B.** A study using water-soluble contrast medium in a steep oblique projection reveals a cervical esophageal perforation *(curved black arrow)* with contrast medium extending inferiorly in the mediastinum *(straight black arrows)* behind the esophagus *(white arrows)*.

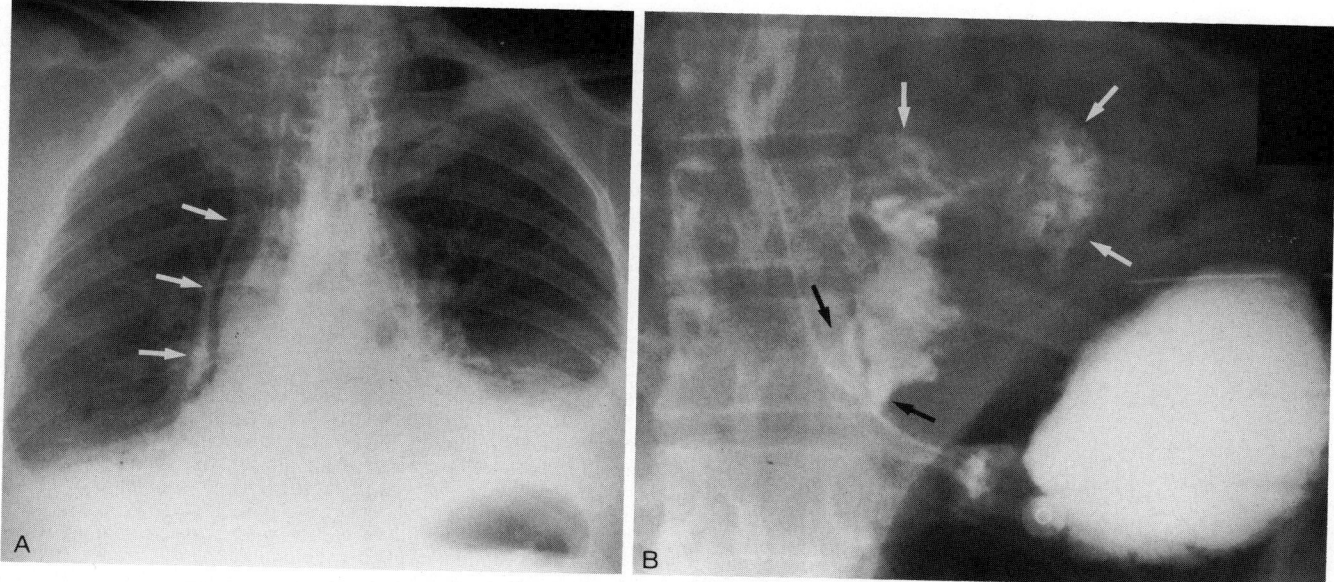

**Figure 31–5. Spontaneous esophageal perforation or Boerhaave's syndrome. A**. A PA chest radiograph shows a right-sided pneumomediastinum *(arrows)* and a left pleural effusion. These findings should be highly suggestive of spontaneous esophageal perforation in a patient (particularly an alcoholic) with vomiting. **B**. A subsequent study using water-soluble contrast medium confirms the presence of a localized perforation of the left lateral wall of the distal esophagus *(black arrows)*, with extension of the leak laterally and superiorly in the mediastinum *(white arrows)*. (**A** and **B** courtesy of Seth N. Glick, M.D., Philadelphia, PA.)

the intra-abdominal segment of the distal esophagus below the diaphragmatic hiatus, however, gas may be detected in the lesser sac or retroperitoneum on abdominal plain films.[34, 40] Such patients may have vague abdominal discomfort without chest pain or any other clinical signs of esophageal perforation. Fortunately, intra-abdominal esophageal perforations are likely to heal spontaneously with conservative treatment, without the need for surgical intervention.[34, 40] As a result, these patients have a more benign clinical course than most patients with thoracic esophageal perforations.

## Contrast Studies

The ideal contrast agent for evaluating a clinically suspected perforation provides diagnostic information about the site and extent of perforation without posing a risk to the patient. It has been shown experimentally that barium is capable of inciting an inflammatory reaction in the mediastinum with subsequent granuloma formation and fibrosis, whereas water-soluble contrast agents such as diatrizoate meglumine and diatrizoate sodium (Gastrografin) are rapidly absorbed from the mediastinum without producing a significant histologic response.[41, 42] The initial radiologic evaluation of a suspected esophageal perforation should therefore be performed with water-soluble contrast medium to avoid this mediastinal reaction. However, Gastrografin is an extremely hypertonic contrast agent that may cause severe pulmonary edema if aspirated into the lungs.[43] Some authors therefore advocate the use of low-osmo-

lality, water-soluble contrast agents such as metrizamide (Amipaque) and iohexol (Omnipaque) to avoid this risk.[44] In any case, water-soluble contrast agents are less radiopaque than barium and tend to disperse quickly in the mediastinum when a perforation is present. As a result, studies using water-soluble contrast agents may fail to detect as many as 15 to 25% of thoracic esophageal perforations and 50% of cervical esophageal perforations.[25, 26, 37] The radiologic examination should therefore be repeated with barium if the initial water-soluble contrast agent fails to demonstrate a leak, as the superior physical properties of barium may permit detection of small leaks not visible on studies using water-soluble contrast agents[41, 42, 45, 46] (Fig. 31–6). In such cases, the deleterious effects of barium in the mediastinum are more than offset by the earlier diagnosis and treatment of a potentially life-threatening condition.

Small perforations may be recognized on esophagrams by relatively localized extravasation of contrast medium from the esophagus into the neck or mediastinum. Because most thoracic esophageal perforations occur near the gastroesophageal junction, contrast medium is usually seen extravasating from the left lateral aspect of the distal esophagus into the adjacent mediastinum. A sealed-off perforation may be manifested by a self-contained extraluminal collection of contrast medium that communicates with the adjacent esophagus (Fig. 31–7). In contrast, larger perforations may result in free extravasation of contrast medium into the mediastinum with extension along fascial planes superiorly or inferiorly from the site of perforation (Fig. 31–8; see Fig. 31–5B).

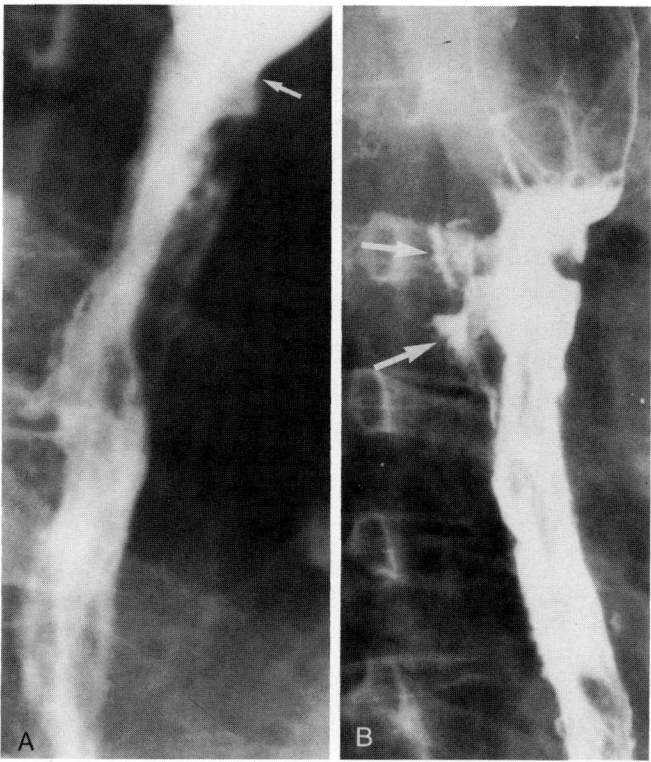

**Figure 31–6. The importance of using barium for the diagnosis of subtle perforations. A.** The initial study using water-soluble contrast medium after an esophagogastrectomy shows an irregular contour below the esophagogastric anastomosis *(arrow).* However, no definite site of perforation is seen. **B.** A second examination performed moments later with barium sulfate shows a sealed-off anastomotic perforation *(arrows)* that was not visible with the water-soluble contrast medium. This case dramatically illustrates how barium should be given to all patients with suspected perforation if the initial study using water-soluble contrast medium fails to demonstrate a leak.

**Figure 31–7. Sealed-off perforations of the thoracic esophagus. A.** There is a self-contained extraluminal collection of contrast medium *(arrows)* adjacent to the left lateral aspect of the distal esophagus after a pneumatic dilatation procedure for achalasia. **B.** A small, sealed-off perforation *(arrows)* is seen at the proximal end of a radiation stricture after endoscopic dilatation of the stricture.

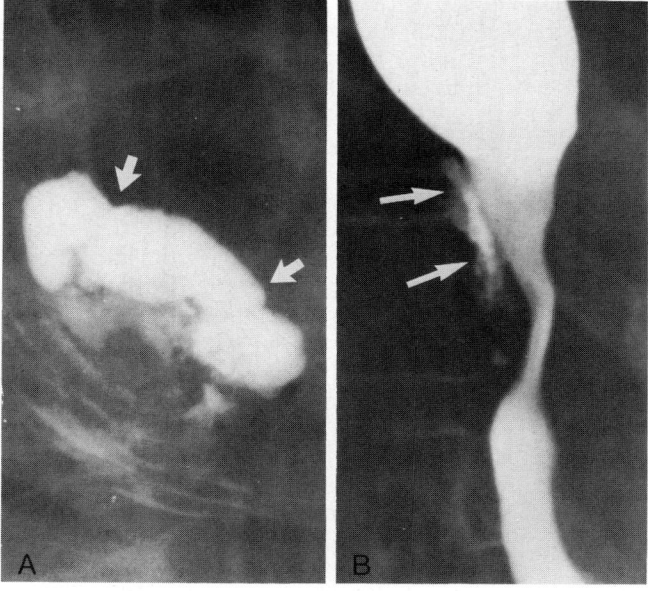

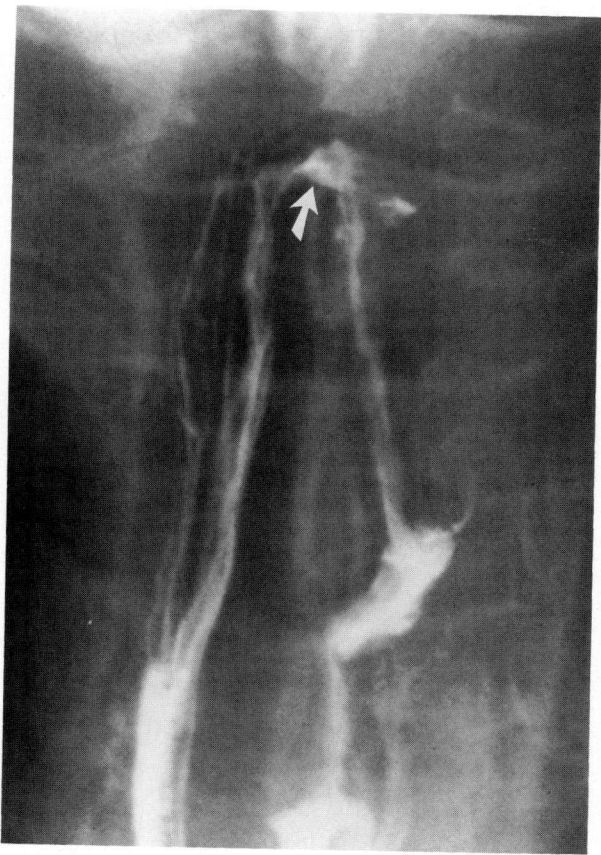

**Figure 31–8. Esophageal perforation by an endotracheal tube.** A water-soluble contrast study shows perforation of the upper esophagus near the thoracic inlet *(arrow)* with an extraluminal track extending inferiorly in the left side of the mediastinum.

# FOREIGN BODY IMPACTION

Nearly 80% of all pharyngeal or esophageal foreign body impactions occur in children who accidentally or intentionally ingest coins, toys, or other foreign objects.[47] In contrast, foreign body impactions in adults are usually caused by animal or fish bones or by unchewed boluses of meat.[47, 48] Bones tend to lodge in the pharynx near the level of the cricopharyngeus, whereas meat usually lodges in the distal esophagus near the gastroesophageal junction.[49] Unlike impactions resulting from sharp foreign bodies, meat impactions are often caused by underlying esophageal rings or strictures. Although 80 to 90% of foreign bodies in the esophagus pass spontaneously, the remaining 10 to 20% require some form of therapeutic intervention.[47]

## Clinical Findings

Animal or fish bones tend to lodge in the pharynx, often near the level of the cricopharyngeus.[49] The patient may complain of pharyngeal dysphagia or of a sensation of a foreign body in the throat, unrelated to swallowing. In contrast, meat bolus impactions tend to occur in the distal esophagus or, less commonly, the midesophagus

and are manifested by the sudden onset of chest pain, odynophagia, or dysphagia.[49] However, some patients with distal foreign body impactions may have dysphagia that is referred to the pharynx, so the subjective site of obstruction is unreliable in determining the level of impaction.

Esophageal perforation occurs in less than 1% of all patients with foreign body impactions.[48] However, the risk of perforation increases significantly if the impaction persists more than 24 hours.[50] Perforation results from transmural esophageal inflammation and subsequent pressure necrosis at the site of impaction. The development of mediastinitis may lead to sudden and rapid clinical deterioration of the patient, manifested by chest pain, sepsis, and shock.[50] Rarely, an impacted foreign body can erode through the wall of the esophagus, producing an aortoesophageal, esophagobronchial, or esophagopericardial fistula (see later section on fistulas).

## Radiographic Findings

### Plain Films

Anteroposterior and lateral films of the neck and chest may occasionally demonstrate bones or other radiopaque foreign bodies in the pharynx or esophagus. Lateral radiographs of the neck are usually more helpful than anteroposterior radiographs in identifying animal or fish bones lodged in the pharynx or cervical esophagus (Fig. 31–9), as these bones are easily obscured by the overlying cervical spine on anteroposterior films. Nevertheless, considerable difficulty may be encountered in differentiating small bone fragments from calcified thyroid or cricoid cartilage.

### Contrast Studies

When a foreign body impaction in the pharynx or esophagus is suspected, an early barium swallow may be performed to determine whether a foreign body is present and whether it is causing obstruction. If the barium study confirms the presence of a foreign body in the esophagus, the radiologist may then attempt to relieve the impaction by performing various therapeutic maneuvers under fluoroscopic guidance (see section on treatment).

Animal or fish bones in the pharynx or cervical esophagus are easily obscured by barium, so that they may be difficult to detect on contrast examinations. However, they can sometimes be recognized as linear filling defects in the vallecula, piriform sinus, or cricopharyngeal region (Figs. 31–10 and 31–11). In some cases, cotton balls or marshmallows soaked in barium may also be helpful for demonstrating small foreign bodies in the pharynx or esophagus.

Foreign body impactions in the thoracic esophagus usually result from a large bolus of unchewed meat lodging above an anatomic or pathologic area of narrowing. The most frequent site of anatomic narrowing is the gastroesophageal junction, but food impactions occasionally occur more proximally, where the esophagus

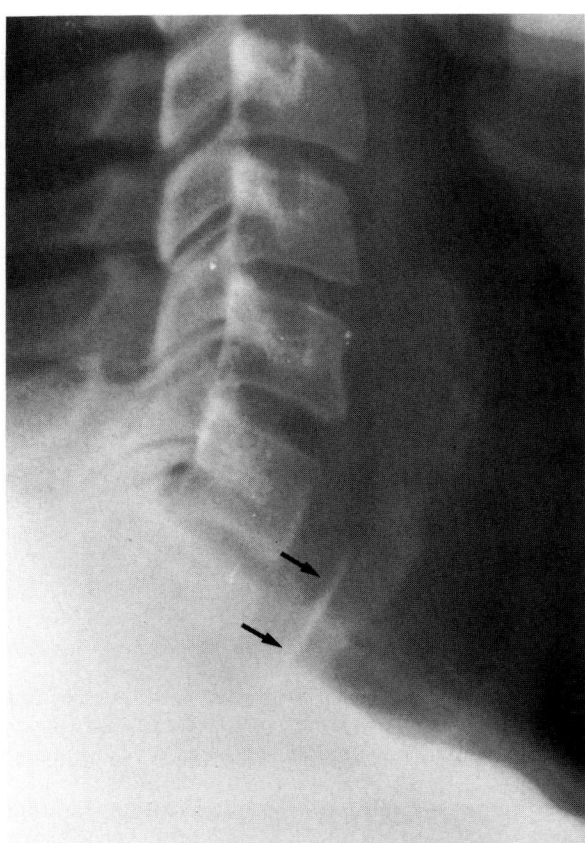

**Figure 31–9. Swallowed pork bone in the neck near the pharyngoesoph-ageal junction.** Note the faintly calcified density *(arrows)* in the region of the cricopharyngeus on a lateral film of the neck.

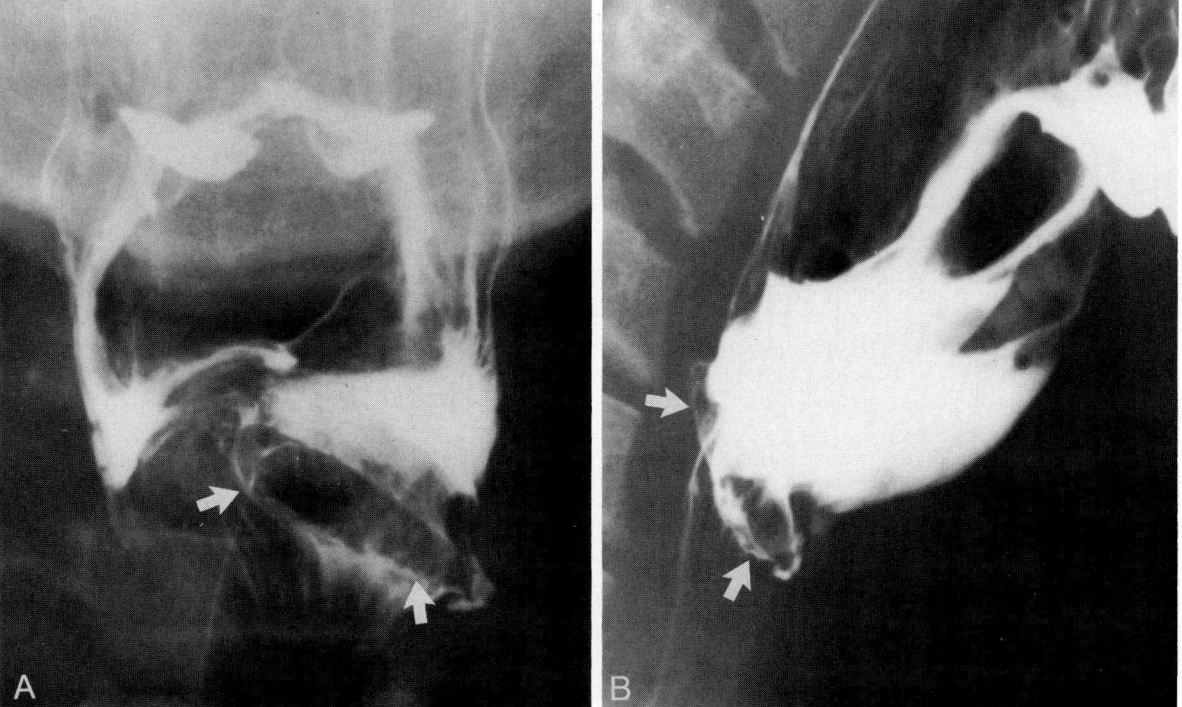

**Figure 31–10. Chicken bone in the piriform sinus.** PA **(A)** and lateral **(B)** views from a barium swallow reveal a linear filling defect *(arrows)* due to an impacted bone in the left piriform sinus.

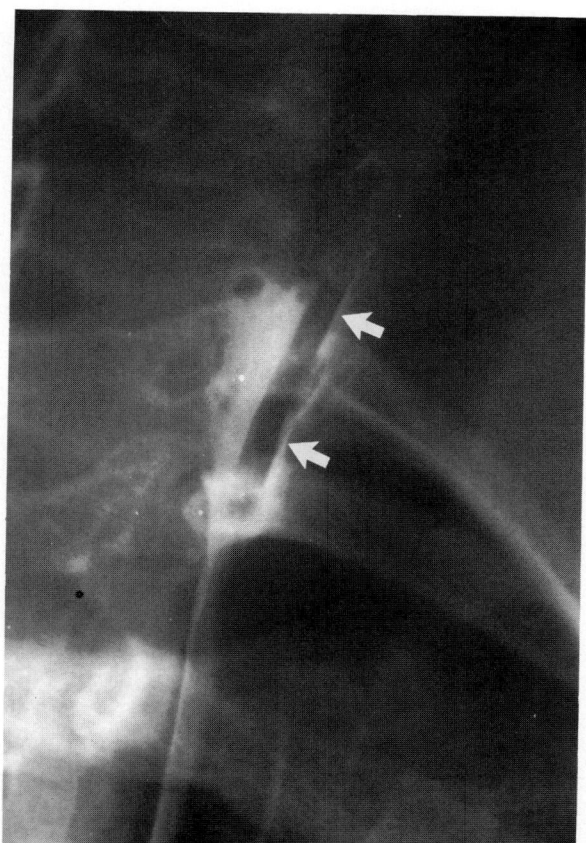

**Figure 31–11 Turkey bone in the cervical esophagus.** A barium swallow reveals a linear filling defect *(arrows)* due to a bone lodged in the cervical esophagus just below the cricopharyngeus.

impaction[47–49] (see Fig. 31–12B). Malignant strictures are a much less common cause of foreign body obstructions in the esophagus.[47] Rarely, food impactions may even result from giant thoracic osteophytes or other structures impinging on the esophagus.[51] Nevertheless, follow-up barium studies often reveal a normal thoracic esophagus without evidence of narrowing or motor dysfunction (Fig. 31–13B).

## Treatment

When swallowed foreign bodies fail to pass spontaneously, some form of therapeutic intervention is required for their removal. Impacted foreign bodies in the pharynx or esophagus may be removed by endoscopy or by the use of a wire basket or a Foley catheter balloon under fluoroscopic guidance.[47–49, 52] These techniques appear to be safe and effective for extracting blunt foreign bodies from the esophagus.

Radiologists may also attempt to relieve esophageal food impactions by several noninvasive maneuvers performed at the time of the initial barium study. One such maneuver is the administration of intravenous glucagon, which facilitates passage of the foreign body by relaxing the lower esophageal sphincter.[53, 54] However, glucagon is unlikely to be effective if an underlying ring or

is extrinsically compressed by the aortic arch or left main bronchus. In other patients, a meat bolus may lodge above a pathologic area of narrowing due to a benign or malignant stricture. However, it is usually not possible to determine whether the underlying esophagus is normal or abnormal, because the foreign body impaction prevents adequate visualization of the esophagus below this level.

When an impacted meat bolus causes complete esophageal obstruction, barium studies may reveal a polypoid filling defect in the esophagus with an irregular meniscus due to barium outlining the superior border of the impacted bolus (Fig. 31–12A). Although the radiographic appearance could be mistaken for a polypoid carcinoma completely obstructing the esophagus, the correct diagnosis is almost always apparent from the clinical history. When the obstruction is incomplete, a small amount of barium may trickle around the impacted meat bolus into the distal esophagus and stomach (Fig. 31–13A). Because the esophagus is incompletely distended below the level of impaction, the radiographic findings may erroneously suggest a stricture in this region.

After an esophageal food impaction has been relieved, another esophagram should be performed to determine if underlying disease is present. Some patients may have Schatzki rings or peptic strictures causing the

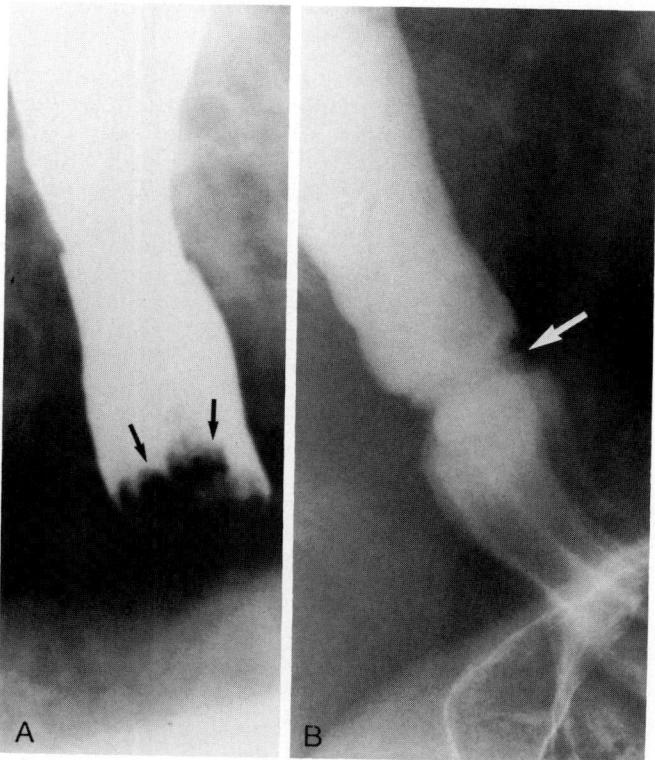

**Figure 31–12. Distal foreign body obstruction that is due to an underlying Schatzki ring. A.** The initial esophagram shows barium outlining the superior border of an impacted bolus of meat *(arrows)* in the distal esophagus, with complete obstruction at this level. **B.** A second esophagram after endoscopic removal of the foreign body shows an underlying Schatzki ring *(arrow)* above a hiatal hernia.

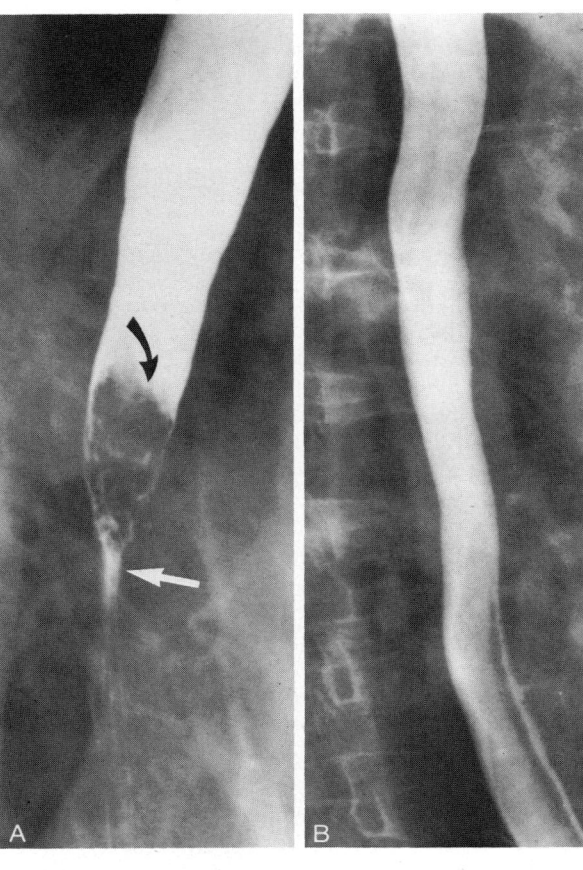

**Figure 31–13. Foreign body obstruction in a normal esophagus. A**. An impacted meat bolus in the midesophagus appears as a polypoid filling defect *(black arrow)*. Note how the incompletely distended esophagus below the impaction *(white arrow)* could be mistaken for a pathologic area of narrowing. **B**. However, a second esophagram after removal of the foreign body shows a normal underlying esophagus.

stricture is present, or if the impaction is located significantly above the lower esophageal sphincter, as glucagon does not affect motor activity in the body of the esophagus.[55]

The use of gas-forming agents (e.g., E-Z-Gas, E-Z-EM Company, Westbury, NY) has also been advocated to distend the esophagus above an obstructing foreign body and facilitate passage of the bolus into the stomach.[56] The combination of intravenous glucagon, an orally administered effervescent agent, and water may also be effective in relieving foreign body obstructions.[57, 58] Rarely, however, abrupt distention of the esophagus by a gas-forming agent may cause esophageal perforation.[57] Thus, there is a theoretic risk of perforating the esophagus by abruptly increasing intraluminal pressure, particularly if the obstructing bolus has been present long enough to cause ischemia or pressure necrosis at the site of impaction. For this reason, gas-forming agents probably should not be used if the obstruction has been present longer than 24 hours.

## FISTULAS

### Esophageal-Airway Fistula

The majority of esophageal-airway fistulas result from direct invasion of the tracheobronchial tree by advanced esophageal carcinomas. Tracheoesophageal or esophagobronchial fistulas (usually involving the left main bronchus) have been reported in 5 to 10% of patients with esophageal cancer.[59, 60] The fistulas tend to occur after radiation therapy, presumably because radiation-induced tumor necrosis accelerates fistula formation. Less commonly, esophageal-airway fistulas may be caused by esophageal instrumentation, foreign bodies, blunt or penetrating injuries to the chest, or, rarely, perforation of an esophageal diverticulum.[61] Esophagobronchial fistulas may also be caused by tuberculosis, histoplasmosis, or other granulomatous diseases in which necrotic, caseating mediastinal lymph nodes erode into the esophagus and tracheobronchial tree.[62] Rarely, esophagobronchial fistulas may be congenital in origin.[63]

Patients with esophageal-airway fistulas often present with paroxysmal coughing after ingestion of liquids.[61] Some patients may have recurrent pneumonitis, hemoptysis, or a productive cough with particles of food in the sputum.[61] However, these fistulas may be difficult to differentiate on clinical grounds from recurrent tracheobronchial aspiration.

When an esophageal-airway fistula is suspected, the radiologic examination should be performed with barium rather than Gastrografin, as hypertonic water-soluble contrast agents may draw fluid into the lungs, causing severe, potentially fatal pulmonary edema.[43] Most fistulas are readily demonstrated on barium studies and are found to arise within advanced, infiltrating esophageal carcinomas (Fig. 31–14). Once barium has entered the trachea or bronchi, however, it can be coughed up into the proximal trachea or larynx, so that delayed

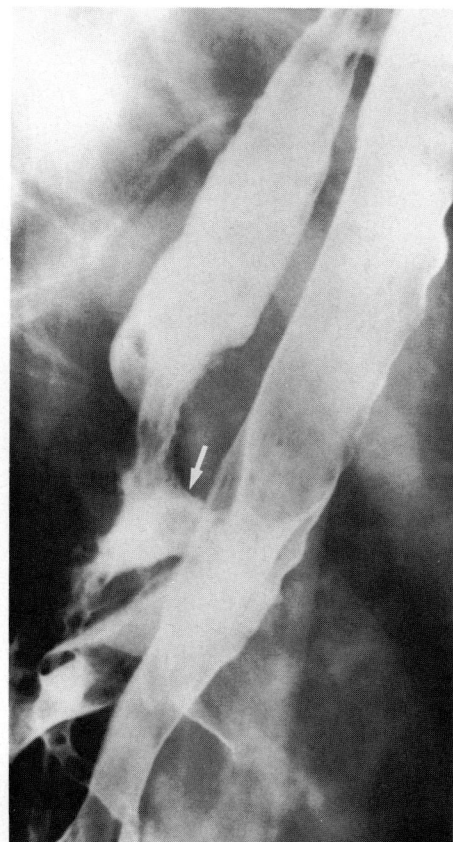

**Figure 31–14. Esophagobronchial fistula (arrow) caused by an advanced, infiltrating esophageal carcinoma.**

overhead radiographs may erroneously suggest tracheo-bronchial aspiration. The initial swallow should therefore be performed in a lateral projection with a video recording of the hypopharynx to differentiate a fistula from aspiration.

## Esophagopleural Fistula

Esophagopleural fistulas are usually caused by previous surgery, esophageal instrumentation, radiation, or advanced esophageal carcinoma directly invading the pleural space.[64] Unlike patients with esophageal-airway fistulas, these individuals may have nonspecific clinical findings such as chest pain, fever, dysphagia, or dyspnea.[64] When an esophagopleural fistula is suspected, the diagnosis can be confirmed by recovery of ingested methylene blue in fluid aspirated during thoracentesis.

Chest radiographs may reveal a pleural effusion, pneumothorax, or hydropneumothorax on the side of the fistula[64] (Fig. 31–15A). However, pneumomediastinum or mediastinal widening is usually not present on chest films, as the mediastinum tends not to be directly involved by the fistula. When an esophagopleural fistula is suspected because of the clinical or plain film findings, a study using water-soluble contrast medium should be performed to confirm the presence of a fistula and to

determine its precise location (Fig. 31–15B). Computed tomography may also be helpful for demonstrating small collections of contrast medium, air, or fluid in the pleural space.[65]

## Aortoesophageal Fistula

Aortoesophageal fistulas are rare but highly lethal fistulas, usually caused by intraesophageal rupture of an atherosclerotic, syphilitic, or dissecting aneurysm of the descending thoracic aorta.[66, 67] These fistulas may also be caused by an infected aortic graft eroding into the esophagus.[68] Rarely, swallowed foreign bodies or advanced carcinomas of the esophagus or lung also produce this complication.

Affected patients may initially present with several small "sentinel" episodes of arterial hematemesis, followed by a symptom-free latent period of hours to weeks and a sudden, final episode of massive hematemesis, exsanguination, and death.[66, 67] This latent period has been attributed to blood clot occluding the fistula, hypotension, and vasoconstriction in response to severe hypovolemia.[66] As a result, early diagnosis of an impending aortoesophageal fistula provides the opportunity for definitive, potentially life-saving surgery with placement of an aortic graft.

Aortoesophageal fistulas should be suspected in patients with arterial hematemesis who have a large atherosclerotic aneurysm of the descending thoracic aorta on chest radiographs. In such cases, studies using water-soluble contrast agents may demonstrate extrinsic compression or displacement of the esophagus by the aneurysm but rarely show leakage of contrast medium into the aorta, because of the flow dynamics of these structures[66] (Fig. 31–16A). When an infected aortic graft has eroded into the esophagus, extravasated contrast medium from the esophagus may occasionally outline the coiled springs of the graft[66, 68] (Fig. 31–16C). The presence of an aortoesophageal fistula may be confirmed by demonstrating extravasation of contrast medium from the aorta into the esophagus by aortography. However, the origin of the fistulous track is often occluded by thrombus, so that aortography may also fail to delineate an aortoesophageal fistula in these patients[67] (Fig. 31–16B).

## Esophagopericardial Fistula

Esophagopericardial fistulas are rare fistulas caused by severe esophagitis, esophageal cancer, swallowed foreign bodies, or prior surgery.[69] These fistulas usually lead to the rapid development of severe pericarditis or cardiac tamponade due to leakage of esophageal contents into the pericardial space. Chest radiographs may reveal pneumopericardium or hydropneumopericardium in 25 to 50% of cases.[69] The diagnosis may be confirmed by having the patient swallow a water-soluble contrast agent to demonstrate the fistulous track or gross filling of the pericardial sac with contrast medium (Fig. 31–17).

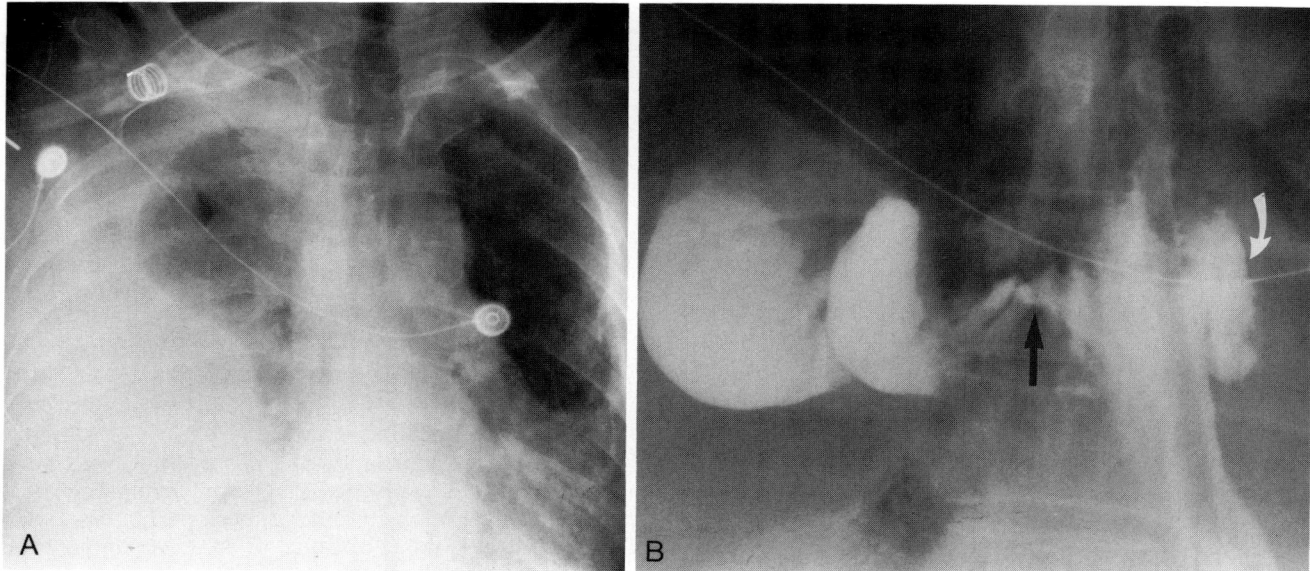

**Figure 31–15. Esophagopleural fistula caused by endoscopic sclerotherapy of esophageal varices. A.** A PA chest radiograph shows a large right pleural effusion. **B.** A study using water-soluble contrast medium reveals an esophagopleural fistula *(black arrow)* with contrast medium extending laterally in the right pleural space. There also is extravasated contrast medium in the mediastinum *(white arrow)*.

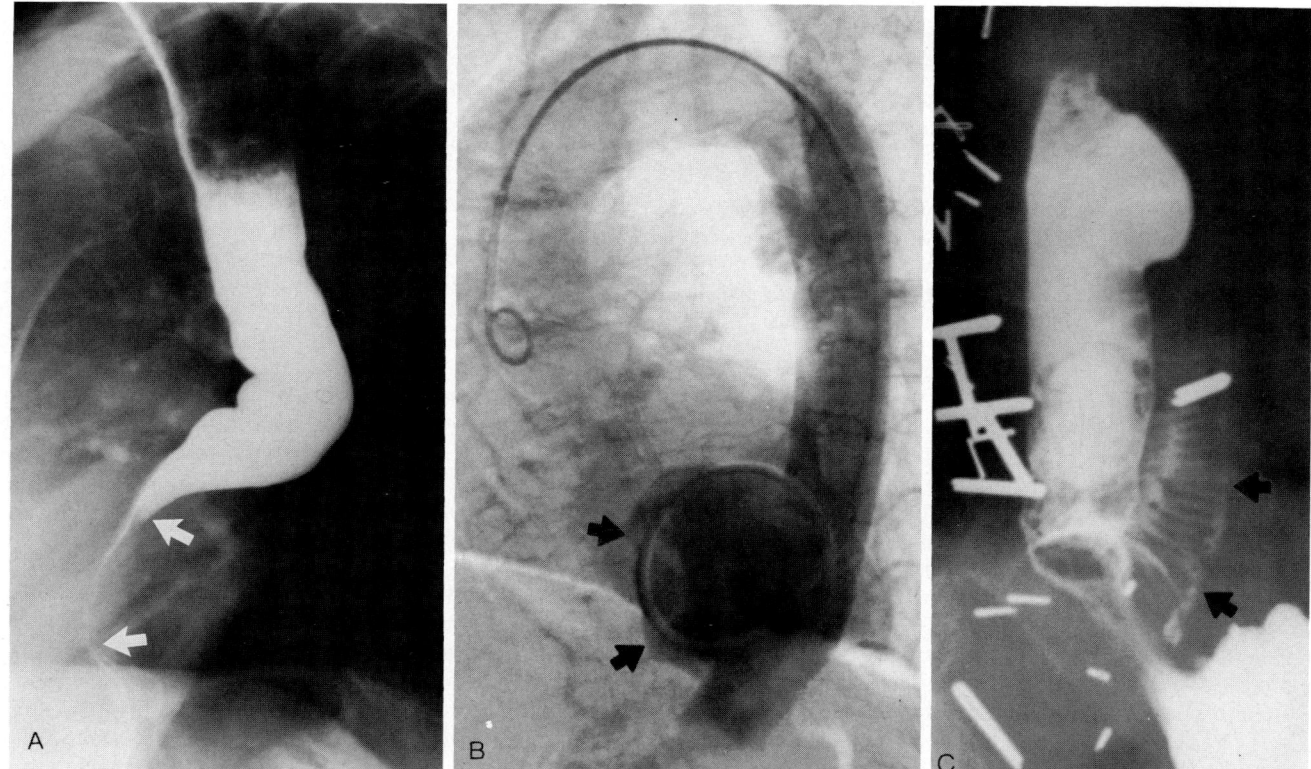

**Figure 31–16. Aortoesophageal fistula caused by an aortic aneurysm. A.** The initial esophagram shows anterior displacement and narrowing of the distal esophagus *(arrows)* by an aneurysm of the descending thoracic aorta. **B.** A subsequent aortogram reveals a saccular aneurysm with intraluminal thrombus *(arrows)* occluding the origin of the fistula. Although radiographic studies failed to demonstrate the fistula, an aortoesophageal fistula was found at surgery. **C.** Another esophagram after placement of a Dacron aortic graft shows a recurrent aortoesophageal fistula with extravasated contrast medium from the esophagus outlining the aortic graft *(arrows)*. This fistula was caused by infection of the graft. (**A** to **C** from Baron RL, Koehler RE, Gutierrez FR, et al: Clinical and radiographic manifestations of aortoesophageal fistulas. Radiology 141:599–605, 1981.)

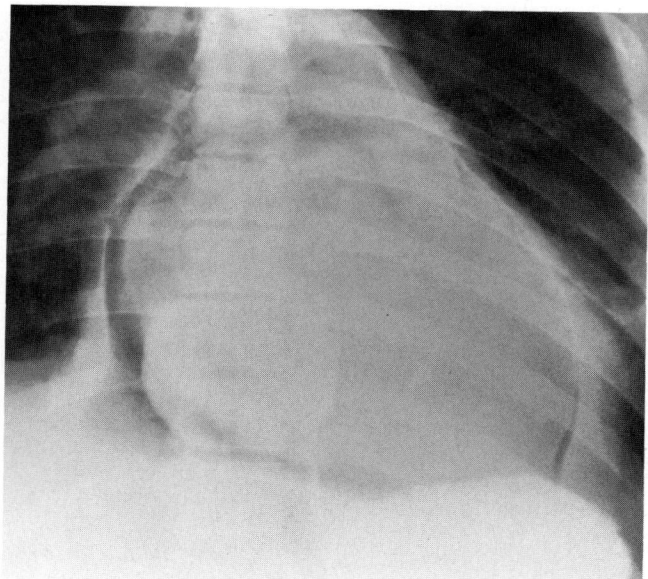

**Figure 31–17. Esophagopericardial fistula caused by a perforated ulcer associated with severe reflux esophagitis.** A PA chest radiograph after oral administration of water-soluble contrast medium reveals a pneumopericardium with free leakage of contrast medium into the pericardial space. Note how air and contrast medium outline the inner aspect of the pericardial sac. Also note how contrast medium is seen faintly in a hiatal hernia. (From D Cyrlak, AJ Cohen, ER Dana, Esophagopericardial fistula: causes and radiographic features, AJR, 141, 1, 177–179, 1983, © by American Roentgen Ray Society.)

## DIVERTICULA

True esophageal diverticula consist of only mucosa without a muscular layer. Diverticula may be classified by their location or by their mechanism of formation. The most common locations include the pharyngoesophageal junction (i.e., Zenker's diverticulum), the midesophagus, and the distal esophagus just above the

esophageal hiatus (i.e., epiphrenic diverticulum). Diverticula may be formed either by pulsion due to increased intraluminal esophageal pressure or by traction due to fibrosis in adjacent periesophageal tissues. Until recently, many midesophageal diverticula were thought to be traction diverticula caused by scarring from tuberculosis or histoplasmosis in perihilar or subcarinal lymph nodes. However, this type of diverticulum has decreased in frequency, so that most midesophageal diverticula are now thought to be of the pulsion variety.[70]

## Clinical Findings

Zenker's diverticulum is discussed in detail in Chapter 17. Pulsion diverticula are usually incidental findings in the esophagus without clinical significance. When symptoms are present, they are almost always related to the patient's underlying esophageal motor disorder.[71] However, some diverticula that are extremely large may cause symptoms. When a large diverticulum fills with food or fluid, it may compress the true lumen of the esophagus, causing dysphagia. Food or fluid that accumulates within a large pulsion diverticulum may also overflow into the esophagus, causing subsequent aspiration. Rarely, these diverticula perforate into the mediastinum or form a fistula to the airway.

## Radiographic Findings

Epiphrenic diverticula may occasionally be recognized on chest radiographs by the presence of a soft tissue mass (often containing an air-fluid level) that mimics a hiatal hernia (Fig. 31–18). However, diverticula are readily detected on esophagrams as barium-filled outpouchings from the esophagus (Figs. 31–19 and 31–20; see Fig. 31–18). They are best seen in profile, but they

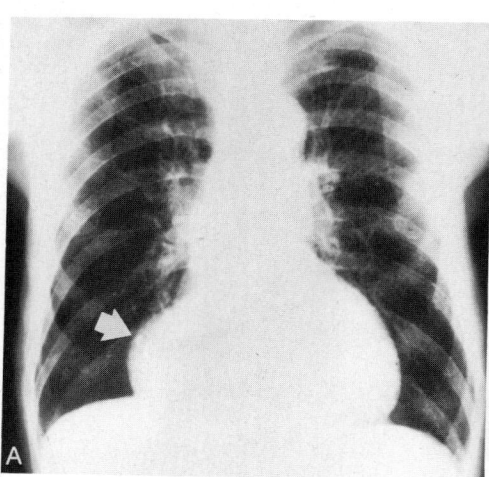
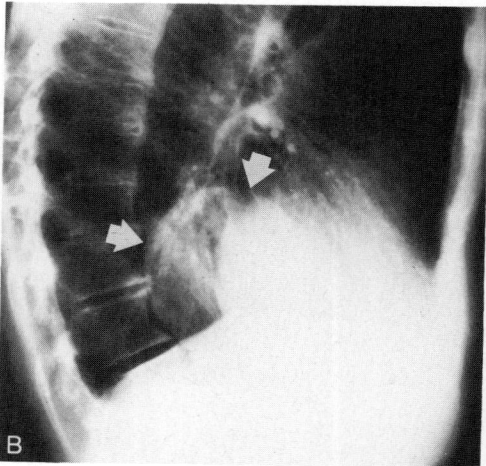
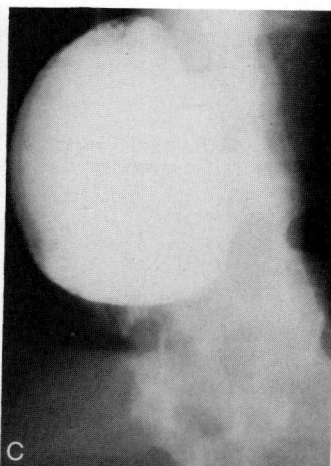

**Figure 31–18. Large epiphrenic diverticulum. A.** A PA chest film shows a prominent bulge along the right border of the heart *(arrow).* **B.** A lateral chest film shows a soft tissue mass *(arrows),* mimicking the appearance of a hiatal hernia. **C.** However, a barium study reveals a large epiphrenic diverticulum.

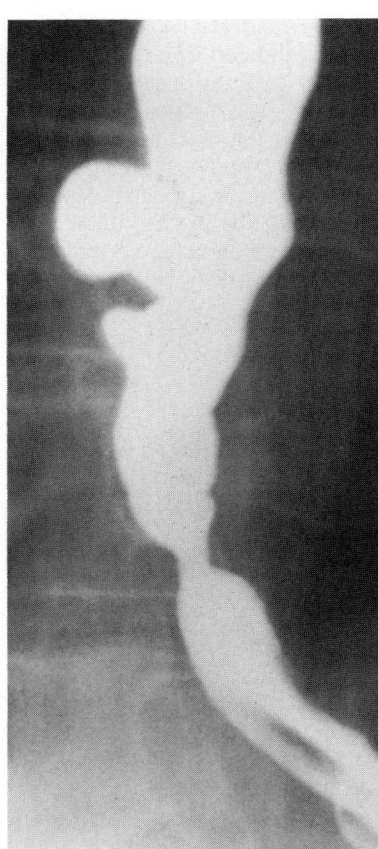

**Figure 31–19. Pulsion diverticula.** Note the smooth contour and wide necks of the diverticula. There also is evidence of diffuse esophageal spasm. Pulsion diverticula are often associated with esophageal motor dysfunction.

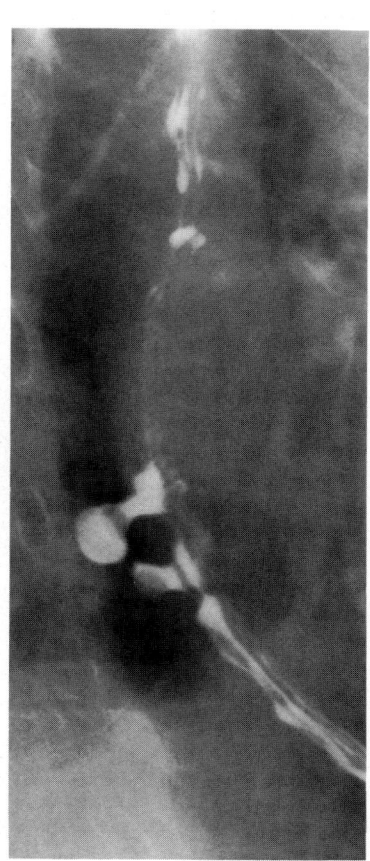

**Figure 31–20. Pulsion diverticula.** The diverticula remain filled after most of the barium has been emptied from the esophagus by peristalsis. Note the rounded contour and wide necks of the diverticula.

may be recognized en face as ring shadows on double contrast studies. Once a diverticulum has been detected, it should be classified as either a pulsion diverticulum or a traction diverticulum. Pulsion diverticula are much more common and are often associated with other radiographic evidence of motor dysfunction (see Fig. 31–19). They usually have a rounded contour and a wide neck and are frequently multiple (see Figs. 31–19 and 31–20). Because they contain no muscle in their wall, they tend to remain filled after the esophagus has emptied of barium (see Fig. 31–20). In contrast, traction diverticula are usually located in the midesophagus and have a tented or triangular configuration as a result of scarring and retraction by granulomatous disease in adjacent subcarinal or perihilar lymph nodes (Fig. 31–21). Traction diverticula contain all layers of the esophageal wall, including muscle, so they tend to empty when the esophagus collapses. Thus, it is usually possible to distinguish pulsion and traction diverticula on radiologic grounds.

## EXTRINSIC IMPRESSIONS

A variety of normal and abnormal structures may cause extrinsic impressions on the esophagus as it courses through the mediastinum. Normal impressions are discussed in Chapter 19. Abnormal impressions are most commonly caused by the heart and great vessels. An enlarged left atrium or ventricle may produce a broad impression on the anterior wall of the distal esophagus. In contrast, a tortuous or ectatic descending thoracic aorta may cause a prominent impression on the posterior wall of the distal esophagus near the esophageal hiatus of the diaphragm (Fig. 31–22). In some

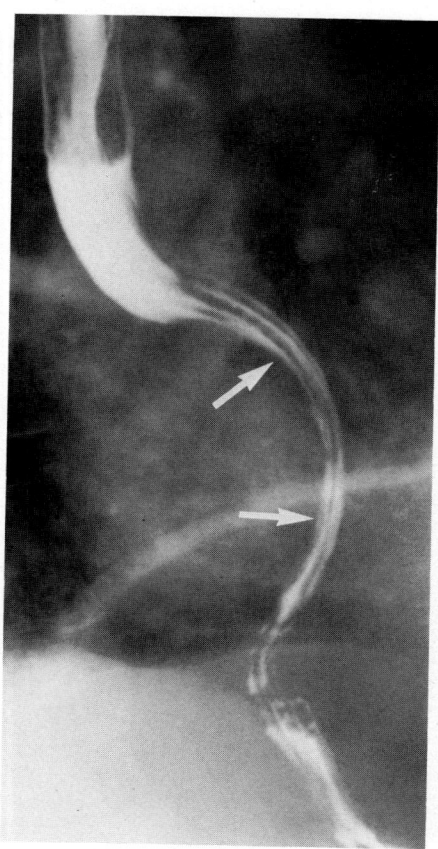

**Figure 31–22. Esophageal impression (arrows) by an ectatic descending thoracic aorta.** The esophagus is narrowed and deviated anteriorly by this structure.

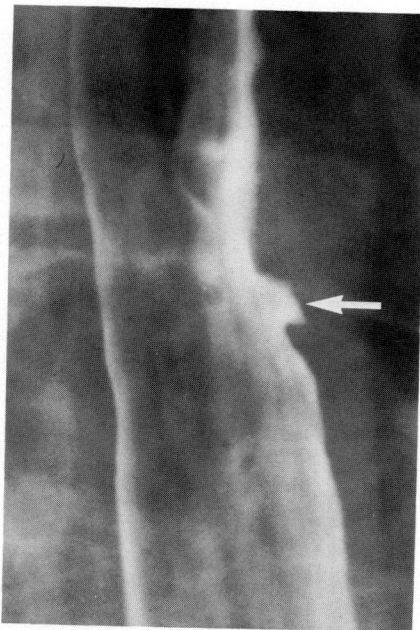

**Figure 31–21. Traction diverticulum (arrow).** The diverticulum has a pointed or triangular tip due to traction from adjacent periesophageal tissues.

patients, compression of the distal esophagus by the aorta may cause dysphagia and weight loss. This condition has been described as "dysphagia aortica."[72] Other congenital abnormalities of the great vessels, such as an aberrant subclavian artery, double aortic arch, and pulmonary sling, may also produce characteristic impressions on the esophagus, as discussed in Chapter 75. The esophagus may also be compressed or displaced by masses in the mediastinum, including substernal thyroid goiters, mediastinal lymphadenopathy, and other benign or malignant neoplasms (Fig. 31–23). In such cases, it is important to differentiate compression or displacement of the esophagus from actual invasion by an adjacent mediastinal mass (see Chapter 29).

Esophageal deviation may also be caused by pulmonary, pleural, or mediastinal scarring, with retraction of the esophagus toward the diseased hemithorax (Fig. 31–24). However, it is usually possible to differentiate esophageal displacement by a benign or malignant mediastinal mass from esophageal retraction by pleuropulmonary scarring, by using the radiologic sign illustrated in Figure 31–25.[73] When the esophagus is displaced or pushed by an extrinsic mass in the mediastinum, it tends to be narrower at this level than above or below the deviated segment (see Figs. 31–22, 31–23, and 31–25A), whereas the esophagus tends to be wider at this level when it is retracted or pulled by pleuropulmonary scar-

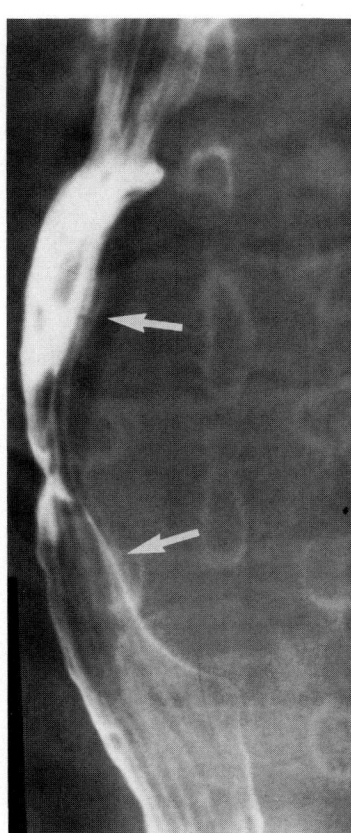

**Figure 31–23. Esophageal impression *(arrows)* by a substernal thoracic goiter.** The esophagus is narrowed and displaced to the right by the goiter.

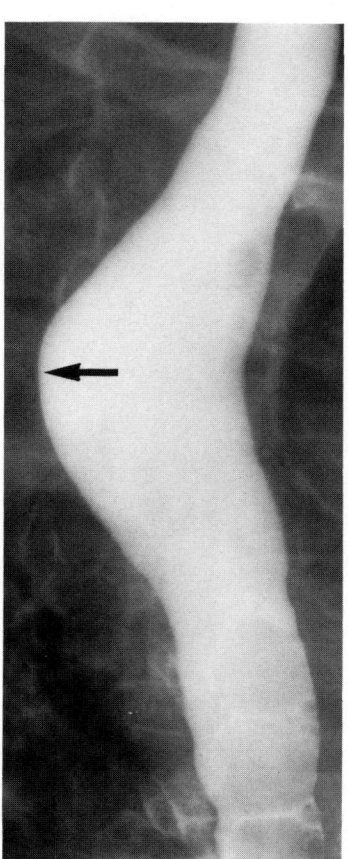

**Figure 31–24. Esophageal retraction by pleuropulmonary scarring.** The esophagus is deviated to the right *(arrow)* because of scarring and volume loss from right upper lobe tuberculosis. Note how the esophagus is widened at the level of deviation. This characteristic widening indicates retraction of the esophagus toward the side of pleuropulmonary scarring rather than displacement by a mass on the opposite side.

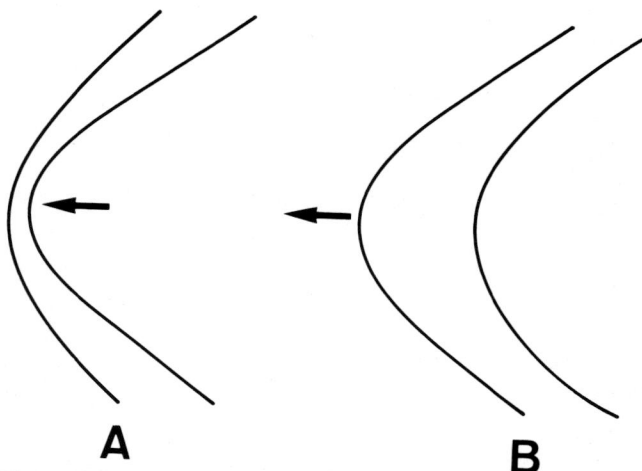

**Figure 31–25. Pushed versus pulled esophagus. A.** When the esophagus is displaced or pushed by an extrinsic mediastinal mass, it tends to be narrower at this level *(arrow)* than above or below the deviated segment. **B.** When the esophagus is retracted or pulled by pleuropulmonary scarring and volume loss, however, it tends to be wider at this level *(arrow)* than above or below the deviated segment. (**A** and **B** from MS Levine, AM Gilchrist, Esophageal deviation: pushed or pulled? AJR, 149, 3, 513–514, 1987, © by American Roentgen Ray Society.)

ring (see Figs. 31–24 and 31–25B). This localized widening or bulging of the esophagus has a characteristic appearance that permits differentiation from an extrinsic mass indenting and displacing the esophagus from the opposite side.[73] When esophageal retraction is suggested by barium studies, chest radiographs should confirm the presence of tuberculosis, radiation damage, postsurgical changes, or other signs of scarring and volume loss in the affected hemithorax. It is important to determine whether the esophagus has been "pushed" or "pulled" from its normal midline position, because esophageal retraction due to pleuropulmonary scarring can be noted and dismissed as an incidental finding, whereas esophageal displacement by a mediastinal mass may require further investigation with computed tomography or magnetic resonance to determine the nature and extent of the mass lesion.

### Acknowledgment

Figures 31–2, 31–3B, 31–4, 31–7A, 31–8 to 31–11, 31–13A and B to 31–15A and B, 31–18 to 31–21, and 31–24 are reproduced from Levine MS: Radiology of the Esophagus. Philadelphia: WB Saunders, 1989.

## References

1. Ansari A: Mallory-Weiss syndrome: revisited. Am J Gastroenterol 64:460–466, 1975.
2. Bubrick MP, Lundeen JW, Onstad GR, et al: Mallory-Weiss syndrome: analysis of fifty-nine cases. Surgery 88:400–405, 1980.
3. Hastings PR, Peters KW, Cohn I: Mallory-Weiss syndrome: review of 69 cases. Am J Surg 142:560–562, 1981.
4. Graham DV, Schwartz JT: The spectrum of the Mallory-Weiss tear. Medicine (Baltimore) 57:307–318, 1977.
5. Baker RW, Spiro AH, Trnka YM: Mallory-Weiss tear complicating upper endoscopy. Gastroenterology 82:140–142, 1982.
6. Hunter TB, Protell RL, Horsley WW: Food laceration of the esophagus: the taco tear. AJR 140:503–504, 1983.
7. Foster DN, Miloszewski K, Losowsky MS: Diagnosis of Mallory-Weiss lesions: a common cause of upper gastrointestinal bleeding. Lancet 2:483–485, 1976.
8. Knaver CM: Mallory-Weiss syndrome: characterization of 75 Mallory-Weiss lacerations in 528 patients with upper gastrointestinal hemorrhage. Gastroenterology 71:5–8, 1976.
9. Wychulis AR, Sasso A: Mallory-Weiss syndrome. Arch Surg 107:868–871, 1973.
10. Clark RA: Intraarterial vasopressin infusion for treatment of Mallory-Weiss tears of the esophagogastric junction. AJR 133:449–451, 1979.
11. Carsen GM, Casarella WJ, Spiegel RM: Transcatheter embolization for treatment of Mallory-Weiss tears of the esophagogastric junction. Radiology 128:309–313, 1978.
12. Thompson NW, Ernst CB, Fry WJ: The spectrum of emetogenic injury to the esophagus and stomach. Am J Surg 113:13–26, 1967.
13. Dallemand S, Amorosa JK, Morris DW, et al: Intramural hematomas of the esophagus. Gastrointest Radiol 8:7–9, 1983.
14. Shay SS, Berendson RA, Johnson LF: Esophageal hematoma: four new cases, a review, and proposed etiology. Dig Dis Sci 26:1019–1024, 1981.
15. Bradley JL, Han SY: Intramural hematoma (incomplete perforation) of the esophagus associated with esophageal dilatation. Radiology 130:59–62, 1979.
16. Steenbergen WV, Fevery J, Broeckaert L, et al: Intramural hematoma of the esophagus: unusual complication of variceal sclerotherapy. Gastrointest Radiol 9:293–295, 1984.
17. Williams B: Oesophageal laceration following remote trauma. Br J Radiol 30:666–668, 1957.
18. Andress M: Submucosal haematoma of the oesophagus due to anticoagulant therapy. Acta Radiol Diagn 11:216–219, 1971.
19. Ashman FC, Hill MC, Saba GP, et al: Esophageal hematoma associated with thrombocytopenia. Gastrointest Radiol 3:115–118, 1978.
20. Chen P, Lebowitz R, Lewicki AM: Spontaneous hematoma of the esophagus. Radiology 100:281–282, 1971.
21. Lowman RM, Goldman R, Stern H: The roentgen aspects of intramural dissection of the esophagus. Radiology 93:1329–1331, 1969.
22. Joffe N, Millan VG: Postemetic dissecting intramural hematoma of the esophagus. Radiology 95:379–380, 1970.
23. Pellicano A, Watier A, Gentile J: Spontaneous double-barreled esophagus. J Clin Gastroenterol 9:149–154, 1987.
24. Campbell TC, Andrews JL, Neptune WB: Spontaneous rupture of the esophagus (Boerhaave's syndrome). JAMA 235:526–528, 1976.
25. Love L, Berkow AE: Trauma to the esophagus. Gastrointest Radiol 2:305–321, 1978.
26. Meyers MA, Ghahremani GG: Complications of fiberoptic endoscopy. I. Esophagoscopy and gastroscopy. Radiology 115:293–300, 1975.
27. Leigh TF, Achord JL: Pharyngeal and esophageal perforations during instrumentation. AJR 91:757–765, 1964.
28. Ghahremani GG, Turner MA, Port RB: Iatrogenic intubation injuries of the upper gastrointestinal tract in adults. Gastrointest Radiol 5:1–10, 1980.
29. O'Connell ND: Spontaneous rupture of the esophagus. AJR 99:186–203, 1967.
30. Panaro VA, Leslie ES: Spontaneous rupture of the esophagus. Radiology 84:252–257, 1965.
31. Rogers LF, Puig W, Dooley BN, et al: Diagnostic considerations in mediastinal emphysema: a pathophysiologic approach to Boerhaave's syndrome and spontaneous pneumomediastinum. AJR 115:495–511, 1972.
32. Christoforidis A, Nelson SW: Spontaneous rupture of the esophagus with emphasis on the roentgenologic diagnosis. AJR 78:574–580, 1957.
33. Wychulis AR, Fontana RS, Payne WS: Instrumental perforations of the esophagus. Dis Chest 55:184–189, 1969.
34. Han SY, Tishler JM: Perforation of the abdominal segment of the esophagus. AJR 143:751–754, 1984.

35. Berry BE, Ochsner JL: Perforation of the esophagus: a 30 year review. J Thorac Cardiovasc Surg 65:1–7, 1973.
36. Maglinte DDT, Edwards MC: Spontaneous closure of esophageal tear in Boerhaave's syndrome. Gastrointest Radiol 4:223–225, 1979.
37. Phillips LG, Cunningham J: Esophageal perforation. Radiol Clin North Am 22:607–613, 1984.
38. Han SY, McElvein RB, Aldrete JS, et al: Perforation of the esophagus: correlation of site and cause with plain film findings. AJR 145:537–540, 1985.
39. Parkin GJS: The radiology of perforated esophagus. Clin Radiol 24:324–332, 1973.
40. Healy ME, Mindelzun RE: Lesser sac pneumoperitoneum secondary to perforation of the intraabdominal esophagus. AJR 142:325–326, 1984.
41. James AE, Montali RJ, Chaffee V, et al: Barium or Gastrografin: which contrast media for diagnosis of esophageal tears? Gastroenterology 68:1103–1113, 1975.
42. Vessal K, Montali RJ, Larson SM, et al: Evaluation of barium and Gastrografin as contrast media for the diagnosis of esophageal ruptures or complications. AJR 123:307–319, 1975.
43. Reich SB: Production of pulmonary edema by aspiration of water-soluble nonabsorbable contrast media. Radiology 92:367–370, 1969.
44. Brick SH, Caroline DF, Lev-Toaff AS, et al: Esophageal disruption: evaluation with iohexol esophagography. Radiology 169:141–143, 1988.
45. Dodds WJ, Stewart ET, Vlymen WJ: Appropriate contrast media for evaluation of esophageal disruption. Radiology 144:439–441, 1982.
46. Foley MJ, Ghahremani GG, Rogers LF: Reappraisal of contrast media used to detect upper gastrointestinal perforations. Radiology 144:231–237, 1982.
47. Webb WA: Management of foreign bodies of the upper gastrointestinal tract. Gastroenterology 94:204–216, 1988.
48. Nandi P, Ong GB: Foreign bodies in the oesophagus: review of 2,394 cases. Br J Surg 65:5–9, 1978.
49. Giordano A, Adams G, Boies L, et al: Current management of esophageal foreign bodies. Arch Otolaryngol 107:249–251, 1981.
50. Barber GB, Peppercorn MA, Ehrlich C, et al: Esophageal foreign body perforation. Am J Gastroenterol 79:509–511, 1984.
51. Underberg-Davis S, Levine MS: Giant thoracic osteophyte causing esophageal food impaction. AJR 157:319–320, 1991.
52. Shaffer HA, Alford BA, de Lange EE, et al: Basket extraction of esophageal foreign bodies. AJR 147:1010–1013, 1986.
53. Ferrucci JT, Long JA: Radiologic treatment of esophageal food impaction using intravenous glucagon. Radiology 125:25–28, 1977.
54. Trenkner SW, Maglinte DDT, Lehman GA, et al: Esophageal food impaction: treatment with glucagon. Radiology 149:401–403, 1983.
55. Hogan WJ, Dodds WJ, Hoke SE, et al: Effect of glucagon on esophageal motor function. Gastroenterology 69:160–165, 1975.
56. Rice BT, Spiegel PK, Dombrowski PJ: Acute esophageal food impaction treated by gas-forming agents. Radiology 146:299–301, 1983.
57. Smith JC, Janower ML, Geiger AH: Use of glucagon and gas-forming agents in acute esophageal food impaction. Radiology 159:567–568, 1986.
58. Kaszar-Seibert DJ, Korn WT, Bindman DJ, et al: Treatment of acute esophageal food impaction with a combination of glucagon, effervescent agent, and water. AJR 154:533–534, 1990.
59. Fitzgerald RH, Bartles DM, Parker EF: Tracheoesophageal fistulas secondary to carcinoma of the esophagus. J Thorac Cardiovasc Surg 82:194–197, 1981.
60. Little AG, Ferguson MK, DeMeester TR, et al: Esophageal carcinoma with respiratory tract fistula. Cancer 53:1322–1328, 1984.
61. Anderson RP, Sabiston DC: Acquired bronchoesophageal fistula of benign origin. Surg Gynecol Obstet 121:261–266, 1965.
62. Vasquez RE, Landay M, Kilman WJ, et al: Benign esophagorespiratory fistulas in adults. Radiology 167:93–96, 1988.
63. Sheiner NM, LaChance C: Congenital esophagobronchial fistula in the adult. Can J Surg 23:489–491, 1980.
64. Weschler RJ, Steiner RM, Goodman LR, et al: Iatrogenic esophageal-pleural fistula: subtlety of diagnosis in the absence of mediastinitis. Radiology 144:239–243, 1982.
65. Weschler RJ: CT of esophageal-pleural fistulae. AJR 147:907–909, 1986.
66. Baron RL, Koehler RE, Gutierrez FR, et al: Clinical and radiographic manifestations of aortoesophageal fistulas. Radiology 141:599–605, 1981.
67. Khawaja FI, Varindani MK: Aortoesophageal fistula: review of clinical, radiographic and endoscopic features. J Clin Gastroenterol 9:342–344, 1987.
68. Seymour EQ: Aortoesophageal fistula as a complication of aortic prosthetic graft. AJR 131:160–161, 1978.
69. Cyrlak D, Cohen AJ, Dana ER: Esophagopericardial fistula: causes and radiographic features. AJR 141:177–179, 1983.
70. Kaye MD: Oesophageal motor dysfunction in patients with diverticula of the mid-thoracic oesophagus. Thorax 29:666–672, 1974.
71. Debas HT, Payne WS, Cameron AJ, et al: Physiopathology of lower esophageal diverticulum and its implications for treatment. Surg Gynecol Obstet 151:593–600, 1980.
72. Birholz JC, Ferrucci JT, Wyman SM: Roentgen features of dysphagia aortica. Radiology 111:93–96, 1974.
73. Levine MS, Gilchrist AM: Esophageal deviation: pushed or pulled? AJR 149:513–514, 1987.

# Gastroesophageal Junction

### Marc S. Levine, M.D.

## INTRODUCTION

The gastroesophageal junction has traditionally been a difficult area to evaluate on barium studies because the physiologic events associated with swallowing produce a dynamic, constantly changing appearance. The use of complicated, often contradictory terminology to describe both normal and abnormal findings at the cardia has also been a source of confusion. Evaluation of the cardia, perhaps more than any other area in the upper gastrointestinal tract, requires meticulous attention to radiographic technique. Although rings, strictures, and hernias are best seen on conventional single contrast barium studies, neoplastic lesions at the cardia are better delineated on double contrast studies. Thus, radiologists must use different techniques during the fluoroscopic examination to evaluate this area optimally.

## RADIOGRAPHIC TECHNIQUE

The gastric cardia is a notoriously difficult area to examine on single contrast barium studies. Because of the overlying rib cage, the fundus is not accessible to manual palpation or compression. If the fundus is not fully distended, crowded gastric folds may obscure surface detail in this region. If larger volumes of barium are used to distend the fundus, however, it becomes relatively opaque, so that only contour abnormalities can be identified. Because of the inherent limitations of single contrast barium studies in examining the cardia and fundus, double contrast techniques have been used to improve radiographic visualization of this area.

The routine double contrast esophagram should include a double contrast examination of the gastric cardia and fundus.[1, 2] After upright double contrast views of the esophagus have been obtained, the patient should be placed in the recumbent right lateral position (i.e.,

right side down) or a slightly prone oblique position to directly visualize the gastric cardia en face. The cardia should be observed for several seconds, and if it appears normal, a single spot film should be obtained. If the cardia appears abnormal, however, additional 2-on-1 or 4-on-1 spot films should be taken as the patient is rotated further to improve mucosal coating in the fundus, so that questionable lesions may be demonstrated both en face and in profile.

After the double contrast portion of the study has been completed, the patient should be placed in the prone right anterior oblique position and instructed to rapidly gulp a thin, low-density barium suspension to achieve optimal distention of the distal esophagus. Single contrast technique is particularly important for evaluating possible rings, strictures, or hernias in this region, as upright double contrast views often fail to produce the degree of distention needed to demonstrate these abnormalities.[3] If necessary, a bolster may be placed beneath the patient's upper abdomen to increase intra-abdominal pressure and improve esophageal distention. When a lower esophageal ring is detected, barium tablets or barium-impregnated marshmallows may also be used to help determine the caliber and obstructive potential of the ring.[4, 5]

## NORMAL RADIOGRAPHIC APPEARANCES

The esophagus is a relatively nondistensible tubular structure with a saccular distal segment that communicates with the stomach. The saccular segment has been called the *phrenic ampulla* or the *vestibule*, as it is the "entrance hall" to the stomach.[6] Manometric studies have shown that the esophageal vestibule corresponds to the location of the lower esophageal sphincter, a 2- to 4-cm high-pressure zone above the gastroesophageal junction that prevents reflux of peptic acid into the esophagus.[7, 8] The vestibule extends inferiorly through the esophageal hiatus of the diaphragm before joining the stomach several centimeters below the hiatus. The short intra-abdominal segment of the esophagus terminates at the gastroesophageal junction or gastric cardia. The left lateral aspect of the cardia is demarcated anatomically by sling fibers that hook around a notch formed between the distal esophagus and gastric fundus (i.e., the cardiac incisura). Important anatomic structures in this region that may be recognized on barium studies include the cardia, Z line, and lower esophageal mucosal and muscular rings. These structures are therefore discussed separately in the following sections.

## Cardia

The cardia may occasionally be visualized on conventional single contrast barium studies as a 1- to 2-cm circular protuberance in the gastric fundus.[9] However, our ability to recognize the normal appearances of the cardia has improved dramatically with the use of double contrast technique. In one study, the normal anatomic landmarks at the cardia were seen on more than 95% of double contrast examinations but on only 20% of single contrast examinations.[10] These structures are often not visualized on single contrast studies because the cardia is obscured by barium in the fundus or by overlying gastric rugae. Thus, double contrast technique is essential for evaluating this area.

The radiographic appearance of the cardia on double contrast studies depends on how firmly it is anchored by the surrounding phrenoesophageal membrane to the esophageal hiatus of the diaphragm. When the cardia is well anchored, protrusion of the distal esophagus into the fundus produces a circular elevation containing four or five stellate folds that radiate to a central point at the gastroesophageal junction (i.e., the cardiac rosette)[10, 11] (Fig. 32–1A). This elevation is demarcated from the adjacent fundus by a curved "hooding" fold that surrounds it laterally and superiorly. In the past, this hooding fold has been called the "sign of the burnoose" because of its resemblance to the cloak-like garment and hood (i.e., the burnoose) worn by Arabs and Moors.[12] Several longitudinal folds are usually seen extending inferiorly from the cardiac rosette along the posterior wall of the lesser curvature. However, it should be recognized that the cardiac rosette and surrounding elevation reflect the closed, resting state of the lower esophageal sphincter, so that these landmarks may be transiently obliterated by relaxation of the lower esophageal sphincter during deglutition.[11]

When the cardia is less firmly anchored to the surrounding phrenoesophageal membrane, the cardiac rosette may be visible without an associated protrusion or circular elevation[11] (Fig. 32–1B). With further ligamentous laxity, the rosette itself may vanish, and the cardia may be characterized by only a single undulant or crescentic line that crosses the area of the esophageal orifice[11] (Fig. 32–1C). Finally, severe ligmentous laxity

may lead to the formation of a hiatal hernia, so that no cardiac structure is identified below the diaphragm. Instead, gastric folds may converge superiorly to a point several centimeters above the esophageal hiatus[11] (Fig. 32–1D). This finding should therefore suggest a sliding hiatal hernia, and a single contrast esophagram should be obtained with the patient in a prone position to confirm the presence of a hernia.

Radiologists should be familiar with the normal radiographic appearances of the cardia, as malignant lesions in this area may be recognized only by distortion, effacement, or obliteration of these landmarks (see later section on carcinoma of the cardia).

## Z Line

The Z line is an irregular, serrated line that demarcates the squamocolumnar mucosal junction.[6, 13] The Z line can sometimes be recognized on double contrast esophagrams as a thin, radiolucent stripe in the distal esophagus with a characteristic zigzag appearance (Fig. 32–2). Occasionally, however, the Z line can be mistaken for superficial ulceration associated with reflux esophagitis, particularly if the esophagus is not completely distended. Because the Z line represents the histologic squamocolumnar junction, it is usually located at or near the gastroesophageal junction. In patients with Barrett's esophagus, however, columnar metaplasia in the distal esophagus may displace the squamocolumnar junction proximally. As a result, an elevated Z line may occasionally be seen radiographically in these patients.

## Mucosal Ring      "B-ring"

A lower esophageal mucosal ring is the most common ring-like narrowing found in the distal esophagus. The ring consists of a membranous ridge that is covered by squamous epithelium superiorly and columnar epithelium inferiorly, so that it corresponds histologically to the squamocolumnar junction.[14, 15] This lower esophageal mucosal ring, also known as a B ring, is manifested radiographically by a thin, web-like area of narrowing at the gastroesophageal junction[13, 15, 16] (Fig. 32–3). The ring has smooth, symmetric margins and a height of 2 to 4 mm.[13, 15, 16] Most asymptomatic mucosal rings have a diameter of more than 20 mm.[13] If the diameter of the ring is less than 20 mm, however, it may cause dysphagia and may therefore represent a pathologic finding (see later section on Schatzki ring).

Lower esophageal mucosal rings are fixed, reproducible structures on barium studies, but the distal esophagus must be adequately distended to visualize these structures. Single contrast technique with the patient in a prone position is particularly well suited for demonstrating lower esophageal rings, as it is the best technique for achieving optimal distention of the distal esophagus. It has been shown that more than 50% of lower esophageal rings seen on prone single contrast

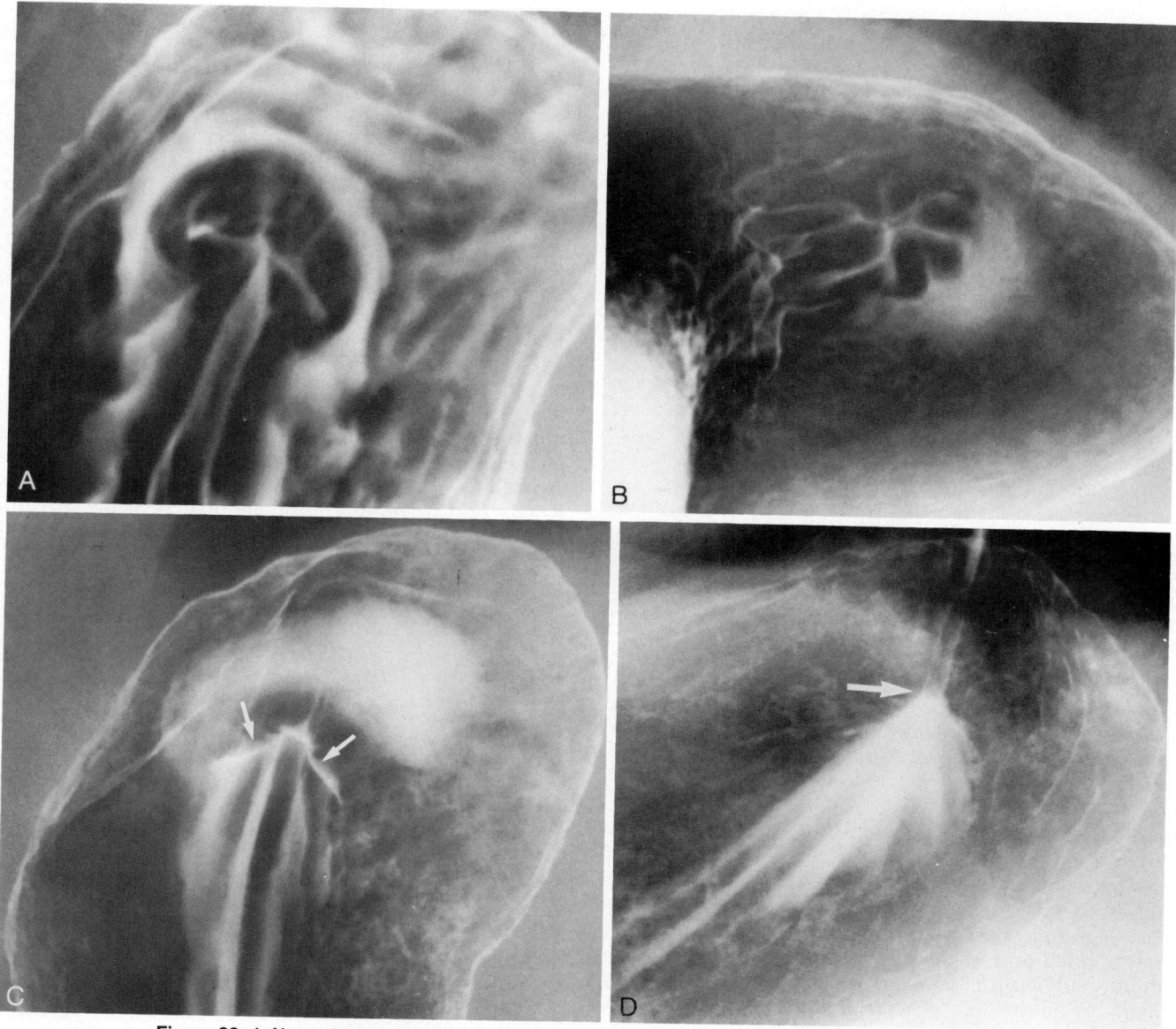

**Figure 32–1. Normal appearances of the gastric cardia. A.** This patient has a well-anchored cardia appearing as a circular protrusion with centrally radiating folds (i.e., the cardiac rosette). **B.** In another patient, there are stellate folds without a surrounding protrusion because of laxity of the ligaments surrounding the cardia. **C.** Further ligamentous laxity has resulted in obliteration of the cardiac rosette. Instead, this patient has a single crescentic line *(arrows)* at the cardia. **D.** In another patient with severe ligamentous laxity, gastric folds in a small hiatal hernia are seen converging superiorly toward a point *(arrow)* several centimeters above the esophageal hiatus of the diaphragm.

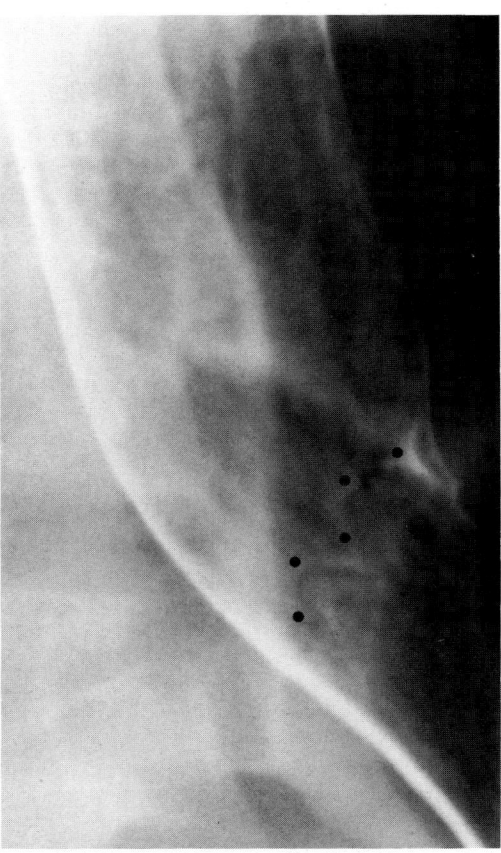

**Figure 32–2. Z line.** The normal Z line is seen as a thin, zigzagging, radiolucent stripe *(dots)* in the distal esophagus near the gastroesophageal junction.

views of the esophagus are not visualized on the double contrast phase of the examination.[3, 17] Thus, biphasic studies are required to demonstrate these structures.

## Muscular Ring       "A ring"

A muscular or contractile ring, also known as an A ring, is found much less frequently in the distal esophagus than a mucosal ring. Muscular rings are located at the proximal end of the esophageal vestibule near the tubulovestibular junction and are completely covered by squamous epithelium.[8] Unlike a mucosal ring, which is a fixed anatomic structure, a muscular ring occurs as a transient physiologic phenomenon due to active muscular contraction in the distal esophagus.

A muscular ring usually appears radiographically as a relatively broad, smooth area of narrowing that changes considerably in caliber and configuration during the fluoroscopic examination[7, 13, 15] (see Fig. 32–3). Because a muscular ring is caused by active muscular contraction, it may vanish completely with esophageal distention and may therefore be observed as a transient finding at fluoroscopy.[7, 13, 15] Not infrequently, both mucosal and muscular rings are visible during the same examination (see Fig. 32–3). In such cases, the fixed nature of the mucosal ring distinguishes it from the dynamic, changing

appearance of the muscular ring above. Rarely, however, a persistent muscular ring is observed in patients with diffuse esophageal spasm.[15]

## SCHATZKI RING

Although some investigators have used the terms *Schatzki ring* and *lower esophageal ring* interchangeably, Schatzki himself originally described this entity as a pathologically stenotic ring that caused dysphagia.[18] Because most lower esophageal rings are asymptomatic, they probably should not be called Schatzki rings. Instead, the term should be reserved for symptomatic, narrow-caliber rings at the gastroesophageal junction. Thus, the diagnosis of a Schatzki ring is made on the basis of clinical and radiographic criteria.

## Pathogenesis

The pathogenesis of a Schatzki ring is uncertain. Some investigators have favored a congenital origin, but the rarity of symptoms before 50 years of age tends to refute this theory.[6] Others have postulated that it results from plication or crinkling of a redundant mucosa in the distal esophagus.[19] However, many investigators believe that a Schatzki ring represents an annular, ring-like structure due to scarring from reflux esophagitis.[6, 15, 20–22] This

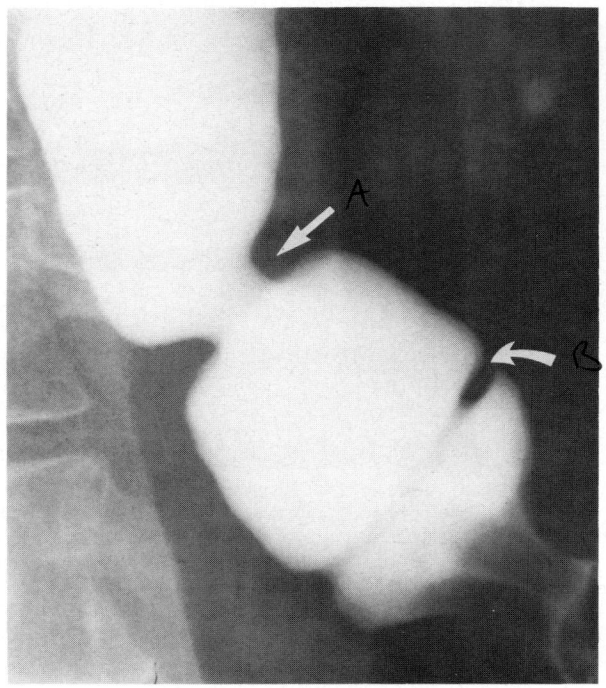

**Figure 32–3. Lower esophageal rings.** The mucosal ring appears on a prone single contrast esophagram as a thin, web-like constriction *(curved arrow)* at the gastroesophageal junction above a small hiatal hernia, whereas the muscular ring appears as a relatively broad area of narrowing *(straight arrow)* near the superior border of the esophageal vestibule. Unlike mucosal rings, muscular rings are often a transient finding at fluoroscopy.

theory is supported by documented cases in which Schatzki rings have undergone progression or transformation into true peptic strictures on serial radiologic examinations.[22] Nevertheless, it is difficult to explain the frequent absence of reflux symptoms in these patients. The data are therefore inconclusive.

## Clinical Findings

Schatzki rings are typically manifested by episodic dysphagia for solids.[13, 15, 23] Affected individuals may have minimal dysphagia or may be asymptomatic until a large bolus of food lodges above the ring. Because the most frequent offending agent is an inadequately chewed piece of meat, this condition has been described as the "steakhouse syndrome."[24] The impacted bolus in the distal esophagus may cause severe chest pain or an uncomfortable "sticking" sensation behind the lower sternum.[25] Resolution of symptoms almost always occurs when the impacted bolus is passed, regurgitated, or removed. Rarely, a prolonged bolus obstruction leads to esophageal perforation.[15]

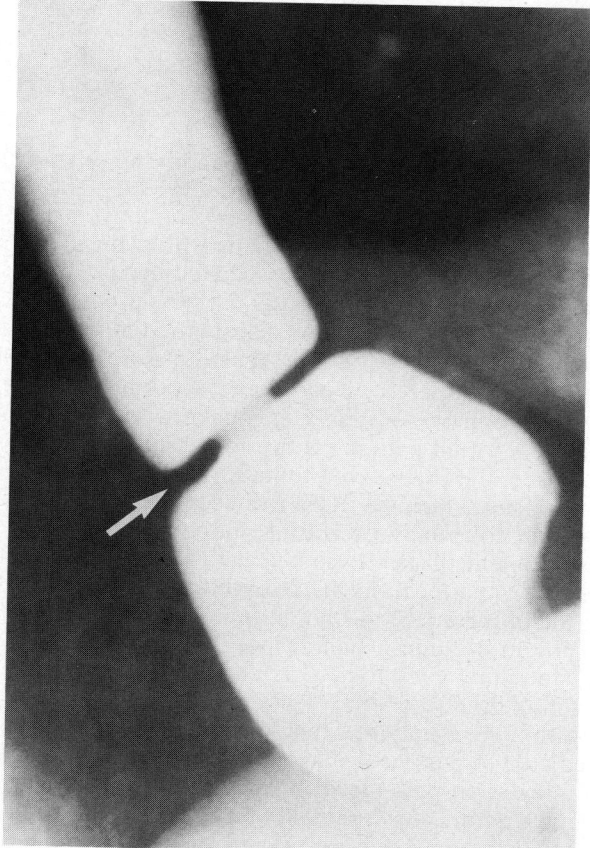

**Figure 32–4. Schatzki ring.** The ring appears on a prone single contrast esophagram as a thin (less than 13 mm in diameter), web-like constriction *(arrow)* at the gastroesophageal junction above a hiatal hernia. Note that except for its smaller caliber, it has the same appearance and location as an asymptomatic mucosal ring. This patient presented with dysphagia.

Relief from symptoms is usually obtained by simply explaining the benign nature of the ring and advising these individuals to eat more slowly and chew their food more carefully. However, some patients with recurrent dysphagia may require mechanical disruption of the ring by direct endoscopic rupture, bougienage, pneumatic dilatation, or, rarely, surgery.[26, 27]

## Radiographic Findings

A Schatzki ring usually appears radiographically as a thin (2 to 4 mm in height), web-like constriction (less than 13 mm in diameter) at the gastroesophageal junction[13, 15–18, 23] (Fig. 32–4). A hiatal hernia is almost always observed below the level of the ring. Except for its smaller caliber, a Schatzki ring therefore has the same appearance and location as an asymptomatic mucosal ring. Almost all rings less than 13 mm in diameter cause dysphagia,[16, 28] so that they may be classified as Schatzki rings on the basis of the radiographic findings. Occasionally, however, rings between 13 and 20 mm in size may also cause symptoms, so that the diagnosis of a Schatzki ring in these patients requires some knowledge of the clinical history.

Like other rings in the lower esophagus, Schatzki rings are visualized on barium studies only if the lumen above and below the ring is distended beyond the caliber of the ring. As a result, single contrast views of the distal esophagus with the patient prone may demonstrate Schatzki rings that are not visible, even in retrospect, on the double contrast phase of the examination[3, 17] (Fig. 32–5). When biphasic studies are performed, esophagography is even more sensitive than endoscopy in diagnosing these structures.[17]

## Differential Diagnosis

A Schatzki ring has such a characteristic appearance that the radiographic findings are virtually diagnostic of this entity. Occasionally, however, other abnormalities such as annular peptic strictures, webs, or localized esophageal cancers may produce similar findings. Annular peptic strictures constitute about 15% of all peptic strictures in the distal esophagus.[13] Annular strictures may resemble Schatzki rings, but they tend to be more irregular and asymmetric and have a greater height than rings.[13, 18] Esophageal webs may occasionally be found in the distal esophagus near the gastroesophageal junction.[29] In such cases, the web can be mistaken for a Schatzki ring, but it tends to be located several centimeters or more above the gastroesophageal junction, so that it can usually be differentiated from a lower esophageal ring by its more proximal location. Rarely, a focally infiltrating esophageal carcinoma produces a localized constriction that superficially resembles a Schatzki ring. However, the presence of asymmetry, irregularity, and shelf-like borders within the narrowed segment should indicate the need for early endoscopy to rule out a malignant lesion.

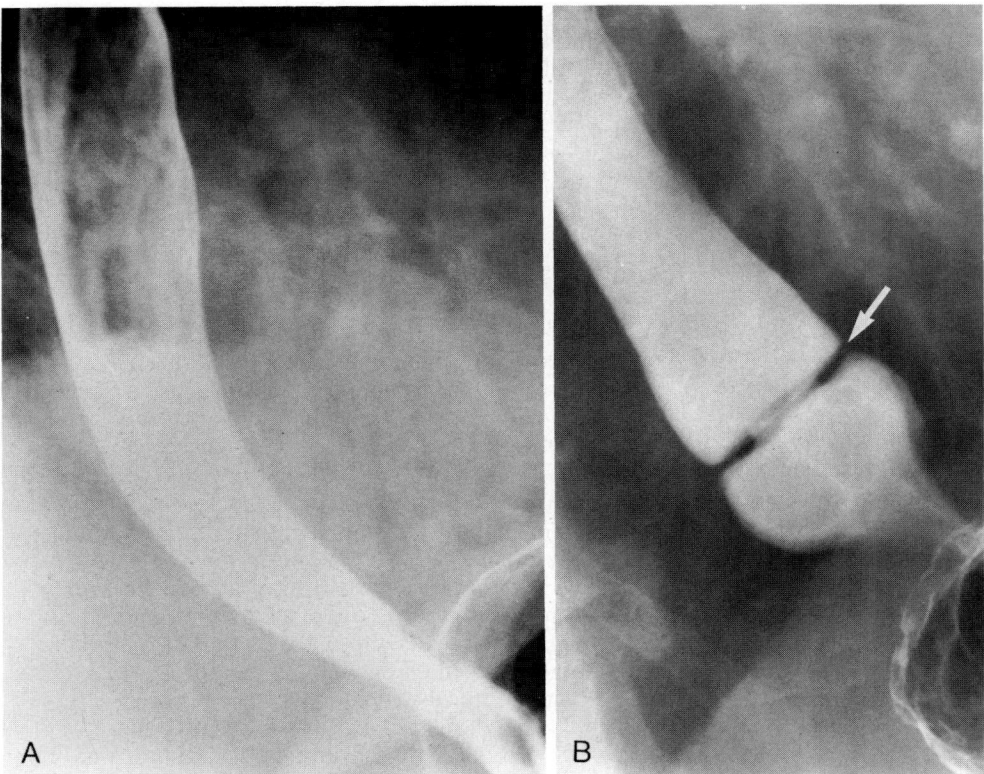

Figure 32–5. Schatzki ring seen only on a prone single contrast esophagram. **A**. An upright double contrast view of the distal esophagus shows no evidence of a lower esophageal ring. **B**. However, a prone single contrast view from the same examination shows a hiatal hernia with an unequivocal Schatzki ring *(arrow)* above the hernia.

## HIATAL HERNIA

Hiatal hernias are classified as either sliding or paraesophageal hernias, depending on the relationship of the cardia to the diaphragm and herniated portion of the stomach. About 99% of all hiatal hernias are sliding, and the remaining 1% are paraesophageal.[30] Despite its rarity, a paraesophageal hernia, unlike a sliding hernia, is considered to be a potentially life-threatening condition because of the risk of volvulus, incarceration, or strangulation of the hernia.

## Sliding Hiatal Hernia

### Pathogenesis

The phrenoesophageal membrane is a firm elastic structure surrounding the gastroesophageal junction that normally tethers the distal esophagus to the diaphragm and prevents the proximal portion of the stomach from herniating through the esophageal hiatus of the diaphragm into the chest. With aging, however, a lifetime of constant swallowing causes progressive wear and tear on the phrenoesophageal membrane, with eventual stretching or rupture of the membrane and axial herniation of the stomach into the chest.[7, 8, 30, 31] As a result, the cardia lies above the diaphragm in these patients. Not unexpectedly, the prevalence of hiatal hernias increases significantly with age. It has been estimated that sliding hiatal hernias are present in about 10% of the adult population of North America.[32]

## Clinical Significance

Considerable controversy exists about the relationship between a sliding hiatal hernia and the subsequent development of gastroesophageal reflux and reflux esophagitis. Because most patients with clinically significant reflux disease have an associated hernia,[33, 34] it has been postulated that a hiatal hernia predisposes to gastroesophageal reflux by disrupting the mechanical integrity of the gastroesophageal junction.[35] A sliding hiatal hernia therefore may have a permissive role in the development of reflux esophagitis. However, only about 5% of all patients with radiographically diagosed hiatal hernias have symptomatic gastroesophageal reflux.[32] Thus, intrinsic dysfunction of the lower esophageal sphincter may be a more important factor in the development of gastroesphageal reflux, independent of the anatomic location of the sphincter above or below the diaphragm.[35, 36] A sliding hiatal hernia is therefore of doubtful clinical significance when it occurs as an isolated finding without other clinical or radiologic signs of reflux disease.

Although a hiatal hernia per se is a relatively poor predictor of gastroesophageal reflux or reflux esophagitis, almost all patients with severe reflux esophagitis or peptic strictures have radiologic evidence of a hernia.[37, 38] It has therefore been postulated that severe inflammation and scarring from reflux esophagitis causes longitudinal esophageal shortening that disrupts the phrenoesophageal membrane and pulls the gastric fundus into the thorax.[30, 35, 37] In such cases, the hiatal hernia may be an effect rather than a cause of the patient's esophagitis.

## Radiographic Diagnosis

A sliding hiatal hernia may be recognized radiographically when the gastroesophageal junction is located above the esophageal hiatus of the diaphragm. Single contrast barium studies with the patient prone are more likely to demonstrate a hiatal hernia than double contrast studies with the patient upright, because the hernia is frequently reduced into the abdomen in the upright position and because the hernia is more difficult to distend adequately when the patient is standing. The subject should therefore be instructed to continuously drink a thin, low-density barium suspension in the prone right anterior oblique position for optimal demonstration of these structures.

Because a lower esophageal mucosal ring demarcates the anatomic location of the gastroesophageal junction, a sliding hiatal hernia may be diagnosed on barium studies obtained with the patient prone when a mucosal ring is observed 2 cm or more above the diaphragmatic hiatus[13] (see Fig. 32–3). Even in the absence of a definite mucosal ring, a hiatal hernia can often be recognized by the presence of gastric folds within the hernia (Fig. 32–6). These folds may continue inferiorly through the diaphragmatic hiatus into the abdominal portion of the stomach. Not infrequently, the hernia may be kinked or narrowed at the esophageal hiatus because of extrinsic

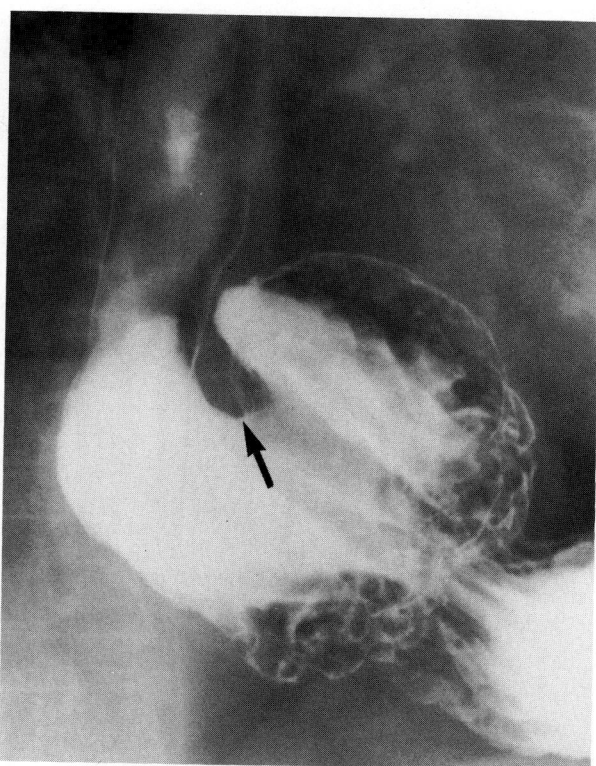

**Figure 32–7. Large hiatal hernia.** There is a prominent diagonal notch *(arrow)* on the superior aspect of the hernia due to crossing gastric sling fibers at the cardiac incisura. This appearance may erroneously suggest a mixed sliding-paraesophageal hernia.

compression by the surrounding diaphragm at this level. Occasionally, a prominent diagonal notch may also be seen on the left lateral and superior aspect of the hernia because of crossing gastric sling fibers at the cardiac incisura[30] (Fig. 32–7).

A sliding hiatal hernia can also be diagnosed on double contrast esophagrams obtained with the patient upright, but this technique is far less reliable than single contrast examinations obtained with the patient prone.[3] A hiatal hernia may be recognized on double contrast radiographs if gastric folds within the hernia are seen extending 2 cm or more above the esophageal hiatus of the diaphragm. Partial collapse of a small hernia may produce a characteristic appearance, with the folds converging toward a point several centimeters above the diaphragm[11] (see Fig. 32–1D). A hiatal hernia can also be diagnosed on double contrast radiographs if an areae gastricae pattern is demonstrated within the herniated portion of the fundus[39] (Fig. 32–8).

When a moderate-sized or large hiatal hernia is present, double contrast views of the stomach obtained with the patient in an upright or lateral recumbent position also permit assessment of the mucosa within the hernia for ulcers, neoplasms, or other abnormalities not easily seen on conventional single contrast barium studies. Ulcers are particularly likely to develop at the hiatal orifice, where the gastric mucosa is repeatedly exposed to trauma on the ridge riding over the hiatus. These ulcers have been described as "riding ulcers."[32]

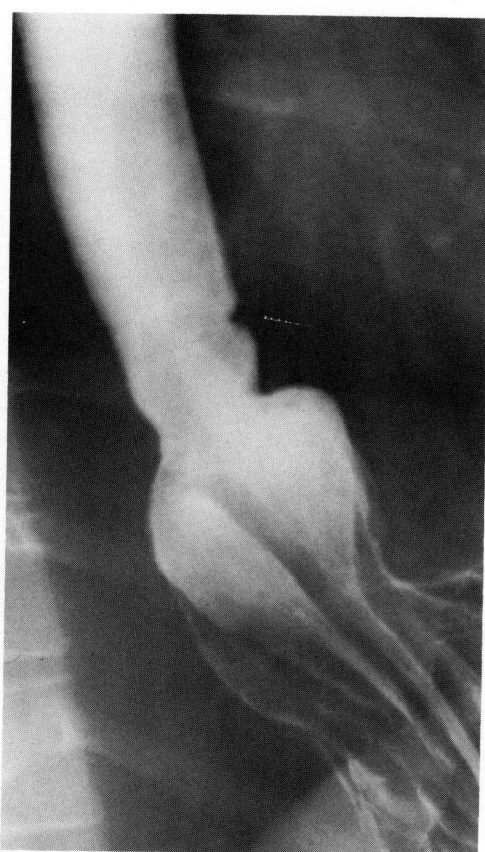

**Figure 32–6. Sliding hiatal hernia.** Gastric rugae are seen in the hernia on this prone single contrast view of the esophagus.

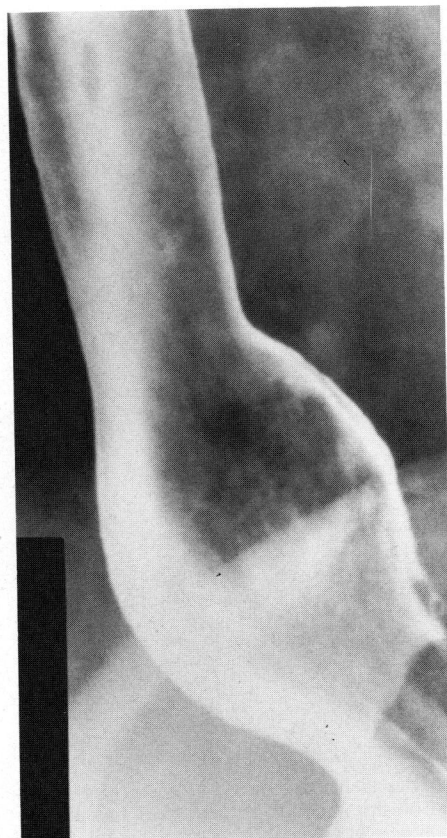

**Figure 32–8. Hiatal hernia seen on an upright double contrast esophagram.** Note how an areae gastricae pattern is present in the hernia.

# Paraesophageal Hernia

## Pathogenesis

In the rare paraesophageal or rolling hernia, a portion of the stomach herniates through the esophageal hiatus into the chest alongside the distal esophagus, and the cardia retains its normal position below the diaphragm. The hernia is thought to occur through a localized weakness or defect in the phrenoesophageal membrane.[32] These patients eventually may develop a mixed sliding-paraesophageal hernia if the gastroesophageal junction also rises above the diaphragm. Rarely, the entire stomach herniates through the esophageal hiatus, producing a gastric volvulus or so-called intrathoracic upside-down stomach.[32]

## Clinical Significance

Most patients with paraesophageal hernias are asymptomatic, and the hernia is an incidental finding on barium studies performed for other reasons. Unlike sliding hiatal hernias, paraesophageal hernias are rarely associated with gastroesophageal reflux or reflux esophagitis. As the hernia enlarges, however, the risk of incarceration, strangulation, and infarction increases.[40, 41] Because these potentially life-threatening complications may occur in previously asymptomatic patients, an argument can be made for surgical repair of all radiographically diagnosed paraesophageal hernias. Otherwise, these hernias may continue to enlarge until a gastric volvulus or other complications have developed at a late stage in life, when the patient is a poor risk for surgery and yet is threatened by a potentially fatal condition.

## Radiographic Diagnosis

A paraesophageal hernia may be diagnosed on single contrast barium studies obtained with the patient prone when a portion of the stomach has herniated through the esophageal hiatus of the diaphragm alongside the distal esophagus (Fig. 32–9). In such patients, the gastric cardia retains its normal position below the diaphragm. In a mixed sliding-paraesophageal hernia, however, the cardia has also herniated above the diaphragm into the

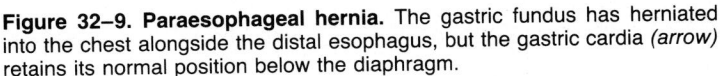

**Figure 32–9. Paraesophageal hernia.** The gastric fundus has herniated into the chest alongside the distal esophagus, but the gastric cardia *(arrow)* retains its normal position below the diaphragm.

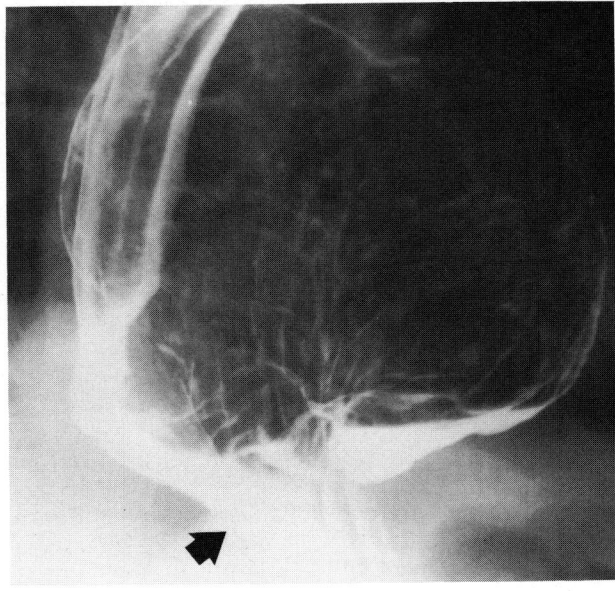

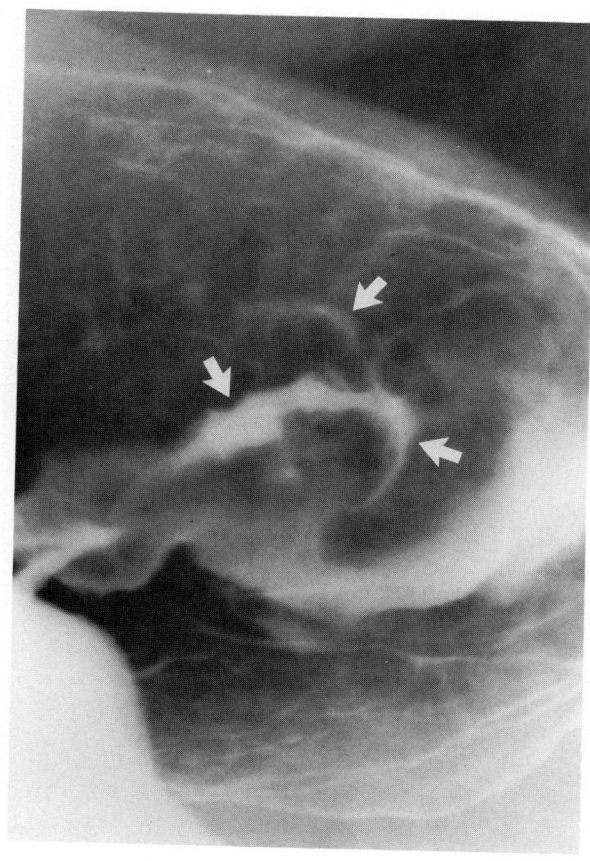

**Figure 32–10. Carcinoma of the gastric cardia.** The normal anatomic landmarks at the cardia have been obliterated and replaced by irregular areas of ulceration *(arrows)* due to tumor in this region.

chest. Occasionally, a sliding hiatal hernia can be mistaken radiographically for a mixed sliding-paraesophageal hernia because of a prominent notch on the superior aspect of the hernia that erroneously suggests a paraesophageal component.[30]

In patients with gastric volvulus or intrathoracic upside-down stomach, almost the entire stomach has herniated through the esophageal hiatus into the chest and has assumed an inverted or upside-down configuration (see Chapter 40). Rarely, traction or torsion of the stomach at or near the level of the hiatus may lead to obstruction, infarction, or perforation of the intrathoracic stomach.[42] These patients often undergo emergency surgery without preoperative barium studies because of their rapidly deteriorating clinical condition.

## CARCINOMA OF THE CARDIA

The clinical and radiographic aspects of carcinoma of the cardia are discussed in detail in Chapter 38. On barium studies, advanced lesions at the cardia may appear as obvious exophytic or infiltrating lesions in the gastric fundus. However, other lesions at the cardia may be recognized only by relatively subtle nodularity, mass effect, or ulceration in this region with distortion, effacement, or obliteration of the normal anatomic landmarks at the cardia[10, 11, 43, 44] (Fig. 32–10). Because these abnormalities at the cardia are extremely difficult to demonstrate on conventional single contrast barium studies, double contrast technique is essential for diagnosing these lesions at the earliest possible stage.

## PROLAPSED ESOPHAGOGASTRIC MUCOSA

Retrograde or anterograde prolapse of mucosa in the esophagogastric region may produce a polypoid filling defect in the distal esophagus or gastric fundus.[45–47] However, mucosal prolapse usually occurs as a transient phenomenon, so that the filling defect intermittently vanishes at fluoroscopy. The distal esophagus may also invaginate into a sliding hiatal hernia or a hiatal hernia may invaginate into the fundus, producing an apparent mass lesion[48] (Figs. 32–11A and 32–12A). However, greater distention of the fundus with barium or gas usually displaces an invaginated hernia above the diaphragm and reduces the invaginated distal esophagus, so that the lesion is a transient finding during the radiologic examination (Figs. 32–11B and 32–12B). Thus, it is usually possible to differentiate prolapsed esophagogastric mucosa or invaginated hernias from true polypoid lesions at the cardia.

## OTHER ABNORMALITIES

Other abnormalities occurring at or near the gastroesophageal junction include peptic strictures (see Chapter 24), inflammatory esophagogastric polyps (see Chapter 27), esophageal or gastric varices (see Chapter 30), primary or secondary achalasia (see Chapters 23 and 29), and squamous cell metastases to the cardia (see Chapter 28).

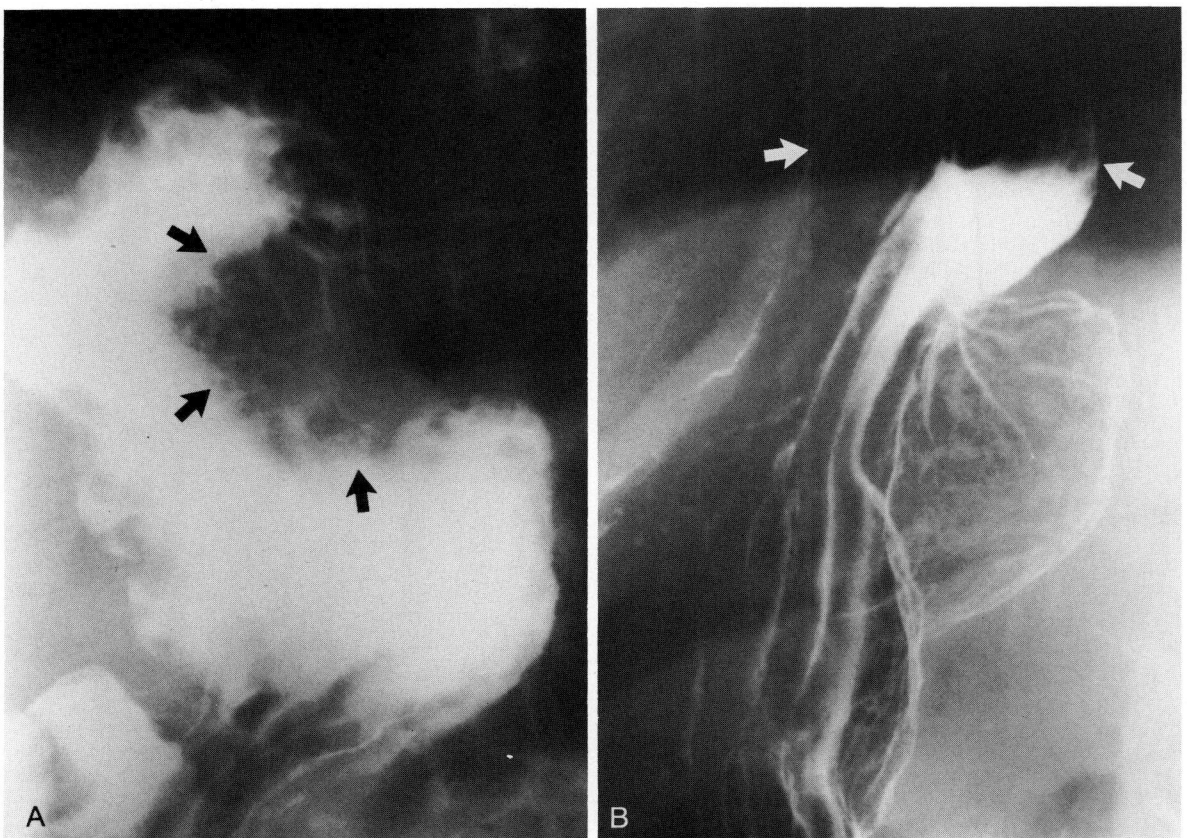

**Figure 32–11. Pseudotumor in the gastric fundus due to an invaginated hiatal hernia. A.** The initial radiograph of the stomach shows an apparent mass lesion *(arrows)* in the fundus. **B.** However, greater gaseous distention of the fundus displaces the hernia above the diaphragm *(arrows)*.

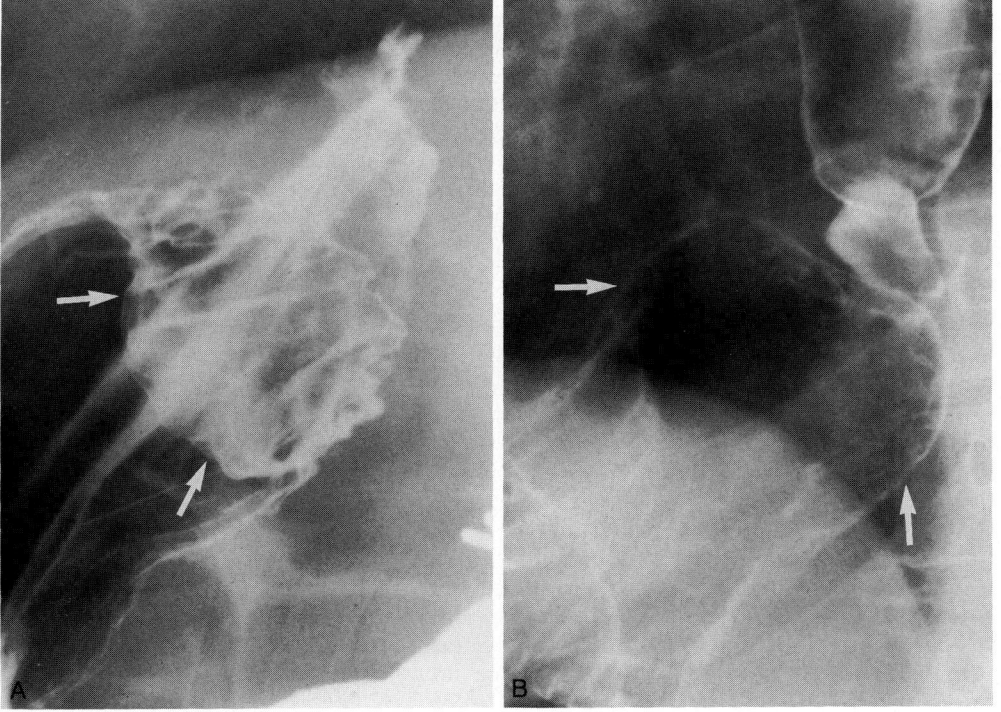

**Figure 32–12. Pseudotumor in the gastric fundus due to an invaginated hiatal hernia. A.** An apparent mass lesion *(arrows)* is seen in the fundus on a double contrast radiograph. **B.** Moments later, the invaginated hernia has risen above the diaphragm *(arrows)*, and the pseudotumor is no longer seen.

## Acknowledgment

Figures 32–1 to 32–3, 32–6, 32–7, and 32–9 to 32–11 are reproduced from Levine MS: Radiology of the Esophagus. Philadelphia: WB Saunders, 1989.

# References

1. Levine MS, Rubesin SE, Herlinger H, et al: Double-contrast upper gastrointestinal examination: technique and interpretation. Radiology 168:593–602, 1988.
2. Levine MS, Rubesin SE: Radiologic investigation of dysphagia. AJR 154:1157–1163, 1990.
3. Chen YM, Ott DJ, Gelfand DW, et al: Multiphasic examination of the esophagogastric region for strictures, rings, and hiatal hernia: evaluation of the individual techniques. Gastrointest Radiol 10:311–316, 1985.
4. Wolf BS: Use of a half inch barium tablet to detect minimal esophageal strictures. J Mt Sinai Hosp 28:80–95, 1961.
5. Ott DJ, Kelley TF, Chen YM, et al: Evaluation of the esophagus with a marshmallow bolus: clarifying the cause of dysphagia. Gastrointest Radiol 16:1–4, 1991.
6. Friedland GW: Historical review of the changing concepts of lower esophageal anatomy: 430 B.C.–1977. AJR 131:373–388, 1978.
7. Wolf BS, Heitmann P, Cohen BR: The inferior esophageal sphincter, the manometric high pressure zone and hiatal incompetence. AJR 103:251–276, 1968.
8. Dodds WJ: Current concepts of esophageal motor function: clinical implications for radiology. AJR 128:549–561, 1977.
9. Hodges FM, Snead LO, Berger RA: A stellate impression in the cardiac end of the stomach simulating tumor. AJR 47:578–583, 1942.
10. Freeny PC: Double-contrast gastrography of the fundus and cardia: normal landmarks and their pathologic changes. AJR 133:481–487, 1979.
11. Herlinger H, Grossman R, Laufer I, et al: The gastric cardia in double-contrast study: its dynamic image. AJR 135:21–29, 1980.
12. Cimmino CV: Sign of the burnous in the stomach. Radiology 75:722–725, 1960.
13. Ott DJ, Gelfand DW, Wu WC, et al: Esophagogastric region and its rings. AJR 142:281–287, 1984.
14. Johnston JR, Griffin JC: Anatomic location of the lower esophageal ring. Surgery 61:528–534, 1967.
15. Goyal RK, Glancy JJ, Spiro HM: Lower esophageal ring. N Engl J Med 282:1298–1305, 1970.
16. Schatzki R, Gary JE: The lower esophageal ring. AJR 75:246–261, 1956.
17. Ott DJ, Chen YM, Wu WC, et al: Radiographic and endoscopic sensitivity in detecting lower esophageal mucosal ring. AJR 147:261–265, 1986.
18. Schatzki R, Gary JE: Dysphagia due to a diaphragm-like localized narrowing in the lower esophagus ("lower esophageal ring"). AJR 70:911–922, 1953.
19. Stiennon OA: The anatomic basis for the lower esophageal contraction ring. AJR 90:811–822, 1963.
20. Rinaldo JA, Gahagan T: The narrow lower esophageal ring: pathogenesis and physiology. Am J Dig Dis 11:257–265, 1966.
21. Scharschmidt BF, Watts HD: The lower esophageal ring and esophageal reflux. Am J Gastroenterol 69:544–549, 1978.
22. Chen YM, Gelfand DW, Ott DJ, et al: Natural progression of the lower esophageal mucosal ring. Gastrointest Radiol 12:93–98, 1987.
23. Ingelfinger FJ, Kramer P: Dysphagia produced by a contractile ring in the lower esophagus. Gastroenterology 23:419–430, 1953.
24. Norton RA, King GD: "Steakhouse syndrome": the symptomatic lower esophageal ring. Lahey Clin Found Bull 13:55–59, 1963.
25. Desai DC, Rider JA, Puletti EJ, et al: Lower esophageal ring. Gastrointest Endosc 15:100–105, 1968.
26. Arvanitakis C: Lower esophageal ring: endoscopic and therapeutic aspects. Gastrointest Endosc 24:17–18, 1977.
27. Som ML, Wolf BS, Marshak RH: Narrow esophagogastric ring treated endoscopically. Gastroenterology 39:634–638, 1960.
28. Schatzki R: The lower esophageal ring: long term follow-up of symptomatic and asymptomatic rings. AJR 90:805–810, 1963.
29. Bjork VO, Charonis CG: Lower oesophageal web. Thorax 22:156–164, 1967.
30. Dodds WJ: Esophagus and esophagogastric region. *In* Margulis AR, Burhenne HJ (eds): Alimentary Tract Radiology (3rd ed). St. Louis: CV Mosby, 1983, pp 529–603.
31. Wolf BS: Sliding hiatal hernia: the need for redefinition. AJR 117:231–247, 1973.
32. Skinner DB: Hernias (hiatal, traumatic, and congenital). *In* Berk JE (ed): Bockus Gastroenterology (4th ed). Philadelphia: WB Saunders, 1985, pp 705–716.
33. Wright RA, Hurwitz AL: Relationship of hiatal hernia to endoscopically proved reflux esophagitis. Dig Dis Sci 24:311–313, 1979.
34. Ott DJ, Gelfand DW, Wu WC: Reflux esophagitis: radiographic and endoscopic correlation. Radiology 130:583–588, 1979.
35. Behar J: Reflux esophagitis: pathogenesis, diagnosis, and management. Arch Intern Med 136:560–566, 1976.
36. Cohen S, Harris LD: Does hiatus hernia affect competence of the gastroesophageal sphincter? N Engl J Med 284:1053–1056, 1971.
37. Ho CS, Rodrigues PR: Lower esophageal strictures, benign or malignant? J Can Assoc Radiol 31:110–113, 1980.
38. Ott DJ, Dodds WJ, Wu WC, et al: Current status of radiology in evaluating for gastroesophageal reflux disease. J Clin Gastroenterol 4:365–375, 1982.
39. Gelfand DW, Ott DJ: Areae gastricae traversing the esophageal hiatus: a sign of hiatus hernia. Gastrointest Radiol 4:127–129, 1979.
40. Shocket E, Neber J, Drosg RE: The acutely obstructed, incarcerated paraesophageal hiatal hernia. Am J Surg 108:805–810, 1964.
41. Hill LD: Incarcerated paraesophageal hernia: a surgical emergency. Am J Surg 126:286–291, 1973.
42. Gerson DE, Lewicki AM: Intrathoracic stomach: when does it obstruct? Radiology 119:257–264, 1976.
43. Freeny PC, Marks WM: Adenocarcinoma of the gastroesophageal junction: barium and CT examination. AJR 138:1077–1084, 1982.
44. Levine MS, Laufer I, Thompson JJ: Carcinoma of the gastric cardia in young people. AJR 140:69–72, 1983.
45. De Lorimier AA, Warren JP: Prolapse of the mucosa at the esophagogastric junction. AJR 84:1061–1069, 1960.
46. Kaye JJ, Stassa G: Mimicry and deception in the diagnosis of tumors of the gastric cardia. AJR 110:295–303, 1970.
47. Rudnick JP, Ferrucci JT, Eaton SB, et al: Esophageal pseudotumor: retrograde prolapse of gastric mucosa into the esophagus. AJR 115:253–256, 1972.
48. Ghahremani GG, Collins PA: Esophago-gastric invagination in patients with sliding hiatus hernia. Gastrointest Radiol 1:253–261, 1976.

# Postoperative Esophagus

**Stephen E. Rubesin, M.D.**

**Ernest F. Rosato, M.D.**

## INTRODUCTION

Radiologic evaluation of the postoperative esophagus requires an understanding of the operative procedures and of the normal postoperative radiologic appearances. The purpose of the radiologic examination is to define the anatomy and to detect complications during the early postoperative period (i.e., less than 4 weeks from surgery) and late postoperative period (i.e., more than 4 weeks from surgery)[1] (Table 33–1). During the early postoperative period, the most common complications include stasis due to adynamic ileus or vagotomy, obstruction due to anastomotic edema, and perforation due to anastomotic breakdown. During the late postoperative period, the most common complications include aspiration, gastroesophageal reflux, anastomotic stricture, and recurrent tumor. Depending on the nature of the surgery and the status of the patient, the postoperative radiologic examination should be tailored to demonstrate suspected complications in these individuals.

## RADIOGRAPHIC TECHNIQUE

Early postoperative complications may be manifested by a variety of findings on plain films of the chest and abdomen (Fig. 33–1). A dilated viscus with air-fluid levels should suggest anastomotic outlet obstruction. Pneumomediastinum, cervical or subcutaneous emphysema, a widened mediastinum, or a rapidly enlarging pleural effusion should suggest anastomotic breakdown and perforation.[2] However, some patients with perfo-

ration may have normal plain films, and others may have no clinical signs of a leak, so that some perforations are discovered unexpectedly on postoperative contrast studies.

Barium and water-soluble contrast agents each have advantages and disadvantages in evaluating patients during the early postoperative period.[3–5] Barium is su-

### TABLE 33–1. COMPLICATIONS OF ESOPHAGEAL SURGERY

**Early Complications**
Common
    Anastomotic or staple-line leak
    Anastomotic narrowing
    Gastric or duodenal atony
    Aspiration
    Gastroesophageal reflux
Uncommon
    Pneumothorax
    Mediastinal hematoma
    Empyema
    Vocal cord paresis
    Chylothorax
    Ischemia of colonic or jejunal bypass
    Delayed bypass emptying

**Late Complications**
Common
    Anastomotic stricture
    Aspiration
    Recurrent carcinoma
    Gastroesophageal reflux and its sequelae
Uncommon
    Delayed conduit emptying
    Tracheoesophageal fistula
    Anastomotic or staple line leak

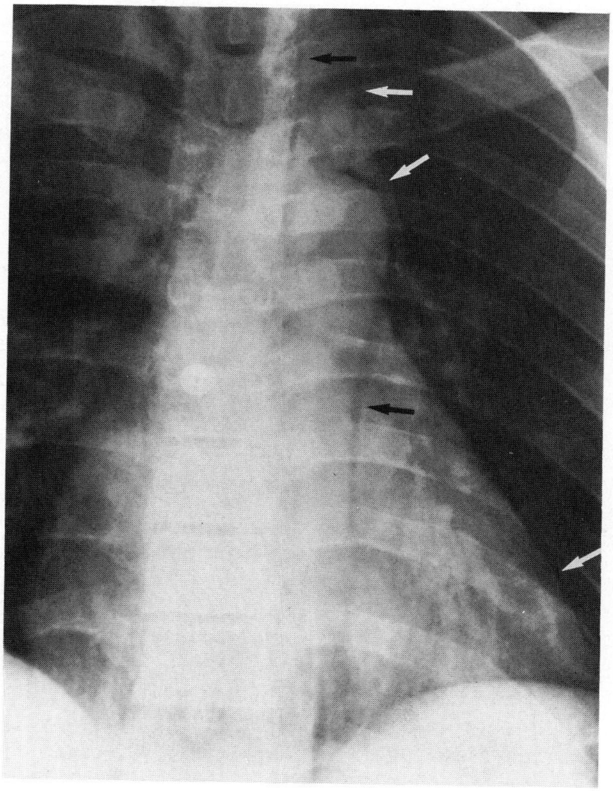

**Figure 33–1. Pneumomediastinum after balloon dilatation of a distal esophageal stricture.** Linear collections of gas *(arrows)* outline the descending thoracic aorta, great vessels, and pericardial sac.

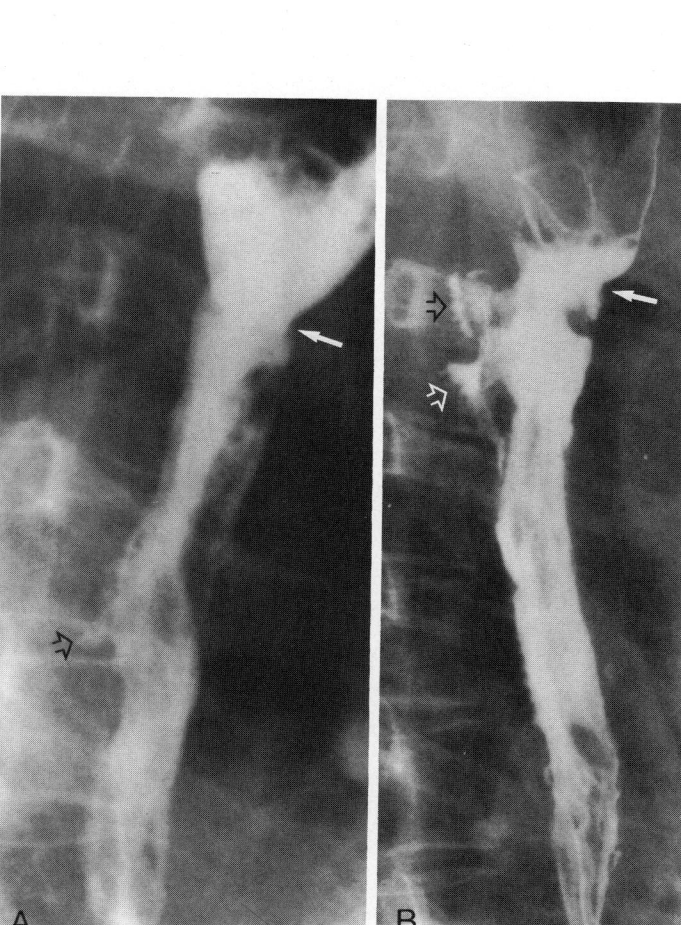

**Figure 33–2. Leak at esophagogastric anastomosis shown better with barium than with water-soluble contrast agent. A.** A Gastrografin study shows an irregular contour below the esophagogastric anastomosis *(solid arrow)*. A questionable leak or ulcer is outlined *(open arrow)*. **B.** A barium swallow performed immediately after the Gastrografin study clearly demonstrates a contained perforation *(open arrows)* below the esophagogastric anastomosis *(solid arrow)*. The stomach is collapsed on both views.

perior to water-soluble contrast agents in demonstrating the postoperative anatomy as well as the presence and extent of extraluminal contrast medium (Fig. 33–2). If there is a perforation, however, extravasated barium in the mediastinum may incite a granulomatous reaction.[4] In contrast, water-soluble contrast agents (i.e., diatrizoate meglumine and diatrizoate sodium [Gastrografin]) in the mediastinum do not cause mediastinitis.[4] Because they are hyperosmolar, however, water-soluble contrast agents may cause severe pulmonary edema if they enter the lungs via aspiration or a tracheoesophageal fistula.[6–8] Nonionic contrast agents are not hyperosmolar and are therefore unlikely to cause pulmonary edema, but their use has been limited by their high cost.[9]

The following approach is suggested for the radiologic evaluation of the postoperative esophagus. Water-soluble contrast agents should be used during the early postoperative period to rule out a perforation or anastomotic leak into the mediastinum or pleural space. If no contrast medium is seen to extravasate from the esophagus on the initial spot films, barium should then be given for a more detailed examination. However, barium should be used as the primary contrast agent if aspiration or an esophageal-airway fistula is suspected. After the early postoperative period, the radiologic examination should be performed as a biphasic study that includes double contrast views with high-density barium and single contrast views with low-density barium.

## GASTROESOPHAGEAL REFLUX AND HIATAL HERNIA

Patients with gastroesophageal reflux may undergo surgery because of intractable reflux esophagitis, peptic strictures, or Barrett's esophagus. The most frequently performed antireflux operations are the Nissen fundoplication, the Belsey Mark IV repair, and the Hill posterior gastropexy.[10] In each of these procedures, the esophagus is mobilized, the hiatal hernia is reduced, and the intra-abdominal esophagus is restored. Preservation of the lower esophageal sphincter and vagus nerve is also essential.

In the Nissen fundoplication, the gastric fundus is wrapped 360 degrees around the intra-abdominal esophagus to create an antireflux valve.[11] In the Belsey Mark IV repair, the gastric fundus is sutured to the intra-abdominal esophagus, creating an acute esophagogastric junction angle (angle of His) and a 240-degree fundoplication wrap around the left lateral aspect of the distal esophagus.[12, 13] In the Hill posterior gastropexy, the gastroesophageal junction is returned to an intra-abdominal location and anchored to the preaortic fascia (median arcuate ligament), thereby accentuating the esophagogastric junction angle and lengthening the segment of intra-abdominal esophagus.[14] However, a fundoplication is not performed. The Belsey Mark IV repair uses a transthoracic approach, whereas the Hill posterior gastropexy uses a transabdominal approach. The Nissen fundoplication is usually performed via a transabdominal

approach, but a transthoracic approach may be required in complicated cases (e.g., patients with recurrent gastroesophageal reflux after an unsuccessful fundoplication).

## Normal Postoperative Appearances

The Nissen fundoplication wrap normally appears as a large fundal mass with a smooth contour and surface[15, 16] (Fig. 33–3). If the patient drinks barium in a recumbent, steep oblique or lateral position, the distal esophagus is shown to curve smoothly through the center of the fundoplication wrap.[17] The smooth, symmetric wrap and its consistent relationship with the distal esophagus readily differentiate a fundoplication wrap from a true tumor in the fundus.

The gastric wrap of the Belsey Mark IV repair produces a smaller defect than the Nissen fundoplication.[18] The esophagus forms two distinct angles as it passes through the 240-degree fundoplication[18] (Fig. 33–4). The intra-abdominal esophagus has a shallow upper angle where the esophagus, fundus, and diaphragm are sutured together and a lower angle where the stomach is pulled upward toward the esophagus.[18]

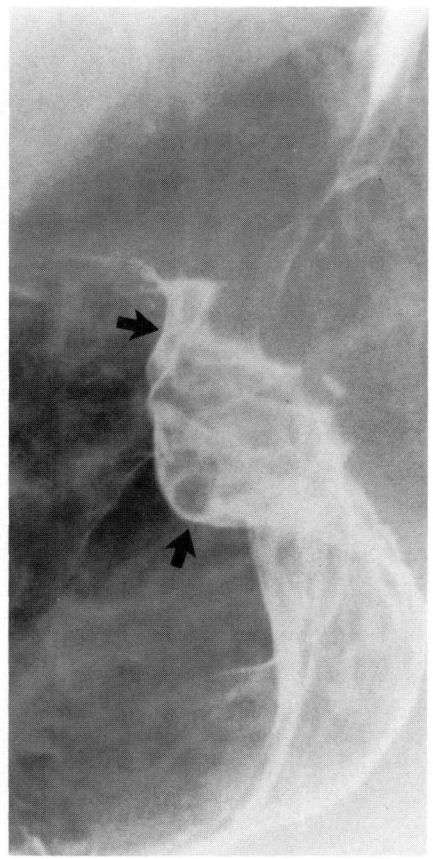

**Figure 33–3. Normal Nissen fundoplication.** The fundoplication wrap is seen as a smooth-surfaced, well-defined mass *(arrows)* in the gastric fundus.

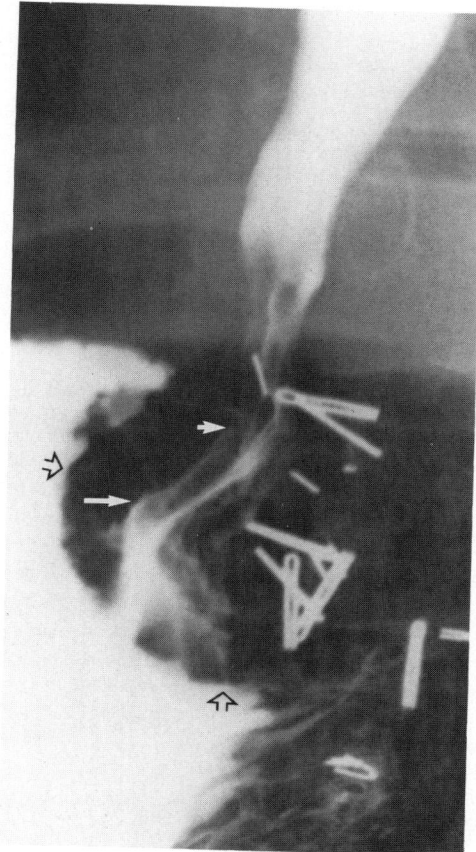

**Figure 33–4. Normal Belsey Mark IV repair.** The fundoplication wrap is seen as a well-circumscribed mass *(open arrows)* in the gastric fundus. As the esophagus passes through the fundoplication wrap, a shallow angle is formed where the esophagus, fundus, and diaphragm are sutured together *(short solid arrow).* A steeper angle *(long solid arrow)* is formed where the stomach is pulled upward toward the esophagus.

In the Hill posterior gastropexy, the intra-abdominal esophagus is lengthened, and the angle of His is accentuated.[19] Whatever antireflux operation is performed, neither gastroesophageal reflux nor a hiatal hernia should be observed after a successful repair.

## Complications

### Obstruction

During the early postoperative period, edema of the fundoplication wrap may cause transient dysphagia. This complication may be manifested on esophagrams by a large, smooth fundal mass associated with smooth, tapered narrowing of the intra-abdominal esophagus and delayed emptying of contrast material.[15] The edema usually subsides within 1 to 2 weeks, and a second esophagram demonstrates a much smaller defect in this region because of the normal fundoplication wrap.

Some patients may have persistent narrowing of the esophagus, causing dysphagia or the "gas bloat" syndrome, with upper abdominal fullness and inability to belch after meals.[10] In such cases, esophagrams may demonstrate fixed narrowing of the distal esophagus due to a tight fundoplication wrap (Fig. 33–5) or to excessive closure of the esophageal hiatus of the diaphragm.[20, 21]

## Recurrent Hiatal Hernia and Gastroesophageal Reflux

Complete disruption of the fundoplication sutures is manifested radiographically by a recurrent hiatal hernia and gastroesophageal reflux without visualization of a fundoplication wrap[22, 23] (Fig. 33–6). Partial disruption of the fundoplication sutures may be manifested by a partially intact wrap associated with one or more outpouchings from the gastric fundus (Fig. 33–7) or by an hourglass appearance of the stomach as the fundus slips through the fundoplication.[22, 23] An hourglass stomach may also be caused by inappropriate placement of the fundoplication around the gastric body. Finally, disruption of the diaphragmatic sutures (but not the fundoplication sutures) may result in a recurrent hiatal hernia with continued demonstration of an intact fundoplication wrap[22] (Fig. 33–8).

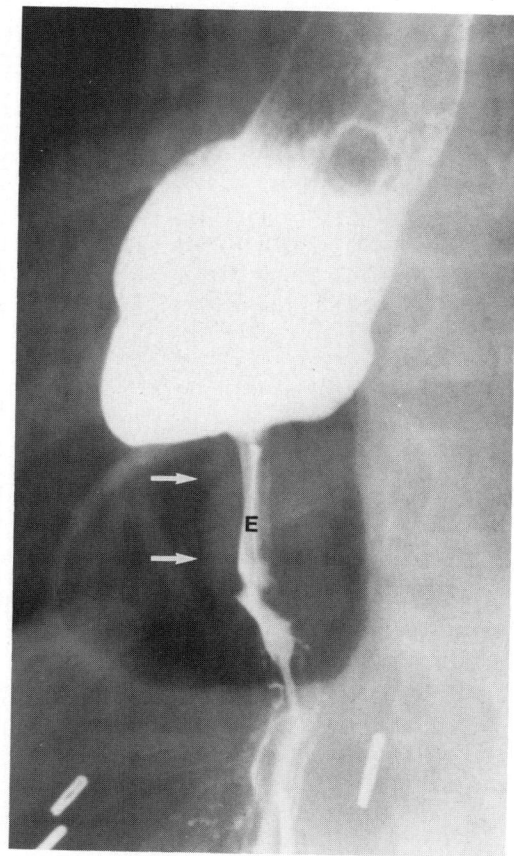

**Figure 33–5. Persistent obstruction of the distal esophagus by a tight Nissen fundoplication wrap.** The esophageal lumen (E) is narrowed by a tight fundoplication wrap *(arrows).* The proximal esophagus is mildly dilated. There was delayed emptying of barium from the distal esophagus.

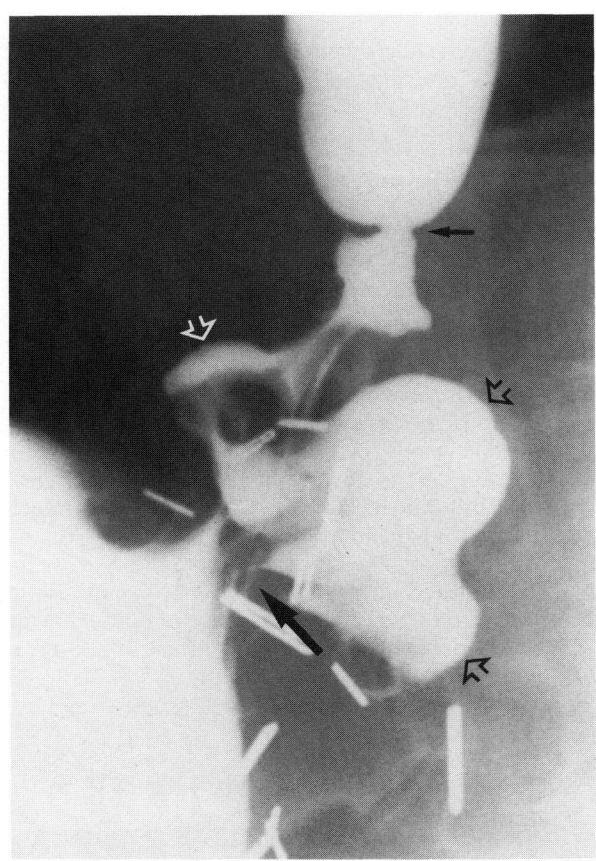

**Figure 33–6. Fundoplication wrap breakdown and recurrent hiatal hernia.** Multiple gastric outpouchings *(open arrows)* are seen above the level of the diaphragm *(large black arrow)*. The expected mass of a fundoplication wrap is not present in the gastric fundus. A focal peptic stricture is also noted at the gastroesophageal junction *(small black arrow)*.

**Figure 33–7. Partial fundoplication wrap breakdown.** The fundal wrap is partially intact *(small arrows)* but does not encircle the distal esophagus. A small fundal outpouching is present *(large arrow)*. Barium is seen in the distal esophagus because of gastroesophageal reflux.

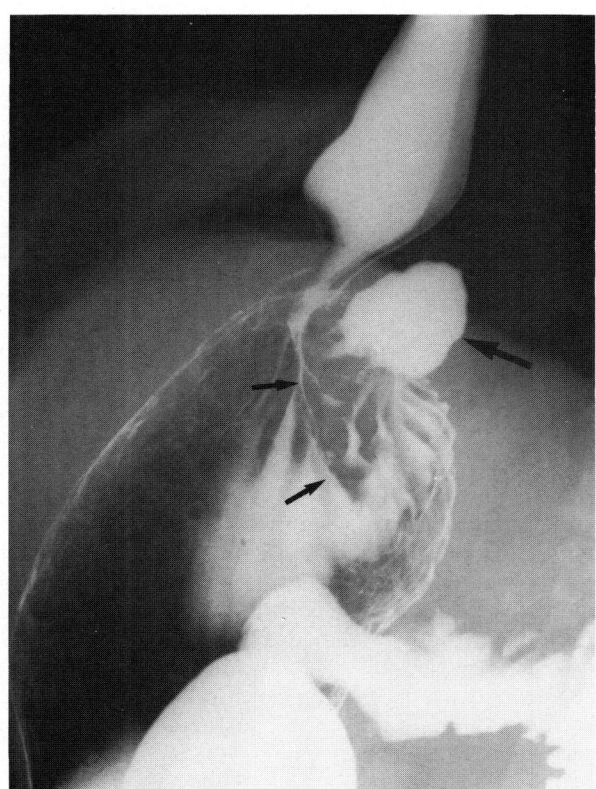

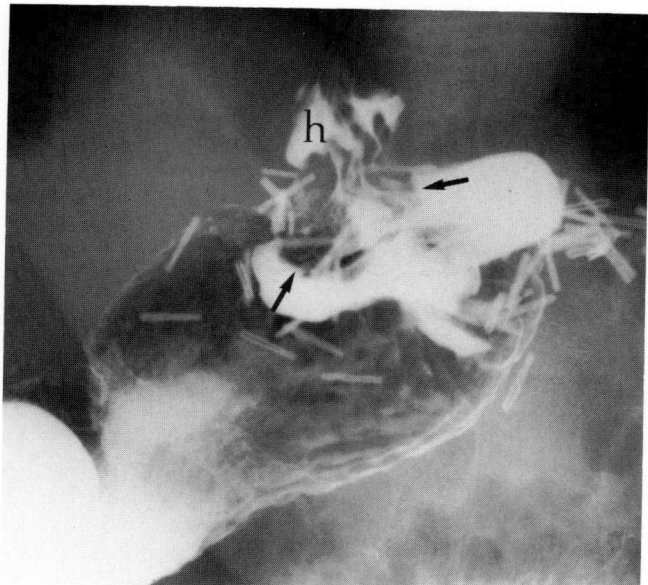

**Figure 33–8. Recurrent hiatal hernia due to disruption of sutures closing the esophageal hiatus of the diaphragm.** A small hiatal hernia (h) lies above the intact fundoplication wrap *(arrows)*.

## Angelchik Prosthesis

In the past, the Angelchik antireflux prosthesis has been used as a surgical alternative for the treatment of gastroesophageal reflux disease. A fundoplication wrap was created by placing a horseshoe-shaped silicon prosthesis around the intra-abdominal esophagus and gastric cardia[24, 25] (Fig. 33–9). Because of a high complication rate, however, the prosthesis is no longer used. Complications included migration of the prosthesis into

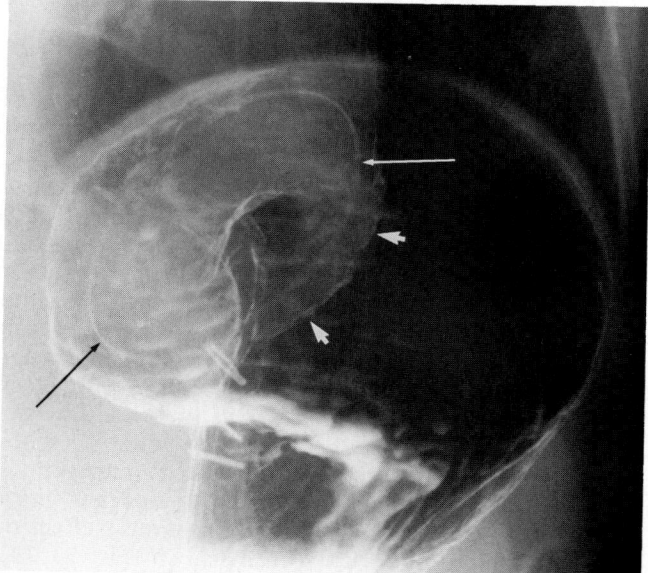

**Figure 33–9. Normal Angelchik prosthesis.** A radiopaque ring *(long arrows)* is embedded in the Angelchik prosthesis. The presence of the prosthesis surrounding the gastric fundus is also manifested as increased radiodensity and a line *(short arrows)*.

the abdominal cavity or mediastinum, slippage of the prosthesis, and erosion of the prosthesis into the stomach.[25-31]

## BENIGN STRICTURES

Benign esophageal strictures may be treated by a variety of surgical and nonsurgical procedures, including esophageal bougienage, fluoroscopically controlled balloon dilatation, and esophageal replacement with a gastric tube, jejunal graft, or colonic interposition. The site, extent, and etiology of the stricture affect the therapeutic choice. Surgery is most frequently required for the treatment of lye strictures. Esophageal replacement surgery may also be performed on patients with intractable strictures due to gastroesophageal reflux disease.

### Balloon Dilatation

Peroral balloon dilatation of strictures under fluoroscopic guidance is an effective alternative to esophageal bougienage.[32, 33] This procedure has a lower risk of perforation and a longer symptom-free interval than bougienage.[34-37]

## CARCINOMA

Because they usually have advanced tumors at the time of diagnosis, patients with esophageal carcinoma continue to have 5-year survival rates of only 5 to 10%, despite advances in radiologic imaging, surgical technique, and treatment with radiation or chemotherapy.[38] As a result, most of these patients undergo palliative therapy to relieve dysphagia and pain and to prevent starvation by restoring the ability to swallow. Palliation of advanced esophageal cancers can be achieved not only by surgery but also by radiation therapy, esophageal intubation, and endoscopic laser therapy. The various surgical and nonsurgical options for palliation or cure of esophageal carcinoma are listed in Table 33–2.

**TABLE 33–2. TREATMENT OF ESOPHAGEAL CARCINOMA**

Surgery
    Esophagogastrectomy
    Gastric interposition
        Mediastinal pull-through with transhiatal esophagectomy
        Substernal bypass with exclusion of esophagus
    Gastric tube
    Colonic interposition
    Jejunal interposition
    Free jejunal graft
Radiation therapy
Percutaneous or endoscopic dilatation
Endoscopic laser resection
Palliative intubation

## Esophagogastrectomy

Esophagogastrectomy is the operation performed most frequently for cure or palliation of carcinoma of the intrathoracic esophagus or gastric cardia. Distant metastases and aortic or tracheobronchial invasion by tumor are relative contraindications to surgery, but local extension of tumor and mediastinal adenopathy are not.[39] A right-sided thoracotomy and abdominal incision are performed on most patients with midthoracic esophageal cancers.[38] However, a left-sided thoracotomy is performed on patients with cancers involving the distal esophagus and cardia or lesions that have extensive nodal metastases near the celiac axis or lesser curvature of the stomach.[38] After resection of the diseased esophagus and cardia, the stomach is mobilized on its vascular pedicle and placed in the thorax with the lesser curvature facing the mediastinum (Fig. 33–10). Whenever possible, an antireflux procedure is performed by invaginating the distal esophagus into the stomach or by creating a fundoplication. Emptying of the denervated stomach is facilitated by pyloromyotomy or pyloroplasty. Left-sided esophagogastrectomies and pylorus-sparing procedures are being performed with increased frequency.

The most common complications during the early postoperative period include anastomotic leaks, obstruction, gastric atony and dilatation, and aspiration into the larynx. A study using water-soluble contrast medium (followed by a barium study if there is no evidence of a

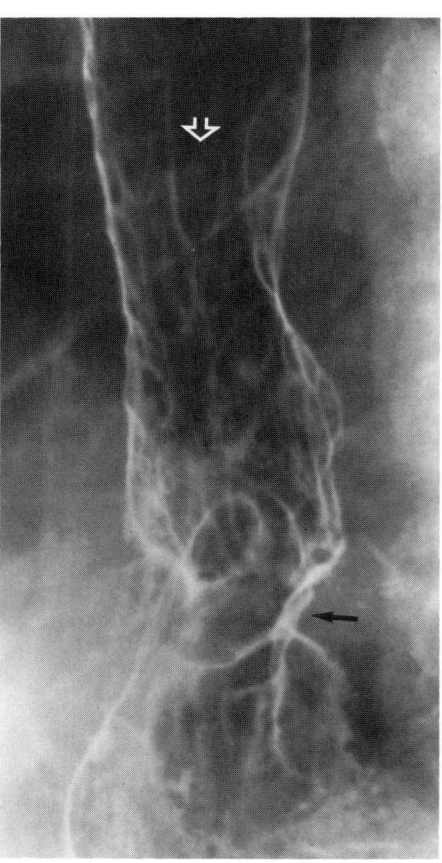

**Figure 33–11. Esophagogastrectomy with reflux esophagitis.** Numerous confluent plaques and pseudomembranes *(open arrow)* cover the esophageal mucosa above the esophagogastric junction *(solid arrow).* Free gastroesophageal reflux was seen at fluoroscopy.

leak) is usually performed within 7 to 10 days of surgery to rule out a leak at the esophagogastric anastomosis or pyloroplasty. Mechanical obstruction may also be an early finding at the esophagogastric anastomosis or pylorus because of edema, hemorrhage, or leak, or at the distal end of the intrathoracic stomach because of gastric volvulus or extrinsic compression of the stomach by the diaphragm.

The most common complications during the late postoperative period include gastroesophageal reflux and its sequelae, anastomotic strictures, fistulas, and recurrent tumor.[39] Acute gastroesophageal reflux may result in aspiration pneumonia. Chronic gastroesophageal reflux may lead to reflux esophagitis (Fig. 33–11), peptic strictures (Fig. 33–12), Barrett's esophagus, and, eventually, esophageal adenocarcinoma (Fig. 33–13). Healing of anastomotic leaks may result in benign anastomotic strictures. Although recurrent tumor in the mediastinum is best demonstrated by computed tomography or magnetic resonance, barium studies may reveal a smooth or spiculated area of extrinsic mass effect on the mediastinal border of the stomach[39, 40] (Fig. 33–14). Recurrent esophageal carcinoma may also be demonstrated by barium studies (Fig. 33–15). Any suspicious area should be further evaluated by endoscopy and biopsy. Delayed perforations may occasionally be

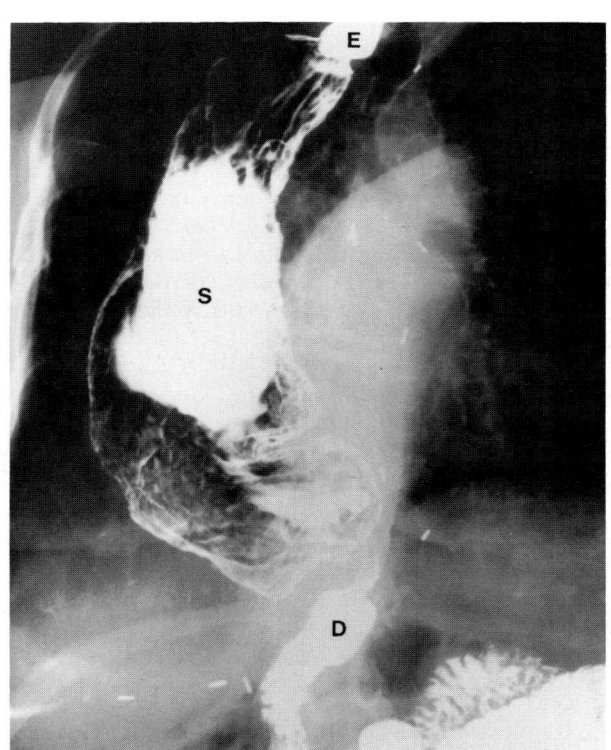

**Figure 33–10. Normal right-sided esophagogastrectomy.** The stomach (S) lies in the right hemithorax with the lesser curvature facing the mediastinum. The proximal duodenum (D) has been elevated and stretched by a Kocher maneuver. Barium is seen in the distal esophagus (E) because of gastroesophageal reflux.

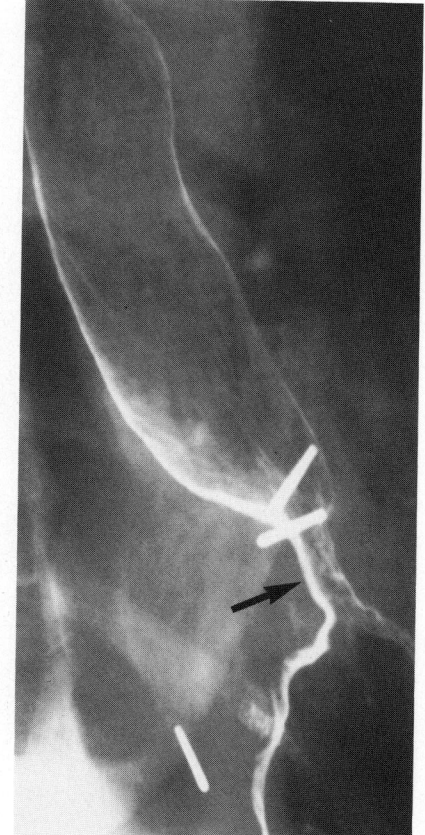

**Figure 33–12. Esophagogastrectomy with peptic stricture.** A smooth, tapered stricture *(arrow)* is seen above the esophagogastric anastomosis.

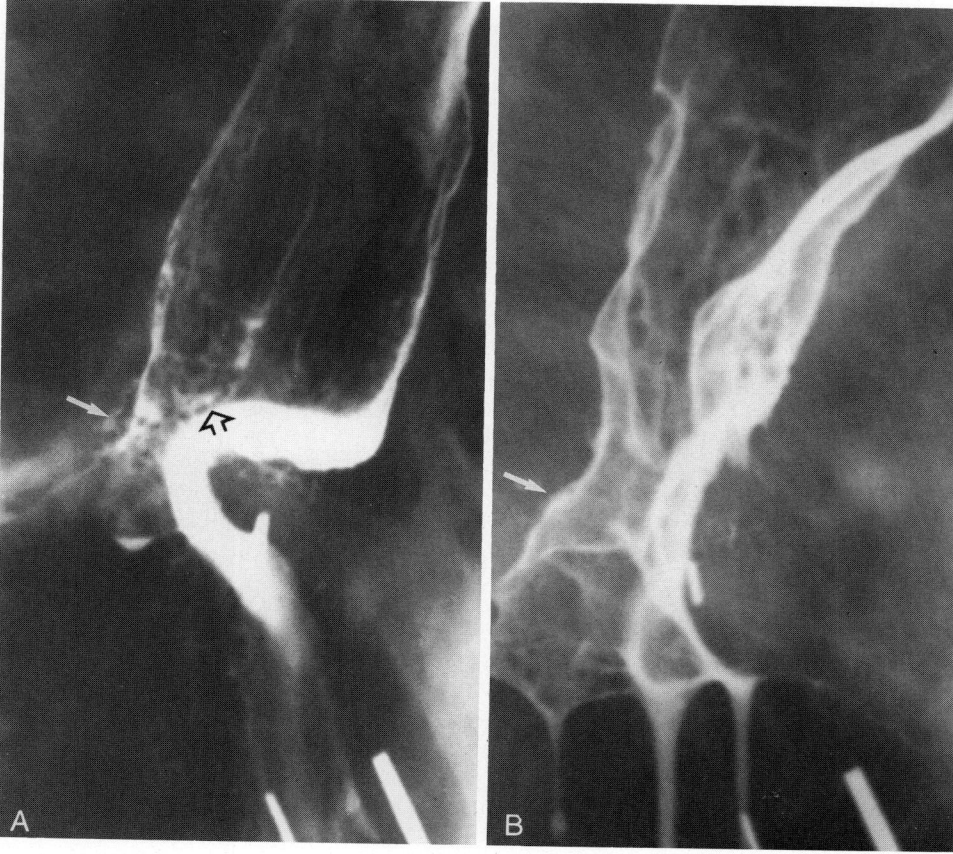

**Figure 33–13. Esophagogastrectomy with a superimposed adenocarcinoma in Barrett's esophagus. A.** Reflux esophagitis after esophagogastrectomy is manifested by a finely nodular mucosa *(open arrow)* just proximal to the esophagogastric anastomosis *(solid arrow)*. **B.** Two years later, an irregular, infiltrating lesion with coarsely nodular mucosa is seen just above the esophagogastric anastomosis *(arrow)*. Surgery revealed an adenocarcinoma arising in Barrett's mucosa.

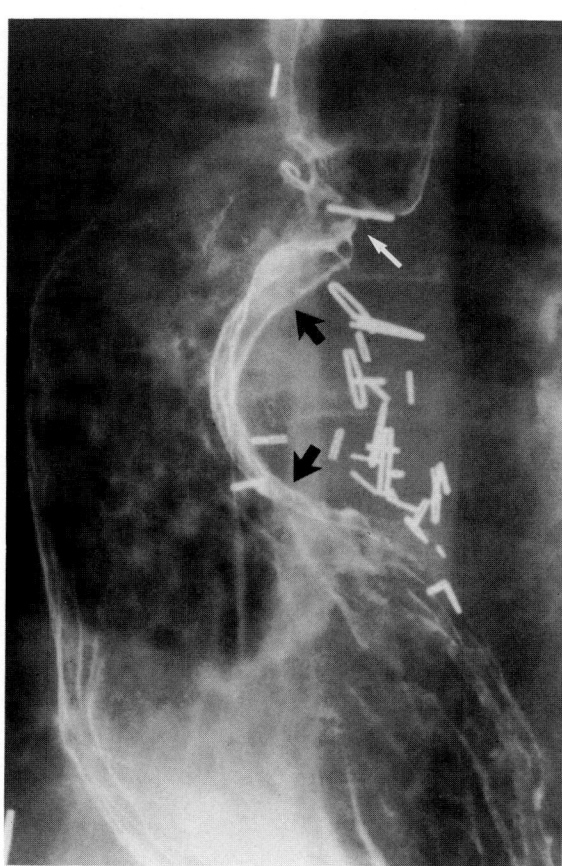

**Figure 33–14. Esophagogastrectomy with recurrent mediastinal tumor.** A smooth, extrinsic area of mass effect *(black arrows)* is seen on the lesser curvature of the intrathoracic stomach below the esophagogastric anastomosis *(white arrow)*.

**Figure 33–15. Esophagogastrectomy with recurrent esophageal carcinoma.** The distal esophagus is diffusely narrowed and irregular *(long arrows)* and has a nodular surface pattern because of recurrent esophageal carcinoma. (The esophagogastric anastomosis is denoted by a short arrow.)

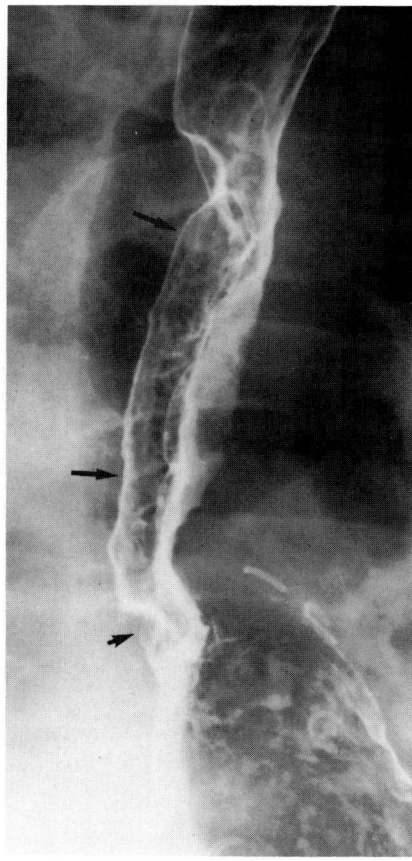

caused by recurrent mediastinal tumor or mediastinal irradiation (Fig. 33–16).

## Gastric Tube and Gastric Bypass Procedures

Conduits created from the greater curvature of the stomach may also be used to replace or bypass a benign or malignant esophageal stricture.[41] The greater curvature conduit is brought superiorly into the anterior or posterior mediastinum or through a subcutaneous tunnel in a reversed or nonreversed direction.[42, 43] The most frequent complications of the use of gastric tubes are leakage and stricture formation at the anastomosis in the neck.

The stomach can also be used as a palliative bypass organ for advanced esophageal carcinoma without resorting to thoracotomy.[44] In such cases, the stomach is brought superiorly through an anterior or posterior

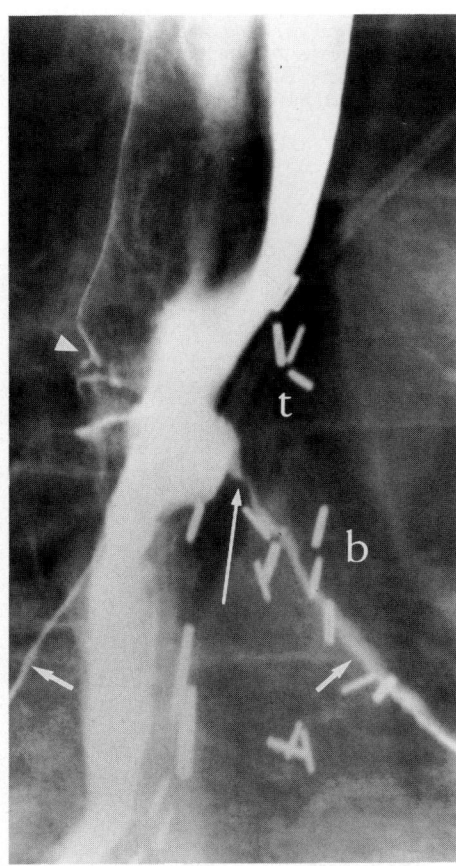

**Figure 33–16. Esophagogastrectomy with a delayed tracheo-esophageal fistula due to mediastinal irradiation.** A tracheoesophageal fistula *(long arrow)* is seen arising at the esophagogastric anastomosis *(arrowhead).* Barium flows into the left and right main bronchi *(short arrows).* There was no evidence of tumor at the anastomosis or in the mediastinum demonstrated by endoscopy or computed tomography. b = left main bronchus; t = air-filled trachea.

mediastinal tunnel into the neck via a transabdominal, transhiatal approach. The fundus is then anastomosed to the pharynx or cervical esophagus. The diseased esophagus may be either resected or excluded. If the stomach has been placed substernally, the medial portion of the clavicle, sternoclavicular joint, and upper portion of the manubrium may also be resected to provide increased space at the thoracic inlet. The major complications of these procedures include tracheobronchial aspiration and anastomotic leak with subsequent stricture formation.[44]

## Colonic Interposition, Jejunal Interposition, and Free Jejunal Graft

Various segments of the colon and jejunum may be used to bypass severe peptic strictures, caustic strictures, or inoperable esophageal cancers. When colonic interposition is performed, the right or transverse colon is placed in an isoperistaltic direction (Fig. 33–17), whereas the left colon is placed in either an isoperistaltic or an antiperistaltic direction.[45] If the colon is placed in the anterior mediastinum, the cologastric anastomosis is usually located on the anterior wall of the stomach.[45] If the colon is placed in the posterior mediastinum, however, the cologastric anastomosis is located on the posterior wall of the upper stomach.[45] A vagotomy and pyloroplasty are also performed. A preoperative barium enema should be performed to rule out significant colonic disease before surgery. A preoperative angiogram should also be obtained to demonstrate the vascular anatomy of the colon and to rule out vascular disease, particularly in patients with suspected atherosclerosis.[46]

Colonic interposition has much higher morbidity and mortality rates than esophagogastrectomy. Anastomotic leaks occur in about 25 to 40% of patients.[46, 47] They are usually located at the proximal anastomosis, leading to abscess and stricture formation[46, 47] (Fig. 33–18). Other postoperative complications include anastomotic edema and obstruction, chylothorax, mediastinal hematoma or abscess, empyema, and intra-abdominal abscess.[46] Ischemia of the transposed colon may be manifested radiographically by spasm, ulceration, loss of haustration, or a nodular mucosa.[47] Occasionally, during the early postoperative period, the mucosal folds in the interposed transverse colon may resemble jejunal folds, but this finding disappears after 1 to 3 months.[45]

Stricture formation at the proximal anastomosis is the most common late postoperative complication, occurring in 20 to 40% of patients[45–47] (see Fig. 33–18). The transposed colon may also become dilated and redundant, leading to the development of delayed graft emptying with bloating, pain, and dysphagia. Other late complications include diverticulitis or carcinoma of the transposed colon, coloesophageal reflux, colobronchial fistulas, gastric outlet obstruction, and small bowel obstruction within the transverse mesocolon defect created at the time of surgery.[48]

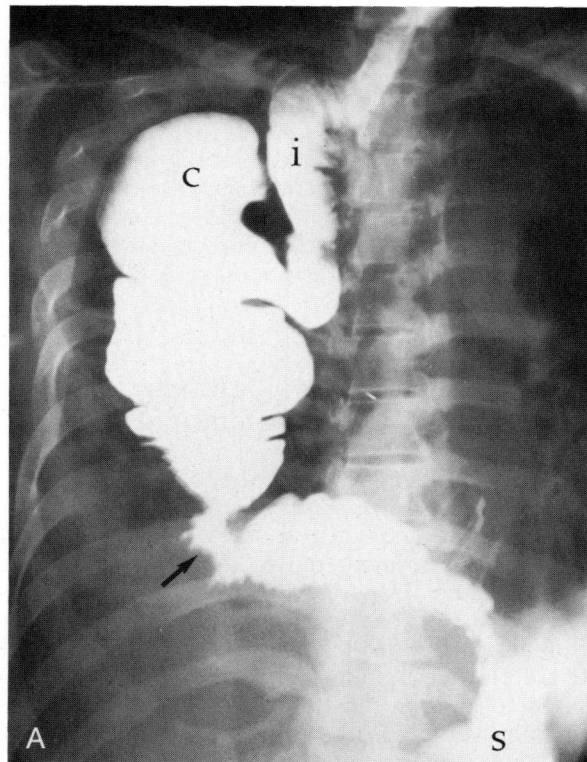

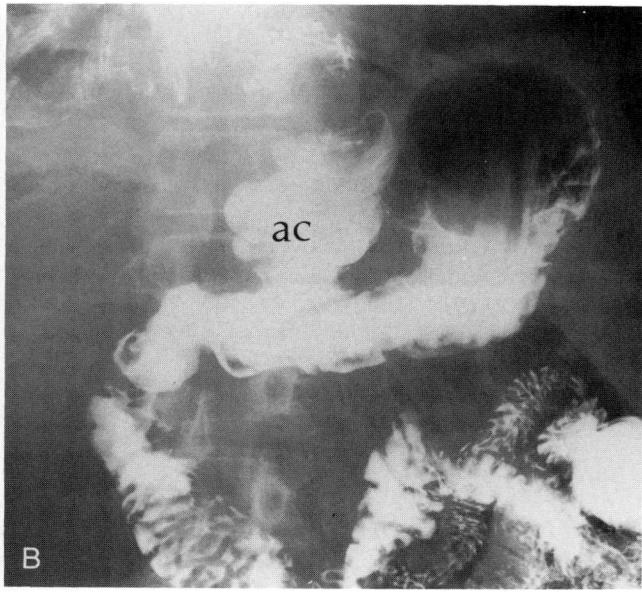

**Figure 33–17. Normal colonic interposition. A.** There is an isoperistaltic right colonic interposition with anastomosis of the terminal ileum (i) to the cervical esophagus. Mild narrowing of the colon occurs as it passes through the diaphragm *(arrow)*. C = cecum; S = stomach. **B.** The ascending colon (ac) is anastomosed to the lesser curvature of the stomach.

**Figure 33–18. Colonic interposition with stricture formation after an anastomotic leak at the esophagocolonic anastomosis.** A tight stricture *(open arrow)* is present at the anastomosis between the esophagus (E) and the colon (C). A short, blind-ending track *(solid arrow)* is seen at the site of a prior anastomotic leak.

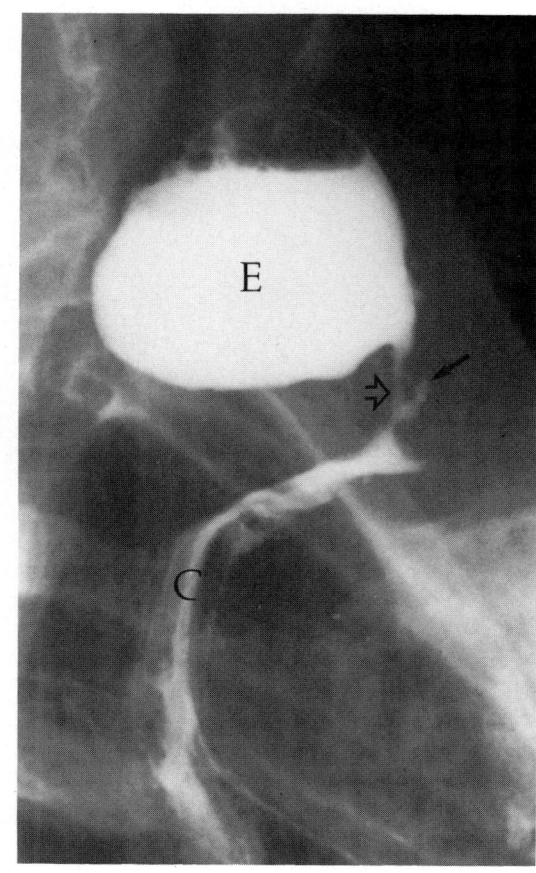

## Palliative Intubation

Palliative esophageal intubation may be performed to allow oral feeding through advanced, obstructive esophageal cancers or to obturate malignant tracheoesophageal fistulas. The Celestin tube is most commonly used. After esophageal bougienage, the tube is positioned by endoscopy or by a combined procedure using endoscopy and a gastrostomy.[49] A study using water-soluble contrast medium is performed after tube placement to evaluate tube position and patency and to rule out esophageal perforation. The Celestin tube should be fixed in position, with its upper tulip-shaped tip proximal to the tumor and its distal tip in the stomach[50] (Fig. 33–19). Contrast medium should flow easily through the lumen of the tube with little, if any, contrast material seen flowing around the outer portion of the tip.[49]

Esophageal perforation is the most serious complication of the use of the Celestin tube. Obstruction of the tube may be caused either by kinking of the tube or by luminal obstruction due to mucosal prolapse, food impaction, or residual or recurrent tumor.[49, 51] In other patients, the tube can migrate proximally above the tumor or distally into the stomach (Fig. 33–20). Reflux of gastric contents through the Celestin tube may lead

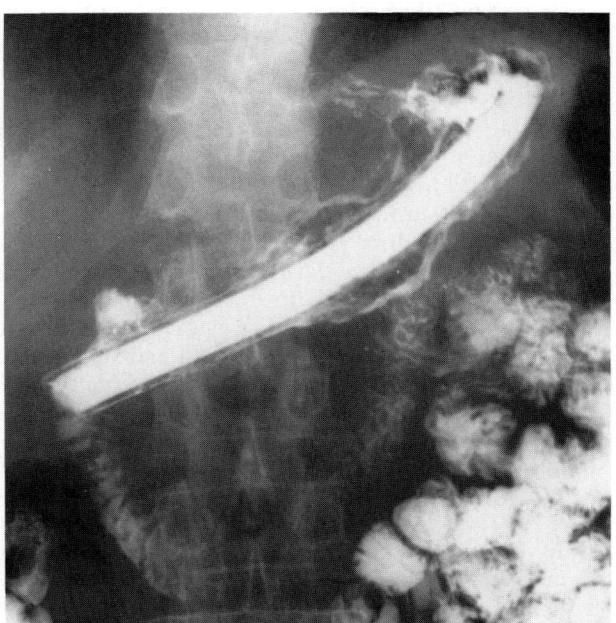

**Figure 33–20. Celestin tube migration.** The entire tube has migrated into the stomach.

to reflux esophagitis or aspiration pneumonia.[52, 53] Rarely, the Celestin tube may cause pressure necrosis of the esophageal wall, resulting in a mediastinal leak or aortoesophageal fistula.

## Laser Therapy

Endoscopic laser therapy is a palliative procedure that provides transient relief from dysphagia in patients with unresectable or obstructive esophageal carcinoma. The intraluminal tumor is coagulated and vaporized, resulting in a widened diameter of the esophageal lumen. This technique allows oral feeding in patients whose average survival after therapy is only 3 to 7 months.[54] Laser therapy has a major advantage over radiation therapy, because no damage occurs to adjacent organs.[55] Furthermore, patients may undergo multiple laser treatments, whereas radiation therapy is limited by the total radiation dose to the mediastinum. Complications of laser therapy include esophageal perforation, tracheoesophageal fistulas, pneumopericardium, and pneumoperitoneum.[54, 55]

## ACHALASIA

Neither medical therapy nor surgery can correct the abnormal esophageal motility and lower esophageal sphincter dysfunction that occur in patients with achalasia. The two major forms of therapy, pneumatic dilatation and cardiomyotomy, are both aimed at improving esophageal emptying by disrupting the high-pressure lower esophageal sphincter.

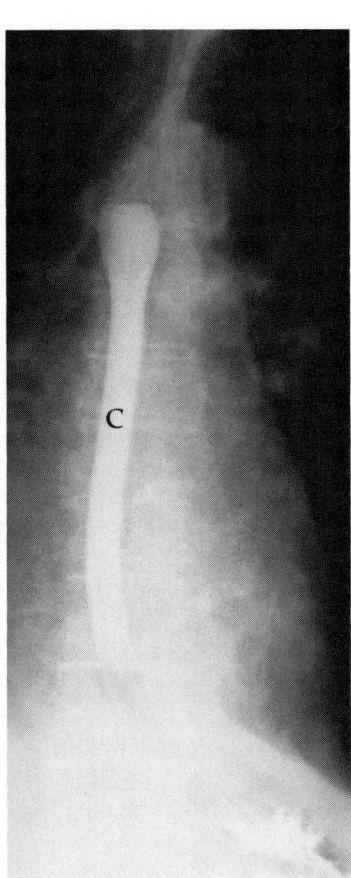

**Figure 33–19. Normal Celestin tube placement.** The Celestin tube (C) filled with contrast medium passes through an obstructive lower esophageal carcinoma into the stomach.

## Pneumatic Dilatation

The most serious complication of pneumatic dilatation is lower esophageal perforation, occurring in 1 to 4% of patients.[56] Although the presence of chest pain or fever after the procedure should suggest this complication, some patients may have clinically silent or delayed perforations.[57] A study using water-soluble contrast medium should therefore be performed after pneumatic dilatation to rule out a perforation, regardless of the patient's symptoms.[58, 59] If no perforation is seen with water-soluble contrast medium, barium should be given to demonstrate greater anatomic detail and subtle leaks. Perforations usually occur on the left posterolateral wall of the distal esophagus just above the diaphragm. Some patients may have small, sealed-off perforations that resemble intramural dissections, whereas others may have free perforations into the mediastinum or pleural space.[60, 61] Increasing symptoms during the early postoperative period may necessitate another esophagram to demonstrate a delayed perforation or a perforation that is not initially visualized because of edema and spasm at the dilatation site. In addition, edema and spasm at the gastroesophageal junction may lead to delayed esophageal emptying despite adequate disruption of the lower esophageal sphincter fibers. Thus, the radiographic appearance immediately after dilatation is also a poor predictor of the efficacy of the procedure.[59]

## Cardiomyotomy

Cardiomyotomy, or Heller myotomy, is an effective form of therapy for patients with untreated achalasia or achalasia that is unresponsive to pneumatic dilatation. The myotomy is performed by surgically dividing the lower esophageal sphincter fibers, thereby disrupting the sphincter. Some surgeons perform a concomitant antireflux procedure. After cardiomyotomy, there should be free flow of contrast medium from the esophagus into the stomach with decreased esophageal dilatation and absence of the beak-like narrowing of the esophagogastric region associated with achalasia.[62] In about 50% of cases, there is eccentric ballooning of the esophagus at the site of Heller myotomy[63] (Fig. 33–21). The most common early postoperative complication is perforation of the distal esophagus. Persistent dysphagia during the late postoperative period may indicate an inadequate myotomy or a tight fundoplication wrap. Conversely, postoperative gastroesophageal reflux, reflux esophagitis, and peptic strictures may indicate the need for an antireflux procedure.

## VARICES

Endoscopic sclerotherapy, transjugular intrahepatic portal-systemic shunts, portal-systemic shunt surgery, and esophageal devascularization procedures are the major forms of therapy for esophageal varices. Endoscopic sclerotherapy is discussed in Chapter 30.

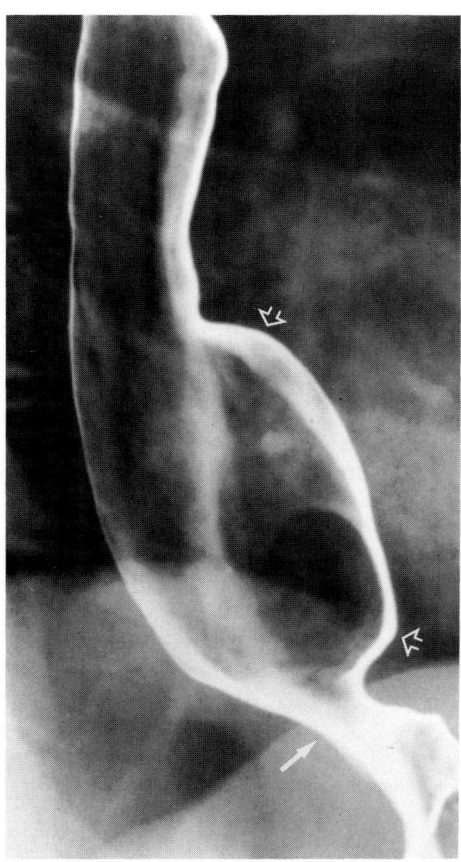

**Figure 33–21. Ballooning of the distal esophagus after cardiomyotomy for achalasia.** There is eccentric outpouching or ballooning of the distal esophageal wall at the cardiomyotomy site *(open arrows).* The gastroesophageal junction *(solid arrow)* is now widely patent.

## Sugiura Procedure

The Sugiura procedure is a popular technique in Japan for surgical devascularization of esophageal varices.[64, 65] Venous collaterals between paraesophageal varices and the wall of the esophagus are ligated from the level of the left inferior pulmonary vein to the esophageal hiatus. The esophagus is then transected at the level of the diaphragm and subsequently reanastomosed. Bridging veins between the abdominal esophagus and proximal stomach as well as the stomach and lesser curvature are also ligated. A splenectomy, selective vagotomy, and pyloroplasty are often performed. The Sugiura procedure does not alter hepatic function or cause hepatic encephalopathy.

A widely patent esophageal lumen should be demonstrated at the transection line after a Sugiura procedure.[66] Varices are found to decrease in size or disappear in more than 90% of patients within several months of surgery. The most common early postoperative complication is suture breakdown, leading to esophageal perforation and mediastinitis.[67] Other patients may develop a hiatal hernia, gastroesophageal reflux, or anastomotic stricture after this procedure.

## Acknowledgment

Figures 33–3 to 33–9, 33–12 to 33–15, and 33–17 to 33–21 are reproduced from Levine MS: Radiology of the Esophagus. Philadelphia: WB Saunders, 1989.

# References

1. Rubesin SE, Levine MS: Postoperative esophagus. *In* Levine MS: Radiology of the Esophagus. Philadelphia: WB Saunders, 1989, pp 267–290.
2. Dodds WJ, Stewart ET, Vlymen WJ: Appropriate contrast media for evaluation of esophageal disruption. Radiology 144:439–441, 1982.
3. Ott DJ, Gelfand DW: Gastrointestinal contrast agents: indications, uses and risks. JAMA 249:2380–2384, 1984.
4. James AE, Montali RJ, Chaffee V, et al: Barium or Gastrografin: which contrast media for diagnosis of esophageal tears. Gastroenterology 68:1103–1113, 1975.
5. Foley MJ, Ghahremani GG, Rogers LF: Reappraisal of contrast media used to detect upper gastrointestinal perforations. Radiology 144:231–237, 1982.
6. Dunbar JS, Skinner GB, Wortzman G, et al: An investigation of effects of opaque media on the lungs with comparison of barium, Lipiodol and Dionosil. AJR 82:902–926, 1959.
7. Reich SB: Production of pulmonary edema by aspiration of water-soluble nonabsorbable contrast media. Radiology 92:367–370, 1969.
8. Chiu CL, Gambach RR: Hypaque pulmonary edema: a case report. Radiology 111:91–92, 1974.
9. Brick SH, Caroline DF, Lev-Toaff AS, et al: Esophageal disruption: evaluation with iohexol esophagography. Radiology 169:141–143, 1988.
10. Bredenburg CE: Gastrointestinal reflux and hiatus hernia. *In* Fromm D (ed): Gastrointestinal Surgery. New York: Churchill Livingstone, 1985, pp 163–205.
11. Nissen R: Gastropexy and "fundoplication" in surgical treatment of hiatal hernia. Am J Dig Dis 6:954–961, 1961.
12. Skinner DB, Belsey RHR: Surgical management of esophageal reflux and hiatus hernia. Long term results with 1030 patients. J Thorac Cardiovasc Surg 53:33–54, 1967.
13. Orringer MB, Skinner DB, Belsey RHR: Long term results of the Mark IV operation for hiatal hernia and analyses of recurrence and their treatment. J Thorac Cardiovasc Surg 63:25–33, 1972.
14. Hill LD: Management of recurrent hiatal hernia. Arch Surg 102:296–302, 1971.
15. Skucas J, Mangla JC, Adams JT, et al: An evaluation of the Nissen fundoplication. Radiology 118:539–543, 1976.
16. Thoeni RF, Moss AA: The radiographic appearance of complications following Nissen fundoplication. Radiology 131:17–21, 1979.
17. Cohen WN: The fundoplication repair of sliding esophageal hiatus hernia: the roentgenographic appearance. AJR 104:625–631, 1968.
18. Feigin DS, James AE, Stitik FP, et al: The radiological appearance of hiatal hernia repairs. Radiology 110:71–77, 1974.
19. Teixidor HS, Evans JA: Roentgenographic appearance of the distal esophagus and the stomach after hiatal hernia repair. AJR 119:245–258, 1973.
20. Demeester TR, Johnson LF, Kent AH: Evaluation of current operations for the prevention of gastroesophageal reflux. Ann Surg 180:511–525, 1974.
21. Polk HC: Fundoplication for reflux esophagitis: misadventures with the operation of choice. Ann Surg 183:645–652, 1976.
22. Saik RP, Greenburg AG, Peskin GW: A study of fundoplication disruption and deformity. Am J Surg 134:19–24, 1977.
23. Hatfield M, Shapir J: The radiologic manifestations of failed antireflux procedures. AJR 144:1209–1214, 1985.
24. Angelchik JP, Cohen R: A new surgical procedure for the treatment of gastroesophageal reflux and hiatal hernia. Surg Gynecol Obstet 148:246–248, 1979.
25. Lewis RA, Angelchik JP, Cohen R: A new surgical prosthesis for hiatal hernia repair. Radiology 135:630, 1980.
26. Peloso OA: Intra-abdominal migration of an antireflux prosthesis. JAMA 248:351–353, 1982.
27. Starling JR, Reichelderfer MO, Pellett JR, et al: Treatment of symptomatic gastroesophageal reflux using Angelchik prosthesis. Ann Surg 195:686–691, 1982.
28. Haney PJ, Gunadi IK, Arnold J, et al: Spontaneous penetration of an antireflux prosthesis into the stomach. Gastrointest Radiol 8:303–305, 1983.
29. Lackey C, Potts J: Penetration into the stomach: a complication of the antireflux prosthesis. JAMA 248:350, 1982.
30. Burhenne LJW, Fratkins LB, Flak B, et al: Radiology of the Angelchik prosthesis for gastroesophageal reflux. AJR 142:507–511, 1984.
31. Curtis DJ, Benjamin SB, Kerr R, et al: Angelchik anti-reflux device: radiographic appearance of complications. Radiology 151:311–313, 1984.
32. London RL, Trotman BW, DiMarino AJ, et al: Dilatation of severe esophageal strictures by inflatable balloon catheter. Gastroenterology 80:173–175, 1981.
33. Owman T, Lunderquist A: Balloon catheter dilatation of esophageal strictures—a preliminary report. Gastrointest Radiol 7:301–305, 1982.
34. Goldthorn JF, Ball WS, Wilkinson LG, et al: Esophageal strictures in children: treatment by serial balloon catheter dilatation. Radiology 153:655–658, 1984.
35. Starck E, Paolucci V, Herzer M, et al: Esophageal stenosis: treatment with balloon catheters. Radiology 153:637–640, 1984.
36. Dawson SL, Mueller PR, Ferrucci JT, et al: Severe esophageal strictures: indications for balloon catheter dilatation. Radiology 153:631–635, 1984.
37. McLean GK, Cooper GS, Hartz WH, et al: Radiologically-guided balloon dilatation of gastrointestinal strictures. Part I—technique and factors influencing procedural success. Radiology 165:35–40, 1987.
38. Meyer JA: Cancer of the esophagus. *In* Fromm D (ed): Gastrointestinal Surgery. New York: Churchill Livingstone, 1985, pp 207–232.
39. Owen JW, Balfe DM, Koehler RE, et al: Radiologic evaluation of complications after esophagogastrectomy. AJR 140:1163–1169, 1983.
40. Agha FP, Orringer MB, Amendola MA: Gastric interposition following transhiatal esophagectomy: radiographic evaluation. Gastrointest Radiol 10:17–24, 1985.
41. Calenoff L, Norfray J: The reconstructed esophagus. AJR 125:864–876, 1975.
42. Heimlich HJ: Esophagoplasty with reversed gastric tube. Am J Surg 123:80–92, 1972.
43. Fetouh SA, Duffner RH, Postlethwait RW, et al: Radiologic aspects of Beck gastric tube in esophageal reconstruction. AJR 129:425–431, 1977.
44. Orringer MB, Sloan H: Substernal gastric bypass of the excluded esophagus for palliation of esophageal carcinoma. J Thorac Cardiovasc Surg 70:836–851, 1975.
45. Agha FP, Orringer MB: Colonic interposition: radiographic evaluation. AJR 142:703–708, 1984.
46. Christensen LR, Shapir J: Radiology of colonic interposition and its associated complications. Gastrointest Radiol 11:233–240, 1986.
47. Larson TC, Shuman LS, Libshitz HI, et al: Complications of colonic interposition. Cancer 56:681–690, 1985.
48. Perlmutter DH, Tapper D, Teele RL, et al: Colobronchial fistula as a late complication of coloesophageal interposition. Gastroenterology 86:1570–1572, 1984.
49. Lipinski JK, Conway SS, Kottler RE, et al: The radiology of oesophageal tubes for malignant strictures. Clin Radiol 33:453–459, 1982.
50. Russell E, Shapiro R, Wilson GL: Radiologic aspects of Celestin tube intubation for incurable obstruction. Radiology 102:531–532, 1972.
51. Giarardet RE, Ransdell HT, Wheat MW: Palliative intubation in the management of esophageal carcinoma. Ann Thorac Surg 18:417–430, 1974.

52. Kairaluoma MI, Kalevi J, Karkola P, et al: Celestin tube palliation of unresectable esophageal carcinoma. J Thorac Cardiovasc Surg 73:783–786, 1977.

53. Haynes JW, Miller PR, Steiger Z, et al: Celestin tube use: radiographic manifestations of associated complications. Radiology 150:41–44, 1984.

54. Wolf EL, Frager J, Brandt LJ, et al: Radiographic appearance of the esophagus and stomach after laser treatment of obstructing carcinoma. AJR 146:519–522, 1986.

55. Fleischer D, Kessler F: Endoscopic Nd:YAG laser therapy for carcinoma of the esophagus: a new form of palliative treatment. Gastroenterology 85:600–606, 1985.

56. Okike N, Payne WS, Neufeld DM, et al: Esophagomyotomy versus forceful dilatation for achalasia of the esophagus: results in 899 patients. Ann Thorac Surg 28:119–125, 1979.

57. Zegel HG, Kressel HY, Levine GM, et al: Delayed perforation after pneumatic dilatation for the treatment of achalasia. Gastrointest Radiol 4:219–221, 1979.

58. Stewart ET, Miller WN, Hogan WJ, et al: Desirability of roentgen esophageal examination immediately after pneumatic dilatation for achalasia. Radiology 130:589–591, 1979.

59. Ott DJ, Wu WC, Gelfand DW, et al: Radiographic evaluation of the achalasic esophagus immediately following pneumatic dilatation. Gastrointest Radiol 9:185–191, 1984.

60. Bradley JL, Han SY: Intramural hematoma (incomplete perforation) of the esophagus associated with esophageal dilatation. Radiology 130:59–62, 1979.

61. Agha FP, Lee HH: The esophagus after endoscopic pneumatic balloon dilatation for achalasia. AJR 146:25–29, 1986.

62. Meyer JA: Nonmalignant disease of the esophagus. *In* Fromm D (ed): Gastrointestinal Surgery. New York: Churchill Livingstone, 1985, pp 113–162.

63. Rubesin SE, Kennedy M, Levine MS, et al: Distal esophageal ballooning following Heller myotomy. Radiology 167:345–347, 1988.

64. Sugiura M, Futagawa S: A new technique for treating esophageal varices. J Thorac Cardiovasc Surg 66:677–685, 1973.

65. Sugiura M, Futagawa S: Further evaluation of the Sugiura procedure in the treatment of esophageal varices. Arch Surg 112:1317–1321, 1977.

66. Greenspan R, Kressel HY, Laufer I, et al: Radiographic findings in the esophagus following the Sugiura procedure. Radiology 144:245–247, 1982.

67. Koyama K, Takagi Y, Ouchi K, et al: Results of esophageal transection for esophageal varices: experience in 100 cases. Am J Surg 139:204–209, 1980.

# Esophagus: Differential Diagnosis

## Marc S. Levine, M.D.

**TABLE 34–1. ULCERATION**

**TABLE 34–2. MUCOSAL NODULARITY**

**TABLE 34–3. SOLITARY MASS LESIONS**

**TABLE 34–4. MULTIPLE SUBMUCOSAL MASSES**

**TABLE 34–5. THICKENED FOLDS**

**TABLE 34–6. STRICTURES**

---

### TABLE 34–1. ULCERATION*

| Cause | Radiographic Findings | Distribution | Comments |
|---|---|---|---|
| **Common** | | | |
| Reflux esophagitis | Shallow, punctate, or linear ulcers; deep ulcers less common | Distal | Reflux symptoms, hiatal hernia, and/or gastroesophageal reflux |
| *Candida* esophagitis | Ulcers associated with diffuse plaque formation (i.e., "shaggy" esophagus) | Variable | Odynophagia in immunocompromised (usually AIDS) patients |
| Herpes esophagitis | Discrete, superficial ulcers | Middle or distal | Odynophagia in immunocompromised patients; occasionally in healthy patients |
| Drug-induced esophagitis | Discrete, superficial ulcers; occasionally giant, flat ulcers | Midesophagus near aortic arch or left main bronchus | Odynophagia in patients taking oral medications (i.e., doxycycline or tetracycline) |
| **Uncommon** | | | |
| Radiation esophagitis | Superficial or deep ulcers | Conform to radiation portal | History of radiation therapy |
| Caustic esophagitis | Superficial or deep ulcers | Variable | History of caustic ingestion |
| Tuberculous esophagitis | Superficial or deep ulcers | Variable | History of pulmonary tuberculosis or AIDS |
| Cytomegalovirus esophagitis | One or more giant, flat ulcers | Variable | AIDS patients |
| HIV esophagitis | One or more giant, flat ulcers | Variable | HIV-positive patients with odynophagia |
| Crohn's disease | Aphthous ulcers | Variable | Advanced Crohn's disease in small bowel or colon |
| Nasogastric intubation | Shallow ulcers or giant, flat ulcers | Distal | History of intubation |
| Alkaline reflux esophagitis | Superficial or deep ulcers | Distal | Total gastrectomy and esophagojejunostomy |
| Behçet's disease | Superficial ulcers | Variable | Oral and genital ulcers and ocular inflammation |
| Epidermolysis bullosa dystrophica | Superficial ulcers or bullae | Variable | Skin disease |
| Benign mucous membrane pemphigoid | Superficial ulcers or bullae | Variable | Skin disease |

*AIDS = acquired immunodeficiency syndrome; HIV = human immunodeficiency virus.

## TABLE 34–2. MUCOSAL NODULARITY

| Cause | Radiographic Findings | Distribution | Comments |
|---|---|---|---|
| **Common** | | | |
| Reflux esophagitis | Nodular or granular mucosa (nodules poorly defined) | Distal one third or one half of thoracic esophagus | Reflux symptoms, hiatal hernia, and/or gastroesophageal reflux |
| *Candida* esophagitis | Discrete plaques | Localized or diffuse | Odynophagia in immunocompromised patients |
| Glycogenic acanthosis | Nodules or plaques | Localized or diffuse | Asymptomatic |
| **Uncommon** | | | |
| Barrett's esophagus | Reticular pattern | Localized | Often adjacent to distal aspect of stricture |
| Superficial spreading carcinoma | Poorly defined, coalescent nodules or plaques | Localized or diffuse | May be asymptomatic |
| Esophageal papillomatosis | Multiple excrescences | Diffuse | Asymptomatic |
| Acanthosis nigricans | Tiny nodules | Diffuse | Skin disease |
| Cowden's disease | Tiny nodules (i.e., hamartomatous polyps) | Diffuse | Hereditary disorder with associated malignant tumors of skin, gastrointestinal tract, and thyroid |
| Leukoplakia | Tiny nodules | Localized or diffuse | Rare |

## TABLE 34–3. SOLITARY MASS LESIONS

| Cause | Radiographic Findings | Distribution | Comments |
|---|---|---|---|
| **Mucosal Lesions** | | | |
| Papilloma | Sessile or slightly lobulated polyp | Variable | Asymptomatic |
| Adenoma | Sessile or pedunculated polyp | Distal | Arises in Barrett's mucosa |
| Inflammatory esophagogastric polyp | Polypoid protuberance with contiguous fold arising near cardia | Distal | Associated reflux esophagitis |
| Carcinoma | Plaque-like, sessile, or polypoid lesion | Variable | Small lesions may be early esophageal cancers |
| **Submucosal Lesions** | | | |
| Leiomyoma | Smooth submucosal mass | Variable | Usually asymptomatic |
| Fibrovascular polyp | Large pedunculated mass with sausage-shaped appearance | Arises in cervical esophagus but extends distally | May be regurgitated into mouth or occlude larynx, causing sudden death |
| Granular cell tumor | Smooth submucosal mass | Usually distal | Associated lesions on skin or tongue |
| Lipoma | Sessile or pedunculated lesion | Variable | Fatty density on computed tomographic scans |
| Hemangioma | Smooth submucosal mass | Variable | Risk of exsanguination |
| Idiopathic varix | Smooth submucosal mass | Variable | Effaced or obliterated with esophageal distention |
| Duplication or retention cysts | One or more submucosal masses | Variable | Asymptomatic |

## TABLE 34–4. MULTIPLE SUBMUCOSAL MASSES

| Cause | Distribution | Comments |
|---|---|---|
| **Benign Lesions** | | |
| Leiomyomas (leiomyomatosis) | Diffuse | Usually asymptomatic |
| Granular cell tumors | Middle or distal | Associated lesions on skin or tongue |
| Hemangiomas | Diffuse | Osler-Weber-Rendu disease |
| Retention cysts (esophagitis cystica) | Distal | Asymptomatic |
| **Malignant Lesions** | | |
| Hematogenous metastases | Middle or distal | Usually malignant melanoma |
| Lymphoma | Diffuse | Usually non-Hodgkin's lymphoma |
| Leukemia | Diffuse | Usually asymptomatic |
| Kaposi's sarcoma | Diffuse | Patients with acquired immunodeficiency syndrome |

## TABLE 34–5. THICKENED FOLDS

| Cause | Radiographic Findings | Distribution | Comments |
|---|---|---|---|
| Varices | Tortuous or serpiginous folds | Uphill: distal Downhill: middle | Effaced or obliterated with esophageal distention; no dysphagia |
| Esophagitis | Smooth, nodular, or scalloped folds | Diffuse | Reflux symptoms or other findings of esophagitis |
| Varicoid carcinoma | Thickened, lobulated folds | Variable | Rigid, fixed appearance at fluoroscopy; dysphagia common |
| Lymphoma | Thickened, lobulated folds | Variable | Usually non-Hodgkin's lymphoma |

## TABLE 34–6. STRICTURES

| Cause | Radiographic Findings | Comments |
|---|---|---|
| **Distal Esophagus** | | |
| Peptic strictures | Symmetric or asymmetric | Associated hiatal hernia |
| Barrett's esophagus | Symmetric or asymmetric (i.e., peptic strictures) | Barrett's mucosa found in 10% of peptic strictures |
| Nasogastric intubation | Long area of narrowing | Rapidly progressive |
| Zollinger-Ellison syndrome | Long area of narrowing | May be initial manifestation of disease |
| Crohn's disease | Short or long | Advanced Crohn's disease in small bowel or colon |
| Alkaline reflux strictures | Short or long | Rapidly progressive; seen after total gastrectomy and esophagojejunostomy |
| Carcinoma (usually adenocarcinoma) | Irregular narrowing with nodularity or ulceration | Arises in Barrett's esophagus; often invades gastric cardia and fundus |
| **Midesophagus** | | |
| Barrett's esophagus | Tapered or ring-like | Hiatal hernia and/or gastroesophageal reflux; adjacent reticular pattern |
| Radiation | Usually tapered | History of radiation therapy |
| Caustic ingestion | Single or multiple; long strictures common | History of caustic ingestion |
| Oral medications | Usually near level of enlarged left atrium | Potassium chloride or quinidine |
| Opportunistic infection (usually candidiasis) | Short or long | History of *Candida* esophagitis |
| Epidermolysis bullosa dystrophica | High strictures or webs | Skin disease |
| Benign mucous membrane pemphigoid | High strictures of webs | Skin disease |
| Eosinophilic esophagitis | Usually tapered | History of allergies and peripheral eosinophilia |
| Chronic graft-versus-host disease | Relatively long | History of marrow transplant |
| Carcinoma (usually squamous cell carcinoma) | Irregular narrowing with nodularity or ulceration | History of smoking and/or alcohol consumption |
| Metastatic tumor | Tapered or irregular narrowing | Usually lung or breast cancer |

# SECTION

# VI

# Stomach and Duodenum

# Peptic Ulcers

Marc S. Levine, M.D.

## INTRODUCTION

Peptic ulcers are thought to occur in about 10% of the adult population in Western countries.[1] The ulcers may be located in the stomach or in the duodenum. Some patients have acute ulcers that heal rapidly with medical therapy, whereas others have chronic ulcers with intermittent relapses and remissions. Peptic ulcers are important not only because of the frequent occurrence of pain or other symptoms but also because of the morbidity and mortality associated with complications such as bleeding and perforation. Although duodenal ulcers are virtually always benign, a small percentage of gastric ulcers are found to be malignant. Thus, gastric ulcers require careful evaluation and follow-up to differentiate benign and malignant lesions.

## EPIDEMIOLOGY

During the late 19th and early 20th centuries, gastric ulcers were much more common than duodenal ulcers.[2] Since that time, there has been a dramatic reversal of this relationship, so that duodenal ulcers are now more common than gastric ulcers.[2] Although duodenal ulcers occur in adults of all ages, gastric ulcers are found predominantly in patients over the age of 40.[1, 2] Regardless of the location of the ulcers, the sex distribution is about equal.[3] Peptic ulcers are thought to be caused by a combination of hereditary and environmental factors. Specific etiologic agents that have been implicated in the development of ulcers include stress, smoking, alcohol, coffee, aspirin, other nonsteroidal anti-inflammatory drugs, and, most recently, *Helicobacter pylori.* However, the precise mechanism of ulcer pathogenesis is uncertain.

## Hereditary Factors

Between 15 and 50% of patients with gastric or duodenal ulcers have a family history of ulcers.[4, 5] This familial aggregation of peptic ulcers is explained primarily by hereditary rather than environmental factors, because studies of twins have found a much greater concordance of ulcers in monozygotic twins than in dizygotic twins.[4] Patients with blood type O also have a higher incidence of ulcers than those with other blood types.[4] Finally, peptic ulcers are more common in patients with genetic syndromes such as multiple endocrine neoplasia type 1, systemic mastocytosis, and tremor-nystagmus-ulcer syndrome.[4] Thus, hereditary factors have clearly been implicated in the development of peptic ulcers.

## Stress

Some investigators believe that emotional stress contributes to the development of peptic ulcers by increasing secretion of peptic acid.[6, 7] However, others have found that stressful life events are no more common in patients with ulcers than in the general population.[8] Thus, the role of stress in the development of peptic ulcers remains uncertain.

## Smoking, Alcohol, and Coffee

Some investigators have found that cigarette smokers are more likely to have ulcers than nonsmokers,[9, 10] but others have found no significant correlation between smoking and peptic ulcers.[11] Although alcohol and coffee are thought to stimulate acid secretion, their role in ulcer pathogenesis is also uncertain.[9]

## Aspirin

Aspirin appears to be a major cause of gastric ulcers, particularly when taken in high doses.[12–15] In one study, gastric ulcers were found in 17% of patients receiving high-dose aspirin therapy for 3 months or longer.[15] It has been shown that salicylates can disrupt the gastric mucosal barrier, permitting back diffusion of hydrogen ions into the mucosa and subsequent mucosal injury.[16] This local effect of aspirin in the pathogenesis of gastric ulcers is supported by the observation that ordinary aspirin tablets are associated with gastric ulcers about four times more frequently than enteric-coated tablets.[15] However, gastric ulcers have also been induced experimentally in cats by intravenous infusion of aspirin.[17] Thus, the development of ulcers may sometimes be mediated by a systemic effect of ingested aspirin. Despite the strong correlation between aspirin and gastric ulcers, this drug does not appear to be related to the development of duodenal ulcers.[12]

## Other Nonsteroidal Anti-inflammatory Drugs

Other nonsteroidal anti-inflammatory drugs such as indomethacin, naproxen, and ibuprofen have also been implicated in the development of gastric ulcers.[18–20] Endoscopic studies of normal volunteers have shown that severe mucosal injury may occur within 24 hours of ingesting these drugs.[18] It has been found experimentally that nonsteroidal anti-inflammatory agents block the formation of cyclooxygenase, an enzyme required for the synthesis of prostaglandins.[20] Because prostaglandins are thought to have cytoprotective properties in the stomach, inhibition of prostaglandin synthesis may lead to mucosal injury. Whatever the explanation, gastric ulcers have been found to occur with increased frequency in patients treated with high doses of nonsteroidal anti-inflammatory drugs.[20]

## Steroids

Some investigators believe that steroids are also an etiologic factor in the development of peptic ulcers, particularly gastric ulcers. This concern often results in discontinuation of steroid therapy in patients with ulcer symptoms or occult gastrointestinal bleeding. In a large double-blind study, however, patients receiving steroids were found to have the same frequency of peptic ulcers as the general population.[21] It is therefore questionable whether steroids have any role in ulcer pathogenesis. Nevertheless, steroids can mask the clinical findings associated with peptic ulcers, so that a large ulcer or even a perforated ulcer may fail to produce symptoms in these patients.

## Helicobacter pylori

*H. pylori* (formerly known as *Campylobacter pylori*) is a gram-negative, spiral-shaped bacillus that was first isolated on endoscopic biopsies in 1983.[22] Since that time, investigators have found that the prevalence of *H. pylori* infection in the stomach ranges from 70 to 95% in patients with chronic antral gastritis.[23] Furthermore, eradication of the organism by antimicrobial therapy usually results in healing of the gastritis.[24] Thus, there is considerable evidence that *H. pylori* has a causal role in the development of antral gastritis (see Chapter 36).

The relationship between *H. pylori* and peptic ulcers is more controversial. Although *H. pylori* infection of the stomach is found in 60 to 80% of patients with gastric ulcers, there is no definite evidence of cause and effect.[24, 25] The relationship between *H. pylori* and duodenal ulcers is also uncertain. Between 85 and 100% of patients with duodenal ulcers have evidence of *H. pylori* gastritis.[24–26] Not infrequently, there is also evidence of gastric metaplasia at the border of the ulcers, with *H. pylori* infection of the metaplastic epithelium.[27] The infected mucosa is thought to be more susceptible to ulceration. As a result, it has been postulated that peptic acid and *H. pylori* have a synergistic effect in the development of duodenal ulcers.[28] A causal role of *H. pylori* is also supported by studies showing that eradication of the organism by bismuth, metronidazole, or other antibiotics results not only in a higher rate of ulcer healing but also in a lower relapse rate.[25, 27] Nevertheless, *H. pylori* is most prevalent in the elderly, whereas duodenal ulcers occur in adults of all ages. Furthermore, hypersecretion of acid can lead to duodenal ulcers in the absence of *H. pylori*, and *H. pylori* gastritis often occurs in the absence of duodenal ulcers.[24] Thus, further investigation is needed to better elucidate the role of *H. pylori* in the development of peptic ulcers.

## PATHOGENESIS AND PATHOPHYSIOLOGY

Although the term *peptic ulcer* encompasses both gastric and duodenal ulcers, clinical and laboratory data suggest that the pathophysiology of these ulcers is related to their site of origin. In general, duodenal ulcers are thought to result from increased secretion of peptic acid, whereas gastric ulcers are thought to result from weakened mucosal resistance in patients who have normal or even decreased acid secretion.

## Duodenal Ulcers

Increased secretion of peptic acid has often been documented in patients with duodenal ulcers.[29–31] These individuals may have not only increased basal secretion of acid but also an increased secretory response to a food stimulus or pentagastrin.[31] It has been postulated that this phenomenon is caused by increased vagal activity, which stimulates secretion of gastrin from the gastric antrum with subsequent parietal cell hyperplasia and increased acid secretion.[30] Gastric hyperacidity may also be related to loss of the normal inhibitory effect of high acid levels in the stomach on gastrin secretion. Whatever the explanation, increased secretion of peptic acid appears to be a major factor in the development of duodenal ulcers.

## Gastric Ulcers

Unlike duodenal ulcers, gastric ulcers are often associated with normal or even decreased secretion of peptic acid.[1, 23] Instead, altered mucosal resistance is thought to be the critical factor in ulcer pathogenesis. The ability of the stomach to resist autodigestion by its own peptic juices is related to the secretion of bicarbonate and a water-insoluble mucous gel, which together constitute the gastric mucosal barrier.[32] In patients with gastric ulcers, the gel structure of this mucosal barrier is significantly weakened.[33] Because prostaglandins have cytoprotective properties that contribute to the integrity of the gastric mucosal barrier, aspirin and other nonsteroidal anti-inflammatory drugs may promote ulcer formation by inhibiting synthesis of prostaglandins.[20]

Other possible factors in the pathogenesis of gastric ulcers include chronic gastritis, duodenogastric reflux of bile, and delayed gastric emptying. Because patients with gastric ulcers often have chronic gastritis in the vicinity of the ulcers, it has been suggested that gastritis is the underlying disease process and that the ulcers occur as a secondary phenomenon.[34] Other investigators have found that patients with gastric ulcers often have an unusually high concentration of bile acids in the stomach, so duodenogastric reflux of bile may be another pathophysiologic factor in the development of these lesions.[35] Finally, Dragstedt found that gastric stasis caused by pyloric stenosis or gastric atony may predispose patients to the development of gastric ulcers by prolonging exposure of the gastric mucosa to acid and pepsin in the stomach.[36] These stasis-induced gastric ulcers have come to be known as *Dragstedt ulcers*.

## CLINICAL FINDINGS

Patients with peptic ulcers usually present with epigastric pain. The pain is often described as a gnawing, aching, or burning discomfort between the xiphoid cartilage and the umbilicus.[37] Ulcer pain also tends to have a rhythmic nature, occurring after meals and at night. Whereas gastric ulcer pain classically occurs less than 2 hours after meals, duodenal ulcer pain occurs 2 to 4 hours after meals and is more likely to waken the patient at night.[37] Nevertheless, there is so much overlap in the timing and quality of the pain that it is difficult to differentiate these ulcers on clinical grounds.

Other patients with peptic ulcers may have right upper quadrant, back, or chest pain or other symptoms such as bloating, belching, nausea, vomiting, anorexia, and weight loss.[37] Depending on the clinical presentation,

the differential diagnosis may include reflux esophagitis, gastritis, duodenitis, cholecystitis, pancreatitis, gastroenteritis, irritable bowel syndrome, ischemic bowel disease, Crohn's disease, and gastric or pancreatic carcinoma.[37]

Still other patients with peptic ulcers may initially present with signs or symptoms caused by complications of their ulcers, such as perforation, obstruction, and bleeding. When ulcers on the posterior wall of the stomach or duodenum penetrate into the pancreas, the normally rhythmic epigastric pain associated with ulcers is replaced by a more constant pain that radiates to the back.[38] In contrast, free perforation of a gastric or duodenal ulcer results in generalized peritonitis with peritoneal guarding and rebound, shock, and prostration. The major factors contributing to mortality resulting from this complication include age over 60 and a delay of more than 24 hours from the time of diagnosis to the time of surgery.[39]

Some ulcers may be associated with considerable edema and spasm or scar formation that results in varying degrees of gastric outlet obstruction, manifested by postprandial nausea and vomiting. Obstructive symptoms are more commonly caused by ulcers in the distal antrum, pyloric channel, or duodenum than by ulcers in the gastric fundus or body. Pyloric channel ulcers are particularly prone to cause vomiting. The latter patients may have a characteristic clinical syndrome (the pyloric channel syndrome), manifested by severe postprandial epigastric pain that is relieved by vomiting.[40, 41]

Upper gastrointestinal bleeding is a serious, potentially life-threatening complication of peptic ulcers. Some patients may have one or more episodes of massive hemorrhage, manifested by hematemesis, melena, or rectal bleeding, whereas others may have chronic, low-grade hemorrhage, manifested by guaiac-positive stool or iron deficiency anemia.[37] Gastric ulcers are more likely to bleed than duodenal ulcers, probably because of the greater size of the ulcers and greater age of the patients.[37]

The diagnosis of peptic ulcer disease is also complicated by the fact that 25 to 50% of patients with proven gastric or duodenal ulcers are asymptomatic.[37, 42] These lesions may be clinically silent until the development of an acute abdominal catastrophe caused by bleeding or perforation of the ulcer. Conversely, patients with classic ulcer symptoms are not always found to have ulcers on radiologic or endoscopic examinations.[43] Thus, peptic ulcer disease remains a challenging clinical diagnosis.

## TREATMENT

The aim of medical therapy for peptic ulcers is to relieve ulcer symptoms and accelerate ulcer healing by decreasing exposure of the ulcer to peptic acid secretions. In the past, high-dose antacids have been used to neutralize existing acid in the stomach and duodenum. More recently, $H_2$ receptor antagonists such as cimetidine and ranitidine have proved to be extremely effective in accelerating healing of both gastric and duodenal ulcers by suppressing acid secretion.[23] Because peptic ulcers tend to recur, some patients may benefit from low-dose maintenance therapy with these drugs to decrease the likelihood of recurrent ulcers. Omeprazole is even more effective than H$_2$ blockers in suppressing acid secretion and accelerating ulcer healing by selectively inhibiting the gastric proton pump that controls the first step in the production of gastric acid.[44, 45]

Because of their cytoprotective properties in the stomach, prostaglandins may also have a role in the treatment of gastric ulcers. Misoprostol, a synthetic prostaglandin analogue, has been shown to be effective in accelerating ulcer healing.[46] Exogenous administration of prostaglandins to patients receiving aspirin or other nonsteroidal anti-inflammatory drugs also seems to prevent the development of gastric ulcers in these individuals.[47] Sucralfate, colloidal bismuth, and carbenoxolone are other drugs that have been used with varying degrees of success in the treatment of gastric ulcers.

Surgical intervention may ultimately be required for recurrent or intractable ulcers that fail to heal with medical therapy or for ulcer complications such as bleeding and perforation. The most common operations include partial gastrectomy, vagotomy and pyloroplasty, and hyperselective vagotomy. These surgical procedures and their complications are discussed in Chapter 41. Because of better diagnosis and medical treatment of peptic ulcer disease, the need for surgery in these patients has decreased dramatically during the past 30 years.[48, 49] Nevertheless, it is often a lifelong disease with periodic exacerbations and remissions, so long-term treatment may be required.[50]

# RADIOGRAPHIC FINDINGS

## Gastric Ulcers

### Examination Technique

The double contrast examination should be performed as a biphasic study that includes double contrast views of the stomach with a high-density barium suspension and prone or upright compression views with a low-density barium suspension (see Chapter 19). Ulcer detection is facilitated by the routine administration of 0.1 mg of glucagon intravenously to induce gastric hypotonia. Ulcers located on the posterior wall or on the lesser or greater curvature of the stomach are usually well seen on double contrast radiographs obtained in supine or oblique projections. However, some ulcers may not be detected if mucosal coating by the high-density barium is inadequate. Depending on the quality of coating, additional rotation of the patient may be required to improve mucosal coating and demonstrate these lesions.

Flow technique can be used to better delineate shallow ulcers on the posterior wall or lesser curvature[51] (Fig. 35–1). By slowly rotating the patient from side to side, it is possible to manipulate the barium pool so that a thin layer of high-density barium gradually flows across the dependent surface of the stomach. This technique is particularly helpful for demonstrating ulcers high on the lesser curvature near the gastric cardia.[51]

Upright compression views are also helpful for evaluating ulcers on the lesser curvature. With the patient in an upright position, the weight of the barium tends to pull the antrum inferiorly and straighten the lesser curvature. As a result, these views are often ideal for assessing features of benign ulcer disease, such as the depth of penetration and the presence of Hampton's line.[52] In patients with a high transverse stomach, the use of prone, right anterior oblique views with 15 to 45 degrees of cephalic tube angulation has also been advocated for demonstrating lesser curvature ulcers that are sometimes missed on the routine examination.[53]

Because of the effects of gravity, ulcers on the nondependent or anterior wall of the stomach may not be filled with barium on double contrast radiographs obtained in the usual supine or oblique projections (Fig. 35–2A). Prone compression views of the gastric antrum and body should therefore be obtained routinely to demonstrate ulcers on the anterior wall (Fig. 35–2B). When ulcers or other lesions are suspected in this location, double contrast views of the anterior wall can also be obtained by placing the patient in a prone Trendelenburg position.[54]

### Shape

Gastric ulcers appear classically as round or ovoid collections of barium (see Figs. 35–1B and 35–2B). However, ulcer craters may have a variety of shapes, appearing as linear, rod-shaped, rectangular, serpiginous, or flame-shaped lesions[55–58] (Fig. 35–3). Linear ulcers constitute about 5% of all gastric ulcers diagnosed on double contrast studies.[57] These linear ulcers probably represent a stage of ulcer healing both in the stomach and in the duodenum.[57, 58]

### Size

The radiographic sensitivity in diagnosing gastric ulcers is related primarily to ulcer size; ulcers greater than 5 mm in size are more likely to be detected on barium studies.[59] However, a major advantage of double contrast technique is its ability to distend the stomach and efface the normal mucosal folds to delineate small ulcers (Fig. 35–4). As a result, the majority of gastric ulcers diagnosed on double contrast studies are less than 1 cm in size.[58] The increasing prevalence of small ulcers may also be related to the aggressive medical treatment these patients often receive before undergoing radiologic investigations.

Large ulcers tend to be located more proximally in the stomach[60] (Fig. 35–5). Occasionally, these ulcers may be recognized on abdominal plain films by the presence of gas in the ulcer crater. Giant gastric ulcers (ulcers greater than 3 cm in size) have a higher risk of complications such as bleeding and perforation.[61] However, the majority of giant ulcers are found to be benign.[61] Thus, the size of the ulcer has no relationship to the presence of carcinoma.

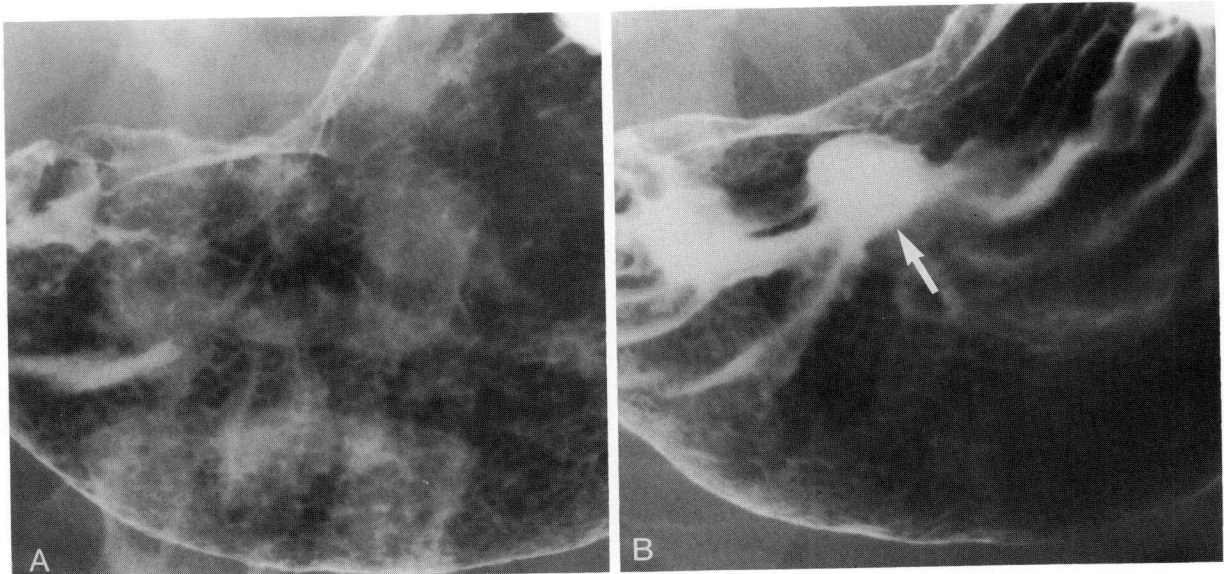

**Figure 35–1. Importance of flow technique for posterior wall ulcers. A**. The initial supine film shows no evidence of an ulcer, even in retrospect. **B**. With flow technique, however, an ulcer *(arrow)* is seen on the posterior wall of the antrum. Note how folds radiate to the edge of the ulcer crater.

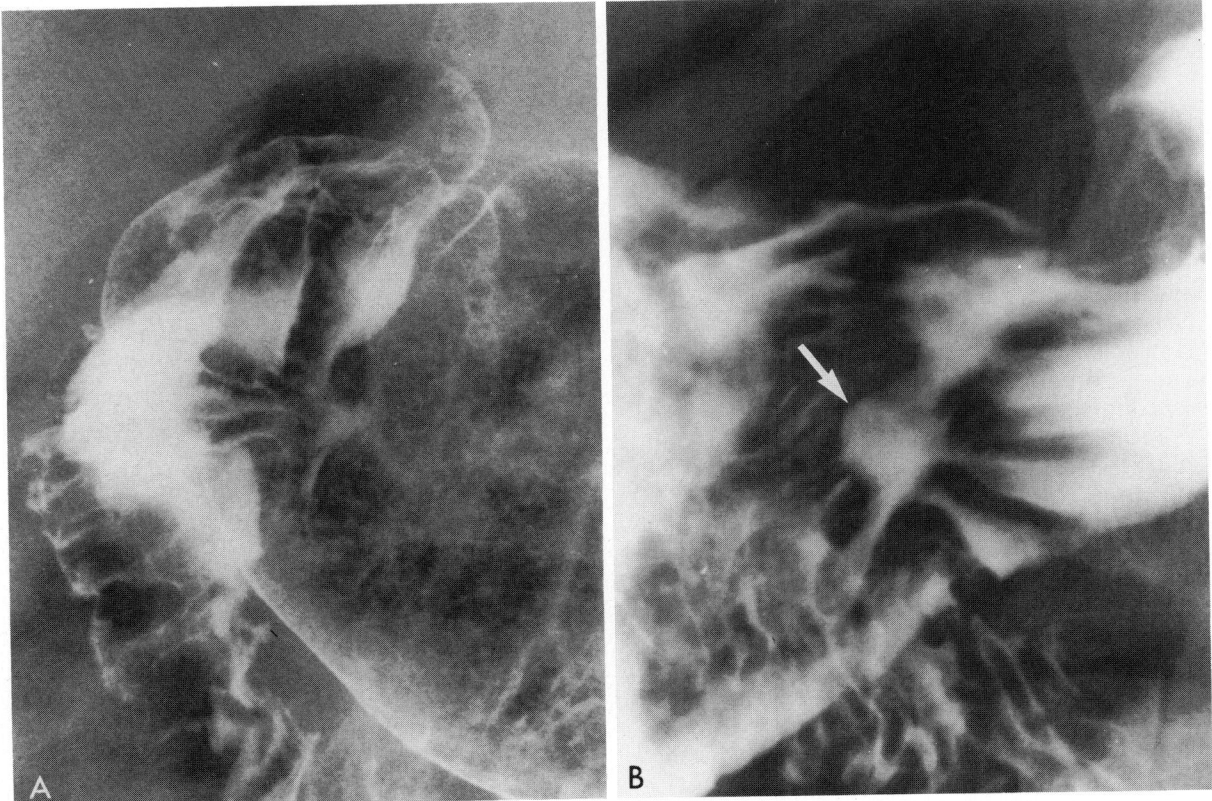

**Figure 35–2. Importance of prone compression for anterior wall ulcers. A**. The initial supine film shows abnormal folds in the antrum without a definite ulcer. **B**. However, a prone compression view shows filling of an anterior wall ulcer *(arrow)*. Note how folds radiate to the edge of the ulcer crater.

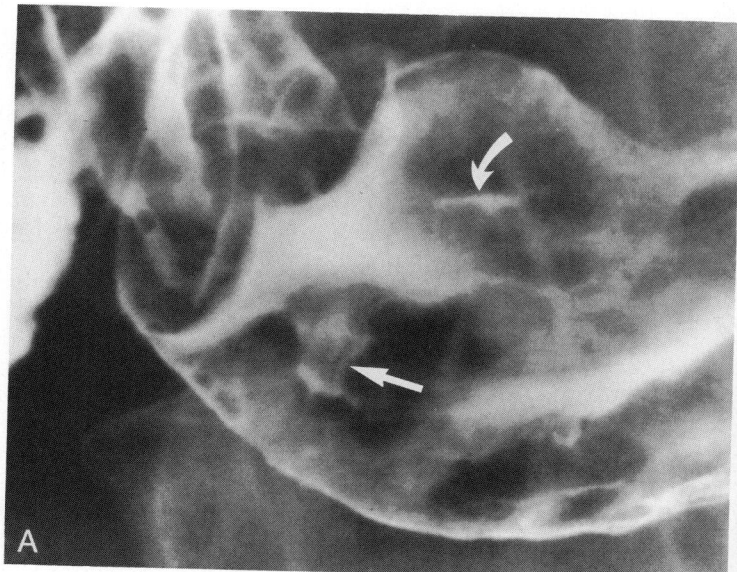

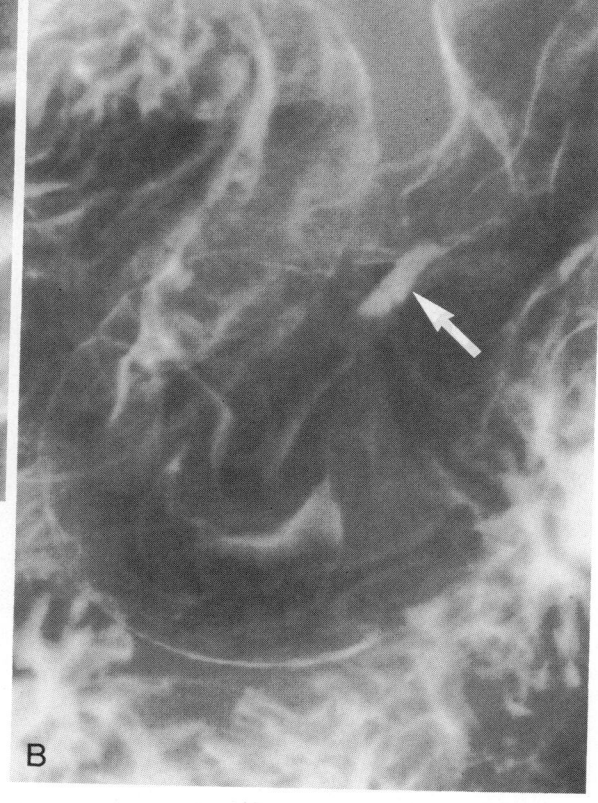

**Figure 35–3. Gastric ulcers of different shapes. A**. This patient has star-shaped *(straight arrow)* and linear *(curved arrow)* ulcers in the antrum. **B**. In another patient, a rod-shaped ulcer *(arrow)* is seen in the stomach.

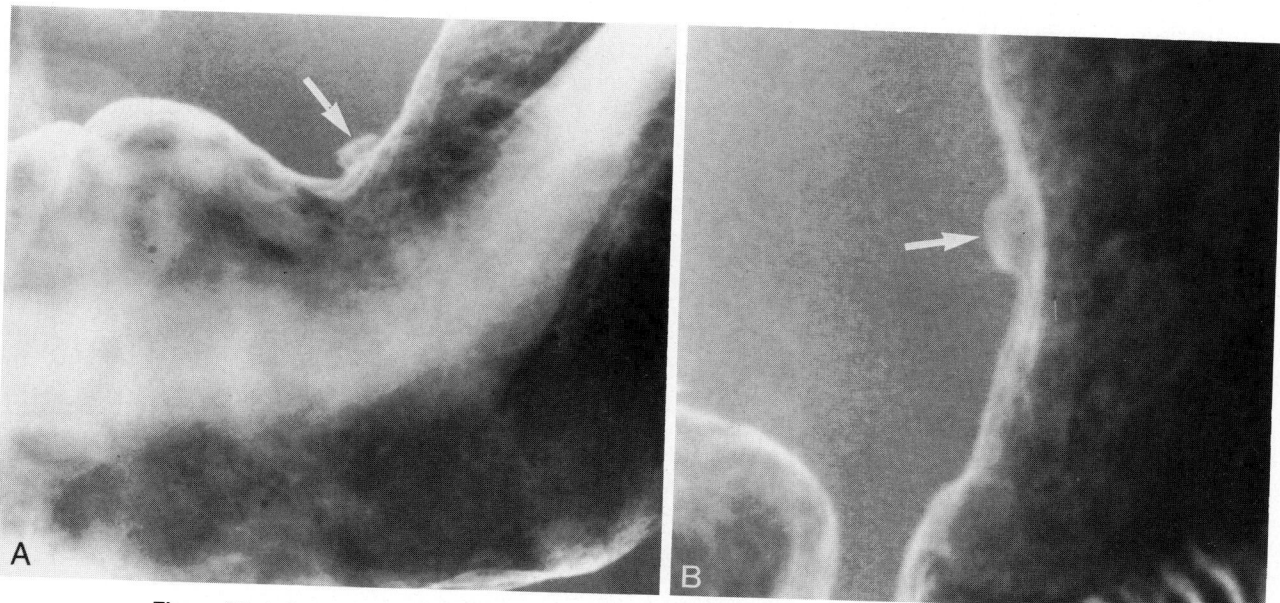

**Figure 35–4. Small gastric ulcers (A and B)**. Despite their small size, these lesser curvature ulcers *(arrows)* are well seen on double contrast radiographs.

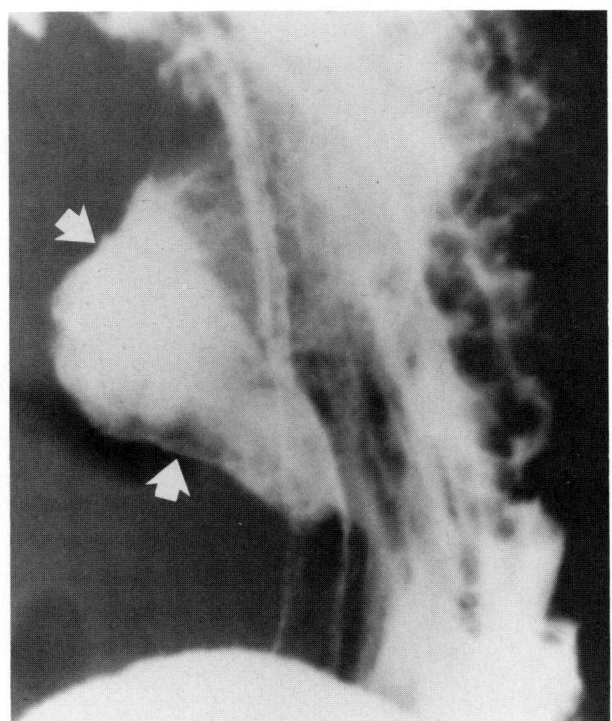

**Figure 35–5. Giant gastric ulcer.** A giant ulcer *(arrows)* is seen projecting from the lesser curvature of the gastric body. Large ulcers tend to be located more proximally in the stomach.

## Location

Most gastric ulcers are located on the lesser curvature or posterior wall of the antrum or body of the stomach.[58, 60, 62, 63] In various studies, only 1 to 7% of gastric ulcers are located on the anterior wall and 3 to 11% on the greater curvature.[58, 60, 62, 64] In younger patients, ulcers tend to occur in the distal part of the stomach, whereas in older patients, they tend to be located more proximally in the stomach, particularly on the lesser curvature.[65, 66] The latter ulcers have been described as "geriatric ulcers."[65] Thus, the distribution of gastric ulcers is influenced by the age of the patients being studied.

Benign greater curvature ulcers are almost always located in the distal half of the stomach.[58, 64, 67] The vast majority are caused by ingestion of aspirin or other nonsteroidal anti-inflammatory drugs.[58, 67] Benign gastric ulcers are much less common in the fundus than in the antrum or body of the stomach and are rarely found on the proximal half of the greater curvature.[58, 64] Thus, any ulcer in this location should be considered malignant until proved otherwise. Except for these ulcers high on the greater curvature, the location of the ulcer has no relationship to the presence of carcinoma.

Gastric ulcers are occasionally found in hiatal hernias.[68] They tend to occur on the lesser curvature aspect of the hernia, where the hernial sac is compressed by the esophageal hiatus of the diaphragm.[68] Because the hernia is inaccessible to palpation, double contrast tech-

nique is particularly helpful for demonstrating these ulcers.

## Morphologic Features

Ulcers on the lesser or greater curvature are readily visualized in profile on barium studies, permitting analysis of the size, shape, and depth of the ulcer crater as well as associated findings such as radiating folds, Hampton's line, or an ulcer mound or collar. However, ulcers on the anterior or posterior wall may be difficult or impossible to visualize in profile, so these lesions must be evaluated on the basis of their en face appearance. In such cases, double contrast technique is particularly helpful in assessing the surrounding mucosa for signs of benign or malignant disease.

### Lesser Curvature Ulcers

Ulcers on the lesser curvature typically appear as smooth, round or ovoid craters that project beyond the contour of the adjacent gastric wall[52, 58, 69] (Fig. 35–6; see Fig. 35–4). However, some ulcers may have a "collar button" or "mushroom" appearance in which the base of the ulcer is wider than the neck.[52] Other ulcers may be associated with Hampton's line as a result of undermining of the mucosa surrounding the orifice of the crater. Hampton's line is often best seen on upright compression views of the lesser curvature as a thin, barely perceptible radiolucent line that separates barium in the ulcer crater from barium in the gastric lumen.[52, 69] Although this finding is virtually pathognomonic of a benign ulcer, it is detected radiographically in only a small percentage of patients with lesser curvature ulcers. Occasionally, the rim of undermined mucosa surrounding the orifice of the crater may become more edematous, producing a wide, radiolucent band or ulcer collar[52] (see Fig. 35–6B). Still other ulcers may be associated with enough inflammation and edema to produce an ulcer mound that is seen in profile as a smooth, bilobed hemispheric mass projecting into the lumen on both sides of the ulcer.[52] Ulcer mounds usually have poorly defined outer borders that form obtuse, gently sloping angles with the adjacent gastric wall.[52] Hampton's lines, ulcer collars, and ulcer mounds are all considered to be classic features of benign gastric ulcers.

Retraction of the gastric wall adjacent to lesser curvature ulcers sometimes leads to the development of smooth, symmetric folds that radiate to the edge of the ulcer crater[58] (see Fig. 35–6A). Occasionally, these ulcers may be associated with retraction of the opposite wall, producing an incisura on the greater curvature. Other lesser curvature ulcers may be associated with enlarged areae gastricae because of inflammation and edema of the surrounding mucosa[58] (see Fig. 35–6A).

### Greater Curvature Ulcers

In the past, almost all ulcers on the greater curvature of the stomach were thought to be malignant.[70] It is now recognized that benign ulcers may occur on the distal

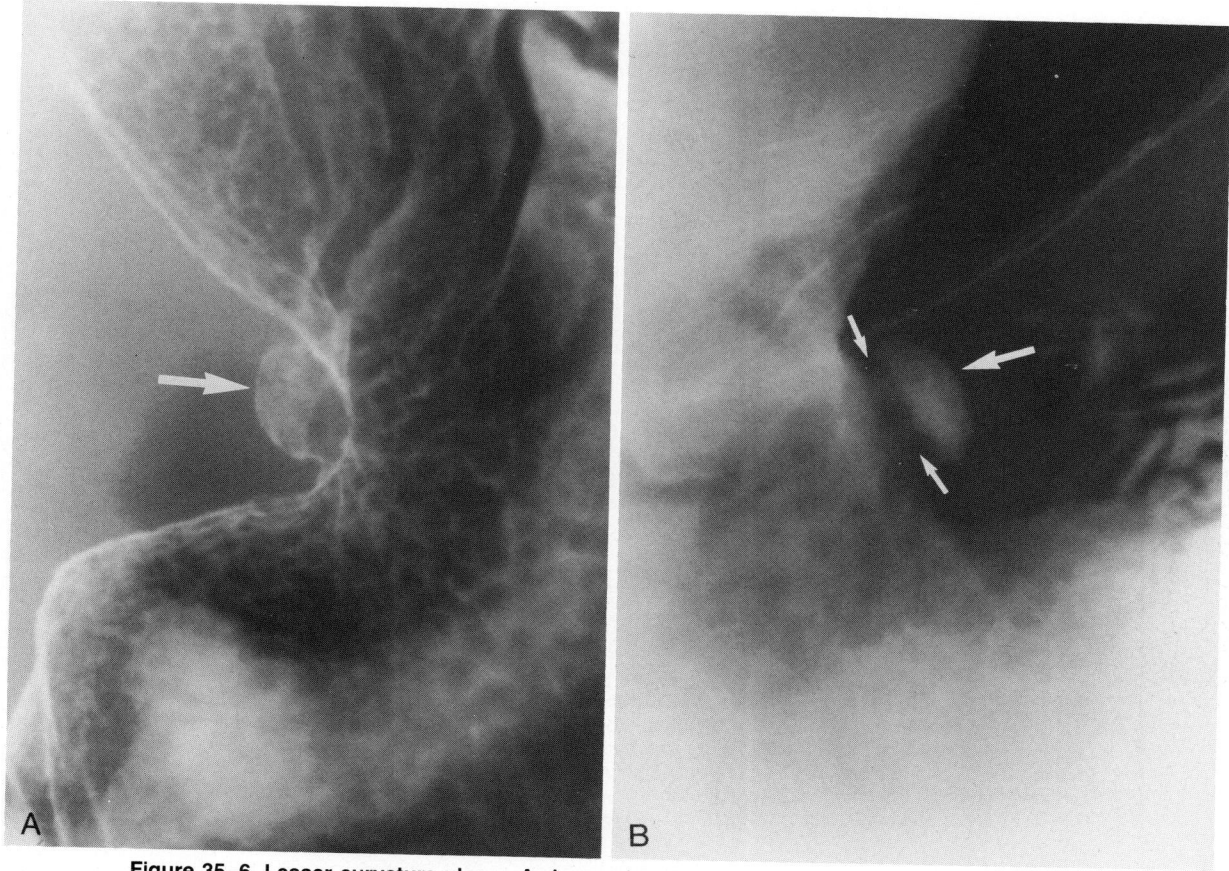

**Figure 35–6. Lesser curvature ulcers. A**. A smooth, round ulcer *(arrow)* is seen projecting beyond the lesser curvature. The radiating folds and enlarged areae gastricae in the adjacent mucosa are due to associated inflammation and edema. (From Levine MS, Creteur V, Kressel HY, et al: Benign gastric ulcers: diagnosis and follow-up with double contrast radiography. Radiology 164:9–13, 1987.) **B**. In another patient, a lesser curvature ulcer *(large arrow)* is demonstrated on a prone compression view. Note the radiolucent band of edema or ulcer collar *(small arrows)* adjacent to the ulcer. Both of these cases demonstrate classic features of benign gastric ulcers.

half of the greater curvature, particularly in patients who have ingested aspirin or other nonsteroidal anti-inflammatory drugs[58, 67] (Figs. 35–7 and 35–8). It has been postulated that these ulcers result from localized mucosal injury as the dissolving aspirin tablets collect by gravity in the most dependent portion of the stomach. Because of their typical location on the greater curvature, these lesions have been described as "sump ulcers."[67] This phenomenon may also account for the frequent finding of linear or serpiginous aspirin-induced erosions on or near the greater curvature (see Chapter 36).[71] Because of their location, greater curvature ulcers have a tendency to penetrate inferiorly into the gastrocolic ligament, occasionally leading to the development of a gastrocolic fistula (see later section on fistulas).

Unlike ulcers on the lesser curvature, greater curvature ulcers often appear to have an intraluminal location because of circular muscle spasm and retraction of the adjacent gastric wall[72] (see Fig. 35–8A). Greater curvature ulcers also tend to be associated with a considerable mass effect and thickened, irregular folds due to marked edema and inflammation surrounding the ulcer[58, 72] (see

Fig. 35–8). Occasionally, the inner margin of the ulcer may be concave toward the lumen because of a large mass of overhanging, edematous tissue, producing the "quarter moon" or "crescent" sign.[52, 73] This edematous tissue may partially occlude the orifice of the crater, leading to incomplete filling of the ulcer.[73] Because of these morphologic features, benign greater curvature ulcers often have a suspicious radiographic appearance, so the usual criteria for differentiating benign and malignant ulcers elsewhere in the stomach are unreliable for ulcers in this location.[58, 72] Thus, endoscopy and biopsy may be required for some greater curvature ulcers despite a history of aspirin ingestion.

### Posterior Wall Ulcers

An ulcer on the dependent or posterior wall of the gastric antrum or body may fill with barium, producing the conventional appearance of an ulcer crater (Fig. 35–9; see Fig. 35–1B). However, shallow ulcers on the posterior wall may be coated by only a thin layer of barium, producing a ring shadow on double contrast

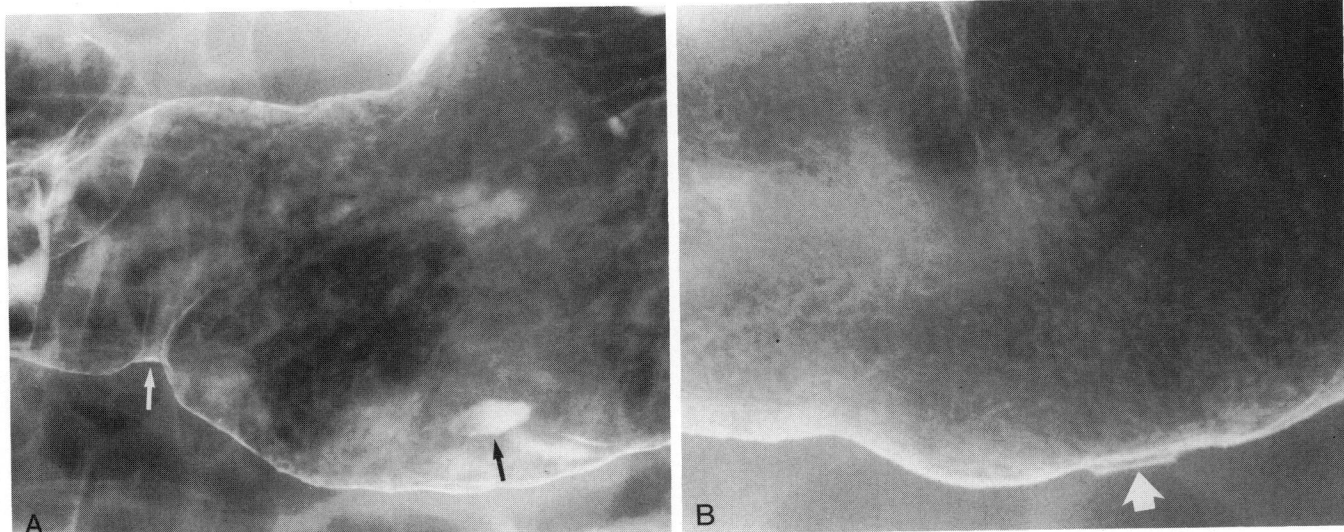

**Figure 35–7. Greater curvature ulcers caused by aspirin and indomethacin. A**. A small aspirin-induced ulcer *(black arrow)* is seen in the gastric body adjacent to the greater curvature. An area of scarring seen more distally on the greater curvature *(white arrow)* is due to a healed ulcer in this location. **B**. In another patient, an extremely shallow ulcer *(arrow)* is seen on the greater curvature due to ingestion of indomethacin. Note the absence of radiating folds or other signs of ulcer disease. This ulcer could easily be missed without optimal radiographic technique.

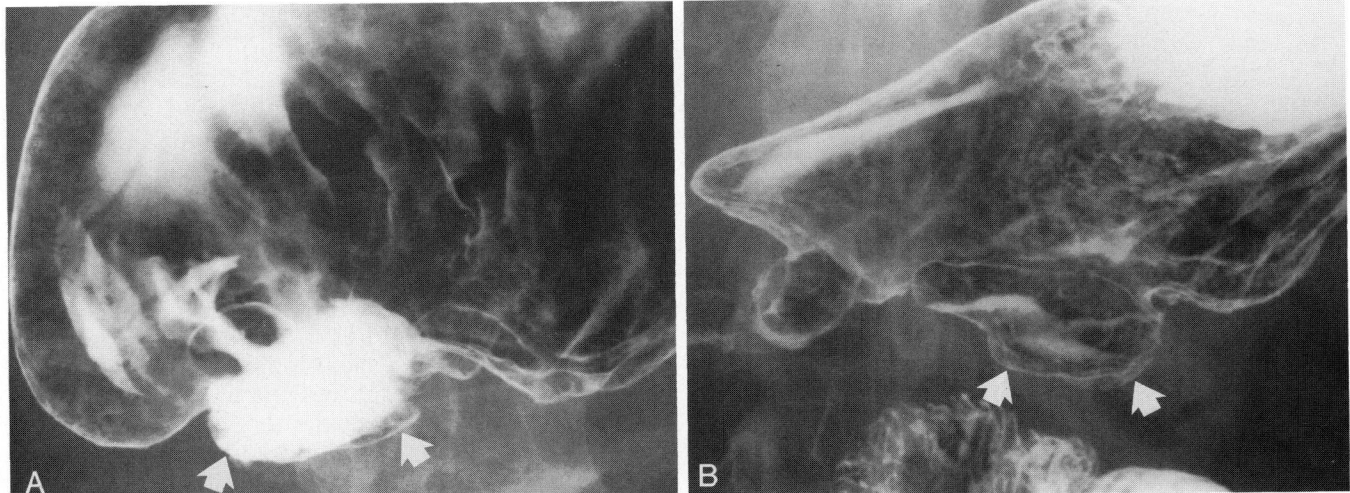

**Figure 35–8. Giant greater curvature ulcers caused by aspirin. A**. This large ulcer *(arrows)* on the greater curvature has an apparent intraluminal location and is associated with thickened, irregular folds and considerable mass effect from an adjacent mound of edema. **B**. In another patient, thickened, irregular folds are seen abutting a large greater curvature ulcer *(arrows)*. In both cases, endoscopic biopsies revealed no evidence of tumor, and follow-up studies after treatment with $H_2$ blockers showed complete healing of the ulcers. Both patients had taken high doses of aspirin.

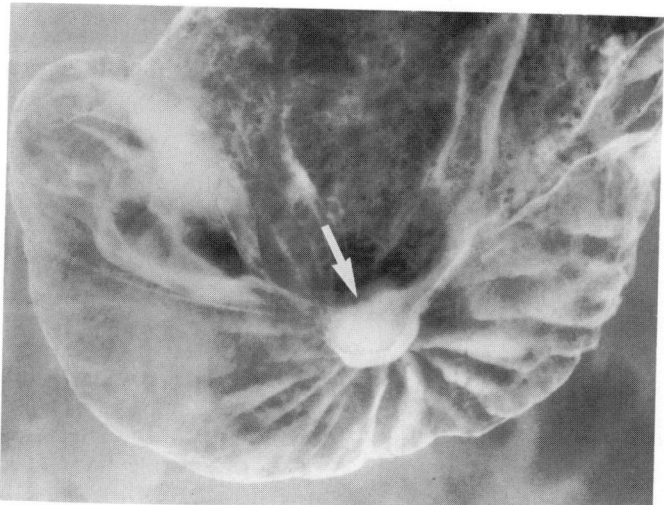

**Figure 35–9. Posterior wall ulcer.** A large ulcer *(arrow)* is present on the posterior wall of the stomach. Multiple folds are seen radiating to the edge of the ulcer crater.

are enlarged or distorted in the region of the ulcer because of inflammation and edema of the adjacent mucosa.[58] An ulcer collar or mound may also be seen en face as a radiolucent halo representing a rim of edematous tissue surrounding the ulcer. Because the ulcer mound gradually decreases in thickness until it merges with the gastric wall, it usually has poorly defined outer borders that fade peripherally into the adjacent mucosa. Posterior wall ulcers may also be associated with a spectacular collection of folds that radiate to the edge of the ulcer crater or adjacent edematous mound.[58] Occasionally, the edema and spasm associated with antral ulcers may cause such severe narrowing and deformity of the distal stomach that it is difficult to evaluate these ulcers by the usual radiologic criteria (Fig. 35–11).

### Anterior Wall Ulcers

An ulcer on the nondependent or anterior wall of the gastric antrum or body may also appear as a ring shadow because of barium coating the rim of the unfilled ulcer crater tangential to the central beam of the x-ray[74] (Fig. 35–12A). In such cases, the ulcer may be demonstrated by turning the patient 180 degrees to the prone position, so that the ulcer is located on the dependent wall and fills with barium (Fig. 35–12B). Prone compression views of the stomach with low-density barium should therefore be obtained routinely to demonstrate these

studies (Fig. 35–10A). In such cases, the use of flow technique to manipulate the barium pool over the surface of the ulcer should result in filling of the ulcer crater[51] (Fig. 35–10B). It is important not only to determine the size and shape of these posterior wall ulcers but also to assess the en face appearance of the surrounding mucosa. Not infrequently, the areae gastricae

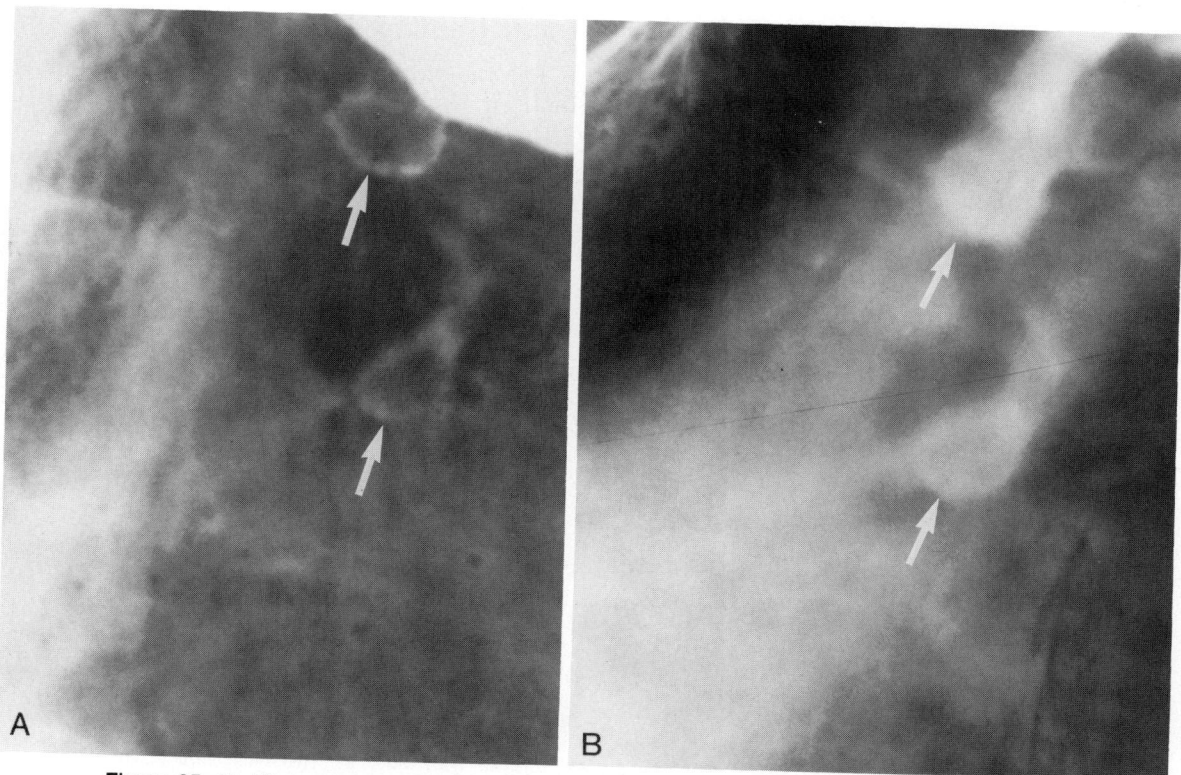

**Figure 35–10. Ring shadows caused by shallow posterior wall ulcers. A.** The initial supine film shows two discrete ring shadows *(arrows)* in the upper body of the stomach where barium coats the rim of shallow, unfilled ulcers on the posterior wall. **B.** The use of flow technique to manipulate the barium pool over the surface of the ulcers results in filling of the craters *(arrows)*.

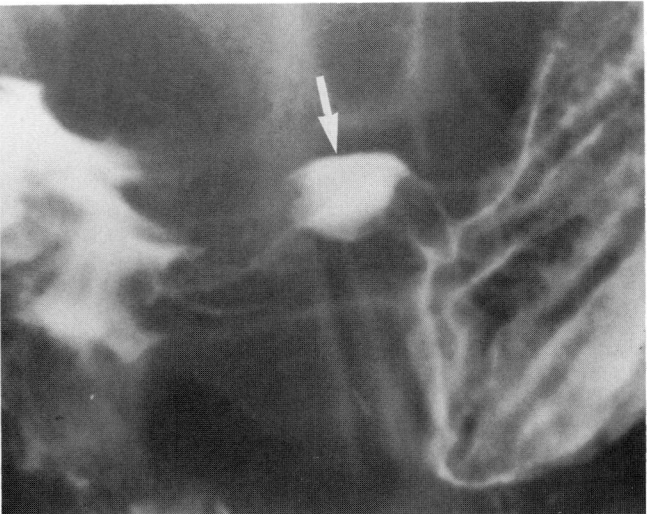

**Figure 35–11. Antral ulcer associated with marked edema and spasm.** A large ulcer _(arrow)_ is seen in the gastric antrum. This ulcer is difficult to evaluate by the usual radiologic criteria because of antral narrowing and deformity due to edema and spasm accompanying the ulcer.

lesions. Double contrast views of the anterior wall may also be helpful in patients with suspected ulcers in this location (see earlier section on examination technique).

## Multiplicity

The frequency of multiple ulcers on conventional single contrast barium studies has ranged from 2 to 8%.[75, 76] With double contrast technique, however, multiple ulcers have been detected in about 20% of patients

with ulcers or ulcer scars.[77] This more closely approximates the 20 to 30% prevalence of multiple ulcers at endoscopy, surgery, and autopsy.[78, 79] The data therefore suggest that double contrast studies are considerably more sensitive than single contrast studies in diagnosing gastric ulcers.

In the past, it has been stated that the presence of multiple gastric ulcers favors benign disease. In one series of 29 patients with multiple ulcers, however, 20% had malignant lesions.[80] It is now recognized that patients may have coexisting benign and malignant ulcers, so each ulcer must be evaluated individually for radiologic signs of a benign or malignant lesion. Occasionally, the combined edema and spasm from adjacent ulcers may produce a conglomerate mass that is mistaken radiographically for a malignant lesion.[77, 80] In such cases, double contrast studies may better delineate individual ulcers by permitting greater distention of the stomach and effacement of rugal folds.[77]

When multiple gastric ulcers are present, they tend to be found in the gastric antrum or body (Fig. 35–13). There is often a marked discrepancy in the size of the ulcers, so a small satellite ulcer may be adjacent to a large ulcer. Multiple gastric ulcers or ulcer scars also tend to occur more frequently in patients who are taking aspirin or other nonsteroidal anti-inflammatory drugs (see Fig. 35–7A). In one study, more than 80% of patients with multiple ulcers had a history of aspirin ingestion.[79] Thus, a careful drug history should be obtained from all patients with multiple gastric ulcers.

## Ulcer Healing and Scarring

The radiologic assessment of ulcer healing is important for evaluating the success or failure of medical

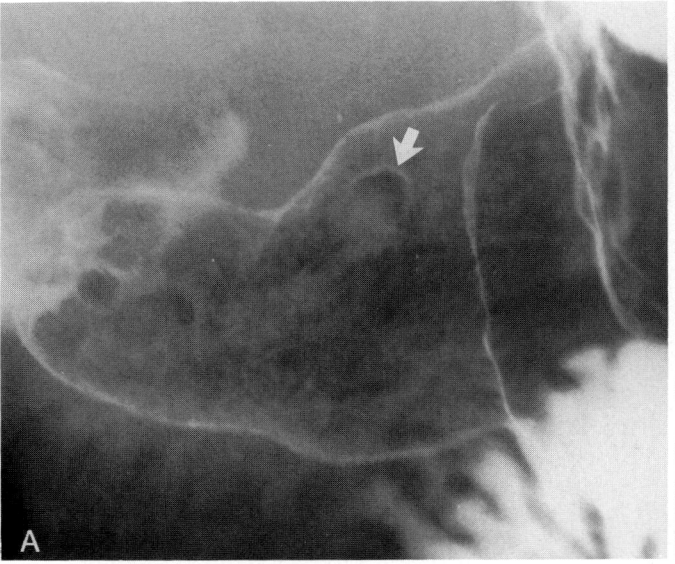
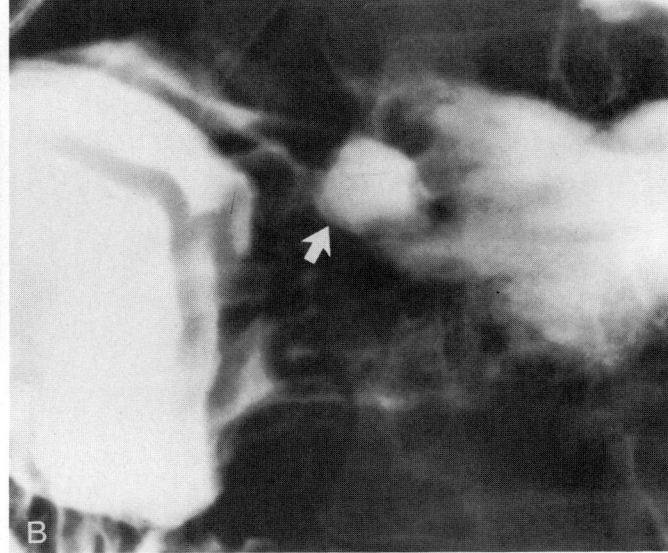

**Figure 35–12. Partial ring shadow caused by an anterior wall ulcer. A.** The initial supine film shows a partial ring shadow _(arrow)_ in the antrum. **B.** A prone compression film shows the anterior wall ulcer _(arrow)_ filling with barium. (**A** and **B** from Levine MS, Rubesin SE, Herlinger H, et al: Double contrast upper gastrointestinal examination: technique and interpretation. Radiology 168:593–602, 1988.)

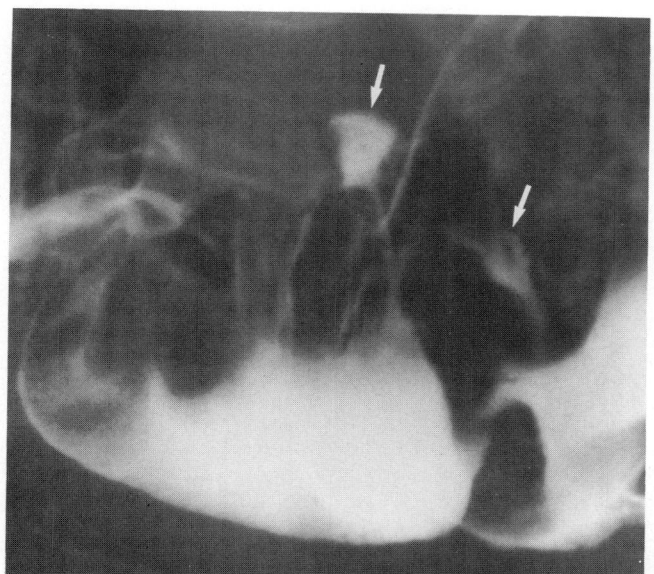

**Figure 35–13. Multiple gastric ulcers.** Two discrete ulcers *(arrows)* are seen on the lesser curvature and posterior wall of the antrum.

may undergo splitting, so that the original crater is replaced by two separate ulcer niches at the periphery of the healing ulcer[58] (Fig. 35–15). This phenomenon probably occurs because healing and re-epithelialization are more rapid in the central portion of the ulcer than in the periphery.

Benign gastric ulcers usually respond dramatically to conservative medical treatment with $H_2$ receptor antagonists. The average interval between the initial barium study showing the ulcer and the follow-up study showing complete healing is about 8 weeks.[58] Follow-up barium studies to demonstrate ulcer healing should therefore be performed after 6 to 8 weeks of medical treatment, because studies performed sooner are unlikely to show complete healing.

In general, complete radiologic healing of a gastric ulcer has been considered a reliable sign that the ulcer is benign. Rarely, complete healing of malignant ulcers may occur with medical therapy.[81, 82] However, nodularity of the ulcer scar or irregularity, clubbing, or amputation of radiating folds should suggest the possibility of an underlying malignancy. The surrounding gastric mucosa therefore must be evaluated carefully after ulcer healing has occurred. If suspicious findings are present, endoscopy and biopsy are still required to rule out a malignant lesion.

Ulcer healing may be associated with the development of an ulcer scar, as granulation tissue generated during healing matures into fibrous tissue. Although ulcer scars are not often detected on single contrast barium studies, 90% of healed gastric ulcers produce a visible ulcer scar on double contrast studies.[58] Double contrast technique is particularly well suited for demonstrating these scars,

therapy and for confirming the presence of benign ulcer disease (see next section on benign versus malignant ulcers). Ulcer healing may be manifested radiographically not only by a decrease in the size of the ulcer crater but also by a change in its shape. Previously round or ovoid ulcers often have a linear appearance on follow-up studies, so linear ulcers presumably represent a stage of ulcer healing[57, 58] (Fig. 35–14). Other ulcers

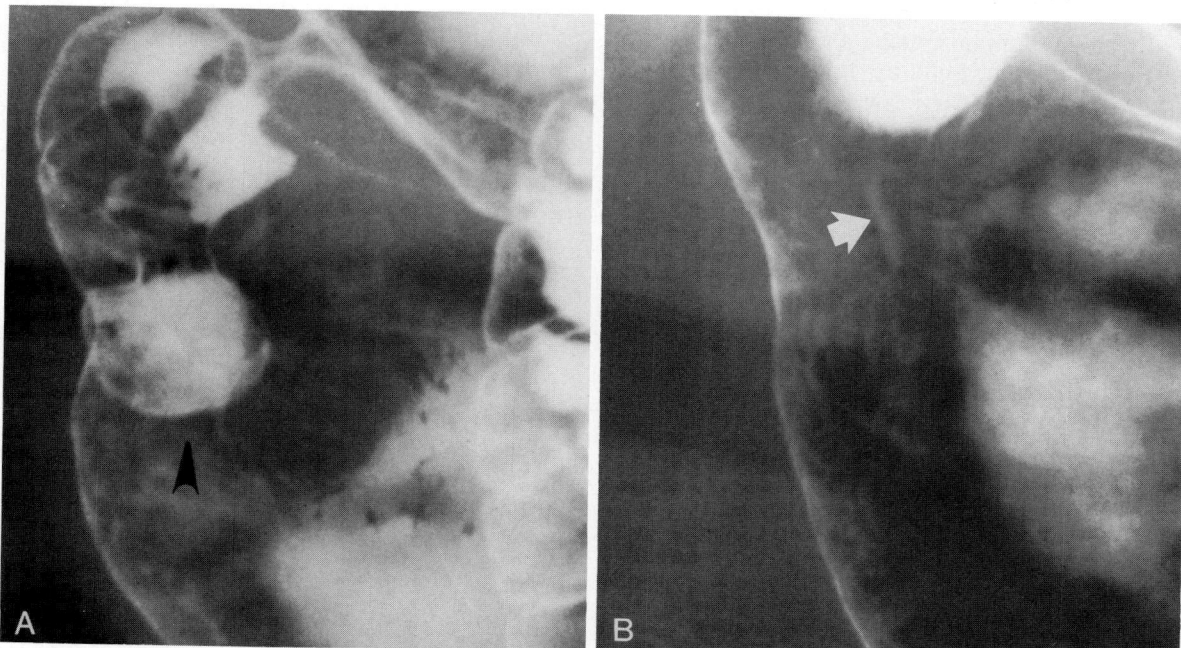

**Figure 35–14. Development of a linear ulcer during healing. A.** A large, round ulcer *(arrowhead)* is seen on the posterior wall of the antrum. **B.** A follow-up study 8 weeks later shows significant ulcer healing with a residual linear ulcer *(arrow)* in this location. (**A** and **B** from Levine MS, Creteur V, Kressel HY, et al: Benign gastric ulcers: diagnosis and follow-up with double-contrast radiography. Radiology 164:9–13, 1987.)

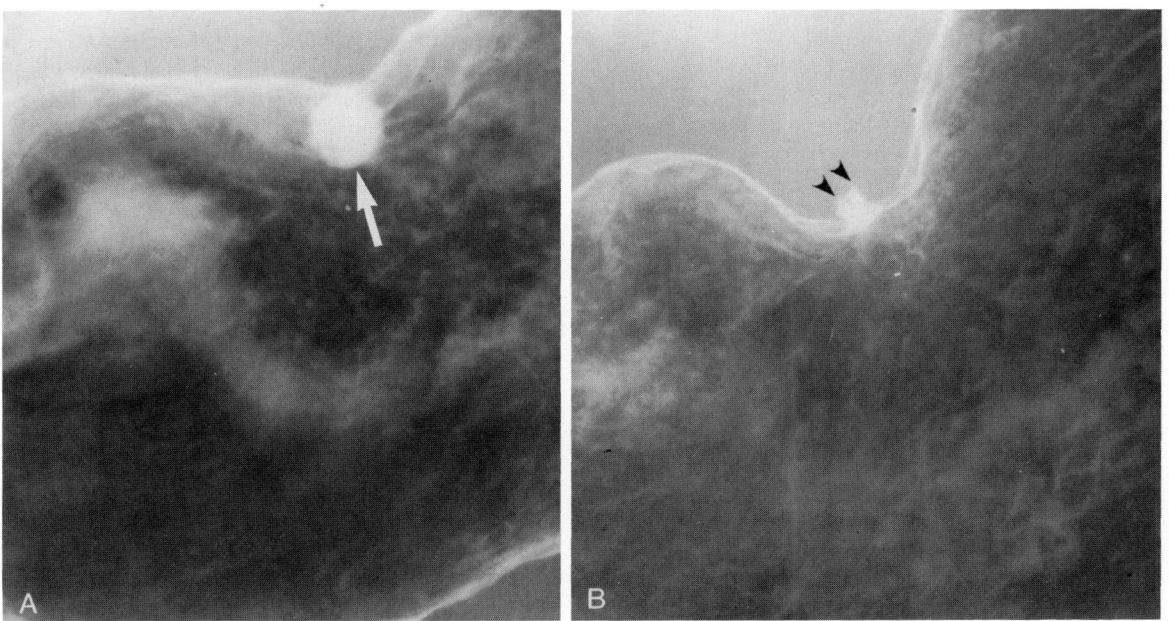

**Figure 35–15. Splitting of an ulcer during healing. A**. A round ulcer *(arrow)* is seen adjacent to the lesser curvature. **B**. A follow-up study several weeks later shows splitting of the ulcer with two closely spaced niches *(arrowheads)* at the site of the original crater.

because gaseous distention of the stomach permits recognition of relatively subtle areas of wall flattening or deformity or of abnormal folds associated with scars. The discovery of an ulcer scar is important because it indicates that the patient has had peptic ulcer disease in the past. Nevertheless, the absence of an ulcer scar in no way excludes the possibility that the patient has had previous ulcers.

Ulcer scars may be manifested radiographically by a central pit or depression, radiating folds, and/or retrac-tion of the adjacent gastric wall.[58, 83, 84] The location of the ulcer is a major determinant of the morphologic features of the scar. Healing of ulcers on the lesser curvature may lead to the development of relatively innocuous scars, manifested by slight flattening or re-traction of the adjacent gastric wall with or without radiating folds[58, 83] (Fig. 35–16). As a result, some ulcer scars on the lesser curvature may be quite subtle.

In contrast, healing of ulcers on the greater curvature or posterior wall of the stomach often leads to the

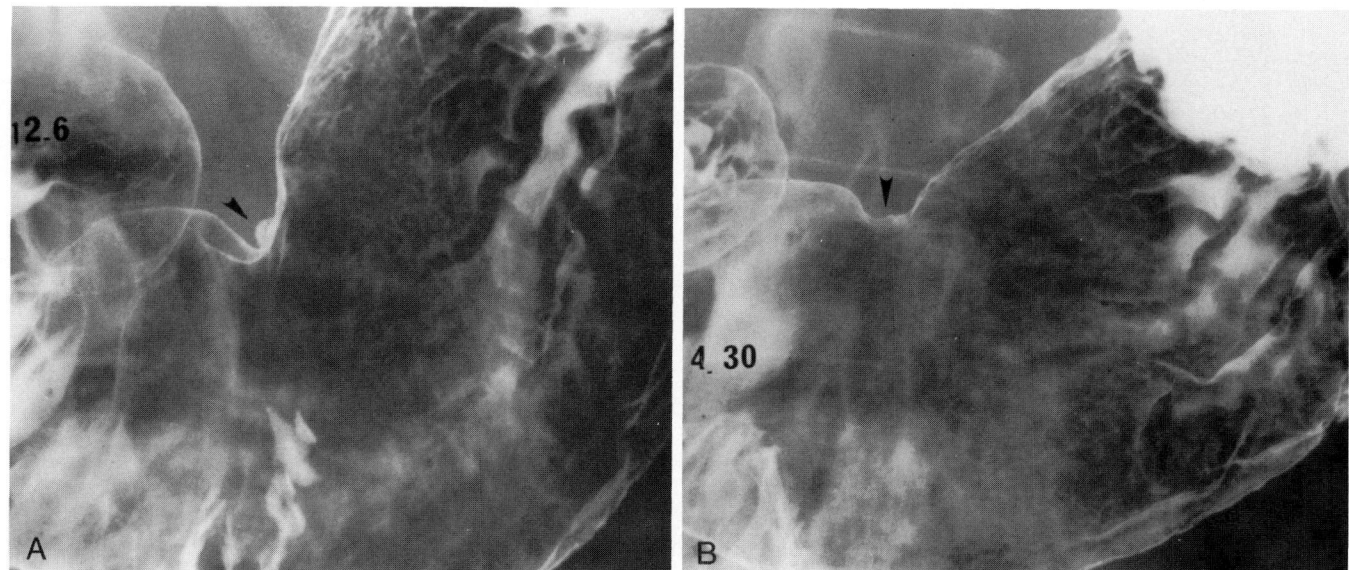

**Figure 35–16. Healing of a lesser curvature ulcer with scarring. A**. A small, benign-appearing ulcer *(arrowhead)* is seen on the lesser curvature. **B**. A follow-up study 5 months later shows complete healing of the ulcer with slight flattening and retraction of the adjacent gastric wall *(arrowhead)*.

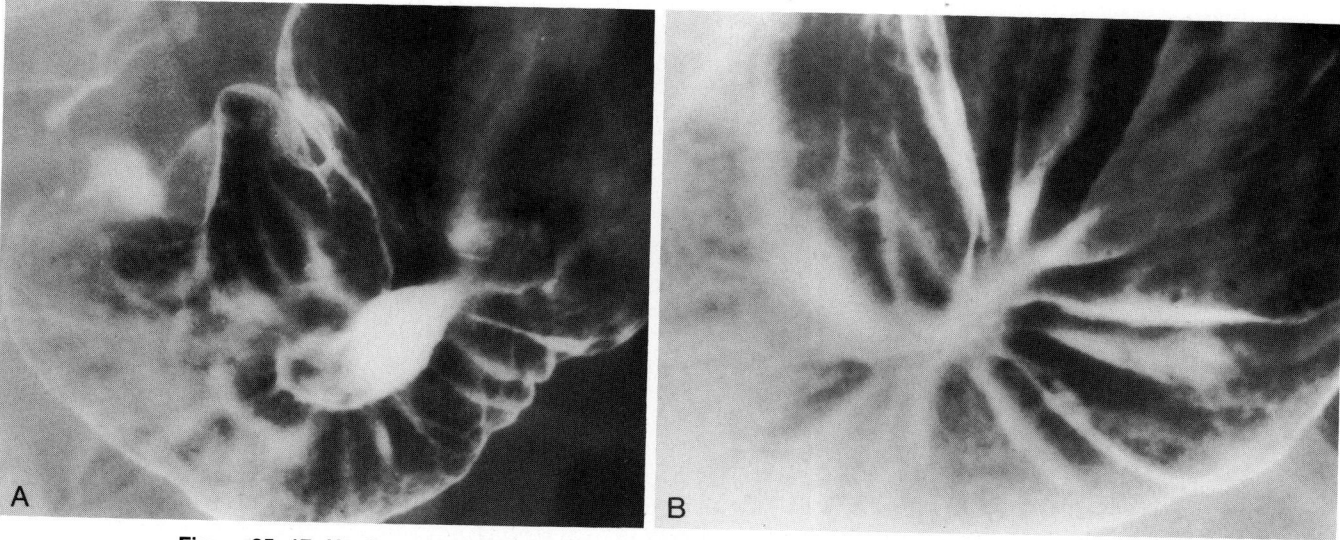

**Figure 35–17. Healing of a posterior wall ulcer with scarring. A.** There is a large posterior wall ulcer with multiple folds seen radiating to the edge of the ulcer crater. **B.** A follow-up study 8 weeks later shows complete healing of the ulcer with spectacular folds radiating to the site of the previous crater.

development of spectacular radiating folds[58, 83] (Fig. 35–17). The folds may converge to a central point or to a circular or linear pit or depression.[58, 83, 84] This central depression can be mistaken radiographically for a shallow, residual ulcer crater. In other cases, this central depression may have a bald, featureless appearance, so that it is unclear whether complete ulcer healing has occurred (Fig. 35–18). However, the central depression of an ulcer scar tends to have more gradually sloping margins than an ulcer crater and should remain unchanged on sequential follow-up studies. A re-epithelialized ulcer scar can also be differentiated radiographically from an active ulcer by the presence of normal

areae gastricae within the central portion of the scar[58] (Fig. 35–19). The latter finding indicates complete ulcer healing, so further radiologic or endoscopic evaluation is unnecessary.

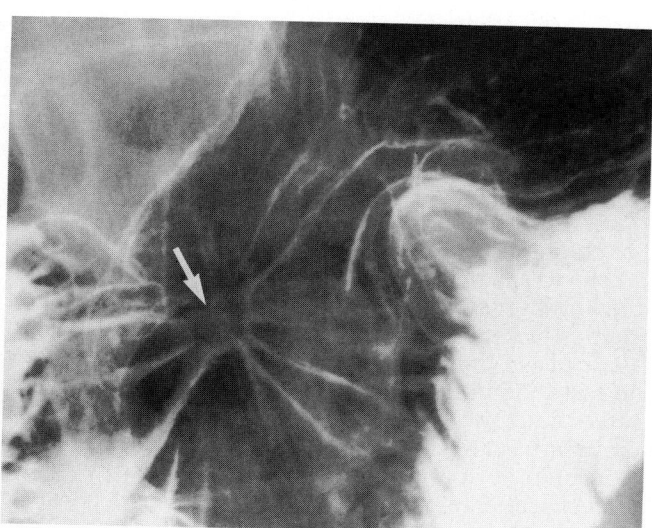

**Figure 35–18. Ulcer scar with folds radiating to a central depression.** Multiple folds are seen radiating to a bald, featureless central area *(arrow)* that could be mistaken for a shallow, residual ulcer crater. (From Levine MS, Creteur V, Kressel HY, et al: Benign gastric ulcers: diagnosis and follow-up with double-contrast radiography. Radiology 164:9–13, 1987.)

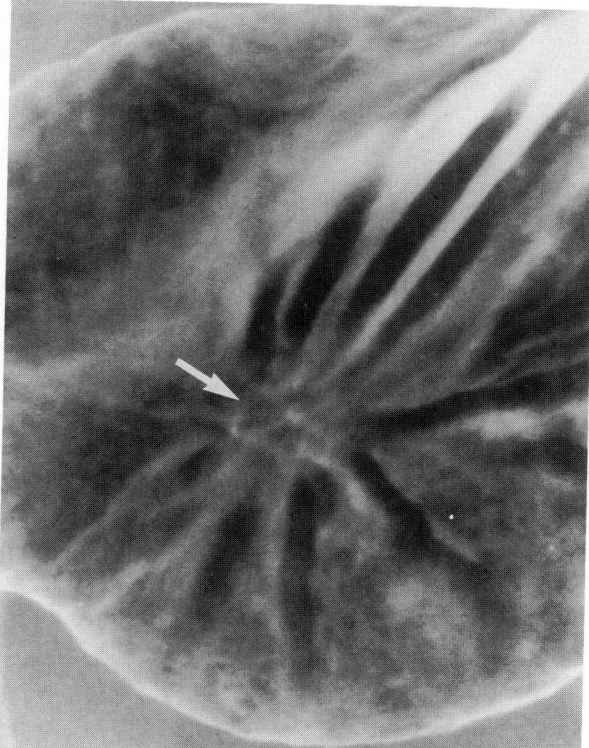

**Figure 35–19. Re-epithelialized ulcer scar with centrally radiating folds.** This scar can be differentiated from an active ulcer by the presence of normal areae gastricae within the central portion of the scar *(arrow)*. (From Levine MS, Rubesin SE, Herlinger H, et al: Double contrast upper gastrointestinal examination: technique and interpretation. Radiology 168:593–602, 1988.)

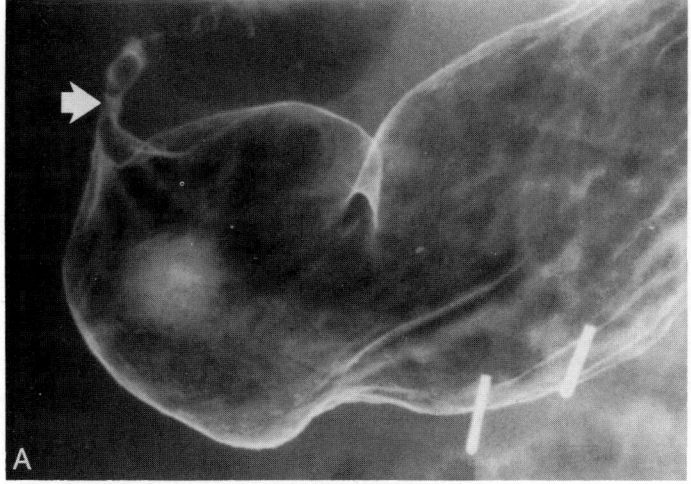

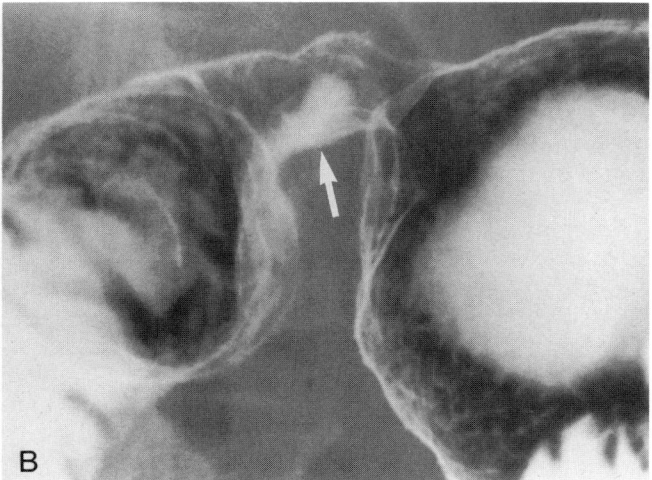

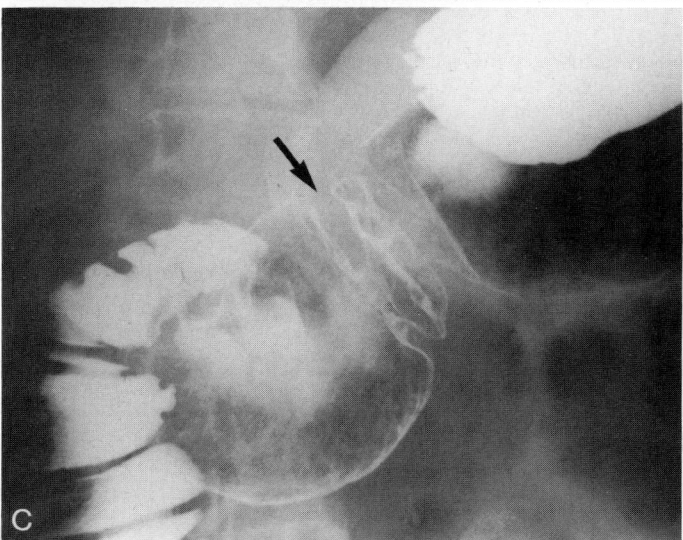

**Figure 35–20. Various types of gastric scarring from ulcer disease. A**. This patient has marked antral narrowing and deformity *(arrow)* caused by scarring from a previous antral ulcer. This degree of narrowing may lead to gastric outlet obstruction. **B**. Another patient has a widened, eccentric pylorus *(arrow)* due to scarring from peptic ulcer disease. **C**. A third patient has an hourglass stomach with focal narrowing of the gastric body *(arrow)* due to severe ulcer scarring.

Healing of antral ulcers may also lead to the development of a prominent transverse fold that can be mistaken for an antral web or diaphragm.[83] In other patients, severe scar formation may be manifested by antral narrowing and deformity (Fig. 35–20A). The narrowed segment usually has a smooth, tapered appearance, but asymmetric scarring may result in flattening and shortening of the lesser or greater curvature, so that the pylorus has an eccentric location in relation to the antrum and duodenal bulb (Fig. 35–20B). Occasionally, an ulcer scar may be associated with such irregular antral narrowing that it mimics the linitis plastica appearance of a primary scirrhous carcinoma of the stomach.[85] When antral scarring cannot be differentiated from a scirrhous carcinoma on radiologic criteria, endoscopy and biopsy are required for a more definitive diagnosis. Healing of ulcers on the lesser curvature of the gastric body may also lead to marked retraction and deformity of the opposite wall, producing a deep incisura on the greater curvature.[83, 84] Rarely, scarring of the gastric body may result in the development of an "hour-glass" stomach with focal narrowing in this region (Fig. 35–20C).

## Benign Versus Malignant Ulcers

More than 95% of gastric ulcers diagnosed in the United States are found to be benign.[52, 86] Nevertheless, radiologic examinations are often thought to be unreliable in differentiating benign ulcers from ulcerated carcinomas. Previous reports indicate that 6 to 16% of gastric ulcers that appear benign on conventional single contrast barium studies are malignant.[87–90] Although these studies were performed between 1955 and 1975, many gastroenterologists have used these data as the justification for performing endoscopy and biopsy on all patients with radiographically diagnosed gastric ulcers to rule out cancer.

With double contrast techniques, however, it is possible to obtain a much more detailed study of the mucosa surrounding the ulcer for signs of malignancy, such as irregular mass effect, nodularity, rigidity, or mucosal destruction. Several studies have found that virtually all gastric ulcers with an unequivocally benign appearance on double contrast studies are in fact benign lesions.[58, 91] In those studies, about two thirds of all benign ulcers had a benign radiographic appearance, so unnecessary endoscopy could be avoided in most patients with gastric ulcers diagnosed on double contrast examinations. This finding has enormous implications for the evaluation of gastric ulcers in general, because barium studies are safer and less expensive than endoscopy.

Unequivocally benign gastric ulcers are characterized en face by a round or ovoid ulcer crater surrounded by a smooth mound of edema or regular, symmetric mucosal folds that radiate to the edge of the crater[58, 91] (see Figs. 35–9, 35–14A, 35–15A, and 35–17A). The areae gastricae adjacent to the ulcer may be enlarged as a result of inflammation and edema of the surrounding mucosa[58] (see Fig. 35–6A). However, the areae gastricae can often be seen to extend to the edge of the ulcer crater without evidence of nodularity, mass effect, or tumor infiltration. When viewed in profile, benign gastric ulcers project outside the gastric lumen and are often associated with a smooth, symmetric ulcer mound or collar or with smooth, straight mucosal folds that radiate to the edge of the ulcer crater (see Figs. 35–4, 35–6, and 35–16A) (see earlier section on morphologic features).

In contrast, malignant ulcers are characterized en face by an irregular ulcer crater eccentrically located in an irregular mass with distortion or obliteration of the normal areae gastricae surrounding the ulcer.[58] Although radiating folds may be present, they tend to be nodular and irregular and may stop well short of the ulcer crater (Fig. 35–21). In addition, the tips of the folds may be fused, clubbed, or amputated.[92] When viewed in profile, malignant ulcers do not project beyond the expected

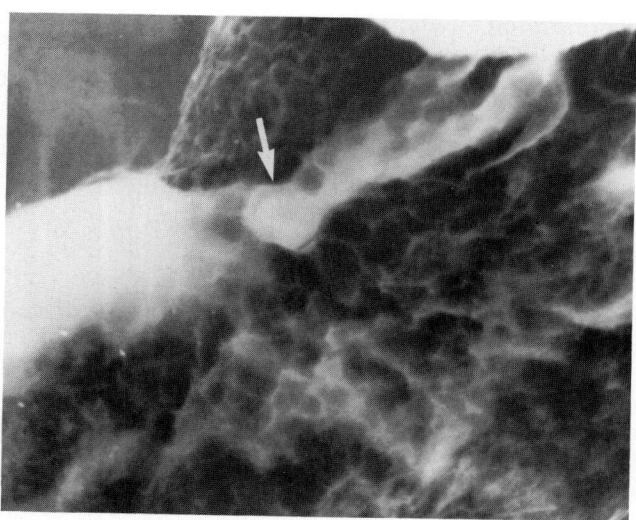

**Figure 35–22. Benign gastric ulcer with an indeterminate radiographic appearance.** A 1-cm ulcer *(arrow)* is seen near the lesser curvature with enlarged, nodular areae gastricae surrounding the ulcer because of inflammation and edema of the adjacent mucosa. Although the radiographic findings are equivocal, endoscopic biopsies revealed no evidence of tumor, and a follow-up study showed complete healing of the ulcer.

gastric contour, and there is often a discrete tumor mass that forms acute angles with the gastric wall rather than the obtuse, gently sloping angles expected for a benign mound of edema. There may also be nodularity of the adjacent mucosa or thickened, lobulated folds radiating to the ulcer because of infiltration by tumor.

Equivocal ulcers are those that have mixed features of benign and malignant disease, so that a confident diagnosis cannot be made on the basis of radiologic criteria. For example, edema and inflammation surrounding an acute ulcer may result in enlarged, distorted areae gastricae, mass effect, or thickened, irregular folds, producing an indeterminate radiographic appearance (Fig. 35–22). Similarly, greater curvature ulcers that have an apparent intraluminal location or considerable associated mass effect and shouldered edges may result in equivocal radiographic findings (see Fig. 35–8). Most ulcers that have an equivocal appearance are ultimately found to be benign. However, it seems prudent to err on the side of caution by suggesting the possibility of malignancy in some benign lesions to avoid missing an early carcinoma.

Gastric ulcers that have an unequivocally benign appearance on double contrast studies can be followed radiographically until complete healing without need for endoscopic intervention.[58] However, ulcers that have an equivocal or suspicious appearance should be evaluated endoscopically for a more definitive diagnosis. Endoscopy is a relatively accurate technique for detecting gastric carcinoma, but false-negative biopsies and brushings have been reported in some patients with malignant lesions.[93] If the radiographic findings raise suspicion of malignancy, negative endoscopic or cytologic findings should not be taken as definitive evidence of a benign ulcer. Instead, follow-up barium studies should be performed at regular intervals until complete healing is

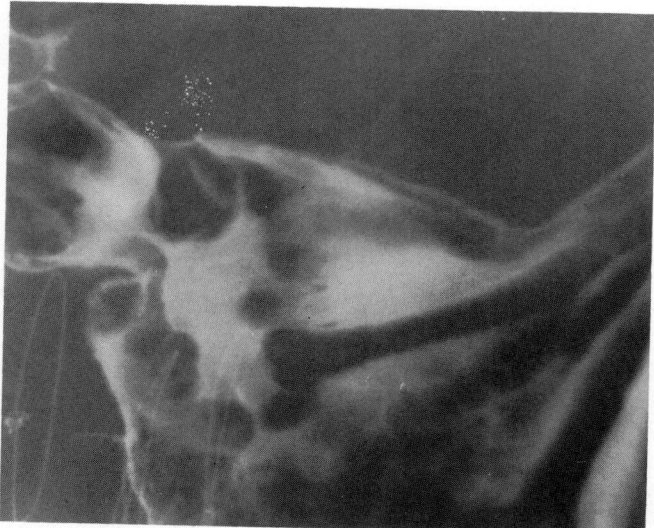

**Figure 35–21. Malignant gastric ulcer.** This patient has an irregular ulcer on the posterior wall of the antrum with scalloped borders and nodular, clubbed folds surrounding the ulcer. These are classic features of a malignant ulcer. (From Levine MS, Creteur V, Kressel HY, et al: Benign gastric ulcers: diagnosis and follow-up with double contrast radiography. Radiology 164:9–13, 1987.)

demonstrated. If the ulcer fails to heal with adequate medical treatment or if it continues to have a suspicious radiographic appearance, subsequent endoscopy may be necessary. Even if results of endoscopic biopsies and brushings remain negative, surgical resection should be considered for some patients who have radiographic findings highly suggestive of malignant disease.

## Duodenal Ulcers

Unlike gastric ulcers, duodenal ulcers are virtually always benign. When these ulcers are detected radiographically, treatment with H$_2$ receptor antagonists can therefore be initiated without need for endoscopy. However, a significant percentage of duodenal ulcers are located on the anterior wall of the duodenal bulb, so a definitive diagnosis is best made with prone compression views of the duodenum. Furthermore, duodenal ulcers may be obscured by edema, spasm, or scarring of the bulb. Conversely, barium trapped in the crevices of a deformed bulb can mimic ulcer craters. Radiologists should therefore be aware of the limitations of barium studies in diagnosing duodenal ulcers and of the need to perform a biphasic examination in these patients.

### Examination Technique

Double contrast views of the duodenum must be complemented by prone compression views to demonstrate ulcers on the anterior wall of the bulb.[94] However, these anterior wall ulcers may be hidden in the barium pool unless adequate compression of the bulb is obtained with an inflatable balloon or other prone compression device (Fig. 35–23). Other duodenal ulcers are best seen on upright compression views. Thus, optimal radiologic evaluation of the duodenum requires a biphasic examination that includes double contrast views of the duodenal bulb with high-density barium and prone or upright compression views with low-density barium.[95]

### Shape

Most duodenal ulcers appear radiographically as round or ovoid collections of barium (Fig. 35–24). However, about 5% of duodenal ulcers diagnosed on double contrast studies have a linear configuration[57, 96] (Fig. 35–25). These linear ulcers tend to be located near the base of the duodenal bulb and often have a transverse orientation in relation to the bulb[96] (see Fig. 35–25A). As in the stomach, linear ulcers are thought to represent a stage of ulcer healing.[55, 96] In fact, they may be indistinguishable from linear ulcer scars.

### Size

The vast majority of duodenal ulcers seen on barium studies are less than 1 cm in size. A major advantage of double contrast technique is its ability to demonstrate small duodenal ulcers, frequently no more than several millimeters in diameter (see Fig. 35–25B and C). Nevertheless, giant ulcers are occasionally detected in the duodenum (see later section on giant duodenal ulcers).

### Location

About 95% of duodenal ulcers are located in the duodenal bulb and the remaining 5% in the postbulbar duodenum.[97] Bulbar ulcers may involve the apex, central portion, or base of the bulb (see Fig. 35–24). Unlike gastric ulcers, which rarely occur on the anterior wall, as many as 50% of duodenal ulcers are located on the anterior wall of the bulb.[66, 98] When they occur, postbulbar ulcers usually are located in the proximal descending duodenum above the papilla of Vater (see later section on postbulbar ulcers). Thus, the presence of one or more ulcers distal to the papilla should raise the possibility of Zollinger-Ellison syndrome (see later section on Zollinger-Ellison syndrome).

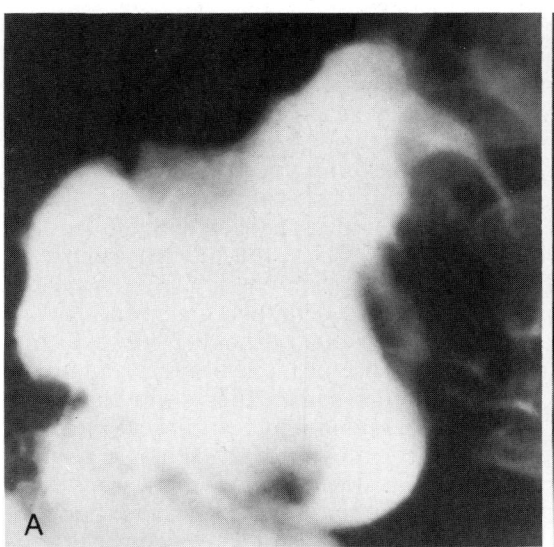
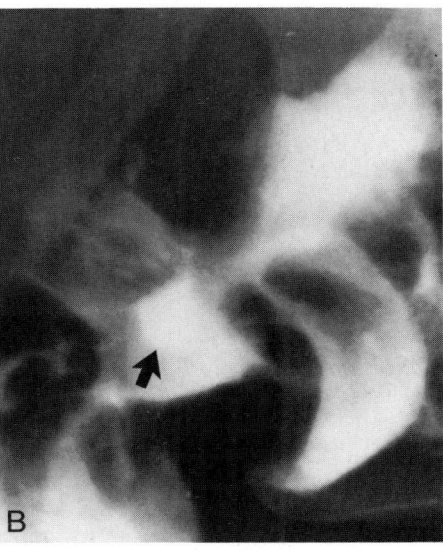

**Figure 35–23. Importance of prone compression for anterior wall duodenal ulcers. A.** The initial prone film shows no evidence of a duodenal ulcer. **B.** Compression of the bulb with an inflatable balloon clearly demonstrates an ulcer crater *(arrow)* on the anterior wall. This ulcer was hidden in the barium pool on the earlier film.

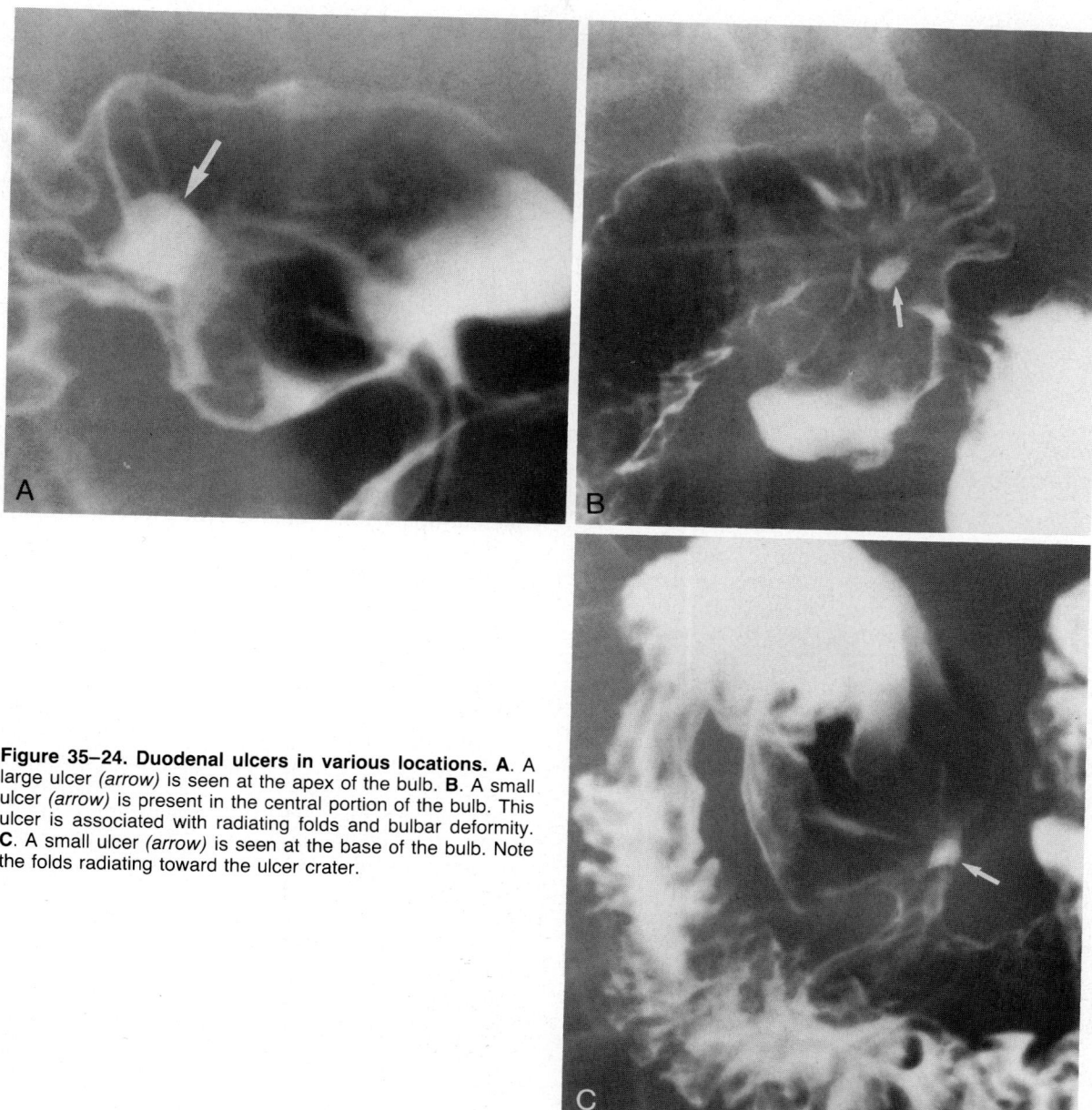

**Figure 35–24. Duodenal ulcers in various locations. A**. A large ulcer *(arrow)* is seen at the apex of the bulb. **B**. A small ulcer *(arrow)* is present in the central portion of the bulb. This ulcer is associated with radiating folds and bulbar deformity. **C**. A small ulcer *(arrow)* is seen at the base of the bulb. Note the folds radiating toward the ulcer crater.

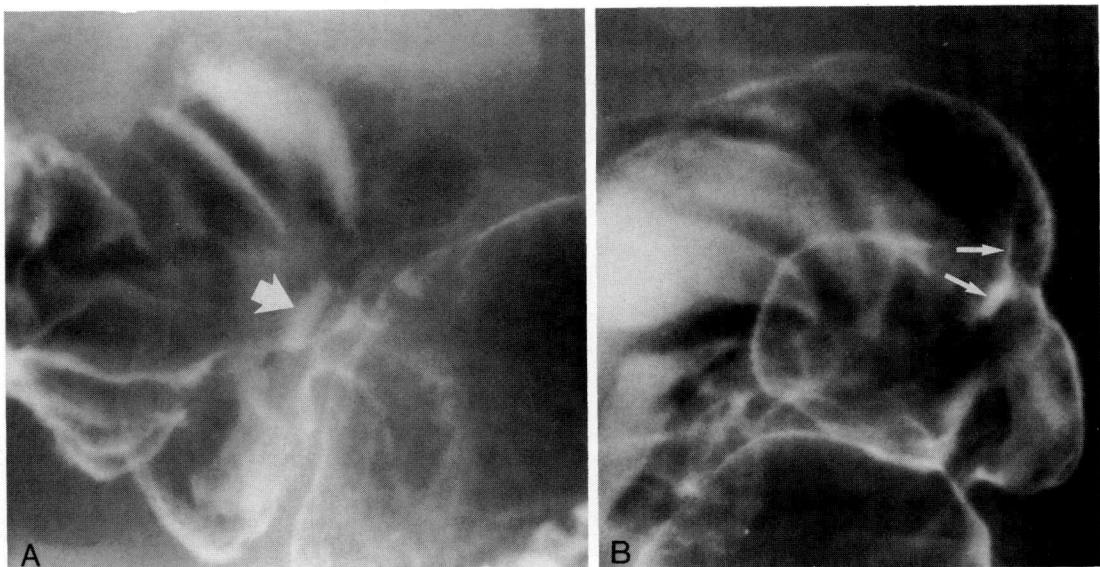

**Figure 35–25. Linear duodenal ulcers. A**. A linear ulcer *(arrow)* is seen at the base of the bulb. The ulcer has a transverse orientation in relation to the bulb. **B**. In another patient, there is a linear ulcer *(arrows)* near the apex of the bulb.

## Morphologic Features

### Bulbar Ulcers

Ulcers in the duodenal bulb usually appear as discrete niches that can be visualized en face or in profile (see Fig. 35–24). The ulcers are often surrounded by a smooth, radiolucent mound of edematous mucosa. Occasionally, the size of the ulcer mound may be quite striking in relation to the central crater (Fig. 35–26B). Bulbar ulcers also tend to be associated with radiating folds that converge centrally at the edge of the crater (see Fig. 35–24B and C). In patients with shallow ulcers or small, healing ulcers, the ulcer crater may be visible only with optimal radiographic technique. Thus, the presence of radiating folds should prompt a careful search for an active ulcer at the site of fold convergence before attributing these folds to an ulcer scar.

As in the stomach, ulcers on the anterior wall of the duodenal bulb may be difficult to detect on routine double contrast views. Other anterior wall ulcers may be manifested by a ring shadow caused by barium coating the rim of the unfilled ulcer crater[74] (Fig. 35–26A). These anterior wall ulcers can be demonstrated by obtaining prone or upright compression views of the bulb to fill the crater with barium (see Fig. 35–26B).

Duodenal ulcers are often associated with significant deformity of the bulb caused by edema and spasm accompanying the ulcer or scarring from a previous ulcer[94] (see Fig. 35–24B). This deformity may obscure small ulcers in the bulb, resulting in a significant number of false-negative examinations. Thus, it is important to recognize the limitations of the radiologic diagnosis of duodenal ulcers in the presence of a deformed bulb. Although a confident diagnosis of peptic ulcer disease can be made in patients with bulbar deformity, it is often unclear whether an active ulcer is present. Nevertheless, symptomatic patients with a deformed bulb on barium studies should probably be treated for an active duodenal ulcer because of the high risk of ulcer disease, whether or not an ulcer is demonstrated with certainty.

### Postbulbar Ulcers

Postbulbar ulcers are usually located on the medial wall of the proximal descending duodenum above the papilla of Vater[97, 99] (Fig. 35–27). These ulcers are notoriously difficult to demonstrate on barium studies, presumably because severe edema and spasm accompanying the ulcer prevent visualization of the ulcer crater. The edema and spasm often result in a smooth, rounded indentation on the lateral wall of the descending duodenum opposite the crater[99] (see Fig. 35–27A). In some cases, this indentation may be the only radiologic sign of a postbulbar ulcer (Fig. 35–28). Other patients may develop a "ring stricture" with eccentric narrowing of the postbulbar duodenum due to scarring and fibrosis from previous ulcers in this location[100] (Fig. 35–29). It may not be possible to differentiate edema and spasm from an ulcer scar in the descending duodenum, but an active postbulbar ulcer should be suspected in patients with right upper quadrant pain or upper gastrointestinal bleeding. Hypotonic duodenography may be performed to better delineate postbulbar ulcers when these lesions are suspected on routine barium studies.[100]

### Giant Duodenal Ulcers

Giant duodenal ulcers are defined as duodenal ulcers greater than 2 cm in size.[101] These ulcers are important

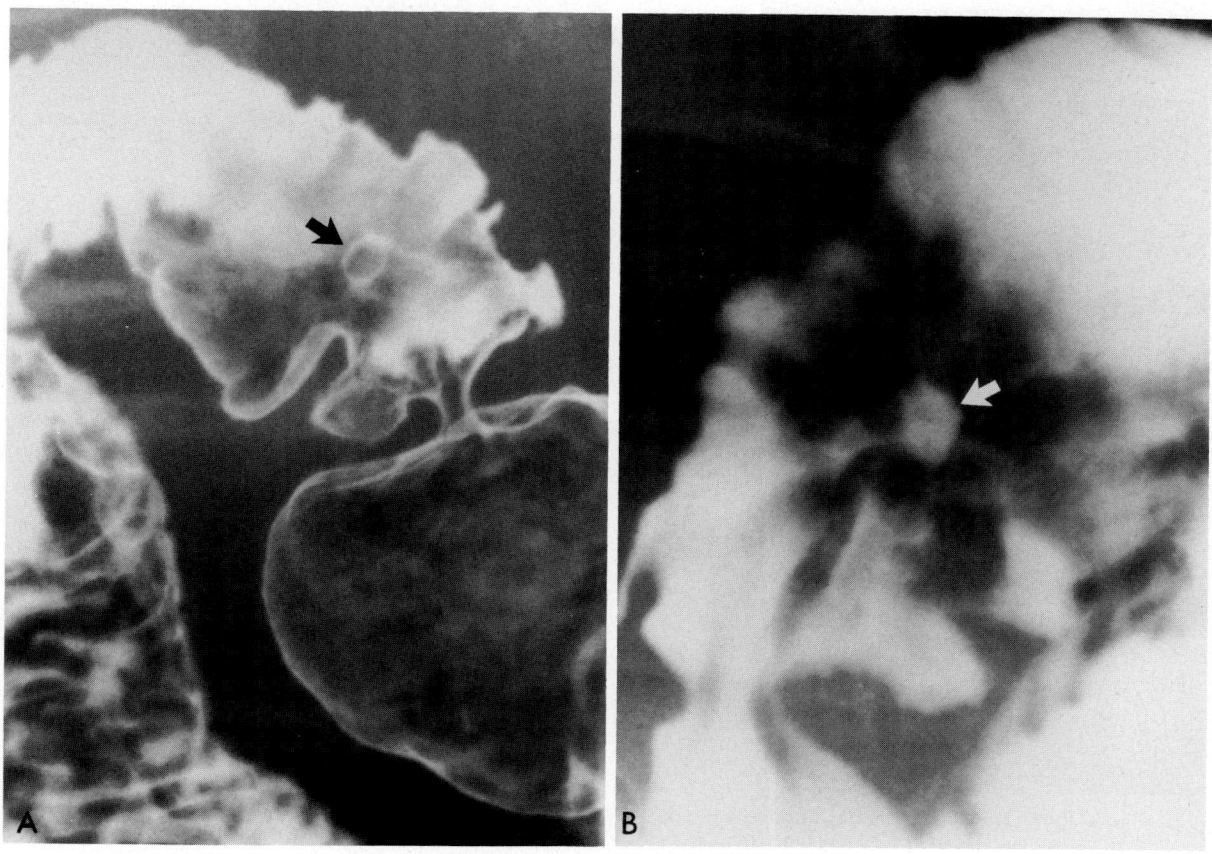

**Figure 35–26. Ring shadow caused by an anterior wall duodenal ulcer. A**. A double contrast view of the duodenum shows a ring shadow *(arrow)* in the bulb due to barium coating the rim of an unfilled ulcer on the nondependent surface. **B**. A prone compression view shows filling of the anterior wall ulcer *(arrow)*. Note the large, radiolucent mound of edema surrounding the ulcer.

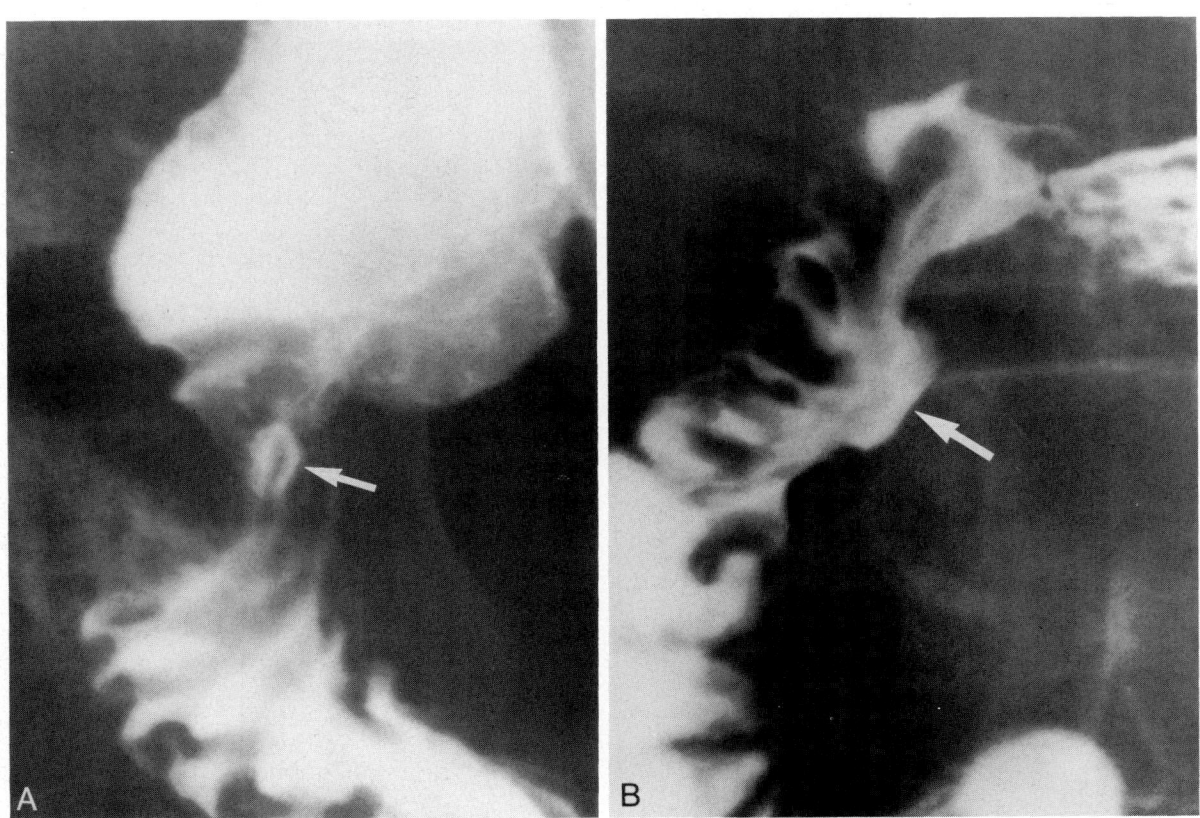

**Figure 35–27. Postbulbar duodenal ulcers. A**. An ulcer *(arrow)* is seen on the medial wall of the proximal descending duodenum. There is also a smooth, rounded indentation of the lateral wall due to associated edema and spasm. **B**. Another patient has a large, relatively flat ulcer *(arrow)* on the medial wall of the postbulbar duodenum above the papilla of Vater. Note the folds radiating toward the ulcer crater.

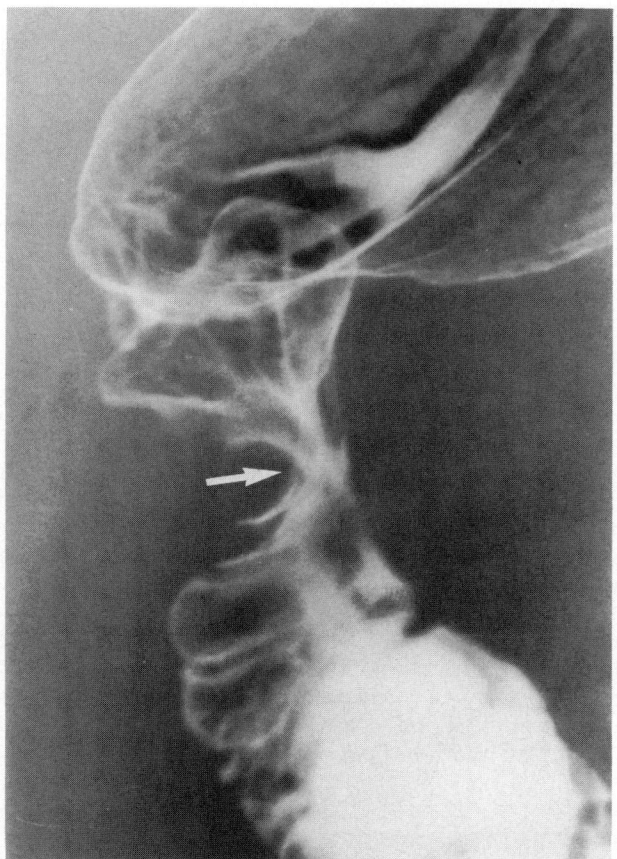

**Figure 35–28. Postbulbar duodenal ulcer.** A prominent indentation is seen on the lateral aspect of the proximal descending duodenum *(arrow)* due to edema and spasm accompanying a postbulbar ulcer that was not visualized on this study.

denal diverticulum and pancreatic pseudocyst. In such cases, a barium study should be performed for a more certain diagnosis.

## Multiplicity

About 15% of patients with duodenal ulcers have multiple ulcers.[106] Most of these ulcers are located in the duodenal bulb. The presence of multiple ulcers should raise the possibility of Zollinger-Ellison syndrome (see later section on Zollinger-Ellison syndrome).

## Ulcer Healing and Scarring

Duodenal ulcers usually heal rapidly during treatment with $H_2$ receptor antagonists. As the ulcers decrease in size, they often have a linear appearance.[55, 96] Ulcer healing may lead to the development of an ulcer scar, manifested by radiating folds or bulbar deformity. When radiating folds are present, they almost always converge at the site of the previous ulcer. In some patients, a residual depression in the central portion of the scar may simulate an active ulcer crater. As a result, it is often difficult to differentiate small, healing ulcers from ulcer scars. Nevertheless, follow-up barium studies to demonstrate ulcer healing are probably unnecessary for patients with uncomplicated duodenal ulcers who have

because of the increased risk of complications such as perforation, obstruction, and upper gastrointestinal bleeding.[102] Nevertheless, treatment with $H_2$ receptor antagonists may lead to dramatic ulcer healing, so these patients can often be managed conservatively without need for surgery.[103] Giant duodenal ulcers are almost always located in the duodenal bulb and may be so large that they replace virtually the entire bulb (Fig. 35–30). Paradoxically, these giant ulcers can be mistaken radiographically for a normal or scarred bulb. However, their constant size and shape at fluoroscopy should help to differentiate these lesions from the changing appearance of the duodenal bulb[101, 103, 104] (Fig. 35–31). Occasionally, giant duodenal ulcers may contain asymmetric areas of deeper ulceration, producing an "ulcer within an ulcer" appearance.[103] In other patients, a radiolucent band of edema may be identified in the duodenum adjacent to the ulcer (see Fig. 35–31). Marked edema and spasm accompanying the ulcer may also cause focal constriction of the duodenum, with varying degrees of gastric outlet obstruction.[101, 103]

Giant duodenal ulcers may occasionally be recognized on ultrasound studies as discrete, hypoechoic cystic lesions anterolateral to the head of the pancreas.[105] The differential diagnosis for these lesions includes a duo-

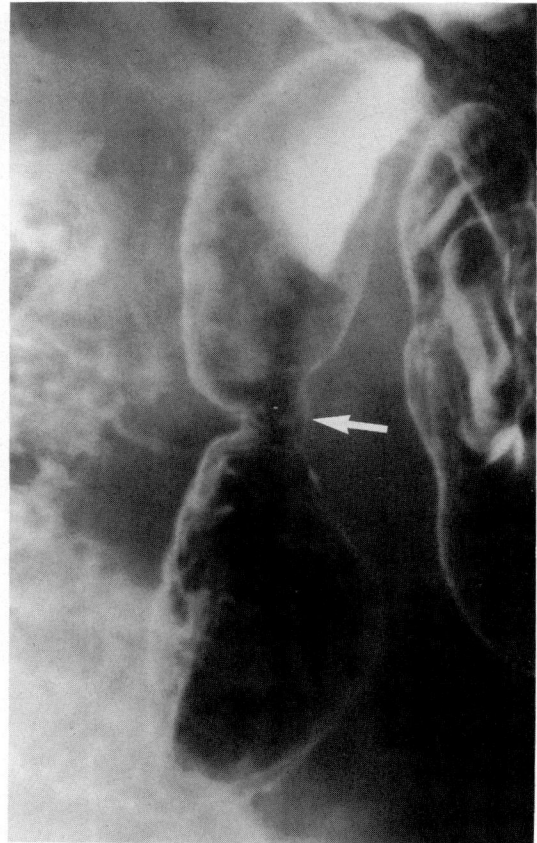

**Figure 35–29. Postbulbar ring stricture.** There is eccentric narrowing *(arrow)* of the postbulbar duodenum due to scarring and fibrosis from a previous ulcer in this location.

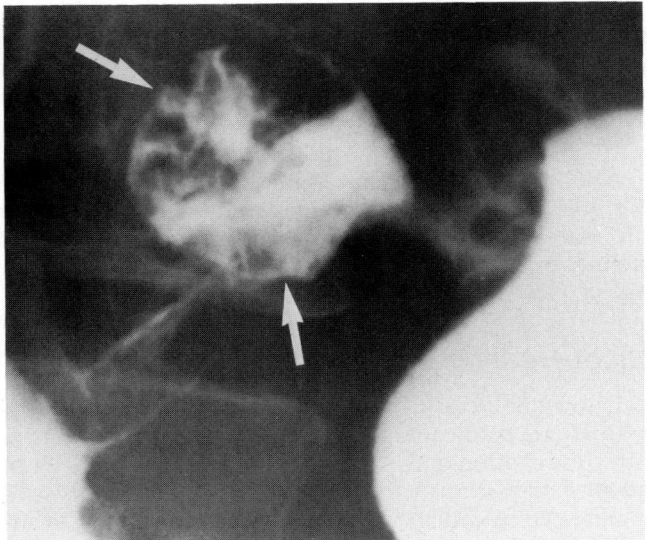

**Figure 35–30. Giant duodenal ulcer.** This giant ulcer *(arrows)* has replaced virtually the entire duodenal bulb. Paradoxically, such ulcers can be mistaken for a normal or scarred bulb.

an adequate clinical response to medical therapy, because these ulcers are virtually always benign. Follow-up studies should therefore be reserved for patients with intractable ulcer symptoms or ulcer complications such as obstruction.

Bulbar deformity results from asymmetric scarring and retraction of the duodenal bulb during ulcer healing. Uninvolved segments of the bulb may balloon out between areas of fibrosis, producing one or more pseudodiverticula. These pseudodiverticula can usually be differentiated from ulcers by their tendency to change in size and shape at fluoroscopy. When multiple pseudodiverticula are present, the duodenal bulb may have a classic "cloverleaf" appearance (Fig. 35–32).

## Pyloric Channel Ulcers

Pyloric channel ulcers should be treated as gastric ulcers rather than duodenal ulcers in terms of the need for aggressive evaluation and follow-up to differentiate these lesions from ulcerated carcinomas. Most pyloric channel ulcers are less than 1 cm in size, and they are usually located on the lesser curvature aspect of the pylorus. They also tend to be located on the anterior wall of the pylorus, so they may appear as ring shadows on double contrast views.[107] However, the ulcer should fill with barium on prone or upright compression views (Fig. 35–33). Some pyloric channel ulcers may cause marked edema and spasm of the pylorus and distal antrum, so that optimal radiologic evaluation of this area is not possible. However, irregularity, angulation,

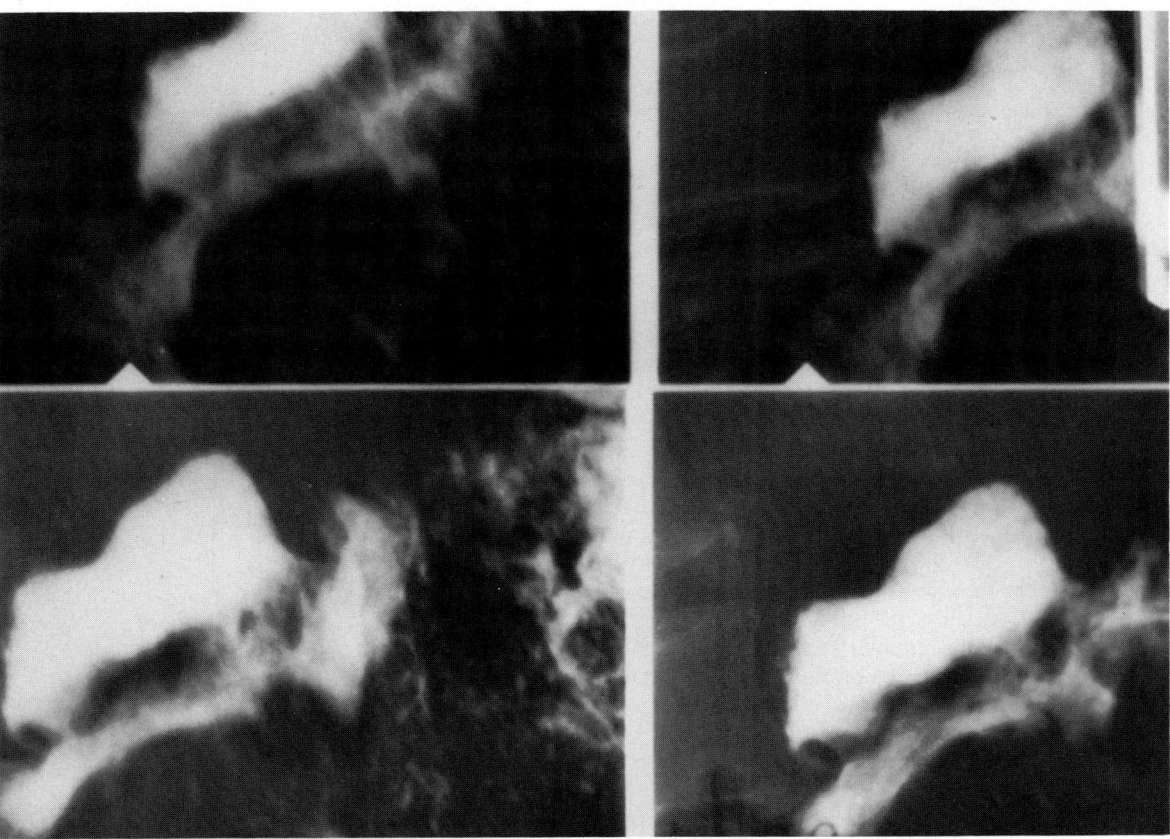

**Figure 35–31. Giant duodenal ulcer.** Four spot films of the bulb show that this giant ulcer has a constant size and shape. In contrast, the duodenal bulb has a changing appearance at fluoroscopy. Also note the large radiolucent band of edema adjacent to the ulcer.

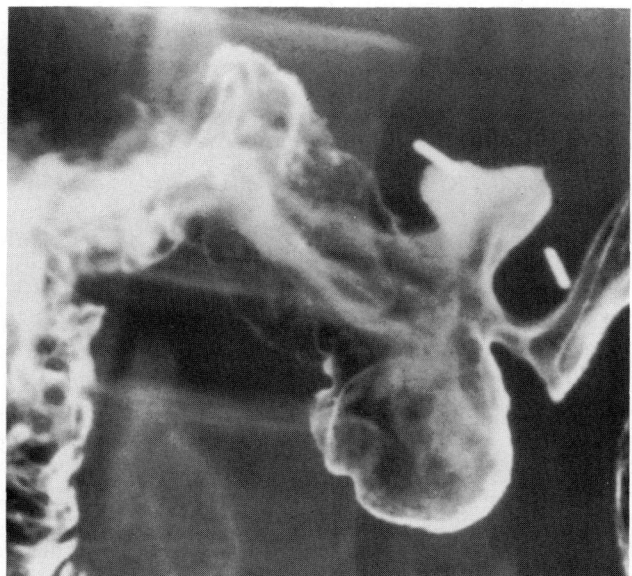

**Figure 35–32. Scarred duodenal bulb.** Marked scarring of the bulb has resulted in the development of multiple pseudodiverticula, producing a cloverleaf appearance.

or distortion of the pylorus should raise the possibility of an ulcer in symptomatic patients.

Pyloric channel ulcers must be differentiated radiographically from pseudodiverticula caused by scarring from previous ulcer disease or a surgical pyloroplasty. However, ulcers usually have a fixed configuration, whereas pseudodiverticula are more likely to change in size and shape at fluoroscopy. The presence of mucosal folds in the region of the outpouching should also suggest a pseudodiverticulum rather than an ulcer. Occasionally, adult hypertrophic pyloric stenosis may be manifested radiographically by a narrowed, elongated pyloric channel with diamond-shaped outpouchings or dimples extending superiorly or inferiorly from this region, but these patients usually have a long-standing history of obstructive symptoms.

Healing of pyloric channel ulcers may lead to narrowing, elongation, or angulation of the pylorus. Depending on the degree of scarring, gastric outlet obstruction may ensue.

## DIFFERENTIAL DIAGNOSIS

Gastric or duodenal ulcers occasionally may be simulated by a variety of double contrast artifacts, including barium precipitates, stalactites, and see-through phenomena (see Chapter 4).[108] An inadequate or poorly prepared barium suspension may result in the development of barium precipitates that resemble tiny ulcers in the stomach or duodenum. However, these precipitates can be differentiated from ulcers by their failure to project beyond the contour of the stomach or duodenum in profile and by the absence of associated findings such as mucosal edema or radiating folds. "Stalactites" are hanging droplets of barium that are sometimes seen on the nondependent or anterior gastric wall.[109] Although a stalactite can be mistaken for a small ulcer on a single radiograph, the transient nature of this finding at fluoroscopy differentiates a stalactite from a true ulcer. Finally, calcified densities (e.g., renal calculi or calcified splenic arteries) or structures containing contrast medium (e.g., colonic diverticula or the subarachnoid space) seen through the stomach or duodenum on double contrast radiographs can be mistaken for ulcers. However, these artifacts are easily recognized by obtaining films in multiple projections.

The most important consideration in the differential diagnosis of a benign gastric ulcer is an ulcerated gastric carcinoma (see earlier section on benign versus malignant ulcers). An ulcer that is surrounded by a discrete mound of edema can also be mistaken radiographically for an ulcerated submucosal mass such as a leiomyoma.[110, 111] However, the edematous mass surrounding an ulcer usually has poorly defined borders that form obtuse angles with the adjacent gastric wall, whereas a submucosal mass has well-defined borders that form right angles with the adjacent gastric wall.[111] When gastric ulcers are associated with massive edema, there may be such narrowing and deformity that the radiographic findings erroneously suggest an infiltrating carcinoma. This problem is more likely to occur with

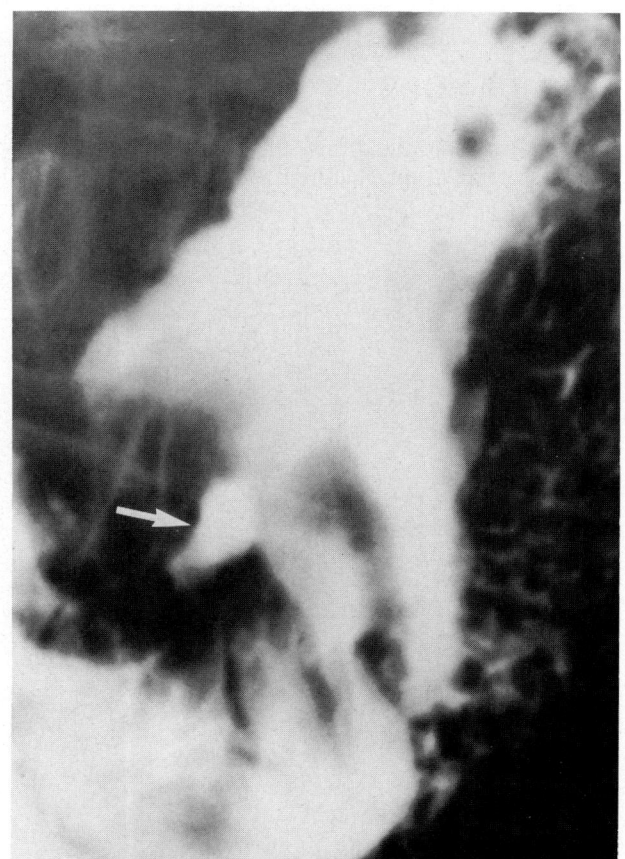

**Figure 35–33. Pyloric channel ulcer.** A prone compression view shows barium filling an ulcer crater *(arrow)* on the anterior wall of the pyloric channel.

prepyloric ulcers causing gastric outlet obstruction, so that it is not possible to assess the distal antrum adequately. If a malignant lesion cannot be excluded on radiologic criteria, endoscopy should be performed for a more definitive diagnosis.

Although multiple gastric or duodenal ulcers may be present in patients with uncomplicated peptic ulcer disease, this finding should raise the possibility of Zollinger-Ellison syndrome, cytomegalovirus infection, caustic ingestion, other granulomatous conditions such as Crohn's disease, tuberculosis, sarcoidosis, or syphilis, and, rarely, lymphoma (see Chapters 36 and 39). In many cases, however, the correct diagnosis is suggested by the clinical history.

Gastric ulcer scars that are manifested by radiating folds must be differentiated from early gastric cancers. Although these tumors may be associated with radiating folds, the folds tend to have a more lobulated, nodular, or irregular appearance.[92] Endoscopy and biopsy should therefore be performed for a more certain diagnosis if the radiographic findings are equivocal. Benign-appearing ulcer scars may also result from healing of lymphomatous gastric lesions treated with chemotherapy (see Chapter 39).[112] Finally, ulcer scars may resemble surgical scars resulting from prior gastrostomy, cystogastrostomy (internal drainage of a pancreatic pseudocyst into the stomach), or wedge resection of the stomach.[84] However, ulcer scars can usually be differentiated from surgical scars on the basis of the clinical history.

## COMPLICATIONS

The major complications of peptic ulcers include upper gastrointestinal bleeding, obstruction, and perforation. These complications are often life threatening, and early treatment is essential for decreasing morbidity and mortality. As in the diagnosis of peptic ulcers, radiologists have a major role in the recognition of these complications.

## Upper Gastrointestinal Bleeding

Bleeding peptic ulcers may be manifested by sudden, massive upper gastrointestinal hemorrhage with hematemesis, melena, or rectal bleeding or by chronic, low-grade hemorrhage with guaiac-positive stool or iron deficiency anemia. Endoscopy has a sensitivity of more than 90% in detecting the bleeding site in these patients.[113] Barium studies are less accurate because of the difficulty of obtaining adequate mucosal coating in the presence of bleeding and the inability to determine whether a radiographically diagnosed lesion is the actual source of bleeding. Nevertheless, double contrast studies have a reported sensitivity of 70 to 80% in detecting the bleeding site in patients with acute upper gastrointestinal hemorrhage.[113, 114]

The most frequent radiologic sign of bleeding in a gastric or duodenal ulcer is a blood clot at the base of the ulcer. The clot may be manifested by one or more smooth or irregular filling defects in the barium-filled ulcer crater[114] (Fig. 35–34). Granulation tissue or debris in the ulcer may produce similar findings. However, the defect usually represents an adherent blood clot in patients who have a history of recent upper gastrointestinal bleeding. Subsequent dislodgment of the clot may lead to recurrent bleeding with potentially catastrophic consequences. These patients should therefore be observed carefully for a period of 24 to 48 hours when a blood clot is detected on barium studies.

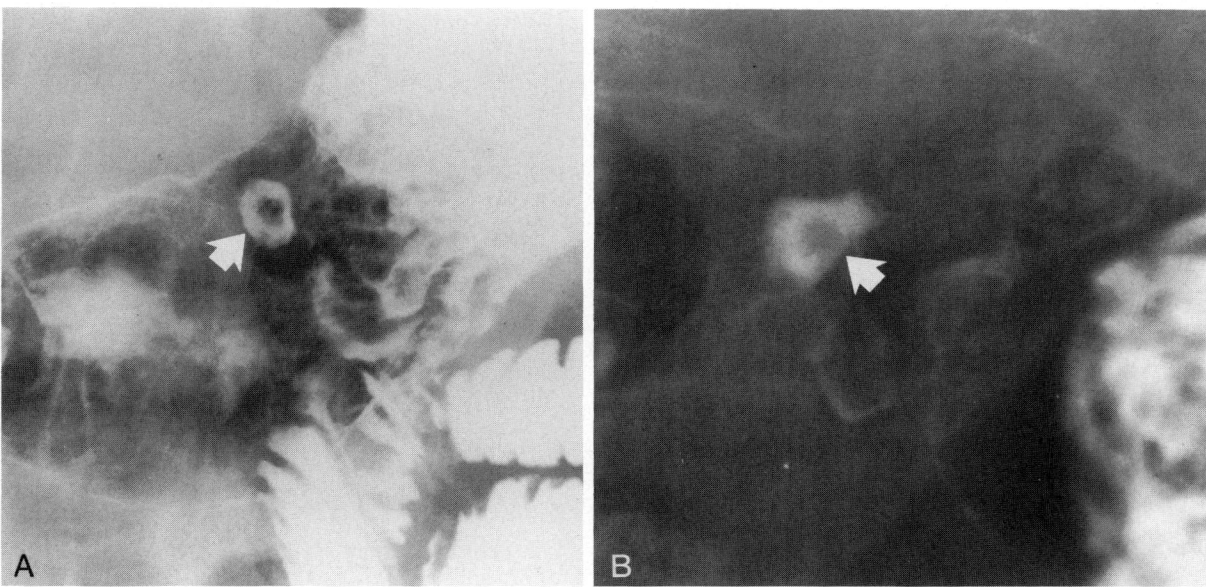

**Figure 35–34. Ulcers with blood clots. A**. A radiolucent filling defect is seen in the central portion of a barium-filled ulcer *(arrow)* on the posterior wall of the stomach. This patient presented with hematemesis 1 day earlier. **B**. A blood clot is faintly seen in the central portion of this duodenal ulcer *(arrow)*.

## Obstruction

Ulcers that are located in the fundus, body, or proximal antrum of the stomach rarely cause obstruction. However, ulcers located in the distal antrum, pyloric channel, or duodenum may cause gastric outlet obstruction as a result of either edema and spasm associated with the acute ulcer or scarring and fibrosis associated with ulcer healing. In patients with severe gastric outlet obstruction, abdominal radiographs may reveal a dilated stomach with retained food and debris (Fig. 35–35). This food or fluid in the stomach may dilute ingested barium so that it is difficult to obtain diagnostic upper gastrointestinal examinations. The stomach should therefore be decompressed with a nasogastric tube before performing barium studies. The patient should also be examined with high-density barium in the upright or semiupright position to facilitate passage of barium to the site of obstruction.

Severe scarring from ulcers in the distal antrum or pyloric channel may be manifested radiographically by a relatively short segment of narrowing with delayed emptying of barium from the stomach (see Fig. 35–20A). Unfortunately, it is sometimes difficult to differentiate these areas of scarring from localized scirrhous carcinomas involving the prepyloric region of the antrum.[115] Irregular narrowing and abrupt, shelf-like proximal borders should favor malignancy (see Fig. 38–11).

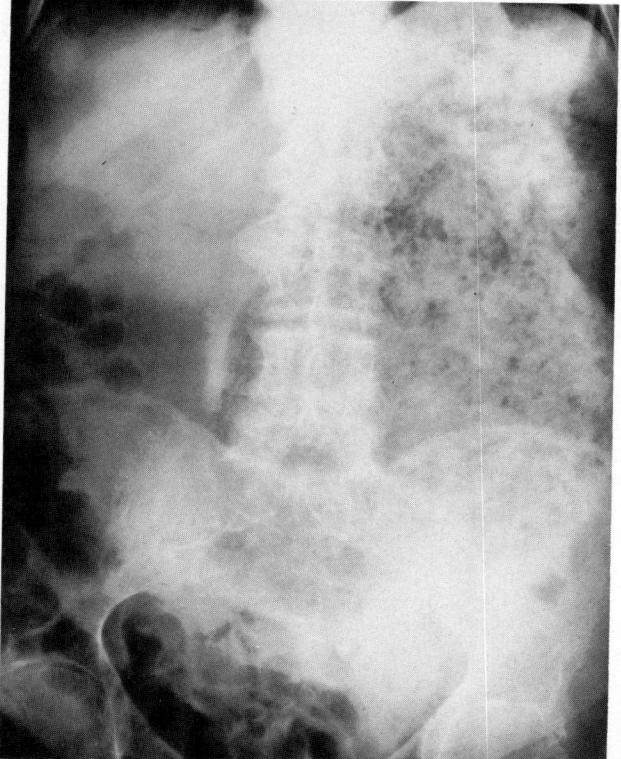

**Figure 35–35. Gastric outlet obstruction caused by a pyloric channel ulcer.** An abdominal radiograph shows a markedly dilated stomach with retained food and debris due to gastric outlet obstruction. After the stomach was decompressed, endoscopy revealed a pyloric channel ulcer causing the obstruction.

However, endoscopy and biopsy may be required for a more certain diagnosis.

Scarring from duodenal ulcers may also lead to gastric outlet obstruction. Although bulbar ulcers rarely cause obstruction, postbulbar ulcers may lead to the development of strictures in the proximal descending duodenum with subsequent obstruction (see earlier section on postbulbar ulcers). Other causes of duodenal narrowing and obstruction include Crohn's disease, tuberculosis, strongyloidiasis, tumors, hematomas, duplication cysts, and extrinsic compression of the duodenum by an annular pancreas, pancreatitis, pancreatic pseudocysts, or pancreatic carcinoma.

## Perforation

Penetrating ulcers on the anterior wall of the stomach or duodenum may perforate directly into the peritoneal cavity, whereas penetrating ulcers on the posterior wall of the stomach or duodenum usually result in a walled-off or "confined" perforation. Some penetrating ulcers may also involve other hollow organs, producing a fistula. The various types of perforations are considered separately in the following sections.

### Free Perforation

Ulcers on the anterior wall of the stomach or duodenum directly abut the peritoneal cavity, so perforation of a penetrating ulcer in this location may result in acute peritonitis with free spillage of gastric and duodenal contents into the peritoneal cavity. Because anterior wall ulcers occur much more frequently in the duodenum than in the stomach, the majority of patients with this complication have perforated duodenal ulcers. Although obstruction, ischemia, toxic megacolon, diverticulitis, and appendicitis are other causes of peritonitis, a perforated duodenal ulcer is the most common cause of peritonitis in the adult population.

The volume of gas that escapes into the peritoneal cavity from a perforated peptic ulcer depends on how quickly the site of perforation becomes sealed off. In one study, free intraperitoneal air was detected on abdominal radiographs in only about two thirds of patients with perforated duodenal ulcers.[116] Thus, the presence of pneumoperitoneum in an acutely ill patient strongly supports the diagnosis of a perforated duodenal ulcer, but the absence of pneumoperitoneum in no way excludes this diagnosis.

If abdominal radiographs reveal pneumoperitoneum in patients with clinical signs of peritonitis, immediate surgery is warranted. If there is no evidence of pneumoperitoneum, studies with water-soluble contrast agents may be performed to determine whether a perforation has occurred. However, only about 50% of patients with perforated duodenal ulcers are found to have extravasation of contrast medium from the duodenum, presumably because the perforation has sealed off before the examination.[117] When extravasation of contrast medium does occur, about half of the patients

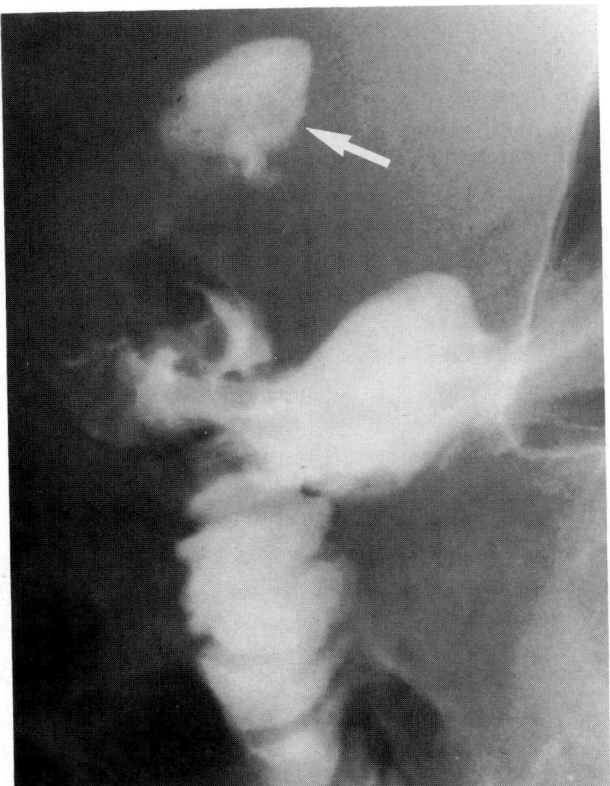

**Figure 35–36. Perforated duodenal ulcer.** Contrast medium is seen tracking superiorly from the region of the duodenal bulb into a walled-off collection *(arrow)*. This patient presented with clinical signs of peritonitis.

delayed diagnosis of retroperitoneal perforations has led to unusually high morbidity and mortality in these patients.[121] Nevertheless, this complication may be suspected when abdominal radiographs demonstrate mottled or linear collections of gas in the retroperitoneum in patients with a known history of peptic ulcer disease. CT is helpful for confirming the presence and extent of retroperitoneal abscess formation. Prompt surgical drainage of the abscess is required.

## Confined Perforation

Penetrating ulcers on the posterior wall of the stomach or duodenum are often associated with the development of a walled-off or confined perforation due to an inflammatory reaction and fibrous adhesions that seal off the perforation site as the ulcer enters adjacent structures. The pancreas is involved in 65 to 75% of patients with confined perforations.[38, 123] Other less common sites of involvement include the lesser omentum, transverse mesocolon, liver, spleen, biliary tract, and colon.[38, 123] If the affected structure is a hollow organ such as the colon or biliary tract, this process may lead to the development of a fistula (see later section on fistulas).

Less than 50% of patients with posterior penetrating ulcers and confined perforations have evidence of extraluminal gas or contrast medium collections on studies with water-soluble contrast agents.[38] However, a posterior penetrating ulcer should be suspected when an unusually deep ulcer crater is seen in profile on the posterior wall of the stomach or duodenum. In such

are found to have a generalized leak into the peritoneal cavity (see Fig. 40–42) and half are found to have a walled-off leak[117] (Fig. 35–36). With a free perforation, contrast medium may be seen leaking from the duodenal bulb into the subhepatic space or elsewhere into the peritoneal cavity. Occasionally, extravasated contrast medium or free intraperitoneal air may be demonstrated by computed tomography (CT) in patients with unsuspected perforations.[118]

Much less frequently, ulcers on the posterior wall of the stomach may perforate into the lesser peritoneal cavity or lesser sac, a potential space between the stomach and pancreas.[119] An abscess in the lesser sac may be manifested by extraluminal gas collections in the left upper quadrant on abdominal radiographs or by an extrinsic mass effect on the posterior wall of the stomach or actual leakage of contrast medium into the lesser sac on studies with water-soluble contrast agents[119] (Fig. 35–37). CT is extremely useful for documenting these fluid collections or abscesses in the lesser sac.[120]

In patients with perforated ulcers on the posterior wall of the stomach or duodenum, extravasated peptic secretions occasionally dissect through the retroperitoneum, causing extensive abscess formation in the anterior pararenal space.[121, 122] Because the inflammatory process is confined to the retroperitoneum, these patients usually have no peritoneal signs or symptoms, so the clinical presentation is often misleading. As a result,

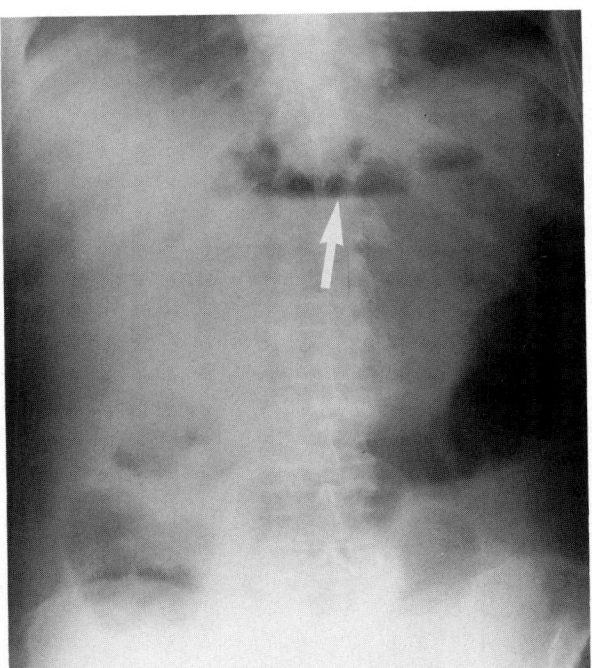

**Figure 35–37. Lesser sac abscess caused by a perforated gastric ulcer.** An upright abdominal plain film shows an air-fluid level *(arrow)* in the lesser sac due to a lesser sac abscess. A subsequent study with a water-soluble contrast agent revealed a perforated posterior wall gastric ulcer with leakage of the contrast agent directly into the lesser sac.

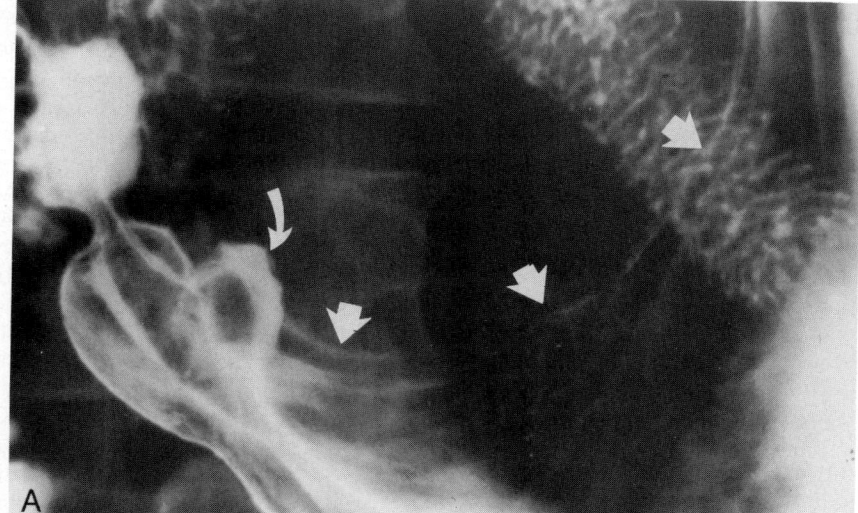

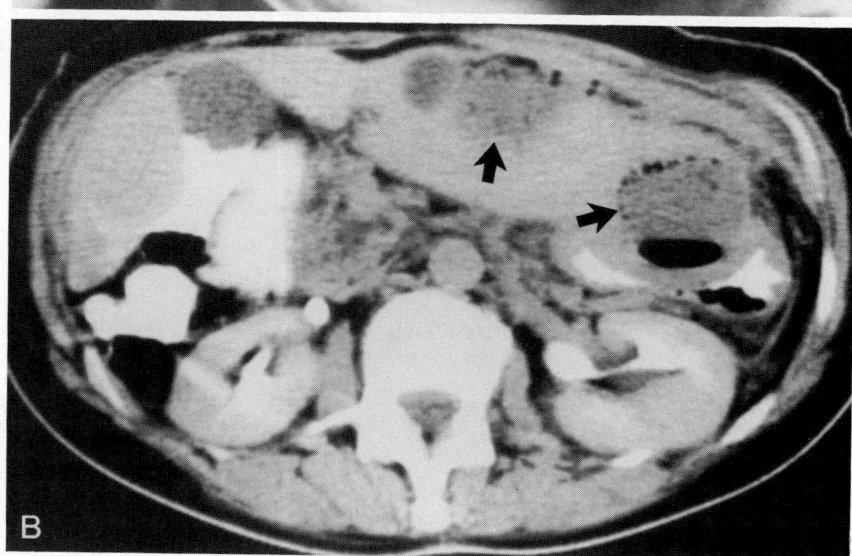

**Figure 35–38. Penetrating lesser curvature ulcer with an associated hepatic abscess. A.** A barium study shows a deep ulcer *(curved arrow)* on the lesser curvature of the distal antrum. Also note the large area of extrinsic mass effect *(straight arrows)* on the adjacent gastric wall. **B.** A CT scan reveals several gas- and fluid-containing abscess cavities *(arrows)* in the left lobe of the liver. These abscesses were caused by penetration of the ulcer into the hepatic parenchyma.

cases, CT may be helpful for demonstrating signs of pancreatic penetration, including loss of fascial planes and the presence of soft tissue bands or low-density sinus tracks between these structures.[124]

Penetrating ulcers on the lesser curvature of the stomach occasionally enter the adjacent hepatic parenchyma, resulting in the development of an abscess in the left lobe of the liver. This complication should be suspected when contrast studies demonstrate a deep ulcer on the lesser curvature associated with an extrinsic mass effect on the adjacent gastric wall (Fig. 35–38A). In such cases, CT can be used to demonstrate the presence of a confined perforation involving the liver (Fig. 35–38B).

Splenic penetration by a gastric ulcer is extremely unusual because of the rarity of benign ulcers on the posterior wall or greater curvature of the gastric fundus. When it occurs, however, it is a potentially life-threatening complication, because rupture of the ulcer into the spleen may lead to sudden, massive gastrointestinal bleeding.[125] Although barium studies are usually nonspecific, transmural penetration by an ulcer high on the greater curvature or posterior wall of the stomach may be suspected if the ulcer extends well beyond the adjacent gastric contour.[126] In such cases, CT may demonstrate extension of the ulcer directly into the substance of the spleen.[125] If CT confirms splenic penetration by a benign gastric ulcer, early surgery is required because of the risk of catastrophic gastrointestinal bleeding in these patients.

## Fistulas

Penetrating ulcers in the stomach or duodenum occasionally erode through the wall of adjacent hollow organs, producing a variety of fistulas, including gastroduodenal, gastrocolic, duodenocolic, choledochoduodenal, duodenorenal, and gastropericardial fistulas. These fistulas are considered separately in the following sections.

### Gastroduodenal Fistulas (Double Channel Pylorus)

The double channel pylorus is an acquired gastroduodenal fistula caused by a penetrating ulcer in the distal antrum that erodes directly into the base of the duodenal bulb.[127-129] These ulcers are usually located on the lesser curvature of the prepyloric antrum but are occasionally located on the greater curvature.[128, 129] Paradoxically, the development of a double channel pylorus may lead to significant relief from ulcer symptoms, possibly because the fistula improves gastric emptying.[129]

Although the double channel pylorus is often difficult to visualize at endoscopy, it is readily detected on barium studies.[128, 129] The double channel pylorus is typically manifested by two discrete tracks extending from the distal antrum into the base of the duodenal bulb (Fig. 35–39). The track on the greater curvature side of the stomach usually represents the true pyloric channel, whereas the track on the lesser curvature side represents the fistula. The barium-filled tracks are often separated by a thin, radiolucent bridge or septum that is best seen on prone compression views. Sequential barium studies occasionally demonstrate progression from a penetrating prepyloric ulcer to a double channel pylorus (Fig. 35–40).

### Gastrocolic Fistulas

In the past, most gastrocolic fistulas have been caused by primary carcinoma of the stomach or transverse colon invading the gastrocolic ligament (see Chapter 40).[130]

With the increasing use of aspirin in this pill-oriented society, however, benign aspirin-induced ulcers on the greater curvature of the stomach have become a more common cause of gastrocolic fistulas than carcinoma of the stomach or transverse colon.[67, 131] Affected individuals typically have a history of ingesting large doses of aspirin or aspirin-containing compounds.[67, 131] As the ulcers enlarge, they may penetrate inferiorly into the gastrocolic ligament, eventually leading to the development of a gastrocolic fistula. This complication may be manifested by the clinical triad of diarrhea, feculent vomiting, and foul-smelling eructations.[130] When a gastrocolic fistula is suspected on clinical grounds, endoscopy is contraindicated because of the risk of perforation and peritonitis.[131] However, barium studies may reveal giant ulcers on the greater curvature of the gastric antrum or body with early filling of the transverse colon via the fistula[131] (Fig. 35–41). Because of the greater pressures generated in a barium enema examination, this technique is also useful for demonstrating fistulas that cannot be visualized on upper gastrointestinal examinations. Both upper and lower gastrointestinal studies may be required to determine whether the fistula has resulted from a benign greater curvature ulcer, gastric or colonic carcinoma, lymphoma, Crohn's disease, tuberculosis, or other unusual causes.

### Duodenocolic Fistulas

Duodenocolic fistulas are usually caused by carcinoma of the ascending colon or hepatic flexure invading the

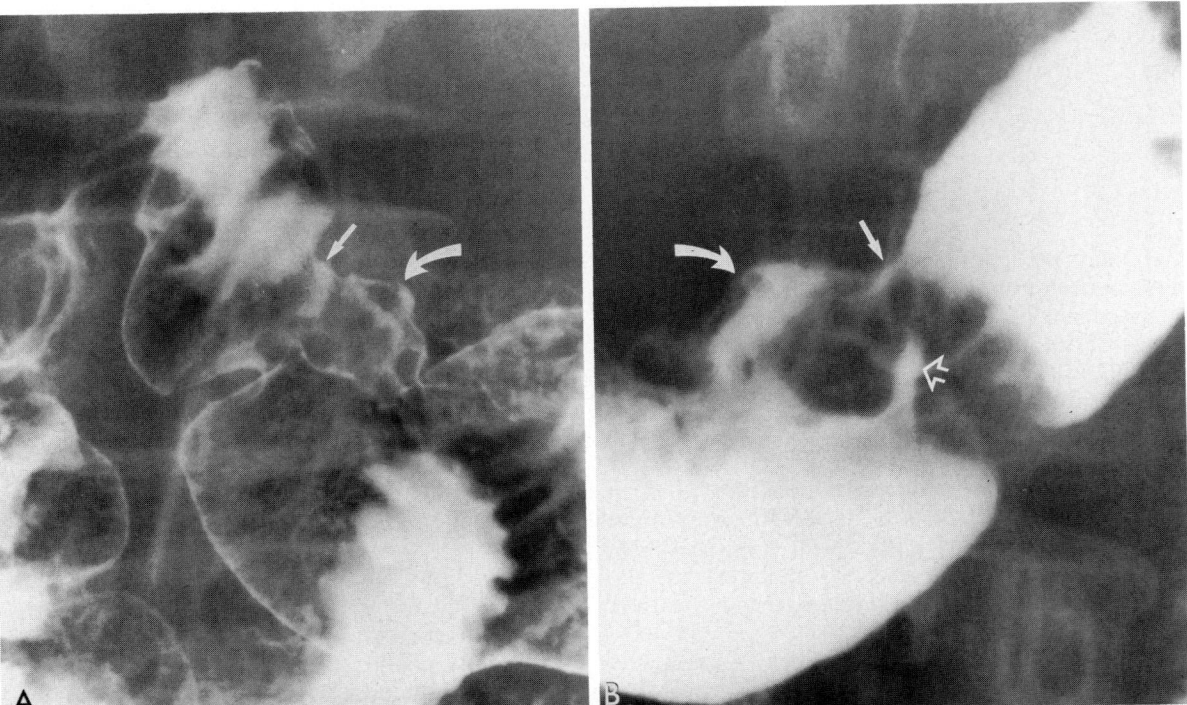

**Figure 35–39. Double channel pylorus. A.** A double contrast view of the antrum shows a prepyloric lesser curvature ulcer *(curved arrow)* that communicates distally with the base of the duodenal bulb *(straight arrow)*. **B.** A prone view of the antrum also delineates the lesser curvature ulcer *(curved arrow)* with a track *(straight arrow)* extending from the ulcer into the duodenum. Note the normal pyloric channel *(open arrow)* inferiorly.

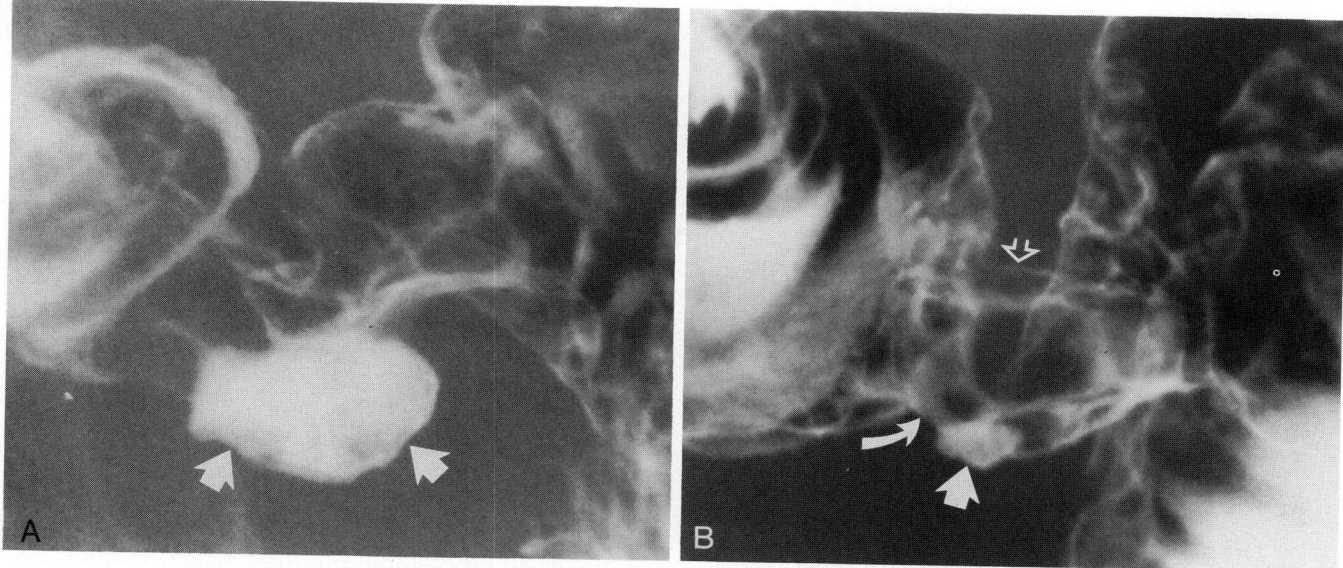

**Figure 35–40. Double channel pylorus. A**. The initial barium study shows a large ulcer *(arrows)* on the greater curvature of the distal antrum. **B**. A follow-up study 4 weeks later shows marked healing of the ulcer *(straight arrow)* after treatment with H₂ blockers. However, a fistulous track *(curved arrow)* is now seen extending from the ulcer into the base of the duodenal bulb. The normal pyloric channel *(open arrow)* is also visualized. This case is unusual, because the double channel pylorus usually results from ulcers arising on the lesser curvature rather than the greater curvature of the distal antrum.

descending duodenum.[132] Occasionally, these fistulas may result from penetrating ulcers in the duodenal bulb or postbulbar duodenum that have eroded into the hepatic flexure of the colon.[133, 134] Affected individuals may present with abdominal pain, diarrhea, feculent vomiting, foul-smelling eructations, or undigested food in the stool.[132] Although upper gastrointestinal studies may fail to demonstrate the fistula, barium enema examinations are almost always successful because of the greater pressures generated by this technique.[134]

### Choledochoduodenal Fistulas

About 90% of enterobiliary fistulas occur as complications of stones in the biliary tract.[135] Only about 5% are caused by peptic ulcer disease.[135] Most of these patients have penetrating duodenal ulcers that rupture into the common bile duct, producing a choledochoduodenal fistula.[135] These patients usually have symptoms related to their underlying ulcers but occasionally present with abnormal liver function tests, jaundice, or

**Figure 35–41. Gastrocolic fistula caused by an aspirin-induced greater curvature ulcer.** A double contrast upper gastrointestinal study reveals a giant ulcer *(large arrow)* on the greater curvature of the stomach with barium entering a wide fistulous track *(small arrows)* that communicates directly with the transverse colon. This patient had been taking high doses of aspirin.

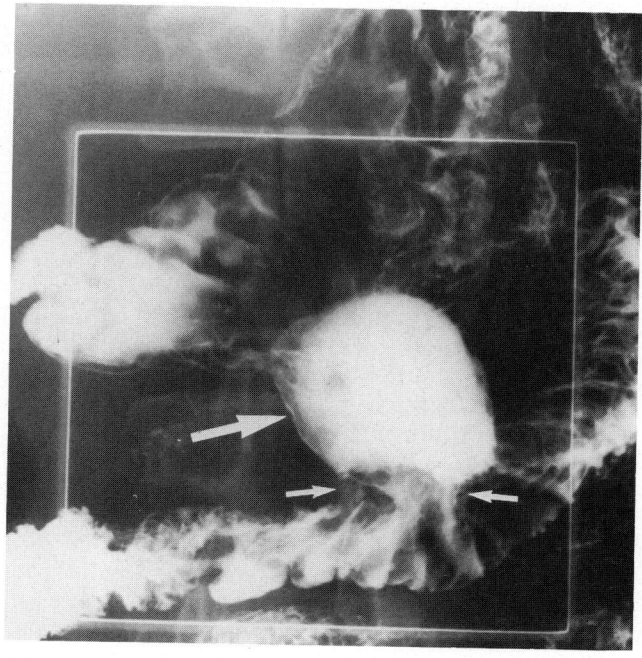

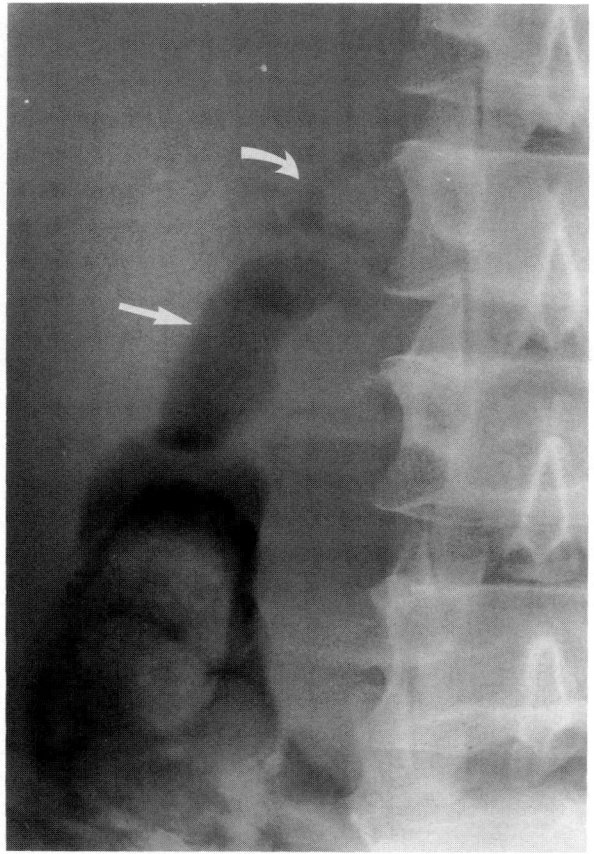

**Figure 35–42. Pneumobilia caused by a choledochoduodenal fistula.** A close-up view from an abdominal plain film shows gas in the gallbladder (*straight arrow*) and bile ducts (*curved arrow*) caused by a choledochoduodenal fistula in a patient with a giant duodenal ulcer.

ascending cholangitis.[136] Abdominal radiographs may reveal pneumobilia with gas in the gallbladder or bile ducts (Fig. 35–42), and barium studies may demonstrate a duodenal ulcer, duodenal scarring, or reflux of barium into the biliary tract.[136–138] However, the inflammatory process may seal off the fistula, so the absence of communication with the biliary tract in no way excludes this diagnosis. Rarely, penetrating ulcers may lead to the development of cholecystoduodenal, cholecystogastric, or choledochogastric fistulas.[135]

### Duodenorenal Fistulas

Penetrating postbulbar duodenal ulcers rarely rupture posteriorly into the pyelocalyceal system of the right kidney, producing a duodenorenal fistula.[139] These fistulas may be demonstrated on barium studies or on retrograde pyelography. Other rare causes of duodenorenal fistulas include malignancy, infection, and trauma.

### Gastropericardial Fistulas

Benign ulcers in the intrathoracic portion of the stomach (either a hiatal hernia or a gastric pull-through after esophagogastrectomy) rarely erode through the pericardium, producing a gastropericardial fistula.[140]

This complication is catastrophic for the patient because it usually leads to the rapid development of purulent pericarditis, cardiac tamponade, and death. The sudden appearance of pneumopericardium on chest radiographs of an acutely ill patient with an intrathoracic stomach should therefore raise the possibility of a gastropericardial fistula. Upper gastrointestinal studies with water-soluble contrast media may document the presence of a fistula by showing extravasation of contrast medium into the pericardial sac.[141] Because of the high mortality associated with this complication, the best hope for survival of the patient is early surgery with drainage of the pericardium and closure of the fistula.[140]

## ZOLLINGER-ELLISON SYNDROME

Since its original description by Zollinger and Ellison in 1955,[142] Zollinger-Ellison syndrome has been recognized as an unusual but life-threatening condition characterized by marked hypersecretion of gastric acid and a severe form of peptic ulcer disease in patients with non–beta islet cell tumors of the pancreas. These tumors not only may cause a devastating ulcer diathesis but also may behave as malignant lesions, metastasizing to the liver or other structures. Nevertheless, the development of potent antisecretory agents for controlling acid secretion as well as sophisticated techniques for localizing these islet cell tumors has greatly improved survival. Although barium studies may reveal typical features of peptic ulcer disease, it is sometimes possible to suggest the diagnosis of Zollinger-Ellison syndrome on the basis of the radiographic findings.

## Pathology

Zollinger-Ellison syndrome is caused by the uncontrolled release of gastrin from autonomously functioning non–beta islet cell tumors known as gastrinomas. About 75% of these tumors are located in the pancreas, 15% in the duodenum, and 10% in other extraintestinal locations, including the liver, ovaries, and lymph nodes.[143, 144] The majority of gastrinomas are thought to be malignant; multiple tumors or metastases are found at the time of diagnosis in 30 to 50% of patients.[144] The liver is the most frequent site of metastatic disease.

Most gastrinomas occur as sporadic tumors. However, about 25% are genetically transmitted as part of the hereditary syndrome multiple endocrine neoplasia type 1.[145] This syndrome is characterized not only by pancreatic tumors but also by parathyroid, pituitary, and adrenal tumors. Interestingly, gastrinomas associated with multiple endocrine neoplasia type 1 tend to have a more benign clinical course than isolated gastrinomas.

## Clinical Aspects

More than 90% of patients with Zollinger-Ellison syndrome have upper gastrointestinal ulcers caused by hypersecretion of gastric acid.[144] The presenting symptoms may be indistinguishable from those associated with ordinary peptic ulcers. However, the possibility of Zollinger-Ellison syndrome should be considered in patients who have multiple ulcers, ulcers in unusual locations, ulcers that are resistant to medical therapy, frequent and early recurrence of ulcers after cessation of therapy, or postoperative recurrence of ulcers.[143, 144]

The second most common clinical problem in Zollinger-Ellison syndrome is diarrhea, which occurs in up to 50% of patients and is the presenting symptom in 35%.[143, 144] This diarrhea is related primarily to the severe volume load caused by the secretion of several liters of acid into the intestines each day. The acidic pH of the small bowel may also damage the intestinal mucosa, resulting in a sprue-like state with villous atrophy, malabsorption, and steatorrhea.[146] Other patients may present initially with reflux symptoms or dysphagia due to the development of severe reflux esophagitis or peptic strictures.[147]

The diagnosis of Zollinger-Ellison syndrome is established by the demonstration of hypergastrinemia and gastric acid hypersecretion in a patient with peptic ulcers, diarrhea, or other clinical features of a gastrinoma. In the appropriate clinical setting, fasting serum gastrin levels greater than 1000 pg/mL should be virtually diagnostic of Zollinger-Ellison syndrome.[144] However, not all patients have such high serum gastrin levels. Furthermore, varying degrees of hypergastrinemia may also occur in patients with atrophic gastritis, gastric outlet obstruction, G cell hyperplasia, and retained antrum. Gastrin provocation tests such as the secretin stimulation test have been used to differentiate Zollinger-Ellison syndrome from other causes of hypergastrinemia. Administration of secretin causes a paradoxical rise in serum gastrin to more than 200 pg/mL above basal levels in more than 90% of patients with Zollinger-Ellison syndrome.[144]

In the past, total gastrectomy has been the treatment of choice for preventing hypersecretion of acid and its complications in patients with Zollinger-Ellison syndrome. However, $H_2$ receptor antagonists such as cimetidine and ranitidine have proved to be extremely effective in suppressing acid secretion and promoting ulcer healing without need for surgery.[144] Omeprazole, a potent inhibitor of acid secretion, has been shown to be particularly safe and efficacious for the long-term treatment of these patients.[148] Thus, total gastrectomy should probably be reserved for individuals who are noncompliant with medical therapy.

As fewer patients succumb to the ulcer diathesis in Zollinger-Ellison syndrome, widespread metastatic disease has been the major cause of morbidity and mortality in these patients. Greater attention has therefore been focused on early detection and excision of the underlying gastrinomas responsible for this syndrome. Unfortunately, these gastrinomas are notoriously difficult to diagnose on preoperative imaging studies; no tumor is found at surgery in about 50% of patients with Zollinger-Ellison syndrome.[149] Nevertheless, successful localization of gastrinomas may be achieved by CT, abdominal angiography, or selective portal venous sampling for gastrin (see Chapters 114 and 117). CT should

probably be the initial procedure of choice for detecting both the primary gastrinoma and liver metastases.[150] If the CT findings are equivocal, however, angiography or selective portal venous sampling may improve the diagnostic yield in these patients.[151, 152]

The most important prognostic factor affecting survival is the extent of tumor at the time of surgery. Patients with no tumor or lesions that are resectable at laparotomy have 5-year survival rates greater than 90%, whereas patients with liver metastases have 5-year survival rates less than 20%.[144] The aim of therapy for patients with Zollinger-Ellison syndrome is therefore to remove the underlying gastrinomas at the earliest possible stage.

## Radiographic Findings

Barium studies of the upper gastrointestinal tract are often performed on patients with Zollinger-Ellison syndrome who present with severe, intractable ulcer symptoms. These studies may demonstrate a characteristic constellation of findings and occasionally reveal abnormalities that are virtually pathognomonic of this syndrome.[153–157] Hypersecretion of acid often results in a large volume of fluid in the stomach, duodenum, and proximal jejunum that dilutes the barium and compromises mucosal coating. Many patients have markedly thickened gastric folds, particularly in the fundus and body of the stomach, not only because of edema and inflammation but also because of gastrin-induced parietal cell hyperplasia (Fig. 35–43A). Duodenal and jejunal folds may also have a grossly thickened, edematous appearance because of a severe inflammatory response to the enormous amount of gastric secretions entering the proximal small bowel. Although thickened folds may be caused by a variety of conditions in the stomach and duodenum (see later section on differential diagnosis), the combination of thickened folds and excessive fluid in the stomach, duodenum, and proximal jejunum should suggest the possibility of Zollinger-Ellison syndrome.[157]

Approximately 75% of the ulcers in Zollinger-Ellison syndrome are located in the stomach or duodenal bulb, so they cannot be differentiated radiographically from ordinary peptic ulcers.[158] However, the remaining 25% are located in the postbulbar duodenum or proximal jejunum.[158] Because peptic ulcers rarely occur distal to the papilla of Vater, the presence of one or more ulcers in the third or fourth portion of the duodenum or in the proximal jejunum should be highly suggestive of Zollinger-Ellison syndrome (Fig. 35–43B). Patients with this syndrome are also more likely to have multiple ulcers than other patients with peptic disease.[158]

## Differential Diagnosis

Markedly thickened gastric folds may be present in a variety of conditions, including hypertrophic gastritis, Ménétrier's disease, and lymphoma. Similarly, thickened duodenal or jejunal folds may be caused by a host

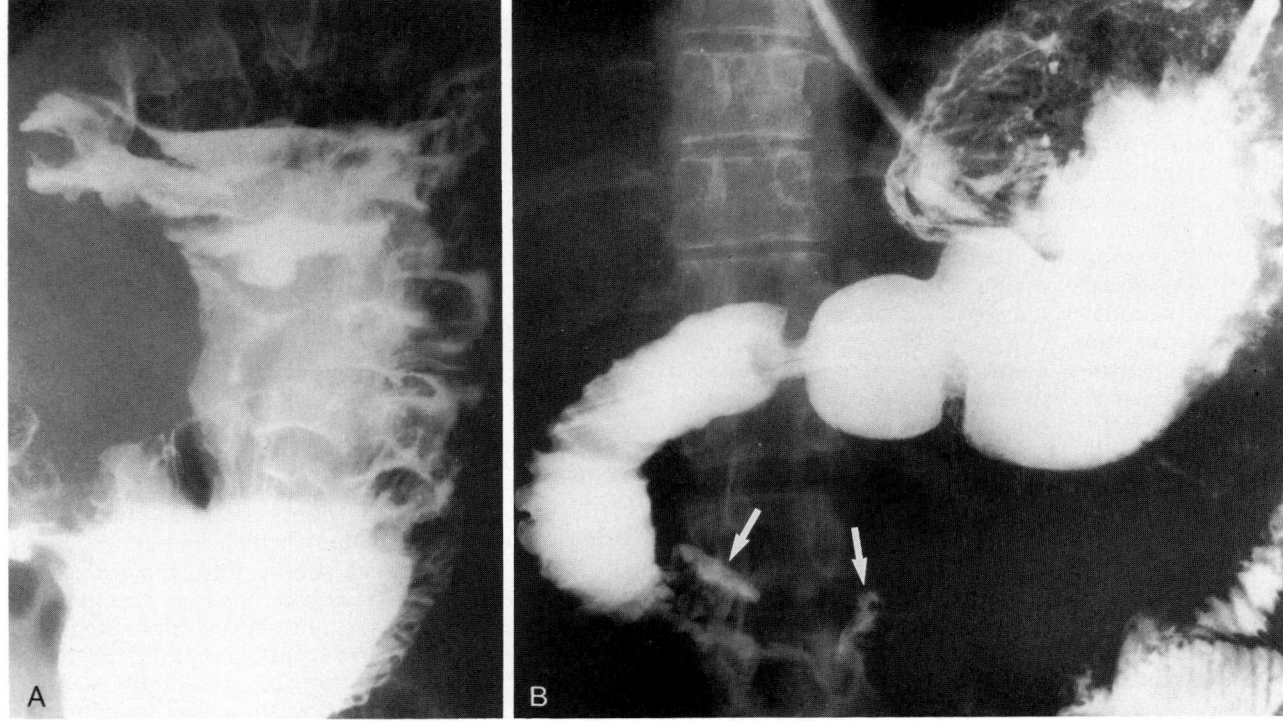

**Figure 35–43. Zollinger-Ellison syndrome. A**. There are markedly thickened folds in the gastric fundus and body. The barium is diluted by excessive fluid in the stomach. **B**. In another patient, two discrete ulcers *(arrows)* are seen in the third and fourth portions of the duodenum. Ordinary peptic ulcers rarely occur distal to the papilla of Vater, so ulcers in this location should suggest the possibility of Zollinger-Ellison syndrome. (**B** courtesy of Stephen W. Trenkner, M.D., Minneapolis, MN.)

of inflammatory or infectious processes. Although thickened folds are a nonspecific finding, the simultaneous presence of increased fluid in the upper gastrointestinal tract and one or more ulcers in unusual locations should strongly suggest Zollinger-Ellison syndrome. If this syndrome is suspected on the basis of the radiographic findings, a fasting serum gastrin level should be obtained for a more definitive diagnosis.

### Acknowledgment

Figures 35–1A and B, 35–2A and B, 35–7A and B, 35–8A, 35–9, 35–16A and B, 35–17A and B, 35–20A and B, 35–24A, 35–25A and B, 35–26A and B, 35–29, 35–32, and 35–34A are reproduced from Laufer I, Levine MS (eds): Double Contrast Gastrointestinal Radiology (2nd ed). Philadelphia: WB Saunders, 1992.

## References

1. Boyd EJS, Wormsley KG: Etiology and pathogenesis of peptic ulcer. *In* Berk JE, Haubrich WS, Kalser MH, et al (eds): Bockus Gastroenterology (4th ed). Philadelphia: WB Saunders, 1985, pp. 1013–1059.
2. Bonnevie O: Changing demographics of peptic ulcer disease. Dig Dis Sci 30(suppl 11):85–145, 1985.
3. Kurata JH, Haile BM, Elashoff JD: Sex differences in peptic ulcer disease. Gastroenterology 88:96–100, 1985.
4. Rotter JI: The genetics of peptic ulcers: more than one gene, more than one disease. Prog Med Genet 4:1–58, 1980.
5. Tarpila S, Samloff IM, Pikkarainen P, et al: Endoscopic and clinical findings in first-degree relatives of duodenal ulcer patients and control subjects. Scand J Gastroenterol 17:503–506, 1982.
6. Peters MN, Richardson CT: Stressful life events, acid hypersecretion, and ulcer disease. Gastroenterology 84:114–119, 1983.
7. Walker P, Luther J, Samloff IM, et al: Life events, stress and psychosocial factors in men with peptic ulcer disease. Gastroenterology 94:323–330, 1988.
8. Thomas J, Greig M, Piper DW: Chronic gastric ulcer and life events. Gastroenterology 78:905–911, 1980.
9. Friedman GD, Siegelaub AB, Seltzer CC: Cigarettes, alcohol, coffee, and peptic ulcer. N Engl J Med 290:469–473, 1974.
10. Piper DW, Nasiry R, McIntosh J, et al: Smoking, alcohol, analgesics, and chronic duodenal ulcer. Scand J Gastroenterol 19:1015–1021, 1984.
11. Wormsley KG: Smoking and duodenal ulcer. Gastroenterology 75:139–142, 1978.
12. Chapman BL, Duggan JM: Aspirin and uncomplicated peptic ulcer. Gut 10:443–450, 1969.
13. Levy M: Aspirin use in patients with major upper gastrointestinal bleeding and peptic-ulcer disease. N Engl J Med 290:1158–1162, 1974.
14. Cameron AJ: Aspirin and gastric ulcer. Mayo Clin Proc 50:565–570, 1975.
15. Silvoso GR, Ivey KJ, Butt JH, et al: Incidence of gastric lesions in patients with rheumatic disease on chronic aspirin therapy. Ann Intern Med 91:517–520, 1979.
16. Davenport HW: Salicylate damage to the gastric mucosal barrier. N Engl J Med 276:1307–1312, 1967.
17. Bugat R, Thompson MR, Aures D, et al: Gastric mucosal lesions produced by intravenous infusion of aspirin in cats. Gastroenterology 7:754–759, 1976.
18. Lanza FL, Royer GL, Nelson RS, et al: The effects of ibuprofen, indomethacin, aspirin, naproxen, and placebo on the gastric mucosa of normal volunteers: a gastroscopic and photographic study. Dig Dis Sci 24:823–828, 1979.
19. Peoples JB: Peptic ulcer disease and the nonsteroidal anti-inflammatory drugs. Am Surg 51:358–362, 1985.

20. Roth SH, Bennett RE: Nonsteroidal anti-inflammatory drug gastropathy: recognition and response. Arch Intern Surg 147:2093–2100, 1987.
21. Conn HO, Blitzer BL: Nonassociation of adrenocorticosteroid therapy and peptic ulcer. N Engl J Med 294:473–479, 1976.
22. Warren JR, Marshall BJ: Unidentified curved bacilli on gastric epithelium in active chronic gastritis. Lancet 2:1273–1275, 1983.
23. Isenberg JI, McQuaid KR, Laine L, et al: Acid-peptic disorders. *In* Yamada T (ed): Textbook of Gastroenterology. Philadelphia: JB Lippincott, 1991, pp 1241–1339.
24. Chamberlain CE, Peura DA: *Campylobacter* (*Helicobacter*) *pylori*: is peptic disease a bacterial infection? Arch Intern Med 150:951–955, 1990.
25. Peterson WL: *Helicobacter pylori* and peptic ulcer disease. N Engl J Med 324:1043–1048, 1991.
26. Yardley JH, Paull G: *Campylobacter pylori*: a newly recognized infectious agent in the gastrointestinal tract. Am J Surg Pathol 12(suppl):89–99, 1988.
27. Marshall BJ, Goodwin GS, Warren JR, et al: Prospective double-blind trial of duodenal ulcer relapse after eradication of *Campylobacter pylori*. Lancet 2:1437–1442, 1988.
28. Dooley CP: *Helicobacter pylori* infection and peptic ulcer disease. Curr Opin Gastroenterol 9:112–117, 1993.
29. Grossman MI, Kirsner JB, Gillespie IE: Basal and histalog-stimulated gastric secretion in control subjects and in patients with peptic ulcer or gastric cancer. Gastroenterology 45:14–26, 1963.
30. Wormsley KG: The pathophysiology of duodenal ulceration. Gut 15:59–81, 1974.
31. Isenberg JI, Grossman MI, Maxwell V, et al: Increased sensitivity to stimulation of acid secretion by pentagastrin in duodenal ulcer. J Clin Invest 55:330–337, 1975.
32. Kauffman GL: The gastric mucosal barrier. Dig Dis Sci 30(suppl II):69s–76s, 1985.
33. Younan F, Pearson J, Allen A, et al: Changes in the structure of the mucous gel on the mucosal surface of the stomach in association with peptic ulcer disease. Gastroenterology 82:827–831, 1982.
34. Gear MWL, Truelove SC, Whitehead R: Gastric ulcer and gastritis. Gut 12:639–645, 1971.
35. Rhodes J, Barnardo DE, Phillips SF, et al: Increased reflux of the bile into the stomach in patients with gastric ulcers. Gastroenterology 57:241–252, 1969.
36. Dragstedt LR: A concept of the etiology of gastric and duodenal ulcers. Gastroenterology 30:208–220, 1956.
37. Roth JLA, Stein GN, Morissey JR, et al: Diagnosis of peptic ulcer. *In* Berk JE, Haubrich WS, Kalser MH, et al (eds): Bockus Gastroenterology (4th ed). Philadelphia: WB Saunders, 1985, pp 1060–1115.
38. Haubrich WS, Roth JLA, Bockus HL: The clinical significance of penetration and confined perforation in peptic ulcer disease. Gastroenterology 25:173–201, 1953.
39. Krippaehne WW, Fletcher WS, Dunphy JE: Acute perforation of duodenal and gastric ulcer: factors affecting mortality. Arch Surg 88:874–882, 1964.
40. Burge H, Gill AM, Lewis RH: The pyloric-channel syndrome and gastric ulceration. Lancet 1:73–75, 1963.
41. Glickman MG, Szemes G, Loeb P, et al: Peptic ulcer of the pyloric region. AJR 113:147–158, 1971.
42. Dunn JP, Etter LE: Inadequacy of the medical history in the diagnosis of duodenal ulcer. N Engl J Med 266:68–72, 1962.
43. Sharma MP, Choudhari G: Nocturnal pain and duodenal ulcer. Br J Clin Pract 42:198–199, 1967.
44. Lind T, Cederberg C, Ekenved G, et al: Effect of omeprazole—a gastric proton pump inhibitor—on pentagastrin stimulated acid secretion in man. Gut 24:270–276, 1983.
45. McFarland RJ, Bateson MC, Green JRB, et al: Omeprazole provides quicker symptom relief and duodenal ulcer healing than ranitidine. Gastroenterology 98:278–283, 1990.
46. Agrawal NM, Saffouri B, Kruss DM, et al: Healing of benign gastric ulcers: a placebo-controlled comparison of two dosage regimens of Misoprostol, a synthetic analogue of prostaglandin E₁. Dig Dis Sci 30(suppl 11):164s–170s, 1985.
47. Gilbert DA, Surawicz CM, Silverstein FE, et al: Prevention of acute, aspirin-induced gastric mucosal injury by 15-R-15 methyl prostaglandin E₂: an endoscopic study. Gastroenterology 86:339–345, 1984.
48. Penn I: The declining role of the surgeon in the treatment of acid-peptic disease. Arch Surg 115:134–135, 1980.
49. Gustavsson S, Kelly KA, Melton LJ, et al: Trends in peptic ulcer surgery: a population-based study in Rochester, Minnesota, 1956–1985. Gastroenterology 94:688–694, 1988.
50. Hirschowitz BI: Natural history of duodenal ulcer. Gastroenterology 85:967–970, 1985.
51. Kikuchi Y, Levine MS, Laufer I, et al: Value of flow technique for double-contrast examination of the stomach. AJR 147:1183–1184, 1986.
52. Nelson SW: The discovery of gastric ulcers and the differential diagnosis between benignancy and malignancy. Radiol Clin North Am 7:5–25, 1969.
53. Gardiner GA, Racker DR: Cephalic angled views for detection of occult lesser curvature ulcers. Gastrointest Radiol 10:153–155, 1985.
54. Goldsmith MR, Paul RE, Poplack WE, et al: Evaluation of routine double contrast views of the anterior wall of the stomach. AJR 126:1159–1163, 1976.
55. Poplack WE, Paul RE, Goldsmith MR, et al: Linear and rod-shaped peptic ulcers. Radiology 122:317–321, 1977.
56. Amaral NM: Radiographic diagnosis of shallow gastric ulcers: a comparative study of technique. Radiology 129:597–600, 1978.
57. Braver JM, Paul RE, Philipps E, et al: Roentgen diagnosis of linear ulcers. Radiology 132:29–32, 1979.
58. Levine MS, Creteur V, Kressel HY, et al: Benign gastric ulcers: diagnosis and follow-up with double-contrast radiography. Radiology 164:9–13, 1987.
59. Ott DJ, Gelfand DW, Wu WC: Detection of gastric ulcer: comparison of single- and double-contrast examination. AJR 139:93–97, 1982.
60. Gelfand DW, Dale WJ, Ott DJ: The location and size of gastric ulcers: radiologic and endoscopic evaluation. AJR 143:755–758, 1984.
61. Barragry TP, Blatchford JW, Allen MO: Giant gastric ulcers: a review of 49 cases. Ann Surg 203:255–259, 1986.
62. Sun DCH, Stempien SJ: The Veterans Administration Cooperative Study on Gastric Ulcer. Site and size of the ulcer as determinants of outcome. Gastroenterology 61:576–584, 1971.
63. Thompson G, Stevenson GW, Somers S: Distribution of gastric ulcers by double-contrast barium meal with endoscopic correlation. J Can Assoc Radiol 34:296–297, 1983.
64. Findley JW: Ulcers on the greater curvature of the stomach. Gastroenterology 40:183–187, 1961.
65. Amberg JR, Zboralske FF: Gastric ulcers after 70. AJR 96:393–399, 1966.
66. Sheppard MC, Holmes GKT, Cockel R: Clinical picture of peptic ulceration diagnosed endoscopically. Gut 18:524–530, 1977.
67. Kottler RE, Tuft RJ: Benign greater curve gastric ulcer: the "sump-ulcer." Br J Radiol 54:651–654, 1981.
68. Hocking BV, Alp MH, Grant AK: Gastric ulceration within hiatus hernia. Med J Aust 2:207–208, 1976.
69. Wolf BS: Observations on roentgen features of benign and malignant ulcers. Semin Roentgenol 6:140–150, 1971.
70. Pack GT: The relationship of gastric ulcer to gastric cancer. Cancer 3:515–522, 1950.
71. Levine MS, Verstandig A, Laufer I: Serpiginous gastric erosions caused by aspirin and other nonsteroidal antiinflammatory drugs. AJR 146:31–34, 1986.
72. Zboralske FF, Stargardter FL, Harell GS: Profile roentgenographic features of benign greater curvature ulcers. Radiology 127:63–67, 1978.
73. Han SY, Witten DM: Benign gastric ulcer with "crescent" (quarter moon) sign. Radiology 113:573–575, 1974.
74. Linbert M, Krause GR: The "ring" shadow in the diagnosis of ulcer. AJR 90:767–773, 1963.
75. Welch CE, Allen AW: Gastric ulcer: study of Massachusetts General Hospital cases during the 10-year period 1938–1947. N Engl J Med 240:277–283, 1949.
76. Smith FH, Boles RS, Jordon SM: Problem of gastric ulcers reviewed. JAMA 153:1505–1508, 1953.
77. Bloom SM, Paul RE, Matsue H, et al: Improved radiologic detection of multiple gastric ulcers. AJR 128:949–952, 1977.

78. Dolphin JA, Smith LA, Waugh JM: Multiple gastric ulcers: their occurrence in benign and malignant lesions. Gastroenterology 25:202–205, 1953.

79. Dagradi AE, Falkner RE, Lee ER: Multiple benign gastric ulcers. Am J Gastroenterol 62:36–45, 1974.

80. Taxin RN, Livingston PA, Seamon WB: Multiple gastric ulcers: a radiographic sign of benignity? Radiology 114:23–27, 1975.

81. Sakita T, Ogura Y, Takasu S, et al: Observations on the healing of ulcerations in early gastric cancer. Gastroenterology 60:835–844, 1971.

82. Kagan RA, Steckel RJ: Gastric ulcer in a young man with apparent healing. AJR 128:831–834, 1977.

83. Keller RJ, Wolf BS, Khilnani MT: Roentgen features of healing and healed benign gastric ulcers. Radiology 97:353–359, 1970.

84. Gelfand DW, Ott DJ: Gastric ulcer scars. Radiology 140:37–43, 1981.

85. Levine MS, Kong V, Rubesin SE, et al: Scirrhous carcinoma of the stomach: radiologic and endoscopic diagnosis. Radiology 175:151–154, 1990.

86. Wenger J, Brandborg LL, Spellman FA: Cancer: Part I. Clinical aspects. Gastroenterology 61:598–605, 1971.

87. Hayes MA: The gastric ulcer problem. Gastroenterology 29:609–620, 1955.

88. Kirsch IE: Benign and malignant gastric ulcers: Roentgen differentiation. Radiology 64:357–365, 1955.

89. Elliott GU, Wald SM, Benz RI: A roentgenologic study of ulcerating lesions of the stomach. AJR 77:612–622, 1957.

90. Schulman A, Simpkins KC: The accuracy of radiological diagnosis of benign, primarily and secondarily malignant gastric ulcers and their correlation with three simplified radiological types. Clin Radiol 26:317–325, 1975.

91. Thompson G, Somers S, Stevenson GW: Benign gastric ulcer: a reliable radiologic diagnosis? AJR 141:331–333, 1983.

92. Ichikawa H: Differential diagnosis between benign and malignant ulcers of the stomach. Clin Gastroenterol 2:329–332, 1973.

93. Segal AW, Healy MJR, Cox AG, et al: Diagnosis of gastric cancer. Br Med J 2:669–672, 1975.

94. Stein GN, Martin RD, Roy RH, et al: Evaluation of conventional roentgenologic techniques for demonstration of duodenal ulcer craters. AJR 91:801–807, 1964.

95. Levine MS, Rubesin SE, Herlinger H, et al: Double contrast upper gastrointestinal examination: technique and interpretation. Radiology 168:593–602, 1988.

96. de Roos A, Op den Orth JO: Linear niches in the duodenal bulb. AJR 140:941–944, 1983.

97. Rodriguez HP, Aston JK, Richardson CT: Ulcers in the descending duodenum: postbulbar ulcers. AJR 119:316–322, 1973.

98. Classen M: Endoscopy in benign peptic ulcer. Clin Gastroenterol 2:315–318, 1973.

99. Ball RP, Segal AL, Golden R: Postbulbar ulcers of the duodenum. AJR 59:90–99, 1948.

100. Bilbao MK, Frische LH, Rosch J, et al: Postbulbar duodenal ulcer and ring-stricture. Radiology 100:27–35, 1971.

101. Mistilis SP, Wiot JF, Nedelman SH: Giant duodenal ulcer. Ann Intern Med 59:155–164, 1963.

102. Eisenberg RL, Margulis AR, Moss AA: Giant duodenal ulcers. Gastrointest Radiol 2:347–353, 1978.

103. Jaazewski R, Crane SA, Cid AA: Giant duodenal ulcers: successful healing with medical therapy. Dig Dis Sci 28:486–489, 1983.

104. Kirsh IE, Brendel T: The importance of giant duodenal ulcer. Radiology 91:14–19, 1968.

105. Parulekar SG, Lubert M: Ultrasound demonstration of giant duodenal ulcer. Gastrointest Radiol 8:29–31, 1983.

106. Kawai K, Ida K, Misaki F, et al: Comparative study for duodenal ulcer by radiology and endoscopy. Endoscopy 5:7–13, 1973.

107. Wills JS: Pyloric channel ulcers and the air-contrast examination. Radiology 130:250–252, 1979.

108. Gobel VK, Kressel HY, Laufer I: Double contrast artifacts. Gastrointest Radiol 3:139–146, 1978.

109. Op den Orth JO, Ploem S: The stalactite phenomenon on double contrast studies of the stomach. Radiology 117:523–525, 1975.

110. Linsman JR: Gastric ulcers simulating intramural, extramucosal tumors. AJR 101:421–424, 1967.

111. Bonfield RE, Mantel W: The problem of differentiating benign antral ulcers from intramural tumors. Radiology 106:25–27, 1973.

112. Fox ER, Laufer I, Levine MS: Radiographic response of gastric lymphoma to chemotherapy. AJR 142:711–714, 1984.

113. Thoeni RF, Cello JP: A critical look at the accuracy of endoscopy and double-contrast radiography of the upper gastrointestinal (UGI) tract in patients with substantial UGI hemorrhage. Radiology 135:305–308, 1980.

114. Fraser GM: The double contrast barium meal in patients with acute upper gastrointestinal bleeding. Clin Radiol 29:625–634, 1978.

115. Balthazar EJ, Rosenberg H, Davidian MM: Scirrhous carcinoma of the pyloric channel and distal antrum. AJR 134:669–673, 1980.

116. Edwards RH, Foster JH: Pneumoperitoneum in perforated duodenal ulcer. Am J Surg 104:551–554, 1962.

117. Jacobson G, Berne CJ, Meyers HI, et al: The examination of patients with suspected perforated ulcer using a water-soluble contrast medium. AJR 86:37–49, 1961.

118. Fultz PJ, Skucas J, Weiss SL: CT in upper gastrointestinal tract perforations secondary to peptic ulcer disease. Gastrointest Radiol 17:5–8, 1992.

119. Feldman M: Lesser peritoneal sac perforation complicating benign peptic ulcer. Gastroenterology 15:689–695, 1950.

120. Jeffrey RB, Federle MP, Wall S: Value of computed tomography in detecting occult gastrointestinal perforation. J Comput Assist Tomogr 7:825–827, 1983.

121. Hashmonai M, Abrahamson J, Erlik D, et al: Retroperitoneal perforation of duodenal ulcers with abscess formation. Ann Surg 173:409–414, 1971.

122. Wulsin JH: Peptic ulcer of the posterior wall of the stomach and duodenum with retroperitoneal leak. Surg Gynecol Obstet 134:425–429, 1972.

123. Cassel C, Ruffin JM, Bone FC: The clinical features of walled off perforated peptic ulcer. South Med J 44:1021–1026, 1951.

124. Madrazo BL, Halpert RD, Sandler MA, et al: Computed tomographic findings in penetrating peptic ulcer. Radiology 153:751–754, 1984.

125. Glick SN, Levine MS, Teplick SK, et al: Splenic penetration by benign gastric ulcer: preoperative recognition with CT. Radiology 163:637–639, 1987.

126. Joffe N, Antonioli DA: Penetration into spleen by benign gastric ulcers. Clin Radiol 32:177–181, 1981.

127. Farack UM, Goresky CA, Jabbari M, et al: Double pylorus: a hypothesis concerning its pathogenesis. Gastroenterology 66:596–600, 1974.

128. Jamshidnejad J, Koehler RE, Narayan D: Double channel pylorus. AJR 130:1047–1050, 1978.

129. Hegedus V, Poulsen PE, Reichardt J: The natural history of the double pylorus. Radiology 126:29–34, 1978.

130. Smith DL, Dockerty MB, Black BM: Gastrocolic fistulas of malignant origin. Surg Gynecol Obstet 134:829–832, 1972.

131. Laufer I, Thornley GD, Stolberg H: Gastrocolic fistula as a complication of benign gastric ulcer. Radiology 119:7–11, 1976.

132. Hershenson LM, Kirsner JB: Duodenocolic fistula. Gastroenterology 19:864–873, 1951.

133. Sasson L, Weiskopf S: Duodenocolic fistula as a complication of peptic ulcer. Am J Gastroenterol 29:51–58, 1958.

134. Starzl TE, Dorr TW, Meyer WH: Benign duodenocolic fistula. Arch Surg 78:611–619, 1959.

135. Berguer LH: Internal biliary fistulas. Am J Gastroenterol 43:11–22, 1965.

136. Constant E, Turcotte JG: Choledochoduodenal fistula: the natural history and management of an unusual complication of peptic ulcer disease. Ann Surg 167:221–228, 1968.

137. McEwan-Alvarada G, Dysart DN: Choledochoduodenal fistulas complicating duodenal ulcer. Am J Dig Dis 12:947–954, 1967.

138. Hoppenstein JM, Medoza CB, Watne AL: Choledochoduodenal fistula due to perforating duodenal ulcer disease. Ann Surg 173:145–147, 1971.

139. Stock FE: Duodenorenal fistula: a complication of peptic ulceration. Br J Surg 42:330–331, 1955.

140. West AB, Nolan N, O'Briain DS: Benign peptic ulcers penetrating pericardium and heart: clinicopathological features and factors favoring survival. Gastroenterology 94:1478–1487, 1988.

141. O'Driscoll J, Hourihane JB: Intrapericardial barium in a case of peptic ulceration. Br J Radiol 49:177–179, 1976.

142. Zollinger RM, Ellison EH: Primary peptic ulcerations of the

jejunum associated with islet cell tumors of the pancreas. Ann Surg 142:709–728, 1955.

143. Wolfe MM, Jensen RT: Zollinger-Ellison syndrome: current concepts in diagnosis and management. N Engl J Med 317:1200–1209, 1987.

144. Del Valle J, Yamada T: Zollinger-Ellison syndrome. *In* Yamada T (ed): Textbook of Gastroenterology. Philadelphia: JB Lippincott, 1991, pp 1340–1352.

145. Ballard HS, Frane B, Havtsock RJ: Familial multiple endocrine adenoma–peptic ulcer complex. Medicine (Baltimore) 43:481–516, 1964.

146. Mausbach CM II, Wilkins RM, Dobbins WO, et al: Intestinal mucosal function and structure in the steatorrhea of Zollinger-Ellison syndrome. Arch Intern Med 121:487–494, 1968.

147. Miller LS, Vinayek R, Frucht H, et al: Reflux esophagitis in patients with Zollinger-Ellison syndrome. Gastroenterology 98:341–346, 1990.

148. Maton PN, Vinayek R, Frucht H, et al: Long-term efficacy and safety of omeprazole in patients with Zollinger-Ellison syndrome: a prospective study. Gastroenterology 97:827–836, 1989.

149. Deveney CW, Deveney KE, Stark D, et al: Resection of gastrinomas. Ann Surg 198:546–553, 1983.

150. Wank SA, Doppman JL, Miller DL, et al: Prospective study of the ability of computerized axial tomography to localize gastrinomas in patients with Zollinger-Ellison syndrome. Gastroenterology 92:905–912, 1987.

151. Maton PN, Miller DL, Doppman JL, et al: The role of selective angiography in the management of patients with Zollinger-Ellison syndrome. Gastroenterology 92:913–918, 1987.

152. Cherner JA, Doppman JL, Norton JA, et al: Selective venous sampling for gastrin to localize gastrinomas: a prospective assessment. Ann Intern Med 105:841–847, 1986.

153. Amberg JR, Ellison EH, Wilson SD, et al: Roentgenographic observations in the Zollinger-Ellison syndrome. JAMA 190:185–187, 1964.

154. Missakian MM, Carlson HC, Huzenga KA: Roentgenographic findings in Zollinger-Ellison syndrome. AJR 94:429–437, 1965.

155. Nelson SW, Christoforidis AJ: Roentgenologic features of the Zollinger-Ellison syndrome; ulcerogenic tumor of the pancreas. Semin Roentgenol 3:254–266, 1968.

156. Zboralske FF, Amberg JR: Detection of the Zollinger-Ellison syndrome: the radiologist's responsibility. AJR 104:529–543, 1968.

157. Nelson SW, Lichtenstein JE: The Zollinger-Ellison syndrome. *In* Marshak RH (ed): Radiology of the Stomach. Philadelphia: WB Saunders, 1983, pp 334–381.

158. Ellison EH, Wilson SD: The Zollinger-Ellison syndrome: reappraisal and evaluation of 260 registered cases. Ann Surg 160:514–530, 1964.

# Inflammatory Conditions

Marc S. Levine, M.D.

## EROSIVE GASTRITIS

Erosions are defined histologically as epithelial defects that do not penetrate beyond the muscularis mucosae. Although erosive gastritis is rarely diagnosed on conventional single contrast barium studies, it has become a relatively frequent finding on double contrast studies, with an overall incidence of 0.5 to 20% reported in the radiologic literature.[1-6] However, not all patients with erosive gastritis are symptomatic. Thus, it is difficult to be certain of the clinical significance of gastric erosions demonstrated on radiologic or endoscopic examinations.

### Pathogenesis

In about 50% of patients with erosive gastritis, there are no apparent predisposing factors.[7] Such cases may occur as a variant of peptic ulcer disease. However, known causes include aspirin, other nonsteroidal anti-inflammatory drugs, alcohol, steroids, stress, trauma, burns, Crohn's disease, viral or fungal infection, and endoscopic heater probe therapy or other iatrogenic trauma.[8-14]

Considerable attention has been focused on the role of aspirin and other nonsteroidal anti-inflammatory drugs in the development of erosive gastritis. Both clinical and laboratory investigations have shown that these agents are capable of disrupting the mucosal barrier in the stomach, causing erosive gastritis and gastric ulcers (see Chapter 35).[8, 9, 15-22] In one study, 40% of patients receiving chronic aspirin therapy for 3 months or longer had endoscopic evidence of erosive gastritis, and 17% had gastric ulcers.[19] Other studies of healthy volunteers have shown that two or more aspirin tablets may cause an acute erosive gastritis that is recognized endoscopically within 24 hours after ingestion of the drug.[20-22] Maximal damage usually occurs by 1 to 3 days, and evidence of healing may be documented endoscopically by 1 week.[22] Thus, gastric erosions may form rapidly after ingestion of aspirin or other nonsteroidal anti-inflammatory drugs and may heal rapidly when these drugs are withdrawn.

## Clinical Findings

Patients with erosive gastritis may present with vague dyspepsia, ulcer-like symptoms, or upper gastrointestinal bleeding.[23] However, other patients with this condition are asymptomatic. Indeed, some erosions may persist for years in the absence of clinical symptoms.[24] Because gastric erosions may be discovered as incidental findings on radiologic or endoscopic examinations, it is important to rule out other abnormalities in the stomach and duodenum before assuming that the erosions are the cause of the patient's symptoms.

## Radiographic Findings

Two types of erosions may be identified on double contrast studies. The most common type is the complete, or "varioliform," erosion in which punctate or slit-like collections of barium representing the epithelial defects are surrounded by radiolucent halos of edematous, elevated mucosa[3, 5, 7] (Fig. 36–1). Varioliform erosions typically occur in the gastric antrum and are often aligned on rugal folds.[3, 5, 23] Because they are shallow lesions, erosions on the dependent or posterior wall may be better delineated by use of flow technique for manipulating a thin layer of barium over the mucosal surface.[25] In some patients, erosive gastritis may be manifested only by scalloped or nodular antral folds (Fig. 36–2A). Depending on the quality of mucosal coating, erosions may be faintly seen on the crest of the folds (Fig. 36–2B). These scalloped antral folds may persist after the erosions have healed. Occasionally, residual epithelial nodules or polyps may also be detected at the site of the healed erosions. These hyperplastic polyps are thought to represent the sequelae of chronic erosive gastritis.[23]

Incomplete or "flat" erosions are epithelial defects without elevation of the surrounding mucosa. They appear radiographically as linear streaks or dots of barium[6, 7] (Fig. 36–3). Because the surrounding mucosa is normal, incomplete erosions are much more difficult to detect than are varioliform erosions and account for less than 5% of all erosions diagnosed on double contrast studies.[6] Occasionally, incomplete erosions may be associated with slight flattening or deformity of the adjacent gastric wall.

Although no etiologic significance is usually attributed to the shape or location of gastric erosions diagnosed on double contrast studies, aspirin and other nonsteroidal anti-inflammatory drugs may produce distinctive linear or serpiginous erosions that tend to be clustered in the body of the stomach, on or near the greater curvature[26] (Fig. 36–4). It has been postulated that these erosions result from localized mucosal injury that occurs as the dissolving tablets collect by gravity in the dependent portion of the stomach. Other patients receiving nonsteroidal anti-inflammatory drugs may have linear erosions in the antrum[26] (Fig. 36–5). Detection of these lesions should therefore lead to careful questioning of the patient about the possibility of nonsteroidal anti-inflammatory drug use. If recent ingestion of these drugs is confirmed in symptomatic patients, withdrawal of the offending agent often produces a rapid clinical response.[26]

Other conditions may also be manifested by erosive gastritis. In some patients, gastric erosions are seen as an early sign of Crohn's disease with multiple "aphthous ulcers" in the stomach.[11, 12] However, these patients almost always have associated Crohn's disease involving the small bowel or colon (see later section on Crohn's disease). Severe erosive gastritis or ulceration may also result from opportunistic infection by cytomegalovirus in patients with acquired immunodeficiency syndrome

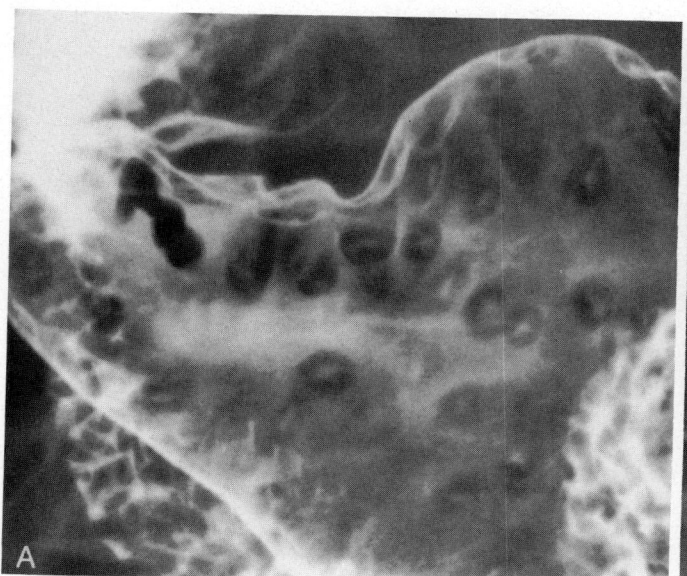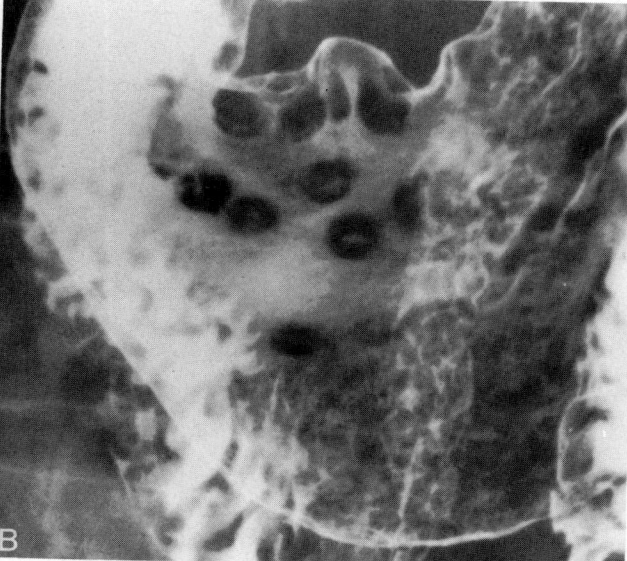

**Figure 36–1. Erosive gastritis. A** and **B**. In both patients, multiple varioliform erosions in the antrum are seen as tiny barium collections with surrounding halos of edematous mucosa.

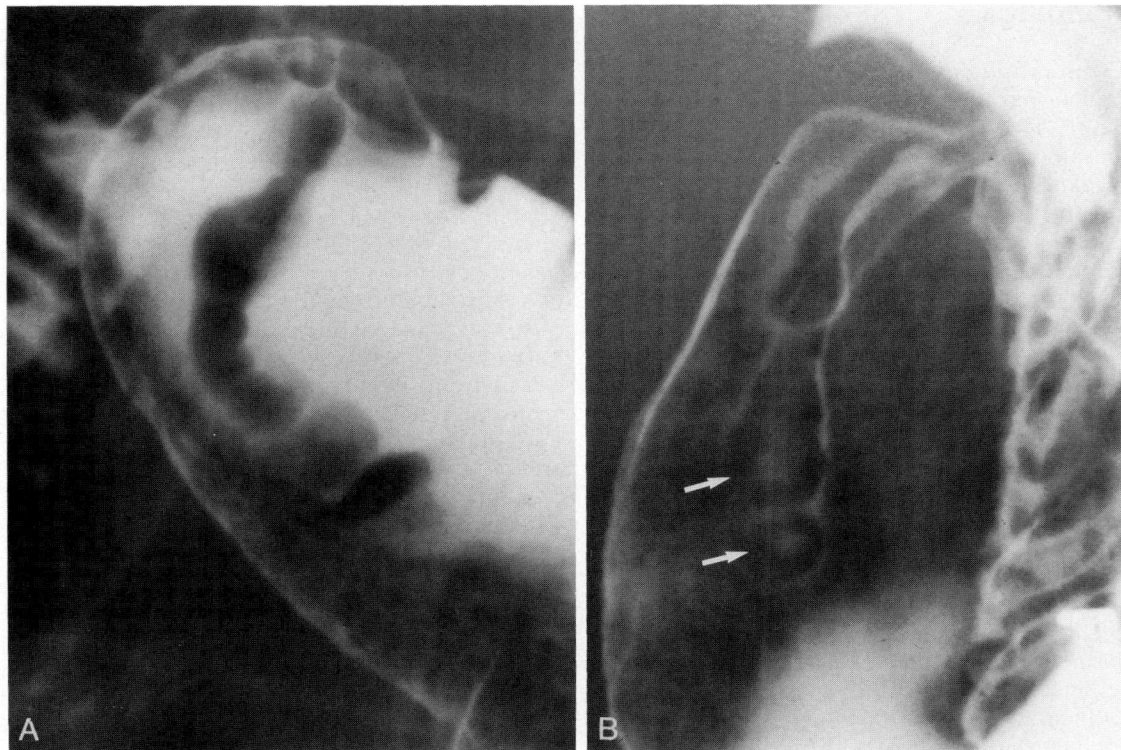

**Figure 36–2. Erosive gastritis with scalloped antral folds. A**. A thickened, lobulated fold is present in the gastric antrum. **B**. In another patient, several erosions *(arrows)* can be seen on the crest of a scalloped fold.

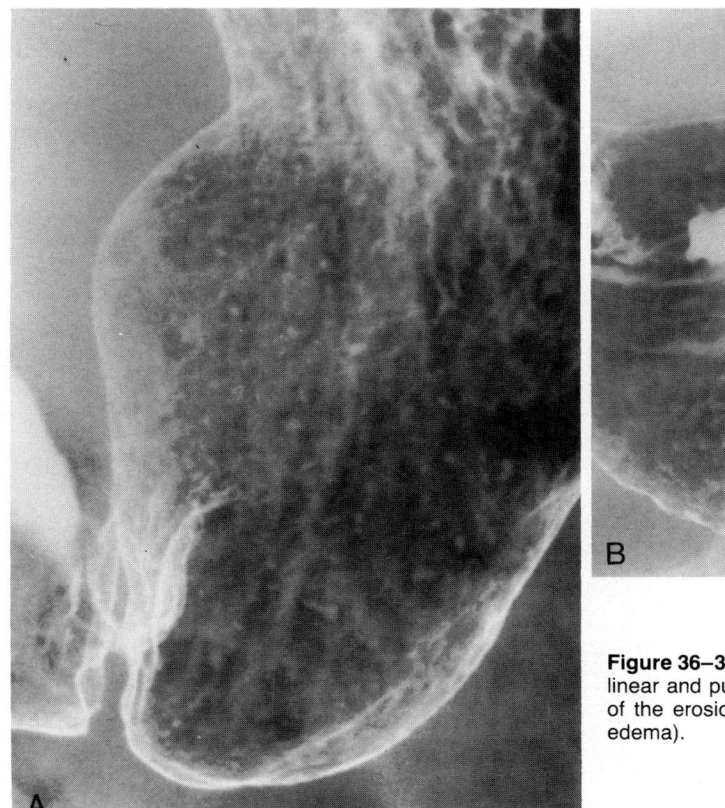

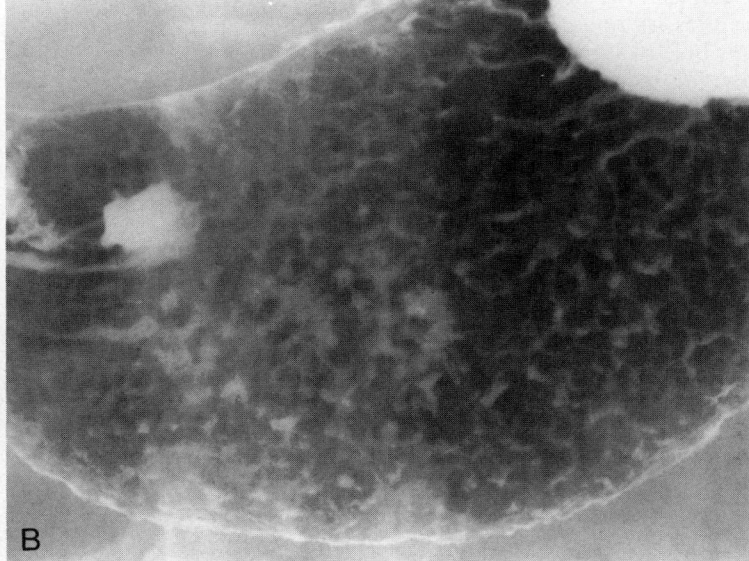

**Figure 36–3. Erosive gastritis. A** and **B**. In both patients, there are numerous linear and punctate erosions in the gastric antrum and body. Note how many of the erosions are incomplete (i.e., they are not surrounded by mounds of edema).

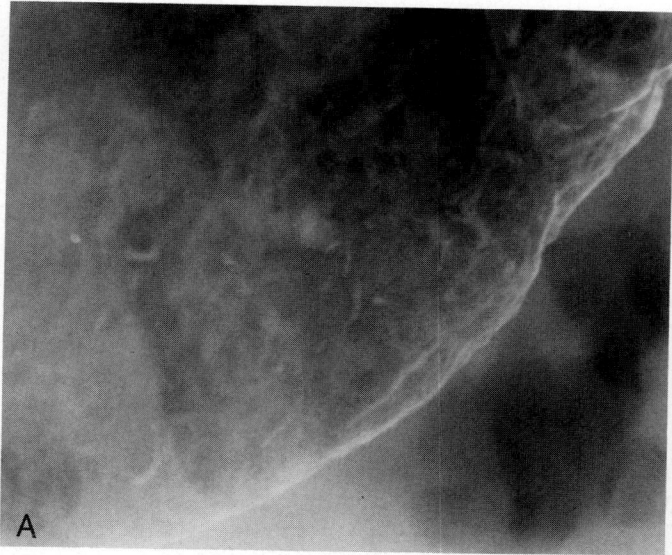

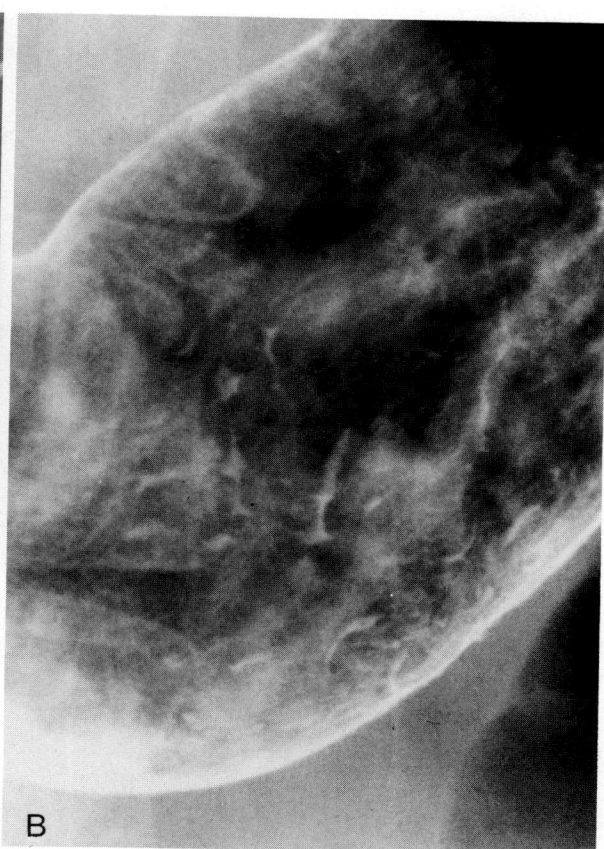

**Figure 36–4. Erosive gastritis caused by nonsteroidal anti-inflammatory drugs. A** and **B**. Distinctive linear and serpiginous erosions are clustered in the body of the stomach near the greater curvature as a result of aspirin **(A)** and indomethacin **(B)** ingestion. (**A** and **B** from MS Levine, A Verstandig, I Laufer, Serpiginous gastric erosions caused by aspirin and other nonsteroidal antiinflammatory drugs, AJR, 146, 1, 31–34, 1986, © by American Roentgen Ray Society.)

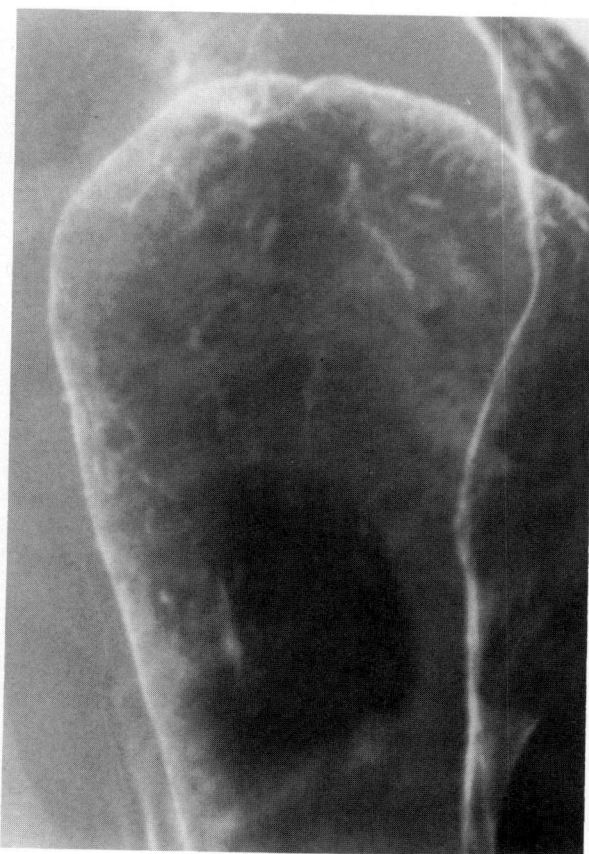

**Figure 36–5. Erosive gastritis caused by a nonsteroidal anti-inflammatory drug.** There are multiple linear erosions in the gastric antrum. This patient was taking naproxen. (From MS Levine, A Verstandig, I Laufer, Serpiginous gastric erosions caused by aspirin and other nonsteroidal antiinflammatory drugs, AJR, 146, 1, 31–34, 1986, © by American Roentgen Ray Society.)

(AIDS).[27] Rarely, erosions or shallow ulcers may occur as a complication of endoscopic heater probe therapy or other iatrogenic trauma[14] (Fig. 36–6).

## Differential Diagnosis

Gastric erosions occasionally may be mistaken radiographically for ulcerated submucosal masses or "bull's-eye" lesions in the stomach. However, the central ulcer of a bull's-eye lesion is considerably larger than an erosion, and the surrounding mass also tends to be larger than the radiolucent mound of edema surrounding an erosion (see Figs. 39–2 and 39–19D). Thus, it is usually possible to distinguish these lesions by radiographic criteria.

Gastric erosions must also be differentiated from barium precipitates in the stomach.[28] However, barium precipitates do not have a radiolucent halo, and when viewed in profile, they appear as small clumps of barium on the mucosal surface that do not project beyond the gastric contour (Fig. 36–7). If an artifact is suspected, additional views of the stomach should be obtained to demonstrate the transient nature of this finding.

## ANTRAL GASTRITIS

Alcohol, tobacco, coffee, and, more recently, *Helicobacter pylori* have been implicated in the development of antral gastritis (see later section on *H. pylori* infec-

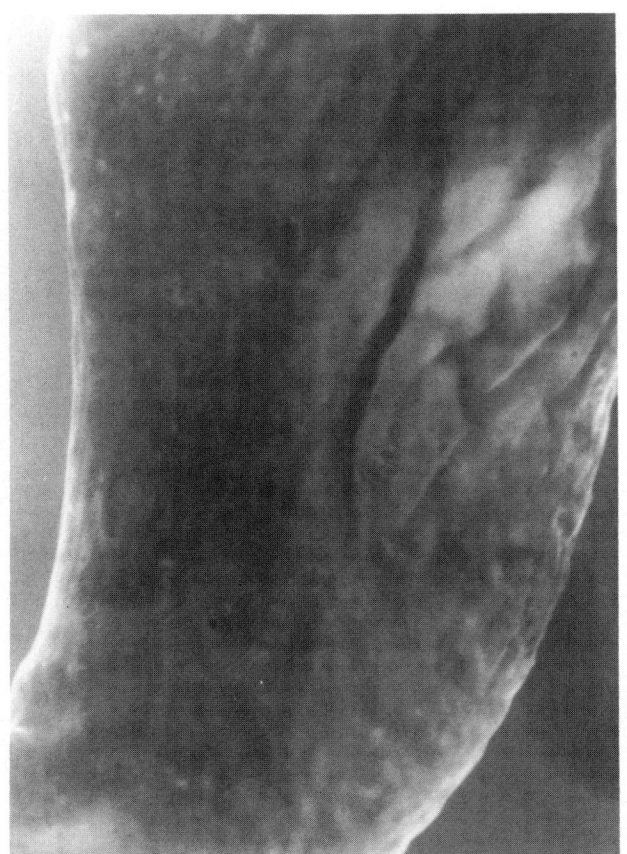

**Figure 36–7. Barium precipitates simulating gastric erosions.** Unlike erosions, however, the precipitates are sharp and distinct and have no surrounding radiolucent halos.

tion).[29] Some patients with this condition also have increased secretion of peptic acid, but others have normal or even decreased acid secretion.[29] Affected individuals may present with dyspepsia, epigastric pain, or other symptoms that are indistinguishable from those of peptic ulcer disease. Treatment is generally aimed at suppressing acid secretion in the stomach by the use of $H_2$ receptor antagonists.

## Radiographic Findings

Antral gastritis may be manifested on barium studies by mucosal crenulation, thickened folds, and spasm or decreased distensibility of the antrum.[29, 30] Crenulation or corrugation of the lesser curvature of the distal antrum may be observed as a transient or persistent finding at fluoroscopy[30] (Fig. 36–8A). Other patients may have thickened, scalloped, or lobulated folds in the antrum that tend to be oriented on its longitudinal axis[29] (Fig. 36–8B). Occasionally, however, these thickened folds may have a transverse orientation (see Fig. 36–8A). Still other patients may have a single lobulated fold that arises on the lesser curvature of the prepyloric antrum and extends into the pylorus or base of the duodenal bulb[31] (Fig. 36–9). This hypertrophied antralpyloric fold is thought to be a sequela of chronic antral

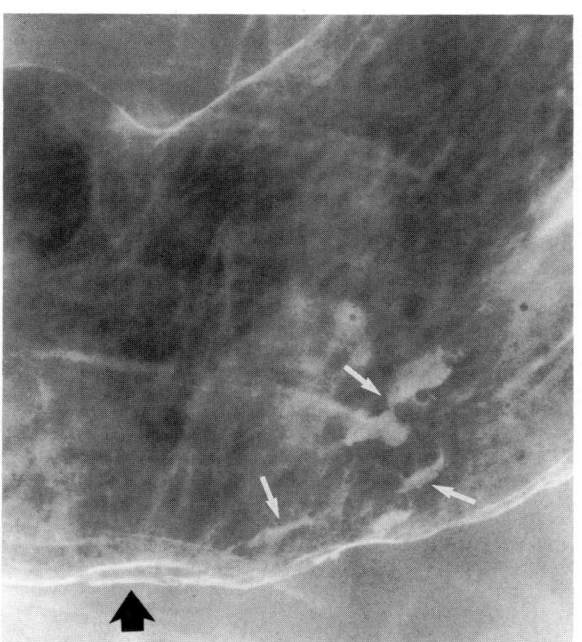

**Figure 36–6. Heater-probe ulcers and erosions.** Shallow, irregular ulcers and linear erosions are seen en face *(white arrows)* and in profile *(black arrow)* on the greater curvature of the stomach. These ulcerations occurred as a direct complication of endoscopic heater probe therapy. (From Rummerman J, Rubesin SE, Levine MS, et al: Gastric ulceration caused by heater probe coagulation. Gastrointest Radiol 13:200–202, 1988.)

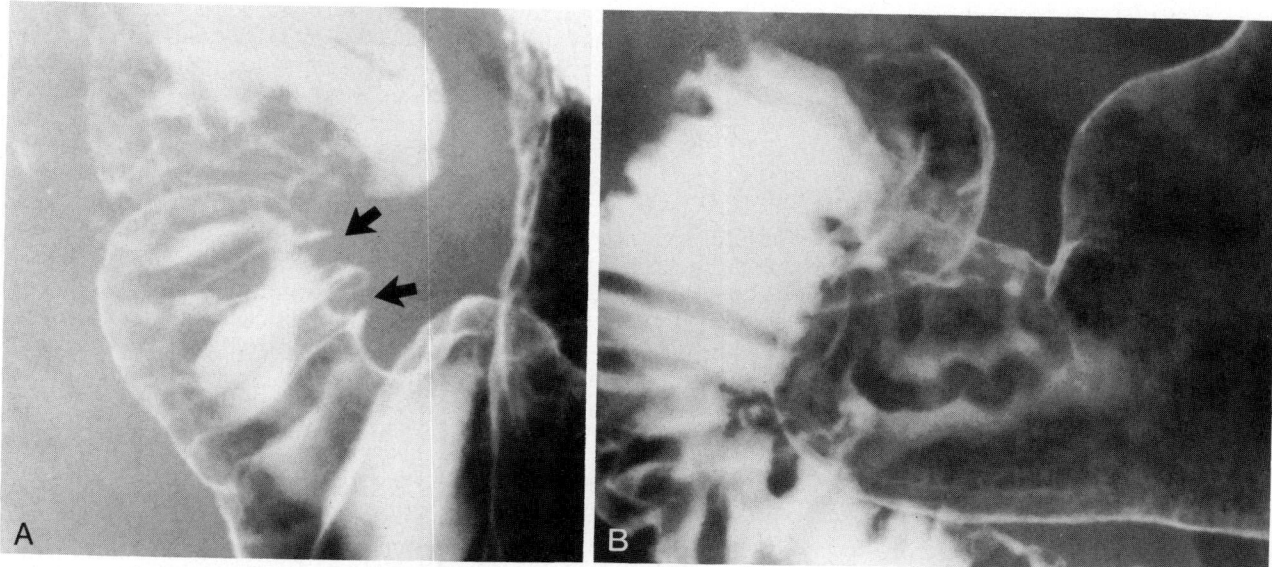

**Figure 36–8. Antral gastritis. A.** There is crenulation *(arrows)* of the lesser curvature of the distal antrum associated with thickened transverse folds. **B.** In another patient, antral gastritis is manifested by thickened, scalloped folds on the long axis of the stomach.

gastritis. Endoscopy probably is unwarranted when a typical hypertrophied antral-pyloric fold is seen on barium studies.[31] Occasionally, however, this fold can be mistaken radiographically for a polypoid or plaque-like carcinoma on the lesser curvature. In such cases, endoscopy and biopsy are required to rule out a malignant lesion.

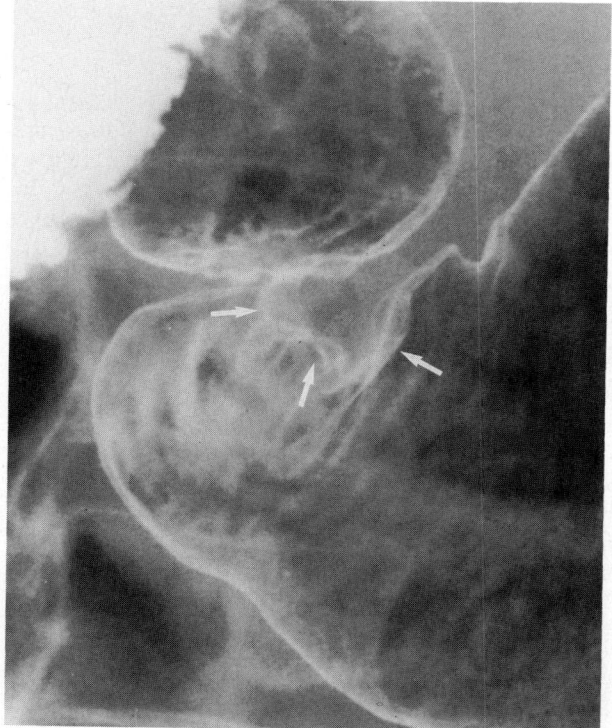

**Figure 36–9. Hypertrophied antral-pyloric fold.** A single lobulated fold *(arrows)* on the lesser curvature of the distal antrum extends into the pylorus. The characteristic location and appearance of this fold should differentiate it from a polypoid or plaque-like antral carcinoma.

## Differential Diagnosis

Severe antral gastritis must be differentiated radiographically from gastric carcinoma. In patients with gastric carcinoma, however, the narrowed antrum tends to have a more abrupt transition with the adjacent stomach and a more fixed, rigid contour with obliteration of peristalsis at fluoroscopy. In contrast, patients with antral gastritis tend to have a more distensible antrum with more gradual transitions and preservation of peristalsis. Thus, it is usually possible to differentiate these conditions by radiographic criteria. When the folds are markedly thickened and lobulated, antral gastritis can also mimic the appearance of lymphoma, varices, or even arteriovenous malformations in the antrum.[32] In such cases, endoscopy may be required for a more definitive diagnosis.

## HYPERTROPHIC GASTRITIS (HYPERTROPHIC HYPERSECRETORY GASTROPATHY)

Hypertrophic gastritis, also known as hypertrophic hypersecretory gastropathy, is characterized by marked glandular hyperplasia and increased secretion of acid in the stomach.[33, 34] Gastric folds may be thickened not only because of glandular hyperplasia but also because of edema and inflammation in the stomach. As many as two thirds of patients with this condition have associated duodenal ulcers, and a smaller percentage have gastric ulcers as a result of increased acid secretion.[34] Although the pathogenesis of hypertrophic gastritis is uncertain, glandular hyperplasia in the stomach may be caused by pituitary, hypothalamic, or vagal stimuli.[33] These patients may present clinically with epigastric pain, nausea and vomiting, or, less frequently, upper gastrointestinal bleeding.[33, 34] If the radiographic or endoscopic findings support the diagnosis of hypertrophic gastritis, treatment with H₂ receptor antagonists is often initiated to suppress acid secretion in the stomach.

## Radiographic Findings

Hypertrophic gastritis is manifested on barium studies by thickened folds, predominantly in the gastric fundus and body, because the acid-secreting portion of the stomach is most affected by this condition (Fig. 36–10). Several studies have shown that there is a significant correlation between the degree of fold thickening and the amount of acid secretion in the stomach.[35, 36] Although mildly or moderately thickened folds are occasionally observed as a normal variant in patients who have normal acid secretion, markedly thickened folds (i.e., folds that are greater than 1 cm in width) should suggest the possibility of hypertrophic gastritis. When enlarged gastric rugae are encountered on barium studies, it is incumbent on the radiologist to search carefully for peptic ulcers because of the high prevalence of ulcers in these patients.

## Differential Diagnosis

Ménétrier's disease and lymphoma are the major considerations in the differential diagnosis of hypertrophic gastritis. Ménétrier's disease tends to be manifested by more dramatic radiographic findings with massively enlarged gastric folds (see later section on Ménétrier's disease). Unfortunately, there is considerable overlap in the degree of fold thickening in Ménétrier's disease and hypertrophic gastritis. However, Ménétrier's disease is characterized by normal or decreased acid secretion and a protein-losing enteropathy, so that the clinical and laboratory findings are extremely helpful for differentiating these conditions. Gastric lymphoma may also be manifested by thickened gastric folds, but the folds tend to have a more lobulated appearance and are often associated with ulcers, masses, or bull's-eye lesions (see Chapter 39). Gastric carcinoma is a less common cause of thickened folds, and it is usually associated with loss of distensibility and decreased or absent peristalsis in the involved portion of the stomach.[37] If the radiographic findings are equivocal, endoscopy and biopsy may be required to rule out malignant lesions. Rarely, other conditions such as Zollinger-Ellison syndrome, eosinophilic gastritis, and varices may be manifested by thickened folds in the stomach, but the correct diagnosis can be suggested on the basis of the clinical history and presentation.

## MÉNÉTRIER'S DISEASE

Since its original description by Ménétrier in 1898, Ménétrier's disease has been recognized as a rare condition of unknown etiology characterized by marked glandular hypertrophy in the stomach, enlarged gastric rugae, hypochlorhydria, and hypoproteinemia. In the past, this condition has also been called cystic gastritis, giant hypertrophic gastritis, giant mucosal hypertrophy, and hyperplastic gastropathy. Ménétrier's disease may cause chronic, disabling symptoms, occasionally necessitating a gastric resection. Despite its rarity, this entity has received considerable attention in the radiologic literature because of its often dramatic appearance on barium studies.

## Pathology

Ménétrier's disease is characterized histologically by thickening and hyperplasia of the mucosa due to cystic dilatation and elongation of gastric mucous glands as-

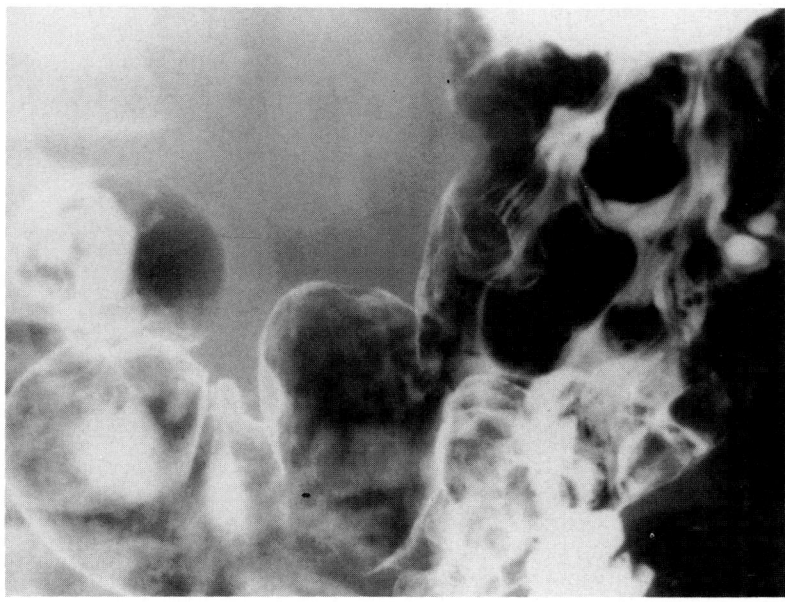

**Figure 36–10. Hypertrophic gastritis.** Thickened, lobulated folds are seen in the body of the stomach. Note how the antrum appears normal.

sociated with deepening of the foveolar pits.[38] This often results in increased secretion of mucus into the gastric lumen. At the same time, gastric acid output is markedly decreased or absent in about 75% of patients.[39] These individuals may also have a protein-losing enteropathy due to loss of protein from the hyperplastic mucosa into the gastric lumen.[40, 41] Inflammatory changes are sometimes present in the stomach in either a patchy or a diffuse distribution.

## Clinical Findings

Ménétrier's disease tends to occur in older patients and is more common in men than in women.[39] Affected individuals may present with epigastric pain, nausea and vomiting, diarrhea, anorexia, weight loss, or peripheral edema.[38, 39, 42] Laboratory studies may reveal hypoalbuminemia due to a protein-losing enteropathy and hypochlorhydria due to decreased acid secretion.[38] For reasons that are unclear, patients with Ménétrier's disease may also develop a hypercoagulable state with an increased risk of deep venous thrombosis.[43] Rarely, the development of gastric carcinoma has been described in patients with pre-existing Ménétrier's disease.[44, 45] However, it is unclear whether Ménétrier's disease is a premalignant condition or whether this association is coincidental.

Some patients with Ménétrier's disease may have spontaneous remission of symptoms, and others may respond to treatment with H₂ blockers, vagotomy, or antibiotics. However, the majority of patients have a prolonged illness with symptoms that persist for a period of years.[42] In patients with intractable symptoms, a total gastrectomy occasionally may be required.[43] However, these patients should undergo surgery only as a last resort.

## Radiographic Findings

Ménétrier's disease is classically manifested on barium studies by grossly thickened, lobulated folds in the gastric fundus and body with relative sparing of the antrum[46] (Fig. 36–11A). In one study, however, the antrum was involved in nearly 50% of patients, so that diffuse thickening of gastric folds does not preclude this

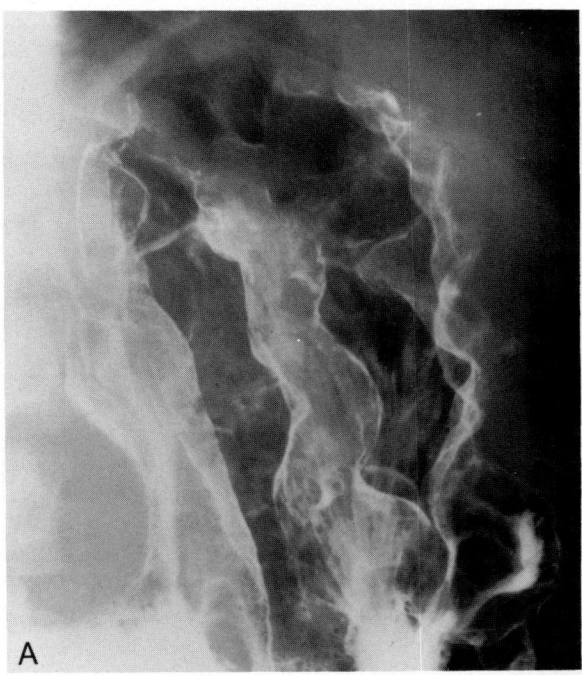
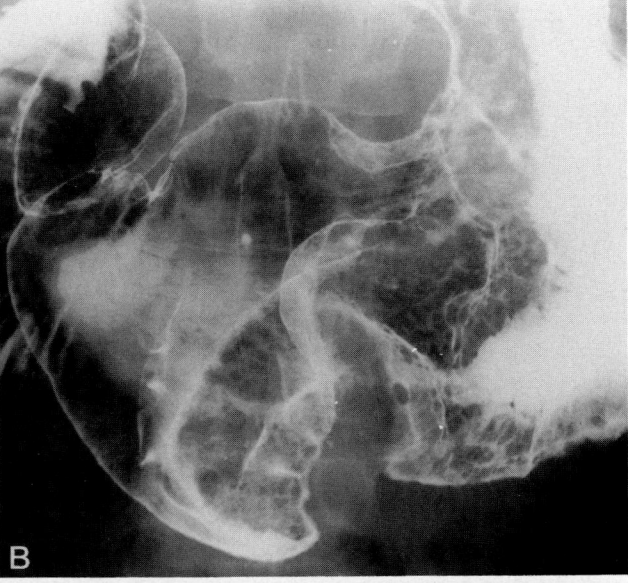
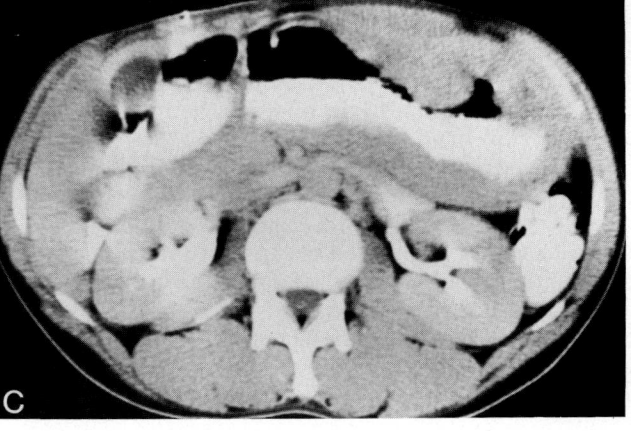

**Figure 36–11. Ménétrier's disease. A.** Grossly thickened folds are present in the gastric fundus. **B.** A giant, mass-like elevation of the folds is seen on the greater curvature of the gastric body. This appearance could be mistaken for a polypoid gastric carcinoma. Note how the distal antrum is relatively spared. **C.** A computed tomographic scan shows massive thickening of the gastric wall with mass-like protrusions into the lumen. Endoscopic biopsy specimens revealed pathologic changes of Ménétrier's disease without evidence of tumor.

diagnosis.[47] The greatest degree of fold thickening often occurs on or near the greater curvature.[46] Focally enlarged folds occasionally can be mistaken radiographically for polypoid carcinomas[46] (Fig. 36–11B). In other patients, excessive mucus in the stomach may dilute the barium and compromise mucosal coating. Ménétrier's disease is characterized on computed tomography by a markedly thickened gastric wall with mass-like elevations representing giant, heaped-up folds protruding into the lumen (Fig. 36–11C). When Ménétrier's disease is suspected radiographically, full-thickness biopsies may be performed to confirm the diagnosis.

## Differential Diagnosis

Although a variety of conditions may be manifested by thickened gastric folds, they rarely produce the degree of fold thickening seen in Ménétrier's disease. Gastric lymphoma may be associated with enlarged folds, but neoplastic infiltration should be suggested by the presence of polypoid masses, ulcers, or bull's eye lesions in these patients (see Chapter 39). Occasionally, gastric carcinoma may also be manifested by thickened folds, but an infiltrating cancer tends to narrow the lumen and obliterate peristalsis, whereas the stomach usually remains pliant and distensible in patients with Ménétrier's disease. Zollinger-Ellison syndrome may also be characterized by thickened folds and increased secretions that impair mucosal coating in the stomach. However, the presence of thickened folds in the duodenum and proximal jejunum and one or more ulcers in the stomach, duodenal bulb, or postbulbar duodenum should suggest the correct diagnosis (see Chapter 35). Gastric varices should also be included in the differential diagnosis, but varices tend to have a more serpiginous appearance and are usually confined to the region of the gastric cardia or fundus (see Chapter 30). Other conditions involving the stomach, such as eosinophilic gastritis, Crohn's disease, sarcoidosis, syphilis, and tuberculosis, may also be manifested by thickened folds. However, the correct diagnosis is often suggested by the clinical history and presentation.

## ATROPHIC GASTRITIS

Atrophic gastritis is important because of its association with pernicious anemia, a megaloblastic anemia caused by decreased synthesis of intrinsic factor and subsequent malabsorption of vitamin $B_{12}$. Pernicious anemia is a disease of the elderly; it accounts for 50 of every 100,000 hospital admissions in the United States.[48] Although the pathogenesis is uncertain, an autoimmune mechanism has been postulated because of the frequent finding of parietal cell or intrinsic factor antibodies in these individuals.[49] More than 90% of patients with pernicious anemia have atrophic gastritis, with atrophy of mucosal glands, loss of parietal and chief cells, thinning of the mucosa, and varying degrees of intestinal metaplasia.[50]

## Pathogenesis

Atrophic gastritis may be classified into two types (type A and type B), which have different histologic, immunologic, and secretory characteristics.[51, 52] In type A gastritis, mucosal atrophy is confined to the gastric fundus and body with antral sparing. This type of atrophic gastritis is thought to result from immunologic injury (i.e., antiparietal cell antibodies) and is usually associated with pernicious anemia.[51] In contrast, type B gastritis is characterized by severe antral atrophy with limited involvement of the fundus and body. This form of atrophic gastritis is more common and usually results from mucosal injury by endogenous or exogenous agents such as bile acids or alcohol.[51, 52]

## Clinical Findings

Although atrophic gastritis rarely causes symptoms, some patients with pernicious anemia may initially present with neurologic symptoms as a result of long-standing vitamin $B_{12}$ deficiency. Early diagnosis of pernicious anemia is therefore important, so that vitamin $B_{12}$ replacement therapy can be initiated before the development of irreversible neurologic sequelae. Because the average adult has a 3- to 6-year body store of vitamin $B_{12}$,[53] the gastric lesion in pernicious anemia may antedate the hematologic and neurologic abnormalities in this condition by several years. The diagnosis of atrophic gastritis on upper gastrointestinal studies therefore might permit these patients to be treated before the fully blown clinical entity of pernicious anemia has developed.

Atrophic gastritis associated with pernicious anemia is also important because of an increased risk of gastric carcinoma. In one study, the risk of developing gastric cancer was found to be about three times greater than that in the general population.[54] Although some investigators advocate endoscopic or radiologic surveillance of patients with known pernicious anemia, others believe that the risk of cancer is not high enough to warrant routine screening.[54–57] Nevertheless, any patient with pernicious anemia who has occult gastrointestinal bleeding should be evaluated aggressively for possible gastric carcinoma.

## Radiographic Findings

The diagnosis of atrophic gastritis in pernicious anemia may be suggested on conventional single contrast barium studies by the presence of a narrowed, tubular stomach with decreased or absent mucosal folds, predominantly in the body and fundus (i.e., the "bald" fundus).[58] In one study, atrophic gastritis was diagnosed on single contrast examinations in about 50% of patients with pernicious anemia, but a false-positive diagnosis was made in about 10% of controls.[58] Thus, the radiologic diagnosis of atrophic gastritis in pernicious anemia has been limited by a lack of criteria that are both sensitive and specific for this condition.

With routine double contrast technique, another study found that about 80% of patients with pernicious anemia have a fundal diameter of 8 cm or less, absent folds in the fundus and body, and small (1 to 2 mm in diameter) or absent areae gastricae in the stomach[59] (Fig. 36–12). Unfortunately, this combination of findings is also present in about 10% of age-matched controls.[59] Because of the low prevalence of pernicious anemia in the general population, routine laboratory studies (e.g., the Schilling test) to screen for pernicious anemia solely on the basis of a suggestive upper gastrointestinal examination are not warranted. Nevertheless, areae gastricae have been observed in the stomach in only about 40% of patients with pernicious anemia, and when present, the areae gastricae have had a small, uniform appearance.[59] It has previously been postulated that variations in the size of the areae gastricae are dependent on parietal cell mass.[60] Thus, the small size and frequent absence of areae gastricae in pernicious anemia may be explained by the loss of parietal cells and associated achlorhydria that occur in these individuals.

Many questions remain about the appearance of the areae gastricae in patients with atrophic gastritis and pernicious anemia. However, focal enlargement of the areae gastricae should raise the possibility of intestinal metaplasia or even a superficial spreading carcinoma. Because intestinal metaplasia may predispose these patients to the development of gastric carcinoma, an abnormal areae gastricae pattern should be evaluated by endoscopy and biopsy.

## Differential Diagnosis

The most important consideration in the differential diagnosis of atrophic gastritis is the scirrhous form of gastric carcinoma (i.e., linitis plastica). However, scirrhous tumors are usually characterized by a nodular, distorted mucosa and thickened, irregular folds;[61] atrophic gastritis is characterized by a smooth, featureless mucosa and decreased or absent mucosal folds. Thus, it is almost always possible to differentiate linitis plastica from atrophic gastritis by radiologic criteria. Scarring from peptic ulcer disease or other conditions may also be characterized by gastric narrowing, but the antrum and body tend to be involved rather than the fundus. The clinical history is also helpful; patients with atrophic gastritis are unlikely to have prior ulcers because of the underlying achlorhydria associated with this condition.

## EOSINOPHILIC GASTRITIS

Eosinophilic gastroenteritis is an unusual condition characterized by eosinophilic infiltration of the stomach and small bowel.[62–64] Rarely, the esophagus may be involved by this disease (see Chapter 26). Almost all patients with eosinophilic gastroenteritis have a peripheral eosinophilia ranging from 10 to 80%.[64] About half the patients have a history of allergic diseases.[62] The clinical symptoms are related to the site and extent of

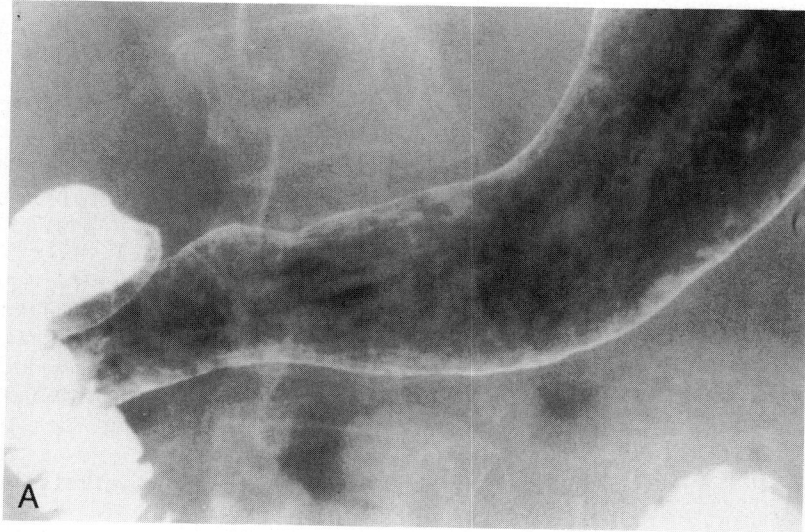

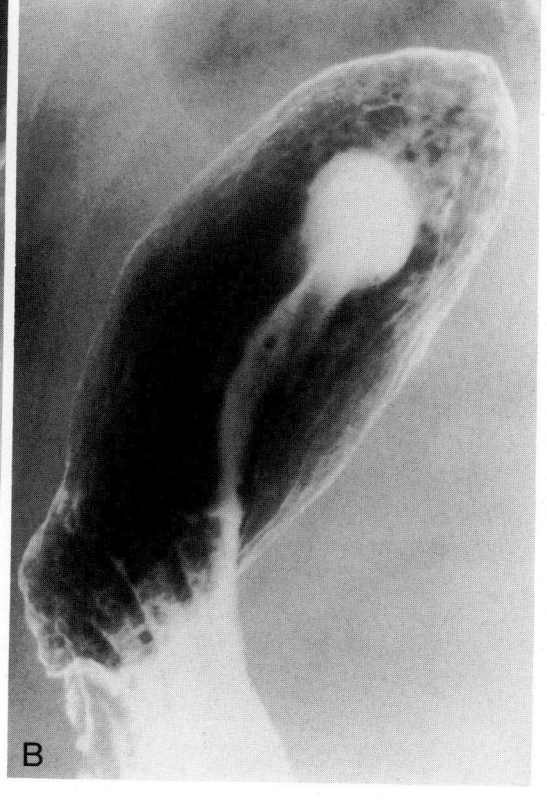

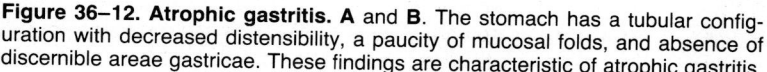
**Figure 36–12. Atrophic gastritis. A** and **B**. The stomach has a tubular configuration with decreased distensibility, a paucity of mucosal folds, and absence of discernible areae gastricae. These findings are characteristic of atrophic gastritis.

gastrointestinal involvement. Patients with eosinophilic gastritis usually present with epigastric pain, nausea and vomiting, or, less frequently, upper gastrointestinal bleeding.[62, 64] In contrast, patients with eosinophilic enteritis may have diarrhea, malabsorption, or a protein-losing enteropathy.[62, 64] Although treatment with steroids often produces a dramatic clinical response, eosinophilic gastroenteritis is a chronic, relapsing disease; exacerbations often occur after long asymptomatic intervals.[62–64]

## Radiographic Findings

Eosinophilic gastritis usually involves the antrum or antrum and body of the stomach.[62, 64, 65] Rarely, however, disease may be confined to the proximal portion of the stomach with antral sparing.[66] Barium studies may demonstrate mucosal nodularity, thickened folds, or narrowing and rigidity of the distal half of the stomach[64, 67] (Fig. 36–13). Occasionally, severe antral narrowing may cause gastric outlet obstruction.[68] About 50% of patients with eosinophilic gastritis have concomitant involvement of the small bowel, which is manifested by diffuse thickening and nodularity of small bowel folds.[67]

## Differential Diagnosis

When eosinophilic gastritis is manifested by thickened folds, the differential diagnosis includes antral gastritis, hypertrophic gastritis, Ménétrier's disease, Zollinger-Ellison syndrome, lymphoma, and other conditions associated with thickened folds. However, the distribution of disease is helpful in differentiating these conditions; hypertrophic gastritis, Ménétrier's disease, and Zollinger-Ellison syndrome tend to involve the proximal por-

tion of the stomach, whereas eosinophilic gastritis predominantly involves the antrum. When eosinophilic gastritis is manifested by antral narrowing, the differential diagnosis includes a primary scirrhous carcinoma of the stomach, metastatic breast cancer, caustic ingestion, radiation, Crohn's disease, and other granulomatous conditions involving the stomach, such as sarcoidosis, tuberculosis, and syphilis. However, the correct diagnosis is often suggested on the basis of the clinical history. When eosinophilic gastritis is suspected on the basis of upper gastrointestinal examination, a small bowel follow-through should be performed to determine whether the small bowel is also involved by this disease.

# GRANULOMATOUS CONDITIONS

## Crohn's Disease

Although Crohn's disease primarily affects the small bowel and colon, early signs of upper gastrointestinal involvement may be detected on double contrast barium studies in more than 20% of patients with granulomatous ileocolitis.[69] Occasionally, the onset of upper gastrointestinal disease coincides with or even precedes the onset of ileal or colonic disease, so that these patients do not necessarily have known Crohn's disease when they seek medical attention. Endoscopic biopsies from the stomach or duodenum may fail to reveal granulomas because of the superficial nature of the biopsies and the patchy distribution of the disease.[70] Thus, the absence of definitive histologic findings should not discourage a diagnosis of gastroduodenal Crohn's disease if the clinical and radiographic findings suggest this condition.

## _Clinical Findings_

Early gastroduodenal involvement by Crohn's disease may be asymptomatic. However, more advanced disease may be manifested by pain, vomiting, and weight loss.[71–73] Some patients may have symptoms indistinguishable from those of peptic ulcer disease with severe epigastric pain or burning relieved by food and antacids.[73] In others, antral or duodenal narrowing may cause gastric outlet obstruction with intractable nausea and vomiting.[71–73] These patients may also present with diarrhea due to associated ileocolic involvement. Gastroduodenal Crohn's disease should therefore be suspected in any patient with abdominal pain, vomiting, and diarrhea.[71]

Other patients with gastroduodenal Crohn's disease may have acute or chronic upper gastrointestinal bleeding with hematemesis, melena, or guaiac-positive stool.[73] However, massive upper gastrointestinal bleeding is rare.[74] The development of a gastrocolic or duodenocolic fistula is classically manifested by feculent vomiting, diarrhea, and weight loss.[75] However, this triad of findings is present in only about 30% of patients, so that gastrocolic fistulas often are not suspected on clinical grounds.[76]

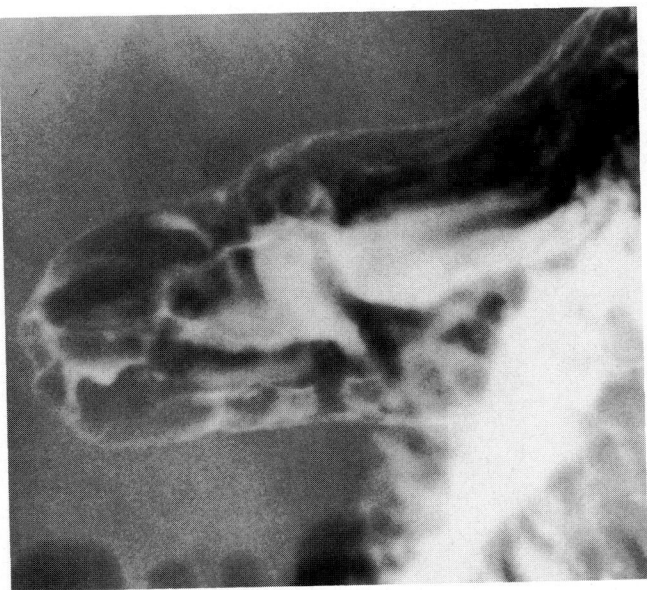

**Figure 36–13. Eosinophilic gastritis.** Thickened, nodular folds are seen in the gastric antrum. Other causes of antral gastritis could produce identical findings.

Early, asymptomatic gastroduodenal Crohn's disease requires no specific treatment. In patients with more advanced disease, sulfasalazine (Azulfidine) or steroids may effectively relieve epigastric pain or other upper gastrointestinal complaints.[73] However, a surgical bypass procedure such as a gastrojejunostomy or duodenojejunostomy is often required to alleviate symptoms of gastric outlet obstruction.[73] Although these operations do not affect the patient's underlying Crohn's disease, they may provide long-term relief from upper gastrointestinal obstruction.

## Radiographic Findings

As in the ileum or colon, gastroduodenal Crohn's disease is characterized by nonstenotic and stenotic phases of involvement. The initial nonstenotic phase is manifested by a spectrum of findings, including aphthous ulcers, larger ulcers, thickened folds, and distorted, effaced, or, rarely, "cobblestoned" mucosa. Subsequent fibrosis and scarring lead to the stenotic phase of involvement with progressive gastric outlet obstruction due to antral, pyloric, or duodenal narrowing and stricture formation. Thus, the radiologic features of gastroduodenal Crohn's disease are virtually identical to those found in the small bowel and colon.

### Gastric Involvement

Gastric Crohn's disease almost always involves the antrum or antrum and body of the stomach.[77, 78] More proximal extension of Crohn's disease is unusual, and isolated fundal involvement is rarely found.[79] When the stomach is affected by Crohn's disease, the duodenum also tends to be involved.[77, 78, 80, 81] Most patients have associated granulomatous ileocolitis, but the diagnosis of Crohn's disease may not be known at the time of clinical presentation. When gastric involvement is suggested by upper gastrointestinal studies, a small bowel follow-through or barium enema should be performed to determine whether there is concomitant ileocolic disease.

Aphthous ulcers, the earliest histologic lesions of Crohn's disease, may be detected in the stomach in more than 20% of patients with granulomatous ileocolitis.[69] As in the colon, these lesions appear radiographically as punctate or slit-like collections of barium surrounded by radiolucent mounds of edema[12, 69, 82] (Fig. 36–14). The aphthous ulcers tend to be clustered in the antrum or antrum and body of the stomach. Unfortunately, these lesions may be indistinguishable from varioliform gastric erosions due to a variety of causes (see earlier section on erosive gastritis). However, Crohn's disease should be suspected when gastric erosions are found in patients with crampy abdominal pain and diarrhea, and a small bowel follow-through should be performed to evaluate the terminal ileum in these individuals.

More advanced gastroduodenal Crohn's disease may be manifested by one or more larger ulcers, thickened folds, and a nodular or cobblestoned mucosa in the

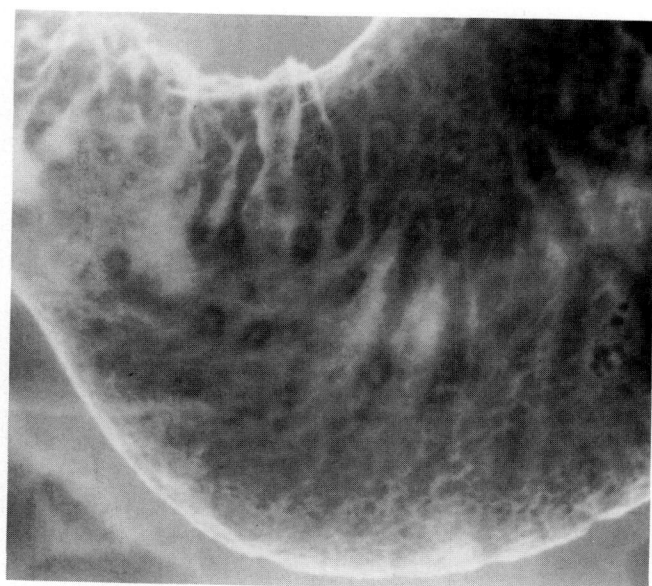

**Figure 36–14. Early gastric Crohn's disease with multiple aphthous ulcers.** These lesions are indistinguishable from varioliform erosions in the stomach. However, this patient had typical findings of Crohn's disease in the terminal ileum. (Courtesy of Robert A. Goren, Philadelphia, PA.)

gastric antrum or body[77, 78, 80] (Fig. 36–15). Other patients may have abnormal gastric motility with decreased peristalsis and increased secretions.[80] Eventually, scarring and fibrosis may lead to the development of a narrowed, tubular, funnel-shaped antrum that has been likened to the sacramental ram's horn, or shofar, used to sound the advent of the Jewish New Year[83] (Fig. 36–16). In

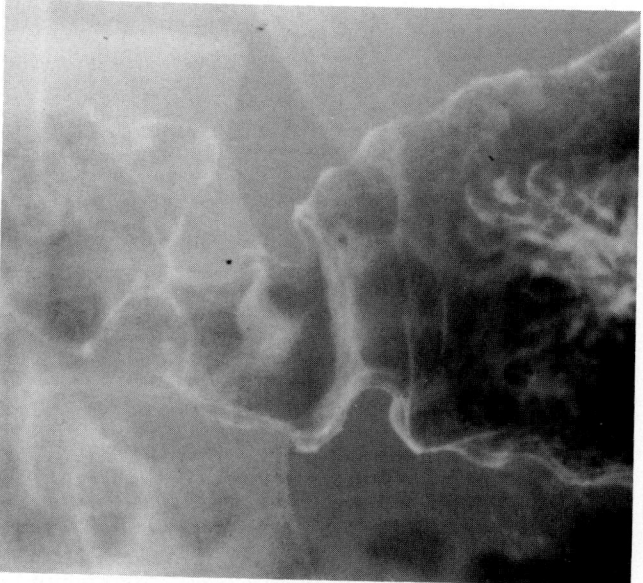

**Figure 36–15. Gastric Crohn's disease.** Thickened, nodular folds are seen in the antrum of the stomach. (From Levine MS: Crohn's disease of the upper gastrointestinal tract. Radiol Clin North Am 25:79–91, 1987.)

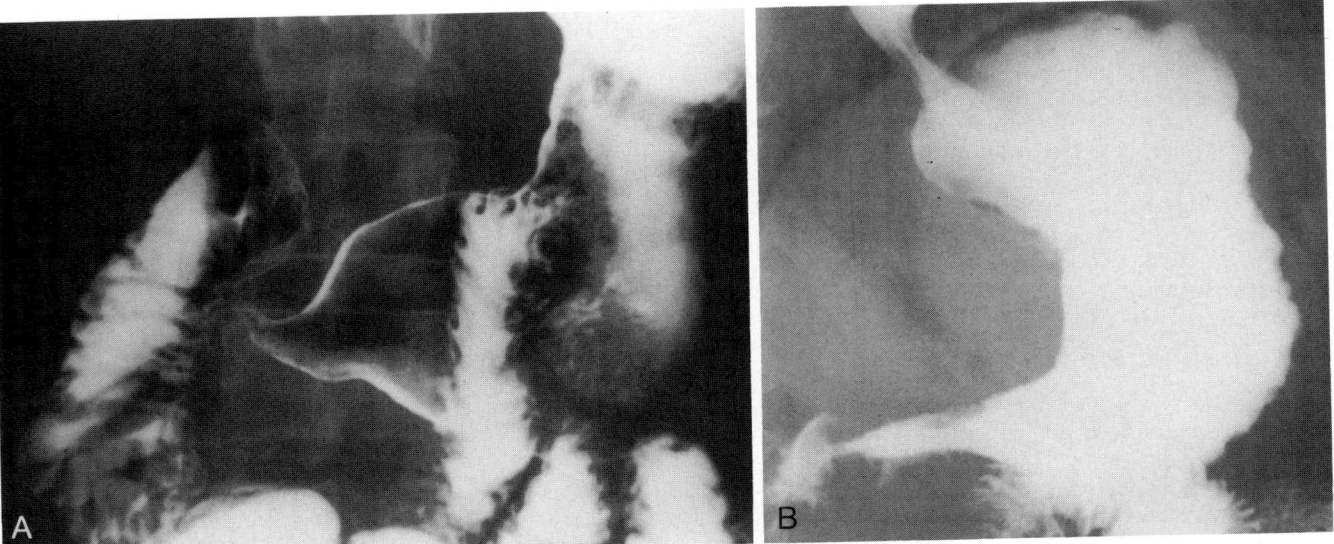

**Figure 36–16. Gastric Crohn's disease with antral narrowing. A** and **B**. In both cases, there is smooth, funnel-shaped narrowing of the antrum, resulting in the classic "ram's horn" sign of gastric Crohn's disease. (**A** from Levine MS: Crohn's disease of the upper gastrointestinal tract. Radiol Clin North Am 25:79–91, 1987. **B** courtesy of Anna S. Lev-Toaff, M.D., Philadelphia, PA.)

other patients, combined gastroduodenal scarring may produce a single, continuous tubular structure involving the antrum and duodenum with obliteration of the normal anatomic landmarks at the pylorus[73, 80] (Fig. 36–17). Because of its resemblance to a postsurgical stomach after a Billroth I gastrectomy, this finding has been described as the "pseudo–Billroth I" sign of gastroduodenal Crohn's disease.[84] Rarely, filiform polyps may be found in the stomach as a sequela of severe granulomatous gastritis[85] (Fig. 36–18).

Patients with Crohn's disease occasionally develop gastrocolic fistulas.[75, 76, 86] These patients usually have underlying Crohn's disease of the transverse colon with extension of a fistula via the gastrocolic ligament to the greater curvature of the stomach. On barium studies, the greater curvature may have a nodular or spiculated appearance with thickened, distorted folds in the region of the fistula. These findings probably represent a nonspecific inflammatory response to the adjoining fistula rather than actual extension of Crohn's disease to the stomach. Gastrocolic fistulas are demonstrated on only about one third of upper gastrointestinal examinations, so barium enemas often are required for diagnosis of these fistulas.[76]

### Duodenal Involvement

Although duodenal involvement by Crohn's disease is usually associated with antral involvement, isolated duodenal Crohn's disease occurs more frequently than isolated Crohn's disease of the stomach.[80] As elsewhere in the gastrointestinal tract, aphthous ulcers represent the earliest morphologic abnormality in the duodenum[12, 82] (Fig. 36–19). With progression of the disease, one or more larger ulcers may be found in the duodenal bulb or postbulbar duodenum[87, 88] (Fig. 36–20). A solitary

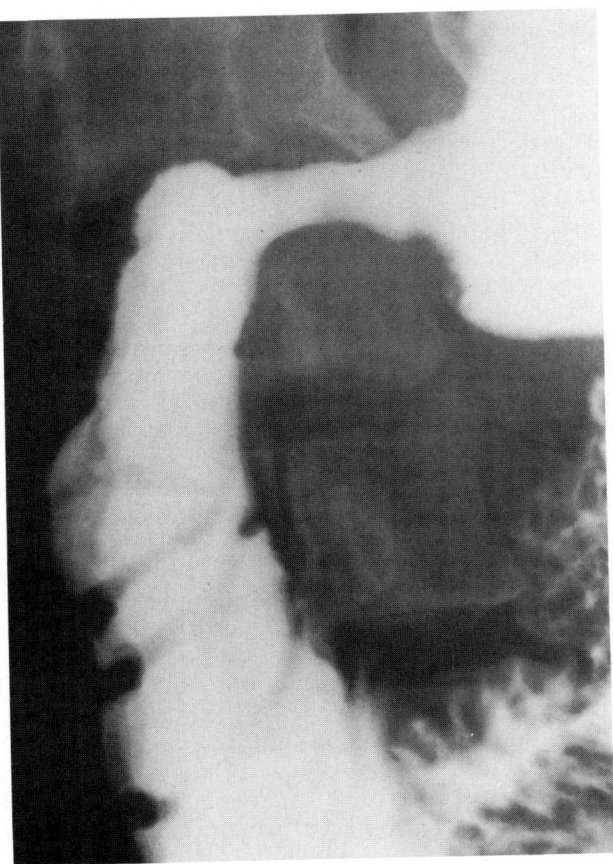

**Figure 36–17. Gastroduodenal Crohn's disease.** There is contiguous narrowing of the antrum and duodenum, with obliteration of the normal anatomic landmarks at the pylorus. Because the antrum and duodenum merge together as a single tubular structure, this finding has been described as the pseudo–Billroth I sign of gastroduodenal Crohn's disease. (From Levine MS: Crohn's disease of the upper gastrointestinal tract. Radiol Clin North Am 25:79–91, 1987.)

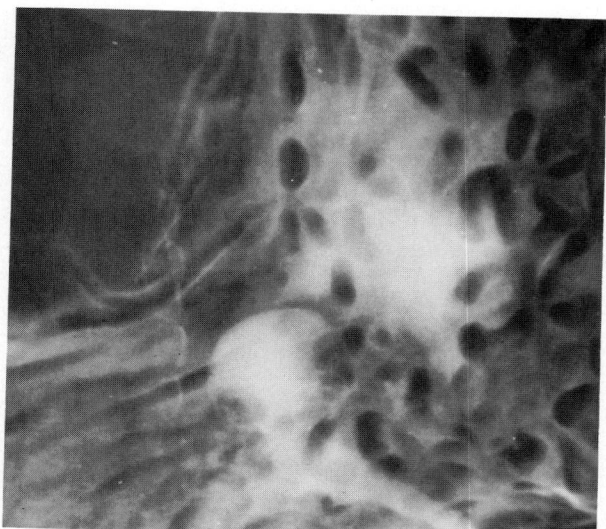

**Figure 36–18. Gastric Crohn's disease with filiform polyps.** Multiple linear and ovoid filling defects are seen in the stomach in a patient with long-standing Crohn's disease. (From Levine MS: Crohn's disease of the upper gastrointestinal tract. Radiol Clin North Am 25:79–91, 1987.)

eccentric, asymmetric nature of this scarring, uninvolved segments of the duodenum may balloon outward between areas of fibrosis, resulting in one or more sacculations.[87, 88] Duodenal strictures often involve the postbulbar duodenum and have a characteristic appearance with smoothly tapered narrowing of the apical portion of the duodenal bulb and adjacent segment of the descending duodenum[84, 88] (Fig. 36–22). As a result, scarring from duodenal Crohn's disease usually can be differentiated radiographically from the puckered, "cloverleaf" type of bulbar deformity associated with scarring from peptic ulcer disease.[84] Other patients may have multiple strictures in the second or third portions of the duodenum with contiguous disease in the proximal jejunum.[84] As expected, multifocal duodenal Crohn's disease may be manifested by skip lesions with intervening segments of normal bowel.[88] In advanced disease, obstructive strictures in the second or third portion of the duodenum may cause massive proximal dilatation, resulting in a megaduodenum[88] (Fig. 36–23).

Primary duodenal Crohn's disease rarely leads to fistula formation. However, duodenocolic fistulas occasionally may result from advanced Crohn's disease in the transverse colon with subsequent fistulization to the third portion of the duodenum[84, 89] (Fig. 36–24). These patients may have thickened, spiculated folds in the duodenum adjoining the fistula as a result of nonspecific inflammatory changes, but there rarely is histologic evidence of Crohn's disease in the duodenum.[89] The fistulas may be difficult to delineate on upper gastrointestinal studies and are more likely to be visualized on barium enemas because of the higher pressures generated with this technique. Because these duodenal changes represent a nonspecific inflammatory response rather than actual involvement of the duodenum by Crohn's disease, follow-up barium studies after resection of the fistula may show a completely normal duodenum.[89]

duodenal ulcer may be indistinguishable from an ordinary peptic ulcer, but the presence of other antral or duodenal findings of Crohn's disease should suggest the correct diagnosis. Duodenal involvement may also be manifested by thickened, nodular folds in the descending duodenum[87, 88] (Fig. 36–21). Eventually, however, the folds may become effaced, and the mucosa may have a nodular or cobblestoned appearance due to shallow, intersecting areas of linear ulceration similar to those found in advanced ileocolitis.[88]

Subsequent scarring and fibrosis may lead to one or more areas of duodenal narrowing. Because of the

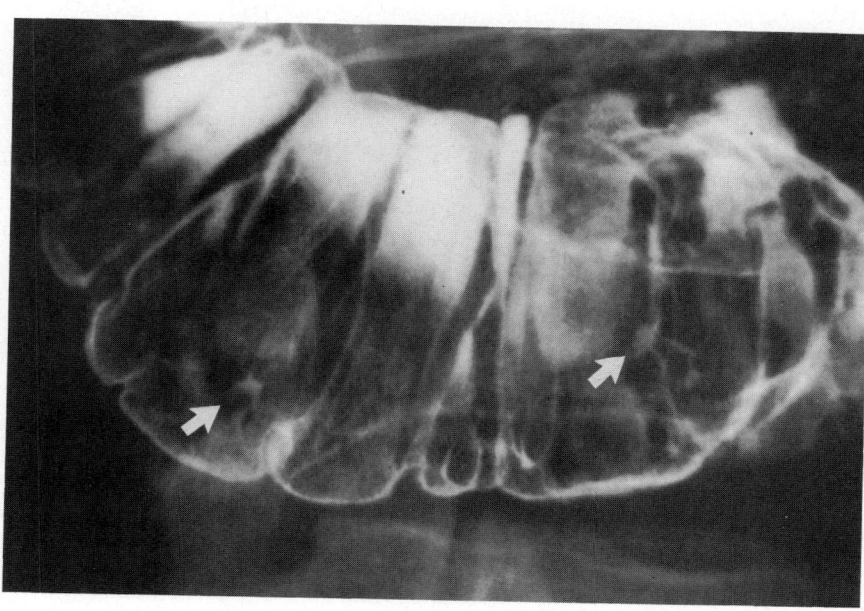

**Figure 36–19. Duodenal Crohn's disease with aphthous ulcers.** Several discrete aphthous ulcers (arrows) are seen in the distal duodenum near the ligament of Treitz. Note the stellate configuration of the ulcers. (Courtesy of Louis Engelhom, M.D., Brussels, Belgium.)

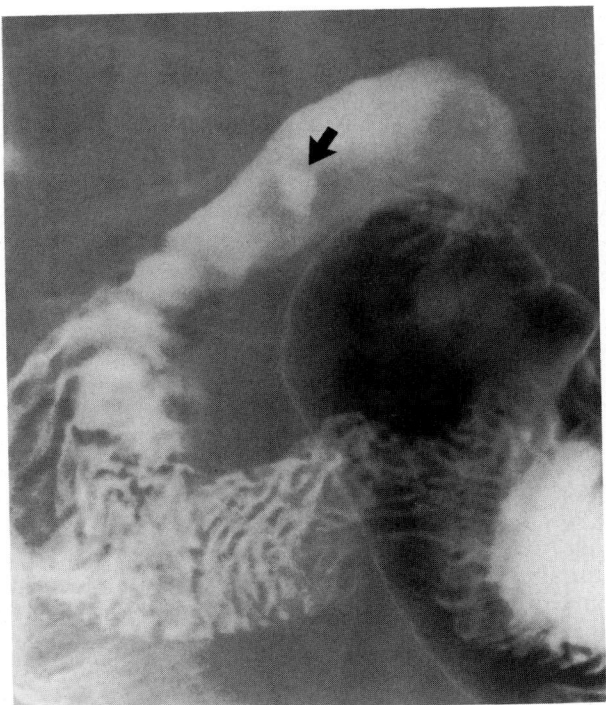

**Figure 36–20. Duodenal Crohn's disease with a postbulbar ulcer (arrow) and narrowing.** An atypical peptic ulcer in the postbulbar duodenum could produce similar findings. (From Levine MS: Crohn's disease of the upper gastrointestinal tract. Radiol Clin North Am 25:79–91, 1987.)

## Differential Diagnosis

### Stomach

Aphthous ulcers in the stomach may be indistinguishable radiographically from gastric erosions due to alcohol, aspirin, other nonsteroidal anti-inflammatory drugs, or other causes. Although gastric involvement by

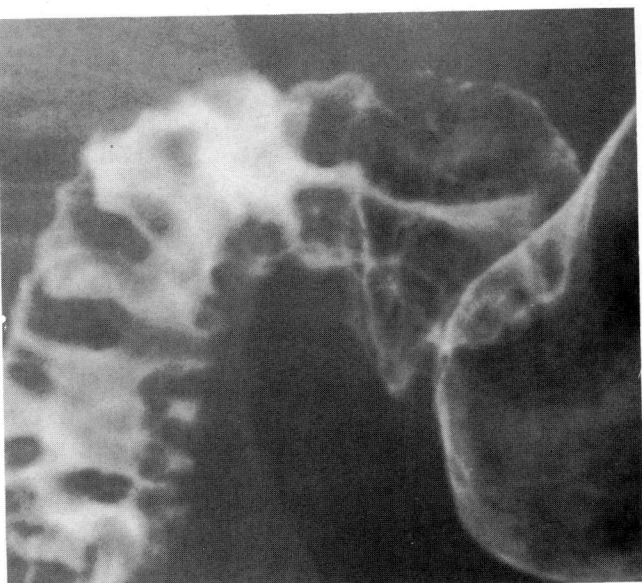

**Figure 36–21. Duodenal Crohn's disease with thickened folds.** Note how the folds have a thickened, nodular appearance in the proximal duodenum. Peptic duodenitis could produce similar findings.

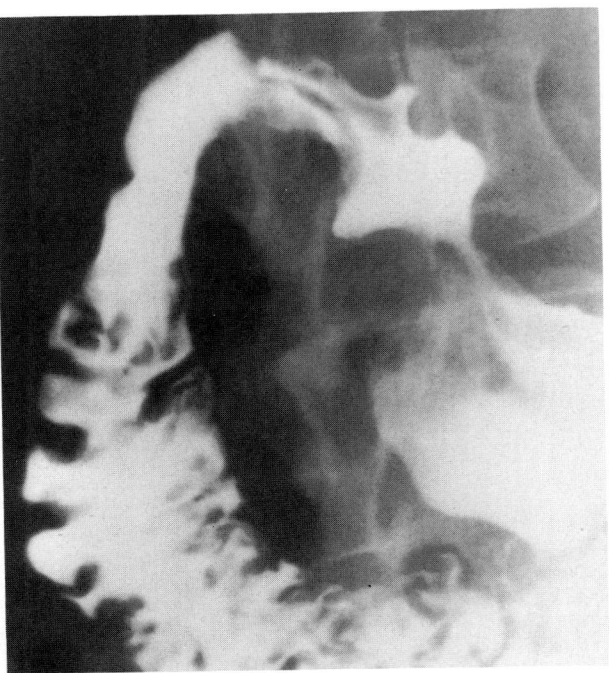

**Figure 36–22. Duodenal Crohn's disease with stricture formation.** There is smooth, tapered narrowing of the apical portion of the bulb and adjacent segment of the descending duodenum. This appearance is characteristic of Crohn's disease.

Crohn's disease is much less common than erosive gastritis, the possibility of Crohn's disease should be suspected in patients who have crampy abdominal pain or diarrhea, and a small bowel follow-through or barium enema should be performed to search for concomitant ileocolitis.

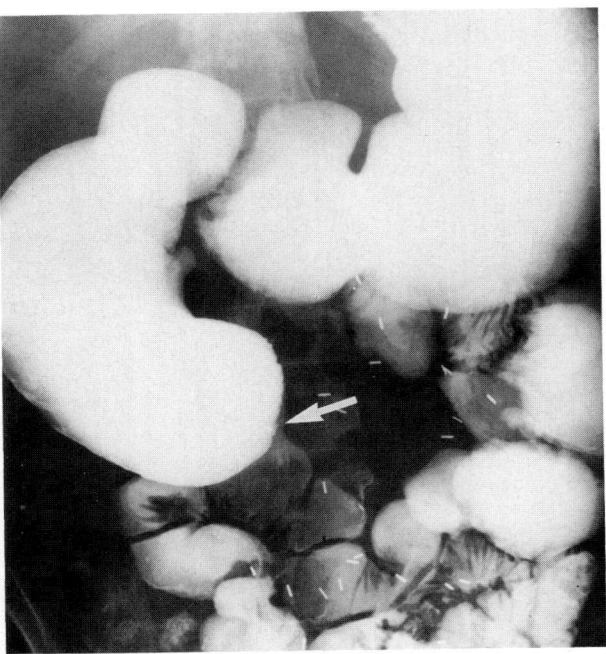

**Figure 36–23. Duodenal Crohn's disease with a megaduodenum.** There is high-grade obstruction (arrow) of the distal duodenum with marked duodenal dilatation above this level. (From Levine MS: Crohn's disease of the upper gastrointestinal tract. Radiol Clin North Am 25:79–91, 1987.)

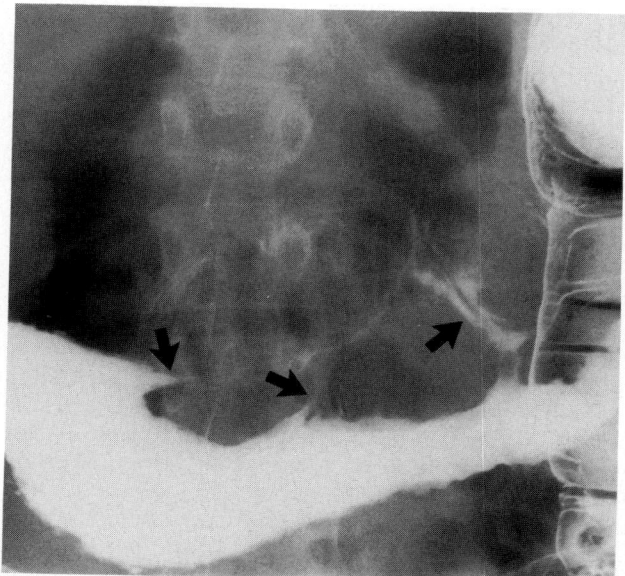

**Figure 36–24. Crohn's disease with duodenocolic fistulas.** A barium enema shows three separate fistulous tracks *(arrows)* extending from the superior border of the transverse colon to the third portion of the duodenum. Note the tubular, severely ulcerated appearance of the transverse colon due to advanced granulomatous colitis. Duodenocolic fistulas almost always result from primary Crohn's disease of the colon with nonspecific inflammatory changes in the duodenum adjoining the fistula. (From Levine MS: Crohn's disease of the upper gastrointestinal tract. Radiol Clin North Am 25:79–91, 1987.)

Although the stenotic phase of gastroduodenal Crohn's disease produces characteristic funnel-shaped antral narrowing, other conditions may produce similar findings. The most important diagnostic consideration is scirrhous carcinoma of the stomach. However, the narrowed antrum of Crohn's disease tends to have a smooth, tubular configuration, whereas scirrhous carcinoma produces a linitis plastica appearance with a distorted, more irregular mucosal contour.[61] Nevertheless, it may be difficult to distinguish Crohn's disease from gastric carcinoma on the basis of radiologic criteria. In one study, about one third of patients with antral narrowing caused by Crohn's disease underwent surgery because the radiographic findings simulated a scirrhous carcinoma.[83] Antral narrowing may also be caused by a variety of other conditions, including peptic ulcer disease, sarcoidosis, tuberculosis, syphilis, eosinophilic gastritis, caustic ingestion, and radiation. However, the correct diagnosis is often suggested by the clinical history and presentation.

Gastrocolic fistulas may result not only from Crohn's disease but also from benign, penetrating ulcers on the greater curvature of the stomach in patients who are taking aspirin.[90] Much less commonly, these fistulas may be caused by carcinoma of the stomach or transverse colon invading the gastrocolic ligament.[86] When Crohn's disease is responsible for the fistula, however, a barium enema examination usually reveals advanced granulomatous colitis in the transverse colon.

### Duodenum

Duodenal Crohn's disease may simulate a variety of other inflammatory conditions. Aphthous ulcers in the duodenum may be indistinguishable from varioliform duodenal erosions. However, erosive duodenitis usually involves the duodenal bulb, whereas the aphthous ulcers of Crohn's disease may be located anywhere in the duodenum from the bulb to the ligament of Treitz. The presence of one or more ulcers in the duodenal bulb or postbulbar duodenum should raise the possibility of Zollinger-Ellison syndrome, but these patients usually have markedly thickened folds and increased secretions in the stomach (see Chapter 35). Thickened, nodular folds may be caused not only by Crohn's disease but also by intrinsic duodenitis, pancreatitis, or other conditions. Scarring from duodenal Crohn's disease most frequently produces strictures in the postbulbar portion of the descending duodenum. However, scarring from postbulbar duodenal ulcers may produce a similar appearance.[91] A focal area of narrowing may also be caused by annular duodenal carcinomas, but these lesions can usually be differentiated by their shelf-like, overhanging borders. As in the stomach, suspected duodenal involvement by Crohn's disease should lead to a careful small bowel follow-through or barium enema for ruling out Crohn's disease in the small bowel or colon.

## Sarcoidosis

Sarcoidosis is a systemic granulomatous disease of unknown origin. It is manifested pathologically by the presence of noncaseating granulomas containing multinucleated giant cells, but other granulomatous diseases may produce identical findings. The majority of patients have thoracic sarcoidosis with bilateral hilar lymphadenopathy or fibronodular pulmonary infiltrates on chest radiographs. About 40% of patients have extrathoracic disease involving the eye, skin, lymph nodes, liver, spleen, heart, and musculoskeletal or nervous system. Although sarcoidosis is rarely thought to affect the gastrointestinal tract, one investigator found noncaseating granulomas in mucosal biopsy specimens from the stomach in 10% of patients with known sarcoidosis.[92] Thus, gastrointestinal involvement by this disease may be more common than is generally recognized.

### Clinical Findings

Sarcoidosis involves the stomach more frequently than any other portion of the gastrointestinal tract. However, most patients with gastric sarcoidosis are asymptomatic.[92] Occasionally, antral narrowing may cause varying degrees of gastric outlet obstruction manifested by epigastric discomfort and bloating, nausea, vomiting, anorexia, and weight loss.[93, 94] Other patients may have abdominal pain or upper gastrointestinal bleeding due to ulceration of the overlying mucosa.[95, 96] When gastric sarcoidosis produces symptoms, treatment with steroids produces a dramatic clinical response in about two thirds of patients, but symptomatic improvement is not necessarily accompanied by pathologic resolution of disease.[94] Occasionally, surgical intervention may be required if there is persistent gastric outlet obstruction, massive bleeding, or a suspicion of malignancy on the basis of the radiographic or endoscopic findings.

### Radiographic Findings

Gastric sarcoidosis may be manifested by a spectrum of radiographic findings. In patients with superficial disease, double contrast upper gastrointestinal studies may demonstrate a localized area of mucosal nodularity or thickened, irregular folds[97] (Fig. 36–25A). Other patients may have benign- or malignant-appearing ulcers in the stomach.[95, 96] More advanced gastric sarcoidosis is characterized by smooth, cone-shaped antral narrowing and deformity[95, 96] (Fig. 36–25B). Similar findings may be caused by scarring from peptic ulcer disease, caustic ingestion, radiation, and a variety of other granulomatous conditions, including Crohn's disease, tuberculosis, syphilis, and fungal disease.[95] However, the possibility of gastric sarcoidosis should be suspected in patients with characteristic changes of sarcoidosis in the thorax. Occasionally, more irregular gastric narrowing may pro-duce a linitis plastica appearance indistinguishable from that of a scirrhous gastric carcinoma.[96, 98] Whether smooth or irregular, antral narrowing results from extensive granulomatous involvement of the stomach. Unfortunately, superficial endoscopic biopsies often fail to demonstrate granulomas when the disease is confined to the submucosa or deeper layers of the gastric wall.

## Tuberculosis

Gastroduodenal involvement occurs in less than 0.5% of all patients with tuberculosis.[99] The stomach and duodenum are rarely involved because of the sparsity of lymphoid tissue in the upper gastrointestinal tract, the high acidity of peptic secretions, and the rapid passage of ingested organisms into the small bowel. Most patients with gastric or duodenal tuberculosis are found to have generalized tuberculosis. Gastroduodenal infection is presumably caused by ingestion of the bacillus or by hematogenous spread to lymphatics in the wall of the stomach or duodenum.[100] Although routine pasteurization of milk has dramatically decreased the incidence of gastrointestinal tuberculosis in the United States, some patients may travel to the United States from other countries such as South Africa or India, where tuberculosis is endemic. Gastric tuberculosis has also been encountered with increased frequency in patients with AIDS, particularly those of Haitian origin.[101]

### Clinical Findings

Patients with gastric or duodenal tuberculosis may present with epigastric pain or upper gastrointestinal bleeding.[102–104] Subsequent scarring may cause nausea and vomiting due to the development of gastric outlet obstruction.[104] Although the clinical findings are nonspecific, the possibility of gastroduodenal tuberculosis should be considered in patients with known pulmonary tuberculosis or in patients who have migrated from areas where tuberculosis is endemic.

Stool cultures for tuberculosis are unreliable; some patients with pulmonary tuberculosis may have positive culture results in the absence of gastrointestinal infection, whereas others may have negative culture results despite gastrointestinal disease.[100] A definitive diagnosis of gastroduodenal tuberculosis can be made when endoscopic biopsies reveal caseating granulomas in the stomach or duodenum. However, biopsies often fail to demonstrate granulomas because of the small size of the sample specimens and the submucosal location of the granulomas.[104] Depending on the severity of disease, gastroduodenal tuberculosis may be treated by antituberculous drug therapy or, if necessary, gastric resection or bypass.

### Radiographic Findings

Gastric tuberculosis may be manifested on barium studies by one or more areas of ulceration, most frequently on the lesser curvature of the antrum or in the

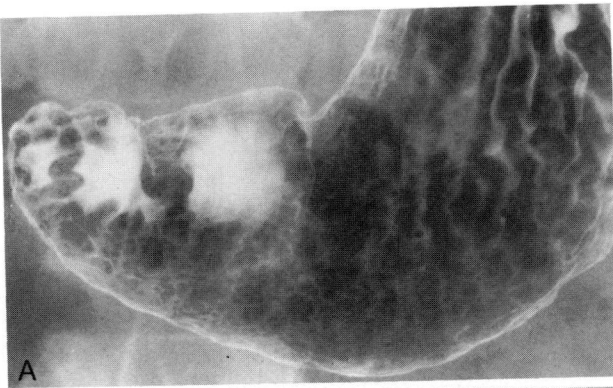

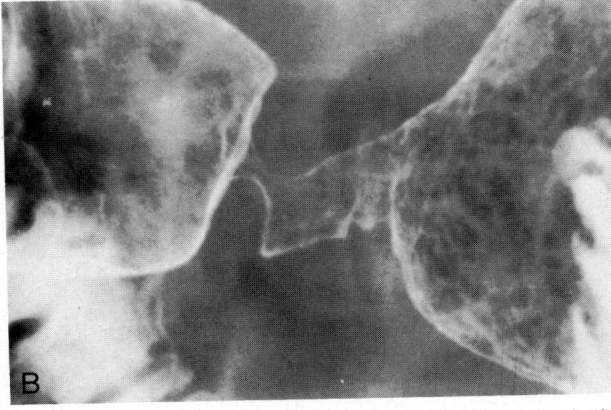

**Figure 36–25. Gastric sarcoidosis. A**. A double contrast study shows considerable nodularity of the mucosa in the gastric antrum. This patient had pulmonary sarcoidosis, and endoscopic biopsy specimens revealed noncaseating granulomas in the stomach. **B**. In another patient, more advanced gastric sarcoidosis is manifested by marked antral narrowing and deformity. (**B** courtesy of Seth N. Glick, M.D., Philadelphia, PA.)

region of the pylorus.[101, 105] Subsequent scarring and fibrosis may cause marked antral narrowing, eventually leading to the development of gastric outlet obstruction.[105] Occasionally, the narrowed antrum may have an irregular contour, simulating the linitis plastica appearance of a primary scirrhous carcinoma of the stomach.[105] As in the ileocecal region, advanced gastric tuberculosis may be associated with the development of multiple fistulous tracks in this region.[105]

Duodenal tuberculosis may also be manifested radiographically by ulcers, thickened folds, narrowing, or fistulas.[106–109] As in Crohn's disease, duodenal tuberculosis is often associated with contiguous involvement of the distal antrum. Enlarged tuberculous lymph nodes adjacent to the duodenum may cause widening, narrowing, or obstruction of the duodenal sweep.[109] Rarely, duodenorenal fistulas have been described in patients with tuberculosis of the right kidney involving the duodenum.[110]

## Syphilis

Gastric syphilis is a rare disease; it occurs in less than 1% of all patients with secondary or tertiary syphilis.[111] Nevertheless, gastric involvement should be suspected in young patients with untreated lues who develop epigastric pain, nausea and vomiting, or upper gastrointestinal bleeding.[112] Occasionally, it is possible to isolate *Treponema pallidum* on endoscopic biopsy specimens and to confirm the diagnosis of gastric syphilis by demonstrating the spirochetes on darkfield microscopy.[113] These patients may have symptomatic relief and objective resolution of their gastric lesions with antiluetic therapy.

### *Radiographic Findings*

Gastric syphilis may be manifested radiographically by mucosal nodularity, erosions, shallow or deep ulcers, and thickened folds, predominantly in the antrum[111, 112, 114] (Fig. 36–26). As the disease progresses, some patients may develop smooth, tubular, funnel-shaped narrowing of the antrum.[111] Occasionally, however, the narrowed antrum may have an irregular contour, mimicking the linitis plastica appearance of a primary scirrhous carcinoma of the stomach.[115] When gastric syphilis is suspected on the basis of the clinical and radiographic findings, endoscopic biopsy specimens are required for a more definitive diagnosis.

## Fungal Diseases

A variety of fungal diseases may rarely involve the stomach. Gastric histoplasmosis may be manifested by thickened folds, ulceration, or narrowing of the stomach.[116, 117] Gastric candidiasis may be associated with the development of large aphthoid ulcerations.[13] Other rare fungal infections of the stomach include actinomycosis and mucormycosis.[118, 119]

## OTHER INFECTIOUS CAUSES

### *Helicobacter pylori* Infection

*H. pylori* (formerly known as *Campylobacter pylori*) is a gram-negative bacillus that was first isolated from the stomach by use of endoscopic biopsy specimens in 1983.[120] Although the relationship between *H. pylori* and peptic ulcers is controversial (see Chapter 35), this organism may have a major role in the development of gastritis. In various studies, the prevalence of *H. pylori* infection in the stomach has ranged from 70 to 75% in patients with histologic evidence of gastritis.[121] Furthermore, eradication of the organism by antimicrobial therapy usually results in healing of the gastritis.[122] These findings support the argument that *H. pylori* may indeed be a cause of chronic gastritis. However, *H. pylori*

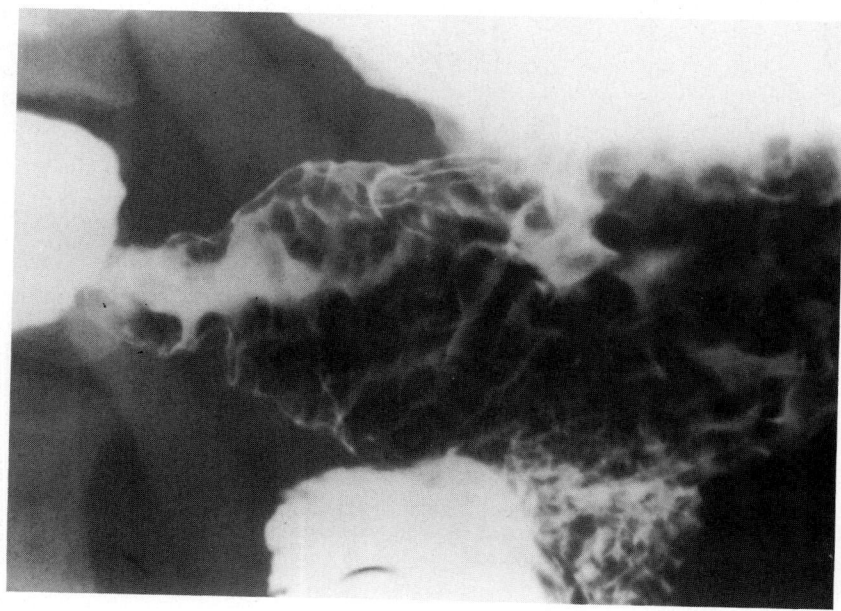

**Figure 36–26. Gastric syphilis.** Mucosal nodularity and thickened folds are seen in the antrum in this patient with proven gastric syphilis.

infection and histologic gastritis often occur in asymptomatic patients, particularly those older than 60 years of age.[123] The clinical significance of *H. pylori* gastritis therefore remains uncertain.

Some patients with *H. pylori* gastritis may have an acute clinical presentation consisting of nausea, vomiting, and epigastric pain.[124] As indicated earlier, however, many patients with this condition are asymptomatic.[123] Triple therapy with bismuth, metronidazole, and other antibiotics is usually effective in eradicating the organism from the stomach. However, it remains unclear whether such therapy is required.

### Radiographic Findings

*H. pylori* gastritis may be manifested on barium studies by thickened folds, most commonly in the gastric antrum or body[125] (Fig. 36–27). The radiographic findings are nonspecific, because enlarged folds may be caused by a variety of inflammatory or neoplastic conditions. Occasionally, patients with *H. pylori* gastritis may have markedly thickened, nodular folds in the gastric fundus and body, mimicking the appearance of Ménétrier's disease or lymphoma.[126] Computed tomographic evaluation of *H. pylori* gastritis may demonstrate circumferential thickening of the antrum or focal thickening of the posterior gastric wall, occasionally simulating a gastric carcinoma.[127]

## Cytomegalovirus Infection

Cytomegalovirus is a member of the herpesvirus group that has been recognized with increased frequency as an opportunistic invader of the gastrointestinal tract in immunocompromised patients, particularly patients with AIDS. The colon is the most common site of infection (see Chapter 63).[128] Much less frequently, patients with

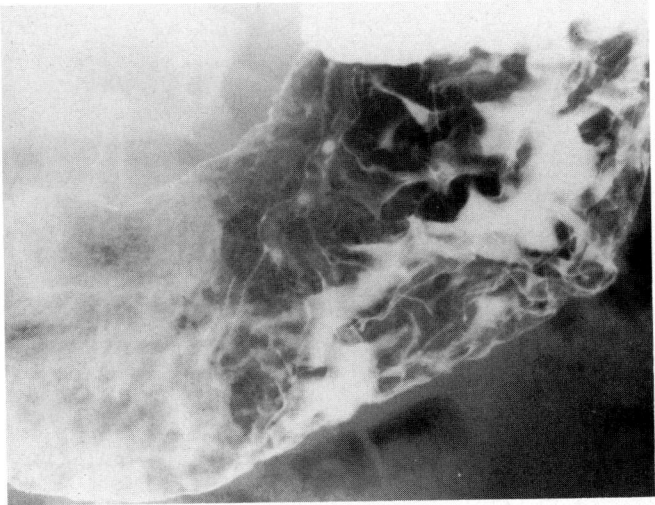

**Figure 36–27.** ***H. pylori* gastritis.** Thickened, irregular folds are present in the body of the stomach. Gastric brushing and biopsy specimens were positive for *H. pylori.*

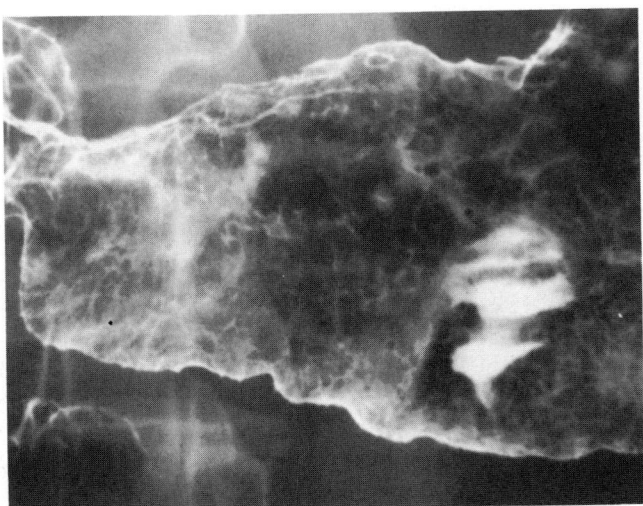

**Figure 36–28. Cytomegalovirus gastritis.** Mucosal nodularity and tiny ulcerations are seen in the gastric antrum. Note the irregular contour of the stomach. This patient had AIDS.

AIDS may develop cytomegalovirus esophagitis or gastritis;[27, 128–133] interestingly, these conditions rarely occur in other immunocompromised patients.

### Radiographic Findings

Cytomegalovirus gastritis may be manifested radiographically by mucosal nodularity; erosions; shallow or deep ulcers; thickened, nodular folds; and, in severe cases, antral narrowing[27, 131, 132] (Fig. 36–28). The narrowed antrum may have a serrated, irregular contour. Ulceration or narrowing of the stomach should therefore suggest the possibility of cytomegalovirus gastritis in patients with AIDS. However, other opportunistic infections such as cryptosporidiosis and toxoplasmosis occasionally produce similar findings in AIDS patients (see later sections on cryptosporidiosis and toxoplasmosis). Rarely, deep ulcers result in the development of fistulas to adjacent structures such as the colon.[133] When cytomegalovirus gastritis is suspected in patients with AIDS, the diagnosis can be confirmed by demonstrating characteristic inclusion bodies on endoscopic biopsy specimens or brushings or by obtaining positive cultures for cytomegalovirus.

## Cryptosporidiosis

*Cryptosporidium*, a protozoan, may infect the small bowel in patients with AIDS, causing a profuse secretory diarrhea (see Chapter 48). Much less frequently, cryptosporidiosis may involve the stomach.[130, 131, 134] In such cases, barium studies may demonstrate antral narrowing and rigidity, occasionally associated with one or more deep areas of ulceration.[130, 131, 134] When computed tomography is performed on these patients, it may confirm the presence of a narrowed lumen with a markedly thickened gastric wall.[135] Cytomegalovirus gastritis should be the major consideration in the differential diagnosis of antral narrowing and ulceration in patients with AIDS (see earlier section on cytomegalovirus infection). When opportunistic gastritis is suspected on the basis of barium studies, endoscopic brushing, biopsy, and culture specimens should be obtained for a more definitive diagnosis.

## Toxoplasmosis

Opportunistic infection of the stomach by toxoplasmosis is a rare cause of antral narrowing in patients with AIDS.[136] The diagnosis may be confirmed by demonstration of the teardrop-shaped trophozoites in histologic specimens from the stomach.[136] Toxoplasmosis should therefore be included in the differential diagnosis of antral narrowing in AIDS patients.

## Strongyloidiasis

*Strongyloides stercoralis* is a parasite of worldwide distribution that causes infection of the stomach, duodenum, and proximal small bowel.[137–139] Cases are occasionally encountered in metropolitan areas of the United States in patients who have emigrated from areas of endemic infection such as Africa, Asia, and South America.[139] Strongyloidiasis may also occur as an opportunistic infection in patients with AIDS. Affected individuals may present with abdominal pain, nausea and vomiting, diarrhea, malabsorption, or hypoalbuminemia due to a protein-losing enteropathy.[138] A peripheral eosinophilia is present in 25 to 35% of patients.[138]

## *Radiographic Findings*

Gastric involvement by strongyloidiasis is occasionally manifested radiographically by antral gastritis or narrowing.[138, 139] The duodenum and proximal jejunum are more commonly involved. Barium studies may demonstrate thickened or effaced mucosal folds, ulceration, and narrowing or dilatation of the duodenum[137–139] (Fig. 36–29A). In advanced cases, the bowel may have a "lead pipe" appearance due to tubular narrowing of the lumen and obliteration of the normal fold pattern (Fig. 36–29B). Occasionally, marked duodenal dilatation results in the development of a megaduodenum (see Fig. 36–29B). Other conditions such as Zollinger-Ellison syndrome, scleroderma, and celiac disease may also be manifested by a dilated duodenum, but these conditions can usually be differentiated from strongyloidiasis by clinical and radiographic criteria. Occasionally, scarring of the duodenal wall may permit reflux of barium into the biliary tree via an incompetent sphincter of Oddi.[138, 139] Although strongyloidiasis is rarely found in the United States, this possibility should be considered when barium studies reveal characteristic findings in patients with AIDS or in patients who have a recent history of travel to endemic areas.

## EMPHYSEMATOUS GASTRITIS

Emphysematous gastritis is a rare type of phlegmonous gastritis in which gas is found in the gastric wall due to infection by gas-forming organisms such as *Escherichia coli*, *Proteus vulgaris*, *Clostridium perfringens*, and *Staphylococcus aureus*.[140–142] This condition is usually

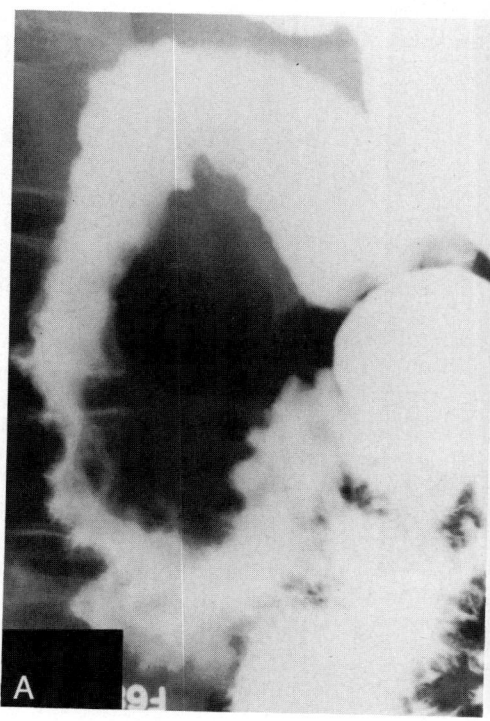
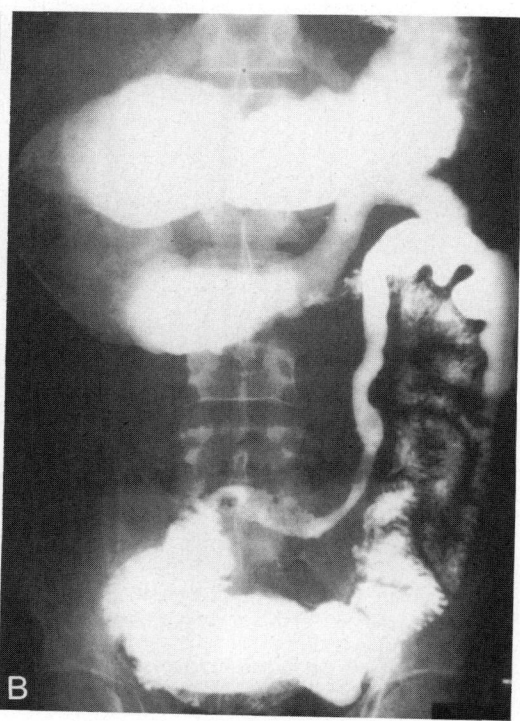

**Figure 36–29. Duodenal strongyloidiasis. A.** Markedly thickened, edematous folds are present in the duodenum. This patient had AIDS. **B.** In another patient with more advanced disease, there is a markedly dilated duodenum (i.e., a megaduodenum) with effaced mucosal folds. Also note the smooth, tubular appearance of the proximal jejunum, producing a lead pipe appearance. This patient had recently immigrated to the United States from an area where strongyloidiasis was endemic. (**B** courtesy of Murray K. Dalinka, M.D., Philadelphia, PA.)

caused by profound insults to the stomach, such as caustic ingestion, gastroduodenal surgery, or gastric volvulus.[140, 141] Subsequent inflammation, ischemia, or necrosis of the stomach may permit gas-forming organisms to enter the gastric wall. These patients may present with an acute, fulminating illness characterized by severe abdominal pain, hematemesis, tachycardia, fever, and shock.[140, 141] Supportive therapy with parenteral fluids and antibiotics should be initiated, but a nasogastric tube should not be placed in the stomach because of the high risk of perforation. Despite intensive treatment, mortality rates as high as 60% have been reported.[141]

## Radiographic Findings

Emphysematous gastritis is characterized on abdominal plain films by multiple streaks, bubbles, or amorphous collections of gas in the wall of the stomach, silhouetting the gastric shadow[140–142] (Fig. 36–30). These intramural gas collections have a constant relationship to the stomach with changes in the patient's position, so that they can be differentiated from residue or food, which shifts to the dependent portion of the stomach on upright or decubitus views.[141] Studies with a water-soluble contrast agent may be performed to confirm the

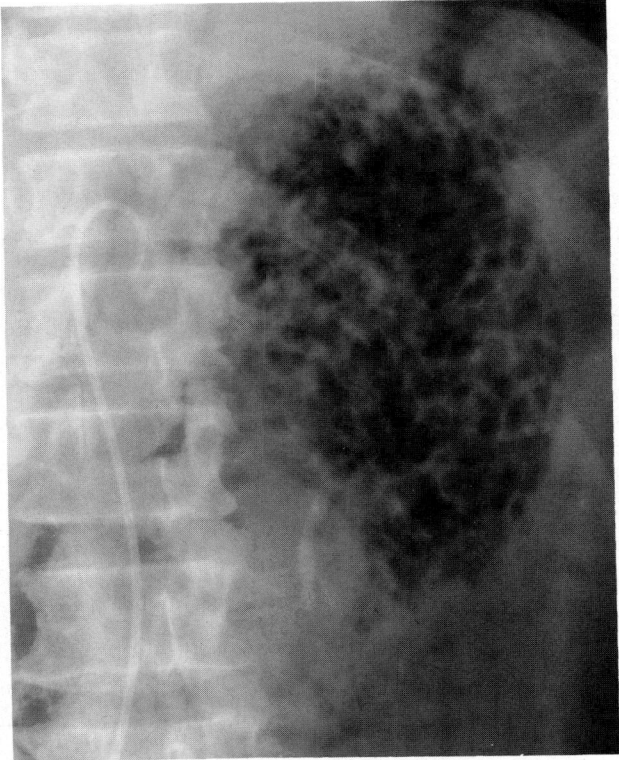

**Figure 36–30. Emphysematous gastritis.** A close-up view from an abdominal plain film shows numerous mottled and bubbly collections of gas in the wall of the stomach. An attempted embolization of a gastric carcinoma led to gastric necrosis and subsequent infection by gas-forming organisms.

extraluminal location of these gas collections. These studies may also demonstrate intramural dissection or actual extravasation of contrast medium from the stomach. Occasionally, computed tomography may demonstrate small collections of gas in the gastric wall that are not recognized on abdominal plain films.[143]

## Differential Diagnosis

Emphysematous gastritis must be differentiated from other rare conditions known as gastric emphysema and gastric pneumatosis. Emphysematous gastritis is typically characterized by bubbly or mottled collections of intramural gas, whereas gastric emphysema is characterized by long, linear collections of intramural gas around the circumference of the stomach[142, 144] (see Fig. 40–45). In gastric emphysema, gas is thought to enter the wall of the stomach via mucosal rents caused by increased intraluminal pressure associated with gastric outlet obstruction or by iatrogenic trauma due to endoscopy or other gastric instrumentation. Although the radiographic findings are dramatic, these patients may be asymptomatic. Thus, gastric emphysema can usually be differentiated from emphysematous gastritis by clinical and radiographic criteria.

Gastric pneumatosis is an extremely rare form of pneumatosis intestinalis in which multiple gas-filled cysts or blebs are found in the wall of the stomach.[142] This condition much more commonly involves the small bowel or colon (see Chapter 13). When present in the stomach, the gas-filled intramural cysts may be indistinguishable from the bubbly gas collections associated with emphysematous gastritis. However, patients with gastric pneumatosis are usually asymptomatic, whereas patients with emphysematous gastritis are acutely ill. Thus, these conditions can be differentiated on the basis of the clinical history and presentation.

## PSEUDOLYMPHOMA

Gastric pseudolymphoma, also known as benign lymphoid hyperplasia or chronic lymphocytic gastritis, is a benign inflammatory condition of unknown etiology characterized by proliferation of lymphoid tissue in the stomach.[145] Unfortunately, this condition may be extremely difficult to differentiate from gastric carcinoma or lymphoma on radiologic or endoscopic examinations.[145] Affected individuals may present with epigastric pain, nausea and vomiting, diarrhea, weight loss, or chronic upper gastrointestinal bleeding.[145] In pseudolymphoma, lymphocytes infiltrating the gastric wall are arranged in follicles, which resemble the germinal centers in reactive lymph nodes.[145] Because germinal centers are rarely found in patients with lymphoma, the diagnosis of pseudolymphoma can be made on the basis of histopathologic criteria. Although gastric pseudolymphoma is a benign condition, surgery is often performed on these patients because of the difficulty in obtaining a definitive preoperative diagnosis. A partial gastrectomy is usually curative.

## Radiographic Findings

Gastric pseudolymphoma may be manifested on barium studies by a spectrum of findings, including benign- or malignant-appearing ulcers, infiltrating or constricting lesions, thickened folds, and multiple, small umbilicated masses in the stomach.[146, 147] As a result, gastric pseudolymphoma may be indistinguishable radiographically from gastric carcinoma or lymphoma.[146] Thus, endoscopy or even surgery may be required to differentiate pseudolymphoma from a true malignant lesion in the stomach.

## CAUSTIC INGESTION

Accidental or intentional ingestion of caustic agents may lead to severe injury of the upper gastrointestinal tract. Although the esophagus is more commonly involved (see Chapter 26), gastroduodenal injury may also occur. The esophagus is classically damaged by strong alkaline agents such as liquid lye (i.e., concentrated sodium hydroxide), whereas the stomach and duodenum are damaged by strong acids such as hydrochloric, sulfuric, acetic, oxalic, carbolic, and nitric acid.[148] However, esophageal injury often occurs in patients who ingest strong acids, and gastroduodenal injury occurs in 5 to 10% of patients who ingest strong alkali.[149] Pathologically, injury to the stomach and duodenum occurs in three phases, including 1) an acute necrotic phase 1 to 4 days after caustic ingestion, 2) an ulceration-granulation phase 5 to 28 days after caustic ingestion, and 3) a final phase of cicatrization and scarring beginning 3 to 4 weeks after caustic ingestion.[149, 150]

Patients with gastroduodenal injury by caustic agents may present with severe abdominal pain, nausea and vomiting, hematemesis, fever, and shock.[150, 151] A study with a water-soluble contrast agent is often performed to assess the extent and severity of injury to the upper gastrointestinal tract. In stable patients who have no evidence of perforation, conservative treatment can be initiated with antibiotics, steroids, and parenteral feedings.[151] After a latent period of 3 to 4 weeks, however, many patients develop rapidly progressive signs of gastric outlet obstruction because of antral scarring and fibrosis.[151] As a result, a gastroenterostomy or partial gastrectomy may still be required to alleviate obstructive symptoms.[150]

## Radiographic Findings

Ingested caustic agents tend to flow down the lesser curvature of the stomach into the antrum, causing severe pylorospasm that delays emptying into the duodenum.[148, 152] As a result, the lesser curvature and distal antrum of the stomach sustain the greatest degree of damage, whereas the duodenum is relatively spared.[148, 152] During the acute phase of injury, studies with water-soluble contrast medium may demonstrate thickened, edematous folds; ulceration; gastric atony; or mural defects due to edema and hemorrhage.[152] In fulminating cases, gastric necrosis may be manifested on abdominal plain films by streaky, bubbly, or mottled gas collections that are unaffected by changes in the patient's position.[153] This appearance may result from passage of intraluminal gas into the gastric wall or from secondary infection by gas-forming organisms.[153] In such cases, studies with water-soluble contrast medium may demonstrate a confined or free perforation with intramural dissection of contrast, extragastric collections, or free extravasation into the peritoneal cavity (Fig. 36–31).

If patients survive the acute illness, barium studies performed 4 weeks or more after caustic ingestion may demonstrate progressive narrowing and deformity of the antrum or antrum and body of the stomach.[152, 154] In some patients, the narrowed antrum may have a smooth, tubular configuration (Fig. 36–32A), whereas in others, it may have a more irregular contour, mimicking the appearance of a primary scirrhous carcinoma of the stomach.[152, 155] Antral narrowing from caustic ingestion may also be indistinguishable from that of peptic ulcer disease, Crohn's disease, sarcoidosis, tuberculosis, or other granulomatous conditions involving the stomach. However, the diagnosis of caustic injury is usually apparent from the clinical history. About 20% of patients with antral scarring from caustic ingestion also have scarring of the esophagus[154] (Fig. 36–32B).

Although pylorospasm tends to protect the duodenum in patients who have ingested caustic agents, occasional

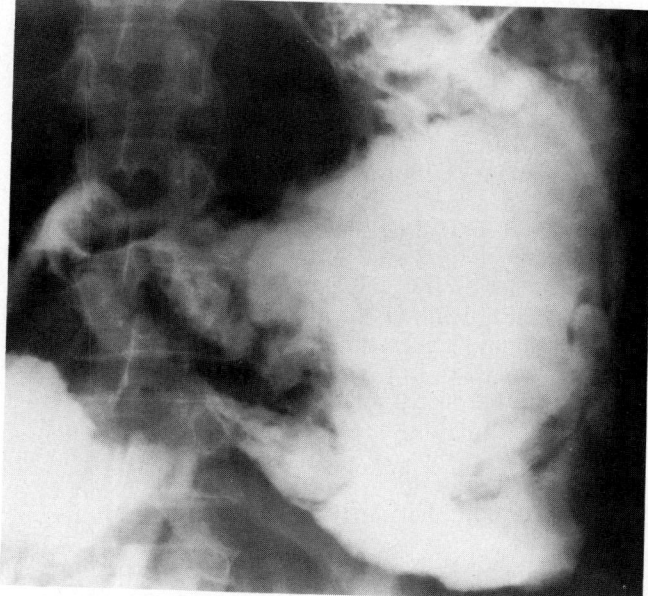

**Figure 36–31. Severe gastric injury caused by caustic ingestion.** A study with water-soluble contrast medium shows a grossly abnormal stomach with intramural dissection of contrast medium and numerous mural defects due to edema and hemorrhage after acid ingestion.

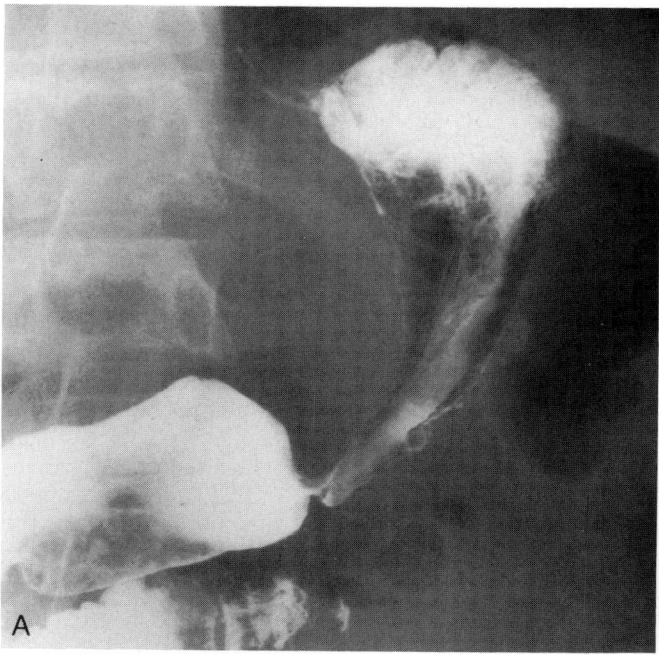
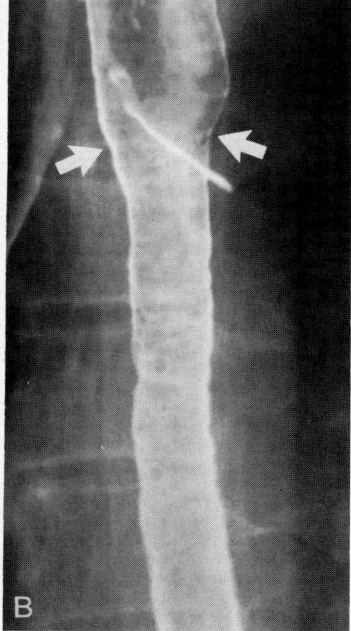

**Figure 36–32. Caustic scarring of the stomach and esophagus.** **A**. A double contrast study of the stomach shows marked antral narrowing and deformity due to scarring from previous lye ingestion. **B**. An esophagram shows an associated stricture in the esophagus, extending distally from the carina *(arrows)* to the gastroesophageal junction. Aspirated barium is also present in both main stem bronchi.

cases of severe duodenal injury have been reported.[156] In such cases, barium studies may demonstrate thickened, edematous folds; spasm; atony; ulceration; and, eventually, strictures in the duodenum anywhere from the bulb to the ligament of Treitz.[152] These patients usually have evidence of associated gastric injury.

## RADIATION

Radiation doses of 5000 rad or more to the upper abdomen may cause significant injury to the stomach and duodenum when these structures are included in the radiation portal.[157, 158] The distal antrum and pyloric region are most commonly affected, but the duodenal sweep may also be involved in patients who have received radiation to the right upper quadrant. Inflammatory changes in the stomach and duodenum typically occur 1 to 6 months after radiation therapy, whereas scarring and fibrosis occur 6 months or more after treatment.[157, 158] Affected individuals may present with dyspepsia, epigastric pain, nausea and vomiting, or upper gastrointestinal bleeding.[157, 158] Although the symptoms may suggest peptic ulcer disease, the possibility of radiation injury should be considered in any patient who has undergone radiation therapy during the past 12 months.

### Radiographic Findings

The acute phase of radiation injury to the stomach may be manifested radiographically by gastroparesis, spasm, thickened folds, or ulceration predominantly involving the distal antrum and pyloric region and, occasionally, the duodenum.[157, 158] Rarely, perforation

of deep ulcers may result in acute peritonitis.[157] Subsequent scarring and fibrosis may lead to the development of antral or, less commonly, duodenal narrowing 6 months or more after completion of radiation therapy.[157] Occasionally, the narrowed antrum may have an irregular contour, simulating a scirrhous carcinoma of the stomach.[159] However, the correct diagnosis is usually apparent from the clinical history.

## FLOXURIDINE TOXICITY

Because floxuridine (5-FUDR) is extracted almost completely by the liver after infusion into the hepatic artery, it is the agent of choice for hepatic artery infusion chemotherapy in patients with unresectable liver metastases. In the past, 5-FUDR has been administered via catheters placed percutaneously into the hepatic artery, but surgically implantable infusion pumps have replaced external catheter systems at many hospitals as the primary means of delivering 5-FUDR into the liver in patients with liver metastases.[160] Unfortunately, gastroduodenal inflammation, ulceration, and bleeding may occur as a direct complication of this form of chemotherapy.

### Pathogenesis

In patients who are receiving 5-FUDR via catheters placed percutaneously into the hepatic artery, gastroduodenal toxicity presumably occurs because the drug is infused directly into vessels supplying the stomach and duodenum, such as the gastroduodenal and right gastric arteries. In patients who have hepatic artery infusion pumps, the gastroduodenal and right gastric arteries are surgically ligated at the time of pump placement to prevent overflow of the drug into these vessels. Nevertheless, gastroduodenal inflammation and ulceration have been documented radiographically and endoscopically in patients receiving 5-FUDR therapy via a hepatic artery infusion pump.[161–163] Gastroduodenal toxicity apparently occurs because of the development of small collateral channels between the hepatic artery and the gastroduodenal or right gastric arteries after these vessels have been ligated. This hypothesis is supported by a study in which gastroduodenal complications did not occur when all of the vessels supplying the superior border of the distal stomach and proximal duodenum were surgically ligated at the time of pump placement.[164] Whatever the explanation, it is important to recognize that severe gastroduodenal inflammation or ulceration may occur as a complication of hepatic artery infusion of 5-FUDR not only via an external catheter system but also via an implantable pump.

## Clinical Findings

Gastroduodenal toxicity should be suspected when patients who are receiving hepatic artery infusion of 5-FUDR develop intractable nausea, vomiting, epigastric pain, or upper gastrointestinal bleeding.[163] Although the possibility of metastatic tumor may be considered in these patients, the temporal relationship between 5-FUDR therapy and the onset of symptoms should suggest the correct diagnosis. In most cases, cessation of chemotherapy leads to a dramatic clinical response.

## Radiographic Findings

Gastroduodenal toxicity resulting from hepatic artery infusion of 5-FUDR may be manifested radiographically by severe gastritis, duodenitis, or gastroduodenal ulceration.[163, 165–167] Some patients may have ulcers or thickened folds in the stomach, whereas others may have severe duodenitis with markedly thickened, edematous folds in the duodenum[163] (Fig. 36–33). Ischemia, bleeding, vasculitis, or other inflammatory or infectious conditions involving the duodenum may produce similar findings. However, the temporal relationship between 5-FUDR therapy and the onset of symptoms should suggest the correct diagnosis. When 5-FUDR toxicity is suspected on the basis of barium studies, cessation of chemotherapy should lead to rapid clinical improvement with dramatic regression of these abnormalities on follow-up studies.

## DUODENITIS

The pathophysiology of duodenitis is controversial. Because this condition is often associated with gastric hyperacidity, it has been postulated that duodenitis represents part of the spectrum of peptic ulcer disease.[168–171] However, gastric acid secretion may be nor-

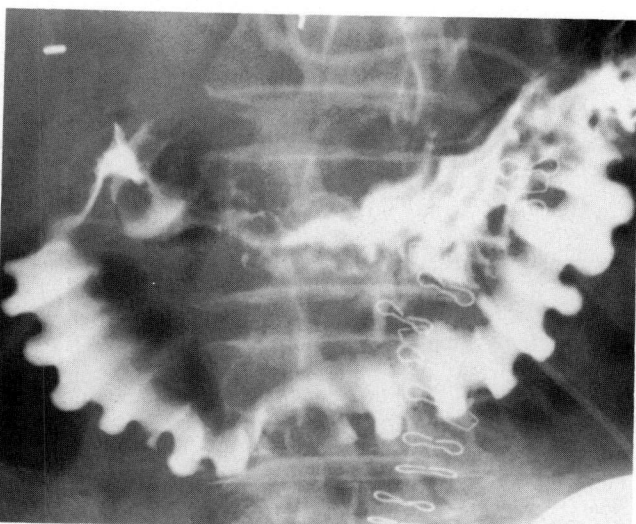

**Figure 36–33. Severe duodenitis caused by 5-FUDR toxicity.** A barium study shows markedly thickened, edematous folds in the duodenum to the level of the ligament of Treitz. This patient was receiving 5-FUDR via a hepatic artery infusion pump. (Reprinted from, by permission of the publisher, Hiehle JF, Levine MS: Gastrointestinal toxicity of 5-FU and 5-FUDR: radiographic findings. Can Assoc Radiol J 42:109–112, 1991.)

mal or even decreased in patients with duodenitis, so that some investigators believe that it is a distinct clinical entity unrelated to peptic ulcer disease.[172–174] Other data suggest that *H. pylori* may also have a role in the development of this condition.[175]

Whatever the pathophysiology, duodenitis is thought to be a significant cause of dyspepsia in the adult population.[168, 169, 173, 176] Dyspepsia may be manifested by vague upper abdominal symptoms, including epigastric pain or distress, nausea, fatty food intolerance, or early satiety. Less frequently, erosive duodenitis may be associated with signs of upper gastrointestinal bleeding, such as hematemesis, melena, or guaiac-positive stool.[173] In some patients, hemorrhagic duodenitis may occur as a complication of myocardial infarction or congestive heart failure.[177] Occasionally, the site of bleeding in the duodenum can be documented by angiography.[178, 179]

## Radiographic Findings

The diagnosis of duodenitis may be suggested radiographically in patients who have a spastic, irritable duodenal bulb or thickened, nodular folds in the proximal duodenum[180] (Fig. 36–34). For reasons that are unclear, patients with chronic renal failure who are undergoing dialysis often have enlarged duodenal folds to a degree rarely encountered in other patients with duodenitis[181, 182] (Fig. 36–35). In most cases, however, thickened folds and spasm are nonspecific findings, so the upper gastrointestinal examination generally has not been considered to be a reliable technique for diagnosing duodenitis.

With double contrast technique, it is possible to demonstrate more subtle signs of inflammatory disease

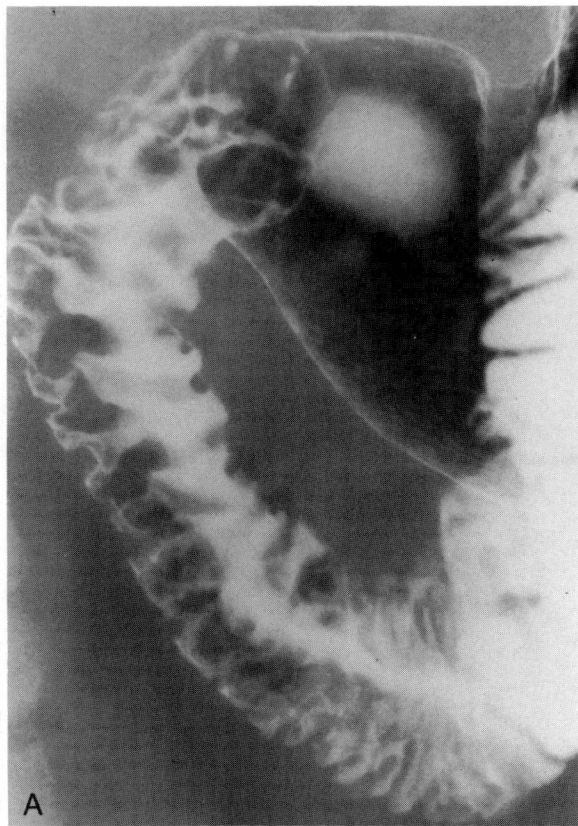

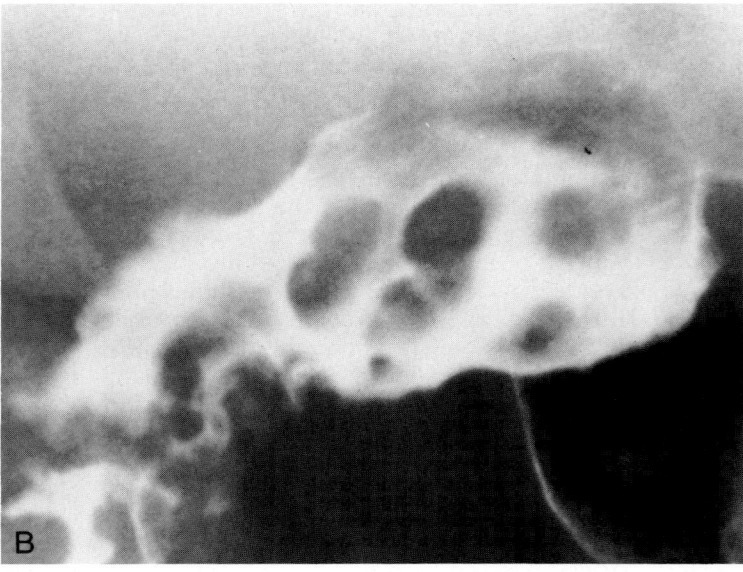

**Figure 36–34. Duodenitis. A**. Thickened, irregular folds are seen in the proximal duodenum. **B**. In another patient, thickened folds and mucosal nodularity are present in the duodenal bulb.

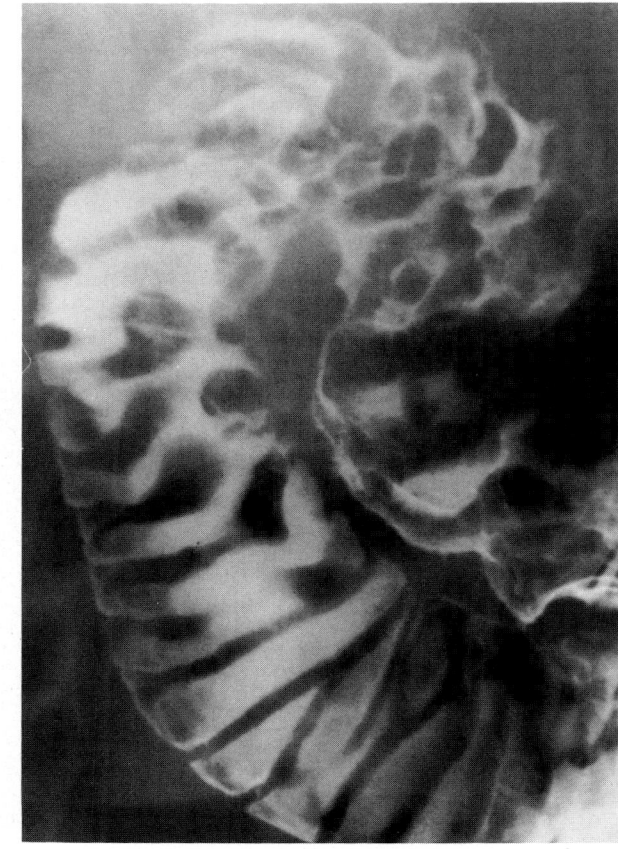

**Figure 36–35. Severe duodenitis associated with chronic renal failure.** Grossly thickened, polypoid folds are seen in the proximal duodenum. This patient was undergoing dialysis for chronic renal failure.

in the duodenum. This inflammation may be manifested by mucosal nodules or nodular folds or by diffuse coarsening of the mucosal surface pattern of the bulb with lucent areas surrounded by barium-filled grooves that resemble the areae gastricae in the stomach.[183–185] With double contrast technique, it is also possible to diagnose erosive duodenitis, a condition previously thought to be solely in the domain of the endoscopist.[6, 184, 185] These erosions may be found in the duodenal bulb or, less commonly, in the descending duodenum. As in the stomach, incomplete erosions appear as tiny flecks of barium in the duodenum, whereas complete or varioliform erosions appear as central barium collections surrounded by radiolucent halos of edematous mucosa[6, 184, 185] (Fig. 36–36). False-positive radiologic diagnoses occasionally may result from normal mucosal pits in the duodenum that are mistaken for incomplete erosions on double contrast studies[186] (Fig. 36–37). Barium precipitates may also simulate incomplete erosions. Thus, a confident diagnosis of erosive duodenitis can be made only when true varioliform erosions are demonstrated.

Some patients with celiac disease (nontropical sprue) may have severe duodenitis with thickened folds or nodular mucosa in the descending duodenum.[187] Others may have small (1 to 4 mm), hexagonal filling defects in the duodenal bulb, which produce a distinctive mosaic pattern or "bubbly" bulb[188] (Fig. 36–38). Unlike heterotopic gastric mucosa, which predominantly involves the juxtapyloric region of the bulb (Fig. 36–39), these nodules tend to be distributed more diffusely throughout the bulb. This finding may reflect the underlying changes of celiac disease in the duodenum or Brunner's gland hyperplasia due to associated duodenitis.[188] In any case, the presence of a bubbly bulb or thickened duodenal folds should suggest the possibility of celiac disease in patients with malabsorption. A small bowel enema or

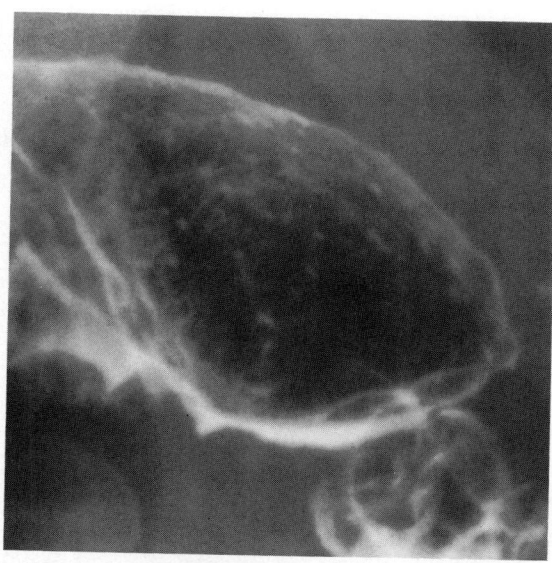

**Figure 36–37. Mucosal pits simulating erosive duodenitis.** Punctate collections of barium trapped in tiny, epithelialized pits can be mistaken for duodenal erosions. However, note that these collections are not surrounded by radiolucent mounds of edema. (From JG Bova, V Kamath, FO Tio, et al, The normal mucosal surface pattern of the duodenal bulb: radiologic-histologic correlation, AJR, 145, 4, 735–738, 1985, © by American Roentgen Ray Society.)

small bowel biopsy may be required for a more definitive diagnosis (see Chapter 49).

Duodenitis may also be caused by Crohn's disease, caustic ingestion, radiation, 5-FUDR toxicity, and infectious processes such as tuberculosis and strongyloidiasis. These conditions and their radiographic findings are discussed elsewhere in this chapter. Finally, duodenitis

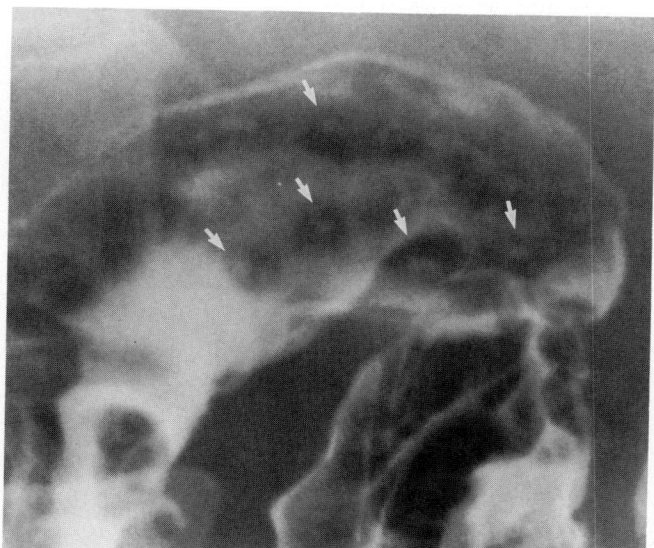

**Figure 36–36. Erosive duodenitis.** Varioliform erosions are seen in the duodenum as tiny flecks of barium surrounded by radiolucent mounds of edematous mucosa *(arrows).* (From Levine MS, Rubesin SE, Herlinger H, et al: Double-contrast upper gastrointestinal examination: technique and interpretation. Radiology 168:593–602, 1988.)

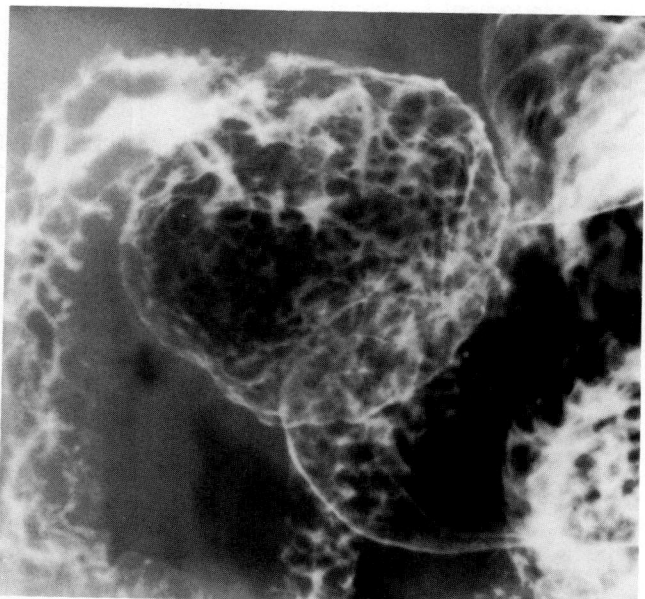

**Figure 36–38. Celiac disease with a bubbly bulb.** There are multiple hexagonal filling defects in the duodenal bulb and thickened, irregular folds in the descending duodenum due to associated duodenitis. (From B Jones, TM Bayless, SR Hamilton, et al, "Bubbly" duodenal bulb in celiac disease: radiologic-pathologic correlation, AJR, 142, 1, 119–122, 1984, © by American Roentgen Ray Society.)

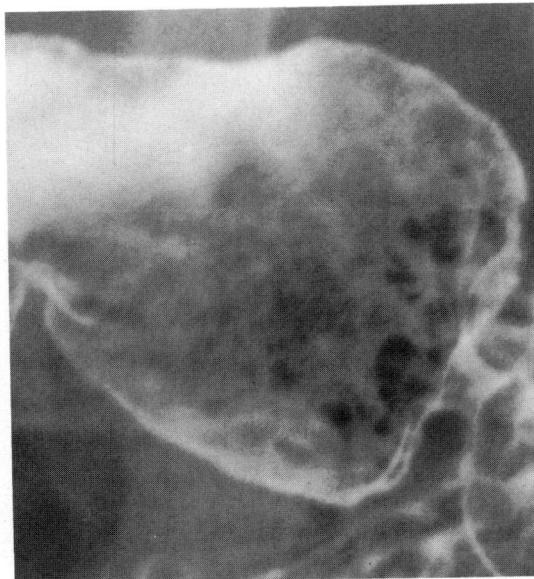

**Figure 36–39. Heterotopic gastric mucosa.** Multiple discrete, angulated filling defects are seen at the base of the duodenal bulb. This appearance is characteristic of heterotopic gastric mucosa in the bulb. (From Levine MS, Rubesin SE, Herlinger H, et al: Double-contrast upper gastrointestinal examination: technique and interpretation. Radiology 168:593–602, 1988.)

may occur in patients with underlying pancreatitis involving the head of the pancreas. In such cases, the correct diagnosis is suggested by thickened, spiculated duodenal folds associated with widening of the duodenal sweep or compression of the medial aspect of the descending duodenum (see Chapter 40).

### Acknowledgment

Figures 36–1A, 36–7, 36–10, 36–11A, and 36–35 are reproduced from Laufer I, Levine MS (eds): Double Contrast Gastrointestinal Radiology (2nd ed). Philadelphia: WB Saunders, 1992.

Figure 36–13 is reproduced from Herlinger H, Maglinte D (eds): Clinical Radiology of the Small Intestine. Philadelphia: WB Saunders, 1989.

Figure 36–32A and B is reproduced from Levine MS: Radiology of the Esophagus. Philadelphia: WB Saunders, 1989.

## References

1. Poplack W, Paul RE, Goldsmith M, et al: Demonstration of erosive gastritis by the double-contrast technique. Radiology 117:519–521, 1975.
2. Laufer, I: An assessment of the accuracy of double contrast gastroduodenal radiology. Gastroenterology 71:874–878, 1976.
3. Op den Orth JO, Dekker W: Gastric erosions: radiological and endoscopic aspects. Radiol Clin (Belg) 45:88–89, 1976.
4. Op den Orth JO, Dekker W: Gastric polyps or erosions. AJR 129:357–358, 1977.
5. Tragardh B, Wehlin L, Ohashi K: Radiologic appearance of complete gastric erosions. Acta Radiol Diagn (Stockh) 19:634–642, 1978.
6. Catalano D, Pagliari U: Gastroduodenal erosions: radiological findings. Gastrointest Radiol 7:235–240, 1982.
7. Laufer I, Hamilton J, Mullens JE: Demonstration of superficial gastric erosions by double contrast radiography. Gastroenterology 68:387–391, 1975.
8. Thorsen WB, Western D, Tanaka Y, et al: Aspirin injury to the gastric mucosa: gastrocamera observations on the effect of pH. Arch Intern Med 121:499–506, 1968.
9. Lanza F, Royer G, Nelson R: An endoscopic evaluation of the effects of non-steroidal anti-inflammatory drugs on the gastric mucosa. Gastrointest Endosc 21:103–105, 1975.
10. Roberts DM: Chronic gastritis, alcohol, and non-ulcer dyspepsia. Gut 13:768–774, 1972.
11. Laufer I, Trueman T: Multiple superficial gastric erosions due to Crohn's disease of the stomach. Radiologic and endoscopic diagnosis. Br J Radiol 49:726–728, 1976.
12. Ariyama J, Wehlin L, Lindstrom CG, et al: Gastroduodenal erosions in Crohn's disease. Gastrointest Radiol 5:121–125, 1980.
13. Cronan J, Burrell M, Trepeta R: Aphthoid ulcerations in gastric candidiasis. Radiology 134:607–611, 1980.
14. Rumerman J, Rubesin SE, Levine MS, et al: Gastric ulceration caused by heater probe coagulation. Gastrointest Radiol 13:200–202, 1988.
15. Davenport HW: Salicylate damage to the gastric mucosal barrier. N Engl J Med 276:1307–1312, 1967.
16. Edman D: Effects of salicylates on the gastric mucosa as revealed by roentgen examination and the gastrocamera. Acta Radiol Diagn (Stockh) 11:57–64, 1971.
17. MacDonald WC: Correlation of mucosal histology and aspirin intake in chronic gastric ulcer. Gastroenterology 65:381–389, 1973.
18. Cameron AJ: Aspirin and gastric ulcer. Mayo Clin Proc 50:565–570, 1975.
19. Silvoso GR, Ivey KJ, Butt JH, et al: Incidence of gastric lesions in patients with rheumatic disease on chronic aspirin therapy. Ann Intern Med 91:517–520, 1979.
20. O'Laughlin JC, Hoftiezer JW, Ivey KJ: Effect of aspirin on the human stomach in normals: endoscopic comparison of damage produced one hour, 24 hours, and 2 weeks after administration. Scand J Gastroenterol 16:211–214, 1981.
21. Lanza FL, Nelson RS, Rack MF: A controlled endoscopic study comparing the toxic effects of sulindac, naproxen, aspirin, and placebo on the gastric mucosa of healthy volunteers. J Clin Pharmacol 24:89–95, 1984.
22. Graham DY, Smith JL, Dobbs SM: Gastric adaptation occurs with aspirin administration in man. Dig Dis Sci 28:1–6, 1983.
23. McLean AM, Paul RE, Philipps E, et al: Chronic erosive gastritis—clinical and radiological features. J Can Assoc Radiol 33:158–162, 1982.
24. McAdam WAF, Morgan AG, Jackson A, et al: Multiple persisting idiopathic gastric erosions. Gut 16:410, 1975.
25. Kikuchi Y, Levine MS, Laufer I, et al: Value of flow technique for double contrast examination of the stomach. AJR 147:1183–1184, 1986.
26. Levine MS, Verstandig A, Laufer I: Serpiginous gastric erosions caused by aspirin and other nonsteroidal anti-inflammatory drugs. AJR 146:31–34, 1986.
27. Balthazar EJ, Megibow AJ, Hulnick DH: Cytomegalovirus esophagitis and gastritis in AIDS. AJR 144:1201–1204, 1985.
28. Gohel VK, Kressel HY, Laufer I: Double contrast artifacts. Gastrointest Radiol 3:139–146, 1978.
29. Berg HM: Antral gastritis. Radiology 59:324–335, 1952.
30. Turner CJ, Lipitz LR, Pastore RA: Antral gastritis. Radiology 113:305–312, 1974.
31. Glick SN, Cavanaugh B, Teplick SK: The hypertrophied antral-pyloric fold. AJR 145:547–549, 1985.
32. Lewis TD, Laufer I, Goodacre RL: Arteriovenous malformation of the stomach: radiologic and endoscopic features. Am J Dig Dis 23:467–470, 1978.
33. Stempien SJ, Dagradi AE, Reingold IM, et al: Hypertrophic hypersecretory gastropathy. Am J Dig Dis 9:471–493, 1964.
34. Tan DTD, Stempien SJ, Dagradi AE: The clinical spectrum of hypertrophic hypersecretory gastropathy. Gastrointest Endosc 18:69–73, 1971.
35. Moghadam M, Gluckmann R, Eyler WR: The radiological assessment of gastric acid output. Radiology 89:888–895, 1967.

36. Press AJ: Practical significance of gastric rugal folds. AJR 125:172–183, 1975.

37. Balthazar EJ, Davidian MM: Hyperrugosity in gastric carcinoma: radiographic, endoscopic, and pathologic features. AJR 136:531–535, 1981.

38. Fieber SS, Rickert RR: Hyperplastic gastropathy. Am J Gastroenterol 76:321–329, 1981.

39. Scharschmidt BF: The natural history of hypertrophic gastropathy (Ménétrier's disease). Am J Med 63:644–652, 1977.

40. Citrin Y, Sterling K, Halsted JA: The mechanism of hypoproteinemia associated with giant hypertrophy of the gastric mucosa. N Engl J Med 257:906–912, 1957.

41. Jarnum S, Jensen KB: Plasma protein turnover (albumin, transferrin, IgG, IgM) in Ménétrier's disease (giant hypertrophic gastritis): evidence of non-selective protein loss. Gut 13:128–137, 1972.

42. Searcy RM, Malagelada JR: Ménétrier's disease and idiopathic hypertrophic gastropathy. Ann Intern Med 100:560–565, 1984.

43. Suudt TM, Compton CC, Malt RA: Ménétrier's disease: a trivalent gastropathy. Ann Surg 208:694–701, 1989.

44. Rubin RG, Fink H: Giant hypertrophy of the gastric mucosa associated with carcinoma of the stomach. Am J Gastroenterol 47:379–388, 1967.

45. Williams SM, Harned RK, Settles RH: Adenocarcinoma of the stomach in association with Ménétrier's disease. Gastrointest Radiol 3:387–390, 1978.

46. Reese DF, Hodgson JR, Dockerty MB: Giant hypertrophy of the gastric mucosa (Ménétrier's disease): a correlation of the roentgenographic, pathologic, and clinical findings. AJR 88:619–626, 1962.

47. Olmsted WW, Cooper PH, Madewell JE: Involvement of the gastric antrum in Ménétrier's disease. AJR 126:524–529, 1976.

48. Maxfield DL, Boyd WC: Pernicious anemia: a review, an update, and an illustrative case. J Am Osteopath Assoc 8:133–142, 1983.

49. Jeffries GH, Sleisenger MH: Studies of parietal cell antibody in pernicious anemia. J Clin Invest 44:2021–2038, 1965.

50. Joske RA, Finckh ES, Wood IJ: Gastric biopsy: a study of 1,000 consecutive successful gastric biopsies. Q J Med 24: 269–294, 1955.

51. Strickland RG, Mackay IR: A reappraisal of the nature and significance of chronic atrophic gastritis. Am J Dig Dis 18:426–440, 1973.

52. Jeffries GH: Pernicious anemia and atrophic gastritis. *In* Samter M (ed): Immunological Diseases. Boston: Little Brown, 1978, pp 1296–1307.

53. Babior BM, Bunn HF: Megaloblastic anemias. *In* Braunwald E, Isselbacher KJ, Petersdorf RG, et al (eds): Harrison's Principles of Internal Medicine (11th ed). New York: McGraw-Hill, 1987, pp 1498–1504.

54. Elsborg L, Mosbech J: Pernicious anaemia as a risk factor in gastric cancer. Acta Med Scand 206:315–318, 1979.

55. Cheli R, Santi L, Ciancamerla G, et al: A clinical and statistical follow-up study of atrophic gastritis. Am J Dig Dis 18:1061–1066, 1973.

56. Siurala M, Lehtola J, Ihamaki T: Atrophic gastritis and its sequelae: results of 19–23 years follow-up examinations. Scand J Gastroenterol 9:441–446, 1974.

57. Borch K: Epidemiologic, clinicopathologic, and economic aspects of gastroscopic screening of patients with pernicious anemia. Scand J Gastroenterol 21:21–30, 1986.

58. Laws JW, Pitman RG: The radiological features of pernicious anaemia. Br J Radiol 33:229–237, 1960.

59. Levine MS, Palman CL, Rubesin SE, et al: Atrophic gastritis in pernicious anemia: diagnosis by double-contrast radiography. Gastrointest Radiol 14:215–219, 1989.

60. Mackintosh CE, Kreel L: Anatomy and radiology of the areae gastricae. Gut 18:855–864, 1977.

61. Levine MS, Kong V, Rubesin SE, et al: Scirrhous carcinoma of the stomach: radiologic and endoscopic diagnosis. Radiology 175:151–154, 1990.

62. Edelman, MJ, March JL: Eosinophilic gastroenteritis. AJR 9:773–778, 1964.

63. Klein NC, Hargrove L, Sleisenger MH, et al: Eosinophilic gastroenteritis. Medicine (Baltimore) 49:299–319, 1970.

64. Goldberg HI, O'Kieffe D, Jenis EH, et al: Diffuse eosinophilic gastroenteritis. AJR 119:342–351, 1973.

65. Burhenne HJ, Carbone JV: Eosinophilic (allergic) gastroenteritis. AJR 96:332–338, 1966.

66. Balfe DM: Eosinophilic gastritis. AJR 152:1322, 1989.

67. Wehunt WD, Olmsted WW, Neiman HL, et al: Eosinophilic gastritis. Radiology 120:85–89, 1976.

68. Freundlich IM, Schaupp R, Lehman JS: Eosinophilic gastroenteritis: a case report with extensive jejunal involvement. Radiology 86:493–495, 1966.

69. Levine MS: Crohn's disease of the upper gastrointestinal tract. Radiol Clin North Am 25:79–91, 1987.

70. Danzi JT, Farmer RG, Sullivan BH, et al: Endoscopic features of gastroduodenal Crohn's disease. Gastroenterology 70:9–13, 1976.

71. Fielding JF, Toye DKM, Beton DC, et al: Crohn's disease of the stomach and duodenum. Gut 11:1001–1006, 1970.

72. Haggitt RC, Meissner WA: Crohn's disease of the upper gastrointestinal tract. Am J Clin Pathol 59:613–622, 1973.

73. Nugent FW, Richmond M, Park SK: Crohn's disease of the duodenum. Gut 18:115–120, 1977.

74. Kim US, Zimmerman MJ, Weiss M: Massive upper gastrointestinal hemorrhage associated with Crohn's disease of the stomach and duodenum. Am J Gastroenterol 59:244–249, 1973.

75. Metzger WH, Ranganath KA: Crohn's disease presenting as a gastrocolic fistula. Am J Gastroenterol 65:258–261, 1976.

76. Kokal W, Pickleman J, Steinberg JJ, et al: Gastrocolic fistula in Crohn's disease. Surg Gynecol Obstet 146:701–704, 1978.

77. Cohen WN: Gastric involvement in Crohn's disease. AJR 101:425–430, 1967.

78. Marshak RH, Maklansky D, Kurzban JD, et al: Crohn's disease of the stomach and duodenum. Am J Gastroenterol 77:340–343, 1982.

79. Gray RR, Grosman H: Crohn's disease involving the proximal stomach. Gastrointest Radiol 10:43–45, 1985.

80. Legge DA, Carlson HC, Judd ES: Roentgenologic features of regional enteritis of the upper gastrointestinal tract. AJR 110:355–360, 1970.

81. Beaudin D, DaCosta LR, Prentice RSA, et al: Crohn's disease of the stomach. Am J Dig Dis 18:623–629, 1973.

82. Kelvin FM, Gedgaudas RK: Radiologic diagnosis of Crohn's disease (with emphasis on its early manifestations). Crit Rev Diagn Imaging 16:43–91, 1981.

83. Farman J, Faegenburg D, Dallemand S, et al: Crohn's disease of the stomach: the "ram's horn" sign. AJR 123:242–251, 1975.

84. Nelson SW: Some interesting and unusual manifestations of Crohn's disease ("regional enteritis") of the stomach, duodenum, and small intestine. AJR 107:86–101, 1969.

85. Zegel HG, Laufer I: Filiform polyposis. Radiology 127:615–619, 1978.

86. Laufer I, Joffe N, Stolberg H: Unusual causes of gastrocolic fistula. Gastrointest Radiol 2:21–25, 1977.

87. Wise L, Kyriakos M, McCown A, et al: Crohn's disease of the duodenum. Am J Surg 121:184–194, 1971.

88. Thompson WM, Cockrill H, Rice RP: Regional enteritis of the duodenum. AJR 123:252–261, 1975.

89. Herlinger H, O'Riordan D, Saul S, et al: Nonspecific involvement of bowel adjoining Crohn's disease. Radiology 159:47–51, 1986.

90. Laufer I, Thornley GD, Stolberg H: Gastrocolic fistula as a complication of benign gastric ulcer. Radiology 119:7–11, 1976.

91. Bilbao MK, Frische LH, Rösch J, et al: Postbulbar duodenal ulcer and ring-stricture. Radiology 100:27–35, 1971.

92. Palmer ED: Note on silent sarcoidosis of the gastric mucosa. J Lab Clin Med 52:231–234, 1958.

93. Allen EH, Batten JC, Jefferson K: Sarcoidosis of the alimentary tract. Br J Radiol 29:56–61, 1956.

94. Chinitz MA, Brandt LJ, Frank MS, et al: Symptomatic sarcoidosis of the stomach. Dig Dis Sci 30:682–688, 1985.

95. Nathan MH, Newman A, Ochsner JL, et al: Sarcoidosis of the upper gastrointestinal tract. AJR 84:275–280, 1960.

96. Dunbar RD: Sarcoidosis and its radiologic manifestations. Crit Rev Diagn Imaging 28:185–220, 1978.

97. Levine MS, Ekberg O, Rubesin SE, et al: Gastrointestinal sarcoidosis: radiographic findings. AJR 153:293–295, 1989.
98. Bellan L, Semelka R, Warren CPW. Sarcoidosis as a cause of linitis plastica. J Can Assoc Radiol 39:72–74, 1988.
99. Chazan BI, Aitchison JD: Gastric tuberculosis. Br Med J 2:1288–1290, 1960.
100. Thoeni RF, Margulis AR: Gastrointestinal tuberculosis. Semin Roentgenol 14:283–294, 1979.
101. Brody JM, Miller DK, Zeman RK, et al: Gastric tuberculosis: a manifestation of acquired immunodeficiency syndrome. Radiology 159:342–348, 1986.
102. Subei I, Attar B, Schmitt G, et al: Primary gastric tuberculosis. Am J Gastroenterol 82:769–772, 1987.
103. Misra D, Rai RR, Nundy S, et al: Duodenal tuberculosis presenting as bleeding peptic ulcer. Am J Gastroenterol 83:203–204, 1988.
104. Nair KV, Pai CG, Rajogopal KP, et al: Unusual presentations of duodenal tuberculosis. Am J Gastroenterol 86:756–760, 1991.
105. Pinto RS, Zausner J, Beranbaum ER: Gastric tuberculosis. AJR 110:808–812, 1970.
106. Balikian JP, Yenikomshian SM, Jidejian YD: Tuberculosis of the pyloro-duodenal area. AJR 101:414–420, 1967.
107. Black GA, Carsky EW: Duodenal tuberculosis. AJR 131:329–330, 1978.
108. Tishler JMA: Duodenal tuberculosis. Radiology 130:593–595, 1979.
109. Gupta SK, Jain AK, Gupta JP, et al: Duodenal tuberculosis. Clin Radiol 39:159–161, 1988.
110. Schwartz DT, Garnes HA, Lattimer JK, et al: Pyeloduodenal fistula due to tuberculosis. J Urol 104:373–375, 1970.
111. Cooley RN, Childers JH: Acquired syphilis of the stomach. Gastroenterology 39:201–207, 1960.
112. Reisman TN, Leverett FL, Hudson JR, et al: Syphilitic gastropathy. Am J Dig Dis 20:588–593, 1975.
113. Sachar DB, Klein RS, Swerdlow F, et al: Erosive syphilitic gastritis: dark-field and immunofluorescent diagnosis from biopsy specimen. Ann Intern Med 80:512–515, 1974.
114. Mitchell RM, Bralow SP: Acute erosive gastritis due to early syphilis. Ann Intern Med 61:933–938, 1964.
115. Anai H, Okada Y, Okubo K, et al: Gastric syphilis simulating linitis plastica type of gastric cancer. Gastrointest Endosc 36:624–626, 1990.
116. Fitzpatrick TJ, Neimay BH: Histoplasma capsulatum infection associated with gastric ulcer and fatal hemorrhage. Arch Intern Med 91:49–55, 1953.
117. Fisher JR, Sanowski RA: Disseminated histoplasmosis producing hypertrophic gastric folds. Am J Dig Dis 23:282–285, 1978.
118. Van Olmen G, Larmuseau MF, Geboes K, et al: Primary gastric actinomycosis. Am J Gastroenterol 79:512–516, 1984.
119. Lawson H, Schmaman A: Gastric phycomycosis. Br J Surg 61:743–746, 1974.
120. Warren JR, Marshall BJ: Unidentified curved bacilli on gastric epithelium in active chronic gastritis. Lancet 2:1273–1275, 1983.
121. Isenberg JI, McQuaid KR, Laine L, et al: Acid-peptic disorders. In Yamada T (ed): Textbook of Gastroenterology. Philadelphia: JB Lippincott, 1991, pp 1241–1339.
122. Chamberlain CE, Peura DA: *Campylobacter (Helicobacter) pylori*: is peptic disease a bacterial infection? Arch Intern Med 150:951–955, 1990.
123. Dooley CP, Cohen H, Fitzgibbons PL, et al: Prevalence of *Helicobacter pylori* infection and histologic gastritis in asymptomatic patients. N Engl J Med 321:1562–1566, 1989.
124. Saita H, Murakami M, Yoo JK, et al: Link between *Helicobacter pylori*–associated gastritis and duodenal ulcer. Dig Dis Sci 38:117–122, 1993.
125. Morrison S, Dahms BB, Hoffenberg E, et al: Enlarged gastric folds in association with *Campylobacter pylori* gastritis. Radiology 171:819–821, 1989.
126. Chaloupka JC, Gay BB, Caplan D: *Campylobacter* gastritis simulating Ménétrier's disease by upper gastrointestinal radiography. Pediatr Radiol 20:200–201, 1990.
127. Urban BA, Fishman EK, Hruban RH: *Helicobacter pylori* gastritis mimicking gastric carcinoma at CT evaluation. Radiology 179:689–691, 1991.
128. Teixidor HS, Honig CL, Norsoph E, et al: Cytomegalovirus infection of the alimentary tract: radiologic findings with pathologic correlation. Radiology 163:317–323, 1987.
129. Balthazar EJ, Megibow AJ, Hulnick DH, et al: Cytomegalovirus esophagitis in AIDS: radiographic features in 16 patients. AJR 149:919–923, 1987.
130. Megibow AJ, Balthazar EJ, Hulnick DH: Radiology of nonneoplastic gastrointestinal disorders in acquired immune deficiency syndrome. Semin Roentgenol 22:31–41, 1987.
131. Falcone S, Murphy BJ, Weinfeld A: Gastric manifestations of AIDS: radiographic findings on upper gastrointestinal examination. Gastrointest Radiol 16:95–98, 1991.
132. Farman J, Lerner ME, Ng C, et al: Cytomegalovirus gastritis: protean radiologic manifestations. Gastrointest Radiol 17:202–206, 1992.
133. Agel NM, Tanner P, Drury A, et al: Cytomegalovirus gastritis with perforation and gastrocolic fistula formation. Histopathology 18:165–168, 1991.
134. Berk RN, Wall SD, McArdle CB, et al: Cryptosporidiosis of the stomach and small intestine in patients with AIDS. AJR 143:549–554, 1984.
135. Soulen MC, Fishman EK, Scatarige JC, et al: Cryptosporidiosis of the gastric antrum: detection using CT. Radiology 159:705–706, 1986.
136. Smart PE, Weinfeld A, Thompson NE, et al: Toxoplasmosis of the stomach: a cause of antral narrowing. Radiology 174:369–370, 1990.
137. Louisy CL, Barton CJ: The radiological diagnosis of *Strongyloides stercoralis* enteritis. Radiology 98:535–541, 1971.
138. Berkman YM, Rabinowitz J: Gastrointestinal manifestations of strongyloidiasis. AJR 115:306–311, 1972.
139. Dallemand S, Waxman M, Farman J: Radiological manifestations of *Strongyloides stercoralis*. Gastrointest Radiol 8:45–51, 1983.
140. Henry GW: Emphysematous gastritis. AJR 68:15–18, 1952.
141. Meyers HJ, Parker JJ: Emphysematous gastritis. Radiology 89:426–431, 1967.
142. Nelson SW: Extraluminal gas collections due to diseases of the gastrointestinal tract. AJR 115:225–248, 1972.
143. Monteferrante M, Shimkin P: CT diagnosis of emphysematous gastritis. AJR 153:191–192, 1989.
144. Schorr S, Marcus M: Intramural gastric emphysema. Br J Radiol 35:641–644, 1962.
145. Orr RK, Lininger JR, Lawrence W: Gastric pseudolymphoma: a challenging clinical problem. Ann Surg 200:185–194, 1984.
146. Perez CA, Dorfman RF: Benign lymphoid hyperplasia of the stomach and duodenum. Radiology 87:505–510, 1966.
147. Bahk YW, Ahn JS, Choi HJ: Lymphoid hyperplasia of the stomach presenting as umbilicated polypoid lesions. Radiology 100:277–280, 1971.
148. Nevin IN, Turner WW, Gardner HT: Early and late roentgenologic findings in corrosive gastritis. AJR 81:603–608, 1959.
149. Franken EA: Caustic damage of the gastrointestinal tract: roentgen features. AJR 118:77–85, 1973.
150. Citron BP, Pincus IJ, Geokas MC, et al: Chemical trauma of the esophagus and stomach. Surg Clin North Am 48:1303–1311, 1968.
151. Goldman LP, Weigert JM: Corrosive substance ingestion: a review. Am J Gastroenterol 79:85–90, 1984.
152. Muhletaler CA, Gerlock AJ, de Soto L, et al: Gastroduodenal lesions of ingested acids: radiographic findings. AJR 135:1247–1252, 1980.
153. Levitt R, Stanley RJ, Wise L: Gastric bullae: an early roentgen finding in corrosive gastritis following alkali ingestion. Radiology 115:597–598, 1975.
154. Poteshman NL: Corrosive gastritis due to hydrochloric acid ingestion. AJR 99:182–185, 1967.
155. Kleinhaus U, Rosenberger A, Adler O: Early and late radiological features of damage to the stomach caused by acid ingestion. Radiol Clin (Belg) 46:26–37, 1977.
156. Herrington JL: Stenosis of the gastric antrum and proximal duodenum resulting from the ingestion of a corrosive agent. Am J Surg 107:580–585, 1964.
157. Roswit B, Malsky SJ, Reid CB: Severe radiation injuries of the stomach, small intestine, colon, and rectum. AJR 114:460–475, 1972.

158. Goldstein HM, Rogers LF, Fletcher GH, et al: Radiological manifestations of radiation-induced injury to the normal upper gastrointestinal tract. Radiology 117:135–140, 1975.

159. Lane D: Irradiation gastritis simulating carcinoma. Med J Aust 2:576–577, 1970.

160. Williams NN, Daly JM: Infusional versus systemic chemotherapy for liver metastases from colorectal cancer. Surg Clin North Am 69:401–410, 1989.

161. Wells JJ, Nostrant TT, Wilson JAP, et al: Gastroduodenal ulcerations in patients receiving selective hepatic artery infusion chemotherapy. Am J Gastroenterol 80:425–429, 1985.

162. Shike M, Gillin JS, Kemeny N, et al: Severe gastroduodenal ulcerations complicating hepatic artery infusion chemotherapy for metastatic colon cancer. Am J Gastroenterol 81:176–179, 1986.

163. Hiehle JF, Levine MS: Gastrointestinal toxicity of 5-FU and 5-FUDR: radiographic findings. J Can Assoc Radiol 42:109–112, 1991.

164. Hohn DC, Stagg RJ, Price DC, et al: Avoidance of gastroduodenal toxicity in patients receiving hepatic arterial 5-fluoro-2'-deoxyuridine. J Clin Oncol 3:1257–1260, 1985.

165. Hall DA, Clouse ME, Gramm HF: Gastroduodenal ulceration after hepatic arterial infusion chemotherapy. AJR 136:1216–1218, 1981.

166. Chuang VP, Wallace S, Stroehlein J, et al: Hepatic artery infusion chemotherapy: gastroduodenal complications. AJR 137:347–350, 1981.

167. Mann FA, Kubal WS, Ruzicka FF: Radiographic manifestations of gastrointestinal toxicity associated with intraarterial 5-fluorouracil infusion. Radiographics 2:329–339, 1982.

168. Thomson WO, Robertson AG, Imrie CW, et al: Is duodenitis a dyspeptic myth? Lancet 1:1197–1198, 1977.

169. Greenlaw R, Sheehan DG, DeLuca V, et al: Gastroduodenitis: a broader concept of peptic ulcer disease. Dig Dis Sci 25:660–662, 1980.

170. Myren J: Gastric secretion in duodenitis. Scand J Gastroenterol 17(suppl):98–101, 1982.

171. Sircus W: Duodenitis: a clinical, endoscopic, and histopathologic study. Q J Med 56:593–600, 1985.

172. Gelzayd EA, Gelfand DW, Rinaldo JA: Nonspecific duodenitis: a distinct clinical entity? Gastrointest Endosc 19:131–133, 1973.

173. Gelzayd EA, Biederman MA, Gelfand DW: Changing concepts of duodenitis. Am J Gastroenterol 64:213–216, 1975.

174. Collen MJ, Loebenberg MJ: Basal gastric acid secretion in nonulcer dyspepsia with or without duodenitis. Dig Dis Sci 34:246–250, 1989.

175. Wyatt JI, Rathbone BJ, Dixon MF, et al: *Campylobacter pyloridis* and acid induced gastric metaplasia in the pathogenesis of duodenitis. J Clin Pathol 40:841–848, 1987.

176. Cheli R: Symptoms in chronic non-specific duodenitis. Scand J Gastroenterol 17(suppl):84–86, 1982.

177. Katz AM: Hemorrhagic duodenitis in myocardial infarction. Ann Intern Med 51:212–218, 1959.

178. Baum S, Ward S, Nusbaum M: Stress bleeding from the mid-duodenum: an often unrecognized source of gastrointestinal hemorrhage. Radiology 95:595–609, 1970.

179. Blakemore WS, Baum S, Nusbaum M: Diagnosis and management of massive hemorrhage from postoperative stress ulcers of the descending duodenum. Surg Clin North Am 50:979–984, 1970.

180. Fraser GM, Pitman RG, Lawrie JH, et al: The significance of the radiological finding of coarse mucosal folds in the duodenum. Lancet 2:979–982, 1964.

181. Wiener SN, Vertes V, Shapiro H: The upper gastrointestinal tract in patients undergoing chronic dialysis. Radiology 92:110–114, 1969.

182. Zukerman GR, Mills BA, Koehler RE, et al: Nodular duodenitis: pathologic and clinical characteristics in patients with end-stage renal disease. Dig Dis Sci 11:1018–1024, 1983.

183. Glick SN, Gohel VK, Laufer I: Mucosal surface patterns of the duodenal bulb. Radiology 150:317–322, 1984.

184. Gelfand DW, Dale WJ, Ott DJ, et al: Duodenitis: endoscopic-radiologic correlation in 272 patients. Radiology 157:577–581, 1985.

185. Levine MS, Turner D, Ekberg O, et al: Duodenitis: a reliable radiologic diagnosis? Gastrointest Radiol 16:99–103, 1991.

186. Bova JG, Kamath V, Tio FO, et al: The normal mucosal surface pattern of the duodenal bulb: radiologic-histologic correlation. AJR 145:735–738, 1985.

187. Marn CS, Gore RM, Ghahremani GG: Duodenal manifestations of nontropical sprue. Gastrointest Radiol 11:30–35, 1986.

188. Jones B, Bayless TM, Hamilton SR, et al: "Bubbly" duodenal bulb in celiac disease: radiologic-pathologic correlation. AJR 142:119–122, 1984.

# Benign Tumors

**Marc S. Levine, M.D.**

## INTRODUCTION

Between 85 and 90% of all neoplasms in the stomach and duodenum are benign.[1] About half are mucosal lesions, and half are submucosal. The majority of benign gastric and duodenal tumors are fortuitous findings on radiologic or endoscopic examinations performed for other reasons. However, tumors that are large or ulcerated may cause upper gastrointestinal bleeding or other symptoms. Depending on their histologic features, some benign tumors are also important because of an associated risk of malignant degeneration. Although gastric and duodenal polyps are not often diagnosed on single contrast barium studies, the use of double contrast technique has led to greater detection of these lesions.

## MUCOSAL LESIONS

Gastric and duodenal polyps are sessile or pedunculated lesions arising from the mucosa and projecting into the lumen of the stomach and duodenum. These polyps account for about 50% of all benign gastric and duodenal tumors.[2, 3] The vast majority are located in the stomach, but duodenal polyps are occasionally found (see later section on duodenal polyps). In the past, gastric polyps were detected infrequently on conventional single contrast barium studies, with a reported incidence of only 0.014 to 0.047%.[4-6] Because the overlying rib cage precludes manual palpation or compression of the proximal stomach, polyps arising in the gastric fundus and body have been particularly difficult to diagnose on single contrast studies. However, the routine use of double contrast technique has dramatically improved our ability to detect gastric polyps, with a reported incidence of 1 to 2% on double contrast studies.[7, 8] Although the majority are small, innocuous hyperplastic polyps, some larger lesions are adenomatous polyps that are capable of undergoing malignant degeneration via an adenoma-carcinoma sequence similar to that found in the colon. The need for endoscopic biopsy or removal of these polyps is directly related to their size and appearance. Radiologists therefore have an important role in the detection of gastric polyps and in subsequent decisions about the management of these lesions.

## Hyperplastic Polyps

Hyperplastic polyps are the most common benign epithelial neoplasms found in the stomach, accounting for 75 to 90% of all gastric polyps.[9] Because hyperplastic polyps are not premalignant, they must be differentiated from adenomatous polyps, which have a known risk of malignant degeneration. Although histologic specimens are required for a definitive diagnosis, hyperplastic polyps have such a characteristic appearance on double contrast barium studies that they can usually be distinguished from adenomatous polyps without need for endoscopic intervention.

### Pathogenesis

Because hyperplastic polyps often develop in patients with chronic erosive gastritis, it has been postulated that the lesions represent healed gastric erosions, with persistent epithelial nodules at the site of the previous erosions.[10-12] They also occur more frequently in patients with atrophic gastritis[13] or bile reflux gastritis.[14] Thus, hyperplastic polyps are probably not true neoplasms but instead are thought to result from excessive regenerative hyperplasia in areas of chronic gastritis.[15]

### Pathology

Hyperplastic polyps consist histologically of elongated, branching, cystically dilated glandular structures lined by a single layer of tall epithelial cells with abundant cytoplasm and small, basal nuclei.[15, 16] The polyps often have an edematous stroma, containing a variable number of chronic inflammatory cells and thin muscle bundles originating from the muscularis mucosae.[15, 16]

Hyperplastic polyps usually appear grossly as one or more small, sessile nodules that have a smooth, dome-shaped contour. As the lesions increase in size, they may assume a nipple-shaped or pedunculated configuration. However, hyperplastic polyps tend to have a self-limited growth pattern, so that the majority are less than 1 cm in size.[7, 15]

Because hyperplastic polyps are not true neoplasms, they have no malignant potential and should not be considered premalignant lesions in the stomach.[15, 17] However, patients with hyperplastic polyps do seem to be at increased risk for harboring separate, coexisting gastric carcinomas. In various series, 8 to 28% of patients with hyperplastic polyps in the stomach have been found to have synchronous gastric carcinomas.[16, 17] This association is probably related to the presence of underlying atrophic gastritis, which predisposes to the development of polyps and cancer.[15] Whatever the explanation, hyperplastic polyps in the stomach are important because of the increased risk of gastric carcinoma in these patients.

Fundic gland polyps appear to be a variant of hyperplastic polyps, consisting histologically of hyperplastic fundic glands that have no malignant potential.[18] Affected individuals almost always have multiple (up to 50) gastric polyps, so this entity has been called *fundic gland polyposis*.[18, 19] Fundic gland polyps are found in the stomach in about 40% of patients with familial polyposis coli[18, 19] (see later section on polyposis syndromes). However, the histopathologic features of fundic gland polyps are identical whether they occur as isolated lesions in the stomach or as part of a diffuse polyposis syndrome.

## Clinical Findings

Most hyperplastic polyps are small, asymptomatic lesions detected as incidental findings on radiologic or endoscopic examinations.[7] However, polyps that have a friable or ulcerated surface may be associated with low-grade upper gastrointestinal bleeding.[20] Rarely, large, pedunculated polyps in the gastric antrum may prolapse through the pylorus into the duodenum, causing obstructive symptoms.[20]

## Radiographic Findings

The majority of hyperplastic polyps in the stomach appear radiographically as smooth, sessile, round or oval lesions, ranging from 5 to 10 mm in size.[7, 15] Most patients have multiple polyps that tend to be clustered in the gastric fundus or body[7] (Fig. 37–1). When multiple polyps are present, they also tend to be the same size.[15]

On double contrast examinations, hyperplastic polyps on the dependent surface of the stomach (the posterior wall) typically appear as smooth, round filling defects in the barium pool, whereas polyps on the nondependent surface (the anterior wall) appear as ring shadows that are etched in white by barium trapped between the edge

of the polyp and the adjacent mucosa (see Fig. 37–1A). Occasionally, a small hanging droplet of barium, or "stalactite," on a nondependent or anterior wall polyp can be mistaken en face for a central area of ulceration[21] (see Fig. 37–1B). However, it should be seen as a transient finding, as the droplet of barium invariably falls off the polyp during fluoroscopic observation. In other patients, hyperplastic polyps may be recognized on double contrast radiographs only by the presence of one or more stalactites on the nondependent wall, because these hanging droplets are observed more frequently on protruded lesions than on a smooth surface.[22] In such cases, careful examination of the area with prone compression views should demonstrate the underlying polyp responsible for this phenomenon.

Although most hyperplastic polyps are less than 1 cm in size, some lesions may be as large as 2 to 6 cm.[20, 23] These atypical hyperplastic polyps may be lobulated or pedunculated lesions[20, 23] (Fig. 37–2). A giant hyperplastic polyp or conglomerate mass of hyperplastic polyps may occasionally be mistaken radiographically for a polypoid gastric carcinoma[20, 23] (see Fig. 37–2B). Rarely, pedunculated polyps in the antrum may prolapse into the duodenum, causing intermittent gastric outlet obstruction[20] (Fig. 37–3).

Fundic gland polyps also appear on double contrast radiographs as multiple small (less than 1 cm in size), sessile lesions in the stomach[18] (see Fig. 37–12). Although confined to the gastric fundus and body, they are otherwise indistinguishable from typical hyperplastic polyps.[18] Rarely, spontaneous regression of fundic gland polyps has been reported.[19, 24]

## Differential Diagnosis

When smooth, sessile lesions less than 1 cm in size are detected radiographically in the stomach, they are almost always found to be hyperplastic polyps. Occasionally, small leiomyomas may produce similar findings.[7] However, smooth muscle tumors of this size are virtually all benign, so it is probably not important to differentiate these lesions.

Hyperplastic polyps that appear as ring shadows on double contrast radiographs must be differentiated from shallow ulcers on the dependent or posterior gastric wall and from unfilled ulcers on the nondependent or anterior wall. With flow technique, however, ulcer craters on the dependent wall should fill with barium, producing a discrete niche or collection.[25] In contrast, ulcers on the nondependent wall should fill with barium on prone compression views of the stomach. Thus, it is usually possible to differentiate these lesions by performing a biphasic examination that includes flow technique and prone compression.

Polyps that appear as ring shadows must also be distinguished from "see-through" artifacts caused by calcified or contrast agent–filled structures overlying the stomach. Such structures can mimic the appearance of anterior wall polyps on a single radiograph (Fig. 37–4A), but their location outside the stomach is readily

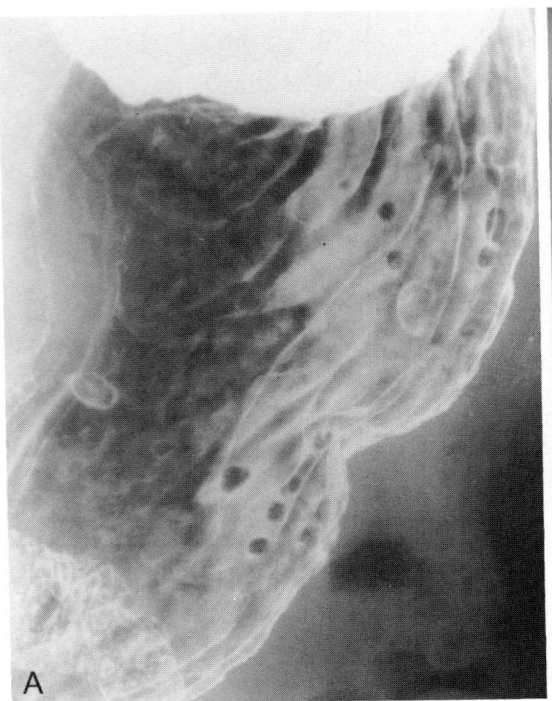

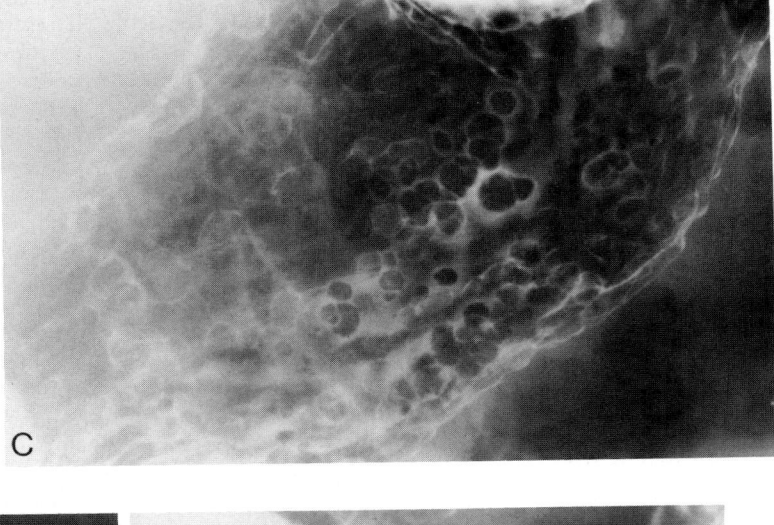

**Figure 37–1. Multiple hyperplastic polyps. A.** Polyps on the dependent surface or posterior wall appear as filling defects in the barium pool, whereas polyps on the nondependent surface or anterior wall are etched in white. **B.** This patient has multiple anterior wall polyps containing hanging droplets of barium, or stalactites, that could be mistaken for central areas of ulceration. **C.** Innumerable hyperplastic polyps are present in the gastric body.

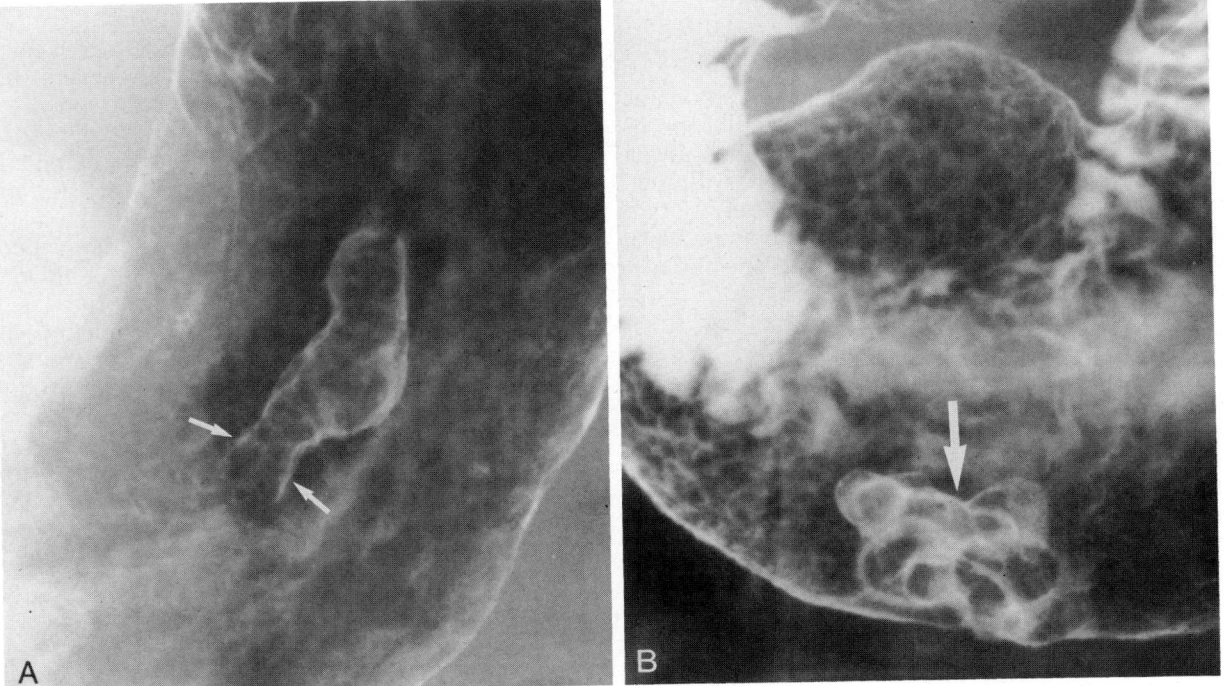

**Figure 37–2. Atypical hyperplastic polyps. A.** A long, pedunculated polyp is present in the gastric body. The polyp has a discrete stalk *(arrows)*. This patient had pernicious anemia. **B.** A giant hyperplastic polyp *(arrow)* is seen in the antrum in another patient. This lesion is quite lobulated and could be mistaken for a polypoid carcinoma.

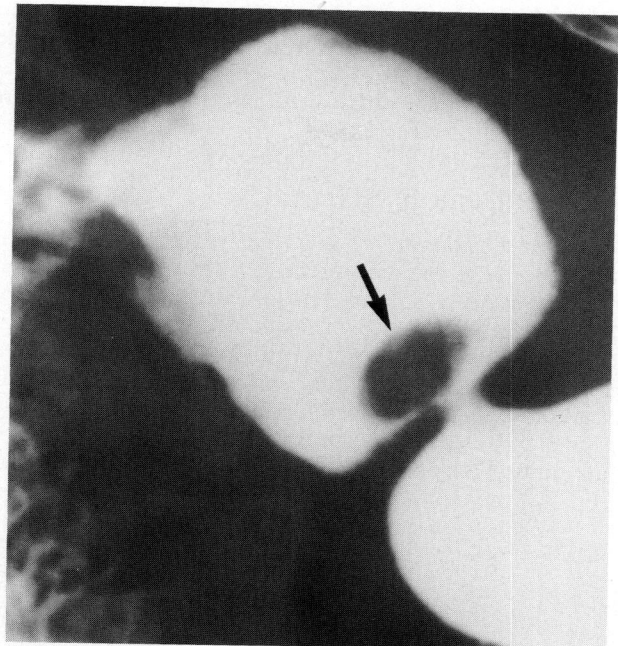

**Figure 37–3. Prolapsed hyperplastic polyp (arrow).** This patient has a pedunculated polyp that has prolapsed from the antrum into the base of the duodenal bulb.

apparent on radiographs obtained in other projections (Fig. 37–4B).

Hyperplastic polyps that have a lobulated appearance or are greater than 1 cm in size cannot be distinguished radiographically from adenomatous polyps in the stom-

ach. Rarely, giant hyperplastic polyps or a conglomerate mass of hyperplastic polyps can mimic the appearance of a polypoid gastric carcinoma[20, 23] (see Fig. 37–2B). Thus, atypical polyps should be examined by biopsy or resected for a definitive diagnosis.

The differential diagnosis for multiple hyperplastic polyps in the stomach includes multiple leiomyomas, multiple adenomatous polyps, or gastric involvement by one of the polyposis syndromes. However, leiomyomas are usually larger and less numerous than hyperplastic polyps and have the radiologic features of submucosal lesions. Adenomatous polyps also tend to be larger and less numerous and have a more lobulated appearance than most hyperplastic polyps. Unfortunately, both types of polyps may occur simultaneously in the same patient.[20] However, an adenomatous polyp should be suspected if one lesion is disproportionately larger than the others, as hyperplastic polyps tend to be the same size.[7] Finally, a generalized polyposis syndrome should be suspected if multiple polyps are also present in the small bowel or colon (see later section on polyposis syndromes).

## Management

Almost all smooth, sessile polyps less than 1 cm in size are hyperplastic polyps with no malignant potential. Thus, small, round or ovoid gastric polyps detected on double contrast studies should be considered innocuous lesions without need for further investigation or treatment. However, endoscopic biopsy or polypectomy should be performed if the polyp is lobulated or pedun-

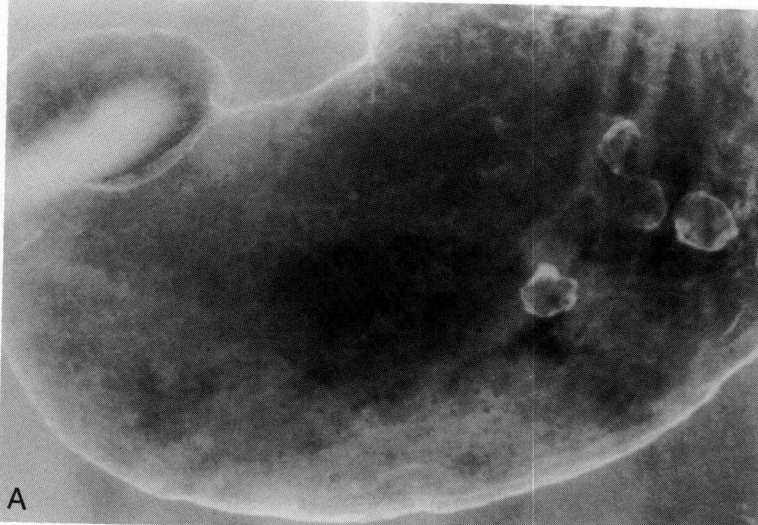

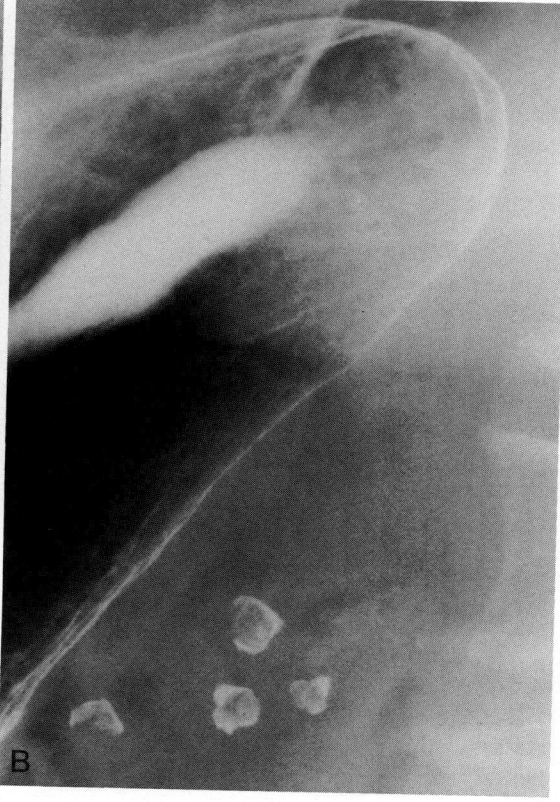

**Figure 37–4. See-through artifacts mimicking hyperplastic polyps in the stomach. A.** Multiple ring shadows are seen in the gastric body. These could represent hyperplastic polyps on the anterior wall that are etched in white. **B.** However, a lateral view shows multiple barium-filled colonic diverticula behind the stomach.

culated, if it is greater than 1 cm in size, or if it has enlarged on follow-up studies.

## Adenomatous Polyps

In the past, adenomatous polyps were thought to account for the majority of benign epithelial neoplasms in the stomach.[6, 26] With greater detection of small hyperplastic polyps on radiologic and endoscopic examinations, it is now recognized that adenomatous polyps constitute less than 20% of all gastric polyps.[7, 8, 17] Nevertheless, adenomatous polyps are important because they are dysplastic lesions that are capable of undergoing malignant degeneration. As a result, these lesions must be treated more aggressively than hyperplastic polyps in the stomach.

### Pathology

Adenomatous polyps are composed of dysplastic epithelium. Depending on the predominant glandular architecture, they may be classified as tubular, villous, or tubulovillous adenomas. Although villous adenomas occur in the stomach (see later section on villous tumors), most gastric adenomas are tubular or mixed tubulovillous adenomas.[16] Unlike hyperplastic polyps, these lesions contain large, hyperchromatic nuclei with frequent mitoses. Malignant degeneration occurs via an adenoma-carcinoma sequence similar to that found in the colon. One or more foci of carcinoma in situ or invasive carcinoma are present in nearly 50% of resected adenomatous polyps greater than 2 cm in size, but malignant changes are rarely found in smaller lesions.[1, 16, 27, 28] As in the colon, the risk of malignancy therefore depends primarily on polyp size. Nevertheless, adenocarcinoma is about 30 times more common than adenomatous polyps in the stomach, so most gastric cancers are thought to originate de novo and not from pre-existing polyps.[15, 17]

Adenomatous polyps are often found in the stomach in patients with pernicious anemia and chronic atrophic gastritis.[29-31] Because of the recognized association between atrophic gastritis and gastric carcinoma (see Chapter 38), the risk of developing a separate, coexisting cancer in the stomach may be greater than the risk of malignant degeneration in an adenomatous polyp.[15, 32] In various series, as many as 30 to 40% of patients with adenomatous polyps in the stomach have been found to have synchronous gastric carcinomas.[15, 17] Thus, detection of an adenomatous polyp in the stomach should lead to a careful search for other lesions.

### Clinical Findings

Because of their greater size, adenomatous polyps in the stomach produce symptoms more frequently than hyperplastic polyps. These patients may present with epigastric pain or bloating, upper gastrointestinal bleeding, or, rarely, gastric outlet obstruction caused by a ball valve effect of polyps arising near the pylorus or prolapse of pedunculated antral polyps into the duodenum.[27, 33, 34] Because of the association between adenomatous polyps and atrophic gastritis, gastric analysis may reveal hypochlorhydria or achlorhydria in as many as 85 to 90% of patients.[32-34]

## Radiographic Findings

Almost all adenomatous polyps seen radiographically in the stomach are greater than 1 cm in size.[6, 15, 28] The majority occur as solitary lesions, most frequently in the antrum[15, 28] (Fig. 37–5). Occasionally, however, multiple adenomatous polyps are found (Fig. 37–6). They may be sessile or pedunculated and tend to have a more lobulated appearance than hyperplastic polyps (see Figs. 37–5 and 37–6). When the lesions are pedunculated, the stalk may be seen en face as an inner ring shadow

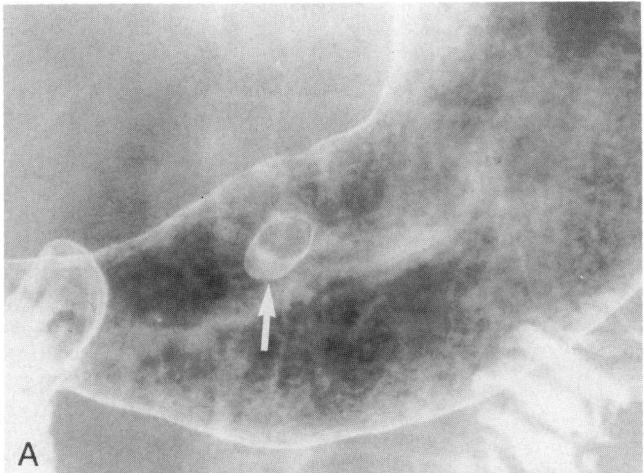

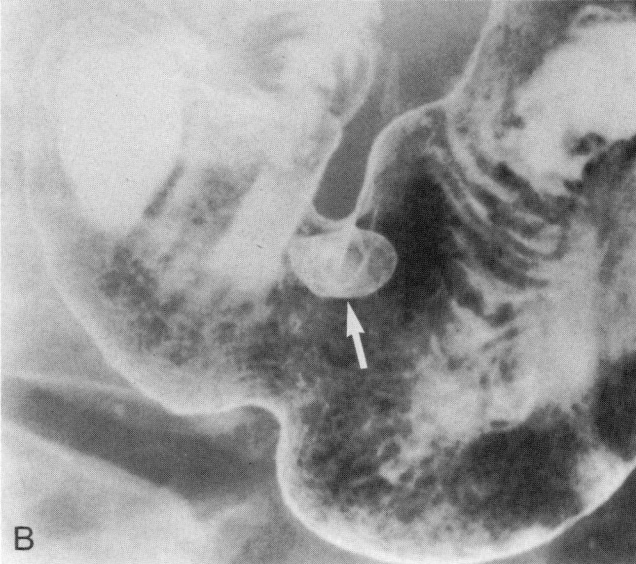

**Figure 37–5. Adenomatous polyps. A.** A sessile polyp *(arrow)* is present in the antrum. **B.** A pedunculated antral polyp *(arrow)* is seen in another patient. Note how the stalk appears as an inner ring shadow overlying the head of the polyp, producing the Mexican hat sign. (**B** courtesy of Dean D. T. Maglinte, M.D., Indianapolis, IN.)

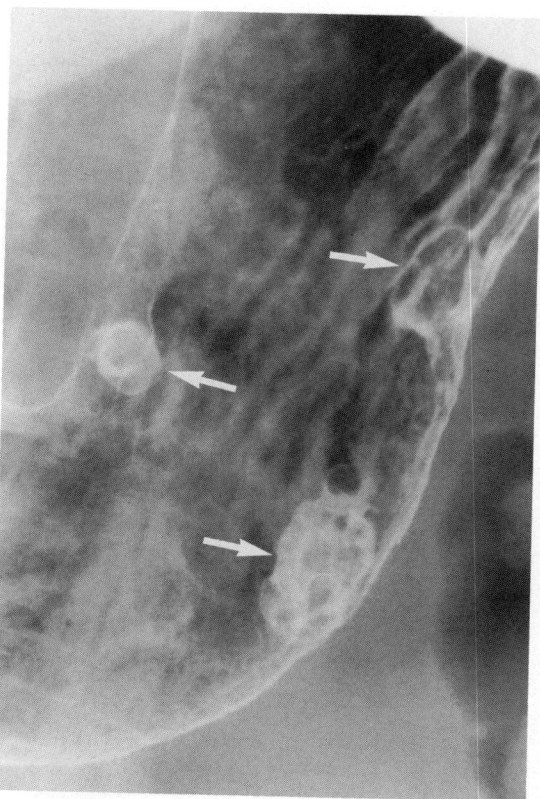

**Figure 37–6. Multiple adenomatous polyps.** The polyps (arrows) are larger and more lobulated than most hyperplastic polyps in the stomach. The most distal lesion on the greater curvature is indistinguishable from a polypoid carcinoma.

overlying the head of the polyp, producing the "Mexican hat" sign classically found with pedunculated polyps in the colon (see Fig. 37–5B). Rarely, pedunculated antral polyps may prolapse through the pylorus, causing intermittent gastric outlet obstruction.[6]

As with hyperplastic polyps, lesions on the nondependent or anterior wall may be etched in white on double contrast radiographs. Occasionally, a hanging droplet of barium or stalactite on these nondependent lesions can mimic the appearance of ulceration.[21] However, actual ulceration of an adenomatous polyp is rarely seen radiographically.

## Differential Diagnosis

Adenomatous polyps in the stomach that appear as smooth, sessile lesions may be difficult to distinguish radiographically from hyperplastic polyps. However, adenomatous polyps are almost always greater than 1 cm in size and tend to occur as solitary lesions, whereas hyperplastic polyps are usually less than 1 cm in size and are often multiple.[7] Adenomatous polyps that have a relatively smooth contour can also be mistaken for leiomyomas or other submucosal lesions. Finally, adenomatous polyps that are larger and more lobulated may be indistinguishable radiographically from polypoid gastric carcinomas (see Fig. 37–6). However, the latter polyps often harbor one or more foci of carcinoma in

situ or invasive carcinoma, so aggressive management of these lesions is warranted.

## Management

When a gastric polyp is detected radiographically, endoscopic biopsies should be performed if the lesion has features of an adenomatous polyp (i.e., is greater than 1 cm in size, is lobulated or pedunculated, or appears larger on follow-up studies). If biopsies confirm the presence of an adenomatous polyp, it should be resected because of the risk of malignant degeneration.[35] Regardless of the endoscopic findings, polyps greater than 2 cm in size should always be resected because of the even greater likelihood that they are adenomatous and the greater risk of malignancy in adenomatous polyps of this size.[6, 8, 17] If invasive carcinoma is present in the resected specimen, a wedge resection of the stomach or partial gastrectomy may be required.[36] As in the colon, a much more aggressive approach is therefore warranted in the management of adenomatous polyps than hyperplastic polyps because of the increased cancer risk in these patients.

## Duodenal Polyps

Duodenal polyps are much less common than gastric polyps. Hyperplastic polyps, which account for 75 to 90% of benign gastric polyps,[9] are rarely found in the duodenum. Instead, most duodenal polyps are adenomatous.[3, 37] The majority of patients are asymptomatic, so the polyps are detected as incidental findings on radiologic or endoscopic examinations. Occasionally, however, they may cause low-grade upper gastrointestinal bleeding or obstructive jaundice.[3, 38]

As with adenomatous polyps in the stomach, the frequency of malignant degeneration is directly related to polyp size. Adenomatous polyps greater than 2 cm should be resected because of the high risk of cancer in these lesions.[3]

## Radiographic Findings

Duodenal polyps usually appear as smooth, sessile lesions in the first or second portion of the duodenum (Fig. 37–7). They tend to be less than 2 cm in size, but giant duodenal polyps have occasionally been described.[39] Most duodenal polyps occur as solitary lesions, but multiple adenomatous, hamartomatous, or inflammatory polyps may be found in the duodenum as part of a diffuse polyposis syndrome (see later section on polyposis syndromes).

## Differential Diagnosis

Sessile polyps in the duodenum may be difficult to distinguish radiographically from leiomyomas, Brunner's gland hamartomas, or other submucosal masses, so endoscopy may be required for a definitive diagnosis. Occasionally, gastric mucosa that has prolapsed into the

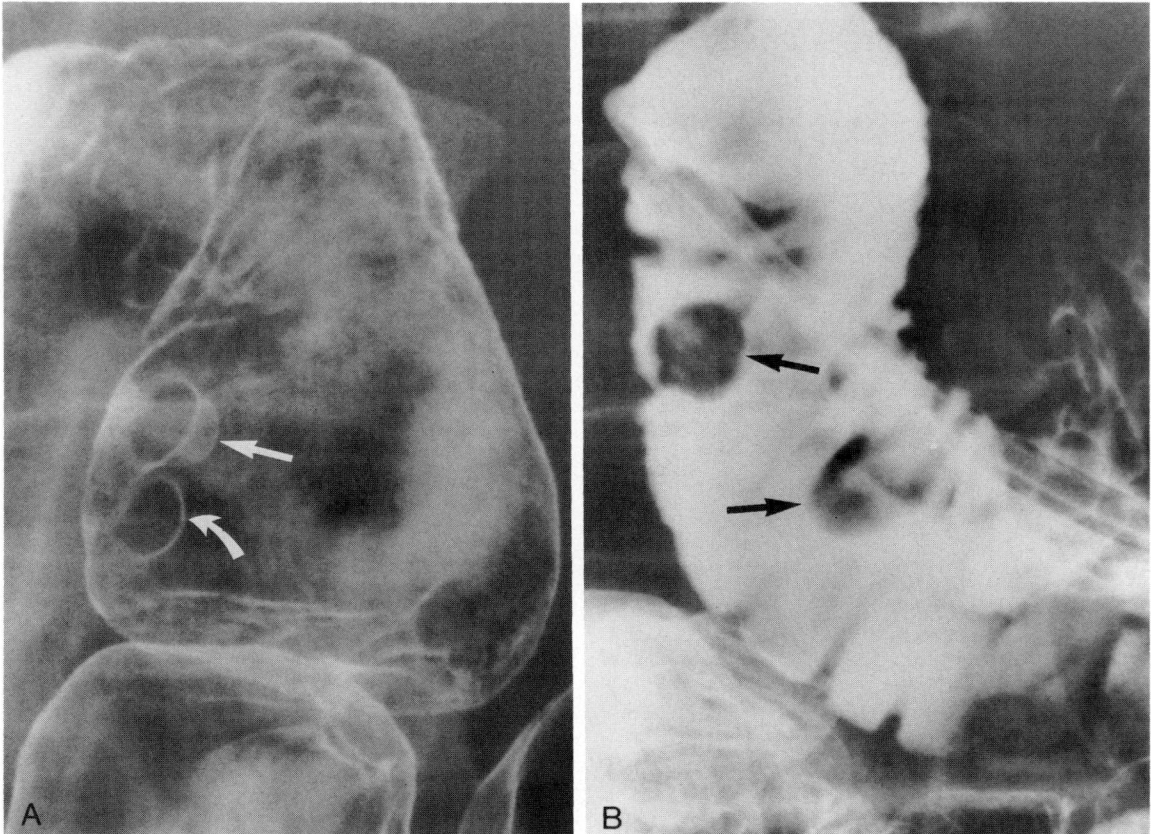

**Figure 37–7. Duodenal polyps. A.** Two polyps are present in the duodenal bulb. The lower polyp is seen as a ring shadow *(curved arrow)* and the higher polyp as a bowler hat *(straight arrow).* **B.** Several adenomatous polyps *(arrows)* are seen in the descending duodenum in another patient. This study was performed through a tube in the proximal duodenum.

duodenum can be mistaken for a polypoid lesion (Fig. 37–8). However, prolapsed gastric mucosa is manifested by a characteristic mushroom-shaped defect at the base of the bulb that often occurs as a transient finding at fluoroscopy.[40, 41] Pedunculated antral polyps that have prolapsed through the pylorus can also be mistaken for polypoid lesions in the duodenum (see Fig. 37–3). However, the latter lesions are often found to migrate between the stomach and duodenum at fluoroscopy. In other patients, apparent polypoid lesions may result from heaped-up areas of redundant mucosa on the inner aspect of the superior duodenal flexure between the first and second portions of the duodenum (Fig. 37–9). However, these "flexural pseudolesions" can usually be differentiated from true polyps by their characteristic location and changeable appearance at fluoroscopy.[42, 43]

## Villous Tumors

Adenomatous polyps in the stomach and duodenum that contain predominantly villous elements have been called villous adenomas, papillary adenomas, papillomas, or adenomatous papillomas.[44] Because of their high malignant potential, however, the term *villous tumors* is probably better, because it avoids the

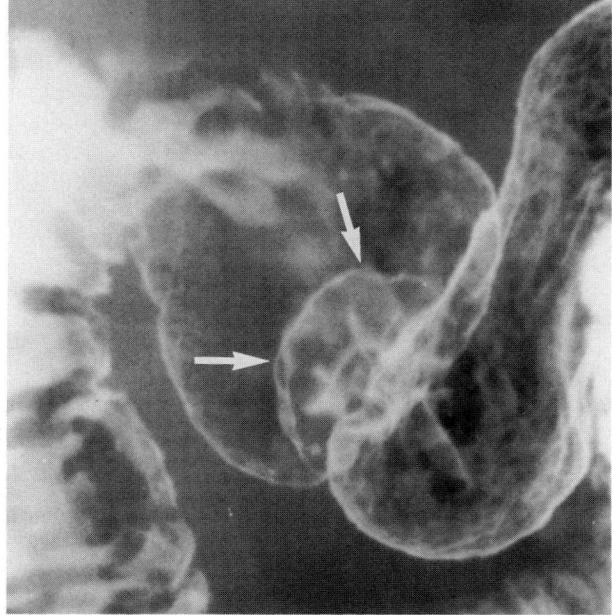

**Figure 37–8. Prolapsed gastric mucosa.** The prolapsed mucosa produces a mushroom-shaped defect *(arrows)* at the base of the bulb. The characteristic appearance and location of the prolapsed antral mucosa should differentiate this finding from a true polypoid lesion.

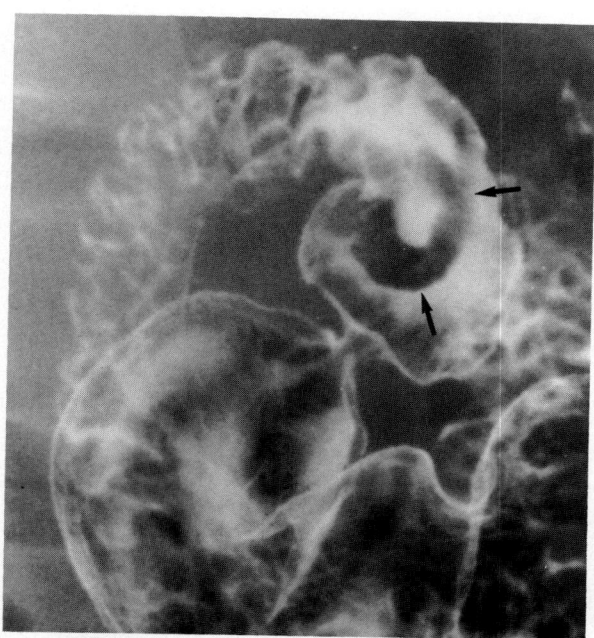

**Figure 37–9. Duodenal pseudolesion.** Redundant mucosa at the superior duodenal flexure simulates an ulcerated mass *(arrows)* at the apex of the bulb. However, the characteristic appearance and location of this finding should suggest a flexural pseudolesion.

erroneous impression that these lesions are always benign.[45–49]

## Pathology

Villous tumors in the stomach and duodenum closely resemble those in the colon, appearing grossly as polypoid masses with numerous frond-like projections. They usually occur as solitary lesions, ranging from 3 to 9 cm in size,[49, 50] but giant villous tumors as large as 15 cm have been reported.[47] Even large villous tumors rarely cause obstruction because of the soft consistency of these lesions.[46, 47] Although villous tumors may be found throughout the stomach, duodenal lesions are usually located in the descending duodenum near the papilla of Vater.[48–51]

Villous tumors in the stomach and duodenum are associated with an even higher risk of malignant change than villous tumors in the colon. The risk of malignancy is directly related to the size of the lesion. In the stomach, malignant changes are found in 50% of lesions 2 to 4 cm in size and in 80% of lesions greater than 4 cm in size.[52] Similarly, malignant changes are found in 30 to 60% of villous tumors in the duodenum, with the highest cancer risk in lesions greater than 4 cm in size.[44, 47, 48, 51] Although villous tumors in the stomach and duodenum have been classified as benign neoplasms in this chapter, they generally should be treated as malignant lesions until proved otherwise.

## Clinical Findings

Nearly 80% of patients with villous tumors in the stomach and duodenum are older than 50 years of age.[51] The majority have low-grade upper gastrointestinal

bleeding, with melena, guaiac-positive stool, and/or iron deficiency anemia.[47–49, 51, 52] Although gastric outlet obstruction is unusual, villous tumors occasionally act as the lead point for a gastroduodenal or duodenojejunal intussusception.[47, 48] Rarely, villous tumors in the upper body or fundus of the stomach prolapse through the cardia into the distal esophagus, causing dysphagia.[49] Because villous tumors in the duodenum are frequently located near the papilla of Vater, some patients present clinically with obstructive jaundice.[48, 49, 51]

Although villous tumors in the colon often cause severe diarrhea and electrolyte depletion, villous tumors in the stomach and duodenum rarely produce these complications.[47–49] Gastric and duodenal lesions seem to have the same secretory abilities as those in the colon, but reabsorption of fluid and electrolytes in the small and large bowel apparently prevents the development of a diarrheal syndrome.[40]

Villous tumors in the stomach and duodenum should be resected because of the high risk of malignancy. Although some benign lesions can be removed endoscopically, those harboring invasive carcinoma require a surgical procedure such as a partial gastrectomy or pancreaticoduodenectomy.[44, 48, 50, 51]

## Radiographic Findings

Villous tumors in the stomach and duodenum usually appear radiographically as polypoid masses, ranging from 3 to 9 cm in size.[49, 50, 53] The lesions often have a reticular or "soap bubble" appearance with serrated, feathery margins because of barium trapped in multiple clefts between the frond-like projections of the tumor[45, 46, 49, 53–56] (Fig. 37–10). Because these lesions are soft and pliable, they may vary considerably in size and shape with manual compression, and the mobile portion of the tumor may flop back and forth in the lumen during the fluoroscopic examination.[40] Although these tumors rarely cause obstruction, malignant degeneration may lead to the development of an annular lesion with shelf-like, overhanging borders.[57] Thus, villous tumors in the upper gastrointestinal tract have the same radiologic features as those in the colon.

Villous tumors in the duodenum are usually located near the papilla of Vater[48–51] (see Fig. 37–10B), but occasional lesions are found as far proximally as the duodenal bulb.[58] Because these lesions are easily obscured by superimposed mucosal folds, they are best seen on double contrast studies with optimal distention of the duodenum. Hypotonic duodenography (after intravenous administration of 1 mg of glucagon) is a particularly effective technique for effacing the overlying folds so that lesions in the periampullary duodenum can be delineated better.[50, 55, 56] If an equivocal or suspicious finding is detected in the duodenum on routine double contrast examinations, a hypotonic duodenogram should therefore be performed for a more detailed examination of this area.

## Differential Diagnosis

Villous tumors in the stomach and duodenum can often be recognized on upper gastrointestinal studies by

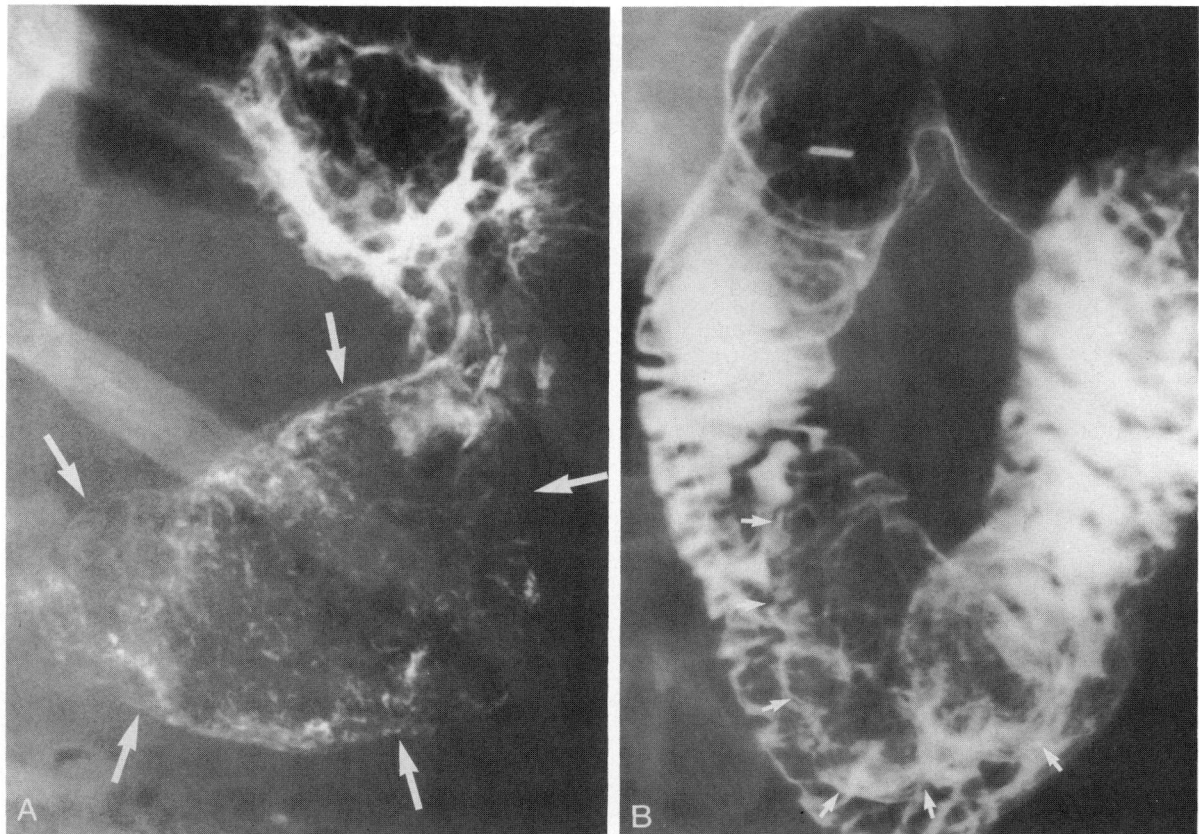

**Figure 37–10. Villous tumors. A.** A giant villous tumor *(arrows)* is present in the gastric antrum and body. The lesion has a characteristic soap bubble appearance because of trapping of barium between the frond-like projections of the tumor. (Courtesy of Abraham Ghiatis, M.D., San Antonio, TX.) **B.** In another patient, a villous tumor of the duodenum appears as a polypoid mass *(arrows)* just below the level of the papilla. Again note the characteristic reticular appearance of the lesion.

their characteristic soap bubble appearance. Occasionally, a large gastric bezoar with barium trapped in its interstices produces similar findings.[49] However, the freely mobile nature of the bezoar with changes in the patient's position should differentiate this entity from a true villous tumor. Although carcinoma or lymphoma of the stomach or duodenum may also be manifested by a bulky intraluminal mass, these lesions rarely produce a soap bubble appearance.

## Polyposis Syndromes

With the widespread use of double contrast radiography and endoscopy, gastroduodenal involvement by the various polyposis syndromes has proved to be far more common than was previously recognized (see Chapter 66). In patients with familial polyposis coli and Gardner's syndrome (sometimes classified together as familial adenomatous polyposis syndrome), detection of adenomatous polyps in the stomach or duodenum is particularly important because of the malignant potential of these lesions and the increased risk of developing gastric or duodenal carcinoma. Some investigators therefore believe that periodic surveillance of the upper

gastrointestinal tract should be performed for all patients with familial polyposis coli or Gardner's syndrome.

### Familial Polyposis Coli

Familial polyposis coli is a hereditary, autosomal dominant disease characterized by the development of innumerable adenomatous polyps throughout the colon.[59] In untreated patients, malignant degeneration of one or more polyps leads to the inevitable development of colonic carcinoma by the age of 50.[59] In the past, gastric and duodenal polyps were detected on single contrast barium studies in less than 5% of patients with this disease.[60] With the use of double contrast radiography and endoscopy, however, gastric and duodenal polyps have been detected in 68 to 92% of patients.[61–65] Most reports showing a high incidence of gastroduodenal polyps have been published in the Japanese literature. This may be partly related to more rigorous upper gastrointestinal screening of patients with familial polyposis coli in Japan than in the West. In any case, the colonic lesions in familial polyposis coli are virtually all adenomatous polyps, whereas the gastric and duodenal lesions may be adenomatous, hyperplastic, or fundic gland polyps.[18, 62, 63, 66, 67]

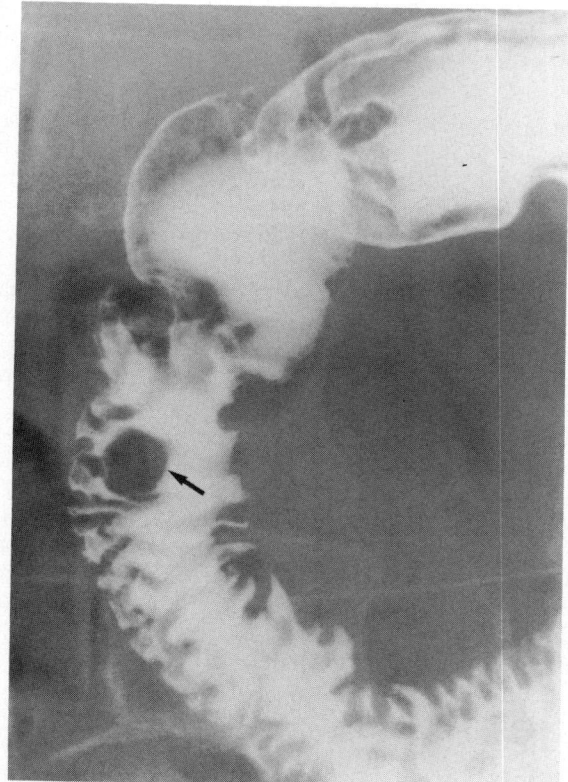

**Figure 37–11. Familial polyposis coli with an adenomatous polyp in the duodenum.** A large, sessile polyp *(arrow)* is seen in the proximal descending duodenum.

For adenomatous polyps in the stomach, the risk of malignant degeneration appears to be less than that of adenomatous polyps in the colon. However, both gastric and duodenal carcinomas have been reported in patients with familial polyposis coli.[59, 63, 67, 68] Adenomatous polyps in the stomach and duodenum rarely cause symptoms, so they are usually detected during routine screening of patients with this syndrome. The polyps may be

solitary or multiple and have the same radiologic features as adenomatous polyps in general (Fig. 37–11). Because of the risk of cancer, some investigators believe that a partial gastrectomy should be performed if multiple adenomatous polyps are found in the stomach.[69] However, most authors favor a more conservative approach, using radiologic or endoscopic surveillance to monitor these lesions.[64, 68, 70]

About 40% of patients with familial polyposis coli also have multiple small, sessile fundic gland polyps in the upper body and fundus of the stomach—so-called fundic gland polyposis.[18, 19, 63] These fundic gland polyps are composed of hyperplastic fundic glands that have no malignant potential.[19] Although fundic gland polyps never involve the antrum, the lesions are otherwise indistinguishable from ordinary hyperplastic polyps on double contrast barium studies[18, 19] (Fig. 37–12).

## *Gardner's Syndrome*

Gardner's syndrome closely resembles familial polyposis coli, as it is characterized by autosomal dominant inheritance, colonic polyposis, and, if untreated, the inevitable development of colonic carcinoma.[59] However, this syndrome has other extracolonic manifestations, including sebaceous cysts, soft tissue tumors, skeletal osteomas, and a marked tendency for excessive proliferation of fibrous tissue, resulting in desmoid tumors, hypertrophic scars, and mesenteric or retroperitoneal fibrosis.[59] These patients also have a 100 to 200 times greater risk of developing periampullary duodenal carcinoma than the general population.[71] It has been postulated that the high frequency of extracolonic manifestations in Gardner's syndrome reflects a different phenotypic expression of the same genetic defect responsible for familial polyposis coli.[65] As a result, the term *familial adenomatous polyposis syndrome* has been used to encompass both familial polyposis coli and Gardner's syndrome.

In the past, gastric and duodenal polyps have been

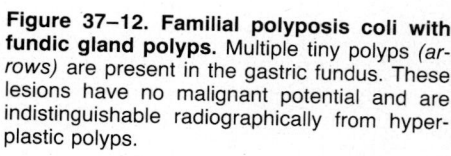

**Figure 37–12. Familial polyposis coli with fundic gland polyps.** Multiple tiny polyps *(arrows)* are present in the gastric fundus. These lesions have no malignant potential and are indistinguishable radiographically from hyperplastic polyps.

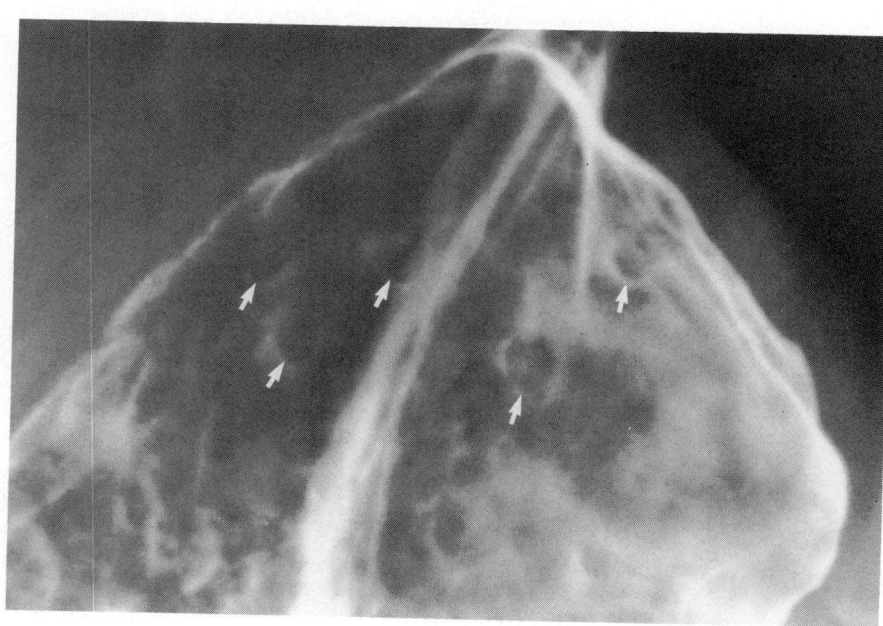

found in less than 5% of patients with Gardner's syndrome.[59] However, this low figure may simply reflect a failure to investigate these patients adequately. Studies with double contrast radiography and endoscopy indicate that gastric or duodenal polyps are present in 50 to 70% of patients with Gardner's syndrome.[65, 67, 72, 73] As with familial polyposis coli, these individuals may have fundic gland polyps in the stomach or adenomatous polyps in the stomach or duodenum.[65, 67, 72, 73]

Because adenomatous polyps are premalignant, patients with Gardner's syndrome are at increased risk for developing gastric or duodenal carcinoma.[71–75] Duodenal malignancies occur more frequently and tend to be located in the periampullary region of the descending duodenum.[71, 73, 74] In a review of the literature, periampullary duodenal carcinomas were found in 2 to 3% of all patients with Gardner's syndrome.[71] Because of this cancer risk and because patients with pre-existing adenomatous polyps are usually asymptomatic, periodic screening of the upper gastrointestinal tract has been advocated for patients with this syndrome.[71, 73]

## *Peutz-Jeghers Syndrome*

Peutz-Jeghers syndrome is a hereditary, autosomal dominant disease characterized by mucocutaneous pigmentation and gastrointestinal polyposis.[59] The abnormal pigmentation is almost always located on the buccal mucosa or lips and, less frequently, on the face or volar surface of the hands and feet. The polyps in Peutz-Jeghers syndrome involve the small bowel in 90% of patients, the colon in 30%, the stomach in 25%, and the duodenum in 15%.[76] The small bowel and gastric polyps are usually hamartomatous malformations without malignant potential.[76, 77] However, the colonic polyps may be adenomatous polyps that are capable of undergoing malignant degeneration.[76, 77] Furthermore, Peutz-Jeghers syndrome may be associated with an increased risk of extraintestinal malignancies, including pancreatic, breast, and uterine carcinomas.[78] Although small bowel and colonic polyps may cause bleeding or intussusception, patients with gastric and duodenal polyps are usually asymptomatic.[77]

Gastric and duodenal polyps in Peutz-Jeghers syndrome usually appear radiographically as one or more sessile or pedunculated lesions, ranging from 0.1 to 3.0 cm in size[77, 78] (Fig. 37–13). Innumerable 1- to 2-mm nodules may be present in the small bowel, but such carpeting is much less likely to occur in the stomach or colon.[77] Rarely, a large polyp or a conglomerate mass of polyps in the stomach may serve as the lead point for a gastroduodenal intussusception.[79]

## *Cronkhite-Canada Syndrome*

Since its original description by Cronkhite and Canada in 1955,[80] Cronkhite-Canada syndrome has been recog-

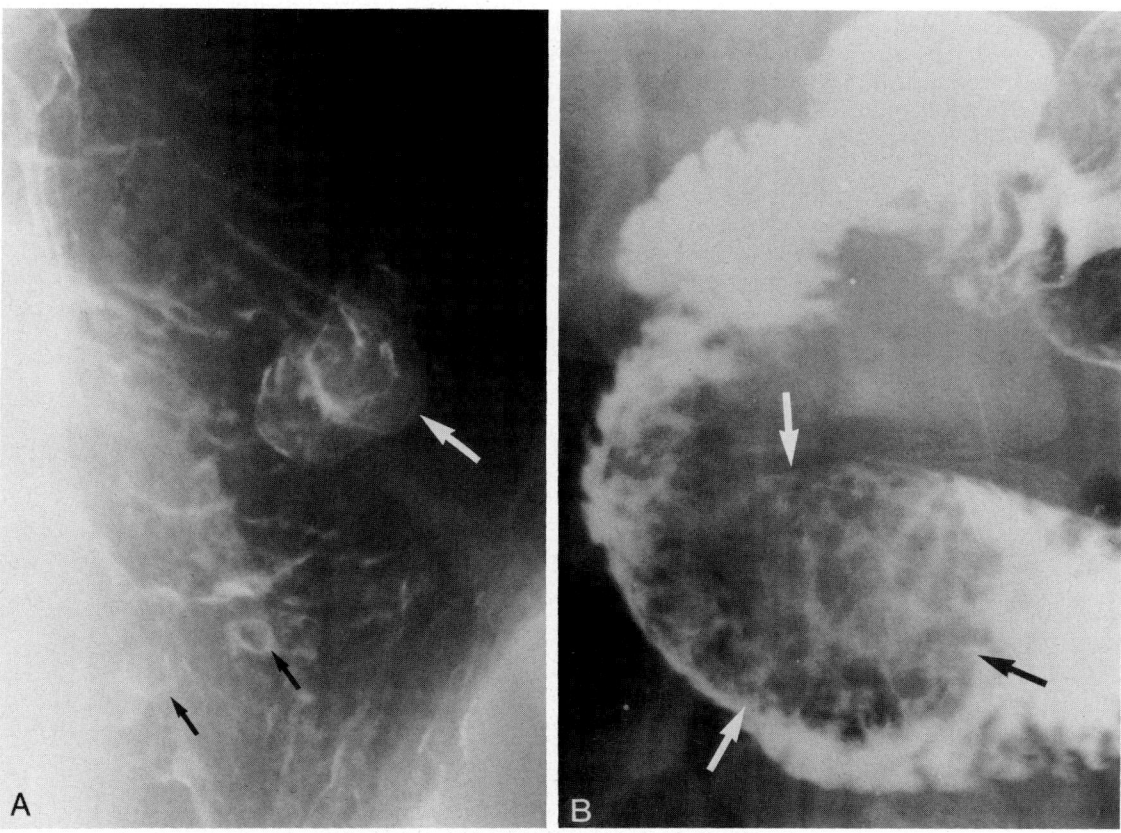

**Figure 37–13. Peutz-Jeghers syndrome with hamartomatous polyps. A.** A large, lobulated polyp *(white arrow)* is present in the gastric body. Other small polyps *(black arrows)* are also visible. **B.** A giant hamartomatous polyp *(arrows)* is seen in the descending duodenum.

nized as a nonfamilial gastrointestinal polyposis associated with a triad of ectodermal abnormalities, including alopecia, onychodystrophy, and hyperpigmentation.[59, 81] The polyps are inflammatory or juvenile-type hamartomatous polyps that have little or no malignant potential (see later section on juvenile polyposis).[81] Nevertheless, Cronkhite-Canada syndrome is a serious, potentially life-threatening disease, occurring in middle-aged or elderly individuals whose clinical condition may deteriorate rapidly because of severe vomiting, diarrhea, weight loss, and electrolyte depletion.[59, 81]

The gastrointestinal polyps in Cronkhite-Canada syndrome almost always involve the stomach and colon and less frequently involve the small bowel.[81, 82] These patients usually have innumerable tiny (3 to 10 mm), sessile polyps in the stomach and colon[81–83] (Fig. 37–14A). A distinctive "whiskering" effect may be observed along the margin of the stomach on single or double contrast examinations because of trapping of barium between these tiny mucosal excrescences and/or en-

larged areae gastricae[82, 83] (Fig. 37–14B and C). When accompanied by characteristic ectodermal findings, this whiskering should be highly suggestive of Cronkhite-Canada syndrome. Some patients also have thickened rugal folds[82] (see Fig. 37–14B). In extreme cases, enlarged gastric rugae can mimic the appearance of hypertrophic gastritis, lymphoma, or Ménétrier's disease.[82, 83] In fact, it has been postulated that Cronkhite-Canada syndrome represents a severe form of Ménétrier's disease and that a continuum exists between these entities.

## Juvenile Polyposis

Juvenile polyps are thought to be hamartomatous. Most juvenile polyps occur as sporadic (i.e., five or fewer) colonic lesions in children.[59] However, numerous juvenile polyps may be present in the colon in patients with juvenile polyposis coli or in the stomach, small bowel, and colon in patients with generalized juvenile gastrointestinal polyposis.[84, 85] Juvenile polyps in the

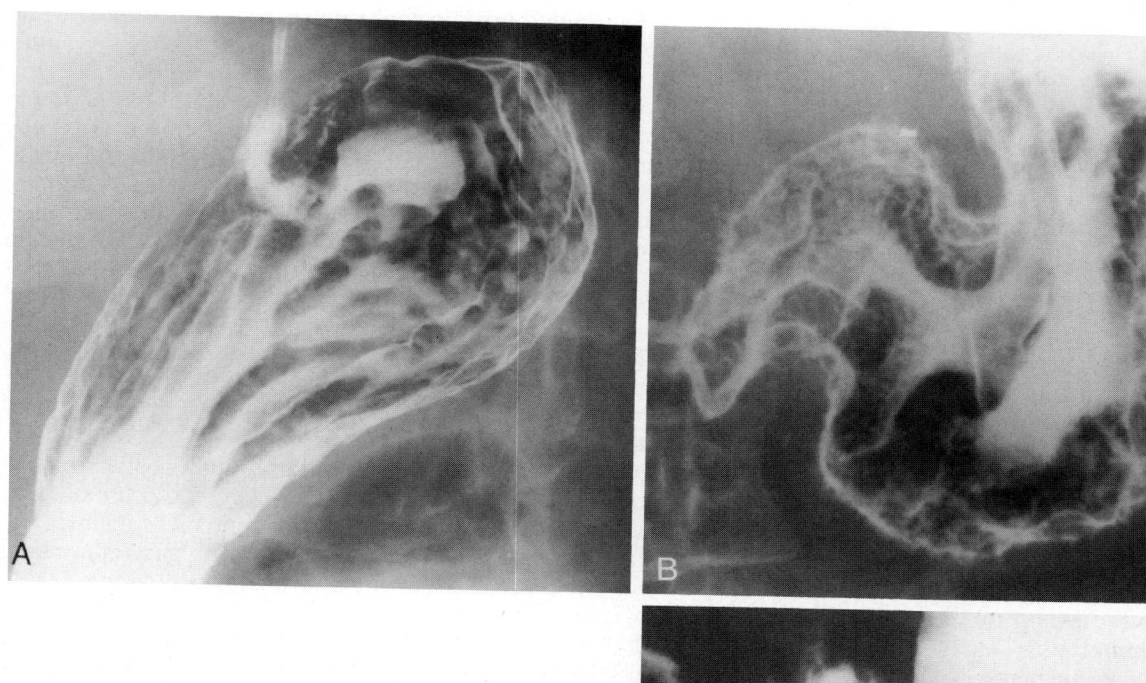

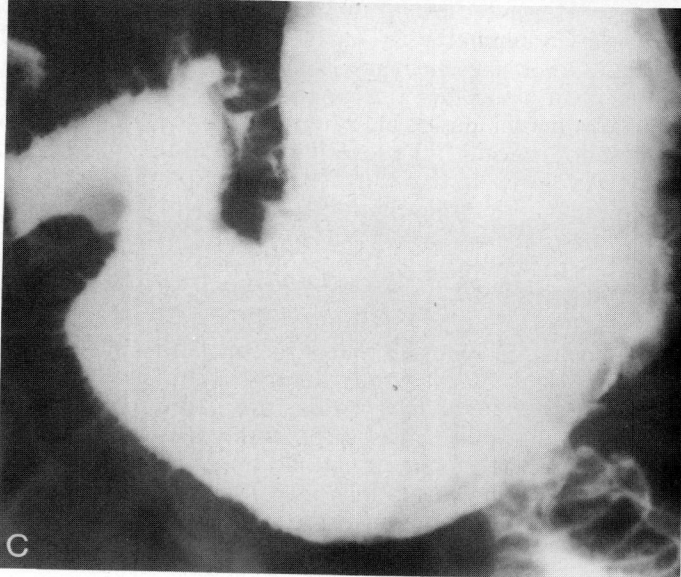

**Figure 37–14. Cronkhite-Canada syndrome involving the stomach. A.** Multiple tiny polyps are present in the gastric fundus. **B.** Thickened folds are seen in the gastric antrum and body. There is also whiskering of the greater curvature. **C.** A single contrast view better delineates this whiskering effect on the greater curvature due to trapping of barium between tiny mucosal excrescences. This finding is characteristic of gastric involvement by Cronkhite-Canada syndrome.

stomach, small bowel, or colon may cause gastrointestinal bleeding or recurrent, transient intussusceptions.[85] Contrary to earlier reports, data also suggest that juvenile polyposis may be a premalignant condition associated with an increased risk of adenocarcinoma.[86]

### Cowden's Disease (Multiple Hamartoma Syndrome)

Cowden's disease or multiple hamartoma syndrome is a rare hereditary, autosomal dominant disease characterized by endodermal, mesodermal, and ectodermal abnormalities; skeletal malformations; and benign or malignant tumors of the skin, breast, thyroid, and gastrointestinal tract.[87, 88] These patients have typical mucocutaneous lesions, including circumoral papillomatosis and nodular gingival hyperplasia.[88] Radiologic or endoscopic examinations of the gastrointestinal tract have rarely been performed on these patients, so the true frequency of gastrointestinal involvement by Cowden's disease is uncertain. However, multiple small, sessile polyps have been documented in the esophagus, stomach, small bowel, and colon in patients with this syndrome.[87, 88] Affected individuals may have hamartomatous, juvenile, or hyperplastic polyps.[88] Although these patients may have a slightly increased risk of developing colonic carcinoma, periodic screening has been advocated primarily to rule out associated breast or thyroid cancer.[87]

## SUBMUCOSAL LESIONS

Mesenchymal tumors arising in the submucosa constitute about half of all benign neoplasms in the stomach and duodenum.[2, 3] Nearly 90% are leiomyomas.[89] Other less common submucosal lesions include leiomyoblastomas, lipomas, hemangiomas, lymphangiomas, glomus tumors, neural tumors, granular cell tumors, inflammatory fibroid polyps, ectopic pancreatic rests, Brunner's gland hamartomas, and duplication cysts. Most benign submucosal tumors are incidental findings at surgery or at autopsy. However, lesions that are large or ulcerated may cause abdominal pain or upper gastrointestinal bleeding. Other mesenchymal tumors are important because of an associated risk of malignancy. Unfortunately, submucosal masses are often difficult to visualize at endoscopy because the overlying mucosa appears normal. As a result, barium studies are particularly helpful in diagnosing these lesions.

### Leiomyomas

Leiomyomas constitute about 90% of mesenchymal tumors and 40% of all benign tumors in the stomach and duodenum.[1, 89, 90] These lesions are important not only because they may cause symptoms but also because a small percentage of smooth muscle tumors are found to be malignant. However, it is often difficult to distinguish leiomyomas from leiomyosarcomas on the basis of radiologic, endoscopic, or histopathologic criteria, so their classification as benign or malignant lesions ultimately depends on the biologic behavior of the tumor.

### Pathology

Leiomyomas consist histologically of intersecting bundles of spindle-shaped cells in a characteristic whorling pattern that distinguishes these tumors from normal smooth muscle.[89, 91] The lesions are sharply circumscribed but not encapsulated. Leiomyomas usually appear endoscopically as smooth submucosal masses bulging beneath a stretched or flattened mucosa. With increasing size, different growth patterns may lead to the development of endogastric, exogastric, or dumbbell lesions.[1] About 80% are endogastric lesions that remain intramural but grow toward the lumen. The latter tumors occasionally develop a pseudopedicle as they elongate into the lumen. Another 15% are exogastric lesions that remain subserosal but grow outward from the stomach toward the peritoneal cavity. The remaining 5% are dumbbell lesions that have both endogastric and exogastric components.

The vast majority of leiomyomas in the stomach and duodenum occur as solitary lesions, but multiple tumors are present in 1 to 2% of patients.[1] Leiomyomas may be found in the antrum, body, or fundus of the stomach or, less frequently, in the duodenum.[91, 92] These tumors are usually less than 3 cm in size, but some giant leiomyomas are as large as 25 cm.[91] As a leiomyoma increases in size, necrosis and ulceration of the central portion of the tumor may occur as it outgrows its blood supply.[93] In other patients, ulceration may result from thinning and stretching of the overlying mucosa as the tumor grows toward the lumen.[94] Whatever the explanation, ulceration occurs in 50 to 70% of gastric leiomyomas greater than 2 cm in size.[1, 93]

About 10% of smooth muscle tumors in the stomach are found to be malignant.[1] However, it is often difficult to distinguish leiomyomas from leiomyosarcomas on the basis of histopathologic criteria.[90, 91] The most commonly accepted microscopic index of malignancy is the degree of mitotic activity in the tumor; lesions containing more than 25 mitotic figures per 25 high-power fields are usually malignant, whereas lesions containing fewer than 25 mitotic figures per 25 high-power fields are usually benign.[91] However, mitotic activity may be increased in only a portion of a malignant smooth muscle tumor, so random biopsy specimens or frozen sections may erroneously suggest a benign lesion. Thus, a definitive diagnosis of malignancy ultimately depends on the tumor's biologic behavior and the demonstration of invasive growth beyond the stomach via direct extension, lymphatic spread, or hematogenous metastases[90] (see Chapter 39).

### Clinical Findings

Gastric and duodenal leiomyomas occur with approximately equal frequency in men and women older than the age of 50.[91, 92] Most patients with lesions less than 3 cm in size are asymptomatic.[92] With increased growth, however, ulceration of the tumor may cause epigastric pain or upper gastrointestinal bleeding, manifested by hematemesis, melena, guaiac-positive stool, and/or iron deficiency anemia.[90–92] Other patients may have nausea, vomiting, weight loss, or a palpable abdominal mass. Pedunculated leiomyomas in the gastric antrum occasionally occlude the pylorus or prolapse into the duodenum, causing intermittent gastric outlet obstruction.[95] Rarely, gastric leiomyomas may act as the lead point for a gastrogastric or gastroduodenal intussusception.[95, 96] Most patients with gastric and duodenal leiomyomas greater than 3 cm in size are symptomatic, but exogastric lesions may grow to enormous size without causing symptoms.[1]

## Radiographic Findings

Although most gastric and duodenal leiomyomas are not diagnosed on abdominal plain films, a large tumor in the stomach is occasionally recognized as a soft tissue mass indenting the gastric air shadow.[2] Rarely, gastric leiomyomas contain irregular streaks or clumps of mot-

tled calcification that are visible on abdominal or chest radiographs[97–99] (Fig. 37–15). Mucinous adenocarcinomas of the stomach may also calcify, but the calcification in these lesions tends to have a punctate, granular, or finely stippled appearance[100] (see Fig. 38–3). The differential diagnosis for left upper quadrant calcification also includes calcified adrenal, renal, or splenic lesions.

Most gastric and duodenal leiomyomas appear radiographically as discrete submucosal masses (Figs. 37–16 to 37–19). They have the same radiologic features as intramural, extramucosal lesions elsewhere in the gastrointestinal tract.[101] When viewed in profile, the lesions have a smooth surface that is etched in white on double contrast radiographs, and their borders form either right angles or slightly obtuse angles with the adjacent gastric or duodenal wall (see Fig. 37–16A). When viewed en face, the intraluminal surface of these tumors has abrupt, well-defined borders (see Fig. 37–16B). Because the overlying mucosa is usually intact, a normal areae gastricae pattern can often be seen overlying these lesions (see Fig. 37–18). The latter finding indicates the intramural location of these tumors, as the areae gastricae are almost always obliterated by mucosal disease.

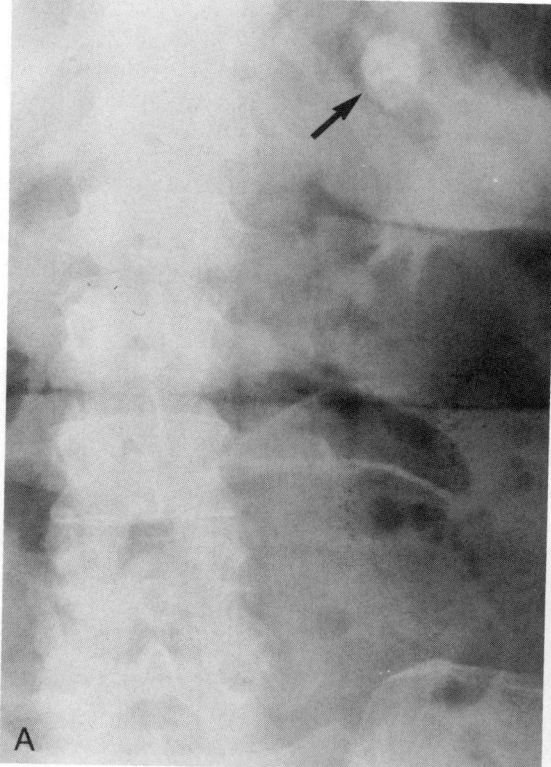

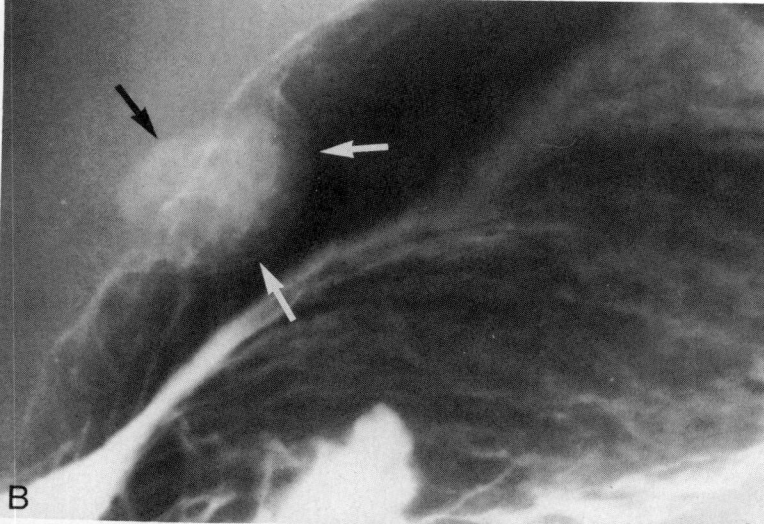

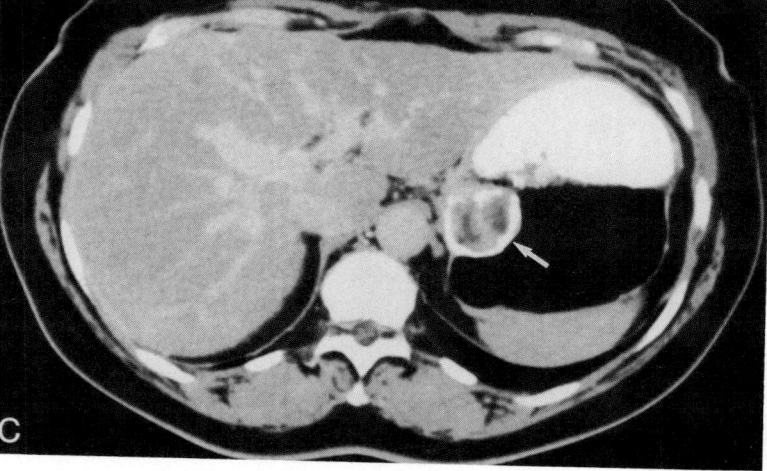

**Figure 37–15. Calcified leiomyomas. A.** A close-up view of an abdominal plain film reveals a dense clump of calcification *(arrow)* in the left upper quadrant. **B.** A barium study shows that this calcification *(black arrow)* is located within a discrete submucosal mass *(white arrows)* in the stomach. This type of calcification is typical of leiomyomas. **C.** In another patient, a peripherally calcified leiomyoma *(arrow)* is shown on a CT scan. (**C** courtesy of Alec J. Megibow, M.D., New York, NY.)

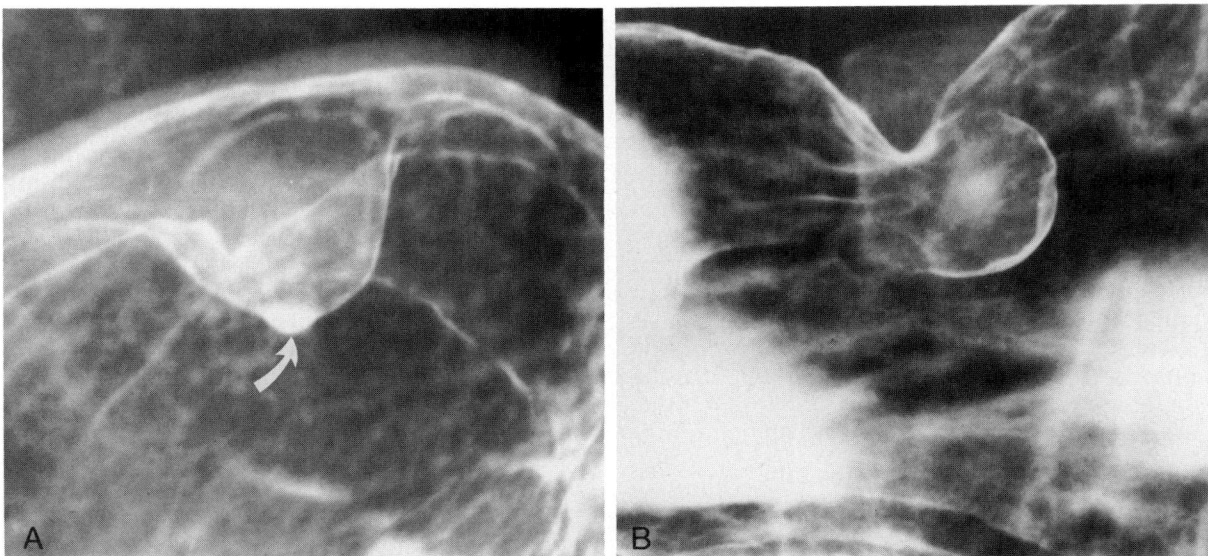

**Figure 37–16. Gastric leiomyomas. A.** A leiomyoma is seen in profile in the gastric fundus. Note how the lesion has smooth borders that form slightly obtuse angles with the adjacent gastric wall. This view was taken with the patient upright, and a barium stalactite *(arrow)* is seen hanging down from the inferior surface of the lesion. **B.** In another patient, a small leiomyoma is seen en face in the gastric body. This lesion also has typical features of a submucosal mass with smooth, well-defined borders. A hanging droplet of barium or stalactite is visible on the surface of this anterior wall lesion.

Gastric leiomyomas may vary in size from tiny lesions of several millimeters to enormous masses that encroach significantly on the lumen (see Fig. 37–17).[91] Tumors greater than 2 cm in size frequently contain areas of ulceration, manifested radiographically by a central barium-filled crater (usually 0.2 to 2.0 cm in size) within a smooth or slightly lobulated submucosal mass (see Figs.

37–18 and 37–19A). Because of their characteristic appearance, ulcerated leiomyomas have been described as "bull's-eye" or "target" lesions. Occasionally, a hanging droplet of barium or stalactite on an anterior wall leiomyoma mimics the appearance of ulceration[21] (see Fig. 37–16B). However, the stalactite can be recognized as a transient finding at fluoroscopy.

Because ulcerated leiomyomas may cause significant upper gastrointestinal bleeding, ulceration is generally considered an indication for surgery.[92] Occasionally,

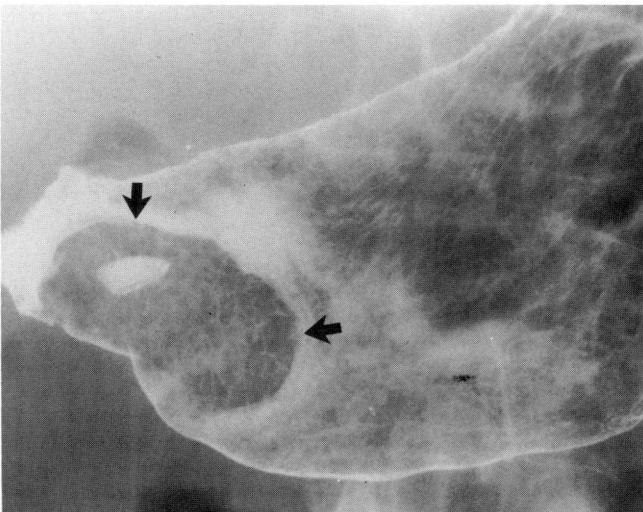

**Figure 37–18. Ulcerated leiomyoma.** A centrally ulcerated submucosal mass *(arrows)* is present in the gastric antrum. An areae gastricae pattern is visualized above the lesion because the overlying mucosa is intact. This is a characteristic feature of submucosal masses.

**Figure 37–17. Giant leiomyoma.** This lesion in the gastric fundus encroaches significantly on the lumen.

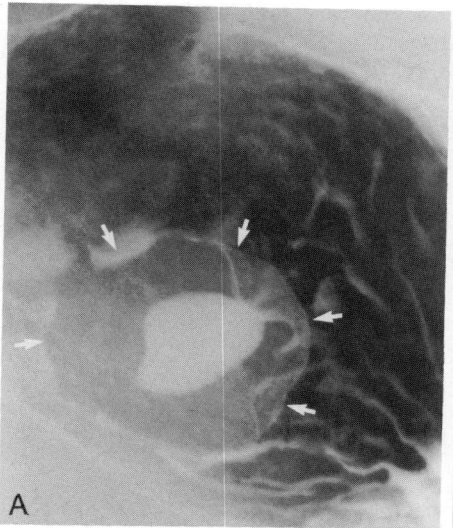 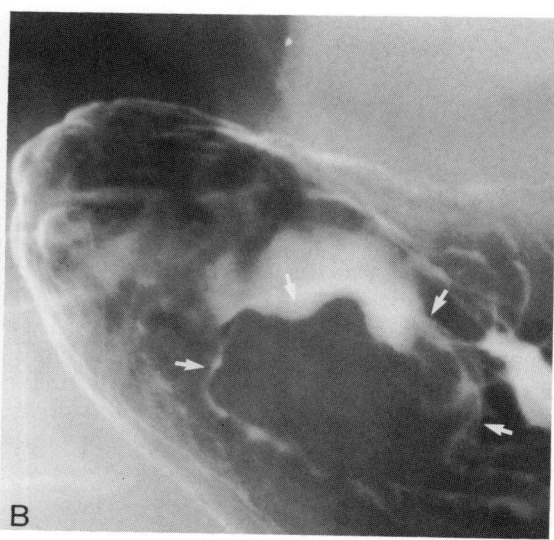

**Figure 37–19. Ulcerated leiomyoma with healing of the ulcer. A.** The initial study reveals a relatively large leiomyoma *(arrows)* in the fundus with a central area of ulceration. **B.** A follow-up study 3½ years later shows complete healing of the ulcer in the leiomyoma *(arrows)*. (**A** and **B** from O'Riordan D, Levine MS, Yeager BA: Complete healing of ulceration within a gastric leiomyoma. Gastrointest Radiol 10:47–49, 1985.)

however, complete healing of ulceration in a gastric leiomyoma has been observed on follow-up barium studies (see Fig. 37–19), so conservative medical treatment may lead to cessation of bleeding when surgery is contraindicated.[102] Alternatively, bleeding can sometimes be controlled angiographically by selective embolization of feeding vessels.[103]

Although most leiomyomas in the stomach have a typical submucosal appearance, exogastric leiomyomas that grow outward from the stomach may be indistinguishable radiographically from extrinsic mass lesions. However, the presence of a central dimple or spicule at the apex of the mass should suggest an intramural rather than an extrinsic lesion.[104] This area of tenting presumably results from traction on the gastric wall by the base or pedicle of the mass as it enlarges. Other leiomyomas that grow intraluminally may become pedunculated lesions. Rarely, pedunculated gastric leiomyomas prolapse into the duodenum or precipitate a gastrogastric or gastroduodenal intussusception.[95, 96]

## Differential Diagnosis

Leiomyomas are the most common benign submucosal tumors found in the stomach and duodenum. However, other intramural lesions such as lipomas, neurofibromas, hemangiomas, Brunner's gland hamartomas, and ectopic pancreatic rests may also be manifested by a discrete submucosal mass in the stomach or duodenum. Occasionally, lipomas can be recognized by their tendency to change in size and shape at fluoroscopy. Similarly, ectopic pancreatic rests can be suggested by their characteristic location on the greater curvature of the stomach adjacent to the pylorus, particularly if a central barium collection is present in the orifice of a primitive ductal system. In most cases, however, these submucosal lesions cannot be distinguished on the basis of radiologic criteria.

Leiomyomas that are ulcerated appear as typical bull's-eye or target lesions. Although a solitary bull's-eye lesion in the stomach or duodenum is most likely to represent an ulcerated leiomyoma on empirical grounds, other benign mesenchymal tumors that are ulcerated could produce identical findings. In contrast, the presence of multiple bull's-eye lesions should suggest a malignant condition such as metastatic disease, lymphoma, or Kaposi's sarcoma, because gastric and duodenal leiomyomas are rarely multiple.[1]

An antral or duodenal ulcer surrounded by a radiolucent mound of edema may also simulate an ulcerated leiomyoma. Conversely, an ulcerated leiomyoma can be misdiagnosed as an ulcer in the stomach or duodenum.[105] However, a leiomyoma usually has discrete borders, whereas the edematous mound surrounding a gastric or duodenal ulcer tends to have a more gradual transition with the adjacent mucosa.

Exogastric leiomyomas are often difficult to distinguish radiographically from extrinsic masses involving the stomach, particularly pancreatic pseudocysts or other pancreatic lesions. Gastric compression by an enlarged liver, spleen, kidney, or other abdominal mass may produce similar findings. As indicated earlier, however, the presence of a central dimple or spicule at the apex of the mass should suggest an exogastric, intramural lesion such as a leiomyoma or leiomyosarcoma[104] (see Fig. 39–28A). When extrinsic mass lesions are suspected, computed tomography (CT) and ultrasound are helpful for establishing the correct diagnosis (see Fig. 39–28B).

## Management

Small, asymptomatic submucosal masses that are detected radiographically in the stomach or duodenum can probably be followed conservatively without need for endoscopic or surgical intervention, as the majority are innocuous leiomyomas. In such cases, follow-up barium studies may be performed at 6-month or yearly intervals to be certain that the tumor is not enlarging. However, lesions greater than 2 cm in size should be resected because of the risk of malignancy and the difficulty in distinguishing benign and malignant smooth muscle tumors by histopathologic criteria.[1, 90] Depending on the size of the lesion, it can be enucleated, locally excised, or, if necessary, removed by partial gastrectomy or duodenectomy.[90, 92]

## Leiomyoblastomas

Leiomyoblastomas are unusual smooth muscle tumors that occur predominantly in the stomach. However, these tumors have also been reported in the small bowel, omentum, retroperitoneum, and uterus.[106] Leiomyoblastomas differ histologically from leiomyomas, but the gross morphologic findings are virtually identical.[91] As with other smooth muscle tumors, leiomyoblastomas are important because of the risk of malignancy in these lesions.

### Pathology

Leiomyoblastomas consist histologically of round, polygonal, or epithelioid cells with eccentric nuclei, perinuclear vacuolization, and a clear or acidophilic cytoplasm.[106–109] Because of the histologic findings, these tumors have also been called epithelioid leiomyomas.[109, 110] Most leiomyoblastomas are benign lesions, but metastases to the liver or other structures occur in about 10% of patients.[111] As with other smooth muscle tumors, malignant lesions usually have increased mitotic activity on microscopic examination.[109] Size is also an important factor in predicting biologic behavior, as metastases rarely occur with lesions less than 6 cm in size.[109] Nevertheless, many authors believe that all leiomyoblastomas should be resected because of the difficulty in distinguishing benign and malignant lesions by histopathologic criteria.[106, 110]

Gastric leiomyoblastomas tend to occur as solitary lesions, most frequently in the antrum, but multiple tumors have been reported.[109, 112] As with leiomyomas, the majority of lesions appear as submucosal masses, often with central necrosis and ulceration.[111, 112] Occasionally, however, they have an exogastric pattern of growth.[112]

### Clinical Findings

Unlike leiomyomas, leiomyoblastomas are more common in men than in women.[109, 111] These patients may be asymptomatic, or they may have pain, vomiting, upper gastrointestinal bleeding, or a palpable abdominal mass.[106, 108, 111, 112] Occasionally, giant exogastric leiomyoblastomas rupture suddenly into the peritoneal cavity, causing catastrophic intraperitoneal bleeding.[113]

### Radiographic Findings

Gastric leiomyoblastomas are indistinguishable radiographically from other smooth muscle tumors (see earlier section on leiomyomas). The majority appear as smooth submucosal masses, often containing a central area of ulceration[108, 112] (Fig. 37–20). Some endogastric

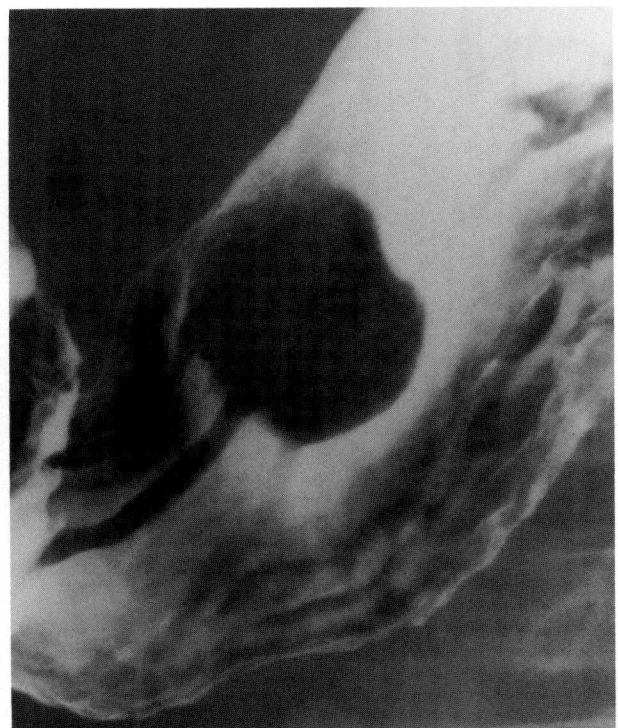

**Figure 37–20. Gastric leiomyoblastoma.** A large submucosal mass is present in the gastric body. This lesion is indistinguishable from a leiomyoma.

lesions can become pedunculated, whereas exogastric lesions can be mistaken for extrinsic masses involving the stomach[112] (Fig. 37–21A). Cystic degeneration of these exogastric leiomyoblastomas is occasionally manifested on CT by a cystic mass abutting the stomach[114] (Fig. 37–21B). The differential diagnosis for these lesions is discussed in detail in the previous section on leiomyomas.

## Lipomas

Lipomas constitute about 2 to 3% of benign gastric tumors.[115–118] Duodenal lipomas are even rarer. The majority are small, asymptomatic lesions that are incidental findings at autopsy. Thus far, no cases of malignant degeneration of gastrointestinal lipomas have been reported. Occasionally, however, lesions that are large or ulcerated cause obstruction or bleeding. Although lipomas usually cannot be differentiated from other submucosal masses in the stomach or duodenum on barium studies, CT has proved to be a valuable technique for diagnosing these lesions.

### Pathology

Lipomas are composed of mature fat cells surrounded by a fibrous capsule. Of all gastrointestinal lipomas, only 5% are located in the stomach or duodenum.[119] They tend to occur as solitary lesions, most frequently

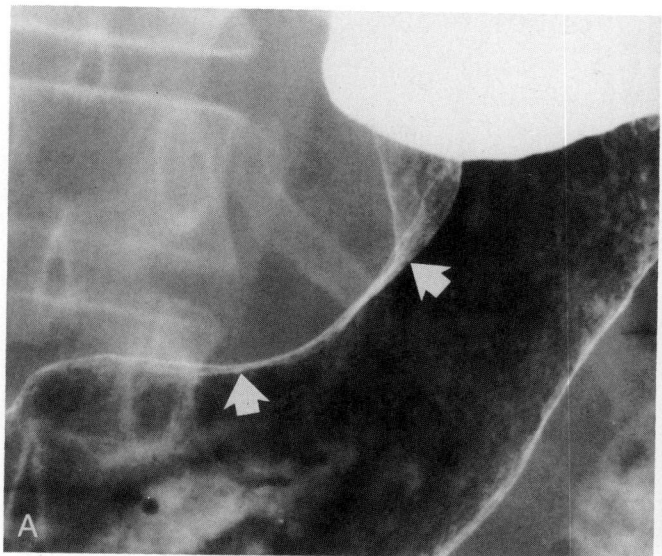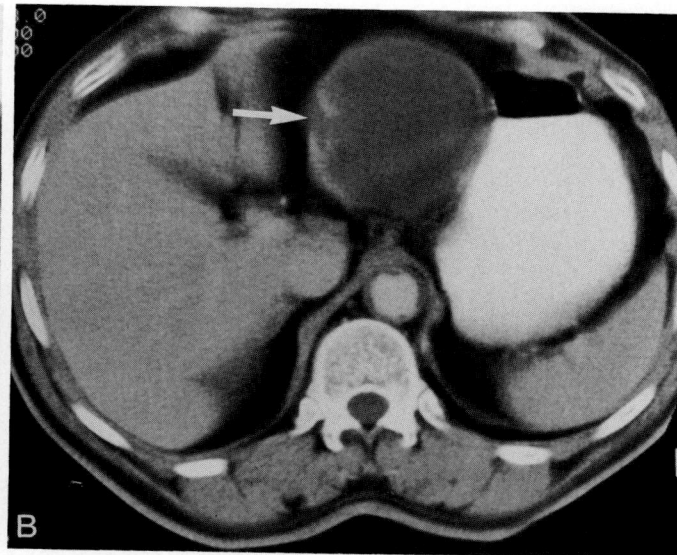

**Figure 37–21. Exogastric leiomyoblastoma. A.** A barium study shows a smooth extrinsic impression *(arrows)* on the lesser curvature of the gastric body. **B.** A CT scan shows a smooth, well-defined cystic mass *(arrow)* abutting the stomach. At surgery, this patient was found to have an exogastric leiomyoblastoma with cystic degeneration of the tumor. (**A** and **B** courtesy of Kyunghee C. Cho, M.D., Newark, NJ.)

in the gastric antrum.[115, 117–119] About 95% are endogastric lesions that arise in the submucosa and grow toward the lumen, whereas the remaining 5% are exogastric lesions that arise in the subserosa and grow outward from the stomach.[117] As lipomas increase in size, they may develop areas of superficial ulceration as a result of pressure necrosis of the overlying mucosa.[118] Lesions that grow intraluminally may become pedunculated and occasionally prolapse into the duodenum or act as the lead point for a gastroduodenal intussusception.[120]

## Clinical Findings

Although small lipomas are usually asymptomatic, larger lesions may undergo ulceration, causing abdominal pain or upper gastrointestinal bleeding.[117, 118, 121] Rarely, pedunculated gastric lipomas that prolapse into the duodenum cause recurrent nausea and vomiting due to intermittent gastric outlet obstruction.[117, 120] Small, asymptomatic lipomas in the stomach or duodenum can be followed conservatively without need for surgical intervention. However, larger lesions that are symptomatic should be resected.[118]

## Radiographic Findings

Large gastric or duodenal lipomas containing a sufficient amount of fat occasionally appear as radiolucent shadows on abdominal plain films.[122] Barium studies typically reveal a smooth submucosal mass or ulcerated bull's-eye lesion indistinguishable from a leiomyoma or other mesenchymal tumors[115, 116] (Fig. 37–22A). Although the majority occur as isolated antral lesions,[115, 117–119] multiple lipomas are occasionally pres-

ent in the stomach and duodenum.[119, 123] Because lipomas have a soft consistency, the correct diagnosis can be suggested if they change in size and shape with peristalsis or manual palpation at fluoroscopy[116, 123] (Fig. 37–22B). Rarely, pedunculated antral lipomas prolapse into the duodenum or act as the lead point for a gastroduodenal intussusception.[120]

CT has proved to be of considerable value in diagnosing gastrointestinal lipomas.[118, 124–126] These lesions are manifested on CT by well-circumscribed areas of uniform fatty density with an attenuation of −80 to −120 Hounsfield units[118, 124] (Fig. 37–22C). In contrast, liposarcomas, which rarely occur in the gastrointestinal tract, appear as heterogeneous lesions containing multiple septa and areas of greater density than fat.[127] Thus, a gastric or duodenal lipoma can be definitively diagnosed by CT and unnecessary endoscopy or surgery can be avoided.

## Hemangiomas

Hemangiomas constitute less than 2% of all benign tumors in the stomach.[128] They are even rarer in the duodenum. The lesions may be classified as capillary hemangiomas composed of numerous tiny vascular structures or, less commonly, as cavernous hemangiomas composed of large blood spaces or sinusoids lined by endothelial tissue. It is uncertain whether these lesions are true neoplasms capable of autonomous growth or congenital malformations.[129] They tend to occur as solitary lesions, but multiple hemangiomas may be present in the stomach, small bowel, and colon. Occasionally, gastrointestinal hemangiomas are associated with telangiectasias of the skin.[130]

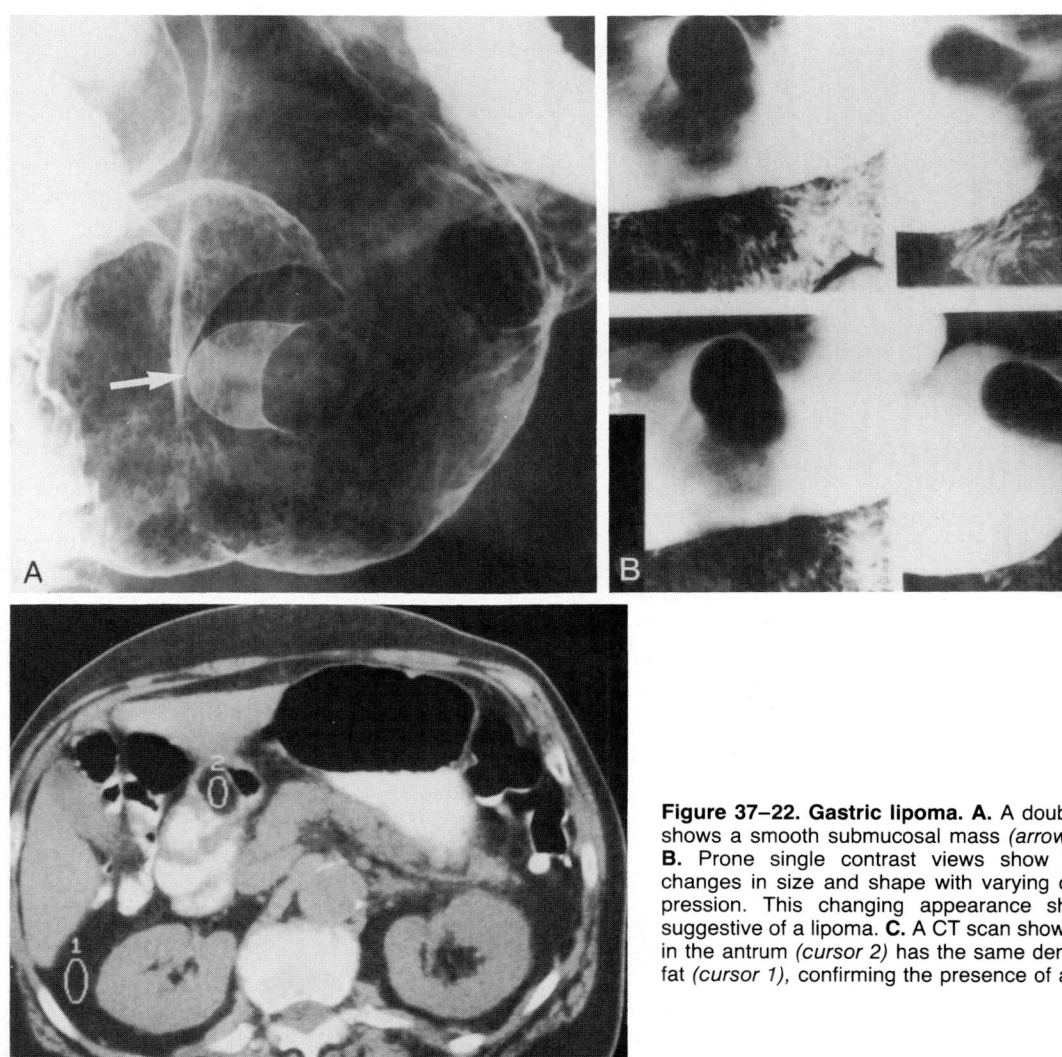

**Figure 37–22. Gastric lipoma. A.** A double contrast view shows a smooth submucosal mass *(arrow)* in the antrum. **B.** Prone single contrast views show how the lesion changes in size and shape with varying degrees of compression. This changing appearance should be highly suggestive of a lipoma. **C.** A CT scan shows how the lesion in the antrum *(cursor 2)* has the same density as perirenal fat *(cursor 1),* confirming the presence of a lipoma.

Although sarcomatous changes are rarely found in gastrointestinal hemangiomas, these highly vascular lesions are dangerous because of the risk of massive upper gastrointestinal bleeding.[129] Endoscopy typically reveals a bluish black submucosal lesion that has been likened to the appearance of a "mass of worms."[131] Surgical resection is usually curative.

## Radiographic Findings

Hemangiomas in the stomach typically appear as smooth submucosal masses indistinguishable from leiomyomas or other mesenchymal tumors.[130, 131] However, the presence of phleboliths within the lesion should be virtually pathognomonic of a hemangioma.[130–132] Such phleboliths are occasionally visible on abdominal plain films and their intimate relationship to the stomach is subsequently confirmed by barium studies.[130–132] The presence of additional hemangiomas on the skin should also suggest the correct diagnosis.

## Lymphangiomas

Lymphangiomas are rare benign tumors of the stomach and duodenum.[133, 134] These lesions consist histologically of irregularly dilated lymphatic channels lined by benign-appearing endothelial cells. Lymphangiomas are thought to be developmental malformations arising from sequestered lymphatic tissue that fails to communicate with the normal lymphatic system.[134] Subsequent accumulation of fluid accounts for the cystic nature of these lesions.

Although they may occur anywhere in the body, lymphangiomas rarely affect the gastrointestinal tract. These lesions are usually incidental findings in asymptomatic patients. Occasionally, however, they are large enough to cause obstruction or intussusception.[134] Gastroduodenal lymphangiomas in symptomatic patients should be resected.

## Radiographic Findings

Lymphangiomas may appear radiographically as smooth intramural masses indistinguishable from leiomyomas or other mesenchymal tumors in the stomach or duodenum.[134] Because of their cystic nature, these lesions may be pliable at fluoroscopy and are occasionally seen to change in shape with manual compression.[134] However, gastroduodenal lipomas may produce identical findings.

## Glomus Tumors

Glomus tumors are derived from glomus bodies, specialized arteriovenous communications that regulate temperature in the skin.[135] Because glomus bodies are particularly abundant in the nail beds and pads of the finger tips and toes, glomus tumors are classically subungual in location. Rarely, however, glomus tumors are found in the stomach.[135–137]

The majority of patients with glomus tumors in the stomach are asymptomatic. However, ulcerated tumors may cause upper gastrointestinal bleeding.[135, 137] Although local excision is usually curative, these highly cellular lesions can appear malignant on frozen sections at the time of surgery, so that an unnecessarily extensive resection is performed.[135, 136]

## Radiographic Findings

Glomus tumors in the stomach usually occur as solitary lesions in the antrum, ranging from 1 to 4 cm in size.[136] These tumors appear radiographically as smooth submucosal masses (with or without ulceration) and therefore are indistinguishable from leiomyomas or other more common mesenchymal tumors in the stomach[138] (Fig. 37–23). Occasionally, glomus tumors contain tiny flecks of calcification.[135] These tumors also have a soft consistency, so they can be mistaken for lipomas because of their tendency to change in size and shape at fluoroscopy.[138]

## Neural Tumors

Neural tumors constitute about 5 to 10% of benign gastric tumors.[1] The majority are nerve sheath tumors (neurilemomas, schwannomas, or neuromas).[139] The tumors are composed histologically of Schwann cells that have elongated nuclei in a palisade arrangement.[139] As they outgrow their blood supply, these lesions may undergo central necrosis and ulceration with subsequent upper gastrointestinal bleeding.[139] Most nerve sheath tumors are benign, but sarcomatous changes in these lesions have occasionally been reported.[1]

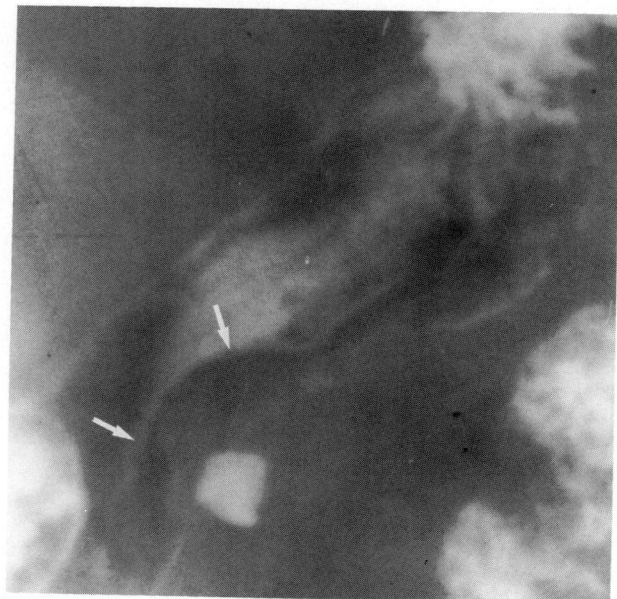

**Figure 37–23. Glomus tumor.** An ulcerated submucosal mass *(arrows)* is seen on the greater curvature of the antrum. This lesion cannot be distinguished from other, more common mesenchymal tumors in the stomach. (Courtesy of Bruce Knox, M.D., Norfolk, VA.)

Neurofibromas are other less common neural tumors in the stomach. These tumors arise from sympathetic nerves of Auerbach's myenteric plexus or, less frequently, Meissner's plexus.[140] Gastric neurofibromas are usually small, asymptomatic lesions that are incidental findings at surgery or at autopsy.[140] Occasionally, however, these tumors cause abdominal pain, nausea and vomiting, or upper gastrointestinal bleeding.[140] They tend to be isolated lesions, but multiple neurofibromas may be present in the stomach and duodenum in patients with generalized neurofibromatosis or von Recklinghausen's disease.[141, 142] The latter condition is characterized by multiple neurofibromas in the spinal, cranial, and sympathetic nerves; cutaneous neurofibromas; skin pigmentation; bone abnormalities; and other congenital malformations. About 10% of neurofibromas in the stomach eventually undergo malignant degeneration.[140] The risk of malignancy seems to be greatest in lesions associated with generalized neurofibromatosis.

## Radiographic Findings

Neural tumors in the stomach usually appear radiographically as discrete submucosal masses (with or without ulceration) that are indistinguishable from leiomyomas or other mesenchymal tumors (Fig. 37–24). However, some exogastric lesions grow outward from the stomach, projecting as lobulated masses into the peritoneal cavity.[140] Others have an hourglass or dumbbell configuration.[140] Although they are rare, gastroduodenal neurofibromas should be suspected when multiple submucosal masses are found in the stomach or

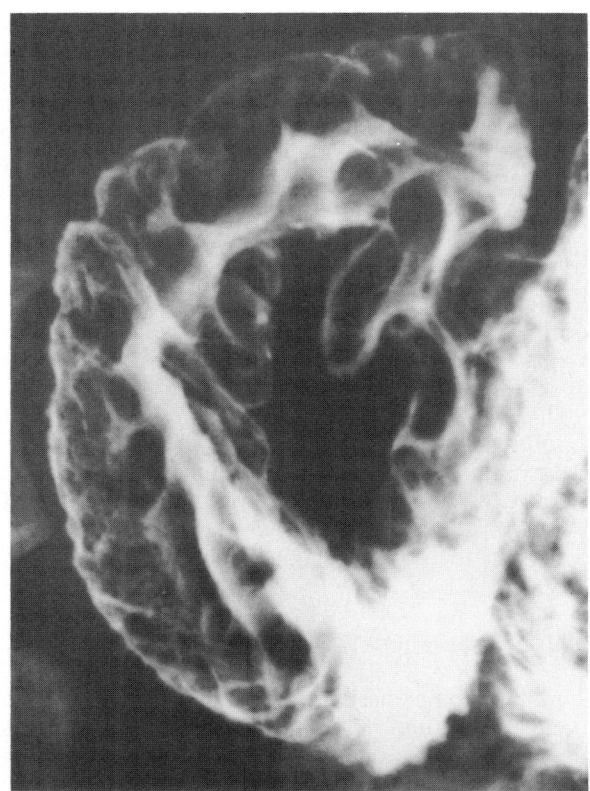

**Figure 37–25. Duodenal neurofibromas in a patient with neurofibromatosis.** Multiple submucosal masses are present in the first and second portions of the duodenum. This patient also had cutaneous neurofibromas and other stigmata of neurofibromatosis. (Courtesy of Seth N. Glick, M.D., Philadelphia, PA.)

duodenum in patients with cutaneous neurofibromas or other stigmata of neurofibromatosis (Fig. 37–25).

## Granular Cell Tumors

Granular cell tumors are rare benign tumors occurring predominantly in the skin, tongue, breast, and subcutaneous tissues.[143] These tumors originally were called granular cell myoblastomas, but more recent histochemical and electron microscopic data suggest that they have a neural derivation, arising from Schwann cells.[144] These lesions are composed of sheets of polygonal tumor cells containing an eosinophilic-staining, granular cytoplasm.[144] About 7% of granular cell tumors are located in the gastrointestinal tract, including the esophagus, stomach, colon, appendix, and biliary tree.[145] Granular cell tumors in the stomach are usually unexpected findings at surgery or at autopsy.[146] Occasionally, however, ulcerated lesions may cause epigastric pain or upper gastrointestinal bleeding.[146, 147] Surgical resection is usually curative.

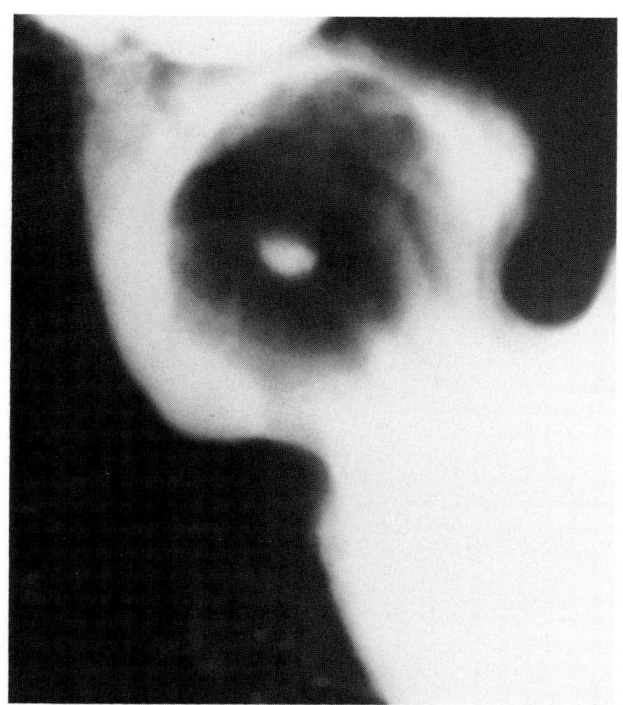

**Figure 37–24. Gastric neurofibroma.** An ulcerated submucosal mass is seen en face in the antrum. This lesion cannot be distinguished radiographically from an ulcerated leiomyoma. (Courtesy of Sat Somers, M.D., Ontario, Canada.)

## Radiographic Findings

Granular cell tumors in the stomach usually appear radiographically as discrete submucosal masses, ranging from 0.5 to 2.5 cm in size.[146] The lesions may be

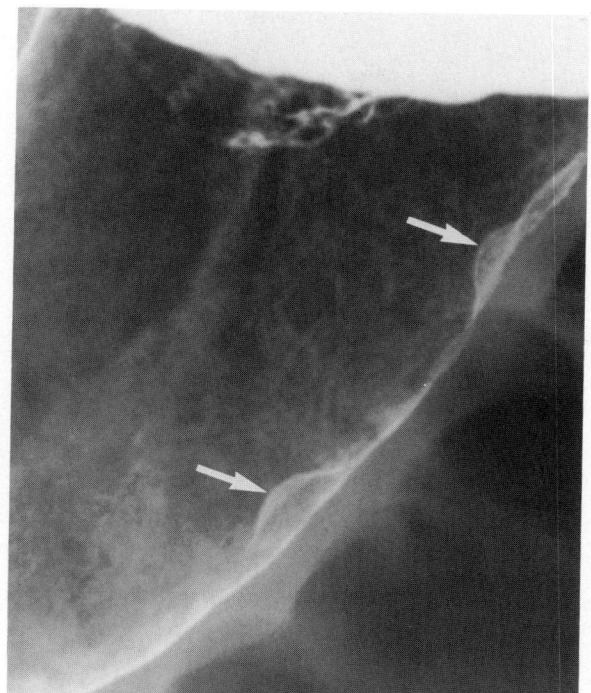

**Figure 37–26. Granular cell tumors.** Several small submucosal masses *(arrows)* are present on the greater curvature of the stomach. This patient had additional granular cell tumors on the tongue.

ulcerated. Occasionally, multiple granular cell tumors are present in the stomach[148] (Fig. 37–26). Despite their rarity, granular cell tumors should be suspected when submucosal lesions are found in the stomach in patients who have additional lesions involving the skin, tongue, or breast.

## Inflammatory Fibroid Polyps

Inflammatory fibroid polyps are uncommon submucosal lesions characterized histologically by whorls of fibrous tissue and blood vessels associated with an inflammatory infiltrate containing a high percentage of eosinophils.[149, 150] They tend to occur in the stomach but are also found in the small bowel and colon.[151] Because of the histologic findings, these lesions have also been called submucosal granulomas with eosinophilic infiltration, eosinophilic granulomas, fibromas, and granulomatous polyps.[152–154] However, inflammatory fibroid polyps are unrelated to eosinophilic granulomas of the lung or bone, which are composed primarily of histiocytes rather than fibroblasts. Nor are these lesions associated with a peripheral eosinophilia as is eosinophilic gastroenteritis, a separate and more diffuse condition.[151]

Although the etiology is uncertain, it has been postulated that inflammatory fibroid polyps have an allergic or inflammatory origin and are therefore not true neoplasms.[149, 152, 155] One theory is that a localized break in the mucosa incites an inflammatory response in the adjacent submucosa, with connective tissue proliferation in the form of a polypoid mass.[155] Whatever their origin,

inflammatory fibroid polyps are benign lesions without any known risk of malignant degeneration.

### Clinical Findings

Inflammatory fibroid polyps may cause epigastric pain or upper gastrointestinal bleeding due to superficial ulceration of the lesions.[150] Pedunculated polyps occasionally prolapse into the duodenum, causing intermittent gastric outlet obstruction.[150] Symptomatic lesions should be resected.

### Radiographic Findings

Inflammatory fibroid polyps in the stomach are usually located in the antrum.[149, 151, 156] They tend to occur as solitary lesions, ranging from 1 to 5 cm in size.[149, 157] They may appear radiographically as sessile or, less frequently, pedunculated polyps with a smooth or slightly lobulated contour[156, 157] (Fig. 37–27). As a result, these lesions may be indistinguishable from adenomatous polyps in the stomach. Inflammatory fibroid polyps that have a submucosal appearance can also be mistaken for leiomyomas or other mesenchymal tumors.[156] When these lesions are pedunculated, they occasionally prolapse through the pylorus, causing gastric outlet obstruction.[153] Rarely, inflammatory fibroid polyps are large, lobulated lesions, mimicking the appearance of polypoid gastric carcinomas.[150]

## Ectopic Pancreatic Rests

Although not true neoplasms, ectopic pancreatic rests are included in this chapter because they are submucosal lesions that are difficult to distinguish from leiomyomas

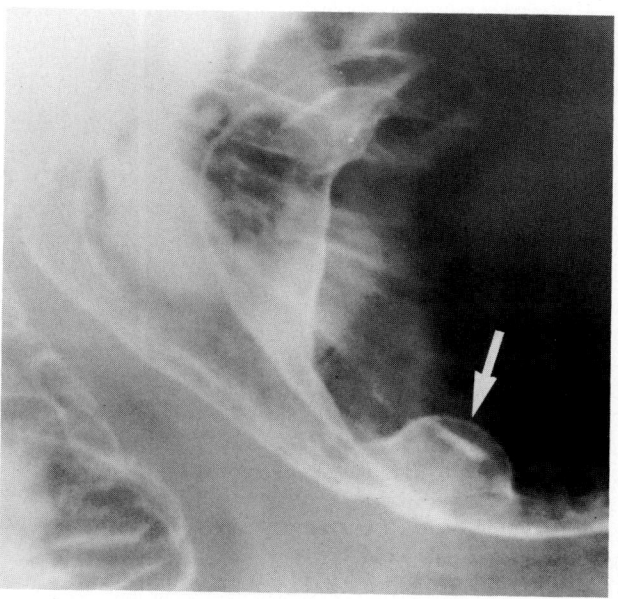

**Figure 37–27. Inflammatory fibroid polyp.** A sessile, slightly lobulated polyp *(arrow)* is seen on the greater curvature of the gastric antrum. This lesion is indistinguishable from an adenomatous polyp in the stomach.

or other mesenchymal tumors in the stomach or duodenum. Most ectopic pancreatic rests are incidental findings in patients seeking medical attention for other reasons. However, it may be necessary to resect these lesions if they cause symptoms or if a neoplastic condition cannot be excluded by radiologic or endoscopic examinations.

## Pathology

Ectopic pancreatic rests consist histologically of all pancreatic elements, including acini, ducts, and islet cells, but ductal structures tend to be arranged more haphazardly in these lesions than in normal pancreatic tissue.[158] Ectopic pancreatic rests are thought to result from abnormal embryologic development in which fragments of the ventral or dorsal pancreatic anlage are implanted in the intestinal wall.[159] These primitive epithelial buds may undergo varying degrees of differentiation toward mature glandular tissue. The term *adenomyosis* has been used to encompass a histologic spectrum of lesions, ranging from undifferentiated glandular epithelium to well-differentiated pancreatic tissue.[160, 161] Lesions consisting of poorly differentiated acinar and ductal structures have been called adenomyomas, whereas well-differentiated nodules of pancreatic tissue have been called ectopic, heterotopic, or aberrant pancreatic rests.[160–162] Because these lesions all contain duct-like structures and smooth muscle in various stages of differentiation, some authors believe that they should all be classified as myoepithelial hamartomas.[163]

Ectopic pancreatic rests occur throughout the gastrointestinal tract, but about 80% are located in the stomach, duodenum, or proximal jejunum.[164, 165] Occasionally, this anomaly is found in the gallbladder, biliary tree, liver, spleen, omentum, mesentery, appendix, mediastinum, or even Meckel's diverticulum.[166]

## Clinical Findings

Ectopic pancreatic rests in the stomach and duodenum are usually small, asymptomatic lesions. However, some patients have epigastric pain or upper gastrointestinal bleeding.[167–169] It has been postulated that these complications result from irritation or ulceration of the adjacent gastric or duodenal mucosa by pancreatic secretions.[159, 164] Occasionally, lesions arising near the pylorus cause gastric outlet obstruction.[170] Rarely, ectopic pancreatic rests develop the same diseases that affect normal pancreatic tissue, including pancreatitis, pseudocysts, and benign or malignant pancreatic tumors.[171, 172] Because upper gastrointestinal symptoms are more likely to be caused by peptic ulcer disease or other unrelated disorders, this anomaly should not be accepted as the source of the patient's symptoms without careful radiologic or endoscopic evaluation of the entire stomach and duodenum. Ectopic pancreatic rests should be resected only if the patient is symptomatic or if a significant neoplasm cannot be excluded nonoperatively.

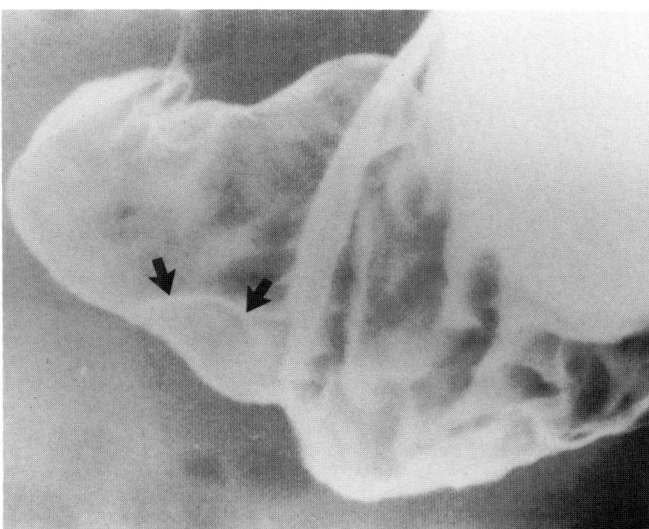

**Figure 37–28. Ectopic pancreatic rest.** The lesion appears as a discrete submucosal mass *(arrows)* on the greater curvature of the distal antrum. This is a characteristic location for ectopic pancreatic rests.

## Radiographic Findings

Ectopic pancreatic rests in the stomach and duodenum usually appear radiographically as smooth, broad-based submucosal masses, closely resembling leiomyomas or other mesenchymal tumors[159, 165, 173–176] (Fig. 37–28). They are almost always solitary lesions, ranging from 1 to 3 cm in size.[159, 174] Ectopic pancreatic rests in the stomach tend to be located on the greater curvature of the antrum 1 to 6 cm from the pylorus[175, 176] (see Fig. 37–28), whereas duodenal lesions are most frequently found in the proximal duodenum between the duodenal bulb and the papilla of Vater.[177] Although they arise in the submucosa, ectopic pancreatic rests occasionally appear as sessile or lobulated lesions indistinguishable from adenomatous polyps or even polypoid carcinomas.[175]

Ectopic pancreatic rests in the stomach and duodenum often contain a central umbilication or dimple, representing the orifice of a primitive ductal system.[173–176] In about 50% of patients, this orifice is manifested radiographically by a central collection of barium that varies from 1 to 5 mm in diameter and 5 to 10 mm in depth.[175] Rarely, a deep umbilication extends outside the contour of the stomach.[175] When viewed en face, these umbilicated lesions have the typical bull's-eye appearance of ulcerated leiomyomas or other mesenchymal tumors. In other patients, barium may reflux into rudimentary ductal structures that terminate in tiny club-shaped pouches.[159, 164] The latter finding should be virtually pathognomonic of ectopic pancreatic rests. However, these structures are rarely visualized spontaneously on barium studies. As a result, some investigators have advocated a combined radiologic-endoscopic technique for diagnosing pancreatic rests in the stomach or duodenum by cannulating the origin of the duct and injecting a small amount of barium at fluoroscopy to demonstrate these ductal structures.[178]

## Differential Diagnosis

The presence of a centrally umbilicated submucosal mass on the greater curvature of the gastric antrum 1 to 6 cm from the pylorus should suggest the possibility of an ectopic pancreatic rest. Leiomyomas or other benign mesenchymal tumors on the greater curvature may have a similar appearance. However, leiomyomas often contain eccentric areas of ulceration, and their location in the stomach is more variable. Although ulcers on the greater curvature of the antrum may produce similar findings, the edematous mound surrounding an ulcer tends to have more gradual borders that fade peripherally into the adjacent mucosa, whereas ectopic pancreatic rests are more sharply delineated. Other conditions such as metastatic disease, lymphoma, and Kaposi's sarcoma may also be manifested by bull's-eye lesions. However, the latter patients usually have multiple lesions in the stomach and duodenum, whereas ectopic pancreatic rests are almost always solitary lesions. If the radiographic findings are equivocal, endoscopy and biopsy should be performed for a more definitive diagnosis.

## Brunner's Gland Hyperplasia (Brunner's Gland Hamartomas)

Brunner's glands in the duodenum normally secrete an alkaline mucus that protects the mucosa from the damaging effects of acidic gastric juices entering the duodenum. Brunner's gland hyperplasia is therefore thought to occur as a response to hypersecretion of acid in the stomach.[179] However, hyperchlorhydria has been documented by gastric analysis in less than 50% of patients with this condition,[180] so a causal relationship between gastric hyperacidity and Brunner's gland hyperplasia has not been proved.

## Pathology

Hyperplastic Brunner's glands may be manifested grossly by diffuse enlargement of Brunner's glands throughout the proximal duodenum or by massive enlargement of a single gland. In the past, solitary lesions have been called Brunner's gland adenomas.[181–183] However, pathologic examination of these lesions has revealed an intimate admixture of ducts, acini, smooth muscle, and adipose tissue without evidence of cellular atypia, so most investigators now believe that they should be classified as hamartomas rather than true neoplasms.[184–186] Their hamartomatous origin is supported by the absence of malignant degeneration in these lesions. Nevertheless, Brunner's gland hamartomas are important because they can be mistaken for neoplastic lesions on radiologic or endoscopic examinations and because they occasionally may cause symptoms.

## Clinical Findings

Except for its association with duodenal ulcers and gastric hypersecretory states,[179] the diffuse form of Brunner's gland hyperplasia has no clinical significance. However, solitary Brunner's gland hamartomas occasionally cause obstructive symptoms, epigastric pain, or upper gastrointestinal bleeding due to ulceration of the overlying mucosa.[181, 186–188]

Although the diffuse form of Brunner's hyperplasia requires no specific treatment, solitary lesions should be resected if they cause significant symptoms or if the pathologic diagnosis is in doubt.[186] An endoscopic polypectomy may be feasible if the lesion is small and sufficiently pedunculated.[186, 188] However, surgery may be required for larger lesions that cannot be removed endoscopically.[186]

## Radiographic Findings

The diffuse form of Brunner's gland hyperplasia is manifested radiographically by multiple small, rounded nodules in the proximal duodenum, producing a characteristic "cobblestone" or "Swiss cheese" appearance[189–192] (Fig. 37–29A). The nodules tend to be most abundant in the duodenal bulb with fewer nodules in the descending duodenum, so the lesions correspond to the normal anatomic distribution of Brunner's glands.[190] Occasionally, central flecks of barium may be identified in the nodules. As a result, it has been postulated that these lesions actually represent chronic duodenal erosions in various stages of re-epithelialization.[193]

Brunner's gland hamartomas may appear as one or more submucosal or sessile lesions, ranging from several millimeters to several centimeters in size[183, 186, 190, 192, 194, 195] (Fig. 37–29B and C). Some patients with enlarged Brunner's glands have markedly thickened, irregular folds in the proximal duodenum because of concomitant duodenitis[195] (Fig. 37–29D). Rarely, large intramural masses cause mechanical obstruction of the duodenum or act as the lead point for a duodenojejunal intussusception.[186, 194, 196]

## Differential Diagnosis

The differential diagnosis for the diffuse form of Brunner's gland hyperplasia includes the various polyposis syndromes, benign lymphoid hyperplasia, heterotopic gastric mucosa, and nodular duodenitis. Although the polyposis syndromes may also be manifested by multiple rounded nodules in the duodenum, these individuals almost always have a generalized intestinal polyposis, whereas Brunner's gland hyperplasia is confined to the duodenum. Similarly, benign lymphoid hyperplasia may be manifested radiographically by multiple small nodules in the duodenal bulb and proximal duodenum[197] (Fig. 37–30). However, these patients may have generalized lymphoid hyperplasia of the small bowel or colon caused by an immunoglobulin deficiency state. Heterotopic gastric mucosa in the duodenum is characterized by angulated or polygonal 1- to 5-mm nodules or plaques

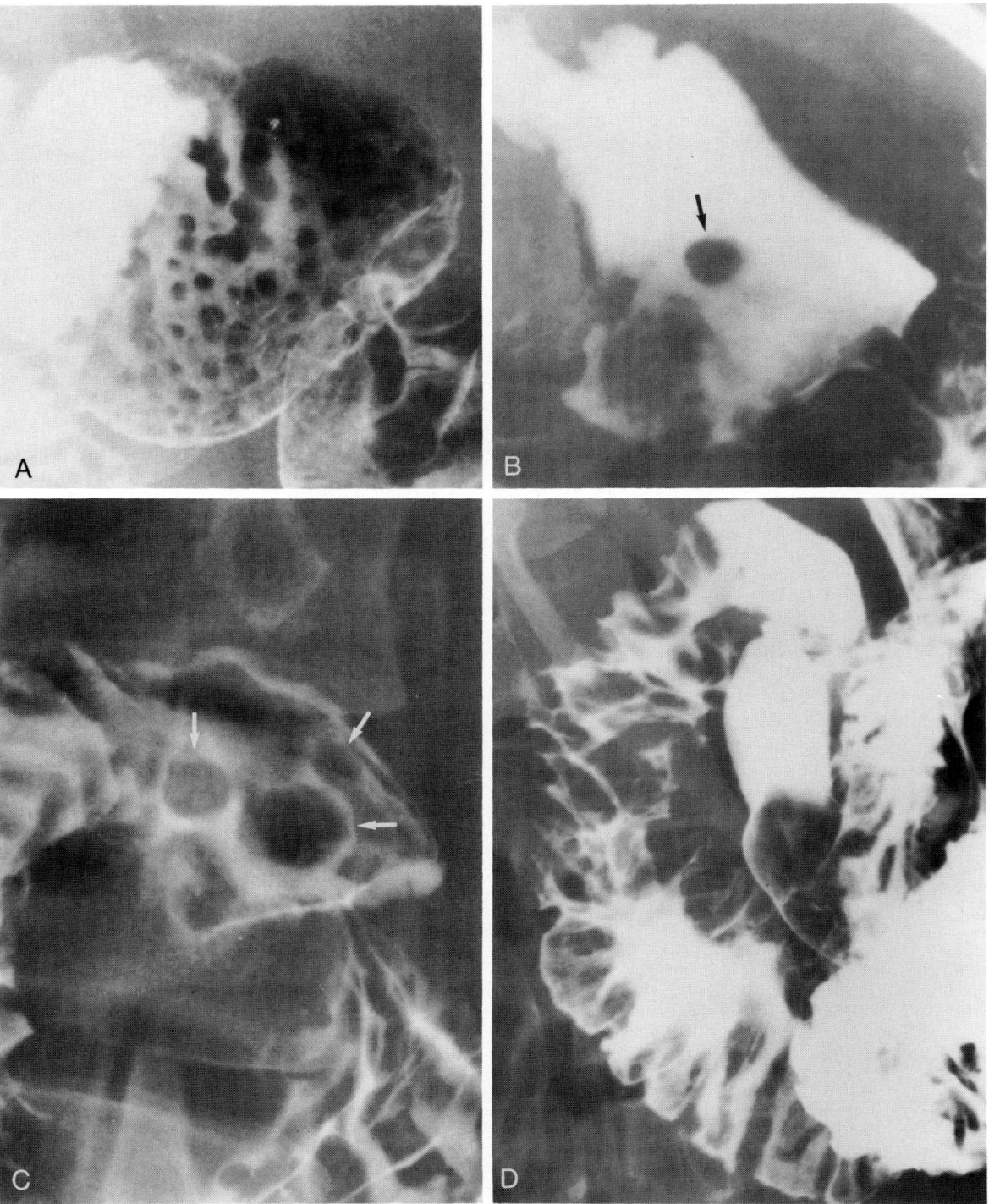

**Figure 37–29. Brunner's gland hyperplasia: spectrum of findings. A.** Multiple tiny, rounded nodules are present in the duodenal bulb in a patient with diffuse Brunner's gland hyperplasia. **B.** A small polyp *(arrow)* is seen in the duodenal bulb in another patient with Brunner's gland hamartoma. **C.** This patient has several Brunner's gland hamartomas in the duodenum, manifested by submucosal masses *(arrows)* in the bulb. **D.** A fourth patient with enlarged Brunner's glands has markedly thickened, disorganized folds in the descending duodenum because of concomitant duodenitis. (**D** courtesy of Dean D. T. Maglinte, M.D., Indianapolis, IN.)

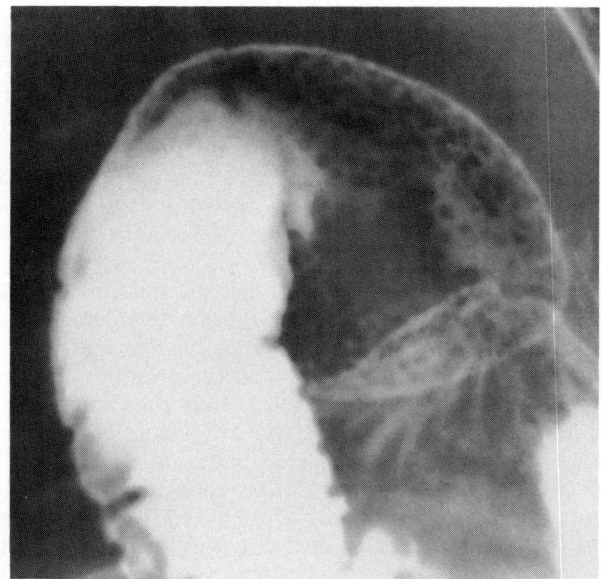

**Figure 37–30. Benign lymphoid hyperplasia.** Innumerable tiny nodules are present in the duodenal bulb. This patient had hypogammaglobulinemia.

that, unlike Brunner's glands, tend to be clustered near the base of the duodenal bulb[198, 199] (Fig. 37–31). Finally, nodular duodenitis may be manifested by thickened, nodular folds that can resemble hyperplastic Brunner's glands. However, the nodular folds tend to coalesce in the inflamed duodenum, whereas enlarged Brunner's glands have more discrete borders.

Solitary Brunner's gland hamartomas are difficult to distinguish radiographically from other polypoid lesions in the duodenum. Depending on their appearance, they

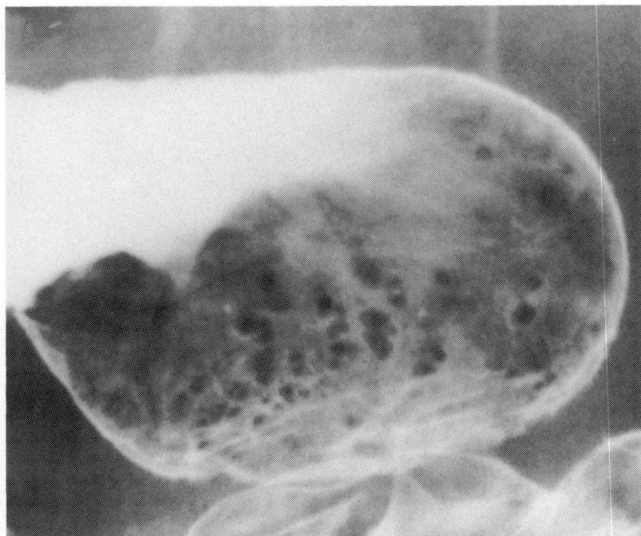

**Figure 37–31. Heterotopic gastric mucosa in the duodenum.** There are discrete, angulated filling defects near the base of the duodenal bulb. This appearance is so characteristic of heterotopic gastric mucosa that a confident diagnosis can be made on the basis of double contrast studies without need for endoscopy.

can resemble mucosal lesions such as adenomatous polyps or submucosal lesions such as leiomyomas. Occasionally, prolapsed gastric mucosa in the duodenal bulb produces similar findings. However, prolapsed mucosa is usually recognized as a mushroom-shaped defect at the base of the bulb that occurs as a transient finding at fluoroscopy[40, 41] (see Fig. 37–8). Rarely, a pedunculated polyp in the gastric antrum that has prolapsed into the duodenum can also be mistaken for a duodenal lesion such as a Brunner's gland hamartoma[6] (see Fig. 37–3).

## Duplication Cysts

Duplication cysts are hollow, epithelium-lined, spherical or tubular structures that are directly attached to some portion of the gastrointestinal tract, most frequently the distal ileum.[200–203] They tend to occur on the mesenteric side of the bowel, often sharing a common blood supply and muscular coat with the adjacent bowel wall. The majority of duplication cysts are spherical duplications that have no direct communication with the normal gastrointestinal tract.[203, 204] However, the rare tubular form of duplication may communicate with the gastrointestinal lumen at its proximal or distal end.[203, 204]

Duplication cysts of the stomach and duodenum are uncommon lesions, making up only 4 to 5% of all intestinal duplications.[204, 205] However, they may be associated with a variety of complications such as bleeding, obstruction, or perforation. These lesions should therefore be surgically repaired or removed whenever feasible.

### *Pathology*

Gastrointestinal duplication cysts are congenital malformations, probably resulting from faulty embryologic budding or defective recanalization of the alimentary tube during early fetal life.[203, 206–208] Histologically, they are fluid-filled cysts containing a well-developed smooth muscle layer and mucous membrane lining. This mucous membrane is usually identical with that of the parent bowel, but duplication cysts occasionally contain gastric, intestinal, pancreatic, or even respiratory epithelium.[203, 209] When ectopic gastric mucosa is present in the cyst, secretion of peptic acid may cause ulceration or bleeding.[209] Otherwise, most duplication cysts are filled with clear, mucinous fluid secreted by the mucous membrane lining. Depending on the volume of secretions, the cysts may vary from 1 to 25 cm in size.[200, 209] Duplication cysts of the stomach usually arise from the greater curvature of the antrum or body,[202, 205, 210] whereas duplication cysts of the duodenum usually arise from the anteromedial aspect of the first or second portion of the duodenum.[204, 206, 209]

Duplication cysts of the stomach and duodenum may be associated with a variety of other congenital anomalies, including intestinal or biliary atresia, malrotation, imperforate anus, double gallbladder, and double uterus.[200] These patients also tend to have duplication cysts elsewhere in the gastrointestinal tract.[210, 211] Unlike mediastinal duplication cysts, however, duplication cysts of the stomach and duodenum are rarely associated with hemivertebrae or other vertebral anomalies.[205, 209]

## Clinical Findings

Gastric duplication cysts are twice as common in women as in men,[211] whereas duodenal duplication cysts have an approximately equal sex distribution.[206] The vast majority of gastric duplications cause symptoms during the first year of life, so they are almost always diagnosed during early childhood.[205, 210, 211] In contrast, duodenal duplications may not cause symptoms early in life, so 35 to 40% of cases are discovered in patients older than 20 years of age.[209, 212]

The most common presenting findings in children or adults with duplication cysts of the stomach or duodenum are a palpable abdominal mass and vomiting.[205, 206, 209–211] The latter symptom results from encroachment on the adjacent stomach or duodenum by the enlarging cyst. In infants with gastric duplication cysts, nonbilious vomiting may erroneously suggest hypertrophic pyloric stenosis.[213, 214] In contrast, duodenal duplication cysts tend to be associated with bilious vomiting.[204] Less frequently, older children or adults may present with abdominal pain, weight loss, fever, and/or upper gastrointestinal bleeding.[204–207, 209–211] Abdominal pain probably results from progressive distention of the cyst by its own secretions.[207] Fever occurs if the cyst becomes infected. Upper gastrointestinal bleeding is caused by

localized pressure necrosis of the adjacent gastric or duodenal wall or by ulceration of a cyst that communicates directly with the stomach or duodenum.[204, 206, 210] Duodenal duplication cysts may also compress the ampulla of Vater or the pancreatic or common bile ducts, causing acute pancreatitis or obstructive jaundice.[206, 209] Rarely, duplication cysts present as surgical emergencies because of torsion or perforation of the cyst with associated peritonitis.[209, 215, 216] A case of carcinoma arising in a gastric duplication cyst has also been reported.[217]

Because of these complications, duplication cysts of the stomach and duodenum should be treated surgically. Gastric duplication cysts can often be excised without difficulty from their attachment to the greater curvature of the stomach.[211, 214] Because of their proximity to the ampulla of Vater, however, duodenal duplication cysts frequently cannot be resected without performing a pancreaticoduodenectomy and reconstructive biliary surgery. Instead of resorting to such a radical procedure, some surgeons prefer to create a window between the cyst and the adjacent duodenum by excising a portion of the common wall between these structures to permit internal drainage and decompression of the cyst.[204, 209]

## Radiographic Findings

Duplication cysts of the stomach and duodenum may occasionally be recognized on abdominal plain films by the presence of a soft tissue mass indenting the gastric or duodenal air shadows. The transverse colon may also be displaced inferiorly by gastric duplications. Rarely,

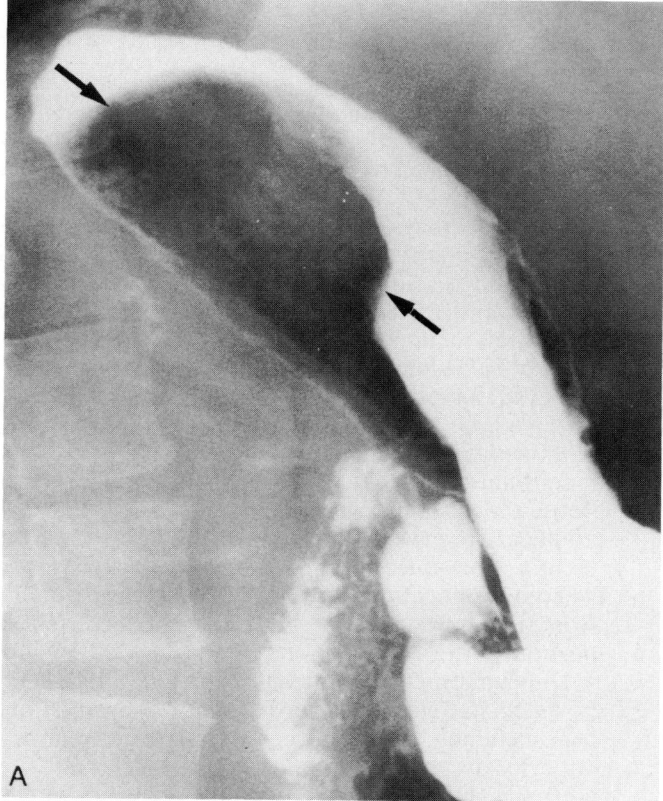

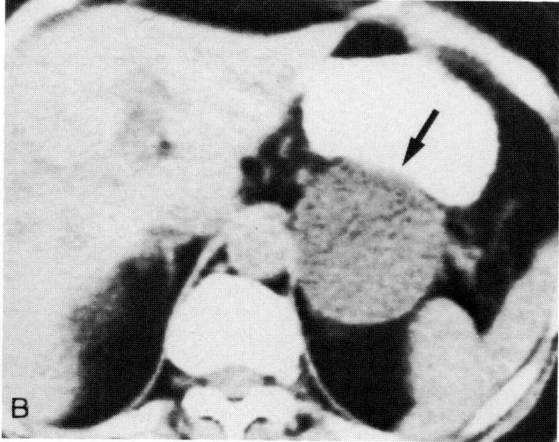

**Figure 37–32. Gastric duplication cyst. A.** A barium study shows a smooth mass *(arrows)* indenting the posterior wall of the gastric fundus. **B.** A CT scan shows a thin-walled, fluid-filled mass *(arrow)* abutting the stomach. (**A** and **B** from BA Thornhill, KC Cho, HT Morehouse, Gastric duplication associated with pulmonary sequestration: CT manifestations, AJR, 138, 6, 1168–1171, 1982, © by American Roentgen Ray Society.)

curvilinear calcification may be identified in the cyst wall.[218, 219] However, calcification is more commonly seen in mesenteric, renal, or adrenal cysts.

Gastric duplication cysts typically appear on barium studies as intramural or extrinsic mass lesions involving the greater curvature or, less commonly, the posterior wall or lesser curvature of the stomach[202, 220] (Fig. 37–32). Similarly, duodenal duplication cysts can be recognized as smooth submucosal or extrinsic masses involving the medial wall of the descending duodenum.[204, 209, 212] Less frequently, they may appear as well-defined, oval filling defects in the duodenum[206, 209, 212] (Fig. 37–33). As gastric and duodenal duplication cysts increase in size, they may encroach significantly on the lumen of the adjacent stomach and duodenum, causing progressive obstruction. Because duplication cysts are fluid-filled structures, manual compression or peristalsis occasionally causes these lesions to change in size and shape at fluoroscopy.[221] Rarely, communicating duplications can be recognized as oval or tubular, barium-filled structures adjacent to the stomach or duodenum because of opacification of the cyst lumen[221, 222] (Fig. 37–34).

Both ultrasound and CT may be helpful in confirming the cystic nature of gastric or duodenal duplications that are visualized indirectly on barium studies. These structures usually appear on ultrasound scans as sonolucent masses with strong posterior wall echoes and through transmission.[221, 223] In some patients, the mucosal lining of the cyst is manifested by an echogenic inner ring surrounded by a relatively hypoechoic muscle layer.[221, 223] Echogenic internal components may occasionally be seen in cysts that are infected or hemorrhagic.[223] These duplications can also be recognized on CT scans as

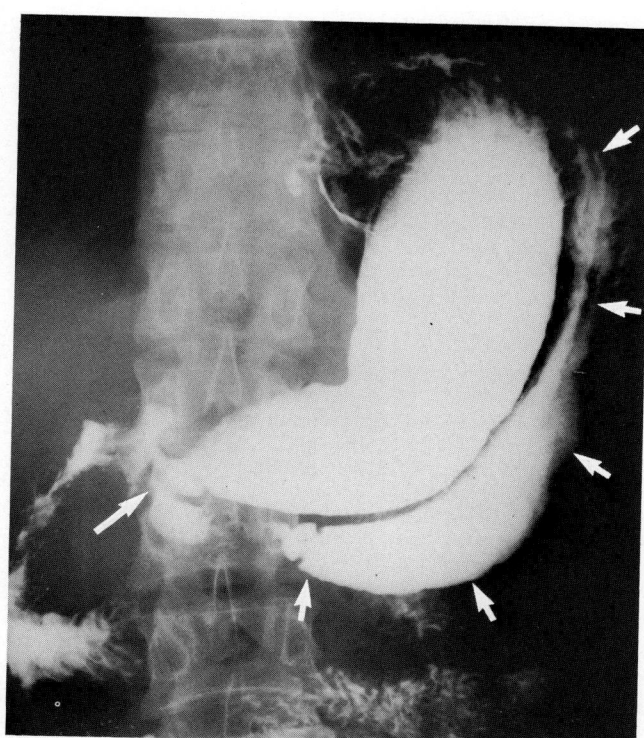

**Figure 37–34. Communicating gastric duplication.** Barium has entered a long, tubular duplication cyst *(short arrows)* on the greater curvature of the stomach. The duplication extends from the fundus to the pylorus, where it communicates with the lumen *(long arrow)*. This form of duplication is extremely uncommon.

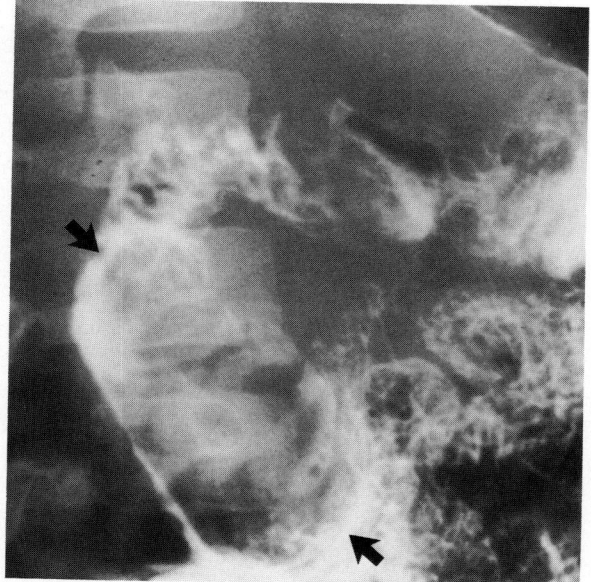

**Figure 37–33. Duodenal duplication cyst.** There is a large intramural mass *(arrows)* in the descending duodenum. Note the smooth contour of the lesion. An intramural hematoma or choledochal cyst could produce similar findings.

discrete, fluid-filled structures abutting the greater curvature of the stomach or medial wall of the descending duodenum[219, 222, 224] (see Fig. 37–32B). Rarely, CT may demonstrate cyst wall calcification[219] or enteroliths within the cyst.[224]

## Differential Diagnosis

The finding on barium studies of a smooth intramural lesion on the greater curvature of the gastric antrum or medial wall of the descending duodenum should suggest the possibility of a duplication cyst, particularly in children. However, other intramural lesions (i.e., leiomyomas, lipomas, or hematomas) or extrinsic lesions (i.e., pancreatic tumors, pancreatic pseudocysts, or choledochal cysts) involving the stomach or duodenum may produce identical radiographic findings. When duplication cysts are suspected on barium studies, ultrasound or CT may be helpful for documenting the cystic nature of these structures. It should be recognized that other cystic lesions in the upper abdomen, such as choledochal cysts, mesenteric cysts, omental cysts, and pancreatic pseudocysts, can resemble duplication cysts on ultrasound or CT studies.[223, 224] Nevertheless, the finding of a cystic mass that is contiguous with the greater curvature of the stomach but separable from the gallbladder, extrahepatic biliary tree, and pancreas should be highly suggestive of a duplication cyst.

### Acknowledgment

Figures 37–1B, 37–4A and B, 37–6, 37–7A, 37–8, 37–10B, 37–16A and B, 37–17, 37–22A to C, 37–28, 37–29A, 37–30, and 37–31 are reproduced from Laufer I, Levine MS (eds): Double Contrast Gastrointestinal Radiology (2nd ed). Philadelphia: WB Saunders, 1992.

Figure 37–34 is reproduced from Marshak RH, Lindner AE, Maklansky D (eds): Radiology of the Stomach. Philadelphia: WB Saunders, 1983.

# References

1. Good CA: Benign tumors of the stomach and duodenal bulb. J Can Assoc Radiol 16:92–104, 1965.
2. Ochsner SF, Janetos GP: Benign tumors of the stomach. JAMA 191:881–887, 1965.
3. Delpy JC, Bruneton JN, Drouillard J, et al: Non-vaterian duodenal adenomas: report of 24 cases and review of the literature. Gastrointest Radiol 8:135–141, 1983.
4. Finesilver EM: Benign tumors of the stomach. Surgery 12:216–235, 1942.
5. Overgaard K: Polyps of the stomach and duodenum. Acta Radiol 30:343–361, 1948.
6. Marshak RH, Feldman F: Gastric polyps. Am J Dig Dis 10:909–935, 1965.
7. Gordon R, Laufer I, Kressel HY: Gastric polyps found on routine double-contrast examination of the stomach. Radiology 134:27–30, 1980.
8. Feczko PJ, Halpert RD, Ackerman LV: Gastric polyps: radiological evaluation and clinical significance. Radiology 155:581–584, 1985.
9. Ming S-C: The classification and significance of gastric polyps. *In* Yardly JH, Morson BC, Abell M (eds): The Gastrointestinal Tract. International Academy of Pathology Monograph. Baltimore: Williams & Wilkins, 1977, pp 149–175.
10. Green PHR, Fevre DI, Barrett PJ, et al: Chronic erosive (verrucous) gastritis: a study of 108 patients. Endoscopy 9:74–78, 1977.
11. McLean AM, Paul RE, Philipps E, et al: Chronic erosive gastritis: clinical and radiological features. J Can Assoc Radiol 33:158–162, 1982.
12. Elta GH, Fawaz KA, Dayal Y, et al: Chronic erosive gastritis: a recently recognized disorder. Dig Dis Sci 28:7–12, 1983.
13. Elsborg L, Andersen D, Myhre-Jensen O, et al: Gastric mucosal polyps in pernicious anaemia. Scand J Gastroenterol 12:49–52, 1977.
14. Joffe N, Goldman H, Antonioli DA: Recurring hyperplastic gastric polyps following subtotal gastrectomy. AJR 130:301–305, 1978.
15. Ming S-C: The adenoma-carcinoma sequence in the stomach and colon. II. Malignant potential of gastric polyps. Gastrointest Radiol 1:121–125, 1976.
16. Tomosulo J: Gastric polyps. Histologic types and their relationship to gastric carcinoma. Cancer 27:1346–1355, 1971.
17. Ming S-C, Goldman H: Gastric polyps. A histogenetic classification and its relation to carcinoma. Cancer 18:721–726, 1965.
18. Iida M, Yao T, Watanabe H, et al: Fundi gland polyposis in patients without familial adenomatosis coli: its incidence and clinical features. Gastroenterology 86:1437–1442, 1984.
19. Iida M, Yao T, Itoh H, et al: Natural history of fundic gland polyposis in patients with familial adenomatosis coli/Gardner's syndrome. Gastroenterology 89:1021–1025, 1985.
20. Joffe N, Antonioli DA: Atypical appearances of benign hyperplastic polyps. AJR 131:147–152, 1978.
21. Op den Orth JO, Ploem S: The stalactite phenomenon on double contrast studies of the stomach. Radiology 117:523–525, 1975.
22. Aronchick J, Laufer I, Glick SN: Barium stalactites: observations on their nature and significance. Radiology 149:588–591, 1983.
23. Smith HJ, Lee EL: Large hyperplastic polyps of the stomach. Gastrointest Radiol 8:19–23, 1983.
24. Iida M, Yao M, Watanabe H, et al: Spontaneous disappearance of fundic gland polyposis: report of three cases. Gastroenterology 79:725–728, 1980.
25. Kikuchi Y, Levine MS, Laufer I, et al: Value of flow technique for double-contrast examination of the stomach. AJR 147:1183–1184, 1986.
26. Marshak RH, Lindner AE: Polypoid lesions of the stomach. Semin Roentgenol 6:151–168, 1971.
27. Hay JL: Surgical management of gastric polyps and adenomas. Surgery 39:114–119, 1956.
28. Op den Orth JO, Dekker W: Gastric adenomas. Radiology 141:289–293, 1981.
29. Elsborg L, Andersen D, Bastrup-Madsen P: Gastrocamera screening in pernicious anaemia. With special reference to the occurrence of gastric polyps and cancer. Scand J Gastroenterol 8:5–8, 1973.
30. Laxen F: Gastric carcinoma and pernicious anaemia in long-term endoscopic follow-up of subjects with gastric polyps. Scand J Gastroenterol 19:535–540, 1984.
31. Borch K: Epidemiologic, clinicopathologic, and economic aspects of gastroscopic screening of patients with pernicious anaemia. Scand J Gastroenterol 21:21–30, 1986.
32. Hay JL: Polyps and adenomas of the stomach. Surgery 33:446–451, 1953.
33. Yarnis H, Marshak RH, Friedman AI: Gastric polyps. JAMA 148:1088–1094, 1952.
34. Bone GE, McClelland RN: Management of gastric polyps. Surg Gynecol Obstet 142:933–938, 1976.
35. Lanza FL, Graham DY, Nelson RS, et al: Endoscopic upper gastrointestinal polypectomy: report of 73 polypectomies in 63 patients. Am J Gastroenterol 75:345–348, 1981.
36. ReMine SG, Hughes RW Jr, Weiland LH: Endoscopic gastric polypectomies. Mayo Clin Proc 56:371–375, 1981.
37. Hancock RJ: An 11-year review of primary tumours of the small bowel including the duodenum. Can Med Assoc J 103:1177–1179, 1970.
38. Griffen WO, Schaeffler JW, Schindler S, et al: Ampullary obstruction by benign duodenal polyps. Arch Surg 97:449–449, 1968.
39. Deutschberger O, Tchertkoff V, Daino J, et al: Benign duodenal polyp: review of the literature and report of a giant adenomatous polyp of the duodenal bulb. Am J Gastroenterol 38:75–84, 1962.
40. Levin EJ, Felson B: Asymptomatic gastric mucosal prolapse. Radiology 57:514–520, 1951.
41. Feldman M, Myers P: The roentgen diagnosis of prolapse of the gastric mucosa into the duodenum. Gastroenterology 20:90–99, 1952.
42. Nelson JA, Sheft DJ, Minagi H, et al: Duodenal pseudopolyp: the flexural fallacy. AJR 123:262–267, 1975.
43. Burrell M, Toffler R: Flexural pseudolesions of the duodenum. Radiology 120:313–315, 1976.
44. Schulten MF, Dyasu R, Beal JM: Villous adenoma of the duodenum: a case report and review of the literature. Am J Surg 132:90–96, 1976.
45. Shauffer IA, O'Connor SJ: Villous tumors of the stomach. Radiology 86:734–735, 1966.
46. Meltzer AD, Ostrum BJ, Isard HJ: Villous tumors of the stomach and duodenum. Report of three cases. Radiology 87:511–513, 1966.
47. Bremer EH, Battaile WG, Bulle PH: Villous tumors of the upper gastrointestinal tract. Clinical review and report of a case. Am J Gastroenterol 50:135–143, 1968.
48. Mir-Madjlessi S-H, Farmer RG, Hawk WA: Villous tumors of the duodenum and jejunum. Report of four cases and review of the literature. Am J Dig Dis 18:467–476, 1973.
49. Miller JH, Gisvold JJ, Weiland LH, et al: Upper gastrointestinal tract: villous tumors. AJR 134:933–936, 1980.
50. Kutim ND, Ranson JHC, Gouge TH, et al: Villous tumors of the duodenum. Ann Surg 181:164–168, 1975.
51. Spira IA, Wolff WI: Villous tumors of the duodenum. Am J Gastroenterol 67:63–68, 1977.
52. Walk L: Villous tumors of the stomach. Clinical review and report of two cases. Arch Intern Med 87:560–569, 1951.
53. Gaitini O, Kleinhaus U, Munichor M, et al: Villous tumors of the stomach. Gastrointest Radiol 13:105–108, 1988.

54. Malmed LA, Levin B. Villous adenoma of the duodenum. AJR 94:362–365, 1965.
55. Ring EJ, Ferucci JT, Eaton SB, et al: Villous adenoma of the duodenum. Radiology 104:45–48, 1972.
56. Dayal Y, Bass AG, Kraft AR, et al: Villous adenoma of the duodenum. Am J Surg 124:394–398, 1972.
57. Dwyer WA, O'Brien RF: Duodenal obstruction due to malignant villous adenoma. J Med Soc NJ 67:477–479, 1970.
58. Boyer CW. Adenoma of the duodenal bulb. A case report. AJR 90:753–755, 1963.
59. Dodds WJ: Clinical and roentgen features of the intestinal polyposis syndromes. Gastrointest Radiol 1:127–142, 1976.
60. Mayo CW, DeWeerd JH, Jackman RJ: Diffuse familial polyposis of the colon. Surg Gynecol Obstet 93:87–96, 1951.
61. Yao T, Iida M, Ohsato K, et al: Duodenal lesions in familial polyposis of the colon. Gastroenterology 73:1086–1092, 1977.
62. Itai Y, Kogure T, Okugama Y, et al: Radiographic features of gastric polyps in familial adenomatosis coli. AJR 128:73–76, 1977.
63. Watanabe H, Enjoji M, Yao T, et al: Gastric lesions in familial adenomatosis coli. Their incidence and histologic analysis. Hum Pathol 9:269–283, 1978.
64. Jarvinen H, Nyberg M, Peltokallo P: Upper gastrointestinal tract polyps in familial adenomatosis coli. Gut 24:333–339, 1983.
65. Tonelli F, Nardi F, Bechi P, et al: Extracolonic polyps in familial polyposis coli and Gardner's syndrome. Dis Colon Rectum 28:664–668, 1985.
66. Denzier TB, Harned RK, Pergam CJ: Gastric polyps in familial polyposis coli. Radiology 130:63–66, 1979.
67. Iida M, Yao T, Itoh H, et al: Natural history of gastric adenomas in patients with familial adenomatosis coli/Gardner's syndrome. Cancer 61:605–611, 1988.
68. Ohsato K, Watanabe H, Itoh H, et al: Simultaneous occurrence of multiple gastric carcinomas and familial polyposis of the colon. Jpn J Surg 4:165–174, 1974.
69. Boley SJ, McKinnon WMP, Marzulli VF: The management of familial gastrointestinal polyposis involving stomach and colon. Surgery 50:691–696, 1961.
70. Hoffman DC, Goligher JC: Polyposis of the stomach and small intestine in association with F.P. coli. Br J Surg 58:126–128, 1971.
71. Pauli RM, Pauli ME, Hall JG: Gardner syndrome and periampullary malignancy. Am J Med Genet 6:205–219, 1980.
72. Burt RW, Berenson MM, Lee RG, et al: Upper gastrointestinal polyps in Gardner's syndrome. Gastroenterology 86:295–301, 1984.
73. Iida M, Yao T, Itoh H, et al: Natural history of duodenal lesions in Japanese patients with familial adenomatosis coli (Gardner's syndrome). Gastroenterology 96:1301–1306, 1989.
74. Jones TR, Nance FC: Periampullary malignancy in Gardner's syndrome. Ann Surg 185:565–573, 1977.
75. Coffey RJ, Knight CD, van Heerden JA, et al: Gastric adenocarcinoma complicating Gardner's syndrome in a North American woman. Gastroenterology 88:1263–1266, 1985.
76. Bartholomew LG, Moore CE, Dahlin DC, et al: Intestinal polyposis associated with mucocutaneous pigmentation. Surg Gynecol Obstet 114:1–16, 1962.
77. Godard JE, Dodds WJ, Phillips JC, et al: Peutz-Jeghers syndrome: clinical and roentgenographic features. AJR 113:316–324, 1971.
78. Buck JL, Harned RK, Lichtenstein JE, et al: Peutz-Jeghers syndrome. Radiographics 12:365–378, 1992.
79. Sheward JD: Peutz-Jeghers syndrome in childhood: unusual radiologic features. Br Med J 1:921–923, 1962.
80. Cronkhite LW, Canada WJ: Generalized gastrointestinal polyposis. An unusual syndrome of polyposis, pigmentation, alopecia, and onychotrophia. N Engl J Med 252:1011–1015, 1955.
81. Daniel ES, Ludwig SL, Lewin KJ, et al: The Cronkhite-Canada syndrome: an analysis of clinical and pathological features and therapy in 55 patients. Medicine (Baltimore) 61:293–309, 1982.
82. Dachman AH, Buck JL, Burke AP, et al: Cronkhite-Canada syndrome: radiologic features. Gastrointest Radiol 14:285–290, 1989.
83. Kilcheski T, Kressel HY, Laufer I, et al: The radiographic appearance of the stomach in Cronkhite-Canada syndrome. Radiology 141:57–60, 1981.
84. Veale AMO, Bussey HJR, Morson BC: Juvenile polyposis coli. J Med Genet 3:5–16, 1966.
85. Sachatello CR, Pickren JW, Grace JT: Generalized juvenile gastrointestinal polyposis. A hereditary syndrome. Gastroenterology 58:699–708, 1970.
86. Jass JR, Williams CB, Bussey HJR, et al: Juvenile polyposis: a precancerous condition. Histopathology 13:619–630, 1988.
87. Hauser H, Ody B, Plojoux O, et al: Radiologic findings in multiple hamartoma syndrome (Cowden disease). Radiology 137:317–323, 1980.
88. Gold BM, Bagla S, Zarrabi MH: Radiologic manifestations of Cowden disease. AJR 135:385–387, 1980.
89. Salmela H: Smooth muscle tumors of the stomach. Acta Chir Scand 134:384–391, 1968.
90. Delikaris P, Golematis B, Missitzis G, et al: Smooth muscle neoplasms of the stomach. South Med J 76:440–442, 1983.
91. Morrissey K, Cho ES, Gray GF, et al: Muscular tumors of the stomach: clinical and pathological study of 113 cases. Ann Surg 178:148–155, 1973.
92. Kavlie H, White TT: Leiomyomas of the upper gastrointestinal tract. Surgery 71:842–848, 1972.
93. Tayiem AK: Recurrent massive gastrointestinal bleeding due to gastric leiomyoma. J Kans Med Soc 81:460–461, 1980.
94. Siegelman SS, Gold JA, Simon M, et al: Ulceration of intramural gastric neoplasms. Am J Dig Dis 14:127–134, 1969.
95. Short WF, Young BR: Roentgen demonstration of prolapse of benign polypoid gastric tumors into the duodenum, including a dumbbell-shaped leiomyoma. AJR 103:317–320, 1968.
96. Grundy A, Rayter Z, Shorthouse AJ: Gastrogastric intussuscepting leiomyomas. Gastrointest Radiol 9:319–321, 1984.
97. Leigh TF: Calcified gastric leiomyoma. Report of a case. Radiology 55:419–422, 1950.
98. Crummy AB, Juhl JH: Calcified gastric leiomyoma. AJR 87:727–728, 1962.
99. Graham JC, Blanchard IT, Scatliff JH: Calcified gastric leiomyoma presenting as a mediastinal mass. AJR 114:529–531, 1972.
100. McGinnis GO: Adenocarcinoma of the stomach with calcification: a case report. Gastroenterology 39:90–93, 1960.
101. Schatzki R, Hawes LE: The roentgenological appearance of extramucosal tumors of the esophagus: analysis of intramural extramucosal lesions of the gastrointestinal tract in general. AJR 48:1–15, 1942.
102. O'Riordan D, Levine MS, Yeager BA: Complete healing of ulceration within a gastric leiomyoma. Gastrointest Radiol 10:47–49, 1985.
103. Cho KJ, Reuter SR: Angiography of duodenal leiomyomas and leiomyosarcomas. AJR 135:31–35, 1980.
104. Herlinger H: The recognition of exogastric tumours. Report of six cases. Br J Radiol 39:25–36, 1966.
105. Stassa G, Klingensmith WC: Primary tumors of the duodenal bulb. AJR 107:105–110, 1969.
106. Lavin P, Hajdu SI, Foote FW: Gastric and extragastric leiomyoblastomas. Clinicopathologic study of 44 cases. Cancer 29:305–311, 1972.
107. Stout AP: Bizarre smooth muscle tumors of the stomach. Cancer 15:400–409, 1962.
108. Abramson DJ: Leiomyoblastomas of the stomach. Surg Gynecol Obstet 136:118–125, 1973.
109. Appelman HD, Helwig EB: Gastric epithelioid leiomyoma and leiomyosarcoma (leiomyoblastoma). Cancer 38:708–728, 1976.
110. Dalaker K, Harket R: Leiomyoblastoma (epithelioid leiomyoma) of the stomach. Acta Chir Scand 146:141–144, 1980.
111. van Steenbergen W, Kojima T, Geboes K, et al: Gastric leiomyoblastoma with metastases to the liver. A 36-year follow-up study. Gastroenterology 89:875–881, 1985.
112. Faegenburg D, Farman J, Dallemand S: Leiomyoblastoma of the stomach. Radiology 117:297–300, 1975.
113. Kelsey JR: Leiomyoblastoma of the stomach presenting as acute intraperitoneal hemorrhage. Gastroenterology 51:539–541, 1966.
114. Choi BI, Ok ID, Im JG, et al: Exogastric cystic leiomyoblastoma with unusual CT appearance. Gastrointest Radiol 13:109–111, 1988.
115. Rogers JV, Adams EK: Gastric lipoma. Radiology 67:84–85, 1956.
116. Culver GJ, Toffolo RR: Criteria for roentgen diagnosis of submucosal gastric lipoma. Radiology 82:254–257, 1964.

117. Turkington RW: Gastric lipoma. Report of a case and review of the literature. Am J Dig Dis 10:719–726, 1965.

118. Maderal F, Hunter F, Fuselier G, et al: Gastric lipomas: an update of clinical presentation, diagnosis, and treatment. Am J Gastroenterol 79:964–967, 1984.

119. Weinberg T, Feldman M: Lipomas of the gastrointestinal tract. Am J Clin Pathol 25:272–281, 1955.

120. Klein N: A prolapsed lipoma in the duodenal bulb. Br J Radiol 23:233–235, 1950.

121. Chu AG, Clifton JA: Gastric lipoma presenting as peptic ulcer: case report and review of the literature. Am J Gastroenterol 78:615–618, 1983.

122. Skorneck AB: Gastric lipoma. Arch Intern Med 89:615–620, 1952.

123. Deeths TM, Madden PN, Dodds WJ: Multiple lipomas of the stomach and duodenum. Dig Dis 20:771–774, 1975.

124. Megibow AJ, Redmond PE, Bosniak MA, et al: Diagnosis of gastrointestinal lipomas by CT. AJR 133:743–745, 1979.

125. Heiken JP, Forde KA, Gold RP: Computed tomography as a definitive method for diagnosing gastrointestinal lipomas. Radiology 142:409–414, 1982.

126. Imoto T, Nobe T, Koga M, et al: Computed tomography of gastric lipomas. Gastrointest Radiol 8:129–131, 1983.

127. Stephens DH, Sheedy PF, Hattery RH, et al: Diagnosis and evaluation of retroperitoneal tumors by computed tomography. AJR 129:395–402, 1977.

128. Gladden JR: Hemangioma of the stomach. Am J Surg 56:495–498, 1942.

129. Marine R, Lattomus WW: Cavernous hemangioma of the gastrointestinal tract. Radiology 70:860–863, 1958.

130. Kerekes ES: Gastric hemangioma. Radiology 82:468–469, 1964.

131. Flannery MG, Caster MP: Hemangioma of the stomach with a roentgenologic diagnostic point. AJR 77:38–39, 1957.

132. Simms SM: Gastric hemangioma associated with phleboliths. Gastrointest Radiol 10:51–53, 1985.

133. Davis JG, Peck H, Gray BL: Lymphangioma of the duodenum. AJR 81:613–615, 1959.

134. Davis M, Fenoglio-Preiser C, Haque AK: Cavernous lymphangioma of the duodenum. Gastrointest Radiol 12:10–12, 1987.

135. Harig BM, Rosen Y, Dallemand S, et al: Glomus tumor of the stomach. Am J Gastroenterol 63:423–428, 1975.

136. Appelman HD, Helwig EB: Glomus tumors of the stomach. Cancer 23:203–213, 1969.

137. Weitzner S: Glomus tumor of the stomach: report of a case and review of the literature. Am J Gastroenterol 51:322–328, 1969.

138. Schneider HJ. Glomus tumor of the stomach. AJR 92:1026–1028, 1964.

139. Canney RL: Neurogenic tumours of the stomach. Br J Surg 36:139–147, 1948.

140. Banks BM: Neurofibroma of the stomach. Gastroenterology 41:158–167, 1950.

141. Perea VD, Gregory LJ: Neurofibromatosis of the stomach. Report of a case associated with von Recklinghausen's disease and review of the literature. JAMA 182:259–263, 1962.

142. Hoare AM, Elkington SG: Gastric lesions in generalized neurofibromatosis. Br J Surg 63:449–451, 1976.

143. Lack EE, Worsham GF, Callihan MD, et al: Granular cell tumor: a clinicopathologic study of 110 patients. J Surg Oncol 13:301–306, 1980.

144. Fisher ER, Wechsler H: Granular cell myoblastoma—a misnomer: electron microscopic and histochemical evidence concerning its Schwann cell derivation and nature (granular cell schwannoma). Cancer 15:936–954, 1962.

145. Johnston J, Helwig EB: Granular cell tumors of the gastrointestinal tract and perianal region: a study of 74 cases. Dig Dis Sci 26:807–816, 1981.

146. Naidech HJ, Axelrod RS, Seliger G: Granular cell tumor (myoblastoma) of the stomach. AJR 113:245–247, 1971.

147. Miranda D: Benign granular cell tumor ("myoblastoma") of the stomach. Am J Gastroenterol 65:344–348, 1976.

148. Schwartz DT, Gaetz HP: Multiple granular cell myoblastomas of the stomach. Am J Clin Pathol 44:453–457, 1965.

149. Helwig EB, Ranier A: Inflammatory fibroid polyps of the stomach. Surg Gynecol Obstet 96:355–367, 1953.

150. Carlson E, Ward JG: Inflammatory gastric polyps (eosinophilic granulomas of the stomach). Am J Surg 99:352–357, 1960.

151. Samter TG, Alstott DF, Kurlander GJ: Inflammatory fibroid polyps of the gastrointestinal tract: a report of 3 cases, 2 occurring in children. Am J Clin Pathol 45:420–436, 1966.

152. Vanek J: Gastric submucosal granuloma with eosinophilic infiltration. Am J Pathol 25:397–407, 1949.

153. Booker RJ, Grant RN: Eosinophilic granuloma of the stomach and small intestine. Surgery 30:388–397, 1951.

154. Salm R: Gastric fibroma with eosinophilic infiltration. Gut 6:85–91, 1965.

155. Bullock WK, Moran ET: Inflammatory fibroid polyps of the stomach. Cancer 6:488–493, 1953.

156. Harned RK, Buck JL, Shekitka KM: Inflammatory fibroid polyps of the gastrointestinal tract: radiologic evaluation. Radiology 182:863–866, 1992.

157. Allman RN, Cavanagh RC, Helwig EB, et al: Inflammatory fibroid polyp. Radiology 127:69–73, 1978.

158. Pearson S: Aberrant pancreas. Arch Surg 63:168–184, 1951.

159. Besemann EF, Auerbach SH, Wolfe WW: The importance of roentgenologic diagnosis of aberrant pancreatic tissue in the gastrointestinal tract. AJR 107:71–76, 1969.

160. Cimmino CV: Gastric adenomyosis vs. aberrant pancreas. Radiology 65:73–77, 1955.

161. Bush WH, Hall DG, Ward BH: Adenomyosis of the gastric antrum in children. Radiology 111:179–181, 1974.

162. Goldberg HI, Margulis AR: Adenomyoma of the stomach. AJR 96:382–386, 1966.

163. Clarke BE: Myoepithelial hamartoma of the gastrointestinal tract. A report of eight cases with comment concerning genesis and nomenclature. Arch Pathol 30:143–151, 1940.

164. Kjellman L: Aberrant pancreas. Acta Radiol 34:225–234, 1950.

165. Copleman B: Aberrant pancreas in the gastric wall. Radiology 81:107–111, 1963.

166. Martinez LO, Gregg M: Aberrant pancreas in the gallbladder. J Can Assoc Radiol 24:234–235, 1973.

167. Tonkin RD, Field TE, Wykes PR: Pancreatic heterotopia as a cause of dyspepsia. Gut 3:135–139, 1962.

168. Abrahams JI: Heterotopic pancreas simulating peptic ulceration. Arch Surg 93:589–592, 1966.

169. Clark RE, Teplick SK: Ectopic pancreas causing massive gastrointestinal hemorrhage. Report of a case diagnosed angiographically. Gastroenterology 69:1331–1333, 1975.

170. Matsumoto Y, Kawai Y, Kimura K: Aberrant pancreas causing pyloric obstruction. Surgery 76:827–829, 1974.

171. Holman E, Wood DA, Stockton AB: Unusual cases of hyperinsulinism and hypoglycemia. Arch Surg 47:165–176, 1943.

172. Green PHR, Barratt PJ, Percy JP, et al: Acute pancreatitis occurring in gastric aberrant pancreatic tissue. Am J Dig Dis 22:734–740, 1977.

173. Littner M, Kirsh I: Aberrant pancreatic tissue in the gastric antrum. Radiology 59:201–211, 1952.

174. Rooney DR: Aberrant pancreatic tissue in the stomach. Radiology 73:241–244, 1959.

175. Kilman WJ, Berk RN: The spectrum of radiographic features of aberrant pancreatic rests involving the stomach. Radiology 123:291–296, 1977.

176. Thoeni RF, Gedgaudas RK: Ectopic pancreas: usual and unusual features. Gastrointest Radiol 5:37–42, 1980.

177. Feldman F, Weinberg T: Aberrant pancreas: a case of duodenal syndrome. JAMA 148:893–898, 1952.

178. Rohrmann CA, Delaney JH, Protell RL: Heterotopic pancreas diagnosed by cannulation and duct study. AJR 128:1044–1045, 1977.

179. Franzin G, Musola R, Ghidini O, et al: Nodular hyperplasia of Brunner's glands. Gastrointest Endosc 31:374–378, 1985.

180. Kaplan EL, Dyson WL, Fitts WT: The relationship of gastric hyperacidity to hyperplasia of Brunner's glands. Arch Surg 98:636–639, 1969.

181. Nelson OF, Whitaker EG, Roberts FM: Adenoma of Brunner's glands. Am J Surg 110:977–980, 1965.

182. Earlam RJ, Cowan WK: Adenoma of Brunner's gland. Br J Surg 53:736–738, 1966.

183. Osborne R, Toffler R, Lowman RM: Brunner's gland adenoma of the duodenum. Am J Dig Dis 18:689–694, 1973.

184. Lempke RE: Intussusception of the duodenum: report of a case due to Brunner's gland hyperplasia. Ann Surg 150:160–166, 1959.

185. ReMine WH, Brown PW, Gomes MMR, et al: Polypoid hamartomas of Brunner's glands. Arch Surg 100:313–316, 1970.

186. Strutynsky N, Posniak R, Mori K: Obstructing hamartoma of Brunner's glands of the duodenum. Dig Dis Sci 27:279–282, 1982.

187. Stephens GL, Harbrecht PJ: Bleeding Brunner gland adenoma of duodenum simulating duodenal ulcer. Ann Surg 148:845–850, 1958.

188. Ponka JL, Shaalan AK: Massive gastrointestinal hemorrhage secondary to tumors of Brunner's glands. Am J Surg 108:51–56, 1964.

189. Erb WH, Johnson TA: Hyperplasia of Brunner's glands simulating duodenal polyposis. Gastroenterology 11:740–745, 1948.

190. Dodd GD, Fishler JS, Park OK: Hyperplasia of Brunner's glands. Report of two cases with review of the literature. Radiology 60:814–823, 1953.

191. Buchanan EB: Nodular hyperplasia of Brunner's glands of the duodenum. Am J Surg 101:253–257, 1961.

192. Weinberg PE, Levin B: Hyperplasia of Brunner's glands. Radiology 84:259–262, 1965.

193. Walk L: Nodular hyperplasia of duodenal Brunner's glands—does it exist? Endoscopy 14:162–165, 1982.

194. Maglinte DDT, Mayes SL, Ng AC, et al: Brunner's gland adenoma: diagnostic considerations. J Clin Gastroenterol 4:127–131, 1982.

195. Merine D, Jones B, Ghahremani GG, et al: Hyperplasia of Brunner glands: the spectrum of its radiographic manifestations. Gastrointest Radiol 16:104–108, 1991.

196. Lempke RE: Intussusception of the duodenum: report of a case due to Brunner's gland hyperplasia. Ann Surg 150:160–166, 1959.

197. Govoni AF: Benign lymphoid hyperplasia of the duodenal bulb. Gastrointest Radiol 1:267–269, 1976.

198. Langkemper R, Hoek AC, Dekker W, et al: Elevated lesions in the duodenal bulb caused by heterotopic gastric mucosa. Radiology 137:621–624, 1980.

199. Agha FP, Ghahremani GG, Tsang TK, et al: Heterotopic gastric mucosa in the duodenum: radiographic findings. AJR 150:291–294, 1988.

200. Gross RE, Holcomb GW, Farber S: Duplications of the alimentary tract. Pediatrics 9:449–468, 1952.

201. Oeconomopoulos CT, Swenson O: Duplications of the gastrointestinal tract. J Pediatr 60:361–368, 1962.

202. Kremer RM, Lepoff RB, Izant RJ: Duplication of the stomach. J Pediatr Surg 5:360–364, 1970.

203. Taft DA, Hairston JT: Duplication of the alimentary tract. Am Surg 42:455–462, 1976.

204. Soper RT, Selke AC: Duplication cyst of the duodenum: case report and discussion. Surgery 68:562–566, 1970.

205. Pruksapong C, Donovan RJ, Pinit A, et al: Gastric duplication. J Pediatr Surg 14:83–85, 1979.

206. Inouye WY, Farrell C, Fitts WT, et al: Duodenal duplication: case report and literature review. Ann Surg 162:910–916, 1965.

207. Leffall LS, Jackson M, Press H, et al: Duplication cyst of the duodenum. Arch Surg 94:30–34, 1967.

208. Agha FP, Gabriele OF, Abdulla FH: Complete gastric duplication. AJR 137:406–407, 1981.

209. Thompson NW, Labow SS: Duplication of the duodenum in the adult. Arch Surg 94:301–306, 1967.

210. Torma MMJ: Of double stomachs. Arch Surg 109:555–557, 1974.

211. Bartels RJ: Duplication of the stomach. Am Surg 33:747–752, 1967.

212. Faegenburg D, Bosniak M: Duodenal anomalies in the adult. AJR 88:642–657, 1962.

213. Kammerer M: Duplication of the stomach resembling hypertrophic pyloric stenosis. JAMA 207:2101–2102, 1969.

214. Parker BC, Guthrie J, France NE, et al: Gastric duplications in infancy. J Pediatr Surg 7:294–298, 1972.

215. Sheppard MD, Gilmour JR: Torsion of a pedunculated gastric cyst. Br Med J 1:874–875, 1945.

216. Kleinhaus S, Boley SJ, Winslow P: Occult bleeding from a perforated gastric duplication in an infant. Arch Surg 116:122, 1981.

217. Mayo HW, McKee EE, Anderson RM: Carcinoma arising in reduplication of the stomach (gastrogenous cyst): a case report. Ann Surg 141:550–555, 1955.

218. Alford BA, Armstron P, Franken EA, et al: Calcification associated with duodenal duplications in children. Radiology 134:647–648, 1980.

219. Omojola MF, Hood IC, Stevenson GW: Calcified gastric duplication. Gastrointest Radiol 5:235, 1980.

220. Bower RJ, Sieber WK, Kiesewetter WB: Alimentary tract duplications in children. Ann Surg 188:669–674, 1978.

221. McAlister WH, Siegel MJ: Duodenal duplication. AJR 152:1328–1329, 1989.

222. Hulnick DH, Balthazar EJ: Gastric duplication cyst: GI series and CT correlation. Gastrointest Radiol 12:106–108, 1987.

223. Kangarloo H, Sample WF, Hansen G, et al: Ultrasonic evaluation of abdominal gastrointestinal tract duplication in children. Radiology 131:191–194, 1979.

224. Bar-Ziv J, Katz R, Nobel M, et al: Duodenal duplication cyst with enteroliths: computed tomography and ultrasound diagnosis. Gastrointest Radiol 14:220–222, 1989.

# Carcinoma

Marc S. Levine, M.D.
Alec J. Megibow, M.D.

## GASTRIC CARCINOMA

There has been a dramatic decline in the incidence of gastric carcinoma during the past 50 years.[1-3] Nevertheless, it remains a deadly disease, with overall 5-year survival rates of less than 20%.[4-9] During the past decade, attention has been focused on the role of double contrast barium studies and endoscopy for the early diagnosis of gastric cancer. The Japanese have had tremendous success in detecting early gastric cancer by mass screening of the adult population with these techniques. However, it is difficult to justify such screening programs outside Japan because of the lower incidence of this malignancy. Thus, the prognosis for gastric carcinoma remains dismal in most parts of the world.

## Epidemiology

Gastric carcinoma has striking geographic variations, with the highest incidences reported in Japan, Chile, Finland, Poland, and Iceland.[3, 10] However, Japanese immigrants and their offspring living in the United States have a significantly lower incidence of gastric cancer than those living in Japan.[10, 11] Such epidemiologic data suggest that environmental factors have a major role in the development of gastric carcinoma. Dietary habits may be particularly important in explaining the observed geographic differences in cancer risk. The high incidence of gastric carcinoma in Japan has been attributed to the heavy consumption of rice and salty foods in the Japanese diet.[12] A high concentration of nitrates in food or drinking water has also been implicated in some parts of the world.[11] Nitrates are converted by bacteria in the stomach to nitrosamines, which have been shown to be carcinogenic agents associated with the development of gastric carcinoma in laboratory rats.[13] Thus, populations with a higher average intake of nitrates probably have a higher gastric cancer risk.

Hereditary factors have also been implicated in gastric cancer patients. For example, these individuals have a higher frequency of blood type A and a lower frequency of blood type O than the general population.[14] Nevertheless, hereditary factors are probably less important than environmental factors in the development of gastric carcinoma.

## Predisposing Conditions

Conditions that are thought to predispose patients to the development of gastric carcinoma include atrophic gastritis, pernicious anemia, gastric polyps, partial gastrectomy, and Ménétrier's disease. However, whether the cancer risk in any of these patients is high enough to warrant routine surveillance is controversial.

### Chronic Atrophic Gastritis and Pernicious Anemia

Atrophic gastritis has been classified into two types, which have different histologic, immunologic, and secretory characteristics. Type A gastritis involves predominantly the gastric fundus and body and is thought to result from immunologic injury by antiparietal cell antibodies, so it is usually associated with pernicious anemia.[15] In contrast, type B gastritis, which is more common, involves predominantly the antrum and usually results from mucosal injury by infectious or toxic agents.[15] Long-term studies indicate that about 10% of patients with type B gastritis develop gastric carcinoma within 10 to 20 years.[16, 17] At surgery, these cancers are often found to arise from pre-existing areas of intestinal metaplasia.[18, 19] Thus, chronic atrophic gastritis and intestinal metaplasia are thought to be important predisposing factors in the development of gastric carcinoma.

Although less common, type A gastritis in patients with pernicious anemia may also be associated with an increased risk of developing gastric carcinoma. In one study, the risk was found to be about three times greater than that in the general population.[20] Most of these cases involved the gastric fundus or body. Although some investigators advocate radiologic or endoscopic surveillance of patients with known pernicious anemia, others believe that the risk of cancer is not high enough to warrant routine screening.[21] Nevertheless, any patient with pernicious anemia who has guaiac-positive stool or other upper gastrointestinal complaints should be evaluated aggressively for possible gastric carcinoma.

## Gastric Polyps

Adenomatous polyps account for less than 20% of all gastric polyps.[22] As in the colon, they are premalignant lesions that are capable of undergoing malignant degeneration via an adenoma-carcinoma sequence.[23] Nearly 50% of adenomatous polyps greater than 2 cm in size are found to harbor carcinomatous foci.[24, 25] All adenomatous polyps should therefore be resected because of the risk of malignant transformation. Nevertheless, adenocarcinoma is about 30 times more common than adenomatous polyps in the stomach, so most gastric cancers are thought to originate de novo and not from pre-existing polyps.[23, 26]

## Partial Gastrectomy

Patients who undergo partial gastrectomy may be at increased risk for the development of gastric carcinoma. A gastric "stump" cancer is defined as a primary carcinoma of the gastric remnant occurring a minimum of 5 years after partial gastrectomy for gastric ulcers or other benign disease.[27] Affected individuals usually have undergone a Billroth II rather than a Billroth I procedure.[28, 29] These tumors tend to be located in the distal portion of the gastric remnant near the gastrojejunal anastomosis. It has been postulated that recurrent bile reflux above the anastomosis causes chronic gastritis, intestinal metaplasia, and, eventually, gastric carcinoma. These cancers usually develop after latent periods of 15 to 25 years from the time of gastric resection. In various studies, the mortality from gastric cancer 15 years or more after partial gastrectomy has been three to seven times greater than that expected for the general population.[29–31] Some authors therefore advocate routine endoscopic surveillance of the gastric remnant starting 15 years after surgery.[30] However, other investigators have found no greater incidence of gastric carcinoma than expected for the general population as long as 25 years after surgery.[32] Thus, the need for surveillance in these patients remains controversial.

Gastric carcinoma has also been reported as a late complication of gastrojejunostomy for benign disease in the absence of partial gastrectomy.[33, 34] As in patients who have undergone a Billroth II procedure, bile reflux gastritis and intestinal metaplasia are thought to be predisposing factors in the development of gastric carcinoma. In any case, patients may be at increased risk for developing gastric carcinoma after gastrojejunostomy without a gastric resection.

## Ménétrier's Disease

Ménétrier's disease is a rare disorder of unknown etiology characterized by a hypertrophic gastropathy associated with decreased gastric acid secretion and protein-losing enteropathy (see Chapter 36). Anecdotal cases of gastric carcinoma have been described in patients with Ménétrier's disease.[35, 36] However, it is unclear whether this association is coincidental or whether Ménétrier's disease is a premalignant condition.

## Pathology

### Gross Features

Most gastric carcinomas are polypoid or ulcerated lesions.[37–39] Polypoid carcinomas may have a plaque-like, lobulated, or fungating appearance. Most such lesions probably arise de novo rather than from pre-existing polyps.[23, 26] Ulcerated carcinomas may contain deep, irregular or broad, shallow areas of ulceration due to necrosis and excavation of the tumor.[37] The ulcer may be surrounded by a thin rind of malignant tissue or by an obvious mass lesion, so that many polypoid tumors have ulcerated components.

Less commonly, gastric carcinomas may be diffusely infiltrative lesions that spread along the gastric wall with relatively little intraluminal growth.[37] These scirrhous tumors may produce a classic linitis plastica appearance due to submucosal thickening and fibrosis incited by the tumor. Other gastric carcinomas may be superficial spreading lesions that are confined to the mucosa or submucosa without invading the deep muscle layers of the gastric wall.[37]

Rarely, patients with gastric carcinoma have multiple primary lesions separated by normal mucosa. In one study, two or more synchronous tumors were present in 2% of 1835 patients with gastric cancer.[40] In such cases, individual lesions may have different morphologic features.

### Histologic Features

More than 95% of malignant tumors in the stomach are adenocarcinomas.[3] The remaining lesions include lymphoma, leiomyosarcoma, Kaposi's sarcoma, carcinoid, and other rare gastric malignancies (see Chapter 39). The majority of adenocarcinomas are of mucous cell origin and are capable of forming glandular structures and secreting mucous substances.[37] Occasionally, excessive mucin accumulates extracellularly in colloid or mucinous adenocarcinomas.[37] Other adenocarcinomas are composed of distinctive signet-ring cells containing large amounts of intracytoplasmic mucin and compressed, eccentric nuclei.[37] As they infiltrate the gastric wall, these signet-ring cells often incite a marked desmoplastic response in the submucosa and muscularis propria, producing the classic pathologic features of a primary scirrhous carcinoma. These scirrhous tumors account for 5 to 15% of all gastric cancers.[7, 9]

Most adenocarcinomas of the stomach are diagnosed at an advanced stage. By definition, advanced lesions have invaded the muscularis propria, and they are usually associated with metastases to regional lymph nodes or other local or distant structures. In contrast, early gastric cancers are defined histologically as cancers in which malignant invasion is limited to the mucosa or submucosa, regardless of the presence of lymph node metastases.[41] The largest number of early gastric cancers has been reported in Japan as a result of mass screening of the adult population. Unlike advanced carcinomas, which have a dismal prognosis, early gastric cancers are curable lesions with 5-year survival rates of more than 90% (see later section on treatment and prognosis).

## Distribution

At one time, most gastric carcinomas were located in the antrum.[42] However, there has been a gradual shift in the distribution of gastric cancer from the antrum proximally to the fundus during the past 50 years.[1, 42, 43] As a result, these lesions now have a relatively even distribution in the stomach, with about 30% located in the antrum, 30% in the body, and 30% in the fundus or cardiac region.[1, 8, 9, 43] The remaining 10% are diffusely infiltrating lesions involving the entire stomach. This changing pattern of disease has important implications for cancer detection, as radiologists and endoscopists must meticulously evaluate the gastric cardia and fundus for signs of malignancy.

## Routes of Spread

Gastric carcinoma may invade local, regional, or distant structures by four pathways: direct extension, lymphatic spread, intraperitoneal seeding, and hematogenous metastases. The various pathways of spread are discussed separately in the next sections.

## Direct Extension

Gastric carcinoma has a marked tendency to involve contiguous structures such as the liver, pancreas, and spleen.[39] Longitudinal spread of tumor along the gastrointestinal tract is also relatively common; the distal esophagus is directly involved by carcinoma of the cardia in about 60% of patients,[44] whereas the duodenum is involved by carcinoma of the antrum in 13 to 18% of patients.[37, 45] Tumor involving the greater curvature of the stomach may spread inferiorly via the gastrocolic ligament to the transverse colon, occasionally resulting in the development of a gastrocolic fistula.[46, 47]

## Lymphatic Spread

Because of the abundant lymphatics in the stomach, lymph node metastases are found in 74 to 88% of patients with gastric carcinoma.[37] These patients may initially have involvement of local (perigastric) nodes and, subsequently, regional (celiac, hepatic, left gastric, and splenic) or distant (left supraclavicular and left axillary) nodes.[10] The frequency of lymphatic metastases is related to the size and depth of penetration of the tumor. Nevertheless, lesions may be classified as early gastric cancers, regardless of the presence of lymph

node metastases, if malignant invasion is confined to the mucosa or submucosa.[41]

## Intraperitoneal Seeding

Patients with gastric carcinoma may have intraperitoneally seeded metastases to the rectosigmoid colon, cecum, small bowel, or other sites in the abdomen. In advanced cases, diffuse carcinomatosis may be associated with small bowel obstruction and ascites. Some patients with signet-ring cell adenocarcinomas may have bilateral drop metastases to the ovaries, known as Krukenberg tumors.[48] Although other malignancies can metastasize to the ovaries, gastric carcinoma is responsible for the majority of cases.[48] Some of these patients may present with bilateral ovarian masses as the initial manifestation of their disease.

## Hematogenous Metastases

Because the stomach is drained by the portal vein, the liver is the most common site of hematogenous or blood-borne metastases from gastric carcinoma.[39] Other less common sites of hematogenous spread include the lungs, adrenals, kidneys, bones, and brain.

## Clinical Aspects

Gastric carcinoma is usually considered a disease of middle and late life, with a peak incidence between 50 and 70 years of age.[10, 38, 49] However, 3 to 5% of patients with gastric cancer are younger than 35 years of age and 1% are younger than 30.[49–52] Furthermore, the percentage of young patients with gastric cancer has more than doubled since 1970.[52] These tumors tend to be more aggressive lesions in young patients, with a worse prognosis than gastric carcinoma in general.[52, 53] It is therefore important not to be lulled into a false sense of security about the possibility of malignancy because of the patient's age.

Gastric carcinoma is twice as common in men as in women.[2, 6, 10] However, carcinoma of the cardia has a much greater predilection for men (7:1) than carcinoma elsewhere in the stomach.[54] The explanation for this discrepancy is unclear.

Most patients with gastric carcinoma are symptomatic only when they have advanced lesions with local or distant metastases.[10, 11] The most common presenting findings include epigastric pain, bloating, early satiety, nausea, vomiting, anorexia, weight loss, a palpable epigastric mass, and signs or symptoms of upper gastrointestinal bleeding, such as hematemesis, melena, guaiac-positive stool, and iron deficiency anemia.[10, 11, 38] However, these findings may be caused by a variety of benign conditions such as ulcers and gastritis. As a result, there is often a considerable lag time between the onset of symptoms and the diagnosis of gastric cancer.

The clinical presentation is also affected by the location and morphologic features of the tumor. Most patients with carcinoma of the cardia present with recent onset of dysphagia, particularly for solids.[55-57] Dysphagia may be caused by tumor obstructing the cardia, whether or not the lesion has invaded the esophagus. Some patients may complain of food sticking behind the lower sternum, but others may have a sensation of blockage referred to the thoracic inlet or pharynx. The gastric cardia and fundus should therefore be carefully evaluated in all patients with dysphagia, regardless of location, to rule out a carcinoma of the cardia masquerading as a pharyngeal or esophageal disorder.

Early satiety is a particularly common complaint in patients with primary scirrhous carcinomas.[58] Nausea and vomiting are also common findings, not because of gastric outlet obstruction but because of the decreased capacity of a stomach that is diffusely infiltrated by tumor.[58] Paradoxically, gastric emptying may be more rapid than normal in these patients.

Other patients with advanced gastric cancer may initially present with signs or symptoms of metastatic disease, such as anorexia, weight loss, abdominal masses, hepatic enlargement, jaundice, ascites, back pain, or neurologic findings.[11] Patients with ovarian metastases may have bilateral pelvic masses (Krukenberg tumors), and patients with drop metastases to the rectosigmoid colon may have a Blumer shelf found on rectal examination. For reasons that are unclear, the anorexia associated with advanced gastric cancer is often characterized by a selective distaste for beef products.[11]

## Endoscopic Findings

When biopsy specimens and brushings are obtained, endoscopy has a reported overall sensitivity of 94 to 98% in diagnosing gastric carcinoma.[59-62] However, multiple biopsy specimens (at least seven) should be taken from suspicious lesions to decrease the risk of sampling error.[61] It should also be recognized that endoscopy is a much less reliable technique for diagnosing scirrhous tumors. In various series, the sensitivity of endoscopy in detecting these lesions has ranged from only 33 to 70%.[63-65] False-negative endoscopic biopsy specimens or brushings may occur not only because scirrhous tumors are located predominantly in the submucosa but also because the tumor cells are often separated by large areas of fibrosis. In some cases, three or more endoscopic examinations may be required for a definitive histologic diagnosis.[65] Thus, excessive reliance on negative endoscopic findings may lead to a significant delay in the diagnosis and treatment of these tumors.

## Radiographic Findings

### Early Gastric Cancer

The double contrast upper gastrointestinal examination has been widely recognized as the best radiologic technique for diagnosing early gastric cancer.[66-69] The Japanese Endoscopic Society has divided these lesions into three basic types.[70] Type I lesions are elevated lesions that protrude more than 5 mm into the lumen. Type II lesions are superficial lesions that are further subdivided into three groups, types IIa, IIb, and IIc, depending on their morphologic features. Type IIa lesions are elevated but protrude less than 5 mm into the lumen. Type IIb lesions are essentially flat. Type IIc lesions are slightly depressed but do not penetrate beyond the muscularis mucosae. Type III lesions are true mucosal ulcerations, with the ulcer penetrating the muscularis mucosae but not the muscularis propria. When early gastric cancers exhibit more than one of these morphologic features, they may have a dual classification, with the most predominant pattern listed first (i.e., type III + IIc).

Type I early gastric cancers typically appear as small, elevated lesions in the stomach.[67, 68] Because adenomatous polyps may undergo malignant degeneration (see earlier section on gastric polyps), the possibility of early gastric cancer should be suspected for any sessile or pedunculated polyps greater than 1 cm in size. Other type I lesions may protrude considerably into the lumen and still be classified histologically as early gastric cancers[68] (Fig. 38-1A). Thus, polypoid carcinomas cannot be definitively diagnosed as early or advanced lesions on the basis of the radiographic findings.

Type II early gastric cancers are superficial lesions with elevated (IIa), flat (IIb), or depressed (IIc) components. These lesions may be manifested by plaque-like elevations, mucosal nodularity, shallow areas of ulceration, or some combination of these findings[66-69] (Fig. 38-1B and C). Occasionally, type II lesions may be quite extensive and involve a considerable surface area of the stomach.

Type III early gastric cancers are typically characterized by shallow, irregular ulcer craters with nodularity of the adjacent mucosa and clubbing, fusion, or amputation of radiating folds[67, 68] (Fig. 38-1D). Careful analysis of the radiographic findings usually allows these lesions to be distinguished from benign gastric ulcers, which have different radiographic features (see Chapter 35). Although some lesions with an equivocal or suspicious appearance are found to be benign ulcers, endoscopy and biopsy should be performed for all lesions with suspicious radiographic findings to avoid missing early cancers.

About 70% of the ulcers in type IIc or III early gastric cancers are reported to undergo significant healing on medical treatment.[71] It has been postulated that these cancers are characterized by a cycle of ulceration, healing, and recurrent ulceration. Rarely, complete healing of malignant ulcers has also been described.[71] However, malignancy may still be suspected on follow-up barium studies if mucosal nodularity or other abnormalities are detected at the site of the previous ulcer.

The Japanese have reported an incidence of early gastric cancer (i.e., the percentage of all gastric cancers that are detected as early lesions) of 25 to 46%[72-75] compared with an incidence of only 5 to 24% in Western countries.[67-69, 76-82] This discrepancy can be attributed to mass screening of the adult population in Japan because of the unusually high prevalence of gastric carcinoma in that country. Occasionally, however, early gastric can-

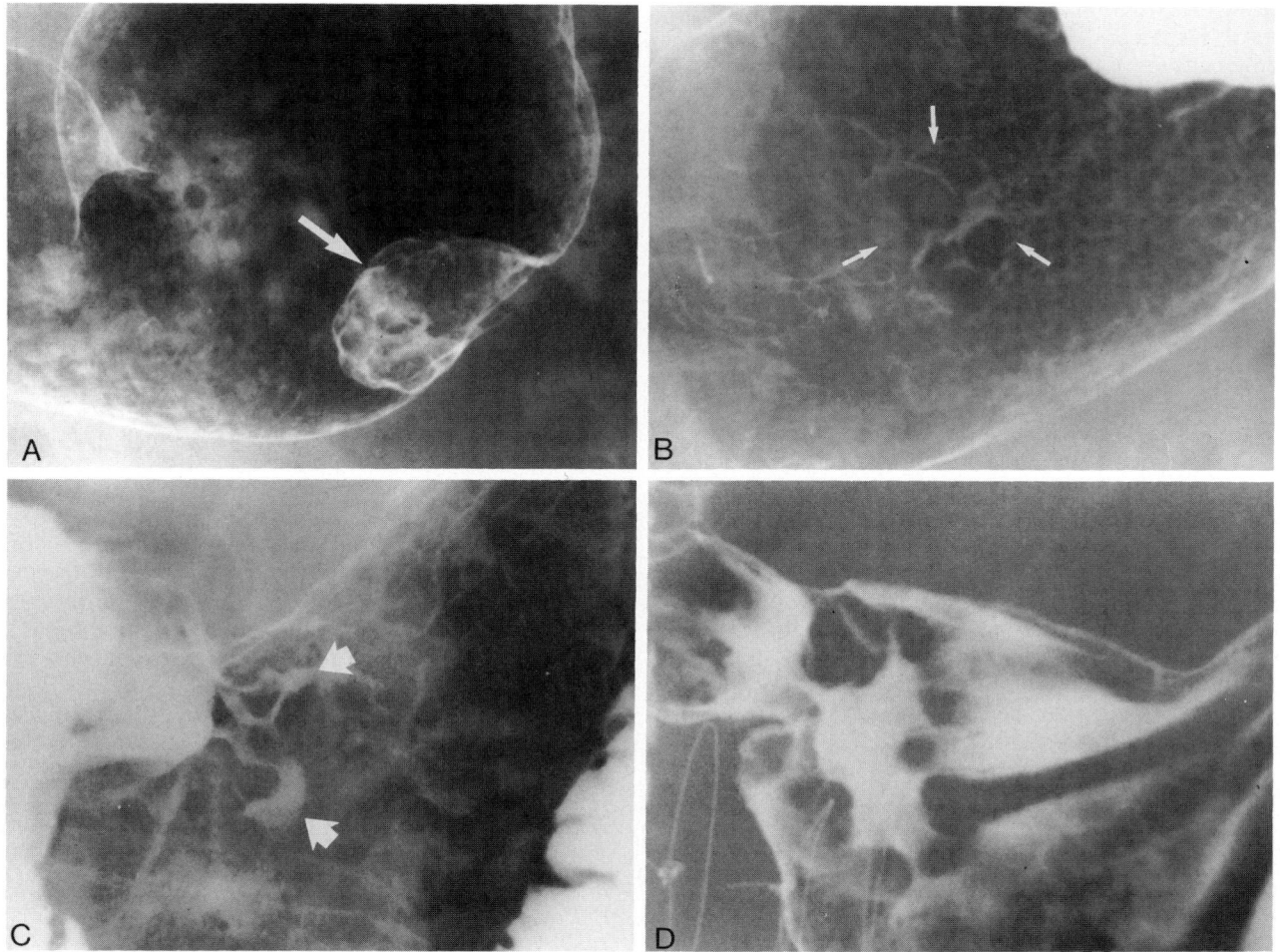

**Figure 38–1. Early gastric cancers. A.** A type I lesion is seen as a polypoid mass *(arrow)* on the greater curvature of the gastric body. Despite its size, this lesion was found to be an early cancer. (Courtesy of Kyunghee C. Cho, M.D., Newark, NJ.) **B.** A type IIa lesion is manifested by a focal cluster of shallow elevations and nodules *(arrows)* in the gastric body. **C.** A type IIc lesion is manifested by shallow, irregular areas of ulceration and nodularity *(arrows)* in the gastric antrum. **D.** A type III lesion is seen as a scalloped, irregular antral ulcer with nodular, clubbed folds surrounding the ulcer crater. (**D** from Levine MS, Creteur V, Kressel HY, et al: Benign gastric ulcers: diagnosis and follow-up with double-contrast radiography. Radiology 164:9–13, 1987.)

cers may be detected in symptomatic patients with epigastric pain, upper gastrointestinal bleeding, or other complaints.[69] Early gastric cancers may also be fortuitous findings in patients who undergo radiologic or endoscopic examinations for other reasons. Nevertheless, radiologists and endoscopists in the West are unlikely to detect a significant number of early gastric cancers as long as these examinations are performed predominantly on symptomatic patients.[69]

## Advanced Carcinoma

### Plain Films

Polypoid gastric carcinomas are occasionally recognized on abdominal plain films by the presence of a soft tissue mass indenting the gastric shadow (Fig. 38–2A). Primary scirrhous carcinomas may also be recognized by a narrowed, tubular configuration of the gas-filled stomach (Fig. 38–2B). Rarely, mucin-producing scirrhous carcinomas contain gross areas of calcification that have a stippled, punctate, or sand-like appearance on abdominal plain films[83–86] (Fig. 38–3A). This calcification is thought to occur in areas of necrosis or mucinous degeneration within the tumor.[84, 85] When abdominal plain films raise suspicion of gastric carcinoma, barium studies should be performed for a more definitive diagnosis (Fig. 38–3B). Computed tomography (CT) is also a particularly sensitive technique for demonstrating calcification in these tumors (Fig. 38–3C).

### Barium Studies

Advanced gastric carcinomas may appear as polypoid, ulcerative, or infiltrating lesions. However, many lesions have mixed morphologic features, so there is considerable overlap in the classification of these tumors. Be-

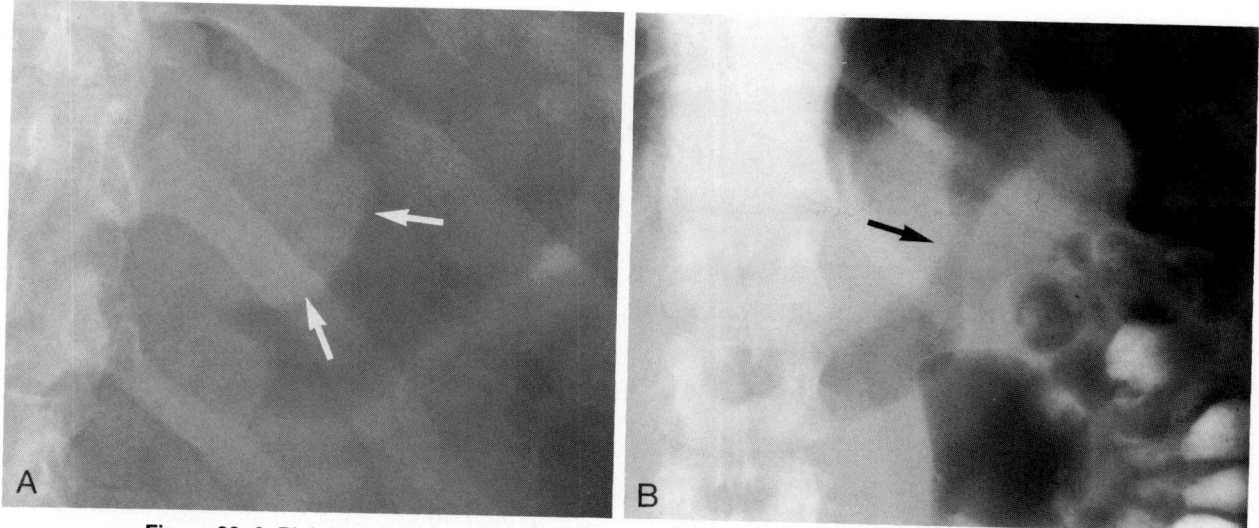

**Figure 38–2. Plain film findings of gastric carcinoma. A.** A close-up view from an abdominal plain film shows a soft tissue mass *(arrows)* indenting the lesser curvature of the gas-filled stomach. This was a polypoid gastric carcinoma. **B.** In another patient, the gas-filled stomach has a narrowed, tubular appearance *(arrow)* due to a scirrhous carcinoma (linitis plastica).

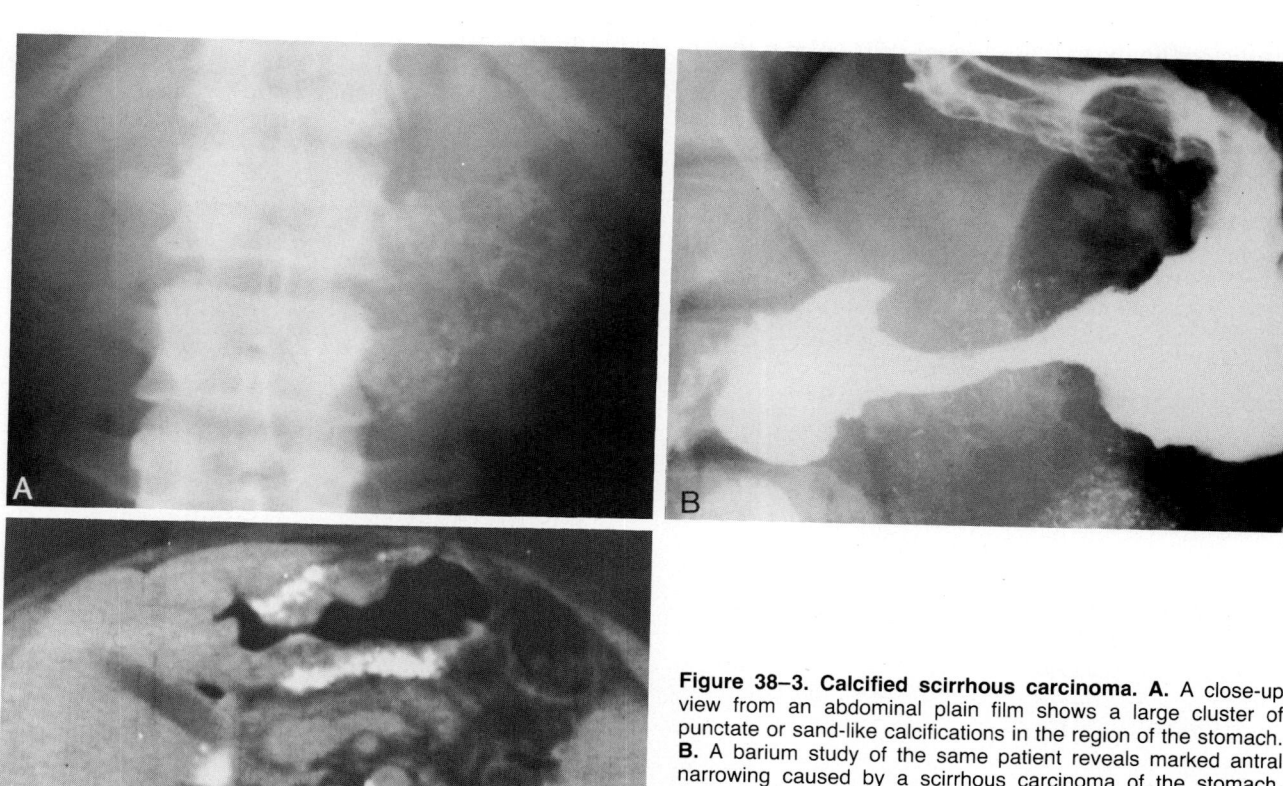

**Figure 38–3. Calcified scirrhous carcinoma. A.** A close-up view from an abdominal plain film shows a large cluster of punctate or sand-like calcifications in the region of the stomach. **B.** A barium study of the same patient reveals marked antral narrowing caused by a scirrhous carcinoma of the stomach. Again note multiple calcifications in this mucin-producing tumor. **C.** A CT scan shows lobulated thickening of the gastric wall with extensive calcification in another patient with scirrhous carcinoma. (**C** courtesy of Eugene Libson, M.D., Jerusalem, Israel.)

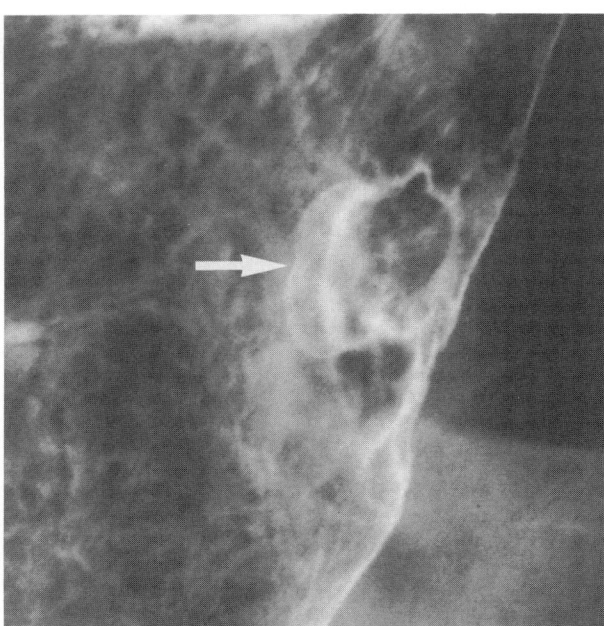

**Figure 38–4. Polypoid gastric carcinoma.** A polypoid mass *(arrow)* is seen on the greater curvature of the stomach.

cause scirrhous carcinomas and cardiac carcinomas lead to distinctive findings, these lesions are considered separately in later sections.

Polypoid carcinomas appear as lobulated or fungating masses that protrude into the lumen (Figs. 38–4 and 38–5). On double contrast studies, lesions on the dependent or posterior wall are seen as filling defects in the barium pool, whereas lesions on the nondependent or anterior wall are etched in white by a thin layer of barium trapped between the edge of the mass and the adjacent mucosa. These tumors often contain one or more irreg-

ular areas of ulceration. Some bulky lesions may encroach significantly on the lumen, but gastric outlet obstruction is an uncommon complication. Rarely, two or more synchronous carcinomas are detected in the stomach[40, 87] (see Fig. 38–5). Polypoid antral carcinomas occasionally prolapse through the pylorus into the duodenum, appearing as mass lesions at the base of the bulb (Fig. 38–6).

Ulcerated carcinomas are those in which the bulk of the tumor mass has been replaced by ulceration (Figs. 38–7 and 38–8). Although these lesions are often called malignant ulcers, the term is a misnomer because it is not the ulcer but the surrounding tumor that is malignant. In general, malignant ulcers are characterized en face by an irregular ulcer crater eccentrically located in a rind of malignant tissue.[88, 89] The ulcers may have scalloped, angular, or stellate borders. Discrete tumor nodules are often seen in the adjacent mucosa. Folds converging to the edge of the ulcer may be blunted, nodular, clubbed, or fused as a result of tumor infiltration.[88, 89] On double contrast studies, malignant ulcers on the nondependent or anterior wall may be etched in white, so a double ring shadow is observed in the stomach, with the outer ring representing the edge of the tumor and the inner ring representing the edge of the ulcer (see Fig. 38–7A). In such cases, prone compression views should demonstrate filling of the ulcer crater within a discrete tumor mass on the anterior wall (see Fig. 38–7B). A biphasic examination is therefore essential for detecting these lesions.

When viewed in profile, malignant ulcers usually have

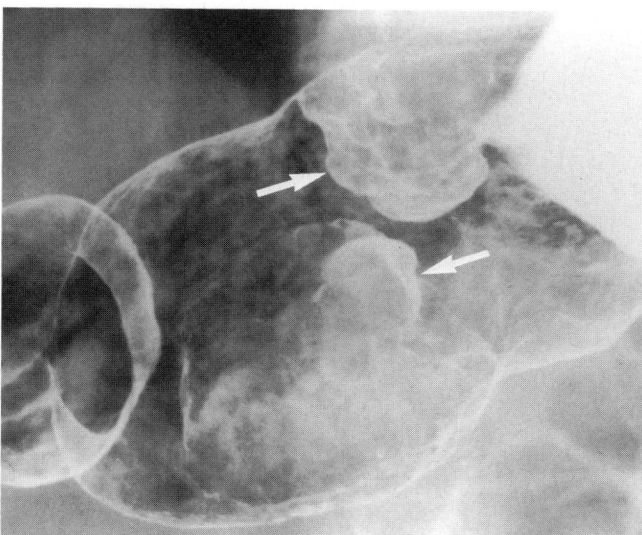

**Figure 38–5. Synchronous gastric carcinomas.** Two discrete polypoid masses *(arrows)* are seen in the stomach due to separate primary gastric carcinomas.

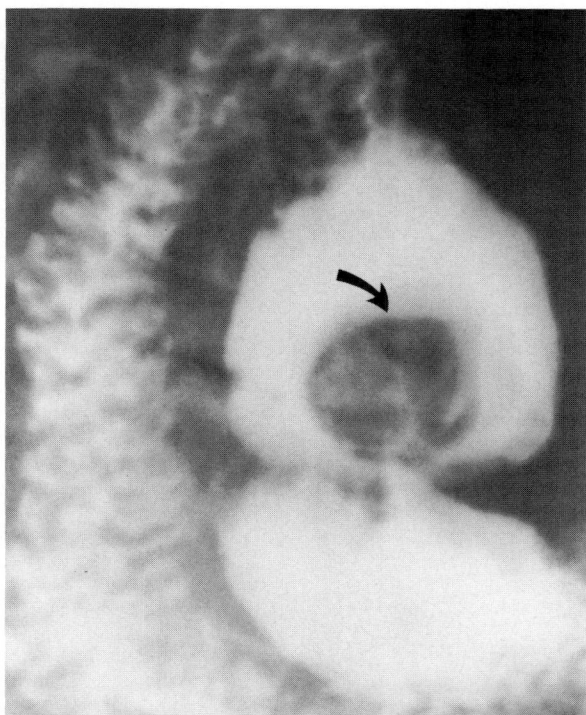

**Figure 38–6. Prolapsed antral carcinoma.** A polypoid mass *(arrow)* is seen at the base of the duodenal bulb. This patient had an antral carcinoma that had prolapsed into the duodenum.

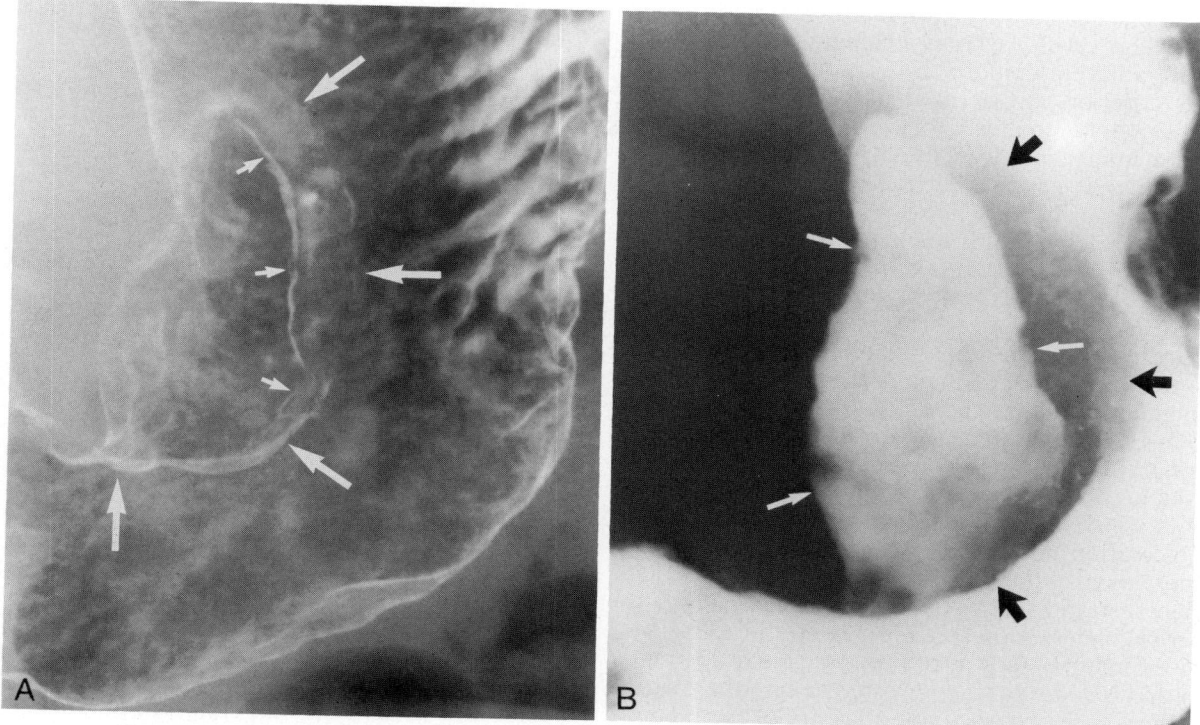

**Figure 38–7. Ulcerated gastric carcinoma. A.** A double contrast view of the stomach shows a relatively large mass that is etched in white *(large arrows)* near the lesser curvature of the gastric body. Also note a second curvilinear density *(small arrows)* due to barium coating the rim of an unfilled central ulcer. **B.** A prone compression view shows the mass as a radiolucent filling defect *(black arrows)* on the anterior wall of the stomach. Note how the central ulcer *(white arrows)* fills with barium when the patient is in the prone position. The ulcer has a convex inner border and an apparent intraluminal location, demonstrating the features of a Carman-Kirkland meniscus complex.

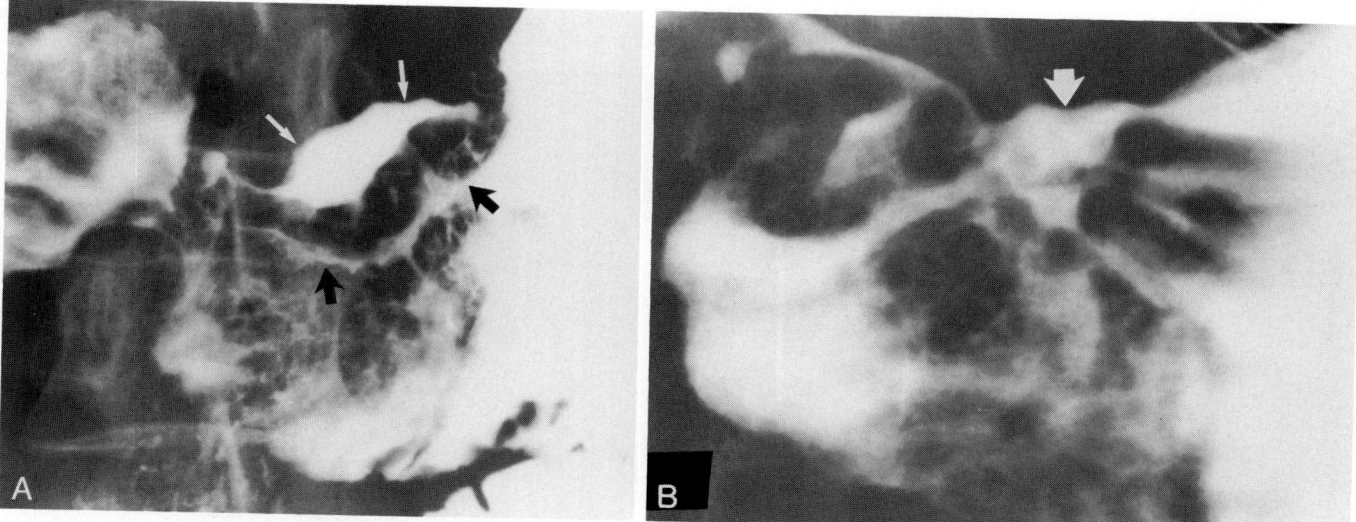

**Figure 38–8. Malignant gastric ulcers. A.** A meniscoid ulcer *(white arrows)* is seen on the lesser curvature of the antrum. Note the rind of malignant tumor *(black arrows)* surrounding the ulcer. **B.** Another malignant ulcer *(arrow)* is seen on the lesser curvature of the antrum. This ulcer has an apparent intraluminal location. Also note how the folds converging to the ulcer have a clubbed, nodular appearance due to infiltration by tumor.

an intraluminal location, often within a discrete tumor mass (see Fig. 38–8), whereas benign ulcers project beyond the adjacent contour of the stomach.[88, 89] However, this criterion can be used only for ulcers on or near the lesser or greater curvature. The tumor mass surrounding malignant ulcers usually forms acute angles with the adjacent gastric wall rather than the obtuse, gently sloping angles expected for a benign mound of edema.[88, 89] Abnormal folds may also be seen radiating to the edge of the ulcer crater or to the edge of the surrounding mass as a result of tumor infiltrating the folds (see Fig. 38–8B).

No sign in gastrointestinal radiology has generated more confusion or disagreement than the meniscus sign of a malignant ulcer, which was originally described by Carman in 1921[90] and refined by Kirkland in 1934.[91] The Carman-Kirkland meniscus complex is caused by a cancer straddling the lesser curvature of the gastric antrum or body in which the tumor is a broad, flat lesion with central ulceration and elevated margins. Manipulation and compression of the lesion at fluoroscopy may result in the demonstration of a discrete ulcer crater that has a meniscoid configuration (see Figs. 38–7B and 38–8A). The convex inner border of the meniscus may be quite irregular and is almost always directed toward the gastric lumen, whereas the concave outer border of the meniscus, representing the base of the broad, shallow ulcer, tends to be smoother and usually does not project beyond the expected gastric contour.[88, 89] A radiolucent halo may be seen adjacent to the meniscus as a result of apposition of the elevated edges of the tumor on the anterior and posterior walls. Although the Carman-Kirkland meniscus complex is a reliable radiologic sign of malignancy, it can be demonstrated in only a small percentage of all malignant ulcers in the stomach. The radiographic criteria for differentiating benign and malignant ulcers are discussed further in Chapter 35.

Infiltrating carcinomas are manifested by irregular narrowing of the stomach with nodularity and spicula-

tion of the mucosa (Fig. 38–9). Some infiltrating lesions may have polypoid or ulcerated components. In advanced cases, these lesions may cause gastric outlet obstruction.

About 15% of antral carcinomas involve the duodenum by direct extension of tumor from the distal antrum.[37, 45] Duodenal involvement may be manifested radiographically by mass effect, nodularity, ulceration, or irregular narrowing of the proximal duodenum. Rarely, advanced gastric carcinomas on the greater curvature of the stomach may spread inferiorly via the gastrocolic ligament to the superior border of the transverse colon, resulting in the development of a gastrocolic fistula.[46, 47] Although these fistulas may occasionally be demonstrated by an upper gastrointestinal study, they are more likely to be demonstrated by a barium enema because of the higher pressures generated during this examination.

### SCIRRHOUS CARCINOMA

Scirrhous gastric carcinomas are almost always thought to involve the distal half of the stomach, arising near the pylorus and gradually extending upward from the antrum into the body and fundus.[58, 92] These tumors are classically manifested radiographically by irregular narrowing and rigidity of the stomach, producing a linitis plastica or "leather bottle" appearance[58, 92] (Fig. 38–10). In advanced cases, the stomach may be diffusely infiltrated by tumor. Other patients may have localized scirrhous tumors that are confined to the prepyloric region of the antrum, appearing as short, annular lesions with shelf-like proximal borders[93] (Fig. 38–11). Surprisingly, it is difficult to find cases in the literature of lesions involving the proximal stomach on upper gastrointestinal examinations. With double contrast technique, however, nearly 40% of patients with these scirrhous tumors have localized lesions in the gastric fundus or body with antral sparing[65] (Figs. 38–12 and 38–13). Detection of these lesions is presumably related

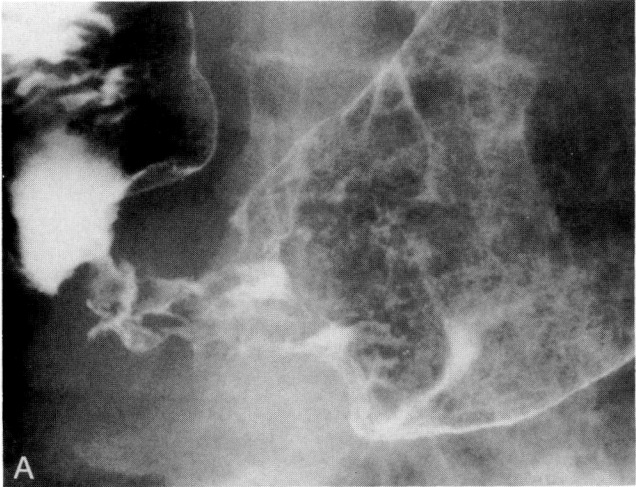
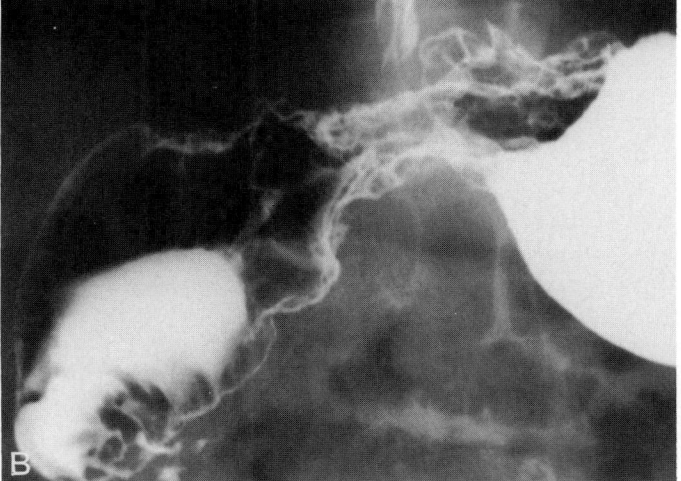

**Figure 38–9. Infiltrating gastric carcinomas. A.** There are irregular narrowing and ulceration of the antrum due to an advanced, infiltrating carcinoma. **B.** In another patient, an infiltrating cancer of the proximal stomach causes marked narrowing and spiculation of the upper body.

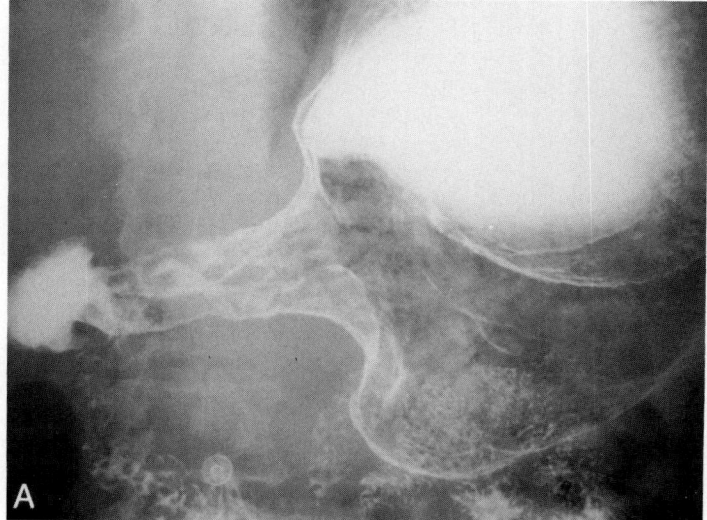

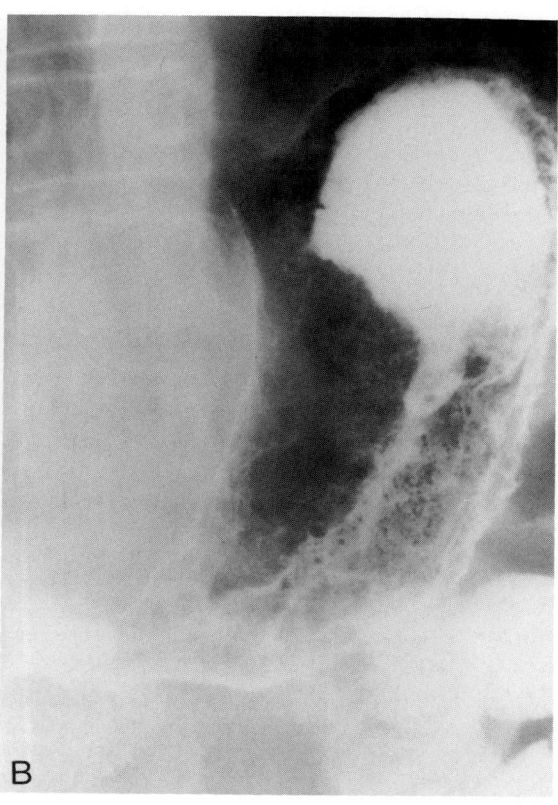

**Figure 38–10. Scirrhous carcinomas of the stomach. A.** There are marked narrowing and rigidity of the antrum due to infiltration of the wall by tumor. **B.** In another patient, there is encasement of the entire stomach by a scirrhous tumor, producing a diffuse linitis plastica appearance.

to gaseous distention of the proximal stomach on double contrast studies. In any case, radiologists should be aware that a significant percentage of patients with scirrhous tumors have localized lesions involving the gastric fundus or body rather than the classic form of linitis plastica involving the distal stomach.

Although scirrhous carcinomas are classically manifested by gastric narrowing and rigidity, some tumors may cause only mild loss of distensibility. Instead, these lesions may be recognized on double contrast studies primarily by distortion of the normal surface pattern of the stomach with mucosal nodularity, spiculation, ulcer-

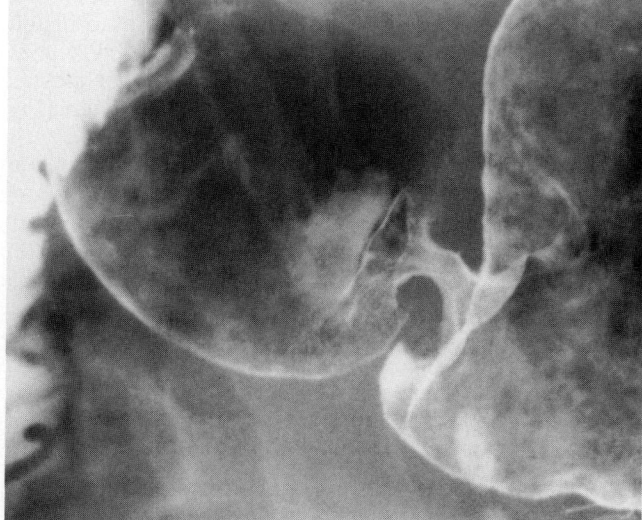

**Figure 38–11. Localized scirrhous carcinoma of the distal antrum.** There is a short, annular lesion in the prepyloric region of the antrum. Note how the lesion has an abrupt, shelf-like proximal border.

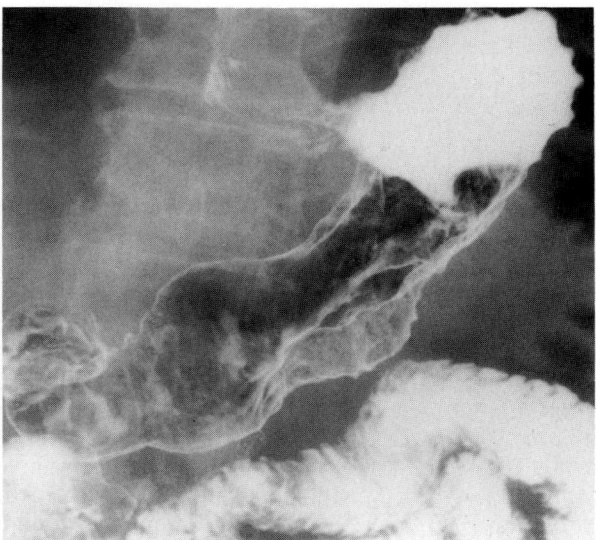

**Figure 38–12. Localized scirrhous carcinoma of the proximal half of the stomach.** There is irregular narrowing of the fundus and body with sparing of the antrum.

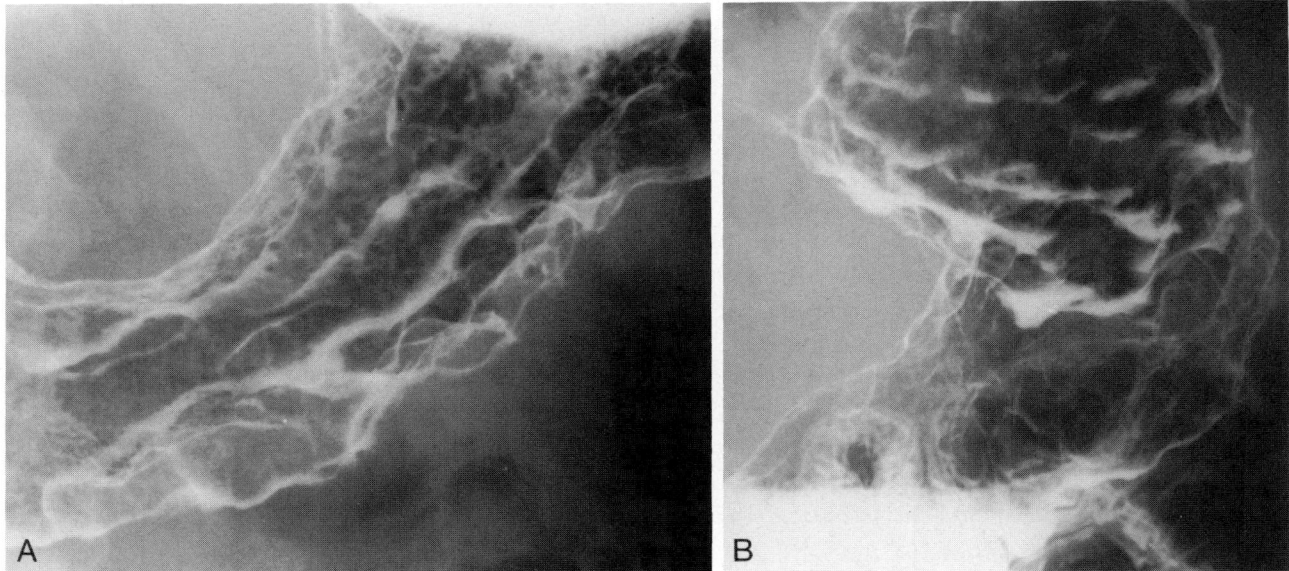

**Figure 38–13. Scirrhous carcinomas of the proximal stomach with thickened folds. A.** This patient has a localized scirrhous carcinoma of the gastric body. The tumor has caused only mild loss of distensibility. However, there is distortion of the normal surface pattern of the stomach with thickened, irregular folds and mucosal nodularity. (From Levine MS, Kong V, Rubesin SE, et al: Scirrhous carcinoma of the stomach: radiologic and endoscopic diagnosis. Radiology 175:151–154, 1990.) **B.** In another patient, a scirrhous carcinoma of the fundus and body is manifested by thickened, lobulated folds without significant narrowing.

ation, or thickened, irregular folds[65] (see Fig. 38–13). Thus, some lesions are likely to be missed if the radiologist relies too heavily on gastric narrowing as the major criterion for diagnosing these tumors.

### CARCINOMA OF THE CARDIA

Tumors arising at the cardia are notoriously difficult to detect on conventional single contrast barium studies. Because the overlying rib cage precludes manual palpation or compression of the fundus, even large lesions at the cardia may be obscured by crowded folds or relatively opaque barium that prevents adequate visualization of this region. With double contrast technique, however, it is possible to evaluate the normal anatomic landmarks at the cardia and surrounding gastric mucosa for signs of malignancy. As a result, double contrast barium studies may detect lesions at the cardia that are missed on conventional single contrast examinations.[94–98]

When viewed en face, the normal cardia often appears on double contrast studies as a circular elevation containing four or five stellate folds that radiate to a central button at the gastroesophageal junction (the cardiac "rosette")[95, 96] (see Fig. 38–22B). Some lesions at the cardia may be recognized only by relatively subtle nodularity, mass effect, or ulceration in this region with distortion, effacement, or obliteration of these landmarks[95–98] (Fig. 38–14). Enlargement or lobulation of the surrounding elevation should also suggest a neoplastic lesion. Finally, the protrusion surrounding a normal cardia should disappear when barium is swallowed, as this landmark is obliterated by relaxation of the lower esophageal sphincter.[96] A lesion should therefore be suspected if the protrusion persists during passage of the barium bolus at fluoroscopy. Conversely, an apparent abnormality at the cardia must be an artifact if it vanishes as the cardia opens.

Advanced carcinomas of the gastric cardia or fundus are usually exophytic or infiltrating lesions. Exophytic tumors appear as bulky, lobulated intraluminal masses in the gastric fundus, often containing irregular areas of ulceration.[98, 99] In contrast, infiltrating lesions are manifested by thickened, nodular folds and decreased distensibility of the fundus.[98, 99] Advanced tumors may completely encase the fundus, producing a linitis plastica appearance with a small, irregular residual lumen (Fig. 38–15).

When an equivocal or suspicious lesion is detected in the region of the gastric cardia or fundus, endoscopy should be performed for a definitive diagnosis. Nevertheless, radiographically demonstrated lesions at the cardia may occasionally be missed on endoscopy.[100] The barium study should therefore be repeated despite a negative endoscopic examination, if the initial study suggests a malignant lesion. Rarely, some patients with continuing radiologic evidence of malignancy may require surgery without preoperative histologic confirmation.

Secondary esophageal involvement by advanced lesions may be manifested radiographically by a polypoid or fungating mass that extends from the fundus into the distal esophagus or by thickened folds or irregular narrowing of the distal esophagus without a discrete

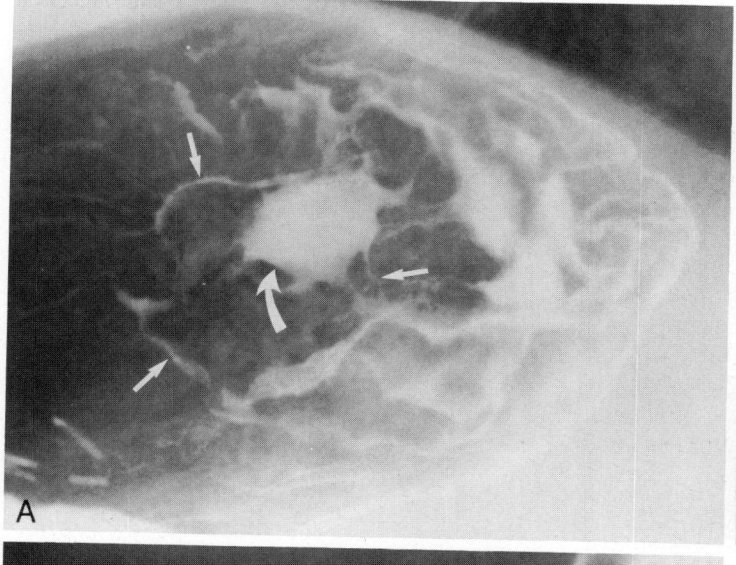

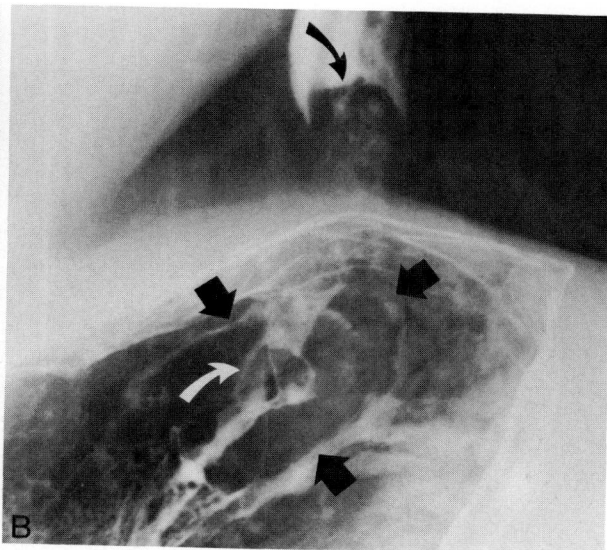

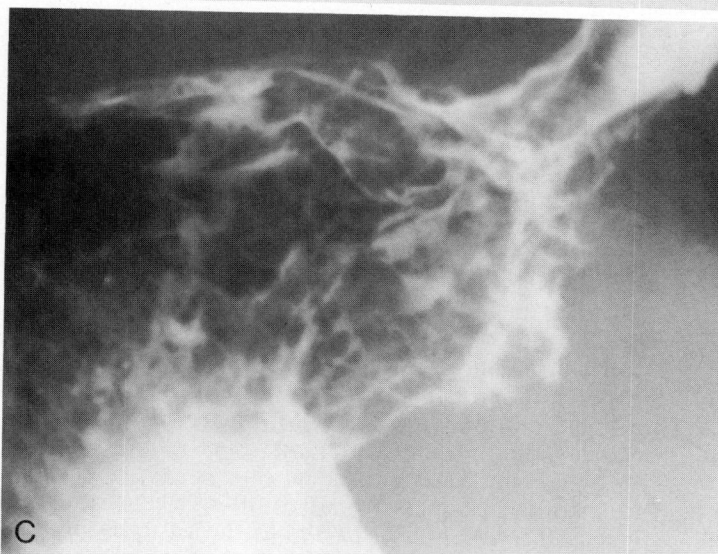

**Figure 38–14. Carcinoma of the cardia. A.** The normal anatomic landmarks at the cardia have been obliterated and replaced by a plaque-like lesion *(straight arrows)* containing a shallow area of ulceration *(curved arrow).* **B.** In another patient, the cardiac rosette has been replaced by a relatively flat mass *(straight black arrows)* with a central ulcer *(white arrow).* The tumor extends into the distal esophagus *(curved black arrow).* (**B** from MS Levine, I Laufer, JJ Thompson, Carcinoma of the gastric cardia in young people, AJR, 140, 1, 69–72, 1983, © by American Roentgen Ray Society.) **C.** In a third patient, there is diffuse nodularity in the fundus with obliteration of the normal cardiac landmarks. Also note involvement of the distal esophagus.

**Figure 38–15. Secondary achalasia caused by gastric carcinoma. A.** There is smooth, tapered narrowing of the distal esophagus, producing the classic beak-like appearance of achalasia. **B.** However, a radiograph of the stomach reveals an advanced, scirrhous carcinoma of the gastric fundus that has invaded the distal esophagus.

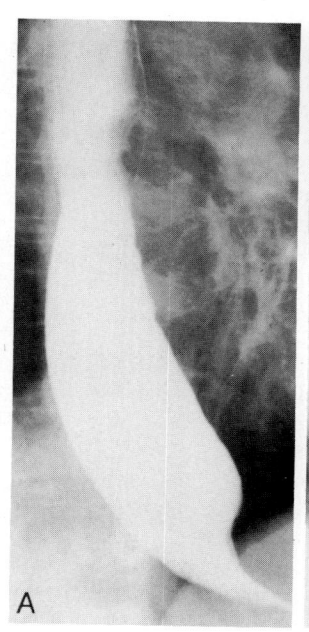

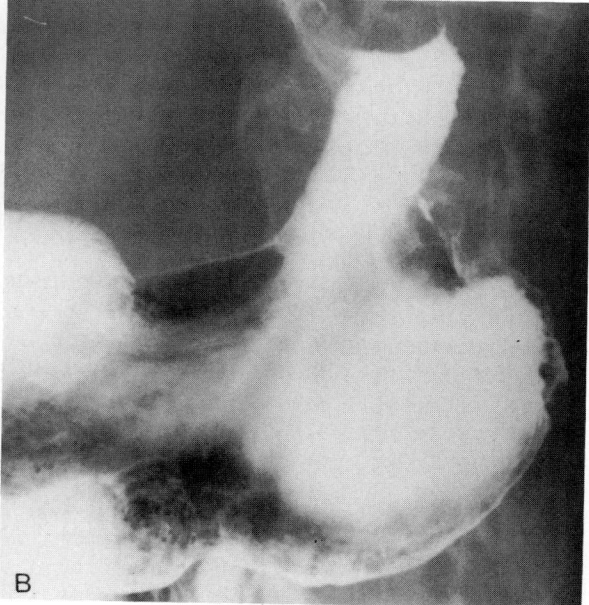

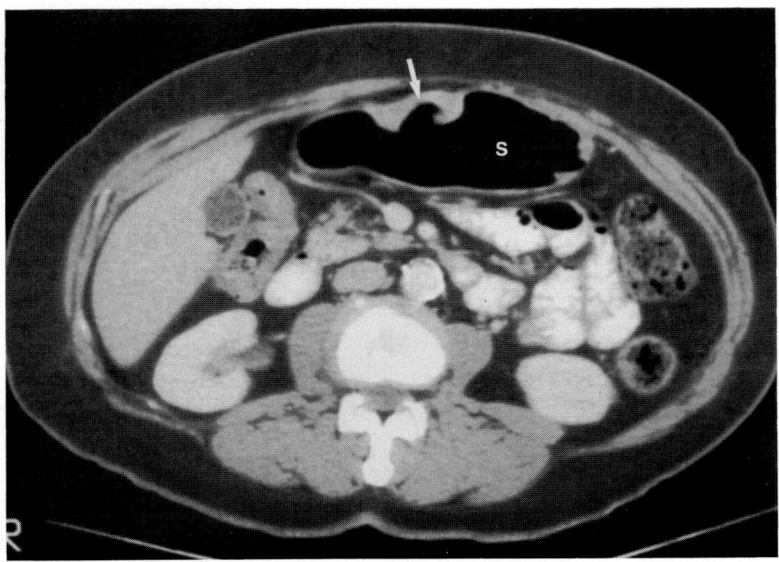

**Figure 38–16. Malignant gastric ulcer.** A CT scan shows an ulcerated mass on the anterior wall of the gastric body. Note how gas enters the ulcer crater *(arrow)*. S = stomach.

lesion[98, 99] (see Fig. 38–14B and C). Esophageal involvement is usually confined to a 4- to 5-cm segment above the gastroesophageal junction but may extend as far proximally as the aortic arch.[99] Submucosal spread of tumor may also result in secondary achalasia with tapered, beak-like narrowing of the distal esophagus at or just above the gastroesophageal junction[99, 101] (see Fig. 38–15) (see Chapter 29). However, certain morphologic features such as asymmetry, abrupt transitions, and mucosal nodularity or ulceration should suggest an underlying malignancy.[101] Secondary achalasia should also be suspected when the narrowed segment extends proximally a discrete distance from the gastroesophageal junction. In such cases, careful radiologic evaluation of the fundus is essential to rule out a carcinoma of the cardia as the cause of these findings.

### Computed Tomography

Polypoid gastric carcinomas are readily detected on CT scans as soft tissue masses protruding into the lumen of the stomach. However, ulcerated carcinomas may be more difficult to demonstrate on CT scans. Recognition of these lesions is facilitated by the use of negative intraluminal contrast agents such as water or gas. When the stomach is distended with gas, an ulcerated carcinoma may appear on a CT scan as a soft tissue mass containing a gas-filled ulcer crater (Fig. 38–16). Infiltrating carcinomas may also be recognized on CT scans by wall thickening and loss of the normal rugal fold pattern when the stomach is distended with negative contrast agents (Fig. 38–17). Some of these tumors may be associated with only minimal (4- to 8-mm) wall thickening. In contrast, scirrhous carcinomas may be characterized by significant wall thickening with marked contrast enhancement on dynamic CT scans (Fig. 38–18). However, these scirrhous tumors are relatively avascular, so the reason for this phenomenon is unclear.

Some mucinous carcinomas may also demonstrate low attenuation because of their high mucin content,[102] whereas other mucinous carcinomas may be calcified (Fig. 38–19).

Carcinoma of the gastric cardia may be difficult to demonstrate on CT scans because of the normal soft tissue thickening that occurs at the gastroesophageal junction due to the reflections of the phrenoesophageal ligament and the attachments of the gastrohepatic ligament on the adjacent lesser curvature of the stomach. Prolapsed hiatal hernias in the fundus may also create the erroneous impression of a soft tissue mass in this region. If a lesion is suspected at the gastroesophageal junction, subsequent scans with the patient in the prone position after administration of an effervescent agent

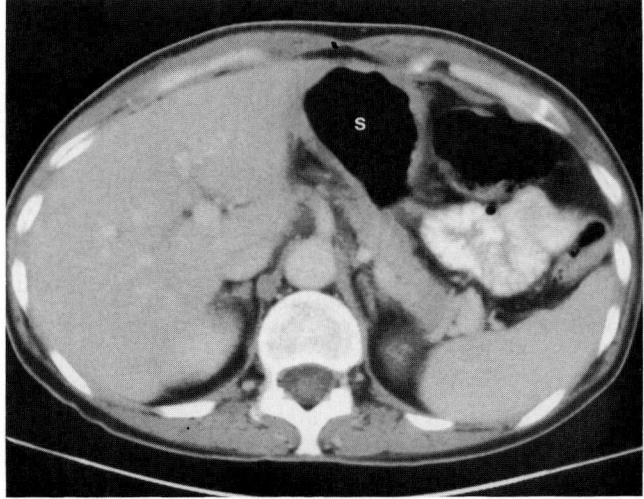

**Figure 38–17. Infiltrating gastric carcinoma.** A CT scan shows a slightly thickened gastric wall with loss of the normal rugal fold pattern. Wisp-like soft tissue stranding adjacent to the stomach indicates extension of tumor into the perigastric fat. S = stomach.

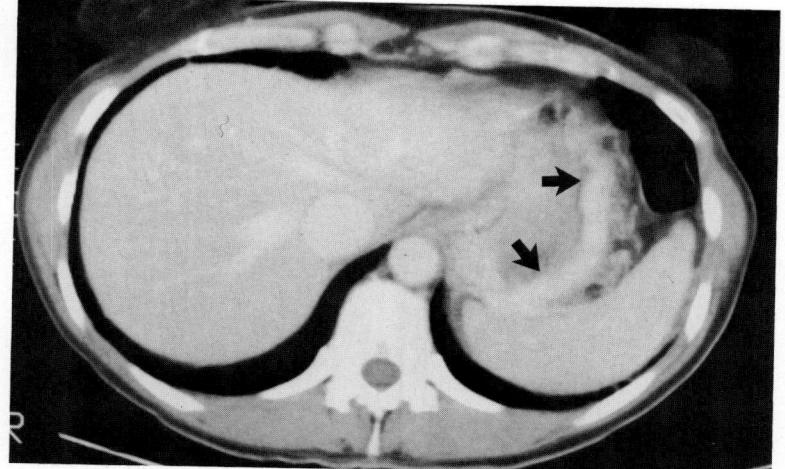

**Figure 38–18. Scirrhous carcinoma of the stomach.** There is a markedly thickened gastric wall *(arrows)* that enhances considerably on a dynamic CT scan.

should result in maximal distention of the gastric fundus for better delineation of neoplastic soft tissue thickening or a true mass lesion at the cardia (Fig. 38–20).

## Differential Diagnosis

### *Early Gastric Cancer*

Early gastric cancers may appear radiographically as depressed (i.e., ulcerated), elevated (i.e., polypoid), or superficial lesions. Ulcerated cancers must be distinguished from benign gastric ulcers (see earlier section on early gastric cancer). Occasionally, early gastric lymphomas may also appear as ulcerated lesions (see Chapter 39). Polypoid cancers must be distinguished from adenomatous or hyperplastic polyps or other benign or malignant tumors in the stomach. Finally, superficial cancers must be distinguished from a focal area of gastritis or intestinal metaplasia. When early gastric cancer is suspected on the basis of barium studies, endoscopy and biopsy are required for a definitive diagnosis.

### *Advanced Carcinoma*

The major consideration in the differential diagnosis of an ulcerated gastric carcinoma is a benign gastric ulcer with a surrounding mound of edema (see Chapter 35). Polypoid or ulcerated carcinomas must also be distinguished from other polypoid or ulcerated malignancies such as lymphoma and leiomyosarcoma (see Chapter 39). Although the latter tumors tend to appear as smooth or slightly lobulated submucosal masses, they occasionally have a polypoid or ulcerated appearance. Thus, histologic specimens are ultimately required to differentiate these lesions.

Most cases of linitis plastica are caused by gastric carcinoma, but metastatic breast cancer involving the stomach may produce identical radiographic findings[65, 103–105] (Fig. 38–21) (see Chapter 39). Omental metastases or carcinoma of the transverse colon invading the stomach via the gastrocolic ligament may also cause circumferential narrowing of the antrum or body, closely resembling the appearance of a primary scirrhous carcinoma.[103, 106] The possibility of metastatic disease should therefore be considered in any patient with linitis plastica who has a history of malignancy, particularly breast carcinoma.

Cone-shaped antral narrowing and deformity may also be caused by scarring from peptic ulcer disease, caustic ingestion, radiation, or a variety of granulomatous diseases, including Crohn's disease, tuberculosis, sarcoidosis, and syphilis[107] (see Chapter 36). Antral narrowing may also occur in elderly patients with a "senile" antrum due to gastric atrophy.[108] In general, a smooth antral contour and lack of nodularity, spiculation, or ulceration should suggest benign disease. Occasionally,

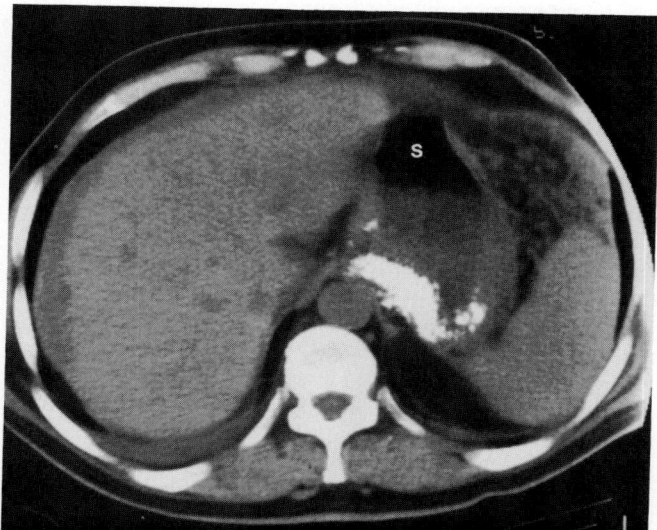

**Figure 38–19. Calcified mucinous carcinoma of the stomach.** There is marked thickening of the gastric wall with multiple areas of calcification in the tumor. S = stomach.

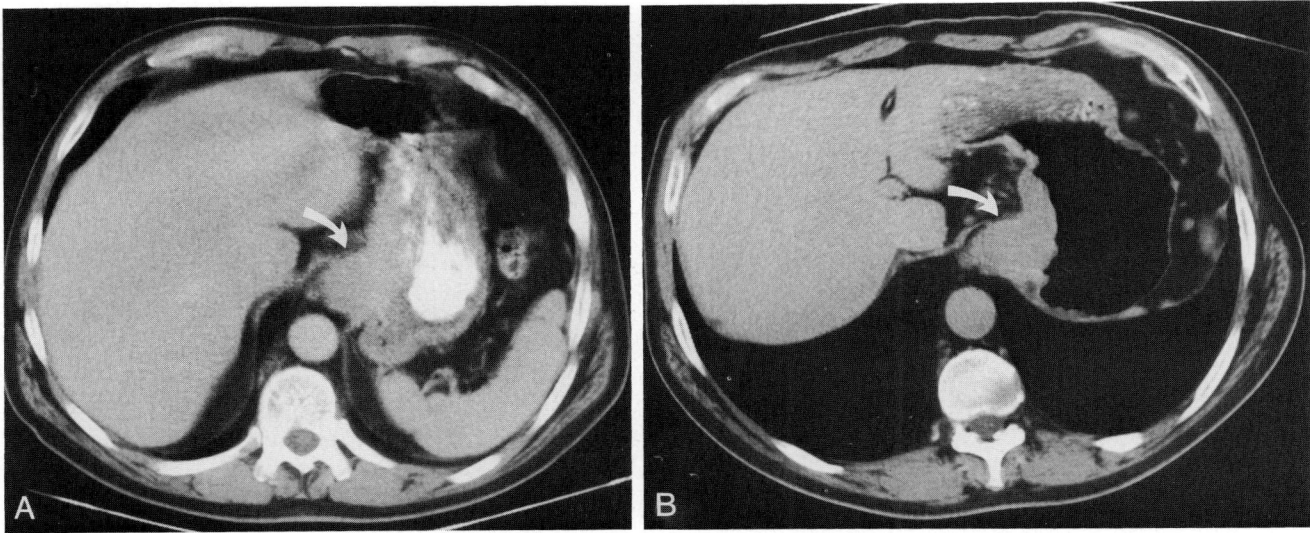

**Figure 38–20. Carcinoma of the cardia. A.** A supine CT scan shows considerable soft tissue thickening *(arrow)* near the gastroesophageal junction. **B.** A prone scan after administration of an oral effervescent agent confirms the presence of a lobulated soft tissue mass *(arrow)* in this location.

however, these conditions may produce more irregular gastric narrowing and a linitis plastica appearance.

Carcinoma of the cardia invading the distal esophagus may be indistinguishable from a primary adenocarcinoma in Barrett's esophagus invading the stomach[109] (see Fig. 28–20). However, carcinoma of the cardia tends to have a greater degree of gastric involvement in relation to that of the esophagus. Squamous cell carcinoma of the esophagus may also spread distally via submucosal esophageal lymphatics to the gastric cardia or fundus, producing a polypoid lesion in the fundus[110, 111] (see Fig. 28–11). Occasionally, a conglomerate of varices in the fundus may be manifested by a single lobulated lesion that closely resembles a polypoid fundal or cardiac carcinoma[112–114] (see Fig. 30–10). Rarely, the distal

esophagus may invaginate into a sliding hiatal hernia or a hiatal hernia may invaginate into the fundus, producing an apparent mass lesion[115] (see Figs. 32–11 and 32–12). However, this retrograde mucosal prolapse usually occurs as a transient finding at fluoroscopy. Finally, inadequate gaseous distention of the fundus can mimic the appearance of an infiltrating fundal tumor on double contrast studies (Fig. 38–22A). However, additional views of the stomach after administration of a second dose of effervescent agent should show that the fundus is normal in these patients (Fig. 38–22B).

## Staging

CT and endoscopic ultrasound have been used for the evaluation and staging of patients with gastric carcinoma. The evolving role of endoscopic ultrasound (i.e., endosonography) in these patients is discussed in Chapter 10. Early reports indicate that it is a promising technique for preoperative staging of gastric carcinoma.[116–118]

Contrary to early claims that CT could prevent unnecessary surgery in patients with unresectable gastric carcinoma, the primary role of CT is to assess the presence and extent of extragastric spread of tumor to facilitate decisions about the feasibility of radical versus palliative surgery.[119, 120] Some patients with apparently resectable cancers who undergo subtotal gastrectomies are subsequently found to have tumor in lymph node groups that are not routinely inspected at the time of surgery. CT may therefore permit surgeons and oncologists to optimize the treatment of gastric cancer patients by better delineating the extent of tumor in these individuals.

CT evaluation of patients with gastric carcinoma requires a thorough understanding of the mechanisms of

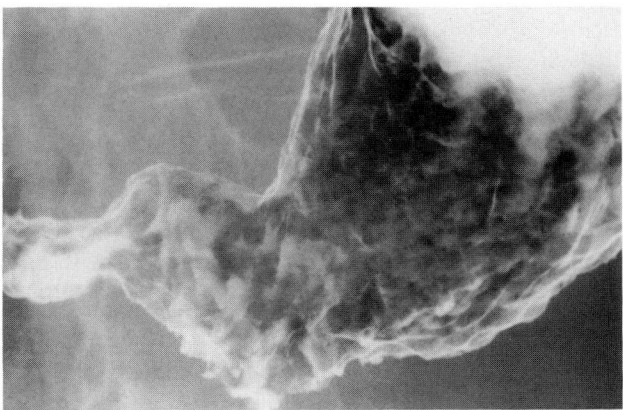

**Figure 38–21. Metastatic breast cancer involving the stomach.** There is antral narrowing with distortion of the normal surface pattern and a nodular, irregular mucosa in this region. A primary scirrhous carcinoma of the stomach could produce identical findings. (From Levine MS, Kong V, Rubesin SE, et al: Scirrhous carcinoma of the stomach: radiologic and endoscopic diagnosis. Radiology 175:151–154, 1990.)

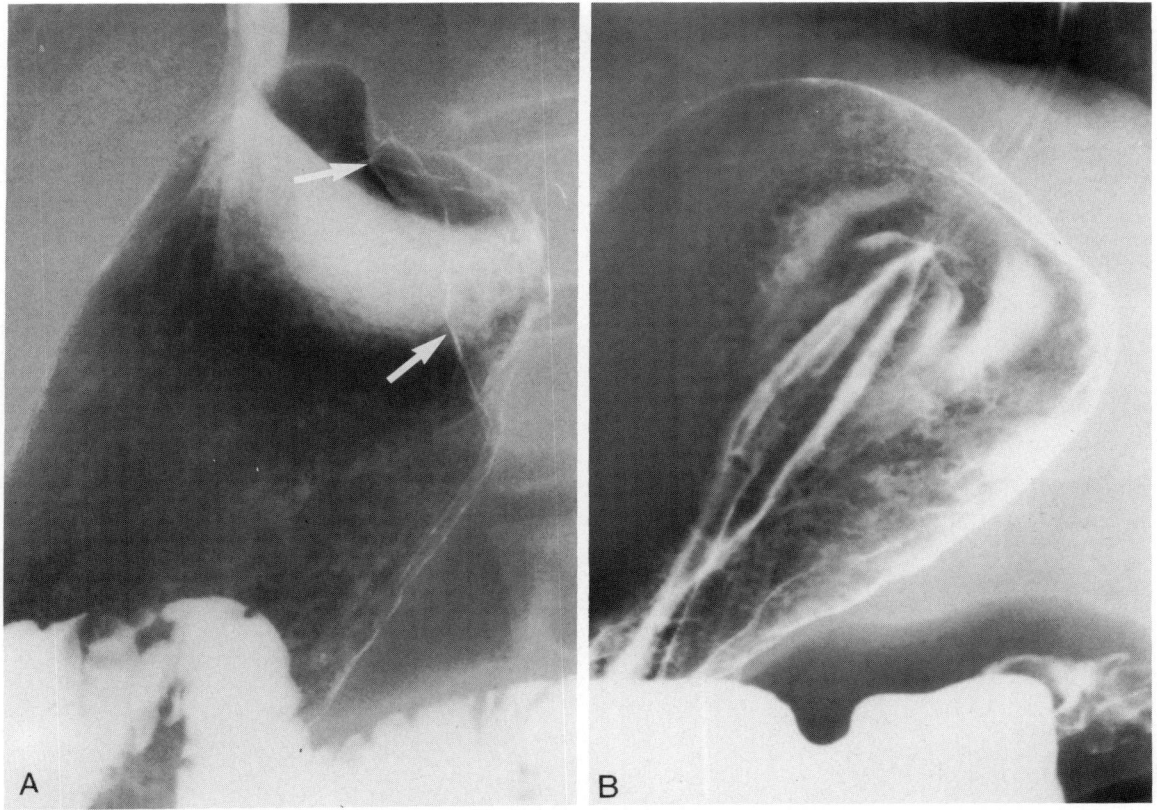

**Figure 38–22. Inadequate gaseous distention mimicking a fundal tumor. A.** A double contrast radiograph of the stomach shows a possible infiltrating lesion on the posterior wall of the fundus *(arrows)*. **B.** After administration of additional effervescent agent, there is better distention of the fundus, eliminating the possibility of tumor. Note how the normal cardiac rosette is now visible.

the spread of tumor, including direct extension, lymphatic spread, intraperitoneal seeding, and hematogenous metastases. The role of CT in detecting these various forms of tumor spread is discussed in the following sections.

## Direct Extension

When gastric carcinoma has extended through the serosa, it can spread along peritoneal reflections from the stomach. Cardiac or lesser curvature lesions may extend into the gastrohepatic ligament; greater curvature lesions may extend into the gastrocolic ligament; anterior wall lesions may extend into the gastroepiploic omentum; and posterior wall lesions may extend into the lesser sac (Fig. 38–23). Tumor may then spread via these ligamentous and peritoneal reflections to adjacent organs. The liver may be invaded via the gastrohepatic ligament, the transverse colon via the gastrocolic ligament, and the pancreas via the lesser sac (Fig. 38–24). Tumors arising at the gastric cardia may also invade the esophagus, diaphragm, aorta, or gastrohepatic ligament (Fig. 38–25).

CT may demonstrate varying degrees of soft tissue stranding due to invasion of the perigastric fat by tumor (see Fig. 38–23B). As the process becomes more exten-

sive, the soft tissue strands may evolve into tiny (4- to 8-mm) nodules that eventually coalesce into sheets of metastatic tumor. The abnormal margin of the stomach in the region of the tumor must be scrutinized to detect these subtle changes.

Using the tumor, node, and metastases (TNM) staging system, tumors extending into the perigastric fat are classified as T3 lesions, whereas tumors that are invading adjacent structures are classified as T4 lesions.[121] In the past, CT has had variable success in predicting local invasion by gastric carcinoma. For example, the accuracy of CT in predicting pancreatic invasion is only about 50%.[122, 123]

## Lymphatic Spread

Gastric carcinoma frequently metastasizes via the lymphatic system to draining lymph nodes. Unfortunately, CT is not able to detect tumor in normal-size nodes or to differentiate reactive changes from tumor in nodes that are enlarged. Enlarged nodes may also be obscured by a bulky, exophytic tumor mass. Although gastric carcinoma initially tends to metastasize to regional lymph nodes, extensive intramural lymphatic communications may result in adenopathy at sites remote from the primary tumor.

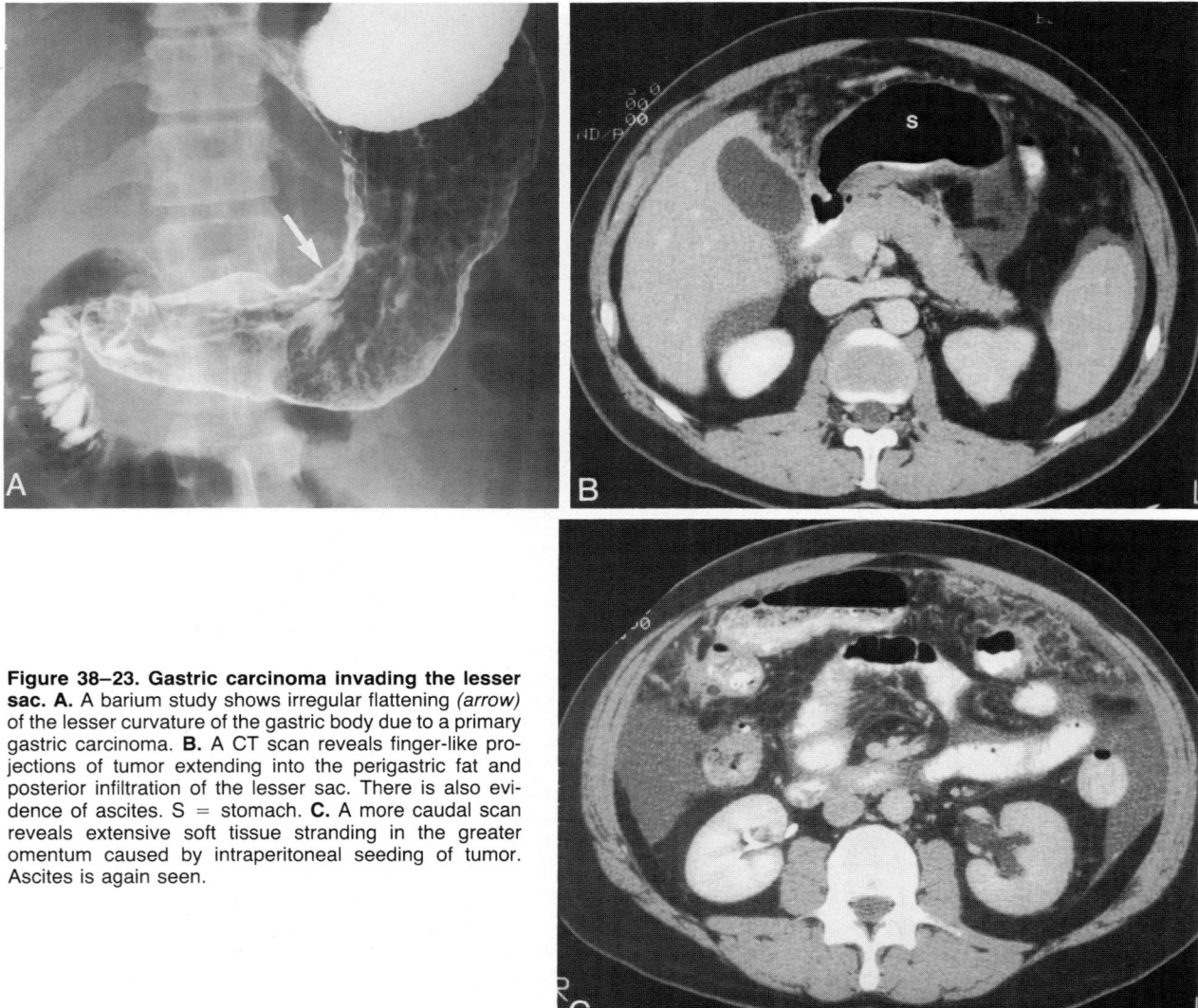

**Figure 38–23. Gastric carcinoma invading the lesser sac. A.** A barium study shows irregular flattening *(arrow)* of the lesser curvature of the gastric body due to a primary gastric carcinoma. **B.** A CT scan reveals finger-like projections of tumor extending into the perigastric fat and posterior infiltration of the lesser sac. There is also evidence of ascites. S = stomach. **C.** A more caudal scan reveals extensive soft tissue stranding in the greater omentum caused by intraperitoneal seeding of tumor. Ascites is again seen.

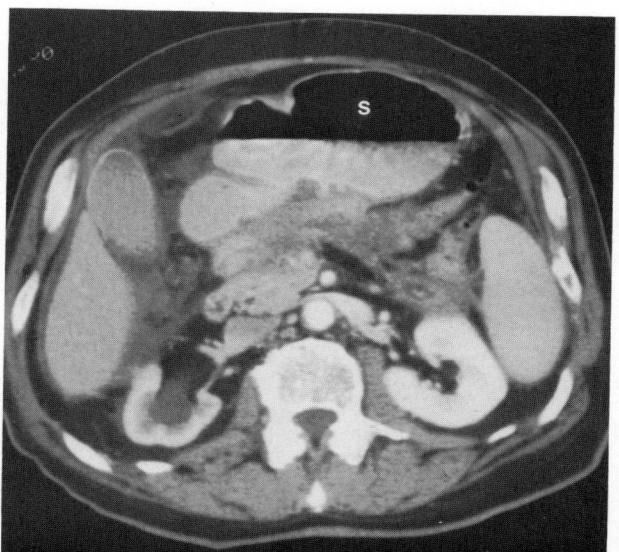

**Figure 38–24. Gastric carcinoma invading the pancreas.** An ulcerated cancer on the posterior wall of the stomach blends imperceptibly with the adjacent pancreas, indicating pancreatic invasion. S = stomach.

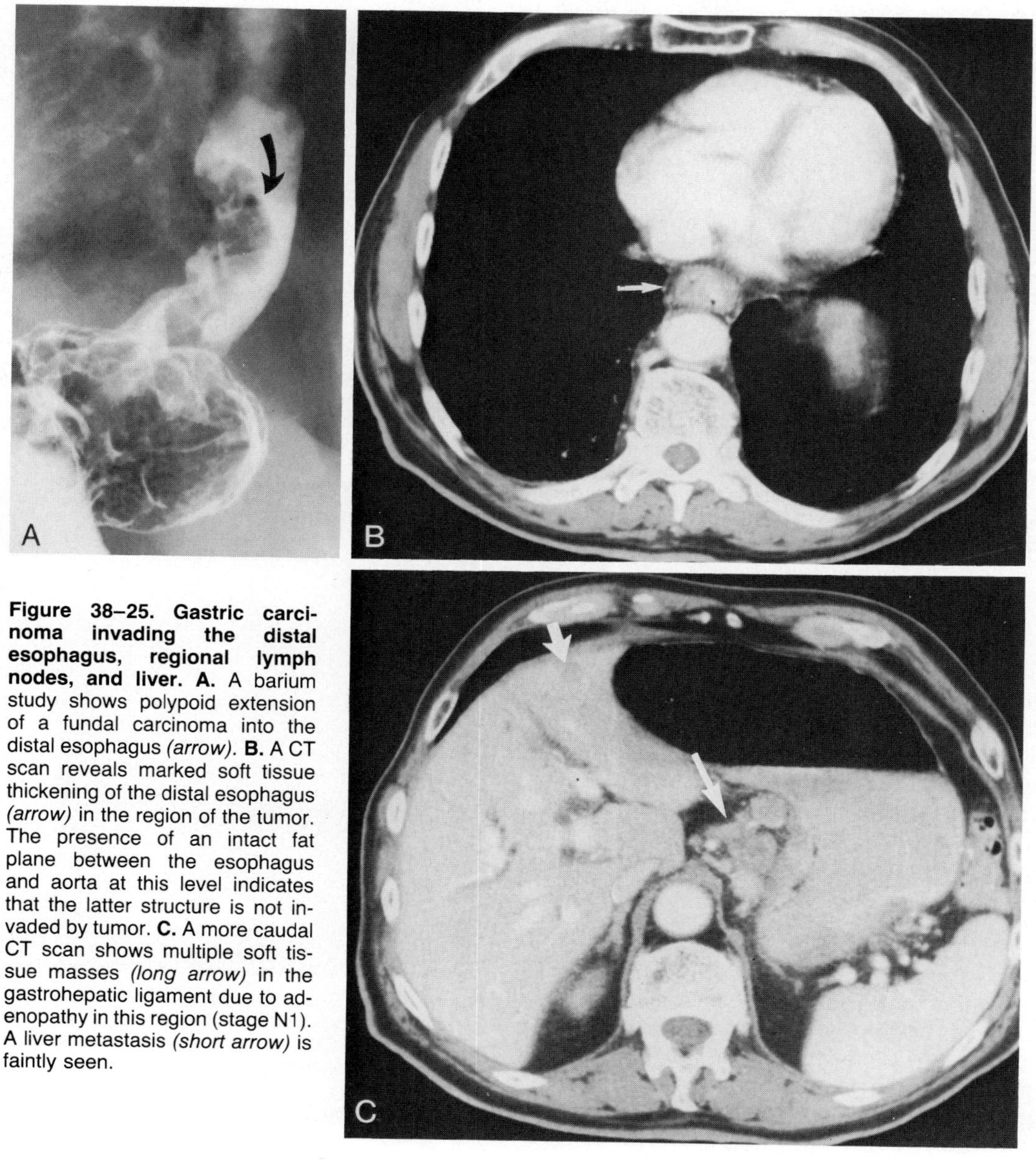

**Figure 38–25. Gastric carcinoma invading the distal esophagus, regional lymph nodes, and liver. A.** A barium study shows polypoid extension of a fundal carcinoma into the distal esophagus *(arrow)*. **B.** A CT scan reveals marked soft tissue thickening of the distal esophagus *(arrow)* in the region of the tumor. The presence of an intact fat plane between the esophagus and aorta at this level indicates that the latter structure is not invaded by tumor. **C.** A more caudal CT scan shows multiple soft tissue masses *(long arrow)* in the gastrohepatic ligament due to adenopathy in this region (stage N1). A liver metastasis *(short arrow)* is faintly seen.

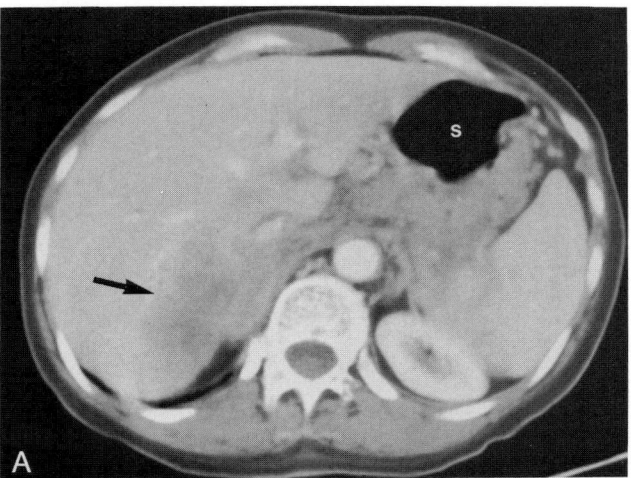

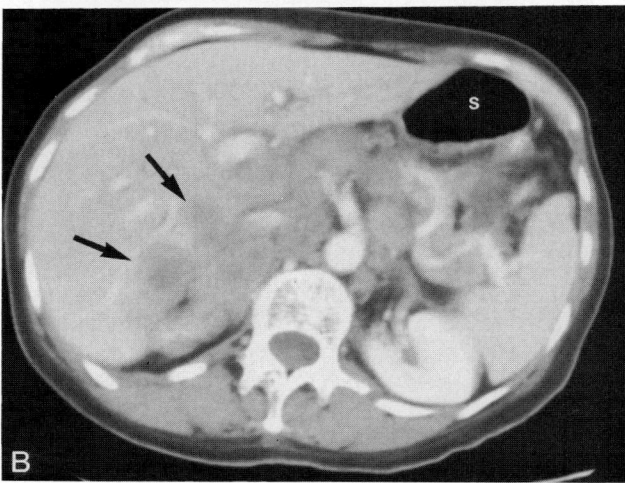

**Figure 38–26. Gastric carcinoma with lymph node and liver metastases. A.** A CT scan of a patient with gastric carcinoma reveals marked thickening of the gastric wall posteriorly. Arrow indicates a metastasis in the liver. **B.** A more caudal scan shows multiple enlarged, confluent lymph nodes surrounding the pancreas and celiac axis. In both scans, metastases are also seen in the liver *(arrows)*. S = stomach.

According to the TNM staging system, adenopathy in the peripyloric region, gastrocolic ligament, or gastrohepatic ligament is considered local (stage N1) (see Fig. 38–25C). The presence of local adenopathy has significant prognostic implications, but, for all practical purposes, recognition of adenopathy in these areas is not critical because these nodes are almost always removed at the time of gastrectomy. Secondary lymphatic drainage sites include the porta hepatis, hepatoduodenal ligament, and peripancreatic region. Involvement of any of these nodal groups places the patient in a more advanced stage (N2) in the TNM system (Fig. 38–26). Demonstration of adenopathy in these patients by CT is facilitated by the routine use of dynamic sequential scanning techniques to differentiate enlarged nodes from the opacified portal vein and mesenteric arterial circulation. Demonstration of involved secondary nodes is far more important than demonstration of local adenopathy, because these nodes are not removed during routine gastric cancer surgery and are therefore responsible for a high percentage of treatment failures. The reported accuracy of CT in detecting adenopathy from gastric carcinoma has ranged from 58 to 75%.[122, 123]

## Intraperitoneal Seeding

The CT appearance of intraperitoneally seeded metastases from gastric carcinoma cannot be distinguished from that of other causes of intraperitoneal dissemination of tumor. These metastases may be manifested on CT scans by nodules, loculated fluid collections (particularly in peritoneal reflections), and irregular, beaded thickening and stranding of the mesentery and omentum (see Fig. 38–23C). Some patients with signet-ring cell gastric carcinomas may have intraperitoneally seeded metastases to the ovaries that are known as *Krukenberg tumors*. These ovarian metastases typically appear on CT scans as relatively uniform soft tissue masses rather than the predominantly cystic lesions expected for primary epithelial neoplasms of the ovaries[124, 125] (Fig. 38–27). Thus, demonstration on CT scans of bilateral, relatively solid-appearing adnexal masses should lead to careful evaluation of the stomach to rule out an unsuspected gastric carcinoma.

## Hematogenous Metastases

In descending order of frequency, the liver, lungs, and adrenals are the most common sites of blood-borne metastases from gastric carcinoma (see Figs. 38–25 and 38–26). The liver should be evaluated by dynamic CT protocols using contrast enhancement. Various CT techniques for examining the liver are discussed in detail in Chapter 101.

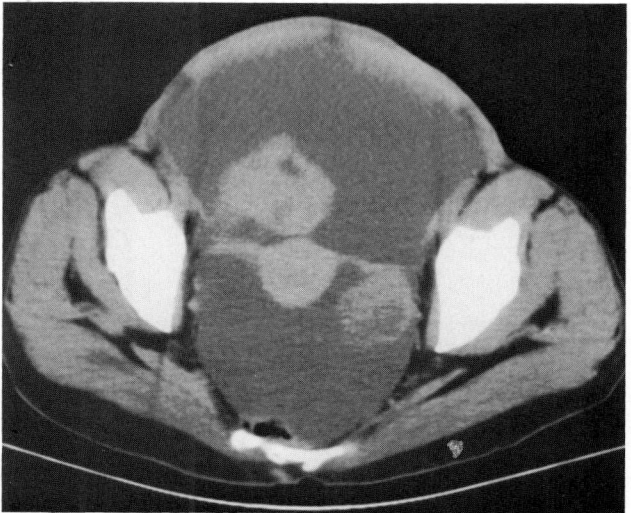

**Figure 38–27. Gastric carcinoma with ovarian metastases (Krukenberg tumors).** This patient was being evaluated for a pelvic mass and ascites. A CT scan demonstrates marked ascites with a right-sided adnexal mass that has a more solid appearance than expected for most primary epithelial neoplasms of the ovaries. Higher scans revealed an unsuspected gastric carcinoma that had metastasized to the ovaries.

## Accuracy of Computed Tomography

There is considerable controversy in the literature about the accuracy of CT for the preoperative staging of gastric carcinoma. In one series of 95 patients, the positive predictive value of CT for assessing the resectability of gastric cancer was 81% and the negative predictive value was 64%.[126] In another series of 32 patients with gastroesophageal junction cancers, however, the positive and negative predictive values for assessing resectability were 91 and 90%, respectively.[127] CT has a reported accuracy of 75 to 90% for detecting pancreatic invasion, 57 to 88% for detecting adenopathy, and 67 to 97% for detecting liver metastases from gastric carcinoma.[122, 126, 128–131] This wide discrepancy reflects the rapid technologic changes in CT that have occurred during the past decade. However, it should be recognized that CT is probably more accurate in detecting distant adenopathy from gastric carcinoma than local adenopathy.[128] This has important implications because locally involved nodes are routinely removed at surgery.

## Treatment and Prognosis

Surgery is the only curative form of therapy in patients with gastric carcinoma. Depending on the location of the tumor, a subtotal or total gastrectomy or an esophagogastrectomy may be performed. Unfortunately, about 60% of patients who undergo surgery are found to have unresectable tumors.[10] Nevertheless, a palliative resection or bypass procedure may still be performed on these patients to prevent complications such as bleeding or obstruction. Radiation therapy has also been advocated for palliation of inoperable lesions. Adjuvant chemotherapy has been used in some patients, but the benefits of this treatment remain uncertain. Laser therapy has also been used to treat patients with obstructive tumors. A detailed discussion of the various operations and postoperative complications is presented in Chapter 41.

Patients with advanced gastric carcinoma have a dismal prognosis, with 5-year survival rates of only 3 to 21%.[4–9] In contrast, patients with early gastric cancer have 5-year survival rates of 85 to 100%.[73, 74, 81, 82] Early detection of these lesions is therefore essential for improving survival of patients. Thus far, most early gastric cancers have been detected in Japan as a result of mass screening of the adult population in that country. However, some symptomatic patients with gastric cancer in the West are also found to have early lesions. Because it is frequently not possible to distinguish early gastric cancer from advanced carcinoma on preoperative studies, an aggressive surgical approach is justified for all patients with resectable lesions.

## DUODENAL CARCINOMA

Duodenal carcinoma is a rare malignancy, accounting for less than 1% of all gastrointestinal neoplasms.[132]

Almost all of these lesions are located in the postbulbar portion of the duodenum at or below the level of the ampulla of Vater.[133, 134] The most common presenting clinical findings include nausea, vomiting, abdominal pain, weight loss, and upper gastrointestinal bleeding. An increased incidence of duodenal carcinoma has been reported in patients with Gardner's syndrome (see Chapter 66) and celiac disease (see Chapter 49), so some form of radiologic or endoscopic surveillance may be warranted for these patients.[135, 136] Duodenal carcinoma has also been associated with Crohn's disease and neurofibromatosis.[137–139]

Duodenal carcinomas usually appear radiographically as polypoid, ulcerated, or annular lesions at or, more commonly, distal to the ampulla of Vater[140] (Fig. 38–28). Some polypoid carcinomas may arise in pre-existing villous tumors (see Chapter 37). Rarely, duodenal carcinomas have a more proximal location, appearing as ulcerated masses in the duodenal bulb.[141] Nevertheless, the vast majority of duodenal ulcers are benign, so endoscopy should be considered only for lesions that have suspicious radiographic features.

Duodenal carcinoma may be manifested on CT scans by a discrete mass or mass-like thickening of the duodenal wall. When local adenopathy is present, it may be difficult to differentiate duodenal carcinoma from an adjacent pancreatic neoplasm. However, this is also a difficult area to explore at surgery, so CT may be helpful in the preoperative assessment of these patients.[142]

Although ampullary and periampullary carcinomas may be confused with primary pancreatic carcinomas, it is important to distinguish these lesions because ampullary tumors have a much better prognosis. Hypotonic

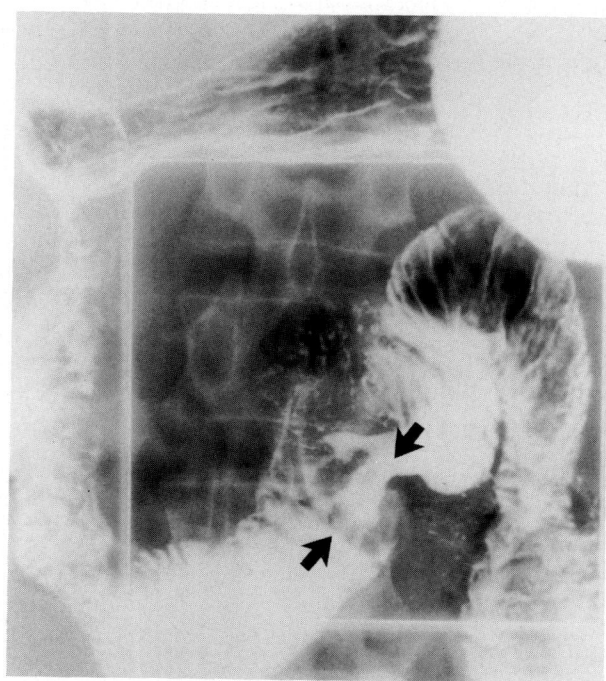

**Figure 38–28. Duodenal carcinoma.** There is an annular lesion with shelf-like borders *(arrows)* in the distal duodenum near the duodenojejunal junction.

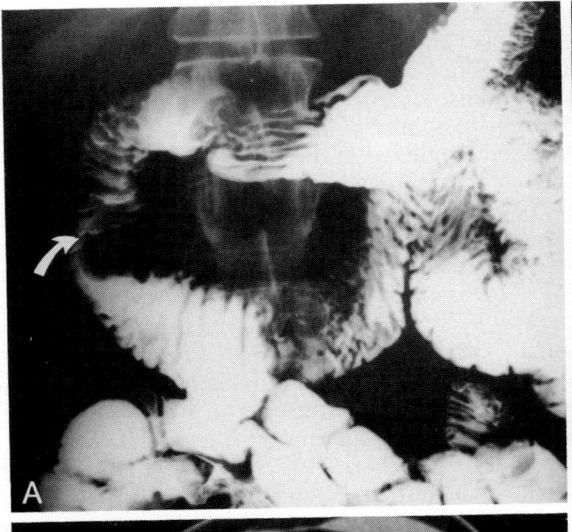

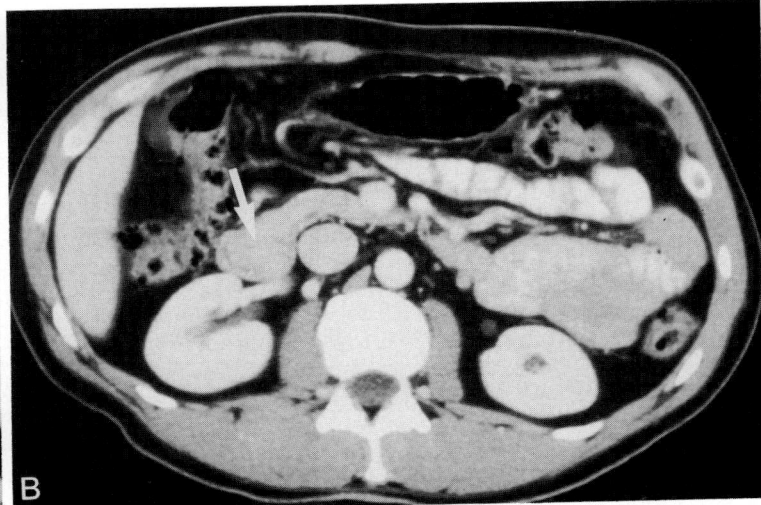

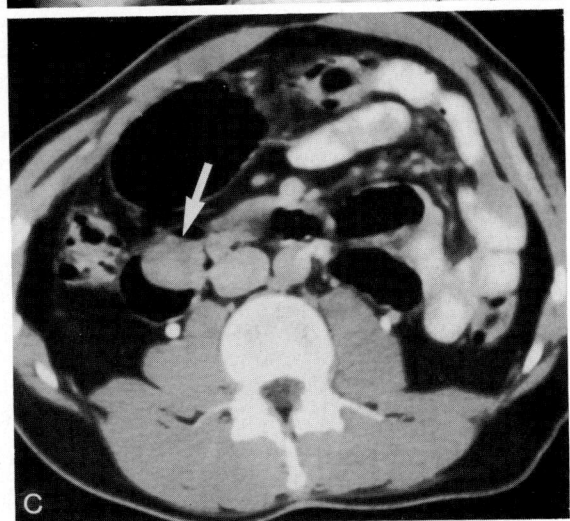

**Figure 38–29. Ampullary carcinoma. A.** A barium study shows a mass *(arrow)* on the medial aspect of the descending duodenum at the level of the papilla. **B.** A CT scan also shows a soft tissue mass *(arrow)* in this region. **C.** After administration of additional effervescent agent and 0.1 mg of intravenous glucagon, a subsequent scan with the patient in the left-side-down decubitus position clearly delineates this intraluminal mass *(arrow)* in the descending duodenum.

CT duodenography may be useful for differentiating these lesions. The examination is facilitated by placing the patient in the left-side-down decubitus position after administration of an effervescent agent and 0.1 mg of intravenous glucagon to obtain scans of the gas-filled duodenal sweep. Both ampullary and periampullary lesions may be well demonstrated with this technique[143] (Fig. 38–29).

### Acknowledgment

Figures 38–1B, 38–7A and B, 38–11, and 38–12 are from Laufer I, Levine MS (eds): Double Contrast Gastrointestinal Radiology (2nd ed). Philadelphia: WB Saunders, 1992.

Figure 38–15A and B is from Levine MS: Radiology of the Esophagus. Philadelphia: WB Saunders, 1989.

## References

1. Cady B, Ramsden DA, Stein A, et al: Gastric cancer: contemporary aspects. Am J Surg 133:423–429, 1977.
 2. Devesa SS, Silverman DT: Cancer incidence and mortality trends in the United States: 1935–74. J Natl Cancer Inst 60:545–571, 1978.
 3. Howson CP, Hiyama T, Wynder EL: The decline in gastric cancer: epidemiology of an unplanned triumph. Epidemiol Rev 8:1–27, 1986.
 4. Dupont JB, Lee JR, Burton GR, et al: Adenocarcinoma of the stomach: review of 1,497 cases. Cancer 41:941–947, 1978.
 5. Ochsner A, Weed TE, Nuessle WR: Cancer of the stomach. Am J Surg 141:10–14, 1981.
 6. Faivre J, Justrabo E, Hillon P, et al: Gastric carcinoma in Côte d'Or (France): a population-based study. Gastroenterology 88:1874–1879, 1985.
 7. Moore JR: Gastric carcinoma: 30-year review. Can J Surg 29:25–28, 1986.
 8. McBride CM, Boddie AW: Adenocarcinoma of the stomach: are we making any progress? South Med J 80:283–286, 1987.
 9. Cady B, Rossi RL, Silverman ML, et al: Gastric adenocarcinoma: a disease in transition. Arch Surg 124:303–308, 1989.
10. Boland CR, Scheiman JM: Tumors of the stomach. *In* Yamada T (ed): Textbook of Gastroenterology. Philadelphia: JB Lippincott, 1991, pp 1353–1379.
11. Kurtz RC, Sherlock P: Carcinoma of the stomach. *In* Berk JE (ed): Bockus Gastroenterology. Philadelphia: WB Saunders, 1985, pp 1278–1304.
12. Oiso T: Incidence of stomach cancer and its relation to dietary

habits and nutrition in Japan between 1900 and 1975. Cancer Res 35:3254–3258, 1975.

13. Tatematsu M, Furihata C, Katsuyama T, et al: Independent induction of intestinal metaplasia and gastric cancer in rats treated with *N*-methyl-*N'*-nitro-*N*-nitrosoguanidine. Cancer Res 43:1335–1341, 1983.

14. Bentall HH, Aird I: A relationship between cancer of stomach and the ABO blood groups. Br Med J 1:799–801, 1953.

15. Strickland RG, Mackay IR: A reappraisal of the nature and significance of chronic atrophic gastritis. Am J Dig Dis 18:426–440, 1973.

16. Walker IR, Strickland RG, Ungar B, et al: Simple atrophic gastritis and gastric carcinoma. Gut 12:906–911, 1971.

17. Cheli R, Santi L, Ciancamerla G, et al: A clinical and statistical follow-up study of atrophic gastritis. Am J Dig Dis 18:1061–1066, 1973.

18. Morson BC: Carcinoma arising from areas of intestinal metaplasia in the gastric mucosa. Br J Cancer 9:377–385, 1955.

19. Sipponen P, Kekki M, Siurala M: Age-related trends of gastritis and intestinal metaplasia in gastric carcinoma patients and in controls representing the population at large. Br J Cancer 49:521–526, 1984.

20. Elsborg L, Mosbech J: Pernicious anaemia as a risk factor in gastric cancer. Acta Med Scand 206:315–318, 1979.

21. Schafer LW, Larson DE, Metton LJ, et al: Risk of development of gastric carcinoma in patients with pernicious anemia: a population-based study in Rochester, Minnesota. Mayo Clinic Proc 60:444–448, 1985.

22. Ming S-C: The classification and significance of gastric polyps. *In* Yardley JH, Morson BC, Abell M (eds): The Gastrointestinal Tract. International Academy of Pathology Monograph. Baltimore: Williams & Wilkins, 1977, pp 149–175.

23. Ming S-C: The adenoma-carcinoma sequence in the stomach and colon. II. Malignant potential of gastric polyps. Gastrointest Radiol 1:121–125, 1976.

24. Tomosulo J: Gastric polyps. Histologic types and their relationship to gastric carcinoma. Cancer 27:1346–1355, 1971.

25. Op den Orth JO, Dekker W: Gastric adenomas. Radiology 141:289–293, 1981.

26. Ming S-C, Goldman H: Gastric polyps. A histogenetic classification and its relation to carcinoma. Cancer 18:721–726, 1965.

27. Feldman F, Seaman WB: Primary gastric stump carcinoma. AJR 115:257–267, 1972.

28. Morgenstein L, Yamakawa T, Seltzer D: Carcinoma of the gastric stump. Am J Surg 125:29–38, 1973.

29. Caygill CPJ, Hill MJ, Kirkham JS, et al: Mortality from gastric cancer following gastric surgery for peptic ulcer. Lancet 1:929–931, 1986.

30. Viste A, Opheim P, Thunold J, et al: Risk of carcinoma following gastric operations for benign disease. Lancet 2:502–504, 1986.

31. Offerhaus GJA, Tersmette AC, Huibregtse K: Mortality caused by stomach cancer after remote partial gastrectomy for benign conditions: 40 years of follow up of an Amsterdam cohort of 2633 postgastrectomy patients. Gut 29:1588–1590, 1980.

32. Schafer LW, Larson DE, Melton LJ, et al: The risk of gastric carcinoma after surgical treatment for benign ulcer disease: a population-based study in Olmsted County, Minnesota. N Engl J Med 309:1210–1213, 1983.

33. Dougherty SH, Foster CA, Eisenberg MM: Stomach cancer following gastric surgery for benign disease. Arch Surg 117:294–297, 1982.

34. Goodman P, Levine MS, Gohil MN: Gastric carcinoma after gastrojejunostomy for benign disease: radiographic findings. Gastrointest Radiol 17:211–213, 1992.

35. Rubin RG, Fink H: Giant hypertrophy of the gastric mucosa associated with carcinoma of the stomach. Am J Gastroenterol 47:379–388, 1967.

36. Williams SM, Harned RK, Settles RH: Adenocarcinoma of the stomach in association with Ménétrier's disease. Gastrointest Radiol 3:387–390, 1978.

37. Ming S-C: Atlas of Tumor Pathology, Fascicle 7, Tumors of the Esophagus and Stomach. Washington, DC: Armed Forces Institute of Pathology, 1973, pp 144–205.

38. Olearchyk AS: Gastric carcinoma: a critical review of 243 cases. Am J Gastroenterol 70:25–45, 1978.

39. Wanke M, Schwan H: Pathology of gastric cancer. World J Surg 3:675–684, 1979.

40. Moertel CG, Bargen JA, Soule EH: Multiple gastric cancers. Gastroenterology 32:1095–1103, 1957.

41. Shirakabe H, Nishizawa M, Maruyama M, et al: Atlas of X-ray Diagnosis of Early Gastric Cancer. New York: Igaku-Shoin, 1982, pp 1–18.

42. Meyers WC, Damiano RJ, Rotolo FS, et al: Adenocarcinoma of the stomach: changing patterns over the last 4 decades. Ann Surg 205:1–8, 1987.

43. Antonioli DA, Goldman H: Changes in the location and type of gastric adenocarcinoma. Cancer 50:775–781, 1982.

44. Dodge OG: The surgical pathway of gastro-oesophageal carcinoma. Br J Surg 49:121–125, 1961.

45. Kakeji Y, Tsujitani S, Baba H, et al: Clinicopathologic features and prognostic significance of duodenal invasion in patients with distal gastric carcinoma. Cancer 68:380–384, 1991.

46. MacMahon CE, Lund P: Gastrocolic fistulae of malignant origin. Am J Surg 106:333–347, 1963.

47. Smith DL, Dockerty MB, Black BM: Gastrocolic fistulas of malignant origin. Surg Gynecol Obstet 134:829–834, 1972.

48. Holtz F, Hart WR: Krukenberg tumors of the ovary: a clinicopathologic analysis of 27 cases. Cancer 50:2438–2447, 1982.

49. Hansen RM, Hanson GA: Gastric carcinoma. Am J Gastroenterol 74:497–503, 1980.

50. Klein EW, Williams SF: Carcinoma of the stomach in young adults. Am J Gastroenterol 38:69–74, 1962.

51. Bloss RS, Miller TA, Copeland EM: Carcinoma of the stomach in the young adult. Surg Gynecol Obstet 150:883–886, 1980.

52. Holburt E, Freedman SI: Gastric carcinoma in patients younger than 36 years. Cancer 60:1395–1399, 1987.

53. Grabiec J, Owen DA: Carcinoma of the stomach in young persons. Cancer 56:388–396, 1985.

54. MacDonald WC: Clinical and pathologic features of adenocarcinoma of the gastric cardia. Cancer 29:724–731, 1972.

55. Block GE, Lancaster JR: Adenocarcinoma of the cardioesophageal junction. Arch Surg 88:852–858, 1964.

56. Fierst SM: Carcinoma of the cardia and fundus of the stomach. Am J Gastroenterol 57:403–409, 1972.

57. Webb JN, Busuttil A: Adenocarcinoma of the oesophagus and of the oesophagogastric junction. Br J Surg 65:475–479, 1978.

58. Raskin MM: Some specific radiological findings and consideration of linitis plastica of the gastrointestinal tract. Crit Rev Diagn Imaging 8:87–105, 1976.

59. Qizilbash AH, Castelli M, Kowalski MA, et al: Endoscopic brush cytology and biopsy in the diagnosis of cancer of the upper gastrointestinal tract. Acta Cytol 24:313–318, 1980.

60. Llanos O, Guzman S, Duarte I: Accuracy of the first endoscopic procedure in the differential diagnosis of gastric lesions. Ann Surg 195:224–226, 1982.

61. Graham DY, Schwartz JT, Cain GD, et al: Prospective evaluation of biopsy number in the diagnosis of esophageal and gastric cancer. Gastroenterology 82:228–231, 1982.

62. Tatsuta M, Iishi H, Okuda S, et al: Prospective evaluation of diagnostic accuracy of gastrofibroscopic biopsy in diagnosis of gastric cancer. Cancer 63:1415–1420, 1989.

63. Winawer SJ, Posner G, Lightdale CJ, et al: Endoscopic diagnosis of advanced gastric cancer: factors influencing yield. Gastroenterology 69:1183–1187, 1975.

64. Evans E, Harris O, Dickey D, et al: Difficulties in the endoscopic diagnosis of gastric and oesophageal cancer. Aust N Z J Surg 55:541–544, 1985.

65. Levine MS, Kong V, Rubesin SE, et al: Scirrhous carcinoma of the stomach: radiologic and endoscopic diagnosis. Radiology 175:151–154, 1990.

66. Koga M, Nakata H, Kiyonari H, et al: Roentgen features of the superficial depressed type of early gastric carcinoma. Radiology 15:289–292, 1975.

67. Montesi A, Graziani L, Pesaresi A, et al: Radiologic diagnosis of early gastric cancer by routine double-contrast examination. Gastrointest Radiol 7:205–215, 1982.

68. Gold RP, Green PH, O'Toole KM, et al: Early gastric cancer: radiographic experience. Radiology 152:283–290, 1984.

69. White RM, Levine MS, Enterline HT, et al: Early gastric cancer: recent experience. Radiology 155:25–27, 1985.

70. Murakami T: Pathomorphological diagnosis. *In* Murakami T (ed): Early Gastric Cancer. Tokyo: University of Tokyo Press, 1971, pp 53–55.

71. Sakita T, Ogura Y, Takasu S, et al: Observations on the healing of ulcerations in early gastric cancer: the life cycle of the malignant ulcer. Gastroenterology 60:835–844, 1971.

72. Kawai K: Diagnosis of early gastric cancer. Endoscopy 1:23–28, 1971.

73. Kaneko E, Nakamura T, Umeda N, et al: Outcome of gastric carcinoma detected by gastric mass survey in Japan. Gut 18:626–630, 1977.

74. Okui K, Tejima H: Evaluation of gastric mass survey. Acta Chir Scand 146:185–187, 1980.

75. Kaibara N, Kawaguchi H, Nishidoi H, et al: Significance of mass survey for gastric cancer from the standpoint of surgery. Am J Surg 142:543–545, 1981.

76. Evans DMD, Craven JL, Murphy F, et al: Comparison of early gastric cancer in Britain and Japan. Gut 19:1–9, 1978.

77. Seifert E, Butke H, Gail K, et al: Diagnosis of early gastric cancer. Am J Gastroenterol 71:563–567, 1979.

78. Ohman U, Emas S, Rubio C: Relation between early and advanced gastric cancer. Am J Surg 140:351–355, 1980.

79. Green PH, O'Toole KM, Weinberg LM, et al: Early gastric cancer. Gastroenterology 81:247–256, 1981.

80. Busuttil A, Webb JN: Early carcinoma of the stomach: a ten-year survey. J R Coll Surg Edinb 26:322–327, 1981.

81. Carter KJ, Schaffer HA, Ritchie WP: Early gastric cancer. Ann Surg 199:604–609, 1984.

82. Green PHR, O'Toole KM, Slonim D, et al: Increasing incidence and excellent survival of patients with early gastric cancer: experience in a United States medical center. Am J Med 85:658–661, 1988.

83. Gemell NI: Calcification within a gastric carcinoma. AJR 91:779–783, 1964.

84. Thomas RL, Rice RP: Calcifying mucinous adenocarcinoma of the stomach. Radiology 88:1002–1003, 1967.

85. Balthazar E, Rosenthal N: Calcifying mucin-producing adenocarcinoma of stomach. N Y State J Med 73:2704–2706, 1973.

86. Lwin TOM, Soodeen TH: A case report of calcified mucinous adenocarcinoma of the stomach. J Can Assoc Radiol 24:370–373, 1973.

87. Brandt D, Muramatsu Y, Ushio K, et al: Synchronous early gastric cancer. Radiology 173:649–652, 1989.

88. Nelson SW: The discovery of gastric ulcers and the differential diagnosis between benignancy and malignancy. Radiol Clin North Am 7:5–25, 1969.

89. Wolf BS: Observations on roentgen features of benign and malignant gastric ulcers. Semin Roentgenol 6:140–150, 1971.

90. Carman RD: A new roentgen-ray sign of ulcerating gastric cancer. JAMA 77:990–992, 1921.

91. Kirklin BR: The value of the meniscus sign in the roentgenologic diagnosis of ulcerating gastric carcinoma. Radiology 22:131–135, 1934.

92. Marshak RH, Lindner AE, Maklansky D: Carcinoma of the stomach. *In* Marshak RH, Lindner AE, Maklansky D (eds): Radiology of the Stomach. Philadelphia: WB Saunders, 1983, pp 108–146.

93. Balthazar EJ, Rosenberg H, Davidian MM: Scirrhous carcinoma of the pyloric channel and distal antrum. AJR 134:669–673, 1980.

94. Kobayashi S, Yamada A, Kawai B, et al: Study on early cancer of the cardiac region: x-ray findings of the surrounding area of the oesophago-gastric junction. Australas Radiol 16:258–270, 1972.

95. Freeny PC: Double-contrast gastrography of the fundus and cardia: normal landmarks and their pathologic changes. AJR 133:481–487, 1979.

96. Herlinger H, Grossman R, Laufer I, et al: The gastric cardia in double-contrast study: its dynamic image. AJR 135:21–29, 1980.

97. Levine MS, Laufer I, Thompson JJ: Carcinoma of the gastric cardia in young people. AJR 140:69–72, 1983.

98. Freeny PC, Marks WM: Adenocarcinoma of the gastroesophageal junction: barium and CT examination. AJR 138:1077–1084, 1982.

99. Balthazar EJ, Goldfine S, Davidian NM: Carcinoma of the esophagogastric junction. Am J Gastroenterol 74:237–243, 1980.

100. Milnes JP, Hine KR, Holmes GKT, et al: Limitations of endoscopy in the diagnosis of carcinoma of the cardia of the stomach. Br J Radiol 55:593–595, 1982.

101. Lawson TL, Dodds WJ: Infiltrating carcinoma simulating achalasia. Gastrointest Radiol 1:245–248, 1976.

102. Miyake H, Maeda H, Kurauchi S, et al: Thickened gastric walls showing diffuse low attenuation on CT. J Comput Assist Tomogr 13:253–255, 1989.

103. Meyers MA, McSweeney J: Secondary neoplasms of the bowel. Radiology 105:1–11, 1972.

104. Joffe N: Metastatic involvement of the stomach secondary to breast carcinoma. AJR 123:512–521, 1975.

105. Cormier WJ, Gaffey TA, Welch JM, et al: Linitis plastica caused by metastatic lobular carcinoma of the breast. Mayo Clin Proc 55:747–753, 1980.

106. Rubesin SE, Levine MS, Glick SN: Gastric involvement by omental cakes. Gastrointest Radiol 11:223–228, 1986.

107. Eisenberg RL: Gastrointestinal Radiology: A Pattern Approach (2nd ed). Philadelphia: JB Lippincott, 1990, pp 205–222.

108. Bryk D, Elguezabal A: Roentgen problems in evaluating the atrophic stomach of the elderly. AJR 123:236–241, 1975.

109. Levine MS, Caroline D, Thompson JJ, et al: Adenocarcinoma of the esophagus: relationship to Barrett mucosa. Radiology 150:305–309, 1984.

110. Allen HA, Bush JE: Midesophageal carcinoma metastatic to the stomach: its unusual appearance on an upper gastrointestinal series. South Med J 76:1049–1051, 1983.

111. Glick SN, Teplick SK, Levine MS, et al: Gastric cardia metastasis in esophageal carcinoma. Radiology 160:627–630, 1986.

112. Belgrad R, Carlson HC, Payne WS, et al: Pseudotumoral gastric varices. AJR 91:751–756, 1964.

113. Kaye JJ, Stassa G: Mimicry and deception in the diagnosis of tumors of the gastric cardia. AJR 110:295–303, 1970.

114. Anderson MF, Dunnick NR: Pseudotumor caused by gastric varices. Am J Dig Dis 22:929–932, 1977.

115. Ghahremani GG, Collins PA: Esophago-gastric invagination in patients with sliding hiatus hernia. Gastrointest Radiol 1:253–261, 1976.

116. Hyder N: Endoscopic ultrasonography of tumors of the esophagus and the stomach. Surg Endosc 1:17–23, 1987.

117. Tio TL, Coene PP, Schouwink MH, et al: Esophagogastric carcinoma: preoperative TNM classification with endosonography. Radiology 173:411–417, 1989.

118. Tio TL, Coene PP, Luiken GJ, et al: Endosonography in the clinical staging of esophagogastric carcinoma. Gastrointest Endosc 36:92–100, 1990.

119. Scatarige JC, DiSantis DJ: CT of the stomach and duodenum. Radiol Clin North Am 27:687–706, 1989.

120. Cook AO, Levine BA, Sirinek KR, et al: Evaluation of gastric adenocarcinoma. Abdominal computed tomography does not replace celiotomy. Arch Surg 121:603–606, 1986.

121. American Joint Committee on Cancer: Manual for Staging of Cancer (3rd ed). Philadelphia: JB Lippincott, 1988, pp 69–71.

122. Halvorsen RA Jr, Thompson WM: Gastrointestinal cancer: diagnosis, staging, and the follow-up role of imaging. Semin Ultrasound CT MR 10:467–480, 1989.

123. Halvorsen RA Jr, Thompson WM: Primary neoplasms of the hollow organs of the gastrointestinal tract. Staging and follow-up. Cancer 67(suppl 4):1181–1188, 1991.

124. Megibow AJ, Hulnick DH, Balthazar EJ, et al: Ovarian metastases: computed tomographic appearances. Radiology 156:161–164, 1985.

125. Cho KC, Gold BM: Computed tomography of Krukenberg tumors. AJR 145:285–288, 1985.

126. Andaker L, Morales O, Hojer H, et al: Evaluation of preoperative computed tomography in gastric malignancy. Surgery 109:132–135, 1991.

127. Rasch L, Brenoe J, Olesen KP: Predictability of esophagus- and cardiatumor resectability by preoperative computed tomography. Eur J Radiol 11:42–45, 1990.

128. Sussman SK, Halvorsen RA Jr, Illescas FF, et al: Gastric adenocarcinoma: CT versus surgical staging. Radiology 167:335–340, 1988.

129. Dehn TCB, Reznek RH, Nocler IB, et al: The preoperative assessment of advanced gastric cancer by computed tomography. Br J Surg 71:413–415, 1984.

130. Halvorsen RA Jr, Thompson WM: Computed tomographic staging of gastrointestinal tract malignancies. Part I. Esophagus and stomach. Invest Radiol 22:2–16, 1987.

131. Kleinhaus U, Militianu D: Computed tomography in the preoperative evaluation of gastric carcinoma. Gastrointest Radiol 13:97–101, 1988.

132. Spira IH, Ghazi A, Wolff WI: Primary adenocarcinoma of the duodenum. Cancer 39:1721–1726, 1977.

133. Cortese AF, Cornell GN: Carcinoma of the duodenum. Cancer 29:1010–1015, 1972.

134. Joesting DR, Beart RW Jr, van Heerden JA, et al: Improving survival in adenocarcinoma of the duodenum. Am J Surg 141:228–231, 1981.

135. Itoh H, Iida M, Kuroiwa S, et al: Gardner's syndrome associated with carcinoma of the duodenal bulb: report of a case. Am J Gastroenterol 80:248–250, 1985.

136. Levine ML, Dorf BS, Bank S: Adenocarcinoma of the duodenum in a patient with nontropical sprue. Am J Gastroenterol 81:800–802, 1986.

137. Meiselman MS, Ghahremani GG, Kaufman MW: Crohn's disease of the duodenum complicated by adenocarcinoma. Gastrointest Radiol 12:333–336, 1987.

138. Slezak P, Rubio C, Blomqvist L, et al: Duodenal adenocarcinoma in Crohn's disease of the small bowel: a case report. Gastrointest Radiol 16:15–17, 1991.

139. McGlinchey JJ, Santer GJ, Haggani MT: Primary adenocarcinoma of the duodenum associated with cutaneous neurofibromatosis. Postgrad Med J 58:115–116, 1982.

140. Nix GAJJ, Wilson JHP, Dees J: Primary malignant tumours of the duodenum. ROFO 142:385–390, 1985.

141. Barloon TJ, Lu CH, Honda H, et al: Primary adenocarcinoma of the duodenal bulb: radiographic and pathologic findings in two cases. Gastrointest Radiol 14:223–225, 1989.

142. Farah MC, Jafri SZ, Schwab RE, et al: Duodenal neoplasms: role of CT. Radiology 162:839–843, 1987.

143. Bree RL, Megibow AJ: Hypotonic CT duodenography in the evaluation of periampullary neoplasms. Radiology 177:251, 1990.

# Other Malignant Tumors

Marc S. Levine, M.D.

Alec J. Megibow, M.D.

## METASTASES

Gastric metastases are found at autopsy in less than 2% of patients who die of carcinoma.[1] Duodenal metastases are even rarer. Nevertheless, metastases to the stomach and duodenum have been encountered more frequently as combined treatment with surgery, radiation, or chemotherapy has led to prolonged survival of patients with widespread metastatic disease. The majority of lesions are hematogenous metastases from malignant melanoma or carcinoma of the breast. Less frequently, the stomach and duodenum may be involved by lymphatic spread of tumor or by direct extension of tumor from neighboring structures or mesenteric reflections such as the gastrocolic ligament, transverse mesocolon, and greater omentum. These various forms of spread produce characteristic radiographic findings that are considered separately in the following sections.

## Clinical Aspects

Most gastroduodenal metastases are unexpected findings at surgery or autopsy.[2, 3] However, ulcerated metastases may cause upper gastrointestinal bleeding with hematemesis, melena, or guaiac-positive stool.[4, 5] Other patients may have epigastric pain, nausea, vomiting, early satiety, anorexia, or weight loss. However, the latter findings are sometimes caused by systemic chemotherapy or the hypercalcemia associated with widespread metastatic disease.[6] As a result, gastroduodenal metastases may not be suspected even if symptoms are present.

Most patients with gastroduodenal metastases have a known underlying malignancy. Occasionally, however, metastases to the stomach and duodenum may be the initial manifestation of an occult primary tumor. Other malignancies such as carcinoma of the breast and kidney can metastasize to the stomach and duodenum many years after treatment of the original lesion.[6, 7] Thus, it is important to ascertain whether there is a history of malignancy for all patients with upper gastrointestinal disease.

## Radiographic Findings

### Hematogenous Metastases

True hematogenous or blood-borne metastases to the stomach and duodenum may be caused by a variety of malignant tumors, including malignant melanoma and carcinoma of the breast or lung. Although malignant melanoma has the highest percentage of gastrointestinal metastases,[2, 8] breast cancer is such a common disease that it rivals melanoma as the most common cause of metastases to the bowel.[6] Much less frequently, the stomach and duodenum may be involved by hematogenous metastases from thyroid or testicular carcinoma or from other remote malignancies.[1]

Hematogenous metastases usually appear radiographically as one or more discrete submucosal masses in the stomach, duodenum, or small intestine[6, 9–12] (Fig. 39–1). When multiple lesions are present, they tend to be of varying sizes because of periodic showers of tumor emboli into the arterial supply of the bowel.[9, 13] As they

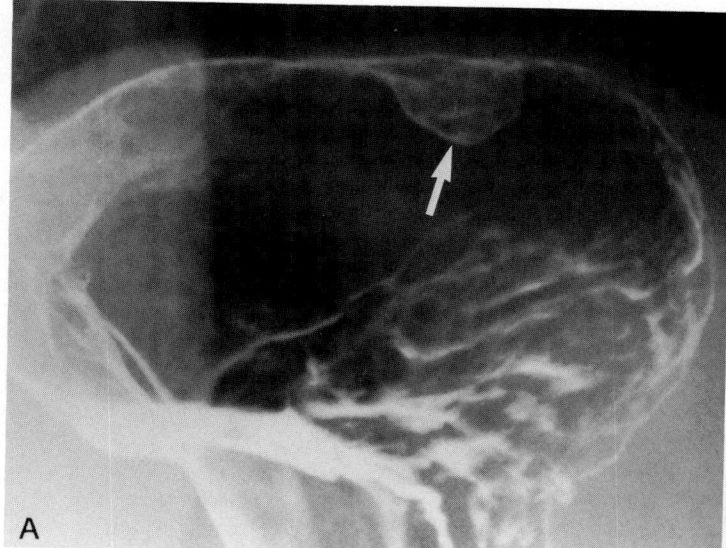

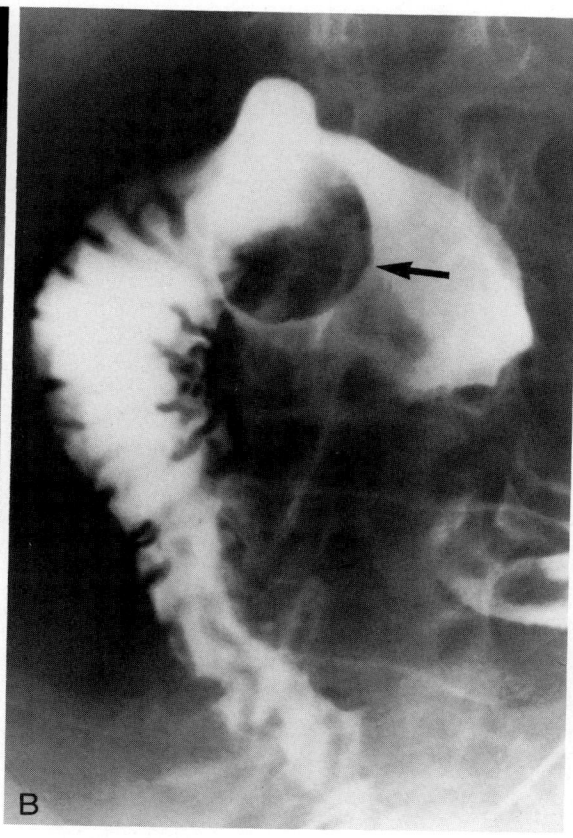

**Figure 39–1. Gastric metastases from malignant melanoma. A.** A discrete submucosal mass *(arrow)* is seen in the gastric fundus. **B.** In another patient, a large submucosal mass *(arrow)* is present in the duodenal bulb.

outgrow their blood supply, these submucosal masses may undergo central necrosis and ulceration, producing classic "bull's-eye" or "target" lesions[9, 11–13] (Fig. 39–2). In general, bull's-eye lesions have large central ulcers in relation to the size of the surrounding mass.[9, 13] Superficial fissures occasionally radiate peripherally from the central ulcer crater, producing a "spoke-wheel" pattern[9] (see Fig. 39–2B). Rarely, bull's-eye lesions undergo spontaneous regression after systemic chemotherapy.[11]

Hematogenous metastases from malignant melanoma, breast or lung cancer, or other malignancies may also appear radiographically as larger, more lobulated masses in the stomach or duodenum (Fig. 39–3). Other patients may develop giant ulcers or cavities as a result of necrosis and excavation of the tumor. These cavitated metastases can be recognized on barium studies as amorphous collections of barium (usually ranging from 5 to 15 cm in size) that communicate with the lumen[12, 14] (Fig. 39–4). Computed tomography (CT) is also well suited for demonstrating these giant, cavitated lesions.[15] Rarely, noncavitated metastases that have a significant exoenteric component can mimic the appearance of extrinsic mass lesions compressing the stomach or duodenum.[11]

Hematogenous metastases from carcinoma of the breast may also be manifested by a narrowed, rigid stomach, producing a linitis plastica or "leather bottle" appearance indistinguishable from that of a primary scirrhous carcinoma[6, 9, 10, 12] (Fig. 39–5). Unlike scirrhous carcinoma, however, metastatic breast cancer involving

the stomach does not elicit a significant desmoplastic response. Instead, this linitis plastica appearance results from highly cellular deposits of metastatic tumor in the gastric wall.[9] The degree of gastric narrowing is variable, so there may be only mild loss of distensibility. Nevertheless, these lesions can be recognized on double contrast studies by distortion of the normal surface pattern of the stomach, with mucosal nodularity, spiculation, ulceration, or thickened, irregular folds[16] (see Fig. 39–5). Furthermore, these lesions may involve the proximal portion of the stomach with sparing of the antrum[16] (see Fig. 39–5B). The possibility of metastatic disease should therefore be considered in any patient with linitis plastica who has a history of breast carcinoma.

The linitis plastica form of metastatic breast cancer involving the stomach is characterized on CT by marked thickening of the gastric wall. With the use of negative intraluminal contrast agents and dynamic scanning techniques, CT often reveals enhancement of the thickened gastric wall with relative preservation of the overlying rugal folds (Fig. 39–6).

## Lymphatic Spread

Gastric metastases are found at autopsy in 2 to 15% of patients who die of squamous cell carcinoma of the esophagus.[17] These metastases are thought to be caused by tumor emboli that seed the gastric cardia or fundus via submucosal esophageal lymphatics extending subdiaphragmatically to paracardiac, lesser curvature, and

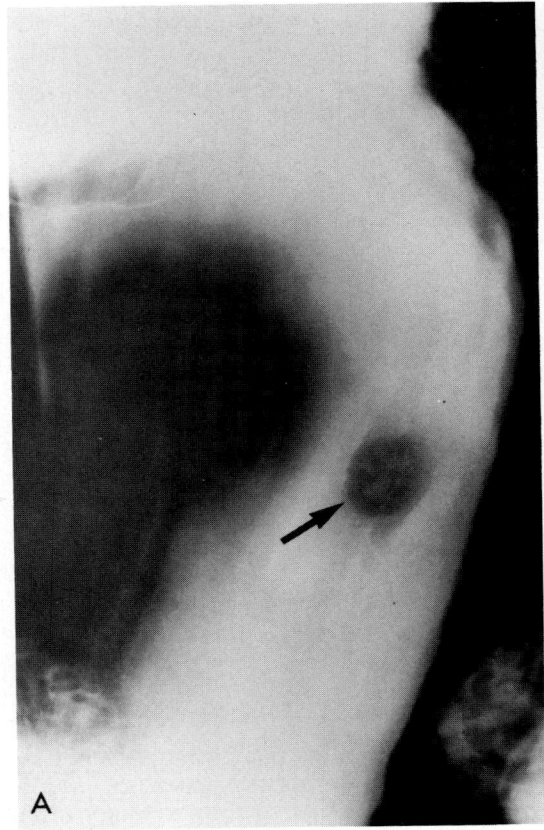

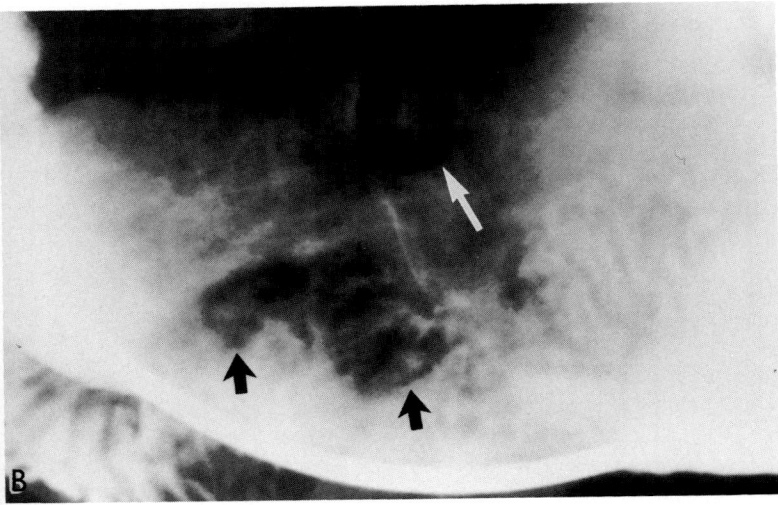

**Figure 39–2. Ulcerated gastric metastases from malignant melanoma. A.** A centrally ulcerated submucosal mass or bull's-eye lesion *(arrow)* is seen in the gastric body. **B.** In another patient, a prone compression view reveals multiple bull's-eye lesions *(black arrows)* in the stomach. Superficial fissures are seen radiating from the central ulcer of a metastasis on the lesser curvature, producing a spoke-wheel appearance *(white arrow).*

**Figure 39–3. Gastric metastasis from malignant melanoma.** There is a large, lobulated mass *(arrows)* on the greater curvature of the stomach. This lesion could be mistaken for a leiomyosarcoma or even an adenocarcinoma.

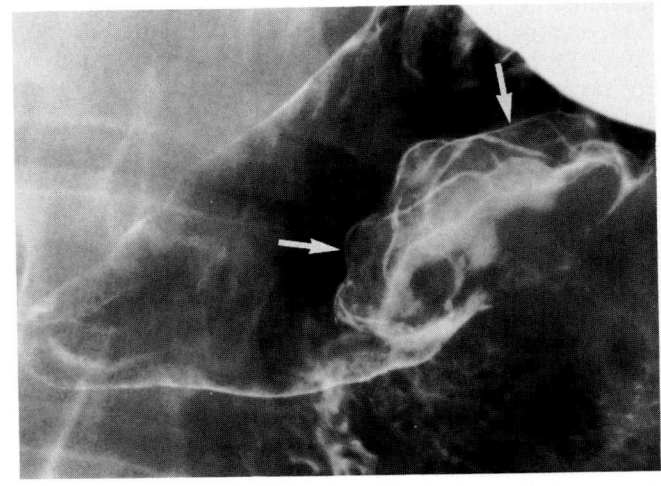

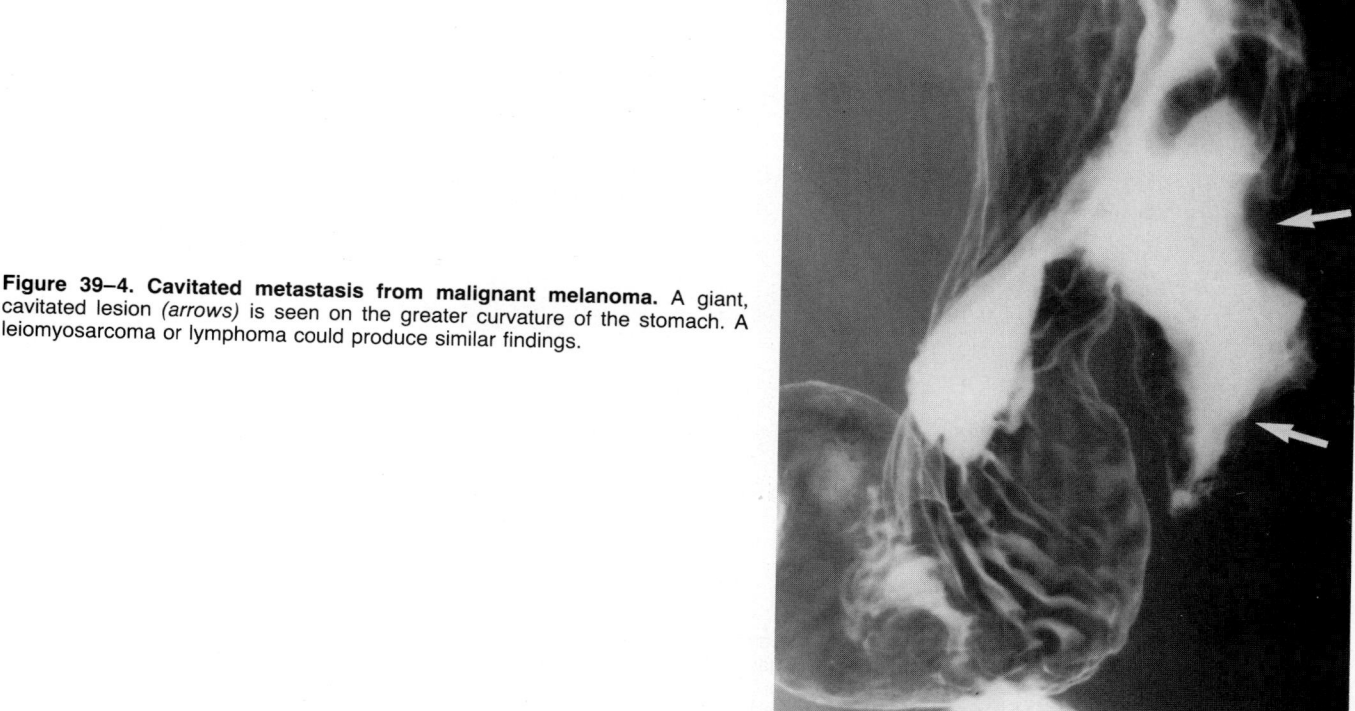

**Figure 39–4. Cavitated metastasis from malignant melanoma.** A giant, cavitated lesion *(arrows)* is seen on the greater curvature of the stomach. A leiomyosarcoma or lymphoma could produce similar findings.

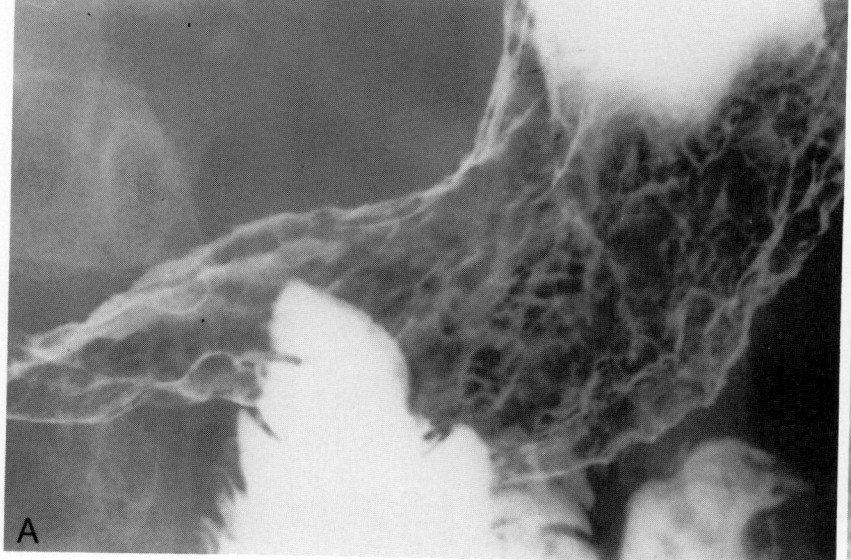

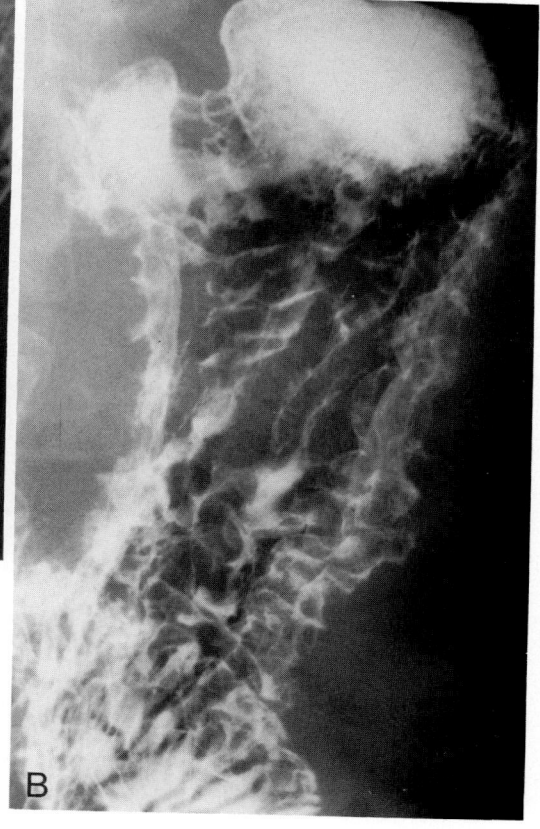

**Figure 39–5. Metastatic breast cancer involving the stomach with a linitis plastica appearance. A.** There is only mild loss of distensibility of the gastric antrum and body, but the mucosa has a nodular, irregular appearance due to infiltration by metastatic tumor. **B.** In another patient, the area of involvement is confined to the proximal half of the stomach. Note that the fundus and body have an irregular contour with thickened, spiculated folds. (**A** and **B** from Levine MS, Kong V, Rubesin SE, et al: Scirrhous carcinoma of the stomach: radiologic and endoscopic diagnosis. Radiology 175:151–154, 1990.)

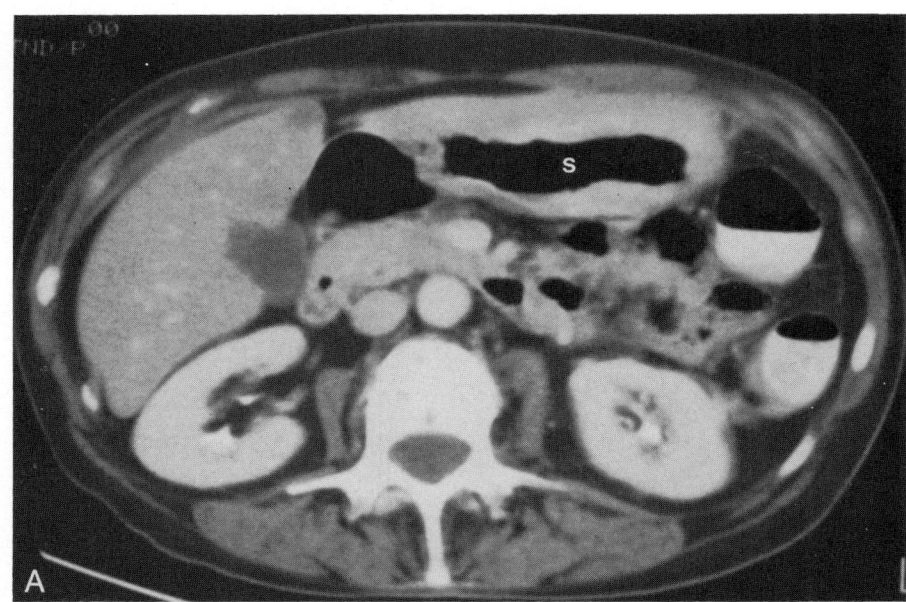

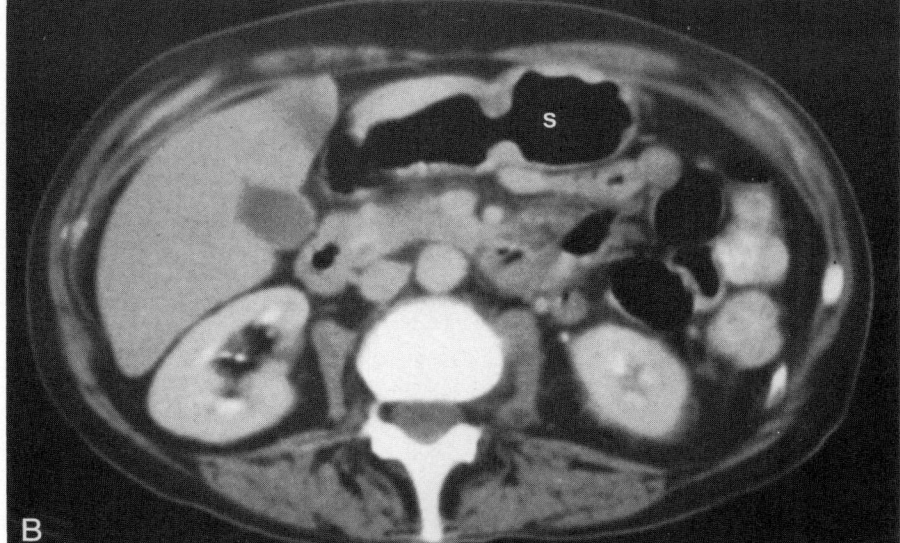

**Figure 39–6. Metastatic breast cancer with a linitis plastica appearance on a CT scan.** Two images (**A** and **B**) from a CT scan reveal a thickened, hyperdense gastric wall with relative preservation of the overlying rugal folds. S = stomach.

celiac nodes. Squamous cell metastases to the gastric fundus usually appear radiographically as large submucosal masses, often containing central areas of ulceration[17, 18] (Fig. 39–7). As a result, these lesions can be mistaken for gastric leiomyomas, leiomyosarcomas, or even adenocarcinomas.[19] Squamous cell metastases to paracardiac or other lymph nodes in the upper abdomen often appear on CT scans as multiple low-attenuation masses relative to skeletal muscle (Fig. 39–8).

The duodenum may occasionally be involved by peripancreatic lymphadenopathy from pancreatic carcinoma, lymphoma, or other malignant tumors. In such cases, barium studies may demonstrate nodular indentations on the medial border of the descending duodenum or widening of the duodenal loop. However, pancreatic carcinoma, pancreatic pseudocysts, and pancreatitis may produce identical radiographic findings. CT is extremely helpful for determining the cause of a pancreatic mass and for differentiating such a mass from adjacent lymphadenopathy.

Malignant tumors that metastasize to retroperitoneal lymph nodes near the superior mesenteric root may be manifested radiographically by an extrinsic mass effect, nodular indentations, ulceration, or, in advanced cases, obstruction of the distal duodenum near the ligament of Treitz[20] (Figs. 39–9 and 39–10). CT is ideally suited for demonstrating retroperitoneal adenopathy as the cause of these abnormalities on barium studies (see Fig. 39–9B). Occasionally, retroperitoneal tumor involving the duodenum may cause delayed gastric emptying and massive gastric dilatation out of proportion to the degree

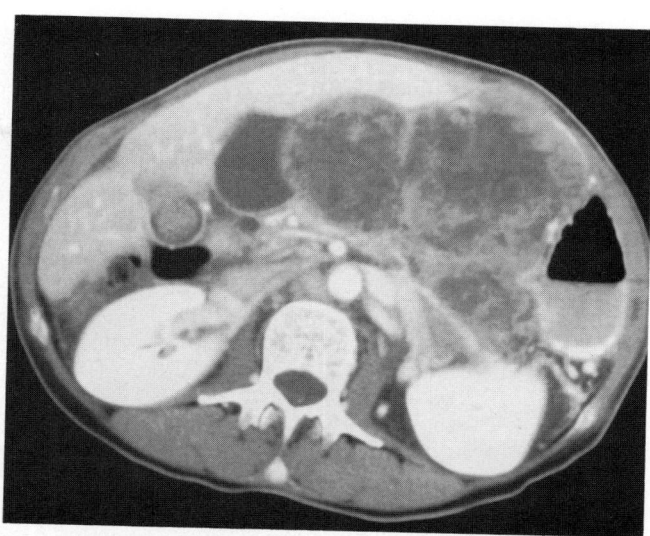

**Figure 39–8. Metastatic adenopathy from squamous cell carcinoma of the esophagus.** A bulky mass of adenopathy is seen in the region of the lesser sac. The low attenuation of the enlarged nodes is characteristic of squamous cell metastases.

of duodenal dilatation[21] (Fig. 39–11). The disproportionate degree of gastric dilatation in these patients may be related to vagal destruction by retroperitoneal tumor, which decreases gastric peristalsis and exacerbates gastric distention. Whatever the explanation, it should be recognized that duodenal obstruction by retroperitoneal tumor can mimic the appearance of acute gastric outlet obstruction.

## Direct Invasion

The stomach and duodenum may be directly invaded by malignant tumors arising in neighboring structures such as the esophagus, pancreas, and kidney. The stomach and duodenum may also be involved by direct extension of colonic carcinoma along mesenteric reflections such as the gastrocolic ligament and transverse mesocolon or by contiguous spread of tumor from the greater omentum. Because the radiographic findings depend on the pathways of spread, the various primary malignancies are discussed separately.

### Esophageal Carcinoma

Unlike squamous cell carcinomas of the esophagus, adenocarcinomas arising in Barrett's mucosa have a marked tendency to invade the gastric cardia or fundus.[22, 23] Gastric involvement may be manifested radiographically by a polypoid or ulcerated mass in the gastric fundus. In other cases, however, double contrast views of the fundus may reveal more subtle findings, with distortion or obliteration of the normal anatomic landmarks at the cardia and irregular areas of ulceration[22] (see Fig. 28–20). It is often difficult to determine whether tumors at the gastroesophageal junction have arisen in the esophagus or in the stomach. However, esophageal adenocarcinomas often have a

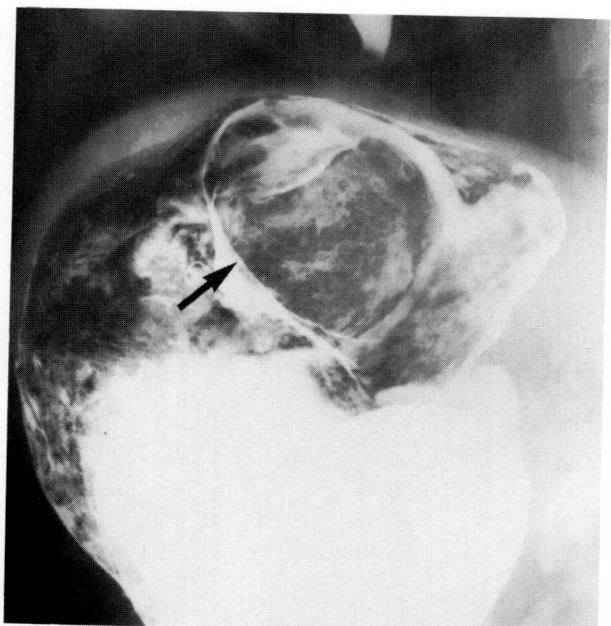

**Figure 39–7. Squamous cell metastasis to the gastric cardia.** There is a giant submucosal mass *(arrow)* in the fundus that could be mistaken for a leiomyoma or a leiomyosarcoma. (From Glick SN, Teplick SK, Levine MS: Squamous cell metastases to the gastric cardia. Gastrointest Radiol 10:339–344, 1985.)

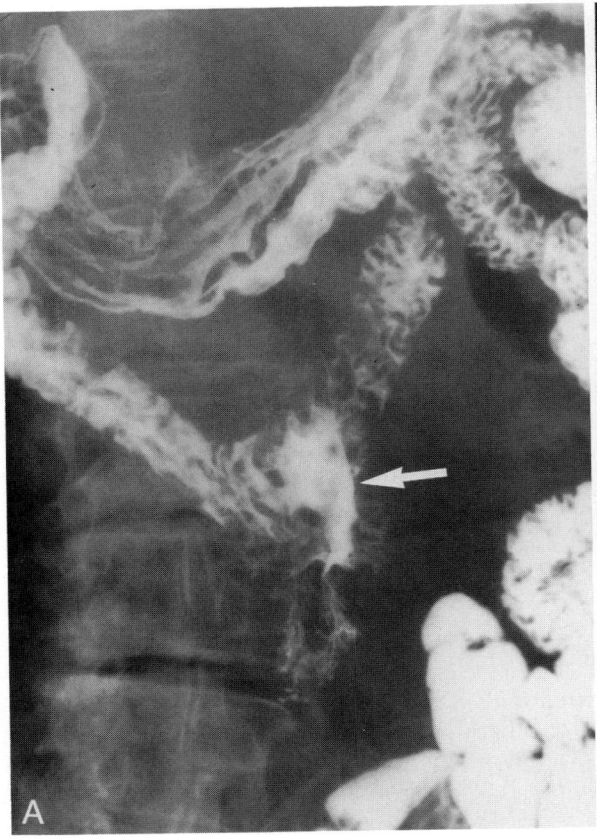

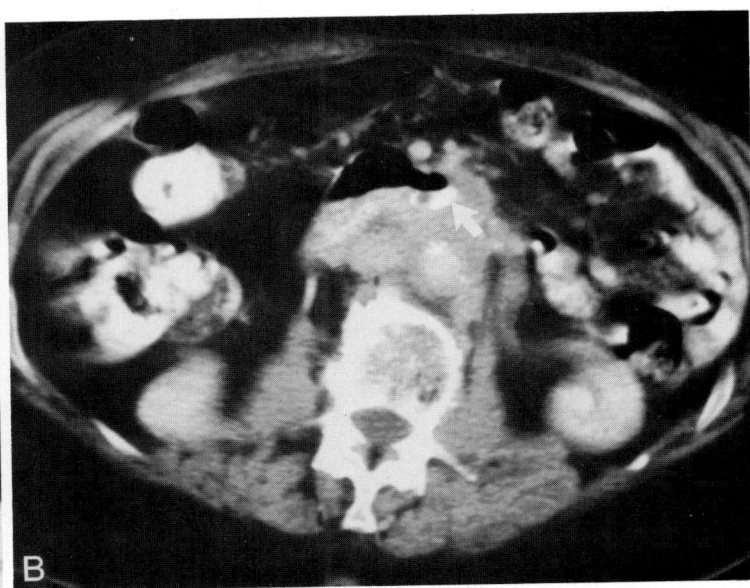

**Figure 39–9. Duodenal invasion by retroperitoneal adenopathy. A.** A barium study shows an ulcerated lesion *(arrow)* at the junction of the third and fourth portions of the duodenum. **B.** A CT scan reveals a conglomerate mass of para-aortic adenopathy engulfing the distal duodenum with associated ulceration *(arrow)*.

**Figure 39–10. Duodenal obstruction by metastatic adenopathy near the superior mesenteric root.** There are focal narrowing and obstruction of the distal duodenum *(arrow)* near the ligament of Treitz due to metastatic ovarian cancer. The duodenum is considerably dilated above this level.

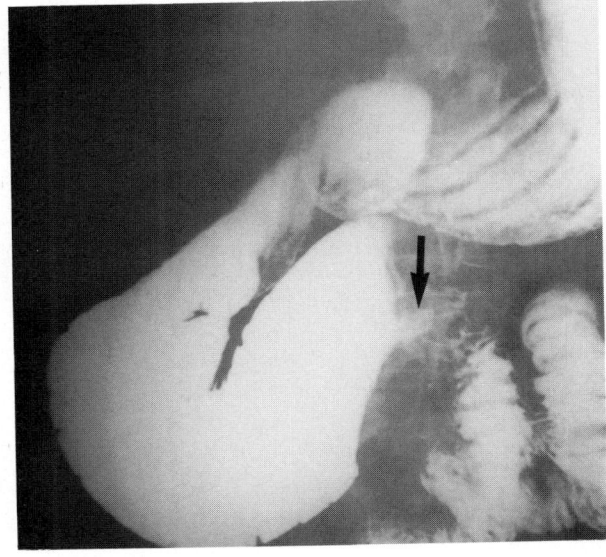

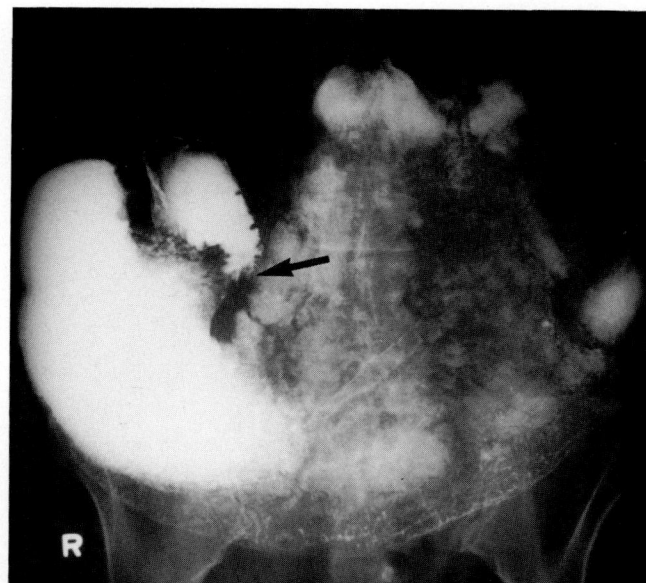

**Figure 39–11. Duodenal obstruction by retroperitoneal metastases.** A delayed overhead radiograph from an upper gastrointestinal study shows abrupt narrowing of the descending duodenum *(arrow)* with massive gastric dilatation out of proportion to the degree of duodenal dilatation. The dilated stomach extends inferiorly into the pelvis. (From Shammash JB, Rubesin SE, Levine MS: Massive gastric distention due to duodenal involvement by retroperitoneal tumors. Gastrointest Radiol 17:214–216, 1992.)

disproportionate degree of esophageal involvement in relation to that of the stomach, whereas gastric or cardiac carcinomas have a greater degree of fundal involvement.

### Pancreatic Carcinoma

The nature and extent of gastroduodenal involvement by pancreatic carcinoma depend on whether the underlying tumor is located in the head, body, or tail of the pancreas. Carcinoma of the pancreatic head may cause widening of the duodenal loop or extrinsic compression of the medial border of the descending duodenum or greater curvature of the gastric antrum, whereas carcinoma of the pancreatic body or tail may cause extrinsic compression of the posterior wall of the gastric fundus and body or the superior border of the distal duodenum near the ligament of Treitz.[24] Actual invasion of the stomach or duodenum may be manifested radiographically by spiculated mucosal folds, nodularity, mass effect, ulceration, or obstruction[24] (Figs. 39–12 to 39–14). Rarely, gastroduodenal invasion by pancreatic carcinoma leads to the development of fistulas between the tumor and the bowel. However, such fistulas may also occur as a complication of severe pancreatitis.

CT is of limited value in predicting duodenal invasion by pancreatic carcinoma, but distention of the duodenum with gas or water may be helpful in some cases.

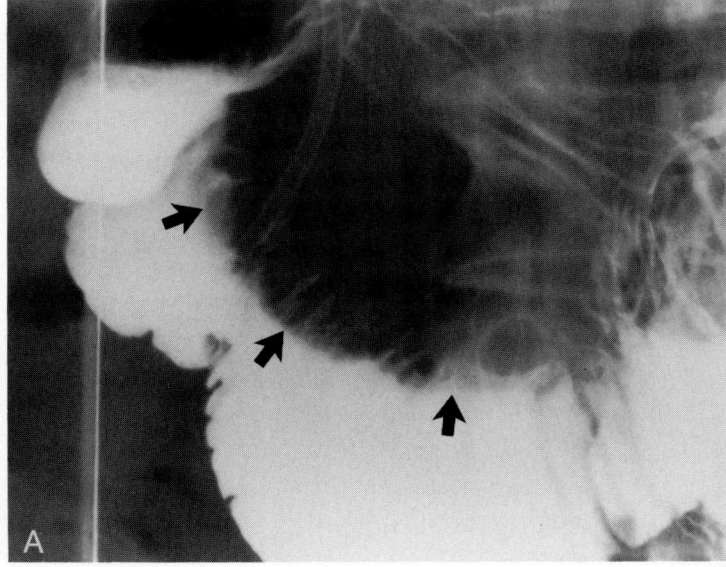

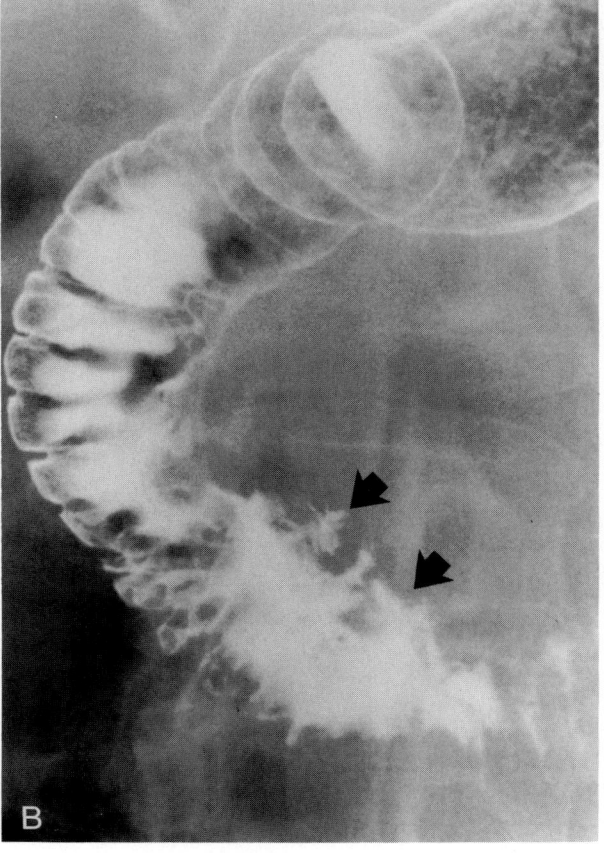

**Figure 39–12. Duodenal invasion by pancreatic carcinoma. A.** Mass effect and spiculated mucosal folds *(arrows)* are seen on the medial aspect of the descending duodenum due to invasion by carcinoma of the head of the pancreas. **B.** In another patient, there is irregular ulceration *(arrows)* of the descending duodenum due to invasion by tumor.

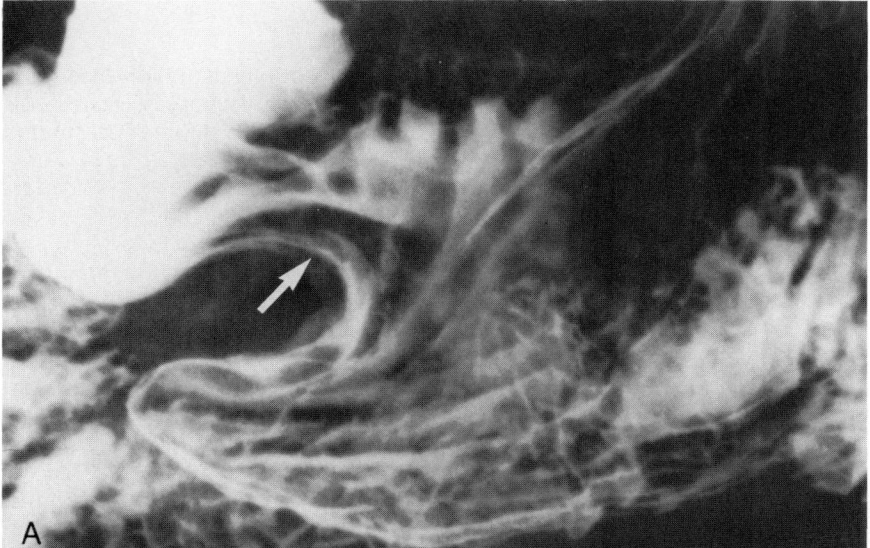

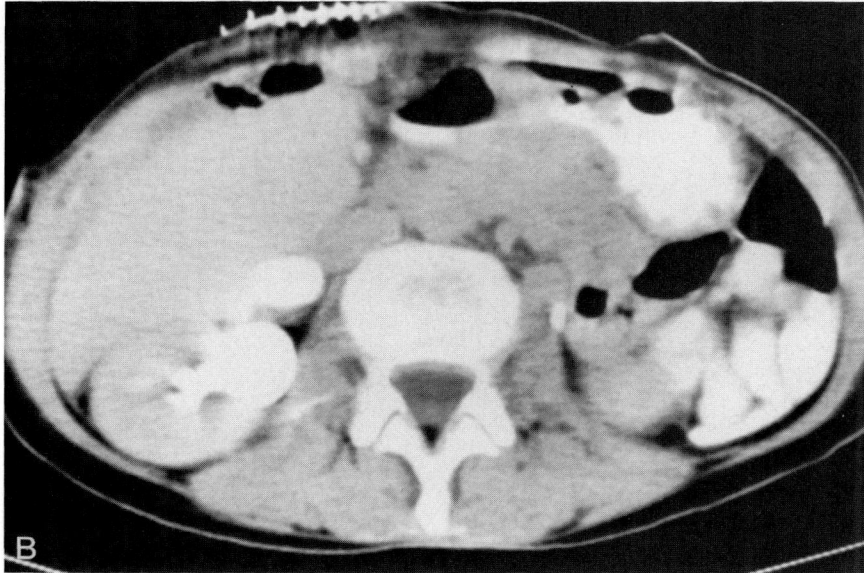

**Figure 39–13. Gastric invasion by pancreatic carcinoma. A.** A barium study shows a focal area of mass effect *(arrow)* on the greater curvature of the stomach. **B.** A CT scan reveals an advanced pancreatic carcinoma invading the stomach.

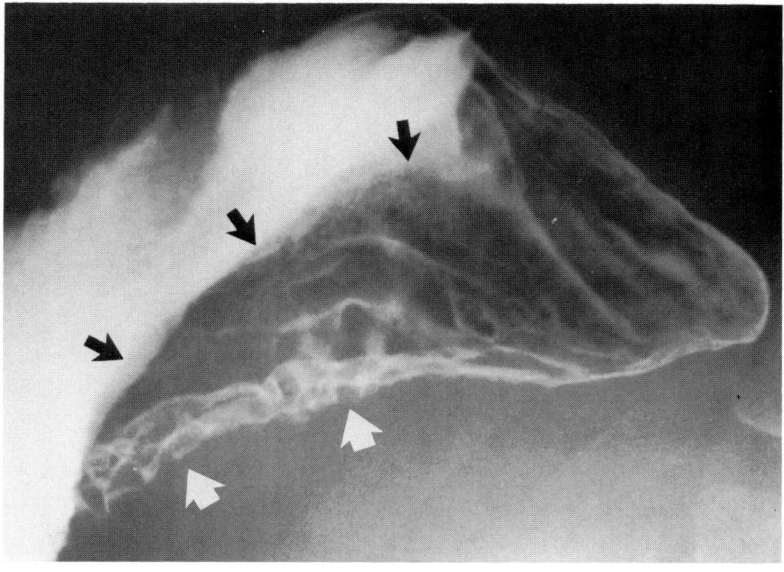

**Figure 39–14. Gastric invasion by pancreatic carcinoma.** There is extrinsic mass effect *(black arrows)* on the posterior wall of the gastric fundus due to an adjacent carcinoma of the pancreatic tail. The spiculated gastric contour *(white arrows)* indicates gastric invasion by tumor.

Most patients with suspected pancreatic neoplasms undergo CT as the initial diagnostic examination, so a barium study should be performed for a more detailed assessment of the duodenum when it appears to be narrowed or obstructed on CT scans. Regardless of the CT findings, a barium study or endoscopy is essential for any patient with melena and an adjacent pancreatic mass. CT is of greater value in determining the cause of an abnormal retrogastric impression, because it can differentiate pancreatic carcinoma from pancreatic pseudocysts, retrogastric varices, or other abnormalities in the retroperitoneum[25, 26] (Fig. 39–15; see Fig. 39–13).

### Renal Cell Carcinoma

Direct invasion of the duodenum by right-sided renal cell carcinomas may be manifested radiographically by mass effect, nodularity, or ulceration of the posterolateral border of the descending duodenum. However,

renal cell carcinoma tends not to elicit a desmoplastic response in the wall of the bowel, so duodenal involvement may also be manifested by a polypoid intraluminal mass, mimicking the appearance of a primary duodenal carcinoma.[7, 9] In patients with advanced renal cell carcinomas, CT is helpful for determining the presence and extent of tumor and its proximity to the duodenum. When a contiguous lesion is identified, however, CT is not a reliable examination for determining whether or not there is duodenal invasion.

### Colonic Carcinoma

Colonic carcinomas may involve the stomach and duodenum by direct extension along mesenteric reflections such as the gastrocolic ligament and transverse mesocolon. The gastrocolic ligament is the proximal portion of the greater omentum that extends superiorly from the anterosuperior border of the transverse colon

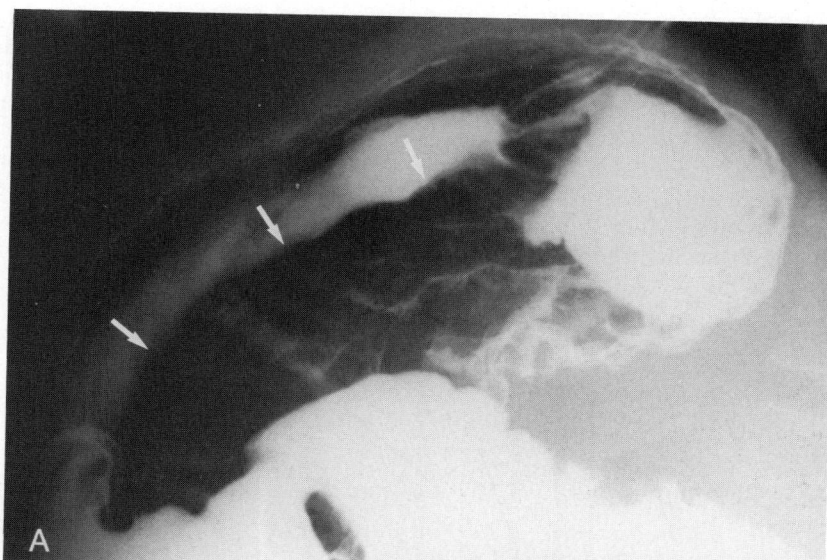

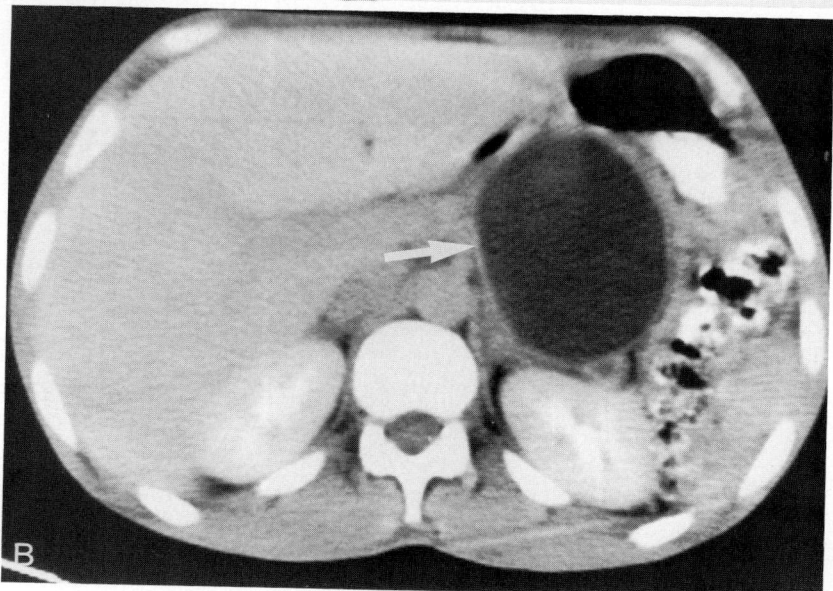

**Figure 39–15. Gastric involvement by a pancreatic pseudocyst. A.** A barium study shows smooth extrinsic compression *(arrows)* of the posterior wall of the gastric fundus. **B.** A CT scan reveals a large pancreatic pseudocyst *(arrow)* as the cause of this finding.

to the greater curvature of the stomach (Fig. 39–16). Because of this anatomic relationship, carcinoma of the transverse colon may invade the stomach via the gastrocolic ligament, producing mass effect, nodularity, and spiculated, tethered mucosal folds on the greater curvature of the gastric antrum or body.[9, 27] In other patients, carcinoma of the ascending colon or hepatic flexure may invade the duodenum via the lateral reflection of the transverse mesocolon, producing mass effect, nodularity, ulceration, or spiculated mucosal folds on the lateral border of the descending duodenum[28, 29] (Fig. 39–17A). When characteristic changes are detected radiographically in the stomach or duodenum, a barium enema examination should be performed to rule out an unsuspected carcinoma of the transverse colon or hepatic flexure as the basis for these findings. CT may also reveal the colonic neoplasm and the mode of spread to the stomach or duodenum (Fig. 39–17B).

Carcinoma of the transverse colon invading the stomach or carcinoma of the hepatic flexure invading the duodenum occasionally leads to the development of gastrocolic (see Fig. 40–40) or duodenocolic fistulas[9, 28, 30, 31] (see Fig. 40–41). Although these fistulas may be demonstrated by an upper gastrointestinal study, they are more likely to be seen in a barium enema examination because of the higher pressures generated.[30, 31] Both gastrocolic and duodenocolic fistulas may be associated with a characteristic clinical syndrome of feculent vomiting, foul-smelling eructations, and undigested food particles in the stool.[31] In the past, the majority of gastrocolic fistulas had a malignant origin. In today's pill-oriented society, however, most such fistulas are probably caused by benign, aspirin-induced greater curvature gastric ulcers that penetrate through the gastrocolic ligament into the transverse colon (see Chapter 35).

### Omental Metastases

Bulky metastatic deposits in the greater omentum or omental "cakes" usually result from widespread intraperitoneal dissemination of ovarian carcinoma or, less frequently, cervical, uterine, bladder, gastric, colonic, pancreatic, or breast carcinoma.[32] These omental deposits may spread superiorly to the stomach via the proximal portion of the greater omentum, also known as the gastrocolic ligament (see Fig. 39–16). Gastric involvement by omental metastases is characterized radiographically by mass effect, nodularity, flattening, or spiculated, tethered mucosal folds on the greater curvature of the gastric antrum or body[33] (Fig. 39–18A). These changes reflect serosal involvement by tumor as well as a desmoplastic response that occurs along the insertion of the gastrocolic ligament on the greater curvature. In advanced cases, there may be circumferential narrowing of the gastric antrum due to encasement by metastatic tumor.[33]

Carcinoma of the transverse colon invading the stomach via the gastrocolic ligament may produce identical radiographic findings (see earlier section on colonic carcinoma).[9, 27] In such cases, however, a barium enema examination should demonstrate the primary colonic

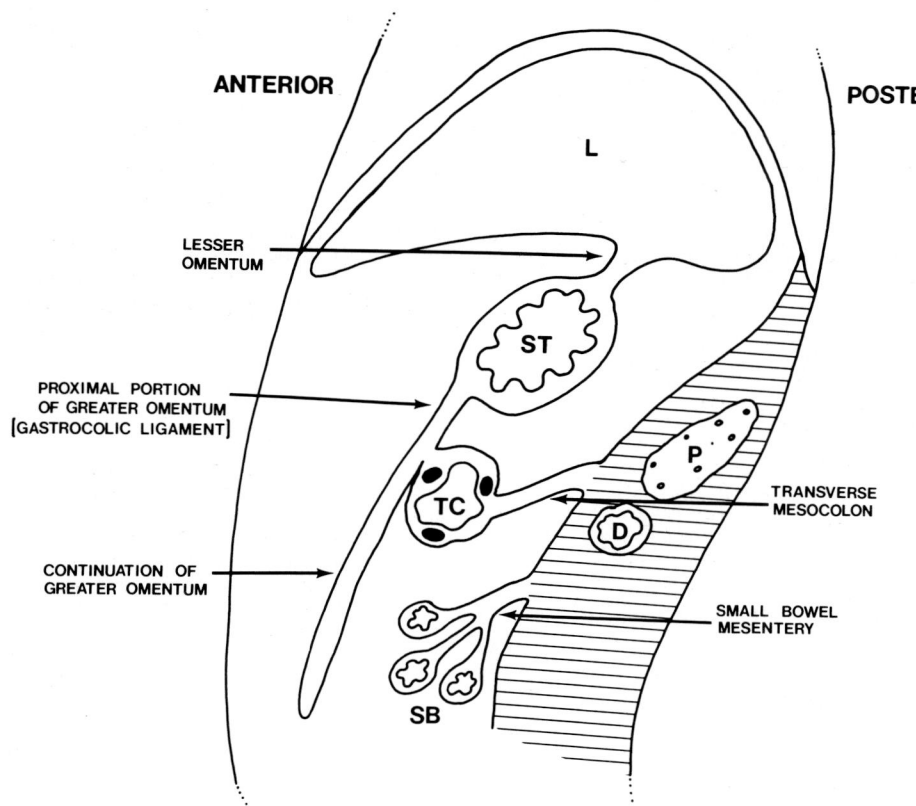

**ANTERIOR**

**POSTERIOR**

L

LESSER
OMENTUM

ST

PROXIMAL PORTION
OF GREATER OMENTUM
[GASTROCOLIC LIGAMENT]

P

TC

D

TRANSVERSE
MESOCOLON

CONTINUATION OF
GREATER OMENTUM

SB

SMALL BOWEL
MESENTERY

**Figure 39–16. Sagittal diagram showing the mesenteric attachments of the stomach, small bowel, and colon.** Because the proximal portion of the greater omentum (i.e., the gastrocolic ligament) inserts along the greater curvature of the stomach, contiguous spread of tumor from the transverse colon or greater omentum affects primarily this region. (From Rubesin SE, Levine MS: Omental cakes: colonic involvement by omental metastases. Radiology 154:593–596, 1985.)

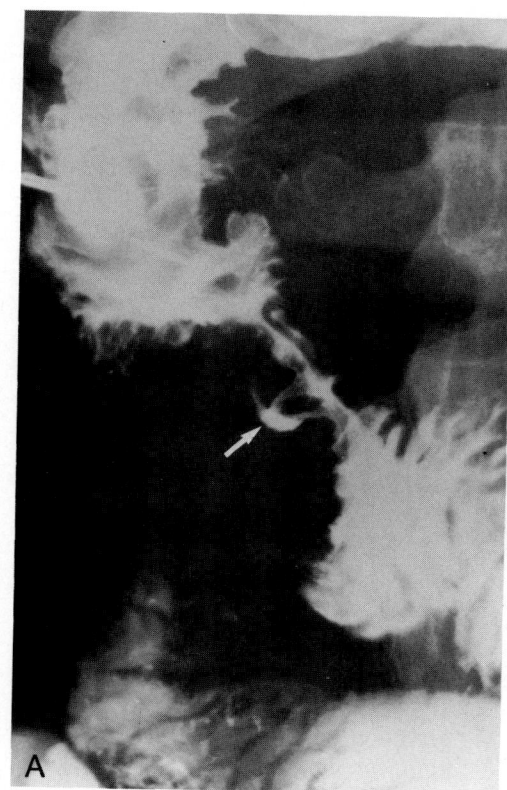

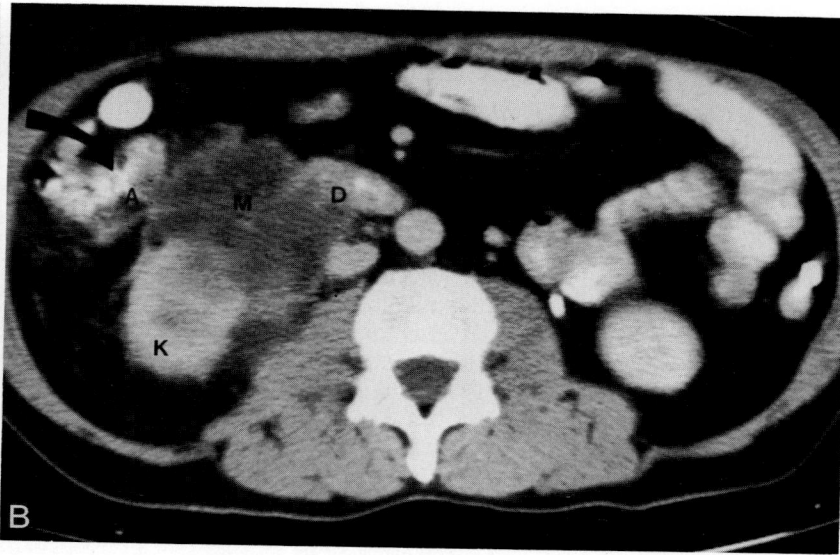

**Figure 39–17. Duodenal invasion by colonic carcinoma. A.** A large area of mass effect is seen on the lateral border of the descending duodenum with associated ulceration *(arrow)*. This finding was caused by carcinoma of the hepatic flexure invading the duodenum. **B.** In another patient, a CT scan shows invasion of the duodenum by recurrent carcinoma arising from the region of an ileotransverse colonic anastomosis (A). A heterogeneous mass (M) is seen invading the duodenum (D) and right kidney (K). Contrast medium is present in the bowel *(arrow)* adjacent to the anastomosis.

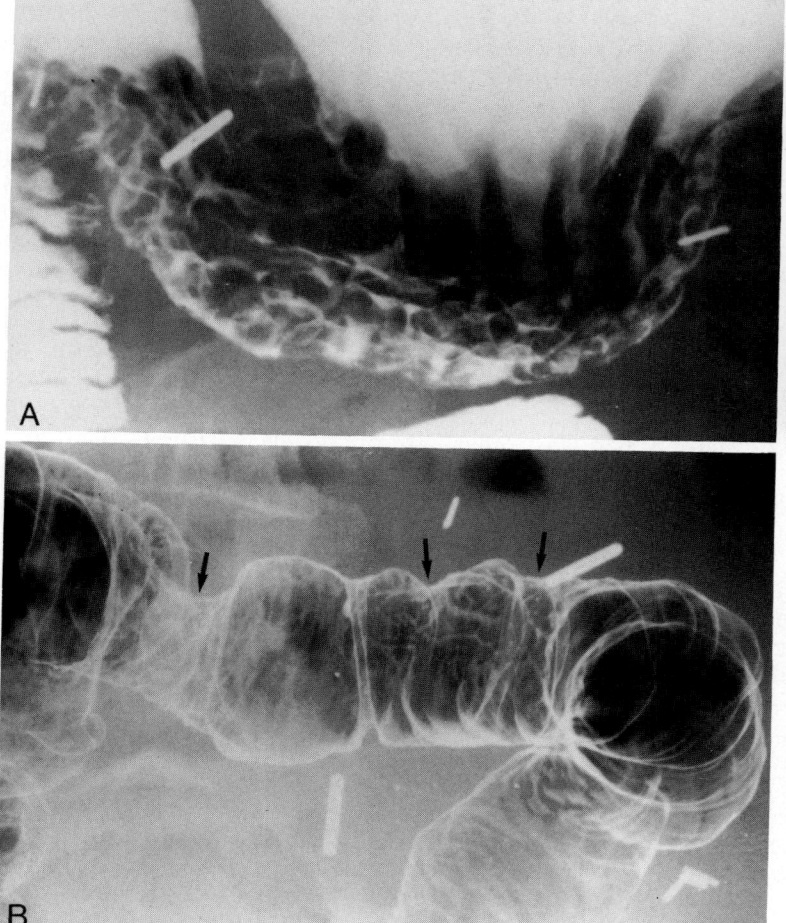

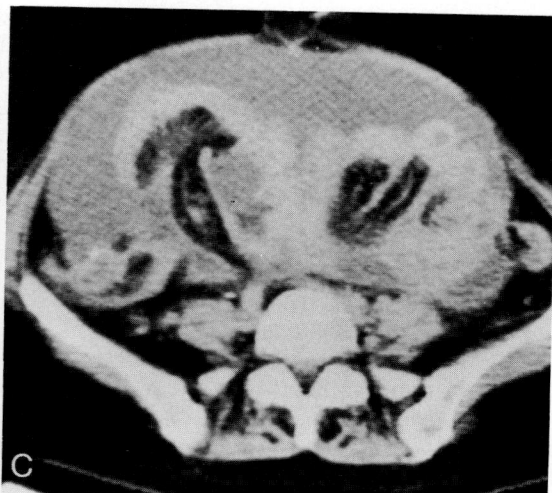

**Figure 39–18. Gastric and colonic involvement by omental metastases from ovarian carcinoma. A.** An upper gastrointestinal study shows spiculated folds and mucosal nodularity on the greater curvature of the gastric antrum and body caused by direct extension of tumor from the greater omentum. **B.** A barium enema shows spiculation and tethering of the superior border of the transverse colon *(arrows)* caused by simultaneous colonic involvement by omental tumor. **C.** In another patient, a CT scan reveals a bulky omental cake separating the small bowel from the anterior abdominal wall.

carcinoma responsible for these findings. In contrast, patients with omental metastases involving the stomach almost always have associated colonic involvement by omental tumor, with mass effect, nodularity, and spiculated mucosal folds on the superior border of the transverse colon or, in advanced cases, circumferential narrowing of the bowel[34] (Fig. 39–18B). These patients also tend to have intraperitoneally seeded metastases to the classic sites described by Meyers, including the anterior border of the rectosigmoid colon, the superior border of the sigmoid colon, the medial border of the cecum or distal ileum, and the lateral border of the ascending colon.[35, 36] A barium enema examination should therefore differentiate omental metastases to the stomach and colon from gastric invasion by a primary carcinoma of the transverse colon. In our experience, gastric involvement by omental metastases is at least 10 times more common than gastric invasion by colonic carcinoma.

When gastric involvement by omental metastases is suspected on barium studies, CT should be performed to better delineate the nature and extent of metastatic tumor. Although conventional barium studies provide indirect evidence of omental disease, CT can reveal omental masses as small as 1 cm.[32] More extensive omental metastases may be manifested on CT scans by a spectrum of findings, ranging from a lacy reticular appearance to bulky masses.[37] When the greater omentum is diffusely infiltrated by tumor, an omental cake may displace the colon or small bowel from the anterior abdominal wall[32, 38] (Fig. 39–18C). Unless the lumen of the bowel is distended with contrast medium or gas, however, it is difficult to determine whether there is actual invasion of the stomach or transverse colon.

## Differential Diagnosis

Hematogenous metastases that appear as small, sessile lesions in the stomach and duodenum may be difficult to differentiate radiographically from multiple hyperplastic or adenomatous polyps. Metastases that have a more typical submucosal appearance can be mistaken for benign intramural lesions such as leiomyomas, lipomas, and ectopic pancreatic rests. However, these benign mesenchymal tumors tend to occur as solitary lesions, whereas metastases are usually multiple. Centrally ulcerated (i.e., bull's-eye) lesions may be caused not only by hematogenous metastases but also by lymphoma, Kaposi's sarcoma, and carcinoid tumors. Although there are no reliable criteria for differentiating metastatic disease and lymphoma, the bull's-eye lesions of lymphoma tend to be the same size, whereas ulcerated metastases are often different sizes because of periodic showers of tumor into the arterial supply of the bowel.[9, 13] Occasionally, varioliform erosions surrounded by unusually prominent mounds of edema can be mistaken for bull's-eye lesions. However, varioliform erosions are rarely greater than 1 cm in size, and the central barium collections tend to be smaller than those seen in ulcerated submucosal masses.

Giant, cavitated lesions in the stomach and duodenum may be caused not only by metastatic disease (particularly malignant melanoma) but also by lymphoma, leiomyosarcoma, and, rarely, adenocarcinoma. However, leiomyosarcoma and adenocarcinoma tend to occur as solitary lesions, so the presence of multiple cavitated masses in the stomach, duodenum, or small bowel should favor a diagnosis of metastatic disease or lymphoma.

The linitis plastica appearance caused by metastatic breast cancer is most often confused radiographically with that of a primary scirrhous carcinoma. Circumferential gastric involvement by pancreatitis, pancreatic carcinoma, colonic carcinoma, omental metastases, lymphoma, or Crohn's disease and scarring from various types of severe gastritis may produce similar findings. Nevertheless, the possibility of metastatic disease should be considered when a linitis plastica appearance is detected in patients who have previously been treated for breast carcinoma.

Direct invasion of the stomach and duodenum by metastatic tumor may be simulated by various benign and malignant conditions in the upper abdomen. Compression or displacement of the greater curvature or posterior wall of the stomach or of the medial border of the descending duodenum may be caused not only by pancreatic carcinoma but also by pancreatitis, pancreatic pseudocysts, peripancreatic lymphadenopathy, abdominal aortic aneurysms, or other retroperitoneal processes (see Fig. 39–15). Various signs of bowel wall invasion (i.e., mass effect, nodularity, and spiculated, tethered mucosal folds) may also result from a nonspecific desmoplastic response to inflammatory conditions involving the stomach. Thus, pancreatitis may produce changes on the greater curvature that are impossible to distinguish radiographically from pancreatic or colonic carcinoma or omental metastases involving the stomach. Other imaging techniques such as CT are helpful for differentiating these conditions.

## LYMPHOMA

Lymphoma involves the stomach more frequently than any other portion of the gastrointestinal tract. Gastric lymphoma accounts for 50% of all gastrointestinal lymphomas, 25% of all extranodal lymphomas, and 3 to 5% of all malignant neoplasms in the stomach.[39–42] More than 50% of patients with gastric lymphoma have localized disease that is confined to the stomach and regional lymph nodes (i.e., primary gastric lymphoma); the remainder have generalized lymphoma with associated gastric involvement (i.e., secondary gastric lymphoma).[42] When it occurs, duodenal lymphoma usually results from contiguous transpyloric spread of lymphoma from the stomach. Because of its rarity, duodenal lymphoma is considered separately in a later section.

Because the gross pathologic findings are nonspecific, gastric lymphoma is often difficult to differentiate from gastric carcinoma by radiologic or endoscopic examinations. However, gastric lymphoma has a much better prognosis than gastric carcinoma, with overall 5-year survival rates of 50 to 60%.[43, 44] Thus, failure to obtain biopsy specimens from an advanced lesion that is assumed to be inoperable gastric cancer may deprive the patient of the opportunity for cure or long-term palliation. Proper staging of the tumor is also important so that a rational decision can be made about treatment options such as surgery, radiation, and chemotherapy.

## Pathology

Using Rappaport's system for the histologic classification of gastric lymphoma, 90 to 95% of patients have histiocytic or lymphocytic lymphomas and the remaining 5 to 10% have Hodgkin's disease. Whatever the cell type, gastric lymphoma is thought to originate in submucosal lymphoid tissue, with subsequent proliferation of lymphomatous cells in the gastric wall. In the majority of patients, the tumor is confined to the stomach or regional lymph nodes at the time of diagnosis. In the Ann Harbor staging system, stage $I_E$ lesions involve the gastric wall, stage $II_E$ lesions involve regional lymph nodes in the abdomen, stage III lesions involve lymph nodes above and below the diaphragm, and stage IV lesions are widely disseminated lymphomas that involve extra-abdominal lymph nodes as well as the omentum, mesentery, peritoneum, liver, spleen, lungs, or brain.[42] The major factors affecting survival of patients with primary gastric lymphoma are the depth of invasion of the gastric wall and the presence or absence of nodal disease.

## Clinical Aspects

Gastric lymphoma occurs more frequently in men than in women, and the average age at the time of diagnosis is 55 to 60 years.[45] The most common presenting clinical findings include abdominal pain, nausea, vomiting, anorexia, weight loss, a palpable epigastric mass, and upper gastrointestinal bleeding.[45] Occasionally, these patients develop an acute abdomen due to spontaneous perforation of an ulcerated gastric lymphoma or perforation complicating systemic chemotherapy.[46] Patients with generalized lymphoma may also have a fever or other signs of systemic disease. Whether or not lymphoma is confined to the stomach, these lesions are often quite extensive in relation to the clinical presentation. Thus, gastric lymphoma should be suspected when a relatively advanced lesion in the stomach is associated with a paucity of clinical complaints.

## Endoscopic Findings

Gastric lymphoma is usually manifested at endoscopy by enlarged rugal folds, infiltrative masses, or one or more nodular, polypoid, or ulcerated lesions in the stomach.[47, 48] Occasionally, endoscopy may reveal a characteristic "volcano crater" in which a discrete ulcer is surrounded by a narrow ridge of tumor.[48] However, lymphoma is often difficult to distinguish from gastric carcinoma at endoscopy. Depending on the endoscopic findings, leiomyomas, metastatic disease, Ménétrier's disease, hypertrophic gastritis, and benign gastric ulcers may also be considered in the differential diagnosis. Cytopathologic specimens are therefore required for histologic confirmation. Unfortunately, superficial biopsies are often nondiagnostic because lymphoma tends to infiltrate the gastric wall beneath an intact mucosa. Whenever possible, multiple biopsy specimens and brushings should therefore be taken from ulcerated or polypoid areas where tumor is likely to be present. Deep biopsy specimens should also be obtained when the overlying mucosa appears normal. With adequate cytologic and biopsy specimens, endoscopy has a sensitivity of 85 to 95% in diagnosing gastric lymphoma.[48–50]

## Treatment and Prognosis

When the diagnosis of gastric lymphoma has been established, proper staging of the tumor is needed to determine the appropriate treatment and assess prognosis. Additional diagnostic examinations include chest radiography, CT scanning of the chest and abdomen, and, possibly, [67]Ga scanning. If there is no evidence of generalized lymphoma, multiple biopsy specimens of celiac, mesenteric, para-aortic, and iliac lymph nodes can be obtained at surgery for definitive staging of the tumor.

Most investigators believe that the best treatment for localized gastric lymphoma with or without regional lymph node involvement (i.e., stage $I_E$ or stage $II_E$ lesions) is a subtotal gastrectomy with postoperative radiation therapy.[42, 45, 51, 52] Adjuvant chemotherapy has also been advocated for patients with stage $II_E$ lesions.[52] Although the role of systemic chemotherapy for localized gastric lymphoma remains controversial, advanced gastric lymphoma (i.e., stage III or stage IV lesions) is sometimes treated by radiation or chemotherapy without a gastric resection.[45] Unfortunately, massive upper gastrointestinal bleeding or even gastric perforation may be a complication of systemic chemotherapy, resulting in treatment failures.[46]

Although lymphocytic lymphoma has a better prognosis than histiocytic lymphoma, long-term survival depends primarily on the stage of the tumor rather than the cell type.[53, 54] In various studies, reported 5-year survival rates range from 62 to 90% for stage $I_E$ lesions and from 29 to 50% for stage $II_E$ lesions, but significantly lower rates are reported for stage III and stage IV lesions.[43, 51, 54] After treatment, some patients may develop recurrent gastric lymphoma, whereas others may have recurrent tumor in distal nodal groups without evidence of gastric disease. Patients with recurrent lymphoma almost always become symptomatic within 2 years of treatment, so the prognosis is excellent for patients who remain asymptomatic for more than 5 years.[55] Gastric lymphoma has a better prognosis then gastric carcinoma because of its inherent growth characteristics and its tendency to remain in the gastric wall for prolonged periods.

## Radiographic Findings

Although 90 to 95% of gastric lymphomas are detected on barium studies, a specific diagnosis of lymphoma is made in less than 20% of cases.[41, 45] The diagnosis of gastric lymphoma is rarely suggested by the radiologist because of its resemblance to gastric carcinoma, a much more common malignant neoplasm in the stomach. In other patients, the radiographic findings may erroneously suggest inflammatory conditions such as hypertrophic gastritis, Ménétrier's disease, or benign gastric ulcers. Although certain morphologic features should favor gastric lymphoma, endoscopy and biopsy are required for a definitive diagnosis.

### *Early Gastric Lymphoma*

Early gastric lymphomas (i.e., lesions confined to the mucosa or submucosa) may occasionally be detected on double contrast barium studies. The tumors have an average size of only 3.5 cm at the time of diagnosis.[56] They are usually depressed lesions, appearing as shallow, irregular areas of ulceration associated with nodular surrounding mucosa due to lymphomatous infiltration of the adjacent gastric wall.[56] Occasionally, early gastric lymphomas may be manifested by small nodules, ulcerated submucosal masses, or enlarged rugal folds.[56] These lesions may be indistinguishable from early gastric cancers, so deep endoscopic biopsies are required for a definitive diagnosis.

### *Advanced Gastric Lymphoma*

Gastric lymphomas are usually advanced lesions with an average diameter of 10 cm or more at the time of diagnosis.[41] Although the entire stomach may be infiltrated by tumor, the majority of cases involve the antrum and body.[57] Depending on their gross pathologic characteristics, gastric lymphomas may be classified radiographically as infiltrative, ulcerative, polypoid, or nodular lesions.[41, 57–59] However, there is considerable overlap between these pathologic types, with many lesions having combined infiltrative, ulcerative, and polypoid features.

Infiltrative gastric lymphomas are characterized by focal or diffuse enlargement of rugal folds due to submucosal spread of tumor[41, 57–59] (Fig. 39–19A). The folds are often massively enlarged and have a distorted, nodular contour, so they can be mistaken for polypoid masses. Even with extensive lymphomatous infiltration, however, the stomach usually remains pliable and distensible without significant narrowing of the lumen.[41, 57] In contrast, Hodgkin's disease often incites a marked desmoplastic response in the gastric wall, so that these lesions may produce a linitis plastica appearance indistinguishable from that of a primary scirrhous carcinoma.[60]

Ulcerative lymphomas are characterized by one or more ulcerated lesions in the stomach[41, 57–59] (Fig. 39–19B). Occasionally, these ulcers may be surrounded by a smooth mound of tumor or symmetric, radiating folds,

mimicking the appearance of benign gastric ulcers.[58] More frequently, however, these ulcers have an irregular configuration associated with nodular surrounding mucosa or thickened, irregular folds due to lymphomatous infiltration of the gastric wall[41, 58, 59] (see Fig. 39–19B). Other gastric lymphomas may appear as giant, cavitated lesions as a result of necrosis and excavation of the tumor.[58]

Polypoid gastric lymphomas are characterized by one or more lobulated intraluminal masses that may be indistinguishable from polypoid carcinomas[41, 57, 58] (Fig. 39–19C). Not infrequently, the polypoid form of gastric lymphoma is associated with the infiltrative or ulcerative forms, so barium studies may also demonstrate thickened folds or ulcers in these patients.

The nodular form of gastric lymphoma is characterized by multiple submucosal nodules or masses, ranging from several millimeters to several centimeters in size.[58, 59] These submucosal masses often undergo central ulceration, producing typical bull's-eye or target lesions[61] (Fig. 39–19D). The central barium collections tend to be relatively large in relation to the surrounding elevations. Other patients may have multiple discrete polyps indistinguishable from those associated with the various polyposis syndromes.

About 10% of patients with gastric lymphoma have contiguous transcardiac spread of tumor from the gastric fundus into the distal esophagus.[62] Esophageal involvement is usually manifested by thickened, irregular folds, luminal narrowing, or, less frequently, a polypoid intraluminal mass in the distal esophagus.[62] Because adenocarcinoma is a much more common malignant tumor in the stomach, however, the findings are more likely to result from distal esophageal involvement by a fundal or cardiac carcinoma.

Gastric lymphoma also tends to involve the duodenum by contiguous transpyloric spread from the distal antrum. In one series, about 30% of patients with gastric lymphoma had concomitant duodenal involvement on barium studies (see later section on duodenal lymphoma).[62] Because gastric carcinoma invades the duodenum in only 5 to 13% of patients,[63, 64] it has been suggested that concomitant involvement of the stomach and duodenum by tumor should suggest lymphoma. However, adenocarcinoma is so much more common than lymphoma that it is still the most likely diagnosis on empirical grounds.

Patients with advanced gastric lymphoma are sometimes treated exclusively with radiation or chemotherapy. Follow-up barium or CT studies are useful in these patients for documenting the response to treatment and for evaluating gastrointestinal bleeding or other symptoms that develop after the initiation of radiation or chemotherapy[65, 66] (Figs. 39–20 and 39–21). Follow-up studies may show dramatic regression or resolution of the lymphomatous lesions. However, subsequent examinations may reveal considerable narrowing and deformity of the stomach due to residual scarring and fibrosis.[66] In other patients, chemotherapy may lead to marked regression of ulcerated mass lesions with the development of benign-appearing ulcers or ulcer scars

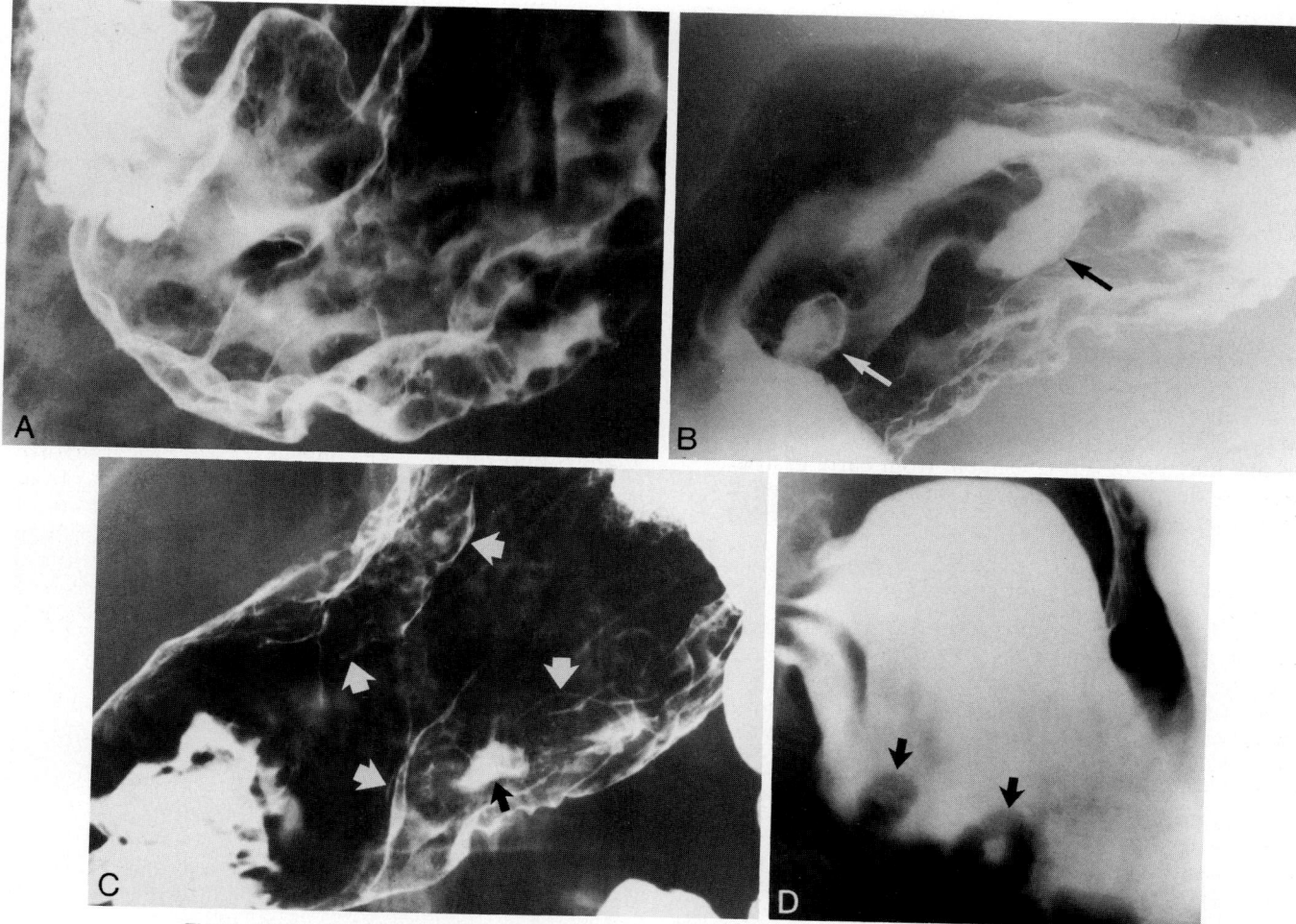

**Figure 39–19. Various forms of gastric lymphoma. A.** Diffusely thickened, irregular folds are present in the stomach due to lymphomatous infiltration of the gastric wall. **B.** Several discrete ulcers *(arrows)* are seen in the fundus. Also note thickened, lobulated folds in the adjacent stomach. **C.** Two separate polypoid masses *(white arrows)* are seen on the lesser and greater curvature of the stomach. The greater curvature mass is ulcerated *(black arrow)*. (**C** courtesy of Duane G. Mezwa, M.D., Royal Oak, MI.) **D.** Two centrally ulcerated submucosal masses or bull's-eye lesions *(arrows)* are present in the gastric antrum.

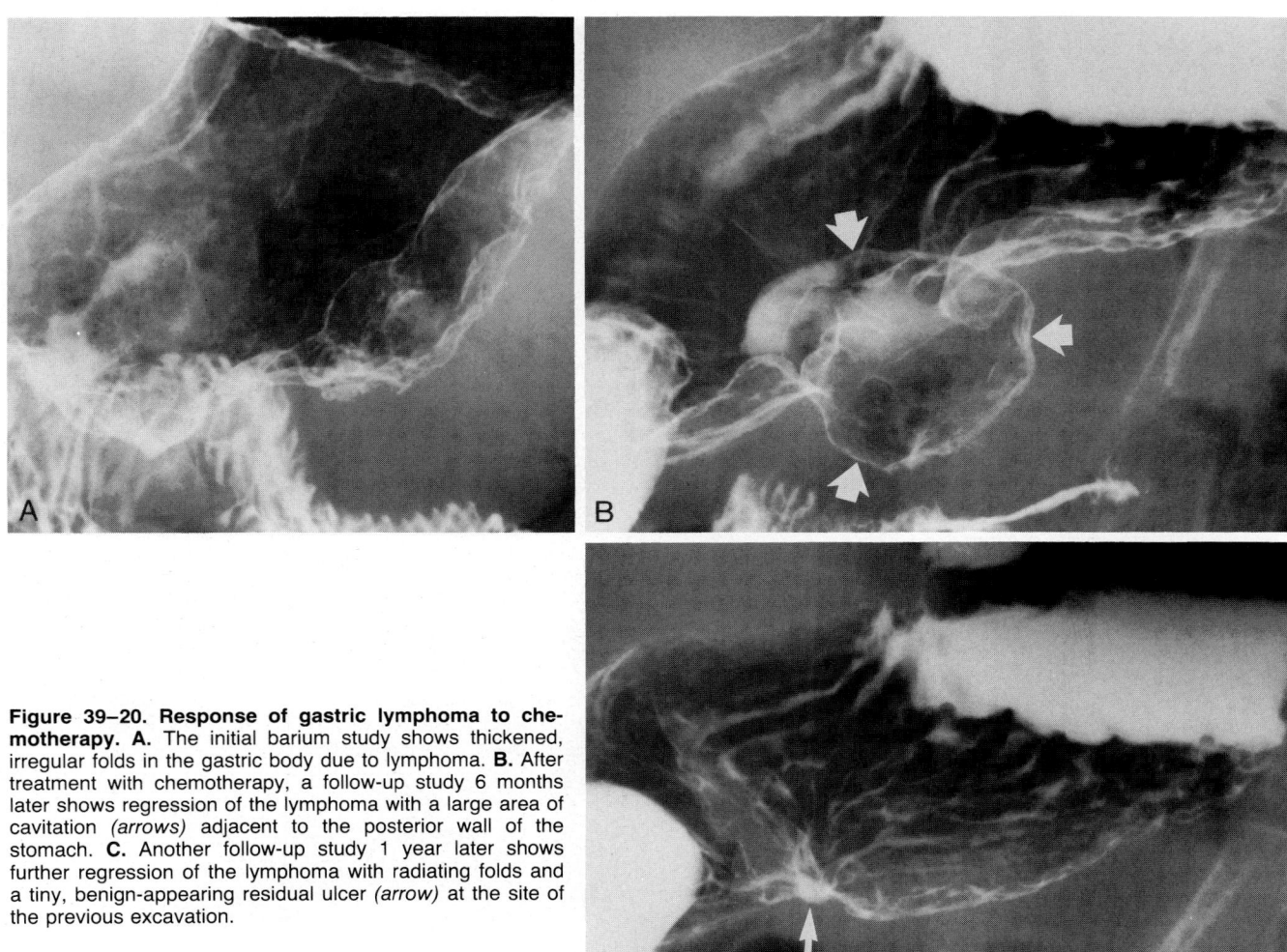

**Figure 39–20. Response of gastric lymphoma to chemotherapy. A.** The initial barium study shows thickened, irregular folds in the gastric body due to lymphoma. **B.** After treatment with chemotherapy, a follow-up study 6 months later shows regression of the lymphoma with a large area of cavitation *(arrows)* adjacent to the posterior wall of the stomach. **C.** Another follow-up study 1 year later shows further regression of the lymphoma with radiating folds and a tiny, benign-appearing residual ulcer *(arrow)* at the site of the previous excavation.

**Figure 39–21. Response of duodenal lymphoma to chemotherapy. A.** A conglomerate mass of adenopathy surrounds the mesenteric vessels. The duodenum is engulfed by this mass. **B.** Another CT scan 1 week after two cycles of chemotherapy shows multiple tiny collections of gas in the duodenal wall as a result of rapid tumor lysis and mural necrosis. A tiny amount of free air *(arrow)* is seen in the peritoneal cavity. This patient had developed clinical signs of peritonitis.

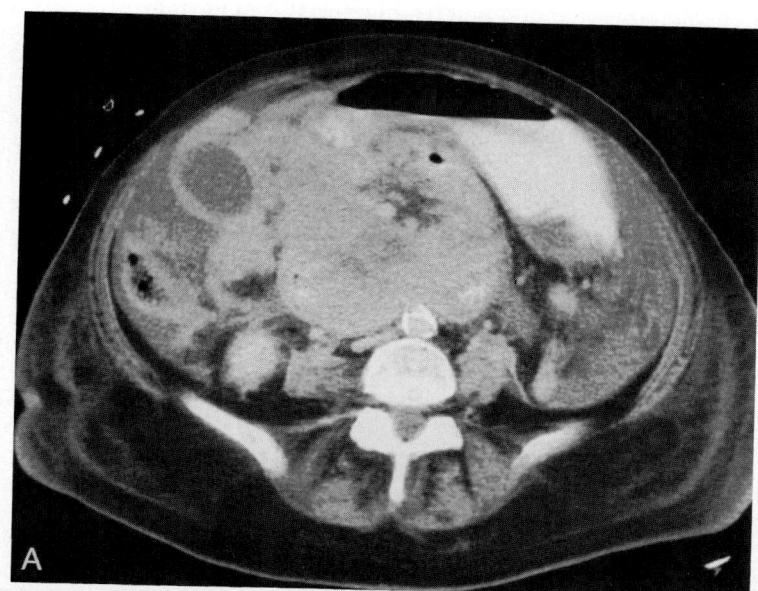
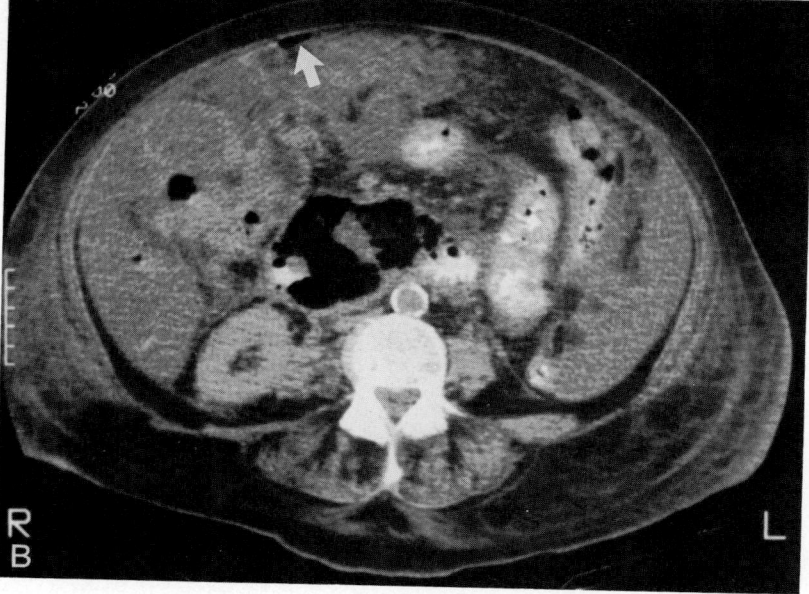

at the site of the previous lesions[65] (see Fig. 39–20C). However, chemotherapy may also lead to further ulceration or perforation of these lymphomatous lesions, with the development of massive upper gastrointestinal bleeding or peritonitis (see Figs. 39–20B and 39–21B).[65]

## Computed Tomography

CT is the primary imaging modality for the pretreatment evaluation of abdominal lymphoma. It is important to recognize gastric involvement at the time of the initial study. Three forms of gastric lymphoma may be demonstrated by CT: polypoid, infiltrating, and hypertrophic[67, 68] (Fig. 39–22). Any portion of the stomach may be involved, and transpyloric spread of lymphoma into the duodenum is a relatively common occurrence (Fig. 39–23). Unfortunately, it is often difficult to distinguish lymphoma from adenocarcinoma on the basis of the CT findings. However, the diagnosis of gastric lymphoma should be suggested by homogeneous thickening of the gastric wall with preservation of the overlying rugal folds[67, 68] (see Fig. 39–22). Adenopathy also tends to be bulkier in lymphoma than in adenocarcinoma, and retroperitoneal involvement is more common.

When gastric lymphoma is suspected on the basis of the CT findings, histologic verification should be obtained before initiating treatment.[69, 70] As stated previously, deep endoscopic biopsies are required for a definitive diagnosis. Endoscopic ultrasound has also been used to characterize the depth of gastric wall involvement by this disease.[71]

## Differential Diagnosis

Infiltrative gastric lymphomas may be difficult to distinguish radiographically from other causes of thickened gastric folds, such as hypertrophic gastritis, Ménétrier's disease, and gastric carcinoma. However, certain morphologic features are helpful for differentiating these conditions. Ménétrier's disease tends to involve the gastric fundus and body with sparing of the antrum, whereas lymphoma tends to involve the distal two thirds of the stomach with sparing of the fundus.[57] Although primary scirrhous carcinomas of the stomach may be manifested by thickened folds, these lesions usually cause luminal narrowing and rigidity.[16] In contrast, luminal narrowing rarely occurs in patients with gastric lymphoma. Thus, lymphoma should be suspected when barium studies demonstrate grossly enlarged folds in a stomach that remains pliant and distensible. Deep endoscopic biopsies may then be obtained for a histologic diagnosis.

Ulcerated gastric lymphomas may be impossible to distinguish radiographically from ulcerated carcinomas. Much less frequently, ulcerated lymphomas that have a relatively innocuous appearance can be mistaken for benign gastric ulcers.[58] When lymphoma is characterized by multiple areas of ulceration, the differential diagnosis includes various inflammatory or infectious conditions involving the stomach, such as Zollinger-Ellison syndrome, Crohn's disease, tuberculosis, syphilis, and cytomegalovirus (see Chapters 35 and 36). However, the correct diagnosis is often suggested by the clinical history.

Polypoid gastric lymphomas may be indistinguishable from polypoid carcinomas. Other lymphomas that appear as submucosal masses can be mistaken for gastric leiomyosarcomas. Although uncommon, giant, cavitated lymphomas may be impossible to differentiate from cavitated leiomyosarcomas or cavitated metastases from malignant melanoma or other tumors. However, leiomyosarcomas usually occur as solitary lesions in the stomach, whereas lymphoma and metastatic disease may be characterized by multiple lesions in the stomach,

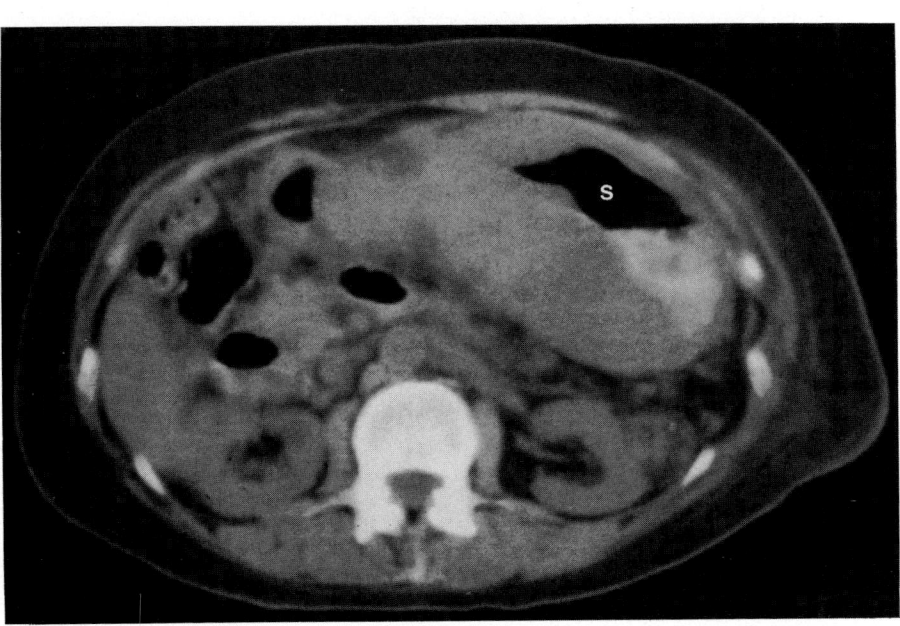

**Figure 39–22. CT demonstration of gastric lymphoma.** A CT scan reveals massive thickening of the wall of the stomach due to the infiltrative form of gastric lymphoma. The homogeneous appearance of this thickened wall is characteristic of lymphoma. S = stomach.

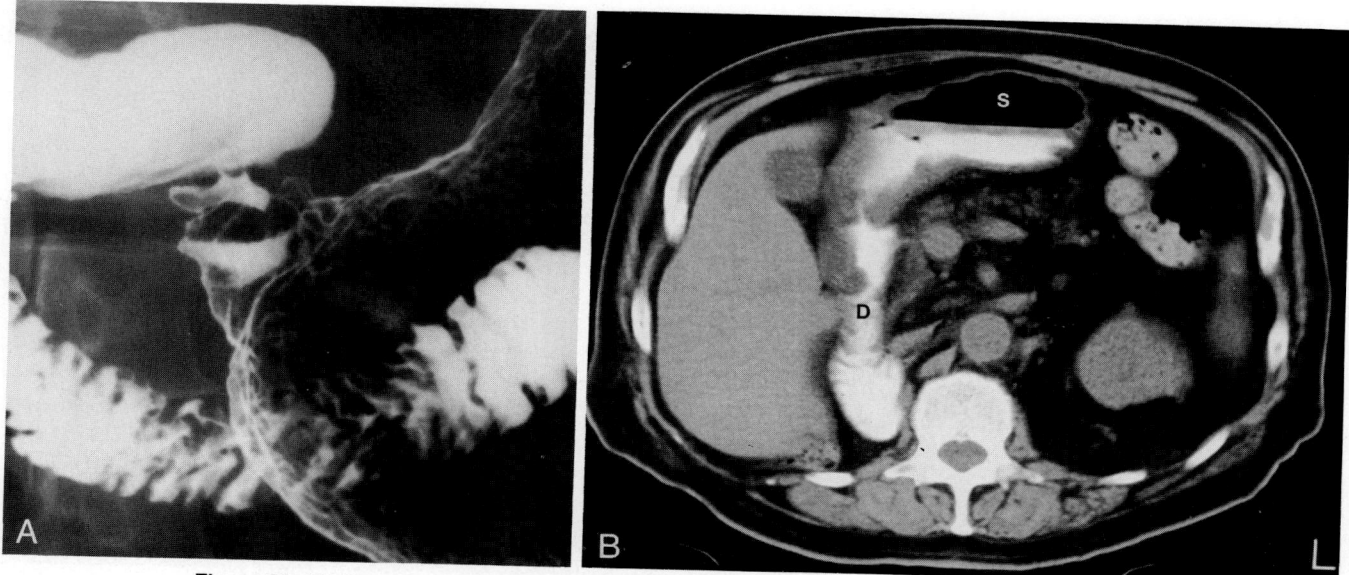

**Figure 39–23. Transpyloric spread of lymphoma into the duodenum. A.** A barium study shows nodularity and deformity of the distal antrum and pyloric region caused by gastric lymphoma. The duodenal bulb appears normal. **B.** However, a CT scan reveals a lymphomatous mass extending from the distal antrum into the proximal duodenum. Even in retrospect, duodenal involvement is not seen on the barium study. S = stomach; D = duodenum. (**A** and **B** courtesy of Edward Lubat, M.D., Ridgewood, NJ.)

duodenum, and small bowel. In patients with gastric lymphoma, exophytic masses usually demonstrate homogeneous attenuation on dynamic CT scans[67, 68] (see Fig. 39–22). In contrast, leiomyosarcomas tend to have a heterogeneous appearance due to areas of liquefactive necrosis (see Figs. 39–28 and 39–29).

Bull's-eye lesions in the stomach may be caused not only by lymphoma but also by Kaposi's sarcoma, carcinoid tumors, and metastases from primary malignant tumors arising in the skin, lung, breast, or other locations. However, lymphomatous lesions tend to be of relatively uniform size, whereas metastases are often of variable size as a result of periodic showers of tumor into the bowel.[9, 13] Leiomyomas and other benign submucosal masses that are ulcerated may also have a bull's-eye appearance, but they almost always occur as solitary lesions in the stomach and duodenum.

In summary, gastric lymphoma is manifested by nonspecific gross pathologic findings, so a specific diagnosis is often not possible on radiologic criteria. Despite this diagnostic dilemma, gastric lymphoma should be suspected when barium studies reveal multiple polypoid or ulcerated lesions, nodular elevations, or thickened folds without significant luminal narrowing. Deep endoscopic biopsy specimens may then be taken from suspicious areas in the stomach for histologic corroboration. If the endoscopic findings are equivocal, however, a laparotomy may ultimately be required for a definitive diagnosis.

## Duodenal Lymphoma

Duodenal involvement by lymphoma usually results from contiguous spread of tumor from the distal stomach or proximal jejunum (see Fig. 39–23) or from encase-ment of the duodenum by a conglomerate mass of lymphomatous nodes in the retroperitoneum[67, 72] (see Fig. 39–21A). Because of the paucity of lymphoid tissue in the duodenum, primary duodenal lymphoma is a rare entity, constituting less than 5% of all small bowel lymphomas.[73] As in the stomach, duodenal lymphoma is characterized radiographically by infiltrative, ulcerative, polypoid, and nodular forms (Fig. 39–24A). CT may reveal nodular masses, cavitated lesions, or long, infiltrated segments with mass-like thickening of the duodenum (Fig. 39–24B). Occasionally, duodenal or small bowel lymphoma may occur as a complication of long-standing celiac disease.[74, 75] Unfortunately, treatment with a gluten-free diet has not been effective in preventing this complication. Thus, periodic radiologic surveillance of the duodenum and small bowel has been advocated to detect these lesions at the earliest possible stage.[75]

## LEIOMYOSARCOMA

Leiomyosarcomas are uncommon neoplasms, constituting only 1 to 3% of all malignant tumors in the stomach.[45, 76, 77] These smooth muscle tumors are often confined to the wall of the stomach for prolonged periods before invading adjacent structures, so they have a better prognosis than gastric adenocarcinomas. Because of their rarity, duodenal leiomyosarcomas are considered separately in a later section.

## Pathology

The majority of leiomyosarcomas involving the gastrointestinal tract arise in the stomach.[78] About 90%

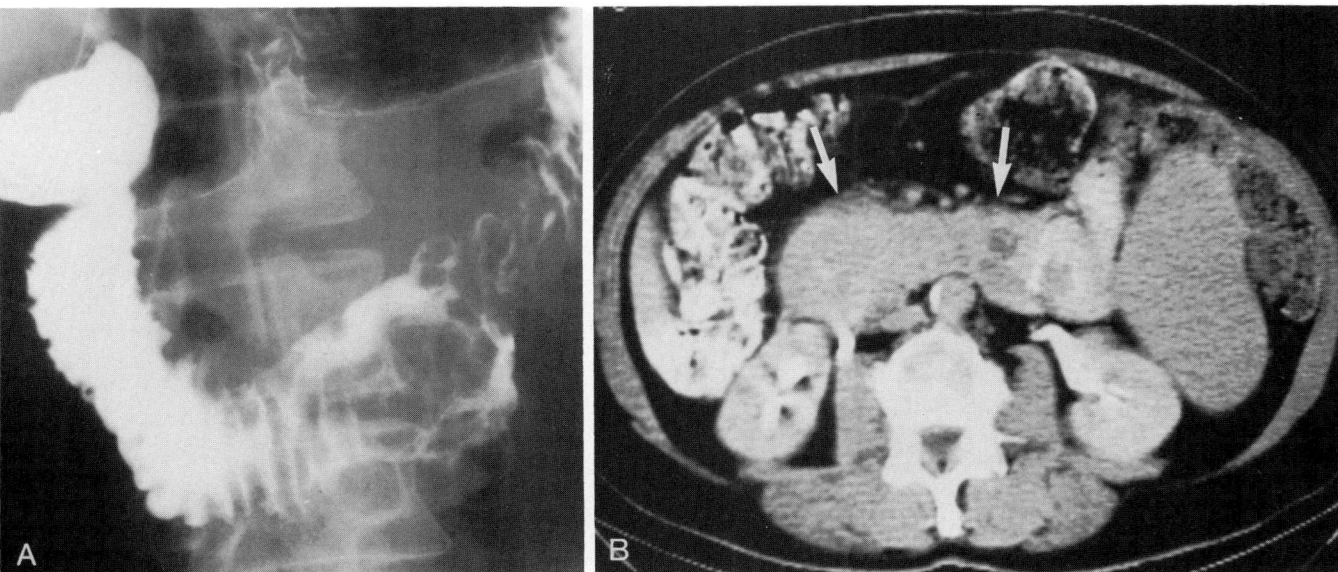

**Figure 39–24. Duodenal lymphoma. A.** A barium study shows a bulky mass lesion and thickened folds in the third and fourth portions of the duodenum. **B.** A CT scan reveals mass-like thickening of the duodenum *(arrows)* due to a long segment of infiltrating lymphoma. (**A** and **B** courtesy of Kyunghee C. Cho, M.D., Newark, NJ.)

involve the fundus and body, and the remaining 10% involve the antrum.[76] These tumors are mesenchymal lesions, originating in the muscularis propria. Most leiomyosarcomas consist histologically of interlacing whorls of spindle-shaped cells with eosinophilic cytoplasm and fusiform nuclei.[78, 79] However, some lesions contain distinctive epithelioid cells with eccentric nuclei and perinuclear vacuolization. The latter tumors are called epithelioid leiomyosarcomas or leiomyoblastomas.[80] Whatever the predominant cell type, gastric leiomyosarcomas tend to be large lesions with an average diameter of 10 cm at the time of diagnosis.[76, 81] They often contain large cystic cavities or ulcers because of hemorrhage or necrosis of the tumor.[81]

Gastric leiomyosarcomas may have endogastric or exogastric patterns of growth, depending on whether they grow toward or away from the lumen.[82, 83] As they enlarge, exogastric lesions may invade adjacent structures such as the pancreas, colon, and diaphragm.[83] Patients with advanced lesions may have widespread intraperitoneal seeding or hematogenous metastases to the liver, lung, or bones.[77, 83] Unlike adenocarcinomas, however, leiomyosarcomas rarely metastasize to regional lymph nodes.[77, 83]

The most commonly accepted index of malignancy is the degree of mitotic activity in the tumor; lesions containing more than 10 mitotic figures per 10 high-power fields are usually thought to be malignant, whereas lesions containing fewer than 2 mitotic figures per 10 high-power fields are thought to be benign.[83, 84] However, the degree of mitotic activity, cellular atypia, and nuclear pleomorphism may vary markedly within the lesion, so histopathologic criteria are unreliable for differentiating benign and malignant smooth muscle tumors. Furthermore, well-differentiated tumors may

have greater mitotic activity than necrotic, aggressive tumors that are more likely to invade adjacent structures. Others believe that gross features of the tumors, such as size and homogeneity, correlate better with the risk of metastases. In any case, a definitive diagnosis of malignancy ultimately depends on the biologic behavior of the lesion.

## Clinical Aspects

Gastric leiomyosarcomas occur more frequently in men than in women by a ratio of approximately 2:1.[76, 81, 85] Affected individuals are usually middle-aged or elderly. The average duration of symptoms at the time of diagnosis is 4 to 6 months.[76, 81, 85] The most common presenting clinical findings include nausea, vomiting, epigastric pain, weight loss, a palpable abdominal mass, and upper gastrointestinal bleeding.[76, 81, 83] Some patients with exogastric lymphomas may be asymptomatic until the lesions have reached enormous sizes.[86]

When leiomyosarcomas are suspected on the basis of barium studies, endoscopy can be performed for a more definitive diagnosis. However, positive biopsy specimens may not be obtained unless the overlying mucosa is ulcerated. Endoscopy therefore has limited value in diagnosing these tumors. CT can also be performed to determine the relationship of suspicious lesions to the gastric wall and to guide needle aspiration biopsies of endoscopically inaccessible lesions.

Gastric leiomyosarcomas generally have a better prognosis than gastric carcinomas, with reported 5-year survival rates ranging from 20 to 55%.[77, 79, 83] Tumors smaller than 5 cm have the best possibility for cure, although it is questionable whether these lesions are all malignant.

In contrast, tumors greater than 8 cm in size are often found to be advanced, unresectable lesions at the time of diagnosis.[85] Surgery is the only curative form of therapy. Depending on the extent of tumor, a wedge resection or a subtotal or total gastrectomy may be required. However, leiomyosarcomas rarely metastasize to regional lymph nodes, so a lymph node dissection is of little therapeutic benefit to these patients.[83] Although the role of radiation or chemotherapy is uncertain, some authors advocate chemotherapy when hepatic metastases are present.[77]

## Radiographic Findings

Abdominal plain films generally have limited value for diagnosing gastric leiomyosarcomas. Occasionally, however, these tumors may be recognized by the presence of a soft tissue mass indenting the gastric bubble.[87] One or more extraluminal gas collections may also be seen in the left upper quadrant as a result of necrosis and cavitation of the tumor.[88] Rarely, leiomyosarcomas may contain mottled areas of calcification (see Fig. 39-27), but CT is a more sensitive technique for demonstrating this finding.[89]

More than 90% of patients with gastric leiomyosarcomas have abnormal barium studies.[77, 90, 91] However, the correct diagnosis is suggested in only about half the cases because of the difficulty in distinguishing these lesions from benign smooth muscle tumors or from other benign or malignant lesions in the stomach.[91] About 50% of leiomyosarcomas are intramural lesions, 35% are exogastric, and 15% are endogastric.[86] Intramural lesions typically appear as large, lobulated submucosal masses in the gastric fundus or body[77, 86, 91] (Fig. 39-25). Some leiomyosarcomas may contain one or more ulcers or, less frequently, giant areas of cavitation[77] (Fig. 39-26). Barium retained within these cavities may be seen on delayed films taken 24 hours later.[88] Exogastric

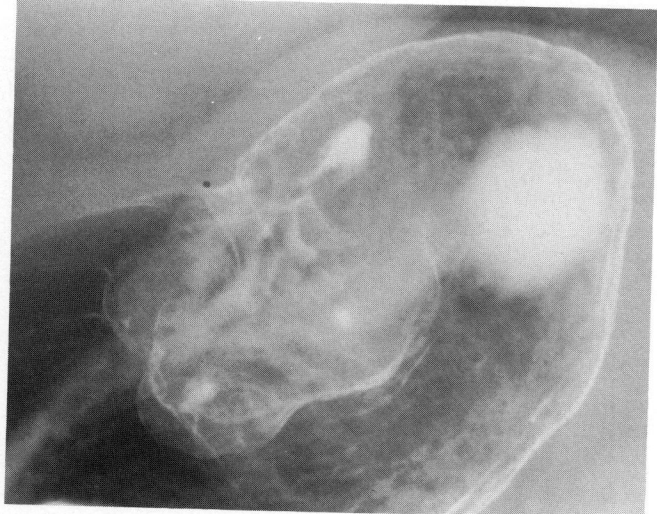

**Figure 39–25. Gastric leiomyosarcoma.** A large, lobulated submucosal mass is seen in the gastric fundus.

lesions may be manifested by giant soft tissue masses that cause extrinsic compression of the adjacent gastric wall[77, 82] (Figs. 39-27 and 39-28). However, an important clue to the diagnosis of an exogastric leiomyosarcoma is the presence of a central dimple or spicule at the site of attachment or pedicle of the mass[92] (see Fig. 39-28A). Finally, endogastric leiomyosarcomas may appear as polypoid intraluminal masses indistinguishable from primary gastric carcinomas.

The diagnosis of a leiomyosarcoma should be suggested on CT scans by the presence of a large exogastric mass[93, 94] (Fig. 39-29; see Fig. 39-28B). CT is particularly helpful for demonstrating the extent of the mass and invasion of adjacent structures.[95-97] Ulceration or cavitation of the mass may also be clearly shown with this technique (see Fig. 39-29A). On dynamic, contrast-enhanced CT scans, leiomyosarcomas often have a heterogeneous appearance with areas of low attenuation due to extensive necrosis of the tumor[89] (see Figs. 39-28B and 39-29). This feature is useful for differentiating a gastric leiomyosarcoma from a gastric lymphoma, which tends to have a more homogeneous appearance on CT scans (see Fig. 39-22). Rarely, leiomyosarcomas may be so necrotic that they appear as water density lesions (see Fig. 39-29C).

In patients with advanced leiomyosarcomas, CT may reveal metastases in the liver or peritoneal cavity. Liver metastases may be hypervascular, so if there is a known history of leiomyosarcoma, both unenhanced and enhanced scans of the liver should be obtained for optimal detection of these lesions. Peritoneal involvement by tumor is indistinguishable on CT scans from other intraperitoneally seeded metastases.

Leiomyosarcomas are characterized on angiograms by relatively well-circumscribed, hypervascular masses with huge feeding arteries and draining veins and intense tumor staining.[98] However, it is not possible to differentiate benign and malignant smooth muscle tumors by angiographic criteria. Angiography is also not able to distinguish leiomyosarcomas from other hypervascular lesions such as carcinoids, neurogenic tumors, and vascular metastases.[98]

## Differential Diagnosis

Some leiomyosarcomas may be as small as 2 cm, so it is not always possible to distinguish benign and malignant smooth muscle tumors by radiologic criteria.[77] In general, however, submucosal masses that are larger and more lobulated or contain areas of ulceration are more likely to be malignant. The major considerations in the differential diagnosis include lymphoma and other benign or malignant tumors of mesenchymal origin. Cavitated leiomyosarcomas may be impossible to distinguish radiographically from lymphoma or metastases from malignant melanoma or other tumors. However, patients with lymphoma or metastatic melanoma often have multiple lesions in the stomach and small bowel, whereas leiomyosarcomas occur as solitary lesions.

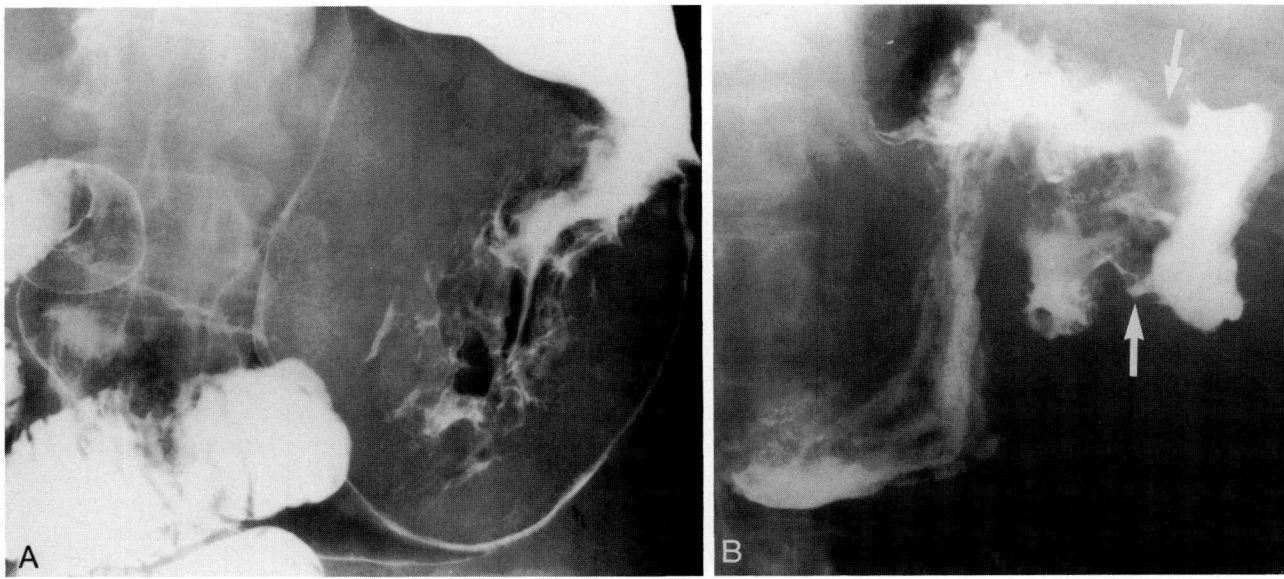

**Figure 39–26. Gastric leiomyosarcomas with cavitation. A.** A giant leiomyosarcoma is present in the stomach. Barium is trapped within irregular cavities in the mass. (Courtesy of Hans Herlinger, M.D., Philadelphia, PA.) **B.** Another cavitated lesion is manifested by a large extraluminal collection of barium *(arrows).*

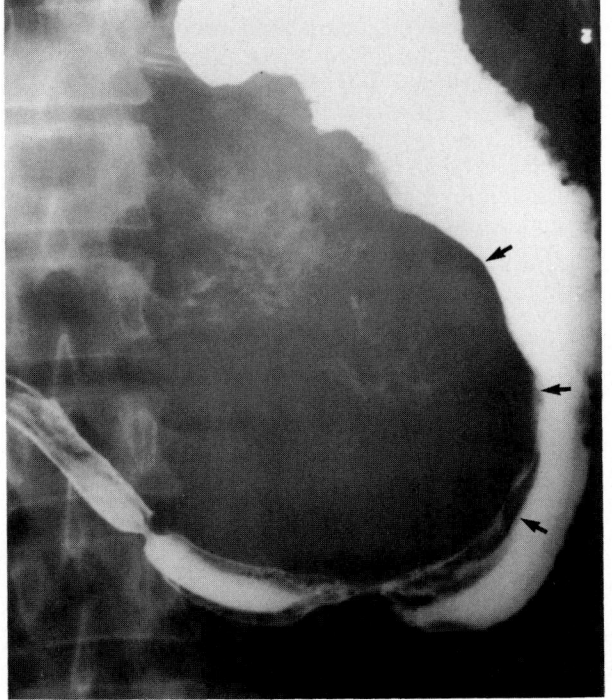

**Figure 39–27. Exogastric leiomyosarcoma with calcification.** A giant exogastric mass causes displacement and compression *(arrows)* of the medial border of the stomach. Mottled areas of calcification are seen in the tumor.

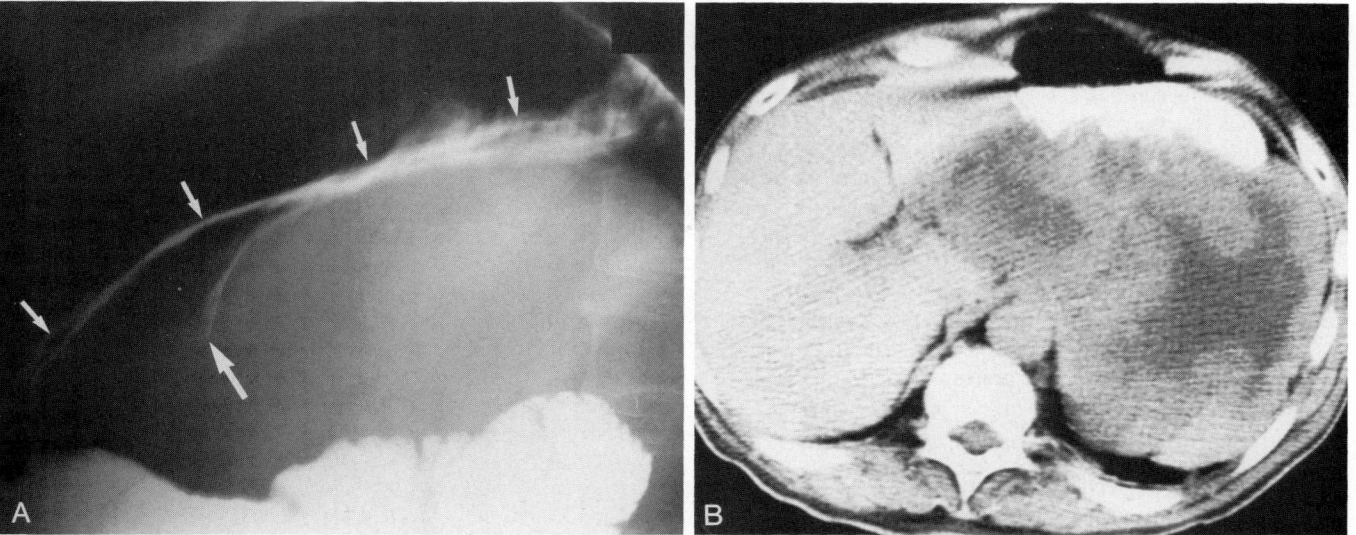

**Figure 39–28. Exogastric leiomyosarcoma. A.** A lateral radiograph of the stomach shows a giant exogastric mass compressing the posterior wall of the gastric fundus *(small arrows)*. However, a central dimple or spicule *(large arrow)* is seen at the site of attachment of the mass. This finding should suggest the possibility of an exogastric leiomyosarcoma. **B.** A CT scan reveals a giant heterogeneous mass with multiple low-density areas due to necrosis of the tumor. This heterogeneous appearance is characteristic of leiomyosarcomas on CT scans. (**A** and **B** courtesy of Hans Herlinger, M.D., Philadelphia, PA.)

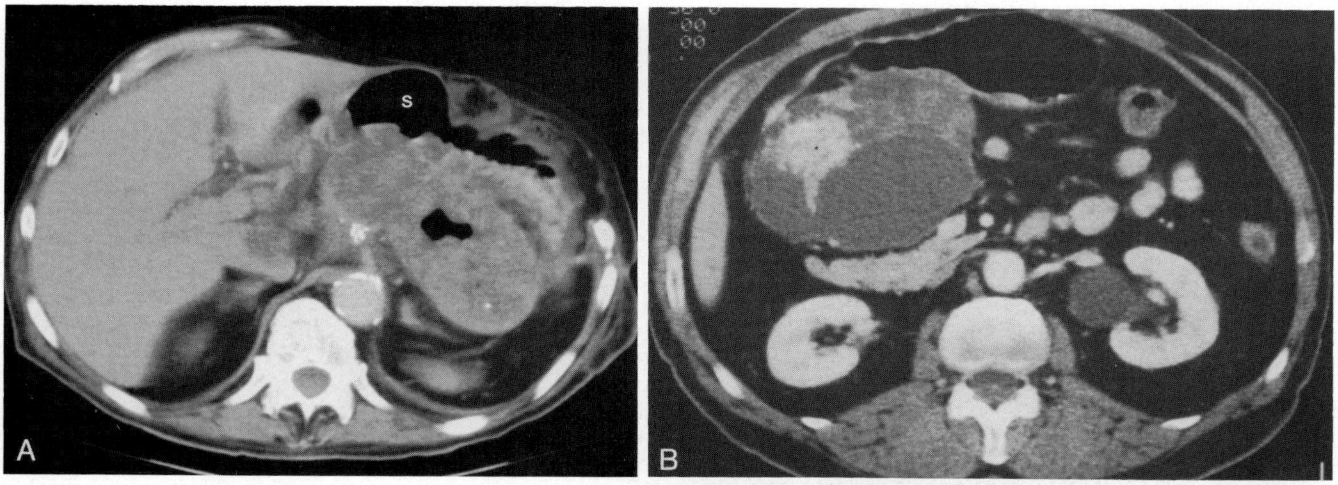

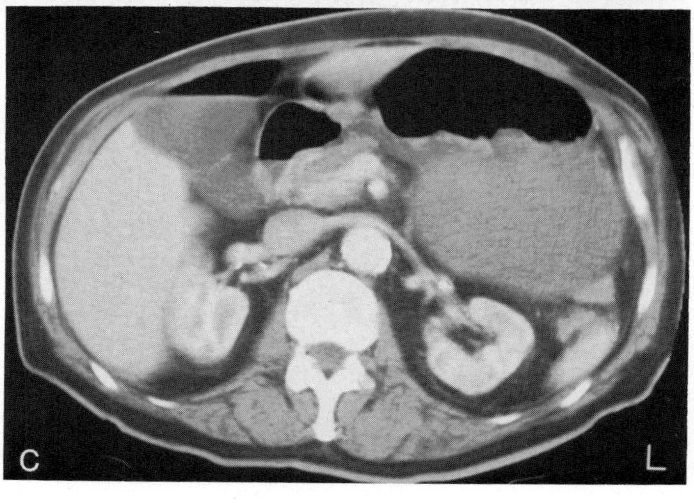

**Figure 39–29. CT demonstration of gastric leiomyosarcomas. A.** A heterogeneous exogastric mass is seen arising from the posterior wall of the stomach (S). Note the large central gas collection due to necrosis and cavitation of the tumor. **B.** In another patient, a heterogeneous exogastric mass is seen insinuating between the stomach and pancreas. **C.** In a third patient, a gas- and fluid-filled mass projects posteriorly from the stomach. Although uncommon, this degree of necrosis may occur in leiomyosarcomas.

Leiomyosarcomas that have an exogastric growth pattern can mimic the appearance of extrinsic mass lesions arising in the liver, pancreas, kidney, or mesentery. In such cases, the typical CT finding of a bulky, heterogeneous mass involving the gastric wall should suggest the correct diagnosis (see Figs. 39–28B and 39–29). Occasionally, water density leiomyosarcomas may be difficult to distinguish from cystic pancreatic neoplasms or pancreatic pseudocysts. Angiography may be helpful in determining the origin of the mass in these patients. Duplication cysts may also appear on CT scans as water density lesions involving the greater curvature of the stomach. However, duplication cysts tend to be smaller and may occasionally communicate with the gastric lumen.[99, 100]

## Duodenal Leiomyosarcoma

Leiomyosarcomas constitute only 10% of all malignant tumors in the duodenum.[101] The sex distribution is approximately equal, unlike that in gastric leiomyosarcomas.[101–103] The most common presenting clinical findings include upper gastrointestinal bleeding, anemia, weight loss, abdominal pain, a palpable mass, or, less frequently, obstructive jaundice.[101, 104] Unfortunately, many patients remain asymptomatic until they have advanced lesions. Aggressive surgical treatment (i.e., duodenectomy or pancreaticoduodenectomy) is often advocated.[101–103] However, duodenal leiomyosarcomas tend to invade adjacent structures or metastasize to the liver, so these patients often have a relatively poor prognosis.[104]

About 80% of duodenal leiomyosarcomas are located in the second or third portion of the duodenum.[101, 102] Intramural lesions may appear radiographically as submucosal masses, often containing areas of ulceration or cavitation[101, 102, 104] (Fig. 39–30A). Despite their large size, they rarely cause duodenal obstruction. Other leiomyosarcomas that have an exoenteric growth pattern may be indistinguishable on barium studies from pancreatic neoplasms, pancreatic pseudocysts, or other extrinsic mass lesions involving the duodenum.[102] CT is particularly useful for demonstrating these exoenteric lesions, which tend to project laterally from the second portion of the duodenum (Fig. 39–30B). Like gastric leiomyosarcomas, lesions in the duodenum often contain areas of low attenuation due to necrosis of the tumor.[104]

## KAPOSI'S SARCOMA

The classic form of Kaposi's sarcoma occurs primarily in elderly men and is manifested by slow-growing violaceous or hemorrhagic lesions on the lower extremities. During the past decade, however, patients with acquired immunodeficiency syndrome (AIDS) have developed a much more aggressive form of Kaposi's sarcoma characterized by widespread visceral lesions, particularly in the gastrointestinal tract. In various series, about 35% of patients with AIDS have Kaposi's sarcoma[105–108] and about 50% with Kaposi's sarcoma have gastrointes-

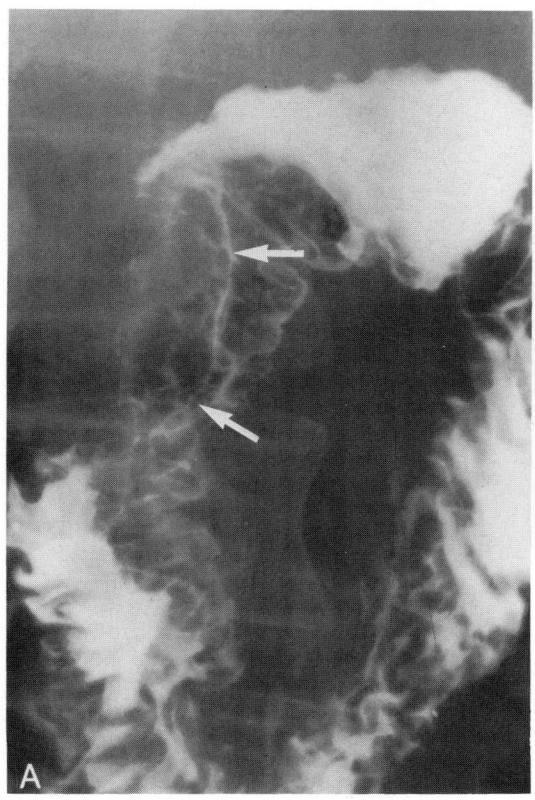

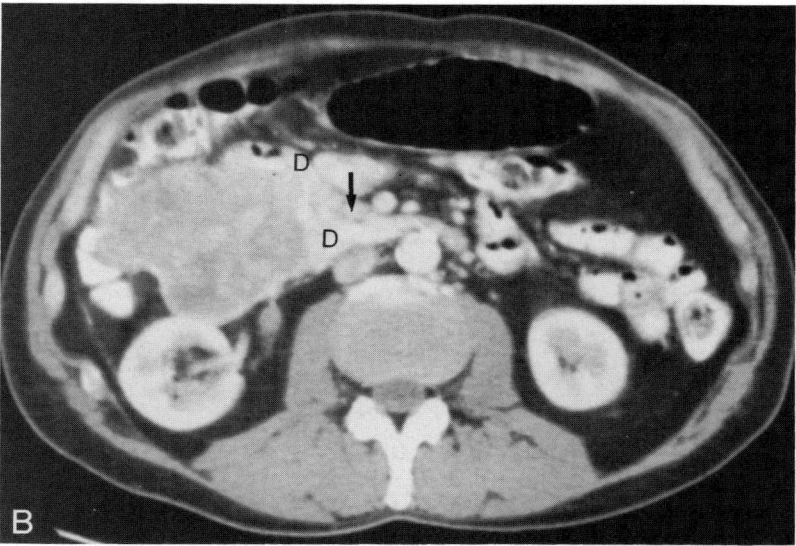

**Figure 39–30. Duodenal leiomyosarcomas. A.** A barium study shows a large intramural mass *(arrows)* on the lateral border of the descending duodenum. **B.** In another patient, a lobulated, heterogeneous mass projects laterally from the duodenum (D). This appearance is characteristic of duodenal leiomyosarcomas on CT scans. (The uncinate process of the pancreas is denoted by an arrow.)

tinal involvement.[106, 109–111] The stomach, duodenum, and small bowel are the most common sites of involvement.[109, 112] The colon is affected less frequently, and the esophagus is rarely involved by Kaposi's sarcoma.[109, 112] Demonstration of these lesions on upper gastrointestinal examinations has important prognostic implications, so optimal radiographic technique is required when barium studies are performed on these patients.

## Clinical Aspects

For reasons that are unclear, most AIDS patients with Kaposi's sarcoma are homosexuals rather than intravenous drug abusers or transfusion recipients.[108, 113] Gastrointestinal involvement by Kaposi's sarcoma is almost always associated with cutaneous disease, but occasional cases have been reported in the absence of skin lesions.[111] Gastroduodenal lesions occasionally cause abdominal pain or upper gastrointestinal bleeding.[107, 108, 112] However, gastrointestinal symptoms usually result from opportunistic infection rather than the underlying lesions of Kaposi's sarcoma. In fact, AIDS patients with Kaposi's sarcoma have a particularly poor prognosis because they develop opportunistic infections even more frequently than other AIDS patients.[107, 108] Chemotherapy is sometimes used to treat gastrointestinal Kaposi's sarcoma, but this form of therapy poses significant risks in patients who are already immunocompromised.

## Pathologic and Endoscopic Findings

Kaposi's sarcoma is probably a lesion of vascular origin, consisting histologically of whorled bundles of spindle-shaped cells in a matrix of vascular clefts containing red blood cells and hemosiderin.[112, 114] Gastroduodenal involvement by Kaposi's sarcoma may be manifested on endoscopy by a variety of findings, including 1) flat, hemorrhagic patches or macular discolorations; 2) raised, reddish purple nodules, often containing central areas of ulceration (i.e., volcano lesions); and 3) coalescent plaques or masses.[109, 110, 112] Although the gross appearance at endoscopy is characteristic, superficial biopsy results are often negative because of the submucosal origin of the lesions.[106, 107, 109, 110]

## Radiographic Findings

Small macular discolorations of the mucosa cannot be shown on barium studies, so endoscopy is a much more sensitive technique for diagnosing the earliest gastrointestinal manifestations of Kaposi's sarcoma.[109, 110, 112] However, elevated lesions can be shown on barium studies, particularly if double contrast technique is used.[106] Gastroduodenal involvement may be manifested radiographically by one or more submucosal defects, ranging from 0.5 to 3.0 cm in size[106, 112, 115, 116] (Fig. 39–31). As these nodules enlarge, they often undergo central ulceration, producing one or more target or bull's-eye lesions[109, 112, 116] (Fig. 39–32). Other patients

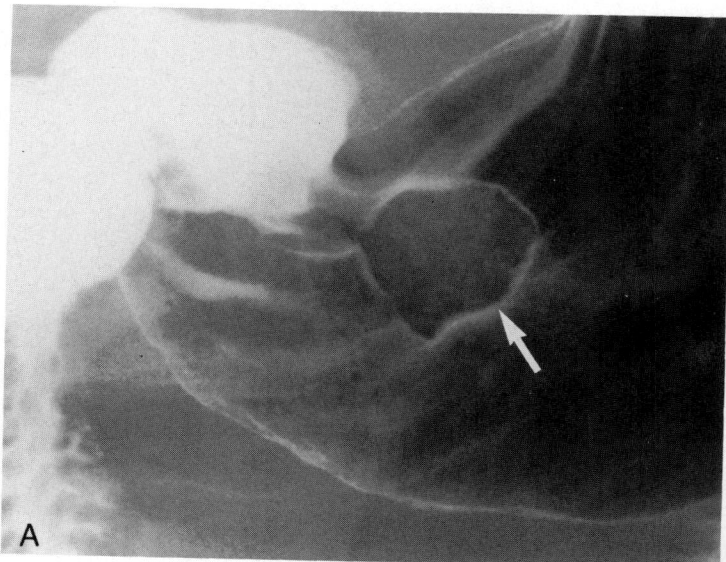

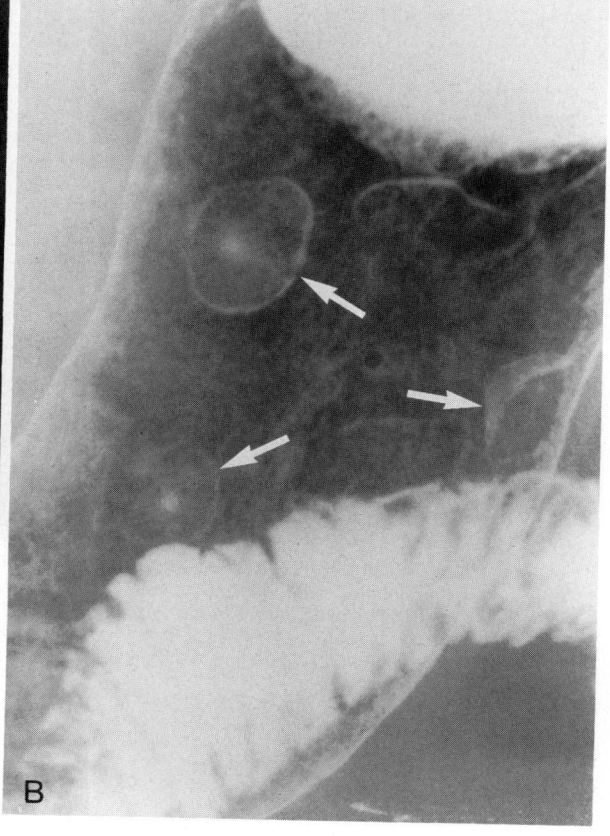

**Figure 39–31. Kaposi's sarcoma with submucosal masses in AIDS patients. A.** A solitary submucosal mass *(arrow)* is seen in the gastric antrum. **B.** In another patient, multiple submucosal masses *(arrows)* are present in the stomach. The tiny collections of barium overlying several anterior wall lesions represent hanging droplets of barium or "stalactites" rather than ulcers. (**B** courtesy of Seth N. Glick, M.D., Philadelphia, PA.)

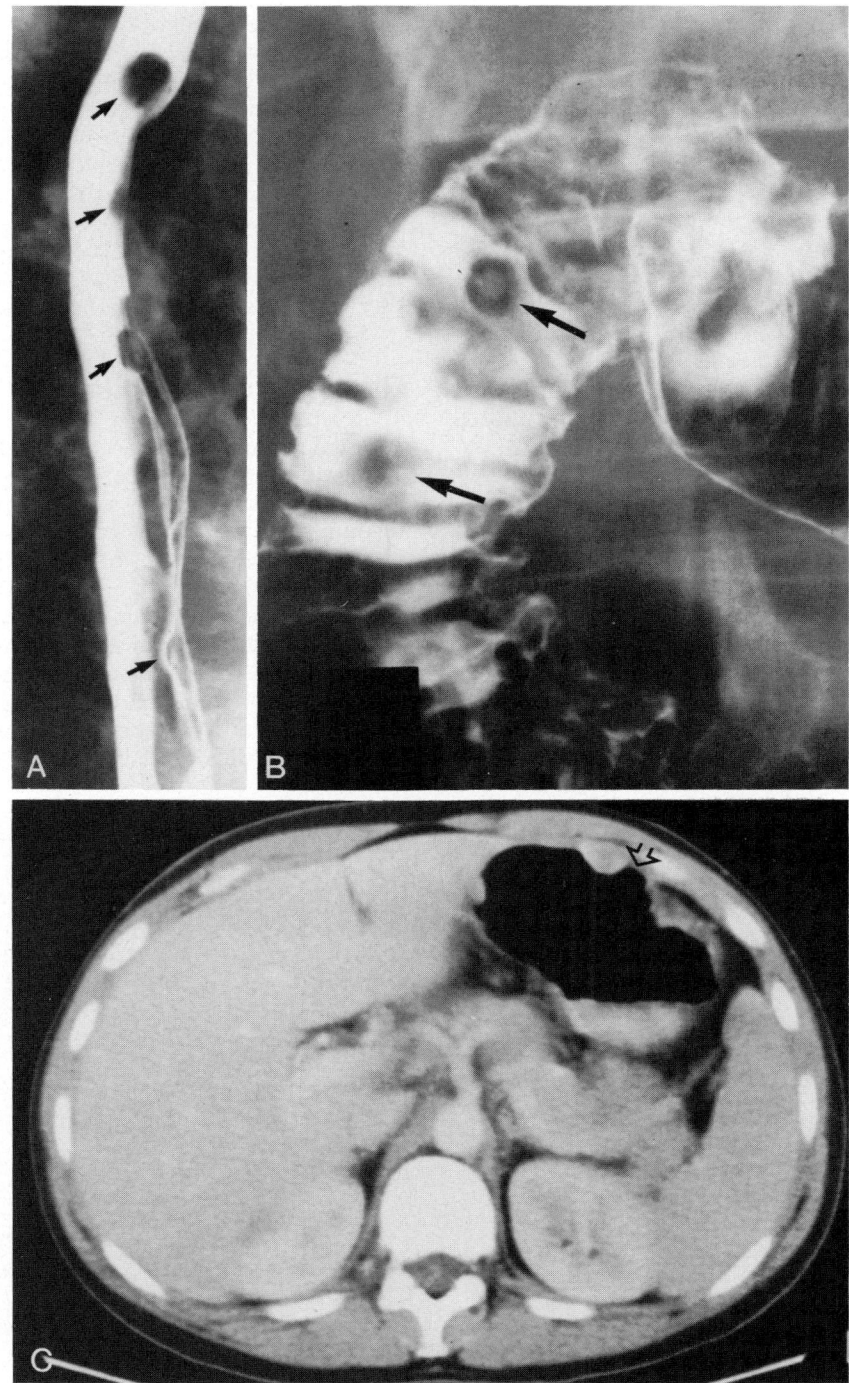

**Figure 39–32. Kaposi's sarcoma with bull's-eye lesions in AIDS patients. A.** Multiple submucosal nodules *(arrows)* are present in the esophagus. **B.** Several bull's-eye lesions *(arrows)* are seen in the duodenum in the same patient. (**A** and **B** courtesy of Robert Goren, M.D., Philadelphia, PA.) **C.** In another patient, a CT scan reveals an ulcerated submucosal mass on the greater curvature of the stomach. Note that gas outlines the ulcer *(arrow).*

may have thickened, nodular folds or polypoid masses in the stomach or duodenum[106, 112] (Fig. 39–33). Rarely, an infiltrating form of Kaposi's sarcoma involving the stomach may produce a linitis plastica appearance indistinguishable from that of a primary scirrhous carcinoma[117] (Fig. 39–34). When suspicious lesions are detected in the stomach or duodenum, a small bowel follow-through may be performed to determine whether additional lesions are present in the small bowel. CT may also be used to determine whether retroperitoneal adenopathy, splenomegaly, or other evidence of Kaposi's sarcoma is present in the abdomen.[118] Occasionally, barium studies or CT may demonstrate tumor nodules in the gastrointestinal tract due to Kaposi's sarcoma in AIDS patients who are being evaluated for opportunistic infection (see Fig. 39–32C). If there is already other evidence of extracutaneous Kaposi's sarcoma, however, the presence of gastrointestinal involvement does not significantly affect the management of these patients.[119, 120]

## Differential Diagnosis

Kaposi's sarcoma and lymphoma are the major considerations in the differential diagnosis of multiple, small nodular elevations in the stomach or duodenum in

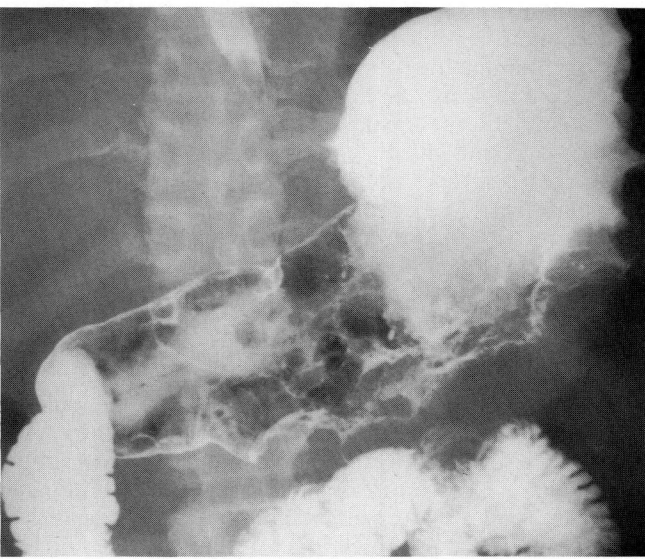

Figure 39–34. Kaposi's sarcoma with a linitis plastica appearance in an AIDS patient. The stomach has a markedly narrowed, irregular appearance caused by the infiltrating form of Kaposi's sarcoma.

patients with AIDS.[106, 112] However, it should be recognized that gastric lymphoma is much rarer than small bowel lymphoma in these individuals. Metastases, leukemic infiltrates, or multiple polyps (i.e., a polyposis syndrome) may produce similar findings. Kaposi's sarcoma and lymphoma are also the major considerations for multiple bull's-eye lesions in patients with AIDS.[106, 112] When ulceration, narrowing, or thickened folds are demonstrated in the stomach, the possibility of opportunistic infections such as cryptosporidiosis, cytomegalovirus infection, or tuberculosis should also be considered.[116] Thus, endoscopic biopsies, brushings, and cultures may be required to differentiate Kaposi's sarcoma or other infiltrative lesions from the various opportunistic infections that occur in these patients.

## CARCINOID TUMORS

Carcinoids are endocrine tumors arising in the gastrointestinal tract that are capable of producing a variety of vasoactive substances. Only about 2 to 3% of all gastrointestinal carcinoids are located in the stomach or duodenum.[121, 122] Nevertheless, these lesions are important because they are slow-growing tumors with a well-recognized malignant potential.

## Pathology

Carcinoid tumors of the stomach and duodenum originate from Kulchitsky cells in the crypts of Lieberkühn. The tumors consist histologically of clusters or ribbons of small, uniform, round or polygonal cells. Because their cytoplasm contains eosinophilic granules that have an affinity for silver stain, these lesions have sometimes

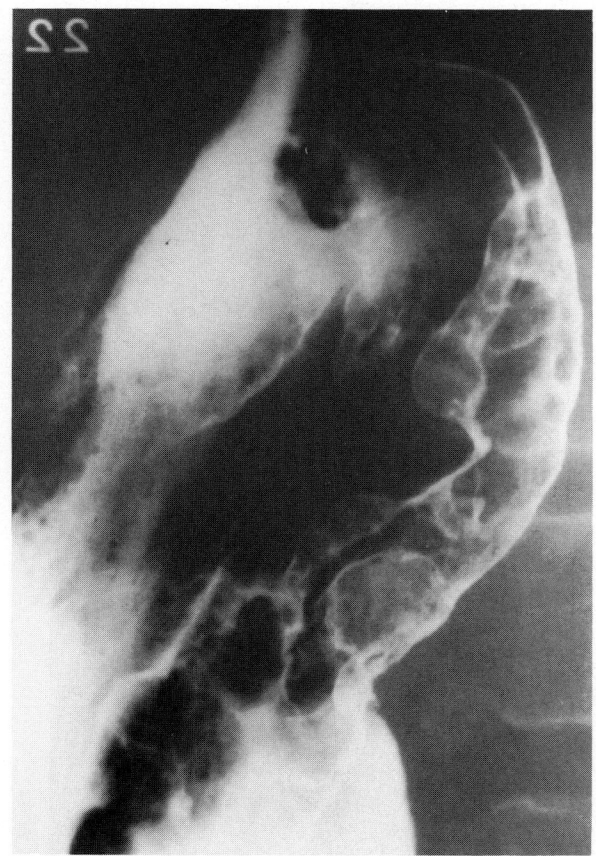

Figure 39–33. Kaposi's sarcoma in an AIDS patient. Multiple polypoid masses are seen on the posterior wall of the fundus.

been called *argentaffinomas*. Gastric carcinoids secrete predominantly 5-hydroxytryptophan rather than 5-hydroxytryptamine (serotonin), so they rarely show evidence of endocrine function.[123] Most gastric carcinoids are located in the distal antrum, often on the lesser curvature,[124] and most duodenal carcinoids are located in the first or, less commonly, second portion of the duodenum.[125]

## Clinical Aspects

Gastric carcinoids have an equal sex distribution and usually occur in patients older than the age of 40.[123] Many patients with carcinoid tumors in the stomach or duodenum are asymptomatic.[126] However, they may present clinically with abdominal pain, nausea, vomiting, weight loss, anorexia, or upper gastrointestinal bleeding.[123–125, 127] Gastric lesions often bleed regardless of size, and massive bleeding of ulcerated lesions as small as 1 cm has been described.[128] Unlike carcinoids arising in the small bowel, gastric and duodenal carcinoids rarely produce the carcinoid syndrome.[123–125] However, they are low-grade malignancies that can eventually metastasize to adjacent structures or the liver. Metastases are found in 20 to 30% of patients with gastric carcinoids at the time of diagnosis,[122] but long-term survival has been reported even when regional or

hepatic metastases are present. These tumors therefore have a much better prognosis than gastric carcinoma.

## Radiographic Findings

Carcinoid tumors of the stomach and duodenum may be manifested by a spectrum of radiographic findings. The majority of patients with gastric carcinoids have one or more submucosal-appearing masses ranging from 1 to 4 cm in size[123, 129] (Fig. 39–35A). Ulceration of the central portion of the tumor may produce a bull's-eye appearance.[123] The differential diagnosis for solitary gastric carcinoids includes leiomyomas, ectopic pancreatic rests, and other submucosal lesions, whereas the differential diagnosis for multiple carcinoids includes metastases, lymphoma, and Kaposi's sarcoma. Other patients may have one or more sessile or even pedunculated lesions that are indistinguishable from hyperplastic or adenomatous polyps.[130, 131] Still other patients may have benign- or malignant-appearing gastric ulcers, which tend to be located on or near the lesser curvature.[123] Finally, advanced carcinoid tumors of the stomach may appear as polypoid intraluminal masses indistinguishable from gastric carcinomas[123, 129, 132] (Fig. 39–35B).

Duodenal carcinoids can be recognized on barium studies as one or more polypoid defects in the duodenal

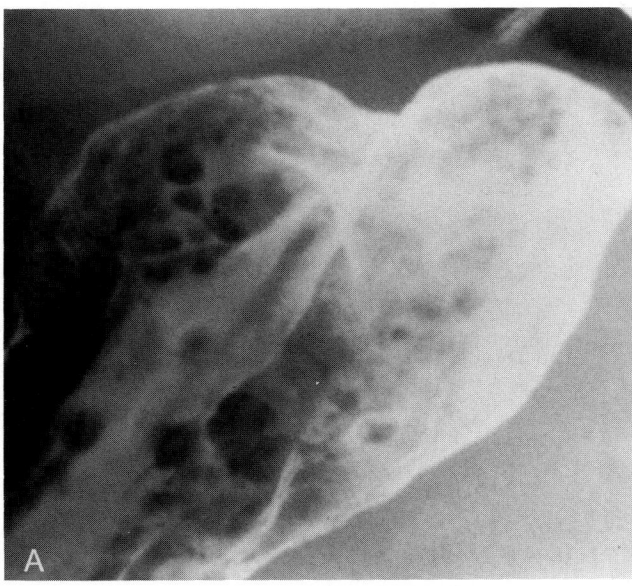

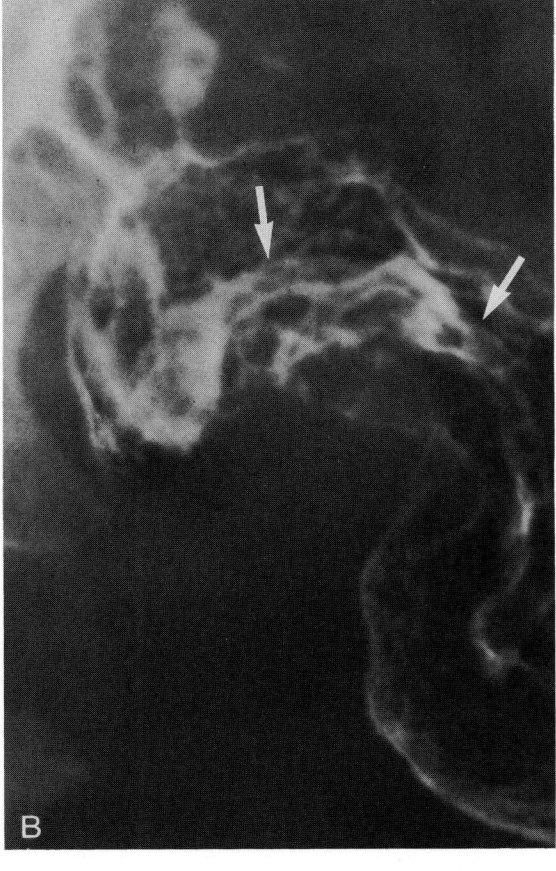

**Figure 39–35. Gastric carcinoid tumors. A.** Multiple submucosal nodules are seen in the gastric fundus. **B.** In another patient, a polypoid mass *(arrows)* is present on the greater curvature of the stomach. This lesion is indistinguishable from other polypoid tumors in the stomach.

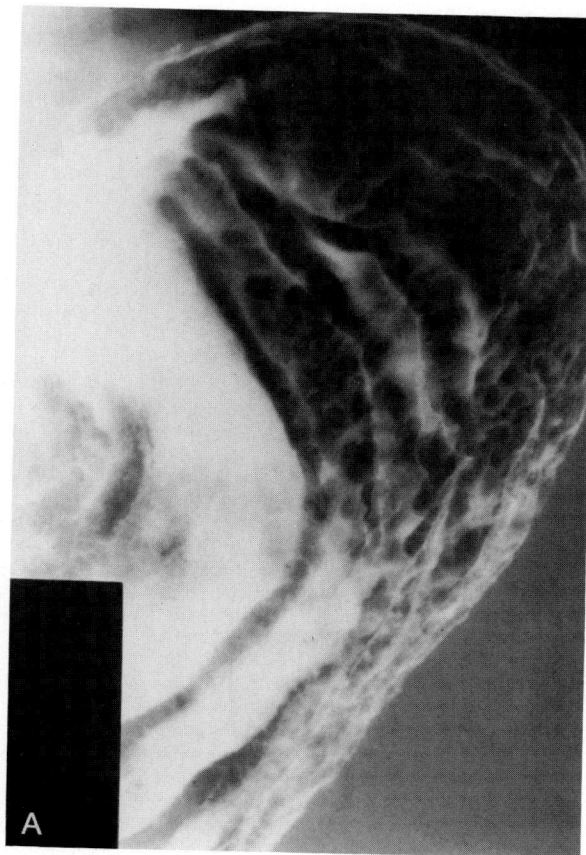
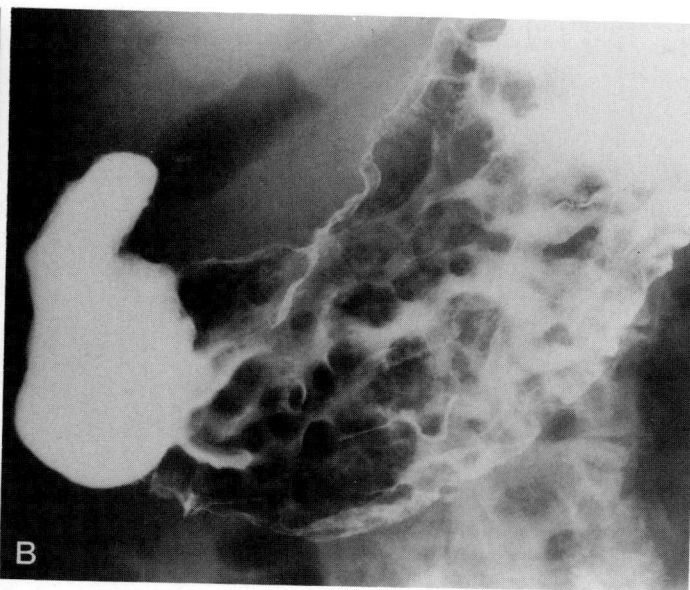

**Figure 39–36. Other malignant tumors involving the stomach. A.** Innumerable tiny nodules are seen in the gastric fundus due to chronic lymphocytic leukemia. **B.** In another patient, multiple submucosal masses are seen in the stomach due to multiple myeloma.

bulb or proximal descending duodenum.[133–135] The lesions may appear as submucosal masses or, less frequently, as polypoid or ulcerated lesions.[133–135] When gastric or duodenal carcinoids are detected radiographically, endoscopic biopsies are required for a definitive diagnosis.

When abdominal CT is performed for patients with known carcinoid tumors, both unenhanced and enhanced scans should be obtained to optimize detection of liver metastases.[136]

## MISCELLANEOUS TUMORS

Other unusual malignancies that have been reported in the stomach and duodenum include liposarcomas, fibrosarcomas, neurofibrosarcomas, hemangioendotheliomas, hemangiopericytomas, plasmacytomas, and choriocarcinomas.[137–139] Rarely, the stomach may be involved by leukemia or multiple myeloma[140] (Fig. 39–36). Squamous cell carcinomas and mixed adenosquamous carcinomas have also been described as rare malignant tumors in the stomach, arising from congenital rests of squamous epithelium or from pre-existing areas of squamous metaplasia.[141, 142]

### Acknowledgment

Figures 39–4, 39–12B, 39–14, 39–18C, 39–19A and D, and 39–20A to C are reproduced from Laufer I, Levine MS (eds): Double Contrast Gastrointestinal Radiology (2nd ed). Philadelphia: WB Saunders, 1992.

## References

1. Menuck LS, Amberg JR: Metastatic disease involving the stomach. Am J Dig Dis 20:903–913, 1975.
2. McNeer G, Das Gupta T: Life history of melanoma. AJR 93:686–694, 1965.
3. Asch MJ, Wiedel PD, Habif DV: Gastrointestinal metastases from carcinoma of the breast: autopsy study and 18 cases requiring operative intervention. Arch Surg 96:840–843, 1968.
4. Pomerantz H, Margolin HN: Metastases to the gastrointestinal tract from malignant melanoma. AJR 88:712–717, 1962.
5. Klein MS, Sherlock P: Gastric and colonic metastases from breast carcinoma. Am J Dig Dis 17:881–886, 1972.
6. Chang SF, Burrell MI, Brand MH, et al: The protean gastrointestinal manifestations of metastatic breast carcinoma. Radiology 126:611–617, 1978.
7. Khilnani MT, Wolf BS: Late involvement of the alimentary tract by carcinoma of the kidney. Am J Dig Dis 5:529–540, 1960.
8. Das Gupta TK, Brasfield RD: Metastatic melanoma of the gastrointestinal tract. Arch Surg 88:969–973, 1964.
9. Meyers MA, McSweeney J: Secondary neoplasms of the bowel. Radiology 105:1–11, 1972.
10. Joffe N: Metastatic involvement of the stomach secondary to breast carcinoma. AJR 123:512–521, 1975.
11. Goldstein HM, Beydonn MT, Dodd GD: Radiologic spectrum of metastatic melanoma to the gastrointestinal tract. AJR 129:605–612, 1977.
12. Lipshutz HI, Lindell MM, Dodd GD: Metastases to the hollow viscera. Radiol Clin North Am 20:487–499, 1982.
13. Felson B: "Bull's eye" lesions: solitary or multiple nodules in

the gastrointestinal tract with large central ulceration. JAMA 229:825–826, 1974.

14. Zornoza J, Goldstein HM: Cavitating metastases of the small intestine. AJR 129:613–615, 1977.

15. Radin DR, Halls JM: Cavitating metastases of the stomach and duodenum. J Comput Tomogr 11:283–287, 1987.

16. Levine MS, Kong V, Rubesin SE, et al: Scirrhous carcinoma of the stomach: radiologic and endoscopic diagnosis. Radiology 175:151–154, 1990.

17. Glick SN, Teplick SK, Levine MS, et al: Gastric cardia metastasis in esophageal carcinoma. Radiology 160:622–630, 1986.

18. Glick SN, Teplick SK, Levine MS: Squamous cell metastases to the gastric cardia. Gastrointest Radiol 10:339–344, 1985.

19. Allen HA, Bush JE: Midesophageal carcinoma metastatic to the stomach: its unusual appearance on an upper gastrointestinal series. South Med J 76:1049–1051, 1983.

20. Smith SJ, Carlson HC, Gisvold JJ: Secondary neoplasms of the small bowel. Radiology 125:29–33, 1977.

21. Shammash JB, Rubesin SE, Levine MS: Massive gastric distention due to duodenal involvement by retroperitoneal tumors. Gastrointest Radiol 17:214–216, 1992.

22. Levine MS, Caroline D, Thompson JJ, et al: Adenocarcinoma of the esophagus: relationship to Barrett mucosa. Radiology 150:305–309, 1984.

23. Keen SJ, Dodd GD, Smith JL: Adenocarcinoma arising in Barrett's esophagus: pathologic and radiologic features. Mt Sinai J Med 51:442–450, 1984.

24. Mani JR, Zboralske F, Margulis AR: Carcinoma of the body and tail of the pancreas. AJR 96:429–446, 1966.

25. Balthazar EJ, Megibow AJ, Naidich DP, et al: Computed tomographic recognition of gastric varices. AJR 142:1121–1125, 1984.

26. Marn CS, Glazer GM, Williams DM, et al: CT-angiographic correlation of collateral venous pathways in isolated splenic vein occlusion: new observations. Radiology 175:375–380, 1990.

27. Bachman AL: Roentgen appearance of gastric invasion from carcinoma of the colon. Radiology 63:814–822, 1954.

28. Treitel H, Meyers MA, Maza V: Changes in the duodenal loop secondary to carcinoma of the hepatic flexure of the colon. Br J Radiol 43:209–213, 1970.

29. Meyers MA, Whalen JP: Roentgen significance of the duodenocolic relationships: an anatomic approach. AJR 117:263–274, 1973.

30. Zanca P: Gastrocolic fistula complicating carcinoma of the colon. Radiology 48:244–248, 1947.

31. Vieta JO, Blanco R, Valentine GR: Malignant duodenocolic fistula: report of two cases with one or more synchronous gastrointestinal cancers. Dis Colon Rectum 19:542–552, 1976.

32. Levitt RG, Koehler RE, Sagel SS, et al: Metastatic disease of the mesentery and omentum. Radiol Clin North Am 20:501–510, 1982.

33. Rubesin SE, Levine MS, Glick SN: Gastric involvement by omental cakes: radiologic findings. Gastrointest Radiol 11:223–228, 1986.

34. Rubesin SE, Levine MS: Omental cakes: colonic involvement by omental metastases. Radiology 154:593–596, 1985.

35. Meyers MA: Distribution of intra-abdominal malignant seeding: dependency on dynamics of flow of ascitic fluid. AJR 119:198–206, 1973.

36. Meyers MA: Intraperitoneal spread of malignancies and its effect on the bowel. Clin Radiol 32:129–146, 1981.

37. Walkey MM, Friedman AC, Radecki PD: Computed tomography of peritoneal carcinomatosis. Radiology 171:152–170, 1989.

38. Levitt RG, Sagel SS, Stanley RJ: Detection of neoplastic involvement of the mesentery and omentum by computed tomography. AJR 131:835–838, 1978.

39. Bush RS, Ash CL: Primary lymphoma of the gastrointestinal tract. Radiology 92:1349–1354, 1969.

40. Freeman C, Berg JW, Cutler SJ: Occurrence and prognosis of extranodal lymphomas. Cancer 29:252–260, 1972.

41. Menuck LS: Gastric lymphoma: a radiologic diagnosis. Gastrointest Radiol 1:157–161, 1976.

42. Brady LW: Malignant lymphoma of the gastrointestinal tract. Radiology 137:291–298, 1980.

43. Dworkin B, Lightdale CJ, Weingrad DN, et al: Primary gastric lymphoma: a review of 50 cases. Dig Dis Sci 27:986–992, 1982.

44. Brooks JJ, Enterline HT: Primary gastric lymphomas: a clinicopathology study of 58 cases with long-term follow-up and literature review. Cancer 51:701–711, 1983.

45. Nelson RS, Lanza FL: Malignant tumors of the stomach. In Berk JE, Haubrich WS, Kalser MH, et al (eds): Bockus Gastroenterology (4th ed). Philadelphia: WB Saunders, 1985, pp 1267–1277.

46. Sandler RS: Primary gastric lymphoma. Am J Gastroenterol 79:21–25, 1984.

47. Grossman E, Winawer SJ: Diffuse gastrointestinal lymphosarcoma: gastroscopic and proctoscopic observations. Gastrointest Endosc 16:202–204, 1970.

48. Nelson RS, Lanza FL: The endoscopic diagnosis of gastric lymphoma: gross characteristics and histology. Gastrointest Endosc 20:183–184, 1974.

49. Cabre-Fiol V, Vilardell F: Progress in the cytological diagnosis of the gastric lymphoma. Cancer 41:1456–1461, 1978.

50. Spinelli P, Gullo CL, Pizzetti P: Endoscopic diagnosis of gastric lymphomas. Endoscopy 12:211–214, 1980.

51. Shin MH, Karas M, Nisce L, et al: Management of primary gastric lymphoma. Ann Surg 195:196–202, 1982.

52. Mittal B, Wasserman TH, Griffith RC: Non-Hodgkin's lymphoma of the stomach. Am J Gastroenterol 78:780–787, 1983.

53. Naqvi MS, Burrows L, Kark AE: Lymphoma of the gastrointestinal tract: prognostic guides based on 162 cases. Ann Surg 170:221–231, 1969.

54. Lim FE, Hartman AS, Tan EGC, et al: Factors in the prognosis of gastric lymphoma. Cancer 39:1715–1720, 1977.

55. Loehr WJ, Mujahed Z, Zahn RD, et al: Primary lymphoma of the gastrointestinal tract: a review of 100 cases. Ann Surg 170:232–238, 1969.

56. Sato T, Sakai Y, Ishiguro S, et al: Radiologic manifestations of early gastric lymphoma. AJR 146:513–517, 1986.

57. Sherrick DW, Hodgson JR, Dockerty MB: The roentgenologic diagnosis of primary gastric lymphoma. Radiology 84:925–932, 1965.

58. Zornoza J, Dodd GD: Lymphoma of the gastrointestinal tract. Semin Roentgenol 15:272–287, 1980.

59. Fork FT, Ekberg O, Haglund U: Radiology in primary gastric lymphoma. Acta Radiol Diagn 25:481–488, 1984.

60. Bloch C: Roentgen features of Hodgkin's disease of the stomach. AJR 99:175–181, 1967.

61. Ounnick NR, Harell GS, Parker BR: Multiple "bull's-eye" lesions in gastric lymphoma. AJR 126:965–969, 1976.

62. Hricak H, Thoeni RJ, Margulis AR, et al: Extension of gastric lymphoma into the esophagus and duodenum. Radiology 135:309–312, 1980.

63. Koehler RE, Hanelin LG, Laing FC, et al: Invasion of the duodenum by carcinoma of the stomach. AJR 128:201–205, 1977.

64. Kakeji Y, Tsujitani S, Baba H, et al: Clinicopathologic features and prognostic significance of duodenal invasion in patients with distal gastric carcinoma. Cancer 68:380–384, 1991.

65. Fox ER, Laufer I, Levine MS: Response of gastric lymphoma to chemotherapy: radiographic appearance. AJR 142:711–714, 1984.

66. Libshitz HI, Lindell MM, Maor MH, et al: Appearance of the intact lymphomatous stomach following radiotherapy and chemotherapy. Gastrointest Radiol 10:25–29, 1985.

67. Buy JN, Moss AA: Computed tomography of gastric lymphoma. AJR 138:859–865, 1982.

68. Megibow AJ, Balthazar EJ, Naidich DP, et al: Computed tomography of gastrointestinal lymphoma. AJR 141:541–547, 1983.

69. Blackledge G, Best JK, Crowther D: Role of computed tomography in staging and management of gastrointestinal lymphoma. J R Soc Med 72:818–822, 1979.

70. Sharma S, Singhal S, Dixit S, et al: Primary gastric lymphoma: role of computed tomography. Trop Gastroenterol 12:31–36, 1991.

71. Tio TL, den Hartog-Jager FC, Tytgat GN: Endoscopic ultraso-

nography of non-Hodgkin lymphoma of the stomach. Gastroenterology 91:401–408, 1986.

72. Meyers MA, Katzen B, Alonso DR: Transpyloric extension to duodenal bulb in gastric lymphoma. Radiology 115:575–580, 1975.

73. Balikian JP, Nassar NT, Shamma'a MH, et al: Primary lymphomas of the small intestine including the duodenum: a Roentgen analysis of twenty-nine cases. AJR 107:131–141, 1969.

74. Holmes GKT, Stokes PL, Sorahan TM, et al: Coeliac disease, gluten-free diet, and malignancy. Gut 17:612–619, 1976.

75. Collins SM, Hamilton JD, Lewis TD, et al: Small-bowel malabsorption and gastrointestinal malignancy. Radiology 126:603–609, 1978.

76. Bedikian AY, Khankhanian N, Vadivieso M, et al: Sarcoma of the stomach: clinicopathologic study of 43 cases. J Surg Oncol 13:121–127, 1980.

77. Nauert TC, Zornoza J, Ordonez N: Gastric leiomyosarcomas. AJR 139:291–297, 1982.

78. Stanley WM, Groshong LE: Leiomyosarcomas of the gastrointestinal tract. Am Surg 35:809–816, 1969.

79. Ranchod M, Kempson RL: Smooth muscle tumors of the gastrointestinal tract and retroperitoneum. Cancer 39:255–262, 1977.

80. Appelman HD, Helwig EB: Gastric epithelioid leiomyoma and leiomyosarcoma (leiomyoblastoma). Cancer 38:708–728, 1976.

81. Appelman HD, Helwig EB: Sarcomas of the stomach. Am J Clin Pathol 67:2–10, 1977.

82. Train JS, Hertz I, Keller RJ: Exogastric smooth muscle tumors. Am J Gastroenterol 76:544–550, 1981.

83. Shin MH, Farr GH, Papachristou DN, et al: Myosarcomas of the stomach: natural history prognostic factors and management. Cancer 49:177–187, 1982.

84. Morrissey K, Cho ES, Gray GF, et al: Muscular tumors of the stomach: clinical and pathological study of 113 cases. Ann Surg 178:148–155, 1973.

85. Bedikian AY, Khankhanian N, Heilbrun LK, et al: Primary lymphomas and sarcomas of the stomach. South Med J 73:21–24, 1980.

86. Berg J, McNeer G: Leiomyosarcoma of the stomach: a clinical and pathological study. Cancer 13:25–33, 1960.

87. Stauber SL, Messer J, Berger HW: Gastric leiomyosarcoma diagnosed on chest roentgenogram: importance of the stomach bubble. Mt Sinai J Med 50:514–516, 1983.

88. Phillips JC, Lindsay JW, Kendall JA: Gastric leiomyosarcoma: roentgenologic and clinical findings. Am J Dig Dis 15:239–246, 1970.

89. Scatarige JC, Fishman EK, Jones B, et al: Gastric leiomyosarcoma; CT observations. J Comput Assist Tomogr 9:320–327, 1985.

90. ReMine WH: Gastric sarcomas. Am J Surg 120:320–323, 1970.

91. Lindsay PC, Ordonez N, Raaf JH: Gastric leiomyosarcoma: clinical and pathological findings of fifty patients. J Surg Oncol 18:399–421, 1981.

92. Herlinger H: The recognition of exogastric tumours: report of six cases. Br J Radiol 39:25–34, 1966.

93. Bruneton JN, Drouillard J, Roux P, et al: Leiomyoma and leiomyosarcoma of the digestive tract—a report of 45 cases and review of the literature. Eur J Radiol 1:291–300, 1981.

94. Stavorovsky M, Morag B, Stavorovsky H, et al: Smooth muscle tumors of the alimentary tract. J Surg Oncol 22:109–114, 1983.

95. McLeod AJ, Zornoza J, Shirkhoda A: Leiomyosarcoma: computed tomographic findings. Radiology 52:133–136, 1984.

96. Megibow AJ, Balthazar EJ, Hulnick DH, et al: CT evaluation of gastrointestinal leiomyomas and leiomyosarcomas. AJR 144:727–733, 1985.

97. Stanley JH, Ravenel D, Parker TH, et al: Exogastric leiomyoblastoma: a rare gastric neoplasm mimicking left hepatic mass on computed tomography. J Comput Tomogr 10:187–190, 1986.

98. Granmayeh M, Jonsson K, McFarland W, et al: Angiography of abdominal leiomyosarcoma. AJR 130:725–730, 1978.

99. Lo J, Sage MR, Paterson HS, et al: Gastric duplication in an adult. J Comput Assist Tomogr 7:328–330, 1983.

100. Hulnick DH, Balthazar EJ: Gastric duplication cyst: GI series and CT correlation. Gastrointest Radiol 12:106–108, 1987.

101. Pujari BD, Deadhare SG: Leiomyosarcoma of the duodenum. Int Surg 61:237–238, 1976.

102. Olurin EO, Solanke TF: Case of leiomyosarcoma of the duodenum and a review of the literature. Gut 9:672–677, 1968.

103. McBrien MP, Garrett PEM: Leiomyosarcoma of the duodenum. Br J Surg 58:685–689, 1971.

104. Kanematsu M, Imaeda T, Iianuma G, et al: Leiomyosarcoma of the duodenum. Gastrointest Radiol 16:109–112, 1991.

105. Hill CA, Harle TS, Mansell PWA: The prodrome, Kaposi sarcoma, and infections associated with acquired immunodeficiency syndrome: radiologic findings in 39 patients. Radiology 149:393–399, 1983.

106. Wall SD, Friendman SL, Margulis AR: Gastrointestinal Kaposi's sarcoma in AIDS: radiographic manifestations. J Clin Gastroenterol 6:165–171, 1984.

107. Friedman SL, Wright TL, Altman DF: Gastroenterology Kaposi's sarcoma with acquired immunodeficiency syndrome. Gastroenterology 89:102–108, 1985.

108. Henderson RG, Rahmatulla TD: An epidemic tumour. Br J Radiol 60:511–512, 1987.

109. Saltz RK, Kurtz RC, Lightdale CJ, et al: Kaposi's sarcoma: gastrointestinal involvement correlation with skin findings and immunologic function. Dig Dis Sci 29:817–823, 1984.

110. Ell C, Matek W, Gramatzki M, et al: Endoscopic findings in a case of Kaposi's sarcoma with involvement of the large and small bowel. Endoscopy 17:161–164, 1985.

111. Lustbader I, Sherman A: Primary gastrointestinal Kaposi's sarcoma in a patient with acquired immune deficiency syndrome. Am J Gastroenterol 82:894–895, 1987.

112. Rose HS, Balthazar EJ, Megibow AJ, et al: Alimentary tract involvement in Kaposi sarcoma: radiographic and endoscopic findings in 25 homosexual men. AJR 139:661–666, 1982.

113. Jaffe HW, Bregman DJ, Selik RM: Acquired immune deficiency syndrome in the United States: the first 1,000 cases. J Infect Dis 148:339–345, 1983.

114. Balthazar EJ, Richman A: Kaposi's sarcoma of the stomach. Am J Gastroenterol 67:375–379, 1977.

115. Frager DH, Frager JD, Brandt LJ, et al: Gastrointestinal complications of AIDS: radiologic features. Radiology 158:597–603, 1986.

116. Falcone S, Murphy BJ, Weinfeld A: Gastric manifestations of AIDS: radiographic findings on upper gastrointestinal examination. Gastrointest Radiol 16:95–98, 1991.

117. Hadjiyane C, Lee YH, Stein L, et al: Kaposi's sarcoma presenting as linitis plastica. Am J Gastroenterol 86:1823–1825, 1991.

118. Jeffrey RB, Nyberg DA, Bottles K, et al: Abdominal CT in acquired immunodeficiency syndrome. AJR 146:7–13, 1986.

119. Leibman AJ, Gold BM: Gastric manifestations of autoimmune deficiency syndrome–related Kaposi's sarcoma on computed tomography. J Comput Tomogr 10:85–88, 1986.

120. Jeffrey RB Jr, Goodman PC, Olsen WL, et al: Radiologic imaging of AIDS. Curr Probl Diagn Radiol 17:73–117, 1988.

121. Godwin JD: Carcinoid tumors: an analysis of 2837 cases. Cancer 36:560–569, 1975.

122. Balthazar EJ: Carcinoid tumors of the alimentary tract. Gastrointest Radiol 3:47–56, 1978.

123. Balthazar EJ, Megibow A, Bryk D: Gastric carcinoid tumors: radiographic features in eight cases. AJR 139:1123–1127, 1982.

124. DeLuca RF, Ferrer JP, Gambescia RA, et al: Gastric carcinoid endoscopically simulating leiomyoma. Am J Gastroenterol 70:163–166, 1978.

125. Warren KW, McDonald WM, Logan CJ: Periampullary and duodenal carcinoid tumors. Gut 5:448–453, 1964.

126. Wengrower D, Fich A: Primary duodenal carcinoid. Am J Gastroenterol 82:1069–1070, 1987.

127. Abrams JS: Multiple malignant carcinoids of the stomach. Arch Surg 115:1219–1221, 1980.

128. Honig LJ, Weingarten G: A gastric carcinoid tumor with massive bleeding. Am J Gastroenterol 61:40–44, 1974.

129. Bluth I: Gastrointestinal carcinoid tumors: Roentgen features. Radiology 74:573–580, 1960.

130. Gueller R, Haddad JK: Gastric carcinoids simulating benign polyps. Gastrointest Endosc 21:153–155, 1975.

131. Syre-Smith G: Polypoid carcinoid tumor of the stomach. J Can Assoc Radiol 28:217–218, 1977.

132. Okeon MM, Bieber WP: Carcinoid tumor of the stomach resembling carcinoma. AJR 103:314–316, 1968.

133. Seymour EQ, Griffin CN, Kurtz SM: Carcinoid tumors of the

duodenal cap presenting as multiple polyploid defects. Gastrointest Radiol 7:19–21, 1982.

134. Clements JL, Roche RR: Carcinoid of the duodenum: a report of six cases. Gastrointest Radiol 9:17–21, 1984.

135. Eschelman DJ, Duva-Frissora AD, Martin LC, et al: Metastatic carcinoid presenting as a duodenal mass. AJR 156:1301–1302, 1991.

136. Bressler EL, Alpern MB, Glazer GM, et al: Hypervascular hepatic metastases: CT evaluation. Radiology 162:49–53, 1987.

137. Godard JE, Fox JE, Levinson MJ: Primary gastric plasmacytoma. Am J Dig Dis 18:508–512, 1973.

138. Pentimone F, Camici M, Cini G, et al: Duodenal plasmacytoma·

a rare extramedullary location simulating a carcinoma. Acta Haematol 61:155–160, 1979.

139. Jindrak K, Bochetto JF, Alpert LI: Primary gastric choriocarcinoma. Hum Pathol 7:595–604, 1976.

140. Feingold ML, Goldstein MJ, Lieberman PH: Multiple myeloma involving the stomach: report of a case with gastroscopic observations. Gastrointest Endosc 16:107–110, 1969.

141. Won OH, Farman J, Krishnan MN, et al: Squamous cell carcinoma of the stomach. Am J Gastroenterol 69:594–598, 1978.

142. Straus R, Heschel S, Fortmann DJ: Primary adenosquamous carcinoma of the stomach. Cancer 24:985–995, 1969.

# Miscellaneous Abnormalities

Ronald L. Eisenberg, M.D.

## VARICES

### Gastric Varices

Fundal gastric varices, which are usually associated with esophageal varices, represent dilated peripheral branches of the short gastric and left gastric veins resulting from portal hypertension. The presence of gastric varices without esophageal varices has classically been considered a sign of isolated splenic vein occlusion, most commonly secondary to pancreatitis or pancreatic carcinoma.[1] Obstruction of the splenic vein forces the large amount of blood normally carried to the spleen by the splenic artery to find a different route to the vena cava. Blood is shunted through the short gastric veins in their course from the splenic hilum over the fundus of the stomach to anastomose with branches of the coronary vein and distal esophageal plexus. If the portal vein is patent, blood can return to the liver through the coronary vein and no esophageal varices are produced.[1] However, although isolated gastric varices often develop in patients with splenic vein obstruction, portal hypertension is so much more common that it is likely to account for most patients with this finding.[2]

Gastric varices appear radiographically as multiple smooth, lobulated filling defects projecting between curvilinear, crescentic collections of barium (Fig. 40–1). Occasionally, a single large gastric varix may appear as a fundal mass, simulating a neoplastic process.[2] Gastric varices must be differentiated from other causes of thickened folds in the fundus of the stomach. The considerable changeability in the size and shape of varices should eliminate the possibility of a neoplastic process. Extension along the lesser curvature makes Ménétrier's disease unlikely. Additional evidence for gastric varices includes the presence of concomitant esophageal varices and an appropriate clinical history. At times, however, it can be impossible to distinguish gastric varices radiographically from Ménétrier's disease or a malignant lesion. In such cases, endoscopy is required for a definitive diagnosis.

Gastric varices appear on computed tomographic (CT) scans as well-defined clusters of rounded or tubular soft tissue densities within the posterior and posteromedial wall of the proximal stomach (see Fig. 30–13). The wall of the stomach is scalloped, and there is no cleavage plane between the gastric lumen and the varicosities. In some patients, CT scans may indicate the

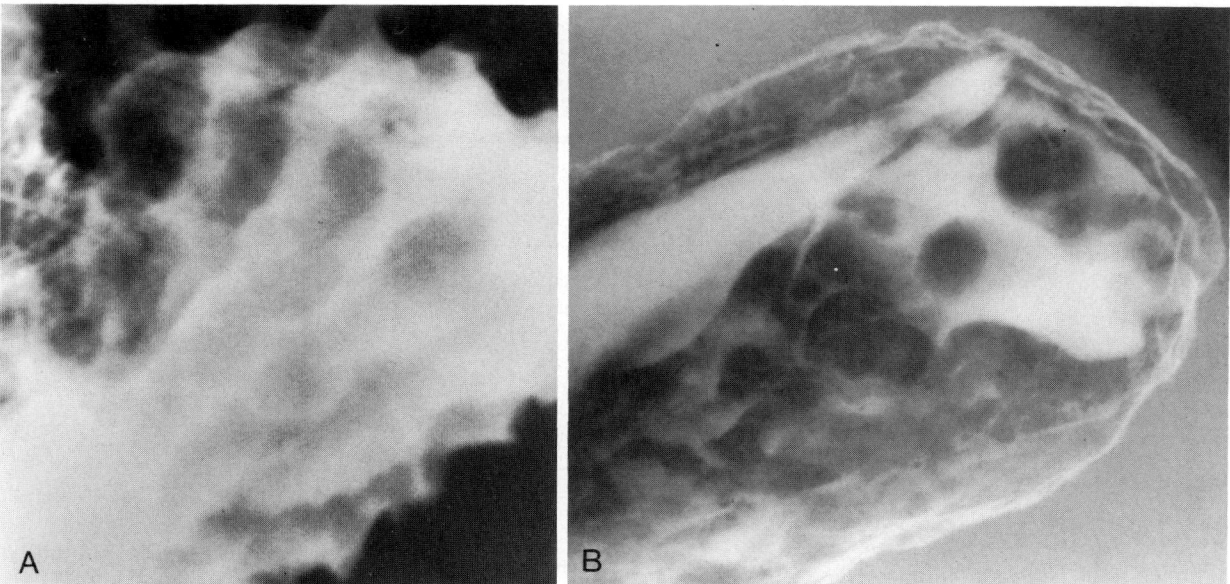

**Figure 40–1. Fundal gastric varices.** Both single contrast **(A)** and double contrast **(B)** barium studies show the varices as multiple smooth, lobulated filling defects in the fundus. (**A** from Eisenberg RL: Gastrointestinal Radiology: A Pattern Approach [2nd ed]. Philadelphia: JB Lippincott, 1990. **B** courtesy of Marc S. Levine, M.D., Philadelphia, PA.)

etiology of the varices by identifying such conditions as hepatic cirrhosis, calcific pancreatitis, and pancreatic carcinoma.

Gastric varices occurring at sites other than the fundus are unusual and may pose a diagnostic dilemma. Varices of the gastric antrum and body, which reflect collateral flow to the liver through a dilated, tortuous gastroepiploic vein in a patient with splenic vein obstruction proximal to a patent coronary vein, produce enlargement of mucosal folds primarily along the greater curvature (Fig. 40–2). This appearance can be differentiated from that of a malignant lesion because of the pliability and variation in size and shape of the varices in response to external compression, change in position, and degree of gastric distention.[3]

## Duodenal Varices

Duodenal varices typically produce diffuse, serpiginous thickening of mucosal folds (Fig. 40–3). They are almost always associated with esophageal varices and can be complicated by gastrointestinal bleeding. Occasionally, an isolated duodenal varix can present as a solitary filling defect.[4]

## DIVERTICULA

### Gastric Diverticula

Gastric diverticula generally arise from the posterior aspect of the fundus. A large gastric diverticulum that fails to fill with gas or barium can mimic a smooth-bordered submucosal mass. On subsequent examina-

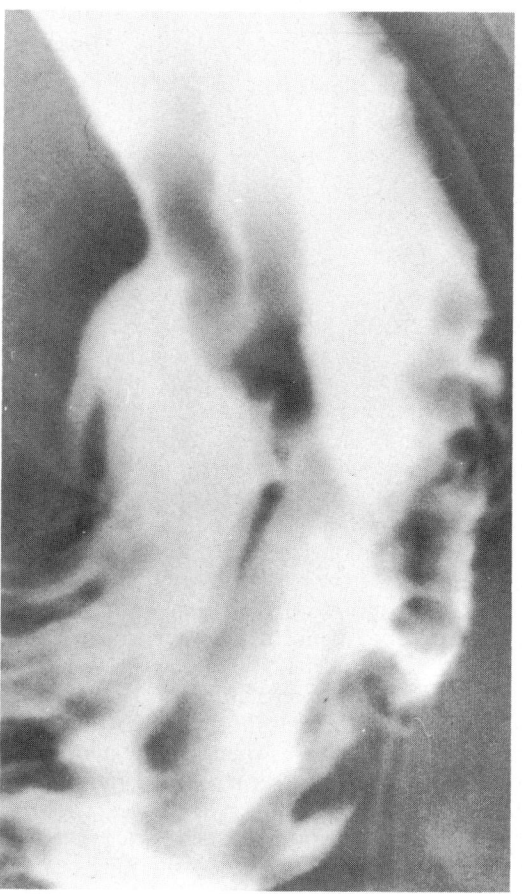

**Figure 40–2. Nonfundal gastric varices.** Thickened, tortuous folds in the body of the stomach are due to a dilated gastroepiploic vein. (From Sos T, Meyers MA, Baltaxe HA: Nonfundic gastric varices. Radiology 105:579–580, 1972.)

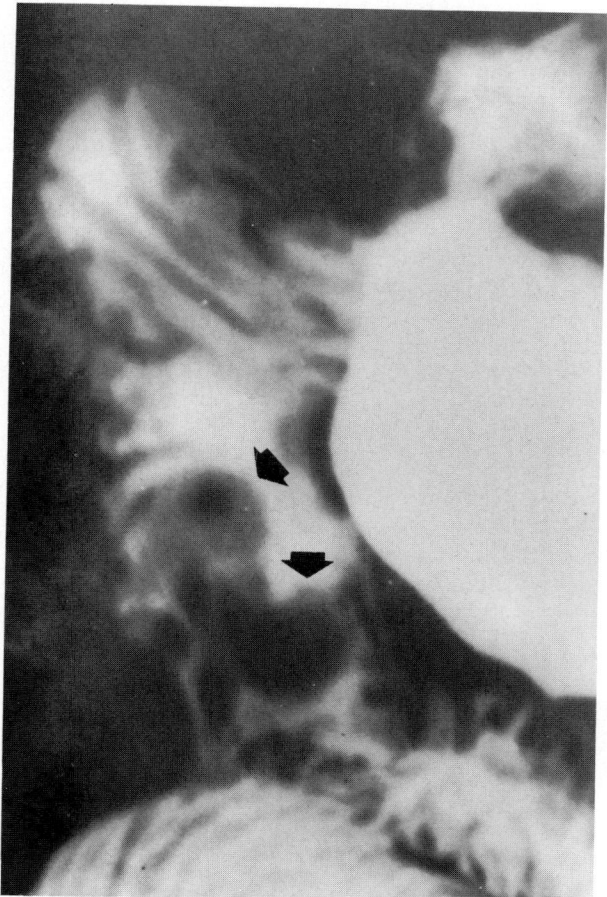

**Figure 40–3. Duodenal varices.** Thickened, serpiginous folds *(arrows)* are present in the descending duodenum. (From Eisenberg RL: Gastrointestinal Radiology: A Pattern Approach [2nd ed]. Philadelphia: JB Lippincott, 1990.)

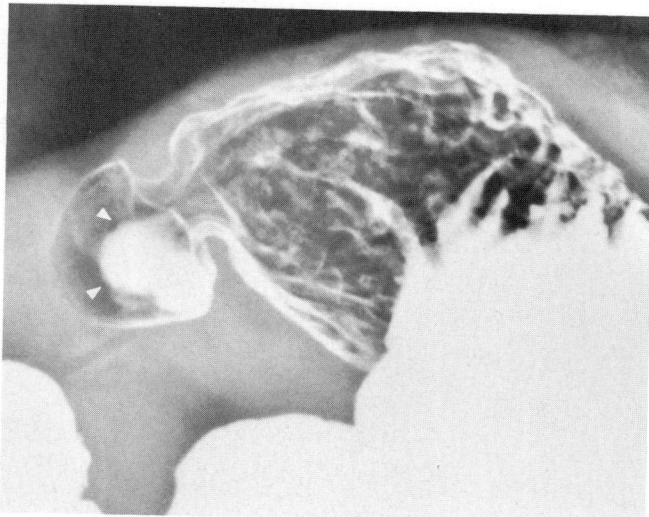

**Figure 40–4. Gastric diverticulum.** A large diverticulum is seen arising from the posterior wall of the fundus. Pooling of barium *(arrowheads)* in the diverticulum could be mistaken for an area of ulceration. (From Eisenberg RL: Gastrointestinal Radiology: A Pattern Approach [2nd ed]. Philadelphia: JB Lippincott, 1990.)

tract. They are acquired lesions, consisting of a sac of mucosal and submucosal layers herniated through a muscular defect, and they fill and empty by gravity as a result of pressure generated by duodenal peristalsis. Although most commonly found along the medial border of the descending duodenum in the periampullary region (Fig. 40–6), diverticula frequently arise in the third and fourth portions of the duodenum (30 to 40%)

tion, barium can usually be demonstrated to enter the diverticulum, establishing the diagnosis (Fig. 40–4). At times, a collection of barium may pool in a gastric diverticulum, mimicking an area of ulceration (see Fig. 40–4). Diverticula rarely occur in the antrum, where they may simulate an ulcer crater.

Intramural or partial gastric diverticulum is a rare anomaly characterized by focal invagination of the mucosa into the muscular layer of the gastric wall.[5] It is usually located on the greater curvature of the distal antrum. The diverticulum may be manifested radiographically by a tiny collection of barium extending outside the contour of the adjacent gastric wall (Fig. 40–5). These structures have no clinical significance, although they can be mistaken for ulcers or ectopic pancreatic rests on the greater curvature.

## Duodenal Diverticula

### *True Diverticula*

Diverticula of the duodenum are incidental findings in 1 to 5% of barium studies of the upper gastrointestinal

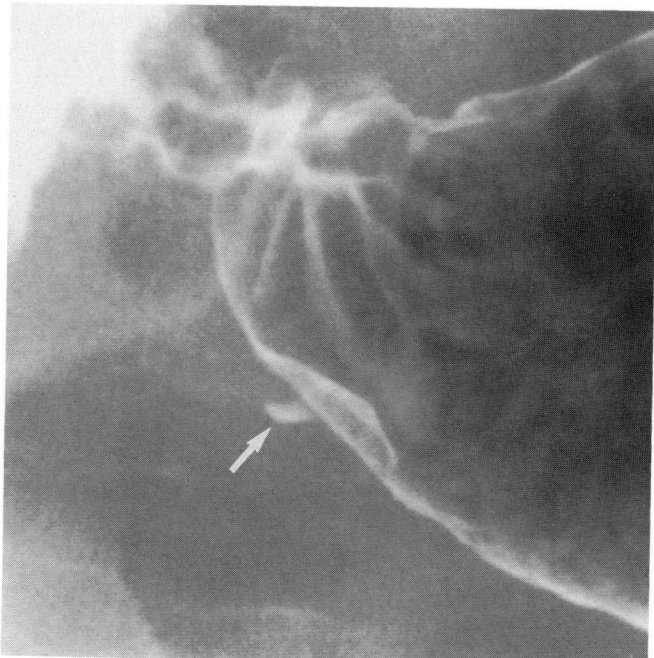

**Figure 40–5. Intramural or partial gastric diverticulum.** A tiny, barium-filled outpouching *(arrow)* is seen on the greater curvature of the distal antrum. There is a heaped-up area overlying the diverticulum, so it could be mistaken for an ectopic pancreatic rest. (Courtesy of Marc S. Levine, M.D., Philadelphia, PA.)

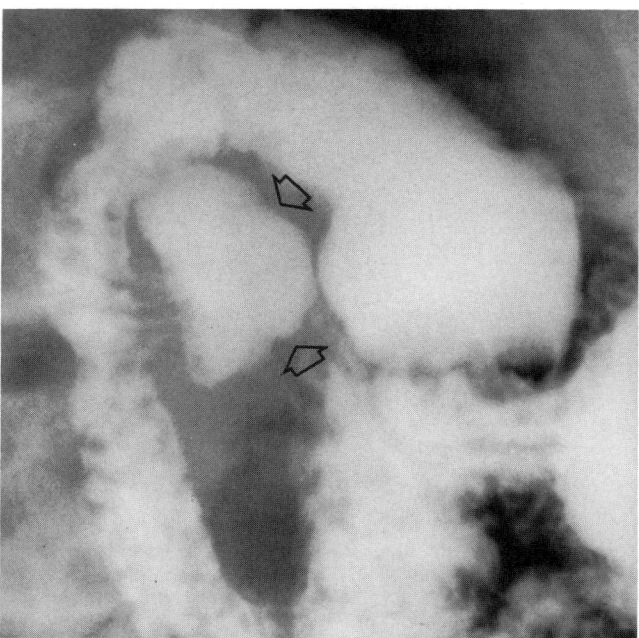

**Figure 40–6. Duodenal diverticulum.** A typical diverticulum *(arrows)* is seen arising from the medial border of the descending duodenum. (From Eisenberg RL: Gastrointestinal Radiology: A Pattern Approach [2nd ed]. Philadelphia: JB Lippincott, 1990.)

and can even occur on the lateral border of the descending duodenum (Fig. 40–7).

On barium examinations, duodenal diverticula typically have a smooth, rounded shape, are often multiple, and generally change configuration during the course of

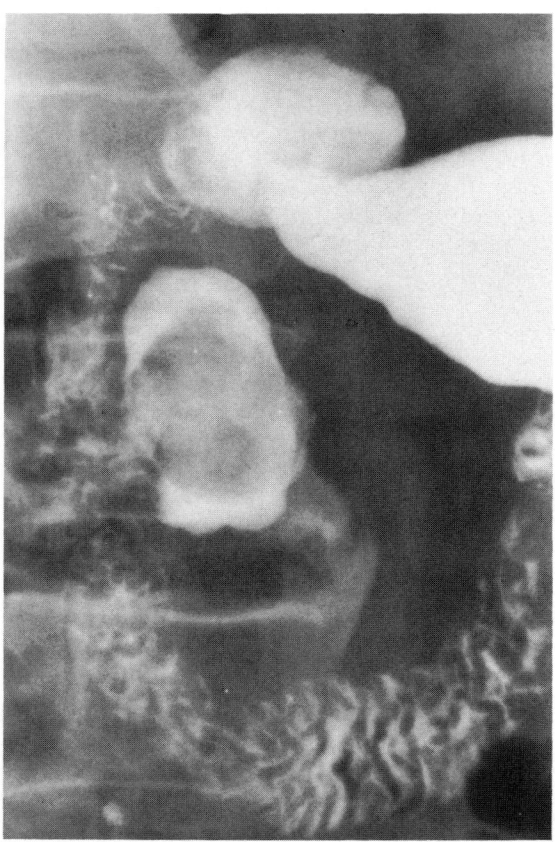

**Figure 40–8. Duodenal diverticulum with a blood clot.** This diverticulum contains a large, irregular filling defect representing a blood clot in a patient with recent upper gastrointestinal bleeding. (From Eisenberg RL: Gastrointestinal Radiology: A Pattern Approach [2nd ed]. Philadelphia: JB Lippincott, 1990.)

the study. The lack of inflammatory reaction (i.e., spasm or edema) permits a duodenal diverticulum to be differentiated from a postbulbar ulcer. Bizarre, multilobulated diverticula occasionally occur.[6] Filling defects representing inspissated food particles, blood clots, or gas can be identified in a duodenal diverticulum (Fig. 40–8). However, these defects are inconstant and may change in appearance or disappear at fluoroscopy.

Although the overwhelming majority of duodenal diverticula are asymptomatic, serious complications can develop. Duodenal diverticulitis mimics numerous abdominal diseases (including cholecystitis, peptic ulcer disease, and pancreatitis) and is a diagnosis of exclusion. Complications of inflamed duodenal diverticula include hemorrhage, perforation, abscesses, and fistulas. Because duodenal diverticula are retroperitoneal structures, perforation occurs without clinical signs of peritonitis or radiographic signs of free intraperitoneal gas. The most common radiographic finding associated with a perforated duodenal diverticulum is retroperitoneal gas localized to the area surrounding the duodenum and the upper pole of the right kidney.[7] A large diverticulum may occasionally cause symptoms of partial obstruction of the upper gastrointestinal tract.

Anomalous insertion of the common bile duct and pancreatic duct into a duodenal diverticulum can be

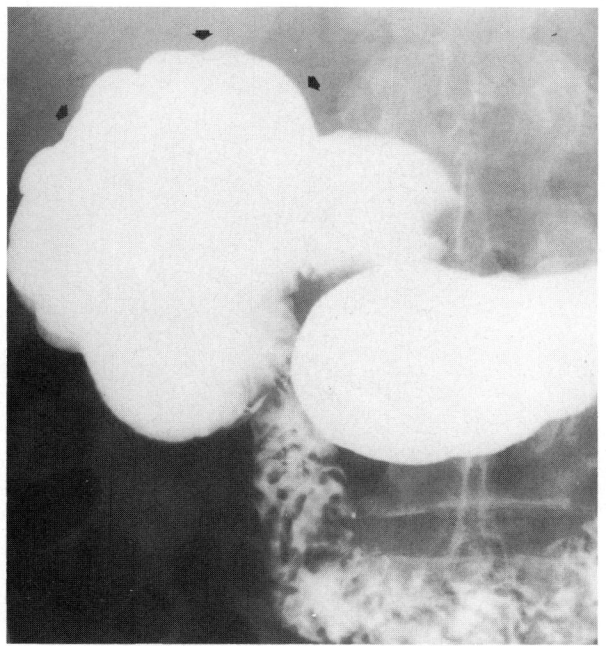

**Figure 40–7. Giant duodenal diverticulum.** A giant diverticulum *(arrows)* is seen arising from the lateral border of the proximal descending duodenum. (From Eisenberg RL: Gastrointestinal Radiology: A Pattern Approach [2nd ed]. Philadelphia: JB Lippincott, 1990.)

demonstrated in about 3% of carefully performed T tube cholangiograms. This anatomic arrangement appears to interfere with the normal emptying mechanisms of the ductal systems and predisposes to obstructive biliary and pancreatic disease. The absence of an ampullary sphincter mechanism permits spontaneous reflux of barium from the diverticulum into the common bile duct, and this can be a cause of ascending infection.[8]

## Pseudodiverticula

Pseudodiverticula are exaggerated outpouchings or sacculations of the inferior and superior recesses of the duodenal bulb. They are usually located at the base of the bulb and are related to duodenal ulcer disease (Fig. 40–9). The sacculations may be caused by edema and circular muscle spasm associated with an active ulcer or by scarring and fibrosis from a previous ulcer. However, the degree of deformity is not directly related to ulcer size; small ulcers may produce large deformities, and large ulcers may produce little alteration in bulb contour.

## Intraluminal Diverticula

An intraluminal duodenal diverticulum is a sac of duodenal mucosa originating in the second portion of the duodenum near the papilla of Vater. The formation of a diverticulum in adults from a congenital duodenal web or diaphragm appears to be due to purely mechanical factors such as forward pressure by food and strong peristaltic activity. When filled with barium, an intraluminal duodenal diverticulum appears as a finger-like sac separated from contrast medium in the duodenal lumen by a radiolucent band representing the wall of the diverticulum (the "halo" sign)[9] (Fig. 40–10). When

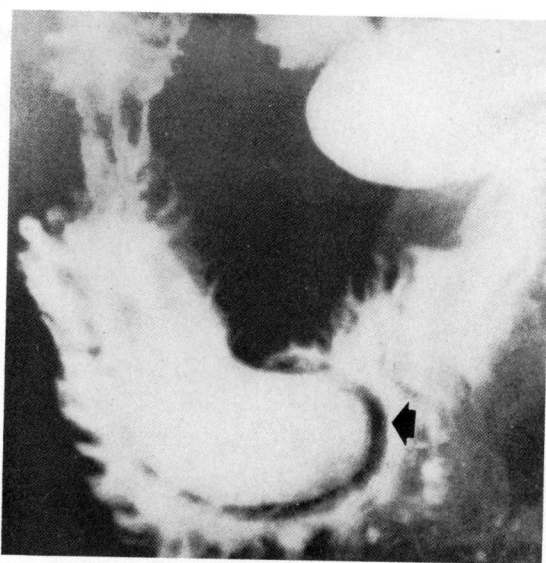

**Figure 40–10. Intraluminal duodenal diverticulum.** Note the characteristic halo sign *(arrow)* and barium filling the diverticulum. (From JCH Laudan, GI Norton, Intraluminal duodenal diverticulum, AJR, 90, 756–760, 1963, © by American Roentgen Ray Society.)

empty of barium, it can simulate a pedunculated polyp. Complications of intraluminal duodenal diverticula include retention of food and foreign bodies and partial duodenal obstruction. Increased intraluminal pressure may cause reflux of duodenal contents into the pancreatic duct and an acute episode of pancreatitis.

Intraluminal duodenal diverticulum and its predecessor, the congenital duodenal diaphragm, frequently occur in association with other anomalies, including annular pancreas, midgut volvulus, situs inversus, choledochocele, congenital heart disease, Down's syndrome, imperforate anus, Hirschsprung's disease, omphalocele, hypoplastic kidneys, and exstrophy of the bladder.

## DIAPHRAGMS AND WEBS

### Antral Mucosal Diaphragms

Antral mucosal diaphragms are thin, membranous septa that are usually located within 3 cm of the pyloric canal and are oriented perpendicular to the long axis of the stomach. Clinical symptoms of partial gastric outlet obstruction (epigastric pain, fullness, and vomiting, particularly after a heavy meal) correlate with the size of the central aperture of the antral mucosal diaphragm. Symptoms of obstruction do not occur if the diameter of the aperture is greater than 1 cm. Even with minute central orifices as small as 2 mm, no obstructive symptoms may be produced until adult life. Infrequently, infants with mucosal diaphragms present with projectile vomiting in the neonatal period. With severe obstruction, gastric emptying is greatly delayed and barium can be seen to pass in a thin stream (jet effect) through the center of the orifice.[10]

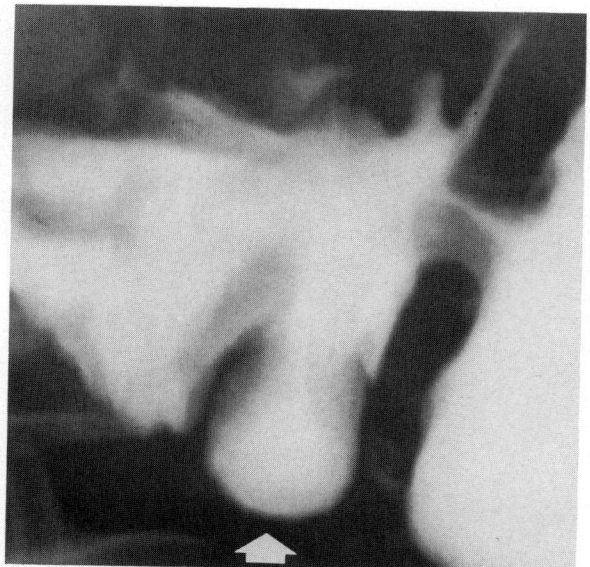

**Figure 40–9. Duodenal pseudodiverticulum.** An exaggerated outpouching *(arrow)* is seen at the base of the bulb due to duodenal ulcer disease. (From Eisenberg RL: Gastrointestinal Radiology: A Pattern Approach [2nd ed]. Philadelphia: JB Lippincott, 1990.)

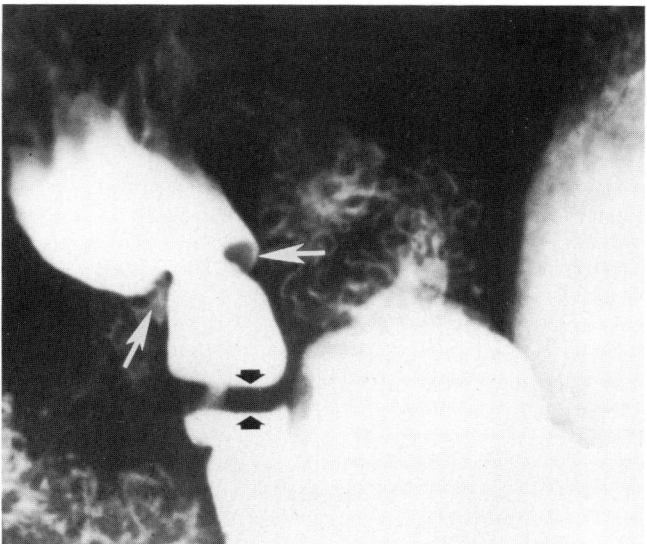

**Figure 40–11. Antral mucosal diaphragm.** A band-like defect *(black arrows)* is seen arising at right angles to the gastric wall. The web is approximately 5 mm thick. The pyloric channel is denoted by white arrows. (From E Bjorgvinsson, C Rudzki, AM Lewicki, Antral web, Am J Gastroenterol, 79, 663–665, 1984, © by The American College of Gastroenterology.)

The nonobstructing antral mucosal diaphragm appears radiographically as a persistent, sharply defined, 2- to 3-cm-wide band-like defect in the barium column that arises at right angles to the gastric wall (Fig. 40–11). Although this appearance can be simulated by a prominent transverse mucosal fold in the antrum, the fold does not extend across the gastric lumen, nor is it generally perfectly straight. The antral mucosal diaphragm is best seen when the stomach proximal and distal to it is distended. The portion of the antrum proximal to the pylorus and distal to the mucosal diaphragm can mimic a second duodenal bulb (Fig. 40–

12). The distal antrum can sometimes even be confused with a gastric diverticulum or ulcer, although on close inspection it clearly lies within the line of the stomach and changes size and shape during the examination.[11]

Because an antral mucosal diaphragm is readily amenable to surgical correction, it is important that the proper diagnosis be made. Radiologists must suggest the possibility of an antral mucosal diaphragm to the endoscopist, because the orifice can closely simulate the pylorus on endoscopy and thus be easily overlooked.

## Duodenal Webs

Congenital duodenal webs or diaphragms are web-like projections of the mucous membrane that occlude the lumen of the duodenum to varying degrees. The majority of reported cases have occurred in the second portion of the duodenum near the ampulla of Vater. Radiographically, the congenital duodenal web appears as a thin, radiolucent line extending across the lumen, often with proximal duodenal dilatation (Fig. 40–13). Because the duodenal obstruction is incomplete, small amounts of gas may be scattered through the more distal portions of the bowel.[12] On rare occasions, a web may balloon out distally, producing a rounded, barium-filled, comma-shaped sac (see earlier section on intraluminal diverticula).

## ADULT HYPERTROPHIC PYLORIC STENOSIS

The histologic, anatomic, and radiographic abnormalities in adult hypertrophic pyloric stenosis are indistinguishable from those in the infantile form.[13] Indeed, the

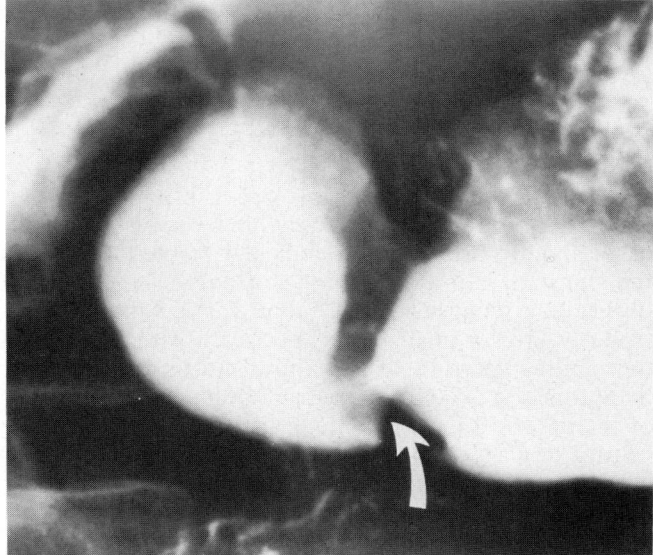

**Figure 40–12. Antral mucosal diaphragm.** The lumen is so narrowed by the diaphragm *(arrow)* that the antrum distal to the diaphragm simulates a second duodenal bulb. (From Eisenberg RL: Gastrointestinal Radiology: A Pattern Approach [2nd ed]. Philadelphia: JB Lippincott, 1990.)

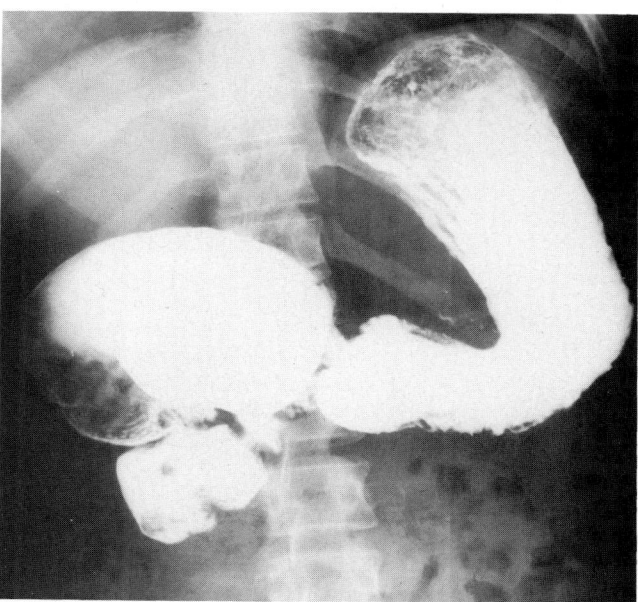

**Figure 40–13. Duodenal web.** There is high-grade stenosis of the second portion of the duodenum. The presence of gas in the bowel distal to the web indicates that the obstruction is incomplete. (From Eisenberg RL: Gastrointestinal Radiology: A Pattern Approach [2nd ed]. Philadelphia: JB Lippincott, 1990.)

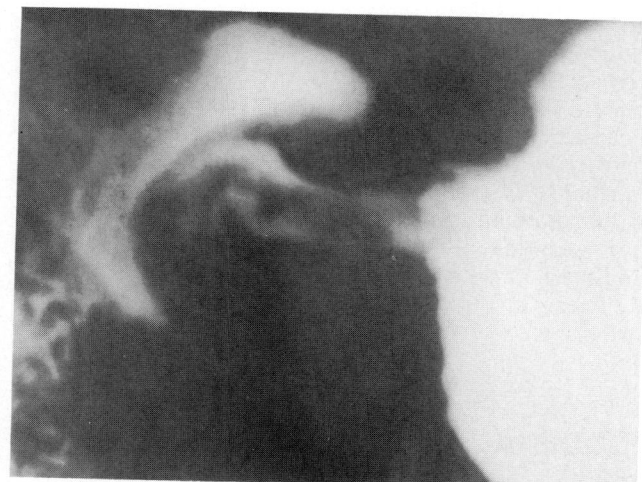

**Figure 40–14. Adult hypertrophic pyloric stenosis.** The pyloric canal is narrowed and elongated with a characteristic concave indentation on the base of the duodenal bulb. (From Eisenberg RL: Gastrointestinal Radiology: A Pattern Approach [2nd ed]. Philadelphia: JB Lippincott, 1990.)

disease in adults may represent a milder form of the same entity observed in infants and children. Most cases of adult hypertrophic pyloric stenosis go unrecognized because the patients are asymptomatic. Some complain of nausea and vomiting, epigastric pain, weight loss, and anorexia. Unlike children, adults infrequently have high-grade gastric outlet obstruction with hypertrophic pyloric stenosis.

About half of all patients with demonstrable pyloric hypertrophy have concomitant gastric ulceration. This probably reflects the development of an ulcer as a result of delayed gastric emptying, which interferes with the passage of semisolid food and results in increased gastrin production and consequent hyperacidity.

Elongation and narrowing of the pyloric canal are characteristic radiographic findings in adult hypertrophic pyloric stenosis (Fig. 40–14). The pylorus is elongated, measuring 2 to 4 cm in length (normal length, ≤1 cm in adults). Hypertrophy of the musculature produces a narrowed segment, the contour of which can be smooth or slightly irregular. Invagination of the mucosa into the narrow pyloric canal produces the characteristic "double track" sign. The proximal end of the narrowed pylorus merges gradually with the contiguous stomach, resulting in a smooth, round juncture without the shoulders expected for a malignant neoplasm. Another classic sign of adult hypertrophic stenosis is a symmetric, concave, crescentic indentation on the base of the duodenal bulb (see Fig. 40–14). This mushroom-shaped defect is presumably due to partial invagination of the hypertrophied muscle mass into the bulb.

A less common and atypical form of muscular hypertrophy has been termed *focal hypertrophy* or *torus hyperplasia*. It occurs as the result of localized muscle hypertrophy on the lesser curvature, at the level where normal muscle fibers usually converge to form a muscular prominence called the torus. Additional uneven hypertrophy of the muscle fibers along the greater curvature leads to the development of a characteristic

radiographic appearance. The distal antrum and pyloric canal are asymmetrically narrowed, the lesser curvature is flattened or concave, and the greater curvature is slightly serrated.

## GASTRIC OUTLET OBSTRUCTION

In adults, peptic ulcer disease is by far the most common cause of gastric outlet obstruction (60 to 65% of cases) (Fig. 40–15). The ulcers are usually located in the duodenum, occasionally in the pyloric channel or prepyloric gastric antrum, and rarely in the body of the stomach. Narrowing of the lumen in peptic ulcer disease can result from spasm, acute inflammation and edema, muscular hypertrophy, or contraction of scar tissue. In most patients, several of these factors combine to produce gastric outlet obstruction.[14]

Most patients with peptic ulcer disease causing pyloric obstruction have a long history of ulcer symptoms. Indeed, gastric outlet obstruction as the initial manifestation of peptic ulcer disease is unusual and should raise the suspicion of gastric malignancy.

An annular, constricting carcinoma of the distal antrum or pylorus is the second leading cause of gastric outlet obstruction (30 to 35% of cases) (Fig. 40–16). Other infiltrative primary malignant tumors or metastatic lesions obliterating the lumen of the distal stomach and proximal duodenum can also produce the radiographic pattern of gastric outlet obstruction. Unlike patients with peptic ulcer disease, about one third of patients with gastric outlet obstruction caused by malignancy have no pain. A large majority have a history of pain of less than 1 year's duration.[15]

Abdominal plain films in patients with gastric outlet

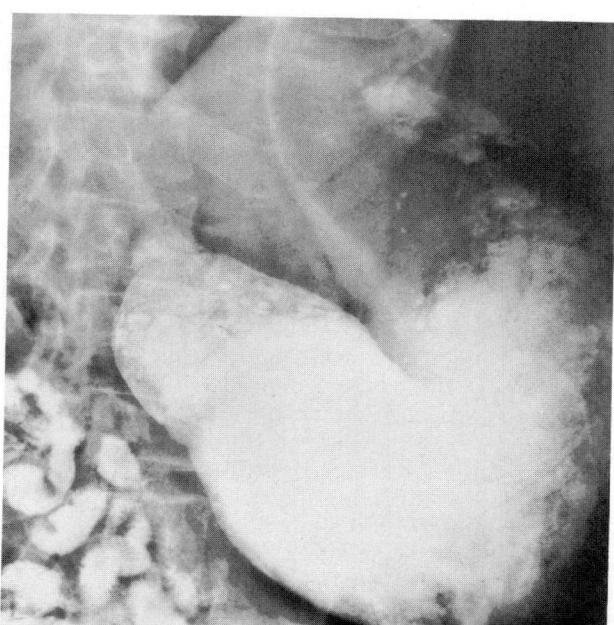

**Figure 40–15. Gastric outlet obstruction caused by peptic ulcer disease.** Note gastric distention and dilution of the barium by retained fluid in the stomach. (From Eisenberg RL: Gastrointestinal Radiology: A Pattern Approach [2nd ed]. Philadelphia: JB Lippincott, 1990.)

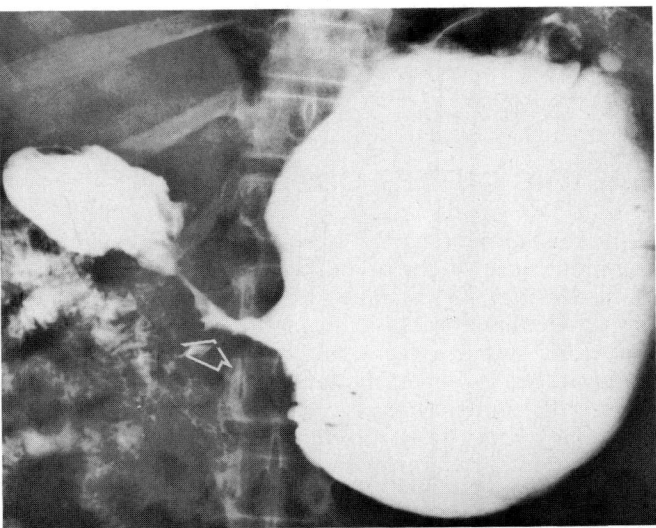

**Figure 40–16. Gastric outlet obstruction caused by an annular carcinoma of the antrum.** There is irregular narrowing of the distal antrum *(arrow)* with proximal dilatation of the stomach. (From Eisenberg RL: Gastrointestinal Radiology: A Pattern Approach [2nd ed]. Philadelphia: JB Lippincott, 1990.)

obstruction often demonstrate the outline of the dilated, gas-filled stomach. On barium examination, a mottled density of nonopaque material represents excessive overnight gastric residual. There is a marked delay in gastric emptying, with barium often retained in the stomach for 24 hours or longer. The stomach may become enormously dilated and, with the patient in the upright position, extend inferiorly into the lower abdomen or pelvis. The critical differential diagnosis is between a benign (primarily peptic ulcer disease) and malignant cause of gastric outlet obstruction. The presence of a persistent fleck of barium in a narrowed pyloric channel suggests peptic ulcer disease. However, a discrete filling defect suggests malignancy, as does nodularity or irregularity of the mucosa proximal to the constricted area. It is essential that every effort be made to express barium into the duodenal bulb. The finding of distortion and scarring of the bulb with the formation of pseudodiverticula makes peptic ulcer disease the most likely etiology. Conversely, a radiographically normal duodenal bulb increases the likelihood of underlying malignancy. In many patients, unfortunately, it is impossible to differentiate confidently on barium studies between a benign and a malignant cause of gastric outlet obstruction. In these cases, endoscopy or surgical exploration is required to exclude the possibility of a malignant lesion.

Gastric outlet obstruction is infrequently caused by other conditions involving the distal stomach and proximal duodenum. Mural infiltration or spasm resulting from inflammatory disorders (Crohn's disease, sarcoidosis, syphilis, and tuberculosis) may cause sufficient thickening of the gastric wall to produce an obstructive appearance (Fig. 40–17). Severe pancreatitis and cholecystitis can incite inflammatory spasm, which leads to obliteration of the lumen of the proximal duodenum

and gastric outlet obstruction.[16] Antral narrowing may also be caused by fibrous scarring after ingestion of corrosive substances. On rare occasions, deposition of amyloid in the stomach wall can be so pronounced that it causes severe luminal narrowing and gastric outlet obstruction (see later section on amyloidosis).

Prolapse of a benign antral polyp into the duodenum can produce intermittent gastric outlet obstruction with an intraluminal filling defect in the duodenal bulb. Other conditions causing gastric outlet obstruction (discussed elsewhere in this chapter) include antral mucosal diaphragm, gastric volvulus, and adult hypertrophic pyloric stenosis.

# DUODENAL OBSTRUCTION

A variety of congenital anomalies, inflammatory disorders, and malignancies can cause obstruction of the duodenum. Many of these conditions are discussed elsewhere in this book.

## Mesenteric Root Syndrome

The transverse portion of the duodenum lies in a fixed position in a retroperitoneal location. It is situated in a closed compartment bounded anteriorly by the root of the mesentery, which carries the superior mesenteric vessel sheath (artery, vein, and nerve), and posteriorly by the aorta and lumbar spine (at the L2-3 level, where lumbar lordosis is most pronounced). Even in normal persons, there is often a transient delay of barium at the point at which the transverse duodenum crosses the

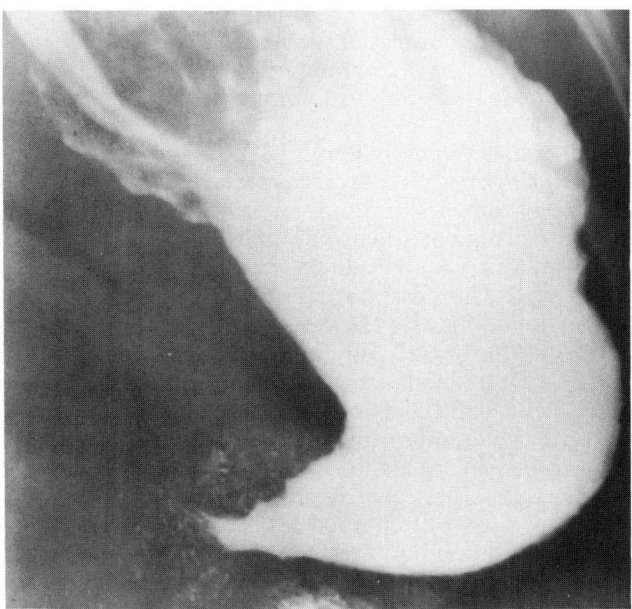

**Figure 40–17. Gastric outlet obstruction caused by Crohn's disease.** There is tapered narrowing of the distal antrum due to Crohn's disease involving the stomach. (From Eisenberg RL: Gastrointestinal Radiology: A Pattern Approach [2nd ed]. Philadelphia: JB Lippincott, 1990.)

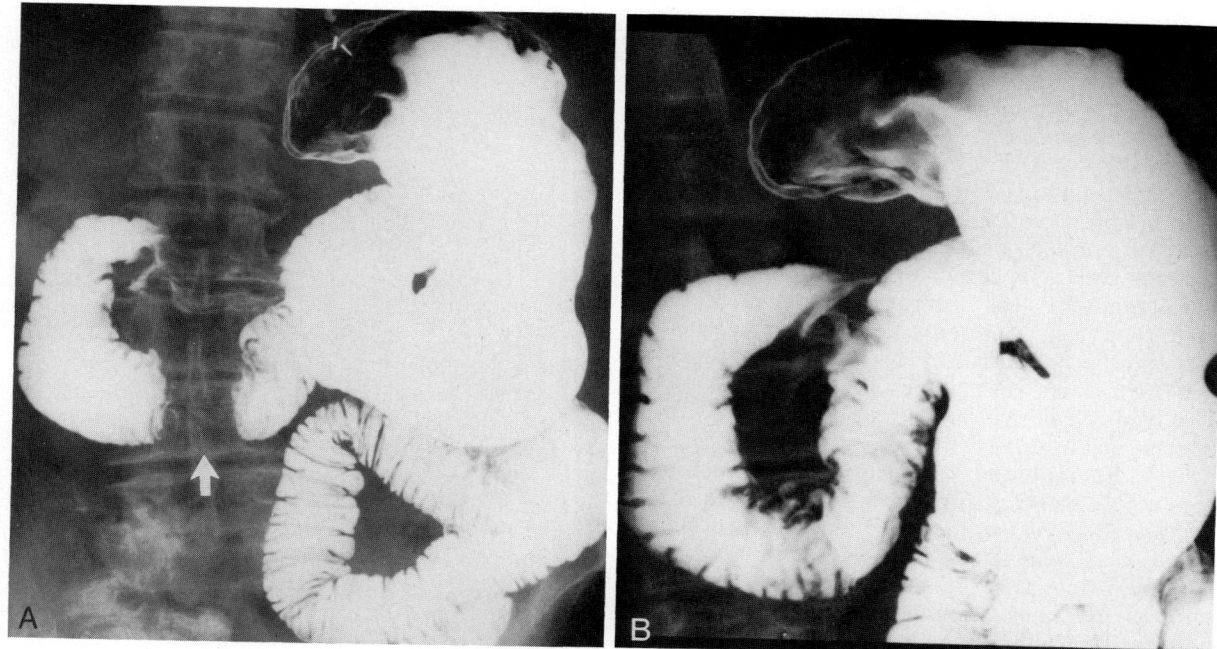

**Figure 40–18. Normal patient with findings mimicking those in mesenteric root syndrome. A.** A frontal projection shows apparent obstruction of the third portion of the duodenum by the mesenteric root *(arrow)*. **B.** However, a right anterior oblique projection obtained moments later shows a normal duodenal sweep without evidence of obstruction.

spine. This can be associated with mild, inconstant proximal duodenal dilatation (Fig. 40–18).

Any process that tends to close the nutcracker-like jaws of the aorticomesenteric angle results in some degree of compression of the transverse portion of the duodenum. It is most common in asthenic persons, especially those who have lost substantial weight. Prolonged bed rest or immobilization in the supine position (patients with body casts or whole body burns or patients who are fixed in a position of hyperextension after spinal injury or surgery) causes the mesenteric root to fall back and compress the anterior aspect of the transverse duodenum, resulting in relative duodenal obstruction.[17, 18] In patients who lose weight and retroperitoneal fat because of debilitating illness, the increased dragging effect of the mesenteric root also narrows the aorticomesenteric compartment. Similarly, conditions leading to relaxation of abdominal wall musculature (e.g., multiple pregnancies) can obstruct the transverse duodenum.[19]

In patients with diseases causing reduced duodenal peristaltic activity, especially when the patients are placed in a supine position, the combination of lumbar spine, aorta, and mesenteric root may constitute enough of a barrier to cause significant obstruction of the transverse duodenum. As a result, the mesenteric root syndrome sometimes occurs in patients with scleroderma, who have a dilated, atonic duodenum caused by smooth muscle atrophy and fibrosis (Fig. 40–19). Other collagen diseases, such as dermatomyositis and systemic lupus erythematosus, may produce the same radiographic pattern. In Chagas' disease, inflammatory destruction of intramural autonomic plexuses by *Trypa-*

*nosoma cruzi* can lead to generalized gastrointestinal aperistalsis and dilatation that most frequently involve the esophagus and colon but can also affect the duodenum. Dysfunction of the vagus nerve can also result in dilatation of the proximal duodenum. This can occur after surgical vagotomy for peptic ulcer disease or after chemical vagotomy due to ingestion of drugs such as atropine, morphine, or diphenoxylate (Lomotil). Dis-

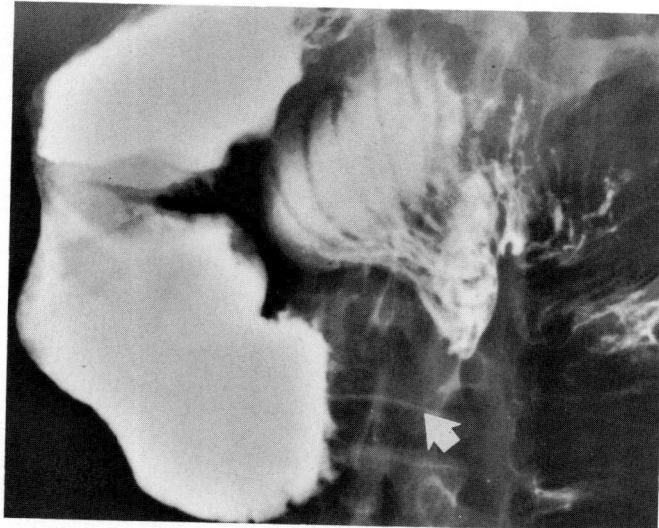

**Figure 40–19. Mesenteric root syndrome caused by scleroderma.** The duodenum is markedly dilated and atonic proximal to the aorticomesenteric angle *(arrow)*. (From Eisenberg RL: Gastrointestinal Radiology: A Pattern Approach [2nd ed]. Philadelphia: JB Lippincott, 1990.)

ordered duodenal motility and dilatation can also be seen in patients with neuropathies secondary to diabetes, porphyria, and thiamine deficiency.

An adynamic ileus caused by any acute upper abdominal inflammatory process may cause relative obstruction and proximal dilatation of the duodenum. This duodenal atony is seen in patients with acute pancreatitis, cholecystitis, and peptic ulcer disease.[20]

Any space-occupying process within the aorticomesenteric angle can also compress the transverse duodenum. Inflammatory thickening of the bowel wall or mesenteric root (e.g., pancreatitis, Crohn's disease, tuberculous enteritis, peptic ulcer disease, and strongyloidiasis) or metastases to the mesentery or mesenteric nodes can lead to relative duodenal obstruction.

Regardless of the underlying pathophysiologic mechanism, the radiographic appearance is almost identical in all patients with the mesenteric root syndrome. Pronounced dilatation of the first and second portions of the duodenum is associated with a vertical, linear extrinsic pressure defect in the transverse portion of the duodenum overlying the spine (see Fig. 40–19). The duodenal mucosal folds are intact but compressed.

## Other Causes

Intramural hematoma, intraluminal duodenal diverticulum, and aortoduodenal fistula (all discussed elsewhere in this chapter) are other causes of duodenal obstruction. Ulceration with stricture formation can also be a complication of radiation therapy of the upper abdomen.[21] A rare cause of duodenal obstruction is the preduodenal portal vein, which crosses in front of rather than behind the duodenum. Although it has been reported that the preduodenal portal vein may cause duodenal obstruction, it is difficult to understand how the low venous pressure within a thin-walled vessel can cause intestinal blockage. Preduodenal portal vein is associated with a high incidence of malformations (e.g., duodenal bands, annular pancreas, and malrotation), which most likely cause the clinical picture of duodenal obstruction and lead to the incidental discovery of the abnormal vessel. The main surgical implication of the preduodenal portal vein is that the anomaly must be recognized to avoid injury to the vessel during operations on the biliary tract and duodenum.[22]

## GASTRIC DILATATION WITHOUT OUTLET OBSTRUCTION

Acute or chronic dilatation of the stomach with prolonged retention of food and barium can occur without any organic gastric outlet obstruction. Gastric retention is defined as vomiting of food eaten more than 6 hours earlier or the presence of food in the stomach at the time of an upper gastrointestinal series (assuming that the patient has not eaten for 8 to 10 hours). It is critical to remember that gastric retention does not necessarily mean gastric outlet obstruction and that "corrective" surgery may be contraindicated.[23]

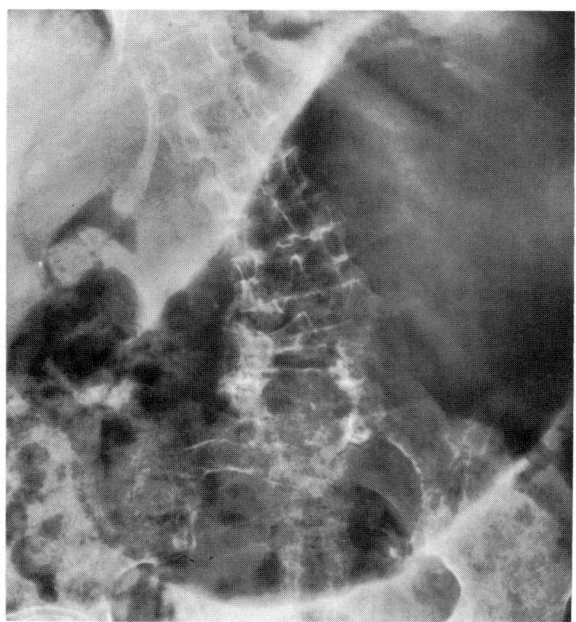

**Figure 40–20. Massive gastric dilatation.** An abdominal plain film shows an enormous quantity of gas filling a markedly dilated stomach that extends inferiorly into the pelvis. (From Eisenberg RL: Gastrointestinal Radiology: A Pattern Approach [2nd ed]. Philadelphia: JB Lippincott, 1990.)

The appearance of gastric dilatation without obstruction is indistinguishable from that of organic gastric outlet obstruction on abdominal plain films. Huge quantities of air and fluid may fill a massively enlarged stomach that can extend even to the floor of the pelvis (Fig. 40–20). Administration of barium usually demonstrates a large amount of solid gastric residue. Peristalsis is irregular, sluggish, and ineffectual. When barium studies demonstrate retained food in the stomach without evidence of gastric outlet obstruction, the various nonobstructive causes of gastric retention must be excluded before accusing the patient of disregarding instructions and eating before the examination.

## Acute Gastric Dilatation

Acute gastric dilatation is characterized by sudden and severe distention of the stomach by fluid and gas, usually accompanied by vomiting, dehydration, and peripheral vascular collapse. Within minutes or hours, a normal stomach can expand into a hyperemic, cyanotic, atonic sac that fills the abdomen. Most cases of acute gastric dilatation occur during the first several days after abdominal surgery (Fig. 40–21). The incidence of this postoperative complication has decreased dramatically with the advent of nasogastric suction, improved anesthetics, close monitoring of acid-base and electrolyte balances, and meticulous care in the handling of tissues at surgery. Acute gastric dilatation can also be a complication of other medical or surgical diseases, including abdominal trauma and peritoneal inflammatory processes.

Acute gastric dilatation may be a fatal condition, if

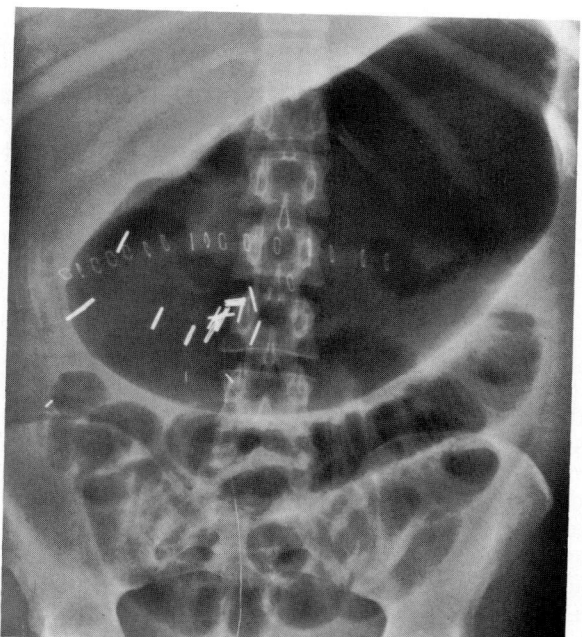

**Figure 40–21. Acute gastric dilatation resulting from abdominal surgery.** (From Eisenberg RL: Gastrointestinal Radiology: A Pattern Approach [2nd ed]. Philadelphia: JB Lippincott, 1990.)

gastric cardia can lead to copious vomiting, aspiration, asphyxiation, and cardiac arrest. Acute gastric dilatation can cause gastric perforation with peritonitis or result in severe fluid and electrolyte disturbances, dehydration, decreased urine output, and shock.[23]

## Chronic Gastric Dilatation

The development of gastric dilatation can be indolent and essentially asymptomatic. Between 20 and 30% of patients with diabetes have a dilated stomach with decreased or absent gastric peristalsis (i.e., diabetic gastroparesis). Most of these patients have long-standing, poorly controlled disease and evidence of peripheral neuropathy or other complications.[24] Patients with neurologic abnormalities (brain tumor, bulbar poliomyelitis, and tabes dorsalis) may also develop chronic gastric retention, although in these conditions, decreased peristalsis and dilatation more commonly involve the esophagus. Pronounced gastric dilatation can also develop in patients with scleroderma, polymyositis, dermatomyositis,[25] and myotonic muscular dystrophy.[26] Other causes include electrolyte and acid-base imbalances, lead poisoning, and porphyria (Fig. 40–22).

untreated. Prompt response to appropriate therapy can usually be achieved if early signs are recognized. Unfortunately, pain is seldom severe until gastric dilatation is pronounced. Distention can progress rapidly because of aerophagia or air sucking. Sudden relaxation of the

## ABNORMAL EXTRINSIC MASSES
### Stomach

Extrinsic impressions on the stomach may be caused by an anomalous lobe of the liver, aberrant position of

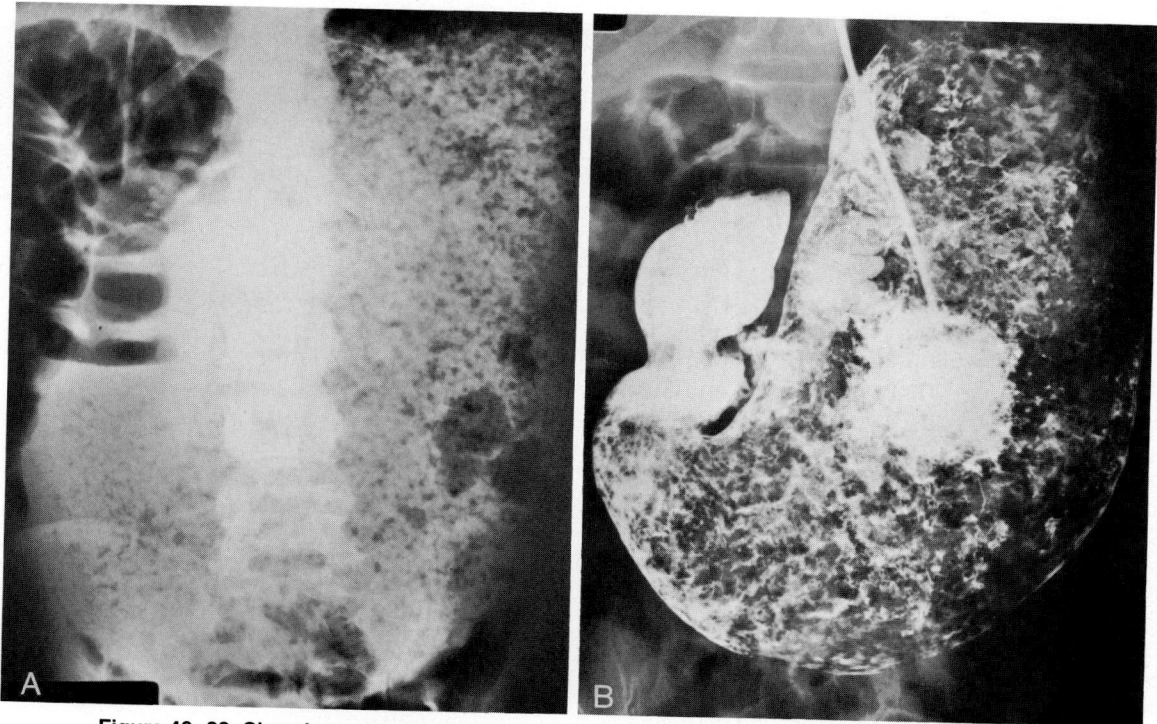

**Figure 40–22. Chronic gastric dilatation caused by severe electrolyte and acid-base imbalance.**
**A.** An abdominal plain film shows a marked amount of particulate material in a dilated stomach. **B.** A contrast study confirms the plain film findings. This patient had poorly controlled diabetes.

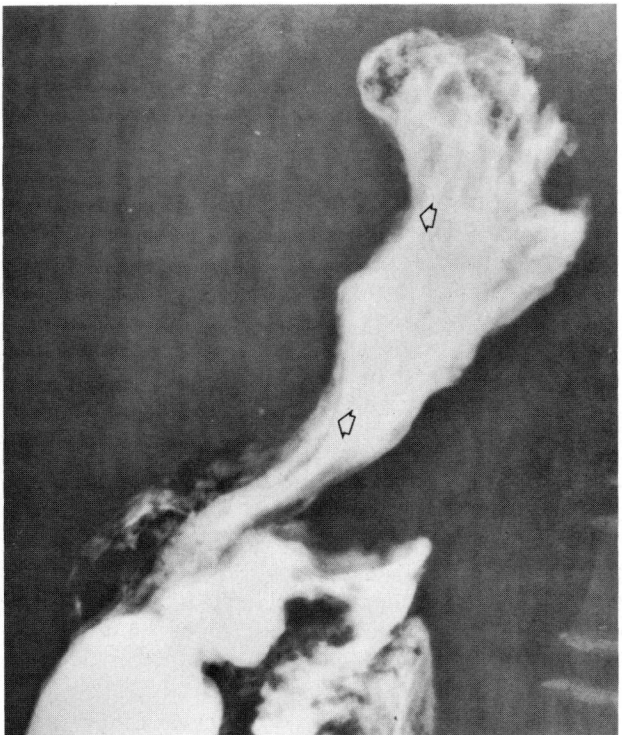

**Figure 40–23. Gastric impressions by a polycystic liver.** Two large extrinsic impressions *(arrows)* on the anterior aspect of the stomach could be mistaken for intramural lesions. (From Eisenberg RL: Gastrointestinal Radiology: A Pattern Approach [2nd ed]. Philadelphia: JB Lippincott, 1990.)

the spleen or left kidney, or pathologic enlargement of these structures (Fig. 40–23). CT can aid in differentiating these extrinsic defects from true intragastric lesions.

## Duodenum

A variety of disease states involving organs in the right upper quadrant may cause displacement of or extrinsic pressure on the duodenal bulb and sweep. Even when normal, the common bile duct can produce a linear or small, rounded impression on the duodenal bulb. A dilated common bile duct tends to cause a large tubular defect that arises superiorly and to the right of the barium-filled duodenum (Fig. 40–24). Extrinsic pressure on the duodenum may also result from any cause of enlargement of the gallbladder (e.g., hydrops, carcinoma, and pericholecystic abscess).

Hepatomegaly or anomalous lobes of the liver may cause marked leftward displacement of the duodenal bulb and sweep.[27, 28] This is especially prominent when there is hypertrophy of the caudate lobe. Hepatic cysts and tumors as well as metastatic lymphadenopathy in the periportal region can also cause an extrinsic impression on the duodenal bulb and sweep.

Masses in the right kidney or adrenal gland can

impress the posterolateral aspect of the duodenal sweep.[29] Generalized renal enlargement (secondary to a bifid collecting system or hydronephrosis), multiple cysts, polycystic disease, or hypernephroma can also impress and displace the duodenum (Fig. 40–25). Anterior displacement of the duodenum can be caused by enlargement of the right adrenal gland in patients with Addison's disease or adrenal carcinoma.

The midportion of the descending duodenum is crossed anteriorly by the transverse colon. In up to 3% of patients, there is a closer than normal positional relationship between these two structures, resulting in a mutual indentation.[30] Carcinoma of the right side of the colon, especially of the hepatic flexure, can result in an extrinsic pressure defect on the outer border of the descending duodenum.[31] This may be caused by lymph node enlargement from metastatic spread or by direct extension of the neoplastic process across the short fascial plane of the lateral reflection of the transverse mesocolon, which attaches the hepatic flexure of the colon to the lower portion of the descending duodenum.

Dilated vessels can produce single or multiple impressions on the outer wall of the duodenal bulb and sweep. These may result from duodenal varices caused by portal hypertension or from dilated arterial collateral pathways resulting from occlusion of the celiac axis or superior mesenteric artery.[32]

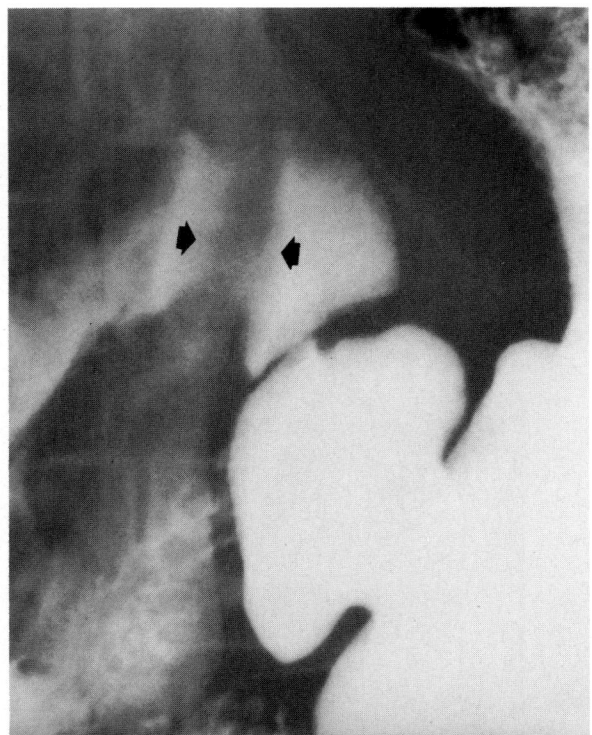

**Figure 40–24. Duodenal impression by a dilated common bile duct.** The dilated duct produces a characteristic tubular impression *(arrows)* on the duodenum near the apex of the bulb. (From Eisenberg RL: Gastrointestinal Radiology: A Pattern Approach [2nd ed]. Philadelphia: JB Lippincott, 1990.)

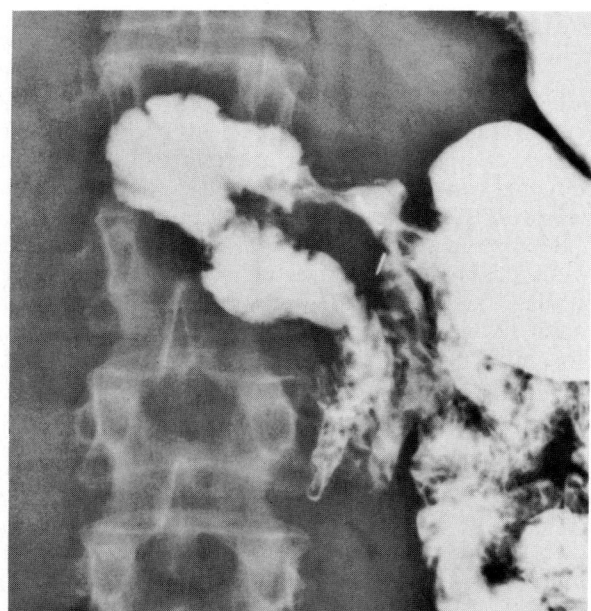

**Figure 40–25. Duodenal impression by a polycystic right kidney.** The duodenum is displaced to the left of the spine by the polycystic kidney. (From Eisenberg RL: Gastrointestinal Radiology: A Pattern Approach [2nd ed]. Philadelphia: JB Lippincott, 1990.)

# WIDENING OF THE DUODENAL SWEEP

Widening of the duodenal sweep is often considered to be suggestive evidence of malignancy or inflammation in the head of the pancreas. However, this finding is not always caused by pancreatic disease, so it must be interpreted with caution. There is great variation in the configuration of the duodenal sweep among normal patients, and slight degrees of widening are difficult to recognize with confidence. In heavy patients, the combination of a high transverse stomach and long vertical course of the descending duodenum can create the illusion of a large sweep, which is actually within normal limits. In addition, widening of the sweep can be related to upward pressure on the duodenal bulb or downward pressure on the third portion of the duodenum rather than an impression by the head of the pancreas on the medial aspect of the second portion of the duodenum.

True widening of the duodenal sweep may be caused by pancreatic neoplasms or by benign pancreatic disease (pancreatitis or pancreatic pseudocysts) (Figs. 40–26 and 40–27) (see next section). Although there are numerous radiographic criteria for distinguishing benign and malignant pancreatic disease involving the duodenum, it is often difficult to make a precise diagnosis on the basis of barium studies.

Enlargement of lymph nodes near the head of the pancreas can also widen the duodenal sweep[33] (Fig. 40–28). The subpyloric lymph nodes lie below the flexure that forms the junction between the first and second portions of the duodenum. The pancreaticoduodenal nodes lie medial to the head of the pancreas in the groove between it and the duodenum. Enlargement of

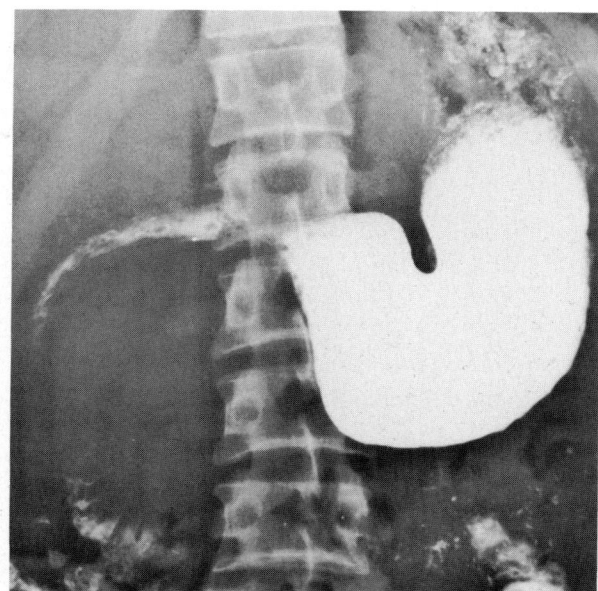

**Figure 40–26. Widening of the duodenal sweep caused by acute pancreatitis.** (From Eisenberg RL: Gastrointestinal Radiology: A Pattern Approach [2nd ed]. Philadelphia: JB Lippincott, 1990.)

these peripancreatic lymph nodes because of lymphoma, metastases, or inflammatory disease can produce the radiographic pattern of a widened duodenal sweep. A similar appearance can be produced by cystic lymphangiomas of the mesentery, which are benign, unilocular or multilocular cystic structures that contain serous or chylous fluid. These structures may result from congenital or developmental displacement and obliteration of draining lymphatics, or they may result from acquired lymphatic obstruction after trauma. Dilated pancreati-

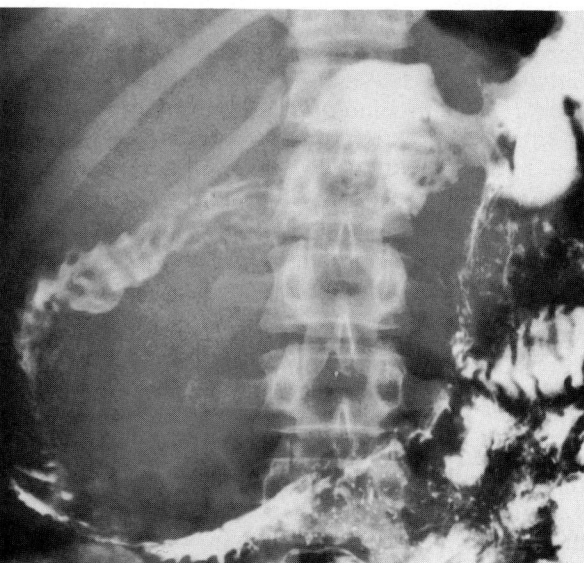

**Figure 40–27. Widening of the duodenal sweep by a pancreatic pseudocyst.** Pancreatitis or pancreatic carcinoma could produce similar findings (see Fig. 40–26). (From Eisenberg RL: Gastrointestinal Radiology: A Pattern Approach [2nd ed]. Philadelphia: JB Lippincott, 1990.)

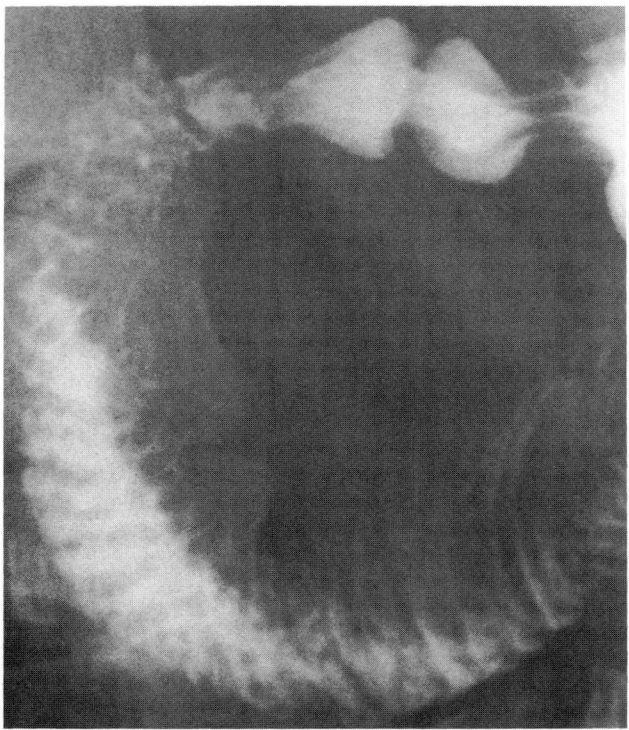

**Figure 40–28. Widening of the duodenal sweep by peripancreatic lymphoma.** Enlarged peripancreatic lymph nodes have produced a double contour on the medial aspect of the duodenum with associated spiculation. Pancreatitis or pancreatic carcinoma could produce similar findings. (From Eisenberg RL: Gastrointestinal Radiology: A Pattern Approach [2nd ed]. Philadelphia: JB Lippincott, 1990.)

coduodenal collateral vessels in patients with occlusion of the celiac axis or superior mesenteric artery infrequently produce a smooth, concave impression on the medial aspect of the descending duodenum that may simulate a mass in the head of the pancreas.

Retroperitoneal masses (primary or metastatic neoplasms or cysts) can also widen the duodenal sweep.[34] Downward displacement of the third portion of the duodenum by an aortic aneurysm can produce a similar radiographic appearance. A choledochal cyst (localized dilatation of the common bile duct) occurring near the ampulla of Vater can result in generalized widening of the duodenal sweep or a localized impression near the papilla (Fig. 40–29).

## PANCREATIC DISEASES AFFECTING THE STOMACH AND DUODENUM

Before the advent of ultrasound and CT, alterations in the configuration and mucosal pattern of the antrum and duodenal sweep on barium studies were the major radiographic findings of inflammatory or neoplastic disease involving the head of the pancreas. Although now primarily of historical interest, radiographic changes on upper gastrointestinal series occasionally suggest otherwise unexpected pancreatic disease.

Enlargement of the head of the pancreas can produce

a mass impression on the inner aspect of the duodenal sweep that creates a double contour effect (Fig. 40–30). This appearance results from differential filling of the duodenum, with the interfold spaces along the inner aspect of the sweep containing less barium than the corresponding spaces along the outer aspect. Localized impressions on the sweep can cause nodular indentations. A nonspecific sign, originally attributed to malignant disease but probably more common in inflammatory disorders, is the "inverted 3" sign of Frostberg[35] (Fig. 40–31). The central limb of the 3 represents the point of fixation of the duodenal wall, where the pancreatic and common bile ducts insert into the papilla. The impressions above and below this point reflect either tumor mass, edema of the minor and major papillae, or smooth muscle spasm and edema in the duodenal wall.

Fine or coarse sharpening and elongation of barium-filled crevices between the duodenal folds (i.e., spiculation) results from mucosal edema and muscular irritation (Fig. 40–32). This appearance can be seen in patients with pancreatitis or pancreatic carcinoma. Displacement or frank splaying of the spikes suggests tumor infiltration of the wall with traction and fixation of folds.

Fold effacement appears as straightening of the upper inner margin of the descending duodenum and flattening of normal interfold crevices, usually with a slight reduc-

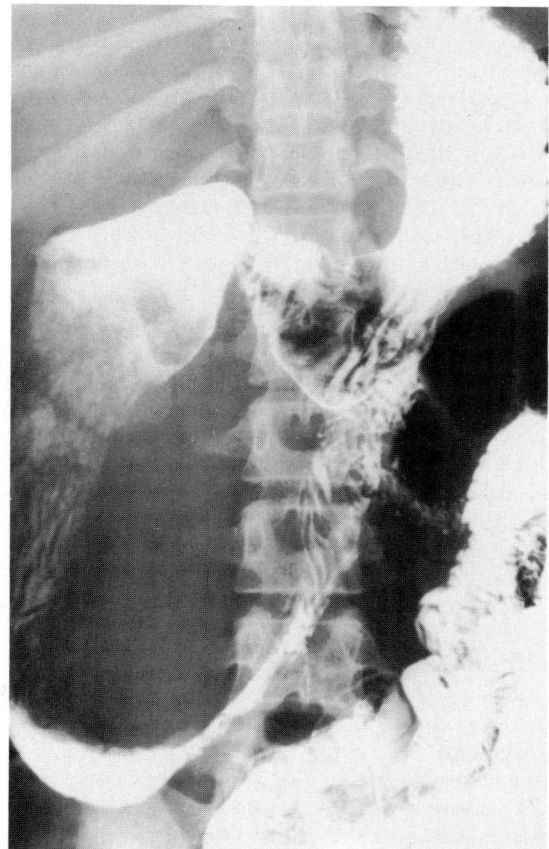

**Figure 40–29. Widening of the duodenal sweep by a choledochal cyst.** (From Eisenberg RL: Gastrointestinal Radiology: A Pattern Approach [2nd ed]. Philadelphia: JB Lippincott, 1990.)

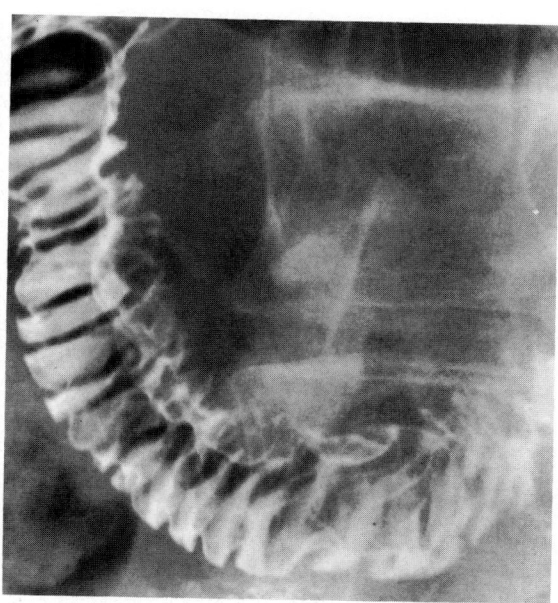

**Figure 40–30. Duodenal involvement by pancreatic carcinoma.** An enlarged pancreatic head produces a double contour on the medial border of the duodenum. (From Eisenberg RL: Gastrointestinal Radiology: A Pattern Approach [2nd ed]. Philadelphia: JB Lippincott, 1990.)

tion in luminal caliber (Fig. 40–33). Although classically attributed to chronic inflammatory change causing fibrosis and rigidity of the duodenal wall, a similar pattern can be seen in patients with pancreatic malignancy.

In advanced disease, duodenal involvement by pancreatitis, pancreatic pseudocysts, or pancreatic carcinoma may be manifested by the development of ulcers, cavities, or even pancreaticoduodenal fistulas. Pancreatitis, pseudocysts, or neoplasms involving the head of the pancreas may be manifested by a smooth area of extrinsic mass effect on the greater curvature of the gastric antrum (i.e., the "antral pad" sign). Further

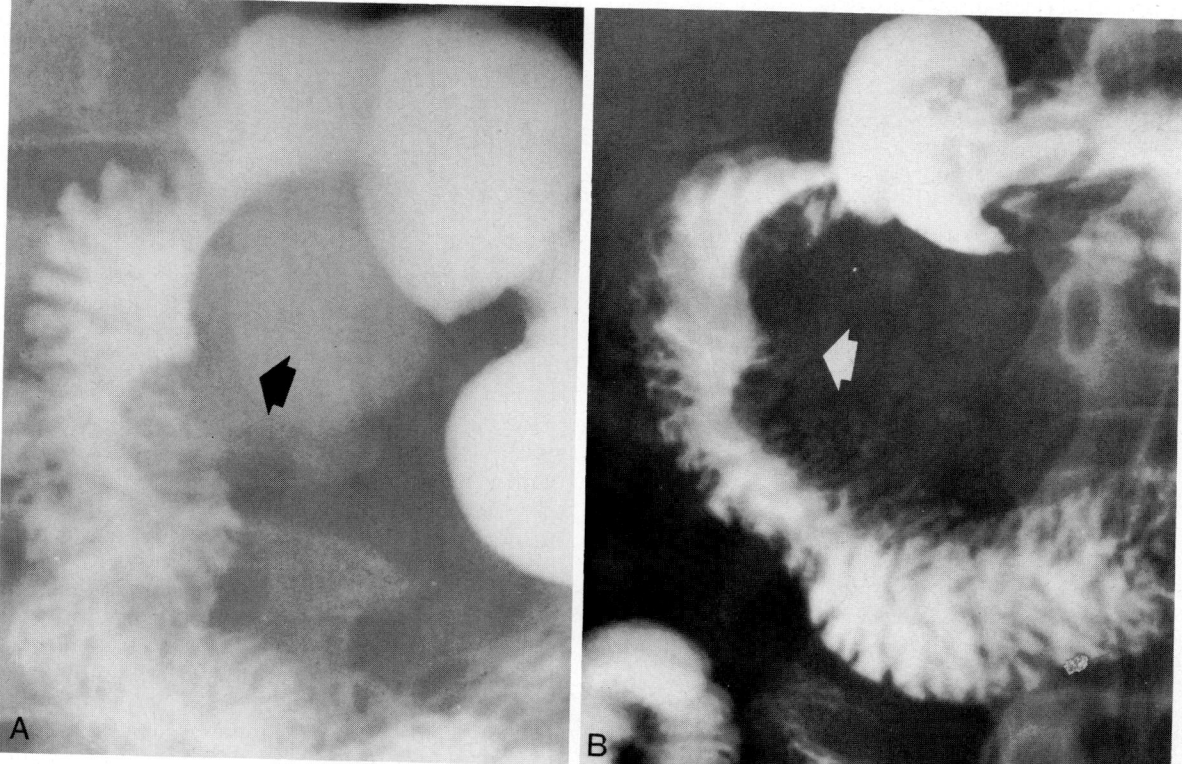

**Figure 40–31. The inverted 3 sign of Frostberg. A** and **B.** Two cases are shown of a widened duodenal sweep with fixation of the duodenal wall at the papilla *(arrows)*, producing the inverted 3 sign. The patient in **A** had pancreatic carcinoma, whereas the patient in **B** had acute pancreatitis, so this sign is nonspecific.

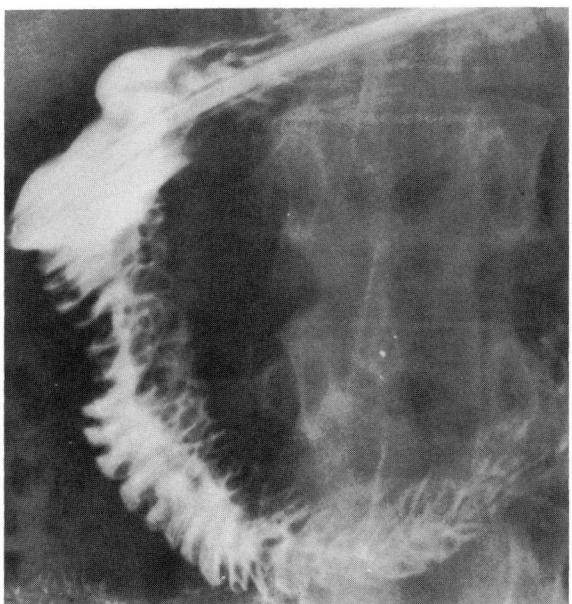

**Figure 40–32. Duodenal involvement by chronic pancreatitis.** There is an extrinsic impression on the medial border of the descending duodenum with associated spiculation of mucosal folds. (From Eisenberg RL: Gastrointestinal Radiology: A Pattern Approach [2nd ed]. Philadelphia: JB Lippincott, 1990.)

infiltration of the stomach by the inflammatory process or tumor may produce an irregular gastric contour with spiculated, tethered mucosal folds on the greater curvature (Fig. 40–34). Similarly, disease involving the

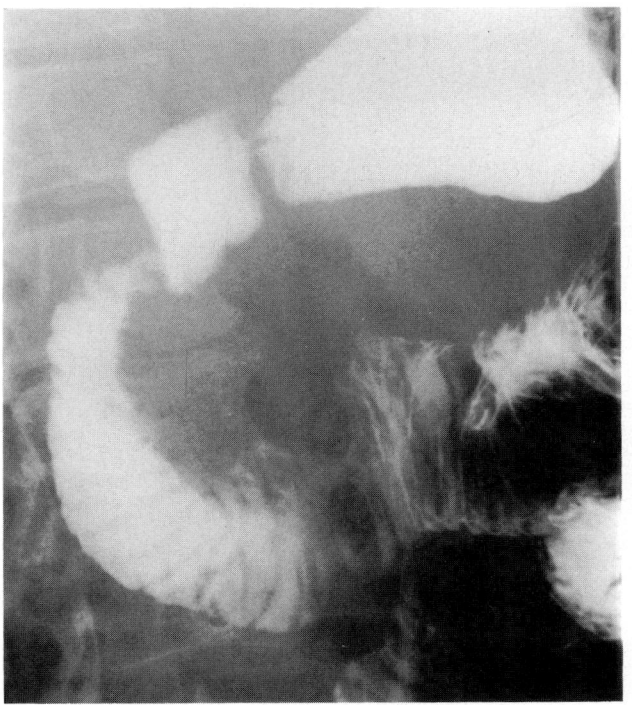

**Figure 40–33. Duodenal involvement by chronic pancreatitis.** There are fold effacement and flattening of the medial border of the second and third portions of the duodenum. (From Eisenberg RL: Gastrointestinal Radiology: A Pattern Approach [2nd ed]. Philadelphia: JB Lippincott, 1990.)

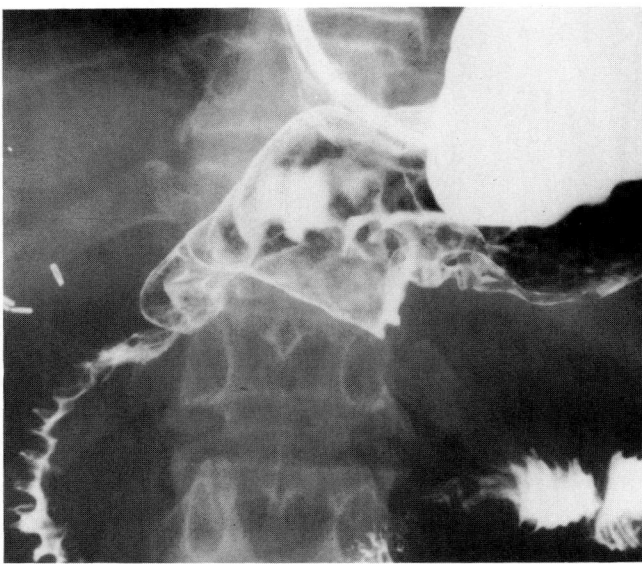

**Figure 40–34. Gastric involvement by pancreatitis.** There are flattening, irregularity, and spiculation of the greater curvature of the antrum due to extension of the inflammatory process to the stomach. Also note involvement of the proximal duodenum. (Courtesy of Marc S. Levine, M.D., Philadelphia, PA.)

body or tail of the pancreas may be manifested by extrinsic compression, flattening, or spiculation of the posterior wall of the gastric fundus or body (Fig. 40–35A and B). When gastric involvement by pancreatic disease is suspected on the basis of barium studies, CT or ultrasound may be performed for a more definitive diagnosis (Fig. 40–35C).

## UNUSUAL FILLING DEFECTS

### Bezoars

A bezoar is an intragastric mass composed of accumulated ingested material. *Phytobezoars,* which are composed of undigested vegetable matter, have classically been associated with the eating of unripe persimmons, a fruit containing substances that coagulate on contact with gastric acid to produce a sticky gelatinous material, which then traps seeds, skin, and other foodstuffs. *Trichobezoars* (composed of hair) occur predominantly in females, especially those with schizophrenia or other mental instability. The accumulated, matted mass of hair can enlarge to occupy the entire lumen of the stomach, often assuming the shape of the organ. A small percentage of bezoars are composed of both hair and vegetable matter and are called *trichophytobezoars.*

Symptoms of gastric bezoars result from the mechanical effects caused by the presence of the foreign body. They include crampy epigastric pain and a sense of dragging, fullness, or heaviness in the upper abdomen. The incidence of associated peptic ulcers is high, especially with the more abrasive phytobezoars. When bezoars are large, symptoms of pyloric obstruction can clinically simulate gastric carcinoma.

Abdominal plain films often show the bezoar as a soft

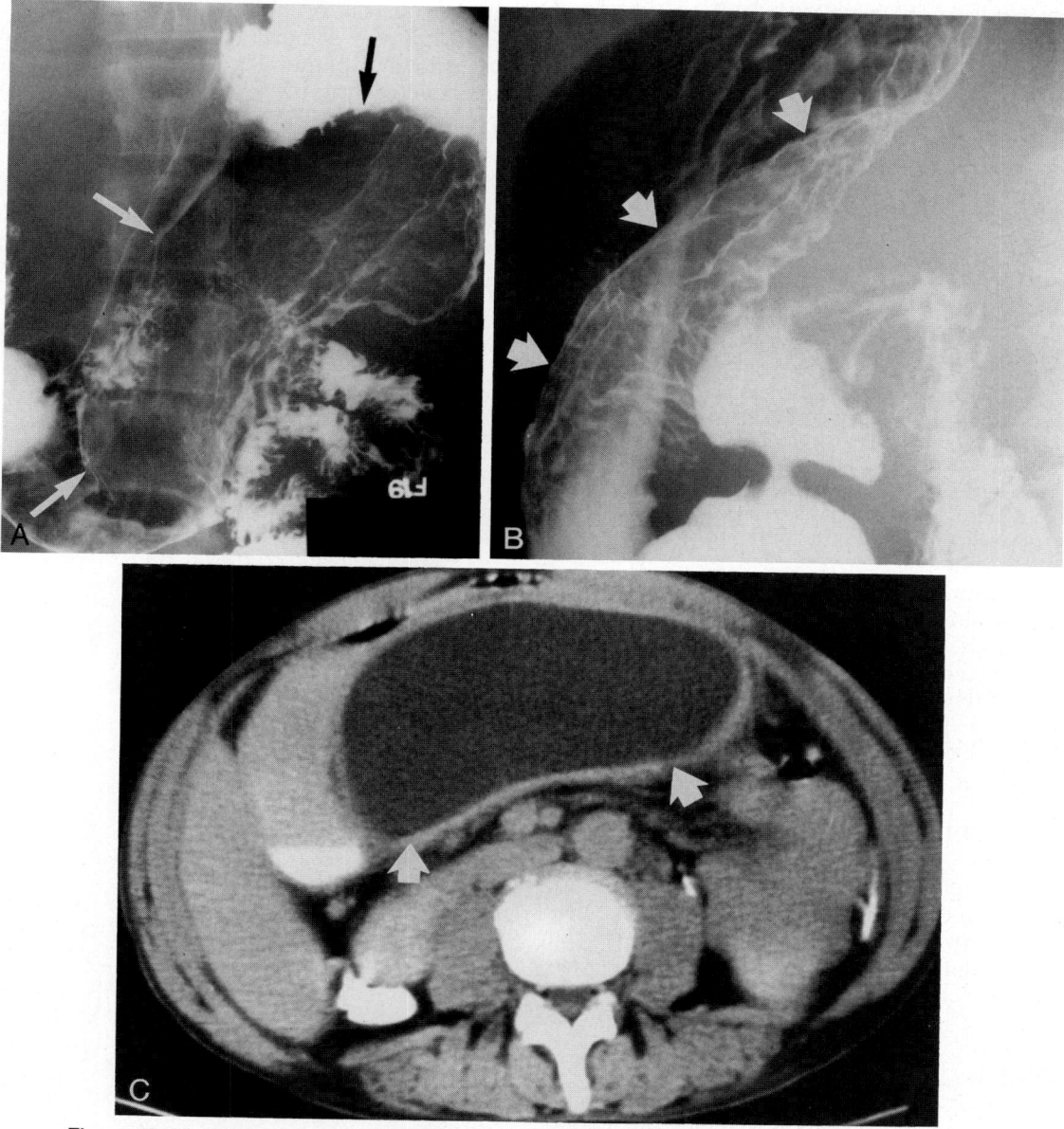

**Figure 40–35. Gastric involvement by a pancreatic pseudocyst. A.** A supine view of the stomach shows a large area of extrinsic mass effect *(arrows)* on the gastric fundus and body. **B.** A lateral view shows the retrogastric mass in profile *(arrows)*. **C.** A CT scan reveals a large pancreatic pseudocyst *(arrows)* compressing and displacing the stomach.

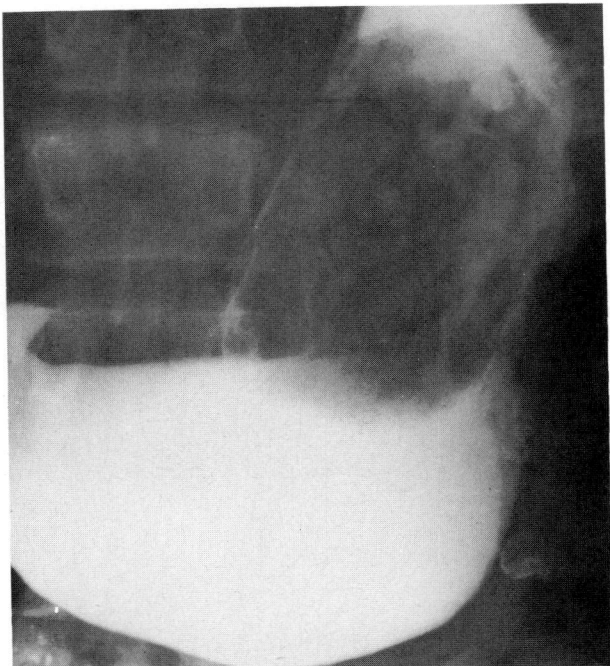

**Figure 40–36. Gastric bezoar.** The bezoar appears as a smooth filling defect in the stomach that could be mistaken for an enormous gas bubble. This patient was a model airplane builder who had been ingesting glue. (From Eisenberg RL: Gastrointestinal Radiology: A Pattern Approach [2nd ed]. Philadelphia: JB Lippincott, 1990.)

tissue mass floating in the stomach at the air-fluid interface. On barium studies, contrast medium entering the interstices of the bezoar may result in a characteristic mottled or streaked appearance. The filling defect is occasionally completely smooth, simulating an enormous gas bubble that is freely movable within the stomach (Fig. 40–36).

## Foreign Bodies

Foreign bodies may appear as radiolucent filling defects in the barium-filled stomach or duodenum. This appearance can be produced by a variety of ingested substances, including food, pills, and nondigestible material.

## Hematomas

In patients with upper gastrointestinal bleeding, blood clots may appear as single or multiple filling defects in the stomach or duodenum. Hemorrhage into the wall of the stomach secondary to a bleeding diathesis, anticoagulant therapy, or trauma can present as a large intramural gastric mass, which most commonly involves the fundus.

Intramural duodenal hematoma is a recognized complication of blunt trauma to the abdomen. More than 80% of reported cases have occurred in children or young adults, and child abuse is a major cause in infants and young children.[36] It is believed that the hematoma results from the bowel's being crushed between the

anterior abdominal wall and the vertebral column. Because the retroperitoneal second and third portions of the duodenum are relatively fixed, these areas are prone to such injury if enough force is applied to the anterior abdominal wall. When the mucosa is separated from the loose submucosa, bleeding leads to dissection along the submucosal compartments. Intramural duodenal hematomas may also be caused by a bleeding diathesis, anticoagulation, or endoscopic trauma.[37]

Intramural duodenal hematomas may appear as circumscribed intramural masses with well-defined margins. Some degree of stenosis and obstruction are usually present (Fig. 40–37A). The right psoas margin can be

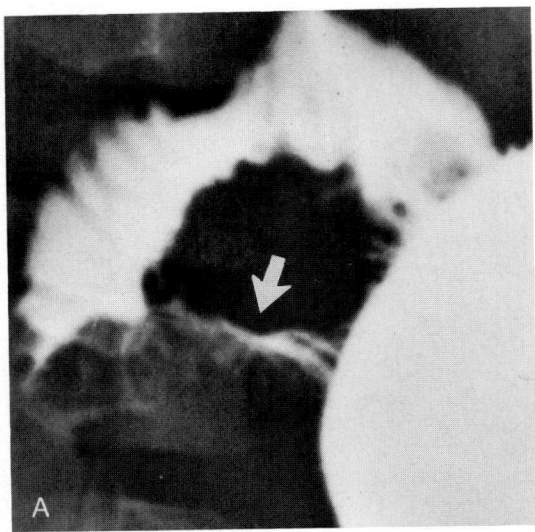

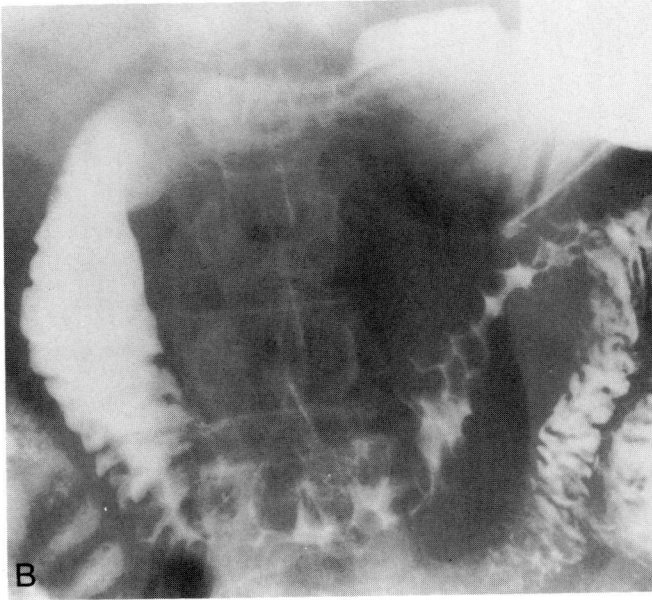

**Figure 40–37. Intramural duodenal hematomas. A.** There is marked narrowing of the distal descending duodenum *(arrow)* due to a large hematoma in a young child who had been kicked in the abdomen by his father. (From Eisenberg RL: Gastrointestinal Radiology: A Pattern Approach [2nd ed]. Philadelphia: JB Lippincott, 1990.) **B.** In another patient who had been undergoing anticoagulant therapy for a prosthetic heart valve, there is thumbprinting of the distal duodenum due to extensive intramural hemorrhage. (Courtesy of Richard L. Baron, M.D., Pittsburgh, PA.)

obliterated because of associated retroperitoneal bleeding. A "coil spring" appearance has been described, and late rupture into the peritoneal or retroperitoneal space may occur. Although some patients have discrete hematomas, others have diffuse hemorrhage in the duodenal wall, manifested by thickened, spiculated folds or thumbprinting (Fig. 40–37B).

## Intragastric and Intraduodenal Gallstones

An extremely rare cause of a filling defect in the stomach is an intragastric gallstone. Gallstones may enter the stomach in patients with cholecystogastric or cholecystoduodenal fistulas. Like other foreign bodies in the stomach, intragastric gallstones may cause mucosal irritation and lead to ulceration, bleeding, perforation, and even gastric outlet obstruction. Erosion of a gallstone into the duodenal bulb may cause gastric outlet obstruction (Bouveret's syndrome), a rare but life-threatening condition.[38]

## GASTRIC VOLVULUS

Gastric volvulus is an uncommon acquired twist of the stomach on itself that can lead to gastric outlet obstruction. It is usually associated with a large esophageal or paraesophageal hernia that permits part or all of the stomach to assume an intrathoracic position. Free upward movement of the stomach is limited by several ligaments that normally anchor the stomach within the abdomen. The most rigid point of attachment is the site at which the second portion of the duodenum assumes a retroperitoneal position and thus becomes fixed to the posterior abdominal wall. The gastrocolic and gastrolienal ligaments also contribute to fixation of the stomach. Because of these points of anatomic fixation, torsion of the stomach may occur with significant degrees of gastric herniation. Gastric volvulus can also be secondary to eventration or paralysis of the diaphragm. Cases of idiopathic gastric volvulus without apparent cause have also been reported.

In small herniations, the proximal portion of the stomach enters the hernia sac first. Obstruction or strangulation almost never occurs at this stage. As herniation progresses, the body and a variable portion of the antrum come to lie above the diaphragm, so that the stomach can become an entirely intrathoracic organ that is prone to a volvulus. *Organoaxial* volvulus refers to rotation of the stomach upward around its long axis (a line connecting the cardia with the pylorus). In this condition, the antrum moves from an inferior to a superior position. In *mesenteroaxial* volvulus, the stomach rotates from right to left or left to right about the long axis of the gastrohepatic omentum (a line connecting the middle of the lesser curvature with the middle of the greater curvature).[39]

Gastric volvulus can be asymptomatic if there is no

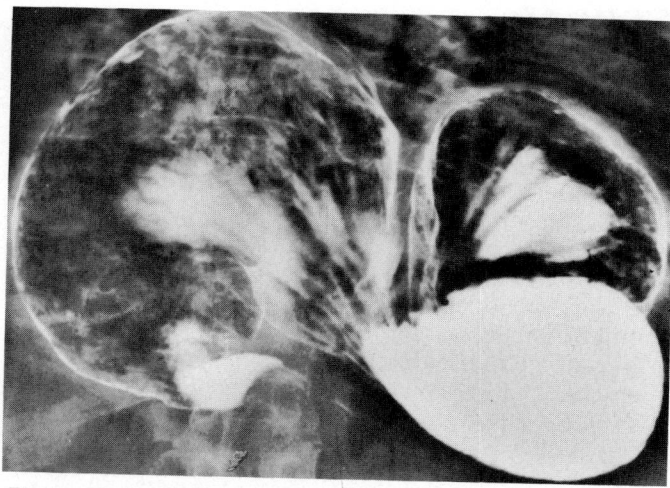

**Figure 40–38. Gastric volvulus.** This patient has an organoaxial volvulus of the stomach causing gastric outlet obstruction. The stomach is located above the diaphragm with inversion of the greater curvature above the lesser curvature and downward pointing of the pylorus. (From Eisenberg RL: Gastrointestinal Radiology: A Pattern Approach [2nd ed]. Philadelphia: JB Lippincott, 1990.)

outlet obstruction or vascular compromise. However, acute volvulus associated with interference with the blood supply is a surgical emergency. The classic clinical triad in this condition consists of violent retching with production of little vomitus, constant severe epigastric pain, and great difficulty in advancing a nasogastric tube beyond the distal esophagus. Vascular occlusion leads to necrosis, shock, and a mortality rate of about 30%.

The radiographic signs of gastric volvulus are characteristic. They include a double air-fluid level on abdominal plain films obtained with the patient upright and inversion of the stomach with the greater curvature above the level of the lesser curvature, positioning of the cardia and pylorus at the same level, and downward pointing of the pylorus and duodenum on contrast studies[40] (Fig. 40–38).

## GASTRODUODENAL AND DUODENOJEJUNAL INTUSSUSCEPTIONS

Gastroduodenal and duodenojejunal intussusceptions are rare entities usually associated with gastric or duodenal tumors that serve as the lead point for the intussusception. In gastroduodenal intussusception, characteristic radiographic signs include foreshortening and narrowing of the distal stomach, converging or telescoping mucosal folds in the distal stomach or duodenum, prepyloric collar-shaped outpouchings, widening of the pyloric channel, a coil spring appearance of duodenal mucosal folds, and widening of the duodenum with an associated filling defect.[41] Similarly, duodenojejunal intussusception produces an intraluminal mass associated with a characteristic coil spring pattern.[42]

# FISTULAS

## Gastrocolic and Duodenocolic Fistulas

Fistulous communications between the stomach and duodenum and other abdominal organs may occur as a complication of benign or malignant disease. Although traditionally gastrocolic fistulas most frequently originated from primary carcinomas of the colon or stomach, the widespread use of aspirin and other nonsteroidal anti-inflammatory drugs that have ulcerogenic properties has made greater curvature gastric ulcers a more common cause of gastrocolic fistula formation than malignancy. As the ulcer penetrates inferiorly, involvement of the gastrocolic ligament permits spread of inflammation to the superior border of the transverse colon, which is almost always the site of the colonic end of the fistula (Fig. 40–39).

Malignant tumors causing gastrocolic (Fig. 40–40) or duodenocolic (Fig. 40–41) fistulas are almost always bulky and infiltrating and are associated with a marked inflammatory reaction. The tumor apparently extends from the serosa of one viscus into the wall of another, followed by lumen-to-lumen necrosis. The presence of growing tumor and fibrous stroma within the wall of a malignant fistula accounts for the length of these tracks and the relative separation of bowel loops.[43]

Malignant gastrocolic fistulas are frequently demonstrated during barium enema examination but are rarely detected on upper gastrointestinal series. This phenomenon is probably related to preferential flow from the colon to the stomach. The higher than usual intraluminal

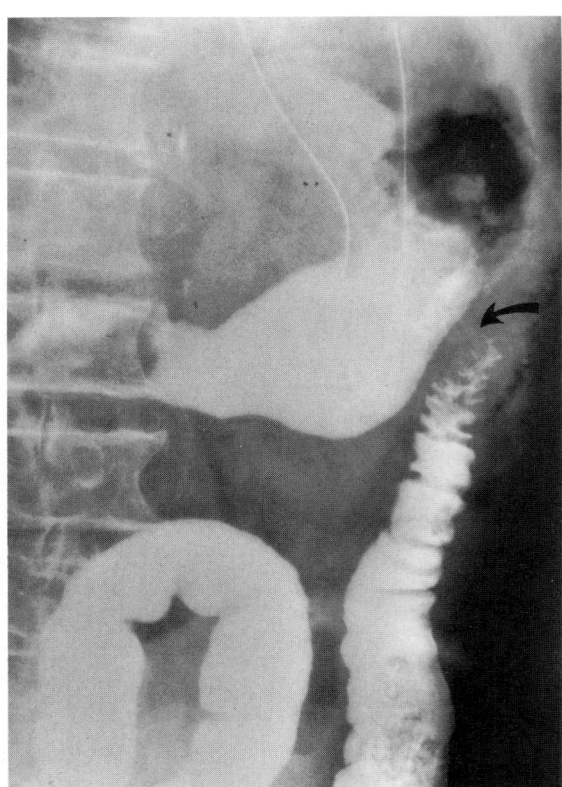

**Figure 40–40. Gastrocolic fistula** *(arrow)* caused by carcinoma of the splenic flexure. (From Eisenberg RL: Gastrointestinal Radiology: A Pattern Approach [2nd ed]. Philadelphia: JB Lippincott, 1990.)

pressure in the colon at the time of a barium enema examination may overcome resistance in the rigid, nondistensible fistula, allowing passage of barium into the stomach. When an upper gastrointestinal series is performed under more physiologic conditions, the intraluminal pressure in the proximal gastrointestinal tract may not be sufficient to overcome this resistance.[44]

A fistulous communication between the stomach, jejunum, and colon (gastrojejunocolic fistula) or directly between the stomach and colon represents a grave complication of marginal ulceration after gastric surgery for peptic ulcer disease[45] (Fig. 40–42). Most patients with this condition have diarrhea and weight loss; pain, vomiting, and bleeding occur in one third to one half of cases. These fistulas may be recognized first during a barium enema examination in which contrast medium is seen to extend directly from the transverse colon into the stomach. These postsurgical fistulas are associated with a high mortality rate, especially if recognized late.

## Cholecystoduodenal Fistulas

Fistulas between the gallbladder and duodenum may be caused by acute cholecystitis (90%) or severe peptic ulcer disease (6%). The remaining cases are caused by trauma or tumor. Acute cholecystitis most commonly results in the development of a cholecystoduodenal fistula, but the inflamed gallbladder can also perforate

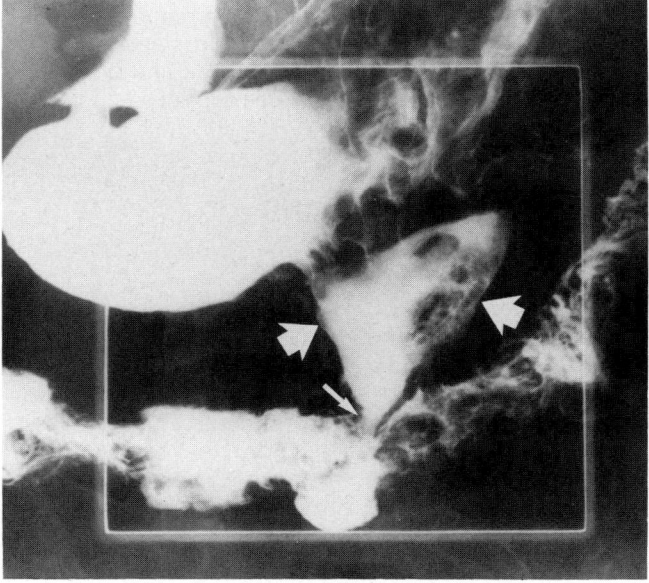

**Figure 40–39. Gastrocolic fistula caused by a benign greater curvature ulcer.** An upper gastrointestinal study shows a giant ulcer *(large arrows)* on the greater curvature of the stomach with barium entering a fistula *(small arrow)* that communicates directly with the transverse colon. (Courtesy of Marc S. Levine, M.D., Philadelphia, PA.)

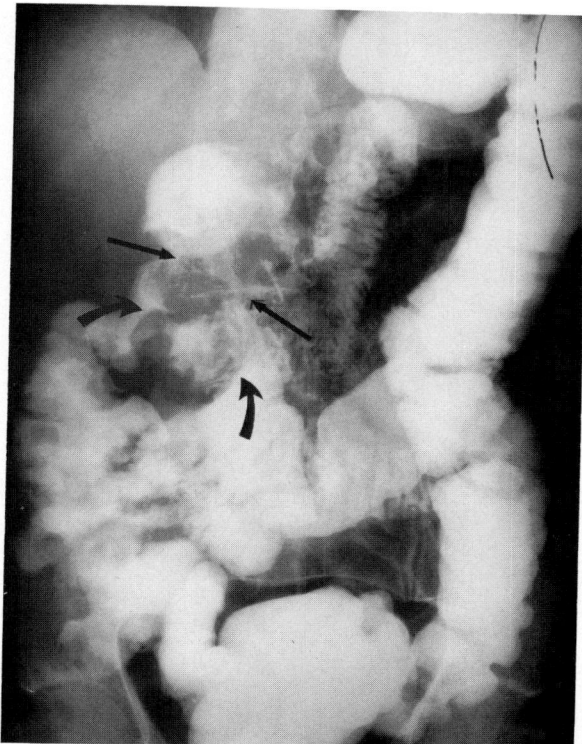

**Figure 40–41. Duodenocolic fistula caused by carcinoma of the proximal transverse colon.** A barium enema examination shows an annular carcinoma *(curved arrows)* of the proximal transverse colon, with barium entering the duodenum via a duodenocolic fistula *(straight arrows)*. (From JO Vieta, R Blanco, GR Valentini: Malignant duodenocolic fistula: report of two cases, each with one or more synchronous gastrointestinal cancers, Dis Colon Rectum, 19, 6, 542–552, 1976, © by American Society of Colon and Rectal Surgeons, Inc.)

the stomach, jejunum, or hepatic flexure of the colon. In patients with severe peptic ulcer disease, a penetrating duodenal or gastric ulcer can perforate the gallbladder or bile duct.[46] Regardless of the etiology, abdominal plain films often demonstrate gas in the biliary tree (see Fig. 35–42). On upper gastrointestinal studies, barium usually fills the cholecystoduodenal fistula.

## Other Fistulas

Aortoduodenal fistulas can occur as a complication of abdominal aortic aneurysms or of prosthetic vascular grafts. Pressure necrosis of the third portion of the duodenum, which is fixed and apposed to the anterior wall of an aortic aneurysm, can lead to digestion of the aortic wall by enteric secretions with the development of an aortoduodenal fistula. Secondary fistulas result from pseudoaneurysm formation with erosion into the adherent duodenum or dehiscence of the suture line caused by infection associated with leakage of intestinal contents through the duodenum, whose blood supply has been compromised at surgery. Aortoduodenal fistula is often a fatal condition, characterized clinically by abdominal pain, gastrointestinal bleeding, and a palpable, pulsatile mass. Barium studies may demonstrate compression or displacement of the third portion of the

duodenum by an extrinsic mass (Fig. 40–43A). On rare occasions, tracking of extraluminal contrast medium along a graft into the paraprosthetic space outlines the wall of the abdominal aorta[47] (Fig. 40–43B).

Fistulas between the duodenum and right kidney rarely develop as a complication of pyelonephritis, particularly tuberculous pyelonephritis. The pathologic mechanism is usually rupture of a perirenal abscess into the duodenum, which is best demonstrated on retrograde pyelography. On rare occasions, a duodenal ulcer may penetrate the tissues surrounding the kidney, producing a duodenorenal fistula.

## GASTRIC AND DUODENAL PERFORATION

The most frequent cause of pneumoperitoneum with peritonitis is perforation of a peptic ulcer, either gastric or, more commonly, duodenal (Fig. 40–44A). However, in about 30% of perforated peptic ulcers, no free intraperitoneal gas can be identified. Thus, failure to demonstrate a pneumoperitoneum is of no value in excluding the possibility of a perforated ulcer. In general, the absence of gas in the stomach and the presence of gas scattered throughout the small and large bowel suggest a gastric perforation as the cause of pneumoperitoneum.

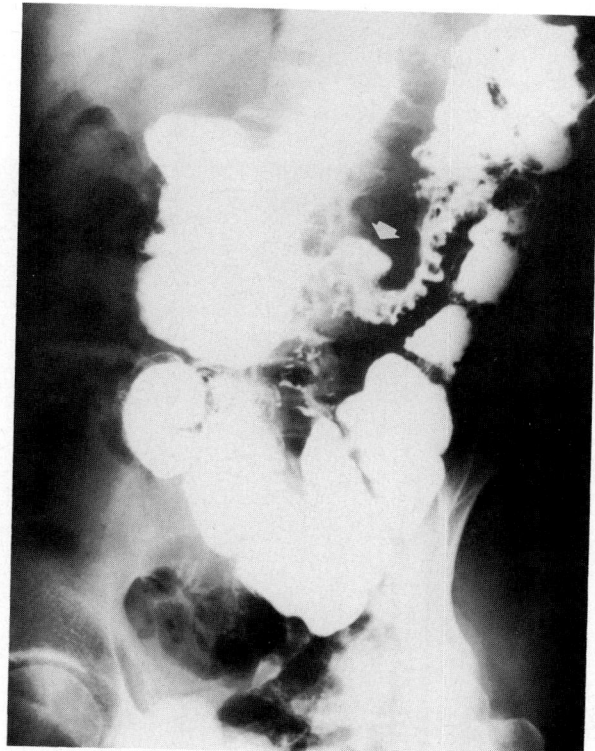

**Figure 40–42. Gastrojejunocolic fistula.** This patient had undergone a partial gastrectomy and gastrojejunostomy. There is a large anastomotic ulcer *(arrow)* at the gastrojejunostomy with filling of the jejunum and transverse colon via a gastrojejunocolic fistula. (From RH Thoeni, JR Hodgson, HH Scudamore, The roentgenologic diagnosis of gastrocolic and gastrojejunocolic fistulas, AJR, 83, 876–881, 1960, © by American Roentgen Ray Society.)

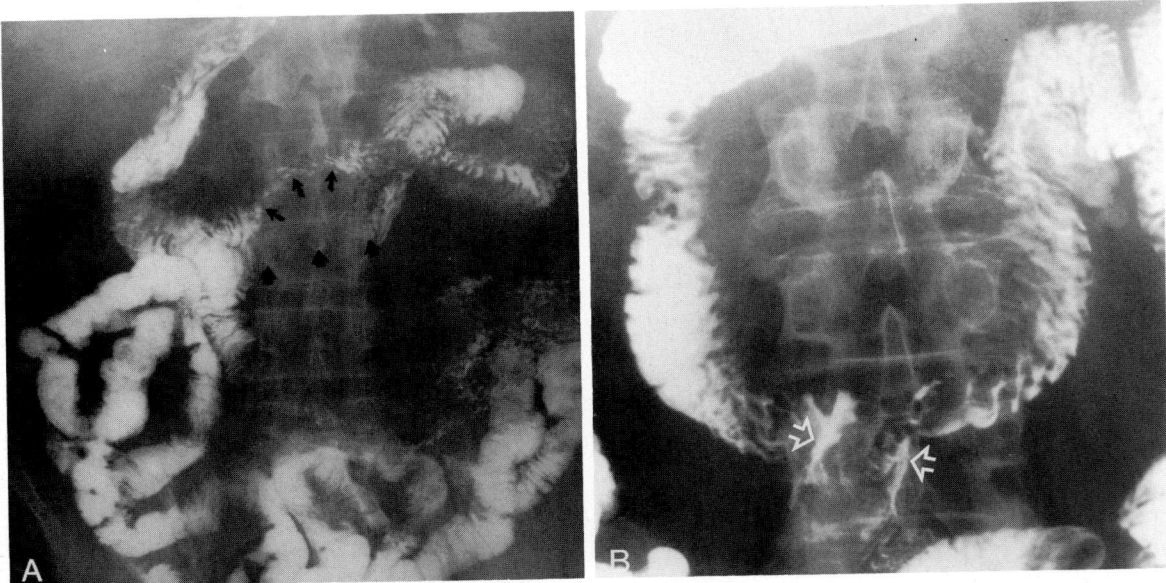

**Figure 40–43. Aortoduodenal fistulas. A.** The fistula causes extrinsic compression of the third portion of the duodenum *(thin arrows)* and displacement of an adjacent loop of jejunum *(thick arrows).* No contrast medium is seen entering the fistula. (From GM Wyatt, MI Rauchway, HB Spitz, Roentgen findings in aorto-enteric fistulae, AJR, 126, 4, 714–722, 1976, © by American Roentgen Ray Society.) **B.** In another patient with an aortic graft, extravasated contrast medium from the distal duodenum is seen tracking between the graft and the aorta *(arrows).* (Courtesy of Marc S. Levine, M.D., Philadelphia, PA.)

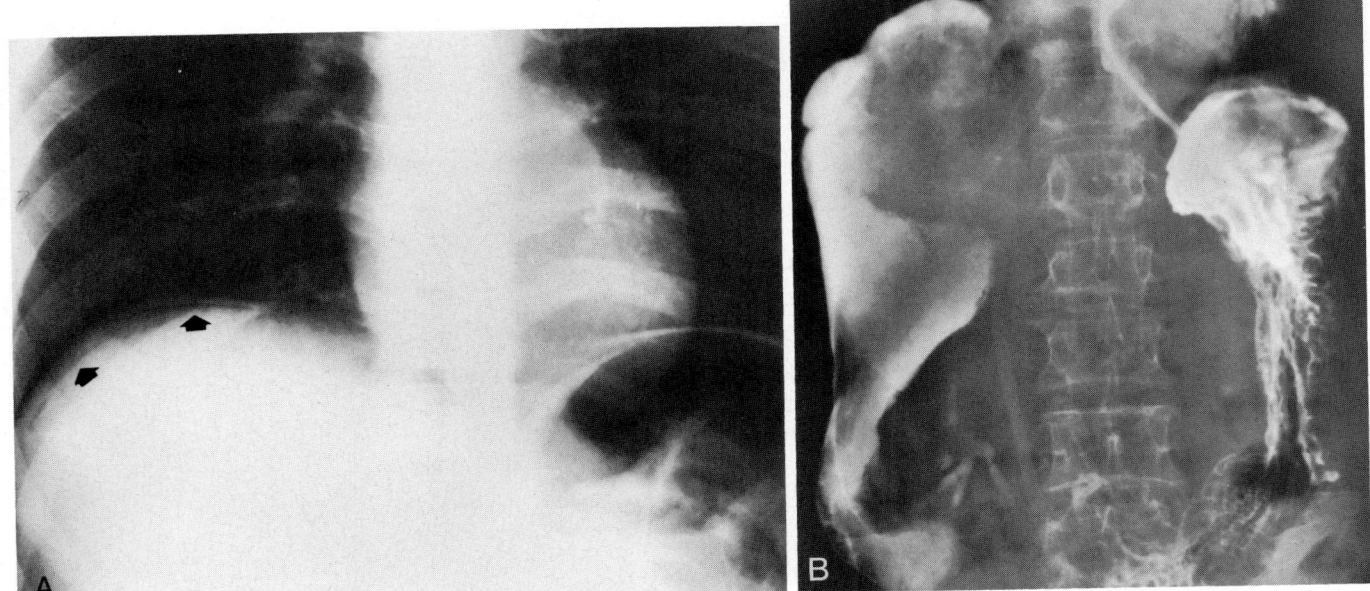

**Figure 40–44. Pneumoperitoneum caused by a perforated duodenal ulcer. A.** Free intraperitoneal air is seen beneath the right hemidiaphragm *(arrows).* **B.** A study using a water-soluble contrast agent shows free extravasation of the contrast agent from the duodenum into the right side of the peritoneal cavity. (From Eisenberg RL: Gastrointestinal Radiology: A Pattern Approach [2nd ed]. Philadelphia: JB Lippincott, 1990.)

Little or no colonic gas in the presence of a gastric air-fluid level and small bowel distention makes a colonic perforation more likely. However, these radiographic findings can be misleading, so a firm diagnosis of the site of perforation requires study with a water-soluble contrast agent[48] (Fig. 40–44B).

## BENIGN GASTRIC EMPHYSEMA

Although usually a sign of infection, ischemia, increased intraluminal pressure, or severe vomiting, gas in the wall of the stomach is occasionally demonstrated in the absence of underlying disease.[49] Pneumatosis intestinalis can affect the wall of the stomach, although far more commonly it involves the small bowel. Nonbacterial gastric emphysema can also result from spontaneous or traumatic rupture of a pulmonary bulla into the areolar tissue surrounding the esophagus. Changes in intrapulmonary pressure force the gas into the upper portion of the esophagus, creating a valve-like mechanism with gradual downward extension of gas into the submucosal or subserosal layers of the gastric wall. When gas is seen radiographically in the wall of the stomach in patients who are asymptomatic, gastric pneumatosis, traumatic emphysema of the stomach secondary to endoscopic perforation, and rupture of a pulmonary bulla into the esophageal wall are the most likely diagnostic possibilities (Fig. 40–45).

## AMYLOIDOSIS

Deposition of the amorphous, eosinophilic, extracellular protein-polysaccharide complex of amyloid in the stomach can produce a broad spectrum of radiographic findings.[50] Amyloid infiltration may cause marked thick-

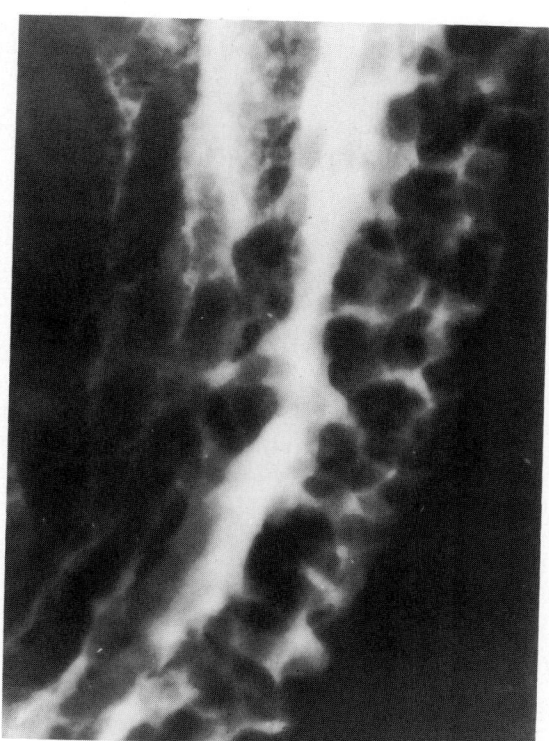

**Figure 40–46. Gastric involvement by amyloidosis.** There are thickened, nodular folds in the stomach due to infiltration of the gastric wall by amyloidosis. (From Eisenberg RL: Gastrointestinal Radiology: A Pattern Approach [2nd ed]. Philadelphia: JB Lippincott, 1990.)

ening and rigidity of the wall of the stomach, especially in the antrum, with luminal narrowing and radiographic findings of linitis plastica. Generalized thickening of gastric folds can also occur (Fig. 40–46). Infrequently,

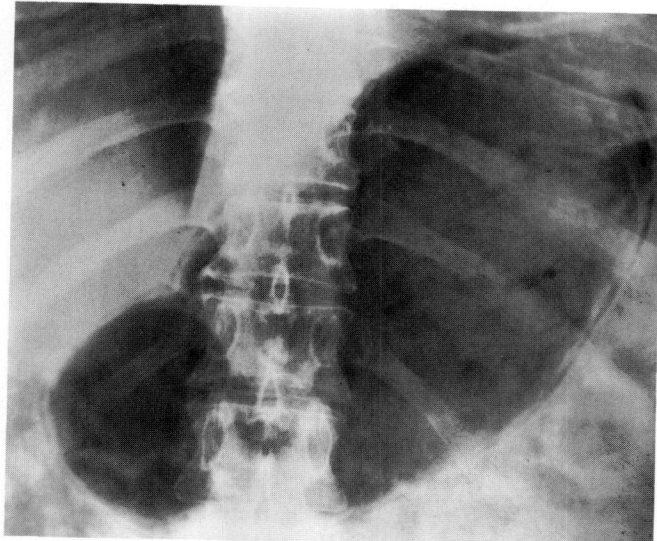

**Figure 40–45. Benign gastric emphysema.** Linear collections of gas are seen in the gastric wall as a complication of endoscopy. (From Eisenberg RL: Gastrointestinal Radiology: A Pattern Approach [2nd ed]. Philadelphia: JB Lippincott, 1990.)

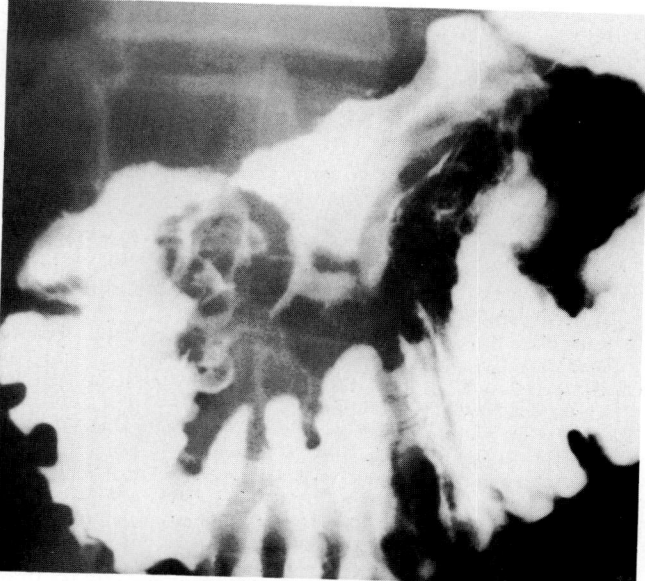

**Figure 40–47. Duodenal involvement by cystic fibrosis.** A thickened, coarse fold pattern is seen in the duodenum in a patient with cystic fibrosis. (From Eisenberg RL: Gastrointestinal Radiology: A Pattern Approach [2nd ed]. Philadelphia: JB Lippincott, 1990.)

localized deposition of amyloid within the wall of the stomach can produce a gastric filling defect that is ulcerated.

## CYSTIC FIBROSIS

A thickened, coarse fold pattern in the duodenum is commonly demonstrated in patients with cystic fibrosis (Fig. 40–47). Associated findings include nodular indentations on the duodenal wall, smudging or poor definition of the mucosal fold pattern, and redundancy, distortion, and kinking of the duodenal contour. These changes are usually confined to the first and second portions of the duodenum, although the thickened fold pattern occasionally extends into the proximal jejunum. The cause of duodenal fold thickening in cystic fibrosis is obscure. It has been postulated that the lack of pancreatic bicarbonate in patients with cystic fibrosis results in inadequate buffering of gastric acid, causing mucosal irritation and muscular contractions that produce the thickened, abnormal mucosal folds.[51]

### Acknowledgment

Figure 40–35A to C is reproduced from Laufer I, Levine MS (eds): Double Contrast Gastrointestinal Radiology (2nd ed). Philadelphia: WB Saunders, 1992.

## References

1. Muhletaler C, Gerlock J, Goncharenko V, et al: Gastric varices secondary to splenic vein occlusion: radiographic diagnosis and clinical significance. Radiology 132:593–598, 1979.
2. Levine MS, Kieu K, Rubesin SE, et al: Isolated gastric varices: splenic vein obstruction or portal hypertension? Gastrointest Radiol 15:188–192, 1990.
3. Sos T, Meyers MA, Baltaxe HA: Nonfundic gastric varices. Radiology 105:579–580, 1972.
4. Bateson EM: Duodenal and antral varices. Br J Radiol 42:744–747, 1969.
5. Treichel J, Gerstenberg E, Palme G, et al: Diagnosis of partial gastric diverticula. Radiology 119:13–18, 1976.
6. Millard JR, Ziter FMH, Slover WP: Giant duodenal diverticula. AJR 121:334–337, 1974.
7. Wolfe RD, Pearl MJ: Acute perforation of duodenal diverticulum with roentgenographic demonstration of localized retroperitoneal emphysema. Radiology 104:301–302, 1972.
8. Nelson JA, Burhenne HJ: Anomalous biliary and pancreatic duct insertion into duodenal diverticula. Radiology 120:49–52, 1976.
9. Loudan JCH, Norton GI: Intraluminal duodenal diverticulum. AJR 90:756–760, 1963.
10. Clements JL, Jinkins JR, Torres WE, et al: Antral mucosal diaphragms in adults. AJR 133:1105–1111, 1979.
11. Bjorgvinsson E, Rudzki C, Lewicki AM: Antral web. Am J Gastroenterol 79:663–665, 1984.
12. Pratt AD: Current concepts of the obstructing duodenal diaphragm. Radiology 100:637–643, 1971.
13. Balthazar EJ: Hypertrophic pyloric stenosis in adults: radiographic features. Am J Gastroenterol 78:449–453, 1983.
14. Dworkin HJ, Roth HP: Pyloric obstruction associated with peptic ulcer. JAMA 180:1007–1010, 1962.
15. Balthazar EJ, Rosenberg H, Davidian MM: Scirrhous carcinoma of the pyloric channel and distal antrum. AJR 134:669–674, 1980.
16. Aranha GV, Prinz RA, Greenlee HB, et al: Gastric outlet and duodenal obstruction from inflammatory pancreatic disease. Arch Surg 119:833–835, 1984.
17. Berk RN, Coulson DB: The body cast syndrome. Radiology 94:303–305, 1970.
18. Wallace RG, Howard WB: Acute superior mesenteric artery syndrome in the severely burned patient. Radiology 94:307–310, 1970.
19. Fischer HW: The big duodenum. AJR 83:861–875, 1960.
20. Simon M, Lerner MA: Duodenal compression by the mesenteric root in acute pancreatitis and in inflammatory conditions of the bowel. Radiology 79:75–81, 1962.
21. Rogers LF, Goldstein HM: Roentgen manifestations of radiation injury to the gastrointestinal tract. Gastrointest Radiol 2:281–291, 1977.
22. Braun P, Collins PP, Ducharme JC: Preduodenal portal vein: a significant entity? Report of two cases and a review of the literature. Can J Surg 17:316–322, 1974.
23. Rimer DG: Gastric retention without mechanical obstruction. Arch Intern Med 117:287–299, 1966.
24. Gramm HF, Reuter K, Costello P: The radiologic manifestations of diabetic gastric neuropathy and its differential diagnosis. Gastrointest Radiol 3:151–155, 1978.
25. Horowitz M, McNeil JD, Maddern GJ, et al: Abnormalities of gastric and esophageal emptying in polymyositis and dermatomyositis. Gastroenterology 90:434–439, 1986.
26. Nowak TV, Ionasescu V, Anuras S: Gastrointestinal manifestations of the muscular dystrophies. Gastroenterology 82:800–810, 1982.
27. Chon H, Arger PH, Miller WT: Displacement of duodenum by an enlarged liver. AJR 119:85–88, 1973.
28. Meyers HI, Jacobson G: Displacements of stomach and duodenum by anomalous lobes of the liver. AJR 79:789–793, 1958.
29. Bluth I, Vitale P: Right renal enlargement causing alterations in the descending duodenum: a radiographic demonstration. Radiology 76:777–784, 1961.
30. Poppel MH: Duodenocolic apposition. AJR 83:851–856, 1960.
31. Treitel H, Meyers MA, Maza V: Changes in the duodenal loop secondary to carcinoma of the hepatic flexure of the colon. Br J Radiol 43:209–213, 1970.
32. Shimkin PM, Pearson KD: Unusual arterial impressions upon the duodenum. Radiology 103:295–297, 1972.
33. Zeman RK, Schiebler M, Clark LR, et al: The clinical and imaging spectrum of pancreaticoduodenal lymph node enlargement. AJR 144:1223–1227, 1985.
34. Leonidas JC, Kopel FB, Danese CA: Mesenteric cysts associated with protein loss in the gastrointestinal tract. AJR 112:150–154, 1971.
35. Frostberg N: Characteristic duodenal deformity in cases of different kinds of perivaterial enlargement of the pancreas. Acta Radiol 19:164–173, 1938.
36. Kleinman PK, Brill PW, Winchester P: Resolving duodenal-jejunal hematoma in abused children. Radiology 160:747–750, 1986.
37. Ghishan FK, Werner M, Vieira P, et al: Intramural duodenal hematoma: an unusual complication of endoscopic small bowel biopsy. Am J Gastroenterol 82:368–370, 1987.
38. Holl J, Sackmann M, Hoffmann R, et al: Shock-wave therapy of gastric outlet syndrome caused by a gallstone. Gastroenterology 97:472–474, 1989.
39. Gerson DE, Lewicki AM: Intrathoracic stomach: When does it obstruct? Radiology 119:257–264, 1976.
40. Scott RL, Felker R, Winer-Muram H, et al: The differential retrocardiac air-fluid level: a sign of intrathoracic gastric volvulus. J Can Assoc Radiol 37:119–121, 1986.
41. Meyers MA: Gastroduodenal intussusception. Am J Med Sci 254:347–355, 1967.
42. Van Beers B, Trigau JP, Pringot J: Duodenojejunal intussusception secondary to duodenal tumors. Gastrointest Radiol 13:24–26, 1988.
43. Smith DL, Dockerty MD, Black BM: Gastrocolic fistulas of malignant origin. Surg Gynecol Obstet 134:829–832, 1972.
44. Martinez LO, Manheimer LH, Casal GL, et al: Malignant fistulae of the gastrointestinal tract. AJR 131:215–218, 1978.
45. Swartz MJ, Paustian FF, Chleborad WJ: Recurrent gastric ulcer with spontaneous gastrojejunal and gastrocolic fistulas. Gastroenterology 44:527–531, 1963.

46. Haff RC, Wise L, Ballinger WF: Biliary-enteric fistulas. Surg Gynecol Obstet 133:84–88, 1971.
47. Wyatt GM, Rauchway MI, Spitz HB: Roentgen findings in aortoenteric fistulae. AJR 126:714–722, 1976.
48. Miller RE: The radiological evaluation of intraperitoneal gas (pneumoperitoneum). Crit Rev Diagn Imaging 4:61–85, 1973.
49. Lee S, Rutledge JN: Gastric emphysema. Am J Gastroenterol 79:899–904, 1984.
50. Carlson HC, Breen JF: Amyloidosis and plasma cell dyscrasias: gastrointestinal involvement. Semin Roentgenol 21:128–138, 1986.
51. Phelan MS, Fine DR, Zentler-Munro L, et al: Radiographic abnormalities of the duodenum in cystic fibrosis. Clin Radiol 34:573–577, 1983.

# Postoperative Stomach and Duodenum

**Claire Smith, M.D.**

## INTRODUCTION

Gastric and duodenal operations are performed to control obesity, resect malignant or benign masses, control complications of ulcer disease, and establish nutritional support. Some 15 to 20% of postsurgical patients present with new or recurrent symptoms related to physiologic, metabolic, or anatomic factors[1, 2] (Table 41–1). A multispecialty team approach is often needed to diagnose and treat these patients. This chapter reviews the range of operations performed on the stomach and duodenum, the spectrum of postoperative complications, available diagnostic tests, and management strategies currently employed.

## TERMINOLOGY

Guidelines describing postoperative changes of the stomach and duodenum have been well established. Radiologic evaluation should include the extent of bowel resection; the type, location, and diameter of the anastomosis; and the speed, direction, and completeness of gastric emptying.[3–5]

Several common eponyms deserve further explanation. The Billroth I procedure (Figs. 41–1 and 41–2) entails partial gastric resection (antrectomy) with gastroduodenostomy. The Billroth II procedure (Fig. 41–3; see Fig. 41–1) involves gastric resection with gastrojejunostomy and either Roux-en-Y or loop-type gastroenteric anastomosis. With the Roux-en-Y anastomosis, the jejunum is divided, the proximal end or side of the small bowel is attached to the stomach, and the distal end of the loop is anastomosed to the side of the distal jejunum (see Fig. 41–1). With a loop-type gastroenterostomy, the stomach is joined to the side of the small bowel. A variable length of duodenum and jejunum forms a proximal or afferent loop, which carries pancreaticobiliary secretions toward the stomach, and a distal or efferent loop, which flows in a downstream direction (see Fig. 41–3). The gastroenterostomy may be anterior to the transverse colon, or the small bowel may be brought up through an opening made in the transverse mesocolon to lie along the posterior wall of the stomach in a retrocolic location. The anastomosis is placed in the dependent portion of the stomach to facilitate gastric emptying.[3, 5]

Further definition of the loop-type configuration describes how the proximal or afferent loop is related to the curvatures of the stomach. In a right-to-left (isoperistaltic) anastomosis (see Fig. 41–3), the proximal loop of small bowel is first attached to the right or lesser curvature portion of the stomach with the distal loop of small bowel on the left or greater curvature area (see Fig. 41–3). A left-to-right (antiperistaltic) anastomosis defines the opposite configuration (see Fig. 41–3B). Choice of configuration depends on the surgeon's preference and the patient's body habitus.

Different terms are used for gastric operations performed for weight control.[6] For gastric stapling operations (Fig. 41–4) without bowel anastomosis, a small proximal gastric pouch and a narrow channel lead to the distal stomach (Fig. 41–5). Gastric bypass operations create a restricted proximal gastric pouch and a narrow anastomosis or channel to the small bowel via the standard loop or Roux-en-Y configuration (Fig. 41–6). The stomach is not resected, but there may or may not be gastric transection between the staple lines.

## DIAGNOSTIC TESTING FOR POSTOPERATIVE COMPLICATIONS

The diagnostic approach to patients with suspected postsurgical complications (Fig. 41–7) depends on the patient's condition, the length of time since surgery, and the type of presenting complaints.[7] The physician directing the examination should gather all pertinent clin-

## TABLE 41–1. COMPLICATIONS OF GASTRIC AND DUODENAL SURGERY

Esophageal dysmotility
    Tissue damage at operation
    After vagotomy
Esophagitis
    Gastroesophageal reflux
    Alkaline reflux
    Alimentary tube use
Gastric emptying problems
    Gastric stasis
    Secondary gastric effects from impaired small bowel motility
    Dumping syndrome
    Generalized bowel ileus
    Bezoar formation
Gastritis and gastric remnant ulcerations
    Technical factors
        Indication for original operation
        Type of operation
        Experience of surgeon
        Adequacy of surgery
        Presence of unabsorbable sutures
    Presence of hypersecretory states
        Incomplete vagotomy
        Gastrinoma with Zollinger-Ellison syndrome
        Antral G cell hyperplasia
        Retained antrum syndrome
        Hyperparathyroidism
    Ulcerogenic substance use
        Cigarette and tobacco products
        Ulcerogenic drugs
    Alkaline reflux
Neoplasm
    Recurrent tumor
    Gastric remnant cancer
Anastomotic leak or bowel perforation
    Abscess
    Fistula
Bowel obstruction
    Narrow anastomotic or channel diameter
        Edema
        Marginal ulcer
        Stricture after ulcer healing
        Prolapse and intussusception
        Bezoar formation
Gastrojejunocolic fistula
Jejunitis
Metabolic effects
    Malabsorption
        Steatorrhea with decreased vitamin D absorption
        Shortened intestinal transit time
        Inadequate mixture of pancreatic juices, bile salts, and food
    Iron deficiency anemia
        Inadequate diet
        Impaired resorption of dietary iron
        Chronic blood loss
    Vitamin $B_{12}$ anemia
        Decrease of gastric intrinsic factor
        Rarely, bacterial overgrowth
    Weight loss and malnutrition
        Insufficient caloric intake
        Incomplete digestion of food
        Inadvertent gastroileostomy
        Diarrhea
Psychologic effects
    Phantom ulcer syndrome
Nutritional support problems
    Intraperitoneal leakage of gastric contents
    Tube malposition, dislodgement, or blockage
    Gastroesophageal reflux and aspiration

Adapted from Smith C, Gardiner R: Postoperative stomach and recurrent abdominal pain. *In* Thompson WM (ed): Common Problems in Gastrointestinal Radiology. Chicago: Year Book Medical Publishers, 1989, pp 202–211.

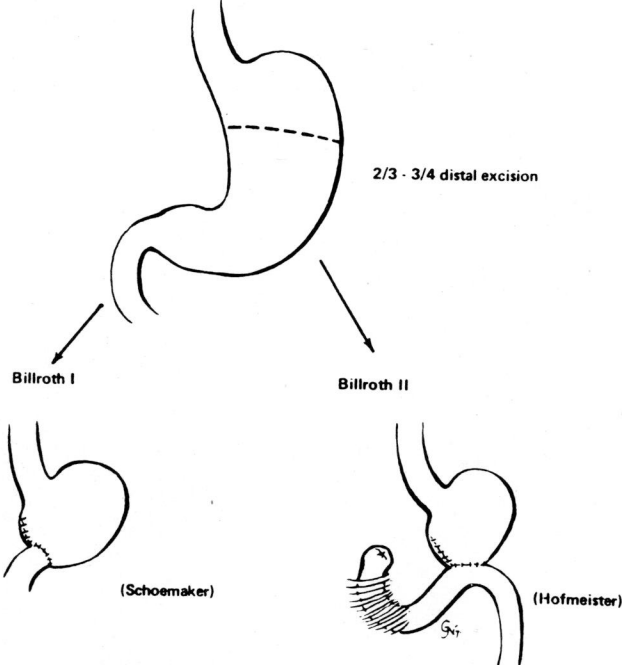

**Figure 41–1. Reconstruction procedures after subtotal gastric resection.** Between 66 and 75% of the distal stomach is resected, excising the antral-gastric mechanism and most of the parietal cell mass. The continuity of the gut is reconstructed with a gastroduodenostomy (a Billroth I) anastomosis or with a gastrojejunostomy (a Billroth II) anastomosis. The Schoemaker and Hofmeister modifications include partial closure of the lesser curvature.

ical details before starting the study to minimize misdiagnosis.[8]

## Contrast Studies

In general, water-soluble contrast agents are used in the immediate postoperative period when anastomotic

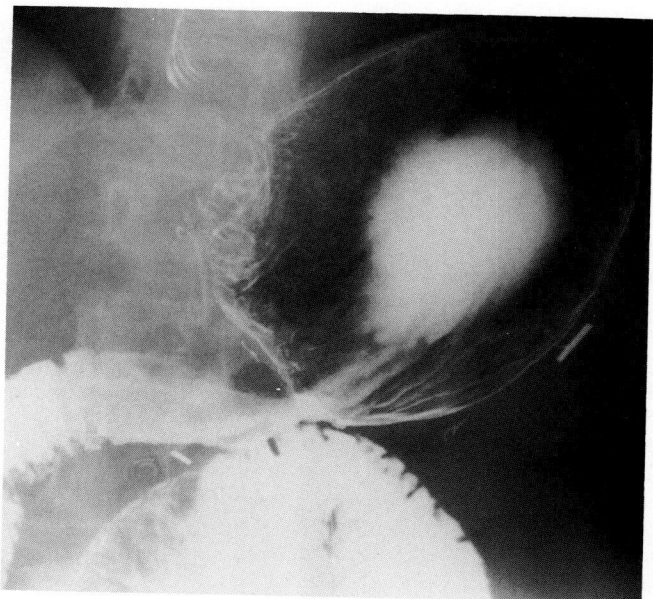

**Figure 41–2. The Billroth I gastroduodenostomy.**

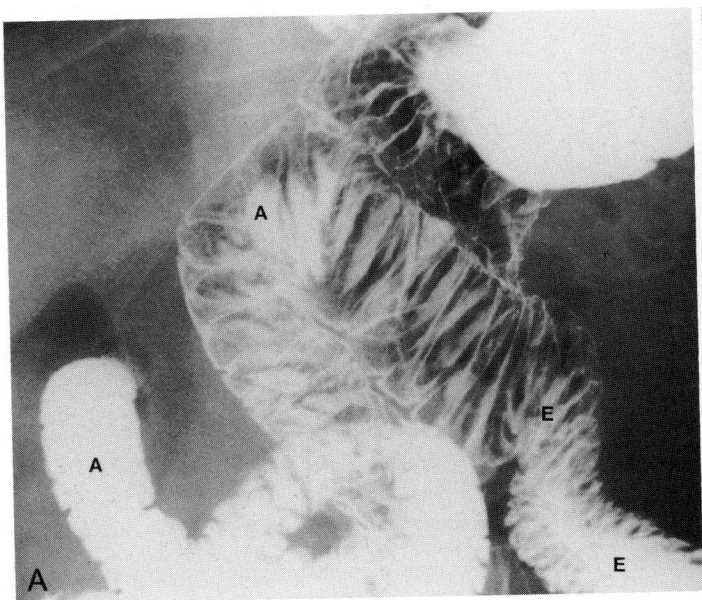

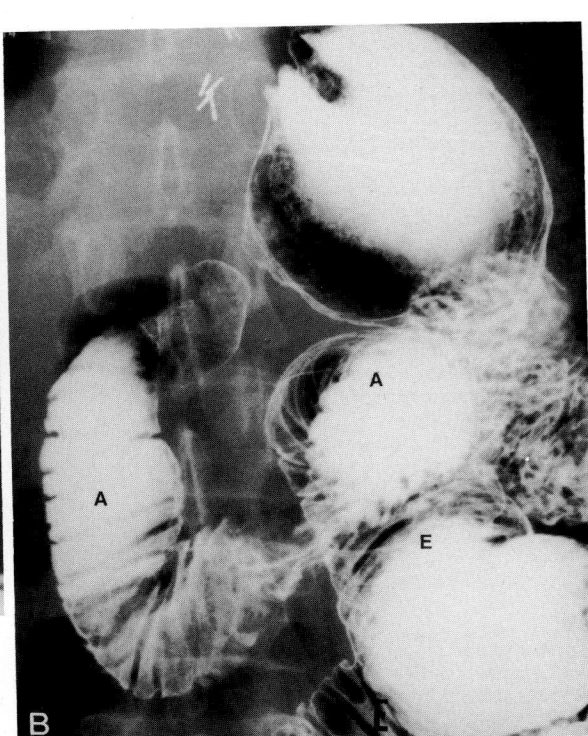

**Figure 41–3. The Billroth II gastrojejunostomy. A.** Isoperistaltic or right-to-left anastomosis. The afferent loop (A) first attaches to the right or lesser curvature portion of the stomach. The efferent loop (E) carries gastric contents more distally. **B.** Antiperistaltic or left-to-right anastomosis. The afferent loop (A) first attaches to the left or greater curvature portion of the stomach. E = efferent loop.

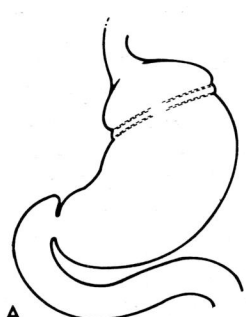

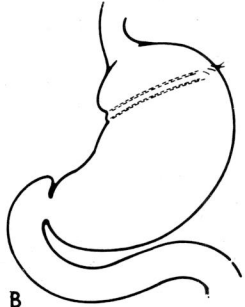

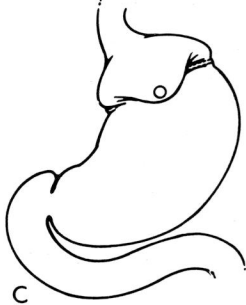

**Figure 41–4. Gastric partition stapling procedures.** These procedures create a small gastric pouch and a narrow channel leading to the distal stomach. **A.** Three central staples are omitted. **B.** Staples along the greater curvature are omitted and the anastomosis is reinforced. **C.** Gastrogastrostomy. Horizontal stapling procedures have a tendency to break down and necrose. (**A** to **C** modified from Pories WJ: Surgery for morbid obesity. *In* Dudley H [ed]: Rob and Smith's Operative Surgery: Alimentary Tract and Abdominal Wall [4th ed]. London: Butterwroth, 1983, pp 316–332.)

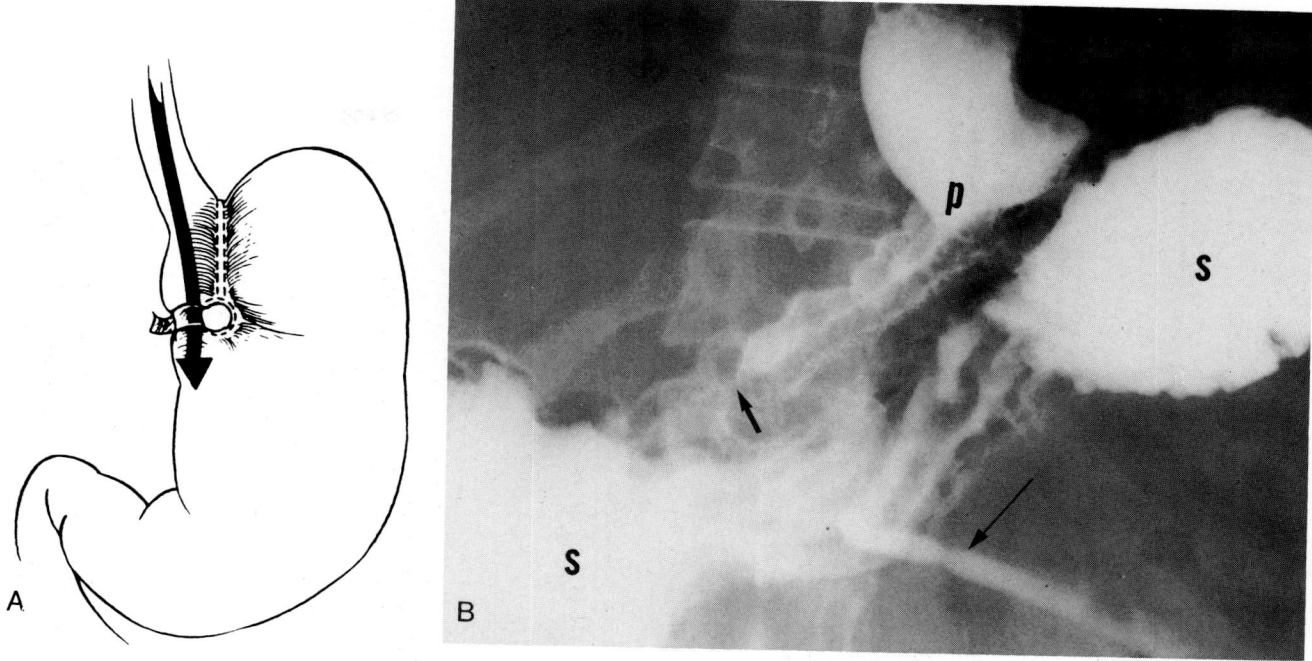

**Figure 41–5. Mason's vertical banded gastroplasty. A.** Diagram depicting the procedure. (Modified from Mason EE: Vertical banded gastroplasty for obesity. Arch Surg 117:701–706, 1982. Copyright 1982, American Medical Association.) **B.** Water-soluble contrast agent demonstrates the proximal gastric pouch (P), the gastric channel *(short arrow)* surrounded by a radiopaque ring, and a gastrostomy tube *(long arrow)* in the distal stomach (S).

leaks, staple line dehiscences, bowel perforations, fistulas, or abscesses are suspected. Plain radiographs must be obtained before all contrast studies. The configuration of surgical staples, clips, and drains helps to determine the type of operation. Foreign bodies or abnormal gas collections may also be found.[5] In morbidly obese patients, fluoroscopic evaluation may be limited or impossible and bowel perforation may be recognized only by seeing surgical drains outlined with contrast material on later films when compared with pre–contrast study radiographs.[6]

Barium studies provide a reliable overview of anatomic alterations not achievable by endoscopic means. Choice of single or double contrast techniques depends on clinical circumstances and the physician's preference. Single contrast examinations are helpful for detecting fistulas, evaluating the rate and direction of liquid flow, and examining debilitated patients who are unable to change position rapidly.[8] Essentials of single column techniques are careful fluoroscopic tracking of contrast material, palpation, and mucosal relief films.

Double contrast techniques afford an excellent view of mucosal detail without the need for extensive palpation.[9] The patient's cooperation is more critical for these studies. Because each patient is unique and surgical variations are numerous, protocols for position changes and film sequences are not readily established. The fluoroscopist must maintain a careful balance between mucosal coating and egress of barium and gas through the anastomosis. This is facilitated by use of glucagon, initial administration of only small amounts of barium, prompt positioning of the patient, and timely elevation

and lowering of the table. Esophageal motility can be evaluated and compression films of the anastomosis obtained by using the same low-density contrast agents as employed in routine biphasic upper gastrointestinal studies.[2, 8–12]

For obese patients whose gastric restrictive procedures have not resulted in weight loss, examination methods must also be altered.[2, 13, 14] Because fluoroscopic evaluation is limited, the first swallow of contrast material must be promptly filmed with the patient in the proper position. This position is determined by staple line geometry demonstrated on the preliminary abdominal radiograph[13] (Table 41–2). Contrast material should be administered slowly to prevent overdistention of the small proximal gastric pouch and vomiting. In patients with gastric bypass procedures, the channel and small bowel loops can be examined reliably but the distal stomach is more difficult to evaluate. Fluoroscopically guided percutaneous injection of contrast material directly into the distal stomach has been used.[14, 15] Endoscopy of the distal stomach using a pediatric colonoscope is the preferred route, particularly in perioperative patients. It is successful in at least 70% of patients after gastric bypass.[16]

Limitations of contrast studies in patients with prior gastric or duodenal surgery include apparent masses caused by postsurgical plication defects, contrast material trapped within deformed perianastomotic folds simulating recurrent ulcers, and edema or suture granulomas mimicking gastric neoplasm[8] (Fig. 41–8). Alternatively, ulcers or masses may be thought to be postsurgical deformities. Also, early mucosal changes of

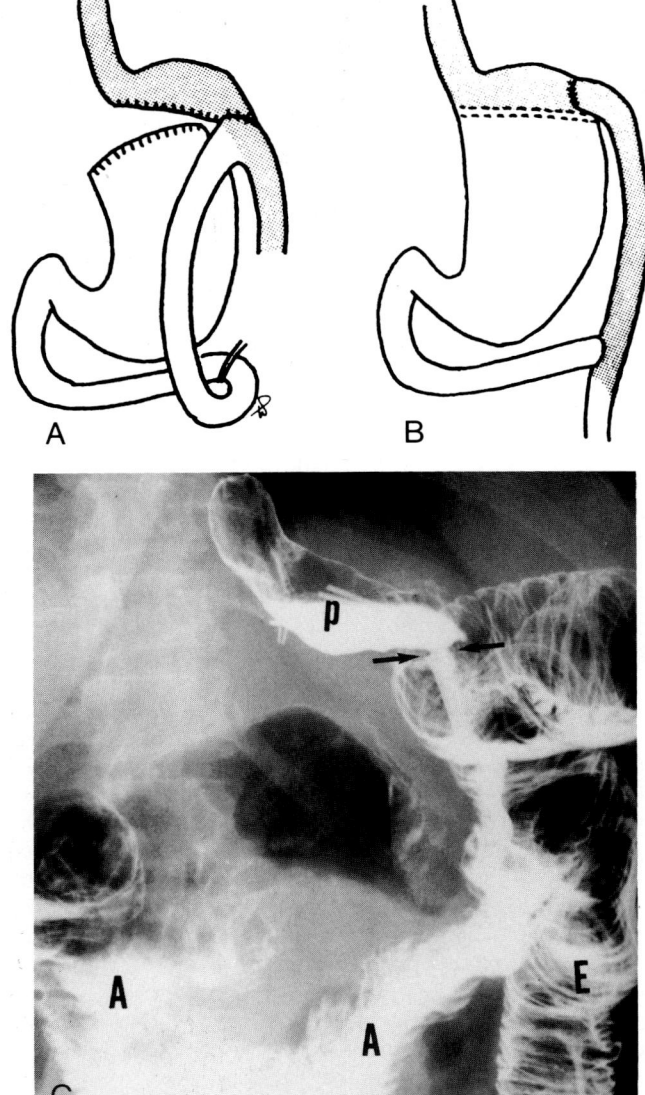

**Figure 41–6. Gastric bypass procedures. A.** Mason's first gastric bypass operation involved gastric transection to form a small pouch, which was anastomosed with a loop of jejunum. **B.** In the current version of this procedure, the stomach is first stapled rather than transected. A Roux-en-Y anastomosis provides intestinal continuity. **C.** The small proximal gastric pouch (P) empties into the small bowel via a narrow channel *(arrows)*. The afferent loop (A) is filled with barium and gas from the effervescent granules administered for this biphasic examination. Gas fills the distal stomach, which has been transected from the proximal gastric pouch. (**C** from Smith C, Gardiner R: Post-operative stomach and recurrent abdominal pain. *In* Thompson WM [ed]: Common Problems in Gastrointestinal Radiology. Chicago: Year Book Medical Publishers, 1989, pp 202–211.)

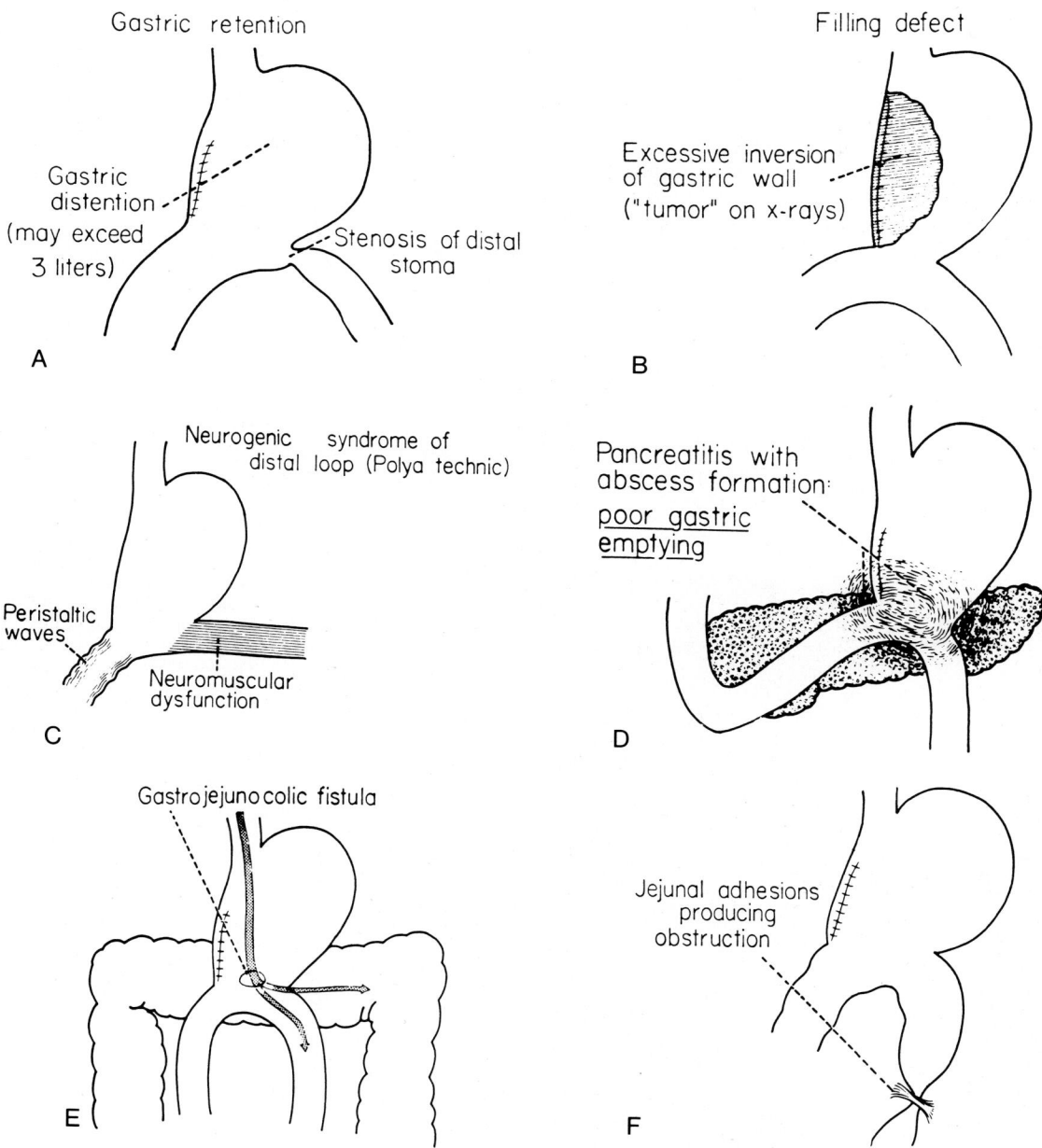

**Figure 41–7. Complications of gastric surgery. A.** Gastric retention. **B.** Inversion of an excessive amount of stomach along the lesser curvature may cause a filling defect on barium studies. **C.** "Neurogenic" syndrome of the distal loop is more common after the Polya than the Hofmeister modification of the Billroth II type of gastric resection. **D.** Postoperative pancreatitis can interfere with gastric emptying. **E.** Gastrojejunocolic fistula. **F.** Fibrous adhesions are an important cause of postoperative alimentary dysfunction.

*Illustration continued on following page*

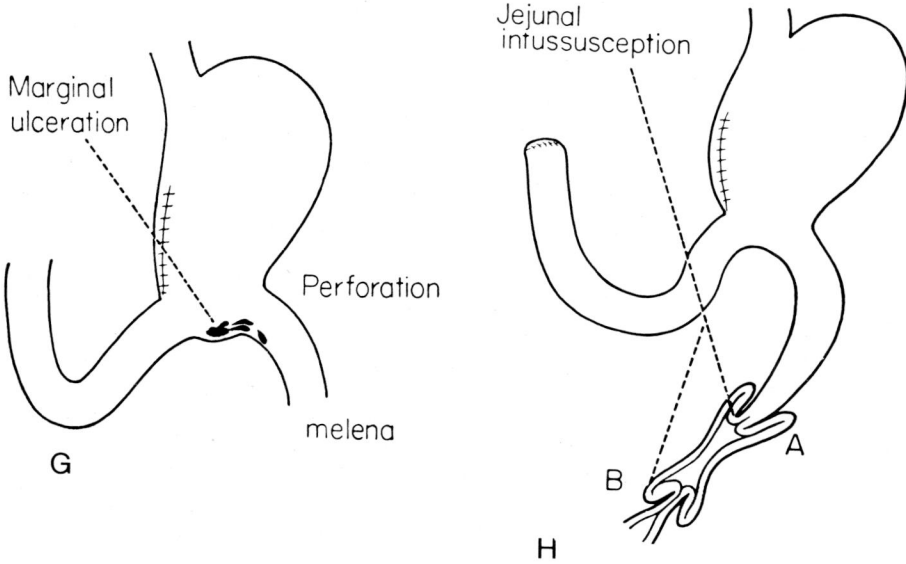

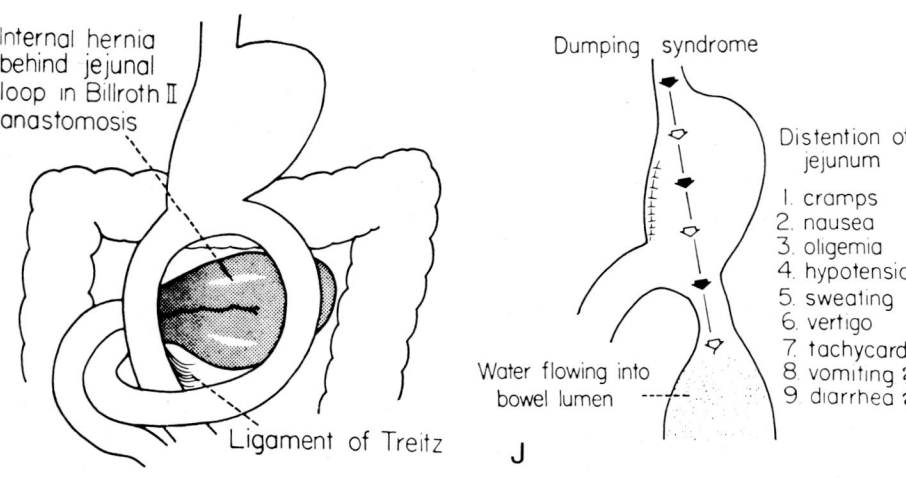

**Figure 41–7** *Continued.* **G.** Marginal ulceration most often develops slightly distal to the stoma. **H.** Jejunal intussusception may also involve the afferent loop with forward intussusception into the stomach or the distal loop with retrograde intussusception into the stomach. **I.** Internal herniation of a jejunal loop. **J.** The dumping syndrome is due to the rapid entrance of food into the small bowel, which causes fluid to enter the gut, resulting in intestinal distention and a reduction of plasma volume.

**TABLE 41–2. STAPLE LINE GEOMETRY PREDICTS OPTIMAL INITIAL EXAMINATION POSITION**

| Staple Geometry | Probable Surgery | Optimal Initial Position |
|---|---|---|
| Vertical | Gastroplasty, lesser curvature channel | Right posterior oblique |
| Horizontal | Gastroplasty, greater curvature channel | Left posterior oblique |
| Mixed or confusing | Gastric bypass | Left posterior oblique |
| | Revision operation | |
| | Unknown anatomy | Left posterior oblique |
| | Vertical gastroplasty | Right posterior oblique |

From Smith C, Gardiner R, Kubicka RA, et al: Gastric restrictive surgery for obesity: early evaluation. Radiology 153:321–327, 1984.

metaplasia associated with alkaline reflux usually escape radiologic detection.[9, 17] Lastly, some anatomic configurations preclude adequate contrast examination despite meticulous fluoroscopic technique.

## Ultrasound

In the immediate postoperative period, ultrasound is usually limited by surgical wounds and bowel gas. For obese patients, technical limitations are amplified. When these limitations are no longer present, the advantages of real-time sonography include multiplanar sections, nonionizing radiation, and little need for preparation, cooperation, or movement of the patient.

## Computed Tomography

Oral, rectal, and intravenous contrast agents are needed to evaluate the postoperative patient.[18] If pa-

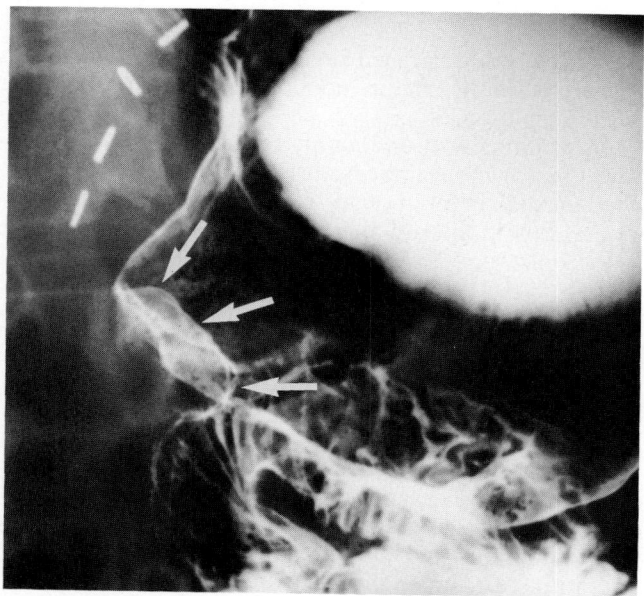

**Figure 41–8. Perianastomotic deformity.** Arrows outline a persistent mass in the stomach near the anastomosis in this patient, who has had a right-to-left loop type of gastrojejunostomy (the Billroth II procedure) for ulcer disease. This mass was secondary to operative deformity.

tients are too ill to drink, contrast agents should be injected via alimentary tubes. In patients who have had gastric bypass procedures for weight control or in patients with long Roux-en-Y or afferent loops, computed tomography may be helpful in evaluating these portions of the gut.[19]

## Nuclear Medicine

Scintigraphic emptying studies are useful for patients with suspected postgastrectomy stasis syndromes, afferent loop dysfunction, motility problems of dumping and diarrhea, and postoperative symptoms of unclear etiology. The tests are easily performed with radiolabeled solids and liquids and can detect and quantitate subtle abnormalities of gastric emptying[20, 21] (Fig. 41–9).

## Magnetic Resonance Imaging

Magnetic resonance imaging of the alimentary tract provides multiplanar images with excellent contrast resolution without the use of intravenous materials or ionizing radiation.[22] Inherent disadvantages include motion of respiration or peristalsis and the isointensity of bowel contents and adjacent organs. In the future, shorter scanning times and better oral contrast materials may overcome these limitations.

## Endoscopy

Endoscopy of the postoperative stomach and duodenum is an excellent diagnostic tool. It is useful in the detection of immediate postoperative problems and the diagnosis and treatment of some chronic complications. Although anatomic arrangements with long Roux-en-Y loops or gastric bypass procedures make endoscopy difficult, significant unexpected pathologic alterations can be detected.[23] In patients with less complicated postoperative anastomoses, experienced endoscopists are able to differentiate precisely between significant perianastomotic disease and normal postoperative deformities.[24]

Endoscopy is needed to define the mucosal changes related to gastritis (Fig. 41–10). Because alkaline reflux is the most common cause of postoperative dyspepsia

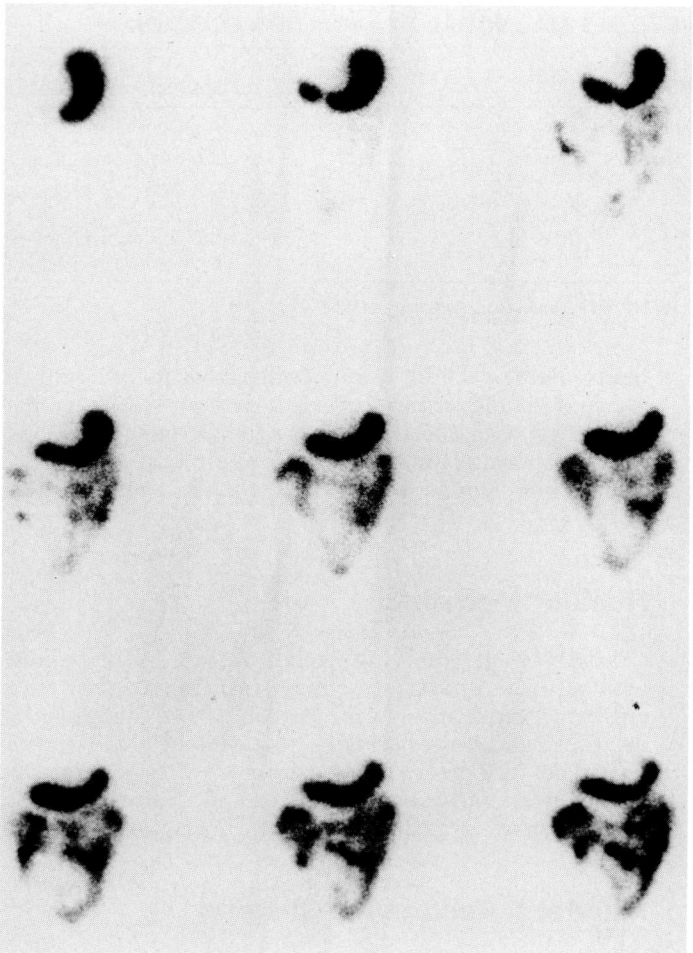

**Figure 41–9. Radionuclide gastric emptying: solid phase.** Serial images of the abdomen obtained at 15-minute intervals for up to 2 hours demonstrate normal emptying of the stomach with greater than 60% of the administered radioactive meal emptied at 2 hours.

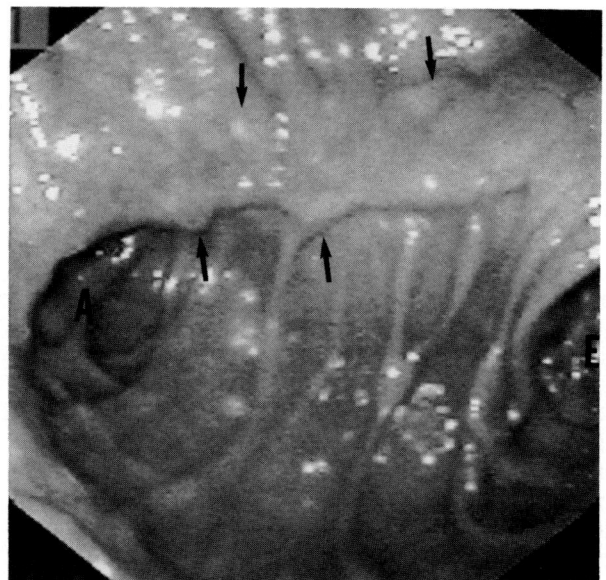

**Figure 41–10. Endoscopic evaluation of a Billroth II gastrojejunostomy.** Afferent (A) and efferent (E) lumina are well seen. Gastric nodularity *(arrows)* adjacent to the anastomosis indicates gastritis.

and may require surgical revision, accurate detection is crucial. Barium examinations do not reliably provide this information.[24–26]

Disadvantages of endoscopy include the possibility of bowel perforation, increased risk in patients with diminished cardiac or pulmonary reserves, and technical factors related to altered anatomy and the expertise of the endoscopist.

## DISEASES AND THEIR OPERATIONS

### Weight Control Surgery

Morbid obesity is associated with excess mortality and a number of therapeutic measures have been developed.[27] Although dietary and behavioral therapy and gastric balloons and bubbles are available, present-day operations are more effective in reducing excess body weight in the morbidly obese patient.[28]

Current gastric operations for weight control create a small gastric pouch with restricted egress, causing early satiety, decreased caloric intake, and weight loss.[29] Many different configurations of the proximal gastric pouch, channel, and distal stomach or small bowel have been devised. Gastrogastrostomies and horizontal stapling procedures performed in the early years have been replaced by other techniques, but there are still patients with intact configurations created by surgical procedures used during the development of bariatric surgery.[14]

## Vertical Banded Gastroplasty

At present, many surgeons prefer vertical stapling.[29, 30] In the vertical banded gastroplasty, the small volume tubular gastric pouch and narrow channel are formed on the lesser curvature side of the stomach. The channel is usually reinforced by an opaque ring or a nonopaque mesh band (see Fig. 41–5).[29]

## Gastric Bypass

In gastric bypass operations, a small proximal gastric pouch is anastomosed to the jejunum via a narrow channel in a standard loop or Roux-en-Y configuration (see Fig. 41–6). The distal stomach is intact but functionally separate from the food pathway.

## Complications of Operations for Weight Control (see Table 41–1)

Gastric physiology is not significantly altered in gastric stapling procedures, and the channel between the stomach and small bowel is narrow in gastric bypass procedures, so physiologic and metabolic complications are rare. Mechanical problems, however, are fairly frequent.

### Outlet Obstruction

Outlet obstruction is not uncommon in the early postoperative period.[30] Vomiting must be controlled because regurgitation can stress the staple lines and cause dehiscence or gastric perforation. Early outlet problems are usually due to edema and symptoms resolve with supportive measures.

Chronic problems appear when the channel lumen is less than 6 to 8 mm wide. The stenosis occurs more than 6 weeks after surgery. Because weight loss is dramatic, patients often do not seek prompt follow-up. Patients return because of symptoms resulting from gastroesophageal reflux or because of accumulation of debris in the proximal gastric pouch (Fig. 41–11). Techniques of balloon dilatation of channel stenoses now provide effective alternatives to reoperation.[31]

### Anastomotic Leak and Abscess Formation

All gastrointestinal operations are associated with a risk of postoperative abscess and anastomotic leak.[7] These risks are greater in morbidly obese patients.[32, 33] If the leakage and abscess are contained, percutaneous abscess drainage with imaging guidance can often spare the patient a second operation.[34]

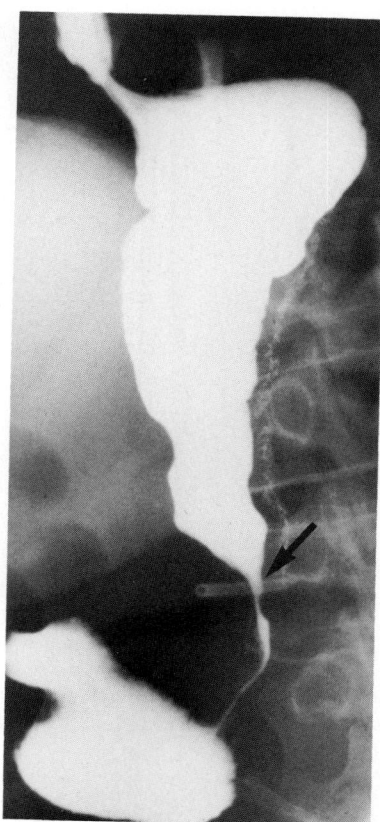

**Figure 41–11. Channel stenosis after vertical banded gastroplasty.** This patient presented with recurrent chest pain. There is severe outlet obstruction at the channel *(arrow)* with overdistention of the proximal gastric pouch and gastroesophageal reflux.

### Staple Line Dehiscence

Because gastric restrictive operations are designed to reduce gastric capacity, the integrity of the staple lines is important. Dehiscence of the staples allows gastric contents to exit through both the surgically created narrow channel and the area of staple line separation (Fig. 41–12).

### Pouch Perforation

Perforation of the proximal gastric pouch may be secondary to ischemia, hyperacidity, or erosion by enteric tubes.[6] In patients who have had gastric bypass, distal stomach perforations can occur as frequently as proximal pouch leakages. If a gastrostomy tube is present, direct injection of contrast material allows easy examination of the distal stomach. Otherwise, percutaneous injection of contrast agents or endoscopy may be attempted.[15, 16]

### Ulcerations

Stress ulcers, suture line ulcerations, and ulcerations at the channel can also occur.[30, 35] Gastritis in the excluded portion of the stomach develops in many patients after gastric bypass surgery.

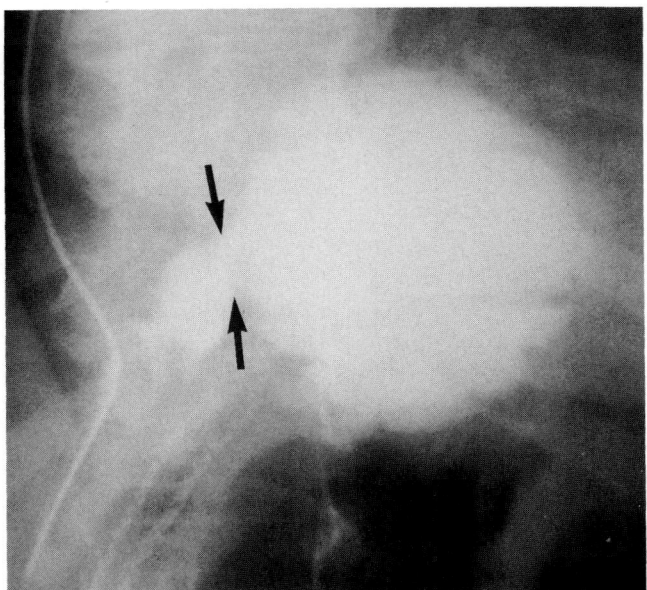

**Figure 41–12. Staple line dehiscence.** Perioperative examination shows contrast medium exiting the proximal pouch through an area of staple line dehiscence *(arrows)* into the gastric fundus. Contrast medium does not outline the nasogastric tube, which is in the proximal pouch just above the channel.

## Surgery for Gastric Cancer and Gastric Masses

Gastric cancer can be cured only if it is found and resected (Fig. 41–13) in its early stages. Before the widespread use of double contrast radiography and endoscopy, less than 5% of gastric cancers were removed in the early stages.[36] Currently, more than 15% of all gastric cancers are either stage I or stage II with a 3-year survival of about 85%.[36] If curative surgery is planned, adequate node dissection includes removing nodes in at least one nodal group remote from the site where the cancer originated. Even with resection for cure, the 5-year survival is 25%[37, 38] (Fig. 41–14).

In patients with unresectable tumor, palliation by laser therapy is useful in relieving outlet obstruction. After palliation, however, 5-year survivors are unusual.[37]

Other benign or malignant gastric or duodenal masses may require surgical removal to alleviate symptoms. After resection, anatomy varies and reflects the amount of bowel resected and the type of anastomosis performed.

## *Postoperative Complications*

Patients' clinical courses after operations for cancer are problematic because resections are extensive and the patients are generally debilitated. The consequences of dumping, diarrhea, weight loss, and malnutrition increase postoperative difficulties.

## *Physiologic and Metabolic Problems*

Subtotal gastric resection, removal of the normal emptying mechanism of the pylorus, and extensive denervation of the stomach can alter gastric and intestinal motility, absorption, and biliary kinetics and cause a variety of physiologic problems.[39] Gastric emptying is often impaired when the normal pyloric channel is altered or when a previously unrecognized motility disorder becomes accentuated postoperatively.[36, 40]

## *Gastric Stasis*

Gastric stasis causes postprandial bloating, vomiting, pain, and weight loss in the absence of mechanical obstruction (Fig. 41–15). Symptoms develop in 1 to 25% of patients, depending on the type of bowel reconstruction.[40] Although the exact pathophysiology of gastric stasis is unknown, ineffective gastric emptying, impaired bowel motility, and alkaline reflux gastritis have been implicated.[40, 41] When severe, gastric stasis may require surgery to fashion the anastomosis into a different configuration or even total gastrectomy.

Nuclear medicine emptying studies are required to quantitate the rate of gastric emptying when the anastomotic diameter is normal.[20, 21]

## *Dumping*

Patients with the dumping syndrome present with vasomotor and cardiovascular symptoms: weakness, dizziness, sweating, nausea, colic, diarrhea, and an urgent desire to lie down after eating.[41, 42] High-carbohydrate foods precipitate the worst attacks. These symptoms are presumably caused by the rapid influx of food into the duodenum or jejunum, where sugars and polysaccharides are degraded. These sugars exert a strong osmotic effect that causes a net influx of fluid into the bowel, resultant distention, cramping, catharsis, and a presumed hormonal effect on the vasomotor system. Dumping has been reported to occur in 5 to 50% of patients depending on the type of operation.[42] Most patients improve with dietary changes. Surgical reconstruction is usually unrewarding.[39, 42]

## *Anemia*

Extensive gastric resection may lead to anemia because of malabsorption, inadequate oral intake, or chronic blood loss.

Iron deficiency anemia after gastric surgery may be related to rapid food passage in the duodenum and proximal jejunum (where iron is absorbed) and decreased levels of acid and pepsin, which help convert organic iron to inorganic iron, which the gut can absorb.[43, 44]

Vitamin $B_{12}$ deficiency is caused by loss of intrinsic factor rather than bacterial overgrowth as previously thought.

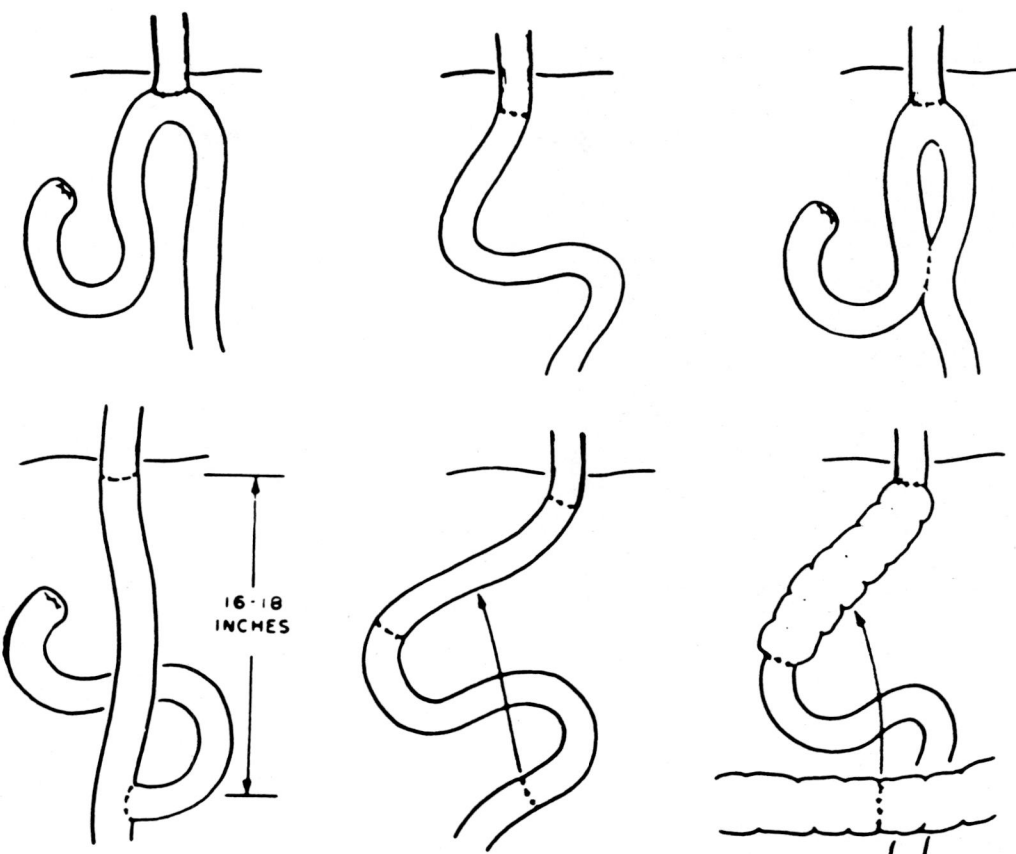

**Figure 41–13. Methods of alimentary tract reconstruction used after total gastrectomy.** (From Scott HW, Gobbel WG, Law DH: Alimentary tract reconstruction after total gastrectomy. Surg Gynecol Obstet 121:1231–1242, 1965. By permission of Surgery, Gynecology & Obstetrics.)

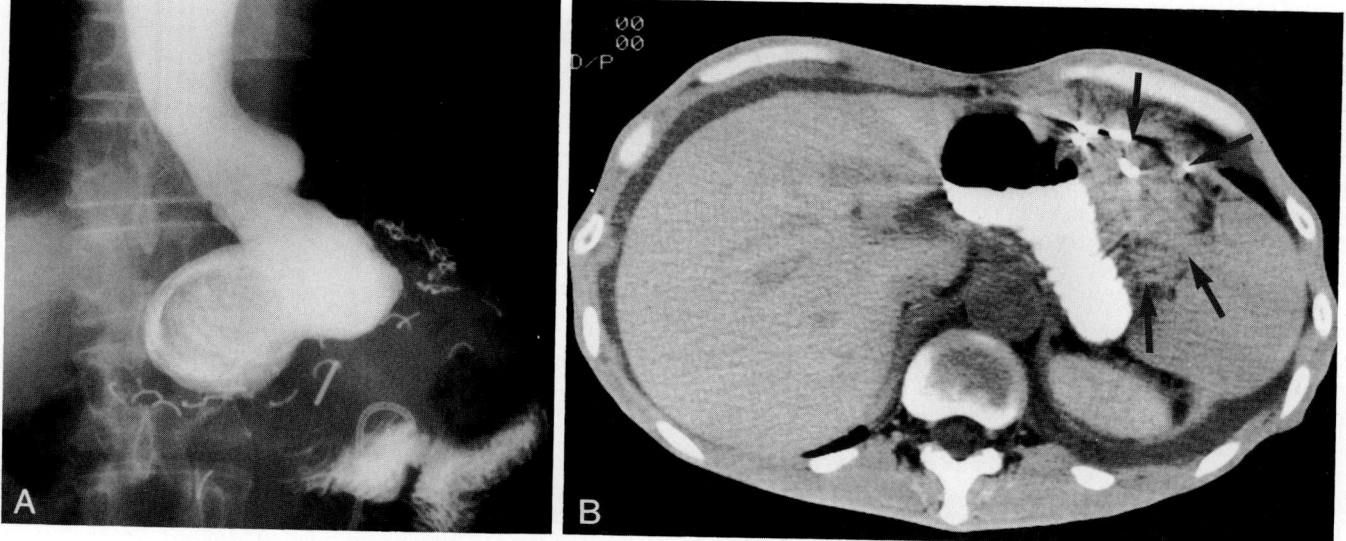

**Figure 41–14. Recurrent gastric neoplasm. A.** There is high-grade obstruction in the proximal small bowel in this patient, who has undergone a gastrectomy for carcinoma. **B.** Computed tomographic scan shows recurrent neoplasm *(arrows)* near the contrast medium–filled proximal bowel.

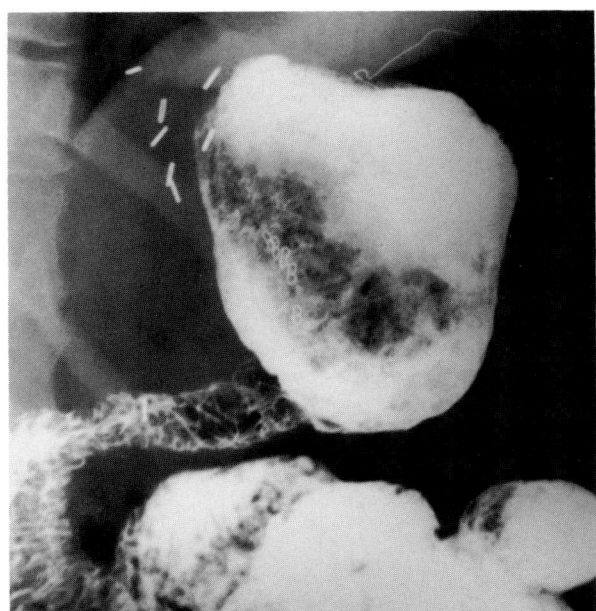

**Figure 41–15. Gastric stasis after a Billroth II gastrojejunostomy.** Abundant retained secretions and food are present within the gastric remnant. The anastomosis was patent, and scintigraphic emptying studies showed significant gastric stasis.

These metabolic deficiencies are accentuated in patients with total gastrectomy. Chronic nutritional problems far outweigh mechanical postgastrectomy syndromes or the rapid weight loss seen in the early postoperative course.[45]

## Peptic Ulcer Disease Surgery

The incidence, presentation, pathophysiology, treatment, and complications of peptic ulcer disease are rapidly changing.[45] The number of operations for ulcers has declined significantly.[47] During the periods 1970 through 1978 and 1974 through 1988, the hospitalization rate for patients with duodenal ulcers decreased by 43%, with a net decrease of 36% for all ulcer-related problems.[48, 49] These trends can be attributed to a number of factors: the development of $H_2$ blockers, although these changes antedate the clinical introduction of these drugs; physician and utilization committee preference for treating ulcers on an outpatient basis; and changing indications for surgery.[47, 50]

During the early 1970s, hospital admissions for patients with gastric ulcer complications remained stable.[48] The difference in rates of admission for gastric and duodenal ulcers reflects the pathogenesis of the diseases.[46] In contrast to duodenal ulcer patients, who have increased secretion of gastric acid and a more pronounced than normal secretory response to meals, patients with gastric ulcers secrete acid at a normal to low rate. Gastroduodenal reflux and defective mucosal defenses may be major mechanisms for gastric ulcers. Surgical approaches reflect these fundamental differences.[46]

## Duodenal Ulcer Surgery

Surgery for duodenal ulcer attempts to alter gastroduodenal physiology so that healing occurs and ulcers do not. Several surgical procedures have been developed and there is considerable controversy over the optimal procedure.

Vagotomy (Fig. 41–16) is central to all surgical procedures for duodenal ulcer diathesis.[46] Acid secretion and parietal cell response to gastrin and other stimulants decrease after vagotomy. Because vagotomy also causes gastric stasis, a drainage procedure must be performed. Ulcers recur in 4 to 27% of patients who have had truncal vagotomy and pyloroplasty.[51, 52] Antral resection is usually performed in conjunction with vagotomy to reduce acid production further by removing the antral source of gastrin and to prevent gastric stasis. Although ulcer recurrence after antrectomy is less than 1%, the side effects of diarrhea, dumping, and weight loss are increased.[53, 54]

Highly selective vagotomy (parietal cell vagotomy) is a procedure in which branches of the vagus nerves that supply the fundic portion of the stomach are sectioned but hepatic, celiac, and motor branches are preserved so that an emptying procedure need not be performed. The operation is less traumatic, does not require anastomosis or creation of a suture line, does not alter gastric emptying, and has no physiologic or metabolic side effects. Ulcer recurrence rates range between 4 and 11%.[53, 55]

## Gastric Ulcers

Surgery for gastric ulcer is more straightforward. Because overproduction of acid is not a fundamental problem, vagotomy is usually not needed. Partial gastric resection to remove the ulcer-bearing mucosa is sufficient to prevent ulcer recurrence in more than 95% of patients.[46, 55]

## Indications for Operation: Complications of Ulcers

At present, the primary indications for surgery in patients with peptic ulcer disease are perforation, ulcer intractability, hemorrhage, and obstruction.[46, 54, 55] Patients with ulcers that fail to heal despite 12 to 15 weeks of controlled medical therapy and patients who have recurrent ulceration despite adequate medical care are also surgical candidates.

### Perforation

In patients with acute perforation, the surgeon must decide whether to oversew the ulcer or perform definitive therapy.[56, 57] Factors that enter into this decision include the chronicity of ulceration, condition of the patient, and experience of the surgeon. In young patients without scarring, simple closure of duodenal ulcers involves a less than 20% chance of recurrence. In older patients, a simple patch is often insufficient.[57] Perforated

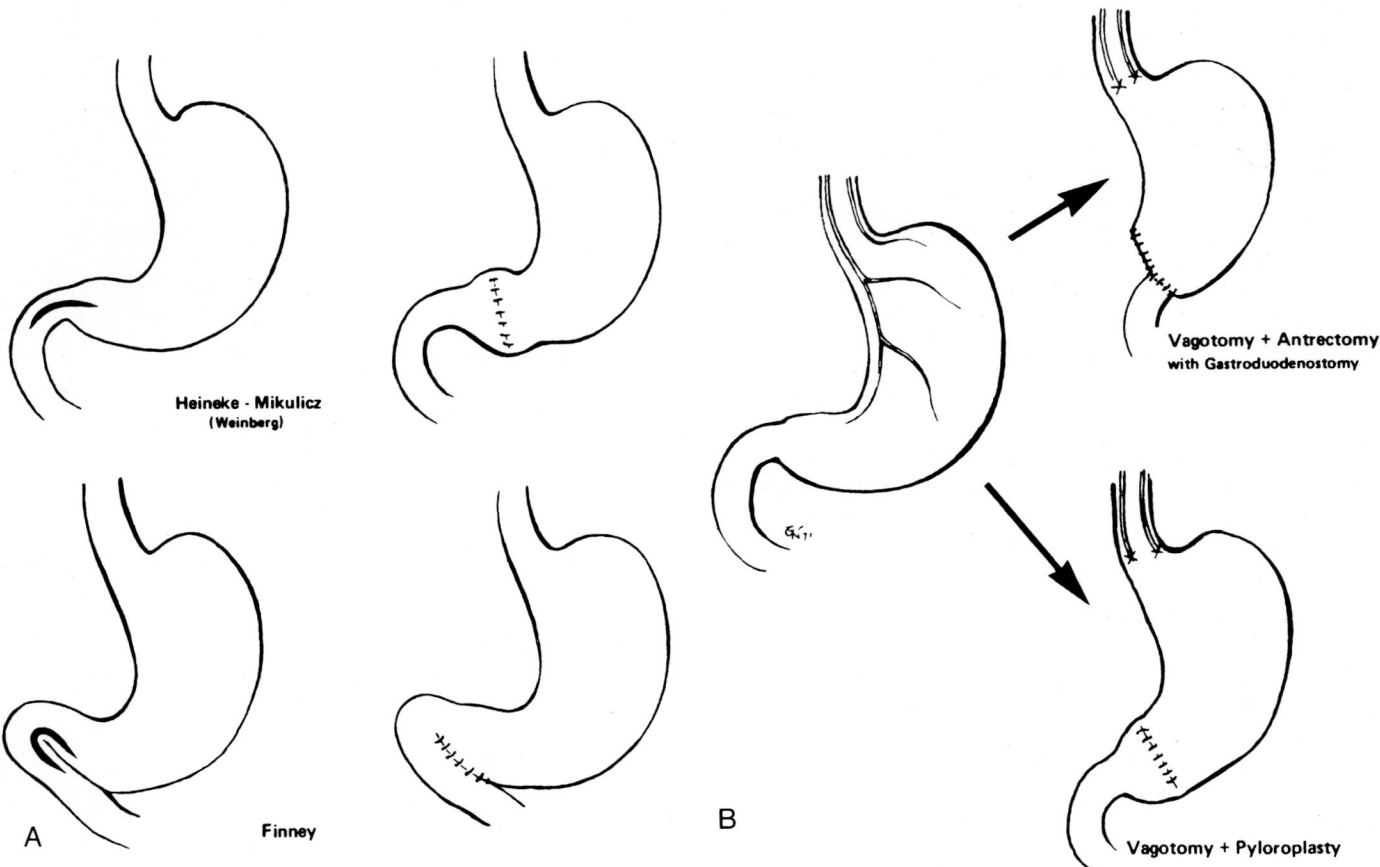

**Figure 41–16. Ulcer surgery. A.** Two types of pyloroplasties are commonly used. The Mikulicz pyloroplasty is created by making a longitudinal incision through the distal stomach, pylorus, and proximal duodenum. The incision is closed in a vertical fashion, which destroys the sphincteric mechanism. In the Finney pyloroplasty, a two-layer anastomosis is made between the stomach and duodenum. **B.** Current operations for duodenal ulcer. Vagotomy is a necessary part of these procedures in order to diminish gastric acid output. The choice lies between vagotomy plus antrectomy and vagotomy plus pyloroplasty.

gastric ulcers are usually treated with partial gastrectomy with or without vagotomy. Parietal cell vagotomy without drainage is an alternative approach.[54]

### Ulcer Intractability

Ulcer intractability is a major indication for surgical resection. Some 10 to 15% of patients with duodenal ulcers do not heal after 6 weeks of high-dose H$_2$ blockers, and 15 to 30% of patients who do heal initially eventually relapse.[46, 58, 59] A high degree of safety and low postoperative recurrence are noted when surgery is performed electively.

### Hemorrhage

Approximately 70% of major bleeding from ulcers stops spontaneously.[57] Surgery is needed when shock occurs and when bleeding continues despite adequate medical endoscopic and radiologic therapy. The optimal operation for duodenal ulcer bleeding is controversial; vagotomy plus pyloroplasty or vagotomy plus antrectomy are acceptable approaches.[46]

### Obstruction from Edema or Fibrosis

Duodenal obstruction occurs in less than 10% of patients with peptic ulcer disease. Acutely, the patient is decompressed with a nasogastric tube and supported parenterally.[46] Vagotomy with gastric resection or drainage is the standard approach. If scarring is marked, a gastrojejunostomy may be needed.

## Postoperative Complications

### Recurrent Ulcers

Factors that influence postoperative ulcer recurrence include the type of original surgery, experience of the surgeon, presence of a hypersecretory state, outlet obstruction, underlying neoplasm, and behavioral risk factors[52, 59–61] (Fig. 41–17). Barium studies are less reliable than endoscopy for evaluating patients for recurrent ulcer. Contrast studies may be needed if the anatomy is distorted and endoscopic visualization is difficult.[61]

### Leakage

Leakage from the duodenal stump or anastomosis occurs in 1 to 5% of patients.[33] Factors that predict the occurrence of stump leakage are not reliable.[7]

### Anastomotic Stricture

After ulcer surgery, anastomotic narrowing can occur even in the absence of recurrent ulceration. Conservative treatment with balloon dilatation may be attempted as an alternative to surgical revision.[31]

### Prolapse

Intussusception of either mucosa alone or full-thickness wall prolapse can occur through the anastomosis in

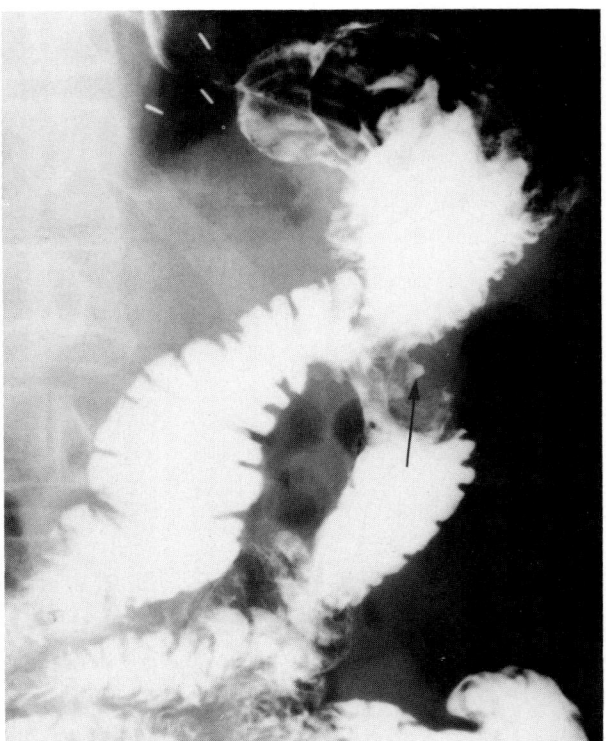

**Figure 41–17. Recurrent ulceration after a Billroth II gastrojejunostomy.** A mound of edema surrounds a perianastomotic ulcer *(arrow)* in the efferent loop of jejunum.

an antegrade direction. This complication is uncommon; symptoms indicate intermittent outlet obstruction.[62]

### Neoplasm After Surgery for Ulcer Disease

At one time it was thought that 3 to 10% of patients who had surgery for benign ulcer disease would develop carcinoma in the gastric remnant 10 to 15 years after surgery.[63] It is now questioned whether these patients have any greater risk than the general population.[64, 65]

## NUTRITIONAL SUPPORT

During the past two decades there have been many advances in enteral and parenteral nutritional support. Enteric routes are preferred when patients have an intact gastrointestinal system. Before 1980, operative gastrostomy was required to establish permanent access. Since then, percutaneous gastrostomy (see Chapter 21), either endoscopically or radiologically placed, has proved successful and popular, with few complications and essentially no mortality.

Contraindications to percutaneous methods include bowel obstruction, gastric ulcers, carcinoma, coagulopathies, ascites, altered postoperative anatomy, and other anatomic abnormalities that interfere with apposition of the stomach to the abdominal wall.

Complications of percutaneous gastrostomy include wound infection, hemorrhage, intraperitoneal leakage, gastrocolic fistula, tube blockage, migration, and

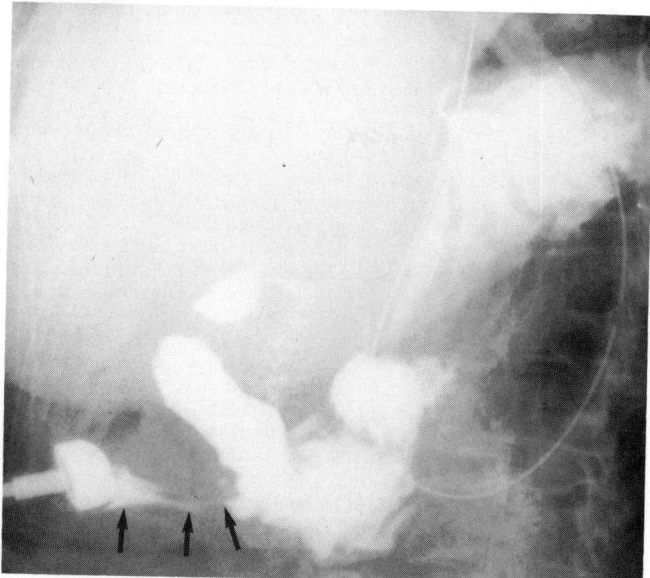

**Figure 41–18. Migration of percutaneous gastrostomy tube.** The bulbous end of this endoscopically placed gastrostomy tube has migrated out of the stomach into the perigastric tissues. A small tract *(arrows)* to the stomach is present.

dislodgement[66, 67] (Fig. 41–18). With radiologic techniques, a gastrostomy tube can be turned into a jejunostomy feeding tube. This method eliminates the risk of aspiration of gastric contents and allows nutrition to be given to patients with gastric atony. Complication rates are low and about equal for the endoscopic and radiologic approaches, so the choice depends on local expertise.

## SUMMARY

Patients with gastric and duodenal operations often present challenging problems to their physicians. A thorough understanding of the complex anatomic and physiologic alterations that occur after surgery, wise use of current technologic advances, and close communication between physician and health care colleagues are essential to ensure accurate diagnosis and effective management strategies.

### Acknowledgment

Figures 41–1 and 41–16A and B are reproduced from Sabiston DC (ed): Textbook of Surgery (14th ed). Philadelphia: WB Saunders, 1991.

Figure 41–6A and B is reproduced from Sabiston DC (ed): Textbook of Surgery (13th ed). Philadelphia: WB Saunders, 1986.

Figure 41–7A to J is reproduced from Hardy JD (ed): Complications in Surgery and Their Management. Philadelphia: WB Saunders, 1981.

## References

1. Moody FG, McGreevy JM: Complications of gastric surgery. *In* Greenfield LJ (ed): Complications in Surgery and Trauma (2nd ed). Philadelphia: JB Lippincott, 1990, pp 449–470.
2. Smith C, Gardiner R: Postoperative stomach and recurrent abdominal pain. *In* Thompson WM (ed): Common Problems in Gastrointestinal Radiology. Chicago: Year Book Medical Publishers, 1989, pp 202–211.
3. Burhenne HJ: Roentgen anatomy and terminology of gastric surgery. AJR 91:731–743, 1964.
4. Gedgaudas-McClees RK, McClees EC: Radiology of the stomach. *In* Gedgaudas-McClees RK (ed): Handbook of Gastrointestinal Imaging. New York: Churchill Livingstone, 1987, pp 33–68.
5. Burhenne HJ: The post-operative stomach. *In* Taveras JM, Ferruci JT (eds): Radiology Diagnosis-Imaging-Intervention. Philadelphia: JB Lippincott, 1986, pp 1–11.
6. Smith C, Gardiner R, Kubicka RA, et al: Radiology of gastric restrictive surgery. Radiographics 5:193–216, 1985.
7. Flint LM: Early postoperative acute abdominal complications. Surg Clin North Am 68:445–455, 1988.
8. Stevenson GW: Technique of examination. *In* Margulis AR, Burhenne HJ (eds): Alimentary Tract Radiology. St. Louis: CV Mosby, 1983, pp 1699–1719.
9. Ominsky SH, Moss AA: The postoperative stomach: comparative study of double-contrast barium examinations and endoscopy. Gastrointest Radiol 4:17–21, 1979.
10. Gold RP, Seaman WB: The primary double-contrast examination of the postoperative stomach. Radiology 124:297–305, 1977.
11. Gohel VK, Laufer I: Double-contrast examination of the postoperative stomach. Radiology 129:601–607, 1978.
12. Odo Op Den Orth J: The postoperative stomach. *In* Laufer I (ed): Double Contrast Gastrointestinal Radiology with Endoscopic Correlation. Philadelphia: WB Saunders, 1979, pp 289–329.
13. Smith C, Gardiner R, Kubicka RA, et al: Gastric restrictive surgery for obesity: early radiologic evaluation. Radiology 153:321–327, 1984.
14. Goodman P, Halpert RD: Radiological evaluation of gastric stapling procedures for morbid obesity. Crit Rev Diagn Imaging 32:37–67, 1991.
15. Barmier EP, Solomon H, Charuzi I, et al: Radiologic assessment of the distal stomach and duodenum after gastric bypass: percutaneous CT-guided transcatheter technique. Gastrointest Radiol 9:203–205, 1984.
16. Freeman JB: The use of endoscopy after gastric partitioning for morbid obesity. Gastroenterol Clin North Am 16:339–347, 1987.
17. Ott DJ, Munitz HA, Gelfand DW, et al: The sensitivity of radiography of the postoperative stomach. Radiology 144:741–743, 1982.
18. Balthazar EJ: CT of the gastrointestinal tract: principles and interpretation. AJR 156:23–32, 1991.
19. Zingas AP, Amin KA, Loredo RD, et al: Computed tomographic evaluation of the excluded stomach in gastric bypass. Comput Tomogr 8:231–236, 1984.
20. Malmud LS, Fisher RS, Knight LC, et al: Scintigraphic evaluation of gastric emptying. Semin Nucl Med 12:116–125, 1982.
21. Mettler FA Jr, Guiberteau MJ: Essentials of Nuclear Medicine. Philadelphia: WB Saunders, 1991, pp 177–207.
22. Wall SD: Magnetic resonance imaging of the alimentary canal. *In* Herlinger H, Megibow A (eds): Gastrointestinal Radiology Reviews. New York: Marcel Dekker, 1990, pp 213–231.
23. Sinar DR, Flickinger EG, Park HK, et al: Retrograde endoscopy of the bypassed stomach segment after gastric bypass surgery: unexpected lesions. South Med J 78:255–258, 1985.
24. Max MH, West B, Knutson CO: Evaluation of postoperative gastroduodenal symptoms: endoscopy or upper gastrointestinal roentgenography? Surgery 86:578–582, 1979.
25. Ott DJ, Munitz HA, Gelfand DW, et al: The sensitivity of radiography of the postoperative stomach. Radiology 144:741–743, 1982.
26. Cotton PB, Shorvon PJ: Analysis of endoscopy and radiography in the diagnosis, follow-up and treatment of peptic ulcer disease. Clin Gastroenterol 13:383–402, 1984.
27. Cole HM (ed): Gastric restrictive surgery: diagnostic and therapeutic technology assessment (DATTA). JAMA 261:1491–1494, 1989.
28. Kirby DF, Wade JB, Mulls PR, et al: A prospective assessment of the Garren-Edwards gastric bubble and bariatric surgery in the treatment of morbid obesity. Am Surg 16:253–272, 1987.

29. Linner JH: Overview of surgical techniques for the treatment of morbid obesity. Gastroenterol Clin North Am 16:253–272, 1987.

30. Buckwalter JA, Herbst CA Jr: Perioperative complications of gastric restrictive operations. Am J Surg 146:613–618, 1983.

31. Gotbert S, Afzelius LE, Hambraeus G, et al: Balloon catheter dilatation of strictures in the upper digestive tract. Radiologe 22:479–483, 1982.

32. Poulos A, Peat K, Lorman JG, et al: Gastric operation for the morbidly obese. AJR 136:867–870, 1981.

33. Burrell M, Curtis AMcB: Sequelae of stomach surgery. Crit Rev Diagn Imaging 10:17–97, 1977.

34. Mishkin JD, Meranze SG, Burke DR, et al: Interventional radiologic treatment of complications following gastric bypass surgery for morbid obesity. Gastrointest Radiol 13:9–14, 1988.

35. Cheung LY: Treatment of established stress ulcer disease. World J Surg 5:235–240, 1981.

36. Welch CE, Malt RA: Surgery of the stomach, duodenum, gallbladder, and bile ducts. N Engl J Med 316:999–1008, 1987.

37. Davis GR: Neoplasms of the stomach. *In* Sleisenger MH, Fordtran JS (eds): Gastrointestinal Disease: Pathophysiology, Diagnosis, Management (4th ed). Philadelphia: WB Saunders, 1989, pp 745–772.

38. Kodama Y, Sugimachi K, Soejima K, et al: Evaluation of extensive lymph node dissection for carcinoma of the stomach. World J Surg 5:241–248, 1981.

39. Koelz HR, Gewertz BL: The stomach. Part I: vagotomy. Clin Gastroenterol 8:305–319, 1979.

40. Fich A, Neri M, Camilleri M, et al: Stasis syndromes following gastric surgery: clinical and motility features of 60 symptomatic patients. J Clin Gastroenterol 12:505–512, 1990.

41. Woodward ER, Hocking MP: Postgastrectomy syndromes. Surg Clin North Am 67:509–520, 1987.

42. Alexander-Williams J, Hoare AM: The stomach. Part II: partial gastric resection. Clin Gastroenterol 8:321–353, 1979.

43. Bradley EL III: The stomach. Part III: total gastrectomy. Clin Gastroenterol 8:354–371, 1979.

44. Schrock TR, Way LW: Total gastrectomy. Am J Surg 135:348–355, 1978.

45. Tovey FI, Godfrey JE, Lewis MR: A gastrectomy population: 25–30 years on. Postgrad Med J 66:450–456, 1990.

46. Mulholland MW, Debas HT: Chronic duodenal and gastric ulcer. Surg Clin North Am 67:489–507, 1987.

47. McConnell DB, Baba GC, Deveney CW: Changes in surgical treatment of peptic ulcer disease within a veterans hospital in the 1970s and the 1980s. Arch Surg 124:1164–1167, 1989.

48. Elashoff JD, Grossman MI: Trends in hospital admissions and death rates for peptic ulcer disease in the United States from 1970 to 1978. Gastroenterology 78:280–285, 1980.

49. Kurata JH, Honda GD, Frankl H: Hospitalization and mortality rates for peptic ulcers: a comparison of a large health maintenance organization and United States data. Gastroenterology 83:1008–1016, 1982.

50. Bardhan KD, Cust G, Hinchliffe RFC, et al: Changing pattern of

51. Sheaff CM, Nyhus LM: Recurrent ulcer. *In* Nyhus LM, Wastell C (eds): Surgery of the Stomach and Duodenum. Boston: Little, Brown, 1986, pp 516–534.

52. Stabile BE, Passaro E Jr: Recurrent peptic ulcer. Gastroenterology 76:124–135, 1976.

53. Jordan PH Jr, Thornby J: Should it be parietal cell vagotomy or selective vagotomy-antrectomy for treatment of duodenal ulcer?—A progress report. Ann Surg 205:572–590, 1986.

54. Jordan PH Jr: Operations for peptic ulcer disease and early postoperative complications. *In* Sleisenger MH, Fordtran JS (eds): Gastrointestinal Disease: Pathophysiology, Diagnosis, Management (4th ed). Philadelphia: WB Saunders, 1989, pp 939–952.

55. Richardson CT: Gastric ulcer. *In* Sleisenger MH, Fordtran JS (eds): Gastrointestinal Disease: Pathophysiology, Diagnosis, Management (4th ed). Philadelphia: WB Saunders, 1989, pp 879–909.

56. Graham DY: Complications of peptic ulcer disease and indications for surgery. *In* Sleisenger MH, Fordtran JS (eds): Gastrointestinal Disease: Pathophysiology, Diagnosis, Management (4th ed). Philadelphia: WB Saunders, 1989, pp 925–938.

57. Jordan PH Jr, Morros C: Perforated peptic ulcer. Surg Clin North Am 68:315–329, 1988.

58. Boyd EJS, Johnston DA, Penston JG, et al: Does maintenance therapy keep duodenal ulcers healed? Lancet 1:1324–1327, 1988.

59. Schirmer BD, Meyers WC, Hanks JB, et al: Marginal ulcer: a difficult surgical problem. Ann Surg 195:653–661, 1982.

60. Thirlby RC, Feldman M: Postoperative recurrent ulcer. *In* Sleisenger MH, Fordtran JS (eds): Gastrointestinal Disease: Pathophysiology, Diagnosis, Management (4th ed). Philadelphia: WB Saunders, 1989, pp 952–962.

61. Mosiman F, Donovan JA, Alexander-Williams J: Pitfalls in the diagnosis of recurrent ulceration after surgery for peptic ulcer disease. J Clin Gastroenterol 7:133–136, 1985.

62. Poppel MH: Gastric intussusceptions. Radiology 78:602–608, 1962.

63. Kobayashi S, Prolla JC, Kirsner JB: Late gastric carcinoma developing after surgery for benign conditions: endoscopic and histologic studies of the anastomosis and diagnostic problems. Dig Dis 15:905–912, 1970.

64. Schafer LW, Larson DE, Melton J III, et al: The risk of gastric carcinoma after surgical treatment for benign ulcer disease: a population-based study in Olmstead County, Minnesota. N Engl J Med 309:1210–1213, 1983.

65. Greene FL: Neoplastic changes in the stomach after gastrectomy. Surg Gynecol Obstet 171:477–480, 1990.

66. McKay MD, Tedesco FJ: Percutaneous endoscopic gastrostomy. *In* Bennett JR, Hunt RH (eds): Therapeutic Endoscopy and Radiology of the Gut (2nd ed). Baltimore: Williams & Wilkins, 1990, pp 207–214.

67. Ho C-S: Percutaneous gastrostomy by radiological technique. *In* Bennett JR, Hunt RH (eds): Therapeutic Endoscopy and Radiology of the Gut (2nd ed). Baltimore, Williams & Wilkins, 1990, pp 215–221.

admissions and operations for duodenal ulcer. Br J Surg 76:230–236, 1989.

# Stomach and Duodenum: Differential Diagnosis

**Marc S. Levine, M.D.**

## TABLE 42–1. GASTRIC ULCERS (NO MASS)

| CAUSE | LOCATION | COMMENTS |
| --- | --- | --- |
| Erosions | | |
| Idiopathic | Antrum or body; often aligned on rugal folds | Varioliform erosions |
| Aspirin or other nonsteroidal anti-inflammatory drugs | Usually on or near greater curvature of body | Linear or serpiginous erosions |
| Crohn's disease | Antrum or body | Associated Crohn's disease in small bowel or colon |
| Ulcers | | |
| Peptic ulcer disease | Usually on lesser curvature or posterior wall of antrum or body | Follow ulcer to healing to confirm benignity |
| Aspirin or other nonsteroidal anti-inflammatory drugs | Distal half of greater curvature | May simulate malignant ulcer |
| Gastritis | Variable | Hypertrophic gastritis, granulomatous conditions, radiation, caustic ingestion, infections |
| Zollinger-Ellison syndrome | Variable | Associated ulcers in atypical locations; hypergastrinemia |
| Pseudolymphoma | Antrum or body | Mimics appearance of malignant ulcer |
| Early gastric cancer | Variable | Nodular or deformed folds surrounding ulcer |

## TABLE 42–2. GASTRIC MASS LESIONS

| CAUSE | RADIOGRAPHIC FINDINGS | COMMENTS |
|---|---|---|
| Benign mucosal lesions | | |
| Hyperplastic polyps | Round, sessile polyps in fundus or body; usually multiple | Not premalignant |
| Adenomatous polyps | Lobulated or pedunculated polyps in antrum; often solitary | Premalignant |
| Polyposis syndromes | Multiple polyps in stomach (also in small bowel or colon) | Familial adenomatosis polyposis, Peutz-Jeghers syndrome, Cronkhite-Canada syndrome, juvenile polyposis, and Cowden's disease |
| Villous tumor | Giant mass with "soap bubble" appearance | Premalignant; rare in stomach |
| Bezoar | Giant mass-like filling defect; freely movable | Unusual eating habits |
| Malignant mucosal lesions | | |
| Carcinoma | Polypoid mass; ulceration common | Usually advanced gastric cancer but occasionally may be early cancer |
| Benign submucosal lesions | | |
| Leiomyoma | Smooth submucosal mass; ulceration common; rarely multiple | May be difficult to differentiate from leiomyosarcoma |
| Leiomyoblastoma | Smooth submucosal mass; ulceration common | Risk of malignancy |
| Lipoma | Submucosal mass with changeable shape at fluoroscopy; fatty density on computed tomographic scan | Usually asymptomatic |
| Hemangioma | Submucosal mass with phleboliths | Risk of massive gastrointestinal bleeding |
| Lymphangioma | Submucosal mass | Rare |
| Glomus tumor | Submucosal mass | Usually asymptomatic |
| Neurofibroma | Solitary or multiple submucosal masses | Von Recklinghausen's disease |
| Granular cell tumor | Solitary or multiple submucosal masses | Associated lesions on skin or tongue |
| Inflammatory fibroid polyp | Sessile or pedunculated polyp in antrum; usually solitary | Usually asymptomatic |
| Ectopic pancreatic rest | Submucosal mass with central umbilication; usually on greater curvature of distal antrum; rarely multiple | Usually asymptomatic |
| Duplication cyst | Submucosal mass on greater curvature of antrum or body; rarely communicates with lumen | Usually symptomatic during first year of life |
| Malignant submucosal lesions | | |
| Leiomyosarcoma | Solitary, lobulated submucosal mass; ulceration or cavitation common | Better prognosis than carcinoma |
| Metastases | One or more submucosal masses; ulceration or cavitation common; "bull's-eye" lesions of varying sizes | Most commonly malignant melanoma or metastatic breast cancer |
| Lymphoma | One or more submucosal masses; ulceration or cavitation common; bull's-eye lesions of similar sizes | Usually non-Hodgkin's lymphoma |
| Kaposi's sarcoma | Multiple submucosal masses or bull's-eye lesions | Homosexuals with acquired immunodeficiency syndrome; usually have Kaposi's sarcoma on skin |
| Carcinoid | Multiple submucosal masses or bull's-eye lesions | Carcinoid syndrome uncommon |
| Leukemia | Multiple submucosal masses or polyps | Rare |
| Multiple myeloma | Multiple submucosal masses | Rare |

## TABLE 42–3. THICKENED GASTRIC FOLDS

| CAUSE | DISTRIBUTION | COMMENTS |
| --- | --- | --- |
| Benign conditions | | |
| Antral gastritis | Antrum | |
| Hypertrophic gastritis | Fundus and body | Ulcer-like symptoms |
| Ménétrier's disease | Fundus and body (massive folds) | Increased acid secretion; frequent duodenal ulcers |
| Zollinger-Ellison syndrome | Fundus and body (increased secretions; ulcers common) | Hypochlorhydria and hypoproteinemia |
| | | Hypergastrinemia due to non–beta islet cell tumors |
| Varices | Fundus and cardia (serpentine folds) | Portal hypertension or splenic vein obstruction |
| Eosinophilic gastritis | Antrum | Peripheral eosinophilia; history of allergic diseases |
| Crohn's disease | Antrum and body | Advanced Crohn's disease in small bowel or colon |
| Sarcoidosis | Antrum | Pulmonary sarcoidosis |
| Tuberculosis | Antrum | History of acquired immunodeficiency syndrome or travel to endemic areas |
| Caustic ingestion | Antrum | History of caustic ingestion |
| Radiation | Antrum | History of radiation therapy (5000 rad or more) |
| Floxuridine (5-FUDR) toxicity | Antrum and body | Hepatic artery infusion chemotherapy |
| Amyloidosis | Antrum | Systemic amyloidosis |
| Pseudolymphoma | Antrum and body | Mimics lymphoma |
| Malignant conditions | | |
| Lymphoma | Localized or diffuse | May have generalized lymphoma |
| Carcinoma | Localized or diffuse | Associated narrowing and rigidity of stomach |

## TABLE 42–4. GASTRIC NARROWING

| CAUSE | RADIOGRAPHIC FINDINGS | COMMENTS |
| --- | --- | --- |
| Benign conditions | | |
| Scarring from peptic ulcer disease | Smooth or asymmetric antral narrowing | History of ulcers |
| Atrophic gastritis | Diffusely narrowed, tubular stomach with decreased or absent folds | Pernicious anemia |
| Eosinophilic gastritis | Antral narrowing | Peripheral eosinophilia; history of allergic diseases |
| Crohn's disease | Funnel-shaped antral narrowing ("ram's horn" or "shofar" sign) | Advanced Crohn's disease in small bowel or colon |
| Sarcoidosis | Cone-shaped antral narrowing | Pulmonary sarcoidosis |
| Tuberculosis | Antral narrowing; fistulas common | History of acquired immunodeficiency syndrome or travel to endemic areas |
| Syphilis | Funnel-shaped antral narrowing | Occurs in less than 1% of patients with syphilis |
| Caustic ingestion | Narrowing of antrum or antrum and body | History of caustic ingestion; esophageal scarring in 20% |
| Radiation | Antral narrowing | History of radiation therapy (5000 rad or more) |
| Cytomegalovirus infection | Antral narrowing and ulceration | Patients with acquired immunodeficiency syndrome |
| Amyloidosis | Antral narrowing | Systemic amyloidosis |
| Pseudolymphoma | Narrowing of antrum or body | Mimics lymphoma or carcinoma |
| Antral diaphragm or web | Transverse, web-like area of antral narrowing | May be asymptomatic |
| Malignant conditions | | |
| Scirrhous carcinoma | Linitis plastica | Antral narrowing classic, but isolated involvement of proximal stomach in 40% |
| Metastatic breast cancer | Linitis plastica | Recent or remote history of breast cancer |
| Omental cake | Mass effect and spiculated folds on greater curvature; occasionally circumferential | Omental metastases from ovarian carcinoma or other malignant neoplasms |
| Hodgkin's disease | Linitis plastica | May have generalized Hodgkin's disease |
| Kaposi's sarcoma | Linitis plastica | Homosexuals with acquired immunodeficiency syndrome; usually have Kaposi's sarcoma on skin |

## TABLE 42–5. GASTRIC OUTLET OBSTRUCTION

| CAUSE | RADIOGRAPHIC FINDINGS | COMMENTS |
|---|---|---|
| Peptic ulcer disease | Antral, pyloric, or duodenal ulcer with spasm, edema, or scarring | Difficult to differentiate from tumor if high-grade obstruction |
| Antral scarring | Antral narrowing | Crohn's disease, sarcoidosis, tuberculosis, syphilis, caustic ingestion, radiation |
| Carcinoma | Infiltrating antral or pyloric channel tumor | Usually advanced lesions |
| Other malignant tumors | Irregular narrowing and/or extrinsic compression of antrum or duodenum | Pancreatic carcinoma, lymphoma, retroperitoneal metastases |
| Hypertrophic pyloric stenosis | Elongated, narrowed pylorus | Uncommon cause of obstruction in adults |
| Antral diaphragm or web | Transverse, web-like area of antral narrowing | Degree of obstruction depends on size of central aperture of web |
| Gastric volvulus | Dilated, upside-down, intrathoracic stomach | Surgical emergency if incarcerated or strangulated |
| Gastroparesis | Flaccid stomach with decreased or absent peristalsis but no mechanical outlet obstruction | History of diabetes or other conditions associated with gastroparesis |

## TABLE 42–6. DUODENAL FILLING DEFECTS

| CAUSE | RADIOGRAPHIC FINDINGS | COMMENTS |
|---|---|---|
| Non-neoplastic conditions | | |
| Prolapsed antral mucosa | Mushroom-shaped defect at base of bulb | Usually asymptomatic |
| Flexural pseudotumor | Filling defect at superior duodenal flexure due to redundant mucosa | May simulate mass or ulcer |
| Heterotopic gastric mucosa | Tiny, polygonal or angulated nodules at base of bulb | No clinical significance |
| Brunner's gland hyperplasia | Multiple rounded nodules in proximal duodenum ("Swiss cheese" appearance) | Associated with duodenitis |
| Benign lymphoid hyperplasia | Multiple tiny, rounded nodules in proximal duodenum | Associated with immunologic disorders |
| Choledochocele | Submucosal mass in region of ampulla | Congenital anomaly |
| Duplication cyst | Submucosal mass on medial wall of descending duodenum | Congenital anomaly |
| Intramural hematoma | Submucosal mass on medial wall of duodenum | Bleeding diathesis, anticoagulation, or trauma |
| Benign tumors | | |
| Polyps | Smooth, sessile elevations; usually solitary | Hyperplastic or adenomatous |
| Polyposis syndromes | Multiple polypoid lesions | Familial adenomatous polyposis, Peutz-Jeghers syndrome, Cronkhite-Canada syndrome, and juvenile polyposis |
| Villous adenoma | Polypoid mass with frond-like projections; usually near ampulla | High malignant potential |
| Mesenchymal lesions | Submucosal mass, often with central ulceration or umbilication | Leiomyoma, lipoma, neurogenic tumor, Brunner's gland hamartoma, ectopic pancreatic rest |
| Malignant tumors | | |
| Duodenal carcinoma | Polypoid mass at or distal to papilla of Vater | Gastrointestinal bleeding or obstruction |
| Ampullary carcinoma | Polypoid mass in region of ampulla | Jaundice common |
| Leiomyosarcoma | Lobulated submucosal mass; ulceration or cavitation common | Better prognosis than carcinoma |
| Metastases | Multiple submucosal masses or bull's-eye lesions | Most commonly malignant melanoma or metastatic breast cancer |
| Lymphoma | Multiple submucosal masses or bull's-eye lesions | Usually non-Hodgkin's lymphoma |
| Kaposi's sarcoma | Multiple submucosal masses or bull's-eye lesions | Occurs in homosexuals with acquired immunodeficiency syndrome; usually have Kaposi's sarcoma on skin |
| Carcinoid | Multiple submucosal masses or bull's-eye lesions | Carcinoid syndrome uncommon |

## TABLE 42–7. THICKENED DUODENAL FOLDS

| CAUSE | RADIOGRAPHIC FINDINGS | COMMENTS |
|---|---|---|
| Duodenitis | Thickened, nodular folds in proximal duodenum; occasionally associated with erosions | Not a reliable diagnosis unless folds grossly thickened |
| Brunner's gland hyperplasia | Thickened, nodular folds in proximal duodenum | Usually associated with duodenitis |
| Chronic renal failure | Markedly thickened, nodular folds, particularly in bulb | Usually on dialysis |
| Pancreatitis | Thickened folds associated with medial compression or widening of duodenal sweep | Elevated serum amylase level; computed tomography or ultrasound for confirmation |
| Zollinger-Ellison syndrome | Thickened folds in stomach, duodenum, and proximal jejunum | Ulcers in atypical locations |
| Crohn's disease | Thickened folds, ulceration, or strictures | Associated Crohn's disease in small bowel or colon |
| Parasitic infection (giardiasis and strongyloidiasis) | Thickened or effaced folds, irritability, and spasm in duodenum and proximal jejunum | Stool cultures or small bowel brushings and biopsies for diagnosis |
| Cryptosporidiosis | Thickened folds in duodenum and small bowel | History of acquired immunodeficiency syndrome; profuse secretory diarrhea |
| Celiac disease | Thickened folds in proximal duodenum | Often associated with "bubbly" bulb |
| Intramural hemorrhage | Thickened, spiculated folds or thumbprinting | History of bleeding diathesis, anticoagulation, or trauma |
| Varices | Serpentine folds in proximal duodenum | Portal hypertension |
| Lymphoma | Thickened folds or thumbprinting | Usually non-Hodgkin's lymphoma |

## TABLE 42–8. DILATED DUODENUM (MEGADUODENUM)

| CAUSE | ASSOCIATED RADIOGRAPHIC FINDINGS | COMMENTS |
|---|---|---|
| Scleroderma | Dilated small bowel with hide-bound appearance | Systemic signs of scleroderma |
| Celiac disease | Dilated small bowel with decreased number of folds in jejunum | Malabsorption |
| Zollinger-Ellison syndrome | Thickened folds and increased secretions in stomach and duodenum; one or more ulcers | Hypergastrinemia |
| Strongyloidiasis | Thickened or effaced folds, ulceration, or "lead pipe" appearance in duodenum and jejunum | History of acquired immunodeficiency syndrome or travel to endemic areas |
| Mesenteric root syndrome | Broad, linear crossing defect on distal duodenum by mesenteric root | Thin or bedridden patients |
| Vagotomy | Dilated small bowel | Appropriate surgical history |
| Obstruction | Benign or malignant narrowing or extrinsic compression of duodenum | Postbulbar ulcer, Crohn's disease, pancreatitis, metastatic disease |
| Ileus | Dilated duodenum without mechanical obstruction | Postoperative ileus, metabolic imbalance, pancreatitis |

## TABLE 42–9. EXTRINSIC IMPRESSIONS ON THE DUODENUM

| CAUSE | LOCATION | RADIOGRAPHIC FINDINGS | COMMENTS |
|---|---|---|---|
| Pancreatic disease | Medial | Widened duodenal sweep | Pancreatitis, pancreatic pseudocyst, or pancreatic carcinoma |
| Peripancreatic adenopathy | Medial | Widened duodenal sweep | Peripancreatic metastases or lymphoma |
| Aortic aneurysm | Medial | Widened duodenal sweep | Aortoduodenal fistula is rare complication |
| Gallbladder disease | Superior | Extrinsic compression of bulb or proximal duodenum | Acute or chronic cholecystitis or hydrops of the gallbladder |
| Liver disease | Superior | Extrinsic compression of bulb or proximal duodenum | Hepatomegaly of any cause |
| Renal disease | Posterolateral | Extrinsic compression of descending duodenum | Polycystic kidney, renal cell carcinoma |
| Colonic disease | Anterolateral | Extrinsic compression of descending duodenum | Carcinoma of the hepatic flexure |

# SECTION
# VII

# Small Bowel

*Section Editor*

Hans Herlinger, M.D.

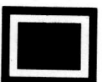

# Barium Examinations

**Hans Herlinger, M.D.**

## HISTORICAL BACKGROUND

Restricted by limitations of equipment and x-ray film, early investigators with interest in the small bowel had to concentrate on function rather than surface anatomy.[1-3] By 1923 it became possible for Forssel[4] to report in greater detail on the types of neuromuscular activity encountered in the gastrointestinal tract. Morse and Cole[5] were soon able to describe the radiologic anatomy of the small intestine. Improvements in x-ray apparatus design and barium suspension stability led to standardization of the follow-through examination. Golden[6] considered a single dose of 280 mL of barium to be sufficient because it would avoid overdistention and reduce overlap of loops. Weltz[7] used a larger amount of barium given in 30-mL aliquots at 5-minute intervals after an initial dose of 200 mL. He believed that the quality of the examination depended on the degree of lumen filling and that larger amounts of barium protected against the deleterious effects of the secretions in the bowel lumen. Marshak[8] recommended the use of a single dose of 480 to 600 mL of a 50% w/v suspension of barium to reduce transit time and obtain more complete and continuous filling of bowel loops.

The introduction of flocculation-resistant barium suspensions in the 1950s contributed significantly to improvements in examination quality. Ardran and colleagues[9] were the first to demonstrate its benefits. Yet, even this form of barium suspension was not completely immune to the adverse effects of secretions, and methods were introduced to accelerate transit and shorten the time of exposure to the secretions. With this purpose in mind, Weintraub and Williams[10] recommended giving glasses of iced water after the initial quantity of barium. Having the patient lie on the right side also promoted earlier and more complete emptying

of barium from the stomach.[11] Of the drugs used for transit acceleration, only metoclopramide has withstood the test of time. Its use was first reported by Grivaux and colleagues[12] and was further described by Howarth and co-workers[13] and Kreel.[14]

## SMALL BOWEL FOLLOW-THROUGH

### Conventional (Radiographic) Follow-through

Despite the many years of keen interest in and clinical research on the development of barium radiology of the small intestine, the technique used by the majority of radiologists is still that usually referred to as the conventional follow-through. This method may commence as a double contrast upper gastrointestinal study, even in patients without symptoms of dyspepsia. A further dose of lower-density barium is then administered and a succession of overhead films is used to monitor its progress. Henceforth, we refer to this as the *radiographic follow-through*. The appearance of barium in the cecum becomes an indication for fluoroscopy to demonstrate the terminal ileum. The various overhead films are inspected for any indication of abnormality, and fluoroscopy is done if any abnormality is seen.

The experience of any physician active in this field includes several examples of lesions that were not detected by inspection of these overhead films (Fig. 43–1). Maglinte and co-workers[15] discussed 45 such conventional studies that missed 48 significant lesions. Radiographic findings of the National Cooperative Crohn's Disease Study involving 13 university hospitals and reported in 1979 also bore testimony to the limitations of this barium technique.[16] There can be no doubt that

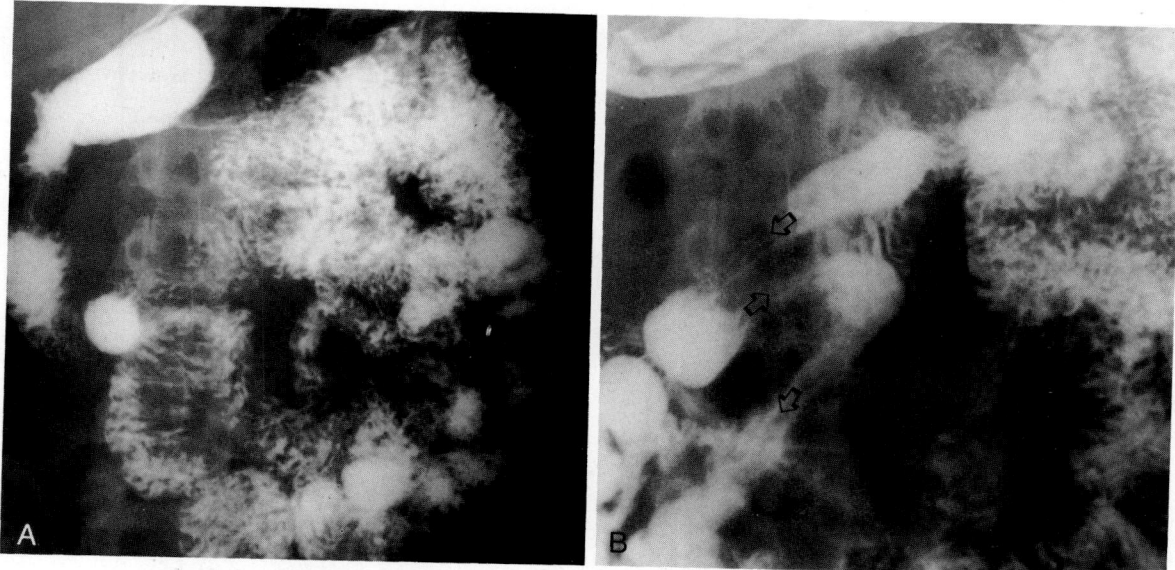

**Figure 43–1. Reliance on overhead films of barium-filled small bowel loops may cause lesions to be missed. A.** An overhead film of a patient with Crohn's disease of the terminal ileum shows apparant normality of the jejunum. **B.** Fluoroscopic spot film with abdominal compression and slight rotation of the patient demonstrates active Crohn's disease involving a long segment of jejunum *(arrows).*

this form of examination is flawed because of the tendency of the sinuous coils of intestine to overlap and hide their lesions. Because of its simplicity, clinicians order it almost routinely, "thinking that they are learning something about the gut—or at least ruling out small bowel disease."[17]

## Fluoroscopic Follow-through

Unlike the radiographic follow-through examination, this method is specifically designed for investigation of the small intestine. The following are the requirements for its successful performance:

1. Preparation and premedication of the patient
2. A barium suspension suitable for the small bowel
3. Where indicated, an abbreviated single contrast examination of esophagus, stomach, and duodenum
4. Fluoroscopic compression spot films of all small bowel loops

**Preparation of the Patient.** This need not be overdone. Cleansing the colon as for a barium enema is not a requirement. It is sufficient to administer a colon-active laxative in the afternoon before the study—for example, three or four tablets of bisacodyl (Dulcolax)—and have the patient abstain from food and drink from 8 PM.

Two tablets of metoclopramide (total dose, 20 mg) are given by mouth about 15 minutes before the examination commences. This is omitted in patients with high-grade small bowel obstruction and in the rare patient with a history of a reaction to this drug.

**Barium Suspension.** A barium suspension of 40 to 50% w/v is recommended. This could be undiluted

EntroBar (Lafayette Pharmacal, Lafayette, IN) or Entero-H (E-Z-EM Company, Westbury, NY) diluted with an equal volume of water. The barium should not contain sorbitol which is hyperosmolar and in higher concentration causes diarrhea and in lower concentration reduces the crispness of the barium outline of mucosal folds. Initially, 300 mL of the suspension is given and the patient is turned to the right side or a single contrast upper gastrointestinal examination is done first. An equal second dose is subsequently sipped by the patient.

**Fluoroscopy.** Proximal loops of jejunum are best viewed with the patient horizontal and turned to the right. One or two compression spot films may be exposed. The patient should return for further fluoroscopy after having taken the second quantity of barium and having spent 10 or 15 minutes in the right lateral decubitus position. In some patients, barium has reached the terminal ileum in this time; others require a further period of right lateral recumbency. It is necessary for all bowel loops to be inspected while pressure is applied by the gloved hand or by a compression device. All loops must be separated from one another and viewed filled as well as flattened. Spot films should be taken of many of the loops using graded compression and virtually always some degree of rotation of the patient (Fig. 43–2A and B). This is continued until the terminal ileum has been studied and recorded on a spot film. Overhead views of the abdomen, with the patient prone, may be taken at intervals or only as a final film that serves for orientation (Fig. 43–2C). The emphasis of the examination must be on fluoroscopy and fluoroscopic spot filming. Attention should also be directed to a study of the mobility and pliability of all small bowel loops during compression.[18] The fluoroscopic follow-through using metoclopramide has been completed in 37.6 minutes in 25 of 50 patients.[19]

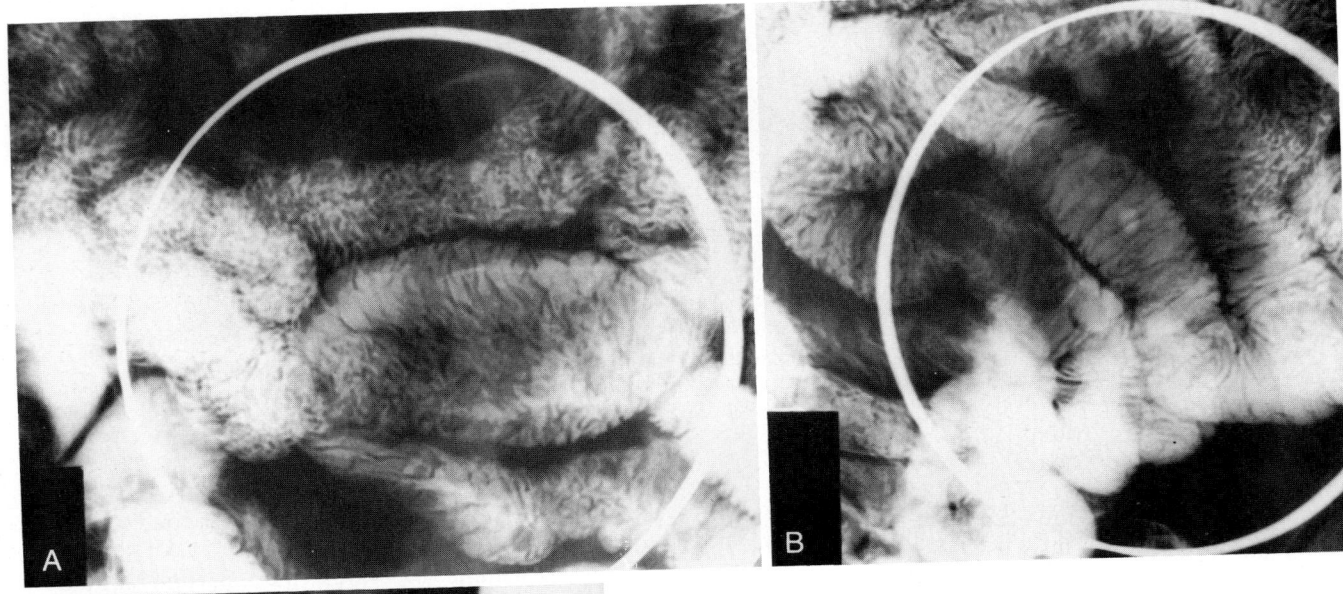

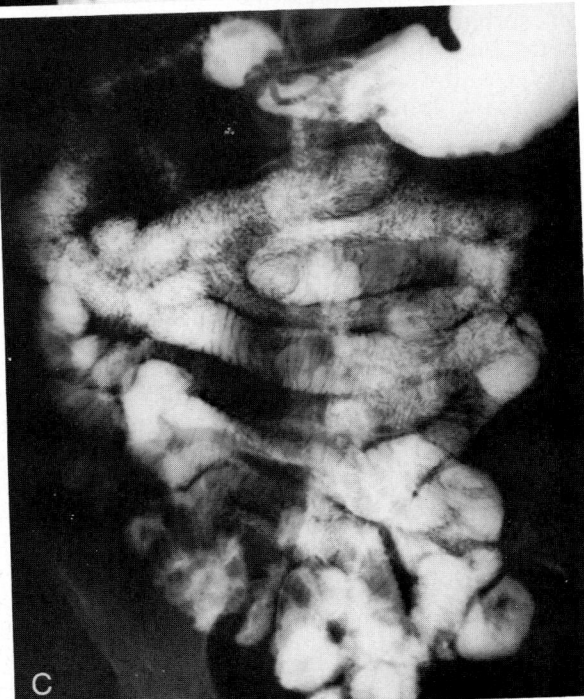

**Figure 43–2. Normal fluoroscopic small bowel follow-through. A.** Compression spot film of jejunal loops. **B.** Compression spot film of loops of proximal ileum. **C.** Final overhead radiograph.

**Premedication.** Metoclopramide serves primarily to speed transit of barium suspension out of the stomach and through the small bowel. It not only increases the amplitude of ring contractions and renders the sweeping action more effective but also increases resting tone and thus reduces lumen diameter. This action is most noticeable in the jejunum, where the mucosal folds have a less chaotic appearance and may assume a herringbone-like pattern[19] in which individual fold thicknesses can be estimated (Fig. 43–3). Occasionally, there may also be an increase of tone in the ileum, especially its pelvic loops. This is helpful because it shortens such loops, tends to elevate them out of the pelvis, and makes them available for compression.[19] The intragluteal injection of ceruletide after most of the barium has left the stomach has been found to cause more pronounced and at times excessive shortening and narrowing of these ileal loops[19] (Fig. 43–4). However, at present ceruletide is not available in the United States.

**Limitations and Indications.** A major limitation of fluoroscopic follow-through is the fact that drug-induced transit acceleration is inevitably associated with narrowing of the bowel lumen. In consequence, mucosal folds appear somewhat crowded and are often difficult to assess. A spurious appearance of nodularity may be produced by the overlap of loops with crowded folds. Furthermore, this technique cannot test the distensibility of the lumen and may miss segments with early mural infiltration.

The dedicated fluoroscopic follow-through adequately demonstrates longer bowel segments with nondistensible walls, such as those in radiation enteropathy, ischemia, and stenotic Crohn's disease. If combined with a pneumocolon, it is the peroral method of choice for investigation of the distal ileum. This additional technique should always be used whenever distal loops of ileum are not adequately outlined during the follow-through examination. It is a worthwhile supplementary procedure and is valuable in definite or questionable distal ileal inflammatory disease.

It has been suggested[20] that a double contrast upper gastrointestinal examination could be done at the end of the small bowel study if these two examinations had to be carried out in the same session. A likely problem of this examination sequence, however, would be an accumulation of barium in the transverse colon obscuring the stomach.

**Fluoroscopic Follow-through After Double Contrast Upper Gastrointestinal Examination.** This sequence of studies should be avoided for several reasons:

1. There is an excessive difference in concentration and viscosity (240% w/v against 40 to 50% w/v) between the barium suspensions used in double contrast study of the upper gastrointestinal tract and those suitable for small bowel passage. These suspensions do not readily mix and may remain largely separate by the time they reach the ileum.
2. The leading, heavier upper gastrointestinal barium suspension would tend to sink into pelvic loops of ileum and may inhibit transradiation. Suboptimal results are likely.
3. The gas or air introduced into the stomach for double contrast study passes rapidly into the small bowel and tends to break up the barium column.

## Double Contrast Follow-through

At the completion of the fluoroscopic small bowel follow-through, effervescent granules are administered with water to produce 700 to 800 mL of $CO_2$ (e.g., two packages of E-Z Gas, E-Z-EM Company). The patient is then positioned to direct the gas into the small intestine. Radiographs are taken with moderate compression during passage of the gas through the gut.

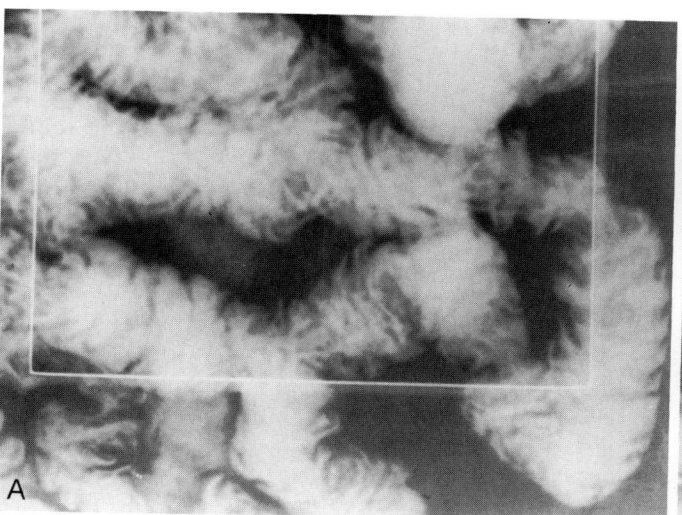
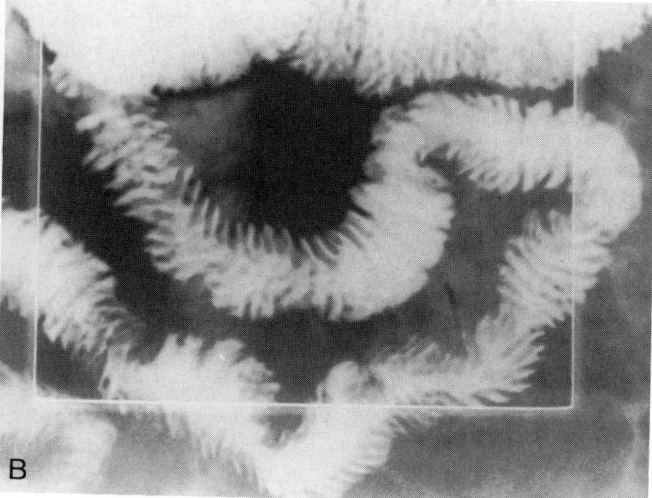

**Figure 43–3. The jejunum after metoclopramide. A.** The jejunum during follow-through examination before an intravenous injection of metoclopramide. **B.** After injection of metoclopramide a fairly regular herringbone pattern may develop. It is now possible to measure the thickness of the circular folds.

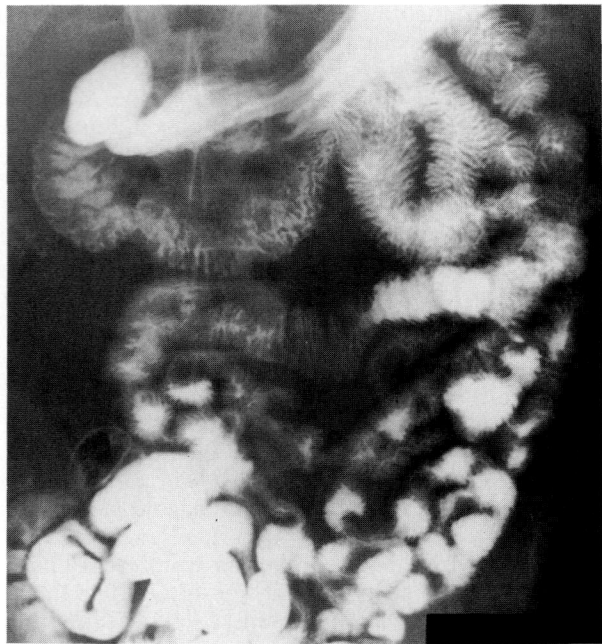

**Figure 43–4. Fluoroscopic follow-through after metoclopramide and ceruletide.** Herringbone patterns are seen in the jejunum. Ileal loops show vigorous contractions and are somewhat shortened and elevated out of the pelvis. The examination was completed in 20 minutes.

Small bowel double contrast was reported to have been attained in 43% of patients of a series.[21] In our experience, this method has not significantly enhanced the quality of fluoroscopic follow-through examinations.

## PERORAL PNEUMOCOLON

This technique is used to obtain double contrast views of the distal ileum and right colon after the oral administration of barium. After the barium has reached the cecum and right colon, 1 mg of glucagon is injected intravenously to promote reflux of air through the ileocecal valve and facilitate its retrograde extension into the ileum. A soft catheter is introduced into the rectum and air insufflation can begin. By rotating the patient, the air is advanced into the right colon and cecum.[22–25] Overdistention of the cecum should be avoided. To direct the air through the valve, it may help to have the patient turn to the left in a semiprone position. The rectal tube is removed as soon as sufficient air has entered the ileum. Spot films are then taken with compression. This technique can produce exquisite double contrast detail of the distal ileum and is able to distinguish clearly a pathologic from a normal appearance (Figs. 43–5 and 43–6). It may also be of value in double contrast imaging of the right colon, provided bowel preparation has been adequate. There is a failure rate of about 10%, however, when gas cannot be induced to reflux through the ileocecal valve.

## RETROGRADE SMALL BOWEL ENEMA

The complete reflux examination described by Miller[26] requires preparation of the colon as for a barium enema. Conscious sedation of the patient (1 to 3 mg of midazolam hydrochloride [Versed] intravenously with the usual safeguards) helps to allay discomfort. Glucagon 1 mg intravenously facilitates backflow through the ileocecal valve. A barium suspension of 20 to 30% w/v is infused, and up to 2 L may be needed. So that barium in the left colon does not hinder visualization of small bowel loops, only tap water at room temperature should be infused through the rectum if required after the 2 L of barium has been used. The colon may be drained after enough barium has refluxed into the small bowel.

This technique is no longer used frequently. Its major application at present is in the investigation of bowel obstruction thought from plain film study to be in either the distal ileum or the right colon. A barium enema should then be used as the first contrast study, to be extended into a reflux small bowel examination if the colon is found to be unobstructed.

## ENTEROCLYSIS (SMALL BOWEL ENEMA)

The terms *enteroclysis* and *small bowel enema* denote either the same intubation-based barium study of the small bowel or studies with minor differences in technique. Small bowel enema is the term most widely used in Europe, and enteroclysis predominates in the United States. Throughout this chapter, enteroclysis refers to several slightly different techniques of intubation-based barium examination of the small bowel, whether single contrast, double contrast, or biphasic.

### Historical Considerations

Passage of tubes into the duodenum was in common use in the 1920s,[27] mainly for aspiration of duodenal contents for the diagnosis of possible gallstone disease. Specialized tubes were designed, including one with an inflatable balloon used to obstruct the lumen of the duodenum for the injection of radiographic contrast medium into the distended duodenum above the balloon.[28] An article on direct visualization of lesions in the small intestine was published by Pesquera in 1929[29] and was the first description of an intubation-based small bowel examination. Ten years elapsed before another significant publication further advanced this method of examination. Gershon-Cohen and Shay[30] coined the term *barium enteroclysis;* they injected air after a barium-water infusion and claimed that the resulting double contrast filling offered a check on the findings in the single contrast phase. A larger series of tube studies was published by Schatzki in 1943.[31] He referred to the small bowel as the "step-child of roentgenology" and stressed

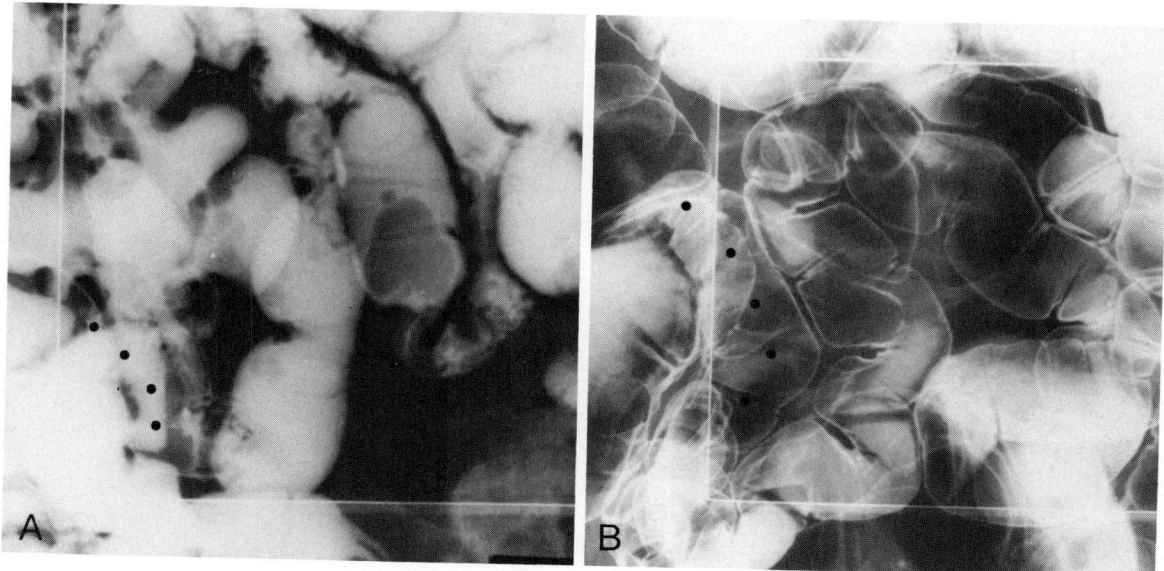

**Figure 43–5. Value of peroral pneumocolon for demonstration of normality. A.** Fluoroscopic follow-through fails to provide sufficient information about the terminal ileum *(dots)*. **B.** The peroral pneumocolon not only ascertains normality of the terminal ileum *(dots)* but also outlines additional normal loops of distal ileum.

the importance of a constant rate of inflow of the small bowel enema fluids. In a discussion after Schatzki's paper, Ross Golden suggested that it might be advantageous to use a tube with a balloon that could be inflated in the duodenum to prevent reflux of contrast materials, which would exit the tube distal to the balloon. Other clinically relevant papers appeared in England in 1960.[32, 33] Of crucial importance to the wider utilization of single contrast enteroclysis was the publi-

cation of a monograph by Sellink in 1971.[34] Trickey and co-workers[35] were the first to infuse a methylcellulose-containing solution as a double contrast agent after barium. This suggestion was taken up by Herlinger,[36] who described a fully standardized methylcellulose double contrast small bowel enema after several years of practice and evaluation. Further stimuli to the more widespread usage and diverse clinical applications of enteroclysis were the publications by Maglinte and

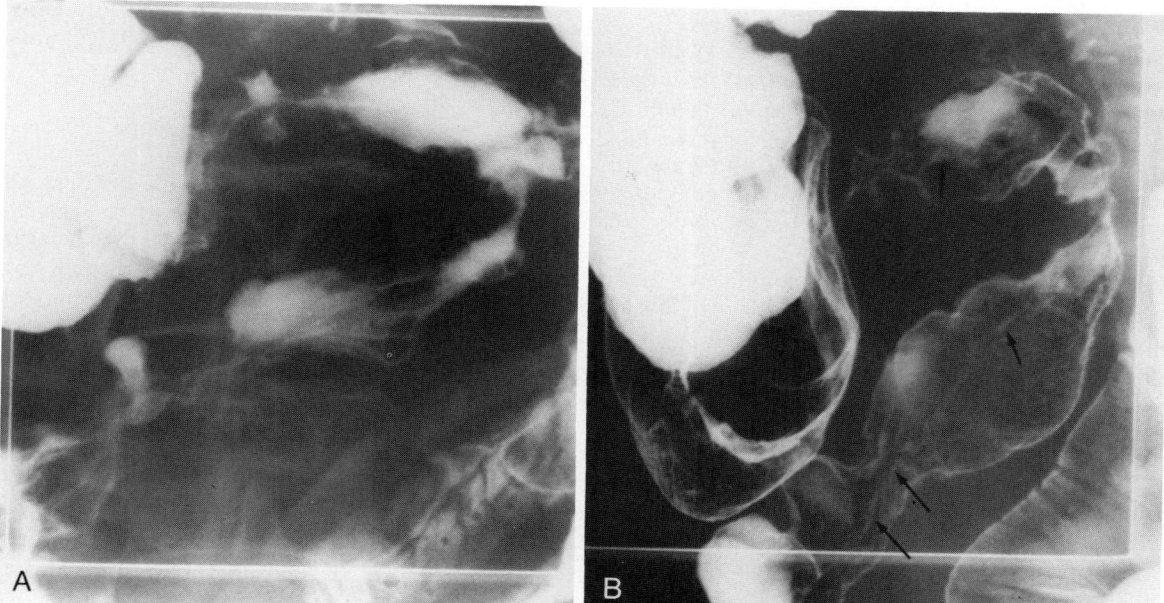

**Figure 43–6. Peroral pneumocolon provides more detailed information in a case of Crohn's disease of the terminal ileum. A.** Spot film in a fluoroscopic follow-through examination shows an abnormal terminal ileum consistent with Crohn's disease. **B.** The peroral pneumocolon demonstrates several linear and focal ulcerations *(arrows)* and confirms the presence of a stricture.

colleagues[37, 38] and Nolan[39] and additional work by Herlinger.[40] Other important papers came from Europe, among them works by Antes and Lissner,[41] Ekberg,[42] Fuchs and Geiter,[43] Salomonowitz and Czembirek,[44] Sanders and Ho,[45] and Fleckenstein and Pedersen.[46] Fleckenstein and Pedersen[46] in 1975 were the first to compare the follow-through examination and enteroclysis. They found the latter significantly better throughout the small bowel except for the terminal ileus, where the two techniques were of equal value.

## Drawbacks of Intubation Studies

The patient's discomfort associated with tube passage is the major disadvantage of enteroclysis. Gershon-Cohen, in a lecture to the Philadelphia Roentgen Ray Society in 1939, placed this in context: "[the] technique depends upon intubation of the duodenum and has the shortcomings inherent in this procedure. The ease and rapidity in which the entire small intestinal tract may be visualized more than compensates for this handicap."[30] The patient's discomfort during passage of the tube, however, must not be taken lightly by the radiologist. Reassurance, experience in the technique, and, when necessary, sedation of the patient are prerequisites.

Enteroclysis should not be undertaken unless there are symptoms or signs that indicate small bowel disease or the need to exclude it. The slightly higher radiation dose to the patient compared with that in follow-through examinations is then justified.[47]

## Advantages

Enteroclysis has the following inherent advantages:

1. By introducing barium beyond the gastric outflow–regulating action of the pylorus, contrast materials can be introduced directly into the small bowel as rapidly as indicated.
2. Lumen distention is controlled by the rate of infusion. By testing lumen distensibility, diseases that produce segments of reduced distensibility are rendered conspicuous.
3. Distention of the jejunum causes relative small bowel hypotonia, making it possible to display all dilated bowel loops simultaneously at the end of the examination.
4. Lumen distention is the most important aspect of enteroclysis; it is more important than double contrast. It causes straightening of the circular folds and makes it possible to determine morphologic normality on the basis of measurable parameters.
5. The examination is normally completed within 20 to 30 minutes.

## Single Contrast

An empty colon is desirable. The tube passed through the mouth should reach the distal duodenum. This is followed by infusion of a barium suspension with a concentration varying from 28% w/v in thin patients to 42% w/v in the obese. About 600 mL of barium suspension is infused at rates between 50 and 75 mL/min. More barium is required if the cecum has not been reached.

Water may be infused after the barium suspension to achieve better filling of the distal ileum, to provide a brief double contrast effect in the jejunum, to produce prestenotic distention, and to outline the colon in patients in whom a barium enema cannot be done.[48]

The Sellink technique has been modified by Nolan and Cadman.[49] Up to 1200 mL of a 19% w/v barium suspension is infused by gravity. Water is added when the terminal ileum has become opacified.

## Biphasic Enteroclysis with Methylcellulose

Before describing the overall technique in detail, it is useful to point to the few differences in the methods used by the chief proponents of enteroclysis. Maglinte[50] infuses 400 to 450 mL of a 50% w/v barium suspension (EntroBar) and usually completes the single contrast examination of all bowel loops before infusing methylcellulose. He may terminate the study with the single contrast examination if he thinks the clinical objective has been achieved. Herlinger[51] infuses 180 to 240 mL of an 80% w/v suspension of barium (Entero-H), filling only about half the small bowel. The infusion of methylcellulose then propels the denser barium toward the terminal ileum, gradually converting single into double contrast. Thus, all bowel loops are studied while lumen distention and transradiance increase. It is possible to terminate the examination before double contrast development has been completed. The following description of barium enteroclysis with methylcellulose applies to both methods.

### Preparation of the Patient

**Bowel Preparation.** I no longer advocate a barium enema–type preparation and do not suggest the use of magnesium citrate. Because a fairly clean right colon is desirable, a colon contact laxative should be administered during the late afternoon of the preceding day. Dulcolax, three or four tablets taken with one or two glasses of water, would be suitable. Nothing further is to be taken by mouth until the time of the examination. Emergency enteroclysis can be done without any bowel preparation.

**Drugs.** All peristalsis-inhibiting drugs should be discontinued, at least on the day of the examination. This applies strongly to morphine-like narcotic analgesics (e.g., Demerol).

Metoclopramide (Reglan) may be given as two tablets (10 mg each) 15 to 20 minutes before the examination. It may facilitate passage of the tube through and out of the stomach and promotes uninterrupted barium flow through the small bowel.[52] A rare complication may be release of catecholamines from a pheochromocytoma.[53]

**Conscious Sedation.** Anxious patients, including accompanied outpatients, should not be denied conscious sedation.[54] Midazolam may be used with care. Vital signs should be recorded at the start and at intervals through the study. Midazolam administration requires individualization of dosage. Midazolam should be injected intravenously as a 1-mg dose over 1 minute. Further 1-mg doses may be administered at intervals of no less than 5 minutes, without exceeding an overall maximum of 3 mg unless skilled personnel and equipment for the maintenance of airway patency are at hand. Respiratory depression is more likely to occur in aged and debilitated patients, in whom a dose of 1 mg should not be exceeded. Midazolam does not significantly affect small bowel peristaltic activity.

Diazepam (Valium), 3 mg injected slowly intravenously, has been found to be an effective anxiolytic agent.[54] Rarely, it is necessary, in younger, generally fit patients, to increase the dose to 5 mg. I advise diluting the diazepam with aspirated blood before injecting it and always injecting it into a vein.

Accompanied outpatients, after sedation, should remain in the department until they are seen by the radiologist and are considered fit to leave.

**Topical Anesthesia for Transnasal Intubation.** Xylocaine viscous, a 2% solution of lidocaine, is used as a surface anesthetic for the nasal passage and nasopharynx. Up to 5 mL can be instilled slowly into one nostril while the other nostril is compressed. The patient is asked to breathe through the mouth during instillation and to swallow when the viscous material is felt at the back of the throat. During instillation the patient's head is tilted back slightly and then angled to one side and the other. Additional surface anesthesia is rarely needed.

**Topical Anesthesia for Peroral Intubation.** Cetacaine spray (Cetylite Industries, Pennsauken, NJ) contains 2% of dose-limiting tetracaine. This rapidly acting surface anesthetic is sprayed to the back of the throat, including the uvula and the posterior wall of the oropharynx. Its flavor is not generally appreciated by patients. A total spraying time of 2 seconds should not be exceeded. Toxic complications are rare.

## Intubation

**Catheters.** Maglinte's catheter with an inflatable balloon[55] near the catheter tip and proximal to its side ports has found widespread acceptance (Maglinte catheter, Cook Inc., Bloomington, IN). A similar catheter with a silicone balloon is produced by E-Z-EM. Both catheters are 12 French in caliber and permit balloon distention with up to 20 mL of air. In the Cook catheter, the portion beyond the balloon is too long and tends to buckle. The side holes are large enough to allow passage of a guidewire, a potential source of damage to the bowel wall. The purpose of the inflated balloon is to prevent or at least greatly reduce reflux into the stomach. This makes it possible to select infusion rates suited to each patient's examination. Occasionally, patients complain of epigastric pain when the balloon has been

fully inflated. Aspiration of about 3 mL of air from the balloon immediately stops the pain.

When a balloon catheter is not required, it is possible to use a catheter of much reduced diameter. An 8 French catheter is now available from Nicholas GmbH (Sulzbach/Ts, Germany). The package includes an oily lubricant for injection into the catheter to avoid problems during withdrawal of the stiffening wire. When this catheter is used for the Herlinger type of enteroclysis, I recommend diluting Entero-H to a 70% w/v suspension.

**Transnasal Catheter Introduction.** With the guidewire some 5 inches short of the tip, the lubricated catheter is gently introduced while the patient's neck is maximally extended. Slight resistance is normally felt at the posterior wall of the nasopharynx. Force must never be used to overcome it. Instead, the catheter should be pulled back slightly, rotated, and advanced again. When the catheter is beyond this point, the patient should be asked to flex the head toward the chest and swallow while the catheter is advanced through the pharynx and esophagus.

**Peroral Catheter Introduction.** With the patient sitting at the edge of the x-ray table and surface anesthetic given as previously described, the catheter is placed over the tongue under vision. The patient is then asked to flex the head toward the chest and to try to swallow without fully closing teeth or lips. The catheter is then inserted rapidly as far as the approximate level of the lower esophageal sphincter. If resistance is encountered at any level of insertion, fluoroscopy is required before further advance. If the catheter tip has doubled over within the esophagus, further insertion should continue under fluoroscopy until the doubled-over segment has entered the stomach. It is easy to straighten out the catheter in the stomach by partly withdrawing it and partly advancing the guidewire.

**Catheter Passage Through the Stomach.** More often than not, the catheter tip is found to have entered the fundal recess. The patient should be turned fully to the right and the catheter taken back to the cardia and reintroduced with slight tip rotation toward the right (Fig. 43–7A and B). In patients with a large fundus and horizontal stomach, the guidewire is held back at the cardia and the catheter advanced over it through almost 360 degrees within the fundal recess until it enters the elevated body of the stomach and passes to the right.

The catheter may readily pass through the antrum into the duodenal bulb. More often it is necessary to determine the position of the bulb first. This is usually achieved by turning the patient to the left. By using a hand-operated device for abdominal compression or by manipulating the curved tip of the torque-controlled guidewire, it should then be possible to direct the catheter into the bulb (Fig. 43–7C).

Passage through the upper duodenal flexure is facilitated with the patient turned to the left. The stomach then shifts toward the left, taking with it the mobile first part of duodenum and thus widening the flexure (Fig. 43–7D). Catheter advance through the lower duodenal flexure may occur spontaneously or be helped by craniad-directed hand pressure. During all these maneuvers,

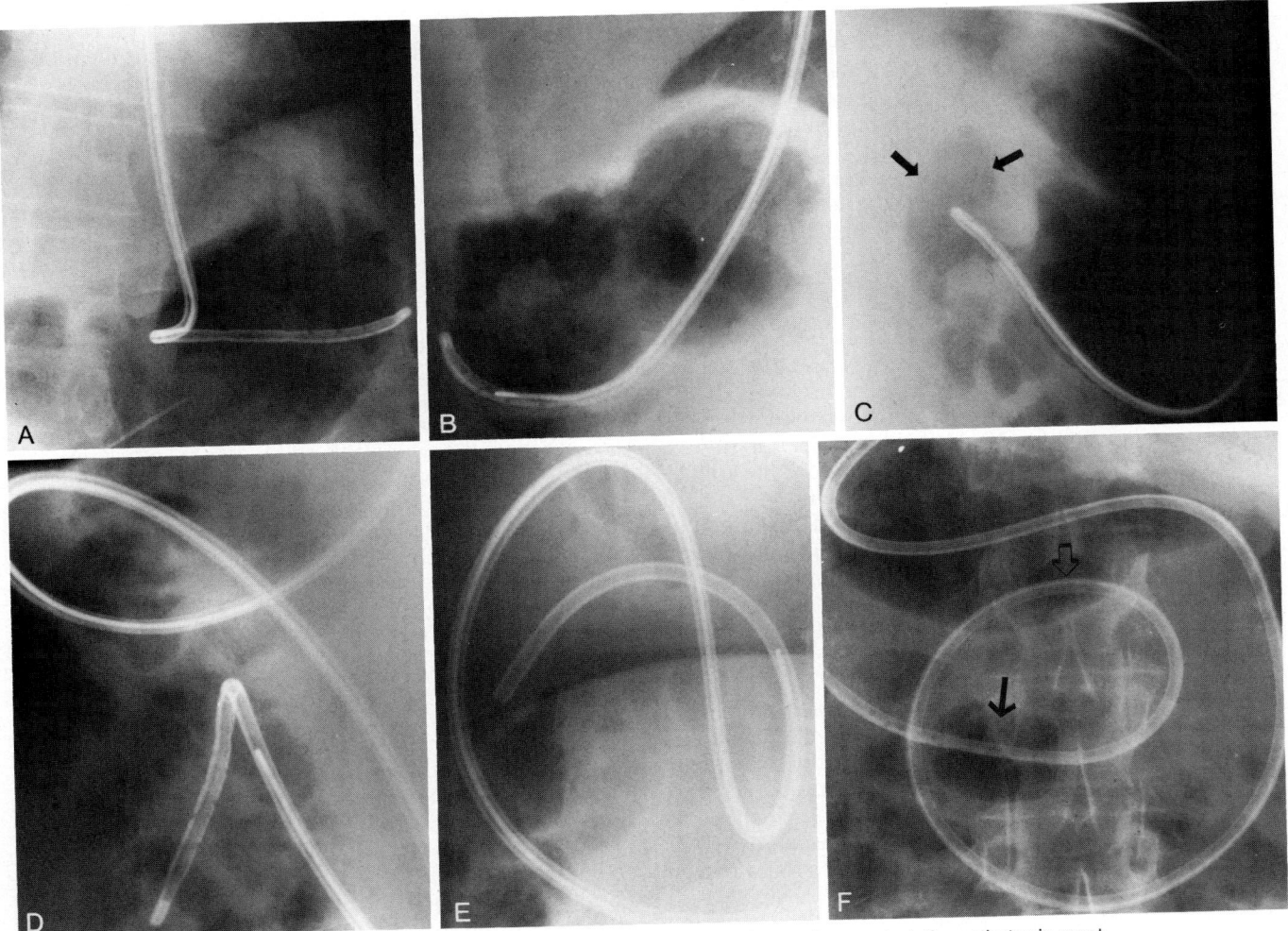

**Figure 43–7. Intubation technique. A.** After intubation with the patient seated, the catheter is most often found to have entered the gastric fundus. **B.** With the patient turned fully right, it is usually simple to rotate the catheter and move it into the body of the stomach. **C.** It may be necessary to turn the patient well to the left to outline the duodenal bulb with gastric air *(arrows).* With the help of the guidewire it is then possible to move the catheter into the bulb. **D.** The patient may have to turn further to the left to widen the upper duodenal flexure, especially if the patient is slim. The catheter is then advanced through it while the wire is held back. **E.** Having taken the catheter into the ascending duodenum, the patient should turn into a semiprone position to widen the duodenojejunal flexure. The catheter is usually advanced into the first loop of jejunum with the wire held back. **F.** The catheter has now entered sufficiently into the jejunum (the patient is prone). The balloon has been inflated *(solid arrow).* (Open arrow indicates ligament of Treitz.)

the curved tip of the guidewire is held back at the nearest curvature and the catheter is advanced over it.

To negotiate the duodenojejunal flexure, it is first necessary to decrease its usually acute angulation. The patient should be turned to one side and then further into a semiprone position. This allows the jejunum on its mesentery to fall away slightly from the retroperitoneal duodenum. The patient is asked to breathe deeply and cough intermittently until the catheter has entered the first loop of jejunum (Fig. 43–7E). During this advance, the curved tip of the guidewire is held at or near the inferior duodenal flexure. If possible, the catheter should be advanced far enough into the jejunum for the inflated balloon to be beyond the ligament of Treitz (Fig. 43–7F). When using a balloon catheter, it is not necessary to take much time to achieve entry into the jejunum. It may suffice to place the balloon in the distal duodenum, just beyond the level of superior mesenteric vessels.

For further details of tube manipulation, the reader should consult reference[55] or, better still, attend an enteroclysis-practicing department of radiology.

**Complications of Intubation.** There is a single report of duodenal perforation during catheter passage.[56] To avoid this, the guidewire must always be kept within the catheter. No force should be used if there is resistance to catheter advance. When the catheter is held up at an unusual site, a small amount of barium should be injected to detect the cause (e.g., possible entry into a diverticulum).

## Infusion of Contrast Materials

**Methods of Infusion.** For occasional enteroclysis, a low-cost, hand-operated plastic pump (Jack Rabbit pump, Black and Decker) may be adequate. However, it provides only an approximate estimate of flow rate. The ideal instrument is an electric peristaltic pump (e.g., RS-7800 Minipump, Renal Systems, Minneapolis, MN). It makes possible an accurately adjustable and continuous rate of flow,[57] suitable especially for infusion of methylcellulose and of the larger amount of lower-density barium used in the Maglinte method. In the Herlinger method it is relevant to know with some accuracy how much of the higher-density barium is being introduced. It has therefore been customary to use 60-mL syringes for the injection of 180 to 220 mL of barium or to use an electric pump to infuse it from a calibrated container (Fig. 43–8).

**Rates of Flow.** Sellink suggested that infusions be started at a flow rate of 75 mL/min for initial evaluation of the motility response.[58] Further adjustment of the flow rate is based on these considerations:

1. Infused barium should advance through the bowel in an uninterrupted column and without causing undue focal lumen distention. Flow rates are adjusted accordingly.
2. Flow rate matters greatly during the infusion of methylcellulose. Higher rates increasingly dilate the proximal jejunum, causing hypotonia throughout the small bowel and slowing progress. Too low

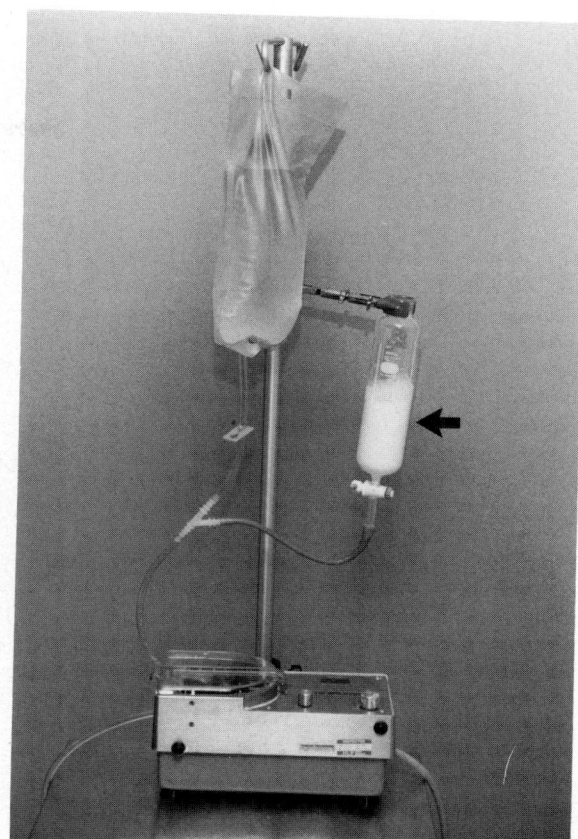

**Figure 43–8. Arrangement of apparatus for pump infusion of barium and methylcellulose by the Herlinger method.** A calibrated container *(arrow)* is used to control the amount of barium infused. The tubing from container through pump and to patient holds 50 mL of barium at the start of the infusion.

a rate causes insufficient lumen distention with accelerated passage. Thus, fluoroscopy is essential for correct selection of the rate of flow.

**Infusion of Barium, the Single Contrast Phase.** Maglinte, who usually infuses up to 450 mL of barium, stops its introduction as soon as the distal ileum has become opacified. He may then terminate the study or proceed with the infusion of methylcellulose to obtain double contrast (Fig. 43–9). For the Herlinger technique, 180 to 220 mL is introduced, depending on the size of the patient. More barium is required for large patients and for those with a dilated bowel and fluid increase (as in obstruction or malabsorption). The single contrast phase continues distally during the initial stages of methylcellulose infusion, which propels the denser barium toward the ileocecal valve (Fig. 43–10). Compression fluoroscopy is important in the single contrast phase. Spot films should be taken when an abnormality is suspected. The jejunum is best imaged with the patient turned to the right, the ileum with the patient supine or turned left. Infusion of methylcellulose follows that of barium, usually without interruption.

**Purpose of Methylcellulose.** Methylcellulose has the following functions in enteroclysis:

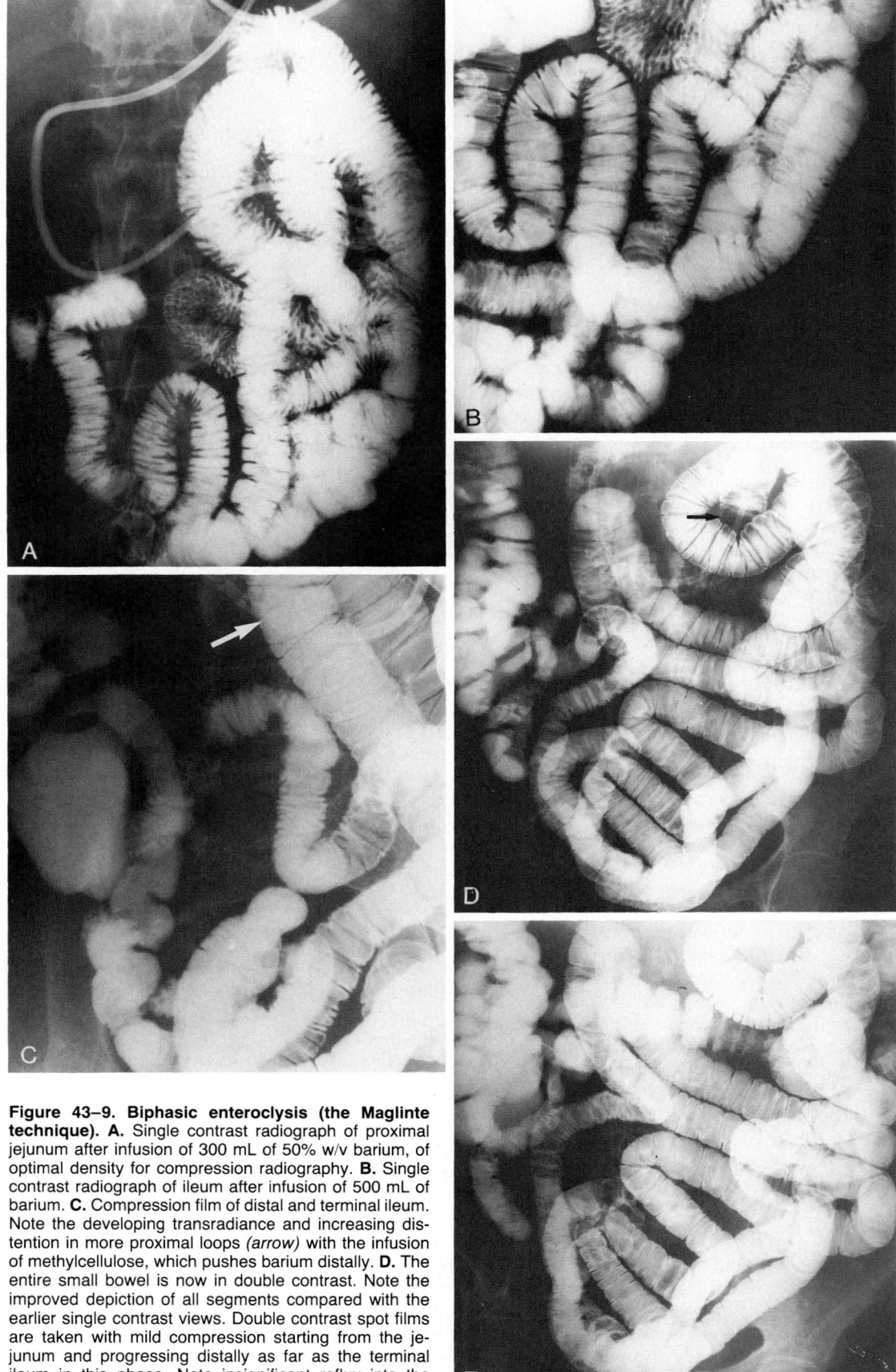

**Figure 43–9. Biphasic enteroclysis (the Maglinte technique). A.** Single contrast radiograph of proximal jejunum after infusion of 300 mL of 50% w/v barium, of optimal density for compression radiography. **B.** Single contrast radiograph of ileum after infusion of 500 mL of barium. **C.** Compression film of distal and terminal ileum. Note the developing transradiance and increasing distention in more proximal loops *(arrow)* with the infusion of methylcellulose, which pushes barium distally. **D.** The entire small bowel is now in double contrast. Note the improved depiction of all segments compared with the earlier single contrast views. Double contrast spot films are taken with mild compression starting from the jejunum and progressing distally as far as the terminal ileum in this phase. Note insignificant reflux into the duodenum proximal to the inflated balloon *(arrow)*. **E.** Radiograph obtained after tube removal. Absence of barium in the sigmoid colon is not unusual in a properly executed enteroclysis. An understanding of the response of the small bowel to changed rates of flow renders the double contrast appearance and the degree of bowel distention reproducible.

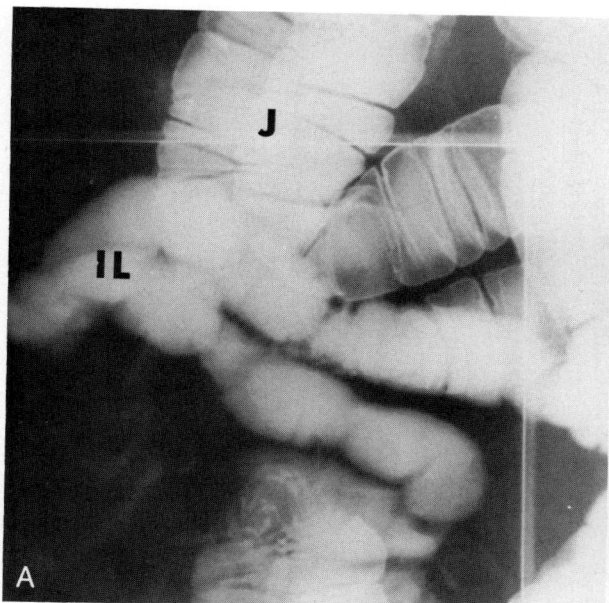
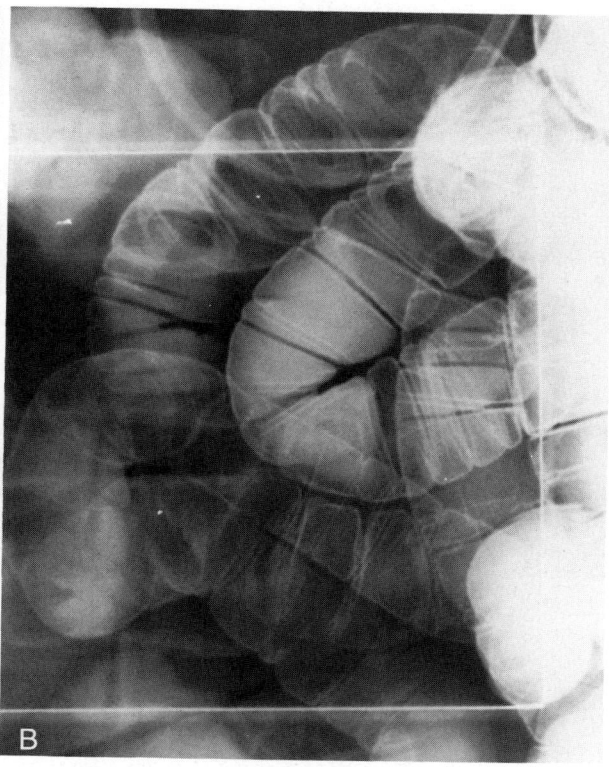

**Figure 43–10. The single contrast phase advances before the developing double contrast. A.** A loop of ileum, as yet nondistended in single contrast, has crossed close to an already distended loop of jejunum in developing double contrast. IL = ileum; J = jejunum. **B.** Later, both loops are imaged in double contrast distention.

1. It propels the barium column into the distal ileum and the colon.
2. It gradually distends the small bowel lumen, straightens the circular folds, and tests the distensibility of individual segments. Nondistended bowel loops can give misleading information (e.g., a false impression of nodulation) (Fig. 43–11).
3. It has low diffusivity with compatible barium suspensions and thus preserves an interface between the density of the barium coating the mucosa and the water density of the distended lumen. Provided that vigorous abdominal compression has been avoided during this stage, double contrast develops throughout the small bowel and persists for 15 to 20 minutes. However, even with the best technique, there is some diffusion of barium into methylcellulose and this becomes more noticeable in the ileum. The double contrast density difference between barium and methylcellulose is therefore greatest in the jejunum.
4. As a result of either double contrast or merely dilution and transradiance, intestinal surface detail can be studied even when two or three bowel loops overlap (see Fig. 43–10B). This is important because lumen distention within the limited space of the peritoneal cavity increases the incidence of overlapping bowel loops.
5. On entry into the colon, methylcellulose promotes evacuation of barium.

**Infusion of Methylcellulose, the Double Contrast Phase.** A 0.5% solution of methylcellulose in water can be prepared from commercially available methylcellulose powder. The details of preparation have been described.[36] Ready-made preparations of hydroxypropyl methylcellulose must be diluted with an equal volume of water to obtain a 0.5% solution. These preparations are hydroxypropyl methylcellulose (Methocel) and Enterocel (Lafayette Pharmacal, Lafayette, IN).

The methylcellulose infusion follows that of barium, usually without delay. A total of 1500 to 2000 mL is needed if good double contrast is to be achieved throughout the small bowel. The infusion rate is related to the rate at which barium has moved through the small bowel. Thus, faster barium flow is usually followed by a faster infusion of methylcellulose (80 to 120 mL/min). It is always important, even with balloon catheters, to avoid significant reflux into the stomach. Such reflux could be dangerous in feeble, elderly patients, in whom esophageal reflux and aspiration of the refluxed material could be a serious complication.

Maglinte, by opacifying all of the small bowel with barium at 50% w/v, emphasizes the single contrast phase and has the option of terminating the examination at that state (see Fig. 43–11). When it is considered relevant to achieve good double contrast in the distended bowel loops by either method, care must be taken during methylcellulose infusion (i.e., the phase of developing double contrast). Abrupt compression of the abdomen and sudden release of compression are to be avoided because they would promote mixing of barium and methylcellulose. Even abrupt movements of the patient should be avoided. When double contrast has fully developed, abdominal compression can be applied more freely.

## Fluoroscopy and Radiography

The conducting radiologist must be present during the entire enteroclysis. There is much to be done when the

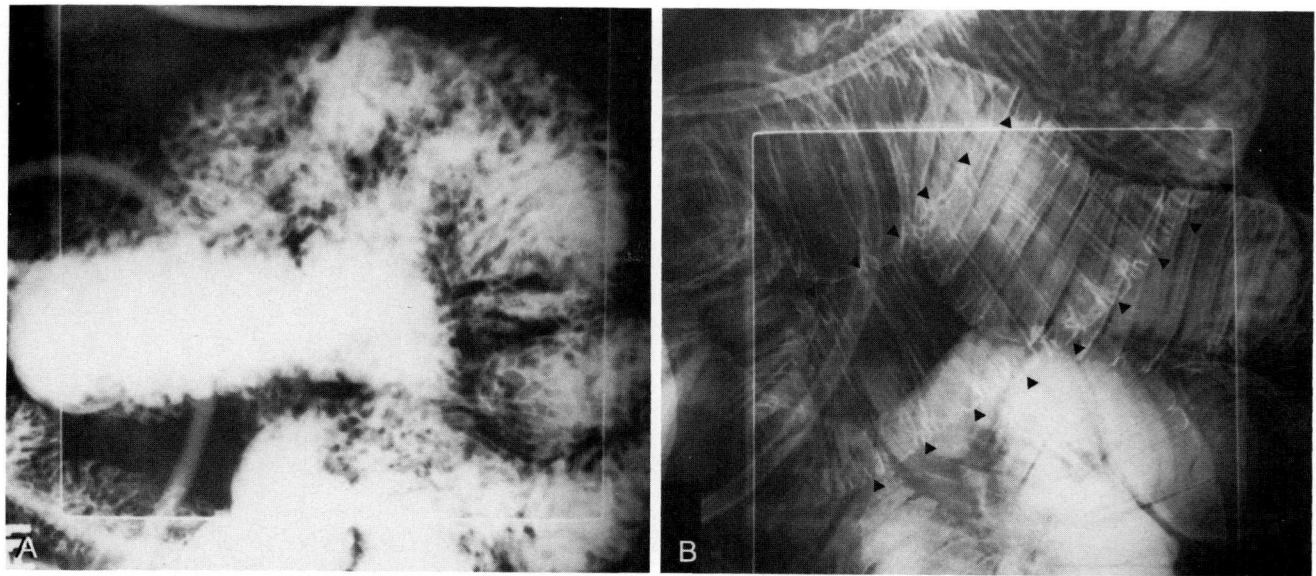

**Figure 43–11. Enteroclysis, proximal jejunum. A.** Single contrast radiograph showing lumen of loops mostly collapsed; superimposition of crisscrossing folds produces a false impression of nodulation. **B.** Same loops in methylcellulose-induced double contrast distention. All folds are normal and straight, with parallel sides. This view also illustrates the ability to visualize surface detail in superimposed loops (crossing loop indicated by arrowheads).

catheter has been positioned and infusions have begun. The sequence of loop opacification should be monitored by intermittent fluoroscopy during the single contrast phase. Individual loops should be examined by compression with the patient suitably rotated. During methylcellulose infusion in the Herlinger method, attention must be given to the gradual dilution and double contrast development proximally and, at the same time, to the further advance of the single contrast phase in distal bowel loops. In the distal ileum, where loops frequently become crowded and may not be accessible to compression, it is useful to take early spot films in single contrast to aid evaluation later (Fig. 43–12).

Several spot films obtained with compression are exposed during all phases of developing double contrast (Figs. 43–13 to 43–15). Final spot films of all segments in double contrast are usually obtained. The infusion of methylcellulose is then stopped. With the tube still in place, the examination is completed by taking an overhead view of the abdomen on a 17 × 14 film with the patient prone (Fig. 43–16). This view demonstrates the entire small bowel in continuing double contrast and is useful for orientation. Often, another overhead film is obtained to demonstrate distal bowel loops. The tube is angled 35 degrees caudad to project more posterior distal loops beyond those lying anteriorly that would otherwise obscure them (see Fig. 43–12C).

The radiologist then deflates the balloon and removes the catheter. It is occasionally useful to bring the patient back after bowel evacuation for further study of the area of the terminal ileum.

**Bowel Prolapsed into the Pelvis.** After hysterectomy or any pelvic exenteration, ileal loops may prolapse extensively into the pelvis and may even be fixed in position by adhesions. The usual compression views with the patient supine are unhelpful. The best possible images are obtained with the patient in a lateral or off-lateral position after all prolapsed loops have become transradiant (Fig. 43–17). The 35-degree angled view with the patient prone is also helpful.

**Practical Pointers.** If in doubt about the amount of barium to be infused by the Herlinger method, it is better to err on the side of too much. In such cases or when flow through the small intestine has been too rapid, barium and methylcellulose may advance into the colon and reach the rectum before distal small bowel double contrast has been achieved. At this stage patients find it difficult not to void. To deal with this problem, I always have available an empty barium enema set. I insert the nozzle into the rectum and allow the contents to drain into the bag while the methylcellulose infusion continues until the entire small bowel has been adequately imaged.

In some cases of small bowel obstruction, proximal loops may become distended with barium and methylcellulose. After taking the films, I now leave the catheter in position, disconnect it from the pump, and promote siphonage of excess fluid (Fig. 43–18). Later, the catheter is removed in the usual way.

For patients referred because of obscure blood loss and for others with malabsorption, I add an examination of the distal duodenum and of the duodenojejunal flexure to the standard enteroclysis. After the overhead filming, the balloon is deflated and the catheter pulled back into the mid-duodenum. The balloon is then reinflated and further injections of barium, often with air double contrast, are made. The purpose is to include an area that is often not visualized during upper endoscopy.

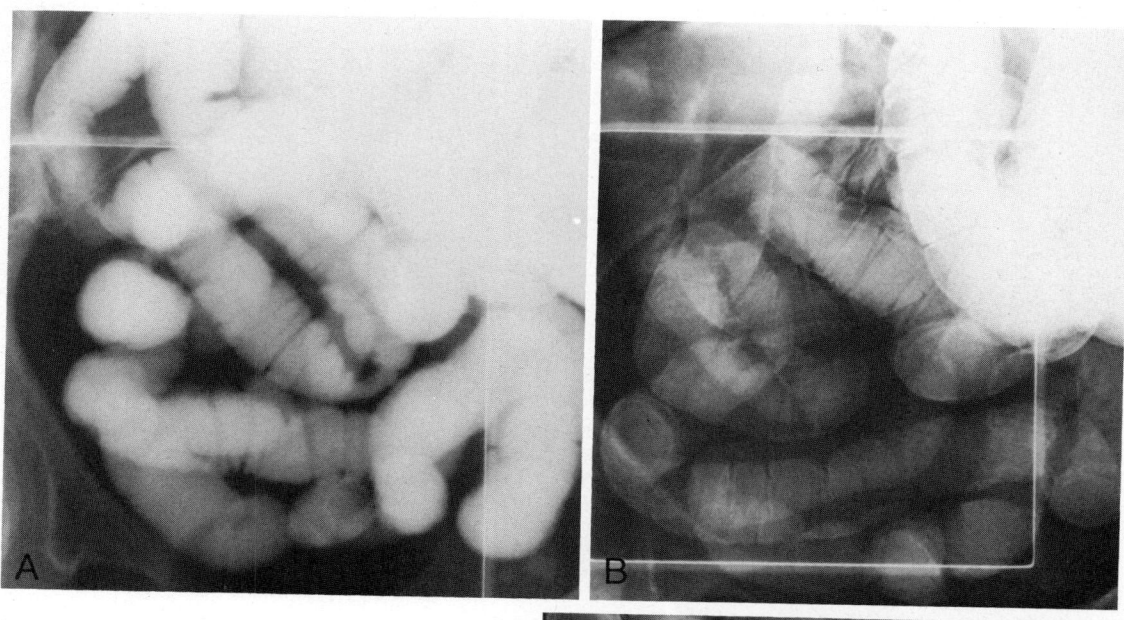

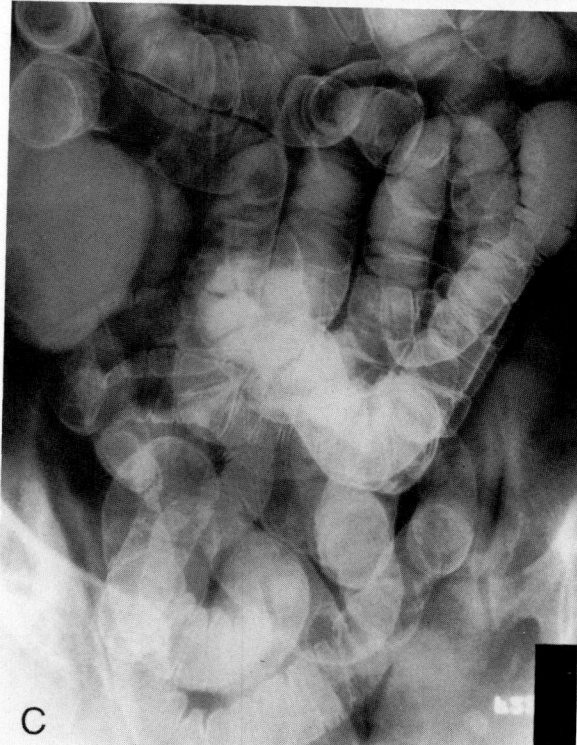

**Figure 43–12. Distal ileal loops.** These loops should be spot filmed in single and double contrast, at times aided by an angled view. **A.** Distal ileum shown in single contrast with compression. There is possible abnormality of the most distal segment. **B.** Same segments seen in double contrast. Normality is still in doubt. **C.** An overhead view with the patient prone and the tube angled 35 degrees caudad clearly demonstrates normal appearance of distal loops of ileum.

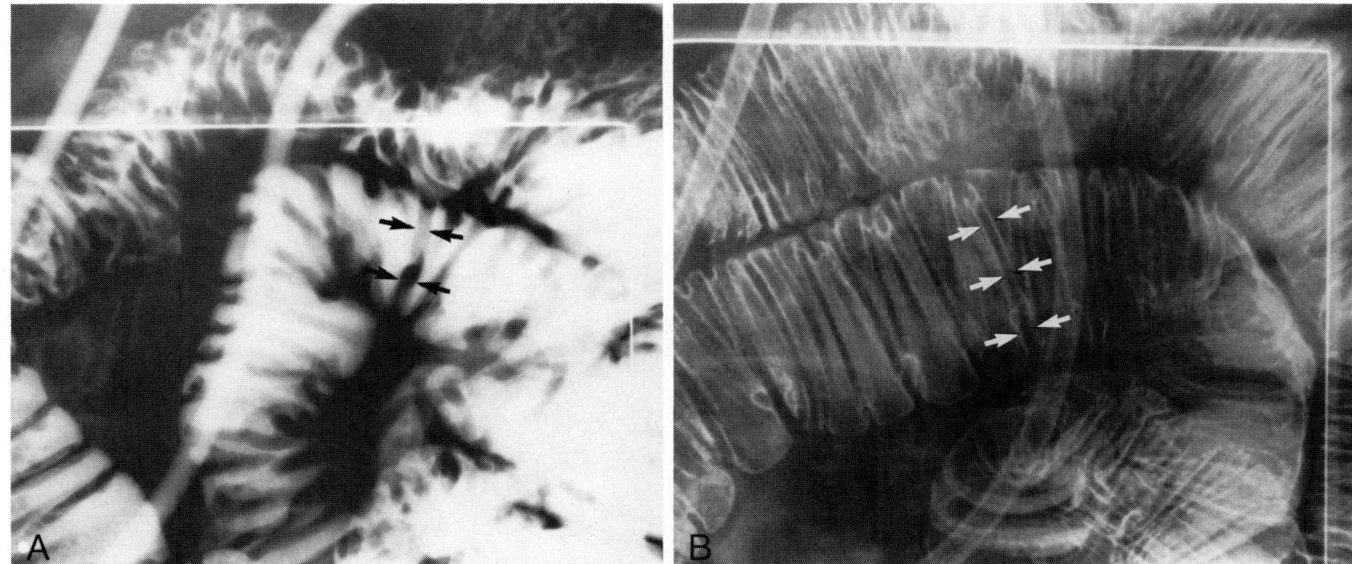

**Figure 43–13. Proximal loops of jejunum in single and double contrast. A.** Single contrast radiograph with insufficient distention. Note the thickness of a jejunal fold *(arrows)*. **B.** The same segments in double contrast with lumen distention. The same fold *(arrows)* now appears less thick and is shown in its fully straightened state, in which measurements of normal values should always be made.

## DOUBLE CONTRAST ENTEROCLYSIS WITH AIR

This has been the standard method of enteroclysis in Japan for many years.[59–61] After intubation, 400 to 500 mL of 60% w/v barium suspension is slowly injected. Injection of air is begun after barium has reached the terminal ileum. Compression spot films of the jejunum are taken. An anticholinergic agent is injected as soon as air reaches the cecum. Further spot films are obtained.[61]

This technique has the advantages over methylcellulose enteroclysis that there is a greater double contrast density difference and that mixing between the two contrast materials is impossible. Yet, I have not found this technique to be consistently successful for the overall demonstration of the small intestine. It is, however, the best way to demonstrate clearly specific small bowel segments, usually as a further study in special cases of inflammatory bowel disease (Fig. 43–19).

## QUANTITATIVE DETERMINATION OF NORMALITY

Morphologic normality can be established with considerable accuracy and is based on observations of Kerckring's folds, lumen diameters, wall thickness, and villi.

*Kerckring's folds* (plicae circulares, valvulae conniventes) are bands of mucosa containing a fibrovascular core of submucosa. The folds are more crowded in the jejunum (four to seven per inch) and gradually become more widely separated to only two to four folds per inch in the ileum. The folds are also deeper and thicker (up

to 2 mm) in the jejunum, shallower and thinner (about 1 mm) in the ileum (Fig. 43–20A and B). It is important to measure these fold thicknesses and number per length during adequate lumen distention (see Fig. 43–13A and B).

*Lumen diameters* decrease gradually from jejunum into ileum. In the lumen-distending enteroclysis, upper limits of normality are somewhat technique dependent and are usually considered to be 4.5 cm for the proximal jejunum and 3.5 cm for the ileum.

*Wall thickness:* When two adjacent bowel loops are found to be strictly parallel to each other over a distance of some 5 cm, the distance between the two barium-coated mucosal surfaces represents the combined wall thickness. This normally gives a reading of 1 to 2 mm for a single wall thickness (Fig. 43–21).

*Villi* are finger-like, submillimeter projections containing a core of lamina propria covered by epithelium. Their projection into a barium layer can produce tiny relative radiolucencies that are better seen on the edge of folds (Fig. 43–22). This appearance should not be confused with the earliest changes of flocculation, which can produce a similar but fine linear radiolucency pattern. It has been claimed that double contrast enteroclysis using a guaran-modified barium suspension would show normal villi consistently.[62]

## ACCURACY OF ENTEROCLYSIS AND SMALL BOWEL FOLLOW-THROUGH

Ideally, enteroclysis and the dedicated small bowel follow-through should be compared prospectively, performing both with the same consecutive patients and

*Text continued on page 785*

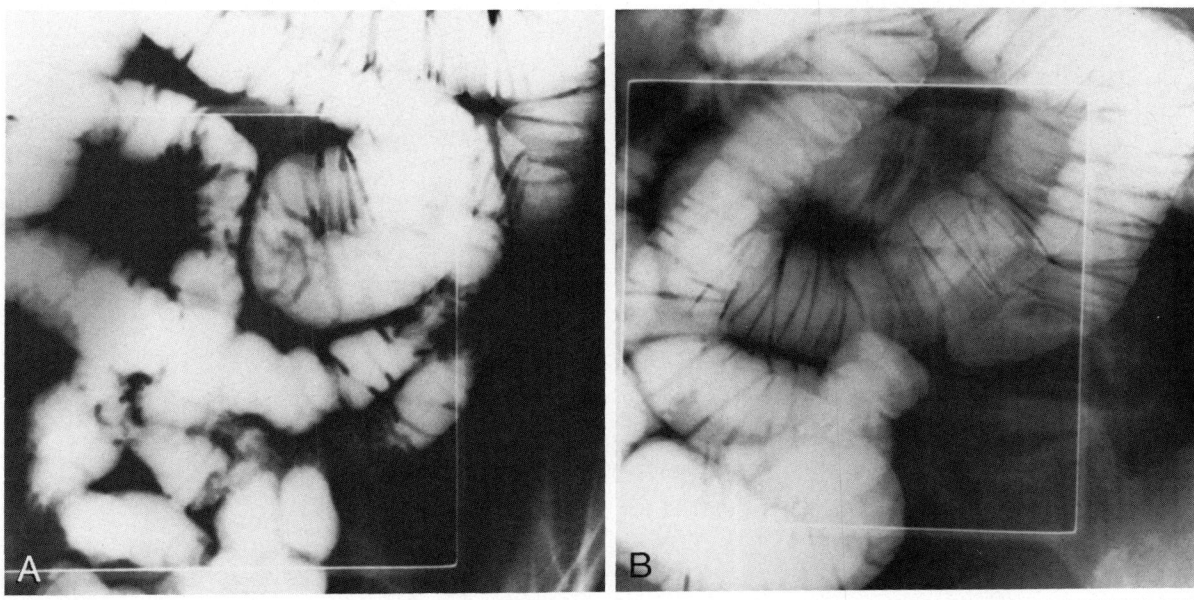

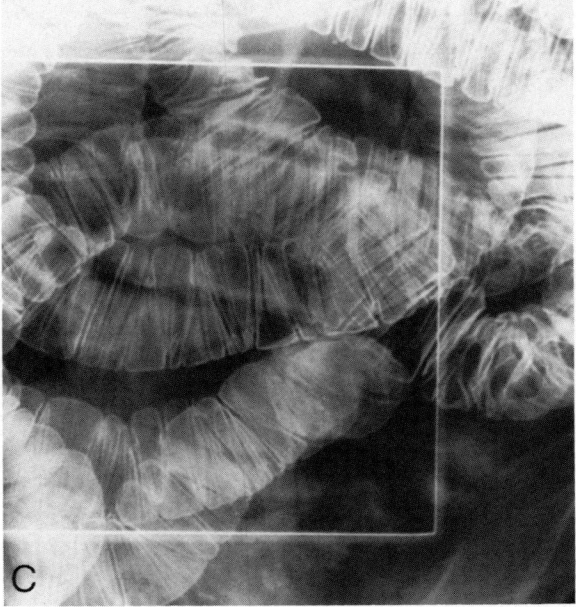

**Figure 43–14. Mid–small bowel in three stages of opacification. A.** Single contrast radiograph, with bowel not yet distended. **B.** Single contrast radiograph, with barium somewhat diluted by methylcellulose, lumen fully distended. Some lesions are shown well at this stage (e.g., melanoma metastases), and further infusions can be halted. **C.** Same segments in double contrast. The shape and distribution of folds appear no better than in the distended single contrast phase **(B)**. However, any finer surface pathologic feature, linear or micronodular, would be identified only in this view.

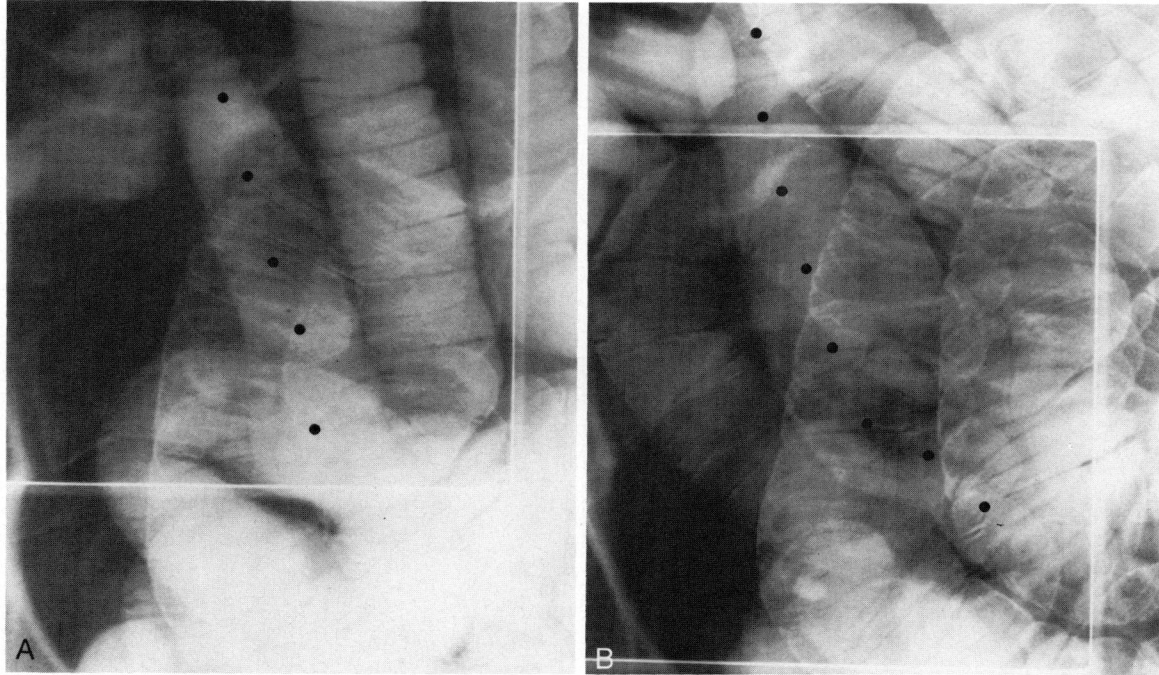

**Figure 43–15. Distal ileum in single and double contrast. A.** Terminal ileum *(dots)* and other distal loops in diluted single contrast, well distended. **B.** Same area in double contrast; more of the terminal ileum is now visible *(dots).* Note the reduced contrast between the barium covering the mucosa and the barium-admixed methylcellulose occupying the lumen.

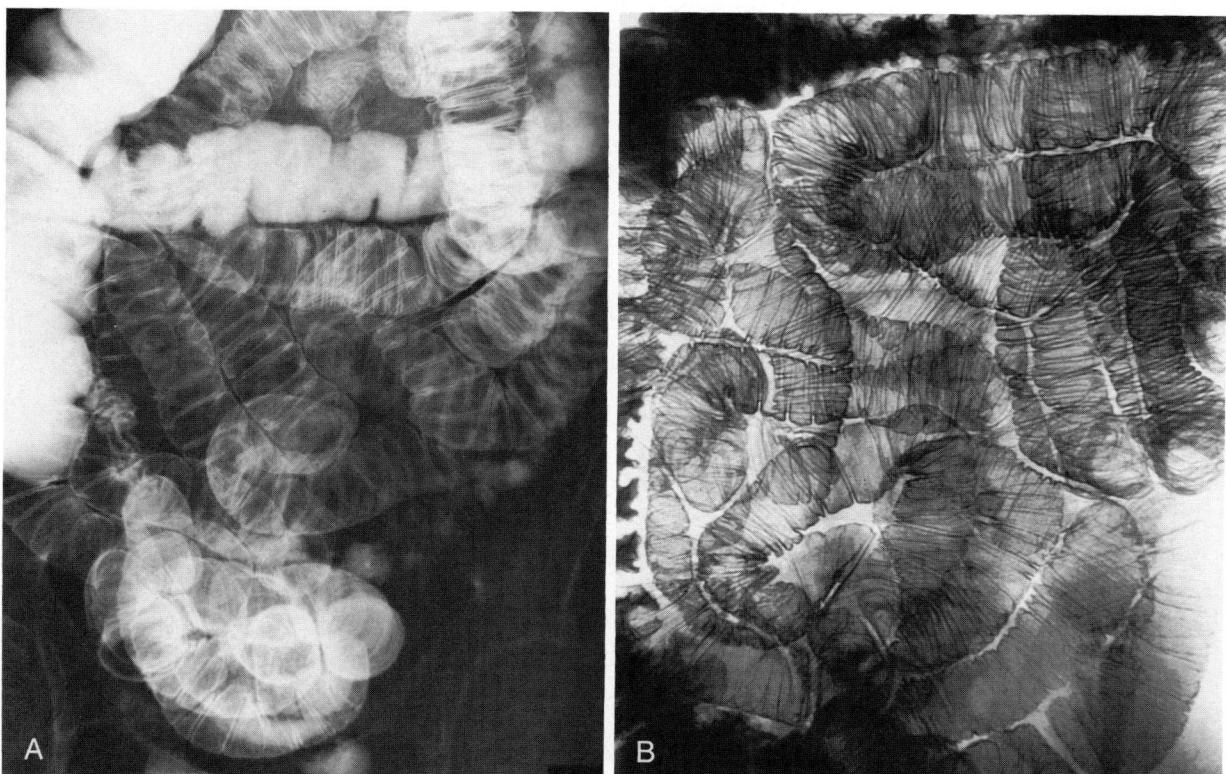

**Figure 43–16. End of enteroclysis, final overhead films with the patient prone. A.** Normal overhead view. Note persisting barium coating of mucosal surfaces and continued distention of the lumen by methylcellulose. Surplus barium has filled the colon as far as the splenic flexure. A prone, caudad-angled view would be obtained in this case to separate the normal-appearing loops of distal ileum. **B.** In another case the final overhead film was digitized and reversed, showing normality in an aesthetically pleasing form.

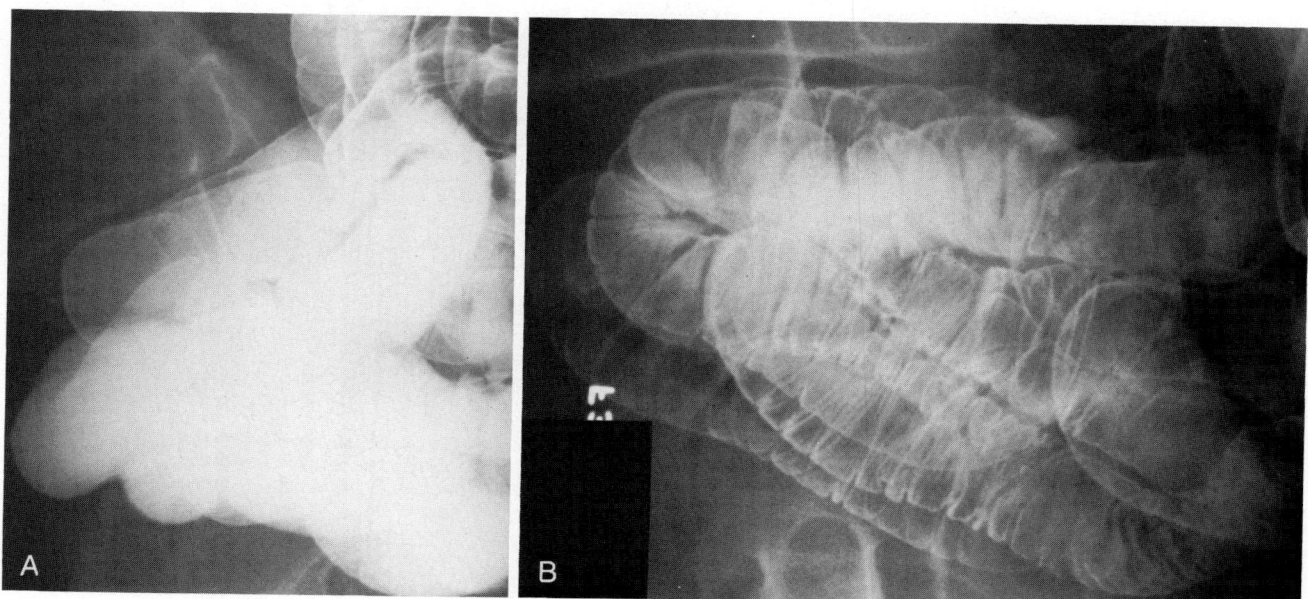

**Figure 43–17. Ileal loops prolapsed into the pelvis.** The patient had a total hysterectomy. Straight prone or supine views are unhelpful. An angled view improves visualization. **A.** Prolapsed loops in a single contrast, lateral view of the pelvis. **B.** When double contrast has been established throughout the prolapsed loops, a lateral or off-lateral film of the pelvis provides the best possible image.

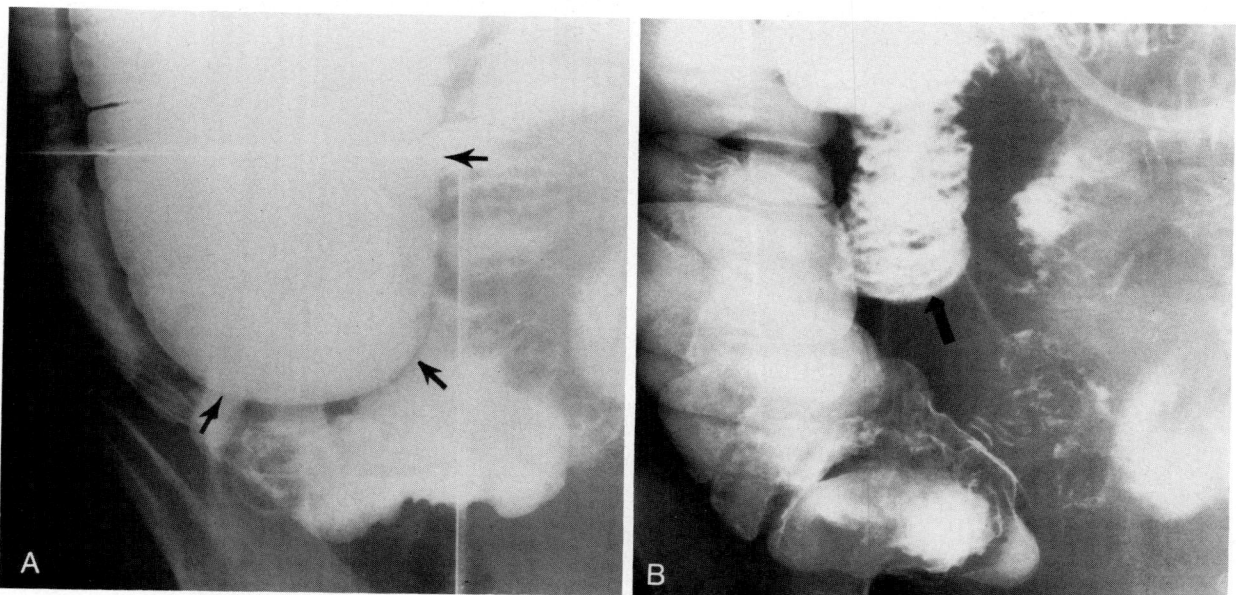

**Figure 43–18. Small bowel obstruction caused by an ileal carcinoid. A.** A grossly dilated loop of distal jejunum *(arrows)* flattens the cecum and ascending colon. It would be a mistake to allow the patient to leave the department in this state. **B.** The enteroclysis tube was left in situ and excess fluid was siphoned off through it. The loop of jejunum *(arrow)* is now collapsed and the cecum and ascending colon are filled.

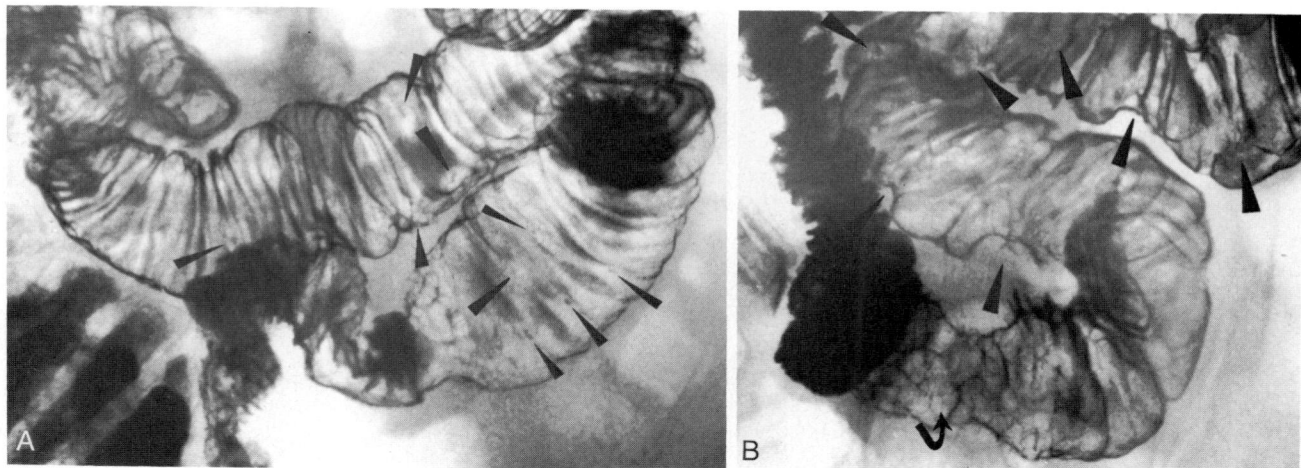

**Figure 43–19. Recurrent Crohn's disease.** Supine, air double contrast views of the distal ileum with manifestations of Crohn's disease recurrence after resection of the terminal ileum. **A.** View taken 12 months after surgery. Multiple tiny ulcerations are indicated by arrowheads. **B.** Air double contrast view 12 months later. Additional, slightly deeper ulcers are now seen *(arrowheads),* and the ulceronodular ("cobblestone") pattern close to the anastomosis has extended transaxially *(arrow).* (**A** and **B** courtesy of Hikoo Shirakabe, M.D., Tokyo, Japan.)

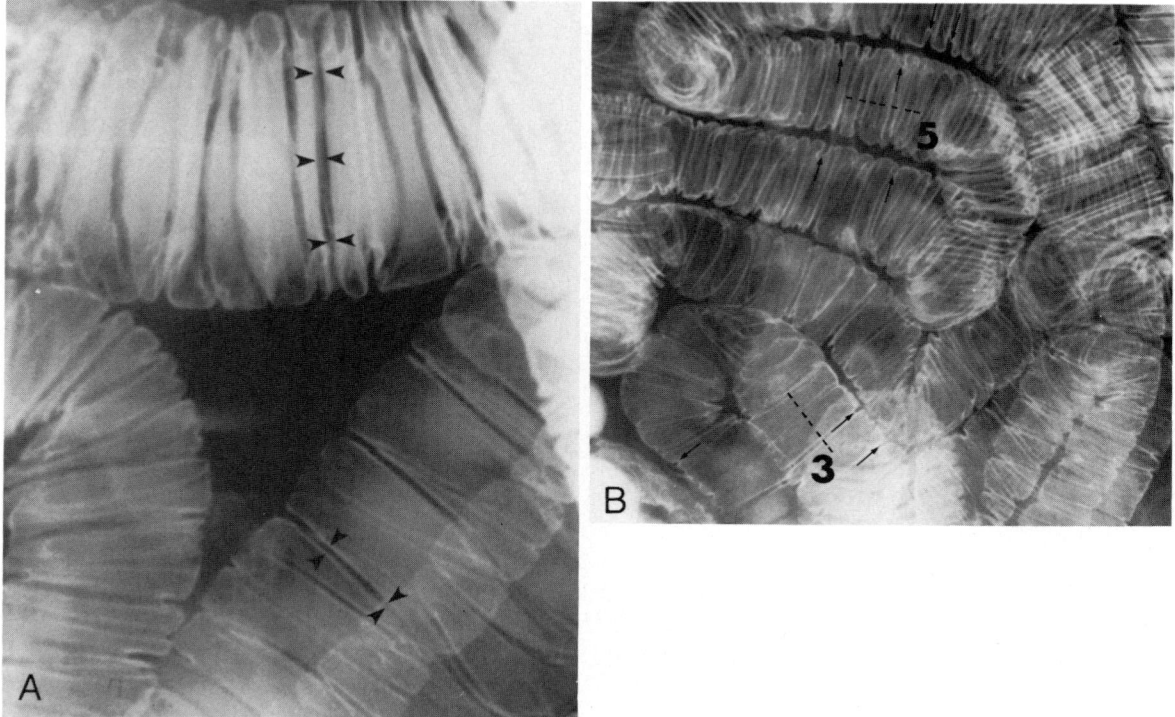

**Figure 43–20. Measurable parameters of morphologic normality. A.** Thickness of folds *(arrowheads).* Jejunal folds are up to 2 mm thick (top); ileal folds are slightly thinner, measuring 1.0 to 1.5 mm (bottom). **B.** Overview film. Folds in the proximal jejunum are closer together than those in the ileum. There are normally four to seven folds per inch in the proximal jejunum (here five folds) and two to four folds per inch in the more distal ileum (here three folds). The height of folds in the jejunum exceeds that in the ileum *(arrows).*

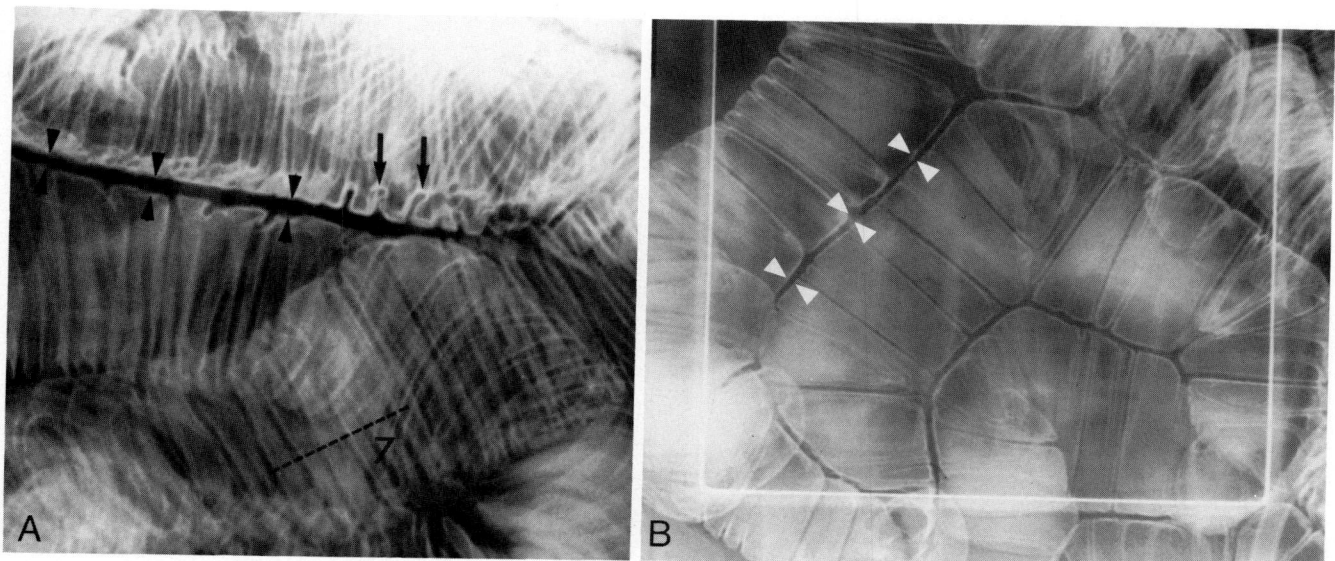

**Figure 43–21. Normal wall thickness.** The combined wall thickness of two adjacent bowel loops can be measured provided the barium-coated mucosal surfaces are parallel to each other over at least 5 cm. **A.** Normal jejunum. Arrowheads indicate the mucosal surfaces of two parallel loops. The combined distance is 3 mm; therefore, a single bowel wall is 1.5 mm thick (normal range 1.0 to 2.0 mm). Note that there are seven folds per inch and that the height of the folds can be seen when shown in profile at the side of the lumen *(arrows).* **B.** Normal, well-distended ileum. Note the thinness and wider separation of the shallower folds and the reduced combined wall thickness *(arrowheads)* of 2.0 mm, or 1.0 mm for each wall.

with equal quality and expertise. Because of the infrequency of small bowel disease, many patients would have to be examined in this way to achieve a meaningful result. Such prospective analysis would be impossible because it would cause excessive radiation exposure of

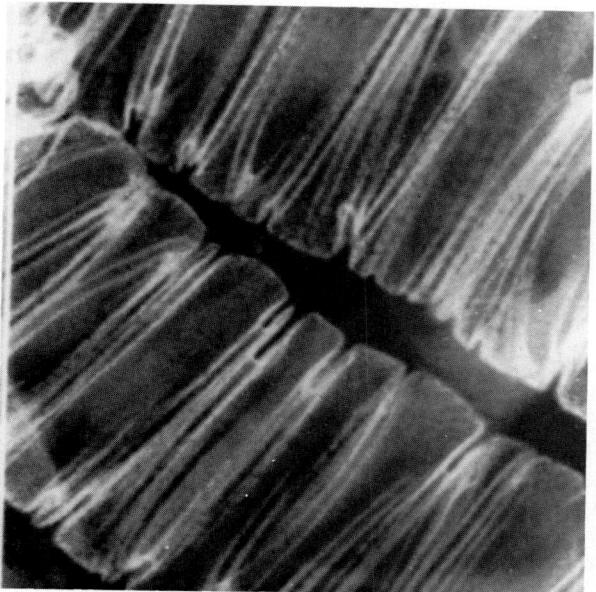

**Figure 43–22. Villous pattern of the small bowel.** Not infrequently, it is possible to identify a pattern of rounded lucencies less than 1.0 mm in diameter in the barium-coated mucosal surface. These are best appreciated tangentially on the sides of mucosal folds or can be seen throughout the surface, as in this illustration. These micronodules represent normal villi protruding into the thin layer of barium.

patients and would be too time-consuming and expensive. However, there has been one limited prospective comparison study involving 200 consecutive patients who were examined by either dedicated follow-through or enteroclysis, in single or double contrast.[63] Because patients with specific small bowel–related problems were mostly assigned to enteroclysis, this series did not lend itself to estimation of relative sensitivity in diagnosing pathology. In the three forms of examination, the measurability of the folds was assessed objectively in the jejunum, the ileum, and the terminal ileum. For the jejunum and ileum, the follow-through showed a statistically significantly lower percentage of fold measurability than enteroclysis. No significant difference in fold measurability was found between the single and double contrast intubation studies, although an estimate of subjective quality favored the double contrast technique. No significant difference in the three methods was found in the terminal ileum. Because the single and double contrast enteroclysis techniques share the ability to distend the bowel lumen and straighten folds, it was not surprising that fold measurability was the same for both.

Retrospective studies, usually targeted to a specific diagnostic problem, are the only other methods available for obtaining numeric estimates of sensitivity for the two techniques—follow-through and enteroclysis. An example concerned the ability to diagnose the presence of primary malignant small bowel tumors.[64] In all the patients in this investigation, a malignant tumor was eventually demonstrated at surgery, and all patients had been referred for small bowel study. Enteroclysis demonstrated 90% of the tumors, the conventional examination only 33%. As in all such comparative retrospec-

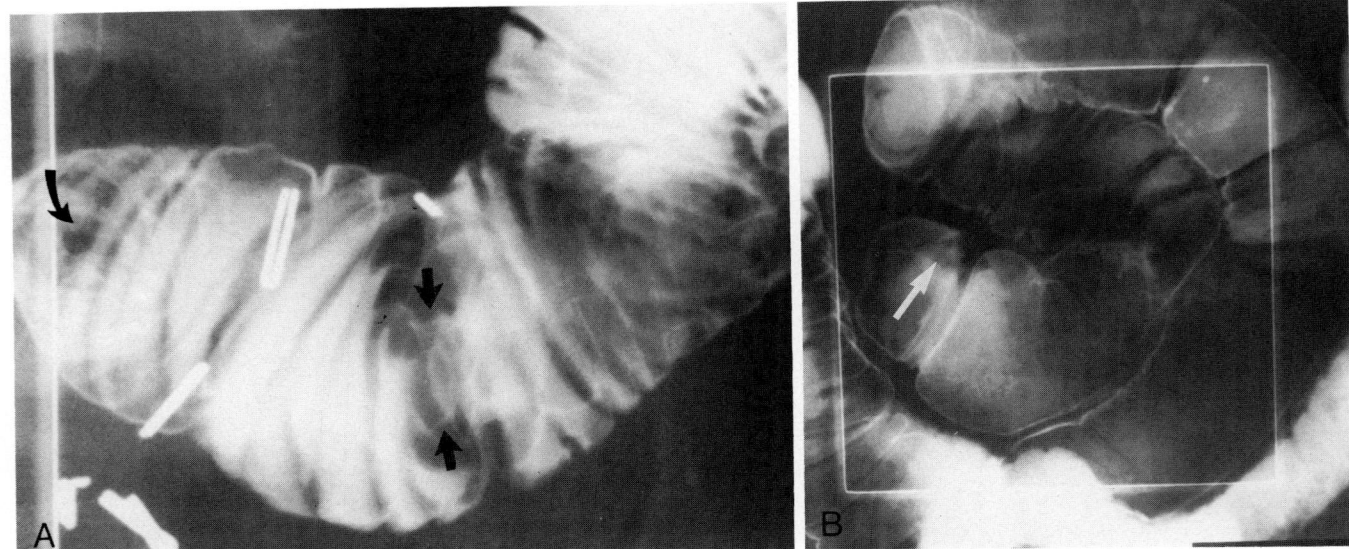

**Figure 43–23. Ileostomy barium examination. A.** Patient with intermittent abdominal distention. Single contrast study using a Foley catheter with minimally inflated balloon *(curved arrow)*. A short, narrowed segment *(straight arrows)* was considered to be due to an adhesion. Surgery confirmed this. **B.** Air double contrast ileostomy examination to rule out Crohn's disease a few months after total colectomy. About 5 ft of normal small bowel was outlined. (Arrow indicates minimally inflated Foley's catheter in ileostomy.)

tive evaluations, like was not compared with like: the enteroclysis was superbly done, but the follow-through was not performed by a dedicated, fluoroscopy-based technique. However, this study reflected the difference between the potentially more accurate enteroclysis and the radiographic follow-through, which is still the primary study in most departments of radiology in the United States.

Thus, for comparisons, one must make do with either careful but limited-scope prospective studies[63] or reports of personal experience in isolated cases in which both techniques had been done, with enteroclysis always providing the more accurate diagnosis. Perhaps common sense should be used to judge the relative merits of enteroclysis and follow-through. I suggest simply examining the films obtained by the two methods and asking which could confidently detect pathologic conditions or determine morphologic normality.

## INDICATIONS FOR ENTEROCLYSIS

In isolated centers in the United States[64] and several radiology departments in Europe, enteroclysis is the primary radiologic technique for investigating the small bowel. I believe there is still a place for the dedicated, fluoroscopic small bowel follow-through. However, enteroclysis should be the primary barium study when the following clinical indications exist:

1. Malabsorption states or a clinical suspicion of their presence.
2. Partial mechanical small bowel obstruction, high grade, low grade, or intermittent, or small bowel obstruction with a history of laparotomy for malignancy and/or radiation treatment of the abdomen.

3. To confirm the presence or absence of Crohn's disease suspected on the basis of prior studies. To show extent of disease and rule out a proximal "skip" lesion in patients needing surgery.
4. Obscure gastrointestinal tract bleeding after a full range of prior investigations has produced negative results. A relevant lesion is more likely to be demonstrated if there is also abdominal pain.
5. Clinical importance of excluding small bowel disease.
6. Small bowel examination in aged and debilitated patients who should not be exposed to the lengthy and physically demanding small bowel follow-through.

## ILEOSTOMY ENEMA

This should be the preferred technique for examining the small bowel when an ileostomy is present. A Foley catheter is introduced and its balloon is inflated no more than is needed to occlude the opening through the fascia when slight traction is applied (usually 3 mL of air). The balloon must not be inflated enough to occlude the bowel lumen itself, which could damage the mucosa. An injection of 1 mg of glucagon facilitates retrograde flow of barium as well as of methylcellulose or air should double contrast be required (Fig. 43–23).

### Acknowledgment

Figures 43–9A to E and 43–23A are reproduced from Herlinger H, Maglinte D (eds): Clinical Radiology of the Small Intestine. Philadelphia: WB Saunders, 1989.

Figures 43–11A and B, 43–14B and C, and 43–20A and B are reproduced from Laufer I, Levine MS (eds): Double

Contrast Gastrointestinal Radiology (2nd ed). Philadelphia: WB Saunders, 1992.

# References

1. Williams FH: The Roentgen Rays in Medicine and Surgery. New York: Macmillan, 1901.
2. Rieder H: Radiologische Untersuchungen des Magens und Darmes beim lebenden Menschen. Muench Med Wochenschr 51:1548, 1904.
3. Hulst H: Skiagraphy of the stomach and intestines. Physicians Surgeons (Detroit and Ann Arbor) 77:391–411, 1905.
4. Forssel G: Studies of the mechanism of movement of the mucous membrane of the digestive tract. AJR 10:81, 1923.
5. Morse RW, Cole LG: The anatomy of the normal small intestine as observed roentgenographically. Radiology 8:149, 1927.
6. Golden R: Technical factors in the roentgen examination of the small intestine. AJR 82:965–972, 1959.
7. Weltz GA: Der kranke Duenndarm im Roentgenbild. ROFO 55:20–40, 1937.
8. Marshak RH: Roentgen findings in lesions of the small bowel. Am J Dig Dis 6:1084–1114, 1961.
9. Ardran GM, French JM, Mucklow EH: Relationship of the nature of the opaque medium to small intestine radiograph pattern. Br J Radiol 23:697–702, 1950.
10. Weintraub S, Williams RG: A rapid method of roentgenologic examination of the small intestine. AJR 61:45–55, 1949.
11. Nice CM: Roentgenographic pattern and motility in small bowel studies. Radiology 80:39–45, 1963.
12. Grivaux M, Cornet A, Wattez E: Le metoclopramide en radiologie digestive. Semin Hop Paris 44:2338–2345, 1964.
13. Howarth FH, Cockel R, Roper BW, et al: The effect of metoclopramide upon gastric motility and its value in barium progress meals. Clin Radiol 20:294–300, 1969.
14. Kreel L: The use of oral metoclopramide in the barium meal and follow-through examination. Br J Radiol 43:31–35, 1970.
15. Maglinte DDT, Burney BT, Miller RE: Lesions missed on small bowel follow-through: analysis and recommendations. Radiology 144:737–739, 1982.
16. Goldberg HI, Carruthers SB, Nelson JA, et al: Radiographic findings of the National Cooperative Crohn's Disease Study. Gastroenterology 77:925–937, 1979.
17. Spiro H: Foreword. *In* Herlinger H, Maglinte D (eds): Clinical Radiology of the Small Intestine. Philadelphia: WB Saunders, 1989, pp ix–x.
18. Herlinger H, Lintott DJ: Standard examination of the small bowel. *In* Margulis AR, Burhenne HJ (eds): Alimentary Tract Radiology (3rd ed). St. Louis: CV Mosby, 1983, pp 907–914.
19. Grumbach K, Herlinger H, Laufer I, et al: Metoclopramide-ceruletide assisted small bowel examination. ROFO 149:47–51, 1988.
20. Bret P, Cuche C, Schmutz G: Radiology of the Small Intestine. New York: Springer-Verlag, 1989, p 9.
21. Fraser GM, Preston PG: The small bowel follow-through enhanced with an oral effervescent agent. Clin Radiol 34:673–679, 1983.
22. Kellett MJ, Zboralske FF, Margulis AR: Peroral pneumocolon examination of the ileocecal region. Gastrointest Radiol 1:361–365, 1977.
23. Kelvin FM, Gedgaudas RK, Thompson WM, et al: The peroral pneumocolon examination: its role in evaluating the terminal ileum. AJR 139:115–121, 1982.
24. Kressel HY, Evers KA, Glick SN, et al: The peroral pneumocolon examination: technique and indications. Radiology 144:414–416, 1982.
25. Fitzgerald EJ, Thompson GT, Somers SS, at al: Pneumocolon as an aid to small bowel studies. Clin Radiol 36:633–637, 1985.
26. Miller RE: Complete reflux examination of the small bowel. Radiology 84:457–462, 1986.
27. Einhorn M: The Duodenal Tube and Its Possibilities (2nd ed). Philadelphia: FA Davis, 1926.
28. Cole LG: Artificial dilatation of the duodenum by radiographic examination. AJR 3:204, 1911.
29. Pesquera GS: Method for direct visualization of lesions in the small intestine. AJR 22:254–257, 1929.
30. Gershon-Cohen J, Shay H: Barium enteroclysis method for direct immediate examination of the small intestine by single and double contrast technique. AJR 42:456–458, 1939.
31. Schatzki R: Small bowel enema. AJR 50:743–751, 1943.
32. Scott-Harden WG: Examination of the small bowel. *In* McLaren JW (ed): Modern Trends in Diagnostic Radiology. London: Butterworth, 1960, pp 84–87.
33. Pygott F, Street DF, Schellshear MF, et al: Radiological investigation of the small intestine by small bowel enema technique. Gut 1:366–370, 1960.
34. Sellink JL: Examination of the Small Intestine by Means of Duodenal Intubation. Lieden: Stenfert Kroese, 1971.
35. Trickey SE, Halls J, Hodson CJ: A further development of the small bowel enema. J R Soc Med 56:1070–1073, 1963.
36. Herlinger H: A modified technique for the double contrast small bowel enema. Gastrointest Radiol 3:201–207, 1978.
37. Maglinte DDT, Elmore MF, Eisenberg M, et al: Meckel diverticulum: radiologic demonstration by enteroclysis. AJR 134:925–932, 1980.
38. Maglinte DDT, Lappas JC, Kelvin FM, et al: Small bowel radiography: how, when and why? Radiology 163:297–305, 1987.
39. Nolan DJ: Radiological Atlas of Gastrointestinal Disease. New York: John Wiley & Sons, 1984.
40. Herlinger H: Small bowel. *In* Laufer I (ed): Double Contrast Gastrointestinal Radiology with Endoscopic Correlation. Philadelphia: WB Saunders, 1979, pp 423–494.
41. Antes G, Lissner J: Die Doppelkontrastdarstellung des Dünndarms mit Barium und Methylzellulose. ROFO 134:10–15, 1981.
42. Ekberg O: Double contrast examination of the small bowel. Gastrointest Radiol 8:51–54, 1977.
43. Fuchs HF, Geiter B: Roentgenolgische Untersuchungen-Duenndarm. *In* Domschke W, Koch H (eds): Diagnostik in der Gastroenterilogie—Methodik und Bewertung. Stuttgart: Thieme, 1979.
44. Salomonowitz E, Czembirek H: Dynamische Doppel Kontrastuntersuchung des Duenndarmes. ROFO 133:274–278, 1980.
45. Sanders DE, Ho CS: The small bowel enema: experience with 150 examinations. AJR 127:743–751, 1976.
46. Fleckenstein P, Pedersen G: The value of the duodenal intubation method (Sellink modification) for the radiological visualization of the small bowel. Scand J Gastroenterol 10:423–425, 1975.
47. Salomonowitz E: Radiation dose of double contrast and single contrast examinations. *In* Herlinger H, Maglinte D (eds): Clinical Radiology of the Small Intestine. Philadelphia: WB Saunders, 1989, pp 147–150.
48. Sellink JL, Miller RE: Radiology of the Small Bowel: Modern Enteroclysis Technique and Atlas. The Hague: Martinus Nijhoff, 1982.
49. Nolan DJ, Cadman PJ: The small bowel enema made easy. Clin Radiol 38:295–301, 1987.
50. Maglinte DDT, Herlinger H: Single contrast and biphasic enteroclysis. *In* Herlinger H, Maglinte D (eds): Clinical Radiology of the Small Intestine. Philadelphia: WB Saunders, 1989, pp 107–118.
51. Herlinger H, Maglinte DDT: The small bowel enema with methylcellulose. *In* Herlinger H, Maglinte D (eds): Clinical Radiology of the Small Intestine. Philadelphia: WB Saunders, 1989, pp 119–137.
52. Schulze-Delrieu K: Metroclopramide drug therapy. N Engl J Med 305:28–33, 1981.
53. Plovin PF, Mennard J, Corrol P: Hypertensive crisis in patients with pheochromocytoma given metroclopramide. Lancet 2:1357–1358, 1976.
54. Maglinte DDT, Lappas JC, Chernish SN, et al: Improved tolerance of enteroclysis by use of sedation. AJR 151:951–952, 1988.
55. Maglinte DDT, Herlinger H: Enteroclysis catheters, intubation, and infusion. *In* Herlinger H, Maglinte D (eds): Clinical Radiology of the Small Intestine. Philadelphia: WB Saunders, 1989, pp 85–105.
56. Diner WC: Duodenal perforation during intubation for small bowel enema study. Radiology 168:39–41, 1988.
57. Maglinte DDT, Miller RE: A comparison of pumps used for enteroclysis. Radiology 152:815, 1984.
58. Sellink JL: Single contrast enteroclysis. *In* Margulis AR, Burhenne

J (eds): Alimentary Tract Radiology. St. Louis: CV Mosby, 1983, pp 871–890.

59. Kobayashi S, Nishizawa M, Mizuno K, et al: X-ray examination of the small intestine. (1). Double contrast method as a routine examination. Jpn J Clin Radiol 19:619–625, 1974 (in Japanese).

60. Kobayashi S, Nishizawa M: X-ray examination of small intestine—double contrast method by duodenal intubation. Stomach Intest 11:157–165, 1976.

61. Shirakabe H, Kobayashi S: Air double contrast barium study of the small bowel. *In* Herlinger H, Maglinte D (eds): Clinical Radiology of the Small Intestine. Philadelphia: WB Saunders, 1989, pp 139–145.

62. Desaga JF: Visualization of the mucosal villi on double-contrast barium studies of the small intestine by using a high molecular fraction of guaran. Gastrointest Radiol 14:25–30, 1989.

63. Taverne PP, van der Jagt EJ: Small bowel radiography. A prospective comparative study of three techniques in 200 patients. ROFO 143:293–297, 1985.

64. Bessette JR, Maglinte DDT, Kelvin FM, et al: Primary malignant tumors in the small bowel: a comparison of the small-bowel enema and conventional follow-through examination. AJR 153:741–744, 1989.

# Cross-sectional Imaging

**44**

Amorino Vecchioli, M.D.

Antonio De Franco, M.D.

Giulia Maresca, M.D.

Richard M. Gore, M.D.

## INTRODUCTION

Barium studies are the primary means of examining patients with suspected small bowel disease. Although these techniques afford exquisite mucosal detail, they cannot reliably detect, characterize, or differentiate the extraluminal component of many neoplastic, infectious, traumatic, and ischemic disorders of the small bowel. This chapter details the applications of cross-sectional imaging in patients with known or suspected small bowel disease.

## ULTRASOUND

In the early development of ultrasound, the small bowel and mesentery were considered detriments and inhibitors of sonographic evaluation of the intra-abdominal organs.[1-4] Technical advances in gray-scale ultrasound, high-resolution real-time sonography, and color flow and duplex Doppler sonography have greatly expanded the applications of ultrasound in evaluating small bowel disease.

Sonography is useful in further characterizing individual bowel loop abnormalities seen on barium studies.

### Scanning Technique

Real-time scanning of the small bowel should be performed with the highest-frequency transducer possible, usually 3.5 or 5 MHz. The bowel loops should be imaged axially and longitudinally and the transducer must be angulated to find the major axis of each major segment.[5]

The following elements must be carefully scrutinized while performing small bowel sonography: mural thickness, mural symmetry, mural homogeneity, peristalsis, and intraluminal contents.[1, 3]

### Normal Sonographic Anatomy

When axially imaged, the small bowel appears as a 2- to 3-cm echogenic structure with a "target" appearance.[5-13] The target represents the various layers of bowel wall (Fig. 44–1): mucosa and lamina propria (echogenic), muscularis mucosae (hypoechoic), submucosa (echogenic), muscularis propria (hypoechoic), and serosa (echogenic).[6, 9, 10] In normal bowel these layers can be differentiated only by high-frequency endoscopic ultrasound. Only two layers, an echogenic center and hypoechoic periphery, can be visualized in nondistended loops on transabdominal scans (Fig. 44–2). The thickness of the intestinal wall measured from the lumen to the outer edge of the hypoechoic layer should be 5 mm or less in nondistended segments and 3 mm or less when the gut is distended. If the bowel wall is thicker than 5 mm or appears asymmetrically thickened, pathology should be suspected.[1, 3, 6]

Normal fluid-filled loops change shape and empty during peristalsis, and an abnormality should be suspected when a bowel segment fails to change configuration over a 30- to 60-second period. Gas-distended

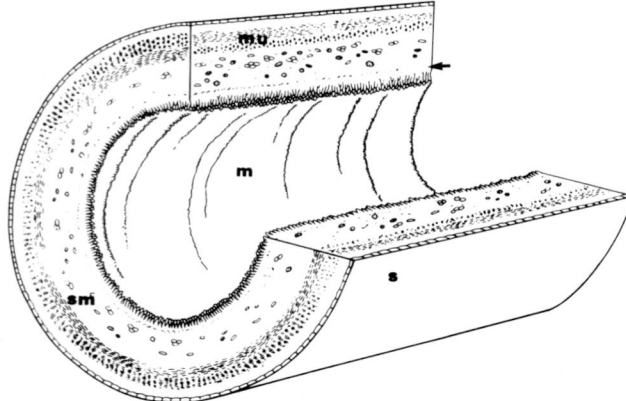

**Figure 44–1. Normal small bowel on cross section.** The carpet-like surface of the mucosa (m) and the areolar tissue of the lamina propria are echogenic. The muscularis mucosae *(arrow)*, when visualized, is hypoechoic. The thick layer of submucosa (sm) contains numerous blood vessels and lymph channels in loose connective tissue that is echogenic. This layer is most susceptible to disease including edema. The muscularis (mu) is composed of two sets of fibers, oriented circularly and longitudinally, that are echogenic. A thin layer of echogenic serosa and mesothelial covering(s) lines the outer surface of the small bowel. (From Pozniak MA, Scanlon KA, Yandow D, et al: Current status of small-bowel ultrasound. Radiologe 30:254–265, 1990.)

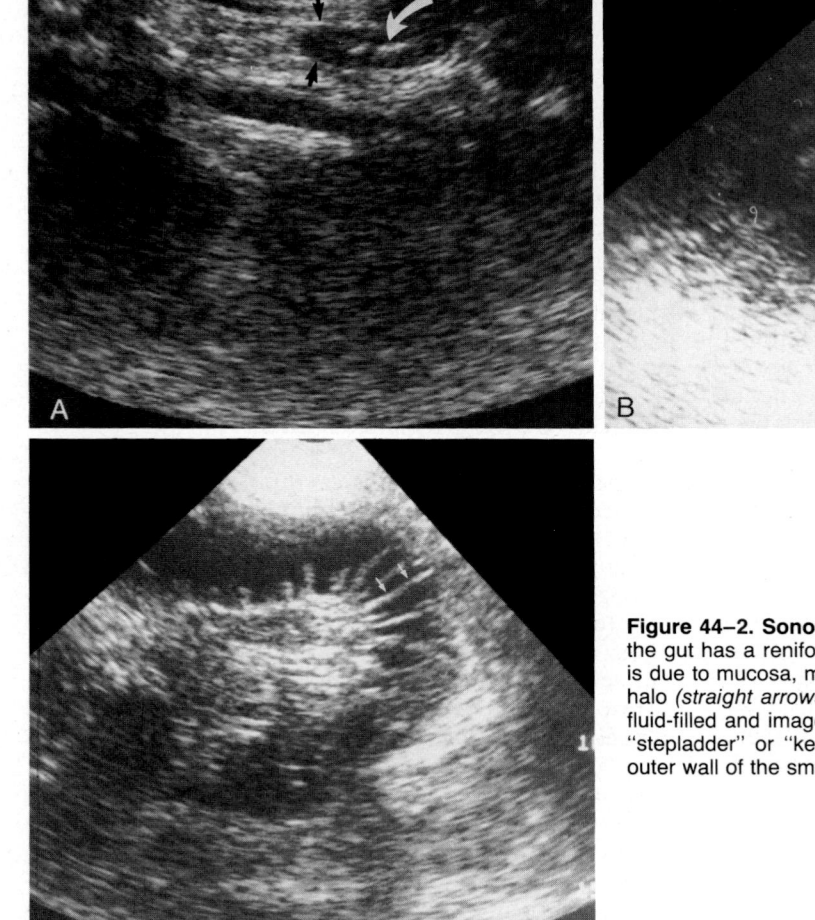

**Figure 44–2. Sonographic appearance of small bowel. A.** When collapsed, the gut has a reniform appearance. The central echogenic line *(curved arrow)* is due to mucosa, mucus, lamina propria, and intraluminal gas; the hypoechoic halo *(straight arrows)* represents the remainder of the small bowel wall. When fluid-filled and imaged axially **(B)** and longitudinally **(C)**, the small bowel has a "stepladder" or "keyboard" appearance. Ascites (A) in **B** clearly outlines the outer wall of the small bowel. Arrows in **B** and **C** indicate valvulae conniventes.

loops are highly reflective, producing distal shadowing and reverberation artifacts. The change in the distribution of gas within a loop during peristalsis or with transducer compression should also be observed.[1, 3, 6]

When the valvulae conniventes are identified, the sonographer can be certain that small bowel is being studied.[1, 3, 6] Valvulae are more difficult to observe in the ileum, where they are fewer and smaller than in the jejunum; in the terminal ileum they can be absent altogether. Evaluation of the small bowel wall is simplified when ascites or intraluminal fluid is present[8] (Fig. 44–3; see Fig. 44–2). Demonstration of the valvulae conniventes is facilitated by the ingestion of fluid to distend the lumen.

## Small Bowel Mesentery

The small bowel mesentery can be visualized sonographically in patients with ascites. It is a series of fan-like echogenic stripes that attach the small bowel to the posterior wall of the abdomen (see Fig. 44–3); its root extends from the right iliac fossa to the duodenojejunal junction.[14] Imaging of the mesentery can be difficult in thin patients.

The mesentery is an elongated structure, about 1.5 cm thick with highly reflective peritoneal surfaces. The middle of the mesentery shows high-level echoes from fat, whereas the periphery shows low-level echoes. Mesenteric leaves show no peristalsis, in contrast to the small bowel loops attached to their distal end. The thickness of the mesentery ranges from 0.7 to 1.2 cm. Within the mesentery, small vascular structures 1 to 2 mm in diameter can be demonstrated and represent the mesenteric vessels. With color Doppler sonography, these vessels can be readily located and studied with

| TABLE 44–1. ETIOLOGIES OF PSEUDOKIDNEY OR ATYPICAL TARGET APPEARANCE OF SMALL BOWEL |
|---|
| Adenocarcinoma |
| Lymphoma |
| Leiomyoma |
| Leiomyosarcoma |
| Crohn's disease |
| Small bowel metastases |
| Intussusception |
| Intramural hematoma |

duplex Doppler sonography to assess small bowel perfusion. The mesentery can be most easily seen by scanning the left lower quadrant, using an oblique scanning plane parallel to the axis of the left iliac vessels.[14]

## Mural Pathology

The most common sonographic finding in small bowel disease is mural thickening, which causes a nonspecific pattern that has been variously called the "pseudokidney," target, "bull's-eye," "doughnut," "cockade," or "ring" sign.[1–13]

Any disorder that produces small bowel thickening can cause the pseudokidney appearance, so named because of its superficial resemblance to a normal kidney. The various etiologies of the pseudokidney sign are listed in Table 44–1, and some of the more important ones are described in the following.[1–13]

## Neoplasms

Intrinsic neoplasms of the small bowel (e.g., adenocarcinoma, leiomyosarcomas, and carcinoids) have a target-like appearance (Fig. 44–4). Compared with inflammatory mural thickening, the wall thickening produced by the tumors is more pronounced, asymmetric, and irregular with interruption of the layers of the wall. Peristalsis is often absent in the affected bowel segment.[6] The small intestine and mesentery can also be involved by metastases and other masses arising in the peritoneum, retroperitoneum, and lymph nodes.

In patients with small bowel lymphoma, the gut and lymph nodes often have a striking hypoechoic appearance. This infiltrative process permeates and thickens the bowel wall[6, 15] (Fig. 44–5). The adjacent mesenteric nodes are often involved as well, producing the "sandwich" sign or mesenteric "cake" sign, consisting of an echogenic band containing the subperitoneal fat and connective tissue of the small bowel mesentery encased by multiple lobulated, hypoechoic masses[16] (Fig. 44–6).

## Obstruction

Sonography, although not a primary means of diagnosing small bowel obstruction, can be useful in inte-

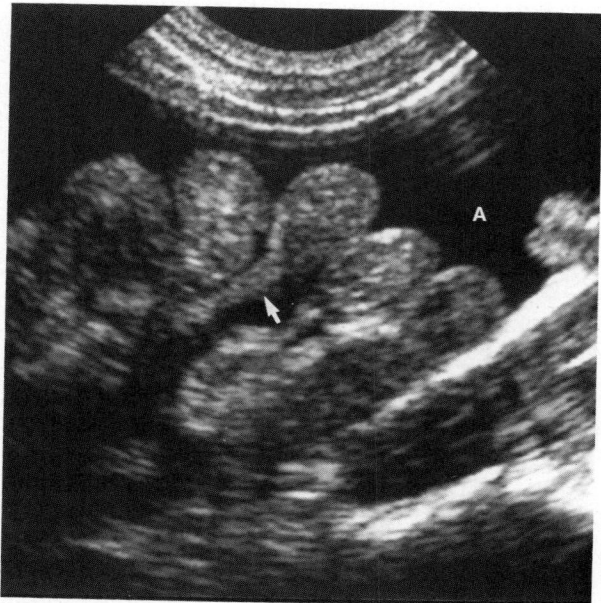

**Figure 44–3. Normal small bowel mesentery.** Ascites (A) outlines individual mesenteric leaves *(arrow)*.

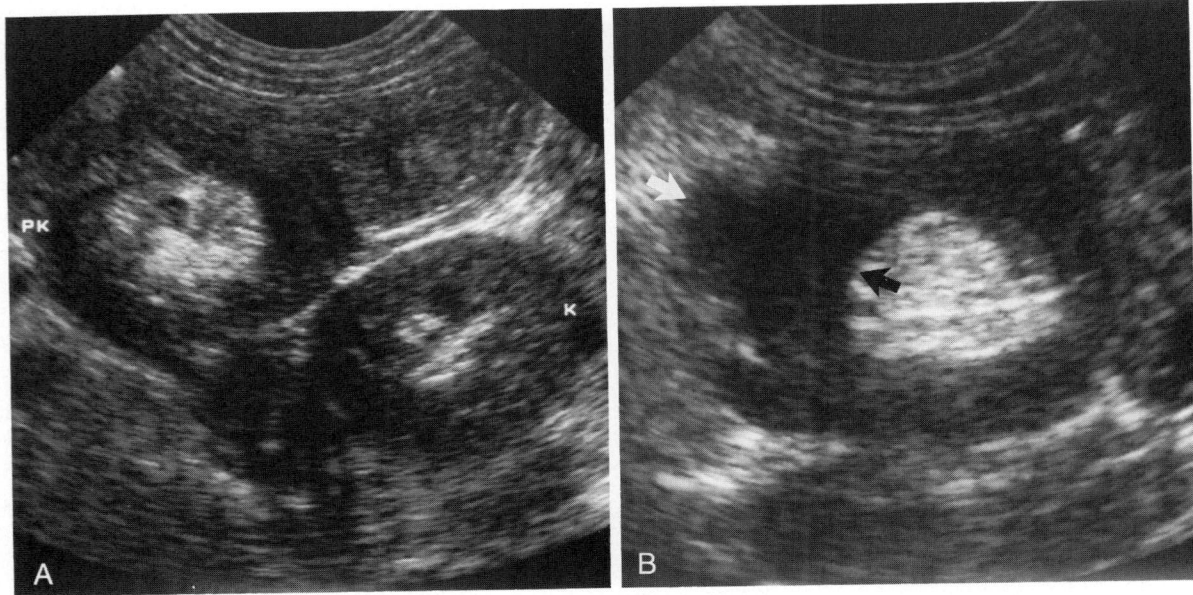

**Figure 44–4. Jejunal adenocarcinoma. A.** Pseudokidney sign (PK) caused by a jejunal adenocarcinoma adjacent to the right kidney (K). **B.** The wall is unevenly thickened *(arrows)*, measuring more than 2 cm.

grating abdominal plain film findings with clinical information.[17] This is particularly true in the 6% of patients with small bowel obstruction who have virtually gasless abdomens.[1, 3, 5]

Small bowel obstruction should be suspected when there are multiple fluid-filled loops of bowel, bowel dilatation greater than 3 cm, prominent valvulae conniventes in the fluid-filled jejunum, and vigorous peristalsis (see Fig. 44–2B and C). In acute obstruction, peristalsis is often vigorous, but as the bowel decompensates

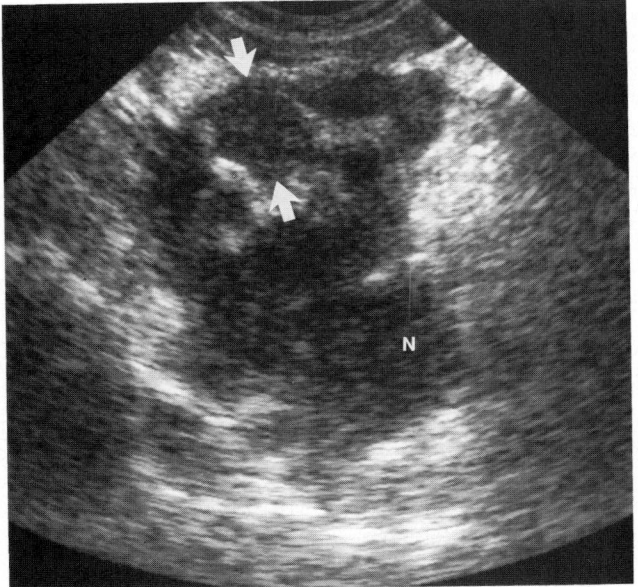

**Figure 44–5. Non-Hodgkin's lymphoma.** There is hypoechoic mural thickening *(arrows)* of a segment of ileum. Low-density nodes (N) are present in the adjacent mesentery.

the degree of peristalsis diminishes. It may then become disordered and produce nonpropulsive to-and-fro or swirling motion of intraluminal echoes. Intraluminal fluid can vary in echogenicity from anechoic to echogenic with internal debris. The cause of obstruction, such as a tumor or hernia, is occasionally visualized.[17–19]

Two specific types of bowel obstruction can be identified by sonography: the afferent loop syndrome and closed loop obstructions. In the former, which occurs after a Billroth II procedure, ultrasound may demonstrate a dilated loop of bowel in the upper abdomen that often has a U shape on coronal views.[20] Peristalsis is often present, the pancreatic head is enlarged and hypoechoic, and there is biliary dilatation.[20]

Closed loop obstructions caused by hernias and adhesions dilate with fluid that can be detected sonographically. If venous pressure is exceeded by the intraluminal pressure, an ischemic infarct and hemorrhage develop. An aperistaltic, isolated U-shaped loop of fluid-filled bowel results. Mural thickening with inhomogeneous echogenicity accompanies the hemorrhage, and extraluminal fluid around the affected loop may also be present. Both of these disorders require immediate surgery.

In patients with ileus (Fig. 44–7), peristalsis is absent and the small bowel is fluid filled.

## Intussusception

Intussusception is common in children but rare in adults.[21, 22] Ultrasound shows a target-like lesion (Fig. 44–8), in which the hypoechoic halo is produced by the mesentery and the edematous wall of the intussuscipiens and the hyperechoic center is produced by multiple interfaces of compressed mucosal, submucosal, and ser-

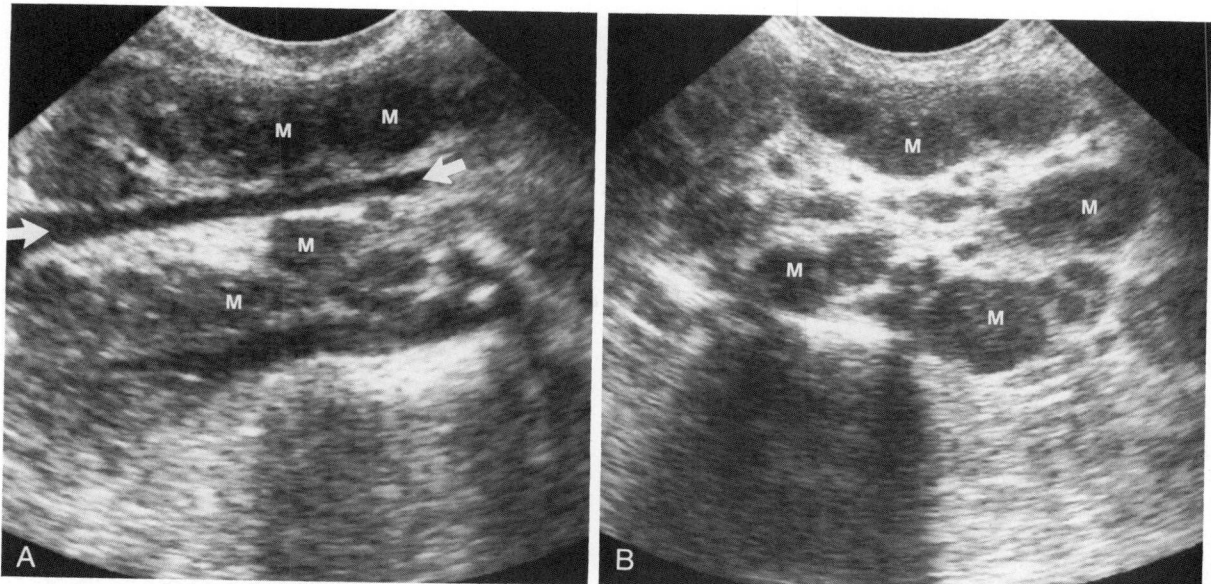

**Figure 44–6. The sandwich or "mesenteric cake" sign of lymphoma infiltrating the mesentery.**
**A.** Longitudinal scan shows the central echogenic band containing the superior mesenteric artery *(arrows)* surrounded by hypoechoic masses (M). **B.** Corresponding transverse scan shows the masses (M) to better advantage.

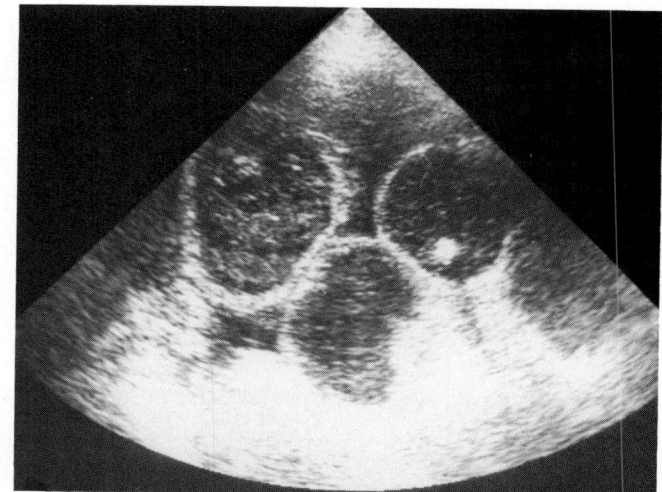

**Figure 44–7. Adynamic ileus.** Fluid-filled loops of small bowel contain echogenic material. They showed no peristalsis at real-time sonography.

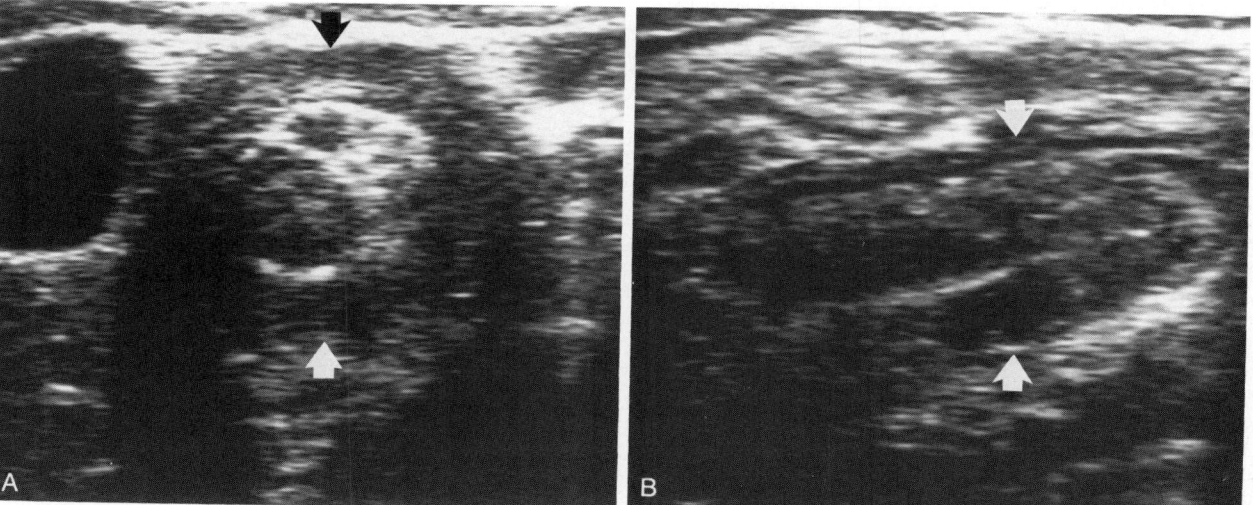

**Figure 44–8. Intussusception.** Transverse **(A)** and longitudinal **(B)** scans of an intussusception *(arrows)*. (Courtesy of G. Fariello, M.D., Rome, Italy.)

osal surfaces of the intussusceptum.[23–25] Multiple concentric rings, best seen on transverse scans, are also characteristic.[18] The corresponding appearance on longitudinal scans is that of multiple, thin, parallel, hypoechoic and echogenic stripes. Some reports suggest that there is a positive relationship between increasing mural thickness of the hypoechoic wall and inability to reduce the intussusception hydrostatically.[18]

## Inflammatory Lesions

Crohn's disease is the most common inflammatory disease of the small bowel in Western countries. The sonographic appearance depends on the duration and severity of disease and the presence of complications.[26–28]

Mural thickening (0.5 to 1.8 cm) is the most common finding, producing an abnormal, pseudokidney appearance (Fig. 44–9). Early in the disease, wall stratification is maintained; later, scarring and fibrosis result in a stiff thickened wall in which the various layers cannot be discerned.[26–28]

Conglomeration is another characteristic sonographic finding in Crohn's disease. Matted, inflamed bowel loops together with thickened mesentery and enlarged lymph nodes produce a primarily hypoechoic abdominal mass containing scattered echo-dense areas (Fig. 44–10). With creeping fat of the mesentery, conglomerations can produce ill-defined and diffuse echoes within the inflammatory mass. Peristalsis is reduced in the affected loop, which appears stiff and fixed during compression, and proximal, often fluid-filled, segments are dilated.

Sonography has a reported sensitivity of 67 to 76% and specificity of 88% in the diagnosis of ileal Crohn's disease.[28–31] Some 88% of patients with Crohn's disease show the target sign, caused by inflammatory, edematous thickening of the small bowel wall. The wall thickness ranges from 0.5 to 1.8 cm and should be measured on transverse scans with and without abdominal compression.[26, 30] The equivalent of the target sign in transverse scans is the sandwich image obtained by longitudinal scanning.[29] When these are combined with other sonographic observations, the sensitivity and specificity of the ultrasound examination in Crohn's disease increase to 88 and 91%, respectively.[28, 30]

Ultrasound cannot replace conventional radiology in the diagnosis of Crohn's disease but often can integrate radiologic data. It is useful in detecting complications such as abscess formation and identifying reduction in bowel wall thickness after successful medical therapy.[26] In addition, ultrasound is helpful in differentiating Crohn's disease and ileal lymphoma; in lymphoma there is more massive and irregular thickening of the bowel wall with displacement of the hyperechoic intraluminal gas. Ultrasound has a sensitivity of 82% and a specificity of 100% in the detection of postsurgical recurrence of Crohn's disease.[32, 33]

## Doppler

Duplex and color flow Doppler sonography can be used to evaluate mesenteric blood flow. The superior mesenteric artery can be interrogated in most patients, and its signal varies depending on the nutritional state of the individual: during fasting, a high-impedance pattern is seen with little diastolic flow. Postprandially, there is vasodilation with marked increases in overall mesenteric circulation and diastolic flow. Initial results of Doppler studies to evaluate the celiac and mesenteric

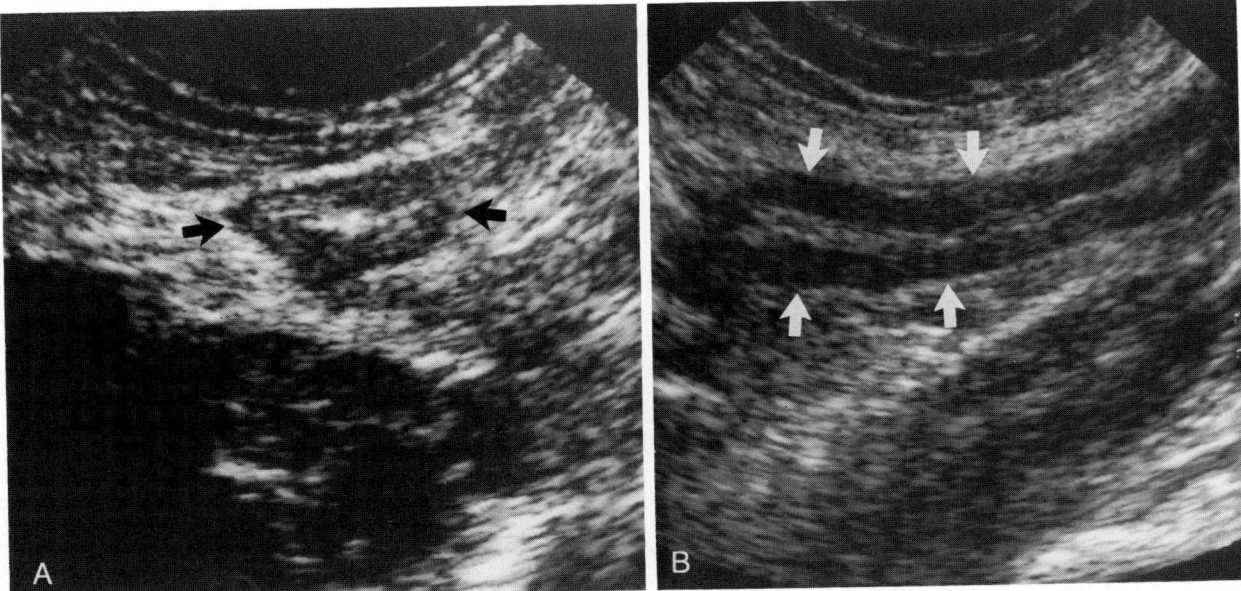

**Figure 44–9. Crohn's disease.** Homogeneous, regular mural thickening *(arrows)* of the involved bowel loop is seen in Crohn's ileitis. **A.** Transverse view has a target appearance. **B.** Longitudinal view.

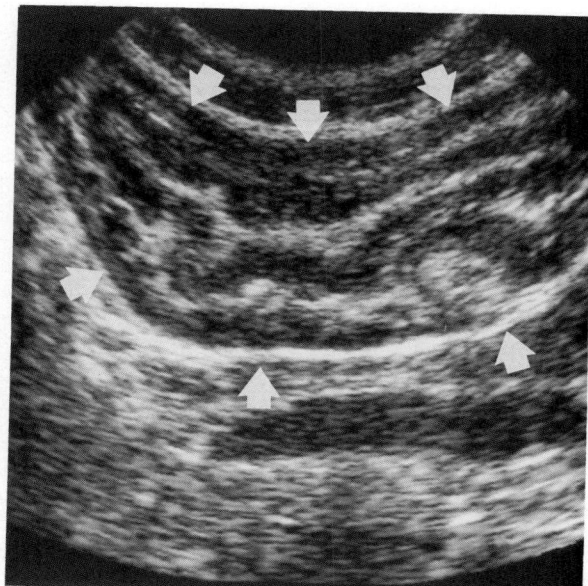

**Figure 44–10. Conglomeration of bowel in Crohn's disease.** Several ileal loops are matted together, producing a "mass" (arrows).

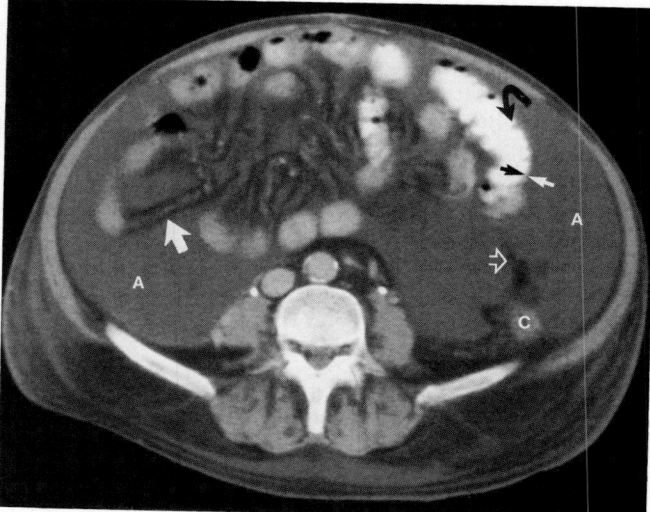

**Figure 44–11. Small bowel loops in ascites.** Contrast medium outlines the inner surface (small black arrow) and ascites (A) outlines the outer surface (small white arrow) of a jejunal loop; mural thickness is 2 mm. Individual valvulae conniventes (curved arrow) are visualized. The ascites also outlines individual mesenteric leaves (large white arrow) containing fat and blood vessels. Open arrow shows appendices epiploicae. C = colon.

arteries in patients with mesenteric angina and the dumping syndrome have been encouraging.[34–39]

## COMPUTED TOMOGRAPHY

Computed tomography (CT) of the small bowel provides extremely useful information concerning the mural, serosal, and mesenteric extent of neoplastic, vascular, inflammatory, and obstructive disorders.[40–45] In certain clinical situations, (ischemia, abscess, obstruction, Crohn's disease), CT should be the initial diagnostic examination.

Preparation of the patient, bowel opacification, and intravascular contrast agent administration are discussed in detail in Chapters 8 and 80.

### Normal Computed Tomographic Anatomy of Small Bowel and Mesentery

The normal small bowel when imaged axially on CT scans should have a wall thickness less than 4 mm (Fig. 44–11). Valvulae conniventes are commonly seen in the jejunum and are usually not visualized in the ileum.[46] The wall should be symmetric and have a homogeneous attenuation. The surrounding mesentery should have a fat density (excluding lymph nodes and blood vessels) measuring less than −75 Hounsfield units.[47]

Neoplastic, inflammatory, and vascular disorders of the small bowel wall are recognized on CT scans by thickening of the bowel wall. It is important to characterize the abnormality as focal, segmental, or diffuse and to determine the degree of mural thickening, symmetry of involvement, pattern of contrast enhancement, and smooth versus irregular or lobulated inner or outer contour. To further narrow the differential diagnosis, associated findings such as abscess, lymphadenopathy, metastases, phlegmon, and adjacent inflammatory response in the mesentery (Table 44–2) should be sought.

### Benign Diseases

Most benign intestinal lesions cause circumferential and symmetric mural thickening, usually less than 1 cm. The bowel wall has either a homogeneous soft tissue density or alternate rings of high and low density called

### TABLE 44–2. SMALL BOWEL PATHOLOGY CATEGORIZED BY COMPUTED TOMOGRAPHIC CRITERIA

| CRITERIA | PATHOLOGIC DIAGNOSIS (%) | | |
| --- | --- | --- | --- |
| | Neoplastic | Inflammatory | Edema |
| Wall > 1.5 cm and/or mesenteric mass > 1.5 cm | 83 | 17 | 0 |
| Wall > 3 mm but ≤ 1.5 cm; mesenteric masses ≤ 1.5 cm | 12 | 82 | 6 |
| Wall > 3 mm but ≤ 1.5 cm; no mesenteric masses; increased number of blood vessels; increased attenuation of mesenteric fat | 14 | 19 | 67 |

Modified from S James, DM Balfe, JKT Lee, et al, Small-bowel disease: categorization by CT examination, AJR, 148, 5, 863–868, 1987, © by American Roentgen Ray Society.

the "double halo" (two rings) or target (three rings) sign (Fig. 44–12). These different densities are best appreciated during the arterial phase of enhancement and are secondary to submucosal edema, inflammation, and/or fat deposition.[40–48] They can be found in Crohn's disease, ischemic enteritis, infectious enteritis, radiation enteritis, eosinophilic gastroenteritis (Fig. 44–13), Henoch-Schönlein purpura, and bowel edema associated with portal hypertension.

In benign disease, the process is usually segmental or diffuse and the adjacent mesenteric fat is often thickened with a streaky, higher-density appearance. With progressive disease, the bowel wall may become thicker (1 to 2 cm) but the symmetric, circumferential involvement and segmental distribution are maintained.[40–48]

## Malignant Disease

The hallmarks of a malignant small bowel lesion are eccentric or asymmetric mural thickening, a lobulated inner and outer contour, and/or a focal soft tissue mass exceeding 2 cm from the lumen to the serosal surface[40, 46, 49, 50] (Fig. 44–14). The lumen is narrowed, the outer contour of the mass is often spiculated, and there is abrupt transition between normal and abnormal gut wall. The presence of mesenteric, retroperitoneal, and liver metastases, regional adenopathy, and/or malignant-appearing ascites confirms the presence of neoplasm.[40, 46, 49, 50]

CT has a detection rate of 80% for small bowel tumors and provides accurate preoperative staging in 61% of cases.[50] Leiomyomas and leiomyosarcomas (Fig. 44–15) have a characteristic pattern of a bulky lesion that grows eccentrically and sometimes calcifies.[51, 52] When larger than 4 cm, they may have a low-attenuation center.[50] Carcinoids present with radiating soft tissue strands in the mesentery with displacement of small bowel loops and a small mesenteric mass in the right lower quadrant.[53–55] Lymphomas typically present with homogene-

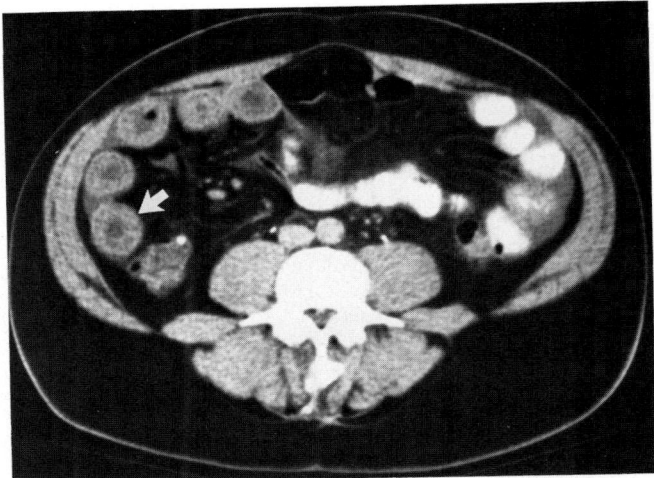

**Figure 44–13. Eosinophilic gastroenteritis.** The ileal loops have a target appearance *(arrow)* characterized by a soft tissue density inner ring, low-density central ring, and soft tissue density outer ring. A small amount of adjacent fluid is identified.

ous mural thickening greater than 2 cm associated with a normal-sized or enlarged lumen[56–58] (Fig. 44–16). Adenocarcinomas typically manifest as solitary soft tissue masses causing lumen narrowing and obstruction. When located in the duodenum, they are often difficult to differentiate from pancreatic tumors.[49, 50]

## Obstruction

The diagnosis of bowel obstruction is traditionally made on the basis of clinical findings, history, plain films of the abdomen, and contrast studies of the gut.[59–61] Megibow and colleagues found that CT had 94% sensitivity, 96% specificity, and 95% accuracy in diagnosing bowel obstruction (Fig. 44–17). Furthermore, CT identified the cause of obstruction in 73% of patients in this series.[60] The authors concluded that CT is the exami-

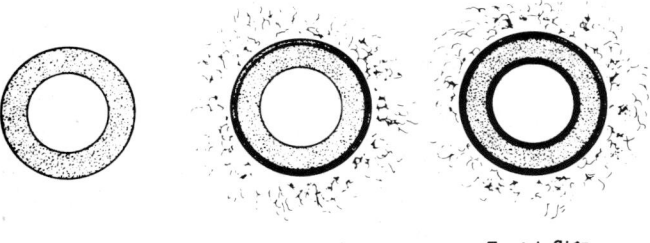

Homogeneous    Double Halo Sign    Target Sign

**Figure 44–12. Benign small bowel disease.** Diagram depicting cross section of small bowel in benign intestinal disease. The scan may exhibit homogeneous enhancing soft tissue density; two concentric rings of low and high attenuation (double halo sign); or three concentric rings of high, low, and high density (target sign). The presence of two or three concentric rings has similar clinical significance. These density differences are due to mucosal hyperemia, the degree of contrast enhancement, and submucosal edema, inflammation, and fat deposition. (From EJ Balthazar, CT of the gastrointestinal tract: principles and interpretation, AJR, 156, 1, 23–32, 1991, © by American Roentgen Ray Society.)

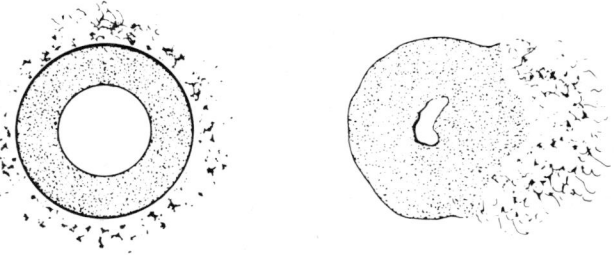

Benign    Malignant

**Figure 44–14. Cross section of abnormal bowel.** In benign disease a CT scan demonstrates modest (0.3 to 1.0 cm) circumferential and symmetric wall thickening associated with an inflammatory response in the adjacent mesentery. Neoplasms produce greater mural thickening (>2 cm), asymmetric involvement, lobulated contour, and lumen narrowing. (From EJ Balthazar: CT of the gastrointestinal tract: principles and interpretation, AJR, 156, 1, 23–32, 1991, © by American Roentgen Ray Society.)

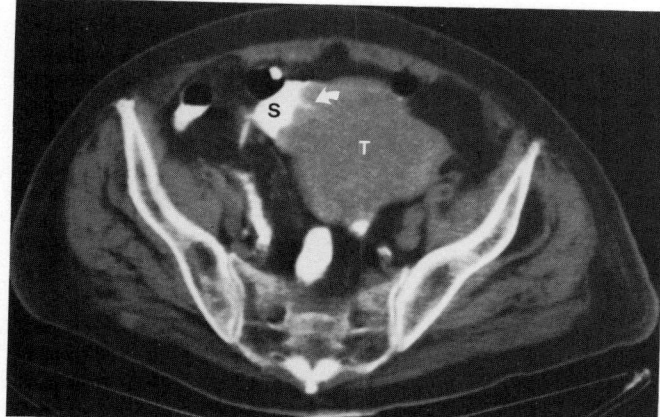

**Figure 44–15. Leiomyosarcoma of the ileum.** This tumor (T) manifested as a large ulcerating *(arrow)* mass that caused partial small bowel obstruction. S = dilated ileum proximal to mass.

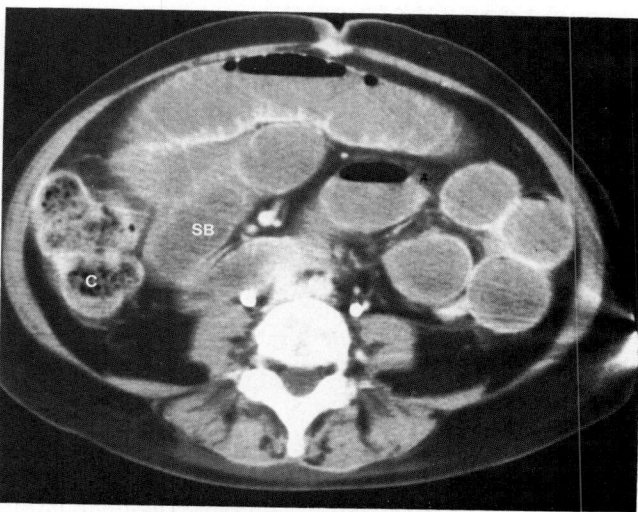

**Figure 44–17. Small bowel obstruction diagnosed on CT.** Note the dilated, fluid-filled small bowel (SB) and the normal-sized, stool-filled cecum (C). The level of obstruction was correctly identified as the terminal ileum by CT. The offending carcinoid neoplasm, however, was not visible.

nation of choice for patients with a history of abdominal malignancy and clinical symptoms suggesting bowel obstruction.[60] CT has a secondary role for patients with a history of abdominal surgery without cancer who most likely have adhesions. In patients without a surgical history, CT is of greatest value when there are systemic signs suggesting infection, bowel infarction, and a palpable abdominal mass.[60]

## Intussusception

Intussusceptions are manifest as three different patterns that reflect their severity and duration: target sign (Fig. 44–18), a sausage-shaped mass with alternating layers of low and high attentuation, and a reniform mass.[62]

Pathophysiologically, the target represents the earliest stage of intussusception. As it progresses, a layering pattern with alternating low-density (mesenteric fat) and high-attenuation (bowel wall) areas develops. If the condition is untreated, edema and mural thickening develop. An intussusception with a reniform appearance is due to severe edema and vascular compromise and constitutes a surgical emergency.[62–64]

Intussusception is almost invariably associated with either acute intestinal obstruction or partial and recurrent obstruction, air-fluid levels, and proximal bowel distention. The mesenteric arcade associated with the intussuscepted loop may show traction as it accompanies this eccentrically placed region of mesentery. If infarction occurs, this mass may be surrounded by intraperitoneal fluid, edema, and hemorrhage in the mesentery and even perforation.[65, 66]

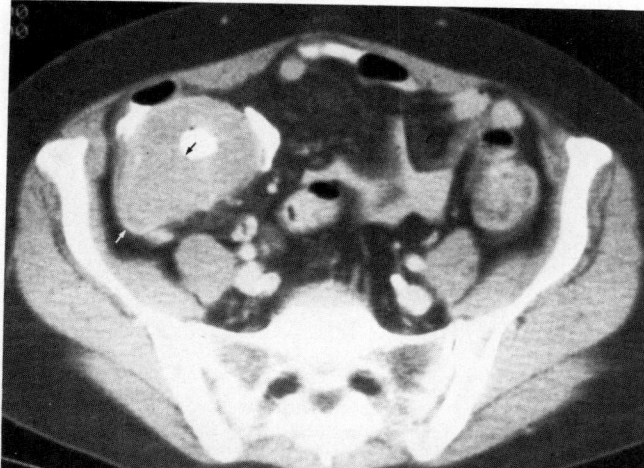

**Figure 44–16. Non-Hodgkin's lymphoma of the terminal ileum.** This neoplasm *(arrows)* has homogeneous mural attenuation with a lobulated posterolateral margin 4.3 cm in thickness. Lumen caliber is preserved.

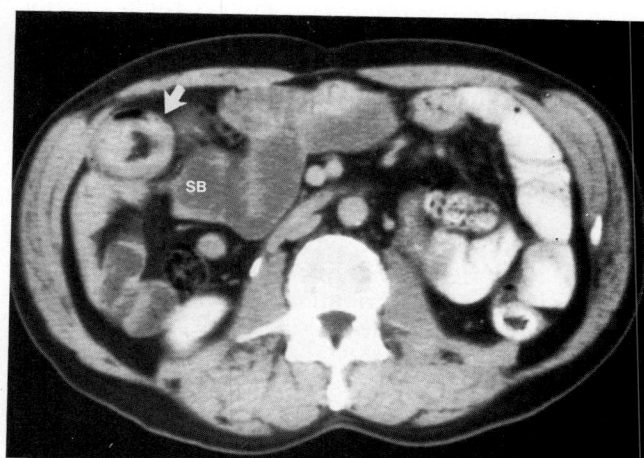

**Figure 44–18. Ileoileal intussusception.** The intussusception *(arrow)* has a target appearance; the low-density central region is the intussuscepted mesenteric fat. There is modest small bowel (SB) dilation proximally. The lead point was an ileal fibroma.

## Closed Loop Obstruction

Closed loop obstruction is indicated on CT scans by a characteristic U-shaped configuration of a distended loop of bowel with collapsed bowel distal to the obstruction. Mural edema and hemorrhage may also be present.[67, 68]

## Afferent Loop Syndrome

When the afferent loop of a Billroth II gastrojejunostomy becomes obstructed, it can appear as a cystic mass in the right upper quadrant and epigastrium.[69, 70]

## Hernias

Hernias are a major cause of mechanical small bowel obstruction, and CT is useful in depicting the precise site and type of hernia and its contents. Inguinal hernias can be distinguished from femoral hernias by locating the hernia sac anterior (inguinal) or posterior (femoral) to the inguinal ligament. Spigelian, obturator, lumbar, and ventral hernias are nicely depicted on CT scans.[71–75] A complete discussion of hernias can be found in Chapter 134.

## Inflammatory Disease

Inflammatory diseases of the gut become manifest on CT scans only when the disease has spread beyond the mucosa and involves full mural thickness. The associated mural thickening is nonspecific because this finding is also common in neoplastic and ischemic disorders. The fat of the adjacent mesentery should also be carefully examined because the edema and cellular infiltrate that accompany small bowel disease increase the density of the normally low-attenuation fat. Accordingly, the involved fat shows a hazy density and linear stranding adjacent to abnormal segments of gut (Fig. 44–19). Phlegmons or frank abscesses may develop.[76–80]

The extramucosal complications of Crohn's disease, such as "creeping fat" of the mesentery, phlegmon, abscess, and fistula, are well depicted on CT scans and are discussed in Chapters 47 and 159.

## Ischemic Disease

Ischemic bowel disease typically produces mild (5 to 10 mm), circumferential, and symmetric mural thickening with segmental distribution. The wall may have a homogeneous or double halo density.[81–85] Mesenteric and intraperitoneal blood and small bowel dilatation with congestive changes in the mesentery may also be present (Fig. 44–20). With proper intravenous contrast techniques, thrombus may be visible in the superior mesenteric and portal vein and rarely, superior mesenteric artery.[86, 87]

With infarction, pneumatosis (Fig. 44–21) and portal venous gas can be identified with greater accuracy than

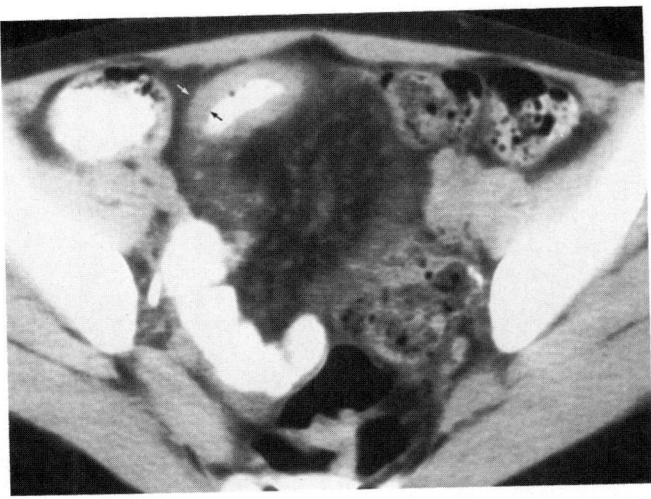

**Figure 44–19. Crohn's disease.** Homogeneous circumferential mural thickening *(arrows)* of the ileum is present. Edematous changes are seen in the adjacent fat posteromedially.

on plain films because overlap of other bowel loops is not a problem and CT is sensitive in identifying gas density.[88–90]

## Hemorrhage

Mural hemorrhage associated with trauma, bleeding diathesis, or ischemia is readily identified on CT scans. The wall is thickened with areas of high density.[43, 83, 91]

## Infectious Disease

Infections of the small bowel can lead to increased secretions, mural thickening, lumen dilation, and fold

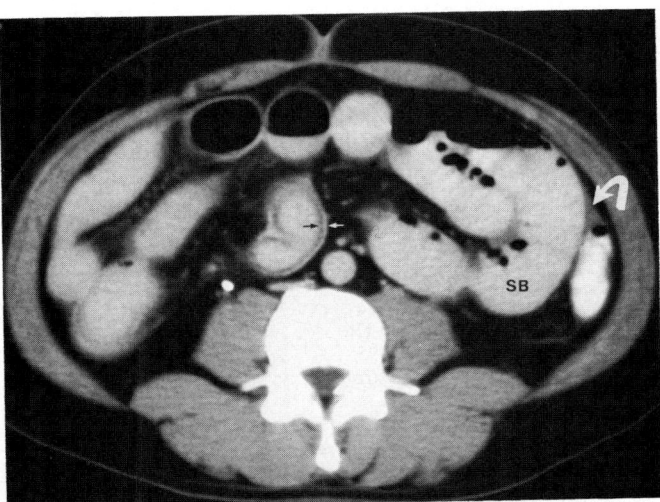

**Figure 44–20. Ischemic enteritis.** This patient with rheumatoid arthritis presented with abdominal pain. The CT scan shows a segment of proximal ileal wall thickening with a double halo appearance *(straight arrows)*. Modest small bowel (SB) dilatation proximally and some intraperitoneal hemorrhage *(curved arrow)* are seen.

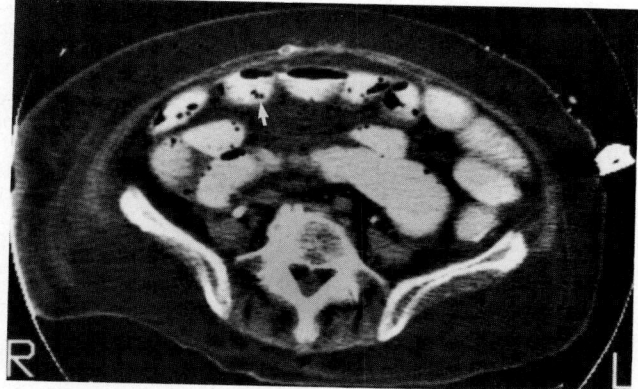

**Figure 44–21. Pneumatosis intestinalis.** A CT scan was obtained to evaluate abdominal pain and modest small bowel distention in this patient with ischemic enteritis. The intramural gas *(arrow)* was not appreciated on plain abdominal films.

thickening. Ancillary findings such as ascites, solid organ disease, adenopathy, and mesenteric changes can help clarify the diagnosis.[92-98]

In patients with the acquired immunodeficiency syndrome, bowel infections are common; *Mycobacterium avium-intracellulare*, *Cryptosporidium*, and *Isospora belli* are the most common organisms. Patients with *M. avium-intracellulare* infection may have marked adenopathy, hepatosplenomegaly, and diffuse mural thickening of the jejunum.[92-98] In patients with graft-versus-host disease, prolonged mucosal coating of the small bowel may be present.

## MAGNETIC RESONANCE IMAGING

Magnetic resonance imaging of the small bowel has been slow to develop for several reasons: the proven efficacy of CT, long acquisition times leading to poor spatial resolution, and the lack of a good magnetic resonance contrast agent for the gut.[99-106] For these reasons, the technique should now be used only as an adjunct to CT and other imaging techniques in evaluating the small bowel. Selective application of magnetic resonance imaging to the small bowel is illustrated in Chapter 9.

## References

1. Dubbins PA: The gastrointestinal tract. *In* Kurtz AB, Goldberg BB (eds): Gastrointestinal Ultrasonography. New York: Churchill Livingstone, 1988, pp 195–236.
2. Carroll BR: US of the gastrointestinal tract. Radiology 172:605–608, 1989.
3. Fleischer AC, Purulekar S, Seibert JJ: Sonography of the small bowel. *In* Herlinger H, Maglinte D (eds): Clinical Radiology of the Small Intestine. Philadelphia: WB Saunders, 1989, pp 153–159.
4. Fleischer AC, Muhletaler CA, James AE: Detection of bowel lesions during abdominal and pelvic sonography. JAMA 244:2096–2099, 1980.
5. Rao BK, Fleischer AC: Sonography of the gastrointestinal tract. Curr Opin Radiol 2:207–212, 1990.
6. Fleischer AC, Muhletaler CA, James AE Jr: Sonographic assessment of the bowel wall. AJR 136:887–891, 1981.
7. Fleischer A, Dowling A, Weinstein M, et al: Sonographic patterns of distended, fluid filled bowel. Radiology 133:681–685, 1979.
8. Weill F, Zeltner F, Rohmer P, et al: Les images gastriques et intestinales en ultrasonographie abdominale. J Radiol 60:579–590, 1979.
9. Wang KY, Kimmey MB: Intestinal ultrasound. Appl Radiol 20:59–66, 1991.
10. Kimmy MB, Martin RW, Haggitt RC, et al: Histologic correlates of gastrointestinal ultrasound images. Gastroenterology 96:433–441, 1989.
11. Bluth EI, Merritt CRB, Sullivan MA: Ultrasonic evaluation of the stomach, small bowel and colon. Radiology 133:677–680, 1979.
12. Fakhry JR, Berk RN: The "target" pattern: characteristic sonographic feature of stomach and bowel abnormalities. AJR 137:969–972, 1981.
13. Morgan CL, Trought WS, Oddison TA, et al: Ultrasound patterns of disorders affecting the gastrointestinal tract. Radiology 135:129–135, 1980.
14. Derchi LE, Solbiati L, Rizzatto G, et al: Normal anatomy and pathologic changes of the small bowel mesentery: US appearance. Radiology 164:649–652, 1987.
15. Miller JH, Hindman BW, Lam AHK: Ultrasound in the evaluation of small bowel lymphoma in children. Radiology 135:409–414, 1980.
16. Mueller PR, Ferrucci JT, Harbin WP, et al: Appearance of lymphomatous involvement of the mesentery by ultrasonography and body computed tomography: the "sandwich sign." Radiology 134:467–473, 1980.
17. Meiser G, Meissner K: Ileus and intestinal obstruction—ultrasonographic findings as a guideline to therapy. Hepatogastroenterology 34:194–199, 1987.
18. Scheible W, Goldberg LE: Diagnosis of small bowel obstruction: the constriction of diagnostic ultrasound. AJR 133:685–688, 1979.
19. Pon MS, Scudamore C, Harrison RC, et al: Ultrasound demonstration of radiographically obscure small bowel obstruction. AJR 133:145–146, 1979.
20. Hopens T, Coggs GC, Goldstein HM, et al: Sonographic diagnosis of afferent loop obstruction. AJR 138:967–969, 1982.
21. Bowerman RA, Silver TM, Jaffe MH: Real-time ultrasound diagnosis of intussusception in children. Radiology 143:527–529, 1982.
22. Morin ME, Blumenthal DH, Tan A, et al: The ultrasonic appearance of ileocolic intussusception. J Clin Ultrasound 9:516–518, 1981.
23. Verbanck JJ, Rutgeerts LJ, Douterlungne PH, et al: Sonographic and pathologic correlation in intussusception of the bowel. J Clin Ultrasound 14:393–397, 1986.
24. Skaane P, Skjennald A: Ultrasonic features for ileocecal intussusception. J Clin Ultrasound 17:590–593, 1989.
25. Alessi V, Salerno G: The "hay-fork" sign in the ultrasonographic diagnosis of intussusception. Gastrointest Radiol 10:177–179, 1985.
26. Gore RM: Cross-sectional imaging of inflammatory bowel disease. Radiol Clin North Am 25:115–129, 1987.
27. Schmutz G, Drape JL, Behnaim M, et al: Aspect echographique de la maladie de Crohn. J Radiol 67:697–706, 1986.
28. Bonnerberg A, Erckenbrecht J, Peter P, et al: Detection of Crohn's disease by ultrasound. Gastroenterology 83:430–436, 1982.
29. Holt S, Samuel E: Grey scale ultrasound in Crohn's disease. Gut 20:590–595, 1979.
30. Dubbins PA: Ultrasound demonstration of bowel wall thickness in inflammatory bowel disease. Clin Radiol 35:227–231, 1984.
31. Kaftori JK, Peri M, Kleinhaus U: Ultrasonography in Crohn's disease. Gastrointest Radiol 9:137–142, 1984.
32. Pedersen BH, Gronvnall S, Dorph S, et al: The value of dynamic ultrasound scanning in Crohn's disease. Scand J Gastroenterol 21:969–972, 1986.
33. Di Candio G, Mosca F, Campatelli A, et al: Sonographic

detection of postsurgical recurrence of Crohn's disease. AJR 146:523–526, 1986.

34. Moneta GI, Taylor DC, Helton WS, et al: Duplex ultrasound measurement of postprandial blood flow. Gastroenterology 95:1294–1301, 1988.

35. Lynch TG, Hobson RW, Kerr JC, et al: Doppler ultrasound, laser Doppler, and perfusion fluorometry in bowel ischemia. Arch Surg 123:483–486, 1988.

36. Bellamy EA, Bassi MC, Cosgrove DO: Ultrasound demonstration of changes in the normal portal venous system following a meal. Br J Radiol 57:147–151, 1984.

37. Taylor KJW: Gastrointestinal duplex Doppler. *In* Kurtz AB, Goldberg BB (eds): Gastrointestinal Ultrasonography. New York: Churchill Livingstone, 1988, pp 261–287.

38. Gill RW: Measurement of the blood flow by ultrasound: accuracy and sources of error. Ultrasound Med Biol 11:626–641, 1985.

39. Hartnell GG, Gibson RN: Doppler ultrasound in the diagnosis of intestinal ischemia. Gastrointest Radiol 12:285–288, 1987.

40. Balthazar EJ: CT of the gastrointestinal tract: principles and interpretation. AJR 156:23–32, 1991.

41. Hulnick DH, Megibow AJ: Computed tomography of the small bowel. *In* Herlinger H, Maglinte D (eds): Clinical Radiology of the Small Intestine. Philadelphia: WB Saunders, 1989, pp 161–200.

42. Bert P, Cuche C, Schmutz G: Radiology of the Small Intestine. Paris: Springer-Verlag, 1989, pp 39–43.

43. Merine D, Fishman EK, Jones B: CT of the small bowel and mesentery. Radiol Clin North Am 27:707–715, 1989.

44. Nemcek AA: CT of acute intestinal disorders. Radiol Clin North Am 27:773–786, 1989.

45. Scatarige JC, Allen HA, Fishman EK: Computed tomography of the small bowel. Semin Ultrasound CT MR 8:403–423, 1987.

46. Desai RK, Tagliabue JR, Wegryn SA, et al: CT evaluation of wall thickening in the alimentary tract. Radiographics 11:771–783, 1991.

47. Silverman PM, Kelvin FM, Korobkin M, et al: Computed tomography of the normal mesentery. AJR 143:953–957, 1984.

48. James S, Balfe DM, Lee JKT, et al: Small-bowel disease: categorization by CT examination. AJR 148:863–868, 1987.

49. Dudiak KM, Johnson CD, Stephens DH: Primary tumors of the small intestine: CT evaluation. AJR 152:995–998, 1989.

50. Laurent F, Raynaud M, Biset JM, et al: Diagnosis and categorization of small bowel neoplasms: role of computed tomography. Gastrointest Radiol 16:115–119, 1991.

51. Megibow AJ, Balthazar EJ, Hulnick DH, et al: CT evaluation of gastrointestinal leiomyomas and leiomyosarcomas. AJR 144:727–731, 1985.

52. McLeod AJ, Zornoza J, Shirkohoda A: Leiomyosarcoma: computed tomography findings. Radiology 152:133–136, 1984.

53. Adolph JM, Kimmig BN, Georgi P, et al: Carcinoid tumors: CT and I-131 meta-iodo-benzylguanidine scintigraphy. Radiology 164:199–203, 1987.

54. Picus D, Glazer HS, Levitt RG, et al: Computed tomography of abdominal carcinoid tumors. AJR 143:581–584, 1984.

55. Cockey BM, Fishman EK, Jones B, et al: Computed tomography of abdominal carcinoid tumor of the gastrointestinal tract. J Comput Assist Tomogr 9:38–44, 1985.

56. Megibow AJ, Balthazar EJ, Naidich DP, et al: Computed tomography of gastrointestinal lymphoma. AJR 141:541–547, 1983.

57. Pagani JJ, Bernardino ME: CT-radiographic correlation of ulcerating small bowel lymphomas. AJR 136:998–1000, 1981.

58. Blackledge G, Best JK, Crowther D: Role of computed tomography in staging and management of gastrointestinal lymphoma. J R Soc Med 78:818–822, 1979.

59. Megibow AJ, Balthazar EJ, Cho KC, et al: Bowel obstruction: evaluation with CT. Radiology 180:313–318, 1991.

60. Rubesin SE, Herlinger H: CT evaluation of bowel obstruction: a landmark article—implications for the future. Radiology 180:307–308, 1991.

61. Schnyder PA, Candarjis: CT detection of benign and malignant abnormalities of the small bowel. Eur J Radiol 3:33–38, 1983.

62. Merine D, Fishman EK, Jones B, et al: Enteroenteric intussusception: CT findings in nine patients. AJR 148:1129–1132, 1987.

63. Bar-Ziv J, Solomon A: Computed tomography in adult intussusception. Gastrointest Radiol 16:264–266, 1991.

64. Jeffrey RB: Computed tomography of acute small bowel abnormalities. *In* Herlinger H, Megibow A: Gastrointestinal Radiology Reviews, Volume I. New York: Marcel Dekker, 1990, pp 231–256.

65. Abiri S, Baer J, Abiri M: Computed tomography and sonography in small bowel intussusception: a case report. Am J Gastroenterol 81:1076–1077, 1986.

66. Knowles MC, Fishman EK, Kuhlman JE, et al: Transient intussusception in Crohn disease: CT evaluation. Radiology 170:814, 1989.

67. Balthazar EJ, Bauman JS, Megibow AJ: CT diagnosis of closed loop obstruction. J Comput Assist Tomogr 9:953–955, 1985.

68. Cho KC, Hoffman-Tretin JC, Alterman DD: Closed-loop obstruction of the small bowel: CT and sonographic appearance. J Comput Assist Tomogr 13:256–258, 1989.

69. Gale ME, Gerzof SG, Kiser LC, et al: CT of afferent loop obstruction. AJR 138:1085–1088, 1982.

70. Swayne LC, Love MG: Computed tomography of chronic afferent loop obstruction: a case report and review. Gastrointest Radiol 10:39–41, 1985.

71. Harkin WP: Computed tomographic diagnosis of internal hernia. Radiology 143:736–737, 1982.

72. Ghahremani GG, Jimenez MA, Rosenfeld M, et al: CT diagnosis of occult incisional hernias. AJR 148:139–142, 1987.

73. Ghahremani GG, Gore RM: CT diagnosis of postoperative abdominal complications. Radiol Clin North Am 27:787–804, 1989.

74. Pyatt RS, Alona BR: Spigelian hernia. J Comput Assist Tomogr 6:643–645, 1982.

75. Megibow AJ, Wagner AG: Case report: obturator hernia. J Comput Assist Tomogr 7:350–352, 1983.

76. Gore RM: CT of inflammatory bowel disease. Radiol Clin North Am 27:717–729, 1989.

77. Gore RM, Goldberg HI: Computed tomographic evaluation of the gastrointestinal tract in diseases other than primary adenocarcinoma. Radiol Clin North Am 20:781–796, 1982.

78. Jones B, Fishman EK, Hamilton SR, et al: Submucosal accumulation of fat in inflammatory bowel disease: CT/pathologic correlation. J Comput Assist Tomogr 10:759–763, 1986.

79. Fishman EK, Jones B: Evaluation of Crohn's disease. *In* Fishman EK, Jones B (eds): Computed Tomography of the Gastrointestinal Tract. New York: Churchill Livingstone, 1988, pp 85–107.

80. Gore RM, Marn CS, Kirby DF, et al: CT findings in ulcerative, granulomatous, and indeterminate colitis. AJR 143:279–284, 1984.

81. Federle MP, Chun G, Jeffrey RB, et al: Computed tomographic findings in bowel infarction. AJR 142:91–95, 1984.

82. Alpern MB, Glazer GM, Francis IR: Ischemic or infarcted bowel: CT findings. Radiology 166:149–152, 1988.

83. Balthazar EJ, Hulnick DH, Megibow AJ, et al: Computed tomography of intramural intestinal hemorrhage and bowel ischemia. J Comput Assist Tomogr 11:67–72, 1987.

84. Clark RA: Computed tomography of bowel infarction. J Comput Assist Tomogr 11:757–762, 1987.

85. Perez C, Leauger J, Puig J, et al: Computed tomographic findings in bowel ischemia. Gastrointest Radiol 14:241–245, 1989.

86. Vogelzang RL, Anshuetz SL, Gore RM, et al: Thrombosis of the splanchnic veins: CT diagnosis. AJR 150:93–96, 1988.

87. Rosen A, Korobkin M, Silverman PM, et al: Mesenteric vein thrombosis: CT identification. AJR 143:83–86, 1984.

88. Kelvin FM, Korobkin M, Rauch RF, et al: Computed tomography of pneumatosis intestinalis. J Comput Assist Tomogr 8:276–280, 1984.

89. Connor R, Jones B, Fishman EK, et al: Pneumatosis intestinalis: role of computed tomography in diagnosis and management. J Comput Assist Tomogr 8:269–275, 1984.

90. Smerud MJ, Johnson CD, Stephens DH: Diagnosis of bowel infarction: a comparison of plain films and CT scans in 23 cases. AJR 154:99–103, 1990.

91. Ploujoux O, Hauser H, Wettstein P: Computed tomography of intramural hematoma of the small intestine. Radiology 144:559–561, 1982.

92. Jones B, Fishman EK: CT of the gut in the immunocompromised host. Radiol Clin North Am 27:763–772, 1989.

93. Kotler DP: Gastrointestinal complications of the acquired immunodeficiency syndrome. *In* Yamada T (ed): Textbook of

Gastroenterology. Philadelphia: JB Lippincott, 1991, pp 2086–2103.

94. Wall SD, Ominsky S, Altman DF, et al: Multifocal abnormalities of the gastrointestinal tract in AIDS. AJR 146:1–5, 1986.

95. Balthazar EJ, Gordon R, Hulnick D: Ileocecal tuberculosis: CT and radiologic evaluation. AJR 154:499–503, 1990.

96. Radin DR: Intraabdominal *Mycobacterium tuberculosis* vs. *Mycobacterium avium-intracellulare* infections in patients with AIDS: distinction based on CT findings. AJR 156:487–491, 1991.

97. Vincent ME, Robbins AH: *Mycobacterium avium-intracellulare* complex enteritis: pseudo-Whipple's disease in AIDS. AJR 144:921–922, 1985.

98. Angus KW: Cryptosporidiosis and AIDS. Baillieres Clin Gastroenterol 4:425–441, 1990.

99. Werthmuller WC, Margulis AR: Magnetic resonance imaging of the alimentary tube. Invest Radiol 26:195–200, 1991.

100. Stark DD, Fahlvik AK, Klaveness J: Abdominal imaging. JMRI 3:285–295, 1993

101. Rubin DL, Muller HH, Sidhu MK, et al: Liquid oral magnetic particles as a gastrointestinal contrast agent for MR imaging: efficacy in vivo. JMRI 3:113–118, 1993.

102. Unger EC, Fritz TA, Palestrant D, et al: Preliminary evaluation of iron phytate (inositol hexaphosphate) as a gastrointestinal MR contrast agent. JMRI 3:119–124, 1993.

103. Rubin DL, Muller HH, Nino-Murcia M, et al: Intraluminal contrast enhancement and MR visualization of the bowel wall: efficacy of PFOB. J Magn Reson Imaging 1:371–380, 1991.

104. Rinck PA, Smevik O, Nilsen G, et al: Oral magnetic particles in MR imaging of the abdomen and pelvis. Radiology 178:775–779, 1991.

105. Mitchell DG, Vinitski S: Principles and protocol optimization for MRI of the abdomen and pelvis. Crit Rev Diagn Imaging 31:117–144, 1990.

106. Boudghène FP, Bach-Gansmo T, Grange J-D, et al: Contribution of oral magnetic particles in MR imaging of the abdomen with spin-echo and gradient-echo sequences. JMRI 3:107–112, 1993.

# Angiography and Interventional Radiology

**Albert A. Nemcek, Jr., M.D.**

**Robert L. Vogelzang, M.D.**

## INTRODUCTION

In addition to general aspects of small bowel angiography, this chapter describes in detail the angiographic features of acute and chronic mesenteric ischemia. Despite the increasing use of computed tomography (CT) and sonography for patients with unexplained abdominal pain, angiography continues to be the test of choice for suspected mesenteric ischemia. In addition, angiography allows selective infusion of pharmacologic agents that may improve the chances for a favorable outcome in cases of mesenteric ischemia; thrombolytic therapy and percutaneous transluminal angioplasty show promise in the treatment of acute mesenteric vascular occlusion and of chronic mesenteric ischemia.

In the section on nonvascular interventions, the indications and techniques for small bowel enterostomy are discussed. The more general topic of management of enteric fistulas is also described.

## ANGIOGRAPHY OF THE SMALL BOWEL

### Diagnosis and Radiologic Management of Acute Mesenteric Ischemia

#### Clinical and Angiographic Features

CT has been increasingly employed in the assessment of patients with acute abdominal pain. Because of the ability of CT to evaluate the bowel wall, the surrounding mesentery, and major vascular structures, this method can often suggest the presence of mesenteric ischemia or infarction, sometimes quite specifically. Despite this, angiography remains the test of choice for studying patients with suspected mesenteric ischemia. Angiography provides detailed anatomic and etiologic information that aids therapeutic planning and directs further diagnostic work-up. In addition, selective catheterization allows the angiographer to initiate various transcatheter therapies when these are appropriate.

Patients with acute mesenteric ischemia are generally elderly and commonly have coexistent medical disorders, especially cardiac disease, hypotension or hypovolemia, or sepsis. Severe abdominal pain is frequently present and in the early stages is characteristically out of proportion to physical findings. Unexplained abdominal distention and gastrointestinal bleeding should also place ischemia high on the list of differential considerations. When significant physical findings have developed, they usually indicate that ischemia has progressed to infarction. On laboratory evaluation, an elevated white blood cell count and metabolic acidosis are frequent findings.[1, 2]

Before angiography, a plain film of the abdomen is important, not so much to identify specific signs of bowel ischemia but mainly to help exclude other diagnostic considerations.[1, 2] Lateral abdominal aortography reveals the status of the proximal mesenteric vessels and should be the initial step in angiographic evaluation of mesenteric ischemia.[1, 3, 4] If the proximal portion of the superior mesenteric artery (SMA) is patent, selective arteriography of this vessel is performed for a detailed study of the superior mesenteric trunk and its branches and of the mesenteric venous drainage. Acute mesenteric ischemia is primarily a disorder of the superior mesenteric territory, and selective celiac and inferior mesenteric injections are not usually necessary. However, these further studies can provide information about the presence and extent of collateral supply to the superior mesenteric territory, particularly when the chronicity of a superior mesenteric occlusion is questioned. These additional angiograms can also be considered if clinical data strongly suggest involvement of the stomach, the duodenum, or the segment of colon supplied by the inferior mesenteric artery.

Major causes of acute mesenteric ischemia are SMA thrombosis or embolism, mesenteric venous thrombosis, and the nonocclusive form of ischemia.[1-4] The relative proportion of each of these categories has differed in reported series. At least part of this disparity reflects a greater understanding and better recognition of possible etiologies, and part reflects improved treatment or the prevention of underlying disorders. Vasculitis, aortic or mesenteric arterial dissection (Fig. 45–1), trauma, bowel strangulation, and other disorders are less common causes of mesenteric ischemia. Involvement of all or most of the superior mesenteric territory typically produces severe and life-threatening mesenteric ischemia. Focal ischemia can result from more limited or segmental forms of the previously mentioned etiologies and causes less severe clinical manifestations.[1]

One review suggested that SMA occlusion (Figs. 45–2 to 45–5) is now the most frequent cause of acute mesenteric ischemia, with embolism more common than thrombosis.[2] The angiographic distinction between these two entities can be difficult.[3, 4] Multiple filling defects, tracking of contrast medium at the lateral aspects of a

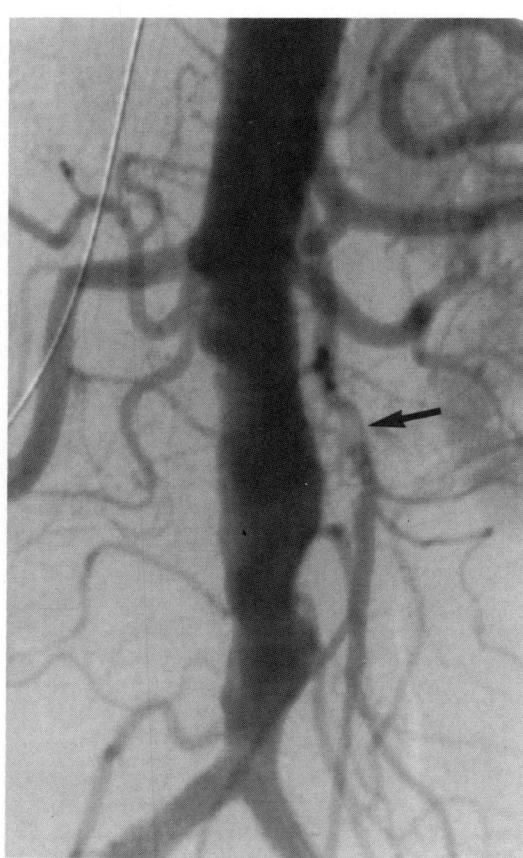

**Figure 45–2. Superior mesenteric embolus.** A nearly occlusive filling defect *(arrow)* is present in the main SMA trunk, with tracking of contrast medium around it and patency of the more distal SMA.

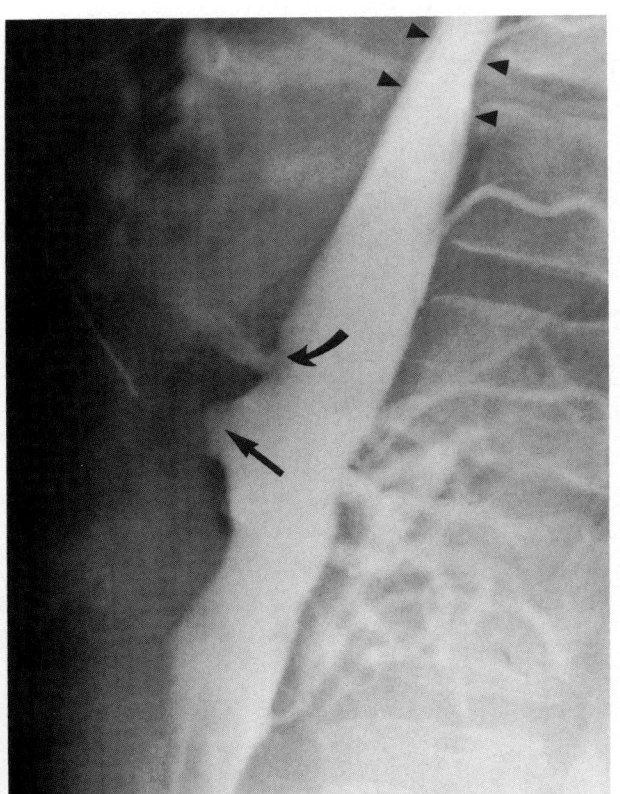

**Figure 45–1. Acute mesenteric ischemia caused by aortic dissection.** The celiac *(curved arrow)* and superior mesenteric *(straight arrow)* arteries are both occluded near their origins because of involvement by dissection flap. Narrowing of the patent true lumen of the upper abdominal aorta is present *(arrowheads)*.

filling defect, and convex menisci protruding into the opacified vascular lumen suggest emboli. Emboli also tend to lodge at vascular branch points and to be sited more distally than occlusive thrombus, which most often forms in the vicinity of a pre-existent atherosclerotic stenosis of the proximal SMA. At times, however, emboli can lodge at proximal stenoses or an embolus can initiate more proximal propagation of a thrombus.

Mesenteric venous thrombosis (Fig. 45–6) accounts for up to 10 to 20% of cases of acute mesenteric ischemia.[3] Causes of this disorder include hypercoagulable states, portal hypertension, abdominal inflammatory disease, previous surgery (particularly splenectomy), and trauma.[1, 2, 5] Often, no predisposing condition is identified. Patients may present with less severe illness than in other forms of acute mesenteric ischemia;[2] recognition that major venous occlusion does not always result in ischemia has increased as more cases of mesenteric venous thrombosis are identified with the use of cross-sectional imaging.[6] On superior mesenteric arteriography,[3, 7, 8] slowing of the arterial flow is noted, with prolonged staining of the bowel wall and of smaller mesenteric arterial branches. Arterial vasoconstriction may be present. Normal mesenteric veins either fail to opacify or show filling defects; venous collaterals may be visualized.

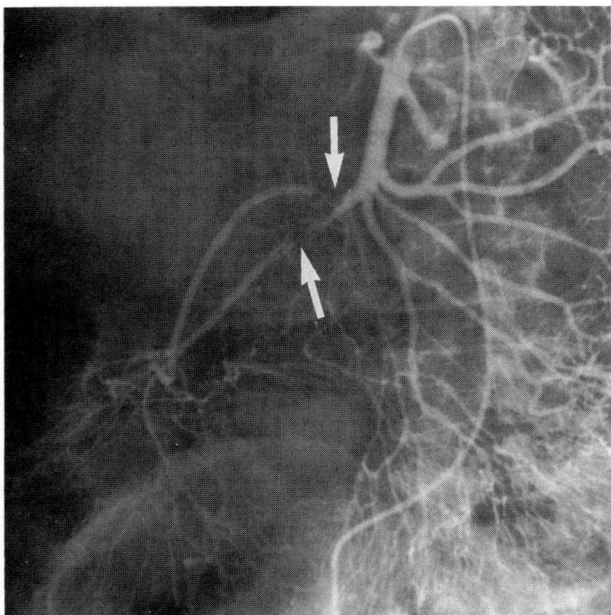

**Figure 45–3. Superior mesenteric emboli.** Multiple filling defects *(arrows)* are present in SMA branches in a patient with atrial fibrillation.

Anatomic vascular obstruction need not be present for mesenteric ischemia and infarction to occur. Diminished cardiac output, systemic hypotension or hypovolemia, and certain pharmacologic agents such as digitalis can all result in severely diminished intestinal blood flow, presumably mediated by vasoconstriction of the mesenteric arteries.[1] Nonocclusive mesenteric ischemia (Fig. 45–7) accounts for a substantial proportion of cases of acute mesenteric ischemia,[3, 9] although its incidence may be decreasing.[2] On angiography, intense vasospasm

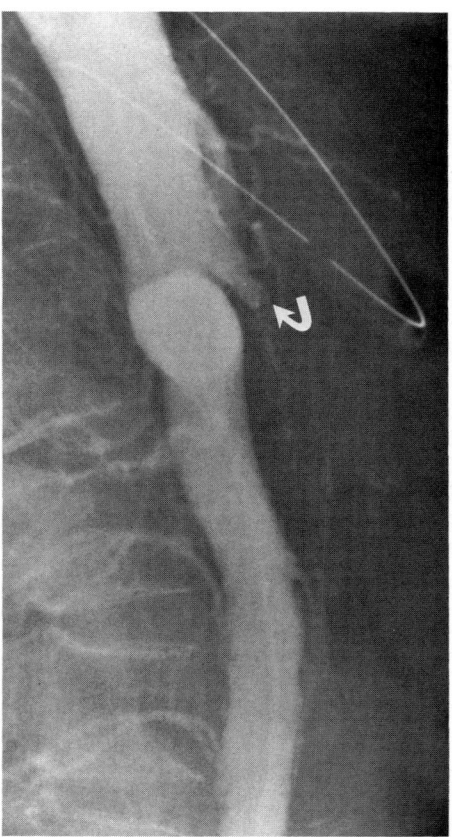

**Figure 45–5. Mesenteric arterial thrombosis.** Abrupt occlusion of the SMA is present just distal to its origin *(arrow)*.

is characteristic.[3, 4, 10, 11] Spasm is frequently irregular or segmental, with more severe areas of narrowing often seen at the origins of arterial branches. Regular and diffuse spasm can also occur. Contrast medium flows sluggishly through mesenteric vessels, causing delayed

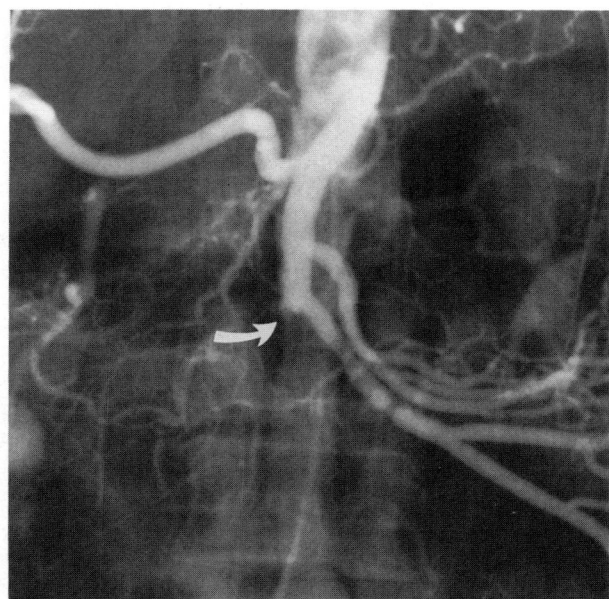

**Figure 45–4. Superior mesenteric embolus.** Abrupt occlusion *(arrow)* of the superior mesenteric trunk is present distal to jejunal branches in a patient with atrial fibrillation.

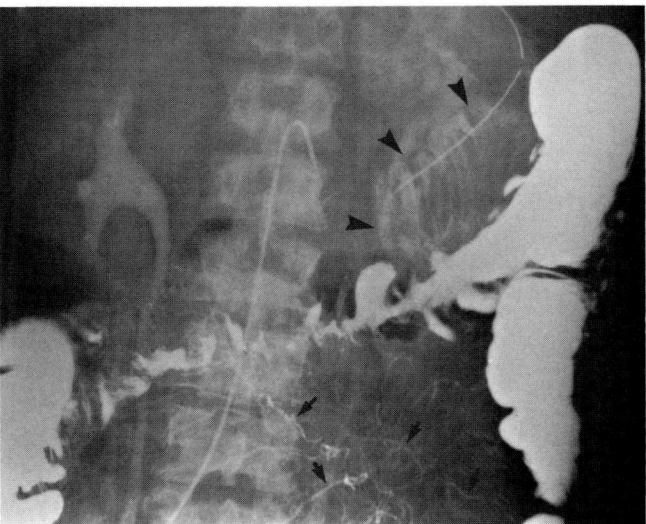

**Figure 45–6. Mesenteric venous thrombosis.** Delayed films after superior mesenteric arterial contrast medium injection show no filling of the mesenteric venous system. Small arterial branches *(arrows)* remain opacified and prolonged staining of the bowel wall *(arrowheads)* is noted. Residual barium is present in the colon.

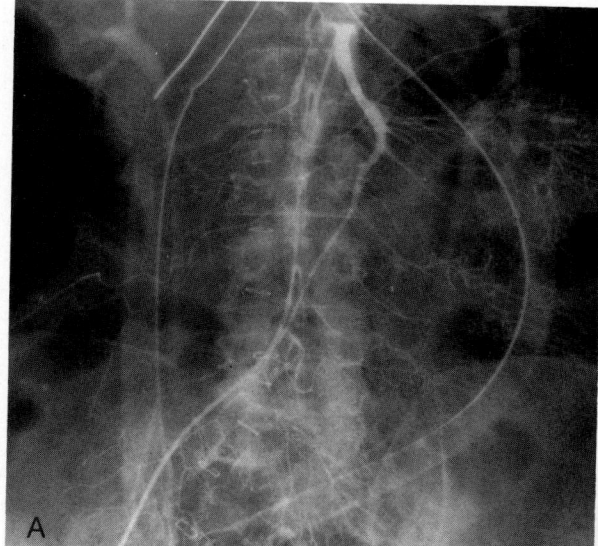

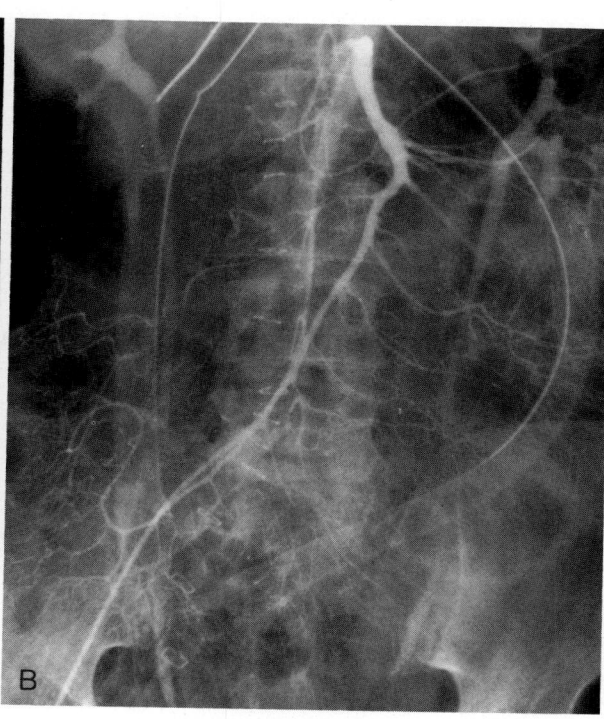

**Figure 45–7. Nonocclusive mesenteric ischemia. A.** Diffuse mesenteric arterial spasm is present, with poor filling of smaller arterial branches. **B.** Improvement in the spasm is noted after initiation of intra-arterial papaverine infusion.

opacification of peripheral and mural branches. In this regard, the findings are similar to those of mesenteric venous thrombosis, although normal veins eventually fill in most cases of nonocclusive ischemia.[7] Increased reflux of contrast medium into the aorta can also be seen,[3] reflecting increased impedance to mesenteric flow. In practice this finding is usually judged subjectively, although more objective and quantitative means of assessing superior mesenteric flow based on aortic reflux have been described.[12, 13]

If angiography fails to confirm the clinical suspicion of acute mesenteric ischemia, it can be followed immediately by other radiologic studies such as barium enema or abdominal CT to help identify alternative abdominal disorders.

Despite improved methods of diagnosis and therapy for acute mesenteric ischemia, this disorder continues to be associated with a high mortality rate. In the late 1970s, Boley and colleagues[14] described their "aggressive approach" to acute mesenteric ischemia. Although even with this approach about half of those afflicted expire, it represents a distinct improvement compared with earlier controlled studies that showed only 10 to 30% survival; in addition, the aggressive approach may allow more bowel to be salvaged in those who have survived.[1–3, 11, 14] Central to this concept is early diagnosis and characterization of mesenteric ischemia by emergency angiography, even if surgical therapy has already been deemed necessary. Hesitation because of reluctance to expose an ill patient to the potential hazards of angiography leads to progressive deterioration of the status of the bowel, and elimination of angiography may result in less than optimal surgical therapy. Another salient feature is the selective infusion of vasodilators (see Fig.

45–7) into the SMA, the rationale for which is the association of vasospasm with both nonocclusive and occlusive mesenteric ischemia. When mesenteric angiography has revealed vasospasm or arterial occlusion, a test dose of a vasodilator should be given. Boley and co-workers[1] favored a 25-mg bolus of tolazoline for this purpose because of its rapid action, although papaverine and other agents can also be used.[11] This initial dose of tolazoline allows improved visualization of peripheral arteries and of the venous phase, may help predict the efficacy of continued vasodilator infusion, and in rare instances[14] may eliminate the signs and symptoms of ischemia. Even if no angiographic response is seen, selective vasodilator infusion is started if possible. Various vasodilators have been tried,[11] but papaverine has been used most extensively, diluted in saline to a concentration of 1.0 mg/mL and administered at a rate of 30 to 60 mg/h.[3, 11, 14] Patients receiving papaverine should be monitored for hypotension and cardiac arrhythmias; the therapy is contraindicated in patients with complete heart block.[1, 11] This agent should not be mixed with heparin or used in alkaline solutions such as lactated Ringer's.[11] In nonsurgical candidates—those without persistent peritoneal signs who have minor arterial occlusions or nonocclusive ischemia—papaverine can be continued as long as no complications develop and until the clinical and angiographic abnormalities improve. In patients who are surgical candidates, papaverine is recommended both pre- and postoperatively to salvage as much bowel as possible. Subsequent angiography helps to assess the further need for papaverine infusion or surgical intervention. Papaverine infusion should be replaced by saline infusion a half-hour before the subsequent study, to evaluate recurrence of vasospasm.[1, 11]

## Thrombolytic Therapy for Mesenteric Vascular Occlusion

The tenuous status of the bowel in most cases of acute mesenteric ischemia with major vascular occlusion and the life-threatening character of resultant bowel infarction usually mandate aggressive surgical therapy. However, a number of anecdotal case reports suggest a potential role for transcatheter thrombolytic therapy in selected cases of recent mesenteric vascular occlusion.[15–20] Candidates for this therapy have included patients deemed unlikely to survive major surgery because of coexistent disease, patients with minor or partial vascular occlusions or mild symptoms (who, it could be argued, might need only observation, conservative therapy, and possibly anticoagulation), and those with extensive portal-mesenteric venous thrombosis precluding surgical thrombectomy or bypass. Patients who develop occlusion of mesenteric arterial grafts might also be considered for referral to interventional radiologists skilled in the use of thrombolytic agents. The presence of peritoneal signs suggesting bowel necrosis, however, is a contraindication to thrombolytic therapy.

Potential limitations of the use of mesenteric thrombolysis include the development of hemorrhagic bowel infarction or of severe bleeding from the mucosa of ischemic bowel, distal embolization of a partially lysed clot, and progressive deterioration of the status of the bowel during the time required to achieve complete lysis.[11, 21] However, these have not been major limitations in the cases published so far. In one report, transient severe pain after discontinuation of streptokinase infusion was postulated to be due to either distal embolization or vasoconstriction after reperfusion, but follow-up angiography and laparotomy revealed bowel that appeared normally perfused.[15]

Both streptokinase and urokinase have been used for mesenteric vascular thrombolysis, with most reports and reviews following the trend in peripheral thrombolysis by favoring urokinase. As with peripheral therapy, dose regimens and exact technical points have varied. Concomitant use of vasodilators may be reasonable, although Morse and Clark[11] cautioned that mixing of urokinase and papaverine can result in precipitation. For SMA thromboembolic occlusion, direct infusion is accomplished via a securely seated selective arterial catheter. If experience with peripheral thrombolysis is any indication, one might expect in such cases to uncover mesenteric arterial stenoses that might be amenable to balloon angioplasty (see later). In patients with thrombosis of the mesenteric veins, a direct infusion is less easily performed. Morse and Clark[11] reported their single attempt at indirect lysis of mesenteric venous thrombi via SMA infusion. Other investigators have reported successful thrombolysis after direct infusion via transhepatic puncture and catheterization of the portal-mesenteric venous system.[17, 20] With sonographic guidance, such a puncture would generally be easy to perform. Theoretically, one could argue that even when bowel viability is not threatened by mesenteric venous thrombosis, thrombolytic therapy may be worthwhile to prevent the development of collateral varices and their complications.

# Diagnosis and Radiologic Management of Chronic Mesenteric Ischemia

## Clinical and Angiographic Features

Patients whose mesenteric circulation cannot respond sufficiently when there is increased demand for blood flow may develop a characteristic array of symptoms that define chronic mesenteric ischemia.[1, 2] Visceral abdominal pain that occurs shortly after meals, when metabolic requirements of the bowel rise, is the hallmark of the disorder. Note that the designation chronic does not imply constant; the pain results from repeated acute (but reversible) episodes of inadequate intestinal perfusion. This pain, termed *abdominal angina*, can be considered the intestinal equivalent of angina pectoris resulting from coronary artery disease and of intermittent lower extremity claudication from peripheral vascular disease. Typically, the pain is epigastric in location and lasts about 1 to 3 hours. During the acute episodes, bowel motility and absorptive function may be impaired. Nausea, vomiting, and diarrhea can occur. As the condition becomes protracted, weight loss is typical and often severe. This results partly from malabsorption and partly from a reluctance to eat that not unexpectedly accompanies the anticipation of abdominal pain and can progress to outright fear of eating (sitophobia).

With few exceptions,[1] chronic intestinal ischemia is the result of atherosclerotic involvement of the splanchnic arteries (Fig. 45–8). It is most often seen in the elderly, is frequently associated with a history of heavy smoking, and affects women more often than men.[1, 2, 22–24]

Confirmation of chronic mesenteric ischemia can be difficult for a number of reasons. Characteristic symptoms such as abdominal pain and weight loss can mimic those of several other disorders. Physical signs such as abdominal bruits, cachexia, or evidence of significant atherosclerotic disease in other locations are also nonspecific. Although newer objective means of assessing intestinal perfusion are being investigated,[2] none have yet proved their value.

Similar difficulties arise with angiographic evaluation. The degree of confidence in the diagnosis of chronic mesenteric ischemia is greatest when classic symptoms combine with the angiographic demonstration of occlusions or high-grade stenoses in at least two of the three mesenteric vessels. When angiography fails to show these findings, the diagnosis should be questioned. Conversely, when these findings are present, the diagnosis must not be based on angiography alone. Both pathologic and radiologic studies have shown that significant atherosclerotic involvement of the splanchnic arteries may be unaccompanied by symptoms,[25, 26] probably attesting to the development of effective mesenteric collateral vessels.

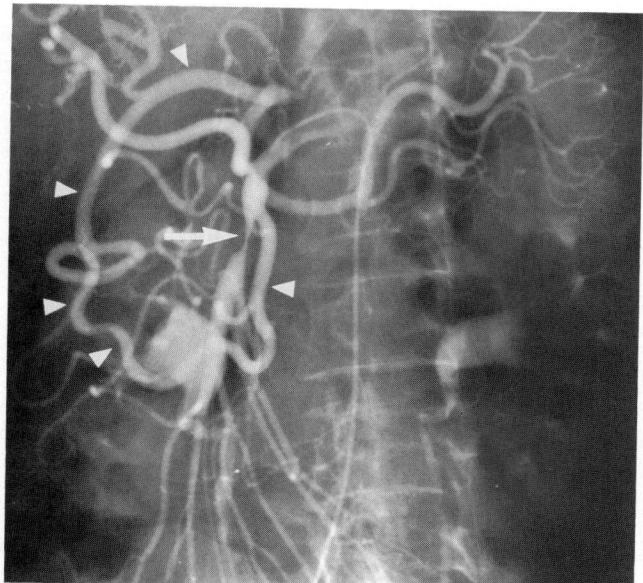

**Figure 45–8. Chronic mesenteric ischemia.** Superior mesenteric arteriogram of a 62-year-old woman with intermittent episodes of abdominal pain reveals a severe SMA stenosis *(arrow)*. There is filling of the celiac territory via an enlarged pancreaticoduodenal arcade *(arrowheads)* (the inferior pancreaticoduodenal artery arises from the SMA proximal to the stenosis). The presence of the collateral flow attests to the occlusion of the celiac origin, as also noted with lateral aortography. Symptomatic relief occurred after patch angioplasty of the SMA and aorta-to–celiac artery bypass with autologous vein.

Angiographic evaluation for chronic mesenteric ischemia should begin with a lateral aortogram, to assess the proximal portions of the celiac, superior mesenteric, and inferior mesenteric arteries. Anteroposterior aortography and selective mesenteric arteriography can be used to provide more detail regarding development of collateral vessels, patterns of flow, and the exact locations of stenoses.

## Celiac Compression Syndrome

Narrowing of the proximal celiac artery can result from extrinsic compression by the median arcuate ligament of the diaphragm or by the celiac ganglion.[1] Because both structures lie superior to the celiac origin, the typical angiographic appearance is of smooth asymmetric narrowing by compression from above and occasional caudad displacement of the proximal segment of the celiac artery[1, 27] (Fig. 45–9). The degree of stenosis may vary with respiration, diminishing during inspiration.[28]

The clinical significance of this anatomic abnormality is controversial.[1, 27, 29] Most patients with characteristic angiographic features of the celiac compression syndrome are asymptomatic. This in itself does not preclude the possibility that the abnormality could give rise to symptoms: many patients with severe atherosclerotic mesenteric stenoses are also asymptomatic. Abdominal pain has occasionally been associated with celiac compression, and in a few patients symptomatic improve-

ment has followed surgical decompression. However, symptoms often fail to fit the typical clinical picture associated with chronic mesenteric ischemia, suggesting that they may reflect a different etiology and perhaps one that would give rise to symptoms even with isolated celiac compression. This still leaves open the question of whether celiac compression can contribute to chronic mesenteric ischemia, especially when associated with atherosclerotic lesions of the other mesenteric arteries. Certainly, the occurrence of collateral filling of the celiac artery in association with celiac compression is convincing evidence that this abnormality can be hemodynamically significant.

## Balloon Angioplasty in the Treatment of Chronic Mesenteric Ischemia

Traditional treatment of chronic mesenteric ischemia has consisted of surgical revascularization. Symptomatic relief after successful surgical repair has been good. Rapp and colleagues[24] reported both short- and long-term relief of symptoms in 56 of 60 patients (93%) in whom visceral endarterectomy or antegrade bypass was performed, with a mean follow-up of 4.4 years. However, surgical therapy has suffered from a relatively high rate of perioperative morbidity and mortality. In the same series,[24] there were 5 perioperative deaths in 67 surgical interventions (7.5%), and even higher rates have been reported for other series.[22, 23] This may reflect a high rate of coexistent medical disease.

Application of balloon angioplasty to mesenteric arterial stenoses has been limited by the relatively uncommon occurrence of symptoms attributable to these lesions and by concern about potentially catastrophic

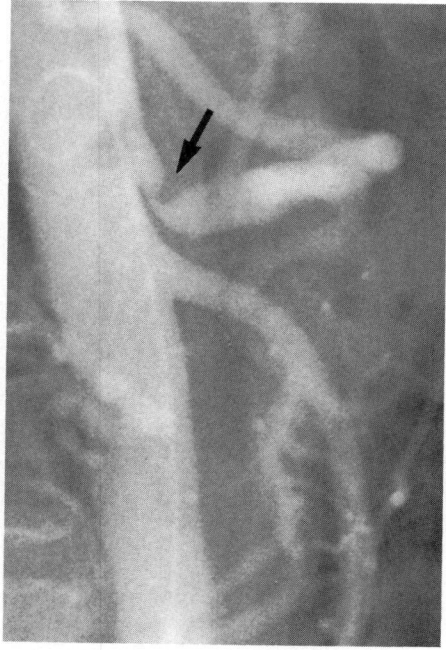

**Figure 45–9. Celiac artery compression *(arrow)*.** Typical appearance shown by a lateral aortogram.

complications, particularly the development of acute mesenteric ischemia and bowel infarction. Nevertheless, this method has been applied both safely and successfully to a number of mesenteric stenoses.[30-39] Many of the reports of its use have referred to single patients, and this could be associated with bias toward favorable results. However, series of up to 10 patients have now been reported.[32] Complications have been few and have included puncture site hematomas and an asymptomatic SMA dissection. No mesenteric vascular emergencies have been reported, nor has periprocedural mortality been a problem despite the fact that many of the reported patients have been poor surgical candidates. After successful angioplasty, relief of symptoms has occurred in the majority of the patients. Most patients have had symptoms of chronic mesenteric ischemia. However, there is one report of angioplasty of an SMA stenosis that resulted in relief of acute pain and signs of peritoneal irritation and guaiac-positive stool in a patient who was considered a poor surgical risk because of cardiopulmonary disease.[39] Most lesions have been atherosclerotic; successful dilatation of mesenteric fibromuscular dysplasia has also been reported.[34, 37] As might be anticipated, stenoses caused by extrinsic celiac compression have responded poorly to balloon angioplasty,[32, 36] although there has been a case of successful dilatation of the celiac artery in a patient with recurrent stenosis after surgery for median arcuate ligament compression.[35] The stenosis in this case was thought to be the result of postoperative scarring. Ostial stenosis, generally the result of atherosclerotic disease of the aortic wall, may be less amenable to angioplasty than stenoses involving only the mesenteric vessels.[31, 32] Up to this point, dilatation of the inferior mesenteric artery has not been performed or deemed necessary. Along these lines, few data exist concerning the relative risk and benefit of limiting angioplasty to one major mesenteric artery when amenable stenoses are found in others (Fig. 45–10). One option made possible by the relative ease of a subsequent procedure is to delay attempts involving other lesions until the clinical response to the initial angioplasty is assessed.

Follow-up has been relatively short in reports published so far, usually of the order of a few months to about 2 years. Recurrence of symptoms has been fairly high in some of the larger series but has frequently responded to a second angioplasty. In the report of Odurny and colleagues,[32] for example, symptoms recurred in five of eight patients who had initially responded for periods of 6 to 24 months; symptomatic relief was again attained after a second dilatation in three of these patients.

Visceral artery angioplasty is often more technically demanding than its peripheral counterpart because the sharp downward angulation of these arteries makes them more difficult to catheterize. In some cases this problem has been solved by using a brachial or axillary puncture approach, although this exposes the patient to slightly higher risks of serious morbidity (see Fig. 45–10). The use of thinner and more flexible angioplasty catheters

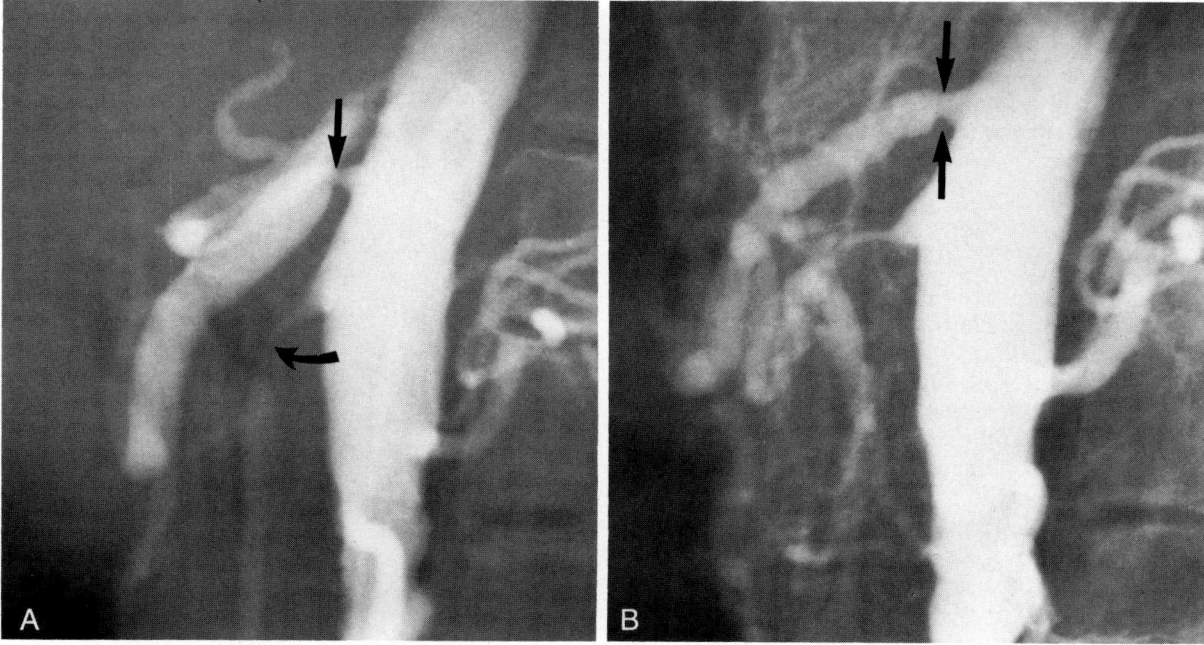

**Figure 45–10. Balloon angioplasty. A.** Lateral aortography shows severe narrowing of celiac *(straight arrow)* and superior mesenteric *(curved arrow)* arteries in a patient with symptoms of chronic mesenteric ischemia. **B.** Improved patency of the celiac artery is noted after balloon angioplasty *(arrows).* The superior mesenteric stenosis could not be catheterized; despite this, there was symptomatic improvement. The case also illustrates a possible complication of this procedure: catheterization via a left axillary puncture site was necessary for celiac angioplasty, and the patient developed a large axillary pseudoaneurysm with a left upper extremity neurologic deficit.

and of torque control guidewires should make catheterization via the femoral route easier to perform.

If systematic evaluation of larger numbers of mesenteric angioplasties affirms the safety and the encouraging results claimed by early reports, this technique may well become the initial method of choice in the treatment of symptomatic mesenteric stenoses.

## Other Vascular Disorders

Aneurysms of the SMA are relatively uncommon compared with splenic artery aneurysms.[40, 41] Etiologies have included medial degeneration, atherosclerosis, and trauma, but the most commonly reported cause is mycotic, representing nearly 60% of SMA aneurysms in one review.[41] Nonmycotic aneurysms may occlude, leading to bowel ischemia, or may rupture.[41] Isolated superior mesenteric branch aneurysms are uncommon but may rupture catastrophically.[41, 42]

Aneurysms of the superior mesenteric vein have also been described.[43] Congenital, traumatic, and inflammatory etiologies have been proposed. Although rare, they may cause abdominal pain, gastrointestinal bleeding, or compression of adjacent structures.

Superior mesenteric arteriovenous fistulas can be congenital[44] or can result from rupture of an SMA aneurysm,[45] from penetrating trauma,[46] or from prior abdominal surgery.[47, 48] Successful transcatheter embolization of fistulas involving the main SMA trunk or SMA branches has been described.[46, 47, 49]

Superior mesenteric arteriovenous malformations have been shown to be a cause of gastrointestinal bleeding; they are seen in younger adults and are thought to be congenital in etiology.[50, 51] On angiography, findings include dilatation of feeding vessels and draining veins, increased vascularity and capillary blush, and early venous drainage.

Various conditions can involve mesenteric vessels. Findings in hereditary hemorrhagic telangiectasia and pseudoxanthoma elasticum are discussed in Chapter 22. Polyarteritis nodosa (Fig. 45–11) and related disorders are associated with small aneurysms of medium and small arteries.[52] The gastrointestinal tract is affected in about half the cases.[53] Similar aneurysms can be seen in the setting of intravenous drug abuse.[54] Although collagen-vascular diseases are among the causes of mesenteric arteritis,[55] arteriographic findings have been reported infrequently. Mesenteric Takayasu's arteritis has been described involving both superior and inferior mesenteric arteries, producing either narrowing or small aneurysms.[56, 57] Mesenteric arterial narrowing can occur in patients receiving ergot preparations, methysergide, and barbiturates;[54] ergotism can also lead to the development of mesenteric aneurysms.[55] Fibromuscular dysplasia may involve mesenteric vessels; it has been stated that the classic "string of beads" appearance of this entity is less common than a tubular stenosis when the celiac artery or SMA is affected.[58] Narrowing and occlusion of visceral arteries are rare manifestations of Behçet's disease.[59]

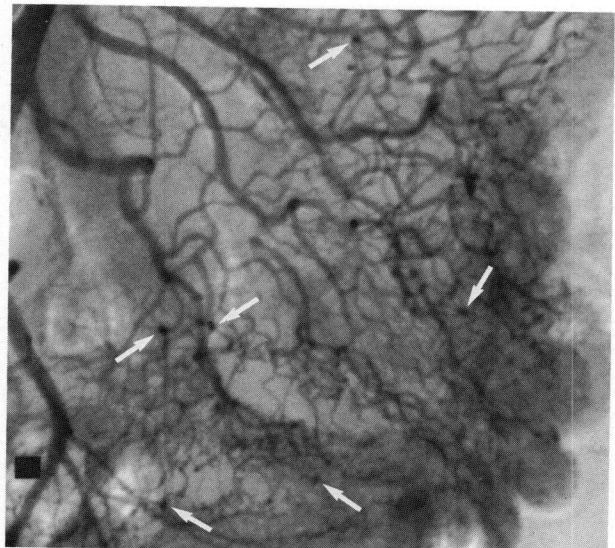

**Figure 45–11. Polyarteritis nodosa.** Multiple small aneurysms, some of which are indicated by arrows, arise from superior mesenteric branches in a patient with polyarteritis nodosa.

## Tumors

Angiography is rarely used in the primary diagnosis of tumors of the small bowel, although it would occasionally be more helpful here than in portions of the gastrointestinal tract more accessible to endoscopy and less prone to overlap on barium studies. Neoplasms may also be identified during the angiographic work-up for gastrointestinal hemorrhage.

Leiomyomas are common small bowel tumors that may bleed. Angiographically, they are highly vascular and well defined (Fig. 45–12); early venous filling is common.[60, 61] Leiomyosarcomas with large necrotic components show less overall vascularity but still show tumor vessels at their margins.[60]

Carcinoid tumors elicit a fibrotic response in the adjacent mesentery that is reflected in a characteristic angiographic appearance of stellate crowding, kinking, and an irregular contour of mesenteric branches. The neoplasm itself is hypovascular but can cause smooth arterial narrowings and occlusions. Venous drainage is typically via multiple collaterals. As might be expected, other processes resulting in mesenteric fibrosis may give a similar appearance.[61–63]

Metastatic lesions of the small bowel vary in appearance depending on their pathologic origin. Adenocarcinomas tend to show signs of encasement without tumor vascularity.[54]

## Inflammatory Conditions

A short discussion of the arteriographic findings in inflammatory bowel disease is given in Chapter 60.

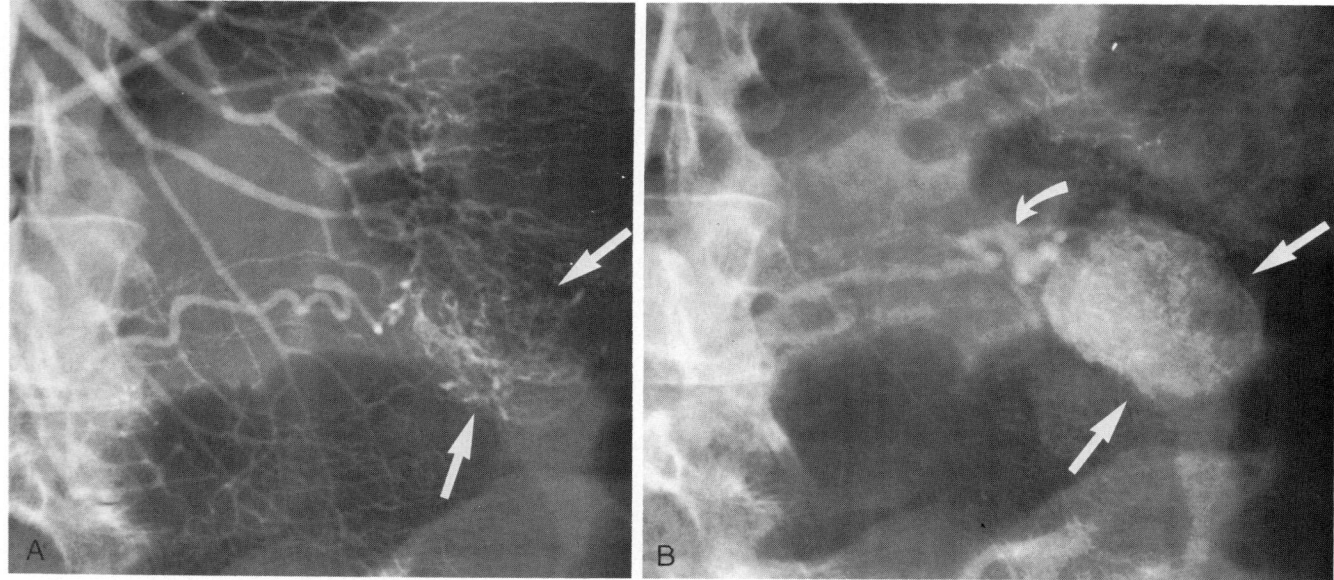

**Figure 45–12. Superior mesenteric arteriography in a patient with intermittent arterial bleeding.**
**A.** Increased vascularity is noted in a portion of the jejunum in the arterial phase *(arrows)*. **B.** In the late arterial phase, a well-defined tumor stain is noted *(straight arrows)*, with a dilated early draining vein *(curved arrow)*. Diagnosis: leiomyoma.

## NONVASCULAR INTERVENTIONAL RADIOLOGY OF THE SMALL BOWEL

### Percutaneous Enterostomy

Direct percutaneous catheterization of the small bowel has been performed much less often than percutaneous gastrostomy.[64–72] The procedure is made difficult by the mobility and compliance of small bowel loops as well as by the difficulty associated with providing and maintaining their distention. Although fluoroscopic guidance has been used in many cases, CT and ultrasonography have also proved useful in localization and puncture of small bowel.

Indications for percutaneous jejunostomy include the need for prolonged enteric feeding in patients in whom a gastrostomy by percutaneous or endoscopic route is not possible. This can occur, for example, when a large hiatal hernia is present or in postsurgical patients after a gastric pull-up procedure or after a partial gastrectomy with a small and high-positioned gastric remnant.[64, 68] Transnasal or transoral intubation of the small bowel can show the location of an appropriate small bowel loop and provide access for distention with air, contrast medium, or supportive balloons. In most cases, C-arm fluoroscopy has been used to identify an anterior loop of proximal jejunum. As with percutaneous gastrostomy, anchoring devices have been used to aid catheterization. Koolpe and colleagues described a unique case in which a CT-guided translumbar retroperitoneal approach was used to puncture the duodenum.[67] An anterior approach was thought to be contraindicated in this case because the patient was receiving peritoneal

dialysis and there was considered to be danger of causing peritonitis with anterior catheter placement.

Even if a gastrostomy can be performed, disease of the gastric antrum or duodenum (such as gastric or invasive pancreatic carcinoma) may preclude placement of a gastrojejunostomy tube. One group,[65] working through a gastrostomy site, was able to manipulate a balloon occlusion catheter through the second portion of the duodenum, the lumen of which was severely compromised by pancreatic carcinoma. The balloon could be fixed manually under the anterior abdominal wall, facilitating the initial puncture for jejunostomy placement.

Direct percutaneous small bowel catheterization has also been used to treat symptoms of enteric obstruction or stasis. Such situations usually require surgery, but percutaneous management can be considered an alternative in patients who are poor surgical candidates. Maneuvers designed to distend or fix the bowel are often not possible, nor are they likely to be necessary because significant intrinsic distention of bowel is present. Acute palliation and long-term prevention of recurrence of closed loop obstruction in a patient with metastatic colon carcinoma have been described.[70] Symptoms of blind or afferent loop stasis have also been relieved by this method.[66, 69] An alternative approach in afferent loop syndromes has been percutaneous management: a drainage tube can be passed percutaneously into the liver or gallbladder and through the biliary tree into the affected bowel limb[73] (Fig. 45–13). A possible benefit of this route is simultaneous drainage of the biliary tree, because these patients may have associated biliary stasis or cholangitis. The occurrence of delayed septic shock

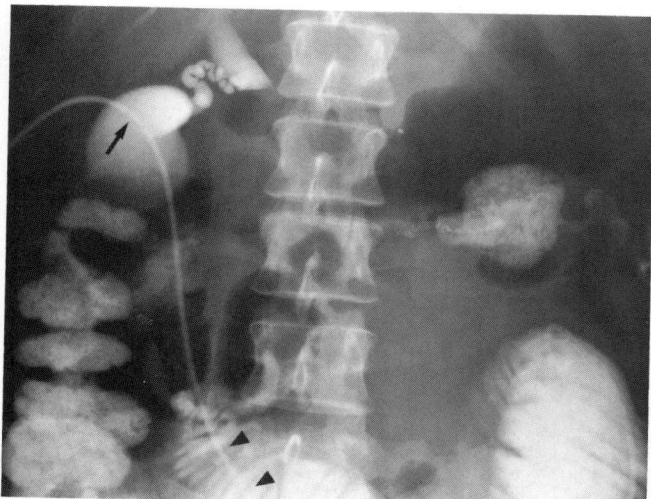

**Figure 45–13. Percutaneous cholecystostomy.** Patient with pancreatic carcinoma, after Roux-en-Y cholecystojejunostomy and gastrojejunostomy, who developed abdominal pain, elevated serum bilirubin level, and septicemia. A CT scan revealed a dilated afferent bowel loop anastomosed to gallbladder. Percutaneous cholecystostomy with passage of catheter via gallbladder *(arrow)* and into jejunal loop *(arrowheads)* resulted in improvement of symptoms.

in one patient in whom transhepatic treatment of an afferent loop was performed suggests that placement of a separate biliary drain may be advisable.[74] In appropriate circumstances, feeding tubes have been placed via a transhepatic biliary route.[75, 76] It is important in such cases to infuse feeding solutions through a tube placed well beyond the native or postsurgical biliary-enteric junction.

One last possible indication for percutaneous jejunostomy is in the treatment of chronic biliary tract disease in patients in whom a biliary-enteric anastomosis had been created. A surgical option to facilitate what may have to be repeated jejunostomies in these patients is the establishment of an easily catheterized entry site by extraperitoneal subcutaneous attachment of a segment of bowel.[72] The site is marked with metallic clips, facilitating localization by fluoroscopy. Multiple punctures of the subcutaneous loop can be performed, allowing simple access to the biliary tree for drainage, stone removal, and stricture dilatation. This obviates the need for multiple and more risky and painful transhepatic catheterizations. The puncture in the bowel closes quickly.

Maroney and Ring[71] considered this approach so worthwhile that they extended it to patients with biliary-enteric anastomoses who had not had specially constructed subcutaneous loops. They performed percutaneous jejunostomy and transjejunal biliary catheterization in 11 patients for a variety of biliary interventions. Initially, they used a transhepatically placed balloon-tipped catheter to guide their puncture. In later cases they found that direct puncture of jejunal loops with a 22-gauge needle was readily performed without this ancillary step, being guided by landmarks provided during CT localization, by fluoroscopy after fine-needle cholangiography with flow of contrast medium into the

loop, and by cutaneous scars from previous jejunal tubes. The authors speculated that postoperative adhesions surrounding the jejunal loop stabilized it, thus facilitating puncture and subsequent manipulations. Catheters were pulled immediately after the interventional procedure in most of the patients, and there were no resultant problems.

## Management of Enteric Leaks

One of the surprising results encountered as experience accumulated with percutaneous abdominal abscess drainage was the fact that abscesses with enteric communication could frequently be cured without the need for surgical intervention.[77] It had been commonly assumed that many such collections would eventually require surgical repair of the site of leakage. Indeed, communication of bowel with an abscess cavity has been repeatedly noted to be a cause for recurrence or failure of cure of abdominal abscesses.[77–81] Similarly, it was thought that enterocutaneous fistulas would require surgical intervention. However, a number of principles have been developed that permit successful management of enteric fistulas (Fig. 45–14), with or without associated abscesses, in the majority of cases.

The first principle is that any associated abscess must be well drained. This is true whether the abscess is drained via percutaneous puncture or is encountered on catheterization of an enterocutaneous fistula. Without drainage, the fistula has little chance of closing. In addition, even if such a fistula cannot be cured by percutaneous means, drainage of an associated abscess improves the patient's condition and provides temporization until the patient becomes better able to tolerate surgery with improved chances of a good surgical result.[81, 82]

Experience with abscesses in fistulous communications with bowel has shown that the fistula is commonly not appreciated at the time of the initial drainage.[78, 81, 83, 84] Frequently, communication with bowel is detected at follow-up sinography (Fig. 45–15). Such demonstration is important for assessment of the cause of the abscess and appropriate planning of subsequent therapy.[84] Clinical signs that an abscess or sinus tract may be communicating with bowel include persistent undiminished drainage, drainage of feculent material, or failure of the abscess cavity to decrease in size.[81,83–85] (Collections may also fail to close if lined by tumor, which may not have been suspected at initial drainage; if no fistula is demonstrated we have occasionally found it worthwhile to analyze biopsy specimens of the wall of a collection that fails to decrease in size.) If there is a suspicion of a fistula but none can be demonstrated with sinography, gentle probing of recesses or "beaks" of the cavity with a guidewire may uncover a tract.[83, 85, 86]

When a fistula is identified, the next aim is control of the tract. This optimally requires manipulating a guidewire followed by a catheter into the tract and taking it close to the site of the leak. If an enterocutaneous fistula is present, we generally perform gentle sinography with

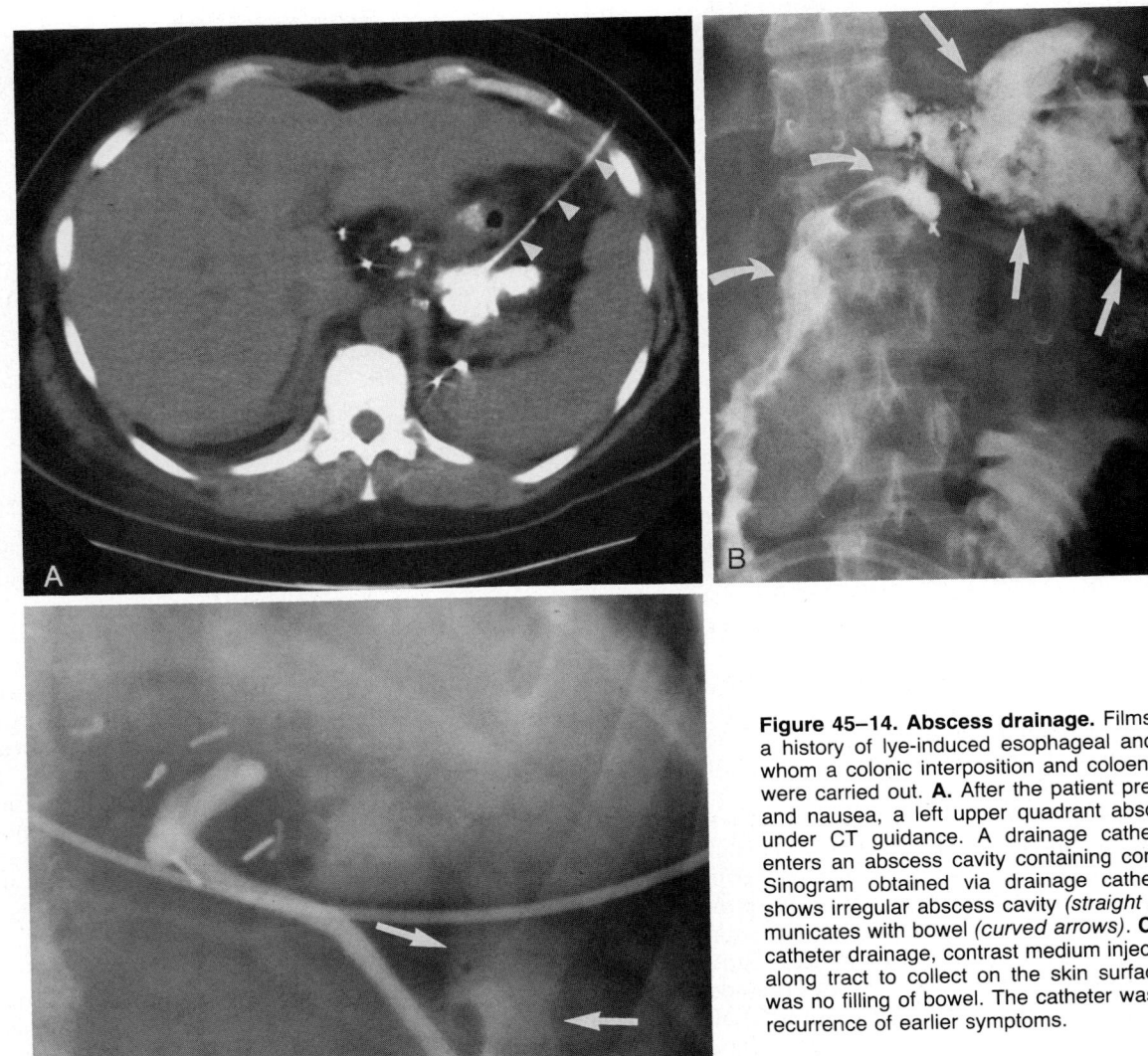

**Figure 45–14. Abscess drainage.** Films of a patient with a history of lye-induced esophageal and gastric injury in whom a colonic interposition and coloenteric anastomosis were carried out. **A.** After the patient presented with fever and nausea, a left upper quadrant abscess was drained under CT guidance. A drainage catheter *(arrowheads)* enters an abscess cavity containing contrast medium. **B.** Sinogram obtained via drainage catheter *(arrowheads)* shows irregular abscess cavity *(straight arrows)* that communicates with bowel *(curved arrows)*. **C.** After 8 weeks of catheter drainage, contrast medium injection results in spill along tract to collect on the skin surface *(arrows)*; there was no filling of bowel. The catheter was removed without recurrence of earlier symptoms.

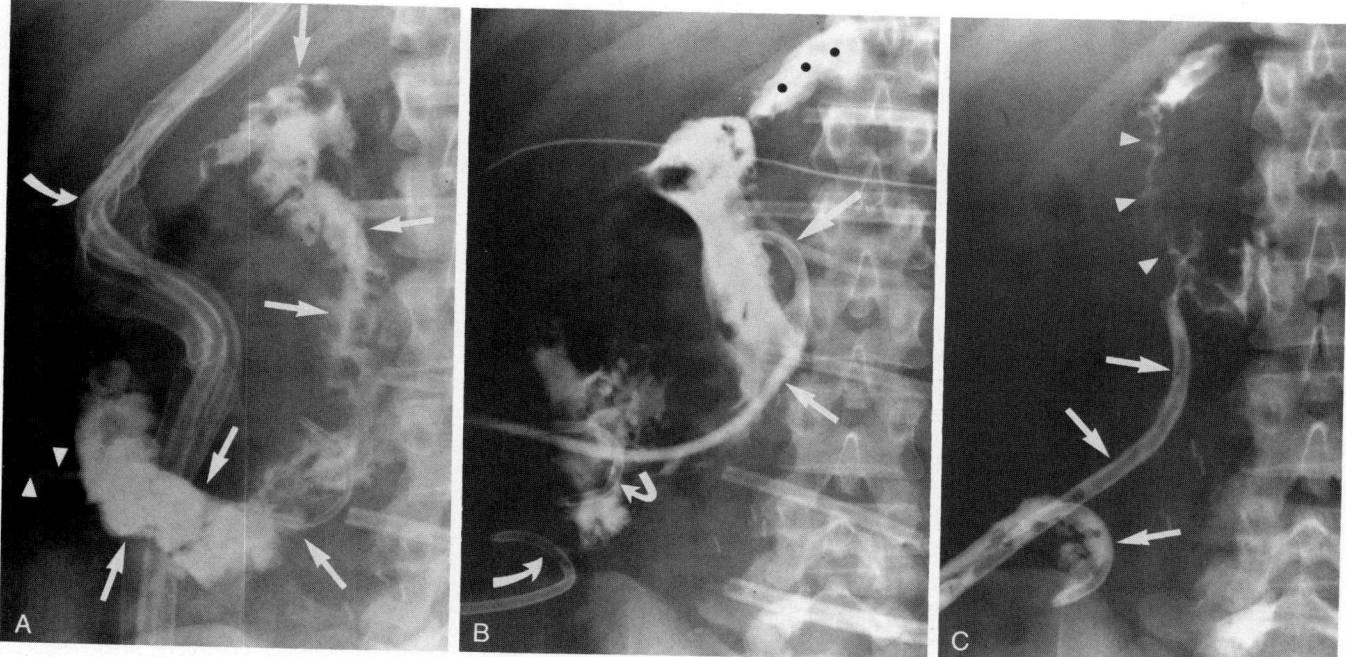

**Figure 45–15. Abscess drainage: multiple catheters.** Bowel injury was discovered at laparotomy in a patient who had abdominal trauma. **A.** Sinogram obtained immediately after abscess drainage. The drainage catheter *(arrowheads)* enters an irregular cavity *(straight arrows)*; no filling of bowel is noted on initial injection. Curved arrow = surgical drain. **B.** Ten days later, three drainage catheters have been placed, two in the lower portion of the abscess cavity *(curved arrows)* and one in its cephalad aspect *(straight arrow)*. Filling of bowel *(black dots)* is now apparent. **C.** Three months later, the abscess cavity has almost completely collapsed, but a fistula to bowel *(arrowheads)* is still present. Two catheters remain in place *(arrows)*. With continued drainage, the fistula eventually closed and the catheters were removed.

a small angiographic dilator or "Christmas tree" adapter attached to a syringe and then attempt to enter the tract with an atraumatic torqueable guidewire or a J-tipped guidewire. Passage of the wire may be difficult because of irregular tissue interfaces, and at no time should the wire be forced ahead. Various techniques have been described to aid catheterization, including use of systems allowing wire manipulation simultaneously with contrast medium injection, use of a balloon to obturate the tract and fill it better, alternate advancement of catheter and guidewire, and initial use of soft-tipped rubber catheters with added end holes.[85–88] For manipulation into a tract extending from an abscess cavity, a variety of curved-tip angiographic catheters can be used, again with J-tipped or soft-tipped torqueable guidewires. When performing such manipulations, a separate safety wire placed within the abscess cavity may be advisable. Ultimately, two or more catheters are often needed, with at least one within any associated abscess cavity and one in the fistulous tract or as close to its orifice as possible (see Fig. 45–15).

The final catheter positions, type of catheters, and catheter management vary according to the character and amount of drainage. A number of investigators stress a distinction between high-output (>200 mL/d) and low-output (<200 mL/d) fistulas,[84–86] although high-output drainage may quickly decrease in volume after appropriate management.[81] For high-output fistulas, we

adopt a method similar to that recommended by McLean and colleagues,[85, 86] who suggested placement of a large drain such as a T tube through the rent in the bowel wall and into the bowel lumen concurrently with sump drainage of the tract adjacent to the T tube. The rationale for this approach is that, despite the fact that placement of a tube through the rent initially retards healing, a desirable outcome should be expedited by the diversion of intestinal contents and resolution of adjacent inflammation. It should be noted that other investigators have not claimed that direct catheterization of the bowel would be imperative in this setting, nor would it seem necessary for low-output fistulas. The degree of benefit from bowel catheterization in the management of both types of enteric fistulas deserves further investigation.

The catheters are managed according to established principles of abscess drainage. If clogging of the tube with thick debris becomes an issue, gentle intermittent irrigation with small aliquots of sterile saline is helpful; however, excessive irrigation may hinder closure of the leak. When catheter output diminishes, tubes can be shortened if desired and gradually pulled. If a tube has been placed into the bowel lumen, it should be clamped before removal; a significant increase in drainage from other catheters suggests that removal would be premature, and it should be reopened to drainage.[85]

As drainage is taking place, efforts should be directed

toward optimizing nutritional status and diverting bowel flow from the site of the leak.[78, 81, 84–86] This can include cessation of oral feeding combined with parenteral nutrition or enteral tube feedings (if the tube can be placed distal to the leak without reflux to the level of the leak), replacement of fluids and attention to electrolyte balance (particularly with high-output fistulas), and possible nasogastric suction.

Drainage of abscesses associated with *Crohn's disease* is a topic especially germane to this discussion. Abscesses are a common complication of Crohn's disease, and when they develop they regularly show communication with bowel. Suboptimal results could almost be assured whenever the underlying bowel causing the abscess is diseased. Nevertheless, a number of reports have suggested that percutaneous drainage has a role in patients with this disorder.[89–92] Percutaneous drainage often leads to abscess resolution and in some cases surgery may be avoided entirely. Although cure is less likely when fistulas are present, palliation of the inflammatory process and improved overall medical status of the patient make it possible to perform single stage surgical resection and bowel anastomosis, which might otherwise not be possible. Development of iatrogenic enterocutaneous fistulas, a complication of surgical abscess drainage, has not been a problem to date. Total parenteral nutrition is advocated as having an important ancillary role in this setting, improving the chances that the inflamed bowel will heal. Whether patients "cured" with percutaneous drainage develop local abscess recurrence over longer periods of follow-up remains to be seen.[81]

The likelihood of cure of enteric leaks is influenced strongly by the success with which the previously noted principles are applied. Bowel that is otherwise normal should generally respond to these endeavors, although drainage may be prolonged for weeks or even months,[78, 81, 84–86, 93] testing the patience of everyone involved in the case. When there is pancreatic involvement associated with the fistula, drainage may be particularly lengthy.[81, 85] In cases in which the bowel is intrinsically diseased—for example, by tumor, previous irradiation, or, as discussed earlier, inflammation—or in cases in which there is unresolved distal bowel obstruction, fistulas may not close at all and require surgical intervention.[78, 81, 85, 86] From the outset, discussion of these points with the patient and the referring physician is essential.

# References

1. Boley SJ, Brandt LJ, Veith FJ: Ischemic disorders of the intestines. Curr Probl Surg 15:1–85, 1978.
2. Reinus JF, Brandt LJ, Boley SJ: Ischemic diseases of the bowel. Gastroenterol Clin North Am 19:319–343, 1990.
3. Clark RA, Gallant TE: Acute mesenteric ischemia: angiographic spectrum. AJR 142:555–562, 1984.
4. Wittenberg J, Athanasoulis CA, Shapiro JH, et al: A radiologic approach to the patient with acute, extensive bowel ischemia. Radiology 106:13–24, 1973.
5. Grendell JH, Ockner RK: Mesenteric venous thrombosis. Gastroenterology 82:358–372, 1982.
6. Vogelzang RL, Gore RM, Anschuetz SL, et al: Thrombosis of the splanchic veins: CT diagnosis. AJR 150:93–96, 1988.
7. Tey PH, Sprayregen S, Ahmed A, et al: Mesenteric vein thrombosis: angiography in two cases. AJR 136:809–811, 1981.
8. Clemett AR, Chang J: The radiologic diagnosis of spontaneous mesenteric venous thrombosis. Am J Gastroenterol 63:209–215, 1975.
9. Ottinger LW: Mesenteric ischemia. N Engl J Med 307:535–537, 1982.
10. Siegelman SS, Sprayregen S, Boley SJ: Angiographic diagnosis of mesenteric arterial vasoconstriction. Radiology 112:533–542, 1974.
11. Morse SS, Clark RA: Management of nonocclusive and occlusive mesenteric ischemia. *In* Kadir S (ed): Current Practice of Interventional Radiology. Philadelphia: BC Decker, 1991, pp 394–400.
12. Anderson JH, Gianturco C, Wallace S: An automated technique for the angiographic "spillover" determination of blood flow. AJR 124:451–457, 1975.
13. Clark RA, Colley DP, Jacobsen ED, et al: Superior mesenteric angiography and blood flow measurement following intra-arterial injection of prostaglandin E$_1$. Radiology 134:327–333, 1980.
14. Boley S, Sprayregen S, Siegelman S, et al: Initial results from an aggressive roentgenological and surgical approach to acute mesenteric ischemia. Surgery 82:848–855, 1977.
15. Vujic I, Stanley J, Gobien RP: Treatment of acute embolus of the superior mesenteric artery by topical infusion of streptokinase. Cardiovasc Intervent Radiol 7:94–96, 1984.
16. Hillers TK, Ginsberg JS, Panju A, et al: Intraarterial low-dose streptokinase infusion for superior mesenteric artery embolus. Can Med Assoc J 142:1087–1088, 1990.
17. Yankes JR, Uglietta JP, Grant J, et al: Percutaneous transhepatic recanalization and thrombolysis of the superior mesenteric vein. AJR 151:289–290, 1988.
18. Pillari G, Doscher W, Fierstein J, et al: Low dose streptokinase in the treatment of celiac and superior mesenteric artery occlusion. Arch Surg 118:1340–1342, 1983.
19. Flickinger EG, Johnsrude IS, Ogburn NL, et al: Local streptokinase infusion for superior mesenteric artery thromboembolism. AJR 140:771–772, 1983.
20. Bilbao JI, Rodriguez-Cabello J, Longo J, et al: Portal thrombosis: percutaneous transhepatic treatment with urokinase—a case report. Gastrointest Radiol 14:326–328, 1989.
21. Klatte EC, Becker GJ, Holden RE, et al: Fibrinolytic therapy. Radiology 159:619–624, 1986.
22. Zelenock GB, Graham LM, Whitehouse WM Jr, et al: Splanchnic atherosclerotic disease and intestinal angina. Arch Surg 115:497–501, 1980.
23. Stanton PE Jr, Hollier PA, Seidel TW, et al: Chronic intestinal ischemia: diagnosis and therapy. J Vasc Surg 4:338–344, 1986.
24. Rapp JH, Reilly LM, Qvarfordt PG, et al: Durability of endarterectomy and antegrade grafts in the treatment of chronic visceral ischemia. J Vasc Surg 3:799–806, 1986.
25. Dick AP, Graff R, Gregg DM, et al: An arteriographic study of mesenteric arterial disease. Gut 8:206–220, 1967.
26. Croft RJ, Menon GP, Marston A: Does "intestinal angina" exist? A critical study of obstructed visceral arteries. Br J Surg 68:316–318, 1981.
27. Colapinto RF, McLoughlin MJ, Weisbrod GL: The routine lateral aortogram and the celiac compression syndrome. Radiology 103:557–563, 1972.
28. Reuter SR: Accentuation of celiac compression by the median arcuate ligament of the diaphragm during deep expiration. Radiology 98:561–564, 1971.
29. Szilagyi DE, Rian RL, Elliot JP, et al: The celiac artery compression syndrome: does it exist? Surgery 72:849–862, 1972.
30. Picetti C, Fuochi C, Moser E, et al: Angina abdominalis: transluminale perkutane Angioplastik der arteria mesenterica superior. Vasa 19:260–262, 1990.
31. Sniderman KW: Angioplasty for treatment of chronic mesenteric ischemia. *In* Kadir S (ed): Current Practice of Interventional Radiology. Philadelphia: BC Decker, 1991, pp 400–408.
32. Odurny A, Sniderman KW, Colapinto RF: Intestinal angina: percutaneous transluminal angioplasty of the celiac and superior mesenteric arteries. Radiology 167:59–62, 1988.

33. Roberts L Jr, Wertman DA Jr, Mills SR, et al: Transluminal angioplasty of the superior mesenteric artery: an alternative to surgical revascularization. AJR 141:1039–1042, 1983.

34. Golden DA, Ring EJ, McLean GK, et al: Percutaneous transluminal angioplasty in the treatment of abdominal angina. AJR 139:247–249, 1982.

35. Saddekni S, Sniderman KW, Hilton S, et al: Percutaneous transluminal angioplasty of nonatherosclerotic lesions. AJR 135:975–982, 1980.

36. Novelline RA: Percutaneous transluminal angioplasty: newer applications. AJR 135:983–988, 1980.

37. Uflacker R, Goldany MA, Constant S: Resolution of mesenteric angina with percutaneous transluminal angioplasty of a superior mesenteric artery stenosis using a balloon catheter. Gastrointest Radiol 5:367–369, 1980.

38. Furrer J, Gruentzig A, Kugelmeier J, et al: Treatment of abdominal angina with percutaneous dilatation of an arteria mesenterica superior stenosis. Cardiovasc Intervent Radiol 3:43–44, 1980.

39. Van Denise WH, Zawacki JK, Phillips D: Treatment of acute mesenteric ischemia by percutaneous transluminal angioplasty. Gastroenterology 91:475–478, 1986.

40. Weidner W, Fox P, Brooks JW, et al: The roentgenographic diagnosis of aneurysms of the superior mesenteric artery. AJR 109:138–142, 1970.

41. Stanley JC, Thomason NW, Fry WJ: Splanchnic artery aneurysms. Arch Surg 101:689–697, 1970.

42. Reuter SR, Fry WJ, Bookstein JJ: Mesenteric artery branch aneurysms. Arch Surg 97:497–499, 1968.

43. Mathias KD, Hoffman J, Krabb HJ, et al: Aneurysm of the superior mesenteric vein. Cardiovasc Intervent Radiol 10:269–271, 1987.

44. Takehara H, Komi N, Hino M: Congenital arteriovenous fistula of the superior mesenteric vessels. J Pediatr Surg 23:1029–1031, 1988.

45. Knox M, Chuang VP, Stewart MT: Superior mesenteric aneurysm and arteriovenous fistula: angiographic and CT features. AJR 145:383–384, 1985.

46. Desai SB, Modhe JM, Aulakh BG, et al: Percutaneous transcatheter steel-coil embolization of a large proximal post-traumatic superior mesenteric arteriovenous fistula. J Trauma 27:1091–1094, 1987.

47. Uflacker R, Saadi J: Transcatheter embolization of superior mesenteric arteriovenous fistula. AJR 139:1212–1214, 1982.

48. Donell ST, Hudson JK: Iatrogenic superior mesenteric arteriovenous fistula. J Vasc Surg 8:335–338, 1988.

49. Kim D, Guthaner DF, Walter JF, et al: Embolization of visceral arteriovenous fistula with a modified steel wire technique. AJR 142:1215–1218, 1984.

50. Sheedy PF II, Fulton RE, Atwell DT: Angiographic evaluation of patients with chronic gastrointestinal bleeding. AJR 123:338–347, 1975.

51. Moore JD, Thompson NW, Appelman HD, et al: Arteriovenous malformations of the gastrointestinal tract. Arch Surg 111:381–388, 1976.

52. Fauci AS, Haynes BF, Katz P: The spectrum of vasculitis: clinical, pathologic, immunologic, and therapeutic considerations. Ann Intern Med 89:660–676, 1978.

53. Capps JH, Klein RM: Polyarteritis nodosa as a cause of perirenal and retroperitoneal hemorrhage. Radiology 94:143–146, 1970.

54. Reuter SR, Redman HC, Cho KJ: Gastrointestinal Angiography. Philadelphia: WB Saunders, 1986.

55. Tupler RH, Bansal SK: Mesenteric aneurysms associated with ergotism. AJR 155:897–898, 1990 (letter).

56. Yamato M, Lecky JW, Hiramatsu K, et al: Takayasu arteritis: radiographic and angiographic findings in 59 patients. Radiology 161:329–334, 1986.

57. Gotsman MS, Beck W, Schrire V: Selective angiography in arteritis of the aorta and its major branches. Radiology 88:232–248, 1967.

58. Luescher TF, Lie JT, Stanson AW, et al: Arterial fibromuscular dysplasia. Mayo Clin Proc 62:931–952, 1987.

59. Park JH, Han MC, Bettman MA: Arterial manifestations of Behçet disease. AJR 143:821–825, 1984.

60. Kaude J, Silseth CH, Tylen U: Angiography in myomas of the gastrointestinal tract. Acta Radiol Diagn 12:691–704, 1972.

61. Boijsen E, Reuter SR: Mesenteric angiography in the evaluation of inflammatory and neoplastic disease of the intestine. Radiology 87:1028–1036, 1966.

62. Seigel RS, Kuhns LR, Borlaza GS, et al: Computed tomography and angiography in ileal carcinoid tumor and retractile mesenteritis. Radiology 134:437–440, 1980.

63. Gold RE, Redman HC: Mesenteric fibrosis simulating the angiographic appearance of carcinoid tumor. Radiology 103:85–86, 1972.

64. Coleman CC, Coons HG, Cope C, et al: Percutaneous enterostomy with the Cope suture anchor. Radiology 174:889–891, 1990.

65. Rosenblum J, Taylor FC, Lu C-T, et al: A new technique for direct percutaneous jejunostomy tube placement. Am J Gastroenterol 85:1165–1167, 1990.

66. Maile CW, Hanna PD: Direct percutaneous drainage of an obstructed afferent loop. AJR 152:521–522, 1989.

67. Koolpe HA, Dorfman D, Kramer M: Translumbar duodenostomy for enteral feeding. AJR 153:299–300, 1989.

68. Gray RR, Ho C-S, Yee A, et al: Direct percutaneous jejunostomy. AJR 149:931–932, 1987.

69. Camunez F, Simo G, Echenagusia A, et al: Percutaneous duodenostomy in blind loop syndrome. AJR 150:1199, 1988 (letter).

70. Bezreh JS: Percutaneous catheter drainage of closed-loop small-bowel obstruction. AJR 141:797–798, 1988.

71. Maroney TP, Ring EJ: Percutaneous transjejunal catheterization of Roux-en-Y biliary-jejunal anastomoses. Radiology 164:151–153, 1987.

72. Russell E, Yrizarry JM, Huber JS, et al: Percutaneous transjejunal biliary dilatation: alternate management for benign strictures. Radiology 159:209–214, 1986.

73. Lee LE, Teplick SK, Haskin PH, et al: Refractory afferent loop problems: percutaneous transhepatic management of two cases. Radiology 165:49–50, 1987.

74. Morita S, Takemura T, Matsumoto S, et al: Septic shock after percutaneous transhepatic drainage of obstructed afferent loop: case report. Cardiovasc Intervent Radiol 12:66–68, 1989.

75. Train JS, Dan SJ, Mitty HA: Percutaneous transhepatic hyperalimentation for patients with biliary drainage catheters. AJR 144:255–256, 1985.

76. McDonald DG, Khalil MF, Vernon JK: Percutaneous transhepatic insertion of a jejunal feeding tube. Radiology 148:309–310, 1983.

77. Gerzof SG, Robbins AH, Johnson WC, et al: Percutaneous catheter drainage of abdominal abscesses. A five year experience. N Engl J Med 305:653–657, 1981.

78. Papanicolaou N, Mueller PR, Ferrucci JT Jr, et al: Abscess-fistula association: radiologic recognition and percutaneous management. AJR 143:811–815, 1984.

79. vanSonnenberg E, Mueller PR, Ferrucci JT Jr: Percutaneous drainage of 250 abdominal abscesses and fluid collections. Part 1: results, failures, and complications. Radiology 151:337–341, 1984.

80. Gerzof SG, Johnson WC, Robbins AH, et al: Expanded criteria for percutaneous abscess drainage. Arch Surg 120:227–232, 1985.

81. Lambiase RE, Cronan JJ, Dorfman GS, et al: Postoperative abscesses with enteric communication: percutaneous treatment. Radiology 171:497–500, 1989.

82. vanSonnenberg E, Wing VW, Casola G, et al: Temporizing effect of percutaneous drainage of complicated abscesses in critically ill patients. AJR 142:821–826, 1984.

83. Kerlan RK Jr, Pogany AC, Jeffrey RB, et al: Radiologic management of abdominal abscesses. AJR 144:145–149, 1985.

84. Kerlan RK Jr, Jeffrey RB Jr, Pogany AC, et al: Abdominal abscess with low-output fistula: successful percutaneous drainage. Radiology 155:73–75, 1985.

85. McLean GK: Interventional radiology of the gastrointestinal tract. Curr Probl Diagn Radiol 19:85–132, 1990.

86. McLean GK, Mackie JA, Freiman DB, et al: Enterocutaneous fistulae: interventional radiologic management. AJR 138:615–619, 1982.

87. Sacks BA, Vine HS, Bartek S, et al: Postoperative abscess drainage in patients with established sinus tracks or drains. Radiology 142:537–538, 1982.

88. Palestrant AM: Cannulation of catheter tracks and narrowed channels. Radiology 143:561–562, 1982.

89. Doemeny JM, Burke DR, Meranze SG: Percutaneous drainage of abscesses in patients with Crohn's disease. Gastrointest Radiol 13:237–241, 1988.

90. Casola G, vanSonnenberg E, Neff CC, et al: Abscesses in Crohn disease: percutaneous drainage. Radiology 163:19–22, 1987.

91. Lambiase RE, Cronan JJ, Dorfman GS, et al: Percutaneous drainage of abscesses in patients with Crohn disease. AJR 150:1043–1045, 1988.

92. Safrit HD, Mauro MA, Jaques PF: Percutaneous abscess drainage in Crohn's disease. AJR 148:859–862, 1987.

93. Beltran J, Grande J, Ferreres I, et al: Percutaneous management of abdominal abscesses with GI tract fistulous communications: report of 2 cases. Gastrointest Radiol 9:65–68, 1984.

# Role of the Small Intestine in Immunity

**Frank P. Brooks, M.D., Sc.D.**

**Hans Herlinger, M.D.**

## INTRODUCTION

The small intestine is an important part of the body's immune system and takes part in both its cellular and humoral components. Although the main purpose of the gastrointestinal tract must be absorption of nutrients, there is need for a parallel mechanism to protect the body from the effects of food and bacterial antigens. This immunologic function has to be carried out without compromising unduly the intake of food substances. Thus, the small intestine has special immune protection–related problems and has had to develop mechanisms that differ from those prevailing in the rest of the body.

Antigens introduced into the gut may initiate an antibody response that not only leads to the production of specialized secretory immunoglobulins at the mucosal surface but also stimulates appropriate cell-mediated immune responses. Moreover, the gut-associated lymphoid tissue is part of a common mucosal immune system that causes effector cells stimulated by antigen challenge at any one site to become distributed to the other mucosal surfaces—respiratory, urogenital, mammary, and ocular.

## STRUCTURE AND PHYSIOLOGY OF GUT-ASSOCIATED LYMPHOID TISSUES

Gut-associated lymphoid tissue is the basis of the gut as an immune organ. Lymphoid cells occur either in the form of aggregates or in a nonaggregated distribution.

### Lymphoid Aggregates

These aggregates consist of Peyer's patches (PPs) lymphoid follicles, and mesenteric lymph nodes.

### Peyer's Patches

PPs are aggregations of cells and lymphoid follicles in the submucosa and lamina propria, mostly of the ileum but also of the jejunum. About 200 PPs are found in humans, a larger number in the young than in those of more advanced years. Of major importance are specialized cells, known as M cells, that overlie the dome of the PPs. These cells are ultrathin, have short microvilli, and are able to transport foreign antigenic macromolecules, bacteria, and viruses to subjacent macrophages and lymphoid cells, some of which invaginate the cytoplasm of the M cells (Fig. 46–1). The purpose seems to be rapid initiation of specific mucosal immune processes. Lymphoid cells in the PPs show preferential specialization for immunoglobulin A (IgA) production.[1] Interaction with helper T cells is required for this differentiation.

**Radiographic Appearance.** Studies of resected specimens[2] showed that PPs were mostly situated at the antimesenteric side of the bowel, in line with the longitudinal axis of the bowel segment. Their surface had a granular appearance and interrupted the normal fold pattern (Fig. 46–2).

### Nonaggregated Lymph Follicles

These structures are scattered throughout the mucosa, and most of them are covered by M cells. Their function resembles that of PPs.

### Lymphocytes in Nonaggregated Tissue

Lymphocytes, both B and T cells, are scattered throughout the bowel wall but are mostly found in the

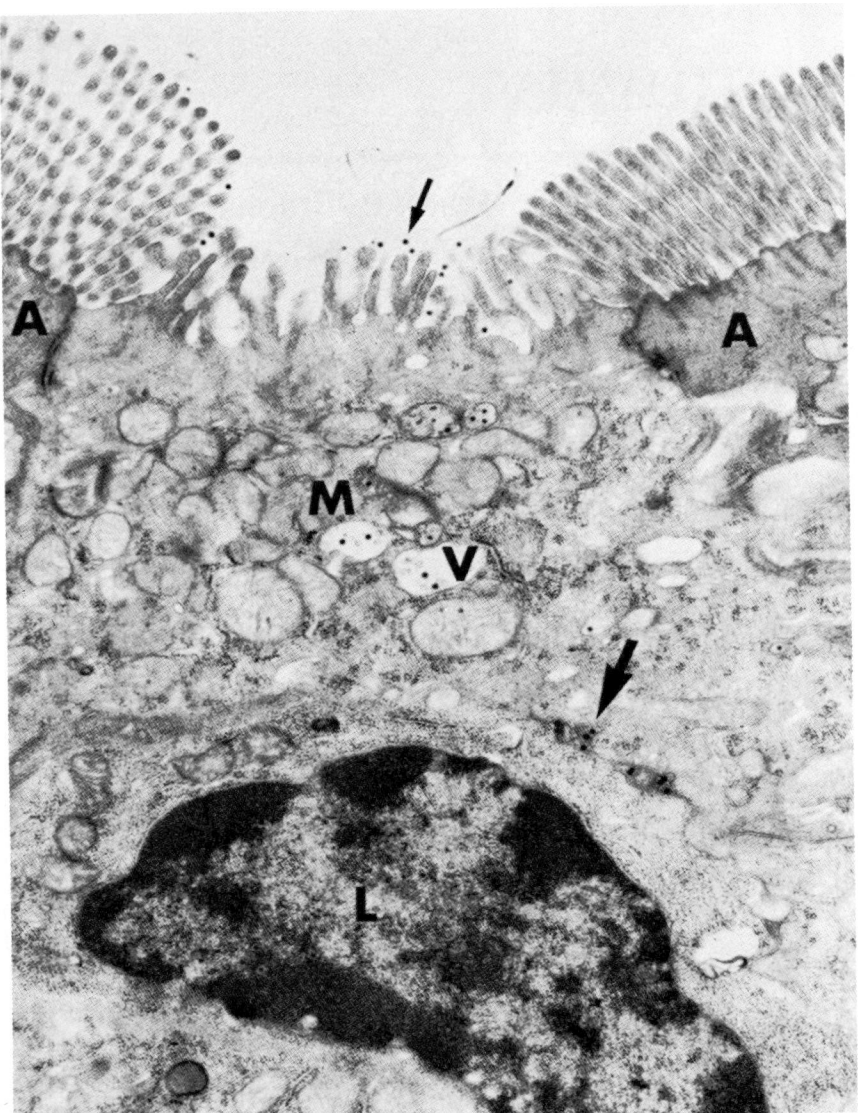

**Figure 46–1. Electron micrograph of ileal mouse epithelium overlying Peyer's patch.** Reovirus was inoculated 30 minutes earlier. Virions adhere to the surface *(small arrow)* and are seen within vesicles (V) of an M cell (M) and in the extracellular space *(large arrow)*. Virions are also seen on the surface of an invaginated lymphocyte (L). The apical surface of adjacent absorptive cells (A) is virtually devoid of adherent virions. (From Wolf JL, Kauffman RS, Finberg R, et al: Determinants of reovirus interaction with intestinal cells and absorptive cells of murine intestine. Gastroenterology 85:291–300, 1983.)

**Figure 46–2. PP on the antimesenteric side of the midileum.** Radiograph of a fixed specimen after resection of a lipoma. A coarse granular pattern covers its surface *(arrows)* and mucosal folds are interrupted. (From Ushio K, Yamada T, Itabashi M, et al: Roentgenologic specimen study of Peyer's patches in the jejunum and proximal ileum. Gastrointest Radiol Rev 1:1–13, 1990.)

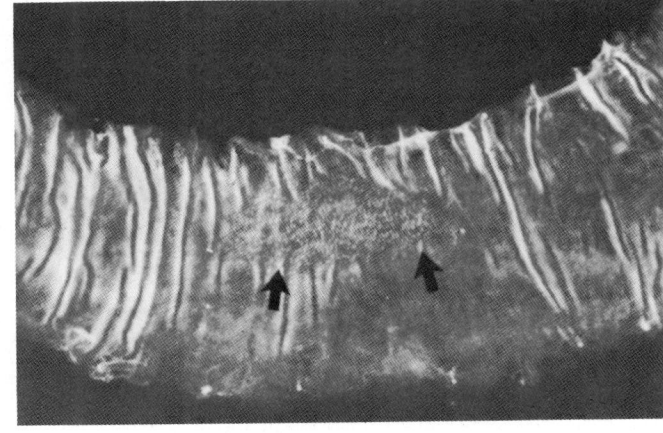

lamina propria. B cells and helper T cells predominate. In addition, there are macrophages and mast cells. Intraepithelial lymphocytes, found between epithelial cells, are mostly T cells (Fig. 46–3).

## Migration of Lymphocytes

Activated lymphocytes leave the PPs and travel through mesenteric nodes and thoracic duct into the blood stream. They leave the blood by binding to specialized venules, the high endothelial venules. During this migration they mature into lymphoblasts of T cell or B cell lineage.[3] They then migrate to mucosal sites, B lymphoblasts having matured to IgA-secreting plasma cells. After antigen activation, lymphocytes tend to acquire a nonmigratory character, settling in sites similar to those where their cognate antigen was encountered. Lymphocytes not only return to the lamina propria of the intestine but also become localized in other parts of the mucosal immune system, such as the mammary glands, genitalia, and bronchi. T lymphoblasts migrate mostly to peripheral lymph nodes.

## THE IMMUNE SYSTEM

The immune system[4] is generally based on humoral immunity, which depends on antibodies produced by plasma cells, and cell-mediated immunity, which involves the ability of lymphocytes to act against antigens and microorganisms to limit their damage to the body. The lymphocytes derive from stem cells and are processed in either the thymus (T cells) or the bone marrow (B cells). Most of the B cells become differentiated into plasma cells that form and release immunoglobulins (Fig. 46–4).

## Humoral Immunity

Humoral antibodies enter the intestinal mucosa from plasma cells in the lamina propria. The principal immunoglobulin in plasma is immunoglobulin G, but in the intestine it is IgA.

### Immunoglobulin A

In the lamina propria of the small intestine, there are 20 to 30 IgA-containing plasma cells for every one cell containing immunoglobulin G. Monomeric IgA, a single Y-shaped molecule, consists of four chains (Fig. 46–5): two long chains known as heavy chains, which are linked by disulfide bonds, and two light chains (kappa and lambda). When exposed to proteolytic enzyme digestion, the immunoglobulin molecule splits at the bonding site. The light chains and part of the heavy chains constitute a fragment known as Fab; it contains the portion of the molecule involved in antigen recognition and binding. The remainder of the molecule consists of heavy chains and is known as the Fc fragment. Fc is concerned with the biologic consequences of binding, such as activation of complement.

Monomeric IgA is found mostly in plasma and in body tissue other than the gut mucosa. Near mucosal surfaces of the gut, the plasma cells produce dimeric IgA, two IgA molecules joined by disulfide bonds, the joining (J) chains. The IgA dimer binds to a receptor on the membrane of an adjacent epithelial cell. The receptor, known as the secretory component, is a glycoprotein with a molecular weight of 70,000.[5] Entry into the epithelial cells occurs by endocytosis, followed by secretion into the gut lumen of the entire secretory IgA molecule with a molecular weight of 385,000. The secretory component reinforces the J chain and renders the secretory IgA more resistant to proteolysis within the

**Figure 46–3. Schematic representation of immune system–related cells in a villus.** (From Kagnoff MF: Immunology of the digestive system. *In* Johnson LR [ed]: The Physiology of the Gastrointestinal Tract. New York: Raven Press, 1981, pp 1337–1359.)

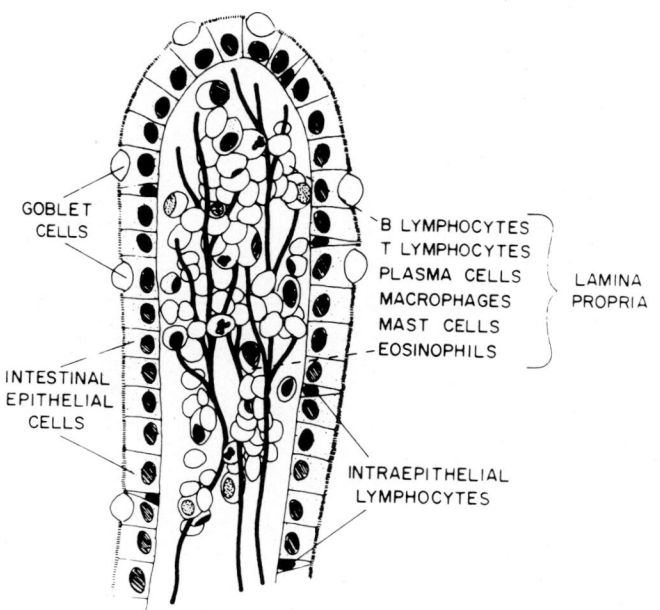

GOBLET CELLS

INTESTINAL EPITHELIAL CELLS

B LYMPHOCYTES
T LYMPHOCYTES
PLASMA CELLS
MACROPHAGES
MAST CELLS
EOSINOPHILS

LAMINA PROPRIA

INTRAEPITHELIAL LYMPHOCYTES

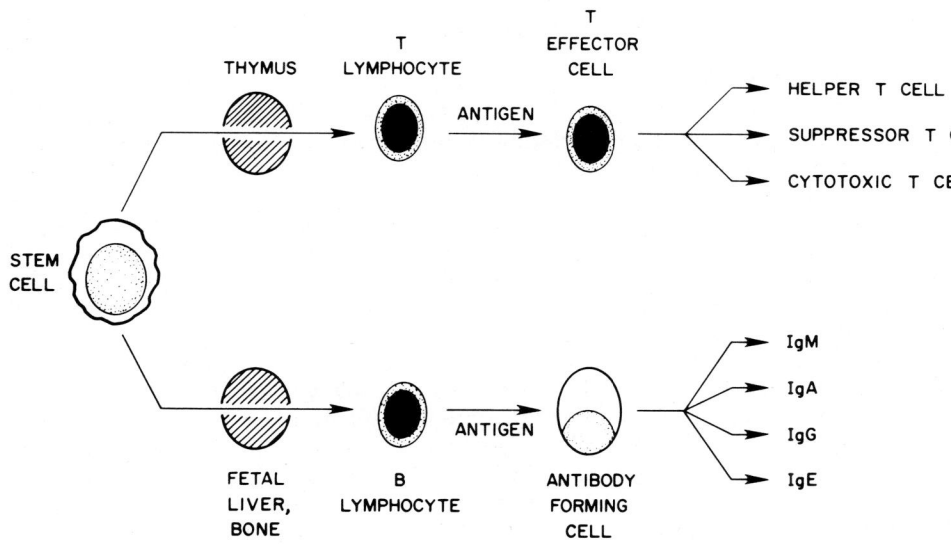

**Figure 46–4. Development of the immune system, schematic representation.** T lymphocytes develop from stem cells in the thymus and B lymphocytes from stem cells in the fetal liver and bone marrow. (From Kagnoff MF: Immunology of the digestive system. *In* Johnson LR [ed]: The Physiology of the Gastrointestinal Tract. New York: Raven Press, 1981, pp 1337–1359.)

gut lumen. Approximately 3 g of secretory IgA enters the gut lumen of an average adult every day.

In the gut lumen, secretory IgA prevents adherence of bacteria to epithelial cells and neutralizes bacterial toxins. IgA has antiviral properties and blocks the absorption of antigens.[6]

## Immunoglobulin M

Immunoglobulin M is a much larger polymeric immunoglobulin than IgA and is secreted into the gut lumen in similar secretory form. Normally occurring in small amounts, it becomes the major immunoglobulin in patients with IgA deficiency.

## Cell-mediated Immunity

**The Lamina Propria.** In the lamina propria, CD4$^+$ T cells outnumber CD8$^+$ T cells. Subpopulations of CD4$^+$ cells include those with helper, suppressor, and memory functions, the last group probably in the majority.[7] Subpopulations of CD8$^+$ cells perform cytotoxic and suppressor functions; a smaller number are natural killer cells.

Cell-mediated immune responses may begin with the ingestion and breakdown of antigens by macrophages. Antigen fragments then interact with major histocompatibility complexes on the surface of the macrophages and are recognized by T cell receptors. In addition to

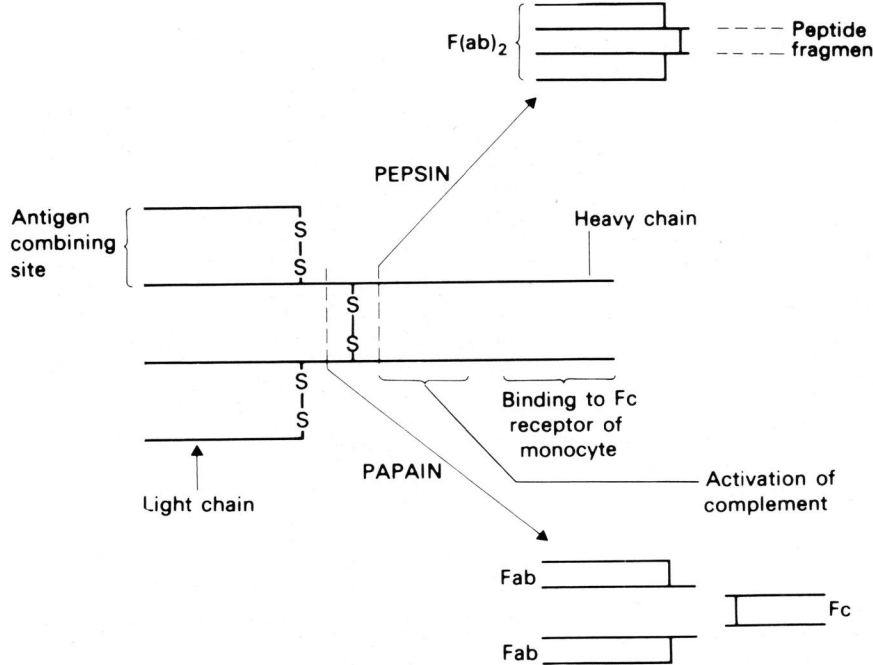

**Figure 46–5. Diagrammatic representation of an IgA molecule.** -S—S- = disulfide bond. (From Thomas HC, Jewell DP: Clinical Gastrointestinal Immunology. Oxford: Blackwell Scientific Publications, 1979, pp 1–37.)

macrophages, epithelial cells and dentritic cells are capable of antigen presentation. Antigen recognition is essential to the function of both helper and cytotoxic T cells. Cytokines such as interleukin stimulate the proliferation of helper T cells. Controlled activation is particularly important for the regulation of cytotoxic T cell function to avoid damage to the surrounding tissue when cytotoxic actions are not needed.

**Intraepithelial Lymphocytes.** These are located between epithelial cells, and 80% of them are capable of mediating several cytotoxic functions. They may also be involved in inducing major histocompatibility complex antigens on epithelial cells. They can neutralize numerous infectious agents and form a first line of defense at the bowel surface. Intraepithelial T cells have been shown to have a stimulating effect on epithelial cell renewal.[8]

**Neuroimmunoregulation.** Increasing importance is given to the ability of T cells and B cells to respond to neuropeptides in the gut. Vasoactive intestinal polypeptide, substance P, and somatostatin can act as regulators of lymphoid cell proliferation and immunoglobulin production and be involved in the recirculation of effector lymphocytes from lymphoid compartments such as PPs.[9]

# IMMUNODEFICIENCIES

## Selective Immunoglobulin A Deficiency

This is the most common immunodeficiency in adults and occurs in 1 in 700 persons. A compensatory increase in immunoglobulin M production causes the majority of affected persons to remain asymptomatic. Other patients may present with malabsorption and a sprue-like syndrome that may respond favorably to gluten exclusion.[10] Precipitating antibodies to cow's milk protein are found in the plasma of more than half the patients. Nodular lymphoid hyperplasia with or without giardiasis may form the radiologic presentation.

IgA deficiency may be associated with numerous other disorders, including pernicious anemia, lactase deficiency, and inflammatory bowel disease. IgA deficiency has been reported in 1 in 40 patients with celiac disease.[11] Malignant tumors are more common in patients with IgA deficiency and other immunodeficiencies.[12]

## Common Variable Immunodeficiency Syndrome

This heterogeneous syndrome includes at least two subtypes, one with mainly immunoglobulin deficiencies and the other with abnormalities of T cell function. There may be defects of macrophage antigen processing, ineffective interaction between macrophages and T cells, and decreased helper T cell function. Immunoglobulin-producing cells are usually reduced in number in the small bowel, and only small amounts of secretory immunoglobulin may appear in the gut lumen. An excess

of suppressor T cells and impairment of helper T cells may exist.

Nodular lymphoid hyperplasia may also be seen in this condition. Nodules formed by lymphoid aggregates may be found in the small intestine or throughout the gastrointestinal tract.[13] In a report of six cases,[14] multiple 1- to 3-mm discrete nodules were shown in the small intestine by barium study and were not often umbilicated (Fig. 46–6). The most commonly associated infection is giardiasis, which causes chronic diarrhea and malabsorption.

# IMMUNOPATHOLOGY OF THE GASTROINTESTINAL TRACT IN HUMAN IMMUNODEFICIENCY VIRUS INFECTION

Human immunodeficiency virus can enter through the gastrointestinal tract. A traumatized rectum in homosexuals, M cells covering lymphoglandular complexes in the distal colon,[15] and tonsillar M cells may provide entry sites. The virus binds to the surface of cells expressing the CD4 antigen. After binding, the viral envelope fuses with the membrane of mostly CD4+ T lymphocytes and the virus becomes internalized.[16] The virus may also enter macrophages.

The migration of mucosa-derived lymphocytes to distant gut-associated lymphoid tissue mucosal sites explains the presence of human immunodeficiency virus–

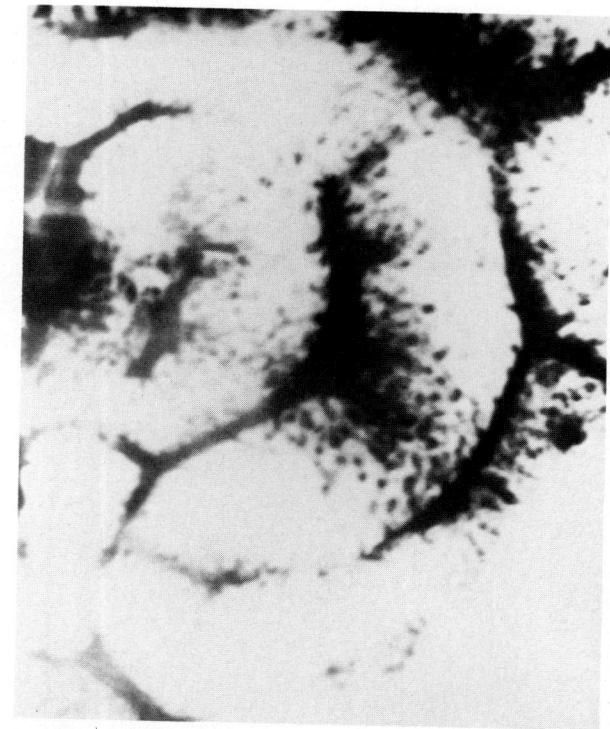

**Figure 46–6. Nodules (about 3 mm) evenly distributed over the small bowel mucosa.** Nodular lymphoid hyperplasia is seen in a patient with common variable immunodeficiency.

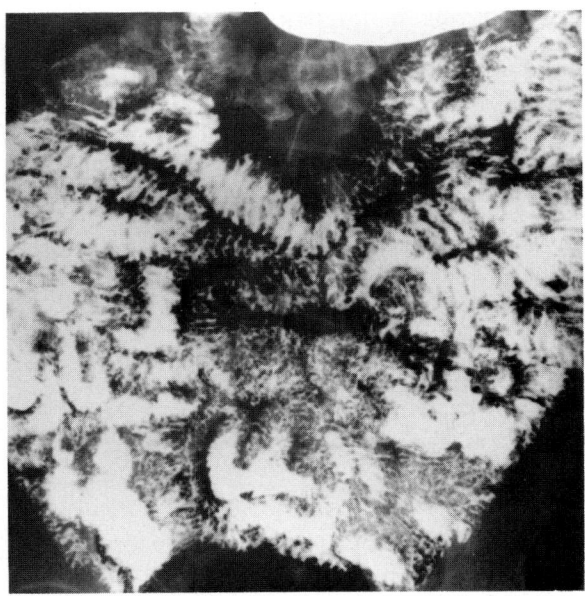

**Figure 46–7. Alpha chain disease.** Barium study in a young patient from Israel. Nodules extend over most of the mucosal surface and folds are thickened. Immunoproliferative small intestinal disease may still be short of the stage of lymphoma. (Courtesy of Eugene Libson, M.D., Jerusalem, Israel.)

infected mononuclear cells throughout the gastrointestinal tract. This leads to a gradual reduction in the number of CD4$^+$ T cells while the number of CD8$^+$ T cells remains virtually constant. Remaining CD4$^+$ T cells show impaired function, limiting the terminal differentiation of IgA-secreting plasma cells and reducing the level of secretory immunoglobulin in the gut lumen. Nonspecific host defenses are also impaired, as are gastric acid secretion and intestinal peristalsis. This contributes to colonization of the gut by an increased number of bacteria.[16]

In this setting, the gastrointestinal tract in human immunodeficiency virus disease becomes more suscep-tible to opportunistic infections (see Chapter 48). Malignant neoplasia supervenes in about 12% of patients with acquired immunodeficiency syndrome.[17] Kaposi's sarcoma is the most common malignant tumor (see Chapter 51). Non-Hodgkin's lymphoma accounts for 35% of malignancies in these patients and may be related to Epstein-Barr virus infection.

## ALPHA CHAIN DISEASE

Alpha chain disease is associated with increased plasma cell infiltration of the small bowel lamina propria

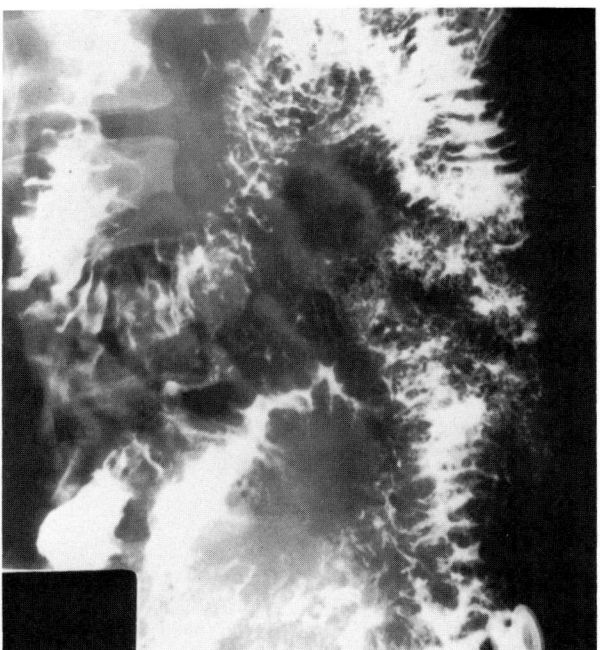

**Figure 46–8. Mediterranean lymphoma.** In another young patient from Israel, barium examination indicates the presence of extramural masses. Mucosal folds are irregularly thickened. (Courtesy of Eugene Libson, M.D., Jerusalem, Israel.)

and presents with malabsorption. In time, lymphoma may develop. Those affected are young people (10 to 30 years) living along the Mediterranean basin in areas of poor hygienic conditions.

Fragments of incomplete IgA heavy chains can be found in the plasma and in secretions. The lamina propria of the small bowel is heavily infiltrated with mature plasma cells and small lymphocytes. Infiltration extends into mesenteric lymph nodes with preservation of their architecture. The term *immunoproliferative small intestinal disease* has been proposed by the World Health Organization. At this stage of the disease, remission after treatment with antibiotics is possible.[18] Barium studies show diffuse fine nodularity throughout the small bowel or confined to more proximal areas (Fig. 46–7).

Eventually, infiltration extends through the submucosa to involve the entire bowel wall. Plasma cells have become atypical and dysplastic and are accompanied by immunoblasts. Lymph node architecture is obliterated. Alpha heavy chain protein is no longer secreted. The condition has developed into an immunoblastic lymphoma. Barium studies at this late stage show irregular, coarse nodularity and separation of bowel loops by larger mass lesions (Fig. 46–8).

# References

1. Owen RL, Jones AL: Epithelial cell specialization within human Peyer's patches: an ultrastructural study of intestinal lymphoid follicles. Gastroenterology 66:189–203, 1974.
2. Ushio K, Yamada T, Itabashi M, et al: Roentgenologic specimen study of Peyer's patches in the jejunum and proximal ileum. Gastrointest Radiol Rev 1:1–13, 1990.
3. Dunkley ML, Husband AJ: Distribution and functional characteristics of antigen-specific helper T cells arising after Peyer's patch immunization. Immunology 61:475–482, 1987.
4. Brooks FP: The role of the small intestine in immunity. *In* Herlinger H, Maglinte D (eds): Clinical Radiology of the Small Intestine. Philadelphia: WB Saunders, 1989, pp 31–38.
5. Ahnen DJ, Brown WR, Kloppel TM: Secretory component: the polymeric immunoglobulin receptor. Gastroenterology 89:667–682, 1985.
6. MacDermott RP, Stenson WF: The immune system. *In* Yamada T (ed): Textbook of Gastroenterology. Philadelphia: JB Lippincott, 1991, pp 85–102.
7. James SP: Mucosal T-cell function. Gastroenterol Clin North Am 20:597–612, 1991.
8. Tagliabue A, Boraschi D, Villa L, et al: IgA dependent cell-mediated activity against enteropathogenic bacteria: distribution, specificity and characterization of the effector cells. J Immunol 133:988–992, 1984.
9. Guillemin R, Cohn M, Melnechuk T (eds): Neural Modulation of Immunity. New York: Raven Press, 1985.
10. Amman AJ, Hong R: Selective IgA deficiency: presentation of 30 cases and review of the literature. Medicine (Baltimore) 50:223–236, 1971.
11. McCarthy DM, Katz SI, Gazze JM, et al: Selective IgA deficiency associated with total villous atrophy of the small intestine and an organ-specific anti–epithelial cell antibody. J Immunol 120:932–938, 1978.
12. Waldman TA, Strober W, Blaese RM: Immunodeficiency disease and malignancy. Ann Intern Med 77:605–628, 1972.
13. Webster ADB, Kenwright S, Ballard J, et al: Nodular lymphoid hyperplasia of the bowel in primary hypogammaglobulinaemia: study of in vivo and in vitro lymphocyte function. Gut 18:364–372, 1977.
14. Crooks DJM, Brown WR: The distribution of intestinal nodular hyperplasia in immunoglobulin deficiency. Clin Radiol 31:701–706, 1980.
15. O'Leary AD, Sweeney EC: Lymphoglandular complexes of the colon: structure and distribution. Histopathology 10:267–283, 1986.
16. Smith PD, Mai UEH: Immunopathophysiology of gastrointestinal disease in HIV infection. Gastroenterol Clin North Am 21:331–345, 1992.
17. Danzig JB, Brandt LJ, Reinus JF, et al: Gastrointestinal malignancy in patients with AIDS. Am J Gastroenterol 86:715–718, 1991.
18. Rambaud J-C, Piel J-L, Galian A, et al: Complete clinical, histological and immunological remission in a patient with alpha-chain disease treated with oral antibiotics. Gastroenterol Clin Biol 2:49–61, 1978.

# Crohn's Disease

Hans Herlinger, M.D.
Dina F. Caroline, M.D.

## INTRODUCTION

Crohn's disease is an idiopathic inflammatory disease that can affect any part of the gastrointestinal tract from the mouth to the anus. The small bowel is the major site of involvement. With the exception of malignant neoplasms, Crohn's disease can be the most devastating disease to involve the gastrointestinal tract. It has a worldwide distribution but is most common in northern Europe, North America, and Japan. Prevalence has increased, mostly in younger age groups, with a peak between 15 and 25 years.[1] What was formerly believed to be a second incidence peak in older patients is now thought to have been due predominantly to ischemic colitis. Both sexes are equally affected. A familial tendency has frequently been described.

The small bowel is involved by Crohn's disease in 80% of patients, with the terminal ileum by far the most common location. Disease is confined to the small bowel in 30% of patients and affects the colon together with the small bowel in 50% of patients. Isolated involvement of the colon occurs in 15 to 20% and isolated perianal disease in 2 to 3%.[2] Upper gastrointestinal tract involvement is recognized with increasing frequency but invariably occurs with small bowel and/or colonic disease.

## CLINICAL CONSIDERATIONS

Although the focus of this chapter is on small intestinal Crohn's disease, differences in presentation from colonic disease must be mentioned. Patients with colonic Crohn's disease are more likely to present with blood loss, perianal disease, toxic megacolon, and extraintestinal complications. Small intestinal Crohn's disease has a slightly better prognosis, although there are apt to be complications such as abscesses, fistulas, and obstruction. Abdominal pain, mild diarrhea, weight loss, and pyrexia are likely clinical presentations. A common clinical finding is that of a right lower quadrant mass that represents the diseased ileum often with the cecum. Delays of 3 to 4 years[3, 4] have been reported between the onset of symptoms and the diagnosis of small bowel Crohn's disease.

Many factors contribute to the development of diarrhea. Inflamed bowel mucosa causes increased secretion of fluid and electrolytes. Extensive terminal ileal disease or resection impairs bile salt reabsorption, leading to malabsorption of fat and fat-soluble vitamins. Bacterial overgrowth secondary to strictures, fistulas to colon, adhesions, or bypassed loops can also cause diarrhea. The combination of decreased food absorption and intermittent obstructions accentuates weight loss.[5]

Depiction of abnormalities of the small bowel, especially early changes of Crohn's disease, requires optimal methods of examination. It is generally appreciated that the traditional small bowel follow-through examination is inadequate for detailed evaluation of the small bowel. This was the case in the large National Cooperative Crohn's Disease Study of 1979, which is still frequently mentioned.[6] By current standards, the radiographic evaluations on which that study was based are considered inadequate.

## RADIOLOGY

Several types of radiologic investigation for the evaluation of small bowel Crohn's disease are in current use. We and others[7, 8] believe that enteroclysis should be the method of choice for the following indications:

1. To demonstrate the early changes of the disease
2. To depict the full extent of involvement and the possible presence of skip lesions should surgery be contemplated
3. To determine the cause of any clinical deterioration in a hitherto stable Crohn's patient
4. To distinguish among spasm, active stenotic disease, and a fibrous stricture
5. To investigate postoperative complications of Crohn's disease
6. To rule out positively the presence of small bowel Crohn's disease

A review of 100 patients referred for enteroclysis for suspected Crohn's disease has shown excellent correlation with the clinical assessment during 2 or more years of follow-up.[9] One third of the patients had normal appearances on enteroclysis and none developed clinical disease. In one third of the patients, enteroclysis demonstrated subtle lesions of early Crohn's disease. Every patient who subsequently required surgery was found to have severe disease by radiographic criteria.[9]

A fluoroscopic small bowel follow-through examination (see Chapter 43) can be adequate for these indications:

1. As a follow-up study in patients known to have small bowel Crohn's disease and whose clinical picture has shown little change (although areas of early disease are likely to be missed).
2. In cases in which Crohn's disease is known to involve predominantly the terminal ileum. The follow-through should then be combined with a peroral pneumocolon. In the experience of Glick,[10] the distal 20 to 50 cm of ileum can be seen in double contrast in 80 to 90% of patients.
3. To investigate (together with peroral pneumocolon) possible recurrence of Crohn's disease after ileocecal resection.

A double contrast barium enema is the best way to examine the anastomosis and the preanastomotic bowel after more extensive colon resection. In patients with an ileostomy, a retrograde small bowel enema is recommended for the demonstration of more distal small bowel loops.

Computed tomography (CT) is an important complement to barium studies, especially for investigating the complications of small intestinal Crohn's disease, abscesses, phlegmons, fistulas, and obstructions. Increasingly, it has become the primary method of investigation when these complications are suspected.

## CLINICAL COURSE

Crohn's disease is a chronic disease that is usually characterized by periods of symptom exacerbation interspersed with periods of clinical quiescence. A subgroup of patients (10 to 20%) experience extended remission lasting 20 years or longer after initial presentation.[11] A continuing problem with the clinical and radiographic assessment of Crohn's disease is that the clinical condition does not necessarily correlate with the radiographic severity of the disease.

## PROGRESSION OF CROHN'S DISEASE

It is possible, by means of enteroclysis, to classify lesions into those associated with early, intermediate, and advanced stages of Crohn's disease and to relate these to changes in histopathology.[12, 13]

### Early Disease[14, 15]

Pathology and radiology correlate well. The earliest changes to be seen histologically are hyperplasia of lymphoid tissue and obstructive lymphedema in the submucosa. Extension of submucosa into the core of mucosal folds then causes folds to thicken, at this stage in regular and symmetric form (Fig. 47–1).

Affected villi contain an excess of mononuclear cells and produce increased amounts of mucous secretions.[16] Thickened villi adhere to one another, producing a

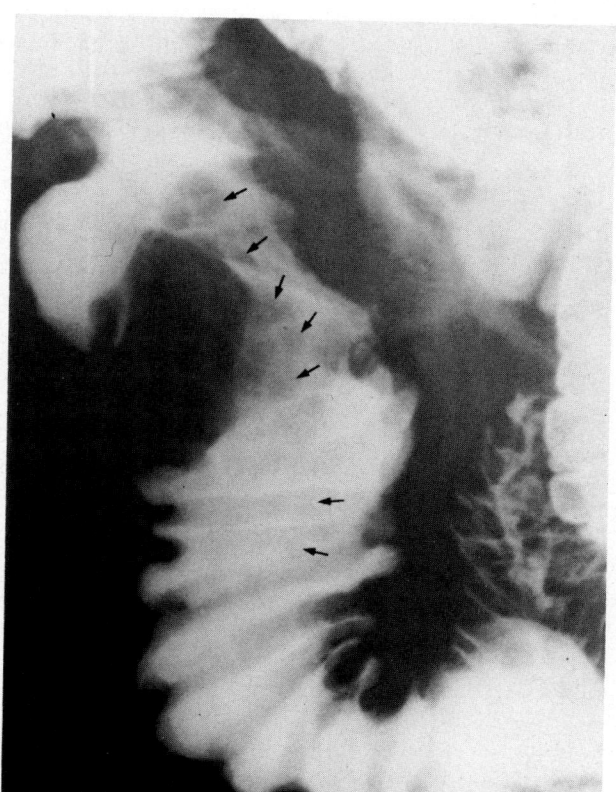

**Figure 47–1. Recurrence of Crohn's disease in the neoterminal ileum.** Smoothly thickened folds, narrowed segment at anastomosis, and numerous aphthoid ulcers are present *(arrows)*.

coarse villous pattern that is readily identified on barium studies[17, 18] (Fig. 47–2A and B).

Hyperplasia of lymph follicles in the lamina propria can be associated with shallow mucosal erosions 1 to 3 mm in size, surrounded by a small halo of edema, the aphthoid ulcers[19] (Fig. 47–3A and B).

None of the three earliest radiologically visible mucosal surface features are specific for the diagnosis of Crohn's disease. However, if two or even three of these signs appear together, the likelihood of early Crohn's disease is high[20] (see Figs. 47–1 and 47–3A and B).

## Intermediate Disease

While the disease process gradually extends transmurally, further changes take place in the mucosa and submucosa. The edema in the submucosa may increase enough to widen the base of some folds sufficiently to cause their partial or total disappearance. This process is akin to the thumbprinting seen in ischemia (Fig. 47–4). However, in patients with ischemia, the fold abnormalities change over a period of days to weeks, whereas in patients with Crohn's disease the fold abnormalities persist and are usually associated with changes of more advanced Crohn's disease elsewhere in the small bowel. The mucosal inflammatory infiltrate tends to show focal variations in intensity. This, together with patchy submucosal fibrosis, leads to distortion and interruption of folds[21] (Fig. 47–5).

Several of the aphthoid ulcers enlarge, deepen, and may present a stellate or rose thorn shape (Fig. 47–6). Other aphthoid ulcers extend and may fuse with ulcers close to them to assume crescentic or linear shapes. A typical finding is that of a long linear ulcer at the mesenteric border,[21–23] which may be separated from the adjacent submucosa by a parallel seam of edema (Fig. 47–7). The mesenteric border ulcer causes thickening, sclerosis, and retraction of the adjacent mesentery and of the mesenteric border of the involved bowel. The transaxially unaffected antimesenteric border becomes redundant and assumes an appearance of pleating or sacculation.

An inflammatory cellular infiltrate with focally pronounced edema and granulation tissue can give rise to localized mucosal elevations, inflammatory polyps.[24] These lesions are common in the colon but infrequent in the small bowel. When present, they are found in small numbers in an area of mucosa that is denuded of folds (Fig. 47–8). Occasionally, a bowel segment contains many inflammatory polyps, all up to 1 cm in diameter and separated from one another by curving lines of barium occupying the crevices between the elevations. Where seen in profile, the polyps appear as notches[25] demarcated by protrusions of barium (Fig. 47–9). The diameter of such bowel segments is not reduced. We refer to this as the *nodular pattern,* stressing its essential difference from the ulceronudular or "cobblestone" pattern of advanced, fissuring ulcer-related disease. Figure 47–10 demonstrates all the intermediate stage alterations in a short segment of terminal ileum.

## Advanced Disease

The transmural advance of the disease has reached the serosa and beyond. Deep linear clefts of ulceration, the fissures,[26, 27] are typical of this stage of the disease (Fig. 47–11). Islands of surviving mucosa surrounded by extensive ulceration would give the appearance of ele-

*Text continued on page 832*

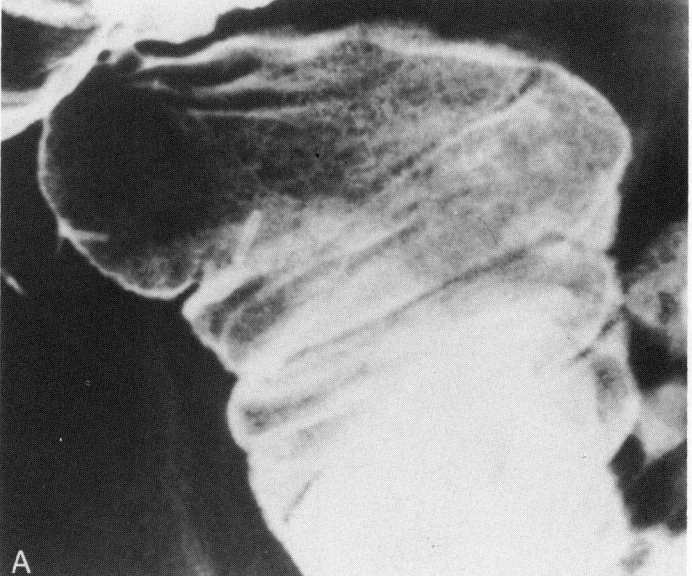
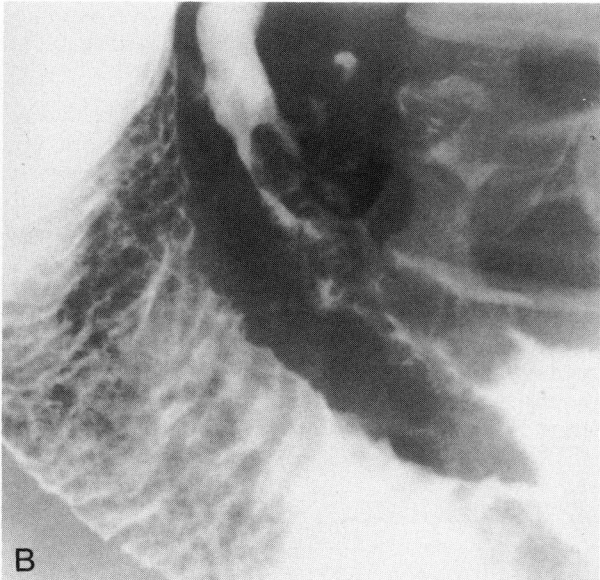

**Figure 47–2. Coarse villous pattern in early Crohn's disease. A.** This pattern is the only abnormality shown; folds are normal. (Courtesy of O. Ekberg, M.D., Malmö, Sweden.) **B.** Fold thickening is seen in addition to the coarse villous pattern (adjacent to more advanced disease).

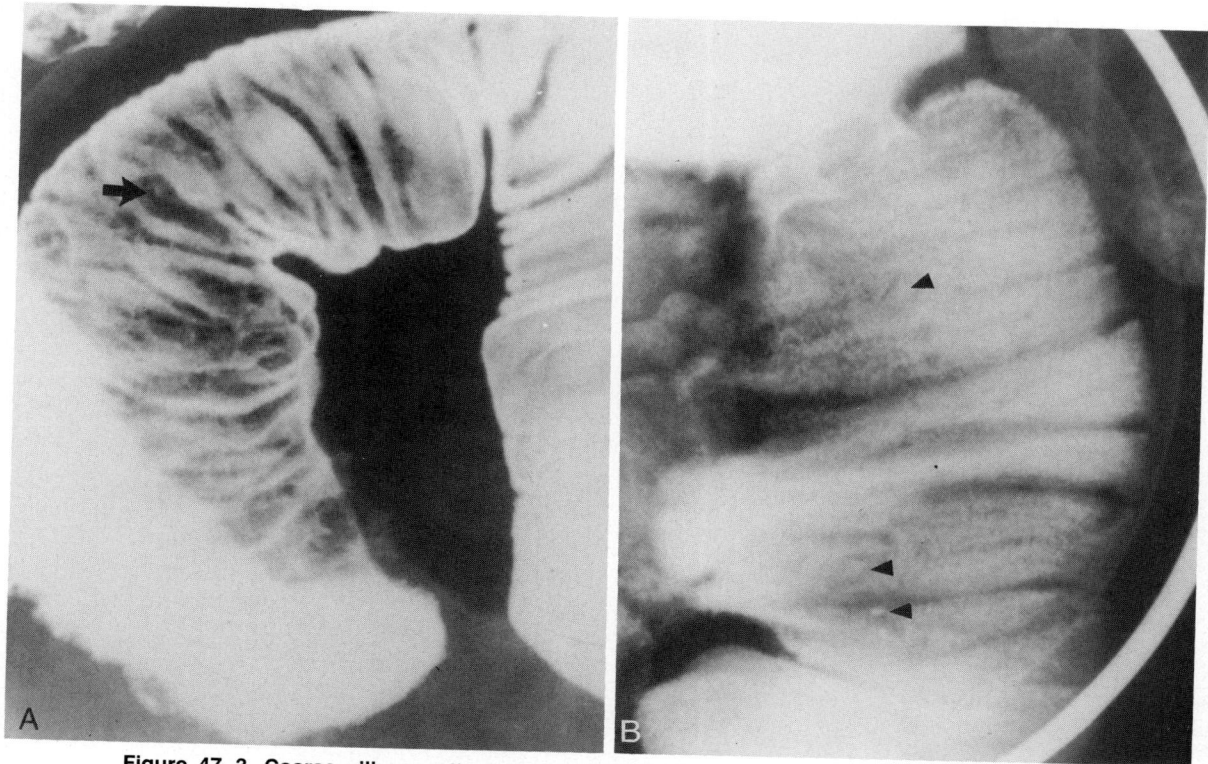

**Figure 47–3. Coarse villous pattern plus aphthoid ulcers. A.** Double contrast view; aphthoid ulcers are well shown *(arrow)*. (Courtesy of Seth Glick, M.D., Philadelphia, PA.) **B.** Coarse villi are shown in single contrast with compression. Aphthoid ulcers are also visible *(arrowheads)*.

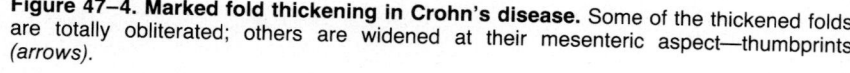

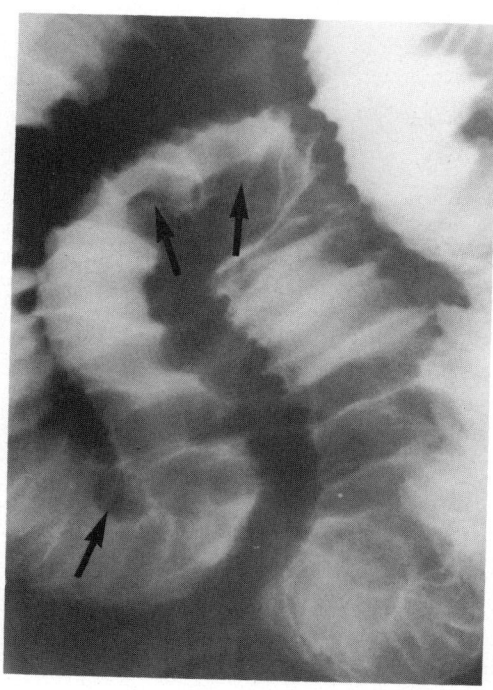

**Figure 47–4. Marked fold thickening in Crohn's disease.** Some of the thickened folds are totally obliterated; others are widened at their mesenteric aspect—thumbprints *(arrows)*.

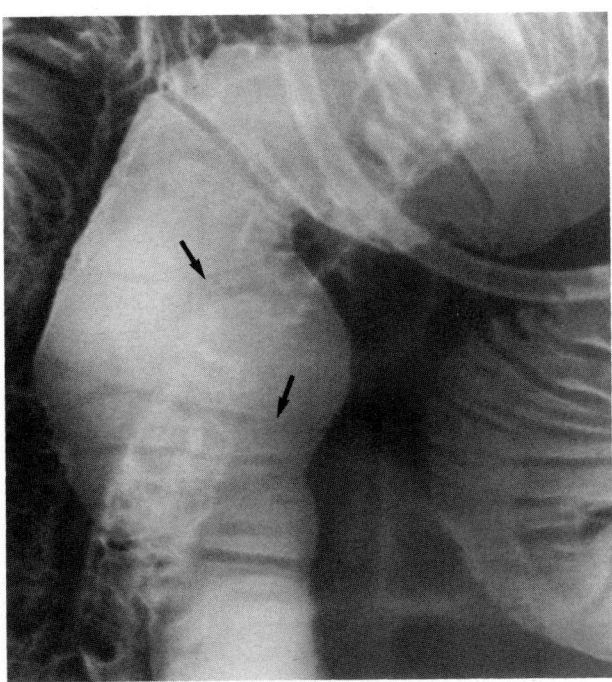

**Figure 47–5. Interruption and distortion of folds.** Few folds are interrupted *(arrows)*; there is an area devoid of folds, associated with lumen widening. A loop with more advanced changes is superimposed.

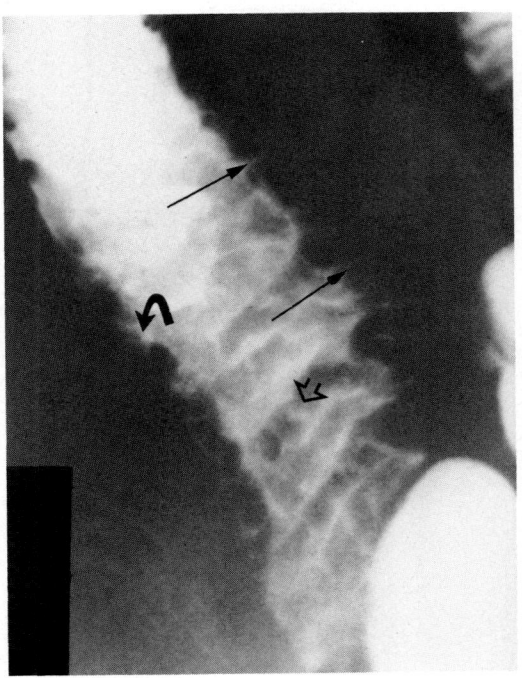

**Figure 47–6. Progression of aphthoid ulcers.** Aphthoid ulcers have enlarged and become more elongated *(open arrow)*. Deepened ulcers are identified in profile view, some of "rose thorn" appearance *(long arrows)* and others more broad based *(curved arrow)*. Folds are unevenly thickened.

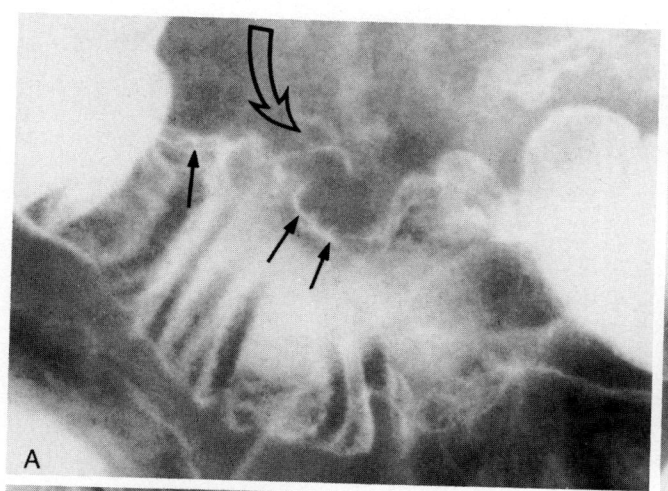

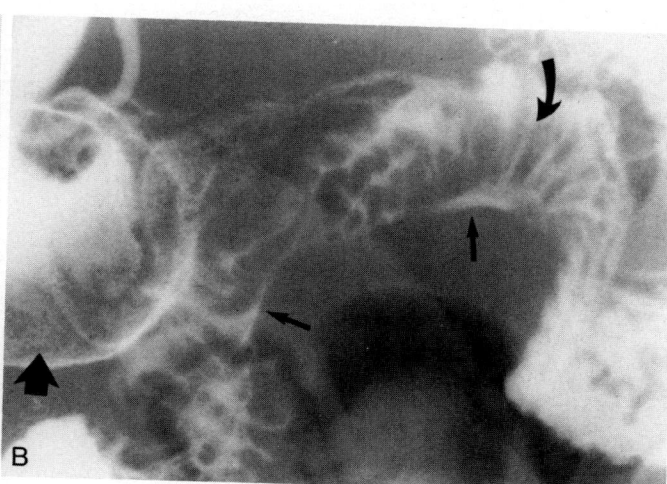

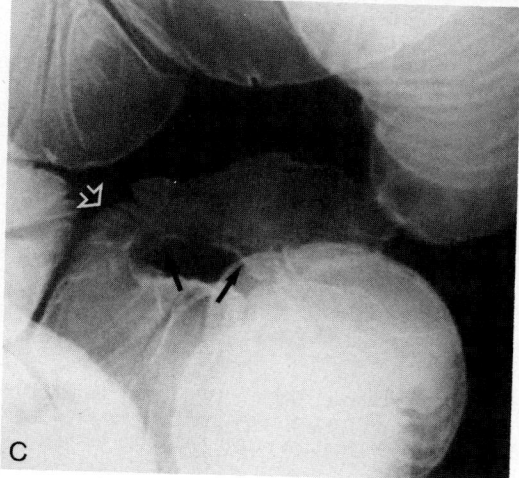

**Figure 47–7. Skip lesions with mesenteric border ulceration. A.** Long, irregular linear ulcer is seen at the mesenteric border *(solid arrows)*, with ulceration extending into the mesentery *(open arrow)*. The antimesenteric border shows pronounced pleating. (From Herlinger H: The small bowel enema and the diagnosis of Crohn's disease. Radiol Clin North Am 20:721–742, 1982.) **B.** Two short linear ulcers are seen at the mesenteric border *(small arrows)*. Thickened folds diverge *(curved arrow)* toward the unaffected antimesenteric side. (The thick arrow to adjacent segment shows a coarse villous pattern.) **C.** A short skip lesion is identified by a linear mesenteric border ulcer *(solid arrows)* and antimesenteric redundancy *(open arrow)*.

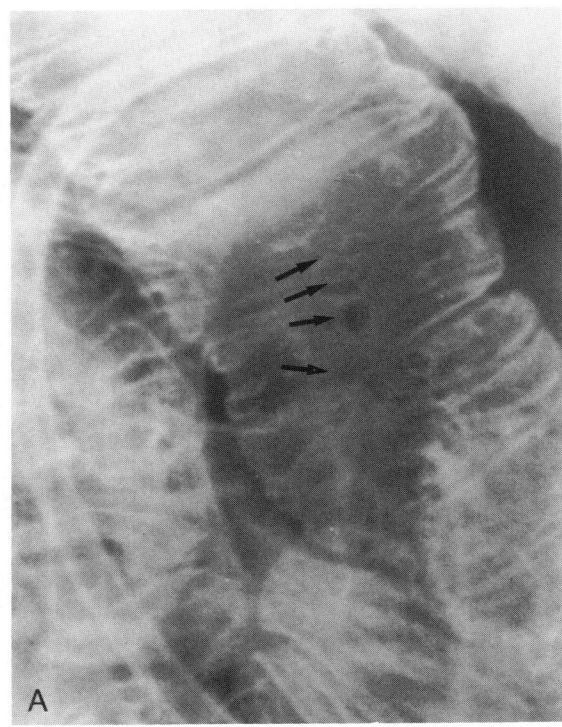

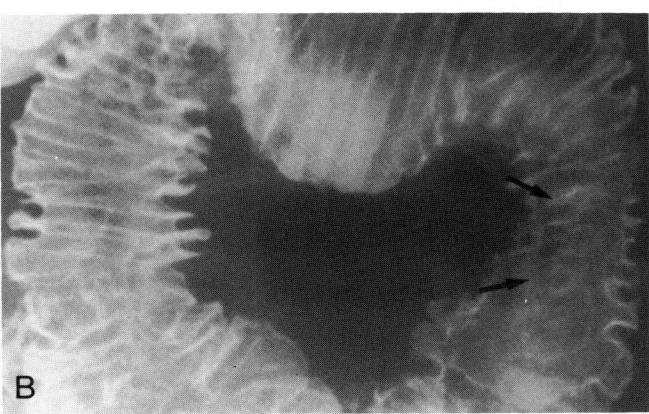

**Figure 47–8. Inflammatory polyps in an area of mucosal fold obliteration. A.** Group of inflammatory polyps of varying sizes *(arrows).* **B.** Several polyps in a short segment of bowel without folds *(arrows).* There are thickened folds in the other bowel segments.

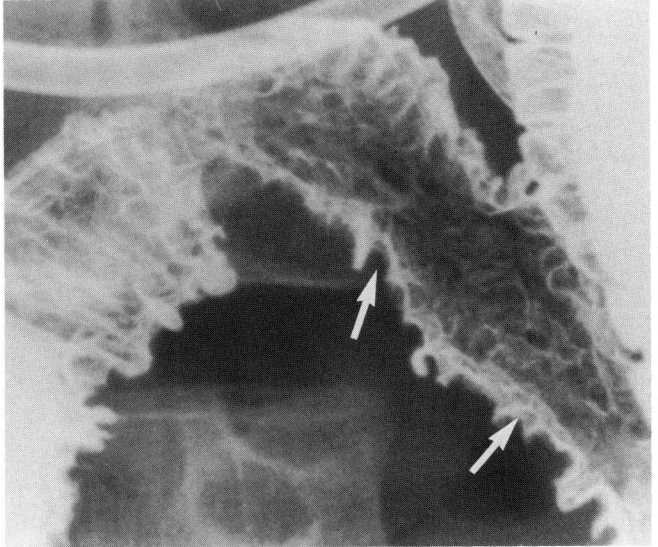

**Figure 47–9. Nodular patterns.** Many inflammatory nodules are separated by curved lines of barium in the crevices between them. These are not linear ulcers. Nodules appear as notches in profile view *(arrows).*

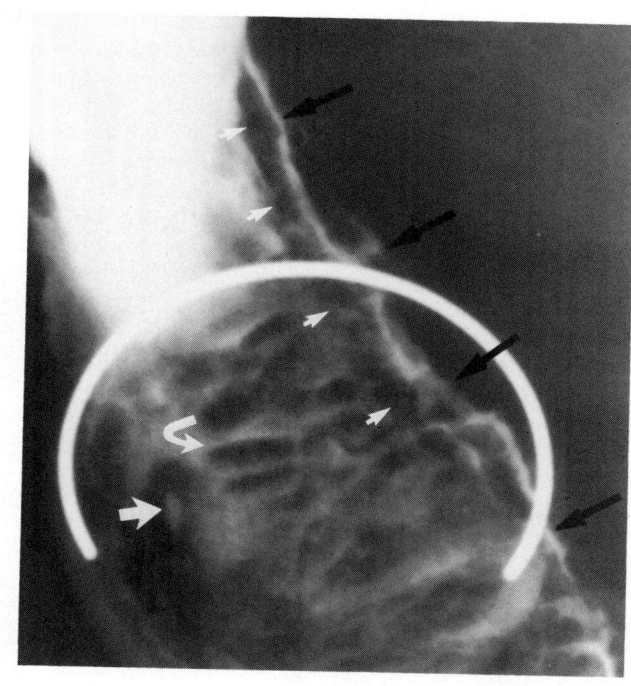

**Figure 47–10. Features of the intermediate stage of Crohn's disease.** There is a long mesenteric border ulcer *(black arrows),* with a line of edema at its luminal side *(small white arrows).* Interrupted, thickened folds *(curved arrow)* are present. Aphthoid ulcers have enlarged and deepened *(thick short white arrow).*

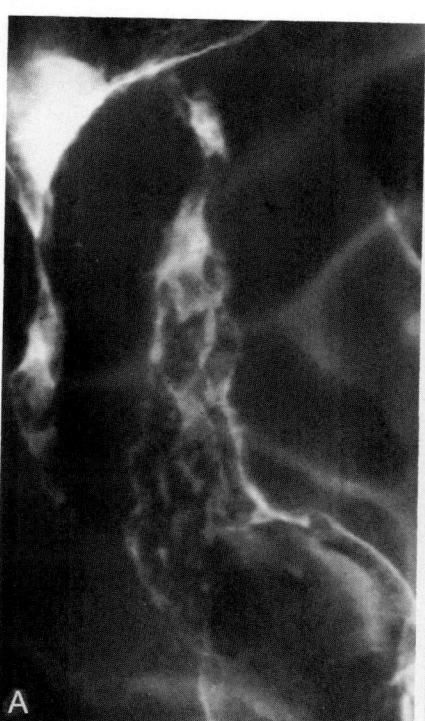

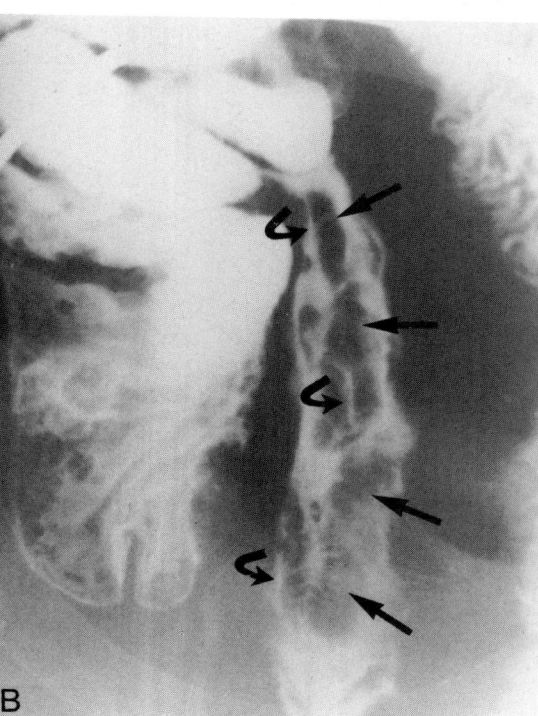

**Figure 47–11. Linear ulcers or fissures with lumen narrowing. A.** Narrowed segment of terminal ileum with numerous fissures. **B.** Terminal ileum with fissures *(curved arrows)* and large inflammatory polyps *(straight arrows).*

vation above the ulcerated background. These islands of mucosa may then be regarded as pseudopolyps.[24] The deep fissures characteristic of this advanced stage may present a combination of fairly regular axial and trans-axial fissuring, separating the pseudopolyps from one another. This pattern is always associated with lumen reduction and is referred to as the ulceronodular or cobblestone pattern[12] (Fig. 47–12). It must not be confused with the nodular pattern of the less advanced stage of the disease. Another feature of advanced disease is the formation of large flat ulcers probably derived from the enlargement of aphthoid ulcers (Fig. 47–13).

Changes associated with the linear mesenteric ulceration advance in a caudad direction as the disease progresses. The antimesenteric redundancy shown earlier gradually disappears, being incorporated in the transaxial extension of Crohn's disease[12] (Fig. 47– 14). The bowel wall is now thickened, more by fibrosis than by inflammatory infiltrate (sometimes referred to as sclerolipomatosis). On palpation, bowel loops are still mobile but no longer pliable. CT demonstrates well the thickened bowel wall and also the inflammatory changes extending into the mesentery.[28]

## COMPLICATIONS

### Strictures

Strictures are caused by collagen deposition, mostly throughout the submucosa. They are a major or a contributing cause of small bowel obstruction and may have to be treated surgically. Strictures or stricture-like findings are reported in 21% of patients with small bowel Crohn's disease.[6] Enteroclysis is valuable because

it makes possible a radiologic distinction of fibrotic strictures from lumen narrowing by spasm (Fig. 47–15), active ulcerated stenotic disease (Fig. 47–16), or narrowing associated with a surrounding inflammatory process (Fig. 47–17). Resistance to lumen distention when tested by enteroclysis can confirm the presence of a fibrous stricture (Fig. 47–18). Obstruction by a fibrous stricture requires surgery. Strictureplasty[29] (Fig. 47–19) rather than resection is increasingly recommended.

Resective surgery in small bowel Crohn's disease is followed by a high degree of disease recurrence. After ileocecal resection, endoscopic evidence of recurrence was noted in the neoterminal ileum of 73% of patients after 1 year; however, only 20% had symptoms. Three years later, there was endoscopic evidence of recurrence in 85% of patients and 34% had symptoms. The same pattern of endoscopically observed and histologically confirmed recurrence was demonstrated after more extensive resection and ileocolic anastomosis.[30] The need for multiple resections has made small bowel Crohn's disease a major cause of the short bowel syndrome. Thus, whenever possible, strictureplasty should replace resection.

### Abscesses or Phlegmons

Inflammatory lesions may remain closely related to a diseased segment (Fig. 47–20) or may extend into the pelvis (Fig. 47–21) or occasionally into the psoas muscle (Fig. 47–22). Barium studies depicting small bowel or colon close to an abscess may demonstrate a nonspecific proximity effect.[31] Barium demonstrates an abscess by outlining a group of several tracts extending into it or by entering a few small spaces in various parts of an

*Text continued on page 838*

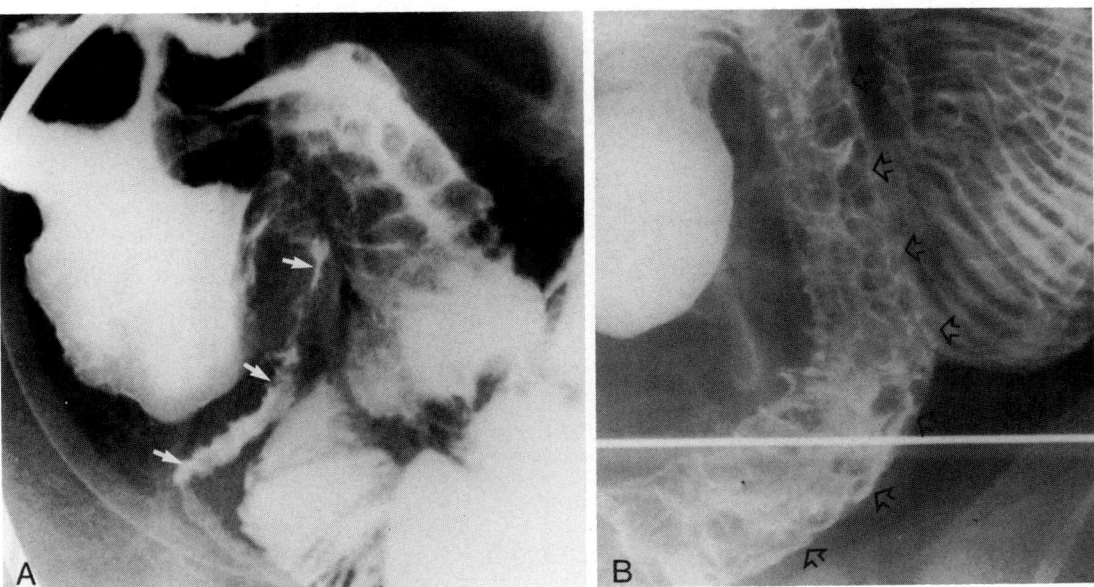

**Figure 47–12. Ulceronodular pattern or cobblestoning. A.** Terminal ileum with longitudinal and transverse fissures separating islands of swollen mucosa. The appendix is narrowed by ulcerated Crohn's disease *(arrows).* **B.** A less regular pattern of fissures surrounds swollen islands of mucosa of varied sizes in a poorly distensible bowel segment *(arrows).*

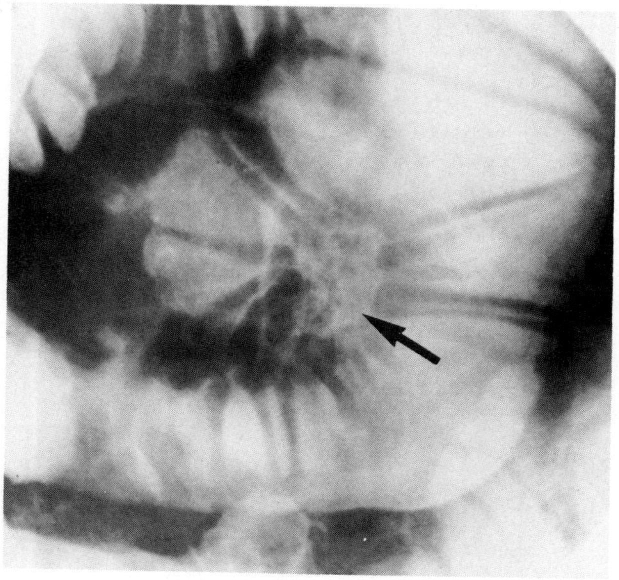

**Figure 47–13. Large Crohn's ulcer.** A large, flat ulcer is seen en face *(arrow)*. It is surrounded by a rim of edema and by converging folds.

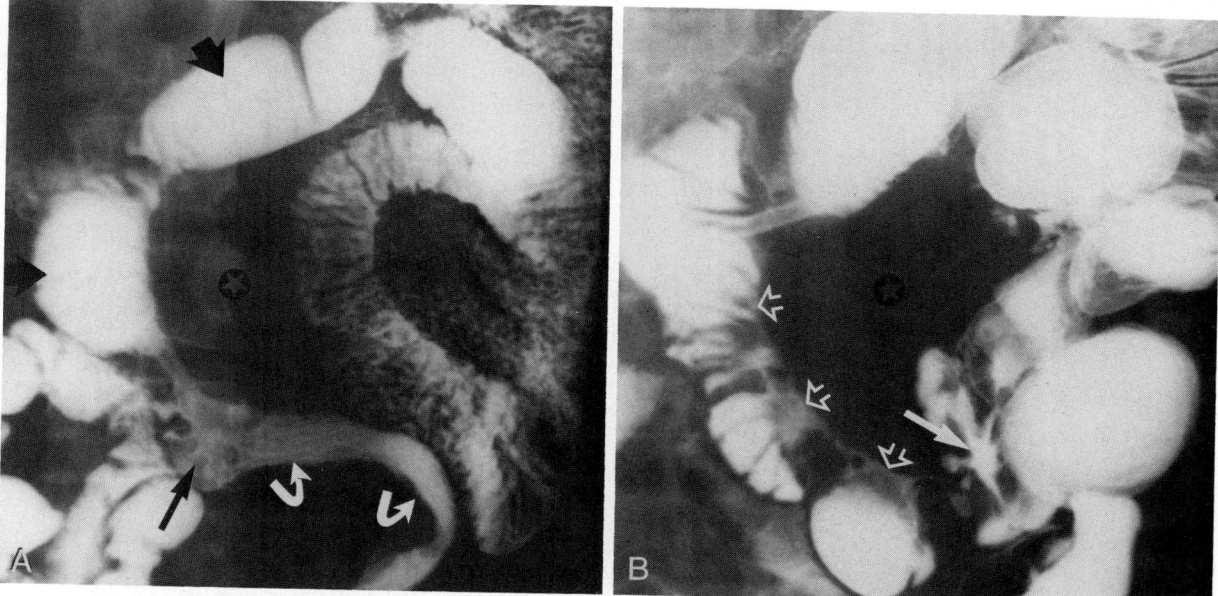

**Figure 47–14. Advancing Crohn's disease in patients with mesenteric border ulceration. A.** In the upper part of the image, the mesenteric border is straight and shortened with the redundant antimesenteric border forming sacculations *(thick arrows)*. Disease intensity progresses in a caudad direction. A more distal saccule *(thin arrow)* has been overtaken by the transaxial progression of Crohn's disease. More distally *(curved arrows)*, bowel is uniformly ulcerated and narrowed. The space near the mesenteric border is occupied by mesentery thickened by sclerolipomatosis *(asterisk)*. **B.** Similar caudad progression of Crohn's disease in a bowel segment with mesenteric border ulceration *(open arrows)*. The antimesenteric side changes from redundancy with pleating to sacculation and is then abruptly incorporated into an area of ulceration and fistulas *(solid arrow)*. Again, see the space occupied by mesenteric sclerolipomatosis *(asterisk)*.

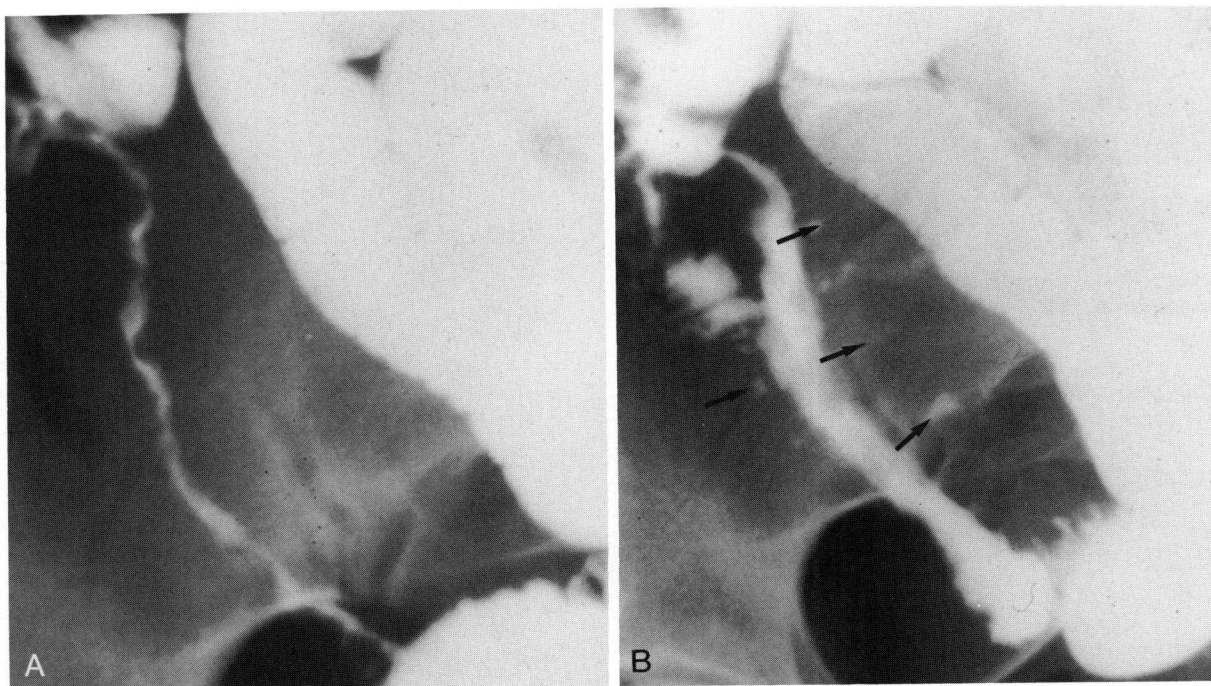

**Figure 47–15. Narrowed terminal ileum, spasm or stricture? A.** Appearance typical of a "string" sign (like a frayed string). **B.** With methylcellulose advancing toward the cecum, the narrowed segment widens and barium-outlined tracks *(arrows)* are seen to extend into a surrounding inflammatory mass. Spasm has caused the string sign.

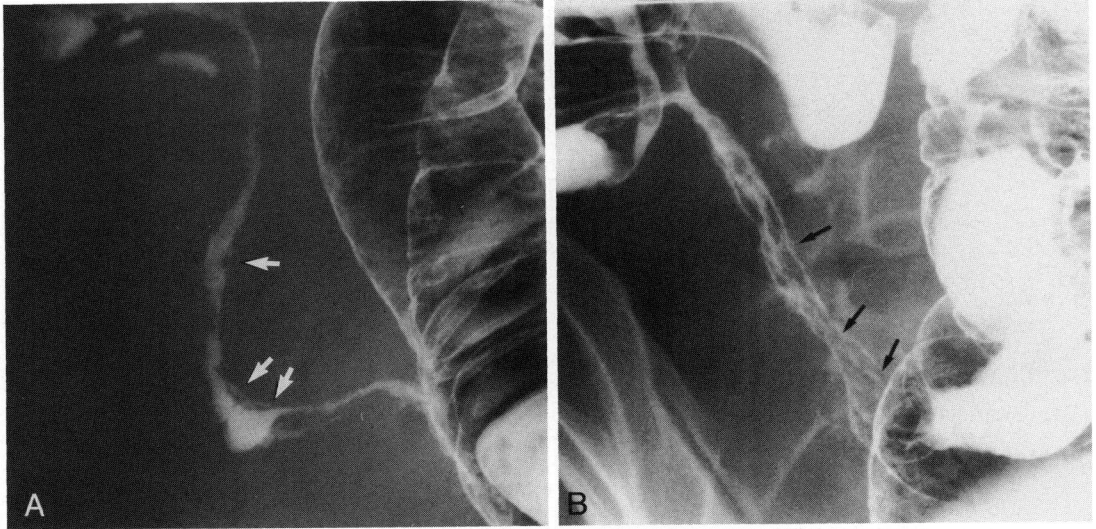

**Figure 47–16. Narrowed terminal ileum caused by active Crohn's disease. A.** Narrowing with a suggestion of ulceration *(arrows)*. **B.** Enteroclysis in double contrast widens the lumen sufficiently *(arrows)* to present an appearance of extensively fissured stenotic stage of Crohn's disease. Medical treatment is indicated.

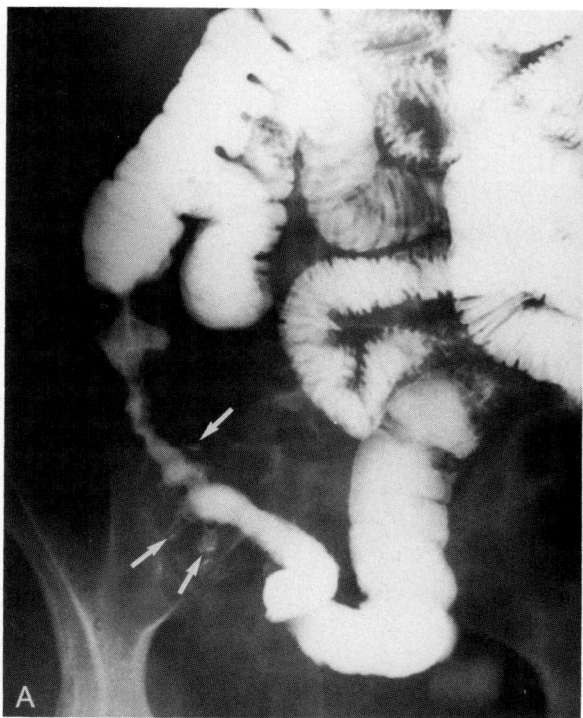

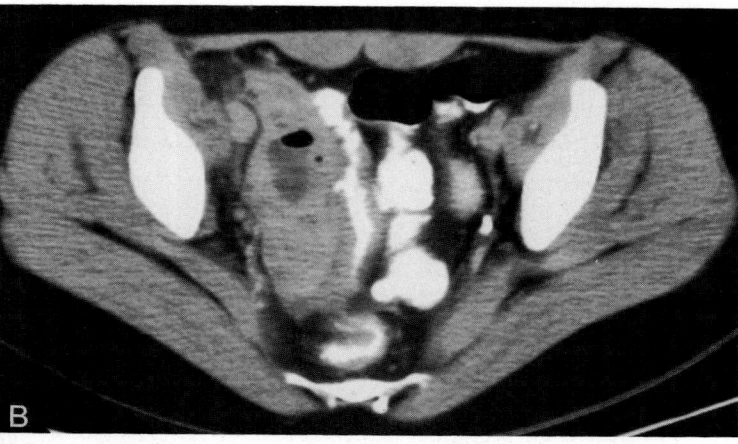

**Figure 47–17. Recurrent Crohn's disease in neoterminal ileum with narrowing caused by adjacent abscess. A.** The neoterminal ileum is narrowed and a few extraluminal collections of barium are seen *(arrows)*. **B.** CT scan demonstrates the contrast medium–filled, narrowed ileum with a large fluid- and gas-containing abscess lateral to it. (Courtesy of D. D. T. Maglinte, M.D., Indianapolis, IN.)

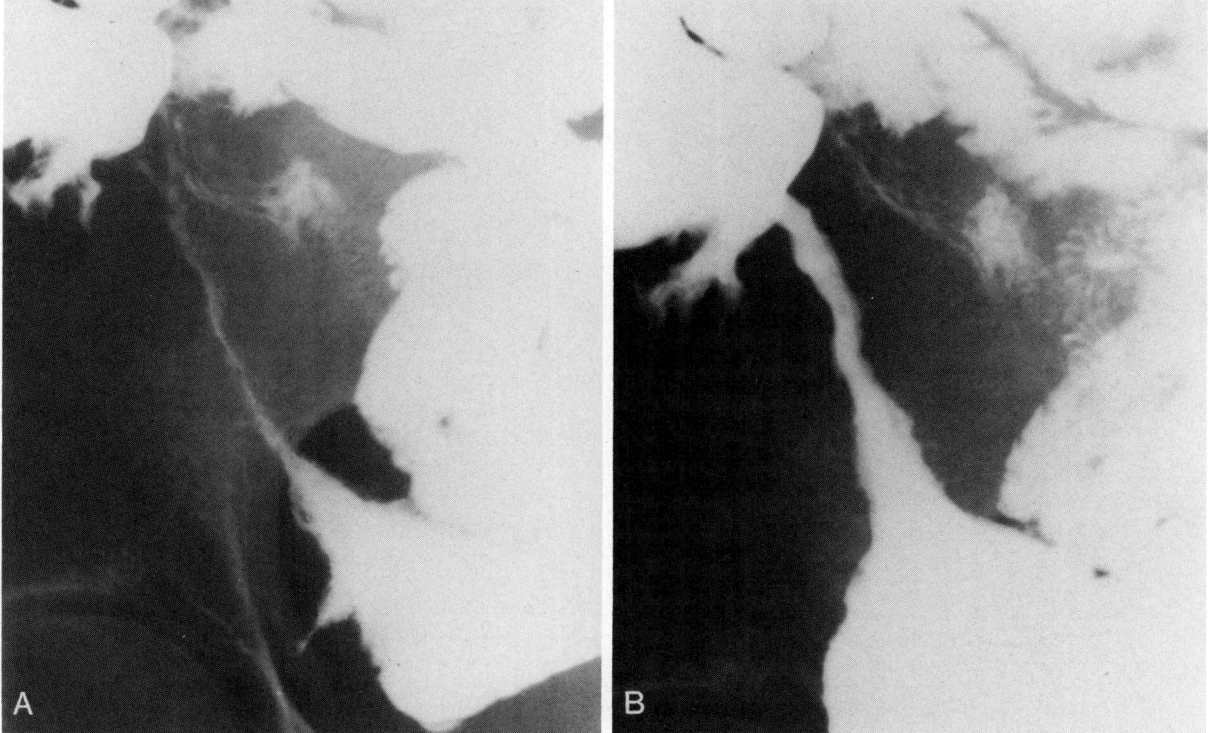

**Figure 47–18. Narrowed terminal ileum, spasm or stricture? A.** Fluoroscopic follow-through demonstrates a featureless narrowing of the terminal ileum in a patient known to have Crohn's disease. **B.** After administration of metoclopramide, the terminal ileum is widened slightly without showing any features of ulcerated stenotic disease. This is a fibrous stricture.

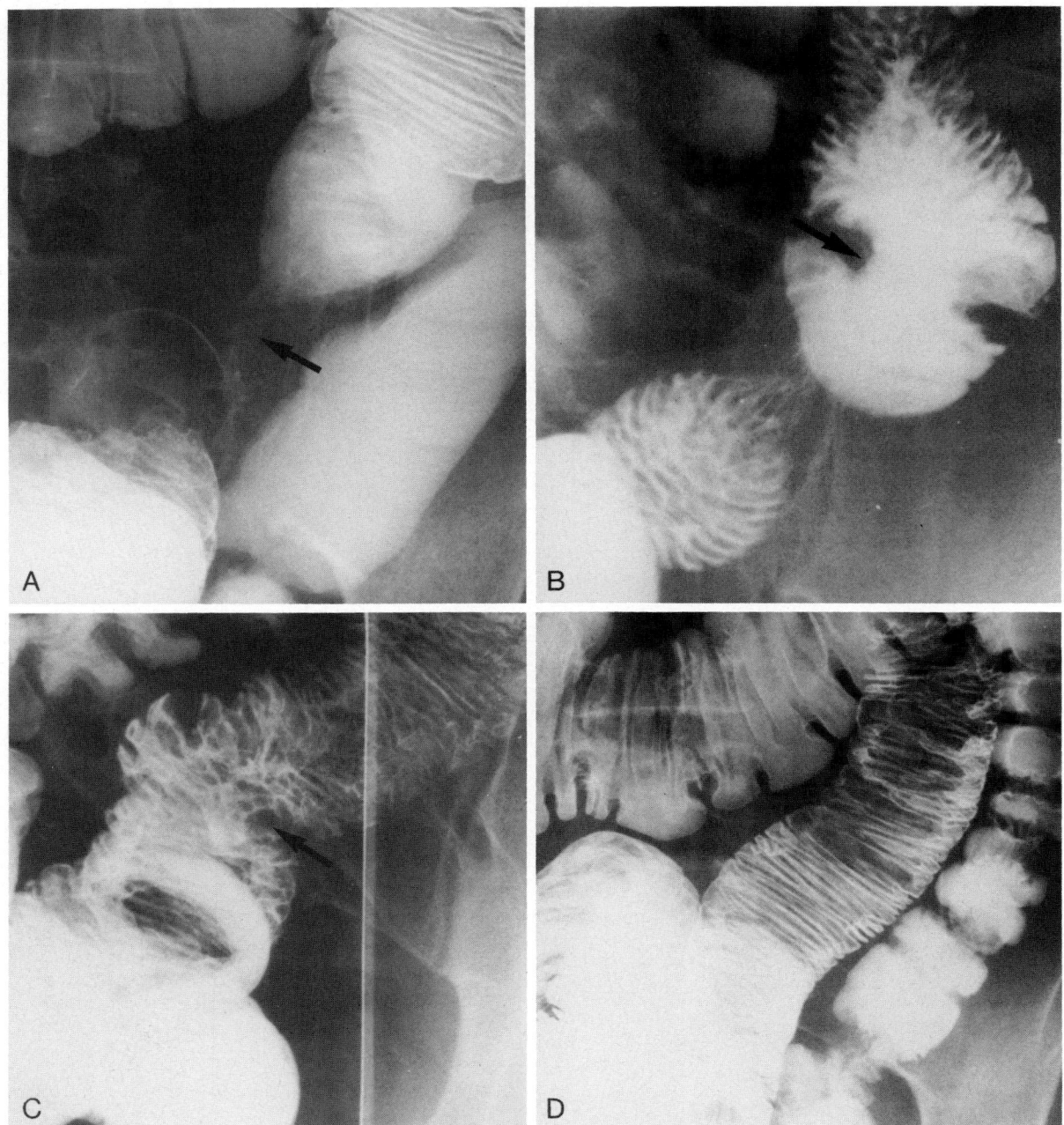

**Figure 47–19. Strictureplasty. A.** Enteroclysis demonstrates a tight, unchanging stricture in distal jejunum *(arrow),* associated with significant obstruction. **B.** A strictureplasty was done and was outlined by enteroclysis *(arrow)* 2 months later. **C.** Appearance of the strictureplasty site *(arrow)* 18 months later. **D.** After a further 6 months, there was virtually no trace of the strictureplasty.

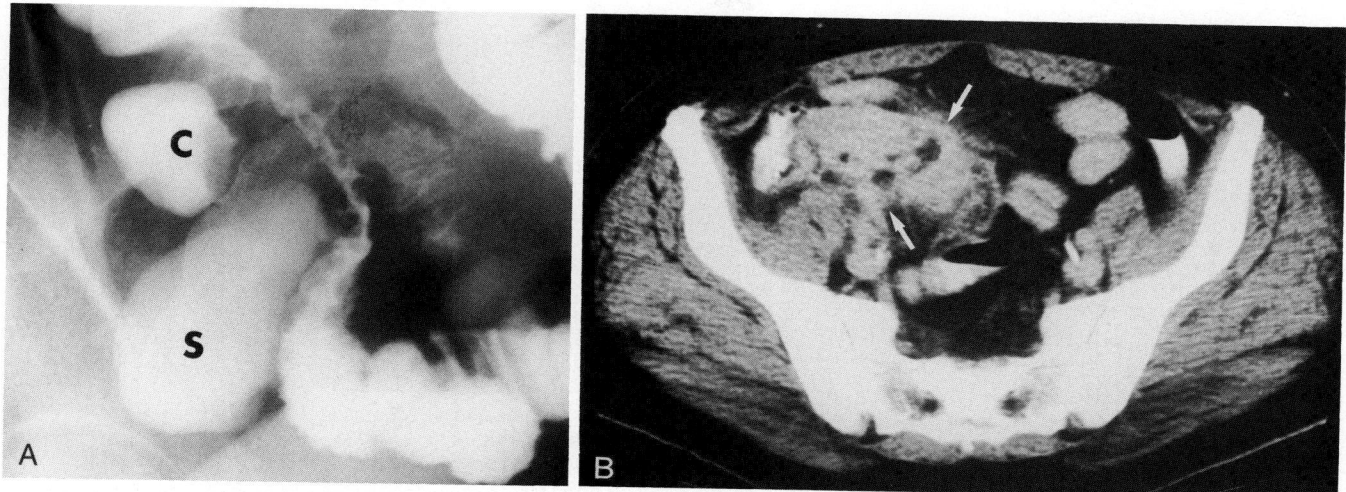

**Figure 47–20. Ileocecal Crohn's disease with an inflammatory mass. A.** Enteroclysis demonstrates an ulceronodular pattern throughout the narrowed terminal ileum together with involvement of the cecum (C). S = sigmoid colon. **B.** Corresponding CT scan demonstrates a surprisingly large inflammatory mass in the right lower quadrant *(arrows)*.

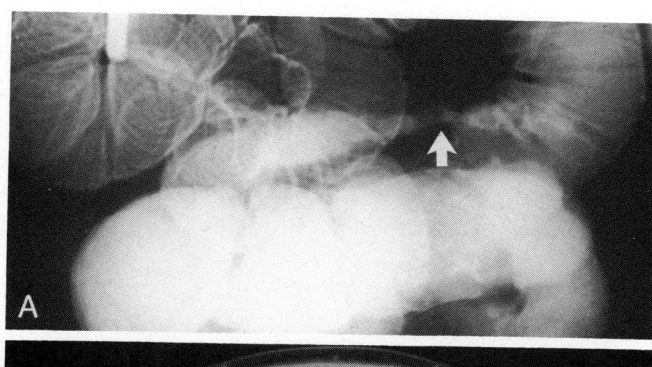

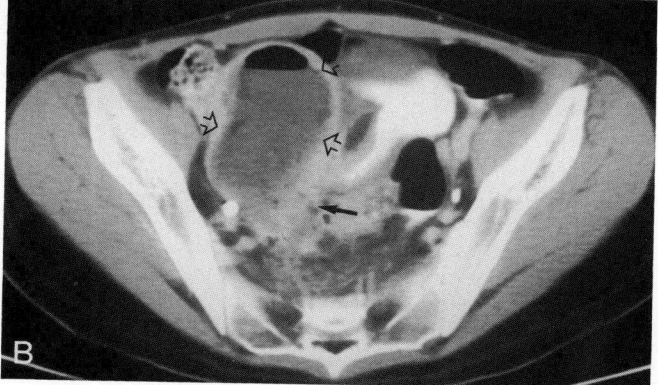

**Figure 47–21. Inflammatory lesion extending toward the pelvis.** This female patient with known Crohn's disease had recently increased right lower quadrant pain. **A.** Enteroclysis outlines a narrowed, ulcerated segment of ileum *(arrow)* that extended toward the pelvic inlet. **B.** A CT scan outlines the contrast medium–filled, thick-walled segment with Crohn's disease leading into an area of extra-mural inflammation *(solid arrow)*. A large cystic mass *(open arrows)* represents a pyosalpinx secondary to tubal obstruction by the Crohn's inflammatory process.

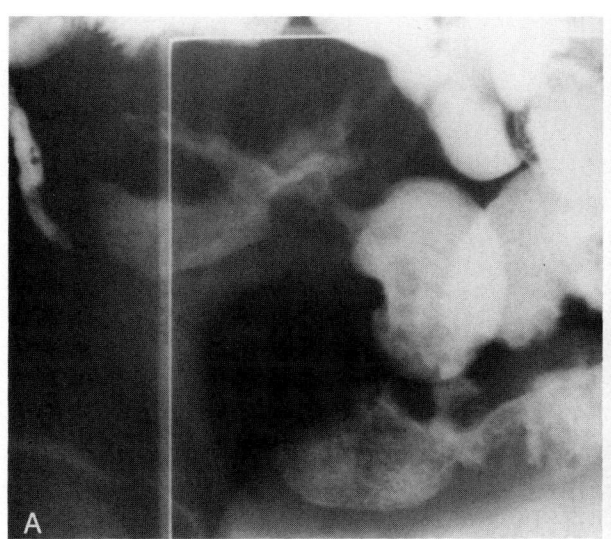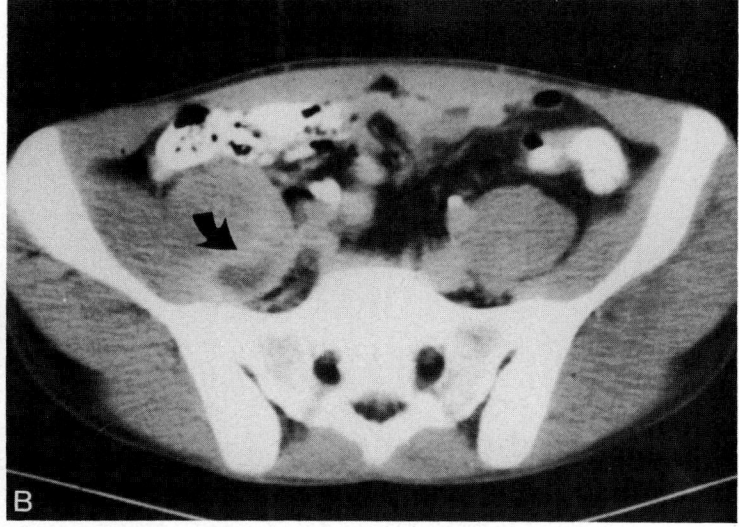

**Figure 47–22. Long-standing ileocecal Crohn's disease with psoas abscess. A.** A film taken during a fluoroscopic follow-through shows advanced ileal disease with a fistula. **B.** CT scan demonstrates a psoas abscess containing fluid *(arrow)*. The actual fistula was not outlined.

inflammatory mass. However, CT[32] and possibly ultrasound are the diagnostic methods of choice. Nevertheless, the CT findings are not specific for Crohn's disease and could also be seen with periappendicitis, diverticulitis, or neoplasms.

In a surgical review, abscesses were diagnosed in 129 of 610 patients with small bowel Crohn's disease (21%).[33] Abscesses were mostly intraperitoneal in location and all were treated surgically. Reoperation was required in 12%, and an external fistula developed in 22%.[33] Percutaneous drainage of Crohn's abscesses is now a well-established nonsurgical method of treatment.[34] Of 50 abscesses drained percutaneously, all were successfully evacuated and none needed surgical drainage or developed a catheterization-related fistula.[34]

## Fistulas

These are abnormal communications between two epithelial surfaces or an epithelial surface and the skin. A wide range of incidence from 6%[35] to 33%[36] is reported. Fistulas are also a consequence of transmural extension of the disease. Those between the terminal ileum and the cecal area are the most common and are often multiple (Fig. 47–23). An enterocolic fistula (Fig. 47–24) may lead to bacterial overgrowth and is one of the causes of malabsorption associated with Crohn's disease.[37] An enterocutaneous fistula is well shown with barium or CT (Fig. 47–25). Enterovesical fistulas are not often outlined with barium (Fig. 47–26), but the presence of barium in the bladder can be demonstrated by CT or by the Bourne test;[38] the presence of a fistula may be confirmed on a CT scan by outlining of air in a bladder in which there is no instrumentation.

Of considerable interest are Crohn's fistulas to the duodenum. Because the attachment of the transverse mesocolon crosses the mid-descending duodenum, fis-

tulization from the transverse colon is not unusual. A recurrence of Crohn's disease in neoterminal ileum after ileotransverse anastomosis may be associated with such a fistula and invariably leaves the duodenum uninvolved by the disease[32] (Fig. 47–27). Ileosigmoid fistulas are also of interest. They often bypass strictured obstructions in the ileocecal area and may serve a useful purpose. In the majority of cases, their entry site into the sigmoid colon shows only minor nonspecific changes (Fig. 47–28). If surgery is to be done, it usually suffices to resect the diseased ileum and the stricture, leaving the sigmoid colon intact.[32, 39]

## Free Perforations

Free perforations are rare because transmural fissures deepen slowly enough for adhesions to neighboring structures to form. Free perforations occur slightly more frequently in the small bowel than in the colon and are more likely to occur in the terminal ileum.[40, 41]

## REMISSION

A combination of mucosal atrophy and fibrosis can result in unmistakeable residual changes of Crohn's disease. Folds are interrupted, distorted, and absent in some areas. Unlike the situation in the colon, postinflammatory polyps, either rounded or filiform, are a rare finding in the small bowel (Fig. 47–29).

## CROHN'S JEJUNOILEITIS

Diffuse jejunoileitis forms a subset of Crohn's enteritis in which the distal ileum may be spared and disease progression may be craniad, toward the duodenum. It

*Text continued on page 843*

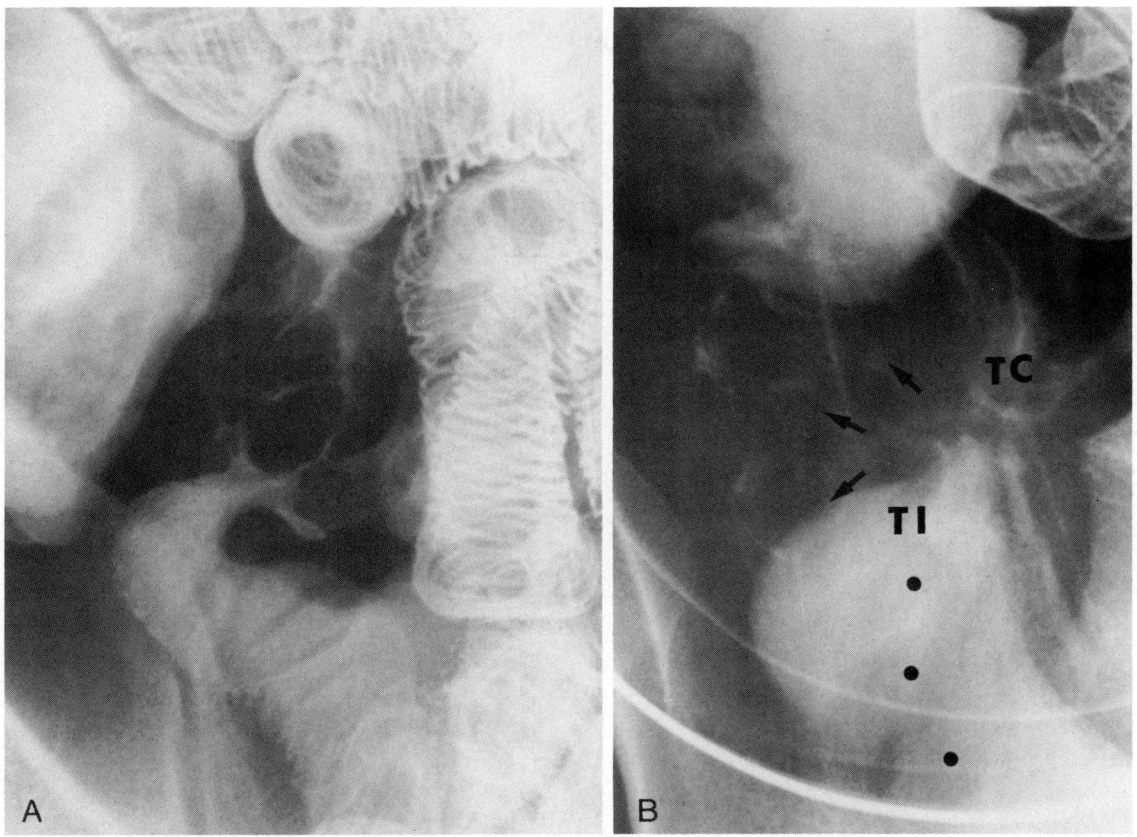

**Figure 47–23. Ileocecal fistulas in Crohn's disease. A.** Several ileocecal fistulas are present in this patient with Crohn's disease limited to the terminal ileum. **B.** In this patient with a severely narrowed ileocecal area, multiple fistulas extend from the terminal ileum (TI, dots) in the direction of the contracted cecum *(arrows)*. A broad fistula reaches the transverse colon (TC), which has come to lie close to this area.

**Figure 47–24. Jejunocolic fistula.** A fistula *(arrow)* extends from diseased jejunum (J) to adjacent transverse colon (TC). This could be a cause of bacterial overgrowth and of malabsorption by bypassing much of the intestinal absorptive surface.

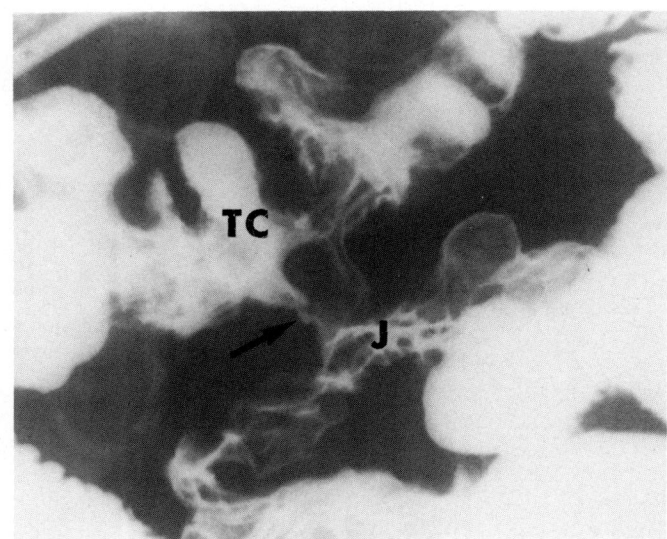

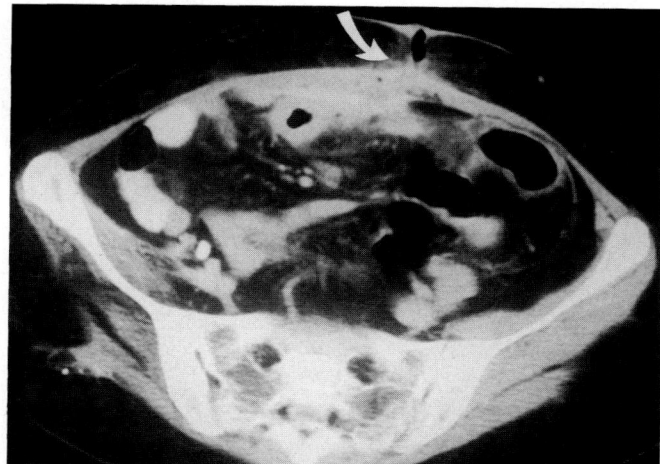

**Figure 47–25. Enterocutaneous fistula.** A CT scan shows an enterocutaneous fistula *(arrow)* extending through the anterior abdominal wall.

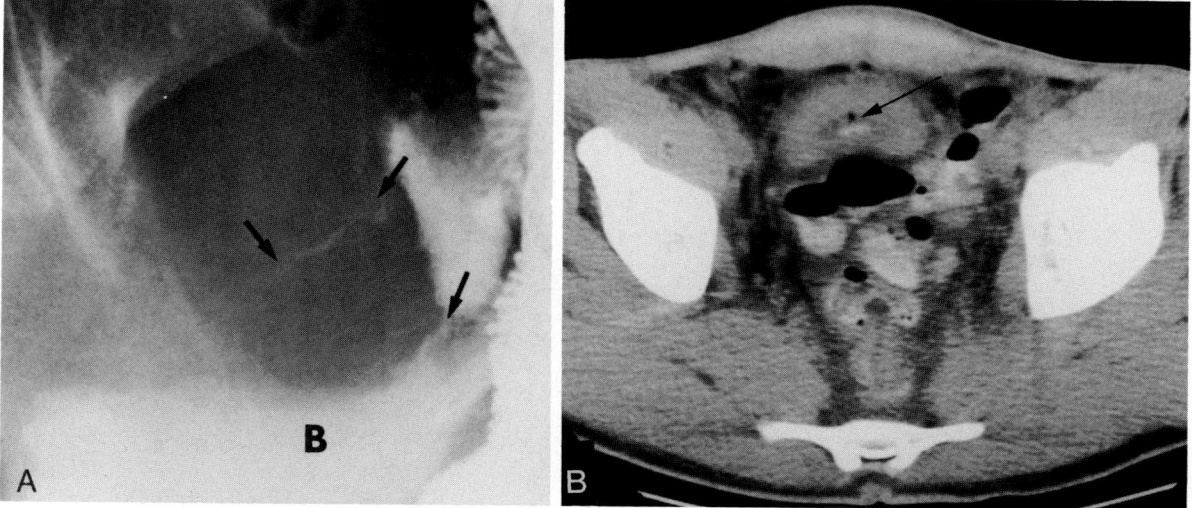

**Figure 47–26. Crohn's fistulas to the bladder. A.** Enteroclysis demonstration of two fistulas *(arrows)* between a segment of ileal Crohn's disease and the bladder (B). (From Herlinger H: The small bowel enema and the diagnosis of Crohn's disease. Radiol Clin North Am 20:721–742, 1982.) **B.** A CT scan without intravenous contrast shows barium and air *(arrow)* in the bladder, which establishes the presence of an enterovesical fistula.

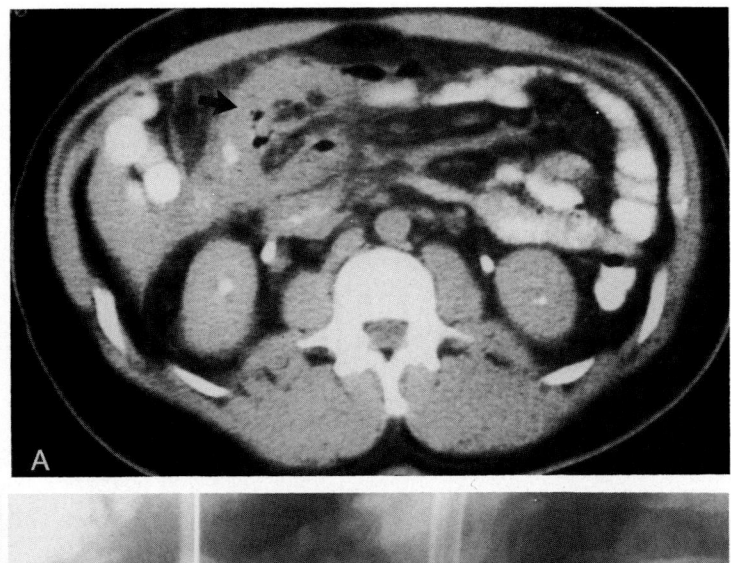

**Figure 47–27. Fistula to duodenum.** This patient with known Crohn's disease had a recent right hemicolectomy with ileotransverse anastomosis and presented with pain, vomiting, and pyrexia. **A.** A CT scan shows an abscess *(arrow)* in the area of the anastomosis. **B.** An enteroclysis film shows partial obstruction close to the anastomosis *(arrow)* with several tracks into the abscess beginning to opacify. **C.** A later enteroclysis film shows the tracks in the abscess well opacified and barium beginning to reach the colon. Note that barium has now outlined the duodenum, through a fistula (not identified). Fistulas to the duodenum from intestinal Crohn's disease do not cause duodenal Crohn's disease.

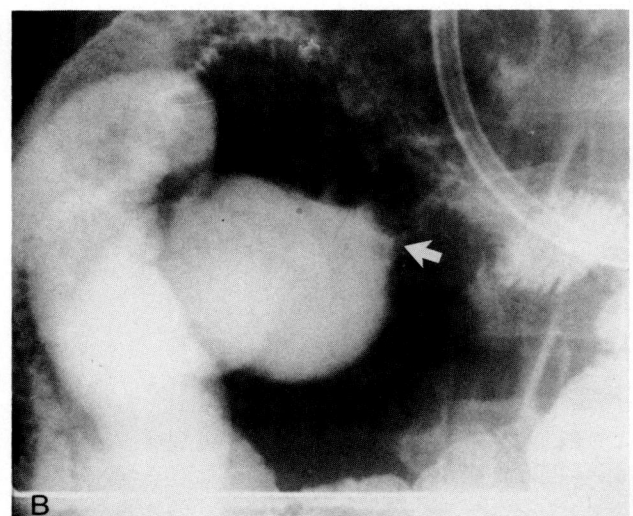

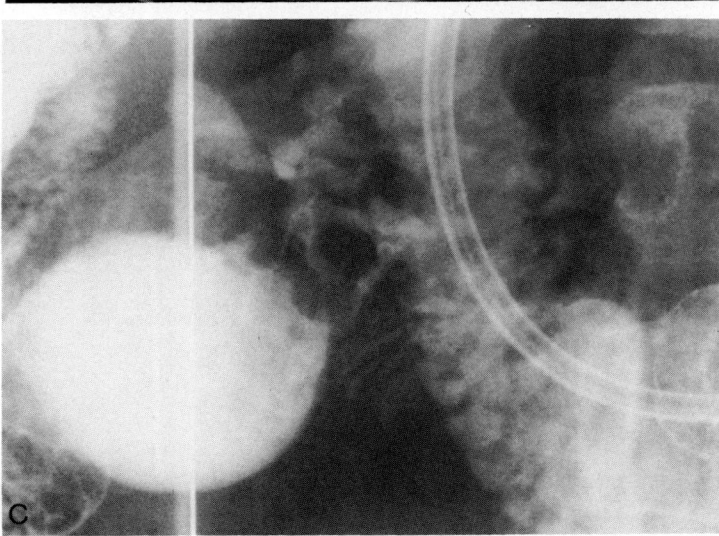

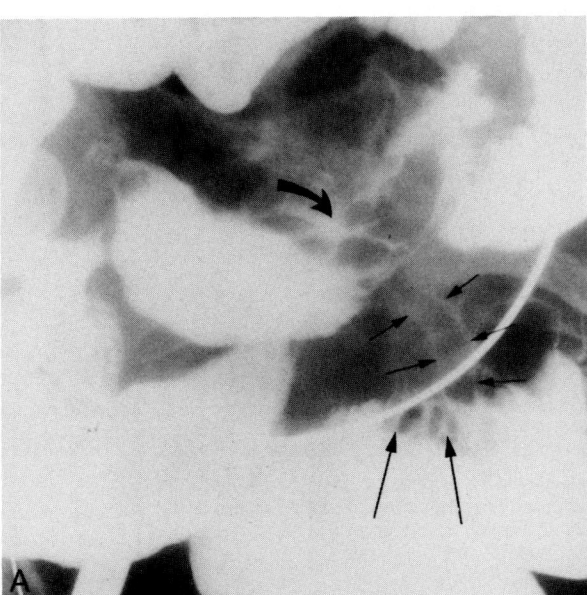

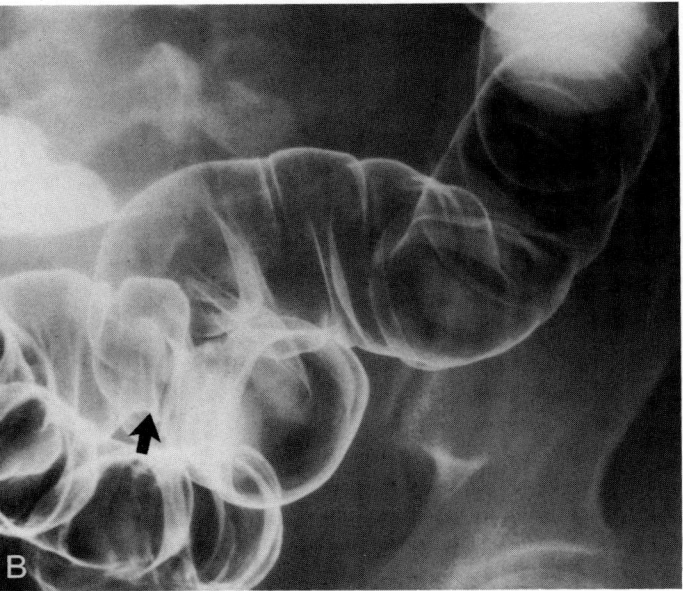

**Figure 47–28. Significance of ileosigmoid fistulas. A.** Two fistulous tracks *(short arrows)* extend from Crohn's diseased ileum *(curved arrow)* to a short segment of sigmoid colon in which thickened folds can be identified *(long arrows).* **B.** Double contrast barium enema done before surgery. The sigmoid colon shows no evidence of Crohn's disease, merely a short segment with slight fold thickening and limitation of distention *(arrow),* a nonspecific finding. Only rarely does Crohn's disease spread from the origin of a fistula to its termination site in the sigmoid colon.

841

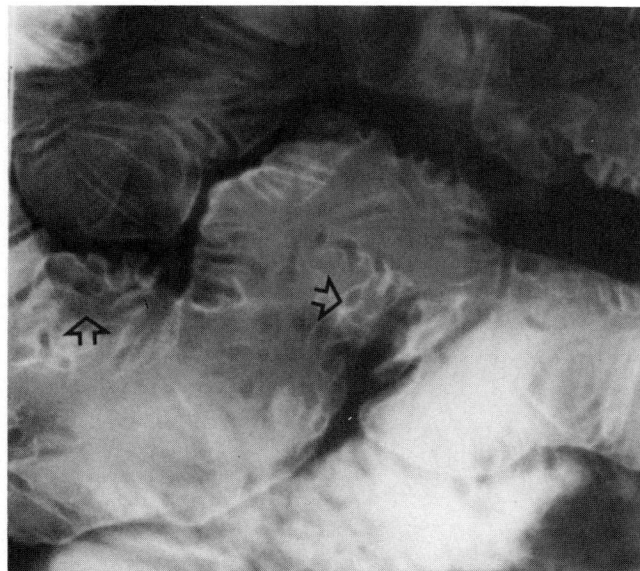

**Figure 47–29. Crohn's disease in remission.** Residual changes are distortion and interruption of folds and the rare presence of postinflammatory polyps of the filiform type *(arrows).*

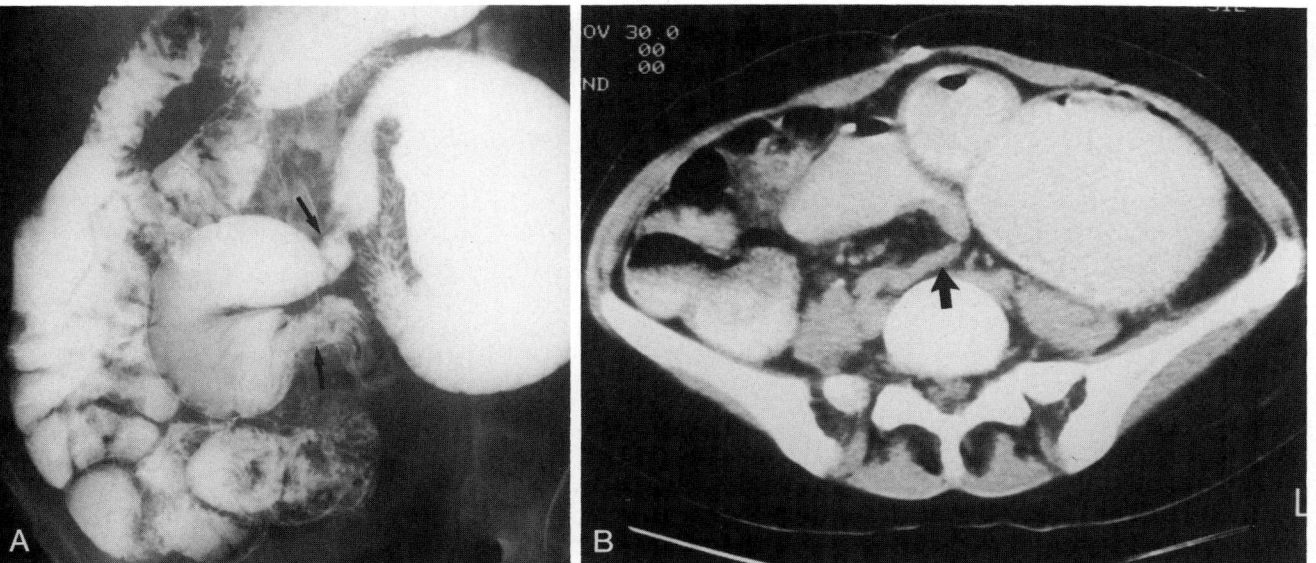

**Figure 47–30. Jejunoileitis.** An infrequent but usually aggressive subset of small bowel Crohn's disease has its location in the jejunum, often with an unaffected terminal ileum. **A.** Small bowel study shows segmental narrowing and ulceration *(arrows)* causing partial obstruction of two segments. **B.** CT scan depicts one of the strictures *(arrow)* causing obstruction.

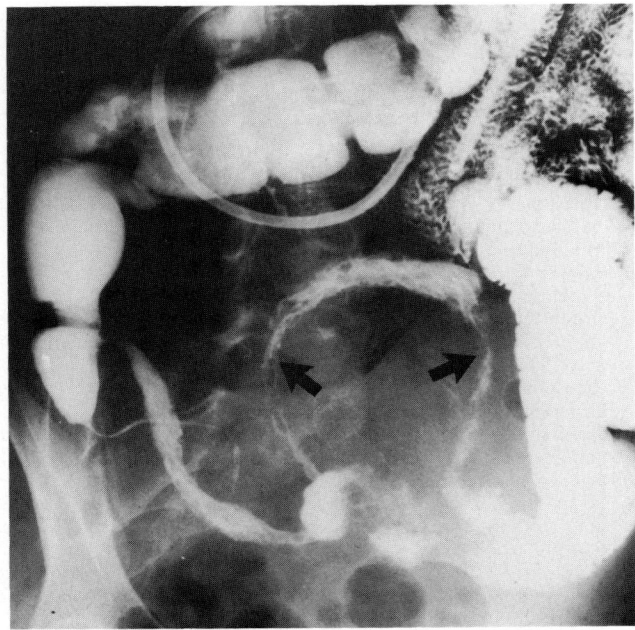

**Figure 47–31. Crohn's carcinoma.** This male patient with long-standing Crohn's disease came to small bowel resection because of obstruction *(arrows)*. Neither the radiologists nor the surgeons had suspected Crohn's cancer. Histology demonstrated multiple sites of primary carcinoma. (Courtesy of Alfeo Montesi, M.D., Ancona, Italy.)

is relatively rare and affected 5.9% of 676 patients with small bowel Crohn's disease reported in one study.[42] It is progressive and not responsive to treatment. Complications include obstruction (Fig. 47–30).

## CROHN'S CARCINOMA

An increased prevalence of carcinoma in patients with small bowel Crohn's disease is usually reported. A survey of patients with long-standing Crohn's disease from central Israel[43] suggested that no increased prevalence existed. Another report[44] considered Crohn's disease to be definitely premalignant. All, however, agreed that Crohn's cancers exhibit special features that are to the disadvantage of the patient.[45, 46] Younger persons are affected (average age 46 years), the distal ileum is the preferred site (76%), and areas of long-standing disease are more likely to be involved, rendering radiologic identification difficult. Surgically bypassed bowel was another likely site at which radiologic identification was difficult; this form of surgery is no longer performed. Fistulas may be sites at which carcinoma arises, and any bleeding from such fistulas should be suspect. A preoperative radiologic diagnosis is almost impossible because of the absence of characteristic features, and this is also the case at laparotomy[45] (Fig. 47–31). It is not surprising that Crohn's carcinoma has a dismal prognosis with survival from the time of diagnosis measured in months.[47]

## Acknowledgment

Figures 47–1 and 47–9 are reproduced with permission from Herlinger H, Maglinte D (eds): Clinical Radiology of the Small Bowel. Philadelphia: WB Saunders, 1989.

Figures 47–4 and 47–15 are reproduced with permission from Laufer I, Levine MS (eds): Double Contrast Gastrointestinal Radiology (2nd ed). Philadelphia: WB Saunders, 1992.

## References

1. Sandler RS, Golden AL: Epidemiology of Crohn's disease. J Clin Gastroenterol 8:160–165, 1986.
2. Mekhjian HS, Switz DM, Melnyk CS, et al: Clinical features and natural history of Crohn's disease. Gastroenterology 58:898–906, 1979.
3. Farmer RG, Hawk WA, Turnbull RB: Clinical patterns in Crohn's disease: a statistical study of 615 cases. Gastroenterology 68:627–635, 1975.
4. Dyer NH, Dawson AM: Diagnosis of Crohn's disease. A continuing source of error. Br Med J 1:735–737, 1970.
5. Ogorek CP, Caroline DF, Fisher RS: Presentation, evaluation, and natural history of inflammatory bowel disease. *In* MacDermott RP, Stenson WF (eds): Inflammatory Bowel Disease. New York: Elsevier, 1992.
6. Goldberg HI, Caruthers SB, Nelson JA, et al: Radiographic findings of the National Cooperative Crohn's Disease Study. Gastroenterology 77:925–937, 1979.
7. Ekberg O: Crohn's disease of the small bowel examined by double contrast technique: a comparison with oral technique. Gastrointest Radiol 1:355–359, 1977.
8. Vallance R: An evaluation of the small bowel enema based on an analysis of 350 consecutive examinations. Clin Radiol 31:227–332, 1980.
9. Maglinte DDT, Chernish SM, Kelvin FM, et al: Crohn disease of the small intestine: accuracy and relevance of enteroclysis. Radiology 184:1–6, 1992.
10. Glick SN: Crohn's disease of the small intestine. Radiol Clin North Am 25:25–45, 1987.
11. Hywel-Jones J, Lennard-Jones JE, Young AC: Reversibility of radiological appearances during clinical improvement in colonic Crohn's disease. Gut 10:738–743, 1969.
12. Engelholm L, DeToeuf MD, Herlinger H, et al: Crohn's disease of the small bowel. *In* Herlinger H, Maglinte D (eds): Clinical Radiology of the Small Intestine. Philadelphia: WB Saunders, 1989, pp 295–334.
13. Rubesin SE, Bronner M: Radiologic-pathologic concepts in Crohn's disease. Adv Gastrointest Radiol 1:27–55, 1991.
14. Ekberg O, Lindstrom C: Superficial lesions in Crohn's disease of the small bowel. Gastrointest Radiol 4:389–393, 1979.
15. Engelholm L, Mainguet P, Potuliege P: Radiology in early Crohn's disease of the small intestine. *In* The Management of Crohn's Disease. Leiden: Excerpta Medica, 1976, p 73.
16. Dvorak AM, Connell AB, Dickers GR: Crohn's disease: a scanning electron microscopic study. Hum Pathol 10:165–177, 1979.
17. Glick SN, Teplick SK: Crohn's disease of the small intestine: diffuse mucosal granularity. Radiology 154:313–317, 1985.
18. Jones B, Hamilton SR, Rubesin SE, et al: Granular small bowel mucosa: a reflection of villous abnormality. Gastrointest Radiol 12:219–225, 1987.
19. Nolan DJ, Gourtsoyannis NC: Crohn's disease of the small intestine: a review of the radiological appearances in 100 consecutive patients examined by a barium infusion technique. Gastrointest Radiol 31:597–603, 1980.
20. Marshak RH, Wolf BS: Roentgen findings in regional enteritis. AJR 74:1000–1014, 1955.
21. Engelholm L, De Toeuf J, Peeters JP: Maladie de Crohn du grêle et du colon. *In* Traité de Radiodiagnostic, Tome VI, Urgences Abdominales. Grêle, Colon. Paris: Masson, 1982, pp 333–383.

22. Carlson HC: Perspective: the small bowel examination in the diagnosis of Crohn's disease. AJR 147:63–65, 1986.
23. Hildell J, Lindstrom C, Wenckert A: Radiographic appearance in Crohn's disease. I. Accuracy of radiographic methods. Acta Radiol Diagn 20:609–625, 1979.
24. Buck JL, Dachman AH, Sobin LH: Polypoid and pseudopolypoid manifestations of inflammatory bowel disease. Radiographics 11:293–304, 1991.
25. Nolan DJ, Piris J: Crohn's disease of the small intestine: a comparative study of the radiological and pathological appearances. Clin Radiol 31:591–596, 1980.
26. Whitehead R: Mucosal Biopsy of the Gastrointestinal Tract. Philadelphia: WB Saunders, 1985, pp 227–233.
27. Herlinger H: The small bowel enema and the diagnosis of Crohn's disease. Radiol Clin North Am 20:721–742, 1982.
28. Nolan DJ: Radiology of Crohn's disease of the small intestine. A review. J R Soc Med 74:294–300, 1981.
29. Dehn TC, Kettlewell MG, Mortensen NJ, et al: Ten-year experience of strictureplasty for obstructive Crohn's disease. Br J Surg 70:338–341, 1989.
30. Rutgeers P, Gegoes K, Vantrappen G, et al: Predictability of the postoperative course of Crohn's disease. Gastroenterology 99:956–963, 1990.
31. Herlinger H, O'Riordan D, Saul S, et al: Nonspecific involvement of bowel adjoining Crohn's disease. Radiology 159:47–51, 1986.
32. Fishman EK, Wolf EJ, Jones B, et al: CT evaluation of Crohn's disease: effect on patient management. AJR 148:537–540, 1987.
33. Ribeiro MB, Greenstein AJ, Yamazaki Y, et al: Intra-abdominal abscess in regional enteritis. Ann Surg 213:32–36, 1991.
34. Casola G, vanSonnenberg E, Neff CC, et al: Abscesses in Crohn disease: percutaneous drainage. Radiology 163:19–22, 1987.
35. Steinberg DM, Cooke WT, Alexander-Williams J: Abscess and fistula in Crohn's disease. Gut 14:865–869, 1973.
36. Brahme F: Roentgenology of Crohn's disease. *In* Regional Enteritis. International Symposium. Stockholm: Nordiska Bokhandeln, 1971, p 81.
37. Rutgeers P, Ghoos Y, Vantrappen G, et al: Ileal dysfunction and bacterial overgrowth in patients with Crohn's disease. Eur J Clin Invest 11:199–206, 1981.
38. Amendola MA, Agha FP, Dent TL, et al: Detection of occult colovesical fistula by the Bourne test. AJR 142:715–717, 1984.
39. Korelitz BI: The ileorectal and ileosigmoidal fistula in Crohn's disease: a clinical radiological correlation. Mt Sinai J Med 51:341–346, 1984.
40. Ferraro V, Hunt PS: Perforation in Crohn's disease of the small bowel. Med J Aust 140:101–102, 1984.
41. Greenstein AJ, Mann D, Sachar DB, et al: Free perforation in Crohn's disease. A survey of 99 cases. Am J Gastroenterol 80:682–689, 1985.
42. Crohn BB, Yarnis H: Regional Enteritis (2nd ed). New York: Grune & Stratton, 1958.
43. Fireman Z, Grossman A, Lilos P, et al: Intestinal cancer in patients with Crohn's disease. A population study in central Israel. Scand J Gastroenterol 24:346–350, 1989.
44. Senay E, Sachar DB, Keohane M, et al: Small bowel carcinoma in Crohn's disease. Distinguishing features and risk factors. Cancer 63:360–363, 1989.
45. Moesgaard F, Knudsen JT, Christensen N: Adenocarcinoma of the small intestine associated with Crohn's disease. Acta Chir Scand 145:577–580, 1979.
46. Fell J, Snooks S: Small bowel adenocarcinoma in patients with Crohn's disease. J R Soc Med 80:51–52, 1987.
47. Hawker PC, Gyde SN, Thompson H, et al: Adenocarcinoma of the small intestine complicating Crohn's disease. Gut 23:188–193, 1982.

# Infections and Other Inflammatory Conditions

Olle Ekberg, M.D.

Bronwyn Jones, M.D.

Hans Herlinger, M.D.

## INTRODUCTION

Parasitic and a number of other infectious diseases of the small bowel are endemic in developing parts of the world, where they constitute a major health problem. Because of the enormous increase in international travel, these diseases are now more commonly encountered in developed countries. The growing number of immunodeficient patients in most parts of the world also contributes to the high incidence of enteric infections. Most of the conditions described in this chapter present a fairly nonspecific radiologic appearance. In addition, other diseases, such as Crohn's disease, lymphoma, or amyloidosis, may enter into the radiologic differential diagnostic consideration. In consequence, the clinical setting and the clinical findings for each such patient become important assets when attempting a radiologic differential diagnosis.

## PARASITIC INFESTATIONS

### Ascariasis

*Ascaris lumbricoides* is the largest nematode found in the human intestine and infests more than a quarter of the world's population. Local prevalence may reach 90%.[1] Infection occurs after ingestion of embryonated eggs. The larvae emerge in the duodenum, penetrate the intestinal mucosa, and enter the portal venous system. Through the liver they pass into the lungs, where they undergo further development. A pulmonary hypersensitivity reaction can ensue with bronchospasm and bronchiolitis. Löffler's syndrome—pulmonary infiltration and eosiniophilia—is a frequent clinical manifestation. Larvae may be found in the sputum at this stage. The larvae then migrate to the pharynx and are swallowed. They become adult worms after reaching the small intestine.

Only minimal tissue reaction occurs when the larvae penetrate the bowel wall. A large worm load may be associated with nutritional deficiencies, especially in children and patients with borderline nutritional status. Occasionally, larvae may perforate the bowel, causing peritonitis. In large numbers they may cause intestinal obstruction. They may migrate into other areas and cause jaundice, pancreatitis, and appendicitis. The more usual symptoms are vague abdominal discomfort, colicky pain, and occasionally diarrhea. Patients may have mild eosinophilia. The diagnosis is based on finding eggs, adult worms, or larvae in the stool.

If present in large numbers, ascarids can be recognized

845

on plain films of the abdomen, usually as longitudinal soft tissue densities outlined by a seam of gas (Fig. 48–1A). A larger bolus of coiled parasites may create a so-called whirlpool effect, often near the ileocecal valve, where obstruction is most likely to occur. Worms may also be seen in the colon. Edema of the intestinal mucosa may also be evident on plain films. On barium examination the worms cause a distinct filling defect that may be up to 35 cm in length (Fig. 48–1B). The identification of an ascaris may be further confirmed by seeing the worm's intestinal tract filled with ingested barium.

## Hookworm Infestation (Ancylostomiasis)

Intestinal hookworm disease in humans is caused by *Ancylostoma duodenale* and *Necator americanus.* Filiform larvae penetrate the skin, usually of the feet, enter venules, and reach the lungs. Pulmonary abnormalities may become evident. The larvae emerge from alveolar capillaries and reach the small bowel after tracheopharyngeal passage. They anchor themselves to the intestinal mucosa and mature. Hookworms secrete an anticoagulant substance that facilitates outflow of blood. Continuous or intermittent suction by each of the many worms and bleeding from the sites of their attachment can cause significant blood loss.[2] Infestation is second in world prevalence after ascariasis. Epigastric discomfort

and tenderness occur when the infection is significant and may mimic peptic ulcer disease. Mild to moderate anemia is common. A mild malabsorption state may occur with a large hookworm load.[3] Eosinophilia and hypoalbuminemia are usually found.

Diagnosis requires the identification of hookworm eggs in the feces. Adult worms are far too small to be seen radiologically. Nonspecific radiographic findings include thickening of the mucosal folds, flocculation of barium, and hypermotility of the duodenum and proximal jejunum.

## Tapeworm (Cestode) Infestation

The cestodes are relatively long, segmented intestinal flatworms. Human infection results from ingestion of larvae that live in the flesh of intermediate hosts.[4] *Diphyllobothrium latum,* the fish tapeworm, is commonly found in northern Europe, northern parts of North America, and Asia. Infection may result from eating raw or inadequately cooked fish. Larvae invade the ileum and may cause vitamin $B_{12}$ deficiency. However, most infected persons remain asymptomatic. *Taenia solium,* the pork tapeworm, is ingested in larval form with inadequately cooked meat. The adult worm inhabits the small intestine, where it remains solitary or lives in small numbers. There may be only a few minor symptoms. Diagnosis requires the identification of ova or proglottids (segments) in the stool. A more serious

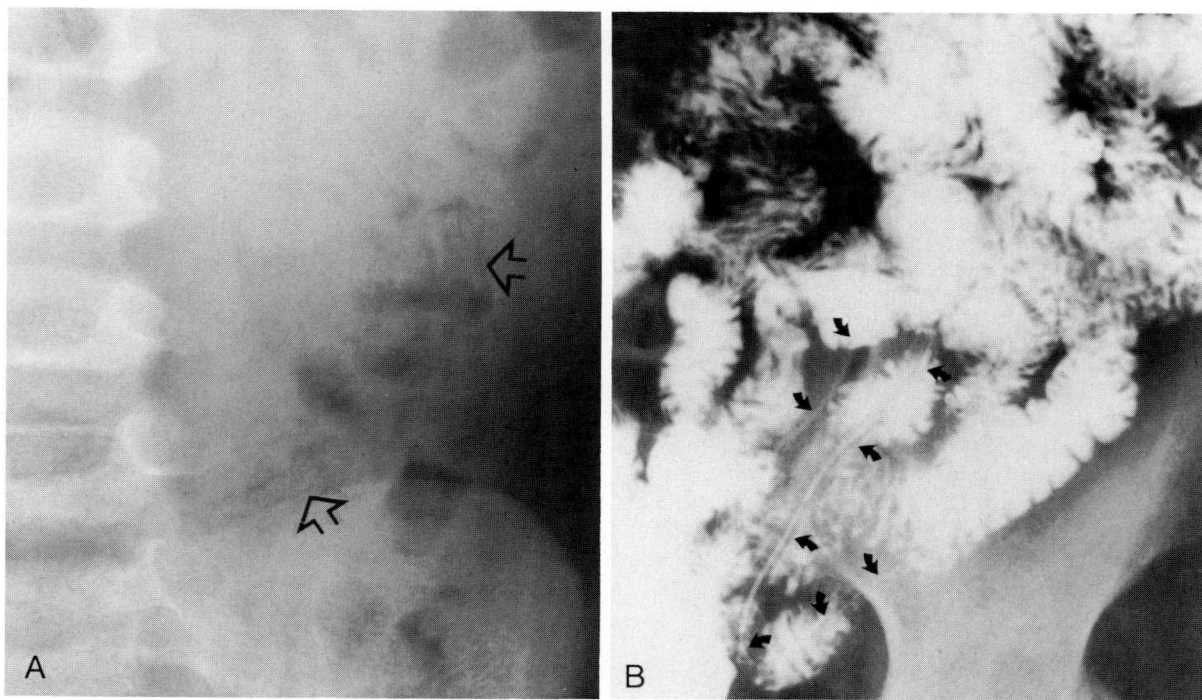

**Figure 48–1. Ascariasis. A**. Plain abdominal film of a child. Longitudinal worm structures are faintly outlined by a seam of air within the transverse colon *(arrows)*. **B**. Barium study. A single ascaris, about 25 cm long, is outlined against surrounding barium and characterized by a thin line of barium within its digestive tract *(arrows)*. (Courtesy of Erich E. Eidenschwank, M.D., New York, NY.)

clinical condition follows the ingestion of the ova of *T. solium.* This can result in cysticercosis with symptoms that result from the invasion of skeletal muscle, brain, and other tissues. *Taenia saginata,* the beef tapeworm, is much larger than *T. solium* and may reach a length of 15 ft. Symptoms may include small bowel obstruction and the effects of toxic metabolites released by the worm. However, most persons remain asymptomatic.

The adult forms of both taeniae may cause mild irritation of the intestinal mucosa near the points of their attachment, and this may be radiologically evident as slight thickening of mucosal folds. In small bowel barium studies and in barium enemas, the worm may be apparent as a long, thin translucent filling defect extending over a considerable length of the intestine. Cysticercosis is revealed by typical calcifications in muscle and brain.

## Strongyloidiasis

*Strongyloides stercoralis* is commonly found in the warm and moist soil of the tropics. The larvae enter through the skin and migrate via the venous system to the lungs. They penetrate alveoli and migrate to the small bowel. Only female parasites invade the superficial part of the mucosa of the duodenum and jejunum. Their ova pass into the bowel lumen, where rhabdoid larvae rapidly emerge. In most circumstances, these larvae are evacuated with the stool and change into infective filariform larvae if deposited in warm, moist soil. Those with light infestation may remain asymptomatic. Autoinfection occurs if the filariform larval stage is reached within the bowel lumen or on the perianal skin; in this way the infestation can persist for as long as 65 years.[5] Immunodeficiency states enhance the rate of change to the filariform larval state within the gut and can result in life-threatening hyperinfection.[6]

Small bowel barium examinations may show increased or decreased motility, narrowing, or dilatation of the lumen. Ulcerations can be seen. Effacement of mucosal folds is usual, producing a "pipe stem" appearance[7] of the proximal bowel (Fig. 48–2). Dilatation of the duodenum has been reported.

## Giardiasis

*Giardia lamblia,* a protozoan intestinal flagellate, is a frequent cause of travelers' diarrhea. It is endemic in many parts of the world. Particularly high infestation rates occur in travelers to Russia, especially St. Petersburg. In the United States, it is the intestinal pathogen most frequently responsible for outbreaks of waterborne diarrheal illnesses. Infection is acquired by ingesting cysts in drinking water contaminated by feces from humans or animals susceptible to *G. lamblia.* Cysts of *G. lamblia* are hardy, and ingestion of a relatively small number causes infection, especially in institutions for the elderly.[7] A lectin on the surface of trophozoites (free-living stage) in the bowel lumen may bind to a

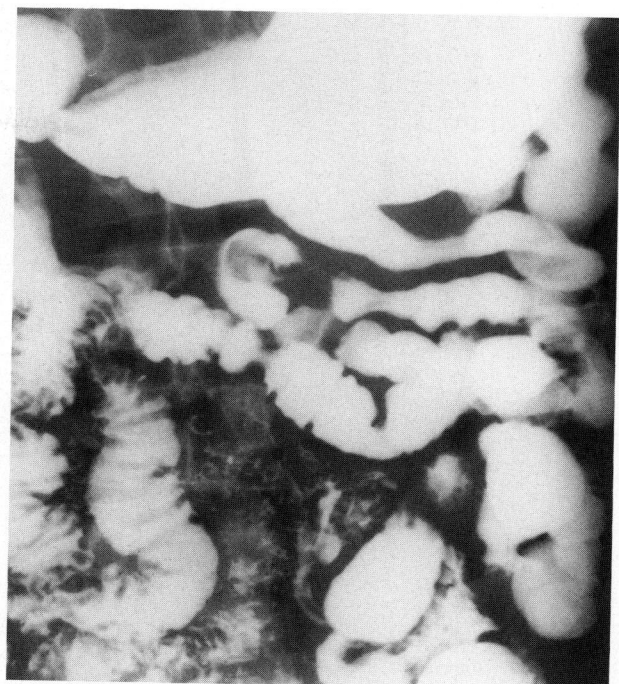

**Figure 48–2. Strongyloidiasis.** The proximal segments of jejunum are slightly narrowed and either featureless or with thickened folds. (Courtesy of Jack Farman, M.D., New York.)

receptor on the brush border of epithelial cells. Injury to the bowel wall is believed to be mediated through cytotoxic T cells.[8] The antibody response that occurs in patients infected with *Giardia* can be used diagnostically. Secretory immunoglobulins are particularly important for control of this mostly intraluminal parasite. There is a relationship between increased immunoglobulin A secretion and clearance and between immunoglobulin A absence and continuing infection.[9]

*Giardia* infection may present as asymptomatic cyst passage, as an acute self-limited diarrhea, or as a chronic state of diarrhea, malabsorption, and weight loss. Lactase deficiency may develop in some patients, and the effects of lactose intolerance may be confused with relapse or reinfection. There is an association between giardiasis and dysgammaglobulinemia and also with isolated immunoglobulin A deficiency.

Duodenal mucosal biopsy or duodenal aspirates provide a more reliable diagnosis of giardiasis. However, examination of stool for ova and trophozoites tends to be the more usual but less productive first method of investigation. Eosinophilia is absent. Radiographic findings are nonspecific, although they can suggest the diagnosis in the right clinical setting. Duodenal and jejunal folds are irregularly thickened and there is hypermotility[10] (Fig. 48–3). These changes are due to widespread infiltration by inflammatory cells and edema. This may be pronounced enough to cause the lumen to be narrowed. Increased secretions are usually found in the duodenum and jejunum. The ileum is normal in appearance.

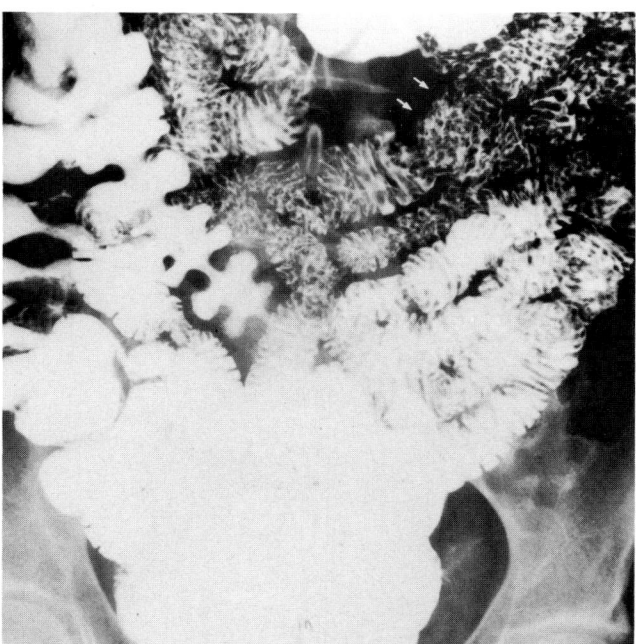

**Figure 48–3. Giardiasis.** The duodenal and jejunal folds are thickened, irregular, and distorted *(arrows)*. There was increased peristalsis. Similar changes were found in the duodenum.

## Coccidiosis

*Isospora belli.* Nearly every domestic or wild animal can carry these parasites. Poultry and especially newborn calves are often infected and may transmit infection to humans. Sporozoites enter the mucosa of the upper small intestine and produce a usually self-limited, mild diarrheal illness. The disease assumes much greater significance when it occurs in patients with disordered immune function, especially those with acquired immunodeficiency syndrome (AIDS).

*Cryptosporidium.* The organisms affect the upper small intestine without penetrating the mucosa. A mild, self-limited diarrheal disease has been described in immunologically competent persons. In the majority of instances, however, cryptosporidia cause opportunistic infections in immunodeficient patients. Diarrhea is then profuse and life threatening. Cryptosporidiosis and isosporiasis are discussed in greater detail later in this chapter and in Chapter 160.

## Anisakiasis

Nematodes of the *Anisakis* genera inhabit the intestinal tracts of marine mammals and piscivorous birds. Eggs are passed in the feces and hatch in the sea. Larvae enter into the marine food chain, are distributed widely, and are ingested by fish such as herring, cod, and salmon. Although they normally reside in the intestine of fish, *Anisakis* larvae migrate into muscle if fish are not filleted promptly after capture. Humans are infected by eating raw or insufficiently cooked contaminated fish or squid.[11] Symptoms of anisakiasis occur when larvae enter the wall of the stomach or intestine. In humans, potentially the final hosts, the development of *Anisakis* is arrested in the fourth larval stage. The 2- to 3.5-cm larvae have been identified—and removed—during gastric endoscopy. The disease is prevalent especially in Japan and The Netherlands but has been encountered in California and Alaska.

Several types of lesions can be produced by *Anisakis* larvae that have burrowed into the wall of the intestine. Ulcers, abscesses, eosinophilic granulomas, and perforations are possible findings. Abdominal pain and pyrexia are among the clinical presentations. Radiologic changes can be pronounced. They include bowel wall thickening, mucosal edema, narrowing of the lumen, and ulceration (Fig. 48–4). In the terminal ileum, there

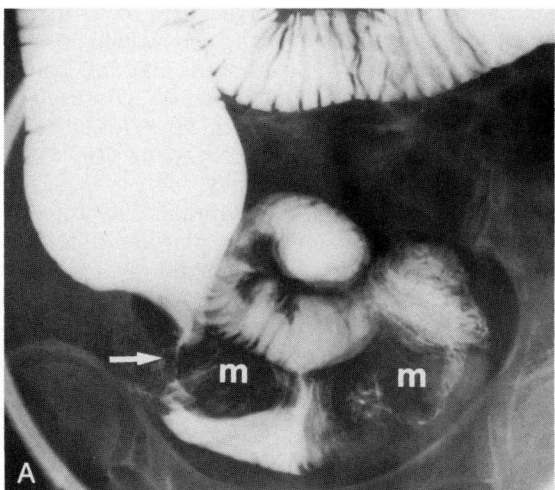
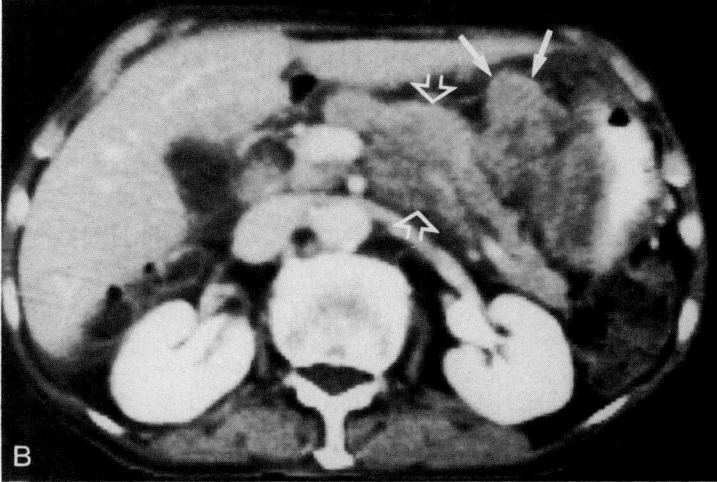

**Figure 48–4. Anisakiasis. A.** Small bowel enema. Marked obstruction of a loop of ileum in the pelvis is due to narrowing caused by fibrotic thickening of the wall *(arrow)*. There is also a mass effect (m) when compression is applied. **B.** A computed tomographic scan demonstrates a large extramural mass extending anteriorly *(solid arrows)*. There is also a mass in the pancreas *(open arrows)*.

may be nodular edema and features of lymph node enlargement. The worm may occasionally be seen as a filling defect on barium studies.[11]

## *Trypanosoma cruzi* Infection

Infection with the South American parasite *Trypanosoma cruzi* can lead to Chagas' disease. The trypanosome is capable of destroying ganglion cells throughout the body and is a well-known cause of achalasia of the esophagus. A similar syndrome is based on autonomic denervation and neuron loss in the small bowel and colon, and affected individuals may present with pseudo-obstruction, abdominal distention, and pain.[12]

Radiologic findings include dilated small bowel loops with transit delay. Methacholine administration produces hyperperistalsis, indicating increased sensitivity to cholinergic agonists, a result of the denervation.

## BACTERIAL INFECTIONS

### Tuberculosis

Intestinal tuberculosis continues to be a major health problem in many underdeveloped countries. In the same areas, Crohn's disease is rarely diagnosed. The previously frequent association between pulmonary and intestinal tuberculosis no longer prevails, and only a minority of patients with abdominal tuberculosis now have an abnormal chest film.[13]

The ileocecal area is the site most commonly involved. Gross pathologic changes can be classified as ulcerative (60%), hypertrophic (10%), or ulcerohypertrophic (30%). Transmural fibrosis, stenosis, and fistulas are

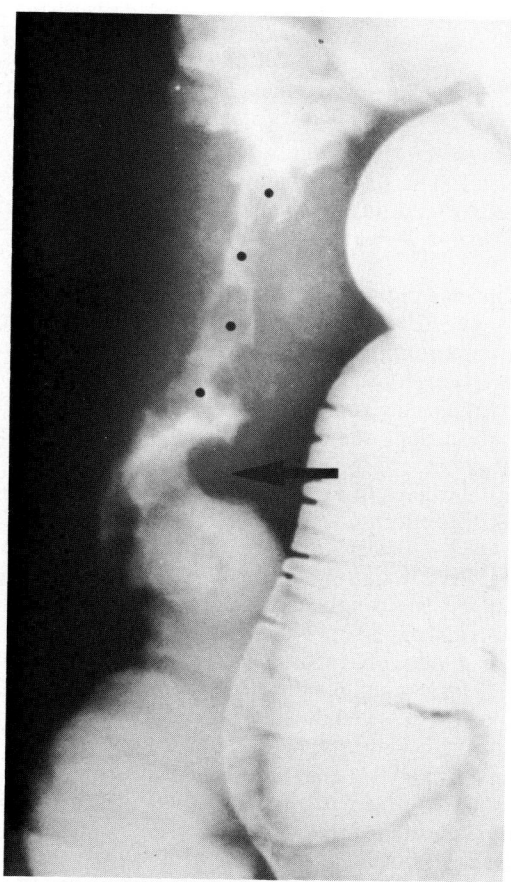

Figure 48–6. Ileocecal tuberculosis in a male patient with a long history of the disease. Active, ulcerating disease is seen in the ascending colon *(dots)*. The cecum cannot be identified. The terminal ileum and the gaping ileocecal valve *(arrow)* are in direct continuation with the ascending colon.

common findings. Patients complain predominantly of abdominal pain, weight loss, and fever. Diarrhea and anal lesions are rare.

A definitive diagnosis should be made before antituberculous treatment is begun. This usually requires obtaining tissue and identifying the organism by culture. X-ray changes merely suggest the diagnosis. Early changes include nodular thickening of mucosal folds, which may become distorted and later effaced. The cecum tends to be more severely involved than the terminal ileum (Fig. 48–5). Ulcerations typically extend transaxially and heal with the formation of short annular strictures.[14] Involvement of the ileocecal area characteristically leads to pronounced shrinkage of the cecum (Fig. 48–6), at times with loss of the ileocecal angle and a widely patent ileocecal valve. In contrast, in Crohn's disease longitudinal ulcers predominate; the terminal ileum tends to be more severely affected than the cecum and the ulceronodular, or "cobblestone," pattern is a characteristic finding.

## Yersiniosis

*Yersinia enterocolitica* is a gram-negative rod with prevalence in Scandinavian and other northern Euro-

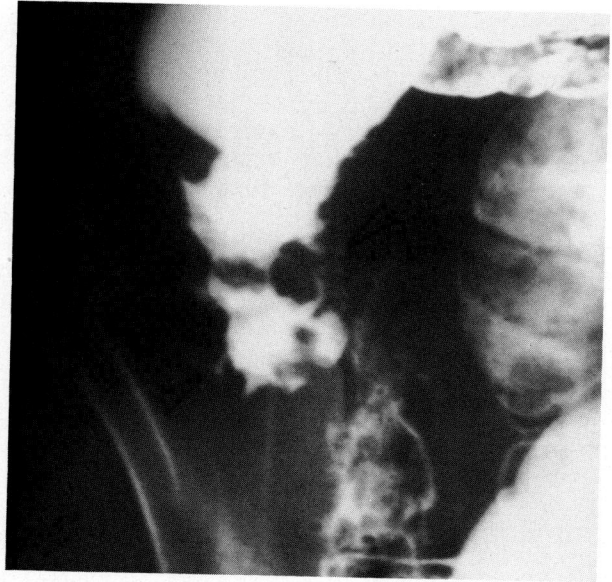

Figure 48–5. Ileocecal tuberculosis in an adult female patient. Nodular thickening of folds is more pronounced in the cecum than in the terminal ileum. (Courtesy of P. Shah, M.D., and R. Ramakantan, M.D., Bombay, India.)

pean countries. Epidemics have been caused by ingestion of contaminated dairy products. In the United States, the incidence of yersiniosis appears to be increasing. Transmission of the disease is chiefly by the fecal-oral route. Persons between the ages of 5 and 20 years are predominantly affected. The disease tends to be self-limited. The organisms invade the epithelium of the ileum and ascending colon, causing small focal ulcerations associated with enlargement of regional lymph tissue.

Abdominal pain, the most frequent symptom, is typically localized to the right lower quadrant and mimics that in appendicitis. At laparotomy the terminal ileum may be edematous and reddened with heaped-up mesenteric fat, while the appendix is normal. The clinical presentation depends on the patient's age. Children and teen-agers are more likely to present with an acute terminal ileitis. Other patients have a more insidious onset, with abdominal pain, diarrhea, and fever for 1 to 2 weeks. The bacteria can be isolated from the feces in the majority of patients. Positive serologic test results also confirm the diagnosis.[15]

Numerous case reports have described arthritides—septic or reactive—in association with *Yersinia* enteritis.[16] *Yersinia*-specific immune complexes have been found in the synovial fluid of patients with reactive arthritis.[17] In patients with an iron overload, a more virulent form of *Y. enterocolitica* septicemia occurs and may be associated with liver abscesses and pronounced mesenteric adenopathy.[18]

Radiologic findings are mostly limited to the terminal ileum, where thickened mucosal folds, nodules, and aphthous ulcers are seen (Fig. 48–7). Lumen narrowing is not part of this pattern. These changes are most pronounced during the first 2 weeks and then subside. Resolution is usually observed within 5 to 8 weeks. It should be noted that the radiologic changes outlast the resolution of symptoms. The radiologic distinction, particularly in the terminal ileum, between Crohn's disease and yersiniosis is important. Transmural Crohn's disease tends to cause lumen narrowing, which would be unusual for yersiniosis. Crohn's disease is characterized by deeper, often transmural ulcerations, whereas ulcerations in *Yersinia* ileitis remain superficial.[19] The cobblestone appearance in Crohn's disease is due to deep fissuring, whereas a somewhat similar nodular pattern in yersiniosis is caused by enlarged lymphoid tissues bulging into the lumen and trapping barium. Transmural Crohn's disease of the terminal ileum does not resolve entirely, but resolution always occurs in *Yersinia* ileitis.

## Nontyphoidal Salmonellosis

Community outbreaks of enteric infection are common and are caused by consumption of infected poultry, meats, eggs, and dairy products. In the United States, 25 to 40% of such outbreaks are caused by nontyphoidal *Salmonella*. In the northeastern United States there was an almost 10-fold increase in infections with *Salmonella enteritidis* during the 1980s, possibly related to methods used in the mass production of eggs.[20]

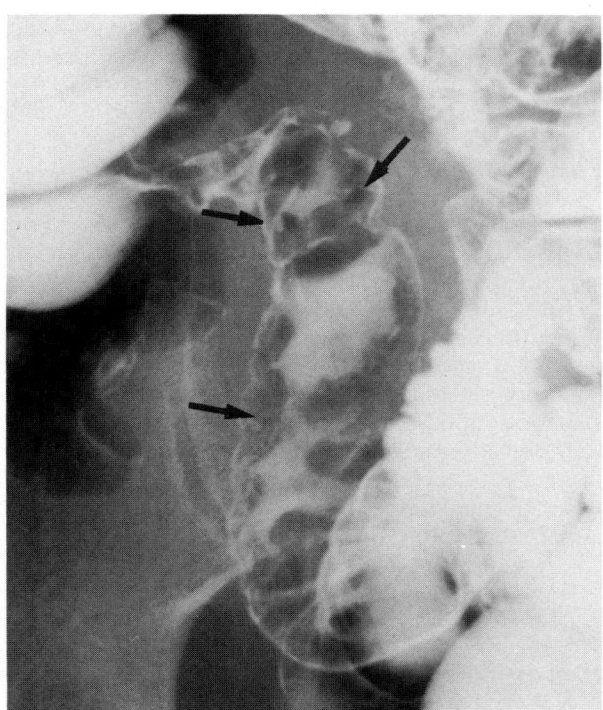

**Figure 48–7. Yersiniosis.** Mucosal folds in the terminal ileum are largely replaced by enlarged lymphatic nodules that appear as multiple submucosal masses. Superficial ulcerations *(arrows)* are also present.

The gram-negative bacteria cause mild mucosal ulcerations in the small bowel, reach the lamina propria, may cause patchy inflammation in the submucosa, and involve draining mesenteric lymph nodes. The bacteria seem to produce a secretory factor, which may be responsible for the diarrhea with its increased fluid and electrolyte secretion into the bowel lumen. Occasionally, nontyphoidal *Salmonella* causes more extensive lesions and gives rise to an intense colitis with small hemorrhages, ulcerations, and microabscesses.

The incubation period has been reported to vary between 6 and 72 hours.[7] The presenting clinical features are diarrhea, fever, and muscle pain.[21] The diarrhea usually resolves after 3 to 4 days. Patients with malignancies, immunodeficiency, and other debilitating states tend to suffer a more severe illness with progressive salmonellosis and bacteremia.[22] A chronic carrier state develops in a small minority of patients.

Plain film radiographs may show signs of enteritis, moderately distended small bowel loops with air-fluid levels. Barium studies may show shallow ulceration in the distal ileum and colon. This self-limited disease is normally diagnosed by stool culture without recourse to barium radiology. Isolation of the bacteria from blood is possible in less than 10% of cases.

## Campylobacteriosis

Another form of infectious diarrhea is caused by *Campylobacter fetus* or *Campylobacter jejuni*. In one study, *Campylobacter* was the most frequent cause of bacterial diarrhea. The most common route of transmission appears to be from infected farm animals and their food products.[23] *Campylobacter* has also been isolated from fresh water and from the sea. Diarrhea, which may be bloody, fever, and abdominal pain are the usual presenting symptoms. Symptoms may last 2 weeks, occasionally longer. A chronic form of infection, often with bacteremia, is a frequent finding in immunocompromised patients, such as those with AIDS.

White blood cells are usually found in stool specimens. The most reliable diagnosis of *Campylobacter* enteritis is by stool culture. Radiographic findings are usually confined to the distal ileum and colon. There is usually marked thickening of the bowel wall associated with irregularity, spiculation, and nodularity.[23, 24] Nodular lymphoid hyperplasia may also be found.

## Histoplasmosis

Histoplasmosis is usually a self-limited pulmonary disease caused by the fungus *Histoplasma capsulatum*. Rarely, the gastrointestinal tract becomes part of a disseminated infection. In such a case, the lamina propria of the small bowel has been reported to contain a large number of *Histoplasma*-laden macrophages. Extension of the lamina propria into villi causes villous enlargement and a radiologic appearance of micronodularity of the mucosa.[25, 26] Radiologic findings resemble those in Whipple's disease.

## VIRAL INFECTIONS

### Cytomegalovirus Infections

Infection resulting from tissue penetration by cytomegalovirus (CMV) is virtually confined to immunodeficient or immunosuppressed patients and is described later in this chapter and in Chapter 160.

### Other Viral Infections

Rotavirus is a segmented RNA virus and is a major cause of severe gastroenteritis in young children.

Enteric adenovirus is second to rotavirus as a cause of gastroenteritis in children younger than the age of 2 years. The illness is generally less severe but tends to last longer than that caused by rotavirus.

Norwalk virus has been obtained from stool in purified form and its structure has been studied. However, it has not been possible to culture it or transmit it to animals. This virus affects older children and adults and has been a cause of outbreaks of gastroenteritis in 40% of members of community groups.[27] Infection is by the fecal-oral route, with an incubation period of 12 to 48 hours. The proximal small intestine is the site of histopathologic lesions.[28] No description of radiologic findings has been reported, nor would radiology be likely to further the diagnosis.

## OTHER INFLAMMATORY DISORDERS

### Nonspecific Ulcers and Stenoses

Known causes of isolated small intestinal ulceration include tuberculosis, potassium chloride tablets, Crohn's disease, Behçet's syndrome, celiac sprue, heterotopic gastric mucosa, previous irradiation, ischemia (including emboli without infarction), vasculitis, trauma, jejunal ulcers in gastrinoma, and arsenic poisoning.[29] Enteric coated potassium chloride, formerly the most frequent cause of isolated small bowel ulcers, is no longer in use, and such ulcers have become rare findings. Rarer still are ulcers that do not fit into any of the foregoing categories, the nonspecific or idiopathic ulcers.

There have been reports of intestinal ulceration, hemorrhage, and even perforation in patients taking nonsteroidal anti-inflammatory drugs, especially indomethacin.[30] This large group of drugs, which includes ibuprofen, is used by millions of people worldwide. Ulceration is believed to be due to depression of prostaglandin synthase. Increased intestinal permeability and small bowel inflammation seem to be associated with prolonged use of nonsteroidal anti-inflammatory drugs, especially if the recommended dose is exceeded. In addition to ulceration, there have been rare instances of obstruction by multiple, short, diaphragm-like strictures, mostly in the distal ileum, not readily shown by barium studies.[31]

Idiopathic ulcers may be single or multiple and may be followed by or associated with stenosis. Some patients have chronic abdominal pain, nausea, and vomiting; others are asymptomatic. The ulcers may be millimeter sized or larger. They are sometimes difficult to identify because there is usually no surrounding inflammatory change. Radiologic features include a short narrowed segment with sharp demarcation to normal bowel (Fig. 48–8). The appearance of the stenosis differs from that associated with many secondary ulcers, such as the stenoses in Crohn's disease and vasculitis, which characteristically have tapered edges and signs of adjacent small bowel edema or infiltration. Multiple ulcers complicating adult celiac disease (chronic stage of ulcerative jejunoileitis) may heal with the formation of short strictures.

### Extrinsic Inflammation

Any inflammatory process in the abdomen may involve adjacent loops of small bowel. Especially prone to do so are periappendiceal and tubo-ovarian abscesses. Peridiverticulitis of sigmoid or other colonic origin can also involve the small bowel.[32] With extensive involvement of small bowel, especially if there is also vascular compromise, symptoms tend to be of increased severity with diarrhea and/or hemorrhage.

Radiologic features include an extrinsic mass effect with displacement and deformity of small bowel loops (Figs. 48–9 and 48–10). Along the concave aspect of

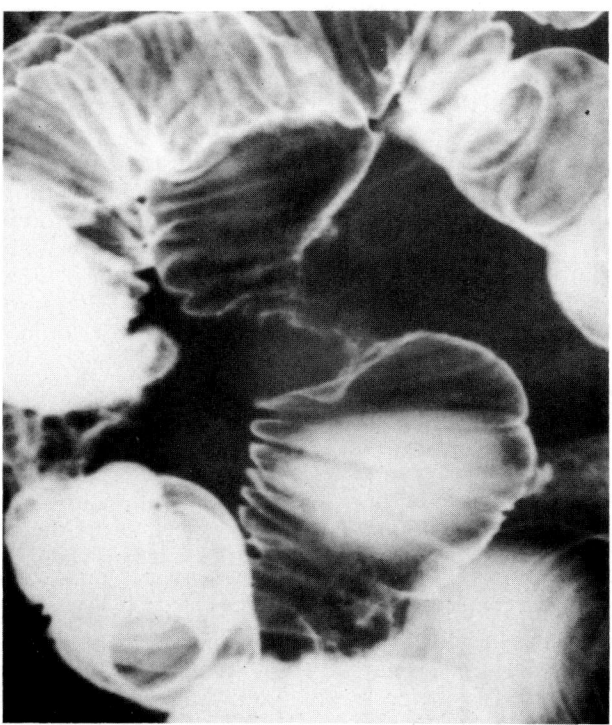

**Figure 48–8. Nonspecific ulceration and stenosis.** Small bowel enema (barium-air) outlines a short stricture in the midileum. The transition to normal bowel is abrupt. At least one shallow ulcer is seen in the stenotic segment.

involved bowel loops there may be swelling and flattening of the folds.[33] An important consequence may be the formation of postinflammatory adhesions, one of the more infrequent causes of small bowel obstruction.

## "Backwash" Ileitis

Based on pathology reports, up to 25% of patients with ulcerative colitis have some degree of involvement

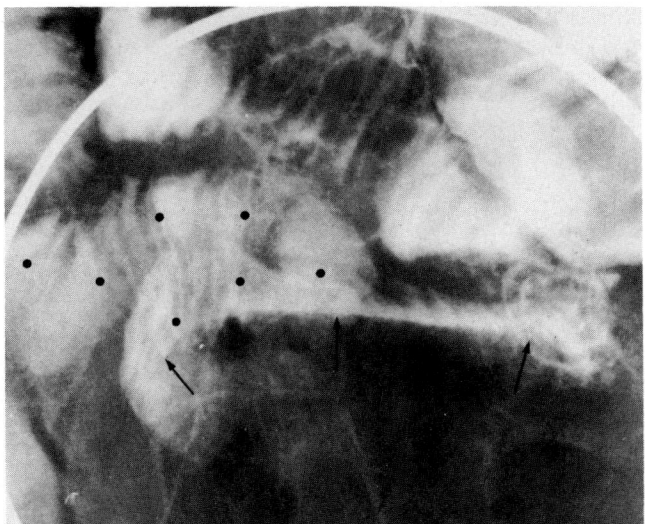

**Figure 48–9. Periappendiceal abscess.** The distal portion of the terminal ileum *(dots)* is unaffected. More proximally, the abscess has displaced and compressed swollen mucosal folds *(arrows)*.

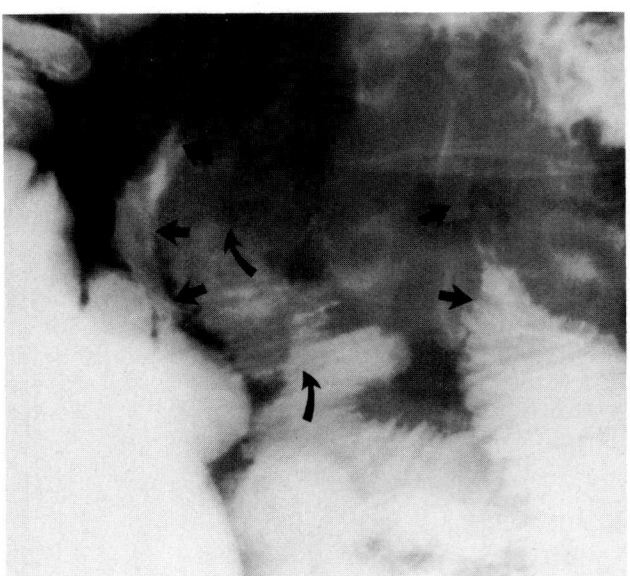

**Figure 48–10. Effect of periappendiceal abscess on small bowel.** A large periappendiceal abscess affects several small bowel segments, which are seen to be displaced *(straight arrows)* or show flattening of swollen folds *(curved arrows)*.

of the terminal ileum. This may be related to incompetence of the ileocecal valve, but this has not been proved. Patients with ulcerative colitis with and without involvement of the terminal ileum have similar symptoms.

Radiologic features consist mostly of a widely open ileocecal valve and either absence of mucosal folds or slight thickening of folds, both caused by submucosal edema (Fig. 48–11). At other times the mucosa has a more nodular appearance. Strictures or ulcerations do not occur.

## Nonspecific Terminal Ileitis

There is disagreement about the significance of a few radiologically shown superficial lesions in the distal ileum in young patients who complain of protracted, crampy abdominal pain, diarrhea, and right lower quadrant tenderness. Do these lesions indicate early Crohn's disease or some other disease? A radiologic examination of the small bowel and colon frequently makes it possible to distinguish between pathology and a normal variant. Crohn's disease may be diagnosed unequivocally by a careful barium study if more extensive transmural lesions are demonstrated. Diagnostic problems arise in patients with superficial lesions confined to a short segment of terminal ileum in the presence of a normal colon. Such lesions can include mucosal nodules that represent either enlargement of lymph follicles or an increase in their number. There may also be blunting, effacement, thickening, and irregularity of mucosal folds (Fig. 48–12). Accumulation of tiny specks of barium, sometimes surrounded by a halo, may be due to aphthoid ulcers. Regional lymph nodes may be slightly enlarged. However, in the given clinical setting and with the lesions confined to a limited portion of the terminal

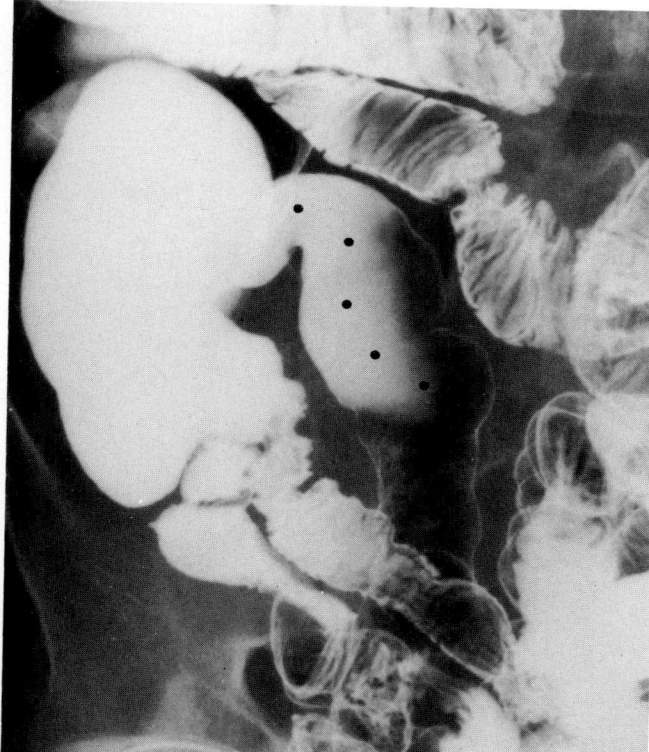

**Figure 48–11. Backwash ileitis in ulcerative colitis.** In the terminal ileum *(dots)*, there is effacement of mucosal folds with a smooth mucosal surface and contour.

ileum, these findings have been shown not to progress to recognizable Crohn's disease.[34] The superficial terminal ileitis might be an abortive form of Crohn's disease. A serologic examination can rule out yersiniosis. It is also possible that these patients suffer from an infection caused by an as yet unidentified virus.

## INFLAMMATORY DISEASE IN IMMUNODEFICIENCY

Infection of the gut by opportunistic organisms (often multiple infections simultaneously) is common in immunocompromised patients. Two main groups of immunodeficient individuals—AIDS patients and post-transplantation patients—are discussed as examples of the immunocompromised population. In addition, other causes of diffuse inflammation, such as graft-versus-host disease (GVHD) after bone marrow transplantation, are briefly presented.

## Gastrointestinal Infections in Acquired Immunodeficiency Syndrome (see also Chapter 60)

Barium studies of patients with human immunodeficiency virus disease often demonstrate multiple abnormalities in the gastrointestinal tract.[35] Multiple organs may be infected by a single opportunistic organism, or

a single organ may be the site of multiple coexistent infections. In one study, involving a group of 66 patients with AIDS and diarrhea, specific infectious agents were found in 36 patients, of whom 22% had multiple infections.[36]

Many of the organisms that infect the gut of immunocompromised patients have specific areas of predilection. For example, *Candida* commonly causes esophagitis but rarely enteritis[37, 38] or colitis, *Cryptosporidium* commonly produces enteritis but rarely colitis, and CMV is more likely to affect the esophagus and colon than the small bowel.

### Cytomegalovirus Infection

CMV is a DNA herpesvirus harbored by 40 to 60% of the general population and by 98% of homosexuals. It occasionally causes self-limited disease in immunocompetent patients.[39] Asymptomatic, CMV-positive blood donors may harbor CMV in leukocytes and transmit the virus to immunodeficient patients, transplant recipients, granulocytopenic cancer patients, and patients undergoing chemotherapy for leukemia or lymphoma.[40]

CMV infection is common in all immunocompromised populations. Biopsies may demonstrate typical eosinophilic round or oval intranuclear or cytoplasmic inclusion bodies in enterocytes, macrophages, fibroblasts, and the endothelial cells of vessels in the submucosa.[41] CMV induces a vasculitis that may lead to focal ischemia and infarction, ulceration, and perforation.[42] Any part of the gastrointestinal tract can be involved but the most frequent sites are the esophagus, stomach, and colon.

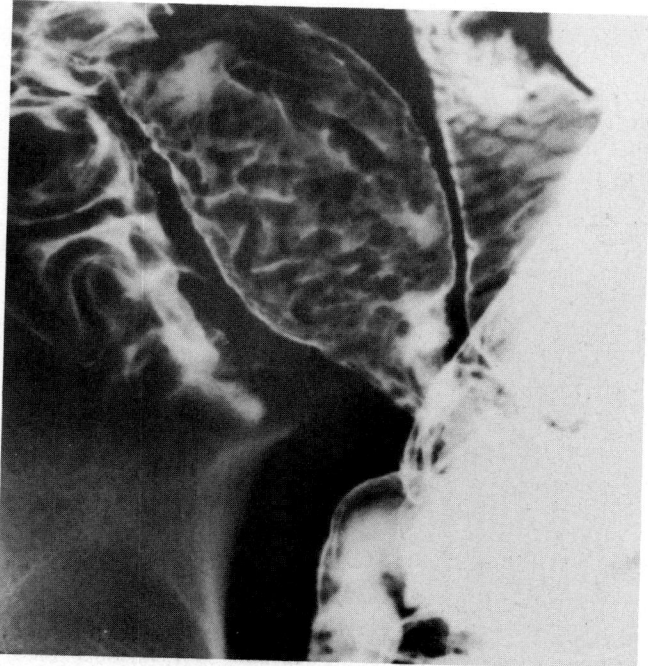

**Figure 48–12. Nonspecific terminal ileitis.** An irregular arrangement of thickened mucosal folds, fine mucosal nodularity, and possible superficial erosions are identified. These changes reverted to normal after a few weeks.

CMV colitis frequently stops on reaching the ileocecal valve. However, in about half of the patients of one series[42] the CMV infection had extended into the terminal ileum. Diffuse CMV enteritis is rare; multiple foci of small bowel disease with ulceration and the danger of bleeding and perforation are more likely. Of interest is the case of a cancer patient undergoing radiation and chemotherapy who developed hematochezia and had an ileocecal resection; a large flat ulcer in the terminal ileum was due to CMV necrotizing vasculitis and CMV infection was also confirmed immunohistochemically.[43]

**Radiologic Findings.** Barium enema changes in CMV colitis may resemble those in ulcerative colitis with diffuse granularity[44] or granulomatous colitis with discrete or aphthous ulcers.[45] Involvement of the terminal ileum shown by barium or computed tomography (CT) was found to be characterized by wall thickening and submucosal nodularity and by often deep ulcerations[42] (Fig. 48–13). An unusual finding is a diffuse CMV enteritis, more pronounced in the ileum, where few ulcers were demonstrated (Fig. 48–14). The presence of jejunoileal or terminal ileal CMV ulcers should be regarded as serious and even potentially fatal, as in a reported case of an AIDS patient.[46]

## Cryptosporidiosis

Cryptosporidia of various subgroups are found in virtually every animal. *Cryptosporidium parvum* affects humans and cattle. It is not unusual for people working with calves to become infected and suffer a self-limited diarrheal illness. Outbreaks of cryptosporidial infection are likely to be transmitted by water and may produce an acute disease limited to 10 to 14 days in immunologically normal persons.[47]

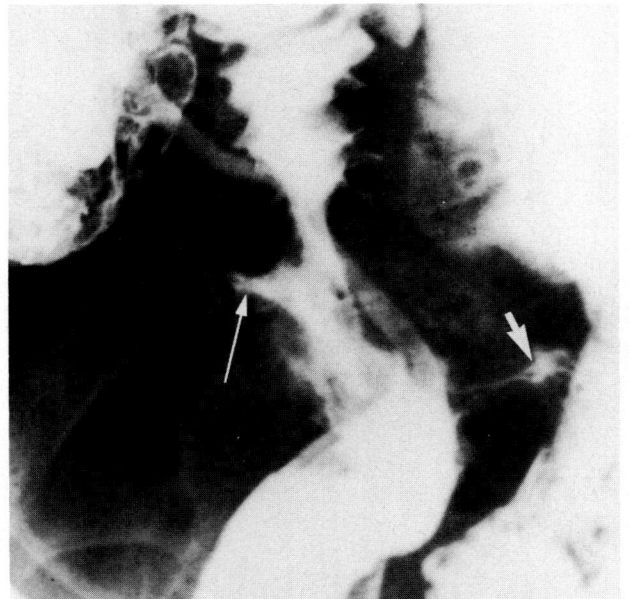

**Figure 48–13. CMV terminal ileitis in AIDS.** The lumen is unevenly narrowed and spiculated. A penetrating ulcer *(long arrow)* and a fistulous tract *(short arrow)* are shown. (From Teixidor HS, Honig CL, Norsoph E, et al: Cytomegalovirus infection of the alimentary canal: radiologic findings with pathologic correlation. Radiology 163:317–323, 1987.)

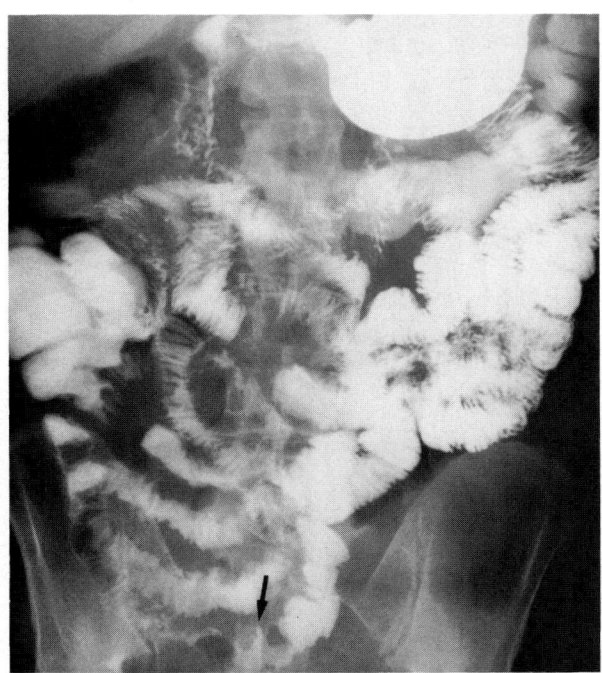

**Figure 48–14. CMV enteritis in AIDS.** Distal ileal loops are separated, and their lumen is narrowed. At least one ulcer is seen in the terminal ileum *(arrow).*

Infection follows the ingestion of thin-walled, sporulated oocysts, which excyst in the proximal small bowel and release sporozoites, which develop further and can autoinfect. Cryptosporidia do not invade the mucosa. The parasite in the endogenous stage nestles between microvilli and is enclosed in a parasitophorous vacuole.[47] How the parasite causes mucosal damage and secretory diarrhea is not clear. Diagnosis is based on finding oocysts in stool (flotation technique) or by mucosal biopsy. However, because the oocysts are minute (3 to 5 µm) and are passed intermittently, they may be missed.

Cryptosporidia are the most common cause of enteritis in patients with AIDS. A severe cholera-like illness develops gradually, with cramping abdominal pain and vomiting. Malabsorption is significant. It may respond to treatment but it tends to recur because of endogenous reinfection.

**Radiologic Findings.** Barium studies have shown thickening of small bowel folds caused by edema (Fig. 48–15), slight separation of bowel loops caused by wall thickening (see Fig. 48–15B), and increased secretions.[48] Fold thickening is generally regular and is seen predominantly in the duodenum and jejunum. Severe mucosal damage may be associated with an amorphous "ribbon bowel." Mucosal atrophy and flattening of the villi may contribute to this pattern. A normal small bowel follow-through examination does not exclude the disease in early cases. CT scans may show small shotty (<0.5 cm) lymph nodes but, unlike the situation in mycobacterial infection, extensive lymphadenopathy is not usually found. One patient with AIDS was reported to have an enterovesical fistula caused by cryptosporidiosis.[49] Interestingly, the fistula was demonstrated by CT, a barium study and cystoscopy having been normal.

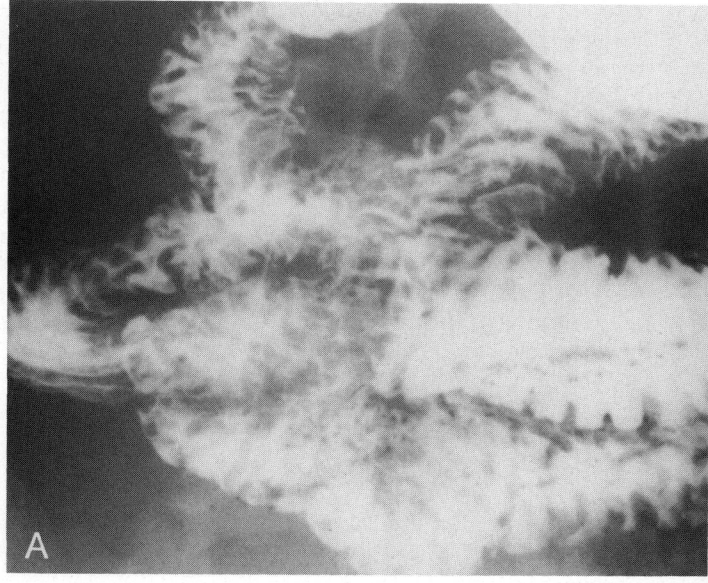
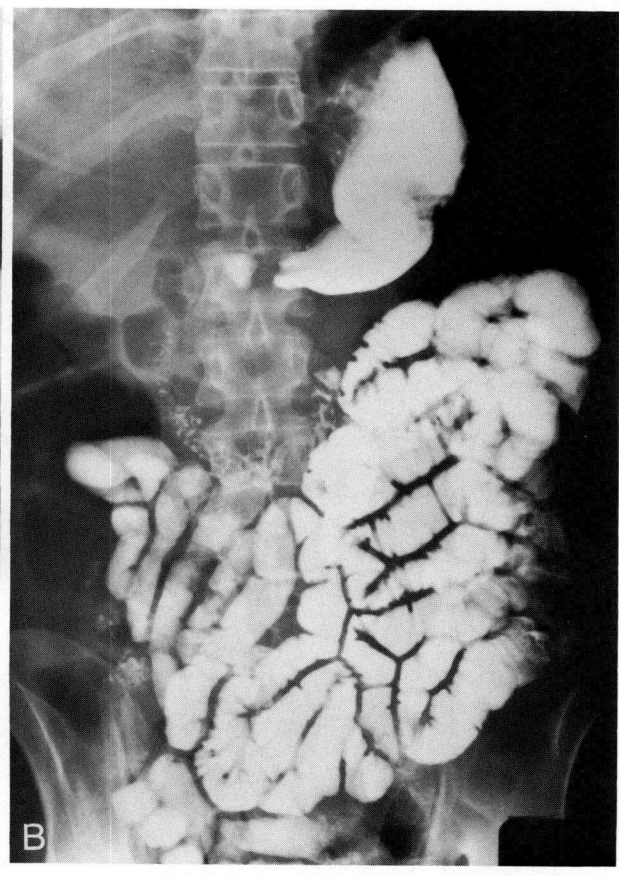

**Figure 48–15. Cryptosporidiosis in AIDS. A.** Follow-through examination shows thickened folds in the jejunum. **B.** A film from a small bowel series of another patient shows diffuse fold thickening and mild flattening of the profile of small bowel loops. Note the slight separation of the loops, indicating wall thickening.

## Isosporiasis

*I. belli,* also a coccidial parasite, resembles *Cryptosporidium* in its wide zoonotic distribution and the occurrence of self-limited infections in immunologically normal persons. However, *Isospora* invades the enterocytes, in which it undergoes its sexual and nonsexual cycles. Its development cannot be completed endogenously, and autoinfection is unlikely. Oocysts are thick walled, oval, and larger than those of *Cryptosporidium.* The prevalence of isosporiasis in AIDS patients in Haiti is 15% and far exceeds that in AIDS patients in the United States.[50] Barium studies show nonspecific changes of fold thickening and widening of the lumen in the proximal small bowel.[51]

## Tuberculosis and Atypical Mycobacterial Infections

The incidence of both typical and atypical tuberculous infections is increased in immunocompromised hosts. Extrapulmonary tuberculosis is currently used by the Centers for Disease Control as an index infection for the diagnosis of AIDS in human immunodeficiency virus–positive individuals.[52, 53] *Mycobacterium tuberculosis* infection occurs more frequently in AIDS patients in Africa and Haiti.

**Tuberculosis.** Tuberculosis may present as peritonitis or focal involvement of the gut, most commonly in the ileocecal area. In barium enema studies, ileocecal tuberculosis is seen as thickening and gaping of the lips of the ileocecal valve and narrowing of the terminal ileum (the Fleischner sign)[54, 55] or as a coned cecum, a result of scarring. Tuberculous peritonitis and mesenteritis may cause ascites, peritoneal or mesenteric thickening, and retroperitoneal and mesenteric adenopathy, all best shown by CT.[56–58]

Balthazar and colleagues compared the CT and barium enema findings in 11 patients with ileocecal tuberculosis, of whom 5 had AIDS and 6 did not.[59] Changes were more pronounced in the AIDS group. Contrast studies showed thickened folds, spasticity with luminal narrowing, and superficial ulceration. One patient presented with distal ileal obstruction, and two patients receiving antituberculous chemotherapy developed partial small bowel obstruction and required surgical resection. CT findings included enlargement of the ileocecal valve and/or wall thickening of the cecum and terminal ileum. Pericecal lymphadenopathy was common, the nodes being either homogeneous or of lower attenuation centrally.[59]

**Mycobacterial Infections.** *Mycobacterium avium* and *Mycobacterium intracellulare* are difficult to differentiate clinically or by microbiological methods. It is customary to refer to them as *Mycobacterium avium-intracellulare* (MAI), or MAI complex. MAI infection is common in AIDS patients. The usual portal of entry is thought to be the small bowel.[60] Although the small bowel may be the most common site of infection, the organisms are ubiquitous in AIDS patients, and a granulomatous hepatitis is frequently present. The paucity of tissue response is striking. Many patients with small bowel infection seem to be asymptomatic, but in 60% of those infected with MAI the organisms could be isolated from the small bowel at autopsy.

In a subgroup of patients with MAI enteritis, large numbers of macrophages filled with the mycobacteria are seen in the lamina propria of the mucosa and distend the villi. This can result in pronounced malabsorption. There is a superficial clinical and radiologic resemblance to Whipple's disease, but the MAI organisms are acid fast and are not Whipple's bacilli.

**Radiologic Findings.** Diffuse and often irregular fold thickening is demonstrated by barium examination of the small bowel (Fig. 48–16A). Enteroclysis may identify micronodularities of the mucosal surface, the results of villous distention by the foamy macrophages in the lamina propria (Fig. 48–16B). CT typically demonstrates bulky mesenteric lymphadenopathy (sometimes of low attenuation) as well as thickening of the small bowel wall (Fig. 48–16C). Usually, the adenopathy is more mesenteric than retroperitoneal.

The demonstration of focal visceral lesions and of low-density lymph nodes by contrast-enhanced CT favors tuberculous infection.[61] On the other hand, marked hepatic and splenic enlargement, diffuse jejunal wall thickening, and enlarged soft tissue density nodal masses suggest MAI infection.[61] However, such differentiation is tentative, and cultures are required. Fine-needle biopsy of enlarged nodes in patients with MAI infection may demonstrate foamy macrophages with acid-fast bacilli. Liver biopsy may be diagnostic.

## Transplantation and the Gastrointestinal Tract

Long-term immunosuppression is necessary after transplantation to prevent rejection of the transplanted organ. The immunosuppressive regimen unfortunately

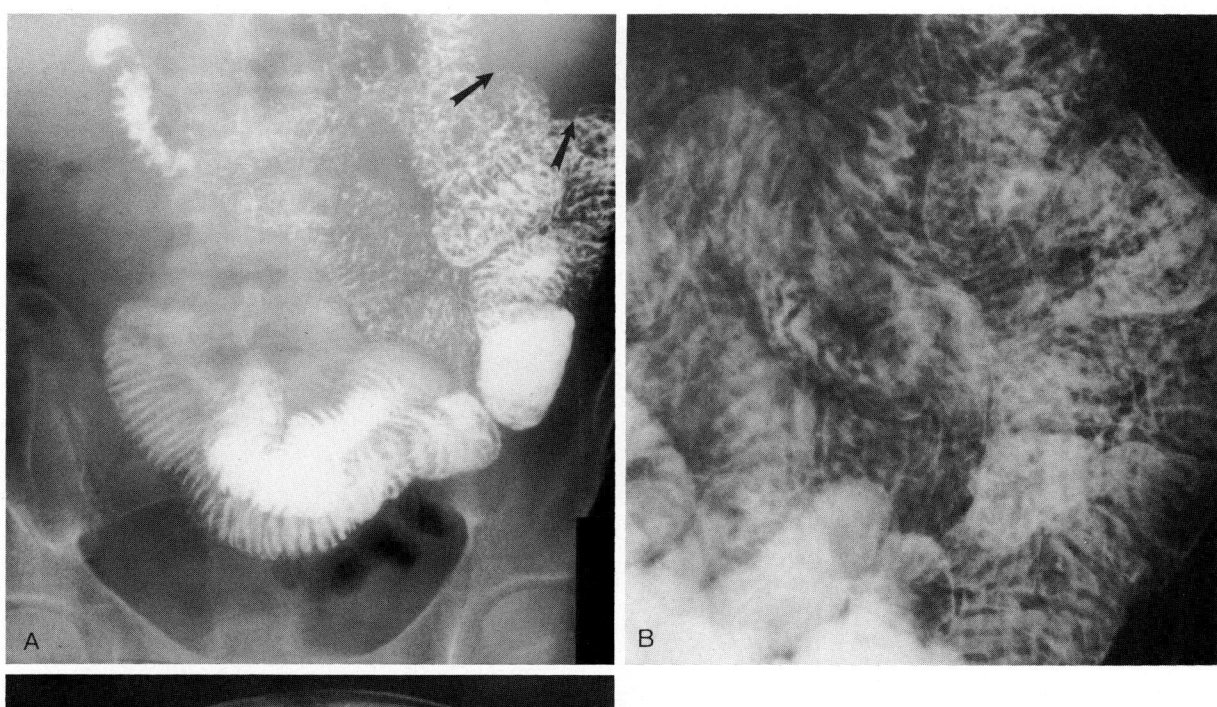

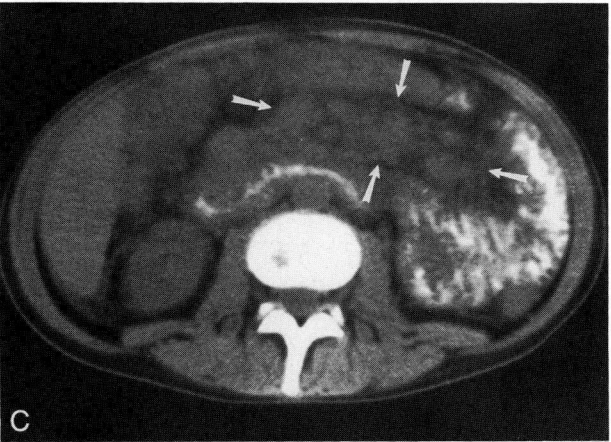

**Figure 48–16. MAI enteritis in AIDS. A.** A film from a small bowel follow-through shows diffuse thickening of the folds with mild distention and splenomegaly *(arrows)*. **B.** In another patient, enteroclysis demonstrates fold thickening with a general micronodular pattern of the mucosa. This pattern is caused by distention of villi. **C.** A CT scan from a third patient demonstrates the minimal distention of the small bowel with moderate fold enlargement. A group of enlarged mesenteric nodes is outlined by arrows. (**C** from Stephens DH [ed]: Gastrointestinal Disease [4th Series], Test and Syllabus. Reston, VA: American College of Radiology, 1991, p 188.)

causes increased susceptibility to infection and the development of cancers. Toxicity and mucositis constitute a further problem.[62] Addition of cyclosporine to the immunosuppressive regimen has produced additional problems.[63]

Many gastrointestinal complications have been reported after transplantation. These include peptic ulcer disease; massive hemorrhage; colon perforation (in association with diverticulitis, CMV infection, or idiopathic); fecal impaction, sometimes leading to obstruction, ileus, or even colonic necrosis; and pancreatitis.[64] Steroids are thought to play a role, especially in ulceration, bleeding, pancreatitis, and colon perforation. Gastrointestinal complications are likely to occur after kidney,[64, 65] liver,[66] cardiac,[67] heart-lung, and bone marrow transplantations.[68, 69] The following discussion is limited to gastrointestinal complications of bone marrow transplantation.

## Gastrointestinal Inflammation After Bone Marrow Transplantation

Leukemia, lymphoma, aplastic anemia, metabolic disorders of the hematopoietic system, and certain metastatic diseases (e.g., metastases from breast cancer) have all been treated with bone marrow transplantation. Before transplantation, the patient's bone marrow is destroyed by high-dose radiation or chemotherapy. The bone marrow is then repopulated by a transplant from a compatible donor. The transplanted marrow (graft) mounts an immunologic response to the patient (host).

The following intestinal complications may occur:

1. The induction protocol of high-dose radiotherapy and/or chemotherapy causes mucositis with oropharyngeal and abdominal pain, vomiting, diarrhea. It may last up to 3 weeks.
2. Impairment of the host's immune status leads to opportunistic bacterial, fungal, viral, and parasitic infections.
3. Acute GVHD develops.

Superinfection with opportunistic organisms is a major problem after bone marrow transplantation.[70-74] Organisms that most frequently cause infection include *Candida,* herpes simplex, CMV, and bacteria, as well as viral organisms: varicella-zoster virus, Epstein-Barr virus, hepatitis viruses, rotavirus, adenovirus, and coxsackieviruses A or B. The enteric viruses may overwhelm the immunodeficient patient and produce profuse bloody diarrhea, rapid clinical deterioration, and a high mortality rate,[70, 72-74] especially if GVHD has already commenced.

The major complication of bone marrow transplantation is intestinal GVHD, in which mucosal surfaces become inflamed and raw. GVHD occurs in acute and chronic forms. Acute GVHD appears soon after transplantation (up to about 100 days post-transplantation) and, until recently, has affected 50 to 70% of those with allogeneic transplants, with a fatal outcome in up to 15%[75-79] (personal communication, G. Vogelzang, M.D., Northwestern University, Chicago, IL). Addition

of cyclosporine, combined with methylprednisolone or methotrexate, to the post-transplantation regimen has decreased the incidence of acute GVHD by about half.[80]

Together with the skin and the liver, the gastrointestinal tract is the major target organ in acute GVHD. A profuse, protein-containing secretory diarrhea; a maculopapular rash over palms, soles, and trunk; and jaundice are hallmarks of the disease.[68, 69, 80, 81] Acute GVHD causes major defects in the normal physiologic barriers to infection of skin and gut. When such patients have superinfections with opportunistic enteric pathogens, the prognosis is especially poor. Furthermore, the therapy for acute GVHD worsens the infection-related clinical course because it further depresses the patient's defective defense mechanisms.

## Radiologic Findings in Enteric Infections and Acute Graft-Versus-Host Disease

Initial reports of the abnormalities found in small bowel follow-through examinations in acute intestinal GVHD stressed predominantly jejunal fold thickening or effacement of folds producing a characteristic, featureless ribbon bowel, once thought to be pathognomonic for acute GVHD.[82-86] It has since been realized that the ribbon or tubular small bowel is not specific for GVHD but simply reflects the severe mucosal damage. This pattern has also been found in other enteric infections[87] (Figs. 48–17 and 48–18A), ischemia, corrosive injury, drug toxicity, infiltrating diseases such as amyloid and mastocytosis, lymphoma, pseudolymphoma, Crohn's disease, radiation damage,[88] and allergic states.[89]

Severe viral enteritis can produce small bowel changes indistinguishable from those of GVHD[87] (see Figs. 48–17 and 48–18A). The same study showed that acute GVHD and viral infection can also cause inflammation in other organs, namely the stomach, duodenum, and colon (Fig. 48–19). Gastric abnormalities seen in a series of 28 patients[87] included dilatation, delayed emptying, antral deformity, and prolonged barium coating. In the duodenum, fold thickening, or effacement, and a tubular or shaggy appearance have been reported. Small bowel changes caused by either acute GVHD or a viral infection (e.g., CMV) were seen in all patients and included fold thickening or effacement, lumen narrowing, and separation of bowel loops. Changes found in the colon were haustral fold thickening, loss of haustration producing a tubular colon, spasm, ulceration, and a granular mucosal pattern reminiscent of ulcerative colitis[87] (see Fig. 48–19).

In four patients, an unusual and prolonged mucosal coating of the small bowel was seen on follow-up plain films of the abdomen taken up to more than 2 days later (see Fig. 48–18). This coating resembled a "cast" of the small intestine and remained unchanged for more than 48 hours in one patient. We have no explanation for this prolonged barium coating. All four patients with this finding had severe mucosal disease and subsequently passed sloughed mucosa in bloody diarrheal stools. The barium may have adhered to the mucosa, the raw surface of the submucosa, or pseudomembranes or may have been trapped between sloughed mucosa and the bare surface of the intestine. On CT scans, the correlates of the prolonged coating in the small intestine[90] are circular collections of contrast medium in bowel shown in cross section or parallel tracks of contrast medium in longitudinal section (see Fig. 48–18C). Other CT findings in acute GVHD and viral enteritis are bowel wall thickening, pericolic inflammation, a "halo" sign compatible with submucosal edema, mesenteric thickening, and small mesenteric nodes.

Chronic GVHD can follow acute GVHD or occur de novo. Although it usually develops more than 100 days after transplantation, it can occur as early as 45 to 50 days. The target organs are the skin and the esophagus. The skin changes resemble those of scleroderma, with dry, tight skin and hyperpigmentation. In the esophagus, chronic GVHD produces a desquamative esophagitis and webs or strictures after healing.[91] Rarely, fibrotic strictures develop in the small intestine. More commonly found in the small bowel are a patchy fibrosis involving lamina propria and submucosa and a stasis-related bacterial overgrowth. Malabsorption and a chronic infection may give rise to diarrhea.

## Preventive Therapy After Allogeneic Bone Marrow Transplantation

It is generally accepted that, of the various organisms contributing to morbidity and mortality in allogeneic bone marrow transplantation patients, CMV plays a major role. Ganciclovir has shown potent activity against CMV. CMV-seropositive patients were tested for CMV excretion after transplantation and, if positive, were given ganciclovir prophylactically for up to 100 days. In a similar group of 35 placebo-treated patients, 15 developed CMV disease. Among 37 patients who were given prophylactic ganciclovir, only 1 developed CMV disease. Hematologic toxicity was caused by ganciclovir but resolved when the drug was stopped.[92]

## Typhlitis

Typhlitis is an inflammatory and/or necrotizing process that involves the cecum and/or the terminal ileum and appendix. It was first reported in leukemic children undergoing chemotherapy. It has now also been found in adults as a complication of leukemia, lymphoma, aplastic anemia, immunosuppressive drug therapy after

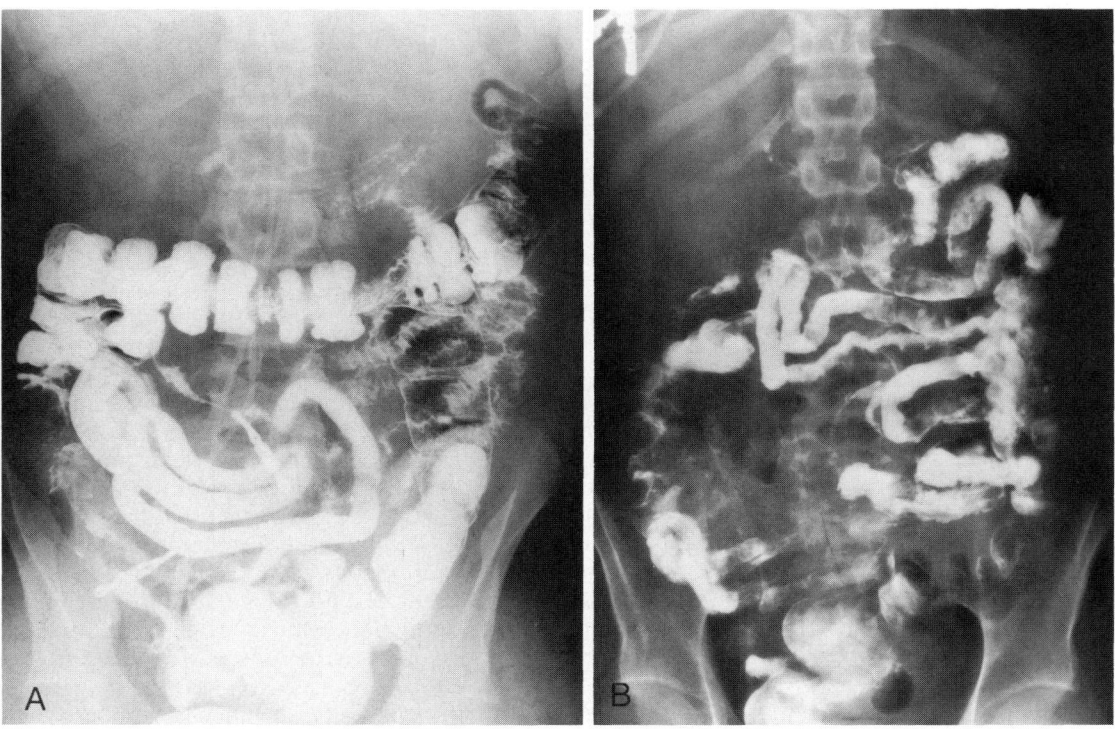

**Figure 48–17. Enteric viral infection.** This 20-year-old man with no evidence of acute GVHD was infected with rotavirus and adenovirus. **A.** Film from a small bowel series shows fold thickening in the jejunum and ribbon-like appearance of the distal small bowel. There is spasm in the proximal ascending colon. **B.** Film from a small bowel series performed 19 days later shows a diffuse amorphous pattern with almost complete effacement of small bowel folds. (From B Jones, SS Kramer, R Saral, et al, Gastrointestinal inflammation after bone marrow transplantation: graft-versus-host disease or opportunistic infection? AJR, 150, 2, 277–281, 1988, © by American Roentgen Ray Society.)

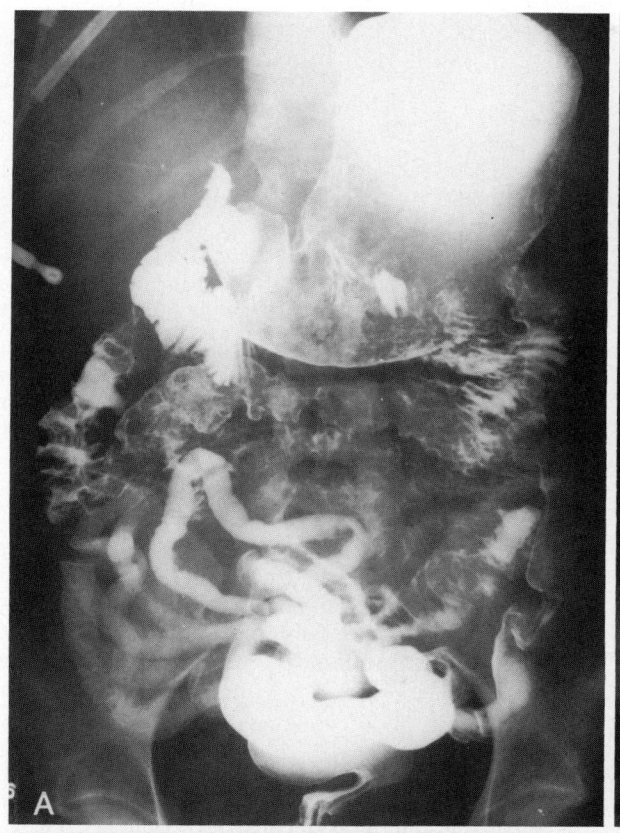

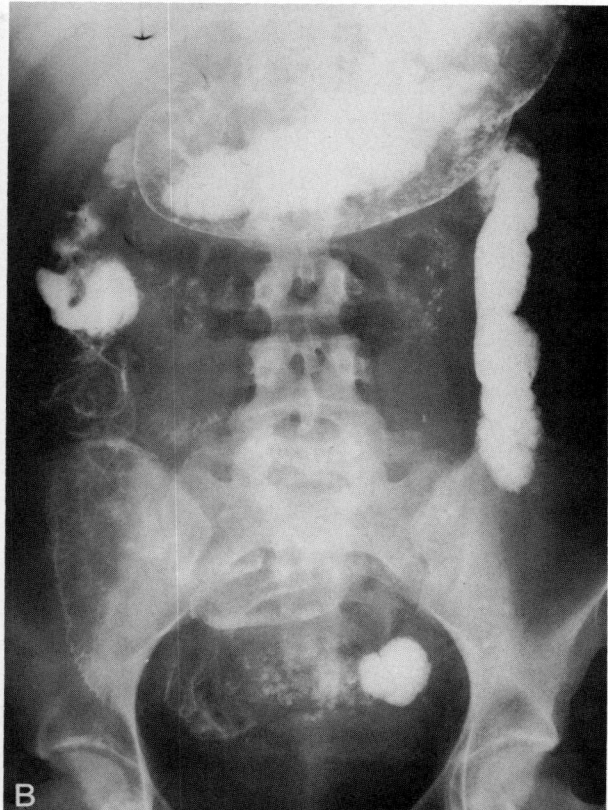

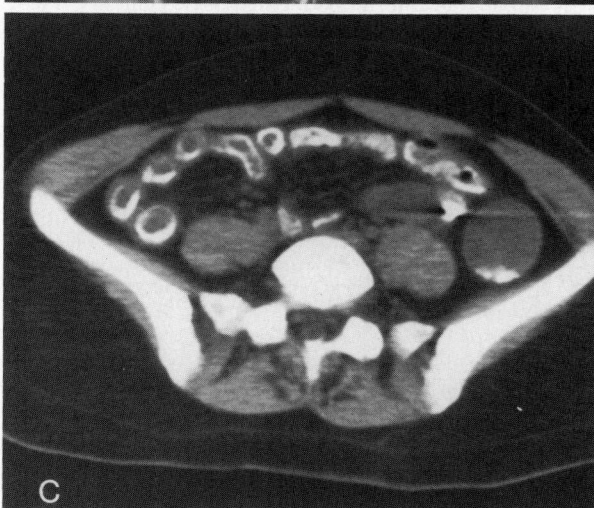

**Figure 48–18. Prolonged barium coating in severe GVHD and adenoviral enteritis. A.** An 8-hour film from a small bowel series demonstrates gastric atony and dilatation. Fold thickening is seen in proximal small bowel and there is ribbon bowel distally. The colon appears spastic and edematous on the right and is ahaustral on the left. (From DJ Winston, RP Gale, DV Meyer, et al, Infectious complications of human bone marrow transplantation, Medicine [Baltimore], 58, 1, 1–31, 1979, © by Williams & Wilkins, 1979.) **B.** A follow-up film taken 24 hours later shows persistent gastric atony with unusual coating of the mucosa. Several abnormal small bowel loops in the right lower quadrant have a cast-like appearance. (Reprinted from Hochhauser L, Thompson G, Somers S: Opportunistic gastritis in graft-versus-host disease, by permission of the publisher, Can Assoc Radiol J 34:316–318, December 1983.) **C.** A CT scan obtained on the same day as the film in **B** reveals abnormal coating of many bowel loops with circles of contrast medium in cross section and parallel tracks in longitudinal section. Slight mesenteric and periaortic adenopathy is also seen. (From Jones B, Fishman EK: Computed tomography and the other inflammatory bowel diseases. *In* Fishman EK, Jones B [eds]: Computed Tomography of the Gastrointestinal Tract. Churchill Livingstone, New York, 1988, pp 109–128.)

organ transplantation, and AIDS.[93–95] Typhlitis was formerly known as neutropenic enterocolitis or as the ileocecal syndrome[96] and is now often referred to as neutropenic typhlitis because of its close association with profound neutropenia. Infections (e.g., with CMV), leukemic or lymphomatous infiltration, or focal ischemia can be associated with typhlitis. Early diagnosis and treatment of typhlitis are essential; untreated typhlitis progresses rapidly to transmural necrosis and perforation and has a high mortality rate. Treatment with high-dose antibiotics and intravenous fluids should be initiated before transmural necrosis has occurred.

Examinations with barium or a water-soluble contrast agent should be carried out with careful fluoroscopy and the lowest possible intraluminal pressures because there is a risk of perforation. Less invasive imaging studies, such as CT studies, may be safer and are useful in diagnosis and in monitoring the course of the disease. CT findings in typhlitis include wall thickening (occasionally with low-attenuation intramural areas consistent with edema or necrosis), pneumatosis, pericolonic fluid, and thickening of fascial planes[97, 98] (Fig. 48–20). Recognition of the transmural inflammatory process on CT scans, in the appropriate clinical setting, is highly suggestive of typhlitis. The specificity of this finding, however, is low; other disorders that can present with bowel wall

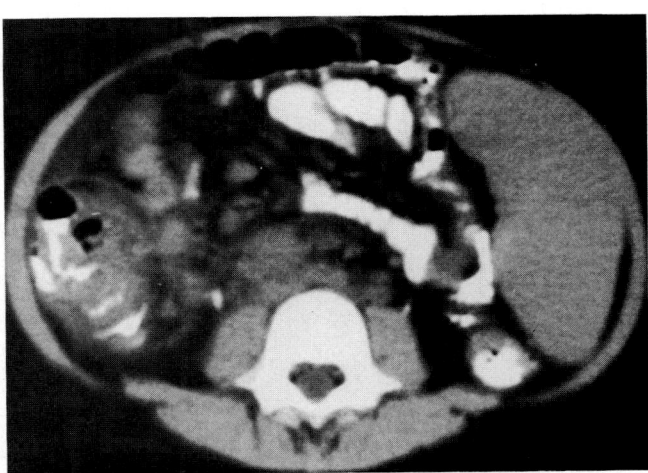

**Figure 48–20. Typhlitis.** A CT scan through the right lower quadrant in a 15-year-old girl with myeloid leukemia reveals diffuse bowel wall thickening in the terminal ileum and cecum with pericolonic inflammation. Also note the marked splenomegaly. (From Jones B, Fishman EK: Computed tomography and the other inflammatory bowel diseases. *In* Fishman EK, Jones B [eds]: Computed Tomography of the Gastrointestinal Tract. Churchill Livingstone, New York, 1988, pp 109–128.)

thickening in this area include leukemic infiltration, intramural hemorrhage, ischemia, segmental pseudomembranous colitis, appendicitis, and even right-sided diverticulitis. In pseudomembranous colitis, however, pericolic inflammation is less pronounced than in typhlitis.[99, 100]

### Acknowledgment

Figures 48–14 and 48–15A are reproduced with permission from Herlinger H, Maglinte D (eds): Clinical Radiology of the Small Intestine. Philadelphia: WB Saunders, 1989.

# References

1. Pawlowski AS: Ascariasis. Clin Gastroenterol 7:157–178, 1978.
2. Mahamood A: Blood loss caused by helminthic infections. Trans R Soc Trop Med Hyg 60:766–769, 1966.
3. Sheehy TW, Meroney W, Cox RS, et al: Hookworm disease and malabsorption. Gastroenterology 42:148–156, 1962.
4. Monroe LS: Gastrointestinal parasites. *In* Berk JE, Haubrich WS, Kalser MH, et al (eds): Bockus Gastroenterology (4th ed). Philadelphia: WB Saunders, 1985, pp 4250–4348.
5. Guerrant RL, Bobak DA: Bacterial and protozoal gastroenteritis. N Engl J Med 325:327–340, 1991.
6. Igra-Siegman Y, Kapila R, Sen P, et al: Syndrome with hyperinfection with *Strongyloides stercoralis*. Rev Infect Dis 3:397–407, 1981.
7. Dallemand S, Waxman M, Farman J: Radiological manifestations of *Strongyloides stercoralis*. Gastrointest Radiol 8:45–51, 1983.
8. Lev B, Ward H, Keusch GT, et al: Lectin activation in *Giardia lamblia* by host protease: a novel host-parasite interaction. Science 232:71–73, 1986.
9. Cevallos AM, Farthing MJG: Parasitic infections of the gastrointestinal tract. Curr Opin Gastroenterol 9:96–102, 1993.
10. Brandon J, Glick SN, Teplick SK: Intestinal giardiasis: importance of serial filming. AJR 144:581–584, 1985.
11. Matsui T, Jida M, Murakami M, et al: Intestinal anisakiasis: clinical and radiologic features. Radiology 157:299–302, 1985.

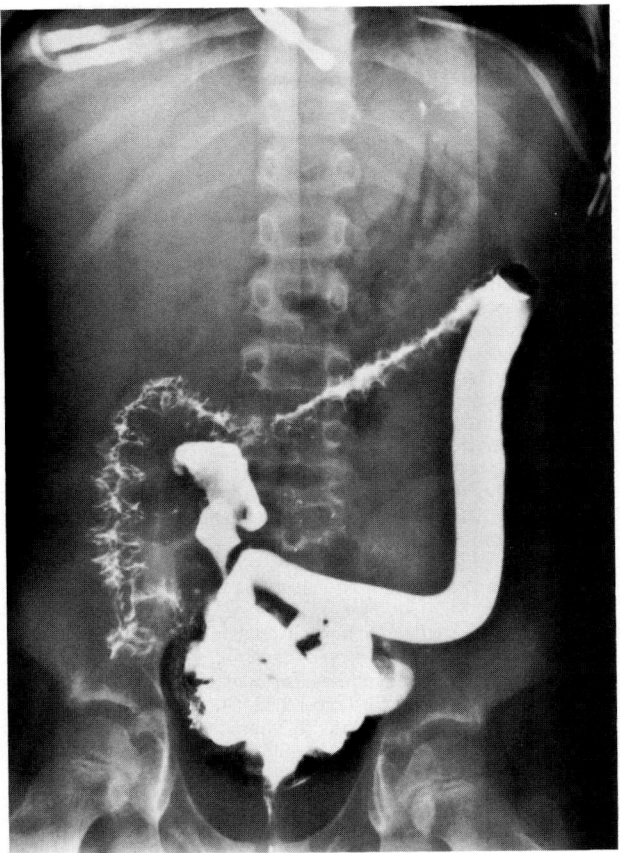

**Figure 48–19. Colonic GVHD.** A film from a barium enema study shows diffuse loss of haustration and shortening of the left colon from the splenic flexure to the rectum. Spasm or edema or both extend from the cecum to the splenic flexure.

12. Smith B: The myenteric plexus in Chagas disease. J Pathol Bacteriol 94:462–463, 1967.
13. Palmer KR, Patil DH, Basran GS, et al: Abdominal tuberculosis in urban Britain—a common disease. Gut 26:1296–1305, 1985.
14. Thoeni RF, Margulis AR: Gastrointestinal tuberculosis. Semin Roentgenol 14:283–294, 1979.
15. VanTrappen G, Agg HO, Ponette E, et al: *Yersinia* enteritis and enterocolitis: gastroenterological aspects. Gastroenterology 72:220–227, 1977.
16. Tripoli LC, Brouillette DE, Nicholas JJ, et al: Disseminated *Yersinia* enterocolitica. Case report and review of literature. J Clin Gastroenterol 12:85–89, 1990.
17. Lahesmaa-Rantala R, Graufors K, Isomaki H, et al: *Yersinia*-specific antibodies in the synovial fluid of patients with *Yersinia* triggered reactive arthritis. Ann Rheum Dis 46:510–514, 1987.
18. Abcarian PW, Demos BE: Systemic *Yersinia enterocolitica* infection associated with iron overload and deferoxamine therapy. AJR 157:773–775, 1991.
19. Ekberg O, Sjostrom B, Brahme F: Radiological findings in *Yersinia* ileitis. Radiology 123:15–19, 1977.
20. Update: *Salmonella enteritidis* infections and shell eggs—United States. MMWR 39:909–912, 1990.
21. Merson MH, Morris GK, Sack DA, et al: Travelers' diarrhea in Mexico. A prospective study of physicians and family members attending a congress. N Engl Med J 294:1299–1305, 1976.
22. Miranda AG, Dupont HL: Small intestine: infections with common bacterial and viral pathogens. *In* Yamada T (ed): Textbook of Gastroenterology. Philadelphia: JB Lippincott, 1991, pp 1447–1472.
23. Mee AS, Shield M, Burke M: *Campylobacter* colitis: differentiation from acute inflammatory bowel disease. J R Soc Med 78:217–223, 1985.
24. Brodey PA, Fertig S, Aron JM: *Campylobacter* enterocolitis: radiographic features. AJR 139:1199–1201, 1982.
25. Bank S, Trey C, Gans I: Histoplasmosis of the small bowel with "giant" intestinal villi and secondary protein-losing enteropathy. Am J Med 39:492–501, 1965.
26. Eisenberg RL: Gastrointestinal Radiology. A Pattern Approach (2nd ed). Philadelphia: JB Lippincott, 1990, p 475.
27. Blacklow NR, Greenberg HB: Viral gastroenteritis. N Engl J Med 325:252–264, 1991.
28. Schreiber DS, Blacklow NR, Trier JS: The mucosal lesion of the proximal small intestine in acute infectious nonbacterial gastroenteritis. N Engl J Med 288:1318–1323, 1973.
29. Bayless TM: Small intestine ulcers and strictures: isolated and diffuse. *In* Sleisenger MH, Fordtran JS (eds): Gastrointestinal Disease: Pathophysiology, Diagnosis, Management (4th ed). Philadelphia: WB Saunders, 1989, pp 1320–1327.
30. Rampton DS: Non-steroidal anti-inflammatory drugs and the lower gastrointestinal tract. Scand J Gastroenterol 22:1–4, 1987.
31. Bjarnason I, Price AB, Zanelli G, et al: Clinicopathological features of nonsteroidal antiinflammatory drug–induced small intestinal strictures. Gastroenterology 94:1070–1074, 1988.
32. Frager D, Wolf EL, Frager JD, et al: Small intestinal complications of diverticulitis of the sigmoid colon. JAMA 256:3258–3261, 1987.
33. O'Riordan D, Herlinger H: Diagnosis of extrinsic abscesses affecting the small intestine. Mt Sinai J Med 51:347–350, 1984.
34. Ekberg O, Baath L, Sjostrom B, et al: Are superficial lesions of the distal part of the ileum early indicators of Crohn's disease in adult patients with abdominal pain? A clinical and radiologic long term investigation. Gut 25:341–346, 1984.
35. Wall SD, Ominsky S, Altman DF, et al: Multifocal abnormalities of the gastrointestinal tract in AIDS. AJR 146:1–5, 1986.
36. Antony MA, Brandt LJ, Klein RS, et al: Infectious diarrhea in patients with AIDS. Dig Dis Sci 33:1141–1146, 1988.
37. Joshi SN, Garvin PJ, Sunwoo YC: Candidiasis of the duodenum and jejunum. Gastroenterology 80:829–833, 1981.
38. Radin DR, Fong TL, Halls JM, et al: Monilial enteritis in acquired immunodeficiency syndrome. AJR 141:1289–1290, 1983.
39. Surawicz C, Myerson D: Self-limited cytomegalovirus colitis in immunocompetent individuals. Gastroenterology 94:194–199, 1988.
40. McDonald GG, Rees GM: Approach to gastrointestinal problems in the immune compromised patient. *In* Yamada T (ed): Textbook of Gastroenterology. Philadelphia: JB Lippincott, 1991, pp 900–927.
41. Balthazar EJ, Megibow AJ, Hulnick D, et al: Cytomegalovirus esophagitis in AIDS: radiographic features in 16 patients. AJR 149:919–923, 1987.
42. Teixidor HS, Honig CL, Norsoph E, et al: Cytomegalovirus infection of the alimentary canal: radiologic findings with pathologic correlation. Radiology 163:317–325, 1987.
43. Weber FH, Frierson HF, Myers BM: Cytomegalovirus as a cause of isolated severe ileal bleeding. J Clin Gastroenterol 14:53–55, 1992.
44. Balthazar EJ, Megibow AJ, Fazzini E, et al: Cytomegalovirus colitis in AIDS: radiographic findings in 11 patients. Radiology 155:585–589, 1985.
45. Caroline DF, Hilpert PL, Russin VL: CMV colitis mimicking Crohn's disease in a patient with acquired immune deficiency syndrome (AIDS). J Can Assoc Radiol 38:227–228, 1987.
46. Kram HB, Shoemaker WC: Intestinal perforation due to cytomegalovirus infection. Dis Colon Rectum 33:1037–1040, 1990.
47. Soave R: Treatment strategies for cryptosporidiosis. Ann N Y Acad Sci 616:442–451, 1990.
48. Berk RN, Wall SD, McArdle CB, et al: Cryptosporidiosis of the stomach and small intestine in patients with AIDS. AJR 143:549–554, 1984.
49. Meyers SA, Kuhlman JE, Fishman EK: Enterovesical fistula in a patient with cryptosporidiosis and AIDS. CT demonstration. Clin Imaging 14:143–145, 1990.
50. DeHovitz JA, Pape JW, Boncy M, et al: Clinical manifestations and therapy of *Isospora belli* infection in patients with the acquired immunodeficiency syndrome. N Engl J Med 315:87–90, 1986.
51. Shein R, Gelb A: *Isospora belli* in a patient with acquired immunodeficiency syndrome. J Clin Gastroenterol 6:525–528, 1984.
52. Sathe SS, Reichman LB: Mycobacterial disease in patients infected with the human immunodeficiency virus. Clin Chest Med 10:445–463, 1989.
53. Buckner CB, Leithiser RE, Walker CW, et al: The changing epidemiology of tuberculosis and other mycobacterial infections in the United States: implications for the radiologist. AJR 156:255–264, 1991.
54. Carrera GF, Young S, Lewicki AM: Intestinal tuberculosis. Gastrointest Radiol 1:147–155, 1976.
55. Gershon-Cohen J, Kremens V: X-ray studies of ileocecal valve in ileocecal tuberculosis. Radiology 62:251–254, 1954.
56. Hulnick DH, Megibow AJ, Naidich DP, et al: Abdominal tuberculosis: CT evaluation. Radiology 157:199–204, 1985.
57. Epstein BM, Mann JH: CT of abdominal tuberculosis. AJR 139:861–866, 1982.
58. Bargallo N, Nicolan C, Luburich P, et al: Intestinal tuberculosis in AIDS. Gastrointest Radiol 17:115–118, 1992.
59. Balthazar EJ, Gordon R, Hulnick D: Ileocecal tuberculosis: CT and radiologic evaluation. AJR 154:499–503, 1990.
60. Vincent ME, Robbins AH: *Mycobacterium avium-intracellulare* complex enteritis: pseudo-Whipple disease in AIDS. AJR 144:921–922, 1985.
61. Radin DR: Intraabdominal *Mycobacterium tuberculosis* vs *Mycobacterium avium-intracellulare* infections in patients with AIDS. Distinction based on CT findings. AJR 156:487–491, 1991.
62. Mitchell EP, Schein PS: Gastrointestinal toxicity of chemotherapeutic agents. Semin Oncol 9:52–64, 1982.
63. Kahan BD: Cyclosporine. N Engl J Med 321:1725–1738, 1989.
64. Thompson WM, Meyers W, Seigler HF, et al: Gastrointestinal complications of renal transplantation. Semin Roentgenol 13:319–328, 1978.
65. Rees JI, Evans C: Imaging after renal transplantation. Clin Radiol 43:4–7, 1991 (editorial).
66. Van Thiel DH, Dindzans VJ, Gavaler JS, et al: The postoperative problems and management of the liver transplant recipient. Prog Liver Dis 9:657–685, 1990.

67. Kirklin JK, Holm A, Aldrete JS, et al: Gastrointestinal complications after cardiac transplantation. Ann Surg 211:538–541, 1990.

68. McDonald GB, Shulman HM, Sullivan KM, et al: Intestinal and hepatic complications of human bone marrow transplantation. Part 1. Gastroenterology 90:460–477, 1986.

69. McDonald GB, Shulman HM, Sullivan KM, et al: Intestinal and hepatic complications of human bone marrow transplantation. Part 2. Gastroenterology 90:770–784, 1986.

70. Hochhauser L, Thompson G, Somers S: Opportunistic gastritis in graft-versus-host-disease. J Can Assoc Radiol 34:316–318, 1983.

71. Navari RM, Sharma P, Deeg HJ, et al: Pneumatosis cystoides intestinalis following allogeneic marrow transplantation. Transplant Proc 15:1720–1724, 1983.

72. Townsend TR, Bolyard EA, Yolken RH, et al: Outbreak of coxsackie A1 gastroenteritis: a complication of bone marrow transplantation. Lancet 1:820–823, 1982.

73. Winston DJ, Gale RP, Meyer DV, et al: Infectious complications of human bone marrow transplantation. Medicine (Baltimore) 58:1–31, 1979.

74. Zahradnik JM, Spencer MJ, Porter DD: Adenovirus infection in the immunocompromised patient. Am J Med 68:725–732, 1980.

75. Beschorner WE: Destruction of the intestinal mucosa after bone marrow transplantation and graft-versus-host disease. Surv Synth Pathol Res 3:264–274, 1984.

76. Moir DH, Turner JJ, Ma DDF, et al: Autopsy findings in bone marrow transplantation. Pathology 1:197–204, 1982.

77. Sale GE, Shulman HM, McDonald GB, et al: Gastrointestinal graft-versus-host disease in man. Am J Surg Pathol 3:291–299, 1979.

78. Slavin RE, Santos GW: The graft versus host reaction in man after bone marrow transplantation: pathology, pathogenesis, clinical features, and implication. Clin Immunol Immunopathol 1:472–478, 1973.

79. Thomas ED, Storb R, Clift RA, et al: Bone-marrow transplantation. N Engl J Med 292:895–902, 1975.

80. Spencer GD, Shulman HM, Myerson D, et al: Diffuse intestinal ulceration after marrow transplantation: a clinicopathologic study of 13 patients. Hum Pathol 17:621–633, 1986.

81. Thorning D, Howard JD: Epithelial denudement in the gastrointestinal tracts of two bone marrow transplant recipients. Hum Pathol 17:560–566, 1986.

82. Fisk JD, Shulman HM, Greening RR, et al: Gastrointestinal radiographic features of human graft-versus-host disease. AJR 136:329–336, 1981.

83. Rosenberg HK, Serota FT, Koch P, et al: Radiographic features of gastrointestinal graft-versus-host disease. Radiology 138:371–374, 1981.

84. Schimmelpenninck M, Zwaan F: Radiographic features of small intestinal injury in human graft-versus-host disease. Gastrointest Radiol 7:29–33, 1982.

85. Schuttevaer HM, Kroon HM, Shaw PC: Graft-versus-host disease of the gastrointestinal tract. Diagn Imaging Clin Med 55:254–261, 1986.

86. Shimkin PM, Delellis RA, Carolla RL, et al: Graft-versus-host disease. Radiology 102:623–624, 1972.

87. Jones B, Kramer SS, Saral R, et al: Gastrointestinal inflammation after bone marrow transplantation: graft-versus-host disease or opportunistic infection? AJR 150:277–281, 1988.

88. Gramm HF, Vincent ME, Braver JM: Differential diagnosis of tubular small bowel. Curr Imaging 2:62–70, 1990.

89. Richards DG, Somers S, Issenman RM, et al: Cow's milk protein/soy protein allergy: gastrointestinal imaging. Radiology 167:721–723, 1988.

90. Jones B, Fishman EK, Kramer SS, et al: Computed tomography of gastrointestinal inflammation after bone marrow transplantation. AJR 146:691–695, 1986.

91. McDonald GB, Sullivan KM, Schuffler MD, et al: Esophageal abnormalities in chronic graft-versus-host disease in humans. Gastroenterology 80:914–921, 1981.

92. Goodrich MJ, Mori M, Gleaves CA, et al: Early treatment with ganciclovir to prevent cytomegalovirus disease after allogeneic bone marrow transplantation. N Engl J Med 325:1601–1607, 1991.

93. Amromin GD, Solomon RD: Necrotizing enteropathy: a complication of treated leukemia or lymphoma patients. JAMA 182:23–29, 1962.

94. Mulholland MW, Delaney JP: Neutropenic colitis and aplastic anemia: a new association. Ann Surg 197:84–90, 1983.

95. Wagner ML, Rosenberg HS, Fernbach DJ, et al: Typhlitis: a complication of leukemia in childhood. AJR 109:341–350, 1970.

96. Bierman HR, Amronin G: The ileo-cecal syndrome in the leukopathic conditions. Clin Res 8:134, 1960.

97. Frick MP, Maile CW, Crass JR, et al: Computed tomography of neutropenic colitis. AJR 143:763–765, 1984.

98. Merine DS, Fishman EK, Jones B, et al: Right lower quadrant pain in the immunocompromised patient. CT findings in 10 cases. AJR 149:1177–1179, 1987.

99. Merine D, Fishman EK, Jones B: Pseudomembranous colitis: CT evaluation. J Comput Assist Tomogr 11:1017–1020, 1987.

100. Fishman EK, Kavuru M, Jones B, et al: Pseudomembranous colitis: CT evaluation of 26 cases. Radiology 180:57–60, 1991.

# Malabsorption

## Hans Herlinger, M.D.

## PATHOPHYSIOLOGY

The term *malabsorption* embraces many diseases. The intake of food substances into the body depends on a complex mix of digestion, absorption, and transport beyond the intestinal mucosa. It is not a purpose of this chapter to review all the digestive processes that render food fit for absorption. However, because steatorrhea is a hallmark of malabsorption, it seems relevant to provide a brief account of the digestion, absorption, and assimilation of dietary fat.

### Digestion and Absorption of Dietary Fat

Between 120 and 150 g of lipids is consumed in developed countries per person each day. Most are long chain triglycerides, with smaller amounts of phospho-lipids and cholesterol. The digestive processes involved are emulsification, lipolysis, and formation of micelles. Initial emulsification occurs in the stomach, under the influence of peristalsis and gastric lipase. Emulsification into tinier fat globules continues in the duodenum. Pancreatic lipase, requiring a pH level between 6.0 and 7.5, digests the fat globules to form monoglycerides and fatty acids for complex micelle formations with bile acids and biliary phospholipids. Fat in micellar form can be transported through the unstirred water layer to reach the surface epithelium. Once in contact with the lipid cell walls of the enterocytes, the dietary lipids enter the cytoplasm rapidly, mostly by passive diffusion.

After the dissolution of the micelles, the bile salts remain outside the cell membranes and re-enter the bowel lumen for solubilization of further lipids. They reach the terminal ileum, where almost 95% are reabsorbed and return to the liver, once again to be secreted into bile. The total 3-g body pool of bile salts passes through the enterohepatic circulation 4 to 12 times per day, making available 12 to 36 g of bile salts for the daily process of lipid digestion and absorption.

## Assimilation (Removal) of Dietary Fat

Within the enterocytes, resynthesized triglycerides are formed into chylomicrons with the aid of apolipoproteins (especially apolipoprotein B). In this form they are transported into lymph and blood.

## Disorders of Lipid Absorption

Lipid absorption can be curtailed or interrupted by malfunction of any one or several components of digestion, absorption, and assimilation.

1. High gastric acid output or reduced bicarbonate secretion by the pancreas and liver renders duodenal pH levels too low for lipase activity.
2. Secretion of pancreatic lipase and colipase may be reduced (as in chronic pancreatitis).
3. Parenchymal liver disease or obstructed bile ducts may deprive the bowel lumen of the bile required for efficient emulsification and absorption of lipids.
4. The enterohepatic recirculation of bile salts may be damaged by bacterial overgrowth or interrupted by extensive disease or resection of the distal ileum.
5. Diminution of the number and maturity of enterocytes (as in celiac disease [CD]) contributes to malabsorption and steatorrhea.
6. Lack of beta-lipoprotein causes accumulation of fat globules within and near enterocytes. Interruption of lymphatic communication between bowel and thoracic duct may also be due to other pathologies.

## Other Factors Responsible for Malabsorption

1. Although a wide range of normal values exists for transit through the small bowel, absorption of nutrients can be adversely affected by excessively rapid or slow passage.
2. The brush borders of mature enterocytes produce enzymes needed for the digestion of disaccharides and peptides. Their disordered function may be one of several factors associated with malabsorption.

## CLASSIFICATION OF MALABSORPTION

1. *Maldigestion.* Chronic pancreatitis, cholestasis, deficiency of disaccharidases, ileitis or ileal resection, and Zollinger-Ellison syndrome (ZES) are common conditions associated with malabsorption.
2. *Malabsorption at the mucosal level.* This is the principal mechanism in diseases including CD, extensive Crohn's disease, tropical sprue, short bowel syndrome, cystic fibrosis (CF), eosinophilic gastroenteritis (EGE), Whipple's disease, amyloidosis, hypogammaglobulinemia, mastocytosis, and parasitoses.
3. *Malassimilation.* This occurs in primary or secondary lymphangiectasia and abetalipoproteinemia.
4. *Malabsorption caused by bacterial overgrowth.* This is mostly stasis related and occurs in conditions including idiopathic pseudo-obstruction, systemic sclerosis, diverticulosis, lumen-obstructing lesions, surgical blind loops, and fistulas.

## CLINICAL RECOGNITION OF A MALABSORPTION STATE

Patients with advanced malabsorption may present with any or several of the following clinical features:

1. Diarrhea
2. Steatorrhea (bulky, greasy, difficult to flush stools)
3. Flatulence, abdominal distention
4. Weight loss

The clinical diagnosis of malabsorption is not a problem when its classic features are present. More often, however, the early stages of malabsorption states are atypical and may remain unrecognized for a long time. Specific deficiencies of nutrient or vitamin absorption may be manifested by features such as paresthesia, bone pain, tetany, glossitis, cheilosis, anemia, and lassitude. Two thirds of patients with CD, for example, presented trivial, unusual, or even misleading symptoms.[1] When a malabsorption state is suspected on clinical grounds, it must be confirmed by a number of tests, at this stage not including radiology.

**Blood Tests.** These include a complete blood count, liver function tests, and estimates of iron, folates, albumin, and vitamins K, D, and $B_{12}$.

**Fecal Fat Estimation.** The cumbersome 72-hour quantitative fecal fat analysis has been replaced by a simple qualitative test that can detect fat malabsorption in 90% of cases.[2] Estimation of $^{14}C$ in the breath after ingestion of radioactive triglyceride equals the accuracy of quantitative fecal fat estimation.[3]

**The D-Xylose Absorption Test.** Once considered reliable for estimation of the intestinal stages of digestion and absorption, this test has fallen into disuse because it is affected by renal function and intake of nonsteroidal anti-inflammatory drugs.

**The D-[$^{14}C$]Xylose Breath Test.** This is the test of choice for detecting bacterial overgrowth. Gram-negative bacteria metabolize D-[$^{14}C$]xylose to $^{14}CO_2$, which is exhaled after absorption and measured.[4]

**Hydrogen Test for Lactase Deficiency.** Basal breath hydrogen levels are measured first, followed by ingestion of lactose, at 1 g/kg body weight. A rise of more than 20 ppm in exhaled hydrogen is diagnostic of lactase deficiency. Lactase deficiency was formerly diagnosed by radiology,[5] but this is no longer done.

# RADIOLOGY IN MALABSORPTION

## Barium Suspensions

Many years ago barium suspensions flocculated readily in the presence of fatty acids, mucin, proteins, and other factors. Excessive fluid with inadequately digested fat in the bowel lumen caused flocculation, seen as various forms of barium clumping, and this was referred to as the *malabsorption pattern.* In many instances, however, this pattern was not due to steatorrhea, often remained unexplained, and was even believed to be related to emotional disturbances.[6] Yet radiologists and many clinicians were ready to accept this finding as an indicator of a possible malabsorption state and as the major purpose of radiology in this group of patients.

## Role of Radiology

The role and purpose of radiodiagnosis in malabsorption states have changed. The recognition of a malabsorption state is based on clinical and biochemical evidence. Only exceptionally should radiology be expected to demonstrate features that suggest this diagnosis. The function of radiology is to provide indications of the cause of malabsorption and, at a later stage, of its possible complications. Radiologic features of some of the causes of malabsorption can be unmistakable, as in certain bacterial overgrowth syndromes. With other pathologies, the changes from normality may be quite subtle and identifiable only by using the best possible technique and avoiding flocculation of barium. When barium begins to form flocs, the aggregated barium particles are no longer capable of fine and uniform adherence to the mucosa to provide a radiologic appearance that mirrors subtle surface alterations.

## Technique

Modern barium suspensions no longer flocculate massively, although a lesser degree of aggregation still occurs, especially in follow-through examinations. In malabsorption states in which increased small bowel fluid may be steatorrheic, the deterioration of barium suspensions is related to the quantity of infused barium versus the amount of luminal fluid and to the time available for their interaction. Thus, the more rapidly a larger amount of barium enters and passes through the small bowel, the less deleterious the effect on the barium suspension. This is the main reason why I consider enteroclysis to be the primary barium study of the small bowel when malabsorption is suspected.

It is necessary to modify enteroclysis somewhat when malabsorption with luminal fluid increase is likely. The catheter should not be advanced too far and the balloon should not be inflated beyond the distal duodenum because it is important to include the duodenojejunal flexure in this examination. A larger amount of barium (about 240 mL) is injected more rapidly, followed by methylcellulose. Because, in severe cases of steatorrhea, barium may not adhere for long near the tip of the catheter, compression spot films of the first loops of jejunum should be taken early, disregarding the possible adverse effect on double contrast formation. All bowel loops should be imaged with compression as soon as the lumen has become distended.

## Potential and Limitations

Many diseases may be associated with malabsorption, but barium radiology can demonstrate only a limited number of deviations from normality. Moreover, some of the diseases to be considered (e.g., amyloidosis) can present in several different ways. Many of the causes of malabsorption are rarities, not always seen in the working life of individual radiologists.

The "gold standard" in the diagnosis of malabsorption-related diseases must be mucosal biopsy and histologic study. Yet, there are conditions that share similar clinical and histologic findings. At such times, clinical differential diagnosis can be helped by enteroclysis. More often, the radiologic differential diagnosis is in difficulty when enteroclysis findings are not specific for any single disease. It is then important for the radiologist to know and evaluate the clinical background of the patient and relate it to the x-ray appearances.

From the viewpoint of the radiologist, causes of malabsorption can be divided into two groups:[7]

1. Those in which an almost specific enteroclysis pattern occurs, although clinical tests including mucosal biopsy are needed for confirmation. This group includes the bacterial overgrowth syndromes, adult CD, adult CF, ZES, and short bowel syndrome.
2. Other diseases in which enteroclysis changes may be subtle and are of low specificity. A radiologic differential diagnosis must then be influenced by the clinical background, the patient's history, and the clinical and radiologic pattern of involvement of other organs. Examples of this group are Whipple's disease, lymphangiectasia, amyloidosis, abetalipoproteinemia, mastocytosis, and macroglobulinemia.

Computed tomography (CT) ideally complements the accurate depiction of the mucosa by enteroclysis, being able to demonstrate the state of the bowel wall and the related mesentery, the lymph nodes in the mesentery or retroperitoneum, and more remote changes such as lesions in liver or spleen.

The following descriptions of malabsorption-related diseases include, in addition to the radiologic changes, relevant clinical features and aspects of value in the radiologic differential diagnosis.

# BACTERIAL OVERGROWTH SYNDROMES

The normal small bowel contains up to $10^4$ organisms/mL in the proximal jejunum, virtually all aerobic. More organisms are found in the distal ileum, a result of the incomplete continence of the ileocecal valve. Restriction of bacterial growth in normal small bowel relies on gastric acid; on small bowel peristalsis, especially the interdigestive migrating motor complexes; on the layer of mucus and the rapid turnover of enterocytes (the entire mucosa is replaced every 2 to 4 days);[1] and on the humoral and cellular immune defenses.[8]

Any malfunction of these defenses leads to an increased number of organisms. It is considered abnormal when a jejunal aspirate yields more than $10^6$ organisms/mL. In addition to the numerical increase, organisms are present that are normally found in the colon (including anaerobic bacteria). Antibacterial defenses can be impaired by malfunction of any or several of the conditions listed in Table 49–1.

A bacterial overload of any cause adversely affects digestion and absorption:

1. Increased deconjugation and dehydroxylation of bile salts by the bacteria reduce the amount of conjugated bile salts available for micelle formation and absorption of lipids. Deconjugated bile salts and hydroxylated fatty acids are mucosal irritants, cause fluid and electrolyte secretion, and may be responsible for patchy villous atrophy.
2. Absorption of amino acids and carbohydrates is reduced.
3. Bacteria bind and utilize vitamin $B_{12}$, rendering it unavailable for absorption. On the other hand, bacteria produce absorbable folic acid.

Several of the diseases that are frequently associated with bacterial overgrowth and its consequences are described in the following sections.

## Jejunal Diverticulosis

The diverticula are found predominantly in the jejunum, usually concentrated over a defined segment, aborally decreasing in size. They are acquired herniations of mucosa and submucosa, often with a cover of longitudinal muscle.[9] The diverticula emerge at the site of the mesenteric attachment and vasa recta entry and protrude into the space between the leaves of the mesentery. They may be hidden from view at laparotomy. The majority are asymptomatic. In many instances their presence has been a marker of disordered intestinal motility. The diverticula can be associated with intestinal pseudo-obstruction syndromes, in some cases with degeneration of the myenteric plexus and in others with vacuolation of the jejunal muscularis.[10] Episodes of acute pseudo-obstruction have been reported in 10 to 25% of cases.[11] Bacterial overgrowth resulting from retention within the diverticula or the associated pseudo-obstruction may cause mild to severe malabsorption in more than one third of the cases.[11] Most of the patients can be managed medically with periodic antibiotics. Surgical intervention has been required in up to 20%.[12, 13] Indications for surgery are hemorrhage,[14] severe malabsorption, obstruction, acute diverticulitis, and perforation with abscess formation.[15]

| TABLE 49–1. PREDISPOSING CAUSES OF BACTERIAL OVERGROWTH | |
|---|---|
| **FACTORS** | **CONDITIONS** |
| Stasis | Structural abnormalities |
| | Strictures |
| | Diverticulosis |
| | Pouches |
| | Blind loops |
| | Bypassed bowel |
| | Pseudo-obstruction* |
| Increased bacterial entry | Impaired gastric acid output |
| | Achlorhydria, hypochlorhydria |
| | Gastrectomy |
| | Atrophic gastritis |
| | Omeprazole |
| | Abnormal source of bacteria |
| | Fistulas (e.g., coloenteric) |
| | Infected bile |
| | Resected ileocecal valve |
| Immunodeficiency | Advanced age |
| | Hypogammaglobulinemia |
| | Malignancies |
| | Acquired immunodeficiency syndrome |

*See Table 49–2.

## Radiology in Jejunal Diverticulosis

Plain films obtained with the patient erect may show numerous fluid levels in the upper abdomen, caused by fluid retained in jejunal diverticula. This may be mistaken for small bowel obstruction. A film obtained with the patient supine may avoid misinterpretation because it demonstrates the diverticula as rounded air spaces without valvulae.

Barium studies, follow-through or enteroclysis, generally outline the diverticula adequately. Enteroclysis, especially when an erect double contrast view is included (Fig. 49–1), is slightly more accurate and has demonstrated jejunal diverticulosis in 2 to 2.3% of adults older than 40 years of age.[16] The length of the diverticula-bearing bowel segment is best shown by enteroclysis, an important consideration before surgical resection.

Of the complications of diverticulosis, active bleeding can be demonstrated by technetium Tc 99m sulfur colloid scanning or by blood pool labeling.[17] Selective superior mesenteric or subselective jejunal arteriography can provide a specific diverticulum-related diagnosis. Barium studies in jejunal diverticulitis show the usually smoothly rounded outpouching deformed, elongated, rigid, and tender on compression.[15] CT would demonstrate peridiverticular edema and inflammatory changes in the adjacent mesentery.[17] Perforation of a diverticulum with sealed-off abscess formation may present features of diverticulitis at barium examination, but CT is required to demonstrate the abscess itself[15] (Fig. 49–2).

## Fabry's Disease

Jejunal diverticulosis with bacterial overgrowth and anemia can be a feature of the rare Fabry's disease. The

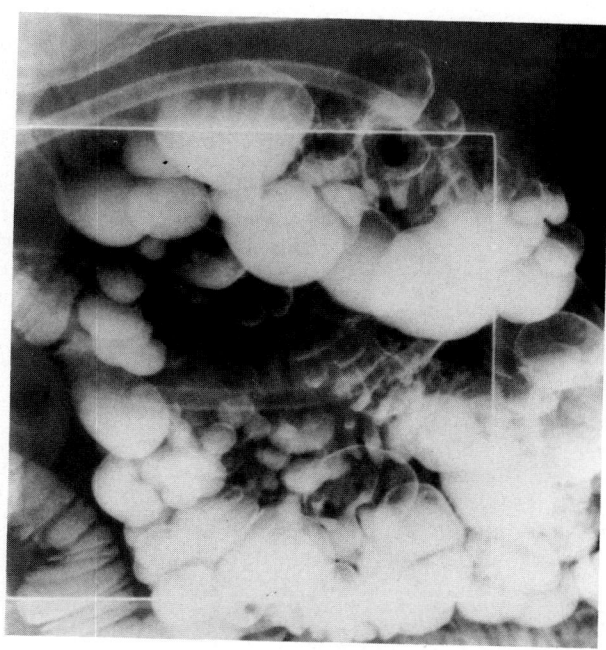

**Figure 49–1. Jejunal diverticulosis.** With the patient almost erect, fluid levels draw attention to the presence of the diverticula.

disease is characterized by glycolipid deposits in most tissues and can be demonstrated by rectal or intestinal biopsy that is not too superficial.[18] Small bowel ischemia may lead to ileal perforation.

## Intestinal Pseudo-obstruction

Pseudo-obstruction is a condition with signs and symptoms of bowel obstruction in the absence of a mechanical cause. The not infrequent association between jejunal

diverticulosis and chronic pseudo-obstruction has already been mentioned. Pseudo-obstructions can be primary or secondary.

### Primary Pseudo-obstruction

This chronic condition may be familial or arise de novo. In both cases the underlying pathologic condition is either a visceral myopathy or a visceral neuropathy. Visceral neuropathy requires full-thickness biopsy and special staining techniques for histologic diagnosis.[19] The

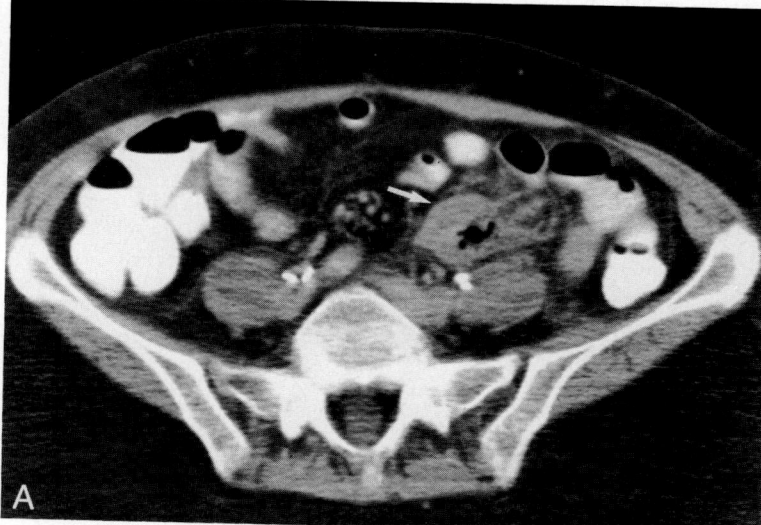

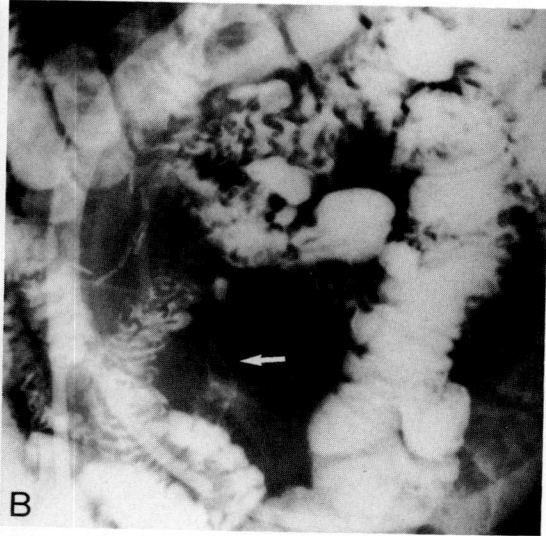

**Figure 49–2. Jejunal diverticulitis.** The patient had acute onset of left paraumbilical pain, chills, and fever. **A.** A CT scan outlines an inflammatory mass involving the jejunum and its mesentery *(arrow).* **B.** Follow-through examination shows multiple jejunal diverticula, one deformed and surrounded by a tender mass *(arrow).* (**A** and **B** from Benya EC, Ghahremani GG, Brosnan JJ: Diverticulitis of the jejunum: clinical and radiologic features. Gastrointest Radiol 16:24–28, 1991.)

myenteric plexus may have been damaged by drugs, viruses, or chemicals. Bowel loops are dilated but show activity, mostly irregular, nonpropulsive contractions. Visceral myopathy is an even rarer disease entity. Dilated bowel loops are virtually aperistaltic and retain an increased amount of fluid and air.

Bacterial overgrowth and malabsorption complicate most of the long-standing cases. An antegrade barium study to exclude a mechanical obstruction should be avoided, if possible. CT examination should take its place. Cisapride, a promising gastrointestinal prokinetic agent, acts selectively on the myenteric plexus[20] and may improve symptoms.

## Secondary Pseudo-obstruction

The pseudo-obstruction syndromes may be associated with a variety of causes, listed in Table 49–2. They have in common the presence of a dilated, flaccid bowel with associated bacterial overgrowth and malabsorption.

## Systemic Sclerosis

Systemic sclerosis is the most frequent cause of chronic intestinal pseudo-obstruction. It is a progressively disabling multisystem disease in which the involvement of kidneys, lungs, and heart threatens survival more than the changes in the gastrointestinal tract. Involvement of the esophagus occurs in most patients. Small bowel changes are reported in about 60% of cases but are not always symptomatic. Malabsorption is seen in one third of the patients and stasis-related bacterial overgrowth is its major cause. However, collagen deposition around vessels in the submucosa and mucosal

### TABLE 49–2. CAUSES OF SECONDARY PSEUDO-OBSTRUCTION

| ABNORMALITY | CAUSES |
|---|---|
| Structural change* | Blind loop |
| | Side-to-side anastomosis |
| | Bypassed bowel |
| | Jejunal diverticulosis |
| | Pouches |
| Smooth muscle disease | Systemic sclerosis |
| | Systemic lupus erythematosus |
| | Mixed connective tissue disease |
| | Muscular dystrophy |
| | Amyloidosis |
| Neurologic disease | Chagas' disease |
| | Carcinomatous visceral neuropathy |
| | Diabetes |

*For further details see Chapter 54.

atrophy are additional factors and reasons for incomplete relief by broad-spectrum antibiotics.

## Radiologic Findings

Aperistalsis in the distal two thirds of the esophagus, a patulous lower esophageal sphincter, and reflux esophagitis possibly leading to Barrett's esophagus have been described in Chapters 23 and 24. Distended, gas- and fluid-containing bowel loops may show irregular activity. The second and third parts of the duodenum and the jejunum are predominantly affected. The pathognomonic finding on barium study is the "hidebound" appearance of the small intestine,[21] a combination of lumen dilatation and crowding of normal circular folds (Fig. 49–3). This is seen in more than 60% of cases of

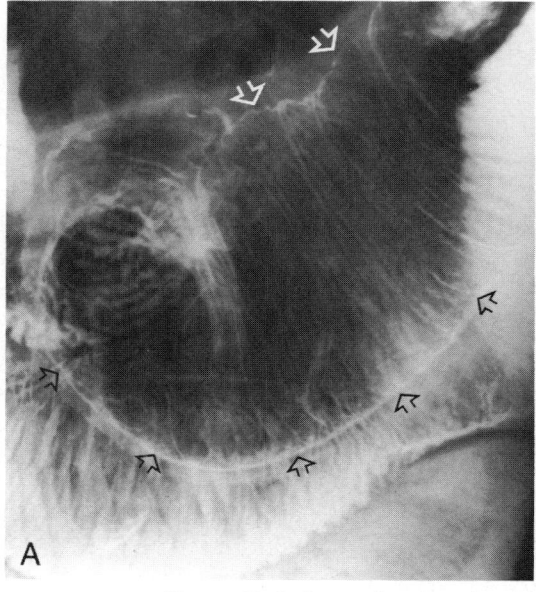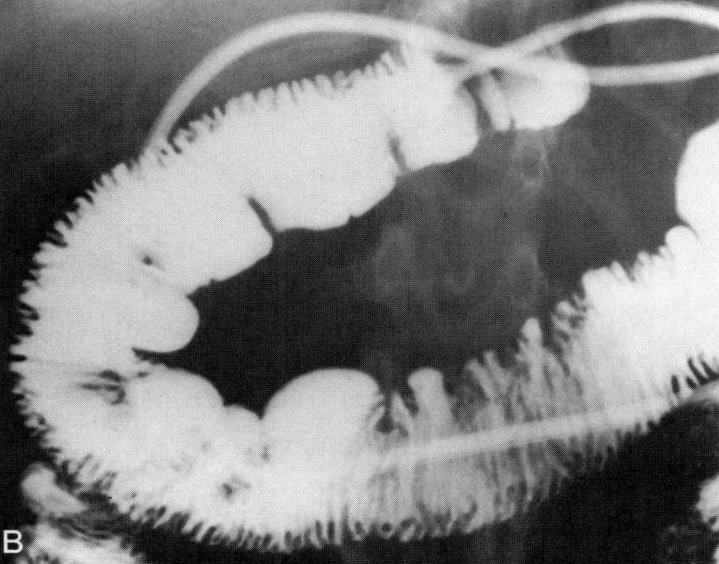

**Figure 49–3. Systemic sclerosis with involvement of the small bowel. A.** Grossly dilated loop of jejunum with crowded folds of normal thickness, the hidebound bowel sign *(arrows).* **B.** Loop of jejunum with crowded folds in a nondistended lumen. Numerous sacculations are seen at the mesenteric border, not at their more usual antimesenteric location.

scleroderma-related pseudo-obstruction and is thought to be due to muscle atrophy and uneven replacement of muscle by collagen, mostly involving longitudinal fibers. Intense fibrosis of the submucosa may contribute to this appearance. Another characteristic finding is sacculation (see Fig. 49–3B), mostly at the antimesenteric border but more often seen in the colon than in the small bowel. (*Note: sacculations* are focal, broad-based, mostly antimesenteric bulges composed of all layers of the wall, usually with weakened muscularis. Acquired *diverticula* are at the mesenteric border, have a narrow neck, and consist of mucosa and submucosa plus some muscle fibers.)

Pneumatosis intestinalis has been described and is prognostically unfavorable. A chronic, benign pneumo-peritoneum may be associated. Transient, nonobstructive intussusceptions have been observed.

## Variants of Systemic Sclerosis

Polymyositis (called dermatomyositis if skin lesions coexist) mostly affects striated muscle. Radiologic changes chiefly affect the pharynx and upper esophagus. In the small bowel, there may be dilatation and delayed transit.

Mixed connective tissue disease, a combination of systemic sclerosis, polymyositis, and systemic lupus erythematosus, is a rare cause of intestinal pseudo-obstruction.

## Amyloidosis

Although it is only infrequently complicated by intestinal pseudo-obstruction, amyloidosis in all its presentations and patterns of involvement of the small bowel is discussed here.

Amyloid is an insoluble, eosinophilic glycoprotein with special staining characteristics.[22] A plasma cell dyscrasia may be responsible for the deposition of amyloid light chain (AL), which contains fragments of monoclonal immunoglobulin light chains (primary or myeloma-associated amyloidosis). Amyloid A (AA) or secondary amyloid affects patients with chronic inflammatory conditions, rheumatoid arthritis, and, rarely, Crohn's disease. The gastrointestinal tract is involved in 70% of cases of primary and 55% of secondary amyloidosis.[23] Apart from the gastrointestinal tract, primary amyloidosis affects kidneys, heart, joints, tongue, and carpal tunnel; secondary amyloidosis affects kidneys, liver, and spleen.

Clinical presentations of intestinal amyloidosis include abdominal pain, diarrhea, obstructive features, and malabsorption of various degrees of severity. Confirmation of clinical or radiologic suspicion requires rectal, gastric, or upper intestinal biopsy.

### Radiology in Intestinal Tract Amyloidosis

Intestinal amyloid can be deposited in the walls of blood vessels, causing ischemia; in the muscularis, caus-

ing muscle atrophy and dysmotility; and in the mucosa and submucosa, producing impairment of absorption.[23] Amyloidosis may remain asymptomatic even with widespread infiltration. Findings of follow-through barium studies include fold thickening, nodularity, lumen narrowing, and separation of loops.

Tada and colleagues[24] studied 26 patients with amyloidosis of the gastrointestinal tract by a combination of enteroclysis, jejunal endoscopy, and biopsy with histology and obtained the following findings:

1. A micronodular mucosal surface pattern in 16 patients together with fold irregularity in 12 of the patients (Fig. 49–4A). Biopsy histologic study showed amyloid deposition in the lamina propria extending into widened villi. The same appearance and its pathologic correlation were described in an earlier case report.[25]
2. Isolated polypoid protrusions into the lumen in three patients (Fig. 49–4B). Histologic study demonstrated massive amyloid deposits in the submucosa.
3. Mucosal 3- to 4-mm nodules shown by enteroclysis (Fig. 49–4C) with shallow ulcers shown by endoscopy in four patients. Histologic examination showed amyloid deposition in the walls of vessels in the submucosa.
4. No radiologic abnormality in three patients.

Earlier barium follow-through examinations of patients with intestinal amyloidosis showed only thickened folds and nodularity. Pseudo-obstruction has been the radiologic feature in 8 of 121 patients with amyloidosis,[26] with only 1 patient surviving more than 3 months.

## Visceral Neuropathy of Carcinomatosis

Intestinal pseudo-obstruction resulting from paraneoplastic visceral neuropathy has been described in small cell carcinoma of the lung.[27] It may precede the demonstration of the tumor. Onset of unexplained pseudo-obstruction in older patients requires exclusion of this possible cause.

## Diabetes and Small Intestinal Dysmotility

Diarrhea and steatorrhea occur in diabetic neuropathy with an incidence of up to 10%.[28] Bacterial overgrowth is the likely cause, but chronic pancreatitis and CD must be ruled out. Plain abdominal films show small bowel dilatation, possibly with features of edema.

## ADULT CELIAC DISEASE

### Introduction

The gold standard for the diagnosis of CD consists of the characteristic, although not specific, changes shown

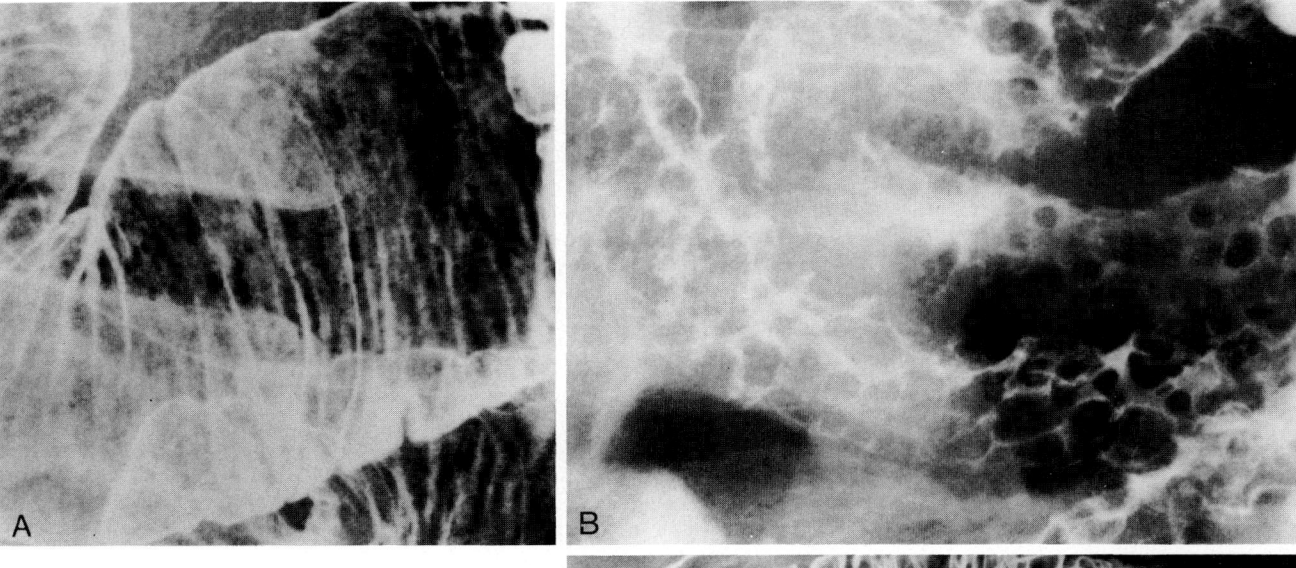

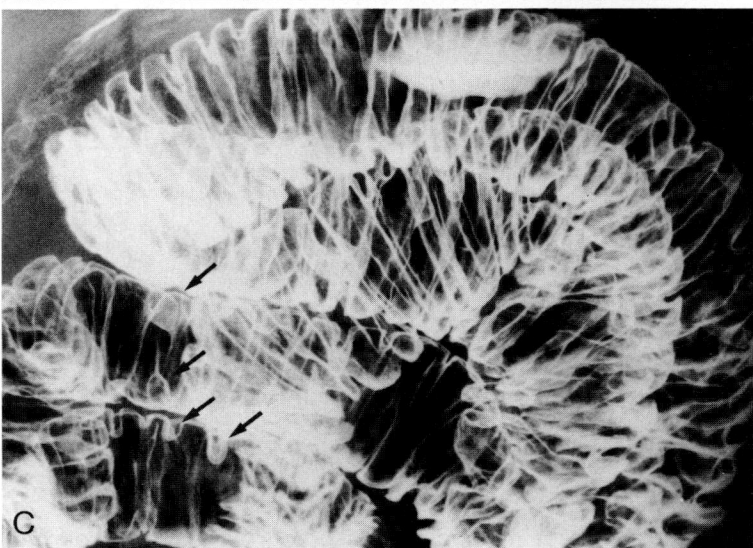

**Figure 49–4. Amyloidosis of the small bowel, enteroclysis. A.** Coarse granularity of the mucosal surface. Histologic examination showed amyloid deposition in the lamina propria extending into wide, blunted villi. **B.** Pattern of coarse nodularities throughout segments of jejunum. Amyloid was deposited in the wall of vessels in the submucosa. **C.** Thickened folds and multiple polyps *(arrows).* Biopsy histologic section showed massive deposition of amyloid in the submucosa. (**A** to **C** from S Tada, M Iida, T Matsui, et al, Amyloidosis of the small intestine: findings on double-contrast radiographs, AJR, 156, 4, 741–744, 1991, © by American Roentgen Ray Society.)

by histologic study of biopsy specimens of duodenal or jejunal mucosa. Their causal relationship to CD must be confirmed by a favorable clinical response to a gluten-free diet and, preferably also, by reversion to near normality on a follow-up mucosal biopsy. Yet this important disease is beset with problems of clinical recognition. Radiology can provide significant help to the clinician because enteroclysis can diagnose or rule out CD in more than two thirds of the patients.

CD appears to be identical in adults and children. Adult CD may be an extension of the childhood disease, separated by years of latency, or it may be a new disease.

## Pathogenesis and Prevalence

Gliadin fractions of gluten are a causative factor. Among genetic factors involved is an association with class II human leukocyte antigens, especially HLA-DR3. Immunologic processes also appear to be in-

volved, with increased production of immunoglobulin A (IgA) and immunoglobulin M (IgM) antigliadin antibodies. Of perhaps overriding importance are an increased number of intraepithelial lymphocytes and activation of T lymphocytes in the lamina propria.[29, 30]

In Europe, prevalence is lowest in the southeast and increases in a northwesterly direction. The highest incidence has been in Ireland, especially in the area surrounding the ancient city of Galway. CD is almost unknown among native Africans, Japanese, and Chinese but does occur on the Indian subcontinent.[30] Adult CD affects women more frequently than men.

## Clinical Diagnosis

Fewer than half of the patients present in typical fashion with steatorrhea, abdominal distention, glossitis, and changes in pigmentation. Atypical presentations are numerous. In one report, hematologic abnormalities led to the diagnosis of CD in 38% of patients.[31] Other patients may complain of neuropathies, even alternating constipation and diarrhea. Of elderly patients with newly developed CD, only 25% presented with typical clinical features.[32] Perhaps the first case report illustrating radiologic features of CD was published in 1935 with the diagnosis of idiopathic adult tetany.[33]

It is a major step from clinical awareness of the possibility of CD and its diagnosis by mucosal biopsy. A screening test for CD would be valuable. Testing for CD-associated antibodies, especially antigliadin IgA, by an enzyme-linked immunosorbent assay, was 100% specific in a selected group of patients.[34] Confirmation of this result in a larger, more mixed group of patients and wider availability of the assay would lead to earlier use of mucosal biopsy.

Mucosal biopsy is now almost universally done during duodenal endoscopy, where it can provide an adequate sample and has the advantage of site selection under vision. Vague dyspepsia is a symptom frequently mentioned by CD patients, and endoscopists rarely hesitate to proceed to gastroduodenal endoscopy. Endoscopists should extend their observations to the appearance of the mucosa in the more distal duodenum. Reduction or absence of duodenal folds is associated with a high incidence of subtotal villous atrophy and mandates biopsies of more distal duodenal mucosa.[35–37]

## Duodenojejunal Mucosa

**The Normal Mucosa.** The entire mucosa, including the folds, is covered by villi. The mucosa is lined by columnar enterocytes, which develop in the depth of crypts and mature as they migrate upward toward the tips of the villi. The height of the villi exceeds the thickness of the lamina propria by a factor of 3 (Fig. 49–5A).

**The Mucosa in Celiac Disease.** Villi are absent or stunted. The lamina propria is considerably thickened, being occupied by hypertrophied crypts and an increased cellular infiltrate (Fig. 49–5B). Enterocytes now migrate and develop more rapidly, not often obtaining full maturity before they are shed into the lumen. As a result of villous atrophy, the available absorptive surface is drastically diminished.

**The Mosaic Pattern.** Duodenojejunal biopsy material in patients with villous atrophy often shows a surface pattern of interlacing grooves separating squares 1 to 3 mm in diameter. This can be seen well through a dissecting microscope. It is also recognized endoscopically, especially when aided by scattering of indigo carmine dye.[38]

**Differential Diagnosis of Villous Atrophy.** Subtotal villous atrophy, as in CD, can be found in the bacterial overgrowth syndromes, immunodeficiency states, ZES, tropical sprue, and parasitoses. Similar grades of villous atrophy may be encountered in EGE, ischemia, and radiation enteropathy.

## Radiologic Findings

### Follow-through in Celiac Disease

**The Moulage Sign.** In 1934[39] "a tendency for barium to clump into smooth, elongated masses in the proximal jejunum" was observed in patients with CD. These clumps represented massive flocculations of the barium suspensions then available. The same appearance was described again 5 years later, named the moulage sign, and claimed to be a specific sign of CD.[40] Some of the illustrations showed elongated, not lumen-imaging clumps of flocculated barium, and others showed barium that depicted a bowel lumen devoid of folds. The

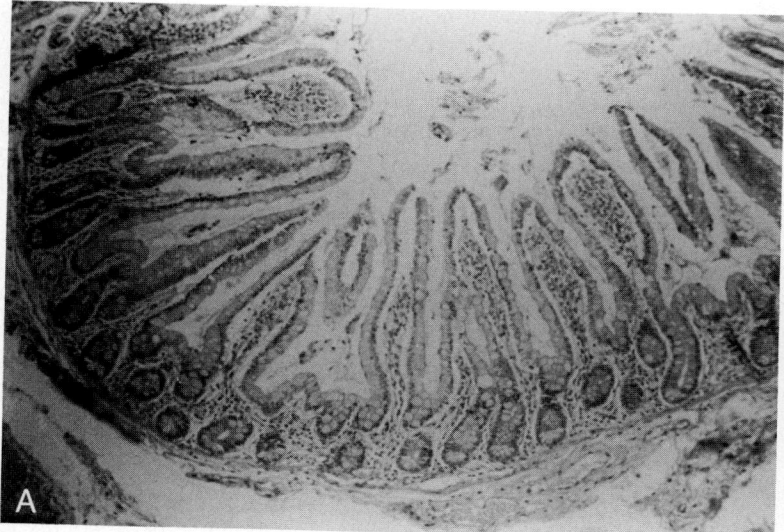
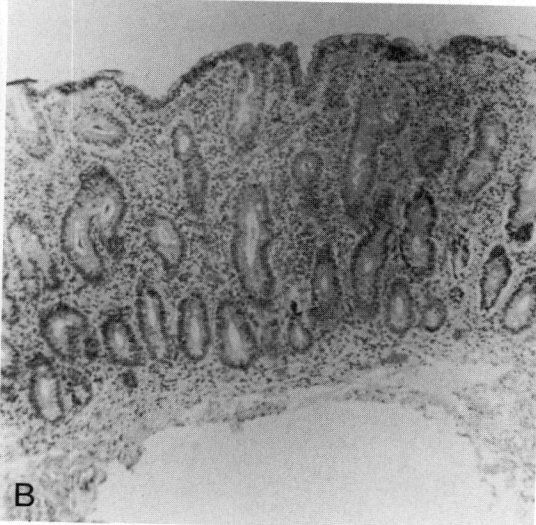

**Figure 49–5. The jejunal mucosa in normality and in CD. A.** Normal jejunal biopsy. Length of the slim villi is three times the thickness of the lamina propria. **B.** Jejunal biopsy in untreated CD. Villous atrophy is total. Lamina propria is considerably thickened with an increased number of crypts and a denser cellular infiltrate.

undescriptive term moulage sign has also been used in more recent publications.[41]

### Other Nonspecific Radiologic Findings

1. Lumen dilatation, mostly of the jejunum, has been defined as more than 30 mm in follow-through examinations. Although lumen dilatation has been correlated with increased fecal fat, it is not specific for CD and can be found in hypoalbuminemia[42] and after gastric resection.

2. Luminal fluid excess can be due to any hypersecretory state, including other conditions associated with malabsorption.

3. Fold thickening, often mentioned as a feature of CD, is not a feature of uncomplicated CD. It occurs only when there is associated edema, as in hypoalbuminemia (Fig. 49–6), or as an artifact, the gradual displacement of the barium coating by mucosal hypersecretion.

4. Painless, transient intussusceptions are often seen in fluoroscopic follow-through examinations. Lumen distention associated with enteroclysis precludes their formation.[43]

## Specific Radiologic Findings

**Jejunal Folds.** Increased separation of the mucosal folds, even their apparent absence, has been mentioned repeatedly.[39–41, 44, 45] With lumen distention achieved by enteroclysis, it became possible to determine degrees of fold separation and their relevance to the diagnosis of CD.[46] Five folds or more per inch is a normal finding (Fig. 49–7A) and renders a diagnosis of CD unlikely. Figure 49–7B shows the distribution of the number of folds in 30 patients and 30 control subjects. In 73% of patients with CD, there were three folds or fewer per inch of distended proximal jejunum (Fig. 49–7C and

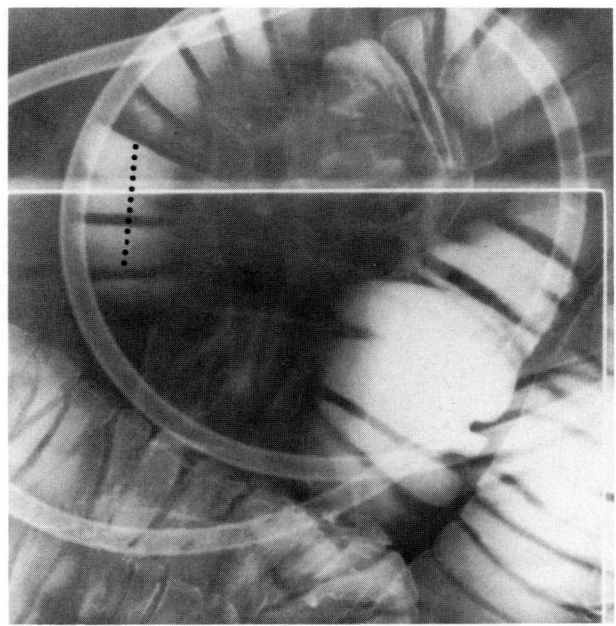

**Figure 49–6. CD.** Thick folds are due to coexistent hypoalbuminemia.

D). A small number of patients in both groups had four folds per inch, a nondiagnostic finding (see Fig. 49–7B).

A small number of follow-through examinations showed essentially the same feature in the jejunum, although in nonmeasurable form. Upper jejunal loops appear flaccid and somewhat distended and remain barium filled for longer than usual. The increased fold separation in the jejunum can also be demonstrated by CT.

**Ileal Folds.** A reversal of the normal fold character between ileum and jejunum is usual in CD. Whereas there are fewer jejunal folds per unit length, those in the ileum increase from the normal number of two to four per inch to four to six per inch. There is also an increase in the thickness of the more closely arranged folds (jejunization).[47] This change is due to the ileum's ability to take on functions normally performed by the jejunum, a process of adaptation.[47] In 30 CD patients it was not always possible to visualize the ileum in adequate distention or before significant flocculation. However, changes in the ileum, especially the increase of fold thickness above the usual 1 mm, were of confirmatory value in some of the patients[46] (Fig. 49–8A and B).

**The Mosaic Pattern.** Radiologic demonstration of this pattern in CD was first reported in 1986.[48] A network of barium-containing grooves separated areas 1 to 3 mm in diameter in 3 of 30 CD patients (Fig. 49–9). Digital image manipulation further improved their visualization.

**Changes in the Duodenum.** Several changes in the appearance of the duodenum in CD were reported at a time when the demonstration of the mesenteric small bowel was less than adequate.[49] Folds can be fewer in number and appear irregular, especially in the distal duodenum. Of 48 patients with dermatitis herpetiformis (DH), 3 with a normal-appearing jejunum had mucosal abnormalities of associated CD confined to the duodenum.[50]

Of particular interest is a report of nodular changes in the duodenum in atypical CD.[51] The three cases described appeared to have, in addition to villous atrophy of the duodenal mucosa, changes expected with increased gastric acid output and an appearance of gastric mucosal metaplasia extending into and beyond the duodenal bulb. Usually in CD there is diminution of gastric acidity, and the mucosal changes associated with villous atrophy commence beyond the duodenal bulb. I also have seen an example of "bubbly duodenum" in a patient with undoubted CD (Fig. 49–10); the significance and explanation of this finding are not yet clear.

## Jejunoileal Fold Pattern Response to a Gluten-free Diet

In an important study in Birmingham, England,[52] the jejunoileal fold pattern and the extent of its response to treatment were investigated by enteroclysis. In patients with a favorable response to gluten withdrawal, the number of folds in the jejunum returned to normal but

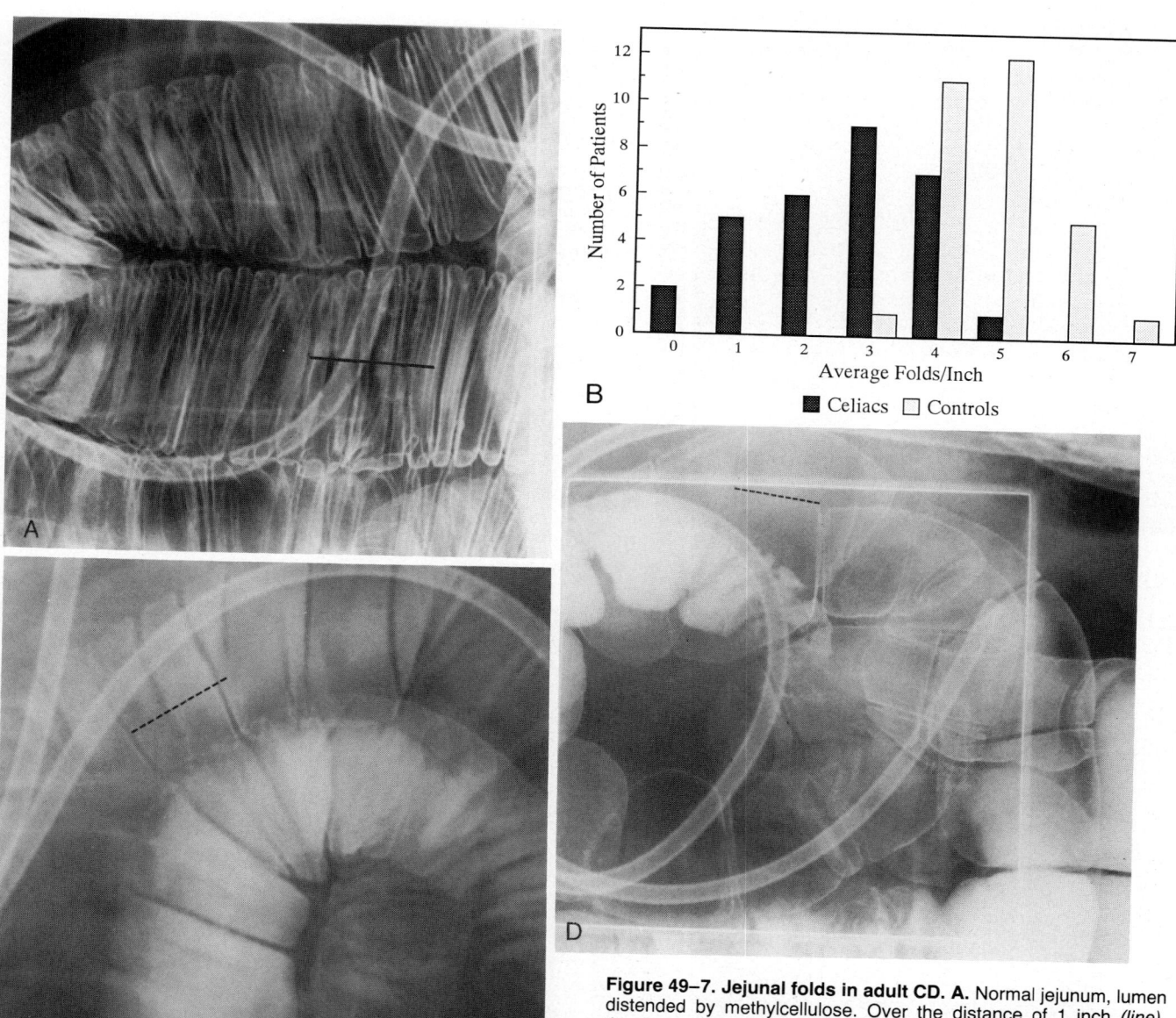

**Figure 49–7. Jejunal folds in adult CD. A.** Normal jejunum, lumen distended by methylcellulose. Over the distance of 1 inch *(line),* there are six to seven folds, a normal number for the proximal jejunum. **B.** Histogram shows the distribution of the number of folds in the distended proximal jejunum in 30 patients with CD and in 30 control subjects. Four folds per inch would be nondiagnostic. Less than four folds per inch is strongly in favor of CD and more than four folds per inch against that diagnosis. **C.** Distended proximal jejunum in CD. Over a distance of 1 inch *(dashed line),* two to three folds can be counted. **D.** Distended proximal jejunum in CD with only one to two folds per inch *(dashed line).*

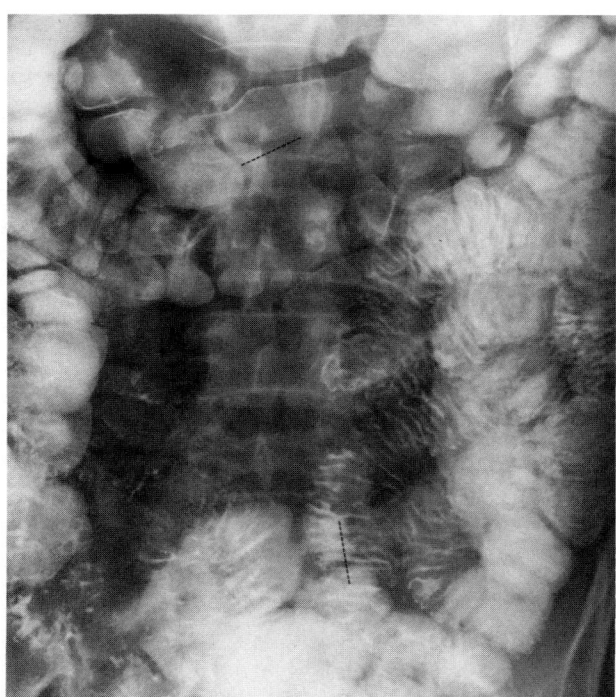

**Figure 49–8. Jejunization of ileum in CD.** Whereas the proximal jejunum shows pronounced fold separation (only one fold per inch), ileal folds are thickened (normally up to 1 mm thick) and crowded with five to six folds per inch *(lines)*.

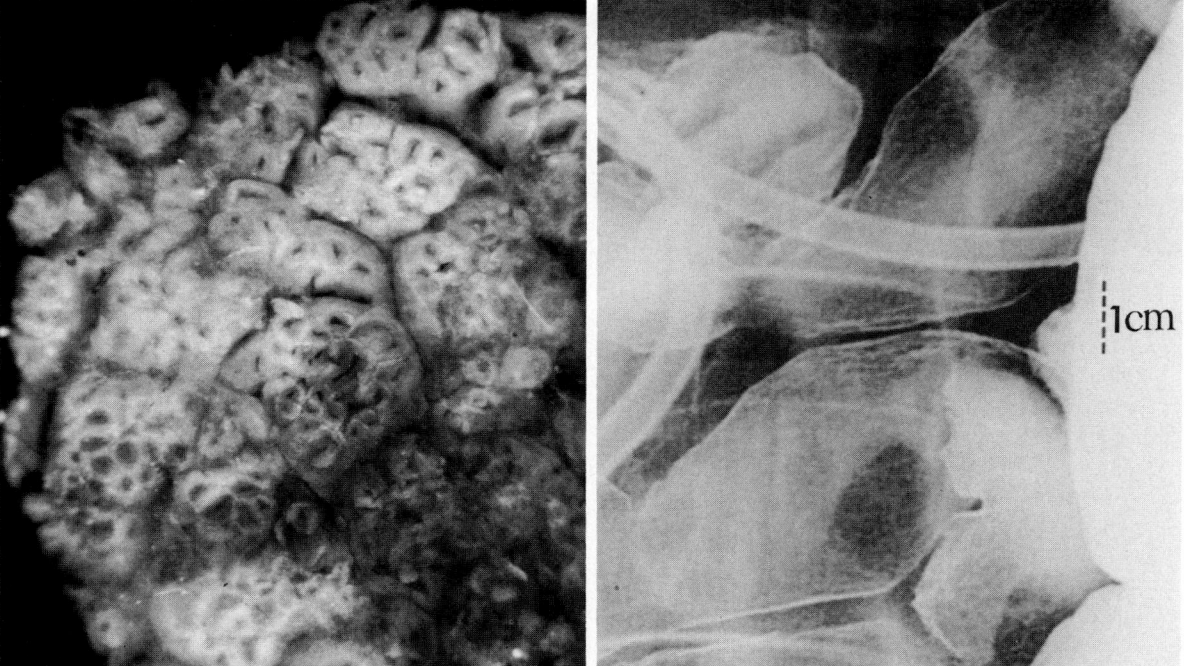

**Figure 49–9. The mosaic pattern in total villous atrophy of CD. A.** Dissecting microscopic appearance of grooves separating a mosaic pattern of islands of mucosa containing numerous crypt openings. (Courtesy of M. S. Losowsky, M.D., Leeds, England.) **B.** Enteroclysis in CD, showing virtual absence of folds. A fine, 1- to 2-mm mesh of barium-filled grooves outlines the mosaic of islands of mucosa.

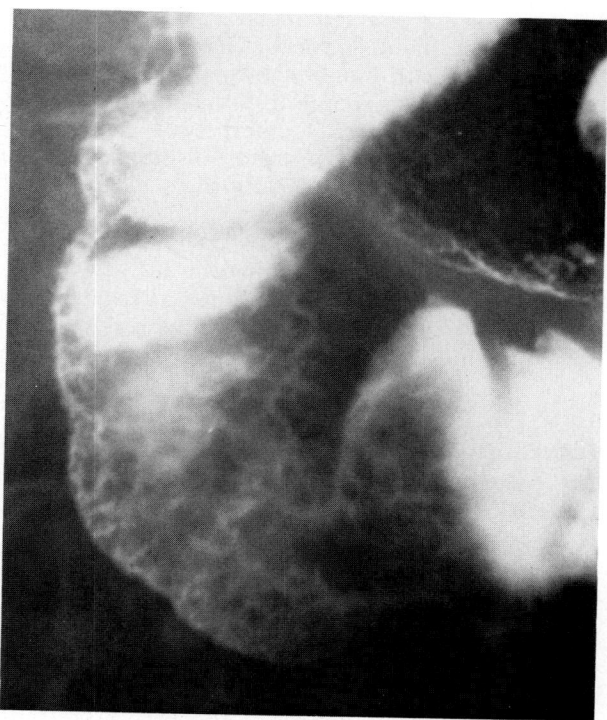

**Figure 49–10. CD showing a nodular pattern in the duodenum (bubbly duodenum).**

there was less improvement in the number of ileal folds per inch. Nonresponders to the gluten-free diet continued to have a decreased number of folds per inch in the proximal jejunum and had even more pronounced crowding of thickened ileal folds. In patients who have intermittent dietary lapses and resume their diet as soon as symptoms recur, enteroclysis may show fold separation over only a limited segment of distended jejunum

with continued fold thickening and crowding in the distal ileum (Fig. 49–11A and B).

## Relevance of Enteroclysis in Celiac Disease

In patients with atypical presentations of CD whose symptoms have some reference to the small bowel

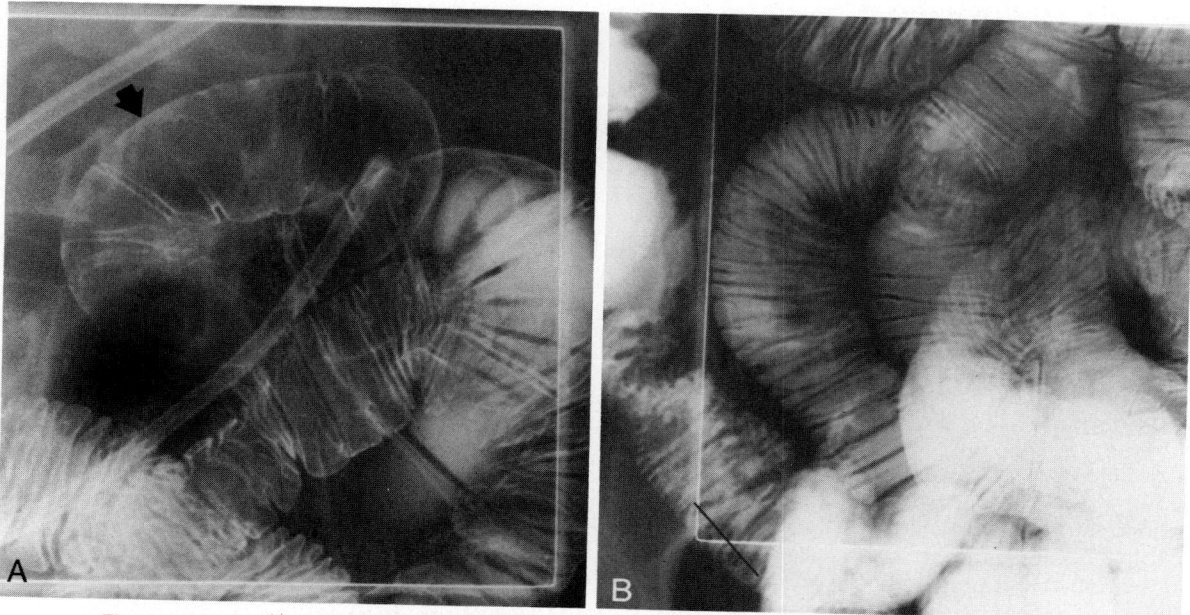

**Figure 49–11. CD in a patient with a history of dietary lapses. A.** Jejunal fold separation is visible only during lumen distention and extends over a limited area. **B.** Crowding of thickened ileal folds persists (line = 1 inch).

(diarrhea or unexplained anemia), enteroclysis can confirm or refute the diagnosis of CD.

In patients with biopsy-shown villous atrophy, crypt hyperplasia, and lamina propria inflammation—the histologic features of CD—enteroclysis can aid in the differential diagnosis from other disorders with similar mucosal abnormality. Such disorders include viral enteritis, bacterial overgrowth, giardiasis, hypogammaglobulinemia, kwashiorkor, and lymphoma.[2]

In CD patients who initially do well with the gluten-free diet and then revert to diarrhea and malabsorption, enteroclysis can demonstrate or help to exclude possible complications.

## Associated Disorders

### Dermatitis Herpetiformis

The papulovesicular rash usually involves limbs, face, and trunk symmetrically. Although the incidence of DH in celiac patients is only about 1%, celiac-type mucosa has been demonstrated in 70% of DH patients.[53] Of 82 patients with DH, most demonstrated either clear-cut evidence of associated CD or abnormalities of small bowel absorptive function in the presence of normal jejunal biopsies.[54] In patients in whom mucosal changes of CD could be demonstrated by biopsy, the distribution of the changes was patchier than is usual in CD itself.[53] On enteroclysis, the appearance of DH-associated CD is the same as that described earlier. A gluten-free diet allows reduction of the dose of dapsone in the treatment of DH and may lead to gradual disappearance of the rash and improvement of the duodenojejunal mucosal abnormalities.

### Selective Immunoglobulin A Deficiency

Deficiency of IgA is generally found in 1 in 500 to 700 persons and occurs with 10 times greater frequency in patients with CD. Some patients remain asymptomatic because IgA deficiency can be masked by an increased output of secretory IgM. It was reported years ago that IgA deficiency may be accompanied by a sprue-like syndrome that tends to respond favorably to gluten withdrawal.[54] Nodular lymphoid hyperplasia can be the radiologic presentation of IgA deficiency, possibly complicated by features of giardiasis.

### Hyposplenism

In 177 patients with untreated CD, hyposplenism was diagnosed in 76% and improved with gluten exclusion.[55] Typical blood film changes diagnostic of hyposplenism (Howell-Jolly bodies, target cells, acanthosis) were found in 29% of 41 patients with CD.[56] The severity of hyposplenism increases with age and the duration of exposure to gluten in the presence of CD. There is no evidence of an associated increased incidence of malignancy.[56]

The size of the spleen correlates well with its function.[57] Spleen size as an indicator of hyposplenism can be measured by scintigraphy or by CT (Fig. 49–12).

### Adenopathy

The demonstration of enlarged mesenteric or retroperitoneal lymph nodes in CD usually implies lymphoma.[58] Occasionally, enlarged nodes may be shown by CT in the absence of malignancy. There are no definite features distinguishing between malignant and benign nodes in CD. However, CD-associated benign adenopathy has been reported to regress with dietary treatment.

### Cavitary Mesenteric Lymph Node Syndrome

This rare CD-associated disease seems to express the effect of hyposplenism on mesenteric lymphadenopathy. The literature contains single case reports of this usually fatal condition, which occurs in long-standing, poorly controlled CD associated with severe hyposplenism.[59, 60] The nodal cavitary masses can occupy a large part of the abdomen and are filled with lipid-rich hyaline material that may produce fat-fluid levels when shown by CT (Fig. 49–13). An association with lymphoma has been reported.[61]

## Variants

### Refractory Sprue

This is a rare entity, assuming that an accurate initial diagnosis of CD was made. The likely cause is noncompliance or inadequate compliance with the exclusion of gluten from the diet. Occasionally it is due to inadvertent exposure to gluten.

### Collagenous Sprue

This is a somewhat dubious entity. Deposition of collagen directly beneath the intestinal epithelium has been regarded by some as a separate entity and an explanation for nonresponse to gluten exclusion.[62] However, a subepithelial band of collagen has also been found in patients with CD who have responded normally to their diet. It is probably not a true entity.

### Unmasked Celiac Disease

Latent CD may be activated by several stimuli. Vagotomy,[63] pregnancy, gastric surgery, respiratory infections,[63] and midgut ischemia are among the factors responsible for activation.

## Complications

### Ulcerative Jejunoileitis

This incompletely understood condition is associated with significant mortality. It may present in acute form

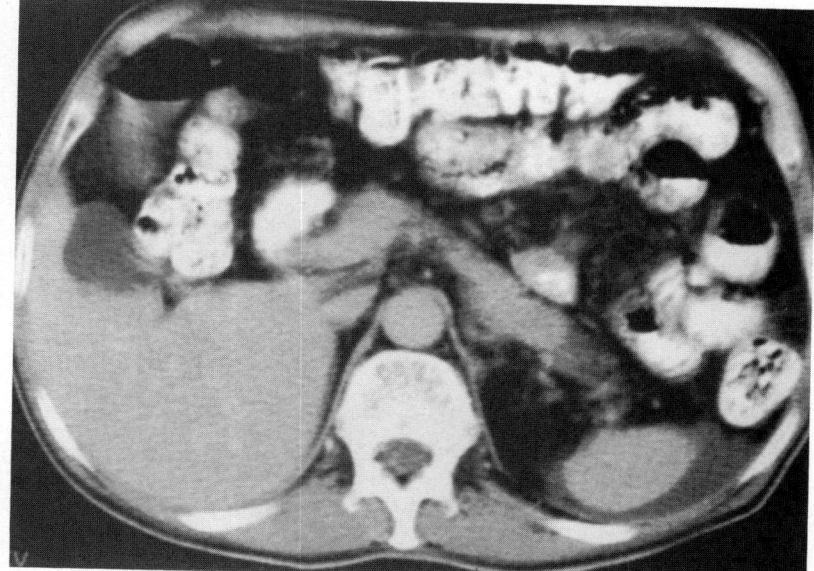

**Figure 49–12. Hyposplenism in CD.** The CT scan demonstrates the small size of the spleen.

or develop gradually. Surgical resection of the involved area of bowel is required. The usual finding is one or several segments of thickened small bowel with irregularly thickened folds and ulceration not readily demonstrated by barium studies (Fig. 49–14A). Other patients have multiple isolated ulcers that tend to penetrate deeply into the bowel wall and, if the patient recovers, leave a residue of multiple, short strictures mostly in the jejunum (Fig. 49–14B).

Ulcerative jejunoileitis bears a distinct relationship to CD. About one third of patients with this relatively rare disease have had a prior diagnosis of CD and early response to gluten withdrawal. A slightly larger group have an inadequately documented history of malabsorption preceding the onset of jejunoileitis; in this group, too, the condition may be related to CD. A much smaller third group present an almost identical condition without any association with CD, which is known as nongranulomatous jejunoileitis.

Careful histologic search of the resected specimen may reveal evidence of lymphoma. In other cases, lymphoma may develop after resection.[64]

## Lymphoma

In 1962 it was shown that lymphoma was a complication of CD and not the primary cause of malabsorption.[65] Small bowel non-Hodgkin's lymphoma is the most common malignancy complicating CD. Most such lymphomas are of T cell derivation. Lymphoma may present in the following ways:

1. With insidious onset in a patient who had been doing well with a gluten-free diet and then developed symptoms of abdominal pain, weight loss,

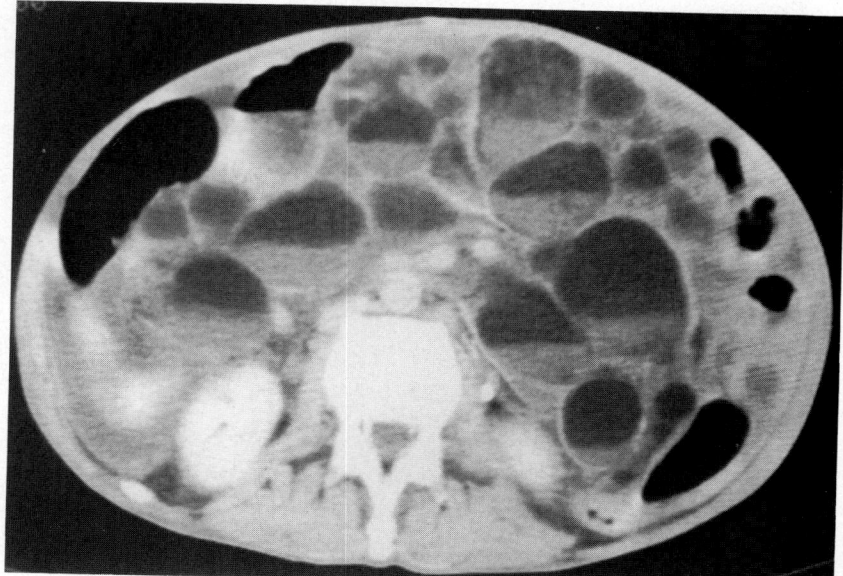

**Figure 49–13. CD complicated by cavitary lymph node syndrome.** The CT scan shows lipid-fluid levels in cavities throughout the mesentery.

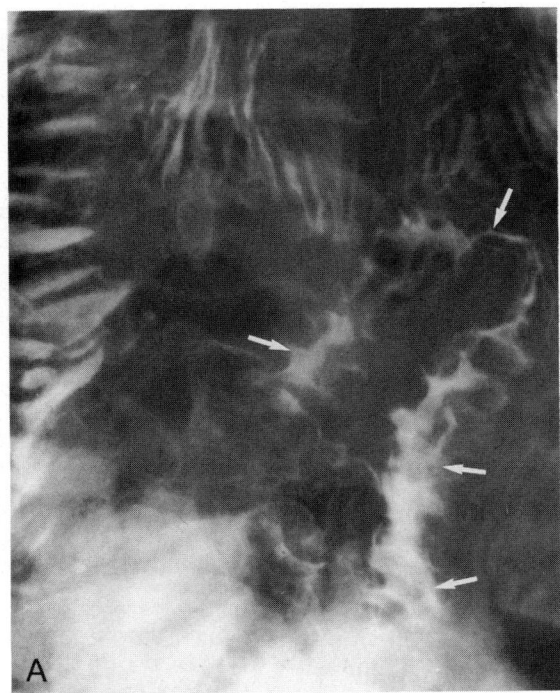

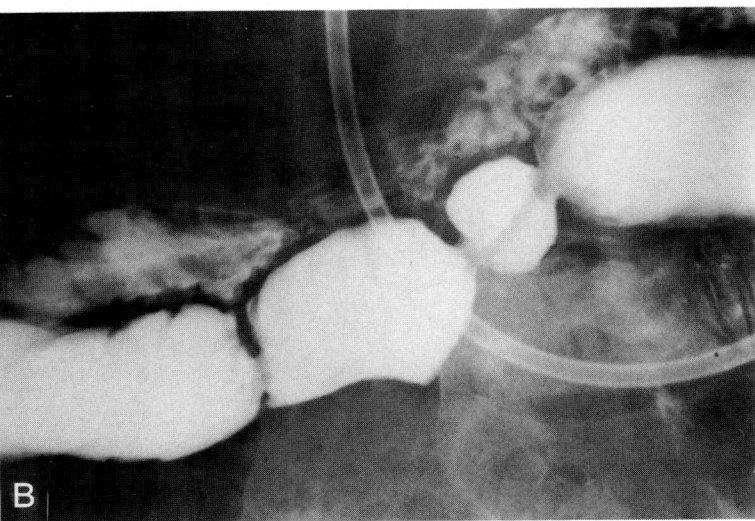

**Figure 49–14. Ulcerative jejunoileitis complicating CD. A.** Active disease. The affected bowel segment *(arrows)* shows nodular filling defects, ulceration, and lumen reduction. Postresection histology showed no evidence of lymphoma. (Courtesy of Fiona M. Stevens, M.D., Galway, Ireland.) **B.** Several short strictures are a result of a discontinuous form of ulcerative jejunoileitis. (Courtesy of M. S. Losowsky, M.D., Leeds, England.)

malabsorption, and perhaps bleeding despite continued adherence to the diet. (*Note:* pain should always raise suspicion of lymphoma in patients with CD.)

2. In a more acute form with perforation, obstruction, or hemorrhage in patients known to have CD.[66] One of my patients presented with bleeding and was shown to have three separate areas of lym-

phoma, one ulcerated (Fig. 49–15A) and the others strictured.

3. Shortly after or concurrent with the appearance of features compatible with CD. This may challenge the doctrine of CD preceding lymphoma and is now referred to as enteropathy-associated T cell lymphoma. In this condition, small bowel involvement by lymphoma is usually widespread and ac-

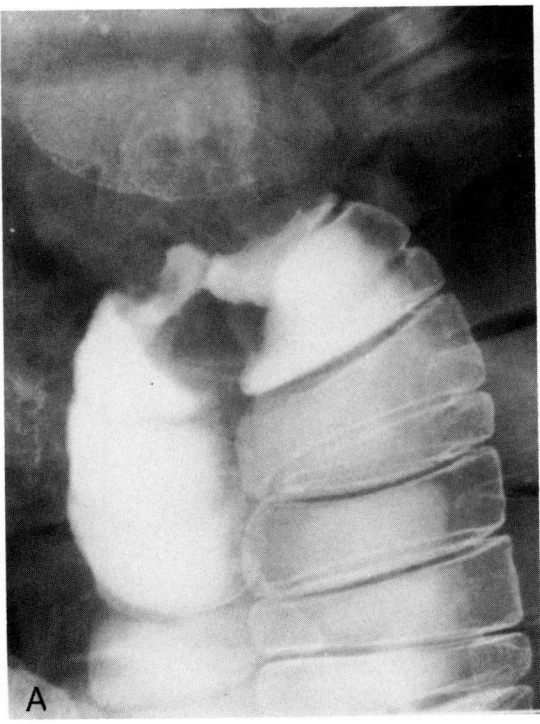

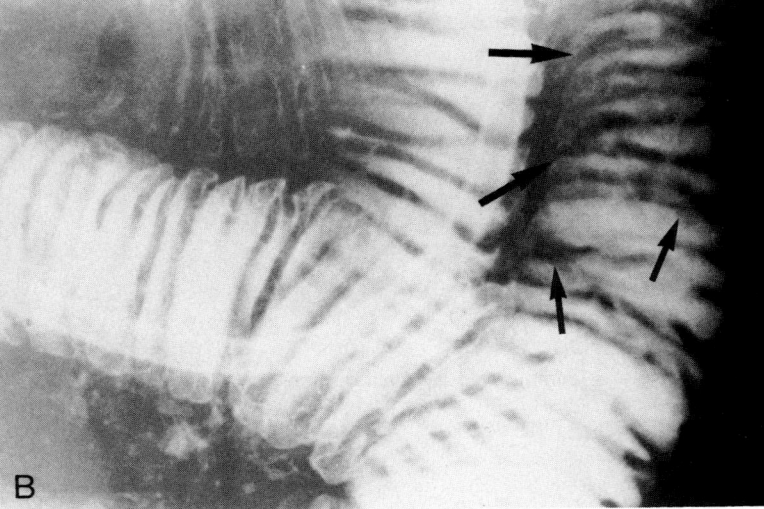

**Figure 49–15. T cell lymphoma complicating CD. A.** Ulcerated apple core–like lesion, one of three T cell lymphomas in this patient with known CD. **B.** Disseminated T cell lymphoma in a patient with a brief history of CD. Arrows indicate the nodular thickening of some of the folds, the only abnormality demonstrated in this patient.

companied by villous atrophy. Indication of associated CD requires the demonstration of subtotal villous atrophy in small bowel segments not involved by lymphoma.[67]

**Radiologic Findings.** Of 15 patients in whom lymphoma was subsequently diagnosed, follow-through barium examinations made this diagnosis in only 4.[32] Only multiple, fairly large polypoid lesions or extrinsic masses could be identified. Demonstration of the subtle features of T cell lymphoma is much more difficult and possible only by enteroclysis (Fig. 49–15B). Limited areas of nodular fold thickening and possibly slight resistance to lumen distention may be the only abnormal findings.[64] Duodenal mucosal biopsies may not be able to confirm this enteroclysis-shown abnormality. Demonstration by CT of wall thickening and enlarged nodes may support the enteroclysis finding and would encourage resort to the (usually only) means of making a definite diagnosis—an open, full-thickness biopsy of the bowel wall.

As already mentioned, ulcerative jejunoileitis is radiologically indistinguishable from lymphoma and requires surgical removal. Radiologic follow-up to identify any later development of lymphoma is essential.

Some reason for optimism is given by a report that strict adherence to gluten exclusion reduces long-term malignancy in CD patients.[68]

## Carcinoma

Deaths resulting from CD are more likely to occur in the early stages of the disease, especially in newly affected elderly patients. Many of these deaths are due to enteropathy-associated T cell lymphoma.

Cancers of the esophagus, pharynx, duodenum (Fig. 49–16), and rectum were found more frequently in patients with CD than in the general population. There

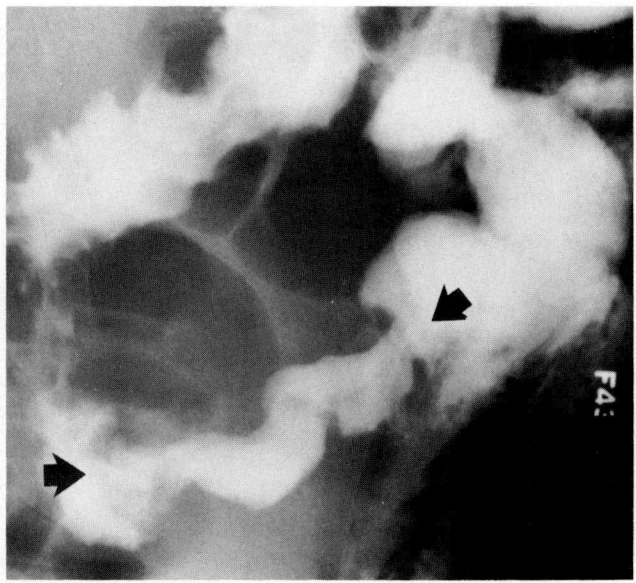

**Figure 49–16. Adenocarcinoma of the ascending duodenum, a complication of CD.**

is also a definite increase of carcinoma of the jejunum.[69–71] Multiple adenocarcinomas of the jejunum and duodenum have been described in a CD patient who had initially done well with a gluten-free diet.[72] Men seem to be at greater risk than women. Again, the clinical picture is that of patients successfully pursuing their dietary restriction, whose earlier symptoms recurred without dietary lapse. Eventually the clinical features of the carcinoma become evident. A radiologic search for the cause of the recurrence of symptoms of CD should be undertaken promptly.

Overall, based on a cohort of 653 patients with CD in Scotland, the total number of deaths from malignant neoplasms was 3.5 times that expected in men and 2.5 times that expected in women. Considering only malignant neoplasms occurring within 5 years of the diagnosis of CD, deaths in males were 6.9 times and those in females were 3.3 times the expected number.[73]

## TROPICAL SPRUE

Tropical sprue is a chronic diarrheal condition found in inhabitants of many tropical countries or individuals returning from a usually prolonged stay in such countries. It is characterized by gastrointestinal symptoms caused by progressive structural abnormalities of the small bowel that may lead to malabsorption. Thus, there are similarities between this condition and nontropical sprue or CD. Identical villous atrophy in the proximal bowel mucosa, similar changes in the lamina propria, anemia, and weight loss may occur in both.

However, the two diseases are essentially different and not only because of their geographic separation. Tropical sprue is likely to manifest with megaloblastic anemia and vitamin $B_{12}$ and folate deficiency; the small bowel is increasingly contaminated with toxicogenic bacteria including coliform organisms. Unlike CD with its proximal predominance, tropical sprue extends throughout the small bowel. The most important distinction is related to treatment. Tropical sprue responds dramatically to broad-spectrum antibiotics and folates. In one report, the patient improved markedly after only 4 days of treatment and was completely well after 6 weeks.[74]

Little has been published about barium radiology in tropical sprue. I am unaware of any enteroclysis having been done. Follow-through studies merely demonstrate lumen dilatation, thickening of folds (Fig. 49–17), and the development of flocculation.[75]

## SHORT BOWEL SYNDROME

Major bowel resections usually follow interruptions of blood supply. Less common reasons for massive resections are volvulus and trauma. In about 25% of cases, this syndrome results from repeated resections, mostly for Crohn's disease and rarely for Peutz-Jeghers syndrome.

The minimal length of small bowel required to sustain life varies. For oral nutritional autonomy, the minimal

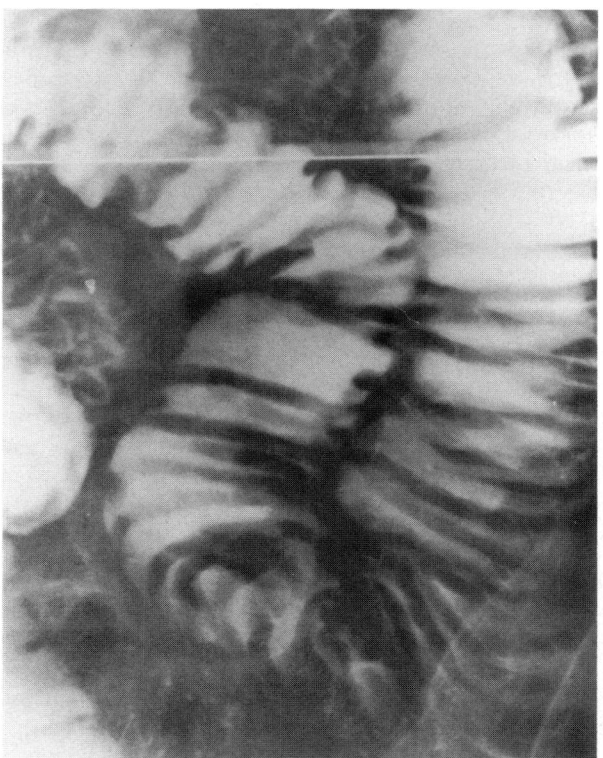

**Figure 49–17. Tropical sprue.** Confirmed case with fold thickening. The patient had resided in Jamaica.

length of normal small bowel with loss of colon has been reported to be 150 cm but with the colon preserved can be only 50 to 70 cm.[76] Normal ileum can take over the functions of the jejunum by a gradual process of adaptation. Total parenteral nutrition, usually undertaken to preserve the patient's nutritional status, adversely affects adaptation and even reduces the residual intestinal mucosal mass. Nutrients within the residual lumen are important stimuli for adaptation. Pectin as a dietary supplement is an example. Pectin is broken down to short chain fatty acids in the colon, and these are readily absorbed by the colonic mucosa.[77]

Lost ileum is metabolically irreplaceable. Resection of more than 100 cm of distal ileum interrupts enterohepatic circulation of bile salts to an extent that can no longer be compensated by the liver. Interference with vitamin $B_{12}$ absorption, hyperoxaluria, and formation of calcium oxalate urinary calculi also occur.

Usually transient increase of gastric acid output and elevated gastrin levels are found in most patients after massive resection of small bowel. This leads to lowering of pH in the proximal residuum of bowel and to further interference with digestion and absorption. Treatment with $H_2$ receptor antagonists is indicated.

Surgical management is aimed mainly at increasing the absorptive area of the short bowel. It includes tapering of dilated segments, use of serosal patches to repair strictures or perforations, and slowing of transit by incorporation of an antiperistaltic segment.[78] These interventions have been beneficial in a small number of

cases. Transplantation of small intestine may eventually become the definitive therapy. (For further discussion see Chapter 54.)

## Radiologic Findings

Barium studies give an indication of the length of the residual bowel and can demonstrate features of adaptation (increased diameters, thickened and more numerous folds, elongation). Any further involvement of bowel by the original disease process (e.g., ischemic change) may be demonstrated (Fig. 49–18).

## EOSINOPHILIC GASTROENTERITIS

This recurrent, mostly self-limited disease tends to affect patients with a history of allergic disorders. The following are required for a diagnosis of EGE:

1. Symptoms related to the gastrointestinal tract
2. Eosinophilic infiltration of the mucosa shown by multiple biopsies of gastric antrum or small bowel—or a characteristic appearance at barium radiology plus peripheral eosinophilia
3. Exclusion of parasitic or extraintestinal disease[79]

Remissions and recurrences are frequent in EGE. In a few cases, specific food sensitivity can be established as the cause of the illness. Most patients respond to corticosteroid therapy. EGE can involve the esophagus and colon, in addition to the stomach and small bowel.

EGE is characterized by three overlapping clinical and radiologic patterns:

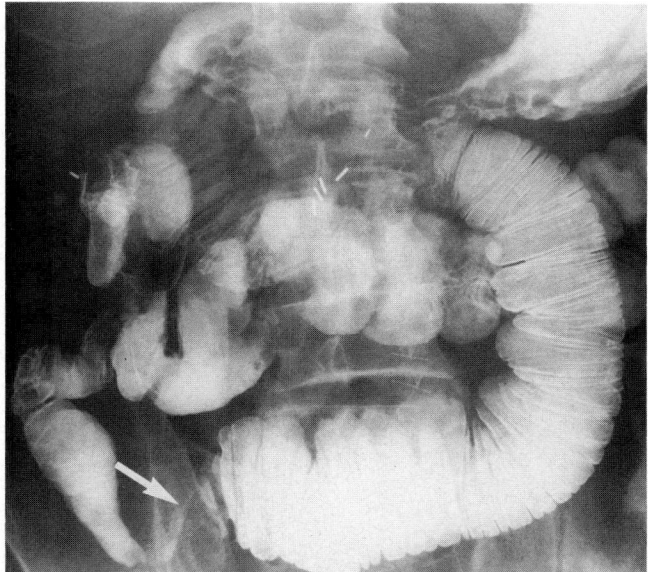

**Figure 49–18. Short bowel syndrome with renewed ischemia.** Massive resection of gangrenous bowel had followed superior mesenteric artery embolism. Ischemia now involves a further segment of bowel *(arrow).*

1. *Mainly mucosal disease.* Nausea, vomiting, diarrhea, and infrequently malabsorption occur; protein loss can be severe, resulting in hypoalbuminemia and reduced immunoglobulin levels. Antral changes are slightly more frequent than those in the small bowel, and antral biopsy often confirms the diagnosis. Gastric antral folds are thickened and may be nodular (Fig. 49–19A). Small intestinal folds are thickened, straight, and rarely nodular and may be more pronounced in the ileum (Fig. 49–19B). These changes may have a patchy distribution with normal intervening bowel. Fold thickening can extend into the colon (Fig. 49–19C).
2. *Predominantly muscularis.* There is focal muscle thickening with narrowing of the lumen. The antrum is a favorite site. This must be distinguished from Ménétrier's disease, carcinoma, lymphoma, and Crohn's disease. Superficial biopsies are likely to be unrewarding. With small bowel involvement, there may be segmental wall thickening and lumen narrowing, not associated with regular fold thickening. (*Note:* eosinophilic granulomas are localized pedunculated or sessile tumors in the distal gastric antrum, rarely in the small bowel. They are not related to EGE or to peripheral eosinophilia.[80])
3. *Predominantly serosal disease.* This rarely occurs without some features of mucosal or muscularis involvement. Eosinophilic ascites and pleural ef-

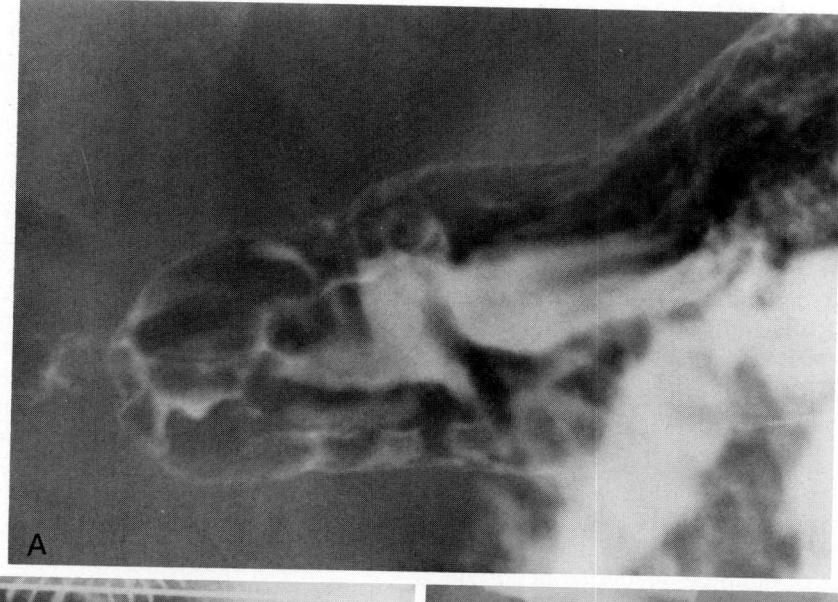

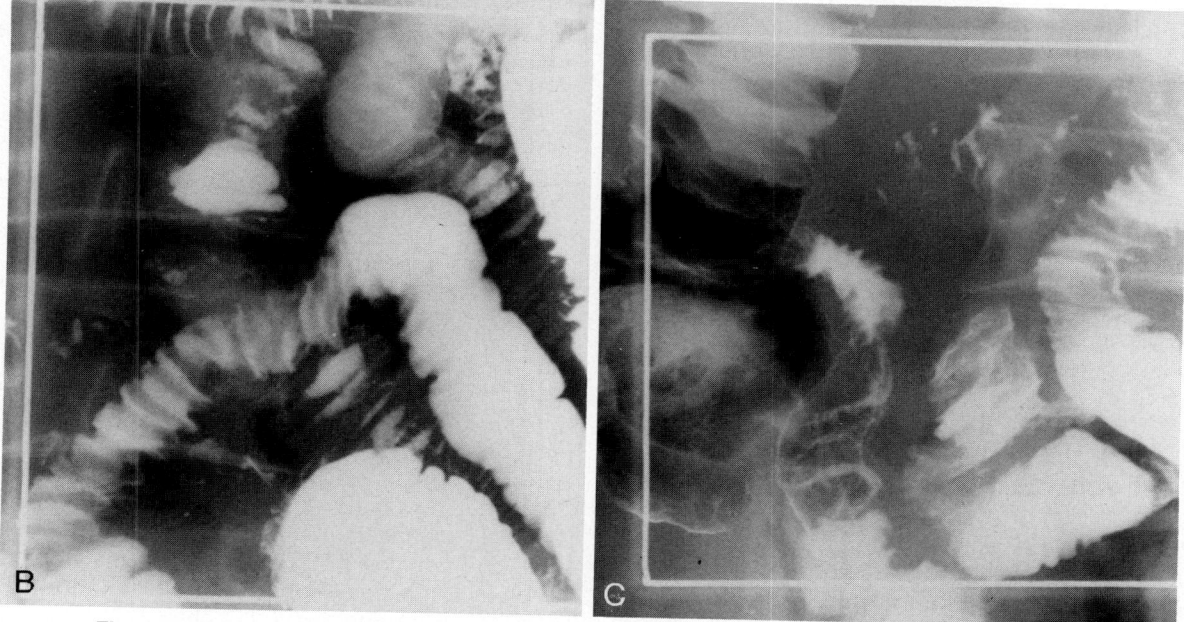

**Figure 49–19. EGE. A.** Nodular thickening of folds in the gastric antrum where an endoscopic biopsy showed eosinophilic infiltration of mucosa and submucosa. **B.** Discontinuous thickening of straight folds in jejunum and ileum. **C.** Fold thickening in terminal ileum and ascending colon.

fusions may be found. Affected small bowel segments show thickening of serosa and subserosa, and there may be lymphadenopathy. CT may be able to reveal these changes before laparotomy.[81]

The radiologic changes in 20 patients with a firm diagnosis of EGE were reported. Twelve of the patients had mainly mucosal disease (more of them with fold thickening in the antrum than in the small bowel). Five had mainly muscle layer involvement, in one of whom tapered narrowing of the esophagus was noted. Ascites was recorded in one of three patients with serosal disease.[79]

## ZOLLINGER-ELLISON SYNDROME

### Pathophysiology

ZES comprises gastric acid hypersecretion, severe peptic ulcer disease, and gastrin-secreting tumors (gastrinomas). The unbridled release of gastrin by a gastrinoma overstimulates acid production by the gastric parietal cells and causes an increase of the parietal cell mass. The maximally stimulated secretion of gastric acid is responsible for the two principal features of ZES: acid peptic disease and diarrhea. An outpouring from the stomach of several liters of highly acidic fluid per day can lead to maldigestion of fat, steatorrhea, and a sprue-like flattening of the damaged jejunal mucosa.[82]

Gastrinomas are located in the pancreas in 75 to 80% of cases, in the duodenum in 15%, and at other sites (stomach, ovaries, lymph nodes) in less than 10%. More than 50% of the tumors are malignant at the time of diagnosis, and metastases, usually to the liver, have already occurred in many. In 20 to 60% of patients with ZES, there are features of multiple endocrine neoplasia type 1, an autosomal dominant disorder with tumors also of the parathyroid glands and anterior pituitary. In eight patients with multiple endocrine neoplasia type 1 and ZES, multiple gastrinomas were demonstrated in the duodenum.[82] In these patients, a Whipple procedure or other pancreatic surgery plus duodenal excision had been carried out. The duodenal gastrinomas were small, 1.0 to 20.0 mm in size. After their removal, four of six patients became normogastrinemic and two were not improved. However, the patients had multiple endocrine tumors, including many microadenomas, in the pancreas. With one exception, immunocytochemical examination failed to demonstrate gastrin in any of the tumors.[82]

### Clinical Features

Most ZES patients present with peptic, mostly duodenal ulcers at some stage of the disease. Infrequently, the ulcers may affect the more distal duodenum or even the jejunum. Underlying ZES is suggested by ulcers refractory to usual therapy, multiple ulcers, recurrent ulceration, ulceration associated with diarrhea, and severe acid reflux esophagitis. Diarrhea is a feature in more than half of the patients, may occur without peptic ulceration, and may precede the diagnosis of ZES by years.[83]

Hypergastrinemia is the hallmark of ZES, but it is also a feature of achlorhydria, pernicious anemia, G cell hyperplasia, and retained antrum. A serum gastrin level of more than 1000 pg/mL is virtually diagnostic of ZES but is not often found. A secretin provocation that produces a paradoxical rise of at least 200 pg/mL is diagnostic of ZES in about 90% of cases. When it is concluded that ZES is the diagnosis, treatment-related considerations require further refinement of the diagnosis. Because many gastrinomas metastasize sooner rather than later, exclusion of any existing mestastases to the liver is the first need. In the absence of metastases, tumor localization and excision are the therapeutic goals.[84]

### Radiologic Findings

Barium studies can show indications of increased gastric acid output, fluid increase, hyper-rugosity, at times exaggerated areae gastricae, and erosions. The duodenal bulb may show fold thickening, erosions, and poor adherence of barium. Peptic ulceration or its scars may be identified. Evidence of pronounced peptic esophagitis is seen in more than 60% of patients. As previously mentioned, peptic ulcer–associated features should suggest consideration of underlying ZES. More specific radiologic findings are related to the effect of high acid output on the duodenum and jejunum:

1. A dilated duodenum with coarse, nodular folds and erosions in some of the nodules (Fig. 49–20); erosive duodenitis has been observed by endoscopy and considered highly suggestive of ZES.[85] The radiologic differential diagnosis includes chronic renal failure and possibly giardiasis or strongyloidiasis.
2. A moderate degree of fold thickening and fluid increase, especially in the proximal jejunum.
3. Duodenal gastrinomas, which are by no means rare and may be shown by double contrast barium radiology. These tumors are usually submucosal and tend to be tiny. Duodenoscopy has occasionally been able to detect them.[86]

Demonstration or exclusion of liver metastases is the further function of radiology. For this purpose, ultrasound was found to be only slightly less sensitive than CT (63% versus 66%); the two tests are complementary, one detecting lesions missed by the other. Invasive, selective angiography had a higher sensitivity of 78%.[87] Magnetic resonance imaging had a sensitivity of 43% for detecting metastatic gastrinoma in the liver, less than that of ultrasound or CT.[88] The performance of magnetic resonance imaging should improve significantly, but at present it is not the method of choice. Ultrasound should probably be used initially for the investigation of possible liver metastases, to be followed by CT. Ultrasound

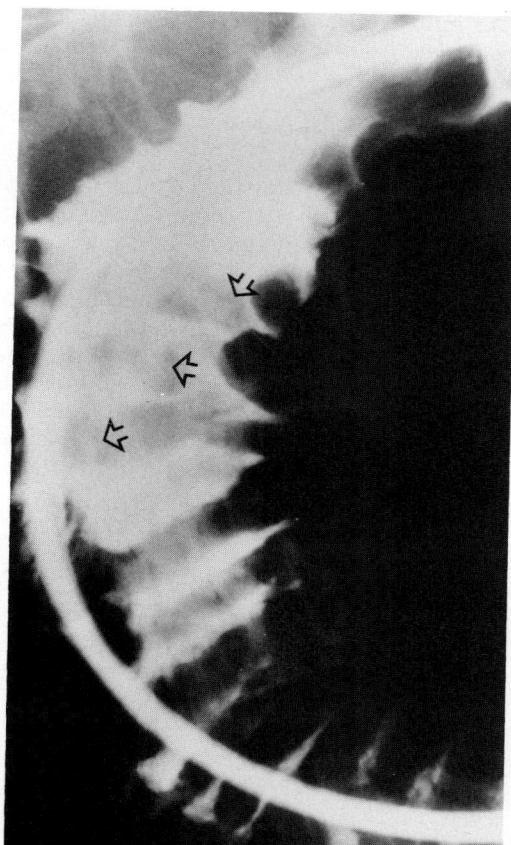

**Figure 49–20. ZES.** The duodenum shows gross thickening of folds, some with nodularities and erosions *(arrows)*. Fold thickening extended into the proximal jejunum.

is also the method of choice for the follow-up of liver metastases.[87]

In the absence of metastatic gastrinoma, the only way to cure ZES patients is to identify the primary tumor or tumors and resect them. In demonstrating the primary tumor, the sensitivities of ultrasound and CT were not far apart (30% versus 46%) and were significantly exceeded by that of selective angiography (64%).[87] The sensitivity of magnetic resonance imaging was only 20%.[88] Future improvements in the radiologic localization of gastrinomas should be made by endoscopic and intraoperative ultrasound. At present, localization of primary gastrinomas by selective arterial injection of secretin is the most accurate method, although it is rather complex.[84] An alternative method, selective venous sampling of portal radicles,[89] is now used less frequently.

With selection of patients for resective surgery and earlier localization of resectable primary gastrinomas, total cure is now reported in 30% of cases.[83]

## Medical Therapy

When surgical removal is not possible or has failed, or during the time needed to investigate suitability for

surgery, there is a need for medical treatment to control gastric acid hypersecretion. $H_2$ receptor antagonists and omeprazole given in adequate dosages do this successfully. This therapy cannot delay the progress of the metastatic disease in the liver. Antineoplastic chemotherapy has resulted in a favorable initial response. Selective hepatic artery embolization of the liver metastases was considered effective in earlier case reports.[90]

## Prognosis

Not all cases of ZES have a malignant course. Five-year survival for all patients with ZES varied between 62 and 75% and 10-year survival between 47 and 58%.[91] Duodenal primary tumors, isolated tumors in lymph nodes, initially small tumors, and those associated with multiple endocrine neoplasia type 1 have a relatively better prognosis.[83]

## ADULT CYSTIC FIBROSIS

One in 2000, usually white, infants is born with the genetic defect that causes CF. Some 50 years ago, four of five such infants died during their first year. It is due to the success of chest medicine that increasing numbers of CF patients survive into adulthood.[92] One third of the more than 15,000 patients on the register of the North American Cystic Fibrosis Foundation are now older than 21 years.[93]

In about 2% of patients, CF is first diagnosed after the age of 18 years.[94] This chapter is concerned mainly with this group of patients. These patients may visit their physician with symptoms of hepatobiliary disease[95] or with symptoms related to the gastrointestinal tract.[94] Of the more typical patients with CF, those diagnosed in infancy or childhood and kept alive by pulmonary care, 85% are found to have malabsorption and steatorrhea.[92] Exocrine pancreatic secretion in patients with CF is commonly viscous and low in bicarbonates and often also in enzymes. Postprandial pH values in the duodenum are frequently below 4.0 in CF patients, who are therefore likely to have evidence of fat malabsorption.[96] Gastric acid output in CF is at normal levels or increased. Reduction of acid output by omeprazole enhances the efficacy of pancreatic enzyme supplements.[97] Characteristic histologic changes are found in the small bowel. Goblet cells contain inspissated mucus and Brunner's glands are dilated with stringy secretions.[94]

## Radiologic Findings

Plain films of the abdomen may show dilated bowel loops and pancreatic calcification. Intestinal impaction and obstruction can occur after childhood, and the term *meconium ileus equivalent* has been applied to it. Insufficient dosage of pancreatic enzyme replacement is the precipitating factor in most cases. A contrast enema is occasionally needed to confirm the diagnosis. In patients with severe constipation or pseudo-obstruction, a diatrizoate meglumine (Gastrografin or Hypaque) enema may draw fluid into the colon and be therapeutic.[98]

A radiologic diagnosis of CF can be suggested in adult patients, whether they are suspected of having CF or hitherto undiagnosed. Such patients may present with features of malabsorption and steatorrhea, and a small bowel barium examination would be requested.

The first unusual finding occurs in the duodenum in 60 to 80% of patients. This was fully described in 1973.[99] Fold thickening, nodular filling defects, flattening of folds, and lumen dilatation with an appearance of sacculation along the lateral border may be observed, mainly in the descending portion (Fig. 49–21A). No ulcerations are seen. There is no accepted explanation for these appearances.

In the small bowel, especially in distal loops, the normal fold pattern is replaced by an irregular network of curving lines, presumably surrounding blobs of inspissated mucus. This pattern extends into the colon (Fig. 49–21B and C).

## ABETALIPOPROTEINEMIA

This rare autosomal recessive disease presents with red blood cell abnormality (acanthosis) and evidence of mild steatorrhea, usually by the age of 2 years. Intestinal biopsy specimens of fasting patients show the enterocytes engorged with lipid droplets. The lamina propria is virtually without lipids and the lymphatics are empty. Long-term complications are related to malabsorption of fat-soluble vitamins, particularly vitamin E. Large-dose supplements of vitamin E may prevent the development of retinopathy and spinocerebellar degeneration.[100] Medium chain triglycerides should replace fat in the patient's diet.

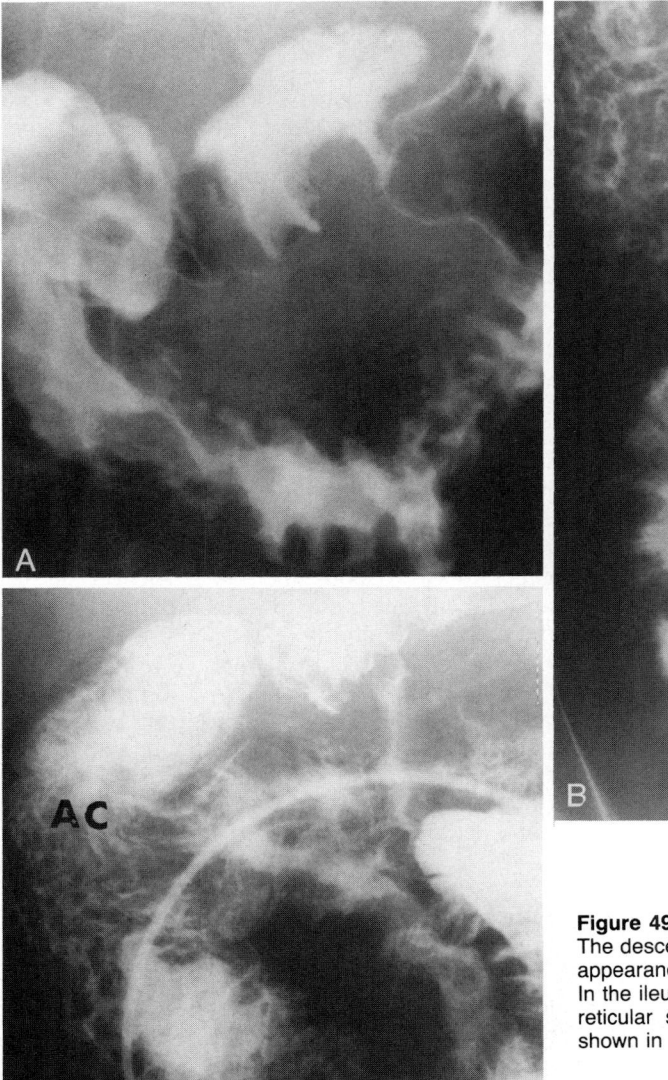

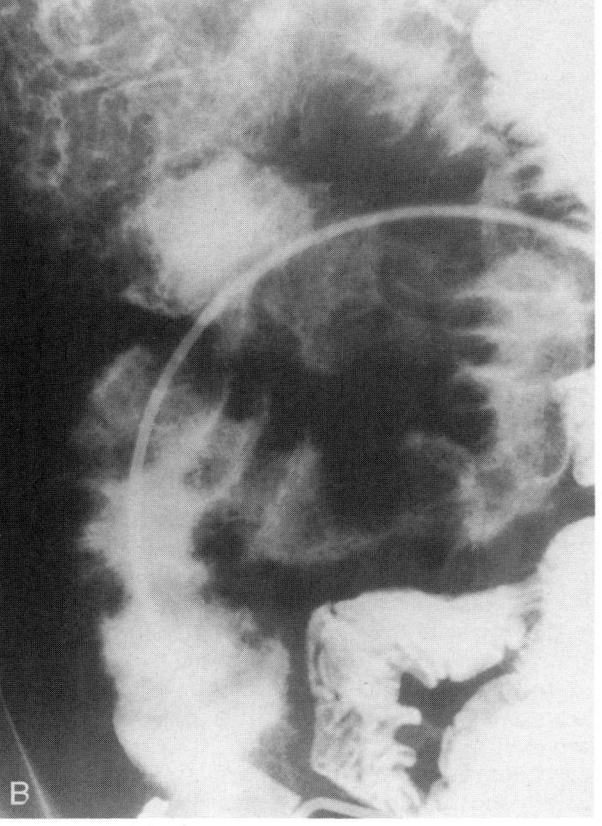

**Figure 49–21. Young adult with newly diagnosed CF. A.** The descending duodenum presents an almost "ram's horn" appearance in its upper part and thickened folds below. **B.** In the ileum there is gross thickening of folds with a vaguely reticular surface pattern. **C.** A coarse reticular pattern is shown in the right colon. AC = ascending colon.

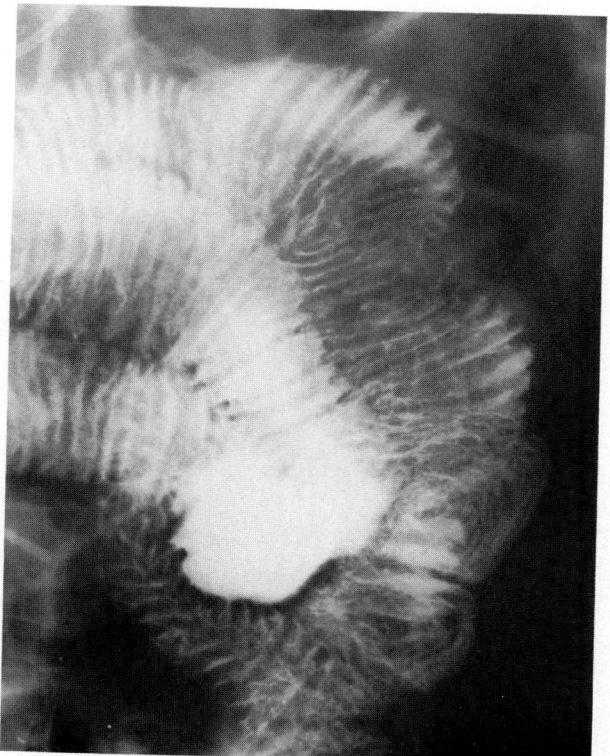

**Figure 49–22. Abetalipoproteinemia.** Folds are moderately thickened and straight. An appearance of fine surface granularity is seen throughout the small bowel.

## Radiologic Findings

Mucosal folds in the duodenum and jejunum are uniformly thickened. Folds are straight, and the lumen may be slightly widened. An appearance of fine graininess of the mucosa may express ballooning of the tips of villi by the accumulation of fat globules within the enterocytes (Fig. 49–22). Radiology is not likely to be required before clinical diagnosis.

# SYSTEMIC MASTOCYTOSIS

Mastocytosis is characterized by accumulation of mast cells, more often confined to the skin (urticaria pigmentosa). Rarely, mast cell infiltration involves other organs (bones, lymph nodes, liver, spleen, gastrointestinal tract), and the condition is then called *systemic mastocytosis.*

Infiltration of the gastrointestinal tract occurs more frequently than was thought in the past. In one study,[101] 12 of 16 consecutive patients were found to have gastrointestinal involvement in the form of mast cell infiltration of the intestinal submucosa and mucosa with local and systemic release of histamine. Increased output of gastric acid at concentrations below that in ZES was associated with duodenal ulceration and duodenitis in 7 of the 16 patients.[101] Diarrhea was the second most frequent symptom, with evidence of malabsorption in 6 of the 16 patients.[101] Diarrhea may be associated with flushing, tachycardia, and hypotension. Drinking even a small amount of alcohol may precipitate symptoms. Treatment with histamine receptor antagonists may give relief.

## Diagnosis

Gastroduodenal endoscopy has confirmed the increased presence of duodenal ulcers and duodenitis.[101] Gastric endoscopic findings include the demonstration of urticaria-like mucosal lesions.[102] Confirmation of the diagnosis relies on jejunal biopsies to demonstrate mast cell infiltration in mucosa and submucosa.[103] Villi are normal or blunted.

Radiologic studies show mild bowel wall thickening and the presence of nodules or even "bull's-eye" lesions.[104, 105] I have found bull's-eye lesions in the duodenum and focal mucosal elevations, believed to be urticarial, in the jejunum (Fig. 49–23).

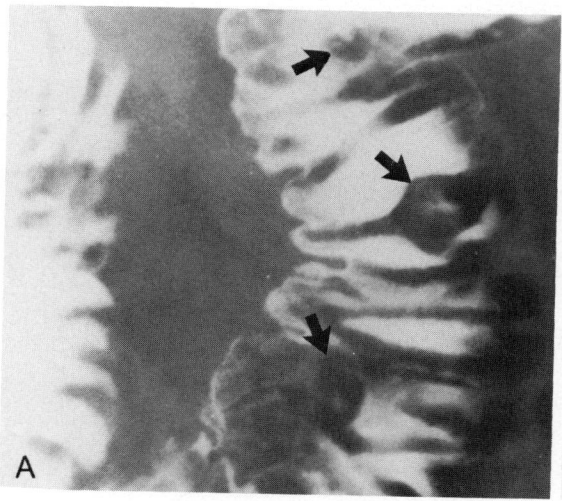
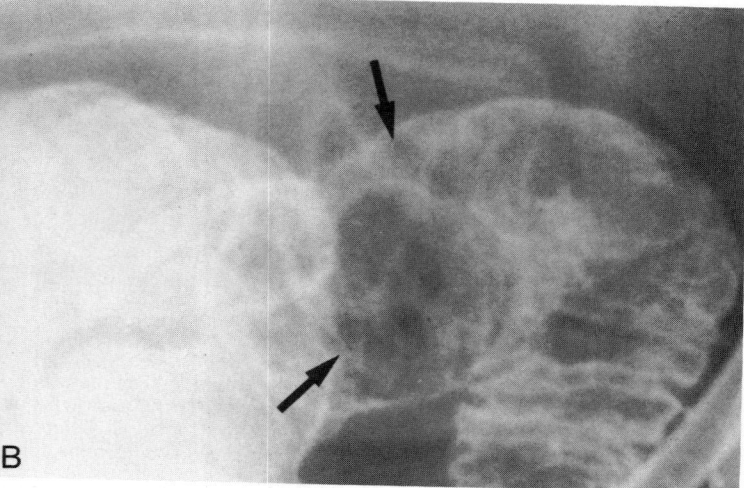

**Figure 49–23. Systemic mastocytosis. A.** A few target lesions are shown in the distal duodenum *(arrows).* **B.** Ill-defined elevations are seen in the jejunum *(arrows)* and may represent urticarial lesions.

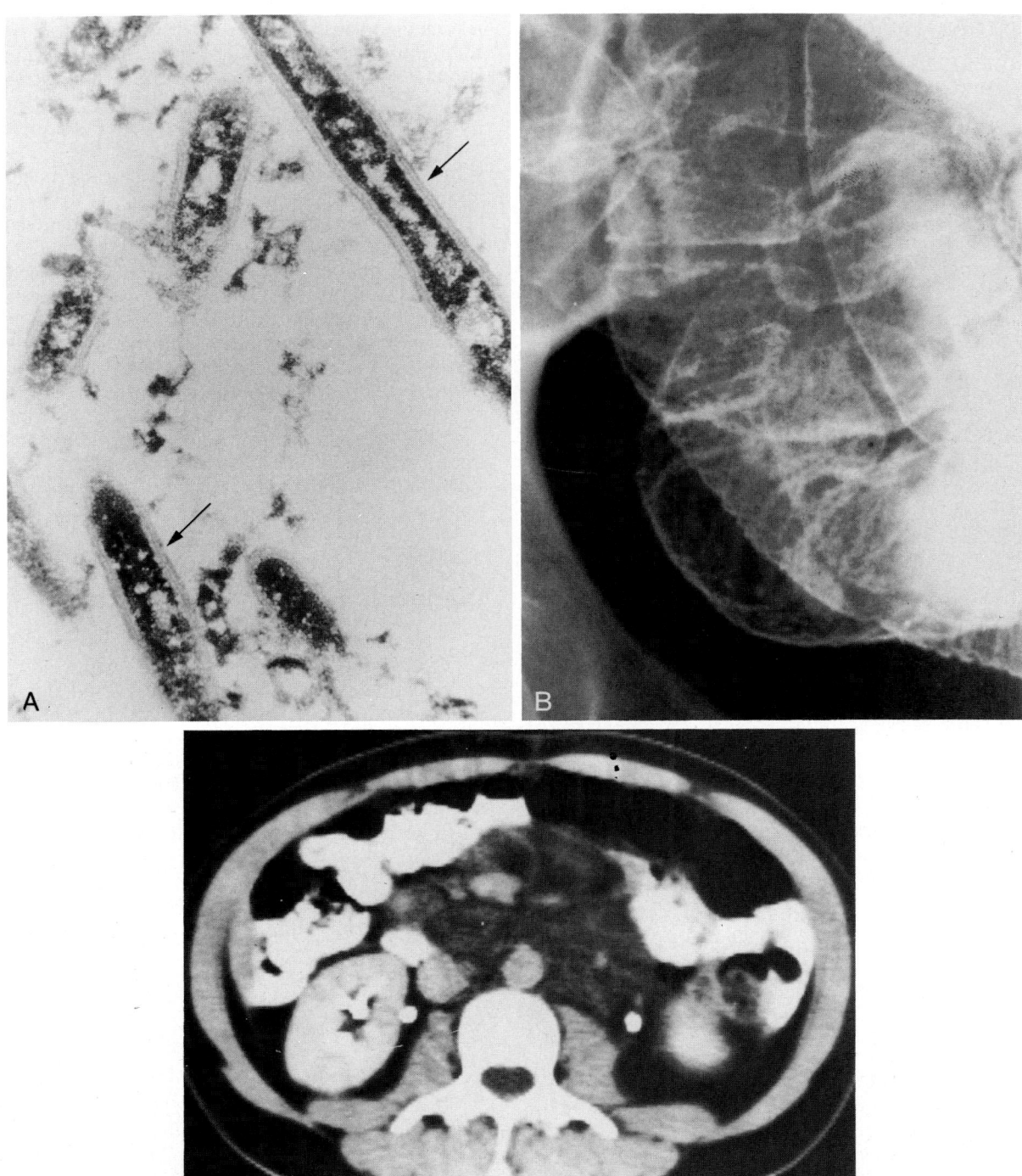

**Figure 49–24. Whipple's disease. A.** Electron microscopic image of a macrophage containing Whipple's bacilli in various stages of disintegration. Note the typical trilaminar outer coat of these bacilli *(arrows)*. **B.** Enteroclysis demonstrates a diffuse 1- to 2-mm micronodular pattern with folds of generally normal thickness. The micronodules represent distended villi filled with a large number of macrophages containing periodic acid–Schiff–positive material (the residue of the bacilli). (**B** courtesy of E. Salomonowitz, M.D., Vienna, Austria.) **C.** Demonstration by CT of a mass of mesenteric and retroperitoneal lymph nodes containing fatty material derived from digested Whipple's bacilli.

# WHIPPLE'S DISEASE

In this rare multisystem disease, glycoprotein-laden, periodic acid–Schiff–positive macrophages can be found in most tissues. There is a predilection for involvement of the small bowel, heart valves, central nervous system, and joint capsules. The disease occurs mostly in middle-aged white men in the United States and northern Europe.[106] It is generally accepted that the bacilli first described by Whipple[107] and called Whipple's bacilli are the cause of the disease. They are consistently and profusely present at diagnosis and disappear after successful antibiotic treatment.[108] Electron microscopy reveals their thick cell wall surrounded by a trilaminar membrane.

## Clinical Features

Onset of the disease is usually insidious and varied, depending on the organs initially affected. Arthralgia, neurologic symptoms, and pyrexia may exist long before intestinal involvement leads to recognition of this protean disease. Diarrhea and steatorrhea, often with occult blood and rarely with melena,[109] may lead to diagnosis by small bowel radiology and duodenoscopy with biopsy. Biopsy specimens from the distal duodenum show the lamina propria filled with a profusion of macrophages containing the periodic acid–Schiff–positive residue of the cell walls of the bacilli and Whipple's bacilli in various stages of disintegration (Fig. 49–24A). Bacilli are also seen in extracellular spaces. The extension of the lamina propria into the villi causes their dilatation, an important feature for radiologic identification of the disease. Lymphatics in the bowel wall and mesentery may be filled with fat globules as a result of Whipple's disease involvement of mesenteric lymph nodes, a usually mild form of secondary lymphangiectasia.

Immune defects are a feature of Whipple's disease. Lymphocytopenia is usual although with a normal T4/T8 ratio. Diminished responsiveness to mitogens and immune tolerance of the massive presence of the bacilli are also observed. Immune dysfunction would be increased in patients with malnutrition caused by delay in the diagnosis of Whipple's disease. There is a superficial resemblance to *Mycobacterium avium-intracellulare* infection in patients with acquired immunodeficiency syndrome. Mucosal biopsy specimens in both cases show foamy periodic acid–Schiff–positive macrophages in the lamina propria. However, the immune defect in acquired immunodeficiency syndrome is more fundamental and the microbacteria are acid-fast, are easily cultured (unlike Whipple's bacilli, which have never been cultured), and have an entirely different electron microscopic appearance.

## Radiologic Findings

Enteroclysis is required for the diagnosis of Whipple's disease by barium examination, which must be con-

firmed by clinical and histologic examinations. The essential feature is diffuse or patchy micronodules 1 to 2 mm in diameter, mostly in the jejunum and at the duodenojejunal junction (Fig. 49–24B). Because the submucosa is not filled with masses of macrophages, it would be expected to appear normal and have folds of normal thickness. However, hypoalbuminemia with albumin levels as low as 1.0 g/mL has been reported and would cause edema of the submucosa and fold thickening.

A useful further radiologic finding is the demonstration by CT of nodal masses in the mesentery and retroperitoneum, typically shown to contain fatty material. At times the entire nodal mass has the Hounsfield values of fat (Fig. 49–24C). A distinctive, highly echogenic mass of retroperitoneal nodes was demonstrated by ultrasound in a patient with Whipple's disease; the echogenicity was due to the high fat content of the mass.[110]

The radiologic differential diagnosis of the micronodular mucosal pattern from that seen in other pathologies is important. The need to interpret radiologic patterns in association with the clinical presentation has already been referred to in the differential diagnosis from *M. avium-intracellulare* infection in acquired immunodeficiency syndrome (Fig. 49–25). CT or ultrasound would also help in differentiation. Although a modest increase of fat may occur in *M. avium-intracellulare* lymphadenopathy, it is not likely to be obvious at CT or ultrasound examination. In lymphangiectasia, diffuse or

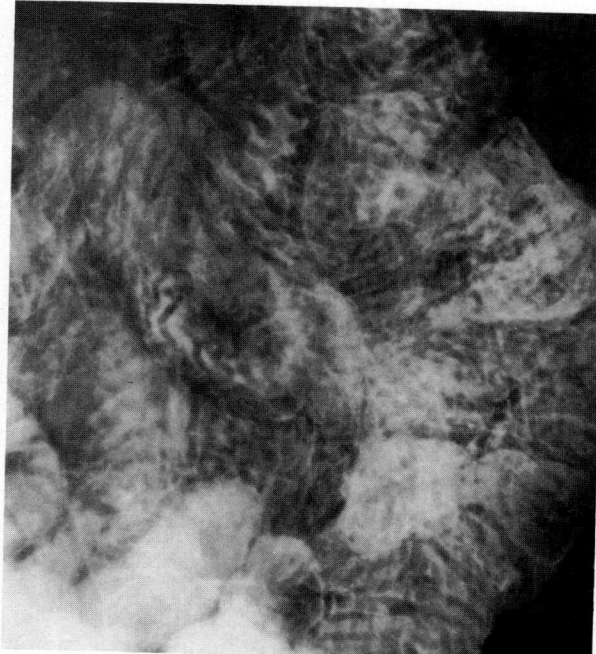

**Figure 49–25. Mycobacterium avium-intracellulare infection in acquired immunodeficiency syndrome.** Follow-through examination demonstrates a nodular pattern with slightly thickened folds. This condition has been called "pseudo-Whipple's" because there is a superficial resemblance. However, the macrophages in *M. avium-intracellulare* infection contain barely digested, acid-fast bacilli, and there is less fatty material in the mesenteric nodal masses.

patchy micronodules 1 to 3 mm in size can also be shown by enteroclysis (see later). However, edematous fold thickening is always associated, and there may be increased fluid in the bowel lumen. Younger patients are affected, and mesenteric nodes are not enlarged except in secondary lymphangiectasia, when the primary pathologic condition may be obvious. Macroglobulinemia rarely involves the small bowel, causing extracellular deposition of macroglobulin in the lamina propria. It is not a diagnosis that could be suggested without some awareness of the hematologic background. Amyloidosis, as mentioned earlier, occasionally manifests with a micronodular pattern. It must be included in the radiologic differential diagnosis. Nodular lymphoid hyperplasia, caused by enlarged lymph follicles bulging into the epithelial layer, is mostly asymptomatic. Nodules are 2 to 4 mm in size, uniformly distributed, and often umbilicated. They are more likely to be found in the distal ileum. If extensively present in adults, they may be related to a viral infection, to an immunodeficiency (e.g., IgA), or rarely to a lymphoproliferative process.

## Prognosis

Whipple's disease was uniformly fatal until the 1960s, when it was shown to respond spectacularly to antibiotics. Antibiotic regimens are usually continued for a year or more, but a shorter period of treatment of 2 to 5 months with clinical follow-up has been suggested.[111] Mucosal biopsies after successful treatment may still show a few periodic acid–Schiff–positive macrophages in the lamina propria, with an otherwise normal appearance. Enteroclysis is indicated in the follow-up of treated patients if intestine-related symptoms recur.

## INTESTINAL LYMPHANGIECTASIA

Intestinal lymphangiectasia occurs in two forms, primary and secondary. Primary lymphangiectasia is part of a congenital malformation of lymphatics that may affect many parts of the body and can become evident at any time between birth and early adulthood. Secondary lymphangiectasia is caused by blockage of lymph drainage in the mesentery, retroperitoneum, or beyond.

## Clinical Features

Impedance of lymph flow from the bowel into the body reduces the intake of chylomicrons and fat-soluble vitamins and raises pressures within peripheral lymphatics, leading to leakage of lymph from the gut surface into the lumen. Lymphenteric fistulas may form and facilitate the escape into the lumen of chylomicrons, proteins, and lymphocytes.[112] The protein-losing enteropathy causes hypoalbuminemia and edema. Lympho-

cytopenia, caused mainly by loss of T lymphocytes into the lumen, impairs cell-mediated immunity.

Lymphangiectasia should be suspected in patients with hypoalbuminemia, lymphocytopenia, diarrhea, and steatorrhea. When found in younger patients, especially with asymmetric edema, it is likely to be primary.

Secondary lymphangiectasia can be part of any condition in which proximal lymphatic pathways are blocked. Extensive abdominal or retroperitoneal carcinoma or lymphoma, retroperitoneal fibrosis, tuberculosis, Whipple's disease, metastatic carcinoid, Crohn's disease, chronic pancreatitis, constrictive pericarditis, and congestive cardiac failure are examples.

## Diagnosis

The demonstration by enteroclysis of micronodules and swollen mucosal folds in lymphangiectasia has already been described and the differential diagnosis has been discussed. A few larger nodules are believed to represent conglomerates of dilated lymphatics in the submucosa. Taken together with the clinical background of the patient, radiology can suggest a diagnosis of lymphangiectasia (Fig. 49–26). Endoscopy extended into the distal duodenum can confirm the diagnosis by identifying the presence of clubbed villi containing whitish material in dilated lacteals. Findings are similar in secondary lymphangiectasia. Endoscopic biopsies are indicated.

CT is important in investigating the causes of secondary lymphangiectasia by demonstrating lymph node enlargement and thickening of the bowel wall and mesentery.

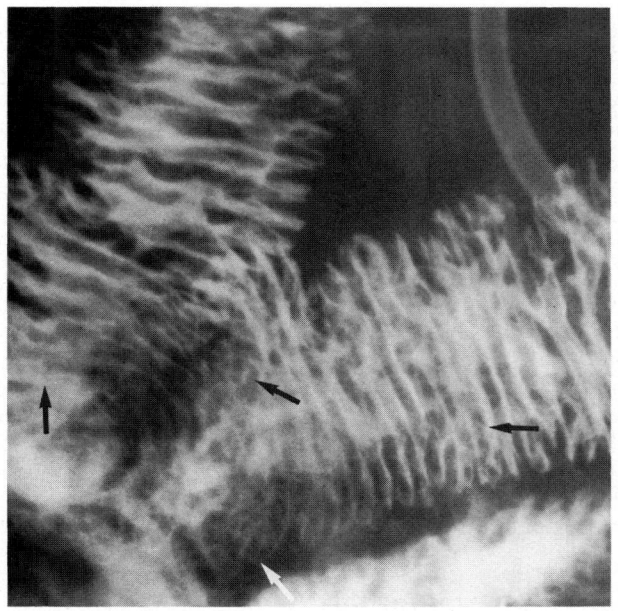

**Figure 49–26. Primary lymphangiectasia.** Enteroclysis shows thickened folds in the jejunum with clusters of about 2-mm micronodules *(arrows)*. They represent villi distended by engorged lacteals.

# WALDENSTRÖM'S MACROGLOBULINEMIA

This disease is characterized by monoclonal IgM protein in the plasma and by lymphadenopathy, hepatosplenomegaly, and anemia. It resembles multiple myeloma but rarely causes osteolytic bone lesions and typically involves a serum IgM spike.[113] Bleeding from mucous membranes is a frequent complication. The development of diarrhea in some patients may be related to lymphoma and retroperitoneal lymphatics obstructing nodal involvement. Lymphatic obstruction can also be caused by massive deposition of IgM protein in the lamina propria, with the occasional appearance of micronodularity on barium studies. It must be stressed that intestinal involvement is an unusual feature of Waldenström's macroglobulinemia.[114]

## Acknowledgment

Figures 49–1, 49–5A and B, 49–7B, 49–9B, 49–13, 49–15B, 49–19A to C, 49–20, 49–22, and 49–24A and C are reproduced from Herlinger H, Maglinte D (eds): Clinical Radiology of the Small Intestine. Philadelphia: WB Saunders, 1989.

# References

1. Losowsky MS: The protean clinical manifestations of celiac disease. *In* Ferguson A (ed): Advanced Medicine. London, Pitman Publishers, 1984, pp 48–60.
2. Rubesin SE, Rubin RA, Herlinger H: Small bowel malabsorption: clinical perspectives. Radiology 184:297–305, 1992.
3. Newcomer AD, Hofmann AF, DiMagno EP, et al: Triolein breadth test: a sensitive and specific test for fat malabsorption. Gastroenterology 76:6–13, 1979.
4. Toskes PP, Donaldson RM Jr: The blind loop syndrome. *In* Sleisenger MH, Fordtran JS (eds): Gastrointestinal Disease: Pathophysiology, Diagnosis, Management (4th ed). Philadelphia: WB Saunders, 1989, pp 1289–1296.
5. Laws JW, Neale G: Radiological diagnosis of disaccharidase deficiency. Lancet 2:139–143, 1966.
6. Golden R: Technical factors in the Roentgen examination of the small intestine. AJR 82:965–972, 1959.
7. Herlinger H: Radiology in malabsorption. Clin Radiol 45:73–78, 1992 (editorial).
8. Haboubi NY, Montgomery RD, Asguith P, et al: Significance of small bowel bacterial overgrowth in the elderly. Gut 31:A1194, 1990 (abstract).
9. Morson BC, Dawson IMP: Gastrointestinal Pathology (2nd ed). Oxford: Blackwell Scientific Publications, 1979, p 242.
10. Krishnamurthy S, Kelly MM, Rohrman CA, et al: Jejunal diverticulosis. Gastroenterology 85:538–547, 1983.
11. Goyal RK: Case records of the Massachusetts General Hospital, case 25-1990. N Engl J Med 322:1796–1806, 1990.
12. Baskin RH, Mayo CW: Jejunal diverticulosis: a clinical study of 87 cases. Surg Clin North Am 32:1185–1196, 1952.
13. Ross CB, Richards WO, Sharp KW, et al: Diverticular disease of the jejunum and its complications. Am Surg 56:319–324, 1990.
14. Wilcox RD, Shatney CH: Surgical implications of jejunal diverticula. South Med J 81:1386–1391, 1988.
15. Benya EC, Ghahremani GG, Brosnan JJ: Diverticulitis of the jejunum: clinical and radiological features. Gastrointest Radiol 16:24–28, 1991.
16. Maglinte DDT, Chernish SM, D'Weese R, et al: Acquired jejunoileal diverticular disease: subject review. Radiology 158:577–580, 1986.
17. Greenstein S, Jones B, Fishman EK, et al: Small bowel diverticulitis: CT findings. AJR 147:271–174, 1986.
18. Sheth KJ, Werlin SL, Freeman ME, et al: Gastrointestinal structure and function in Fabry's disease. Am J Gastroenterol 76:246–251, 1991.
19. Schuffler MD, Jonak Z: Chronic idiopathic intestinal pseudo-obstruction caused by a degenerative disorder of the myenteric plexus: the use of Smith's method to define the neuropathology. Gastroenterology 82:476–486, 1982.
20. Camilleri LJ, Brown AR, Zinsmeister AR, et al: Cisapride corrects the impaired small bowel transit of chyme in chronic intestinal pseudo-obstruction. Gastroenterology 88:1340, 1985 (abstract).
21. Horowitz AL, Meyers MA: The "hide-bound" small bowel of scleroderma: characteristic mucosal fold pattern. AJR 119:332–334, 1973.
22. Gilat T, Revach M, Sohar E: Deposition of amyloid in gastrointestinal tract. Gut 10:98–104, 1969.
23. Yamada M, Hatakeyama S, Tsukagoshhi H: Gastrointestinal amyloid deposition in AL (primary or myeloma associated) and AA (secondary) amyloidosis: diagnostic value of gastric biopsy. Hum Pathol 16:1206, 1985.
24. Tada S, Iida M, Matsui T, et al: Amyloidosis of the small intestine: findings on double-contrast radiographs. AJR 156:741–744, 1991.
25. Smith TR, Cho KC: Small intestine amyloidosis producing a stippled punctate mucosal pattern: radiological-pathological correlation. Am J Gastroenterol 81:477–479. 1986.
26. Legge DA, Wollaeger AE, Carlson HC: Interstinal pseudo-obstruction in systemic amyloidosis. Gut 11:764–767, 1970.
27. Schuffler MD, Baird HW, Flemming CR, et al: Interstinal pseudo-obstruction as the presenting manifestation of small-cell carcinomas of the lung. Ann Intern Med 98:129–134, 1983.
28. Sack TL, Sleisinger MH: Effects of systemic and extraintestinal disease on the gut. *In* Sleisinger MH, Fortran JS (eds): Gastrointestinal Disease: Pathophysiology, Diagnosis, Management (4th ed). Philadelphia: WB Saunders, 1989, pp 488–528.
29. Marsh MM: Gluten, major histocompatibility complexes, and the small intestine. A molecular and immunobiologic approach to the spectrum of gluten sensitivity (celiac sprue). Gastroenterology 102:330–354, 1992.
30. Trier JS: Celiac sprue. Review article, medical progress. N Engl J Med 325:1709–1719, 1991.
31. Paré P, Douville P, Caron D, et al: Sprue: changes in the pattern of clinical recognition. J Clin Gastroenterol 10:395–400, 1988.
32. Cooke WT, Holmes GKT: Coeliac Disease. Edinburgh: Churchill Livingstone, 1984.
33. Comroe B, Pendergrass E: Roentgen study of the gastrointestinal tract in chronic idiopathic adult tetany. AJR 33:647–656, 1935.
34. McMillan SA, Haughton DJ, Biggart JD, et al: Predictive value for celiac disease of antibodies to gliadan, endomysium and jejunum in patients attending for jejunal biopsy. Br Med J 303:1163–1166, 1991.
35. Corazza GR, Brocchi E, Caletti G, et al: Loss of duodenal folds allows diagnosis of unsuspected coeliac disease. Gut 31:1080–1081, 1990.
36. Shanahan F, Weinstein WM: Extending the scope in celiac disease. N Engl J Med 319:782–783, 1988 (editorial).
37. Saverymuttu SH, Sabbat J, Burke M, et al: Impact of endoscopic duodenal biopsy on the detection of small interstinal villous atrophy. Postgrad Med J 67:47–49, 1991.
38. Stevens FM, McCarthy CF: Endoscopic dye-scattering in coeliac disease. Gut 18:398, 1977.
39. Snell AM, Kent JD: Chronic idiopathic steatorrhea, roentgenologic observation. Arch Intern Med 53:615–629, 1934.
40. Kantor JL: The roentgenologic diagnosis of idiopathic steatorrhea and allied conditions. Practical value of the "moulage" sign. AJR 41:758–778, 1939.
41. Marshak RH, Lindner AE: Radiology of the Small Intestine (2nd ed). Philadelphia: WB Saunders, 1976.
42. Farthing NJG, McLean AM, Bartram CI, et al: Radiological features of the jejunum in hypoalbuminemia. AJR 136:883–886, 1981.
43. Cohen MD, Lintott DJ: Transient small bowel intussusceptions in adult coeliac disease. Clin Radiol 29:529–534, 1978.
44. Cooke WT, Holmes GKT: Gluten-induced enteropathy (celiac

disease). *In* Berk JE (ed): Bockus Gastroenterology (4th ed). Philadelphia, WB Saunders, 1985, pp 1719–1757.

45. Muller WSH: Adult celiac disease. *In* Sellink JL, Miller RE (eds): Radiology of the Small Bowel. The Hague: Martinus Nijhoff, 1982, pp 369–379.

46. Herlinger H, Maglinte DDT: Fold patterns in celiac disease. Gastrointest Radiol 10:300, 1985 (abstract).

47. Bova JG, Friedman AC, Weser E, et al: Adaptation of the ileum in nontopical sprue: reversal of the jejunoileal fold pattern. AJR 144:299–302, 1985.

48. Herlinger H, Maglinte DDT: Jejunal fold separation in adult celiac disease: relevance of enteroclysis. Radiology 158:605–611, 1986.

49. Knauer CM, Monroe LS: The roentgenographic abnormalities of the duodenum in celiac sprue. Digestion 101:129–136, 1964.

50. Gillberg R, Kestrup W, Mobacken T, et al: Endoscopic duodenal biopsy compared with biopsies with the Watson capsule from the upper jejunum in patients with dermatitis herpetiformis. Scand J Gastroenterol 17:305–308, 1982.

51. Jones B, Bayless TM, Hamilton SR, et al: "Bubbly" duodenal bulb in celiac disease: radiologic-pathologic correlation. AJR 142:119–122, 1984.

52. Mike N, Udeshi U, Asquith P, et al: Small bowel enema in nonresponsive coeliac disease. Gut 31:883–885, 1990.

53. Brow JR, Parker F, Weinstein WM, et al: The small intestinal mucosa in dermatitis herpetiformis. I. Severity and distribution of the small intestinal lesions and associated malabsorption. Gastroenterology 60:355–361, 1971.

54. Amman AJ, Hong R: Selective IgA deficiency: presentation of 30 cases and a review of the literature. Medicine (Baltimore) 50:223–236, 1971.

55. O'Grady JG, Stevens FM, Harding B, et al: Hyposplenism and gluten-sensitive enteropathy. Gastroenterology 87:1326–1331, 1984.

56. Robertson DAF, Swinson CN, Hall R, et al: Coeliac disease, splenic function and malignancy. Gut 23:666–669, 1982.

57. Robinson PJ, Bullen AW, Hall R, et al: Splenic size and function in adult coeliac disease. Br J Radiol 53:532–537, 1980.

58. Jones B, Bayles STM, Fishman EK, et al: Lymphadenopathy in celiac disease: computed tomographic observations. AJR 142:1127–1132, 1984.

59. Matuchansky C, Colin R, Hemet J: Cavitation of mesenteric lymph nodes, splenic atrophy and a flat small intestinal mucosa. Report of 6 cases. Gastroenterology 87:606–614, 1984.

60. Holmes GKT: Mesenteric lymph node cavitation in coeliac disease. Gut 27:728–733, 1986.

61. Friedman HJ, Chiu BK: Small bowel malignant lymphoma complicating celiac sprue and the mesenteric lymph node cavitation syndrome. Gastroenterology 90:2008–2012, 1986.

62. Weinstein WM, Saunders DR, Tytgat GN, et al: Collagenous sprue: an unrecognized type of malabsorption. N Engl J Med 283:1297–1301, 1970.

63. Losowsky MS, Walker BE, Kelleher J: Malabsorption in clinical practice. Edinburgh: Churchill Livingstone, 1974, pp 191–196.

64. Herlinger H, Maglinte DDT: Malabsorption and immune deficiencies. *In* Herlinger H, Maglinte D (eds): Clinical Radiology of the Small Intestine. Philadelphia: WB Saunders, 1989, pp 349–398.

65. Gough KR, Read AE, Naish JM: Interstinal reticulosis as a complication of idiopathic steatorrhea. Gut 3:232–239, 1962.

66. Cagnoff MF: Celiac disease. *In* Yamada T (ed): Textbook of Gastroenterology. Philadelphia: JB Lippincott, 1991, pp 1513–1514.

67. Wright BH, Jones DB, Clark H, et al: Is adult-onset coeliac disease due to a low-grade lymphoma of intraepithelial lymphocytes? Lancet 337:1373–1374, 1991.

68. Holmes GKT, Pryor P, Lane MR, et al: Malignancy in coeliac disease: effect of a gluten free diet. Gut 30:333–338, 1989.

69. Holmes GKT, Dunn GI, Cockel R, et al: Adenocarcinoma of the upper small bowel complicating coeliac disease. Gut 21:1010–1016, 1980.

70. O'Brien CJ, Saverymuttu S, Hodgson HJF, et al: Coeliac disease, adenocarcinoma of jejunum and in situ squamous carcinoma of oesophagus. J Clin Pathol 36:62–67, 1983.

71. Dannenberg A, Godwin T, Raybourn J, et al: Multifocal ade-

nocarcinoma of the small intestine in a patient with celiac sprue. J Clin Gastroenterol 11:73–76, 1989.

72. Straker RJ, Gunasekaren S, Brady PG: Adenocarcinoma of the jejunum in association with celiac sprue. J Clin Gastroenterol 11:320–323, 1989.

73. Logan RFA, Rifkind EA, Turner ID, et al: Mortality in celiac disease. Gastroenterology 97:265–271, 1989.

74. Trier JS: Case records of the Massachussets General Hospital, case 15-1990. N Engl J Med 322:1067–1075, 1990.

75. Caldwell Vl, Bayles TM: The importance and reliability of the roentgenographic examination of the small bowel in tropical sprue. Radiology 84:227–240, 1965.

76. Gouttebel MC, Saint Aubert B, Colette C, et al: Intestinal adaptation in patients with short bowel syndrome. Dig Dis Sci 34:709–715, 1989.

77. Koruda NJ, Rolandelli RH, Settle RG, et al: Effect of parenteral nutrition supplemented by short-chain fatty acids on adaptation to massive small bowel resection. Gastroenterology 95:715–720, 1988.

78. Thompson JS: Surgical therapy for the short bowel syndrome. J Surg Res 39:81–91, 1985.

79. MacCarty RL, Talley NJ: Barium studies in diffuse eosinophilic gastroenteritis. Gastrointest Radiol 15:183–187, 1990.

80. Schulman A, Morton PCG, Dietrich BE: Eosinophilic gastroenteritis. Clin Radiol 31:101–104, 1980.

81. Smith TR, Schmiedeberg P, Flax H, et al: Nonmucosal predominantly serosal eosinophilic enteritis. A case report. Clin Imaging 14:235–238, 1990.

82. Pipeleers-Marichal M, Somers G, Willems G, et al: Gastrinomas in the duodenums of patients with multiple endocrine neoplasia type 1 and the Zollinger-Ellison syndrome. N Engl J Med 322:723–727, 1990.

83. Valle J, Yamada T: Zollinger-Ellison syndrome. *In* Yamada T (ed): Textbook of Gastroenterology. Philadelphia: JB Lippincott, 1991, pp 1340–1352.

84. Dachman JL, Miller DL, Chang R, et al: Gastrinomas: localization by means of selective intraarterial injection of secretin. Radiology 174:25–29, 1990.

85. Matsui T, Iida M, Fujishima M, et al: Linear erosions on Kerckring's folds may be diagnostic of Zollinger-Ellison syndrome. J Clin Gastroenterol 11:278–281, 1989.

86. Gilholl WJ: Endoscopic diagnosis and removal of a duodenal wall gastrinoma. J Gastroenterol 79:679–683, 1984.

87. London JF, Shawker TH, Doppman JL, et al: Zollinger-Ellison syndrome: prospective assessment of abdominal ultrasound in the localization of gastrinomas. Radiology 178:763–767, 1991.

88. Frucht H, Dachman JL, Norton JA, et al: Gastrinomas: comparison of MR imaging with CT, angiography and ultrasound. Radiology 171:713–717, 1989.

89. Wolfe MM, Jensen RT: Zollinger-Ellison syndrome. Current concepts in diagnosis and management. N Engl J Med 317:1200–1209, 1987.

90. Carrasco CH, Chuang DP, Wallace C: Apudomas metastatic to the liver: treatment by hepatic artery embolization. Radiology 149:79–83, 1983.

91. Maton PN, Gardner JD, Jensen RT: Diagnosis and management of Zollinger-Ellison syndrome. Endocrinol Metab Clin North Am 18:519–543, 1989.

92. Hodson ME: Managing adults with cystic fibrosis. Chest medicine success story. Br Med J 298:471–472, 1989 (editorial).

93. Colten HR: Screening for cystic fibrosis. Public policy and personal choices. N Engl J Med 322:328–329, 1990 (editorial).

94. Park RW, Grand RJ: Gastrointestinal manifestations of cystic fibrosis: a review. Progress article. Gastroenterology 81:1143–1161, 1981.

95. Gaskin KJ, Waters DLM, Howman-Giles R, et al: Liver disease and common bile duct stenosis in cystic fibrosis. N Engl J Med 318:340–346, 1988.

96. Robinson PJ, Smith AL, Sly PD: Duodenal pH in cystic fibrosis and its relationship to fat malabsorption. Dig Dis Sci 35:1299–1304, 1990.

97. Heijerman HG, Lamers CB, Bakker W: Omeprazole enhances the efficacy of pancreatin in cystic fibrosis. Ann Intern Med 114:200–201, 1991.

98. Matseshe J, Go V, Di Magno E: Meconium ileus equivalent

complicating cystic fibrosis in post neonatal children and young adults. Gastroenterology 72:732–736, 1977.

99. Taussig L, Saldino R, di Sent'Agnese P: Radiographic abnormalities of the duodenum and small bowel in cystic fibrosis of the pancreas (mucoviscidosis). Radiology 106:369–376, 1973.

100. Lloyd ML, Olsen WA: Specific mucosal protein deficiency states. *In* Yamada T (ed): Textbook of Gastroenterology. Philadelphia: JB Lippincott, 1991, pp 1520–1529.

101. Cherner JA, Jensen RT, Dubois A, et al: Gastrointerstinal dysfunction in systemic mastocytosis. A prospective study. Gastroenterology 95:657–667, 1988.

102. Borda F, Uribarrena R, Rivero-Puente A: Gastroscopic findings in systemic mastocytosis. Endoscopy 15:342–343, 1983.

103. Barriere H, Dreno B, Pecquet C, et al: Systemic mastocytosis and intestinal malabsorption. Semin Hop Paris 59:2925–2931, 1983.

104. Quinn SF, Shaffer HA Jr, Willard MR, et al: Bull's eye lesions: a new gastrointestinal presentation of mastocytosis. Gastrointest Radiol 9:13–15, 1984.

105. Huang T-Y, Yam LT, Li C-Y: Radiological features of systemic mast-cell disease. Br J Radiol 60:765–770, 1987.

106. Dobbins WO III: Current concepts of Whipple's disease. J Clin Gastroenterol 4:205–208, 1982 (editorial).

107. Whipple GH: A hitherto undescribed disease characterized anatomically by deposits of fat and fatty acids in the intestinal and mesenteric lymphatic tissues. Bull Johns Hopkins Hosp 18:382, 1907.

108. Dobbins W III, Kawanishi H: Bacillary characteristics in Whipple's disease: an electron microscopic study. Gastroenterology 80:1468–1475, 1981.

109. Feldman M, Price G: Intestinal bleeding in patients with Whipple's disease. Gastroenterology 96:1207–1209, 1989.

110. Davis SJ, Patel A: Case report: distinctive echogenic lymphadenopathy in Whipple's disease. Clin Radiol 42:60–62, 1990.

111. Bi JC, Crosetti EE, Maurino EC, et al: Short-term antibiotic treatment in Whipple's disease. J Clin Gastroenterol 13:303–307, 1991.

112. Rubin W: Small intestine: anatomy and structural anomalies. *In* Yamada T (ed): Textbook of Gastroenterology. Philadelphia: JB Lippincott, 1991, pp 1409–1423.

113. Alexanian R: Plasma cell neoplasm. Curr Probl Cancer 3:1–60, 1978.

114. Amrein PC: Case records of the Massachusetts General Hospital, case 3-1990. N Engl J Med 322:183–192, 1990.

# Benign Tumors

### John C. Lappas, M.D.

## CLINICAL CONSIDERATIONS

Primary neoplasms of the small bowel are uncommon, constituting only 2 to 6% of the tumors of the gastrointestinal tract.[1, 2] In some series,[3] benign tumors are outnumbered by malignancies by a ratio of at least 1:1.2; however, such statistics vary depending on the nature of the survey. Benign tumors predominate in most autopsy studies because they are frequently asymptomatic and are therefore common incidental findings. Conversely, when only patients with clinical evidence of disease are investigated, there is significant predominance of malignant tumors. In a 40-year experience at the Massachusetts General Hospital, benign tumors represented 35% of the surgically resected small bowel neoplasms and 74% of the small bowel tumors detected at autopsy.[4] Regardless of the relative incidence of benign and malignant tumors, the apparent immunity of the small bowel to neoplasia is interesting, especially when one considers its length, total mucosal surface area, and diversity of structural elements. Among the factors often associated with the low incidence of epithelial small bowel tumors are the alkalinity and relative sterility of the liquid content of the intestine, the absence of stasis, a high level of immunoglobulin A, protective microsomal enzymes, and rapid cell turnover.[5]

Benign small bowel tumors are usually discovered in persons between the ages of 50 and 80 years and occur with equal infrequency in men and women. Symptomatic neoplasms manifest primarily with obstructive features, inciting intermittent abdominal pain, or, occasionally, signs of complete bowel obstruction. Constitutional symptoms such as anorexia, malaise, and weight loss are uncommon, as is the ability to palpate the tumor at clinical examination. Significant degrees of obstruction can be caused by neoplastic intussusception, and benign tumors are involved in the majority of adult cases.[6]

Bleeding from benign tumors, usually occult, occurs in about 30 to 40% of patients.[6, 7] Gastrointestinal bleeding may develop by ulceration of an epithelial adenoma or in the mucosa overlying an intramural tumor. In reported series in which enteroclysis was used to evaluate occult gastrointestinal blood loss, small bowel neoplasms accounted for one half of the positive findings and there was nearly equal detection of benign and malignant tumors.[8, 9] On occasion, benign tumors bleed severely and require emergency therapy.[6] Less commonly, an exoenteric benign tumor induces intestinal volvulus or compromises the lumen by a simple mass effect.

## IMAGING CONSIDERATIONS

It has been difficult for any institution to gain sufficient experience in the management of benign small bowel neoplasms. Delay and inaccuracy in the diagnosis of these tumors are commonly recognized and are related not only to the infrequency of their occurrence and the vagueness and paucity of their early symptoms and physical findings but also to the generally poor performance of radiologic small bowel follow-through studies.[10] Radiologists have to assume responsibility for the preoperative imaging and diagnosis of small bowel neoplasms, and they should use optimal barium contrast techniques. For this reason, several investigators have advocated enteroclysis with its improved sensitivity and specificity, noting that technical factors inherent in small bowel follow-through studies have accounted for most false-negative diagnoses.[10, 11] Reported series have shown enteroclysis to be more reliable in the demonstration of small bowel tumors,[12, 13] as well as in the evaluation of occult gastrointestinal bleeding[8, 9] and of intestinal obstruction.[12, 14, 15] Imaging modalities such as ultrasonography, computed tomography (CT), and magnetic resonance complement barium studies. CT in particular has been increasingly used for the evaluation of patients with vague abdominal symptoms and may provide the initial opportunity to detect and characterize tumors of the small bowel. The recognition of certain patterns of CT findings now allows a reasonable distinction to be made between benign and malignant small bowel tumors and, in cases of certain benign tumors such as lipoma and leiomyoma, may make it possible to suggest the specific diagnosis.[16, 17] In cases of acute gastrointestinal hemorrhage arising from benign neoplasms, angiographic techniques provide precise localization of the bleeding site and allow therapeutic transcatheter control of the hemorrhage. Angiographic demonstration of tumor neovascularity without contrast agent extravasation may also be of diagnostic importance, especially in patients with chronic occult bleeding when other diagnostic studies, endoscopy and barium contrast, have been negative.[18] Small bowel enteroscopy continues to be developed and will find applications in the evaluation of obscure bleeding and the diagnosis of tumors undetected by radiologic imaging.

Numerous benign tumors can be found in the small bowel, but approximately 90% of them are adenomas, leiomyomas, lipomas, and hemangiomas. Reports of benign tumors arising from virtually all other mesenchymal cell types have appeared sporadically in the literature.[19] Benign small bowel tumors commonly display similar morphologic characteristics on barium contrast studies. A specific histologic diagnosis is only rarely possible, but a useful differential diagnosis can be obtained by observing the location of the tumor, the number of tumors, and certain diagnosis-suggesting radiographic features.

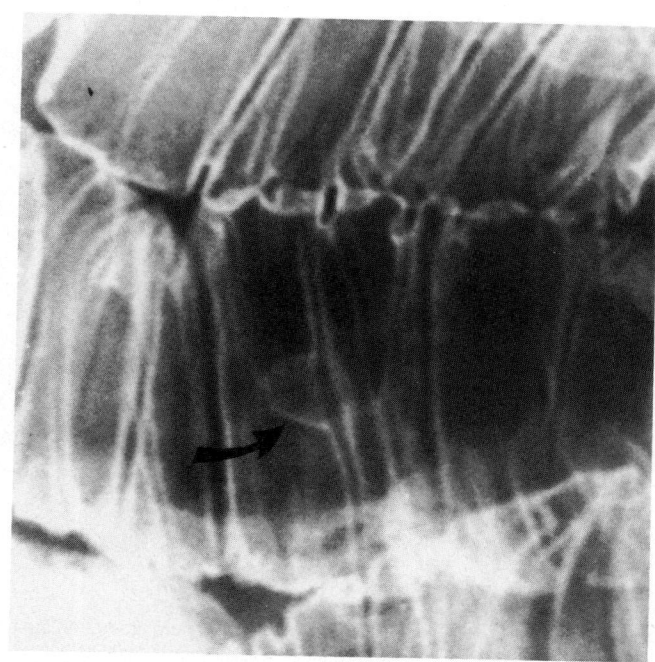

**Figure 50–1. Jejunal adenoma.** Enteroclysis demonstrates a small (8-mm) jejunal adenoma appearing as a smooth sessile mucosal nodule *(arrow).*

## SPECIFIC TUMORS

### Adenoma

Adenomas are proliferative epithelial neoplasms without the gross or histologic characteristics of malignancy. These epithelial tumors are subclassified in a manner similar to colonic adenomas. However, some 40% are villous (papillary) adenomas, relatively more common in the small bowel than in the colon. The remainder are tubular or predominantly tubular adenomatous polyps. Typical adenomas are small (1 to 3 cm), smooth or lobulated polypoid lesions. On barium studies they appear as either sessile or pedunculated intraluminal defects (Fig. 50–1). Although they usually occur singly, on rare occasions these tumors are multiple, especially when they are manifestations of familial polyposis or Gardner's syndrome.[3] Villous adenomas are generally larger than the usual adenomatous polyp and have a strong predilection for duodenal location.[20] They are invariably sessile, multilobulated, and more likely to exhibit symptoms of malignant change.

Brunner's gland adenomas differ from other small bowel adenomas in that they arise from specific mucussecreting glands. Brunner's gland enlargement may be caused by the accumulation of secreted mucin, by diffuse hyperplasia, or by the formation of a discrete polypoid adenoma. These lesions are found most frequently in the duodenum but may also be noted in the proximal jejunum or ileum.[19]

Adenomas are usually asymptomatic, although they may cause low-grade bleeding and occasionally may bleed profusely. If pedunculated, they may intussuscept and present with intestinal obstruction. Some data indicate that small bowel adenomas are premalignant. Of nine patients with adenomas detected in the mesenteric small bowel, five had invasive carcinoma within the resected adenoma.[21] Malignant change is more likely to be observed in symptomatic adenomas, in large adenomas, and in those with villous architecture.

### Leiomyoma

Leiomyomas are the most common benign small bowel tumors, occurring throughout the bowel with a slight predilection for the jejunum.[1–3] Of smooth muscle origin and generally arising in the muscularis propria, they are firm, well-circumscribed but not encapsulated neoplasms. The gross morphology of leiomyomas, as of other tumors of mesenchymal tissue origin, depends on the growth pattern relative to the lumen and the consistency and surface texture of the tumor. Leiomyomas grow slowly as a contiguous mass in either an inward (endoenteric), outward (exoenteric), or bidirectional (dumbbell) fashion.

On barium contrast examinations, endoenteric neoplasms are recognized as oval or round intraluminal defects (Fig. 50–2). Exoenteric leiomyomas, unless of larger size, may be more difficult to detect. They show mild luminal protrusion together with displacement of adjacent bowel loops by the extrinsic tumor. Compromise of the vascular supply to the tumor leads to surface ulceration, which may extend into the center of the tumor. Gastrointestinal bleeding, therefore, is the usual

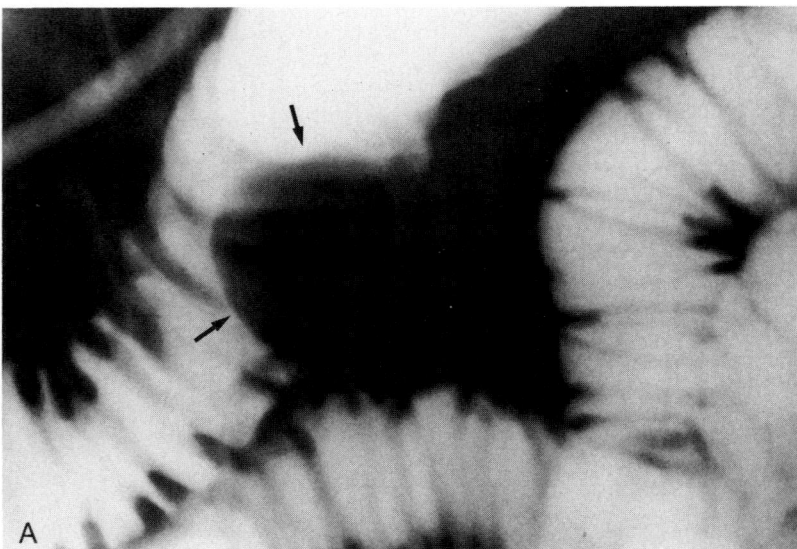

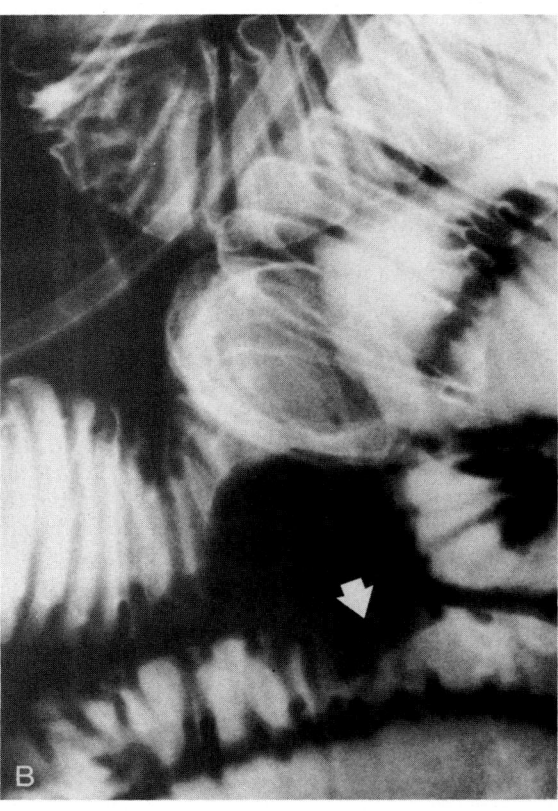

**Figure 50–2. Leiomyoma of jejunum. A.** On barium study, the submucosal nature of the tumor creates a characteristic semicircular mass effect within the lumen *(arrows)*. Smooth surface results from stretching of the overlying normal mucosa. **B.** Compression spot film in the same patient demonstrates a bidirectional growth effect *(arrow)* against an adjacent bowel loop.

symptom associated with leiomyomas. In about half the acute or chronic bleeding episodes associated with small bowel tumors, leiomyomas are responsible.[6, 9] Angiography can demonstrate small bowel leiomyomas, even if performed in the absence of active bleeding.[22] Although vascularity of smooth muscle tumors is variable, they are usually hypervascular with intense capillary opacification and with early visualization of draining veins. Even relatively hypovascular tumors tend to have prominent vessels in their periphery.

Megibow and colleagues[23] reported the usefulness of CT in depicting the nature and extent of small bowel leiomyomas. Cross-sectional images of these tumors correlate with the diagnostic features seen on barium contrast studies. On CT scans, leiomyomas are sharply defined spheric masses, ranging from 1 to 10 cm in size, and display homogeneous tissue density and uniform contrast enhancement (Fig. 50–3). Dense focal calcifications are occasionally noted within the tumor.

Leiomyomas have malignant potential. Malignant change is related to the size and biologic behavior of the tumor and less clearly to its histology. Large size and extensive tumor cavitation are more common in the presence of malignancy. Experience with CT also suggests that malignant smooth muscle tumors are larger than benign tumors, less uniform in shape, and of variable attenuation.[23]

## Lipoma

Lipomas are among the more common benign small bowel neoplasms, being second in frequency to leiomy-omas in most published series.[3, 7, 19] They arise as well-circumscribed submucosal proliferations of fat and usually grow intraluminally, because outward extension tends to be deflected by the firmness of the muscularis propria. Lipomas are characteristically solitary, relatively avascular, and of variable size (1 to 6 cm). More than 50% of these tumors occur in the ileum. Clinical manifestations are infrequent and consist of intermittent intestinal obstruction, usually caused by intussusception (Fig. 50–4), or, less commonly, bleeding from the overlying ulcerated mucosa.

Barium contrast studies demonstrate a sharply demarcated, often pedunculated tumor that tends to conform to the contour of the small bowel lumen (Fig. 50–5). The configuration of the tumor may change during

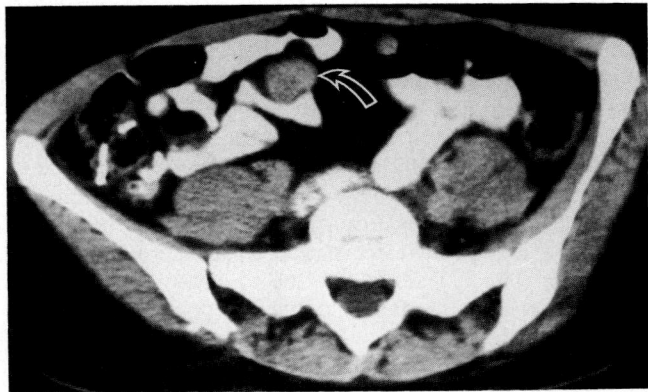

**Figure 50–3. Leiomyoma.** A CT scan shows a homogeneous soft tissue mass *(arrow)* representing an exoenteric small bowel tumor.

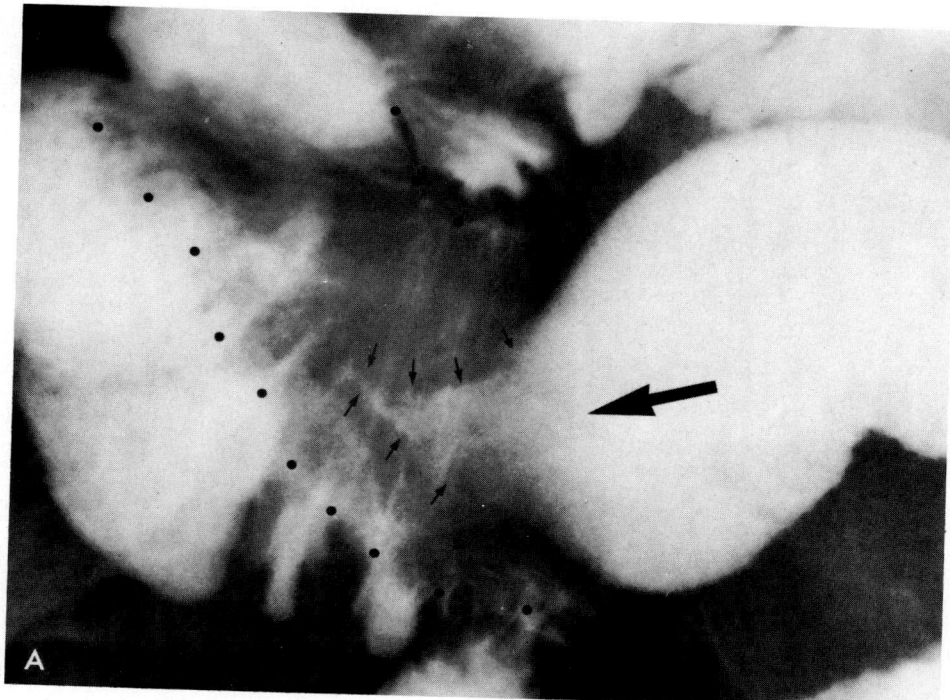

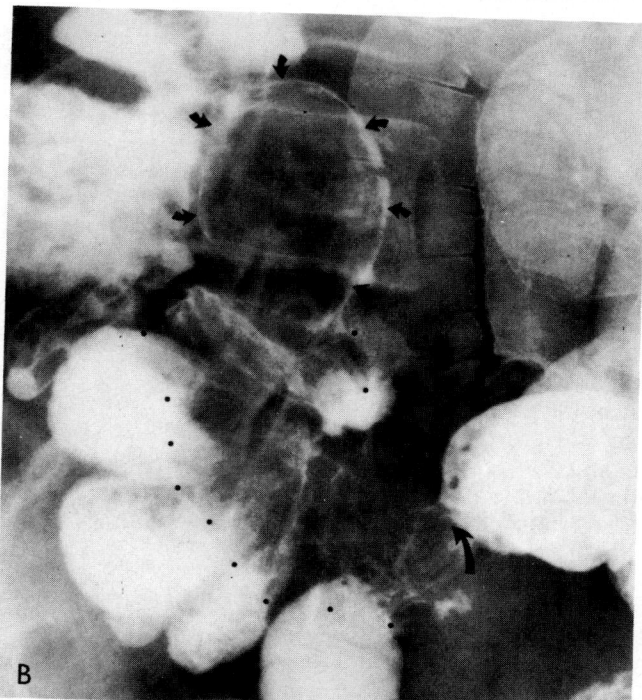

**Figure 50–4. Intussusception of a lipoma of terminal ileum. A.** Beak-shaped narrowing at entry into the intussusception *(arrows)*. Barium flowing back from beyond the intussusception outlines its soft tissue mass *(dots)* and faintly shows the stretched "coil spring" pattern of folds. **B.** Lipoma outlined by barium at the apex of the intussusception *(arrows)*.

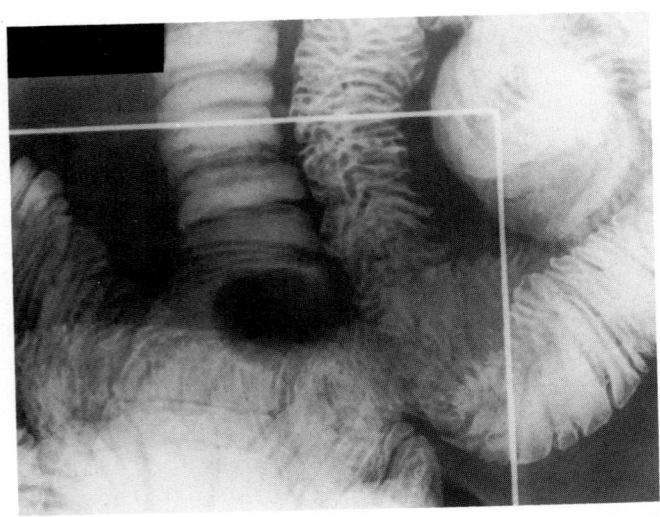

**Figure 50–5. Lipoma.** Enteroclysis demonstrates a lipoma protruding into the bowel lumen. Compression has caused slight flattening of the soft tumor.

compression or peristalsis.[24] CT can establish the diagnosis of small bowel lipoma by showing its attenuation values to be consistent with fat.[25] A homogeneous mass with Hounsfield units between −80 and −120 is considered pathognomonic. Identification of soft tissue strands within an otherwise uniform lipoma on CT scans has been attributed to fibrovascular changes associated with ulceration within the tumor.[25]

## Hemangioma

Benign angiomatous tumors include two principal forms: the capillary hemangioma and the cavernous hemangioma. The latter predominates in the small bowel and occurs either as a simple polypoid tumor or in a diffusely expansive form.[3] Microscopically, these submucosal neoplasms consist of variably enlarged vascular channels or sinuses, lined by endothelium and surrounded by minimal stromal tissue. Hemangiomas may be single or multiple and, although usually a few millimeters in size, may enlarge and protrude into the lumen. Direct invasion of the mucosa or penetration beyond the serosa is uncommon. Multiple phlebectasia refers to the small (1 to 5 mm) cavernous hemangiomas that predominate in the jejunum but may occur throughout the gastrointestinal tract.

In contrast to other small bowel tumors, which are more often asymptomatic, 80% of hemangiomas produce significant symptoms.[6] Gastrointestinal bleeding is the usual manifestation. Hemorrhage in association with a hemangioma is often acute, severe, and intermittent in nature. Anemia and occult fecal blood loss are also common clinical presentations.

The diagnosis of small bowel hemangioma is infrequently established before surgery. Small hemangiomas are rarely demonstrated by barium studies. They must be of sufficient size to be seen as intraluminal or intramural nodular defects (Fig. 50–6). The plain film dem-

onstration of calcified phleboliths, although rare, can also contribute to the diagnosis. Such abnormalities, seen in combination with vascular cutaneous lesions or with syndromes including tuberous sclerosis, Turner's syndrome, and Osler-Weber-Rendu disease, should increase the level of suspicion for intestinal hemangiomas. In selected patients, superior mesenteric arteriography can detect an intestinal vascular abnormality, although differentiation from other vascular tumors or malformations is seldom possible.

## Uncommon Tumors

Neurogenic tumors arise from the intramural neural plexus of the small bowel. Neurofibromas are the more frequently encountered nerve tumors and are composed of all cell types found in peripheral nerves, including Schwann cells.[26] Neurofibromas may occur as single tumors or, more commonly, as multiple lesions with or without systemic neurofibromatosis. Although rare in the general population, neural tumors of the small bowel are reported in 11 to 25% of patients with neurofibromatosis.[24, 26] Malignant transformation is seen in 10 to 15% of cases of neurofibromatosis. Neurilemomas consist entirely of Schwann cells, are encapsulated, and almost never become malignant. Infrequently, neurogenic tumors project intraluminally, but they can also be found in a subserosal position along the antimesenteric border of the intestine. Radiographic findings on barium contrast studies are often nonspecific or nondiagnostic. Identification of these tumors is im-

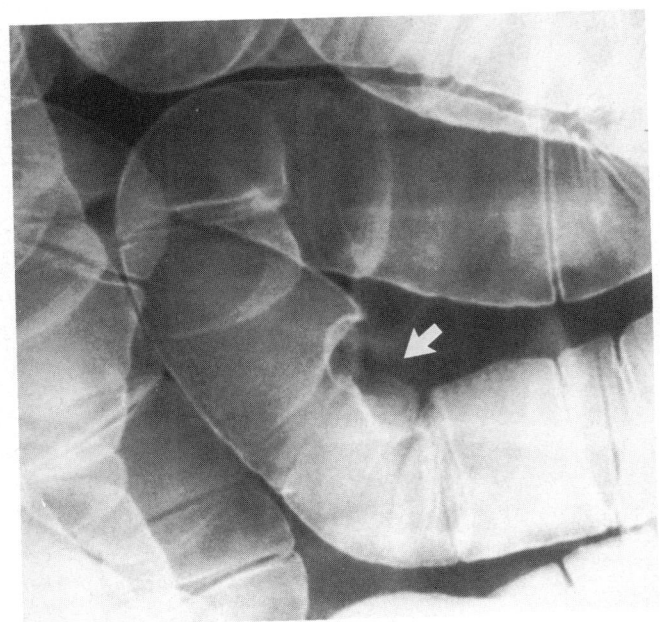

**Figure 50–6. Hemangioma.** Double contrast phase of enteroclysis demonstrates a 1.5-cm, slightly lobulated mural nodule *(arrow)* in a patient with occult gastrointestinal bleeding. Hemangioma was confirmed at surgery. (From Maglinte DDT, Lappas JC, Kelvin FM, et al: Small bowel radiography: how, when, and why? Radiology 163:297–305, 1987.)

portant because bleeding can be substantial and sarco-matous degeneration may occur.[27] Angiography has been suggested as an effective modality for diagnosis of small bowel neurofibromas, because they are often ex-oenteric and are hypervascular with angiographic char-acteristics similar to those of leiomyomas.[27]

Ganglioneuromas are made up of ganglion cells and of cell types seen in neurofibromas. Ganglioneuroma-tosis forms part of the syndrome of multiple endocrine neoplasia type 2B. These lesions are usually invisible macroscopically.

Inflammatory fibroid polyps are occasionally encoun-tered in elderly patients and occur almost exclusively in the ileum. They are usually solitary and are composed of a vascular fibrous stroma with a diffuse inflammatory infiltrate. Their etiology remains uncertain.[28] Contrast studies may demonstrate a smooth, rounded mass in the distal small bowel. In their clinical presentation, inflam-matory fibroid polyps are commonly associated with intussusception.

Myoepithelial hamartoma is a rare developmental tumor consisting of varied amounts of pancreatic tissue, smooth muscle, and epithelial structures. Predominance of pancreatic acinar tissue confers the designation ec-topic pancreas. Most myoepithelial hamartomas occur in the gastric antrum or duodenum, although some are reported in the mesenteric small bowel.[19] Lesions are solitary and usually under 3 cm in size. A smooth, nonpedunculated mass with occasional umbilication can be seen radiographically.

Heterotopic gastric mucosa may be found in the mesenteric small bowel, either as isolated lesions or in association with malformations such as Meckel's diver-ticulum or an enteric duplication. Occasionally, the heterotopic mucosa presents as a polypoid lesion, either sessile or pedunculated.

# POLYPOSIS SYNDROMES

## Peutz-Jeghers Syndrome

The Peutz-Jeghers syndrome is an uncommon disor-der characterized by mucocutaneous melanotic pigmen-tation and multiple hamartomatous polyps. The polyps present a smooth, lobulated, fronded surface, are sessile or pedunculated, and may be several centimeters in diameter. Histologically, the polyps are benign hamar-tomas containing a proliferative smooth muscle core and are lined by normal intestinal epithelium.[19]

Evidence of an autosomal dominant pattern of inher-itance with strong penetrance exists in most cases. No particular sex or racial predilection is observed. These hamartomas grossly resemble adenomatous polyps ex-cept for their variation in size (1 to 5 cm) and their multiplicity. Peutz-Jeghers polyps are more commonly found in the jejunum than the ileum but may also occur in the stomach or colon. In association with Peutz-Jeghers syndrome, there is a slightly increased incidence of carcinoma involving the stomach, duodenum, or colon. Small bowel malignancy is extremely rare.[29] Ex-

traintestinal malignancy, however, has been observed in a significant proportion of patients with the syndrome.[30]

Clinically, small pigmented macules are found on the lips, buccal mucosa, and volar surfaces of the hands and feet. Cutaneous lesions appear in early life, often pre-dating the formation of gastrointestinal polyps. They typically fade during adolescence, with only the buccal lesions persisting into adulthood. Characteristically, the polyps become manifest during the second or third decade. Episodes of intermittent abdominal pain caused by transient intussusception of the small bowel are common. Gastrointestinal bleeding is also a frequent mode of presentation and may be severe. Because Peutz-Jeghers polyps continue to develop throughout the life of the patient, a conservative approach to surgical inter-vention is recommended.[6]

Radiographically, barium contrast studies of the small bowel demonstrate luminal polyps of various sizes. Larger polyps typically present a lobulated contour (Fig. 50–7); pedunculated lesions with broad-based attach-ment may also be detected. Diffuse proliferation of intestinal polyps would be atypical for Peutz-Jeghers syndrome. Usually, uninvolved small bowel segments alternate with others that contain several hamartomas. Small bowel polyps discovered in children younger than 10 years old are commonly Peutz-Jeghers hamartomas. On CT scans, single and multiple Peutz-Jeghers polyps can be detected as soft tissue masses within the contrast medium–filled intestinal loops.[31] Polyps may also be found in the stomach and colon.

## Cowden's Disease

Cowden's disease, or multiple hamartoma syndrome, is an inherited condition of mucocutaneous lesions as-

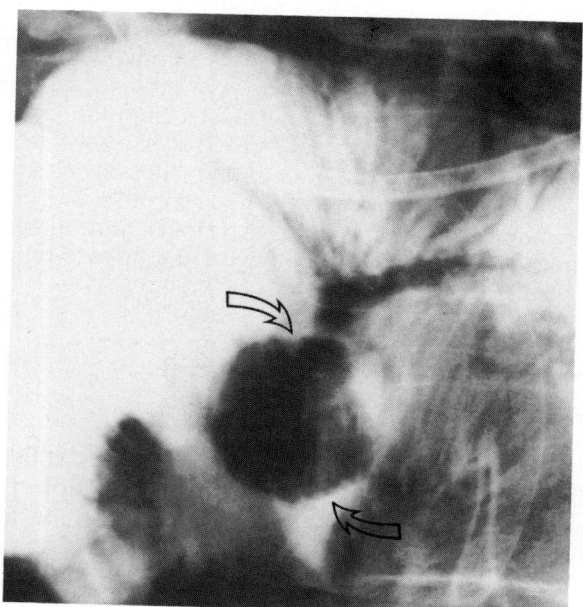

**Figure 50–7. Peutz-Jeghers syndrome.** Typical 2-cm lobulated, jejunal polyp *(arrows).*

sociated with hamartomata and other abnormalities of the breast, thyroid, and gastrointestinal tract. Characteristic papular hyperkeratoses of the skin and mucous membranes serve as markers of the disease. Although gastrointestinal polyposis is a typical feature of Cowden's disease, its true prevalence among individuals affected with this rare condition is difficult to establish. In a 1987 review of published cases of Cowden's disease, Chen and co-workers[32] determined that the small bowel was involved in 14 of 32 patients. The pathologic spectrum of polyps reported in Cowden's disease has included hamartomatous, hyperplastic, lymphomatous, and occasionally adenomatous types. Involvement of any gastrointestinal segment, especially the colon, or of the entire alimentary tract may occur. Enteroclysis has demonstrated multiple small bowel polyps that produced a nodular mucosal surface pattern in a patient with diffuse gastrointestinal tract disease.[32] The occurrence of gastrointestinal polyps in combination with skin, thyroid, and breast lesions should suggest the possible diagnosis of the multiple hamartoma syndrome.

## Cronkhite-Canada Syndrome

Clinical manifestations in combination with diffuse gastrointestinal polyposis define the unique, nonfamilial Cronkhite-Canada syndrome. Symptoms of abdominal pain, diarrhea, and anorexia precede or occur together with the development of the ectodermal changes, alopecia, hyperpigmentation, and dystrophy of nails. The onset is usually gradual, and older adults are affected. Intestinal malabsorption and protein loss can be severe and the clinical course is potentially fatal. Polyps occur in the stomach and colon in virtually all patients, with the small bowel involved in more than half of the cases. The polyps are inflammatory in nature and consist of dilated cystic interstitial glands, closely resembling the hamartoma-like juvenile polyps. Dachman and colleagues[33] classified the patterns of involvement according to radiographic studies as 1) innumerable small polyps carpeting large areas (most common), 2) scattered polyps of various sizes, and 3) sparse involvement with few small polyps. In addition, small bowel studies may show findings related to malabsorption and hypoproteinemia including thickened folds and increased luminal secretions. The etiology of the disease remains obscure.

## Predominantly Extraintestinal Syndromes

Adenomatous polyps in familial polyposis coli typically involve the entire colon. On rare occasion, there may be a lesser degree of involvement of the small bowel. Small bowel adenomas have also been reported to develop in the ileum after colectomy for familial polyposis coli.[34] Tumors of the small bowel, including jejunoileal adenomas and ileal lymphoid polyps, have been reported to occur somewhat more frequently in

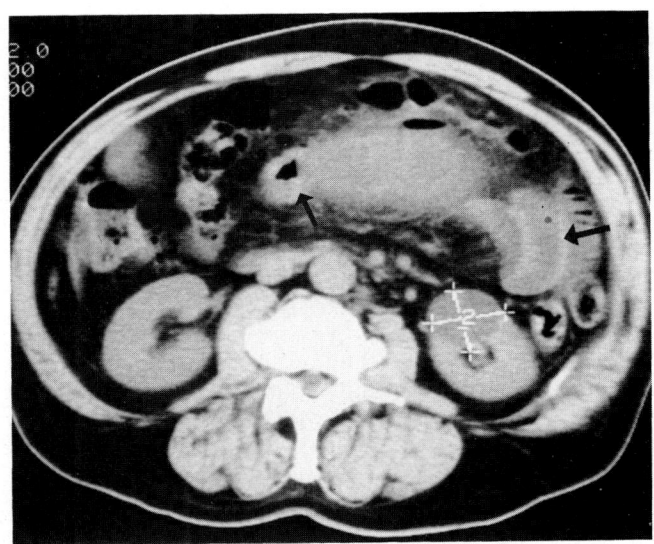

**Figure 50–8. Desmoid tumor.** CT scan showing a mass in the mesentery with mostly lower attenuation than muscle. There is evidence of infiltration into the mesentery and of involvement of two adjacent bowel loops seen here to have thickened walls *(arrows)*. At surgery a desmoid tumor was resected. The adjacent bowel was edematous and viable.

patients with Gardner's syndrome, a variant of familial polyposis.[6, 35] There is a distinct association between Gardner's polyposis and the finding of intra-abdominal desmoids.

Desmoid tumors are usually classified as benign because they do not metastasize, although they have a strong tendency toward local recurrence and focal invasion. Their preferred site is the small bowel mesentery. Most desmoids reported in the radiologic literature have been associated with Gardner's syndrome. However, among a large number of desmoids reported by the Armed Forces Institute of Pathology,[36] only 13% were related to Gardner's syndrome. CT is an ideal imaging method for the demonstration of desmoids as it can also show the extent of invasion of the mesentery and of the small bowel.[37, 38] A CT scan of an unusual mesenteric desmoid tumor with extensive necrosis and without association with Gardner's syndrome is shown in Figure 50–8.

Juvenile polyposis affects predominantly the colon, but small bowel polyps may occasionally occur. The mostly familial syndrome presents in children and can cause significant gastrointestinal bleeding. Polyps are hamartomatous, similar histologically to Cronkhite-Canada polyps, and are generally fewer in number than in the familial polyposis coli. Patients with juvenile polyposis and their relatives have increased risk for the development of gastrointestinal carcinoma.

### Acknowledgment

Figure 50–4A and B is reproduced from Laufer I, Levine MS (eds): Double Contrast Gastrointestinal Radiology (2nd ed). Philadelphia: WB Saunders, 1992.
Figure 50–5 is reproduced from Herlinger H, Maglinte D (eds): Clinical Radiology of the Small Intestine. Philadelphia: WB Saunders, 1989.

# References

1. Gupta S, Gupta S: Primary tumors of the small bowel: a clinico-pathological study of 58 cases. J Surg Oncol 20:161–167, 1982.
2. Good CA: Tumors of the small intestine. AJR 89:685, 1963.
3. Garvin PJ, Herrmann V, Kaminski DL, et al: Benign and malignant tumors of the small intestine. *In* Hickey RC (ed): Current Problems in Cancer. Chicago: Mosby–Year Book, 1979, pp 1–46.
4. Darling RC, Welch CE: Tumors of the small intestine. N Engl J Med 260:397–406, 1959.
5. Sinar DR, O'Brien TF Jr: Benign neoplasms and vascular malformations of the large and small intestine. *In* Sleisenger MH, Fordtran JS (eds): Gastrointestinal Disease: Pathophysiology, Diagnosis, Management (4th ed). Philadelphia: WB Saunders, 1989, pp 1359–1369.
6. Dial P, Cohn I Jr: Tumors of the jejunum and ileum. *In* Scott HW, Sawyers JL (eds): Surgery of the Stomach, Duodenum, and Small Intestine (2nd ed). Boston: Blackwell Scientific Publications, 1992, pp 859–871.
7. Wilson JM, Melvin DB, Gray G, et al: Benign small bowel tumors. Ann Surg 181:247–250, 1975.
8. Maglinte DDT, Elmore MF, Chernish SM, et al: Enteroclysis in the diagnosis of chronic unexplained gastrointestinal bleeding. Dis Colon Rectum 28:403–405, 1985.
9. Rex DK, Lappas JC, Maglinte DDT, et al: Enteroclysis in the evaluation of suspected small intestinal bleeding. Gastroenterology 97:58–60, 1989.
10. Maglinte DDT, Burney BT, Miller RE: Lesions missed on small bowel follow-through: analysis and recommendations. Radiology 144:737–739, 1982.
11. Maglinte DDT, Lappas JC, Kelvin FM, et al: Small bowel radiography: how, when, and why? Radiology 163:297–305, 1987.
12. Maglinte DDT, Hall R, Miller RE, et al: Detection of surgical lesions of the small bowel by enteroclysis. Am J Surg 127:225–229, 1984.
13. Antes G, Lissner J: Double contrast small bowel examination with barium and methylcellulose: result in 300 cases. Radiology 148:37–40, 1983.
14. Nolan DJ, Marks CG: The barium infusion in small intestinal obstruction. Clin Radiol 32:651–655, 1981.
15. Maglinte DDT, Peterson LA, Vahey TN, et al: Enteroclysis in partial small bowel obstruction. Am J Surg 147:325–329, 1984.
16. Dudiak KM, Johnson CD, Stephen DH: Primary tumors of the small intestine: CT evaluation. AJR 152:995–998, 1989.
17. Laurent F, Raynaud M, Biset JM, et al: Diagnosis and categorization of small bowel neoplasms: role of computed tomography. Gastrointest Radiol 16:115–119, 1991.
18. Rollins ES, Picus D, Hicks ME, et al: Angiography is useful in detecting the source of chronic gastrointestinal bleeding of obscure origin. AJR 156:385–388, 1991.
19. Olmsted WW, Ros PR, Hjermstad BM, et al: Tumors of the small intestine with little or no malignant predisposition: a review of the literature and report of 56 cases. Gastrointest Radiol 12:231–239, 1987.
20. Mir-Madjlessi S, Farmer RG, Hawk WA: Villous tumors of the duodenum and jejunum. Report of four cases and a review of the literature. Am J Dig Dis 18:467–476, 1973.
21. Perzin KH, Bridge MF: Adenomas of the small intestine: a clinicopathologic review of 51 cases and a study of their relationship to carcinoma. Cancer 48:799–819, 1981.
22. Uflacker R, Amarat NM, Lima S, et al: Angiography in primary myomas of the alimentary tract. Radiology 139:361–369, 1981.
23. Megibow AJ, Balthazar EJ, Hulnick DH, et al: CT evaluation of gastrointestinal leiomyomas and leiomyosarcomas. AJR 144:727–731, 1985.
24. Herlinger H, Maglinte DDT: Tumors of the small intestine. *In* Herlinger H, Maglinte D (eds): Clinical Radiology of the Small Intestine. Philadelphia: WB Saunders, 1989, pp 399–451.
25. Taylor AJ, Stewart ET, Dodds WJ: Gastrointestinal lipomas: a radiologic and pathologic review. AJR 155:1205–1210, 1990.
26. Sivak MV, Sullivan BH, Farmer RG: Neurogenic tumors of the small intestine: review of the literature and report of a case with endoscopic removal. Gastroenterology 68:374–380, 1975.
27. Uflacker R, Alves MA, Diehl JC: Gastrointestinal involvement in neurofibromatosis: angiographic presentation. Gastrointest Radiol 10:163–165, 1985.
28. Shimer GR, Helwig EB: Inflammatory fibroid polyps of the intestine. Am J Clin Pathol 81:708–713, 1984.
29. Perzin KH, Bridge MF: Adenomatous and carcinomatous changes in hamartomatous polyps of the small intestine (Peutz-Jeghers syndrome): report of a case and review of the literature. Cancer 49:971–983, 1982.
30. Giardiello FM, Welsh WB, Hamilton SR, et al: Increased risk of cancer in the Peutz-Jeghers syndrome. N Engl J Med 316:1511–1514, 1987.
31. Sener RN, Kumcuoglu Z, Elmas N, et al: Peutz-Jeghers syndrome: CT and US demonstration of small bowel polyps. Gastrointest Radiol 16:21–23, 1991.
32. Chen YM, Ott DJ, Wu WC, et al: Cowden's disease: a case report and literature review. Gastrointest Radiol 12:325–329, 1987.
33. Dachman AH, Buck JL, Burke AP, et al: Cronkhite-Canada syndrome: radiologic features. Gastrointest Radiol 14:285–290, 1989.
34. Hamilton SR, Bussey HJR, Mendelsohn G, et al: Ileal adenomas after colectomy in nine patients with adenomatous polyposis coli/Gardner's syndrome. Gastroenterology 77:1252–1257, 1979.
35. Nayler EW, Lebenthal E: Gardner's syndrome: recent developments in research and management. Dig Dis Sci 25:945–959, 1980.
36. Burke AP, Sobin LH, Shekitka KM, et al: Intraabdominal fibromatosis: a pathologic analysis of 130 tumors with comparison of clinical subgroups. Am J Surg Pathol 144:335–341, 1990.
37. Einstein DM, Tagliabue JR, Desai RK: Abdominal desmoids: CT findings in 25 patients. AJR 157:275–279, 1991.
38. Casillas J, Sais GJ, Greve JL, et al: Imaging of intra- and extraabdominal desmoid tumors. Radiographics 11:959–968, 1991.

# Malignant Tumors

## 51

Dean D. T. Maglinte, M.D.

## GENERAL CONSIDERATIONS

### Incidence

Although the small intestine represents 75% of the length and 90% of the mucosal surface of the alimentary tract, it is a relatively rare site for primary malignant tumors. Primary tumors of the small intestine constitute less than 2% of all gastrointestinal tumors, and primary malignancies of the small intestine, less than 3% of all gastrointestinal malignant tumors.[1, 2] Precise numbers expressing the prevalence and distribution of the many forms of malignant neoplasms involving the small intestine differ among reports in the medical literature. In some reports, the duodenum is included. Others confine themselves to the mesenteric small intestine (i.e., jejunum and ileum). Carcinoid tumors may be classified among malignancies or may be listed as a separate category. Some reports are based on autopsy material; others represent findings at laparotomy.

### Etiologic Factors

Several factors contribute to the low incidence of neoplasms in the small intestine.[1, 3] Carcinogens may be diluted by the alkaline constituent fluids of the small intestine and exposure of intestinal mucosa to carcinogens may be reduced by the rapid transit of the contents. The number of bacteria is much smaller than in the colon and the high concentration of immunoglobulin A may result in increased neutralization of potentially carcinogenic viruses. Enzymes such as benzopyrene hydroxylase, which can detoxify potential carcinogens, are present in greater quantities in the small intestine than in the colon.

With regard to metastases, however, the small intestine has its full share in accordance with its length and large surface area. Malignant mesenchymal tumors occur with equal infrequency throughout the alimentary tract.

## Clinical Presentation

Abdominal pain is the most common presenting symptom, found in 69% of 77 patients with histologically confirmed primary malignancies of the small intestine.[4] Gastrointestinal bleeding has been noted in 52%, nausea and/or vomiting in 49%, weight loss (more than 5 lb) in 45%, and diarrhea in 29%. In 4% of patients, an abdominal mass was palpable. In the same review, obstruction was stated to be the presentation in 36% of the patients.[4] Most patients were 50 to 69 years old. At the time of surgery, the majority of patients have had local extension of the tumor and/or distant tumor spread.

## Delays in Diagnosis: Contribution of Clinician and Radiologist

Despite significant improvements in diagnostic technology and operative mortality, the survival of patients with primary malignancies of the small intestine has not changed in four decades. One reason for the failure to improve prognosis has been the considerable delay before the diagnosis is made, resulting in an advanced stage of disease at the time of surgery (Table 51–1). An analysis of the contributions to this delay in diagnosis showed that responsibility was shared by patients who failed to report symptoms, physicians who failed to order the appropriate diagnostic tests, and radiologists who did not arrive at a correct diagnosis.[4] It could be shown that the major delay in diagnosis occurred after medical help was sought by the patient. The delay before medical contact (patient's delay) was only one seventh of the delay after medical contact (physician's delay). Although radiologists were responsible for a minority of the physicians' errors, radiologic errors caused the longest periods of delay of diagnoses (Fig. 51–1). The report concluded that only greater awareness of the small intestine as a potential source of unexplained abdominal

### TABLE 51–1. EXTENT OF METASTASES AT SURGERY (BY HISTOLOGY)*

| TUMOR | INTRAMURAL | LOCAL SPREAD | DISTANT SPREAD | TOTAL |
|---|---|---|---|---|
| Adenocarcinoma | 7 (18.4%) | 13 (34.2%) | 18 (47.4%) | 38 |
| Carcinoid | 6 (33.3%) | 6 (33.3%) | 6 (33.3%) | 18 |
| Leiomyosarcoma | 6 (66.7%) | 1 (11.1%) | 2 (22.2%) | 9 |
| Lymphoma | 1 (10.0%) | 7 (70.0%) | 2 (20.0%) | 10 |
| Total | 20 (26.7%) | 27 (36.0%) | 28 (37.3%) | 75 |

*These data as well as results from other reviews show that more than 70% of patients with primary malignant tumors of the small intestine have local or distant spread at the time of surgery.

Modified from DDT Maglinte, K O'Connor, J Bessette, et al, The role of the physician in the late diagnosis of primary malignant tumors of the small intestine, Am J Gastroenterol, 86, 3, 304–308, 1991, © by The American College of Gastroenterology.

symptoms would lead to prompter use of sensitive methods of radiologic examination and thus to improvement of the patient's prognosis.[4]

ative demonstration of a tumor of the small bowel depends on contrast radiology, primarily a barium examination.

## IMAGING CONSIDERATIONS

### Plain Film Radiography

Plain film radiography may provide information aiding diagnosis if it is done during an obstructive episode or if an ulcerating or necrotic tumor has perforated. The soft tissue outline of a tumor, its displacement of adjacent, gas-filled structures, or the presence of tumor calcification can be a means of positive identification by plain film radiography.

Except for the proximal jejunum, which can sometimes be reached during upper gastrointestinal panendoscopy, and the distal part of the terminal ileum, which can often be entered by the colonoscope, the preoper-

### Barium Studies: Sensitivity, Tumor Demonstration

Barium studies do not have a good record in the surgical literature. The reported sensitivity for the detection of malignant small bowel tumors by the small bowel follow-through (SBFT) examination, the most commonly used method in most institutions, varies widely. Most studies have accepted indirect as well as direct evidence of a tumor as being diagnostic. An abnormality shown by the SBFT has been reported in 53 to 83% of primary malignant tumors,[5–7] although direct evidence of a tumor was noted in only 30 to 44% of the cases. In a study comparing the sensitivity and tumor detection rate of the small bowel enema (enter-

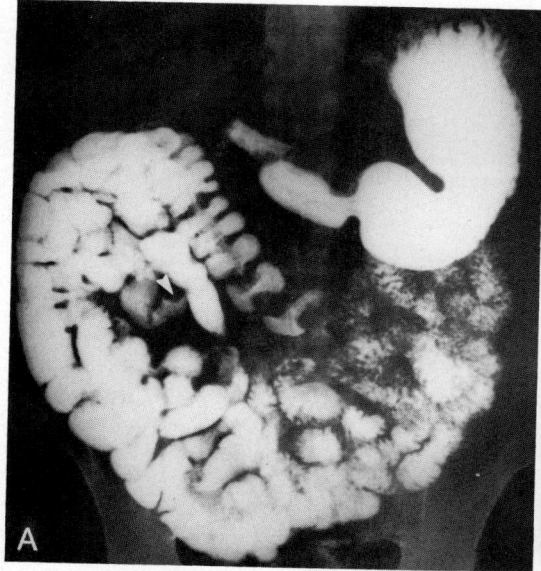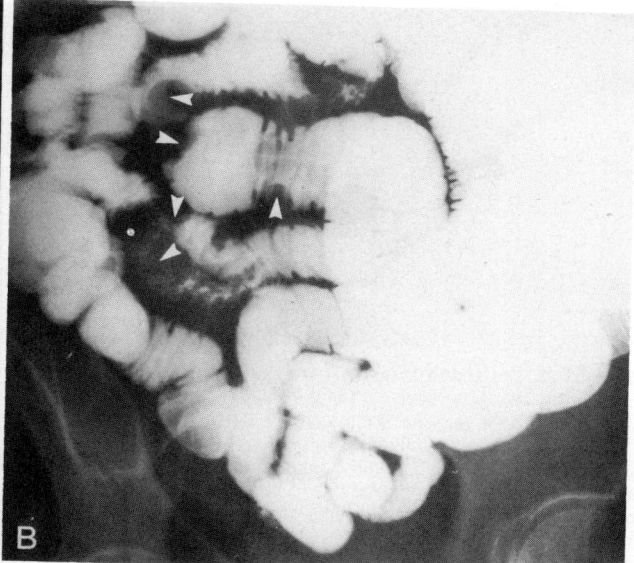

**Figure 51–1. Radiologic delay in diagnosing malignant tumors of the small intestine.** False-negative SBFT in an elderly female patient with unexplained recurrent abdominal pain and anemia. **A.** Overview SBFT radiograph of prone patient, obtained in another institution, does not show an apparent abnormality. Compression films of terminal ileum were unremarkable. In retrospect, there is a suggestion of a small polypoid defect *(arrowhead)* in a loop of ileum in the right hemiabdomen. **B.** After referral to a gastroenterologist, enteroclysis was done 6 months later for similar indications. It shows multiple intramural defects *(arrowheads)*, with partial obstruction of one segment by the largest mass. Surgery revealed multifocal carcinoid with extension to mesenteric nodes.

oclysis) and the SBFT, the SBFT showed abnormalities in 11 of 18 patients for a sensitivity of 61% and enteroclysis showed abnormalities in 19 of 20 patients for a sensitivity of 95%.[8] The actual tumor detection rate was 33% (6 of 18 patients) for the SBFT and 90% (18 of 20 patients) for enteroclysis. Four patients had both types of examination, with normal findings on conventional SBFT followed by demonstration of a tumor by enteroclysis. This clinicoradiologic study shows that the intubation method of barium examination is significantly more sensitive than the oral method of examination for detection of primary malignancies of the small bowel.

## Other Imaging Methods

Arteriography has had limited applications in the primary radiologic diagnosis of malignant small bowel tumors. Its principal use has been in the evaluation of

bleeding of possible small intestinal origin and selective catheterization for transcatheter therapy.

Of the cross-sectional imaging methods, computed tomography (CT) has been increasingly applied to the evaluation of the small intestine.[9–11] It more accurately defines the true extent of barium-demonstrated small bowel lesions by revealing their transmural extension, mesenteric involvement, and distant disease. The imaging methods, however, cannot replace the demonstration of fine mucosal detail that is possible only by adequate barium technique (Fig. 51–2). Clinically effective imaging of the small bowel should be able to demonstrate early and subtle mucosal and mural structural alterations or provide reliable evidence of normality. CT and ultrasound have not been able to exclude diseases of the small intestine, an important deficiency in the work-up of an organ in which disease prevalence is low and symptoms may be referred to or from other organs.[12] There is little experience to date with magnetic

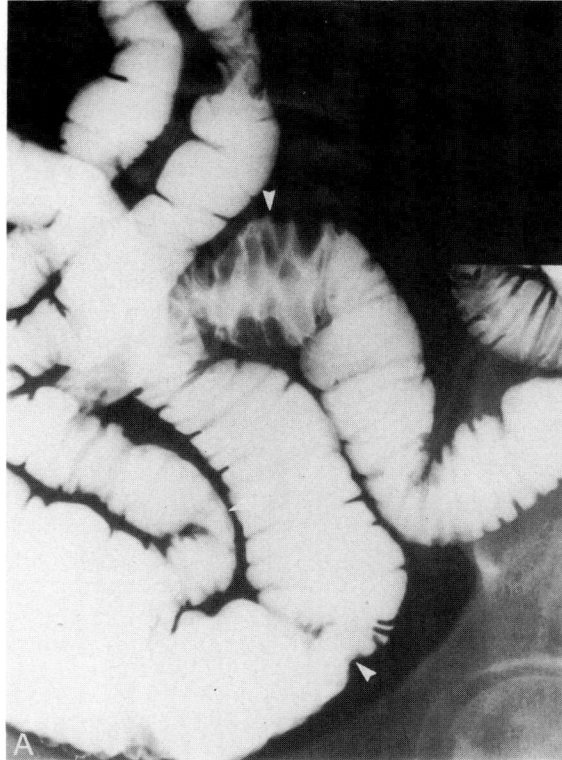
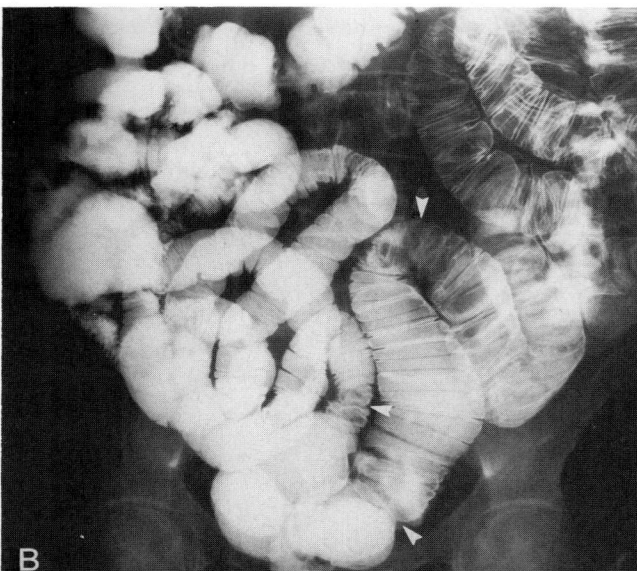
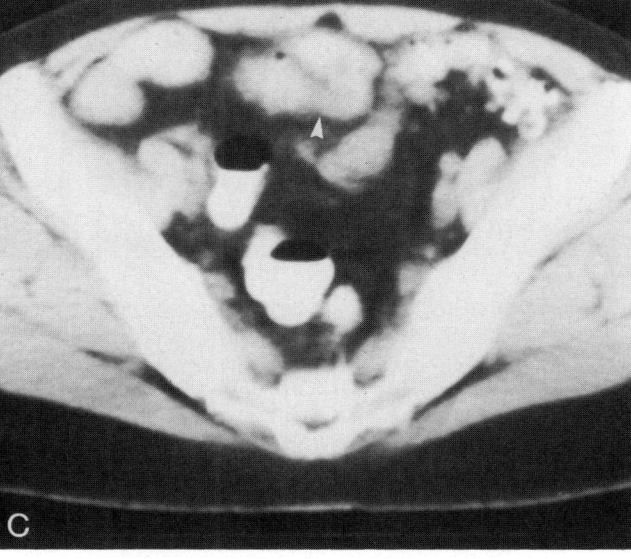

**Figure 51–2. Localized intestinal wall lesions shown by enteroclysis.** A 52-year-old female patient had unexplained weight loss, anemia, and gastrointestinal bleeding. **A.** Enteroclysis shows multifocal segmental nodular thickening of folds *(arrowheads)* with decreased distensibility. Surgery and histology confirmed this to be non-Hodgkin's lymphoma. **B.** Double contrast phase of enteroclysis confirms the abnormalities shown in the single contrast phase *(arrowheads)*. Note positive demonstration of normal thickness and number of folds in uninvolved segments. **C.** CT examination 2 days after enteroclysis for staging of the lymphoma does not show extraluminal or mesenteric involvement. The segmental intestinal wall abnormalities are difficult to appreciate. The folds of the distal small intestine are usually poorly shown on CT scans even when the lumen is opacified by contrast medium. Arrowhead points to one of the abnormal segments.

resonance imaging of the small bowel, and it is not yet possible to predict its role in this field of diagnosis.

# PRIMARY MALIGNANCIES: SPECIFIC TUMORS

## Carcinoid Tumors

The small intestine is the second most common site for carcinoid tumors, and the ileum, the most common site for malignant carcinoids. Almost 50% of carcinoids occur in the appendix and 33% in the small bowel, mostly the distal ileum. They account for 25% of all small bowel tumors.

Carcinoids are slow-growing tumors that arise from enterochromaffin cells at the base of the crypts of Lieberkühn. All carcinoid tumors are potentially malignant and have been called "malignant neoplasms in slow motion."[13] The extent of invasion is a function of time, anatomic location, and size. There are no distinct histologic differences between benign and malignant carcinoid tumors. The malignant status is confirmed if local invasion or distant metastases are observed. Carcinoids less than 1 cm in diameter are rarely invasive, and those greater than 2 cm in diameter are frequently malignant. Although they are slow growing, between 30 and 67% of ileal carcinoids are found to have extended beyond the bowel wall when diagnosed.[14] Even appendiceal carcinoids, which are considered benign, have shown microscopic invasion of the muscularis.

Carcinoid tumors arise from cellular elements that originate in the ectodermal component of the fourth germ layer, the neural crest. They belong to the group of amine precursor uptake and decarboxylation cells. Thus, carcinoid tumors may originate at any site where these cells are located, including the gastrointestinal, pancreatic, biliary, respiratory, and genitourinary tracts and the thymus. Initially, carcinoids grow toward the submucosa as well as the mucosal surface, bulge into the small bowel lumen, and may even become pedunculated and be the lead point of an intussusception. The overlying mucosa may ulcerate, and bleeding may be an early manifestation. Further growth extends into and through the muscularis and then into the serosa. By this time, the effects of hormonal substances produced by the tumor have begun to assert themselves.

## Pathophysiology

Hormonally active substances such as 5-hydroxytryptamine, kallikrein, bradykinin, and histamine are secreted by carcinoid tumors and are generally metabolized in the liver. The major biomedical product of carcinoid tumors is serotonin.[15] Tryptophan is required for its synthesis and must be derived from food. Normally, only about 1% of tryptophan is converted to serotonin, but carcinoid tumors can utilize as much as 60%. Serotonin released by the tumor is bound to platelets in the plasma. Deamination by monoamine oxidase in the liver and the lungs converts serotonin to

5-hydroxyindoleacetic acid (5-HIAA), which is then excreted in the urine in increased amounts. In a normal adult, less than 10 mg of 5-HIAA is excreted in the urine during 24 hours. Output of 5-HIAA is mildly increased in patients taking serotonin-containing foods or drugs like phenothiazines and in patients with malabsorption states or prolonged intestinal obstruction. Kallikrein is related to the production of bradykinin, high levels of which appear in the plasma of patients with carcinoid tumors.[15]

When the tumor has invaded the muscle coat, the local action of serotonin provokes an intense desmoplastic effect. The tumor mass and the associated fibrosis may produce fixation and kinking of a bowel loop, sometimes leading to obstruction. With further tumor growth into the mesentery and invasion of mesenteric lymph nodes, desmoplastic changes extend into that vital area. The masses that develop can exceed the primary tumor in size and in the production of endocrine substances. Gradually, fibrotic changes emanating from these mesenteric masses extend through the mesentery in the form of thick strands that draw in adjacent bowel loops in a spoke-wheel arrangement. Desmoplastic changes involve blood vessels in the mesentery and near the bowel wall, causing ischemia. This is compounded by the development of a special form of elastic fibrosis that causes thickening of mesenteric arteries and veins over a wide area and may lead to vascular occlusions. Ischemic changes ranging from edema to gangrene can affect loops involved in the spoke-wheel arrangement.

Eventually, tumor may spread via the portal stream to the liver to produce further and possibly larger carcinoid metastases. In their presence, vasoactive substances are released directly into the systemic venous flow, giving rise to the carcinoid syndrome. The carcinoid syndrome, however, occasionally occurs without hepatic involvement.[15] It has been suggested that vasoactive products may be absorbed from the peritoneal surface and taken into the systemic circulation by draining lymphatics, thus bypassing the usual metabolic degradation by the liver. In the case of the rare ovarian carcinoid, the chemical mediator is secreted directly into systemic veins.[16] Carcinoids are multiple in about 30% of cases and are associated with other malignant neoplasms, either synchronous or metachronous, in 30 to 40% of patients.[17]

## Clinical Features

Carcinoids, even those in the ileum, produce no symptoms in their early development and do not present specific symptoms for 5 to 7 years. Vague symptoms, such as abdominal pain, occur during these intervening years. More specific but late clinical features are intermittent obstruction, diarrhea, and blood loss. Urinary 5-HIAA levels should be elevated by this time. The carcinoid syndrome is a late and infrequent presentation. It consists of periodic cutaneous flushing, diarrhea, and, less frequently, bronchospasm. The carcinoid syndrome is always associated with elevated blood levels of serotonin, which can occur only if the liver has failed to deaminate serotonin. In 95% of patients with the carcinoid syndrome, there are extensive hepatic carcinoid metastases, virtually always derived from an ileal primary tumor. The entry of serotonin into the right side of the heart produces a special form of subendothelial fibrosis. The left side of the heart is unaffected, being protected by monoamine oxidase in the lung. The presence of liver metastases need not always be associated with clinical carcinoid syndrome.[15]

## Radiology

Carcinoid tumors are at least 10 times more common in the ileum than in the jejunum and most occur in the last 2 ft of ileum. Ileal carcinoids show the highest rate of invasiveness. In addition to location, the size of the primary tumor influences the likelihood of invasion. Of tumors that exceed 2 cm in diameter, 90% were found to have metastasized.[13]

Primary carcinoid tumors are rarely detected by radiology before they reach the size of 2 cm. The inherent limitations of the SBFT make it difficult to demonstrate small submucosal nodules. Whatever the nonspecific symptoms of the patient may be, the demonstration by enteroclysis of a smoothly rounded, mucosal elevation 1 to 2 cm in size located in the distal or terminal ileum must place a carcinoid tumor at the top of the list of differential diagnoses (Fig. 51–3). The tumor may seem to be submucosal or mucosal in origin and is indistin-

guishable from other possible lesions, such as leiomyoma, lipoma, or adenoma. An exoenteric component of a carcinoid should not yet be present, nor should desmoplastic changes have occurred. The presence of one or two additional polyps of similar appearance further strengthens the suspicion of carcinoid[18] (see Fig. 51–1). Drawing attention to the likely presence of a carcinoid at this early stage when curative removal is possible can be regarded as a major success of radiology.

With further tumor growth and extension into the mesentery, specific radiographic features can be detected even though clinical signs may still be nonspecific. There may be crowding of folds surrounding the tumor edge, kinking of the bowel wall with narrowing of the lumen, and occasionally an annular stenosis. An exoenteric mass may become obvious by displacement of adjacent bowel loops (Fig. 51–4). At this stage, CT becomes mandatory. The characteristic CT pattern is that of a small or larger mesenteric mass with curvilinear strands beginnig to extend through the mesentery toward surrounding bowel loops (Fig. 51–5). These mesenteric densities with their characteristic lines of retraction represent metastases that have become larger than the primary tumor.[9, 19, 20] In one report, typical mesenteric metastases were shown by CT in 8 of 10 patients and contained calcifications in 2.[20] CT may not be successful in outlining the primary tumor (Fig. 51–6).

With the carcinoid syndrome fully developed, it is necessary to determine the full extent of metastatic

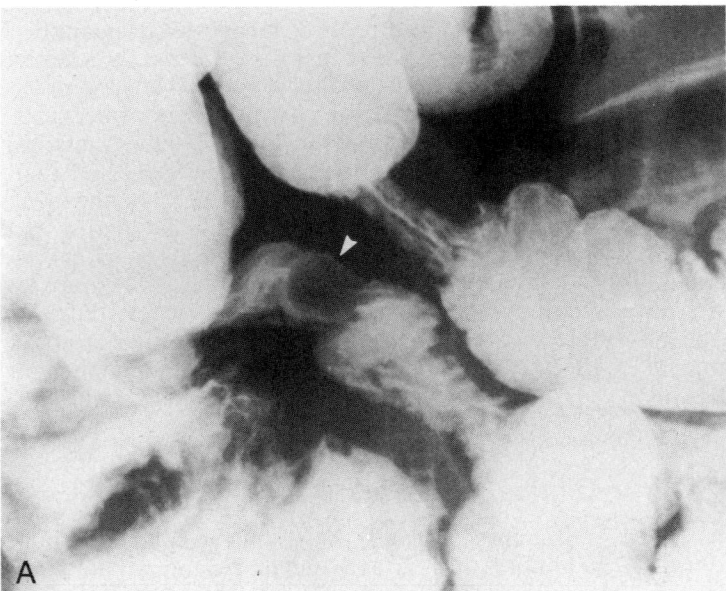

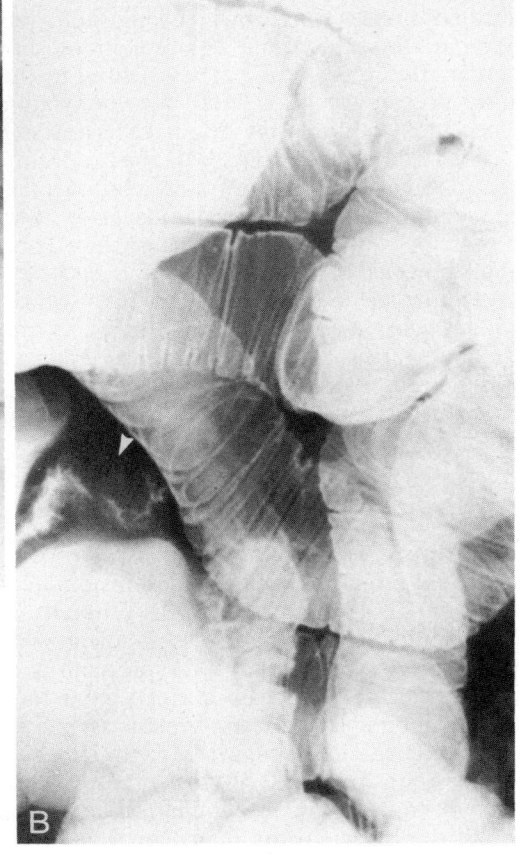

**Figure 51–3. Carcinoid tumor shown by enteroclysis. A.** Enteroclysis done for recurrent lower gastrointestinal bleeding in a 41-year-old woman demonstrates a well-defined, 10-mm submucosal defect *(arrowhead)* in the terminal ileum. Surgery confirmed a small carcinoid tumor. Adjacent nodes were negative for metastases. Prior radionuclide scintigram, visceral arteriography, and abdominal CT did not diagnose the tumor, nor did multiple endoscopic examinations; the first colonoscopy was stated to have included the terminal ileum. **B.** In another patient, larger, broad-based intramural defect (approximately 18 mm—*arrowhead*) was demonstrated by enteroclysis done because of heme-positive stools and abdominal pain. This was shown at surgery to be a carcinoid tumor with involvement of adjacent nodes.

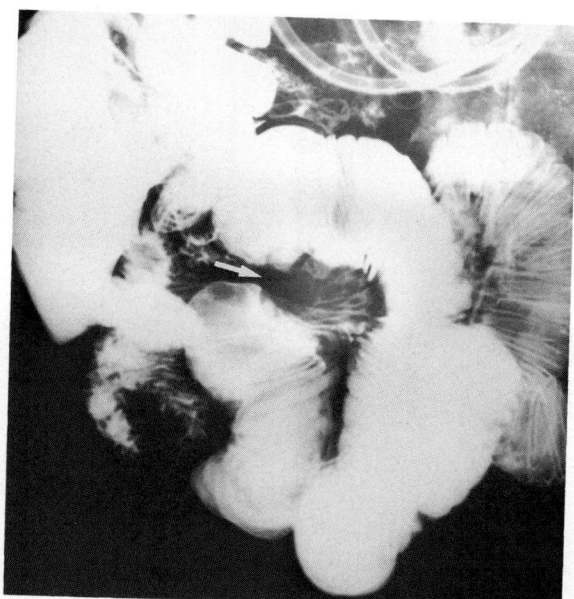

**Figure 51–4. Carcinoid of slightly larger size *(arrow)* with predominant extraluminal mass effect.** The bowel segment involved is fixed and the folds, which are crowded at the tumor edge, are thickened. Surgery revealed a large mesenteric component.

involvement, particularly of the liver. These are shown to best advantage by CT. The metastases are commonly well demarcated, less often diffuse, and usually of low attenuation. They opacify during contrast medium administration.[21] In one report, 3 of 30 patients were found to have pseudocystic metastases.[22]

The angiographic findings of an infiltrating carcinoid are distinctive. Typical are a stellate arterial configuration at the tumor periphery, poor to moderate accumulation within the tumor, nonfilling of major draining veins, and irregular narrowing of mesenteric artery branches.[23] Angiography, however, is not considered necessary if findings obtained by a combination of barium study and CT are typical. Occasionally, however, there may be problems of interpretation of the CT features of mesenteric retraction.[24] Retractile mesenteritis, Hodgkin's disease, extensive radiation damage, and advanced metastatic disease (e.g., from the ovaries) can produce similar appearances. Angiography may then be helpful by demonstrating the primary carcinoid tumor and the changes brought about by its infiltration into the mesentery. It may also demonstrate the usually hypervascular liver metastases.

## Treatment

**Surgical.** All carcinoid tumors identified in the small bowel must be considered potentially malignant and should be resected with a clear margin together with any accessible regional nodes. In the presence of small bowel obstruction, surgical intervention is necessary, preferably by extensive resection. It has been suggested that surgical occlusion of hepatic artery branches for debulking of liver metastases may be performed in patients who already require surgery for small bowel obstruction.[25]

**Interventional Radiology.** Subselective catheterization with small particle embolization of the arterial bed of a metastasis in the liver can produce dramatic clinical improvement and a reduction of 5-HIAA levels.[26, 27]

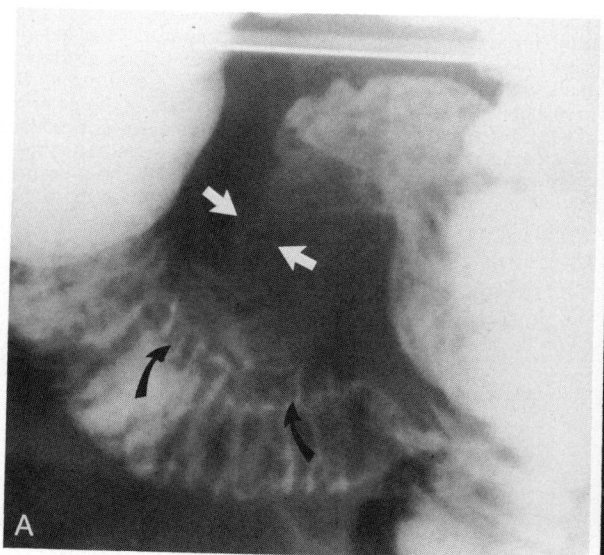
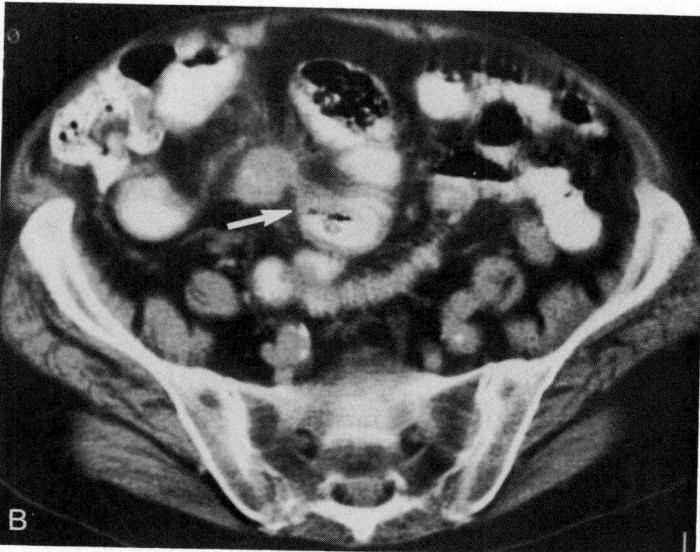

**Figure 51–5. CT of carcinoid. A.** An 80-year-old male patient presented with increasing abdominal distention and anemia. Enteroclysis confirmed small bowel obstruction and demonstrated features highly suggestive of ileal carcinoid as its cause (narrowed segment with crowded folds indicated by straight arrows, leading to curved segment with drawn-out folds shown by curved arrows). **B.** A CT scan is essential at this stage. A large, faintly calcified mesenteric mass is demonstrated. Multiple fibrous strands retract surrounding bowel loops toward the mass. Note wall thickening of affected bowel loops, indicating edema and/or ischemia. The site of obstruction is incorporated in the desmoplasia produced by the hormonally active mesenteric metastatic mass *(arrow)*.

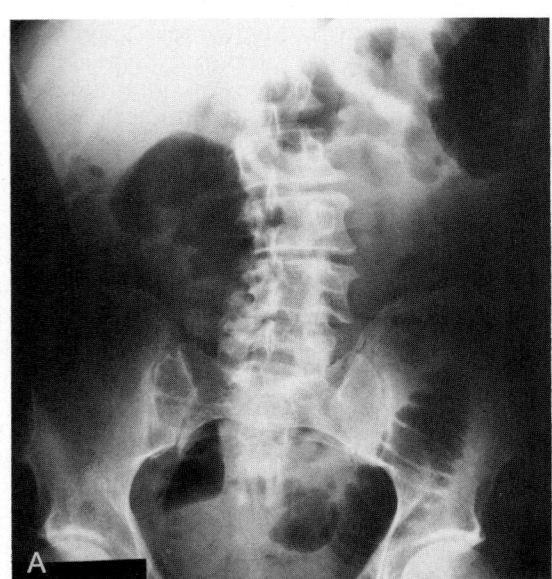

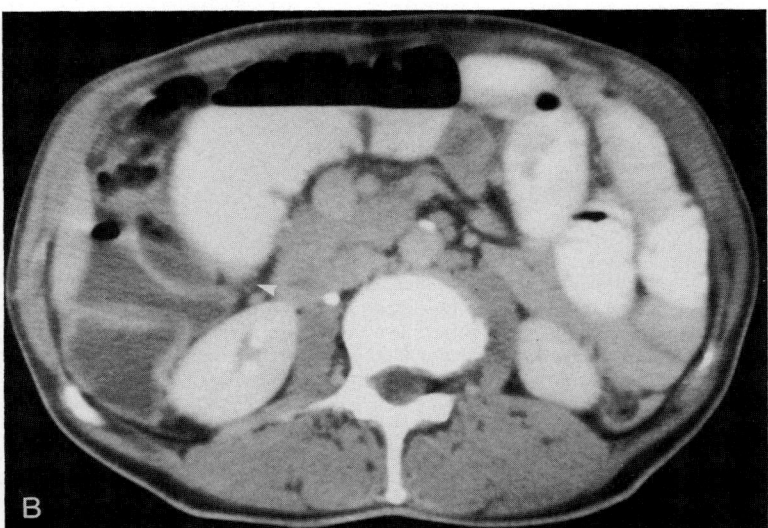

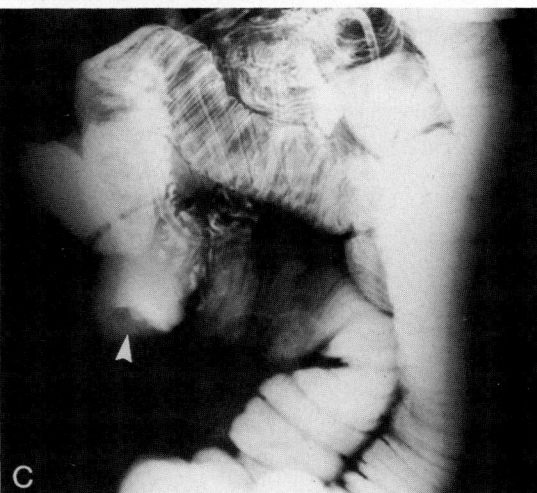

**Figure 51–6. Partial intussusception of a carcinoid tumor.** This elderly patient had abdominal pain and vomiting. **A.** Plain abdominal radiograph shows dilated loops of small bowel consistent with partial mechanical obstruction. **B.** CT scan confirms mechanical obstruction. No mass is apparent at the point of obstruction *(arrowhead)*. No enlarged nodes were seen. Adhesive obstruction was the primary consideration. **C.** Enteroclysis demonstrates a partially intussuscepting mass *(arrowhead)* causing a high-grade obstruction. The pressure of infusion probably initiated the intussusception. Surgery confirmed the presence of an intussuscepting carcinoid. Adjacent nodes were involved.

Symptomatic improvement may even continue during a later rise of 5-HIAA excretion.[26] Embolization is generally preferred to surgical ligation of hepatic artery branches because ligation would be followed by early revascularization through the many available collaterals and would preclude further embolization. Although there is agreement that embolization improves the quality of life of the patient, its effect on survival is less clear. Taken from the first appearance of flushing, the mean life span of patients treated by small particle embolization has been reported to be twice the 3.2-year average of patients who have not been treated in this way.[28] Another report, however, has shown no significant difference in the survival of carcinoid syndrome patients, embolized or not.[29]

Chemotherapy may have a place in support of embolization or when embolization is contraindicated, as with portal vein occlusion. Radiotherapy is generally ineffective except for the patient with occasional, painful bone metastases.

## Adenocarcinoma

### Epidemiology

In the United States, there are approximately 650 new primary adenocarcinomas of the mesenteric small intestine each year.[30] If the duodenum is included, primary adenocarcinomas are the most common primary malignancy in the small intestine and the duodenum is the most frequent site.[31] Worldwide, the prevalence of carcinoma of the small intestine is 0.5 to 3 per 100,000 population and is slightly higher for males than for females. Adenocarcinomas of the small intestine are associated with an increased incidence of primary malignant tumors in other locations. In one series there were additional primary neoplasms outside the small intestine in 17.7% of the patients.[32]

### Pathology

Adenocarcinoma occurs more frequently in the jejunum than in the ileum[7] (Table 51–2). Most jejunal tumors are found in the first 30 cm beyond the ligament of Treitz.[33] Carcinomas of the small intestine seem to be well differentiated even when metastases have developed.[34] A mucin-producing columnar epithelium can frequently be identified.[35] Lymphatic spread to the re-

gional nodes and spread to the liver via the portal venous system are the expected further developments. There may also be peritoneal implants and direct extension into adjacent structures.[36] Multiple adenocarcinomas must be distinguished from metastases. For a tumor to be considered a primary carcinoma, a transition from normal epithelium through severe dysplasia to frank malignancy must be demonstrated at its edge.[37]

## Precancerous Conditions

Adult celiac disease, alpha chain disease, Crohn's disease, and Peutz-Jeghers syndrome are considered to be potentially precancerous.

**Celiac Disease.** There is evidence that adult celiac disease is associated with a higher than expected incidence of carcinoma of the gastrointestinal tract (especially of the esophagus).[38] The mean duration of symptoms of celiac disease before the diagnosis of carcinoma of the gastrointestinal tract has been calculated to be 38½ years. There is also an increased risk of development of adenocarcinomas of the small intestine.[39] Up to 1982, a total of 21 carcinomas of the small intestine attributable to celiac disease had been reported.[40] A survey of a larger group of patients in the United Kingdom found 19 celiac disease–related carcinomas of the small intestine, compared with 0.23 carcinomas expected for the same number of patients without celiac disease.[39] The cause of the increased malignancy associated with celiac disease is unclear, but loss of immune surveillance and viral oncogenesis are possible explanations. An obvious change in the patient's condition, from being well controlled with a gluten-free diet to rapid clinical deterioration during continued dietary restriction, should raise the possibility of superimposed malignancy.

**Crohn's Disease.** The first case report of a carcinoma in the jejunum in a patient with Crohn's disease of the small intestine appeared in 1956.[41] There is an increased prevalence of adenocarcinoma of the small intestine in patients with long-standing Crohn's disease, although accurate figures are not available.[42–46] Crohn's carcinoma differs in several aspects from de novo cancers.[43] Younger patients are affected (46 versus 64 years of age), and there is preferential involvement of the ileum (76 versus 27%). Patients in whom loops of diseased bowel are bypassed, a form of surgery no longer undertaken, are at special risk.[41] It has been suggested that 36% of carcinomas complicating Crohn's disease have

**TABLE 51–2. HISTOLOGY AND SITE DISTRIBUTION OF PRIMARY MALIGNANT TUMORS OF SMALL INTESTINE**

| TUMOR | DUODENUM | JEJUNUM | ILEUM | TOTAL |
|---|---|---|---|---|
| Adenocarcinoma | 19 | 16 | 4 | 39 (50%) |
| Carcinoid | 2 | 1 | 16 | 19 (25%) |
| Leiomyosarcoma blastoma | 2 | 2 | 5 | 9 (12%) |
| Lymphoma | 0 | 3 | 7 | 10 (13%) |
| Total | 23 (30%) | 22 (29%) | 32 (41%) | 77 (100%) |

Modified from DDT Maglinte, K O'Connor, J Bessette, et al, The role of the physician in the late diagnosis of primary malignant tumors of the small intestine, Am J Gastroenterol, 86, 3, 304–308, 1991, © by The American College of Gastroenterology.

developed in bypassed bowel.[41a] Crohn's carcinoma is often diffuse and may not be apparent macroscopically. The diagnosis is more often made after resection and by histology. Preoperative clinical suspicion may be aroused when recrudescence of symptoms after prolonged quiescence or delayed development of a mass, stricture, or obstruction are seen.[44] Barium studies rarely permit a preoperative diagnosis to be made. More often there may be a smooth, benign-appearing stricture.[45] Because of the difficulty and lateness of the diagnosis, the prognosis is generally dismal. Survival from the time of diagnosis is between 7.9 and 11.4 months.[43, 46]

**Peutz-Jeghers Syndrome.** An increased incidence of carcinoma in the stomach, jejunum, and colon has been reported in patients with Peutz-Jeghers syndrome.[34] Of the 380 cases of Peutz-Jeghers syndrome in the literature until 1972, 13 were associated with malignancy but only 1 involved the small intestine.[47] Among 72 patients with Peutz-Jeghers syndrome, subjects of a further report, malignant tumors had developed in 16 (22%), of whom all but 1 had died; nine of the cancers were in the gastrointestinal tract and seven occurred elsewhere.[48] There is also a report of extraintestinal malignancy developing in 15 of 31 patients with Peutz-Jeghers syndrome,[49] suggesting that the gene locus involved is relevant to the development of malignancy in general.

## Radiology

Although CT and sonography can demonstrate the extent of bowel wall and mesenteric involvement as well as regional and distant metastases, these modalities have a limited role in the initial detection of smaller malignant tumors or in the exclusion of their presence. Barium examinations done by an interested and experienced radiologist appear to be best tests for the early diagnosis or confident exclusion of adenocarcinomas of the small intestine.[8–10] Some authors have reported the sensitivity of a combined upper gastrointestinal study and SBFT for adenocarcinoma to be as high as 85 to 90%.[37, 50] These reports, however, include a large percentage of duodenal lesions that were detected during the upper gastrointestinal study. A 1989 report showed that the SBFT had a sensitivity of 61% and enteroclysis or small bowel enema had a sensitivity of 95%.[8] Because of the usual location of adenocarcinomas within 25 cm of the duodenojejunal junction, a patient referred for an upper gastrointestinal examination for pain, vomiting, or anemia should have an evaluation not only of the duodenum but also of the proximal loop of jejunum (Fig. 51–7). A dilated proximal jejunum observed in this extended upper gastrointestinal examination should alert the radiologist to a possible obstructive neoplasm and should be an indication to continue the procedure as a fluoroscopic small bowel study. Suspicion should be high when the dilated distal duodenum or proximal jejunum contains fluid (Fig. 51–8).

The usual radiologic abnormality of a primary adenocarcinoma of the mesenteric small bowel on barium examination is the "apple core" lesion, the same as that found in the rest of the gastrointestinal tract. This is an

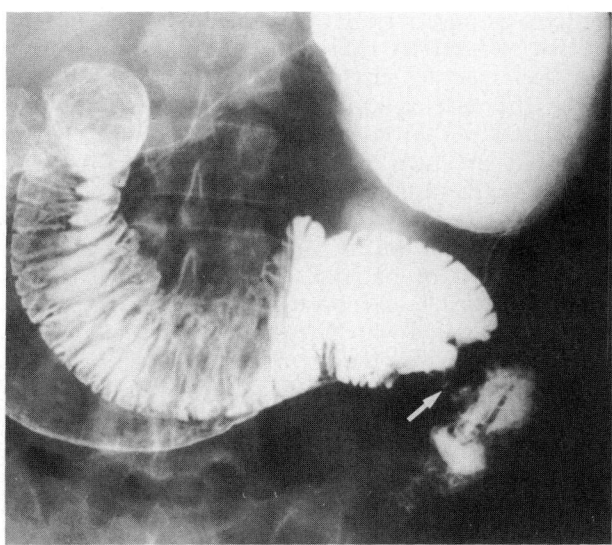

**Figure 51–7. Jejunal carcinoma.** Adenocarcinoma just distal to ligament of Treitz *(arrow)*. The duodenojejunal region should be well outlined in all upper gastrointestinal barium examinations.

annular lesion, a somewhat short, circumferentially narrowed segment with features of mucosal destruction, frequently ulcerated and separated from normal bowel above and below it by overhanging edges (Fig. 51–9). The malignant stricture is usually central in position, rigid, and without change of shape during compression.[51] On occasion, a lymphoma or leiomyosarcoma has a similar appearance. Both of those tumors, however, show alterations of shape with compression because they are usually softer. Carcinoids rarely present as annular lesions. It has been reported that 55% of annular, apple core–type lesions of the small bowel are caused by metastases, mostly from a carcinoma of the colon.[52] These lesions are often longer and cause more pronounced narrowing and obstruction because they are frequently associated with desmoplasia. Ulceration of the metastasis, if present, tends to produce a more irregular cavity. Rarely, a carcinoma is observed as a short, narrow lesion incorporating a sizable ulcer (Fig. 51–10).

In their CT presentation, adenocarcinomas are proximal solitary soft tissue masses causing lumen narrowing and obstruction[9, 11] (Fig. 51–11). The narrowed lumen is shown to be either concentric or asymmetric. The lesions may be heterogeneous in attenuation and show moderate enhancement after intravenous contrast medium administration. Occasionally, the lesion may be observed as a large, well-defined mass without bowel obstruction. Forty-five percent of adenocarcinomas have been found to have atypical CT presentations, especially when ulcerated or located in the duodenum.[11] Local lymph nodes, liver, peritoneal surfaces, and ovaries may be involved secondarily. Intussusception of a carcinoma is also unusual (Fig. 51–12). A patient with several primary adenocarcinomas of the distal ileum manifesting different stages of development on small bowel enema study has been reported.[53]

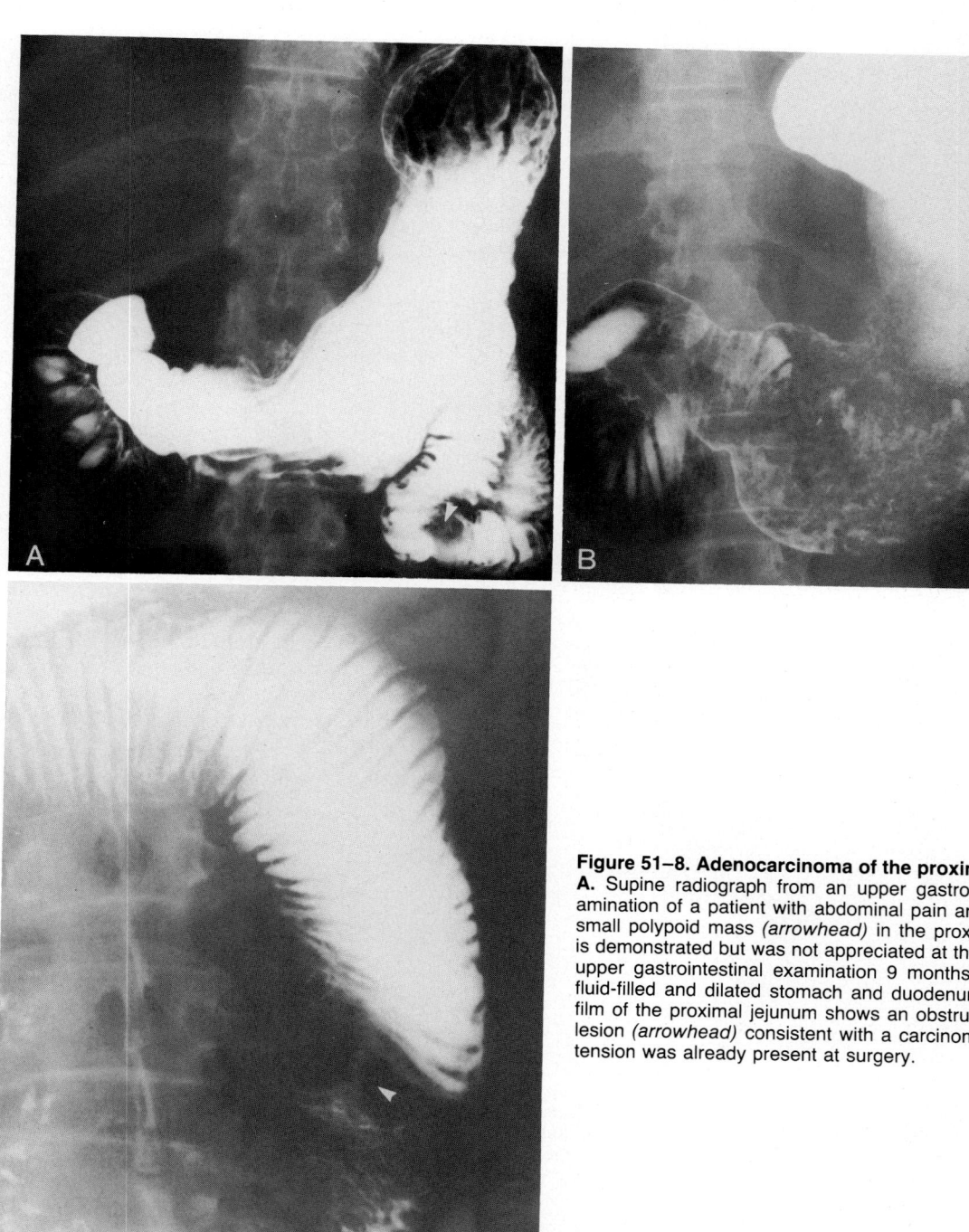

**Figure 51–8. Adenocarcinoma of the proximal jejunum.**
**A.** Supine radiograph from an upper gastrointestinal examination of a patient with abdominal pain and anemia. A small polypoid mass *(arrowhead)* in the proximal jejunum is demonstrated but was not appreciated at the time. **B.** An upper gastrointestinal examination 9 months later shows fluid-filled and dilated stomach and duodenum. **C.** A spot film of the proximal jejunum shows an obstructive annular lesion *(arrowhead)* consistent with a carcinoma. Local extension was already present at surgery.

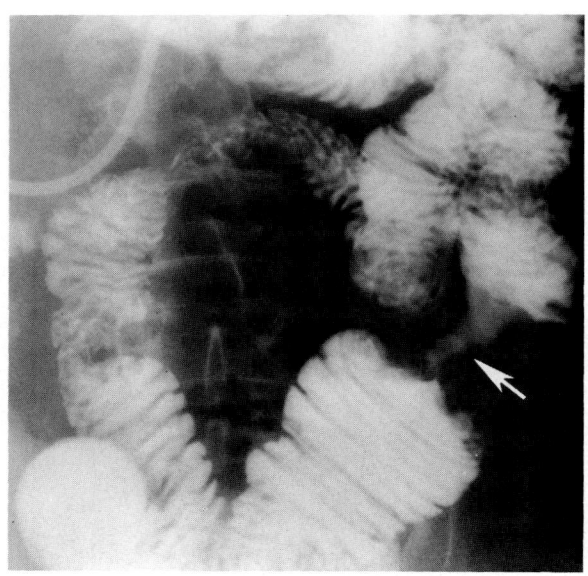

**Figure 51–9. Apple core carcinoma of the jejunum.** The typical apple core lesion is highly suggestive of adenocarcinoma. Enteroclysis reveals a short, circumferentially narrowed segment of proximal jejunum with mucosal destruction and overhanging edges *(arrow)*. An earlier SBFT did not demonstrate the lesion. (From DDT Maglinte, K O'Connor, J Bessette, et al, The role of the physician in the late diagnosis of primary malignant tumors of the small intestine, Am J Gastroenterol 86, 3, 304–308, 1991, © by The American College of Gastroenterology.)

Angiography shows carcinomas as mostly hypervascular tumors that displace unencased feeding arteries. The sonographic appearance of small bowel neoplasms is similar to that of thickened bowel wall in other conditions, such as intramural hemorrhage or inflammatory states.[12]

Differentiation of adenocarcinoma from Crohn's disease is occasionally difficult.[54] The mostly single and short stricture of the carcinoma is a helpful distinguishing feature but can be mimicked by a Crohn's stricture. Characteristic radiographic findings in Crohn's disease—

"cobblestone" appearance, mesenteric border shortening, and ulceration—are not produced by small bowel carcinoma.

## Treatment and Prognosis

The only way to cure carcinoma of the small intestine is by early resection. Major advances in surgical and diagnostic imaging techniques in the 40 years before 1986 did not have an impact on the survival of patients with carcinoma of the small intestine.[7] The lateness of

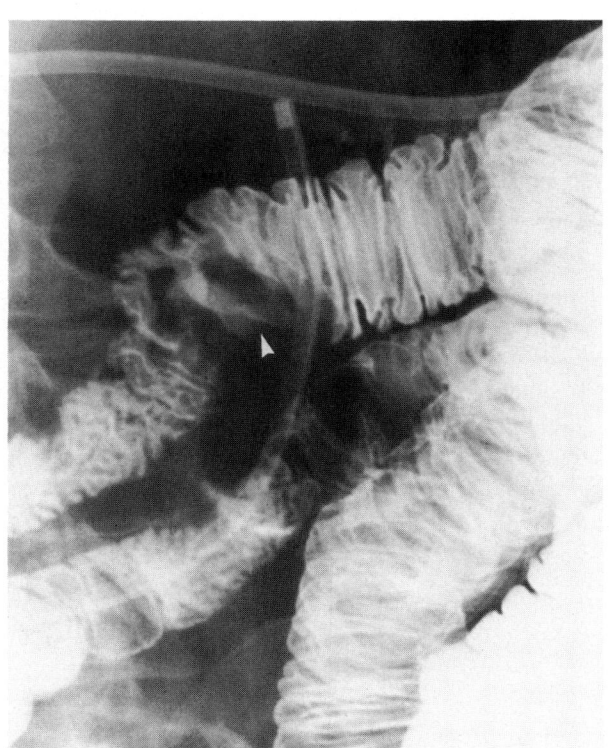

**Figure 51–10. Ulcerated atypical adenocarcinoma of the proximal jejunum.** An annular lesion is not present in this case. A large irregular ulceration in the eccentric mass *(arrowhead)* is the primary finding.

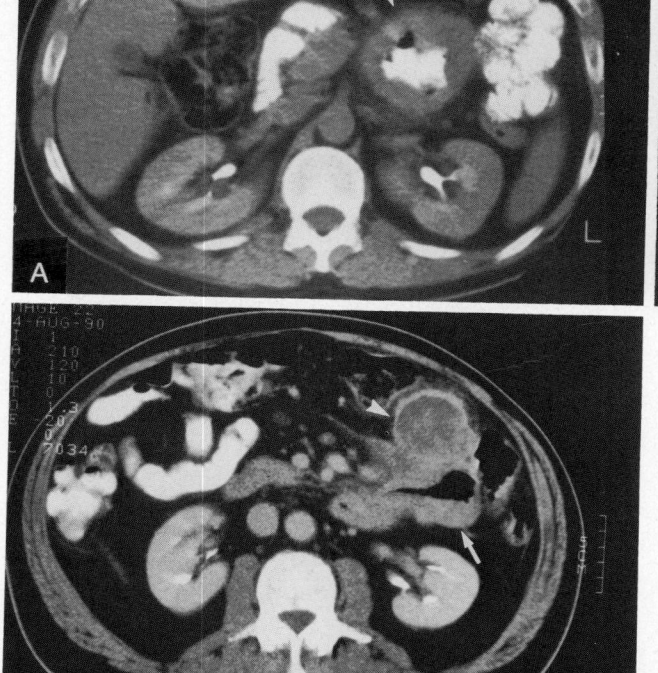

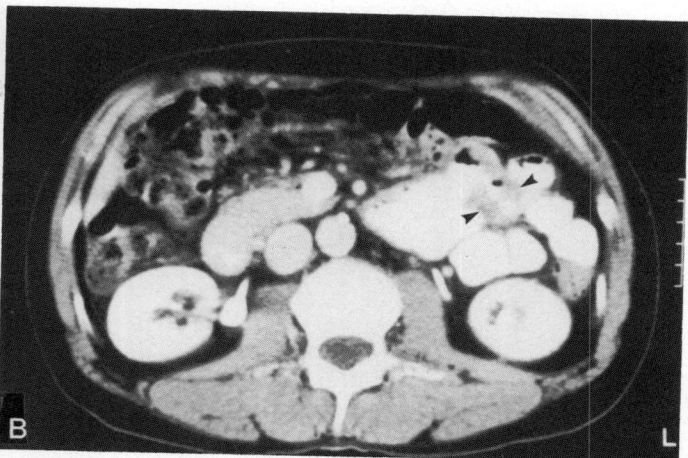

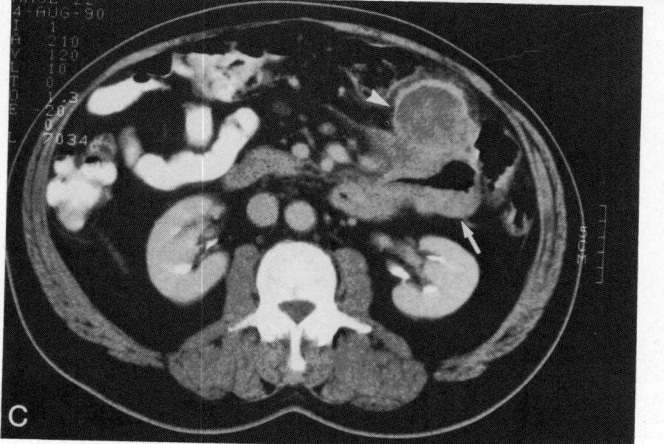

**Figure 51–11. CT of adenocarcinoma of the small intestine. A.** Concentric thickening of a short segment of intestinal wall with irregular narrowing of the lumen *(arrowhead)* is highly suggestive of an adenocarcinoma. **B.** Short stenotic segment with surrounding mass *(arrowheads)* is suggestive of adenocarcinoma. The lesion was not appreciated on the CT scan of this elderly patient evaluated for abdominal pain, vomiting, and anemia. Initial upper gastrointestinal panendoscopy was unremarkable, probably because the lesion was not reached by the scope. Enteroclysis outlined the adenocarcinoma. **C.** Demonstration of a large mesenteric mass *(arrowhead)* with heterogeneous attenuation and associated asymmetric narrowing of the bowel wall *(arrow)*. This finding should suggest an adenocarcinoma with extension into the mesentery.

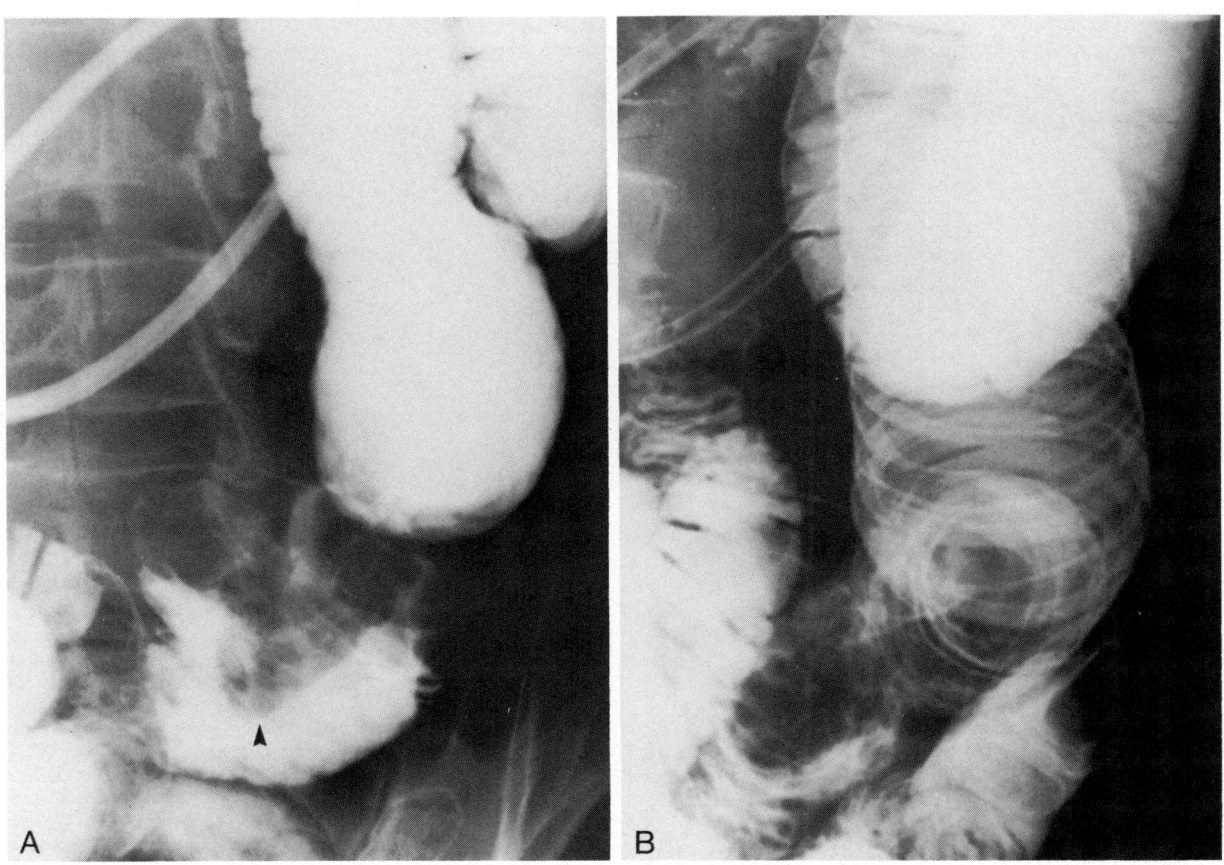

**Figure 51–12. Intussuscepting adenocarcinoma. A.** Single contrast phase of enteroclysis shows an intraluminal polypoid mass *(arrowhead)* with features of intussusception. **B.** Double contrast phase of the same study shows further intussusception of the mass, induced by the infusion.

diagnosis militates against a favorable outcome. The proximity of the invaded nodes to major vessels often prevents a truly radical resection. Five-year survival has been reported to be 46% for carcinoma in the jejunum and 20% for carcinoma in the ileum.[55] In comparison, patients with malignant carcinoids have a better overall survival rate of approximately 64%. Radiation and chemotherapy have little to offer.

## Leiomyosarcoma

It is not clear whether leiomyosarcomas arise de novo or from pre-existing benign smooth muscle tumors. Leiomyosarcomas account for 9% of all primary malignant tumors in the small intestine, with about a half in the ileum and a third in the jejunum.[1] Reliable differentiation between a benign leiomyoma and a leiomyosarcoma cannot be made radiographically. However, smooth muscle tumors that are large or show significant ulceration are usually malignant.

### Pathology

The determination of tumor malignancy can also be a problem for the pathologist. The demonstration of five or more mitotic figures per 10 high-power fields may signify malignancy, especially if associated with nuclear atypia or pleomorphism. But even tumors without mitotic figures have been known to metastasize.[56] A further problem of histology can be the distinction between a neurogenic sarcoma and a leiomyosarcoma. The demonstration by immunoperoxidase staining of S-100 protein favors the former diagnosis. Sarcomas grow more slowly than adenocarcinomas. Sixty-five percent of leiomyosarcomas of the small intestine are reported to be of the exoenteric growth type.[57] They can become extremely large and develop central necrotic and cystic changes. A connection between the tumor cavity and the intestinal lumen may not always be identified. Spread is usually via direct extension into the adjacent parts of the peritoneal cavity or via the hematogenous route to the liver, lungs, or bones. Extension to lymph nodes is infrequent.

### Clinical Features

Patients are often anemic and may complain of abdominal discomfort or pain. The peak incidence is in the sixth decade and males are more often affected than females. Obstruction is not a frequent presentation, although an endoenteric tumor may intussuscept and a large exoenteric mass may compress the intestinal lumen. A mass, often large, soft, and mobile, may be palpated clinically. These large exocenteric tumors may bleed profusely into the peritoneal cavity.

### Radiology

Plain films occasionally show a large soft tissue mass or collections of air representing tumor excavation if in communication with the intestinal lumen. On a contrast study, the cavity fills with barium and several tracts may be outlined (Fig. 51–13). Occasionally, calcifications similar to those often seen in uterine fibroids are present.[58] Because of the predominantly extraluminal growth, leiomyosarcomas usually appear as an extrinsic mass displacing small bowel loops. Barium studies demonstrate a deformity of the small bowel segment from which the tumor originates, with flattening, stretching, and possible ulceration of the mucosa (Fig. 51–14). Adjacent loops may adhere to the mass as a result of infiltration or tethering by the considerable saprophytic blood supply. Leiomyosarcomas alter in shape during compression because they are generally soft. On CT scans, smaller lesions have a nondescript appearance of homogeneous density, associated with the intestinal wall.[9] The more characteristic CT pattern of a leiomyosarcoma is that of a bulky lesion, growing eccentrically and sometimes calcified. Because of the exoenteric growth type of smooth muscle tumors, the manifestations on barium studies tend to be more subtle than the CT findings (Fig. 51–15). The soft tissue component of the tumor usually shows significant enhancement with intravenous contrast medium. Necrosis is seen as a low-density central area rendered more obvious by surrounding contrast enhancement. Calcifications, when present, are more readily detected by CT. Local extensions are demonstrated in a minority of cases. Metastatic disease

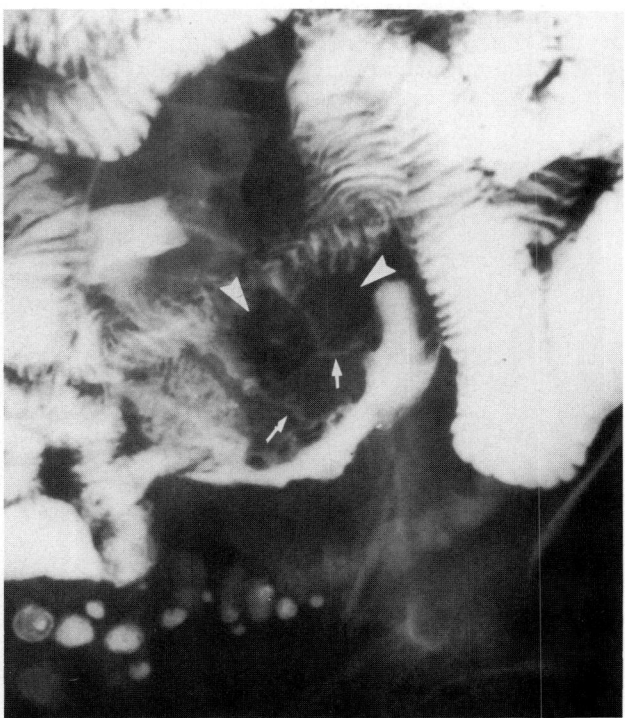

**Figure 51–13. Leiomyosarcoma.** Ulcerated, gas-containing mesenteric mass *(arrowheads)*. Multiple tracts are shown *(arrows)* within the mass. This should not be confused with lymphoma. Barium has entered the necrotic portions of the mass and may remain there for more than 24 hours. Surgery and histologic examination revealed leiomyosarcoma.

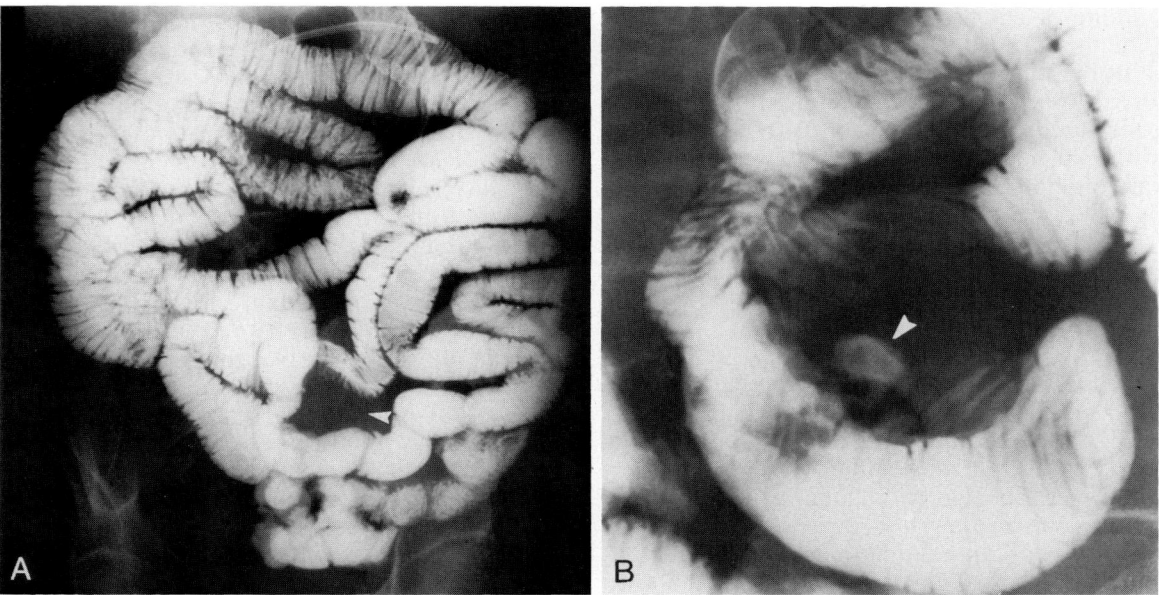

**Figure 51–14. Predominant exoenteric growth of leiomyosarcoma. A.** Enteroclysis demonstrates a loop of intestine displaced and fixed by a mass *(arrowhead)*. **B.** Compression radiograph in the same examination shows intestinal ulceration *(arrowhead)* associated with the mass. This appearance is suggestive of an ulcerating mesenchymal mass with predominance of extraluminal growth, consistent with a leiomyosarcoma.

tends to involve the liver, often with cystic or low-density deposits associated with solid tumor nodules.[59] Peritoneal metastatic masses, occasionally accompanied by masses in the omentum, are well outlined by CT. They are discrete lesions with smooth outer margins, at times containing necrotic areas.[60] Bolus injection of contrast medium can usually differentiate a highly vas-

cular leiomyosarcoma from hypovascular lymphoma.[9] Satellite masses throughout the abdomen indicate peritoneal seeding. Angiography demonstrates characteristic features such as hypervascularity of the sharply demarcated mass, tumor vessels, and early venous return.[61]

Sarcomas of other histologic types are rare and are radiologically indistinguishable from leiomyosarcomas.

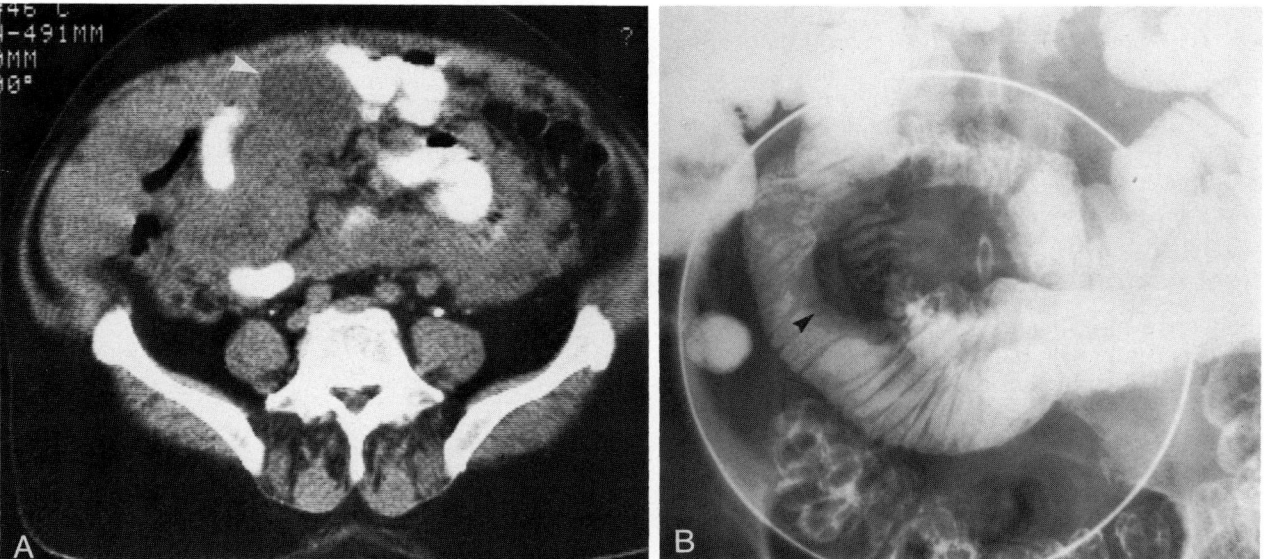

**Figure 51–15. Leiomyosarcoma: CT and enteroclysis. A.** CT scan shows a large mass compressing loops of adjacent bowel. A necrotic portion of the mass is indicated by decreased attenuation *(arrowhead)*. Other sections showed satellite metastases, indicating peritoneal seeding. **B.** Enteroclysis shows the mostly extraluminal component of the tumor by displacement and moderate flattening of the involved bowel loop *(arrowhead)*. The findings at enteroclysis were disproportionate to the large mass shown on CT scans.

## Treatment and Prognosis

The 5-year survival rate may approach 50% with successful surgery, but this figure may be too high because some benign leiomyomas are likely to have been included.[56] Successful surgery requires removal with clear margins of the primary tumors with any contiguous extension into the mensentery. Leiomyosarcomas are resistant to radiotherapy.[33] Limited success has been claimed for systemic chemotherapy.

## Non-Hodgkin's Lymphoma

In contrast to adenocarcinoma and leiomyosarcoma, which produce a focal or segmental lesion, lymphoma tends to originate at multiple sites and to extend along the axis of the small intestine.[62] Primary or secondary lymphoma may occur in any portion of the gastrointestinal tract. In general, primary lymphomas have a better prognosis than carcinomas, with survival rates varying from 30 to 55%.[63] For a diagnosis of primary gastrointestinal lymphoma the following criteria should be fulfilled: 1) no palpable superficial lymph nodes; 2) normal chest roentgenogram (no adenopathy); 3) normal white blood cell count (total and differential); 4) at laparotomy, a predominantly alimentary tract lesion and lymph node involvement, if any, confined to the drainage area of the involved segment of gut; and 5) no involvement of the liver or spleen.[63] Secondary gastrointestinal lymphoma usually affects multiples sites; at autopsy, gross or microscopic evidence of gastrointestinal involvement has been found in up to 51% of cases of disseminated lymphoma.[64] In both the primary and secondary forms, the stomach is most commonly involved (51%), followed by the small intestine (33%), the colon (16%), and the esophagus (less than 1%).[65] Small bowel lymphoma varies in frequency with geographic location, constituting 8.7% of all gastrointestinal tumors in the Middle East, compared with 0.9 to 1% in the United States.[66] The duodenum is less frequently involved than the jejunum or ileum, and the largest number of lymphomas is reported to occur in the distal ileum.

## Classification and Staging

Classification refers to the histologic composition of a non-Hodgkin's lymphoma. Whereas Hodgkin's disease is a single entity and extends in an orderly manner and by contiguity, non-Hodgkin's lymphoma may comprise several diseases, typically with noncontiguous spread. Histologic classification forms the basis for the identification of the subgroups with their different natural histories and responses to treatment. The modified Rappaport classification of non-Hodgkin's lymphoma has been applied for more than 20 years.[67] Its validity has been questioned for a number of reasons, including the fact that lymphocytes, after histologic classification, can transform into other usually larger and more aggressive cell forms.[68] Several other methods of classification have emerged, and a working formulation for clinical usage has been devised by an international study group sponsored by the National Cancer Institute.[69] Cell types are grouped into categories according to their aggressiveness as low grade, intermediate grade, and high grade.[69] Immunohistochemical methods are increasingly added to purely histologic determination. Most of the non-Hodgkin's lymphomas of the small intestine and about 60 to 70% of those elsewhere in the gastrointestinal tract are now classified as high grade and of the large cell or immunoblastic cell type.[70] Fewer are of the diffuse, small, noncleaved cell type, also considered high grade by the working formulation.[71] Burkitt's lymphoma (small, noncleaved) occurs mostly in children, tends to involve the ileocecal area, and is highly aggressive.[72] It has also been found to occur in immunodepressed individuals.[73] Most gastrointestinal non-Hodgkin's lymphomas are of B cell derivation.[74]

Staging refers to the distribution and extent of lymphoma within the body. The Ann Arbor staging system for Hodgkin's disease has been adapted to the staging of non-Hodgkin's lymphoma. The subscript E is used to designate disease of extranodal sites, in this context the small intestine. Stage $I_E$ means disease confined to a single extranodal site. Stage $II_{E1}$ indicates associated involvement of a group of regional lymph nodes. More extensive subdiaphragmatic node involvement is identified as stage $II_{E2}$. Stage $III_E$ refers to small intestinal lymphoma with extension to structures below and above the diaphragm. Stage IV implies widespread dissemination.[73]

The relative influence of classification and staging on the selection of treatment and the patient's prognosis has not been fully agreed.[73] Some authors have considered staging to be the more important determinant.[75, 76] The histologic classification seems to be of less practical clinical relevance than staging because most non-Hodgkin's lymphomas of the small bowel are known to be of large cell type and high-grade aggressiveness. Staging is related directly to treatment options in every patient. Cases of stage $I_E$ small bowel lymphoma are rare; nearly half of the small bowel lymphomas are stage $II_E$. Patients in both groups must have surgery before additional treatment is instituted. Complete excision improves survival.[77]

## Clinical Features

The most frequent clinical presentation is that of abdominal pain,[78] often associated with nausea or vomiting, anemia, weight loss, and pyrexia.[75] A palpable abdominal mass or small bowel obstruction or both may be present. A presentation with bleeding, pyrexia, or obstruction is associated with a reduced life expectancy.[79]

Malabsorption and diarrhea are rare presenting features in the so-called Western form of lymphoma.[80] This sequence of clinical findings can characterize Mediterranean lymphoma and the lymphoma complicating adult celiac disease. The former is discussed later, the latter in Chapter 49.

Patients with systemic lupus erythematosus and with

other diffuse connective tissue diseases have a higher than expected incidence of non-Hodgkin's lymphoma.[81] In most of the cases, immunosuppressive drugs have not been administered.[82] A 1990 report describing 25 patients with small bowel lymphoma included 2 with associated lupus erythematosus.[83] The possibility of non-Hodgkin's lymphoma should be considered in a patient with systemic lupus erythematosus who develops an abdominal mass or adenopathy.

## Radiology

The diverse radiologic appearances on barium study reflect the gross morphology of the disease.[84] The principal radiologic features of lymphoma of the small bowel, as described by Marshak and colleagues,[85] were multiple nodular defects, an infiltrating form, a polypoid form (intussuscepting), an endoexenteric form with excavation and fistula formation, and a predominantly mesenteric invasive form with extraluminal masses (Fig. 51–16). Aneurysmal dilatation has been considered the major radiologic finding in some reports.[86] In a study in which 25 cases of non-Hodgkin's lymphoma of the small intestine were evaluated, the infiltrating form was the most frequent radiologic finding, closely followed by the cavitary form.[83]

Circumferentially infiltrating non-Hodgkin's lymphoma involves a variable length of small intestine with thickening and later effacement of folds.[87] The lumen is more often widened than narrowed; rarely a stricture is formed. Multiple shallow ulcers are not infrequently present but are not well shown by the barium examination. On CT scans, a sausage-shaped mass of relatively homogeneous tissue density can be demonstrated (Fig. 51–17). Thickening of the intestinal wall causes separation from adjoining bowel loops. Contrast enhancement shown by CT is minimal, less than that for leiomyosarcomas or carcinomas.

Replacement of the muscularis and destruction of the autonomic nerve plexus by lymphoma may cause the bowel wall to give way and bulge focally, not necessarily in a circular fashion. Aneurysmal dilatation tends to involve predominantly the unsupported, antimesenteric side of a small bowel segment (see Fig. 51–16D). The contour may revert to normal after treatment; however, perforation is a life-threatening complication. For this reason, complete resection should be attempted whenever possible before chemotherapy.[77]

Focal infiltration may lead to localized perforation into a sealed-off space, usually between the leaves of the mesentery (Fig. 51–18). This cavitary form of non-Hodgkin's lymphoma usually denotes a primary small bowel origin. The site of extravasation is readily shown by enteroclysis, and sites of additional fistulas into the lymphoma cavity are indicated by focally thickened mucosal folds. The irregular contour of the excavation, its relation to the mesenteric border of a small bowel loop, the fact that it contains air and debris, and the generally thin soft tissue space separating it from adjacent bowel distinguish cavitary lymphoma from a barium-containing cavity within an exoenteric leiomyosarcoma. An aneurysmal dilatation or sacculation may

superficially resemble the lymphomatous cavity; it is, however, likely to involve the antimesenteric side of a bowel segment and to be in continuity with the bowel lumen proximally and distally. Cavitary lymphoma requires surgical excision, at times of a considerable extent of involved bowel.

The nodular pattern occurs less often than previously reported. This pattern is seen when the lymphomatous proliferation is extensively submucosal (see Fig. 51–1). Two types can be demonstrated by barium examination. One consists of polypoid lesions 2 cm or more in diameter that may be ulcerated, forming target lesions without extramural extension. This form may be associated with intussusception and secondary obstruction. The second type consists of small, diffuse, nodular lesions, only a few millimeters in diameter, that may occur anywhere in the small intestine but more often in the distal ileum. This form is reported to be seen more frequently in patients with lymphoma of the Mediterranean type.

A lymphomatous tumor may develop in the mesenteric lymph nodes. As it grows, it causes secondary involvement of small bowel. Barium examination may show abutment initially and later displacement and compression of small bowel loops indicating the presence of an extrinsic mass (Fig. 51–19A). The mass eventually infiltrates the compressed bowel wall and may then cause obstruction.[87] The mesenteric mass is best outlined by CT (Fig. 51–19B) when its lobulated contour seems to encase adjacent bowel or produce a classic "sandwich" appearance.[88] Calcification of the mesenteric lymphomatous tumor is rare and is more likely to occur after radiotherapy or chemotherapy.

It is not possible, on the basis of barium studies, to make a firm distinction between extranodal lymphoma of primary small bowel origin and lymphoma secondarily involving small bowel.[89] However, certain enteroclysis-based guidelines can be recognized. The segmentally infiltrating form and the cavitary lymphoma tend to be expressions of primary small intestinal origin, whereas the nodular type denotes dissemination.[90] For a more complete radiologic diagnosis of this entity, enteroclysis and CT are needed to define the location and extent of the tumor and guide needle biopsy.

## Radiologic Differential Diagnosis

In most cases, there is no difficulty in differentiating small bowel lymphoma from Crohn's disease. Thickening of the valvulae conniventes may be an early feature in both conditions and is rarely the only radiologic abnormality in either condition.[91] Fistulas may occur in both diseases, but in Crohn's disease they are associated with other typical alterations. Ulcers in lymphoma are usually more broad-based than the fissured or longitudinal ulcers seen in Crohn's disease.[92]

The apple core deformity typical of adenocarcinoma is unusual in non-Hodgkin's lymphoma. When present, it tends to involve a longer segment, does not show overhanging edges, and may be multiple. Furthermore, lymphoma produces a softer lesion that may show outline change with abdominal compression. CT demon-

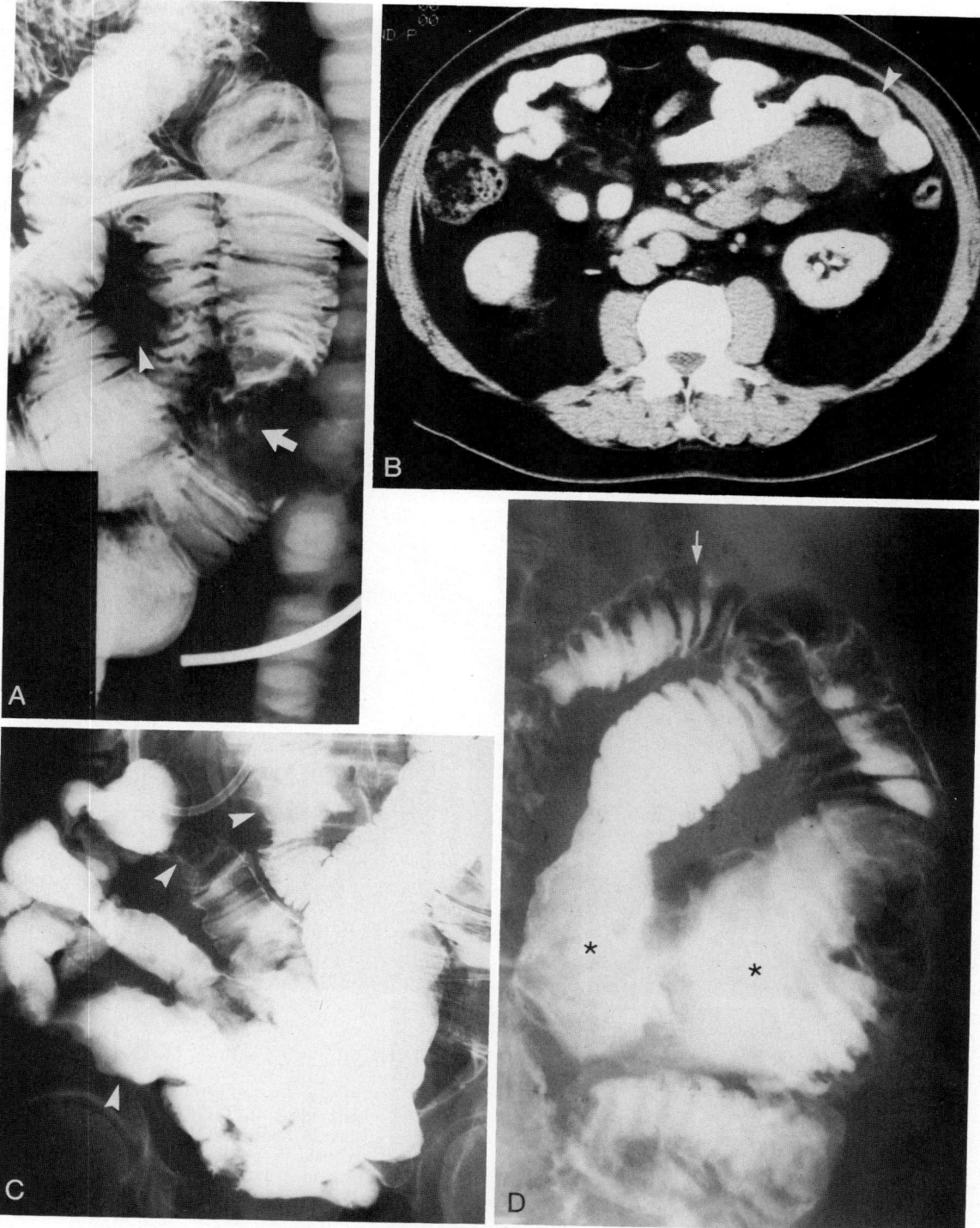

**Figure 51–16. Barium studies in non-Hodgkin's lymphoma involving the small intestine. A.** A solitary tumor infiltrates a bowel segment in nonconcentric fashion *(arrow)*. The mucosa is not destroyed and the appearance of the lesion changed with compression. A mesenteric component is suggested by separation of two adjacent segments *(arrowhead)*. The finding, however, is subtle. **B.** CT scan of the same patient shows an ulcerated mass protruding into the lumen *(arrowhead)*. Additional large mesenteric masses are present and had been difficult to appreciate on enteroclysis. (**A** and **B** courtesy of Jack Scatarige, M.D., Norfolk, VA.) **C.** A diffuse lymphoma involves multiple long segments and presents as numerous polypoid lesions and/or ulcerated segments *(arrowheads)*. The lumen of the most proximal and distal lesions is dilated (aneurysmal). **D.** Aneurysmal dilatation in lymphoma. Spot radiograph in an SBFT shows focal effacement of folds and dilatation of lumen *(asterisks)* extending mostly into the convex, antimesenteric aspect. The dilatation is due to replacement of muscularis propria by the lymphoma. Arrow points to the duodenojejunal junction.

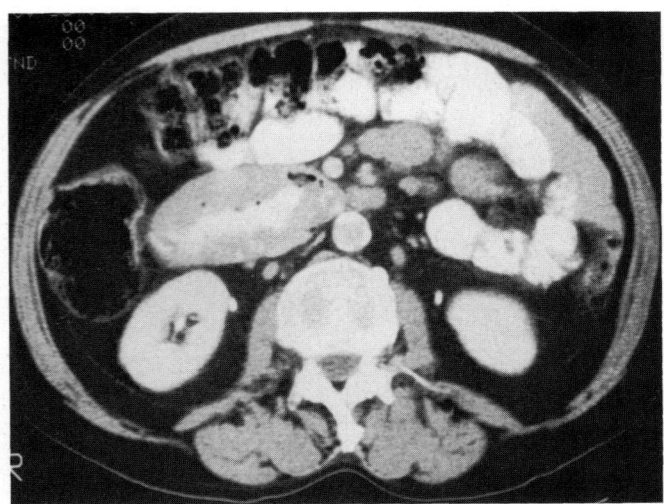

**Figure 51–17. CT appearance of focally infiltrating lymphoma.** There is a sausage-shaped mass concentrically involving a fairly long segment of bowel wall. The attenuation of the thickened wall is relatively homogeneous. This finding should suggest the diagnosis of lymphoma.

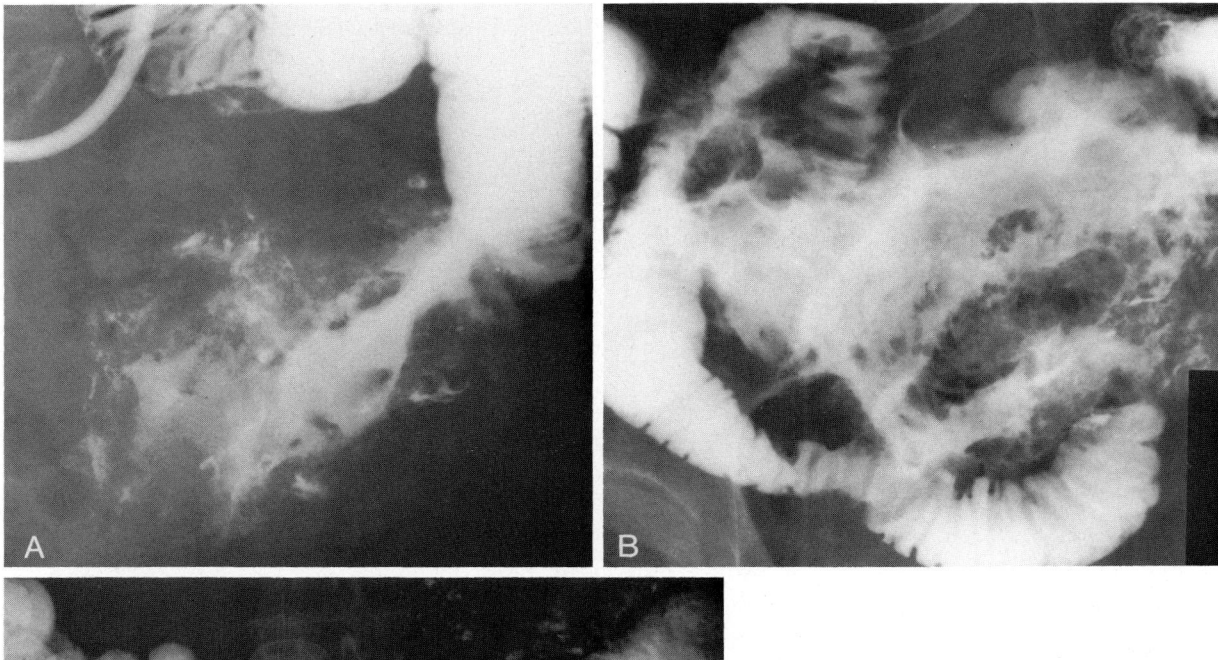

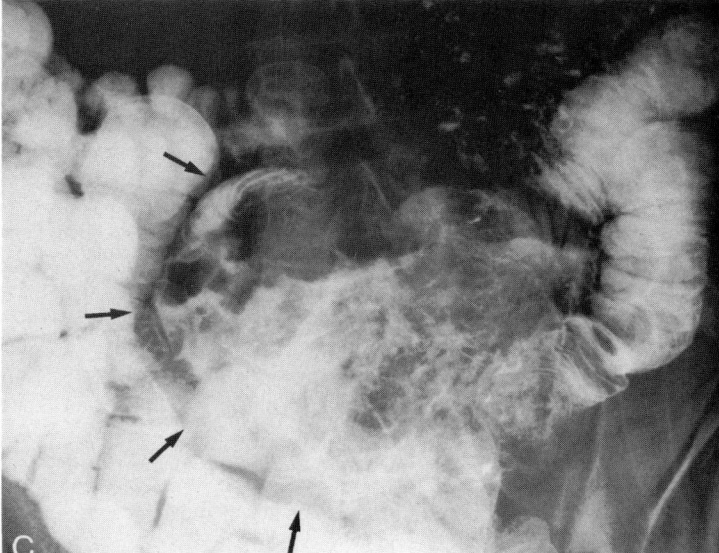

**Figure 51–18. Cavitary non-Hodgkin's lymphoma.** A 74-year-old female patient with a history of abdominal pain and weight loss for 5 months. A mass was palpated in the abdomen. **A.** Barium extravasates into an exoenteric space. **B.** Later film during the enteroclysis outlines the large barium- and air-filled cavity occupying the mesenteric border of several bowel loops. **C.** A final overview film shows that only a thin rim of soft tissue *(arrows)* separates the cavity from surrounding loops. The cavity within a leiomyosarcoma would be surrounded by a thicker residual tumor mass. (**A** to **C** from Fishman EK, Kuhlman JE, Jones RC: CT of lymphoma: spectrum of disease. Radiographics 11:647–669, 1991.)

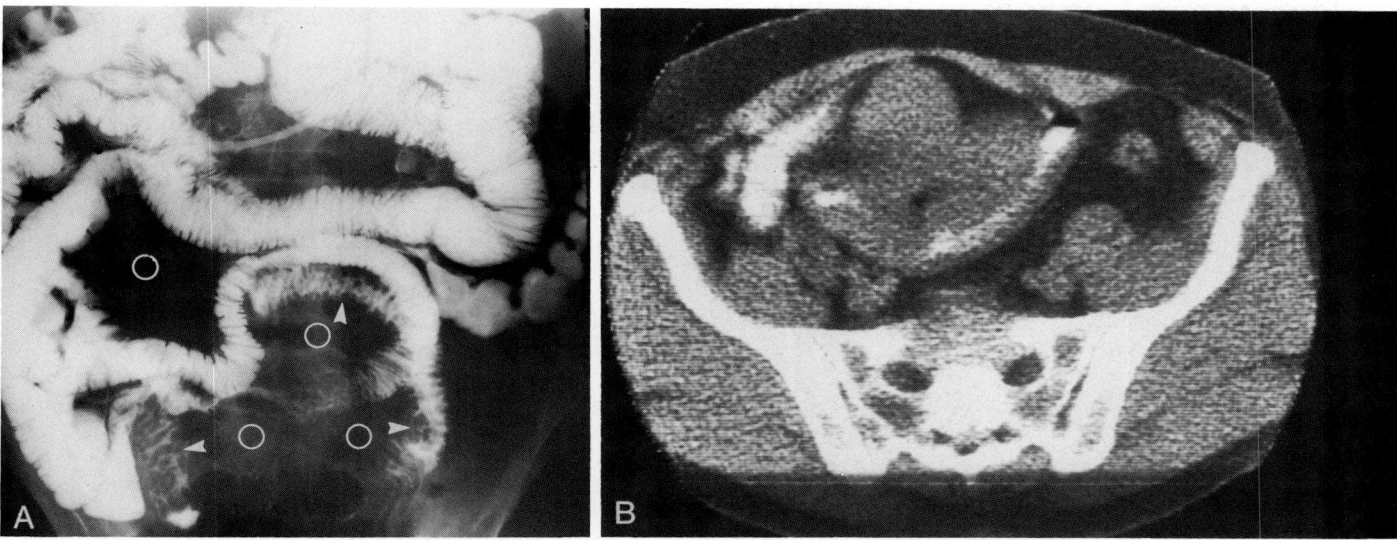

**Figure 51–19. Mesenteric invasive form of lymphoma. A.** Multiple loops of small intestine are displaced by mesenteric masses *(open circles)*. The involved folds are thickened and nodular *(arrowheads)*. There is no evidence of obstruction. **B.** CT done after the enteroclysis **(A)** shows large mesenteric masses displacing and compressing loops of ileum.

stration of more bulky mesenteric node involvement favors lymphoma[93] (see Fig. 51–16A and B).

Nodular lymphoid hyperplasia is characterized by the presence of smaller, evenly distributed nodules of uniform size. The infrequently seen nodules of small bowel lymphoma are larger, variable in size, and irregular in distribution.

### Needle Biopsy for Classification

Percutaneous fine-needle biopsy for a histologic diagnosis of non-Hodgkin's lymphoma can be guided by the barium-outlined lesion.[94] Core biopsies for histology rather than cytology are generally preferred. Use of an 18-gauge biopsy gun gives more accurate placement, fewer crush artifacts, and less discomfort for the patient.[95] However, many still prefer full-thickness biopsy specimens obtained at laparotomy,[96] in the belief that they are more accurate and supply sufficient material for immunologic characterization.

### Staging by Computed Tomography

CT can show involvement of periaortic, celiac, and retrocrural nodes that may be missed during a staging laparotomy.[97] However, CT may fail to identify nodes 1 to 2 cm in size and is of limited reliability in the recognition of hepatic or splenic involvement. This is an important consideration because the presence of lymphoma in the liver changes an otherwise $I_E$ or $II_E$ stage into stage $IV_E$ with its related effect on the patient's prognosis.[98]

### Treatment and Prognosis

Misdiagnosis has delayed the start of correct treatment for more than 6 months in nearly half of patients.[77] Deaths could be grouped into those within 6 months of

diagnosis and those occurring much later. The early deaths were related to complications of chemotherapy, namely bleeding and perforation.[77] Chemotherapy can be hazardous for patients with transmural disease, and surgical excision has been recommended before treatment is begun. Alternatively, cautiously administered, relatively low-dose chemotherapy may have to be employed, always with close observation for any early signs of bleeding or perforation. For advanced disease, after a palliative resection, multidrug chemotherapy appropriate for the histologic type of the non-Hodgkin's lymphoma has been given intermittently for a long time and has been supplemented by radiotherapy for residual disease.[99]

### Other Forms of Non-Hodgkin's Lymphoma

The uncommon American form of Burkitt's lymphoma usually presents with primary intestinal involvement, mostly of the ileocecal area and with an abdominal mass. It has one of the most rapid doubling times of any tumor and mostly affects children. Like the more common Burkitt's lymphoma endemic in Africa, which affects the jaw and retroperitoneal nodes of children, it is associated with Epstein-Barr virus.[100] Gallium 67 radionuclide studies can define the bulk of the abdominal mass and may outline other sites of tumor involvement, including bone.[101] Ultrasound can efficiently outline the usually large and acoustically homogeneous abdominal masses.[102] Barium studies can produce evidence of displacement and infiltration of distal small bowel. Involved loops of bowel show irregular fold thickening, lumen narrowing, and ulceration plus necrosis (Fig. 51–20). Lymph nodes are rarely affected. Combination chemotherapy can produce fairly rapid lysis of tumor masses, but this may be accompanied by serious metabolic disturbances.

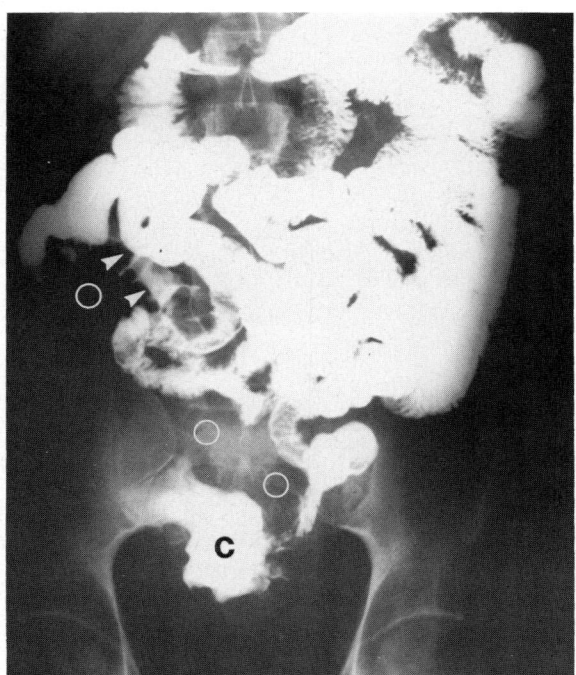

**Figure 51–20. Burkitt's lymphoma.** Large tumor masses *(open circles)* compress and infiltrate distal small intestine and cecum (C). Infiltrated folds are flattened and nodular *(arrowheads)*. This uncommon form of lymphoma should be suspected in a young patient with these findings.

Mediterranean lymphoma forms the end stage of a spectrum of changes termed *immunoproliferative small intestinal disease* by the World Health Organization. Mature plasma cells and pleomorphic lymphocytes proliferate in the mucosa, predominantly of the duodenum and jejunum. In alpha chain disease, another part of the spectrum, the intestinal infiltrate is associated with the presence of alpha heavy chains in the serum. The condition is premalignant and can progress to the diffuse and multifocal Mediterranean lymphoma.

This entity was first reported from Lebanon and the Near East. It affected young adults of Arab and Mediterranean Jewish origin but has now also been found among South African blacks and Mexican Americans and occasionally among adults of most countries.[103] Three distinct stages have been described. In stage A, the plasmacytic infiltrate is confined to the small bowel mucosa, expanding villi. Enteroclysis at this stage would show a micronodular pattern in the proximal small intestine. In stage B, the infiltrate extends into the submucosa, producing lymphoid nodules and atypical lymphocytes. Barium studies would now show thickening of folds and nodularity. Stage C consists of multiple lymphomatous tumors without a dominant mass. The histologic picture has become that of an immunoblastic non-Hodgkin's lymphoma. Spread beyond the intestinal tract is a late feature.[104] In stage A, patients with immunoproliferative small intestinal disease may benefit from treatment with tetracycline and prednisone and further progression may be halted.[105]

Mediterranean lymphoma differs from Western lymphoma in a number of aspects. In Mediterranean lymphoma the average age of patients is the mid-20s, the proximal small bowel is mostly involved, and malabsorption and diarrhea are presenting features. In the Western type of lymphoma, the average age exceeds 40 years, there is some predilection for the distal small bowel, and malabsorption is a rare feature except when associated with celiac disease.

## Immunosuppression and Non-Hodgkin's Lymphoma

Allograft transplant recipients have a 45 to 100 times higher prevalence of non-Hodgkin's lymphoma than the population in general.[106] The lymphoma is usually of the aggressive large cell type and may affect the small intestine in the course of dissemination. Patients receiving conventional immunosuppressive drugs may develop lymphoma with a predilection for the central nervous system. Cyclosporine, now commonly used for immunosuppression, also influences the development of lymphoma and that of other lymphoproliferative disorders. Cyclosporine-associated lymphomas occur early, on average after only 8 months of treatment; the central nervous system tends to be spared; the gastrointestinal tract is the site most commonly affected; and there may be regression of the tumor with decrease or stoppage of the drug.[107] The risk of malignant lymphoma development increases with high dosages of immunosuppressive agents or the use of multiple agents.[108] Most patients show evidence of an associated Epstein-Barr virus infection, which tends to provoke intense proliferation of B lymphocytes, normally controlled by cytotoxic T cells, a mechanism interrupted by cyclosporine suppression.[107]

## Malignant Tumors Complicating Acquired Immunodeficiency Syndrome

**Non-Hodgkin's Lymphoma.** Patients with the acquired immunodeficiency syndrome (AIDS) have an increased likelihood of developing non-Hodgkin's lymphoma, histologically mostly an aggressive, small non–cleaved cell Burkitt's or non-Burkitt's lymphoma or the large cell immunoblastic type.[109] At first, the specific relationship with AIDS was not accepted by the Centers for Disease Control because of the well-known association between lymphoma and any form of immunodeficiency. However, the link between lymphoma and AIDS is no longer in doubt. The prognosis is dismal even after a temporary response to chemotherapy. Of 869 AIDS patients, 108 (12%) developed malignant neoplasms.[110] Lymphoma accounted for 35%, Kaposi's sarcoma for 60%, and miscellaneous tumors for 6.5%.[110]

**Kaposi's Sarcoma.** Of the 65 AIDS patients in whom Kaposi's sarcoma was diagnosed,[110] 78% were male homosexuals and 32% were intravenous drug users, heterosexual or homosexual. Of the tumors found in

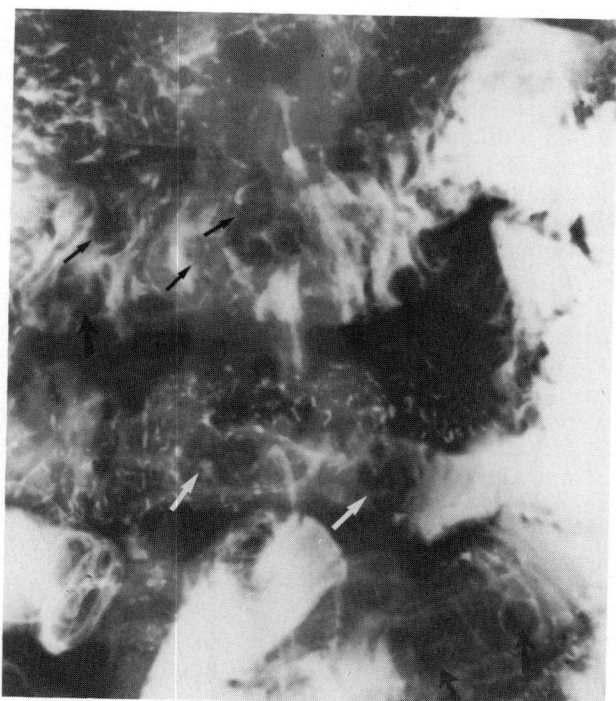

**Figure 51–21. Kaposi's sarcoma and cryptosporidiosis in AIDS.**
The patient had severe diarrhea and weight loss. The barium follow-through examination shows features compatible with cryptosporidiosis (irregularly thickened folds in the proximal jejunum, fluid increase) and with the presence of multiple lesions of Kaposi's sarcoma *(arrows)*—rounded filling defects, some with a central barium collection. (Courtesy of R. Goren, M.D., Philadelphia, PA.)

the gastrointestinal tract, the oropharynx was the site in 13 patients, the esophagus and stomach in 3 patients each, the colon in 1, and the small bowel and liver in 4 patients each. Mean survival from the time of diagnosis was 4.7 months.

Kaposi's sarcomas are frequently multicentric, and violaceous skin lesions usually accompany visceral tumors. The sarcomas are often clinically silent until they become a source of bleeding or concurrent infections occur. Barium studies may show rounded nodules, often with central umbilication. When the sarcomas occur in the small bowel, there are often associated infections, such as cryptosporidiosis (Fig. 51–21). CT is important because it outlines the related lymphadenopathy in the form of retroperitoneal, mesenteric, or pelvic clusters. CT-guided needle biopsy of lymph nodes may be required to confirm the diagnosis of Kaposi's sarcoma and distinguish the adenopathy from that in AIDS-related complex, lymphoma, or *Mycobacterium avium-intracellulare* infection. Associated hepatosplenomegaly favors a diagnosis of Kaposi's sarcoma.[111]

## Hodgkin's Disease

Involvement of the gastrointestinal tract is now considered to be exceptional. If a patient is known to have had Hodgkin's disease and radiologic findings suggest intrinsic involvement of the gastrointestinal tract in keeping with lymphoma, a review of the histology is indicated. If the presence of lymphoma is confirmed, the existence of a second disease process would be a more likely explanation.[112] The development of non-Hodgkin's lymphoma after treatment of Hodgkin's disease has been fully documented.[113] A correct histologic diagnosis is relevant to clinical management, as non-Hodgkin's lymphoma would not respond to chemotherapeutic combinations used in Hodgkin's disease.

### Radiology

Hodgkin's disease has been reported to incite fibrosis of the bowel wall with tapered, eccentric narrowing of the involved segment but without the overhanging edges seen in carcinoma.[113] There may be displacement of noninvolved small bowel by an adjacent nodal mass (Fig. 51–22). Now that Hodgkin's disease is known to involve small bowel only exceptionally, a diagnosis of small intestinal Hodgkin's disease should never be made on a purely radiologic basis.

## SECONDARY MALIGNANCIES

Occasionally, the small intestine may be the only site of metastasis. Frequently, it is an incidental finding in a patient with known abdominal carcinomatosis.[114, 115] The mechanism of tumor spread determines its radiographic appearance. Tumor cells involve the small intestine via different pathways: intraperitoneal spread, hematogenous dissemination, or extension from an adjacent tumor mass either directly or through the lymphatic

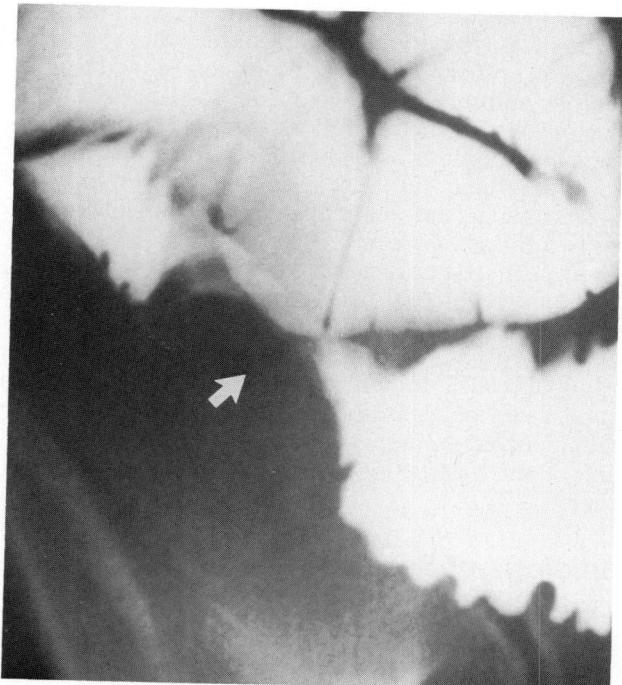

**Figure 51–22. Hodgkin's disease.** There is a smooth impression on a loop of distal small bowel. An extrinsic nodal mass may be the cause of the deformity in this patient *(arrow)*.

chain.[116, 117] Intraperitoneal spread occurs more frequently than hematogenous dissemination and is more likely to pose a problem of radiologic differential diagnosis.[118]

## Anatomic Considerations

The natural pattern of flow of ascitic fluid within the peritoneal recesses influences the serosal implantation of cancer cells.[116] Areas where ascitic fluid accumulates and stagnates before overflowing to an adjacent space are preferred sites for malignant cell deposition. Such sites are the ileocecal region, the numerous pools within the ruffles of the small bowel mesentery, and the depth of the pelvic cavity. The anatomy of the peritoneal space should be understood for proper interpretation.

## Intraperitoneal Seeding of Metastases

Malignant cells deposited on serosal surfaces may adhere through fibrinous exudation. Deposits coalesce and grow into metastatic masses implanted on the serosa of a segment of bowel or on the peritoneal surface between loops. The neoplastic implants (most often from tumors of gastrointestinal origin in men and tumors of ovarian or uterine origin in women) tend to grow in relation to the concave or mesenteric border of bowel loops and can incite fibrosis.

### Clinical Aspects

The primary tumor is known in most cases. Occasionally, the pattern of distribution of the seeded metastases and associated features may indicate the site of an unknown primary tumor. A problem for diagnostic radiology and surgical management is the patient whose small bowel obstruction follows surgery for abdominal malignancy because adhesion, metastases, or radiation enteropathy may be responsible.[119] An enteroclysis-based radiologic differential diagnosis is possible in more than two thirds of cases.[120]

Seeded metastases cause obstruction by protrusion into the bowel lumen, by associated desmoplasia, or by the combined effect of their multiplicity. Blood loss, other than occult, is unusual in seeded metastases. An additional consideration in patients with obstruction secondary to metastases is the radiologic demonstration of noninvolved segments of small bowel proximal to the point of an obstruction for possible palliative bypass surgery.

### Radiology of Seeded Metastases

Only lesions that are large enough to produce focal alterations of the lumen contour or of the mucosal surface pattern can be recognized by barium contrast studies. Interloop metastases must grow to a larger size before their impingement on a segment of bowel can be recognized by radiology. Enteroclysis excels in demonstrating radiologically identifiable seeded metastases and in determining the degree and sites of obstruction caused by them. Metastases are often multiple. Ascites, minimal or pronounced, is almost always present. CT can be of complementary value in determining the full extent of metastatic disease.

When metastases are deposited on the serosal surface of a segment of the small bowel, rounded protrusions toward the lumen of lesions at least 1 cm in diameter can be demonstrated by carefully performed contrast examination. With distention of the small bowel lumen by contrast medium infusion, involvement of a bowel segment becomes more obvious. The folds may assume a curved appearance at the periphery of a metastasis or may seem stretched and "tacked down." When shown predominantly in profile, metastatic infiltration and fixation of folds at the affected bowel edge are accentuated by a divergence of folds toward the unaffected side.[120, 121] Angulation and tethering of folds are features of frequently associated fibrous reaction. Resultant small bowel obstruction can then be of considerable severity (Fig. 51–23). The significance of obstruction can often be better appreciated by delayed filming. Mucosal ulceration is a late feature.[122]

Loops of small bowel that prolapse into the pelvis after a hysterectomy or pelvic exenteration are frequently sites of seeded metastases (Fig. 51–24). Enteroclysis with films taken in oblique or lateral projections is the best method for recognition of metastatic involvement of these segments. Interloop peritoneal metastases produce shallow indentations often with loop fixation and mucosal tethering. They tend to involve the mesenteric border of several small bowel loops, usually in the lowest part of the right infracolic space. The presence of several peritoneal deposits involving adjacent loops of small intestine has been termed *palisading*[122] (Fig. 51–25).

CT plays an important role in the radiologic demonstration of metastatic lesions in the mesentery and lymph nodes as well as in the bowel wall.[13] With advanced and aggressive metastatic disease, the mesentery is extensively involved in addition to multiple serosal deposits. Barium studies may demonstrate multiple areas of small bowel narrowing, often with intervening distention. Small bowel folds in areas of narrowing appear nodular and distorted but are not destroyed or ulcerated. The desmoplastic effect produces shortening of the mesentery with apparent reduction of the length of small bowel loops, which show crowded folds and an abnormal configuration.[123]

### Radiologic Differential Diagnosis

By means of enteroclysis, a preoperative diagnosis of the cause of an obstruction can be made in most patients.[119, 120] Preoperative radiologic differentiation between adhesions, radiation enteropathy, and metastases was previously considered to be only rarely possible.[124] Adhesive bands cause linear compression defects across the lumen, mostly with straight margins. Multiple adhe-

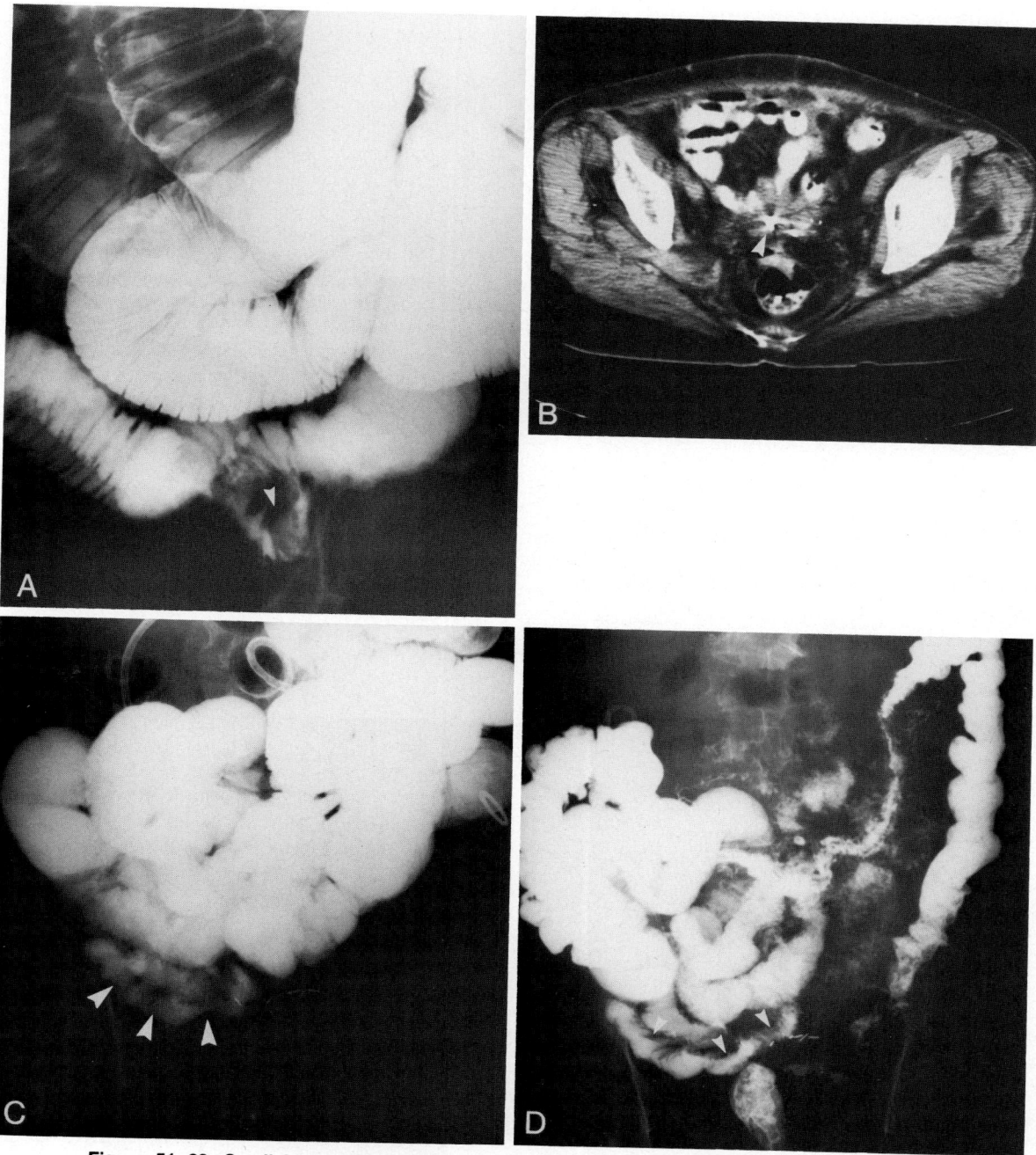

**Figure 51–23. Small bowel obstructions by seeded metastases. A.** Partial obstruction by a seeded metastasis from ovarian carcinoma. Enteroclysis shows focal obstruction involving a pelvic segment of ileum. The obstruction is due to fixation and deformity of a short segment along its mesenteric margin by a mass *(arrowhead)*. This appearance is readily differentiated from that of simple adhesions. **B.** CT scan of pelvic seeded metastases in patient with known ovarian malignancy who presented with symptoms of intestinal obstruction. This CT section shows multiple loops of distal small intestine fixed to a poorly defined mass. The streak artifact in the posterior aspect of the mass is from a right ureteral stent *(arrowhead)*. Note the absence of distention of the small intestine proximal to the fixed segments. **C.** Enteroclysis of the patient in **B** shows moderate distention of the jejunum and proximal ileum proximal to fixed bowel loops in right upper pelvis *(arrowheads)*, consistent with significant obstruction. **D.** Delayed radiograph (24 hours) shows retention of barium in the dilated small intestine. The focal mass effects and tethering along the mesenteric margin of involved loops *(arrowheads)* are better shown than in **C.** Note contrast medium in the normal-caliber colon.

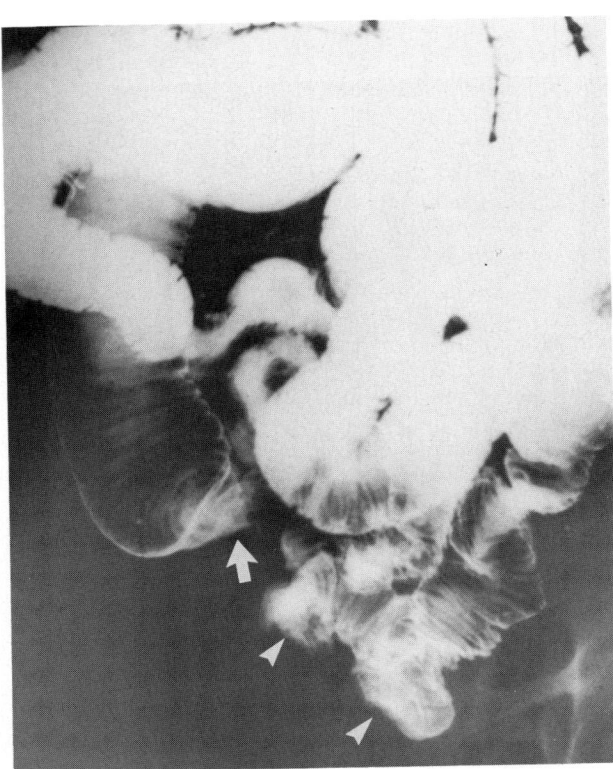

**Figure 51–24. Pelvic seeding of metastases from an ovarian carcinoma.** Multiple fixed loops with nodular defects *(arrowheads)* are involved pelvic segments of ileum. A larger mass causes partial obstruction *(arrow).*

**Figure 51–25. Palisading in seeding metastases.** Lumen and surface pattern alterations are shown in several loops of small intestine that are centrally positioned and fixed. The involved folds are tethered and nondistensible. Mass effects are seen along the mesenteric margins. Enteroclysis was done for possible bypass surgery. Note the short uninvolved proximal jejunum. Massive ascites is apparent. The patient had prior gastrectomy for malignancy.

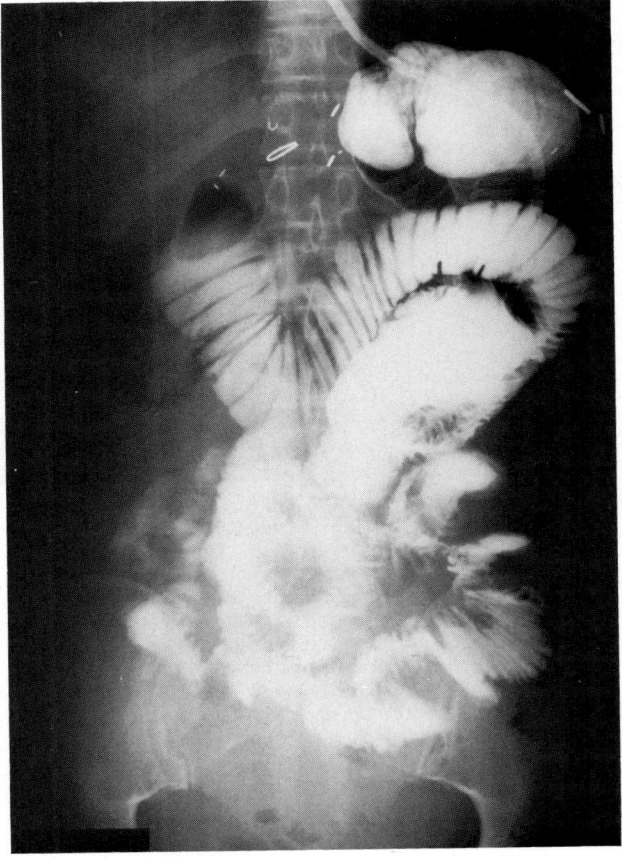

sions are grouped together and usually fixed anteriorly to an abdominal scar. Neither tethering of folds nor nodular defects are observed. Chronic radiation enteropathy produces diffuse thickening of folds with a decreased distance between them, producing a corrugated outline of the involved segments. The distribution of these changes corresponds to the site of the radiation portal.[123] Advanced forms of radiation damage, however, can be associated with the presence of metastases, and the differential diagnosis by contrast radiography can be difficult. Only positive cytology of specimens obtained by needle biopsy can then provide a diagnosis before surgery. Extensive infiltrating metastases involving the right lower quadrant can superficially resemble Crohn's disease.[125] Folds involved, whether displaced, distorted, nodular, or angulated, do not show ulceration or a cobblestone pattern and the presence of fistulas would be unusual. Endometrial implants may seed in the lower right quadrant through reflux of endometrial tissue through the fallopian tubes. The ectopic endometrium continues to be hormonally responsive and may be a site of bleeding and fibrosis. Asymptomatic involvement has also been reported.[126] A plaque-like serosal deposit in the terminal ileum has been shown by small bowel enema.[118] It is frequently seen in association with the more typical radiologic changes affecting the anterior wall of the rectosigmoid.

## Hematogenous Dissemination

The most common hematogenous metastases of the small intestine are from malignant melanoma and bronchogenic carcinoma. Embolic melanoma metastases, although encountered less often than metastases by intra-peritoneal spread, show an affinity for localization in the small intestine and are the most often demonstrated form of hematogenous dissemination. Carcinomas of the lung and breast found at postmortem examination may be small and may not be seen radiologically. Metastases from carcinoma of the breast or from malignant melanoma may come to clinical notice many years after removal of the primary tumor. With carcinoma of the lung, there is no lag time and the clinical features of the primary tumor usually overshadow the symptoms caused by the metastases. The clinical presentations are blood loss and deterioration of the patient's general condition more often than small bowel obstruction.

The early radiologic changes in hematogenous metastases are usually multiple nodules, mostly seen along the antimesenteric border, where the vasa recta arborize into the rich submucosal plexus. The lesions arise at different times and may be grouped into stages of development. Depending on the desmoplastic character or cellularity of the deposits as well as their vascularity, patterns may be produced that suggest the site of the primary carcinoma.

**Metastatic Melanoma.** Although the small bowel is the most frequently affected part of the gastrointestinal tract, the liver bears the highest incidence of metastases within the abdomen, second only to a 70% incidence of deposits to the lung.[127] In an autopsy series, melanoma metastases to the small intestine were found in 58% of cases but came to clinical notice in only 8.9%.[128] Malignant melanoma accounts for almost 3% of all malignant neoplasms and tends to disseminate widely.[127] When a primary melanoma becomes invasive, tumor cells leave its periphery for regional nodes, where they grow to threshold size. Tumor cells then enter the venous circulation and are initially trapped in the pulmonary bed.

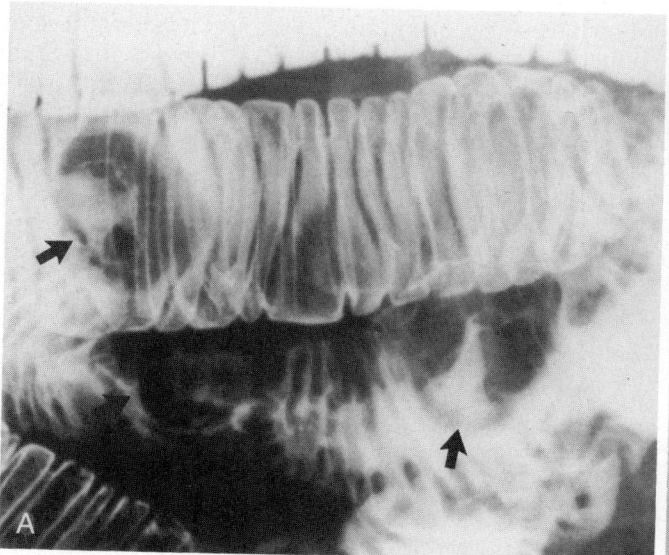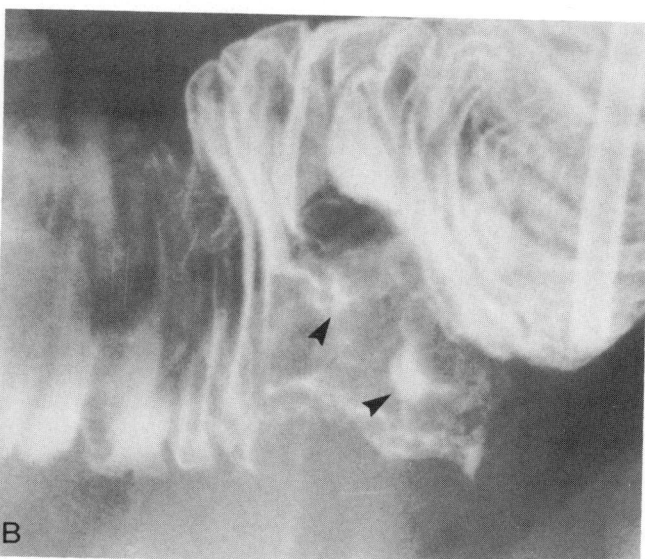

**Figure 51–26. Hematogenous metastases from malignant melanoma. A.** At least three target lesions *(arrows)* are present in a loop of jejunum in a patient with a known history of malignant melanoma. Note the large size of the ulcers in two of the lesions. **B.** A larger polypoid melanoma metastasis contains two ulcers *(arrowheads)*, each with radiating linear ulcerations forming the spoke-wheel pattern typical of melanoma metastases. Also note the absence of obstruction.

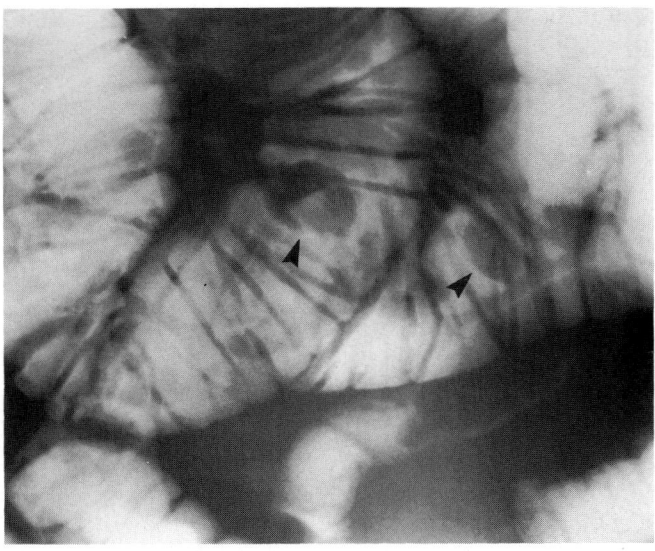

**Figure 51–27. Multiple discrete metastases from lung carcinoma.** Rounded polypoid intramural masses *(arrowheads)* with and without ulceration. The enteroclysis was done because of unexplained anemia. A scar carcinoma was subsequently diagnosed.

Smoothly rounded polypoid lesions of different sizes are the usual appearance of early melanoma metastases to the small bowel (Fig. 51–26). "Target" lesions—nodules with central ulcerations that are frequently found in the stomach and duodenum—occur less often in the mesenteric small intestine.[129, 130] Larger polypoid masses often ulcerate and may show a spoke-wheel pattern of fissuring extending from the ulcer edge to the periphery of the mass (see Fig. 51–26B). The metastases, even when occupying virtually the entire bowel lumen, do not cause significant obstruction. This is due to the softness of the highly cellular mass, which contains little stroma. The demonstration on contrast examination of a nonobstructive large intraluminal mass favors the diagnosis of melanoma metastasis. Such intraluminal masses of melanoma may cause transient intussusceptions or, less often, a high-grade obstruction caused by complete intussusception. Large masses of melanoma deposits may grow through the small bowel wall, expand into the mesentery, and cavitate.[130] Melanoma deposits in exoenteric locations can enlarge considerably before involving a segment of bowel by displacement or compression. Patients with a history of melanoma should have contrast examination if they present with frank or occult bleeding. CT has been successful in outlining melanoma deposits in small bowel; it is the method of choice for demonstrating the totality of metastatic distribution of melanoma throughout the abdominal cavity.[131] Bulky retroperitoneal masses are unusual.

With surgical treatment and chemotherapy, overall survival of patients with disseminated melanoma is reported to be 17.3 months from diagnosis, somewhat improved compared with that in the past.[132]

**Metastases from Bronchogenic Malignancy.** Symptoms do not draw attention to the gastrointestinal tract unless significant bleeding or a perforation occurs. The autopsy incidence of metastases to small bowel was reported to be 11% but was higher (39%) for primary large cell bronchial carcinoma.[133] Metastases may be shown as single or multiple discrete intramural lesions, either flat or polypoid (Fig. 51–27). They are frequently ulcerated. An associated desmoplastic effect may cause constriction and obstruction. The pronounced tendency for the metastasis to penetrate the bowel wall can lead to localized extravasation, rarely to free perforation.[134]

**Breast Metastases.** The stomach, duodenum, and co-

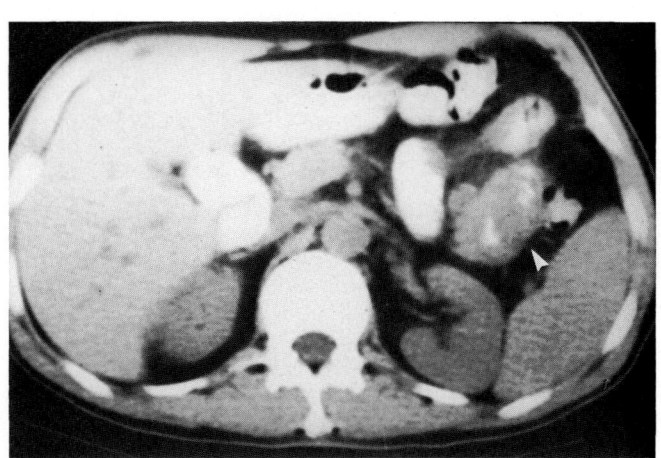

**Figure 51–28. Metastasis to the jejunum from a carcinoma of the descending colon.** CT scan demonstrates a concentrically thickened bowel loop *(arrowhead).* Metastatic disease should be diagnosed when proximal jejunal loops are involved in a patient with a known malignancy of the left colon.

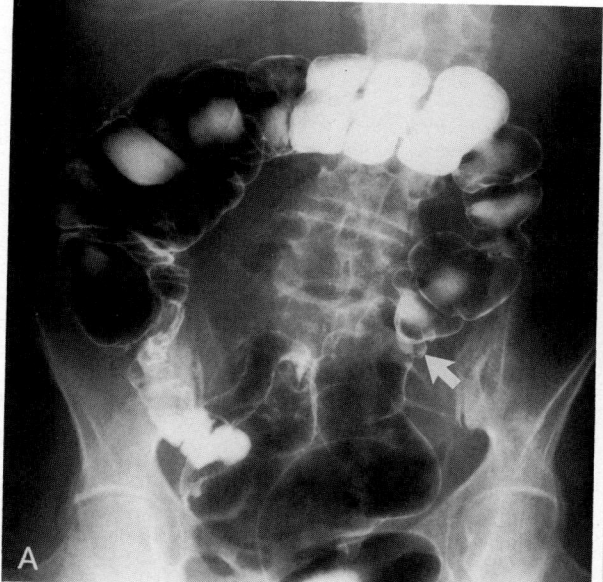

**Figure 51–29. Metastatic involvement of small intestine adjacent to an anastomotic site. A.** Double contrast barium enema done because of lower gastrointestinal bleeding shows end-to-end anastomosis between transverse colon and sigmoid colon *(arrow)* after segmental colectomy for carcinoma. **B.** Enteroclysis after colon examination shows large ulcerating mass *(arrow)* in the small bowel adjacent to the sigmocolic anastomosis. Surgery confirmed metastatic disease.

lon are more often involved than the mesenteric small bowel. It has been claimed that treatment of the primary tumor with corticosteroids increases the likelihood of metastases.[135] Secondary metastases from breast cancer typically form highly cellular masses that spread through the submucosa. The rare metastases to the small bowel have been described as multiple strictures with intervening dilatations or as an intussuscepting ulcerated mural lesion.[136]

## Other Metastatic Pathways

**Direct Extension and Lymphatic Spread.** Lymph node metastases from a left-sided colon carcinoma can invade the proximal jejunum near the ligament of Treitz via lymphatic vessels that parallel the arterial supply. Those draining the distal transverse and the descending colon are near the ascending left colic branch of the inferior mesenteric artery, which courses lateral to the distal horizontal duodenum. The adjacent jejunum is not infrequently involved by this mode of spread (Fig. 51–28). Residual tumor after resection of a cecal malignancy or of a gynecologic malignancy can involve the distal ileum by direct extension via the subperitoneal space.[117] This is also not an infrequent method of involvement of the more proximal mesenteric small bowel.

Blockage of a proximal lymph node by tumor may lead to retrograde flow of lymph and of tumor emboli and to involvement of an adjacent segment of bowel.[137]

After resection for colon carcinoma, this mechanism may be responsible for the metastatic involvement of small bowel near a colocolic anastomotic site (Fig. 51–29).

### Acknowledgment

Figure 51–26B is reproduced from Herlinger H, Maglinte D (eds): Clinical Radiology of the Small Intestine. Philadelphia: WB Saunders, 1989.

## References

1. Barclay THC, Shapira DV: Malignant tumors of the small intestine. Cancer 51:878–881, 1983.
2. Han-ji D, Shi-zhang H, Shu-wei H: Tumors of the small intestine. Report of 131 cases and review of 1024 cases in the literature. Chin Med J 99:91–96, 1986.
3. Lowenfels AB: Why are small bowel tumors so rare? Lancet 1:24–26, 1982.
4. Maglinte DDT, O'Connor K, Bessette J, et al: The role of the physician in the late diagnosis of primary malignant tumors of the small intestine. Am J Gastroenterol 3:304–308, 1991.
5. Vuori JVA, Vuorio MK: Radiological findings in primary malignant tumors of the small intestine. Ann Clin Res 3:16–21, 1971.
6. Eckbert O, Ekholm S: Radiography in primary tumors of the small bowel. Acta Radiol Diagn (Stockh) 21:79–84, 1980.
7. Zollinger RM, Sternfield WC, Schreiber H: Primary neoplasms of the small intestine. Am J Surg 151:654–658, 1986.
8. Bessette JR, Maglinte DDT, Kelvin FM, et al: Primary malignant

tumors in the small bowel: a comparison of the small bowel enema and conventional follow-through examination. AJR 153:741–744, 1989.

9. Hulnick DH, Megibow AJ: Computed tomography of the small bowel. *In* Herlinger H, Maglinte D (eds): Clinical Radiology of the Small Intestine. Philadelphia: WB Saunders, 1989, pp 161–200.

10. Dudiak KM, Daniel-Johnson C, Stevens DH: Primary tumors of the small intestine: CT evaluation. AJR 152:995–998, 1989.

11. Laurent F, Raynaud M, Biset JM, et al: Diagnosis and categorization of small bowel neoplasms: role of computed tomography. Gastrointest Radiol 16:115–119, 1991.

12. Fleischer AC, Paruleker S, Seibert JJ: Sonography of small bowel. *In* Herlinger H, Maglinte D (eds): Clinical Radiology of the Small Intestine. Philadelphia: WB Saunders, 1989, pp 153–159.

13. Moertel CJ, Sauer WG, Dockerty MB, et al: Life history of the carcinoid tumor of the small intestine. Cancer 14:901–912, 1961.

14. Balthazar EJ: Carcinoid tumors of the alimentary tract. I. Radiographic diagnosis. Gastrointest Radiol 3:47–56, 1978.

15. Warner RRP: Carcinoid tumor. *In* Berk JE (ed): Bockus Gastroenterology (4th ed). Philadelphia: WB Saunders, 1985, pp 1874–1886.

16. Hossain J, Al-Mofleh I, Tandon R, et al: Carcinoid syndrome without liver metastases. Postgrad Med J 65:597–599, 1989.

17. Kothari T, Mangla JC: Malignant tumors associated with carcinoid tumors of the gastrointestinal tract. J Clin Gastroenterol 3:43–46, 1981.

18. Jeffree MA, Nolan DJ: Multiple ileal carcinoid tumors. Br J Radiol 60:402–403, 1987.

19. Cockey BM, Fishman EK, Jones B, et al: Computed tomography of abdominal carcinoid tumor. J Comput Assist Tomogr 9:38–42, 1985.

20. Gould M, Johnson RJ: Computed tomography of abdominal carcinoid tumor. Br J Radiol 59:881–885, 1986.

21. Picus D, Glazer HS, Levitt RG, et al: Computed tomography of abdominal carcinoid tumors. AJR 143:581–584, 1984.

22. Dent GA, Feldman J: Pseudocystic liver metastases in patients with carcinoid tumors: report of three cases. Am J Clin Pathol 82:275–279, 1984.

23. Reuter SR, Boijsen E: Angiographic findings in two ileal carcinoid tumors. Radiology 87:836–840, 1966.

24. Seifel RS, Kuhns LR, Borlaza GS: Computed tomography and angiography in ileal carcinoid tumor and retractile mesenteritis. Radiology 134:437–440, 1980.

25. Moertel CJ: Therapy of metastatic carcinoid tumor and the carcinoid syndrome. *In* Boettino JC, Opfell RW, Muggia FM (eds): Liver Cancer. Boston: Martinus Nijhoff, 1985.

26. Allison DJ: Additional experience with hepatic embolization of endocrine metastases. *In* Herlinger H, Lunderquist A, Wallace S (eds): Clinical Radiology of the Liver. New York: Marcel Dekker, 1983.

27. Odurny A, Birch SJ: Hepatic arterial embolization in patients with metastatic carcinoid tumors. Clin Radiol 36:597–602, 1985.

28. Mittey HA, Warner RRP: Control of carcinoid syndrome with hepatic artery embolization. Radiology 155:623–626, 1985.

29. Coup M, Hemingway A, Hodgson HJF, et al: Effect of hepatic artery embolization on survival in carcinoid syndrome. Abstracts of the Jubilee Meeting of the British Society of Gastroenterology, 1987, p 36.

30. Arthaud JB, Guienee VF: Jejunal and ileal adenocarcinoma. Am J Gastroenterol 72:638–646, 1979.

31. Brookes VS, Waterhouse JAH, Powell DJ: Malignant lesions of the small intestine. A 10 year survey. Br J Surg 55:405–410, 1968.

32. Reyes EL, Talley RW: Primary malignant tumors of the small intestine. Am J Gastroenterol 54:30–43, 1970.

33. Herbsman H, Wetstein L: Tumors of the small intestine. Curr Probl Surg 17:121–182, 1980.

34. Morson BC, Dawson IMP: Gastrointestinal Pathology (2nd ed). Oxford: Blackwell Scientific Publications, 1979.

35. Wilson JM, Melvin DB, Gray GF, et al: Primary malignancies of the small bowel. A report of 96 cases and review of the literature. Ann Surg 180:175–179, 1974.

36. Lightdale CJ, Sherlock P: Small intestinal tumors (other than

lymphoma and carcinoid). *In* Berk JE (ed): Bockus Gastroenterology (4th ed). Philadelphia: WB Saunders, 1985, pp 1887–1899.

37. Ouriel K, Adams JT: Adenocarcinoma of the small intestine. Am J Surg 47:66–71, 1984.

38. Harris OD, Cooke WT, Thomason H, et al: Malignancy in adult celiac disease and idiopathic steatorrhea. Am J Med 42:899–912, 1967.

39. Swinson CM, Slevin G, Cole SRC, et al: Coeliac disease and malignancy. Lancet 1:111–115, 1983.

40. Cooke WT, Homes GKT: Coeliac Disease. Edinburgh: Churchill Livingstone, 1984, pp 180–183.

41. Ginzberg L, Schneider KM, Drezin DH: Carcinoma of the jejunum occurring in a case of regional enteritis. Surgery 39:347–351, 1956.

41a. Feczko PJ: Malignancy complicating inflammatory bowel disease. Radiol Clin North Am 25:157–174, 1987.

42. Fell J, Snooks S: Small bowel adenocarcinoma complicating Crohn's disease. JR Soc Med 80:51–52, 1987.

42a. Hamilton SR: Colorectal carcinoma in patients with Crohn's disease. Gastroenterology 89:398–407, 1985.

43. Fresko D, Lazarus S, Dotan J, et al: Early presentation of carcinoma of the small bowel in Crohn's disease ("Crohn's carcinoma"). Case reports and review of the literature. Gastroenterology 82:783–789, 1982.

43a. Church JM, Weakley FL, Fazio VW: The relationship between fistulas and Crohn's disease and associated carcinoma. Dis Colon Rectum 28:361–366, 1985.

44. Kerber GW, Frank PH: Carcinoma of the small intestine and colon as a complication of Crohn's disease: radiologic manifestations. Radiology 150:639–645, 1984.

45. Miller TL, Skucas J, Guder D: Bowel cancer characteristics in patients with regional enteritis. Gastrointest Radiol 12:45–52, 1987.

46. Hawker PC, Guide SN, Thompson H, et al: Adenocarcinoma of the small intestine complicating Crohn's disease. Gut 23:188–193, 1982.

47. Schier J: Diagnostic and therapeutic aspects of tumors of the small bowel. Int Surg 57:789–792, 1972.

48. Spigelman AD, Murday V, Phillips RKS: Cancer and the Peutz-Jeghers syndrome. Gut 30:1588–1590, 1989.

49. Giardiello FM, Welsh SB: Increased risk of cancer in the Peutz-Jeghers syndrome. N Engl J Med 316:1511–1514, 1987.

50. Bruneton JN, Drouillard J, Bourry J, et al: L'adenocarcinome de l'intestin grêle. État actuel du diagnostic et du traitement. Étude de 27 cas et revue de la littérature. J Radiol 64:117–123, 1983.

51. Papadopoulos VD, Nolan DJ: Carcinoma of the small intestine. Clin Radiol 36:409–413, 1985.

52. Levine MS, Droos AT, Herlinger H: Annular malignancies of the small bowel. Gastrointest Radiol 12:53–58, 1987.

53. Wagner KM, Thompson J, Herlinger H, et al: Thirteen primary adenocarcinoma of the ileum and appendix, a case report. Cancer 49:797–801, 1982.

54. Milmann PG, Gold BM, Bagla S, et al: Primary ileal adenocarcinoma simulating Crohn's disease. Gastrointest Radiol 5:55–58, 1980.

55. Johnson AM, Harman PK, Hanks JD: Primary small bowel malignancy. Am Surg 51:31–36, 1985.

56. Ranchod M, Kempson RL: Smooth muscle tumors of the gastrointestinal tract and retroperitoneum: a pathologic analysis of 100 cases. Cancer 39:255–262, 1977.

57. Dodds WJ, Goldberg HI, Margulis AR: Leiomyosarcoma of the small intestine. AJR 107:142–149, 1969.

58. Herlinger H: The recognition of exogastric tumors. Br J Radiol 39:25–36, 1966.

59. Megibow AJ, Balthazar EJ, Hulnick DH, et al: CT evaluation of gastrointestinal leiomyomas and leiomyosarcomas. AJR 144:727–731, 1985.

60. Choi BI, Lee WJ, Chi JG, et al: CT manifestations of peritoneal leiomyosarcomatosis. AJR 155:799–801, 1990.

61. Uflacker R, Amaret NM: Angiography in primary myomas of the alimentary tract. Radiology 139:361–369, 1981.

62. Marshak RH, Lindner AE: Radiologic features of diagnostic importance—cancer of the gastrointestinal tract. JAMA 229:1498–1499, 1974.

63. Dawson IMP, Cornes JS, Morson BC: Primary malignant tumors of the intestinal tract. Br J Surg 49:80–89, 1961.
64. Ehrlich AN, Stalder G, Geller W: Gastrointestinal manifestations of malignant lymphoma. Gastroenterology 54:1115–1118, 1968.
65. Berg JW: Primary lymphomas of the gastrointestinal tract. Nat Cancer Inst Monogr 32:211–215, 1969.
66. Al-Khatech AK: Primary malignant lymphoma of the small intestine. Int Surg 54:295–298, 1970.
67. Rappaport H: The lymphoreticular system. *In* Atlas of Tumor Pathology, Fascicle 8, Section 3. Washington, DC: Armed Forces Institute of Pathology, 1966.
68. Jaffe ES: An overview of the classification of non-Hodgkin's lymphomas. *In* Jaffe ES (ed): Surgical Pathology of the Lymph Nodes and Related Organs. Philadelphia: WB Saunders, 1985, pp 135–145.
69. National Cancer Institute: The non-Hodgkin's lymphoma pathologic classification project (summary and description of a working formulation for clinical usage). Cancer 48:2112–2135, 1982.
70. Lewin KJ, Ranchod M, Dorfman RF: Lymphomas of the gastrointestinal tract. Cancer 42:693–707, 1978.
71. Drogosic SB, Bauer P, Radaszkiewicz T: Primary gastrointestinal non-Hodgkin's lymphomas: a retrospective clinicopathologic study of 150 cases. Cancer 55:1060–1073, 1985.
72. Weinberg DS: Pathology of lymphomas: 1985. Semin Ultrasound CT MR 6:352–361, 1985.
73. Jaffe ES: Relationship of classification to biologic behavior of non-Hodgkin's lymphoma. Semin Oncol 13:3–9, 1986.
74. Papadimitriou CS, Papacharalampous NX, Kittas C: Primary gastrointestinal malignant lymphoma: a morphologic and immunohistochemical study. Cancer 55:870–879, 1985.
75. Weingrad DN, Decosse JJ, Sherlock P, et al: Primary gastrointestinal lymphoma. A 30 year review. Cancer 49:1258–1265, 1982.
76. Fitsch DD, Wilson JAP: Primary gastrointestinal lymphoma. South Med J 78:909–913, 1985.
77. Baildam AD, Williams GT, Schofield PF: Abdominal lymphoma—the place for surgery. J R Soc Med 82:657–660, 1989.
78. Bäck H, Gustavson B, Ridell B, et al: Primary gastrointestinal lymphoma. Incidence, clinical presentation and surgical approach. J Surg Oncol 33:234–238, 1986.
79. Randall J, Obeid ML, Blackledge GRP: Hemorrhage and perforation of gastrointestinal neoplasms during chemotherapy. Ann R Coll Surg Engl 68:286–289, 1986.
80. Konar A, Brown CB, Hancock BW, et al: Protein-losing enteropathy as a sole manifestation of non-Hodgkin's lymphoma. Postgrad Med J 62:399–400, 1986.
81. Agudelo CA, Schumacher HR, Glick JH, et al: Non-Hodgkin's lymphoma in systemic lupus erythematosus. Report of four cases with ultrastructural studies in two. J Rheumatol 8:69–78, 1981.
82. Green JA, Dawson AA, Walker W: Systemic lupus erythematosus and lymphoma. Lancet 2:753–758, 1978.
83. Gilchrist AM, Herlinger H, Carr RF, et al: Small bowel lymphoma, a radiologic pathologic correlation. *In* Herlinger H, Megibow A (eds): Gastrointestinal Radiology Review, Volume 1. New York: Marcel Dekker, 1990, pp 187–211.
84. Gourtsoyiannis NC, Nolan DJ: Lymphoma of the small intestine: radiological appearances. Clin Radiol 39:639–645, 1988.
85. Marshak RH, Lindner AE, Maklansky D: Lymphoreticular disorders of the gastrointestinal tract: roentgenographic features. Gastrointest Radiol 4:103–120, 1978.
86. Craig O, Gregson R: Primary lymphoma of the gastrointestinal tract. Clin Radiol 32:63–71, 1981.
87. Mueller PR, Ferrucci JT: Appearance of lymphomatous involvement of the mesentery by ultrasonography and body computed tomography: the "sandwich" sign. Radiology 134:467–473, 1980.
88. Fishman EK, Kuhlman JE, Jones RJ: CT of lymphoma: spectrum of disease. Radiographics 11:647–669, 1991.
89. Dodd GD: Lymphoma of the hollow abdominal viscera. Radiol Clin North Am 28:771–783, 1990.
90. Rubesin SE, Gilchrist AM, Bronner M, et al: Non-Hodgkin lymphoma of the small intestine. Radiographics 10:985–998, 1990.
91. Sartoris DJ, Harell GS, Anderson MF, et al: Small bowel lymphoma and regional enteritis: radiographic similarities. Radiology 152:291–295, 1984.
92. Nolan DJ, Gourtsoyiannis NC: Crohn's disease of the small intestine. A review of the radiological appearances in 100 consecutive patients examined by a barium infusion technique. Clin Radiol 30:397–603, 1980.
93. Pagani JJ, Bernardino ME: CT-radiographic correlation of ulcerating small bowel lymphomas. AJR 136:998–1000, 1981.
94. Lunderquist A: Percutaneous biopsy of small bowel lesions. *In* Herlinger H, Maglinte D (eds): Clinical Radiology of the Small Intestine. Philadelphia: WB Saunders, 1989, pp 235–236.
95. Parker SH, Hopper KD, Yakes WF, et al: Image-directed percutaneous biopsies with a biopsy gun. Radiology 171:663–669, 1989.
96. Barr LC, Glees JP, Gazet J-C: Diagnostic laparotomy in suspected malignant lymphoma. Ann R Coll Surg Engl 66:402–404, 1984.
97. Blackledge G, Best JK, Crowther D: Role of computed tomography in staging and management of gastrointestinal lymphoma. J R Soc Med 72:818–822, 1979.
98. Bragg DG, Colby TV, Ward GH: New concepts in the non-Hodgkin's lymphomas. Radiologic implications. Radiology 159:289–304, 1986.
99. Brady LW, Asbell SD: Malignant lymphoma of the gastrointestinal tract. Radiology 137:291–298, 1980.
100. Collins J, Caton R, Harty-Goulder B: Burkitt's lymphoma presenting with gastroduodenal involvement. Gastroenterology 85:425–429, 1983.
101. Glass RBJ, Fernbach SK, Conway JJ, et al: Gallium scinitigraphy in American Burkitt lymphoma. AJR 145:671–676, 1985.
102. Shawker TH, Dunnick NR, Head GL, et al: Ultrasound evaluation of American Burkitt's lymphoma. J Clin Ultrasound 7:279–283, 1979.
103. Falchuk KR, Harris NL: Case records of the Massachusetts General Hospital—case 14-1985. N Engl J Med 312:905–914, 1985.
104. Wright DH, Isaacson PG: Gut associated lymphoid tumors. *In* Whitehead R (ed): Gastrointestinal and Oesophageal Pathology. London: Churchill Livingstone, 1989, pp 643–661.
105. Lewin KJ, Kahn LB, Novis BH: Primary intestinal lymphoma of "Western" and "Mediterranean" type, alpha chain disease and massive plasma cell infiltration. Cancer 38:2511–2528, 1976.
106. Penn I: Malignant lymphomas in organ transplant recipients. Transplant Proc 13:736–738, 1981.
107. Honda H, Barloon TJ, Franken EA Jr, et al: Clinical and radiologic features of malignant neoplasms in organ transplant recipients: cyclosporine-treated vs untreated patients. AJR 154:271–274, 1990.
108. Kirkman RI: Case records of the Massachusetts General Hospital, case 29-1991. N Engl J Med 325:183–195, 1991.
109. Ziegler JL, Bragg K, Abrams D, et al: High-grade non-Hodgkin's lymphoma in patients with AIDS. Ann N Y Acad Sci 437:412–419, 1984.
110. Danzig JB, Brandt LJ, Reinus JF, et al: Gastrointestinal malignancy in patients with AIDS. Am J Gastroenterol 86:715–718, 1991.
111. Moon KL, Federle MP, Abrams DI, et al: Kaposi sarcoma and lymphadenopathy syndrome. Limitations of abdominal CT in acquired immunodeficiency syndrome. Radiology 150:479–483, 1984.
112. Castellino RA: Hodgkin disease: Practical concepts for the diagnostic radiologist. Radiology 159:305–311, 1986.
113. Krikorian JG, Burke GS, Rosenberg SA, et al: The occurrence of non-Hodgkin's lymphoma following therapy for Hodgkin's disease. N Engl J Med 300:452–458, 1979.
114. Marshak RH, Lindner AE: Radiology of the Small Intestine (2nd ed). Philadelphia: WB Saunders, 1976.
115. Meyers MA, McSweeney J: Secondary neoplasms of the bowel. Radiology 105:1–11, 1972.
116. Meyers MA: Dynamic Radiology of the Abdomen. Normal and Pathologic Anatomy (3rd ed). New York: Springer-Verlag, 1988.
117. Oliphant M, Berne AS, Meyers MA: Imaging the direct bidirectional spread of disease between the abdomen and the female

pelvis via the subperitoneal space. Gastrointest Radiol 13:285–298, 1988.

118. Herlinger H, Maglinte D: Tumors of the small intestine. *In* Herlinger H, Maglinte D (eds): Clinical Radiology of the Small Intestine. Philadelphia: WB Saunders, 1989, pp 399–451.

119. Caroline DF, Herlinger H, Laufer I, et al: Small bowel enema in the diagnosis of adhesive obstructions. AJR 142:1133–1139, 1984.

120. Herlinger H, Maglinte D: Small bowel obstruction. *In* Herlinger H, Maglinte D (eds): Clinical Radiology of the Small Intestine. Philadelphia: WB Saunders, 1989, pp 479–507.

121. Zboralske FF, Bessolo RJ: Metastatic carcinoma to the mesentery and gut. Radiology 88:302–310, 1967.

122. Marshak RH, Khilnani MT, Eliasoph J, et al: Metastatic carcinoma of the small bowel. AJR 94:385–394, 1965.

123. Wittich G, Salomonowitz E, Szepesi T, et al: Small bowel double-contrast enema in stage III ovarian cancer. AJR 142:299–304, 1984.

124. Osteen RT, Guyton S, Steele G Jr, et al: Malignant intestinal obstruction. Surgery 87:611–615, 1980.

125. Meyers MS, Oliphant M, Teixidor H, et al: Metastatic carcinoma simulating inflammatory colitis. AJR 123:74–83, 1975.

126. Aronchick CA, Brooks FP, Dyson WL, et al: Ileocecal endometriosis presenting with abdominal pain and gastrointestinal bleeding. Dig Dis Sci 28:566–572, 1983.

127. Oddson TA, Rice RP, Seigler HB: The spectrum of small bowel melanoma. Gastrointest Radiol 3:419–423, 1978.

128. Das Gupta T, Brasfield R: Metastatic melanoma—clinicopathological study. Cancer 17:1323–1339, 1969.

129. Goldstein HM, Beydoun MT, Dodd GD: Radiologic spectrum of melanoma metastatic to the gastrointestinal tract. AJR 129:605–612, 1977.

130. Zornoza J, Goldstein HM: Cavitating metastases of the small intestine. AJR 129:613–615, 1977.

131. Fishman EK, Kuhlman JE, Schuchter LM, et al: CT of malignant melanoma in the chest, abdomen and musculoskeletal system. Radiographics 10:603–620, 1990.

132. Reintgen DS, Thompson W, Garbutt J, et al: Radiologic, endoscopic and surgical considerations of malignant melanoma metastatic to the small intestine. Curr Surg 41:87–89, 1984.

133. McNeill PM, Wagman LD, Neifeld JP: Small bowel metastases from primary carcinoma of the lung. Cancer 59:1486–1489, 1987.

134. Joffe N: Symptomatic gastrointestinal metastases secondary to bronchogenic carcinoma. Clin Radiol 29:217–225, 1978.

135. Hartman WH, Sherlock P: Gastroduodenal metastases from carcinoma of the breast. An adrenal steroid–induced phenomenon. Cancer 14:426–431, 1961.

136. Chang SF, Burrell MI, Brand MH, et al: The protean gastrointestinal manifestations of metastatic breast carcinoma. Radiology 126:611–617, 1978.

137. Grinnel RS: Lymphatic block with atypical and retrograde lymphatic metastasis and spread in carcinoma of the colon and rectum. Ann Surg 163:272–280, 1986.

# Obstruction

## 52

Hans Herlinger, M.D.
Stephen E. Rubesin, M.D.

## INTRODUCTION

A diagnosis of intestinal obstruction is made in about 20% of patients admitted to a hospital with an acute abdomen.[1] The small bowel is the usual site of the obstruction. Small bowel obstructions (SBOs) of lower grades of severity are more frequent and include those that occur intermittently, ease spontaneously, and do not require hospital admission.

## PATHOPHYSIOLOGY

### Distention and Fluid Increase

Fluid and electrolytes accumulate above an obstructed small bowel where the small intestinal mucosa reduces their absorption and increases their secretion into the lumen. Swallowed air adds to the degree of distention. In simple obstruction, distention can become pronounced without necessarily interfering with the blood supply. In closed loop obstructions, distention causes a greater amount of secretion and increasingly severe distention. Obstructed closed loops may become ischemic and progress to necrosis (strangulation).[2]

## Strangulation

Strangulation implies mechanical obstruction, impairment of the circulation and, eventually, infarction. Strangulation is particularly likely to occur in a closed loop obstruction, usually a loop of bowel entrapped by a postoperative adhesion. Less often, strangulation obstruction occurs within a hernia or results from severely increased intraluminal pressures sufficient to interfere with venous return. Venous congestion can lead to intramural, intraluminal, and intraperitoneal seepage of blood. This may be aggravated by arterial constriction, resulting in necrosis and possible perforation.[3] Even in simple obstructions, proliferation of bacteria accompanies stasis of intestinal contents. During infarction, with blood loss into the lumen and bowel wall, the bacterial population increases rapidly, now including anaerobic organisms.[4] Toxic metabolites derived from necrotic parts of the bowel wall enter the bowel lumen, perfuse into the peritoneal cavity, and are absorbed into the blood stream.

## CLINICAL PRESENTATION
### Symptoms

Pain, vomiting, and constipation are the classic presenting features of an SBO. Clinical findings vary with the degree and level of SBO and with the vascular status of the obstructed segment. In typical mechanical obstruction, abdominal pain is crampy and gradually increases in intensity, only to abate and recur. With time, increasing bowel distention inhibits motility and the pain tends to subside. Vomiting is more pronounced in proximal SBOs and abdominal distention in distal obstructions.

Intestinal strangulation is suspected when the intermittent crampy pain becomes continuous and increases in severity. Abdominal tenderness and guarding, leukocytosis, pyrexia, and tachycardia in excess of 100 beats per minute are useful but not reliable indicators of a strangulating obstruction.

## Physical Examination

The quality of peristaltic sounds heard during auscultation of the abdomen may be helpful. A silent abdomen may be found in the early postoperative period, in cases of adynamic ileus, or with infarction. High-pitched, tinkling bowel sounds of increasing intensity accompanied by crampy pain indicate hyperactive peristalsis in mechanical SBO. In bowel obstructions in which dilated loops contain little air or are entirely fluid filled, bowel sounds are not heard.[5]

Features of dehydration may be present because fluid secreted into distended bowel loops is unavailable to the circulation.[6] Resultant dehydration and electrolyte imbalance may be accompanied by oliguria, azotemia, hemoconcentration, and circulatory disturbances. A palpable mass in the abdomen may be a feature of a closed loop obstruction. The possible presence of an incarcerated external hernia should always be investigated, but it may escape detection in obese patients or at unusual sites.

## SURGICAL PROBLEMS

### Complete Obstructions

A clinical and plain film diagnosis of SBO can be reliably made in most patients with complete SBO. In acute and complete SBO, early surgery is required, although sufficient time should be allowed to restore the patient's fluid and electrolyte balance. Early surgery in 51 such patients with complete SBO revealed 21 strangulation obstructions (42%), of which 6 contained still viable obstructed bowel.[7] In this entire group of patients, a preoperative diagnosis of strangulation could not be made or excluded reliably. A similar finding was reported in 128 patients with complete mechanical SBO caused by adhesions.[8] Early surgery discovered strangulation obstruction in 53 patients (41.5%), with still viable bowel in 37 of the patients.[8] In the same group of patients, even including the large number of strangulations, early surgery only minimally increased operative mortality, to 5.5%[8] from the 4.6% reported in cases of simple obstructions.

## Developing Strangulation

A major problem is the sufficiently early recognition of strangulation developing in patients with incomplete SBO. Delayed recognition precipitously increases surgical mortality. Closed loop obstructions, so often associated with strangulation, may go through a preliminary period of partial obstruction and still reversible deprivation of the blood supply. Clinical recognition of the prestrangulation stage of a closed loop obstruction is virtually impossible, and only radiology may be able to provide a diagnosis at this stage.[9-11] Clinical recognition of a strangulating obstruction has not improved over the years. In 40% of cases of strangulation, none or only one of the signs of strangulation—pain, pyrexia, absent bowel sounds, leukocytosis, and/or tachycardia—was present.[12] At a fairly early stage, the constancy of the abdominal pain, which previously had been intermittent or colicky, may be the only feature to direct clinical suspicion to the presence of strangulation.[13] Estimation of the serum isoenzyme creatine kinase $CK_1$ (BB) has shown promise for the detection of intestinal infarction.[14] A possible but not yet fully determined advantage of this test could be its greater sensitivity in the early stage of the infarction, which would significantly improve survival.

A further diagnostic problem is that clinical features of strangulation may underemphasize the underlying intestinal obstruction and lead to a false diagnosis of acute mesenteric venous thrombosis.[13]

The plain film of the abdomen has often been considered unhelpful. In a series of obstructions with strangulation, plain films reportedly showed merely SBO in 48%, were equivocal in 35%, and were normal in 17% of patients.[15] On the other hand, a comparison of plain films and computed tomography (CT) in 23 patients with small bowel infarction showed specific plain film findings in 7 patients and specific CT findings in 9 patients.[16] Because plain films and CT scans together provided the diagnosis in only one patient, the overall, separate contributions of the two techniques to clinical diagnosis were of diagnostic value in 15 of the 23 patients (65%).

## Obstruction After Laparotomy for Cancer

In this group of patients, the causes of obstruction include postoperative adhesions, a focal malignant deposit suitable for resection or bypass, extensive carcinomatosis, or radiation enteropathy. Between 21 and 38% of such patients have a benign, adhesive cause of the SBO rather than metastases.[15, 17, 18] Although surgeons differ on the value of an intervention in this group of obstructed patients, they generally agree that the cause of these obstructions cannot be determined preoperatively.[18] In one report,[15] palliative surgery for SBO after laparotomy for malignancy was considered a questionable option even though obstructions were found to be caused by postoperative adhesions in 21% of the cases. Another surgical team, discussing intestinal obstruction caused by metastatic cancer, favored palliative surgery after trial tube decompression; carried out resection and reanastomosis for localized metastatic disease and enteroenterostomies for more advanced disease; and stressed the unexpected finding of adhesions as a cause of obstruction of these patients.[19] The surgeon has the difficult task of weighing the operative morbidity against the opportunity to allow the patient to return home for what may be a short time.[18] A reliable preoperative radiologic diagnosis of the cause of obstruction in this group of patients would make it possible for the surgeon to tailor management decisions to the specific problem of each patient.

Radiology has an important role in demonstrating the site, degree, and cause of an SBO; in recognizing closed loop obstructions; and in preoperatively assessing the cause of SBO in patients previously operated on for abdominal cancer.[20] Concerning the last group of patients, a survey by our department of cases examined by enteroclysis and subsequently taken to laparotomy showed that a diagnosis of obstruction by metastases was correct in 88% and false-negative in 12%. In the same group of patients, 70% of obstructions by adhesions were correctly diagnosed and a false-positive diagnosis was made in 30%. There is, therefore, a tendency for radiology to overdiagnose metastases.

In addition to plain films of the abdomen and the use of barium contrast studies (where indicated), investigations by CT and ultrasound have become increasingly effective.

## RADIOLOGIC IMAGING

### Plain Films of the Abdomen

A more complete discussion has been presented in Chapter 13. Only a few aspects of the interpretative limitations and difficulties in SBO are mentioned here.

Plain abdominal films were compared with enteroclysis and laparotomy for 117 patients with suspected SBO.[21] In blinded retrospective analysis, plain films were categorized as 1) normal, 2) abnormal nonspecific, 3) probable SBO, or 4) definite SBO. In patients with normal or abnormal nonspecific plain films, enteroclysis later showed varying degrees of SBO in 22% (15 of 67). These false-negative interpretations may have been due to long tube decompression or vomiting, proximal obstructions, predominantly fluid-filled loops, or films taken too early in the illness. More frequent still were false-positive diagnoses of obstruction. Of 50 patients with plain film reports of probable or definite obstructions, 21 (42%) were found to have surgically insignificant adhesions or were unobstructed (including 9 cases of adynamic ileus). The authors concluded that plain films are frequently misleading and tend to overdiagnose obstruction and that the practice of serial plain filming in suspected SBO may be of questionable value.[21, 22]

When plain films of the abdomen show features of SBO, they can be a guide to the level of the obstruction.

Proximal and mid–small bowel obstructions tend to show air-fluid levels mostly in the left upper quadrant. A larger number of dilated air-fluid–containing loops, arranged in the line of the mesenteric root, may indicate distal SBO or possibly cecal obstruction. Although distal accumulation of fluid without air in distended loops can give the false impression of more proximal obstruction, prediction of the level of obstruction was correct for 79% of plain films.[21] It is important to be aware of the likely level of SBO when planning a barium study. Distal obstructions should first be investigated by barium enema examination, either to identify an obstructing colonic lesion or, in its absence, to use barium reflux into the ileum for a retrograde demonstration of the obstruction site.

Of over-riding importance is the plain film demonstration of features of a strangulation obstruction, namely edematous folds, pneumatosis, a suggestion of a closed loop obstruction (Fig. 52–1), and occasionally gas in the portal vein.

## Barium Studies

Barium does not inspissate above a small bowel obstruction and can be administered safely in this situation.[23, 24] However, barium filling of dilated bowel loops is unwelcome to the surgeon when early laparotomy is required. Barium should therefore not be used, by mouth or intubation, in patients with complete obstructions. Nor should water-soluble iodinated contrast medium be given to patients with complete SBO. Water-soluble contrast medium is hyperosmolar and stimulates the outpouring of considerable amounts of fluid from the bowel wall. The medium is also diluted by the accumulated fluid above an obstruction, so little radiographic detail is seen.[25] However, if a bowel perforation is suspected, which would contraindicate the use of barium, water-soluble contrast medium may have to be employed, although with questionable radiographic success.

Details of the fluoroscopic small bowel follow-through have been given in Chapter 43. A major limitation to its use in SBO is the fact that lumen distensibility cannot be assessed. As a result, the presence and site of low-grade or intermittent obstructions may not be revealed. This technique may be more successful for higher grades of obstruction but may have to be followed up for many hours in cases in which prolonged obstruction has reduced peristaltic activity. It has been claimed that the peroral method, by revealing gastric atony and dilatation, would draw attention to a strangulating obstruction of small bowel.[26]

Per ileostomy small bowel enema has also been described in Chapter 43. Introduction of barium through an ileostomy is the preferred method for investigating disease assumed to involve more distal ileum. This technique can demonstrate the site and cause of higher-grade distal ileal obstructions. However, it may miss lesser, barely obstructing lesions because distention of the lumen above an obstruction, essential for the rec-

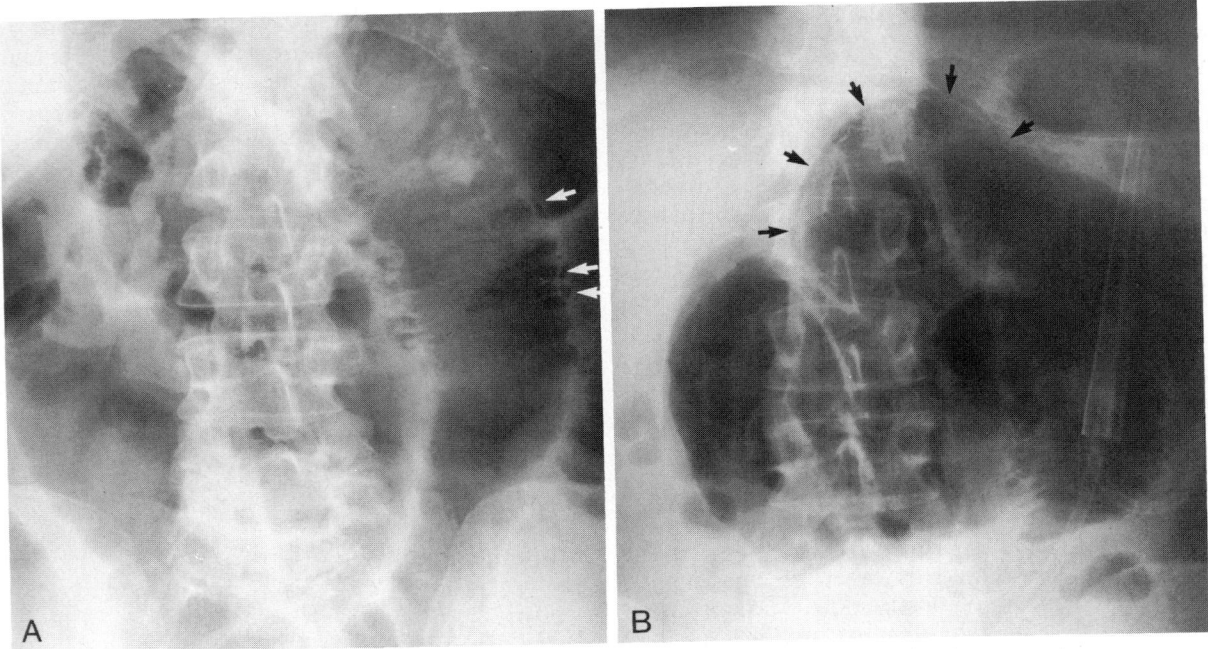

**Figure 52–1. SBO with vascular compromise. A.** Plain film of the abdomen with patient in a supine position shows dilatated bowel loops with evidence of fold thickening and slight pneumatosis *(arrows)*. **B.** Plain film with patient in an erect position shows linear pneumatosis *(arrows)* and pronounced dilatation of loops with fluid levels.

ognition of minor grades of obstruction, cannot be achieved by the retrograde method.

## Enteroclysis

Although fully described in Chapter 43, the use of enteroclysis in SBO offers specific advantages, has special indications, and requires certain modifications of the technique; thus it needs to be discussed further.

### Advantages

Injection of boluses of barium directly into the small bowel reduces dilution by retained fluid and facilitates propulsion toward the site of obstruction even with diminished peristalsis in prolonged higher-grade obstructions. Lumen distention by barium and methylcellulose solution accentuates the flattening effect of a minimally obstructing adhesive band. Enteroclysis accurately demonstrates the level of an obstruction and, especially with methylcellulose-produced double contrast, is highly reliable in determining its cause.

### Contraindications

Enteroclysis is contraindicated 1) in patients with acute and complete SBO, 2) in patients likely to have a strangulating obstruction, and 3) in patients with suspected perforation. Enteroclysis is not the best technique for studying the terminal ileum when this is the only area of clinical interest. A follow-through study with peroral pneumocolon is then preferred. Enteroclysis should be avoided in adynamic ileus.

## Modifications of Technique

No bowel preparation is needed. We do not give the usual oral premedication of 20 mg of metoclopramide to patients with high-grade obstructions. Preliminary films of the abdomen with the patient supine and erect can be of value. They may indicate the level of obstruction and may show features of possible strangulation or even show free air in the peritoneal cavity, both contraindications to barium use.

An already inserted Miller-Abbott or Cantor tube may be used for the infusion of barium and methylcellulose provided the side holes are positioned well beyond the duodenojejunal flexure. If the plain film of the abdomen has shown much residual fluid in distended loops, aspiration of fluid should be arranged before contrast medium is infused. If the decompression tube has not passed far enough into the jejunum, an attempt should be made to advance it sufficiently or, if this is unsuccessful, an enteroclysis catheter should be inserted perorally to extend beyond the ligament of Treitz, to be used for the examination. A three-channel, 14 French, 155-cm-long tube for nasogastric and/or nasoenteric decompression is now available (Maglinte's Decompression Tube, Cook Inc., Bloomington, IN). The main channel is used for decompression and the infusion of contrast materials. Another channel acts as a sump, and the third is used for inflation of a silicone balloon. Nasogastric insertion for decompression would normally be done at the bedside. If enteroclysis is required, the further advance into the jejunum is carried out under fluoroscopy.[27]

In partial SBO of higher grades of severity, when distended bowel loops contain an excess of fluid, an increased amount of barium must be infused—250 to 400 mL and occasionally more. Methylcellulose infusion should follow the barium unless a large amount of retained fluid has been encountered and further introduction of significant amounts of fluid would be unwise and unnecessary. During fluoroscopy, obstructions are identified by a site of abrupt lumen caliber change, from distended to collapsed bowel. Spot films obtained with varying grades of compression should explore this site to determine the causative pathologic change. It must be remembered that obstructions may occur at multiple levels. An external hernia may be the clinically unsuspected cause of obstruction in obese patients. Hernias may become distended during straining with the patient erect and should be filmed using suitable rotation (Fig. 52–2).

The inflated balloon of the enteroclysis catheter may not eliminate reflux in patients with distended proximal bowel. It is important to beware of substantial reflux of methylcellulose into the stomach and of possible vomiting and aspiration, especially in elderly and enfeebled patients. Further infusion must then be stopped and gastric contents siphoned off through the enteroclysis tube. It is also advisable to drain excess fluid from significantly dilated bowel at the end of the enteroclysis by leaving the catheter in place for as long as siphonage continues (Fig. 52–3).

In prolonged obstructions, dilated loops tend to become atonic with gradually decreasing peristalsis. Intraluminal propulsion by the enteroclysis technique can overcome less severe degrees of bowel hypotonia. With more pronounced bowel atony it may take too long to reach the site of obstruction. The enteroclysis catheter must be withdrawn (after deflation of the balloon) and the examination continued as intermittent fluoroscopic follow-through. It may also be necessary to recall the patient for further films and/or fluoroscopy 12 to 24 hours later.

## Ultrasonography

Ultrasound can distinguish dilated small bowel from dilated colon in clinically suspected obstructions. Fluid-filled dilated loops can be identified as proximal small bowel by the demonstration of valvulae conniventes. Peristaltic activity and aperistalsis can be distinguished by sonography. A combination of aperistalsis, fluid-filled distention, and wall thickening shown by ultrasound would support a diagnosis of infarction.[3] Ultrasound could also identify a gallstone ileus when the stone was not seen on plain films.[28]

## Computed Tomography

CT used in the diagnosis of certain types of SBO has several advantages over enteroclysis: 1) no opaque intraluminal contrast medium is required because retained fluid can serve as the CT contrast agent; 2) the examination does not depend on propulsion by small bowel peristalsis; 3) the use of intravenous contrast medium can provide information on the state of the bowel wall; and 4) relevant extramural information can be obtained.

There have been no prospective comparative studies of enteroclysis and CT when applied with the same high quality to a sufficient number of SBOs of different pathologies and grades of severity. However, limited and tentative conclusions are now possible, based mainly on our experience and that of others.[29, 30]

## Enteroclysis or Computed Tomography?

CT may be the method of choice in these forms of SBO:

1. Acute, complete SBO, because it does not require the use of barium and surgeons do not welcome barium-filled bowel at laparotomy. However, many of these patients go to surgery without CT being required.
2. Adynamic ileus. CT readily identifies small bowel dilatation continuing far into the colon and the absence of an abrupt lumen caliber change.
3. Prolonged, high-grade SBO in which propulsive motility has greatly decreased. Enteroclysis would take many hours to advance the barium, which may be retained too long (Fig. 52–4).
4. Suspicion of strangulation in medically managed patients with SBO. CT, when used with intravenous contrast medium, can demonstrate features of vascular compromise ("halo" sign, pneumatosis).[29]

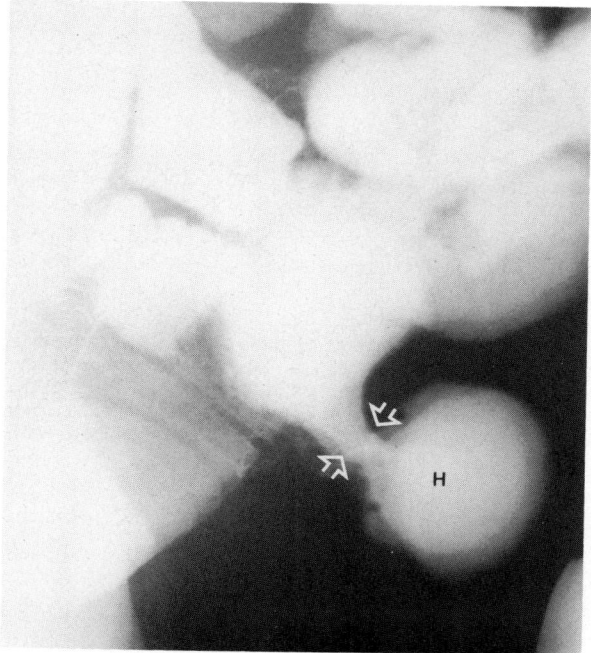

**Figure 52–2. Obese female patient with high-grade SBO and a ventral hernia.** A clinically unsuspected incisional hernia (H) situated below a known ventral hernia was found to be the cause of the obstruction (open arrows indicate the neck of the hernia).

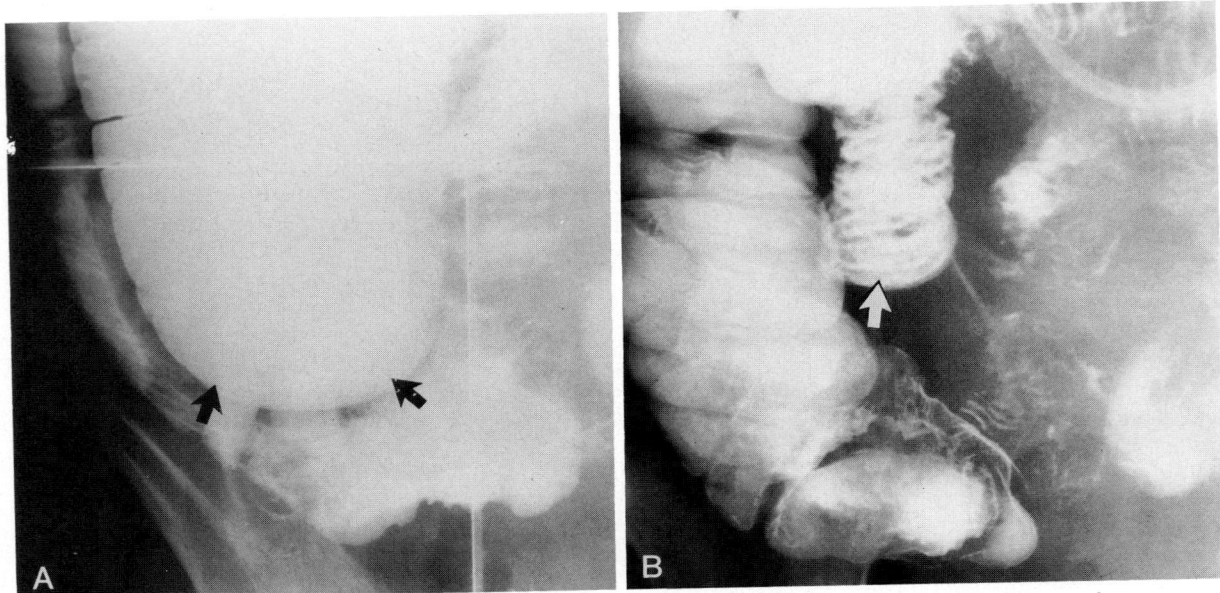

**Figure 52–3. Metastatic carcinoid causing high-grade obstruction. A.** At end of enteroclysis, a grossly dilated loop of jejunum *(arrows)* was found to extend into the lower abdomen, compressing the cecum and ascending colon. The enteroclysis catheter was left in the proximal jejunum and as much as possible of the methylcellulose solution was siphoned off. **B.** Postsiphonage film. The loop of jejunum is now collapsed *(arrow)* and the cecum and ascending colon have expanded.

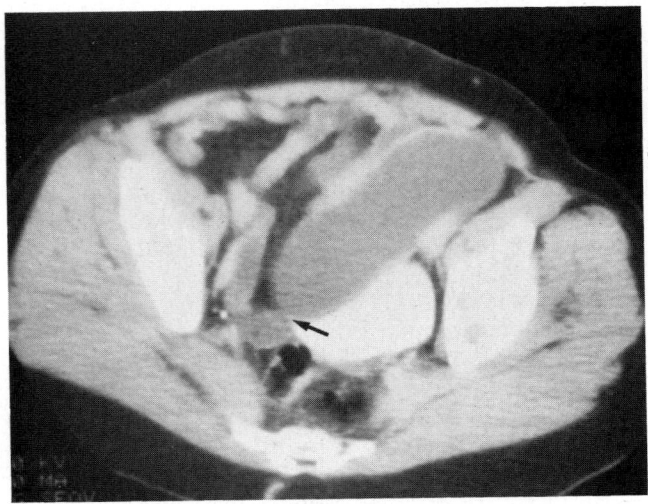

**Figure 52–4. CT demonstration of high-grade SBO caused by adhesions.** No masses are seen at the transition zone *(arrow)* between the dilated bowel anteriorly and the collapsed bowel below. Adhesions are therefore favored as the cause of the obstruction, and this was confirmed by surgery. (Courtesy of Alec J. Megibow, M.D., New York, NY.)

CT and enteroclysis may be complementary in these forms of SBO:

1. Carcinoids presenting with obstruction. CT (or magnetic resonance imaging) demonstration of a typical mesenteric metastatic mass would confirm the enteroclysis diagnosis of a primary ileal carcinoid (Fig. 52–5). (See also Chapter 51.)
2. Peritoneal metastases causing SBO. Diagnosis of obstruction by a carcinoma metastasis shown by enteroclysis would be supported by the CT demonstration of additional metastases and ascites.
3. An enteroclysis-shown extrinsic mass related to an obstruction can be further defined by CT.[30]

Enteroclysis is the likely method of choice in these cases of SBO:

1. Low-grade or intermittent SBO caused by adhesions. Enteroclysis-associated lumen distention can identify minor grades of adhesive band compression (Fig. 52–6).
2. The site of fixation resulting from an adhesive obstruction can be clearly determined, which is important for possible laparoscopic lysis.
3. In the course of investigating partial obstructions, enteroclysis can identify features of a closed loop obstruction.
4. Adhesions as possible causes of obstruction in patients with a history of surgery for abdominal malignancy. Only enteroclysis can provide a positive diagnosis of adhesive band obstruction in these patients. CT, in the presence of nonobstructing metastatic disease, would lead to consideration of the adhesive obstruction as caused by malignancy.
5. Obstruction by advanced radiation enteropathy. Enteroclysis depicts the extent of uninvolved small bowel for bypass surgery (Fig. 52–7).
6. Narrowed segments causing obstruction in Crohn's disease are well assessed by distention during enteroclysis, with fibrous strictures being distinguished from active stenotic disease.

## MAJOR CATEGORIES OF SMALL BOWEL OBSTRUCTION

The causes of SBO can be grouped in three major categories: extrinsic, intrinsic, and intraluminal (Table

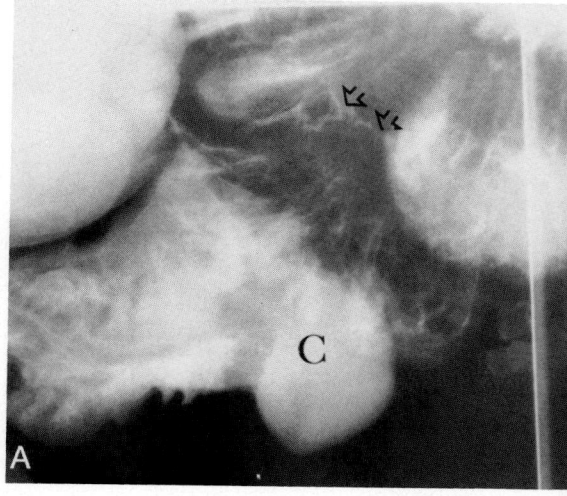

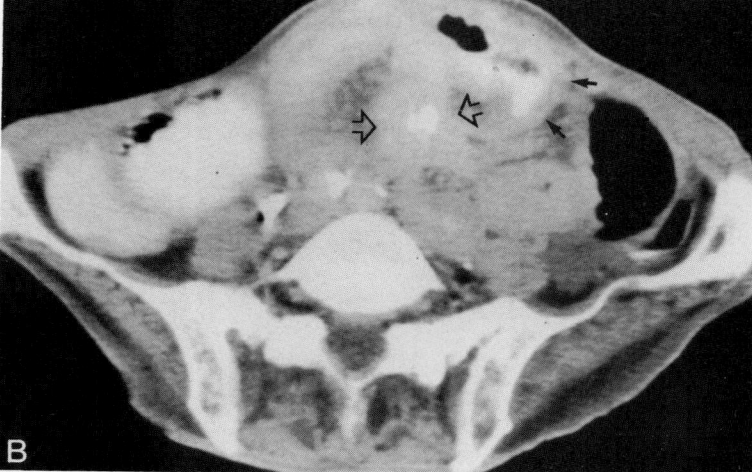

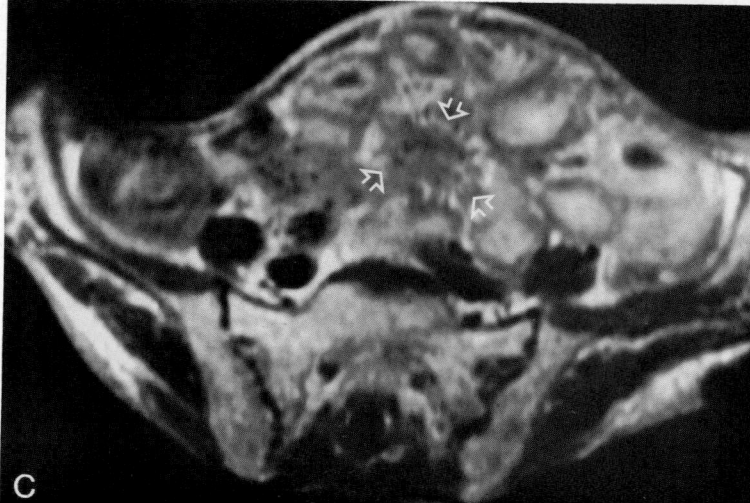

**Figure 52–5. Metastatic carcinoid presenting with high-grade SBO. A.** Enteroclysis. The ileal carcinoid primary *(arrows)* is surrounded by desmoplastically deformed bowel loops. C = colon. **B.** CT scan through the lower abdomen. Dilated bowel loops surround a large mesenteric mass *(open arrows)* containing calcium. The mesentery between mass and surrounding bowel loops contains little fat and appears edematous. In one bowel loop, wall thickening could be demonstrated *(solid arrows)*. **C.** Magnetic resonance. The mesenteric mass is well shown *(arrows)*. Wall thickening is seen in surrounding dilated bowel loops. Mesenteric metastases of carcinoids frequently contain calcium. Desmoplastic retraction caused by the mesenteric mass draws surrounding bowel loops closer and causes interference with venous drainage.

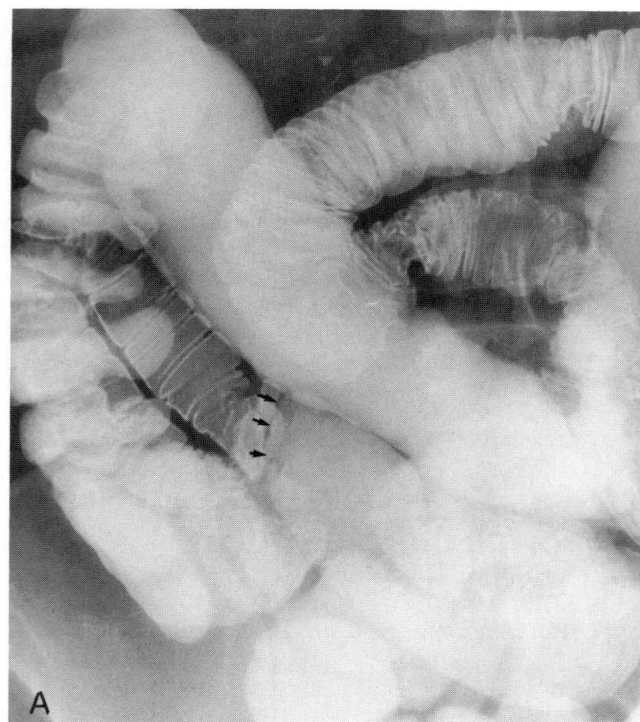

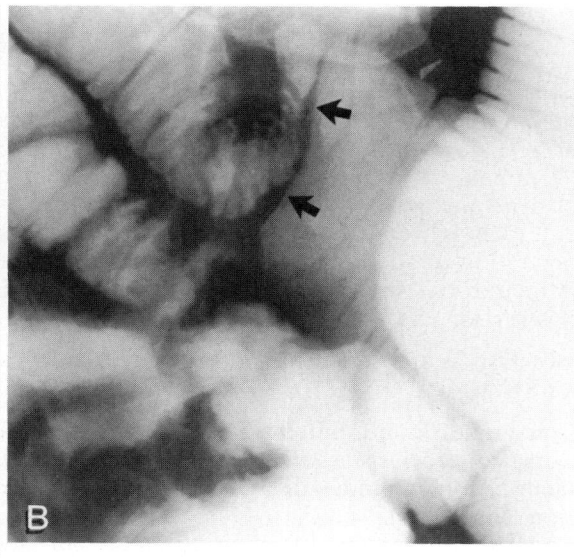

**Figure 52–6. Low-grade SBO by an adhesive band demonstrated by enteroclysis. A.** Film taken before lumen distention. The narrow adhesive band *(arrows)* is barely seen. **B.** Lumen distention accentuates the disproportionate distention of bowel proximal to the obstruction and renders the band *(arrows)* clearly visible.

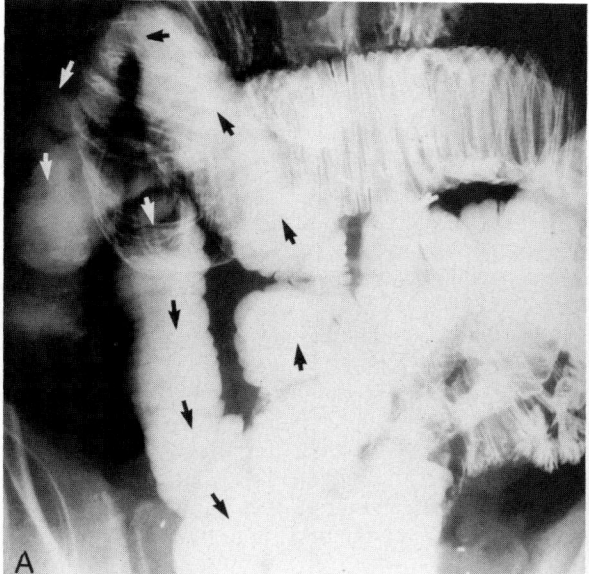

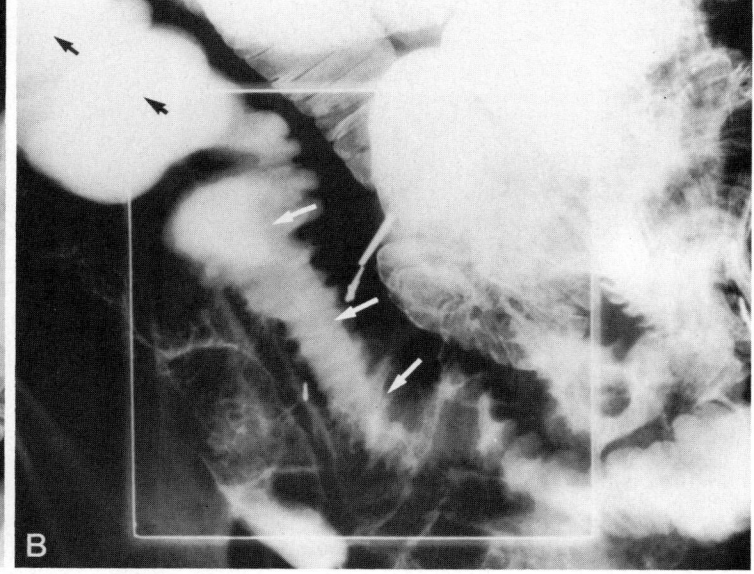

**Figure 52–7. SBO by severe radiation damage in the lower abdomen.** Enteroclysis was performed to determine the extent of still normal proximal bowel suitable for bypass surgery. **A.** A loop of ileum that extends upward and to the right *(arrows)* might appear suitable for bypass at laparotomy. **B.** However, the loop originated *(black arrows)* in the area of radiation damage *(white arrows)*; it is important to draw the surgeon's attention to this.

52–1). Most extrinsic causes obstruct by flattening, twisting, or kinking the small bowel; by circumferentially constricting a hernial opening; or by narrowing the lumen by mass impression and desmoplastic reaction from extrinsic mesenteric tumors, abscesses, or endometriosis.[20, 31] Instrinsic lesions constrict the lumen primarily by thickening of the bowel wall by tumor, fibrosis, or blood. Intraluminal causes obturate the bowel lumen. Intussusception, although usually of intrinsic etiology, obturates the lumen by pushing the proximal small bowel loop into the distal loop.

## OBSTRUCTION BY ADHESIONS

In patients who have undergone at least one laparotomy, subsequent surgery identifies adhesions in more than 90%.[32] The adhesions occupy either the area of surgical intervention or the undersurface of the abdominal scar.[32] However, only a minority of the adhesions produce symptoms. Adhesions are now responsible for at least 60% of SBOs; more than 80% of them arise after surgery, 15% are due to inflammation, and the remaining few are due to congenital or unexplained causes.

### Formation of Adhesions

Fibrin deposition and fibrinous adherence between intraperitoneal surfaces may occur within hours of even mild surgical trauma. It was shown in 1969[33] that mesothelial cells of the peritoneum were capable of promoting fibrinolysis by activation of plasminogen to plasmin. A later report[34] found reduced levels of plasminogen activator in the presence of trauma or ischemia. In these circumstances, fibrinous adhesions can become organized, forming fibrous adhesions by the ingrowth of fibroblasts and new vessels.[35]

Much of the fibrous adhesion formation is related to efforts to close surgically produced peritoneal defects. This tends to be associated with vascular damage caused by crushing, suturing, and ligating tissue.[35] As already mentioned, focal ischemia reduces the availability of plasminogen activator[34] and stimulates the ingrowth of new vessels and the conversion of fibrinous to fibrous adhesions. To prevent this type of adhesion formation, even large peritoneal defects can be left open and bleeding because they heal within days with the formation of a glistening new serosa.[35, 36] Another approach to preventing fibrous adhesions has been the direct application of plasminogen activator to tissue likely to become the site of such adhesions. This has been shown to be successful in animal studies.[32]

### Radiology of Small Bowel Obstruction by Adhesions

Adhesive obstructions have been divided into those caused by a single band, by multiple bands, or by extensive adhesions.[37]

The most important radiographic finding in the diagnosis of adhesive obstructions is an abrupt change in

### TABLE 52–1. SMALL BOWEL OBSTRUCTION IN ADULTS

| | |
|---|---|
| Extrinsic lesions | Intrinsic lesions |
|   Adhesions |   Tumors infiltrating wall of |
|   Hernias |     small intestine |
|     External |     Adenocarcinoma |
|       Inguinal |     Carcinoid tumor |
|       Femoral |     Lymphoma (rare) |
|       Obturator |     Leiomyosarcoma (rare) |
|       Sciatic |   Inflammatory conditions |
|       Perineal |     Crohn's disese |
|       Supravesical |     Tuberculosis |
|       Spigelian |     Potassium chloride stricture |
|       Lumbar |     Eosinophilic gastroenteritis |
|       Incisional |   Vascular |
|       Umbilical |     Radiation enteropathy |
|     Internal |     Ischemia |
|       Paraduodenal |     Hematoma |
|       Epiploic foramen |       Post-traumatic hematoma |
|       Diaphragmatic (traumatic) |       Thrombocytopenia |
|       Transomental |       Anticoagulants |
|       Transmesenteric |       Henoch-Schönlein purpura |
|       Iliac fossa |   Intussusception |
|   Masses |     Adhesions |
|     Extrinsic tumors in |     Tumor |
|       mesentery |     Duplication |
|       Lymphoma |     Inverted Meckel's |
|       Peritoneal metastasis |       diverticulum |
|       Carcinoid |   Intraluminal causes |
|       Desmoid |     Obturation |
|     Abscess |       Gallstone |
|       Diverticulitis |       Bezoar |
|       Pelvic inflammatory disease |       Foreign body |
|       Crohn's disease |       *Ascaris* |
|     Aneurysm |       Meconium |
|     Hematoma | |
|     Endometriosis | |

lumen caliber from dilated bowel proximal to the adhesion to collapsed bowel distal to it (Fig. 52–8). A sharp, straight or slightly curved edge is seen where the band crosses the bowel lumen (Fig. 52–9). Smooth, stretched mucosal folds extend to the edge of the dilated and obstructed proximal lumen (Fig. 52–10). A narrow band-like radiolucency may be seen crossing the bowel between dilated proximal and collapsed distal segments (Fig. 52–11). Because of the lumen distention associated with enteroclysis, a narrow adhesive band that causes only low-grade obstruction can be readily identified (see Fig. 52–6). Compression by broader bands is seen to narrow and flatten a bowel segment that is sharply demarcated from the obstructed and dilated bowel proximal to it (Fig. 52–12). Depending on the duration of the obstruction, exaggerated, normal, or reduced peristalsis can be observed fluoroscopically to extend to the level of the obstructing band. The transition point between bowel compressed by the band and collapsed bowel distal to the obstruction is not well demarcated, except with narrow bands.

### Differentiation of Small Bowel Obstruction by Bands from Metastases

With seeded peritoneal metastases, tumor deposition on small bowel loops occurs preferentially in the depen-

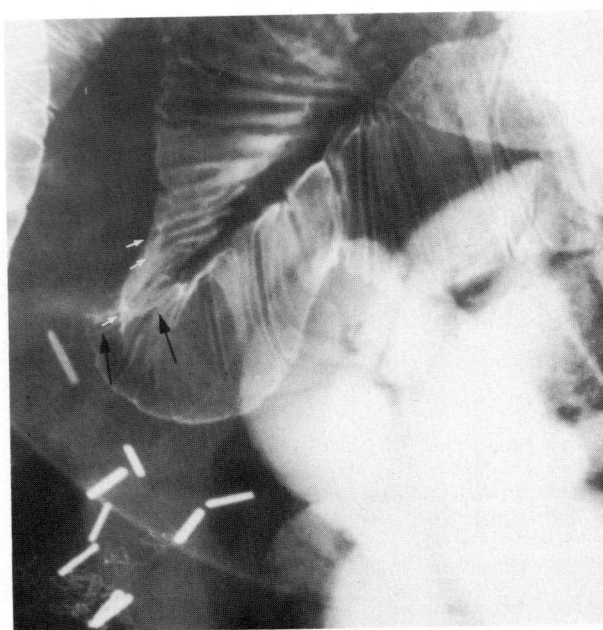

**Figure 52–8. Low-grade SBO caused by adhesions resulting from adjacent, earlier Crohn's disease surgery.** Normal folds are seen extending to the edge of a slightly dilated proximal segment *(black arrows)*. Tethering of folds *(white arrows)* is seen in the narrowed, adhesion-affected segment, which merges almost imperceptibly into normal bowel beyond.

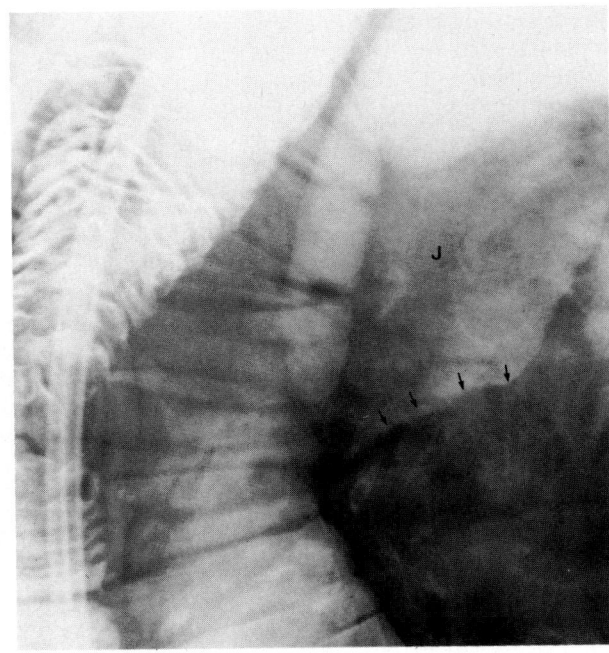

**Figure 52–9. High-grade obstruction by an adhesive band.** A slightly curved edge *(arrows)* crosses the dilated jejunum (J) at the site of adhesive band compression. Retained fluid prevents definition of mucosal folds to the edge of obstruction. The severe degree of obstruction precludes imaging of features distally.

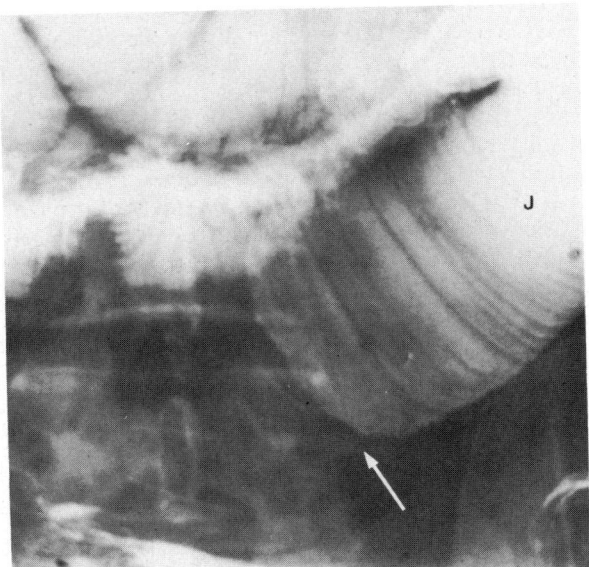

**Figure 52–10. High-grade SBO by an adhesive band.** Sharp cutoff *(arrow)* of a loop of distal jejunum (J) with little barium passing through. In this patient, stretched and otherwise normal mucosal folds can be followed to the edge of the obstruction.

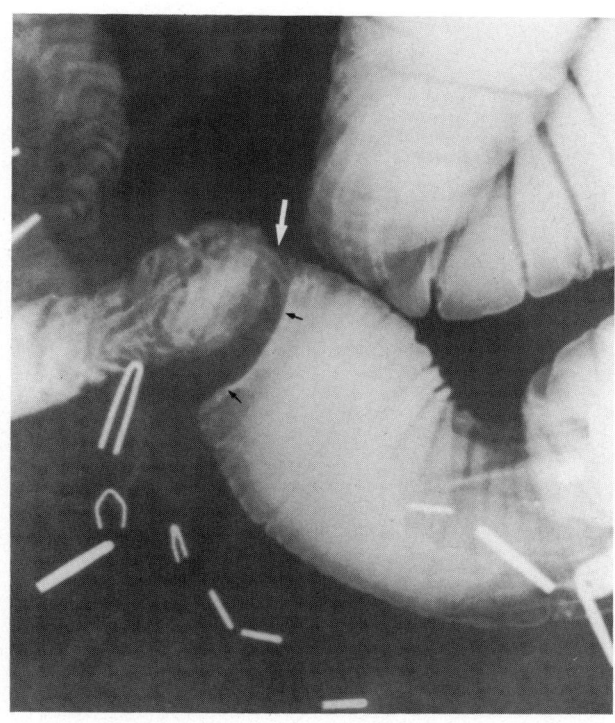

**Figure 52–11. Partial obstruction by a narrow adhesive band.** A lumen-crossing radiolucency *(white arrow)* represents the narrow, partially obstructing adhesive band. A sharp, slightly curved cutoff in the moderately dilated proximal bowel *(black arrows)* pinpoints the site of the obstruction. Normal folds extend to the edge of the cutoff. Slightly twisted folds are visible in the narrow, compressed segment. The difference between the degree of lumen distention proximally and lumen reduction distally expresses the grade of the obstruction.

dent part of the mesenteric cavity and in relation to the ruffles of the mesentery. Thus, tumor deposits are most often seen in the right lower quadrant, where they involve the mesenteric border of distal ileal loops and the medial border of the cecum. The radiographic findings express the mass effect produced by each implant on the serosa of a bowel segment and the frequently associated desmoplastic effect. Direct tumor infiltration

of the bowel wall exaggerates the radiographic findings. In metastatic obstruction there is an extrinsic type of mass effect, predominantly along the mesenteric border of bowel, with tethering of mucosal folds in and near the narrowed segment (Fig. 52–13). With further bowel invasion, the narrowing may become circumferential, still with tethering of folds at its edge[20, 38, 39] (Fig. 52–14). In contrast to the sharp, smooth edge proximally

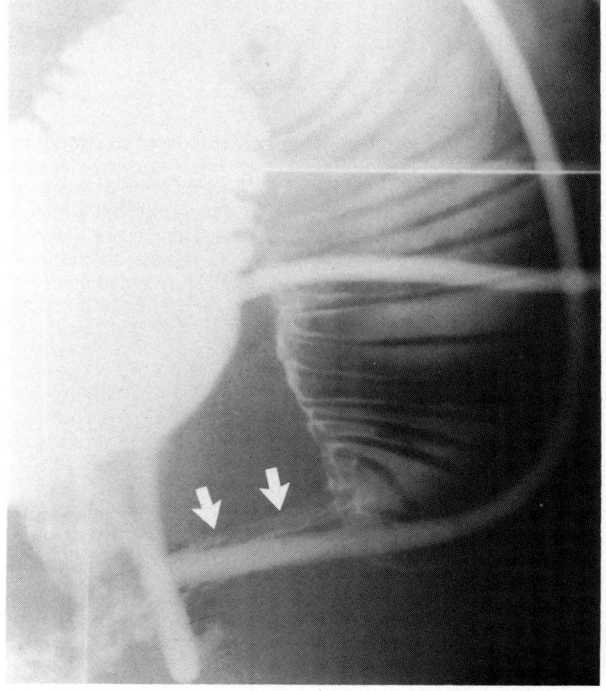

**Figure 52–12. High-grade obstruction by a broad adhesive band.** Crowded longitudinal folds are visible in the narrowed segment compressed by the wide adhesive band *(arrows)*. Mucosal folds extend to the edge of the obstructed segment; cutoff is more gradual.

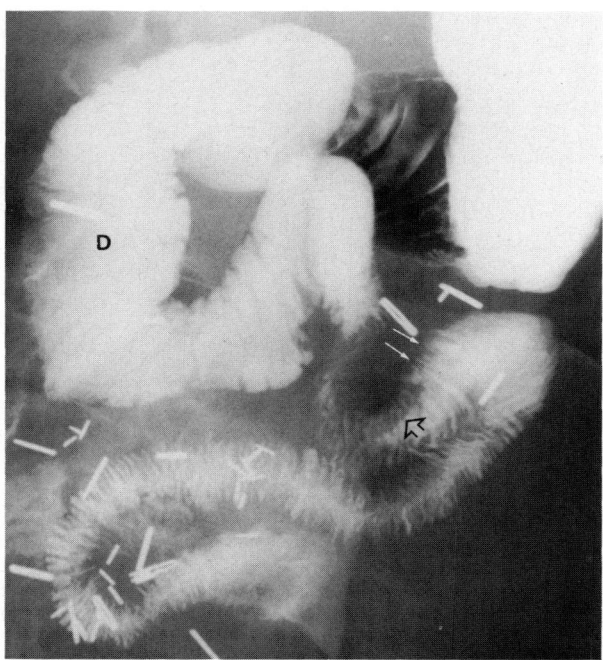

**Figure 52–13. Obstructive metastasis from transitional cell carcinoma.** The tumor extended through the subperitoneal space of the root of the small bowel mesentery. An overhead film from a small bowel follow-through shows dilatation of the duodenum (D). Just beyond the ligament of Treitz is an extrinsic mass effect *(open arrow)* on the mesenteric border of a loop of proximal jejunum with tethering of mucosal folds *(solid arrows)*. Partial SBO is indicated by the disproportionate distention of the duodenum. This is a typical site for retroperitoneally arising metastases, especially from transitional cell carcinoma of the urinary bladder.

**Figure 52–14. Intraperitoneal metastasis from ovarian carcinoma.** Spot film from the single contrast phase of enteroclysis shows extrinsic mass effect *(open arrow)*, angulation of the bowel loop, and tethering of mucosal folds *(small solid arrows)*. Focal, smooth narrowing is caused by the circumferential growth of the metastasis *(large solid arrow)*. The findings are typical for an intraperitoneally seeded metastasis. A further metastatic obstruction was found more distally. Exceptionally, a carcinoid tumor may present with these radiographic findings.

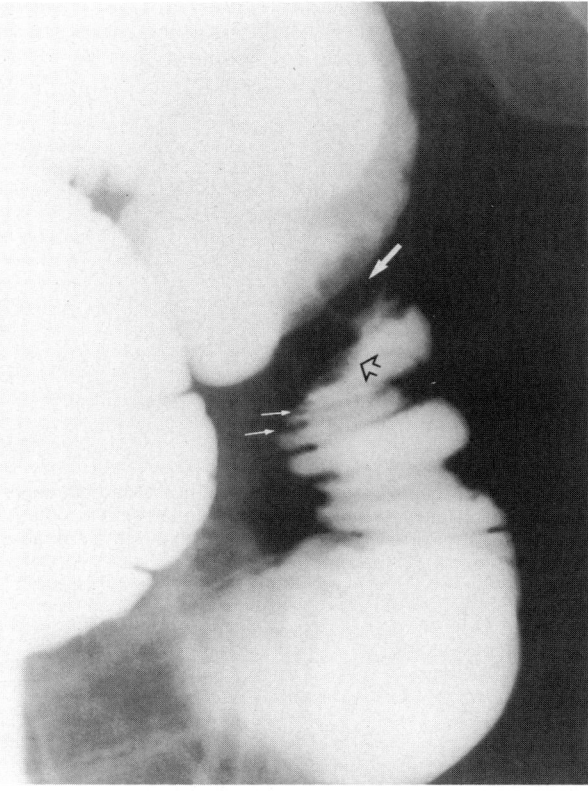

produced by obstructing adhesive bands, obstructions by metastases are characterized by a more rounded and somewhat irregular demarcation against the proximal dilated segment; the narrowed segment may appear frayed and often indented on its mesenteric border (Fig. 52–15A). Mucosal folds in the dilated segment may be interrupted by nodules near the edge of the metastasis (Fig. 52–15B). In contrast to the ill-defined distal demarcation of an adhesive obstruction, the distal margin in a metastatic obstruction is usually well demarcated, rounded, and associated with tethered mucosal folds (Fig. 52–16). Segments of metastatic obstruction tend to be longer than those caused by adhesive bands; mucosal folds may be narrowed by a mass effect against the mesenteric border (see Fig. 52–16A) or flattened and ill-defined by a metastatic mass effect exerted in a vertical plane (see Fig. 52–16B). With an advanced metastasis, annular narrowing can be pronounced. The lumen can be reduced to a tight, string-like channel associated with desmoplastic kinking and angulation (Fig. 52–17); this may be better appreciated on a delayed film (see Fig. 52–17B). Annular narrowing by metastases must be distinguished from primary adenocarcinomas. Primary adenocarcinomas usually involve the proximal small bowel, are not associated with desmoplastic distortion, and therefore produce less severe obstruction. CT can be of value not only for confirmatory examination when a diagnosis of metastatic obstruction based on enteroclysis is uncertain but also for a more successful study in distal obstructions, even in the cecum (Fig. 52–18).

## Closed Loop Obstructions

Closed loop obstructions are most often caused by entrapment of a bowel loop by a single adhesive band, less often by incarceration in an external or internal hernia.[11] The partially obstructed closed loops are in imminent danger of becoming significantly deprived of blood flow, and prompt surgical intervention is essential. Enteroclysis can demonstrate characteristic features of an incomplete closed loop obstruction. A bowel loop of varying length exhibits a single band pattern of occlusion affecting two adjacent fixed points representing the base of the closed loop (Fig. 52–19). Fluoroscopy can identify inflow into the proximal limb and outflow through the distal limb at a rate related to the degree of band obstruction. Compression by the single band can cause focal necrosis and associated extravasation and abscess formation (Fig. 52–20). Clinically unsuspected abdominal wall herniations (e.g., paraileostomy hernias) can be examples of closed loop obstruction. The intraperitoneal segregation of a usually tightly obstructed bowel loop representing an internal hernia (e.g., through a post-traumatic mesenteric defect) is difficult to distinguish from an adhesive band–related closed loop.

CT can demonstrate the rounded configuration of the closed loop and can indicate the site of the twin luminal compression (Fig. 52–21). In addition, CT can provide evidence of vascular compromise. The plain film of the abdomen occasionally suggests the presence of a closed loop obstruction (see Fig. 52–2).

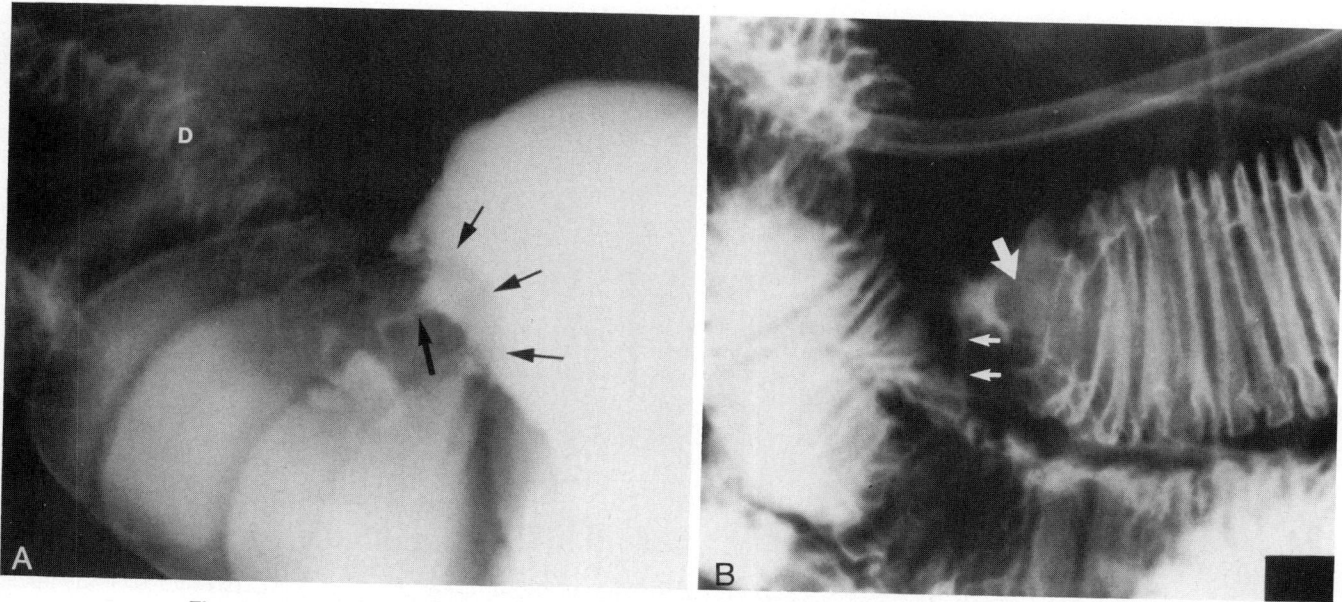

**Figure 52–15. Significantly obstructing annular metastases in patients with a history of cancer.** **A.** Previous colon cancer. The rounded proximal margin of the obstruction is irregular *(thin arrows)* and the gradually narrowing constricted segment shows fraying of its edges *(thick arrow)*. Unaffected distal bowel (D) is sharply demarcated from the annular metastasis. **B.** History of endometrial carcinoma. A nodular mass *(large arrow)* flattens and obliterates folds proximal to a tight annular constriction *(small arrows)*.

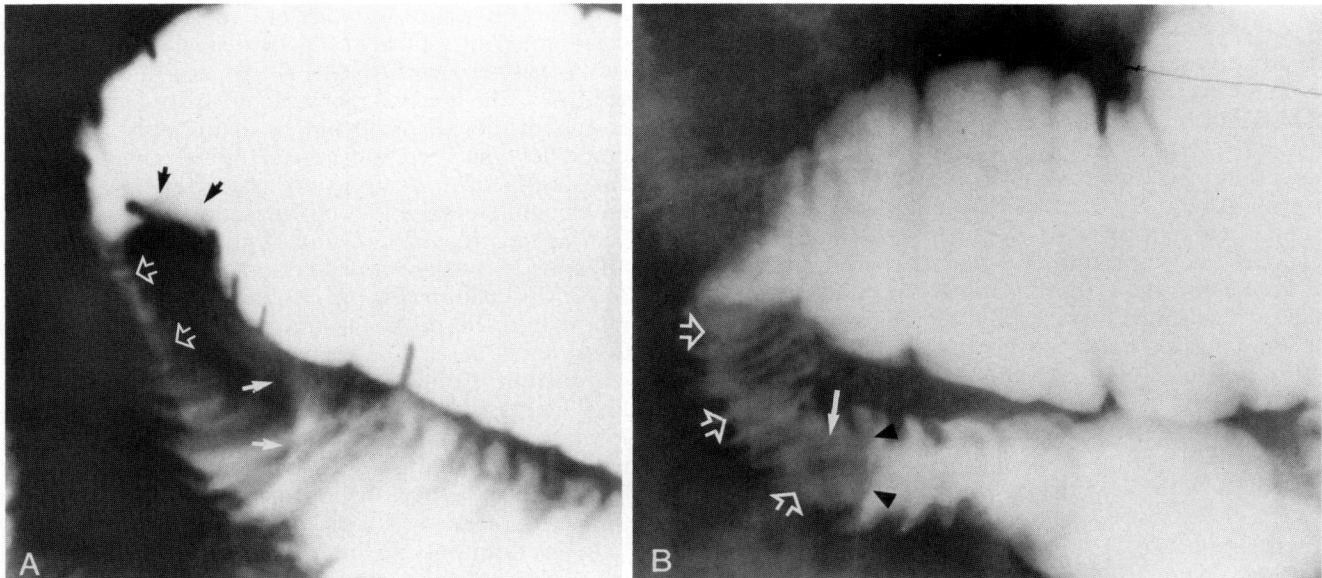

**Figure 52–16. SBO by peritoneal metastases. A.** Fallopian tube carcinoma. Enteroclysis demonstrates partial obstruction of distal jejunum. A small mass effect *(black arrows)* is seen on the mesenteric side of the gradually narrowing, dilated bowel. The narrowed segment shows some displacement and compression of its mesenteric border *(open arrows)*. The distal margin of the obstruction is sharply demarcated, with a rounded configuration *(white arrows)*. These features provide conclusive evidence for a diagnosis of obstruction by a metastasis. This was confirmed by surgery. **B.** Carcinoma of the cervix. The proximal, dilated segment narrows gradually. The obstructing segment *(open arrows)* shows flattening of the lumen, indicated by the decreased barium density. Distally, in the flattened lumen, mucosal fold detail is barely seen, possibly because of infiltration *(solid arrow)*. Distal demarction is abrupt, with a curved contour *(arrowheads)*.

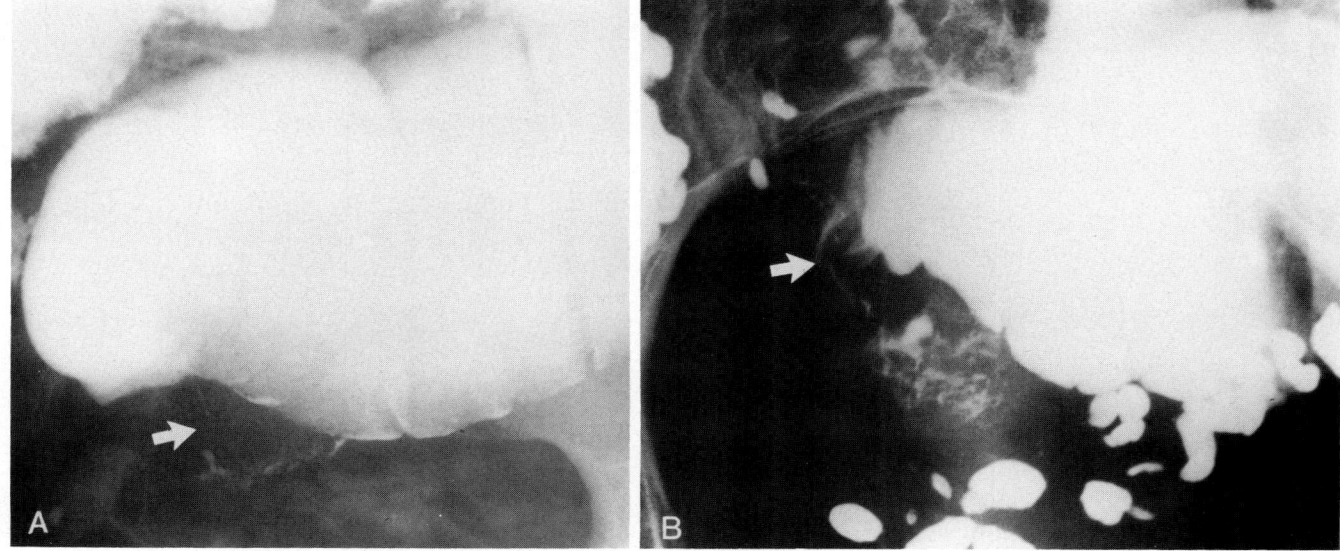

**Figure 52–17. High-grade obstruction of ileum by a metastasis from an endometrial carcinoma.**
**A.** A tight annular constriction *(arrow)* is seen. The distortion, asymmetric mass effect, and severity of obstruction favor a metastatic cause. **B.** Another film was taken 24 hours later. Barium is still retained above the obstruction. The whole length of the narrow and distorted channel through the annular metastasis is now more clearly displayed *(arrow)*. Delayed films often give additional information in high-grade SBOs.

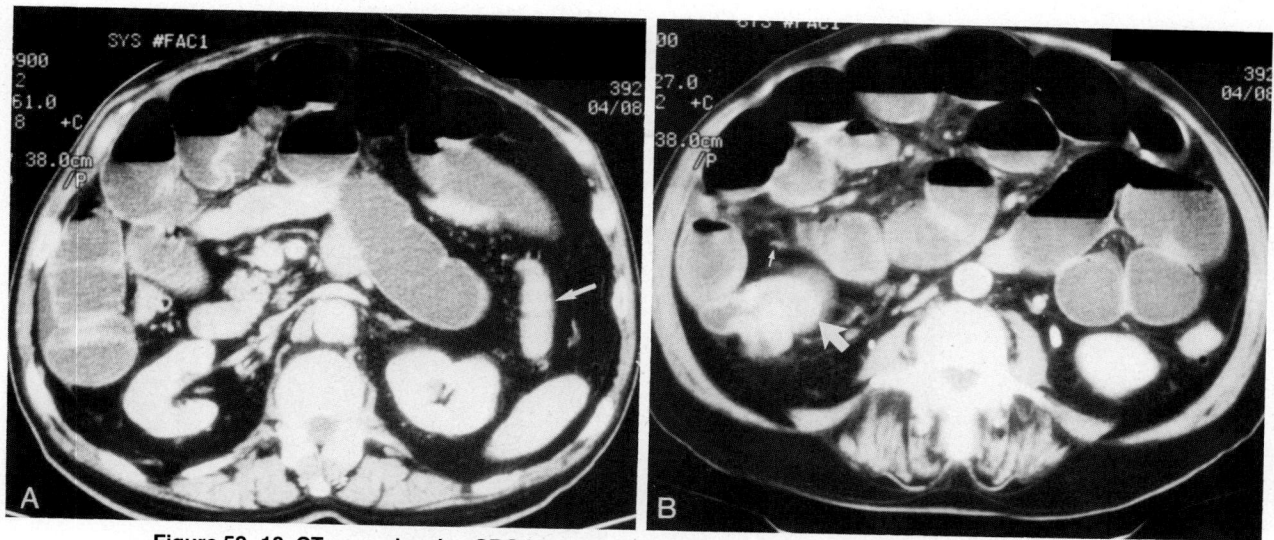

**Figure 52–18. CT scan showing SBO by a carcinoma of the cecum. A.** Distal SBO was suspected, and conservative treatment was unsuccessful. CT scan with intravenous contrast medium shows numerous dilated, air-fluid–filled small bowel loops. A collapsed left colon is seen *(arrow)*. **B.** A larger number of dilated small bowel loops is outlined. A soft tissue mass is seen on the right side, in the position of the cecum *(large arrow)*. Anterior to it, a dilated bowel loop shows incipient, somewhat irregular narrowing *(small arrow)*. A carcinoma of the cecum was diagnosed and subsequently resected. (Courtesy of Alec J. Megibow, M.D., New York, NY.)

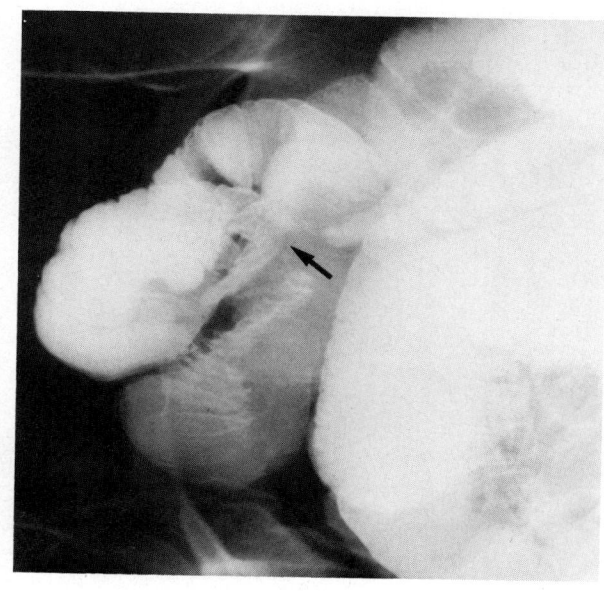

**Figure 52–19. Closed loop obstruction with viable bowel shown by enteroclysis.** A loop of ileum has protruded under an adhesive band. Constriction of the closely apposed entering and exiting limbs is demonstrated *(arrow)*. The adhesive band was lysed by surgery, and the bowel was found to be viable.

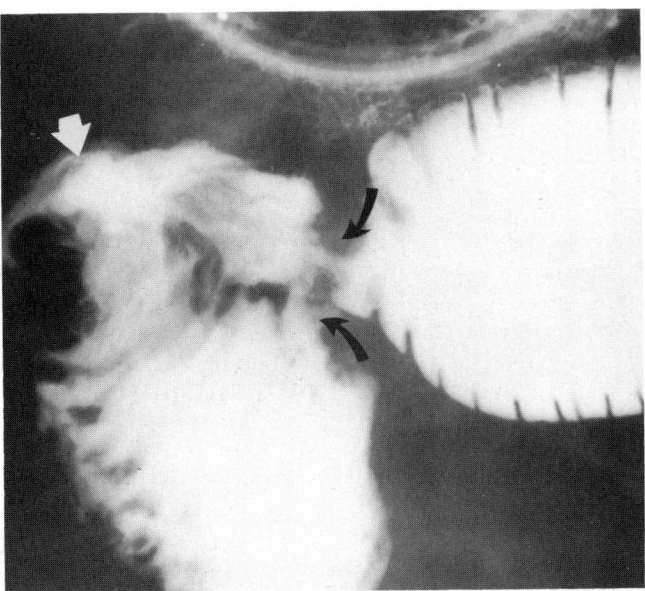

**Figure 52–20. Closed loop obstruction with tight band compression.** Both limbs of the closed loop *(black arrows)* are tightly compressed by a crossing adhesive band. Focal pressure necrosis causes extravasation of barium *(white arrow)* into an abscess space that surrounded the obstructed loop. The patient was subsequently treated by surgical resection and enteroenterostomy.

## *Volvulus Complicating a Closed Loop Obstruction*

As a partially closed loop continues to accumulate fluid by both inflow and secretion, the narrowness of its fixed base becomes more significant relative to the increasing size of the obstructed loop. In this situation, twisting may develop into a secondary form of volvulus and a surgical emergency. Enteroclysis can demonstrate intertwining of the two limbs or twisting of the folds of the closed loop obstruction at the dual fixation site, indicating developing volvulus (Fig. 52–22). A consid-

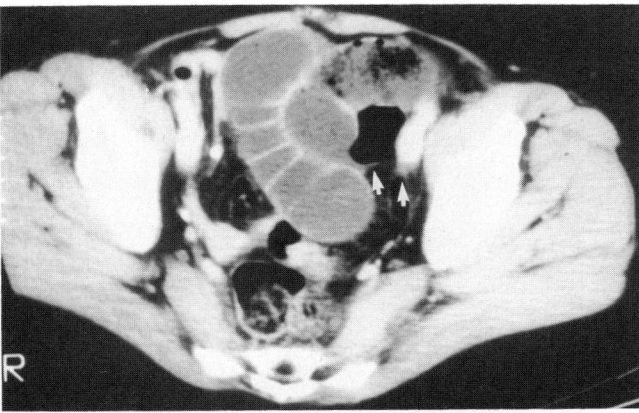

**Figure 52–21. Closed loop obstruction shown by CT scan.** Horseshoe-shaped loop of dilated bowel contains mostly fluid and little air. An area of narrowing that involves both limbs at the base of the loop *(arrows)* is due to an adhesive band. Collapsed ileum is seen to the right of the obstruction. (Courtesy of Alec J. Megibow, M.D., New York, NY.)

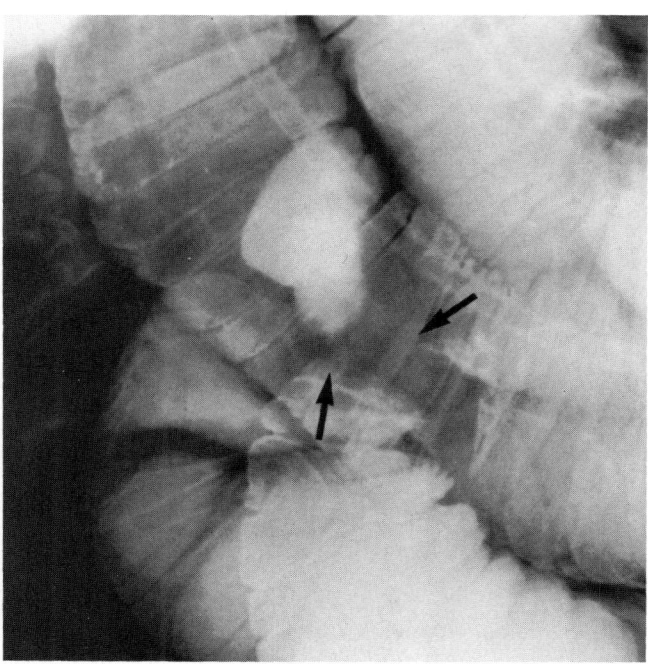

**Figure 52–22. Closed loop obstruction with impending torsion.** The entering and exiting limbs of the closed loop *(arrows)* are seen to cross one another, suggesting incipient torsion. The obstructed bowel loop was resected.

erable reduction in the through-flow of contrast medium is usually seen at this stage. CT is the method of choice if a volvulus is suspected on clinical grounds. CT can demonstrate mesenteric edema, a characteristic "whirl" sign of the rotated mesentery and dilated bowel loops surrounding the twisted and edematous mesentery.[40]

Primary volvulus occurs mostly in children with intestinal malrotation and is occasionally reported in young adults.[41] A generally higher prevalence of primary volvulus occurs in Middle Eastern countries and reaches its peak during the month of Ramadan.[42]

## *Obstruction at an Enterectomy Site*

Occasionally, the lumen of an enteroenteric anastomosis narrows during the first few weeks after surgery and may cause significant obstruction. Barium studies can demonstrate the site and degree of the anastomotic stricture (Fig. 52–23).

## *Obstruction by Multiple Bands*

Multiple bands causing obstruction are found infrequently, always follow abdominal surgery, and adhere to the scar in the abdominal wall. Obstruction by multiple bands is twice as likely to be of low grade as of higher grade. Volvulus or the development of gangrene is unusual. Enteroclysis demonstrates several narrow constrictions, often close together. Various oblique images are needed to bring most of the constrictions into profile view (Fig. 52–24).

Distinction of obstruction by multiple bands from multiple metastases is not difficult. Seeded metastases

**Figure 52–23. High-grade obstruction by a tight stricture at a side-to-side enteroenterostomy *(arrows).* **Surgery and reanastomosis followed.

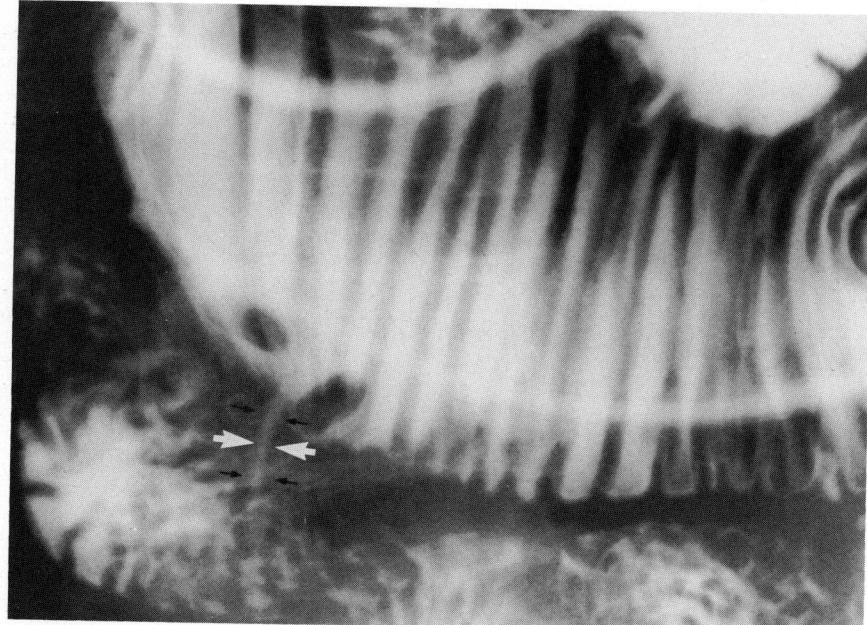

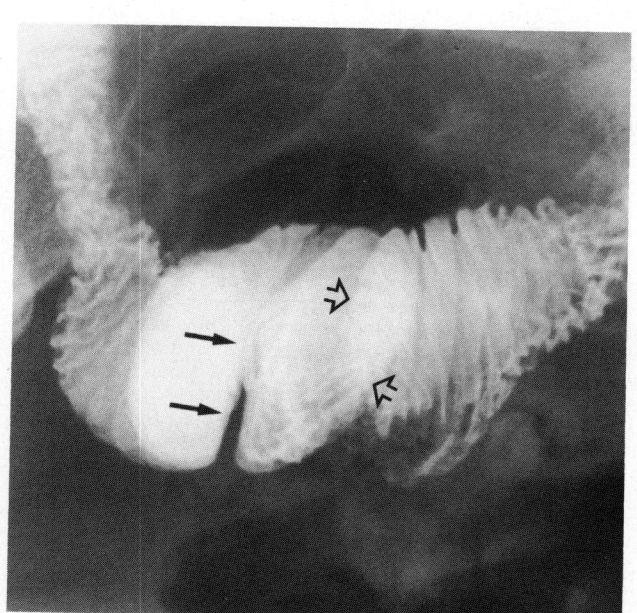

**Figure 52–24. Multiple adhesive bands, low-grade obstruction.** Four adhesive compressions were close to one another. One of these is seen in tangential projection *(solid arrows).* Another is shown obliquely, its anterior and posterior terminations indicated by open arrows. Further adhesive band effects were seen in other projections. The lesions adhered to the anterior abdominal wall and peritoneal scar.

extend over a wider area, tend to congregate in the ileocecal region, and produce rounded extrinsic mass impressions on the bowel wall, usually on the mesenteric border (Fig. 52–25). Infiltration of the mucosa or major focal lumen reduction is rare. Obstruction is the result of multiplicity (Fig. 52–26).

## Extensive Adhesions

Unlike adhesive bands, extensive adhesions enclose and immobilize longer segments of bowel, usually posteriorly in the peritoneal cavity. These adhesions produce mostly low-grade obstruction, a result of lumen narrowing and ineffective peristalsis. Kinking and interference with blood supply do not seem to occur. Aortic bypass surgery and para-aortic lymph node dissection are possible causes of extensive adhesion formation.

Enteroclysis shows a mild and uneven reduction of lumen caliber and fixation of a bowel segment crossing the midabdomen (Fig. 52–27).

## Nonobstructive Adhesions

Minor forms of adhesions do not in themselves cause obstruction, although they may be part of a more extensive adhesive process and may be a source of abdominal pain. Enteroclysis demonstrates adherence between adjacent bowel loops without lumen reduction (Fig. 52–28). Nonobstructive adhesions are also identified by abrupt angulation replacing the normally rounded change of direction of a bowel loop, by fixation between loops as shown during palpation, or by a tent-like deformity of the edge of bowel, rendered more obvious by abdominal compression (Fig. 52–29).

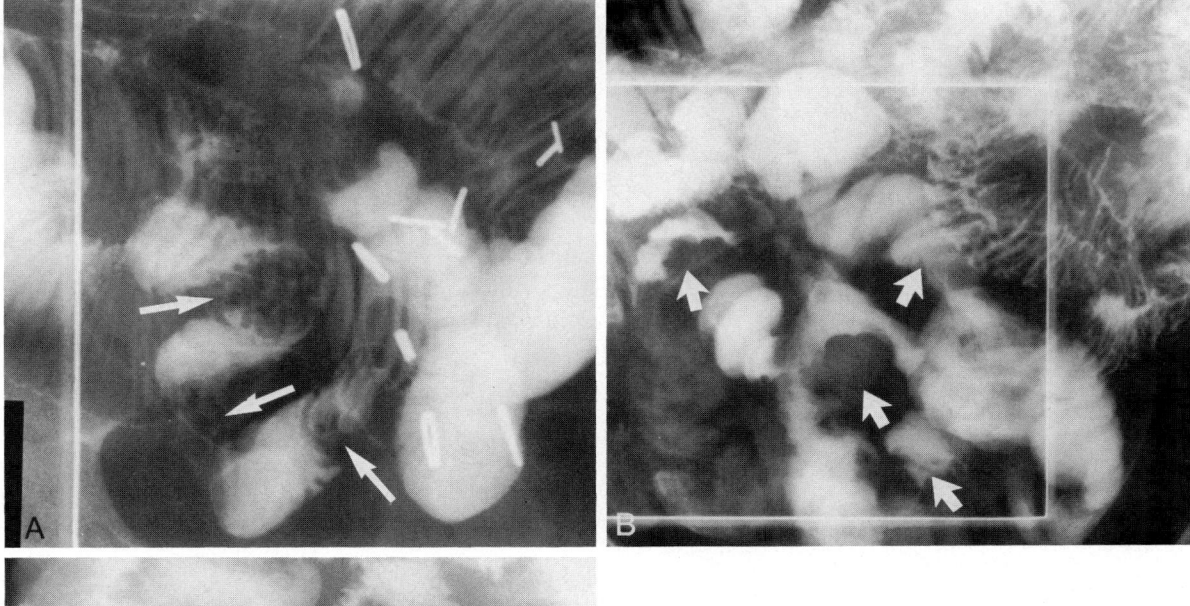

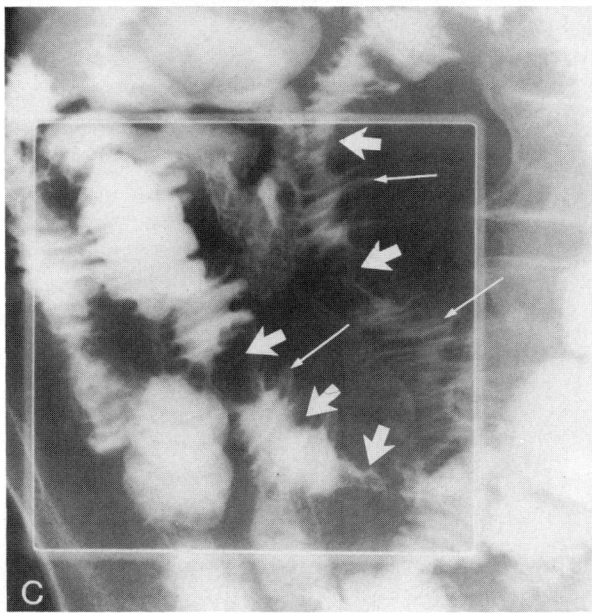

**Figure 52–25. Examples of multiple, seeded peritoneal metastases. A.** Metastases from carcinoma of stomach. Three metastases are indicated by arrows. They all show rounded impressions into the lumen, mostly from the mesenteric border, with tethering of mucosal folds. **B.** Metastases from carcinoma of the cervix. Fluoroscopic follow-through examination with oral metoclopramide before barium. Several rounded protrusions with nodular surfaces *(arrows)* indent the bowel lumen from the mesenteric border side. Some tethering of folds is seen. **C.** Metastases from ovarian carcinoma. The mesenteric border of several bowel loops is almost confluently deformed by metastatic deposits on their peritoneal surfaces *(thick arrows)*, associated with a drawing out of several folds *(thin arrows)* in the direction of the mesenteric root. Also note the mass effect over the course of the root of the small bowel mesentery.

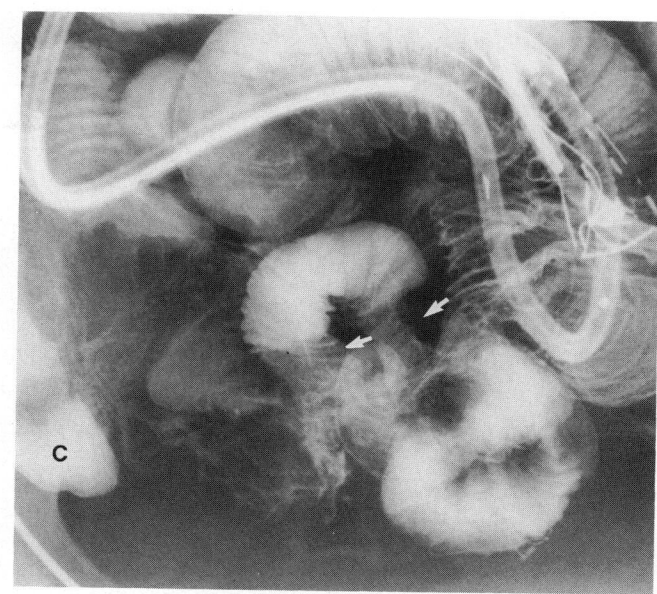

**Figure 52–26. High-grade SBO by multiple seeded metastases in the ileocecal area.** The combination of numerous rounded filling defects with pronounced tethering *(arrows)*, annular involvement, and mass effect in the area medial to the cecum (C) accounts for the severity of the obstruction.

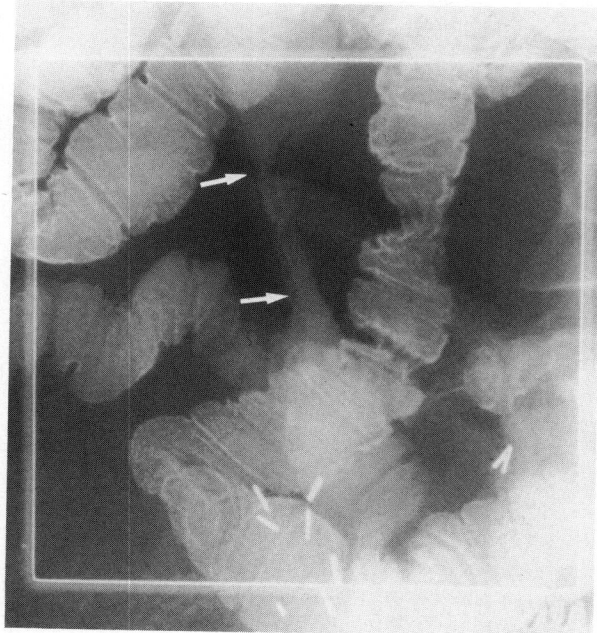

**Figure 52–27. Extensive adhesion after aortic bypass surgery.** Enteroclysis shows a straightened bowel segment with moderate lumen narrowing *(arrows)*, fixed in the area of the surgery. Obstruction is minimal.

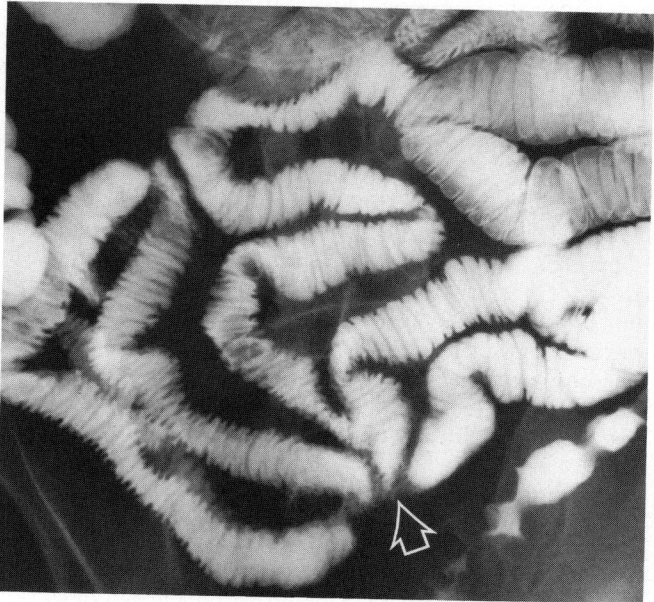

**Figure 52–28. Nonobstructive adherence between bowel loops.** At fluoroscopy, such an adherence *(arrow)* is identified by nonseparation of loops during abdominal compression or by acute angulations, best shown when compression is applied.

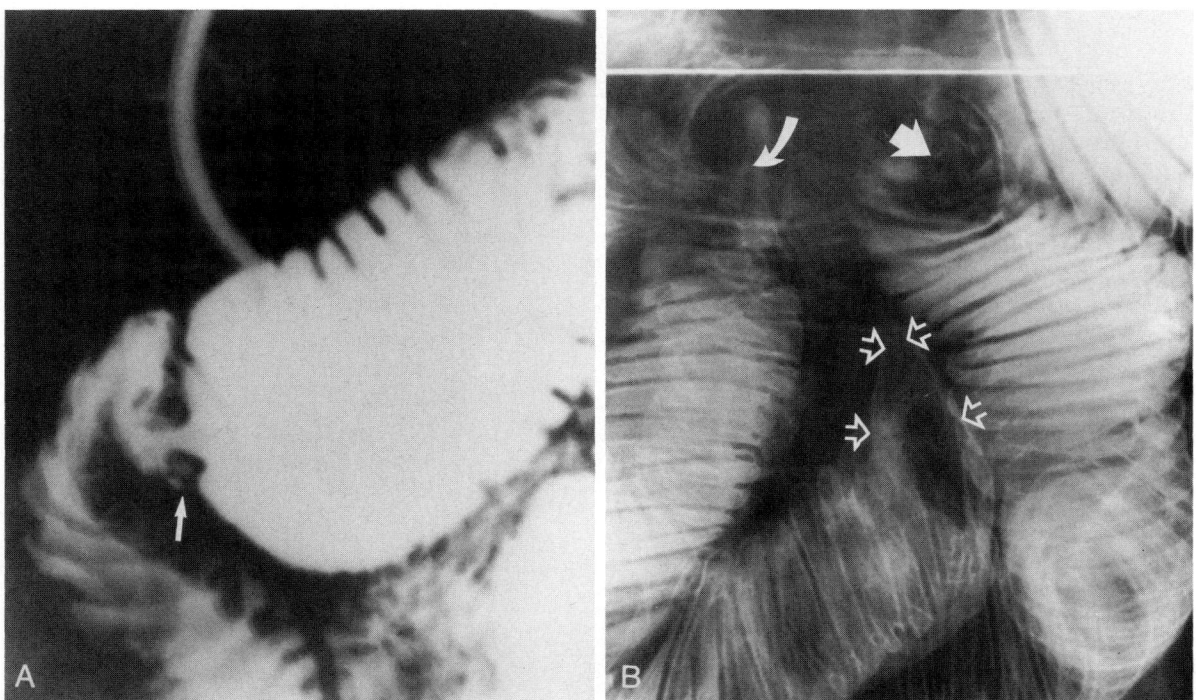

**Figure 52–29. Nonobstructive adhesions associated with an adhesive obstruction. A.** A medium-grade obstruction by a single band *(arrow)* affects a loop of jejunum, shown here in the single contrast phase of enteroclysis. **B.** The same area in the double contrast phase. The crossing single band is now indicated by the straight solid arrow. A tent-like deformity caused by an adhesion involving one side of a nonobstructed bowel segment extends toward and into the adjacent adhesive process *(open arrows)*. A further bowel loop is also affected *(curved solid arrow)* by the adhesion formation that included the obstructing single band.

## OTHER EXTRINSIC CAUSES OF SMALL BOWEL OBSTRUCTION

Extrinsic lesions constitute the vast majority of causes of small bowel obstruction. The most common causes, apart from adhesions, are hernias, peritoneal metastases, carcinoid tumors, and peritonitis (see Table 52–1). Internal hernias are confined within the abdomen and can be herniations of small bowel through a developmental defect or protrusions into a peritoneal reflection or surgically created defect in the peritoneum or mesentery; more frequent is the prolapse of a bowel loop under an adhesive band. External hernias constitute 95% of obstructing hernias and are classified as external because they are often visible or palpable. However, clinically, many external hernias are not obvious, even in thin patients (Fig. 52–30). Only when barium study, CT, ultrasound, magnetic resonance, or peritoneography is performed do some external hernias become evident. The most frequent sites of external herniation are the inguinal (Fig. 52–31) and femoral canals, the periumbilical region, and the sites of surgical incisions.

As with most SBOs, the radiologist usually studies patients with relatively low to moderate grades of obstruction. Patients with painful, tender swellings or suddenly enlarging or irreducible hernias are usually operated on without the benefit of barium studies.

## Internal Hernias

Internal hernias are uncommon causes of SBO, usually occurring near the ligament of Treitz (paraduodenal), the epiploic foramen, or the iliac fossa or through a postsurgical or post-traumatic rent in the diaphragm, omentum, or mesentery.[43–45] Internal and external hernias have similar radiographic features. One or many small bowel loops are crowded together in an abnormal location, encapsulated in the hernial sac. The loops do not usually change position over time. Fluoroscopically, the small bowel loops can be seen to enter into or return from the hernial orifice. At the neck of the hernia, there is smooth, symmetric, tapered narrowing of the lumen of its two adjacent limbs (Fig. 52–32). There may be delayed emptying of barium from loops contained in a hernial sac. Occasionally, a Meckel diverticulum herniates through the inguinal fossa, the so-called hernia of Littre (Fig. 52–33).

## Extrinsic Masses

Extrinsic masses obstructing the small bowel encompass a wide variety of neoplastic, inflammatory, and vascular etiologies (see Table 52–1). These extrinsic masses obstruct by two main mechanisms: compression of the lumen by the mass and distortion of the lumen

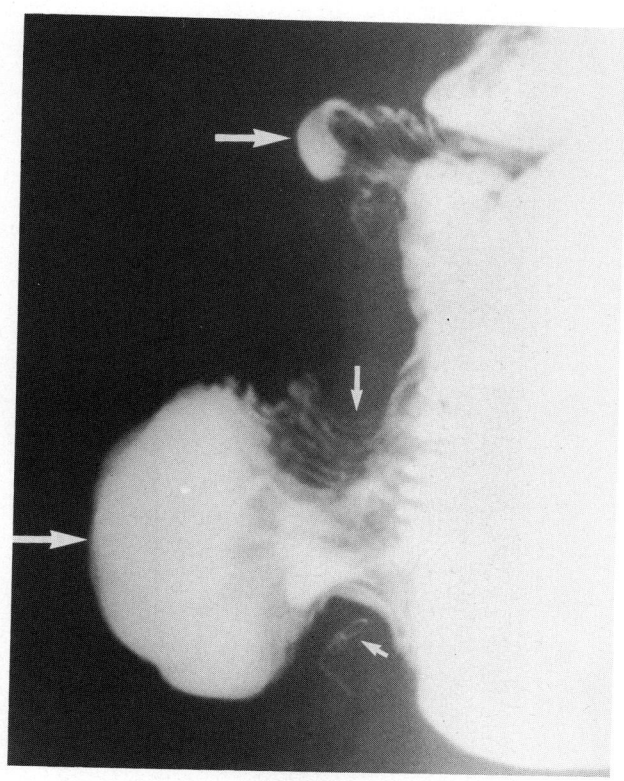

**Figure 52–30. Incisional hernias.** Spot film obtained with the patient in a lateral position shows two contrast medium–filled small intestinal loops *(large arrows)* protruding through the anterior abdominal wall (identified by wire sutures—*small arrow*). Note the mild, smooth compression of the small bowel with preservation of normal folds *(medium-sized arrow)* at the neck of the hernial sac.

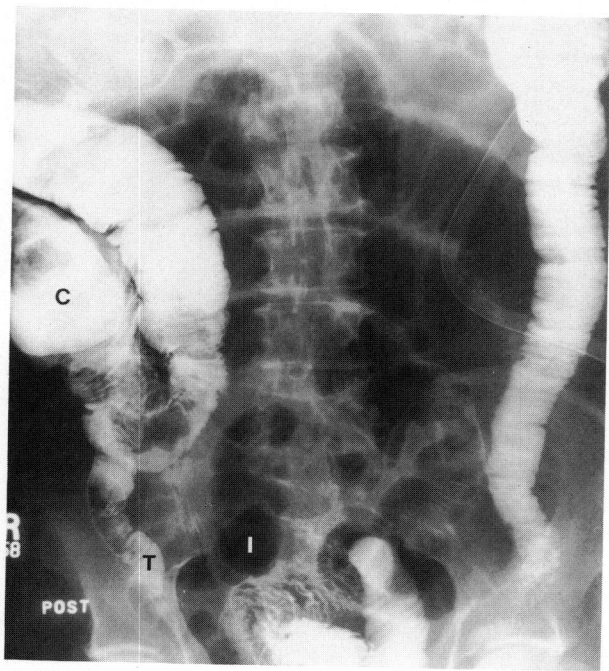

**Figure 52–31. Right inguinal hernia causing SBO and strangulation.** A barium enema was performed to rule out a colonic cause of a distal SBO. The postevacuation film shows diffuse dilatation of the air-filled small bowel (I) to the level of the right inguinal canal. Reflux of barium into the nondistended terminal ileum (T) shows it coursing toward the inguinal ligament. C = cecum. A spot film (not included) showed air in the scrotum. At surgery, the incarcerated loop of distal ileum was obstructed in the inguinal canal, was ischemic, and had perforated.

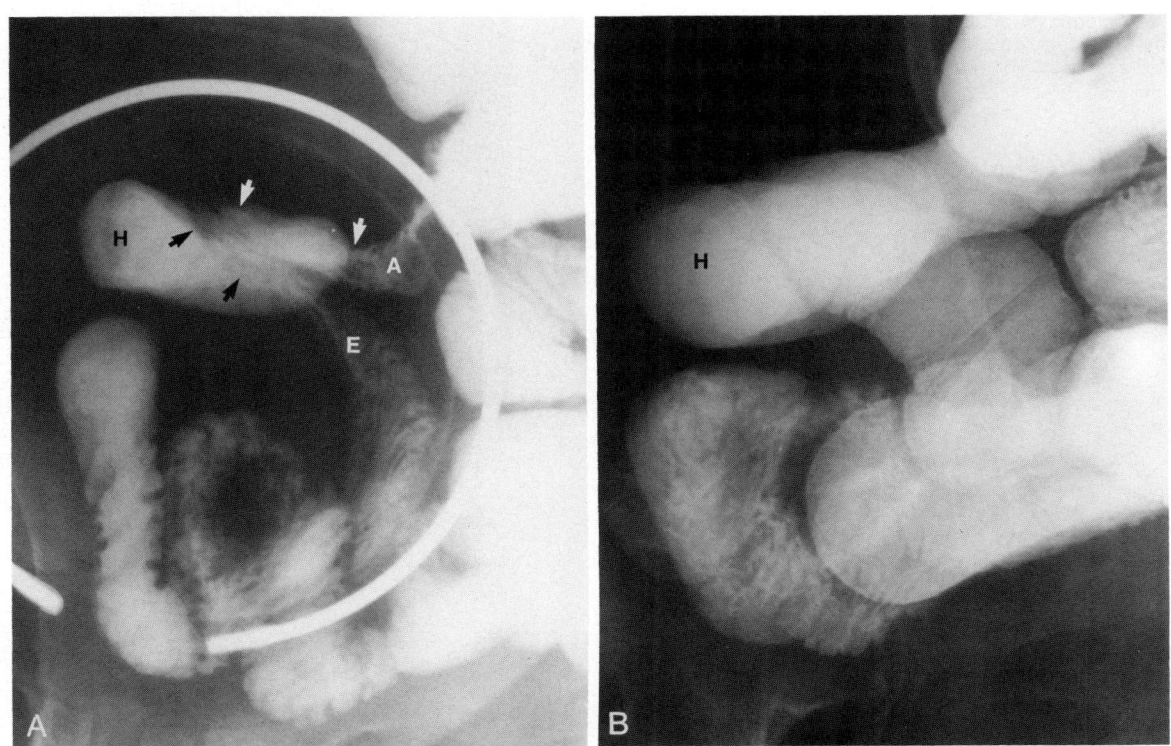

**Figure 52–32. Internal hernia with partial SBO. A.** Spot film from the early, single contrast phase of enteroclysis shows tapered narrowing of the afferent limb as it enters the hernial sac (A, *white arrows*) and of the efferent loop (E, *black arrows*) as it exits from the internal hernial sac (H). The hernia contains a mildly dilated loop of small intestine. Small bowel distal to the hernia is relatively collapsed compared with proximal small bowel. **B.** Spot film in the double contrast phase of the enteroclysis shows distended bowel loops. Both afferent and efferent loops of the internal hernia (H) are now distended.

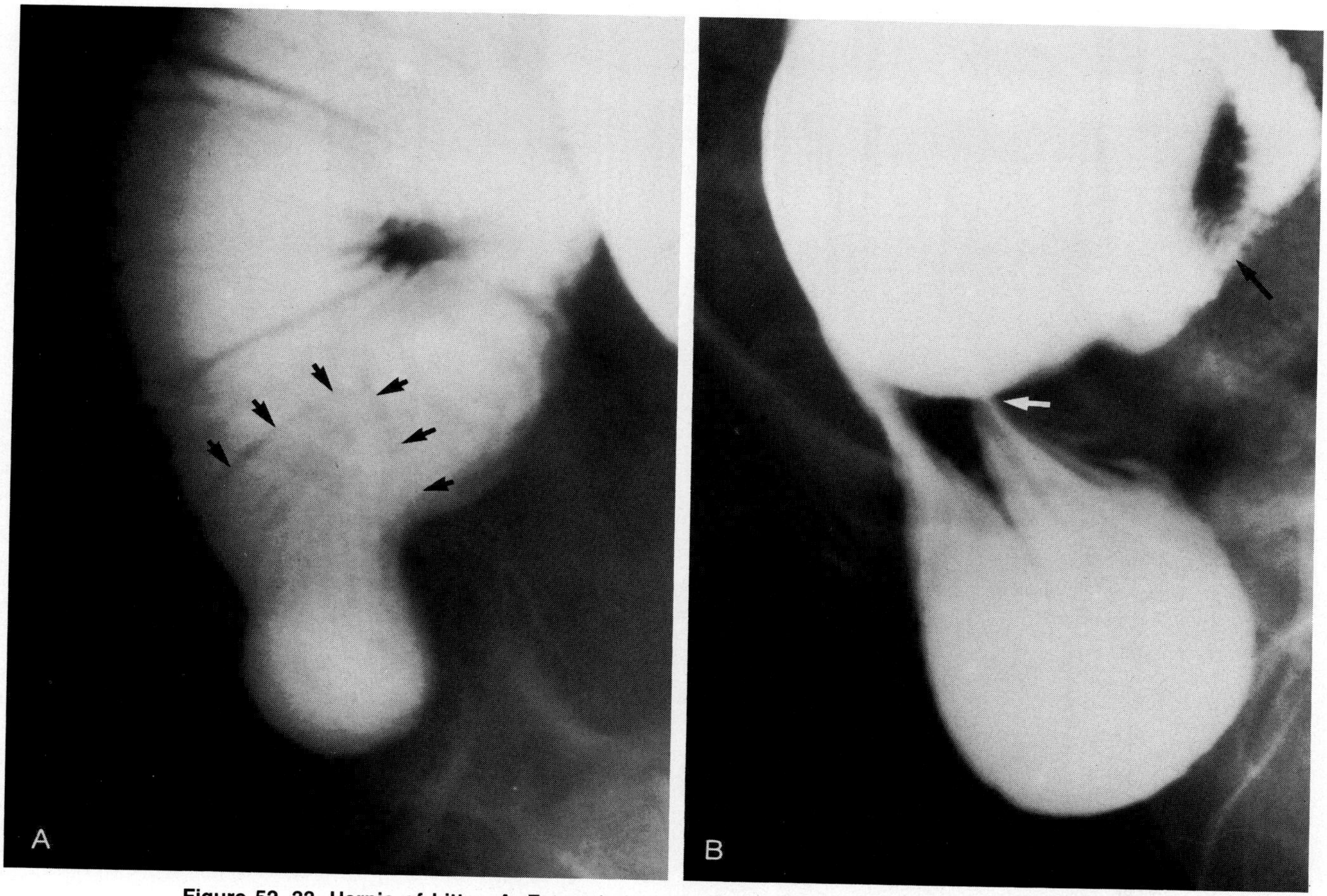

**Figure 52–33. Hernia of Littre. A.** Enteroclysis in a patient with intermittent SBO shows a Meckel diverticulum, identified by the triradiate fold pattern at its base *(arrows)*. **B.** A high-grade obstruction occurred 2 months later and enteroclysis was repeated. The Meckel diverticulum and the adjacent loop of ileum were found incarcerated in a left inguinal hernia (the hernia of Littre) with pronounced narrowing of its exiting limb *(arrow)*.

by a desmoplastic process that affects the small bowel serosa and mesentery.

Advanced mesenteric carcinomatosis, most often from ovarian carcinoma, produces desmoplasia in the mesentery and serosa with secondary effects of bowel loop angulation, crowding, and distortion (Fig. 52–34). Any peritoneally spread process that elicits a desmoplastic reaction in the small bowel serosa or mesentery may have a radiographic appearance similar to that of peritoneal metastases. Carcinoid tumor, tuberculous peritonitis (Fig. 52–35), and desmoid tumors are among the desmoplastic peritoneal conditions that may mimic peritoneal metastases.

Although carcinoid tumors are primarily intrinsic lesions of the ileum, SBO, one of their major clinical presentations, is largely due to desmoplastic mechanisms operating in the mesentery. Small carcinoids may appear as 1- to 2-cm-diameter, relatively smooth-surfaced submucosal masses or broad-based polyps. When carcinoid tumors have infiltrated the deeper layers of the bowel wall, they give rise to lesions with radiographic findings similar to those for peritoneal metastases. Early desmoplastic reaction results in kinking and angulation of the bowel wall with luminal narrowing. Mucosal folds are crowded at the edge of the lesions, similar to those

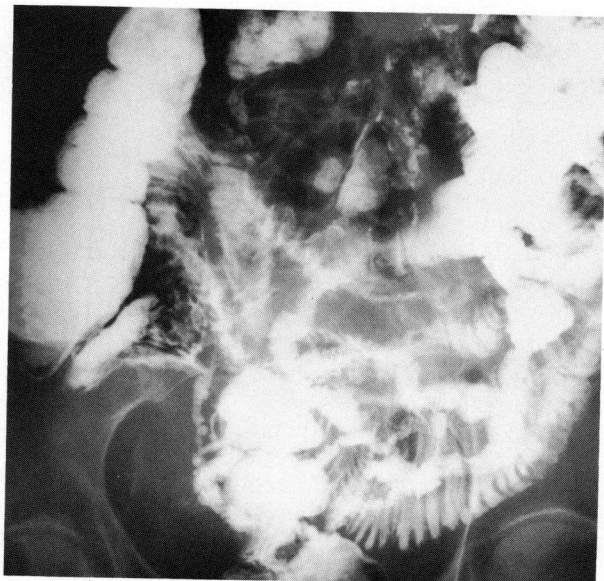

**Figure 52–34. Mesenteric carcinomatosis, primary tumor in pancreas.** Virtually all small bowel loops show distortion, lumen narrowing, tethering of folds, and general retraction toward the root of the mesentery. Severe radiation damage, advanced metastatic carcinoid, and mesenteric fibrosis can produce similar appearances.

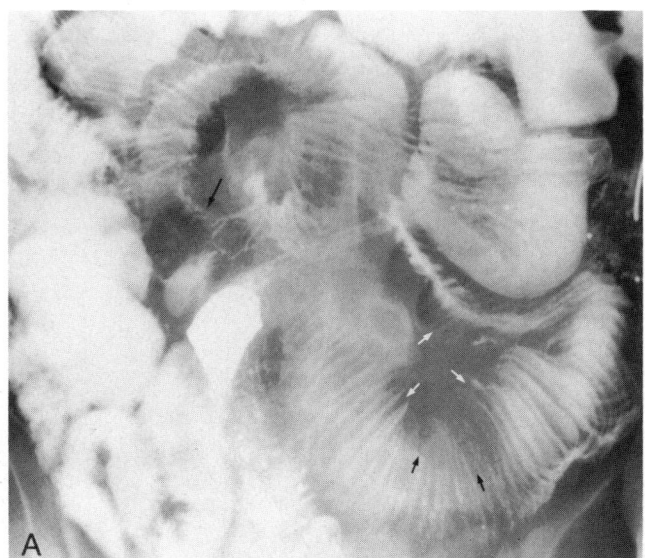

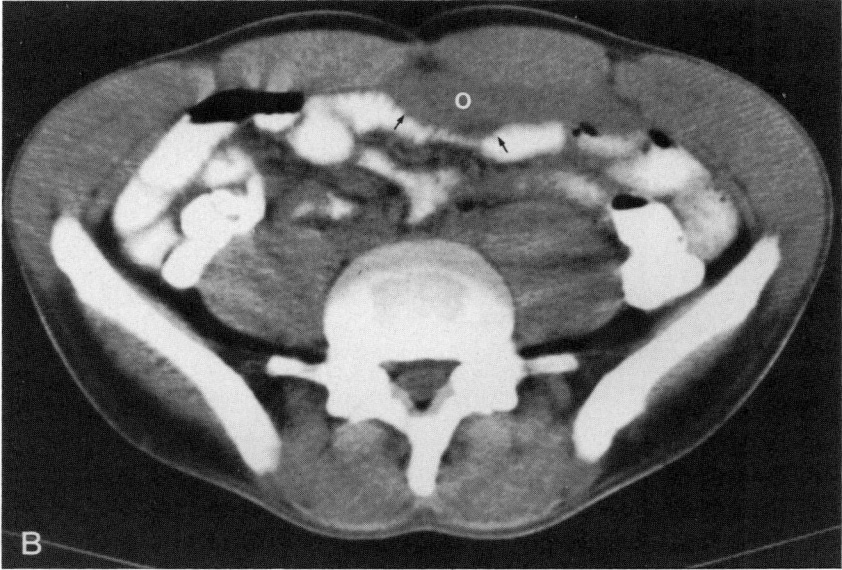

**Figure 52–35. Tuberculous peritonitis causing partial SBO in a young man with acquired immunodeficiency syndrome. A.** Overhead view from an enteroclysis shows disproportionate distention of proximal small bowel. Two loops in the left abdomen show a rounded mass effect on their mesenteric borders *(black arrows)* and crowding and tethering of smooth, normal folds *(white arrows)*. **B.** Axial image from a CT scan shows an omental mass (O) extrinsically impressing a small bowel loop *(arrows)*. The radiographic findings in both **A** and **B** resemble those caused by peritoneal metastases that involve and mildly obstruct the small bowel.

in peritoneal metastases. Carcinoid tumors are usually solitary lesions but may be multiple in up to 30% of cases.[20, 46, 47] Rarely, carcinoids present as annular tumors resembling an annular metastasis.[47] Location of the tumor is of no value in the differentiation from metastases because both lesions predominate in the distal ileum. When carcinoid tumors extensively infiltrate the mesentery, segments of bowel are pulled toward the mesenteric metastatic mass (Fig. 52–36A). Barium-outlined mucosal folds are tethered, producing spiculation of the contour of the mesenteric border (Fig. 52–36B).

Primary non-Hodgkin's lymphomas of the small bowel hardly ever cause SBO even when annular because they are soft lesions that infiltrate the bowel wall[48] and tend to develop early cavitation (Fig. 52–37). However, nodal non-Hodgkin's lymphomas may arise in the mesentery and grow to invade small bowel segments, causing obstruction by compression, kinking, and infiltration (Fig. 52–38). The radiographic findings for mesenteric

lymphoma invading the small bowel are those of a mass separating bowel loops, with fixation, angulation, and narrowing of the loops and tethering of folds (Fig. 52–39). CT scans demonstrate the growing mesenteric mass and its adjacency to and infiltration of bowel loops (see Fig. 52–39B). Non-Hodgkin's lymphoma arising in the mesentery is a more frequent cause of SBO than mesenteric nodal Hodgkin's disease.[20] Leiomyosarcoma, a stromal tumor only rarely seen with annular involvement of a small bowel segment, is also soft and changes shape during compression; it does not cause significant bowel obstruction. (See also Chapter 51.)

## Duplications

Enteric duplications present as extrinsic lesions obstructing the small bowel by compression. Duplications occupy the mesenteric border, primarily of the distal

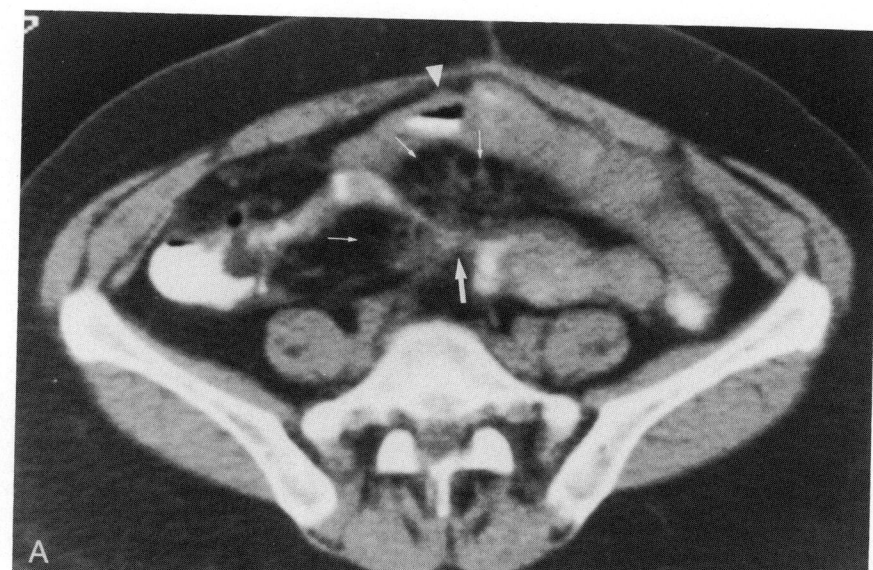

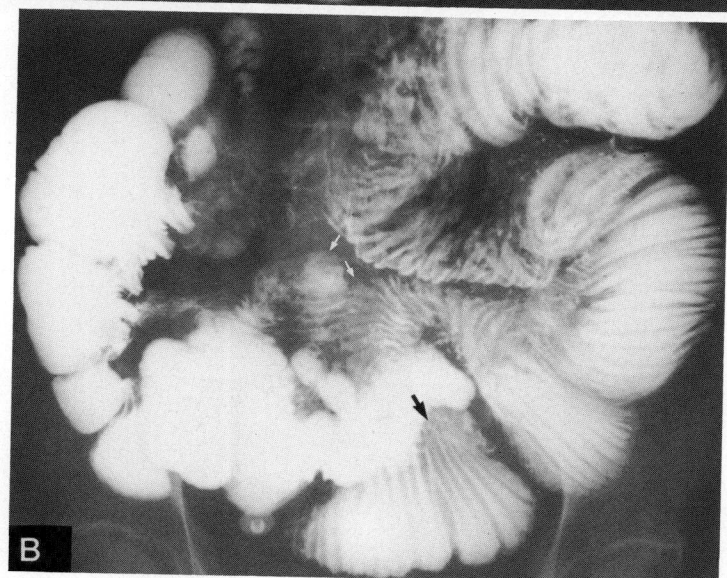

**Figure 52–36. Carcinoid tumor with metastasis to the mesentery causing partial SBO. A.** Axial image from a CT scan demonstrates the mesenteric metastasis as a nodular mass in the root of the small bowel mesentery *(large arrow)*. Linear stranding extends from the mesenteric mass into the mesenteric fat *(small arrows)*. Also note mural thickening of a small bowel loop *(arrowhead)*. **B.** Overhead view from a small bowel follow-through examination shows dilatation of proximal loops. The loops are generally pulled and angulated toward the center of the abdomen, in the direction of the root of the small bowel mesentery *(white arrows)*. The smooth folds are mildly tethered *(black arrow)*. Note crowding of folds along the mesenteric border of many small bowel loops.

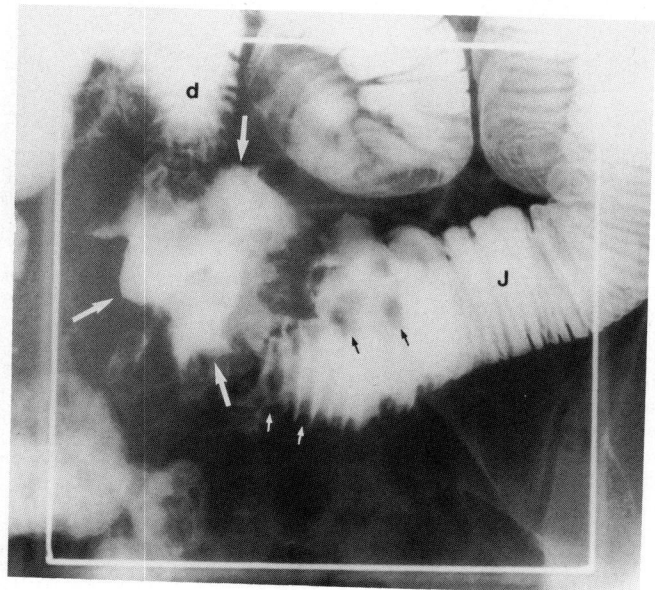

**Figure 52–37. Primary small bowel non-Hodgkin's lymphoma causing mild obstruction.** Spot film from an enteroclysis shows a large cavitary lesion related to the jejunum (J), associated with mild dilatation compared with distal small bowel (D). The patient presented with bleeding, not distention or pain. The cavitation is manifested by an irregular barium collection *(large arrows)* extending beyond the expected confines of the lumen. The primary site of this small bowel lymphoma is indicated by segmental infiltration, coarse nodules *(small black arrows)* and thickened folds *(small white arrows)*. Cavitation represents a later development and was preceded by ulceration.

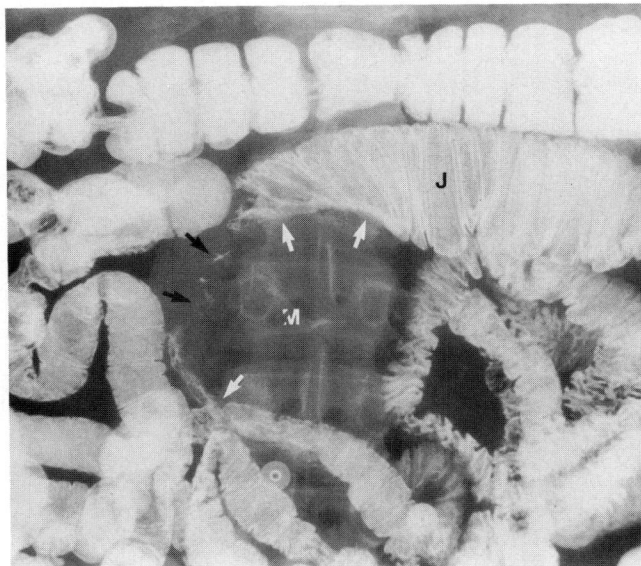

**Figure 52–38. Non-Hodgkin's lymphoma partially obstructing small intestine.** Final overhead view of an enteroclysis shows splaying of a small bowel loop by a mass in the mesentery (M). Extrinsic impression on the mesenteric border of the jejunum *(white arrows)* culminates in irregular lumen narrowing of one segment *(black arrows)*, indicating encirclement and invasion by the tumor. Disproportionate distention of the proximal jejunum (J) indicates partial SBO.

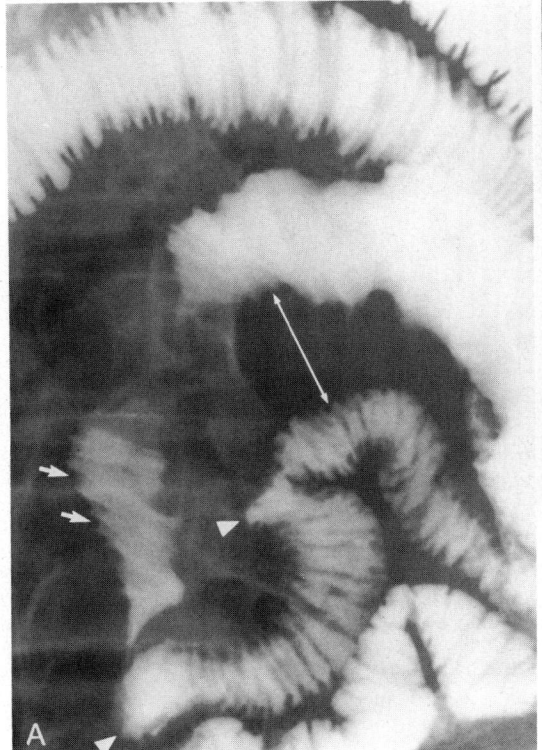

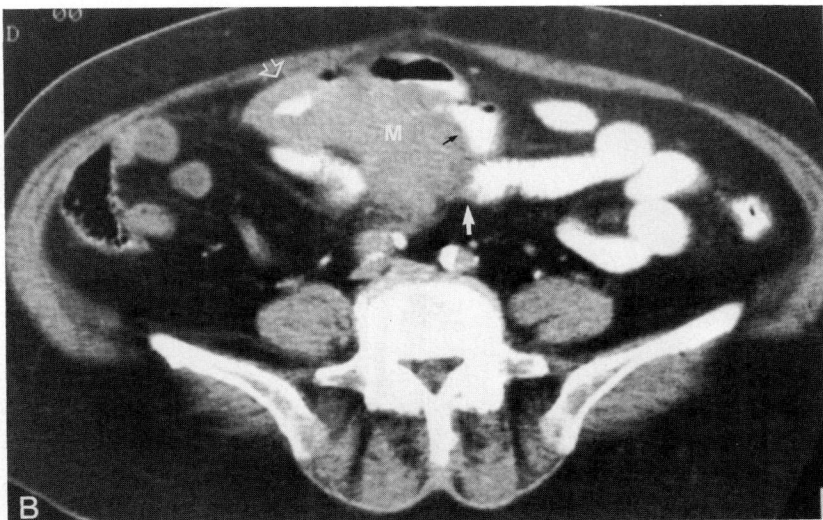

**Figure 52–39. Mass of large cell non-Hodgkin's lymphoma in the small bowel mesentery causes partial SBO. A.** Overhead radiograph shows disproportionate distention of proximal small bowel, separation of bowel loops *(double arrow)*, angulation of bowel loops *(arrowheads)*, and tethering of mucosal folds *(arrows)*. (From Rubesin SE, Gilchrist AM, Bronner M, et al: Non-Hodgkin lymphoma of the small intestine. Radiographics 10:985–998, 1990.) **B.** Axial image from a CT scan shows the mesenteric mass (M) compressing and infiltrating the mesenteric border of a small bowel loop *(black arrow)*. The site of partial obstruction is identified *(white arrow)*. Encasement of a small bowel loop by the tumor is seen *(open arrow)*.

ileum. They may or may not communicate with the small bowel lumen. On barium studies, an extrinsic mass impression is seen on the mesenteric border of the distal ileum. CT better demonstrates the size and nature of the lesion.

## INTRINSIC LESIONS

Intrinsic small intestinal diseases that obstruct the lumen depend on circumferential thickening of the bowel wall, with infiltration of the submucosa and muscularis propria by tumor or inflammation. Because small intestinal contents are liquid, a significant amount of luminal narrowing is necessary to obstruct the small bowel by an intrinsic constricting lesion. The most frequent lesions with the potential for intrinsic obstruction are adenocarcinoma, Crohn's disease, and radiation enteropathy (see Table 52–1). Smaller polypoid tumors of the small intestine usually obstruct by the mechanism of intussusception.

## Adenocarcinoma

Adenocarcinoma of the small intestine is seen more frequently in the duodenum and proximal jejunum than in the ileum. When adenocarcinoma presents with signs of obstruction, the tumor is usually at an advanced stage. Radiographically, a short, annular narrowing is well demarcated by abrupt, nodular, shelving margins. The mucosa in the center of the lesion is replaced by

tumor, manifested as nodular or ulcerated mucosa (Figs. 52–40 and 52–41). The tumor is rigid and does not change shape with either compression or peristalsis. With a severely narrowed lumen, it may be difficult to distinguish an annular carcinoma from a circumferential metastasis because the mucosa cannot be examined. The location of the lesion is a clue to the more likely diagnosis because an obstructing, proximal jejunal, annular infiltrating lesion, unless close to the ligament of Treitz, is more likely to be an adenocarcinoma. The absence of desmoplastic distortion also favors a diagnosis of adenocarcinoma. Because peritoneal metastases usually involve the distal small bowel, an annular infiltrative lesion in the distal ileum is more likely to be a metastasis, especially in the setting of a known primary malignancy.[49] (See also Chapter 51.)

## Crohn's Disease

In the advanced, stenotic phase of Crohn's disease, patients frequently present with recurrent episodes of partial SBO (Figs. 52–42 and 52–43). High-grade obstructions are rare. Narrowing in Crohn's disease may be due to edema, spasm, an inflammatory mass, a fibrous stricture, or rarely a carcinoma. The radiologist must examine stenotic areas carefully and patiently to assess the true luminal diameter. Segments of advanced stenotic disease are usually rigid and narrowed with an irregular contour;[50] the normal small bowel mucosa has been destroyed and has been replaced by ulcerated and nodular tissue. On barium studies, thickening of the

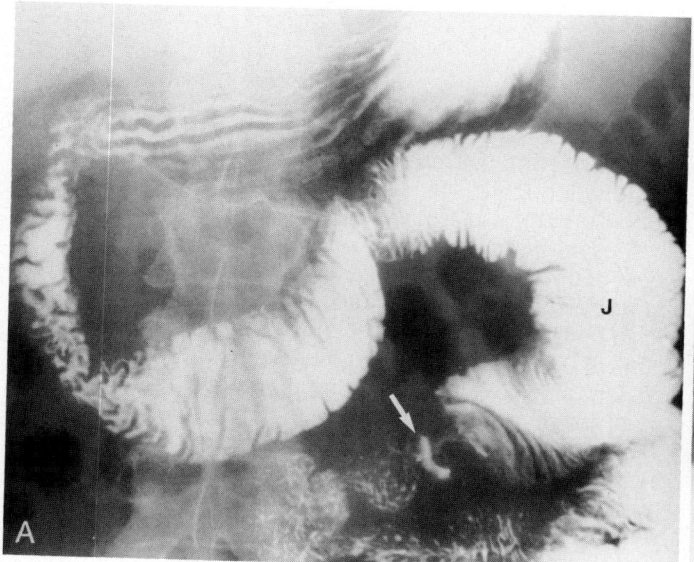
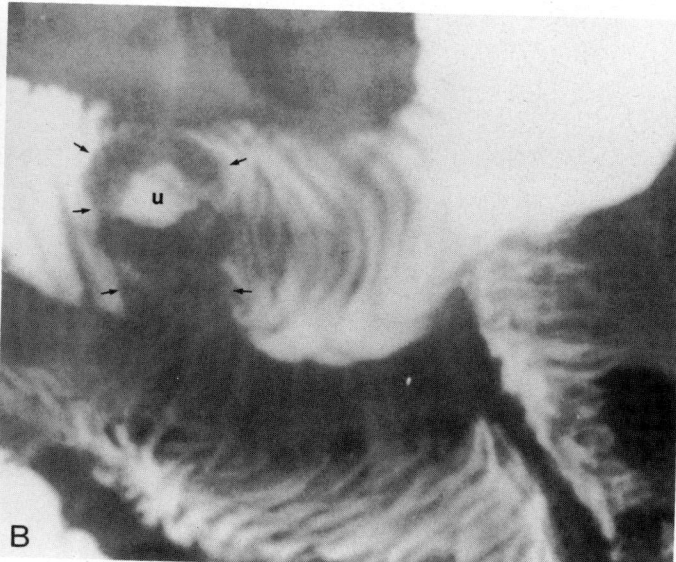

**Figure 52–40. Adenocarcinoma of jejunum with partial SBO. A.** When distention of the duodenum is demonstrated near the ligament of Treitz during an upper gastrointestinal examination, the barium study must be extended into the proximal small bowel, especially in a patient, such as this, with guaiac-positive stool. A circumferential, centrally ulcerated *(arrow)* lesion was found in the first segment of jejunum (J). **B.** Coned-down view using compression shows a well-circumscribed *(arrows)* annular mass with central ulceration (u). Such a finding is typical for an adenocarcinoma in the small bowel.

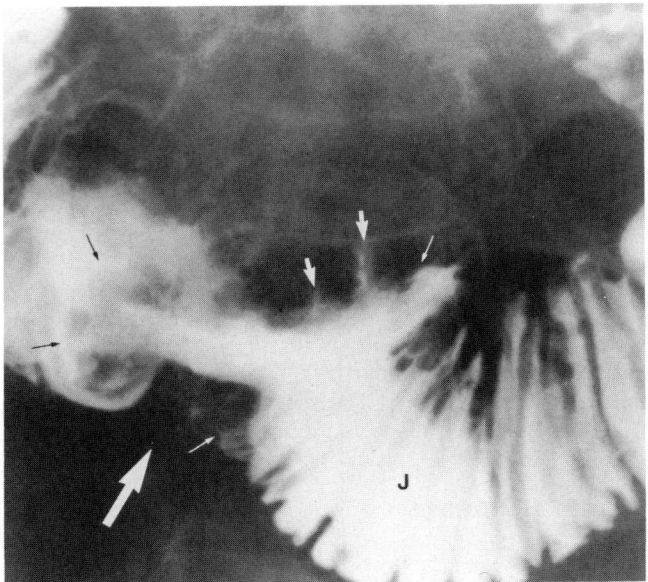

**Figure 52–41. Adenocarcinoma of the small bowel with partial SBO.** Spot film from the single contrast phase of an enteroclysis shows a 4-cm-long annular lesion *(large arrow)*. The proximal jejunum (J) is mildly distended. Note abrupt, "shelving" margins seen in profile *(small white arrows)* and en face *(small black arrows)*. The mucosal contour is irregular *(medium-sized white arrows)*.

bowel wall and mesentery is implied by wide separation of bowel loops. The ability of enteroclysis to distend loops or the use of a promotility agent such as metoclopramide may show that a string-like narrowing can open,

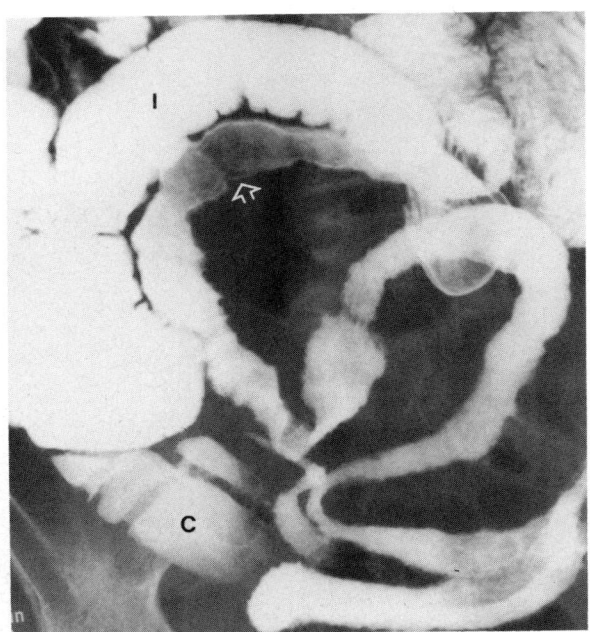

**Figure 52–42. Crohn's disease with low-grade SBO.** Overhead view from a small bowel follow-through shows diffuse narrowing of the distal small bowel. Dilatation of the ileum (I) proximal to the area affected by Crohn's disease indicates mild obstruction. Flow into the cecum (C) is present. Also note the nodular appearance of the ileal mucosa *(arrow)* and the separation of ileal loops because of fibrofatty proliferation in the mesentery.

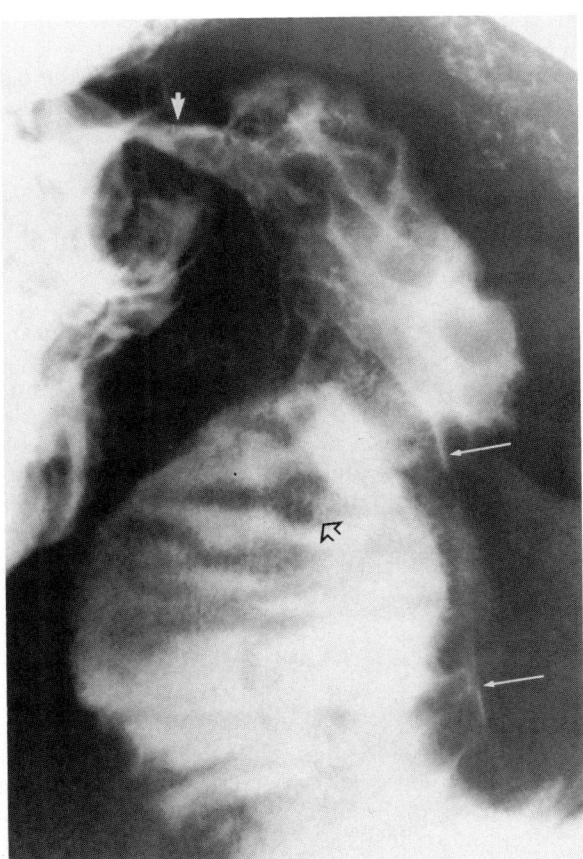

**Figure 52–43. Crohn's disease of the terminal ileum with partial SBO.** Spot film image from a small bowel follow-through examination shows narrowing of the most distal part of the terminal ileum and of the lumen of the ileocecal valve *(short solid arrow)*. Also note a linear mesenteric border ulcer *(long solid arrows)*, nodular mucosa *(open arrow)*, and mucosal granularity.

indicating that the luminal narrowing is due to transient spasm. CT, however, is superior to barium studies in demonstrating an abscess, fibrofatty proliferation, or lymphadenopathy as a cause of separation of bowel loops.[51] (See also Chapter 47.)

Most other primary inflammatory causes of SBO are rare. Tuberculosis is unusual in Western countries but may be seen, especially in immigrants from Southeast Asia.[52] The clue to the diagnosis of tuberculosis is the clinical history and the radiographic finding that the cecum and ascending colon are proportionally more involved than the terminal ileum. Tuberculosis may have "skip" lesions similar to those in Crohn's disease. Diagnosis relies on culture and biopsy results showing mycobacterial organisms. Acute infectious disorders such as *Yersinia* infections rarely cause SBO because significant fibrosis is unlikely to occur. (See also Chapter 48.) Other mimics of Crohn's disease causing SBO include Behçet's disease and carcinoma of the cecum invading the terminal ileum (Fig. 52–44). Strictures may develop as an end stage of ulcerative jejunoileitis complicating celiac disease. These strictures usually occur in the proximal jejunum (Fig. 52–45).

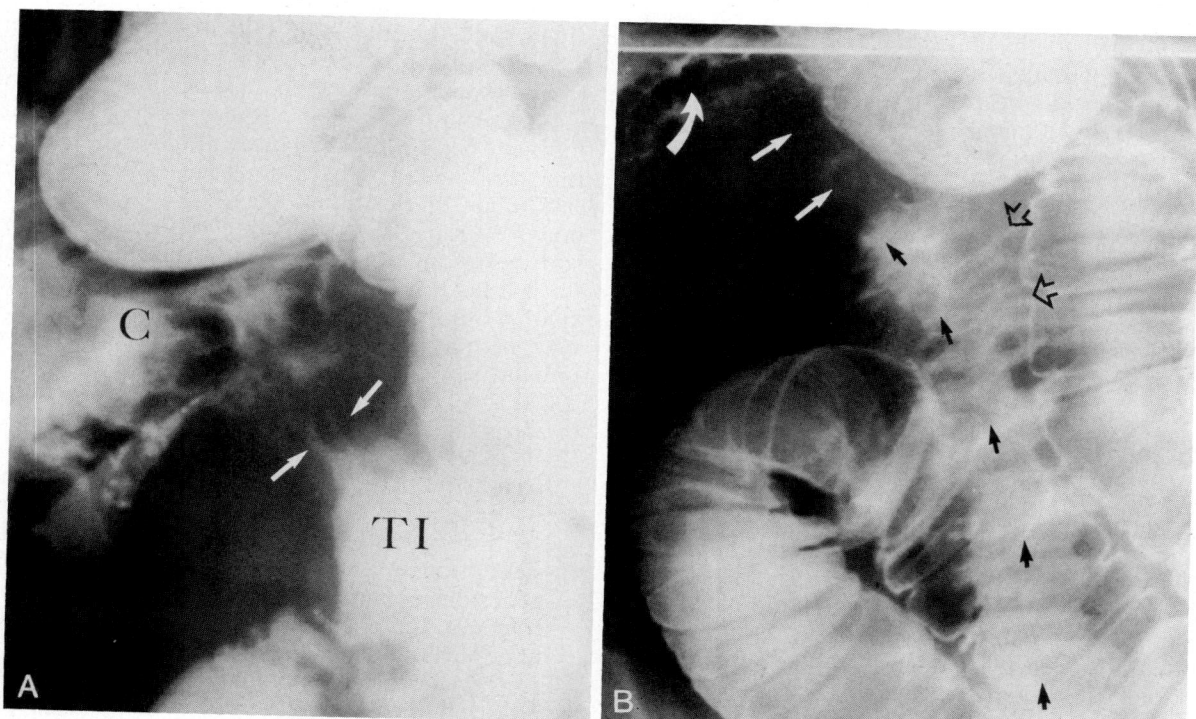

**Figure 52–44. Carcinoma of cecum extending into terminal ileum, mimicking Crohn's disease: enteroclysis. A.** Nodularity of the mucosa of the cecum (C) and ileocecal valve extends into the most distal, narrowed *(arrows)* part of the terminal ileum (TI). A low-grade SBO is present. **B.** In the double contrast phase of enteroclysis, the terminal ileum *(black arrows)* shows fold thickening with drawn-out spiky interspaces *(open arrows)* near the narrowed segment *(white arrows)*. Nodularity of cecal mucosa is seen *(curved arrow)*. The radiographic findings mimic those of Crohn's disease. However, the mucosal nodularity without ulceration extending into the terminal ileum suggests malignancy. The thickened folds of the terminal ileum represent edema, frequently seen proximal to an obstructing malignancy.

**Figure 52–45. Focal strictures associated with celiac disease.** Abrupt, smooth, multiple ring-like narrowings *(arrows)* are seen in the proximal jejunum of a patient with celiac disease. The strictures are probably the sequelae of ulcerative jejunoileitis. Also note loss of folds in the affected jejunum, indicating atrophy of small bowel mucosa typical of celiac disease. (Courtesy of M. S. Losowsky, M.D., Leeds, England.)

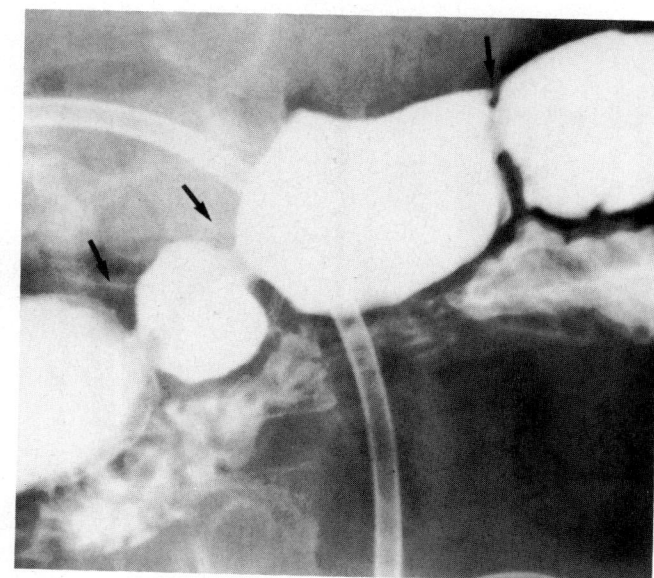

## Radiation Enteropathy

Radiation enteropathy and other vascular lesions may cause mild to moderate SBO. In radiation damage, SBO is caused by adhesions related to radiation serositis and, to a lesser extent, luminal narrowing and dysmotility. Occasionally, smooth, tapered strictures may develop at least 6 months after radiotherapy (Fig. 52–46A). Submucosal edema and fibrosis are the most common findings in radiation enteropathy and are manifested radiographically as smooth, straight, parallel, thick folds that cross the small bowel lumen. Barium fills the compressed interstices between folds, forming the so-called interspace spikes. Separation of bowel loops suggests bowel wall thickening. The changes are localized to the radiation portal, usually in the pelvis. Fixation, kinking, and angulation of small bowel loops suggest coexisting radiation-induced adhesions (Fig. 52–46B). Not infrequently, adhesions form at the entry edge of the radiation portal and may become a cause for adhesive obstruction (Fig. 52–47). Distortion and kinking of diffusely narrowed bowel loops with spiculation of their luminal contour suggest the possibility of peritoneal metastases superimposed on radiation enteropathy. More often, however, these metastases-like appearances are due solely to radiation damage. (See also Chapter 53.)

## INTUSSUSCEPTION

Various extrinsic, instrinsic, and intralumenal processes result in intussusception of small bowel (see Table 52–1). The final common pathway is invagination of an entire proximal small bowel loop and part of its mesentery into the lumen of a small bowel segment distal to it. The inner, advancing proximal segment is termed the intussusceptum and the distal, outer, receiving segment the intussuscipiens. Radiographically, a narrow, tapered, barium-filled channel outlines the intussusceptum (Fig. 52–48). If barium refluxes retrogradely into the lumen of the intussuscipiens, a "coil spring" sign may be seen. The coil spring represents the mucosal surface of the intussuscipiens, depicted as stretched, thick folds representing edema caused by lymphatic or venous obstruction. Polyps causing the intussusception may be outlined distal to the tapered lumen of the intussusceptum.

CT is an effective alternative to barium studies for the diagnosis of an intussusception and of its cause (Fig. 52–49).

Nonobstructive, transient intussusceptions may be seen in any small bowel disorder that is associated with dysmotility, such as celiac disease or scleroderma. Intussusceptions may occur with extrinsic disorders such as adhesions or duplications.

Polypoid tumors, benign or malignant, are the most common cause of small bowel intussusception in the adult. No specific radiographic findings distinguish the benign and malignant tumors that cause intussusceptions. Although a histologic diagnosis cannot be made by radiologic means, a guarded differential diagnosis can be based on the clinical history, location of the tumor, and specific radiographic features. Clinical history is of importance in the diagnosis of Peutz-Jeghers

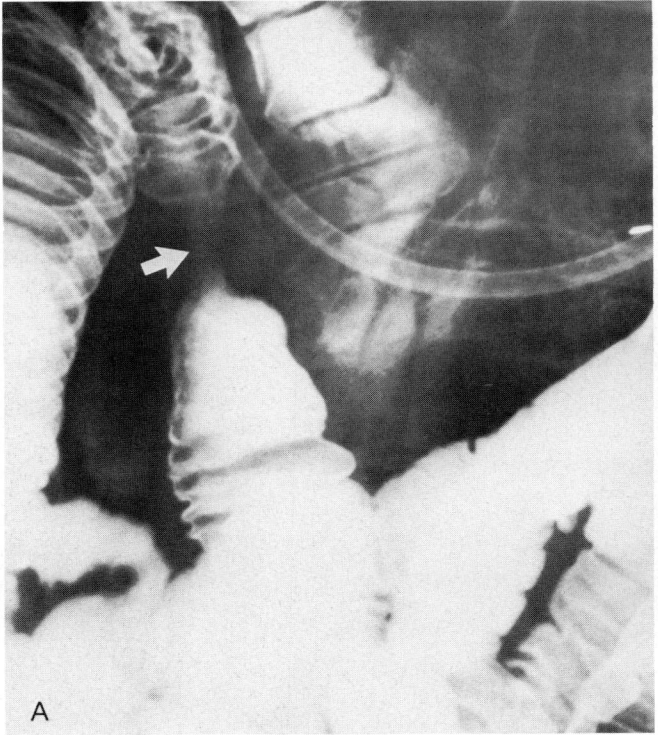 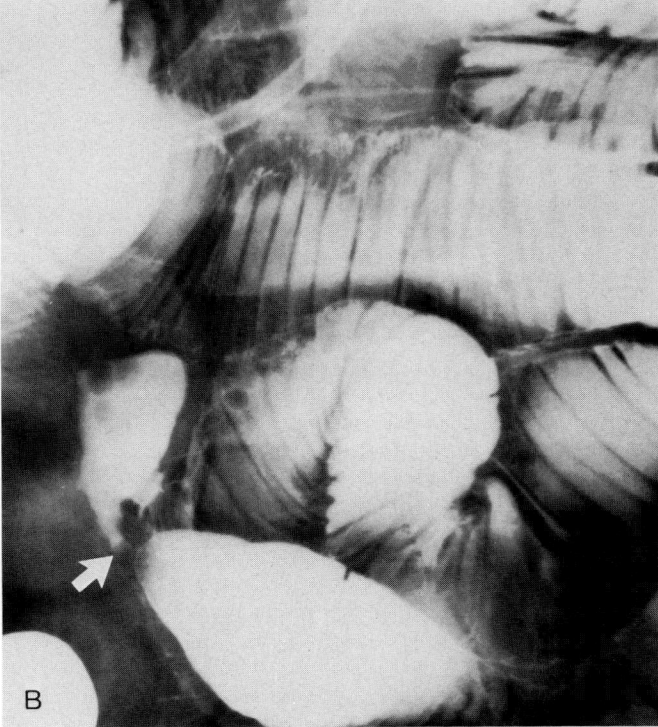

**Figure 52–46. Radiation stricture. A.** Smooth stricture *(arrow)* after radiation for carcinoma of cervix and bladder. Only mild obstruction is caused. Thickening of folds is seen on both sides of the stricture. (Courtesy of Dina Caroline, M.D., Philadelphia, PA.) **B.** Radiation-induced adhesions with fixation, kinking and stricture formation *(arrow)*.

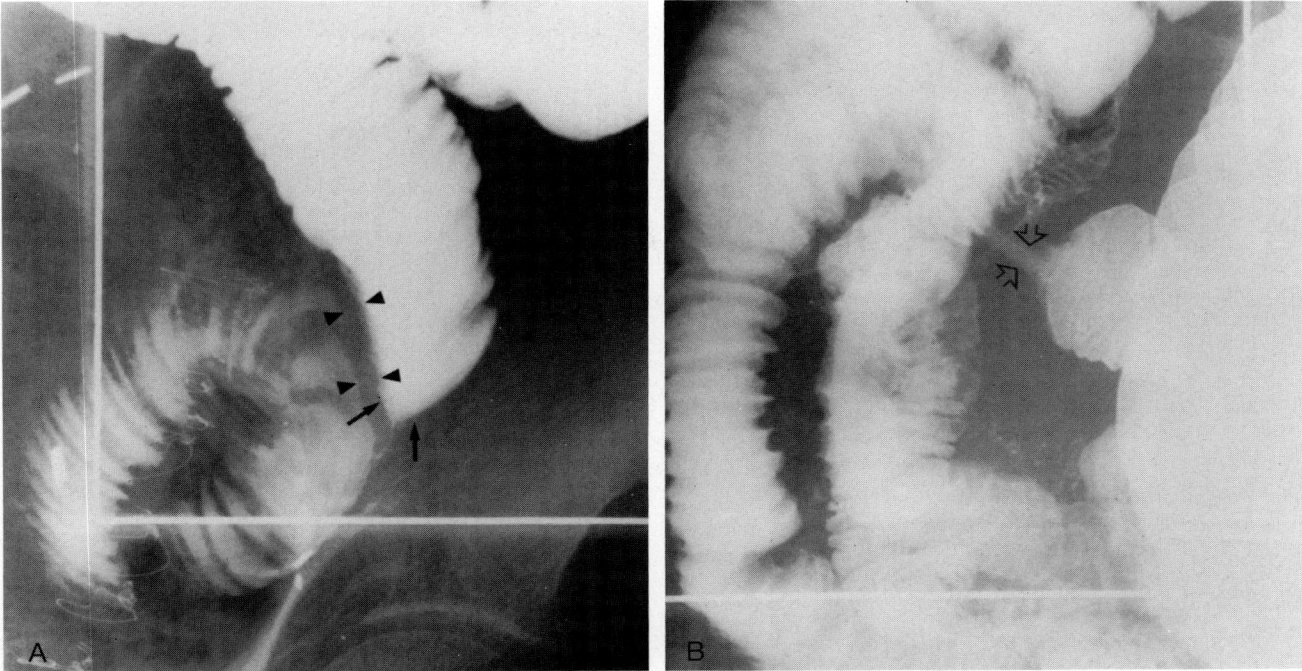

**Figure 52–47. Obstruction of small bowel at entry into an area of radiation enteropathy.** Abrupt lumen narrowing *(arrows)* of dilated and otherwise normal bowel is seen at the site of entry into the sharply marginated area of radiation damage. The mechanism of obstruction appears to be kinking of normal bowel where it joins the radiation-damaged intestine, which is tied down by adhesions. Note the crowded and thickened folds and the thickened wall *(arrowheads)* of the radiation-damaged distal bowel.

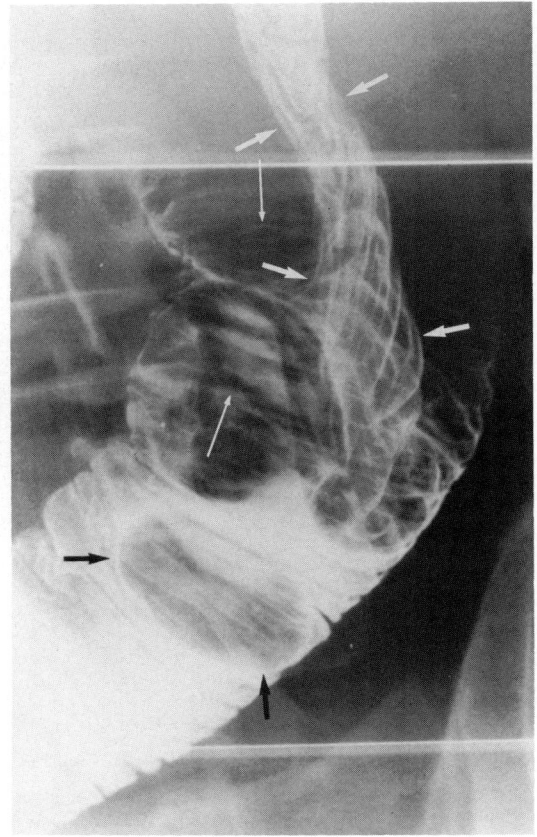

**Figure 52–48. Intussusception of metastatic melanoma with partial SBO.** Spot film from an enteroclysis shows the lumen of the intussusceptum as a narrow, tubular structure lined by twisted mucosal folds *(thick white arrows)*. Retrograde reflux of barium partly coats the mucosa of the intussuscipiens, resulting in a coil spring appearance *(thin white arrows)*. Note that the folds of the intussuscipiens are thickened by edema. The cause of the intussusception is a large, lobulated, smooth-surfaced polyp, etched in white by barium *(black arrows)*.

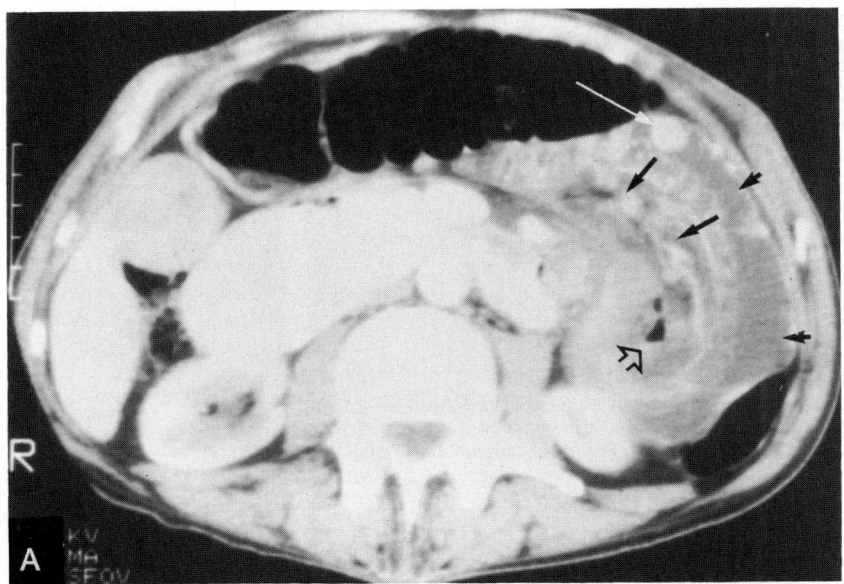

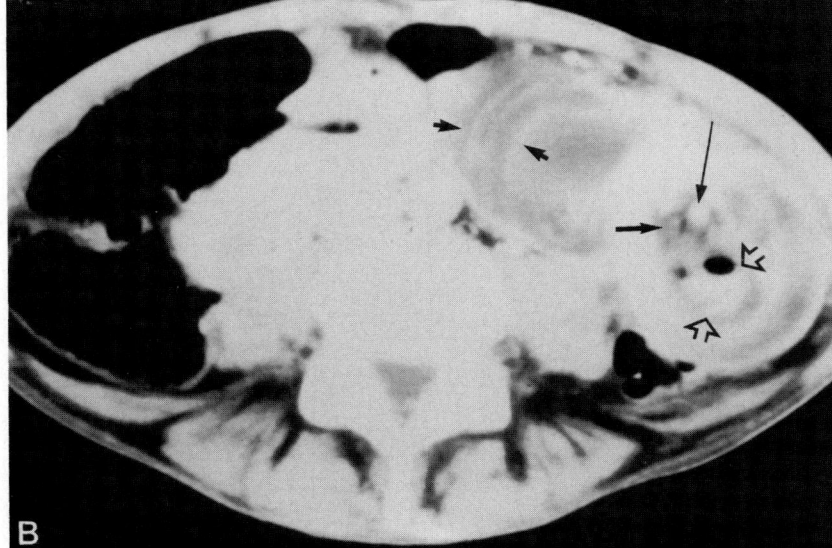

**Figure 52–49. CT scan of an intussusception caused by melanoma metastases. A.** Axial image from a CT scan shows radiographic findings typical of intussusception. The crescentic outline of fat and vascular structures in the small bowel mesentery *(large black arrows)* is partly superimposed on the intussusceptum *(open arrow)*. At least one melanoma metastasis *(white arrow)* is outlined in the wall of the fluid-containing intussuscipiens *(small black arrows)*. **B.** Axial image from a CT scan through the intussusception demonstrates the coil spring pattern of the intussuscipiens *(short arrows)*. The gas-containing intussusceptum is demarcated by a fat seam *(open arrows)*; near it is the invaginated mesentery containing fat and vessels *(medium-sized arrow)*. A melanoma deposit is shown *(long arrow)*. (Courtesy of Alec J. Megibow, M.D., New York, NY.)

polyps or metastatic melanoma complicated by intussusception. Most patients with metastatic melanoma have a clinical history of surgical removal of a skin tumor. However, a small percentage of patients with metastatic melanoma have SBO with intussusception as the initial presentation of their disease.[53] Most patients with Peutz-Jeghers syndrome, an autosomal dominant disorder, have a family history of this syndrome. Some cases are due to spontaneous mutations, but the syndrome is heralded by pigmented lesions near the lips and on the oral mucosa, face, or extremities.[54] These lesions may be overlooked, especially in patients of African or Asian origin, who may first present with bleeding or abdominal pain caused by intussusception (Fig. 52–50). Location of the intussusception is of limited value in distinguishing between the polyps of different histologies. Peutz-Jeghers polyps are most frequently located in the proximal jejunum, and so are adenomas. Stromal tumors (leiomyomas) and lipomas have a relatively uniform distribution in the small bowel.

Radiographic findings are of somewhat greater value. Multiple polypoid tumors suggest a diagnosis of metastases, especially from malignant melanoma, or Peutz-Jeghers syndrome. Peutz-Jeghers polyps usually have a short, broad-based stalk. Barium filling the interstices of a lesion suggests a diagnosis of a mucosal lesion, such as a Peutz-Jeghers polyp or an adenoma. Centrally umbilicated or ulcerated polypoid lesions that intussuscept are usually submucosal tumors such as a leiomyoma or metastatic melanoma. Melanoma metastases have a central umbilication or ulceration in one half of lesions.[55] Intussusception by the soft melanoma metastases is frequently without significant obstruction and may be intermittent. Soft, polypoid lesions also include lipomas, Peutz-Jeghers polyps, and inflammatory fibroid polyps. Pedunculated polyps with long stalks that intussuscept

are usually inflammatory fibroid polyps, lipomas, or invaginated Meckel's diverticulum[56, 57] (Fig. 52–51). Hemangiomas, not infrequent small intestinal lesions, usually present with bleeding and do not intussuscept. Other causes of intussusception described in the literature include Henoch-Schönlein purpura, lymphoma, hematomas, and mesenteric lymphadenopathy. (See also Chapters 50 and 51.)

## INTRALUMINAL CAUSES

Gallstones, bezoars, foreign bodies, meconium, or tangles of *Ascaris* worms may obturate the small bowel lumen, resulting in obstruction. Gallstone-induced SBO, inappropriately termed gallstone ileus, usually occurs in elderly patients, especially women. The classic triad of a calcified gallstone, gas in a shrunken gallbladder or biliary tree, and SBO is seen in a minority of patients.[58, 59] Calcified gallstones are seen on plain films or barium studies in only approximately 15% of patients. CT and ultrasound may better reveal calcified gallstones as the cause of an SBO.[30, 60]

Blunt abdominal trauma, often a seat belt injury, may be followed by the formation of obstructive strictures, usually on the basis of a bowel wall hematoma. The majority of hematomas resolve or leave only minor lumen narrowing after about 2 weeks of conservative treatment. Occasionally, it is necessary to intervene surgically to resect a fibrous stricture.[61]

Medication-related strictures have most often been associated with slow-release potassium preparations and focal ischemic necrosis followed by fibrotic repair. A few cases of intestinal obstruction were caused by multiple concentric diaphragm-like structures with central openings down to pinhole size.[62] These strictures were

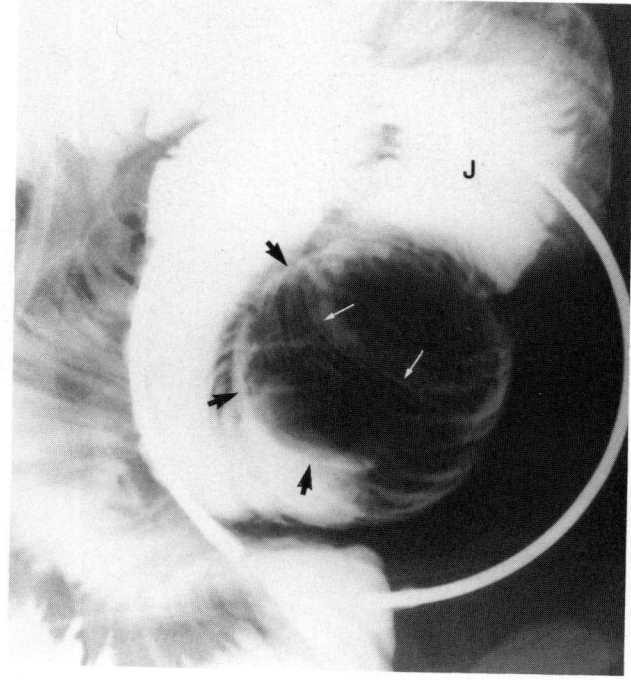

**Figure 52–50. Peutz-Jeghers hamartoma causing intussusception.** Spot film from the single contrast phase of an enteroclysis shows a smooth-surfaced polypoid mass *(black arrows)*. The coil spring pattern of the mucosa of the intussuscipiens is superimposed *(white arrows)*. Dilatation of the proximal jejunum (J) indicates mild obstruction. This 37-year-old black man had never before been diagnosed as having Peutz-Jeghers syndrome. Pigmented lesions were barely visible on his lips and oral mucosa.

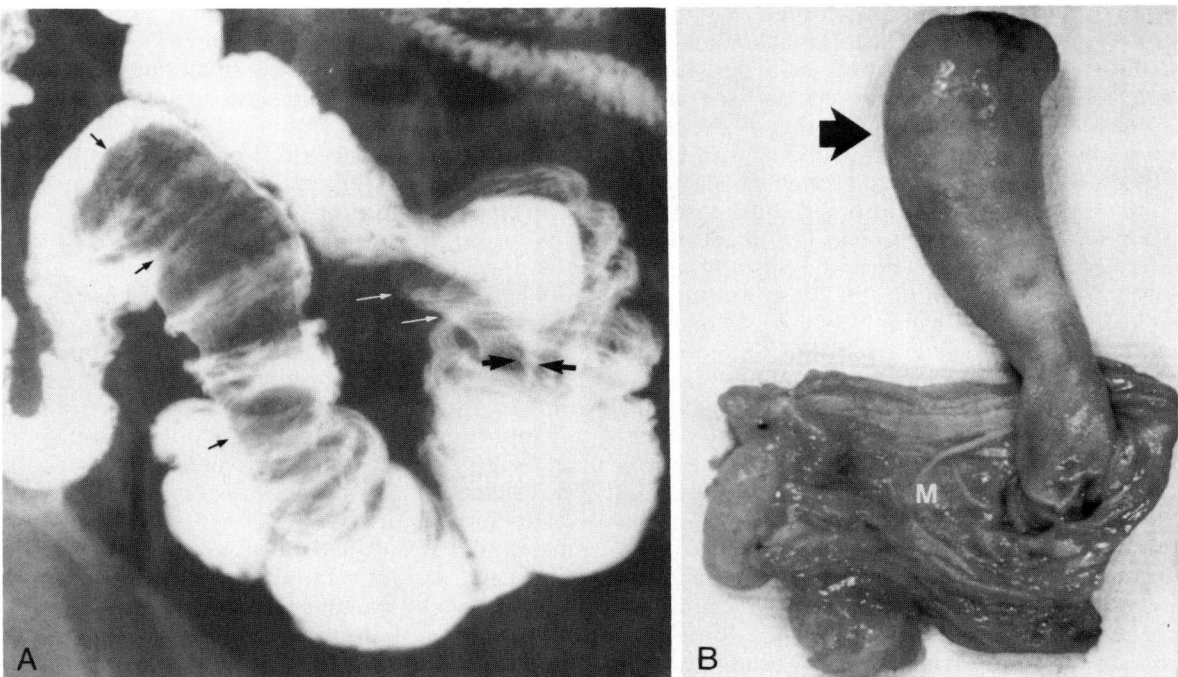

**Figure 52–51. Intussusception of an inverted Meckel diverticulum. A.** Spot film from a follow-through examination shows tapered narrowing of the small bowel *(large black arrows)* representing the intussusceptum. Barium refluxing into the intussuscipiens coats the mucosa, resulting in a coil spring appearance *(white arrows)*. Note the long, polypoid, intraluminal filling defect representing the invaginated Meckel diverticulum *(small black arrows)*. **B.** The surgically resected specimen shows the invaginated Meckel diverticulum as a long polypoid projection *(arrow)* protruding from the mucosal surface (M). (From Rubesin SE, Herlinger H, DeGaeta L: Interlude: test your skills. Radiology 176:636–644, 1990.)

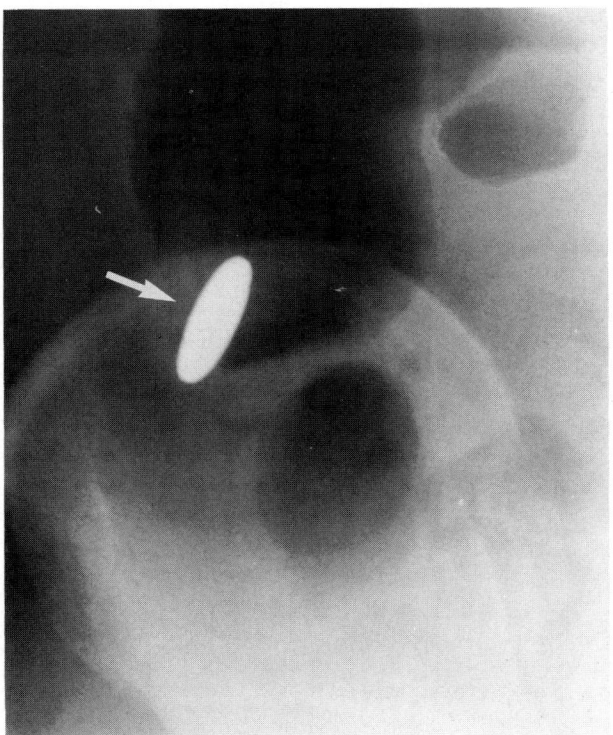

**Figure 52–52. Coin arrested in small intestine.** A coned-down view from an overhead "scout" radiograph before a barium enema shows a coin *(arrow)* overlying the right iliac bone. The air-distended viscus above it was later shown to be dilated small bowel, not cecum. According to the patient, the coin had been in his abdomen for more than 20 years. Subsequent enteroclysis showed a focal stricture in relation to the arrested coin.

shown to be induced by nonsteroidal anti-inflammatory agents.

Only a small percentage of foreign bodies lodge in the ileum (Fig. 52–52) compared with the esophagus, stomach, and colon.[63] SBO by foreign bodies in adults usually occurs in mentally disturbed or retarded patients. A few people who eat indigestible food substances such as persimmons develop small bowel bezoars, mostly in association with a partial gastrectomy or a gastroenterostomy. If a small bowel foreign body or bezoar is detected, the radiologist should search carefully for an underlying obstructive lesion.[64] (See also Chapter 55.)

Meconium ileus equivalent in adults with cystic fibrosis is an SBO related to inspissation of bowel contents and a history of negligent intake of pancreatic enzyme supplements.

## Acknowledgment

Figure 52–33A and B is reproduced from Herlinger H, Maglinte D (eds): Clinical Radiology of the Small Intestine. Philadelphia: WB Saunders, 1989.

Figure 52–47A and B is reproduced from Laufer I (ed): Double Contrast Gastrointestinal Radiology with Endoscopic Correlation. Philadelphia: WB Saunders, 1979.

# References

1. Schwartz SI, Storer EH: Manifestations of gastrointestinal diseases. In Schwartz SI, Shires GT, Spencer FC, et al (eds): Principles of Surgery. New York: McGraw-Hill, 1978, pp 1039–1079,
2. Summers RW, Lu CC: Approach to the patient with ileus and obstruction. In Yamada T (ed): Textbook of Gastroenterology. Philadelphia: JB Lippincott, 1991, pp 715–731.
3. Cho KC, Hoffman-Tretin JC, Alterman DD: Closed-loop obstruction of the small bowel: CT and sonographic appearance. J Comput Assist Tomogr 13:256–257, 1989.
4. Sykes PA, Boulter KH, Schofield PF: The microflora of the obstructed bowel. J Surg 63:721–725, 1976.
5. Cohn I Jr: Intestinal obstruction. In Berk JE, Haubrich WS, Kalser MH, et al (eds): Bockus Gastroenterology (4th ed). Philadelphia: WB Saunders, 1985, pp 2056–2080.
6. Wangensteen OH: Understanding the bowel obstruction problem. Am Surg 135:131–149, 1978.
7. Sarr MG, Bulkley GB, Zuidena GD: Preoperative recognition of intestinal strangulation obstruction. Prospective evaluation of diagnostic capability. Am J Surg 145:176–182, 1983.
8. Otamiri T, Sjoedahl R, Ihse I: Intestinal obstruction with strangulation of the small bowel. Acta Chir Scand 153:307–310, 1987.
9. Price J, Nolan DJ: Post-loop obstruction: diagnosis by enteroclysis. Gastrointest Radiol 14:251–254, 1989.
10. Maglinte DDT, Nolan DJ, Herlinger H: Preoperative diagnosis by enteroclysis of unsuspected closed-loop obstruction in medically managed patients. J Clin Gastroenterol 13:308–312, 1991.
11. Maglinte DDT, Herlinger H, Nolan DJ: Radiologic features of closed loop obstruction: analysis of 25 confirmed cases. Radiology 179:383–387, 1991.
12. Silen W, Hein MF, Goldman I: Strangulation obstruction of the small bowel. Arch Surg 85:121–129, 1962.
13. Glotzer DJ: Differential diagnosis in case records of the Massachusetts General Hospital, case 7–1987. N Engl J Med 316:394–403, 1987.
14. Fried MW, Murthy UK, Hassig SR, et al: Creatine kinase isoenzymes in the diagnosis of intestinal infarction. Dig Dis Sci 36:1589–1593, 1991.
15. Mucha P Jr: Small intestinal obstruction. Surg Clin North Am 67:597–620, 1987.
16. Smerud MJ, Johnson CD, Stephens DH: Diagnosis of bowel infarction: a comparison of plain films and CT scans in 23 cases. AJR 154:99–103, 1990.
17. Ketcham AS, Hoye RC, Pilch YH, et al: Delayed intestinal obstruction following treatment for cancer. Cancer 25:406–410, 1970.
18. Osteen RT, Guyton S, Steele G Jr, et al: Malignant intestinal obstruction. Surgery 87:611–615, 1980.
19. Arenha GV, Folk FA, Greenlee HB: Surgical evaluation of small bowel obstruction due to metastatic carcinoma. Am Surg 47:99–102, 1981.
20. Herlinger H, Maglinte DDT: Small bowel obstruction. In Herlinger H, Maglinte D (eds): Clinical Radiology of the Small Intestine. Philadelphia: WB Saunders, 1989, pp 479–507.
21. Shrake PD, Rex DK, Lappas JC, et al: Radiographic evaluation of suspected small bowel obstruction. Am J Gastroenterol 86:175–178, 1991.
22. Han SY, Laws HL, Aldrete JS: How and when to use barium for diagnosis of small bowel obstruction. South Med J 147:1519–1523, 1979.
23. Frimann-Dahl J: The administration of barium only in acute obstruction. Advantages and results. Acta Radiol 42:285–295, 1954.
24. Nelson SW, Christoforides AJ: The use of barium sulphate suspensions in the study of suspected mechanical obstruction of the small intestine. AJR 101:367–378, 1967.
25. Nelson SW, Christoforides AJ, Roenigh DVM: Dangers and fallibilities of iodinated radiopaque media in obstruction of the small bowel. Am J Surg 109:546–559, 1965.
26. Hunter TB, Fajardo LL, Jarvis JL, et al: Altered gastric and duodenal motility in intestinal obstruction. Gastrointest Radiol 15:193–196, 1990.
27. Maglinte DDT, Steven LH, Hall RC, et al: Dual purpose tube for enteroclysis and nasogastric/nasoenteric decompression. Radiology 185:281–282, 1992.
28. Davies RJ, Sandrasagra FA, Joseph AEA: Ultrasound demonstration of gallstone ileus. Clin Radiol 43:282–284, 1991.
29. Megibow AJ, Balthazar EJ, Cho KC, et al: Bowel obstruction: evaluating with CT. Radiology 180:313–318, 1991.
30. Fukuya T, Hawes DR, Lu CC, et al: CT diagnosis of small-bowel obstruction: efficacy in 60 patients. AJR 158:265–269, 1992.
31. Rennell C, McCort JJ: Bowel gas and fluid. In McCort JJ, Mindelzun RE, Filpi RG, et al (eds): Abdominal Radiology. Baltimore: Williams & Wilkins, 1981, pp 97–180.
32. Menzies D, Ellis H: Intra-abdominal adhesions and their prevention by topical tissue plasminogen activator. J R Soc Med 82:534–535, 1989.
33. Myrhe-Jensen O, Larsen SB, Astrup T: Fibrinolytic activity in serosal and synovial membranes. Arch Pathol 88:623–630, 1969.
34. Raftery AT: Effect of peritoneal trauma on peritoneal fibrinolytic activity and intraperitoneal adhesions formation. An experimental study in the rat. Eur Surg Res 13:397–401, 1981.
35. Ellis H: The causes and prevention of intestinal adhesions. Br J Surg 69:241–243, 1982.
36. Buckman RF, Buckman PD, Hufnagel HV, et al: A physiologic basis for the adhesion-free healing of deperitonealized surfaces. J Surg Res 21:67–76, 1976.
37. Caroline DF, Herlinger H, Laufer I, et al: Small-bowel enema in the diagnosis of adhesive obstruction. AJR 142:1133–1139, 1984.
38. Marshak RH, Khilnani MT, Eliasoph J, et al: Metastatic carcinoma of the small bowel. AJR 94:385–394, 1965.
39. Zboralske FF, Bessolo RJ: Metastatic carcinoma to the mesentery and gut. Radiology 88:302–310, 1967.
40. Goodman P, Raval B: CT diagnosis of acquired small bowel volvulus. Am Surg 56:628–631, 1990.
41. Pole AB, Dean DM: Computed tomography in volvulus of the midgut. Br J Radiol 63:893–894, 1990.
42. Duke JH, Yer MS: Primary small bowel volvulus. Arch Surg 112:685–688, 1977.
43. Ghahremani GG, Meyers MA: Internal abdominal hernias: current problems in radiology. Radiology 5:1–30, 1975.
44. Newsom BD, Kukora JS: Congenital and acquired internal hernias: unusual causes of small bowel obstruction. Am J Surg 152:279–285, 1986.

45. Stankey R: Intestinal herniation through the foramen of Winslow. Radiology 89:929–932, 1967.
46. Moertel CJ, Sauer WG, Dockerty MB, et al: Life history of the carcinoid tumor of the small intestine. Cancer 14:901–912, 1961.
47. McDonald RA: A study of 356 carcinoids of the gastrointestinal tract. Report of four new cases of the carcinoid syndrome. Am J Med 21:867–878, 1956.
48. Rubesin SE, Gilchrist AM, Bronner M, et al: Non-Hodgkin lymphoma of the small intestine. Radiographics 10:985–998, 1990.
49. Levine MS, Drooz AT, Herlinger H: Annular malignancies of the small bowel. Gastrointest Radiol 12:53–58, 1987.
50. Marshak RH, Wolf BS: Roentgen findings in regional enteritis. AJR 74:1000–1014, 1955.
51. Greenstein-Orel S, Rubesin SE, Jones B, et al: Computed tomography vs barium studies in the acutely symptomatic patient with Crohn's disease. J Comput Assist Tomogr 11:1009–1016, 1987.
52. Palmer KR, Patil DH, Basran GS, et al: Abdominal tuberculosis in urban Britain—a common disease. Gut 26:1296–1305, 1985.
53. Das Gupta T, Brasfield R: Metastatic melanoma—clinicopathological study. Cancer 17:1323–1339, 1969.
54. Dormandy TL: Gastrointestinal polyposis with mucocutaneous pigmentation (Peutz-Jeghers syndrome). N Engl J Med 256:1093–1103, 1957.
55. Oddson TA, Rice RP, Seigler HF, et al: The spectrum of small bowel melanoma. Gastrointest Radiol 3:419–423, 1978.
56. Ghahremani GG: Radiology of Meckel's diverticulum. Crit Rev Diagn Imaging 26:1–43, 1986.
57. Rubesin SE, Herlinger H, DeGaeta L: Interlude: test your skills. Radiology 178:636–644, 1990.
58. Eisenman JI, Fink EJ, O'Laughlin BJ: Gallstone ileus. A review of the roentgenographic findings and report of a new roentgen sign. AJR 101:361–365, 1967.
59. Balthazar EJ, Schechter LS: Gallstone ileus: the importance of contrast examinations in the roentgenographic diagnosis. AJR 125:374–378, 1975.
60. Grumbach K, Levine MS, Wexler JA: Gallstone ileus diagnosed by computed tomography. J Comput Assist Tomogr 10:146–148, 1986.
61. Czyrko C, Weltz CR, Markowitz RI, et al: Blunt abdominal trauma resulting in intestinal obstruction: when to operate? J Trauma 30:1567–1571, 1990.
62. Bjarnason I, Price AB, Zanelli G, et al: Clinicopathological features of nonsteroid antiinflammatory drug–induced small intestinal strictures. Gastroenterology 94:1070–1074, 1988.
63. Bloom RR, Nakano PH, Gray SW, et al: Foreign bodies of the gastrointestinal tract. Am J Surg 52:618–621, 1986.
64. Pice JE, Michawl SL, Morgenstein L: Fruit pit obstruction. The propitious pit. Arch Surg 111:773, 1976.

# Vascular Disorders

## 53

Daniel J. Nolan, M.D.

Hans Herlinger, M.D.

## MESENTERIC ISCHEMIA AND INFARCTION

### Introduction

A state of mesenteric vascular insufficiency exists when reduced blood flow can no longer supply the nutritional requirements of an organ, the small bowel in this context. Ischemia of mild to more severe grades and infarction are the consequences. Mesenteric ischemia can be classified as occlusive or nonocclusive. Arterial occlusion may be caused by embolus, thrombus, trauma, compression, or infiltration. Mesenteric venous occlusion is usually due to thrombosis.[1] Nonocclusive mesenteric ischemia may result from splanchnic vasoconstriction, usually as a result of hypovolemic shock. Ischemic changes and infarction usually involve the entire small intestine when there is interruption of the superior mesenteric arterial blood supply. In more peripheral occlusions, the ischemic changes may be localized to a shorter segment of the intestine.

The ischemic process causes a gradient of injury of the bowel wall. Initially, there is increased permeability of mucosal capillaries and mucosal epithelium. Further damage leads to shedding of epithelial cells and then to necrosis of the mucosa. Within 12 to 24 hours, necrosis may have become transmural. Postischemic reperfusion can exacerbate the injury caused by the hypoxia. The eventual survival or recovery of ischemic bowel depends to a large extent on the residual patency of its microvasculature.[2]

### Acute Intestinal Ischemia

#### Major Artery Occlusion

Sudden occlusion of the superior mesenteric artery results in acute ischemia of all or a large part of the intestine and frequently progresses to infarction. The right colon may also be affected. Embolic occlusion of the superior mesenteric artery may result from rheumatic mitral valve disease, the onset of atrial fibrillation, left ventricular thrombus after myocardial infarction, left atrial myxoma, or deep venous thrombosis with the embolus passing into the arterial circulation via a patent foramen ovale. Occlusion by thrombus usually results from arteriosclerotic disease that preferentially affects the origin of the superior mesenteric artery. Thus, occluding emboli are usually located somewhat more distally than thrombi in the superior mesenteric artery. Abdominal trauma, blunt or penetrating, may severely damage or transect the superior mesenteric artery. A midgut volvulus may cause vascular interruption of a considerable length of small intestine. However, the prognosis is less dismal because younger persons are more likely to be affected and the diagnosis can be made at an early stage by computed tomography (CT) by demonstrating characteristic whorls of narrowed bowel around the superior mesenteric artery.[3]

Acute mesenteric ischemia can manifest with the clinical triad of sudden onset of abdominal pain, preexisting cardiac disease, and spontaneous diarrhea and vomiting. These symptoms are nonspecific and frequently result in delayed diagnosis and treatment.[4] Leukocytosis is usual, but laboratory tests are generally not helpful. Mesenteric infarction is associated with a high mortality of up to 80 to 90%, largely because of the difficulty and delay in diagnosis.

Plain radiographs are important in the diagnosis of intestinal infarction. Gas-filled, slightly dilated loops of small intestine with multiple fluid levels may be seen at the time of presentation. Specific radiologic signs on plain abdominal radiographs are found in about 60% of patients. These include mucosal surface irregularity and thickening of the bowel wall. Intramural gas (Fig. 53–1), a grave sign of intestinal necrosis, may be seen as

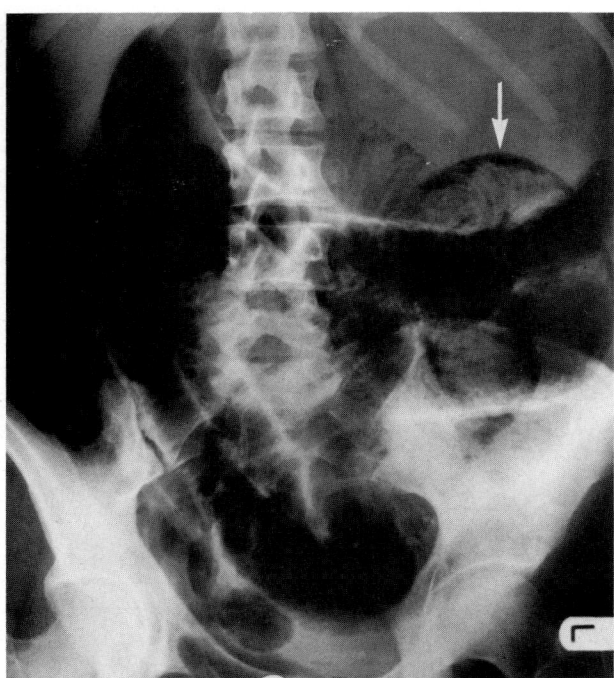

**Figure 53–1. Plain film evidence of intestinal infarction.** Gas in the bowel wall is shown as crescentic shadowing *(arrow)* and as widespread, small, slightly irregular shadows. (From Radin DR, Siskind BN, Alpert S, et al: Small-bowel varices due to mesenteric metastasis. Gastrointest Radiol 11:183–184, 1986.)

long linear streaks, irregular streaks, a localized speckled appearance, and small crescentic shadowing.[5] Intrahepatic portal air is uncommon. Arteriography is only occasionally performed in cases of suspected acute mesenteric ischemia and infarction.

## *Localized Ischemia*

Ischemia of acute onset involving a limited segment of bowel is more likely to result from embolism than from thrombosis; it may also be due to strangulation in a hernia or by a band or may be secondary to trauma. The most common cause is strangulation in an external or internal hernia, the latter often related to an adhesive band.[6] A closed loop obstruction of bowel herniated beneath a band-like adhesion does not necessarily imply that the bowel segment is already devitalized. Early recognition by enteroclysis (Fig. 53–2) has made surgical treatment possible at a time when the herniated bowel is still viable.[7, 8] In localized ischemia, prognosis is generally better than when a large portion of bowel is affected.

**Radiologic Findings.** Plain radiographs sometimes show the localized, air-filled ischemic segment with obvious thickening of the valvulae conniventes. On barium examination, thickening of the valvulae is characteristic (Figs. 53–3 and 53–4). A hallmark of localized ischemic lesions is fairly rapid change of their radiographic appearance, more often to normality than to features of deterioration.[9] CT may be preferred to barium study if gangrene is suspected clinically (Fig. 53–

5). When CT scans were evaluated together with plain abdominal films in 23 subsequently proven cases of infarction, specific changes were found in 15 (65%) of the patients.[10] A rarely demonstrated cause of extensive small bowel ischemia has been infiltration and gradual occlusion of the superior mesenteric artery by an advanced carcinoma of the pancreas (Fig. 53–6).

Blunt trauma to the abdomen may lead to stricture formation by two separate mechanisms.[11] The strictures are likely to occur near the proximal or distal extremes of the small intestine, where mesenteric mobility commences. A tear in the mesenteric attachment causes focal deprivation of blood supply. Alternatively, bowel may be crushed against the spine, usually as part of a seat belt injury. There may be an interval of months or years between the injury and the appearance of the ischemia-related stricture, shown on barium examination as a short, narrowed segment, sometimes with dilatation of bowel proximal to it (Fig. 53–7).

## Mesenteric Vein Thrombosis

Mesenteric vein thrombosis may result from portal hypertension, including that associated with schistosomiasis caused by *Schistosoma japonicum* or *Schistosoma mekoni*, abdominal or pelvic inflammation, abdominal surgery, trauma, renal and cardiac disease, oral contraceptive use, hematologic abnormalities, or a "hypercoagulable" state.[12] In more than 50% of cases, no cause is identified. The superior mesenteric vein is involved in 95% of cases.

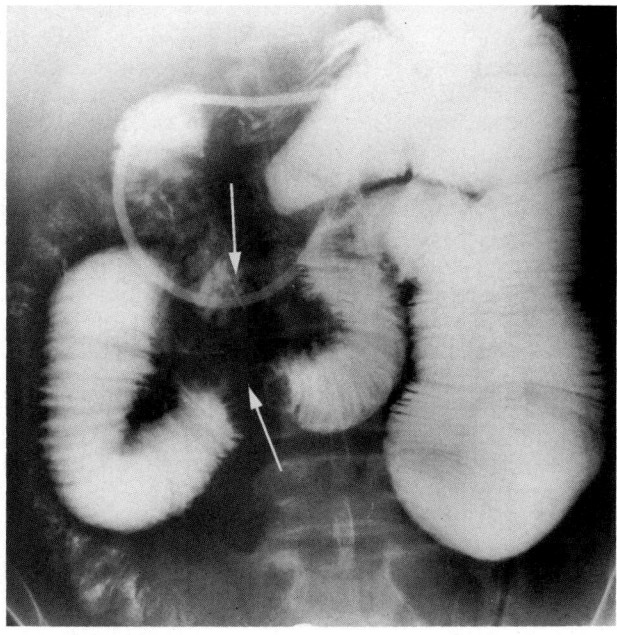

**Figure 53–2. Band obstruction with ischemia of the closed loop.** Note the slightly thickened valvulae in the closed loop, whereas other valvulae are normal. The arrows show the sites of band compression of the segments entering into and exiting from the closed loop obstruction. (From Price J, Nolan DJ: Closed loop obstruction: diagnosis by enteroclysis. Gastrointest Radiol 14:251–254, 1989.)

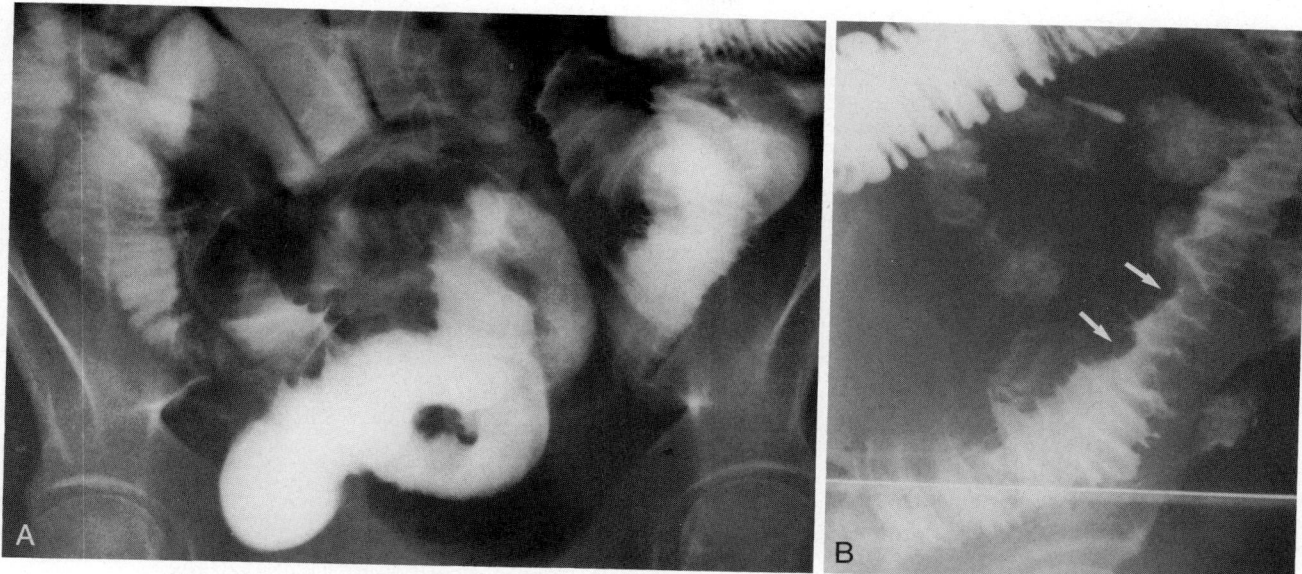

**Figure 53–3. Acute segmental intestinal ischemia. A.** Thickening of the valvulae conniventes is seen throughout much of the ileum. This 39-year-old female experienced acute abdominal pain 6 months after hemicolectomy for cecal volvulus. Symptoms resolved rapidly, and an examination 3 weeks later showed return to normal. (From Nolan DJ: Radiological Atlas of Gastrointestinal Disease. New York: John Wiley & Sons, 1983, p 209.) **B.** Segmental ischemia in a male diabetic. Thumbprinting along the mesenteric border *(arrows)* continues across the lumen as fold interruptions. Changes are most pronounced in the central part of the affected segment. The patient recovered fully.

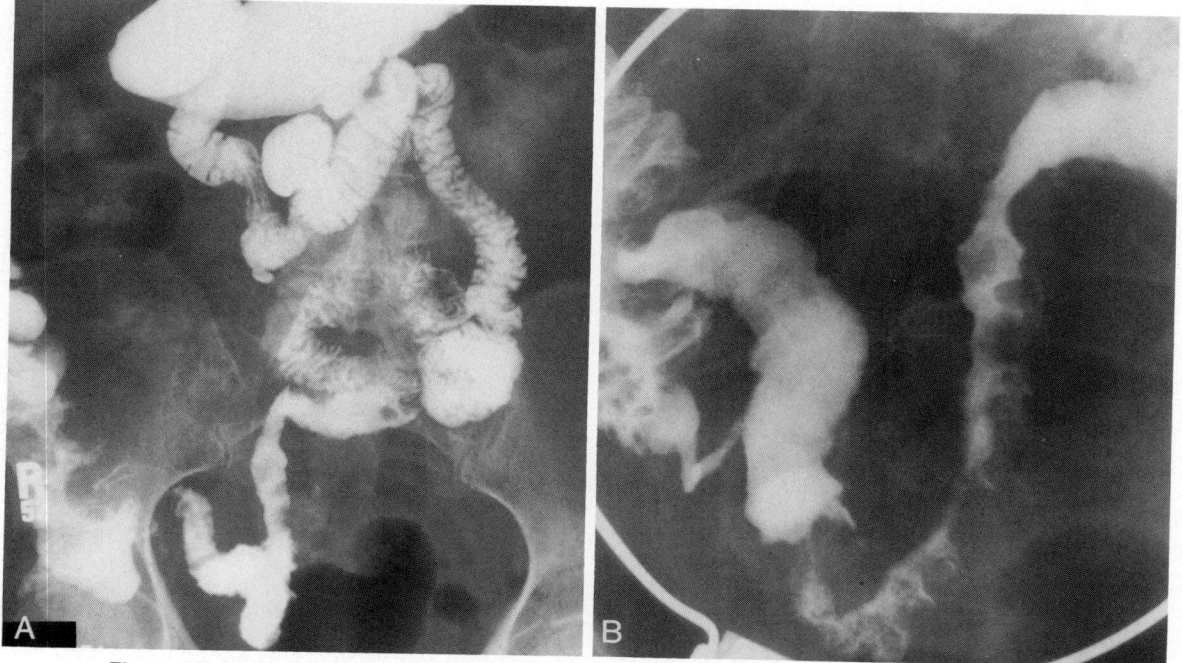

**Figure 53–4. Short bowel after massive resection because of infarction. A.** Overview with evidence or irregular narrowing distally. **B.** Compression spot film of narrowed segment provides evidence of renewed ischemia with lumen reduction and replacement of folds by thumbprint-like filling defects.

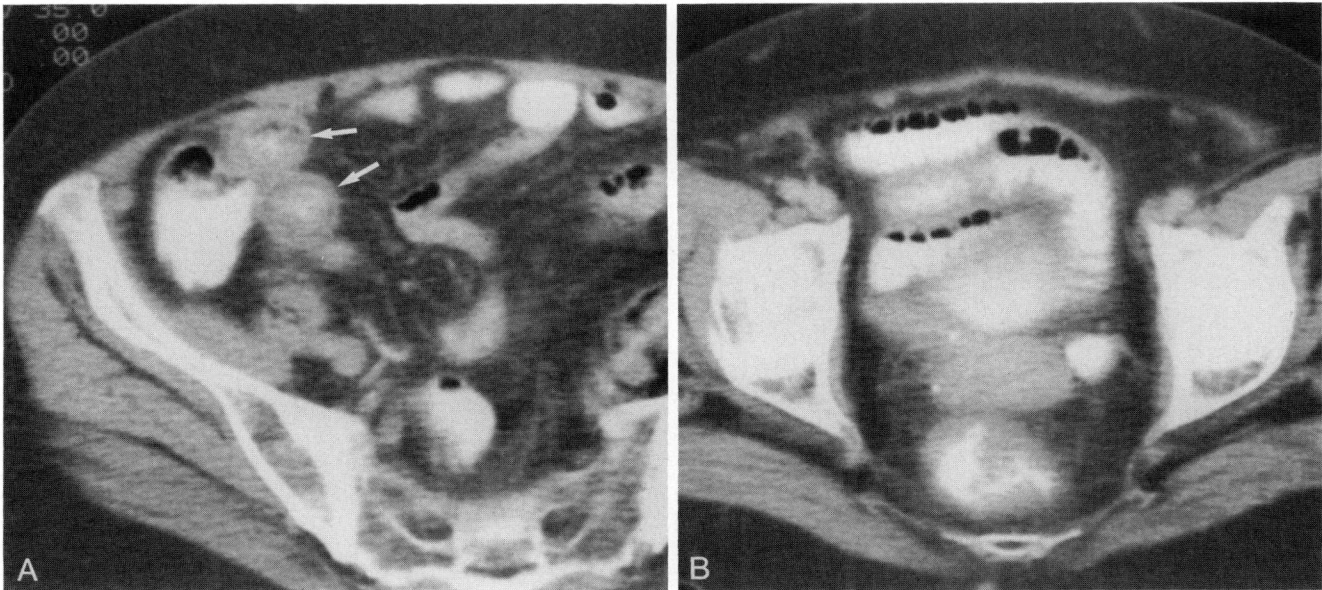

**Figure 53–5. Superior mesenteric artery thrombosis: CT scan. A.** Two dilated, thick-walled bowel loops show the "double halo" sign *(arrows)*. The mesenteric vessels appear congested. **B.** Loop of ileum filled with contrast medium. The bowel wall and valvulae conniventes are thickened. (**B** courtesy of Stephen E. Rubesin, M.D., Philadelphia, PA.)

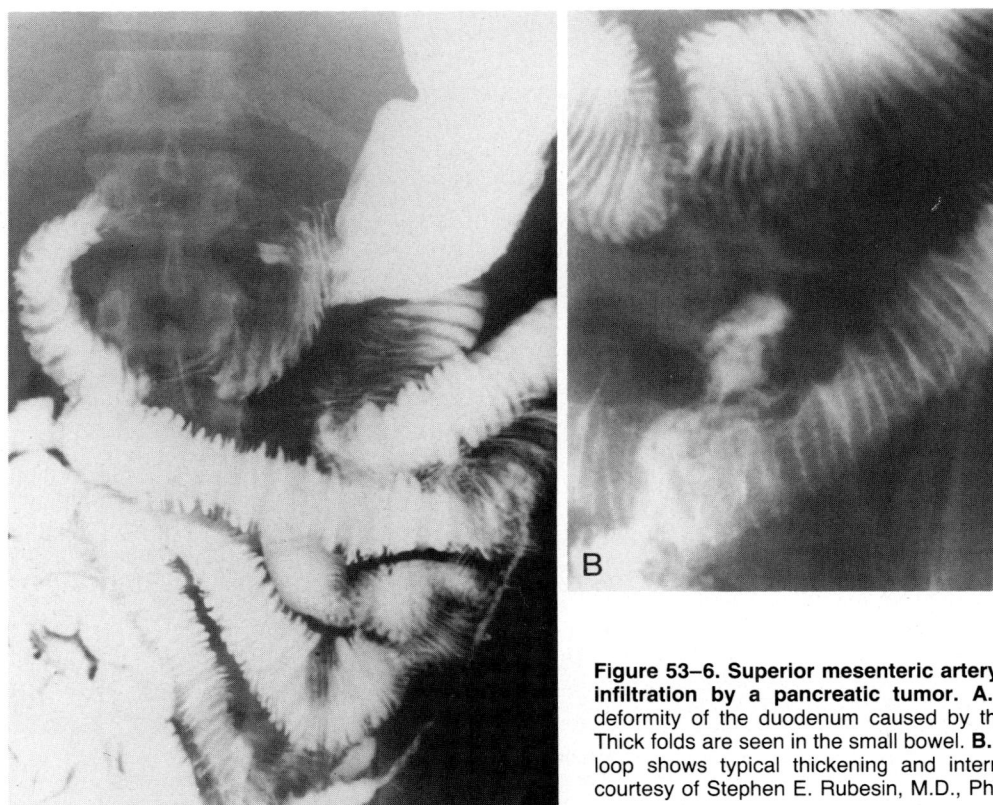

**Figure 53–6. Superior mesenteric artery compression and infiltration by a pancreatic tumor. A.** Displacement and deformity of the duodenum caused by the pancreatic mass. Thick folds are seen in the small bowel. **B.** A more distal bowel loop shows typical thickening and interruption of folds. (**B** courtesy of Stephen E. Rubesin, M.D., Philadelphia, PA.)

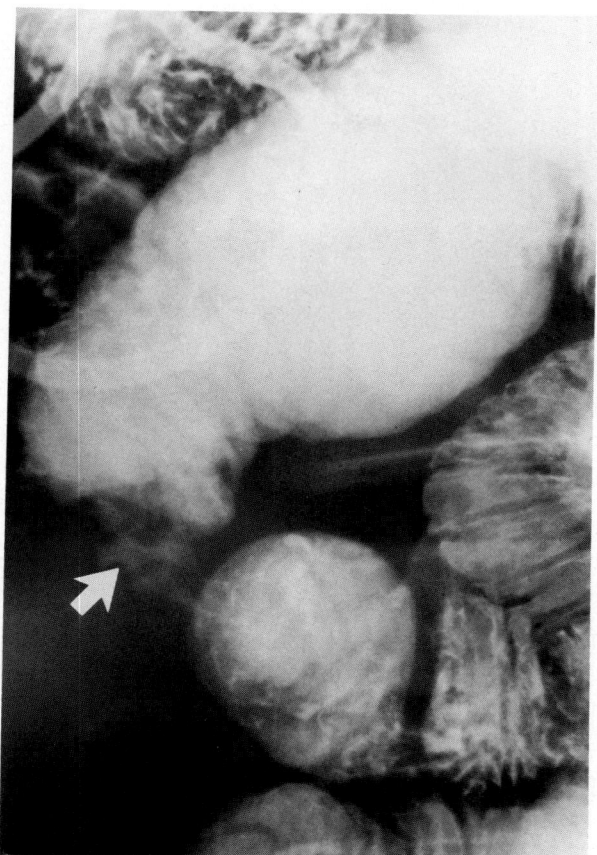

**Figure 53–7. Ischemic stricture caused by trauma.** A short stricture of the jejunum *(arrow)* causes partial obstruction and dilatation proximally. The patient had a history of crushing injury to the abdomen 3 months earlier. Histologic study showed ischemic damage of the circular muscle with contraction and fibrosis. (From Nolan DJ: Radiological Atlas of Gastrointestinal Disease. New York: John Wiley & Sons, 1983, p 221.)

## Clinicopathologic Features

Acute mesenteric vein thrombosis causes hyperemia, edema, and subserosal bleeding into the affected bowel segment, the appearances of a hemorrhagic infarct. Accumulation of blood in tissue and in the bowel lumen is more pronounced than in arterial occlusions. However, arterial thrombosis may be a secondary event in extensive venous occlusions, and it may then be difficult to determine the primary lesion. Rarely, thrombosis develops slowly enough for collateral venous drainage to develop and mitigate the damage to the affected bowel.[13] The symptoms have a more gradual onset than in arterial ischemia but again include severe and intensifying abdominal pain, usually intermittent and colicky, and bloody diarrhea and vomiting.

## Radiologic Findings

Plain abdominal radiographs show ominous, but nonspecific, dilated and gas-filled loops of intestine with pronounced thickening of the intestinal wall and mucosal

irregularity. An edematous bowel segment may appear as a gas-containing structure, straight or gradually curving because of wall thickening and not changing in shape between upright and decubitus views.[14] Not infrequently, thumbprinting may be identified along the mesenteric margin of a distended bowel loop (Fig. 53–8). Occasionally, as a late finding, air may be seen in the intestinal wall. CT is capable of demonstrating wall- or vessel-contained gas that is not yet visible on plain films.

In barium studies, prominently thickened valvulae conniventes are the invariable finding in the acute stage. The intramural accumulation of blood may distend the submucosa to such a degree that folds, because of their core of submucosa, become focally flattened, especially along the mesenteric border. This causes the thumbprinting, which is, however, not specific for infarction or ischemia. It can also occur with inflammatory infiltrates, as in Crohn's disease. The mesenteric border filling defects and the fold thickening are maximal in the center of the ischemic segment. With a large amount of intramural blood, the lumen becomes narrowed and only shallow mesenteric border indentations remain. Because of wall thickening, there is always separation from adjacent bowel loops. Often, even with radiologic changes that appear severe, recovery and a return to normal appearance are likely (Fig. 53–9).

CT scans, after bolus injection of intravenous contrast medium, may establish the diagnosis of venous thrombosis noninvasively. A low-density clot within the superior mesenteric vein may be seen surrounded by a

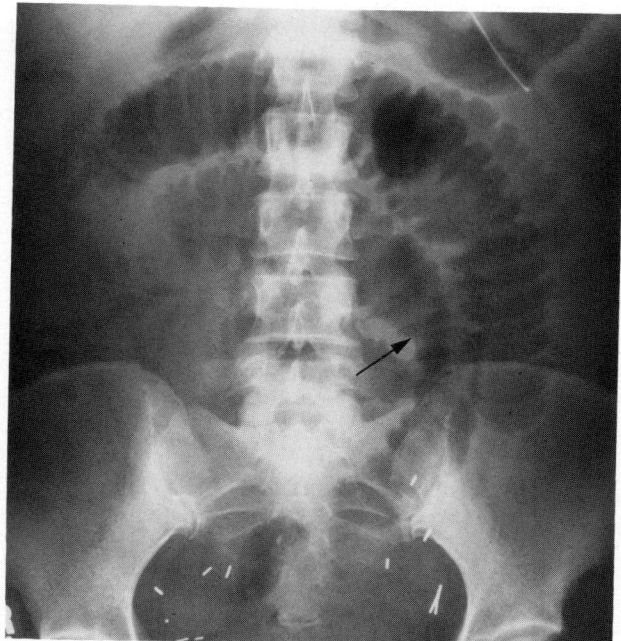

**Figure 53–8. Thumbprinting seen on a plain film of the abdomen.** Plain abdominal film 1 week after total abdominal hysterectomy. Dilated small bowel loops with thick folds are seen. There is also evidence of thumbprinting *(arrow)*. Laparotomy showed that a fibrous adhesion in the right broad ligament area was the cause of twisting and ischemia in viable bowel. (Courtesy Stephen E. Rubesin, M.D., Philadelphia, PA.)

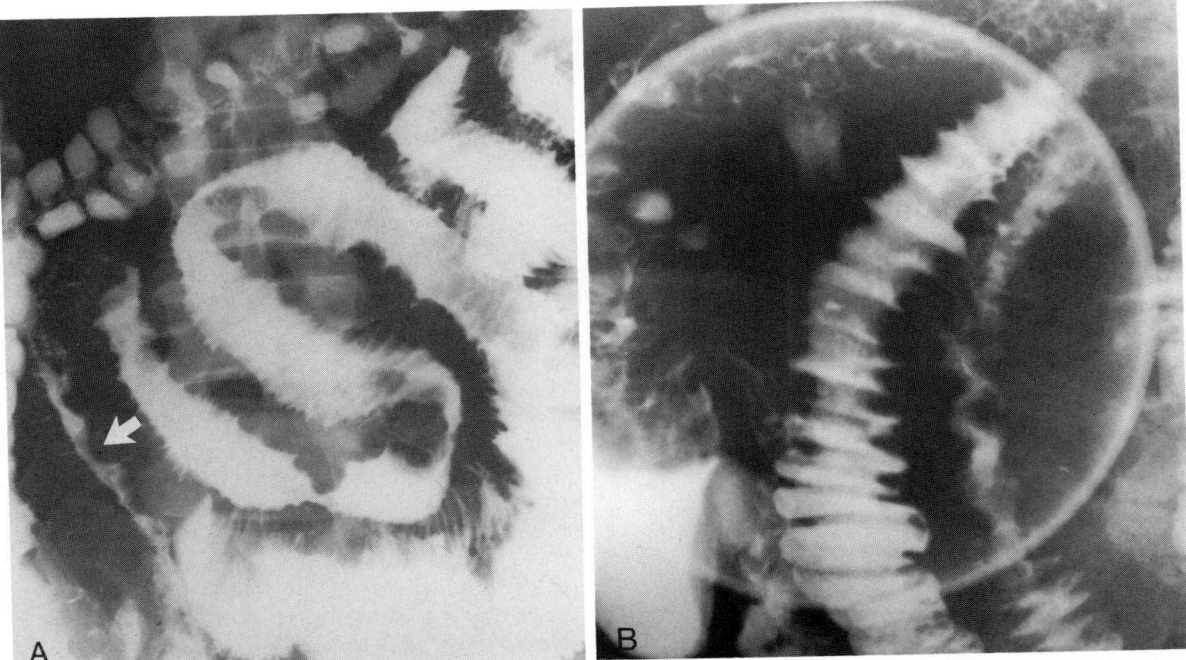

**Figure 53–9. Two cases of mesenteric vein thrombosis. A.** This young woman taking oral contraceptives complained of severe abdominal pain. The follow-through examination shows ileum with thick walls (see separation of loops), mildly thickened folds, pronounced thumbprinting along mesenteric borders, and severe compression of a distal segment *(arrow)* by massive accumulations within the bowel wall. A further examination 10 days later showed virtual normality. **B.** Chronic ischemia caused by mesenteric venous obstruction. Marked thickening of the valvulae conniventes and narrowing of the lumen are seen in this segment of the ileum. At operation a carcinoid tumor mass was found infiltrating the root of the mesentery, obstructing the mesenteric veins. (**B** from Nolan DJ: Radiological Atlas of Gastrointestinal Disease. New York: John Wiley & Sons, 1983, p 210.)

ring of relative contrast enhancement.[15] Magnetic resonance imaging is an alternative method for demonstrating stagnant flow in the superior mesenteric–portal vein complex (Fig. 53–10).

Patients with segmental venous thrombosis may recover spontaneously; others have benefited from anticoagulant therapy. At times it is considered advisable to proceed to surgery. Resection should be done beyond the apparent limits of infarction to avoid leaving behind thrombosed veins. Results of surgery are generally better than with arterial infarction.

## Nonocclusive Mesenteric Ischemia

The underlying mechanism is splanchnic vasoconstriction severe enough to overwhelm the normal autoregulatory processes at the intestinal microvascular level. This may occur in states of severe physiologic stress when the blood supply is diverted to more vital organs. The real incidence of significant nonocclusive ischemia is probably 10 to 20% of cases of acute mesenteric ischemia.

Diagnosis and distinction from occlusive disease can be difficult. Plain abdominal films are not helpful. The radiographic diagnosis is made by superior mesenteric angiography demonstrating nonobstructed vasculature with overall narrowing of vessels and reduced opacification of the bowel parenchyma. Tolazoline or papav-

erine is injected through the mesenteric catheter, followed by continuous infusion with the catheter left in place. A control contrast agent injection may be done. Surgery is done later, if needed. (For detailed information see Chapter 45.)

## *Drugs as a Cause of Ischemia*

Digitalis is a potentially powerful vasoconstrictive agent. It not only reduces splanchnic flow but also causes precapillary sphincters in the intestinal mucosa to contract. Dopamine and vasopressin are other cardiac drugs likely to have a vasoconstrictive effect. Cocaine increases catecholamine stimulation of alpha receptors in the splanchnic bed, causing intense vasoconstriction. "Body packers," persons who ingest packages of cocaine, are at risk. Ergotamines used in the treatment of migraine may cause mesenteric artery spasm.

## Chronic Mesenteric Ischemia

Intestinal angina is the clinical expression of chronic intermittent mesenteric ischemia. Patients present with pain after eating, often associated with nausea, vomiting, diarrhea, and weight loss. The pain may be sufficiently intense for the patient to fear eating (sitophobia). However, this is a rare condition because an effective collateral vascular supply system exists for both colon

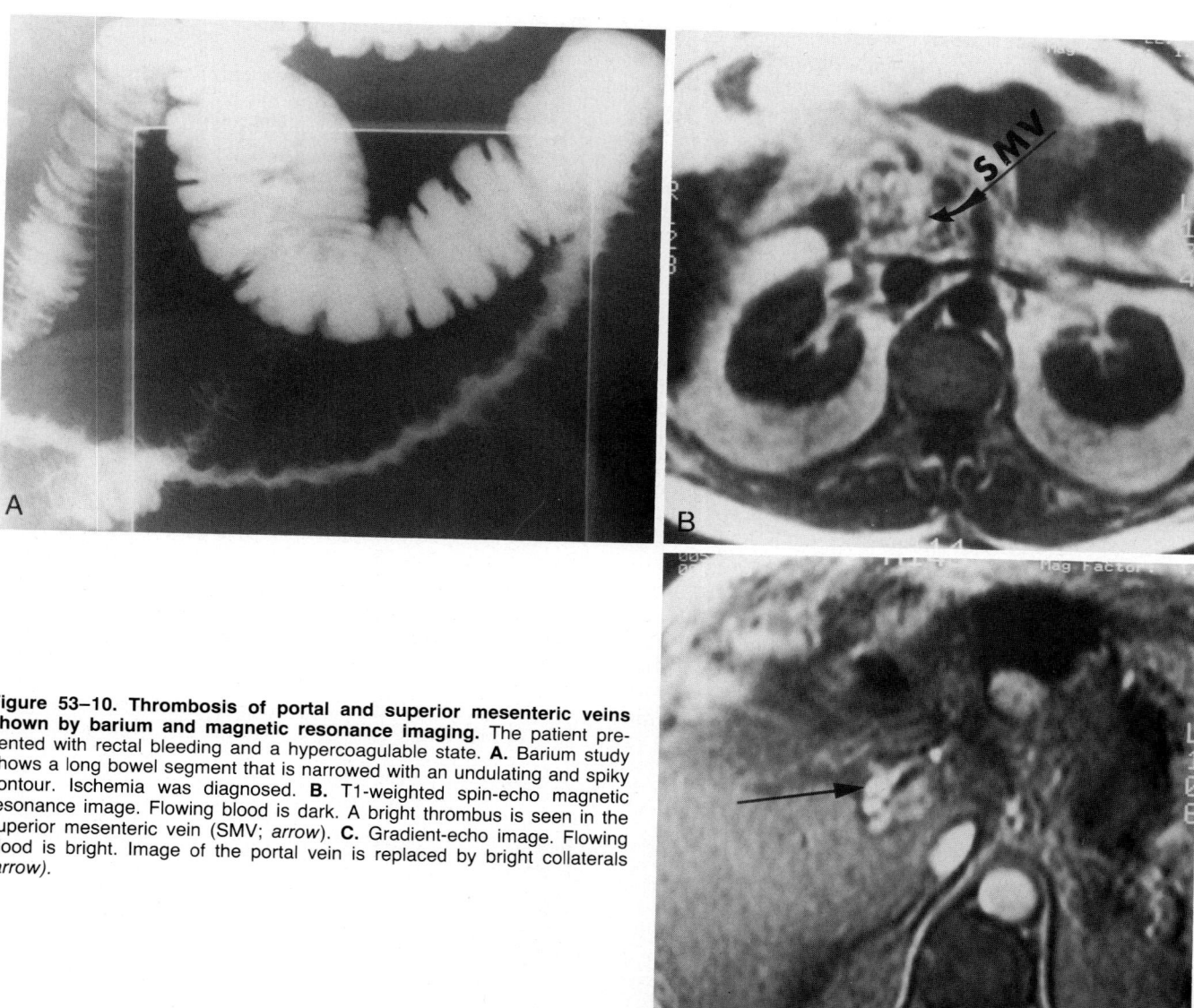

**Figure 53–10. Thrombosis of portal and superior mesenteric veins shown by barium and magnetic resonance imaging.** The patient presented with rectal bleeding and a hypercoagulable state. **A.** Barium study shows a long bowel segment that is narrowed with an undulating and spiky contour. Ischemia was diagnosed. **B.** T1-weighted spin-echo magnetic resonance image. Flowing blood is dark. A bright thrombus is seen in the superior mesenteric vein (SMV; *arrow*). **C.** Gradient-echo image. Flowing blood is bright. Image of the portal vein is replaced by bright collaterals (*arrow*).

and small bowel. Thus, a diagnosis of intestinal angina would be justified only if at least two of the major mesenteric arteries are shown to be occluded and the third artery narrowed by atheroma. A noninvasive alternative to angiography is duplex Doppler ultrasound for the measurement of blood flow in targeted vessels.

When the diagnosis is confirmed, percutaneous transluminal angioplasty may successfully recanalize occluded major arteries.[16] (See Chapter 45.)

## RADIATION ENTERITIS

### Introduction

Chronic radiation enteritis, although an infrequent sequela to abdominopelvic radiation therapy, is a signif-

icant cause of morbidity in patients who survive malignant disease. The underlying pathologic process is an endarteritis obliterans, and compromise of the microvascular circulation is an important factor in the natural history of radiation changes in the intestine.[17]

There is no relationship between the severity of gastrointestinal symptoms during radiotherapy and the subsequent development of chronic radiation enteritis. In one series,[17] about half of the patients who developed chronic radiation enteritis reported diarrhea during radiotherapy. The latent period between radiotherapy and the onset of symptoms varies considerably. Occasionally, gastrointestinal symptoms experienced during radiotherapy may merge imperceptibly into those of chronic radiation enteritis, whereas in other patients symptoms of radiation damage may occur as long as 25 years later. In most cases, features of radiation enteritis appear within 12 years of radiotherapy.

Factors that predispose to the development of chronic radiation enteritis include prior abdominal surgery with adhesive anchoring of bowel loops, peritonitis before the radiotherapy, hypertension, atherosclerosis, diabetes, and a high radiation dose given over a short time. Associated chemotherapy lowers the patient's threshold for radiation damage. Characteristic presenting symptoms include colicky abdominal pain, diarrhea, malabsorption, and small intestinal obstruction.

## Pathophysiology

An acute stage of radiation damage, concurrent with or shortly after radiation, is associated with reduction of crypt cell mitoses. With fewer epithelial cells available, villi become shorter and the mucosa becomes thinner. Mucosal and submucosal edema, hyperemia, inflammatory cell infiltration, and even ulceration occur in this acute stage. Later, in a subacute stage 2 to 12 months after treatment, the mucosa heals and obliterative changes affect arterioles in the submucosa and may lead to thrombosis. The submucosa begins to show fibrotic thickening. Ischemia-related changes merge into the chronic phase. Fibrosis involves the muscularis, ulcerations are seen, the serosa undergoes a diffuse hyaline change, and there are adhesions to other bowel loops. Progressive fibrosis may cause stricture formation.

## Radiologic Appearances

Patients with acute radiation enteritis are not usually referred for a barium examination because temporary interruption of treatment is usually effective. In a patient referred for enteroclysis, bowel loops appeared spastic with thickened folds. With methylcellulose infusion the lumen became distended and folds showed a normal thickness (Fig. 53–11). This would be the expected sequence of findings in mucosal or submucosal edema, an expected feature of acute radiation damage.

In chronic radiation enteritis, a variety of radiologic signs may be present, including thickened valvulae conniventes, wall thickening, later effacement of the mucosal fold pattern, ulceration, stenosis, adhesions, and occasionally sinuses and fistulas.[18, 19] Thickening of valvulae conniventes results from submucosal edema and/or fibrosis. Folds are not only thickened but also held in fairly close approximation to one another so that the fold thickness exceeds the distance between folds. Therefore, barium between the folds may have a spiky appearance (Fig. 53–12). The thickened folds tend to be straight and parallel, whereas in Crohn's disease the thickening is irregular and folds often show fusion and may be distorted. Mural thickening is usual and can be estimated if two adjacent loops are arranged with their mucosal surfaces parallel. Peristaltic activity is decreased or absent in the affected segments. Adherent, featureless pelvic loops cannot be separated, even with com-

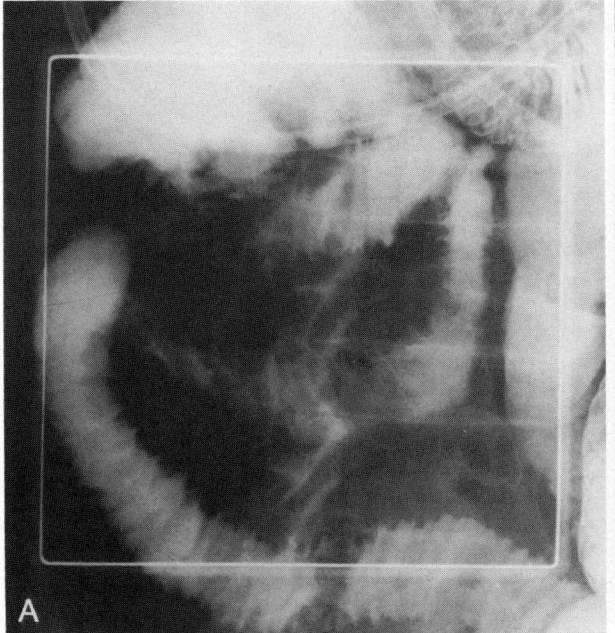
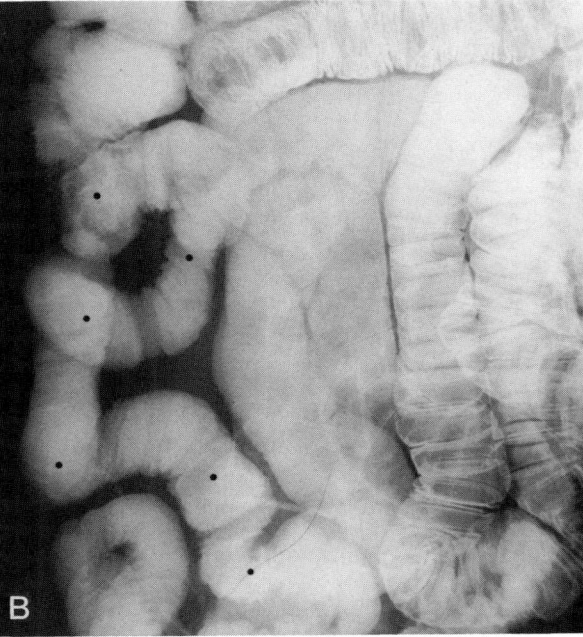

**Figure 53–11. Acute radiation enteritis.** Radiotherapy was given after resection of a cecal carcinoma. Near the end of the course of radiotherapy, the patient complained of diarrhea and abdominal pain. Enteroclysis was requested. **A.** Enteroclysis, single contrast phase. The neoterminal ileum shows thickened folds and a reduced lumen diameter. **B.** After methylcellulose infusion, the lumen of the neoterminal ileum *(dots)* distended normally and folds were no longer thickened. Disappearance of fold thickening is usually seen when edema is present. A diagnosis of acute radiation enteritis was made.

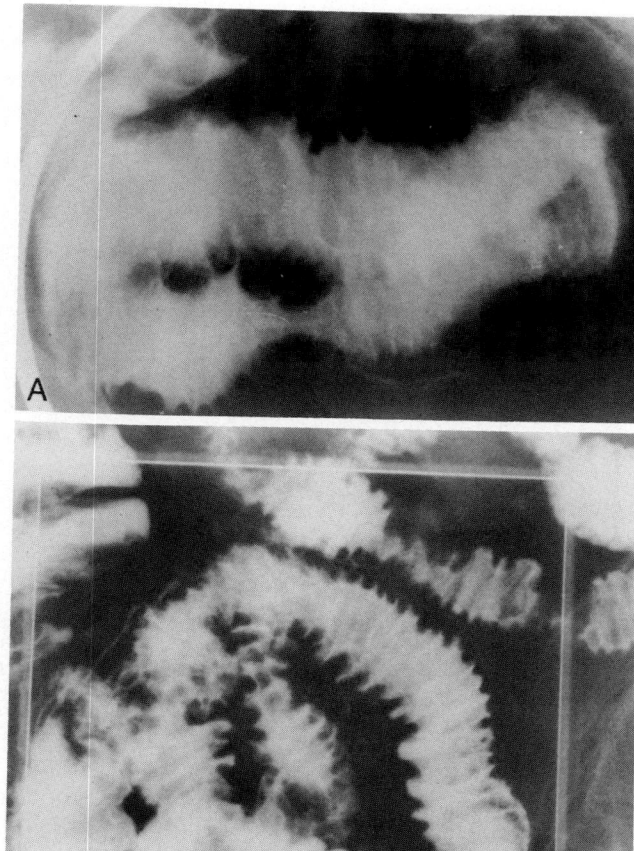

**Figure 53–12. Radiation enteritis. A.** A spot compression view shows thickening of the valvulae conniventes localized to a pelvic loop of ileum. Note the mucosal tacking. The region of apparent narrowing was not constant. (From Mendelson RM, Nolan DJ: The radiological features of radiation enteritis. Clin Radiol 36:141–148, 1985.) **B.** Extensive radiation damage after therapy for carcinoma of the cervix. Bowel loops are narrowed, folds are thickened, and interfold spaces are compressed with a spiky appearance of the edges of the loops. A coarse mucosal villous pattern is seen in most areas.

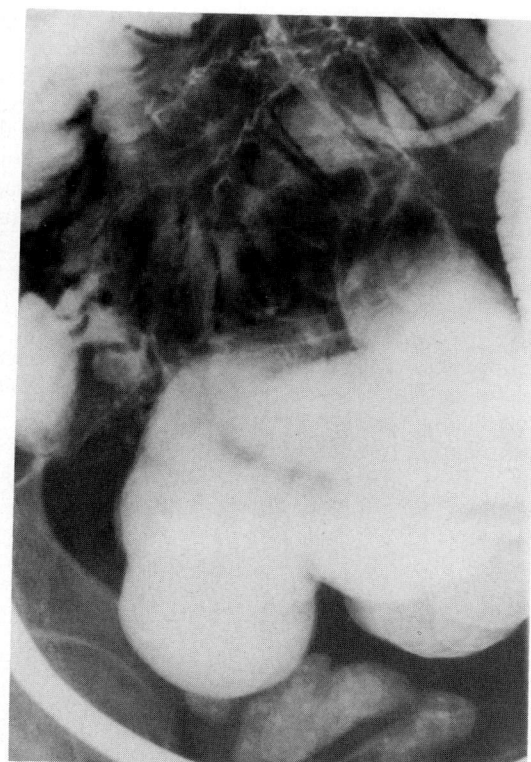

**Figure 53–13. Radiation enteritis.** Adherence between pelvic loops of ileum makes it difficult to identify individual loops and their mucosal pattern, the characteristic pool of barium appearance. (From Mendelson RM, Nolan DJ: The radiological features of radiation enteritis. Clin Radiol 36:141–148, 1985.)

tients with radiation-damaged intestine. Strictures are the cause in a minority of cases. More often, obstruction is due to the combined effect of length of gut involved, lumen narrowing, and reduced or absent peristalsis.

Adhesions between involved segments of intestine are usual and may be revealed by persistent angulation between adjacent loops, relative fixity of the loops, or a characteristic appearance of the mucosal pattern that has been termed *mucosal tacking*. The mucosal tacking

pression, which may result in the characteristic "pool of barium"[18, 20] appearance, making it difficult to distinguish individual segments (Fig. 53–13).

Ulceration is a common advanced feature of chronic radiation enteritis. Most of the ulcers are shallow and not appreciated on barium examination. Occasionally deep ulcers may be seen.[21] Large ulcers may occur in isolation but are more likely to be associated with strictures.

Narrowing of the intestinal lumen and stenosis are frequently found, and there may be dilatation of proximal bowel segments, indicating the presence of low-grade obstruction. Stenoses may be single or multiple and vary in length, from a short, narrowed segment (Fig. 53–14) to a stricture several centimeters long. Small bowel obstruction is a frequent problem in pa-

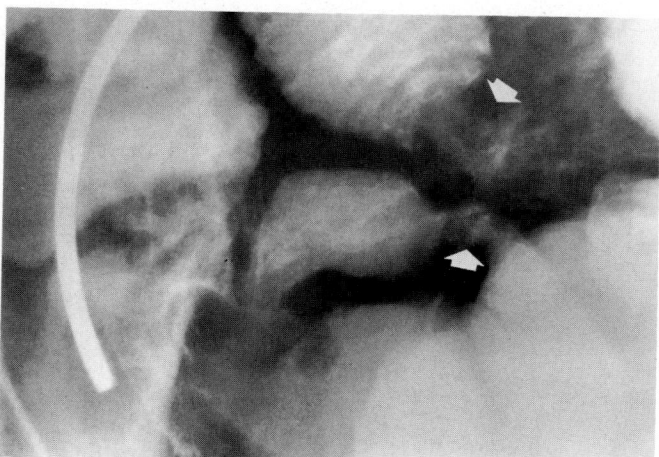

**Figure 53–14. Radiation enteritis.** Two short radiation strictures are seen in adjacent loops of ileum *(arrows).*

is seen as angulation, spiking, and distortion of mucosal folds at the antimesenteric edge of the intestine (Fig. 53–15; see Fig. 53–12). In this way, the folds differ from the usually regular and perpendicular arrangement in most cases of radiation enteropathy. Sinuses and fistulas are uncommon findings; they originate in a segment of radiation-damaged intestine (Fig. 53–16) and are particularly likely to develop at the site of a surgical anastomosis. Effacement of the valvulae conniventes is a gradually appearing, late feature, often associated with shallow ulceration, malabsorption, and bleeding (Fig. 53–17).

CT can provide useful information regarding radiation damage to the small bowel.[22] With high-grade radiation change causing small bowel obstruction, CT demonstrates the extent of wall thickening and of the surrounding fibrosis (Fig. 53–18A). With milder radiation change, CT outlines the affected bowel loop as accurately as enteroclysis (Fig. 53–18B and C).

## INTRAMURAL HEMORRHAGE

Bleeding into the wall of the small intestine may occur in 10 to 35% of patients receiving anticoagulant therapy.[23] Bleeding into the gastrointestinal tract is not always the result of anticoagulation alone; an associated focal lesion is a likely cause and should be looked for.[24] Hematomas are more often found in the jejunum.

Bleeding disorders that characteristically cause intra-

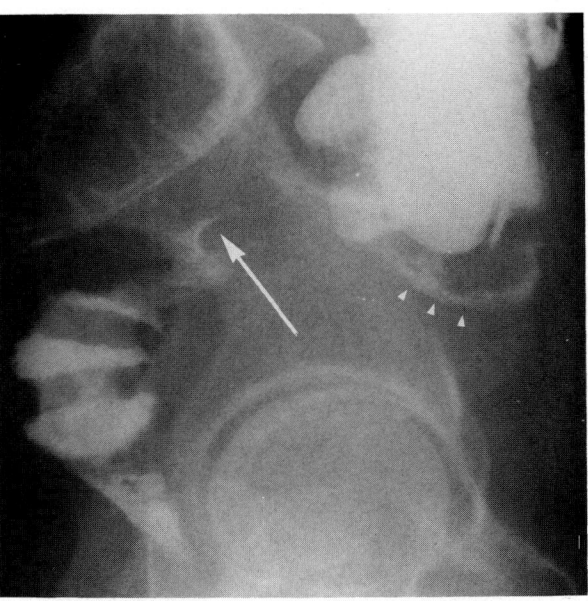

**Figure 53–16. Radiation enteritis with fistulas.** An ileorectal fistula *(arrow)* and an ileocutaneous fistula *(arrowheads)* are seen in a lateral view of the pelvis. (From Meagher T, Nolan DJ: The radiology of irradiated gut. *In* Galland RB, Spencer J [eds]: Radiation Enteritis. London: Edward Arnold, 1990, pp 88–102. Reproduced by permission of Edward Arnold [Publishers] Limited.)

mural hemorrhage include idiopathic thrombocytopenic purpura, leukemia, Henoch-Schönlein purpura, and, rarely, hemophilia.[25] Henoch-Schönlein purpura is described in the following section on vasculitis.

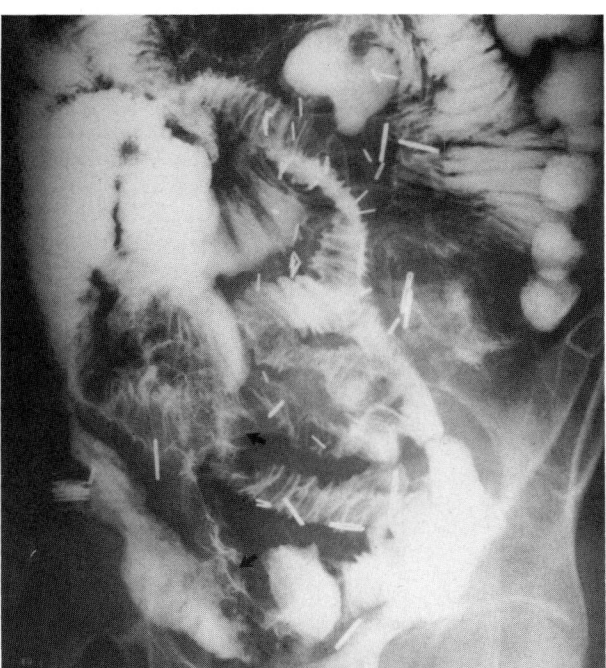

**Figure 53–15. Severe damage from radiation for carcinoma of cervix.** In most of the ileum, bowel segments are narrowed, mostly adherent and aperistaltic, with thick folds and spiky protrusions between folds. Radiation-related obstruction causes lumen distention of a few unaffected loops. A few thumbprints in pelvic loops *(arrows)* may be ischemic because of mesenteric fibrosis. A pelvic exenteration was required.

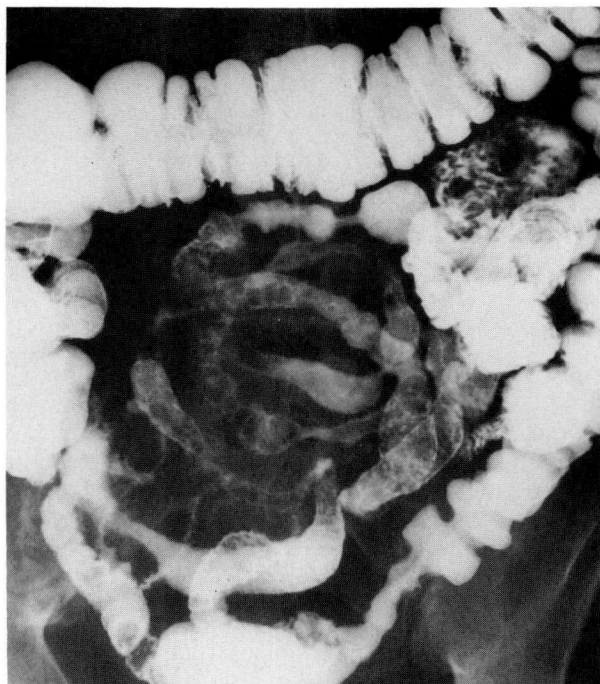

**Figure 53–17. Radiation enteritis involving all of the ileum several years after therapy of carcinoma of the cervix.** Late, atrophic stage of postradiation fibrosis. Loops are fixed in position, are aperistaltic, have barely visible shallow ulcers, and may bleed. Radiation also damaged the rectum and distal sigmoid colon.

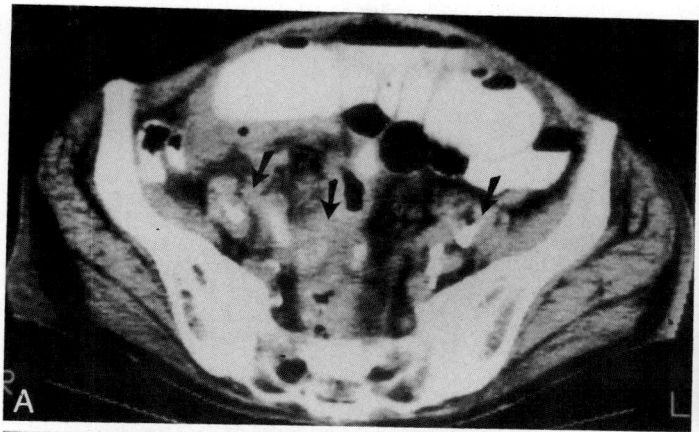
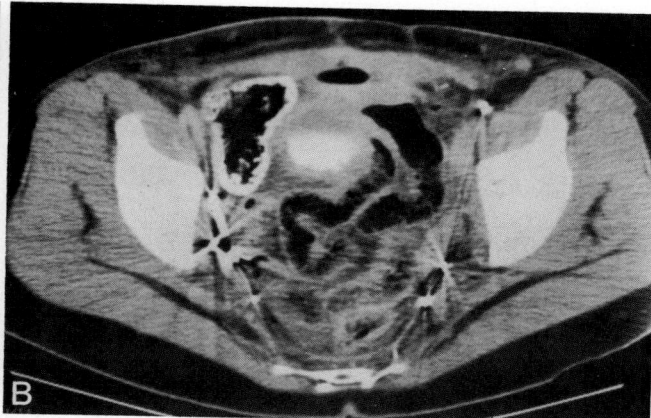

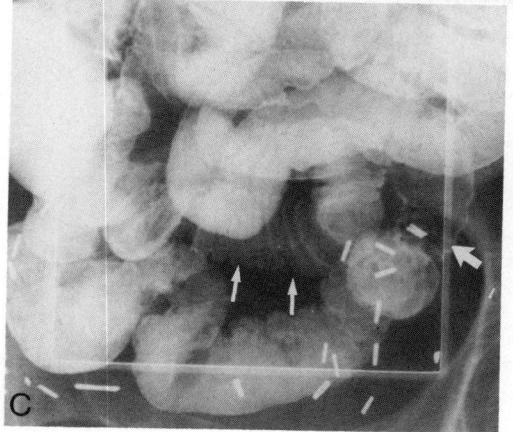

**Figure 53–18. CT scans of two patients irradiated for carcinoma of the cervix. A.** Chronic stage radiation enteritis. Many ileal loops are seen to be narrowed with thickened walls and much surrounding fibrosis *(arrows)*. These changes caused obstruction of proximal bowel loops. (Courtesy of Jill E. Langer, M.D., Philadelphia, PA.) **B.** Mild degree of chronic radiation damage. CT demonstrates fold thickening and slight thickening of the wall of a pelvic loop of ileum. (Streak artifacts result from surgical clips.) **C.** Enteroclysis in the patient in **B.** There is evidence of limited radiation damage to a pelvic loop of ileum *(arrows)*.

Intramural bleeding resulting from blunt trauma is more likely to involve the descending duodenum and occasionally causes intramural hemorrhage in the jejunum or ileum.

Patients with intramural hemorrhage characteristically present with abdominal pain, melena, intestinal obstruction, and/or an abdominal mass. Barium examination of the small intestine shows the changes to be segmental, diffuse, or localized. Uniform, regular thickening of the valvulae conniventes with a symmetric, spike-like configuration simulating a stack of coins may be seen[25] (Fig. 53–19A). In some cases, the thickening of the valvulae is so pronounced that the usual bowel margin is replaced by an undulating contour (Fig. 53–19B). A more localized intramural hemorrhage can manifest as an intramural mass (Fig. 53–20).

## VASCULITIS

An inflammatory occlusive process characterizes the large group of generally rare, systemic conditions that are associated with vasculitis affecting the intestine. Vasculitides can be distinguished by the associated extraintestinal pattern of involvement and by the type of mesenteric vessels they affect. As an example, Churg-Strauss vasculitis affects larger vessels and patients give a history of allergy and have eosinophilia.

In polyarteritis nodosa more than 50% of patients have been found to have visceral vasculitis at autopsy. Because medium-sized to smaller arteries are involved, the resulting bowel lesions can vary from extensive infarction to segmental ischemia.[26] Renal and liver involvement and hypertension are frequent. Hepatitis B virus infection has been associated with half of the cases of polyarteritis nodosa. Angiographic findings are small aneurysms on branches of the superior mesenteric artery.

Lupus erythematosus can cause gastrointestinal involvement by small vessel arteritis in 10 to 60% of cases. Segmental lesions may progress to necrosis and perforation.

Rheumatoid vasculitis usually takes the form of a polyarteritis nodosa. Initial fibrinoid necrosis of the wall of small arteries can progress to thrombosis and cause infarction. The resulting small bowel stricture has been demonstrated in a case report by radiology and pathology[27] (Fig. 53–21).

Henoch-Schönlein purpura affects children and young to middle-aged adults. The clinical presentation may be a triad of palpable purpura (nonthrombocytopenic), arthritis, and abdominal pain. The gastrointestinal tract is involved in more than half of the patients, and there may be hematuria. A postcapillary venulitis is the immediate cause of the intestinal changes, and vessel wall deposition of immunoglobulin A can be shown by direct

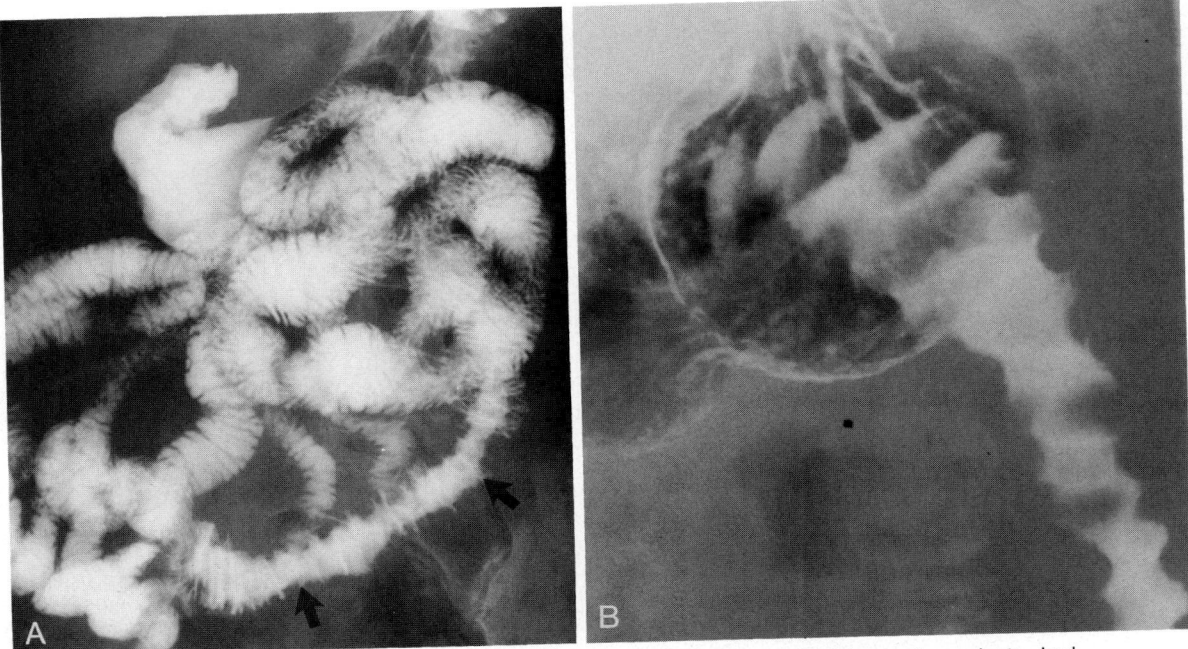

**Figure 53–19. Intramural hemorrhage. A.** The patient, who was receiving anticoagulants, had intramural bleeding into a segment of ileum. Note the stack of coins appearance of straight, thickened folds and reduced lumen diameter *(arrows)*. **B.** The valvulae conniventes are almost completely effaced by pronounced swelling of the submucosa. The bowel lumen is restricted. View of the proximal jejunum in a patient who had taken an excessive amount of anticoagulants.

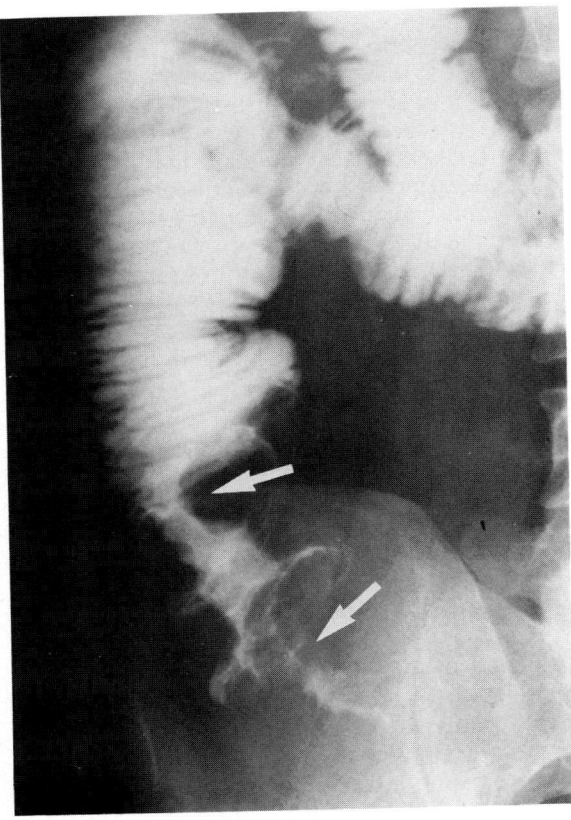

**Figure 53–20. Intramural hemorrhage.** Large, concentric submucosal filling defects *(arrows)* are seen in a short segment of small intestine in a patient receiving anticoagulant therapy. The patient presented with intestinal obstruction. (Courtesy of W. J. Norman, M.D., Shrewsbury, England.)

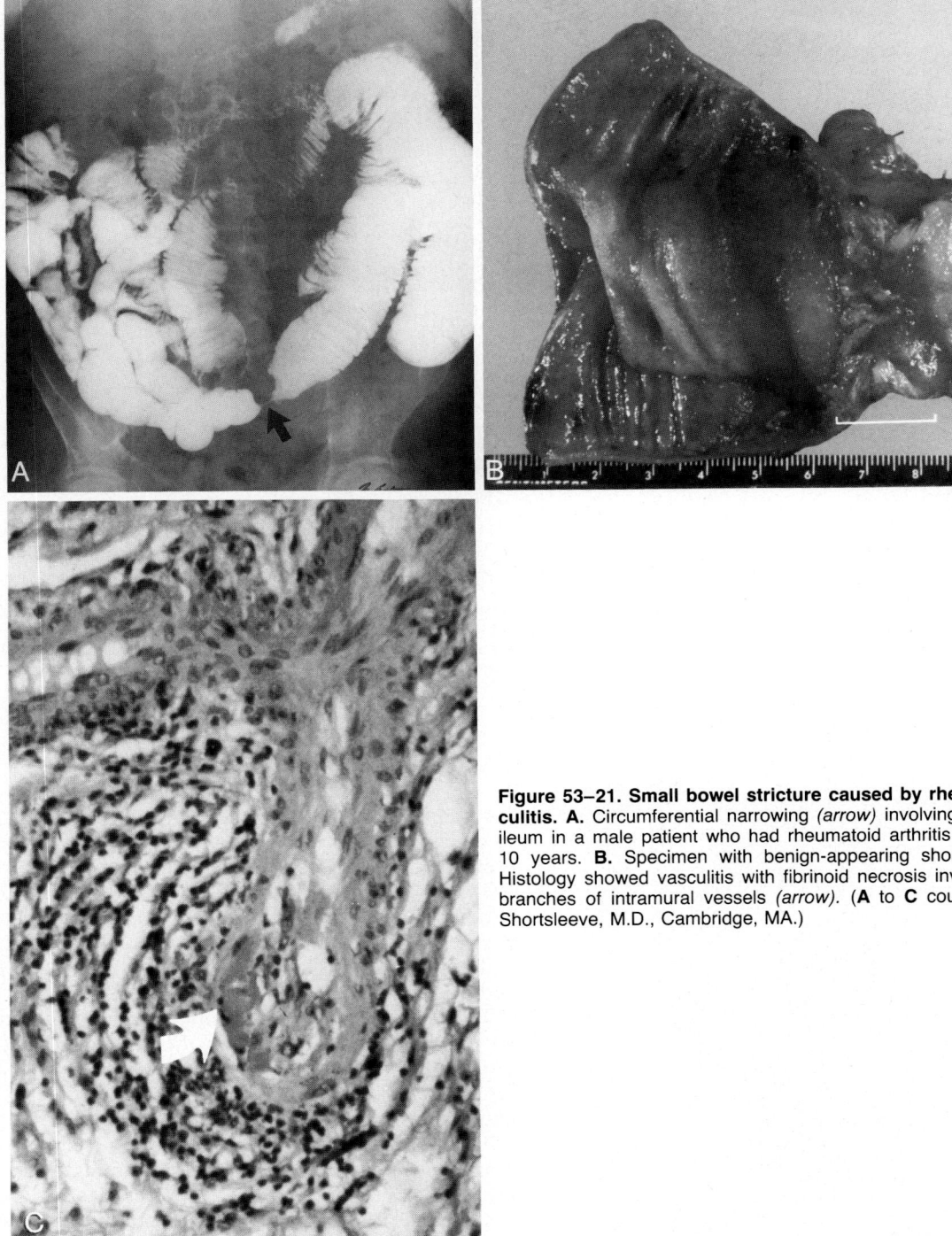

**Figure 53–21. Small bowel stricture caused by rheumatoid vasculitis. A.** Circumferential narrowing *(arrow)* involving 4 cm of mid-ileum in a male patient who had rheumatoid arthritis for more than 10 years. **B.** Specimen with benign-appearing short stricture. **C.** Histology showed vasculitis with fibrinoid necrosis involving several branches of intramural vessels *(arrow)*. (**A** to **C** courtesy of M. J. Shortsleeve, M.D., Cambridge, MA.)

immunofluorescence.[28] Full-thickness necrosis and perforation are rare. Bowel contents are likely to be bloody and the mucosa edematous with features of congestion and hemorrhage. Hemorrhage is mostly confined to the mucosa and submucosa. Erosions and even ulcers are found. Larger vessels are unaffected. Intussusceptions are likely to occur in the childhood form of Henoch-Schönlein purpura but are unusual in adults.[29]

Barium studies show straight, thick folds, usually with a widened lumen and involving a lengthy segment of proximal intestine (Fig. 53–22). Unlike patients with polyarteritis nodosa, for whom early steroid therapy is indicated to reduce renal injury, patients with Henoch-Schönlein purpura tend to recover spontaneously and heal without sequelae, although scarring and stenosis may develop in some cases. However, there may be belated renal involvement, which in few cases can progress to chronic renal disease.

Involvement of the gastrointestinal tract is seen in 10 to 15% of patients with Behçet's disease, a chronic systemic condition with diverse symptoms that mostly affects males between 11 and 30 years of age.[30] Orogenital ulceration is a characteristic feature, although many systems may be involved. Esophageal ulcerations are frequent and may cause bleeding, stricture, and even perforation.[31] The histopathologic basis of the disorder is a nonspecific necrotizing vasculitis. Symptoms may show a pattern of exacerbations and remissions. During the acute phase, patients with gastrointestinal involvement may complain of abdominal pain, vomiting, diarrhea, or constipation. The small and large intestine and, in particular, the ileocecal area may show changes resembling those in Crohn's disease (Fig. 53–23).

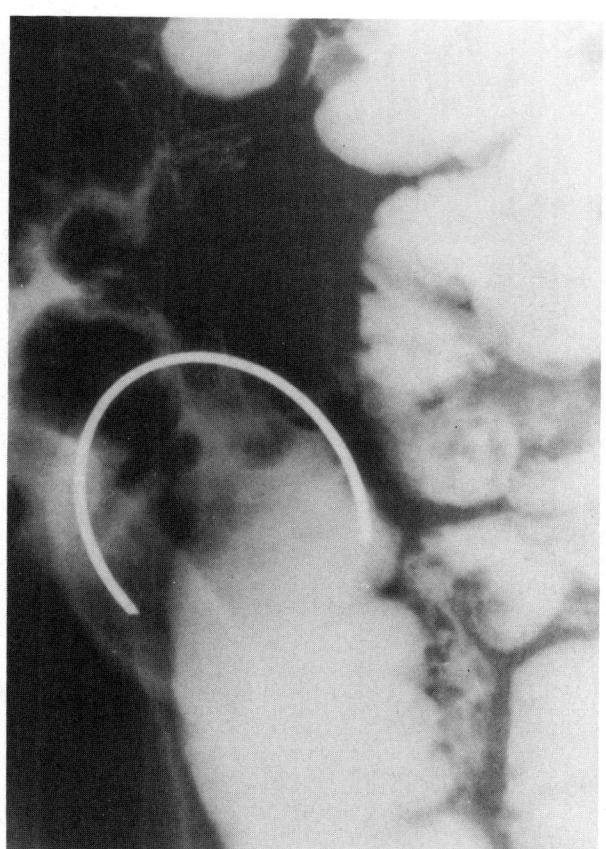

**Figure 53–23. Behçet's disease.** Narrowing and irregularity of the terminal ileum with slight dilatation more proximally are seen in a patient with known Behçet's disease. Note that the ileocecal valve is enlarged. (Courtesy of D. J. Allison, M.D., London.)

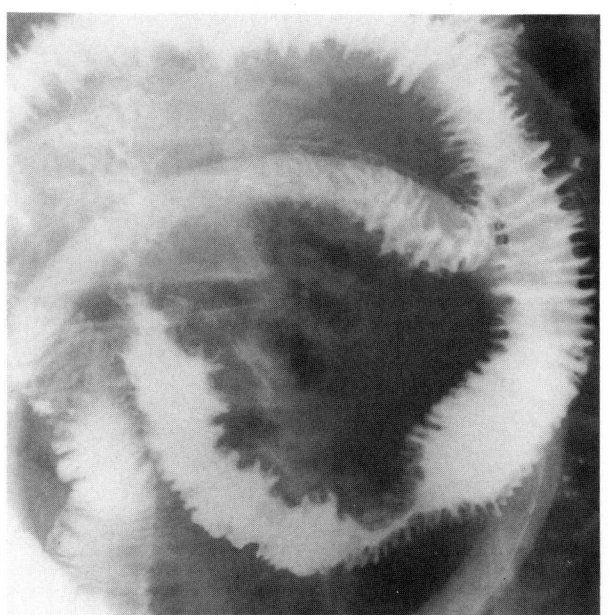

**Figure 53–22. Barium study of a young adult with Henoch-Schönlein purpura.** Fold thickening in partly widened lumen involves about 18 inches of proximal jejunum. The patient recovered without steroids.

## VASCULAR MALFORMATIONS

Vascular ectasias may be congenital or acquired.[32] The classification proposed by Moore and colleagues[33] remains most applicable to real situations:

Type I lesions are found mostly in the right colon of patients older than 55 years of age. They are acquired angiodysplasias and can be identified by angiography[34] and colonoscopy. However, they are frequently identified and have bled in only half of those demonstrated.

Type II lesions occur in younger patients, about 30 to 50 years old, and occur most often in the stomach and proximal small bowel. They are probably congenital arteriovenous malformations (AVMs) and are slightly larger than type I lesions and potentially visible.

Type III lesions occur in families with an autosomal dominant inheritance pattern. They are associated with skin and mucous membrane telangiectasias and also with angiectasias throughout the gastrointestinal tract and liver. Frequent episodes of bleeding characterize these lesions of hereditary telangiectasia or Osler-Weber-Rendu disease. The tiny, multiple ectasias in the jejunum can be shown by meticulous angiography (Fig. 53–24) but not by barium studies.

Angiomatous malformations in the small bowel (type

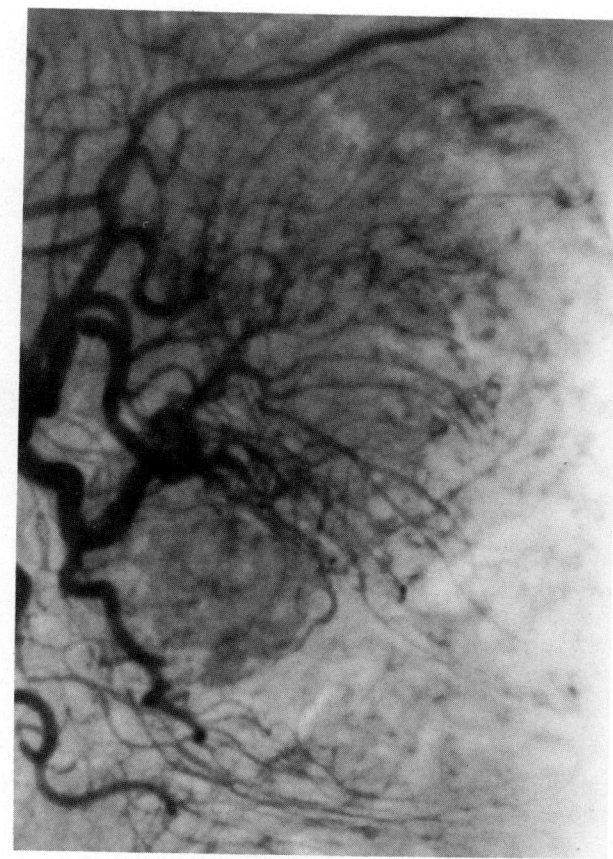

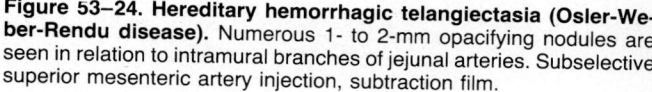

**Figure 53–24. Hereditary hemorrhagic telangiectasia (Osler-We-ber-Rendu disease).** Numerous 1- to 2-mm opacifying nodules are seen in relation to intramural branches of jejunal arteries. Subselective superior mesenteric artery injection, subtraction film.

II) are a not infrequent cause of obscure bleeding—that is, significant blood loss leading to anemia, often with repeated hospitalizations and blood transfusions, that remains undiagnosed after barium studies and endoscopy of the esophagus, stomach, duodenum, and colon. Should the next investigation be enteroscopy, angiography, or enteroclysis? At this stage, enteroscopy is laborious, time-consuming, and uncomfortable for the patient. However, a few interesting reports have appeared.

Lewis and Waye[35] used a sonde-type small intestinal fiberscope to investigate obscure bleeding in 60 patients. It required an average of 6 hours to reach the ileum in 46 of the 60 patients. It was possible to identify a source of bleeding in 20 of the 46 patients, and 16 of the 20 lesions were AVMs. In another report[36] dealing with obscure bleeding, push enteroscopy with a 160-cm colonoscope was employed. Only the distal duodenum and proximal jejunum were reached during the 50-minute procedure. AVMs were found in 12 of 39 patients, and 11 lesions could be cauterized at the same time. AVMs appear to be the most frequent cause of obscure bleeding from the small bowel. Nevertheless, in these studies, 66 and 59%, respectively, of the cases of obscure bleeding remained obscure. In a comment on the report of Fouch and colleagues,[36] Krevsky[37] suggested that negative results of upper endoscopy and of colonoscopy extended into the distal ileum should be followed by enteroclysis before enteroscopy. In replying, Foutch stated that

AVMs would be missed by barium radiology and probably also by angiography.[37]

As far as we know, there is up to now no published report of an AVM having been demonstrated by enteroclysis. In a patient with a long history of obscure blood loss, enteroclysis could demonstrate a $4 \times 11$ mm AVM in the proximal jejunum. The lesion was confirmed by intraoperative endoscopy and resected[38] (Fig. 53–25). Enteroclysis has demonstrated other causes of obscure bleeding in almost 10% of a reported series[39] and, in our experience, in almost 15% of patients in whom obscure bleeding occurred together with abdominal pain.

## HEMANGIOMAS

Hemangiomas are tumor-like lesions, usually considered to be hamartomas. In capillary hemangiomas, vascular channels are tightly packed; cavernous hemangiomas consist of larger vascular spaces. They can be single or multiple but all, sooner or later, bleed. Malignancy is exceptional.

There is a relationship to cutaneous syndromes. Blue rubber bleb nevus syndrome is revealed by multiple cavernous hemangiomas of skin and gastrointestinal tract with repeated bleeding.[40] Klippel-Trenaunay syndrome consists mostly of cutaneous hemangiomas and varicosities, bone hypertrophy, and absence of deep

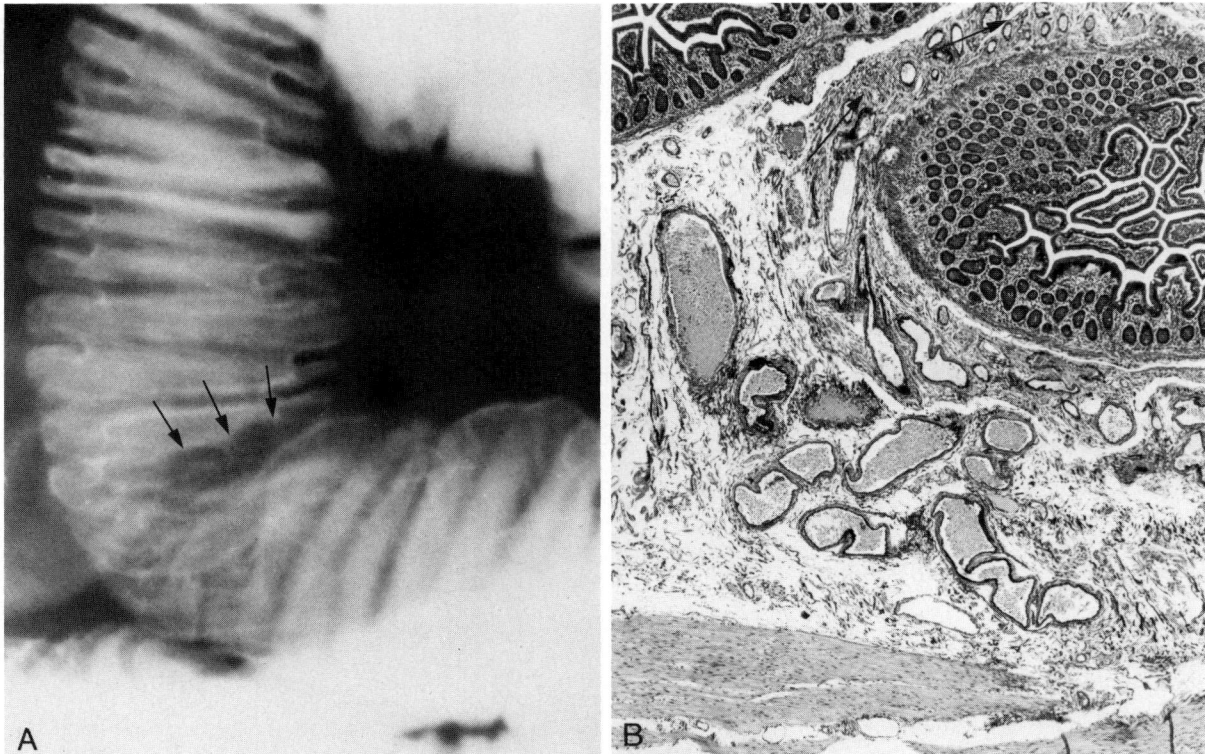

**Figure 53–25. AVM shown by enteroclysis.** This 69-year-old male patient had repeated passage of blood from the rectum. He was fully investigated, but no cause was found. **A.** Enteroclysis demonstrated a 0.4 × 1.4 cm lobulated expansion of part of one fold *(arrows)* in the proximal jejunum. This was thought to be a submucosal process extending up into the fold, possibly an AVM. **B.** An AVM was confirmed surgically and resected. Histologic study shows dilated venous channels in the submucosa that extend into the submucosal core of a fold *(arrows).*

veins. Bleeding is more often from the rectum than the small bowel. However, there are case reports of bleeding from the small bowel; large, tortuous draining veins can be shown angiographically and by CT.[41]

## MESENTERIC VARICES

Mesenteric varices may extend into the small intestine in patients with portal hypertension and occasionally manifest with bleeding. Many such patients also have a history of abdominal surgery, mostly proctocolectomy with ileostomy. The varices may be demonstrated by superior mesenteric angiography or by catheterization of the right ovarian vein via the inferior vena cava.[42] Mesenteric varices may be seen on barium studies as serpiginous filling defects extending under the mucosa.[43, 44] Occasionally, they occur without portal hypertension, in relation to venous occlusion by a metastatic tumor.[45]

### Acknowledgment

Figures 53–3B and 53–9A are reproduced from Herlinger H, Maglinte D (eds): Clinical Radiology of the Small Intestine. Philadelphia: WB Saunders, 1989.

## References

1. Hildebrand HD, Zierler RE: Mesenteric vascular disease. Am J Surg 139:188–192, 1980.
2. Amano H, Bulkley GB, Gorey T, et al: The role of microvascular patency in the recovery of small intestine from ischemic injury. Surg Forum 31:157–161, 1980.
3. Paul AB, Dean DM: Computed tomography in volvulus of the midgut. Br J Radiol 63:893–894, 1990.
4. Wilson C, Gupta R, Gilmour DC, et al: Acute superior mesenteric ischaemia. Br J Surg 74:279–281, 1987.
5. Scott JR, Miller WT, Urso M, et al: Acute mesenteric infarction. AJR 113:269–279, 1971.
6. Raf LE: Ischaemic stenosis of the small intestine. Acta Chir Scand 135:253–259, 1969.
7. Price J, Nolan DJ: Closed loop obstruction: diagnosis by enteroclysis. Gastrointest Radiol 14:251–254, 1989.
8. Maglinte DDT, Herlinger H, Nolan DJ: Radiologic features of closed loop obstruction: analysis of 25 confirmed cases. Radiology 179:383–387, 1991.
9. Ghahremani GG, Meyers MA, Farman J, et al: Ischemic disease of the small bowel and colon associated with oral contraceptives. Gastrointest Radiol 2:221–228, 1977.
10. Smerud MJ, Johnson CD, Stephens DH: Diagnosis of bowel infarction: a comparison of plain films and CT scans in 23 cases. AJR 154:99–103, 1990.
11. Marks CG, Nolan DJ, Piris J, et al: Small bowel strictures after blunt abdominal trauma. Br J Surg 66:663–664, 1979.
12. Grendel JH, Ockner RK: Mesenteric venous thrombosis. Gastroenterology 82:358–372, 1982.

13. Kaplan LM: Case records of the Massachusets General Hospital, case 9–1991. N Engl J Med 324:613–623, 1991.

14. Nelson SW, Egglston W: Findings on plain roentgenograms of the abdomen associated with mesenteric vascular occlusion with a possible new sign of mesenteric venous thrombosis. AJR 83:886–894, 1960.

15. Volgelzang RL, Gore RM, Anschuetz SL, et al: Thrombosis of the splanchnic veins: CT identification. AJR 150:93–96, 1988.

16. Warnock NG, Gaines PA, Beard JD, et al: Treatment of intestinal angina by percutaneous transluminal angioplasty of a superior mesenteric artery occlusion. Clin Radiol 45:18–19, 1992.

17. Carr ND, Pullen BR, Hasleton PS, et al: Microvascular studies in human radiation bowel disease. Gut 25:448–454, 1984.

18. Mendelson RM, Nolan DJ: The radiological features of radiation enteritis. Clin Radiol 36:141–148, 1985.

19. Meagher T, Nolan DJ: The radiology of irradiated gut. In Galland RB, Spencer J (eds): Radiation Enteritis. London: Edward Arnold, 1990, pp 88–102.

20. Mason GR, Dietrich P, Friedland GW, et al: The radiological findings in radiation-induced enteritis and colitis. A review of 30 cases. Clin Radiol 21:232–247, 1970.

21. Halls JM: Radiation damage of the small intestine. Clin Radiol 16:173–176, 1965.

22. Rishman EK, Zinreich ES, Jones B, et al: Computed tomographic diagnosis of radiation ileitis. Gastrointest Radiol 9:149–152, 1984.

23. Hughes CE 3d, Conn J Jr, Sherman JO: Intramural hematoma of the gastrointestinal tract. Am J Surg 133:276–279, 1977.

24. Jaffin BW, Bliss CM, Lamont JT: Significance of occult gastrointestinal bleeding during anticoagulation therapy. Am J Med 83:269, 1987.

25. Khilnani MT, Marshak RH, Eliasoph J, et al: Intramural intestinal hemorrhage. AJR 92:1061–1071, 1964.

26. Lopez LR, Schocket AL, Stanford RE, et al: Gastrointestinal involvement in leukocytoclastic vasculitis and polyarteritis nodosa. J Rheumatol 7:677, 1980.

27. Kuehne SE, Gauvin GP, Shortsleeve MJ: Small bowel stricture due to rheumatoid vasculitis. Radiology 184:215–216, 1992.

28. Kelsey PB, Compton CC: Case records of the Massachusets General Hospital, case 35–1991. N Engl J Med 325:643–651, 1991.

29. Handel J, Schwartz S: Gastrointestinal manifestations of Schön-lein-Henoch syndrome; roentgenologic findings. AJR 78:643–652, 1957.

30. Rosenberger A, Adler OB, Haim S: Radiological aspects of Behçet disease. Radiology 144:261–264, 1982.

31. Anti M, Marra G, Rappaccini GL, et al: Esophageal involvement in Behçet syndrome. J Clin Gastroenterol 8:514–519, 1986.

32. Fataar S, Morton P, Schulman A: Arteriovenous malformations of the gastrointestinal tract. Clin Radiol 32:623–628, 1981.

33. Moore JD, Thompson NW, Appelman HD, et al: Arteriovenous malformations of the gastrointestinal tract. Arch Surg 111:381–389, 1976.

34. Baum S, Athanasoulis CA, Waltman AC, et al: Angiodysplasia of the right colon. AJR 129:789–794, 1977.

35. Lewis BS, Waye JD: Chronic gastrointestinal bleeding of obscure origin: role of small bowel enteroscopy. Gastroenterology 94:1117–1120, 1988.

36. Foutch PG, Sawyer R, Sanowski RA: Push-enteroscopy for diagnosis of patients with gastrointestinal bleeding of obscure origin. Gastrointest Endosc 36:337–341, 1990.

37. Krevsky B: Enteroscopy: exploring the final frontier. Selected summary. Gastroenterology 100:838–839, 1991.

38. Herlinger H, Firth B, Moonka D, et al: Arteriovenous malformation shown by enteroclysis. Case report. AJR (in press).

39. Rex DK, Lappas JC, Maglinte DDT, et al: Enteroclysis in the evaluation of suspected small intestinal bleeding. Gastroenterology 97:58–60, 1989.

40. Golitz LE: Heritable cutaneous disorders that affect the gastrointestinal tract. Med Clin North Am 64:829–846, 1980.

41. Brown R, Ohri SK, Ghosh P, et al: Case report: jejunal vascular malformation in Klippel-Trenaunay syndrome. Clin Radiol 44:134–136, 1991.

42. Gray RK, Grollman JH: Acute lower gastrointestinal bleeding secondary to varices of the superior mesenteric venous system. Radiology 111:559–561, 1974.

43. Fleming RJ, Seaman WB: Roentgenographic demonstration of unusual extra-esophageal varices. AJR 103:281–190, 1968.

44. Agarwal D, Scholz F: Small bowel varices demonstrated by enteroclysis. Radiology 140:350, 1981.

45. Radin DR, Siskind BN, Alpert S, et al: Small-bowel varices due to mesenteric metastasis. Gastrointest Radiol 11:183–184, 1986.

# Postoperative Small Intestine

John C. Lappas, M.D.

Dean D. T. Maglinte, M.D.

## INTRODUCTION

Surgical intervention for lesions in the small intestine requires the use of relatively few techniques, most of them applicable to any segment of the small bowel from the duodenojejunal junction to the ileocecal valve. These techniques include enterotomy for removal of polyps or foreign bodies; enteroplasty to resolve a stricture; enterectomy for the resection of obstructed, traumatized, neoplastic, or necrotic segments; plication to prevent small intestinal obstruction; and the creation of ostomies or mucous fistulas for feeding or drainage purposes.[1] In addition, the small intestine is used for the construction of reservoirs after gastrectomy and proctocolectomy and for reconstitution of biliary or pancreatic flow into the gastrointestinal tract. Surgical bypass of the small intestine has also been performed in an attempt to control morbid obesity or lower serum cholesterol.

Postoperative radiologic studies are rarely performed as a routine baseline follow-up; rather, they are done to investigate complications. In patients with a history of small bowel surgery who present with gastrointestinal symptoms, the postoperative anatomy and site of any anastomosis must be evaluated by carefully performed small bowel radiologic studies (Fig. 54–1).

## SMALL BOWEL AFTER GASTRIC SURGERY

Significant alterations may occur in gastrointestinal physiology after operations on the stomach. Often grouped together as the postgastrectomy syndrome, various pathophysiologic disorders result from the destruction of the pyloric sphincter mechanism or from sequelae of truncal vagotomy. Rapid influx of hyperos-motic gastric contents into the small bowel may become clinically manifest as the dumping syndrome with postprandial cramping and urgent diarrhea. Mild dilatation of the efferent jejunum can be observed. Serotonin, bradykinin, and enteroglucagon are released systemically by the small intestine in response to lumen distention and are in part responsible for the vasomotor component of dumping.[2, 3] Postvagotomy diarrhea may be associated with small bowel dysmotility and impaired pancreatic and biliary function. Malabsorption with changes in the intestinal mucosa and increased bacterial colonization of the proximal small bowel are contributing factors.[3, 4] Latent celiac disease has been activated by gastric surgery, presumably by providing more direct access for gluten.[5] Vagotomy may also render evident previously silent adult celiac disease.[6]

## Afferent Loop Syndrome

Afferent loop obstruction is an uncommon complication of subtotal gastrectomy with a Billroth II gastrojejunostomy and occurs with variable severity, acuteness, or chronicity. Causes include internal hernia, kinking of the anastomosis, an adhesive band, stomal stenosis, neoplasms, and inflammatory disease.[7, 8] An internal hernia is commonly responsible for the onset of an acute syndrome in the immediate postoperative period. Improved surgical techniques incorporating a shortened afferent loop and closure of the retroanastomotic space have reduced the incidence of the syndrome to 0.3%.[8]

Clinically, the diagnosis may be difficult to establish. Patients may present vague symptoms of nausea, cramps, and postprandial fullness or classic features of bilious vomiting with relief of abdominal pain. Acute obstruction of the afferent loop with elevation of serum amylase level can mimic acute pancreatitis. Chronic

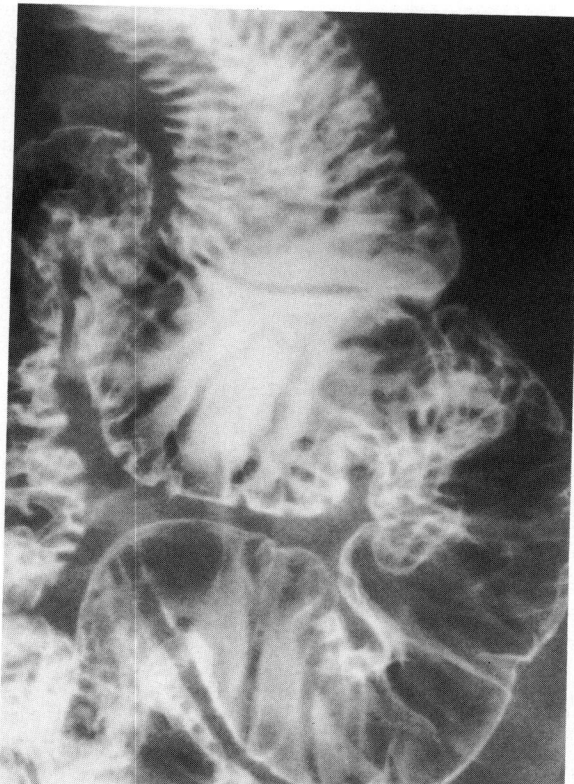

**Figure 54–1. Enteroenteric anastomosis.** End-to-side jejunal anastomosis demonstrated during enteroclysis. Control of intestinal distention achieved by enteroclysis infusion facilitates the radiographic delineation of postoperative small bowel anatomy.

progression of the syndrome can result in malabsorption, intestinal hemorrhage, or perforation.

When the obstruction is located distally, the afferent loop is fluid filled and gasless and abdominal radiographs are often normal. Studies done with barium may suggest the diagnosis by either nonfilling of the afferent loop or preferential filling of a distended proximal loop in association with stasis and delayed emptying. Efficacy of barium studies is controversial because the afferent loop fails to become opacified in 20% of normal patients.[9] Radionuclide studies with [99m]Tc–diisopropyl-iminodiacetic acid may show persistent activity in the afferent loop.[10] Ultrasonography and computed tomography (CT) permit direct visualization of the obstructed afferent loop and are preferred methods for diagnostic imaging.[11–13] CT demonstrates two or more thinly marginated round cystic structures adjacent to the pancreas, which on sequential scans can be traced to represent the U-shaped afferent loop (Fig. 54–2). Nonopacification of the afferent loop is usual after oral contrast agent administration. Transmitted intraluminal pressure from the obstruction may be sufficient to distend the gallbladder and bile ducts, creating additional cystic masses.[12] Ultrasonography similarly demonstrates the dilated afferent loop as a cystic tubular structure in continuity with the gastric anastomosis and biliary system.[13] Uniform size of the obstructed afferent loop and anterior displacement of the superior mesenteric artery may be

useful clues in differentiating this syndrome from pancreatic pseudocysts.[12, 13]

## Jejunogastric Intussusception

Jejunogastric intussusception is a rare but potentially lethal complication after simple gastrojejunostomy or any of the modifications of a Billroth II partial gastrectomy. Intussusception may occur early after operation but is generally a late complication, occurring, on the average, 6 years postoperatively. Retrograde peristalsis without associated abnormality is the most widely mentioned causative factor.[14] Invagination of the efferent loop accounts for 75% of jejunogastric intussusceptions and that of the afferent loop, alone or in combination with the efferent loop, constitutes the remainder.

Clinically, the acute form is associated with the triad of high intestinal obstruction, left upper quadrant abdominal mass, and hematemesis. Chronic intussusception is more difficult to diagnose because of its intermittent nature and vague symptoms.

Radiographically, the diagnosis is typically made with barium studies because abdominal plain films are usually unremarkable. Contrast medium characteristically outlines concentric stretched and edematous jejunal folds that are associated with the mass defect of the intussusceptum within the gastric remnant (Fig. 54–3). Distinction between anatomic types of intussusception is suggested by normal opacification of one postsurgical limb, implying abnormality of the other. Examination during symptomatic periods optimizes the diagnosis of the chronic intermittent forms of jejunogastric intussusception.

## Inadvertent Gastroileostomy

Gastroileostomy represents a surgical misadventure in which an inadvertent anastomosis is performed between

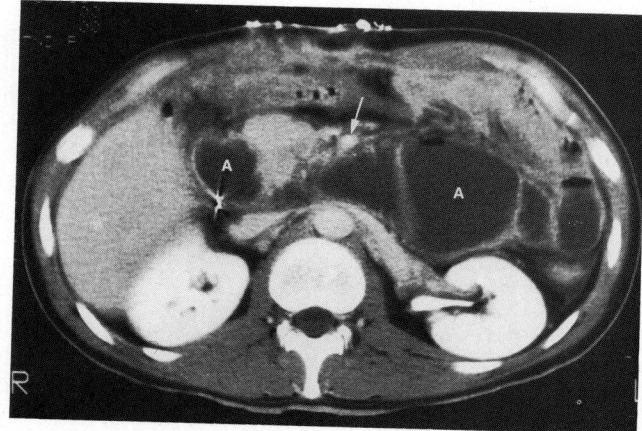

**Figure 54–2. CT scan of afferent loop obstruction.** The abnormally dilated afferent loop (A) is represented by multiple thin-rimmed cystic spaces seen adjacent to the pancreas and causing anterior displacement of the superior mesenteric artery *(arrow)*. Oral contrast medium typically opacifies normal distal efferent loops while the obstructed afferent loop remains nonopacified.

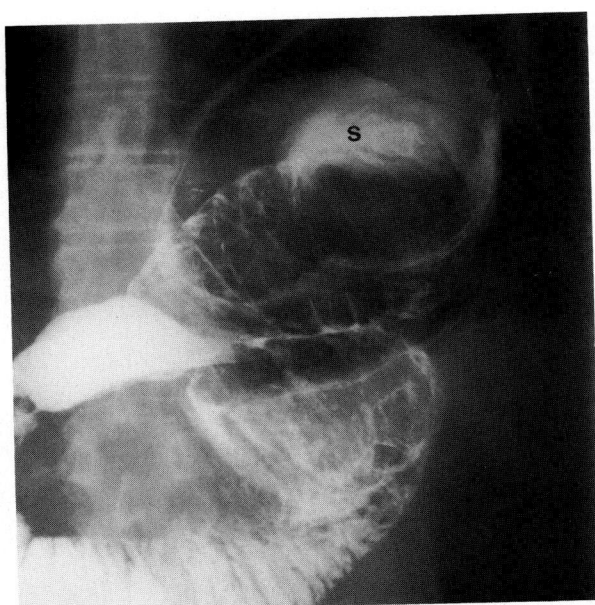

**Figure 54–3. Jejunogastric intussusception.** Retrograde intussusception of the efferent loop into the gastric remnant (S) creates a characteristic coil spring mass defect and obstruction of efferent loop flow.

the stomach and ileum instead of the jejunum. It usually occurs during a difficult operation complicated by the presence of dense adhesions and is the result of improper identification of the ligament of Treitz. Intestinal malrotation and obesity may be contributing factors. Symptoms of diarrhea and weight loss, often extreme, occur shortly after operation. Varying degrees of malabsorption with anemia and electrolyte imbalance result from the short-circuiting of the small bowel. The symptoms of gastroileostomy frequently mimic those associated with postgastrectomy diarrhea or gastrojejunocolic fistula.

Correct preoperative diagnosis requires an accurate interpretation of radiographic studies done with contrast medium.[15] The essential diagnostic feature is recognition of an efferent loop that crosses directly to the right lower quadrant and rapidly opacifies the normal cecum (Fig. 54–4). In gastroileostomy without prior partial gastric resection, recycling of intestinal contrast medium through the stomach, although more confusing, is also diagnostic.[15]

# ENTEROSTOMY AND ENTERECTOMY

Enterostomy refers to a surgically made intestinal opening that is designed to communicate with the skin and function either temporarily or permanently. To prevent a leak from the bowel lumen, an enterostomy is made in bowel segments that are sufficiently mobile to be brought in contact with the anterior abdominal wall. A low enterostomy or ileostomy is used for evacuation of intestinal contents and is discussed later. Jejunostomy, which is also useful for small bowel de-

compression, is an ideal route for administering nutritional support when pathologic lesions exist more proximally and the remainder of the gastrointestinal tract is functional.[1] Advantages of a feeding jejunostomy over gastrostomy include reduced nausea, vomiting, and risk of pulmonary aspiration via gastroesophageal reflux. Intubated jejunostomies satisfy temporary nutritional requirements, whereas long-term jejunal feeding is best accomplished by a Roux-en-Y type of jejunostomy. Various complications can be associated with any of the jejunostomy methods. Enterogastric reflux of the alimentation fluid, stomal necrosis, dislodgement of the catheter with subsequent intra-abdominal leak, and small bowel obstruction at or near the jejunostomy site are reported.[1, 16] Placement of the jejunostomy at least 70 cm from the duodenojejunal junction and fixation of the jejunal loop to the parietal peritoneum are common precautions used during surgical construction. Injecting the jejunostomy catheter with water-soluble contrast medium before initiating enteric feeding is advocated to ascertain proper catheter position and avoid misdirected infusion (Fig. 54–5).

Enterectomy refers to surgical excision of bowel and its related mesentery as indicated by a wide variety of clinical conditions. Segmental resection of the small bowel is generally followed by some form of primary anastomosis, although in some instances an external ostomy is created in conjunction with either closure of

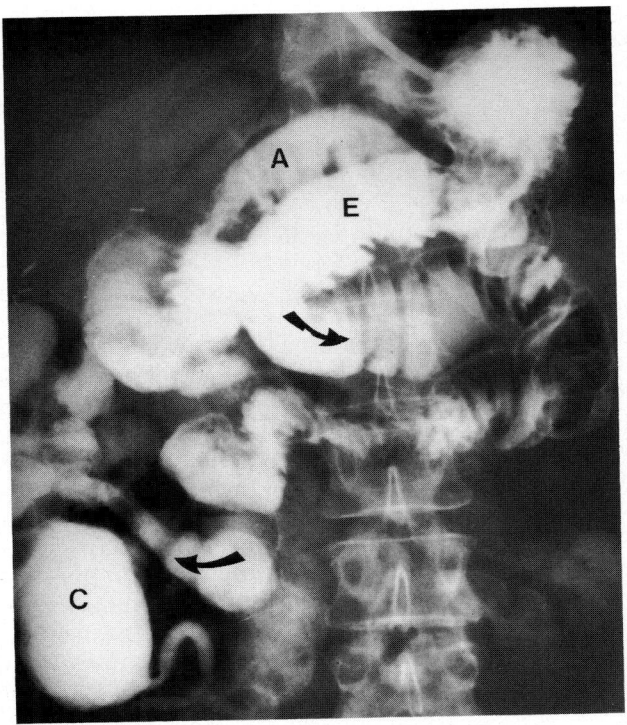

**Figure 54–4. Inadvertent gastroileostomy after subtotal gastrectomy and a planned Billroth II gastroenterostomy.** Enteroclysis infusion into the efferent loop (E) demonstrates its abnormal shortened course *(arrows)* to the right lower quadrant with prompt filling of cecum (C). Progressive barium reflux into the long proximal afferent loop (A) became increasingly apparent during the course of examination.

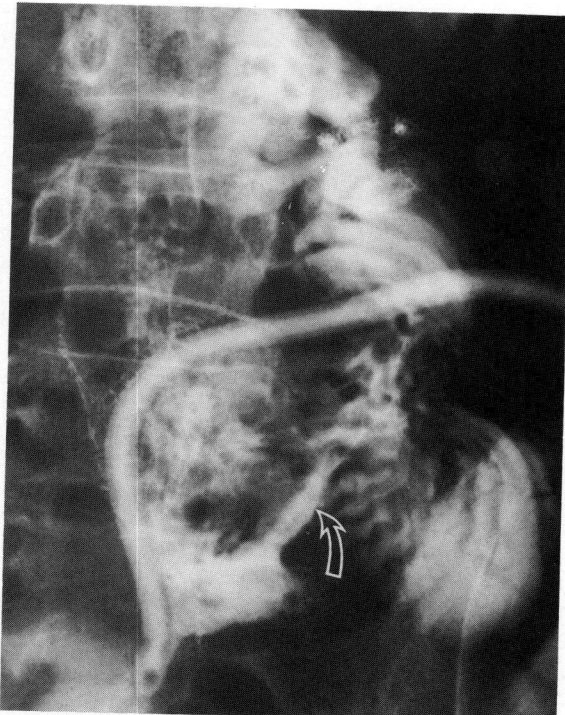

**Figure 54–5. Jejunostomy catheter dislodgment.** Water-soluble contrast medium demonstrates dislodgment of the jejunal catheter with focal contrast medium extravasation and filling of the original tract *(arrow)*. Successful repositioning can often be accomplished by catheter and guidewire manipulations performed under fluoroscopic guidance.

the distal bowel segment or formation of a mucous fistula. Intestinal anastomoses can be constructed end to end, end to side, or side to side. End-to-end anastomosis is preferred whenever possible to avoid small bowel stasis syndromes. An end-to-side anastomosis is used to compensate for disproportionate proximal and distal luminal sizes, and side-to-side anastomosis is indicated in unusual clinical situations that require expeditious bypass of an intestinal obstruction, as with extensive neoplastic disease of the small bowel. When an end-to-side anastomosis is performed, the end of the proximal lumen is anastomosed to the side of the distal intestinal segment. This maneuver ensures that peristalsis within the blind (distal) segment is directed antegradely toward and beyond the anastomotic opening, thereby preventing stasis.[1]

Dehiscence of small bowel anastomoses can occur despite careful preoperative preparation of the patient and meticulous surgical technique. Aside from technical considerations, several factors may adversely affect success of an anastomosis, including sepsis, tissue hypoxia, malignancy, and advanced age of the patient. Intestinal perforation from an anastomotic dehiscence may be detected by the presence of free intraperitoneal air on abdominal plain films. Studies performed with a water-soluble medium may demonstrate the intestinal leak. Similar findings can be detected by CT, which also has the advantage of identifying contaminated peritoneal fluid and imaging the complication of abscess formation

(Fig. 54–6). Localized perianastomotic inflammation arising from suture dehiscence can result in partial intestinal obstruction (Fig. 54–7).

## Blind Pouch Syndrome

Although end-to-end surgical anastomoses have essentially replaced side-to-side anastomoses to restore bowel continuity, the latter procedure was once popular, and blind pouches may occasionally be encountered. Dilatation of blind intestinal segments develops late in the postoperative course, some 5 to 15 years after surgery. Division of the circular muscle during formation of the side-to-side anastomosis results in stasis secondary to motility disturbances with subsequent dilatation of the proximal segment and formation of a blind pouch. The condition occurs with either enteroenteric or enterocolic anastomoses and, although infrequent, focal dilatation of both proximal and distal bowel segments is reported.[17] An incorrectly performed end-to-side anastomosis (side of proximal segment of intestine sutured to the end of the distal intestine) creates a similar anatomic abnormality because of blind end–directed peristalsis.

Hypertrophy of the pouch with inflammation and ulceration may occur in addition to the intestinal stasis. Symptoms of episodic diarrhea, abdominal pain, and weight loss, together with a history of previous intestinal anastomosis, suggest the diagnosis. Blind pouches may be a source of gastrointestinal bleeding.[18] Segmental resection and end-to-end anastomosis are corrective and eliminate late complications.

Radiographically, blind pouches may appear on abdominal films as either fluid-filled soft tissue masses or gas-filled structures of variable size and shape. Small

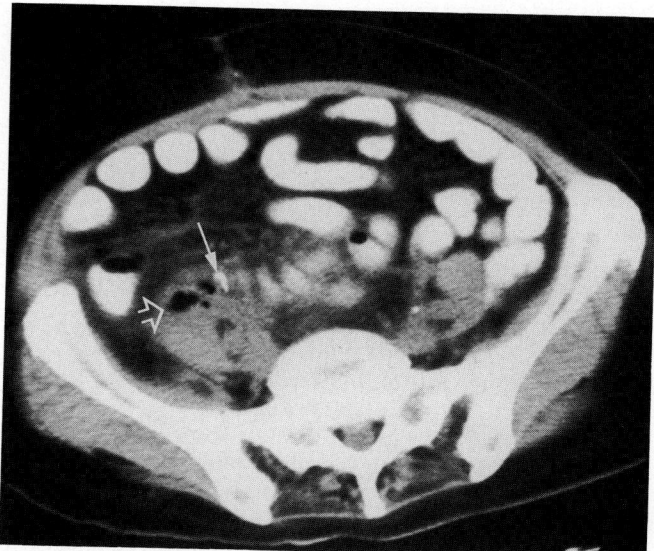

**Figure 54–6. CT scan of perianastomotic abscess.** Breakdown of an enteric anastomosis results in right lower quadrant abscess depicted as a heterogeneous mass. Focal accumulation of extravasated contrast medium *(solid arrow)* and extraluminal gas *(open arrow)* are contained within the abscess.

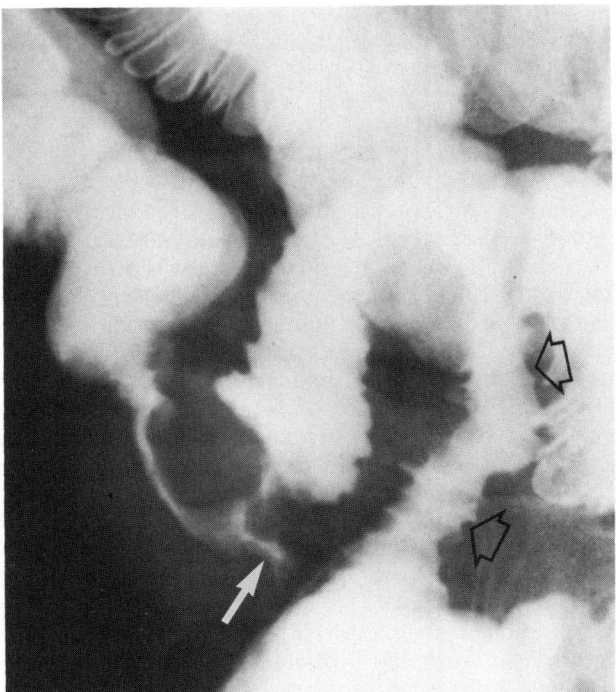

**Figure 54–7. Perianastomotic phlegmon with intestinal narrowing.** Symptoms of mild obstruction ensued in this patient 10 days after segmental ileal resection with end-to-end anastomosis for a benign tumor. Enteroclysis shows short segment of luminal narrowing with small contained leak *(solid arrow)*. Note the mildly narrowed proximal ileal loop with thickened folds *(open arrows)*. At surgery, ischemic dehiscence of the anastomosis was associated with a localized circumferential inflammatory reaction (phlegmon) and submucosal edema of the proximal bowel segment.

bowel studies done with barium, particularly enteroclysis, demonstrate the pouches and their anastomotic location (Fig. 54–8).

## Blind Loop Syndrome

In classic blind loop syndrome, a segment of small intestine has been completely bypassed by an enteroanastomosis. Stagnation of small bowel contents leads to bacterial overgrowth, which in the most severely affected patients can resemble the composition of normal colonic flora in both quantity and complexity of organisms. Bacterial overgrowth in the small intestine may result in profound disturbances of absorptive function, malabsorption of lipids and vitamin $B_{12}$ being most notable.[19] Symptoms and clinical signs of the syndrome include diarrhea, steatorrhea, anemia, abdominal pain, and vitamin deficiencies. Although some of the clinical features are shared with the blind pouch syndrome, the anatomic abnormality associated with the blind loop syndrome is distinctly different. In addition to surgically created blind loops, other anatomic variants may contribute to the development of the syndrome. Chronic small bowel strictures with intervening areas of dilatation such as those that occur in Crohn's disease or radiation enteritis, congenital duplications, jejunoileal

diverticulosis, and intestinal scleroderma are among other causative pathologic conditions. In each case, studies done with barium accurately demonstrate the associated anatomic abnormality.

## Short Bowel Syndrome

The short bowel syndrome is characterized by malnutrition, steatorrhea, and massive acidic diarrhea that result from surgical resection of large portions of the small intestine. Recognition of the metabolic consequences of massive intestinal resection and aggressive correction of fluid and electrolyte deficits have decreased the mortality in the immediate postoperative period.[20]

Some of the more common conditions leading to extensive or repeated intestinal resection are acute mesenteric ischemia with infarction, strangulated internal hernias, volvulus, inflammatory bowel disease, and widespread intraperitoneal malignancy. The resulting degree of malabsorption and fluid loss varies with the length and location of bowel resected, the residual amount of colon, and the nature of the disease process. A jejunal length of less than 200 cm, especially if no colon remains, may necessitate nutritional supplements.[21] Adaptive response of villous hypertrophy and mucosal cellular hyperplasia in the ileum can compensate for resection of a large part of the jejunum. However, the unique ability of the distal ileum to transport selectively intrinsic factor–vitamin $B_{12}$ complex and bile

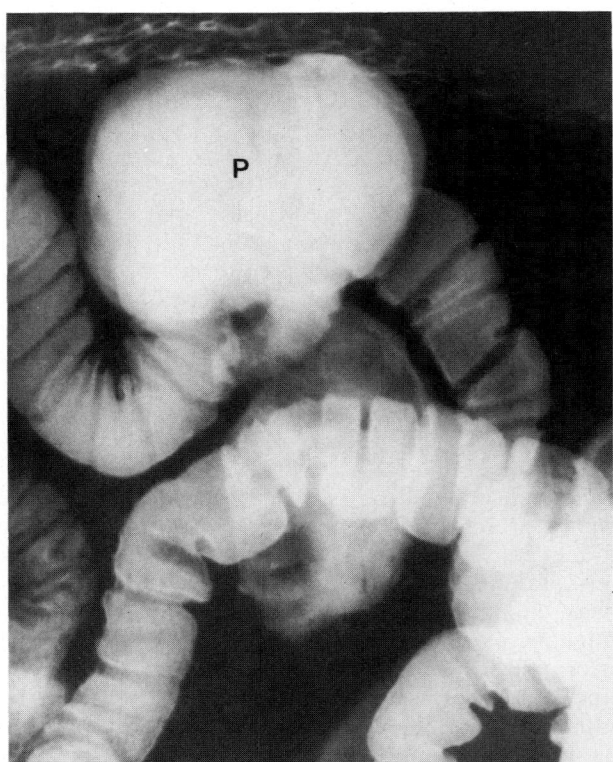

**Figure 54–8. Blind pouch.** Enteroclysis demonstrates saccular blind pouch (P) formation associated with prior side-to-side jejunal anastomosis.

salts cannot be effectively restored after a resection of more than 100 cm (50%) of its length. Increased small bowel motility and effects of gastric hypersecretion are other factors cited as contributing to the physiologic abnormalities after massive small bowel resection.[20]

Assessment of the length of residual small bowel is important in planning nutritional therapy and affects surgical policy should further resection appear necessary. Radiographic measurements of shortened (<200 cm) small bowel as derived from barium contrast studies are comparable to those obtained at operation and sufficiently accurate for use in management decision making.[21] Barium studies also indicate the degree of ileal adaptation, as shown by thickening of an increased number of mucosal folds and an increased luminal diameter. Continuing or recurrent disease for which the resection was performed can also be assessed.

## Jejunoileal Bypass

Although small intestinal bypass is most often performed for palliation of obstructing nonresectable gastrointestinal cancer or radiation damage, the surgical procedure has also been used in the treatment of morbid obesity and control of hyperlipidemia. The rationale supporting jejunoileal bypass for morbid obesity was that weight loss derived from nutrient malabsorption could be achieved by reducing the amount of intestinal mucosa available for digestion and by decreasing the transit time of food within the gastrointestinal tract. In effect, the operation produced an obligatory short bowel malabsorptive state through bypassing small intestine. Initially proposed by Payne and colleagues[22] and modified by Scott and colleagues,[23] jejunoileal bypass connects a 20- to 35-cm length of jejunum to 10 to 30 cm of distal ileum as an end-to-end or end-to-side anastomosis (Fig. 54–9). The end-to-end procedures require decompression of the bypassed small intestine into the transverse or sigmoid colon.

The jejunoileal bypass is associated with numerous early and late complications, despite the production of initial weight loss and other beneficial effects.[24, 25] Chronic diarrhea, metabolic acidosis, fluid and electrolyte imbalances, calcium and magnesium deficiencies, anemia, hyperoxaluria with renal calculi, cholelithiasis, and progressive liver failure develop to a distressing degree postoperatively. These complications are related to unpredictable absorption of nutrients by the surgically shortened gut and to the toxic side effects of bacterial overgrowth in the bypassed bowel. Mechanical complications include small bowel obstruction and intussusception of the bypassed intestine. Obstruction of bypassed segments may also occur by herniation of bowel through mesenteric defects or by volvulus at the ileocolic anastomosis.

Radiologic evaluation of the abdomen after jejunoileal bypass can often be difficult because of the confusing abdominal plain film patterns and residual obesity in some patients. Multiple air-fluid levels with varying degrees of distention in the mainstream small bowel are common postoperative radiographic observations. Bypass enteritis, characterized clinically by episodic abdominal distention with tenderness and fever, also presents multiple gas-distended loops of the bypassed intestine on abdominal radiographs.[26] Pneumatosis intestinalis may occur in conjunction with bypass enteritis. Differentiating such complications as enteritis or mechanical bowel obstruction generally requires barium examination, performed either from an antegrade direction for evaluation of the functional small bowel or by retrograde barium enema for study of the bypassed intestinal segment via its ileocolic anastomosis. Depending on the specific operation performed, bypassed segments of bowel may not be visualized on studies done with contrast medium, and ultrasonography or CT scanning is required. Ultrasonography has been shown to diagnose intussusception of the bypassed segment by demonstrating the pattern of a mass containing strong central echoes surrounded by a sonolucent rim.[27] CT,

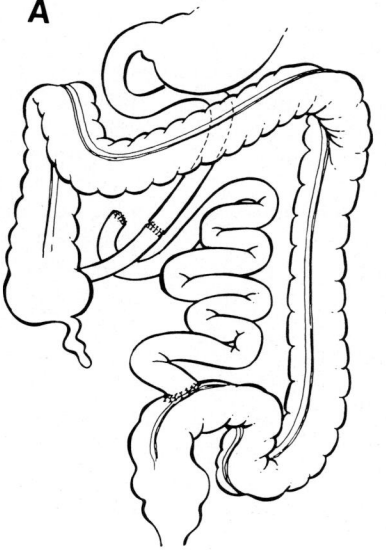 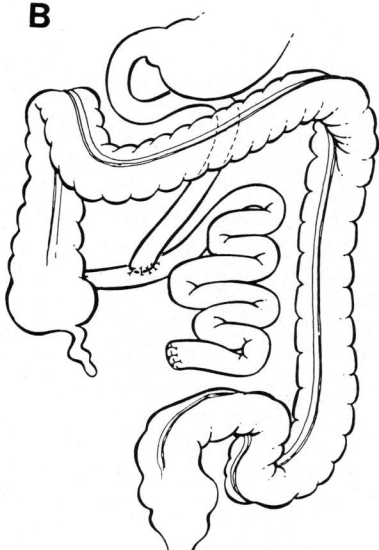

**Figure 54–9. Jejunoileal bypass.** Variations in small bowel bypass procedure for morbid obesity. **A.** Scott's adaptation with end-to-end jejunoileal anastomosis and decompression of the bypassed small bowel into the sigmoid colon. **B.** Small bowel bypass with end-to-side jejunoileostomy (Payne's procedure).

with its ability to evaluate abdominal pathology without interference by gas, appears to be a more reliable modality. A CT "doughnut" indicates intussusception of the bypassed intestine.[28]

The inevitable complications accompanying jejunoileal bypass, the infrequent need to revise or disassemble an intestinal bypass because of progressive liver disease, and excessive mortality have made the surgical procedure unacceptable in the management of morbid obesity.[25] Gastric restriction has replaced jejunoileal bypass.

Partial ileal bypass is performed to manage severe hyperlipidemia. In this procedure, the bowel is transected 200 cm proximal to the ileocecal valve so that only the distal one third of the small intestine is excluded by surgical bypass. Partial ileal bypass does not produce substantial weight loss and is associated with far fewer complications than is jejunoileal bypass for morbid obesity. For hyperlipidemia, partial intestinal bypass appears to produce a significant and sustained reduction of total and low-density lipoprotein cholesterol levels.[29] Long-term results of the surgical procedure are being investigated in a multicenter trial called the Program on the Surgical Control of the Hyperlipidemias.

## ILEOSTOMY AND ILEAL POUCHES

### Conventional Ileostomy

Conventional ileostomy still plays a role in the surgical management of intestinal disease despite newer advances such as the ileal pouch and ileoanal anastomosis. An ileostomy is traditionally performed in clinical situations that preclude normal use of the colon or require its surgical removal. Typical conditions include familial polyposis, inflammatory bowel disease, and diffuse intraabdominal malignancy. Creation of a Brooke ileostomy involves transection of the ileum with mobilization of a 5 cm ileal segment through an abdominal wall defect and specific suturing technique to allow ileostomy maturation.[30]

Malfunction of an ileostomy may occur for a variety of reasons including adhesions, prestomal narrowing of the ileal lumen, paraileostomy herniation, and recurrent neoplastic or inflammatory bowel disease. These abnormalities can present early or late after operation and usually occur at or near the ileostomy site. Symptoms often produced are diarrhea and those of small bowel obstruction.

Management of patients with an ileostomy and suspected complication or ileostomy dysfunction requires good radiologic evaluation of the small intestine. Barium studies including enteroclysis infusion can be safely performed in retrograde fashion in patients with an ileostomy.[31, 32] Specific techniques for adapting enteroclysis catheters, small Foley's catheters, and externally applied ostomy cones for ileostomy intubation have been described.[32] Glucagon may be given to abolish peristalsis and promote retrograde flow of contrast medium. Although infusion per ileostomy is well tolerated by patients and is the preferred approach for diagnostic study,

some authors have had good results with an antegrade small bowel enteroclysis.[33] Retrograde examination, however, allows greater control over visualization of the distal small bowel, where most abnormalities are found. Indentation of bowel, abrupt angulation or caliber change, or fixation of bowel to the abdominal wall or other loops indicates the presence of postoperative adhesions. In cases of mild small bowel obstruction, antegrade enteroclysis may be needed to better demonstrate the hydrodynamic significance of adhesions.[31] Fascial scarring with narrowing of the prestomal segment of ileum as it passes through the abdominal wall may be a cause of partial intestinal obstruction and resulting ileostomy dysfunction.[32] Recurrent Crohn's disease in the distal small bowel can result in radiologic findings and symptoms similar to those of obstructive ileostomy dysfunction. In cases of parastomal herniation, barium studies can demonstrate the herniated bowel and any associated obstruction provided that lateral radiographs are routinely obtained (Fig. 54–10). In one study, CT determined a higher incidence of paraileostomy herniation than was previously reported on the basis of clinical examination—36 versus 10%, respectively.[34] Herniation was associated with large (>3 cm) defects in the anterior abdominal wall at the stomal site and was common lateral to the stoma[34] (Fig. 54–11). Because CT can accurately detect paraileostomy hernia, it is recommended for evaluation of patients with unexplained persistent stoma-related or abdominal symptoms and negative clinical findings.

### Continent Ileostomy

The concept of an internal reservoir associated with a postcolectomy ileostomy was introduced by Kock and later improved after the adaptation of a valve mechanism.[35] Successful surgery obviates the use of an external ileostomy appliance, because the contents of the ileal pouch are evacuated by intubation several times a day. The advantages of this continence-preserving surgical procedure are mainly cosmetic and psychologic.

Creation of a Kock pouch requires the use of the distal 45 cm of ileum, with the most proximal 30 cm segment fashioned into an antiperistaltic reservoir. Suturing of bowel into either an S configuration or, classically, a U shape by joining two 15 cm loops allows formation of the common small bowel pouch after surgical incision of the antimesenteric borders of the adjacent loops. By design, opposing directions of peristalsis in each wall of the pouch serve to prevent propulsive activity from emptying the pouch. Continence is further maintained by intussuscepting the terminal 13-cm segment of ileum into the pouch to form the valve mechanism; the end of the ileum creates the abdominal wall stoma. Suturing of the Kock pouch to the anterior abdominal wall provides stability and prevents volvulus of the pouch and peripouch herniation.

Complications with the valve mechanism, primarily extrusion with incontinence, have been reported in 22% of patients, mostly within 1 year of pouch creation.[36]

**Figure 54–10. Paraileostomy hernia. A.** Retrograde enteroclysis per ileostomy suggests complete intestinal obstruction *(arrow)* in this patient with intermittent symptoms. **B.** Subsequent antegrade study shows several herniated small bowel loops with mild compression *(arrows)* at the site of the abdominal wall defect. Hernia is clearly demonstrated on the lateral view, and antegrade infusion more accurately depicts the functional degree of obstruction. S = ileostomy stoma.

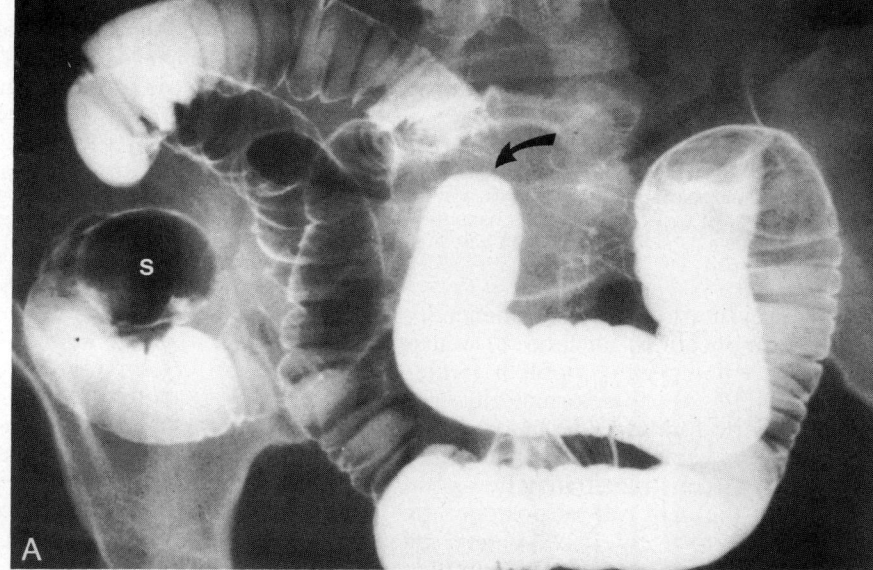

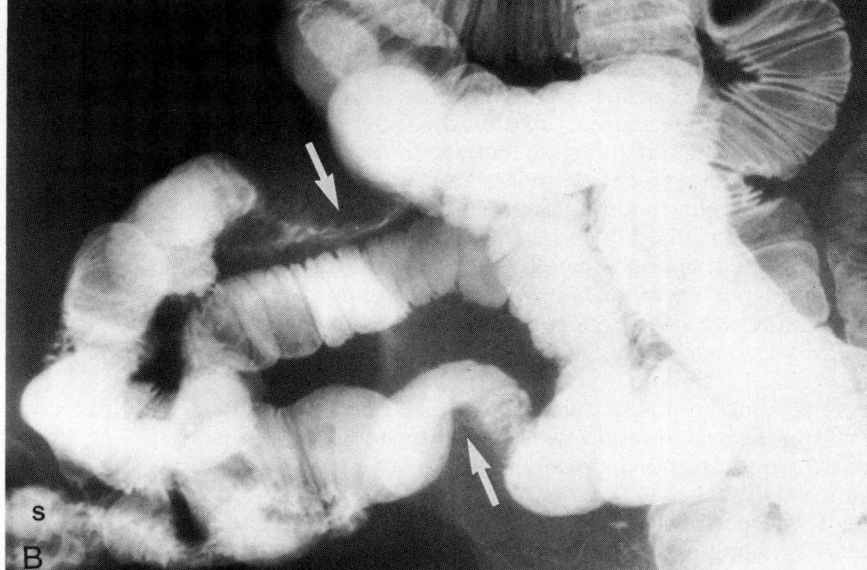

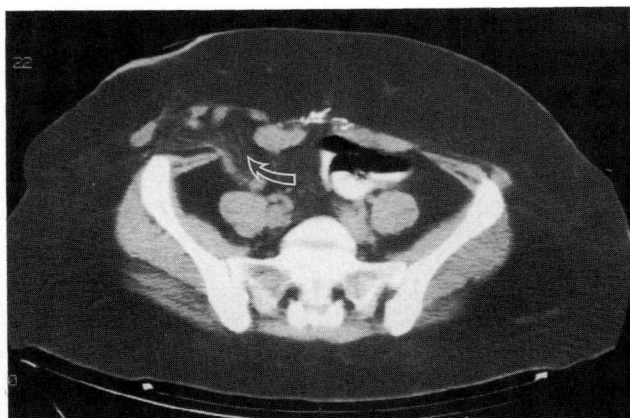

**Figure 54–11. CT scan of paraileostomy hernia.** The CT scan demonstrates a large anterior abdominal wall defect *(arrow)* and herniation of multiple small bowel loops and mesentery. Diagnosis requires review of several scan slices because herniated loops and cutaneous ileostomy stoma are often in different axial planes.

Surgical revision restored continence in 95% of cases.[36] Other complications include a nonspecific ileitis or pouchitis, a temporary problem treated with drainage and antibiotics. Fistula formation, orifice stenosis, abscess, and perforation of the pouch can occur during intubation.[37] Continent ileal and ileoanal reservoirs should not be constructed in patients with Crohn's colitis because of the high rate of postoperative recurrence of this disease.

Radiologic evaluation of the continent ileostomy can be performed by retrograde infusion of contrast medium through the ileostomy drainage tube. Infusion of 150 to 300 mL is usually sufficient to cause adequate pouch distention and barium reflux into the afferent small bowel.[37] The invaginated valve mechanism is seen as a round or lobulated filling defect, and the suture line between the two ileal segments is represented by an oblique straight mucosal ridge. Normal mucosal fold patterns within the pouch become thickened and spiculated when there is pouchitis. Formation of multiple enteroliths in an established Kock's pouch and resulting pouchitis have been reported.[38] Extrusion of the valve from the pouch can lengthen the outlet conduit, render it tortuous, and hinder intubation.[37] Complete extrusion results in incontinence. Radiography in a steeply oblique or lateral view is required to visualize adequately the outlet conduit and ileostomy stoma. Any suspicion of suture dehiscence in the immediate postoperative period or pouch perforation after intubation should be evaluated by using a water-soluble contrast agent instead of barium.

## Ileoanal Pouches

Creation of an ileal reservoir with ileoanal anastomosis after colectomy and rectal mucosectomy has become an important surgical alternative for patients requiring total proctocolectomy. In primary colonic mucosal disease, including ulcerative colitis and the poly-

posis syndromes, this operation removes the entire potentially disease-bearing mucosa while preserving anal continence and the normal defecatory pathway. Two principal forms of pouch construction are used: the S-shaped pouch introduced by Parks and colleagues[39] and the smaller J-shaped pouch of Utsunomiya and co-workers.[40] Construction of an S-shaped pouch requires the folding of a 50-cm segment of ileum into an S configuration, with the distal end allowed to protrude to form an efferent conduit. The folded loops are opened and sutured to create a wide, single pouch (Fig. 54–12). An ileal J pouch is constructed from the distal 15 to 20 cm of ileum, fashioned into a J shape and secured by side-to-side anastomosis of the adjacent loops (Fig. 54–13). After rectal transection and mucosectomy, the constructed ileal pouch is brought down within the rectal cuff and is anastomosed to the dentate line of the anal mucosa. In both methods a proximal diverting ileostomy is established for a 6- to 8-week period to allow healing of the extensive anastomoses. Closure of the protective ileostomy results in functionalization of the ileoanal pouch. Currently, the J pouches are preferred because of the greater simplicity of their construction, adequate reservoir capacity, ease of emptying, and absence of a potentially obstructing efferent limb.[41]

Radiographic evaluation of the ileoanal reservoir is required to exclude anastomotic leakage from the reservoir and to assess other potential complications and function postoperatively.[42] With demonstration of an

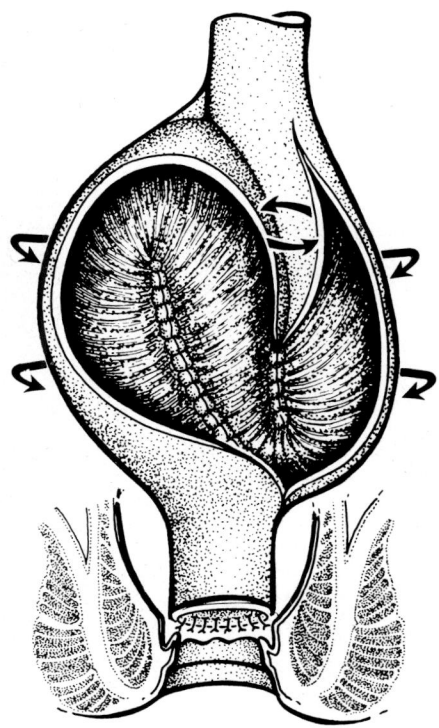

**Figure 54–12. Schematic representation of S-shaped ileoanal pouch.** An S-shaped ileal loop is used to create a reservoir by opposing three segments of terminal ileum *(arrows).* The S pouch has the relatively elongated efferent limb sutured to the dentate line.

**Figure 54–13. J-shaped ileoanal pouch. A.** Schematic representation showing side-to-side anastomosis of adjacent ileal loop and direct anastomosis of inferior apex of the reservoir to the dentate line. (From PW Kremers, FJ Scholz, DJ Schoetz Jr, et al, Radiology of the ileoanal reservoir, AJR, 145, 3, 559–567, 1985, © by American Roentgen Ray Society.) **B.** Normal single contrast pouchogram with characteristic vertical raphe *(solid arrows)* from the anastomotic line and transverse ileal folds. Traces of contrast medium *(open arrow)* often enter a small cuff in the reservoir formed during creation of the pouch and should not be confused with anastomotic leak.

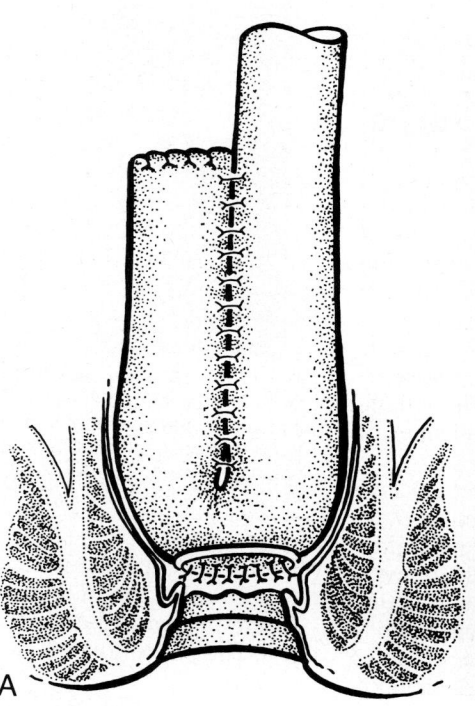

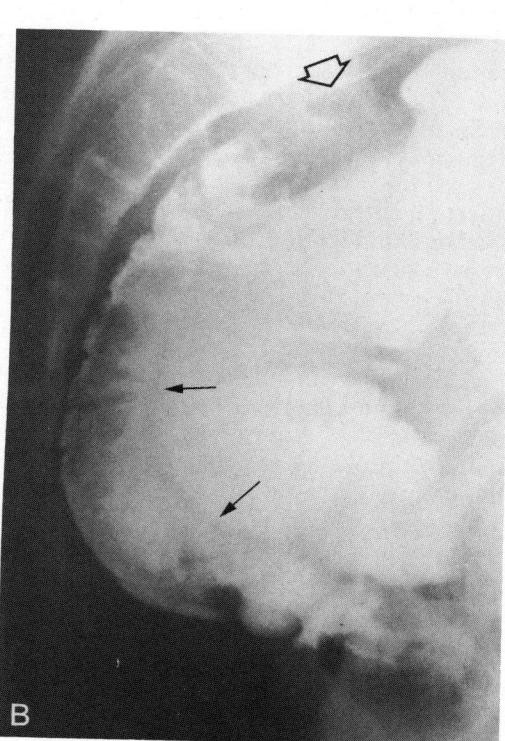

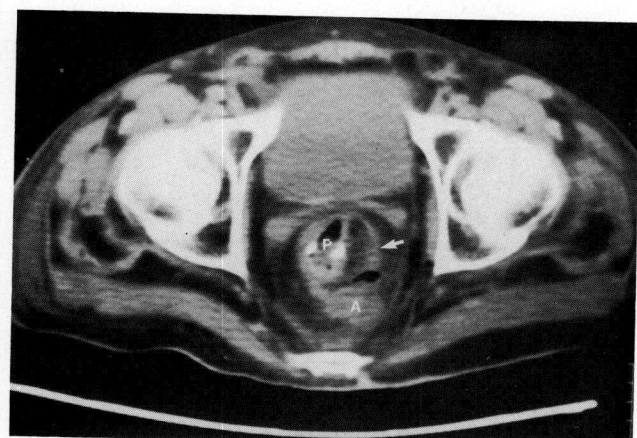

**Figure 54–14. CT scan of peripouch abscess.** An abscess (A) is seen as an abnormal collection with a small amount of gas, posterior to the ileoanal pouch (P). A thickened rectal cuff wall *(arrow)* surrounds the pouch mesentery. The abscess arises from the peripouch region and extends to involve the rectal wall and perirectal fat.

intact anastomosis and no sign of intrapelvic sepsis or fistula, the diverting ileostomy can be closed and intestinal continuity re-established at a second operation. Ileograms (pouchograms) done with contrast medium are performed retrogradely via soft catheter to visualize the reservoir, efferent limb, and ileoanal anastomosis. Further films may be obtained to demonstrate evacuation of the pouch and its postevacuation state.[42] In patients with suspected anastomotic dehiscence and pelvic sepsis, ileograms may demonstrate abnormal findings such as contrast agent extravasation, extraluminal gas, abnormal pouch fold patterns (thickening, spiculation), or extrinsic mass effects. CT scans of patients with infections demonstrate abnormal pouch and rectal wall thickness in addition to inflammatory infiltration of the peripouch and perirectal fat.[43] Abscesses are identified on CT scans, characteristically in the peripouch region between the ileal mesenteric fat and the adjacent rectal muscularis (Fig. 54–14). It has been reported that in patients with infectious complications after ileoanal pouch surgery the ileographic findings are often nonspecific , whereas CT more accurately delineates the inflammatory process and can also direct therapeutic intervention.[43, 44]

Pouchitis, or inflammation of the ileal pouch, occurs in 10 to 20% of patients undergoing restorative proctocolectomy and clinically presents with abdominal cramping, watery stools, and occasional malaise and fever. Pouchograms done with barium demonstrate spasm and thickened ileal pouch folds. Radionuclide scintigraphy showing increased pouch uptake of indium-111–labeled leukocytes can be particularly sensitive for determination of the diagnosis.[44]

Other complications less commonly encountered are stricture of the ileoanal anastomosis and obstruction of the efferent segment, especially with S-shaped pouch construction (Fig. 54–15). Complications related to the diverting ileostomy have been reported and include high ileostomy output, leading to dehydration, and intestinal obstruction after closure of the loop ileostomy[41] (Fig. 54–16). Some patients may develop abdominal distention and associated mild dilatation of small bowel loops on abdominal plain films (Fig. 54–17). Enteroclysis studies are typically normal, and stasis caused by neuromuscular dysmotility in the anastomotic region, similar to the motor disturbances in blind pouch syndrome, is suspected.

## SMALL BOWEL TRANSPLANTATION

Small bowel transplantation is on the verge of becoming an accepted clinical option for treatment of selected patients with intestinal failure in whom total parenteral nutrition is no longer feasible. In small bowel transplantation, the proximal end of the donor bowel is placed in continuity with the native jejunum, and a distal ileostomy is created. The superior mesenteric arterial supply to the transplanted intestine is maintained through a transplanted aortic conduit that is anastomosed to the side of the abdominal aorta. The donor portal vein, providing venous drainage of the small

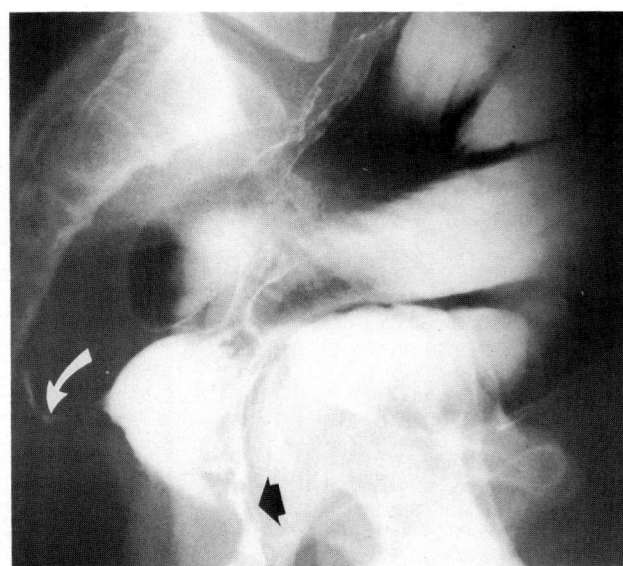

**Figure 54–15. S-shaped ileoanal pouch with abnormal efferent limb.** A pouchogram demonstrates a stenotic segment *(black arrow)* proximal to the anal anastomosis. A small residual sinus tract *(white arrow)* extends posteriorly from the efferent limb into a thickened presacral space, the site of chronically indurated tissue from a prior peripouch abscess. Note anterior displacement of the efferent limb from the sacrum.

bowel allograft, is anastomosed to the side of the native portal vein. Small bowel transplantation can be performed as an isolated surgical procedure or in conjunction with liver transplantation.[45]

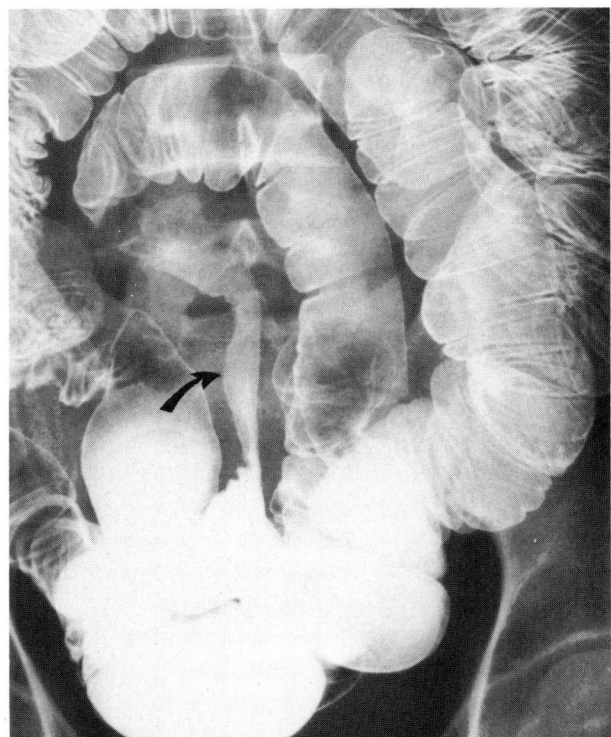

**Figure 54–16. Partial intestinal obstruction in a patient with ileoanal J pouch and prior diverting ileostomy.** Enteroclysis demonstrates narrowing of the distal ileal lumen *(arrow)*, which was adherent to the anterior abdominal peritoneum after closure of the loop ileostomy.

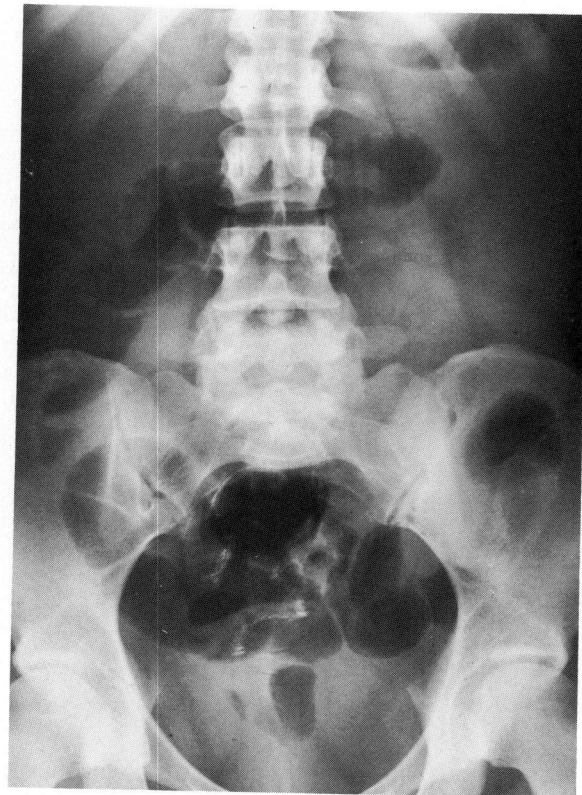

**Figure 54–17. Dysmotility after ileoanal pouch.** Supine plain film of a patient with chronic abdominal distention and functional ileoanal pouch. Despite the presence of several gas-filled ileal loops, enteroclysis showed no evidence of mechanical intestinal obstruction. Dysmotility of the ileoanal pouch is thought to be responsible for the patient's symptoms.

Radiographic evaluation of small bowel transplants involves frequent abdominal radiographs, obtained primarily to follow the postoperative bowel gas patterns or to assess the position of tubes.[46] Examinations of the transplanted small intestine with contrast medium, antegrade or via ileostomy, are useful for excluding surgical complications such as strictures, anastomotic leaks, or perforations. Mucosal fold thickening resulting from submucosal lymphedema is a common finding in the early postoperative period, and normal intestinal peristalsis has been observed as early as 14 days after transplantation.[46] Studies with contrast medium appear to be relatively insensitive for recognition of allograft rejection.[46]

# References

1. Liu KJM, Walker FW: Surgical procedures on the small intestine. *In* Zuidema GD (ed): Shackelford's Surgery of the Alimentary Tract, Volume V (3rd ed). Philadelphia: WB Saunders, 1991, pp 264–285.
2. Wang PY, Talamo RC, Babior BM, et al: Kallikrein-kinin system in postgastrectomy dumping syndrome. Ann Intern Med 80:577–581, 1974.
3. Sawyers JL, Scott HJ: Postgastrectomy sequelae and remedial operations. *In* Scott HJ, Sawyers JL (eds): Surgery of the Stomach, Duodenum, and Small Intestine. Boston: Blackwell Scientific Publications, 1987, pp 767–776.
4. Ballinger WF: Postvagotomy changes in the small intestine. Am J Surg 114:382–387, 1967.
5. Hedburg CA, Melnyk CS, Johnson CF: Glutenopathy appearing after gastric surgery. Gastroenterology 50:796–804, 1966.
6. Moss AA: Postvagotomy unmasking of nontropical sprue. Gastrointest Radiol 1:173–175, 1976.
7. Mitty WF Jr, Grossi C, Nealon TF Jr: Chronic afferent loop syndrome. Ann Surg 172:996–1001, 1970.
8. Jordan GL: Surgical management of postgastrectomy problems. Arch Surg 102:251–259, 1971.
9. Op Den Orth JO: Tubeless hypotonic examination of the afferent loop of the Billroth II stomach. Gastrointest Radiol 2:1–5, 1977.
10. Thomas JL, Cowan RJ, Maynard CD, et al: Radionuclide demonstration of small bowel anatomy in the efferent loop syndrome. J Nucl Med 18:896–897, 1977.
11. Gale ME, Gerzof SG, Kiser LC, et al: CT appearance of afferent loop obstruction. AJR 138:1085–1088, 1982.
12. Swayne LC, Love MB: Computed tomography of chronic afferent loop obstruction: a case report and review. Gastrointest Radiol 10:39–41, 1985.
13. Lee DH, Lim JH, Ko YT: Afferent loop syndrome: sonographic findings in seven cases. AJR 157:41–43, 1991.
14. Waits JO, Baert PW, Charboneau JW: Jejunogastric intussusception. Arch Surg 115:1449–1452, 1967.
15. Katz I, Karp FL: Inadvertent gastroileostomy. AJR 99:162–174, 1967.
16. Matino JJ: Feeding jejunostomy in patients with neurologic disorders. Arch Surg 116:169–171, 1981.
17. Schlegel DM, Maglinte DDT: The blind pouch syndrome. Surg Gynecol Obstet 155:541–544, 1979.
18. Maglinte DDT: Blind pouch syndrome: a cause of gastrointestinal bleeding. Radiology 132:314, 1979.
19. Goldstein F: Bacterial populations of the gut in health and disease: clinical aspects. *In* Bockus HL (ed): Gastroenterology, Volume 2 (3rd ed). Philadelphia: WB Saunders, 1976, pp 152–173.
20. Imbembo AL, Bohrer S, Loeff DS: Small-intestinal insufficiency and the short-bowel syndrome. *In* Zuidema GD (ed): Shackelford's Surgery of the Alimentary Tract, Volume V (3rd ed). Philadelphia: WB Saunders, 1991, pp 330–371.
21. Nightingale JMD, Bartram CI, Lennard-Jones JE: Length of residual small bowel after partial resection: correlation between radiographic and surgical measurements. Gastrointest Radiol 16:305–306, 1991.
22. Payne JH, DeWind L, Schwab CE, et al: Surgical treatment of morbid obesity: sixteen years of experience. Arch Surg 106:432–437, 1973.
23. Scott HW, Dean R, Shull HJ, et al: New considerations in use of jejunoileal bypass in patients with morbid obesity. Ann Surg 177:723–735, 1973.
24. Hocking MP, Duerson MC, O'Leary JP, et al: Jejunoileal bypass for morbid obesity: late follow-up in 100 cases. N Engl J Med 308:995–999, 1983.
25. McFarland RJ, Gazet JC, Pilkington RE: A 13-year review of jejunoileal bypass. Br J Surg 72:81–87, 1985.
26. Moss AA, Goldberg HI, Koehler RE: Radiographic evaluation of complications after jejunoileal bypass surgery. AJR 127:737–741, 1976.
27. Sarti DA, Zablen MA: The ultrasonic findings in intussusception of the blind loop in jejunoileal bypass for morbid obesity. JCU 7:50–52, 1979.
28. Lo G, Fish AE, Brodey PA: CT of the intussuscepted excluded loop after intestinal bypass. AJR 137:157–159, 1981.
29. Campos CT, Matts JP, Santilli SM, et al: Predictors of total and low-density lipoprotein cholesterol change after partial ileal bypass. Am J Surg 155:138–146, 1988.
30. Kock NG, Parle N, Hulten L: Ileostomy. Curr Probl Surg 14:1–52, 1977.
31. Maglinte DDT, Lappas JC, Kelvin FM, et al: Small bowel radiography: how, when, and why? Radiology 163:297–305, 1988.
32. Zagoria RJ, Gelfand DW, Ott DJ: Retrograde examination of the small bowel in patients with an ileostomy. Gastrointest Radiol 11:97–101, 1986.
33. Kay VJ, Nolan DJ: The small bowel enema in the patient with an ileostomy. Clin Radiol 39:418–422, 1988.

34. Etherington RJ, Williams JG, Hayward MWJ, et al: Demonstration of paraileostomy herniation using computed tomography. Clin Radiol 41:333–336, 1990.

35. Kock NG: Continent ileostomy. Progr Surg 12:180–201, 1973.

36. Dozois RR, Kelly KA, Beart RW, et al: Continent ileostomy: the Mayo Clinic experience. *In* Dozois RR (ed): Alternatives to Conventional Ileostomy. Chicago: Year Book Medical Publishers, 1985, pp 180–196.

37. Diner WC, Cockrill HH: The continent ileostomy (Kock pouch): roentgenologic features. Gastrointest Radiol 4:65–73, 1979.

38. Fox ER, Chung T, Laufer I: Case report. Enteroliths in a continent ileostomy. AJR 150:105–106, 1988.

39. Parks AG, Nicholls RJ, Bellieveau P: Proctocolectomy with ileal reservoir and anal anastomosis. Br J Surg 67:533–538, 1980.

40. Utsunomiya J, Iwama T, Imajo M, et al: Total colectomy, mucosal proctectomy and ileoanal anastomosis. Dis Colon Rectum 23:459–466, 1980.

41. Beart RW Jr: Ileostomy and its alternatives. *In* Zuidema GD (ed): Shackelford's Surgery of the Alimentary Tract, Volume IV (3rd ed). Philadelphia: WB Saunders, 1991, pp 172–178.

42. Kremers PW, Scholz FJ, Schoetz DJ, et al: Radiology of the ileoanal reservoir. AJR 145:559–567, 1985.

43. Brown JJ, Balfe DM, Heiken JP, et al: Ileal J pouch: radiologic evaluation in patients with and without postoperative infectious complications. Radiology 174:115–120, 1990.

44. Thoeni RJ, Fell SC, Engelstad B, et al: Ileoanal pouches: comparison of CT, scintigraphy, and contrast enemas for diagnosing postsurgical complications. AJR 154:73–78, 1990.

45. Grant D, Wall W, Mimeault R, et al: Successful small bowel–liver transplantation. Lancet 335:181–184, 1990.

46. Bach DB, Hurlbut DJ, Romano WM, et al: Human orthotopic small intestine transplantation: radiologic assessment. Radiology 180:37–41, 1991.

# Miscellaneous Disorders

Hans Herlinger, M.D.

## ABNORMALITIES OF SMALL BOWEL DEVELOPMENT

### Intestinal Tract Rotation in the Normal Fetus (Fig. 55–1)

Herniation of the lengthening bowel into the yolk sac together with the superior mesenteric artery occurs between weeks 5 and 8 of fetal life. The first stage of rotation, 90 degrees in the anticlockwise direction, of the still-extruded bowel takes place before week 10. The second stage of rotation commences at week 10 and proceeds during re-entry of bowel into the abdomen. The pre-arterial portion enters first. Further small bowel loops extend toward the left, passing behind the superior mesenteric artery. The descending colon occupies the left abdomen. To complete the second stage of rotation, the transverse colon extends to the right side in front of the superior mesenteric artery and the cecum reaches the right upper quadrant. The second stage involves 180 degrees of anticlockwise rotation, giving an overall total rotation of 270 degrees.[1] In the third stage, the cecum and terminal ileum descend into the right iliac fossa. The root of the small bowel mesentery now extends from left of the second lumbar vertebra to the right iliac fossa at the level of the fourth or fifth lumbar vertebra. Mesenteries of the cecum and the ascending and descending colon become obliterated.

### Malrotation

The term malrotation can be applied to any form of rotational abnormality. In a more restricted sense, it indicates various grades of incompleteness of the second stage of rotation.

In nonrotation, a lax umbilical ring makes it possible for the 90-degree-rotated bowel to re-enter the abdomen as a whole without further rotation. The first and second parts of the duodenum are normally placed. From there, small bowel descends vertically to the right of the superior mesenteric artery and occupies most of the right hemiabdomen. Inferiorly, the terminal ileum crosses the abdomen to reach the left-sided cecum (Fig. 55–2). The midgut—small bowel, cecum, ascending colon, and hepatic flexure—may remain mobile and may share a common mesentery. The shortness of the root of such a mesentery makes volvulus a frequent complication.

In situs inversus, the otherwise normal midgut rotation occurs in the clockwise direction, producing a mirror image of the normal distribution of the small bowel and colon. A combination of situs inversus and nonrotation is shown in Figure 55–3.

Malrotation, or mixed rotation, is the most frequently encountered anomaly of the second stage of rotation. Various combinations of incomplete counterclockwise re-entry rotation are possible. The terminal ileum may enter the abdomen first so that the ileum comes to lie in its normal position; the more proximal portion of the prearterial segment, however, may fail to rotate so that the jejunum occupies the right abdomen in downward continuation of the duodenum (Fig. 55–4).

In the third stage, premature fixation or nondescent of the cecum may be associated with the presence of mesenteric bands (Ladd's bands) extending to the cecum from the posterolateral wall of the abdomen.[2] These bands may compress and obstruct the small bowel, usually the duodenum (Fig. 55–5). Cecal fixation may be associated with a normally elongated ascending colon that loops toward the pelvis and causes an inverted appearance of the cecum[3] (Fig. 55–6).

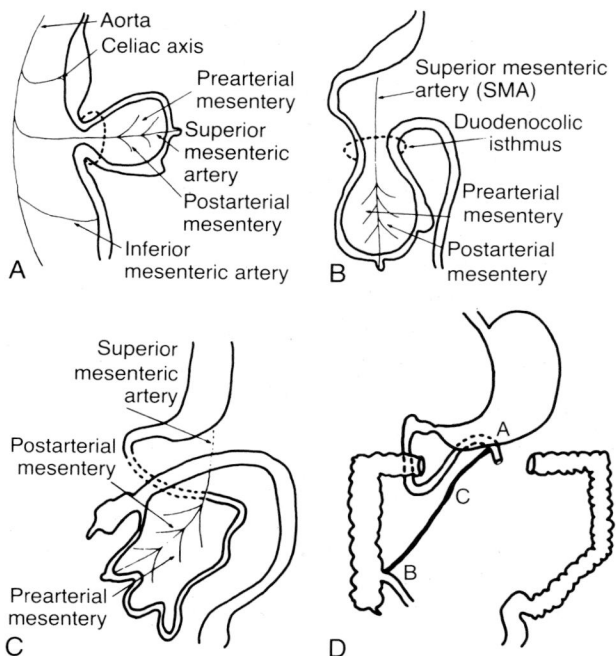

**Figure 55–1. Diagram of small bowel development in a normal fetus.**
**A.** Extruded gut at fifth to eighth fetal week. **B.** Counterclockwise 90-degree rotation, eighth fetal week. **C.** Eleventh fetal week. Re-entry with 180-degree anticlockwise rotation. The proximal jejunum has entered first and has passed from right to left behind the superior mesenteric artery. Later descent of cecum with terminal ileum. **D.** At birth. Stage of fixation has occurred. Root of mesentery (C) extends from ligament of Treitz (A) to ileocecum (B). (**A** to **D** from Houston CS, Wittenborg MH: Roentgen evaluation of anomalies of rotation and fixation of the bowel in children. Radiology 84:1–17, 1965.)

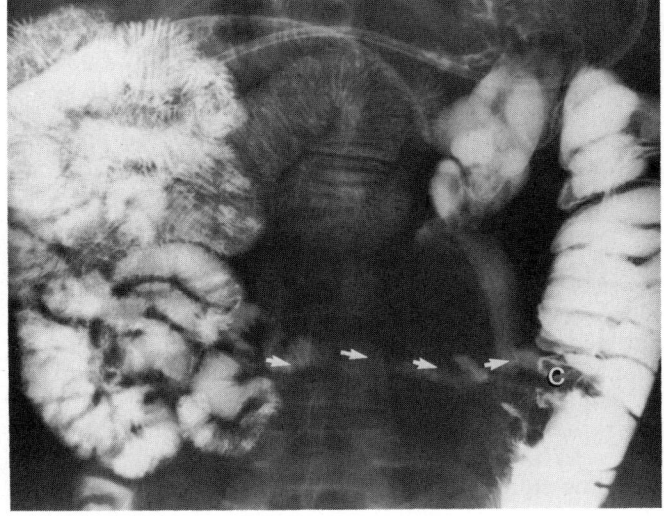

**Figure 55–2. Nonrotation.** The entire small bowel is in the right abdomen. The terminal ileum crosses *(arrows)* to reach the left-sided colon. c = cecum.

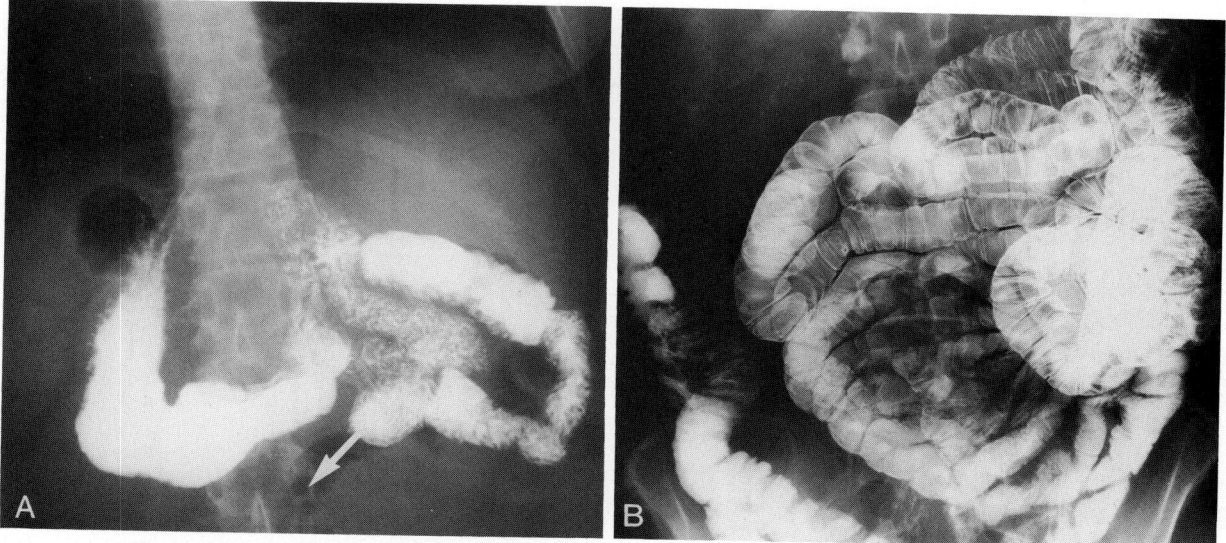

**Figure 55–3. Nonrotation with situs inversus. A.** Dextrogastria. Absence of ligament of Treitz. Air-outlined loop *(arrow)* descends toward left-sided jejunum. **B.** Entire small bowel mostly occupies the left half of the abdomen. The colon is right sided. This is a mirror image of Figure 55–2.

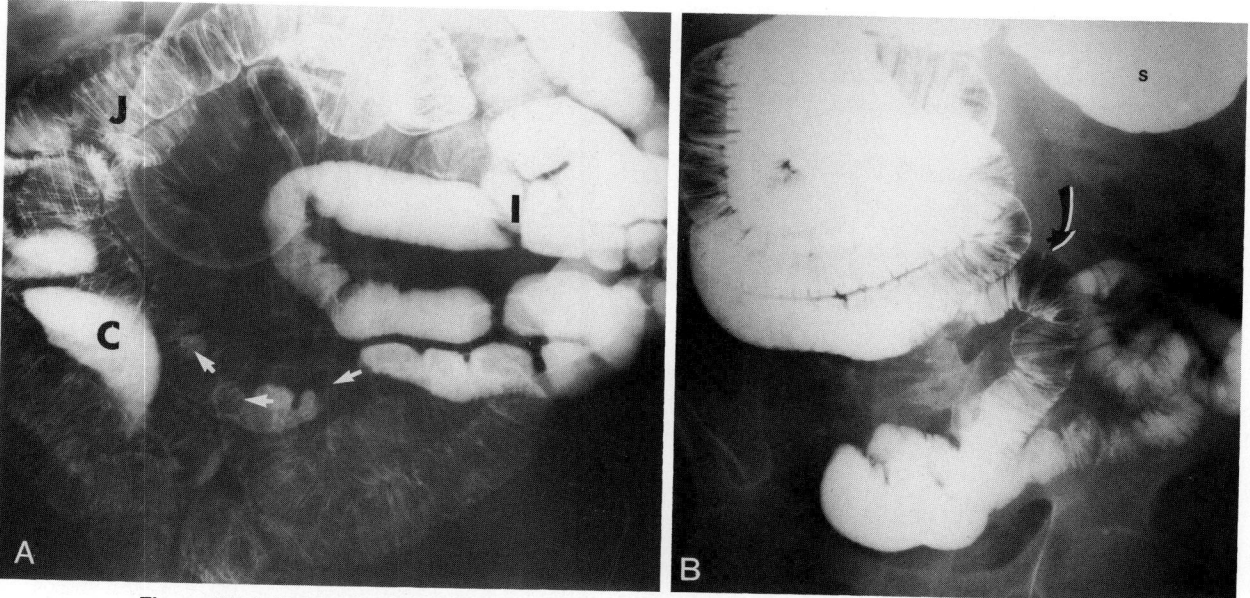

**Figure 55–4. Malrotation during second stage of rotation. A.** The jejunum (J) occupies the entire right abdomen. The ileum (I) is left sided and the terminal ileum crosses to the right *(arrows)* to reach the normally situated cecum (C). **B.** The jejunum appears crowded in the right upper abdomen, being in direct continuation with the descending duodenum. The ligament of Treitz is not present. A bowel segment *(arrow)* emerges to continue as the left-sided ileum. s = stomach.

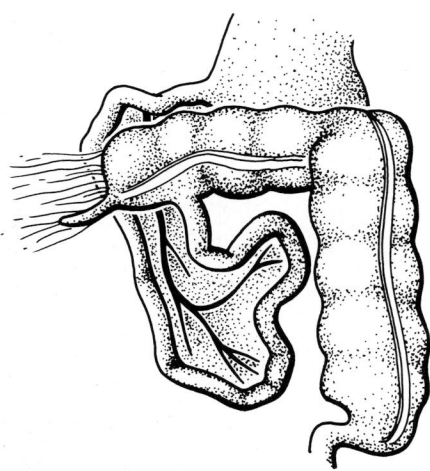

**Figure 55–5. Mixed rotation or malrotation.** The terminal ileum re-entered first. The 180-degree rotation was incomplete. Here, the cecum lies in front of the duodenum; Ladd's bands are present and may compress the duodenum or upper jejunum.

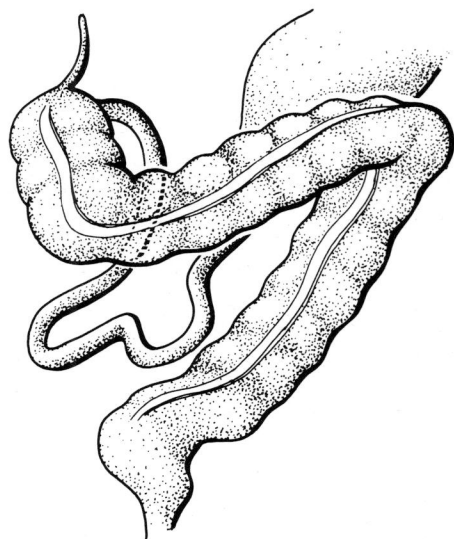

**Figure 55–6. Premature fixation of cecum.** Elongation of transverse colon has caused cecal inversion with appendix directed upward. (From Maglinte DDT, Herlinger H: Congenital and developmental anomalies in adolescents and adults. *In* Herlinger H, Maglinte D [eds]: Clinical Radiology of the Small Intestine. Philadelphia: WB Saunders, 1989, pp 249–273, as adapted from Gray SW, Skandalakis JE: Embryology for Surgeons. Philadelphia: WB Saunders, 1972.)

Reverse rotation is a rare form of malrotation in which the postarterial segment has entered the abdomen first and the colon comes to lie behind the superior mesenteric artery.

## Mesocolic (Paraduodenal) Hernias

These hernias may be regarded as developmental anomalies caused by trapping of bowel loops in colonic mesentery before completion of its fixation and obliteration. The hernial sacs are thus formed by mesocolon. The opening into the left mesocolic hernia is the fossa of Landzert, the anterior edge of which contains the inferior mesenteric vein and left colic artery. The opening into the right mesocolic hernial sac is known as the fossa of Waldeyer and contains the superior mesenteric vessels in its anterior edge.[4]

A right mesocolic (paraduodenal) hernia lies behind the ascending colon or hepatic flexure. Entering and exiting bowel segments are in close proximity (Fig. 55–7). Isolated malrotations of the prearterial segment can

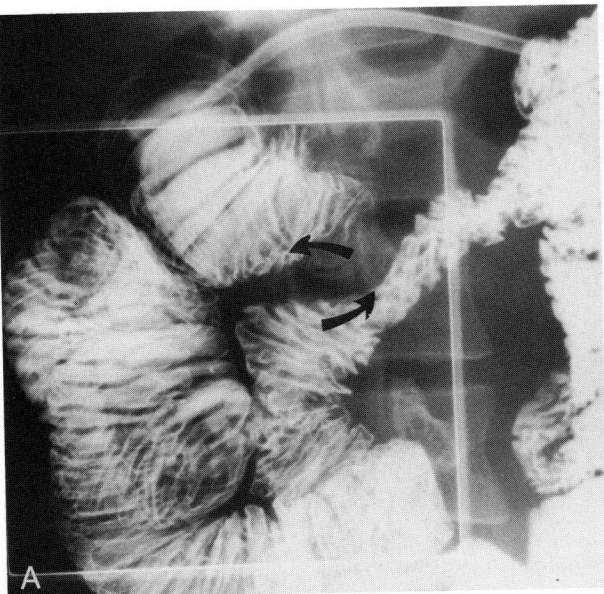
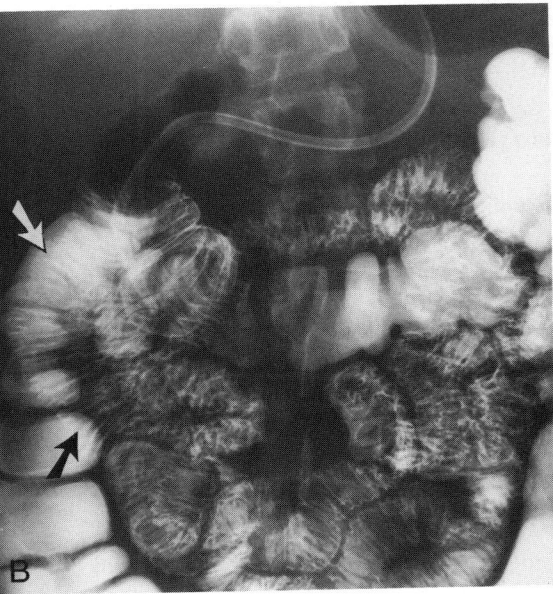

**Figure 55–7. Right mesocolic (paraduodenal) hernia. A.** A few loops of jejunum occupy a right-sided space with entry into it from the descending duodenum *(top arrow)*. The exiting segment *(bottom arrow)* is close to the entering segment and continues in the direction of the left upper abdomen. **B.** Overview. The jejunal loops shown above *(arrows)* were situated behind the hepatic flexure and ascending colon. The patient was asymptomatic at the time of study but gave a history of intermittent partial small bowel obstruction.

superficially resemble a right mesocolic hernia. However, the entering and exiting limbs are widely separated and the jejunal loops are found anterior to the right colon (see Fig. 55–4B). A right mesocolic hernia may be associated with premature fixation of the cecum and the presence of Ladd's bands.

A left mesocolic (paraduodenal) hernia presents as a circumscribed group of jejunal loops that form a convex margin inferiorly. The hernia is enclosed in a sac formed by left mesocolon and extends to the left and caudad. The afferent bowel loop enters the hernial sac posteriorly as a continuation of the duodenum (Fig. 55–8). The exiting limb passes through the hernial orifice, often well below the entering segment. The stomach and the splenic flexure and descending colon may be displaced by the hernia.

Computed tomographic (CT) demonstration can be characteristic. In a right mesocolic hernia, jejunal branches of the mesenteric artery and vein loop behind these vessels and curve to the right. Grouped or crowded loops of jejunum may be seen on the right side.[5] In a left mesocolic hernia, herniated loops of bowel may displace the stomach or be situated behind the pancreas.

Mesocolic hernias are the most frequent of the internal abdominal hernias and account for more than half of the reported cases. It has been claimed that left

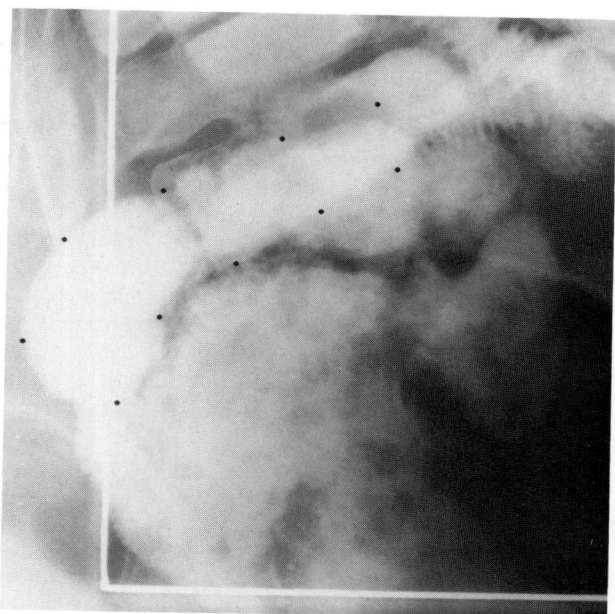

Figure 55–9. Paracecal hernia. A loop of ileum (outlined by dots) has herniated through a defect in the cecal mesentery and extends beyond the right cecal margin.

mesocolic hernias occur three times more often than those on the right side.[4] However, it now appears that right mesocolic hernias are not as rare as was previously suggested. Mesocolic hernias, especially those on the left side, tend to increase in size with time and may then take in greater lengths of bowel. The hernias frequently result in symptoms because they cause varying degrees of intermittent bowel obstruction. Radiologic recognition and surgical repair usually follow several years of unexplained symptoms.[6]

## Other Internal Abdominal Hernias Involving Small Bowel

Paracecal hernias arise during the third stage of rotation when a loop of ileum protrudes behind the cecum at the time of its descent and fixation. Paracecal hernias can also be acquired and pass through congenital or postsurgical defects in a cecal or appendiceal mesentery. Barium studies show a loop of ileum in fixed position behind the cecum and protruding beyond its lateral margin (Fig. 55–9). Paracecal hernias have been reported to account for 13% of internal hernias.[7]

Lesser sac hernias constitute 8% of internal abdominal hernias.[7] Most enter the lesser sac via the foramen of Winslow. In rare cases they protrude through defects in the gastrohepatic omentum[8] or the transverse mesocolon. Normally, the barrier of the transverse colon and greater omentum prevents small bowel access to the foramen of Winslow. Anomalies of development are considered to be necessary for herniation to occur. Such anomalies include a persistent common mesentery, nonfusion of the cecum and ascending colon to the posterior

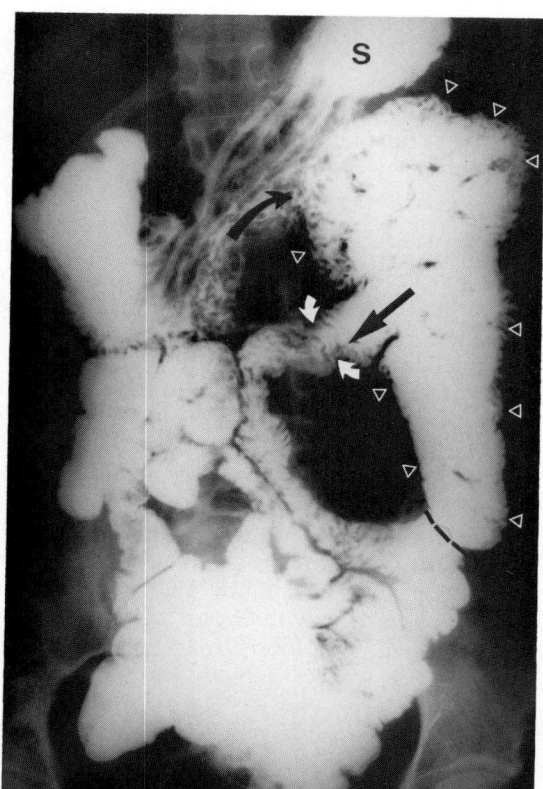

Figure 55–8. Left mesocolic (paraduodenal) hernia. Crowded bowel loops (arrowheads) occupy the left upper abdomen and displace the stomach (S) craniad. The afferent loop enters posteriorly (curved black arrow) as continuation of the duodenum. The efferent loop emerges more distally (straight arrow) and shows a slight reduction of its caliber at the hernial orifice (curved white arrows). (Courtesy of A. Friedman, M.D., Bethesda, M.D.)

wall of the abdomen, an unusually long mesentery, and a larger than normal foramen of Winslow.[9, 10]

Plain films obtained with the patient erect and supine may be valuable. A circumscribed collection of bowel loops with air-fluid levels high up in the left abdomen, usually medial to the displaced stomach and above the transverse colon, favors this diagnosis in the clinical setting of acute bowel obstruction. The recognition of mucosal fold patterns distinguishes this finding from a lesser sac abscess.[11] CT may be used to localize bowel loops within the lesser sac. The hernia contains loops of small bowel more often than cecum (Fig. 55–10) or other parts of the colon.[12]

Intersigmoid and transmesenteric hernias each account for about 6% of internal hernias.[7] Transomental hernias are rare.

## Meckel's Diverticulum

This is the most frequent congenital anomaly involving the intestinal tract. The incidence at autopsies has been reported to be up to 3%.[13] This is a true diverticulum because it contains all the layers of the bowel wall and, unlike pseudodiverticula, arises from the antimesenteric border. The diverticulum is usually situated within 100 cm of the ileocecal valve and is formed by incomplete obliteration of the ileal end of the vitelline duct. A fibrous band, representing the obliterated part of the vitelline duct, may connect the apex of the diverticulum to the umbilicus.

**Clinical Features.** Most Meckel's diverticula do not cause symptoms. Of those that give rise to symptoms, two thirds present before the age of 2 years. It was observed that symptomatic diverticula are three to four times more frequent in males than in females, whereas asymptomatic diverticula affect both sexes equally.[14] A lining of acid-secreting gastric mucosa can be responsible for peptic ulceration within or close to the diverticulum and can cause bleeding, the most frequent clinical presentation, especially during childhood. Diverticulitis,

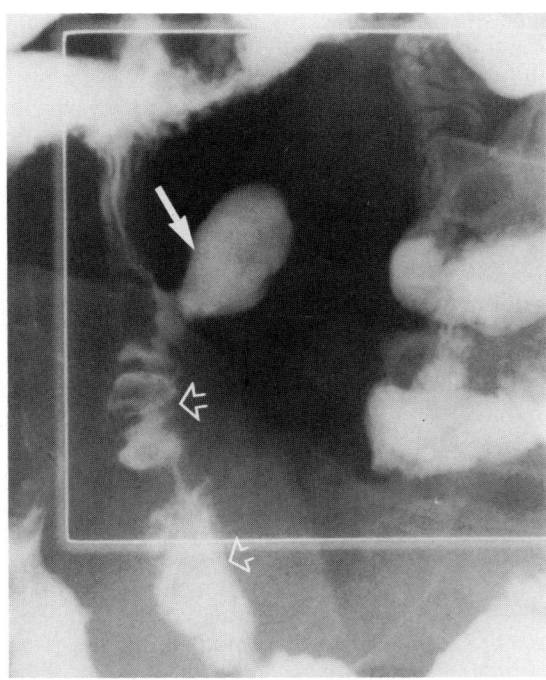

**Figure 55–11. Meckel's diverticulum.** On the follow-through barium examination a Meckel diverticulum is outlined *(solid arrow)*. Separation of bowel loops caused by Crohn's disease *(open arrows)* has facilitated the demonstration of the diverticulum.

mimicking appendicitis, may be caused by obstruction of the diverticular orifice (e.g., by a tumor) or by the presence of an enterolith within the diverticulum. Small bowel obstruction is another important form of presentation. Its causes include torsion in relation to a persistent vitelline band, internal herniation of the diverticulum, or extrusion of the diverticulum into an inguinal hernia (hernia of Littre) (see Fig. 55–12B). Another cause of obstruction is intussusception of an inverted diverticulum.

**Radiologic Diagnosis.** Plain films of the abdomen may demonstrate features of mechanical small bowel obstruction, usually without revealing a Meckel diverticulum as its cause. Occasionally, a large diverticulum may contain sufficient gas to draw attention to this possible diagnosis. An enterolith may lodge in a Meckel diverticulum, but this relationship must be confirmed by barium study. A conventional follow-through examination rarely demonstrates a Meckel diverticulum.[15] However, if the diverticulum is associated with Crohn's disease, the wider separation of distal ileal loops by the disease facilitates demonstration[16] even by follow-through examination (Fig. 55–11).

Enteroclysis is the most reliable barium method for the diagnosis of a Meckel diverticulum.[17–19] The blind-ended sac arises at the antimesenteric border of the ileum with either a broad base or a narrow neck. When it is broad based, enteroclysis in the stage of lumen distention can show a distinctive junctional fold pattern at the site of origin.[17] Typically, this is shown as a triangular arrangement of folds at the base (Fig. 55–12A) or, when not fully distended, as a triradiate fold

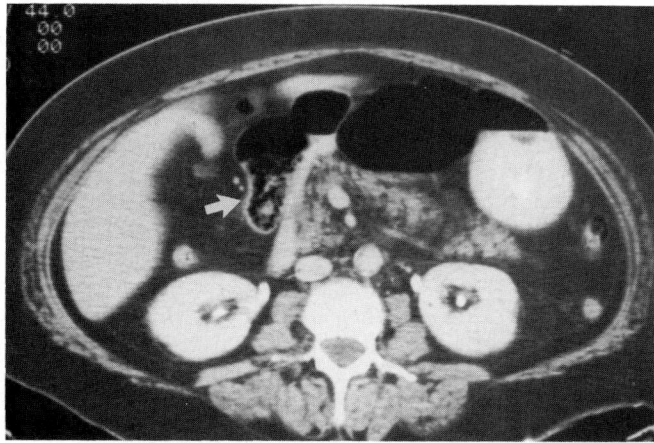

**Figure 55–10. Hernia of cecum through the foramen of Winslow.** On the CT scan the herniated cecum *(arrow)* is outlined as it displaces the stomach and duodenum.

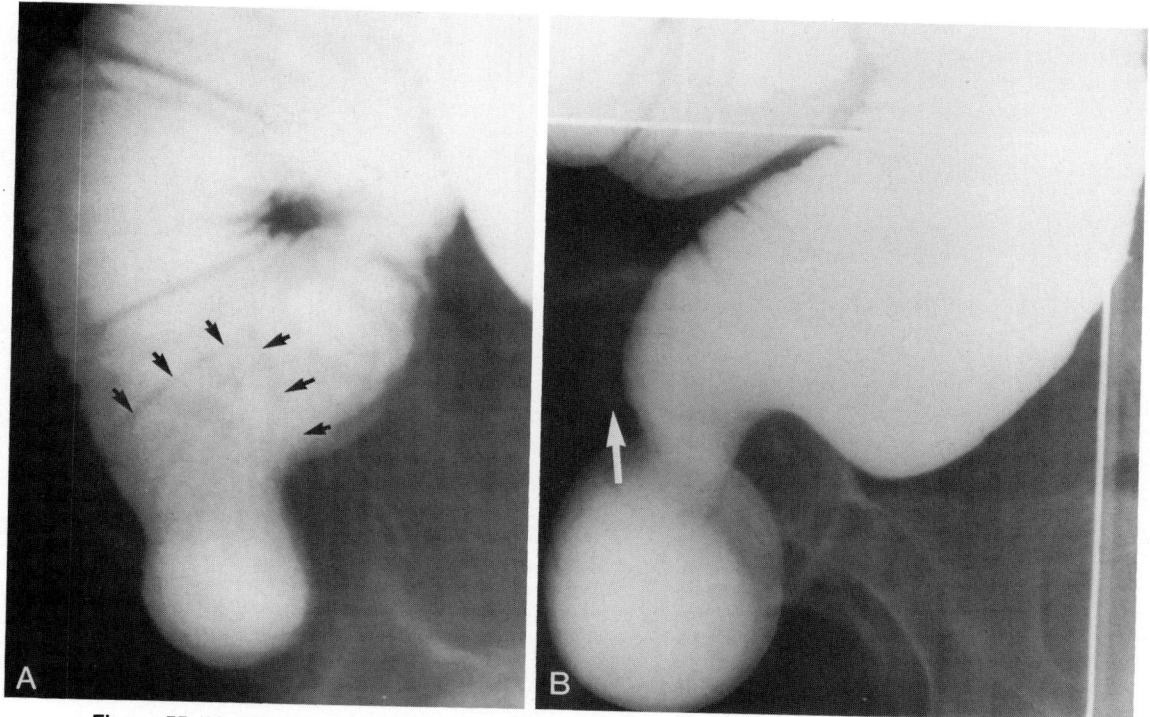

**Figure 55–12. Meckel's diverticulum and hernia of Littre. A.** At its broad-based origin there is a triangular arrangement of folds, the mucosal plateau *(arrows)*. **B.** Two months later, because of a high-grade small bowel obstruction, another enteroclysis was done. An irreducible inguinal hernia of the Meckel diverticulum was found (hernia of Littre). Its exiting limb was severely narrowed and is barely seen on this image *(arrow)*.

pattern.[17, 20] Origin with a narrow neck is seen more rarely (Fig. 55–13). The diagnosis then depends on the clear demonstration of its blind termination and antimesenteric origin. Even with enteroclysis, Meckel's diverticula are not usually identified without a careful search through the distal loops of ileum. Such intermittent fluoroscopic search must be done with compression during both the single and double contrast stages of the enteroclysis. The diverticulum may initially appear small and unremarkable but, with increasing lumen distention,

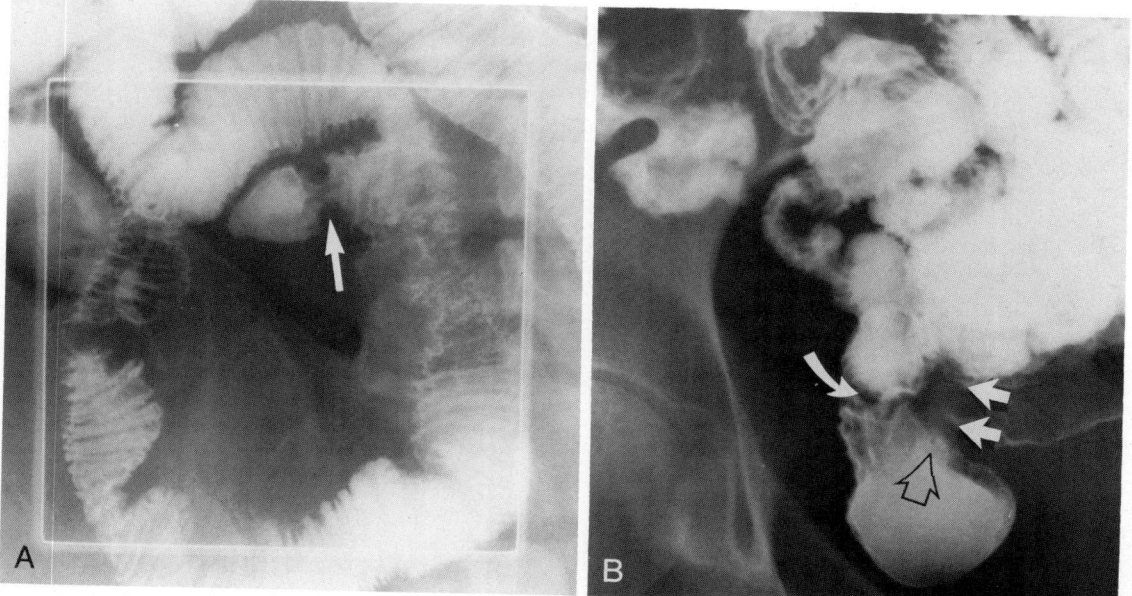

**Figure 55–13. Narrow-necked Meckel's diverticula. A.** Simple Meckel's diverticulum with a narrow origin *(arrow)*. **B.** Short, narrow origin *(curved arrow)* of a Meckel diverticulum. From its apex *(open arrow)* a short, straight lumen *(solid arrows)* extends into the vitelline ligament.

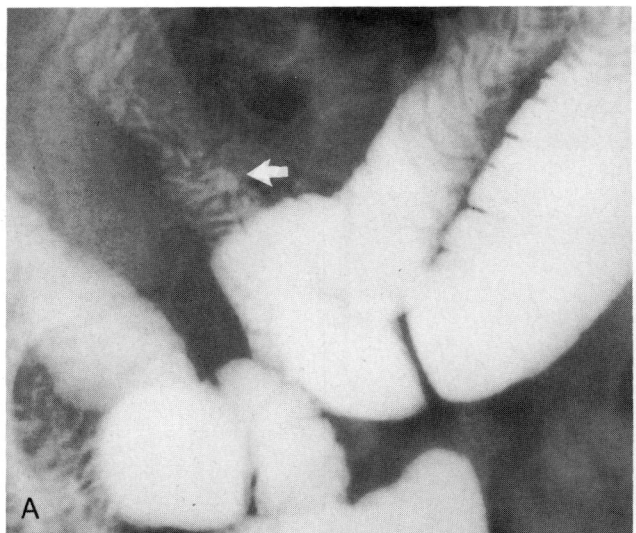 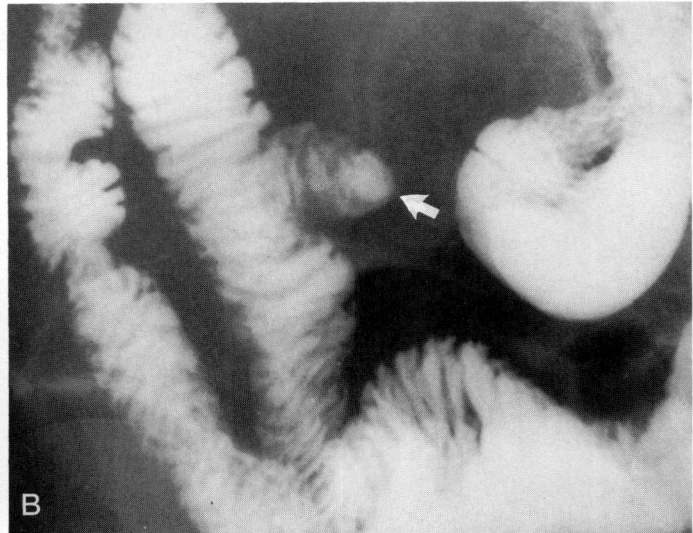

**Figure 55–14. Difficult identification of a Meckel diverticulum. A.** An unremarkable partially filled structure is seen during initial compression *(arrow).* **B.** With further filling and compression during barium infusion the diverticulum becomes obvious *(arrow).* (From DDT Maglinte, MF Elmore, M Isenberg, et al, Meckel diverticulum: radiologic demonstration by enteroclysis, AJR, 134, 5, 925–932, 1980, © by American Roentgen Ray Society.)

may fill more completely (Fig. 55–14), rendering confident diagnosis possible.[21] Mistaking a superimposed bowel loop for a Meckel diverticulum can be avoided if compression views are taken with different obliquities.[22] It is possible for the less experienced to fail to identify even a typical Meckel diverticulum. Occasionally, a Meckel diverticulum is demonstrated by reflux into the ileum during a double contrast barium enema (Fig. 55–15). An inverted, intussuscepting Meckel's diverticulum can be demonstrated by enteroclysis (Fig. 55–16).

**The Meckel Scan.** Because gastric mucosal heterotopia is usually associated with bleeding from a Meckel diverticulum, technetium Tc 99m pertechnetate, which is taken up by gastric mucosa, can be used for scanning. Both false-positive and false-negative results are re-

ported with this test, which is more likely to be successful in children.[23] Enteroclysis can demonstrate features that suggest the presence of ectopic gastric mucosa in a Meckel diverticulum,[21] to be confirmed later by surgery (Fig. 55–17).

## Midgut Duplications

Enteric duplications are either cystic or tubular. When related to the small bowel, they occur more often in the ileum.

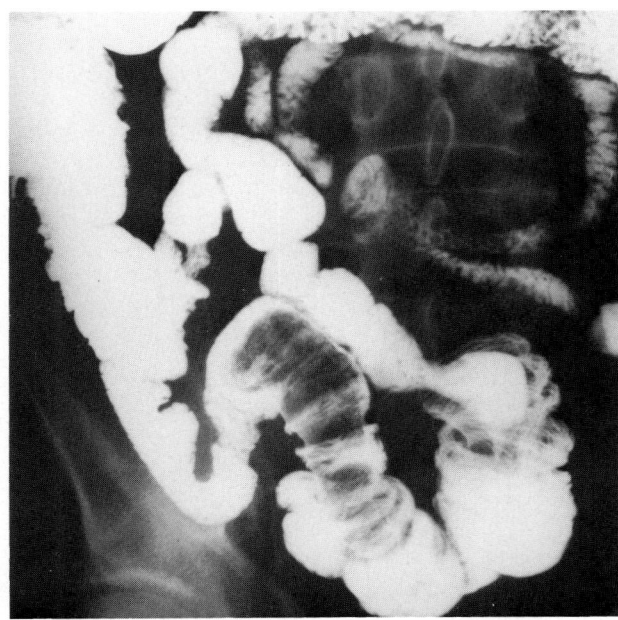

**Figure 55–16. Invaginated Meckel's diverticulum.** The patient presented with gastrointestinal bleeding and episodes of abdominal pain, probably caused by recurring intussusception. At laparotomy the inverted diverticulum was found to contain ulcerated ectopic gastric mucosa.

**Figure 55–15. Meckel's diverticulum *(arrow)* demonstrated by reflux during a double contrast barium enema.** The groove at its origin and the absence of any fold pattern within it suggest aberrant mucosal lining.

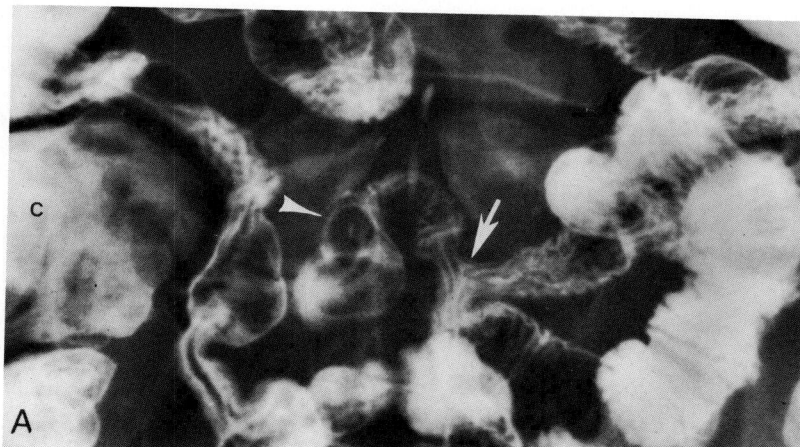
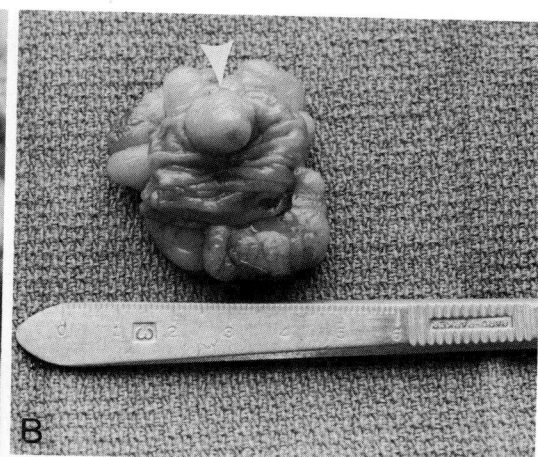
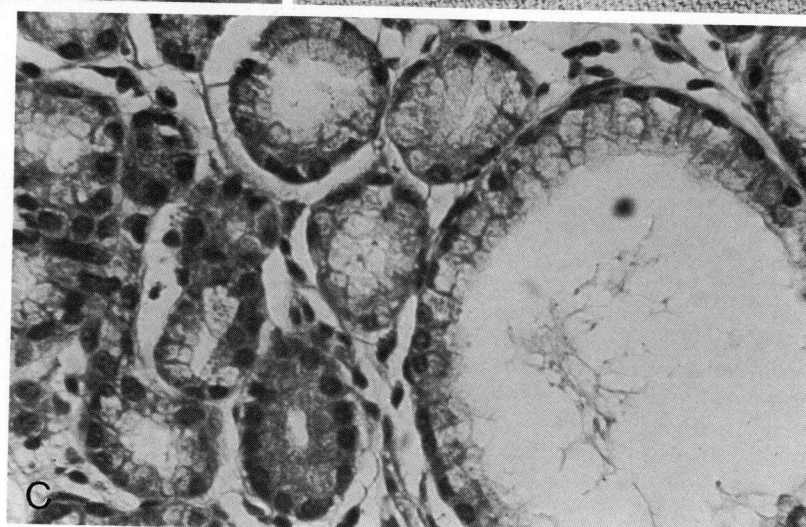

**Figure 55–17. Ectopic mucosa in a Meckel diverticulum. A.** Triradiate fold pattern at the origin of the diverticulum *(arrow)*. An umbilicated filling defect is seen within the diverticulum *(arrowhead)*. **B.** Longitudinally opened diverticulum. A polypoid nodule that represents the filling defect shown in **A** is indicated by an arrowhead. **C.** Histology of nodule revealed gastric epithelium. (**A** to **C** from DDT Maglinte, MF Elmore, M Isenberg, et al, Meckel diverticulum: radiologic demonstration by enteroclysis, AJR, 134, 5, 925–932, 1980, © by American Roentgen Ray Society.)

Enteric duplication cysts can be small and intramural and may cause obstruction. Others are larger, forming unilocular, noncalcified, thick-walled masses adjacent to or at some distance from the mesenteric border of a bowel segment.[24] They are lined with enteric mucosa and, if adjacent to bowel, may share the muscularis. The cysts are likely to cause symptoms during childhood or adolescence. They must be differentiated from lymphangiomas, which have the same age incidence. Lymphangiomas tend to be larger, are multiloculated, contain fluid of varying echogenicity, and are more aggressive.[24]

Tubular enteric duplications occur more infrequently than cystic duplications. They are found on the mesenteric side of the bowel and share its muscle coat. Their lumen may be in communication with the normal bowel at both ends or only at one end. Occasionally there is no communication. When they present with gastrointestinal tract bleeding, they are likely to be lined with gastric mucosa and to communicate with the normal gut. Multiple small bowel–related duplications have been reported in 3 to 6% of cases.[25]

The ectopic gastric mucosal lining can be useful in the diagnosis. $^{99m}$Tc scintigraphy has been reported to have 86% sensitivity.[26] Barium studies show mostly extrinsic-type displacement and deformity of a segment of bowel or opacification of a communicating tubular duplication.

## Segmental Dilatation

A probably congenital neuromuscular disorder is believed to be the cause of isolated dilatation of a segment of small intestine. The condition presents predominantly during childhood, although the diagnosis is also made in a smaller number of adults. Only 33 cases were reported up to 1989.[27] When identified in the neonatal period, it may be overshadowed by other congenital abnormalities like exomphalos. The segmental dilatation found in children is associated with normal peristalsis. Clinical presentation may be anemia associated with ulceration in the dilated segment or a volvulus.

Segmental dilatation found in adults affects the distal ileum and is also known as ileal dysgenesis. It, too, is probably of developmental origin, a supposition supported by the presence of ectopic gastric mucosa or other aberrant mucosal linings.[28] There is focal atonicity, which acts as a peristaltic barrier, and obstructive symptoms are usual.

Barium radiology outlines the flaccid and dilated segment of ileum and occasionally also an ulcer (Fig. 55–18).

## ENDOMETRIOSIS AND THE SMALL BOWEL

Endometriosis is defined as the presence of endometrial tissue outside the myometrium. Endometrial deposition may follow retrograde menstruation. It is a frequently occurring disorder, affecting about 15% of women between menarche and menopause. The bowel is a site of involvement in up to 37% of the patients, with the rectosigmoid area affected in almost 95% of patients.[29] The small bowel, mostly the terminal ileum, becomes a site of endometrial deposition in up to 7% of cases.[30]

The serosal implants of endometrial material are under the influence of ovarian hormones, which cause bleeding into tissue to occur at the end of the menstrual cycle. This produces an inflammatory and desmoplastic response and gradual extension of the implant to involve but not often invade the mucosa. Mucosal ulceration caused by endometriosis is rare. Thus, bleeding into the intestinal lumen would be unusual unless caused by associated ischemia, which may be secondary to the fibrosis or to intussusception. The endometriosis-related desmoplasia continues to be a factor after menopause. However, postmenopausal endometrial activity is unlikely without intake of exogenous estrogens.

**Radiology.** Barium follow-through examinations have not been able to identify endometrial deposits in the

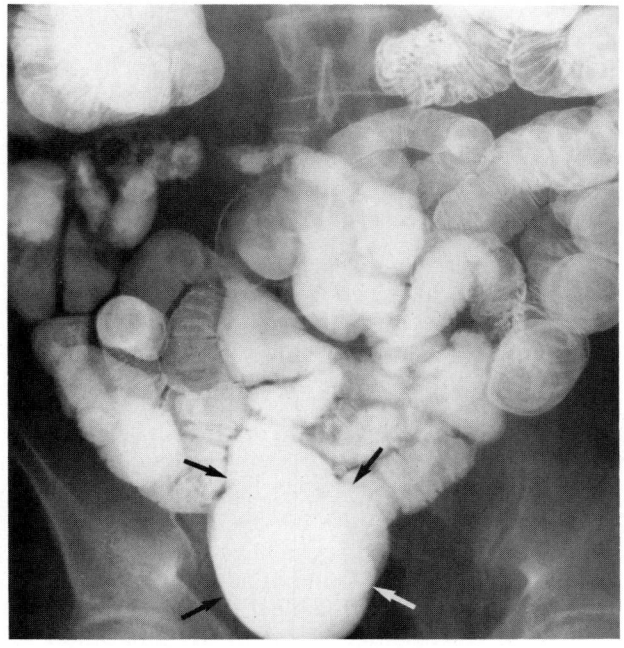

**Figure 55–18. Ileal dysgenesis.** Localized dilatation of ileum *(arrows).* The aperistaltic segment acted as a peristaltic barrier. The condition was probably congenital, an ileal dysgenesis. Resection gave temporary relief. Adhesive obstructions developed later.

small bowel.[31] Enteroclysis has been able to outline and characterize endometrial deposits in terminal ileum (Fig. 55–19). The findings resemble the endometriosis-related changes frequently seen in the rectosigmoid, that is, crinkling of the mucosa and a plaque-like deformity of the lumen. Small bowel obstruction, acute or of lower grade, may be produced by the endometrial deposits.[32] Obstruction is produced by fibrosis-associated kinking, only rarely by intussusception headed by the deposit.[33] Radiologic differentiation from a seeded metastasis is not always possible. Laparoscopy or sigmoidoscopy may then be indicated.

## RETRACTILE MESENTERITIS (LIPODYSTROPHY)

This rare disease of unknown etiology is due primarily to degeneration of mesenteric fat, at times related to excessive fat deposition (panniculitis). Fibrosis follows fat degeneration and necrosis. The massively thickened mesentery contracts, adhesions are formed, and small bowel loops are drawn toward the root of the mesentery. However, nodular masses in the thickened mesentery focally resist retraction and displace some of the loops from their more central position.

Abdominal pain is the most frequent clinical presentation. There may also be fever, nausea, constipation, and even bowel obstruction. However, in 43% of a series of patients the condition was asymptomatic at the time of its incidental discovery.[34] Mesenteric vein thrombosis is a rare complication. Palpation of the abdomen gives the vague impression that an abdominal mass is present. Surgical treatment is not indicated, although surgery may be required for definitive diagnosis. Prednisone and azathioprine are effective provided that treatment is given before fibrosis has become advanced.[35]

**Radiologic Diagnosis.** Barium studies show a combination of loop crowding and loop displacement (Fig. 55–20). Similar appearances can be found in patients with carcinomatosis, especially from ovarian cancer. However, there should always be evidence of indentations and fold changes caused by associated seeding of metastases. Extensive radiation damage may involve the mesentery and cause fibrosis. Evidence of radiation enteropathy would aid differential diagnosis. Ileal carcinoids with extention into the mesentery can produce pronounced loop retraction and may even cause ischemia. Recognition of the typical changes in the mesentery on CT scans facilitates the diagnosis of carcinoid (see Chapter 51). As with many other conditions in the abdomen, the synergistic effect of CT and barium is valuable. CT demonstrates the mesenteric thickening and its fatty composition, thus supporting and advancing the barium-based findings.

**Mesenteric Fibromatosis (Desmoid).** This rare tumorous condition has been reported in 17% of patients with Gardner's syndrome.[36] Occasionally, desmoids occur in the absence of familial polyposis (see Chapter 50).

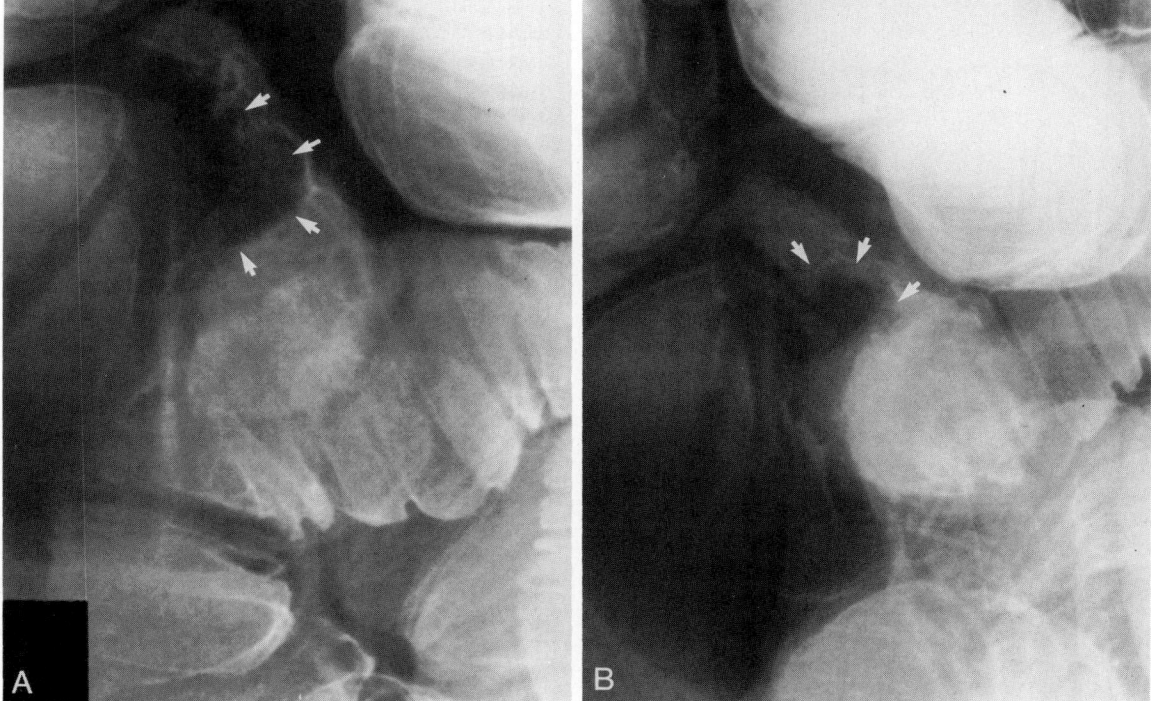

**Figure 55–19. Endometrial implants in terminal ileum. A.** Enteroclysis demonstrates an endometrial deposit in the terminal ileum. This view shows the proximal portion of a plaque-like defect *(arrows)* with irregular crinkling of the mucosa. **B.** Distal termination of the implant *(arrows)* short of the ileocecal valve.

## SCLEROSING ENCAPSULATING PERITONITIS

Practolol, a beta-adrenergic antagonist formerly used in England and unavailable in the United States, has been a cause of sclerosing peritonitis ("practolol peritonitis").[37] Although the now widely used beta-antago-

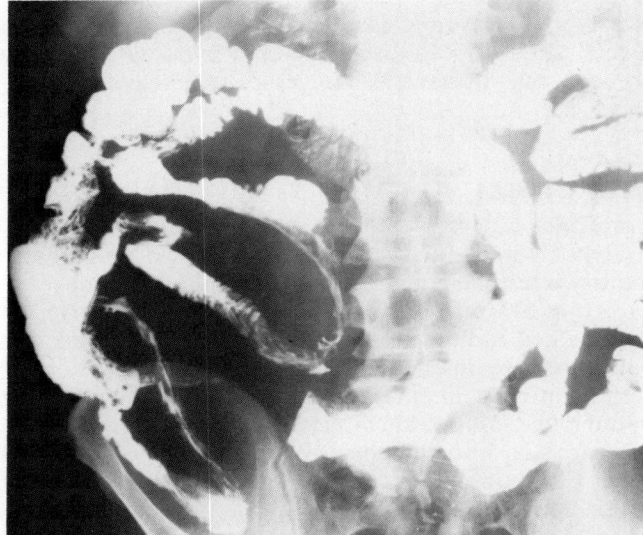

**Figure 55–20. Mesenteric lipodystrophy.** Bowel loops in the left abdomen appear drawn together; those on the right side are separated by fibrous mesenteric masses.

nist propranolol is generally free of this complication, there have been reports of occasional association.[38] However, this association has been challenged and no further reports could be found.

Two distinct entities are often referred to as sclerosing peritonitis:[39]

1. A developmental anomaly, in itself of no clinical significance. An accessory membrane covers the small bowel and attaches to the ascending, transverse, and descending colon, leaving an opening above and below. *Peritoneal encapsulation* is a better term for it (Fig. 55–21).
2. The other entity is also known as the abdominal cocoon syndrome. A densely sclerotic collagenous covering of the peritoneal surface of the small bowel results in obstruction. It is an uncommon but serious complication of chronic ambulatory peritoneal dialysis.[40] Repeated low-grade infections are a likely etiologic factor. If a diagnosis is made before bowel obstruction has occurred, surgical removal of the thickened membrane may be possible. With delayed diagnosis, death occurs within 4 months in 60% of patients. Other possible associations are the presence of a LeVeen shunt and, although unproved, asbestosis.

**Radiology of the Cocoon Syndrome.** In established disease there are characteristic findings. Plain films of the abdomen show centrally located, sometimes dilated loops, with persistence of their position and appearance on serial films. Barium studies show dilatation of prox-

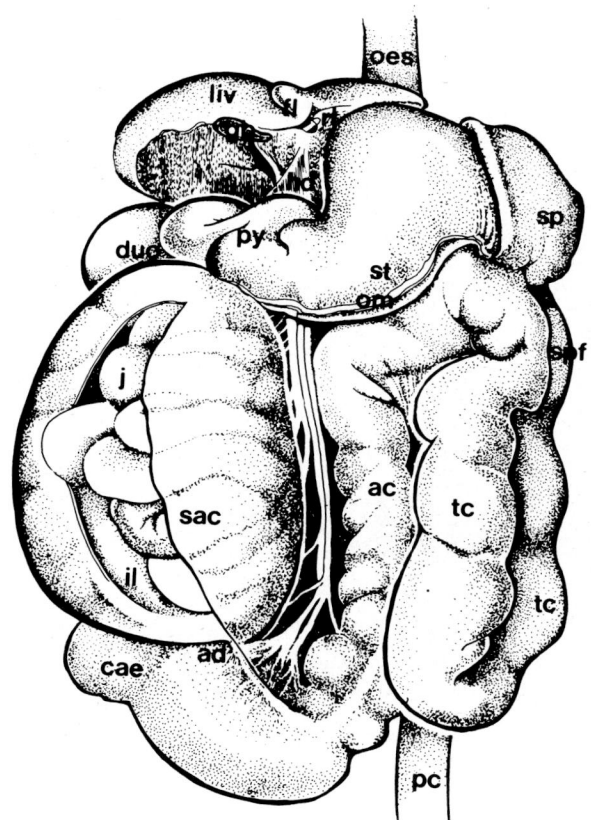

**Figure 55–21. Congenital intestinal encapsulation.** The jejunum and ileum are enclosed in an avascular sac that represents the embryonic coelom. Abnormal placement of the colon. oes = esophagus; liv = liver; fl = falciform ligament; gb = gallbladder; hd = hepatoduodenal ligament; duo = duodenum; py = pylorus; sp = spleen; st = stomach; om = omentum (cut edge); spf = splenic flexure; j = jejunum; sac = avascular sac; ac = ascending colon; tc = transverse colon; il = ileum; cae = cecum; ad = adhesions; pc = pelvic colon. (From Papez JW: A rare anomaly of embryonic origin. Anat Rec 54:197–214, 1932. Copyright © 1932 Wiley-Liss. Reprinted by permission of Wiley-Liss, a division of John Wiley and Sons, Inc.)

imal loops changing to a reduced caliber and loop crowding when encapsulated bowel is reached. Mucosal folds may be crowded with features of sacculation. The cocooned loops are usually low in the abdomen, rigid, and inseparable. Peristaltic activity is reduced and ineffective.[40]

# PNEUMATOSIS CYSTOIDES INTESTINALIS

Cystic or arcuate collections of gas are located in the subserosa or submucosa, more often in the jejunum. These radiolucencies can be identified on plain films of the abdomen, although it may occasionally be difficult to distinguish pneumatosis from fat or intraluminal gas. A barium study may then confirm the extraluminal, intramural location of the pneumatosis.

Although pneumatosis cystoides may cause no symptoms or may be clinically submerged in symptoms of its underlying causes, another more serious type of pneumatosis accompanies ischemic or inflammatory disorders, more often in children. Pneumatosis, in such cases, is more likely to be of linear configuration, possibly associated with gas in the portal venous system. Severe ulcerative colitis has been reported to be accompanied by colonic pneumatosis demonstrated by CT.[41] Of three patients with advanced Crohn's disease, one had pneumatosis of the terminal ileum, also shown by CT.[42] The pneumatosis itself did not contribute to the clinical problem.

The benign form of pneumatosis cystoides has two major groups of etiologies:

1. Gas dissection from the lung in patients with obstructive airway disease. Gas is believed to derive from ruptured alveoli and to dissect along vessels and bronchi into the mediastinum and then along major vessels into the retroperitoneum, from which it moves via the mesentery to the subserosa of bowel loops.
2. Gas entry into the bowel wall from the lumen, either through a mucosal defect (ulcer, tear) or as a result of increased intraluminal pressure and distention but without an obvious mucosal defect. Numerous pathologies can cause this form of pneumatosis. Included are collagen diseases (scleroderma), surgery or endoscopy, inflammatory conditions (Crohn's disease, parasites), intestinal obstruction, jejunal diverticulosis, and blunt trauma.[43] Jejunostomy feeding catheter placement has been another cause of jejunal pneumatosis cystoides[44] (Fig. 55–22). Further associations are bone marrow transplantation[45] and injection sclerotherapy for esophageal varices.[46]

A well-documented complication of pneumatosis is spontaneous rupture of a gas cyst and formation of an often asymptomatic pneumoperitoneum. Treatment is usually unnecessary. Because the cysts contain high levels (70 to 75%) of nitrogen,[47] hyperbaric oxygen therapy can be beneficial in cases of persistent pneumatosis.[48]

# INTESTINAL EDEMA

Hypoalbuminemia is a frequent cause of noninflammatory intestinal edema. Serum albumin levels must fall to 2.0 g/100 mL or less for intestinal edema to be appreciated radiologically. The decreased capillary oncotic pressure in the bowel wall causes an outflow of serum into the interstitial compartment. The resulting volume increase mostly affects the submucosa, including its extension into the core of the small bowel mucosal folds. Hypoalbuminemia may result from malabsorption (e.g., celiac disease, malnutrition), protein loss (lymphangiectasia, Ménétrier's disease, extensive Crohn's disease), the nephrotic syndrome, and cirrhosis. Of interest in radiology is the finding of a lumen diameter

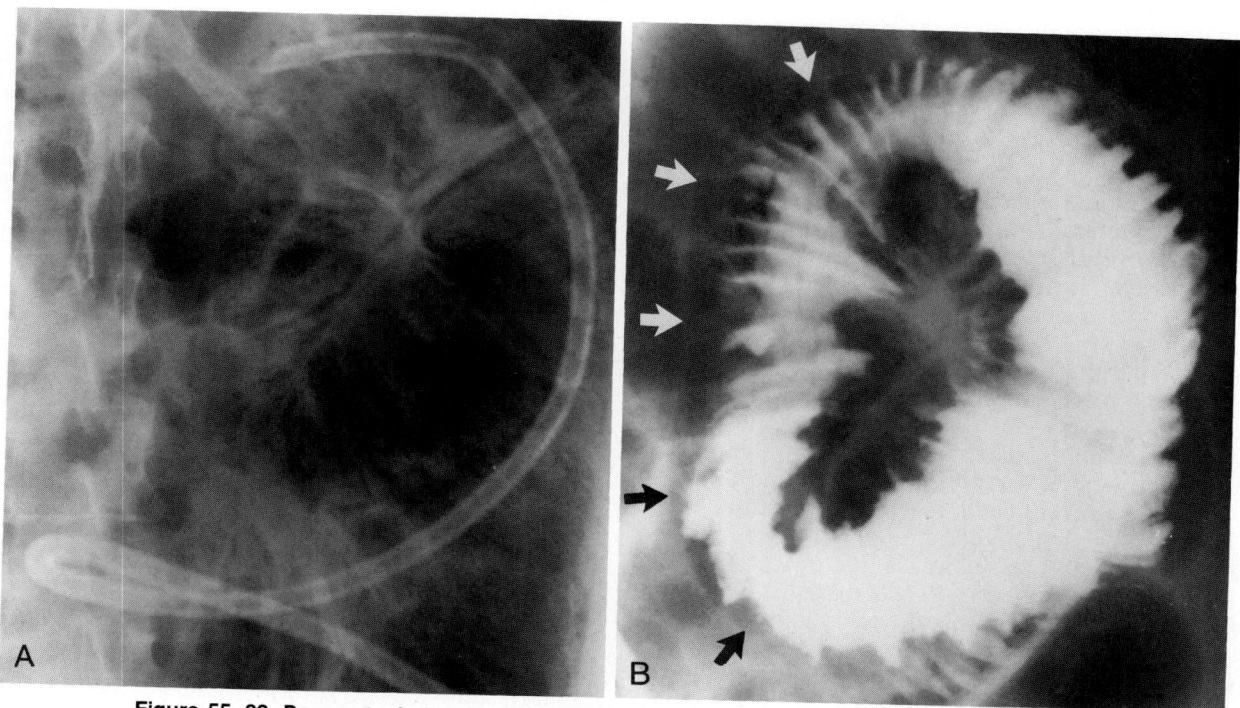

**Figure 55–22. Pneumatosis intestinalis from surgical placement of a jejunal feeding tube. A.** Plain film shows extraluminal, intramural air. **B.** Barium study done in the absence of free intraperitoneal air clearly demonstrates the intramural and extraluminal location of the air *(arrows)*.

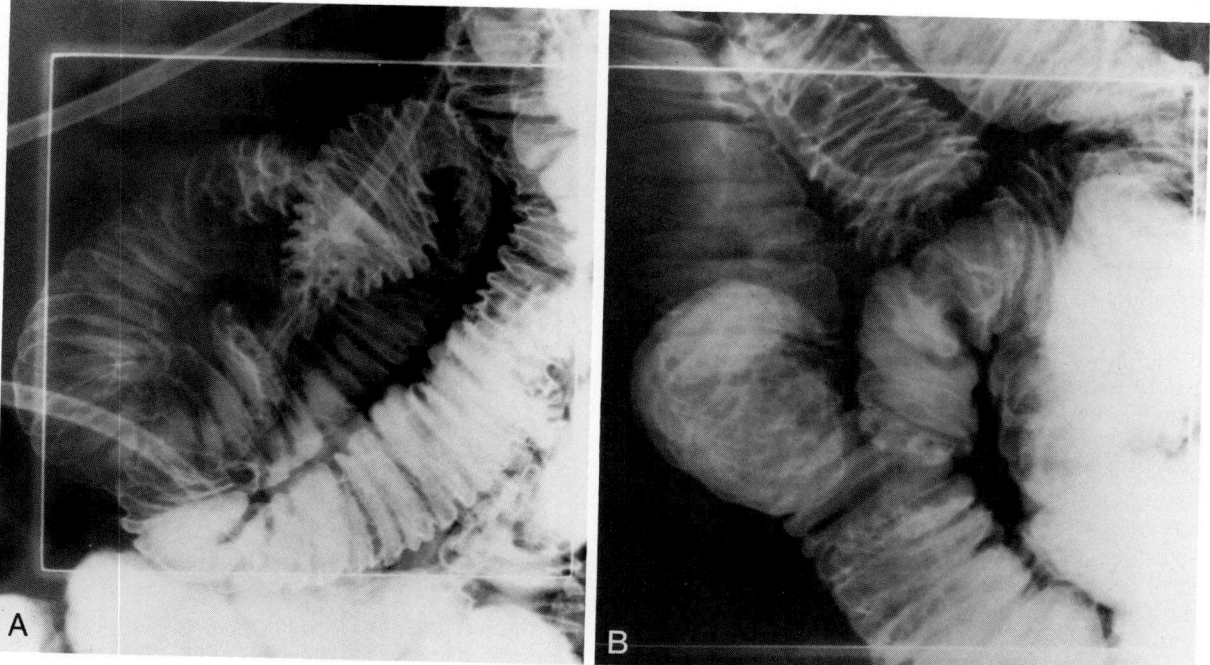

**Figure 55–23. Intestinal edema.** The patient had portal hypertension, portal vein thrombosis, and hepatic cirrhosis. Enteroclysis was done. **A.** Jejunal loops are slightly dilated with obviously thickened mucosal folds. **B.** Fold thickening and lumen diameter increase extend toward the ileum. Ascites was present.

increase in the jejunum in some patients with hypoalbuminemia with values below 2.7 g/100 mL.[49]

Increased venous pressure in the portal area is another frequent cause of intestinal edema. In cirrhotic patients with portal hypertension, intestinal edema is a frequent finding. Several causative factors are involved. They include hypoalbuminemia resulting from decreased liver synthesis of albumin, excess formation of hepatic and mesenteric lymph, and elevated capillary mesenteric hydrostatic pressure.[50] Ascites virtually always accompanies this form of intestinal edema. Systemic venous congestion as in heart failure and sodium and water retention as in renal failure are further etiologic factors in the formation of edema and ascites.

**Radiology.** Although intestinal edema occurs frequently, it is not often an indication for a barium study. Appearances shown by barium are characteristic. Smooth, regular fold thickening is found throughout the small intestine and is often best shown in the jejunum (Fig. 55–23). In severe cases there may be intraluminal fluid increase. The lumen of the jejunum may be slightly widened, there may be a minor degree of wall thickening, and motor activity may be decreased.[51] The right colon may also show features of edema with deformed haustra. Ascites may be demonstrated by plain film or ultrasound.

# ENTEROLITHS, FOREIGN BODIES, BEZOARS

True enteroliths are formed within the small intestine, usually in an area of stasis, a diverticulum or above a stricture (e.g., Crohn's disease). However, they are a rare finding. If composed of bile constituents, enteroliths have usually formed in the duodenum. Enteroliths consisting predominantly of mineral salts—calcium or magnesium—may be found in the ileum.[52] They may contain a foreign body nidus.

A Meckel diverticulum is a possible site for an enterolith. About 25% of Meckel's enteroliths are calcified, and their recognition on a plain film should lead to a barium study for their localization (Fig. 55–24). An enterolith in a Meckel diverticulum may become a cause of diverticulitis and perforation or of pressure erosion of the mucosa and bleeding.

Foreign bodies are mostly ingested by psychiatric patients, children, or prisoners who wish to be transferred to a hospital. Virtually all such foreign bodies, after traversing the stomach, pass through the small bowel without causing damage. Only some 3% are retained in the small bowel.[53]

"Body packers" are smugglers of ingested narcotic substances. This method of illegal importation is used for personal consumption and is not used by major importers. A single abdominal film of the supine individual is required by customs if there is ground for suspicion and informed consent has been obtained. Heroin or other substances contained in condoms or tape-wrapped packages may be demonstrated in the small bowel, colon, or rectum.[54]

Phytobezoars (vegetable residue) and trychobezoars (hair) form in the stomach and can pass into small bowel in the presence of a gastroenterostomy or after pyloroplasty. Occasionally, there has been no prior surgery. Of interest especially in Israel are phytobezoars that form after ingestion of the persimmon fruit, which contains tannin and forms a coagulum with gastric acid.[55] Patients present with small bowel obstruction. Studies with barium or diatrizoate meglumine (Gastrografin) outline the bezoar as an unattached intraluminal mass with a finely lobulated, villous-like surface[56] (Fig. 55–25).

# DRUG-INDUCED DISORDERS

**Fluorinated Pyrimidines.** Floxuridine and fluorouracil are representative of this group of chemotherapeutic agents. They are frequently administered in combination with other agents, either systemically or by intra-arterial hepatic infusion, at times by means of an implanted infusion pump. Toxic reactions are dose related. Among the most infrequent effects is reversible damage affecting the ileum.[57] In patients with severe diarrhea and abdominal pain, a barium examination of the small bowel may demonstrate narrowed ileal loops with thickened or effaced mucosal folds. Much or all of the ileum is affected and its loops are widely separated (Fig. 55–26). Reduction of the dose of pyrimidine or interruption of treatment causes symptoms and radiologic changes to abate. Identical changes in the ileum have followed the administration of flucytosine.[58]

**Cytarabine Chemotherapy.** This drug is used in the treatment of acute leukemia and non-Hodgkin's lymphoma. Lumen distention and thickening of mucosal folds and of the bowel wall have been demonstrated on plain abdominal radiographs. These changes were dose related and were associated with granulocytopenia, diarrhea, and abdominal pain and tenderness.[59]

**Terminal Ileum in "Cathartic Colon."** Colon-irritating cathartics used habitually may cause ahaustral dilatation and atony of the right colon with similar atonic dilatation extending into the terminal ileum.[60] Colon-active cathartics include phenolphthalein, bisacodyl, senna, and cascara. Plain abdominal films and barium studies may show the right colon and terminal ileum to be featureless and dilated. The mucosal surface itself is not abnormal.

Drug-related small bowel ulceration is described in Chapter 48.

# SEAT BELT SYNDROME

Since it became obligatory for front seat car passengers to wear a three-point seat belt, road accident fatalities have decreased significantly. The number of injuries caused by road accidents has also decreased, but seat belt wearers have sustained a changed pattern of these injuries. A marked reduction has occurred in injuries to brain, facial bones, long bones, and abdominal solid organs.[61] Instead, whiplash neck injuries and

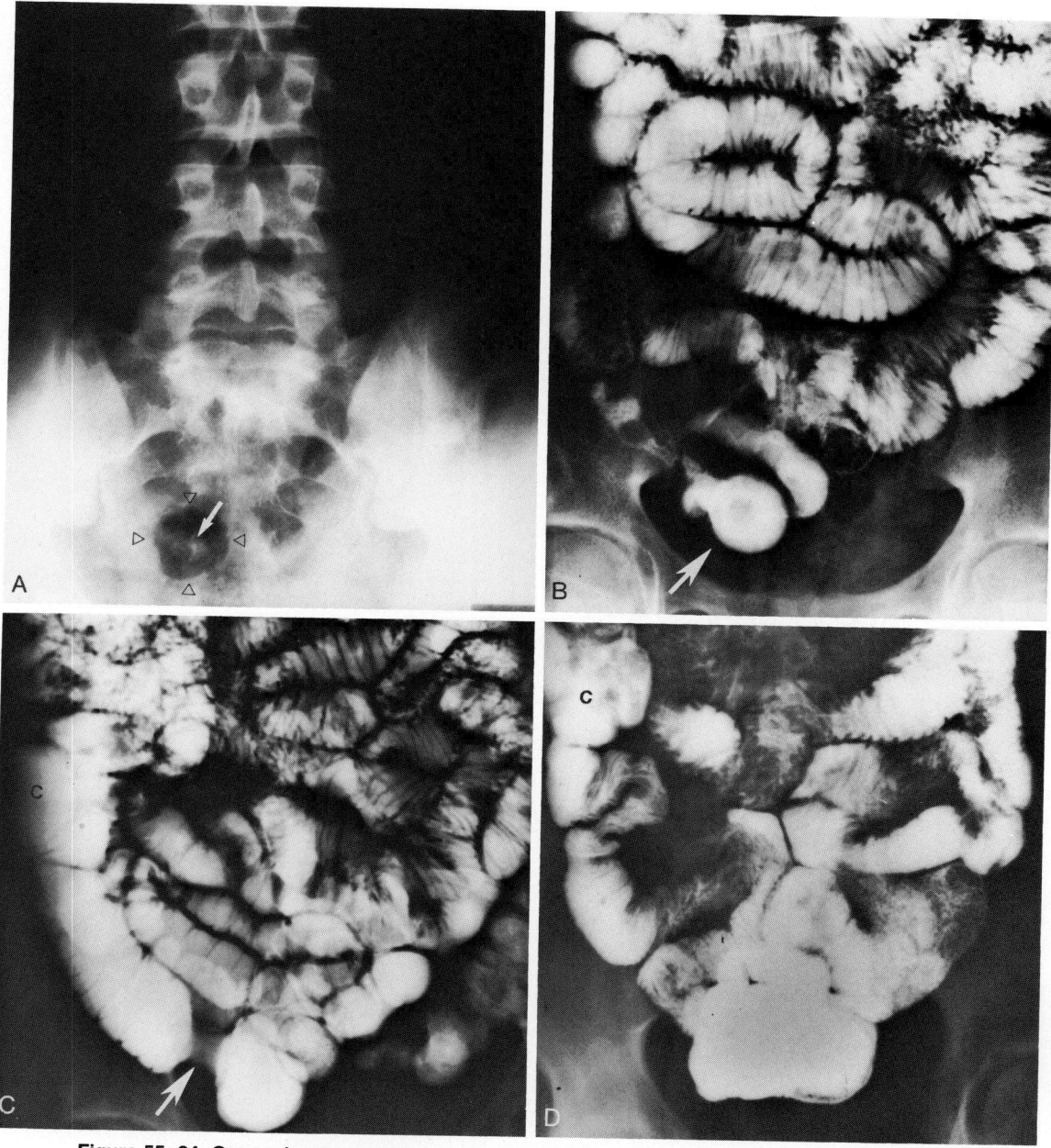

**Figure 55–24. Gas and an enterolith in a Meckel diverticulum. A.** Plain film of abdomen shows a round collection of gas *(arrowheads)* and a small density within it *(arrow).* **B.** Early film of an enteroclysis shows the previously gas-containing space now filled with barium *(arrow).* A filling defect within it corresponds to the density seen earlier, a likely enterolith. **C.** Further barium filling demonstrates a Meckel diverticulum with a narrow neck *(arrow).* The enterolith is obscured by the increased barium filling. The effacement of the fold pattern within the diverticulum was shown at surgery to represent ulcerated ectopic mucosa. **D.** A follow-through examination done 1 month before missed the diverticulum in the barium-overloaded distal ileum. c = cecum. (**B** to **D** from DDT Maglinte, MF Elmore, M Isenberg, et al, Meckel diverticulum: radiologic demonstration by enteroclysis, AJR 134, 5, 925–932, 1980, © by American Roentgen Ray Society.)

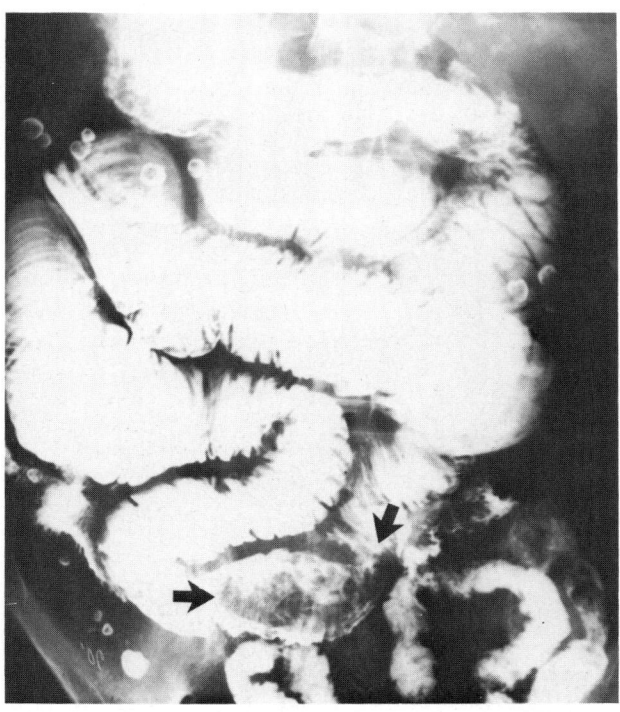

**Figure 55–25. Persimmon phytobezoar.** Prone view of a barium study in a patient with high-grade small bowel obstruction of the distal jejunum. An intraluminal mass *(arrows)* without a point of attachment to the wall was shown, its interstices filled with barium. Because this patient also had a wide gastroenterostomy and lived in Israel, the likely diagnosis was a persimmon phytobezoar. (Courtesy of Anthony G. Verstandig, M.D. From Verstandig AG, Klin B, Bloom RA, et al: Small bowel phytobezoars: detection with radiography. Radiology 172:705–707, 1989.)

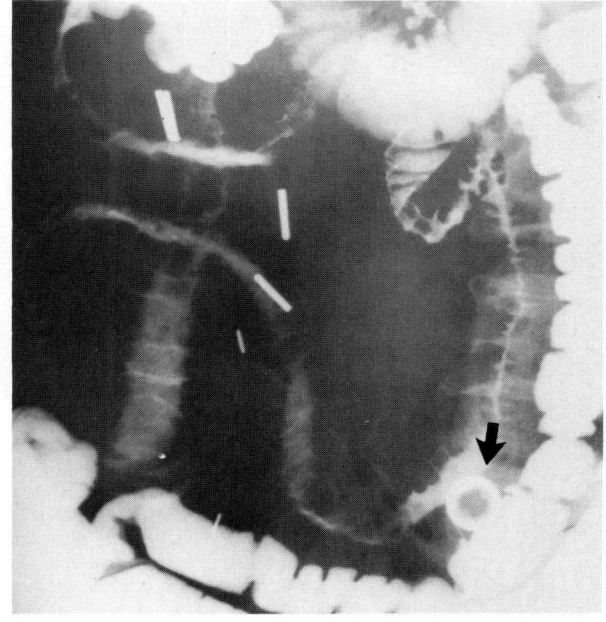

**Figure 55–26. Floxuridine enteritis.** The patient had metastatic colon cancer. Hepatic artery infusion of floxuridine by implanted pump *(arrow)* was complicated by diarrhea, pain, and occult blood. Enteroclysis shows severe narrowing, fold thickening, and loop separation of the ileum. The jejunum is normal. This is a reversible lesion. (Courtesy of Steven E. Rubesin, M.D., Philadelphia, PA.)

injuries to the thoracolumbar spine and the intra-abdominal hollow viscera have increased and are seen in characteristic patterns.

The function of the seat belt during collisions is to prevent ejection from the car and to reduce the severity of impact with the interior of the car.[62] Three mechanisms have been suggested for seat belt–related injuries to bowel and mesentery.[63] Rapid deceleration can cause transection of the jejunum within 20 cm of the ligament of Treitz. A shearing force operates between the relatively fixed proximal and more mobile distal jejunum. A mesenteric tear or, occasionally, an avulsion of the transverse colon and splenic flexure can also be produced in this way. An impact injury is more likely to result if the lap belt has been incorrectly placed to cross the abdomen above the protecting iliac bones. Small bowel, especially if limited in mobility, and its mesentery may be crushed between seat belt and spine. A hematoma and a transverse tear of the mesentery may be produced. Delayed infarction of small bowel has been reported.[64] Transmitted forces from the anterior abdominal wall may significantly increase intraluminal pressures within small bowel loops, especially if they are dilated postprandially or by disease. A single perforation or multiple punctate perforations usually involve the antimesenteric border.[65]

**Management of Patients.** Diagnostic peritoneal lavage is a simple procedure and sensitive in detecting bleeding into the peritoneal cavity.[66] However, it does not distinguish significant from minor bleeds and has caused unnecessary laparotomies. CT has largely taken its place and has become the main tool for the triage of hemodynamically stable patients in major accident units.[67]

Several CT signs suggest bowel and/or mesenteric injury. Extraluminal air is seen in only half of those with bowel perforation.[68] The amount of air may be small and the images must be carefully evaluated (Figs. 55–27A and 55–28A). The smallness of the amount of air may be due to the usual shortness of a tear in the bowel wall, the virtual absence of gas in normal gut, and the fact that the omentum tends to act as a barrier to escape of air. Prior diagnostic peritoneal lavage may introduce air and cause a false-positive reading; thus, CT should always be done before it. Intraperitoneal fluid is seen in all cases of bowel perforation but is not a specific finding (Fig. 55–27C); however, bowel or

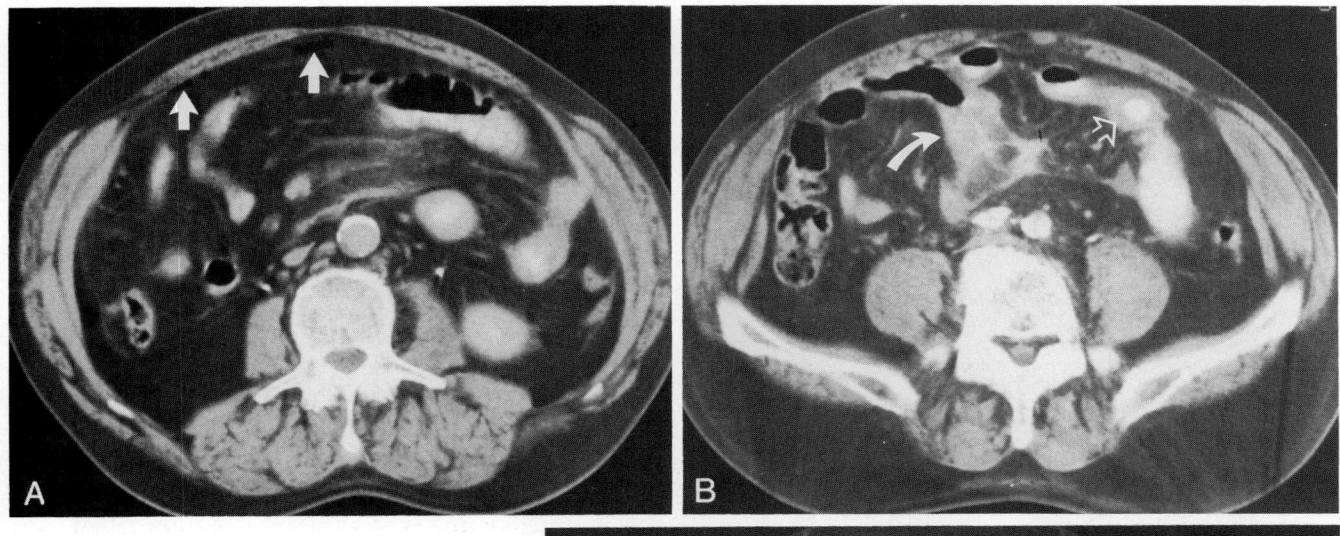

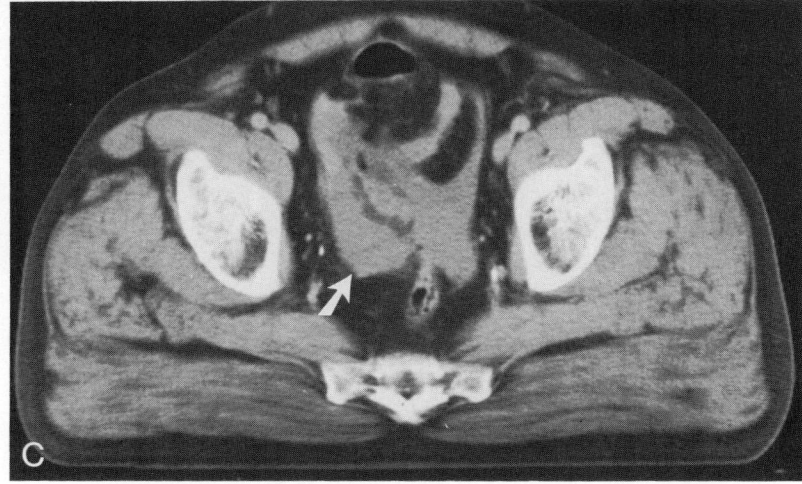

**Figure 55–27. Seat belt trauma, small bowel perforation.** CT scan with oral and intravenous contrast medium. **A.** There is a small amount of extraluminal gas *(arrows)*. **B.** Mesenteric thickening of increased density, probably representing a hematoma *(curved arrow)*, and thickened bowel wall *(open arrow)* are seen. **C.** Free fluid in pelvis *(arrow)* is seen. (Courtesy of Curtis W. Hayes, M.D. From Hayes CW, Conway WF, Walsh JW, et al: Seat belt injuries: radiologic findings and clinical correlation. Radiographics 11:23–36, 1991.)

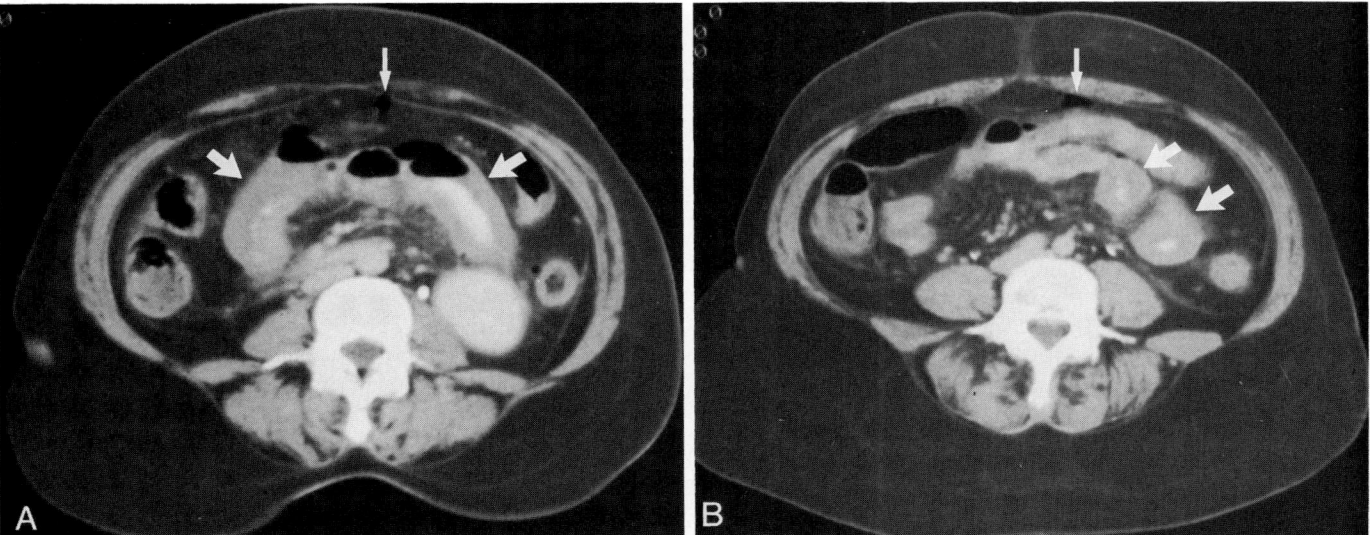

**Figure 55–28. Seat belt trauma, hematoma and perforation.** CT scan with oral and intravenous contrast medium. **A.** Thickened bowel loops are shown in longitudinal section *(large arrows).* **B.** The same thickened loops are shown in transverse section *(large arrows).* Small arrows in **A** and **B** indicate a small amount of free gas, sufficient to make a diagnosis of bowel perforation. (Courtesy of Curtis W. Hayes, M.D. From Hayes CW, Conway WF, Walsh JW, et al: Seat belt injuries: radiologic findings and clinical correlation. Radiographics 11:23–36, 1991.)

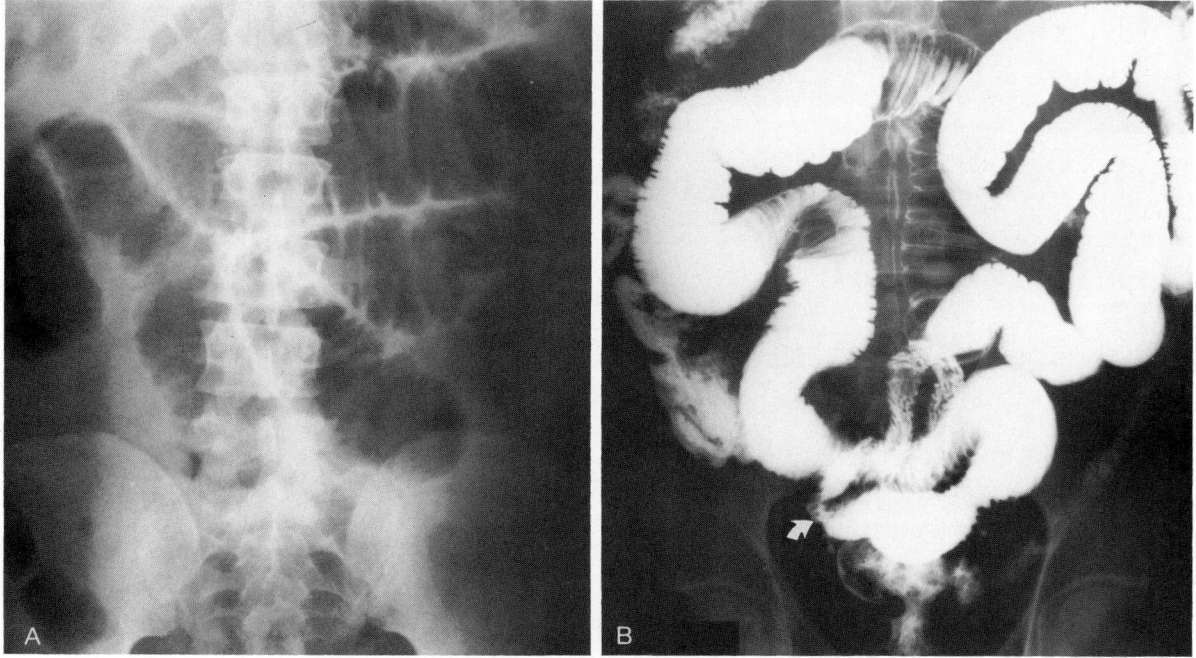

**Figure 55–29. Post-traumatic stricture.** The patient complained of abdominal pain, distention, and vomiting 6 weeks after blunt trauma sustained in a car accident. **A.** Plain film with features of small bowel obstruction. **B.** Enteroclysis shows an area of fixation with lumen narrowing *(arrow)* in a pelvic segment of ileum. Surgery demonstrated an organized mesenteric hematoma and a sealed perforation of ileum at the site of obstruction.

mesenteric injury should be suspected in patients with the appropriate history.[62, 67] A hematoma may be shown as a focal or more diffuse thickening of increased density (sentinel clot) and serves to confirm and localize the injury to the mesentery (Fig. 55–27B) or the bowel wall (see Fig. 55–28). Unenhanced scans were considered slightly better for the recognition of small hematomas,[69] but this has not been the experience of others who routinely use contrast enhancement.[62] Early CT examinations are also useful for inspecting the retroperitoneum and identifying any solid organ lesions. Urgent surgery rather than CT is usual in hemodynamically unstable patients.

Plain films of the abdomen are of limited value. Peroral contrast studies may be indicated in cases of low-grade trauma and in the follow-up of conservatively treated patients in whom postischemic strictures may develop 3 weeks or more later[70] (Fig. 55–29).

### Acknowledgment

Figures 55–4B, 55–5, 55–10, 55–12A, 55–19A and B, 55–24A, and 55–29A and B are reproduced from Herlinger H, Maglinte D (eds): Clinical Radiology of the Small Intestine. Philadelphia: WB Saunders, 1989.

# References

1. Houston CS, Wittenborg MH: Roentgen evaluation of anomalies of rotation and fixation of the bowel in children. Radiology 84:1–17, 1965.
2. Ladd WF: Surgical diseases of the alimentary tract in infants. N Engl J Med 215:705–708, 1936.
3. Louw JH, Cywes S: Embryology and anomalies of the intestine. In Berk JE, Haubrich WS, Kalser MH, et al (eds): Bockus Gastroenterology (4th ed). Philadelphia: WB Saunders, 1985, pp 1439–1473.
4. Meyers MA: Paraduodenal hernias. Radiologic and arteriographic diagnosis. Radiology 95:29–37, 1970.
5. Warshauer DM, Mauro MA: CT diagnosis of paraduodenal hernia. Gastrointest Radiol 17:13–15, 1992.
6. Maglinte DDT, Herlinger H: Congenital and developmental anomalies in adolescents and adults. In Herlinger H, Maglinte D (eds): Clinical Radiology of the Small Intestine. Philadelphia: WB Saunders, 1989, pp 249–273.
7. Hansmann GH, Morton SA: Intraabdominal hernia. Report of a case and review of the literature. Arch Surg 39:973–986, 1939.
8. Tran TL, Regan F, Al-Kutoubi MAO: Computed tomography of lesser sac hernia through the gastrohepatic omentum. Br J Radiol 64:372–374, 1991.
9. Cook JL: Bowel herniation through the foramen of Winslow. Am Surg 36:241–247, 1970.
10. Erskine JM: Hernia through the foramen of Winslow. Surg Gynecol Obstet 125:1093–1109, 1967.
11. Tran TL, Pitt PCC: Hernia through the foramen of Winslow. A report of two cases with emphasis on plain film interpretation. Clin Radiol 40:264–266, 1989.
12. Meyers MA: Internal abdominal hernias. In Meyers MA (ed): Dynamic Radiology of the Abdomen. Normal and Pathologic Anatomy (3rd ed). New York: Springer-Verlag, 1988, pp 424–435.
13. Maglinte DDT, Hall R, Miller RE, et al: Detection of surgical lesions of the small bowel by enteroclysis. Am J Surg 147:225–229, 1984.
14. Margolies MN: Case records of the Massachusetts General Hospital, Case 3–1989. N Engl J Med 320:171–178, 1989.
15. Meguid MM, Wilkinson RH, Canty T, et al: Futility of barium sulfate in diagnosis of bleeding Meckel's diverticulum. Arch Surg 108:361–362, 1974.
16. Glick SN, Maglinte DDT, Herlinger H: Association of Meckel's diverticulum and Crohn's disease. Gastrointest Radiol 13:67–71, 1988.
17. Maglinte DDT, Elmore MF, Isenberg M, et al: Meckel diverticulum: radiologic demonstration by enteroclysis. AJR 134:925–932, 1980.
18. Salomonowitz E, Wittich G, Hajek P, et al: Detection of intestinal diverticula by double contrast small bowel enema: differentiation from other intestinal diverticula. Gastrointest Radiol 8:271–278, 1983.
19. Ho CS, Shewchun J, Greenberg GR: Diagnosis of Meckel's diverticulum in adults. Mt Sinai J Med 51:378–381, 1984.
20. Ghahremani GG: Radiology of Meckel's diverticulum. Crit Rev Diagn Imaging 26:1–43, 1986.
21. Maglinte DDT, Jordan LG, Van Hove ED, et al: Chronic gastrointestinal bleeding from Meckel's diverticulum: radiologic considerations. J Clin Gastroenterol 3:47–52, 1981.
22. Dalinka MK, Wunder JF: Meckel's diverticulum and its complications, with emphasis on roentgen demonstration. Radiology 106:295–298, 1973.
23. Fries M, Mortensen W, Robertson B: Technetium pertechnetate scintigraphy to detect ectopic gastric mucosa in Meckel's diverticulum. Acta Radiol Diagn 25:417–422, 1984.
24. Ros PR, Olmsted WW, Moser RP Jr, et al: Mesenteric and omental cysts: histologic classification with imaging correlation. Radiology 164:327–332, 1987.
25. Gilchrist AM, Sloan JM, Logan CJH, et al: Case report: gastrointestinal bleeding due to multiple ileal duplication diagnosed by scintigraphy and barium studies. Clin Radiol 41:134–136, 1990.
26. Sfakianakis GN, Conway JJ: Detection of ectopic gastric mucosa in Meckel's diverticulum and in other aberrations by scintigraphy. Indications and methods—a 10 year experience. J Nucl Med 22:647–654 (part I), 732–738 (part II), 1981.
27. Ratcliffe J, Tait J, Lisle D, et al: Segmental dilatation of the small bowel: report of three cases and literature review. Radiology 171:827–830, 1989.
28. Morewood DJ, Cunningham ME: Case report: segmental dilatation of the ileum presenting with anemia. Clin Radiol 36:267–268, 1985.
29. Earnest DL, Schneiderman DJ: Other diseases of the colon and rectum. In Sleisenger MH, Fordtran JS (eds): Gastrointestinal Disease: Pathophysiology, Diagnosis, Management (4th ed). Philadelphia: WB Saunders, 1989, pp 1592–1631.
30. McAfee CH, Greer HL: Intestinal endometriosis: a report of 29 cases and a review of the literature. J Obstet Gynecol 67:539–555, 1960.
31. Nitsch B, Ho C-S, Cullen J: Barium study of small bowel endometriosis. Gastrointest Radiol 13:361–363, 1988.
32. Martinbeau PW, Pratt JH, Gaffy TA: Small bowel obstruction secondary to endometriosis. Mayo Clin Proc 50:239–243, 1975.
33. Aronchik CA, Brooks FP, Dyson WL, et al: Ileocecal endometriosis presenting with abdominal pain and gastrointestinal bleeding. Dig Dis Sci 28:566–572, 1983.
34. Kipfer RE, Moertel CF, Dahlin DC: Mesenteric lipodystrophy. Ann Intern Med 80:582–588, 1974.
35. Tytgat GN, Roozendaal K, Winter W, et al: Successful treatment of a patient with retractile mesenteritis with prednisone and azathioprine. Gastroenterology 79:352–356, 1980.
36. Shaffman MA: Familial multiple polyposis associated with soft-tissue and hard-tissue tumors. JAMA 179:514–522, 1962.
37. Marshall AJ, Baddeley H: Practolol peritonitis. Q J Med 181:135–149, 1977.
38. Harty RF: Sclerosing peritonitis and propranolol. Arch Intern Med 140:1124–1126, 1978.
39. Whitehead R: Pathology of the peritoneum and mesentery. In Whitehead R (ed): Gastrointestinal and Oesphageal Pathology. Edinburgh: Churchill Livingstone, 1989, p 824.
40. Holland P: Sclerosing encapsulating peritonitis in chronic ambulatory peritoneal dialysis. Clin Radiol 41:19–23, 1990.
41. Solomon A, Bar-Ziv J, Stern D, et al: Computed tomographic demonstration of intramural colonic air (pneumatosis coli) as a feature of severe ulcerative colitis. Gastrointest Radiol 12:169–171, 1987.
42. John A, Dickey K, Fenwick J, et al: Pneumatosis intestinalis in patients with Crohn's disease. Dig Dis Sci 37:813–817, 1992.

43. Olmstead WW, Madewell JE: Pneumatosis cystoides intestinalis: a pathological explanation of the Roentgen signs. Gastrointest Radiol 1:171–181, 1976.

44. Strain JD, Rudikoff JC, Moore EE, et al: Pneumatosis intestinalis associated with intracatheter jejunostomy feeding. AJR 139:107–109, 1982.

45. Bates FT, Gurney JW, Goodman LR, et al: Pneumatosis intestinalis in bone-marrow transplantation patients: diagnosis on routine chest radiographs. AJR 152:991–994, 1989.

46. DeMarino GB, Sumkin JH, Leventhal R, et al: Pneumatosis intestinalis and pneumoperitoneum after sclerotherapy. AJR 151:953–954, 1988.

47. Dodds WJ, Stewart ET, Goldberg HI: Pneumatosis intestinalis associated with hepatic portal venous gas. Dig Dis 21:992–995, 1976.

48. Masterson JS, Fratken LB, Osler TR, et al: Treatment of pneumatosis cystoides with hyperbaric oxygen. Ann Surg 187:245–247, 1978.

49. Farthing MJG, Madewell JE, Bartram CI, et al: Radiologic features of the jejunum in hypoalbuminemia. AJR 136:883–888, 1981.

50. Balthazar EJ, Gade MF: Gastrointestinal edema in cirrhotics. Radiographic manifestations with emphasis on colonic involvement. Gastrointest Radiol 1:215–223, 1976.

51. Marshak RH: Intestinal edema. *In* Marshak RH, Lindner AE (eds): Radiology of the Small Intestine (2nd ed). Philadelphia: WB Saunders, 1976, pp 72–89.

52. Javors BR, Bryk D: Enterolithiasis: report of four cases. Gastrointest Radiol 8:359–362, 1983.

53. Bloom RR, Nakano PH, Gray SW, et al: Foreign bodies of the gastrointestinal tract. Am J Surg 52:618–621, 1986.

54. Horrocks AW: Abdominal radiography in suspected "body packers." Clin Radiol 45:322–325, 1992.

55. Kaplan O, Klausner JM, Lelcuk S, et al: Persimmon bezoars as a cause of intestinal obstruction: pitfalls in their surgical management. Br J Surg 72:242–243, 1985.

56. Verstandig AG, Klin B, Bloom RA, et al: Small bowel phytobezoars: detection with radiography. Radiology 172:705–707, 1989.

57. Kelvin FM, Gramm HF, Gluck WL, et al: Radiologic manifestations of small bowel toxicity due to floxuridine therapy. AJR 146:39–43, 1977.

58. White CA, Traube J: Ulcerating enteritis associated with flucytosine therapy. Gastroenterology 83:1127–1129, 1982.

59. Tjon A Tham RTO, Vlasveld LT, et al: Gastrointestinal complications of cytosine-arabinoside chemotherapy: findings on plain abdominal radiographs. AJR 154:95–98, 1990.

60. Herlinger H, Maglinte DDT: Miscellaneous disorders. *In* Herlinger H, Maglinte D (eds): Clinical Radiology of the Small Intestine. Philadelphia: WB Saunders, 1989, pp 509–540.

61. Simson JNL: Seat belts—six years on. J R Soc Med 82:125–126, 1989 (editorial).

62. Hayes CW, Conway WF, Walsh JW, et al: Seat belt injuries: radiologic findings and clinical correlation. Radiographics 11:23–36, 1991.

63. Christoph C, McDermott FT, McVey I, et al: Seat belt induced trauma to the small bowel. World J Surg 9:794–797, 1985.

64. Winton TL, Girotti MJ, Manby PN, et al: Delayed intestinal perforation after nonpenetrating abdominal trauma. Can J Surg 28:347–391, 1985.

65. Andrews EW: Pneumatic rupture of the intestine. Surg Gynecol Obstet 12:63–72, 1911.

66. Gomez GA, Alvarez R, Plasencia G, et al: Diagnostic peritoneal lavage in the management of blunt abdominal trauma: a reassessment. J Trauma 27:1–5, 1987.

67. Wolfman NT, Bechtold RE, Scharling ES, et al: Blunt upper abdominal trauma: evaluation by CT. AJR 158:493–501, 1992.

68. Rizzo MJ, Federle MP, Griffiths BG: Bowel and mesenteric injury following blunt abdominal trauma: evaluation with CT. Radiology 173:143–148, 1989.

69. Kelly J, Raptopoulos V, Davidoff A, et al: The value of non–contrast-enhanced CT in blunt abdominal trauma. AJR 152:41–46, 1989.

70. Bryner UM, Longerbeam JK, Reeves CD: Post-traumatic ischemia of the small bowel. Arch Surg 115:1039–1040, 1980.

# Small Bowel: Differential Diagnosis

**William W. Olmsted, M.D.**

## INTRODUCTION

As radiologists and clinicians understand, the radiologic diagnosis of abnormalities of the small intestine is frequently difficult because signs are often nonspecific and there is a fair amount of sign overlap. Diffuse diseases are best suited for a pattern approach, which is more difficult to apply to the diagnosis of small bowel tumors.

Many approaches have been advocated to simplify the differential diagnosis of diffuse small bowel diseases.[1–8] The most logical involve pattern recognition and description of fold abnormalities and the linking of abnormal findings to the pathophysiology of specific diseases.[1, 2, 6, 8] Reliance on other signs of excess fluid or bowel dilatation is hazardous because they are often nonspecific and misleading. In the end, good clinical, radiologic, and pathologic correlation usually makes the specific diagnosis. The role of the radiologist is frequently descriptive—making the correct observation of fold abnormality and then suggesting a reasonable differential diagnosis. The radiologist should always corroborate his or her findings with the pathologist and gastroenterologist so that pathologic diagnoses that do not correlate well with radiographs can be avoided.

The problems associated with correct identification and description of radiologic patterns are affected by the rarity of the disease processes and by problems of examination technique. There is no question that the diffuse diseases discussed in this chapter are extremely rare. In a review of the archives of the Radiologic Registry at the Armed Forces Institute of Pathology, for instance, there were only 20 cases of Whipple's disease and only 4 cases of Waldenström's macroglobulinemia. It is obvious that lack of experience with many of these diseases makes their inclusion on differential diagnostic lists more difficult. In addition, conventional small bowel radiographic techniques are frequently suboptimal in depicting fold abnormality with accuracy. The enteroclysis techniques popularized in the United States by Herlinger and Maglinte, on the other hand, demonstrate fold abnormality well and can be useful in suspected cases of diffuse small bowel disease.[7] The enteroclysis technique, however, should not be used indiscriminately when a conventional small bowel series would suffice. The examination is expensive and uncomfortable for the patient and utilizes a great deal of radiation. Subjects should be well selected for this method of study and should be properly premedicated; good technique is also essential. Images must be of high quality and the radiologist should spend sufficient time in analyzing the images to justify the use of the technique.

## THE PATTERN APPROACH

Application of a pattern approach to the diagnosis of diffuse small bowel diseases produces a differential diagnostic list that is usable and can be remembered. For effective use of the pattern approach, one must limit the parameters as much as possible and simplify. Table 56–1 presents a list of diseases that should be mentioned in a discussion of diffuse small bowel fold abnormality. It is not all-inclusive. Diseases that do not normally affect the structure of individual folds (e.g., celiac disease and lactase deficiency) are not included (see Chapter 49). Diseases or conditions that mainly affect other organs (e.g., pancreatic insufficiency, Zollinger-Ellison syndrome) are also excluded.

Once the differential choices have been limited to diseases that primarily affect the small bowel folds, anatomic understanding of the normal and abnormal small bowel fold becomes essential. Figures 56–1 to 56–4 demonstrate normal, symmetrically thickened, nodularly thickened, and micronodular small bowel folds. The submucosa extending underneath the muscularis mucosae gives rise to the normal fold pattern seen grossly, histologically, and radiologically.[1] This submucosa gives permanence to the fold. Abnormal folds are

---

**TABLE 56–1. DIFFERENTIAL DIAGNOSIS OF DISEASES CAUSING FOLD ABNORMALITY**

Crohn's disease
Lymphoma (primary and secondary)
Amyloidosis
Lymphangiectasia
Whipple's disease
Waldenström's macroglobulinemia

---

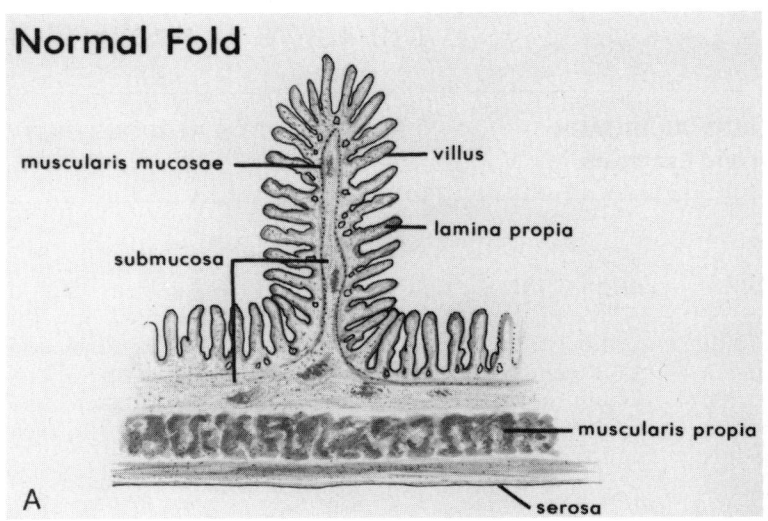

## Normal Fold

- muscularis mucosae
- villus
- lamina propia
- submucosa
- muscularis propia
- serosa

A

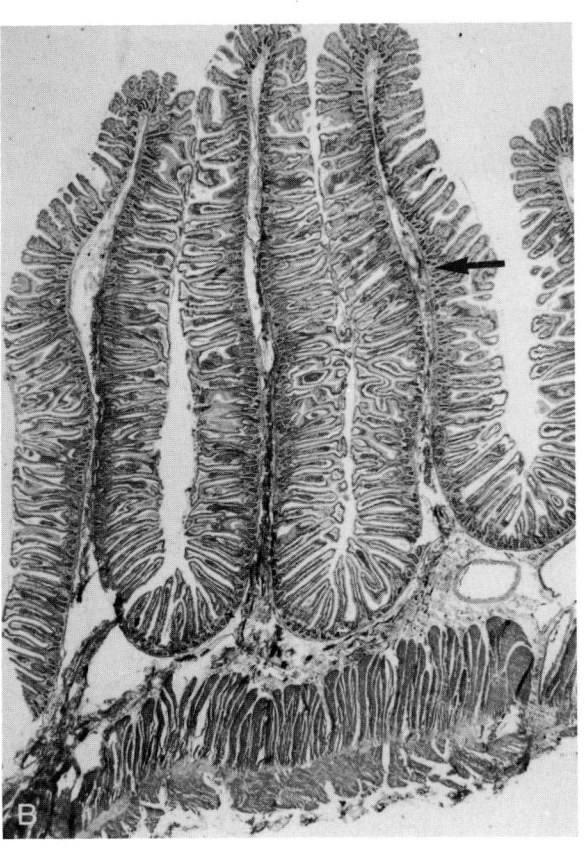

B

**Figure 56–1. Normal small bowel fold. A.** Diagram of low-power histology. **B.** Hematoxylin-eosin, ×125. The submucosa extends into the core of the fold *(arrow)* and gives the fold permanence. Note its normal thin configuration.

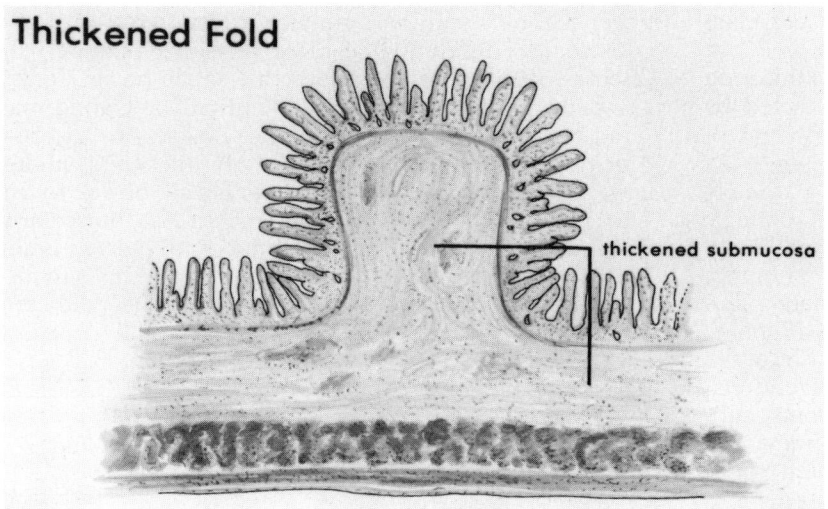

## Thickened Fold

- thickened submucosa

**Figure 56–2. Symmetrically thickened fold.** Thickening is caused by expansion (by cells and/or other substances) of the normally thin submucosal space.

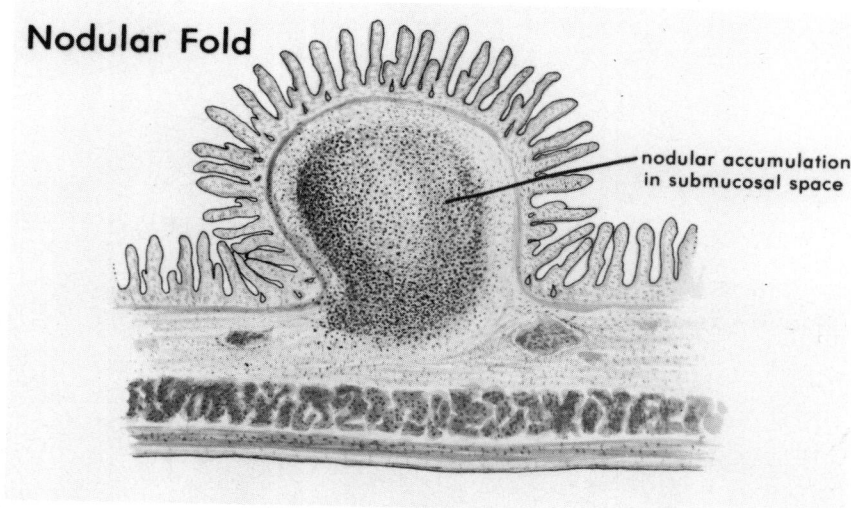

# Nodular Fold

nodular accumulation in submucosal space

**Figure 56–3. Nodularly thickened fold.** These differ in configuration from symmetrically thickened folds because of the circular or oval pattern of accumulation of cells and/or substances.

caused by expansion of the submucosal space by deposition of certain cells and/or substances. If the cells or substances are deposited in a symmetric fashion, a symmetrically thickened fold results (see Fig. 56–2). Oval or circular accumulations in the submucosal space create a nodular fold (see Fig. 56–3). Micronodularity is caused by a completely different process: expansion of the lamina propria of the villus (above the muscularis mucosae) by cells and/or substances (see Fig. 56–4). Frequently, symmetrically thickened, nodular, and micronodular folds coexist, further confusing the analysis of the abnormal small bowel series.

After the radiologist has a thorough understanding of the pathophysiology of normal and abnormal folds, it is necessary to further simplify the pattern approach for better use. Diseases and conditions that occur commonly and enlarge small bowel folds must first be excluded: edema, hemorrhage, and ischemia. However, these conditions may also complicate many of the primary small bowel diseases that cause thickened folds.

## Utilization and Examples

As previously mentioned, all of the diseases and conditions that primarily affect small bowel folds can cause similar radiographic signs. Therefore, most of the diseases and conditions listed in Table 56–1 should be considered when presented with diffuse fold abnormality. By using clinical correlation and, perhaps, some of the secondary and more subtle signs seen on the small bowel series or enteroclysis study, a more specific diagnosis can sometimes be offered.

## *Crohn's Disease and Lymphoma*

Crohn's disease and lymphoma (primary or secondary) are recognized as the great imitators of other diffuse diseases of the small bowel. This is probably because both diseases are transmural and frequently affect mucosa, submucosa, and muscular layers, resulting in multiple radiographic signs. Figure 56–5 shows an

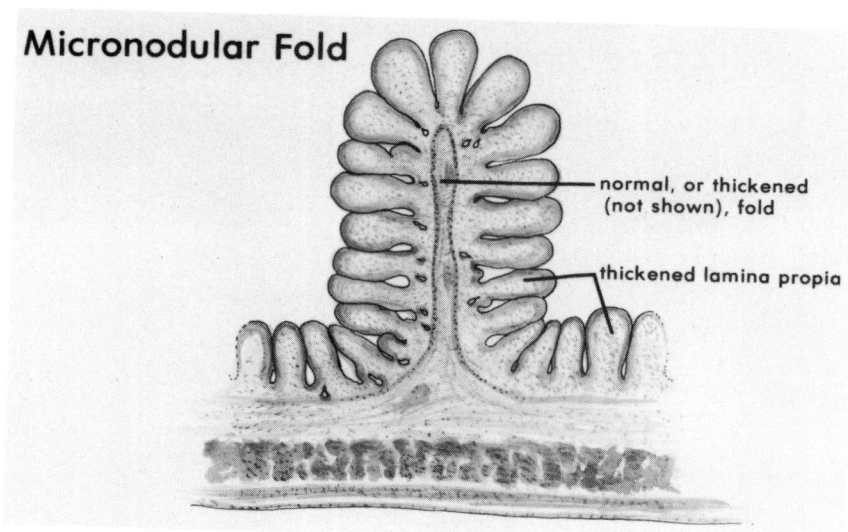

# Micronodular Fold

normal, or thickened (not shown), fold

thickened lamina propia

**Figure 56–4. Micronodular fold.** These are caused by expansion of the lamina propria of the villi. They may or may not be superimposed on thickened or nodular folds. These folds have a micronodular or irregular surface architecture.

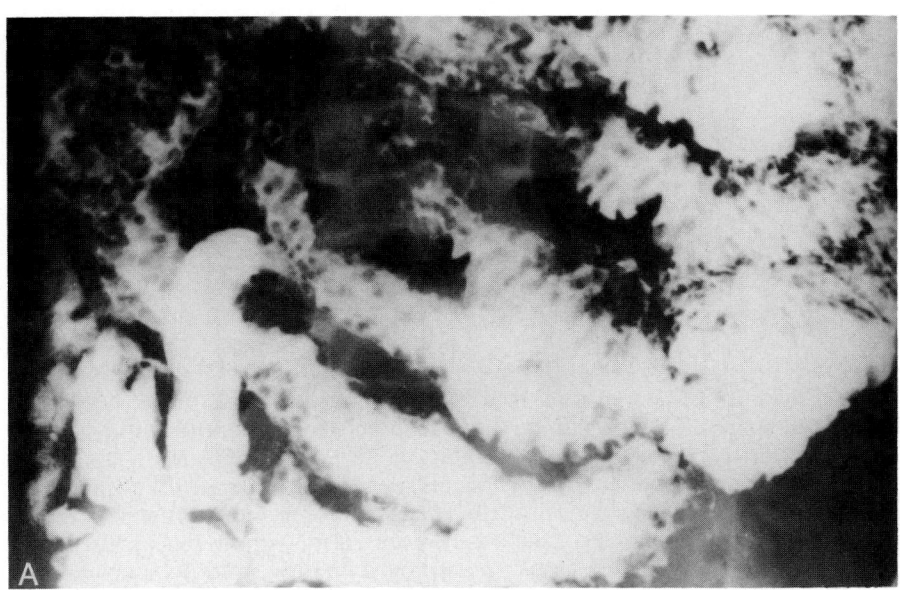

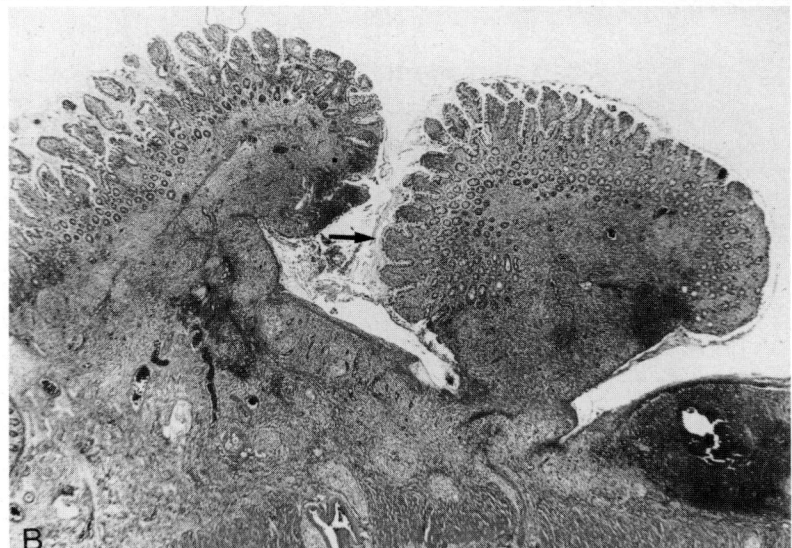

**Figure 56–5. Crohn's disease. A.** Radiographic wall thickening, nodularity, and fold thickening. **B.** Fold thickening (fold on left) and nodularity (fold on right) are obvious histologically. Hematoxylin-eosin, ×130. Note the submucosal inflammatory response, which is partially responsible for wall thickening. Villi blunted by acute and chronic inflammatory infiltrate result in micronodularity *(arrow)* not seen in this example radiographically. (**A** and **B** from WW Olmsted, DE Reagin, Pathophysiology of enlargement of the small bowel fold, AJR, 127, 3, 423–428, 1976, © by American Roentgen Ray Society.)

unusual example of Crohn's disease manifesting with transmural involvement, thickened folds, and inflammatory polyps. Wall thickening is caused by acute and chronic inflammatory tissue bridging submucosal and muscular layers and extending to the serosal surface. The inflammatory polyps (and thickened folds) are the result of this inflammatory reaction extending into the submucosal space beneath the muscularis mucosae giving rise to permanently abnormal folds (see Fig. 56–5B). Frequently, in Crohn's disease the inflammatory exudate involves the individual villus and its lamina propria. This was not seen radiologically in the case in Figure 56–5, but it could result in clubbed villi causing a micronodular fold.[9]

The findings in primary and secondary lymphoma are similar[1, 2] (Fig. 56–6). Transmural and mesenteric involvement is frequently seen with thickened or nodular folds caused by lymphomatous cells extending up into the submucosal space. (Further information can be found in Chapter 51.)

## Amyloidosis

Amyloidosis (especially the primary form) can affect the small bowel fold, usually causing symmetric thick-

ening and occasional micronodularity[10, 11] (Fig. 56–7). Defined broadly as tissue accumulation of insoluble proteins deposited in the submucosa, amyloidosis is a rare cause of small bowel fold abnormality. In a review of the files of the Radiologic Registry of the Armed Forces Institute of Pathology, there were eight cases of primary amyloidosis presenting with small bowel abnormalities. When amyloid involves the small intestine, it is first deposited around the small capillaries in the submucosa. This deposition results in an ischemic small intestine with edema fluid accumulating in small bowel folds and resulting in thickening. Later on, amyloid is deposited in the submucosal space that extends underneath the muscularis mucosae (see Fig. 56–7B). This may result in further symmetric thickening but can also lead to nodularity resulting from patchy deposition of the amyloid. Amyloid deposition in the lamina propria of individual villi has resulted in micronodularity that is recognized radiologically.[11]

## Lymphangiectasia

Both primary and secondary lymphatic abnormalities can distort the small bowel fold. Lymphangiectasia is a rare condition (15 cases in the files of the Radiologic

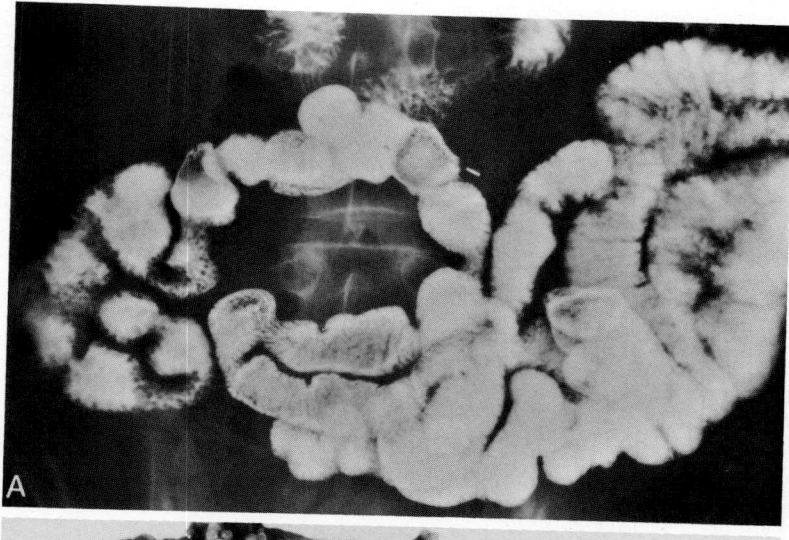

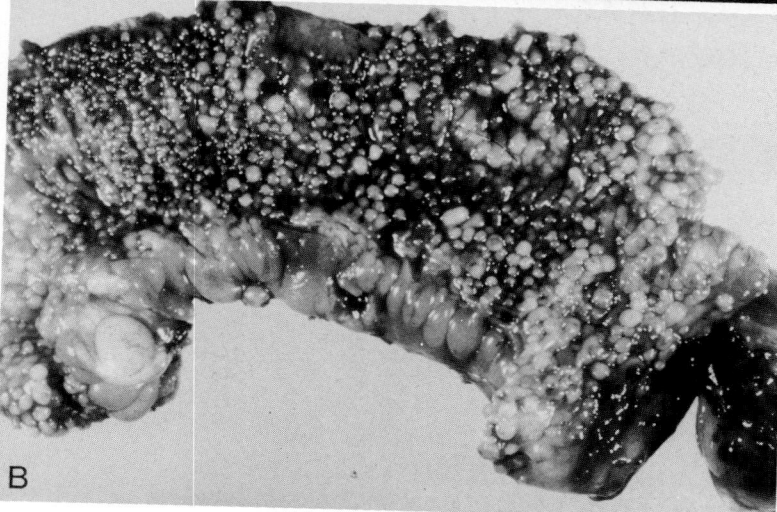

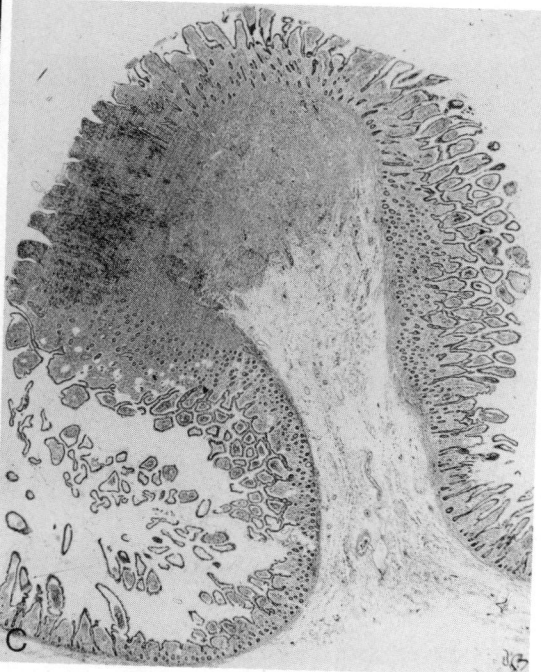

**Figure 56–6. Primary follicular non-Hodgkin's lymphoma. A.** Diffuse small bowel nodularity throughout jejunum. **B.** Gross specimen with nodules projecting into the jejunal lumen. **C.** Low-power histologic section (hematoxylin-eosin, × 10) in another case shows cellular infiltrate in tip of fold's submucosal space resulting in nodular fold. Base of fold is thickened by edema. Edema frequently compounds fold abnormality. (**C** from WW Olmsted, DE Reagin, Pathophysiology of enlargement of the small bowel fold, AJR, 127, 3, 423–428, 1976, © by American Roentgen Ray Society.)

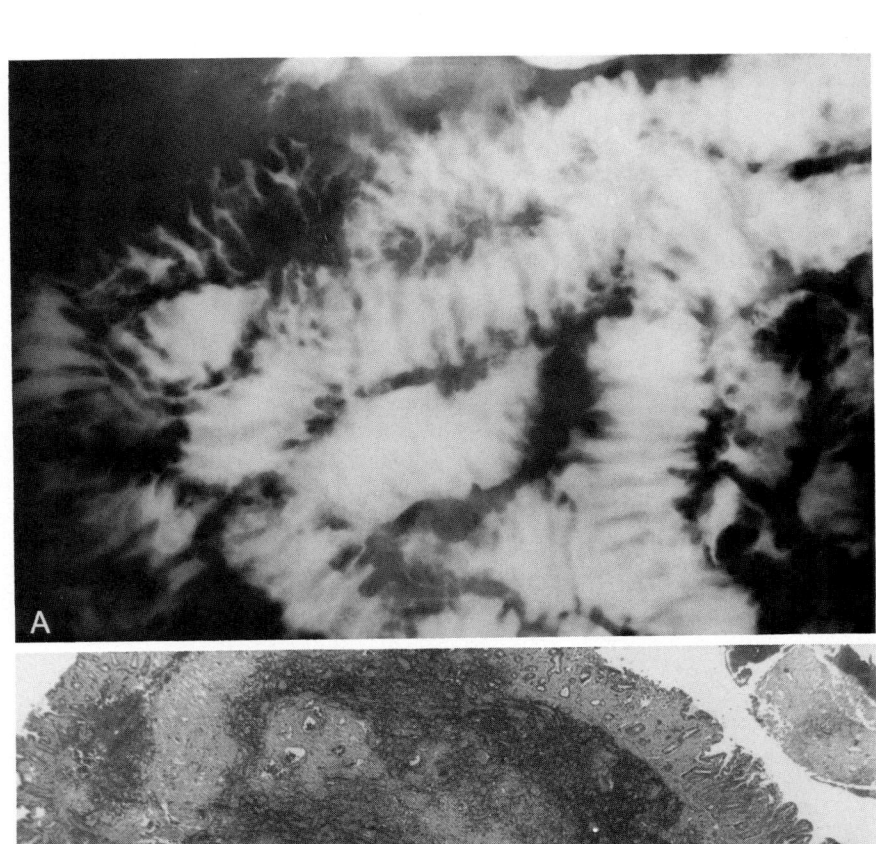

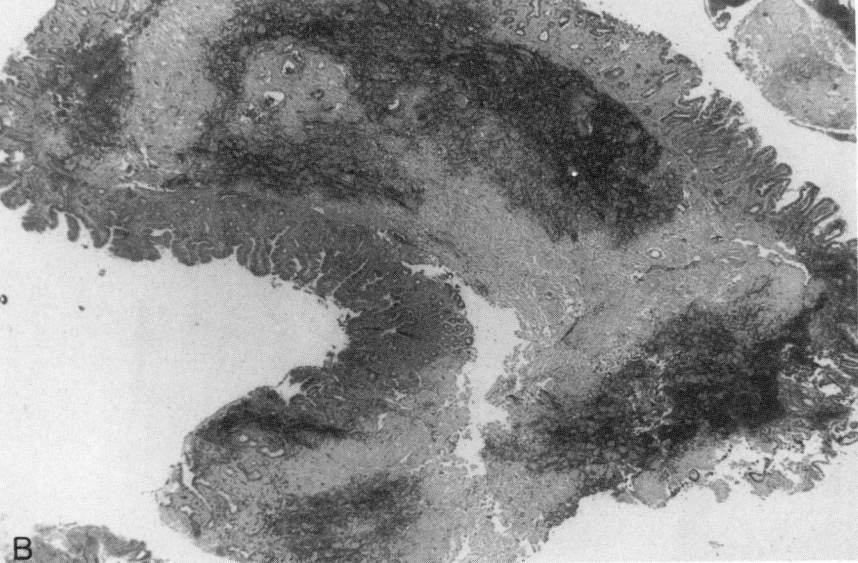

**Figure 56–7. Amyloidosis. A.** Diffuse symmetric fold thickening is seen on conventional small bowel examination. **B.** Low-power histologic section (hematoxylin-eosin, ×12) shows an infiltrated fold.

Registry of the Armed Forces Institute of Pathology). When the small bowel is involved, lymphatics in the submucosa as well as in the mucosal layers are dilated. Thickened, nodular, and micronodular folds result[12, 13] (Fig. 56–8). Primary lymphangiectasia is congenital. Secondary blockage of the lymphatics (e.g., from tuberculosis, lymphoma, or other infiltrating neoplasm) can also cause small bowel fold abnormalities (secondary lymphangiectasia). Because the lymphatics in primary and secondary lymphangiectasia continue to dilate as the disease progresses, they can eventually rupture and spill their lymph content into the small intestinal lumen. This results in excess fluid (chyle) in the intestinal lumen, which may cause dilution of the barium column (excess fluid, hypersecretion), resulting in hazy or dispersed barium. This secondary sign may be helpful in narrowing the differential diagnostic list of small bowel diffuse diseases.

## Disease Affecting the Villus and Resulting in Micronodularity

Whipple's disease and Waldenström's macroglobulinemia are two diseases that involve predominantly the lamina propria of the villus and result in a micronodular fold pattern. However, in addition to the micronodular fold pattern there may occasionally be fold thickening. In the older literature, from the time before enteroclysis was used and micronodularity could not be demonstrated radiologically, both diseases were described as

causing fold abnormality.[14–16] In fact, histology shows that the deposition of the glycoprotein-laden macrophages in Whipple's disease is primarily in the individual villus (Fig. 56–9). The macroglobulin of Waldenström's macroglobulinemia, which is linked with a phospholipid (further increasing the molecular size), tends to be similarly deposited (Fig. 56–10). Radiographs in these diseases reveal the typical irregular or micronodular fold pattern (Fig. 56–11). The abnormality in these cases may be one of fold surface texture rather than fold submucosal space abnormality. Both of these diseases are quite rare (Armed Forces Institute of Pathology Radiologic Registry: Whipple's disease, 20 cases; Waldenström's macroglobulinemia, 4 cases) but should be considered when a micronodular-only or mostly micronodular fold pattern is recognized. A similar pattern is seen in pseudo-Whipple's disease (small bowel enteritis secondary to *Mycobacterium avium-intracellulare* infection).[17]

## RADIOLOGIST'S RESPONSIBILITY

The author believes that the radiologist's responsibility in the evaluation of diffuse diseases of the small intestine is to recognize an abnormality and list an appropriate differential diagnosis. The abnormality can usually be recognized easily as symmetric or asymmetric fold thickening with diffuse or patchy nodularity or with micronodularity. The use of enteroclysis can be crucial

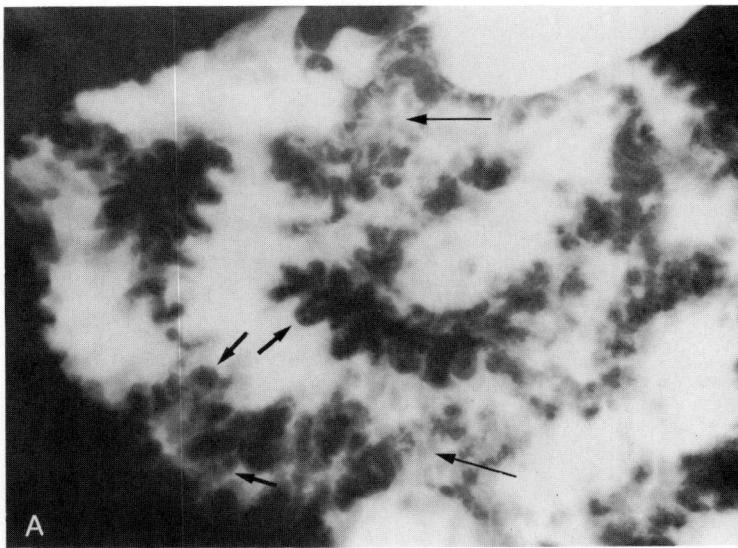

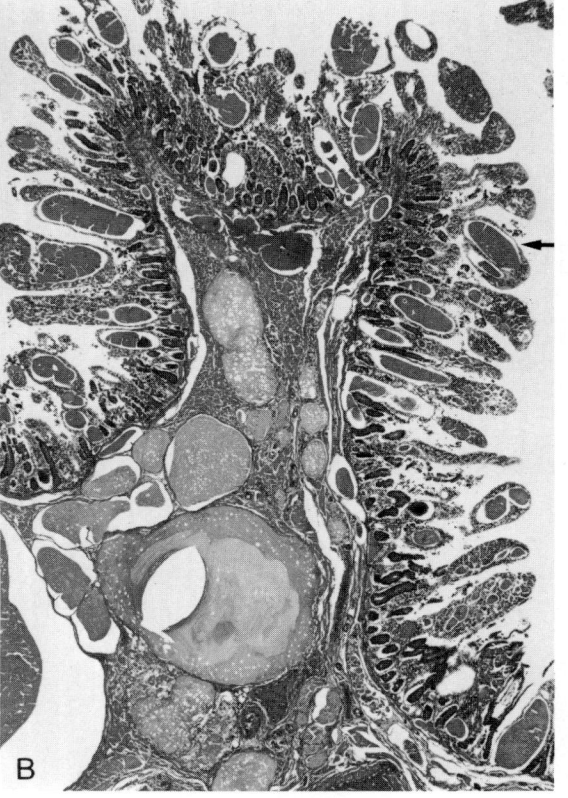

**Figure 56–8. Primary lymphangiectasia. A.** Radiograph shows thick, nodular *(short arrows)*, and micronodular *(long arrows)* folds. **B.** Fold abnormality is caused by dilated submucosal and villous lymphatics *(arrow)*. Hematoxylin-eosin, × 125. Villous abnormality accounts for micronodularity.

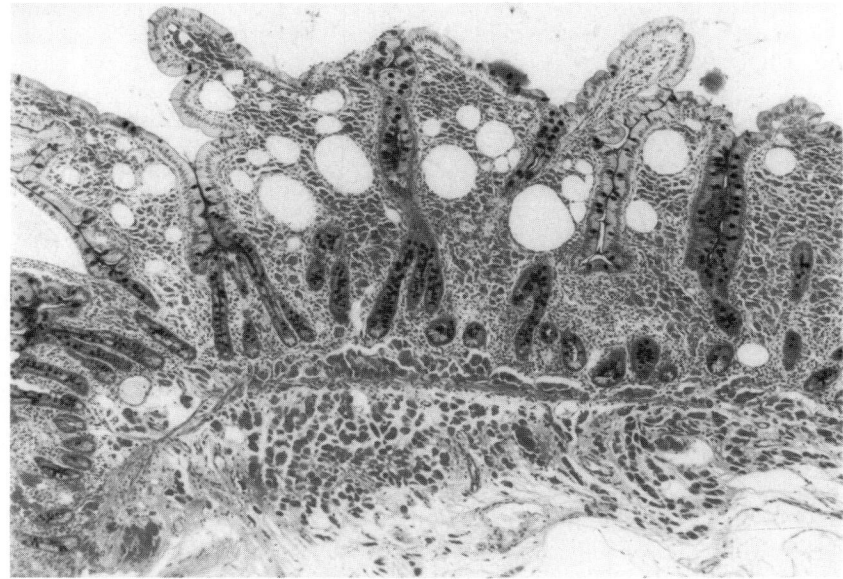

**Figure 56–9. Whipple's disease.** Histologic section of a fold demonstrates deposition of abnormal macrophages in lamina propria of villi. Note limited involvement of submucosal space. Periodic acid–Schiff, ×100.

**Figure 56–10. Waldenström's macroglobulinemia.** Histologic section shows deposition of macroglobulin-phospholipid complex in lamina propria of villi. Note the normal submucosal space and additional secondary lymphangiectasia. Clubbed villi cause micronodular folds. Fold-proper involvement is absent, because the submucosal space is normal. Hematoxylin-eosin, ×40.

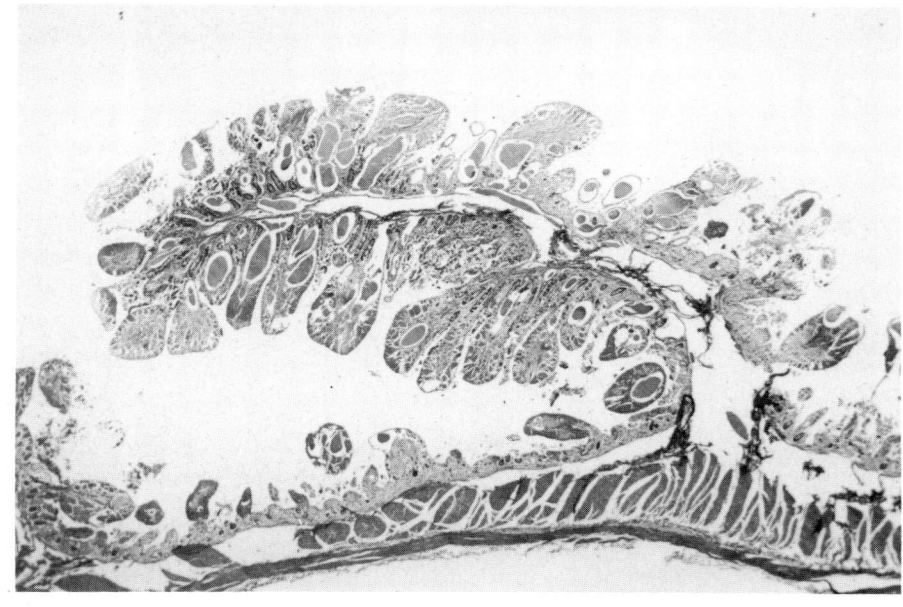

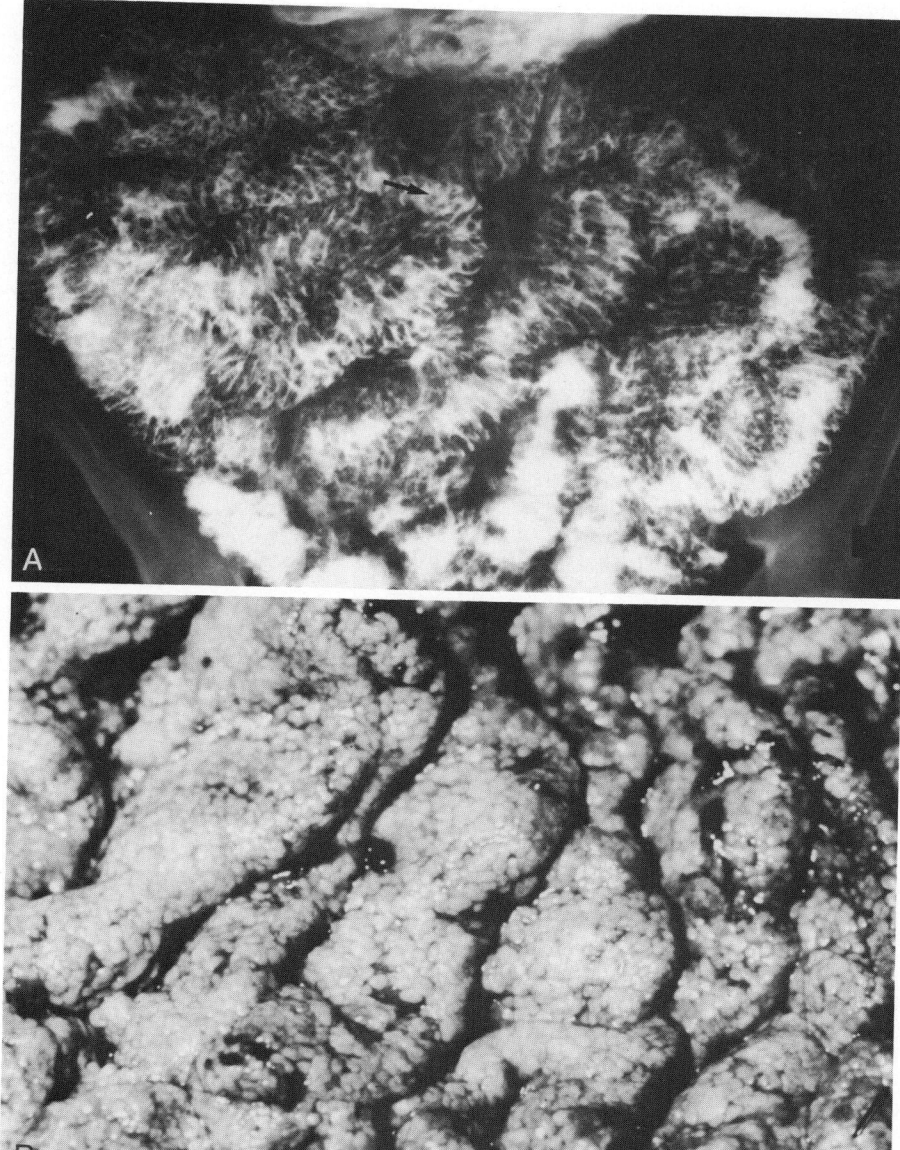

**Figure 56–11. Waldenström's macroglobu-linemia.** Radiograph **(A)** and accompanying gross specimen **(B)** show micronodularity (arrow in **A**) superimposed on normal-sized folds. Folds could also be called wild, feathery, or irregular.

in recognizing fold abnormalities. The differential diagnostic list should be limited. Diseases and conditions that occur frequently (e.g., edema, hemorrhage, and ischemia) should be considered first and possibly eliminated. In considering infrequently occurring diseases and conditions, an understanding of their pathophysiology may be of significant help. Clinical correlation and appropriate pathologic confirmation are critical in management of patients to "triangulate" to a specific diagnosis.

## References

1. Olmsted WW, Reagin DE: Pathophysiology of enlargement of the small bowel fold. AJR 127:423–428, 1976.
2. Olmsted WW, Lichtenstein JE: A pathophysiologic approach to nontumorous small-bowel disease. Mt Sinai J Med 51:360–367, 1984.
3. Marshak R, Hazzi C, Lindner A, et al: Small bowel in immunoglobulin deficiency syndromes. AJR 122:227–240, 1974.
4. Tulley TE, Feinberg SB: A roentgenographic classification of diffuse diseases of the small intestine presenting with malabsorption. AJR 121:283–290, 1974.
5. Marshak RH, Lindner AE: Radiology of the Small Intestine (2nd ed). Philadelphia: WB Saunders, 1976, pp 11, 42–51, 62–68.
6. Goldberg HI, Sheft DJ: Abnormalities in small intestine contour and caliber: a working classification. Radiol Clin North Am 14:461–475, 1976.
7. Herlinger H, Maglinte D (eds): Clinical Radiology of the Small Intestine. Philadelphia: WB Saunders, 1989, pp 349–398.
8. Chen MYM, Ott DJ, Gelfand DW: Radiologic interpretation of diffuse small bowel diseases. Appl Radiol 19:30–37, 1990.
9. Glick SN, Teplick SK: Crohn's disease of the small intestine: diffuse mucosal granularity. Radiology 154:313–317, 1985.
10. Pear B: Radiographic studies of amyloidosis. Crit Rev Radiol Sci 3:425–452, 1972.
11. Smith TR, Cho KC: Small intestine amyloidosis producing a stippled punctate mucosal pattern: radiological-pathological correlation. Am J Gastroenterol 81:477–479, 1986.
12. Olmsted WW, Madewell JE: Lymphangiectasia of the small intestine. Description and pathophysiology of the roentgenographic signs. Gastrointest Radiol 1:241–243, 1976.
13. Fakhri A, Fishman EK, Jones B, et al: Primary intestinal lymphangiectasia: clinical and CT findings. J Comput Assist Tomogr 9:767–770, 1985.
14. Clemett AR, Marshak RH: Whipple's disease. Roentgen features and differential diagnosis. Radiol Clin North Am 7:105–111, 1969.
15. Comer GM, Brandt LJ, Abissi CJ: Whipple's disease: a review. Am J Gastroenterol 78:107–114, 1983.
16. Brandt LJ, Davidoff A, Bernstein LH, et al: Small-intestinal involvement in Waldenström's macroglobulinemia. Case report and review of the literature. Dig Dis Sci 26:174–180, 1981.
17. Vincent ME, Robbins AH: *Mycobacterium avium-intracellulare* complex enteritis: pseudo-Whipple disease in AIDS. AJR 144:921–922, 1985.

# Colon

# Barium Studies

## Igor Laufer, M.D.

## INTRODUCTION

Barium examination of the colon is designed primarily for the detection of mucosal lesions. In this regard, it competes directly with colonoscopy. Although colonoscopy has an advantage in the ability to detect change in color and the ability to obtain biopsy specimens, a properly performed barium contrast study should be fully competitive in the detection of gross as well as subtle colonic lesions.

Barium contrast studies are also suitable for the detection of intramural lesions in the colon. For this purpose, barium examination is clearly superior to endoscopy. Its competitors in this arena are computed tomography and, in selected areas, magnetic resonance imaging and endoscopic ultrasound.

Extrinsic lesions affecting the colon can also be clearly demonstrated by barium study. However, the extramural component of the lesion is much better demonstrated by computed tomography.

## SINGLE VERSUS DOUBLE CONTRAST TECHNIQUE

There remains considerable controversy, especially in the United States, regarding the relative value of single and double contrast techniques. It is generally agreed that the double contrast method is superior at least for the detection of small polypoid lesions and of the early changes of inflammatory bowel disease. In addition, the double contrast method is acknowledged to be superior for the examination of the rectum. There are, in addition, some specific signs, such as mucosal crinkling in endometriosis or metastatic disease, that are much more clearly demonstrated on double contrast study (see Chapter 5).

The single contrast method is preferred for particular indications, including mechanical problems such as obstruction or fistulas and in cases in which control of the barium column is required, as in suspected diverticulitis or intussusception. In addition, in cases of suspected ischemic colitis, the single contrast method is preferred because double contrast study may efface the thumbprinting that is characteristic of ischemia.[1]

Details of the single contrast method are discussed in Chapter 6. The remainder of this chapter deals more specifically with the double contrast enema.

## DOUBLE CONTRAST ENEMA

### Preparation of the Patient

Although a wide variety of preparation regimens are used,[2] most entail the following basic components:
- A clear liquid diet is followed for 24 hours.
- One or preferably two sets of laxatives are taken on the afternoon and evening before the examination.
- A suppository is taken on the morning of the examination.

This basic preparation is effective in most patients when it is followed. However, noncompliance with the prescribed preparation remains a major problem. We make a point of asking the patients when they arrive in the department whether they have in fact taken the preparation and whether it has been effective in producing a clear, watery bowel movement. If there is doubt about the adequacy of the preparation, a preliminary film is exposed. If the film shows indisputable evidence of fecal residue in the colon, the patient is rescheduled for a further 24 hours of preparation.

**TABLE 57–1. ROUTINE DOUBLE CONTRAST ENEMA**

| POSITION | VIEWS |
|---|---|
| Prone | Rectum |
| Left posterior oblique | Sigmoid colon |
| Left lateral | Rectum |
| Supine | Cecum |
| Upright | Flexures |
| Overhead | |
|    Vertical beam | Posteroanterior, left posterior oblique, right posterior oblique |
|    Angled (prone) | Rectosigmoid |
|    Horizontal beam | Right and left lateral, decubitus Cross-table lateral, rectum |

Cleansing enemas certainly improve the cleanliness of the colon. However, they are difficult to perform on outpatients from a logistical viewpoint. Furthermore, they tend to result in significant residual fluid within the colon, and this deteriorates the quality of mucosal coating. The same may be said of oral lavage regimens using solutions such as GoLYTELY.[3]

## Materials

The choice of barium suspension is critical. We prefer a suspension of medium viscosity at approximately 100% w/v (liquid Polibar, E-Z-EM Company, Westbury, NY). The barium suspension must coat the mucosal surface well and for a prolonged period so that artifacts do not develop as the examination proceeds.

The Miller air enema tip is ideal for double contrast studies because it allows barium infusion and air insufflation at the end of the enema tip.[4] Although a retention balloon is attached to the end of the tip, it is not inflated routinely. It is inflated only after the patient has demonstrated that he or she is unable to retain the barium or air. When required, the retention balloon should be inflated under direct fluoroscopic control with no more than 100 mL of air. The balloon need not fill the lumen of the rectum. It should be pulled distally against the anal verge to act as a plug.

A hypotonic drug such as glucagon 1 mg intravenously can be used routinely to improve the quality of the examination and decrease discomfort for the patient. We tend to use glucagon selectively in those patients who are experiencing abdominal discomfort during the procedure, are incontinent of barium and air, or are shown to have a stricture of uncertain cause.

As with the double contrast upper gastrointestinal studies, films are exposed on a 400 speed system at 105 kV(p). We rely primarily on fluoroscopy and spot films for diagnostic purposes, but these are supplemented by a series of routine overhead radiographs as outlined in Table 57–1. These include a series of horizontal beam films that are particularly valuable in patients whose preparation is less than perfect (Fig. 57–1). The quality of these films can be improved by the use of a wedge filter, which evens out the density over the entire film.[5, 6]

## ROUTINE EXAMINATION

A routine sequence of films is summarized in Table 57–1, and selected views are illustrated in Figure 57–2. Several key points are worth mentioning. We start with the patient in the prone or left lateral position so that the sigmoid colon and descending colon are in the dependent position and are easier to fill. It is important to be certain that barium has passed around the splenic

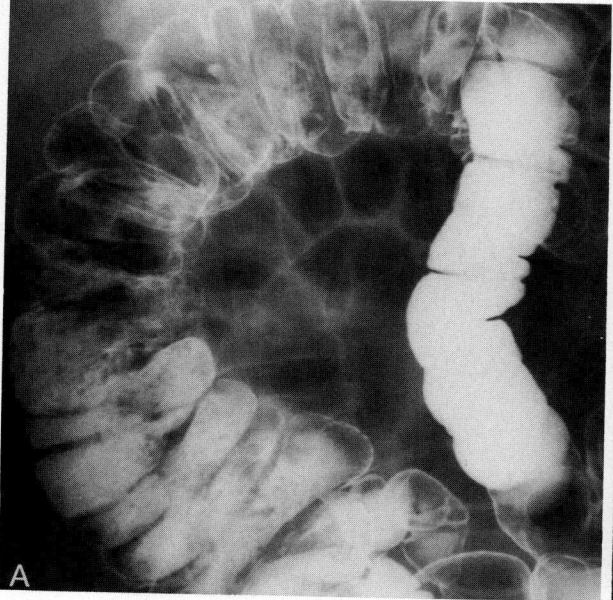
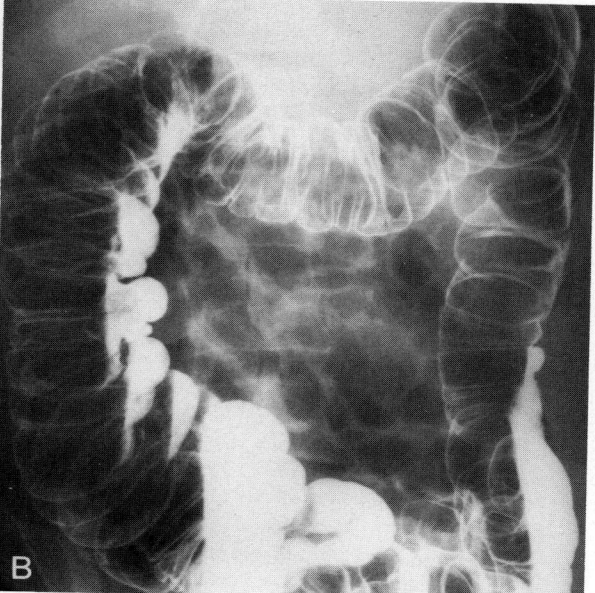

**Figure 57–1. Importance of the decubitus film with imperfect bowel preparation. A.** The oblique film shows considerable fecal residue in the right colon. **B.** The left lateral decubitus film shows the fecal debris layered out with the barium. A clear view is obtained of most of the right colon.

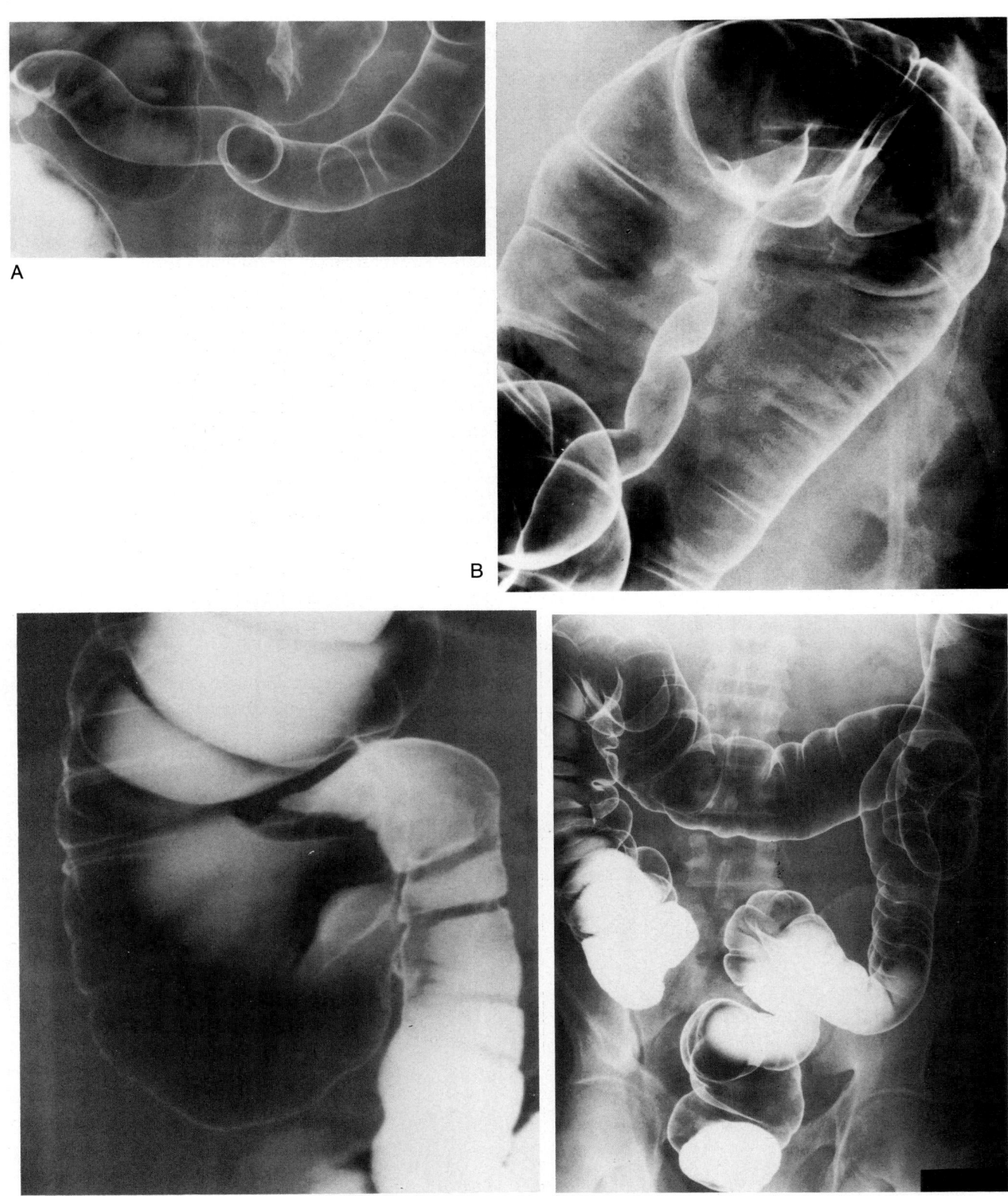

**Figure 57–2. Selected films from normal examinations. A.** Spot film of the sigmoid colon in the left posterior oblique projection. **B.** Upright spot film of the splenic flexure in the right posterior oblique projection. **C.** Spot film of the cecum and terminal ileum in the supine position. **D.** Overhead radiograph in the prone position.

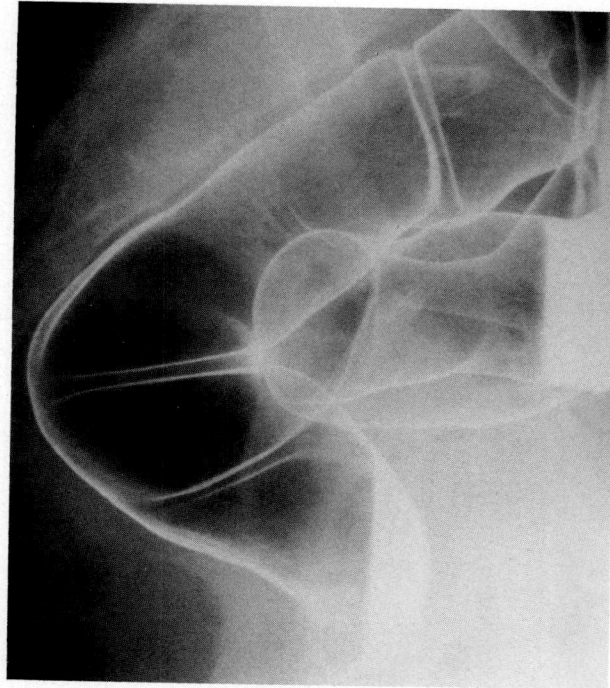

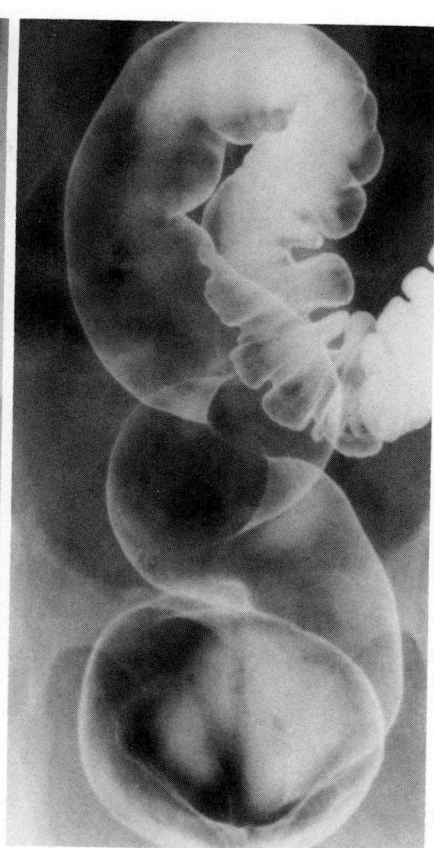

E

**Figure 57–2** *Continued* **E.** Prone, angled view of the recto-sigmoid colon. **F.** Prone, cross-table lateral view of the rectum.

F

flexure before the insufflation of air is started. The air is used to drive the barium across the transverse colon and into the right colon. At several points during the procedure, barium is drained from the rectum by dropping the enema bag on the floor. As the patient turns, it is useful to watch the flow of barium across the mucosal surface because this "flow technique" may be valuable for demonstrating superficial lesions.

## NORMAL APPEARANCES

### Surface Pattern

On most studies, the mucosal surface of the colon has a smooth, featureless appearance (Fig. 57–3A). In some patients, a fine network pattern is seen on the mucosal surface. This has been referred to as the innominate grooves or areae colonicae[7] (Fig. 57–3B). Occasionally, a pattern of pits rather than grooves is seen[8] (Fig. 57–3C). These patterns may be seen en face with the double contrast method or in profile in the barium-filled colon that is partially collapsed[9] (Fig. 57–3D). This is a normal appearance that should not be mistaken for superficial ulceration. The fine network pattern is seen more frequently in countries such as Japan where a barium suspension of lower density and lower viscosity is routinely used. In other patients, fine, transverse striations

are seen as a transient phenomenon that is probably due to contraction of the muscularis mucosae (Fig. 57–3E).

## Lymphoid Follicles

In some patients, a pattern of fine 1- to 3-mm nodules is seen on the mucosal surface. These represent lymphoid follicles (Fig. 57–4A). They are regularly seen in children[10] but may also be seen in older individuals.[11] As long as the lymphoid follicles are less than 2 to 3 mm in diameter, we consider them a normal phenomenon. Enlargement of these lymphoid follicles may be associated with various diseases including inflammation, Crohn's disease, lymphoma, and immune deficiency.[12] In addition, Bronen and colleagues[13] have reported that the presence of unusually prominent lymphoid follicles in an older individual may be associated with colonic tumors and should promote a vigorous search for the presence of an underlying colonic tumor (Fig. 57–4B).

## Terminal Ileum

Lymphoid follicles are typically seen in the terminal ileum, particularly in younger patients (Fig. 57–4C). This is a normal appearance, but the lymphoid follicles may become enlarged and are particularly prominent in

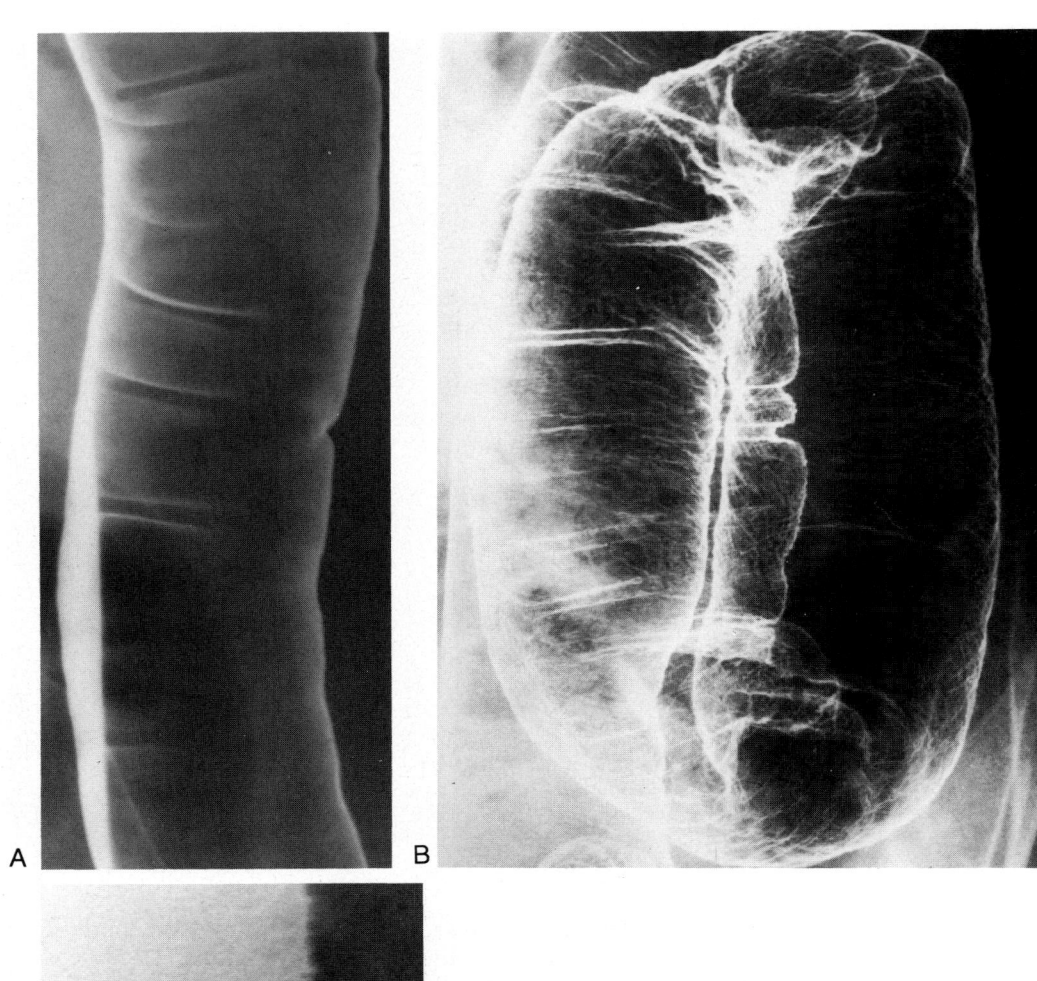

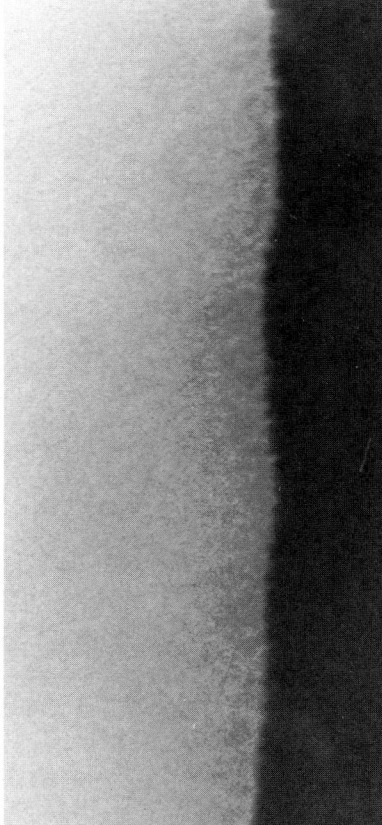

**Figure 57–3. The normal mucosal surface. A.** The smooth, featureless surface usually seen on double contrast study. **B.** Innominate grooves on the surface of the colon. **C.** A single contrast film shows the profile appearance of the innominate lines. These lines should not be mistaken for ulcers.

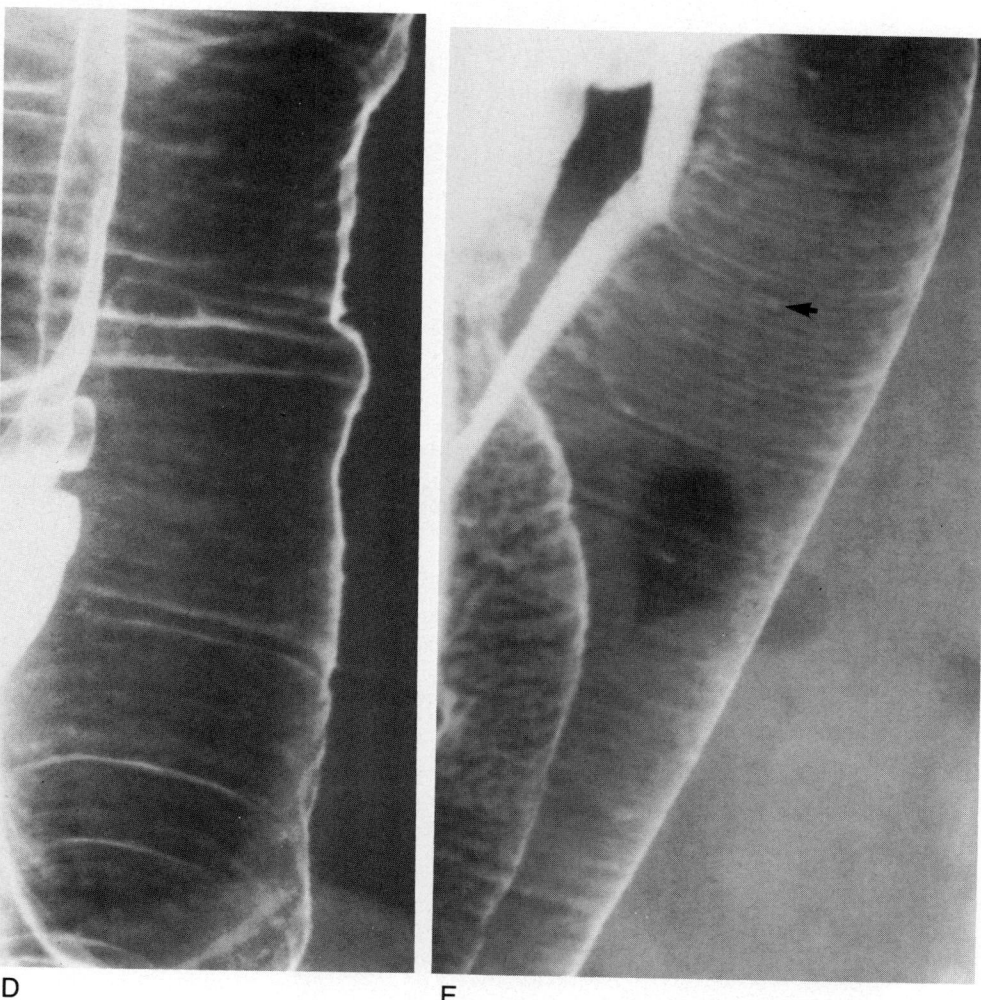

**Figure 57–3** *Continued* **D.** Surface pattern in a normal adult showing pinpoint barium collections en face and in profile. **E.** Transient striation in the transverse colon is due to contraction of the muscularis mucosae. There are also punctate barium collections representing tiny diverticula *(arrow).*

D

E

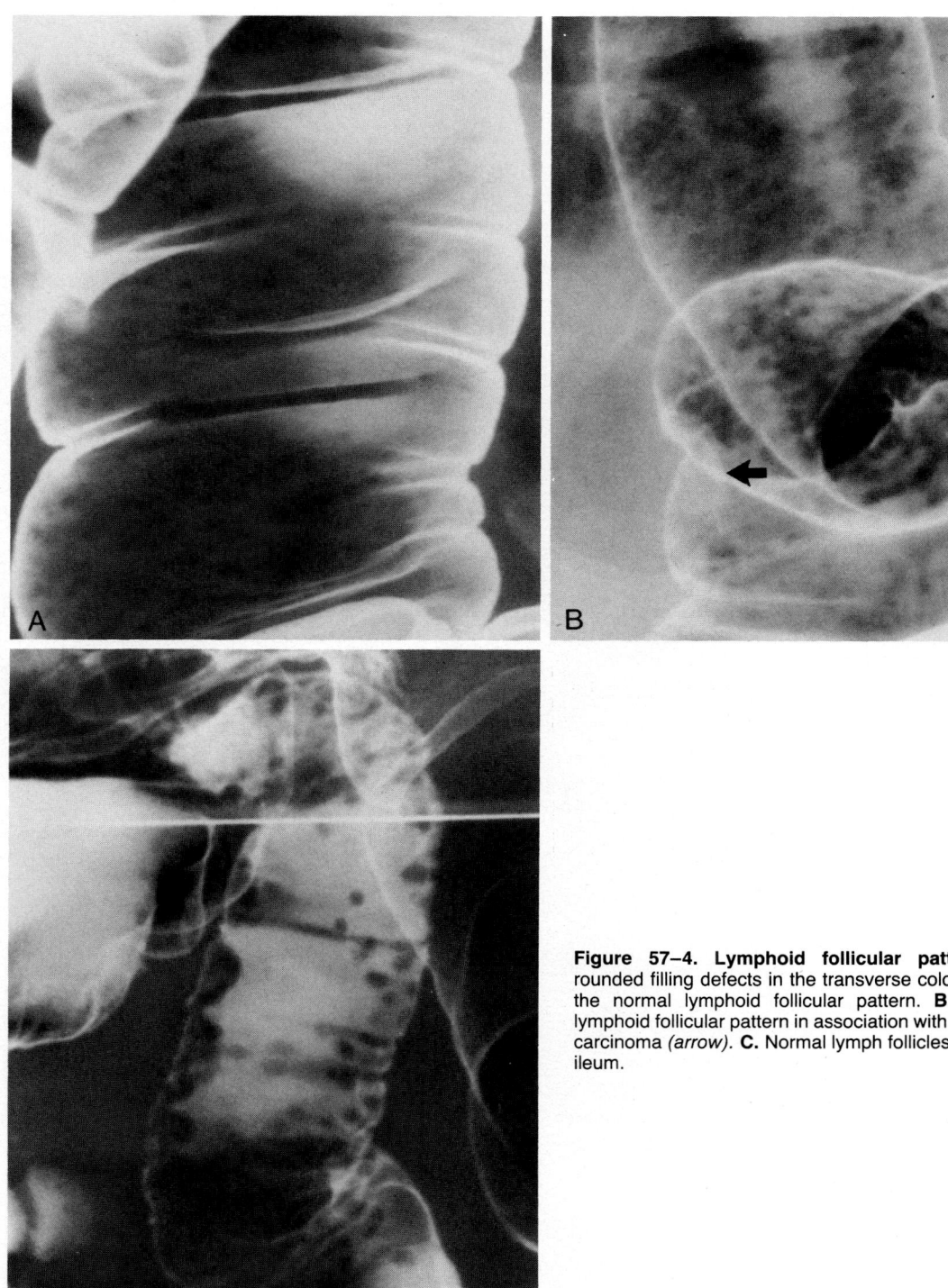

**Figure 57–4. Lymphoid follicular pattern. A.** Tiny rounded filling defects in the transverse colon representing the normal lymphoid follicular pattern. **B.** A prominent lymphoid follicular pattern in association with a small colonic carcinoma *(arrow)*. **C.** Normal lymph follicles in the terminal ileum.

patients with conditions such as *Yersinia* enteritis or lymphoma.

## TECHNICAL PROBLEMS

### Poor Preparation

Poor colonic preparation remains a major obstacle to diagnostic studies. Poor preparation can simulate pathologic conditions such as inflammatory bowel disease (Fig. 57–5). Nevertheless, with the use of horizontal beam radiography (upright and lateral decubitus views), relatively small lesions can still be detected in the presence of fecal debris. In this regard, it is important to keep in mind the distinction between protrusions on the dependent and nondependent surfaces; fecal residue will invariably be found only on the dependent surface, whereas, with appropriate manipulation, true polypoid lesions can be imaged as "etched in white" lesions on the nondependent surface (Fig. 57–6) (see Chapter 4).

### Diverticulosis

The presence of marked sigmoid diverticulosis poses a diagnostic risk because it may be difficult to detect a polypoid mass in the presence of air-filled diverticula. In such cases, it may be necessary to re-examine the sigmoid colon by the single contrast method[14] (Fig. 57–7) or to recommend flexible sigmoidoscopy to clear the sigmoid colon.

### Incontinence

The patient's incontinence may be a limiting problem. An intravenous injection of glucagon will help relax spasm, and inflation of the retention balloon as described previously, under direct visualization, may also overcome this problem.

### Nonfilling of the Right Colon

For various reasons, it may be difficult or impossible to fill the right colon. In some cases, if the patient is asked to evacuate, barium and air will be propelled into the right colon and will provide perfectly adequate views. If this fails, it may be necessary to convert to the single contrast method for adequate filling of the right colon.[15]

## COMPLICATIONS[16]

Many patients experience gas pains during and after the procedure. These can be minimized by using carbon dioxide instead of air for gaseous distention.[17] The most serious complication is perforation of the bowel.[18] In most cases, the perforation occurs in the rectum and is related to the inflation of a retention balloon usually in a diseased rectum. A contrast study with water-soluble contrast agent will show the contrast medium dissecting into the wall of the rectum, and this may extend into the retroperitoneum (Fig. 57–8A). Less frequently, there is a perforation of the intraperitoneal portion of the colon, almost always at the site of diseased bowel (Fig. 57–8B). In patients with diverticulosis, air alone may extravasate during contrast enema and will be recognized as retroperitoneal or intraperitoneal air on the film (Fig. 57–8C).

A barium enema examination should never be performed immediately after sigmoidoscopic biopsy of normal or inflamed rectal mucosa with large biopsy forceps. This sequence is a major predisposing cause of rectal perforation.[19, 20] If a deep rectal biopsy has been done, a barium examination should be postponed for at least 5 days. On the other hand, biopsies of tumors or biopsies performed with the small forceps through flexible endoscopes need not force such long postponements.

Allergic complications are rare but have become more prominent in the last few years.[21] These may represent reactions to the barium, latex of the rectal catheters, or glucagon. In the past few years, the latex of the retention balloons has been replaced by silicone because it was thought to be the source of several severe allergic reactions.[22, 23]

Transient bacteremia has been reported in some studies after barium enema, although clinical problems have not been reported.[24] Nevertheless, in patients with high-risk cardiac lesions such as artificial heart valves, it may be prudent to use antibiotic prophylaxis as recommended by the American Heart Association.[25] This consists of amoxicillin, 3 g by mouth 1 hour before the study and 1.5 g 6 hours after.

In patients with severe ulcerative disease of the bowel, air and contrast medium may enter the perirectal veins, and gas may be seen in the portal vein.[26] This is often, but not always, a fatal occurrence.

## VARIATIONS IN TECHNIQUE

### Suspected Perforation

When perforation of the large bowel is suspected, the study should be done with a water-soluble contrast agent such as diatrizoate meglumine (Gastrografin). If extravasation is not demonstrated, it may be prudent to follow with barium for better definition. In patients with cystic fibrosis, a water-soluble enema can be administered for diagnostic and therapeutic purposes.[27] The hyperosmolar agent draws fluid into the bowel to liquefy the viscid stool with a therapeutic result.

### Peroral Pneumocolon[28]

When the primary diagnostic interest is in the terminal ileum and cecum, an excellent examination can be achieved by use of the peroral pneumocolon. The pa-

*Text continued on page 1040*

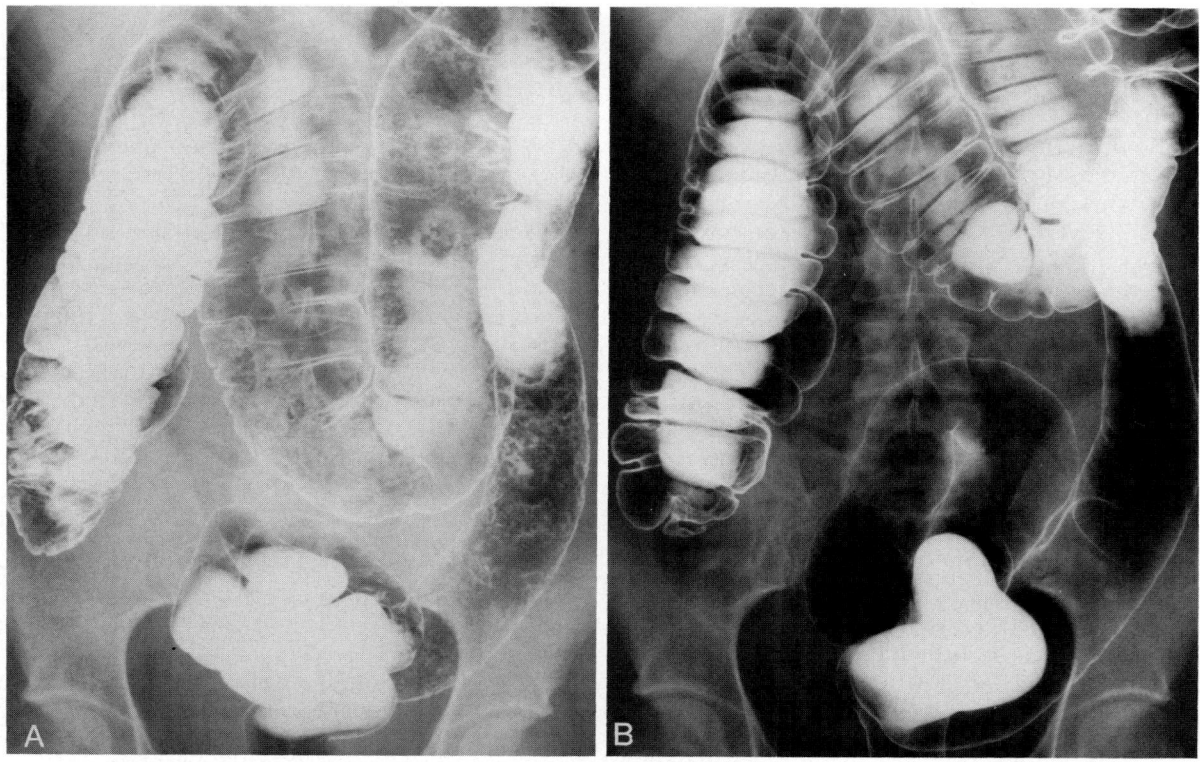

**Figure 57–5. Poor preparation simulating inflammatory bowel disease. A.** The initial study suggests that the mucosa is abnormal throughout the colon. **B.** Another examination with adequate preparation shows that the mucosal surface is normal.

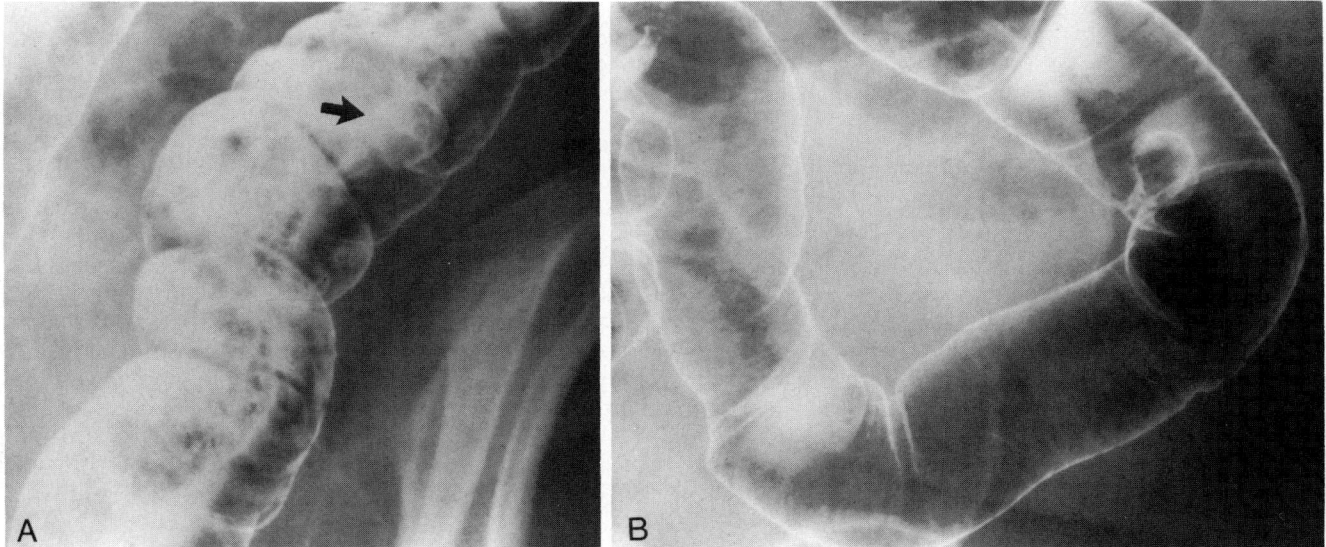

**Figure 57–6. Polyp detection despite fecal debris. A.** There is considerable fecal material in the left colon. Nevertheless, a polyp can be recognized as an etched in white lesion *(arrow).* **B.** A subsequent film, with the fecal material cleared away, shows the pedunculated polyp.

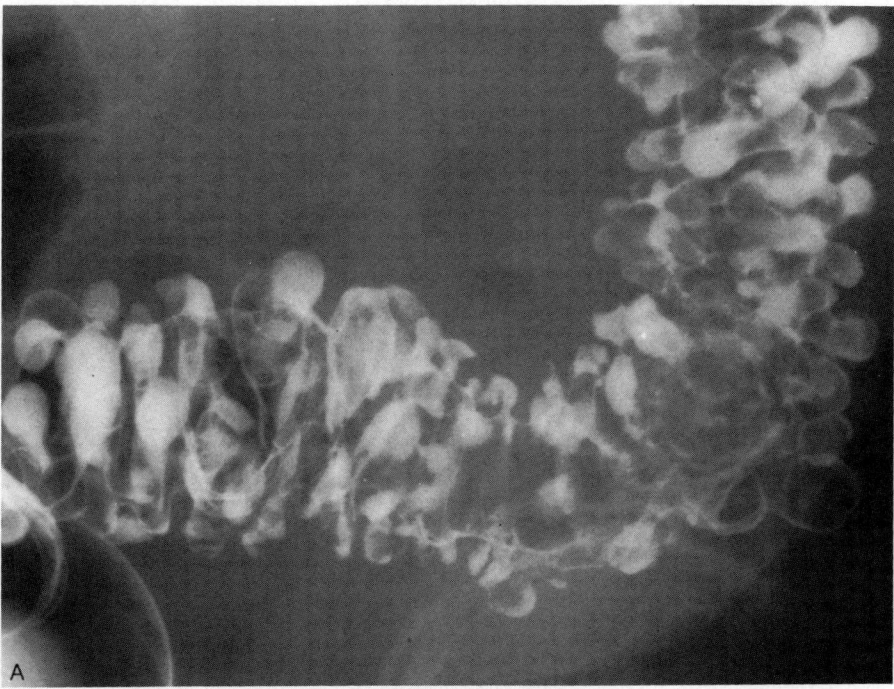

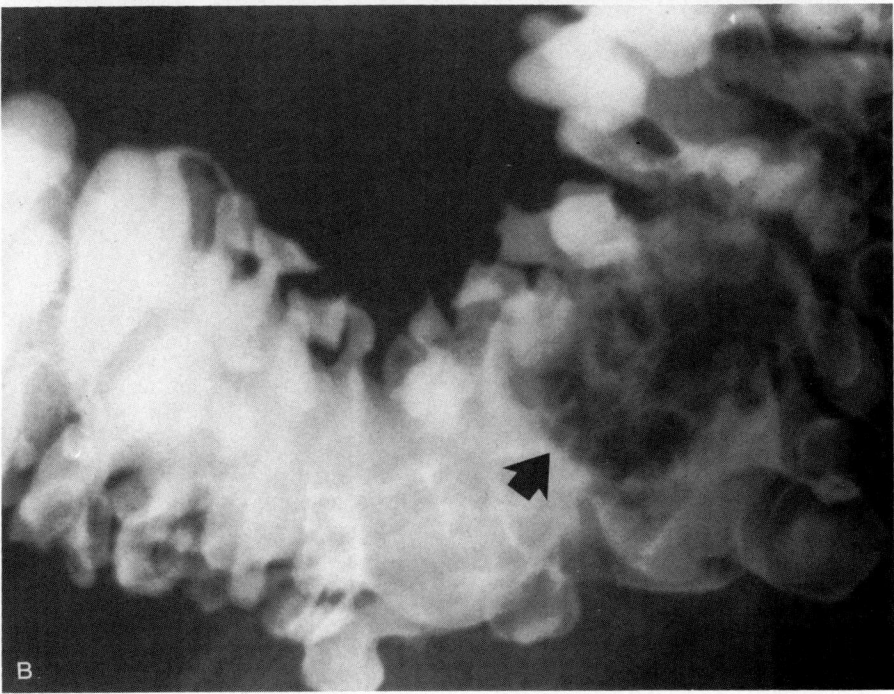

**Figure 57–7. Diverticulosis with sigmoid flush. A.** On the double contrast film, the diverticula are obvious, but a polypoid cancer cannot be identified. **B.** After refilling with single contrast barium, the polypoid cancer *(arrow)* is seen.

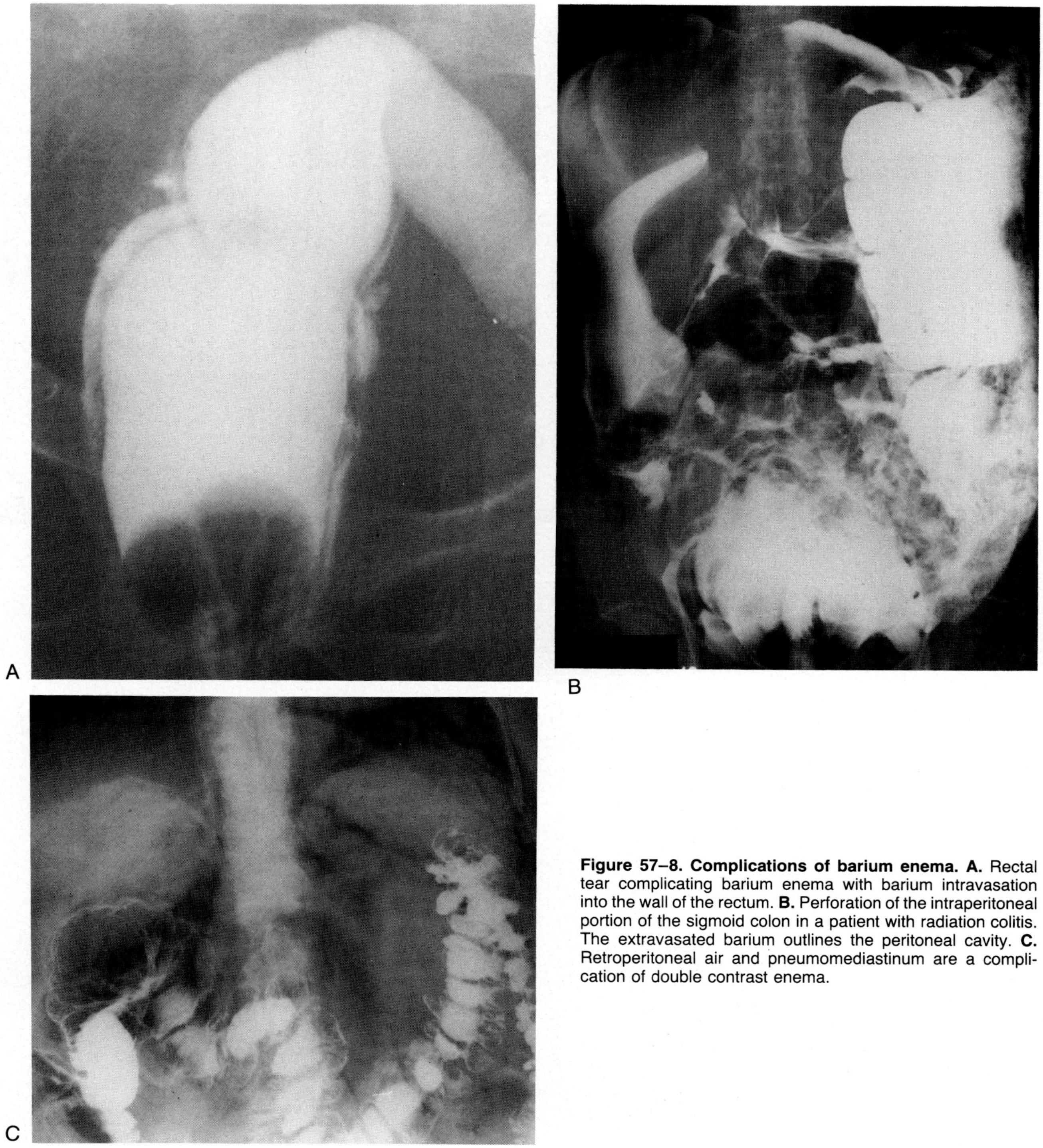

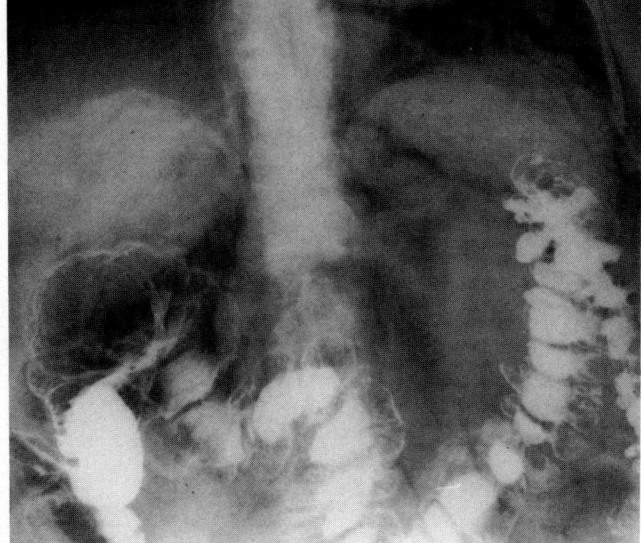

Figure 57–8. Complications of barium enema. A. Rectal tear complicating barium enema with barium intravasation into the wall of the rectum. B. Perforation of the intraperitoneal portion of the sigmoid colon in a patient with radiation colitis. The extravasated barium outlines the peritoneal cavity. C. Retroperitoneal air and pneumomediastinum are a complication of double contrast enema.

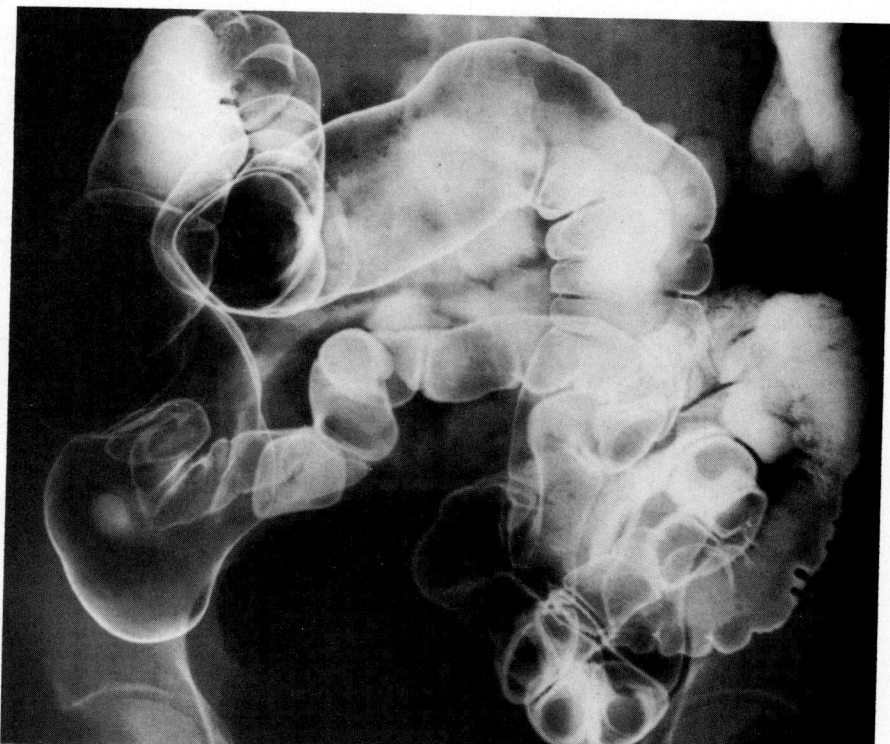

**Figure 57–9. Peroral pneumocolon.** Excellent visualization of the right colon and distal small bowel.

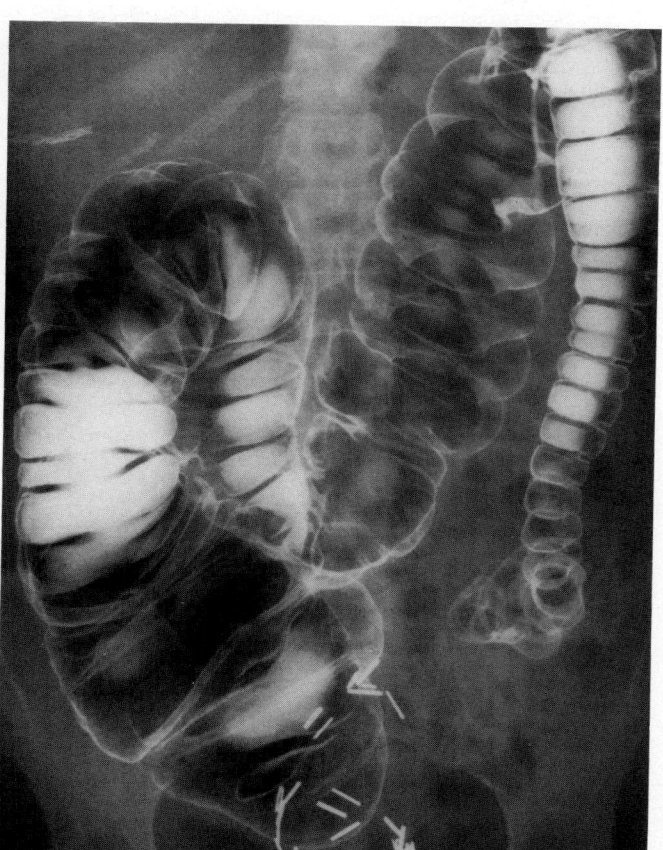

**Figure 57–10. Colostomy enema.** Excellent visualization of the residual colon after colostomy.

tient should undergo preparation of the colon as for a barium enema. After the orally administered barium has reached the right colon, 1 mg glucagon is administered intravenously, and air is insufflated through the rectum. This provides excellent double contrast views of the right colon, cecum, and terminal ileum (Fig. 57–9) (see also Chapter 43).

## Colostomy Enema

Double contrast examinations of excellent quality can be performed through a colostomy. This is particularly important in patients who are being followed after the resection of a previous rectal carcinoma because they have a significant risk of developing a second primary colon cancer. Although a variety of devices have been described, we prefer the technique described by Goldstein and Miller,[29] with a Foley catheter inserted through a nipple that is held against the colostomy (Fig. 57–10).

### Acknowledgment

Figures 57–2B and D, 57–3C and D, 57–7A and B, 57–9, and 57–10 are reproduced from Laufer I, Levine MS (eds): Double Contrast Gastrointestinal Radiology (2nd ed). Philadelphia: WB Saunders, 1992.

Figure 57–3B is reproduced from Laufer I: Double Contrast Gastrointestinal Radiology with Endoscopic Correlation. Philadelphia: WB Saunders, 1979.

Figure 57–8A to C is reproduced from Berk JE, Haubrich WS, Kalser MH, et al (eds): Bockus Gastroenterology, Volume 1 (4th ed). Philadelphia: WB Saunders, 1985.

## References

1. Bartram CI: Obliteration of thumbprinting with double contrast enemas in acute ischemic colitis. Gastrointest Radiol 4:85–88, 1979.
2. Fork ET, Ekberg O, Nilsson G, et al: Colon cleansing regimens. Gastrointest Radiol 7:383–389, 1982.
3. Bakran A, Bradley JA, Breshnihan E, et al: Whole gut irrigation: an inadequate preparation for double contrast barium enema examination. Gastroenterology 73:28–30, 1977.
4. Miller RE: A new enema tip. Radiology 92:1492, 1969.
5. De Lacey G, Wignall B, Ambrose J, et al: The double contrast barium enema: improvements to lateral decubitus views including the use of a wedge filter. Clin Radiol 29:197–199, 1978.
6. Olson DL, Dodds WJ, Stewart ET, et al: Efficacy of an intracassette filter for improved pneumocolon decubitus radiographs. AJR 148:547–549, 1987.
7. Matsuura K, Nakata H, Takeda N, et al: Innominate lines of the colon. Radiology 123:581–584, 1977.
8. Frank DF, Berk RN, Goldstein HM: Pseudoulcerations of the colon on barium enema examination. Gastrointest Radiol 2:129–131, 1977.
9. Williams I: Innominate grooves in the surface of the mucosa. Radiology 84:877–880, 1965.
10. Laufer I, deSa D: The lymphoid follicular pattern: a normal feature of the pediatric colon. AJR 130:51–55, 1978.
11. Kelvin FM, Max RJ, Norton GA, et al: Lymphoid follicular pattern of the colon in adults. AJR 133:821–825, 1979.
12. Glick SN, Teplick SK, Goren RA: Small colonic nodularity and the double contrast barium enema. Radiographics 1:73–86, 1981.
13. Bronen RA, Glick SN, Teplick SK: Diffuse lymphoid follicles of the colon associated with colonic carcinoma. AJR 142:105–109, 1984.
14. Lappas JC, Maglinte DDT, Kopecky KK, et al: Diverticular disease: imaging with post–double-contrast sigmoid flush. Radiology 168:35–37, 1988.
15. Levine MS, Gasparaitis AE: Barium filling for glucagon-resistant spasm on double-contrast barium enema examinations. Radiology 160:264–265, 1986.
16. Gelfand DW: Complications of gastrointestinal radiologic procedures: I. Complications of routine fluoroscopic studies. Gastrointest Radiol 5:293–315, 1980.
17. Bessette JR, Maglinte DDT: Double-contrast barium enema study: simple conversion to $CO_2$. Radiology 162:274–275, 1987.
18. Gelfand DW, Ott DJ, Ramquist NA: Pneumoperitoneum occurring during double-contrast enema. Gastrointest Radiol 4:307–308, 1979.
19. Maglinte DDT, Strong RC, Strate RW, et al: Barium enema after colorectal biopsies: experimental data. AJR 139:693–697, 1982.
20. Harned RK, Consigny PM, Cooper NB: Barium enema examination following biopsy of the rectum or colon. Radiology 145:11–16, 1982.
21. Schwartz EE, Glick SN, Foggs MB, et al: Hypersensitivity reactions after barium enema examination. AJR 143:103–104, 1984.
22. Smith HJ: Performance of barium examination after acute myocardial infarction: report of a survey. AJR 149:63–65, 1987.
23. Gelfand DW: Barium enemas, latex balloons and anaphylactic reactions. AJR 156:1–2, 1991.
24. Butt J, Hentges D, Pelican G, et al: Bacteremia during barium enema study. AJR 130:715–718, 1978.
25. Dajani AS, Bisno AL, Kyung J, et al: Prevention of bacterial endocarditis: recommendations by the American Heart Association. JAMA 264:2919–2922, 1990.
26. Stein MG, Crues JV III, Hamlin JA: Portal venous air associated with barium enema. AJR 140:1171–1172, 1983.
27. Glick SN, Kressel HY, Laufer I, et al: Meconium ileus equivalent: treatment with Hypaque enema. Diagn Imaging 49:149–152, 1980.
28. Kressel HY, Evers KA, Glick SN, et al: The peroral pneumocolon examination. Technique and indication. Radiology 144:414–416, 1982.
29. Goldstein HM, Miller RH: Air contrast colon examination in patients with colostomies. AJR 127:607–610, 1976.

# Evacuation Proctography

**Sat Somers, M.D.**

## INTRODUCTION

The number of patients presenting with disorders affecting the pelvic floor and defecation is increasing. This increase can be attributed to a greater clinical understanding of this problem and of the therapeutic alternatives available. Females constitute 80% of the population presenting with defecation problems. In my practice, 70% of these patients are aged 35 to 55 years.

## PRESENTING SYMPTOMS

**Constipation.** Patients may present with difficulty in initiating defecation, with incomplete defecation, or with the requirement of considerable straining with defecation. In patients with incomplete defecation, mechanical abnormalities such as intussusception and prolapse may be clinically suspected. Some patients may need to resort to digital or positional maneuvers to assist defecation.

**Incontinence.** The clinical presentation of incontinence ranges from constant soiling of clothes that is due to slow intermittent leakage to the inability to hold any stool. The latter group of patients must empty their bowels constantly to prevent accidents, because once they have a desire to defecate they cannot hold the stool.

Other patients who may be referred for evacuation proctography include those with painful defecation and rectal bleeding. The solitary rectal ulcer syndrome is usually suspected in patients with rectal bleeding.[1]

## TECHNIQUE

The dynamic assessment of defecation was first described by Burhenne in 1964.[2] Since then, reports on the technique have been published by several other investigators.[3-7] Most investigators use a modification of the examination as described by Mahieu and colleagues.[3] This modified examination consists of opacifying the rectum and having the patient sit on a commode and go through a series of maneuvers including defecation. In female patients, the vagina is also opacified. The whole procedure is recorded on spot films and videotape. The study is usually completed in about 15 minutes.

The entire examination must be explained to the patient before beginning evacuation proctography. It is helpful to ask the patient to practice such maneuvers as squeezing the buttocks to demonstrate lift while the patient is sitting on the side of a stretcher before the instillation of contrast medium. Doing so ensures that the patient understands all the instructions during the actual procedure.

## Vaginal Opacification

In the female patient, the vagina is first opacified. The agent used for opacification varies. A vaginal tampon soaked with a water-soluble contrast agent used to be the standard vaginal marker that my colleagues and I used until we noted that the tampon can act as a pelvic strut and obscure diagnostic information.[8] Therefore, we now routinely use a radiopaque gel as a vaginal marker. The gel is made with equal parts of Aci-Jel (a low-pH sterile gel for vaginal use) and high-density water-soluble contrast medium. A combination of 12.5 g of Aci-Jel and 12.5 mL of diatrizoate meglumine plus diatrizoate sodium (Hypaque-76) or iohexol (Omnipaque) is instilled into the vagina with a bladder irrigation syringe to which a pediatric enema tip has been attached (Fig. 58–1). The patient is placed in the lithotomy or left lateral decubitus position, the tip of the enema tube is inserted into the vaginal vault, and the contrast medium is injected as the tip is withdrawn. A gauze soaked with barium can also be used as a marker; however, it is more difficult to insert into the vagina.

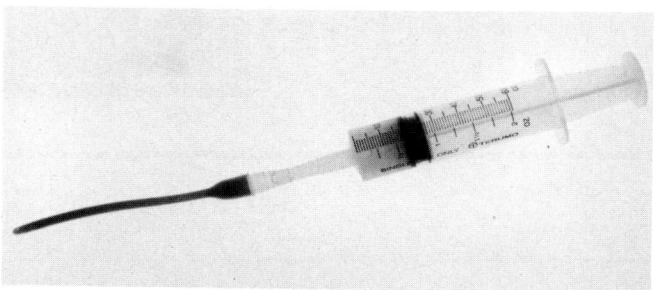

**Figure 58–1. Vaginal opacification device.** Pediatric enema tip attached to a bladder irrigation syringe filled with Aci-Jel and high-density water-soluble contrast medium.

## Rectal Opacification

The next step is opacification of the rectum. A barium paste with a consistency similar to that of stool is preferred. Liquid barium is not physiologic and stresses even a normal continence mechanism. It may also result in abnormal contraction of the pelvic floor and anal muscles at rest, obscuring visualization of deficiencies of muscular resting tone.[5]

A barium paste prepared with barium and potato starch has the appropriate consistency.[3] Commercial preparations such as Evac-U-Paste (E-Z-EM Company, Westbury, NY), although they are slightly less viscous, also work well. A disadvantage of the barium and potato starch mixture is that it does not coat the walls of the lumen well. This problem can be overcome by instilling 30 to 50 mL of high-density liquid barium (e.g., liquid Polibar, E-Z-EM Company) before introducing the barium-starch mixture. The barium-starch mixture is also difficult to instill into the rectum with a regular caulking gun. An orthopedic glue gun, although more expensive, is much easier to use, as it is geared, and it lasts for years. If an orthopedic glue gun is used, a 50-cm half-inch tube that is filled with high-density liquid barium and is attached to the glue gun at one end and to a wide bore enema tip at the other is ideal for the introduction of both rectal contrast agents.

Contrast medium is introduced until the patient reports the sensation of rectal fullness and the desire to evacuate. The position of the anal orifice is marked with a radiopaque paste. The paste is made up with 50 g of petroleum jelly mixed with 50 g of Ultra-R barium sulfate (E-Z-EM Company). The marker facilitates measurement of the anal canal. The patient is then led to the commode for the dynamic study.

## Commode

The defecography commode needs to fulfill the following requirements: it must be sturdy so that the patient is not afraid to sit on it, it must be radiolucent, and it must be designed to allow both lateral and frontal projections as well as safe attachment to the fluoroscopic table. Attachment to the fluoroscopic table allows movement of the commode with the table movement control buttons. Commodes can be built with a personal design or a published design, or they may be purchased from commercially available sources.[9] My colleagues and I use a commode designed by Bernier and associates[9] (Fig. 58–2). It has a centimeter ruler in the midline for exact and direct measurements of the midline sagittal structures on the films (Fig. 58–3).

## Documentation

The radiation dose needed to record this examination should be as low as possible. Therefore, many investigators use videofluoroscopy only. However, the resolution is insufficient to detect subtle radiographic changes and spot films are recommended. Therefore, videofluoroscopy should be performed during the entire examination, with spot 100- or 105-mm films of key events. If stimulable phosphors or digital radiography is used for the spot films, the radiation dose can be reduced even further.

To make the patient feel more comfortable with the procedure, it is preferable to use a remote control fluoroscopy room that has subdued lighting and is cleared of all personnel. Comfort of the patient can sometimes be extremely important in obtaining an accurate assessment of the defecation process.

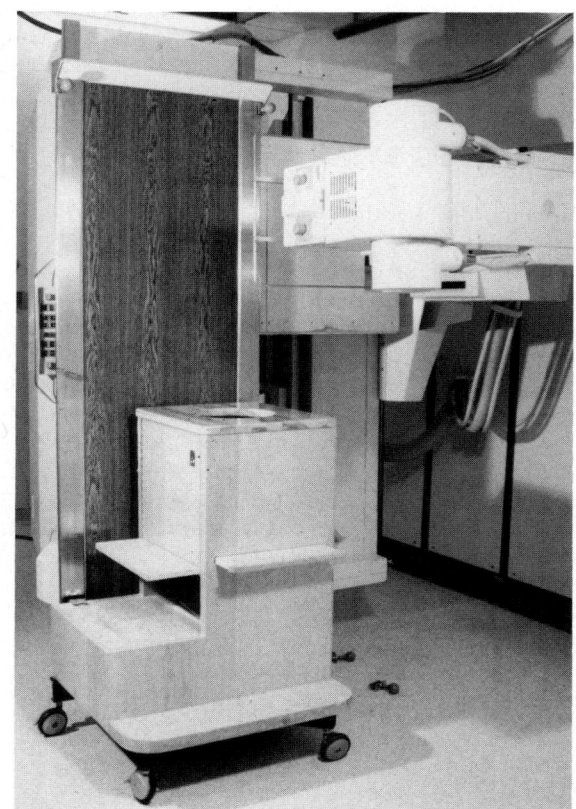

**Figure 58–2. Defecography commode.** The commode is shown attached to a remote control fluoroscopic table. The anterior and lateral footrests have been withdrawn. The footrests on two sides facilitate filming in both the lateral and the anteroposterior projections.

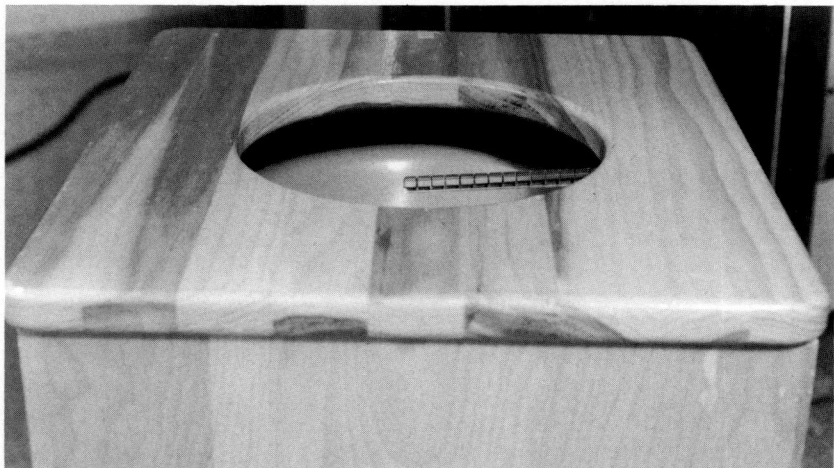

**Figure 58–3. Midline radiopaque centimeter ruler.** The ruler permits direct measurements of midline sagittal structures that have been filmed.

Filming is done in the lateral projection with the patient responding to requests to rest, lift, cough, strain, defecate, and strain after defecation. At rest, there is no conscious contraction of any of the pelvic musculature (Fig. 58–4). On lifting, the patient maximally contracts the pelvic floor musculature and elevates the entire pelvic floor[10] (Fig. 58–5). The muscles involved are the puborectalis and the levator ani. As a result, the anorectal angle becomes acute, and the anal canal lengthens. These changes can be measured and are indicators of the continence mechanism. In the request to cough, the patient is asked to produce a powerful cough at the rest position (Fig. 58–6). This action simultaneously increases intra-abdominal pressure and contraction of the anal and pelvic floor muscles. In normal individuals, there is minimal or no descent of the pelvic floor and total continence. In the request to strain, the patient is asked to strain downward maximally without evacuating

(Fig. 58–7). This stresses the continence mechanism and gives a measure of pelvic floor descent. The anal canal shortens during straining in most women (mean change, 2 mm).[10] Although nearly all patients demonstrate some perineal descent, this portion of the examination is the least reliable, because some patients paradoxically contract the pelvic floor muscles, perhaps for fear of incontinence. Defecation and postdefecation straining are the final parts of this procedure (Figs. 58–8 and 58–9). These films give a measurement of pelvic floor descent and an estimate of the completeness of emptying. Morphologic abnormalities such as intussusception and rectoceles are often visualized at this time, and the changes contributing to the symptoms of patients with difficulty in defecation can be analyzed. Rectoceles are outpouch-

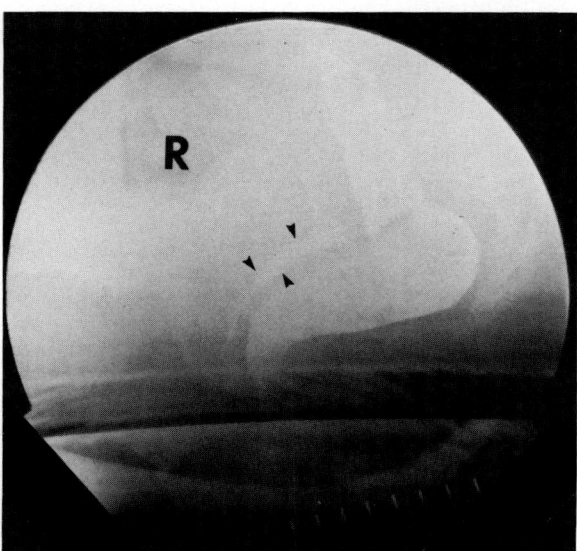

**Figure 58–4. Normal appearance of proctogram during rest** (R). Note the opacified vagina *(arrows)* and its close relationship to the anterior rectal wall.

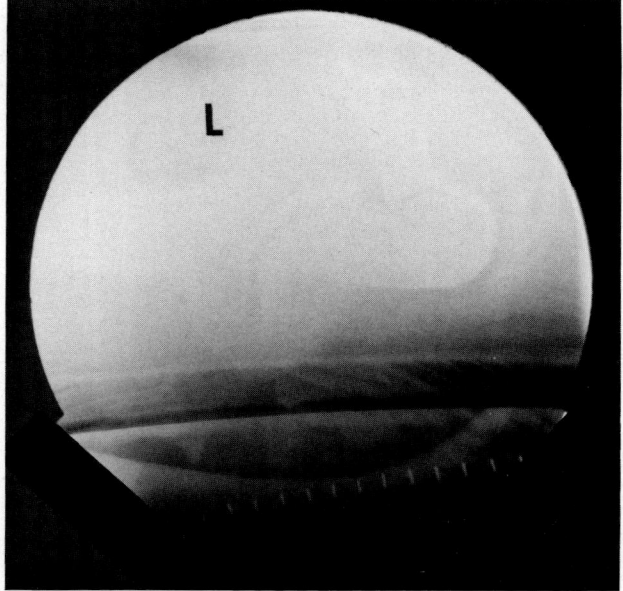

**Figure 58–5. Normal appearance of proctogram during lift** (L). There is good contraction of the puborectalis and the levator ani. The anorectal junction level is raised well above the level of the ischial tuberosities.

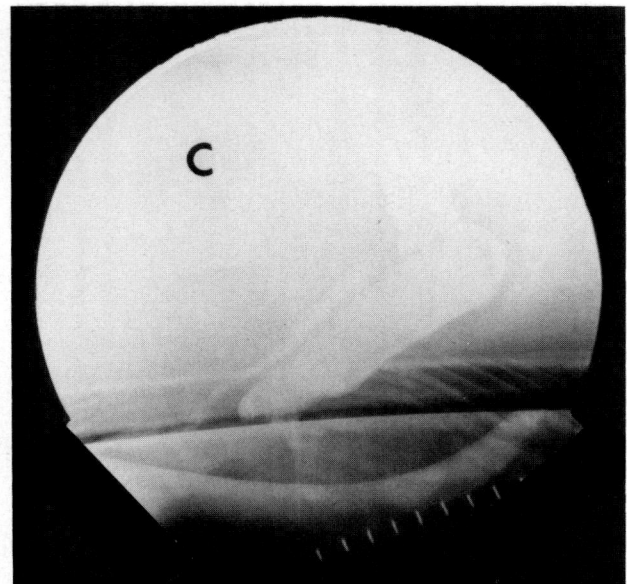

**Figure 58–6. Normal appearance of proctogram during coughing**
(C). There is minimal descent of the anorectal junction compared with
the resting position.

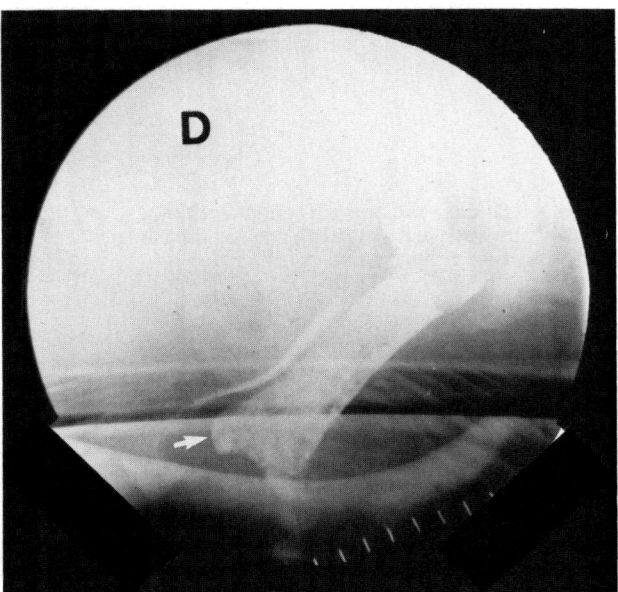

**Figure 58–8. Normal appearance of proctogram during defeca-
tion** (D). The anorectal angle has increased considerably in comparison with the resting position, the anterior rectocele *(arrow)* has
become slightly larger, and the anal canal is open with evacuation in
progress. Note the centimeter marker at the bottom of the film.

ings of the rectum beyond the line of the rectal wall
(Fig. 58–10). They are often normal and are more
common in women.[10] If the rectocele does not empty
completely during defecation, it may produce a feeling
of incomplete evacuation of the rectum.

## Measurements

The measurements taken from the spot films are the
anorectal angle, the anal canal length, the position of

the anorectal junction, and the descent and elevation of
the anorectal junction (Fig. 58–11).

## *Anorectal Angle*

The anorectal angle is measured between the axis of
the anal canal and the tangent to the posterior wall of
the rectum. It can be difficult to measure, for often the
posterior wall of the rectum is not clearly delineated
and the angle becomes highly subjective.[11] Caution

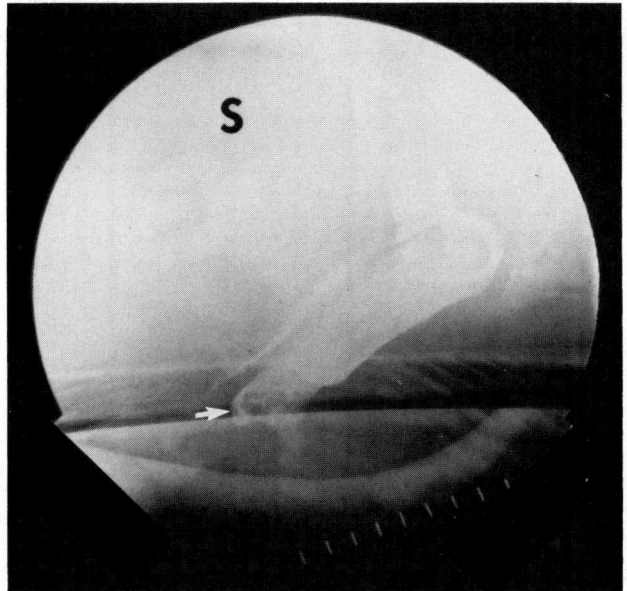

**Figure 58–7. Normal appearance of proctogram during straining**
(S). The anorectal angle shows an increase, and the anorectal junction
level has descended in comparison with the resting position. A small
anterior rectocele *(arrow)* is noted.

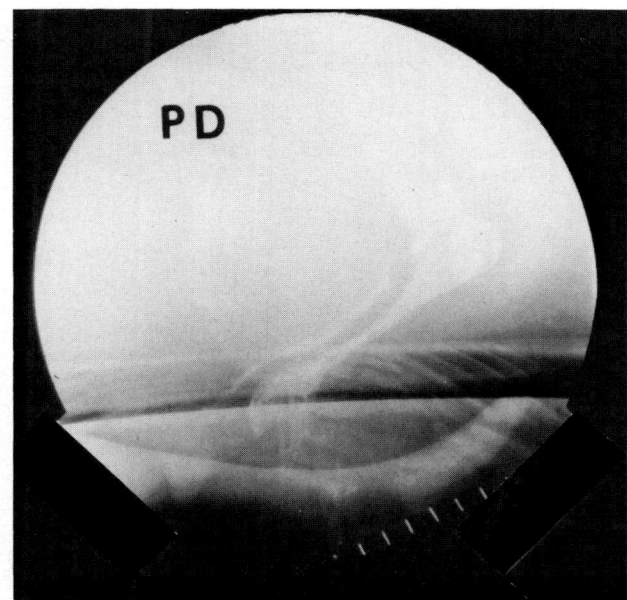

**Figure 58–9. Normal appearance of proctogram during post-
defecation straining** (PD). The rectum is almost completely empty,
and the anterior rectocele has become distorted with the straining.

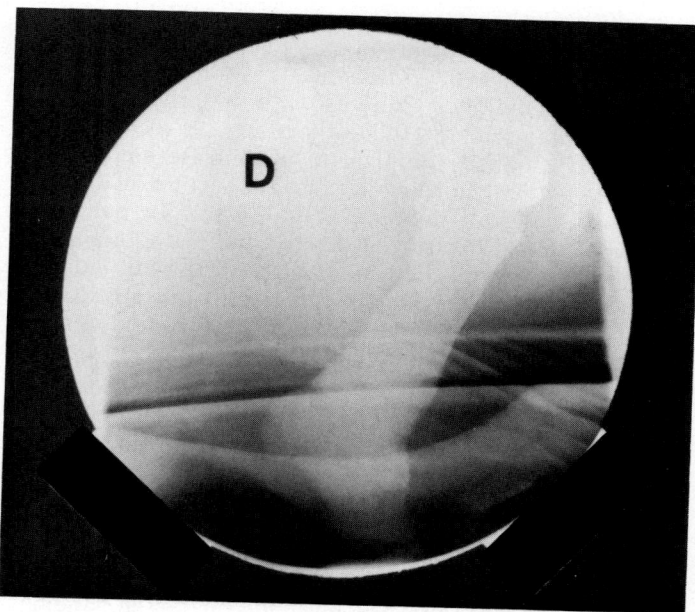

**Figure 58–10. Anterior rectocele**. An outpouching is seen at the anterior wall of the rectum. Anterior rectoceles of moderate size are normal in young females. D = defecation.

should therefore be exercised in assessing its significance. At rest, this angle is usually not greater than 120 degrees in normal control subjects. The normal range, however, is between 70 and 134 degrees, with a mean of about 95 degrees.[10] When the individual squeezes or lifts the buttocks, the anorectal angle decreases to a mean of 19 degrees (range, 6 to 26 degrees) in females, and a mean of 28 degrees (range, 12 to 45 degrees) in males.[10] This angle increases on straining and defecation.

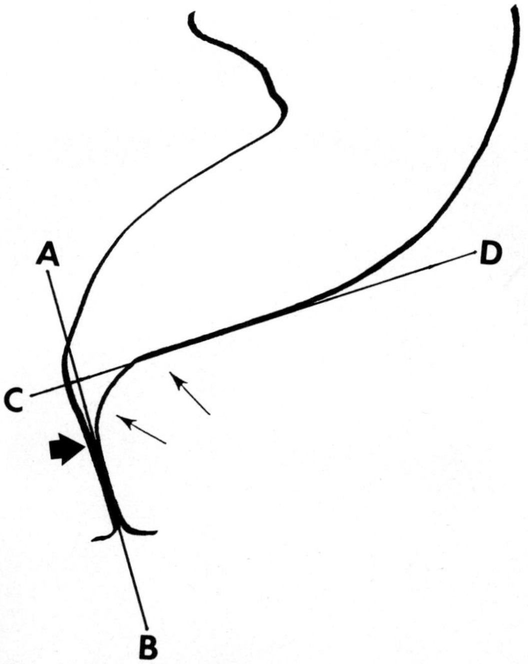

**Figure 58–11. Anorectal angle determination**. The lines AB and CD subtend the posterior anorectal angle. The position of AB is easily determined. CD can be much more difficult to draw. The wide arrow shows the position of the anorectal junction. Below it are the two parallel lines that form the anal canal. The thin arrows point to the puborectalis impression.

The mean anorectal angle on straining in normal young women is 103 degrees, with a range of 75 to 108 degrees. In men, the mean is slightly lower at 98 degrees, with a range of 67 to 123 degrees.[10]

## Anal Canal Length

The anal canal length is easily measured and is the distance covered by the parallel sides of the anal canal before they convert to the diverging walls of the distal rectum. At rest, the mean length of the anal canal is 16 mm (range, 6 to 26 mm) in women and 22 mm (range, 10 to 38 mm) in young men. On lifting (squeezing), the anal canal lengthens to a mean of 19 mm (range, 9 to 26 mm) in women and 28 mm (range, 12 to 45 mm) in men. On straining, the canal shortens slightly and has mean length of 14 mm (range, 6 to 20 mm) in young females and 17 mm (range, 9 to 27 mm) in young males.[10]

## Level of Anorectal Junction

The anorectal junction is the uppermost point of the canal. Its position is measured from an easily visualized fixed point, the ischial tuberosity. A positive measurement indicates a position above the ischial tuberosity, whereas a negative value is a position below it. In normal young males at rest, the mean level of the anorectal junction is 16 mm and increases to 28 mm during lifting (squeezing). It drops to −4 mm during defecation. In the young female, the mean values for the same maneuvers are 4 mm at rest, 14 mm on lifting (squeezing), and 16 mm on defecation.[10] These measurements are significantly different from those of normal young males.

Occasionally, unusual or unexplained features are seen on the lateral projection, and an anteroposterior or oblique view is needed for further clarification. Some patients have a history of using a variety of maneuvers to facilitate evacuation. These patients should be encouraged to go through these maneuvers during the examination, and the mechanisms aiding evacuation should be identified. Patients with a large anterior rectocele that remains full even after the rectum has completely emptied complain of incomplete emptying. They empty the rectocele back into the rectum by digital perineal or vaginal pressure (Fig. 58–12). In patients with a history of obstructed defecation, it is sometimes helpful to perform the examination first with liquid barium, which makes expulsion easier. If this approach is successful, the examination should be repeated in the usual way with one of the thick barium pastes.

## PATHOLOGY

### Enterocele and Sigmoidocele

As shown by the vaginal marker, the vagina may separate from the anterior wall of the rectum during defecation (Fig. 58–13), which usually causes the patient to feel pressure in the perineum. Whenever this separation is seen, the examination should be repeated after the small bowel has been opacified.[4, 10] This repeated examination is usually performed during another visit, and the patient is requested to arrive about 1 hour before the evacuating proctogram to consume 400 to 600 mL of small bowel meal barium. The evacuation proctogram is then repeated. If the gap between the vagina and rectum is due to an enterocele, the opacified small bowel is observed descending (herniating) into a deep pouch of Douglas (Fig. 58–14). If rectal prolapse is also present, the small bowel may invaginate the anterior rectal wall and prolapse along with the rectum through the anal canal (Fig. 58–15). A sigmoidocele can give the same appearance so that the proximal sigmoid

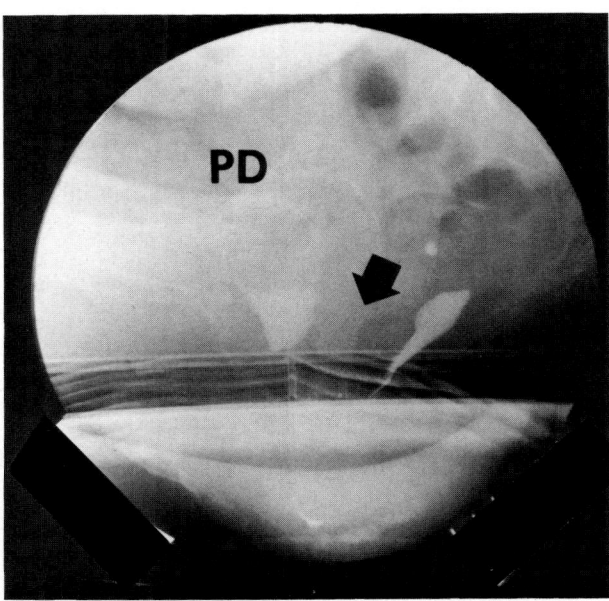

**Figure 58–13. Wide separation of the vagina from the anterior rectal wall.** This separation *(arrow)* could be due to the descent of either an enterocele or a rectocele into the pouch of Douglas. This finding is accentuated by postdefecation straining (PD).

colon must be opacified to allow differentiation (Fig. 58–16). Occasionally, an enterocele and a sigmoidocele are present in the same patient (Fig. 58–17).

### Anterior Wall Prolapse and Rectocele

In anterior wall prolapse, the anterior rectal wall prolapses toward the external anal orifice during the final stages of evacuation. This prolapse is a frequent

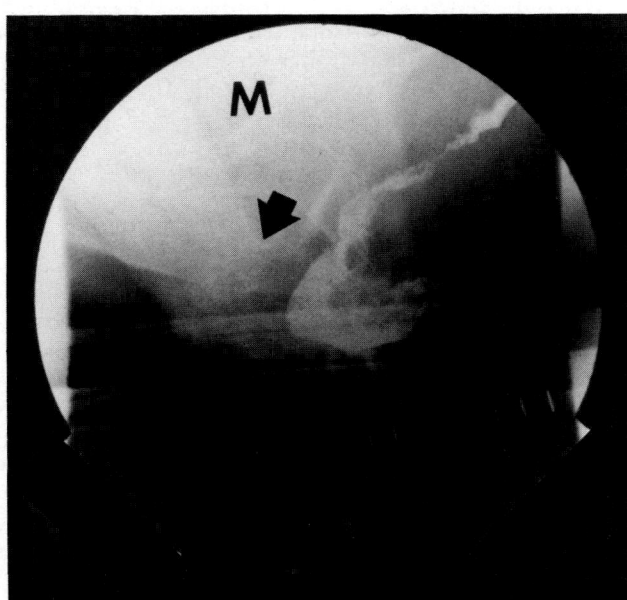

**Figure 58–12. Rectocele manipulation** (M). The arrow points to the digits of the hand that are being used to empty the anterior rectocele into the rectum by pushing it upward.

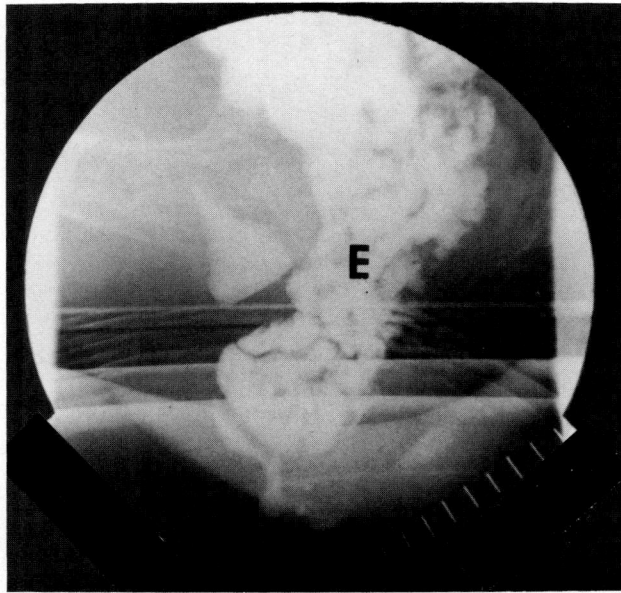

**Figure 58–14. Enterocele.** Opacified small bowel (E) is seen in the pouch of Douglas. The vagina has been pushed anteriorly, and a rectocele is also present.

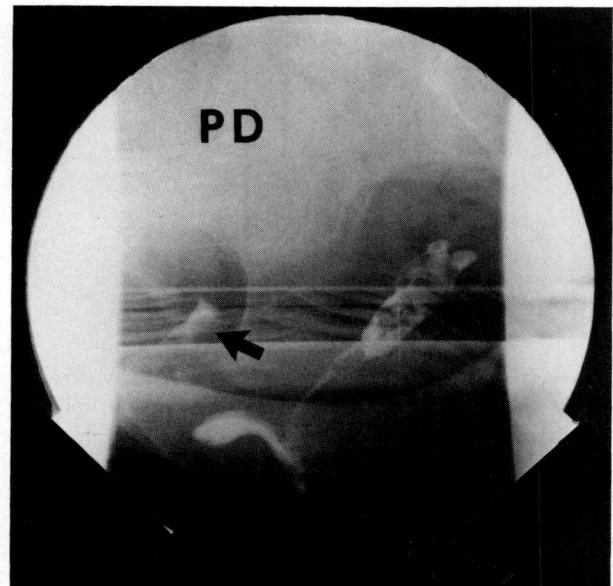

**Figure 58–15. Enterocele and rectal prolapse**. There is separation of the vagina *(arrow)* and rectum, suggesting the presence of an enterocele. In addition, there is prolapse of the rectum into the anal canal. This finding is not uncommon in patients who perform continued straining. The findings are accentuated by postdefecation straining (PD).

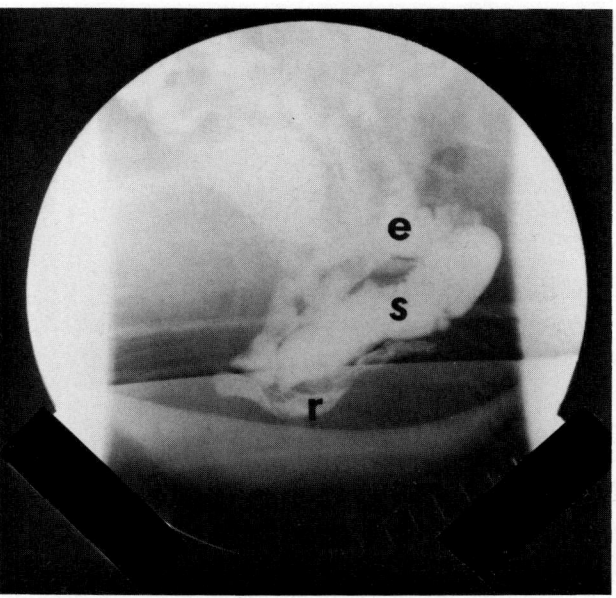

**Figure 58–17. Sigmoidocele and enterocele**. A sigmoidocele (s) and an enterocele (e) are present. There is posterior displacement of the rectum (r). Complete emptying of the rectosigmoid is often impaired.

finding in females and may be responsible for isolating an anterior rectocele. As mentioned earlier, rectoceles are outpouchings of the rectal wall. They are usually anterior and reflect a relative weakness of the rectovaginal septum. Rectoceles are often accompanied by an intussusception, which may obstruct defecation by occluding both the anal canal and the neck of the rectocele[12] (Fig. 58–18). The anterior wall prolapse may precede an intussusception.

## Rectal Intussusception

Rectal intussusception is a concentric invagination of the whole rectal wall that progresses toward the anal canal[13] (Fig. 58–19). It is thought to cause rectal pro-

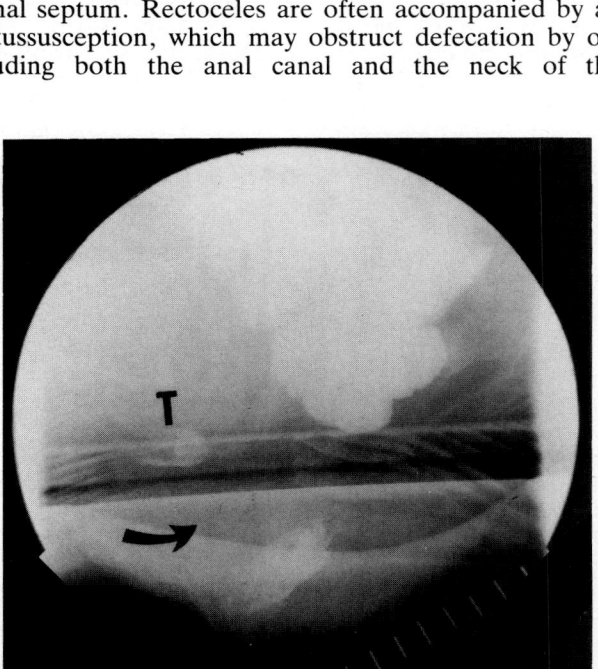

**Figure 58–16. Sigmoidocele**. The vaginal marker (T) has been separated from the anterior rectal wall. As the small bowel has already been opacified, the separation *(arrow)* must be the result of a sigmoidocele, which can be proved by opacifying the distal colon.

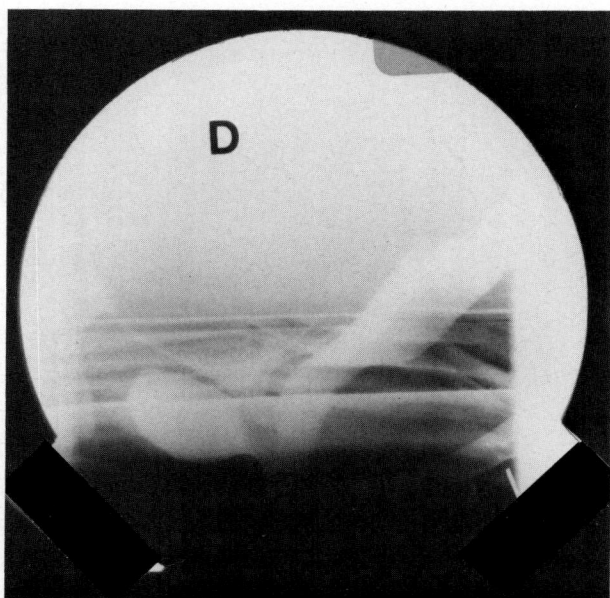

**Figure 58–18. Anterior wall prolapse**. A pronounced anterior wall prolapse occludes the anal canal and the neck of the anterior rectocele. D = defecation.

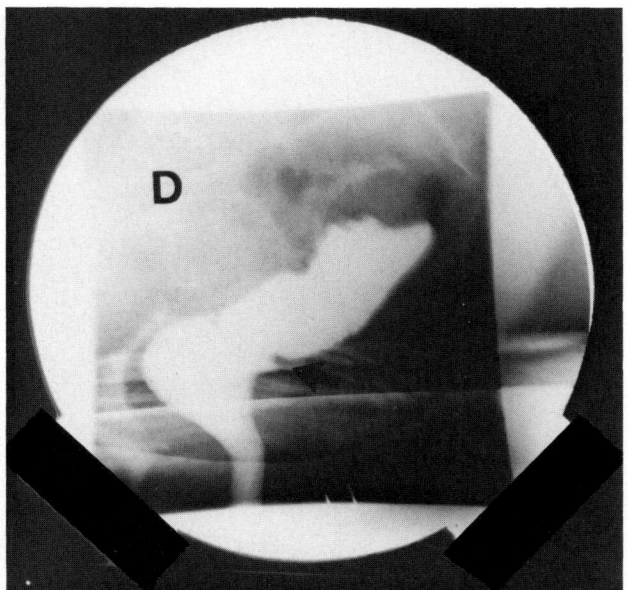

**Figure 58–19. Intussusception.** The concentric invagination of an intussusception is demonstrated during defecation (D).

lapse. The intussusception usually begins about 6 to 8 cm above the anal canal and can commence as an invagination of one of the valves of Houston.[14] The infolding of the intussusception is anterior in the vast majority (62%) of patients. It is annular in 32% and posterior in only 6%. Minor degrees of infolding of less than 3 mm represent mucosal prolapse and are probably not significant. However, inferior extension of the intussusception into the anal canal is abnormal. When an intussusception plugs the anal canal, the symptoms of obstructed defecation[15] and solitary rectal ulcer[1] may be experienced. The patient sometimes learns to relieve the obstruction by pushing the "intussusception plug"

back with a finger placed in the anal canal. Internal prolapse, as seen with an intussusception plug, is revealed only by evacuation proctography. Occasionally, it is demonstrated only at the end of defecation and sometimes only with straining. Therefore, the view depicting postdefecation straining is important (Fig. 58–20). Complete or external prolapses are clinically obvious.

## Posterolateral Rectal Pouches

Posterolateral rectal pouches are herniations of rectal mucosa through the pelvic floor. They are often suspected only on a lateral view but are confirmed in the anteroposterior projection with straining. These pouches are most often found in patients who have difficulties with rectal evacuation, requiring excessive straining. This group of patients who demonstrate excessive straining may have paradoxical contraction of the puborectalis sling or a nonrelaxing anal sphincter.

## Dysfunction of the Puborectalis

In patients with paradoxical contraction of the puborectalis, defecography shows either an increased or an unchanged anorectal angle during straining and defecation (Fig. 58–21). The puborectalis impression is usually prominent because of persistent contraction and increases with the decrease in anorectal angle. This syndrome is fairly common in patients with normal colonic transit and chronic constipation. Bartolo and co-workers found this syndrome in 11 of 49 patients who were examined by proctography.[16] This entity has also been called anismus and spastic floor syndrome.[17]

In some patients, the puborectalis relaxes, but the internal or the external anal sphincter muscle fails to

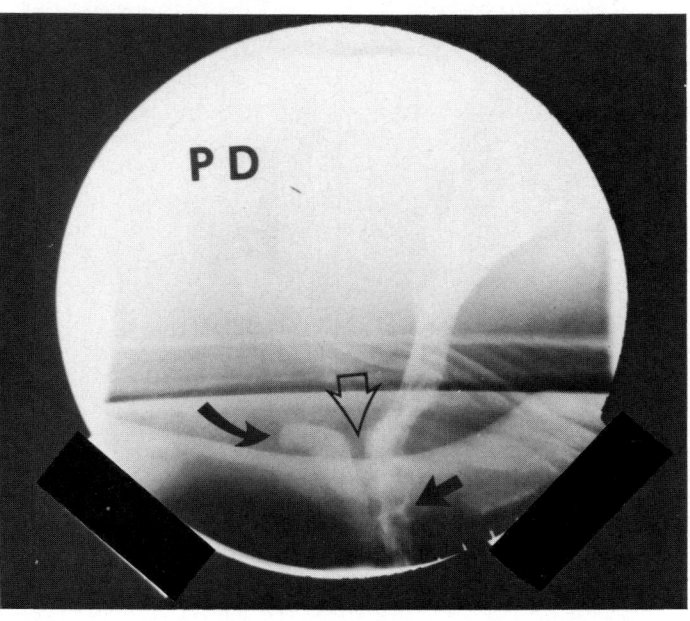

**Figure 58–20. External prolapse.** External prolapse is shown during postdefecation straining (PD). Curved arrow = vagina; straight solid arrow = external prolapse; open arrow = low perineum.

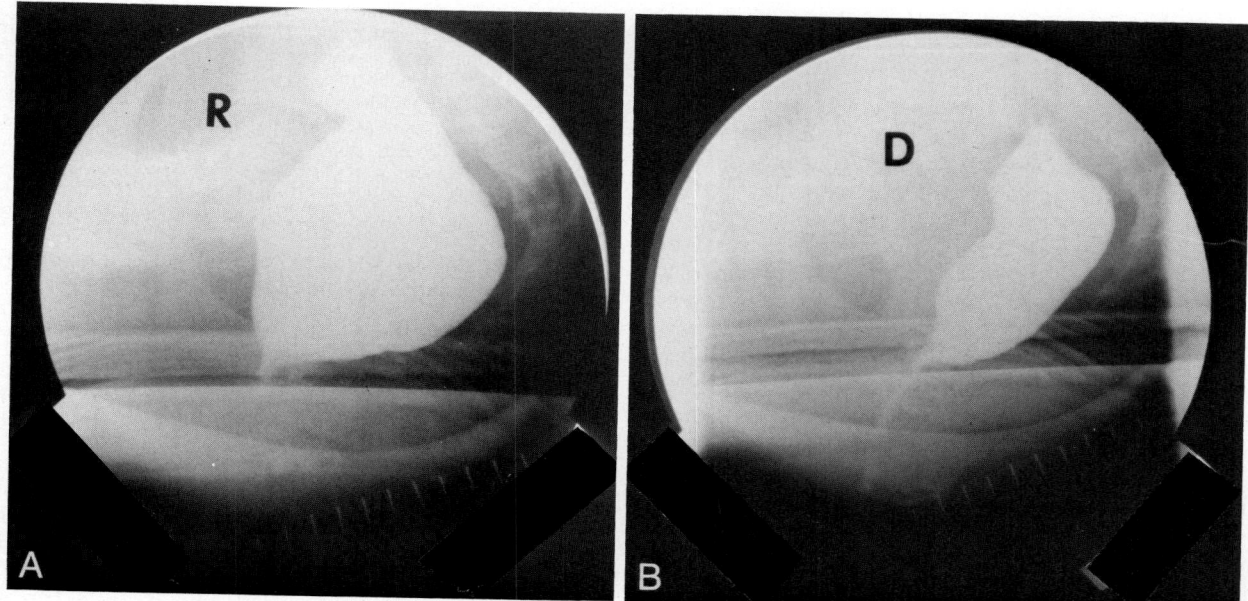

**Figure 58–21. Poor relaxation of anal sphincter.**The anorectal angle is virtually unchanged between rest (R) in **A** and defecation (D) in **B**.

open, or both sphincter muscles fail to open. This failure occurs presumably because of nonrelaxation. The non-relaxing sphincter may be associated with an anal fissure, spinal cord tumors, and painful hemorrhoids.

## Descending Perineum Syndrome

Patients with the descending perineum syndrome also have difficulty defecating. This syndrome entails ballooning of the perineum below the plane of the ischial tuberosities on straining. The perineal descent is usually less than that of the pelvic floor and can be measured with a perineometer.[18] Proctography is, however, a more reliable method of assessing pelvic floor descent.[19] This syndrome may be seen in other disorders involving obstructed defecation and may subsequently lead to injury of the pudendal nerve.

## Constipation and Incontinence

Continuous straining stretches the pudendal nerve by the ballooning of the pelvic floor. The stretching has been shown to increase motor latency of the pudendal nerve.[20] Continued straining can ultimately lead to permanent pudendal nerve damage and incontinence.

Normal control subjects have an anorectal junction level above the ischial tuberosity and an excursion of about 3 cm with straining and defecation. Constipated patients have a low anorectal junction level and good lift, but little or no movement on straining and defecation. The lift excursion is similar to that of normal individuals. Patients with fecal incontinence have a low anorectal junction level (not unlike constipated patients), a small increase on lift, and a large excursion on straining and defecation. Given that the constipated and incontinent patients both have low anorectal junction levels, it seems reasonable to speculate that such low levels are due to constant straining and that the constipated patients will eventually become incontinent as a result of a pudendal neuropathy. Because lift in the constipated group is still satisfactory, it may be possible to prevent incontinence in this group with a perineal support device such as the Lesaffer seat (Defecom, Aalst, Belgium).[21] The Lesaffer perineal support device is designed to prevent excessive descent of the perineum, permit normal relaxation and expulsion, and prevent or minimize nerve damage.

Evacuation proctography in incontinence is of value only in patients with prolapse, anal sphincter trauma, or neurogenic (idiopathic) incontinence. In rectal prolapse, patients are partially incontinent because the intussusception dilates the internal sphincter. When detected by proctography, rectopexy or a postanal repair can be performed.[22] In neurogenic or idiopathic incontinence, if the anorectal angle is widened, a postanal repair can restore this angle and continence.[23] In sphincteric trauma, proctography is useful in assessing the extent of the damage to the pelvic musculature and in monitoring healing.

## NORMAL VARIATIONS

The abnormal findings in evacuation proctography, as described earlier, are much easier to characterize than the normal findings. This greater difficulty in defining normal characteristics arises because there are few data on normal subjects in different age groups[24] and only one study of normal volunteers.[10] This latter study showed that the range of normal characteristics is much greater than originally reported. Authors of several studies agreed that the normal mean anorectal angle is between 90 and 100 degrees.[3, 4, 25, 26] The study of normal young volunteers indicated a range of greater than 60 degrees around this mean. The same study showed a mean pelvic descent of 2 cm; however, values greater than 5 cm in some females and greater than 4 cm in some males were observed. Many investigators believe that a pelvic descent of 3 to 3.5 cm between rest and defecation is abnormal, and this belief has been confirmed by clinical estimates.[27] This discrepancy may be due to the fact that clinical estimates are obtained with the patient lying on a couch in a horizontal lateral position. In this position, the patient may be inhibited from maximal straining for fear of incontinence. In addition, the added weight of the rectal contents contributing to the downward pull of the pelvic floor is absent. Furthermore, the proximal radiographic anal canal probably becomes incorporated into the distal rectum during evacuation as it forms a "cone" configuration. This change increases the apparent descent during evacuation proctography. Another major surprising finding in the study by Shorvon and colleagues was rectal intussusception occurring in normal subjects.[10] However, none of these patients had external prolapse.

In conclusion, evacuation proctography often can provide a unique perspective of disorders of defecation, particularly those relating to constipation and obstructed defecation. Some of the problems depicted by this examination are amenable to surgery. However, because there is considerable overlap between normal and abnormal appearances, it is important to take into account anal manometry, electromyography, colon transit studies, and the patient's clinical findings before making any management decisions.

## References

1. Womack NR, Williams NS, Holmfield JHM, et al: Pressure and prolapse—the cause of the solitary rectal ulcer syndrome. Gut 28:1228–1233, 1987.
2. Burhenne HJ: Intestinal evacuation study: a new roentgenologic technique. Radiol Clin North Am 33:79–84, 1964.
3. Mahieu P, Pringot J, Bodart P: Defecography: 1. Description of a new procedure and results in normal patients. Gastrointest Radiol 9:247–251, 1984.
4. Ekberg O, Nylander G, Fork F-T: Defecography. Radiology 155:45–48, 1985.
5. Shorvon PJ, Stevenson GW: Defaecography: setting up a service. Br J Hosp Med 41:460–466, 1989.
6. Bartram CI, Turnbull GK, Lennard-Jones JE: Evacuation proctography: an investigation of rectal expulsion in 20 subjects without defecatory disturbance. Gastrointest Radiol 13:72–80, 1988.
7. Goei R, van Engelshoven J, Schouten H, et al: Anorectal function: defecographic measurement in asymptomatic subjects. Radiology 173:137–141, 1989.
8. Archer BD, Somers S, Stevenson GW: Technical note: vaginal contrast for defaecography. Radiology 182:278–279, 1992.
9. Bernier P, Stevenson GW, Shorvon P: Defecography commode. Radiology 166:891–892, 1988.
10. Shorvon PJ, McHugh S, Diamant NE, et al: Defecography in normal volunteers: results and implications. Gut 30:1737–1749, 1989.
11. Penninckx F, Debruyne C, Lestar B, et al: Observer variation in the radiological measurement of the anorectal angle. Int J Colorectal Dis 5:94–97, 1990.
12. Mahieu P, Pringot J, Bodart P: Defecography: II. Contribution to the diagnosis of defecation disorders. Gastrointest Radiol 9:253–261, 1984.
13. Hoffman MJ, Kodner IJ, Fry RD: Internal intussusception of the rectum. Dis Colon Rectum 19:435–441, 1984.
14. Broden B, Snellman B: Procidentia of the rectum studied with cineradiography: a contribution to the discussion of causative mechanism. Dis Colon Rectum 11:330–347, 1968.
15. Bartolo DCC, Rose AM, Virjee J, et al: Evacuation proctography in obstructed defaecation and rectal intussusception. Br J Surg 72(suppl):1161–1166, 1985.
16. Bartolo DCC, Roe AM, Virjee J, et al: An analysis of rectal morphology in obstructed defecation. Int J Colorectal Dis 3:17–22, 1988.
17. Kuijpers HC, Bleijenberg G: The spastic pelvic floor syndrome: a cause of constipation. Dis Colon Rectum 28:669–672, 1985.
18. Henry MM, Parks AG, Swash M: The pelvic floor musculature in the descending perineum syndrome. Br J Surg 69:470–472, 1982.
19. Oettle GJ, Roe AM, Bartolo DCC, et al: What is the best way of measuring perineal descent? A comparison of radiographic and clinical methods. Br J Surg 72:999–1001, 1985.
20. Vernava AM, Longo WE, Daniel GL: Pudendal neuropathy and the importance of EMG evaluation of fecal incontinence. Dis Colon Rectum 36:23–27, 1993.
21. Lesaffer LPA: Perineal support device. *In* Smith LE (ed): Practical Guide to Anorectal Testing. New York: Igaku-Shoin, 1990, pp 205–208.
22. Penninckx FM (moderator): Faecal incontinence: symposium. Int J Colorectal Dis 2:173–186, 1987.
23. Henry MM: Pathogenesis and management of fecal incontinence in the adult. Gastroenterol Clin North Am 16:35–45, 1987.
24. McHugh SM, Diamant NE: Anal canal pressure profile: a reappraisal as determined by rapid pull-through technique. Gut 28:1234–1242, 1987.
25. Kelvin FM, Maglinte DDT, Hornback JA, et al: Pelvic prolapse: assessment with evacuation proctography (defecography). Radiology 184:547–551, 1992.
26. Skomorowska E, Hegedus V: Sex difference in anorectal angle and perineal descent. Gastrointest Radiol 12:353–355, 1987.
27. Parks AG, Porter NH, Hardcastle J: The syndrome of the descending perineum. Proc R Soc Med 59:477–482, 1966.

# Cross-sectional Imaging

**59**

Richard M. Gore, M.D.

## INTRODUCTION

The colon can be evaluated by barium enema, colonoscopy and cross-sectional imaging. Although both colonoscopy and barium enema allow superb examination of the mucosa, they cannot directly depict the mural and extraluminal extent of benign and malignant disorders of the large bowel. In this chapter, the applications of ultrasound, computed tomography (CT), and magnetic resonance (MR) in the imaging of patients with known or suspected colonic disease are discussed.

## ULTRASOUND

### Scanning Technique

#### Transabdominal Scans

In specific sonographic assessment of colonic disease, linear array or curvilinear array transducers of the highest possible frequency (5 to 7 MHz) should be used. These transducers help trap the loop in question, minimize the sound path, and displace overlying structures (Fig. 59-1). Imaging in several planes, including the transverse and longitudinal planes, is important.[1-3]

#### Transrectal Ultrasound

A number of different probes are available for transrectal sonography, including single-element transducer, linear, and curvilinear arrays. Scans should be obtained in both the transverse plane (Fig. 59-2) and the longitudinal plane, after a cleansing enema. A latex condom inflated with water is placed over the transducer for protection; for isolation; for displacement of rectal air, which improves acoustic coupling; and for positioning of the region of interest in the focal zone of the transducer (see Chapter 10).[4-6]

### Normal Anatomy

As in other portions of the gastrointestinal tract, up to five layers are visible sonographically[1-4] (Fig. 59-3). The compressed colon should not have a transverse diameter of more than 3 to 4 mm. When filled with fluid, haustra are usually visible, particularly in the right colon[1-3] (Fig. 59-4).

When observed over a 1-minute period, fluid- and stool-filled colon should change configuration because of peristalsis. These changes are best seen in the ascending colon.

### Mural Pathology

As in other portions of the gut, most diseases of the colon cause mural thickening, producing a nonspecific "target" appearance, called the *target sign*. This sign has also been called the "pseudokidney," "bull's-eye," "doughnut," "cockade," or "ring" sign.[1-4] The various causes of the target sign are listed in Table 59-1, and the more important ones are discussed later.

### Neoplasms

Although most cancers are not visualized by standard sonography, large intraluminal, exophytic, and annular tumors (Fig. 59-5) are detectable.[1, 7-11] Polypoid intraluminal tumors predominate in the right colon, and annular constricting lesions are most often seen in the descending and sigmoid colon. These neoplasms are usually hypoechoic. When they cause obstruction, the proximal lumen shows dilatation, hyperperistalsis, and increased intraluminal fluid. When a mass is discovered, the patient should be evaluated for evidence of direct tumor invasion, regional lymph node involvement, and liver metastases.[9-11]

Some authors have reported that ultrasound provides highly accurate diagnosis of colon polyps and carcinoma

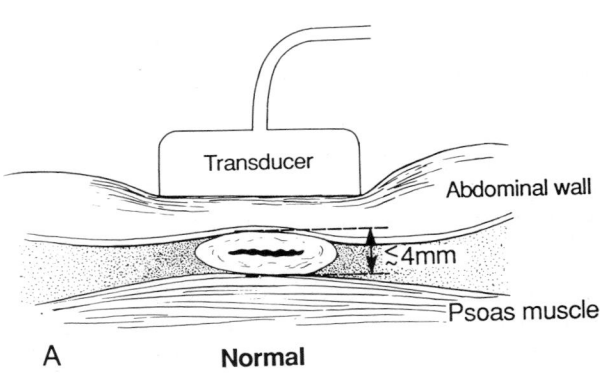

A **Normal**

**Figure 59–1. Compression sonography of the colon.** Diagram **(A)** shows that compression helps trap the colonic segment in question, minimizes the sound path, and displaces overlying structures. Thickness of the compressed colon should be 4 mm or less. (From Wilson SR: The gastrointestinal tract. *In* Rumack CM, Wilson SR, Charboneau JW [eds]: Diagnostic Ultrasound. St. Louis: Mosby–Year Book, 1991, pp 181–207. Modified from Pylaert JBCM: Acute appendicitis: ultrasound evaluation using graded compression. Radiology 1986; 158:355–360.) Transverse noncompression **(B)** and compression **(C)** scans of the cecum in a patient with typhlitis show mural thickening and compressibility. The latter feature is usually seen in benign, acute colitides.

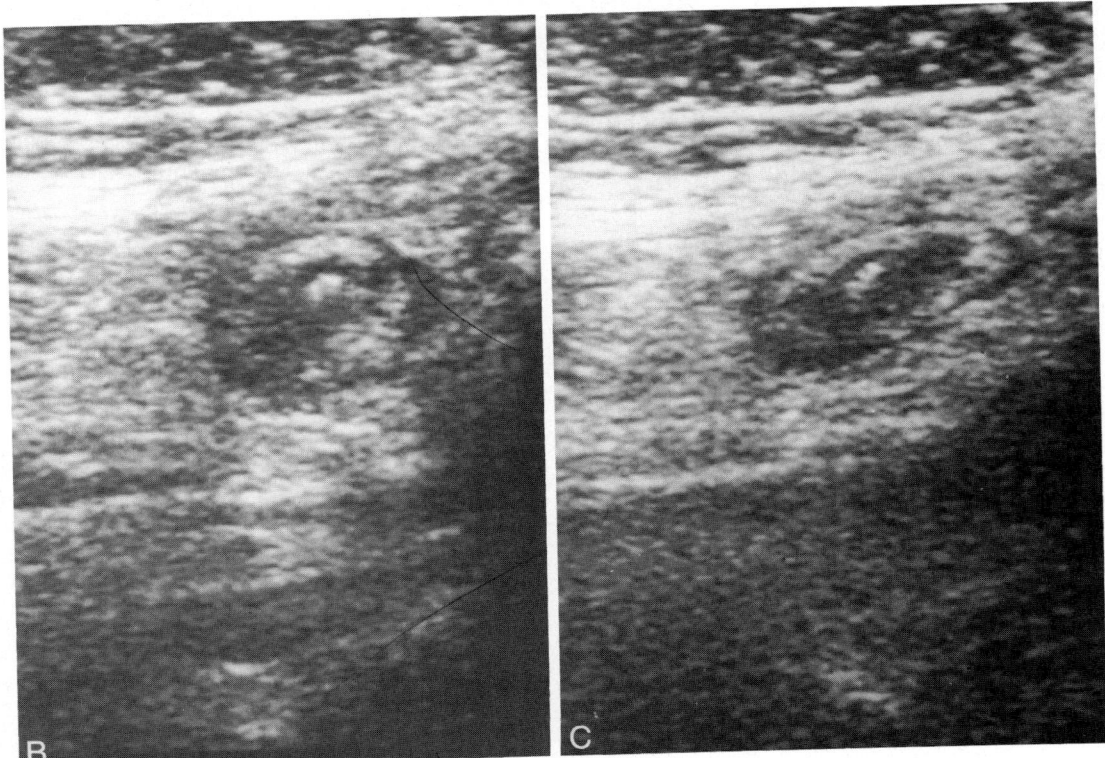

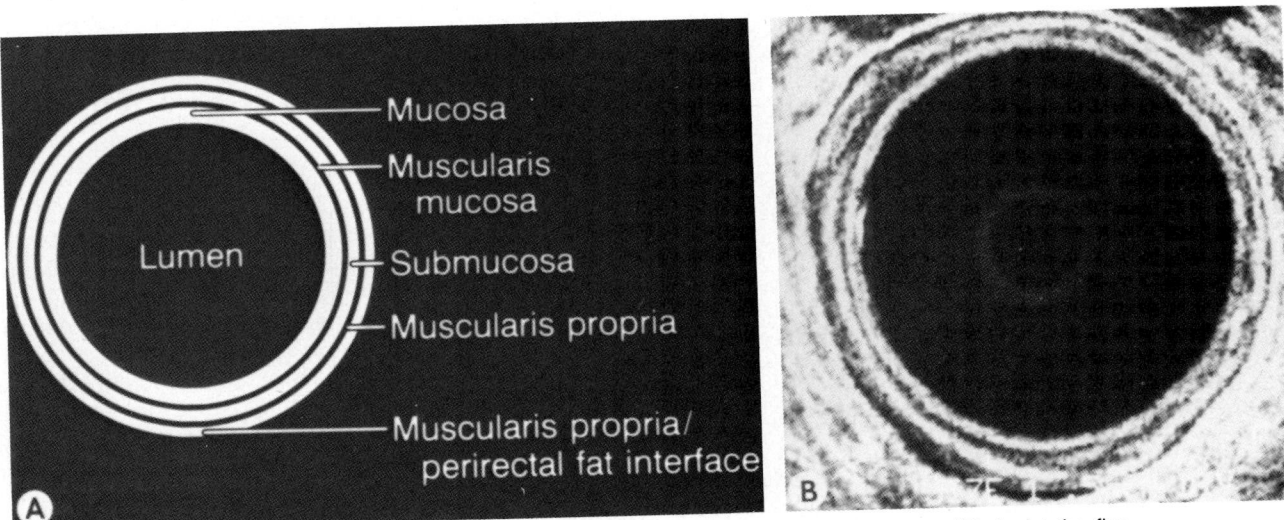

**Figure 59–2. Transrectal ultrasound.** Diagram **(A)** and axial ultrasound scan **(B)** depict the five sonographically visualized layers of rectal wall. (**A** and **B** from Jochem RJ, Reading CC, Dozois RR, et al: Endorectal ultrasonographic staging of rectal carcinoma. Mayo Clin Proc 65:1571–1577, 1990.)

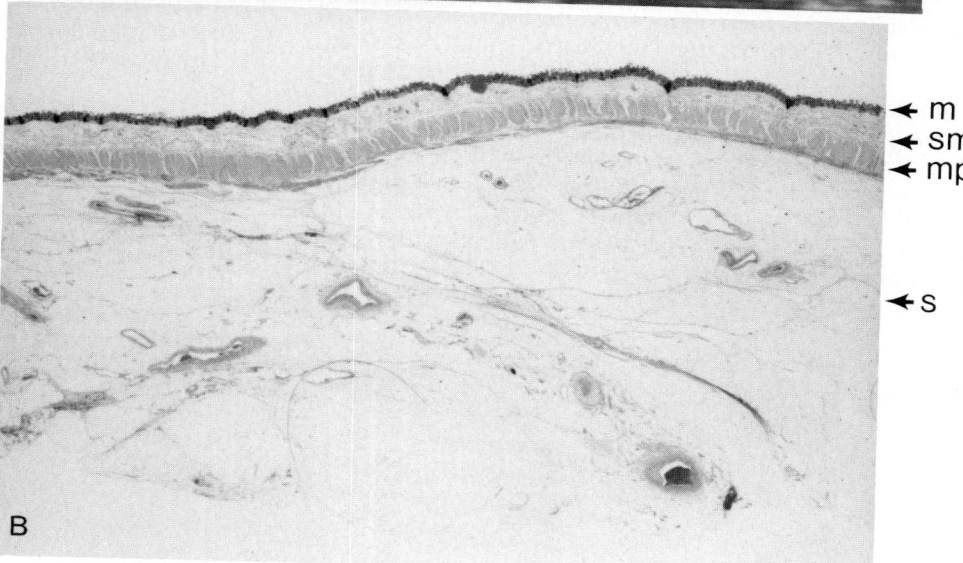

Figure 59–3. Normal colon: sonographic-histologic correlation. The specimen sonogram (A) and corresponding histologic section (B) show that layers 1 (echogenic) and 2 (hypoechoic) correspond to the mucosa (m) and muscularis mucosae (hypoechoic), layer 3 (echogenic) represents the submucosa (sm), layer 4 (hypoechoic) represents the muscularis propria (mp), and layer 5 (echogenic) corresponds to the serosa and subserosal fat (s). (A and B from Kimmey MB, Wang KY, Haggitt RC, et al: Diagnosis of inflammatory bowel disease with ultrasound: an in vitro study. Invest Radiol 25:1085–1090, 1990.)

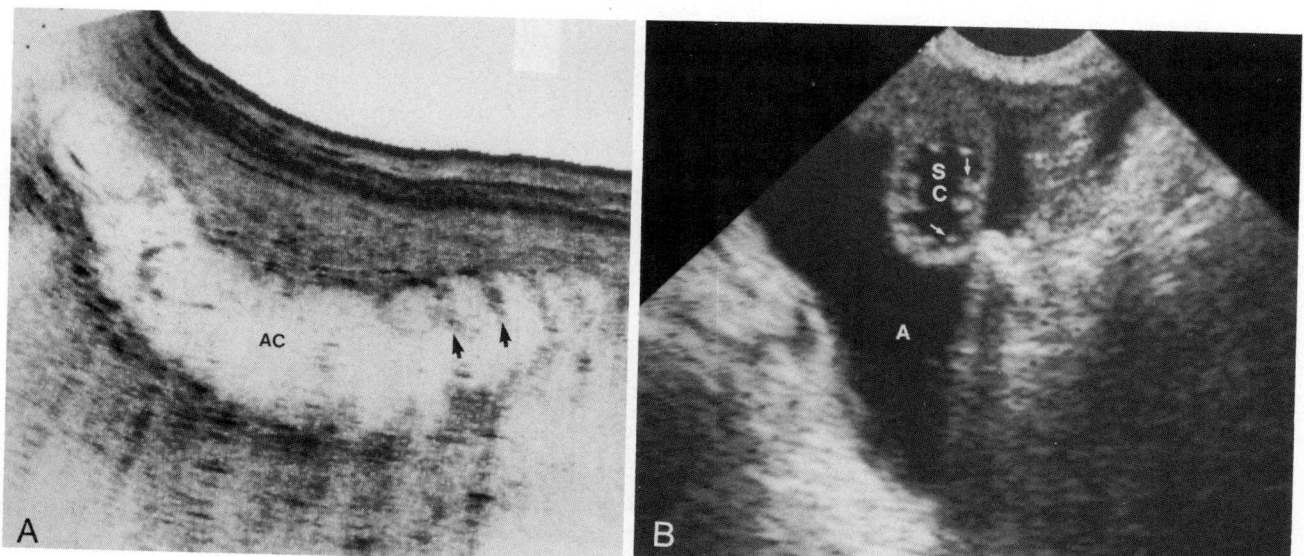

Figure 59–4. Colonic haustra. Sagittal scan (A) of a dilated fluid-filled ascending colon (AC) and axial scan (B) through the fluid-filled sigmoid colon (SC) demonstrate haustra (arrows). A = ascites.

### TABLE 59–1. CAUSES OF TARGET SIGN OF COLON

| BENIGN CAUSES | MALIGNANT CAUSES |
| --- | --- |
| Crohn's disease | Carcinoma |
| Ulcerative colitis | Lymphoma |
| Ischemia | Leiomyosarcoma |
| Typhlitis | |
| Pseudomembranous colitis | |
| Amebic colitis | |
| Hematoma | |
| Low-albumin states | |
| Diverticulitis | |
| Intussusception | |
| Radiation | |

when it is performed after administration of a water enema or a large amount of ingested water.[12]

Lymphoma of the colon can cause hypoechoic mural thickening. Often, enlarged mesenteric lymph nodes can be visualized as well. A more complete discussion of sonography of gastrointestinal lymphoma can be found in Chapters 44 and 151.

By virtue of its ability to depict the various layers of the rectal wall, endorectal ultrasound is a valuable means of determining depth of mural invasion and extension into the perirectal tissue in patients with rectal carcinoma[4–6, 13–21] (Figs. 59–6 and 59–7). This technique

has an accuracy of 80%, a sensitivity of 92%, and a specificity of 76% for detection of invasion of perirectal fat.[6] Endorectal sonography is also valuable in the detection of perirectal lymphadenopathy but is not specific in distinguishing benign from malignant lymph nodes (see Chapters 10 and 68).[13–21]

## Obstruction

Ultrasound is not a primary means of diagnosing large bowel obstruction, but it can be useful in integrating abdominal plain film findings with clinical information, particularly in the small subset of patients with obstruction who have absence of abdominal gas. Indeed, in one series, ultrasound findings were abnormal in 25% of patients with bowel obstruction who had "normal" findings on plain films.[22–24] (See Chapter 44 for a discussion of the sonographic features of volvulus, intussusception, and obstruction.)

## Inflammatory Lesions

Sonography is accurate in differentiating normal from inflamed colon, with thickening of the submucosa or total wall being the most reliable indicator of dis-

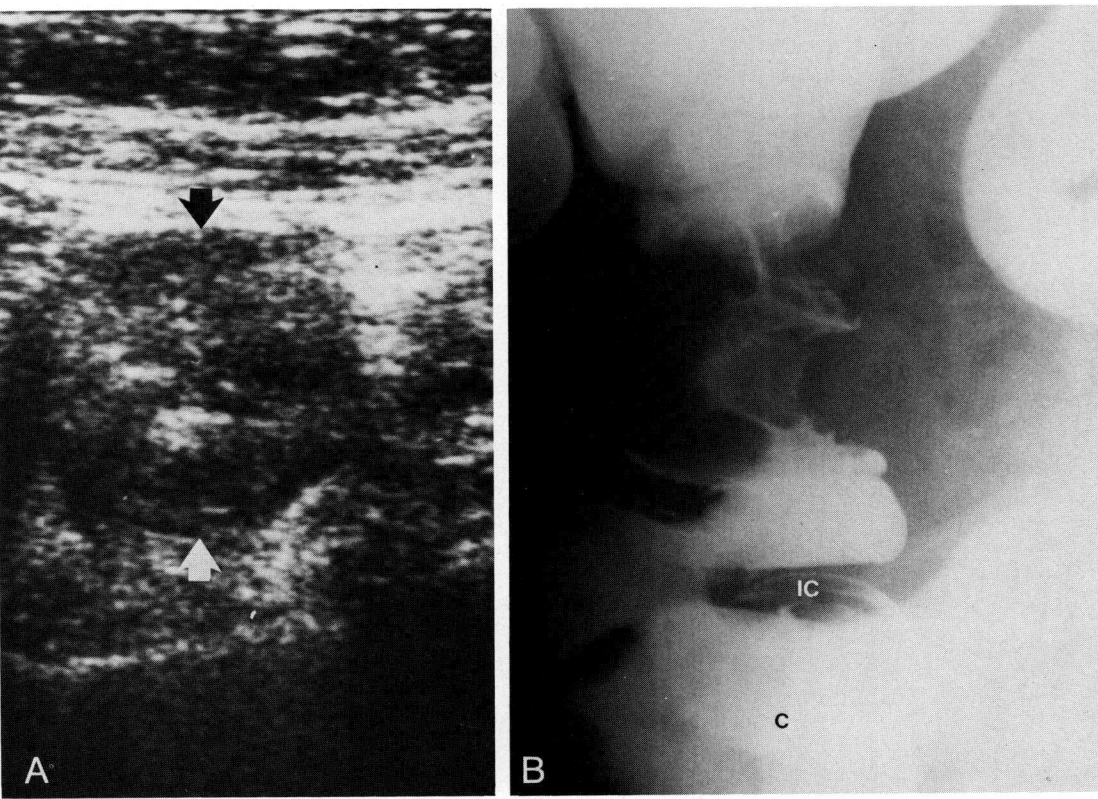

**Figure 59–5. Carcinoma of the ascending colon. A.** Transverse compression sonogram of a patient who presented with right lower quadrant pain shows an incompressible 3-cm mass *(arrows)* with the target sign. **B.** Barium enema confirms the presence of an annular constricting carcinoma *(arrows)* of the ascending colon. C = cecum; IC = ileocecal valve.

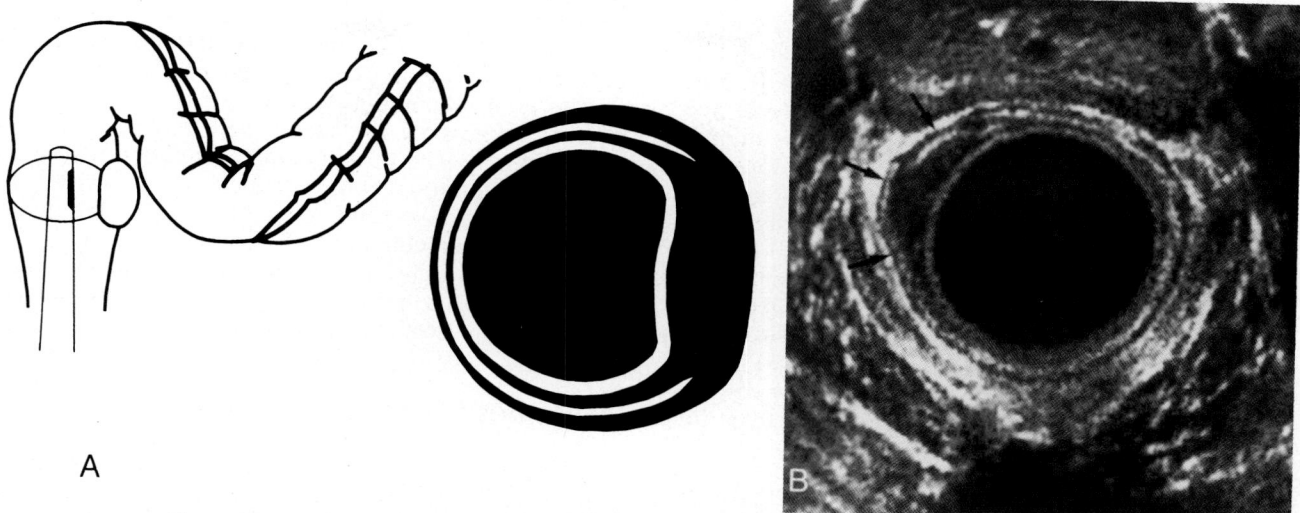

**Figure 59–6. Carcinoma of the rectum: endosonographic findings.** Schematic diagram **(A)** and axial sonogram **(B)** of a stage B1 rectal cancer with an intact muscularis propria/perirectal fat interface *(arrows)*. (From Jochem RJ, Reading CC, Dozois RR, et al: Endorectal ultrasonic staging of rectal carcinoma. Mayo Clin Proc 65:1571–1577, 1990.)

ease.[1–3, 25–27] In ulcerative colitis, the degree of thickening may be mild, and the wall stratification is usually preserved.[28–30] In Crohn's disease, the degree of mural thickening may be moderate to severe, and the wall stratification is often lost. The echogenic innermost luminal layer of the bowel may become hypoechoic (see Chapter 44).[4, 15, 30, 31] Some authors report a high degree of accuracy in differentiating ulcerative colitis from Crohn's colitis on the basis of the sonographic appearance of the colon wall.[9]

The sonographic features of diverticulitis and appendicitis are presented in Chapters 61 and 69, respectively.

## COMPUTED TOMOGRAPHY

CT has proved helpful in the assessment of the mural, serosal, and mesenteric extent of neoplastic, vascular, inflammatory, and obstructive disorders of the colon. Indeed, in certain clinical situations such as appendicitis, Crohn's disease, obstruction, abscess, and diverticulitis, CT should be the initial diagnostic examination.

Preparation of the patient, bowel opacification, and administration of intravascular contrast medium are discussed in detail in Chapters 8 and 80.

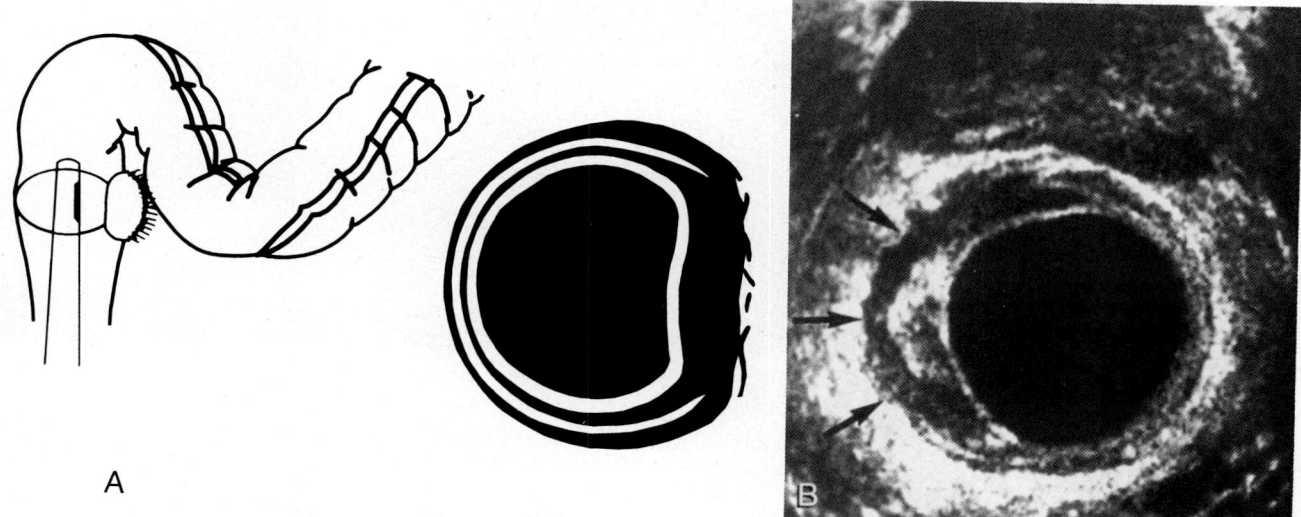

**Figure 59–7. Carcinoma of the rectum: endosonographic findings.** Schematic diagram **(A)** and axial sonogram **(B)** of a stage B2 rectal cancer invading through the muscularis propria/perirectal fat interface *(arrows)*. (Reprinted with permission from Reading CC: Endorectal sonography. Crit Rev Diagn Imaging 33:1–28, 1992. Copyright CRC Press, Inc. Boca Raton, FL.)

## Normal Anatomy

The colon is identified on CT scans by its anatomic location and haustral morphology[32–35] (Fig. 59–8). Visualization is improved by contrast medium, stool, and air within its lumen.[36–39] The colon appears as a ring-like structure (ascending colon, descending colon, and rectum) or tubular structure (transverse colon and sigmoid colon), depending on the position and orientation of bowel loops relative to the scanning plane.[35] Recognition of the cecum is facilitated by visualization of the ileocecal valve and of the terminal ileum filled with contrast medium. The appendix can often be visualized on high-resolution CT images as a small ring-like structure or a tubular structure, either of which may contain air. The pericolic fat is usually homogeneous except for a few thin, enhanced vascular channels.[33, 34]

The normal rectum is between 12 and 15 cm long (Fig. 59–9). The peritoneum reflects on the anterior wall of the proximal rectum, and the floor of the pouch of Douglas is usually situated about 2.5 cm above the prostate and 7.5 cm above the anal orifice. The portion of the rectum beneath the peritoneal reflection and the levator ani muscles lies in the subperitoneal space. Here it is surrounded by perirectal fat, which is surrounded by perirectal fascia, which in turn is surrounded by pararectal fatty tissue. The perirectal space (capsula adiposa rectalis) has a homogeneous fatty density and contains the superior hemorrhoidal vessels. The slightly less homogeneous pararectal space contains more collagen and the middle hemorrhoidal vessels. Fascial thickening and increased density in the fat suggest neoplastic or inflammatory disease.[40]

The thickness of the colon wall can be accurately measured only when the lumen is distended with air or contrast medium. When distended, the normal colon wall has a thickness ranging from 0.9 to 2.6 mm with a 4-mm SD. When collapsed, the colon wall should be no thicker than 0.5 cm. The normal colon wall also has a homogeneous attenuation and does not show the wall stratification observed with ultrasound.[1–2]

## Malignant Disease

Although CT is not a primary diagnostic tool in the evaluation of epithelial and mesenchymal tumors of the colon, it can provide valuable staging information in the preoperative assessment and postoperative search for recurrent or metastatic tumor.[41–54] Primary colon cancer appears on CT scans as a localized soft tissue mass that can be discrete and focal or show semicircular or circumferential mural thickening (Fig. 59–10). The lumen is usually narrowed, and the serosal contour of the mass is often spiculated with abrupt transition between normal and abnormal gut wall. The neoplasm usually has a

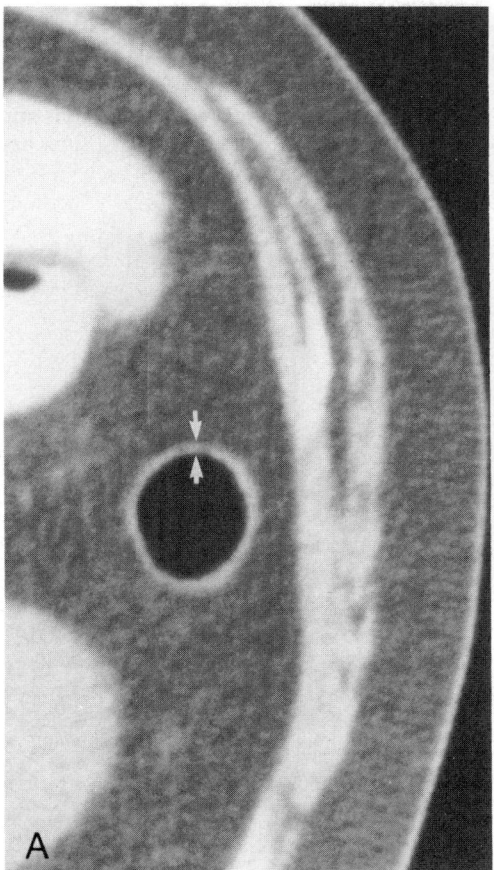

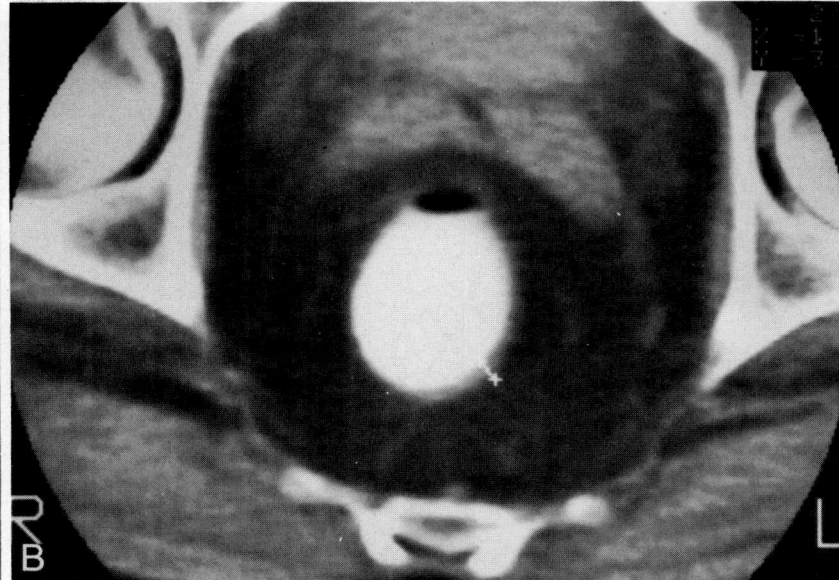

**Figure 59–8. Normal colon and rectum: CT appearance. A.** Air-distending colon has a mural thickness of 2 mm *(arrows)*. The pericolic fat has a homogeneous low density. **B.** Rectum distended by contrast medium. The rectal wall is 4 mm thick. Some definition of the colonic wall is lost when positive contrast agents are used to distend the colon.

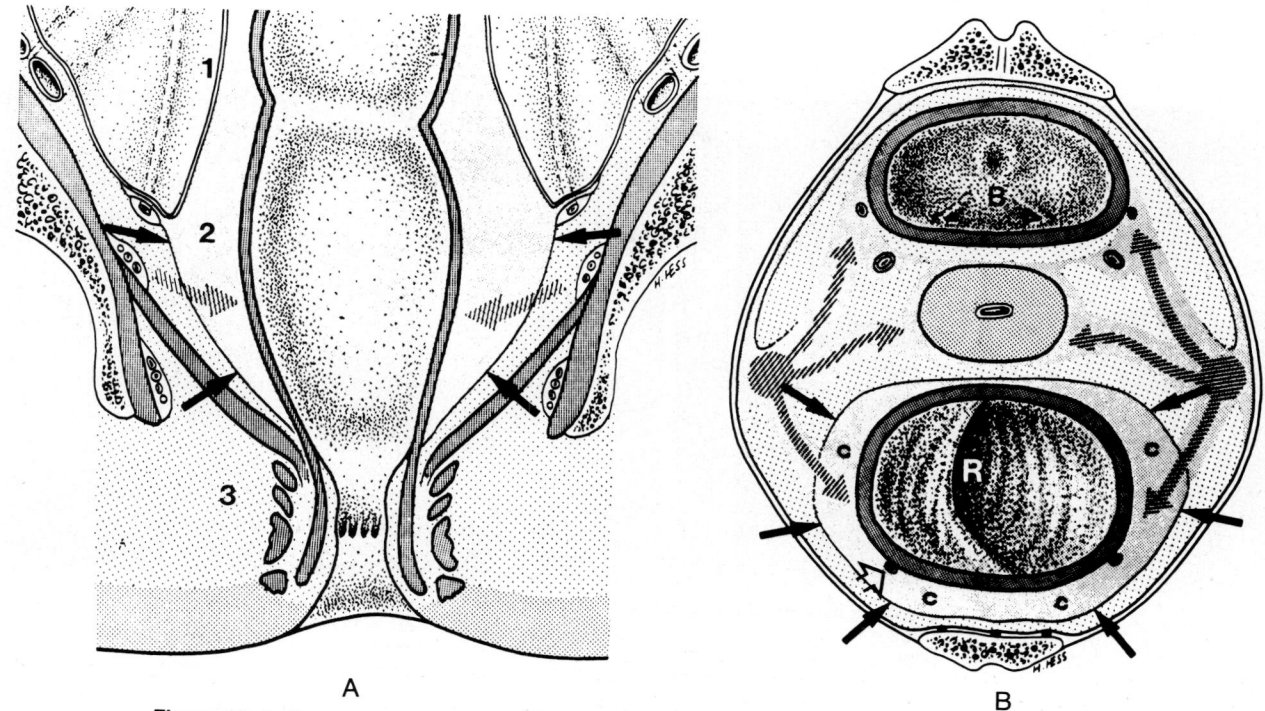

**Figure 59–9. Diagram of the rectal and perirectal compartments.** Coronal **(A)** and transverse **(B)** planes of section. The capsula adiposa rectalis (c) is enclosed by perirectal fascia *(straight arrows)*. Curved shaded arrows depict the subperitoneal space (2) of the paraproctium. The superior hemorrhoidal artery *(open arrow)*, peritoneal cavity (1), and ischiorectal fossa (3) are indicated. B = bladder; R = rectum. (From Grabbe E, Lierse, W, Winkler R: The perirectal fascia: morphology and use in staging of rectal carcinoma. Radiology 149:241–246, 1983.)

homogeneous density, but larger tumors may show low-density necrotic areas centrally. The frond-like masses of villous colonic tumors and psammomatous calcifications of mucinous neoplasms can sometimes be identified (Fig. 59–11).

CT is most useful clinically in the identification of patients with distant metastases. CT is less accurate in patients with malignant disease in lower stages. It cannot

determine extension through the bowel wall (Dukes' B1 versus B2 and T2 versus T3) or detect tumor in normal-sized nodes (Dukes' B2 versus C and TN0 versus TN1).[42–54] CT can also be extremely useful in the follow-up of patients with rectal cancer who have had abdominoperineal resections, because the rectal bed cannot be assessed by colonoscopy or barium studies (Fig. 59–12). In patients with low anterior resections, CT may show a completely exophytic recurrence at the suture line (see Chapter 68).[55–64]

## Benign Disease

As in the small bowel, most benign lesions in the colon cause circumferential and symmetric mural thickening that is usually less than 1 cm in diameter.[34, 41] The bowel wall either shows homogeneous soft tissue density or demonstrates alternate rings of high and low density (Fig. 59–13). Two such alternate rings are called the *double halo sign;* three rings represent the target sign, discussed earlier. This mural inhomogeneity is best appreciated during the arterial phase of enhancement and may result from submucosal edema with inflammation or from fatty deposition, or from both processes. Mural inhomogeneity can be seen in ulcerative and Crohn's colitis, pseudomembranous colitis, radiation colitis, ischemic colitis, and bowel edema associated with portal hypertension.[34, 41]

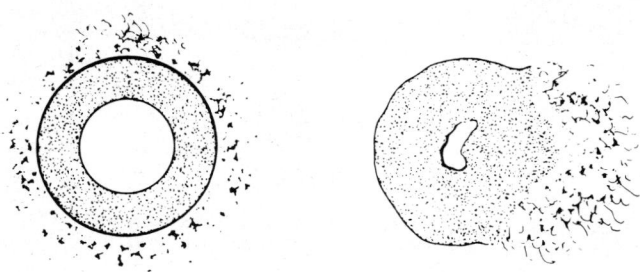

Benign                    Malignant

**Figure 59–10. Diagram of benign versus malignant disease on CT scan.** Benign disease typically shows mild (0.3- to 1.0-cm), circumferential, and symmetric wall thickening and an inflammatory response in the pericolic fat. Neoplasms usually exhibit a thicker bowel wall, asymmetric involvement, lobulated contour, narrowing of the intestinal lumen, and invasion of adjacent structures. (From EJ Balthazar, CT of the gastrointestinal tract: principles and interpretation, AJR, 156, 1, 23–32, 1991, © by American Roentgen Ray Society.)

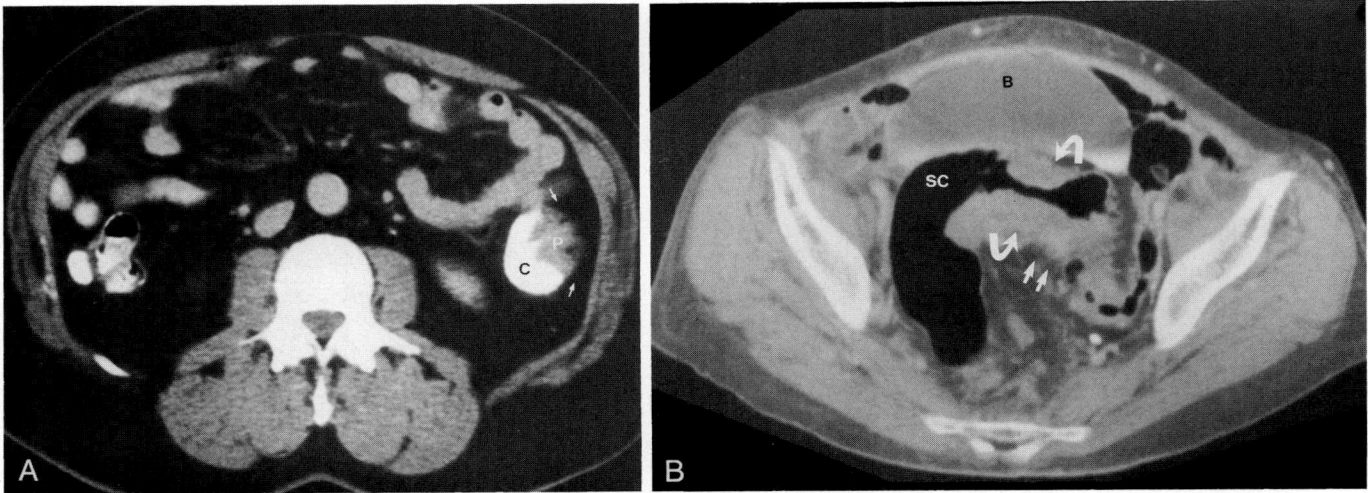

**Figure 59–11. Colorectal cancer: CT appearance. A.** Descending colon (C) distended by contrast medium demonstrates a 4-cm polypoid carcinoma (P). The pericolic fat *(arrows)* is normal, indicating that there is no extramural extension of tumor. **B.** Carcinoma *(curved arrows)* of the sigmoid colon (SC) narrows the lumen and invades *(straight arrows)* the fat of the sigmoid mesocolon. B = bladder.

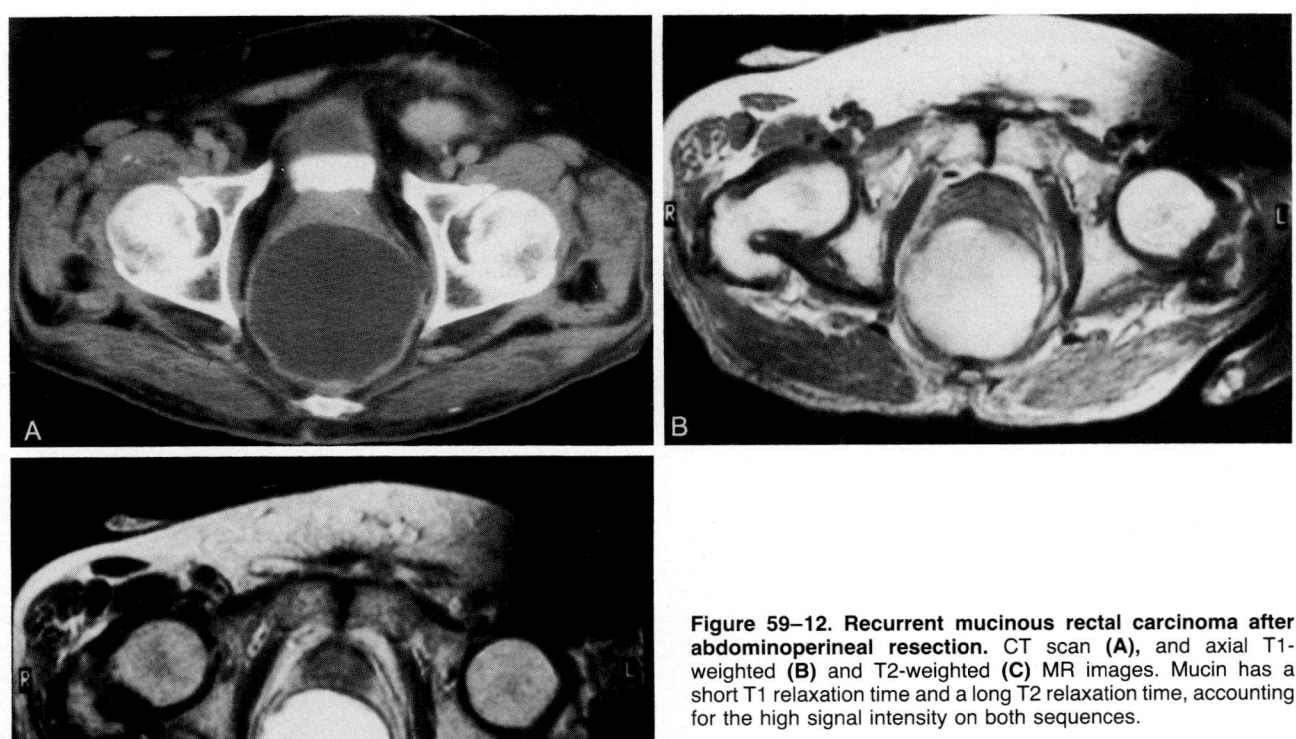

**Figure 59–12. Recurrent mucinous rectal carcinoma after abdominoperineal resection.** CT scan **(A)**, and axial T1-weighted **(B)** and T2-weighted **(C)** MR images. Mucin has a short T1 relaxation time and a long T2 relaxation time, accounting for the high signal intensity on both sequences.

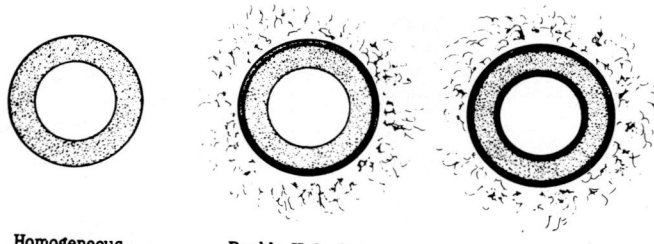

Homogeneous     Double Halo Sign     Target Sign

**Figure 59–13. Diagram of CT findings in benign colonic disease.** The wall of the involved segment may show a homogeneously enhanced soft tissue density, two concentric rings of low and high attenuation (double halo sign), or three concentric rings of high, low, and high density (target sign). The degree of difference in density is related to the severity of mucosal hyperemia, submucosal edema, inflammation, and fat deposition, and to the quality of the CT examination. (From EJ Balthazar, CT of the gastrointestinal tract: principles and interpretation, AJR, 156, 1, 23–32, 1991, © by American Roentgen Ray Society.)

In benign disease, adjacent mesenteric fat is often thickened and has increased attenuation with a number of streaky areas of increased density. With progression of disease, the bowel wall may become thicker (by 1 to 2 cm), but the symmetric, circumferential involvement and segmental distribution are maintained.[34, 41]

## Inflammatory Diseases

Crohn's colitis and ulcerative colitis are manifested by mural thickening on CT scans. The wall tends to be thicker and more homogeneous in Crohn's disease, and the same appearance is associated with small bowel disease, abscesses, fistulas, and "creeping fat" of the mesentery. Chronic ulcerative colitis is typically associated with a target sign because of enlargement and fatty infiltration of the submucosa and thickening of the muscularis mucosae (see Chapters 62 and 159).[65–68] The CT findings of diverticulitis are discussed in Chapter 61, and the CT manifestations of appendicitis are presented in Chapter 69.

## Vascular Diseases

Mural thickening of the colon is the hallmark of ischemic colitis. It may be homogeneous or inhomogeneous with symmetric or lobulated wall thickening. Hemorrhage may be seen in the adjacent mesentery, or fluid may be seen in the peritoneal cavity. If infarction intervenes, curvilinear collections of gas can develop in the colon wall, in the superior mesenteric vein, and in the portal vein, and clot may be present within the superior mesenteric artery or vein. CT is more sensitive than plain film radiography in detecting intramural and intravascular air.[33, 34, 41, 69–72] More complete discussions of ischemic colitis are presented in Chapters 63 and 161.

The changes of radiation colitis are similar to those of ischemic colitis but develop primarily in the rectum. The wall becomes thick, a target sign develops because of mural edema, perirectal fat proliferates, the perirectal

fascia thickens, and fibrous tissue increases (see Chapters 63 and 162).[73]

## Infectious Colitis

Inhomogeneous mural thickening can be seen in patients with infectious colitides. Neutropenic colitis (typhlitis) associated with leukemia typically causes mural thickening of the cecum and may be associated with pneumatosis, pericolic fluid, thickening of fascial planes, and areas of low attenuation within the wall that are due to edema or necrosis.[74, 75] In pseudomembranous colitis (Fig. 59–14), the colon has an irregular contour, transverse haustra, and inhomogeneous mural thickening.[76, 77]

## Obstruction

Megibow and associates have reported that CT has a 94% sensitivity, a 96% specificity, and a 95% accuracy in diagnosing bowel obstruction and that CT allows identification of the cause of obstruction in 73% of cases.[78] The authors concluded that CT is the examination of choice in patients with suspected bowel obstruction and a history of malignant neoplasms of the abdomen (see Chapter 67). CT has a secondary role in the examination of patients having a history of abdominal surgery without cancer, who most likely have adhesions. In patients who have no surgical history, CT is of greatest value when detecting infection, bowel infarction, or a palpable mass.[78]

Intussusception is manifested on CT scans by one of three different patterns, which reflect severity and duration: 1) the target sign; 2) a sausage-shaped mass with alternating layers of high and low attenuation; and 3) a uniform mass (see Chapter 44).[79–83]

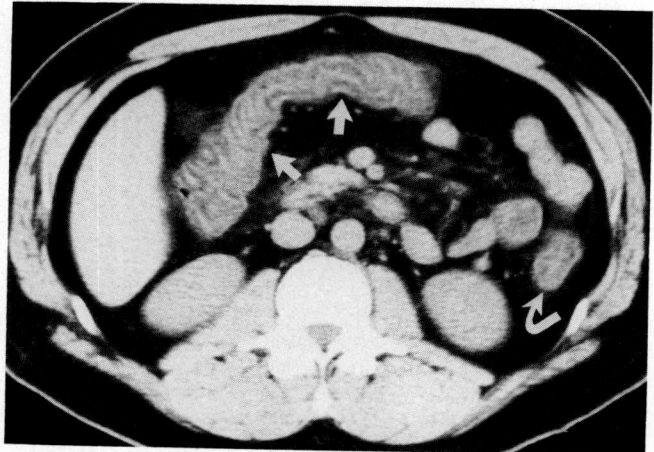

**Figure 59–14. Pseudomembranous colitis: CT appearance.** There is mural thickening of the transverse colon *(straight arrows)* and descending colon *(curved arrow)*. Regions of high and low attenuation are seen within the bowel wall.

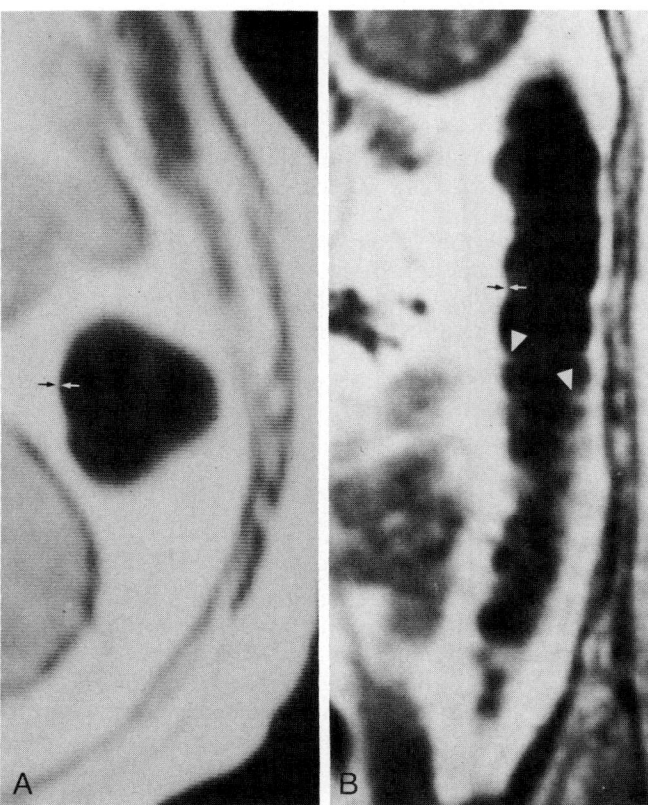

**Figure 59–15. Normal colon: MR appearance.** Axial **(A)** and coronal **(B)** T1-weighted images show normal ascending colon. The wall *(straight arrows)* outlined by fat is difficult to perceive on these T1-weighted images. Arrowheads in **B** indicate haustra.

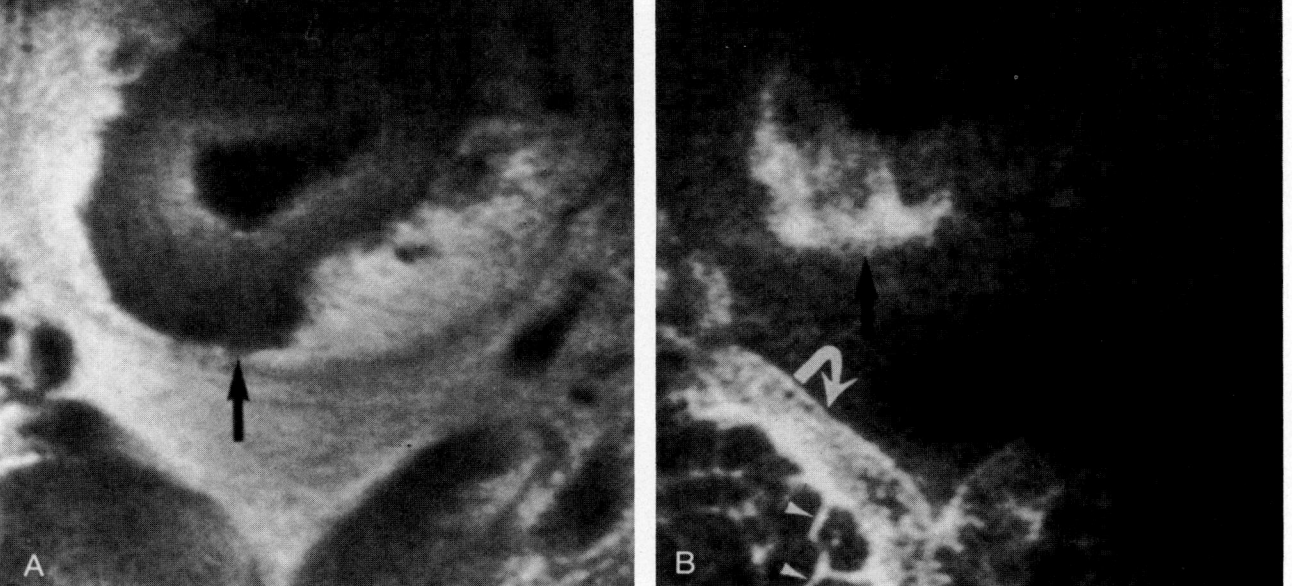

**Figure 59–16. Rectal carcinoma: endorectal MR appearance. A.** Coronal, nonenhanced T1-weighted (600/17) image shows the lesion with nodular extension into the perirectal fat *(arrow).* **B.** Coronal, gadolinium-enhanced, T1-weighted (400/17) image with fat saturation shows enhancement of the lesion and its extension into the perirectal fat *(straight arrow).* The walls of the seminal vesicles *(arrowheads)* and vas deferens *(curved arrow)* are also enhanced. (From Chan TW, Kressel HY, Milestone B, et al: Rectal carcinoma: staging at MR imaging with endorectal surface coil. Radiology 181:461–467, 1991.)

# MAGNETIC RESONANCE IMAGING

MR is not a primary imaging test in the diagnosis of colonic disease. It is restricted by motion artifact caused by respiration, peristalsis, and cardiac pulsation; inferior spatial resolution; lack of suitable luminal contrast agents; and most important, cost and availability. Although gradient-echo imaging permits images to be obtained with a single breath hold, and echo-planar imaging can produce images with subsecond scanning times, the data provided about the colonic wall (Fig. 59–15) have been disappointing.[84–87]

## Neoplasms

The variable course of most of the colon has limited the applicability of MR imaging in the staging of colon cancer. Because of its straight course and protected location deep in the pelvis, the rectum is well suited to conventional and local coil MR imaging. When imaging a rectal cancer for staging, the patient should have a cleansed bowel and be placed in the prone position to promote air retention, which distends the lumen and enhances visualization of the primary tumor. The rectum is insufflated with air as well. Mild distention of the urinary bladder is useful in displacing small bowel out of the pelvis and limiting respiratory motion of the pelvic organs. A vaginal tampon should be inserted in female patients.[86–90]

Axial, sagittal, and coronal T1-weighted images are obtained. Tumor has a longer T1 value than perirectal fat, so that extramural extension is exhibited as strands of low attenuation. When conventional body coils are used, MR, like CT, cannot assess the depth of mural invasion, nor can it distinguish benign from malignant causes of perirectal lymph node enlargement or detect tumor in normal-sized lymph nodes. MR is most useful in detecting metastases and spread to the pelvic sidewalls. In addition, sagittal and coronal scans beautifully depict the relationship of the tumor to the levator ani and external sphincter muscles, which represents vital information in the decision between an operation to save the low anterior sphincter muscle and abdominoperineal resection.[91–93]

MR imaging using an endorectal local coil (Fig. 59–16) shows great promise in staging early rectal cancer because it can depict the various layers of colon wall and because the improved resolution can more easily show extramural tumor extension and perirectal lymph nodes (see Chapter 68).[94]

Initially, it was believed that MR could allow differentiation of fibrosis from recurrent tumor in patients who had undergone anorectal cancer resection and subsequently presented with a presacral mass in the rectal bed. Fibrosis usually produces low signal intensity on T1- and T2-weighted images, and tumor usually produces low signal intensity on T1-weighted images and high signal intensity on T2-weighted images; however, there is considerable overlap in the MR appearances of fibrosis and tumor.[95–97] Positron emission tomography combined with either MR or CT may be the most specific means of differentiating cancer from scar tissue.[98]

## References

1. Wilson SR: The gastrointestinal tract. *In* Rumack CM, Wilson SR, Charboneau JW (eds): Diagnostic Ultrasound. St. Louis: Mosby–Year Book, 1992, pp 181–207.
2. Carroll BR: US of the gastrointestinal tract. Radiology 172:605–608, 1989.
3. Rao BK, Fleischer AC: Sonography of the gastrointestinal tract. Curr Opin Radiol 2:207–212, 1990.
4. Wang KY, Kimmey MB: Intestinal ultrasound. Appl Radiol 20:59–68, 1991.
5. Reading CC: Endorectal sonography. Crit Rev Diagn Imaging 33:1–28, 1992.
6. Jochem RJ, Reading CC, Dozois RP, et al: Endorectal ultrasonographic staging of rectal carcinoma. Mayo Clin Proc 65:1571–1577, 1990.
7. Hulsmans FH, Tio TL, Mathus-Vliegen EMH, et al: Colorectal villous adenoma: transrectal US in screening for invasive malignancy. Radiology 185:193–196, 1992.
8. Holdsworth PJ, Johnston D, Chalmers AG, et al: Ultrasonographic diagnosis of clinically non-palpable primary colonic neoplasms. Br J Radiol 61:190–195, 1988.
9. Limberg B: Diagnosis of inflammatory and neoplastic colonic disease by sonography. J Clin Gastroenterol 9:607–611, 1987.
10. Limberg B: Diagnosis of large bowel tumors by colonic sonography. Lancet 335:144–146, 1990.
11. Limberg B: Diagnostik von Dickdarmtumoren durch Kolonsonographie. Ultraschall Med 2:127–131, 1990.
12. Hirooka N, Ohno T, Misonoo M, et al: Sonoenterocolonography by oral water administration. J Clin Ultrasound 17:585–589, 1989.
13. Saitoh M, Okui K, Sarashina H, et al: Evaluation of echographic diagnosis of rectal cancer using intrarectal ultrasonic examination. Dis Colon Rectum 29:234–242, 1986.
14. Biber BP, Caputo MG, Colby JM: Transrectal ultrasound. Appl Radiol 20:47–51, 1991.
15. Wang KY, Kimmey MB, Nyberg DA, et al: Colorectal neoplasms: accuracy of US in demonstrating the depth of invasion. Radiology 165:827–829, 1987.
16. Hildebrandt U, Feifel G: Preoperative staging of rectal cancer by intrarectal ultrasound. Dis Colon Rectum 28:42–46, 1985.
17. DiCandio G, Mosca F, Campatelli A, et al: Endoscopic staging of rectal carcinoma. Gastrointest Radiol 12:289–295, 1987.
18. Rifkin MD: Endorectal ultrasound of the rectal wall. Semin Ultrasound CT MR 8:424–431, 1987.
19. Goldman S, Arvidsson H, Norming U, et al: Transrectal ultrasound and computed tomography in pre-operative staging of lower rectal adenocarcinoma. Gastrointest Radiol 16:259–263, 1991.
20. Zainea GG, Lee F, McLeary RD, et al: Transrectal ultrasonography in the evaluation of rectal and extrarectal disease. Surg Gynecol Obstet 169:153–156, 1989.
21. Cytron S, Kessler OJ, Baniel J, et al: Incidental finding of rectal carcinoma during transrectal US for prostatic diseases. Radiology 185:197–199, 1993.
22. Meiser G, Meissner K: Ileus and intestinal obstruction—ultrasonographic findings as a guideline to therapy. Hepatogastroenterology 34:194–199, 1987.
23. Verbanck JJ, Rutgeerts LJ, Douterlungne PH, et al: Sonographic and pathologic correlation in intussusception of the bowel. J Clin Ultrasound 14:393–397, 1986.
24. Meiser G, Meissner K: Sonographic differential diagnosis of intestinal obstruction: result of a prospective study of 48 patients. Ultraschall Med 6:39–45, 1985.
25. Hulsman FJH, Tio TL, Reeders JWAJ, et al: Transrectal US in the diagnosis of localized colitis cystica profunda. Radiology 181:201–203, 1991.
26. Hussain S, Dinshaw H: Ultrasonography in amebic colitis. J Ultrasound Med 9:385–388, 1990.
27. Bolondi L, Ferrentino M, Trevisani F, et al: Sonographic appear-

ance of pseudomembranous colitis. J Ultrasound Med 4:489–492, 1985.

28. Kimmey MB, Wang KY, Haggitt RC, et al: Diagnosis of inflammatory bowel disease with ultrasound: an in vitro study. Invest Radiol 25:1085–1090, 1990.

29. Dubbins PA: Ultrasound demonstration of bowel wall thickness in inflammatory bowel disease. Clin Radiol 35:227–231, 1984.

30. Limberg B: Diagnosis of acute ulcerative colitis and colonic Crohn's disease by colonic sonography. J Clin Ultrasound 17:25–31, 1989.

31. Kimmey MB, Wang KY, Haggitt RC, et al: Diagnosis of inflammatory bowel disease with ultrasound: an in vitro study. Invest Radiol 25:1085–1090, 1990.

32. Johnson CD, Stephens DH: Computed tomography of the large bowel and appendix. Mayo Clin Proc 64:1276–1283, 1989.

33. Balthazar EJ: Colon. *In* Megibow AJ, Balthazar EJ (eds): Computed Tomography of the Alimentary Tract. St. Louis: CV Mosby, 1986, pp 279–386.

34. Balthazar EJ: CT of the gastrointestinal tract: principles and interpretation. AJR 156:23–32, 1991.

35. Fischer JK: Normal colon wall thickness on CT. Radiology 145:415–418, 1982.

36. Mitchell DG, Bjorgvinsson E, terMeulen D, et al: Gastrografin versus dilute barium for colonic CT examination: a blind random study. J Comput Assist Tomogr 9:451–453, 1985.

37. Solomon A, Michowitz M, Papo J, et al: Computed tomographic air enema. Gastrointest Radiol 11:194–196, 1986.

38. Koehler RE, Balfe DM, Stanley RJ: Gastrointestinal tract. *In* Lee JKT, Sagel SS, Stanley RJ (eds): Computed Body Tomography (2nd ed). New York: Raven Press, 1989, pp 477–519.

39. Angelelli G, Macarini L: CT of the bowel: use of water to enhance depiction. Radiology 169:848–849, 1988.

40. Grabbe E, Lierse W, Winkler R: The perirectal fascia: morphology and use in staging of rectal carcinoma. Radiology 149:241–246, 1983.

41. Balthazar EJ, Chako AC: Computed tomography in acute gastrointestinal disorders. Am J Gastroenterol 85:1445–1452, 1992.

42. Freeny PC, Marks WM, Ryan JA, et al: Computed tomography of colorectal carcinoma: Preoperative staging and detection of recurrence. Semin Ultrasound CT MR 8:432–445, 1987.

43. Cance WG, Cohen AM, Enker WE, et al: Predictive value of a negative computed tomographic scan in 100 patients with rectal carcinoma. Dis Colon Rectum 34:748–751, 1991.

44. Zanbauer W, Haertel M, Fuchs WA: Computed tomography in carcinoma of the rectum. Gastrointest Radiol 6:79–84, 1981.

45. Ellert J, Kree L: The value of CT in malignant colonic tumors. Comput Tomogr 4:225–249, 1980.

46. Mayes GB, Zornoza J: CT of colon carcinoma. AJR 135:43–46, 1980.

47. Acunas B, Rozanes I, Acunas G, et al: Preoperative CT staging of colon carcinoma (excluding the rectosigmoid region). Eur J Radiol 11:150–153, 1990.

48. Thompson WM: Computed tomographic staging of gastrointestinal malignancies. *In* Najarian JS, Delaney JP (eds): Progress in Gastrointestinal Surgery. Chicago: Year Book Medical Publishers, 1989, pp 333–350.

49. Rotte KH, Klüh S, Kleinau H, et al: Computed tomography and endosonography in the preoperative staging of rectal carcinoma. Eur J Radiol 9:187–190, 1989.

50. Thoeni RF, Moss AA, Schnyder P, et al: Detection and staging of primary rectal and rectosigmoid cancer by computed tomography. Radiology 141:135–138, 1981.

51. vanWaes PFGM, Koehler PR, Feldberg MAM: CT of rectal cancer: its accuracy and effect on patient management. Radiographics 4:801–819, 1984.

52. Thompson WM, Trenkner S: Staging colon cancer and other gastrointestinal neoplasms. *In* Gore RM (ed): Syllabus for Categorical Course on Gastrointestinal Radiology. Reston, VA: American College of Radiology, 1991, pp 55–64.

53. Thompson WM, Halvorsen RA: Computed tomographic staging of gastrointestinal malignancies. Part II. The small bowel, colon and rectum. Invest Radiol 22:96–105, 1987.

54. Balthazar EJ, Megibow AJ, Hulnick D, et al: Carcinoma of the colon: detection and preoperative staging by CT. AJR 150:301–306, 1988.

55. Moss AA, Thoeni RF, Schnyder P, et al: Value of computed tomography in the detection and staging of recurrent rectal carcinomas. J Comput Assist Tomogr 5:870–874, 1981.

56. Butch RJ, Wittenberg J, Mueller PR, et al: Presacral masses after abdomino-perineal resection for colorectal cancer: the need for needle biopsy. AJR 144:309–312, 1985.

57. Freeny PC, Marks WM, Ryan JA, et al: Colorectal carcinoma evaluation with CT: preoperative staging and detection of postoperative recurrence. Radiology 158:347–353, 1986.

58. Lee JKT, Stanley RJ, Sagel SS, et al: CT appearance of the pelvis after abdomino-perineal resection for rectal carcinoma. Radiology 141:737–741, 1981.

59. Thompson WM, Halvorsen RA, Foster WL, et al: Preoperative and postoperative CT staging of rectosigmoid carcinoma. AJR 146:703–710, 1986.

60. McCarthy SM, Barnes D, Deveney K, et al: Detection of recurrent rectosigmoid carcinoma: prospective evaluation of CT and clinical factors. AJR 144:577–579, 1985.

61. Husband JE, Hodson NJ, Parsons CA: The use of computed tomography in recurrent rectal tumors. Radiology 134:677–682, 1980.

62. Thoeni RF: Colorectal cancer: cross-sectional imaging for staging of primary tumor and detection of local recurrence. AJR 156:909–915, 1991.

63. Amato A, Pescatori M, Butti A: Local recurrence following abdominoperineal excision and anterior resection for rectal carcinoma. Dis Colon Rectum 34:317–322, 1991.

64. Reznek R, Husband JE: CT of colorectal carcinoma. *In* Fishman EK, Jones B (eds): Computed Tomography of the Gastrointestinal Tract. New York: Churchill Livingstone, 1988, pp 179–204.

65. Thoeni RF: CT evaluation of carcinomas of the colon and rectum. Radiol Clin North Am 27:731–742, 1989.

66. Gore RM: CT of inflammatory bowel disease. Radiol Clin North Am 27:717–730, 1989.

67. Gore RM, Marn CS, Kirby DF, et al: CT findings in ulcerative, granulomatous, and indeterminate colitis. AJR 143:279–284, 1984.

68. Gore RM: Cross-sectional imaging of inflammatory bowel disease. Radiol Clin North Am 25:115–129, 1987.

69. Alpern MB, Glazer GG, Francis IR: Ischemic or infarcted bowel: CT findings. Radiology 166:144–152, 1988.

70. Balthazar EJ, Hulnick DH, Megibow AJ, et al: Computed tomography of intramural intestinal hemorrhage and bowel ischemia. J Comput Assist Tomogr 11:67–72, 1987.

71. Smerud MJ, Johnson CD, Stephens DH: Diagnosis of bowel infarction: a comparison of plain films and CT scans in 23 cases. AJR 154:99–103, 1990.

72. Nemcek AA: CT of acute gastrointestinal disorders. Radiol Clin North Am 27:773–786, 1989.

73. Doubleday LC, Bernardino ME: CT findings in the perirectal area following radiation therapy. J Comput Assist Tomogr 4:634–638, 1980.

74. Frick MP, Maile CW, Crass JR, et al: Computed tomography of neutropenic colitis. AJR 143:763–765, 1984.

75. Adams GW, Rauch RF, Kelvin FM, et al: CT detection of typhlitis. J Comput Assist Tomogr 9:363–365, 1985.

76. Megibow AJ, Streiter ML, Balthazar EJ, et al: Pseudomembranous colitis: diagnosis by computed tomography. J Comput Assist Tomogr 8:281–283, 1984.

77. Jones B, Fishman EK: CT and other inflammatory bowel diseases. *In* Fishman EK, Jones B (eds): Computed Tomography of the Gastrointestinal Tract. New York: Churchill Livingstone, 1988, pp 109–128.

78. Megibow AJ, Balthazar EJ, Chok C, et al: Bowel obstruction: evaluation with CT. Radiology 180:313–318, 1991.

79. Pottmeyer A, McDowell J, Lang EK: CT findings of a rectal intussusception. AJR 156:870, 1991.

80. Iko BO, Teal JS, Siram SM, et al: Computed tomography of adult colonic intussusception: clinical experimental studies. AJR 143:769–772, 1984.

81. Hodgman CG, Lantz EJ, Maustr FL, et al: Computed tomography of intussusception due to colon lipoma. J Comput Assist Tomogr 11:740–741, 1987.

82. Iko BO, Teal JS, Siram SM, et al: Computed tomography of adult colonic intussusception: clinical and experimental studies. AJR 143:769–772, 1984.

83. Lorigan JG, DuBrow RA: The computed tomographic appearances and clinical significance of intussusception in adults with malignant neoplasms. Br J Radiol 63:257–263, 1990.
84. Werthmuller WC, Margulis AR: Magnetic resonance imaging of the alimentary tube. Invest Radiol 26:195–200, 1991.
85. Stark DD, Fahluik AK, Klaveness J: Abdominal imaging. JMRI 3:285–295, 1993.
86. Guinet C, Buy JN, Sezeur A, et al: Preoperative assessment of the extension of rectal carcinoma: correlation of MR, surgical and histopathologic findings. J Comput Assist Tomogr 12:209–214, 1988.
87. Stark DD: Biliary system, pancreas, spleen, and alimentary tract. *In* Stark DD, Bradley WG (eds): Magnetic Resonance Imaging (2nd ed). St. Louis: Mosby–Year Book, 1992, pp 1838–1853.
88. deLange EE, Fechner RE, Edge SB, et al: Preoperative staging of rectal carcinoma with MR imaging: surgical and histopathologic correlation. Radiology 176:623–628, 1990.
89. Moss AA: Imaging of colorectal carcinoma. Radiology 170:308–310, 1989.
90. Butch RJH, Stark DD, Wittenberg J, et al: Staging rectal cancer by MR and CT. AJR 146:1155–1160, 1986.
91. Plattner V, Leborgne J, Heloury Y, et al: MRI evaluation of the levator ani muscle: anatomic correlations and practical applications. Surg Radiol Anat 13:129–131, 1991.
92. Guinet C, Buy JN, Sezeur A, et al: Preoperative assessment of the extension of rectal carcinoma: correlation of MR, surgical and histopathologic findings. J Comput Assist Tomogr 12:209–214, 1988.
93. Ito K, Kato T, Tadokoro M, et al: Recurrent rectal cancer and scar: differentiation with PET and MR imaging. Radiology 182:549–552, 1992.
94. Chan TW, Kressel HY, Milestone B, et al: Rectal carcinoma: staging at MR imaging with endorectal surface coil. Radiology 181:461–467, 1991.
95. deLange EE, Fechner RE, Wanebo HJ: Suspected recurrent rectosigmoid carcinoma after abdominoperineal resection: MR imaging and histopathologic findings. Radiology 170:323–328, 1989.
96. Rafto SE, Amendola MA, Gefter WB: MR imaging of recurrent colorectal carcinoma versus fibrosis. J Comput Assist Tomogr 12:521–523, 1988.
97. Krestin GP, Steinbrich W, Friedman G: Recurrent rectal cancer: diagnosis with MR imaging versus CT. Radiology 168:307–311, 1988.
98. Schlag P, Lehner B, Strauss LG, et al: Scar or recurrent rectal cancer: positron emission tomography is more helpful for diagnosis than immunoscintigraphy. Arch Surg 124:197–200, 1989.

# Angiography and Interventional Radiology

### Albert A. Nemcek, Jr., M.D.
### Robert L. Vogelzang, M.D.

## ANGIOGRAPHY OF THE COLON

### Colonic Ischemia

Colonic ischemia is the most common vascular disorder of the intestines. Many cases are due to nonocclusive causes; in a minority of cases, embolism or thrombosis is responsible.[1, 2] Obstructive colonic lesions are found in up to 20% of cases, with the ischemic segment being proximal to the obstruction.[1, 2] Most cases of colonic ischemia occur in elderly patients, who typically present with mild, crampy, left-sided abdominal pain and melena. More severe cases can lead to colonic gangrene or perforation. However, the changes of colonic ischemia are usually reversible and include a spectrum of pathologic alterations termed *ischemic colitis* (see Chapter 161).

Patients with suspected colonic ischemia should be evaluated by barium enema or colonoscopy rather than angiography.[1, 2] Barium enema findings depend on the stage of the disease and include thumbprinting, ulceration, bowel wall thickening, and stricture formation.[1, 3, 4] The portion of the colon supplied by the inferior mesenteric artery is most frequently involved, accounting for 80% of cases.[3] Angiography is usually unhelpful. In one review of 1024 cases of ischemic colitis, only 96 (9%) involved evidence of occlusion.[5] This finding suggests that colonic ischemia usually results from underlying low-flow states and/or from degenerative changes in the vasa recta, too small to discern by standard angiography.[1, 5] Although mesenteric vessels show stenoses in about 45% of cases, this finding is common in elderly patients and has no prognostic significance in patients with colonic ischemia.[3, 5] In some patients, the inferior mesenteric branches may actually show hypervascularity, which is similar to the appearance noted in inflammatory conditions of the bowel.[5, 6]

### Angiodysplasia of the Colon

Angiodysplasia (vascular ectasia) of the colon is a vascular disorder that usually affects the right colon in elderly individuals.[7, 8] It has a number of characteristic angiographic features, which depend on the stage and size of the lesion: intense and prolonged opacification of a dilated and tortuous mural colonic vein (the earliest sign), vascular "tufts" (small, densely staining clusters of vessels), tortuous feeding vessels, contrast staining of the bowel wall, and early dense opacification of enlarged draining veins[7–10] (Fig. 60–1). To ensure that the early opacification of the draining vein is not simply the result of prolonged arterial injection, the duration of injection of contrast medium should be shorter than 4 seconds.[8]

The lesions are a major cause of significant gastrointestinal hemorrhage but may be found incidentally (see Chapter 147). Angiography is critical to the diagnosis; the lesions cannot be seen on barium studies and are difficult to identify at surgery and colonoscopy.

Although the exact cause is unknown, angiodysplasia may be the result of a degenerative process in which intermittent intramural venous obstruction leads to venous dilatation and, later, to direct arteriovenous communication[7] (Fig. 60–2). There is an association of colonic vascular ectasia and aortic stenosis.[11]

### Miscellaneous Vascular Disorders

Vascular malformations associated with hereditary hemorrhagic telangiectasia and the small aneurysms seen in polyarteritis nodosa can involve the colon. Colonic varices can develop as a result of portal hypertension or mesenteric venous occlusion.[12] Congenital malformations can affect the colonic vasculature, either as solitary lesions or in combination with more generalized disor-

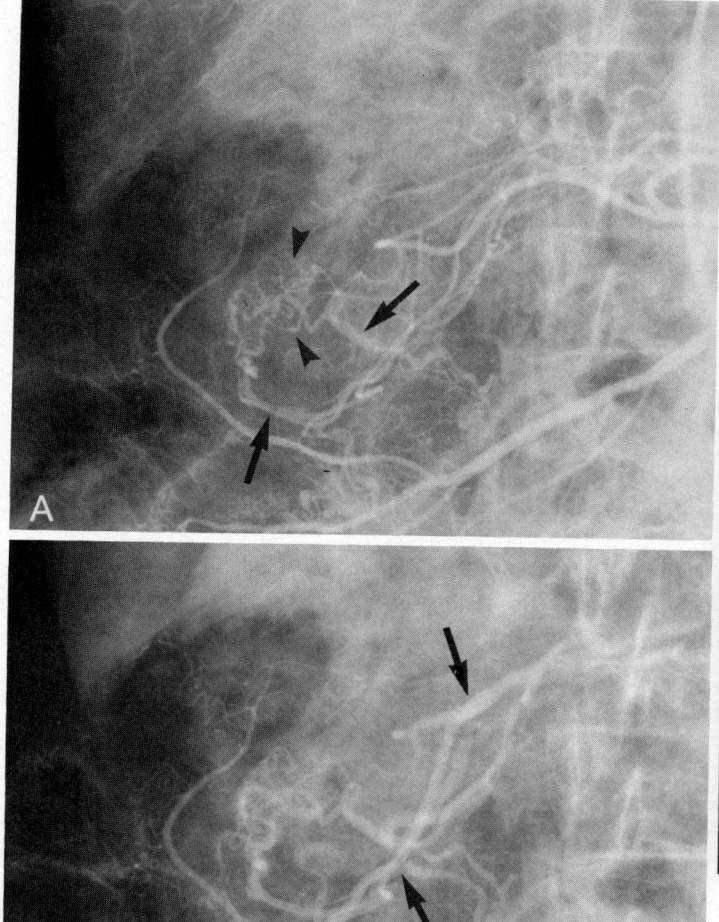

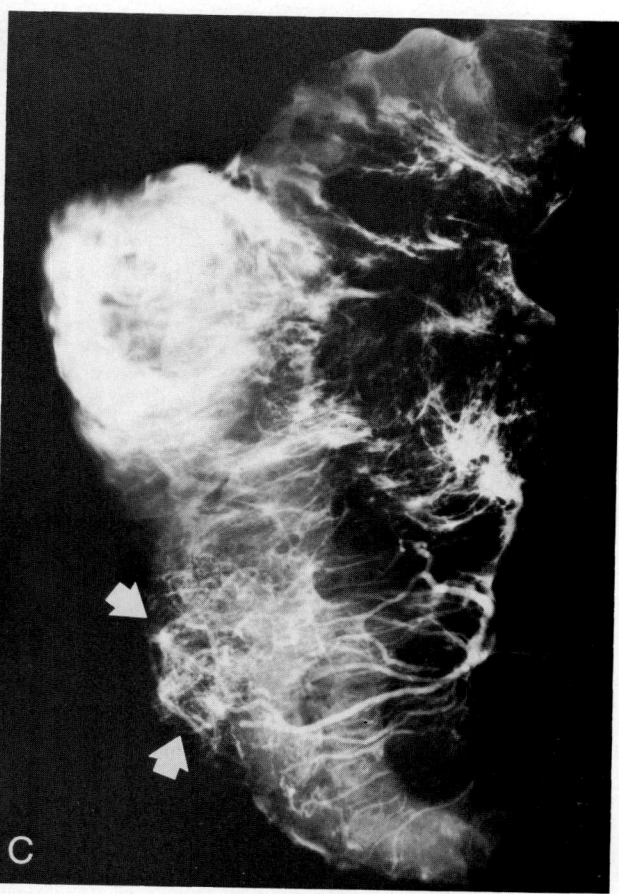

**Figure 60–1. Angiodysplasia of the right colon. A.** Angiogram in a patient with intermittent lower gastrointestinal hemorrhage demonstrates a vascular tuft *(arrowheads)* and paired vessels *(arrows)* indicating early draining veins adjacent to colonic arterial branches. **B.** Prominent draining veins *(arrows)* are opacified later in the angiogram. **C.** Injected specimen radiograph from a different patient demonstrates the abnormal tuft of vessels *(arrows)* characteristic of angiodysplasia.

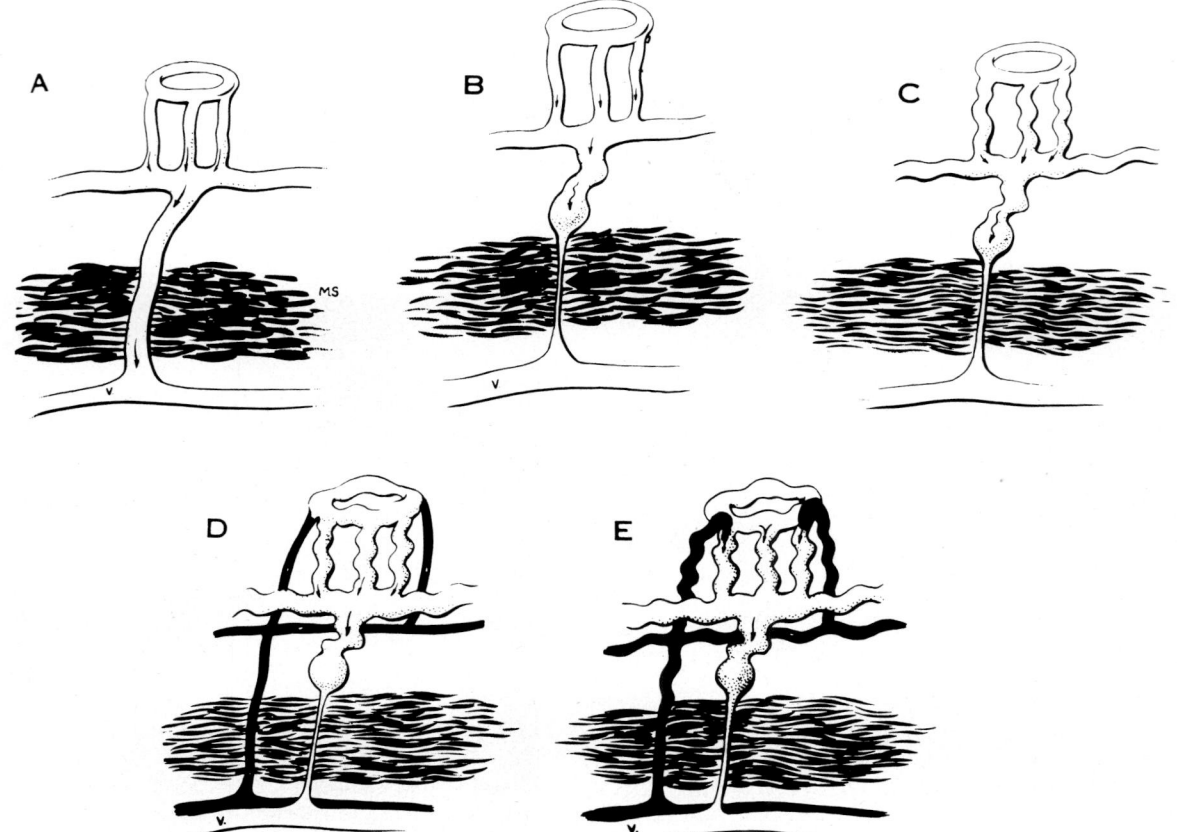

**Figure 60–2. Angiodysplasia of the colon: proposed etiology.** Diagram depicts the proposed mechanism for the development of angiodysplasia. **A.** Normal mucosal and submucosal drainage. **B.** Partial obstruction occurs because of muscular contraction or increased intraluminal pressure. **C.** After recurrent episodes over years, the submucosal vein becomes dilated and tortuous. **D.** The veins and venules draining into the abnormal submucosal vessel subsequently become ectatic. **E.** Eventually, the capillary ring dilates, the precapillary sphincter becomes incompetent, and a small arteriovenous communication is present through the lesion. (**A** to **E** from Boley SJ, Sammartano R, Adams A, et al: On the nature and etiology of vascular ectasias of the colon. Degenerative lesions of aging. Gastroenterology 72:650–659, 1977.)

ders, such as Klippel-Trenaunay-Weber syndrome.[13–17] Acquired arteriovenous fistulas have also been reported.[18]

## Tumors

Angiography is rarely indicated in the work-up of colonic neoplasms. Abnormalities related to tumors, however, may be noted incidentally or on angiograms performed for the work-up of colonic bleeding. Adenocarcinoma varies in appearance because of the variable response of and effect on adjacent tissues and organs.[8, 19] Adenomatous polyps are hypovascular in most instances.[8] Villous adenomas are vascular lesions, with enlarged feeding arteries and draining veins and contrast staining in the parenchymal phase.[20]

## Inflammatory Bowel Disease

Angiography is seldom used in the work-up of inflammatory lesions such as ulcerative colitis, Crohn's disease, or diverticulitis. Acute inflammation usually produces nonspecific findings: increased vascularity with enlargement of feeding arteries, dense capillary blush of the bowel wall, and enlargement and sometimes early opacification of draining veins.[8, 19, 21–23] These findings overlap with those found in early ischemic colitis and may even be normal in the postprandial state.[8] As Crohn's disease progresses, arterial occlusions, irregular arterial narrowing, and hypovascularity may develop in the involved segment.[8, 23, 24]

## NONVASCULAR INTERVENTIONAL RADIOLOGY OF THE COLON

### Drainage of Diverticular Abscess

Percutaneous drainage (Fig. 60–3) of diverticular abscesses is performed to diminish the number of stages necessary for safe and effective surgical treatment (see Chapter 61).[25] In two series, 25 of 40 (63%) patients with diverticulitis and percutaneously drained abscesses

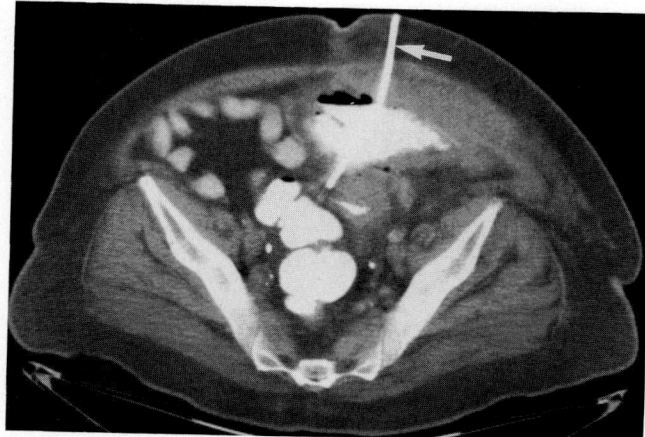

**Figure 60–3. Percutaneous drainage of diverticular abscess.** A drain *(arrow)* courses through the anterior abdominal wall and enters the abscess, which has been opacified with contrast medium. The patient underwent a single stage surgical resection after successful abscess drainage.

or fluid collections had successful single stage procedures (resection and primary anastomosis performed in the same operation) after catheter drainage.[26–28] Catheters were removed before surgery according to standard criteria. In six patients, surgery was deferred, either because it was declined by the patient or because of increased surgical-anesthetic risk. Interestingly, four of these patients remained symptom free for follow-up periods of 10 to 30 months, suggesting that drainage may have a role as the sole therapy in debilitated individuals who are high surgical risks. Of the patients who required more than a single stage operation, inflammatory changes persisted, but the abscess itself was frequently well drained, clinical response to abscess drainage was good, and no complications occurred as a result of the abscess drainage. Fistulas to bowel were reported in 43% of patients in the series, a finding that was associated with a longer period of catheter drainage.

It should be noted that small pericolic abscesses (<3 cm) can usually be treated by resection of the abscess with the diseased bowel and primary colonic anastomosis, or in some cases by antibiotics alone. In addition, catheter placement in such small collections is difficult, so that radiologic intervention in this setting is usually not indicated.

## Drainage of Appendiceal Abscess

Experience with percutaneous drainage of periappendiceal abscesses has been similarly encouraging, with success rates approaching 90% in multiple series.[29–34] The impressive rate of success has prompted some debate about the need for interval appendectomy. Although a number of patients have been percutaneously managed without subsequent appendectomy, some recurrences have been described. This question also confronts surgeons who must decide whether to perform an elective interval appendectomy after successful surgical

drainage of abscess.[31] Multiloculated or ill-defined abscesses, or abscesses associated with diffuse phlegmon, do not respond as well to drainage. Demonstration of fistula to the gut lumen by sinography is common and, as in diverticulitis, is associated with a longer period of catheter drainage.

The improved definition of the periappendiceal inflammatory process by cross-sectional imaging has also raised some interesting questions regarding the need for either surgical or percutaneous intervention in certain patients. In one series, 88% of patients with severe periappendiceal phlegmons or abscesses appearing smaller than 3 cm on computed tomographic scans responded to antibiotic therapy alone.[30]

## Balloon Dilatation of Colonic Strictures

Balloon dilatation of the colon (Fig. 60–4), under either fluoroscopic or colonoscopic control, is becoming increasingly popular.[35–41] Dilatation is reserved for strictures secondary to anastomotic narrowing, necrotizing enterocolitis, Crohn's disease, and healed ischemic colitis. Balloon dilatation can also be used to help develop the capacity of the neorectum in patients who have had a colonic resection and ileoanal anastomosis.[41]

Distal colonic and rectal strictures and strictures near or at colostomy sites are readily catheterized under fluoroscopic guidance. For lesions farther from an external point of access, combined endoscopy and fluoroscopy may be helpful.[36, 42] Because of the risk of fecal soilage, preprocedural antibiotic coverage is essential, even when a defunctionalized bowel loop is to be dilated.[36, 42] One procedural caveat: standard (20-mm-diameter) enteric dilatation balloons may be too small for dilating the distal colon in adults, and the simultaneous use of two or three balloons may be necessary.[35, 36, 42]

## Percutaneous Cecostomy

In nonobstructive colonic distention, the cecum is usually the most severely involved segment. This finding demonstrates Laplace's law, whereby the portion of colon with the greatest diameter (the cecum) responds first with further distention once intraluminal pressure begins to increase.[43] Cecal ileus refers to the situation in which cecal distention develops out of proportion to that of the remainder of the colon.[44] These patients have a mobile cecum suspended on a mesentery. When the patient is in the supine position, the cecum can rotate anteriorly, leading to progressive distention.

Massive colonic distention, when left untreated, may lead to colonic perforation, ischemia, peritonitis, and death. Once massive distention (9 cm or greater) of the cecum occurs, the risk of perforation seems less related to the absolute degree of distention than to the duration of distention.[44] Therefore, early recognition and therapy of this condition are critical.

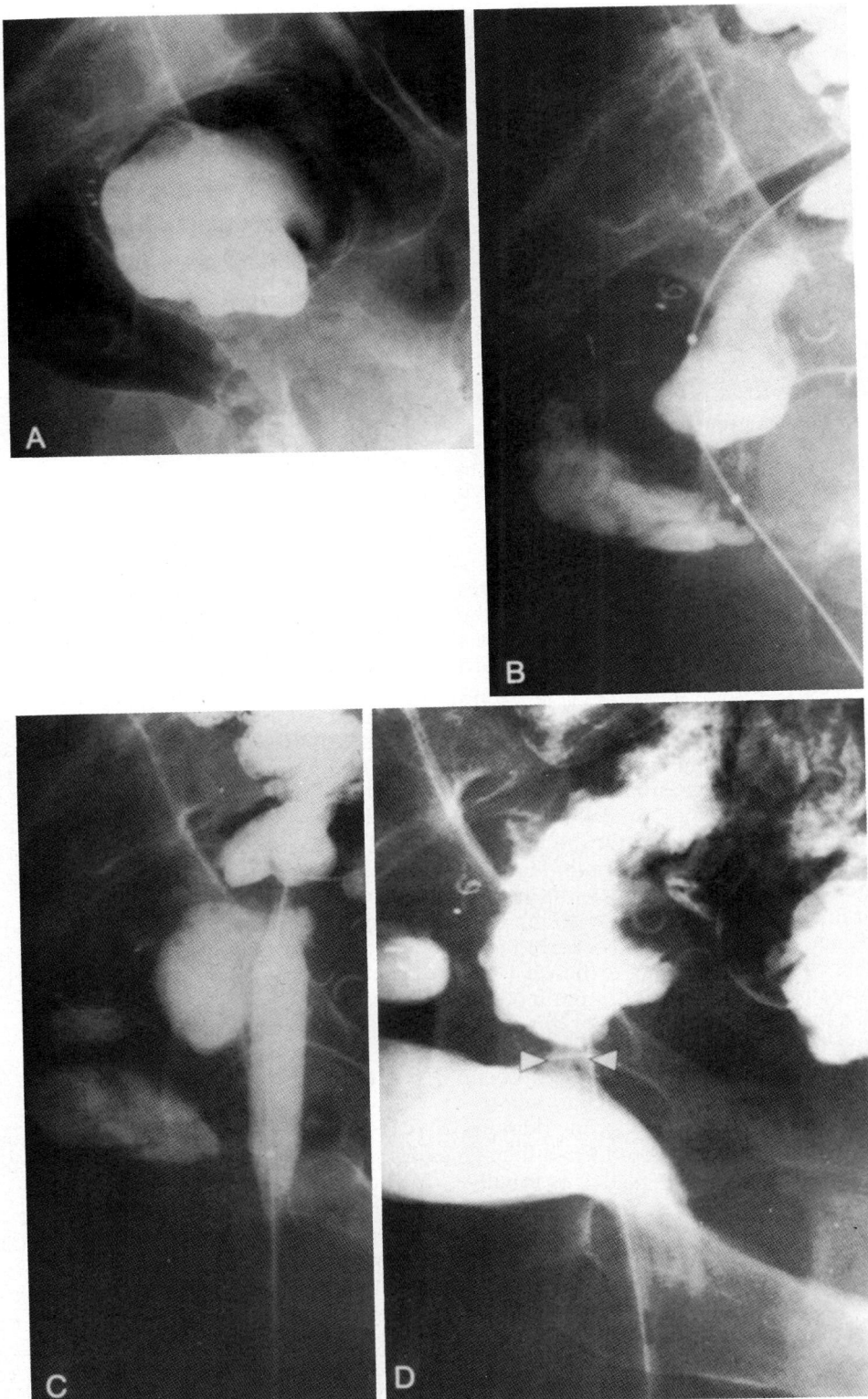

**Figure 60–4. Balloon dilatation of anastomotic stricture. A.** Markedly dilated colon is proximal to a colorectal anastomosis after surgery for carcinoma of the left colon. The barium present is from oral ingestion rather than a barium enema, indicating a significant degree of obstruction. **B.** After insertion of a red rubber catheter, a guidewire was placed in the rectum, and a cobra catheter was used to traverse the stenosis. A heavy-duty exchange guidewire was then placed, and an angioplasty balloon was inserted through the anastomotic region. **C.** The balloon was then inflated and the stricture was dilated. **D.** Postdilatation contrast study demonstrates a greatly increased luminal diameter *(arrowheads)*. (**A** to **D** from Cope C, Burke DR, Meranze SG: Atlas of Interventional Radiology. New York: Gower Medical Publishing, 1990, p 12.15.)

The initial treatment of nonobstructive colonic distention is conservative and includes placement of a nasogastric tube, withholding of oral intake, and treatment of underlying metabolic and other medical disorders. If the distention fails to improve, colonoscopy and colonic decompression tube placement should be attempted.[43, 45, 46] These methods, however, may prove ineffective because of thick retained stool. Distention may recur after initial colonoscopic success.

After unsuccessful colonoscopic decompression, surgical cecostomy has been the next therapeutic approach. However, surgery in these patients, who are often seriously ill, can be risky. Consequently, a number of investigators have attempted percutaneous decompression of the massively dilated but unobstructed cecum.[47–51] Successful decompression has been achieved both with simple aspiration and with drainage tube placement. Reports of percutaneous decompression of the mechanically obstructed colon have also appeared.[52, 53]

A variety of approaches (Fig. 60–5), methods, and tube sizes (Fig. 60–6) have been used for percutaneous cecostomy. Usually, fluoroscopy provides sufficient guidance, although computed tomography may be helpful if there are questions about the approach. Both the trocar and the Seldinger methods of tube placement are feasible for these patients. Although some authors have advocated a retroperitoneal approach to minimize peritoneal contamination, authors of most reports have successfully and safely used a transperitoneal approach.[51] VanSonnenberg and colleagues have noted that a retroperitoneal approach may often be difficult or nearly impossible because the peritoneal reflection in the majority of patients extends far posteriorly, necessitating

an extreme posterior approach, which may be hindered by superimposed bony structures.[47] They have also observed that a retroperitoneal approach is anatomically impossible in patients with the cecum on the mesentery.[47] Others have noted that it can be difficult to predict the site of the peritoneal reflection on the basis of imaging studies obtained with the patient supine.[52]

As with punctures of other hollow viscera, there are theoretic advantages of using anchoring devices to help create secure fixation of the cecum to the anterior abdominal wall, theoretically limiting peritoneal spill and helping to prevent catheter or guidewire dislodgment.[48]

Although further experience with percutaneous cecostomy is necessary to assess risks fully and to evaluate optimal technique and indications, this procedure is an alternative method of colonic decompression in severely ill and debilitated patients.

## Percutaneous Biopsy of Bowel Lesions

Several investigators have assessed the utility of sonography- and fluoroscopy-guided direct biopsy of primary bowel wall lesions. Indications for this approach include 1) lesions that yielded no tissue diagnosis when endoscopic biopsy was performed (a common problem with submucosal lesions); 2) lesions in patients who are poor candidates for endoscopy or open exploration; 3) lesions that because of their location cannot be approached endoscopically; and 4) lesions that, if proved

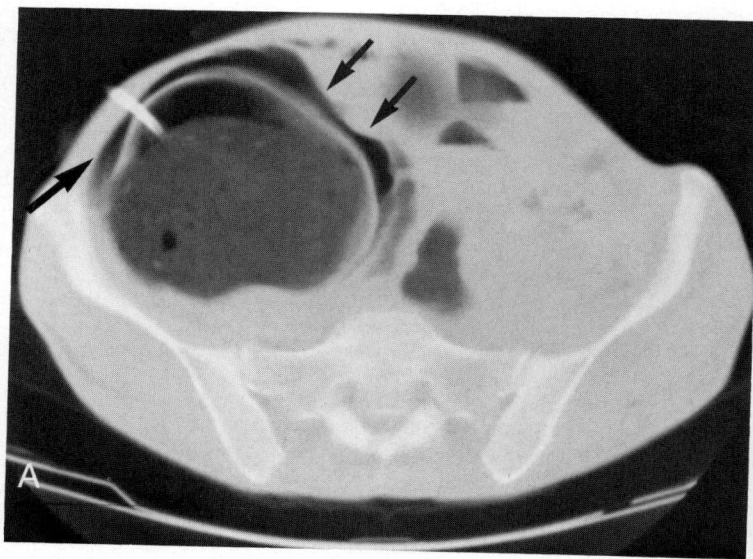
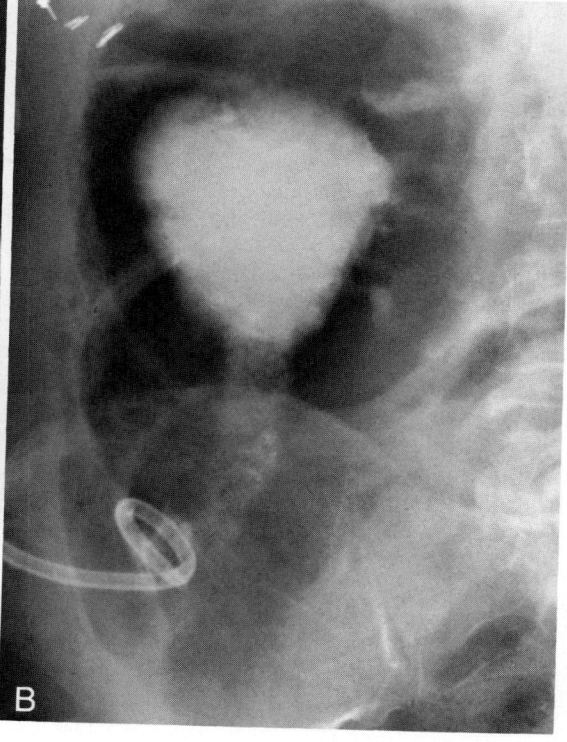

**Figure 60–5. Percutaneous cecostomy.** A transperitoneal approach was used. **A.** Computed tomographic scan. **B.** Abdominal plain film. Air (*arrows*) was introduced into the peritoneal cavity during the procedure.

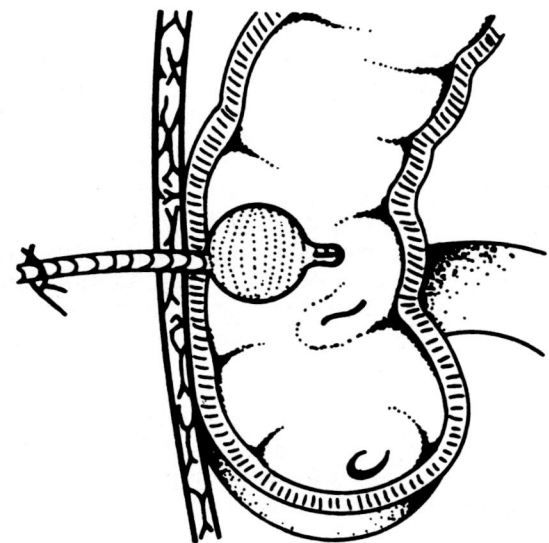

**Figure 60–6. Percutaneous cecostomy catheter.** The balloon holds the cecum against the anterior abdominal wall, minimizing migration and spillage into the peritoneal cavity. (From Casola G, Withers C, vanSonnenberg E, et al: Percutaneous cecostomy for decompression of the massively distended cecum. Radiology 158:793–794, 1986.)

malignant, will stop further investigation or change therapy.[54-57]

In the largest of these series, 78 patients with sonographic evidence of gastrointestinal mass lesions that showed a typical "target" sign were studied by biopsy using 23-gauge needles.[50] These lesions included 18 gastric, 3 small intestinal, and 40 colorectal lesions. Biopsy results that were positive for malignancy were obtained in 50 of 61 (82%) patients later proved to have malignant lesions, and biopsy results read as nonmalignant were obtained in 16 of 17 (94%) patients later proved to have benign lesions, with one biopsy yielding material insufficient for diagnosis. There were no false-positive biopsy results for malignancy. A predictive value for malignant cytology of 100% was obtained, and for nonmalignant cytology, 67%. No complications occurred.

With the use of 20-gauge needles and with guidance provided by barium examination, Owman and Idvall performed biopsies of 47 gastrointestinal lesions.[57] This method has the potential benefit of allowing guidance into extremely small lesions. Their overall accuracy was 78%, with no false-positive or false-negative cytologic reports of malignancy. Excluding cases in which insufficient material was obtained, cytologic accuracy was 98%. Similar diagnostic results have been noted by Solbiati and associates[54] (24 bowel lesions) and Ennis and MacErlean[55] (5 bowel lesions), with no biopsy-related complications.

## References

1. Boley SJ, Brandt LJ, Veith FJ: Ischemic disorders of the intestines. Curr Probl Surg 15:1–85, 1978.
2. Reinus JF, Brandt LJ, Boley SJ: Ischemic diseases of the bowel. Gastroenterol Clin North Am 19:319–343, 1990.
3. Wittenberg J, Athanasoulis CA, Williams LF, et al: Ischemic colitis: radiology and pathophysiology. AJR 123:287–300, 1975.
4. Iida M, Matsui T, Fuchigami T, et al: Ischemic colitis: serial changes in double-contrast barium enema examination. Radiology 159:337–341, 1986.
5. Reeders JWAJ, Tytgat GNJ, Rosenbusch G, et al: Ischaemic Colitis. The Hague: Martinus Nijhoff Publishing, 1984.
6. Athansoulis CA: Angiography of the colon. *In* Dreyfuss JR, Janower ML (eds): Radiology of the Colon. Baltimore: Williams & Wilkins, 1980, pp 317–353.
7. Boley SJ, Sprayregen S, Sammartano RJ, et al: The pathophysiologic basis for the angiographic signs of vascular ectasia of the colon. Radiology 125:615–621, 1977.
8. Reuter SR, Redman HC, Cho KJ: Gastrointestinal Angiography (3rd ed). Philadelphia: WB Saunders, 1986.
9. Baum S, Athanasoulis CA, Waltman AC, et al: Angiodysplasia of the right colon: a cause of gastrointestinal bleeding. AJR 129:789–794, 1977.
10. Baer JW, Ryan S: Analysis of cecal vasculature in the search for vascular malformations. AJR 126:394–405, 1976.
11. Galloway SJ, Casarella WJ, Shimkin PM: Vascular malformations of the right colon as a cause of bleeding in patients with aortic stenosis. Radiology 113:11–15, 1974.
12. Lopata HI, Berlin L: Colon varices: a rare cause of lower gastrointestinal bleeding. Radiology 87:1048–1050, 1966.
13. Phillips GH, Gordon DH, Martin EC, et al: The Klippel-Trenaunay syndrome: clinical and radiologic aspects. Radiology 128:429–434, 1978.
14. Kadir S: Diagnostic Angiography. Philadelphia: WB Saunders, 1986.
15. Ghahremani GG, Kangarloo H, Volberg F, et al: Diffuse cavernous hemangioma of the colon in the Klippel-Trenaunay syndrome. Radiology 118:673–678, 1976.
16. Bell GA, McKenzie AD, Emmons H: Diffuse cavernous hemangioma of the rectum: report of a case and review of the literature. Dis Colon Rectum 15:377–382, 1972.
17. Servelle M: Klippel and Trenaunay's syndrome. Ann Surg 201:365–373, 1985.
18. Peer A, Slutski S, Abrahmsohn R, et al: Transcatheter occlusion of inferior mesenteric arteriovenous fistula: a case report. Cardiovasc Intervent Radiol 12:35–37, 1989.
19. Boijsen E, Reuter SR: Mesenteric angiography in the evaluation of inflammatory and neoplastic disease of the intestine. Radiology 87:1028–1036, 1966.
20. Riba PO, Lunderquist A: Angiographic findings in villous tumors of the colon. AJR 117:287–291, 1973.
21. Brahme F, Hidell J: Angiography in Crohn's disease revisited. AJR 126:941–951, 1976.
22. Lunderquist A, Lunderquist A: Angiography in ulcerative colitis. AJR 99:18–23, 1967.
23. Lunderquist A, Lunderquist A, Knutsson H: Angiography in Crohn's disease of the small bowel and colon. AJR 101:338–343, 1976.
24. Brahme F: Mesenteric angiography in regional enterocolitis. Radiology 87:1037–1042, 1966.
25. Rodkey GV, Welch CE: Changing patterns in the surgical treatment of diverticular disease. Ann Surg 200:466–478, 1984.
26. Mueller PR, Saini S, Wittenburg J, et al: Sigmoid diverticular abscesses: percutaneous drainage as an adjunct to surgical resection in 24 cases. Radiology 164:321–325, 1987.
27. Saini S, Mueller PR, Wittenberg J, et al: Percutaneous drainage of diverticular abscess: an adjunct to surgical therapy. Arch Surg 121:475–478, 1986.
28. Neff CC, vanSonnenberg E, Casola G, et al: Diverticular abscesses: percutaneous drainage. Radiology 163:15–18, 1987.
29. Jeffrey RB Jr, Tolentino CS, Federle MP, et al: Percutaneous drainage of periappendiceal abscesses: review of 20 patients. AJR 149:59–62, 1987.
30. Jeffrey RB Jr, Federle MP, Tolentino CS: Periappendiceal inflammatory masses: CT-directed management and clinical outcome in 70 patients. AJR 149:59–62, 1988.

31. vanSonnenberg E, Wittich G, Casola G, et al: Periappendiceal abscess: percutaneous drainage. Radiology 163:23–26, 1987.

32. Nunez D Jr, Huber JS, Yrizarry JM, et al: Nonsurgical drainage of appendiceal abscesses. AJR 146:587–589, 1986.

33. Barakos JA, Jeffrey RB Jr, Federle MP, et al: CT in management of periappendiceal abscess. AJR 146:1161–1164, 1986.

34. Bagi P, Dueholm S: Nonoperative management of the ultrasonically evaluated appendiceal mass. Surgery 101:602–605, 1987.

35. de Lange EE, Shaffer HA Jr: Rectal stricture: treatment with fluoroscopically guided balloon dilation. Radiology 178:475–479, 1991.

36. McLean GK, Meranze SGL: Interventional radiologic management of enteric strictures. Radiology 170:1049–1053, 1989.

37. McLean GK, Cooper GS, Hartz WH, et al: Radiologically guided balloon dilation of gastrointestinal strictures. Part II. Results of long-term follow-up. Radiology 165:41–43, 1987.

38. McLean GK, Cooper GS, Hartz WH, et al: Radiologically guided balloon dilation of gastrointestinal strictures. Part I. Technique and factors influencing procedural success. Radiology 165:35–40, 1987.

39. Ball WS Jr, Seigel RS, Goldthorn JF, et al: Colonic strictures in infants following intestinal ischemia: treatment by balloon catheter dilation. Radiology 149:469–472, 1983.

40. Skreden K, Wiig JN, Myrvold HE: Balloon dilation of rectal strictures. Acta Chir Scand 153:615–617, 1987.

41. Telander RL, Perrault J, Hoffman AD: Early development of the neorectum by balloon dilations after ileoanal anastomosis. J Pediatr Surg 16:911–916, 1991.

42. McLean GK: Interventional radiology of the gastrointestinal tract. Curr Probl Diagn Radiol 19:87–132, 1990.

43. Vanek VW, Al-Salti M: Acute pseudo-obstruction of the colon (Ogilvie's syndrome): an analysis of 400 cases. Dis Colon Rectum 29:203–210, 1986.

44. Johnson CD, Rice RP, Kelvin FM, et al: The radiologic evaluation of gross cecal distension: emphasis on cecal ileus. AJR 145:1211–1217, 1985.

45. Harig JM, Fumo DE, Loo FD, et al: Treatment of acute nontoxic megacolon during colonoscopy: tube placement versus simple decompression. Gastrointest Endosc 34:23–27, 1988.

46. Strodel WE, Nostrant TT, Eckhauser FE, et al: Therapeutic and diagnostic colonoscopy in nonobstructive colonic dilation. Ann Surg 197:416–421, 1983.

47. vanSonnenberg E, Varney RR, Casola G, et al: Percutaneous cecostomy for Ogilvie syndrome: laboratory observations and clinical experience. Radiology 175:679–682, 1990.

48. Morrison MC, Lee MJ, Stafford SA, et al: Percutaneous cecostomy: controlled transperitoneal approach. Radiology 176:574–576, 1990.

49. Haaga JR, Bick RJ, Zollinger RM Jr: CT-guided percutaneous catheter cecostomy. Gastrointest Radiol 12:166–168, 1987.

50. Casola G, Withers C, vanSonnenberg E, et al: Percutaneous cecostomy for decompression of the massively distended cecum. Radiology 158:793–794, 1986.

51. Crass JR, Simmons RL, Frick MP, et al: Percutaneous decompression of the colon using CT guidance in the Ogilvie syndrome. AJR 144:475–476, 1985.

52. Quinn SF, Jones EN, Maroney T: Percutaneous cecostomy in the management of cecal volvulus: report of a case. J Intervent Radiol 2:127–139, 1987.

53. Patel D, Ansari E, Berman MD: Percutaneous decompression of cecal volvulus. AJR 148:747–748, 1987.

54. Solbiati L, Montali G, Croce F, et al: Fine-needle aspiration biopsy of bowel lesions under ultrasound guidance: indications and results. Gastrointest Radiol 11:172–176, 1986.

55. Ennis MG, MacErlean DP: Biopsy of bowel wall pathology under ultrasound control. Gastrointest Radiol 6:17–20, 1981.

56. Torp-Pedersen S, Grønvall S, Holm HH: Ultrasonically guided fine-needle aspiration biopsy of gastrointestinal mass lesions. J Ultrasound Med 3:65–68, 1984.

57. Owman T, Idvall I: Percutaneous fine needle biopsy guided by barium examinations of the GI tract. Gastrointest Radiol 7:327–333, 1982.

# Diverticular Disease

**61**

## Emil J. Balthazar, M.D.

## INTRODUCTION

Colonic diverticula are acquired herniations of the mucosa and of portions of the submucosa through the muscularis propria.[1-3] Diverticular disease of the colon represents a continuum from an initial, prediverticular phase of marked muscular thickening of the colon wall (myochosis) to frank outpouchings (diverticulosis), and finally to diverticular perforation (diverticulitis). Disease progression from the initial phase to the advanced phases does not necessarily occur.[4-7] This chapter discusses the natural history of this disease and focuses on radiologic diagnosis and intervention.

## DIVERTICULOSIS

### Epidemiology

Diverticular disease is the most common colonic disease in the Western world. Interestingly, this disease was a pathologic curiosity before the 20th century. Its modern development is attributable to the introduction of the roller milling process in 1880, which removes most of the fiber from flour (see later). This process results in a low-residue diet producing low-volume, tenacious stools that require a high degree of propulsive effort for expulsion.[8-10]

In Western countries, colonic diverticula occur in 5% of the population by 40 years of age, in 33 to 50% of the population after 50 years of age, and in more than 50% of the population after 80 years of age. These findings contrast sharply with the prevalence rate of less than 0.2% in underdeveloped areas of Asia and Africa. In individuals from low-prevalence areas who migrate to Western communities, the frequency of diverticula increases within 10 years.[4-11]

The sigmoid colon is involved in up to 95% of patients; the cecum is involved in 5% of patients. Japan is an interesting exception to other developed countries in that patients with right-sided diverticulosis outnumber those with left-sided disease by a ratio of 5:1.[12, 13]

Approximately 4 to 5% of all patients who harbor diverticula and 20% of those whose diverticula are clinically recognized will develop some complication; 1 to 2% will require hospitalization and 0.5% will need surgical intervention or radiologic intervention, or both.[14]

### Etiology

The two fundamental factors contributing to the development of sigmoid diverticula are 1) a pressure gradient between the lumen and serosa, and 2) areas of relative weakness in the bowel wall. The first factor can best be appreciated by considering the tendency of the colon to function not as a tube but as small compartments (Fig. 61–1) created by the haustra (segmentation). The sigmoid is the narrowest portion of the colon and generates the highest intrasegmental pressures. In addition, stool is most dehydrated in the sigmoid colon, further increasing segmentation and motor activity.[15-20]

The colon wall is weakest where the intramural vasa recta penetrate to the submucosal layers. These points are on either side of the taenia mesocolica, and the mesenteric side of the taenia libera and taenia omentalis[15-21] (Fig. 61–2). Diverticula do not usually occur on the haustral row between the taenia omentalis and taenia libera[15-21] (see Fig. 61–2).

### Pathologic Findings

Most colonic diverticula are false diverticula, or pseudodiverticula, because they contain mucosa and sub-

1) **Segmentation**

a c d b e f

a } relax    irregularly
b }          segmenting
c }          in alternating fashion
d } contract
e }
f }

2) **Retropulsion at rectosigmoid sphincter-like action and poor propulsion**

3) **Resistance to forward movement high pressure in compartments delayed transit**

4) **Fibre speeds transit, widens lumen, lessens intraluminal pressure moister bulkier stool**

A

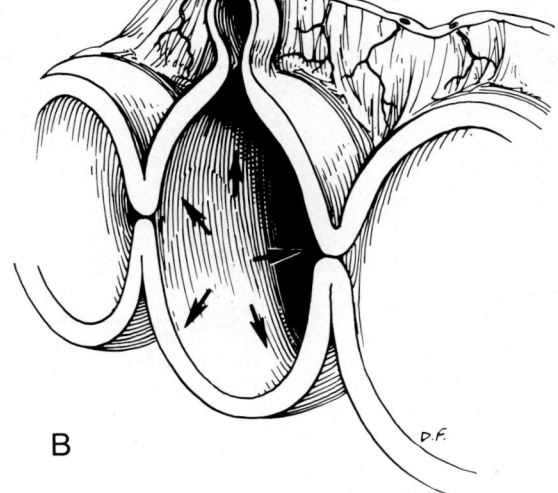

B

**Figure 61–1. The role of colonic segmentation in the development of pulsion diverticula. A.** This diagram illustrates how the haustra compartmentalize the sigmoid colon. Normally, there is alternating contraction of the haustra and intrahaustral nodal points (triangles in 1). In diverticular disease, the haustra are thickened, exaggerated, nonrelaxing, and partially obstructive, leading to increased segmentation. (From Smith A: Diverticular disease of the colon. *In* Phillips SF, Pemberton JH, Shorter RG [eds]: The Large Intestine: Physiology, Pathophysiology, and Disease. New York: Raven Press, 1991, pp 549–577.) **B.** This increase in segmentation causes back pressure effects to occur as both the intrahaustral and haustral sections contract simultaneously, leading to elevated pressures and extrusion of diverticula. (From Dietzen CD, Pemberton JH: Diverticulitis. *In* Yamada T [ed]: Textbook of Gastroenterology. Philadelphia: JB Lippincott, 1991, pp 1734–1748.)

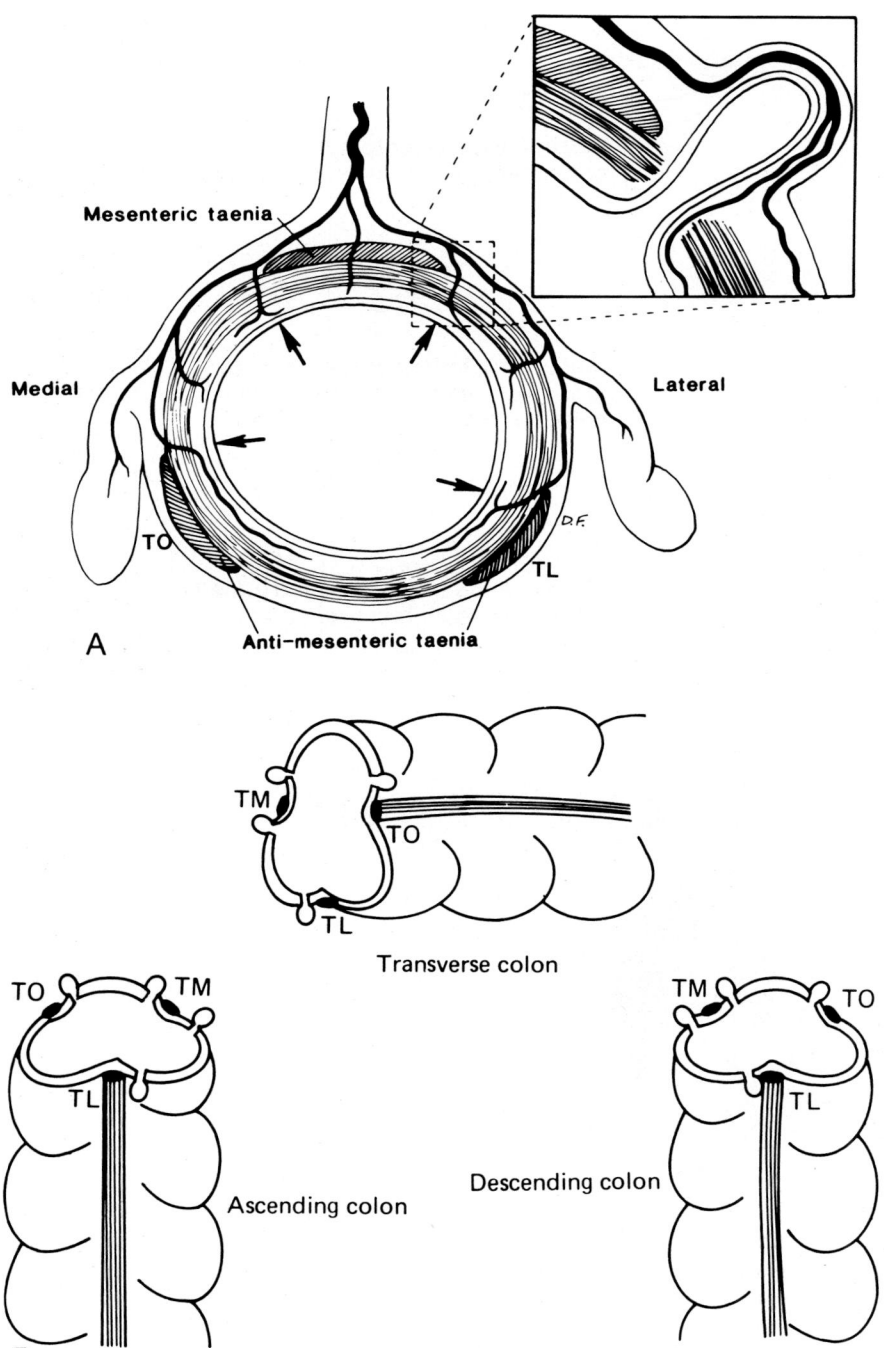

**Figure 61–2. Sites of origin of colonic diverticula. A.** The diverticula develop on either side of the mesenteric taenia (TM) and on the mesenteric side of the antimesenteric taeniae, the taenia omentalis (TO), and taenia libera (TL). These are at sites *(arrows)* where the vasa recta perforate the muscularis propria and penetrate the submucosa (see insert). (From Dietzen CD, Pemberton JH: Diverticulitis. *In* Yamada T [ed]: Textbook of Gastroenterology. Philadelphia: JB Lippincott, 1991, pp 1734–1748.) **B.** The antimesenteric TO-TL haustral row does not give rise to diverticula. TM = mesenteric taenia. (From Meyers MA, Volberg F, Katzen B, et al: Haustral anatomy and pathology: a new look. II. Roentgen interpretation of pathologic alterations. Radiology 108:505–512, 1973.)

mucosa, but not the muscularis propria (Fig. 61–3). They are usually 0.5 to 1.0 cm in size and penetrate the clefts between bundles of circular muscle fibers at points where nutrient arteries pass through the submucosa. The proximity of the diverticula to the arteries is considered key in the development of hemorrhage.[1–3, 22–26]

In the uninflamed state, diverticula are elastic and compressible but have a tendency to empty poorly and, as a result, to fill with inspissated stool. This tendency may account for the increased number of lymphoid follicles found in the lining mucosa.

Most patients with sigmoid diverticula have myochosis, a disorder in which there is thickening of the circular muscle layer, shortening of the taeniae, and narrowing of the lumen. The circular muscle is often corrugated, and its appearance has been likened to that of a concertina.[17–19]

Diverticula of the rectum are rare, because the taeniae become fused at this level, forming a completely encircling, supporting coat.[4–6]

## Clinical Findings

In most patients, diverticulosis is an incidental finding. Patients may complain of symptoms of irritable bowel

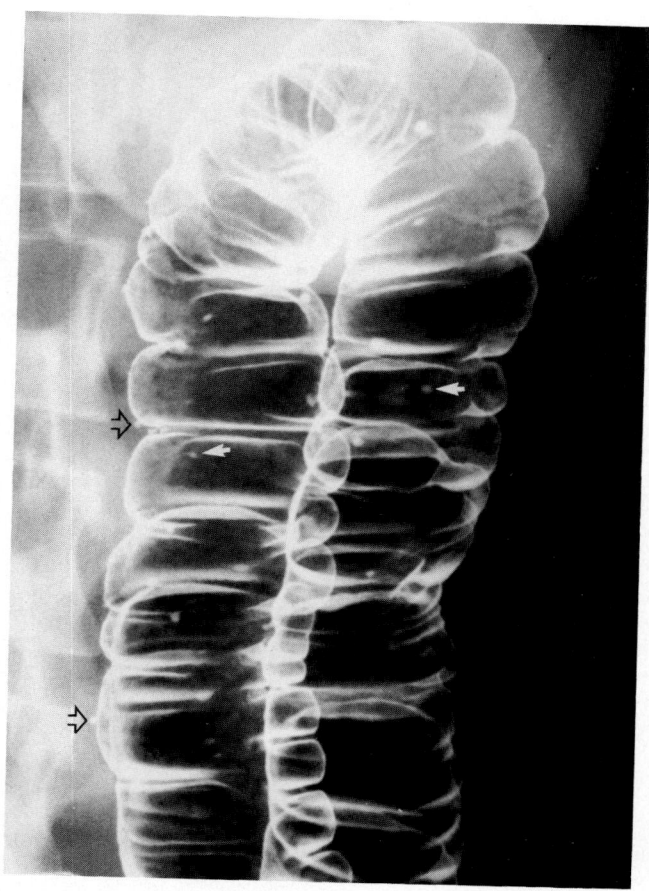

**Figure 61–4. Intramural diverticula.** When small and intramural, diverticula viewed en face *(solid arrows)* can resemble aphthae. Their true nature is best appreciated in profile *(open arrows)*.

syndrome such as chronic or intermittent postprandial lower abdominal pain that is relieved by defecation (see Chapter 144).

## Radiologic Findings

### Plain Films

More than 50% of patients with significant diverticular disease demonstrate a distinctive "bubbly" appearance of the sigmoid colon on routine abdominal radiographs.[27] When pelvic phleboliths are present, there is a statistical correlation between their number and size and the degree of diverticular disease.[28] It is postulated that both of these common disorders are due to the long-term effects of a low-fiber diet and straining while defecating.

### Barium Studies

Diverticulosis is detected more often by double contrast studies than by single contrast studies because of the greater colonic distention and the improved visualization of intramural diverticula. When viewed en face, these immature diverticula may simulate aphthae (Fig. 61–4). Their true nature is established when they are viewed in profile, when they are conical or triangular and 1 to 2 mm high.[29–34]

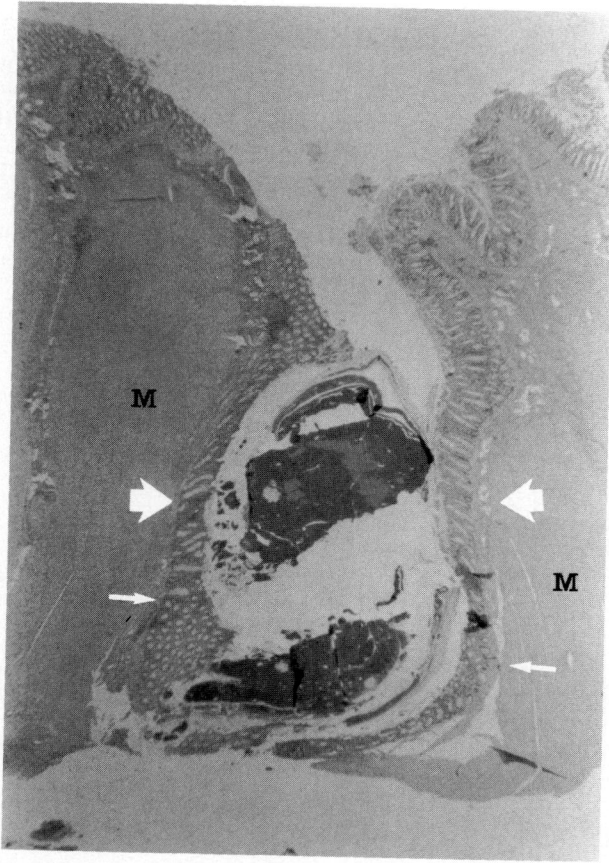

**Figure 61–3. Intramural diverticulum of the sigmoid colon.** There is herniation of the mucosa layer within the muscle coat, forming an intramural diverticulum *(wide arrows)*. There is considerable muscular hypertrophy (M) around a normal mucosal lining *(narrow arrows)*. Residual debris is present in the diverticulum, but there are no inflammatory changes (hematoxylin-eosin, × 4).

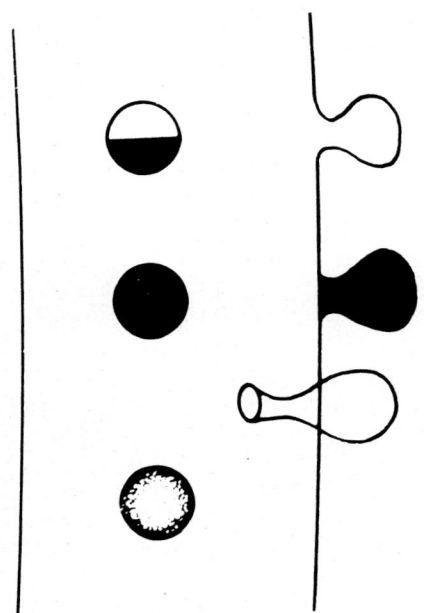

**Figure 61–5. Variable appearance of diverticula on double contrast barium enema.** Their appearance depends on the angle from which they are viewed and on how much barium or air they contain. (From Bartram CI, Kumar P: Clinical Radiology in Gastroenterology. Oxford: Blackwell Scientific Publications, 1981, p 130.)

The mature diverticulum has several characteristic appearances (Fig. 61–5) which depend on the angle with which it is viewed and the degree of barium filling. In profile, the diverticulum appears as a flask-like protrusion measuring several millimeters to several centimeters in length, joined to the wall by a fairly long, large neck. En face, it may appear as a ring shadow or a well-marginated barium collection or may resemble a bowler hat (Fig. 61–6). The size and form of diverticula vary

from one moment to the next, depending on the degree of colonic distention. The alignment of diverticula along the taeniae is usually apparent.[29–34]

Diagnostic difficulties may arise if the diverticulum inverts into the lumen, and a number of diverticular "polypectomies" have been described in the endoscopic literature.[35–38] Also, if feces obstruct the diverticulum, the diverticular orifice may bulge into the lumen, resulting in a ring shadow or filling defect. In profile, only the neck may be visible. If the obstruction is incomplete, a fine linear strand of barium may penetrate the diverticulum, simulating a spur. Because this strand of barium appears outside the lumen, its presence usually allows the correct diagnosis to be made.[30] For this reason, careful attention to the appearance of polyps and diverticula from film to film is necessary.[36, 38]

A diverticulum with a large neck may resemble a sessile polyp, one with a narrow neck may resemble a pedunculated polyp, and an obstructed diverticulum may resemble a polyp or adherent fecal material.[30, 39] In addition, both polyps and diverticula can produce the "bowler hat" sign (Fig. 61–7). If the bowler hat points toward the center of the long axis of the colon, it represents a polyp. If it points away from the center of the long axis of the bowel, it represents a diverticulum. If the bowler hat is located in the midline of the bowel, or is directly parallel to the long axis of the bowel, it cannot be confidently classified as representing either a polyp or a diverticulum.[40] Some authors suggest that when these difficulties arise, particularly in a redundant sigmoid colon with multiple diverticula, the patient should be given a 500- to 750-mL sigmoid enema with water, or a 1.5% w/v suspension of barium as an adjunctive sigmoid contrast medium. This enema is administered after filming the double contrast study and allowing evacuation of air via the enema tube. This technique improves visualization of the sigmoid colon

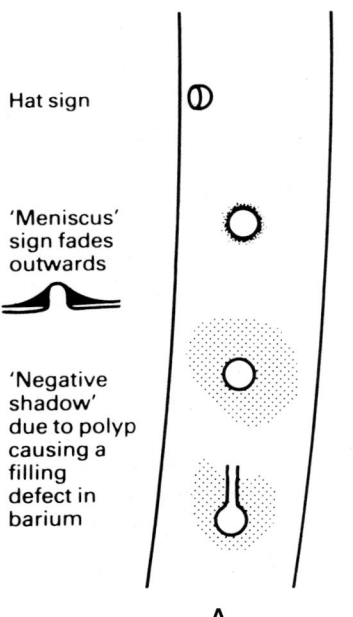

Hat sign

'Meniscus' sign fades outwards

'Negative shadow' due to polyp causing a filling defect in barium

**A**

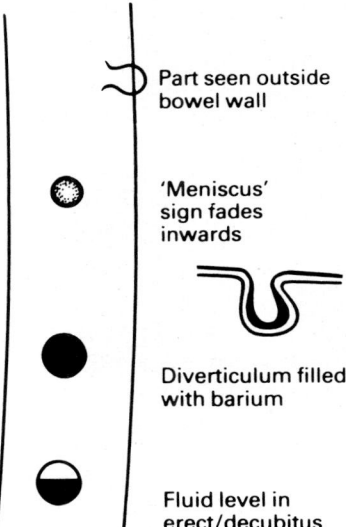

Part seen outside bowel wall

'Meniscus' sign fades inwards

Diverticulum filled with barium

Fluid level in erect/decubitus

**B**

**Figure 61–6. Distinguishing features of polyps and diverticula. A.** Polyps. **B.** Diverticula. (**A** and **B** from Bartrum CI, Kumar P: Clinical Radiology in Gastroenterology. Oxford: Blackwell Scientific Publications, 1981, p 131.)

**Figure 61–7. Principle of bowler hat sign for differentiating polyps from diverticula.** A plastic foam cup with chewing gum, used to simulate a polyp, and the cut end of a plastic test tube, serving as a model for a diverticulum, are coated with high-density barium. **A.** The superior bowler hat *(white arrow)* points towards the center of the cup (i.e., a polyp), and the inferior bowler hat *(black arrow)* points away from the center of the cup (i.e., a diverticulum). **B.** Radiograph obtained after slight rotation shows the simulated polyp and diverticulum in profile. (**A** and **B** from Miller WT, Levine MS, Rubesin SE, et al: Bowler-hat sign: a simple principle for differentiating polyps from diverticula. Radiology 173:615–617, 1989.)

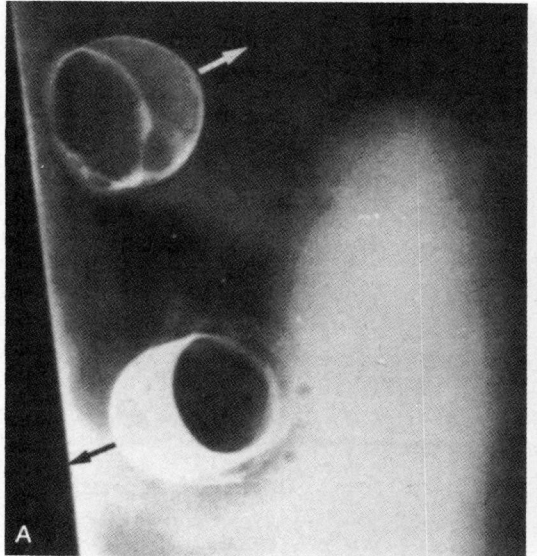
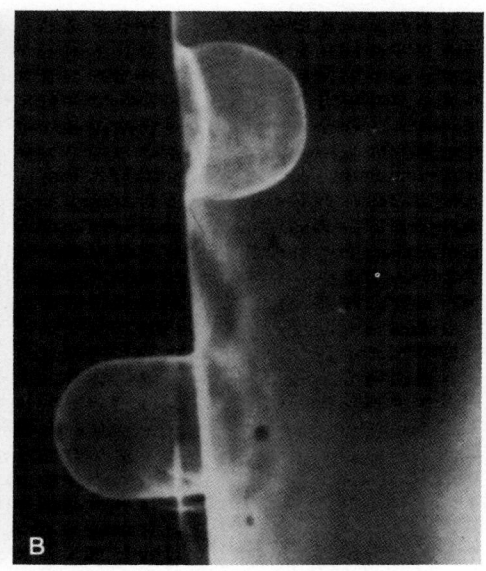

and allows more confident detection of polyps in the presence of multiple diverticula.[41]

Caliber and haustral abnormalities (Fig. 61–8) usually accompany and often antedate the appearance of diverticula, particularly in the sigmoid colon. Haustral clefts usually are symmetric and face one another in the sigmoid; however, in diverticular or prediverticular disease, they indent alternately from one border to another, creating a staggered effect. The circular muscle is hypertonic and thickened, and the taeniae contract.[30] Diverticula originate at the top of the haustra. With progressive disease, the circular muscle continues to undergo hypertrophy, and a "concertina" or zigzag appearance develops. This appearance is due to the alternated, highly compact, deep, and uniform haustra that separate and segment the haustral cul-de-sacs.[30]

## Computed Tomography

Computed tomography (CT) reveals mural thickening of the colon (>4 mm) in myochosis and in most cases of diverticulosis. The diverticula appear as outpouchings that contain air (Fig. 61–9) and that can usually be differentiated from pneumatosis.[42]

# DIVERTICULITIS

## Epidemiology

Diverticulitis is the most common complication of diverticulosis, occurring in 10 to 20% of patients with *known* diverticulosis. In one longitudinal study, clinical

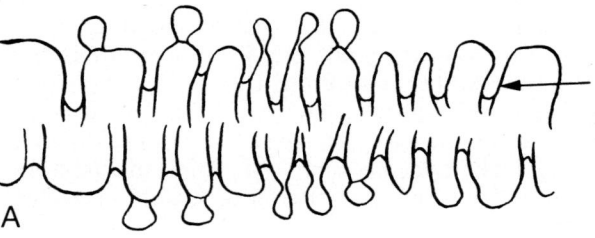
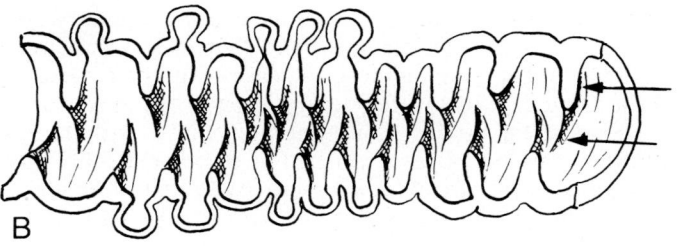

**Figure 61–8. Colonic myochosis. A.** The thickened circular muscle *(arrow)* and shortened taeniae lead to a concertina appearance. **B.** Longitudinal section of the same sigmoid segment shows narrowing of the lumen and prominent haustra *(arrows),* which are staggered in configuration. (**A** and **B** from Weissman A, Clot M, Grellet J: Double Contrast Examination of the Colon. Berlin: Springer-Verlag, 1985, p 150.)

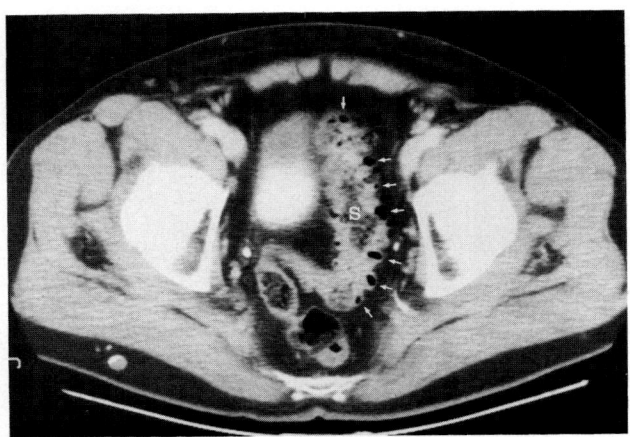

**Figure 61–9. Diverticulosis of the sigmoid colon: CT appearance.** The sigmoid (S) colon demonstrates multiple outpouchings filled with air *(arrows).* No inflammation is seen in the surrounding fat.

diverticulitis was evident in 10% of those patients followed for 5 years and in 37% of those followed for 11 to 18 years. The chance of developing diverticulitis increases if the diverticula are widely distributed, are more numerous than average, and have been present for more than one decade.[4–6, 43–45]

## Pathologic Findings

The stagnation of nonsterile inspissated fecal material within the diverticulum can cause inflammatory erosion of the mucosal lining in early, subclinical stages of diverticulitis. Subsequently, the muscular wall of the diverticulum is eroded. This perforation is the essential feature of diverticulitis.[46–47]

This sequence of events can involve an intramural diverticulum, leading to the formation of an intramural abscess (Fig. 61–10). More commonly, it occurs extramurally within the pericolic fat, leading to fibrinous exudate, abscess formation, local adhesions, or peritonitis. During surgery and pathologic examination, many juxtacolic abscesses are small and difficult to find in the mass of indurated fat and fibrous tissue. It is important to emphasize that the inflammation begins at the apex of the diverticulum, and that it may spread rapidly into the soft pericolic and mesocolic fat. The inflammatory changes in diverticulitis are therefore mainly pericolic, adjacent but outside the bowel wall.[1–4, 46, 47]

The colonic mucosa is not affected in diverticulitis except in the region of the erosion. Fleischner and Ming[17] and Fleischner[20] showed that most inflammatory complications of clinical significance are secondary to the rupture of a diverticulum, and that they occur in a pericolic location in almost all cases. In their series, these complications were present in 65% of the surgical specimens examined. Consequently, these pathologic changes may be better described as peridiverticulitis or pericolitis. True diverticulitis, with inflammation limited to the diverticular lining, was present in 10% of pathologic specimens, and muscular hypertrophy with distor-

tion alone and without inflammation accounted for the remaining 25% of cases.[17, 20]

The consequences of diverticular rupture depend on the host response and virulence of the bacterial contamination. Most patients develop sealed-off abscesses or contained sinus tracts and fistulas. Free perforations are uncommon but can lead to localized pelvic or generalized peritonitis. Fistulas involve adjacent structures, such as small bowel, urinary bladder, vagina, and anterior abdominal wall. Occasionally, several adjacent diverticula communicate with each other along the outer aspect of the deep muscular layers, forming an intramural fistulous tract (Fig. 61–11). In other cases, fistulas extend deeply into the fatty tissue at the site of the attachment of the sigmoid mesocolon.

## Clinical Findings

The classic clinical features of sigmoid diverticulitis are left lower quadrant pain, tenderness, fever, and leukocytosis. Because of this clinical constellation, sigmoid diverticulitis has been called "left-sided appendicitis." Diverticulitis occurring in other colonic locations is more difficult to diagnose clinically. In one review,

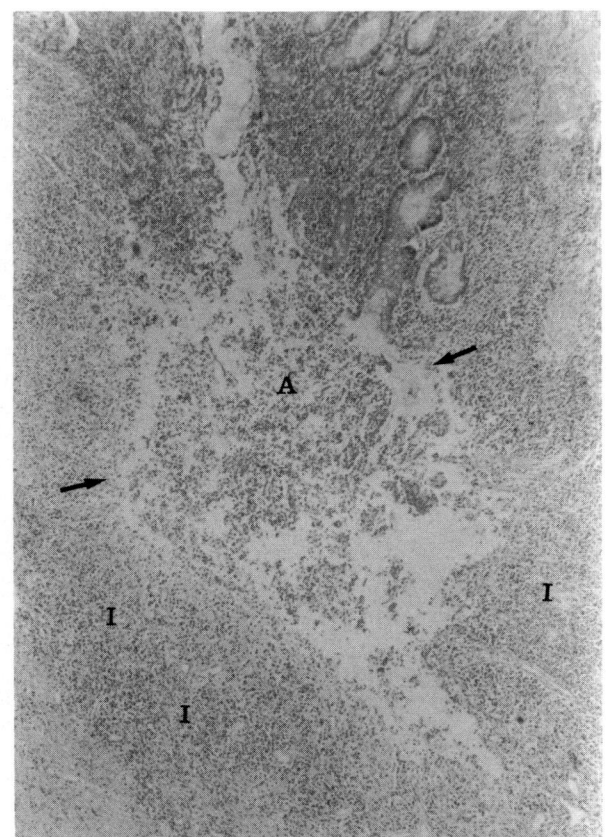

**Figure 61–10. Acute intramural diverticulitis.** This intramural diverticulum is replaced by an abscess (A) that destroys and replaces the herniated mucosal layer *(arrows).* Extensive inflammatory infiltration (I) is present around the abscess (hematoxylin-eosin, × 100).

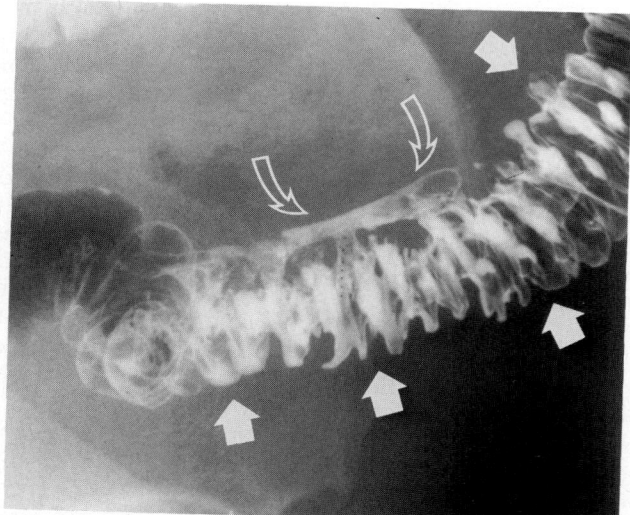

**Figure 61–11. Pericolic fistulous tract in diverticulitis.** Sigmoid colon shows diverticula and a serrated irregular contour consistent with myochosis *(solid arrows)*. A long fistulous tract connecting several ruptured diverticula *(open arrows)* is parallel to the sigmoid colon at the site of the sigmoid mesocolon attachment.

the following clinical features were noted: pain in the left iliac fossa in 85% of patients; palpable mass, tenderness, and muscle guarding in 48%; fever in 30%; vomiting in less than 50%; and partial obstruction in 20%. Mild bleeding occurred in 25% of patients, and about one third of patients had a history of recurrent episodes of similar attacks. Surgical evaluation of this group of 258 patients showed a 20% incidence of pericolic abscess, an 8% incidence of fistulas, and an 18% incidence of peritonitis (Fig. 61–12). The initial clinical diagnosis was sigmoid carcinoma in 32% of patients, but carcinoma was found in only 2% of patients. The occurrence of malignancy was entirely coincidental, but it highlights the clinical difficulties of diagnosing and evaluating patients with suspected acute diverticulitis.[46] These difficulties are further documented by large surgical series of patients with a clinical diagnosis of acute diverticulitis, in whom 25 to 33% of the resected surgical specimens showed no active inflammation, abscess, or fistulas.[18, 47]

Severe diverticulitis can occur in certain groups of patients and produce only minimal or unremarkable clinical symptoms: debilitated elderly patients; patients who have renal failure, are undergoing dialysis, or have had renal transplantation, and patients receiving corticosteroids. Disease in these patients may progress to free perforation, and the diagnosis is often made only when free intra-abdominal air is detected on abdominal films.[48–53]

Younger individuals (<40 years old) often develop severe forms of diverticulitis. In the study of 17 young patients by Freischlag and colleagues, 15 (88%) required emergency surgery for acute complications, and in 13 (76%) of the patients, surgery was required during the first attack.[54] The reasons for this clinical presentation are obscure. Several other observers have also empha-

sized that in young people, the initial attack of colonic diverticulitis is frequently severe.[55–57]

The clinical management of patients with acute diverticulitis depends on the severity, type, and extent of the pericolic inflammatory changes. Mild forms of disease are managed medically with antibiotic therapy. In more severe forms, surgical resection is indicated, either at the time of the diagnosis or after a "cooling-off" interval of antibiotic therapy and percutaneous abscess drainage. Surgery is performed in about 20% of patients admitted to the hospital for diverticulitis and is indicated for the management of abscess, colonic obstruction, perforation and fistula, and hemorrhage that cannot be treated by interventional radiologic methods.[4–6]

Close clinical and radiologic evaluation is crucial in the triage of patients to conservative, radiologic, or surgical management. The radiologic investigation of these patients has two objectives: 1) to confirm the clinical suspicion of diverticulitis and rule out other colonic or pelvic disease, and 2) to evaluate and stage the severity of the inflammatory disease. Sigmoidoscopy is usually contraindicated and serves no useful purpose except in patients who have more chronic forms of disease and present with bleeding, or in patients in whom polyps or sigmoid carcinoma is suspected.

## Radiologic Findings

### Plain Films

Abdominal films taken with the patient supine and upright are usually diagnostic only in the most severe forms of diverticulitis, in which the patient presents with free intraperitoneal air or sealed-off perforations and

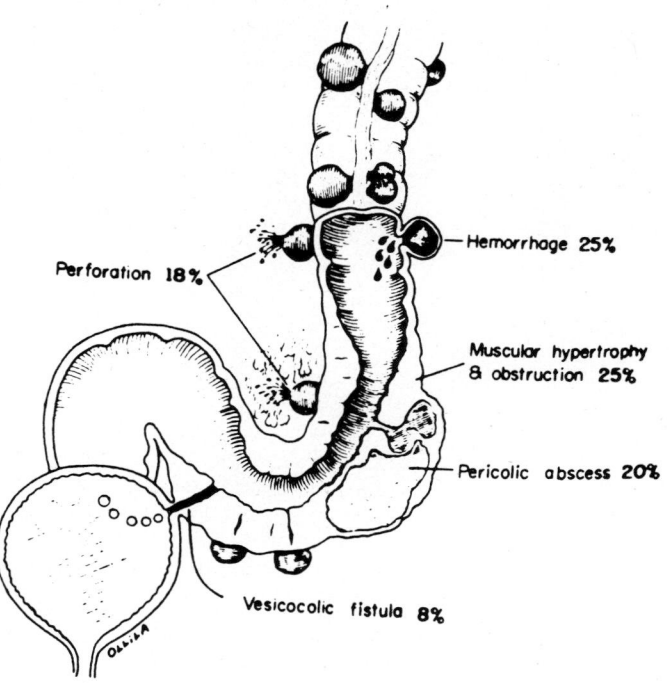

**Figure 61–12. The complications of diverticulitis.**

pelvic extraluminal air. The detection of an ill-defined, left-sided pelvic mass, localized ileus, and fluid in the pelvis suggests the diagnosis in the appropriate clinical setting. In most patients with acute diverticulitis, however, abdominal plain films are unremarkable and do not contribute to the diagnosis.[31, 34, 58–61]

## Contrast Enema Examination

Contrast enema (CE) examination has traditionally been the primary method of examining patients with suspected diverticulitis.[62, 63] It superbly depicts diverticula, the colonic mucosa and lumen, spasm, muscle hypertrophy, and sacculations. These findings, however, are indicative of diverticular disease but not diagnostic of acute diverticulitis. Because this procedure primarily evaluates the colonic lumen and mucosal surface, the pericolic inflammatory process present in most patients with diverticulitis can only be indirectly inferred (Fig. 61–13).

A specific diagnosis of perforated diverticulitis can be made only when there is extravasation of contrast material from a diverticulum into a walled-off abscess, sinus tract, or fistula (see Fig. 61–11), or free extravasation of contrast material into the peritoneal cavity.

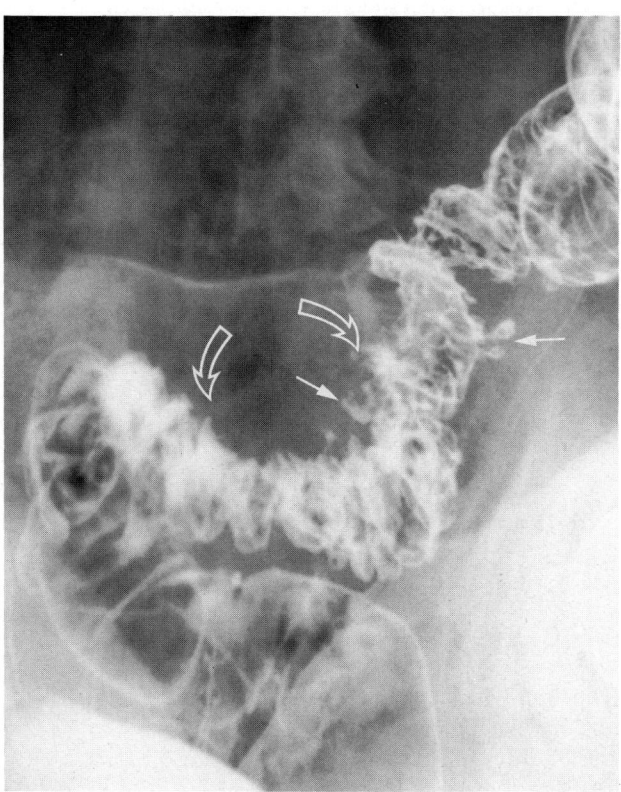

**Figure 61–13. Barium enema in sigmoid diverticulitis.** Multiple small diverticula are present in the sigmoid colon *(solid arrows)*. The sigmoid colon is fixed in the pelvis, has an asymmetric contour, and appears to be compressed by an extrinsic mass *(open arrows)*. The severity, extracolic extension, and chronicity of the inflammatory process cannot be evaluated.

These extraluminal collections of contrast medium vary in size, are usually located adjacent to the colon, compress and displace the colonic wall, and are detected in less than 50% of cases of diverticular perforation.[30–34, 62, 63]

Narrowing of the sigmoid lumen, extrinsic compression, and spasm are present in more than 80% of patients, but these findings are less specific (see Fig. 61–13). Similarly, an altered mucosal pattern is present in 68% of patients, but it is not a reliable indicator of acute inflammation (see Fig. 61–13). Lack of mobility with fixation of the sigmoid colon and narrowing, pointing, and distortion of individual diverticula are indirect signs consistent with either acute or chronic diverticulitis.

A contour defect that is smooth, well defined, and associated with adjacent sigmoid diverticula represents an intramural inflammatory mass (Fig. 61–14). The contents of the intramural mass, whether pus, organized abscess, or merely mural fibrosis, are more difficult to characterize (see Fig. 61–14).

Tracts filled with contrast material passing from ruptured diverticula into the pericolic tissues are commonly seen.[64] They may be single or multiple, end blindly (sinuses) (Figs. 61–15 and 61–16), or connect with an adjacent hollow viscus or abdominal wall (fistulas) (Fig. 61–17). The most common fistulas are colovesical and coloenteric. Colocutaneous fistulas are less frequent and are clinically associated with subcutaneous abscess, emphysema, or fasciitis. Fistulas to the vagina, ureter, appendix, hip, perineum, and soft tissues of the thigh have also been reported.[65–68] With CE, the fistulous tract between the colon and urinary bladder is visualized in only 20% of patients who have colovesical fistulas.[65, 68]

Longitudinal intramural fistulous tracts represent ruptured diverticula that communicate with each other (see Fig. 61–11). Although this sign has also been reported in carcinoma of the colon and Crohn's disease, longitudinal intramural fistulous tracts most often are due to diverticulitis unless there is a previous history or radiographic evidence of Crohn's disease in the remainder of the colon or terminal ileum.[69–72]

### Differentiation of Diverticulitis from Carcinoma

The detection of partial colonic obstruction with sigmoid narrowing, a gradual zone of transition, preservation of the mucosal folds, and associated diverticula are other CE findings indicating diverticulitis (see Fig. 61–17). Abrupt transition at the site of obstruction, a rigid, narrowed lumen, destruction of mucosa, and "apple core" configuration are diagnostic for carcinoma of the colon. CE is valuable in differentiating diverticulitis from carcinoma of the sigmoid colon in most cases. The presence of sigmoid diverticula, however, is not helpful in the differential diagnosis, because 28% of sigmoid cancers involve coincidental diverticula.[72] When the retrograde flow of contrast medium is impeded and the obstructed sigmoid lumen cannot be well visualized, the differentiation of an inflammatory lesion from a malignant lesion cannot be made (Fig. 61–18).

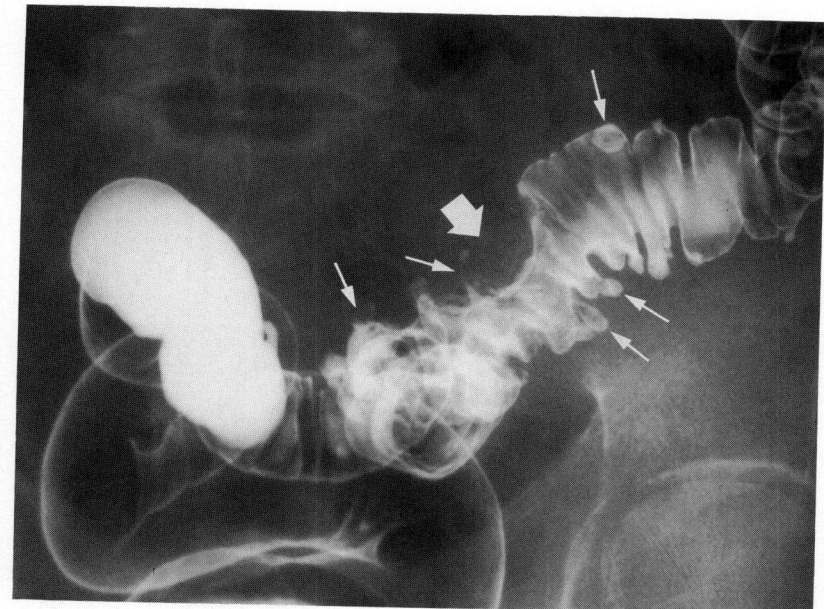

**Figure 61–14. Intramural abscess in sigmoid diverticulitis.** Several diverticula are visualized in a distorted sigmoid colon *(narrow arrows)* that has an irregular contour. A smooth contour defect is present along its superior border *(wide arrow)*, secondary to abscess formation.

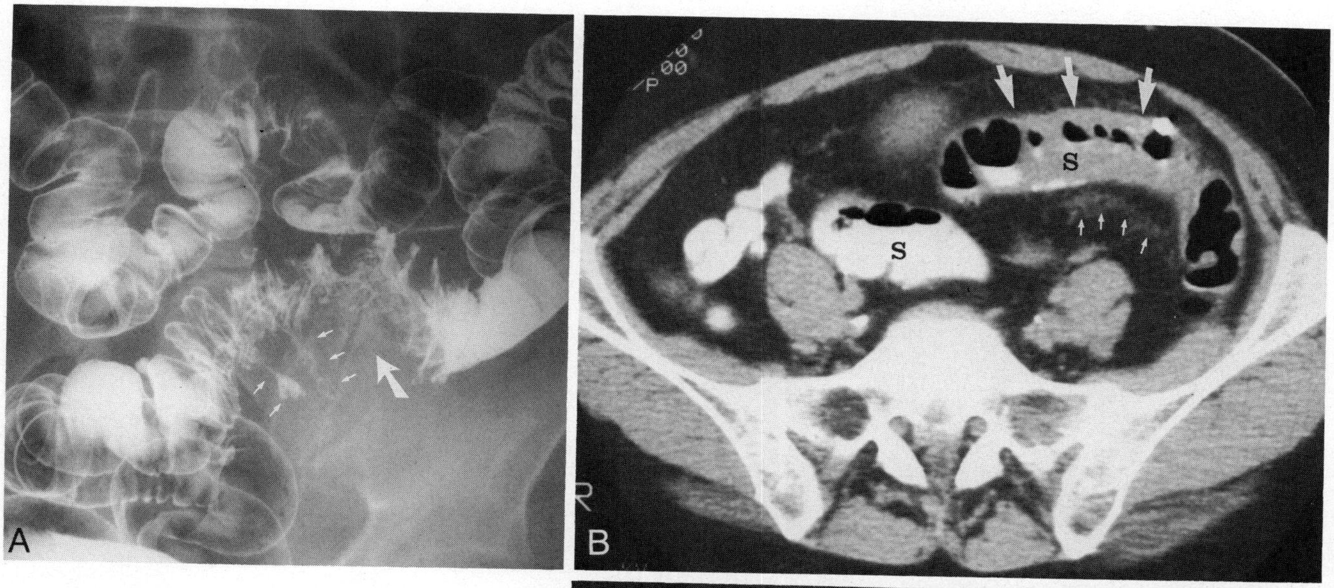

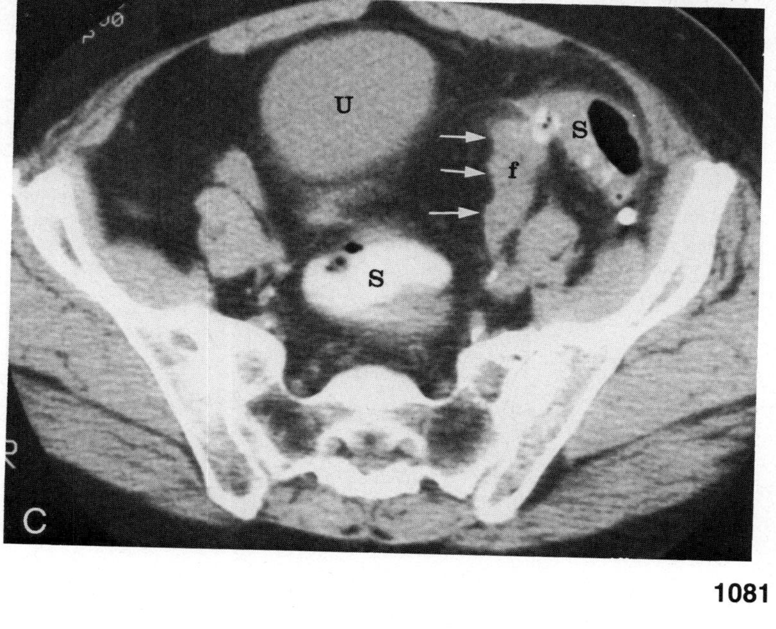

**Figure 61–15. Diverticulitis with sinus tract. A.** The sigmoid colon shows several diverticula and a normal mucosal surface on this barium enema. There is suggestion of an extrinsic mass compressing and displacing the inferior wall of the sigmoid colon *(large arrow)*. Note the narrow sinus tracts *(small arrows)* extending inferiorly. The chronicity or severity of the inflammatory process cannot be characterized. **B.** CT reveals symmmetric mural thickening of the sigmoid colon *(large arrows)* and only mild chronic inflammation in the sigmoid mesocolon *(small arrows)*. Sigmoid lumen (S) is filled with residual barium and air. **C.** CT scan obtained at a slightly lower level shows a thick, fluid-filled fistulous (f) tract *(arrows)*. There is no acute inflammation or abscess. The CT findings were documented at surgery. S = sigmoid; U = urinary bladder.

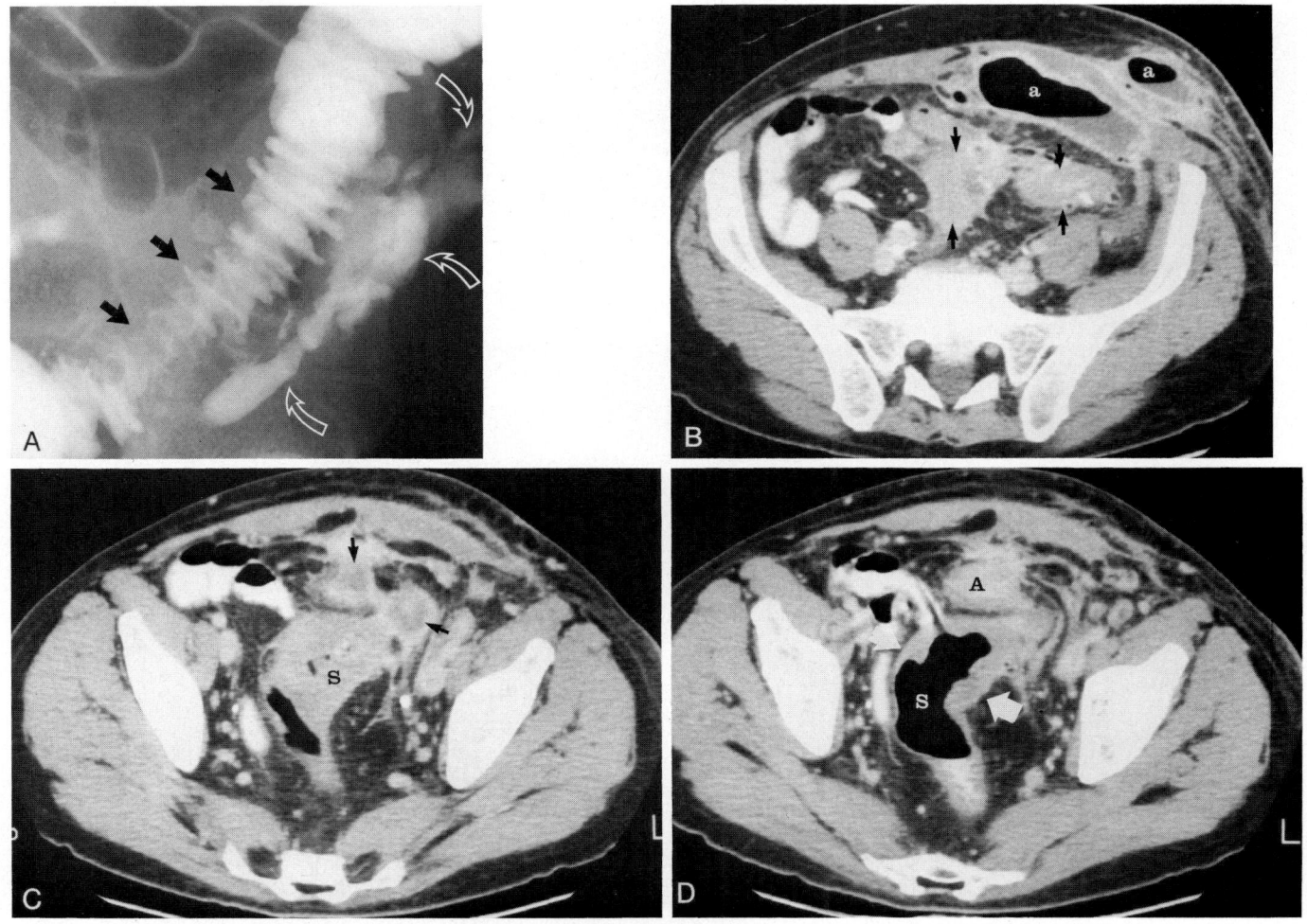

**Figure 61–16. Diverticulitis with sigmoid-cutaneous fistula and pelvic abscess. A.** Diatrizoate meglumine (Hypaque) enema shows myochosis *(solid arrows)* and sigmoid diverticula typical for diverticular disease. There is gross extravasation of contrast material adjacent to the sigmoid colon *(open arrows).* **B.** CT reveals a subcutaneous abscess communicating with an adjacent, anterior pelvic abscess (a). In addition, poorly encapsulated fluid collections (abscesses) are present in the midpelvis *(arrows).* **C.** Other poorly encapsulated abscesses *(arrows)* are adjacent to the thick-walled sigmoid colon (S). The lumen of the sigmoid is not well visualized and the degree and the cause of mural thickening are not certain. **D.** Thickening of the wall of the sigmoid colon (S) is secondary to inflammation and muscle hypertrophy *(arrows).* The abscesses (A) were percutaneously drained, and the patient underwent a one-stage surgical resection.

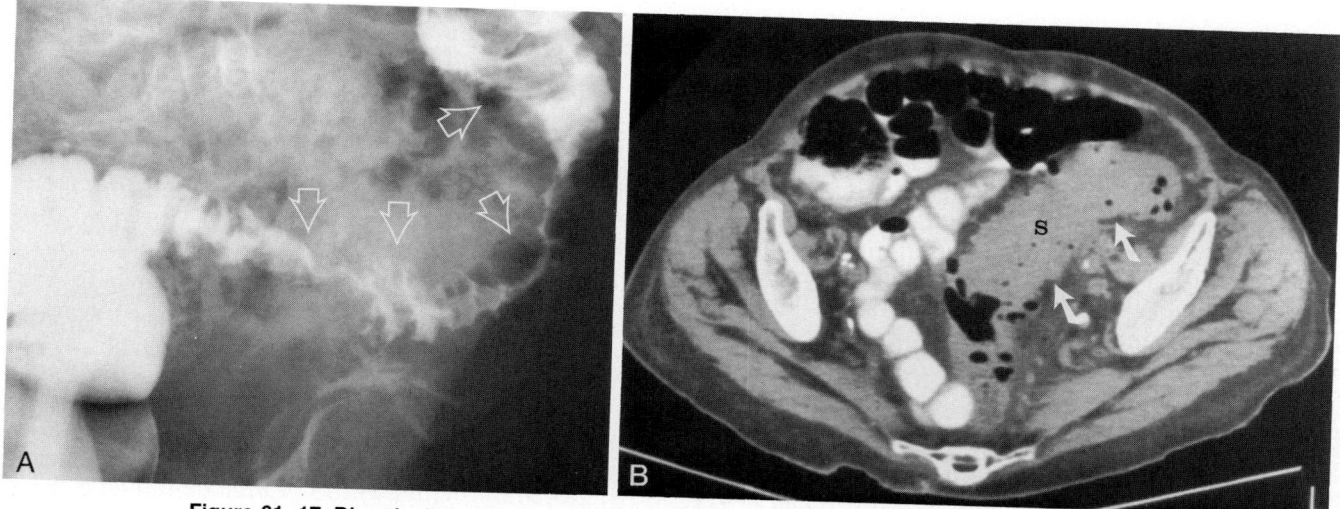

**Figure 61–17. Diverticulitis diagnosed with CE. A.** The sigmoid colon is narrowed and spastic but shows preservation of the mucosal pattern *(arrows)*. The extent of extracolic inflammation is uncertain. **B.** CT reveals mural thickening *(arrows)* of the sigmoid colon (S). The sigmoid lumen is not visualized, and the degree and nature of wall thickening cannot be determined without sigmoid distention by contrast medium or air. No abscess is visualized in the pelvis.

### Advantages and Limitations

Advantages of CE in the diagnosis of diverticulitis are its widespread availability, relatively low cost, and high accuracy in differentiating inflammatory from neoplastic colonic lesions. Other disorders, including Crohn's disease, ulcerative or ischemic colitis, intussusception, and volvulus, can be diagnosed in individuals with similar complaints.

The limitations of CE are related to its low sensitivity in diagnosing mild to moderate forms of acute diverticulitis. Particularly disappointing is its inability to evaluate the presence, type, and extent of the pericolic inflammatory process, which is the hallmark of acute diverticulitis (see Figs. 61–5 and 61–7 to 61–9).

### Ultrasound

Although CT is the primary cross-sectional imaging study for patients with suspected diverticulitis, ultrasound may be the first study ordered for nondescript abdominal pain.[73]

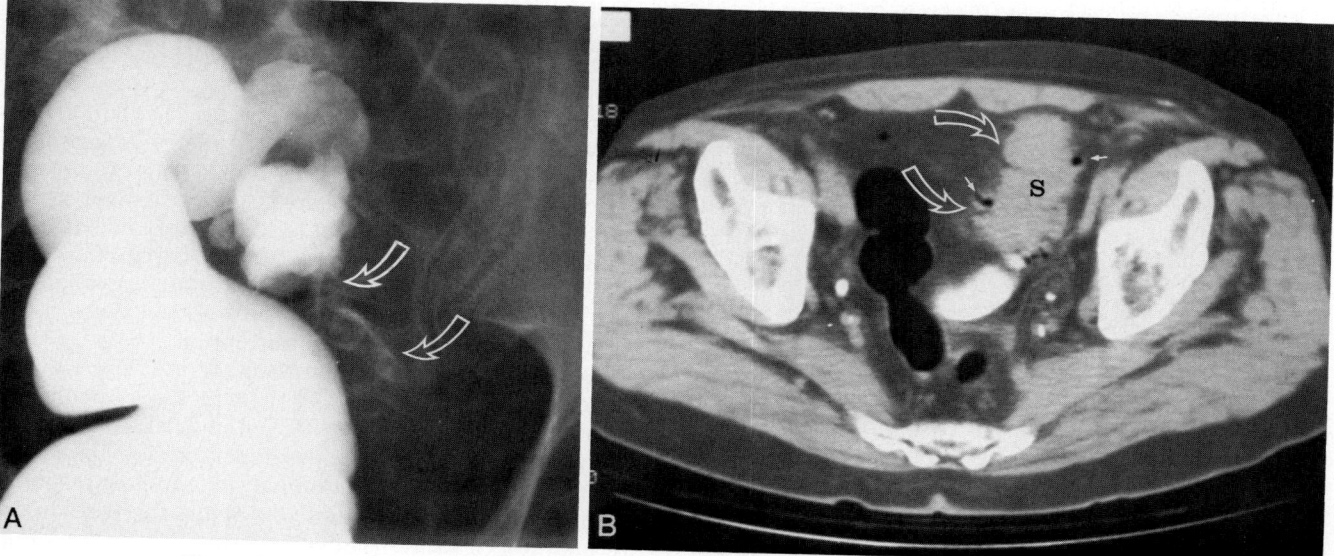

**Figure 61–18. Colonic obstruction in sigmoid diverticulitis. A.** Hypaque enema shows sigmoid obstruction with an abrupt zone of transition between normal lumen and stricture *(arrows)*. These findings mimic sigmoid carcinoma. **B.** CT reveals several air-filled sigmoid diverticula *(small arrows)* and mural thickening of the sigmoid (S), simulating a mass *(large arrows)*. The sigmoid lumen is not visualized, and carcinoma cannot be excluded. Pathologic evaluation revealed chronic diverticulitis with muscle hypertrophy.

The segmental concentric thickening of the gut wall commonly found in patients with diverticular disease manifests as a hypoechoic segment that reflects the predominant thickening of the muscular layer (Fig. 61–19). Inflamed diverticula are brightly echogenic reflectors with acoustic shadowing or ring-down artifact in or beyond the thickened gut wall. Inflammatory changes in the mesocolon are seen as poorly defined, hypoechoic zones without obvious gas or fluid. Intramural sinus tracts appear as high-amplitude linear echoes that often have ring-down artifact within the colon wall. Abscesses appear as loculated, thick-walled fluid collections that may contain gas.[73–76]

## Computed Tomography

Abdominal CT has dramatically improved the diagnosis and management of patients with diverticulitis. CT is ideally suited for evaluating both the intramural component of the inflammatory process and its intraperitoneal or retroperitoneal extension. CT is particularly useful in the evaluation of patients with sepsis who present with left lower quadrant pain, fever, leukocytosis, and a tender palpable pelvic mass.[77–83]

### Technique

Bowel preparation and opacification for abdominal CT are discussed in detail in Chapter 8. The following is a modification of these procedures that is useful in patients with suspected diverticulitis. Unless contraindication exists, patients receive a rapid bolus of intravenous injection of 50 mL of 43% iodinated contrast material at a rate of 1.5 mL/s followed by 150 mL at 0.8 mL/s. Dynamic, sequential, transaxial 10 × 10 mm sections are obtained over the entire abdomen. Approx-

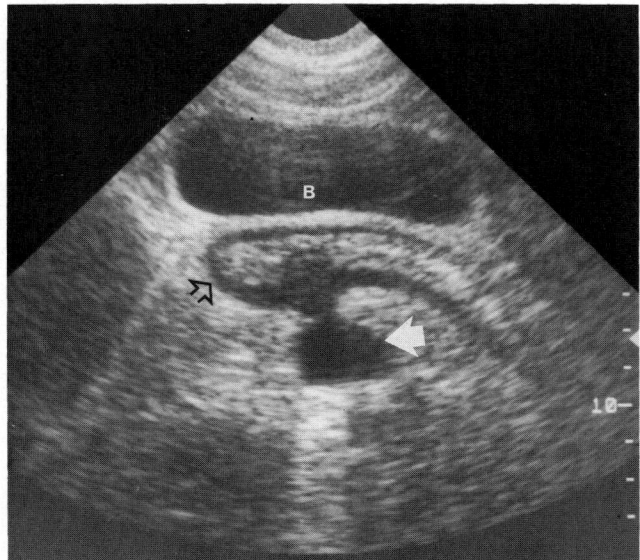

**Figure 61–19. Diverticulitis: ultrasound appearance.** A hypoechoic collection *(solid arrow)* adjacent to the thick-walled sigmoid colon *(open arrow)*. This appearance represents a small, pericolic abscess. B = bladder.

### TABLE 61–1. COMPUTED TOMOGRAPHIC FINDINGS IN DIVERTICULITIS

Detection of sigmoid diverticula
Inflammatory reaction, phlegmon, or abscess in pericolic fat
Circumferential slight thickening of colonic wall
Pericolic sinuses or fistulas
Inflamed sigmoid colon with associated pelvic abscess or peritonitis
Intramural abscess and/or intramural fistulous tract
Induration with thickening of the root of the sigmoid mesocolon

imately 60 minutes before scanning, 800 to 1000 mL of 2% dilute barium (E-Z-Cat) or water-soluble contrast medium (diatrizoate meglumine [Gastrografin]) is administered orally. If there are no peritoneal signs, air insufflation of the rectum is performed after 0.5 mL of glucagon is intravenously administered. Patients are monitored during the entire examination, and if the CT findings are equivocal, pelvic scans that are 5 mm thick and spaced 5 mm apart are repeated over the region of interest. At this time, rectal air insufflation may be repeated for better visualization and distention of the sigmoid lumen. Elective CT scanning is performed after an adequate 24-hour preparation of the colon, which is similar to that used in barium enema examination. Patients with acute symptoms receive no prior preparation, and small bowel opacification is achieved with a 1 to 2% solution of Gastrografin.

### Findings

CT findings in acute diverticulitis are listed in Table 61–1.[78] Diverticula are identified on CT scans at the site of the perforation or at a site adjacent to it in more than 80% of cases of acute diverticulitis. They appear as small outpouchings filled with air, barium, and/or fecal material projecting through the colonic wall (see Fig. 61–9). Symmetric thickening of the colonic wall in excess of 4 mm is seen in about 70% of cases. The thickened wall has a homogeneous density, and its diameter usually measures less than 1 cm in the distended colon (Fig. 61–20). When there is significant muscular hypertrophy, the wall of the colon can measure up to 2 or 3 cm in thickness (Fig. 61–21). In diverticulitis, significant hypertrophy of muscle primarily occurs in the sigmoid segment, and this can mimic carcinoma of the colon (see Fig. 61–17B). It is important to remember that accurate assessment of colon wall thickness is possible only with proper lumen distention.

The hallmark of acute diverticulitis on CT scans is the presence of inflammatory change in the pericolic fat. This sign is seen in 98% of patients. The degree of inflammatory reaction varies, depending on the size of perforation, bacterial contamination, and host response. In mild cases, there is only a slight increase in the attenuation of fat adjacent to the involved colon (Figs. 61–22 to 61–24). Fine linear strands, small fluid collections, and several bubbles of extraluminal air may be present (see Figs. 61–22 to 61–24). In more severe cases, pericolic heterogeneous soft tissue densities representing phlegmons and/or partially loculated fluid col-

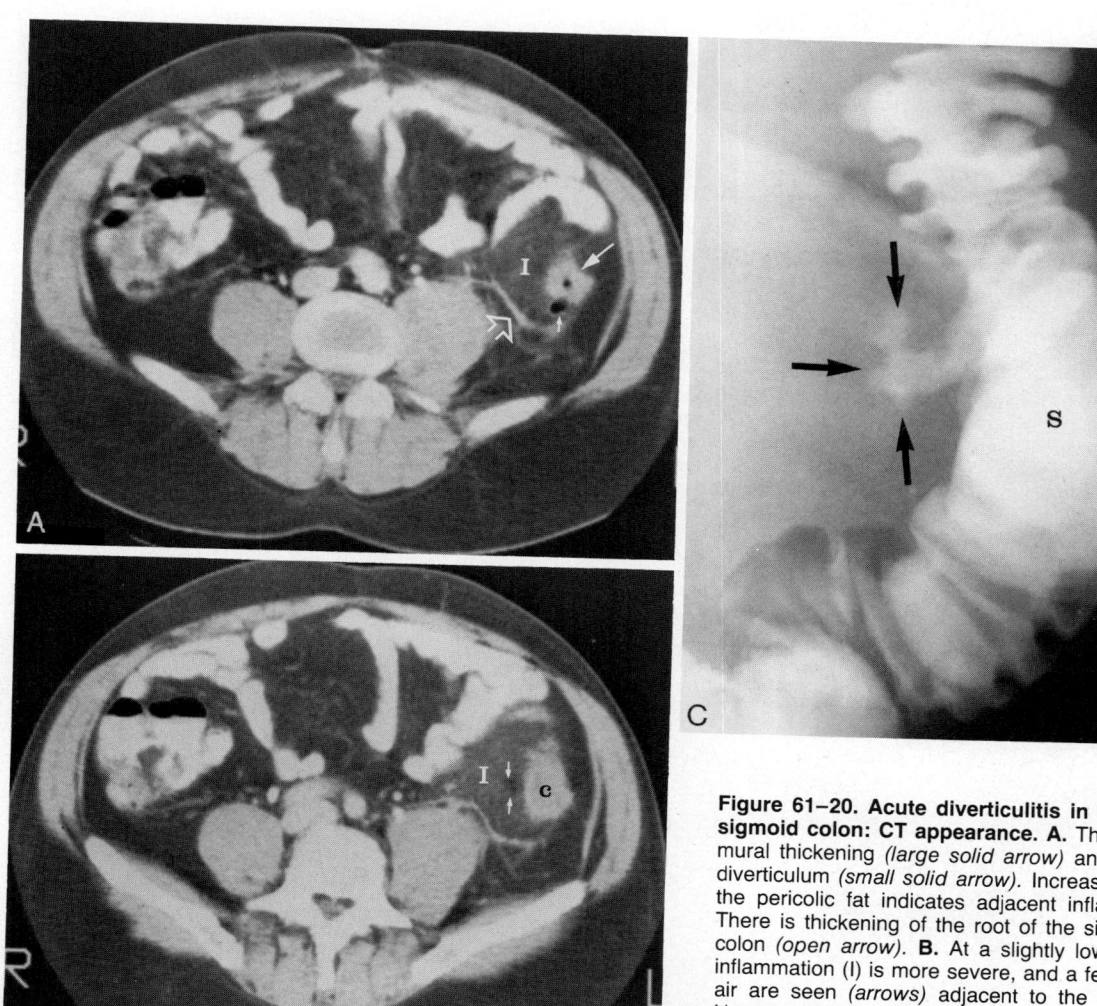

**Figure 61–20. Acute diverticulitis in the proximal sigmoid colon: CT appearance. A.** There are slight mural thickening *(large solid arrow)* and an air-filled diverticulum *(small solid arrow)*. Increased density of the pericolic fat indicates adjacent inflammation (I). There is thickening of the root of the sigmoid meso-colon *(open arrow)*. **B.** At a slightly lower level, the inflammation (I) is more severe, and a few bubbles of air are seen *(arrows)* adjacent to the colon (c). **C.** Hypaque enema confirms the diagnosis of a ruptured, sealed-off, sigmoid (S) diverticulum *(arrows)*.

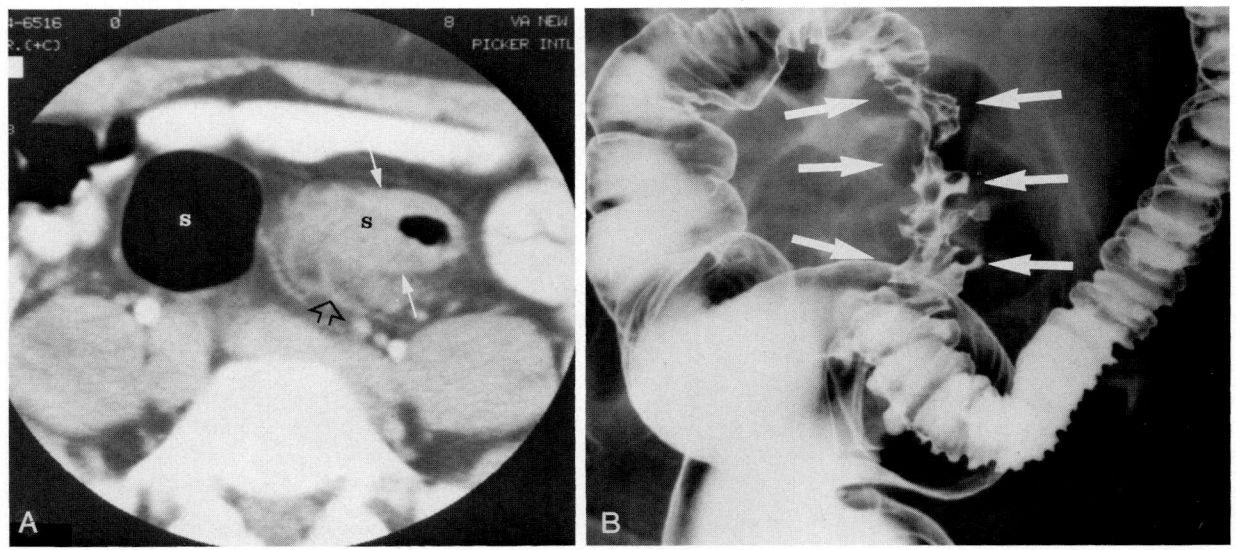

**Figure 61–21. Diverticulitis with significant muscular hypertrophy. A.** CT scan shows circumferential thickening of the left limb of the sigmoid (black s) colon *(solid arrows)*. There is only mild juxtacolic inflammation *(open arrow)*. The right limb of sigmoid colon (air filled and distended) has a normal, thin wall (white s). **B.** Barium enema confirms the CT findings. Narrowing, distortion, and diverticula are present only in the left limb of the sigmoid colon *(arrows)*. The distal sigmoid colon is normal.

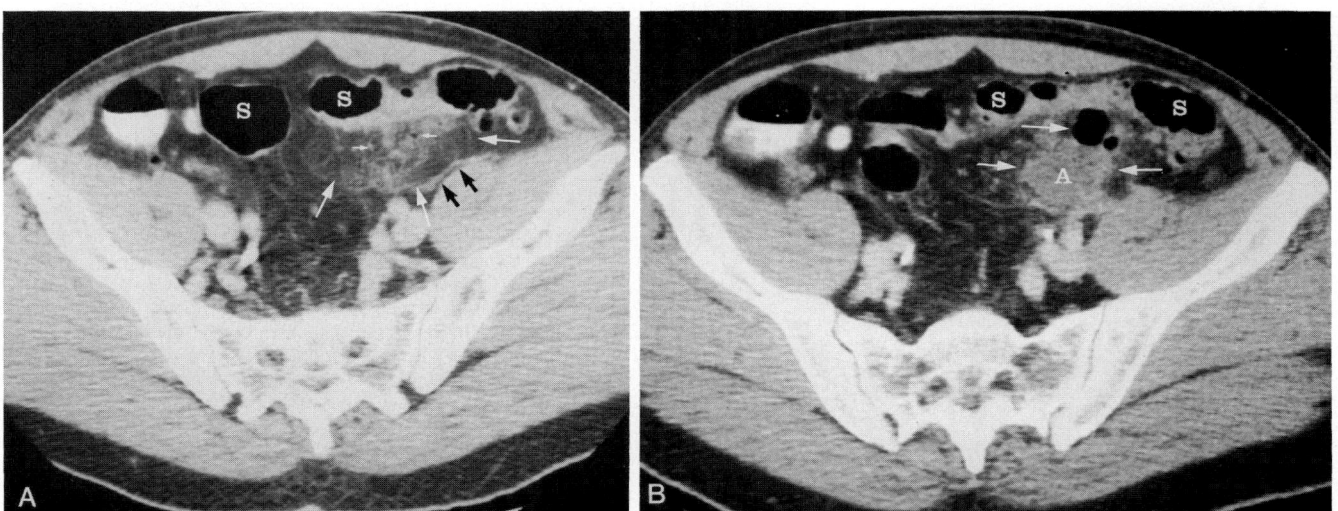

**Figure 61–22. CT of acute diverticulitis: progression to abscess. A.** Initial CT examination reveals inflammatory changes in the sigmoid mesocolon *(large white arrows)*. Induration of the root of the mesocolon is seen *(black arrows)*. Several air bubbles *(small white arrows)* are adjacent to a slightly thick-walled sigmoid colon (S). **B.** Follow-up CT examination 10 days after antibiotic therapy reveals the development of an air- and fluid-filled abscess (A) in the mesocolon *(arrows)*. These findings were confirmed at surgery. S = sigmoid colon.

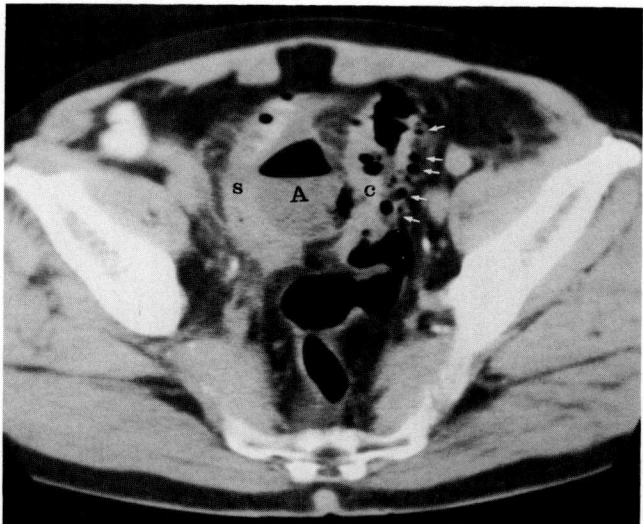

**Figure 61–23. Pelvic abscess secondary to sigmoid diverticulitis.** CT reveals an air- and fluid-filled pelvic abscess (A) sealed off by the sigmoid colon (c) and a small bowel loop (s). Multiple air-filled diverticula are visualized *(arrows).*

lections representing abscess can occur (see Figs. 61–22 and 61–23).

On CT scans, abscesses appear filled with fluid and may contain bubbles of air or air-fluid levels (see Fig. 61–23). These collections can form at a distance from the involved segment of colon. They may form at the flank, groin, thigh, psoas muscle, subphrenic space, or liver. Most abscesses are contained within the sigmoid mesocolon (see Fig. 61–22) or are sealed off by the sigmoid colon and adjacent small bowel loops (see Fig. 61–23).

Acute or chronic inflammation of the sigmoid mesocolon causes induration and thickening of the root,

which results in an oblique, linear density in the left side of the pelvis on CT scans (see Figs. 61–22 and 61–24). Although not pathognomonic, this finding is highly suggestive of sigmoid diverticulitis.

Free diverticular perforation results in extravasation of air and fluid into the pelvis and peritoneal cavity. On CT scans, fluid-containing floating bubbles of air are seen adjacent to the perforated sigmoid colon (see Fig. 61–24). These CT findings signify peritonitis and represent a surgical emergency.

When high-resolution CT techniques are used, small, 1 to 2-cm intramural fluid collections representing intramural abscesses can be detected (Fig. 61–25). Intramural or pericolic fistulas can be recognized as linear fluid-filled tracts within or parallel to the thickened colonic wall. Blind sinus tracts and fistulas manifest as linear or tubular branching structures in the pericolic tissues (see Fig. 61–15). They can communicate with adjacent organs or terminate in an abscess cavity. Although CT has limited value in the detection of coloenteric fistulas, it is extremely useful in the evaluation of patients with suspected colovesical fistulas. In these patients, the pericolic inflammatory mass involves the bladder wall, and the presence of intraluminal air confirms the diagnosis[84–87] (Fig. 61–26).

## Surgical and Computed Tomography Staging

Diverticulitis can be staged both surgically and by CT scanning. Familiarity with the following staging system helps in directing therapy and assessing prognosis[88–93] (Figs. 61–27 to 61–31).

*Stage 0 diverticulitis* is the most common form of diverticulitis, in which the inflammation is contained within the serosa. This mural inflammation usually re-

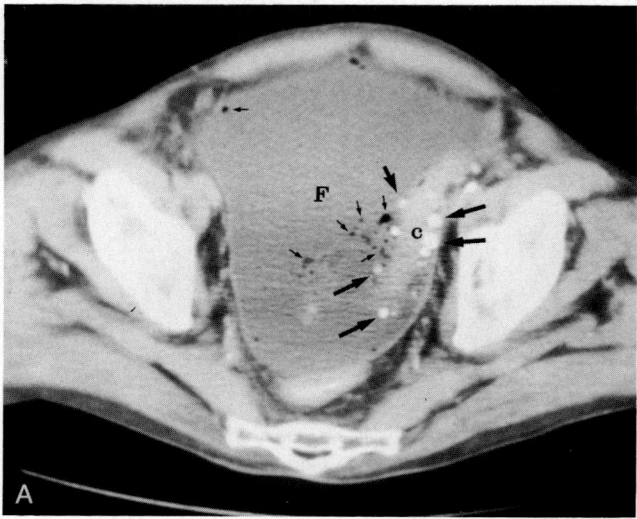 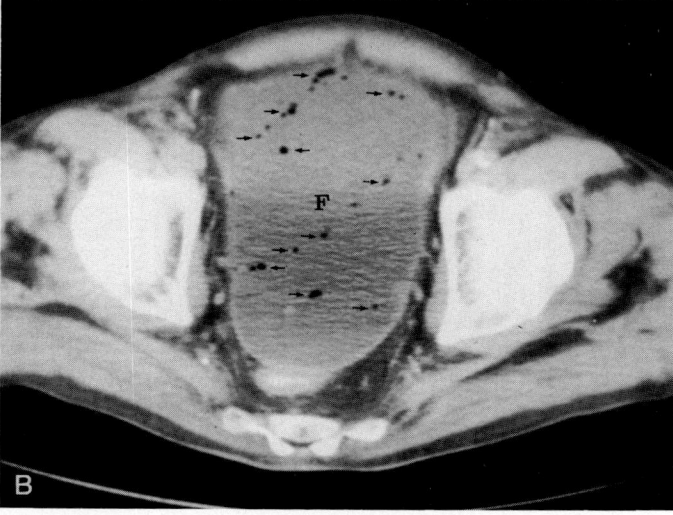

**Figure 61–24. Peritonitis secondary to diverticulitis.** Frank perforation into the peritoneal cavity is present in this 44-year-old male undergoing hemodialysis. **A.** Sigmoid colon (c) contains diverticula filled with contrast medium *(large arrows)*. F = fluid in peritoneal cavity; small arrows = multiple air bubbles. **B.** A large amount of free fluid (F) containing multiple air bubbles *(arrows)* is present in the pelvis.

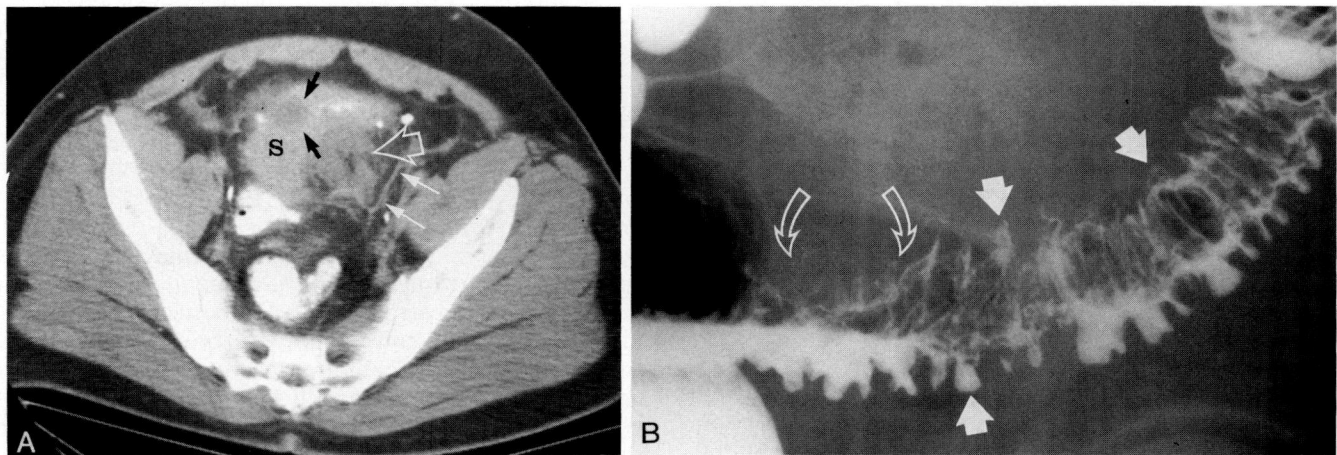

**Figure 61–25. Intramural abscess in sigmoid diverticulitis. A.** CT scan shows an ill-defined fluid collection *(black arrows)* within the wall of the sigmoid colon (S). Associated phlegmon is posterior to the sigmoid colon *(open arrow)*. In addition, there is thickening of the root of the sigmoid mesocolon *(white arrows)*. **B.** Barium enema reveals diverticula *(solid arrows)* and a contour defect along the superior border of sigmoid colon that represents the intramural abscess *(open arrows)*.

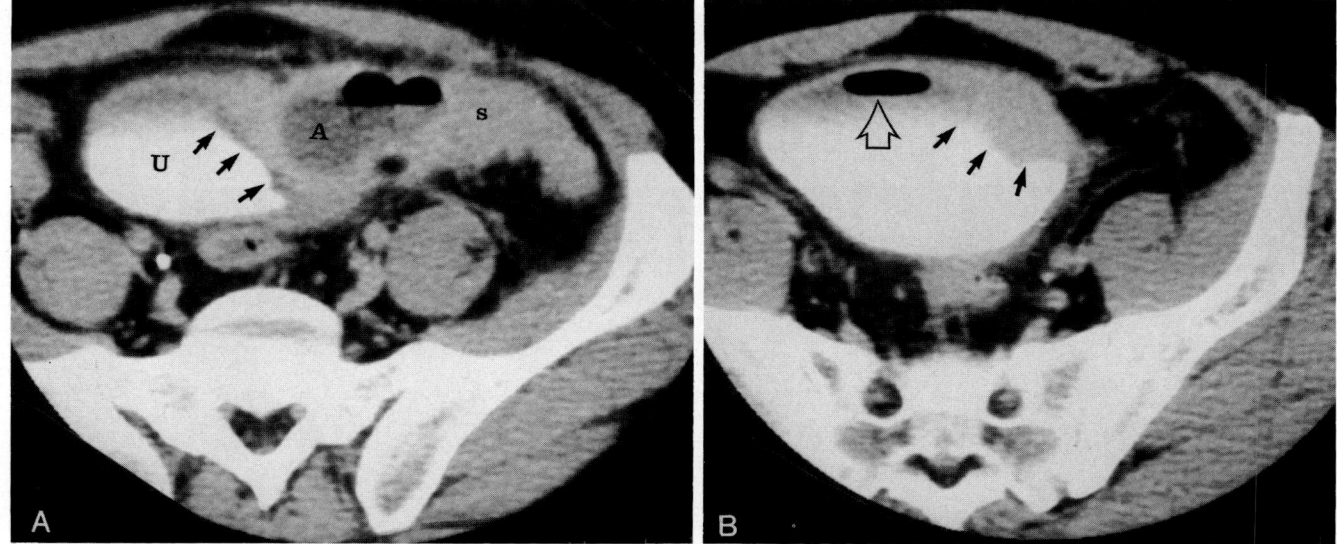

**Figure 61–26. Sigmoid–urinary bladder fistula in acute diverticulitis. A.** CT scan reveals a large air- and fluid-filled abscess (A) between the sigmoid colon (s) and urinary bladder (U). The wall of the urinary bladder (U) is infiltrated and compressed by the inflammatory mass *(arrows)*. **B.** Inflammatory mass is seen in the wall of the bladder *(solid arrows)*. The urinary bladder is filled with contrast material and contains air *(open arrow)*.

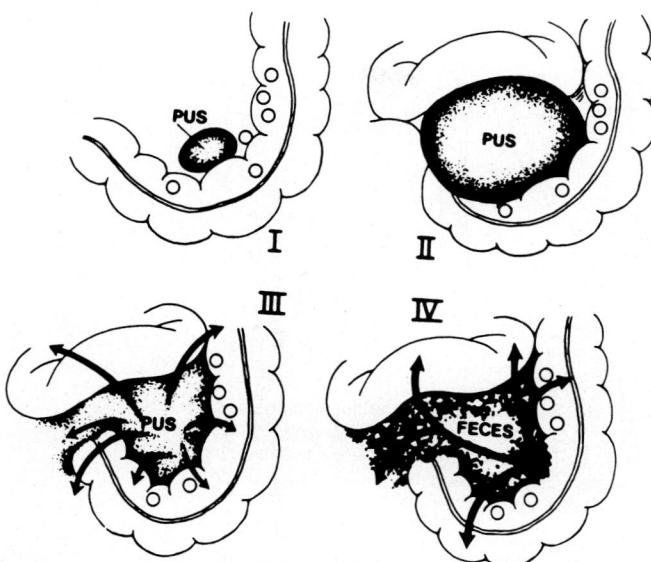

**Figure 61–27. Surgical staging of diverticular abscesses.** Stage I: small (<3 cm) pericolic abscess is contained within the sigmoid mesocolon. Stage II: pelvic abscess has broken out of sigmoid mesocolon but is contained by the pelvic organs. Stage III: the large pelvic abscess has spread into the rest of the peritoneal cavity. Stage IV: large diverticular perforation occurs with fecal contamination of the peritoneal cavity. (From Hinchley EJ, Schaal PGH, Richards GK: Treatment of perforated diverticular disease of the colon. Adv Surg 12:85–109, 1978.)

sponds well to antibiotics. On CT scans, it appears primarily as mural thickening with little inflammatory change in the surrounding fat. Follow-up CT scans are usually not needed in these patients.

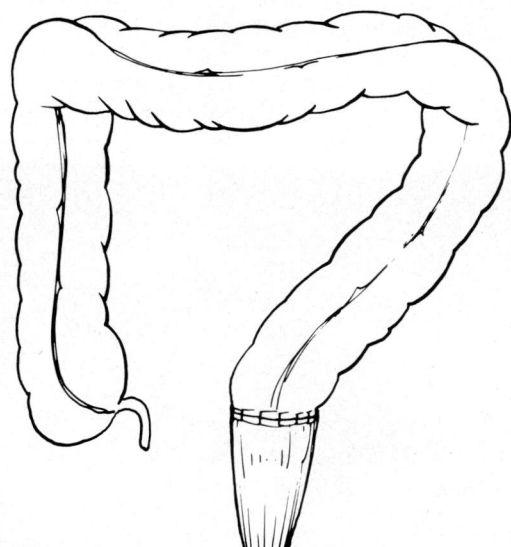

**Figure 61–28. One-stage resection for diverticulitis.** The involved segment is resected, and a primary anastomosis is performed. This procedure is performed for patients with uncomplicated diverticular disease and patients with abscesses (stages II and III) that have been "downgraded" by CT-directed, percutaneous abscess drainage. (From Dietzen CD, Pemberton JH: Diverticulitis. *In* Yamada T [ed]: Textbook of Gastroenterology. Philadelphia: JB Lippincott, 1991, pp 1734–1748.)

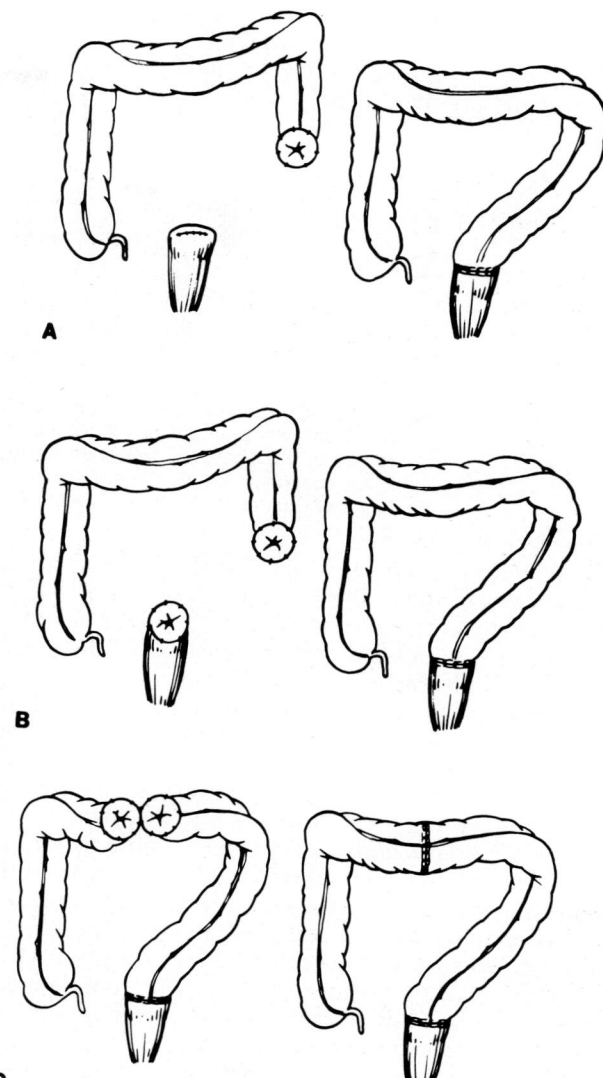

**Figure 61–29. Two-stage approaches to the resection for diverticulitis.** The diseased segment of colon is resected at the first operation in all of these approaches. **A.** Stage I: the fecal stream is diverted, the diseased sigmoid is resected, and the rectum is over-sewn, creating a Hartmann pouch. Stage II: continuity is re-established by a descending colorectostomy. **B.** Stage I: the diseased segment is resected, and both ends of colon are brought to the surface as stomas. Stage II: intestinal continuity is re-established as in **A. C.** Stage I: the diseased sigmoid is resected, and a colorectostomy is constructed and protected by a diverting colostomy. Stage II: the transverse colostomy is closed. (**A** to **C** from Dietzen CD, Pemberton JH: Diverticulitis. *In* Yamada T [ed]: Textbook of Gastroenterology. Philadelphia: JB Lippincott, 1991, pp 1734–1748.)

*Stage I diverticulitis* denotes an abscess or phlegmon that is less than 3 cm in diameter and is confined to the mesocolon. Inflammatory infiltration of pericolic fat and abscess are the major CT findings of this stage. These patients do quite well with 7 to 10 days of antibiotic therapy and seldom progress to stage II or III disease. A follow-up CT scan is recommended, because a wide mouth perforation may not heal.

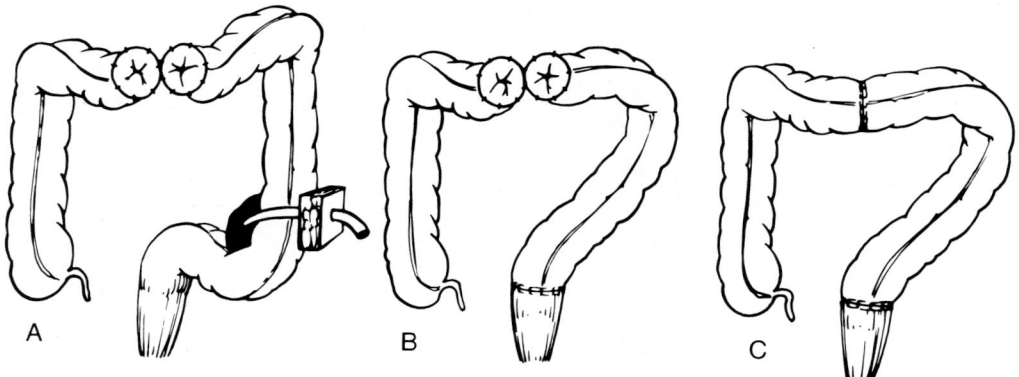

**Figure 61–30. Three-stage resection for diverticulitis. A.** The abscess is drained, and the fecal stream is diverted by a double-barreled colostomy (stage I). **B.** The diseased sigmoid and abscess are resected, and a colorectostomy is constructed (stage II). **C.** The colostomy is closed re-establishing intestinal continuity. (**A** to **C** from Dietzen CD, Pemberton JH: Diverticulitis. *In* Yamada T [ed]: Textbook of Gastroenterology. Philadelphia: JB Lippincott, 1991, pp 1734–1748.)

*Stage II diverticulitis* signifies that the pericolic abscess has broken through the sigmoid mesocolon and has become walled off by the small bowel, greater omentum, fallopian tubes, or other pelvic structures. This stage is associated with abscesses 5 to 15 cm in diameter that are well suited to percutaneous drainage (see Fig. 61–31). With percutaneous drainage, many operative procedures for diverticulitis with abscess can be downgraded from a two- or three-stage operation to a one-stage operation (see Figs. 61–28 to 61–30).

*Stage III diverticulitis* signifies pelvic abscess that has spread beyond the confines of the pelvis to involve other portions of the peritoneal cavity. Fortunately, this form of diverticulitis is relatively infrequent, because the body's defenses usually contain the perforation. At this stage, the patient requires surgery, but percutaneous catheters may allow surgery to be deferred until the patient's status is optimized.

*State IV diverticulitis* is defined as fecal spread into the peritoneal cavity. The CT appearance may be similar to that of stage III, but these patients have acute peritonitis with life-threatening sepsis, so that they usually undergo immediate exploratory laparotomy.[94–101]

### Differentiation of Diverticulitis from Carcinoma

In approximately 10% of patients, diverticulitis cannot be differentiated from colon carcinoma on the basis of CT scans. Most patients with diverticulitis exhibit only mild circumferential wall thickening in the range of 4 to 5 mm. Excessive thickening of the colonic wall, either concentrically or focally, suggests colonic neoplasm. Although most colon cancers are greater than 2 cm thick, neoplastic lesions less than 1 cm in diameter may be seen. These facts account for a significant overlap in colonic wall thickness in diverticulitis and carcinoma, particularly with lesions that are between 1 and 3 cm in thickness. In these cases, it is most helpful to distend the colonic lumen and use high-resolution CT techniques. An abrupt zone of transition with overhanging

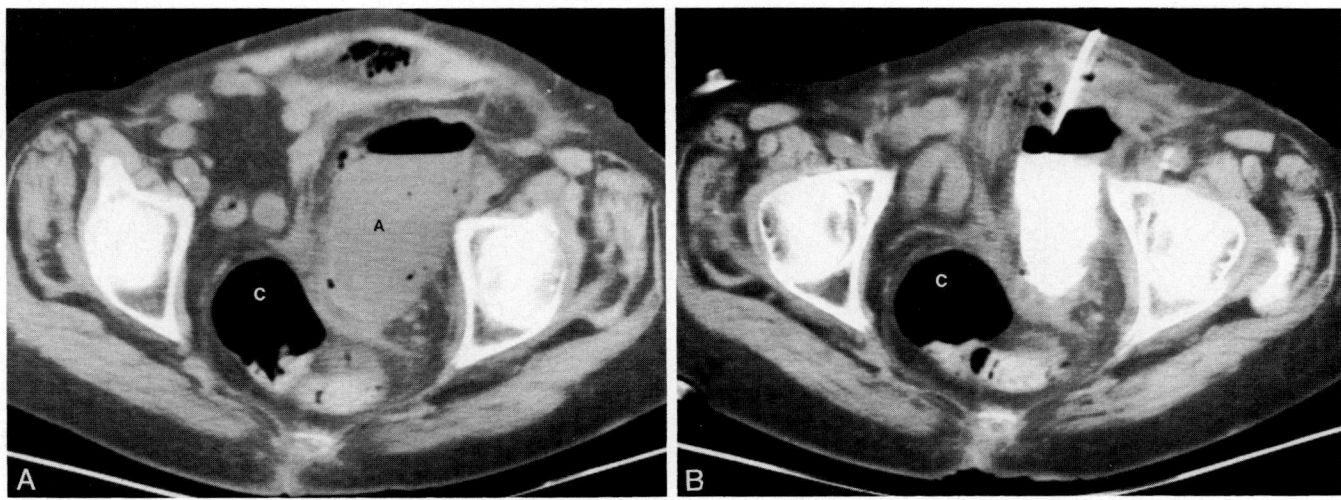

**Figure 61–31. Drainage of diverticular abscess. A.** A large abscess (A) with an air-fluid level lies lateral to the rectosigmoid junction (C). **B.** The abscess cavity is injected with contrast medium after CT-directed percutaneous drainage.

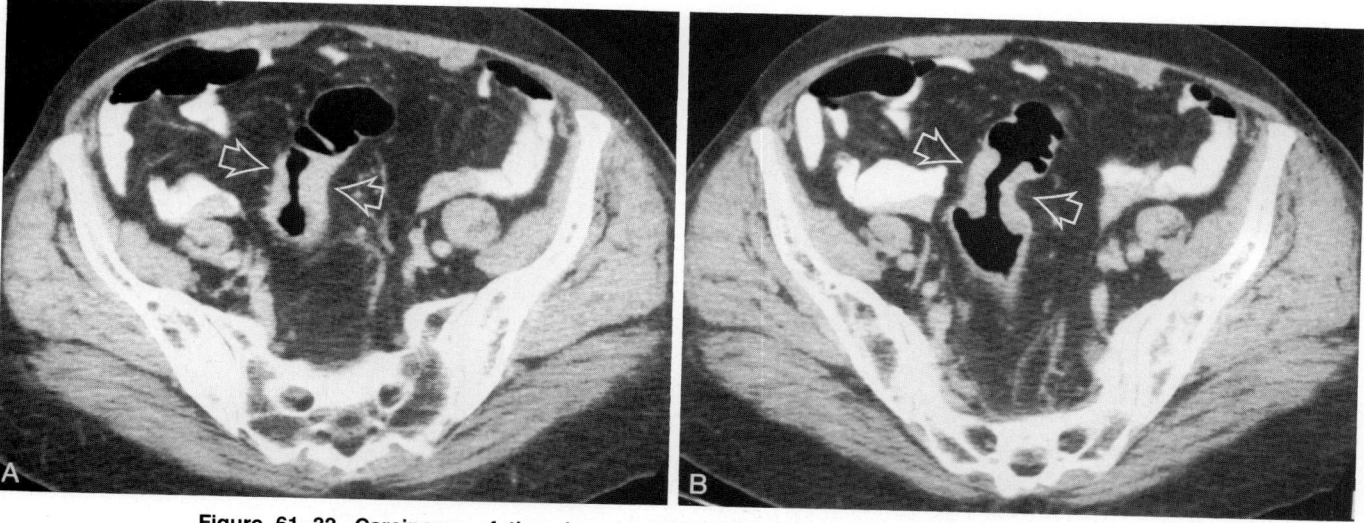

**Figure 61-32. Carcinoma of the sigmoid colon: CT appearance. A.** Initial CT scan shows nonspecific thickening of the wall of the sigmoid colon *(arrows)*. **B.** A second high-resolution CT scan (with 5-mm slice thickness) with better distention of the colonic lumen demonstrates a typical "apple core" lesion *(arrows)*.

edges and a narrow, rigid lumen indicates carcinoma (Fig. 61–32); a tethered or saw-toothed luminal configuration suggests diverticular disease (Fig. 61–33).

The differential diagnosis of cancer versus diverticulitis is extremely difficult in patients presenting with perforated colon carcinoma associated with pericolic inflammation or abscess. An abruptly altered lumen caliber with an asymmetric and lobulated soft tissue mass is diagnostic of perforated sigmoid carcinoma (Fig. 61–34).

With high-quality CT studies, the diagnosis of perforated colon cancer can be made in most patients. When the CT findings are uncertain or equivocal, CE should be used liberally as an important complementary ex-

amination. If the patient improves and immediate surgical resection is not needed, sigmoidoscopy or a barium enema should routinely be performed to confirm the CT diagnosis and exclude sigmoid carcinoma.

### Accuracy, Advantages, and Limitations of Computed Tomography Examination

The frequency of false-negative results of CT examinations in patients with acute diverticulitis has been variously reported in the literature as 2, 7, and 21%.[78, 80, 82] In the series of Johnson and associates, CT examination was diagnostic in only 41% of patients and was consistent with diverticulitis in 38% of patients, in

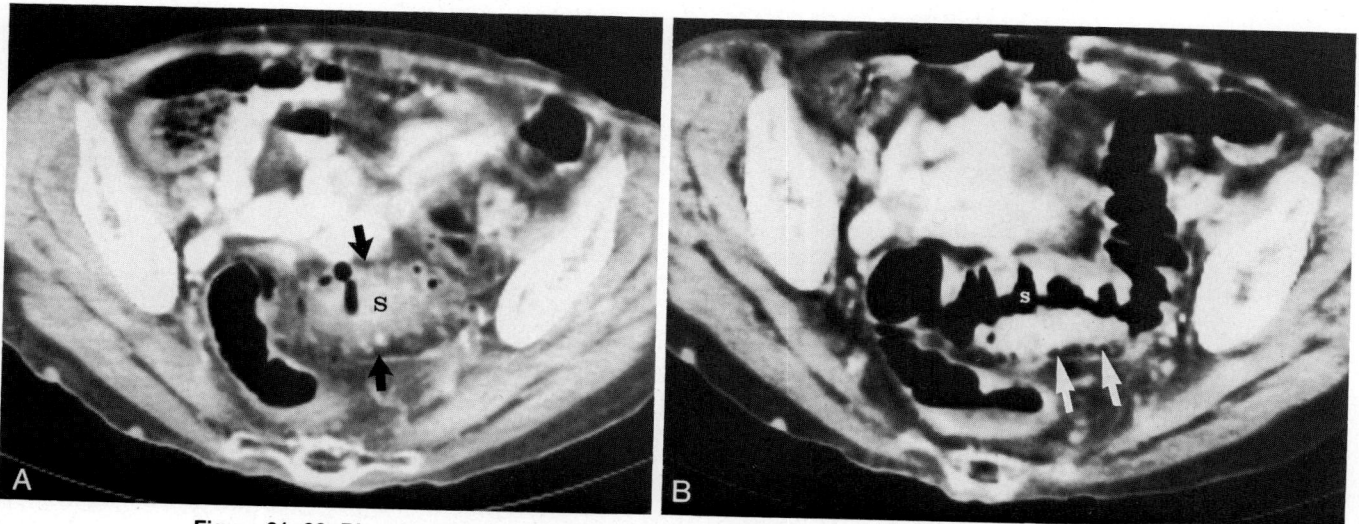

**Figure 61-33. Diverticulitis of the sigmoid colon: CT appearance. A.** Initial CT scan suggests a soft tissue mass *(arrows)* in the sigmoid colon (S). **B.** A second high-resolution CT scan obtained after air insufflation shows significant wall thickening *(arrows)* and a typical saw-toothed configuration of the sigmoid lumen (S).

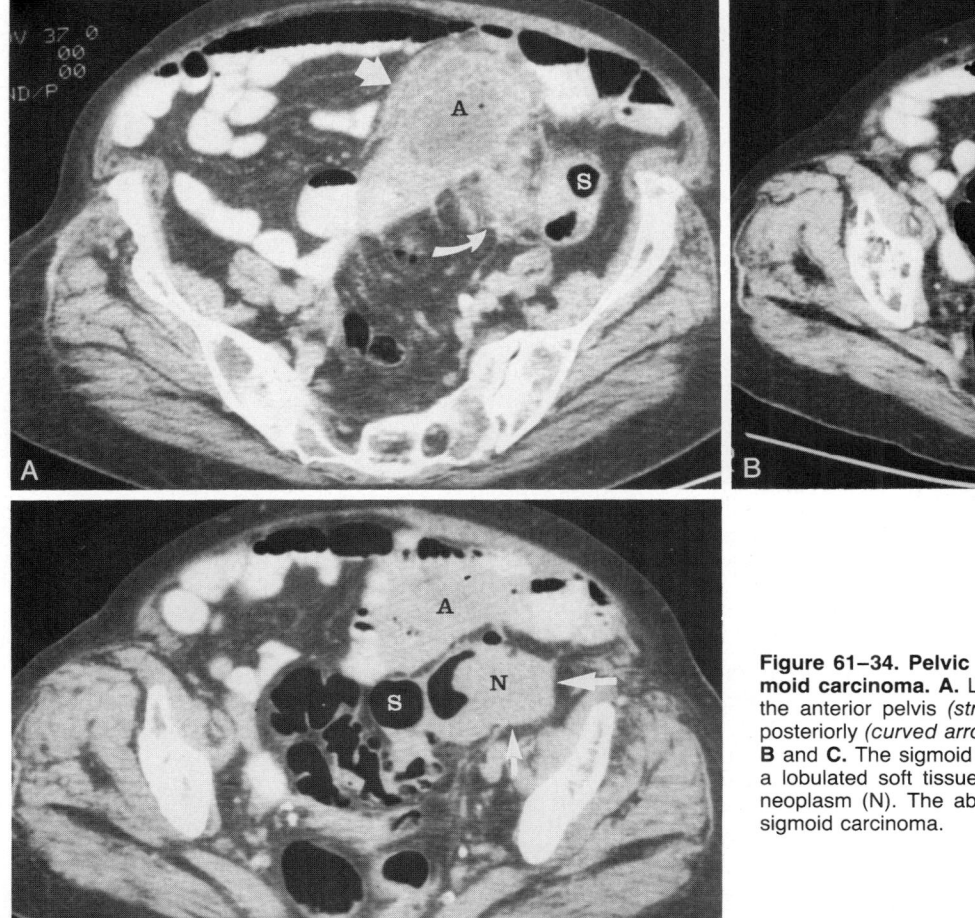

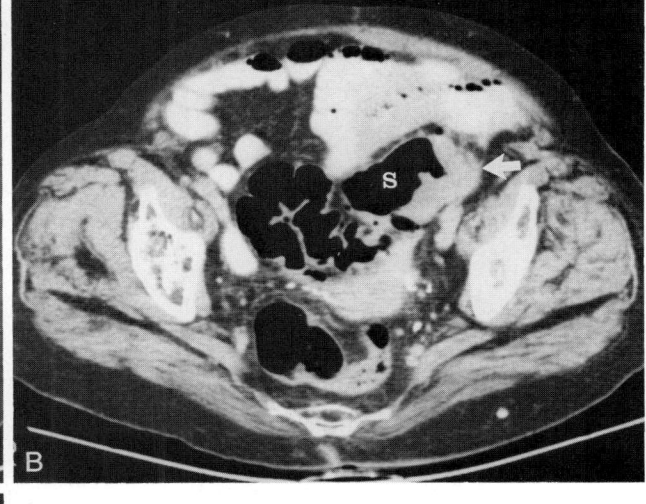

**Figure 61–34. Pelvic abscess secondary to perforated sigmoid carcinoma. A.** Large ill-defined fluid collection is seen in the anterior pelvis *(straight arrow)*. This abscess (A) extends posteriorly *(curved arrow)*, in proximity to the sigmoid colon (S). **B** and **C.** The sigmoid colon (S) is distended with air, revealing a lobulated soft tissue mass *(arrows)* compatible with colonic neoplasm (N). The abscess (A) lies anterior to the perforated sigmoid carcinoma.

contrast with the CE examination, which had 77% sensitivity.[80] On the other hand, the prospective series of Cho and co-workers showed a 93% sensitivity for CT, compared with 80% sensitivity for CE.[82] These discrepancies are explained by differences in the CT technique used, in interpretative experience and criteria, and in the severity of the inflammatory process present in the groups of patients studied.

CT offers several advantages over CE in the evaluation of patients with suspected diverticulitis: 1) CT is less invasive than CE and can be performed in acutely ill patients; 2) CT allows evaluation of the presence and severity of the pericolic inflammatory process, which is not visualized by CE examinations; 3) CT allows detection of extension of disease (abscess, peritonitis) that is distant from the colon and is not visualized by CE studies; 4) CT can visualize a variety of intra-abdominal conditions that explain the patient's symptoms and that cannot be diagnosed by means of CE.[82] In addition, foreign body perforations are better visualized by CT.

Limitations of CT scanning are the higher cost of the examination, limited availability of modern equipment, difficulties in performing emergency CT scanning, and pitfalls in the differential diagnosis of colon carcinoma

in about 10% of cases. In addition, diverticulosis, enteroenteric fistulas, intramural tracking, blind sinus tracts, and associated polyps are better detected by CE studies.

## Cecal Diverticulitis

Cecal diverticulitis is a relatively rare pathologic entity in which patients present with protean clinical manifestations that are often clinically misdiagnosed as appendicitis. Cecal diverticula are classified as true (congenital) or false (acquired). The congenital variety is usually larger and solitary and is characterized by the presence of a well-developed muscle coat. Most cecal diverticula are acquired and are similar to diverticula present in the remainder of the colon. They are usually multiple, involve the cecum and ascending colon, are formed by herniated mucosa and serosa, and lack a muscular coat. Unless perforation is suspected, barium examination remains the primary means of preoperative diagnosis. It allows a correct diagnosis in most cases and ruling out of appendicitis and carcinoma, the other major concerns in the differential diagnosis. The characteristic findings of the barium enema examination include a filling defect with an irregular contour, cecal spasm, fixation and spiculation of the cecal wall, visualization of diverticula, and a normal appearance of the appendix.[102–104]

The CT findings consist of focal pericolic inflammatory changes, slight thickening of the wall of the colon, demonstration of diverticula, and occasionally an intramural or pericolic fluid collection representing an abscess (Fig. 61–35). If the appendix is not seen, findings similar to those of appendicitis or perforated cecal carcinoma make the CT diagnosis uncertain. In general, I advocate initial use of CT scanning in all patients suspected of harboring an intra-abdominal inflammatory process. When CT scanning shows focal pericecal inflammation but the findings are not sufficiently specific, a CE study should be performed promptly.[76, 105, 106]

## Computed Tomography Versus Contrast Enema in the Diagnosis of Diverticulitis

CT and CE are complementary, not competitive, imaging tests used in the diagnosis and evaluation of patients suspected of having diverticulitis. Because of the unique and superior imaging characteristics of CT, I advocate its use as the initial and primary method of radiologic diagnosis, as well as for evaluation of complications. When the CT findings are equivocal or when the acute inflammatory process subsides and surgical resection is not contemplated, the CT diagnosis should be confirmed by CE study.

## DIVERTICULAR HEMORRHAGE

Some 30% of patients with diverticulosis have eventual hemorrhage of the lower gastrointestinal tract, ranging from an occasional guaiac-positive stool to life-threatening rectal bleeding. Diverticular disease is the most common identifiable cause of major rectal bleeding in adults and is responsible for 43% of major rectal bleeding and 35% of minor bleeding occurring in patients older than 65 years of age.[47, 107]

## Pathologic Findings

Although diverticula predominate in the sigmoid and descending colon, severe hemorrhage originates from the right colon in two thirds of patients. The source is typically a single diverticulum, which, in 80% of cases, is not inflamed. There is minute rupture of one of the vasa recta asymmetrically placed, in the wall adjacent to the lumen of the diverticulum (Fig. 61–36). An eccentric focus of media thickening, intramural thickening and duplication, and fragmentation of the internal elastic lamina in the wall of the involved artery at the point of its disruption occur. Some traumatic factor within the lumen of the diverticulum, possibly inspissated stool, induces this eccentric intimal thickening, which eventually weakens and ruptures the vasa recta (Fig. 61–37). The wider-domed necks of right-sided colonic diverticula may expose these vessels to injury over a greater length, explaining the strikingly high incidence of right-sided hemorrhage.[22–26]

## Clinical Findings

Most patients with massive diverticular hemorrhage are elderly, with severe coexistent cardiovascular and pulmonary disease, and they present with sudden onset of mild abdominal cramps and the urge to defecate. Soon after, a large volume of bright red blood or clots, or both, or dark red, maroon, or, least commonly, black stool is passed rectally. Bleeding ceases spontaneously in approximately 80% of patients, but the bleeding may

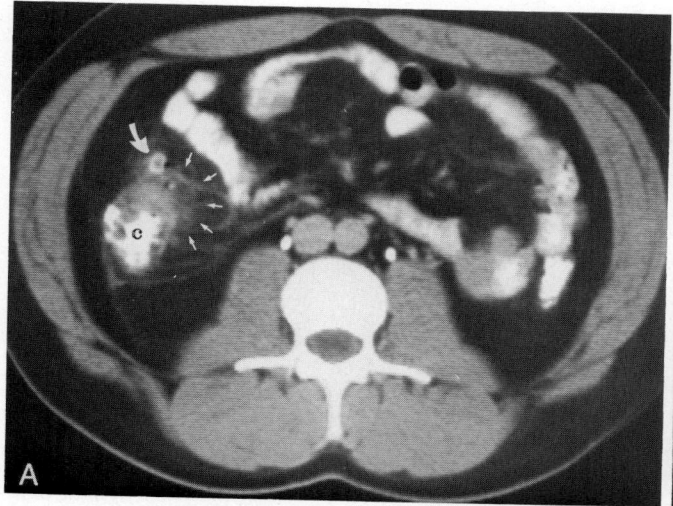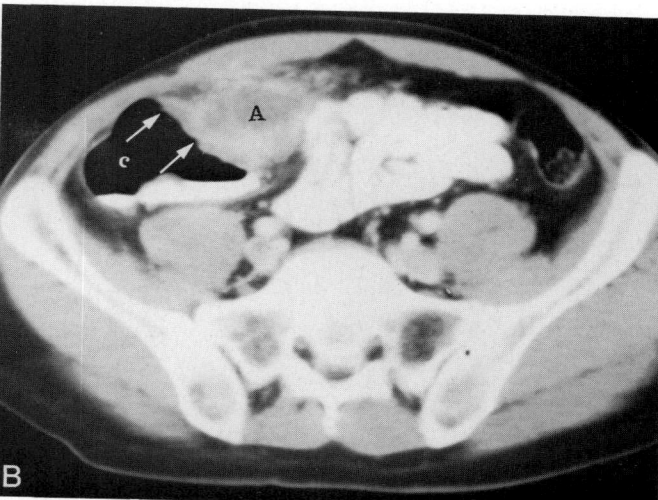

**Figure 61–35. Cecal diverticulitis: CT appearance. A.** Inflammatory reaction *(small arrows)* is present around the cecum (c). A barium-coated diverticulum *(large arrow)* is also seen. **B.** Pericecal abscess in another patient with cecal diverticulitis. The poorly encapsulated abscess (A) is compressing the medial wall of the cecum (c) *(arrows).*

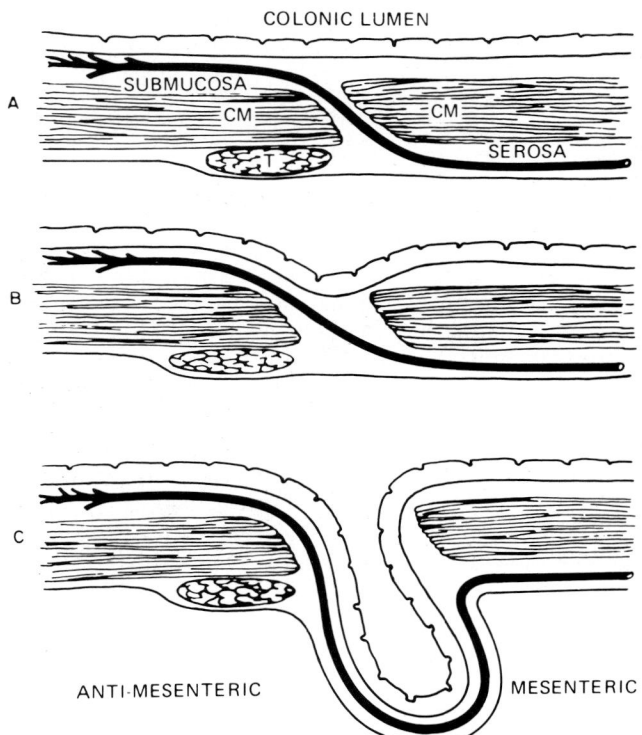

**Figure 61–36. Diverticulum formation and vascular relationships. A.** The vas rectum penetrates the colon wall from the serosa to the submucosa through an obliquely oriented connective tissue septum in the circular muscle (CM). This penetration occurs near the mesenteric side of the taenia (T). **B.** The diverticulum develops through and widens this connective tissue cleft. The mucosal protrusion begins to elevate the artery. **C.** As the diverticulum extends transmurally, the vas rectum is placed over its dome, penetrating to the submucosa on the antimesenteric border of its neck and orifice. (From Meyers MA, Volberg F, Katzen B, et al: Angioarchitecture of colonic diverticula: significance in bleeding diverticulosis. Radiology 108:249–261, 1973.)

be continuous or intermittent. Nearly 25% of patients rebleed in the near or distant future, and if rebleeding does occur, the chance of further rebleeding increases to 50%.[4–7] The differential diagnosis, radiology (Fig. 61–38), and treatment of diverticular hemorrhage are discussed in Chapter 147.[4–7]

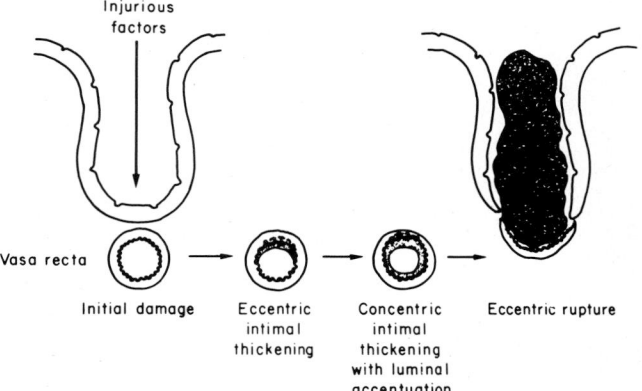

**Figure 61–37. Pathogenesis of colonic diverticular hemorrhage.** Progressive eccentric changes weaken the wall of the vas rectum, which eventually ruptures into the lumen of the diverticulum. (From Meyers MA, Alonso DR, Gray GF, et al: Pathogenesis of bleeding colonic diverticulosis. Gastroenterology 71:577–583, 1976.)

# GIANT SIGMOID DIVERTICULUM

## Etiology

Giant sigmoid diverticulum is a rare complication of diverticulitis. It is believed to result from subserosal perforation and inflammation of a diverticulum, with subsequent air trapping and eventual formation of a large cyst, which is caused by elevated intraluminal pressure of the colon working in tandem with a ball valve mechanism. In time, inflammatory and granulation tissue replaces the mucosal lining of the cyst wall. The trapped air in the cyst increases during defecation and is vented irregularly.[108–114]

## Clinical and Pathologic Findings

Most patients are elderly and have a history of chronic vague abdominal discomfort or acute symptoms suggesting diverticulitis. A palpable mass is detected in 71% of cases, and anatomic communication between the cyst and lumen is present in 82%. The cysts range in size between 6 and 27 cm, with a mean diameter of 13 cm. The cyst may be hyperresonant on percussion.[111–115]

## Radiologic Findings

The barium enema and plain film findings in giant sigmoid diverticulum are striking. Plain films demonstrate a large gas-filled structure in the lower to middle pelvis that can have an air-fluid level. The gas collections may change in size on interval studies.

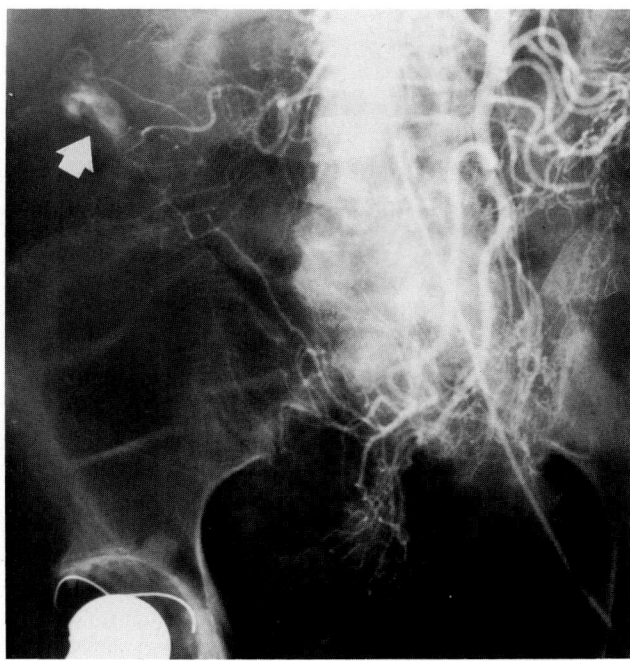

**Figure 61–38. Diverticular hemorrhage: angiographic appearance.** Contrast medium extravasation *(arrow)* into a diverticulum of the ascending colon is identified.

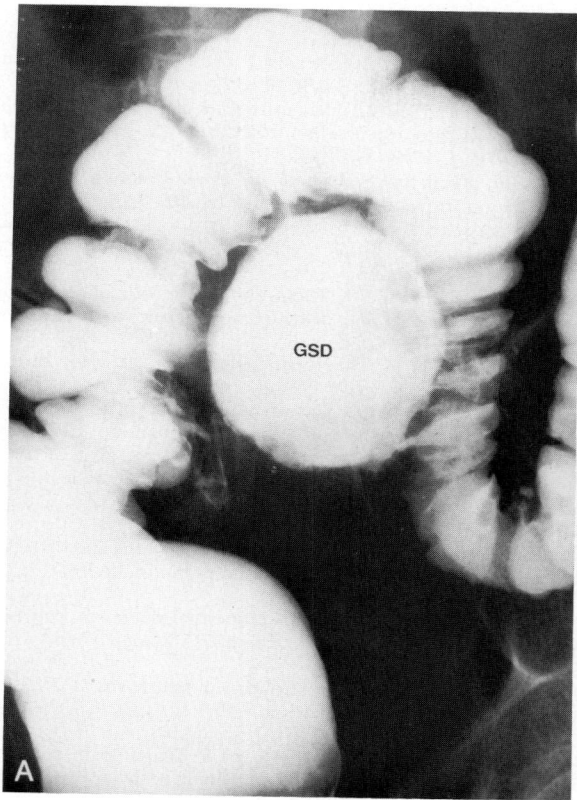
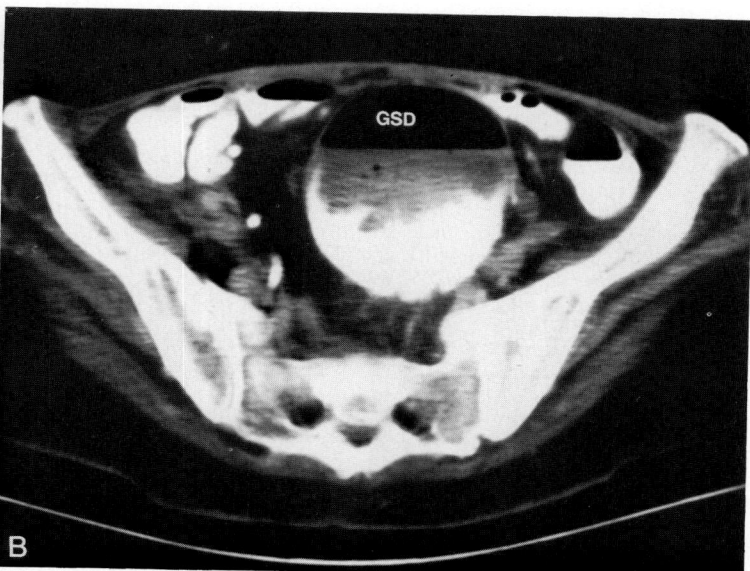

**Figure 61–39. Giant sigmoid diverticulum.** Giant sigmoid diverticulum (GSD) is demonstrated in two different patients on a barium enema study **(A)** and a CT scan **(B)**.

Barium enters these collections on contrast studies in two thirds of patients (Fig. 61–39), and diverticula are seen elsewhere in the colon in 82% of patients. The differential diagnosis of these large collections includes volvulus, giant Meckel's or other small bowel diverticulum, tubo-ovarian abscess, cystitis, emphysematous cholecystitis, infected pancreatic pseudocyst, and vesicoenteric fistula.[111–115]

## Therapy

Giant sigmoid diverticula have the potential for perforation, infarction, or torsion and should be surgically removed to avoid these complications.[116, 117]

### Acknowledgment

Figure 61–12 is reproduced from Davis L (ed): Christopher's Textbook of Surgery (9th ed). Philadelphia: WB Saunders, 1968.

## References

1. Morson BC: Pathology of diverticular disease of the colon. Clin Gastroenterol 4:37–52, 1975.
2. Slack WW: The anatomy, pathology, and some clinical features of diverticulitis of the colon. Br J Surg 50:185–194, 1962.
3. Cotran RS, Kumar V, Robbins SL: Robbins Pathologic Basis of Disease (4th ed). Philadelphia: WB Saunders, 1989, pp 884–886.
4. Roberts PL, Veidenheimer MC: Diverticular disease. *In* Zuidema GD (ed): Shackelford's Surgery of the Alimentary Tract (3rd ed). Philadelphia: WB Saunders, 1991, pp 95–107.
5. Smith AN: Diverticular disease of the colon. *In* Phillips SF, Pemberton JH, Shorter RG (eds). The Large Intestine: Physiology, Pathophysiology, and Disease. New York: Raven Press, 1991, pp 549–577.
6. Naitove A, Almy TP: Diverticular disease of the colon. *In* Sleisenger MH, Fordtran JS (eds): Gastrointestinal Disease: Pathophysiology, Diagnosis, Management (4th ed). Philadelphia: WB Saunders, 1989, pp 1419–1434.
7. Steinhagen RM, Aufses AH: Diverticular disease. *In* Moody FG (ed): Surgical Treatment of Digestive Disease (2nd ed). Chicago: Year Book Medical Publishers, 1990, pp 740–753.
8. Parks TG: Natural history of diverticular disease of the colon. Clin Gastroenterol 4:53–69, 1975.
9. Painter NS, Burkitt DP: Diverticular disease of the colon: a 20th century problem. Clin Gastroenterol 4:3–21, 1975.
10. Painter NS, Burkitt DP: Diverticular disease of the colon: a deficiency disease of Western civilization. Br Med J 2:450–459, 1971.
11. Manousos ON, Truelove SC, Lumbsden K: Prevalence of colonic diverticulosis in general population of Oxford area. Br Med J 3:762–763, 1967.
12. Hughes LE: Postmortem survey of diverticular disease of the colon. I. Diverticulosis and diverticulitis. Gut 10:336–344, 1969.
13. Sugihara K, Muto T, Morioka Y, et al: Diverticular disease of the colon in Japan: review of 615 cases. Dis Colon Rectum 27:531–537, 1984.
14. Dietzen CD, Pemberton JH: Diverticulitis. *In* Yamada T (ed): Textbook of Gastroenterology. Philadelphia: JB Lippincott, 1991, pp 1734–1748.
15. Painter NS: The aetiology of diverticulosis of the colon with special reference to the action of certain drugs on the behaviour of the colon. Ann R Coll Surg Engl 34:98–119, 1965.
16. Painter NS, Truelove SC, Ardan GM, et al: Segmentation and localization of intraluminal pressures in the human colon, with special reference to pathogenesis of colonic diverticula. Gastroenterology 49:169–177, 1965.
17. Fleischner FG, Ming SI-C: Revised concepts on the diverticular disease of the colon. Radiology 84:599–609, 1965.

18. Morson BC: The muscle abnormality in diverticular disease of the sigmoid colon. Br J Radiol 36:385–392, 1963.

19. Williams I: Diverticular disease of the colon without diverticula. Radiology 89:401–412, 1967.

20. Fleischner FG: Diverticular disease of the colon. Gastroenterology 60:316–324, 1971.

21. Meyers MA: Dynamic Radiology of the Abdomen (3rd ed). New York: Springer-Verlag, 1988, pp 407–422.

22. Meyers MA, Volberg F, Katzen B, et al: The angioarchitecture of colonic diverticula. Radiology 108:249–261, 1973.

23. Boley SJ, DiBiase A, Brandt LJ, et al: Lower intestinal bleeding in the elderly. Am J Surg 137:57–64, 1979.

24. Baum S: Angiography and the gastrointestinal bleeder. Radiology 143:569–772, 1982.

25. Meyers MA, Alonso DR, Baer JW: Pathogenesis of massively bleeding colonic diverticulosis. New observations. AJR 127:901–908, 1976.

26. Meyers MA, Alonso DR, Gray FG, et al: Pathogenesis of bleeding colonic diverticulosis. Gastroenterology 71:577–583, 1976.

27. Russin LD: Plain film recognition of air within colonic diverticula. AJR 134:176–177, 1980.

28. Hunter TB, Merkley R, Pitt MJ: Relation between pelvic phleboliths and diverticular disease of the colon. AJR 143:105–107, 1984.

29. Laufer I, Levine M (eds): Double Contrast Gastrointestinal Radiology (2nd ed). Philadelphia: WB Saunders, 1992.

30. Weissman A, Clot M, Grellet J: Double Contrast Examination of the Colon. Berlin: Springer-Verlag, 1985, pp 147–161.

31. Gelfand DW: Gastrointestinal Radiology. New York: Churchill Livingstone, 1984, pp 318–324.

32. Farman J: Gastrointestinal Radiology. Philadelpha: JB Lippincott, 1991.

33. Meyers MA: Diverticular disease. *In* Marshak RH, Lindner AE, Maklansky D (eds): Radiology of the Colon. Philadelphia: WB Saunders, 1980, pp 401–466.

34. Ferrucci JT: Diverticular disease. *In* Dreyfuss JR, Janower ML (eds): Radiology of the Colon. Baltimore: Williams & Wilkins, 1980, pp 160–183.

35. Freeny PC, Walker JH: Inverted diverticula of the gastrointestinal tract. Gastrointest Radiol 4:57–59, 1979.

36. Htoo AM, Bartram CI: The radiological diagnosis of polyps in the presence of diverticular disease. Br J Radiol 52:263–267, 1979.

37. Baker SR, Alterman DD: False-negative barium enema in patients with sigmoid cancer and coexistent diverticula. Gastrointest Radiol 10:171–173, 1985.

38. Glick SN: Inverted colonic diverticulum: air contrast barium enema findings in six cases. AJR 156:961–964, 1991.

39. Keller CE, Halpert RD, Feczko PJ, et al: Radiologic recognition of colonic diverticula simulating polyps. AJR 143:93–97, 1984.

40. Miller WT, Levine MS, Rubesin SE, et al: Bowler-hat sign: a simple principle for differentiating polyps from diverticula. Radiology 173:615–617, 1989.

41. Lappas JC, Maglinte DDT, Kopecky KK, et al: Diverticular disease: imaging with post–double-contrast sigmoid flush. Radiology 168:35–37, 1988.

42. Balthazar EJ: Colon. *In* Megibow AJ, Balthazar EJ (eds): Computed Tomography of the Gastrointestinal Tract. St. Louis: CV Mosby, 1986, pp 279–386.

43. Pohlman T: Diverticulitis. Gastroenterol Clin North Am 17:357–385, 1988.

44. Christie PM, Shaw JHF: Diverticular disease in Auckland. Aust N Z J Surg 58:795–799, 1988.

45. Almy TP, Howell DA: Diverticular disease of the colon. N Engl J Med 302:324–330, 1980.

46. Brown DB, Toomey WF: Diverticular disease of the colon: a review of 258 cases. Br J Surg 47:485–493, 1960.

47. Ming S-C, Fleischner FG: Diverticulitis of sigmoid colon: reappraisal of the pathology and pathogenesis. Surgery 58:627–633, 1965.

48. Galbraith P, Bagg MN, Schabel SI, et al: Diverticular complications of renal failure. Gastrointest Radiol 15:259–262, 1990.

49. Alexander-Williams J: Management of the acute complications of diverticular disease: the dangers of colostomy. Dis Colon Rectum 19:289–292, 1976.

50. Puglisi BS, Kauffman HM, Stewart ET, et al: Colonic perforation in renal transplant patients. AJR 145:555–558, 1985.

51. Canter JW, Shorb PE Jr: Acute perforation of colonic diverticula associated with prolonged adrenocorticosteroid therapy. Am J Surg 121:46–51, 1971.

52. Carson SD, Krom RAF, Uchida K, et al: Colon perforation after kidney transplantation. Ann Surg 188:109–113, 1978.

53. Warshaw AL, Welch JP, Ottinger LW: Acute perforation of the colon associated with chronic corticosteroid therapy. Am J Surg 131:442–446, 1976.

54. Freischlag J, Bennison RS, Thompson JE Jr: Complications of diverticular disease of the colon in young people. Dis Colon Rectum 29:639–643, 1986.

55. Ouriel K, Schwartz SI: Diverticular disease of the colon in the young patient. Surg Gynecol Obstet 156:1–5, 1983.

56. Simonowitz D, Paloyan D: Diverticular disease of the colon in patients under 40 years of age. Am J Gastroenterol 67:69–72, 1977.

57. Chodak GW, Rangel DM, Passaro E Jr: Colonic diverticulitis in patients under age 40: need for earlier diagnosis. Am J Surg 141:699–702, 1981.

58. Wold BS, Khilnani M, Marshak RH: Diverticulosis and diverticulitis: Roentgen findings and their interpretation. AJR 77:726–743, 1957.

59. Schatzki R: The roentgenologic differential diagnosis between cancer and diverticulitis of the colon. Radiology 34:651–660, 1940.

60. Greenall MJ, Levine AW, Nolan DJ: Complications of diverticular disease: a review of the barium enema findings. Gastrointest Radiol 8:353–358, 1983.

61. Nicholas GG, Miller WE, Fitts WE, et al: Diagnosis of diverticulitis of the colon: role of the barium enema in defining pericolic inflammation. Ann Surg 176:205–209, 1972.

62. Kourtesis GJ, Williams RA, Wilson SE: Acute diverticulitis: safety and value of contrast studies in predicting need for operation. Aust N Z J Surg 58:801–804, 1988.

63. Gore RM, Calenoff L: Roentgenographic manifestations of diverticulitis. Ill Med J 159:293–297, 1979.

64. Loeb PN, Berk RN, Saltzstein SL: Longitudinal fistula of the colon in diverticulitis. Gastroenterology 67:720–724, 1974.

65. Smith HJ, Berk RN, Janes JO, et al: Unusual fistulae due to colonic diverticulitis. Gastrointest Radiol 2:387–392, 1978.

66. Lipsit ER, Lewici AM: Subcutaneous emphysema of the abdominal wall from diverticulitis with necrotizing fasciitis. Gastrointest Radiol 4:89–92, 1979.

67. Mayo CW, Blunt CP: Vesicosigmoidal fistulae complicating diverticulitis. Surg Obstet Gynecol 91:612–616, 1950.

68. Geier GR, Ujiki GT, Shields TW: Colovesical fistula. Arch Surg 105:347–351, 1972.

69. Marshak RH, Linder AE, Pochaczeusky R, et al: Longitudinal sinus tracts in granulomatous colitis and diverticulitis. Semin Roentgenol 11:101–110, 1976.

70. Ferrucci JT, Ragsdale BD, Barrett PJ, et al: Double tracking of the sigmoid colon. Radiology 120:307–312, 1976.

71. Marshak RH, Janowitz HD, Present DH: Granulomatous colitis in association with diverticula. N Engl J Med 283:1080–1084, 1970.

72. Ponka JL, Fox JD, Brush C: Coexisting carcinoma and diverticula of the colon. Arch Surg 79:373–384, 1959.

73. Wilson SG: The gastrointestinal tract. *In* Rumack CM, Wilson SR, Charboneau JW (eds): Diagnostic Ultrasound. St. Louis: Mosby–Year Book, 1991, pp 181–208.

74. Suhas SG: Sonography of colonic diverticulitis. J Ultrasound Med 4:659–666, 1985.

75. Wilson SR, Toi A: The value of sonography in the diagnosis of acute diverticulitis of the colon. AJR 154:1199–1201, 1990.

75a. Schwerk WB, Schwarz S, Rothmund M: Sonography in acute colonic diverticulitis. Dis Colon Rectum 35:1077–1084, 1992.

76. Wada M, Kikuchi Y, Doy M: Uncomplicated acute diverticulitis of the cecum and ascending colon: sonographic findings in 18 patients. AJR 155:283–287, 1990.

77. Lieberman JM, Haaga JR: Computed tomography of diverticulitis. J Comput Assist Tomogr 7:431–433, 1983.

78. Hulnick DH, Megibow AJ, Balthazar EJ, et al: Computed tomography in the evaluation of diverticulitis. Radiology 152:481–495, 1984.

79. Jeffrey RB: CT and Sonography of the Acute Abdomen. New York: Raven Press, 1989, pp 234–260.

80. Johnson CD, Baker ME, Rice RP, et al: Diagnosis of acute colonic diverticulitis: comparison of barium enema and CT. AJR 148:541–546, 1987.

81. Balthazar EJ, Megibow A, Schinella RA, et al: Limitations in the CT diagnosis of acute diverticulitis: comparison of CT, contrast enema, and pathologic findings in 16 patients. AJR 154:281–285, 1990.

82. Cho CK, Morehouse HT, Alterman DD, et al: Sigmoid diverticulitis: diagnostic role of CT—comparison with barium enema studies. Radiology 176:111–115, 1990.

83. Lutat E, Balthazar EJ: The current role of computerized tomography in inflammatory disease of the bowel. Am J Gastroenterol 83:107–113, 1988.

84. Goldman SM, Fishman EK, Gatewood OMB: CT demonstration of colovesical fistulae secondary to diverticulitis. J Comput Assist Tomogr 8:462–468, 1984.

85. Kanehann LB, Caroline DF, Friedman AC, et al: CT findings in venous intravasation complicating diverticulitis. J Comput Assist Tomogr 12:1047–1049, 1988.

86. Raval B, Lamki N, St. Ville E: Role of computed tomography in diverticulitis. CT 11:144–150, 1987.

87. Scatarige JC, Fishman EK, Crist DW, et al: Diverticulitis of the right colon: CT observations. AJR 148:737–739, 1987.

88. Hinchley EJ, Schaal PGH, Richards GK: Treatment of perforated diverticular disease of the colon. Adv Surg 12:85–109, 1978.

89. Neff CC, vanSonnenberg E: CT of diverticulitis:diagnosis and treatment. Radiol Clin North Am 27:743–752, 1989.

90. Neff CC, vanSonnenberg E, Casola G, et al: Diverticular abscess: percutaneous drainage. Radiology 163:15–18, 1987.

91. Ambrosetti P, Robert J, Witzig JA, et al: Incidence, outcome, and proposed management of isolated left-sided diverticulitis. Dis Colon Rectum 35:1072–1076, 1992.

92. Mueller PR, Saini S, Wittenberg J, et al: Sigmoid diverticular abscesses: percutaneous drainage an adjunct to surgical resection in 24 cases. Radiology 164:321–325, 1987.

93. Saini S, Mueller PR, Wittenberg J, et al: Percutaneous drainage of diverticular abscess. Arch Surg 121:475–478, 1986.

94. Alanis A, Papanicolaou GK, Tadros R, et al: Primary resection and anastomosis for treatment of acute diverticulitis. Dis Colon Rectum 32:933–934, 1989.

95. Peoples JB, Vilk DR, Maguire JP, et al: Reassessment of primary resection of the perforated segment for severe colonic diverticulitis. Am J Surg 159:291–293, 1983.

96. Eisenstat JE, Rubin RJ, Salvati EP: Surgical management of diverticulitis. Dis Colon Rectum 26:429–432, 1983.

97. Hackford AW, Schoetz DJ, Coller JA, et al: Surgical management of complicated diverticulitis. Dis Colon Rectum 28:317–321, 1985.

98. Wolff BG, Ready Rl, MacCarty RL, et al: Influence of sigmoid resection on progression of diverticular disease of the colon. Dis Colon Rectum 27:645–647, 1984.

99. Klompjen G, Kapusta GR: Options in the treatment of diverticular disease in the colon. Curr Probl Surg 7:479–485, 1990.

100. Asch MJ, Markowitz AM: Diverticulitis coli: a surgical appraisal. Surgery 62:239–247, 1967.

101. Zollinger RW: The prognosis in diverticulitis of the colon. Arch Surg 97:418–421, 1968.

102. Fischer MG, Farkas AM: Diverticulitis of the cecum and ascending colon. Dis Colon Rectum 27:454–458, 1984.

103. Berenbaum SL, Zausner J, Lane B: Diverticular disease of the right colon. AJR 115:334–348, 1972.

104. Gougs TH, Coppa GF, Eng K, et al: Management of diverticulitis of the ascending colon. 10 years experience. Am J Surg 145:387–391, 1983.

105. Townsend RR, Jeffrey RB, Laing FC: Cecal diverticulitis differentiated from appendicitis using graded-compression sonography. AJR 152:1229–1230, 1989.

106. Puylaert JBCM: Ultrasound of Appendicitis. Berlin: Springer-Verlag, 1990.

107. Jeffrey RB: Sonography and CT of acute right lower quadrant pain. *In* Gore RM (ed): Syllabus for the Categorical Course in Gastrointestinal Radiology. Reston, VA: American College of Radiology, 1991, pp 133–137.

108. Moss AA: Giant sigmoid diverticulum: clinical and radiographic features. Dig Dis 20:676–683, 1975.

109. Muhletaler CA, Berger JL, Robinette CL: Pathogenesis of giant colonic diverticula. Gastrointest Radiol 6:217–222, 1981.

110. Westein L, Camera A, Trillo RA, et al: Giant sigmoid diverticulum: report of a case and review of the literature. Dis Colon Rectum 21:110–112, 1978.

111. Gallagher JJ, Welch JP: Giant diverticula of the sigmoid colon: a review of differential diagnosis and operative management. Arch Surg 114:1079–1083, 1979.

112. Kricun R, Stasik JJ, Reither RD, et al: Giant sigmoid diverticulum. AJR 135:507–512, 1980.

113. Rabinowitz JG, Farman J, Dallemand S, et al: Giant sigmoid diverticulum. AJR 121:338–343, 1974.

114. Rosenberg RF, Naidick JB: Plain film recognition of giant colonic diverticulum. Am J Gastroenterol 76:59–69, 1981.

115. Telepack RJ, Huggins TJ, Bova JG: Tuboovarian abscess simulating giant colonic diverticulum. Gastrointest Radiol 9:369–371, 1984.

116. Scerpella PR, Bodensteiner JA: Giant sigmoid diverticula. Arch Surg 124:1244–1246, 1989.

117. Levi DM, Levi JU, Rogers AI, et al: Giant colonic diverticulum: an unusual manifestation of a common disease. Am J Gastroenterol 88:139–142, 1993.

# Ulcerative and Granulomatous Colitis: Idiopathic Inflammatory Bowel Disease

Richard M. Gore, M.D.

Igor Laufer, M.D.

## INTRODUCTION

The term *inflammatory bowel disease* encompasses two forms of chronic, idiopathic intestinal inflammation: ulcerative colitis and Crohn's disease. Although many other inflammatory diseases affect the gut, most are distinguished either by a specific identifiable etiologic agent or process or by the nature of the inflammatory activity. The cause of ulcerative colitis and Crohn's disease is unknown, so these disorders are empirically defined by their typical pathologic, radiologic, clinical, endoscopic, and laboratory features.[1-4]

This chapter summarizes the features that usually permit an operational distinction to be made between ulcerative colitis and Crohn's disease. It must be remembered, however, that the fundamental validity of this classification is uncertain and will so remain until the cause and pathogenesis of these disorders are better understood.[1]

## ULCERATIVE COLITIS

Ulcerative colitis is a diffuse inflammatory disease that principally involves the mucosa of the rectum and colon. The diagnosis is usually made on the basis of clinical symptoms and the presence of inflamed mucosa on sigmoidoscopy and confirmed by the findings on barium enema and mucosal biopsy.[5-7]

## Historical Perspective

Although Hippocrates was aware that diarrhea was not a single disease, it required more than two millenia before ulcerative colitis was distinguished from the all too common infectious enteritides.

In 1859, Wilks described the case of Mrs. Isabella Banks, who had "inflammation of the large intestine" and was "affected by discharge of mucus and blood, where, after death, the whole internal surface of the colon presented a highly vascular soft, red surface covered with tenacious mucus, adherent lymph. . . ."[8] By the turn of the century, ulcerative colitis was fully characterized in terms of its clinical and pathologic criteria.[8, 9]

## Epidemiology

Epidemiologic data have yielded some important clues concerning the etiology of ulcerative colitis. The salient epidemiologic features of ulcerative colitis are listed in Table 62–1 and discussed more fully in the following.

**Incidence.** Ulcerative colitis is more common than Crohn's disease with an annual incidence of 2 to 10 cases per 100,000 population. The worldwide prevalence ranges from 35 to 100 cases per 100,000 population. This wide range is probably due to true differences in disease distribution as well as differences in reporting, diagnostic criteria, and availability of medical care.[10–14]

**Geographic Distribution.** Ulcerative colitis is most prevalent in the developed countries of northern Europe, Scandinavia, the British Isles, the United States, and Israel. The incidence of ulcerative colitis in high-prevalence areas has leveled off, whereas the incidence of Crohn's disease is increasing. In low-prevalence geographic areas, the incidence of ulcerative colitis has been increasing.[15, 16]

**Race and Sex.** Ulcerative colitis is four times more common in whites than in nonwhites, and there is a slight female preponderance.[10–12]

**Religion.** There is a two- to fourfold increase of ulcerative colitis among Jewish persons. The incidence of ulcerative colitis is much lower among Israeli than American and European Jewish individuals. Furthermore, the incidence of disease is lower in Sephardic than in Ashkenazi Jewish persons in Israel. These disparate rates suggest that a hereditary predisposition may be altered by environmental factors.[10–12]

**Age.** The peak age at onset of ulcerative colitis is between 15 and 25 years of age, with a smaller peak at ages 55 to 65 years. Ulcerative colitis is more common than Crohn's disease in children younger than 10 years of age.

**Urban-Rural Distribution.** Ulcerative colitis is more common in urban than in rural populations.[10–12]

**Familial Pattern.** The incidence of ulcerative colitis among first-degree relatives is 30 to 100 times greater than that of the general population. Approximately 15% of patients with ulcerative colitis have a similarly affected first-degree relative. The lifetime risk of developing ulcerative colitis among first-degree relatives is 8.9% for offspring, 8.8% for siblings, and 3.5% for parents. Familial ulcerative colitis seems to follow a polygenic inheritance pattern.[17, 18]

**Smoking.** The risk of developing ulcerative colitis for current smokers compared with lifetime nonsmokers is 59% less, but the risk is elevated by 64% for former smokers. Smoking is not therapeutic, however, and there is no strong evidence of a beneficial effect of smoking on the clinical course of ulcerative colitis. On the other hand, patients who quit smoking before the onset of disease have more frequent hospitalizations and colectomies. This raises the possibility that smoking cessation may lead to more severe illness.[19–21]

**Mortality.** The mortality rate of ulcerative colitis has significantly improved during recent years, and this can be attributed to improvements in diagnosis and management. In the past, ulcerative colitis was responsible for 90% of deaths attributable to inflammatory bowel disease. More recently, the proportion of ulcerative colitis and Crohn's disease deaths is about equal, 1 per 100,000 aged 20 to 29 years, and 3 to 4 per 100,000 for ages 50 to 59 years.[22, 23]

## Pathogenesis and Etiology

Despite exhaustive work by a large number of investigators, the cause of ulcerative colitis is still unknown. Although the participation of genetic, environmental, neural, hormonal, infectious, immunologic, and psychologic factors in the pathogenesis of this disease is well established, none of the mechanisms has proved to be the primary etiologic agent (Fig. 62–1). In addition, it now appears that distal ulcerative proctitis may have a cause different from that of pancolitis.[1–4, 24–28]

**Genetic and Familial Factors.** As stated earlier, familial aggregation of ulcerative colitis is well recognized. The postulated mode of inheritance of susceptibility to ulcerative colitis is through polygenes. The disease occurs with greatest frequency in monozygotic twins. Human leukocyte antigen (HLA) phenotypes B5, BW52, and DR2 also have a significant association with ulcerative colitis. Ulcerative colitis is often associated with the autoimmune disorders sacroiliitis, ankylosing spondylitis, enteropathic oligoarthritis, and anterior uveitis, which are associated with HLA-B27 antigen.[29, 30]

Possibly genes related to ulcerative colitis may encode products that contribute to functional or structural abnormalities in the colon, which render it more susceptible to attack by infection, toxins, and autoimmune actions.[1]

**Anatomic and Physiologic Factors.** Patients with ulcerative colitis have abnormal mucin production, which may permit various intraluminal bacterial products and toxins to attack the mucosa. It is uncertain whether this defect is a cause or an effect of the disease.[31, 32]

**Infectious Factors.** *Chlamydia,* mycobacteria, gut anaerobes, cytomegalovirus, *Yersinia,* and bacterial cell wall components have all been implicated in the etiology of ulcerative colitis. It is also possible that bacteria that normally constitute normal flora may be pathogenic in a susceptible host.[26, 28]

**Enteric Nervous System and Gut Hormones.** In ulcerative colitis, the enteric nervous system and nerves containing substance P and vasoactive intestinal polypeptide become straight, thick, and highly immunoreactive. Substance P and vasoactive intestinal polypeptide

## TABLE 62–1. EPIDEMIOLOGY OF ULCERATIVE COLITIS

| | |
|---|---|
| Worldwide prevalence | 35–100 cases/100,000 population |
| Annual incidence | 2–10 cases/100,000 population |
| Bimodal age distribution | Peak 15–25 y; smaller peak 50–80 y |
| Risk factors | White (2–5 × risk) |
| | Jewish (2–4 × risk) |
| | Live in developed country |
| | Urban dweller |
| | Family history (30–100 × risk) |
| | Sibling with disease (8.8% incidence) |
| | Single |
| | Nonsmoker |

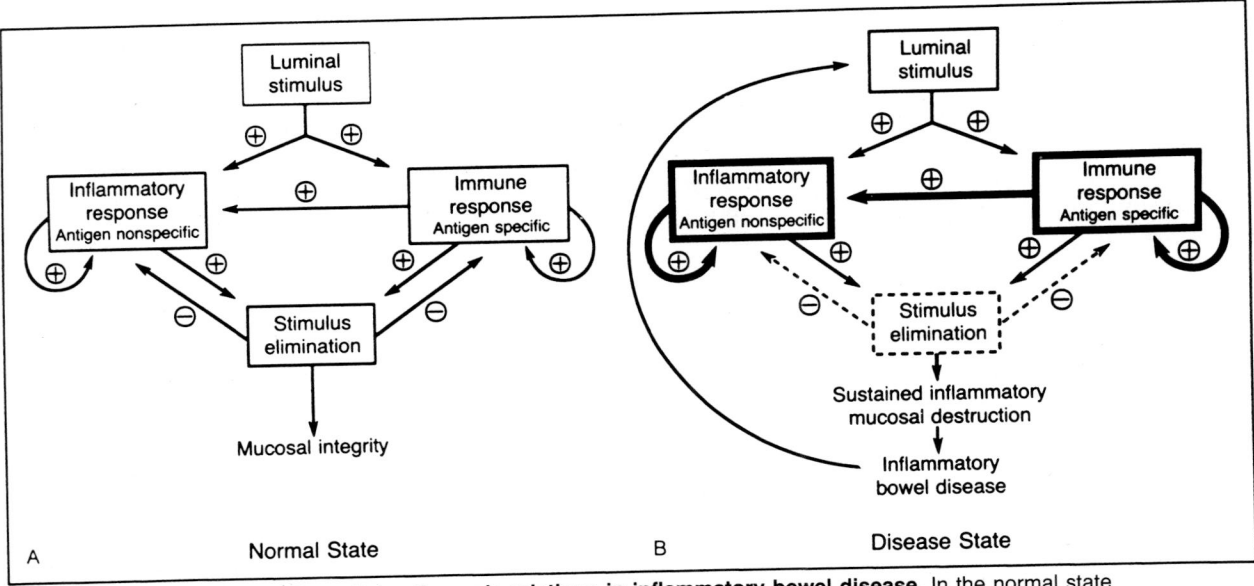

**Figure 62–1. Potential pathogenic relations in inflammatory bowel disease.** In the normal state **(A)**, the lumen of the intestine is confronted by a variety of substances (e.g., dietary antigens and microbial agents) that may stimulate specific immune responses by elements of the mucosal immune system, the production of inflammatory mediators by recruitment and activation of cellular constituents of nonspecific inflammatory responses (e.g., chemotactic formulated bacterial peptides), or both activities. This potentially autoamplifying stimulatory process is counterbalanced by the mucosal barrier that limits the access of luminal constituents and by feedback mechanisms for the down-regulation of immune and inflammatory responses after the elimination of activating stimuli that breach the mucosal barrier. In the presence of disease **(B)**, one or several fundamental alterations in the intestinal defense mechanisms may contribute to sustained inflammation, which ultimately results in tissue destruction and subsequently inflammatory bowel disease. Specific or generalized luminal stimuli (e.g., a persistent infectious agent or general intrinsic defect in the mucosal barrier) may lead to tonic stimulation of immune and inflammatory responses. Alternatively, regulation of immune and inflammatory responses may be intrinsically abnormal, with either exaggerated activation in response to "normal" stimuli or defective feedback mechanisms for down-regulation. Altered regulation of immune and inflammatory responses could also occur in the absence of specific extrinsic activating stimuli. Products of the immune and inflammatory cellular constituents—such as lymphocytes, tissue macrophages, neutrophils, mast cells, eosinophils, and fibroblasts—include a wide variety of cytokines, eicosanoids, and oxygen free radicals that damage tissue. (**A** and **B** from Podolsky DK: Inflammatory bowel disease. Reprinted, by permission of the New England Journal of Medicine, 325; 928–937, 1992.)

are powerful mediators in neurogenic induced inflammation and cause vasodilatation, plasma extravasation, and watery diarrhea. All these factors may have a role in the pathophysiology of inflammatory bowel disease.[26, 28]

**Psychologic and Stress Factors.** Psychologic factors appear to influence the clinical course of ulcerative colitis, although the mechanism is uncertain. Perhaps neurotransmitters and neurohumoral peptides from the brain and gut may play a role. It is unclear whether there is an ulcerative colitis type of personality (neurotic, introverted) that is vulnerable to stress or whether chronic, debilitating disease leads to psychologic changes.[33, 34]

**Immunologic Factors.** The immune system provides an important contribution to the pathogenesis of ulcerative colitis either because of failure to clear a microbial or toxic agent or because of an inappropriate response to it. The immune system probably mediates the tissue injury as well, regardless of the trigger. This is the basis of therapy with corticosteroid and other immunosuppressive agents.[35, 36] The colonic inflammation of ulcerative colitis may merely be an exaggerated "physiologic"

response that is always present within the lamina propria of the colon. There is an alteration of the relative representation of macrophages and T cell and B cell populations and an increase in the numbers of immunoglobulin G–bearing cells. This may be the result of an altered pattern of cytokines that control the differentiation of B cells. The disease is also characterized by a fundamental alteration in antigen-presenting activity associated with a reduction of intestinal suppressor T cells and elevated levels of cytotoxic Leu-7$^+$ cells. Increased levels of specific antibodies to antigens in the gut lumen are also found.[28, 35–37]

**Chemical Mediators.** In acute ulcerative colitis, there is activation of the arachidonic cascade with increased release of chemical mediators, superoxide radicals, prostaglandins, leukotrienes, and thromboxane, which are potent inflammatory and vasoactive mediators.[1, 28]

**Environmental Factors.** As stated earlier, smoking appears to protect against ulcerative colitis, perhaps by correcting the defect in the production of mucus or altering prostaglandin synthesis. Oral contraceptives can disturb the intestinal microcirculation and produce clinical and endoscopic features identical to ulcerative colitis. Some studies suggest a close link between oral contraceptives and ulcerative colitis.[38]

**Diet.** Cow's milk protein, lactose intolerance, and chemical food additives such as carrageenan have been implicated in the development of ulcerative colitis.[39, 40]

Clearly, ulcerative colitis is a complex disease consisting of interactions among initiating organisms or antigens, the host's immune response, and immunologic, environmental, and hereditary influences.

## Clinical Findings

Ulcerative colitis is highly variable in clinical course, severity, and prognosis. Disease activity waxes and wanes and is characterized by acute exacerbations of bloody diarrhea that resolve either spontaneously or after therapy. The most common clinical findings (Table 62–2) are diarrhea, abdominal pain, rectal bleeding, weight loss, and tenesmus; vomiting, fever, constipation, and arthralgias occur less commonly.[1–5, 41]

Ulcerative colitis usually behaves as a chronic low-grade illness in most patients. In 15% of patients, this disease has an acute and fulminating course with explosive diarrhea, hematochezia, and hypotension. Most patients (60 to 75%) have intermittent attacks with complete symptomatic remission between attacks; 4 to 10% have one attack and no subsequent symptoms; 5 to 15% are troubled by continuous symptoms without remission.[1–5, 41, 42]

Patients with ulcerative proctitis have disease of mild severity, and the disease usually remains distal. There is extension to the proximal colon in 15% of patients over a 10-year period and extension to the hepatic flexure in 7%. At presentation, 30% of patients have disease limited to the rectum, 40% have disease extending above the rectum but not beyond the hepatic flexure (so-called substantial disease), and the remaining 30% have pancolitis. Extraintestinal manifestations are present in fewer than 10% of patients at initial presentation: arthralgias, a mild arthritis, eye inflammation, and rash.[1–5, 41, 42]

### TABLE 62–2. ULCERATIVE COLITIS VERSUS CROHN'S DISEASE: CLINICAL FINDINGS*

| CLINICAL FINDING | ULCERATIVE COLITIS | CROHN'S DISEASE |
|---|---|---|
| Diarrhea | + + + + | + + + + |
| Rectal bleeding | + + + + | + + + |
| Abdominal pain | + + + | + + + + |
| Weight loss | + + | + + + + |
| Fever | + | + + + |
| Tenesmus | + + | + + + + |
| Vomiting | 0 | + + + |
| Abdominal mass | 0 | + + + + |
| Perianal disease | 0 | + + + + |
| Malnutrition | + | + + + |
| Pyoderma gangrenosum | + + | + |
| Uveitis | + + | + |

*0 = very rare; + = rare; + + = occasional; + + + = common; + + + + = very common.

### TABLE 62–3. DIFFERENTIATING COLONOSCOPIC AND GROSS PATHOLOGIC FEATURES: ULCERATIVE COLITIS VERSUS CROHN'S DISEASE

| FEATURE | ULCERATIVE COLITIS | CROHN'S DISEASE |
|---|---|---|
| Continuous disease | Always | Exceptional |
| Distribution | Symmetric | Asymmetric |
| Patchiness | Absent | Frequent |
| Rectal disease | Almost always | Often absent |
| Profuse bleeding | Common | Rare |
| Granularity | Common | Less common |
| Cobblestoning | Absent | Characteristic |
| Erythema | Characteristic | Less pronounced |
| Edema (blunted haustra) | Present | Present |
| Friability | Common | Uncommon |
| Spontaneous petechiae | Common | Uncommon |
| Superficial to small ulcers | Occasional | Frequent |
| Large (>1 cm) ulceration | Severe disease | Common |
| Deep longitudinal ulceration | Rare | Common |
| Linear ulceration | Rare | Common |
| Aphthoid ulceration | Absent | Characteristic |
| Serpiginous ulceration | Rare | Common |
| Pseudopolyps | Occasional | Occasional |
| Bridging | Occasional | Occasional |
| Mucosa surrounding ulcer | Abnormal | Normal |

From Silverstein FE, Tytgat GNJ: Atlas of Gastrointestinal Endoscopy. New York: Gower Medical Publishers, 1992, p 11.18.

Physical examination discloses fever, prostration, dehydration, and postural hypotension in the most severe cases. The abdomen may be protuberant because of colonic atony and distention. Abdominal tenderness over the colon and absent bowel sounds are ominous signs suggesting toxic megacolon or early perforation. Milder involvement is manifested as pallor, low-grade fever, evident weight loss, and mild abdominal tenderness.[41–44]

## Endoscopic Findings

Sigmoidoscopy is helpful in establishing the diagnosis of ulcerative colitis because the distal colon and rectum are involved in 90 to 95% of cases (Table 62–3). Early, the mucosa is edematous, with loss of the normal vascular pattern, and friable with bleeding when touched by the endoscope or rubbed with a cotton swab. With disease progression, granular, spontaneously hemorrhagic mucosa is found, associated with a mucopurulent exudate. The haustra are thick and blunted, the lumen seems narrowed and straightened, and the normal thin (<2 mm) mucosal folds are lost. In severe disease, the mucosa is diffusely hemorrhagic, and frank ulceration with loss of mucosal irregularity is seen.[45]

## Radiologic Findings

### Plain Film

Considerable information can be gained by carefully scrutinizing the plain abdominal films of patients with ulcerative colitis. Although attention should be focused on the colon, other abnormalities such as renal calculi, sacroiliitis, ankylosing spondylitis, and avascular necrosis of the femoral heads must also be excluded.[46-51]

Although the extent of ulcerative colitis is generally measured by barium enema and colonoscopy, these procedures carry a higher risk in severely ill patients. The following plain film features can be used to assess the severity and extent of the colitis: 1) the extent of formed fecal residue; 2) the appearance of the mucosal edge; 3) alterations of the haustra; 4) colonic width; and 5) mural thickness.[46]

**Colonic Fecal Residue.** The distal extent of formed fecal residue gives a good indication, although not absolute, of the proximal extent of the colitis (Fig. 62–2). This approach sometimes overestimates but does not underestimate the extent of disease. The following conclusions can be drawn from the extent of residue: 1) if no residue is visible, the patient probably has active pancolitis; 2) if the residue extends down into the sigmoid colon, proctitis is present (this may be indistinguishable from normal); 3) if residue is present only in the proximal colon, the colitis most likely extends to this level but could be more distal.[46-51]

**Mucosa.** The colonic mucosal edge is normally smooth. In active colitis, the line is granular, indistinct, and somewhat fuzzy (Fig. 62–3). With frank ulceration, the mucosal line is disrupted, which causes an irregular edge. With extensive ulceration, only edematous mucosal islands remain. Intramural, mottled-appearing gas shadows may be present in fulminating colitis with necrosis of the bowel wall. Linear pneumatosis suggests either extremely deep ulceration or extraperitoneal perforation with gas trapped adjacent to the bowel wall.[46-54]

**Haustration.** Normal haustral clefts run in parallel, about 2 to 4 mm apart, across one third of the diameter of the colon. Widening of the haustral clefts (see Fig. 62–2) with loss of the parallel lines is an early manifestation of ulcerative colitis and is more obvious on plain films than is the mucosal granularity it accompanies. The haustra may be completely absent as well. Blunting can be confused with underdistention, so it should not be diagnosed if only a small amount of gas is present within the colon.[46-54]

**Colon Diameter.** The upper limit of normal for the diameter of the transverse colon is 5.5 cm. In chronic, "burned out" ulcerative colitis, the colon becomes tubular and narrowed and is considerably less than 5 cm in diameter. In these patients, if the colon is greater than 5 cm in diameter, the inflammation has become transmural, which indicates a fulminant colitis at risk for perforation or toxic megacolon.[52-54]

**Mural Thickness.** In the normal colon, the distance between the line of pericolic fat and gas-filled lumen is less than 3 mm. In chronic ulcerative colitis, it increases to greater than 3 mm in thickness[55] (see Fig. 62–3).

In a study assessing these findings, a combination of four features was pathognomonic for disease proximal to the hepatic flexure: irregularity of the mucosal edge, loss of haustral clefts, increased thickness of the colon wall, and an "empty" right colon.[50]

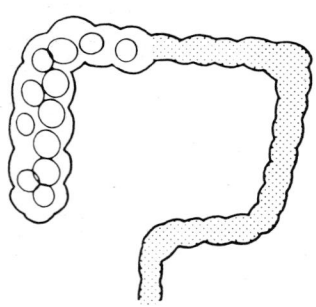

Distal extent residue = proximal active ulcerative colitis

A

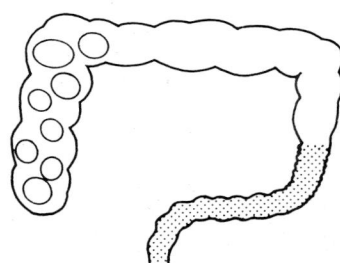

Distal extent residue more proximal than colitis — overestimates extent of disease

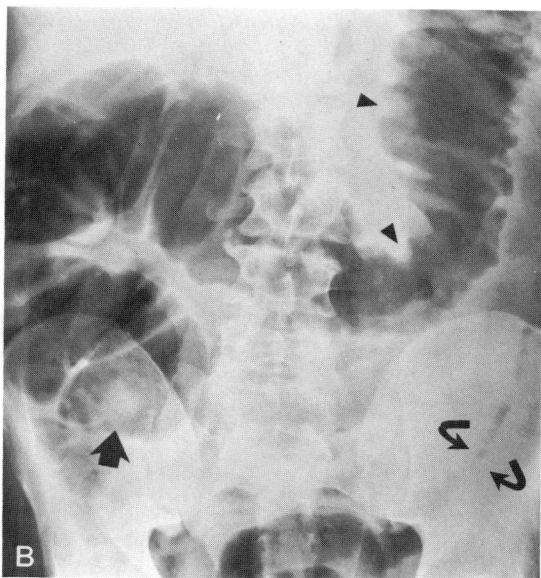

B

**Figure 62–2. Ulcerative colitis: plain film estimation of active disease. A.** The distal extent of fecal residue may overestimate but seldom underestimates the proximal extent of active disease. (From Bartram C, Kumar P: Clinical Radiology in Gastroenterology. Oxford: Blackwell Scientific Publications, 1981, p 135.) **B.** This patient with clinically suspected toxic megacolon demonstrates fecal residue in the cecum *(straight arrow)*. Note the dilatation of the transverse colon and blunted haustral clefts *(arrowheads)* distally. There is narrowing of the sigmoid colon lumen *(curved arrows)* with apparent mural thickening. This patient recovered from fulminant colitis, and disease was found only distal to the midtransverse colon.

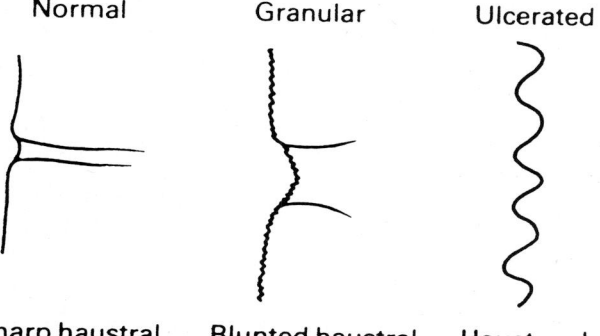

Normal                Granular                Ulcerated

Sharp haustral       Blunted haustral       Haustra absent, coarse
cleft,               clefts, fine           irregular edge
smooth edge          irregular edge
A

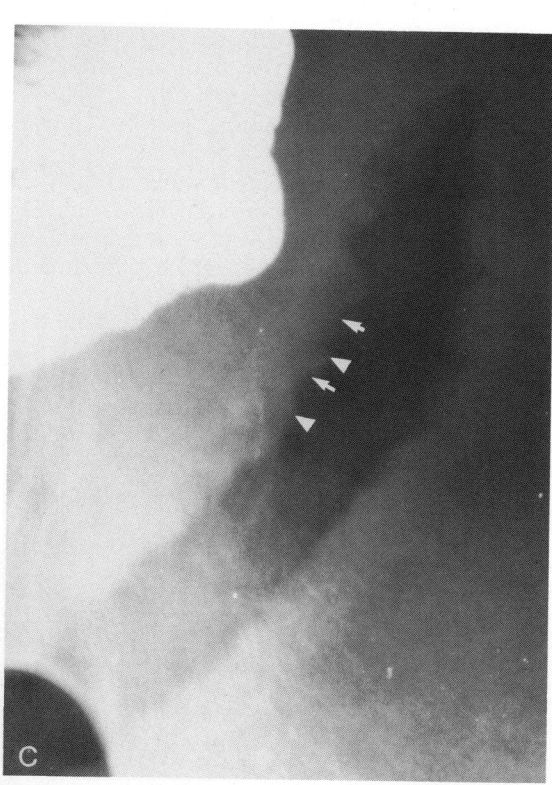

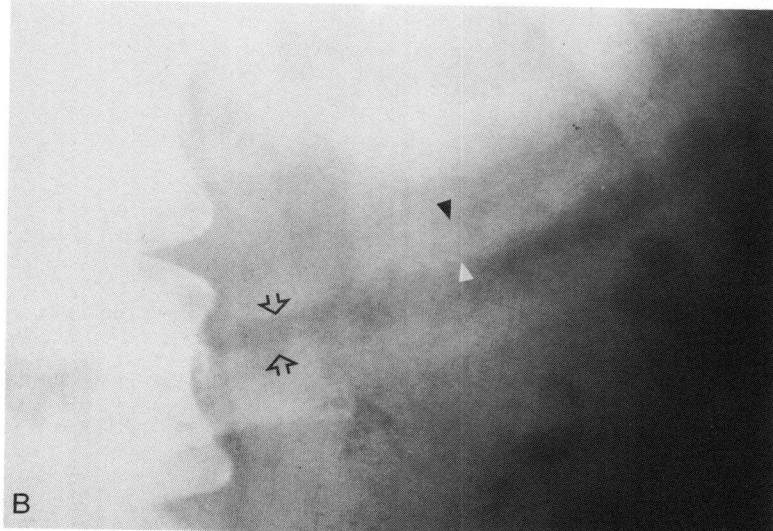

**Figure 62–3. Ulcerative colitis: plain film assessment of mural and mucosal disease. A.** With progressive disease, the normally sharp, well-defined haustra become blunted and then lost. (From Bartram CI, Kumar P: Clinical Radiology in Gastroenterology. Oxford: Blackwell Scientific Publications, 1981, p 135.) **B.** Magnified view of the transverse colon reveals loss of haustration, mural thickening *(arrowheads),* and lumen narrowing *(open arrows).* **C.** Magnified view of the sigmoid colon demonstrates mural thickening and ulceration *(arrows)* and residual islands of edematous mucosa *(arrowheads).*

## *Scintigraphy*[56–61]

Although the diagnosis and disease activity assessment of ulcerative colitis are made primarily by radiographic and endoscopic techniques, both gallium citrate Ga 67 and [111]In-labeled leukocyte scans have proved useful in patients with inflammatory bowel disease. Scintigraphic techniques are useful when there is danger of bowel perforation and the extent and degree of disease activity must be assessed.[56–61]

## *Ultrasound*

Inflammatory bowel disease alters the thickness and echogenicity of the gut wall or individual layers, the integrity of mural stratification, the appearance of surrounding tissues, and bowel motility and compressibility[62–67] (Table 62–4).

Edema is a prominent feature of acute intestinal inflammation. Edema results in thickening of the colon wall and preservation of wall stratification (Fig. 62–4). On transverse section, alternate hyperechoic and hypoechoic layers give rise to a target appearance. In ulcerative colitis, the mucosa becomes thickened and hypoechoic as a result of edema. The submucosa also thickens, yet colonic motility is maintained. With progressive disease, haustral septations are lost. In patients with well-established disease, bowel wall thickness is approximately 0.6 ± 0.2 cm.[62–67] In one series, these changes were seen in all patients with pancolitis, in 94% of those with left-sided colitis, but in only 50% of patients with rectosigmoiditis. If there is extensive pseu-

### TABLE 62–4. ULCERATIVE COLITIS VERSUS CROHN'S COLITIS: SONOGRAPHIC FINDINGS

**ULCERATIVE COLITIS**
Moderately thick, hypoechoic wall
Typical wall stratification maintained
Loss of haustration
Absent peristaltic motion

**CROHN'S COLITIS**
Clearly thickened, hypoechoic wall
Loss of typical wall stratification
Loss of haustration
Diminished compressibility
Absent peristaltic motion

dopolyposis, the thickness of the wall may increase up to 1.5 cm, and this is often accompanied by loss of wall stratification.[66–71]

## *Computed Tomography*

When active disease is limited to the mucosa, without significant narrowing, computed tomography (CT) findings are usually normal in ulcerative colitis. With chronic disease and thickening of the mucosa and submucosa, both mural thickening and lumen narrowing are identified (Table 62–5). The mural thickening is inhomogeneous, having a "target" appearance (Fig. 62–5) with 1) an inner ring of soft tissue density (mucosa, lamina propria, enlarged muscularis mucosae); 2) a middle ring

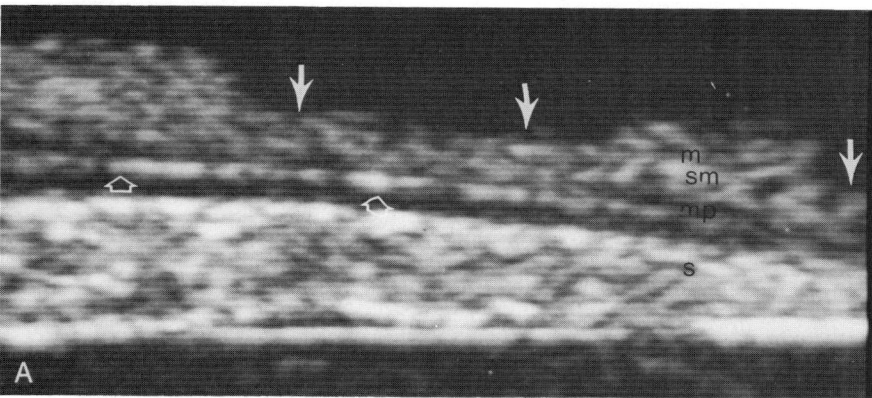

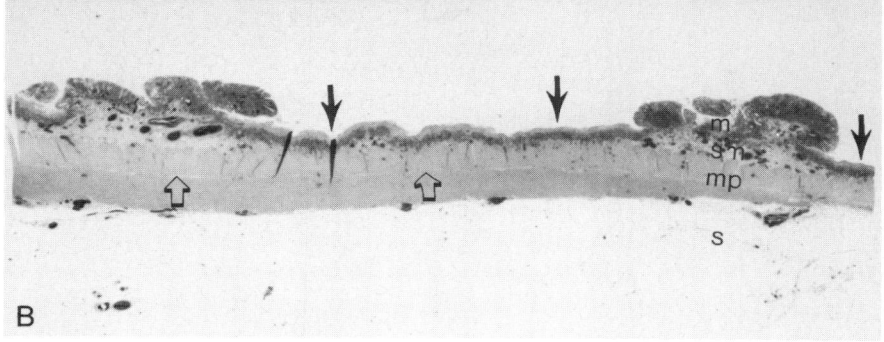

**Figure 62–4. Ulcerative colitis: sonographic findings.** Ultrasound image **(A)** and corresponding histologic section **(B)** of a specimen of ulcerative colitis are shown. Wall stratification is maintained on the sonogram in areas that are not ulcerated. An echogenic line is present that corresponds to the connective tissue between the inner circular and outer longitudinal components of the muscularis propria *(open arrows)*. Solid arrows = areas of ulceration; m = mucosa; sm = submucosa; mp = muscularis propria; s = serosa and subserosal fat. (**A** and **B** from Kimmey MB, Wang KY, Haggitt RC, et al: Diagnosis of inflammatory bowel disease with ultrasound: an in vitro study. Invest Radiol 25:1085–1090, 1990.)

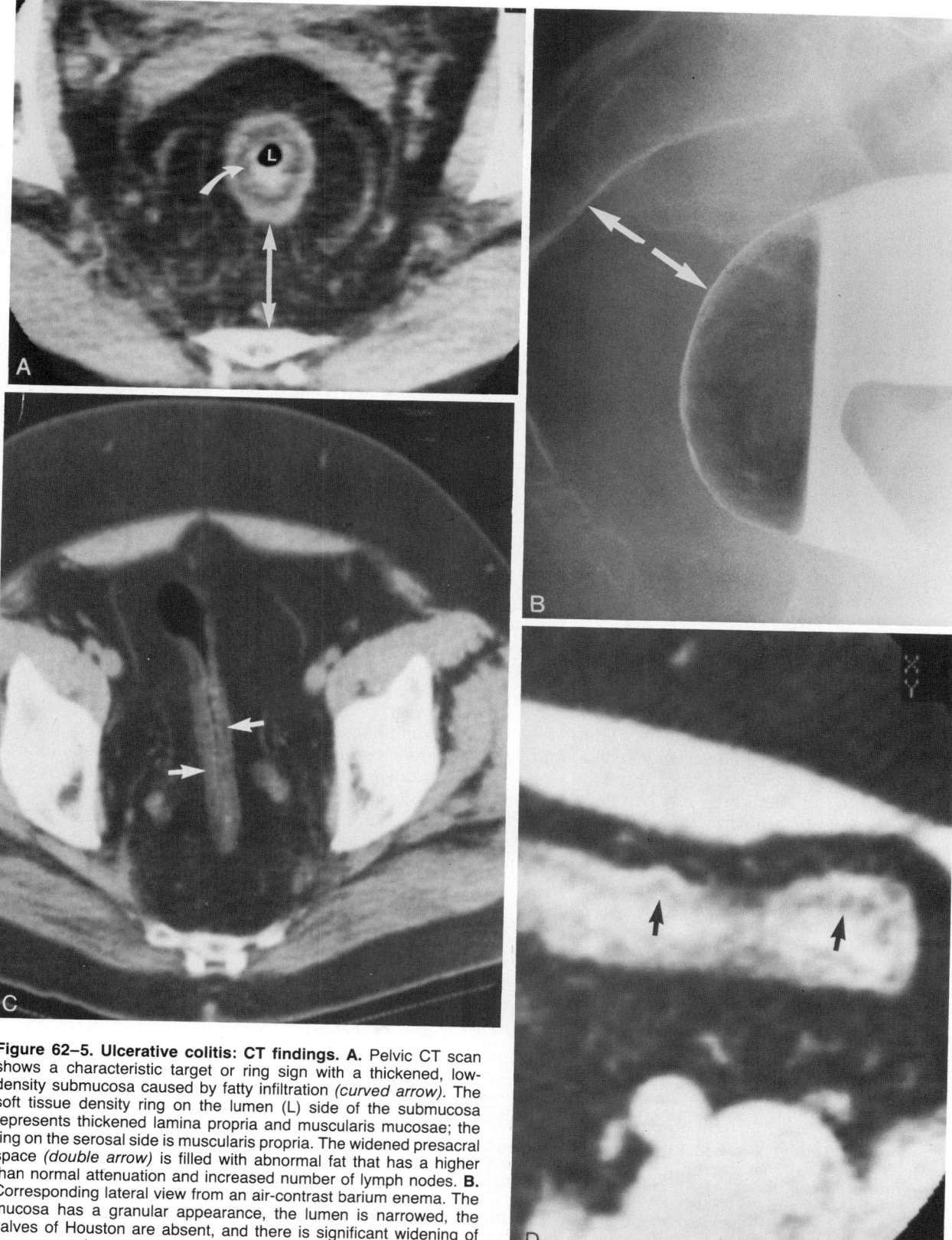

**Figure 62–5. Ulcerative colitis: CT findings. A.** Pelvic CT scan shows a characteristic target or ring sign with a thickened, low-density submucosa caused by fatty infiltration *(curved arrow)*. The soft tissue density ring on the lumen (L) side of the submucosa represents thickened lamina propria and muscularis mucosae; the ring on the serosal side is muscularis propria. The widened presacral space *(double arrow)* is filled with abnormal fat that has a higher than normal attenuation and increased number of lymph nodes. **B.** Corresponding lateral view from an air-contrast barium enema. The mucosa has a granular appearance, the lumen is narrowed, the valves of Houston are absent, and there is significant widening of the presacral space *(arrows)*. **C.** Fatty deposition is demonstrated in the wall of these different patients with chronic ulcerative colitis. Linear lucencies *(arrows)* are seen within the wall. **D.** Magnified view of the sigmoid colon in a different patient shows similar lucencies *(arrows)*. The lumen of the rectosigmoid colon is narrowed despite air insufflation.

## TABLE 62–5. ULCERATIVE COLITIS VERSUS CROHN'S DISEASE: COMPUTED TOMOGRAPHY FINDINGS

**ULCERATIVE COLITIS**
Mural thickening < 1.5 cm
Inhomogeneous CT density of wall
Target appearance of rectum
Increased perirectal and presacral fat

**CROHN'S DISEASE**
Mural thickening > 2 cm
Homogeneous CT density of wall
Mural thickening of small bowel
Abscesses, fistulas, sinus tracts
Mesenteric changes (abscess, phlegmon, fibrofatty proliferation)
Perianal disease

**COMMON FINDINGS**
Mural thickening
Narrowed lumen
Increased lymph node size and number

## TABLE 62–6. ULCERATIVE COLITIS: BARIUM ENEMA FINDINGS

**ACUTE CHANGES**
Mucosal granularity
Mucosal stippling
Collar button ulcers
Haustral thickening or loss
Inflammatory polyps
Confluent, contiguous, circumferential disease

**CHRONIC CHANGES**
Haustral loss
Lumen narrowing
Loss of rectal valves
Widened presacral space
Backwash ileitis
Postinflammatory pseudopolyps

of low attenuation (−10 to −15 Hounsfield units [HU]) resulting from widening and fatty infiltration of the submucosa; and 3) an outer, soft tissue density ring representing the muscularis propria.[72–77]

Thinning of the colonic wall and dilatation of the lumen can be seen in toxic megacolon. Pneumatosis intestinalis is often better appreciated on CT scans than on conventional barium studies.[72–76]

## Barium Enema

The barium enema has the following role in patients with ulcerative colitis: 1) to confirm the clinical diagnosis; 2) to assess the extent and severity of disease; 3) to differentiate ulcerative colitis from Crohn's disease and other colitides; 4) to follow the course of disease; and 5) to detect complications. The major radiographic findings on the barium enema examination in ulcerative colitis are listed in Table 62–6; their anatomic-pathologic origin (Fig. 62–6) and significance are discussed in the following section.[78–84]

## Double Contrast Barium Enema Findings and Their Anatomic-Pathologic Basis

### Granular Pattern

The earliest pathologic changes of ulcerative colitis are hyperemia and the accumulation of inflammatory cells in the mucosa.[85, 86] These changes are manifested by a loss of normal mucosal translucency and obscuration of the submucosal pattern on endoscopy.[87, 88] Subtle thickening of the mucosa or haustral edema may be present radiographically, but these findings are often appreciated only in retrospect.[89] With progressive edema and hyperemia, the mucosa develops a granular pattern[46, 81, 89] (Fig. 62–7A). The smooth, sharp, and distinct appearance of the colonic margin seen on normal double contrast studies is replaced by an amorphous, thickened, and indistinct mucosal line. There is a gradual transition between the normal and abnormal mucosa that extends for several centimeters.[46, 90] This granularity should be distinguished from the granular appearance of chronic ulcerative colitis (Fig. 62–7B). In chronic ulcerative colitis, the mucosal surface pattern is coarser, and there are significant changes in colonic contour.

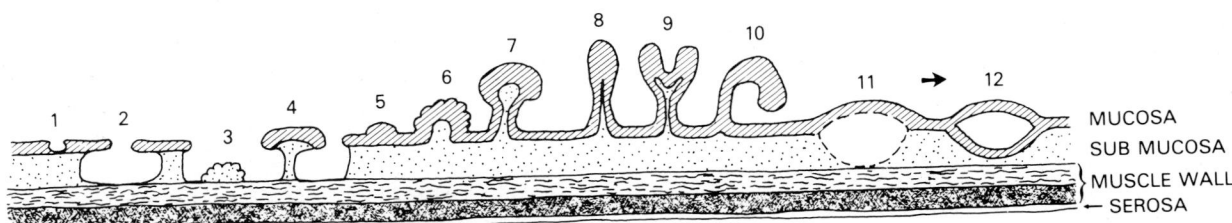

**Figure 62–6. Spectrum of mucosal abnormalities in ulcerative colitis.** 1 = punctate mucosal ulcer–crypt abscess; 2 = collar button ulcer; 3 = polypoid accumulation of granulation tissue; 4 = mucosal remnant forming inflammatory pseudopolyp; 5 and 6 = sessile mucosal polyps (similar morphologic features are seen in hyperplasia, adenoma, and carcinoma); 7 = pedunculated polyp (typically hyperplastic or low-grade adenomas); 8, 9, and 10 = postinflammatory pseudopolyps of various configurations; 11 = mucosal remnant bridging area of active undermining ulceration; 12 = mucosal bridge in quiescent state with previously denuded surfaces covered with new epithelium. (From Lichtenstein JE: Radiologic-pathologic correlation of inflammatory bowel disease. Radiol Clin North Am 25:3–24, 1987.)

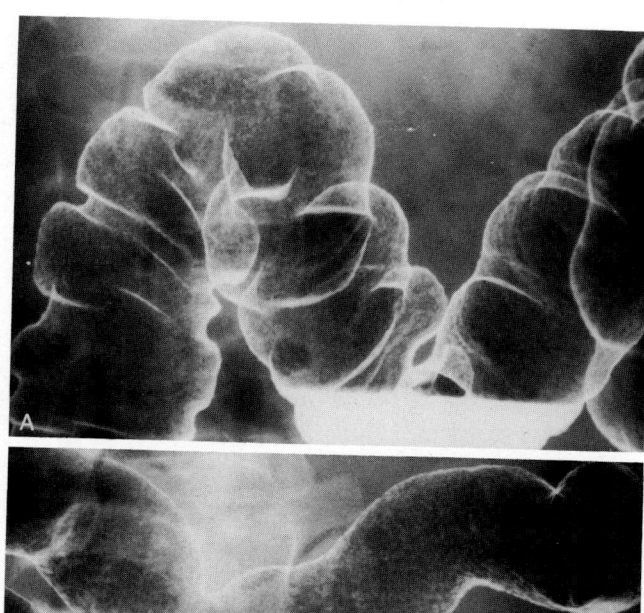

**Figure 62–7. Ulcerative colitis: granular mucosal pattern. A.** Early ulcerative colitis. Notice the blunted haustral clefts on this spot film of the hepatic flexure. The mucosal granularity, attributable to abnormal quantity and quality of mucin, is contiguous, circumferential, and symmetric. **B.** Chronic ulcerative colitis. This spot film of a short, tubular, ahaustral transverse colon shows a coarser surface pattern than that seen in acute disease. TI = terminal ileum; AC = ascending colon.

The granular pattern is primarily a result of abnormalities in the quality and quantity of mucus produced by the involved mucosa.[86] On histologic examination, there is a reduction in the number of goblet cells, which contain less than the normal complement of mucin.[6, 86, 91] Normal mucus is essential to normal barium coating of the gut. Any process, whether benign or malignant, infectious or inflammatory, that alters mucin production will affect mucosal coating and visualization.[86]

## Mucosal Stippling

During the granular phase of ulcerative colitis, inflammatory cells accumulate at the base of the mucosal crypts.[6, 91, 92] Cellular debris tends to block the crypts of Lieberkühn, which leads to the formation of microabscesses, better known as crypt abscesses (Fig. 62–8A). These crypt abscesses eventually erode into the lumen.[6, 91, 92] The ulcers deepen, and barium flecks become adherent to them, producing mucosal stippling[86] (Fig. 62–8B). This stippling resembles white paint applied by dabbing a surface with the end of a fairly dry paintbrush.[81]

## Collar Button Ulcers

With disease progression, the ulcers of the crypt abscess breach the lamina propria and muscularis mucosae and cause undermining of the less resistant areolar tissue of the submucosa.[81] The involved submucosa becomes necrotic, and the ulcers extend laterally, causing further undermining. This undermining is contained by the muscularis propria on the serosal side and by the muscularis mucosae on the lumen side of the colon.[93, 94] The ulcers are frequently related to the taeniae. The mucosal defect is small relative to the degree of undermining and produces a flask-like, "collar button" ulcer[86] (Fig. 62–9).

As these ulcers enlarge and interconnect, the collar button ulcer configuration is lost; a network of residual islands of mucosa and inflammatory pseudopolyps is produced.

## Polyps

A variety of different mucosal protrusions may occur in patients with inflammatory bowel disease and may be seen on barium studies.[86] Their appearance and significance depend on the stage of disease and pathologic origin (Fig. 62–10).

**Inflammatory Pseudopolyps.** In patients with severe ulcerative colitis, there is extensive mucosal and submucosal ulceration in which only small islands of mucosa and submucosa may survive. The inflamed edematous mucosa protrudes above the surrounding areas of ulceration, which gives a polypoid appearance[6, 91] (Fig. 62–11). Because these "polyps" represent merely the remnants of pre-existing mucosa and submucosa rather than new growths, they are termed *pseudopolyps*.[95, 96] Inflammatory pseudopolyps are the natural progression of

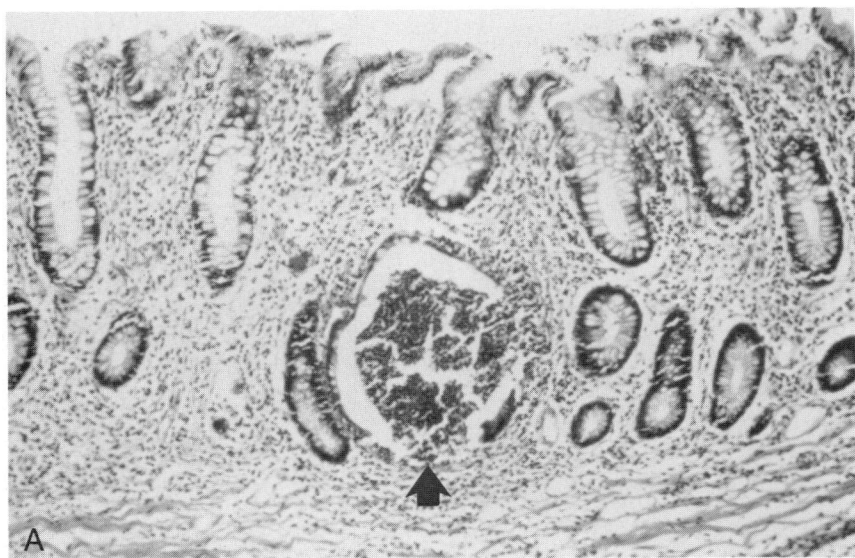

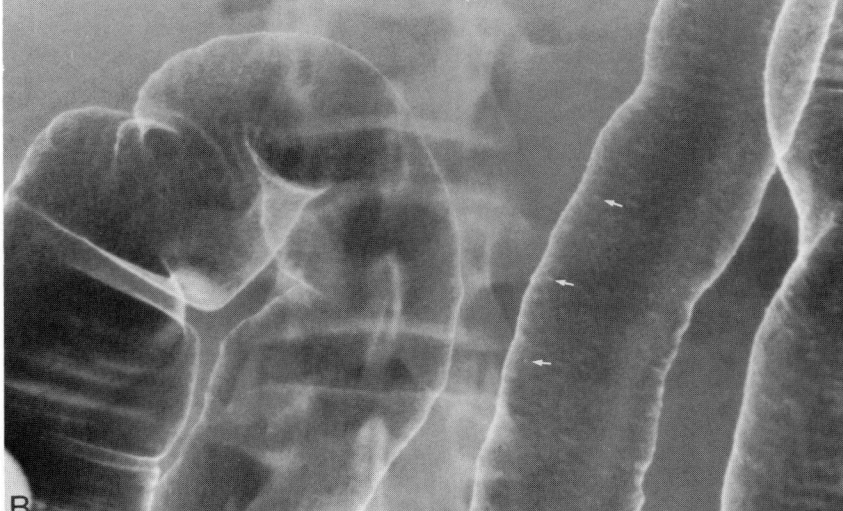

**Figure 62–8. Ulcerative colitis: crypt abscess causing mucosal stippling. A.** A crypt abscess *(arrow)* is seen at the base of a crypt of Lieberkühn. **B.** When these abscesses erode into the lumen, they accumulate punctate collections of barium *(arrows),* which produces mucosal stippling.

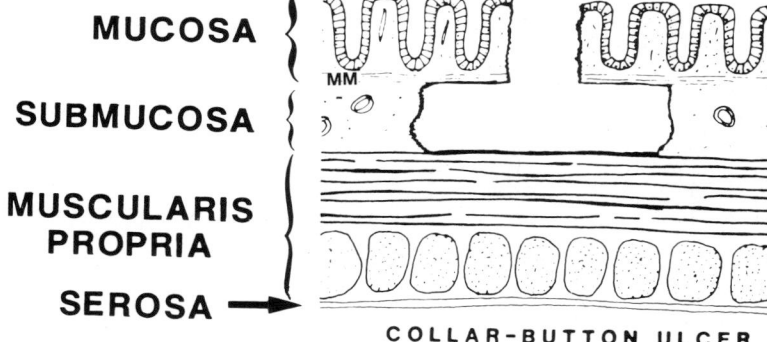

MUCOSA

SUBMUCOSA

MUSCULARIS
PROPRIA

SEROSA

MM

COLLAR-BUTTON ULCER

A

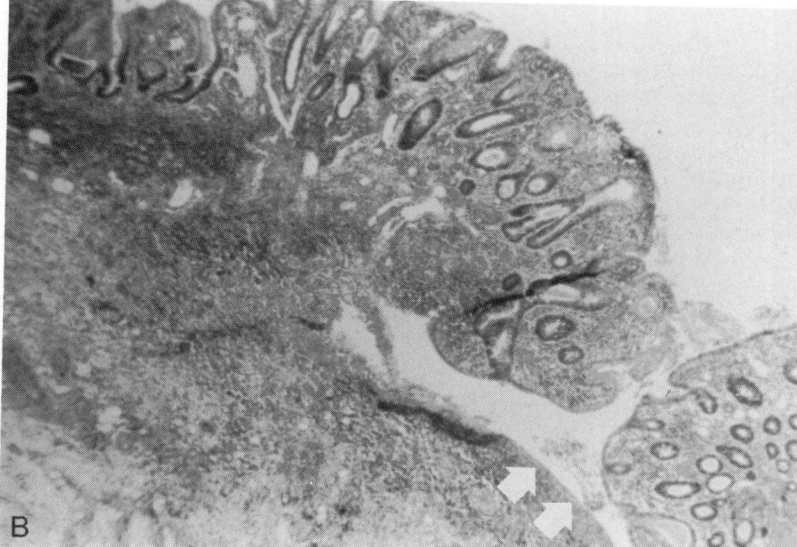

B

C

**Figure 62–9. Ulcerative colitis: collar button ulcers.**
**A.** Diagram showing the narrow neck of the crypt abscess that erodes through the muscularis mucosae (MM) into the submucosa. The ulcer spreads laterally through the submucosa and is contained with a flat base by the resistant inner circular layer of the muscularis propria. (From Lichtenstein JE: Radiologic-pathologic correlation of inflammatory bowel disease. Radiol Clin North Am 25:3–24, 1987.) **B.** Low-power photomicrograph shows characteristic undermining with a flat base *(arrows)*. **C.** Spot film of the splenic flexure shows multiple flask-like ulcers *(arrows)* with a flat base. The ulceration is limited to the layers superficial to the muscularis propria.

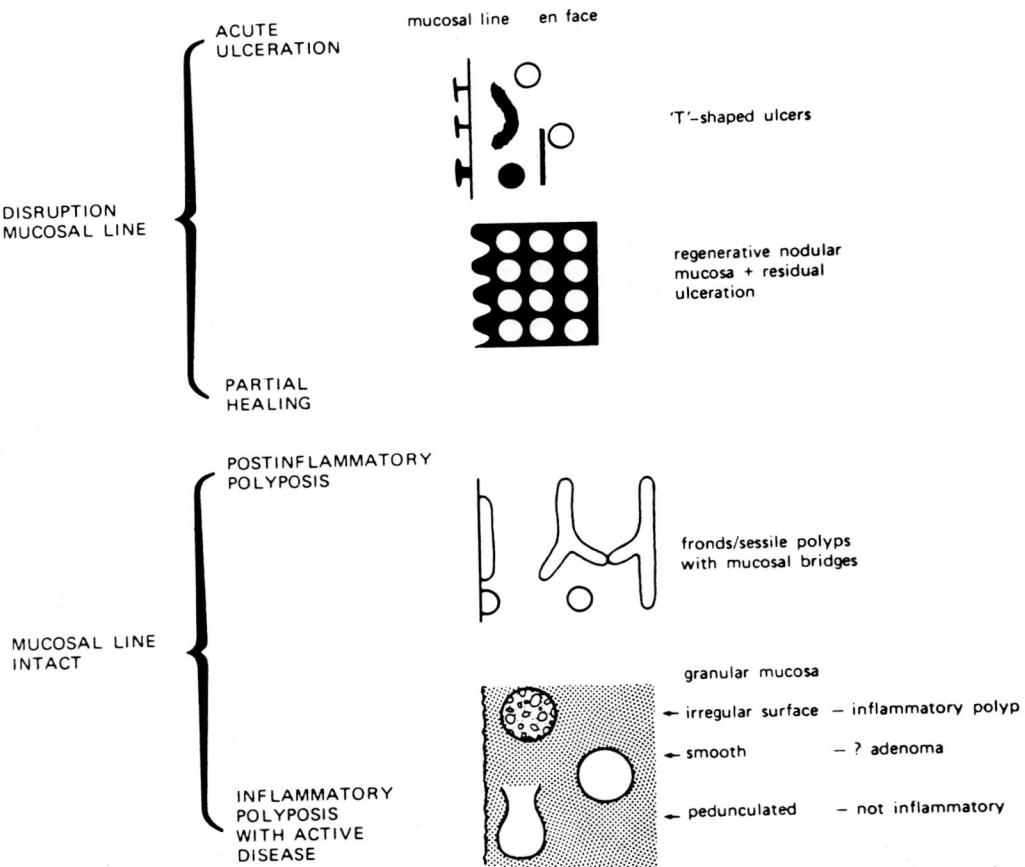

**Figure 62–10. Diagram depicting the causes of polypoid mucosa in ulcerative colitis.** (Reprinted from Bartram CI: Radiology in Inflammatory Bowel Disease. New York: Marcel Dekker, 1983, p 102 by courtesy of Marcel Dekker Inc.)

collar button ulcers: the ulcers extend and interconnect so that the pseudopolyp rather than the ulcers becomes the major radiographic finding.[86, 97–103] Inflammatory pseudopolyps usually occur in ulcerative colitis but may also be seen in Crohn's disease. The cobblestoning pattern seen in Crohn's disease is another type of pseudopolyp in which larger islands of preserved mucosa are surrounded by linear and transverse ulcerations.[86]

**Postinflammatory Pseudopolyps.** When inflammatory bowel disease goes into remission, the denuded mucosa heals and is covered by granulation tissue that has a granular appearance similar to that observed in the early stages of ulcerative colitis.[6, 86, 91] In some patients, the regenerated mucosa has a tendency to overgrow (Fig. 62–12A to C). This overgrowth often results in polypoid lesions that may be small and rounded, be long and filiform, or proliferate into a bush-like structure simulating a villous adenoma. Because the regenerating mucosa is cytologically normal, it is not a true neoplasm but a pseudopolyp. Because this occurs during mucosal healing, it is called a postinflammatory pseudopolyp.[97–103] These polyps represent the aftermath of a severe attack of colitis and may be the only sign of previous disease.

Mucosal bridges (Fig. 62–12D) are also postinflammatory pseudopolyps in which a bridge of mucosa sur-

vives between islands of mucosa surrounded by ulceration. With remission, the underside of the mucosal bridge and the underlying ulcer re-epithelialize.[86, 104, 105]

Postinflammatory pseudopolyps can also be seen after ischemia, after severe infection, and in Crohn's disease. Filiform polyps have also been described in the stomach and small bowel in patients with Crohn's disease.[86]

## Backwash Ileitis

In 10 to 40% of patients with chronic ulcerative pancolitis, the distal 5 to 25 cm of ileum is inflamed (Fig. 62–13). This ileitis occurs only in the presence of pancolitis and usually resolves 1 to 2 weeks after colectomy.[46, 89] Although small ulcerations may be present, this is not a primary inflammation of the ileum. Indeed, the distal ileum can be used to form an ileostomy or pouch. The pathogenesis of this disorder is uncertain but may relate to the reflux of colonic contents into the small bowel, hence the term *reflux* or *backwash* ileitis.[46]

Barium studies reveal a chronic pancolitis associated with a patulous and fixed ileocecal valve that easily refluxes and persistent dilatation of the terminal ileum.[79–81] The normal fold pattern is absent, and the mucosa is granular.

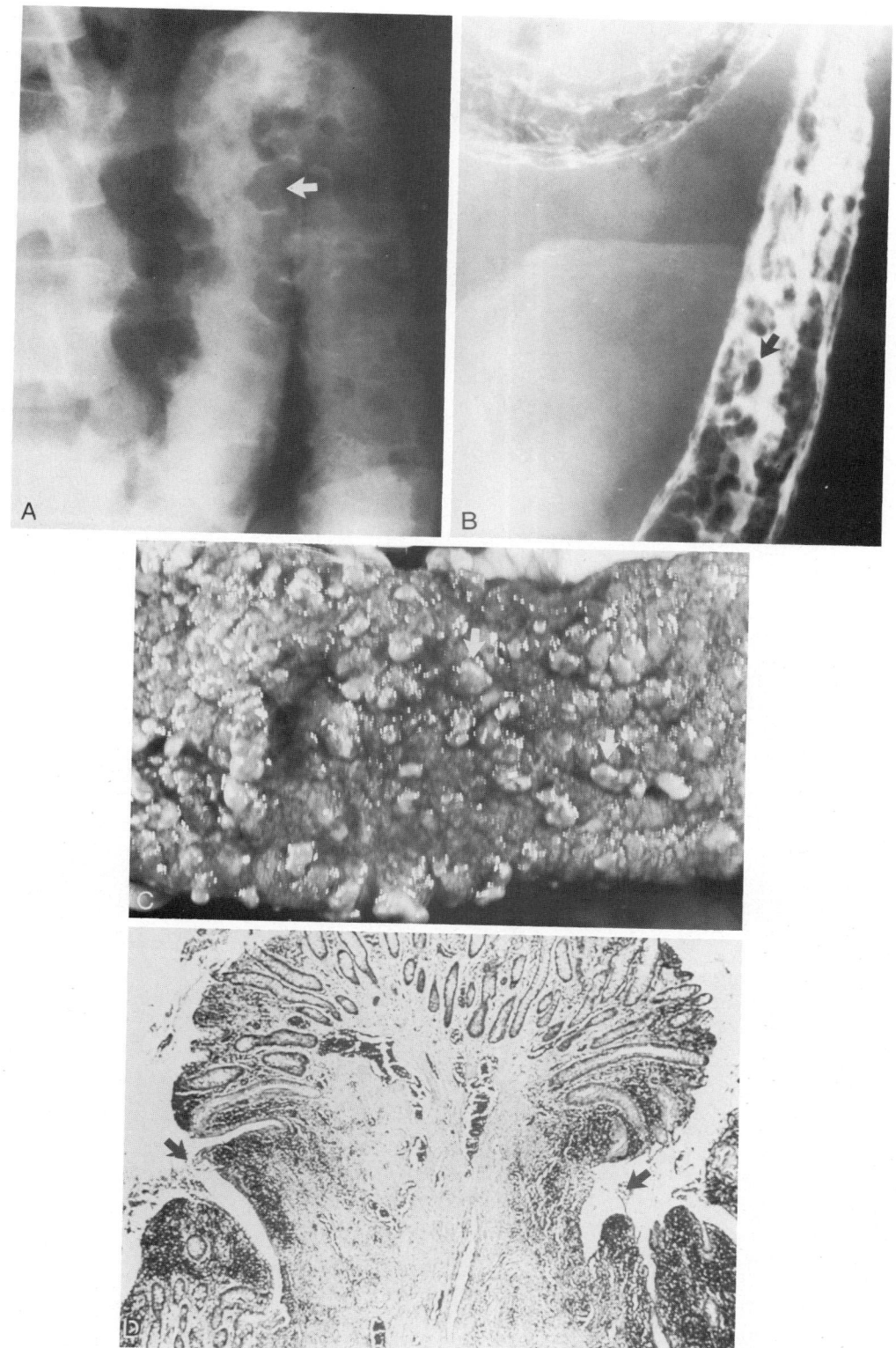

**Figure 62–11. Ulcerative colitis: inflammatory pseudopolyps.** Inflammatory pseudopolyps *(arrows)* are identified on single contrast **(A)** and double contrast **(B)** barium enema studies. These pseudopolyps are seen when extensive mucosal and submucosal ulceration leaves only small residual islands of surviving mucosa and submucosa. Thus, they represent remnants of pre-existing mucosa and submucosa rather than new growths. **C.** Specimen radiograph shows residual islands of intact hyperemic mucosa *(arrows)*. **D.** Photomicrograph shows an inflammatory pseudopolyp. Extensive ulceration has left an island of mucosa undermined on both sides *(arrows)*, attached to the submucosa by a stalk.

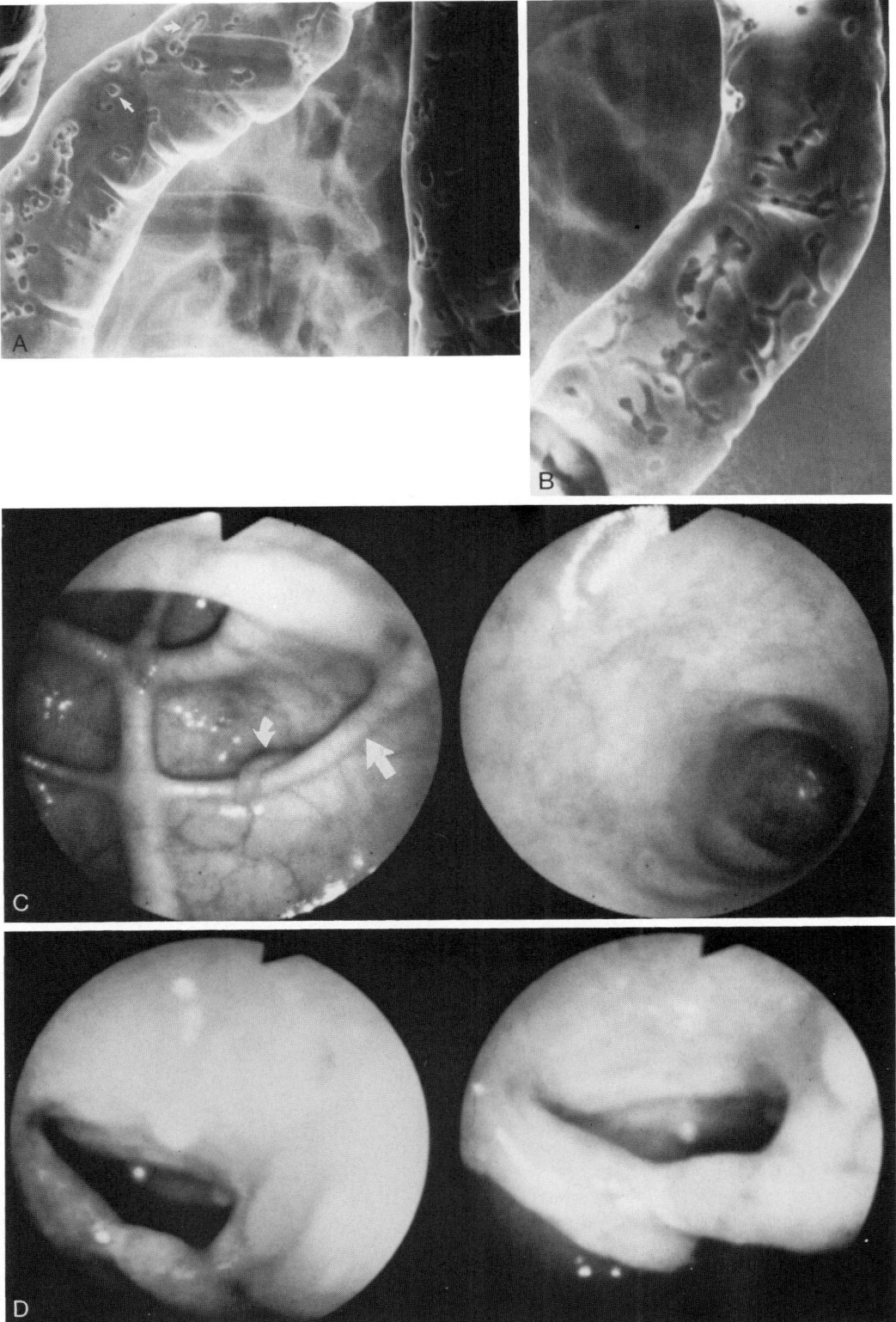

**Figure 62–12. Ulcerative colitis: postinflammatory pseudopolyps.** These pseudopolyps are a manifestation of mucosal healing in which normal tissue elements overgrow. Lesions may be small and round or long and filiform. **A.** Both rounded *(straight arrow)* and filiform *(curved arrow)* pseudopolyps are seen in the distal transverse colon. **B.** The postinflammatory pseudopolyps of this patient are more uniform and filiform. **C.** Colonoscopic view of a filiform polyp *(curved arrow)* on top of a haustrum *(straight arrow).* **D.** Mucosal bridge, an unusual form of postinflammatory pseudopolyp.

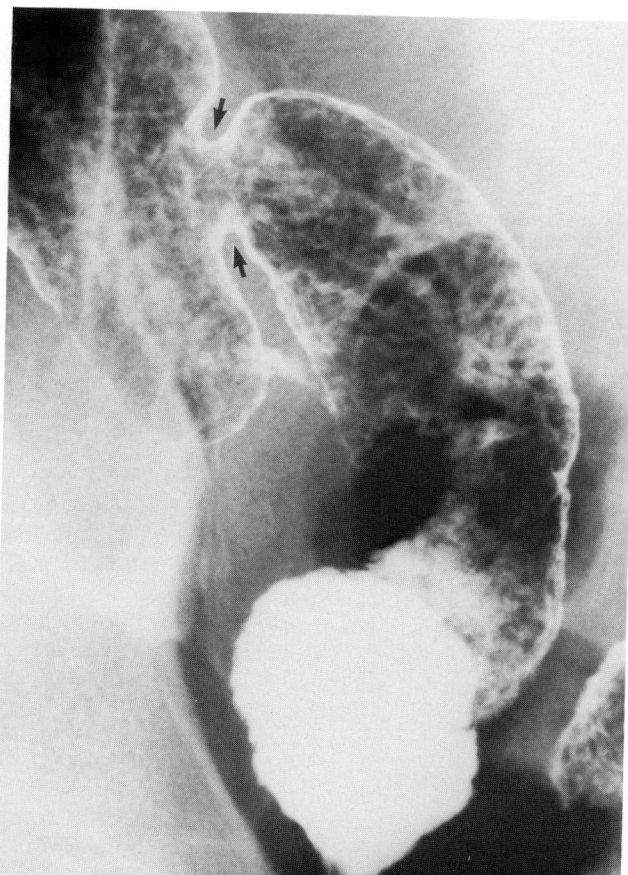

**Figure 62–13. Ulcerative colitis: backwash ileitis.** Backwash ileitis is demonstrated on this spot film of a patient with chronic panulcerative colitis. Notice the patulous ileocecal valve *(arrows)* and dilated, granular-appearing terminal ileum.

## Blunting and Lost Haustra

In the course of ulcerative colitis, the haustral folds undergo two major changes (Figs. 62–14 and 62–15): 1) early in the disease, they are edematous and thickened; 2) with chronic disease, they become blunted or may be completely lost.[46] This evolution of haustral changes can be understood by a brief review of haustral formation.

At birth, colonic haustra are usually absent, which explains why it is difficult to differentiate colonic from small bowel gas in neonates. As the colon grows, the circular muscle of the muscularis propria outgrows the longitudinal muscle, the taeniae coli. This differential growth rate causes the taeniae to "shorten" the colon in an accordion-like fashion, with production of the saccular haustra that usually are first seen by the age of 3 years.

Haustra are fixed anatomic landmarks in the proximal colon because the circular muscle is fused to the taeniae. In the distal colon, haustra are created by active contraction of the taeniae. Consequently, the colon can normally be devoid of haustra distal to the midtransverse colon; loss of haustra in the proximal colon is always abnormal.[81]

In early ulcerative colitis, the haustra are deformed

and thickened owing to edema and may produce a corrugate outline to the colon that has been termed the "indenture" sign.[106, 107]

In chronic ulcerative colitis, the haustra are often lost for two reasons: alterations in the muscle tone of the taeniae[106] and the fact that the colon is foreshortened. In this disease, the taeniae coli become relaxed for some unknown reason. This is associated with abolition of the haustral pattern. With healing, the haustra may reappear as they gain tone. A second major factor is also at work in chronic ulcerative colitis—massive hypertrophy and fixed contraction of the muscularis mucosae (see later), which causes foreshortening of the colon. Thus, the normal accordion-like array of colon on the relatively shorter taeniae is lost.[106, 107]

It is interesting to note that similar findings are seen on radiographs in patients with cathartic colon.[108] Indeed, cathartic colon may simulate chronic, burned out ulcerative colitis radiographically and pathologically. Apparently, cathartics such as senna stimulate the submucosal plexus of Meissner, which in turn stimulates the deeper intermuscular myenteric plexus. With prolonged laxative abuse, abnormal neural pathways regulating colonic motility are established, which leads to

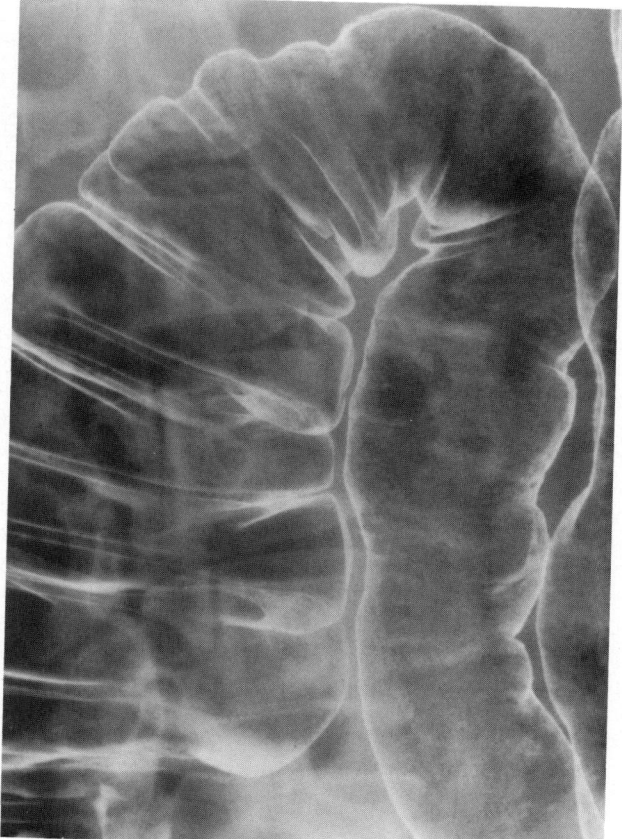

**Figure 62–14. Acute ulcerative colitis: loss of haustra.** Haustra distal to the hepatic flexure are absent, and the taeniae coli are relaxed. The mucosa is granular in appearance. The colon is not shortened at this point because enlargement and contraction of the muscularis mucosae have not yet developed at this early stage of disease.

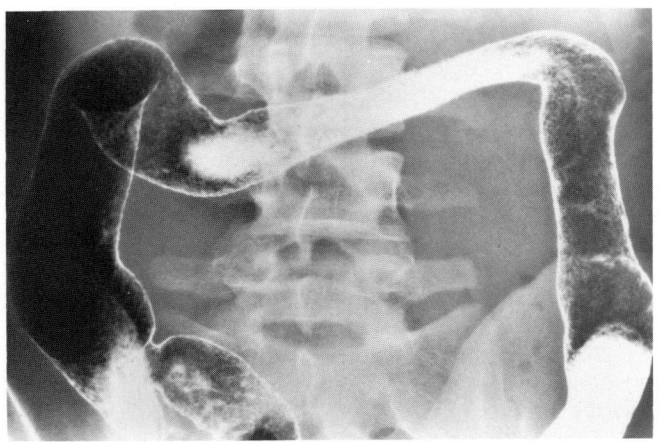

**Figure 62–15. Chronic ulcerative colitis with backwash ileitis: loss of haustra.** The colon is shortened, tubular, ahaustral, and narrow. At this stage of the disease, the muscularis mucosae is hypertrophied and chronically contracted.

neuromuscular incoordination. Perhaps similar events occur in ulcerative colitis. On pathologic examination, the mucosa is atrophic, the submucosa is thickened with fatty deposition, the circular and longitudinal muscles of the colon are minimally thinned, and the muscularis mucosae tends to be somewhat thickened in the cathartic colon, albeit not to the extent seen in chronic ulcerative colitis.[109–111] The return of haustra has been reported in cathartic colon as well.

### Widened Presacral Space

When the rectum is distended, the retrorectal space as projected on true lateral films obtained during barium enema is usually 7.5 mm or less.[112] A distance of 1 to 1.5 cm is considered a moderate increase of this space, and a distance greater than 1.5 cm is abnormal. These values are obtained by measuring the shortest distance between the posterior edge of the barium column and the anterior edge of the fifth sacral segment. The presacral space is frequently widened in chronic ulcerative and Crohn's colitis but may also be seen in obese patients, pelvic lipomatosis, pelvic carcinomatosis, radiation fibrosis, inferior vena cava thrombosis, sacral and rectal tumors, chlamydial infection (lymphogranuloma venereum), and other infectious proctitides.[113–115]

In patients with ulcerative colitis, two processes account for the abnormal presacral space: 1) narrowing of the rectal lumen and its associated mural thickening; and 2) proliferation, inflammation, and infiltration of perirectal fat (see Fig. 62–5A and B). These changes are well demonstrated by CT and correlate with the edematous adipose tissue and enlarged perirectal lymph nodes that are commonly observed at the time of abdominoperineal resection in patients with ulcerative colitis. In patients with Crohn's disease, perirectal abscesses may also contribute to this widening.[72, 73, 116]

### Rectal Valve Abnormalities

At least one rectal valve should be visible on lateral rectal views of double contrast enemas. The fold is usually seen at the level of S-3 and S-4 and should be less than 5 mm thick. The rectal valves are an important

indicator of proctitis and should be interpreted with the size of the presacral space. Two situations are indicative of proctitis: 1) the presacral space is greater than 1.5 cm, with the valve thicker than 6.5 mm or absent; and 2) the presacral space is normal, but the valve thickness is greater than 6.5 mm. Absence of the rectal valves in the presence of a normal presacral space can be a normal variant.[46]

### Mural Thickening

Mural thickening is a common finding in Crohn's disease and chronic ulcerative colitis on cross-sectional imaging.[62–71, 73, 117–121] It is less frequently seen on plain film and barium studies. Because Crohn's disease is characterized by transmural inflammation and fibrosis, it is easy to understand why this thickening occurs. Its pathogenesis is not intuitively obvious in ulcerative colitis, which is predominantly a mucosal disease. In chronic ulcerative colitis (Fig. 62–16), the bowel wall is thickened because of marked hypertrophy of the muscularis mucosae, often by a factor of 40.[123, 124] Forceful contraction of this hypertrophied muscular layer may pull the mucosa away from the longitudinal coat, which produces lumen narrowing.[123, 124] Thickening of the lamina propria with round cell infiltration and extensive fat deposition in the submucosa also significantly contribute to thickening of the bowel wall.[72, 77, 117]

On CT scans, these changes may produce a target appearance (see Fig. 62–5A) of the colon when it is axially imaged: the lumen is surrounded by a ring of soft tissue density (mucosa, lamina propria, hypertrophied muscularis mucosae), which is surrounded by a low-density ring (fatty infiltration of the submucosa), which in turn is surrounded by a ring of soft tissue density (muscularis propria).[72, 77, 117]

The fact that the layers of the bowel wall are still organized and not transmurally diseased accounts for the fact that sonographically, the colon wall maintains its typical wall stratification in ulcerative colitis but is lost in Crohn's disease.[62, 63, 121, 122] Similarly, the ring appearance of the axially imaged colon wall is typical of ulcerative colitis; in Crohn's disease, the wall has a more homogeneous appearance. The thickening is usually

**Figure 62–16. Cause of contour changes in chronic ulcerative colitis.** The diagram depicts the marked hypertrophy of the muscularis mucosae. This muscle, oriented along the long axis of the colon, is chronically contracted even after the intravenous administration of glucagon and in formalin-impregnated specimens. This contraction shortens and narrows the involved colon. The submucosa also widens and shows various degrees of fatty infiltration, further narrowing the lumen. The taeniae coli are relaxed, which abolishes the haustral folds. (From RM Gore, Colonic contour changes in chronic ulcerative colitis: reappraisal of some old concepts, AJR, 158, 1, 59–61, 1992, © by American Roentgen Ray Society.)

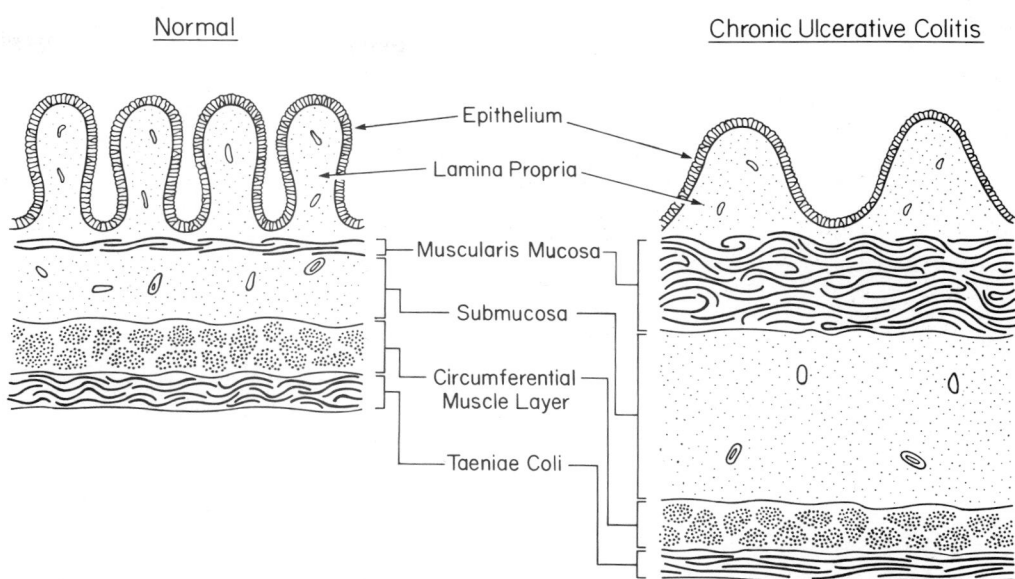

more impressive in Crohn's disease (2.7 cm) than in ulcerative colitis (1.2 cm).[72]

## Strictures

Benign strictures are local sequelae of ulcerative colitis that occur in approximately 10% of patients.[46] They are usually localized and smoothly tapering (Fig. 62–17)

and are only rarely sufficiently narrow to cause obstruction. They are sometimes reversible and are found more commonly in the distal colon. Strictures that are not reversible and are located more proximally in the colon should be viewed with suspicion for a neoplasm.[123–127] The strictures have been attributed to the previously described changes of the muscularis mucosae and are almost invariably associated with mural thickening on cross-sectional imaging.[74]

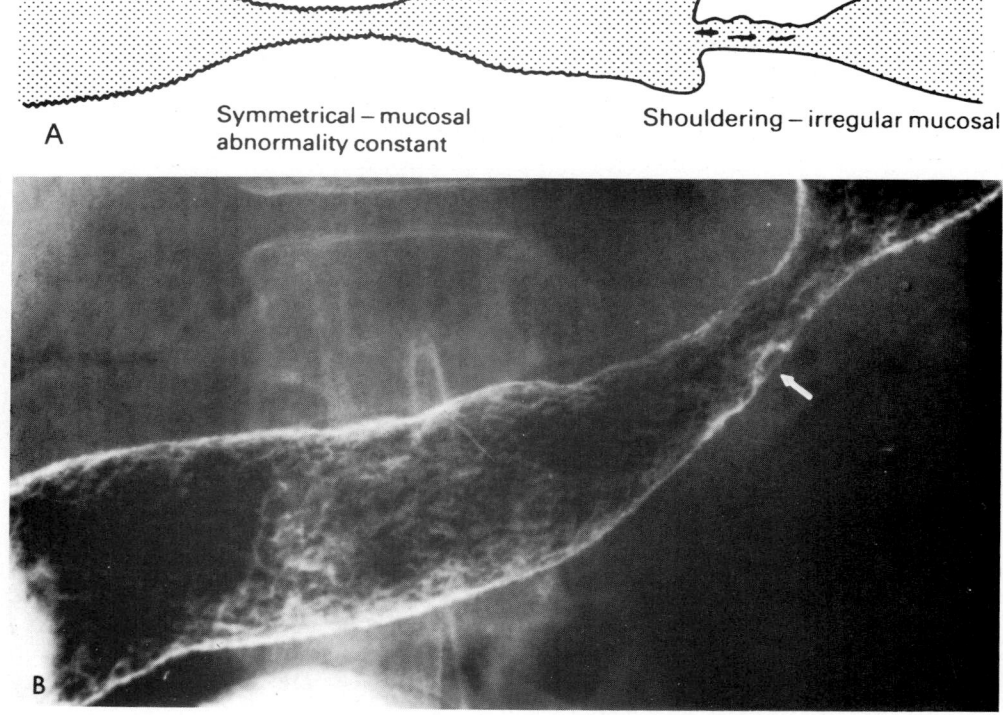

**Figure 62–17. Ulcerative colitis: benign and malignant strictures.** **A.** Benign strictures are often difficult to differentiate from carcinomas in patients with chronic ulcerative colitis. (From Bartram CI, Kumar P: Clinical Radiology in Gastroenterology. Oxford: Blackwell Scientific Publications, 1981, p 137.) **B.** Benign stricture of the distal transverse colon. The mucosa within the strictured segment is granular and identical to the mucosa distally and proximally. There are also inflammatory pseudopolyps *(arrow).*

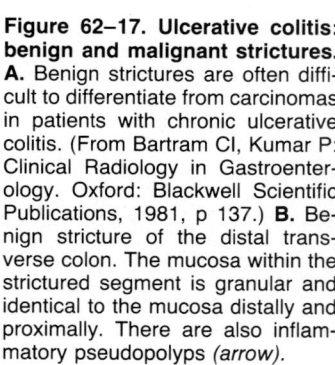

## Distribution

Ulcerative colitis originates in the rectum and extends proximally in a continuous fashion. There is often a fairly sharply defined margin between diseased and normal bowel. The affected mucosa is diffusely, contiguously, confluently, circumferentially, and symmetrically involved without intervening normal mucosa. The rectum is almost invariably involved but may be spared in patients treated with steroid enemas.

## Colonic Complications

Patients with ulcerative colitis are subject to a variety of intestinal complications, which are listed in Table 62–7 and discussed more fully in the following.

## Cancer

The risk of developing colorectal cancer is significantly higher in patients with ulcerative colitis than in the general population, although the precise magnitude of this risk is uncertain. Early reports suggested a 50% cumulative risk at 30 years, whereas more recent studies suggest an annual incidence of 10% after the first decade of colitis. The risk of colorectal cancer also increases with increasing extent of disease; 75 to 80% of patients who develop cancer have pancolitis. Patients with only left-sided colitis still have an increased risk of cancer, but malignancy usually develops a decade later than in patients with universal colitis. Patients with only ulcerative proctitis probably have no greater risk for colon cancer than does the general population.[128–132]

Carcinomas associated with ulcerative colitis differ from those of the general population in that 1) poorly

differentiated glands are seen in 50% of tumors, 2) multiple synchronous neoplasms are seen in nearly 25% of cases, and 3) the lesions are more often flat and scirrhous than in patients without colitis and thus harder to detect[128–132] (Fig. 62–18).

Patients with ulcerative colitis and their managing physicians are thus faced with a life-threatening complication. Of course, proctocolectomy will prevent cancer, but this is not a desirable alternative. Cancer screening has become a popular and controversial issue in this group of patients.[133–135] Since the 1960s, mucosal dysplasia has been considered a precursor of colon cancer or at least a marker of colons at risk for developing cancer.[136] Mucosal dysplasia is often detected near or remote from the neoplasm in ulcerative colitis patients with carcinoma.[137] Dysplasia, however, is patchy, inconsistent, and unpredictably distributed in the colon. Accordingly, colonoscopy with multiple random biopsies as well as biopsies from masses or raised areas is recommended. Flow cytometry searching for aneuploidy has been advocated as a means of increasing the specificity and prognostic significance of the histologic results.[138]

Several studies have shown that certain dysplastic lesions (Fig. 62–19) are radiologically visible. When the dysplasia is elevated and plaque-like or multinodular, it manifests en face as irregular nodular areas with sharply angulated borders, having a "mosaic tile" appearance. Tangentially, these lesions project only 1 to 2 mm above the adjacent normal mucosa. When the dysplasia assumes a more polypoid form, it is indistinguishable from an adenomatous polyp. Unfortunately, most dysplasias occur in flat mucosa and therefore are not detectable on double contrast barium studies.[139, 140]

The management of high-risk patients with panulcerative colitis requires regular radiologic and endoscopic surveillance for detecting the presence of dysplasia, particularly when young patients are involved. The role of the radiologist is to determine the extent of the colitis and the configuration of the colon to aid the endoscopist and to draw attention to any area suggestive of dysplasia or carcinoma.[128–140]

## Toxic Megacolon

Toxic megacolon is the most severe, life-threatening complication of ulcerative colitis; it occurs in 1.6 to 13% of patients. Development is usually during the fourth decade of life and can be the initial manifestation of ulcerative colitis. It is the most common cause of death directly related to ulcerative colitis and is an indication for emergency surgery.[52, 54, 104, 140–142]

### Pathologic Findings

On pathologic examination, there is transmural inflammation with deep fissuring ulcers into the muscularis propria, often with extension to the serosa. These inflammatory changes may be so extensive that large areas of denuded mucosa are seen. The colon undergoes disintegration of normal tissue cohesion, an appearance

**TABLE 62–7. RELATIVE FREQUENCY OF GASTROINTESTINAL COMPLICATIONS IN INFLAMMATORY BOWEL DISEASE**

| COMPLICATION | ULCERATIVE COLITIS | CROHN'S DISEASE |
|---|---|---|
| Anorectal lesions | <20% | 20–80% |
| Fissure in ano | <15% | 25–30% |
| Perianal abscess | <10% | 20–25% |
| First symptom | Very infrequent | 20–25% |
| Fistula in ano | <6% | 20–25% |
| Multiple and complex | Never | Common |
| Multiple anorectal complications | Very infrequent | 20% |
| Massive hemorrhage | | |
| Colon | 3% | <3% |
| Small bowel | Never | <2% |
| Intra-abdominal abscess | Very rare | 15–25% |
| Internal fistulas | Very rare | 20–40% |
| Free perforation | Uncommon | Very uncommon |
| Toxic megacolon | 2–10% | <8% |
| Pseudopolyposis | 15–30% | Less common |
| Strictures | 11–15% | Very common |

From JB Kirsner, RG Shorter: Inflammatory Bowel Disease, 3rd edition. Philadelphia, Lea & Febiger, 1988, pp 257–280. Reprinted with permission.

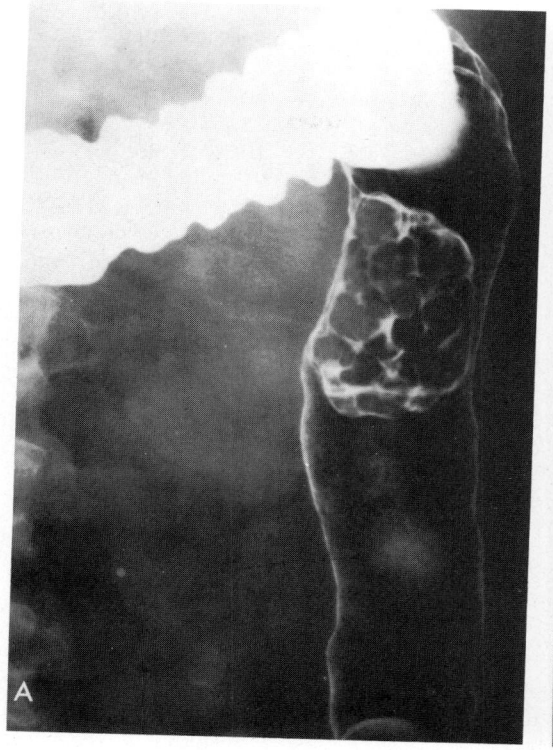
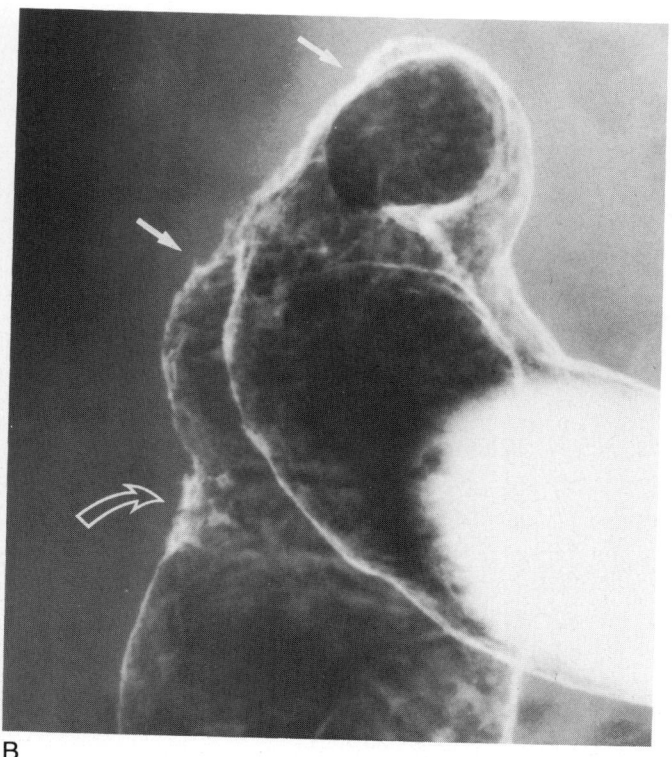

**Figure 62–18. Ulcerative colitis: carcinoma.** Colitic carcinomas often have an atypical appearance. **A.** Unusual polypoid carcinoma in the proximal descending colon. **B.** There is an infiltrative plaque-like carcinoma of the hepatic flexure *(solid arrows)*. A small macrodysplastic lesion *(open arrow)* is present proximal to the carcinoma.

that surgeons have likened to having the consistency of wet tissue paper on handling. The inflammatory exudate seeps through the serosa and may lead to signs of peritonitis even without frank perforation. The external surface of the colon shows intense serositis, and the greater omentum and gastrocolic ligament are edematous and inflamed. These changes are accompanied by vasculitis of the small arterioles and inflammation and destruction of the ganglion cells of the myenteric and submucosal plexuses; there is myocytolysis in the muscularis propria.[143–146] Although the bowel wall appears thickened and nodular on plain abdominal films, the specimen often shows a mural thickness of only 2 to 3 mm in areas of denuded mucosa.

A number of factors further contribute to high intraluminal pressures and decreased muscle tone that can lead to colonic distention in toxic megacolon: antidiarrheal drugs (codeine, morphine, tincture of opium), aerophagia, and hypokalemia. The barium enema has also been implicated as a precipitating factor in toxic megacolon, but this is controversial. Certain evidence suggests that the relationship may be temporal more than a cause-and-effect phenomenon. Nevertheless, the interdiction concerning barium enema studies in patients who are severely ill with ulcerative colitis is probably still valid.[147–150]

Toxic megacolon can also complicate other forms of colitis such as ischemic colitis, Crohn's disease, pseudomembranous colitis, and amebiasis.

## Radiologic Findings

Toxic megacolon (Fig. 62–20) is one of the few life-threatening conditions in which an abdominal plain film is all that is required to establish a firm diagnosis.[151–153]

Dilatation is the hallmark of toxic megacolon; mean diameters of the most dilated segments are between 8.2 and 9.2 cm. Dilatation greater than 5 cm indicates ulceration to the muscle layer and should be considered the threshold for dilatation in fulminating colitis. In the past, the transverse colon was considered the focus of disease, but this is only a reflection of the fact that the transverse colon is the least dependent portion of the large intestine on supine view radiographs. Initially, only a short segment of colon may be involved.[153]

Mucosal islands are a common finding in toxic megacolon and indicate severe disruption of the mucosa. This appearance can be simulated in patients with inflammatory polyps during an acute attack. As stated before, although the colon wall is thin pathologically, it appears thickened radiologically, presumably owing to subserosal or omental edema. A radiolucent stripe may be noted running parallel to the colon, and this probably represents the pericolic fat line.

The profound inflammation and extensive ulceration of toxic megacolon always abolish the haustral pattern, so the presence of normal haustra excludes the diagnosis. Long fluid levels can be seen in the colon as well as small bowel distention, in keeping with an ileus.[153]

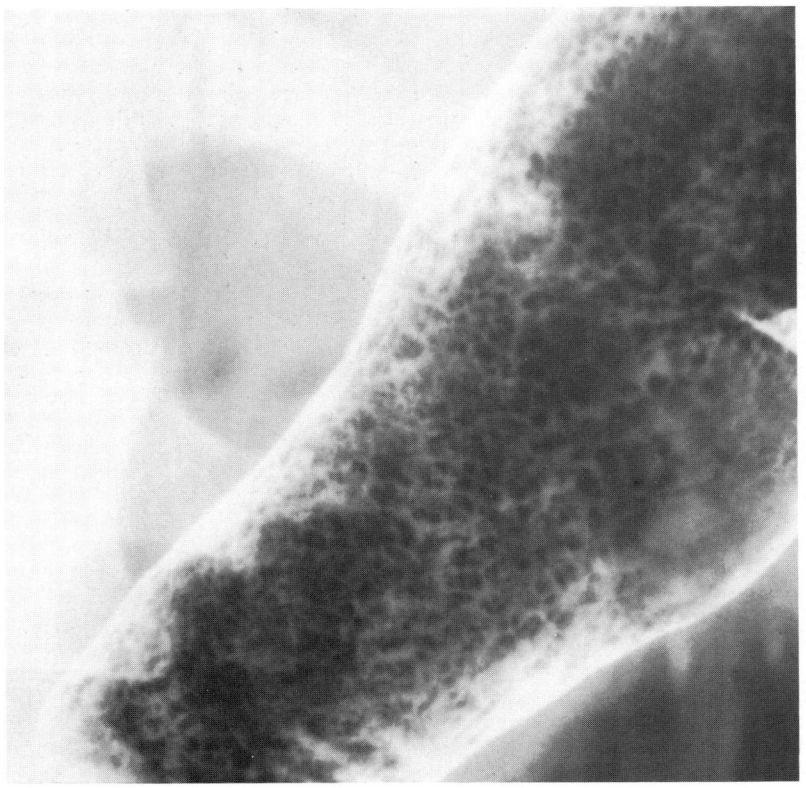

A

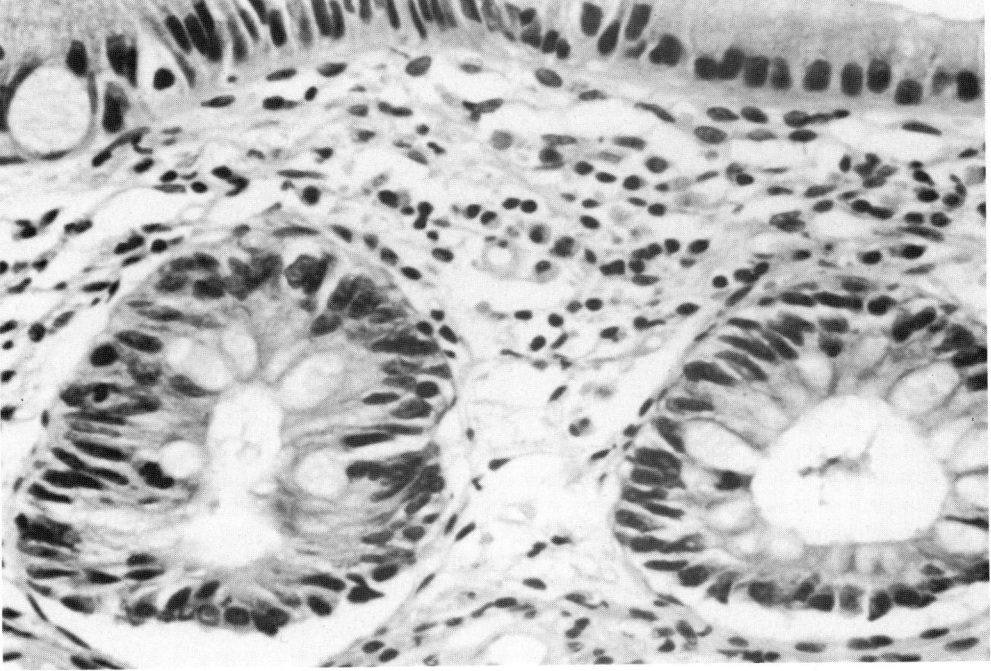

B

**Figure 62–19. Ulcerative colitis: dysplasia. A.** The mucosa of the distal transverse colon is covered by a raised polygonal pattern characteristic of mucosal dysplasia. **B.** Dystrophic (upside-down) goblet cells, some of which have become rounded up, resembling signet ring cells and losing their nuclear polarity as well. (**B** courtesy of Peter J. Feczko, M.D., Royal Oak, MI.)

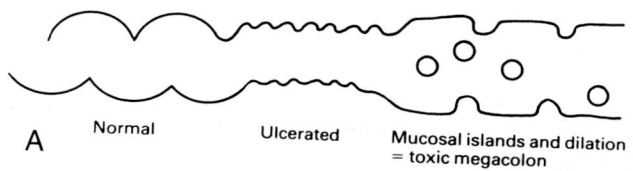

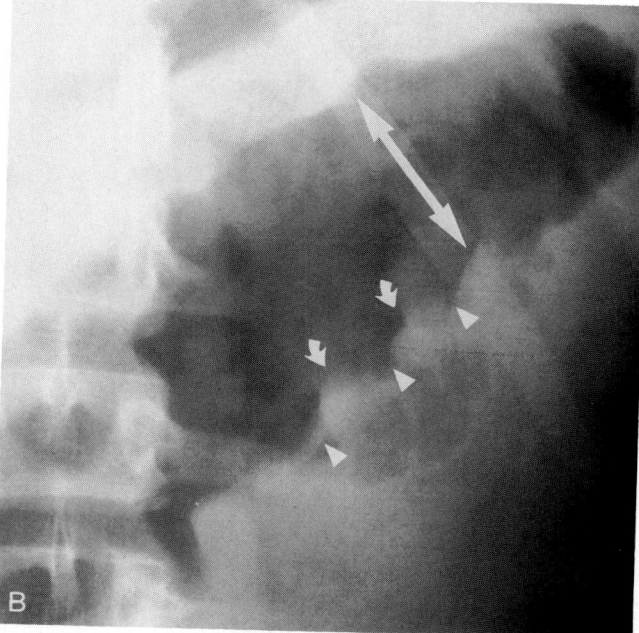

**Figure 62–20. Intestinal complications of ulcerative colitis: toxic megacolon. A.** Toxic megacolon is diagnosed from the presence of dilatation and severe mucosal disease. Dilatation itself may result from many other causes, so deep ulcerations as well as dilatation must be demonstrated. (From Bartram CI, Kumar P: Clinical Radiology in Gastroenterology. Oxford: Blackwell Scientific Publications, 1981, p 136.) **B.** Mucosal islands *(curved arrows),* deep ulcerations *(arrowheads),* and dilatation *(double arrow)* establish the diagnosis.

## Extraintestinal Manifestations

Ulcerative colitis is associated with a wide variety of extraintestinal manifestations (Table 62–8) that can be divided into two major categories: 1) those in which the clinical activity parallels the activity of the bowel disease, and 2) those whose course is independent of the underlying bowel disease, preceding the onset of bowel symptoms or occurring after colectomy.[154–159]

### Hepatobiliary Disease

Approximately 7% of patients with ulcerative colitis have some evidence of liver disease on the basis of clinical and laboratory data. Fatty livers are seen in up to 50% of patients with ulcerative colitis, but these patients are usually asymptomatic in terms of hepatic symptoms. Steatosis probably is a direct complication of the underlying bowel disease (malnutrition, protein depletion, steroids) rather than a true extraintestinal manifestation.[160]

Pericholangitis is found in 35 to 50% of liver specimens obtained from patients with ulcerative colitis and

is more common in patients with pancolitis than in those with only distal disease. Biopsy reveals portal triaditis with inflammatory changes involving connective tissue surrounding branches of the portal vein, hepatic artery, and bile ductules. Pericholangitis usually causes no symptoms; jaundice is rare, but certain evidence suggests that it may represent the early phase of progressive sclerosing cholangitis. Chronic active hepatitis occurs in up to 1% of patients with ulcerative colitis. Cirrhosis develops in approximately 1.5% of patients with ulcerative colitis and is usually secondary to chronic active hepatitis, sclerosing cholangitis, and pericholangitis.[161–163]

Sclerosing cholangitis (Fig. 62–21) is one of the most serious complications of ulcerative colitis; it occurs in 1 to 4% of patients. This "complication" has an independent course unrelated to disease activity or colectomy.[164–167] Studies suggest that primary sclerosing cho-

**TABLE 62–8. EXTRACOLONIC MANIFESTATIONS OF ULCERATIVE COLITIS**

**HEPATOBILIARY**
Nonspecific reactive hepatitis
Sclerosing cholangitis
Pericholangitis
Chronic active hepatitis
Cholangiocarcinoma
Fatty infiltration

**MUSCULOSKELETAL**
Arthritis
Ankylosing spondylitis
Sacroiliitis
Hypertrophic osteoarthropathy
Avascular necrosis

**OCULAR**
Uveitis and iritis
Episcleritis
Conjunctivitis

**MUCOCUTANEOUS**
Pyoderma gangrenosum
Erythema nodosum
Cutaneous vasculitis
Stomatitis

**RENAL**
Uro- and nephrolithiasis
Amyloidosis
Drug-related disease

**BRONCHOPULMONARY**
Pulmonary vasculitis
Pleuropericarditis

**HEMATOLOGIC AND VASCULAR**
Anemia from blood loss
Autoimmune hemolytic anemia
Thrombocytosis
Thromboembolic disease
Increased factors V and VIII
Accelerated thromboplastin III levels
Arteritis of aorta and subclavian artery

**PANCREAS**
Drug-related pancreatitis

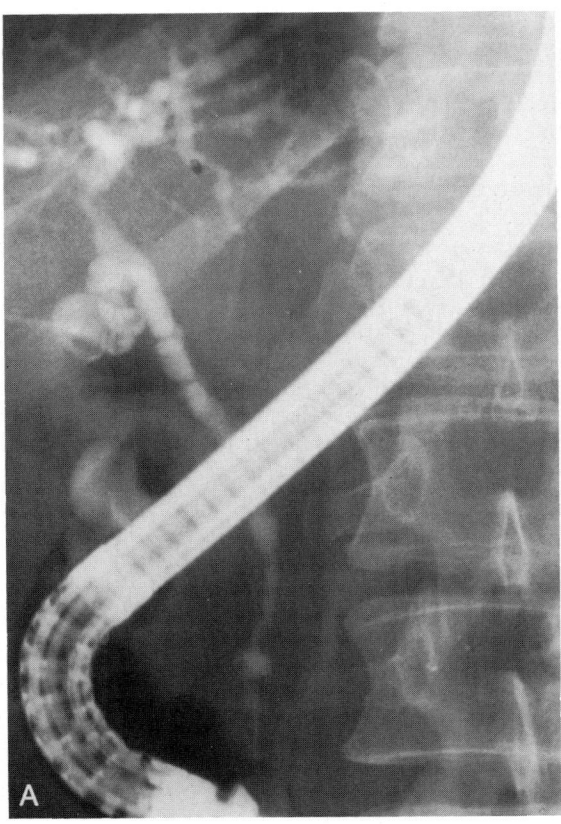

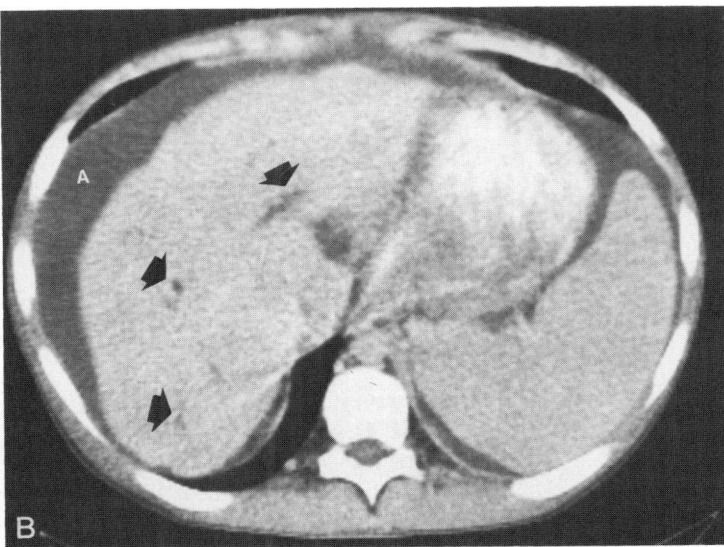

**Figure 62–21. Extraintestinal complications of ulcerative colitis: sclerosing cholangitis. A.** Multiple areas of stricture, beading, and sacculation of the intra- and extrahepatic bile ducts are identified on this endoscopic retrograde cholangiopancreatography examination. **B.** CT scan in a different patient with ulcerative colitis, sclerosing cholangitis, and secondary biliary cirrhosis shows focal areas of intrahepatic ductal dilatation *(arrows)*, a nodular hepatic contour, and ascites (A). (**A** and **B** from Gore RM: Cross-sectional imaging of inflammatory bowel disease. Radiol Clin North Am 25:115–131, 1987.)

langitis and ulcerative colitis are pathophysiologically related in that both colonic and biliary epithelial surfaces have shared antigenic epitopes, and antineutrophil cytoplasmic antibody is present in the serum of patients with either disorder.[168] Indeed, the prevalence of inflammatory bowel disease is so high in patients with sclerosing cholangitis that the colon should be evaluated even in patients without intestinal symptoms.

A complete discussion of sclerosing cholangitis is presented in Chapter 97, but briefly, there is progressive sclerosis of the intra- and extrahepatic bile ducts that can lead to secondary biliary cirrhosis, hepatic failure, and death.[169, 170]

Adenocarcinoma of the gallbladder or bile ducts occurs in 0.4 to 1.4% of patients with ulcerative colitis, which is 10 to 20 times the incidence found in the normal population (see Chapter 96). This complication of sclerosing cholangitis is not associated with chronic cholelithiasis.[156, 157, 171]

### Renal Complications

Patients with ulcerative colitis can develop renal amyloidosis as a manifestation of systemic disease. Some 5% of patients develop nephrolithiasis and urolithiasis because of the dehydration of chronic diarrhea, the inactivity of the patient that leads to calcium mobilization, and changes in urine composition that predispose the patient to stone formation.[172, 173]

### Musculoskeletal Complications

The most common symptomatic extraintestinal manifestation of ulcerative colitis is arthritis: "colitic arthritis" and ankylosing spondylitis (Fig. 62–22). The colitic peripheral arthritis is a seronegative migratory arthritis that affects knees, hips, ankles, wrists, and elbows. Deformity with radiographic change occurs in less than 25% of cases. Joint pain, swelling, and stiffness parallel the course of colonic disease. Erythema nodosum, uveitis, arthritis, and ulcerative colitis often occur together.[174–180]

There is a 30-fold increased incidence of ankylosing spondylitis in patients with ulcerative colitis. Some 80% of patients with both ulcerative colitis and ankylosing spondylitis are HLA-B27–positive. Unlike colitic arthritis, which is episodic and usually nondeforming, ankylosing spondylitis is often inexorable in course and crippling, independent of the activity or extent of colonic disease.[176–179]

The incidence of sacroiliitis is higher than that of ankylosing spondylitis in patients with ulcerative colitis.[174–180] Patients receiving long-term steroid therapy may develop avascular necrosis of the femoral heads.[180]

### Thromboembolic Complications

Patients with ulcerative colitis are at risk for developing deep venous thrombosis and pulmonary emboli. Patients with severe, active ulcerative colitis have the

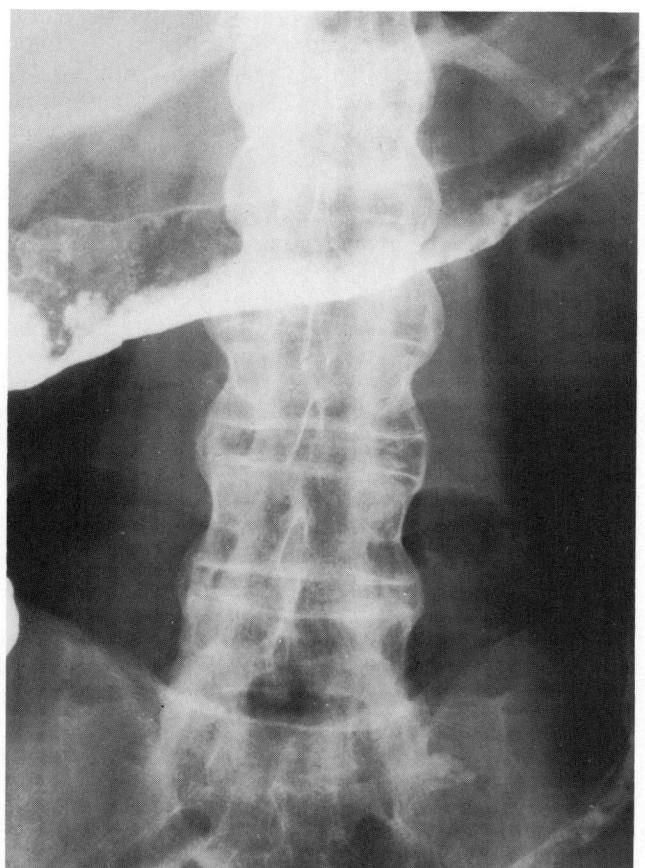

**Figure 62–22. Extraintestinal complications of ulcerative colitis: ankylosing spondylitis.** Fusion of the sacroiliac joints and a "bamboo spine" are demonstrated in this patient with a tubular, ahaustral transverse colon.

following hematologic abnormalities: thrombocytosis; increased levels of factor V, factor VIII, and fibrinogen; and reduced levels of circulating antithrombin III.[181, 182]

## Dermatologic and Ocular Complications

Pyoderma gangrenosum (Fig. 62–23) affects 2 to 5% of patients with ulcerative colitis. This lesion is a discrete cutaneous ulcer with a necrotic base, usually found on the lower extremities. These lesions are usually seen in patients with pancolitis and appear during a bout of active colitis. The skin usually heals after control of the colitis, but occasionally colectomy may be needed to control the disease.[183, 184]

Erythema nodosum develops in 2 to 4% of patients with ulcerative colitis and appears as raised, tender, erythematous swellings, 2 to 5 cm in diameter, along the extensor surface of the arms and legs. Cutaneous disease activity more closely mirrors the colonic disease activity than in pyoderma gangrenosum. Most patients will have only a single episode of erythema nodosum.[183, 184]

Uveitis and episcleritis are the two major ocular complications of ulcerative colitis. They parallel colonic disease activity and usually respond to steroid therapy.[155]

## Therapy

### Medical Management

The treatment of ulcerative colitis depends on the severity, extent, and distribution of disease. Sulfasalazine, a congener of 5-aminosalicylic acid and sulfapyridine, is effective in the treatment of acute ulcerative colitis and in reducing both the frequency and the severity of recurrent attacks. Sulfasalazine attenuates the bowel inflammation by a number of actions: 1) it reduces production of prostaglandins; 2) it diminishes leukotriene production, which activates neutrophils and other constituents of the inflammatory response; 3) it blocks the chemotactic activity of formulated bacterial peptides that help recruit neutrophils to the bowel; and 4) it acts as a scavenger of oxygen free radicals.[185–191] Many patients develop hypersensitivity or less specific forms of intolerance; efforts are now being made to deliver the active component 5-aminosalicylic acid without the sulfapyridine moiety, which apparently causes the hypersensitivity.[185–191]

Corticosteroids are effective in patients with moderate to severe ulcerative colitis. They do not affect the rate or timing of disease recurrence in patients in remission. Topical hydrocortisone in the form of a foam enema is the mainstay of therapy for distal proctocolitis.[185–191]

Azathioprine, 6-mercaptopurine, chloroquine, hydroxychloroquine sulfate (Plaquenil), methotrexate, and cyclosporine are alternative therapies in patients with refractory disease. Bowel rest and nutritional therapy also have beneficial effects on this disease.[185–195]

### Surgery

Although proctocolectomy is always curative for ulcerative colitis, this procedure carries an operative risk,

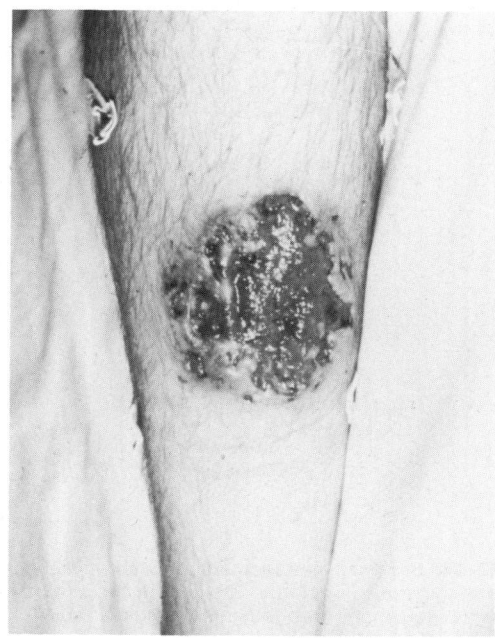

**Figure 62–23. Extraintestinal complications of ulcerative colitis: pyoderma gangrenosum.**

and not all patients are willing to accept an ileostomy. Consequently, colectomy is not indicated for patients who are easily managed medically. There are several major indications for surgery in ulcerative colitis: 1) massive, unremitting colonic hemorrhage; 2) toxic megacolon with impending or frank perforation; 3) fulminant colitis that is unresponsive to antibiotic, supportive, and steroid therapy; 4) obstruction from a stricture; and 5) suspicion or demonstration of colon cancer. Less immediate and definite indications for colectomy are 1) intractable, chronic disease that becomes a physical and social burden to the patient; 2) failure of children to mature at an acceptable rate; and 3) high-grade dysplasia in a patient with pancolitis.[196-202] Fulminant acute disease accounts for approximately 13 to 25% of colectomies in patients with ulcerative colitis. Many of the extraintestinal complications of ulcerative colitis, such as uveitis and pyoderma gangrenosum, will also be eliminated by colectomy. The course of hepatobiliary disease and ankylosing spondylitis, however, is usually not altered by surgery.[196-201]

In the past two decades, tremendous advances have been made in the surgical approach to ulcerative colitis that offer the patient and surgeon a variety of options.

**Proctocolectomy with a Brooke Ileostomy.** This is the standard procedure in which a proctocolectomy is performed, followed by passing the end of the ileum through an opening in the midaspect of the right rectus muscle at a point beneath the umbilicus (Fig. 62–24)

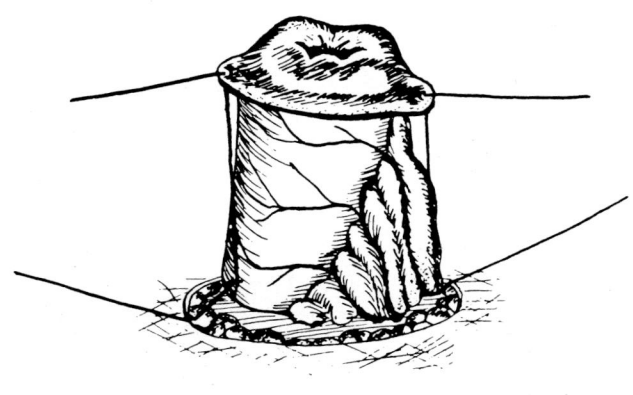

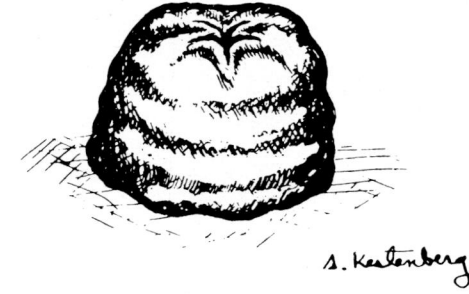

**Figure 62–24. Surgical management of ulcerative colitis: construction of a Brooke ileostomy.** The ileum is brought 5 cm through an abdominal defect and then everted and sutured to the dermis to "mature" the ileostomy.

that allows convenient placement of the forepiece of an ileostomy bag. This procedure is curative and requires one operation, but the patient must constantly wear an external ileostomy appliance that needs to be emptied four to eight times per day. Perineal wound problems, stoma revision, and small bowel obstruction occur in approximately 10 to 25% of patients. Nevertheless, this is the fastest, safest operation but dramatically alters body image in many, particularly younger, patients.[202-204]

**Proctocolectomy with Continent Ileostomy (Kock's Pouch).** In this procedure, a continent ileostomy is made by creating a pouch out of terminal ileum (Fig. 62–25) to hold the intestinal contents, an ileal conduit that leads from the pouch to the stoma, and an intervening intestinal valve. Patients empty the pouch by passing a tube through the valve via the stoma. The ileostomy is continent, so an external appliance is not needed. The nipple valve is created by intussuscepting the terminal ileum in a retrograde manner into the pouch for 3 to 4 cm. Anatomic complications requiring reoperation develop in 40 to 50% of these patients.[202-205]

**Total Colectomy with Ileorectal Anastomosis.** This procedure is no longer popular because of a fairly high complication rate and unpredictable functional result.[202-205]

**Total Proctocolectomy, Rectal Mucosal Stripping, and Ileal Pouch Formation with Anastomosis to the Sphincter.** This procedure involves an abdominal colectomy and a mucosal proctectomy. A J pouch or W pouch is fashioned out of ileum (Fig. 62–26). This reservoir is then anastomosed to the anus (Fig. 62–27). The endorectal ileal pouch–anal anastomosis is given 8 weeks to heal by diverting the gut through a conventional ileostomy.[201, 206-210]

The advantages of this procedure are that no stoma is required and fecal continence is usually maintained, albeit with bowel movements four to eight times per day. This is a technically demanding procedure that requires two operations. Complications include postoperative abscess, pouch fistulas, stenosis, small bowel obstruction, and pouchitis. Some 15% of patients require reoperation, and some ultimately require a conventional ileostomy.[206-210]

Pouchitis is an inflammatory process that can cause tenesmus, bloody diarrhea, and constitutional symptoms similar to those of ulcerative colitis.[211, 212]

## Prognosis

In recent years, the prognosis in ulcerative colitis has improved dramatically. Most patients have mild to moderate disease, and only 15 to 25% require a colectomy. Mortality associated with ulcerative colitis occurs in the first 2 years of disease, primarily in patients older than 40 years: one third attributable to the colonic disease itself, one third caused by complications of the disease (colorectal cancer, sclerosing cholangitis, thromboembolic disease, medical and surgical therapy), and the remainder attributable to unrelated causes. Excess mor-

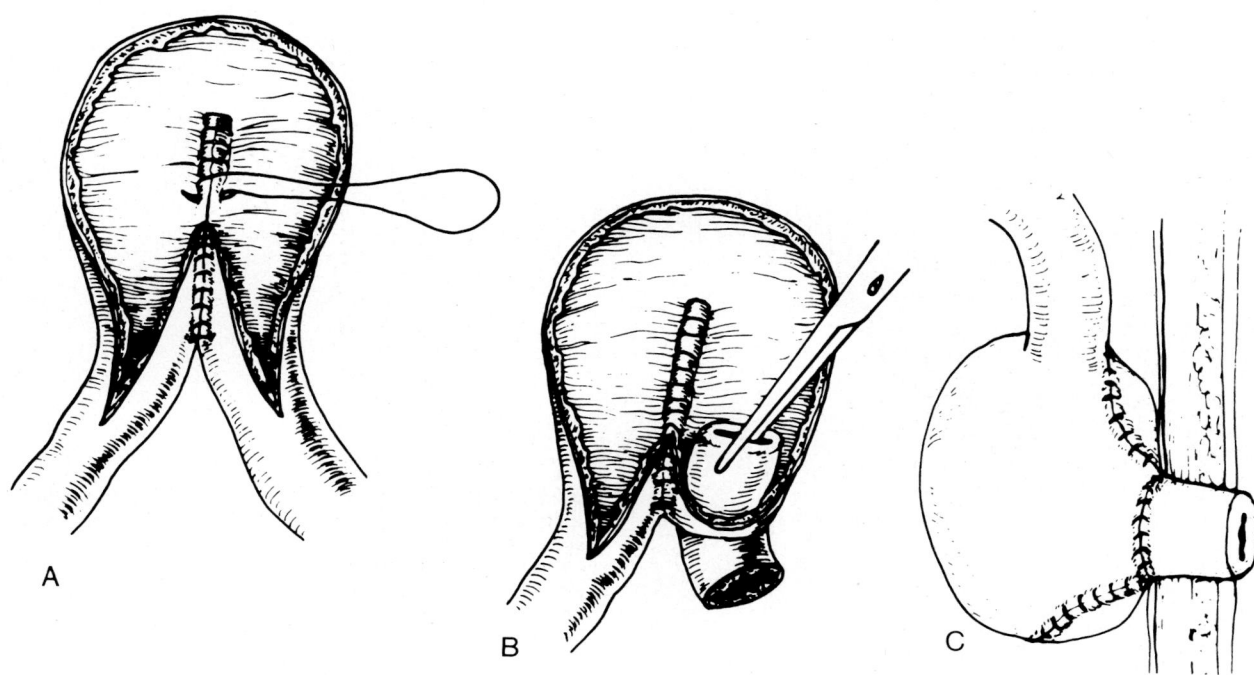

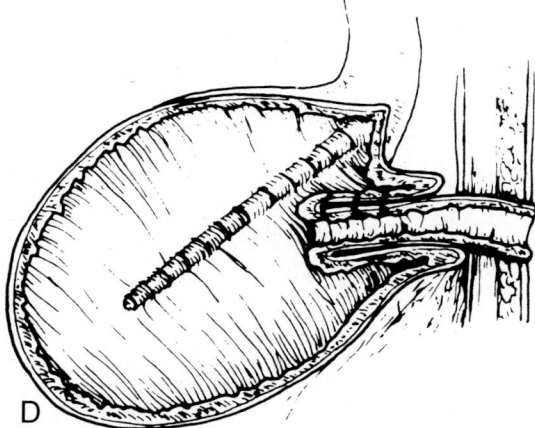

**Figure 62–25. Surgical management of ulcerative colitis: Kock's pouch construction. A.** A 30-cm loop of ileum is sewn together, leaving a 10-cm afferent limb; the loop is opened. **B.** A one-way valve is created by intussuscepting the afferent limb back into the pouch. **C.** The pouch is folded together and sewn closed. The pouch is brought through the abdominal wall and left flush with the skin surface. **D.** Detailed view of the pouch valve in functional, intussuscepted position. (**A** to **D** from Smith LE: Surgical therapy in ulcerative colitis. Gastroenterol Clin North Am 18:99–110, 1989.)

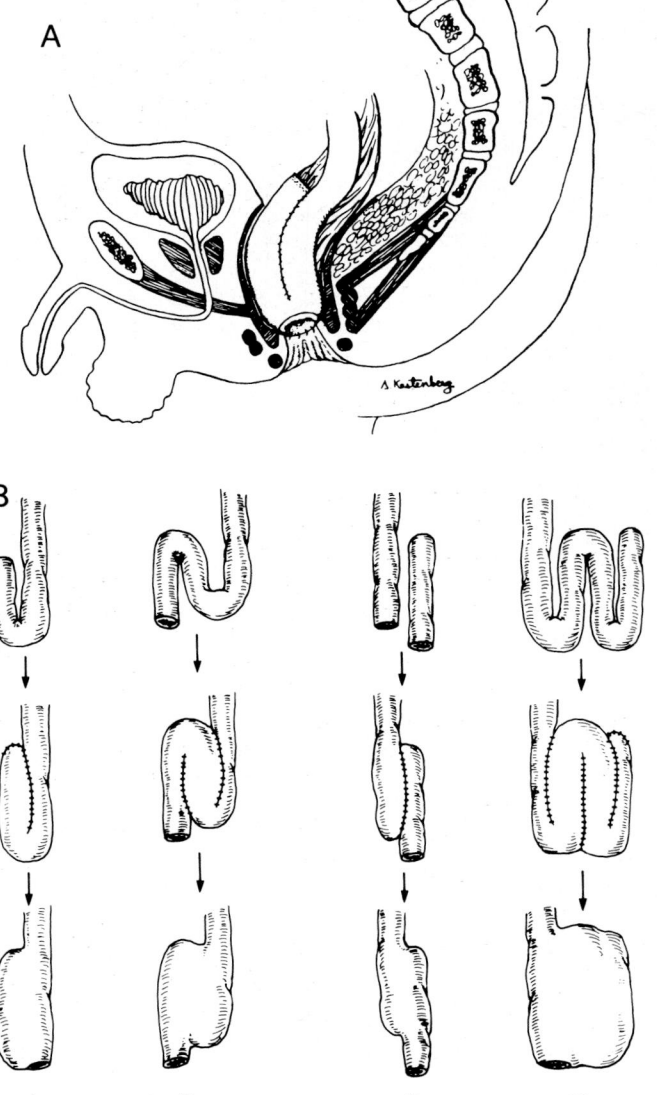

**Figure 62–26. Surgical management of ulcerative colitis: ileal pouch–anal anastomosis. A.** The two-loop ileal J pouch shown in this diagram is simple to construct, provides adequate storage capacity, and is evacuated spontaneously and fully. **B.** The four commonly used configurations for pouches employed in pull-through to the anus procedures. (**B** from Smith LE: Surgical therapy in ulcerative colitis. Gastroenterol Clin North Am 18:99–110, 1989.)

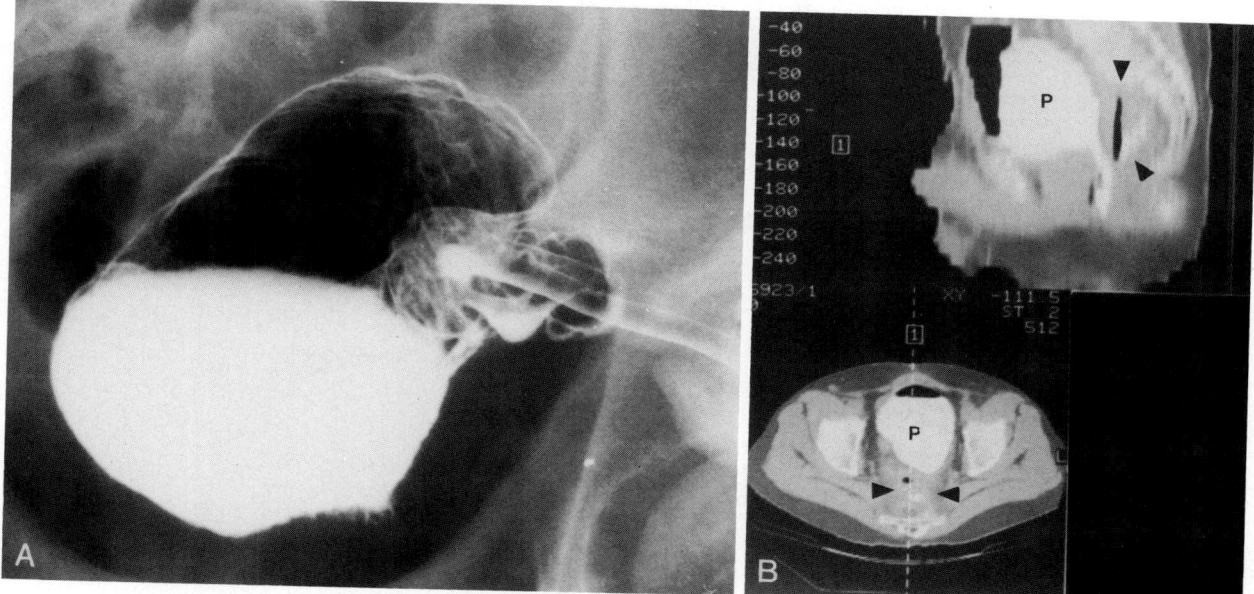

**Figure 62–27. Ileal pouch: radiologic appearance. A.** Normal double contrast examination of an ileal pouch studied before reanastomosis with the remainder of the gut. **B.** Contrast and air are identified in the pouch (P) on this CT scan. Postoperative abscess containing air *(arrowheads)* is identified on both sagittal reformation and axial image.

tality of 2.1% for men and 1.5% for women has been reported, but only for the first 2 years of disease.[213–215]

The majority of patients with ulcerative colitis are able to cope with their disease and achieve what is subjectively interpreted as a relatively acceptable lifestyle.[213–215]

## CROHN'S DISEASE

Crohn's disease is a chronic, cicatrizing disorder of the alimentary tract characterized by granulomatous inflammation of the mucosa, bowel wall, and surrounding mesentery. Any portion of the alimentary tract may be involved, but the terminal ileum and proximal colon are most frequently diseased.[1–5]

The epidemiology, clinical findings, therapy, prognosis, and intestinal and extraintestinal manifestations of Crohn's disease are discussed in Chapter 159. In this chapter, the radiology of Crohn's colitis is emphasized (Fig. 62–28).

## Endoscopic Findings

The major colonoscopic features of Crohn's colitis are summarized in Table 62–3. Aphthoid lesions, cobblestoning, and ulcers in an area of otherwise apparently normal mucosa are diagnostic of Crohn's disease versus ulcerative colitis but can be seen in other colitides. Mucosal granularity and friability are common in early ulcerative colitis but may be a late finding in Crohn's colitis. The rectum is often grossly normal and asymmetric, and discontinuous disease is common.[45]

## Radiologic Findings

### Plain Film

When confined to the colon, Crohn's disease (Fig. 62–29) has features similar to those of ulcerative colitis on plain films. An extended gas-filled stricture of the colon is suggestive of granulomatous colitis but can also be seen in ulcerative colitis, carcinoma, and healing ischemic colitis.[47, 52, 153]

Small bowel obstruction can be seen on plain films in patients with Crohn's disease of the small bowel. It is uncommon, however, to identify stenotic small bowel segments on plain films because gas is not present in the small bowel as often as is found in the colon. Occasionally, a markedly dilated segment of small bowel, reminiscent of a dilated loop of small bowel volvulus or Meckel's diverticulum, can be seen between two stenotic areas.[153]

Evidence of nephrolithiasis, gallstones, ankylosing spondylitis, sacroiliitis, avascular necrosis of the femoral heads, and disorders associated with Crohn's disease and its therapy should also be sought on abdominal plain films.

### Barium Enema

The barium enema features of Crohn's colitis are listed in Table 62–9, summarized in Figure 62–28, and discussed more fully in the next section.

### Ultrasound

In acute, severe Crohn's colitis (see Table 62–4), the normal stratified appearance of the colon wall is lost

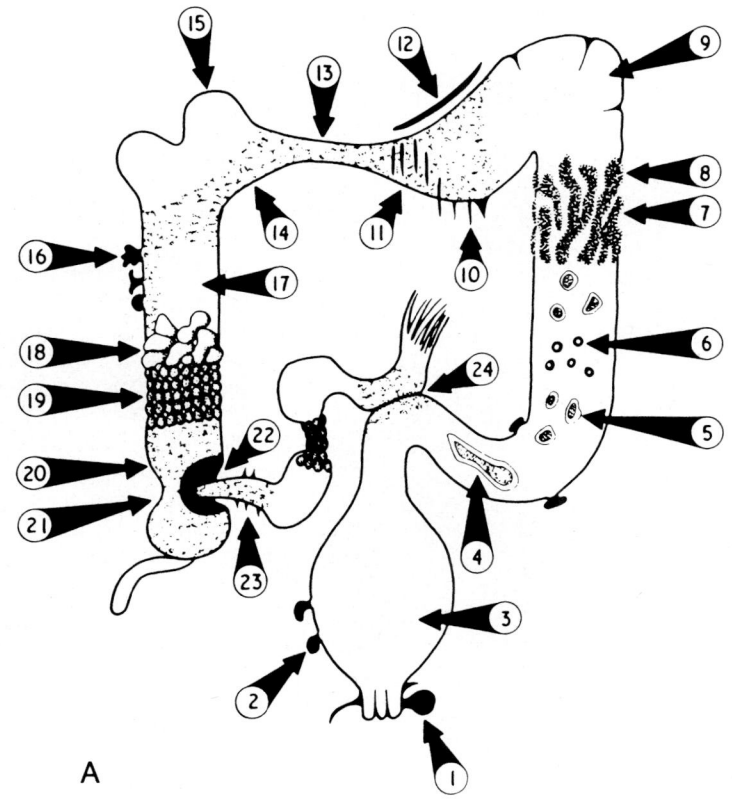

A

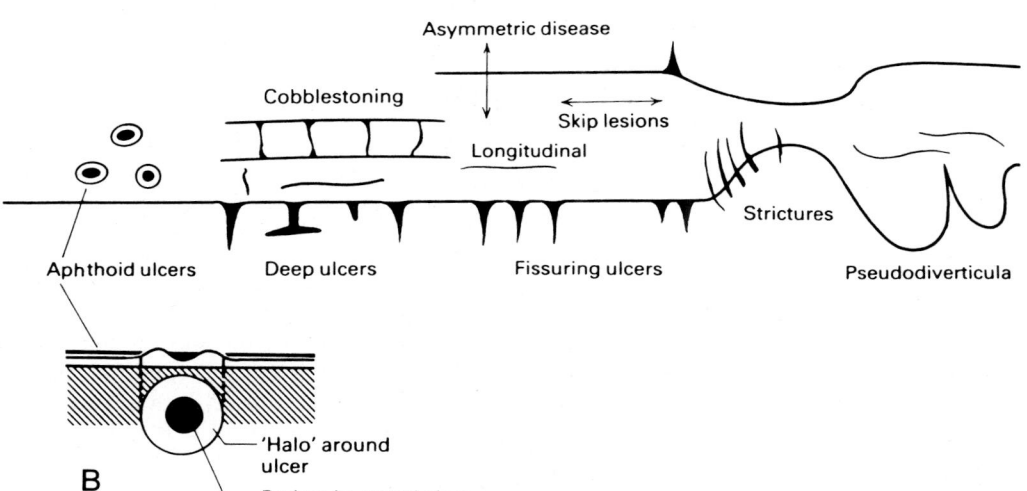

B

**Figure 62–28. Spectrum of radiologic changes in Crohn's colitis on double contrast barium enema examinations. A.** 1 = perianal disease: ulcers, abscess, fissures, anocutaneous fistula; 2 = deep rectal ulcers; 3 = normal rectum in 50% of cases; 4 = island ulcer; 5 = circular discrete ulcers; 6 = aphthoid ulcers; 7 = serpiginous ulceration formed by coalition in a longitudinal form of circular and island ulcers; 8 = thickening of the bowel wall; 9 = normal skip areas; 10 = rose thorn–shaped fissures; 11 = transverse stripes of Welin (en face fissures or crevices between adjacent swollen mucosal folds); 12 = linear confluent intramural ulceration, "double tracking"; 13 = stricture (25% of cases); 14 = eccentric disease, not involving the entire circumference; 15 = pseudosacculations, produced by fibrosis of the opposite wall; 16 = deep pleomorphic ulcers: composite, horned, saccular; 17 = a normal patch surrounded by disease, and patches of disease surrounded by normal mucosa also occur; 18 = inflammatory and postinflammatory pseudopolyps; 19 = cobblestone mucosa—islands of residual swollen mucosa bounded by intersecting linear ulcers; 20 = right-sided disease with normal rectum and distal colon; 21 = contracted, cone-shaped cecum; 22 = enlarged ileocecal valve usually associated with involvement of the terminal ileum; 23 = small bowel disease in 60% of cases; 24 = ileocolic fistula. (From Simpkins KC: Inflammatory bowel disease: ulcerative and Crohn's colitis. *In* Simpkins KC [ed]: A Textbook of Radiological Diagnosis, Volume 4, The Alimentary Tract: The Hollow Organs and Salivary Glands. London: H.K. Lewis, 1988, pp 473–498.) **B.** Diagram further depicting mucosal abnormalities in Crohn's colitis. (From Bartram CI, Kumar P: Clinical Radiology in Gastroenterology. Oxford: Blackwell Scientific Publications, 1981, p 138.)

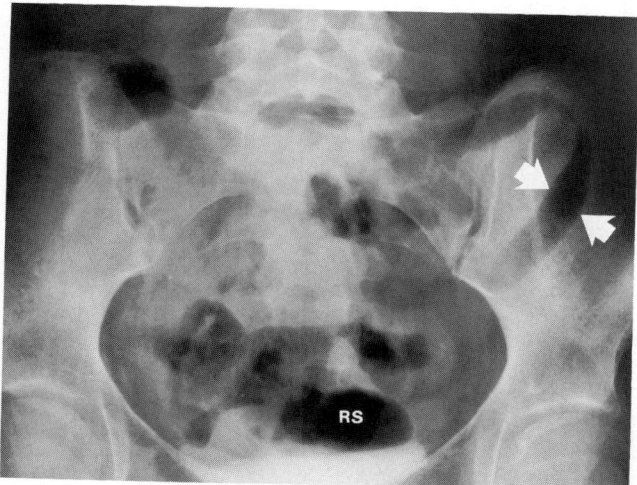

**Figure 62–29. Crohn's disease: plain film finding.** The splenic flexure *(arrows)* is tubular and ahaustral. Note the normal appearance of the rectosigmoid colon (RS).

(Fig. 62–30); the colon wall thickness increases to 1.0 ± 0.3 cm and becomes hypoechoic, and the haustra are lost.[62-71] On real-time sonography, the involved colonic segments are rigid, and peristalsis is absent. With use of these parameters in one series, sonography enabled a correct assessment in 92.5% of patients with isolated small bowel involvement, 91% of patients with ileocolitis, and 89.5% of patients with Crohn's colitis.[66] Sonography can demonstrate reduction in mural thickness in treated Crohn's disease as well.[67-71]

## Computed Tomography

### Mural Disease

With progressive transmural disease, the bowel wall is thickened by edema, fibrosis, inflammation, and lymphangiectasis. On CT scans, these changes are manifested by bowel wall thickening (Fig. 62–31) ranging between 1 and 3 cm, often reaching 10 to 15 times normal thickness. These changes, which occur in up to 83% of patients, are most frequently observed in the terminal ileum, but other portions of the small bowel, colon, duodenum, stomach, and esophagus may be similarly affected. The mural thickening is often discontinuous, and the skip areas correlate well with abnor-

malities seen on barium studies. This does not suggest, however, that all patients with Crohn's disease have mural thickening demonstrable by CT. As previously stated, in early Crohn's disease with superficial ulcerations, the CT scan may appear normal. Conversely, in patients with quiescent disease, the mucosa may be normal, whereas CT shows wall thickening. Rarely, mural changes may antedate mucosal changes seen on barium enema studies.[72-75]

Depending on the chronicity and level of disease activity, the presence of sinus tracts, and corticosteroid intake, the thickened bowel wall may have a homogeneous or, less frequently, an inhomogeneous appearance. A "double halo" appearance of the small bowel and colon has been described in Crohn's disease. An inner low-density ring with an attenuation near that of water (corresponding to severe submucosal edema) or fat (corresponding to submucosal fat deposition) can be seen surrounded by a higher-density ring of muscularis propria and serosa.[77]

This double halo appearance, originally described as specific for Crohn's disease, has been reported in ulcerative colitis, radiation enteritis, ischemic colitis, mesenteric venous thrombosis, acute pancreatitis, and pseudomembranous colitis. Inflamed mucosa and bowel wall may show significant contrast enhancement after bolus intravenous administration of contrast medium, and the intensity of enhancement has been reported to correlate with the clinical activity of disease.[75]

### Lumen

Strictures and lumen narrowing are hallmarks of advanced Crohn's disease. The lumen may appear obliterated—the CT equivalent of the "string" sign. These abnormalities, however, are well demonstrated by conventional means. CT can be helpful in delineating the cause of narrowing: mural thickening or extrinsic compression produced by an abscess or mesenteric mass. In addition, CT can be used to evaluate reduction in bowel wall thickness in patients undergoing medical management for partial obstruction. Before the onset of fibrosis, edema and inflammation are reversible causes of mural thickening and lumen obstruction. A decrease in wall thickness often produces a dramatic increase in lumen cross-sectional area and resolution of the patient's symptoms.[74, 84]

### Mesenteric Disease

The palpation of an abdominal mass or separation of bowel loops on a small bowel series in a patient with Crohn's disease evokes a large differential diagnosis with significantly different prognostic and therapeutic implications: abscess, phlegmon, "creeping fat" or fibrofatty proliferation of the mesentery, thickening of the bowel wall, and enlarged mesenteric lymph nodes. This diagnostic dilemma is further complicated by the fact that many of these patients are receiving immunosuppressive therapy that may mask signs and symptoms, and there may be a significant psychologic overlay.

---

### TABLE 62–9. CROHN'S COLITIS: BARIUM ENEMA FINDINGS

| EARLY CHANGES | LATE CHANGES |
| --- | --- |
| Nodular lymphoid hyperplasia | Fissures |
| Aphthoid ulcerations | Fistulas |
| Deep ulcerations | Haustral loss |
| Confluent ulcerations | Sacculations |
| Cobblestone appearance | Postinflammatory pseudopolyps |
| Asymmetric involvement | Intramural abscess strictures |
| Inflammatory pseudopolyps | |
| Segmental distribution | |
| Skip lesions | |

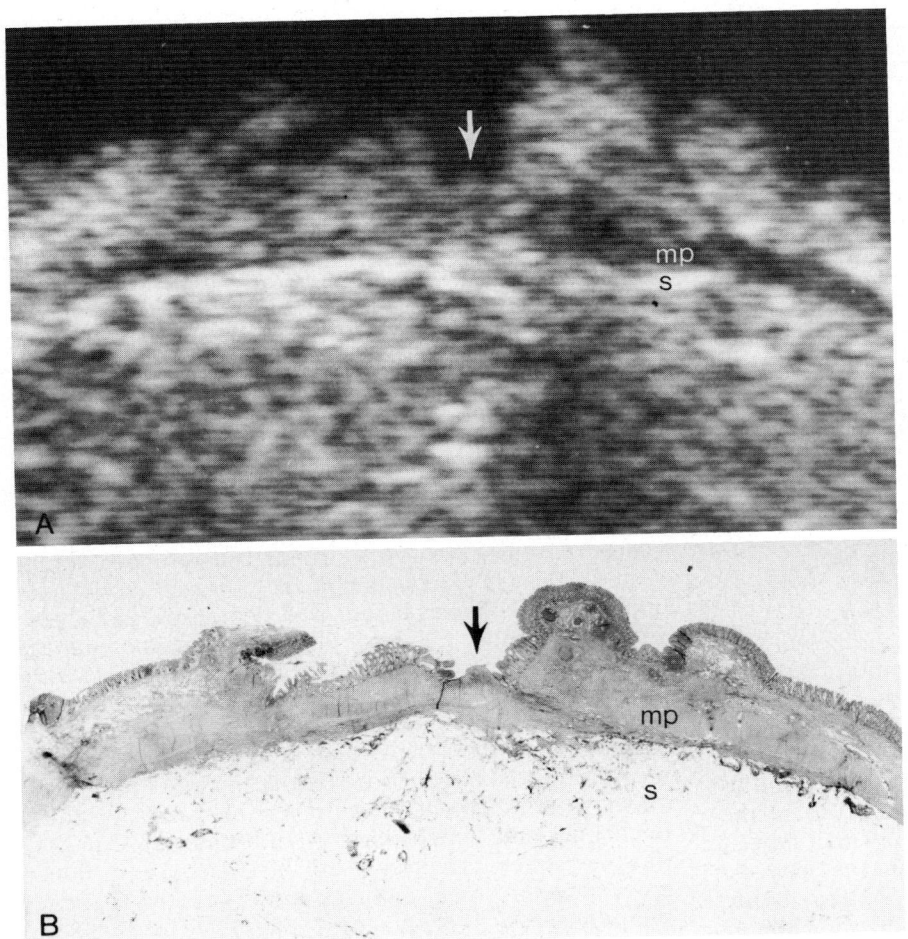

**Figure 62–30. Crohn's disease: sonographic findings.** Ultrasound image **(A)** and corresponding histologic section **(B)** of a specimen of colonic Crohn's disease. Areas of deep ulceration *(arrow)* are present. Note the absence of mural stratification on the sonogram. The only clear layers seen correspond to the muscularis propria (mp) and to the serosa and subserosal fat (s). (**A** and **B** from Kimmey MB, Wang KY, Haggitt RC, et al: Diagnosis of inflammatory bowel disease with ultrasound: an in vitro study. Invest Radiol 25:1085–1090, 1990.)

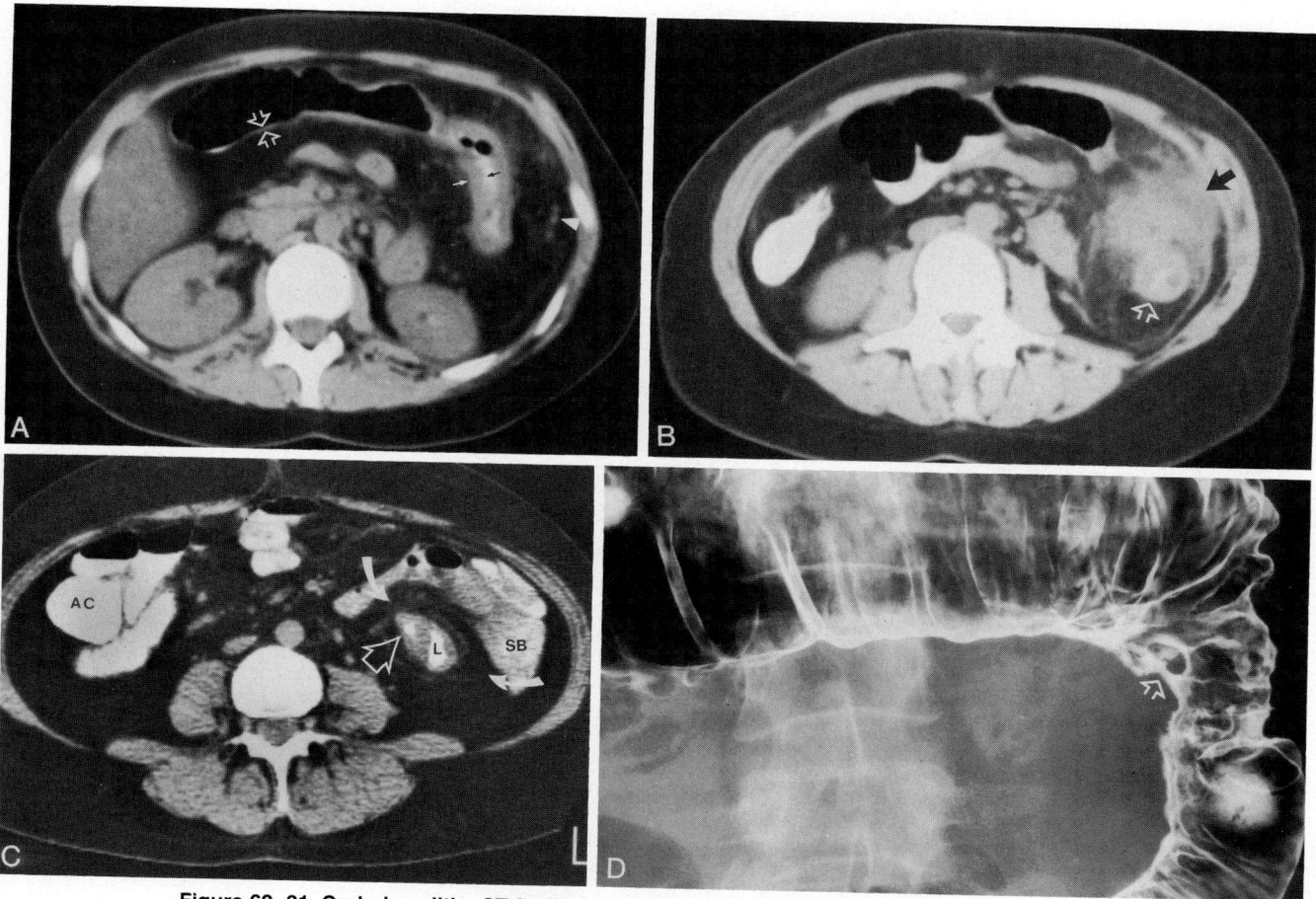

**Figure 62–31. Crohn's colitis: CT findings. A.** There is homogeneous mural thickening of the distal transverse colon *(solid arrows)*. Note the normal mural thickness of the proximal transverse colon *(open arrows)*. The pericolic fat of the involved segment shows increased attenuation and an increased number of lymph nodes *(arrowhead)*. **B.** Phlegmon is demonstrated *(solid arrow)* anterior to the thickened descending colon *(open arrow)*. Note the increased density of the pericolic fat and fascial thickening. No pus could be aspirated from this region. CT **(C)** and corresponding double contrast barium enema **(D)** in a patient with a previous resection of the transverse colon show a paracolic fistula *(open arrows)*. Note the abnormal fat *(curved arrows)* between the colon and small bowel (SB). AC = ascending colon; L = lumen.

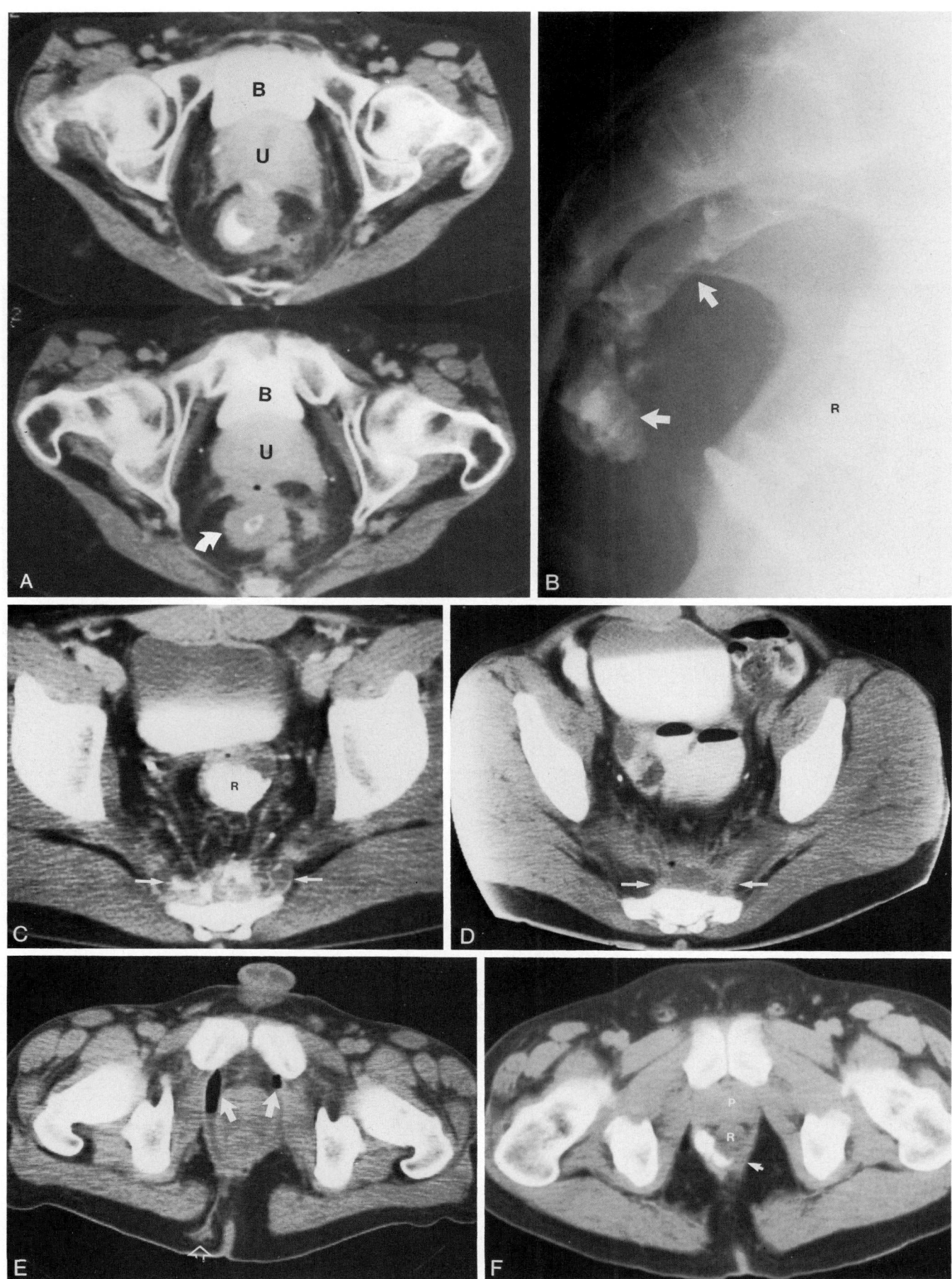

**Figure 62–32** See legend on opposite page

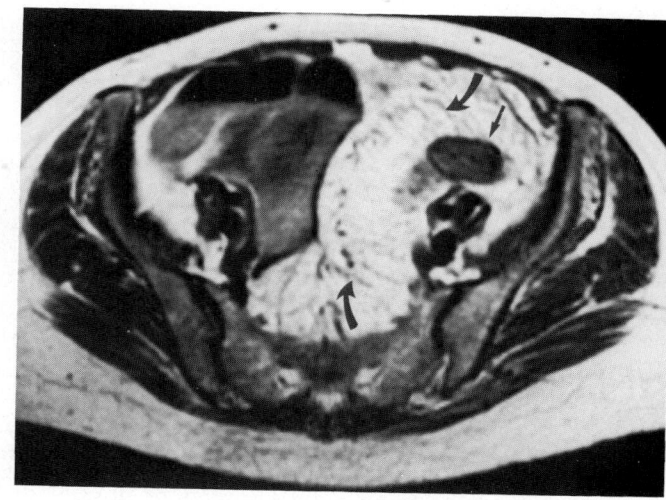

**Figure 62–33. Crohn's colitis: magnetic resonance findings.** Axial T1-weighted magnetic resonance scan shows that the fat of the sigmoid mesocolon *(curved arrows)* is thickened and has several strands of low attenuation corresponding to creeping fat of the mesentery. The wall of the sigmoid colon *(straight arrow)* is thickened as well. (Case courtesy of Martin I. Cohen, M.D., West Hills, CA.)

These extraluminal complications of Crohn's disease can readily be differentiated by CT examination.[72–74]

Fibrofatty proliferation, or creeping fat, of the mesentery is the most common cause of bowel loop separation seen on CT studies in patients with regional enteritis. The sharp interface between bowel and mesentery is lost, and the attenuation value of the fat, usually between −90 and −130 HU, is elevated by 20 to 60 HU owing to the influx of inflammatory cells and fluid (see Fig. 62–31). With more advanced disease, abscess or phlegmon may form. Mesenteric adenopathy with lymph nodes ranging in size between 3 and 8 mm may also occur (see Fig. 62–31). If these lymph nodes become larger than 1 cm in diameter, the presence of lymphoma or small bowel carcinoma (both of which occur with greater frequency in regional enteritis) should be excluded.[72–74]

## Rectal and Anal Pathology

Perianal disease is quite common (see Table 62–7) in patients with Crohn's disease. Unfortunately, this area is often poorly evaluated by barium studies because the enema tip may be inserted too cephalad or because exquisite anal tenderness may preclude adequate retrograde distention and evaluation. In one study, CT proved a sensitive means of evaluating these patients; CT abnormalities (Fig. 62–32) were observed in the perirectal, perianal region in 82% of patients. Pathologic findings included inflammation of fat planes in the perirectal region and ischiorectal fossa (73%), rectal wall thickening (30%), fistulas or sinus tracts (22%), and abscesses (14%). The plane of scanning must continue caudal to the symphysis to include the entire perineum because significant disease was found beneath the symphysis in more than one third of patients.[215]

## Magnetic Resonance

In one study, magnetic resonance proved useful in evaluating fistulas and sinus tracts in patients with Crohn's disease.[216] Magnetic resonance was particularly helpful in patients with anorectal disease because of its ability to show the relationship of the tract to the levator muscles in the coronal plane. Magnetic resonance can also show the mural and mesenteric changes of this disease (Fig. 62–33).

# Double Contrast Barium Enema Findings and Their Anatomic-Pathologic Basis

## Lymphoid Hyperplasia

Lymphoid follicles are a normal component of gut-associated lymphatic tissue. They are aggregates of lymphocytes surrounding germinal centers that straddle the muscularis mucosae. Lymphoid follicles have an

---

**Figure 62–32. Crohn's disease—anorectal pathology: CT findings. A.** Marked homogeneous mural thickening of the rectal wall *(curved arrow)* and narrowing of the lumen are identified in this patient with Crohn's colitis. There is an abscess in the left perirectal space. B = bladder; U = uterus. **B.** In a different patient, a contrast-filled presacral abscess *(arrows)* is identified posterior to the rectum (R). **C** and **D.** Corresponding CT sections. The extent of the abscess *(arrows)* is better appreciated. R = rectum. **E.** In a different patient, a perirectal sinus tract *(open arrow)* extends through the fat of the right ischiorectal fossa into the right buttock. Perirectal abscesses containing air *(solid arrows)* are seen lateral to the rectum. **F.** In a different patient, the course and full extent of a rectocutaneous fistula *(arrow)* medial to the right levator ani muscle are better appreciated on this CT sinogram. P = prostate; R = rectum; arrow = left levator ani muscle.

average macroscopic density of 3.8 per centimeter of adult human colon.[86, 217] They are seen in 50% of barium studies performed on children and 13% of air-contrast barium enemas in adults. Lymphoid follicles appear as 1- to 3-mm elevations in the mucosa without a ring shadow.[217–220]

Lymphoid follicles may enlarge in a wide variety of infectious, neoplastic, immunologic, and inflammatory diseases of the gut, including Crohn's disease.[221] Prominent lymphoid follicles have also been observed in older patients with colonic adenomas and carcinomas.[222]

### Aphthoid Ulcerations

As the lymphoid follicles enlarge, the overlying mucosa may ulcerate with production of the aphthous lesion. These small, superficial ulcers have erythematous margins and are seen on a background of normal or near-normal mucosa.[86] This is in direct contrast to ulcerative colitis, in which ulceration invariably occurs against a background of heavy inflammation.[223, 224] Aphthae are recognized radiographically as punctate central collections of barium surrounded by a radiolucent halo about 1 mm in diameter that produces a target or "bull's-eye" appearance[225–228] (Fig. 62–34). Aphthae may be isolated, be found in clusters, or involve the entire colon.[229]

Aphthoid lesions are found in 44 to 72% of patients with Crohn's disease and may be the only abnormality found in an otherwise normal colon.[230] These ulcers are nonspecific and occur in amebiasis, salmonellosis, shigellosis, herpes, cytomegalovirus infection, Behçet's disease, ischemic colitis, and *Yersinia* enterocolitis.[229, 230]

### Cobblestoning

The aphthous lesions may regress, remain stable, or more commonly enlarge and deepen.[227, 228] As the aphthae expand, they become irregular in outline and lose their surrounding lucent halo. Adjacent ulcers may coalesce, forming a network of longitudinal linear ulceration and transverse fissuring, with edematous intervening mucosa producing a raised, cobbled appearance.[46, 229] As mentioned earlier, this is actually one of many forms of inflammatory pseudopolyposis.

### Transverse Contrast Stripes

Multiple straight white lines measuring more than 1 cm long and up to 1 mm wide have been reported as a fairly specific sign of Crohn's disease. These are produced by barium that lies in narrow furrows between adjacent mucosal folds. It is not certain whether these represent fissures, ulcers, or merely folds in contraction.[231]

### Deep Ulcerations

Fissuring ulcers (Fig. 62–35) are a distinctive feature of Crohn's disease. They typically penetrate beyond the submucosa, with resultant knife-shaped or "rose thorn" fistulas.[86] These fissures and fistulas do not cause pneumoperitoneum because the surrounding serosa is inflamed and involved bowel loops become adherent to one another and to adjacent peritoneal surfaces.[86, 104, 105]

### Pericolic Sinus Tracts

Long interconnecting fistulas are common in Crohn's colitis and occur in the muscularis mucosae or subserosa paralleling the bowel lumen. When not associated with neoplasia or diverticula, pericolic sinus tracts are suggestive of Crohn's disease.[81, 86]

### Sinus Tracts, Fissures, and Fistulas

Sinuses, fissures, and fistulas (Fig. 62–36) are a hallmark of Crohn's disease.[85, 91] Sinuses and fissures represent blind-ended inflammatory tracts that penetrate through the full thickness of the muscle coat later in the disease course. Fistulas communicate with other structures. Anatomic evidence suggests that mechanical factors such as elevated intraluminal pressure rather than any intrinsic pathologic change of Crohn's disease are responsible for these fissures and fistulas.[85, 91] This is based on the facts that there is a significant coincidence of sinuses and strictures and that sinuses arise proximal to the point of maximal stricture. In addition, fissures, sinuses, and fistulas are not constantly associated with myocytolysis, a seemingly necessary process if only the Crohn's inflammation is required for the fissuring.[85, 91]

### Mural Thickening

The mural thickening that occurs in Crohn's disease is more impressive than that found in ulcerative colitis. It is due to transmural inflammation and fibrosis. The submucosa may also accumulate fat in Crohn's disease as well but less commonly than in ulcerative colitis. CT nicely demonstrates mural thickening of the esophagus, stomach, duodenum, small bowel, and colon when these areas are involved by Crohn's disease.[72–75]

### Lumen Narrowing and Strictures

Crohn's disease is a transmural inflammatory process that produces gut wall thickening and fibrosis leading to narrowing of the lumen and shortening of the gut as well.[6, 7] In ulcerative colitis, narrowing results from thickening and contractions of the muscularis mucosae rather than from fibrosis. Strictures are asymmetric in Crohn's disease and tend to be less smooth and circumferential than those seen in ulcerative colitis. Strictures occur in 21% of patients with small bowel disease and 8% of patients with Crohn's colitis.[6, 7, 83, 85]

### Sacculations

The transmural fibrosis of Crohn's disease is often asymmetric (Fig. 62–37). It occurs predominantly on the mesenteric side of the gut, where it is often accompanied by creeping fat of the mesentery. The relatively

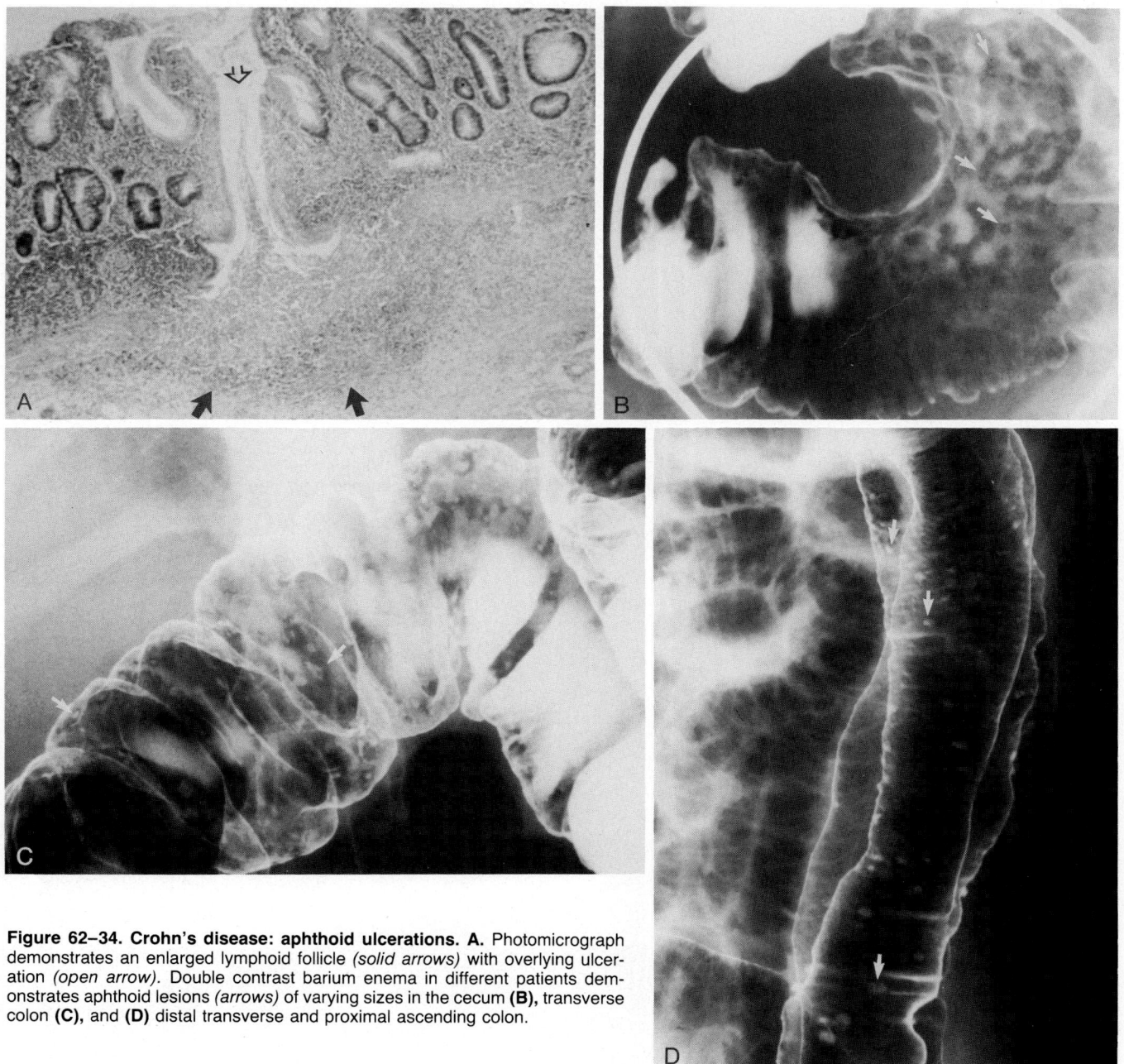

**Figure 62–34. Crohn's disease: aphthoid ulcerations. A.** Photomicrograph demonstrates an enlarged lymphoid follicle *(solid arrows)* with overlying ulceration *(open arrow).* Double contrast barium enema in different patients demonstrates aphthoid lesions *(arrows)* of varying sizes in the cecum **(B),** transverse colon **(C),** and **(D)** distal transverse and proximal ascending colon.

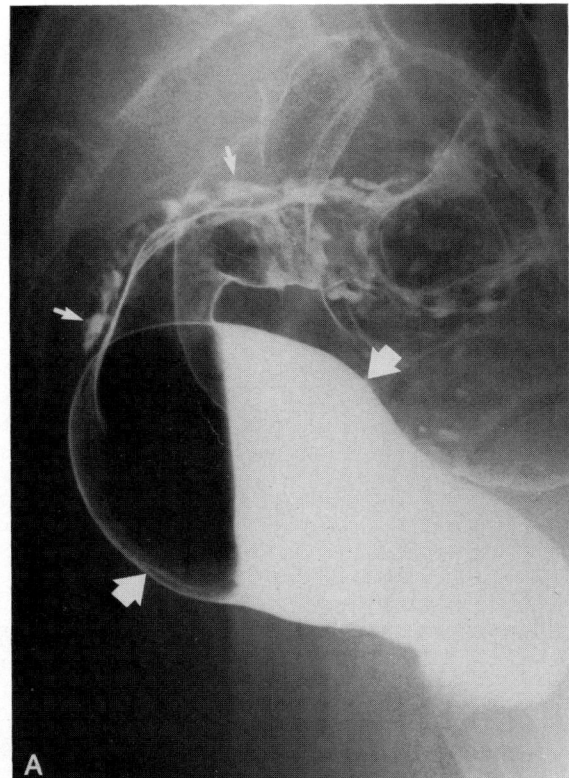

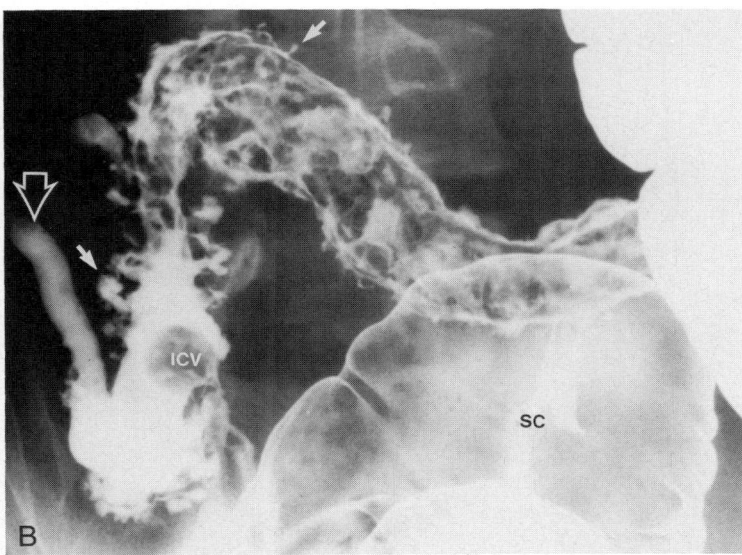

**Figure 62–35. Crohn's disease: deep ulcerations. A.** Lateral film of the rectum from a double contrast barium enema shows deep ulcerations *(small arrows)*. Note the sparing of the distal rectum *(large arrows)*. **B.** Spot film of the splenic flexure demonstrates deep ulcers *(solid arrows)*, a large ileocecal valve (ICV), and sparing of the sigmoid colon (SC). Open arrow = subhepatic appendix.

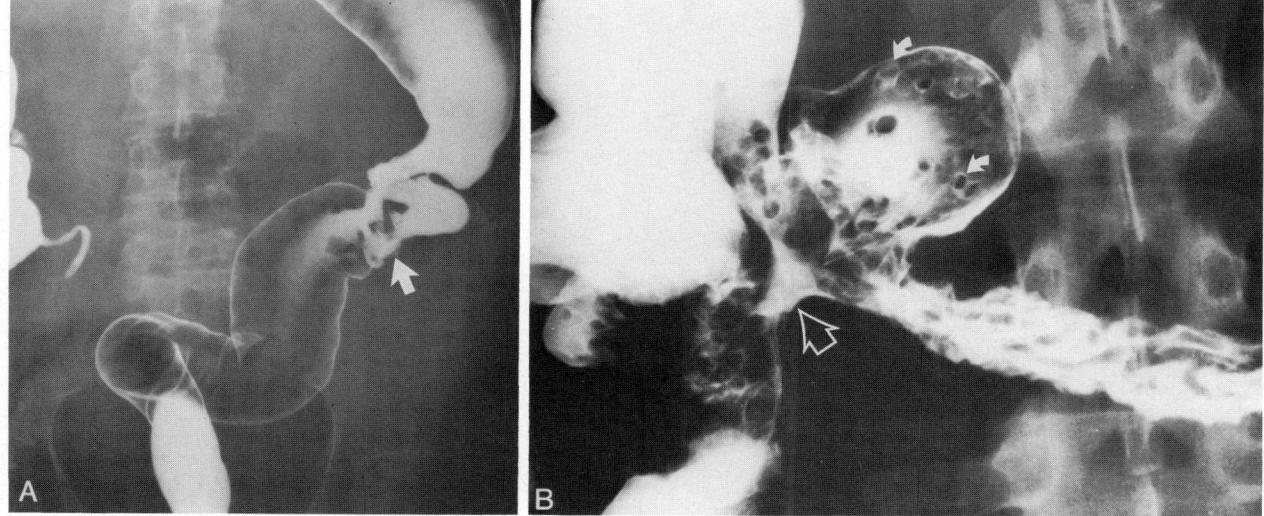

**Figure 62–36. Crohn's disease: strictures and fistulas. A.** The lumen of the proximal sigmoid colon is narrowed, and a colocolic fistula *(arrow)* is present. **B.** Double contrast barium enema shows considerable deformity of the hepatic flexure with a colocolic fistula *(open arrow)* and postinflammatory pseudopolyps *(arrows)*.

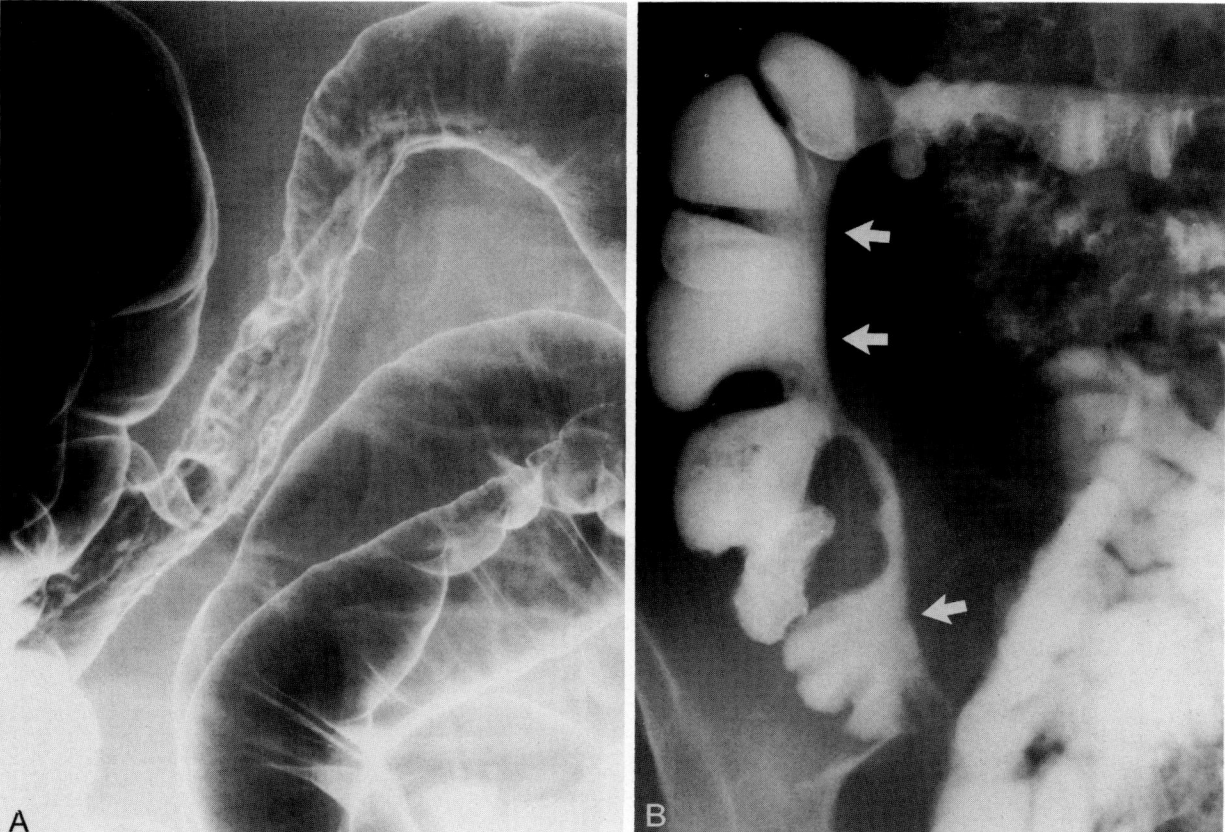

**Figure 62–37. Crohn's disease: distribution. A.** Crohn's disease isolated to the distal transverse colon. The colon proximal and distal to this segment is normal. **B.** Crohn's disease involves primarily the mesenteric side *(arrows)* of the gut, leading to fibrosis and "ballooning" of the antimesenteric border. Crohn's disease is typically discontinuous, patchy, and asymmetric.

unaffected side (usually antimesenteric) remains pliable and tends to bulge when luminal pressure increases owing to peristalsis. Outpouchings may eventually develop. The outpouchings are similar to the so-called pseudosacculations or pseudodiverticula seen in scleroderma.[81, 83, 86]

## Anorectal Disease

Anorectal complications are common in patients with Crohn's disease and include anal fissures, ulcers, abscess, internal hemorrhoids, and stenosis with induration; skin lesions such as erosion, skin tags, ulceration, maceration, external hemorrhoids, and abscess; and fistulas—anal canal to skin, rectum to skin, and rectovaginal. Anal disease develops in 36% of all patients with Crohn's disease, 25% of those with only small bowel involvement, 67% of patients with colonic disease, and nearly all patients with rectal disease.[2, 4, 85, 91, 232]

In approximately one fourth of patients, the anal disease may antedate overt intestinal disease often by as many as 4 years. Accordingly, development of these anorectal disorders warrants radiologic investigation of the entire gastrointestinal tract.[2, 4, 82, 91]

## Distribution

Any portion of the gut, from the mouth to the anus, may be involved by Crohn's disease. Twenty percent of cases are isolated to the colon, 20% are restricted to the small bowel, and 60% involve the colon and small bowel simultaneously. In 5 to 10% of these patients, upper gastrointestinal tract involvement is seen. It is unusual to see isolated esophageal or gastroduodenal Crohn's disease, however. Regardless of location, similar radiographic-pathologic findings obtain: there is discontinuous, patchy, and asymmetric disease involvement (see Fig. 62–37).[2, 4, 224]

## DIFFERENTIATING ULCERATIVE COLITIS FROM CROHN'S COLITIS

The differentiation of Crohn's colitis and ulcerative colitis is important because each disease has different therapeutic and prognostic implications. Patients with ulcerative colitis have a higher risk of developing cancer. They can also have a curative colectomy and are candidates for sphincter-preserving surgery. Patients with

Crohn's disease, however, are not candidates for ileal reservoirs because disease may recur in the ileum.

The following double contrast barium enema features enable the correct diagnosis to be made in most patients. 1) Ulcerative colitis is a contiguous, confluent, circumferential, and symmetric disease that begins in the rectum and extends proximally. 2) Crohn's disease is a patchy, discontinuous disease with asymmetric involvement that can lead to pseudodiverticula. 3) The following types of ulcerations are characteristic of Crohn's disease: aphthoid, discrete, deep (>3 mm), fissure, and rose thorn. 4) A granular mucosa is typical in ulcerative colitis but not in Crohn's colitis. 5) Severe anal and perianal disease is characteristic of Crohn's disease but is exceptionally rare in ulcerative colitis. 6) Spontaneous fistula and sinus tracts are a hallmark of Crohn's disease.[233-241]

Differentiation between these two diseases can be made on radiologic grounds (Table 62-10) in 90 to 95% of patients. This distinction is easier to make in the early stages of disease, because the early manifestations are

### TABLE 62-10. INFLAMMATORY BOWEL DISEASE: RADIOLOGIC DIFFERENTIAL DIAGNOSIS

| FEATURE | COMMONLY FOUND IN | MAY OCCUR IN |
|---|---|---|
| Granular mucosa | Ulcerative colitis | Early Crohn's colitis (rare) |
| Ulceration | | |
| Discrete | Crohn's colitis | Amebiasis |
| | *Yersinia* infection | Ischemia |
| | Behçet's disease | Tuberculosis |
| Confluent (shallow) | Ulcerative colitis | Crohn's disease |
| | | Amebiasis |
| Confluent (deep) | Crohn's disease | Ischemia |
| | | Amebiasis |
| | | Tuberculosis |
| | | *Strongyloides* infection |
| Stricture | | |
| Symmetric | Ulcerative colitis | Tuberculosis |
| | Lymphogranuloma venereum | |
| Asymmetric | Crohn's disease | |
| | Ischemia | |
| | Tuberculosis | |
| Fistula | Crohn's disease | Tuberculosis |
| | Lymphogranuloma venereum | Actinomycosis |
| Inflammatory polyps | Ulcerative colitis | Ischemia (rare) |
| | Crohn's disease | |
| | Schistosomiasis | |
| | Colitis cystica profunda | |
| Small bowel disease | Crohn's disease | Ulcerative colitis (backwash ileitis) |
| | *Yersinia* infection | |
| | Tuberculosis | Behçet's disease |
| | Pseudomembranous enterocolitis | Ischemia |
| Skip lesions | Crohn's disease | Lymphogranuloma venereum |
| | Tuberculosis | |
| | Amebiasis | |
| Toxic megacolon | Ulcerative colitis | Crohn's disease |
| | | Ischemia |
| | | Amebiasis |

From Bartram CI, Laufer I: Inflammatory bowel disease. *In* Laufer I, Levine MS (eds): Double Contrast Gastrointestinal Radiology (2nd ed). Philadelphia: WB Saunders, 1992, pp 579-645.

### TABLE 62-11. INFLAMMATORY BOWEL DISEASE: CLINICAL DIFFERENTIAL DIAGNOSIS

| ULCERATIVE COLITIS | CROHN'S DISEASE |
|---|---|
| Pancolitis | Ileal and jejunal |
| *Campylobacter* infection | *Yersinia* enterocolitis |
| Shigellosis | Salmonellosis |
| Salmonellosis | Tuberculosis |
| Cytomegalovirus infection | *Strongyloides* infection |
| *Escherichia coli* infection | Lymphoma |
| *Clostridium difficile* infection | Radiation enteritis |
| Amebiasis | Carcinoid |
| Behçet's disease | Eosinophilic enteritis |
| Graft-versus-host disease | Carcinoma (rare) |
| Radiation colitis | Ileocecal |
| Diverticular disease | Tuberculosis |
| Ischemic colitis | Typhlitis |
| Proctosigmoiditis | Amebiasis |
| Herpes simplex infection | Graft-versus-host disease |
| Gonorrhea | Appendicitis |
| *Chlamydia* infection | Carcinoma |
| | Colonic |
| | Ischemia |
| | Diverticulitis |
| | Carcinoma |
| | Amebiasis |
| | Tuberculosis |
| | Ischemic colitis |
| | Radiation colitis |
| | *Chlamydia* infection |

From Shanahan F, Targan SR: Inflammatory bowel disease. *In* Kelley WN (ed): Textbook of Internal Medicine (2nd ed). Philadelphia: JB Lippincott, 1992, pp 489-502.

particularly distinctive. When the disease is chronic or when there have been numerous exacerbations and remissions, the distinction may be more difficult. For example, ulcerative colitis in remission may become discontinuous, whereas granulomatous colitis may involve the entire colon.[233-241]

Colitis indeterminate is the term used for cases that show maximal overlap of the pathologic features of ulcerative colitis and Crohn's disease.[233-241]

## DIFFERENTIAL DIAGNOSIS OF INFLAMMATORY BOWEL DISEASE

Because inflammatory bowel disease has such protean clinical manifestations, it is often considered in the differential diagnosis of patients with a wide range of gastrointestinal complaints. Establishing the diagnosis of inflammatory bowel disease depends on integrating a composite of clinical, endoscopic, histologic, and radiographic features over time and excluding infections and other disorders. Diseases that can mimic inflammatory bowel disease, clinically and radiologically, are listed in Tables 62-10 and 62-11.

### Acknowledgment

Figures 62-17B, 62-18A and B, and 62-19A are reproduced from Laufer I, Levine MS (eds): Double Contrast Gastrointestinal Radiology (2nd ed). Philadelphia: WB Saunders, 1992.

Figures 62-24 and 62-26A are reproduced from Sabiston D Jr (ed): Textbook of Surgery (14th ed). Philadelphia: WB Saunders, 1991.

# References

1. Podolsky DK: Inflammatory bowel disease. Part 1. N Engl J Med 325:928–937, 1991.

2. Stenson WF, MacDermott RP: Inflammatory bowel disease. *In* Yamada T (ed): Textbook of Gastroenterology. Philadelphia: JB Lippincott, 1991, pp 1588–1645.

3. Cello JP, Schneiderman DJ: Ulcerative colitis. *In* Sleisenger MH, Fordtran JS (eds): Gastrointestinal Disease: Pathophysiology, Diagnosis, Management (4th ed). Philadelphia: WB Saunders, 1989, pp 1435–1477.

4. Shanahan F. Targan SR: Inflammatory bowel disease. *In* Kelley WN (ed): Textbook of Internal Medicine (2nd ed). Philadelphia: JB Lippincott, 1992, pp 489–502.

5. Bartram C: Introduction. *In* Bartram C (ed): Radiology in Inflammatory Bowel Disease. New York: Marcel Dekker, 1983, pp 1–3.

6. Sommer SC: Ulcerative and granulomatous colitis. AJR 130:817–823, 1977.

7. Price AB, Morson BC: Inflammatory bowel disease: the surgical pathology of Crohn's disease and ulcerative colitis. Hum Pathol 6:7–29, 1987.

8. Kirsner JB: Historical aspects of inflammatory bowel disease. J Clin Gastroenterol 10:286–297, 1988.

9. Myron J: Inflammatory bowel disease: A historical perspective. *In* de Dombal FT, Myren J, Bouchier IAD (eds): Inflammatory Bowel Disease. Oxford: Oxford University Press, 1986, pp 7–28.

10. Mendeloff AI, Calkins BM: The epidemiology of idiopathic inflammatory bowel disease. *In* Kirsner JB, Shorter RG (eds): Inflammatory Bowel Disease (3rd ed). Philadelphia: Lea & Febiger, 1988, pp 3–34.

11. Ekbom A, Adami H-O: The epidemiology of inflammatory bowel disease. Curr Opin Gastroenterol 7:649–663, 1991.

12. Sandler RS: The epidemiology of inflammatory bowel disease. Curr Opin Gastroenterol 6:531–535, 1990.

13. Sonnenberg A, Wasserman IH: Epidemiology of inflammatory bowel disease among US military veterans. Gastroenterology 101:122–130, 1991.

14. Ekbom A, Helmick C, Zack M, et al: The epidemiology of inflammatory bowel disease: a large population-based study in Sweden. Gastroenterology 100:350–358, 1991.

15. Sonnenberg A: Geographic variation in the incidence of and mortality from inflammatory bowel disease. Dis Colon Rectum 19:854–861, 1986.

16. Sonnenberg A, McCarty DJ, Jacobsen SJ: Geographic variation of inflammatory bowel disease within the United States. Gastroenterology 100:143–149, 1991.

17. Orholm M, Munkholm P, Langholz E, et al: Familial occurrence of inflammatory bowel disease. N Engl J Med 324:84–88, 1991.

18. Bennett RA, Rubin PH, Present DH, et al: Frequency of inflammatory bowel disease in offspring of couples both presenting with inflammatory bowel disease. Gastroenterology 100:1638–1643, 1991.

19. Boyko EJ, Koepsell TD, Perera DR, et al: Risk of ulcerative colitis among former and current cigarette smokers. N Engl J Med 316:707–710, 1987.

20. Lorusso D, Misciagna L, Guerra V: Cigarette smoking and ulcerative colitis: a case control study. Hepatogastroenterology 36:202–204, 1989.

21. Calkins BM: A meta-analysis of the role of smoking in inflammatory bowel disease. Dig Dis Sci 34:1841–1854, 1992.

22. Sonnenberg A: Mortality from Crohn's disease and ulcerative colitis in England-Wales and the United States from 1950 to 1983. Dis Colon Rectum 19:624–629, 1986.

23. Bayless TM: Prognosis of inflammatory bowel disease. *In* Kirsner JB, Shorter RG (eds): Inflammatory Bowel Disease (3rd ed). Philadelphia: Lea & Febiger, 1988, pp 747–764.

24. Maratka Z: Pathogenesis and etiology of inflammatory bowel disease. *In* de Dombal FT, Myren J, Bouchier IAD (eds): Inflammatory Bowel Disease. Oxford: Oxford University Press, 1986, pp 29–65.

25. Singleton JW: Epidemiology and etiology of inflammatory bowel disease. Curr Opin Gastroenterol 5:501–505, 1989.

26. Gibson PR: Etiology of inflammatory bowel disease. Curr Opin Gastroenterol 7:642–648, 1991.

27. Geller AJ, Das KM: Etiology of inflammatory bowel disease. Curr Opin Gastroenterol 6:561–564, 1990.

28. Jayanthi V, Probert CSJ, Sher KS, et al: Current concepts of etiopathogenesis of inflammatory bowel disease. Am J Gastroenterol 86:1566–1572, 1991.

29. Cottone M, Bunce M, Taylor CJ, et al: Ulcerative colitis and HLA phenotype. Gut 26:952–954, 1985.

30. Mielants H, Veys EM, Curvelier C, et al: HLA-B27 related arthritis and bowel inflammation. J Rheumatol 12:294–298, 1985.

31. Pullman WE, Elsbury S, Kobayashi M, et al: Enhanced mucosal cytokine production in inflammatory bowel disease. Gastroenterology 102:529–537, 1992.

32. Gibson PR, van de Pole, Barratt PJ, et al: Ulcerative colitis—a disease characterized by the abnormal colonic epithelial cell? Gut 29:516–521, 1988.

33. Helzer JE, Stillings WA, Chammas S, et al: A controlled study of the association between ulcerative colitis and psychiatric diagnosis. Dig Dis Sci 27:513–518, 1982.

34. Drossman DA: Psychosocial aspects of ulcerative colitis and Crohn's disease. *In* Kirsner JB, Shorter RG (eds): Inflammatory Bowel Disease (3rd ed). Philadelphia: Lea & Febiger, 1988, pp 209–226.

35. MacDermott RP, Stenson WF: Alterations of the immune system in ulcerative colitis and Crohn's disease. Adv Immunol 42:285–328, 1988.

36. Deusch K, Reich K: Immunological aspects of inflammatory bowel disease. Endoscopy 24:568–577, 1992.

37. Matsuura T, West GA, Youngman KR, et al: Immune activation genes in inflammatory bowel disease. Gastroenterology 104:448–458, 1993.

38. Lashner BA, Kane SV, Hanauer SB: Oral contraceptives and inflammatory bowel disease. Gastroenterology 89:1032–1036, 1990.

39. Lerner L, Rossi TM, Park B, et al: Serum antibodies to cow's milk proteins in pediatric inflammatory bowel disease: Crohn's disease vs. ulcerative colitis. Acta Paediatr Scand 78:81–86, 1989.

40. Kirschner BS, De Favoro MV, Jensen W: Lactose malabsorption in children and adolescents with inflammatory bowel disease. Gastroenterology 81:829–837, 1981.

41. Lichtenstein GR, Rothstein RD: Clinical inflammatory bowel disease. Curr Opin Gastroenterol 7:628–634, 1991.

42. Singleton JW: Clinical features, course, and laboratory features in ulcerative colitis. *In* Kirsner JB, Shorter RG (eds): Inflammatory Bowel Disease (3rd ed). Philadelphia: Lea & Febiger, 1988, pp 167–174.

43. Peppercorn MA: Inflammatory bowel disease. *In* Taylor MB (ed): Gastrointestinal Emergencies. Baltimore: Williams & Wilkins, 1992, pp 402–414.

44. de Dombal FT, Myren J, Bouchier IAD, et al: Diagnosis of patients with inflammatory bowel disease—the value of clinical features. *In* de Dombal FT, Myren J, Bouchier IAD (eds): Inflammatory Bowel Disease. Oxford: Oxford University Press, 1986, pp 94–110.

45. Silverstein FE, Tytgat GNJ: Atlas of Gastrointestinal Endoscopy (2nd ed). New York: Gower Medical Publishing, 1991, pp 11.2–11.17.

46. Bartram CI: Ulcerative colitis. *In* Bartram CI (ed): Radiology in Inflammatory Bowel Disease. New York: Marcel Dekker, 1983, pp 31–62.

47. Bartram CI: Plain abdominal x-ray in acute colitis. Proc Soc Med 69:617–618, 1976.

48. Bartram CI: Radiology in the current assessment of ulcerative colitis. Gastrointest Radiol 1:383–392, 1977.

49. Gabrielsson N, Grandvist S, Sundelin P, et al: Extent of inflammatory lesions in ulcerative colitis assessed by radiology, colonoscopy, and endoscopic biopsies. Gastrointest Radiol 4:395–400, 1979.

50. Prantera C, Lorenzetti R, Cerro P, et al: The plain abdominal film accurately estimates extent of active ulcerative colitis. J Clin Gastroenterol 13:231–234, 1991.

51. Rice RP: Plain abdominal film roentgenographic diagnosis of ulcerative disease of the colon. Radiology 104:544–550, 1968.

52. Simpson SA, Lewis JR: Plain roentgenography in diagnosis of chronic ulcerative colitis and terminal ileitis. Radiology 84:306–315, 1960.

53. McConnell F, Hanelin J, Robbins LL: Plain film diagnosis of fulminating ulcerative colitis. Radiology 71:674–682, 1958.

54. Caprilli R, Vernia P, Latella G, et al: Early recognition of toxic megacolon. J Clin Gastroenterol 9:160–164, 1987.

55. Bartram CI, Herlinger H: Bowel wall thickness as a differentiating feature between ulcerative colitis and Crohn's disease of the colon. Clin Radiol 30:15–19, 1979.

56. Hotze AL, Biersack HJ: Nuclear medicine in inflammatory bowel diseases. *In* Biersack HJ, Cox PH (eds): Nuclear Medicine in Gastroenterology. Dordrecht: Kluwer Academic Publishers, 1991, pp 169–176.

57. Saverymuttu S: Role of 111-indium white cell scanning in the assessment and management of inflammatory bowel disease. Inflamm Bowel Dis News 11:1–3, 1990.

58. Stein DT, Gray GN, Gregory PB, et al: Location and activity of ulcerative colitis by indium 111 leukocyte scan. Gastroenterology 84:388–393, 1983.

59. Saverymuttu SH, Camilleri M, Rees H, et al: Indium 111 granulocyte scanning in the assessment of disease extent and disease activity in inflammatory bowel disease. Gastroenterology 90:1121–1128, 1986.

60. Froelich JW, Field SA: The role of indium-111 white blood cells in inflammatory bowel disease. Semin Nucl Med 18:147–152, 1988.

61. Froelich JW: Nuclear medicine imaging of inflammatory bowel disease. Radiol Clin North Am 25:133–141, 1987.

62. Limberg B: Diagnosis of inflammatory and neoplastic large bowel diseases by conventional abdominal and colonic sonography. Ultrasound Q 6:151–156, 1988.

63. Kimmey MB, Wang KY, Haggitt RC, et al: Diagnosis of inflammatory bowel disease with ultrasound. Invest Radiol 25:1085–1090, 1990.

64. Limberg B: Diagnosis of inflammatory and neoplastic colonic disease by sonography. J Clin Gastroenterol 9:607–611, 1987.

65. Hata J, Haruma K, Suenga K, et al: Ultrasonographic assessment of inflammatory bowel disease. Am J Gastroenterol 87:443–447, 1992.

66. Schwerk WB, Beckh K, Raith M, et al: A prospective evaluation of high resolution sonography in the differential diagnosis of inflammatory bowel disease. Eur J Gastroenterol Hepatol 4:173–182, 1992.

67. Dubbins PA: Ultrasound demonstration of bowel wall thickness in inflammatory bowel disease. Clin Radiol 35:227–331, 1984.

68. Sonnenberg A, Erckenbrecht, Peter P, et al: Detection of Crohn's disease by ultrasound. Gastroenterology 83:430–434, 1982.

69. Worlicek H, Lutz H, Heyder N, et al: Ultrasound findings in Crohn's disease and ulcerative colitis. A prospective study. JCU 15:153–163, 1987.

70. Pera A, Cammarota T, Comino E, et al: Ultrasonography in the detection of Crohn's disease and in the differential diagnosis of inflammatory bowel disease. Digestion 41:180–184, 1988.

71. Hojlund PB, Gronvall S, Dorph S, et al: The value of dynamic ultrasound scanning in Crohn's disease. Scand J Gastroenterol 21:969–972, 1986.

72. Gore RM: Cross-sectional imaging of the inflammatory bowel disease. Radiol Clin North Am 25:115–131, 1987.

73. Gore RM, Marn CS, Kirby DF, et al: CT findings in ulcerative, granulomatous, and indeterminate colitis. AJR 143:279–282, 1983.

74. Gore RM: CT of inflammatory bowel disease. Radiol Clin North Am 27:717–730, 1989.

75. Hulnick DH: Small intestine. *In* Megibow AJ, Balthazar EJ (eds): Computed Tomography of the Gastrointestinal Tract. St. Louis: CV Mosby, 1986, pp 217–278.

76. Fisher JK: Normal colon wall thickness on CT. Radiology 145:415–418, 1982.

77. Jones B, Fishman EK, Hamilton SR, et al: Submucosal accumulation of fat in inflammatory bowel disease: CT/pathologic correlation. J Comput Assist Tomogr 10:759–763, 1986.

78. Marshak RH, Linder AE, Maklansky D: Radiology of the Colon. Philadelphia: WB Saunders, 1980, pp 64–119.

79. Shaffer HA: Double contrast techniques in the diagnosis of inflammatory bowel disease. Curr Probl Diagn Radiol 7:3–52, 1983.

80. Thoeni RF, Margulis AR: The radiology of inflammatory disease of the colon. Postgrad Radiol 1:187–212, 1981.

81. Simpkins KC: Inflammatory bowel disease: ulcerative and Crohn's colitis. *In* Simpkins KC (ed): A Textbook of Radiological Diagnosis, Volume 4, The Alimentary Tract: The Hollow Organs and Salivary Glands. London: HK Lewis, 1988, pp 473–498.

82. Kelvin FM, Gardiner RH: Clinical Imaging of the Colon and Rectum. New York: Raven Press, pp 64–119, 1987.

83. Bartram CI, Laufer I: Inflammatory bowel disease. *In* Laufer I, Levine MS (eds): Double Contrast Gastrointestinal Radiology (2nd ed). Philadelphia: WB Saunders, 1992, pp 580–645.

84. Gore RM: Inflammatory bowel disease: anatomic-pathologic basis of radiographic findings. *In* Gore RM (ed): Syllabus for Categorical Course on Gastrointestinal Radiology. Reston, VA: American College of Radiology, 1991, pp 77–87.

85. Mitros FA: Atlas of Gastrointestinal Pathology. New York: Gower Medical Publishing, 1992, pp 7.16–7.25.

86. Lichtenstein JE: Radiologic-pathologic correlation of inflammatory bowel disease. Radiol Clin North Am 25:3–24, 1987.

87. Pera A, Bellando P, Caldera D, et al: Colonoscopy in inflammatory disease. Gastroenterology 92:181–185, 1987.

88. Waye JD: Endoscopy in idiopathic inflammatory bowel disease. *In* Kirsner JB, Shorter RG (eds): Inflammatory Bowel Disease (3rd ed). Philadelphia: Lea & Febiger, 1988, pp 353–376.

89. Laufer I, Mullens JE, Hamilton J: Correlation of endoscopy and double-contrast radiography in the early stages of ulcerative and granulomatous colitis. Radiology 118:1–5, 1988.

90. Laufer I: The radiologic demonstration of early changes in ulcerative colitis by double contrast techniques. J Can Assoc Radiol 26:116–121, 1975.

91. Riddell RH: Pathology of idiopathic inflammatory bowel disease. *In* Kirsner JB, Shorter RG (eds): Inflammatory Bowel Disease (3rd ed). Philadelphia: Lea & Febiger, 1988, pp 329–350.

92. Lewin KJ, Riddell RH, Weinstein WM: Gastrointestinal Pathology and its Clinical Implications. New York: Igaku-Shoin, 1992, pp 838–902.

93. Lichtenstein JE, Madewell JE, Feigen DS: The collar button ulcer. Gastrointest Radiol 4:79–84, 1979.

94. Suekane H, Iida M, Matsui T, et al: Radiographic demonstration of longitudinal ulcers in patients with ulcerative colitis. Gastrointest Radiol 4:103–112, 1980.

95. Buckell NA, Williams GT, Bartram CI, et al: Depth of ulceration in acute colitis. Gastroenterology 79:19–25, 1980.

96. Kelly JK, Gabos S: The pathogenesis of inflammatory polyps. Dis Colon Rectum 30:251–254, 1987.

97. Bozna JP, Fisher RL, Barwick KW: Filiform polyposis: an unusual complication of inflammatory bowel disease. J Clin Gastroenterol 7:451–458, 1985.

98. Zegel H, Laufer I: Filiform polyposis. Radiology 127:615–619, 1978.

99. Bray JF: Filiform polyposis of the small bowel in Crohn's disease. Gastrointest Radiol 8:155–156, 1983.

100. Gardiner GA: "Backwash ileitis" with pseudopolyposis. AJR 129:506–507, 1977.

101. Kirks DR, Currarino G, Berk RN: Localized giant pseudopolyposis of the colon. Am J Gastroenterol 69:609–614, 1978.

102. Kelly JK, Langeuin JM, Price KM: Giant and symptomatic inflammatory polyps of the colon and idiopathic inflammatory bowel disease. Am J Surg Pathol 10:420–428, 1986.

103. Hammerman AM, Shatz BA, Susman N: Radiographic characteristics of colonic "mucosal bridges": sequelae of inflammatory bowel disease. Radiology 127:611–614, 1978.

104. Bartram CI: Complications of ulcerative colitis. *In* Bartram CI (ed): Radiology in Inflammatory Bowel Disease. New York: Marcel Dekker, 1983, pp 63–118.

105. Bartram CI: Complications of Crohn's disease. *In* Bartram CI (ed): Radiology in Inflammatory Bowel Disease. New York: Marcel Dekker, 1983, pp 169–202.

106. Gore RM: Colonic contour changes in chronic ulcerative colitis: reappraisal of some old concepts. AJR 158:59–61, 1992.

107. Poppel MH, Beranbaum SL: The indenture sign in acute exudative colitis. Am J Dig Dis 1:382–388, 1957.

108. Campbell WL: Cathartic colon: reversibility of roentgen changes. Dis Colon Rectum 23:445–449, 1983.
109. Smith B: Pathologic changes in the colon produced by anthaquinone purgatives. Dis Colon Rectum 16:455–458, 1973.
110. Urso FP, Urso MJ, Lee CH: The cathartic colon: pathological findings and radiological/pathological correlation. Radiology 116:557–559, 1975.
111. Kim SK, Gerle RD, Rozanski R: Cathartic colitis. AJR 131:1079–1081, 1978.
112. Kattan KR, King AY: Presacral space revisited. AJR 132:437–439, 1979.
113. Krestin GP, Beyer D, Steinbrich W: Computed tomography in the differential diagnosis of the enlarged retrorectal space. Gastrointest Radiol 11:364–369, 1986.
114. Edling NPG, Eklof O: The retrorectal soft tissue space in ulcerative colitis. Radiology 80:949–953, 1963.
115. Eklof O, Gierup J: The retrorectal soft tissue space in children: normal variations and appearance in granulomatous colitis. AJR 108:624–627, 1970.
116. Guillaumin E, Jeffrey RB, Shea WJ, et al: Perirectal inflammatory disease: CT findings. Radiology 161:153–157, 1986.
117. Goldberg HI, Gore RM, Margulis AR, et al: Computed tomography in the evaluation of Crohn's disease. AJR 140:277–282, 1983.
118. Fishman EK, Jones B: Evaluation of Crohn's disease. *In* Fishman EK, Jones B (eds): Computed Tomography of the Gastrointestinal Tract. New York: Churchill Livingstone, 1988, pp 85–107.
119. Balthazar EJ: Colon. *In* Megibow AJ, Balthazar EJ (eds): Computed Tomography of the Gastrointestinal Tract. St. Louis: CV Mosby, 1986, pp 279–386.
120. Gore RM, Goldberg HI: Computed tomographic evaluation of the gastrointestinal tract in disease other than primary adenocarcinomas. Radiol Clin North Am 20:781–796, 1982.
121. Limberg B: Sonographic features of colonic Crohn's disease: comparison of in vivo and in vitro studies. J Clin Ultrasound 18:161–166, 1990.
122. Limberg B: Diagnosis of acute ulcerative colitis and colonic Crohn's disease by colonic sonography. J Clin Ultrasound 17:25–31, 1989.
123. Goulston SJM, McGovern VJ: The nature of benign strictures in ulcerative colitis. N Engl J Med 281:290–295, 1969.
124. Kolodny M: Reversible right colonic strictures in chronic ulcerative colitis. Radiology 97:83–84, 1970.
125. Dombal FT, Watts JM, Watkinson G, et al: Local complications of ulcerative colitis: stricture, pseudopolyposis, and carcinoma of the colon and rectum. Br Med J 1:1442–1447, 1966.
126. Mark MD, Foley MT, Banks PA: Multiple strictures in Crohn's disease of the small bowel: a benign variant. Am J Gastroenterol 84:1047–1050, 1989.
127. Marshak RH, Boch C, Wolf BS: The roentgen findings in strictures of the colon associated with ulcerative and granulomatous colitis. AJR 90:709–716, 1963.
128. Lashner BA: Cancer in inflammatory bowel disease. Curr Opin Gastroenterol 7:622–627, 1991.
129. Bröstrom O, Löfberg R, Nordenvall B, et al: The risk of colorectal cancer in ulcerative colitis. Scand J Gastroenterol 22:1193–1199, 1987.
130. Sachar DB: Cancer in inflammatory bowel disease. Curr Opin Gastroenterol 6:543–546, 1990.
131. Ekbom A, Helmick C, Zack M, et al: Ulcerative colitis and colorectal cancer. N Engl J Med 323:1228–1233, 1990.
132. Lightdale CJ, Sherlock P: Neoplasia and gastrointestinal malignancy in inflammatory bowel disease. *In* Kirsner JB, Shorter RG (eds): Inflammatory Bowel Disease (3rd ed). Philadelphia: Lea & Febiger, 1988, pp 281–298.
133. Nugent FW, Haggitt RC, Gilpin PA: Cancer surveillance in ulcerative colitis. Gastroenterology 100:1241–1248, 1991.
134. Gyde S: Screening for colorectal cancer in ulcerative colitis: dubious benefits and high costs. Gut 31:1089–1092, 1990.
135. Lashner BA: Recommendations for colorectal cancer screening in ulcerative colitis: a review of research from a single university-based surveillance program. Am J Gastroenterol 87:168–175, 1992.
136. Löfberg R, Bröstrom O, Karlen P, et al: Colonoscopic surveillance in long-standing total ulcerative colitis: a 15 year follow-up study. Gastroenterology 99:1021–1031, 1990.
137. Lennard-Jones JE, Melville DM, Morson BC, et al: Precancer and cancer in extensive ulcerative colitis; findings among 401 patients over 22 years. Gut 31:800–806, 1991.
138. Löfberg R, Bröstrom O, Karlen P, et al: DNA aneuploidy in ulcerative colitis: reproducibility, topographic distribution, and relation to dysplasia. Gastroenterology 102:1149–1154, 1992.
139. Hooyman JR, MacCarthy RL, Carpenter RL: Radiographic appearance of mucosal dysplasia associated with ulcerative colitis. AJR 149:47–51, 1987.
140. Stevenson GW, Goodacre R, Jackson R, et al: Dysplasia to carcinoma transformation in ulcerative colitis. AJR 143:108–110, 1984.
141. Feczko PJ: Malignancy complicating inflammatory bowel disease. Radiol Clin North Am 25:157–174, 1987.
142. Grant CS, Dozois RR: Toxic megacolon: ultimate fate of patients after successful medical management. Am J Surg 147:106–109, 1984.
143. Truelove SC, Marks CG: Toxic megacolon. Part I. Pathogenesis, diagnosis and treatment. Clin Gastroenterol 10:107–114, 1981.
144. Greenstein AJ, Aufses AH: Differences in pathogenesis, incidence and outcome of perforation in inflammatory bowel disease. Surg Gynecol Obstet 160:63–69, 1985.
145. Huizenga KA, Schroeder KW: Gastrointestinal complications of ulcerative colitis and Crohn's disease. *In* Kirsner JB, Shorter RG (eds): Inflammatory Bowel Disease (3rd ed). Philadelphia: Lea & Febiger, 1988, pp 257–280.
146. Strauss RJ, Flint GW, Platt N, et al: The surgical management of toxic dilatation of the colon. Ann Surg 184:682–688, 1976.
147. Wrable LD, Brownstein MW: Toxic dilatation of the colon following barium enema examination during the quiescent stage of ulcerative colitis. Am J Dig Dis 13:918–922, 1968.
148. Caprilli R, Vernia P, Colaneri O, et al: Risk factors in toxic megacolon. Dig Dis Sci 25:817–822, 1980.
149. Goldberg HI: The barium enema and toxic megacolon: cause-effect relationship? Gastroenterology 68:617–618, 1975.
150. Fazio VW: Toxic megacolon in ulcerative colitis and Crohn's disease. Clin Gastroenterol 9:389–407, 1980.
151. Halpert RD: Toxic dilatation of the colon. Radiol Clin North Am 25:147–155, 1987.
152. Kramer P, Wittenberg J: Colonic gas distribution in toxic megacolon. Gastroenterology 80:433–437, 1981.
153. Baker SR: The Abdominal Plain Film. East Norwalk, CT: Appleton & Lange, 1990, pp 155–242.
154. Podolsky DK: Inflammatory bowel disease. Part 2. N Engl J Med 325:1008–1016, 1991.
155. Danzi JT: Extraintestinal manifestations of idiopathic inflammatory bowel disease. Arch Intern Med 148:297–302, 1988.
156. Mayer L, Janowitz H: Extraintestinal complications of inflammatory bowel disease. *In* Kirsner JB, Shorter RG (eds): Inflammatory Bowel Disease (3rd ed). Philadelphia: Lea & Febiger, 1988, pp 299–318.
157. Smith JN, Winship DH: Complications and extraintestinal problems in inflammatory bowel disease. Med Clin North Am 64:1611–1631, 1980.
158. Kirsner JB: The local and systemic complications of inflammatory bowel disease. JAMA 242:1177–1183, 1979.
159. Monsen U, Sorstad J, Heller G, et al: Extracolonic diagnoses in ulcerative colitis: an epidemiological study. Am J Gastroenterol 85:711–716, 1990.
160. Schrumpf E, Fausa O, Elgjo K, et al: Hepatobiliary complications of inflammatory bowel disease. Semin Liver Dis 8:201–209, 1988.
161. Williams SM, Harned RK: Hepatobiliary complications of inflammatory bowel disease. Radiol Clin North Am 25:175–188, 1987.
162. Wewer V, Gluud C, Schlichting P, et al: Prevalence of hepatobiliary dysfunction in a regional group of patients with inflammatory bowel disease. Scand J Gastroenterol 26:97–102, 1991.
163. Wee A, Ludwig J: Pericholangitis in chronic ulcerative colitis: primary sclerosing cholangitis of the small bile ducts? Ann Intern Med 102:581–587, 1985.
164. Thorpe MEC, Scheuer PJ, Sherlock S: Primary sclerosing cholangitis, the biliary tree and ulcerative colitis. Gut 8:435–448, 1967.
165. Fleming KA: The hepatobiliary pathology of primary sclerosing cholangitis. Eur J Gastroenterol Hepatol 4:261–265, 1992.

166. Cangemi JR, Wiesner RH, Beaver SJ, et al: Lack of effect of proctocolectomy on the natural history of primary sclerosing cholangitis. Gastroenterology 96:790–794, 1989.
167. Olsson R, Danielsson A, Jarnerot G, et al: Prevalence of primary sclerosing cholangitis in patients with ulcerative colitis. Gastroenterology 100:1319–1323, 1991.
168. Das KM, Vecchi M, Sakamaki S: A shared and unique epitope(s) in human colon: skin and biliary epithelium detected by a monoclonal antibody. Gastroenterology 98:464–469, 1990.
169. Olsson R, Danielsson A, Jarnerot G, et al: Prevalence of primary sclerosing cholangitis in patients with ulcerative colitis. Gastroenterology 100:1319–1323, 1991.
170. Crippin JS, Lindor KD: Primary sclerosing cholangitis: etiology and immunity. Eur J Gastroenterol Hepatol 4:261–265, 1992.
171. Lindor KD, Wiesner RH, MacCarty RL, et al: Advances in primary sclerosing cholangitis. Am J Med 89:73–80, 1990.
172. Fukushima T, Ishiguro N, Matsude Y, et al: Clinical and urinary characteristics of urolithiasis in ulcerative colitis. Am J Gastroenterol 77:238–242, 1982.
173. Banner MP: Genitourinary complications of inflammatory bowel disease. Radiol Clin North Am 25:199–204, 1987.
174. Gravallese EM, Kantrowitz FG: Arthritic manifestations of inflammatory bowel disease. Am J Gastroenterol 83:703–709, 1988.
175. Björkengren AG, Resnick D, Sartoris DJ: Enteropathic arthropathies. Radiol Clin North Am 25:189–198, 1987.
176. Schorr-Lesnick B, Brandt LJ: Selected rheumatologic and dermatologic manifestations of inflammatory bowel disease. Am J Gastroenterol 83:216–223, 1988.
177. DeVos M: Articular diseases and the gut: evidence for a strong relationship between spondyloarthropathy and inflammation of the gut in man. Acta Clin Belg 45:20–24, 1990.
178. Gravallese EM, Kantrowitz FG: Arthritic manifestations of inflammatory bowel disease. Am J Gastroenterol 83:703–709, 1988.
179. Arlat IP, Maier W, Leupold D, et al: Massive periosteal new bone formation in ulcerative colitis. Radiology 144:507–508, 1982.
180. Vakil N, Sparberg M: Steroid-related osteonecrosis in inflammatory bowel disease. Gastroenterology 96:62–67, 1989.
181. Novotny DA, Rubin RJ, Slezak FA, et al: Arterial thromboembolic complications of inflammatory bowel disease. Dis Colon Rectum 35:193–196, 1992.
182. Johns DR: Cerebrovascular complications of inflammatory bowel disease. Am J Gastroenterol 86:367–370, 1991.
183. Mir-Madjlessi SH, Taylor JS, Farmer RG: Clinical course and evolution of erythema nodosum and pyoderma gangrenosum in chronic ulcerative colitis: a study of 42 patients. Am J Gastroenterol 80:615–620, 1985.
184. Thornton JR, Teague RH, Low-Beer TS, et al: Pyoderma gangrenosum and ulcerative colitis. Gut 21:247–248, 1980.
185. Hanauer SB, Kirsner JB: Medical therapy in ulcerative colitis. *In* Kirsner JB, Shorter RG (eds). Inflammatory Bowel Disease (3rd ed). Philadelphia: Lea & Febiger, 1988, pp 431–476.
186. Pena S: Medical treatment of inflammatory bowel disease. Curr Opin Gastroenterol 5:487–494, 1989.
187. Campieri M, Brignola C, Miglioli M, et al: Medical management of inflammatory bowel disease. Curr Opin Gastroenterol 7:607–616, 1991.
188. Markowitz JM, Grancher K, Mandel F, et al: Immunosuppressive therapy in pediatric inflammatory bowel disease. Am J Gastroenterol 88:44–48, 1993.
189. Ginsberg AI, Davis ND, Nochomovitz LE: Placebo-controlled trial of ulcerative colitis with oral 4-aminosalicylic acid. Gastroenterology 102:448–452, 1992.
190. Steinhart AH, Baker JP, Brzezinski A, et al: Azathioprine therapy in chronic ulcerative colitis. J Clin Gastroenterol 12:271–275, 1990.
191. Korelitz BI: Where do we stand on drug treatment for ulcerative colitis? Ann Intern Med 116:692–694, 1992.
192. Stenson WF, Cort D, Rodgers J, et al: Dietary supplementation with fish oil in ulcerative colitis. Ann Intern Med 116:609–614, 1992.
193. Present DH, Meltzer SJ, Krumholz MP, et al: 6-Mercaptopurine in the management of inflammatory bowel disease: short- and long-term toxicity. Ann Intern Med 111:641–649, 1991.
194. Present DH: Sulfasalazine and antibiotics. *In* Korelitz BI, Sohn N (eds): Inflammatory Bowel Disease: Experience and Controversy. Orlando, FL: Grune & Stratton, 1985, pp 125–132.
195. Present DH: 6-Mercaptopurine and other immunosuppresive agents in the treatment of Crohn's disease and ulcerative colitis. Gastroenterol Clin North Am 18:57–72, 1989.
196. Becker JM, Moody FG: Ulcerative colitis. *In* Sabiston D Jr (ed): Textbook of Surgery (14th ed). Philadelphia: WB Saunders, 1991, pp 927–940.
197. Milsom JW: Surgery of cancer and inflammatory bowel disease. Curr Opin Gastroenterol 7:30–35, 1991.
198. Rombeau JL: Operative and perioperative treatment of patients with inflammatory bowel disease. Curr Opin Gastroenterol 7:635–641, 1991.
199. Sedgwick DM, Barton JR, Hamer-Hodges DW, et al: Population-based study of surgery in juvenile onset ulcerative colitis. Br J Surg 78:176–178, 1991.
200. Cohen Z: Surgery in inflammatory bowel disease: Curr Opin Gastroenterol 5:514–519, 1989.
201. Nivatvongs S: Ulcerative colitis. *In* Gordon PH, Nivatvongs S (eds): Principles and Practice of Surgery for the Colon, Rectum and Anus. St. Louis: Quality Medical Publishing, 1992, pp 667–718.
202. Milsom JW: Surgery of colorectal cancer and inflammatory bowel disease. Curr Opin Gastroenterol 9:42–48, 1993.
203. Phillips SF: Conventional and alternative ileostomies. *In* Sleisenger MH, Fordtran JS: Gastrointestinal Disease: Pathophysiology, Diagnosis, Management (4th ed). Philadelphia: WB Saunders, 1989, pp 1477–1480.
204. Kohler LW, Pemberton JH, Zinsmeister AR, et al: Quality of life after proctocolectomy. Gastroenterology 101:679–684, 1991.
205. Smith LE: Surgical therapy in ulcerative colitis. Gastroenterology 6:547–555, 1990.
206. Wexner SD, Wong WD, Rothenberger DA, et al: The ileoanal reservoir. Am J Surg 159:178–185, 1990.
207. Santos MC, Thompson JS: Late complications of the ileal pouch–anal anastomosis. Am J Gastroenterol 88:3–10, 1993.
208. McLeod RS, Churchill DN, Lock AM, et al: Quality of life of patients with ulcerative colitis preoperatively and postoperatively. Gastroenterology 101:1307–1313, 1991.
209. Keighley MRB, Kmiot W: Surgical options in ulcerative colitis: role of ileoanal anastomosis. Aust N Z J Surg 60:835–848, 1990.
210. Galandiuk S, Scott NA, Dozois RR, et al: Ileal pouch–anal anastomosis: reoperation for pouch related complications. Ann Surg 212:445–446, 1990.
211. Brown JJ, Balfe DM, Heiken JP, et al: Ileal J pouch: radiologic evaluation in patients with and without postoperative complications. Radiology 174:115–120, 1990.
212. Kremers PW, Scholz FJ, Schoetz DJ, et al: Radiology of the ileoanal reservoir. AJR 145:559–567, 1985.
213. Love JR, Irvine EJ, Fedorak RN: Quality of life in inflammatory bowel disease. J Clin Gastroenterol 14:15–19, 1992.
214. Drossman DA, Leserman J, Mitchell CM, et al: Health status and health care use in persons with inflammatory bowel disease. Dig Dis Sci 36:1746–1755, 1991.
215. Yousem DM, Fishman EK, Jones B: Crohn disease: perirectal and perianal findings at CT. Radiology 167:331–334, 1988.
216. Koelbel G, Schmiedl U, Majer MC, et al: Diagnosis of fistulae and sinus tracts in patients with Crohn disease: value of MR imaging. AJR 152:999–1003, 1989.
217. Langerman JM, Rowland R: The number and distribution of lymphoid follicles in the human large intestine. J Anat 194:189–194, 1986.
218. Kelvin FM, May RJ, Norton GA: Lymphoid follicular pattern of the colon in adults. AJR 133:831–835, 1979.
219. Colorian J, Calzada R, Jaszewski R: Nodular lymphoid hyperplasia of the colon in adults: is it common? Gastrointest Endosc 36:421–422, 1990.
220. Laufer I, Desa D: Lymphoid follicular pattern: a normal feature of the pediatric colon. AJR 130:51–55, 1978.
221. Kenney PJ, Koehler RE, Shackelford GD: The clinical significance of large lymphoid follicles of the colon. Radiology 142:41–46, 1982.

222. Bronen RA, Glick SN, Teplick SH: Diffuse lymphoid follicles of the colon. Radiology 142:41–46, 1982.

223. Laufer I, Costopoulous L: Early lesions of Crohn's disease. AJR 130:307–311, 1978.

224. Marshak RH: Granulomatous disease of the intestinal tract (Crohn's disease). Radiology 114:3–22, 1975.

225. Simpkins KC: Aphthoid ulcers in Crohn's colitis. Clin Radiol 28:601–604, 1977.

226. Ekberg O, Lindstrom C: Superficial lesions in Crohn's disease of the small bowel. Gastrointest Radiol 4:389–392, 1979.

227. Degrysa HRM, DeSchepper AMAP: Aphthoid esophageal ulcers in Crohn's disease of ileum and colon. Gastrointest Radiol 9:197–201, 1984.

228. Ni X-Y, Goldberg HI: Aphthoid ulcers in Crohn's disease: radiographic course and relationship to bowel appearance. Radiology 158:589–592, 1986.

229. Carlson HC: Radiology of inflammatory bowel disease. *In* Kirsner JB, Shorter RG (eds): Inflammatory Bowel Disease (3rd ed). Philadelphia: Lea & Febiger, 1988, pp 377–428.

230. Kelly JK, Sutherland LR. The chronological sequence in the pathology of Crohn's disease. J Clin Gastroenterol 10:28–33, 1988.

231. Welin S, Welin G: Experience with the Welin modification. *In* Welin S (ed): The Double Contrast Examination of the Colon. Stuttgart: Georg Thieme Verlag, 1976, pp 65–111.

232. Williams WS: Histology of Crohn's syndrome. Gut 5:510–516, 1964.

233. Price AB: Overlap in the spectrum of non-specific inflammatory bowel disease—"colitis indeterminate." J Clin Pathol 31:567–577, 1978.

234. Kirsner JB: Problems in the differentiation of ulcerative colitis and Crohn's disease of the colon: the need for repeated diagnostic evaluation. Gastroenterology 68:187–191, 1975.

235. Margulis AR, Goldberg HI, Lawson TI, et al: The overlapping spectrum of ulcerative and granulomatous colitis: a roentgenographic-pathologic study. AJR 113:325–334, 1970.

236. Kent TH, Ammon RK, Den Besten L: Differentiation of ulcerative colitis and regional enteritis of colon. Arch Pathol Lab Med 89:20–29, 1970.

237. Lennard-Jones JE, Lockhart-Mummery HE, Morson BC: Clinical and pathological differentiation of Crohn's disease and proctocolitis. Gastroenterology 54:1162–1170, 1986.

238. Lewin KJ, Riddel RH, Weinstein WM: Gastrointestinal Pathology and Its Clinical Implications. New York: Igaku-Shoin, 1992, pp 834–927.

239. Stanley P, Fry IK, Dawson AM, et al: Radiological signs of ulcerative colitis and Crohn's disease of the colon. Clin Radiol 22:434–442, 1971.

240. Laufer I, Hamilton J: The radiological differentiation between ulcerative and granulomatous colitis by double contrast radiology. Am J Gastroenterol 66:259–269, 1976.

241. Nugent FW, Kolack PF: Differential diagnosis of chronic ulcerative colitis and Crohn's disease of the colon. *In* Kirsner JB, Shorter RG (eds): Inflammatory Bowel Disease (3rd ed). Philadelphia: Lea & Febiger, 1988, pp 185–208.

# Other Inflammatory Conditions

Seth N. Glick, M.D.

## INTRODUCTION

In daily practice, idiopathic inflammatory bowel disease accounts for the majority of cases of colonic inflammation encountered by the radiologist. However, a number of other causes of colonic inflammation occur with variable frequency. Some, such as ischemic colitis, radiation colitis, and *Clostridium difficile* colitis, are relatively common, whereas the others are either rare or seldom require imaging studies in their management. In many instances, the information derived from the imaging studies in conjunction with the patient's history, symptoms, and laboratory and pathologic findings may result in a specific diagnosis or produce a limited differential diagnosis. It is not uncommon that the appropriate diagnostic studies are repeated or ordered on the basis of the weighted considerations of the radiologist. Even when the diagnosis is established, radiology may have a role in assessing the severity of the process, monitoring the course of the disease, and determining the presence of complications.

The bowel has a limited response to a wide variety of insults, and the findings are nonspecific. In most inflammatory diseases, the changes observed in each entity may be characterized by the usual distribution in the colon, the magnitude of injury, the sequential changes with or without permanent sequelae, and, to an extent, the nature of the superficial mucosal alterations. Abnormalities in other gastrointestinal viscera or nongastrointestinal sites may be associated. For the purpose of diagnostic approach, it is helpful to classify these entities into those that radiologically resemble ulcerative colitis and those that may be confused with Crohn's colitis.

Some may fall into either category. At times, some may present with an appearance that simulates colonic carcinoma, having a palpable mass and a short, narrowed colonic segment.

Anatomic distribution, particularly the presence or absence of rectal involvement, is an important discriminating feature. When the rectum is spared, the likelihood of ulcerative colitis is extremely low, and the number of diagnostic possibilities under consideration can be reduced. The presence of diffuse or segmental changes may also represent differentiating features. In segmental processes, the specific site, the presence of multiple sites, and the nature of the radiologic appearance may provide clues. Diseases that involve the rectum may be divided into those that are confined to the rectum and those that extend to the colon, either continuously as in ulcerative colitis or in a skip manner as in Crohn's colitis. In the case of isolated proctitis or continuous proctocolitis, specific features such as fistula, asymmetry, and mucosal alterations often assist in determining the type of idiopathic inflammatory bowel disease in the differential diagnosis. On rare occasion, some colitides have unique features that are not consistent with either of these two diseases.

Although at times the radiologic appearance may suggest the presence of a process other than inflammatory bowel disease, it is ancillary clinical information that usually indicates this probability. The patient's age, duration of symptoms, rapidity of onset, and failure to respond to or deterioration after standard therapy for idiopathic inflammatory bowel disease are common features that prompt consideration of diagnostic alternatives. Historical information that may contribute significantly includes drug history (particularly antibiotics or chemotherapeutic agents, hormonal preparations), previous radiation therapy, immunosuppression, and pertinent details relating to travel, diet, and sexual activities. In most instances, the combination of this information along with the radiologic description is sufficient to suggest the diagnosis. Thus, the radiologist should be familiar with these entities, their range of appearances, and their related clinical characteristics.

## BACTERIAL INFECTIONS

Infectious colitis may be secondary to bacterial, viral, fungal, and parasitic organisms.[1-4] In Western countries, bacterial colitis represents the most common form of colonic infection, whereas in underdeveloped countries, parasitic infestation occurs most frequently. Imaging studies are not usually performed for patients with bacterial colitis because the diagnosis is readily achieved with routine stool cultures.

The typical presentation of acute onset of dysenteric symptoms consisting of fever, crampy abdominal pain and tenderness with or without vomiting, tenesmus, and small volume diarrhea (frequently bloody) suggests the diagnosis. Furthermore, in most cases, the process is self-limited, and appropriate therapy is supportive. On occasion, routine cultures may be falsely negative, or specialized cultures are required for the organism in question. In this setting, a contrast study may be performed. Barium studies are most likely to be performed in patients with infectious colitides; chronic infections, although they may be diagnosed by biopsy or serologic studies, not uncommonly require laparotomy for diagnosis. It is difficult to make categoric statements concerning the radiologic appearance of these infections because of the paucity of radiologic descriptions (usually scattered case reports). In many cases, the reports are found in older literature before the availability of precise mucosal detail from air-contrast studies or colonoscopy, and the interpretation of the nature and extent of the morphologic alterations may not necessarily be accurate.

## Salmonellosis

*Salmonella* is a gram-negative rod that is ingested with contaminated food or water.[1-4] Colonic involvement occurs in two settings—during the course of typhoid fever or as an acute dysentery. Typhoid fever is secondary to *Salmonella typhi* or *Salmonella paratyphi*. The patient presents initially with high temperature, arthralgia, malaise, headache, and right lower quadrant pain. The organism initially involves the reticuloendothelial system; there is a predilection for Peyer's patches of the terminal ileum, spleen, and mesenteric lymph nodes. The spleen may enlarge after 1 week. Evidence of gastrointestinal involvement occurs in about half the cases and does not manifest until the second or third week of illness, and it is often obscured by the other symptoms. Pain and tenderness in the right lower quadrant are most common. Colonic involvement on barium

enema examination consists of edema and spasm, which produce narrowing and haustral loss in the cecum in conjunction with ileal fold thickening and ulceration. Aphthous ulcers in the ascending colon have been reported.[5] Whereas the ileum is invariably involved, the incidence of colonic changes is unknown. Hemorrhage and perforation may occur at this stage in about 1 to 3% of cases. The symptoms begin to resolve in the fourth week, but relapses can occur. Blood cultures are positive in 90% during the first week, and the organism may be found in the stool during the second and third weeks. Chloramphenicol is the treatment of choice.

A wide variety of *Salmonella* serotypes (e.g., *enteritidis, typhimurium*) may be responsible for sudden onset diarrhea, fever, abdominal pain, nausea, and vomiting.[1-4] The incubation period is 8 to 48 hours. The disease tends to occur in outbreaks, particularly in the summer when food tends to spoil. Homosexuals also appear to be at greater risk than the general population. *Salmonella* has been cultured during initial presentation and relapse of ulcerative colitis, but its pathogenic role in these cases is unclear. In most cases, the small bowel, particularly the ileum, is involved, but not uncommonly a colitis is present. The rectum and sigmoid colon are almost always inflamed; the endoscopic appearance simulates ulcerative colitis.

The barium enema in most reported examples demonstrates a pancolitis with loss of haustra.[6, 7] Areas of ulceration, usually superficial but occasionally deep (and even "collar button" type), are frequently present (Fig. 63–1). Thumbprinting has also been noted. Extensive small bowel thickening and effacement have been described in association with a pancolitis. A segmental ulcerating colitis in the left colon is rare.[8] Fulminant disease and even toxic megacolon may occur, particularly in elderly and debilitated persons. Bacteremia is common, and spread to the gallbladder, bones, lungs, and kidneys can occur.

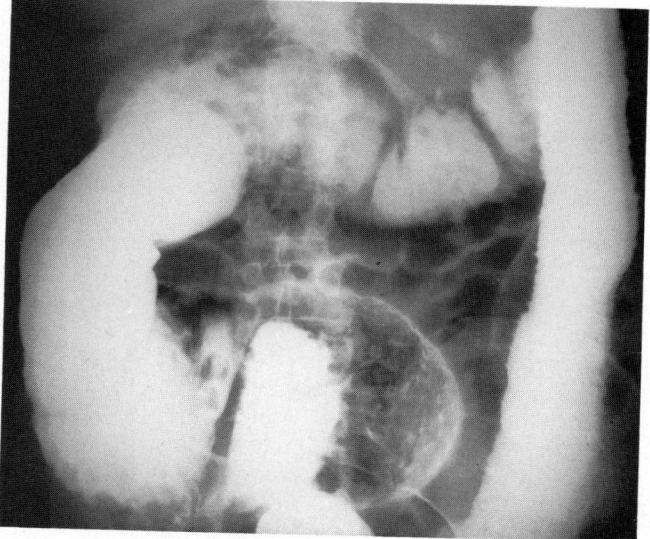

**Figure 63–1. *Salmonella* colitis.** A diffuse colitis with ulcerations is particularly well seen in the descending colon.

Stool cultures, although frequently positive, may need to be repeated to confirm the diagnosis. Serial elevation of febrile agglutinins may help. The disease is self-limited and lasts 1 to 2 weeks. Oral antibiotics are ineffective, and they, as well as antidiarrheal agents, may prolong the illness. In severe cases, parenteral chloramphenicol can be administered.

## Shigellosis

Infection with *Shigella*, a gram-negative rod, may be caused by three species: *S. flexneri*, *S. dysenteriae*, and *S. sonnei*.[1-4] In the United States, *S. sonnei* is the offending organism in 70% of cases, whereas in Mexico and in Asia, *S. dysenteriae* is most common. As with salmonellosis, infection may occur in outbreaks, particularly in warm weather, and there is a greater prevalence in homosexuals than in the general population. The incubation period is 1 to 3 days, and presentation is usually similar to that of *Salmonella* infection. However, a toxin is produced that may cause increased small bowel secretion and watery diarrhea, which lasts a few days and then progresses to dysenteric symptoms. Systemic absorption of the toxin may also produce arthritis, pneumonitis, seizures, peripheral neuropathy, microangiopathy, and hemolytic-uremic syndrome. Bacteremia is rare but can cause vascular collapse. Stool cultures are positive within 1 day of onset and may remain so for months. The possibility of toxic megacolon has been reported. The clinical course is usually self-limited and lasts 7 to 10 days, but it can last as long as a month.

The mortality is 10 to 20% in immunocompromised patients or if there is bacteremia. Treatment is with ampicillin; antispasmodics are contraindicated because they may aggravate the patient's condition.

Sigmoidoscopy almost always shows an inflammatory process simulating ulcerative colitis that may vary from mild granularity and erythema to ulceration.[9, 10] Ulceration is more commonly seen than in salmonellosis. Ulcers are usually superficial and of varying size and shape. They are predominantly stellate but may be linear, serpiginous, or aphthous and are superimposed on a diffusely friable mucosa. A colonoscopic series[10] in patients with *S. dysenteriae* infection demonstrated the ulcerative phase to be most marked in the second and third weeks of the disease, with erythema and edema the most prominent features in the first week. In many cases, the ulcerations are most marked distal to the splenic flexure. Healing then occurs with gradually decreasing erythema. The process is initially continuous, and all cases involved the full extent of the colon. During recovery, involvement may become patchy. Whereas healing is complete in most cases, residual strictures, inflammatory polyps, and even persistent colitis may occur.

Barium enema findings in most reports have demonstrated a predominantly left-sided colitis with deep ulcers that may have a collar button appearance[7] (Fig. 63-2A, and B). Edema of the sigmoid colon has been reported in one case. Aphthous ulcers may also be seen (Fig. 63-3). Another patient with *S. flexneri* infection and discrete flat ulcers in the sigmoid colon and inflammatory polyps in the transverse colon and descending

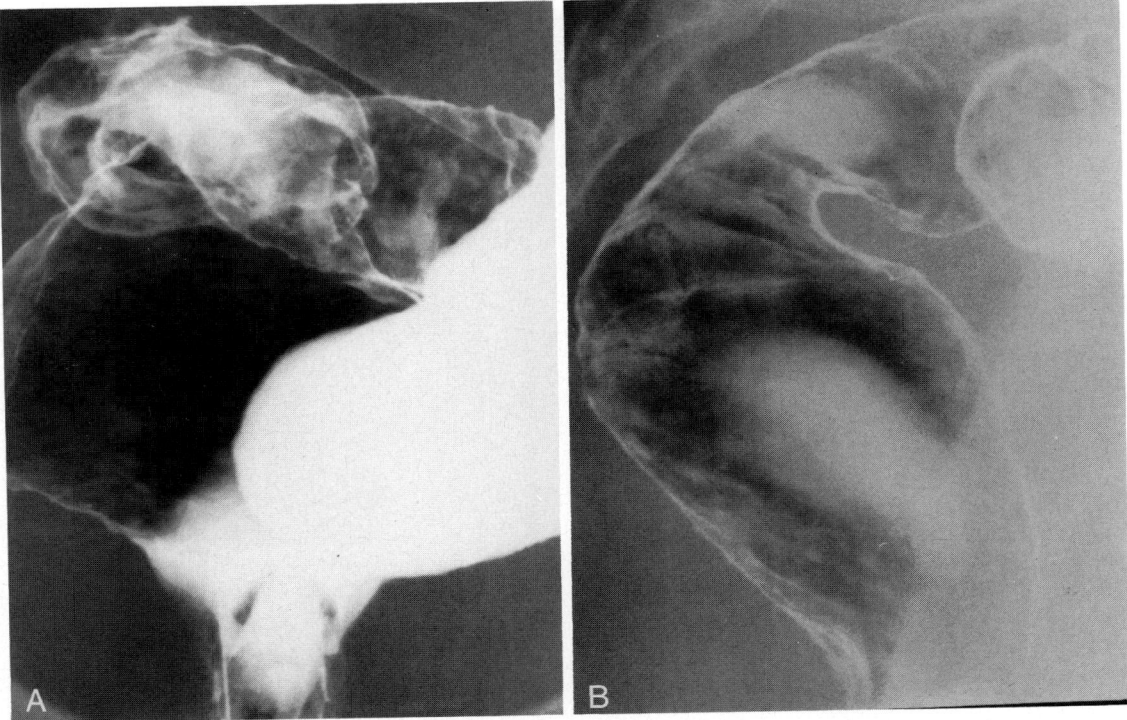

**Figure 63–2. *Shigella* proctocolitis. A.** The frontal view shows granularity of the rectum with deeper ulcers along the superior aspect of the sigmoid colon. **B.** The lateral view shows the granularity of the rectal mucosa with superficial ulceration.

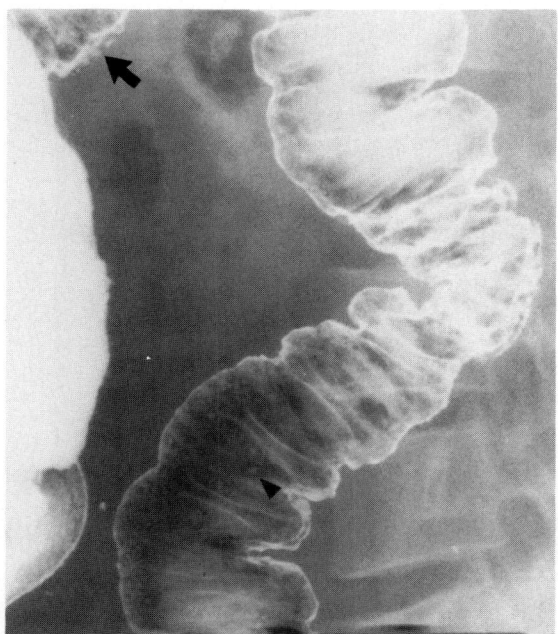

**Figure 63–3. Shigellosis.** An oblique view shows aphthous ulcers in the descending colon *(arrowhead)*. In the transverse colon, deeper, collar button ulcers are seen *(arrow)*.

colon has been described.[11] In this patient, stenosis and inflammatory polyps were present in the sigmoid colon 9 months later. The rectum was normal on the initial barium enema, but this was performed 3 weeks into the disease.

## Campylobacteriosis

*Campylobacter* is the most common of all bacterial pathogens producing colitis; it has been isolated in 7 to 10% of stool cultures performed for diarrhea.[1-4] The offending agent is *C. fetus* subspecies *jejuni*. The disease is usually self-limited within 7 days, but symptoms may persist as long as a month. Recurrence may occur in as many as 25% of patients if the infection is untreated. Approximately half of the patients have a 24-hour prodrome of headache, nausea and vomiting, and arthralgia that progresses to watery and then bloody diarrhea. Both the small and large bowel may be involved, although colitis is most common. Radiologic findings have consisted of some cases demonstrating pancolitis with diffuse granularity and haustral loss simulating ulcerative colitis; others have described scattered aphthous ulcers resembling Crohn's disease.[12-15] The left colon is consistently involved. Hemorrhage, perforation, and toxic megacolon have all been reported as complications. Diagnosis requires culture on selective media, and serologic study may also be helpful for confirmation.

## *Yersinia* Enterocolitis

Infection by this gram-negative rod tends to be more common in certain regions such as Japan, Canada, and Scandinavia.[1-4, 16-19] Specific strains may be endemic to each of these locations, and there may be variations in the clinical and pathologic manifestations. In patients younger than 5 years of age, the predominant symptoms are those of acute right lower quadrant pain and fever simulating appendicitis. In adults, the presentation may be acute or more protracted with fever, pain, and diarrhea evolving during 4 to 6 weeks. Arthralgia or arthritis and rashes such as erythema nodosum or erythema multiforme may be associated.

On barium examination, the terminal ileum is invariably involved; the appearance depends on the stage of the disease.[16] This may consist of scattered small nodules from lymphoid enlargement, discrete punctate aphthous or larger oval ulcers, or a combination of these. The lymphoid nodules predominate in the early and late stages. Folds may also be thickened, but unlike the situation in regional enteritis, stenosis is not a feature. Colonic changes are manifested by aphthous ulcers that are predominantly located in the right colon, but left-sided colonic involvement is occasionally noted[19-21] (Fig. 63–4). Evolution and resolution of the clinical and radiologic features may require several months. Perforation is rare, but hepatic abscess and septicemia are well-documented complications. Diagnosis requires special culture media or serologic studies. However, there is no proven effective treatment, and diagnosis is primarily for the purpose of excluding other entities.

## Colitis Attributable to *Escherichia coli* O157:H7

*E. coli* strains are the most common cause of traveler's diarrhea and are usually self-limited. However, the subtype O157:H7 has drawn increased recognition because it causes high morbidity and mortality. Outbreaks of this infection have been noted in Canada, and residents of nursing homes have been particularly susceptible. The symptoms begin as watery diarrhea without fever and progress over days to a hemorrhagic colitis. The most serious complication is the high association with the hemolytic-uremic syndrome as a result of the toxin. The overall mortality may be as high as 33%. The radiographic findings are similar to those of ischemia with thumbprinting, narrowing, and spasm (Fig. 63–5). Low-density thickening of the wall attributable to edema has been identified on computed tomographic (CT) scans. The transverse colon has been involved in most reported cases with extension to the right, left, or both sides of the colon.[22-24] The morphologic changes are predominantly due to ischemia, and histologic specimens may resemble pseudomembranous colitis. Treatment is supportive, but recognition is also important for isolation procedures to be instituted.

## Tuberculosis

Although once considered rare in Western countries, tuberculosis has been increasing in incidence. As a

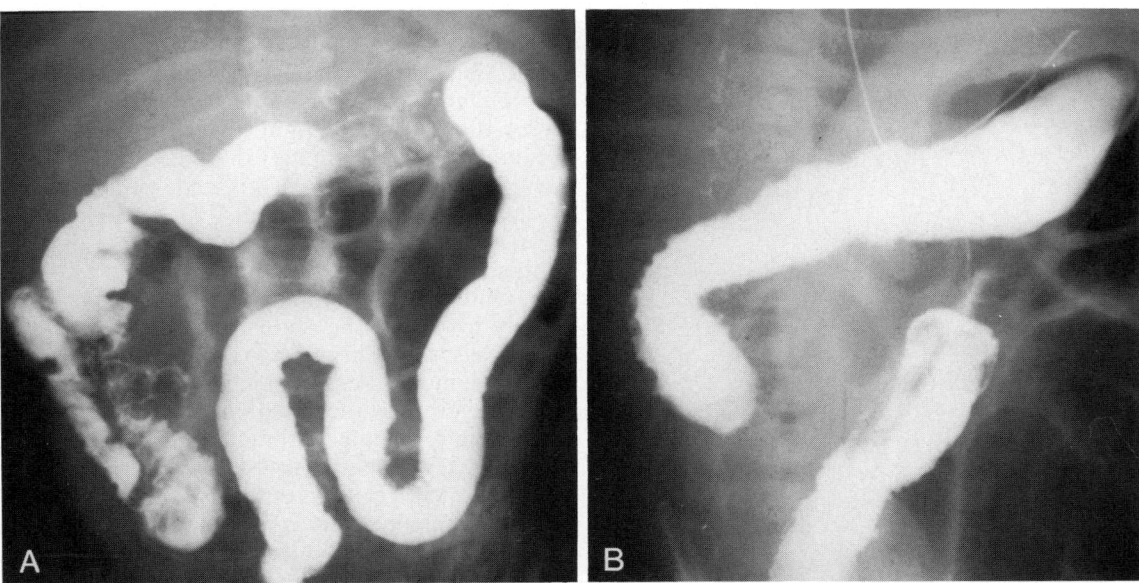

**Figure 63–4.** *Yersinia* **enterocolitis. A.** There is a pancolitis with involvement of the terminal ileum. Note the aphthous ulcers in the distal transverse colon and the thickened folds in the distal ileum. **B.** The entire colon is involved with deep ulcers seen particularly well in the right colon.

result, reports of gastrointestinal tract involvement have became more common. Patients with acquired immunodeficiency syndrome have been noted to be at greater risk than the general population.[25] Most cases are secondary to a pulmonary source, but in the majority there is no evidence of acute or previous pulmonary tuberculosis on chest x-ray examination. In endemic areas of Asia, the cause is usually ingestion of the bovine bacillus. Colonic involvement is most often associated with

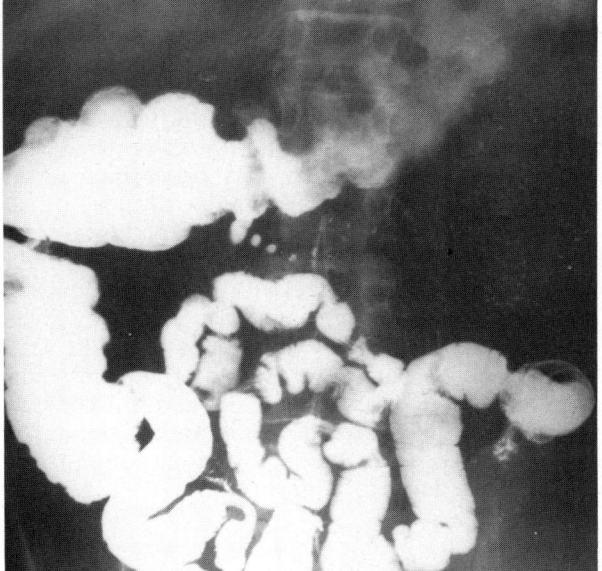

**Figure 63–5. Colitis attributable to** *Escherichia coli* **O157:H7.** This perioral pneumocolon study shows a pancolitis characterized by thumbprinting, best seen in the transverse colon. The changes resemble those seen in ischemic colitis.

ileal disease. Symptoms are usually chronic with combinations of weight loss, fever, pain, palpable mass, and diarrhea. The last appears to be less dominant a feature than in Crohn's disease.

Radiologic changes are usually noted in the ascending and proximal transverse colon and are indistinguishable from those of Crohn's disease[26] (Fig. 63–6A). It has been suggested that certain abnormalities are characteristic, such as oval or circumferential transverse ulcers, loss of anatomic demarcation between the ileum and right colon (Stierlin's sign), and a right-angle intersection between the ileum and cecum with marked hypertrophy of the ileocecal valve (Fleischner's sign) (Fig. 63–6B). These changes represent the exuberant mural thickening, which tends to be greater than in Crohn's disease. Other suggestive features include extremely short segments of involvement of the ileum or cecum (Fig. 63–6C); markedly enlarged lymph nodes, particularly with low density on CT scan; and ascites. However, the most frequent observations consist of some combination of narrowing, deep ulceration, and mucosal granulation producing nodularity and inflammatory polyps. Less common findings include scattered aphthous erosions (Fig. 63–6D), diffuse colitis (Fig. 63–7), segmental colitis distal to the hepatic flexure, and short stricture simulating carcinoma.[26–32] Fistula and sinus tracts are also rare.

Diagnosis can be made with colonoscopic biopsy, which may reveal caseating granulomas or produce positive cultures of acid-fast bacilli.[33] However, the yield from this procedure has been variable. In the absence of confirmatory findings, surgical specimens are necessary. The importance of recognition cannot be overemphasized because steroid therapy in this setting is potentially catastrophic.

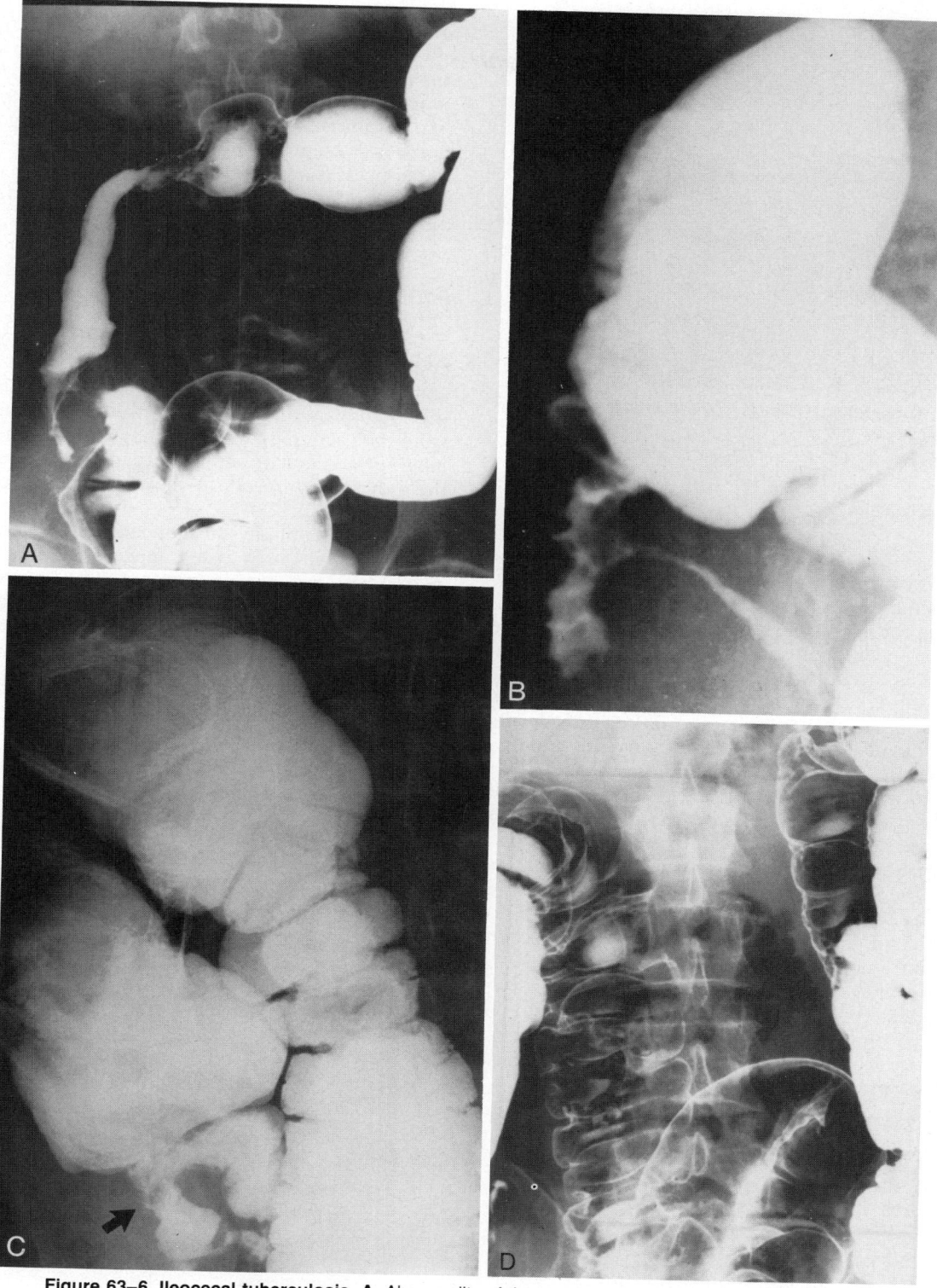

**Figure 63–6. Ileocecal tuberculosis. A.** Abnormality of the terminal ileum and right colon is similar to that seen in Crohn's disease. **B.** Typical abnormality at the ileocecal valve is seen, with narrowing of the terminal ileum and hypertrophy of the ileocecal valve. **C.** Typical lesion of tuberculosis is seen, with short area narrowing in the cecum *(arrow).* **D.** Scattered aphthous ulceration throughout the entire colon is due to tuberculosis. (**D** courtesy of Gary Ghahremani, M.D., Evanston, IL.)

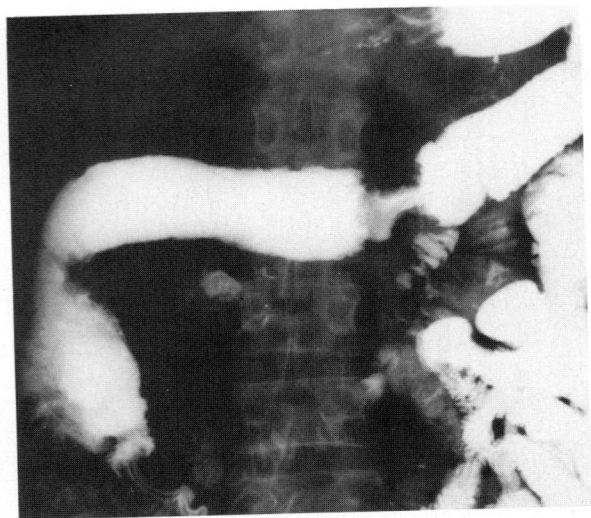

**Figure 63–7. Tuberculosis.** Diffuse colitis proximal to the splenic flexure.

## Actinomycosis

*Actinomyces israelii* is an anaerobic bacterium that may be part of the normal flora of the bowel, but when there is contact with tissues not normally exposed, a pathologic process ensues. Involvement of the bowel occurs after the mesenteric and peritoneal tissues are infected. This occurs after penetrating trauma, after abdominal surgery, or in the presence of a long-standing intrauterine device. Inflammatory masses invade the colon, and fistulas develop. Symptoms include a palpable mass, vague abdominal pain, and diarrhea.

On barium enema examination, extrinsic masses with reactive change or distortion and stricture with or without fistula are noted.[34–36] Fistulas can extend to the skin, where characteristic colonies of sulfur granules may be identified. The ileocecal region is the most common site, often with an antecedent history of appendectomy. The rectosigmoid colon is the usual site in those cases secondary to an intrauterine device. Ultrasound and CT scans may also reveal the large inflammatory mass. Surgery is often necessary for diagnosis and distinction from neoplasm. However, appropriate microbiologic studies are performed on the resected tissue only if the possibility of actinomycosis is considered.

## PARASITIC INFECTIONS

### Anisakiasis

Infestation by larvae of the nematode *Anisakis* within 12 to 24 hours after the ingestion of raw fish can produce a syndrome of abdominal pain, usually severe, occasionally accompanied by fever, nausea and vomiting, or diarrhea.[37–39] The stomach and small intestine are the most common sites, but occasionally the colon may be the dominant location. Eosinophilia is not often present in the serum but is invariably identified on biopsy. The

ascending colon and less commonly the transverse colon are usually involved; the changes are segmental and manifested as marked thumbprinting on barium enema studies. On air-contrast studies, a specific diagnosis is often obtained by demonstration of the larva as a thin linear filling defect 12 to 20 mm long and 0.7 mm wide at the proximal portion of the diseased segment.[39] Serologic studies may also confirm the diagnosis. The worm is present in the stool in less than 25% of cases. The process is self-limited within 7 to 10 days and should not be confused with other entities such as ischemia or carcinoma.

## Amebiasis

Colonic amebiasis is rare in the United States. The cysts are ingested and develop into the invasive trophozoite. Twenty percent of the world population harbors this organism. Infestation by this protozoan may vary from the carrier state to fulminant colitis, and symptoms may be indolent or acute. Spread to the liver and then the lungs may result in abscesses in either of these organs.

Colonic amebiasis is usually an acute ulcerative colitis (95%) that in most cases appears as skip lesions, although the intervening segment may be involved to a much lesser extent[40–42] (Fig. 63–8). At times, the segments appear as short regions of involvement with marked granulation (ameboma).[43] These are seen in 10% of cases and are most often located in the right colon (Fig. 63–9). Diffuse colitis, however, is not unusual (Fig. 63–10A), but the right colon tends to be more

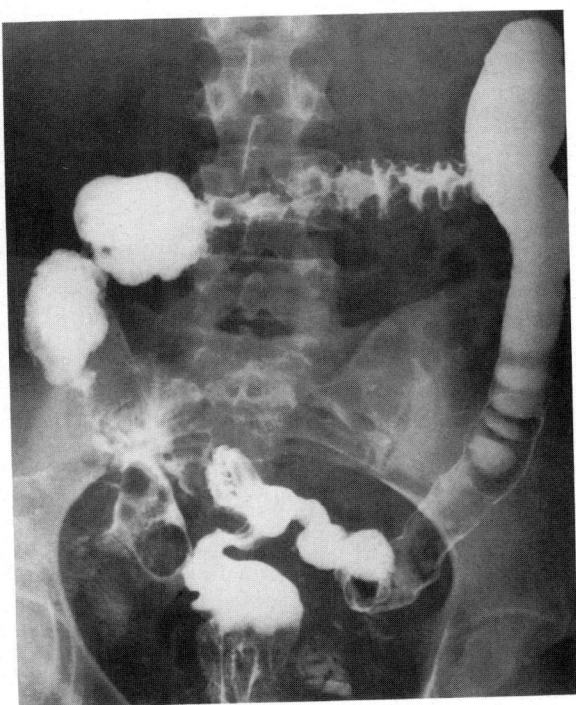

**Figure 63–8. Amebiasis.** There is inflammation of the entire colon with skip areas.

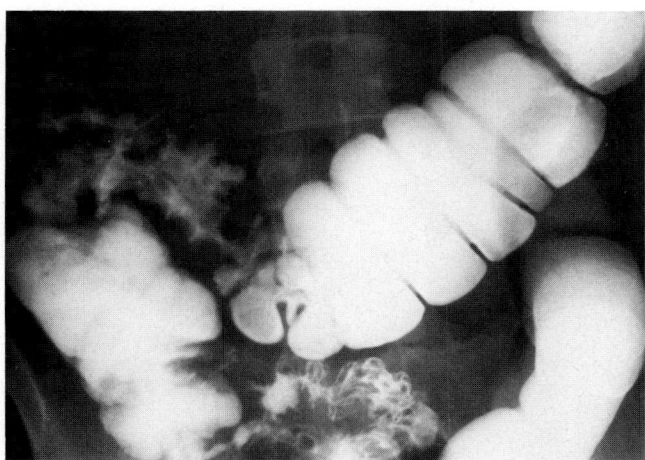

**Figure 63–9. Ameboma.** There is an inflammatory lesion with narrowing of the proximal transverse colon. This type of focal involvement often resembles a tumor and is referred to as an ameboma.

severely involved. Although these changes usually appear as deep ulcers and/or edema, the mucosal surface may contain any combination of aphthous ulcers (Fig. 63–10B), discrete ulcers that may appear as marginal defects, or granularity with barium flecks.[44] The terminal ileum is invariably spared. The coned cecum is suggestive but not specific. Residual deformity and stricture may occur even after appropriate therapy.[45] Less than 1% of patients present with toxic megacolon, and approximately 3% present with typhloappendicitis.

Diagnosis is usually readily apparent by the presence of trophozoites in the stool or on rectal smear. Serologic studies are also quite sensitive. When amebiasis is suspected, a trial of therapy is warranted even after failure to confirm the diagnosis, because steroid therapy may result in severe progression.

## Schistosomiasis

This parasite belongs to the trematode or fluke group of worms, and different strains are endemic to specific geographic areas. *Schistosoma mansoni* is found in the United States, Puerto Rico, and the tropics.[3] *Schistosoma haematobium* is the primary form in Africa and southern Asia, and *Schistosoma japonicum* is usually identified in eastern Asia. Mixed infection with *S. mansoni* and *S. haematobium* is not uncommon, particularly in Egypt. The larva penetrates the skin, where it enters the systemic circulation. It reaches the liver, where it matures into the adult form. Upstream migration occurs through the portal venous system to the colon, where the worms invade the bowel wall and lay eggs. Portal hypertension with secondary hepatosplenomegaly is frequently associated. Whereas total colonic involvement can occur, *S. mansoni* has a predilection for the inferior mesenteric vein and left colon, *S. japonicum* for the superior mesenteric vein and right colon, and *S. haematobium* for the hemorrhoidal veins and rectum and urinary tract. However, exceptions to these tendencies are common. The terminal ileum may also be involved. Bloody diarrhea is the usual presentation, but chronic abdominal pain with intermittent diarrhea and a palpable mass may be seen.

The barium enema examination shows nonspecific colitis involving a variable extent of colon with narrowing, haustral loss, and ulceration.[46] However, a hallmark of this disease is the presence of inflammatory polyps attributable to granulation reaction to the deposition of eggs in the bowel wall[46, 47] (Fig. 63–11A). Colitis may be absent at times, and schistosomiasis (or bilharziasis) may produce a focal polyp of variable size simulating an adenoma[48] (Fig. 63–11B). Another suggestive finding is calcification of the bowel wall or liver, which is most often associated with *S. haematobium* but may also be

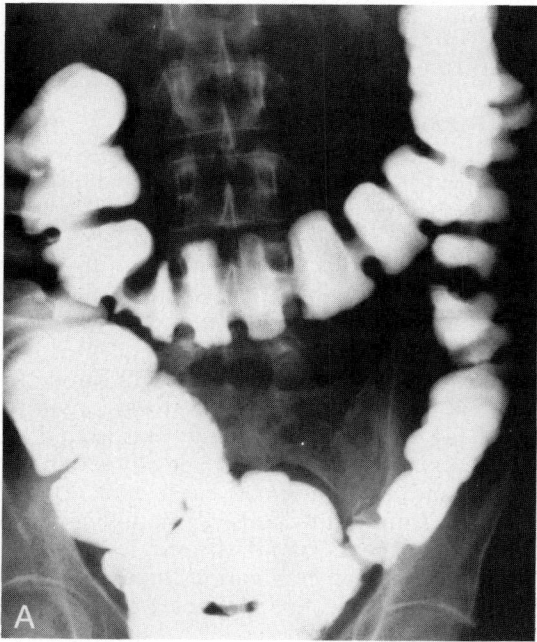

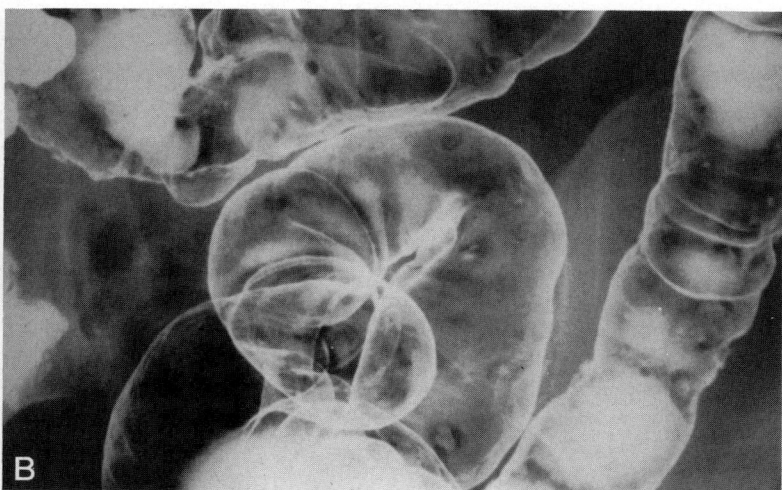

**Figure 63–10. Acute amebiasis. A.** There is diffuse haustral thickening with thumbprinting throughout the colon. **B.** Multiple aphthous ulcers are seen throughout the colon. (**B** courtesy of Harvey Goldstein, M.D., San Antonio, TX.)

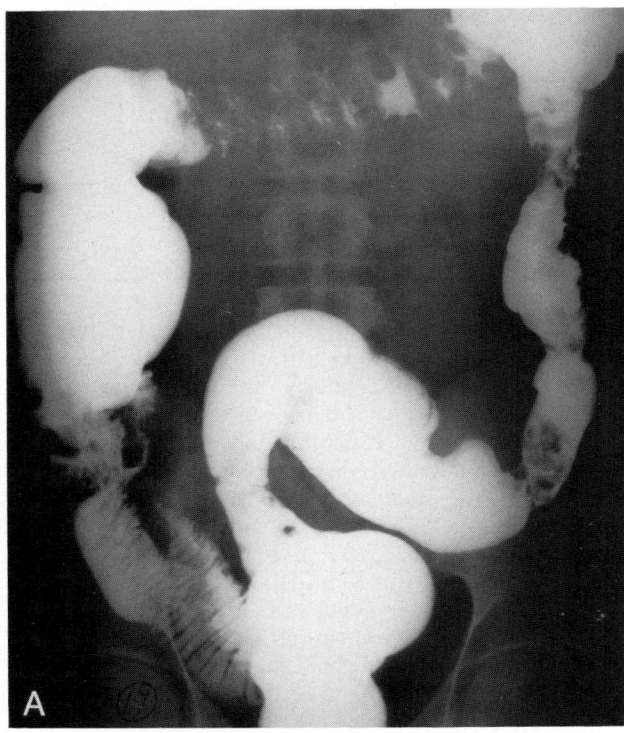

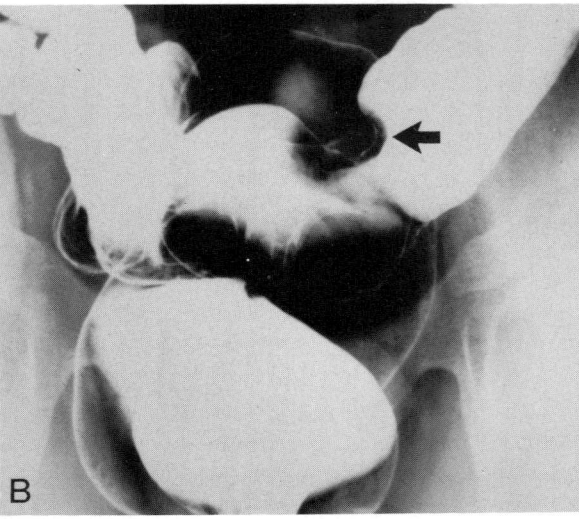

**Figure 63–11. Schistosomiasis. A.** Inflammatory changes are seen throughout the colon, although some polypoid changes are noted in the left colon as well. **B.** A large inflammatory polyp *(arrow)* in a patient with schistosomiasis. (**B** courtesy of Frank Scholz, M.D., Boston, MA.)

seen with *S. japonicum.*[47] CT scanning is particularly sensitive to these changes. Diagnosis can be made by the demonstration of eggs in biopsy specimens or in the stool. Eosinophilia is frequently associated with helminthic infection.

## Strongyloidiasis

The nematode *Strongyloides stercoralis* also gains entrance through the skin. It spreads to the lungs, ruptures into the tracheobronchial tree, and is subsequently ingested. The primary site of involvement is the stomach, duodenum, and proximal small bowel, and a chronic host-parasite relationship is obtained. In most cases, eggs are passed into the stool. However, in circumstances of decreased immunity, the eggs progress to the filariform larval stage and invade the portal system which produces a repeated cycle or autoinfection. The excess parasite load results in a distal accumulation of filariform larvae with subsequent colonic involvement. In view of the setting of severe debilitation, this is often fatal. Radiologic findings are those of a diffuse ulcerative colitis.[49–51] Aphthous ulcers may be identified.[52] Fistulas and sinus tracts may be present. Eosinophilia is the rule, and diagnosis is dependent on the identification of cysts, larvae, or both in the stool.

## Trichuriasis

The whipworm *Trichuris trichiura* predominantly involves children in tropical areas. The worm is minimally invasive but invades the mucosa, with resultant bleeding,

anemia, diarrhea, malaise, and cramps. Intussusception and rectal prolapse are common; the adherent worms serve as the lead point. Eosinophilia is usually present. The barium enema shows clumping and granularity of the barium because of excessive production of mucus.[53, 54] The worms are identified as wavy and then linear lucencies 3 to 5 cm in length, some of which terminate in a ring shape with a central barium collection, simulating an aphthous ulcer or lymph follicles (Fig. 63–12). A pear-shaped cecum, probably caused by edema or spasm, has been described.

## FUNGAL INFECTIONS

### Histoplasmosis

*Histoplasma capsulatum* is a fungus endemic to river basin areas. The lung and skin are the usual sites of involvement, but the gastrointestinal tract may be predominantly involved.[55] This usually occurs in the setting of a chronic debilitating illness in which the intestinal symptoms are overlooked. Anemia and leukopenia may be present. Perforation, obstruction, or hemorrhage may direct attention to the alimentary tract. The ileocecal region is the most common site, but any organ can be involved (Fig. 63–13). Commonly associated are mesenteric adenopathy, hepatosplenomegaly (often with calcifications), and an abnormal chest film. Barium studies may vary from right-sided colonic filling defects to one or more segments of nonspecific inflammation (i.e., narrowing, mucosal granulation, sinus tracts, ulcers) or stricture, diffuse colitis, pericecal mass simulating appendicitis, and rectal polyps.[55–57] Mucosal biopsy

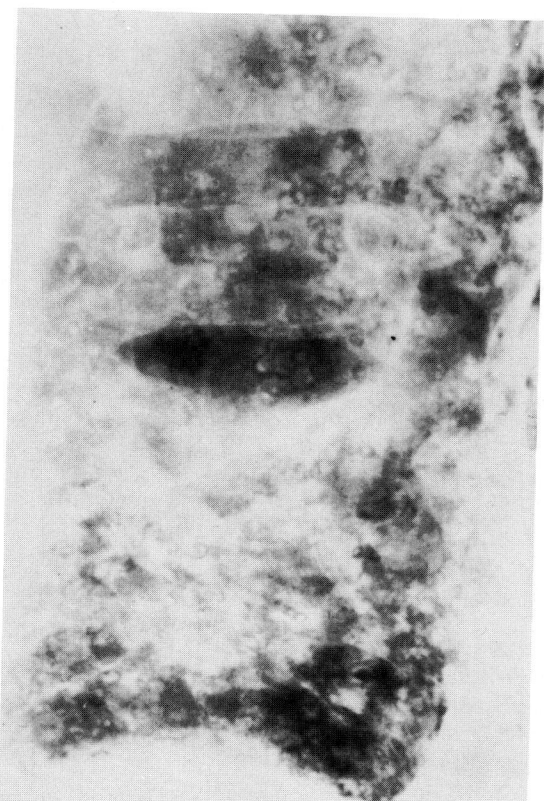

**Figure 63–12. Trichuriasis.** A close-up view of the sigmoid colon shows multiple ring-like lucencies with central barium collection.

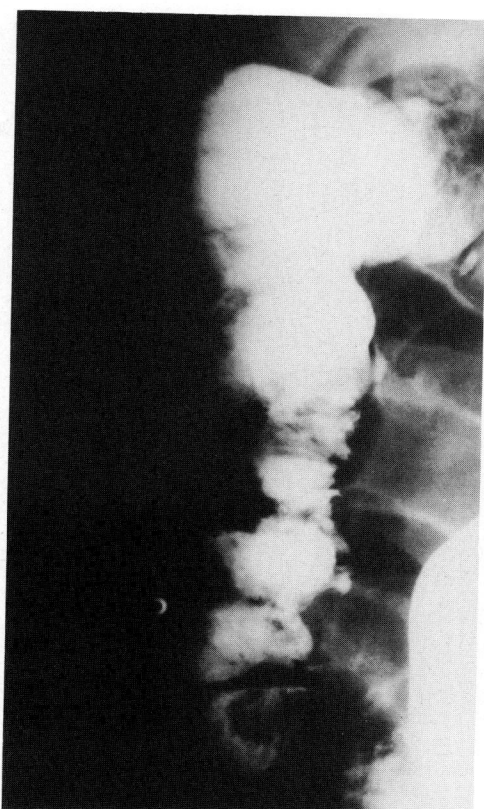

**Figure 63–14. Mucormycosis.** A severe ulcerating colitis involves the ascending colon and cecum. (Courtesy of Ellen Wolf, M.D., New York, NY.)

may yield the fungus, which stains with methenamine silver.

## Mucormycosis

Colonic involvement by this fungus is invariably in a setting of immunosuppression. Diagnosis is rarely made

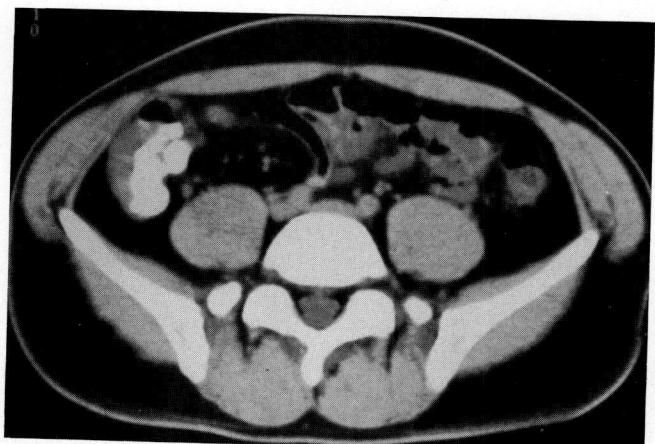

**Figure 63–13. Histoplasmosis.** CT scan shows marked thickening of the cecal wall caused by histoplasmosis. (Courtesy of Bronwyn Jones, M.D., Baltimore, MD.)

preoperatively, and almost all cases have been fatal. The sinuses, lungs, and central nervous system are the usual sites of involvement. Colonic involvement may be isolated or associated with abnormalities elsewhere in the gastrointestinal tract.[58, 59] The right colon is most often affected; the changes consist of a polypoid mass or focal segmental inflammation with or without sinus tracts (Fig. 63–14). Rarely, colitis is present throughout the colon.

## NONINFECTIOUS COLITIS

### Nonspecific Ulcer

Nonspecific colonic ulcer is of unknown etiology. More than half are located in the right colon near the ileocecal valve, and approximately 20% are multiple.[60] The clinical presentation may mimic appendicitis or carcinoma. The ulceration may be superficial or deep and occurs on the antimesenteric border. The most common radiologic abnormality is that of a focal mass with or without ulceration and less commonly a short stricture or segmental colitis[60–64] (Fig. 63–15). The CT scan may show a colonic mass with mesenteric stranding. Preoperative diagnosis is rare but may be suspected after colonoscopy with negative biopsy results.

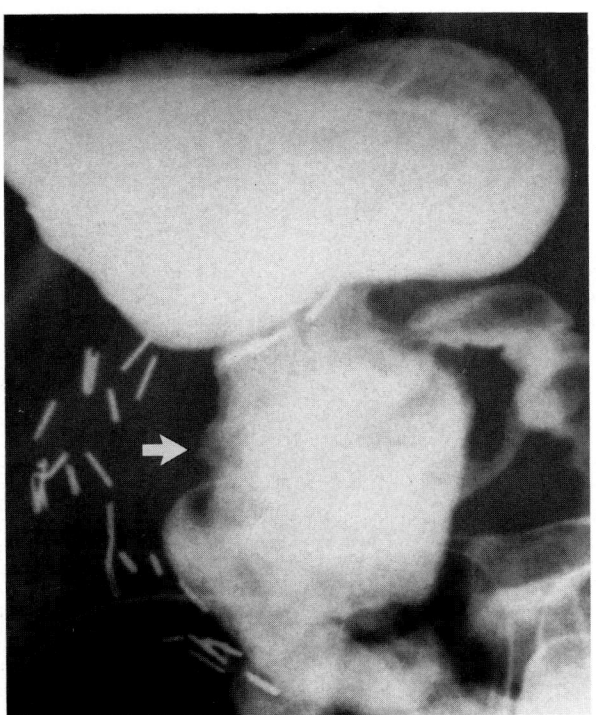

**Figure 63–15. Nonspecific ulcer of the cecum.** There is narrowing of the cecum with an ulcer on the lateral wall *(arrow).*

## Typhlitis

Patients with agranulocytosis, either idiopathic or most commonly after chemotherapy for hematologic malignancy, are at increased risk for development of acute inflammation of the cecum with or without extension to the ascending and even transverse colon. The exact pathogenesis has not been clarified, but infection plays a dominant role. A variety of organisms, particularly clostridia, have been isolated from surgical specimens. Symptom complexes include fever, right lower quadrant pain, and diarrhea.

Plain film findings include ileocecal dilatation with air-fluid levels[65–68] and small bowel obstruction secondary to the inflammation. A soft tissue mass and pneumatosis have been reported in a number of instances. The diagnosis may first be suspected on CT scan on the basis of marked low-density mural thickening predominantly in the right colon in the appropriate clinical setting[69, 70] (Fig. 63–16A). Pneumatosis may be identified. When performed, the barium enema study shows thumbprinting, narrowing, and shallow or deep ulcerations (Fig. 63–16B). The most important differential diagnosis is colitis secondary to *C. difficile* infection. The diagnosis is based on the combination of clinical and imaging findings as well as the exclusion of other entities. Medical treatment is usually satisfactory, although surgery may be necessary in severe cases.

## Microscopic (Collagenous) Colitis

Microscopic (collagenous) colitis is a clinicopathologic entity characterized by a history of variable, but usually long duration, intermittent or chronic watery diarrhea. This occurs predominantly in middle-aged and elderly women. Many of the cases have been associated with arthritis, and there has been speculation that analgesic therapy may play an etiologic role. Laboratory studies and diagnostic procedures, including endoscopy, are usually normal. Diagnosis is achieved by endoscopic biopsy, which reveals increased lymphocytes in the surface epithelium and, in the variant collagenous colitis, an increase in the width of the subepithelial collagen band. The changes are readily distinguished from other forms of inflammatory bowel disease.

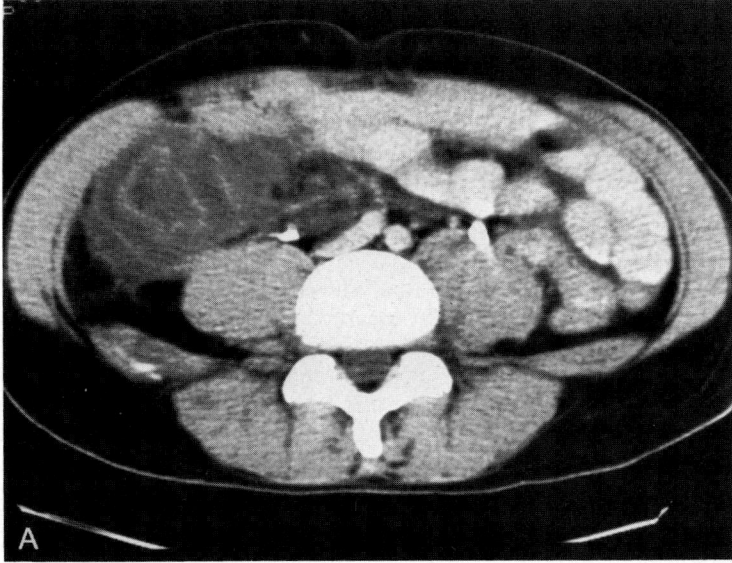
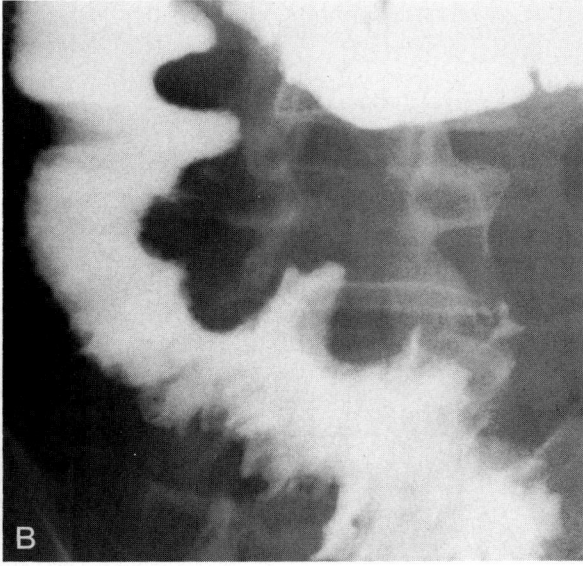

**Figure 63–16. Typhlitis. A.** CT scan shows extensive mural edema involving the right colon. **B.** A barium enema shows thumbprinting and ulceration of the right colon.

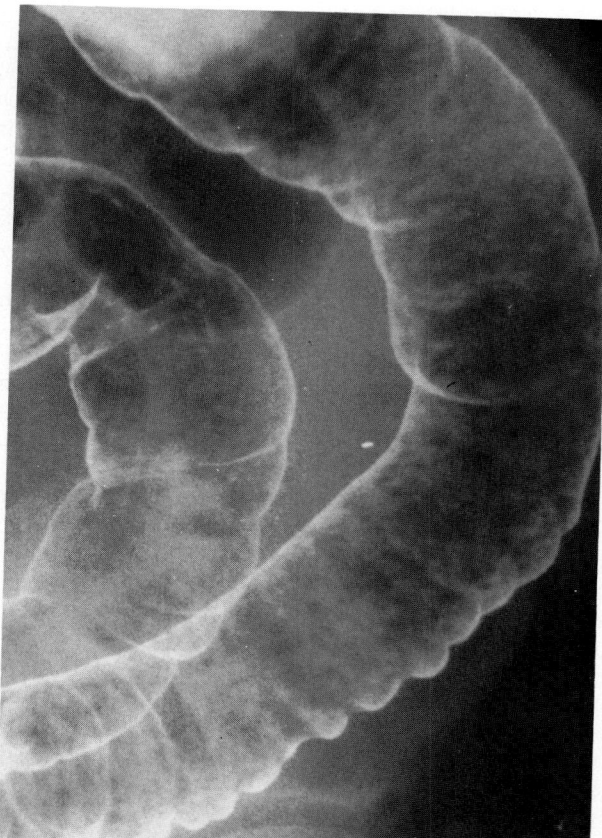

**Figure 63–17. Microscopic colitis.** There is extremely fine granularity involving the sigmoid mucosa.

Whereas the barium enema had been considered incapable of detecting any changes, there have been a few reported cases of nonspecific inflammatory surface abnormalities predominantly in the rectosigmoid region[71, 72] (Fig. 63–17). In the appropriate clinical setting, the diagnostic possibility should be suggested and biopsy performed. Many of these cases have been misdiagnosed as functional bowel disease. Sulfasalazine or steroids may be of benefit in the control of symptoms.

## Eosinophilic Colitis

Eosinophilic gastroenteritis is a disease of unknown etiology that invariably involves the stomach or small bowel. Antral narrowing and focal or diffuse thickening of the small bowel folds, with or without stenosis, are characteristic. Ascites is also frequent, and peripheral eosinophilia is usually present. On occasion, the colon, particularly the right side, may be involved. Thumbprinting, spasm, and narrowing are the primary features on barium study[75] (Fig. 63–18). These may be reversible after the initiation of steroid therapy.

## Sarcoidosis

The precise prevalence of colonic noncaseating granulomas in patients with sarcoidosis is unknown. Clinical

and radiographic abnormalities are rare. Anecdotal reports have consisted of segmental construction in the sigmoid colon or rectum simulating diverticulitis or carcinoma.[74] Another barium enema revealed diffuse small nodules consistent with lymphoid follicles.[75] A segmental nonspecific granular surface alteration may also be observed.

## Graft-Versus-Host Disease

One of the complications of bone marrow transplantation is that the donor immune cells may recognize the host tissue as foreign and stimulate an inflammatory response. The small intestine is invariably involved with the appearance of mural thickening and fold thickening or complete loss of mucosal features ("ribbon" bowel). A significant number of these patients have colonic abnormalities involving the entire colon or less commonly selective right-sided colonic disease.[76] The changes are those of nonspecific colitis (i.e., haustral loss or thickening, spasm, and ulceration) and at times a granular surface pattern (Fig. 63–19). However, in the appropriate clinical setting, these changes may be associated with graft-versus-host disease, combined graft-versus-host disease and viral infection, or viral infection alone. The presence of colitis does not provide distinguishing information for determining which of these diagnostic possibilities are present.

Viral colitis, particularly cytomegalovirus colitis in patients with acquired immunodeficiency syndrome, is discussed in Chapter 160.

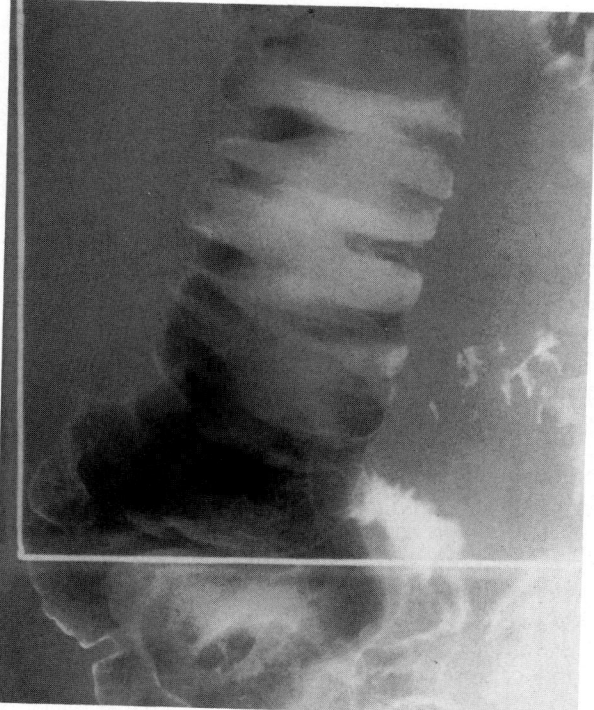

**Figure 63–18. Eosinophilic colitis.** Generalized thickening and thumbprinting of folds in the ascending colon are seen. Note also the presence of considerable ascitic fluid.

density within the mesentery with or without discrete fibrotic masses of soft tissue density. Ultrasound may also reveal solid masses with hypoechoic areas that may resemble a sarcoma, hematoma, or abscess.[78] Surgery is often performed to relieve obstructive symptoms, but steroid therapy may be beneficial.

## Reactive Inflammation

Secondary inflammation may occur in the colon as a response to extension from primary inflammatory processes in other organs or from adjacent abscesses. The site of colonic disease closely correlates with its anatomic contiguity and mesenteric relationships with these structures. The appearance may vary from an extrinsic mass effect with reactive spiculation to long segments of concentric narrowing and spiculation with or without evidence of an adjacent soft tissue mass that may fix and distort the segment (Fig. 63–20). Appendicitis may involve the ascending colon or sigmoid colon (depending on the location of the appendix), and pancreatitis tends to involve a variable length of the transverse colon up to the junction with the descending colon (phrenocolic ligament). In pancreatitis, obstruction (colon cutoff), fistula, necrosis and perforation, and residual stricture may all be associated. Both of these entities may present as primary colitis with pain and diarrhea, with the true cause being obscure.[81] Careful interpretation of the barium enema may allow the radiologist to suggest these possibilities, and a CT scan in conjunction with appropriate laboratory studies may allow an accurate diagnosis. Less commonly, inflammatory disease in the kidneys produce reactive changes in the proximal descending or ascending colon, and acute cholecystitis may have a similar effect on the proximal transverse colon, particularly on the superior aspect.

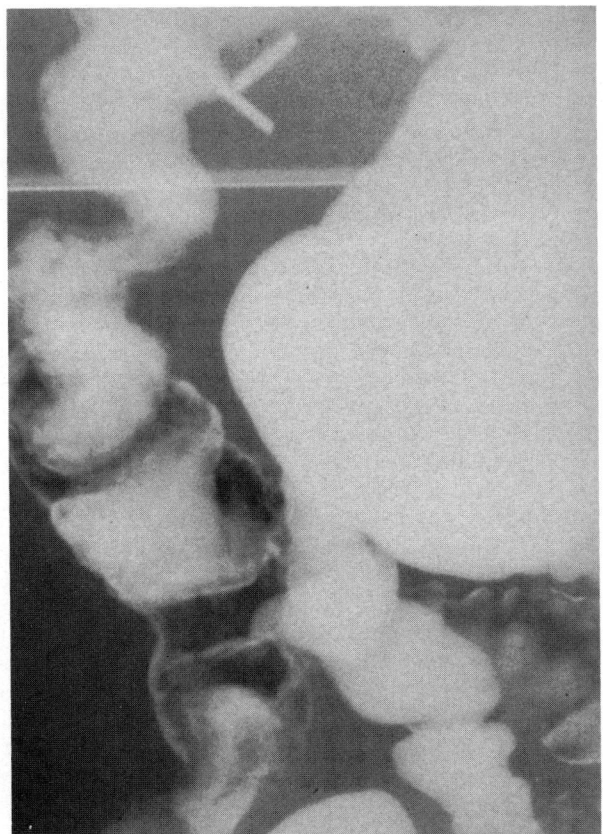

**Figure 63–19. Graft-versus-host disease.** Edema and narrowing of the right colon are present in this bone marrow graft recipient.

## Retractile Mesenteritis

Retractile mesenteritis is a disease of unknown etiology in which a spectrum of inflammatory and fibrotic pathologic changes occur in the mesenteric fat but can extend to the intestinal wall. This may be associated with a similar process in other anatomic regions, particularly retroperitoneal fibrosis. Autoimmune factors have been postulated that may result in ischemia. The patient's age may range from the second to eighth decade, and there is a slight male predominance. Symptoms consist of a combination of abdominal pain, diarrhea, and weight loss. The small bowel is the usual site of involvement, but colonic abnormalities are not uncommon. The sigmoid colon and transverse colon are most prone to these changes because these represent the segments of bowel intimately related to a mesentery.

Barium enema findings may be secondary to ischemia as a result of occlusion of the mesenteric vessels or direct extension of the fibroinflammatory process.[77–80] Thus, long segments of mild to moderate narrowing with thumbprinting, strictures of variable length simulating carcinomatosis or diverticulitis, or an extrinsic mass with reactive changes on the contiguous margin of the bowel wall may be seen. The CT scan is complementary in that it will demonstrate marked increased

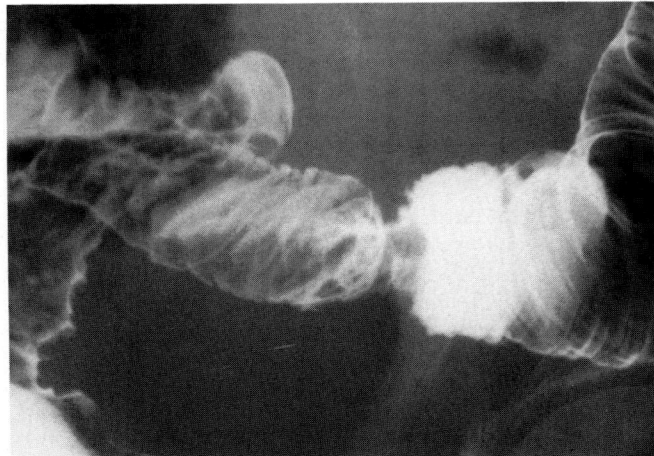

**Figure 63–20. Reactive colitis in the sigmoid colon from adjacent appendicitis.** Deformity, narrowing, and spiculation of the rectum and sigmoid colon are due to the adjacent inflammation from the complications of appendicitis.

# NEUTROPHIL AND MACROPHAGE DYSFUNCTION

## Chronic Granulomatous Disease of Childhood

In patients with conditions associated with neutrophil dysfunction, a colitis that may be segmental or pancolonic and indistinguishable from Crohn's disease has been reported.[82] Fistulas and sinuses may be features. This is seen predominantly in the pediatric population. Chronic granulomatous disease of childhood is an inherited defect of leukocyte function characterized by the inability of phagocytes to kill catalase-positive microorganisms. The ingested bacteria survive within granulocytes, and the clinical result is multifocal abscesses and granuloma. The presence of lipid-bearing histiocytes in the mucosa is highly suggestive. Some degree of colonic involvement is frequent in these patients, but clinically significant involvement is rare. Gastric antral narrowing and even outlet obstruction are more often described and may be present in association with colonic abnormalities.

## Glycogen Storage Disease

Glycogen storage disease Ib is also associated with neutropenia and a metabolic defect in neutrophil activity. Recurrent pyogenic infections are a significant clinical problem. Colonic involvement in the limited number of cases consisted of long or short strictures involving predominantly the colon proximal to the splenic flexure and even the terminal ileum.[83] Granulomas were identified in one case.

## Malacoplakia

Malacoplakia is a granulomatous process that most commonly involves the genitourinary tract. The colon is the most common extraurinary site.[84] Distinctive macrophages that contain pathognomonic intracytoplasmic calcifications (Michaelis-Gutmann bodies) are present on biopsy. The etiology is unknown, but a macrophage defect is most likely. Unlike the urinary tract changes that tend to occur in elderly women, colonic disease shows a wide age distribution. Abnormalities may occur segmentally or diffusely as small polyps or bulky masses. A less frequent manifestation is diffuse nonspecific colitis resembling Crohn's disease (Fig. 63–21). Rectal bleeding, diarrhea, and abdominal pain are the common symptoms in this setting.

# EXOGENOUS CAUSES OF COLITIS

## Caustic Colitis

Direct contact between the colorectal mucosa and caustic substances induced through the rectum by enema

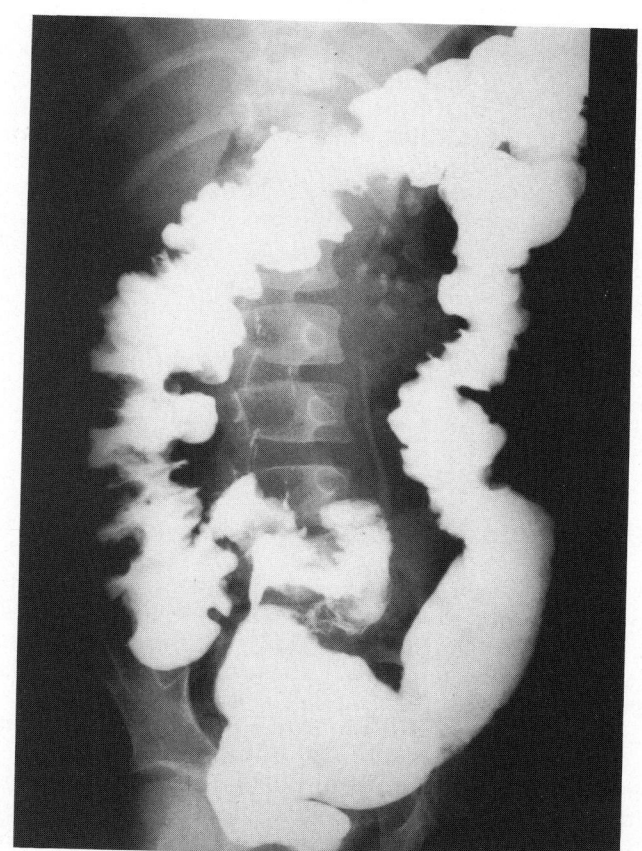

**Figure 63–21. Malacoplakia.** There is a diffuse colitis with thickening of the folds, more severe on the right.

may produce colitis that is transient or may result in complete mucosal slough with subsequent stricture. The most commonly reported agents are detergent or soapsuds enema employed as laxatives or herbal (ritual) enemas practiced in Third World countries as a form of medical therapy.[85–88] In some cases, the injury has been thermal as a result of the high temperature of the liquid.[89] The changes are seen predominantly in the distal colon because of the route of entry. However, skip lesions or transverse and right-sided colonic alterations can occur owing to spasm and prolonged contact. Bloody diarrhea is the usual presenting symptom. The barium study may demonstrate thumbprinting or severe mucosal necrosis and ulceration that may progress to deformity or stricture. A number of patients have required colectomy and colostomy.

## Drug-Induced Colitis

A variety of pharmaceutical agents may be directly or indirectly responsible for colitis through a number of mechanisms.[90] Cancer chemotherapeutic agents may result in ulceration and inflammation secondary to their inhibitory effect on mucosal epithelial cells. In addition, neutropenia may result, as mentioned in typhlitis. Almost all antibiotics may cause *C. difficile* colitis. Vasoconstrictive drugs, antihypertensive medications, and oral contraceptives may result in ischemia-related inflammation. In addition, some therapeutic agents may be associated with hypersensitivity reaction. Penicillin, ampicillin, amoxicillin, and erythromycin have been reported to cause a right-sided hemorrhagic colitis that subsides spontaneously on drug withdrawal.[90, 91] Nonsteroidal anti-inflammatory drugs have been described as responsible for colonic injury, possibly as a result of inhibition of prostaglandin synthesis.[92] Findings have ranged from diffuse or segmental colitis (including isolated proctitis) to scattered discrete ulcers involving any segment, particularly the cecum. Perforation has been reported in several cases, and it has been suggested that these medications may be associated with an increased risk of diverticulitis.

## Clostridium difficile Colitis

*C. difficile* colitis is often considered synonymous with pseudomembranous colitis and antibiotic-induced colitis.[93, 94] Although this is often the case, these associations are not universal. Almost all antibiotics may produce diarrhea, but only a small percentage of these cases are related to *C. difficile*. Of these patients with *C. difficile* colitis, only some will demonstrate pseudomembranes at endoscopy or radiography. Finally, some instances of *C. difficile* colitis may not be associated with antibiotics because immunosuppression (e.g., cancer chemotherapy) may also be responsible. To further complicate the subject, a significant number (20%) of asymptomatic hospitalized patients may show *C. difficile* on stool culture.

Nevertheless, in the clinical setting of a patient receiving antibiotics with sudden onset of watery diarrhea often with some combination of fever, abdominal tenderness, and leukocytosis, this is the probable diagnosis. Less commonly, fever or abdominal distention is the only presenting symptom. Many of the patients are hospitalized and are postoperative. Whereas onset is usually within 2 days to 2 weeks after the introduction of antibiotic therapy, symptoms may begin as late as 8 weeks after the drugs are discontinued. The relationship with the antibiotics becomes obscure, and the history must be elicited. In patients in whom fever predominates, the working diagnosis may be abscess, and a CT scan may be the initial diagnostic investigation. This study may show marked low-density mural thickening with the swollen haustra projecting into the lumen with thin streaks of contrast medium trapped between them[95] (Fig. 63–22A). These changes are pancolonic in the majority, but a significant number are confined to the right colon and less commonly the left.

The majority of cases of pseudomembranous colitis are diagnosed by proctosigmoidoscopy in conjunction with a positive cytotoxicity test for toxin B. However, in approximately 40% of cases, the rectum may be normal or the changes nonspecific.[96] The assay for toxin B requires 48 hours to perform. In severe cases, the plain film of the abdomen may be diagnostic, demonstrating massive thumbprinting throughout the colon that at times may reveal a shaggy margin[97, 98] (Fig. 63–22B). Megacolon may be present. In such instances, a

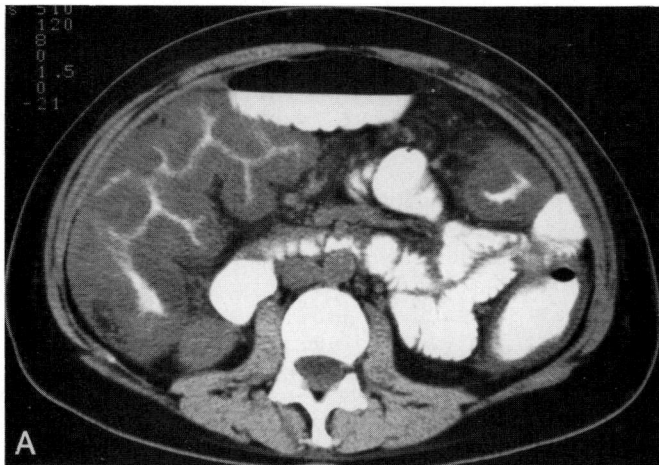
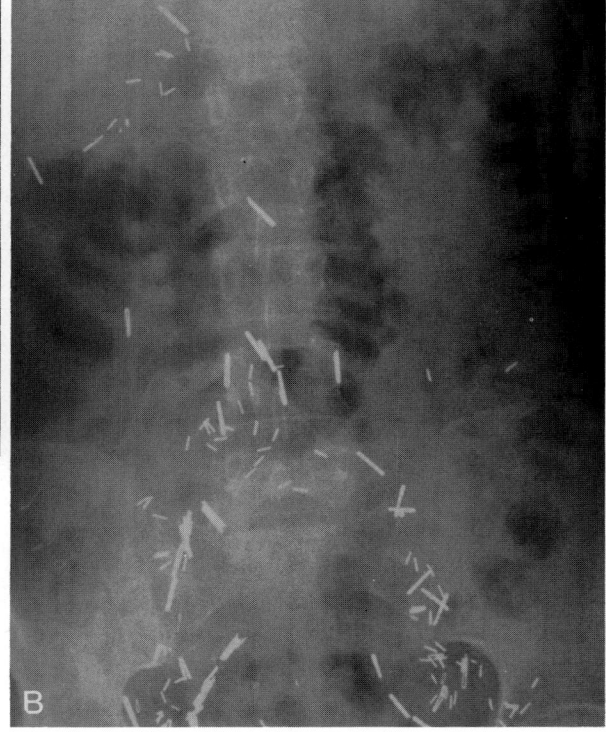

**Figure 63–22. *C. difficile* colitis. A.** CT scan shows extensive thickening of the wall of the colon. (Courtesy of Harvey Goldstein, M.D., San Antonio, TX.) **B.** In another patient, a plain film shows extensive haustral thickening and thumbprinting throughout the colon.

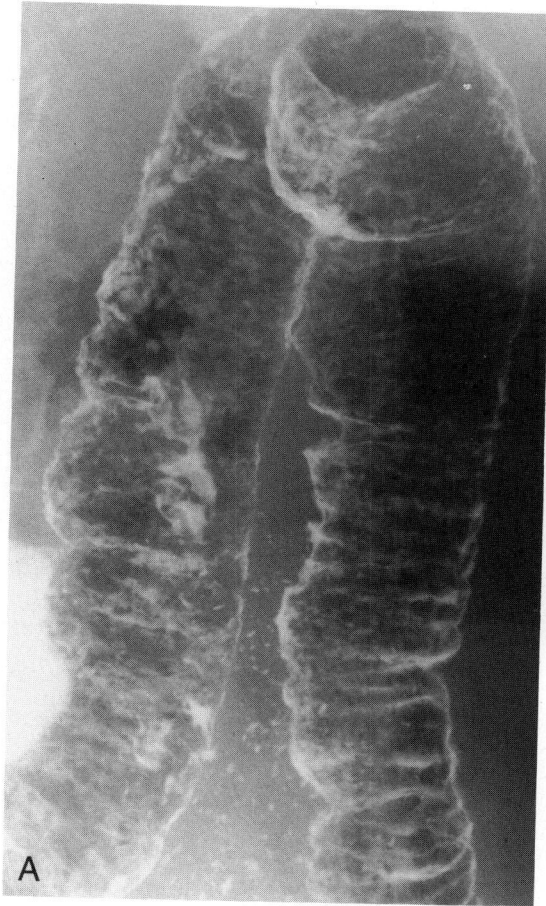

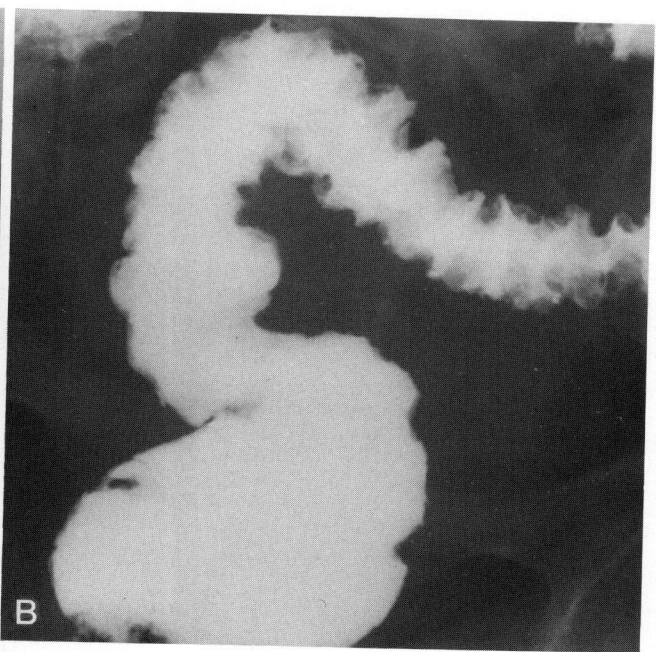

**Figure 63–23.** **C. difficile colitis. A.** The double contrast study shows small, irregular plaques on the mucosal surface representing the pseudomembrane. **B.** Single contrast barium study in another patient shows irregular thumbprinting with barium undermining the plaques.

contrast enema is contraindicated. However, the findings on barium enema in most cases consist of small, subtly elevated round nodules or small, irregular plaque filling defects that may be discrete or confluent and are best seen on air-contrast study[99] (Fig. 63–23). In more advanced cases, a full column study will show coarse polypoid defects or shaggy marginal irregularities.[97, 98] Barium between the plaques may simulate ulcerations; on occasion, barium may undermine the plaques, suggesting intramural tracking. In rare cases, true ulceration caused by plaque sloughing and even intramural air have been described. The diagnosis can be readily made on the barium study. Discontinuation of the drug is often sufficient, but in more severe cases, vancomycin is the treatment of choice. However, relapse may occur in 10 to 39% of treated patients.

# References

1. Griffiths JK: Colonic infections. Curr Opin Gastroenterol 9:83–87, 1993.
2. Rutgeerts P, Geboes K, Ponette E, et al: Colitis caused by endemic pathogens in Western Europe: endoscopic features. Endoscopy 14:212–219, 1982.
3. Tedesco FJ, Moore S: Infectious diseases mimicking inflammatory bowel disease. Am Surg 6:243–249, 1982.
4. Tedesco FJ, Hardin RD, Harper RN, et al: Infectious colitis endoscopically simulating inflammatory bowel disease: a prospective evaluation. Gastrointest Endosc 29:195–197, 1983.
5. Grundy A, Gilks CF: Typhoid: an unusual cause of gastrointestinal bleeding. Br J Radiol 57:344–346, 1984.
6. Saffouri B, Bartolomeo RS, Fuchs B: Colonic involvement in salmonellosis. Dig Dis Sci 24:203–208, 1979.
7. Farman J, Rabinowitz JG, Meyers MA: Roentgenology of infectious colitis. AJR 119:375–381, 1973.
8. Vender RJ, Marignani P: *Salmonella* colitis presenting as a segmental colitis resembling Crohn's disease. Dig Dis Sci 28:848–851, 1983.
9. Speelman P, Kabir I, Islam M: Distribution and spread of colonic lesions in shigellosis: a colonoscopic study. J Infect 150:899–903, 1984.
10. Khuroo MS, Mahajan R, Zargar SA, et al: The colon in shigellosis: serial colonoscopic appearances in *Shigella dysenteriae* I. Endoscopy 22:35–38, 1990.
11. Zalev AH, Warren RE: *Shigella* colitis with radiological and endoscopic correlation: case report. J Can Assoc Radiol 40:328–330, 1989.
12. Lambert JR, Tischler ME, Karmali MA, et al: *Campylobacter* ileocolitis: an inflammatory bowel disease. Can Med Assoc J 121:1377–1379, 1979.
13. Brodey PA, Fertig S, Aron JM: *Campylobacter* enterocolitis: radiographic features. AJR 139:1199–1201, 1982.
14. Tielbeek AV, Rosenbusch G, Muytjens HL, et al: Roentgenologic changes of the colon in *Campylobacter* infection. Gastrointest Radiol 10:358–361, 1985.
15. Kollitz JPM, Davis GB, Berk RN: *Campylobacter* colitis: a common infectious form of acute colitis. Gastrointest Radiol 6:227–229, 1981.

16. Vantrappen G, Agg HO, Ponette E, et al: *Yersinia* enteritis and enterocolitis: gastroenterological aspects. Gastroenterology 72:220–227, 1977.

17. Matsumoto T, Iida M, Matsui T, et al: Endoscopic findings in *Yersinia enterocolitica* enterocolitis. Gastrointest Endosc 36:583–587, 1990.

18. Simmonds SD, Noble MA, Freeman HJ: Gastrointestinal features of culture-positive *Yersinia enterocolitica* infection. Gastroenterology 92:112–117, 1987.

19. Shrago G: *Yersinia enterocolitica* ileocolitis findings observed on barium examination. Br J Radiol 49:181–183, 1976.

20. Atkinson GO, Gay BB, Ball TI, et al: *Yersinia enterocolitica* colitis in infants: radiographic changes. Radiology 148:113–116, 1983.

21. Lachman R, Soong J, Wishon G, et al: *Yersinia* colitis. Gastrointest Radiol 2:133–135, 1977.

22. Kawanami T, Bowen A, Girdany BR: Enterocolitis: prodrome of the hemolytic-uremic syndrome. Radiology 151:91–92, 1984.

23. Peterson RB, Meseroll WP, Shrago GG, et al: Radiographic features of colitis associated with the hemolytic-uremic syndrome. Radiology 118:667–671, 1976.

24. Shortsleeve MJ, Wilson ME, Finklestein M, et al: Radiologic findings in hemorrhagic colitis due to *Escherichia coli* O157:H7. Gastrointest Radiol 14:341–344, 1989.

25. Balthazar EJ, Gordon R, Hulnick D: Ileocecal tuberculosis: CT and radiologic evaluation. AJR 154:499–503, 1990.

26. Vaidya MG, Sodhi JS: Gastrointestinal tract tuberculosis: a study of 102 cases including 55 hemicolectomies. Clin Radiol 29:189–195, 1978.

27. Ehsannulah M, Isaacs A, Filipe MI, et al: Tuberculosis presenting as inflammatory bowel disease: report of two cases. Dis Colon Rectum 27:134–136, 1984.

28. Tishler JM: Tuberculosis of the transverse colon. AJR 133:229–232, 1979.

29. Peh WC: Filiform polyposis in tuberculosis of the colon. Clin Radiol 39:534–536, 1988.

30. Downey DB, Nakielny RA: Aphthoid ulcers in colonic tuberculosis. Br J Radiol 58:561–562, 1985.

31. Carr-Locke DL, Finlay DBL: Radiological demonstration of colonic aphthoid ulcers in a patient with intestinal tuberculosis. Gut 24:453–455, 1983.

32. McDonald JB, Middleton PJ: Tuberculosis of the colon simulating carcinoma. Radiology 118:293–294, 1976.

33. Bhargava DK, Tandon HD, Chawla TC, et al: Diagnosis of ileocecal and colonic tuberculosis by colonoscopy. Gastrointest Endosc 31:68–70, 1985.

34. Maloney JJ, Cho SR: Pelvic actinomycosis. Radiology 148:388, 1983.

35. Fowler RC, Simpkins KC: Abdominal actinomycosis: a report of three cases. Clin Radiol 34:301–307, 1983.

36. Thompson JR, Watts R, Thompson WC: Actinomycetoma masquerading as an abdominal neoplasm. Dis Colon Rectum 25:368–370, 1982.

37. Higashi M, Tanaka K, Kitada T, et al: Anisakiasis confirmed by radiography of the large intestine. Gastrointest Radiol 13:85–86, 1988.

38. Matsui T, Iida M, Murakami M, et al: Intestinal anisakiasis: clinical and radiologic features. Radiology 157:299–302, 1985.

39. Matsumoto T, Iida M, Kimura Y, et al: Anisakiasis of the colon: radiologic and endoscopic features in six patients. Radiology 183:97–99, 1992.

40. Cardoso JM, Kimura K, Stoopen M, et al: Radiology of invasive amebiasis of the colon. Am J Roentgenol 128:935–941, 1977.

41. Balikian JP, Uthman SM, Khouri NF: Intestinal amebiasis: a roentgen analysis of 19 cases including 2 case reports. AJR 122:245–256, 1974.

42. Kolawole TM, Lewis EA: Radiologic observations on intestinal amebiasis. AJR 122:257–265, 1974.

43. Cevallos AM, Farthing MJG: Parasitic infections of the gastrointestinal tract. Curr Opin Gastroenterol 9:96–102, 1993.

44. Matsui T, Iida M, Tata S, et al: The value of double-contrast barium enema in amebic colitis. Gastrointest Radiol 14:73–78, 1989.

45. Martinez CR, Gilman RH, Rabbani GH, et al: Amebic colitis: correlation of proctoscopy before treatment and barium enema after treatment. AJR 138:1089–1093, 1982.

46. Medina JT, Seaman WB, Guzman-Acosta C, et al: The roentgen appearance of schistosomiasis mansoni involving the colon. Radiology 85:682–688, 1965.

47. Lehman JS, Farid Z, Bassily S, et al: Colonic calcification and polyposis. Radiology 98:379–380, 1971.

48. Zuckerman MJ, Goldfarb JP, Cho KC, et al: An unusual pedunculated polyp of the colon: association with schistosomiasis. J Clin Gastroenterol 5:169–172, 1983.

49. Yoshida T, Nozaki F, Tanaka K, et al: *Strongyloides stercoralis* hyperinfection: sequential changes of gastrointestinal radiology after treatment with thiabendazole. Gastrointest Radiol 6:223–225, 1981.

50. Dallemand S, Waxman M, Farman J: Radiological manifestations of *Strongyloides stercoralis*. Gastrointest Radiol 8:45–51, 1983.

51. Drasin GF, Moss JP, Cheng SH: *Strongyloides stercoralis* colitis: findings in four cases. Radiology 126:619–621, 1978.

52. Stoopack PM, Raufman JP: Aphthoid ulceration of the colon in strongyloidiasis. Am J Gastroenterol 86:639–642, 1991.

53. Reeder MM, Astacio JE, Theros EG: Case of the month from the AFIP. Radiology 90:382–387, 1968.

54. Fisher RM, Cremin BJ: Rectal bleeding due to *Trichuris trichiura*. Br J Radiol 43:214–215, 1970.

55. Cappell MS, Mandell W, Grimes MM, et al: Gastrointestinal histoplasmosis. Dig Dis Sci 33:353–360, 1988.

56. Haws CC, Long RF, Caplan GE: *Histoplasma capsulatum* as a cause of ileocolitis. Am J Roentgenol 128:692–694, 1977.

57. Dietz MW: Ileocecal histoplasmosis. Radiology 91:285–289, 1968.

58. De Feo E: Mucormycosis of the colon. AJR 86:86–90, 1961.

59. Agha FP, Lee HH, Boland CR, et al: Mucormycoma of the colon: early diagnosis and successful management. AJR 145:739–741, 1985.

60. Shallman RW, Kuehner M, Williams GH, et al: Benign cecal ulcers. Dis Colon Rectum 28:732–737, 1985.

61. Huded FV, Posner GL, Tick R: Nonspecific ulcer of the colon in a chronic hemodialysis patient. Am J Gastroenterol 77:913–916, 1982.

62. Brodey PA, Hill RP, Baron S: Benign ulceration of the cecum. Radiology 122:323–327, 1977.

63. Gardiner GA, Bird CR: Nonspecific ulcers of the colon resembling annular carcinoma. Radiology 137:331–334, 1980.

64. Marn CS, Yu BFB, Nostrant TT, et al: Idiopathic cecal ulcer; CT findings. AJR 153:761–763, 1989.

65. Del Fava RL, Cronin TG: Typhlitis complicating leukemia in an adult: barium enema findings. Am J Roentgenol 129:347–348, 1977.

66. Abramson SJ, Berdon WE, Baker DH: Childhood typhlitis: its increasing association with acute myelogenous leukemia. Radiology 146:61–64, 1983.

67. Archibald RB, Nelson JA: Necrotizing enterocolitis in acute leukemia: radiographic findings. Gastrointest Radiol 3:63–65, 1978.

68. Taylor AJ, Dodds WJ, Gonyo JE, et al: Typhlitis in adults. Gastrointest Radiol 10:363–369, 1985.

69. Frick MP, Maile CW, Crass JR, et al: Computed tomography of neutropenic colitis. AJR 143:763–765, 1984.

70. Adams GW, Rauch RF, Kelvin FM, et al: CT detection of typhlitis. J Comput Assist Tomogr 9:363–365, 1985.

71. Glick SN, Teplick SK, Amenta PS: Microscopic (collagenous) colitis. AJR 153:995–996, 1989.

72. Feczko PJ, Mezwa DG: Nonspecific radiographic abnormalities in collagenous colitis. Gastrointest Radiol 16:128–132, 1991.

73. MacCarty RL, Talley NJ: Barium studies in diffuse eosinophilic gastroenteritis. Gastrointest Radiol 15:183–187, 1990.

74. Levine MS, Ekberg O, Rubesin SE, et al: Gastrointestinal sarcoidosis: radiographic findings. AJR 153:293–295, 1989.

75. Ell SR, Frank PH: Spectrum of lymphoid hyperplasia: colonic manifestations of sarcoidosis, infectious mononucleosis, and Crohn's disease. Gastrointest Radiol 6:329–332, 1981.

76. Jones B, Kramer SS, Saral R, et al: Gastrointestinal inflammation after bone marrow transplantation: graft-versus-host disease or opportunistic infection? AJR 150:277–281, 1988.

77. Han SY, Koehler RE, Keller FS, et al: Retractile mesenteritis

involving the colon: pathologic and radiologic correlation. AJR 147:268–270, 1986.

78. Periz-Fontan FJ, Soler R, Sanchez J, et al: Retractile mesenteritis involving the colon: barium enema, sonographic, and CT findings. AJR 147:937–940, 1986.

79. Williams RG, Nelson JA: Retractile mesenteritis: initial presentation as colonic obstruction. Radiology 126:35–37, 1978.

80. Thompson GT, Fitzgerald EF, Somers SS: Retractile mesenteritis of the sigmoid colon. Br J Radiol 58:266–267, 1985.

81. Picus D, Shackelford GD: Perforated appendix presenting with severe diarrhea. Radiology 149:141–143, 1983.

82. Werlin SL, Chusid MJ, Caya J, et al: Colitis in chronic granulomatous disease. Gastroenterology 82:328–331, 1982.

83. Couper R, Kapelushnik J, Griffiths AM: Neutrophil dysfunction in glycogen storage disease Ib: association with Crohn's-like colitis. Gastroenterology 100:549–554, 1991.

84. Radin DR, Chandrasoma P, Halls JM: Colon malacoplakia. Gastrointest Radiol 9:359–361, 1984.

85. Kim SK, Cho C, Levinsohn EM: Caustic colitis due to detergent enema. AJR 134:397–398, 1980.

86. Pike BF, Phillippi PJ, Lawson EH: Soap colitis. N Engl J Med 285:217–218, 1971.

87. Segal I, Solomon A, Mirwis J: Radiological manifestations of ritual-enema-induced colitis. Clin Radiol 32:657–662, 1981.

88. Young WS: Herbal-enema colitis and stricture. Br J Radiol 53:248–249, 1980.

89. Jackson KR, Ott DJ, Gelfand DW: Thermal injury of the colon due to colostomy irrigation. Gastrointest Radiol 6:231–233, 1981.

90. Fortson WC, Tedesco FJ: Drug induced colitis: a review. Am J Gastroenterol 79:878–883, 1984.

91. Rimmer MJ, Freeman AH, Low FM: The barium enema diagnosis of penicillin associated colitis. Clin Radiol 33:529–533, 1982.

92. Gibson GR, Whitacre EB, Ricotti CA: Colitis induced by nonsteroidal anti-flammatory drugs. Arch Intern Med 152:625–632, 1992.

93. Gerding DN, Olson MM, Peterson LR, et al: *Clostridium difficile*-associated diarrhea and colitis in adults. Arch Intern Med 146:95–100, 1986.

94. Gebhard RL, Gerding DN, Olson MM, et al: Clinical and endoscopic findings in patients early in the course of *Clostridium difficile*-associated pseudomembranous colitis. Am J Med 78:45–48, 1985.

95. Fishman EK, Kavuru M, Jones B, et al: Pseudomembranous colitis: CT evaluation of 26 cases. Radiology 180:57–60, 1991.

96. Rubesin SE, Levine MS, Glick SN, et al: Pseudomembranous colitis with rectosigmoid sparing on barium studies. Radiology 170:811–813, 1989.

97. Cho KJ, Ting YM, Chuang VP, et al: Roentgenographic features in antibiotic-associated pseudomembranous colitis. Australas Radiol 20:38–41, 1976.

98. Stanley RJ, Melson GL, Tedesco FJ: The spectrum of radiographic findings in antibiotic-related pseudomembranous colitis. Radiology 111:519–524, 1974.

99. Strada M, Meregaglia D, Donzelli R: Double-contrast enema in antibiotic-related pseudomembranous colitis. Gastrointest Radiol 8:67–69, 1983.

# Polyps and Cancer

**Ruedi F. Thoeni, M.D.**
**Igor Laufer, M.D.**

## INTRODUCTION

### Epidemiology

Colorectal cancer is the most common cancer in the U.S. population and is the second most common cause of cancer mortality. It ranks second to lung cancer in males and second to breast cancer in females.[1] The distribution of this disease varies widely throughout the world. It is common in North America, Europe, and New Zealand, and the incidence is low in South America, Africa, and Asia. The United States has one of the highest incidences of colorectal cancer in the world. However, even within the United States the rates vary considerably, being higher in the North, among the urban white population, and among Jewish persons.[2]

The distribution of cancer in the large bowel is of considerable importance because it affects the diagnostic approach. Approximately one half of the cancers are in the rectum and sigmoid colon within reach of the short flexible sigmoidoscope.[3] The remainder are scattered throughout the proximal colon. Some authors suggest that there has been a shift to the right, rendering fewer cancers diagnosable by digital and short sigmoidoscopic examination.[4]

It is estimated that approximately 160,000 new cases of colorectal cancer and more than 60,000 deaths caused by this disease occur annually in the United States. Viewed in a personal way, American adults have approximately 1 chance in 20 of developing colorectal cancer during their lifetime and 1 chance in 40 of dying with this disease. Thus, the problem with colorectal cancer not only concerns us as physicians trying to maintain the health of our patients but also raises concerns about our personal health.

## Etiology[2]

The wide variation and distribution of colorectal cancer throughout the world are probably related to dietary differences. In general, diets low in fiber and high in fat and animal protein are associated with a higher prevalence of colorectal cancer, and this is inversely related to the incidence of gastric cancer. However, these conclusions are based on population studies, and a direct link between diet and colon cancer has not been demonstrated.

## Hereditary Factors[5]

The role of heredity in colorectal cancer has been a subject of interest. Heredity probably plays a role in 5 to 6% of all cases of colorectal cancer. Adenomatous polyposis coli (see Chapter 66) is transmitted by the classic mendelian dominant inheritance pattern, and almost all patients with this condition eventually develop colorectal carcinoma. These patients account for approximately 1% of colorectal cancers. Another 5% arise in patients with hereditary nonpolyposis colorectal cancer. The hereditary nonpolyposis colorectal cancers are subdivided into those in which colorectal cancer is clustered in families (type I) and those in which there is a familial clustering of colorectal cancer with other malignancies such as carcinomas of the endometrium, ovary, and breast (type II). In all these syndromes, carcinomas tend to occur in the proximal part of the colon and are found at a relatively young age.

It has been suggested that an abnormality in the genetic material may be associated with the development of colorectal cancer.[6] In the future, such a biologic marker may allow the identification of patients who are at higher than normal risk of developing this disease.

## Risk Factors

Although colorectal cancer is common in the U.S. population, several factors place individuals at higher than normal risk. These include age, a personal or family history of colorectal polyps or cancer, and chronic ulcerative colitis. The onset of colorectal cancer is clearly related to age. The incidence increases markedly in those older than the age of 50 and peaks in those about 70 years of age. First-degree relatives of patients with colon cancer have a two- to threefold increase in cancer risk, as do patients who have previously been treated for colon cancer.

Patients with chronic ulcerative colitis also have a higher incidence of colorectal cancer. The incidence starts to increase after the disease has been present for about 10 years, and approximately 10% develop cancer for every decade after 10 years of disease activity.[7] These cancers tend to be more uniformly distributed through the colon and often have a scirrhous appearance. It is predominantly patients with pancolitis who are affected.

## PATHOGENESIS

In the past, there was considerable controversy regarding the adenoma-carcinoma sequence. However, it is now believed that most colorectal carcinomas start as benign adenomas that undergo malignant transformation into adenocarcinomas[8] (Fig. 64–1). Larger adenomas (>1 cm) may pose a more significant cancer risk.[9] Thus, it is of clinical importance to detect and remove polypoid lesions larger than 1 cm. First, they are probably adenomas that carry a significant risk of malignant transformation and their removal may prevent the subsequent development of cancer. Second, the polypoid lesion may already have become a colon cancer and the earlier it is removed the less likely it is to have spread.

In patients with chronic ulcerative colitis, carcinoma probably develops through a sequence of inflammation, dysplasia, and carcinoma.[10] Therefore, in the surveillance of patients with chronic ulcerative colitis, "blind" biopsy specimens are often taken throughout the colon in an attempt to detect severe and persistent dysplasia.

The frequency of de novo colon carcinoma—that is, carcinoma developing in normal mucosa without an antecedent adenoma—is unknown. Some Japanese studies have shown small, aggressive, ulcerated tumors that appear to represent de novo carcinomas.[11] It is not yet clear how significant a fraction of colorectal cancers they represent in the world population.

## CLINICAL ASPECTS

Colorectal cancer is a slow-growing malignancy. In most cases, the lesions start as benign adenomas, and during a period of 7 to 10 years malignant transformation may take place in some but certainly not all adenomas. The malignancy grows relatively slowly. Ideally, the disease should be detected before it becomes symptomatic. Colorectal cancer is sufficiently common in the Western world that routine screening is recommended. The American Cancer Society recommends annual digital rectal examination starting at age 40, annual fecal occult blood tests starting at age 50, and, also starting at age 50, sigmoidoscopy every 3 to 5 years.[12] In addition, the American College of Radiology recommends periodic (approximately every 5 years) double contrast barium enema study, especially for patients at higher than normal risk of developing colorectal cancer.[13]

Symptomatic colorectal cancer most often presents with evidence of bleeding. The severity of bleeding may range from the presence of occult blood in the stool to the passage of bright red blood per rectum to the development of iron deficiency anemia. The latter is particularly likely to occur with large tumors in the cecum. Other frequent symptoms of colorectal cancer include abdominal pain, which may be related to the development of obstruction or to tumor invasion of adjacent tissues. Patients may also present with a change in bowel habit or with nonspecific symptoms such as weight loss or fever.

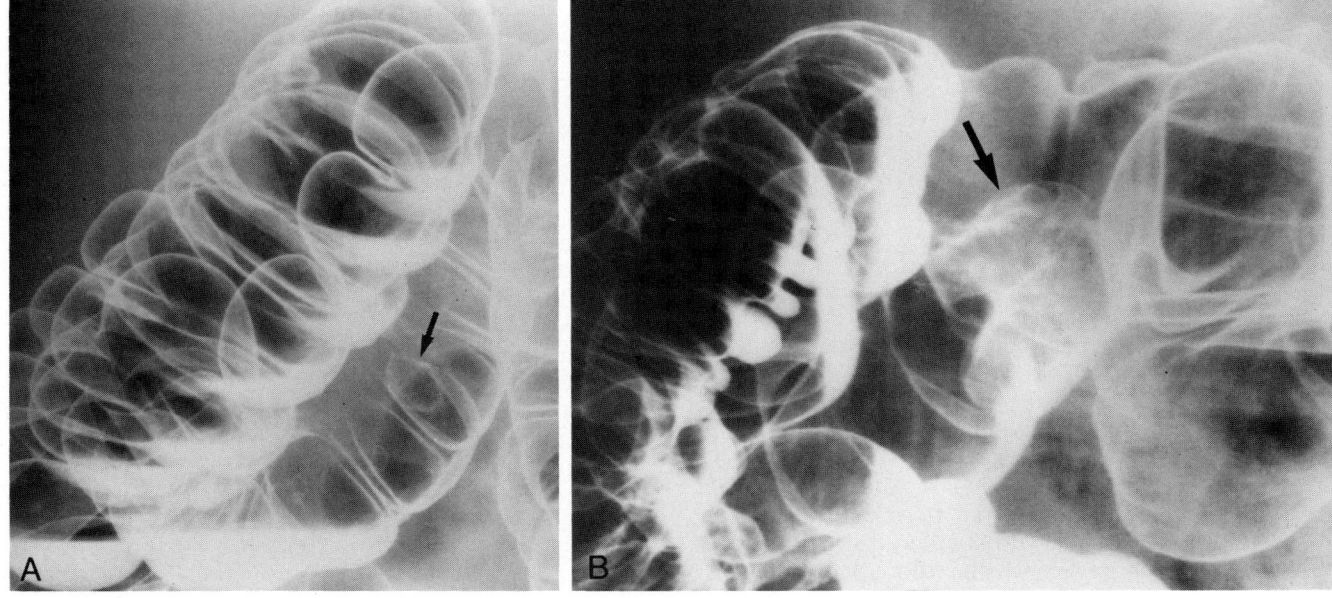

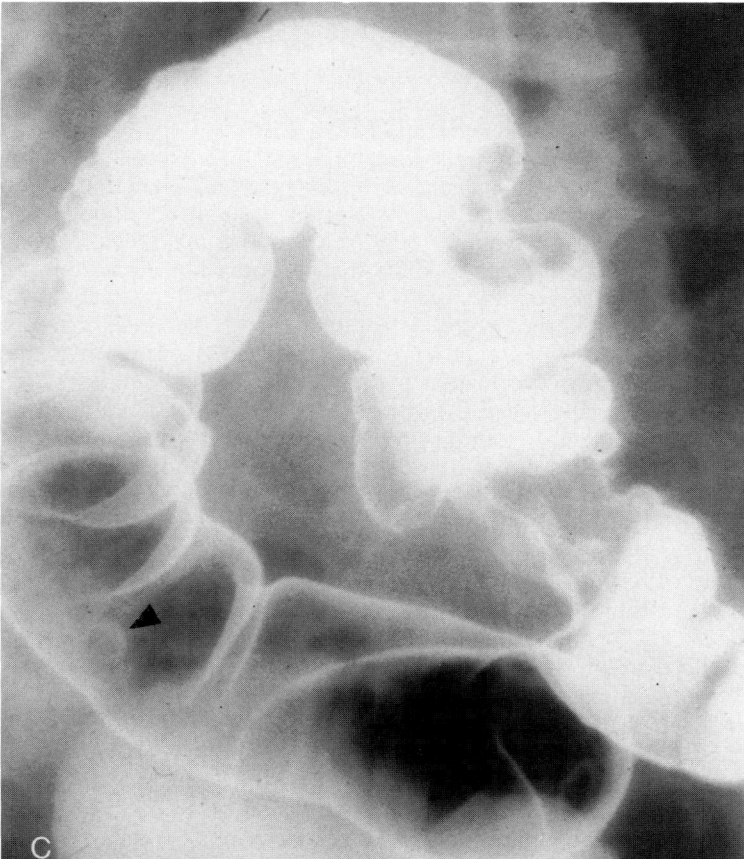

Figure 64–1. The evaluation of colon cancer. A. In 1973, a 1-cm polyp *(arrow)* is demonstrated in the proximal transverse colon. B. Seventeen years later, the small polyp has grown into a full-blown polypoid carcinoma *(arrow)*. C. In another patient, the evolution of colon cancer is demonstrated with adenomas in the distal sigmoid *(arrowhead),* a polypoid carcinoma near the apex of the sigmoid, and an annular carcinoma more proximally in the sigmoid colon.

## Role of Radiology

Radiology plays a critical role in the diagnosis and management of patients with colorectal cancer. The double contrast barium enema may be used for screening, especially for patients who are at higher than normal risk.[13] It is also the primary method for diagnosing symptomatic colorectal cancer and particularly for detecting complications such as obstruction or perforation. Radiology also plays an important role for staging of the tumor in selected cases.

The patient's symptoms are usually related to the location of the tumor. Approximately one third of carcinomas are in the rectum and can be reached by the examining finger or a rigid proctoscope. About one half of large bowel cancers are in the left half of the colon and can be reached with the flexible sigmoidoscope. These tumors on the left side often present with either bright red rectal bleeding or constipation caused by obstruction. The remaining tumors are scattered throughout the colon. Cecal carcinomas constitute about 10% of the entire group and are most likely to present with iron deficiency anemia caused by chronic blood loss. Radiology also plays an important role after treatment for colorectal cancer in the detection of recurrent disease, local and distant metastasis, and metachronous colon tumors.

## DIAGNOSTIC METHODS

### Contrast Enema

The radiologic examination of the colon can be performed with either single or double contrast technique. In most cases the double contrast enema is superior for the examination of the rectum[14] and the detection of small lesions.[15] In most series of double contrast studies, polyps are demonstrated in 10 to 13% of all patients,[16] whereas in single contrast studies polyps are found in 7% of patients.

### Colonoscopy

Many studies have claimed to show that colonoscopy is superior to contrast enema for the detection of polypoid lesions. However, most of these studies do not compare state-of-the-art techniques with operators of similar interest and experience. It is important to realize that there is an error rate inherent in colonoscopy. Part of this error rate derives from failure to reach the cecum in up to 25% of cases.[17] In addition, there are blind spots within the colon. Generally, these are behind folds or around flexures, and polyps or even large cancers in this regions are easily missed[18] (Fig. 64–2). If there are significant radiologic-endoscopic discrepancies, they should be resolved by consensus or by further examinations and it should not be assumed that the endoscopy result was correct.[19]

Colonoscopy and double contrast enema examination have comparable overall accuracy, with detection of approximately 90% of all polypoid lesions. However, the cost and complications of colonoscopy are considerably higher,[20] and we believe that this technique should be used selectively. Colonoscopy or flexible sigmoidoscopy should certainly be used to evaluate suggestive findings in contrast enema studies, particularly in patients with marked diverticular disease. It should also be used for biopsy of lesions and removal of polypoid lesions.

## Cross-sectional Imaging

Computed tomography (CT) has been used to reveal and stage many tumors, including primary and recurrent colorectal neoplasms,[21, 22] and has been joined by magnetic resonance (MR) imaging,[23, 24] transrectal sonography,[25, 26] scintigraphy with monoclonal antibody (MoAb) imaging,[27, 28] and positron emission tomography (PET).[29, 30]

Few studies present an in-depth assessment of the value of the various techniques. A review of the large body of literature on this topic reveals many conflicting reports on the effectiveness of the various methods and opposing recommendations for their use. In many instances, this is due to early, overly enthusiastic conclusions about high success rates with each new imaging technique and underestimation of their pitfalls. Also, some reports in the literature contained incomplete proof of pathology or neglected to include all factors necessary for complete staging of colon neoplasms.

This chapter includes the radiographic features of colorectal tumors as seen by CT, MR imaging, and transrectal ultrasound; assesses the accuracy of each imaging method; and defines the role of these techniques in detecting and staging colon neoplasms at the present time.

## BENIGN EPITHELIAL POLYPS

### Incidence

Benign tumors of the colon are extremely common and usually do not cause symptoms. These polyps have been reported in 10 to 12.5% of patients studied with double contrast techniques, and the incidence rises dramatically with increasing age (Fig. 64–3A). The polyps occur most frequently in the left colon and are scattered throughout the remainder of the transverse and right colon (Fig. 64–3B). It has been reported that, with increasing age of the population, there is a shift in the incidence of polyps to the right side of the colon coinciding with a shift in the distribution of colon carcinoma to the right.[31]

### Pathology

In most cases, the role of radiology is to detect the presence of a polyp. The term *polyp* refers only to a focal, protruded lesion within the bowel. In general

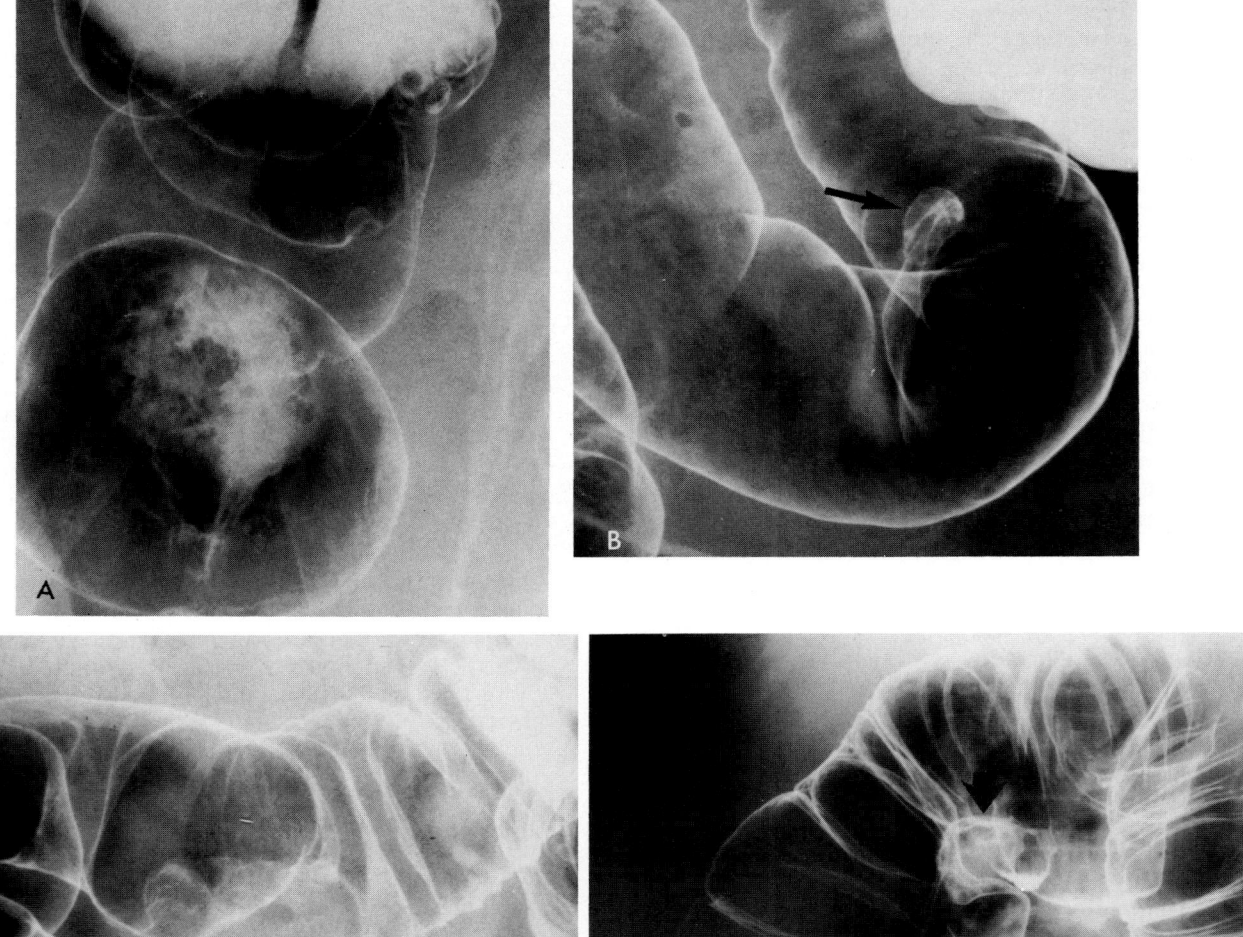

**Figure 64–2. Lesions missed at endoscopy. A.** There is a small sessile polyp behind a fold at the rectosigmoid junction. This lesion was missed twice on sigmoidoscopy and was finally detected at the third sigmoidoscopic examination. **B.** A small polyp situated behind a fold at an area of angulation at the junction of the sigmoid and the descending colon. This polyp was missed on two colonoscopic examinations and was found on the third. (**B** from Laufer I, Smith NC, Mullens JE: The radiological demonstration of colorectal polyps undetected by endoscopy. Gastroenterology 70:167–170, 1976.) **C.** Polypoid carcinoma just proximal to the rectosigmoid junction. This lesion was missed on several sigmoidoscopic and colonoscopic examinations and was confirmed only at surgery. **D.** Polypoid carcinoma at the hepatic flexure missed on initial colonoscopy.

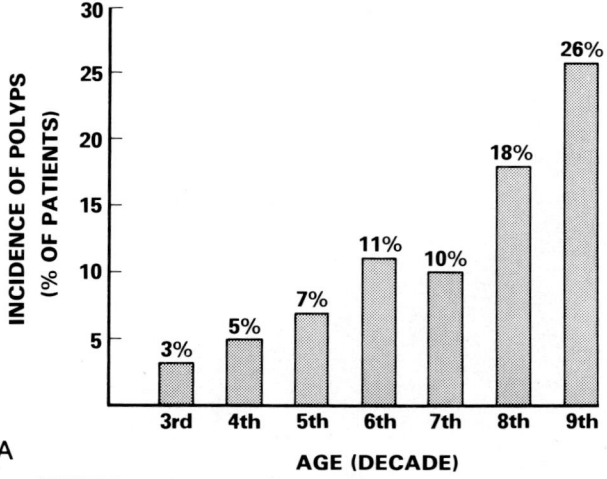

A

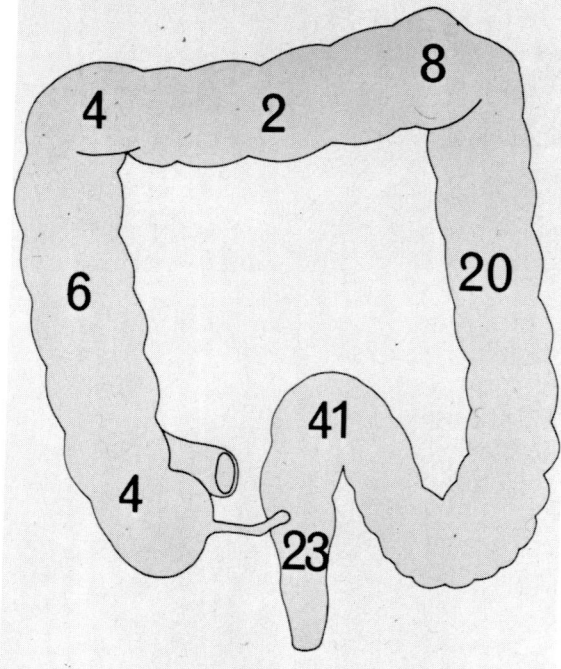

B

**Figure 64–3. Incidence and distribution of colorectal polyps. A.** Incidence of colonic polyps related to age (based on 800 consecutive double contrast enemas). There is an increasing incidence of colonic polyps, ranging from 3% in the third decade of life to 26% in the ninth decade. (From Laufer I: The double contrast enema: myths and misconceptions. Gastrointest Radiol 1:19–31, 1976.) **B.** Distribution of colorectal polyps (based on 108 consecutive polyps). Approximately 60% of the polyps are in the rectum and sigmoid colon.

terms, a polyp may be neoplastic or non-neoplastic. Most non-neoplastic polyps are either inflammatory or hyperplastic. They are generally small and occur most frequently in the distal colon. Neoplastic polyps may represent true neoplasms of any component of the bowel wall. However, epithelial neoplasms—adenomas—are of the most interest because of their relationship to colorectal carcinoma. It is emphasized that the demonstration of a polypoid lesion does not necessarily give information regarding its pathologic nature. Whenever

possible, polyps more than 1 cm in diameter must be removed, preferably by endoscopic polypectomy (Fig. 64–4).

Most colonic adenomas are tubular adenomas. However, tubular adenomas have various degrees of villous change, and as a polyp becomes larger the degree of villous change increases. At the other end of the spectrum, some polyps are villous adenomas because the surface consists of frond-like structures arising from the base of the mucosa. Thus, there may be a transition from tubular adenoma to tubulovillous adenoma to villous adenoma. It has been suggested that any adenoma with more than 75% villous change should be referred to as a villous adenoma.[32] In general, the risk of carcinoma is related to the proportion of villous change in an adenoma.

In small adenomas, it maybe impossible to distinguish villous change radiologically. However, as the adenoma becomes larger and the proportion of villous change increases, a reticular or granular mucosal surface may be seen[33] (Fig. 64–5A). Large villous adenomas have an atypical radiologic appearance.[34] They are large, bulky polypoid masses with barium caught between the frond-like protrusions producing a lacy surface pattern (Fig. 64–5B). Large villous tumors should be removed in toto because malignant degeneration may occur in only a portion of the tumor and random biopsy sampling is unreliable for the detection of malignant change.

Other non-neoplastic polyps may also be found in the colon. These include juvenile polyps, which may be single or multiple and may be found in adults and in children. Hamartomatous polyps are found in patients with Peutz-Jeghers syndrome and inflammatory polyps in patients with Cronkhite-Canada syndrome (see Chapter 66).

## Polyp Detection

A polyp is simply a protrusion of the mucosa into the bowel lumen. Therefore, it may be demonstrated as a radiolucent filling defect, as a contour defect, or as a ring shadow (see Chapter 4). The greatest and most frequent difficulty arises in distinguishing polyps from fecal residue. In general, fecal residue is mobile and is usually found on the dependent surface in the barium pool. In addition, several features may suggest that the filling defect represents a true polyp. These include the "bowler hat" sign (Fig. 64–6A) and the "Mexican hat" sign (Fig. 64–6B). Although the bowler hat sign can also be produced by a diverticulum, the direction of the dome of the bowler hat distinguishes a polyp and a diverticulum.[35] When the dome of the hat points away from the axis of the bowel, the lesion is a diverticulum; when the dome points toward the lumen of the bowel, it is a polyp. These signs are illustrated and discussed in detail in Chapter 4.

Rubesin and co-workers used the term *carpet lesion* to describe a flat, lobulated lesion that is manifest primarily as an alteration in the surface texture of the bowel[36] (Fig. 64–7A). These lesions may be quite large and are mostly tubular adenomas with varying degrees

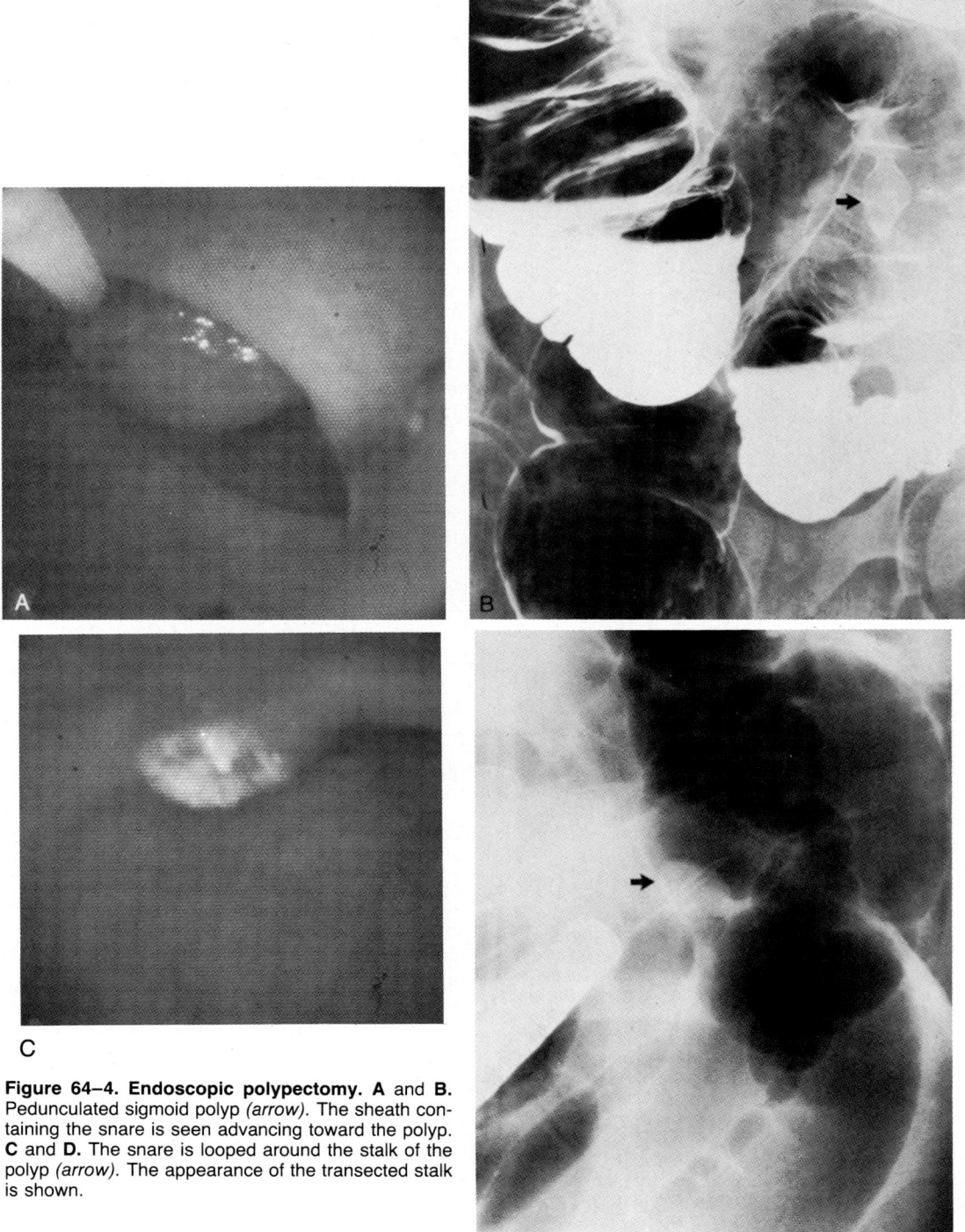

**Figure 64–4. Endoscopic polypectomy. A** and **B.**
Pedunculated sigmoid polyp *(arrow).* The sheath containing the snare is seen advancing toward the polyp.
**C** and **D.** The snare is looped around the stalk of the
polyp *(arrow).* The appearance of the transected stalk
is shown.

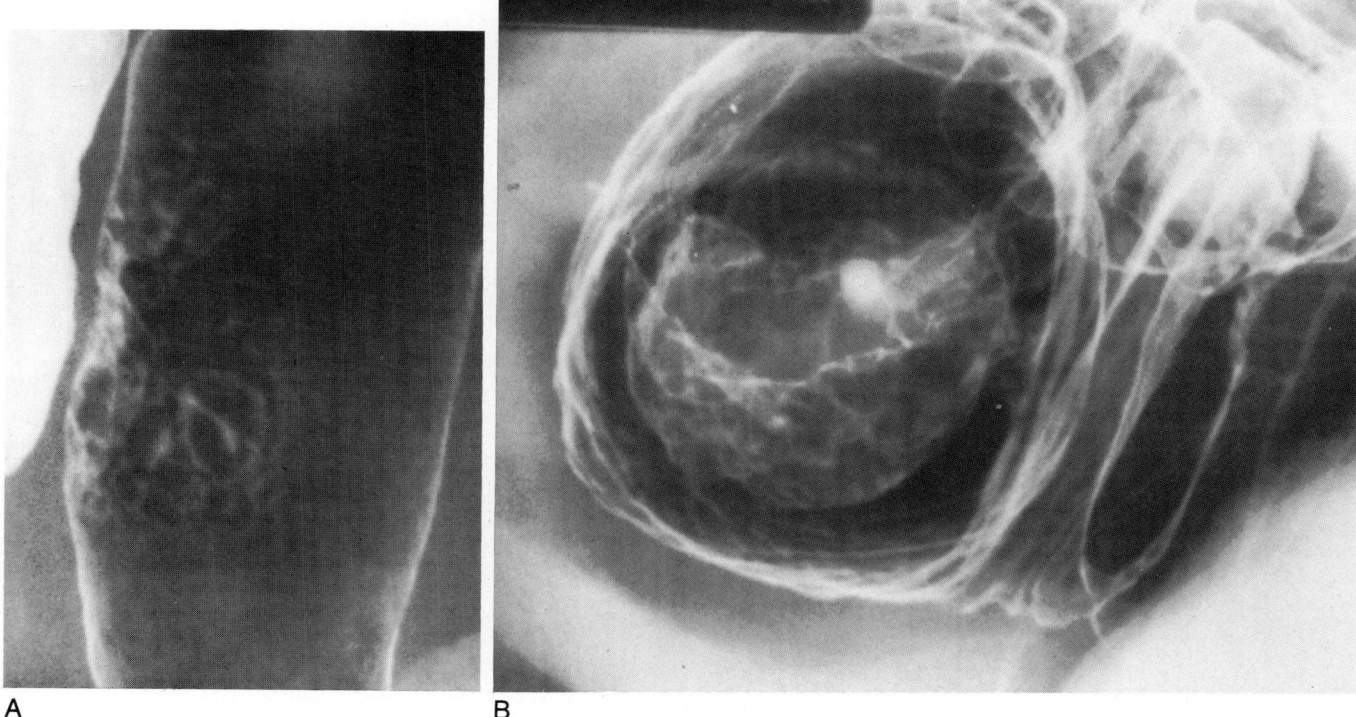

A
B

**Figure 64–5. Villous tumors. A.** A flat tumor in the descending colon with an irregular surface suggestive of a villous adenoma. This was a villoglandular polyp. **B.** Typical villous tumor in the sigmoid colon. This tumor exhibits the typical, irregular, frond-like surface of a villous tumor. It was a malignant villous adenoma.

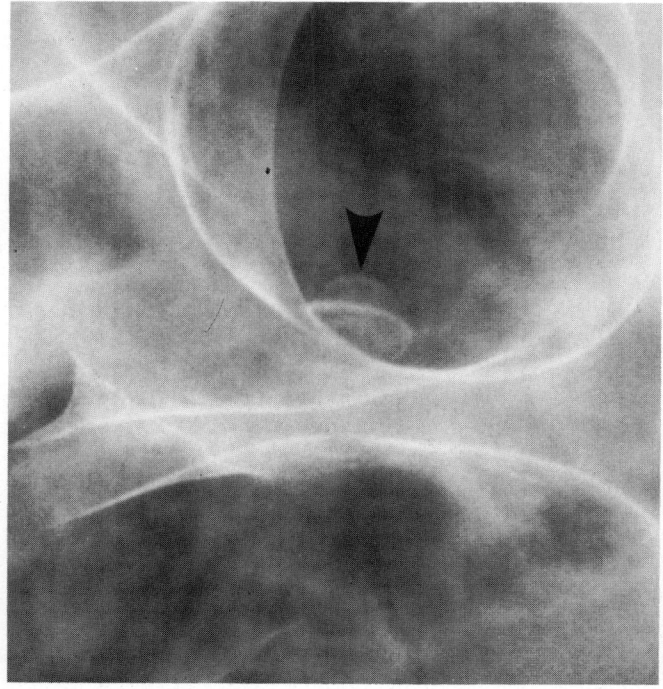

A

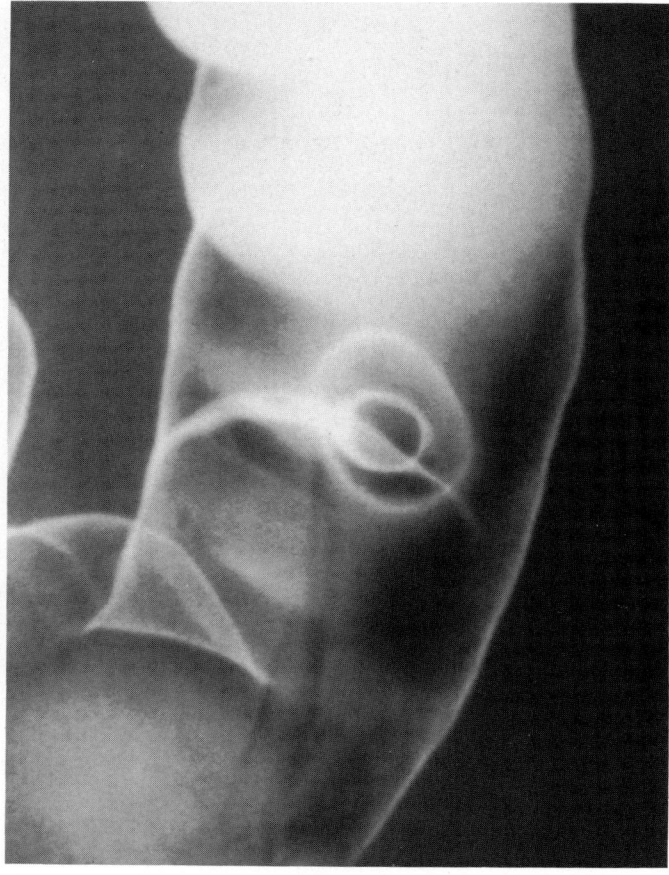

B

**Figure 64–6. Features of polyps. A.** The bowler hat sign representing a sessile polyp. **B.** Mexican hat sign. This is the typical appearance of a pedunculated polyp seen end-on. The outer ring represents the head of the polyp and the inner ring represents the stalk.

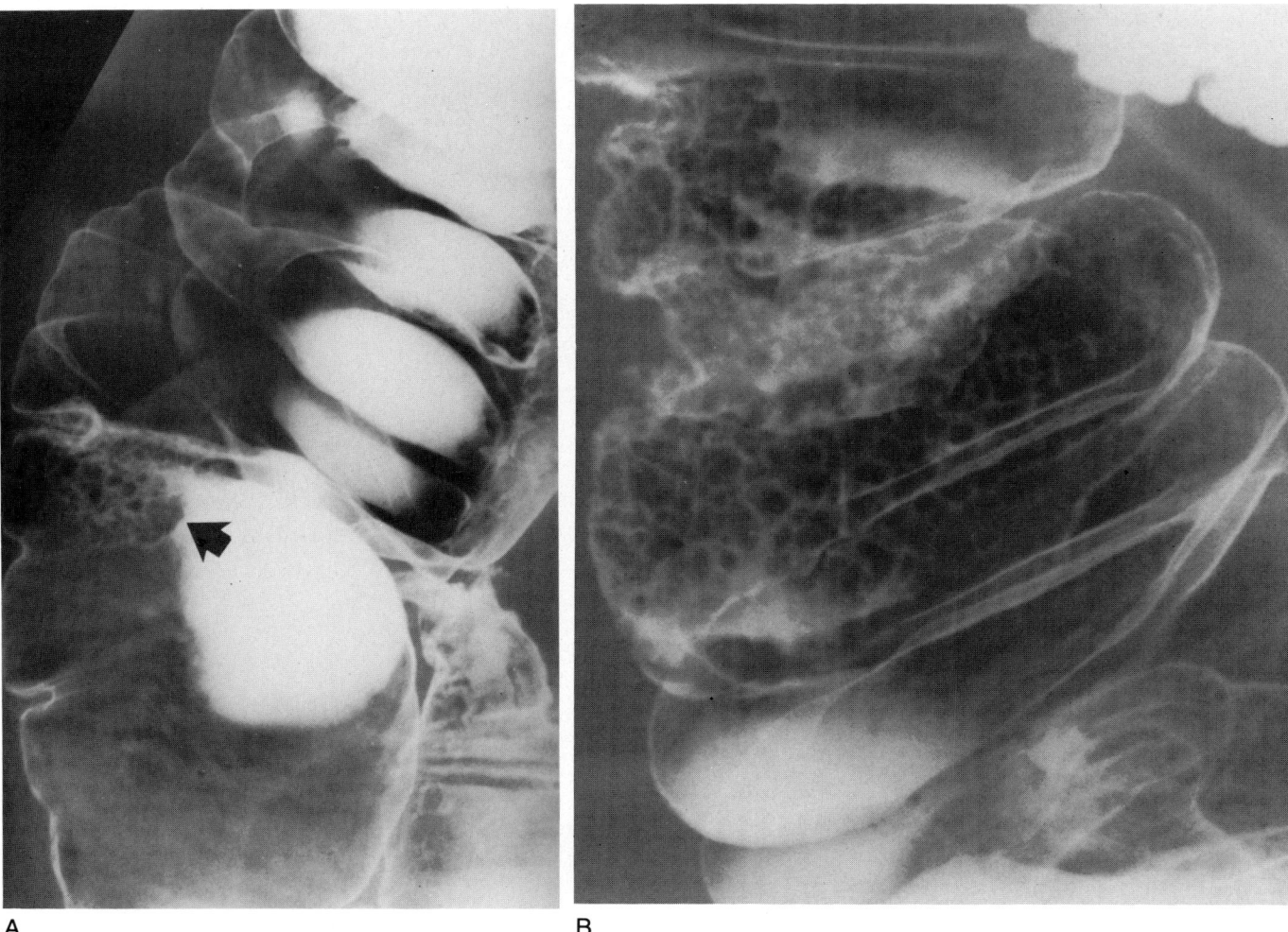

A                  B

**Figure 64–7. Carpet lesions. A.** Typical carpet lesion *(arrow)* in the cecum. **B.** Malignant transformation in a carpet lesion. An obvious polypoid carcinoma is seen in the ascending colon. Surrounding the polypoid lesion is the mucosal change representing the underlying adenoma.

of villous change. In some cases of colorectal carcinoma, the background of a benign carpet lesion can be recognized (Fig. 64–7B).

## Cross-sectional Imaging

Benign lesions of the colon such as hyperplastic polyps or adenomatous polyps are usually not examined by CT or MR imaging. They are demonstrated by barium examinations or by one of the endoscopic techniques and are seen during CT or MR examinations only incidentally. These techniques are used only if these benign tumors become large enough to have a high likelihood of harboring a malignancy. Benign polyps appear as sessile soft tissue masses that protrude into the lumen of the bowel (Fig. 64–8). They are usually detected only if the patient has undergone colonic cleansing or if the polyp is large. If the polyp is pedunculated, CT scans may demonstrate a large polypoid mass that represents the combined polyp and stalk.

Coscina and colleagues suggested that villous adeno-

mas have a characteristic CT appearance based on their high mucus content.[37] The CT features of villous adenomas include homogeneous water density (<10 Hounsfield units) occupying more than half of the lesion and located eccentrically on the luminal side of the mass. No air-fluid level is seen, and the lesion should not have a round cystic configuration. Opaque oral or rectal contrast material should not be used to diagnose a suspected villous adenoma because it obscures the lesion. In these cases, insufflation of air or oily substance administered per rectum may be of help. Because of their malignant potential, larger villous adenomas should always be staged by CT.

On MR images, benign polyps appear as low-density structures on T1-weighted spin-echo sequences and as masses of intermediate or high signal intensity on T2-weighted spin-echo sequences. If there are many mucin-producing cells, the signal intensity of the polypoid mass increases on T1-weighted sequences. Transrectal ultrasound is used for assessment of sessile polyps large enough to have an increased risk for malignancy. In these cases, transrectal ultrasound can be used to deter-

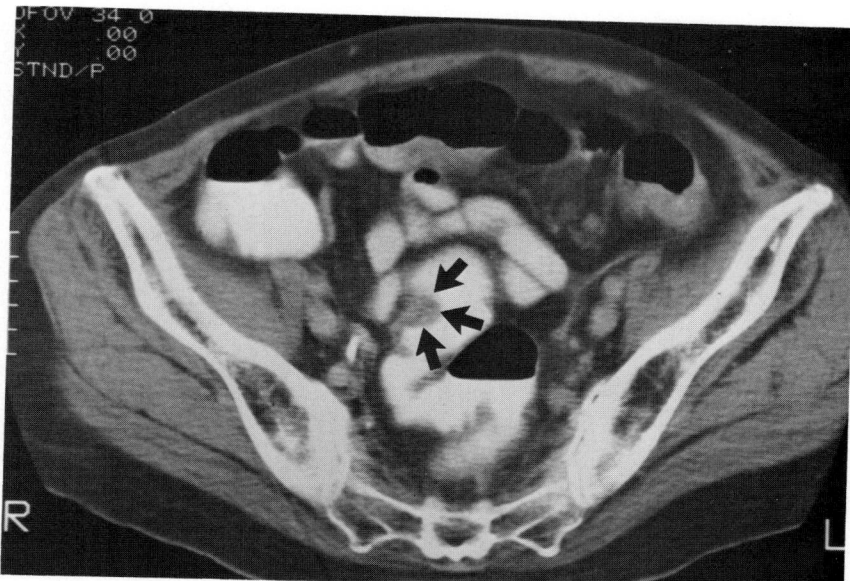

**Figure 64–8. CT scan of benign polyp.** A sessile polyp *(arrows)* identified on the right wall of the sigmoid colon was confirmed by colonscopy in a patient with carcinoma of the rectosigmoid junction.

mine the depth of invasion by a sessile mass that protrudes into the lumen. The depth of invasion is best assessed by transrectal ultrasound because it is the only method that can demonstrate the various layers of the colonic wall. If the intraluminal component is large, false tumor measurements and erroneous depiction of the surface of the mass can occur because of compression of the tumor by the transrectal probe (see also Chapter 10).

## ADENOCARCINOMA

### Early Cancer

The radiologic detection of early colorectal cancer is basically an exercise in the detection of polyps. The typical early colon cancer is a flat, sessile lesion that may produce a contour defect (Fig. 64–9). Although most polyps detected radiologically should be removed if they are more than 5 mm in diameter, a number of radiologic criteria have been used for the detection of malignancy in colorectal polyps.[38] The size of the polyp is the most important criterion. Carcinoma is virtually nonexistent in polyps smaller than 5 mm. The incidence of cancer is approximately 1% in the 5- to 10-mm range (Fig. 64–10), and polyps larger than 2 cm have a 50% chance of being malignant.[39]

Malignant polyps tend to grow more quickly than benign polyps, although there is considerable overlap between the two groups.[40] If there is definite evidence of polyp growth on serial examinations, malignancy should be suspected.

The presence of a long thin stalk is generally a sign of a benign polyp. However, rarely, such polyps harbor malignancy.[41] As a rule, the stalk associated with carcinoma is short and thick (Fig. 64–11).

If the head of the polyp is irregular or lobulated, the probability of malignancy is greater, although some benign polyps may have an irregular or lobulated surface.

### Advanced Cancer

The majority of patients with symptomatic colorectal carcinoma have advanced lesions. These lesions are generally annular or polypoid tumors seen as filling defects in the barium column or as contour defects. In addition, plaque-like lesions can produce abnormal lines on double contrast study (Figs. 64–12 and 64–13).

Advanced cancers are often associated with "sentinel" polyps or additional polyps elsewhere in the colon. Approximately 5% of patients who have a colon carcinoma have additional, synchronous carcinomas in the

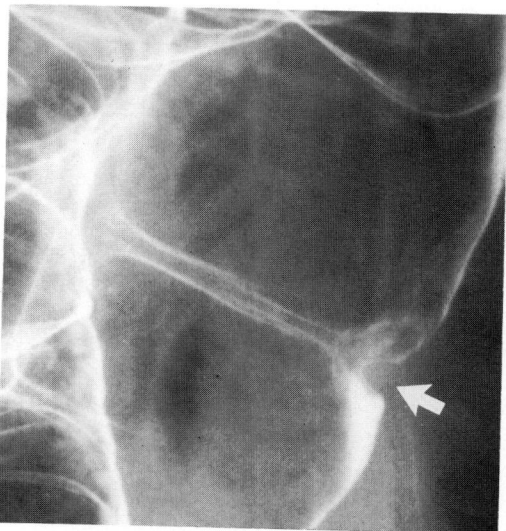

**Figure 64–9. Typical early colon cancer.** A 1-cm polypoid mass with a contour defect *(arrow)* is seen along the lateral wall.

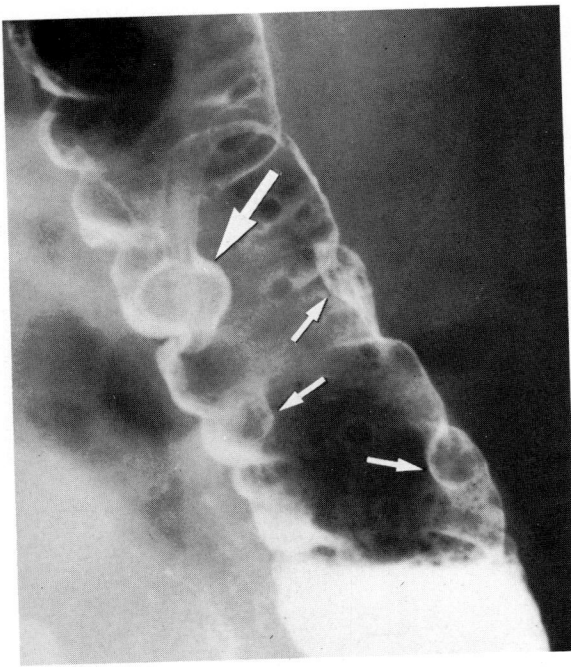

**Figure 64–10. Early colon cancers.** Polypoid carcinoma with a pedicle in a 29-year-old male with rectal bleeding. A pedunculated polyp in the descending colon *(large arrow)* has a typically benign appearance. This was removed at colonoscopy and was found to be a carcinoma with invasion of the stalk. The smaller lesions *(small arrows)* were hyperplastic polyps. (From Laufer I: The double contrast enema: myths and misconceptions. Gastrointest Radiol 1:19–31, 1976.)

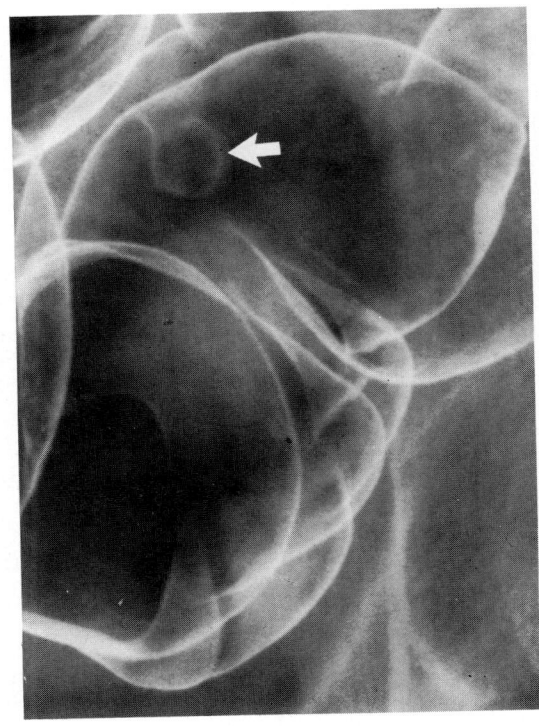

**Figure 64–11. Pedunculated early cancer.** Early carcinoma *(arrow)* with a short, thick stalk.

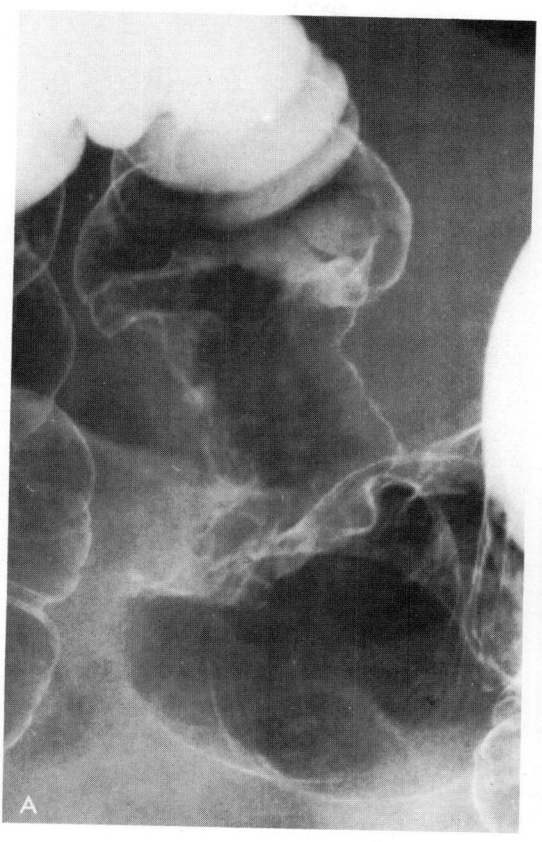

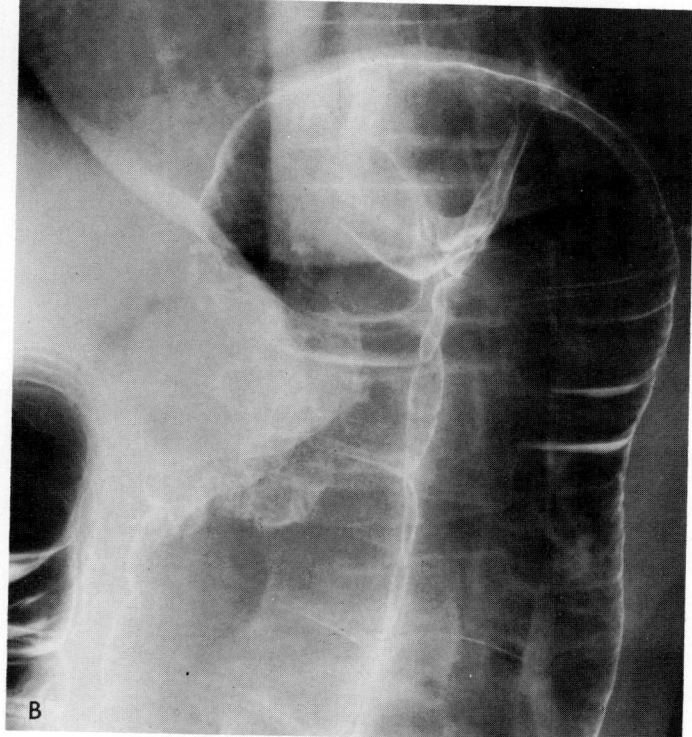

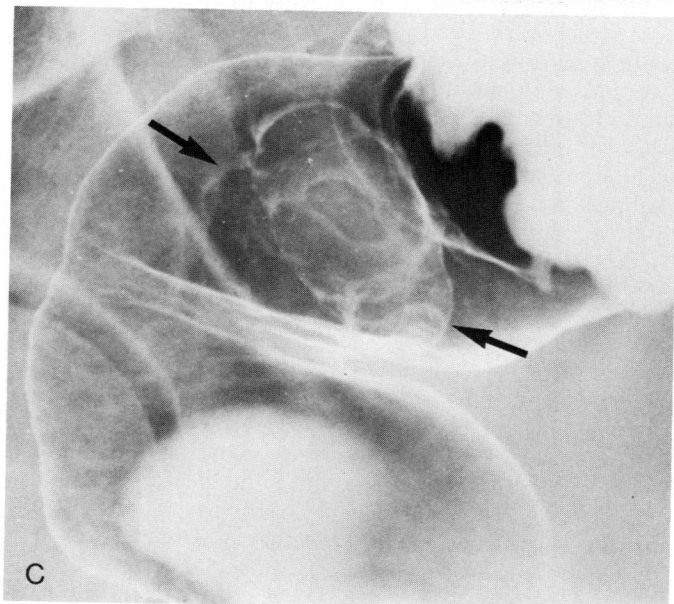

**Figure 64–12. Advanced colon cancers. A.** Typical advanced colon carcinoma. **A.** Annular, "apple core" lesion. **B.** Large polypoid carcinoma at the splenic flexure. **C.** Lateral view shows an ulcerated plaque-like carcinoma etched in white *(arrows)* at the recto-sigmoid junction.

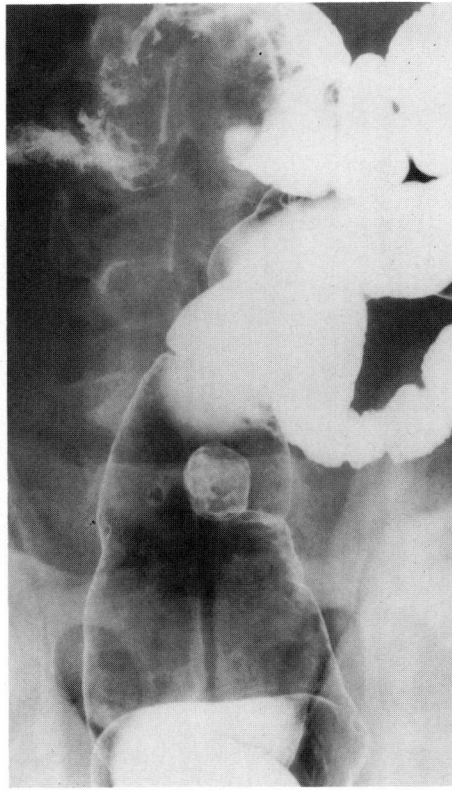

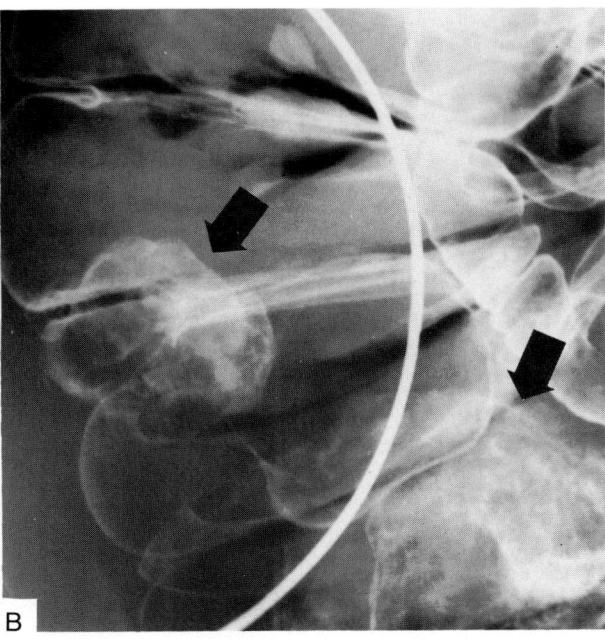

**Figure 64–13. Synchronous tumors. A.** A nearly obstructing polypoid carcinoid is seen in the transverse colon and a second adenoma is seen in the sigmoid colon. **B.** Multiple polypoid carcinomas *(arrows)* in the ascending colon.

colon[42] (see Fig. 64–13). Therefore, whenever possible, the entire colon should be examined even when a carcinoma is encountered in the distal bowel.

Carcinomas are particularly difficult to detect in patients with extensive diverticular disease of the sigmoid colon (Fig. 64–14). If the radiologic examination leaves any doubt regarding the presence of a carcinoma, flexible sigmoidoscopy should be recommended to confirm or exclude lesions in the sigmoid colon.

Advanced carcinoma may have an atypical appearance. The linitis plastica type of carcinoma has predominant submucosal infiltration and fibrous reaction.[43] The radiologic appearance may be suggestive of an inflammatory stricture. This type of carcinoma is particularly likely to develop in patients with ulcerative colitis (see Chapter 62).

## Complications

The most important complications of colorectal cancer include bleeding, bowel obstruction, and perforation. Massive rectal bleeding caused by colon carcinoma is rare; the bleeding is more often manifest as occult blood in the stool or as chronic anemia. Colorectal cancer is one of the major causes of large bowel obstruction (see Chapter 67). Obstruction may be caused by encroachment of the tumor mass on the lumen of the bowel (Fig. 64–15A). Antegrade obstruction and retrograde obstruction tend to be poorly correlated. Frequently, during the barium enema examination, there is a high-grade

obstruction of the retrograde flow of barium when the patient has few or no symptoms of clinical obstruction. In the case of polypoid tumors, obstruction may also be caused by colocolic intussusception (Fig. 64–15B). In patients with long-standing obstruction and colon distention, mucosal ischemia may result in an ulcerative form of colitis affecting the colon proximal to the obstruction.

Advanced cancer may result in perforation of the

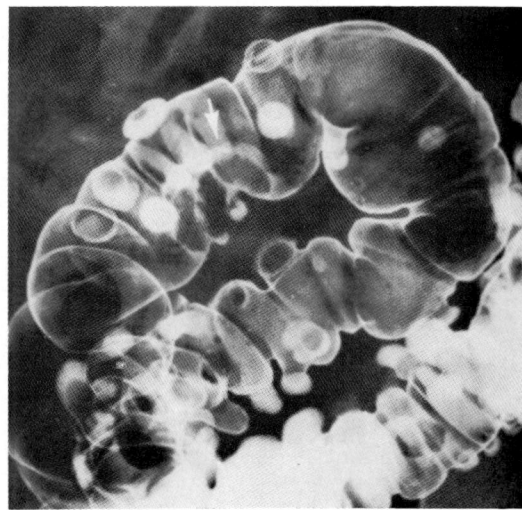

**Figure 64–14. Carcinoma in a patient with diverticulosis.** The polypoid carcinoma *(arrow)* is more difficult to recognize in the presence of extensive diverticulosis.

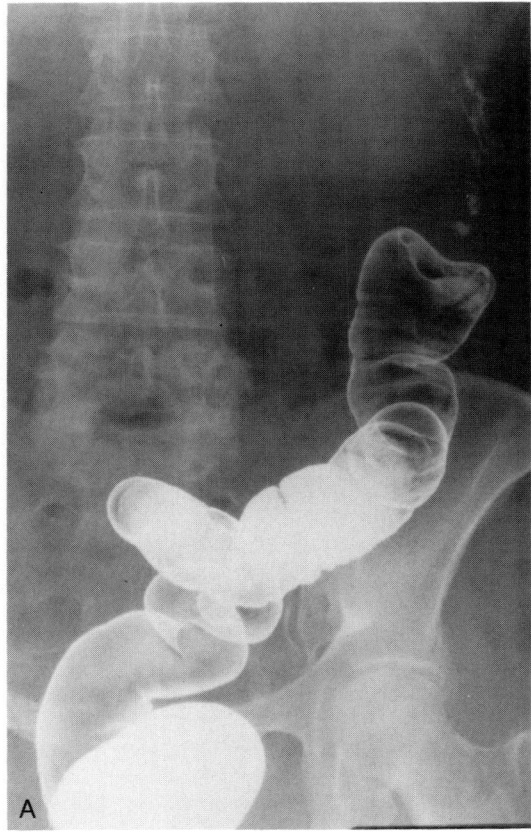

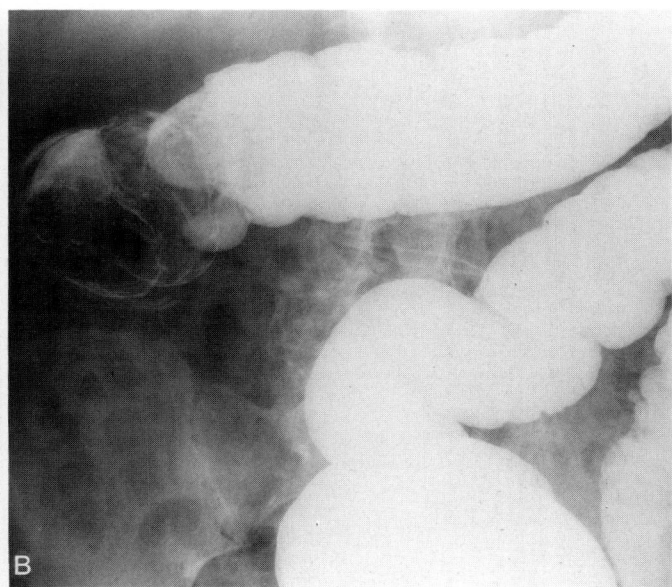

**Figure 64–15. Bowel obstruction by colon carcinoma. A.** An annular carcinoma in the mid-descending colon completely obstructs the retrograde flow of barium. **B.** Cecal carcinoma with colocolic intussusception extending into the midtransverse colon.

colon and a pericolic abscess (Fig. 64–16A). The signs and symptoms and even the radiologic appearances may be difficult to distinguish from those of a pericolic abscess associated with diverticulitis (Fig. 64–16B). However, evidence of gastrointestinal blood loss makes a malignant origin much more likely.[44] Perforation of the colon may lead to a fistula to adjacent organs such as the stomach (Fig. 64–17A), duodenum (Fig. 64–17B), bladder, or vagina. The fistulous communication can be demonstrated by barium study or by the extracolonic presence of gas or contrast medium on CT scans.

## COMPUTED TOMOGRAPHY

### Primary Colorectal Carcinoma

CT and transrectal sonography are better for evaluation of tumor stage than manual examination, barium enema, or fiberoptic techniques. Both CT and sonography may image a colorectal cancer as a discrete mass or focal wall thickening (Fig. 64–18), but this is a nonspecific finding and requires further exploration. This wall thickening may involve the entire circumference of the large bowel section without or with extension beyond the bowel wall (Fig. 64–19). If the tumor is contained within the wall of the colon or rectum, the outer margins of the large bowel appear smooth. However, cross-sectional methods such as CT are not sensitive enough to detect microscopic invasion of the fat

surrounding the colon or rectum (Fig. 64–20). Local adenopathy may or may not be visualized, depending on the size and separability from the main mass (Fig. 64–21A).

Extension of tumor beyond the bowel wall is manifest on cross sections as a mass with irregular borders with or without strands of soft tissue extending from the outer rectal-colonic margin into the perirectal or pericolonic fat. Extracolonic tumor spread is also suggested by loss of tissue fat planes between the large bowel and surrounding muscles—levator ani, obturator internis, piriformis (Fig. 64–21B), coccygeal, and gluteus maximus. However, invasion is definite only when a tumor mass extends directly into an adjacent muscle, obliterating the fat plane and enlarging the individual muscle. Spread to contiguous organs in the pelvis can be simulated by absence of tissue planes between the viscera and the tumor mass without actual invasion. Obliteration of fat planes can be caused by vascular or lymphatic congestion, inflammation, or actual absence of fat because of severe cachexia. Therefore, invasion should be diagnosed cautiously and considered definite only if a major portion of the viscus is enveloped or if an obvious mass also involves an adjacent organ (Fig. 64–22). Distinction between tumor infiltration of adjacent muscle and simple absence of fat separating normal structures is particularly difficult in the area of lower rectum and anal verge.

In our experience, CT results can be improved through the use of a large and rapidly delivered bolus and dynamic scanning with thin sections (3- to 5-mm

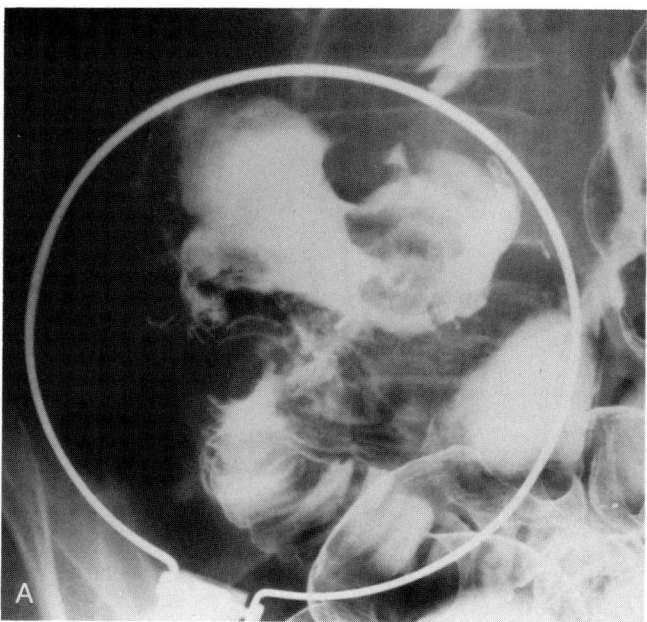

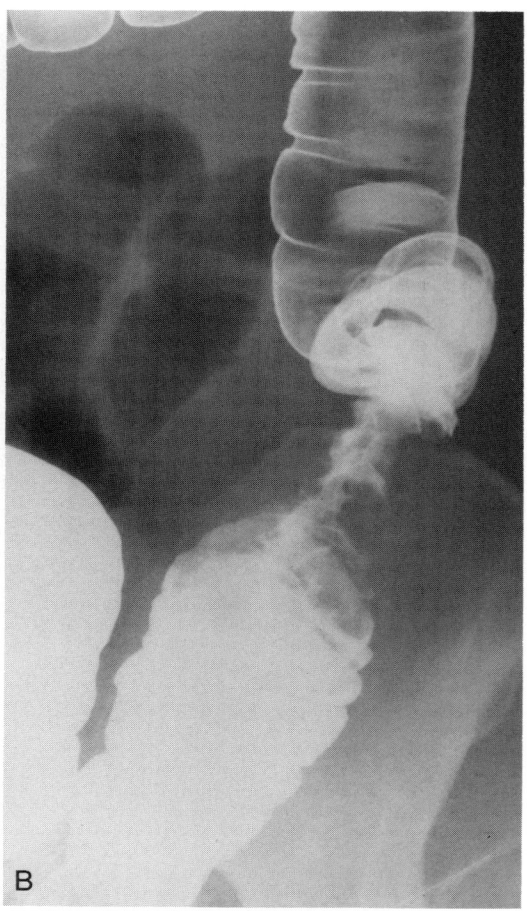

**Figure 64–16. Perforated carcinoma of the colon. A.** Barium filling of a perforation caused by recurrent carcinoma of the colon at the hepatic flexure. **B.** In another patient, a tapered narrowing in the sigmoid colon is due to a pericolic abscess resulting from perforation of a sigmoid carcinoma. The appearance may be difficult to distinguish from that of diverticulitis.

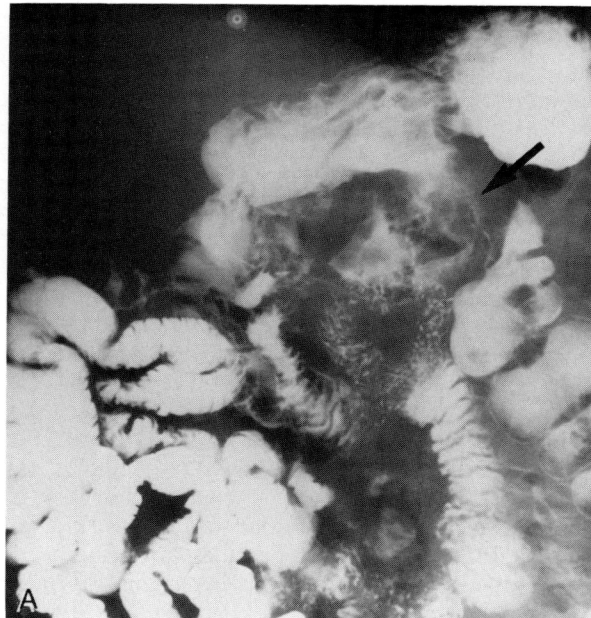

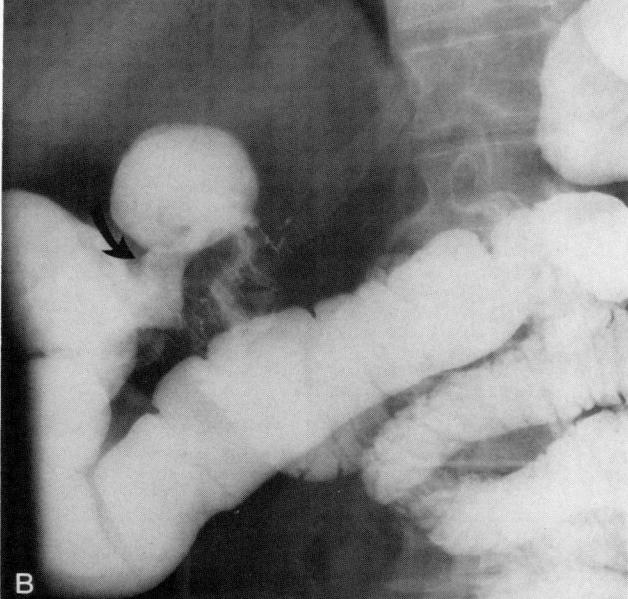

**Figure 64–17. Fistulas complicating carcinoma of the colon. A.** Gastrocolic fistula arising from a carcinoma at the splenic flexure *(arrow)*. **B.** A carcinoma of the transverse colon giving rise to a fistula to the duodenum *(arrow)*.

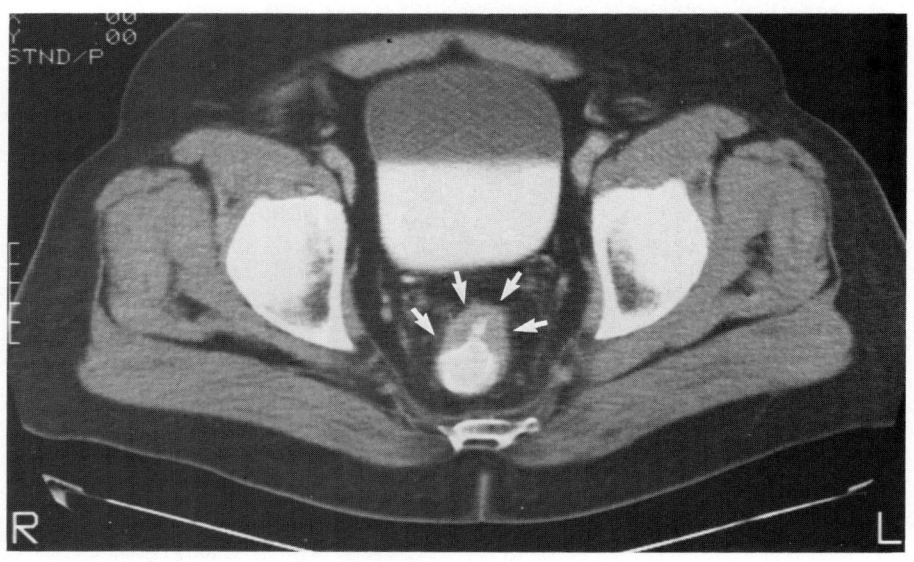

**Figure 64–18. Rectal carcinoma infiltrating the submucosa.** TNM stage T1, N0, M0 (Dukes' stage A). Focal thickening of the anterior rectal wall *(arrows)* is seen with extension to both lateral rectal walls. The outer margin of the rectum is well preserved and no adenopathy is identified. (CT stage II.)

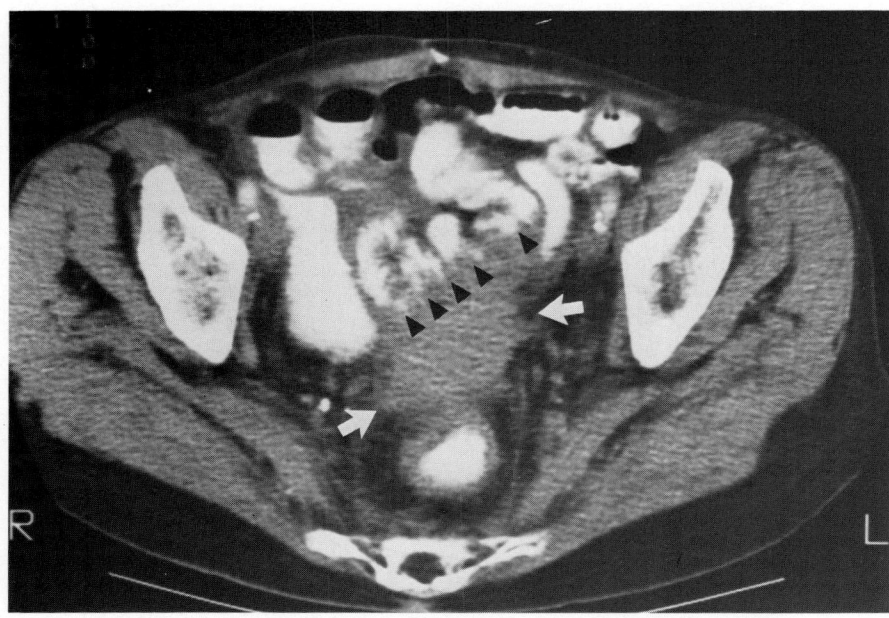

**Figure 64–19. CT scan of invasive sigmoid adenocarcinoma.** TNM stage T3, N0, M0 (Dukes' classification B2). A large tumor mass *(arrows)* invades the adjacent small bowel *(arrowheads)* as evidenced by partial encasement and spiculation of folds in this well-opacified jejunal loop (CT stage IIIA).

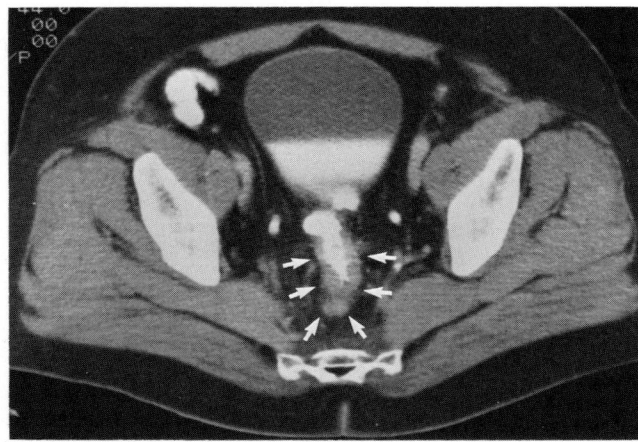

**Figure 64–20. CT scan of rectal tumor with microscopic invasion of fat.** TNM stage T3, N0, M0 (Dukes' stage B2). Thickening of the posterior and both lateral walls of the rectum is seen *(arrows)*. No definite soft tissue stranding is noted in the perirectal fat. (Understaged as CT stage II because of inability to detect microinvasion of tumor into fat.)

**Figure 64–21. Extension of tumor beyond the bowel wall. A.** Rectal carcinoma with invasion of perirectal fat *(solid arrows)* and focal adenopathy *(open arrows)*. TNM stage T3, N1, M0 (Dukes' stage C2). **B.** Rectal carcinoma with direct extension into the piriformis muscles, sacrum, and uterus. TNM stage T3, N0, M0 (Dukes' stage B2). A large soft tissue mass *(open arrows)* is seen invading the piriformis muscles *(solid arrows)*. Invasion of the body of the uterus is also seen *(curved arrows)* with complete obliteration of the rectal lumen (CT stage IIIB).

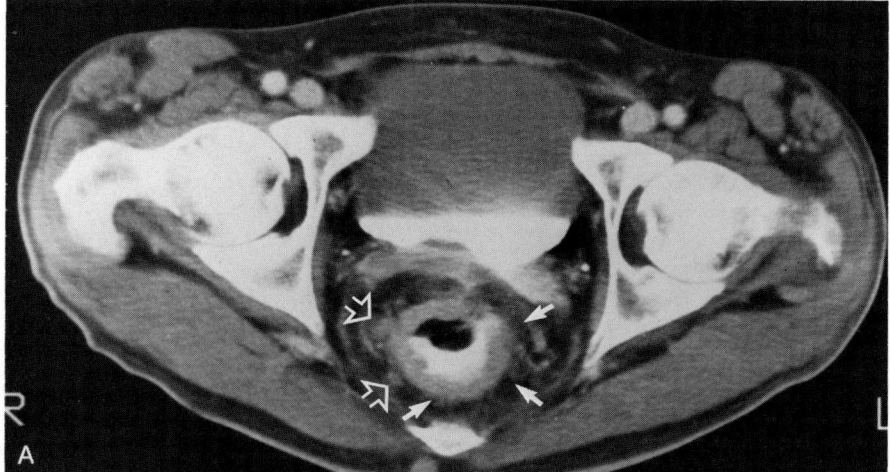

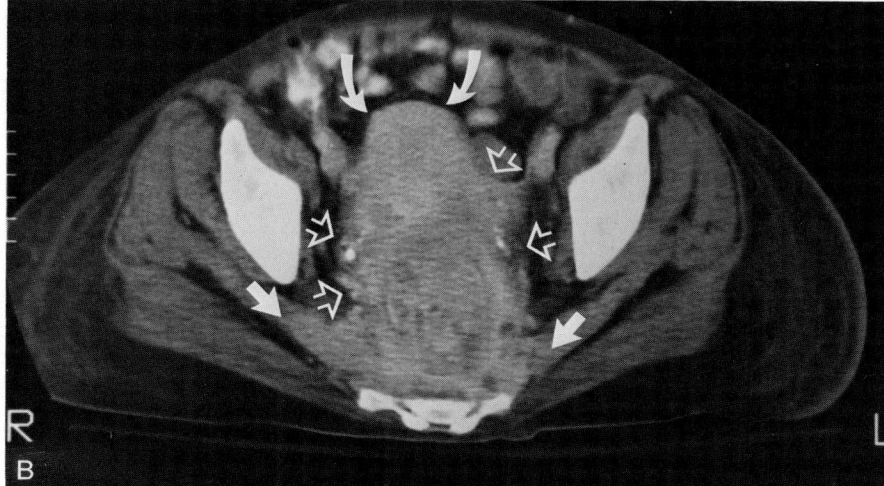

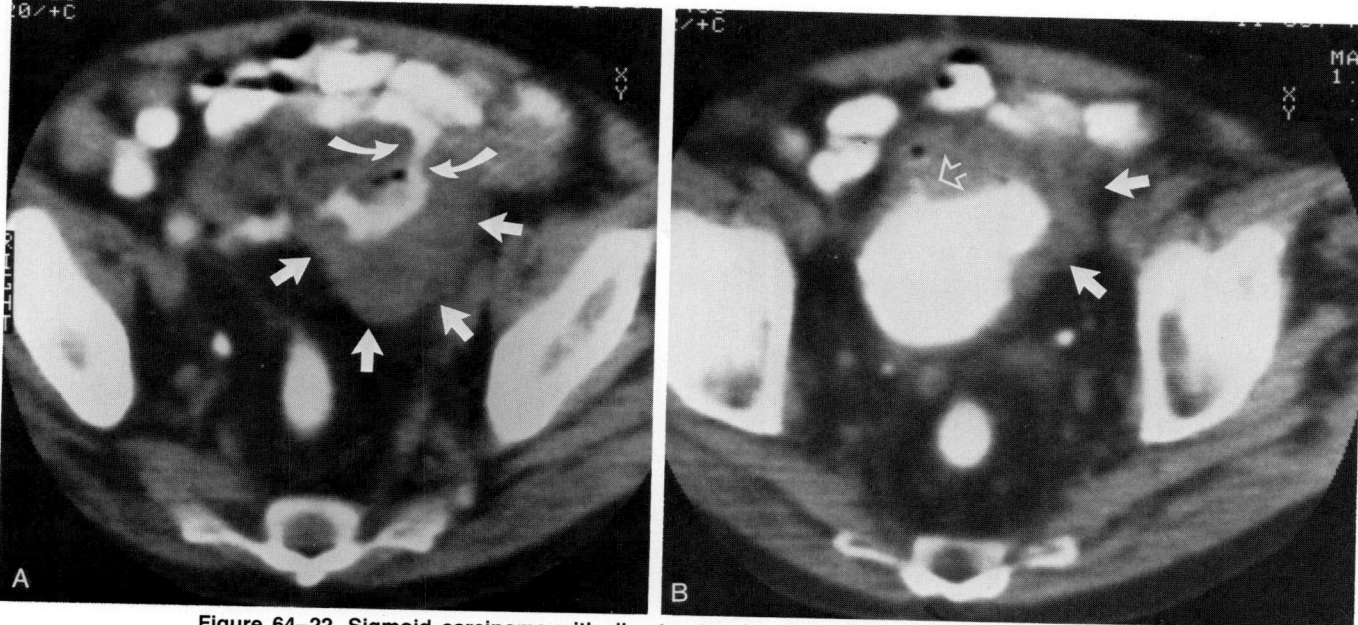

**Figure 64–22. Sigmoid carcinoma with direct extension into bladder.** TNM stage T3, N0, M0 (Dukes' stage B2). **A.** A large tumor mass *(straight arrows)* is seen with contiguous thickening of bladder wall and a fistulous tract *(curved arrows)* (CT stage IIIA). **B.** At a level 2 cm below, thickening of the bladder wall *(solid arrows)* and a small fistulous tract *(open arrow)* are seen.

slices). With the advent of fast CT scanners using either electron beam or helical scanning (slip ring) technology, results can be further improved. Nevertheless, CT appears to have a hard time matching or even surpassing the resolution of soft tissue density differences that MR imaging can provide in the pelvis with or without fat suppression and with or without gadolinium enhancement.

Primary and recurrent colon cancer can invade the seminal vesicles, prostate, bladder (see Fig. 64–22), uterus, ovaries, small bowel (see Fig. 64–19), and sciatic nerves and can produce hydronephrosis by obstructing the ureters. Occasionally, tumors of the prostate, uterus, or ovaries that invade or are contiguous with the rectum or sigmoid colon can be indistinguishable from an invasive colon neoplasm. Tumor necrosis is suggested by areas of low attenuation within the mass, and tumor calcifications indicate a mucinous adenocarcinoma. Occasionally, a fistulous tract can be visualized between the rectum and the bladder by demonstrating air in the tract and air in the bladder. After administration of an intravenous contrast agent, the wall of the tract may be enhanced or a jet of rectal contrast material can be seen to enter the bladder when the patient is scanned in the prone position. Fistulous tracts can also extend into the uterus or vagina and sinus tracts may be seen in the fat of the ischiorectal fossa.

Colon tumors can destroy adjacent bone. Destruction most frequently involves the sacrum and coccyx (Fig. 64–23), but large tumors can involve the ilium. When advanced, invasion of bone is easily diagnosed by identifying bone destruction and evidence of a soft tissue mass adjacent to and within bone. However, minor invasion of bone can be diagnosed only if cortical destruction is seen. Careful analysis of the pelvis using a bone "window" is essential in these cases.

Liver metastases are usually recognized as areas of low attenuation before enhancement, although foci of calcification can be seen within metastatic mucinous adenocarcinomas (Fig. 64–24). After a bolus injection of contrast material, the CT density of hepatic colonic metastasis can change rapidly. The metastatic deposits

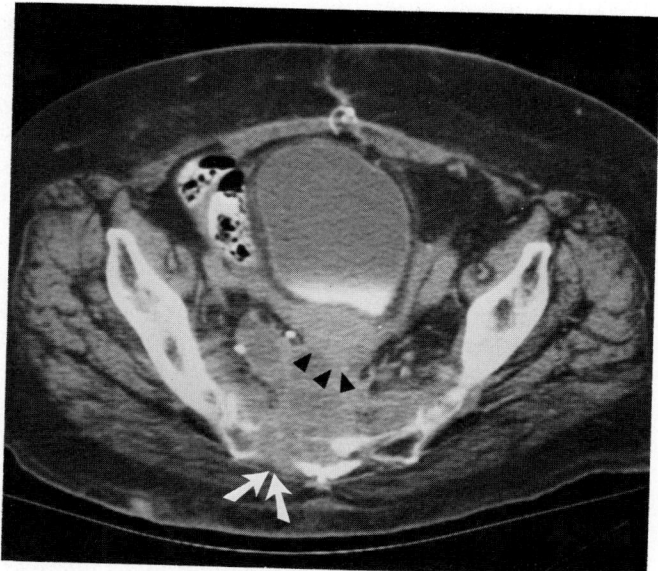

**Figure 64–23. Rectal tumor with adenopathy and direct invasion of bone.** TNM stage T3, N1, M0 (Dukes' classification C2). A large presacral mass extends into the sacrum with destruction of bone *(arrows)*. Note direct extension of mass into uterus *(arrowheads)*. Nodes are inseparable from mass.

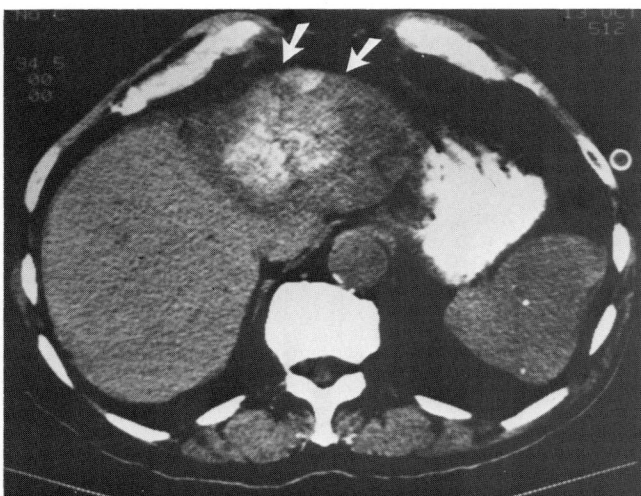

**Figure 64–24. Calcified metastasis to liver in a patient with known metastatic colon carcinoma.** Stippled calcifications *(arrows)* in the left lobe of liver are highly suggestive of mucinous tumor. This patient was studied without intravenous contrast agent because of a severe iodine allergy. (CT stage IV.)

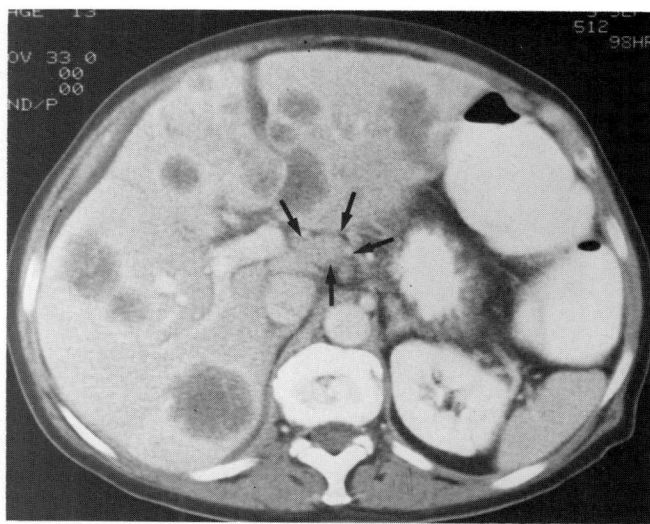

**Figure 64–25. CT with arterial portography showing diffuse liver metastases from invasive mucinous colon carcinoma.** TNM stage T3, N1, M1 (Dukes' stage D). Multiple low-density lesions with peripheral enhancing rims are seen in all segments of the liver. Portal adenopathy *(arrows)* is also seen. (CT stage IV.)

often show early rim enhancement or become uniformly hyperdense, go through an isodense phase, and finally again become low-density lesions. Optimal bolus technique is necessary to avoid false-negative results with metastases that have become isointense with normal liver parenchyma. Such isointensity often occurs with small (<2 cm) lesions. If only one to four hepatic metastases are detected, an aggressive approach appears warranted becasue improved 5-year survival has been demonstrated after removal of isolated metastatic foci.[45] When a screening CT scan shows lesions in only one lobe of the liver, resection of the involved lobe is often considered as long as no other lesions are present in the normal-appearing lobe, the lobe without lesions shows normal function, no focal adenopathy is identified, and no distant spread is evident. In these patients, CT with arterial portography (Fig. 64–25) is the most accurate means of excluding additional lesions in the normal-appearing lobe. For this purpose, at present, CT with arterial portography is superior to MR imaging in revealing lesions in the liver. Intraoperative ultrasound is often used as the "gold standard" with which truth of radiographic diagnosis is determined in the absence of resection and pathologic evaluation of the resected liver segments. In patients for whom resection is not an option, selective catheterization and intra-arterial chemotherapy of liver are often used but only if there is no evidence of tumor spread to other sites. Local or distant adenopathy, adrenal metastases, peritoneal carcinomatosis, metastases to other areas of the gastrointestinal tract, and lung metastases are some of the findings that preclude resection or chemoembolization of liver lesions. Adrenal metastasis occurs in up to 14% of patients with colon carcinoma, producing enlarged, often inhomogeneous adrenal glands.

Generally, rectal or rectosigmoid carcinoma metastasizes to lymph nodes along the external iliac arteries and to the inguinal and para-aortic chains. Low rectal or anal tumors also drain into the inguinal nodes. Metastases may be found in nodes in the retroperitoneum Fig. 64–26) and porta hepatis. In other areas of the colon, lymph node metastases follow the normal pattern of lymph drainage from the involved area.

Lymph node more than 1.0 cm in diameter in the abdomen and in the pelvis are considered abnormal, but although asymmetry and size can be used to determine lymph node abnormality, the pathologic nature of the enlargement cannot be determined absolutely by

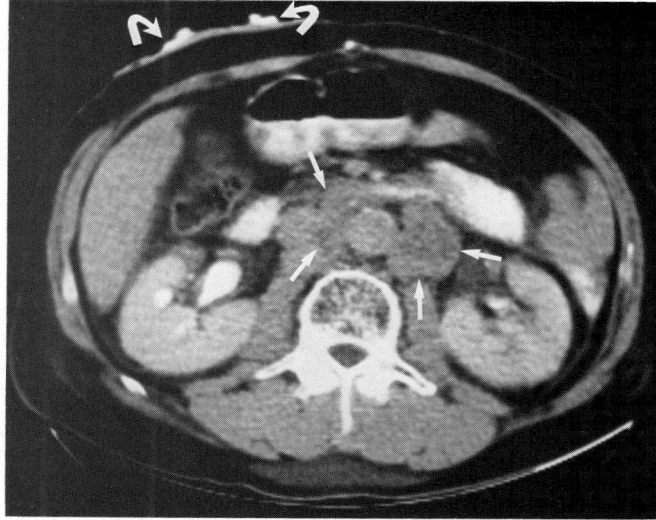

**Figure 64–26. Transmural adenocarcinoma of the sigmoid colon with retroperitoneal adenopathy *(straight arrows)*.** TNM stage T3, N1, M1 (Dukes' stage D). CT scan shows aortocaval and periaortic adenopathy. The patient had a bypass colostomy for inoperable carcinoma. The colostomy adhesive *(curved arrows)* is shown on the anterior abdominal wall.

CT.[46] Benign as well as malignant disease can produce lymphadenopathy, and only lymphangiography or guided biopsy can give a definitive diagnosis. Many metastatic foci are found in normal-sized lymph nodes (<1 cm) that cannot be considered abnormal by CT criteria. Because hyperplastic or inflammatory nodes are extremely rare in the perirectal area, demonstration of nonenhanced small (less than 1 cm) round or oval soft tissue densities suggests the presence of malignant adenopathy.

Although interpretation of CT scans of patients with colon tumors is usually not difficult, there are potential pitfalls to accurate interpretation.[47] CT scans obtained during or soon after surgery or irradiation can demonstrate edema or hemorrhage of the pelvic structures that simulates recurrent neoplasm. Chronic radiation changes in the pelvis[48–50] may be difficult or impossible to distinguish from colon tumors without CT-guided biopsies. It is therefore essential to determine the tumor stage by CT or MR imaging before giving radiation. Benign bone defects can simulate metastatic foci, and nonopacified bowel loops can be mistaken for a tumor mass. Perforation of a colon cancer can result in an inflammatory mass or abscess, which makes diagnosis of the underlying cancer difficult[51] (Fig. 64–27).

## Preoperative Staging by Computed Tomography

The staging of colon tumors has been most frequently based on Dukes' classification[52] or a modification thereof[53, 54] (Table 64–1). Because CT cannot determine whether a tumor is localized to the mucosa or submucosa or extends to the muscularis or even to the serosa, CT staging is based on an analysis of the thickness of the colon wall and the presence or absence of tumor spread to adjacent and distant organs.[55] The size of a recurrent

### TABLE 64–1. SURGICAL-PATHOLOGIC STAGING (MODIFIED DUKES' CLASSIFICATION)

| STAGE | DESCRIPTION |
| --- | --- |
| A | Limited to mucosa |
| B1 | Extension into but not through the muscularis propria |
| B2 | Extension through muscularis, no nodes |
| C1 | Limited to bowel wall, positive nodes |
| C2 | Extension through bowel wall, positive nodes |
| D | Distant metastases |

or primary colon tumor can be measured and the tumor assigned to one of four stages depending on the CT findings (Table 64–2).

More and more surgeons have been using the tumor, node, metastases (TNM) classification (Table 64–3) for staging colon neoplasms.[56] It has the advantage of more precise definition of the depth of infiltration in the bowel wall. Because of the inability of CT to determine depth of invasion to or through the various layers of the colon, CT findings cannot be correlated easily with the TNM classification. For example, tumor limited to mucosa or submucosa (T1, N0, M0) cannot be distinguished from tumor invading the muscularis or infiltrating to but not through the serosa, if present (T2, N0, M0 or T3, N0, M0). Generally, lesions extending beyond bowel wall (T3, N0, M0; T3, N1, M0; or T3, N1, M1) are correctly identified unless microinvasion by tumor is present. Of course, to the assessment of the depth of invasion must be added the presence or absence of positive local nodes or of distant metastases.

Early reports suggested that CT findings related to local extent and regional spread of tumor correlated well with surgical and histopathologic findings, and accuracy rates between 77 and 100% were reported.[47, 55, 57–59] The high accuracy rates of these reports were due

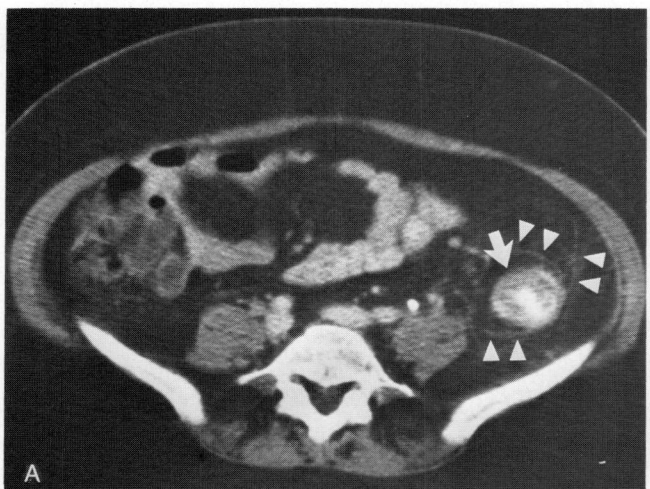
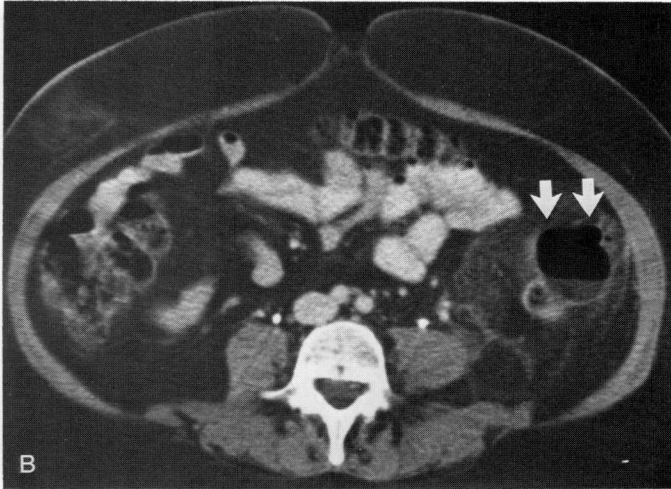

**Figure 64–27. Perforated adenocarcinoma in descending colon. A.** Almost circumferential thickening of wall of the descending colon *(arrow)* is seen. Note minimal soft tissue stranding *(arrowheads)* in the area surrounding the tumor. **B.** A large abscess with an air-fluid level *(arrows)* is seen 3 cm above the tumor. Soft tissue stranding represented an inflammatory reaction.

## TABLE 64–2. COMPUTED TOMOGRAPHIC STAGING OF PRIMARY OR RECURRENT COLORECTAL TUMOR

| STAGE | DESCRIPTION |
|-------|-------------|
| I | Intraluminal mass without thickening of wall |
| II | Thickened wall (>0.6 cm) or pelvic mass, no invasion or extension to sidewalls |
| IIIa | Thickened wall or pelvic mass with invasion of adjacent structures but not to pelvic sidewalls or abdominal wall |
| IIIb | Thickened wall or pelvic mass with extension to pelvic sidewalls and/or abdominal wall without distant metastases |
| IV | Distant metastases with or without local abnormality |

largely to the more advanced cases in these series. For primary colon cancer, CT is more accurate in showing extensive invasion of surrounding tissue and distant metastases such as those in liver and adrenals than in demonstrating local adenopathy or minimal tumor extension.

CT frequently understages patients with microinvasion of pericolonic or perirectal fat or small tumor foci in normal-sized nodes. In one study, the sensitivity and specificity for detecting local extension of tumor were 61.2 and 80.6%, respectively, and for detecting lymph node metastases were 25.9 and 96%, respectively.[22] Other studies showed lower accuracy rates (41 to 64%), largely because of low sensitivity for detection of lymph node metastases (22 to 73%) and of local tumor extent (53 to 77%).[21, 22, 25, 26, 60–62] Lymph node metastases were not analyzed separately in some of the earlier studies. One study found that staging accuracy increased from 17% for Dukes' B lesions to 81% for Dukes' D lesions.[61] Insufficient spatial resolution to detect small perirectal or pericolonic tumor infiltration and a high incidence of

## TABLE 64–3. SURGICAL-PATHOLOGIC STAGING (TUMOR, NODE, METASTASES CLASSIFICATION)

| CLASSIFICATION ASTLER-COLLER (MODIFIED FROM DUKES') | TNM CLASS | DESCRIPTION | APPROXIMATE 5-YEAR SURVIVAL (%) |
|---|---|---|---|
| A | T1, N0, M0 | Nodes (−), limited to submucosa | 80 |
| B1 | T2, N0, M0 | Nodes (−), limited to muscularis | 70 |
| B2 | T3, N0, M0 | Nodes (−), lesion transmural | 60–65 |
| C1 | T2, N1, M0 | Nodes (+), lesion into muscularis | 35–45 |
| C2 | T3, N1, M0 | Nodes (+), lesion transmural | 25 |
| D | M1 | Distant metastases | <25 |

metastatic foci in lymph nodes smaller than 1.5 cm in diameter caused these lower detection rates.

Refinement of CT techniques, such as by colon preparation, prone positioning of the patient, and air distention of the rectum,[63] has increased the accuracy of assessing local tumor extent by CT. Also, lowering the threshold for diagnosing lymph node metastases improved sensitivity for detecting lymph node metastases, but such an approach decreased specificity.

Little information is available about the detection and staging of tumors in the cecum or ascending, transverse, and descending colon. Most tumors in these areas are easily demonstrated (Figs. 64–28 and 64–29), but no investigation has analyzed these lesions in detail.

## MAGNETIC RESONANCE IMAGING

MR imaging, like CT, can be used to detect and stage rectosigmoid tumors more accurately than tumors in the other areas of the colon because of the fixed position of the rectosigmoid colon in relation to the pelvis. For correct depiction of the intraluminal component of tumors, particularly smaller ones, preparation of the colon to avoid confusion with feces, air insufflation, and prone positioning are necessary (Fig. 64–30). On T1-weighted spin-echo images, rectosigmoid tumors appear as wall thickening with signal intensity similar to or slightly higher than that of skeletal muscle (long T1) (see Fig. 64–30A). Because perirectal fat has high signal intensity (short T1), air no signal intensity, and tumor moderate signal intensity (long T1), tumors are shown with high contrast. For the same reasons, extension of tumor beyond the colon wall is seen well on T1-weighted images (Fig. 64–31). On T2-weighted spin-echo images, the signal intensity of tumor increases relative to that of muscle (see Fig. 64–30B); however, the contrast between tumor and perirectal fat decreases because both tissues have long T2 relaxation times. Therefore, T2-weighted images are not as useful as T1-weighted images, particularly for determining extracolonic tumor extension (see Fig. 64–31C). However, if uterine or pelvic sidewall invasion is suspected, T2-weighted sequences are useful because of the differences in signal intensity between tumor and muscle. In general, perirectal tumor invasion is better seen by MR imaging than by CT because of the higher contrast between tumor and fat.[23]

Both CT and MR are unable to distinguish between tumors localized to mucosa (stage I) and those that infiltrate the entire colon wall (stage II). Also, microinvasion cannot be detected by MR and tumor foci in normal-sized nodes go unrecognized.[64] As with CT, the MR diagnosis of lymph node abnormality is based on the size of the nodes.[46, 64] In one series,[23] in five of six cases in which lymph nodes were seen, the nodes were normal in size but contained tumor and in the one case with enlarged nodes (>15 mm in diameter) reactive hyperplasia was present. With a medium magnetic field (0.35 T), lymph nodes are well seen on T1-weighted images but are difficult to detect on T2-weighted images

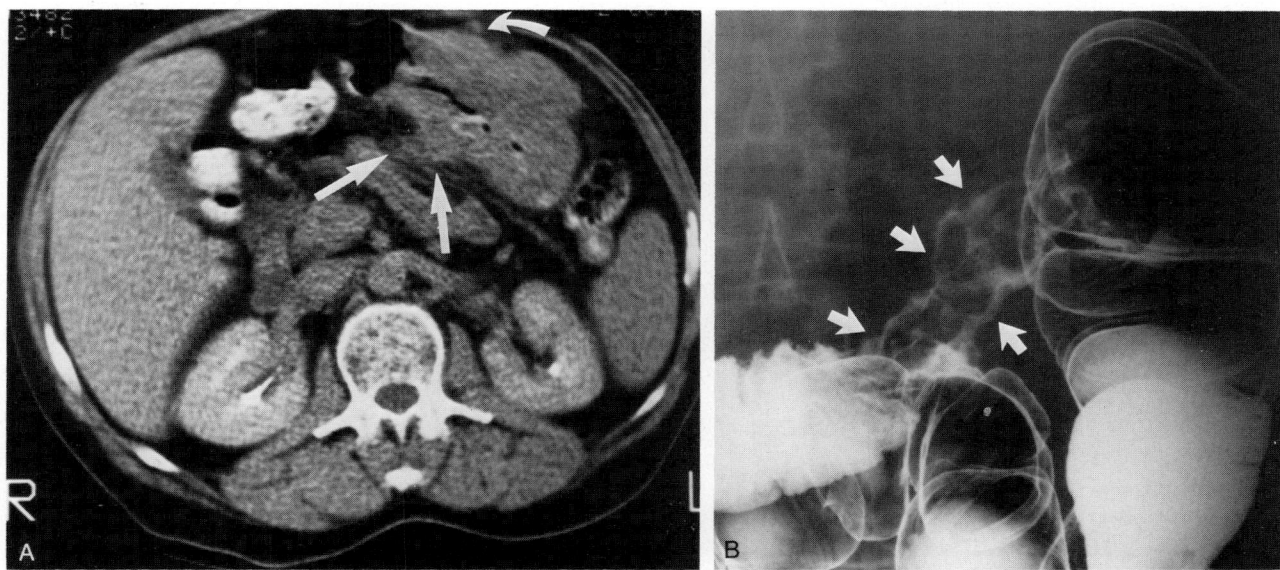

**Figure 64–28. Adenocarcinoma in the transverse colon with invasion of the stomach. A.** The bulky mass extends into surrounding fat through strands *(straight arrows)* of soft tissue reaching into the pericolonic fat. Note the small local node *(curved arrow)* anterior to the transverse colon. **B.** Double contrast barium enema examination demarcates a large, irregular mass *(arrows)*, but extension beyond the colon cannot be determined.

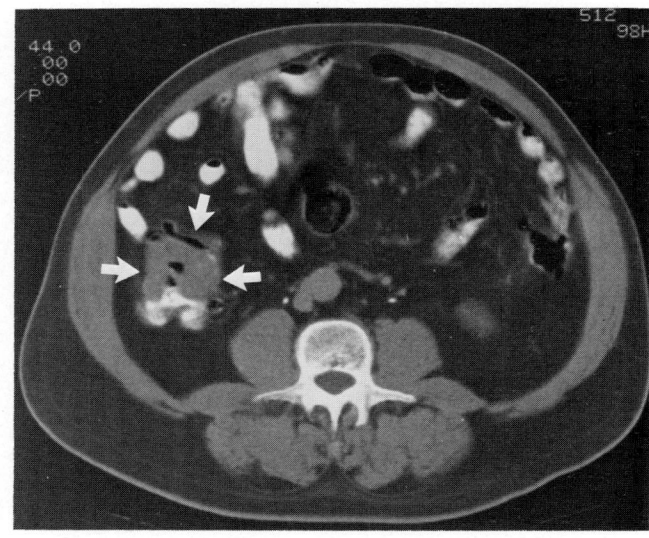

**Figure 64–29. Cecal adenocarcinoma.** A large mass *(arrows)* near the ileocecal valve is confined to the bowel wall.

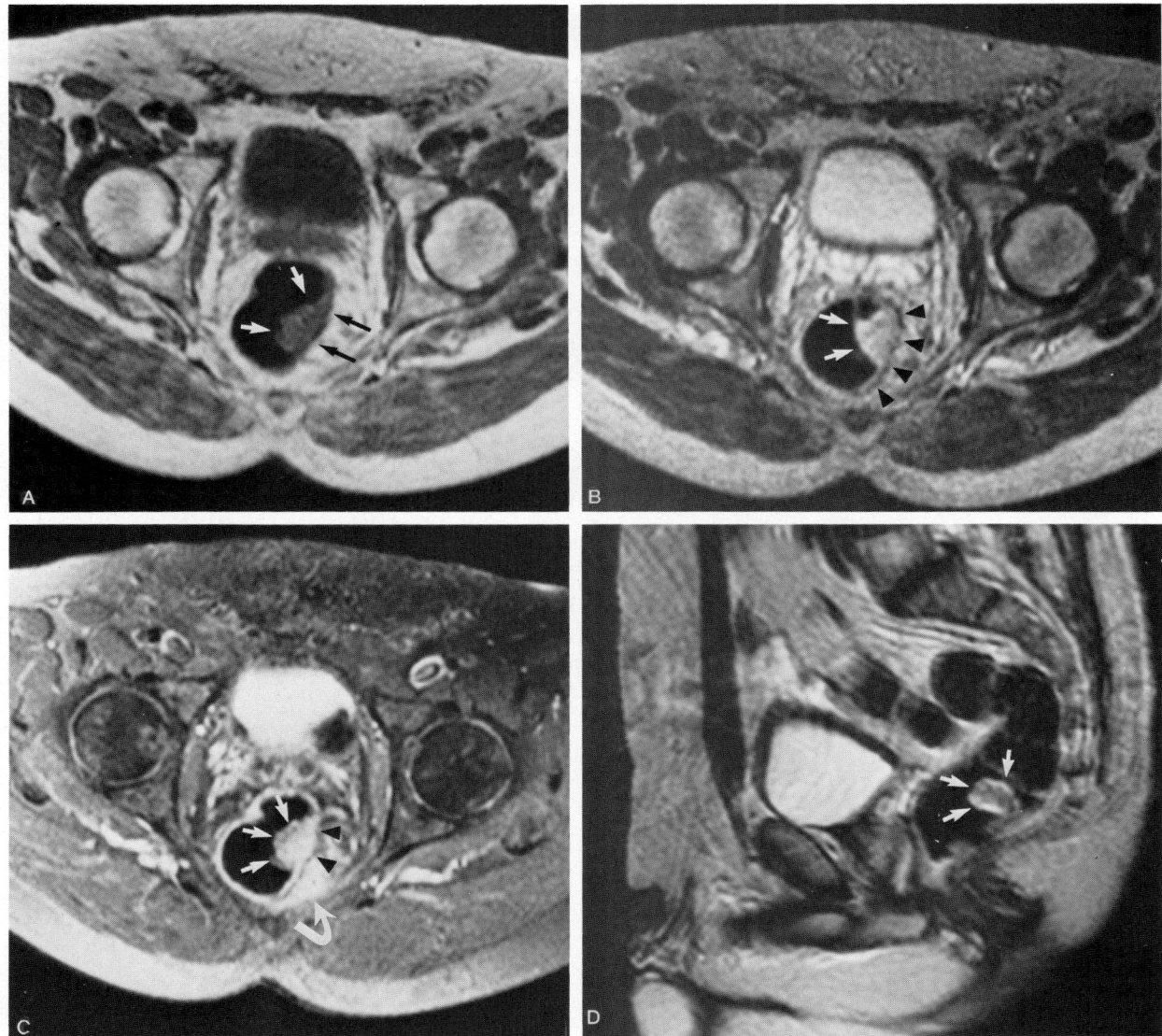

**Figure 64–30. MR image of adenocarcinoma of rectum.** TNM stage T2, N0, M0 (Dukes' stage B1). **A.** T1-weighted transaxial spin-echo image (600/11). The intraluminal component of this rectal adenocarcinoma *(white arrows)* appears as a mass of low signal intensity similar to that of muscle and is clearly outlined against the signal void of air introduced rectally before scanning. Note the well-defined, sharp outer margin *(black arrows)* of this tumor. **B.** T2-weighted transaxial spin-echo image (2500/80). The mass in the left lateral wall of rectum has high signal intensity *(arrows)* and well-defined outer margins *(arrowheads)*. Note that the tissue margins on this T2-weighted image are not as well depicted as on the T1-weighted image. **C.** T1-weighted spin-echo image with gadolinium and fat suppression technique. After administration of gadolinium, the mass appears bright *(straight arrows)* but the margins remain sharply defined *(arrowheads)*, which excludes invasion of perirectal fat. Some edema is noted posterior and slightly lateral to the rectum *(curved arrow)* and may represent mild congestion or inflammation. At surgery, the tumor was confined to the bowel wall. **D.** Sagittal T2-weighted fast spin-echo image. The rectal lesion *(arrows)* is well outlined in the optimally distended rectal ampulla. Scans were obtained with the patient in the prone position.

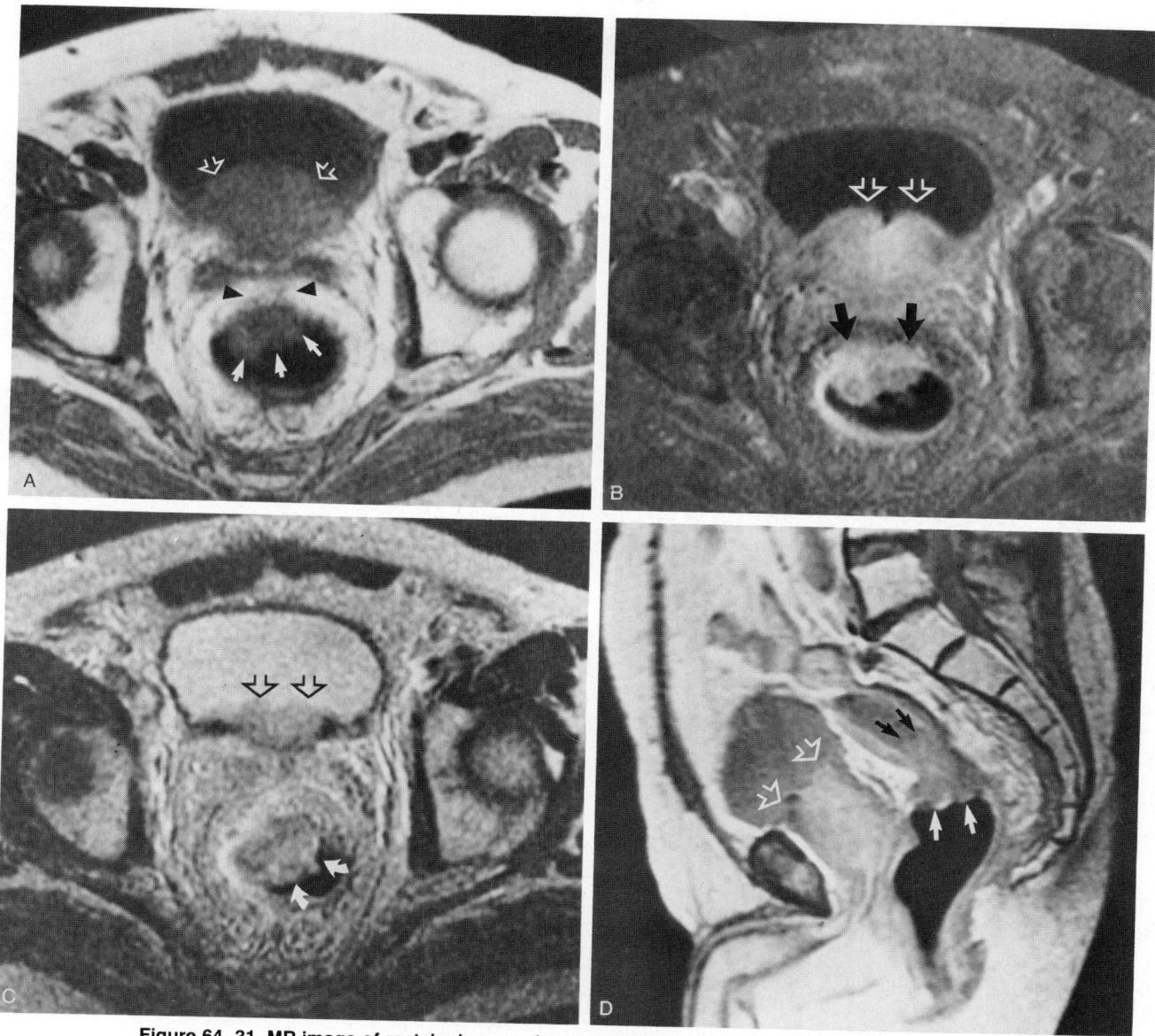

**Figure 64–31. MR image of rectal adenocarcinoma with extension beyond the bowel wall.** TNM stage T3, N0, M0 (Dukes' stage B2). **A.** T1-weighted transaxial spin-echo image (600/11). A mass *(solid arrows)* protrudes from the anterior wall of the rectum into the lumen. Strands of dark signal intensity extending from the outer margin of the rectum into perirectal fat *(arrowheads)* represent invasion of tumor into fat. Enlarged prostate is seen *(open arrows)*. **B.** T1-weighted spin-echo image with gadolinium and fat suppression technique. Extension of tumor beyond the bowel wall *(solid arrows)* is clearly demonstrated. Enlarged prostate is seen *(open arrows)*. **C.** T2-weighted transaxial spin-echo image (2500/80). Although the rectal mass *(solid arrows)* is clearly seen on the T2-weighted spin-echo image, extension of tumor beyond the bowel wall cannot be definitely identified. Enlarged prostate is seen *(open arrows)*. **D.** Sagittal view of the first echo of the T2-weighted spin-echo sequence: proton density image. The sagittal image not only outlines the tumor with protruding edges at superior and inferior margins *(solid arrows)* but also shows slightly thickened wall of sigmoid colon caused by edema. Enlarged prostate is seen *(open arrows)*.

because their high signal intensity is similar to that of fat. With a high magnetic field, nodes can also be detected on T2-weighted images because with high field strength the signal intensity of fat decreases and that of lymph nodes increases, resulting in better image contrast. For demonstration of liver and adrenal metastases, MR and CT are comparable if an optimal CT bolus technique is used. Final comparison of CT and MR is not available yet, but it appears that some liver lesions, particularly in the left lobe, are better seen on MR images, particularly if gating is used. MR imaging with an intravenous contrast agent (e.g., manganese dipyridoxyl-ethylenediamine-diacetate-(bis)phosphate) may render MR superior to CT, particularly for small lesions.

Invasion of adjacent organs is best demonstrated on transverse or coronal MR images, and MR is superior to CT in demonstrating invasion of levator ani. Lateral extension of tumor is difficult to detect on sagittal MR images. Extension into prostate, seminal vesicles, vagina, and cervix can be shown, but extension into bladder may be missed if the bladder is not well distended.

Overall, CT and MR are equally good for staging rectosigmoid tumors, but perirectal disease is better delineated by MR. In the detection of lymph node abnormalities, MR and CT demonstrate lymphadenopathy equally well but both fail to distinguish between benign hyperactive hyperplasia, metastatic adenopathy, and lymphoma. For normal-sized nodes (<10 mm), CT is better than MR because of its superior spatial resolution.[64] MR readily distinguishes nodes from vessels without injection of intravenous contrast material; however, CT offers shorter examination times and better delineation of the gastrointestinal tract because of the well-established use of oral contrast materials. After surgery, MR may be helpful in examining patients with large surgical clips, for whom CT results are inadequate because of artifacts.

## Preoperative Staging by Magnetic Resonance Imaging

At present, MR imaging appears to have the same overall limitations as CT,[23, 65–67] but multiplanar imaging may offer special advantages. An early investigation showed that CT and MR imaging were equally effective in staging. In particular, local tumor extent was well shown on T1-weighted spin-echo images.[23, 67] Direct invasion of tumor into bone or muscles such as the levator ani may be better shown by MR imaging.[23, 24] However, depth of tumor infiltration in bowel wall and presence of metastatic foci in lymph nodes cannot be determined accurately by MR imaging. An overall staging accuracy of 74 to 79% was found, but only small MR imaging series have been reported.[23, 24, 66, 67] Also, preliminary results for 10 patients indicated that endorectal coils have promise for assessment of local tumor extension, but their ability to detect lymphadenopathy, even though superior to that of imaging with a body coil, was limited[68] (see Chapter 68).

## TRANSRECTAL SONOGRAPHY

### Primary Tumor

The major advantage of transrectal ultrasonography is that it can demonstrate the various layers of the colon wall, which enables determination of depth of tumor penetration into the wall. Usually, a colon tumor is visualized as a hypoechoic mass whose margins can be outlined and related to the layers in the colon wall or rectal wall. The depth of infiltration can be assessed from evidence of disruption of the different segments of the rectal or colon wall. On images produced with a radial rotating transducer placed in the rectum, the elements of the rectal wall appear as rings of different echogenicities. The transducer is covered with a balloon filled with water, and often the rectal cavity is also filled with water. The innermost ring is hyperechoic and represents the interface of the balloon and mucosa, the second ring from the center is hypoechoic and is produced by the mucosa and the muscularis mucosae, the third ring is hyperechoic and consists of the submucosa, the fourth ring is again hypoechoic and is formed by the muscularis propria, and the fifth ring is hyperechoic and caused by the perirectal fat or, if it is in an area with peritoneal reflection, by the serosa.

If the examination is performed carefully, even the intraluminal component can be clearly demonstrated as a polypoid or exophytic mass. Filling of the balloon attached to the transducer and the colorectal lumen with water allows optimal visualization of mural and nodal abnormalities. Pericolonic or perirectal abnormalities can also be seen, but depth of penetration beyond the colon wall is limited. Whenever possible, the transducer is passed beyond the tumor into the colon proximal to the lesion for more complete assessment of mural as well as nodal pathology. Peritumoral inflammation and irradiation may simulate more advanced tumor changes because these abnormalities often have a hypoechoic pattern that may not be distinguishable from the echo pattern of tumor, which leads to overestimation of the size of the neoplasm.

Usually, the system for ultrasonographic staging is based on the TNM classification. Three stages are distinguished by ultrasonography: a uT1 tumor is confined to the mucosa and submucosa and does not interrupt the middle echogenic interface, a uT2 lesion is confined to the rectal wall and the outermost echogenic interface is kept intact, and a uT3 tumor penetrates into the perirectal fat and is visualized as a disruption of the outermost hyperechoic ring (Fig. 64–32).

With transrectal ultrasonography, normal lymph nodes are hyperechoic and thus are not routinely seen within the echogenic perirectal fat. Involvement of lymph nodes by tumor is diagnosed on the basis of a hypoechoic pattern of the lymph node with distinct margins, whereas the normal, uninvolved node has a hyperechoic pattern with indistinct boundaries. Not all lymph nodes can be visualized; for example, lymph nodes along the inferior mesenteric artery often cannot be demonstrated. Depiction of direct extension of tumor

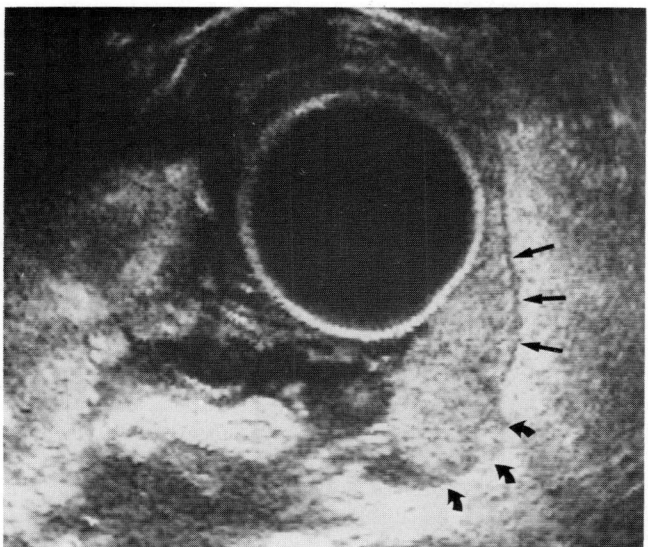

**Figure 64–32. Transrectal sonogram of rectal tumor, stage uT3.** A large mass *(straight arrows)* in the wall of the rectum markedly thickens the muscularis propria. Minimal extension into the perirectal fat *(curved arrows)* is also demonstrated.

into adjacent lymph nodes is considered pathognomonic of a malignant character of lymph nodes.

Smaller probes that can be introduced through the biopsy channel of an endoscope and can pass even through a severe luminal stenosis allow more accurate staging of tumors because the maximal extent of the tumor can be visualized. The echoendoscope has become the instrument of choice for visualization of proximal colon neoplasms because the transducer can be maneuvered into the proximal segments of the colon. The combination of endoscope and endoluminal ultrasound allows demonstration of the surface of the mucosa. With this combination it is possible to obtain a biopsy specimen, visualize the depth of a lesion within the bowel wall, and determine the presence or absence of adjacent lymphadenopathy in one procedure for accurate diagnosis and staging of local tumor extent. However, abdominal ultrasound is needed for assessment of distant metastases, and CT or MR imaging should be added for even more complete evaluation.

## Preoperative Staging by Transrectal Sonography

Although transabdominal sonography may be used to assess the presence or absence of liver metastases, transrectal sonography is increasingly used to detect the depth of tumor infiltration and local adenopathy in patients with rectal carcinomas. As mentioned earlier, its ability to distinguish the normal layers of the bowel wall and to visualize disruption of one or more of these layers by tumor leads to accurate staging of local tumor extent. With this method, sensitivities of 67 to 96% have been reported for assessing perirectal spread, but the presence of regional lymph node metastases is less

well detected (sensitivity 50 to 57%).[25, 26, 65, 66, 69] Another study based on the TNM staging classification showed that results were less accurate with T2 carcinomas, which were often accompanied by peritumoral inflammation or abscesses.[70] Abscesses are fluid-filled structures, usually in the perianal space, and may contain internal echoes but should exhibit good posterior acoustic enhancement. In this study of transcolorectal endosonography, the authors achieved an accuracy of 81% for rectal and 93% for colon carcinomas, with overstaging in 13% and understaging in 2%. However if the lymph nodes were analyzed separately, the sensitivity was 94% and specificity 55% for an overall accuracy of 70%. When transcolorectal ultrasound was compared with Dukes' classification, the overall accuracy was 67%.

The broad range of sensitivities of transrectal sonography for detection of tumor extent in and through bowel wall emphasizes the dependence of this method on the operator. Endoscopic sonography has expanded the application of ultrasonographic methods to the entire colon.[71, 72] Although sonography of colon and rectum appears promising, valid and comprehensive clinical trials remain necessary.

## IMMUNOSCINTIGRAPHY WITH MONOCLONAL ANTIBODIES

### Detection of Primary Colorectal Neoplasm

Since the mid-1970s MoAbs have been used in vivo as tumor-localizing agents and in vitro as diagnostic markers with gamma camera imaging to differentiate tumor cell types.[27, 73] Agents that have been used include anti–carcinoembryonic antigen (anti-CEA) MoAb with iodine 123, anti-CEA MoAbs conjugated with diethylenetriaminepentaacetic acid (DTPA) and labeled with indium 111 and MoAbs B72.3-GYK-DTPA designated as CYT-103 (MoAb B72.3-glycyl-tyrosyl-[N-ε-DTPA]-lysine). Tumor detection was not influenced by the level of serum CEA. MoAb B72.3 targets the high molecular weight tumor-associated glycoprotein 72, which is expressed in 80% of colon cancers and reacts with various mucin-producing adenocarcinomas but has practically no reaction to normal tissues. Some patients had to be given cathartic agents before imaging because of prominent radioactivity in the large bowel. In general, lesion detection is performed 3 to 4 days after MoAb infusion with planar imaging. Single photon emission CT is usually performed 5 to 7 days after MoAb infusion, and its better anatomic definition and determination of approximate size result in improved tumor detection.[28]

Primary adenocarcinomas of the colon and metastatic foci in liver or lymph nodes are seen as areas of increased radioactivity ("hot spots"). Depending on the size and degree of necrosis of the liver metastases, neoplastic deposits in the liver may be visualized as areas of intense accumulation of radioactivity, areas with no accumulation of radioactivity surrounded by normal liver uptake, and intermediate lesions with uptake identical to that of normal liver. In one study using indium 111–labeled CYT-103, "cold" defects in the liver shown by immunoscintigraphy were found to represent areas with moderate to severe necrosis, whereas lesions with normal MoAb uptake had only minor degrees of necrosis.[28] The same study revealed a low incidence of human antimouse antibody formation (16%) and an even lower incidence of adverse reactions (3.5%).[28]

## Preoperative Staging of Primary Colorectal Neoplasm

Several reports have appeared on the use and value of isotope-labeled MoAb immunoscintigraphy for the detection of primary colorectal carcinoma and its metastases.[73–79] Sensitivity ranged from 65 to 86% and specificity from 77 to 92% for the detection of primary tumor, local recurrences, and distant metastases. The major uses of immunoscintigraphy are in detecting occult tumor lesions and in establishing absence of distant disease in patients with isolated, resectable metastases. In one study using indium 111–labeled CYT-103, extrahepatic lesions were confirmed by surgery but not detected by CT or other diagnostic tests in over 10% of the patients, and immunoscintigraphy contributed beneficially to the management of 27% of patients.[78] In another study using indium 111–labeled MoAb ZCE-025,[79] occult recurrences missed by CT and other diagnostic tests were found in 65% of 20 patients, and immunoscintigraphy was beneficial for the management of these patients. It therefore appears feasible to use these agents for accurate immunoscintigraphy in patients with suspected primary, recurrent, or metastatic colorectal neoplasms. However, the validity of this test and the low incidence of adverse reactions must be confirmed in larger series before a final conclusion can be drawn.

## POSITRON EMISSION TOMOGRAPHY

### Primary Colorectal Neoplasm

PET was initially used for detection of functional abnormalities in brain and heart, but its use has been expanded to other applications, such as the detection of primary and recurrent tumors with or without metastases to distant sites. For these tumor studies, fluorine 18–labeled deoxyglucose (18-FDG) has been used and a remarkably close correlation has been found between tumor grade and glucose utilization. Rapid 18-FDG uptake was observed in glioma of rats[80] and in canine osteosarcomas and mammary carcinomas.[81] The new generation of PET scanners has adequate resolution to provide high-quality images of any area of the human body, and it is possible to use this method to detect distant, residual, or recurrent disease in patients with colorectal carcinomas.

For the purpose of identifying tumor tissue, PET images are evaluated quantitatively in regions of interest and time-activity curves are calculated. Tracer uptake is expressed as a differential absorption ratio that is calculated as the tissue concentration ($\mu$Ci/g) divided by injected dose ($\mu$Ci)/body weight (g). After intravenous injection of 18-FDG, PET images show significant uptake by malignant tumors. Quantitative analyses demonstrate rapid uptake of 18-FDG by the tumor, followed by a slight decrease in the differential absorption ratio for up to 40 minutes after 18-FDG administration. In comparison, the 18-FDG concentration is low in nonmalignant lesions and in soft tissue. To determine the optimal time of imaging, ratios of tumor to soft tissue and of tumor to nonmalignant lesions are determined as a function of time. The tumor/soft tissue ratio is highest shortly after injection of 18-FDG, but the tumor/nonmalignant lesion ratio is highest approximately 1 hour after administration of the tracer. In general, 18-FDG accumulation in tumors 1 hour after tracer injection is more than twice as high as in normal tissue or nonmalignant lesions. Therefore, tumor delineation is best performed at that time.

## Staging of Primary Colorectal Neoplasm

Most investigations of the use of PET for colorectal tumors have focused on the detection of recurrent or residual disease.[29, 30] However, PET has also been used to identify distant metastatic foci in patients with primary colorectal neoplasms. Only anecdotal reports or small series are available, and it remains to be seen how accurate results based on PET with 18-FDG are in the staging of colorectal tumors. Metastases have been shown in lymph nodes remote from the primary tumor site and in liver, but the resolution of the PET scanner is limited and detection of tumor should be confined to lesions 1.5 cm or more in diameter.

## ROLE OF CROSS-SECTIONAL IMAGING IN PRIMARY COLORECTAL NEOPLASM

The prognosis for patients with colorectal cancer is closely related to the extent of tumor at the time of diagnosis. The overall 5-year survival rate is about 50% (stage A, 81 to 85%; stage B, 64 to 78%; stage C, 27 to 33%; stage D, 5 to 14%).[82–84] There is a consensus that the most important prognostic factor is the presence or absence of lymph node invasion, but malignant fixation of colorectal tumor through direct invasion also appears to be an important sign. In one study, the 5-year survival of patients with fixed Dukes' B rectal carcinoma was 44%, whereas that of patients with mobile C lesions was 63%.[85]

Accurate noninvasive preoperative assessment of tumor stage based on one or a combination of radiographic techniques would allow appropriate treatment to be planned in each case. Also, precise determination of possible tumor recurrence would permit effective monitoring of success of therapy and surgical intervention for recurrent disease before widespread metastases are present. Such an aggressive approach has been shown to improve survival even in patients with recurrent disease.[86] The following paragraphs analyze the effectiveness of the various imaging techniques for detecting local extent of primary and recurrent colorectal neoplasms. They do not consider distant metastases such as those to the liver.

Based on the available results, routine CT staging is not recommended for primary colorectal tumors. Wall thickening alone is a nonspecific finding in many different diseases (Table 64–4). CT should be reserved for patients suspected of having locally extensive or widespread disease. If CT shows extensive local spread of tumor, these patients can be treated with radiation therapy alone or with radiation and later tumor resection, if feasible. Lymphadenopathy is not a significant clinical problem, but if a colon resection is planned, the decision to use local tumor excision by surgery or colonoscopy cannot be based on CT because of its poor sensitivity to adenopathy. CT may be used to guide fine-needle aspiration for suspected metastases and assess complications such as perforation with abscess formation. Transrectal sonography may be used to determine local tumor extent, but it is doubtful that ultrasonographic diagnosis can be used for management of patients[25] because up to 14% of patients with primary tumors confined to the rectal wall have regional lymph node metastases. Transrectal sonography can frequently detect regional lymph nodes and is superior to CT in this respect, but it cannot indicate the histology of the visualized lymph nodes. MR imaging with coronal views and gadolinium-enhanced images may be beneficial in determining involvement of the levator ani. If involvement is demonstrated, an anterior resection is not indicated and an abdominoperineal (AP) resection is needed. Use of endorectal coils and enhanced MR imaging, particularly MR imaging lymphangiography, might improve staging of colorectal tumors. Whether MR imaging has other advantages over CT in primary colorectal cancer is uncertain, and more comprehensive studies are needed.

The role of MoAb immunoscintigraphy and PET in the evaluation of patients with primary colorectal tumors is still uncertain. Results with immunoscintigraphy are encouraging, and it is expected that addition of this test

will lead to more accurate assessment of distant disease. Nevertheless, in one study only 60% of liver metastases were detected when both cold and hot lesions were considered, and the detection of lymph node metastases was correct in only one of nine patients even when single photon emission CT was used.[28] This dims the hope of achieving acceptable detection rates in the near future. Likewise, for PET to become an acceptable method for staging colorectal neoplasms, the resolution of PET scanners must be improved to the point where detection of metastases of 5 mm or less becomes a reality.

However, an aggressive diagnostic approach that includes pretherapy staging of advanced colon malignancies can enable the most appropriate treatment regimen to be planned. Pretherapy staging is useful when resection of the tumor is not immediately feasible but may become possible after radiation, when advanced disease is suspected and a decision for or against extensive abdominal surgery must be made, and when patients may benefit from local endocavitary radiation.[55, 87]

## POSTOPERATIVE FOLLOW-UP

### Postoperative Colon

Patients who have had surgery for colorectal carcinoma undergo frequent postoperative examinations because of their relatively high risk of developing a second metachronous carcinoma[88] and because of the need to assess postoperative symptoms. Ileocolic (Fig. 64–33) and colocolic anastomoses can be demonstrated in detail by double contrast enema examination, particularly with the use of intravenous glucagon. Plication defects are frequently identified. In some patients, a filling defect resulting from a stitch granuloma may be seen in the early postoperative period (Fig. 64–34). However, this defect regresses and becomes less prominent on follow-up studies.[89] It is important to obtain a postoperative study within approximately 3 months of surgery to establish the baseline appearance of the anastomosis for comparison with subsequent studies.

With the availability of modern surgical staple guns, low anterior resections are being performed with increasing frequency.[90] The surgical anastomoses are beautifully demonstrated by double contrast technique (Fig. 64–35). Radiologic examination of the postoperative colon is discussed in detail in Chapter 70.

### Follow-up for Colorectal Cancer

Patients who have been treated for colorectal cancer undergo follow-up study to detect recurrent disease and metachronous tumors. CT is the examination of choice for the detection of recurrence remote from the anastomotic line and the detection of distant metastases (see later).[91, 92] However, the double contrast enema is the primary diagnostic procedure for the detection of local and anastomotic recurrences (Fig. 64–36) as well as

---

**TABLE 64–4. DIFFERENTIAL DIAGNOSIS
OF COLONIC WALL THICKENING**

Neoplasm (primary and secondary)
Muscular hypertrophy (particularly sigmoid colon)
Crohn's disease
Infectious colitis
Diverticulitis
Intramural abscess (trauma)
Perforation with inflammation
Ischemia or hemorrhage
Vasculitis
Plication defects after surgery

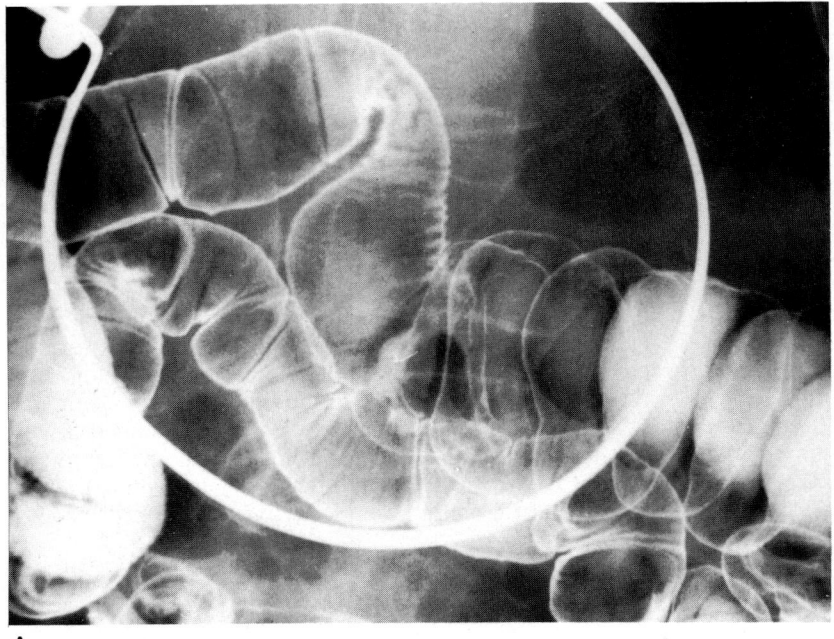

A

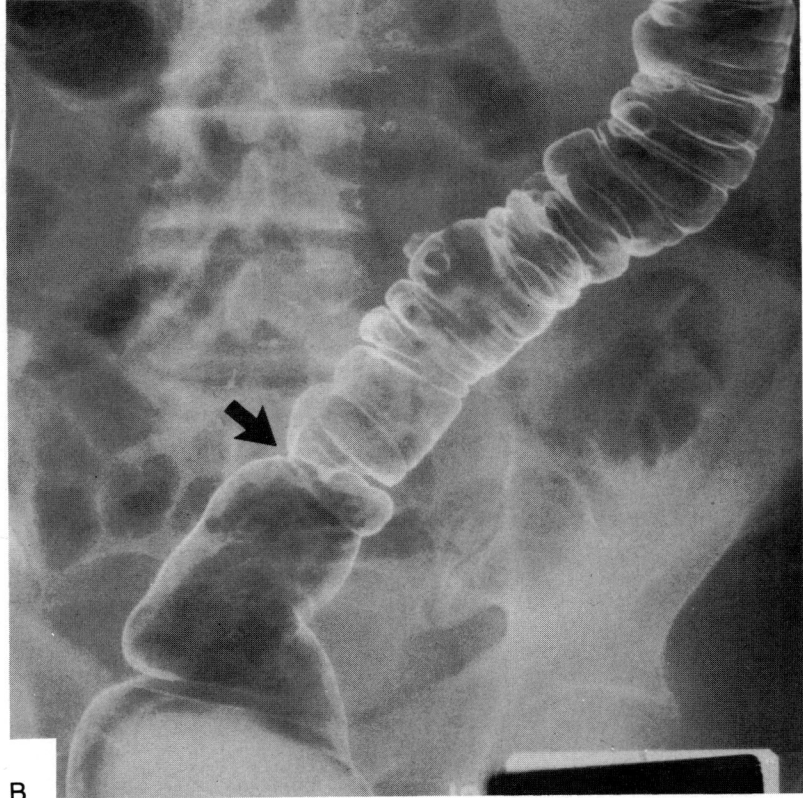

B

**Figure 64–33. Normal postoperative appearances. A.** Normal ileocolic anastomosis in the transverse colon. **B.** Example of a normal colocolic anastomosis *(arrow).*

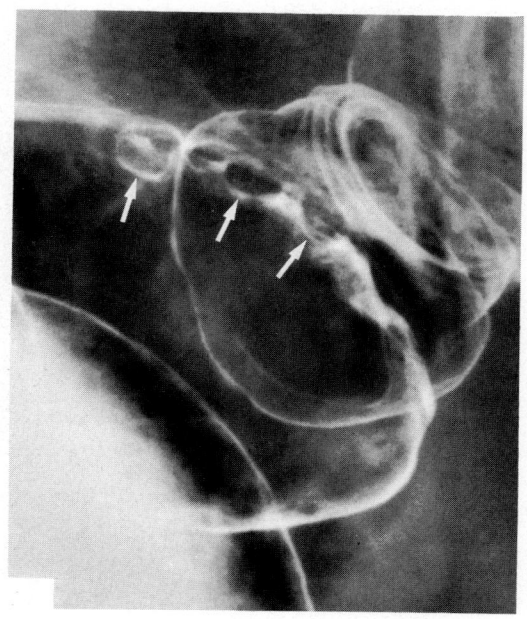

**Figure 64–34. Stitch granuloma.** Colocolic anastomosis with identifiable plication defects caused by sutures *(arrows)*.

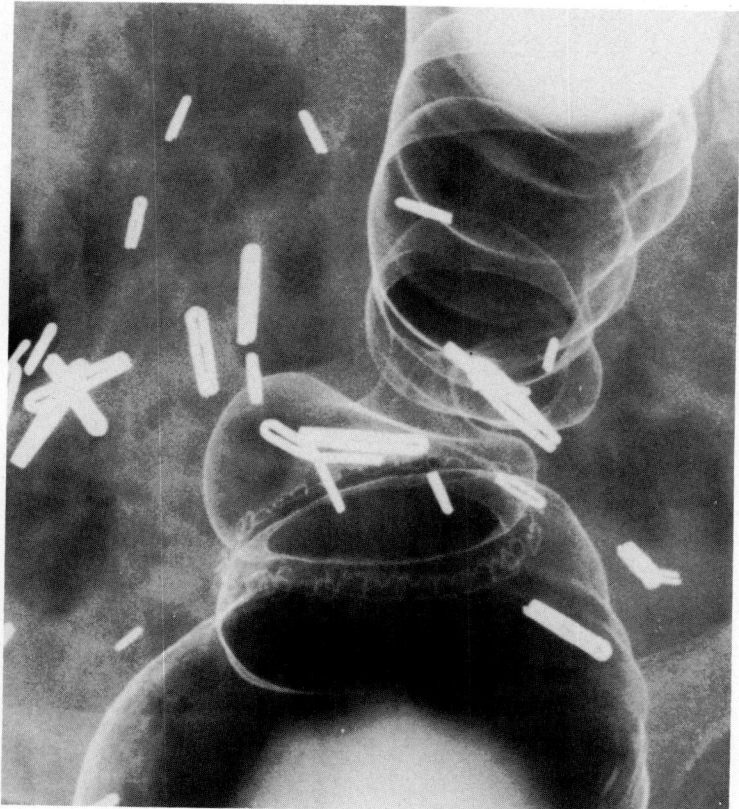

**Figure 64–35. Low anterior resection.** A double contrast examination shows the normal appearance of a low anterior resection using the staple gun.

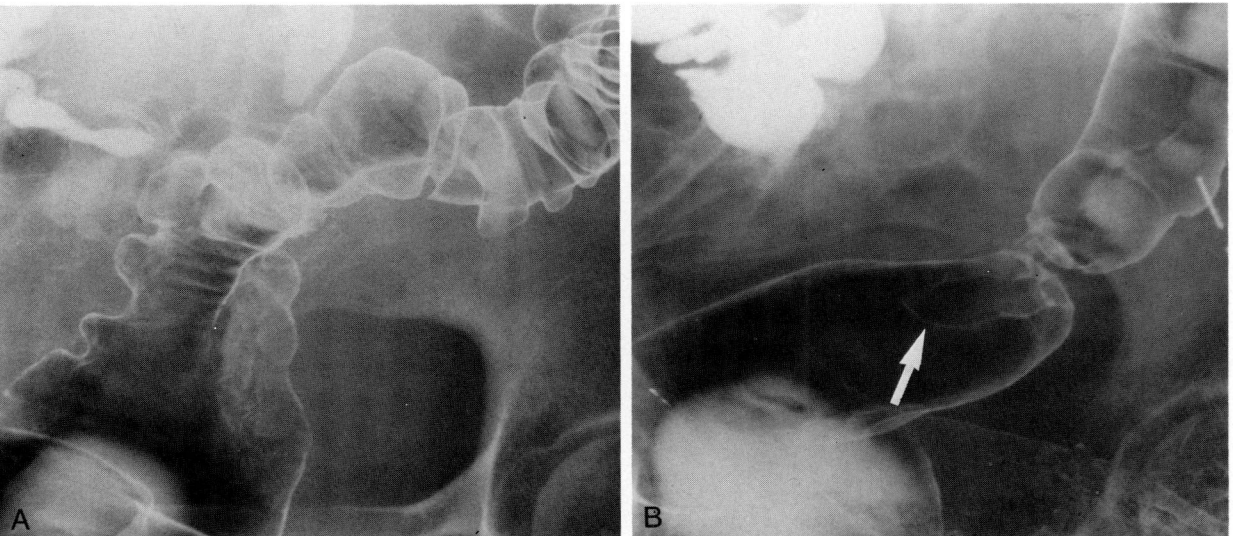

**Figure 64–36. Local recurrence of colon carcinoma. A.** A soft tissue mass represents recurrent colon carcinoma invading the rectosigmoid. **B.** Anastomotic recurrence of colon cancer. Narrowing of the anastomosis with a plaque-like extension of recurrent tumor is seen proximally *(arrow).*

metachronous lesions (Fig. 64–37). It is particularly important to examine the anastomotic site because metastatic deposits tend to be implanted there.[93, 94] Welch and Donaldson have shown that 20% of recurrences after colon resection and anastomosis were found at the anastomotic site.[95] When the anastomotic site appears eccentric or irregular or has nodular filling defects, recurrent tumor should be suspected. Colonoscopy may be helpful, although in some instances it may be misleading because recurrent tumor may be submucosal and biopsy findings may be negative for malignancy. CT and CT-guided biopsy may be useful for determining the presence and nature of an extracolonic mass.

Patients who have undergone abdominoperineal resection with colostomy must also be examined regularly because of the possibility of developing a second tumor. Double contrast examination of the residual colon can usually be performed through the colostomy (see Fig. 64–37 and Chapter 70). CT and MR imaging are of particular value for the detection of pelvic recurrence of tumor in patients who have had abdominoperineal resection.

## IMAGING OF RECURRENT COLORECTAL CARCINOMA

CT and MR imaging have been used extensively to detect recurrent colorectal cancer, and both methods enable detection of recurrence at a time when CEA titers are normal and/or symptoms are absent.[96, 97] Their value is particularly great for patients who have had total AP resection and colostomy. Anastomotic recurrences may be discovered by contrast enema or by colonoscopy. Follow-up studies of patients with potentially curative resection of recurrent tumor demonstrated an average symptom-free period of 38 months, compared with an average survival of 8 months for patients without resection of recurrent tumor.[98–100] Because co-

lorectal carcinoma often recurs outside the bowel lumen, CT and MR imaging are accepted methods for detection of recurrent colorectal tumor. A debate on the appropriate timing of these imaging tests is ongoing and has

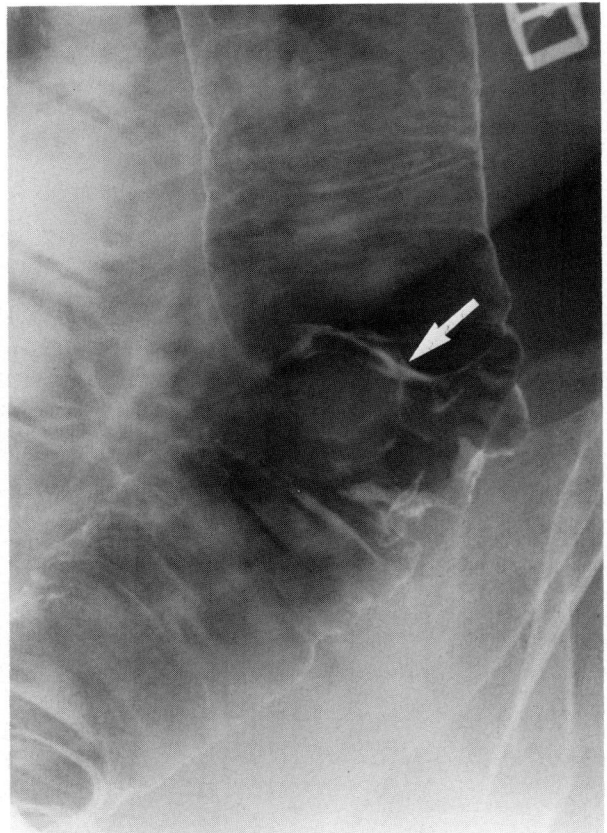

**Figure 64–37. Metachronous carcinoma.** A colostomy enema study performed after total proctectomy for carcinoma shows a new primary carcinoma *(arrow)* in the descending colon.

gained importance because of the high cost of frequent imaging.

The stage, histology, and site of primary tumor at the time of diagnosis have been found most predictive of eventual relapse.[100, 101] Anastomotic recurrence occurs mostly after anterior resection and is usually related to residual tumor outside the colorectal wall that grows into the suture site. Because recurrence may be seen in 30 to 50% of patients who had apparently curative resection and in up to 80% of these patients within the first 2 years,[102] early and frequent follow-up studies have been recommended. The most commonly recommended sequence of follow-up studies consists of a baseline CT or MR imaging study at 3 to 4 months with subsequent imaging examinations at 6-month intervals for 2 to 3 years and then at yearly intervals for up to 5 years.

## Computed Tomography

Early studies established the usefulness of CT in detecting local recurrence and metastases to lymph nodes, liver, peritoneal cavity, and retroperitoneum.[103, 104] As with primary tumors, high rates were reported initially for detection of locally recurrent tumor (sensitivity 93 to 95%),[105, 106] but later investigations indicated accuracy rates ranging from 69 to 88%.[107, 108] Most diagnostic errors are due to inability to detect microscopic invasion of perirectal or pericolonic fat, to assess presence or absence of metastatic foci in normal-sized lymph nodes (even if a diameter of 1 cm or less was used for normal), and to visualize local tumor at the anastomotic site.

In patients who had resection of primary colorectal tumor and reanastomosis, the CT features of recurrent tumor are similar to those described for primary tumors but the recurrence tends to be largely extrinsic to the anastomosis (Fig. 64–38). In these patients, wall thickening might also be caused by plication defects. Some studies of patients who had abdominoperineal resection suggested that streaky densities or a clean operative bed suggests fibrosis whereas the presence of a mostly globular mass favors the diagnosis of tumor recurrence.[49] However, other studies indicated that a mass of soft tissue density representing granulation tissue, hemorrhage, edema, and/or fibrosis could be present in the early postoperative period[55] (Fig. 64–39 and Table 64–5). Changes caused by radiation can also produce the appearance of streaky densities or a presacral mass.[105, 109, 110] Serial CT scans obtained within 28 months after operation showed that persistence of a mass for up to at least 24 months after AP resection may be normal.[110] A baseline CT study 2 to 4 months after surgery frequently demonstrates the presence of a mass. A study at 4 to 9 months often reveals a decrease in size and better definition of margins. In the absence of symptoms and elevated CEA titers, such a change of a mass should not cause concern about local tumor recurrence. How-

### TABLE 64–5. DIFFERENTIAL DIAGNOSIS OF COLORECTAL MASS WITH SOFT TISSUE STRANDING

Neoplasm (primary and secondary)
Focal colitis (e.g., ameboma, Crohn's disease)
Abscess
   Diverticulitis
   Pelvic inflammatory disease with contiguous colorectal
     inflammation
   Rectal perforation and inflammation
   Prostatitis, with contiguous inflammation and/or abscess
Following radiation
Endometriosis
Pancreatitis in either transverse colon or splenic flexure
Transplants of pancreas and kidney with rejection or pancreatitis
   and contiguous involvement of colon or rectum
Peritonitis with infected fluid in pouch of Douglas

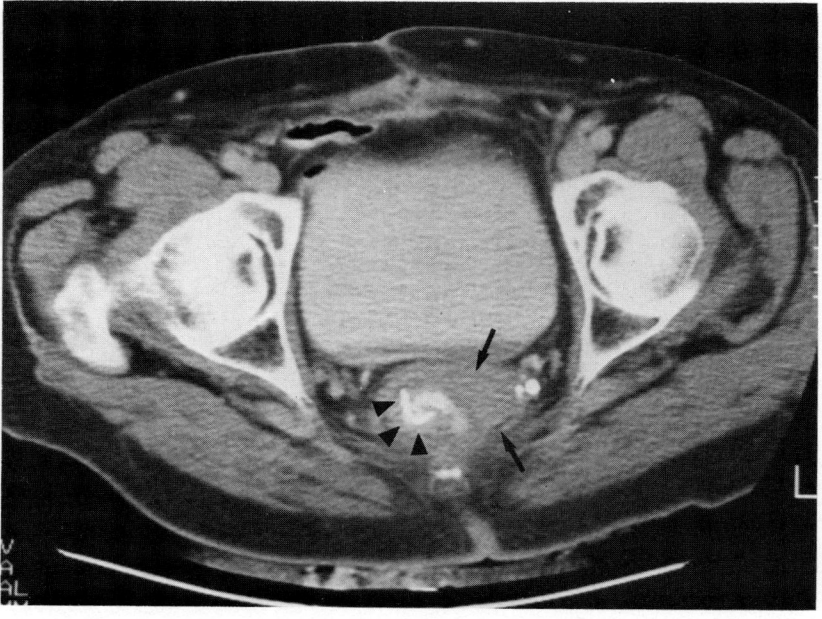

**Figure 64–38. Recurrent rectal carcinoma with extension into perirectal fat.** TNM stage T3, N0, M0. Thickening of the rectal wall is seen on the left side *(arrows)*. There is also extension into the perirectal fat. Staples *(arrowheads)* outline the area of anastomosis. Note the largely extrinsic component of this recurrence.

ever, any increase in size of a mass, with or without invasion of adjacent structures and with or without appearance of lymphadenopathy or perineal soft tissue density, should suggest recurrence, and percutaneous biopsy is indicated[109, 110] (Fig. 64–40). Biopsy results may be negative if the recurrent tumor incites a substantial fibrous reaction.

At present, CT is the best modality for detecting and staging recurrent rectal or rectosigmoid carcinomas because almost all recurrent tumors in patients who had sphincter-saving resection of rectal and rectosigmoid carcinomas develop extraluminally, infiltrating the suture lines secondarily with tumor extension beyond the bowel confines in one fourth of cases. For accurate staging, CT is superior to endoscopy and barium examinations, both of which permit the diagnosis of recurrence and show mucosal detail better than CT. However, without careful distention of colon using rectal contrast material and glucagon, some of the local recurrences may be missed by CT.[108] Although colonoscopy and barium enemas provide information on local disease, CT is the only method that accurately shows recurrence remote from the anastomotic side. In patients with complete AP resections, CT is the only modality

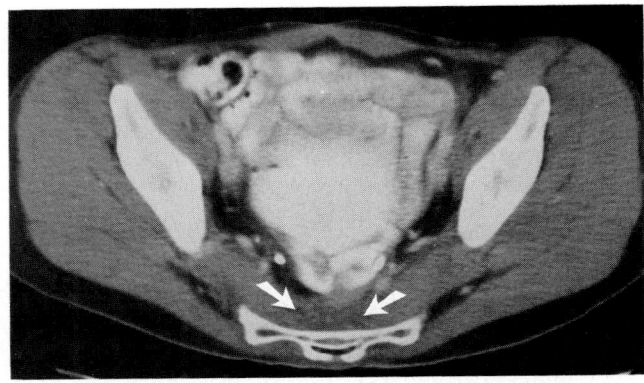

**Figure 64–39. Postsurgical scar in a patient with total AP resection.** A small area of soft tissue density *(arrows)* is seen in the presacral region.

for evaluating recurrent tumor (Fig. 64–41). Therefore, barium enema and CT are complementary methods for evaluating patients with suspected recurrent colon tumor. Definition of the full extent of disease, particularly to distant sites, is necessary if another resection is contemplated. Several studies have demonstrated that

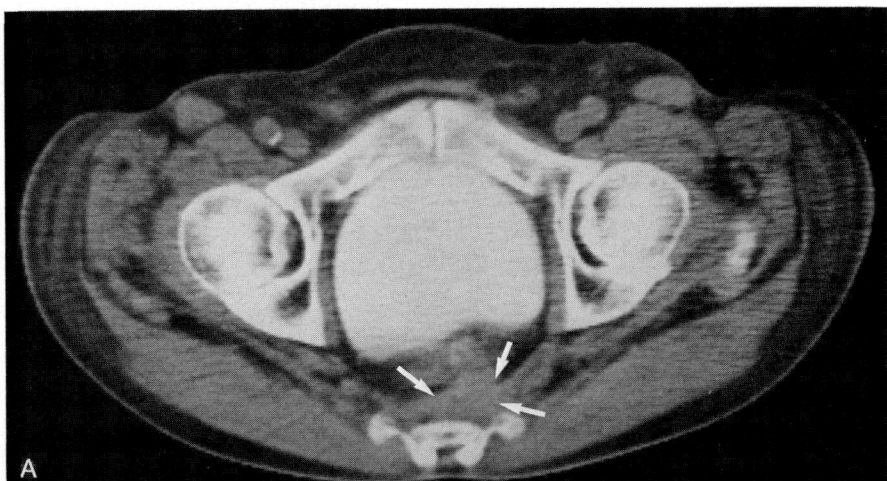

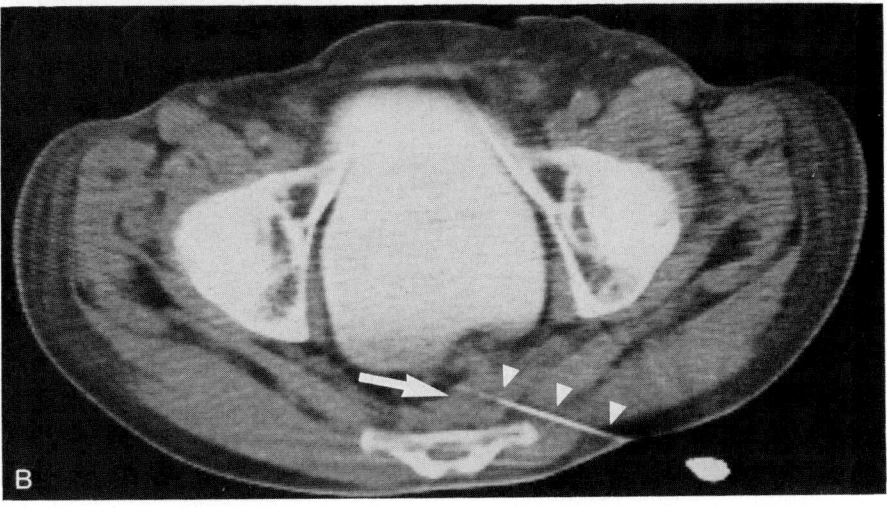

**Figure 64–40. CT scan of recurrent rectal mass in patient with total AP resection. A.** An irregular soft tissue mass *(arrows)* is identified in the area formerly occupied by the rectum. The size of this mass had increased slightly compared with a baseline CT study 1 year before the present examination. **B.** A percutaneous biopsy confirmed the presence of recurrent tumor. Arrowheads outline the needle with its tip in the mass of recurrent tumor *(arrow)*.

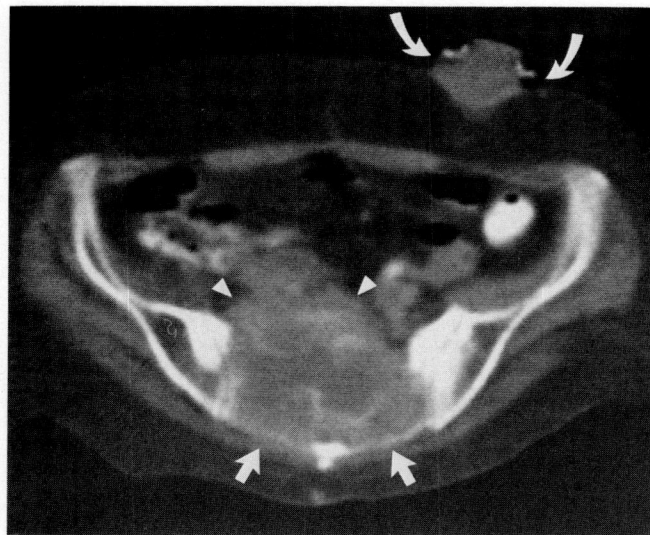

**Figure 64–41. Large recurrent tumor mass in a patient with a colostomy.** The mass *(arrowheads)* extends to the pelvic sidewalls with clear evidence of partial destruction of bone in the sacrum *(straight arrows)*. Colostomy *(curved arrows)* is seen anteriorly.

liver function tests and CEA levels were reported to be unreliable indicators of recurrent disease[22] unless a sudden increase in the CEA level is observed and other causes of the increase can be excluded.

## Magnetic Resonance Imaging

In patients with rectal cancer who had a low anterior resection or a transanal local excision, CT and MR results are similar. In some instances, large clips reduce the quality of CT images, but MR images may also be difficult to analyze when clips are present at an anastomotic site or in an area of lymphadenectomy. After total resection of the rectum, presacral masses are readily detected and staged with MR imaging. Initial reports on patients with total abdominoperineal resection suggested that fibrosis after surgery with or without radiation had a low signal intensity on both T1- and T2-weighted sequences, whereas tumor recurrence had a high signal intensity on T2-weighted images.[111–115] MR imaging was considered superior to CT in distinguishing between fibrosis and recurrent tumor, and the hope was raised that MR imaging could eliminate the need for percutaneous biopsies. However, it appears doubtful that MR imaging can distinguish among recurrent tumor, fibrosis, and inflammation.[116, 117]

One study, using long repetition time (TR), long echo time (TE) (T2-weighted) sequences, examined the value of MR imaging in distinguishing among early fibrosis (1 to 6 months after first treatment), tumor or late fibrosis (more than 12 months), and recurrent tumor. On T2-weighted images, tumor recurrence is diagnosed on the basis of high signal intensity, whereas scar or fibrosis has low signal intensity (Fig. 64–42). The authors found higher signal intensity values for early fibrosis after treatment than for late fibrosis, probably because of increased vascularity, edema, and the presence of immature mesenchymal cells in granulation tissue. Radiation-induced necrosis and postsurgical inflammatory reaction can also contribute to an increase in signal intensity on T2-weighted images. The increase in tissue fluids seen in granulation tissue and necrosis caused by radiation renders distinction between early fibrosis and tumor recurrence difficult or even impossible (Fig. 64–43). However, late fibrosis and tumor recurrence could be clearly distinguished from one another[116] (see Fig. 64–42). Other studies found similar results,[63, 114, 117] but

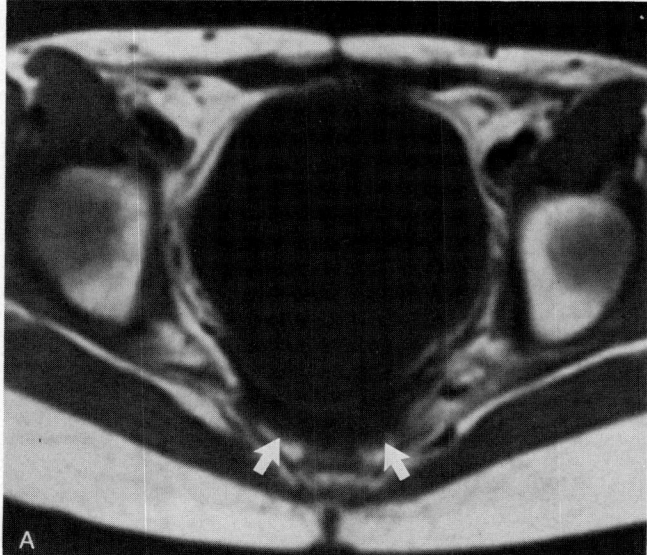

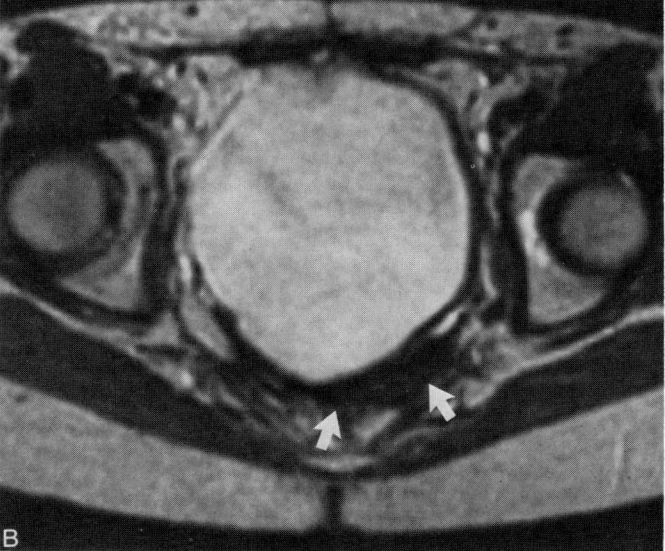

**Figure 64–42. MR image of a postsurgical scar in a patient with total colectomy. A.** T1-weighted spin-echo image (600/20). An area posterior to the bladder has low signal intensity *(arrows)*. **B.** T2-weighted spin-echo image (2500/70). The area of low signal intensity on T1-weighted images remains dark *(arrows)* on a T2-weighted scan, which suggests fibrosis in the surgical bed.

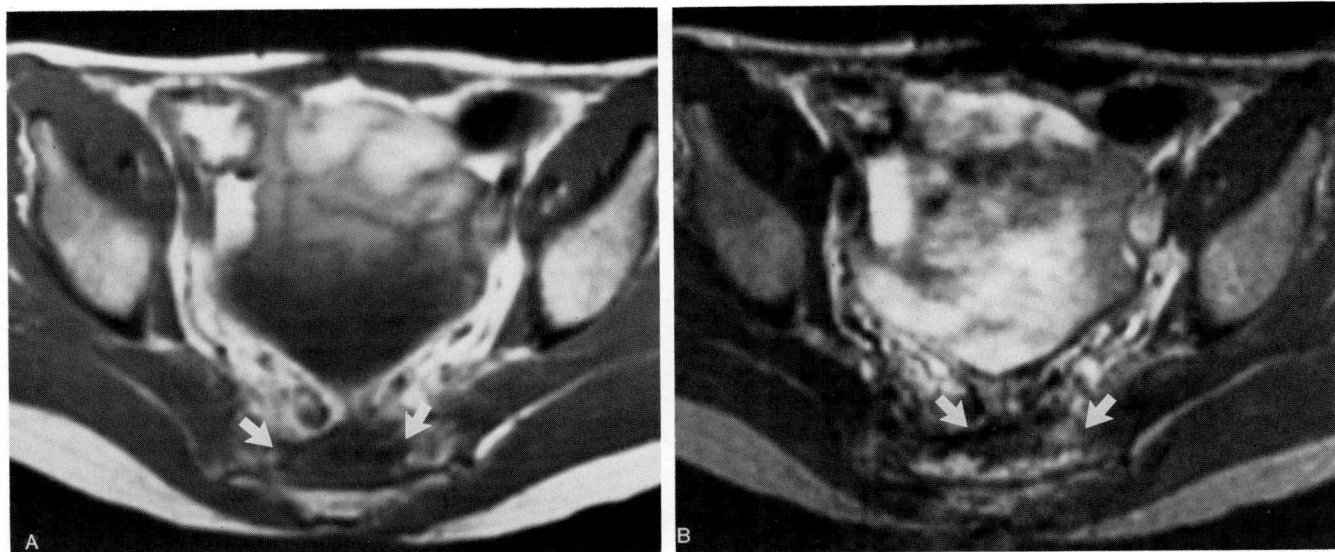

**Figure 64–43. Indeterminate MR image of recurrent carcinoma after total colectomy. A.** T1-weighted spin-echo image (700/20). An area of low signal intensity mixed with some intermediate signal intensity *(arrows)* is seen in the presacral space. **B.** T2-weighted spin-echo image (2500/70). The presacral soft tissue mass has intermediate signal intensity on T2-weighted scans *(arrows)*. This is an indeterminate result and could represent recurrent viable tumor with a moderate amount of fibrous stroma, mild tumor necrosis, inflammation, or granulation tissue after surgery and/or radiation.

one study showed that the accuracy of MR imaging in differentiating between radiation damage and residual or recurrent tumor varied with the primary site: it was excellent for cervical carcinoma but suboptimal for rectal carcinoma.[118] de Lange and colleagues compared MR imaging results with histologic sections from tissue obtained during radical pelvic exenteration or extensive partial resection of a mass in patients with suspected recurrent rectosigmoid carcinoma.[119] They found that the signal intensities on T2-weighted images do not permit prediction of the histologic diagnosis of a lesion. High signal intensity was found in areas of viable tumor (Fig. 64–44), tumor necrosis, benign inflammation, and edematous tissue. Because desmoplastic reaction is a common response to many benign and malignant processes, including tumors of the colon and rectum, areas

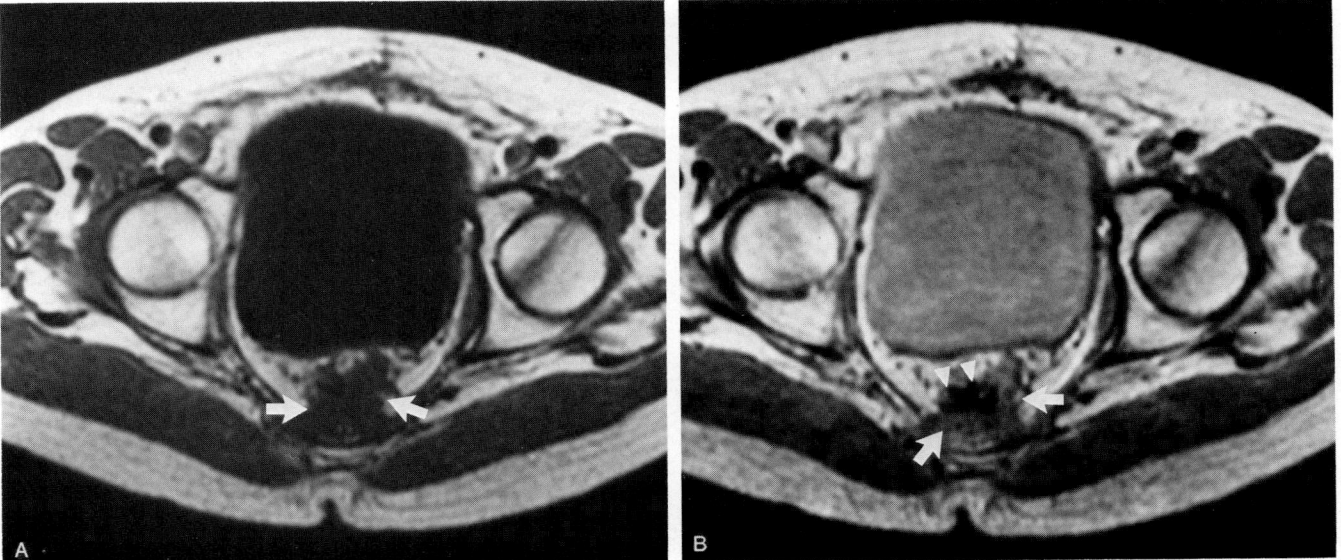

**Figure 64–44. MR image of recurrent rectal carcinoma. A.** T1-weighted spin echo sequence (700/20). An irregular mass of low signal intensity *(arrows)* is seen in the presacral space. **B.** T2-weighted spin-echo image (2500/70). The mass identified on the T1-weighted image increases in signal intensity on the T2-weighted image *(arrows)*, indicating recurrent tumor. Low signal intensity in the center *(arrowheads)* represents tumor necrosis.

of low signal intensity on T2-weighted images were also nonspecific and the differential diagnosis included tumor-induced fibrosis and non-neoplastic, benign fibrotic tissue. However, MR imaging can reveal a presacral mass accurately and demonstrate its extent well. If such a mass consists mainly of desmoplastic tissue with only small strands of interspersed tumor tissue, even a percutaneous biopsy may show only fibrous tissue and no malignant cells. In these cases, a definitive diagnosis must be made by surgical removal of mass or biopsy at laparotomy.

Like CT, MR imaging is a sensitive method for detecting masses after colorectal surgery, but its specificity is not better than that of CT. In these patients, benign and malignant processes cannot be distinguished on the basis of attenuation coefficients and morphologic appearance on CT scans or on the basis of signal intensity on MR images. CT may be more helpful in evaluating anastomoses in patients with suture material or multiple clips from lymphadenectomies because susceptibility artifacts may be prominent in the high magnetic field. However, large clips are also problematic for CT. For overall screening to detect nonlocal recurrence, CT may be more valuable than MR imaging, but more studies are needed to determine the efficacy of these procedures and their possibly complementary natures. A multi-institutional, multimodality prospective study on the use and effectiveness of these imaging techniques is eagerly awaited.[120]

Advances such as enhanced sequences, endoluminal coils, and fast imaging may improve results with MR imaging. However, newer techniques such as MoAb immunoscintigraphy and PET after intravenous injection of 18-FDG are promising and may hold the key to accurate detection of tumor stage and distinction of recurrent rectal cancer from scar.[121]

## Transrectal Sonography

The findings and results of transrectal ultrasound for recurrent colorectal malignancy are similar to those for primary carcinoma, but the examination can be done only for patients who had a transanal local excision, a low anterior resection, or (in women) an abdominoperineal resection. In patients with total AP resection and colostomy, the recurrent tumor should be assessed by CT, MR imaging, PET, or scintigraphy with MoAbs.

Endosonography has enabled highly accurate assessment of local recurrence. In one study, endosonography revealed all 15 recurrences of rectal neoplasm.[122] In four cases, CEA titers were not elevated and rectal or vaginal digital examination, rigid rectoscope examination, and pelvic CT scans were negative. In these four patients, endosonography was the only method that detected recurrence. Therefore, transrectal sonography or endosonography should be used for evaluation of patients when recurrence is suspected or the patients had a tumor grade or stage with a high prognostic factor for recurrence, even if the results of initial tests in routine followup examinations are negative.

## Immunoscintigraphy

Most results of MoAb immunoscintigraphy have been for patients with primary colorectal tumors. Only a small number of patients with recurrent or residual tumor were included in these series. However, there is no reason to believe that results for patients with recurrent disease should be different from those for patients with primary colorectal tumors (Fig. 64–45). Therefore, the reader is asked to consult the earlier section on immunoscintigraphy.

## Positron Emission Tomography

PET has been employed extensively for assessing patients with suspected recurrence or residual tumor from colorectal neoplasms. In several studies, the distinction between neoplasm and scar tissue was made with a high degree of accuracy. In one study, all 21 recurrent tumors had high 18-FDG uptake with lesion/soft tissue ratios between 1.19 and 4.94.[29] However, based on the 18-FDG differential absorption ratio values, one patient was misclassified because of low 18-FDG uptake. All scars in the pelvis after AP resection were correctly identified. In another study, in five patients whose CT and PET results were similar, three recurrences and two scars were correctly identified.[30] In four patients with negative or equivocal CT scans, PET correctly identified all tumors, and in three patients whose CT scans raised suspicion of recurrence, PET correctly excluded recurrence. It appears that PET is an accurate method for detection of recurrence of colorectal neoplasms and may offer an alternative to biopsy because it successfully excludes recurrence in patients with suspicious masses in the surgical bed. Nevertheless, larger series are needed to confirm these results, and

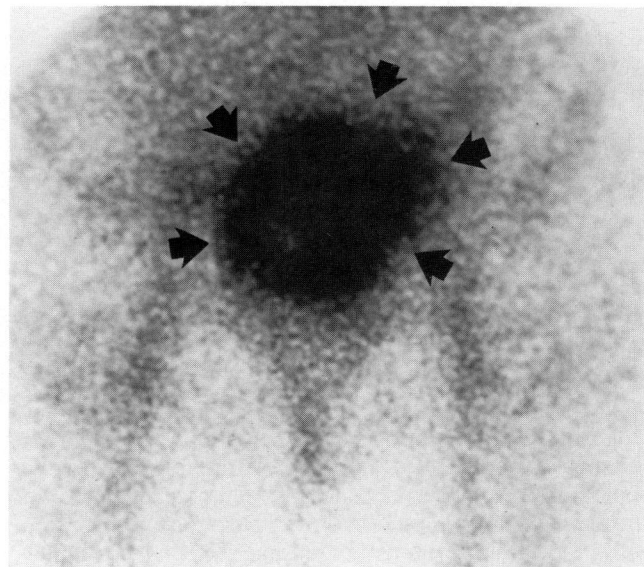

**Figure 64–45. Immunoscintigraphy of recurrent rectal carcinoma.** A large mass of high radioactivity *(arrows)* is seen in the pelvis of a patient with recurrent rectal tumor.

improvements in PET scanners may increase the reliability of the technique in distinguishing between scar and recurrent or residual tumor.

## ROLE OF CROSS-SECTIONAL IMAGING IN RECURRENT COLORECTAL CARCINOMA

It is difficult to compare CT and MR imaging, used alone or in combination, for detection of primary and recurrent disease, mainly because of the great variations for both techniques in the types of scanners used, the scanning methods, and the methods of administering the contrast agent. Even the diagnostic criteria, the study population, and the analysis of the data vary greatly.

After surgery, evaluation of the surgical site is important because local recurrence of colon carcinoma after surgery is not uncommon. In a study of 280 patients who had complete resection of primary adenocarcinoma of the colon, Cass and associates found that 105 patients (37%) had recurrence of the tumor within the first 2 years after surgery.[102] Of these 105 patients, 60% had local recurrence alone, 14% had concomitant local recurrence and distant metastases, and 26% had isolated distant metastases. In 92% of the patients with local recurrences, the recurrent tumor was contiguous to the area of the incision. After surgery, CT has proved a valuable tool in assessing the success of therapy, determining the presence or absence of recurrence, and designing radiation ports for patients with unresectable recurrent tumors.

Because of the high frequency of tumor recurrence in the first 24 months after surgery, a series of follow-up CT examinations is obtained to detect early tumor recurrence. In addition, a CT scan is obtained whenever a patient has a rising CEA titer. Because local recurrence of cancer occurs in 50% within the first year and in 80% within the second year, patients with suspected recurrence should have a baseline study 3 to 4 months after initial surgery, when postsurgical acute changes such as edema and hemorrhage have cleared, and follow-up examinations every 6 months during the first 2 years and then at yearly intervals. The results of the follow-up examinations should be compared with those of the baseline study to avoid unnecessary biopsies. A study is considered positive if a mass or nodes are detected that were not seen on the baseline study or have become larger since the original study. Any new mass or nodes should be biopsied using a transgluteal percutaneous approach in the case of rectosigmoid tumor masses.[123]

Although CT should not be used as the primary modality for examining patients with suspected colon tumors, it is a good method, short of surgery, for assessing presence or absence of recurrent colon tumors with a high degree of reliability, particularly in patients with abdominoperineal resections. This is particularly important for men, in whom a recurrent mass cannot be easily palpated after complete AP resection of a rectal tumor. In women, recurrent masses can frequently be examined by a vaginal approach.

MR imaging cannot distinguish reliably between recurrence and scar on the basis of signal intensity because of the desmoplastic nature of rectal tumors and changes in signal characteristics in the surgical bed caused by hemorrhage and edema immediately after surgery and granulation tissue and edema after radiation. For distinguishing between recurrence and scar, MR imaging has no significant advantage over CT. However, because it can distinguish between soft tissue components of many pelvic organs and detect tissue planes between organs in the pelvis based on even a small amount of fat and improved visualization of these planes with imaging in coronal and sagittal planes, MR imaging often can better determine whether a rectal neoplasm has invaded neighboring organs. However, like CT, MR imaging is poor in assessing microinvasion and metastases to lymph nodes. Whether MR imaging with a lymphangiographic contrast agent that selectively accumulates in lymph nodes becomes a useful and accurate test remains to be seen.

In patients who had low anterior resection, transanal local excision, or (in women) abdominoperineal resection, endosonography has had excellent results in detecting local recurrence and should become an important adjunct to CT arterial portography, PET, and immunoscintigraphy for complete and accurate assessment of patients with suspected recurrence of colorectal neoplasms.

Since the introduction of MoAb immunoscintigraphy, CT results have been challenged and in many instances immunoscintigraphy has surpassed CT in distinguishing scars from recurrent neoplasms. However, metastases to lymph nodes and liver are not detected with acceptable accuracy by this method. Whether PET can improve these results remains to be seen.

As various imaging methods are used more frequently for follow-up study of patients with resected colon tumors, even small tumor recurrences will probably be detected. It is not yet known whether the detection and staging of these recurrent tumors will ultimately improve the overall 5-year survival rate of these patients.

### Acknowledgment

Figures 64–1C; 64–2A, C, and D; 64–3B; 64–4A to D; 64–5A and B; 64–6A and B; 64–7A and B; 64–9; 64–11; 64–12A and B; 64–13A and B; 64–14; 64–33A and B; 64–34; and 64–35 are reproduced from Laufer I, Levine MS (eds): Double Contrast Gastrointestinal Radiology (2nd ed). Philadelphia: WB Saunders, 1992.

## References

1. Boring CC, Squires TS, Tong T: Cancer statistics, 1993. Cancer 43:7–26, 1993.
2. Luk GD: Epidemiology, etiology, and diagnosis of colorectal neoplasia. Curr Opin Gastroenterol 9:19–27, 1993.
3. Smart CR: Cancer of the colon and rectum in the United States: the scope of the problem. *In* Beahrs OH, Higgins JA, Weinstein

JJ (eds): Colorectal Tumors. Philadelphia: JB Lippincott, 1986, pp 3–8.

4. Schub R, Steinheber FU: Rightward shift of colon cancer. J Clin Gastroenterol 8:630–634, 1986.
5. Lynch HT, Lanspa SJ, Lynch JF: Hereditary colon cancer syndromes: polyposis and non-polyposis (Lynch syndromes I and II) variants. *In* MacDonald JS (ed): Gastrointestinal Oncology. Boston: Martinus Nijhoff, 1987, pp 93–148.
6. Vogelstein B: A model of colorectal tumorigenesis. Adv Oncol 7:2–6, 1991.
7. Ransohoff DF: Colon cancer and ulcerative colitis. Gastroenterology 94:1089–1091, 1988.
8. Lane N, Fenoglio CM: The adenoma-carcinoma sequence in the stomach and colon. I. Observations on the adenoma as precursor to ordinary large bowel carcinoma. Gastrointest Radiol 1:111–119, 1976.
9. Winawer SJ, Zauber AG, O'Brien MJ, et al: The national polyp study. Design, methods, and characteristics of patients with newly diagnosed polyps. Cancer 70:1236–1245, 1992.
10. Levin B: Inflammatory bowel disease and colon cancer. Cancer 70:1313–1316, 1992.
11. Maruyama M: Recent trends in gross pathology of early colorectal cancer. Ito Cho (Stomach and Intestine) 22:879–883, 1987.
12. Eddy D: Cancer of the colon and rectum. CA 30:208–215, 1980.
13. Eddy DM, Nugent FW, Eddy JF, et al: Screening for colorectal cancer in a high-risk population. Gastroenterology 92:682–692, 1987.
14. Levine MS, Laufer I: Rectum. *In* Laufer I, Levine MS (eds): Double Contrast Gastrointestinal Radiology (2nd ed). Philadelphia: WB Saunders, 1992, pp 647–686.
15. Ott DJ, Chen YM, Gelfand DW, et al: Single-contrast vs. double-contrast barium enema in the detection of colonic polyps. AJR 146:993–996, 1986.
16. Fork FT, Lindstrom C, Ekelund GR: Reliability of routine double-contrast examination (DCE) of the large bowel in polyp detection: a prospective clinical study. Gastrointest Radiol 8:163–172, 1983.
17. Anderson ML, Heigh RI, McCoy GA, et al: Accuracy of assessment of the extent of examination by experienced colonoscopists. Gastrointest Endosc 38:560–563, 1992.
18. Miller RE, Lehman G: Polypoid colonic lesions undetected by endoscopy. Radiology 129:295–297, 1978.
19. Weyman PJ, Koehler RE, Zuckerman GR: Resolution of radiographic-endoscopic discrepancies in colon neoplasms. J Clin Gastroenterol 3:89–93, 1981.
20. Habr-Gama A, Waye JD: Complications and hazards of gastrointestinal endoscopy. World J Surg 13:193–201, 1989.
21. Thompson WM, Halvorsen RA, Foster WL, et al: Preoperative and postoperative CT staging of rectosigmoid carcinoma. AJR 146:703–710, 1986.
22. Freeny PC, Marks WM, Ryan JA, et al: Colorectal carcinoma evaluation with CT: preoperative staging and detection of postoperative recurrence. Radiology 158:347–353, 1986.
23. Butch RJ, Stark DD, Wittenberg J, et al: Staging rectal cancer by MR and CT. AJR 146:1155–1160, 1986.
24. Guinet C, Buy JN, Ghossain MA, et al: Comparison of magnetic resonance imaging and computed tomography in the preoperative staging of rectal cancer. Arch Surg 125:385–388, 1990.
25. Holdsworth PJ, Johnston D, Chalmers AG, et al: Endoluminal ultrasound and computed tomography in the staging of rectal cancer. Br J Surg 75:1019–1022, 1988.
26. Rifkin MD, Ehrlich SM, Marks G: Staging of rectal carcinoma: prospective comparison of endorectal US and CT. Radiology 170:319–322, 1989.
27. Abdel-Nabi HH, Schwartz AN, Goldfogel G, et al: Colorectal tumors: scintigraphy with In-111 anti-CEA monoclonal antibody and correlation with surgical, histopathologic, and immunohistochemical findings. Radiology 166:747–752, 1988.
28. Abdel-Nabi H, Doerr RJ, Chan HW, et al: In-111 labeled monoclonal antibody immunoscintigraphy in colorectal carcinoma: safety, sensitivity, and preliminary clinical results. Radiology 175:163–171, 1990.
29. Strauss LG, Clorius JH, Schlag P, et al: Recurrence of colorectal tumors: PET evaluation. Radiology 170:329–332, 1989.
30. Gupta NC, Boman BM, Frank AR, et al: PET-FDG imaging for follow-up evaluation of treated colorectal cancer. Radiology 181:199, 1991 (abstract).
31. Bernstein MA, Feczko PJ, Halpert RD, et al: Distribution of colonic polyps: increased incidence of proximal lesions in older patients. Radiology 155:35–38, 1985.
32. Rubesin SE, Levine MS, Laufer I, et al: Villous adenomas: the scientific and the practical. Radiology 167:869–870, 1988.
33. Iida M, Iwashita A, Yao T, et al: Villous tumor of the colon: correlation of histologic, macroscopic, and radiographic features. Radiology 167:673–677, 1988.
34. Delamarre J, Descombes P, Marti R, et al: Villous tumor of the colon: double-contrast study of 47 cases. Gastrointest Radiol 5:69–73, 1980.
35. Miller WT Jr, Levine MS, Rubesin SE, et al: Bowler hat sign: a simple principle for differentiating polyps from diverticula. Radiology 173:615–617, 1989.
36. Rubesin SE, Sul SH, Laufer I, et al: Carpet lesions of the colon. Radiographics 5:537–552, 1985.
37. Coscina WF, Arger PH, Herlinger H, et al: CT diagnosis of villous adenoma. J Comput Assist Tomogr 10:764–766, 1986.
38. Youker JE, Welin S, Main G: Computer analysis in the differentiation of benign and malignant polypoid lesions of the colon. Radiology 90:794–797, 1968.
39. Morson BC: The polyp-cancer sequence in the large bowel. Proc R Soc Med 67:451–457, 1974.
40. Welin S, Youker J, Spratt JS Jr: The rates and patterns of growth of 375 tumors of the large intestine and rectum observed serially by double contrast enema study (Malmö technique). AJR 90:673–687, 1963.
41. Smith TR: Pedunculated malignant colonic polyps with superficial invasion of the stalk. Radiology 115:593–596, 1975.
42. Fischel RE, Dermer R: Multifocal carcinoma of the large intestine. Clin Radiol 26:495–498, 1975.
43. Raskin MM, Viamonte M, Viamonte M Jr: Primary linitis plastica carcinoma of the colon. Radiology 113:17–22, 1974.
44. Laufer I, Joffe N: Some roentgenologic aspects of chronic perforating carcinoma of the colon. Dis Colon Rectum 16:127–135, 1973.
45. Wilson SM, Adson MA: The surgical treatment of hepatic metastases from colorectal cancers. Arch Surg 111:330–334, 1976.
46. Lee KT, Stanley RJ, Sagel SS, et al: Accuracy of CT in detecting intra-abdominal and pelvic lymph node metastases from pelvic cancers. AJR 131:675–679, 1978.
47. Zaunbauer W, Haertel M, Fuchs WA: Computed tomography in carcinoma of the rectum. Gastrointest Radiol 6:79–84, 1981.
48. Frommhold W, Hübener KH: The role of computerized tomography in the after care of patients suffering from a carcinoma of the rectum. Comput Tomogr 5:161–168, 1981.
49. Lee JKT, Stanley RJ, Sagel SS, et al: CT appearance of the pelvis after abdomino-perineal resection for rectal carcinoma. Radiology 141:737–741, 1981.
50. Doubleday LC, Bernardino ME: CT findings in the perirectal area following radiation therapy. J Comput Assist Tomogr 4:634–638, 1980.
51. Colley DP, Farrell JA, Clark RA: Perforated colon carcinoma presenting as a suprarenal mass. Comput Tomogr 5:55–58, 1981.
52. Dukes CE: The classification of cancer of the rectum. J Pathol 35:323–332, 1932.
53. Astler VB, Coller FA: The prognostic significance of direct extension of carcinoma of the colon and rectum. Ann Surg 139:846–851, 1954.
54. Turnbull RB Jr: The no-touch isolation technique of resection. JAMA 231:1181–1182, 1975.
55. Thoeni RF, Moss AA, Schnyder P, et al: Detection and staging of primary rectal and rectosigmoid cancer by computed tomography. Radiology 141:135–138, 1981.
56. Denoix PF: Monograph 4, Paris, French Ministry of Public Health National Institute of Hygiene, 1954.
57. Dixon AK, Fry IK, Morson BC, et al: Preoperative computed tomography of carcinoma of the rectum. Br J Radiol 54:655–659, 1981.
58. Grabbe E, Lierse W, Winkler R: The perirectal fascia: morphology and use in staging of rectal carcinoma. Radiology 149:241–246, 1983.

59. van Waes PF, Koehler PR, Feldberg MA: Management of rectal carcinoma: impact of computed tomography. AJR 140:1137–1142, 1983.

60. Cohan RH, Silverman PM, Thompson WM, et al: Computed tomography of epithelial neoplasms of the anal canal. AJR 145:569–573, 1985.

61. Balthazar EJ, Megibow AJ, Hulnick D, et al: Carcinoma of the colon: detection and preoperative staging by CT. AJR 150:301–306, 1988.

62. Adalsteinsson B, Gilmelius B, Graffman S, et al: Computed tomography in staging rectal carcinoma. Acta Radiol Diagn 26:45–50, 1985.

63. Megibow AJ, Zerhouni EA, Hylnick DH, et al: Air insufflation of the colon as an adjunct to computed tomography of the pelvis. J Comput Assist Tomogr 8:797–800, 1984.

64. Dooms GC, Hricak H, Crooks LE, et al: Magnetic resonance imaging of the lymph nodes: comparison with CT. Radiology 153:710–738, 1984.

65. Hodgman CG, MacCarty RL, Wolff BG, et al: Preoperative staging of rectal carcinoma by computed tomography and 0.15T magnetic resonance imaging: preliminary report. Dis Colon Rectum 29:446–450, 1986.

66. Guinet C, Buy J-N, Sezeur A, et al: Preoperative assessment of the extension of rectal carcinoma: correlation of MR, surgical, and histopathologic findings. J Comput Assist Tomogr 12:209–214, 1988.

67. de Lange EE, Gechner RE, Edge SB, et al: Preoperative staging of rectal carcinoma with MR imaging: surgical and histopathologic correlation. Radiology 176:623–628, 1990.

68. Chan TW, Milestone B, Kressel HY, et al: MR imaging of rectal carcinoma using an endorectal coil. Society of Magnetic Resonance in Medicine, 9th Annual Scientific Meeting and Exhibition, 1990, p 305 (abstract).

69. Herzog U, von Flüe M, Tondelli P, et al: How accurate is endorectal ultrasound in the pre-operative staging of rectal cancer? Dis Colon Rectum 36:127–134, 1993.

70. Tio TL, Coene PPL, Van Delden OM, et al: Colorectal carcinoma: preoperative TNM classification with endosonography. Radiology 179:165–170, 1991.

71. Fukuda M: Endoscopic sonography. Ultrasound 8:141–170, 1986.

72. Takemoto T, Aibe T, Fuji T, et al: Endoscopic ultrasonography. Clin Gastroenterol 15:305–319, 1986.

73. Delaloye B, Bischof-Delaloye A, Buchegger F, et al: Detection of colorectal carcinoma by emission computerized tomography after injection of I-123 labeled Fab or F(ab′)₂ fragments from monoclonal anti-carcinoembryonic antigen antibodies. J Clin Invest 77:301–311, 1986.

74. Mach JP, Buchegger F, Forni M, et al: Use of radiolabeled monoclonal anti-CEA antibodies for the detection of human carcinomas by external photoscanning and tomoscintigraphy. Immunol Today 2:239–249, 1981.

75. Abdel-Nabi HH, Schwartz AN, Higano CS, et al: Colorectal carcinoma detection with indium-111 anticarcinoembryonic antigen monoclonal antibody ZCE 025. Radiology 164:617–621, 1987.

76. Lamki LM, Patt YZ, Murra JL, et al: Scintigraphic findings of colonic cancer using indium-labeled anti-CEA monoclonal antibody ZCE 025 combined with unlabeled antibody. J Nucl Med 27:1021, 1986 (abstract).

77. Carroll RH, Harwood SJ, Sinni BJ: In-111–labeled anti ZCE 025 monoclonal antibody SPECT in abdominal colorectal cancer. J Nucl Med 28:604, 1987 (abstract).

78. Collier BD, Abdel-Nabi H, Doerr R, et al: Detection of colorectal cancer with In-111–labeled CYT-103. Radiology 177:258, 1990 (abstract).

79. Lamki LM, Patt YZ, Murray JL, et al: Superiority of In-111–monoclonal antibody to CT and other conventional imaging studies in the diagnosis of occult recurrence of colorectal cancer. Radiology 177:258, 1990 (abstract).

80. Goodman MM, Elmaleh DR, Merk L, et al: F-18-2 and 3-fluorodeoxy-D-glucose as potential diagnostic tracers for tumors. J Nucl Med 21:37, 1981 (abstract).

81. Paul R, Johansen R, Kurur A, et al: Imaging of canine cancers with 18-F-2-fluoro-2-deoxy-D-glucose (FDG) suggests further applications for cancer imaging in man. Nucl Med Commun 5:641–646, 1984.

82. Kelvin FM, Maglinte DT: Colorectal carcinoma. A radiologic and clinical review. Radiology 164:1–8, 1987.

83. Zinkin LD: A critical review of the classifications and staging of colorectal cancer. Dis Colon Rectum 26:37–43, 1983.

84. Nauta R, Stablein D, Holyoke D: Survival of patients with stage B2 colon carcinoma: the gastrointestinal tumor study group experience. Arch Surg 124:180–182, 1989.

85. Durdey P, Williams NS: The effect of malignant and inflammatory fixation of rectal carcinoma on prognosis after rectal excision. Br J Surg 71:787–790, 1984.

86. Sugarbaker PH, Kemeny N: Management of metastatic cancer to the liver. Adv Surg 22:1–56, 1989.

87. Hamlin DF, Burgener FA, Sischy B: New techniques to stage early rectal carcinoma by computed tomography. Radiology 141:539–540, 1981.

88. Enker WE, Dragacevic S: Multiple carcinomas of the large bowel: a natural experiment in etiology and pathogenesis. Ann Surg 187:8–11, 1978.

89. Shauffer IA, Sequeira J: Suture granuloma simulating recurrent carcinoma. AJR 128:856–857, 1977.

90. Daly BD, Crowley BM: Radiological appearances of colonic ring staple anastomoses. Br J Radiol 62:256–259, 1989.

91. Chen YM, Ott DJ, Wolfman NT, et al: Recurrent colorectal carcinoma: evaluation with barium enema examination and CT. Radiology 163:307–310, 1987.

92. McCarthy SM, Barnes D, Deveney K, et al: Detection of recurrent rectosigmoid carcinoma: prospective evaluation of CT and clinical factors. AJR 144:577–579, 1985.

93. Sharpe M, Golden R: End-to-end anastomosis of the colon following resection: a Roentgen study of 42 cases. AJR 64:769–777, 1950.

94. Fleischner FG, Berenberg AL: Recurrent carcinoma of the colon at the site of anastomosis. Radiology 66:540–547, 1956.

95. Welch JP, Donaldson GA: Detection and treatment of recurrent cancer of the colon and rectum. Am J Surg 135:505–511, 1978.

96. Thoeni RF, Moss AA: The gastrointestinal tract. In Moss AA, Gamsu G, Genant H (eds): Computed Tomography of the Body. Philadelphia: WB Saunders, 1992, pp 643–734.

97. Kelvin FM, Korobkin M, Breiman RS, et al: Recurrent rectal carcinoma in an asymptomatic patient. J Comput Assist Tomogr 6:186–188, 1982.

98. Bühler H, Seefeld U, Dehyle P, et al: Endoscopic follow-up after colorectal cancer surgery. Cancer 54:791–793, 1984.

99. Barkin JS, Cohen ME, Flaxman M, et al: Value of routine follow-up endoscopy program for the detection of recurrent colorectal carcinoma. Am J Gastroenterol 88:1355–1360, 1988.

100. Stulc JP, Petrelli NJ, Herrera L, et al: Anastomotic recurrence of adenocarcinoma of the colon. Arch Surg 121:1077–1080, 1986.

101. Olson RM, Perencevich P, Malcolm AW, et al: Patterns of recurrence following curative resection of adenocarcinoma of the colon and rectum. Cancer 45:2969–2974, 1980.

102. Cass AW, Million RR, Pfaff W: Patterns of recurrence following surgery alone for adenocarcinoma of the colon and rectum. Cancer 37:1861–1865, 1976.

103. Husband JE, Hodson NJ, Parsons CA: The use of computed tomography in recurrent rectal tumors. Radiology 134:677–682, 1980.

104. Ellert J, Kreel L: The value of CT in malignant colonic tumors. J Comput Tomogr 4:225–240, 1980.

105. Moss AA, Thoeni RF, Schnyder P, et al: Value of computed tomography in the detection and staging of recurrent rectal carcinomas. J Comput Assist Tomogr 5:870–874, 1981.

106. Adalsteinsson B, Glimelius B, Graffman S, et al: Computed tomography of recurrent renal carcinoma. Acta Radiol Diagn 22:669–672, 1981.

107. McCarthy SM, Barnes D, Deveney K, et al: Detection of recurrent rectosigmoid carcinoma: prospective evaluation of CT and clinical factors. AJR 144:577–579, 1985.

108. Chen YM, Ott DJ, Wolfman N: Recurrent colorectal carcinoma: evaluation with barium enema examination and CT. Radiology 163:307–310, 1987.

109. Reznek RH, White FE, Young JW, et al: The appearances on computed tomography after abdomino-perineal resection for carcinoma of the rectum: a comparison between the normal

appearances and those of recurrence. Br J Radiol 56:237–240, 1983.

110. Kelvin FM, Korobkin M, Heaston DK, et al: The pelvis after surgery for rectal carcinoma: serial CT observations with emphasis on nonneoplastic features. AJR 141:959–964, 1983.

111. Blum L, Kressel HY, de Roos A, et al: MR imaging differentiation of fibrosis versus recurrent colorectal carcinoma in the pelvis: quantitative assessment. Radiology 169:167, 1988 (abstract).

112. Gomberg JS, Friedman AC, Radecki PD: MRI differentiation of recurrent colorectal carcinoma from postoperative fibrosis. Gastrointest Radiol 11:361–363, 1986.

113. Glazer HS, Lee JKT, Levitt RG, et al: Radiation fibrosis: differentiation from recurrent tumor by MR imaging. Radiology 156:721–726, 1985.

114. Johnson RH, Jenkins JPR, Isherwood I, et al: Quantitative magnetic resonance imaging in rectal carcinoma. Br J Radiol 60:761–764, 1987.

115. Heiken JP, Lee JKT: MR imaging of the pelvis. Radiology 166:11–16, 1988.

116. Ebner F, Kressel HY, Mintz MC, et al: Tumor recurrence versus fibrosis in the female pelvis: differentiation with MR imaging at 1.5T. Radiology 166:333–340, 1988.

117. Rafto SE, Amendola MA, Gefter WB: MR imaging of recurrent colorectal carcinoma versus fibrosis. J Comput Assist Tomogr 12:521–523, 1988.

118. Sugimura K, Carrington BM, Quivey JM, et al: Postirradiation changes in the pelvis: assessment with MR imaging. Radiology 175:805–813, 1990.

119. de Lange EE, Fechner RE, Wanebo HJ: Suspected recurrent rectosigmoid carcinoma after abdominoperineal resection: MR imaging and histopathologic findings. Radiology 170:323–328, 1989.

120. Moss AA: Imaging of colorectal carcinoma. Radiology 170:308–310, 1989.

121. Schlag P, Lehner B, Strauss LG: Scar or recurrent cancer. Arch Surg 124:198–200, 1989.

122. Tschmelitsch J, Glaser K, Schwarz C, et al: Endosonography (ES) in the diagnosis of recurrent cancer of the rectum. J Ultrasound Med 11:149–153, 1992.

123. Butch RJ, Wittenberg J, Mueller PR, et al: Presacral masses after abdominoperineal resection for colorectal carcinoma: the need for needle biopsy. AJR 144:309–312, 1985.

# Other Tumors

Stephen E. Rubesin, M.D.

Emma E. Furth, M.D.

## INTRODUCTION

This chapter discusses a variety of benign and malignant tumors of the colon as separate entities. Although these tumors have a wide range of clinical and radiologic manifestations, they may have typical radiologic features suggestive of their diagnosis.

## LYMPHOMA

### Pathologic Findings

Malignant lymphomas involve the gastrointestinal tract either as primary neoplasms or as part of disseminated disease. The colon is the third most common primary site of lymphoma involving the gastrointestinal tract (after stomach and small bowel), occurring in 6 to 12% of cases.[1-3] Primary lymphoma of the colon is rare, constituting 0.4% of primary colonic malignancies.[4, 5] Colonic involvement by systemic lymphoma is relatively common, with microscopic evidence of tumor in up to 44% of cases at autopsy.[3] However, patients with disseminated lymphoma involving the colon are usually asymptomatic and are not studied with barium techniques. Non-Hodgkin's lymphoma accounts for almost all colonic lymphomas; Hodgkin's disease involving the colon is extremely rare.[1, 6, 7] Large cell lymphoma is the most common primary non-Hodgkin's lymphoma sub-

type.[2] A more complete discussion about the pathology of lymphomas is presented in Chapter 151.

## Clinical Findings

Primary non-Hodgkin's lymphoma of bowel is usually seen in middle-aged or elderly persons.[2] Males are more frequently affected than females by a ratio of 2:1.[6, 8] The signs and symptoms of colonic lymphoma are nonspecific. The average duration of symptoms is 4 to 6 months.[6, 9] Abdominal pain, weight loss, and changing bowel habits occur in 60 to 90% of patients.[6, 9] Rectal bleeding or diarrhea is seen in one fourth of patients.[6] Long-standing ulcerative colitis may be a predisposing condition of colonic lymphoma.[6, 8, 10, 11] A palpable abdominal mass is the most frequent physical finding.[6]

## Radiographic Findings and Differential Diagnosis

The primary form of colonic lymphoma usually involves the cecum or rectum.[12, 13] Systemic lymphoma usually involves the entire colon or long segments of bowel.[7, 13-15] The localized form of colonic lymphoma has a wide variety of radiographic types, including a polypoid mass, a circumferential mural lesion, and a cavitary mass.

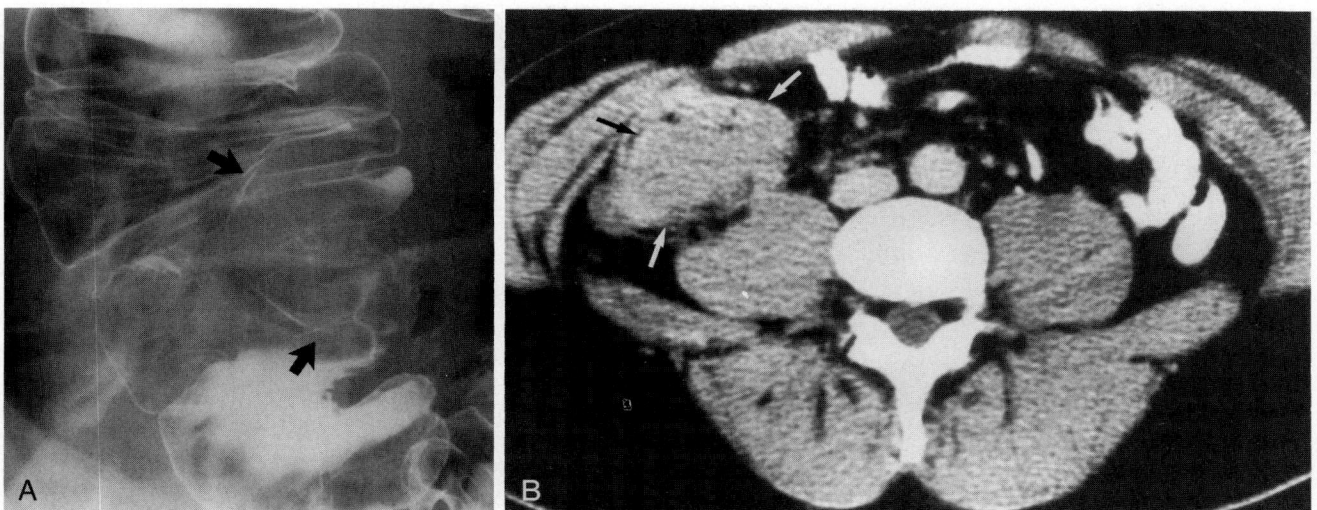

**Figure 65–1. Lymphoma of the ileocecal valve. A.** Spot film from a double contrast barium enema shows a smooth-surfaced mass replacing the ileocecal valve *(arrows).* **B.** Computed tomographic scan shows a right lower quadrant soft tissue mass filling and expanding the cecum *(arrows).*

Bulky, polypoid masses are the most frequent form of primary colonic lymphoma.[5, 9, 12, 15, 16] These lesions vary from 4 to 20 cm in size and are most frequently located near the ileocecal valve[12] (Fig. 65–1). Extension of cecal lymphoma into the terminal ileum is not uncommon (Fig. 65–2).

The annular infiltrating form usually involves a long segment (9 cm) of colon as a concentric narrowing (Fig. 65–3) or cavitary mass[5] (Fig. 65–4). Although the colonic lumen may be narrowed, obstruction is uncommon. The infiltrating lesion is discrete, with thick, irregular, rigid haustral folds and a nodular surface pattern. Although the contour is irregular, the mucosal surface is smooth, suggesting submucosal infiltration rather than mucosal ulceration (Fig. 65–5). Thus, the main differential diagnosis of the annular infiltrating form is submucosal hemorrhage and edema caused by ischemia or bleeding diathesis, as well as an unusual colonic carcinoma.[5]

Large infiltrating tumors may extend into the mesentery or exhibit central cavitation, resulting in the radio-

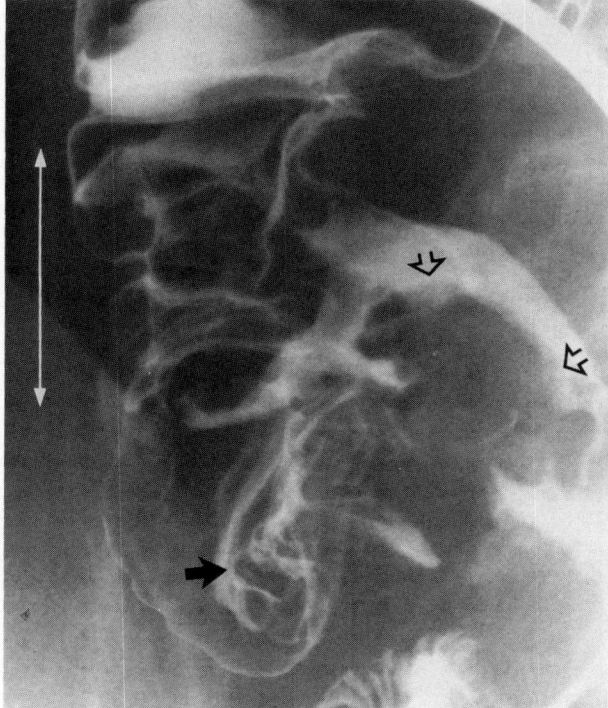

**Figure 65–2. Lymphoma of the ileocecal valve and terminal ileum.** A spot film from a double contrast barium enema shows thick, lobulated, but smooth folds encircling the cecum and proximal ascending colon *(double arrow).* Nodular mucosa *(solid arrow)* is seen near the insertion of the appendix into the cecum. A lobulated mass *(open arrows)* encroaches on the lumen of the terminal ileum.

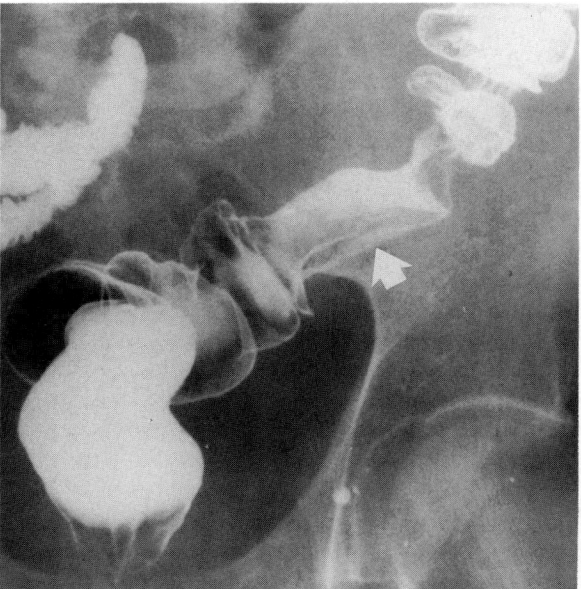

**Figure 65–3. Lymphoma of the sigmoid colon.** A relatively smooth-surfaced concentric lesion is seen in the sigmoid colon *(arrow).* The distal margin is abrupt, the proximal margin tapered. The amount of luminal narrowing is mild for the size and length of the lesion. (Courtesy of Seth N. Glick, M.D., Philadelphia, PA.)

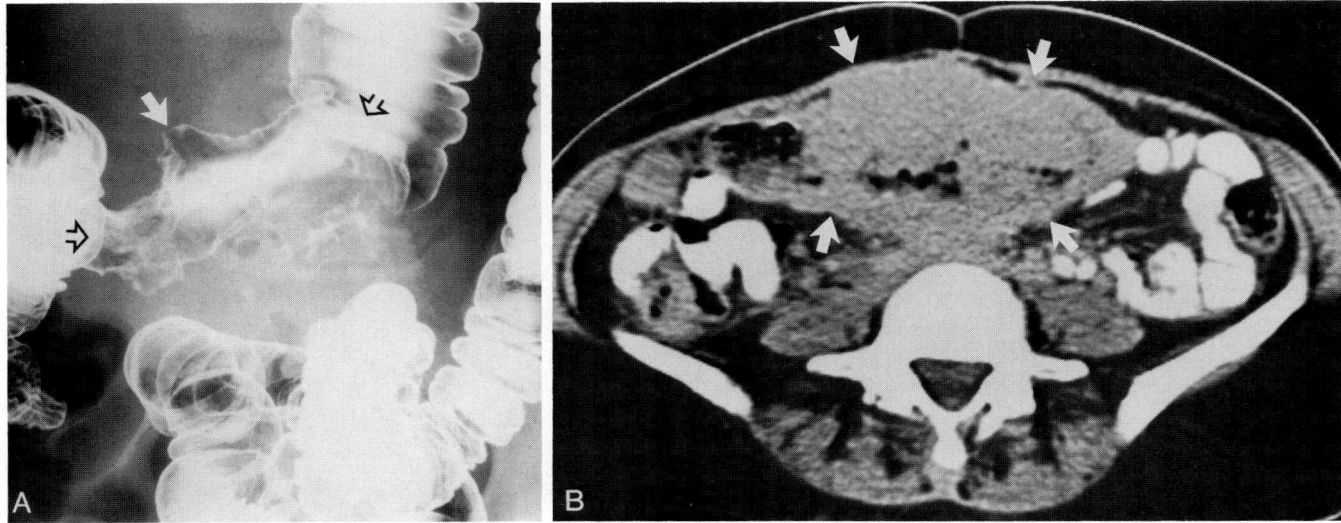

**Figure 65–4. Lymphoma of the transverse colon. A.** A spot film from a double contrast barium enema shows a long (limits shown by open arrows), concentric lesion with an irregular contour involving the midtransverse colon. On the superior surface, protrusion of the contour outside the expected lumen of the bowel *(white arrow)* indicates cavitation into the mass. **B.** On computed tomographic scan, a large soft tissue mass is seen as a lobular thickening of the walls *(arrows)* of the transverse colon.

graphic appearance of a bulky, cavitary mass lesion. The main differential diagnosis of this cavitary form is an unusual perforated colonic carcinoma or a mesenchymal tumor such as a stromal tumor (leiomyosarcoma).

The diffuse form of colonic lymphoma is almost always associated with disseminated disease and involves either long segments or the entire colon. More than 100 nonuniform, smooth, sessile nodules varying from 2 to 25 mm in size carpet the colonic surface[12, 16] (Fig. 65–6). The nodules are occasionally elongated, pedunculated, umbilicated, or filiform.[16] A conglomerate, discrete cecal mass is seen in almost half of the patients.[16] The multinodular form of colonic lymphoma may be confused radiologically with familial polyposis, lymphoid hyperplasia, cystic fibrosis, inflammatory bowel disease, or infectious diseases such as pseudomembranous colitis or schistosomiasis. In contrast to the pseudopolyposis of inflammatory bowel disease, in colonic lymphoma the haustral pattern is preserved and ulceration is uncommon.[7, 12] Conglomerate cecal masses are more frequent in disseminated lymphoma than in the polyposis syndromes.[7, 16] The nodules of colonic lymphoma are nonuniform and large compared with the uniform, 1- to 2-mm nodules of lymphoid hyperplasia. Rarely, diffuse colonic lymphoma may be associated with acute toxic dilatation or pneumatosis coli.[12]

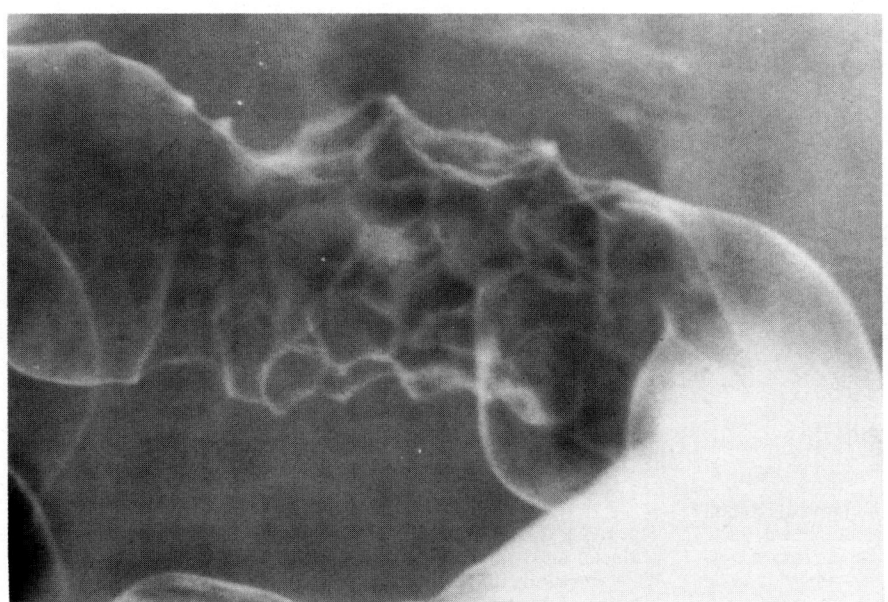

**Figure 65–5. Lymphoma of sigmoid colon.** A spot film from a double contrast barium enema shows an irregular, lobulated contour and mucosal surface pattern, yet the overlying mucosa is smooth. This appearance is typical of a submucosal infiltrating lesion such as a lymphoma or hemangioma.

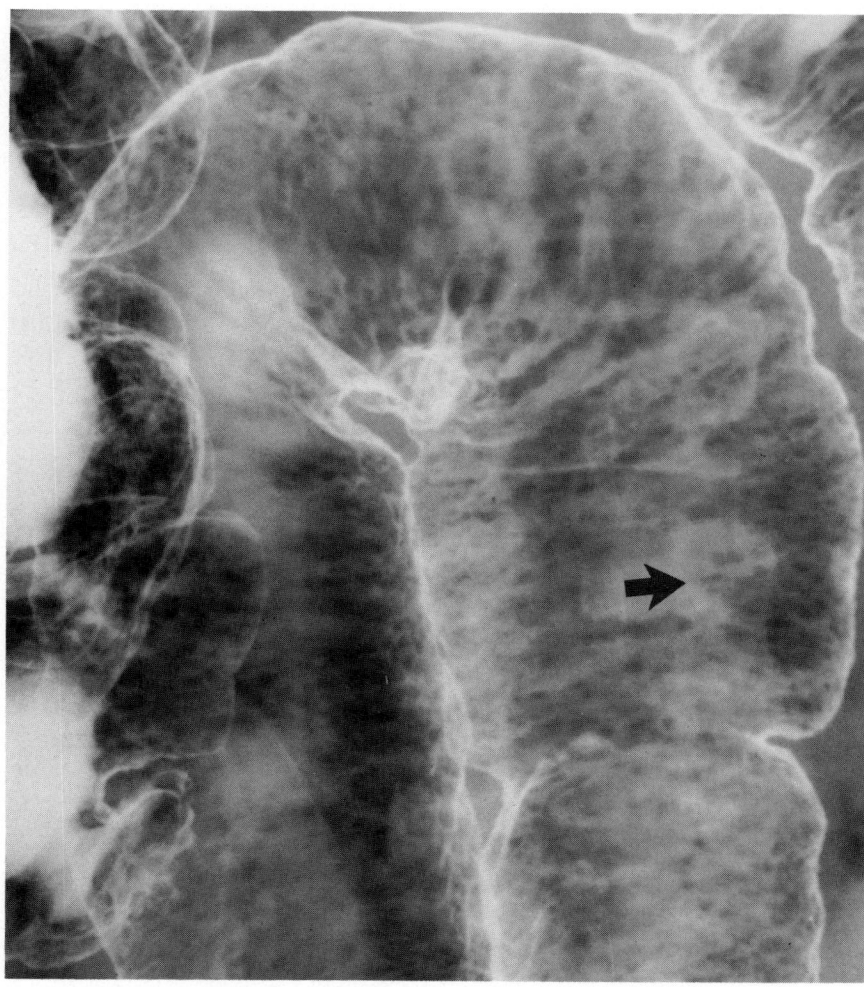

**Figure 65–6. Disseminated lymphoma involving the colon.** A spot film from a double contrast barium enema shows many small, 1- to 3-mm nonuniform nodules (representive area shown by arrow) carpeting the surface of the sigmoid colon. This is an unusual form of diffuse nodules in disseminated lymphoma. Usually these nodules are larger and nonuniform.

In summary, primary colonic lymphoma usually presents with acute abdominal symptoms similar to those of colonic carcinoma but is radiographically dissimilar from colonic carcinoma, appearing as a discrete polypoid, infiltrating, or cavitary mass lesion. Disseminated lymphoma involving the colon is much more common although frequently asymptomatic and is rarely imaged by a barium enema. When seen on barium enema examination, disseminated lymphoma usually appears as long segments of multiple, irregular, large nodules.

## VASCULAR LESIONS

### Hemangioma

#### Clinical and Pathologic Findings

Although hemangiomas of the colon are rare, the radiologic diagnosis is important because these lesions are frequently misdiagnosed at endoscopy and are associated with a high mortality rate.[17] Patients with colonic hemangiomas usually present at a young age with acute, recurrent, painless rectal bleeding or chronic rectal bleeding.[18, 19] The rectal bleeding may be so severe

as to be life threatening,[19] and mortality rates have approached 50%.[20] Obstructive symptoms and diarrhea are uncommon, occurring in 15 to 20% of patients.[18, 21] Patients with anorectal lesions may also complain of tenesmus or constipation.

It is unknown whether colonic hemangiomas are hamartomatous or neoplastic lesions. Cavernous hemangiomas are the most common form; capillary hemangiomas are second in number.[21, 22] Cavernous hemangiomas are unencapsulated lesions usually arising in the submucosa (Fig. 65–7 [see Color Plate I]). They are composed of large, multiloculated thin-walled vessels[20] separated by loose connective tissue (see Fig. 65–7). Cavernous hemangiomas most commonly occur in the rectum and sigmoid colon.[23] Cavernous hemangiomas may be discrete polypoid submucosal masses[21] or, more frequently, diffuse, infiltrative lesions.[19] Polypoid tumors may intussuscept, causing obstruction, and infiltrative lesions usually undergo ulceration and hemorrhage.[18]

Capillary hemangiomas are usually asymptomatic, solitary, sharply circumscribed submucosal masses. The tumors are composed of small vessels lined by well-differentiated, although sometimes hyperplastic, endothelial cells.[20] The vessels are packed together, separated by a scant amount of connective tissue. These tumors

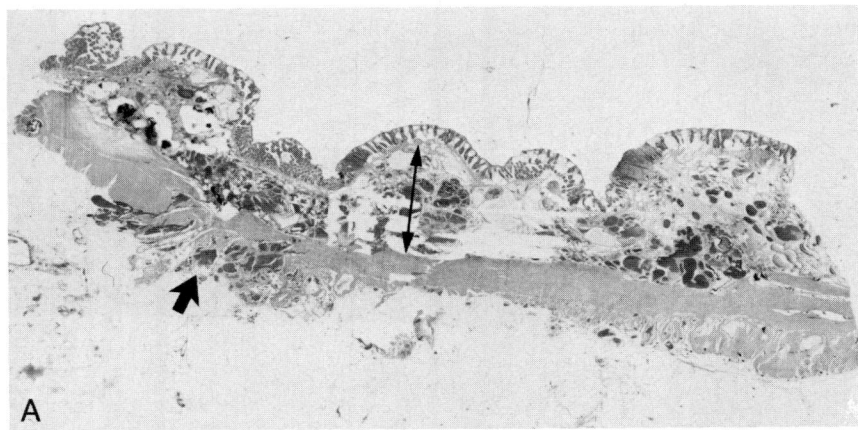

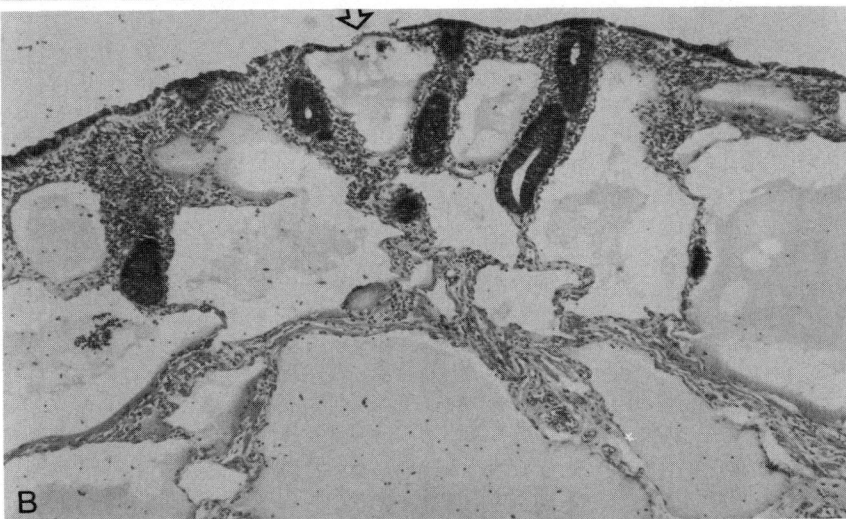

**Figure 65–7. Hemangioma of the colon. A.**
Low-power view of rectosigmoid colon shows an
undulating mucosal surface caused by widening
of the submucosa *(double arrow)*. At this power,
the submucosa is seen to be expanded by blood-
filled spaces. The blood-filled spaces extend to
the subserosal fat in one area *(thick arrow)*. **B.**
Medium-power view of the mucosa from the same
lesion shows many large, almost cystic, spaces
lined by endothelial cells. The spaces are separated by loose connective tissue. The cavernous
spaces extend to the mucosal surface *(arrow)*.
(See Color Plate I.)

are occasionally associated with cutaneous or visceral
hemangiomas.[19, 24] Hemangiomas may occur in the Klippel-Trenaunay syndrome, which consists of the triad of
cutaneous hemangiomas, soft tissue hypertrophy of the
involved lower extremity, and congenital varicose
veins.[23]

## Radiographic Findings and Differential Diagnosis

Rectal hemangiomas are frequently misdiagnosed endoscopically as hemorrhoids or proctitis.[20, 25] Thus, the
radiologist is often the first physician to suggest the
correct diagnosis. Plain films of the abdomen demonstrate phleboliths following the course of the bowel in
50% of cases.[19, 20, 24] Whenever plain films demonstrate
1) phleboliths in a young patient with gastrointestinal
bleeding or 2) phleboliths occurring in clusters, in an
atypical location, or along the expected course of the
rectosigmoid colon, a diagnosis of hemangioma should
be suspected.

Barium enema examination usually shows a circumferential lesion with scalloped contours and a nodular
mucosal surface pattern[19] (Fig. 65–8 [see Color Plate
I]). The colonic lumen is narrowed in one half of
patients. If the tumor is in its usual rectosigmoid loca-

tion, a wide retrorectal space may be seen. If phleboliths
are visible, they are seen in relation to the colonic
tumor.[23] The polypoid forms of hemangioma appear as
smooth, sessile, broad-based submucosal masses.

Although these tumors are usually vascular at angiography, they may be hypovascular or avascular because
of vessel thrombosis and sclerosis.[17] Computed tomography (CT) better demonstrates the true dimensions of
the mass and involvement of the adjacent structures,
such as the urinary bladder.[24]

Hemangioma is included in the differential diagnosis
of polypoid submucosal masses, most frequently lipoma.
It is also included in the differential diagnosis of infiltrative submucosal rectosigmoid lesions such as those in
solitary rectal ulcer syndrome or lymphoma. The clinical
history and phleboliths are the clue to the preoperative
diagnosis.

## Lymphangioma

Lymphangiomas of the colon are extremely rare benign lesions of either neoplastic or hamartomatous origin.[26] Patients with a colonic lymphangioma usually
present in the fourth to sixth decade with abdominal
pain, rectal bleeding, or altered bowel habit.[27] Lym-

phangiomas appear radiographically as 1) a solitary, 2- to 4-cm, often pedunculated polypoid lesion[28] or 2) a smooth, submucosal mass.[26, 29] Thus, the diagnosis of lymphangioma for some resected pedunculated polyps or submucosal mass lesions may come as a surprise to the radiologist.

## Angiodysplasia

### Clinical and Pathologic Findings

Angiodysplasia is a common cause of chronic low-grade gastrointestinal bleeding or acute massive lower gastrointestinal bleeding in elderly patients.[30, 31] These lesions are acquired vascular ectasias that may be due to chronic low-grade colonic obstruction.[30] Angiodysplasias are composed of clusters of dilated, tortuous, thin-walled veins, venules, and capillaries localized in the mucosa and submucosa of the colon (Fig. 65–9 [see Color Plate I]). The mucosal layer overlying the vascular tuft may be thinned or ulcerated. These lesions are single or multiple in number, small (usually less than 5 mm in size), and usually found in the cecum or ascending colon.[30]

Angiodysplasias may coexist with other causes of gastrointestinal bleeding. They were found in 2% of asymptomatic elderly patients at autopsy and, in one series, in 12 of 15 colons removed because of carcinoma.[30] Angiodysplasias are not associated with angiomatous lesions of the skin or other viscera.[30]

### Radiographic Findings

Angiodysplasias are usually detected during the work-up of patients with severe or recurrent lower gastrointestinal bleeding after normal examination of the colon by barium enema or colonoscopy.[31] During the arterial phase of an angiogram, an angiodysplasia appears as a tangle of small vessels at the end of a cecal or right colonic artery (see Chapters 53 and 60). Early filling of draining veins with contrast medium is present. Extravasation of contrast medium rarely occurs.[32] During the venous phase of the angiogram, dense contrast medium is seen filling draining veins. The radiologist is critical to the diagnosis of angiodysplasia, because the surgeon is unable to see or palpate these lesions during surgery. The decision to operate is made on the basis of the radiographic findings and the clinical history of recurrent or severe lower gastrointestinal bleeding.

## Kaposi's Sarcoma

This malignancy is discussed in Chapter 160.

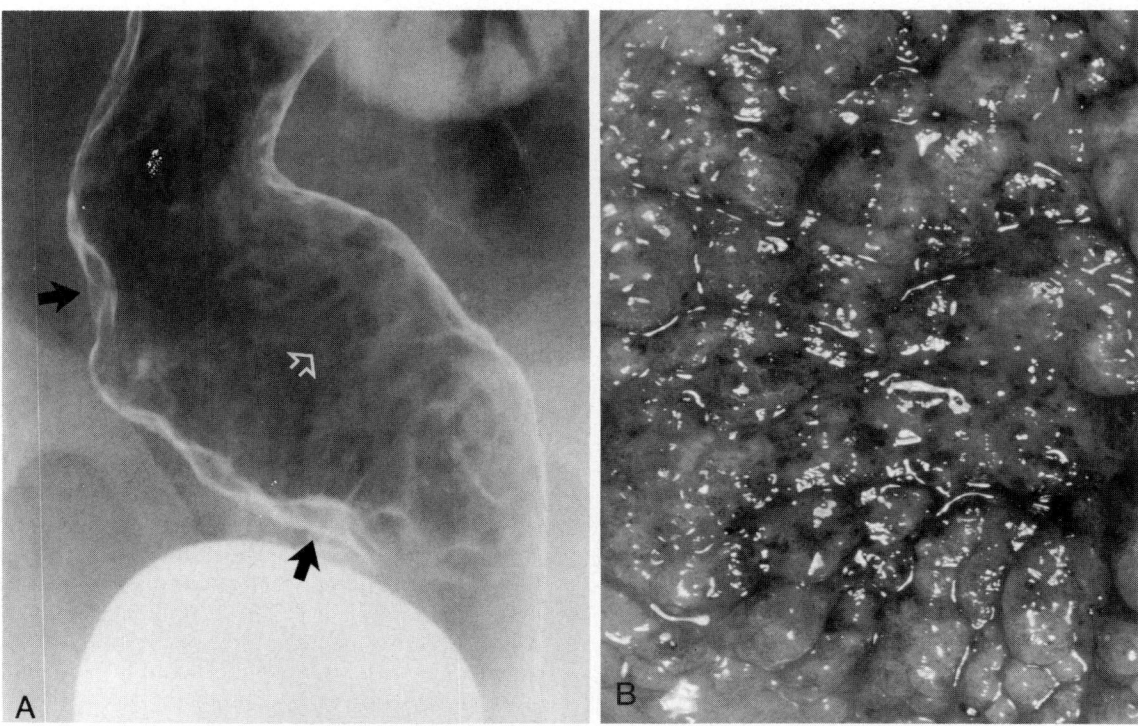

**Figure 65–8. Hemangioma of colon. A.** A prone, angled view of the rectosigmoid junction shows a subtle, circumferential lesion with a lobulated contour *(solid arrows)* and a finely lobulated mucosal surface *(open arrow)*. (From Margulis AR: Case: cavernous hemangioma of the rectum. Gastrointest Radiol 6:363–364, 1981.) **B.** Close-up photograph of the mucosal surface of the hemangioma shows a lobulated surface with areas of focal hemorrhage. This corresponds to the subtle, smooth surface lobulation seen on the radiograph. (See Color Plate I.)

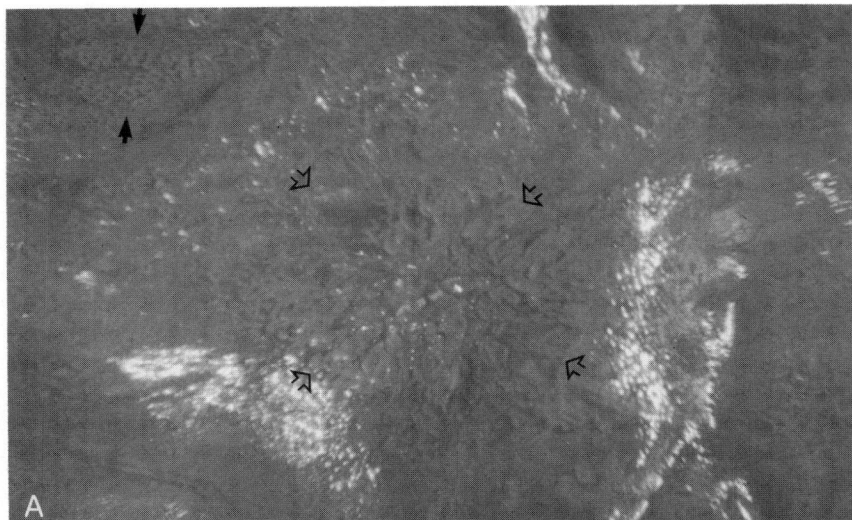
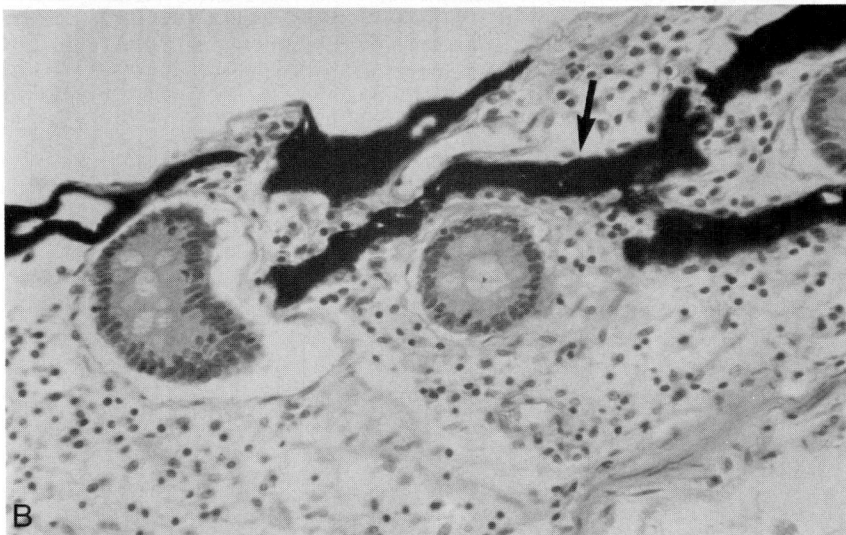

**Figure 65–9. Angiodysplasia of the right colon. A.** Dissecting photomicrograph shows distortion of the surface pattern *(open arrows)* of the colonic mucosa by an underlying tangle of vessels. The normal surface pattern and glandular openings of the colon are marked for comparison *(solid arrows).* **B.** Medium-power view of the colonic mucosa shows thin-walled, endothelium-lined spaces *(arrow)* in the lamina propria. The spaces were filled with a black-staining dye from a prior injection study. (See Color Plate I.)

## CARCINOID TUMORS

### Pathologic Findings

The most common sites of carcinoid tumors are the appendix (35%), ileum (16%), lung (14%), and rectum (13%).[33] Colonic carcinoids exclusive of the rectum constitute only 2 to 3% of all carcinoid tumors.[33, 34] Appendiceal carcinoids are usually discovered during surgery for appendicitis or in normal appendixes removed incidentally as part of other abdominal surgery.[35] Appendiceal carcinoids are discussed in Chapter 69.

The most common sites of colonic carcinoids are the rectum and cecum. Carcinoids involving the cecum and the ascending and transverse colon are of midgut origin. These midgut lesions may synthesize, store, and secrete serotonin. Midgut lesions are composed of insular groups of monomorphic cells of neuroendocrine origin, which usually form tubular structures or cystic formations.[36] These tumors usually stain positively with argentaffin stains, indicating serotonin production.[37] The serotonin is stored in pleomorphic, electron-dense

secretory granules seen during electron microscopy.[36] Although serotonin may be produced, carcinoid syndrome is rare.[38] If carcinoid syndrome is present, it is usually associated with liver metastases.

Hindgut carcinoids involve the descending and sigmoid colon and the rectum. Hindgut tumors are usually formed of monomorphic neuroendocrine cells arranged in trabecular, solid, or tubular patterns[36] (Fig. 65–10 [see Color Plate I]). They mainly synthesize and store a variety of polypeptide hormonal substances such as gastrin, somatostatin, glucagon, and vasoactive intestinal polypeptide.[34, 39] These polypeptides are found in electron-dense pleomorphic secretory granules, which may stain with argyrophil techniques or may be unstained with silver techniques. These tumors do not usually produce serotonin or cause carcinoid syndrome, unless liver metastases are present.

### Rectal Carcinoids

Rectal carcinoids are usually small, smooth, submucosal polypoid lesions less than 2 cm in diameter located

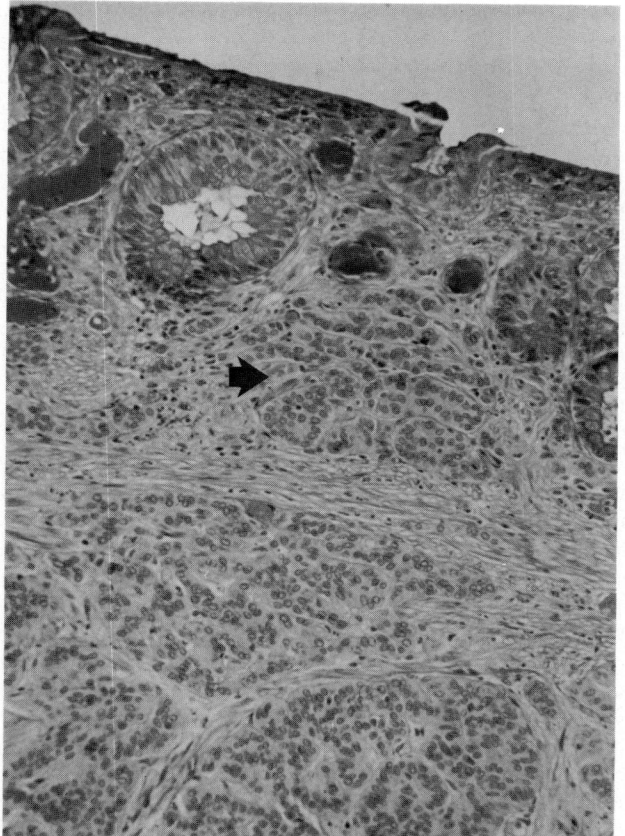

**Figure 65–10. Rectal carcinoid.** Medium-power photomicrograph shows a predominantly trabecular pattern of tumor infiltrating the lamina propria *(arrow)* and submucosa. The tumor is composed of small, uniform, monomorphic cells with typical "salt-and-pepper" nuclei. (See Color Plate I.)

in the lower two thirds of the rectum. They are usually discovered incidentally during a screening barium enema examination or endoscopy or during work-up for rectal pain or bleeding.[40, 41] Small rectal carcinoids have low malignant potential and are cured by simple excision. Large rectal carcinoids have a much greater incidence of metastasis at the initial time of diagnosis.[41] Large rectal carcinoids are seen as irregular ulcerated masses with a nodular edge.[41] Overall, patients with rectal carcinoids have an 83% 5-year survival.[33, 41]

## Colonic Carcinoids (Exclusive of the Rectum)

Carcinoids of the remainder of the colon have a much different clinical history, morphology, and prognosis than rectal carcinoids. Colonic carcinoids exclusive of the rectum are usually large, aggressive lesions with a poor prognosis. Patients usually present in the sixth decade with symptoms similar to those of colonic adenocarcinoma: abdominal pain, distention, and palpable abdominal mass. Rectal bleeding and diarrhea are seen in approximately one third of patients.[42]

Colonic carcinoids exclusive of the rectum are most frequently located in the cecum or right colon.[38, 42]

Radiographically, right colonic carcinoids are 1) bulky, larger than 5 cm, sessile, fungating intraluminal masses or 2) irregular annular lesions[35, 38, 43] (Fig. 65–11). These forms of colonic carcinoid are indistinguishable from colonic adenocarcinoma. Occasionally a smooth, polypoid submucosal mass is seen.

At diagnosis, 50 to 60% of patients have metastases to lymph nodes, liver, mesentery, and peritoneum.[33, 38, 42] Five-year survival is approximately 50%.[33] Thus, colonic carcinoids exclusive of the rectum are large lesions with signs, symptoms, and radiographic findings similar to those of colonic adenocarcinoma.

## FATTY LESIONS

### Lipoma

#### *Clinical Findings*

Although the colon is the most frequent site of gastrointestinal lipoma, colonic lipomas are uncommon, occurring in 0.32% of autopsies.[44, 45] Most patients are asymptomatic, and their tumors are detected at autopsy or during endoscopy or barium enema performed for symptoms attributed to a coexistent lesion.[44, 46] In symptomatic patients, the peak incidence is in the sixth and seventh decades. Abdominal pain and discomfort are

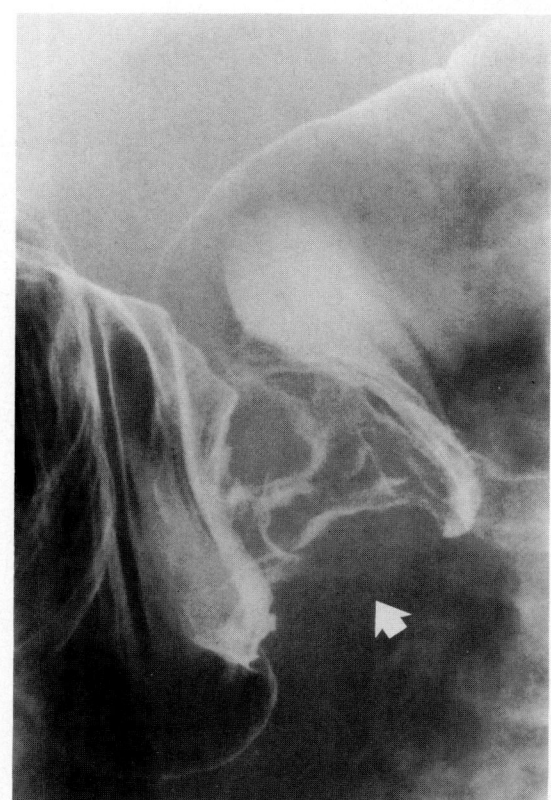

**Figure 65–11. Colonic carcinoid.** Spot film from a double contrast barium enema shows a short, annular lesion *(arrow)* with shelving margins in the hepatic flexure. These radiographic findings are similar to those for a colonic carcinoma; however, the mucosa is smoother than in a typical colonic carcinoma. (Courtesy of Seth N. Glick, M.D., Philadelphia, PA.)

the two most frequent symptoms.[46] Rectal bleeding or pain related to obstructive intussusception is less frequent.

## Pathologic Findings

Most (70%) colonic lipomas are found in the right colon, 90% originating in the submucosa.[44, 46] The remaining 10% of colonic lipomas arise in the appendices epiploicae. Multiple tumors are found in up to 25% of patients.[46] Lipomas are usually less than 3 cm in diameter. Colonic lipomas causing symptoms are usually larger lesions.

A colonic lipoma is an encapsulated mass of mature adipose tissue, usually confined to the submucosa (Fig. 65–12 [see Color Plate II]). Approximately two thirds of tumors are pedunculated, with a broad-based pedicle covered by normal colonic mucosa. These tumors are composed of mature fat cells with varying degrees of fibrous stroma.[47] Focal ulceration, necrosis, calcification, or pseudosarcomatous change may be seen.[47, 48]

## Radiographic Findings

On barium enema, a lipoma appears as a sessile submucosal mass or as a polypoid lesion on a broad-based pedicle[49] (Fig. 65–13). Lipomas are usually round, ovoid, or pear shaped. They are sharply demarcated masses with obtuse angulation with the colonic wall.[50] Although the contour of the tumor may be lobulated, the mucosal surface is smooth (see Fig. 65–13B). Because of the pliable nature of fat, lipomas change shape with palpation, position of the patient (see Fig. 65–13B), or varying degrees of colonic distention.[45, 50] These tumors may elongate during colonic spasm or after colonic evacuation (Fig. 65–14). Lipomas may cause colocolic intussusception or intussusception during barium enema (Fig. 65–15).

Before the advent of CT, barium enemas were considered relatively accurate in the diagnosis of lipoma.[50, 51] However, CT may allow a definitive diagnosis of lipoma.[52, 53] On a CT scan, a colonic lipoma appears as a mass of uniform fat density ($-80$ to $-120$ Hounsfield units) without septa or other large areas of nonfatty tissue[52] (see Fig. 65–14). With the CT diagnosis of lipoma, surgery may not be needed in a patient without symptoms or complication or in a patient who is a poor operative risk.[52, 53] However, a tailored CT scan must be performed. The tumor is surrounded with dilute contrast medium to minimize the potential partial volume effect of air in the colonic lumen. Thus, demonstration of uniform fat in a colonic mass is diagnostic of lipoma. Of further help to the radiologist is the fact that colonic liposarcomas are extremely rare, if nonexistent.[54] In fact, liposarcomas arising in the colon had not been reported as of 1989.[54]

## Fatty Infiltration of the Ileocecal Valve

### Pathologic, Clinical, and Radiographic Findings

Fatty infiltration of the ileocecal valve (lipohyperplasia, lipomatous infiltration) is a localized massive accumulation of submucosal fat in the ileocecal valve. Pathologically, the lack of a capsule differentiates this fatty proliferation from a lipoma.[22] The diagnosis is suggested radiographically when there is a large ileocecal valve with smooth or lobulated contours and a smooth mucosal surface without a discrete polypoid mass. Although rigid measurements are not reliable in distinguishing a normal-sized ileocecal valve from an enlarged valve, some investigators have suggested 4 cm as the upper limit of size for a normal ileocecal valve.[55] In addition, 1.5 cm is considered the upper limit of normal thickness for one "lip" of an ileocecal valve.[56] A normal ileocecal valve has stellate folds radiating toward its center.[56]

### Differential Diagnosis

The radiologist must first decide whether the polypoid projection in the cecum arises on or near the ileocecal valve or is the ileocecal valve. The normal ileocecal valve is at the level of the first complete haustral fold on the medial or posterior colonic wall at the junction

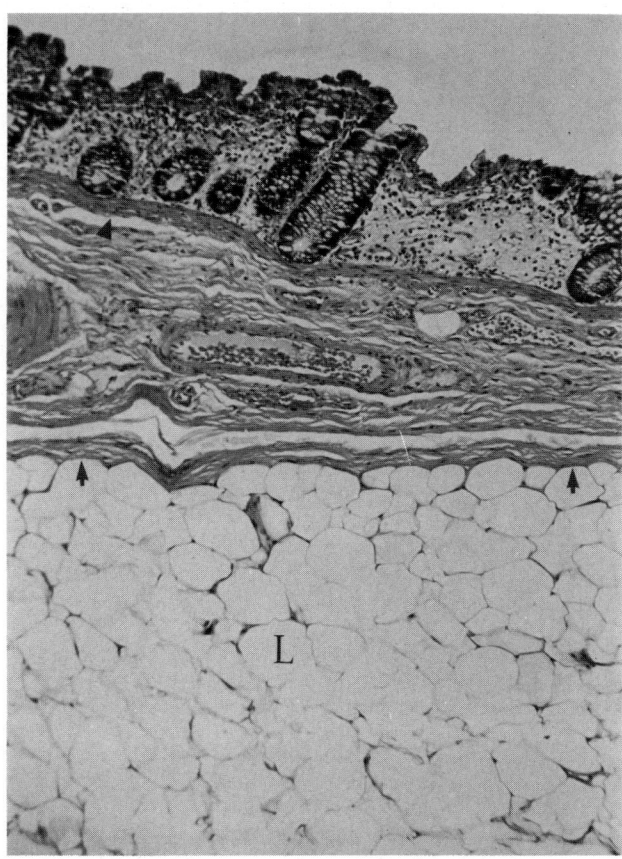

**Figure 65–12. Lipoma of colon.** Medium-power photomicrograph shows mature adipose tissue (L) expanding the submucosa. A fibrous capsule *(arrows)* is seen. Muscularis mucosae is identified by the arrowhead. (See Color Plate II.)

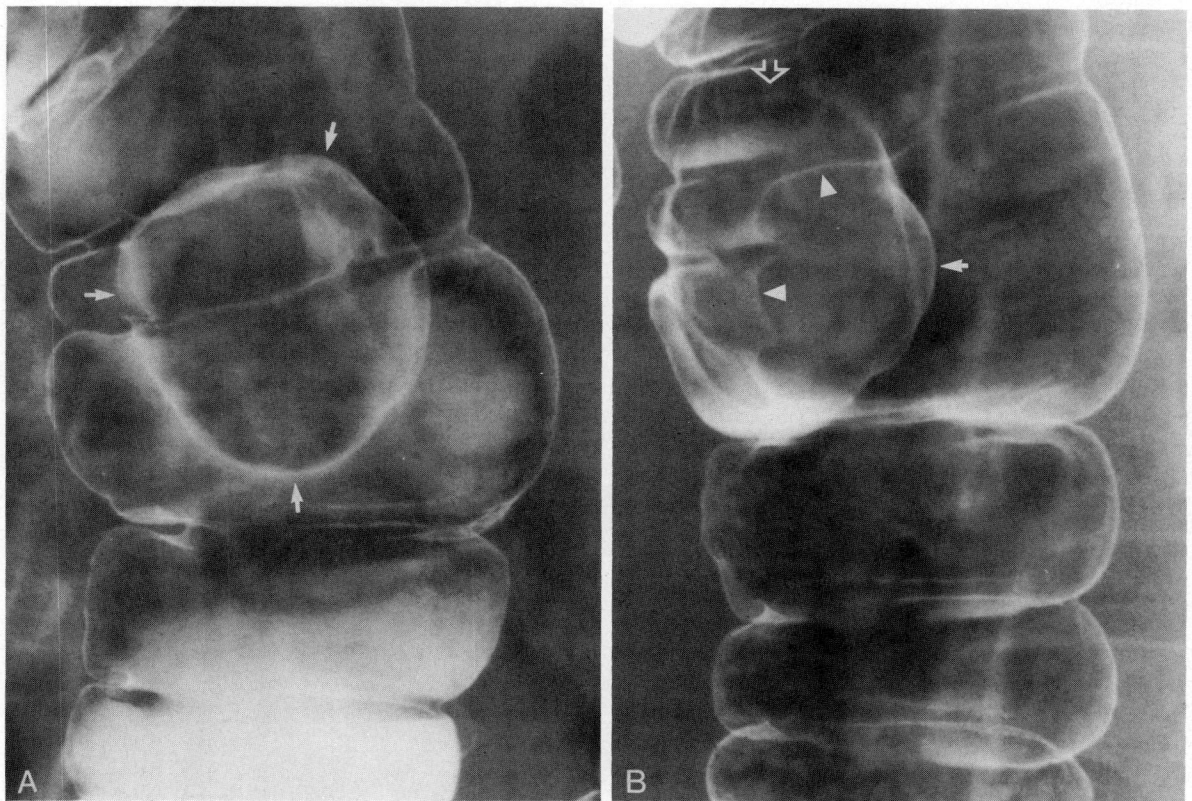

**Figure 65–13. Lipoma of descending colon. A.** Supine spot film from a double contrast barium enema shows a 3-cm-diameter, smooth-surfaced polypoid mass *(arrows)* with a slightly lobulated contour. **B.** Erect spot film shows that the tumor has a broad-based pedicle *(open arrow)*. Note that the lesion has elongated in the erect position. Also, the lobulated contours have become more pronounced *(solid arrow)*. A "kissing" artifact caused by coaptation of the normal colonic wall with the tumor is seen *(arrowheads)*.

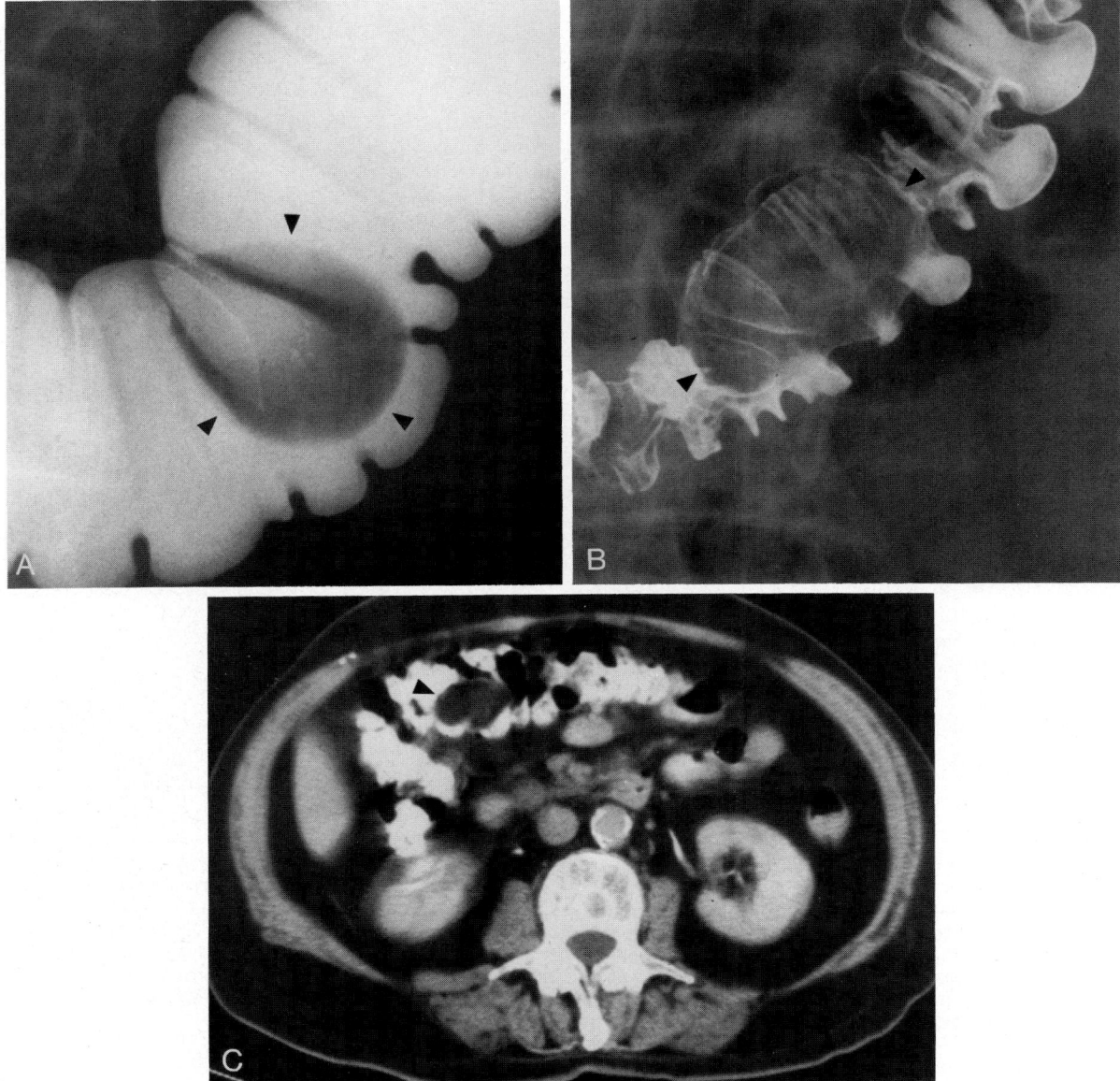

**Figure 65–14. Lipoma of transverse colon. A.** Spot film from a single contrast barium enema shows a smooth-surfaced, pear-shaped filling defect *(arrowheads)* in the barium-filled transverse colon. **B.** Close-up from a postevacuation film shows elongation of the smooth-surfaced filling defect *(arrowheads)* in the collapsed transverse colon. **C.** A CT scan shows a lobulated filling defect *(arrowhead)* in the transverse colon with the same attenuation value as nearby mesenteric fat.

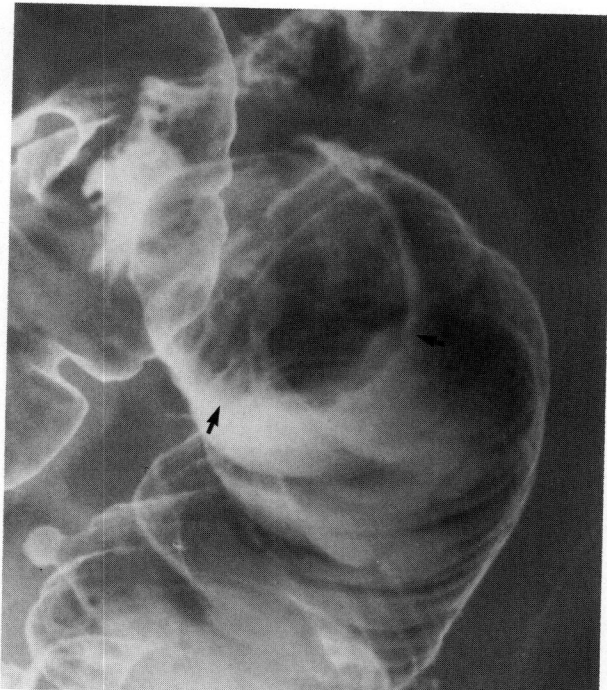

**Figure 65–15. Intussusception of a lipoma during barium enema.** Spot film from a double contrast barium enema shows a smooth-surfaced mass in the distal descending colon *(arrows)*. The proximal descending colon is collapsed.

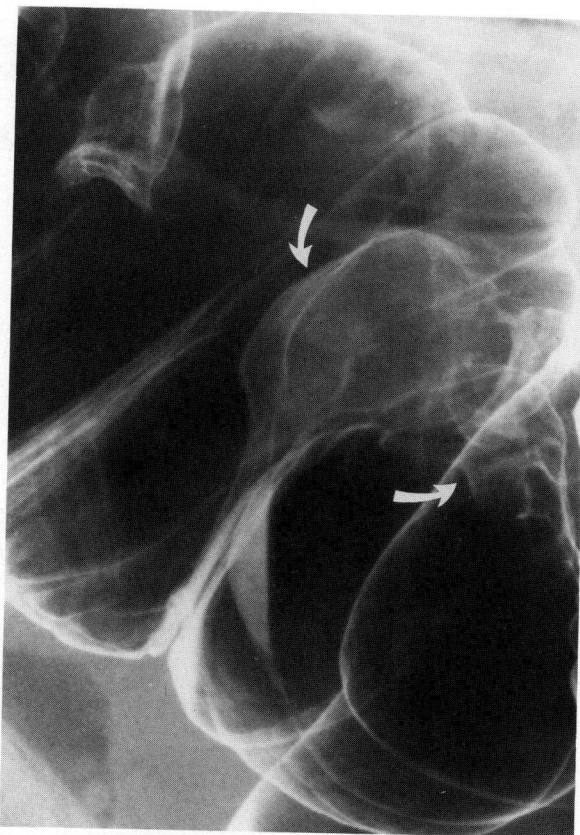

**Figure 65–16. Fatty infiltration of ileocecal valve.** Close-up from a right-side-down decubitus view of the colon shows smooth, slightly lobulated enlargement of the ileocecal valve *(arrows)*. Fatty infiltration was confirmed at colonoscopy performed for other reasons.

of the cecum and the ascending colon. Terminal ileum filling with barium confirms the location of the ileocecal valve. If an ileocecal valve is mildly enlarged (>3 cm), with a smooth or slightly lobulated contour and a smooth mucosal surface, the most likely diagnosis is fatty infiltration (Fig. 65–16). A focal polypoid projection from the ileocecal valve may represent a tumor such as an adenoma or lipoma (Fig. 65–17). Any mucosal surface irregularity of the ileocecal valve suggests a tumor involving the valve, such as an adenocarcinoma. More than a gentle undulating contour with a smooth mucosa suggests the possibility of an infiltrating process such as a lymphoma or Crohn's disease. In Crohn's disease there is fatty hypertrophy of the ileocecal valve, usually associated with radiologic changes of Crohn's disease in the terminal ileum and ileocecal fistulas. In lymphoma, the ileocecal valve is moderately enlarged with a lobulated contour. Lymphoma of the ileocecal valve frequently involves the terminal ileum.

# STROMAL TUMORS

## Pathologic Findings

Although spindle and epithelioid cell lesions of the gastrointestinal tract have traditionally been termed smooth muscle cell lesions (leiomyoma or leiomyosarcoma), most of these tumors are undifferentiated stromal neoplasms.[57–59] Only a minority of these tumors are recognized as arising from smooth muscle cells by

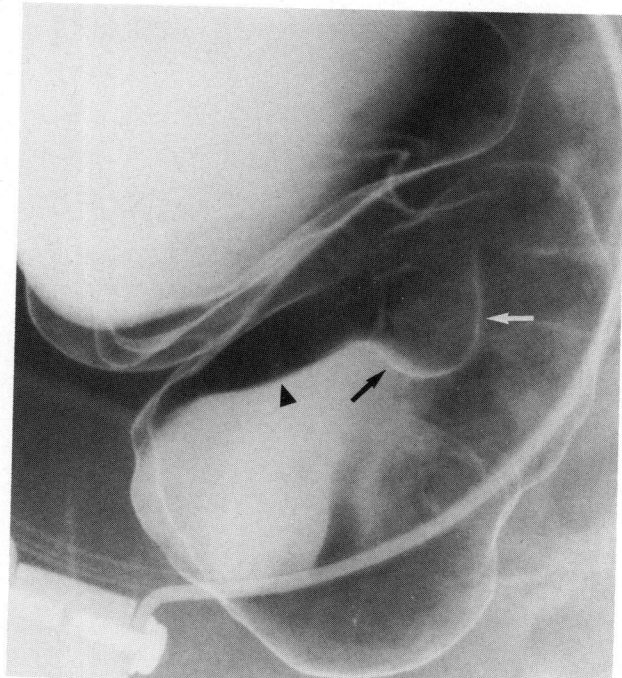

**Figure 65–17. Lipoma on the ileocecal valve.** A small, smooth-surfaced, sessile polyp *(arrows)* with abrupt angulation is seen on the inferior surface of the ileocecal valve *(arrowhead)*.

ultrastructural or immunohistochemical means.[58, 59] A few spindle cell lesions have ultrastructural and immunohistochemical features suggestive of nerve cell sheath origin. The behavior of these tumors is difficult to predict by site or macroscopic or microscopic features. Size is the best predictor of malignant potential.

## Small Stromal Tumors

Only 1% of all gastrointestinal tumors are of stromal origin, and these occur least frequently in the colon.[60] Colonic stromal tumors most frequently occur in the rectum.[61] In general, there are two macroscopic types of colonic stromal tumors—small polypoid lesions and large, bulky masses. Some patients with small polypoid rectal lesions complain of rectal discomfort, pain, and bleeding. Some patients are asymptomatic and the lesions are discovered incidentally during barium enema or endoscopy. Small polypoid lesions are either sessile or pedunculated (Fig. 65–18 [see Color Plate II]), probably arise from the muscularis mucosae, are histologically benign, and do not recur after excision.[62] These small polypoid lesions arising from the muscularis mucosae are the "true" leiomyomas of the colon because they always demonstrate smooth muscle differentiation by their desmin positivity and ultrastructural characteristics. Radiographically, the small rectal lesions are sessile or pedunculated polyps with a smooth or slightly irregular surface. Many small polypoid neurofibromas may be seen in neurofibromatosis (Fig. 65–19).

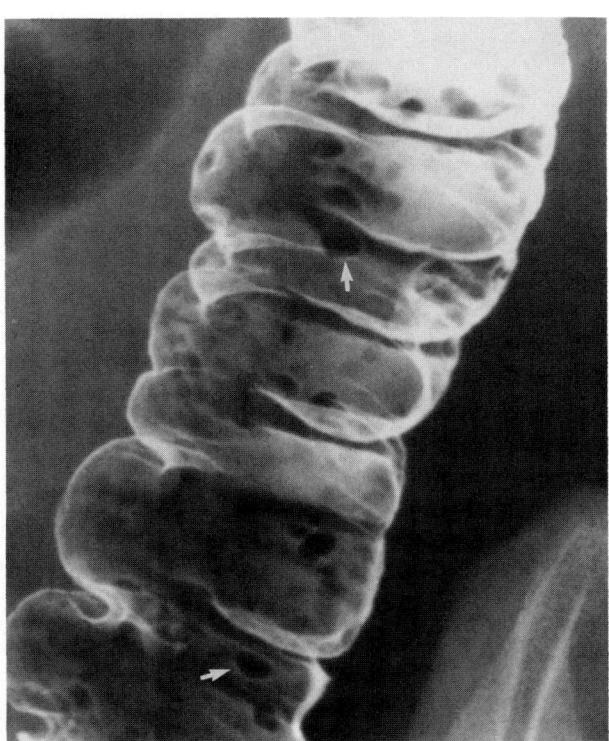

**Figure 65–19. Neurofibromatosis of the colon.** Spot film from a double contrast barium enema shows numerous small, smooth-surfaced filling defects *(arrows)* and hemispheric lines in the descending colon. Neurofibromatosis is a rare cause of colonic polyposis.

## Large Stromal Tumors

Large colonic gastrointestinal stromal tumors present with pain, bleeding, and change of bowel habit but rarely obstruction.[61] These large (>2 cm) lesions probably arise in the muscularis propria. They have a high rate of local recurrence (60%) regardless of histologic differentiation and have a poor prognosis.[62] These bulky lesions are most frequently found in the rectum, with the remainder evenly distributed throughout the colon. Radiographically, a large stromal tumor appears as a large annular lesion with irregular mucosa, a cavitating mass with a prominent extraluminal component, or a submucosal mass with or without central ulceration (Fig. 65–20). Cavitation may lead to superimposed infection and/or perforation with abscess formation.[60] Radiographically, these lesions are confused with colonic lymphomas or perforated colonic carcinomas.

## SQUAMOUS CELL CARCINOMAS

Squamous cell carcinomas of the colon are extremely rare tumors. Most squamous cell carcinomas arise in the rectum and have symptoms identical to those of rectal adenocarcinoma.[63] Squamous cell carcinomas are usually large, bulky, ulcerated masses grossly identical to rectal adenocarcinoma.[63] Colonic squamous cell carcinomas must be distinguished from squamous cell carcinomas

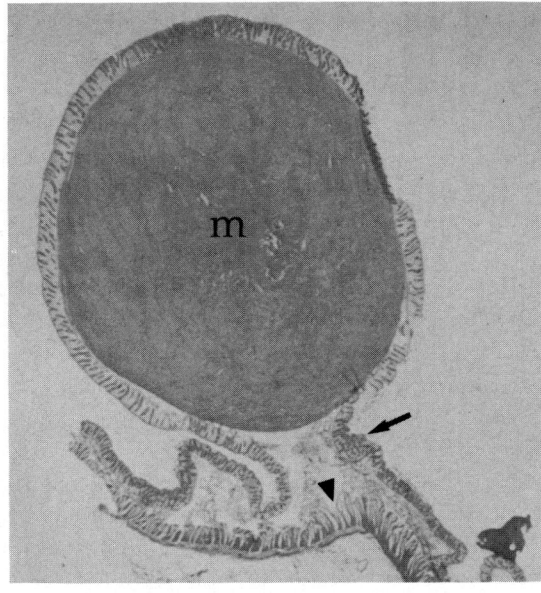

**Figure 65–18. Pedunculated stromal tumor.** Low-power photomicrograph shows a polyp on a short stalk. Normal colonic mucosa overlies a mass (m) lying between the epithelial layer and the muscularis propria *(arrowhead)*. The mucosa of the stalk *(arrow)* is normal. This was a true leiomyoma, probably arising in the muscularis mucosae. (See Color Plate II.) (Courtesy of Scott H. Saul, M.D., West Chester, PA.)

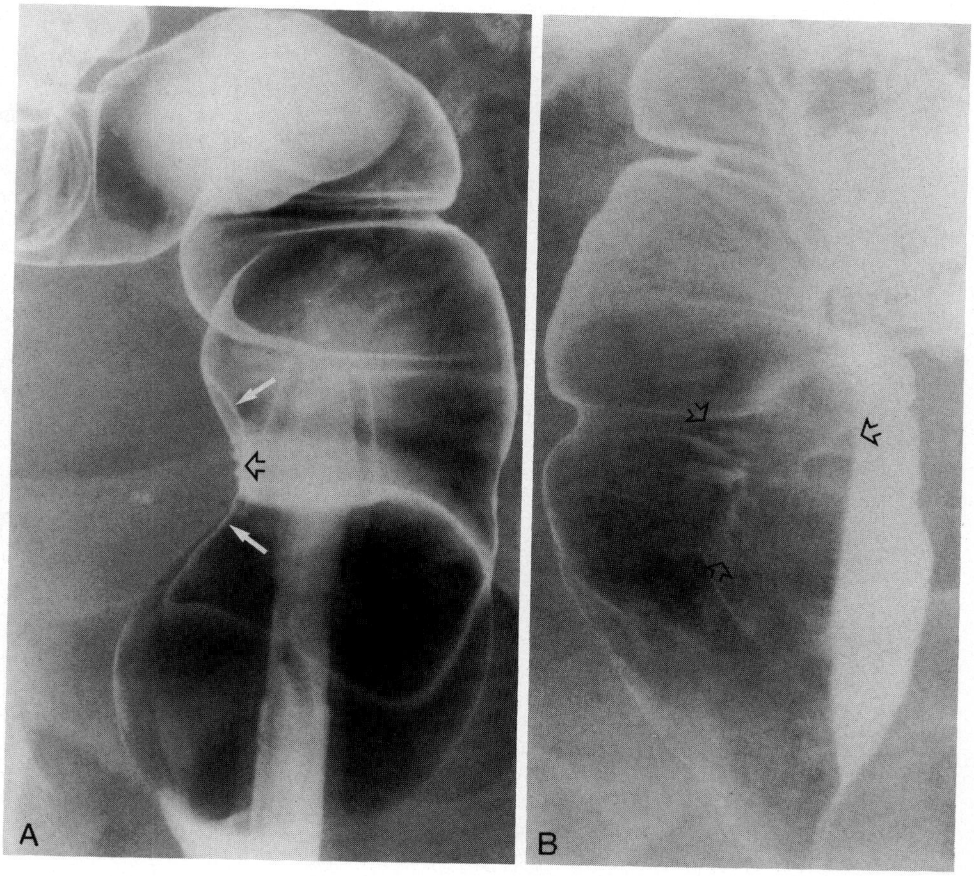

**Figure 65–20. Stromal tumor of rectum. A.** Steep oblique spot film of the rectum from a double contrast barium enema shows a relatively broad-based mass *(arrows)* with focal spiculation of the contour *(arrowhead)*. **B.** Close-up from a left-side-down decubitus overhead view shows focal nodularity of the mucosa *(arrows)* corresponding to the area of spiculation on the oblique view.

that invade the colon from either the anal canal or squamous mucosa–lined fistulas. These lesions must also be distinguished from squamous cell tumors that have metastasized to the colon or poorly differentiated adenocarcinomas that show focal squamous differentiation.

Squamous cell carcinomas are discussed in detail in Chapter 68.

## METASTASES

The radiologist must be thoroughly familiar with the broad spectrum of metastatic disease involving the colon. Metastases to the colon are not uncommon.[64] It is not rare for symptoms produced by gastrointestinal metastases to be the initial manifestation of a primary malignancy.

Colonic metastases can be classified by their mode of dissemination:[65]

1. Direct invasion, from contiguous primary tumor or noncontiguous primary tumor
2. Intraperitoneal seeding
3. Embolic metastases

The radiologic features often identify the lesion as a metastasis, identify the mode of dissemination, and may indicate the most likely primary site of tumor.[66] Radiologic recognition of metastases is also important because

localized embolic metastases may undergo resection for cure or resection to control a complication such as bleeding or obstruction. Recognition of tumor directly invading the colon prepares surgeons for wider excision or the need to perform a colostomy with bypass.[67]

## Direct Invasion from Contiguous Primary Tumor

The most common tumors that directly invade the colon arise in the ovary, uterus, kidney, prostate, cervix (Fig. 65–21), and gallbladder.

### Prostatic Carcinoma

Prostatic carcinoma may spread across Denonvilliers' fascia to invade the rectum anteriorly or circumferentially.[68] Rectal involvement by prostatic carcinoma occurs in 0.5 to 11.5% of patients.[69, 70] A patient's symptoms mimic those arising from rectal carcinoma: obstruction, constipation, and rectal bleeding.[71] The diagnosis of prostatic cancer invading the colon is often unknown at the time of initial barium enema, surgery, or autopsy.[68, 72]

Although the normal prostate abuts the distal rectum, most patients with prostatic carcinoma involving the colon show rectosigmoid junction involvement with dis-

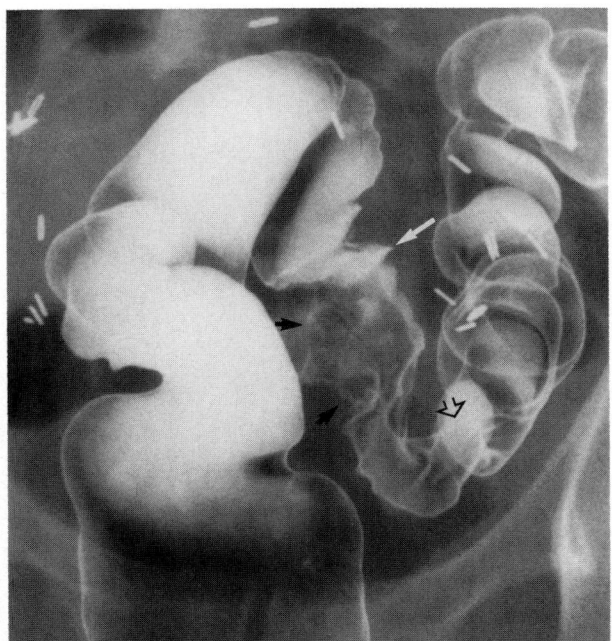

**Figure 65–21. Recurrence of cervical carcinoma invades the sigmoid colon.** Close-up from a prone overhead view of the recto-sigmoid colon shows circumferential involvement of the sigmoid colon. A relatively abrupt margin is seen distally and a smooth, tapered margin proximally *(open arrow)*. The colonic contour is focally spiculated *(white arrow)* and markedly irregular in other regions *(black arrows)*.

tal rectal sparing.[68, 73] Prostatic carcinoma usually spreads cranially to involve the seminal vesicles before it invades posteriorly (Fig. 65–22). Thus, on barium enema examination, early cases show an extrinsic mass effect on the rectosigmoid junction. With colonic invasion, mucosal pleating and tethering are seen en face and a spiculated contour is seen in profile. In advanced cases, the rectum is circumferentially narrowed with a wide presacral space and a spiculated contour [68–70, 73] (Fig. 65–23). In some cases, prostatic carcinoma invades posteriorly to involve the lower rectum (Fig. 65–24). The main differential diagnosis is pelvic malignancy such as carcinoma of the cervix or urinary bladder directly invading the colon. When the radiologic diagnosis is suggested, work-up may include magnetic resonance imaging (Fig. 65–25A), CT (Fig. 65–25B), or transrectal sonography. Endoscopic biopsies with stains for prostatic specific antigen or prostatic acid phosphatase[74, 75] can confirm the radiologic diagnosis.

## Ovarian Carcinoma

When left ovarian carcinoma directly invades the colon, it first involves the inferior border of the sigmoid colon (see Chapter 150).[76] Colonic wall invasion is indicated by angulation of the sigmoid loops, spiculation of the colonic contour, and tethering and angulation of mucosal folds en face (Fig. 65–26). Rarely, a fistula to the sigmoid colon may be seen.[77]

## Renal Cell Carcinoma

Renal carcinoma may be seen to invade the colon directly at the time of initial diagnosis. Occasionally, colonic invasion can be seen with recurrent retroperitoneal tumor, even many years after resection of the primary lesion.[65, 76, 78] Left renal cell carcinomas invade the distal transverse or proximal descending colon.[65] Right renal cell carcinomas invade the second (descending) part of the duodenum. Invasive renal cell carcinoma usually appears as a bulky intraluminal mass without significant signs of obstruction.[65]

## Direct Invasion from Noncontiguous Primary Tumor

Malignancies may spread in the subperitoneal space or by lymphatic permeation (see Chapter 131).[65] Examples of this mode of dissemination include colonic carcinomas spreading to the stomach via the gastrocolic ligament,[79] pancreatic carcinoma invading the transverse colon via the transverse mesocolon, and gastric carcinoma invading the colon via the gastrocolic ligament.[65] The gastrocolic ligament (proximal part of the greater omentum) is the anatomic bridge between the greater curvature of the stomach and the superior border of the transverse colon[76] (Fig. 65–27). Therefore, when gastric carcinoma spreads to the colon, mass effect, fixation, and fold irregularity are seen initially along the superior

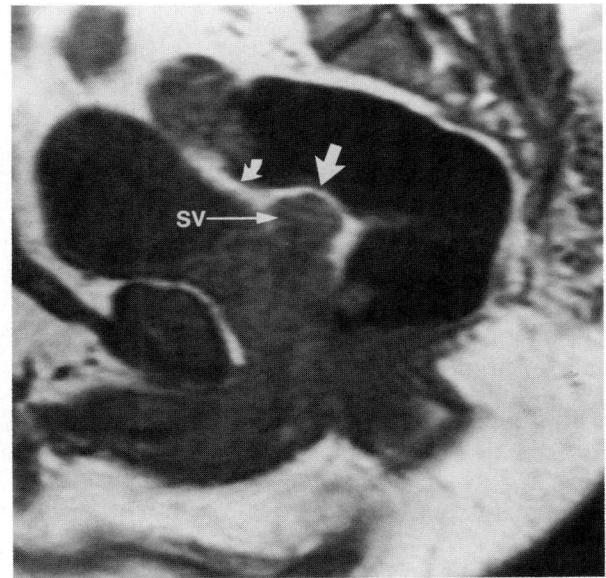

**Figure 65–22. Seminal vesicle invasion by prostatic carcinoma.** T1-weighted sagittal magnetic resonance scan of pelvis shows a mild extrinsic mass effect *(straight arrow)* on the air-filled rectosigmoid junction by an enlarged seminal vesicle (SV). The peritoneal reflection has been lifted cranially and anteriorly *(curved arrow)* because of prostatic and seminal vesicle enlargement. This sagittal scan is a correlate of the smooth extrinsic mass impression of the rectosigmoid junction seen on barium enema examination. (From SE Rubesin, MS Levine, M Bezzi, et al, Rectal involvement by prostatic carcinoma, AJR, 152, 1, 53–57, 1989, © by American Roentgen Ray Society.)

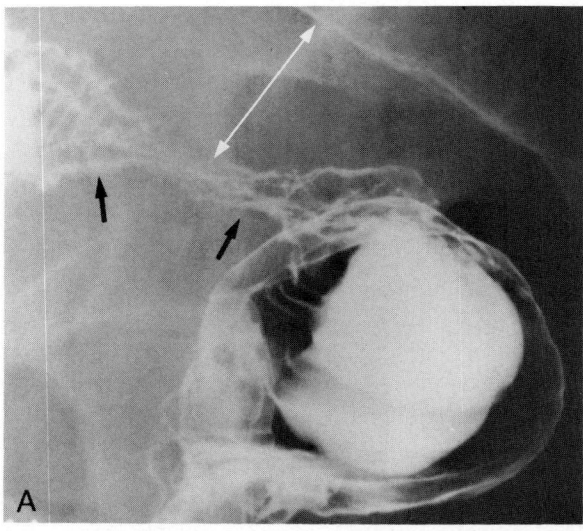

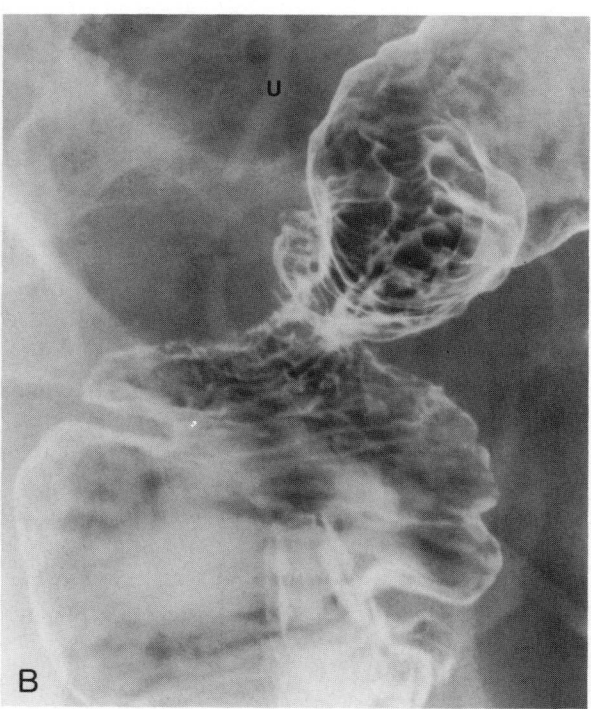

**Figure 65–23. Direct invasion of rectosigmoid colon by prostatic carcinoma. A.** Lateral view of the rectum shows a circumferential mass effect, especially on the anterior wall of the distal sigmoid colon *(single arrows)*. Note the spiculated colonic contour and widening of the presacral space *(double arrow)*. **B.** Frontal view of the rectum shows a spiculated colonic contour and, en face, pleating of the mucosa of the rectosigmoid colon. U = ureter.

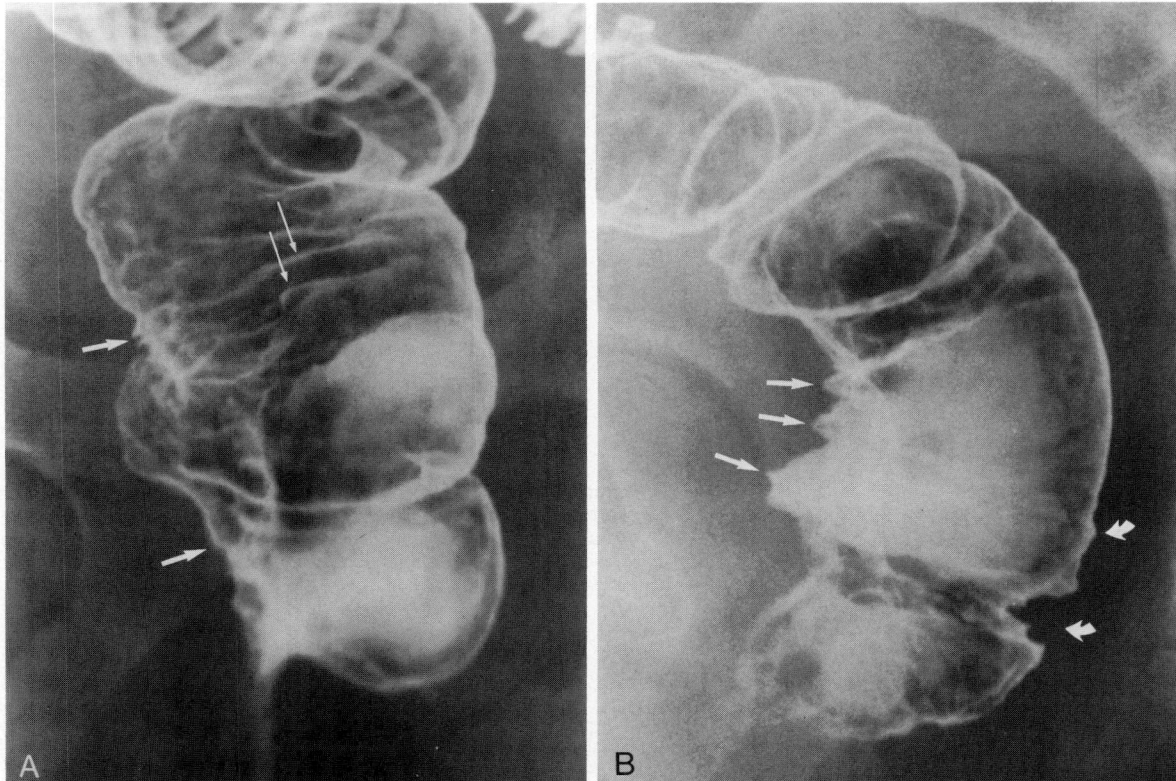

**Figure 65–24. Rectal invasion by prostatic carcinoma. A.** Anteroposterior spot film shows mass effect and spiculation predominantly along the right lateral wall of the rectum *(thick arrows)* and, en face, pleating of the mucosa *(thin arrows)*. Invasion of the mucosa and submucosa was confirmed on rectal biopsy of the mucosa of the right lateral rectal wall. **B.** Lateral spot film of the rectum shows a mass effect along the anterior rectal wall and spiculation of the mucosal contour *(straight arrows)*. Mild circumferential extension is seen distally *(curved arrows)*. (**A** and **B** from SE Rubesin, MS Levine, M Bezzi, et al, Rectal involvement by prostatic carcinoma: radiographic findings, AJR, 152, 1, 53–57, 1989, © by American Roentgen Ray Society.)

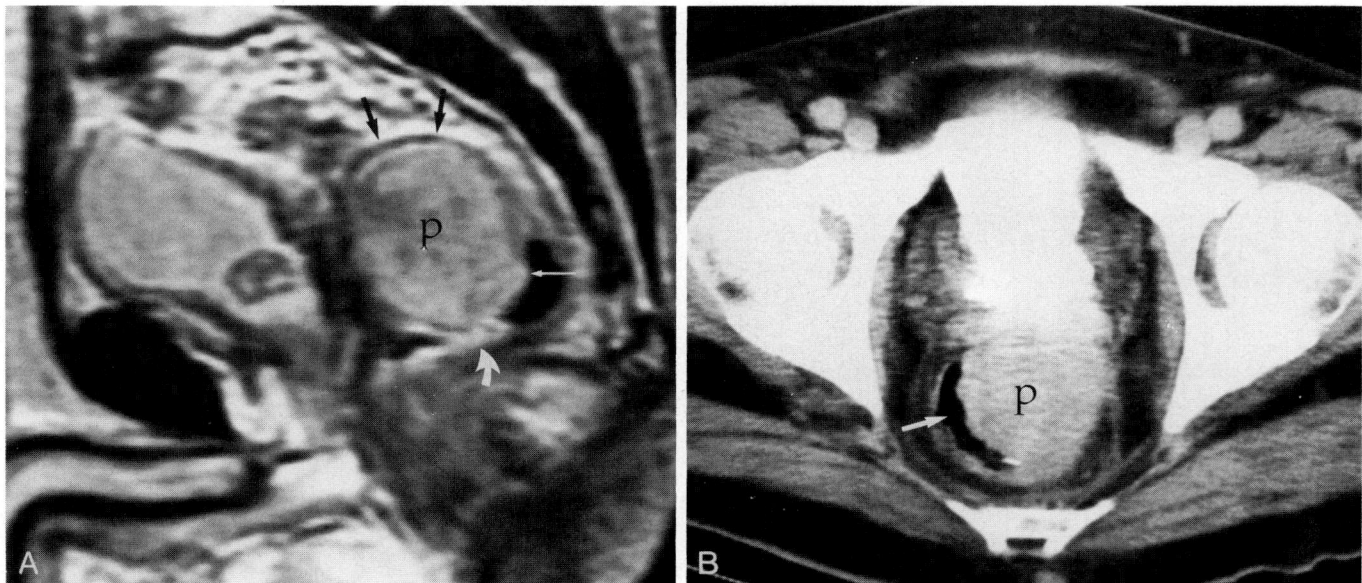

**Figure 65–25. Rectal invasion by prostatic carcinoma. A**. A T2-weighted sagittal magnetic resonance scan of the pelvis shows a huge prostatic mass (p) obliterating the lumen of the rectosigmoid colon *(straight black arrows)* and rectum *(curved white arrow)*. The original rectosigmoid junction is shown *(thin white arrow)*. (From SE Rubesin, MS Levine, M Bezzi, et al, Rectal involvement by prostatic carcinoma: radiographic findings, AJR, 152, 1, 53–57, 1989, © by American Roentgen Ray Society.) **B**. CT scan through the pelvis shows a large prostatic mass (p) displacing and invading the rectum *(arrow)*.

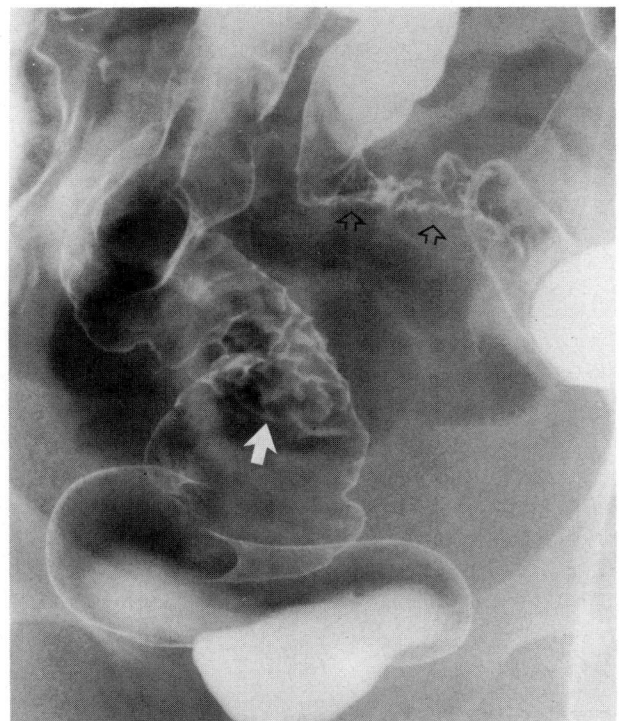

**Figure 65–26. Direct colonic invasion by left ovarian carcinoma.** An overhead view from a double contrast barium enema examination shows spiculation and mass effect along the inferior border of the sigmoid colon *(open arrows)* and, en face, pleating of the mucosa of the rectosigmoid junction *(solid arrow)*.

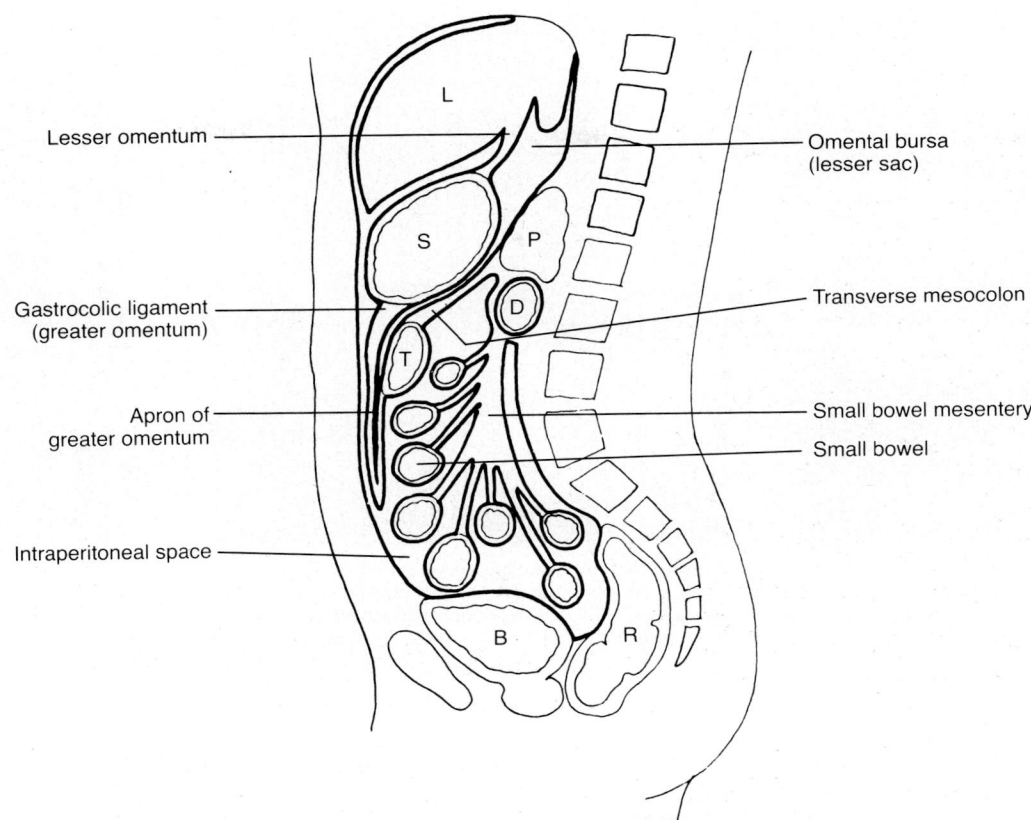

Lesser omentum

Omental bursa
(lesser sac)

Gastrocolic ligament
(greater omentum)

Transverse mesocolon

Apron of
greater omentum

Small bowel mesentery

Small bowel

Intraperitoneal space

**Figure 65–27. Sagittal line drawing of abdomen.** The proximal part of the greater omentum (the gastrocolic ligament) bridges the greater curvature of the stomach (S) with the anterosuperior border of the transverse colon (T). Thus, when gastric or omental processes directly invade the colon, the superior border of the transverse colon is involved first. The transverse mesocolon suspends the transverse colon from the retroperitoneum overlying the pancreas (P). L = colon; D = duodenum; R = rectum; B = bladder. (From Rubesin SE, Fishman EK: Peritoneal metastasis. *In* Fishman EK, Jones B [eds]: Computed Tomography of the Gastrointestinal Tract. Churchill Livingstone, New York, 1986.)

border of the transverse colon, with sacculation of the uninvolved inferior border (Fig. 65–28). Rarely, a cobblestone-like pattern is seen that is confused with Crohn's disease. The main radiographic differential diagnosis is gastric carcinoma, gastric ulcer, or omental cake from peritoneal metastasis secondarily invading the transverse colon.[80]

The transverse mesocolon courses from the retroperitoneum overlying the pancreas to the inferior border of the transverse colon.[66] Therefore, when pancreatic carcinoma invades the transverse colon via the transverse mesocolon, the initial radiographic changes occur on the inferior border of the transverse colon.[65] In some cases, however, pancreatic carcinoma may spread to the superior border of the transverse colon (Fig. 65–29). Pancreatic tail carcinomas may extend along the phrenicocolic ligament to invade the medial border of the splenic flexure.[66]

## Intraperitoneal Seeding

The most common primary tumors that seed the peritoneal cavity are ovarian carcinoma in the female

and gastric, pancreatic, and colonic carcinomas in the male. Occasionally, lymph node metastases to the retroperitoneum and/or mesentery may seed the peritoneal cavity, especially from metastatic breast carcinoma. Other tumors that rarely spread peritoneally are uterine, bladder, and cervical carcinomas.

The distribution of neoplasms in the peritoneal cavity results from directed flow of ascitic fluid by the peritoneal reflections (see Chapters 131 and 132).[81] The peritoneal reflections and mesenteries divide the peritoneal cavity into compartments[81] (Fig. 65–30). The transverse mesocolon divides the abdomen into the supramesocolic and inframesocolic spaces.[81, 82] The small bowel mesentery divides the inframesocolic space into small right and large left regions.[82] The phrenicocolic ligament partially separates the left subphrenic space from the left paracolic gutter, extending from the splenic flexure of the colon to peritoneum overlying the 11th rib.[81] These peritoneal reflections direct the flow of intraperitoneal fluid, affecting the distribution and deposition of peritoneally seeded infections and metastases. Directed flow results in characteristic sites of tumor deposition (see Fig. 65–30). As the most dependent portion of the peritoneal cavity in both the supine and erect positions,

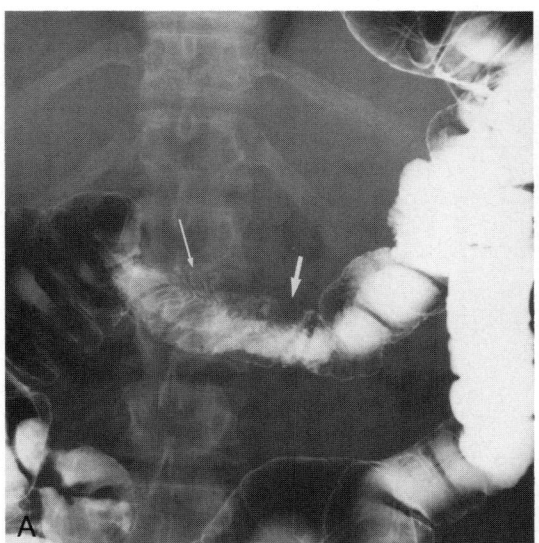
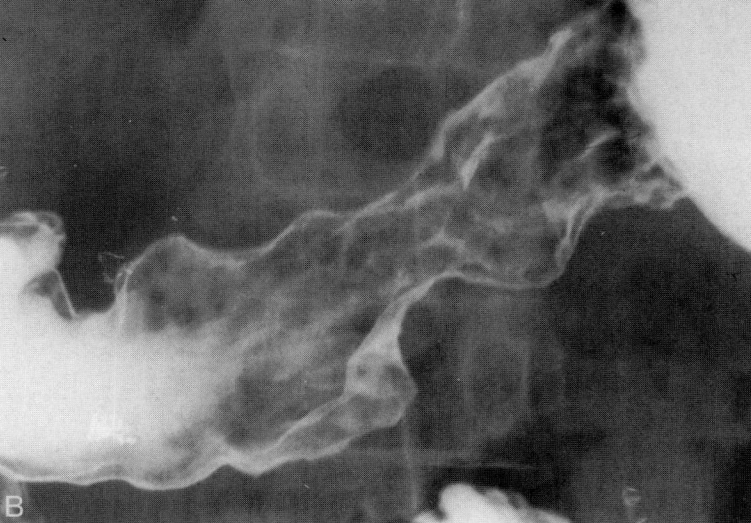

**Figure 65–28. Gastric carcinoma invading the transverse colon. A.** Overhead view from a double contrast barium enema examination shows flattening and extrinsic mass effect *(thick arrow)* involving the superior border of the transverse colon and pleating of mucosal folds en face *(thin arrow)*. **B.** Spot film from a double contrast upper gastrointestinal study shows circumferential narrowing of the gastric antrum with an irregular contour and nodular mucosa, findings compatible with a linitis plastica appearance.

the pouch of Douglas or rectovesicular space is the most common site for peritoneal metastasis (occurring in 56%)[81] (Fig. 65–31). Other sites include the right lower quadrant small bowel loops and medial border of the cecum (41%),[81] the superior border of the sigmoid colon (21%)[81] (Fig. 65–32 [see Color Plate II]), and the right paracolic gutter (18%)[81] (Fig. 65–33).

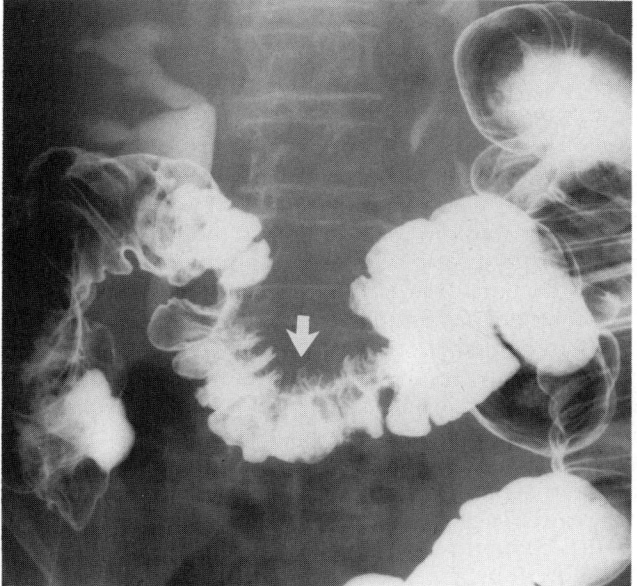

**Figure 65–29. Pancreatic carcinoma invading the transverse colon.** Overhead view from a double contrast barium enema examination shows extrinsic mass effect and spiculation along the superior border of the transverse colon *(arrow)*. Contrast medium in the renal collecting systems is from a prior intravenous urogram.

## Radiographic Findings

Independent of the site of seeded metastasis, the radiographic findings are similar. Initially, there may be an extrinsic mass effect along the side of the bowel wall bathed in peritoneal fluid. With direct invasion of the serosa and/or muscular layers, a desmoplastic reaction occurs. This reaction is manifested radiographically in profile as spiculation of the luminal contour and en face as tethering and pleating of mucosal folds in a fixed, parallel or angulated pattern.[80, 83] Angulation of bowel loops occurs predominantly in the sigmoid colon and small bowel. The differential diagnosis of serosal desmoplastic disease in the pouch of Douglas includes endometriosis (Fig. 65–34), prostatic or cervical carcinoma invading the rectum, an inflammatory process in the pouch of Douglas such as a tubo-ovarian abscess (Fig. 65–35), or abscess caused by diverticulitis, appendicitis, or Crohn's disease. The clinical history, physical findings, and age of the patient contribute to differentiating the various causes. Further work-up may include pelvic ultrasound, CT, or magnetic resonance imaging.

Cecal metastases are invariably accompanied by small bowel changes.[76] Scalloping along the mesenteric border of right lower quadrant ileal loops, fixation and angulation of loops, and spiculation of the luminal contour are seen.

When peritoneal metastases invade the greater omentum, they may secondarily abut and invade the serosa of the transverse colon. These omental cakes initially involve the superior border of the transverse colon at the site of attachment of the greater omentum[80] (Fig. 65–36). Radiographically, a mass effect is seen on the superior border of the transverse colon (see Fig. 65–36), with spiculation of the luminal contour and pleating

# PLATE I

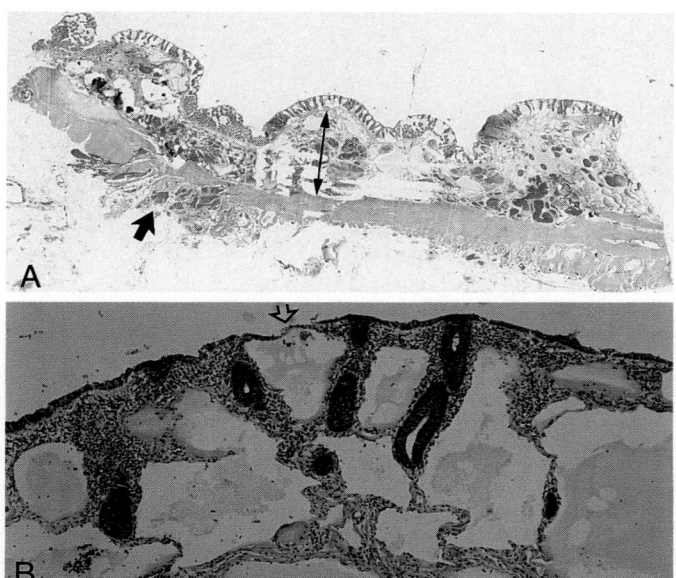

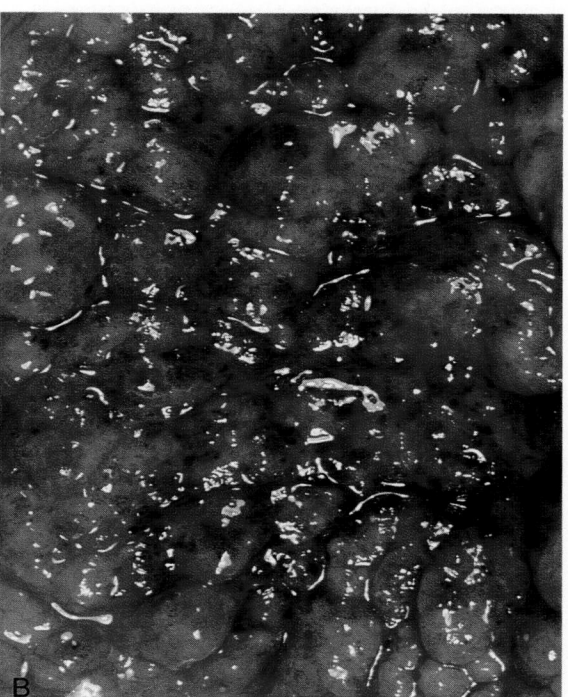

**Figure 65–7. Hemangioma of the colon. A.** Low-power view of recto-sigmoid colon shows an undulating mucosal surface caused by widening of the submucosa *(double arrow)*. At this power, the submucosa is seen to be expanded by blood-filled spaces. The blood-filled spaces extend to the subserosal fat in one area *(thick arrow)*. **B.** Medium-power view of the mucosa from the same lesion shows many large, almost cystic, spaces lined by endothelial cells. The spaces are separated by loose connective tissue. The cavernous spaces extend to the mucosal surface *(arrow)*.

**Figure 65–8. Hemangioma of colon. B.** Close-up photograph of the mucosal surface of the hemangioma shows a lobulated surface with areas of focal hemorrhage. This corresponds to the subtle, smooth surface lobulation seen on the radiograph (Fig. 65–8A).

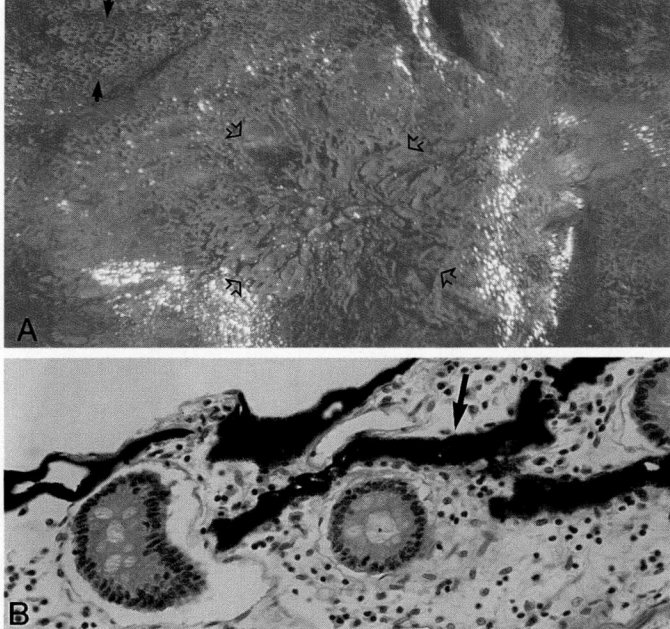

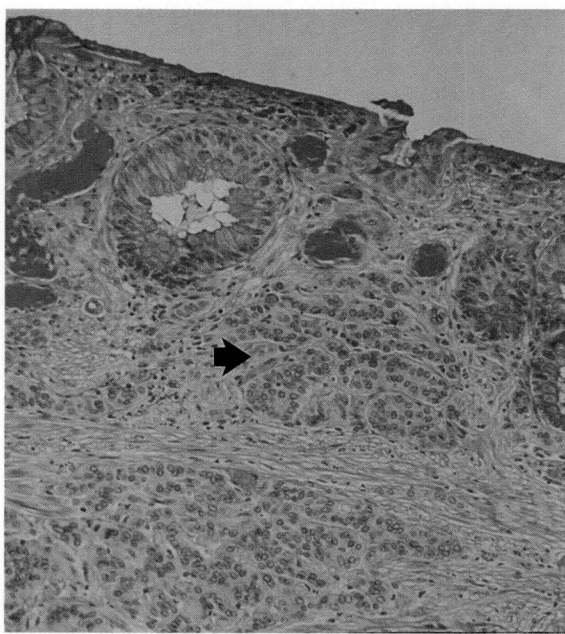

**Figure 65–9. Angiodysplasia of the right colon. A.** Dissecting photomicrograph shows distortion of the surface pattern *(open arrows)* of the colonic mucosa by an underlying tangle of vessels. The normal surface pattern and glandular openings of the colon are marked for comparison *(solid arrows)*. **B.** Medium-power view of the colonic mucosa shows thin-walled, endothelium-lined spaces *(arrow)* in the lamina propria. The spaces were filled with a black-staining dye from a prior injection study.

**Figure 65–10. Rectal carcinoid.** Medium-power photomicrograph shows a predominantly trabecular pattern of tumor infiltrating the lamina propria *(arrow)* and submucosa. The tumor is composed of small, uniform, monomorphic cells with typical "salt-and-pepper" nuclei.

# PLATE II

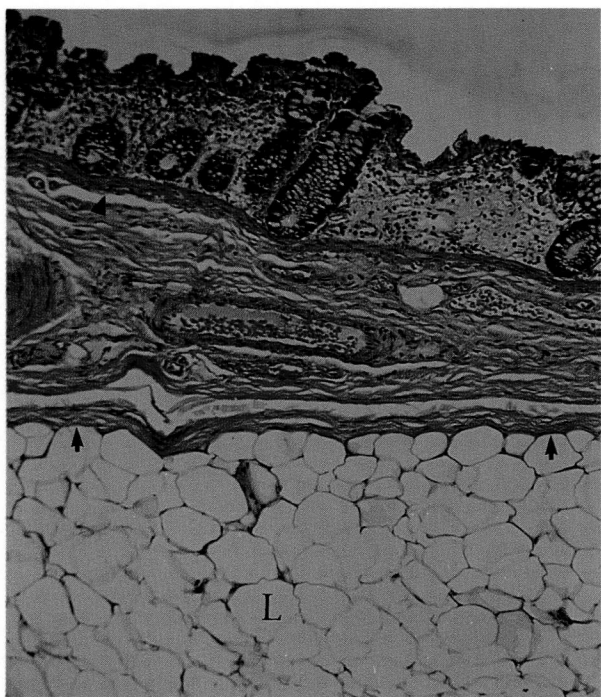

**Figure 65–12. Lipoma of colon.** Medium-power photomicrograph shows mature adipose tissue (L) expanding the submucosa. A fibrous capsule *(arrows)* is seen. Muscularis mucosae is identified by the arrowhead.

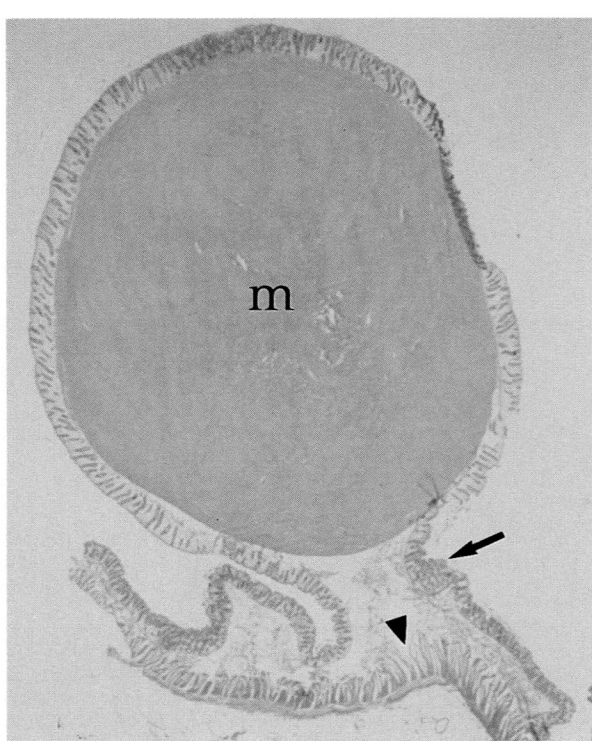

**Figure 65–18. Pedunculated stromal tumor.** Low-power photomicrograph shows a polyp on a short stalk. Normal colonic mucosa overlies a mass (m) lying between the epithelial layer and the muscularis propria *(arrowhead)*. The mucosa of the stalk *(arrow)* is normal. This was a true leiomyoma, probably arising in the muscularis mucosae. (Courtesy of Scott H. Saul, M.D., West Chester, PA.)

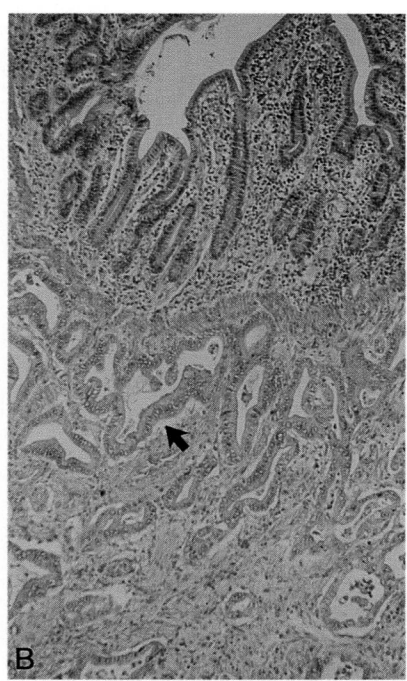

**Figure 65–32. Intraperitoneal spread of pancreatic carcinoma to superior border sigmoid colon. B.** Medium-power photomicrograph of resection specimen shows pancreatic cancer invading the submucosa (representative nest of tumor indicated by arrow).

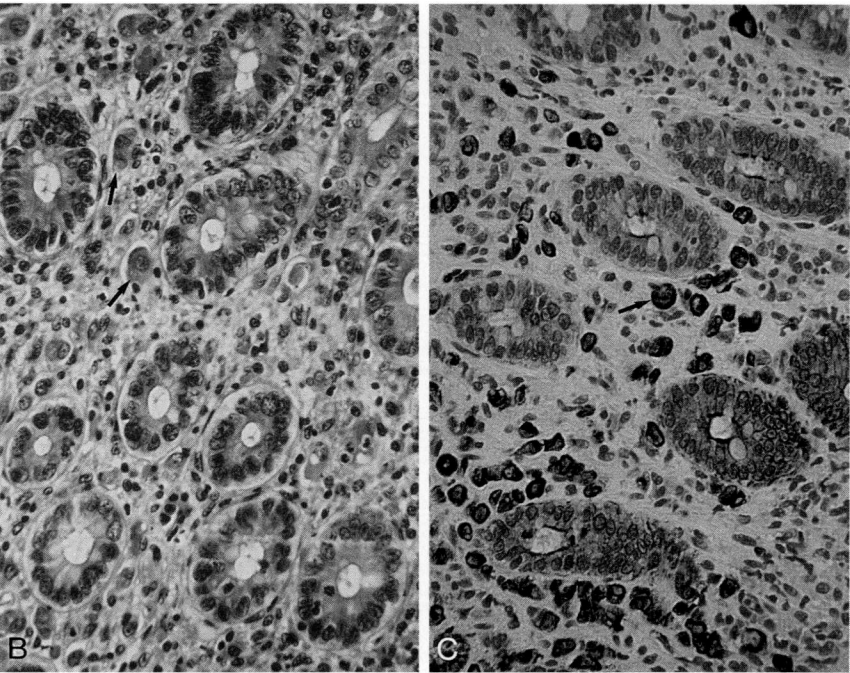

**Figure 65–39. Breast metastases to transverse colon. B** and **C.** Medium-power photomicrographs show individual malignant cells infiltrating the lamina propria (**B,** hematoxylin-eosin; **C,** immunohistochemistry for epithelial membrane antigen). Representative malignant cells are marked with arrows.

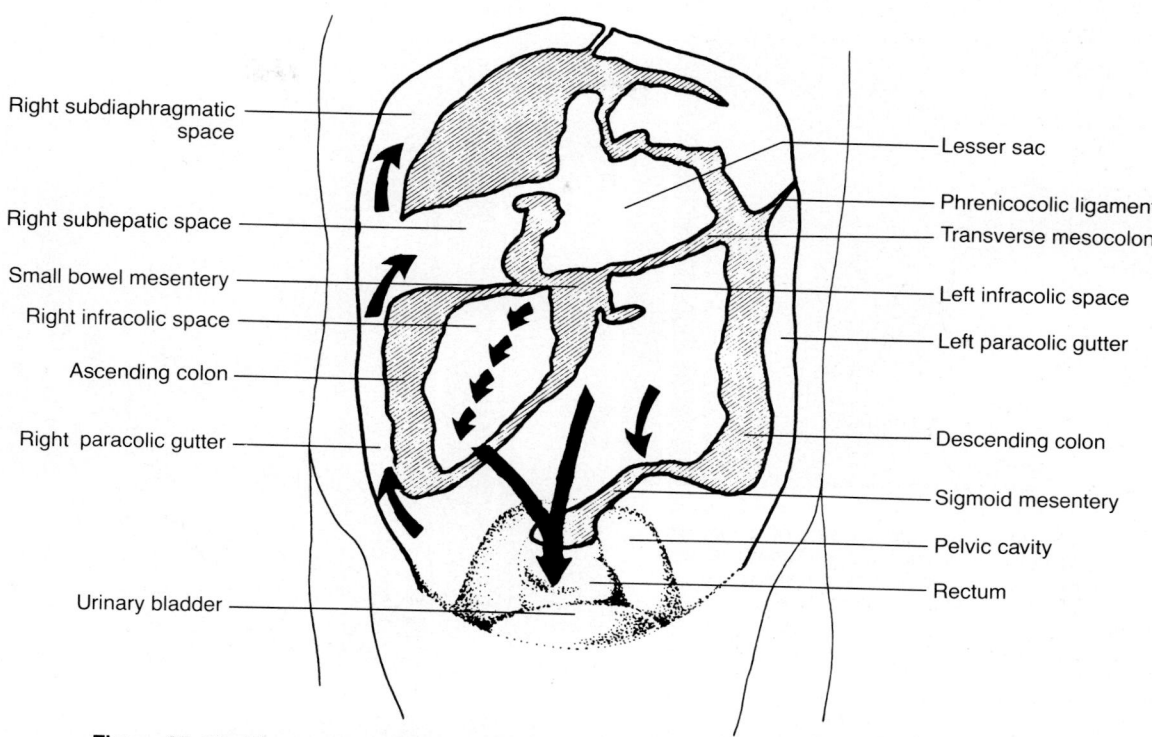

Right subdiaphragmatic space

Right subhepatic space

Small bowel mesentery

Right infracolic space

Ascending colon

Right paracolic gutter

Urinary bladder

Lesser sac

Phrenicocolic ligament

Transverse mesocolon

Left infracolic space

Left paracolic gutter

Descending colon

Sigmoid mesentery

Pelvic cavity

Rectum

**Figure 65–30. Directed flow of intraperitoneal fluid.** The peritoneal reflections direct the flow of intraperitoneal fluid within the peritoneal cavity. Flow from the left inframesocolic space pools in the sigmoid mesentery along the superior border of the sigmoid colon and then courses into the pelvic cavity (rectovesicular space in male, pouch of Douglas in female, and pararectal spaces). Flow in the right inframesocolic space courses down the ruffles of the small bowel mesentery into the right lower quadrant along distal small bowel loops and the medial border of the cecum. Flow then courses into the pelvic cavity from this region. Fluid from the pelvic cavity then courses up the right paracolic gutter to the right subhepatic space and right subdiaphragmatic space. Thus, the sites of pooling (the superior border of the sigmoid colon, the pouch of Douglas or retrovesicular space, the medial border of the cecum, the mesenteric border of the distal small bowel, and the right paracolic gutter) are the predominant sites for intraperitoneal seeding by tumor.

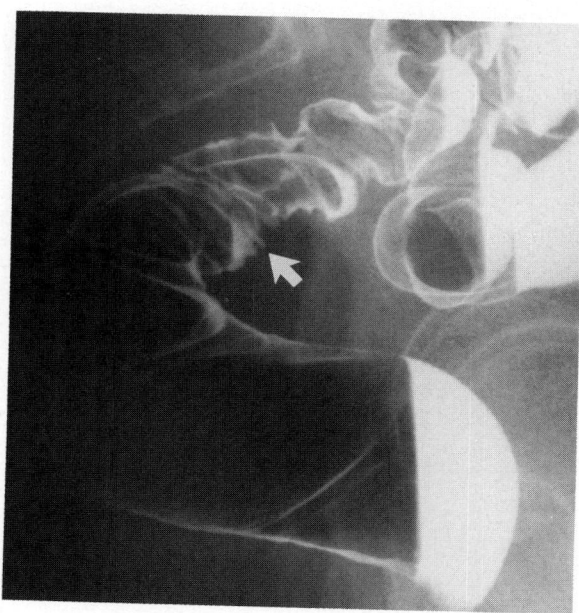

**Figure 65–31. Ovarian carcinoma with intraperitoneal metastases to the rectosigmoid junction.** Prone cross-table lateral view of the rectosigmoid junction shows spiculation *(arrow)* and tethering of folds along the anterior wall of the rectosigmoid junction. En face pleating of the mucosa is seen.

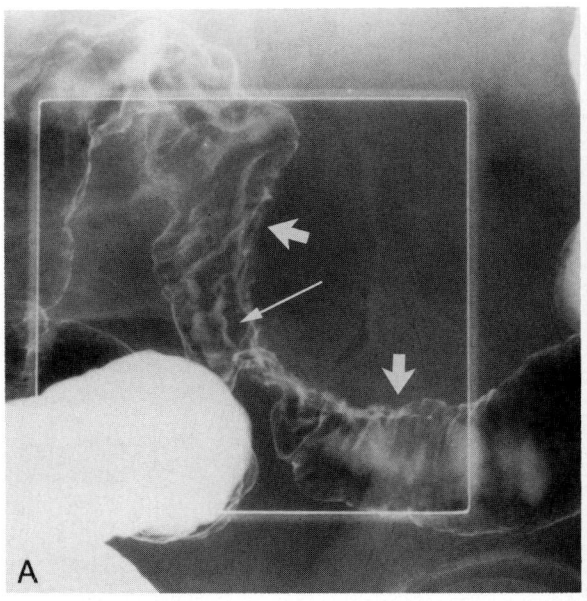

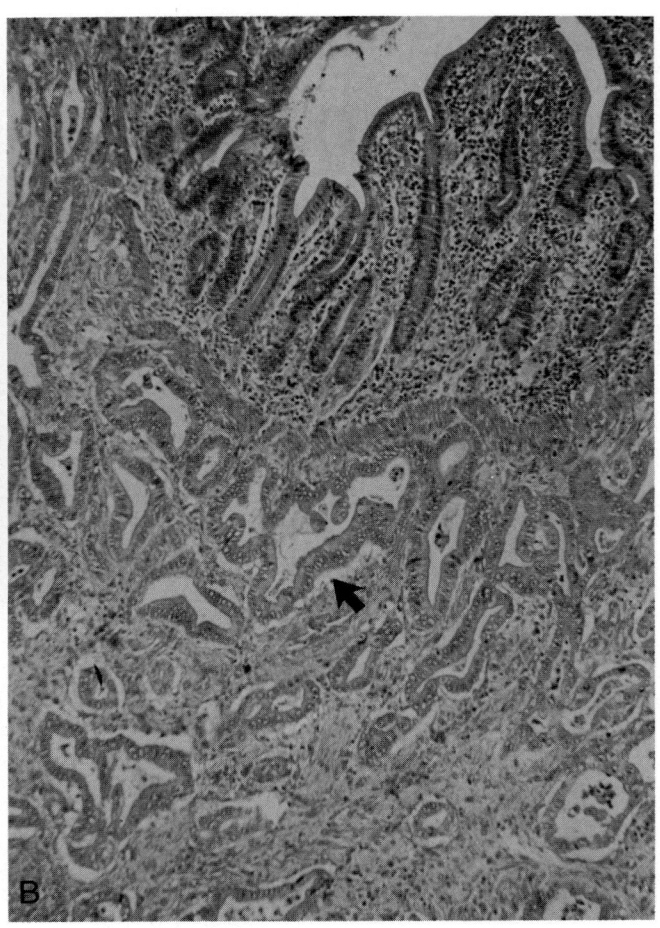

**Figure 65–32. Intraperitoneal spread of pancreatic carcinoma to superior border sigmoid colon. A.** Spot film from a double contrast barium enema shows a broad-based extrinsic mass effect along the superior border of the sigmoid colon *(thick arrows)*, spiculation of the contour, smooth sacculation of the wall opposite the mass effect, and focal nodularity of the mucosa *(thin arrow)*. **B.** Medium-power photomicrograph of resection specimen shows pancreatic cancer invading the submucosa (representative nest of tumor indicated by arrow). (See Color Plate II.)

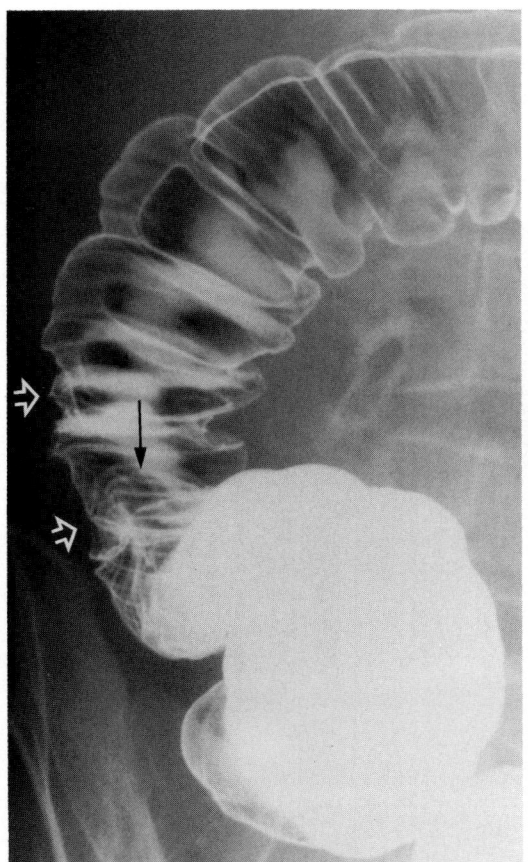

**Figure 65–33. Ovarian carcinoma with intraperitoneal metastases to the right paracolic gutter.** Spot film from a double contrast barium enema shows extrinsic mass effect along the right lateral border of the ascending colon *(open arrows)*, spiculation of the contour, and, en face, pleating of the colonic mucosa *(solid arrow)*.

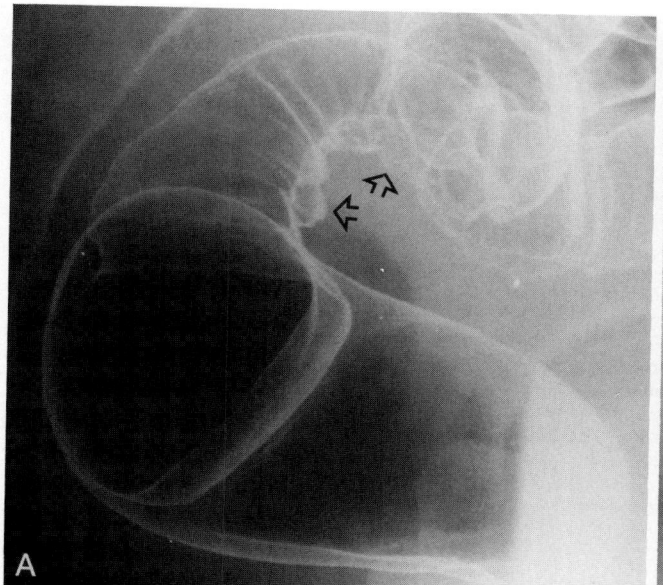

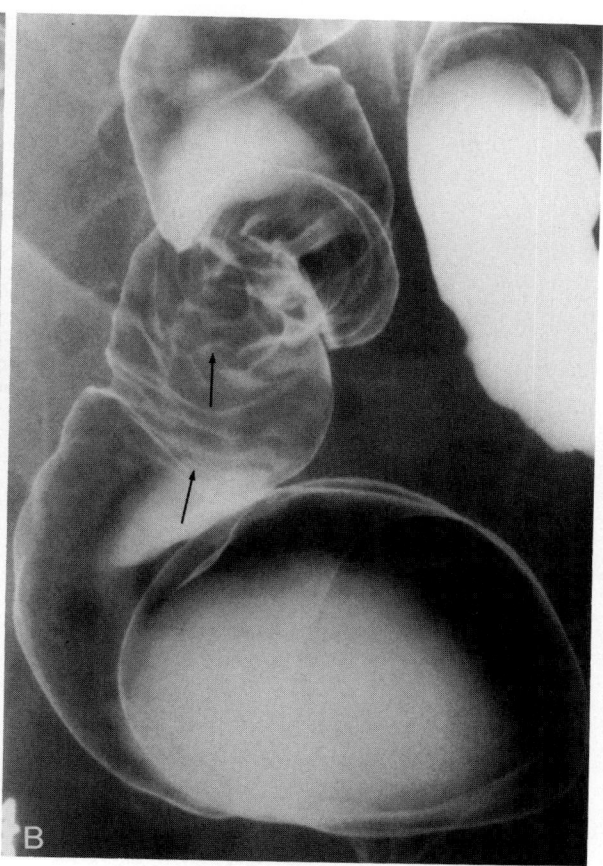

**Figure 65–34. Endometriosis involving the rectosigmoid junction. A.** Prone, cross-table lateral view of the rectum shows extrinsic mass effect along the anterior wall of the rectosigmoid junction *(arrows)* with irregularity of the colonic contour. **B.** Slightly oblique view of the rectosigmoid junction shows smooth pleating of the colonic mucosa *(arrows)*. These findings are identical to those for intraperitoneal metastases invading the rectosigmoid junction. The key to the diagnosis lies in the clinical history and age of the patient.

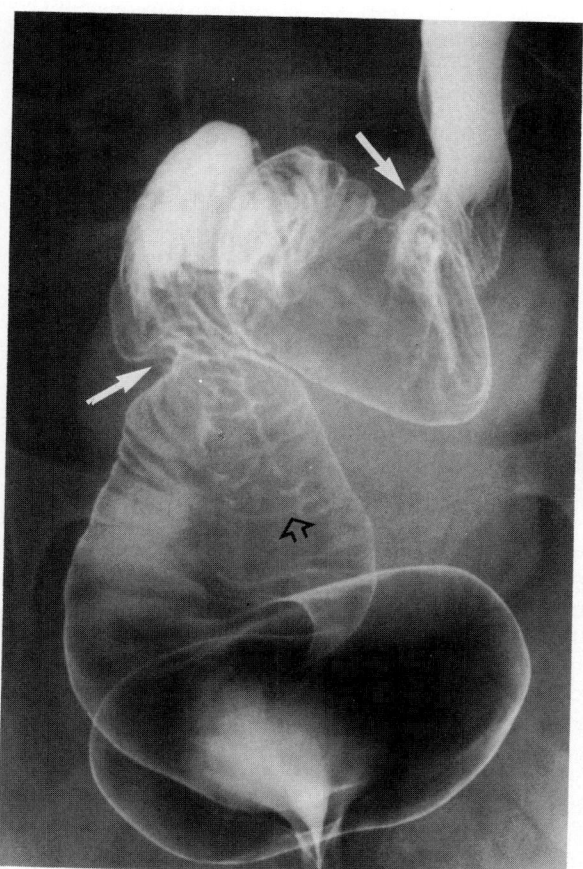

**Figure 65–35. Tubo-ovarian abscess invading the sigmoid and rectosigmoid colon.** Overhead view from a double contrast barium enema shows, en face, pleating of the mucosa of the rectosigmoid junction *(open arrow)*, angulation, focal narrowing, and mucosal pleating of the sigmoid colon *(solid arrows)*.

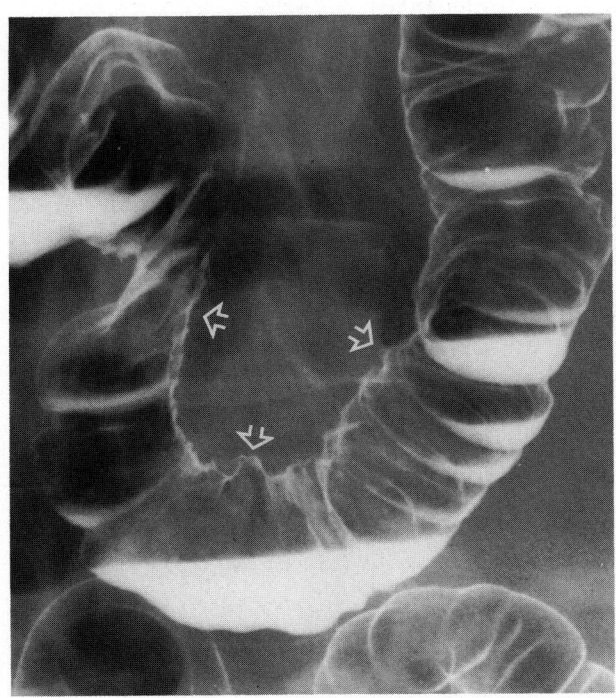

**Figure 65–36. Omental cake from ovarian carcinomatosis invading the transverse colon.** Spot film from a double contrast barium enema of a patient with known ovarian carcinoma with interperitoneal metastases to the greater omentum shows a mass effect along the superior border of the transverse colon *(arrows)*, spiculation of the superior contour, and sacculation of the opposite uninvolved wall. (From Rubesin SE, Levine MS: Omental cakes: colonic involvement by omental metastases. Radiology 154:593–596, 1985.)

and tethering of mucosal folds (Fig. 65–37). The radiographic differential diagnosis is predominantly gastric carcinoma invading the transverse colon or gastrocolic fistula. The clinical history and radiographic finding of metastases involving other portions of colon suggest the correct diagnosis.[80, 84] Inflammatory processes in the gastrocolic ligament such as cholecystitis, pancreatitis (Fig. 65–38), or diverticulitis may have identical radiographic appearances.

## Embolic Metastases

Embolic metastases may manifest with rectal bleeding or incomplete obstruction, often many years after treatment of the primary lesion. The most common primary tumors resulting in embolic metastasis to the colon are melanoma, lung carcinoma, and breast carcinoma.

### Melanoma

Melanoma involves the small intestine more frequently than the colon. Metastatic melanoma usually appears as an umbilicated or ulcerated submucosal mass or as a bulky, polypoid intraluminal mass. Linear fissures may radiate toward the central ulcer of the submucosal mass, giving a "spoke-wheel" appearance.[65] The differential diagnosis of an umbilicated ("target") lesion in the colon includes lymphoma, Kaposi's sarcoma, carcinoid tumor, or gastrointestinal stromal tumor.

### Carcinoma of the Breast

Although carcinoma of the breast is the most common primary malignancy that spreads to the colon, colonic breast metastases are usually small and asymptomatic. At autopsy, almost 6.4% of those who died of metastatic breast carcinoma have metastases to the colon.[85] Radiographically, breast metastases may appear as mural nodules (Fig. 65–39 [see Color Plate II]), eccentric strictures, or irregular circumferential narrowings (linitis plastica)[66] (Fig. 65–40). Occasionally, hematogenous metastases simulate Crohn's disease of the colon.

### Carcinoma of the Lung

Lung carcinoma metastases to the colon are usually asymptomatic, small serosal deposits.[66] Occasionally, however, lung metastases cause obstruction, bleeding, or anemia.[86] These metastases appear radiographically as ulcerated submucosal masses (target lesions), short excentric or annular narrowings, or large mesenteric masses with secondary desmoplastic serosal change.[66]

## SUMMARY

The goal of barium studies is detection of lesions followed by graded differential diagnosis based on morphologic appearances.[87] The clinical history, symptoms, and age of the patient are minor factors.

Most polyps, whether sessile or pedunculated, are adenomatous or hyperplastic. The radiologist assumes a worst-case scenario, that a polyp detected on barium enema examination is within the spectrum of adenomatous change, with the potential for in situ carcinoma or the future development of carcinoma. By far the most important radiographic criterion of malignant potential is the size of the lesion. In the spectrum of adenomas, approximately 1% of 6- to 10-mm tumors

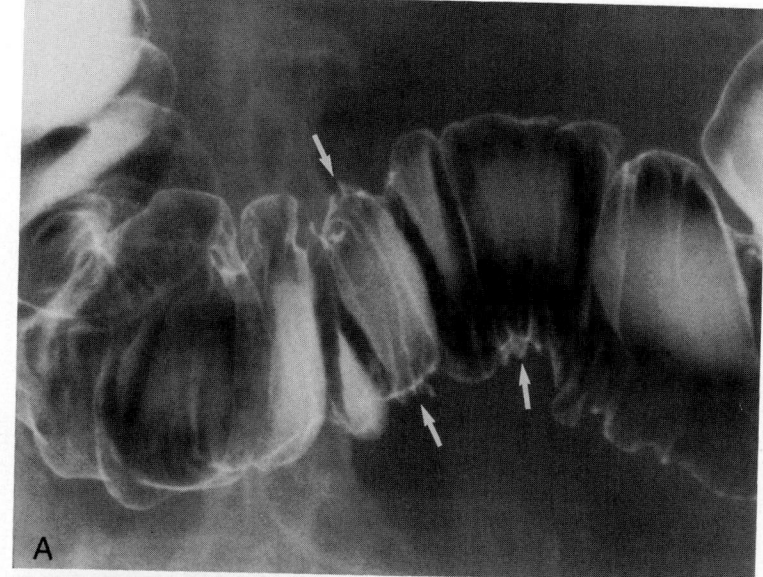

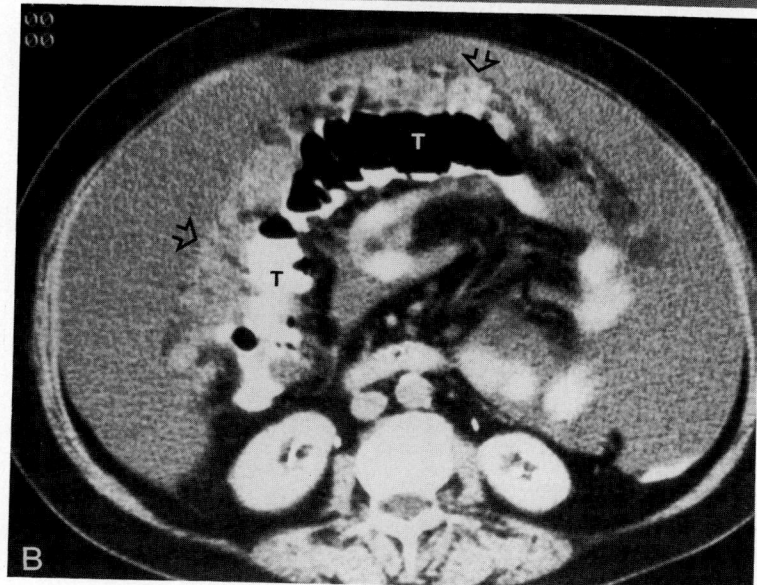

**Figure 65–37. Omental cake from ovarian carcinomatosis invading the transverse colon: barium enema–CT correlation. A.** Spot film from a double contrast barium enema shows spiculation of the colonic contour *(arrows)* and thin transverse stripes crossing the colon as a result of pleating of the mucosa. **B.** CT scan shows enlargement and increased attenuation of greater omentum caused by omental cake *(arrows)* along the anterior border of the transverse colon (T). A large amount of malignant ascites deviates the colon and small bowel loops medially. At surgery, intraperitoneal and greater omental metastases from ovarian carcinoma were found.

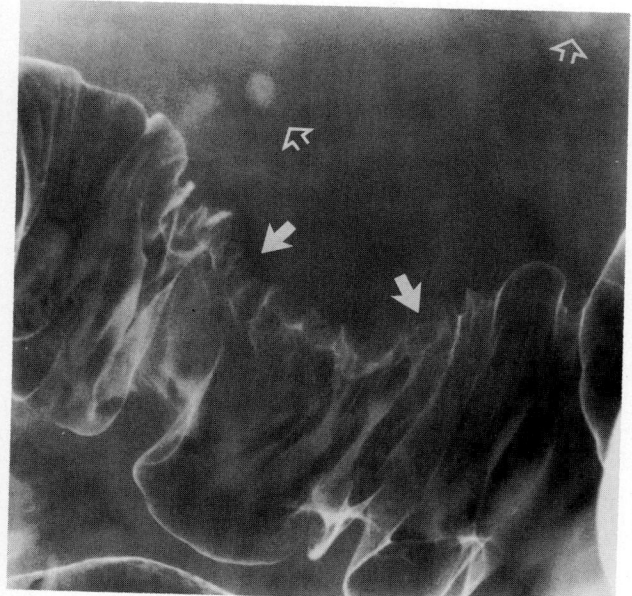

**Figure 65–38. Pancreatitis with inflammatory process spreading to the transverse colon.** Spot film from a double contrast barium enema examination shows mass effect along the superior border of the transverse colon *(solid arrows)*, spiculation of the colonic contour, and opposite wall sacculation. Also note soft tissue calcifications resulting from chronic pancreatitis *(open arrows)*.

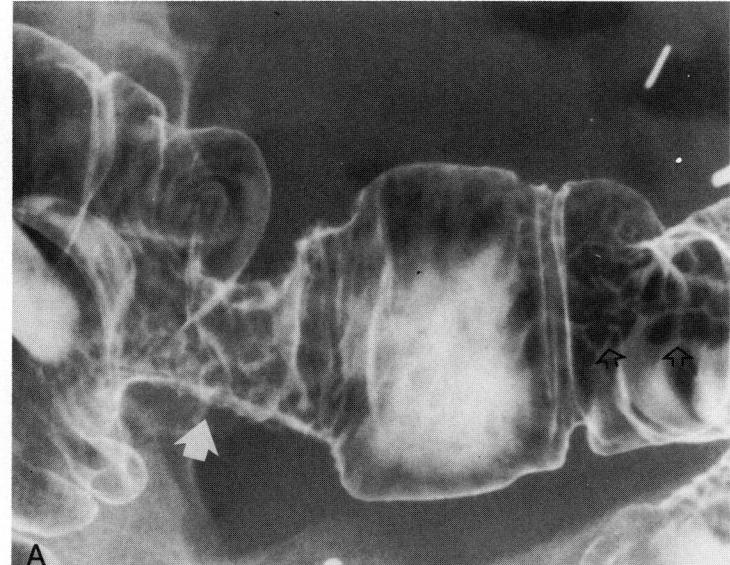

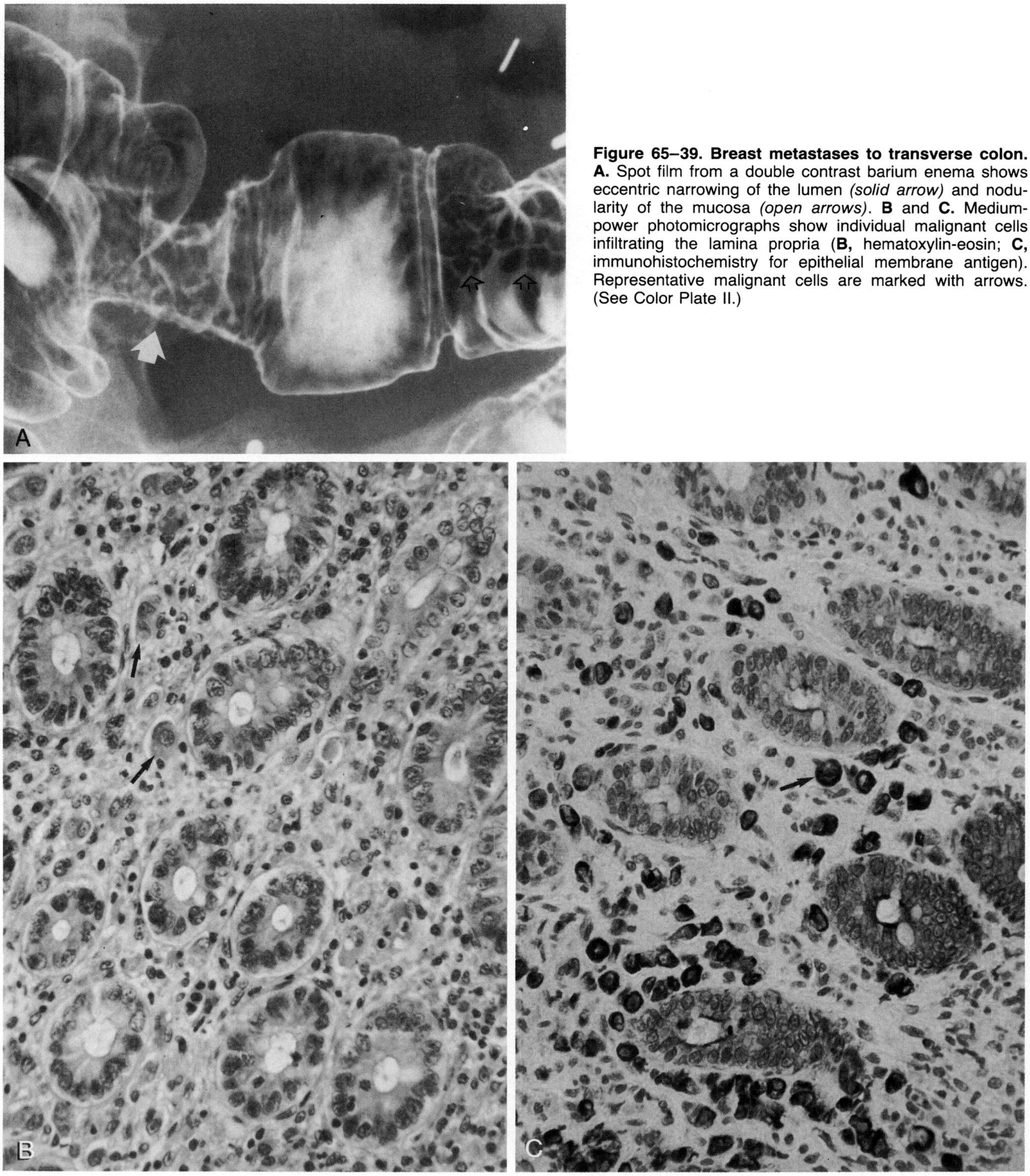

**Figure 65–39. Breast metastases to transverse colon. A.** Spot film from a double contrast barium enema shows eccentric narrowing of the lumen *(solid arrow)* and nodularity of the mucosa *(open arrows)*. **B** and **C.** Medium-power photomicrographs show individual malignant cells infiltrating the lamina propria (**B,** hematoxylin-eosin; **C,** immunohistochemistry for epithelial membrane antigen). Representative malignant cells are marked with arrows. (See Color Plate II.)

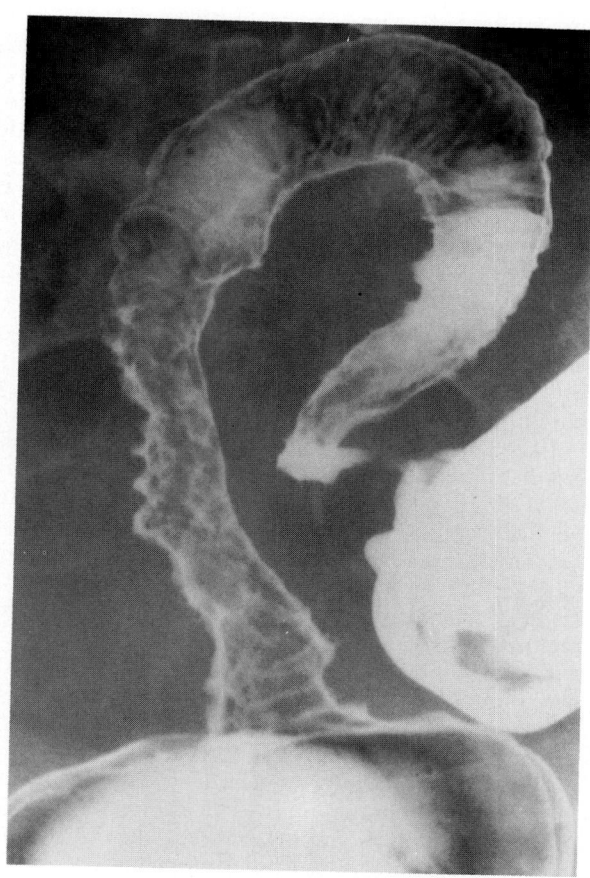

**Figure 65–40. Linitis plastica of the colon caused by hematogenous breast metastases.** Spot film from a double contrast barium enema shows diffuse narrowing of the distal sigmoid colon with spiculation of the contour and mild nodularity of the colonic mucosa. Differential diagnosis includes primary linitis plastica of the colon or granulomatous colitis.

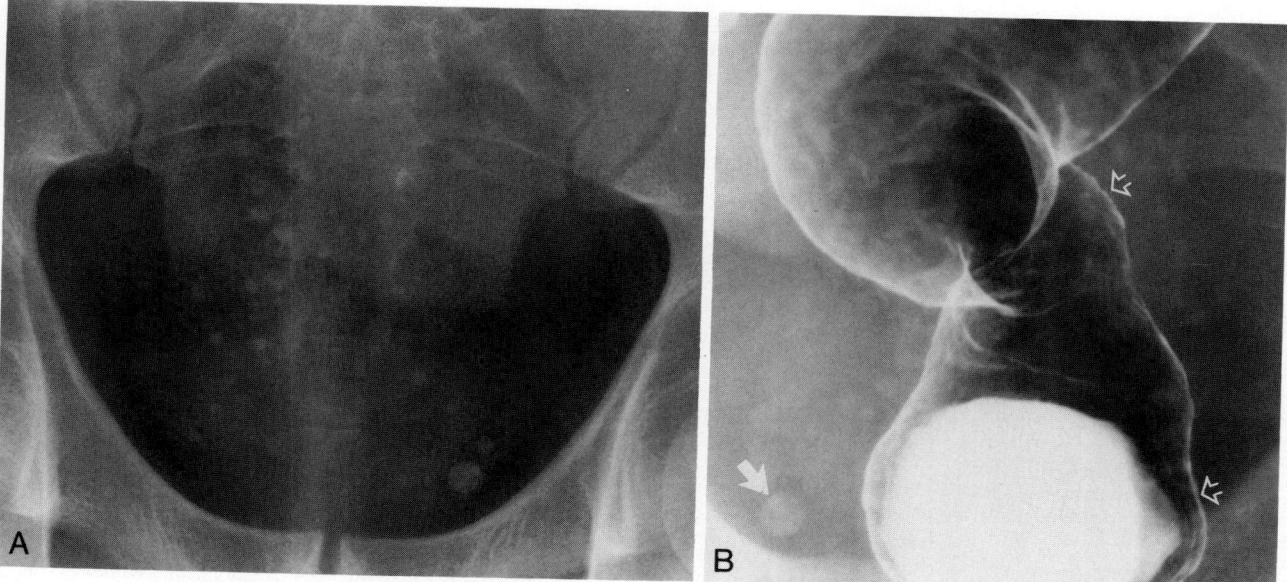

**Figure 65–41. Rectal hemangioma. A.** Scout film of the abdomen in a young man who presented with rectal bleeding shows multiple phleboliths in an unusual distribution, extending vertically in the pelvis. A preliminary diagnosis of rectal hemangioma should be suggested. **B.** Spot film from a double contrast barium enema shows mild narrowing of the rectum and slight irregularity of the rectal surface pattern *(open arrows)*. Phleboliths are seen outside the rectum *(solid arrow)*. A rectal hemangioma was found.

1226

are malignant. Approximately 10% of 1- to 2-cm adenomas are malignant, and approximately 45% of tumors larger than 2 cm are malignant.[88]

A smooth surface is not a helpful criterion for distinguishing a small mucosal or submucosal lesion. Both mucosal and polypoid submucosal masses may have smooth surfaces. A finely granular or villous surface pattern may indicate tubulovillous or villous change.[89–91] Other radiographic signs such as inbowing of contour near the polyp are not specific signs of malignancy.

Radiographically, a polyp is a polyp. The radiologist should not be surprised when a sessile polyp, especially in the rectum, is diagnosed as a hyperplastic polyp, carcinoid, or gastrointestinal stromal tumor.

Large, sessile, polypoid submucosal masses must first be distinguished from polypoid carcinomas. Any mucosal irregularity in a bulky polypoid mass suggests adenocarcinoma. Smooth-surfaced, bulky polypoid masses include lipomas, lymphomas, and hemangiomas. Change in size and shape of a lesion and a pear shape suggest a lipoma. The diagnosis of lipoma may be confirmed by CT.

Cavitary, bulky lesions include perforated colonic carcinomas, lymphomas, and stromal tumors. Rarely, these tumors must be distinguished from Crohn's disease or diverticulitis with abscess formation.

The radiologist may suggest a specific diagnosis with lipomas and hemangiomas. The radiographic diagnosis of hemangioma is important because this lesion may easily be misdiagnosed endoscopically as colitis. In young patients with rectal bleeding, a rectal surface lesion with underlying phleboliths (Fig. 65–41) is typical of hemangioma.

Thus, the majority of the tumors presented in this chapter are significant for their pathologic interest rather than their radiologic basis. Nevertheless, the radiologist should be familiar with the varying clinical histories and appearances of these unusual tumors.

### Acknowledgment

Figures 65–5 and 65–40 are reproduced from Laufer I, Levine MS (eds): Double Contrast Gastrointestinal Radiology. Philadelphia: WB Saunders, 1992.

# References

1. Weinsrad D, DeCosse JJ, Sherlock P, et al: Primary gastrointestinal lymphoma. Cancer 49:1258–1265, 1982.
2. Lewin KJ, Ranchod M, Dorfman RF: Lymphomas of the gastrointestinal tract. A study of 117 cases presenting with gastrointestinal disease. Cancer 42:693–707, 1978.
3. Herrman R, Panahon AM, Barcos MP, et al: Gastrointestinal involvement in non-Hodgkin's lymphoma. Cancer 46:215–222, 1980.
4. Dragosics B, Bauer P, Radaszkiewicz T: Primary gastrointestinal non-Hodgkin's lymphomas: a retrospective clinicopathologic study of 150 cases. Cancer 55:1060–1073, 1985.
5. Messinger NH, Bobroff LM, Beneventano TC: Lymphosarcoma of the colon. AJR 117:281–286, 1973.
6. Wychulis AR, Beahrs OH, Woolner LB: Malignant lymphoma of the colon. Arch Surg 93:215–225, 1966.
7. Wolf BS, Marshak RH: Roentgen features of diffuse lymphosarcoma of the colon. Radiology 75:733–740, 1960.
8. Cornes JS, Wallace MH, Morson BC: Benign lymphomas of the rectum and anal canal. J Pathol Bacteriol 82:371–382, 1961.
9. Marshak RH, Lindner AE, Maklansky D: Lymphoreticular disorders of the gastrointestinal tract: roentgenographic features. Gastrointest Radiol 4:103–120, 1979.
10. Renton P, Blackshaw AJ: Colonic lymphoma complicating ulcerative colitis. Br J Surg 63:542–545, 1976.
11. Sataline LR, Mobley EM, Kirkham W: Ulcerative colitis complicated by colonic lymphoma. Gastroenterology 44:342–347, 1963.
12. O'Connell DJ, Thompson AJ: Lymphoma of the colon. The spectrum of radiologic changes. Gastrointest Radiol 2:377–385, 1978.
13. Zornoza J, Dodd GD: Lymphoma of the gastrointestinal tract. Semin Roentgenol 15:272–287, 1980.
14. Bragg DG, Colby TV, Ward JH: New concepts in the non-Hodgkin lymphomas: radiologic implications. Radiology 159:289–304, 1986.
15. Pochaczevsky R, Sherman RS: Diffuse lymphomatous disease of the colon: its roentgen appearance. AJR 87:670–684, 1962.
16. Williams SM, Berk RN, Harned RK: Radiologic features of multinodular lymphoma of the colon. AJR 143:87–91, 1984.
17. Harned RK, Doby CA, Farley GE: Cavernous hemangioma of the rectum and appendix. Dis Colon Rectum 17:759–762, 1974.
18. Gentry RW, Dockerty MB, Glagett OT: Collective review: vascular malformations and vascular tumors of the gastrointestinal tract. Int Abstr Surg 88:281–323, 1949.
19. Dachman AH, Ros PR, Shekitka KM, et al: Colorectal hemangioma: radiologic findings. Radiology 167:31–34, 1988.
20. Lyon DT, Mantea AG: Large-bowel hemangiomas. Dis Colon Rectum 27:404–414, 1984.
21. Allred HW Jr, Spencer RJ: Hemangiomas of the colon, rectum, and anus. Mayo Clin Proc 49:739–741, 1974.
22. Morson BC, Dawson IMP: Gastrointestinal Pathology. Oxford: Blackwell Scientific Publications, 1979, pp 648–680.
23. Ghahremani GG, Kangarloo H, Volberg F, et al: Diffuse cavernous hemangioma of the colon in the Klippel-Trenaunay syndrome. Radiology 118:673–678, 1976.
24. Perez C, Andreu J, Llauger J, et al: Hemangioma of the rectum: CT appearance. Gastrointest Radiol 12:347–349, 1987.
25. Margulis AR: Selected cases from the film interpretation session of the Society of Gastrointestinal Radiologists. Case 1: hemangioma of the rectum. Gastrointest Radiol 6:363–364, 1981.
26. Lawson JP, Myerson PJ, Myerson DA: Colonic lymphangioma. Gastrointest Radiol 1:85–89, 1976.
27. Camilleri M, Satti MB, Wood CB: Cystic lymphangioma of the colon. Dis Colon Rectum 25:813–816, 1982.
28. Arnet NL, Friedman PS: Lymphangioma of the colon: Roentgen aspects, a case report. Radiology 67:882–885, 1956.
29. Agha FP, Francis IR, Simms SM: Cystic lymphangioma of the colon. AJR 141:709–710, 1983.
30. Boley SJ, Sammartano R, Adams A, et al: On the nature and etiology of vascular ectasias of the colon: degenerative lesions of aging. Gastroenterology 72:650–660, 1977.
31. Baum S, Athanasoulis C, Waltman A, et al: Angiodysplasia of the right colon: a cause of gastrointestinal bleeding. AJR 129:789–794, 1977.
32. Galloway SJ, Casarella WJ, Shimkin PM: Vascular malformations of the right colon as a cause of bleeding in patients with aortic stenosis. Radiology 113:11–15, 1974.
33. Godwin DJ: Carcinoid tumors. An analysis of 2837 cases. Cancer 36:560–569, 1975.
34. Martensson H, Nobin A, Sundler F: Carcinoid tumours in the gastrointestinal tract—an analysis of 156 cases. Acta Chir Scand 149:607–616, 1983.
35. Shulman H, Giustra P: Invasive carcinoids of the colon. Radiology 98:139–143, 1971.
36. Wilander E: Endocrine cell tumours. In Whitehead R (ed): Gastrointestinal and Oesophageal Pathology. Edinburgh: Churchill Livingstone, 1989, pp 629–641.
37. Wilander E, Portela-Gomes G, Grimelius L, et al: Argentaffin and argyrophil reaction of human gastrointestinal carcinoids. Gastroenterology 73:733–736, 1977.

38. Balthazar EJ: Carcinoid tumors of the alimentary tract. Gastrointest Radiol 3:47–56, 1978.
39. Fioca R, Capella C, Bufta R, et al: Glucagon-like, glicentin-like and pancreatic polypeptide–like immunoreactivities in rectal carcinoids and related colorectal cells. Am J Pathol 100:81–92, 1980.
40. Jetmore AB, Ray JE, Gathright JB, et al: Rectal carcinoids: the most frequent rectal tumor. Dis Colon Rectum 35:717–725, 1992.
41. Sato T, Sakai Y, Sonoyama A, et al: Radiologic spectrum of rectal carcinoid tumors. Gastrointest Radiol 9:23–26, 1984.
42. Berardi RS: Carcinoid tumors of the colon (exclusive of the rectum). Review of the literature. Dis Colon Rectum 15:383–391, 1972.
43. Crittenden JJ, Byllesby J, Dodds W: Carcinoid tumor presenting as an annular lesion in the ascending colon. Radiology 97:85–86, 1970.
44. Haller JD, Roberts TW: Lipomas of the colon: a clinicopathologic study of 40 cases. Surgery 55:773–781, 1964.
45. Hurwitz MH, Redleaf PD, Williams HJ, et al: Lipomas of the gastrointestinal tract. AJR 99:84–89, 1967.
46. Castro DB, Stearns MW: Lipomas of the large intestine. Dis Colon Rectum 15:441–444, 1972.
47. Berk RN, Werner LG: The radiology corner: lipoma of the colon. Am J Gastroenterol 61:145–150, 1974.
48. Snover DC: Atypical lipomas of the colon. Dis Colon Rectum 27:485–488, 1984.
49. Kawamoto K, Motooka M, Hirata N, et al: Colonic submucosal tumors: a new classification based on radiologic characteristics. AJR 160:315–320, 1993.
50. Margulis AR, Jovanovich A: The roentgen diagnosis of submucous lipomas of the colon. AJR 84:1114–1120, 1960.
51. Deeths TM, Dodds WJ: Lipoma of the colon. Am J Gastroenterol 58:326–331, 1972.
52. Heiken JP, Forde KA, Gold RP: Computed tomography as a definitive method for diagnosing gastrointestinal lipomas. Radiology 142:409–414, 1982.
53. Megibow AJ, Redmond PE, Bosniak MA, et al: Diagnosis of gastrointestinal lipomas by CT. AJR 133:743–745, 1979.
54. Geboes K: Rare and secondary (metastatic) tumours. *In* Whitehead R (ed): Gastrointestinal and Oesophageal Pathology. Edinburgh: Churchill Livingstone, 1989, pp 779–786.
55. Hinkel CL: Roentgenological examination and evaluation of the ileocecal valve. AJR 68:171–182, 1952.
56. Lasser EC, Rigler LC: Ileocecal valve syndrome. Gastroenterology 28:1–16, 1955.
57. Hendrickson MR, Kempson RL: Smooth muscle tumours. In Whitehead R (ed): Gastrointestinal and Oesophageal Pathology. Edinburgh: Churchill Livingstone, 1989, pp 619–627.
58. Appelman HD: Smooth muscle tumors of the gastrointestinal tract. What we know now that Stout didn't know. Am J Surg Pathol 10(suppl 1):83–89, 1986.
59. Saul SH, Rast ML, Brooks JJ: The immunohistochemistry of gastrointestinal stromal tumors. Evidence supporting an origin from smooth muscle. Am J Surg Pathol 11:464–473, 1987.
60. Rao BK, Kapur MM, Roy S: Leiomyosarcoma of the colon: a case report and review of literature. Dis Colon Rectum 23:184–190, 1980.
61. Akwari OE, Dozois RR, Weiland LH, et al: Leiomyosarcoma of the small and large bowel. Cancer 42:1375–1384, 1978.
62. Walsh TH, Mann CV: Smooth muscle neoplasms of the rectum and anal canal. Br J Surg 71:597–599, 1984.
63. Williams GT, Blackshaw AJ, Morson BC: Squamous carcinoma of the colorectum and its genesis. J Pathol 129:139–147, 1979.
64. Wigh R, Tapley N duV: Metastatic lesions to the large intestine. Radiology 70:222–228, 1958.
65. Meyers MA, McSweeney J: Secondary neoplasms of the bowel. Radiology 105:1–11, 1972.

66. Meyers MA: Dynamic Radiology of the Abdomen: Normal and Pathologic Anatomy (3rd ed). New York: Springer-Verlag, 1988.
67. Gedgaudas RK, Kelvin FM, Thompson WM, et al: The value of preoperative barium enema in the assessment of pelvic masses. Radiology 146:609–613, 1983.
68. Becker JA: Prostatic carcinoma involving the rectum and sigmoid colon. AJR 94:421–428, 1965.
69. Gengler L, Baer J, Finby N: Rectal and sigmoid involvement secondary to carcinoma of the prostate. AJR 125:910–917, 1975.
70. Winter CC: The problem of rectal involvement by prostatic cancer. Surg Gynecol Obstet 105:136–140, 1957.
71. Fry DE, Amin M, Harbrecht PJ: Rectal obstruction secondary to carcinoma of the prostate. Ann Surg 189:488–492, 1979.
72. Aigen AB, Schapira HE: Metastatic carcinoma of prostate and bladder causing intestinal obstruction. Urology 21:464–456, 1983.
73. Rubesin SE, Levine MS, Bezzi M, et al: Rectal involvement by prostatic carcinoma: radiographic findings. AJR 152:53–57, 1989.
74. Huang TY, Yam LT, Li Cy: Unusual radiologic features of metastatic prostatic carcinoma confirmed by immunohistochemical study. Urology 23:218–223, 1984.
75. Li CY, Lam WKW, Yam LT: Immunohistochemical diagnosis of prostatic cancer with metastasis. Cancer 46:706–712, 1980.
76. Meyers MA: Intraperitoneal spread of malignancies and its effect on the bowel. Clin Radiol 32:129–146, 1981.
77. Honda H, Lu CH, Barloon TT, et al: Sigmoid colon fistula complicating ovarian cystadenocarcinoma—a rare finding. Gastrointest Radiol 15:78–81, 1990.
78. Khilnani MT, Wolf BS: Late involvement of the alimentary tract by carcinoma of the kidney. Am J Dig Dis 5:529–540, 1960.
79. Bachman AL: Roentgen appearance of gastric invasion from carcinoma of the colon. Radiology 63:814–822, 1954.
80. Rubesin SE, Levine MS: Omental cakes: colonic involvement by omental metastases. Radiology 154:593–596, 1985.
81. Meyers MA: Distribution of intra-abdominal malignant seeding: dependency on dynamics of flow of ascitic fluid. AJR 119:198–206, 1973.
82. Meyers MA: The spread and localization of acute intraperitoneal effusions. Radiology 95:547–554, 1970.
83. Ginaldi S, Lindell MM, Zornoza J: The striped colon: a new radiographic observation in metastatic serosal implants. AJR 134:453–455, 1980.
84. Krestin GP, Beyer D, Lorenz R: Secondary involvement of the transverse colon by tumors of the pelvis: spread of malignancies along the greater omentum. Gastrointest Radiol 10:283–288, 1985.
85. Asch MJ, Wiedel PD, Habif DV: Gastrointestinal metastases from carcinoma of the breast: autopsy study and 18 cases requiring operative intervention. Arch Surg 96:840–843, 1968.
86. Smith HJ, Vlask MG: Metastasis to the colon from bronchogenic carcinoma. Gastrointest Radiol 2:393–396, 1978.
87. Rubesin SE, Levine MS, Laufer I, et al: Villous adenomas: the scientific and the practical. Radiology 167:869–870, 1988.
88. Muto T, Bussey HJR, Morson BC: The evolution of cancer of the colon and rectum. Cancer 36:2251–2270, 1975.
89. Wolf BS: Roentgen diagnosis of villous tumors of the colon. AJR 84:1093–1104, 1960.
90. Iida M, Iwashita A, Yao T: Villous tumor of the colon: correlation of histologic, macroscopic, and radiographic features. Radiology 167:673–677, 1988.
91. Thompson JJ, Enterline HT: The macroscopic appearance of colorectal polyps. Cancer 48:151–160, 1981.
92. Rubesin SE, Saul SH, Laufer I, et al: Carpet lesions of the colon. Radiographics 5:537–552, 1985.
93. Laufer I, Levine MS (eds): Double Contrast Gastrointestinal Radiology (2nd ed). Philadelphia: WB Saunders, 1992.

# Polyposis Syndromes

Roger K. Harned, M.D.
James L. Buck, M.D.

The polyposis syndromes are rare but fascinating conditions. A thorough knowledge of the clinical and radiographic presentations of these conditions and their complications is required to provide optimal care for these patients and their families.

## FAMILIAL ADENOMATOUS POLYPOSIS SYNDROME

Traditionally, this subject is divided into three broadly overlapping diseases: familial polyposis coli, Gardner's syndrome, and Turcot's syndrome. However, there is mounting evidence that these conditions are varying expressions of the same disease. As a result, the term *familial adenomatous polyposis syndrome* (FAPS) has increasingly been used to refer to the entire spectrum of diseases.

### Genetic Considerations

FAPS is a relatively rare condition, but it is the most common of the polyposis syndromes.[1] Males and females are equally affected. It is inherited as an autosomal dominant trait, although spontaneous mutations occasionally occur.[2] Penetrance is generally thought to be in the range of 80 to 100%, although in one series it was calculated to be less than 60%.[3] Much progress has been made in the past several years toward identification of the responsible gene. The gene has now been localized to a small region on the long arm of chromosome 5, a region where other genes responsible for colorectal carcinoma have been found.[4–6] In the near future, DNA testing may be able to identify those patients at risk for colorectal carcinoma attributable to both FAPS and other causes.

### Colonic Manifestations

As the name implies, FAPS is associated with the development of adenomas. In the colon, where the polyposis is most severe, the adenomas are usually tubular or tubulovillous types. Occasionally, villous adenomas are seen. In the study of colectomy specimens of St. Mark's Hospital in London, which has maintained a polyposis registry since 1925, the mean number of colonic polyps was 1000, with a range of 150 to 5000 polyps. A convention was thereby established by which the presence of 100 or more adenomas was required for the diagnosis of FAPS.[7] However, this criterion should not be applied too strictly. This is especially true in young patients studied by screening examinations. Also, members of certain FAPS families may exhibit only one or several adenomas and still carry the gene and develop colorectal carcinoma.[8]

The adenomas of FAPS are usually small (80% are less than 5 mm in diameter) and sessile.[7] The polyps involve all portions of the colon but may first appear distally. In the St. Mark's series, all patients were found to have rectal polyps, but subsequent series have shown that rectal sparing may occur.[7]

The most common symptoms encountered in FAPS are rectal bleeding and diarrhea, which occur in more than 75% of patients. Abdominal pain and mucous discharge are less frequently seen.[9] However, many FAPS patients are asymptomatic. Unfortunately, if the disease is allowed to take its natural course, colonic adenocarcinoma will develop in virtually every patient and at a much younger age than in the general population. Cancer is particularly likely to be present if gastrointestinal symptoms have already developed.[2] Thus, screening by proctosigmoidoscopy (and colonoscopy or barium enema if adenomas are found) of all family members at risk for the disease is required. Because the polyps do not usually develop until puberty, screening is delayed until 10 years of age.

Formerly, patients with FAPS were treated by colectomy and ileorectal anastomosis. Interestingly, after colectomy, adenomas in the remaining rectum regressed in up to one third of patients.[10] However, even with frequent proctoscopic examinations and fulguration of any persistent or recurrent adenomas, rectal carcinoma

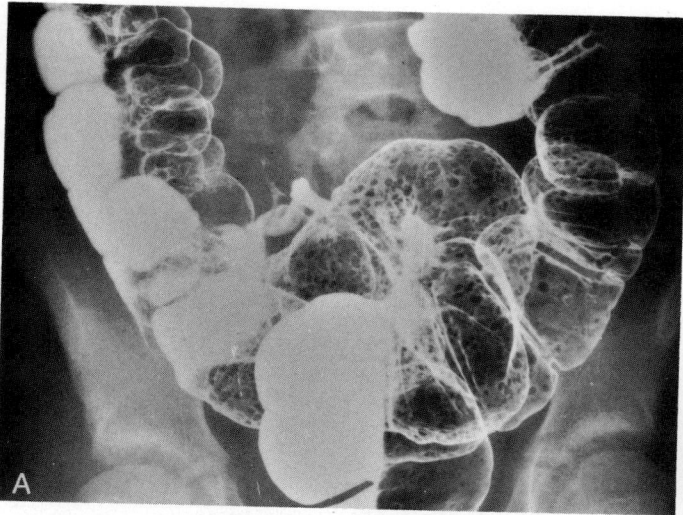
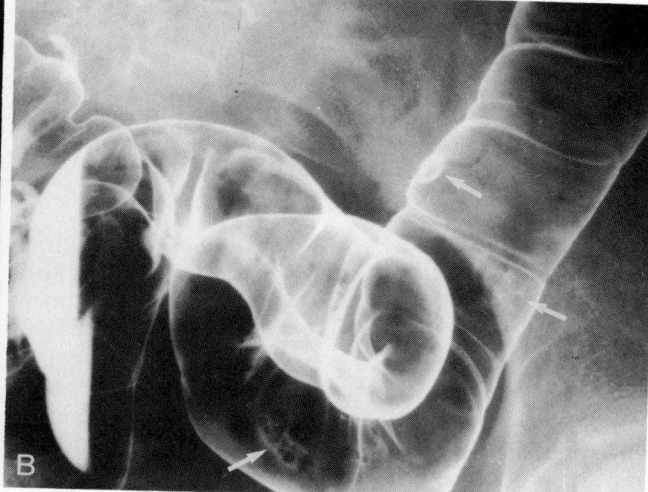

**Figure 66–1. Various appearances of colonic involvement by FAPS. A.** In a 10-year-old boy, a double contrast barium enema demonstrates innumerable small polyps in the colon, particularly carpeting the rectosigmoid region. **B.** In a 17-year-old girl, a double contrast barium enema shows scattered, small to moderate-sized polyps *(arrows)* in the sigmoid colon.

developed in 5 to 40% of cases.[11] A total proctocolectomy and cutaneous ileostomy was therefore recommended at many institutions. More recently, colectomy with mucosal proctectomy and ileoanal anastomosis has become the procedure of choice.[11] This procedure avoids the risk of development of rectal carcinoma without need for a cutaneous ileostomy.

The radiographic appearance of the colon in FAPS varies. Classically, innumerable small or moderate-sized filling defects carpet the entire colon (Fig. 66–1A). However, particularly in younger patients, the polyps may be more widely scattered (Fig. 66–1B). Correlation with colectomy specimens has shown that barium enemas significantly underestimate the number of polyps, especially in young patients whose polyps are usually less than 3 mm in diameter.[12] Unfortunately, despite more vigorous screening efforts in recent years, carcinomas are still found during the work-up of patients with FAPS. Carcinomas may present as a dominant polyp, a saddle lesion, or a typical infiltrating ("apple core") lesion (Fig. 66–2). As in the general population, carcinomas are more commonly found in the left side of the colon.

## Extracolonic Gastrointestinal Manifestations

Although the colon is the primary area of involvement by FAPS, all portions of the gastrointestinal tract lined by columnar epithelium are at risk for the development of adenomas. In certain portions of the bowel, other types of polyps also occur. Originally, these extracolonic gastrointestinal manifestations were considered to be part of the stigmata of Gardner's syndrome.[2] Currently, however, the presence of extracolonic gastrointestinal disease is generally thought to be independent of extraintestinal manifestations of the syndrome.[13–15]

## *Gastric Involvement*

Reported series have documented gastric involvement in more than 50% of patients with FAPS.[15–20] Two distinct types of polyps have been recognized: the fundic gland (hamartomatous) polyp and adenoma.

Fundic gland polyps were first recognized in the setting of FAPS[21] and are the most common gastric manifestation of FAPS in Western countries. However,

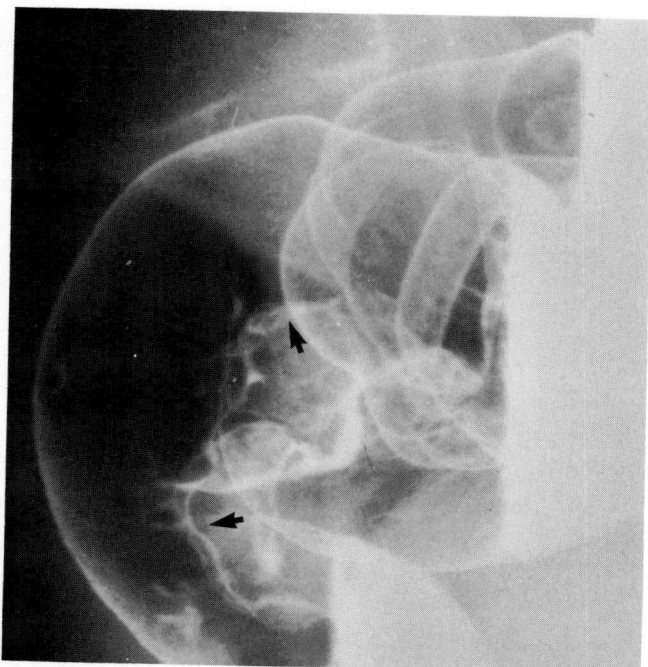

**Figure 66–2. Colon carcinoma in a 32-year-old woman with FAPS.** A saddle carcinoma is seen on the anterior wall of the rectum *(arrows)*. Scattered small polyps are also present.

fundic gland polyps have also been reported in non-FAPS patients.[22-25] Unlike hyperplastic polyps in the stomach, fundic gland polyps are generally not associated with chronic nonspecific gastritis or an increased risk of carcinoma.[26] In FAPS, both sexes are involved, and the polyps are frequently discovered in asymptomatic patients at an average age of 25 to 30 years.[14, 24, 27] The patients without FAPS are typically women; the average age is 50 years.[22]

Fundic gland polyps are almost invariably multiple and appear as small, sessile lesions measuring 1 to 5 mm in diameter in FAPS patients and up to 8 mm in diameter in non-FAPS patients.[2, 17, 19, 21] These polyps are confined to the fundic zone of the stomach (the region including the fundus and body of the stomach, where rugal folds are most prominent). With rare exceptions, the antrum is spared unless coexisting adenomas are present.[2, 14, 24, 27] The radiographic appearance of fundic gland polyposis is characteristic (Fig. 66–3), although endoscopic biopsies should still be obtained. On serial examinations, the polyps may progress, remain stable, or actually resolve.[28]

Tubular and villous adenomas are also seen in the stomach in patients with FAPS. In Japan, the incidence of gastric adenomas in FAPS ranges from 40 to 50%,[16, 21] whereas in Europe and North America, the incidence is less than 15%.[14, 17, 19, 20] The higher incidence of adenomas associated with FAPS in Japan may be related to the higher frequency of adenomas and adenocarcinomas in the general population of that country.[16, 29]

Gastric adenomas are typically sessile polyps ranging from 5 to 10 mm in diameter and are multiple in over half of the reported cases.[21, 27] The adenomas are usually

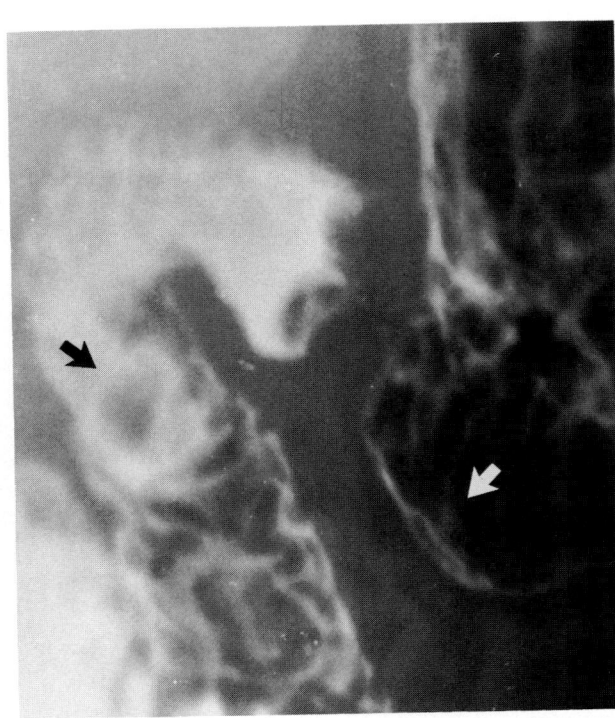

**Figure 66–4. Gastric and duodenal adenomas in a 53-year-old woman after a colectomy for FAPS.** A double contrast study demonstrates polyps in the antrum *(white arrow)* and descending duodenum *(black arrow).*

located in the distal stomach[27] (Fig. 66–4). Unlike fundic gland polyps of the stomach, these adenomas are premalignant lesions. However, the likelihood of malignant transformation is small. Even in Japan, the risk of malignant transformation of gastric adenomas is probably less than 10% in FAPS patients.[21] Regular screening of the stomach by endoscopy or radiology is required, but prophylactic gastrectomy is not recommended for these patients.

## Duodenal Involvement

The duodenum, particularly the periampullary region, is the second most common site of gastrointestinal disease in FAPS. Endoscopic examinations of asymptomatic patients in Japan have revealed tubular adenomas in more than 90% of cases.[15, 30] Subsequently, screening studies from Western countries have revealed adenomas in 47 to 72% of cases.[4, 14, 17-20] The adenomas range from microscopic sizes to 2 cm in diameter, with a majority being 5 mm in diameter or less. The polyps are usually found in the second portion of the duodenum clustered around the papilla (see Fig. 66–4). This differs from the typically bulbar distribution of adenomas in non-FAPS patients.[31, 32] Villous adenomas are commonly seen, and as in non-FAPS patients, they tend to be found in the periampullary region. Villous adenomas are typically large and are more likely to undergo malignant degeneration.

The actual risk of malignant transformation of small

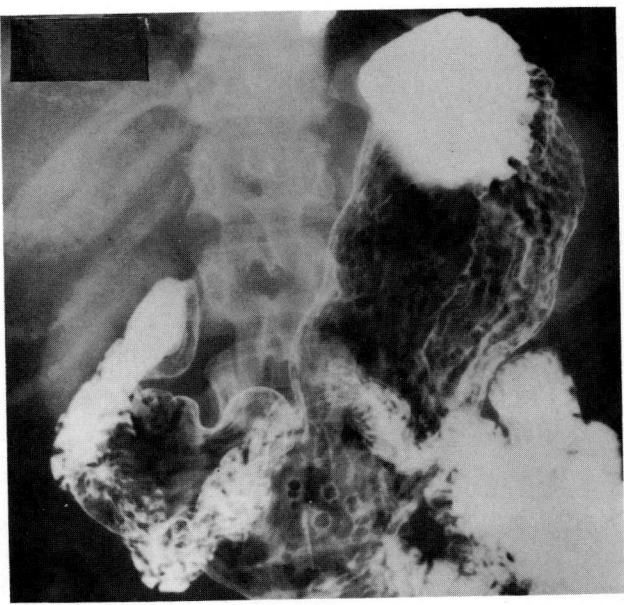

**Figure 66–3. Fundic gland polyposis of the stomach in a 25-year-old woman with FAPS.** A double contrast upper gastrointestinal study demonstrates multiple small filling defects in the fundus and body of the stomach. The antrum is not involved. The gallbladder is faintly opacified from a prior oral cholecystogram.

tubular adenomas has not been determined. None of the small adenomas detected in the above-mentioned series was complicated by carcinoma.[14, 15, 17–20] However, large, symptomatic lesions may contain carcinoma in situ,[33] and duodenal carcinomas are almost always found to coexist with adenomas.[14, 32, 34] This evidence suggests an adenoma-carcinoma sequence similar to that found in the colon.[32, 33] The duodenal-periampullary region is the most frequent site of adenocarcinoma outside the colon in patients with FAPS. The St. Mark's data indicate that 4% of patients will develop periampullary carcinoma less than 5 years after colectomy.[35] This poses difficult problems regarding the management of FAPS patients with significant duodenal disease.

The tiny tubular adenomas seen endoscopically in asymptomatic patients may or may not be detected radiographically,[19, 30] but larger lesions are likely to be detected on upper gastrointestinal series. In general, the polyps appear smooth, but larger lesions may have a villous appearance. Both adenomas and carcinomas typically arise from the medial wall of the duodenum.[32] The carcinomas appear as fungating masses that may extend into the distal common bile duct and produce irregular filling defects on cholangiography[34] (Fig. 66–5).

### Jejunal and Ileal Involvement

Adenomas in the jejunum and ileum have been identified in the majority of FAPS patients in Japan who have undergone intraoperative small bowel endoscopy.[36, 37] Small bowel endoscopy performed through a

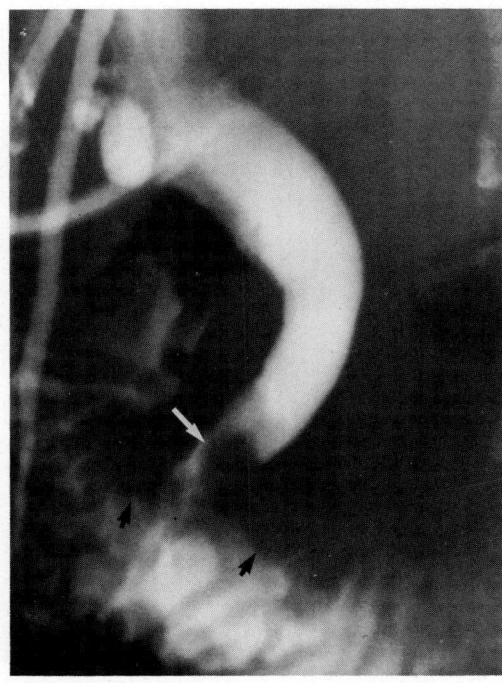

**Figure 66–5. Ampullary carcinoma in a 48-year-old woman with FAPS.** A T tube cholangiogram demonstrates a filling defect *(white arrow)* in the distal common bile duct associated with a mass on the medial wall of the adjacent duodenum *(black arrow).*

cutaneous ileostomy or ileoproctostomy has revealed adenomas in approximately 20% of FAPS patients in Western countries.[17, 20] As in the duodenum, these lesions are typically small and numerous. The significance of these adenomas is unclear. A few cases of adenocarcinoma of the jejunum or ileum have been reported, and in all cases, coexisting adenomas have been found.[38–40] However, the need for routine screening of the small bowel has not been established.

Ileal lymphoid hyperplasia occurs more frequently in patients with FAPS than in the general population. The gross and endoscopic appearance of these lesions is identical to that of adenomas. However, lymphoid hyperplasia has no apparent clinical significance in these patients.

### Biliary Involvement

In a series of 14 patients with FAPS studied by serial endoscopic retrograde cholangiopancreatography, 6 patients developed polyps in the distal common bile duct.[18] Cholangiocarcinoma and gallbladder carcinoma have occasionally been reported in FAPS.[41–44]

## Extraintestinal Manifestations

It was not until the 1950s that the extraintestinal manifestations of FAPS became well known. Gardner and Richards initially described a kindred of patients affected with adenomatous polyps of the colon, sebaceous cysts, and osteomas.[45] Later, fibrous tumors and dental abnormalities were added to the list of lesions included in Gardner's syndrome.[46] Numerous reports have subsequently confirmed the occurrence of these and other extraintestinal manifestations. However, these visible extraintestinal manifestations are uncommon, and even in "Gardner's syndrome" families, it is unusual to see all manifestations in the same patient.[47–50]

### Skin Lesions

Epidermoid cysts (also called sebaceous cysts or epidermal inclusion cysts) are the skin lesions most frequently encountered and the extraintestinal manifestation most likely to be seen on physical examination of patients with FAPS. Epidermoid cysts tend to be located on the face and scalp but may be found at any site. The age at onset varies, but in FAPS, they often appear in childhood before colonic polyps develop.[51] However, other than being an indicator of FAPS, the lesions have no clinical significance. They are completely benign and cause only cosmetic problems, if any. Lipomas and small fibrous tumors of the skin are also seen in FAPS patients.[52]

### Bone Lesions

Osteomas are a well-known manifestation of FAPS. Like epidermoid cysts, they are entirely benign and usually insignificant except for being a possible early

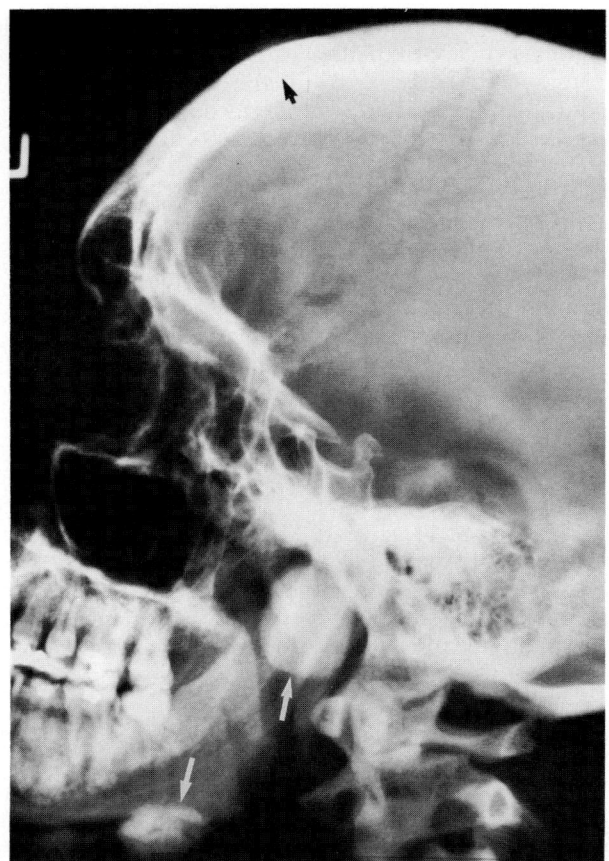

**Figure 66–6. Multiple osteomas in a 23-year-old man with FAPS.**
A lateral view of the face and skull demonstrates two dense bony lesions *(white arrows)* arising from the mandible. A subtle lesion *(black arrow)* is also seen in the frontal bone.

indicator of the disease. In FAPS patients, these dense cortical lesions are most commonly seen in the angle of the mandible, the sinuses, and the outer table of the skull[53] (Fig. 66–6). Other flat bones and long bones are also involved. In an often cited paper in 1975, Utsunomiya and Nakamura reported a high incidence of small densities, which they termed osteomas, in the mandible and maxilla. These lesions, which were typically located near the apices of the teeth, were detected by Panorex examinations in 93% of patients without other signs of Gardner's syndrome.[54] On the basis of these data, they and other authors concluded that most patients with familial polyposis coli actually had Gardner's syndrome.[54, 55] However, subsequent investigators have questioned the sensitivity and specificity of these findings.[56]

In one radiology series, localized or diffuse cortical thickening of the long bones was the most commonly identified bone abnormality in FAPS. Dental abnormalities, particularly impacted or supernumerary teeth, are also commonly found.[57, 58]

## Fibrous Lesions

Fibrous proliferation is a less common but more important feature of FAPS. An increased incidence of

postoperative peritoneal adhesions occurs in FAPS,[48] and retroperitoneal fibrosis has also been reported.[48, 59] More commonly, fibrous tumors, particularly desmoid tumors of the abdominal wall and mesenteric fibromatosis, occur (Fig. 66–7). In the setting of FAPS, these tumors are usually seen postoperatively. They most commonly occur in women of childbearing age, and they may grow rapidly or may first appear during pregnancy.[60] These tumors recur locally after resection, and invasion of bowel is common. Rarely, death may result from intestinal or vascular obstruction, but these tumors should not be considered fibrosarcomas because metastases do not occur.[61]

## Eye Lesions

Congenital pigmented lesions of the retina occur frequently in FAPS patients.[62–64] Although similar lesions are occasionally seen in the general population, the presence of large, multifocal, or bilateral pigmented lesions on funduscopic examination is a strong indicator of FAPS. These lesions may occur before the development of colonic polyposis and may serve as a marker of FAPS, but the absence of such lesions does not exclude this disease.[65, 66]

## Malignant Tumors of the Central Nervous System

The association of malignant tumors of the central nervous system and familial adenomatous polyposis was described by Crail in 1949,[67] but the condition is commonly referred to as Turcot's syndrome because of Turcot's report of two cases in 1959.[68] More than 60 cases have now been reported in the world's literature. The syndrome was initially thought to be inherited in

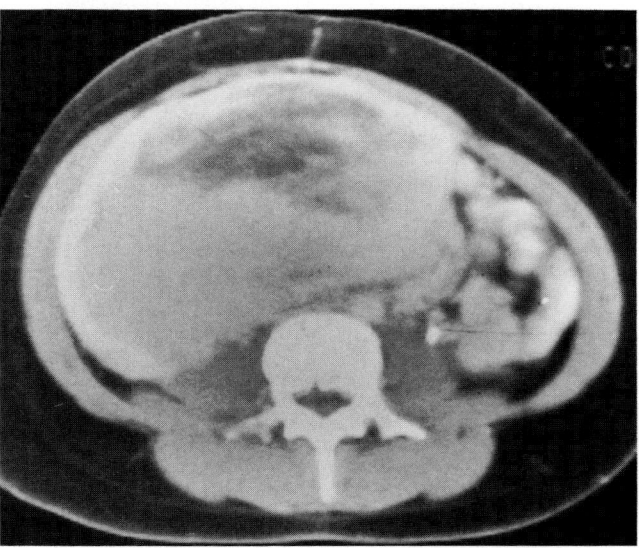

**Figure 66–7. Mesenteric fibromatosis in a 17-year-old girl with FAPS.** A computed tomographic scan (same patient as in Fig. 66–1B) reveals a large mass in the right side of the abdomen, displacing bowel. The ileum was found to be involved at surgery. The low-attenuation area within the mass is due to mucoid degeneration.

an autosomal recessive mode,[69] but subsequent reports have strongly suggested an autosomal dominant inheritance.[70, 71] The colonic adenomas may be identical to those found in other FAPS patients, but in some families, a smaller number of polyps (20 to 100) that are larger than usual (often greater than 3 cm in diameter) have been described.[69, 70] The smaller number of polyps may be due to the younger age of some patients at the time of presentation. Colon carcinoma develops at an even earlier age in these patients (usually the second or third decades) than in other FAPS patients.[72]

Glioblastoma multiforme and other gliomas of the brain were initially the most commonly reported central nervous system tumors. (The condition has been termed the glioma-polyposis syndrome.) Most of these tumors are supratentorial, but posterior fossa and even spinal cord gliomas have been reported.[73, 74] Medulloblastomas have been described more frequently in more recent reports.[70] The colonic disease generally presents first, but in approximately 25% of cases, the central nervous system lesions are detected as the initial manifestation of this syndrome.[75] Because children may die of these brain tumors before the development of colonic disease, the frequency of brain tumors in patients carrying the gene for FAPS is likely to be underestimated.

Although extracolonic gastrointestinal polyps are seen, the stigmata of Gardner's syndrome are usually not present in these patients. However, other extraintestinal manifestations, such as café au lait spots of the skin and focal nodular hyperplasia of the liver, are often identified.[76]

### Thyroid Carcinoma and Other Malignant Neoplasms

At least 35 cases of thyroid carcinoma have been reported in FAPS patients. (The prevalence of thyroid carcinoma in FAPS is calculated to be 160 times greater than that in the general population.[77]) Almost all of the thyroid carcinomas are papillary, and they are frequently multifocal. The patients are, with few exceptions, girls or young women, and the thyroid carcinoma is usually detected before the colonic disease becomes apparent. FAPS should be suspected in any young woman with papillary carcinoma of the thyroid.[78]

Many other endocrine tumors, including multiple endocrine neoplasia type 2, carcinoid tumors, and adrenocortical adenomas and carcinomas, have been reported in FAPS patients.[79–83] Hepatoblastoma has also been reported with increased frequency in patients with a family history of FAPS.[84, 85] It presumably represents another manifestation of the disease, although these children may die of the liver tumor before colonic polyposis develops. Other malignant neoplasms have also been reported; in some cases, these may simply represent a coincidental association. During the past century, however, many lesions that were originally thought to be coincidental have now been recognized as legitimate manifestations of FAPS. In the future, other manifestations of this generalized growth disorder may also be recognized.

## HAMARTOMATOUS POLYPOSIS SYNDROMES

The dominant gastrointestinal lesion in this group of syndromes is the hamartomatous polyp. Hamartomas of the Cronkhite-Canada, multiple hamartoma, and juvenile polyposis syndromes have similar histologic features. However, the Peutz-Jeghers hamartoma has a distinctive morphologic appearance. Mucocutaneous lesions and extraintestinal manifestations are common. Accurate diagnosis of these syndromes is important because of the frequent association with both gastrointestinal and nongastrointestinal malignant neoplasms.

### Peutz-Jeghers Syndrome

Peutz-Jeghers syndrome (PJS) is an inherited disease characterized by gastrointestinal hamartomatous polyps, mucocutaneous pigmentation, extra-alimentary tract neoplasms, and an increased prevalence of malignant neoplasms of the gastrointestinal tract. It has an autosomal dominant inheritance pattern, affecting both sexes equally. Approximately 40 to 50% of cases are sporadic. There is no racial predilection, and the average age at the time of diagnosis is 24 years. One third of patients are diagnosed before the age of 15 years.[86–88]

#### Pathology

The Peutz-Jeghers polyp is composed of an abnormal mixture of smooth muscle and mucosa and is considered to be a hamartoma. The smooth muscle component consists of muscularis mucosae arranged in arborizing, branching bands. The mucosal component is composed of the mucosa characteristic for the site of origin in the gastrointestinal tract.[89] At the base of the polyp, there are often islands of mucosa within bundles of muscle, simulating invasion. This pseudoinvasive appearance may be mistaken for carcinoma.[89, 90] Dysplasia occurs rarely in the PJS polyp, and even more rarely, carcinoma may develop.[89, 91, 92]

#### Clinical Features

**Pigmentation.** Mucocutaneous pigmentation is one of the most characteristic features of PJS. Small, brown, or bluish black macules most commonly occur on the lips and buccal mucosa and less commonly on the dorsal surfaces of the fingers, palms of the hands, and soles of the feet (Fig. 66–8). The pigmentation is rarely present at birth and usually appears after the first or second year of life. The skin and lip pigmentation tends to fade in adulthood, whereas the buccal macules remain unchanged.[86, 93, 94] Less than 5% of PJS patients have no characteristic pigmentation.[95]

**Intussusception.** The majority of PJS patients present with recurrent episodes of abdominal pain and intestinal obstruction caused by intussuscepting intestinal polyps.[94, 96, 97] The intussusceptions may be transient and reduce spontaneously (Fig. 66–9). However, obstruction commonly necessitates surgical intervention.

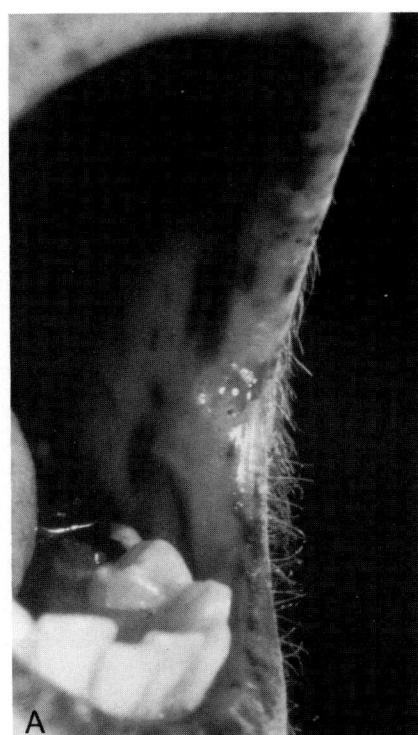

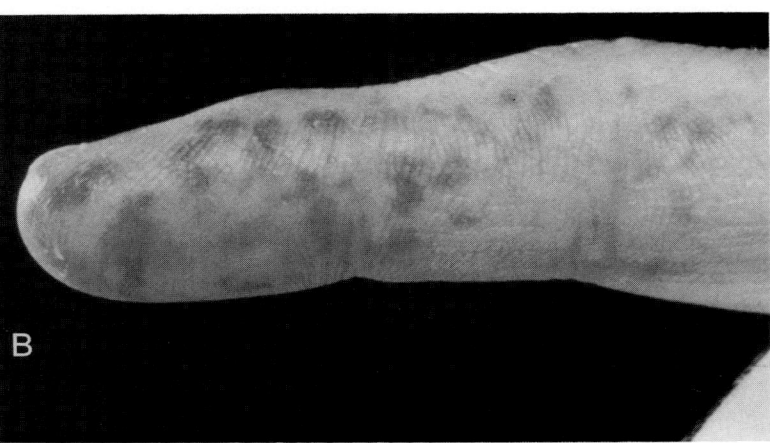

**Figure 66–8. Classic mucocutaneous pigmentation of PJS. A.** Bluish black macules are seen on the lips and buccal mucosa. **B.** Similar pigmentation is present on the palmar surface of the fingers.

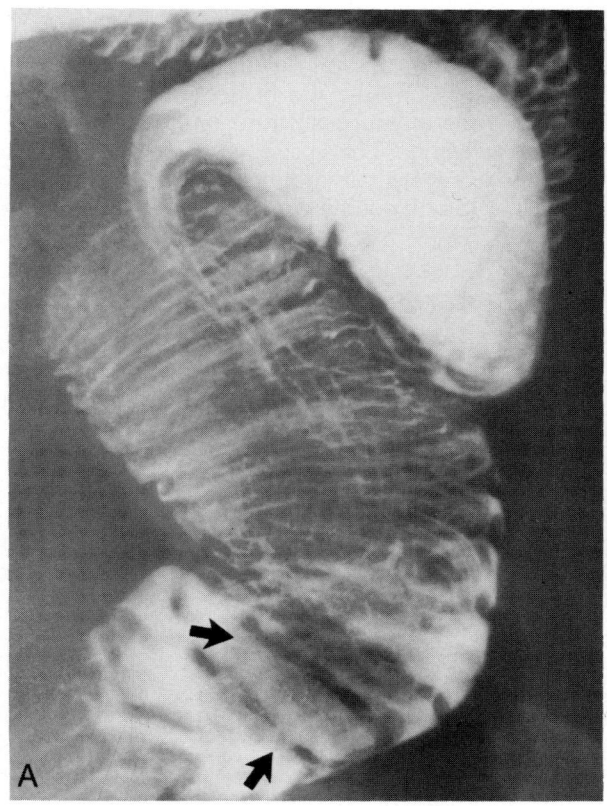

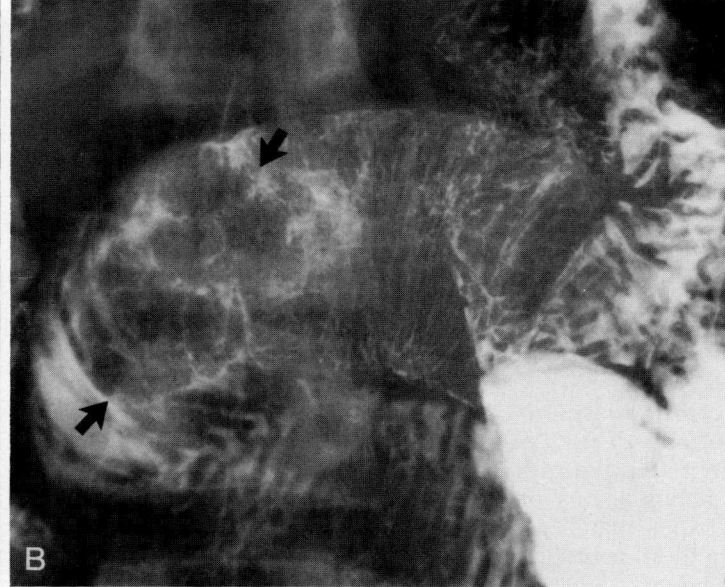

**Figure 66–9. Intussuscepting small bowel hamartomas** *(arrows)* **in a patient with PJS.** Spot films **(A** and **B)** from a small bowel series demonstrate transient intussusceptions that formed and reduced spontaneously.

**Gastrointestinal Bleeding.** Less frequently, patients may present with rectal bleeding, melena, or evidence of anemia.[94, 98] Massive gastrointestinal bleeding is rare.

**Gastrointestinal Carcinoma.** The reported prevalence of malignant neoplasms of the gastrointestinal tract in PJS ranges from 2 to 16%.[91, 92, 96, 99–102] Most carcinomas are located in the gastroduodenal area or colon[96, 103, 104] (Fig. 66–10). These adenocarcinomas in PJS could arise from coexisting adenomas or from foci of dysplasia within the hamartomas. Adenomas coexisting with hamartomatous polyps in PJS patients with intestinal carcinoma have been reported.[96, 103, 105] Several carcinomas arising in areas of dysplasia within hamartomatous polyps of PJS have also been documented.[91, 105–108]

**Extraintestinal Neoplasms.** In a study of 31 PJS patients, Giardiello and colleagues found that cancer developed in 15 (49%). However, only four cancers (13%) occurred in the gastrointestinal tract. Eleven (35%) were nongastrointestinal carcinomas, including four in the pancreas, two in the breast and lungs, one in the uterus and ovary, and one case of multiple myeloma.[99] Relative risk analysis indicated that the observed development of cancer in these patients was 18 times greater than that expected in the general population.[99] Linos and associates reported similar findings in an earlier investigation, which showed that 29% of PJS patients had nongastrointestinal cancers.[88] Spiegelman and colleagues found that malignant tumors developed in 22% of 72 patients. Thirteen percent had gastrointestinal tumors, and 10% had nongastrointestinal malignant neoplasms.[92]

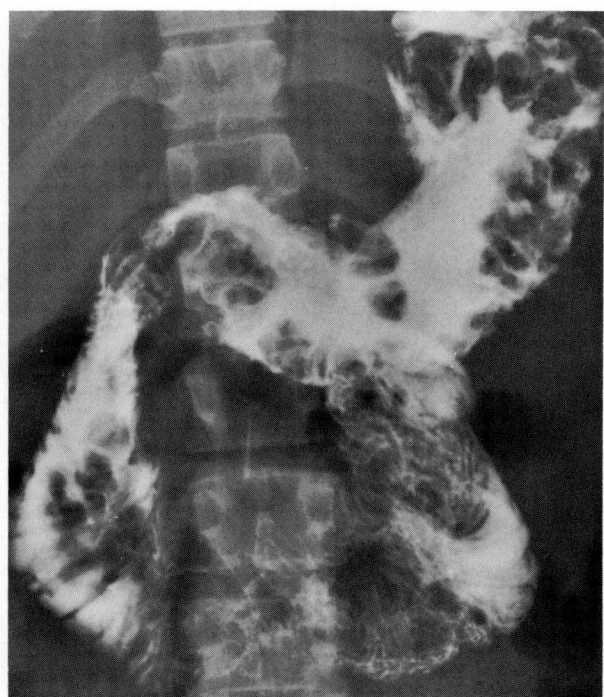

**Figure 66–10. Gastric adenocarcinoma in a 22-year-old woman with a 10-year history of PJS.** The upper gastrointestinal study shows a large, lobulated mass involving most of the stomach. Hamartomatous polyps are also present in the stomach and duodenum.

In addition to the four cases of pancreatic carcinoma in Giardiello's series, several other cases have been reported in the literature, which suggests that PJS patients are at increased risk for developing this neoplasm.[109–111]

A variety of unusual gynecologic neoplasms are common in PJS. An example, present in almost all female PJS patients, is the ovarian sex cord tumor with annular tubules.[112, 113] The tumor is benign, asymptomatic, and quite small and tends to be bilateral. It contains both granulosa and Sertoli cells. A second type of ovarian sex cord stroma tumor appears to be unique to PJS. It has morphologic features suggesting a Sertoli cell nature and produces isosexual precocity.[114, 115] Another unusual lesion seen in PJS is "adenoma malignum," a well-differentiated adenocarcinoma of the uterine cervix.[113, 116–119] This tumor has a relatively benign histologic appearance but aggressive biologic behavior. It may be associated with an increased incidence of benign and malignant mucinous ovarian tumors.[120] Feminizing Sertoli cell testicular tumors have been reported in males with PJS, an indication that gonadal neoplasms involving both sexes are an important part of the syndrome.[121–124]

There is also a tendency in female PJS patients to develop bilateral breast carcinoma.[124–126] At least six cases have been reported in the literature, but the exact prevalence is unknown.[125] These carcinomas may be stimulated by estrogen from the ovarian tumors common to PJS patients.

Other tumors that have occasionally been described in PJS include polyps of the gallbladder, nose, paranasal sinuses, ureter, and urinary bladder and one case of gallbladder carcinoma.[86, 93, 127–131] It is uncertain whether these lesions are true components of PJS or whether they represent random events.[132]

## Radiographic Findings

Hamartomatous polyps are distributed throughout the alimentary tract from the stomach to the rectum (Fig. 66–11). The small bowel is the most common site of involvement; approximately 95% of PJS patients have small intestinal polyps. The polyps vary in size, are usually multiple, and may be sessile or pedunculated. They can be isolated but usually occur in clusters. Carpeting of the bowel with polyps, as is commonly seen with other polyposis syndromes, does not generally occur.[87, 93, 94, 98, 103, 133] Double contrast examinations of the alimentary tract are the most accurate radiographic studies for diagnosing these polyps. Enteroclysis is recommended for the diagnosis of small bowel polyps or obstruction.

Cross-sectional imaging modalities may be helpful for the diagnosis of extraintestinal abnormalities. Ultrasound is particularly useful for detection of ovarian tumors in females and testicular tumors in males. Because of the increased risk of bilateral breast carcinoma, mammography should be employed at an earlier age than for the general population.

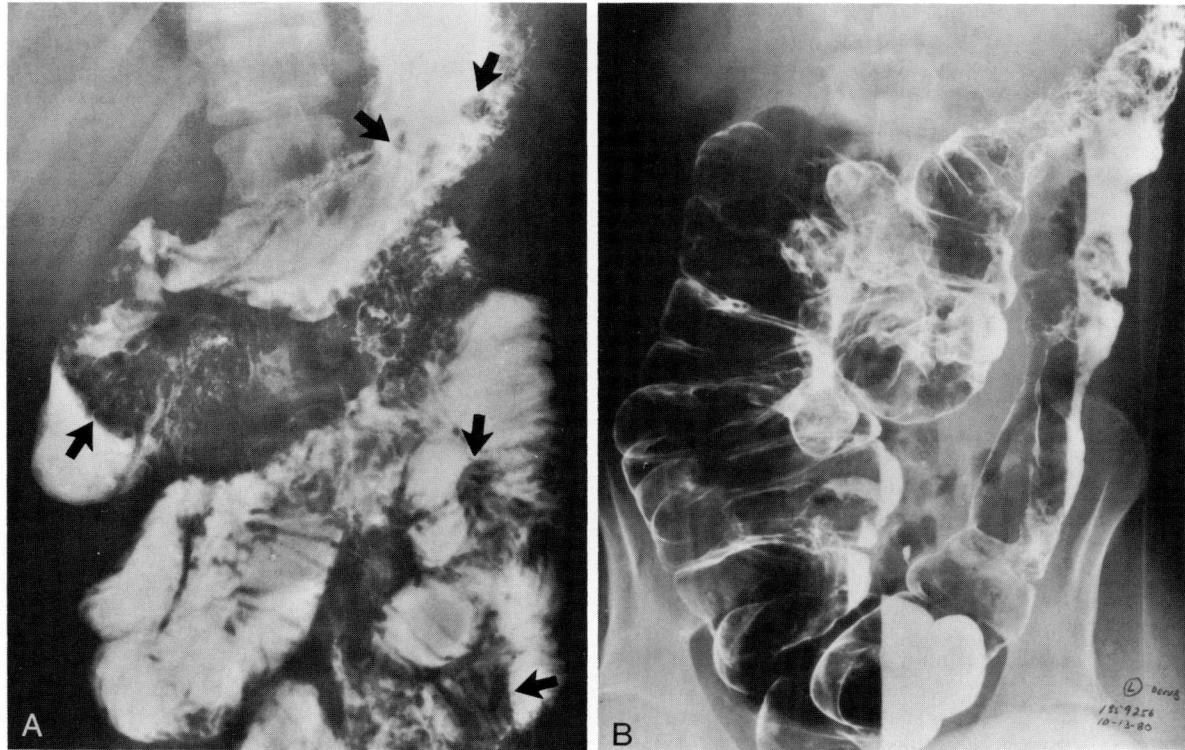

**Figure 66–11. Fourteen-year-old boy with multiple hamartomas throughout the gastrointestinal tract attributable to PJS. A.** An upper gastrointestinal study shows hamartomatous polyps *(arrows)* in the stomach, duodenum, and jejunum. **B.** A double contrast barium enema shows large hamartomas in all segments of the colon.

## Treatment

Because many segments of the gastrointestinal tract are commonly involved, it is usually impossible to remove all polyp-bearing tissue completely. Endoscopic biopsy of polyps will identify dysplastic changes or carcinoma. Endoscopic polypectomy is the recommended procedure for polyps that can be safely resected, particularly those in the colon and duodenum. Surgery is usually required for removal of large polyps causing symptoms such as obstruction or bleeding. When surgery is necessary, intraoperative endoscopy with polypectomy may prevent the need for a more excessive bowel resection.[91]

## Differential Diagnosis

Accurate histologic evaluation of a representative polyp is essential to help differentiate PJS from other gastrointestinal polyposis syndromes. Patients with FAPS do not have the characteristic mucocutaneous pigmentation of PJS, and the polyps are adenomas in contrast to the hamartomas of PJS. The other hamartomatous polyp syndromes (juvenile polyposis, Cronkhite-Canada syndrome, and multiple hamartoma syndrome) can usually be differentiated by the age of the patient, the type and distribution of mucocutaneous lesions, and the histologic features of the hamartomas.

## Multiple Hamartoma Syndrome (Cowden's Disease)

The multiple hamartoma syndrome (MHS) is an uncommon disease characterized by multiple hamartomas and neoplasms of ectodermal, mesodermal, and endodermal origin.[134] In 1963, Lloyd and Dennis reported a case of unusual complex lesions and were the first to recognize that these lesions represented a new syndrome, which they named Cowden's disease after the propositus, Rachel Cowden.[135, 136] In 1972, Weary and associates suggested the name *multiple hamartoma syndrome* as a more accurate designation that reflected the salient features of the disease.[137] There have been approximately 103 cases reported in the English literature.[134–179] The major clinical features are mucocutaneous lesions associated with a variety of thyroid gland abnormalities, breast carcinoma, and hamartomatous polyposis of the gastrointestinal tract. MHS is inherited as an autosomal dominant genetic trait with high penetrance in both sexes.[134] It occurs chiefly in white persons and is uncommon in black and Asian individuals.[167] The mean age at the time of diagnosis is 41 years, with a range of 2 to 78 years.[134, 136]

### Mucocutaneous Lesions

Mucocutaneous lesions occur in all patients and are the hallmark of the disease. They are often the earliest findings of the syndrome, becoming evident at 20 to 30 years of age.[136, 137] Facial papules, oral mucosal papillomatoses, and acral keratoses are the most characteristic lesions and serve as external markers for the syndrome.[134, 136, 137, 167, 175]

Small facial papules, the most distinctive lesions, occur in 83 to 95% of cases. They have a centrofacial and perioral distribution and are considered to be hamartomas of the outer root sheath of the hair follicle.[134, 136, 143, 167, 180]

Oral mucosal lesions also are sensitive indicators of MHS; these consist of smooth papules that usually are benign fibromas located on the gingival, labial, and palatal surfaces.[134, 136, 170, 180, 181] The tongue may have a pebbly or fissured appearance.[137, 167, 170] Other lesions involving the oral cavity include macroglossia, high arched palate, and hypoplasia of the soft palate and uvula.[167, 170]

Less characteristic lesions of MHS are keratoses located on the dorsum of the hands and feet or proximally on the extremities.[136, 180] Other rare dermatologic lesions include squamous cell carcinomas and angiomas.[134, 142, 174, 180, 182, 183]

## Thyroid Abnormalities

The most frequent extracutaneous abnormality in MHS is some form of thyroid disease.[134, 157] The most common lesions are goiters and adenomas.[134, 167] Thyroiditis, thyroglossal duct cysts, and hyper- or hypothyroidism also occur less frequently. Follicular adenocarcinoma of the thyroid gland occurs in 3 to 12% of patients—all cases have been in women.[134, 136, 137]

## Breast Abnormalities

Seventy percent of women with MHS have breast lesions. Fibrocystic disease is the most common, occurring in at least 50% of cases. Anatomic abnormalities of the nipple and areola and virginal hypertrophy of the breast occur with less frequency.[134, 145, 175, 183] Carcinoma of the breast has a prevalence of 30%.[134, 136, 167] The approximate age at onset is 30 to 40 years. The malignant neoplasm is most often ductal carcinoma and tends to be bilateral. Metastases to regional lymph nodes is common at the time of diagnosis.[134] Because carcinoma of the female breast is the most significant lesion in MHS, early detection is essential. Therefore, mammography should be implemented at an earlier age in women with MHS than in the general population. Benign gynecomastia has been recognized in men, but cancer of the male breast has not been reported.[134, 175, 183]

## Genitourinary Abnormalities

A small number of significant genitourinary abnormalities have been reported in MHS, including uterine carcinoma,[144, 161, 167] cervical carcinoma,[149, 167] and transitional cell carcinoma of the bladder.[144, 167]

## Miscellaneous Abnormalities

Many MHS patients have structural facial or skeletal abnormalities. Craniomegaly with a high, broad forehead is one of the most characteristic features.[134] Kyphoscoliosis, pectus excavatum, and structural abnormalities of the hands and feet have all been reported. Eye and nervous system abnormalities described in MHS include angioid streaks of the optic fundus, neuromas of cutaneous nerves, neurofibromas, and meningiomas.[134, 137, 149, 150, 167, 183] A wide range of other organ abnormalities have been reported, but their relationship to this syndrome remains to be determined.

## Gastrointestinal Abnormalities

Multiple nonadenomatous polyps of the gastrointestinal tract are an important feature of MHS and occur in at least 35% of patients.[134, 136, 137, 183] The reported histopathologic appearance of these polyps is confusing. They have variously been called lymphoid, hyperplastic, inflammatory, juvenile, and lipomatous polyps.[137, 140, 154, 165, 175, 178, 184] However, the majority of these polyps are now recognized as hamartomas with little or no malignant potential.[134, 136, 165, 185] The MHS hamartoma differs from the hamartoma of PJS. It is smaller and sessile and is characterized by a less exophytic and arborizing proliferation of the muscularis mucosae.[165, 185] Glycogenic acanthosis of the esophagus has also been reported in two cases.[154, 184]

The gastrointestinal polyps usually have a segmental distribution and are most commonly located in the rectosigmoid colon, followed in decreasing frequency by the stomach, duodenum, small bowel, and esophagus.[134, 136, 165, 175] Diffuse involvement of the gastrointestinal tract occurs less frequently.[175, 178] Characteristically, the polyps are multiple, small, and sessile.[165, 175, 178] Meticulous double contrast radiographic technique is mandatory for detecting these small lesions in the esophagus, stomach, and colon (Fig. 66–12). However, endoscopy may be required for diagnosis of tiny polyps less than 5 mm in diameter. Enteroclysis is the procedure of choice for diagnosing polyps in the jejunum and ileum.

In the majority of patients, gastrointestinal polyps cause no symptoms and are found incidentally or during screening for the syndrome. Three cases of colon carcinoma have been described,[140, 144, 172] but an actual association between colon carcinoma and the syndrome is doubtful and probably fortuitous.[186] Malignant neoplasms of the upper gastrointestinal tract and small bowel have not been reported. Rectosigmoid polyps are clinically important because they can be readily detected; biopsy, therefore, helps identify MHS, so that surveillance for thyroid and breast carcinoma can be initiated. Radiologists should consider MHS in the differential diagnosis for any patient with gastrointestinal polyps, particularly if they are found to be hamartomas. Further examination of such patients for the characteristic mucocutaneous lesions will aid in confirming the diagnosis.[178]

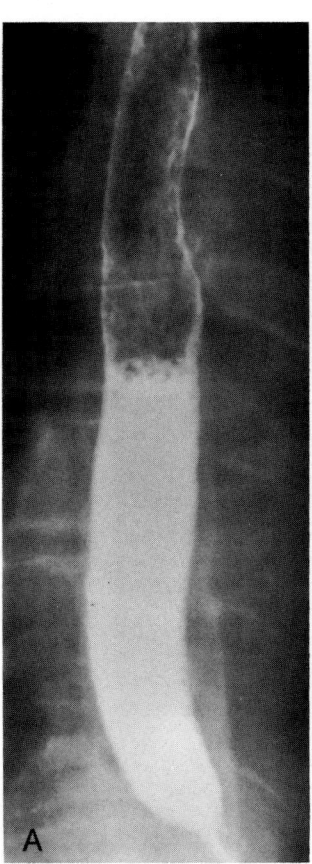
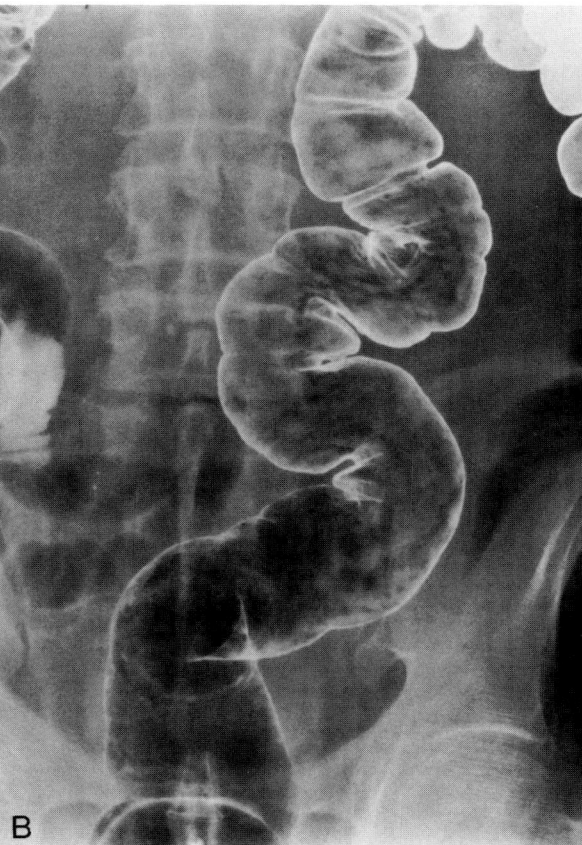

Figure 66–12. **Multiple hamartoma syndrome involving the esophagus and colon in a 53-year-old man.** Tiny, sessile hamartomatous polyps are present in the esophagus **(A)** and rectosigmoid colon **(B)**.

## Cronkhite-Canada Syndrome

A generalized polyposis syndrome associated with characteristic ectodermal changes was first described in a report of two cases by Cronkhite and Canada in 1955.[187] Approximately 100 cases have been reported since that time.[188] Unlike other polyposis syndromes, Cronkhite-Canada syndrome occurs sporadically, and affected patients are usually older adults with an average age of nearly 60 years.[189] (A condition termed *Cronkhite-Canada syndrome of infancy* is usually considered to be a form of juvenile polyposis.[190]) The polyps are found in the stomach, small bowel, and colon in almost all patients. No convincing case of esophageal involvement has been reported.[189] On histologic examination, these hamartomatous polyps closely resemble juvenile polyps, and it is difficult or impossible for pathologists to differentiate them on the basis of histologic criteria.[191] Cronkhite-Canada polyps are usually small (0.5 to 1.5 cm in diameter) and are typically sessile in configuration. Pedunculation is rare.[192]

### Clinical Features

Patients with Cronkhite-Canada syndrome typically present with abdominal pain, anorexia, weight loss, and diarrhea. The diarrhea is complicated by fluid, mineral, blood, and protein loss; electrolyte abnormalities, anemia, and hypoproteinemia ensue. Typically, these gastrointestinal symptoms are followed by the development of abnormalities of the skin, hair, and nails. Multiple brown macules or confluent areas of hyperpigmentation are seen on the skin, particularly involving the hands and feet. Occasionally, vitiligo is also demonstrated. Hair loss involving the scalp or all body hair occurs abruptly. Various dystrophic changes in the nails, sometimes leading to complete nail loss, are also demonstrated.[189] In approximately 10% of cases, the ectodermal changes precede the onset of gastrointestinal disease.[189]

The course of the disease is variable. An analysis of cases reported before 1982 reveals that 20 of 55 patients with Cronkhite-Canada syndrome died of the malnutrition resulting from their disease. Unfortunately, because the disease diffusely involves the gastrointestinal tract, partial resection (e.g., colectomy) is usually ineffective. These debilitated patients also tend to be poor surgical candidates. The condition is therefore managed with vigorous supportive therapy. Some patients have responded to administration of corticosteroids and anabolic steroids, but this is not recommended as initial therapy. Antibiotics are required when patients develop bacterial overgrowth in the bowel or other infectious complications. Clinical remissions, including sustained remissions, occur with or without steroid therapy. It should be noted that the ectodermal changes and even the polyps themselves may completely regress when clinical remission occurs.[193–197]

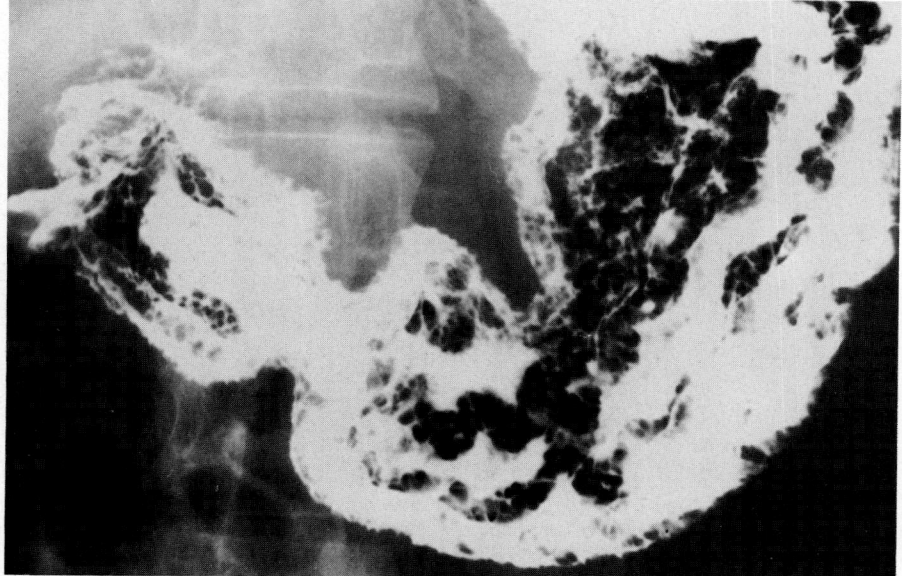

**Figure 66–13. Gastric involvement by Cronkhite-Canada syndrome.** Innumerable small polyps carpet the mucosal surface of the stomach. Thickened rugal folds are also present.

## Radiographic Findings

The disease is best demonstrated radiographically with use of double contrast techniques.[188, 197] In the stomach, innumerable small to moderate-sized polyps carpet the mucosal surface, usually in its entirety. The polyps tend

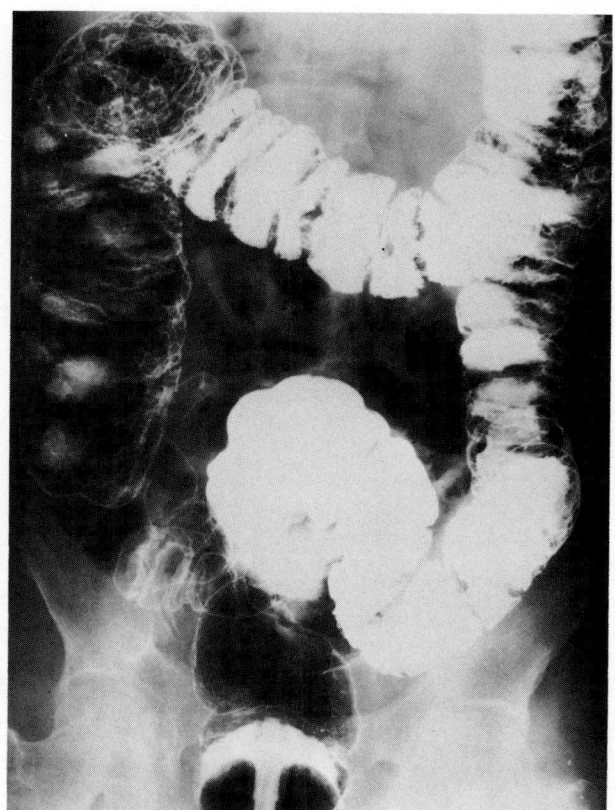

**Figure 66–14. Cronkhite-Canada syndrome in a 53-year-old man.** A double contrast barium enema demonstrates tiny polyps throughout the colon.

to be superimposed on a pattern of thickened rugal folds reminiscent of Ménétrier's disease, except that the thickened folds often involve the antrum (Fig. 66–13). This appearance is characteristic of but not specific for Cronkhite-Canada syndrome. It may also occur in patients with generalized juvenile polyposis and Cowden's disease. The small bowel, particularly the duodenum and terminal ileum, may contain multiple small polyps. The colon (including the rectum) is usually diffusely involved but not to the extent seen in the stomach (Fig. 66–14). Carpeting of the mucosa by polyps is less often seen in the colon.

Despite the fact that the polyps are non-neoplastic, approximately 15% of reported patients have developed malignant neoplasms, including both gastric and colonic adenocarcinoma.[189, 198, 199] However, age- and sex-matched control studies are unavailable, so the relative risk for malignancy in these patients cannot be determined.

## Juvenile Polyposis

Historically, there has been controversy regarding juvenile polyps and their associated syndromes. Recent information has contributed to a better understanding of this complex subject. Jass and colleagues have suggested a classification of the juvenile polyposis syndromes based on genetics, histology, and natural history.[200] They group these syndromes into two main categories: 1) isolated juvenile polyps of childhood and 2) juvenile polyposis of the colon or the entire gastrointestinal tract. The latter category has a subgroup, juvenile polyposis of infancy. The following discussion, with modifications, is based on this classification.

### Pathology

The isolated juvenile polyp of childhood is considered to be a hamartoma with a low risk of malignant

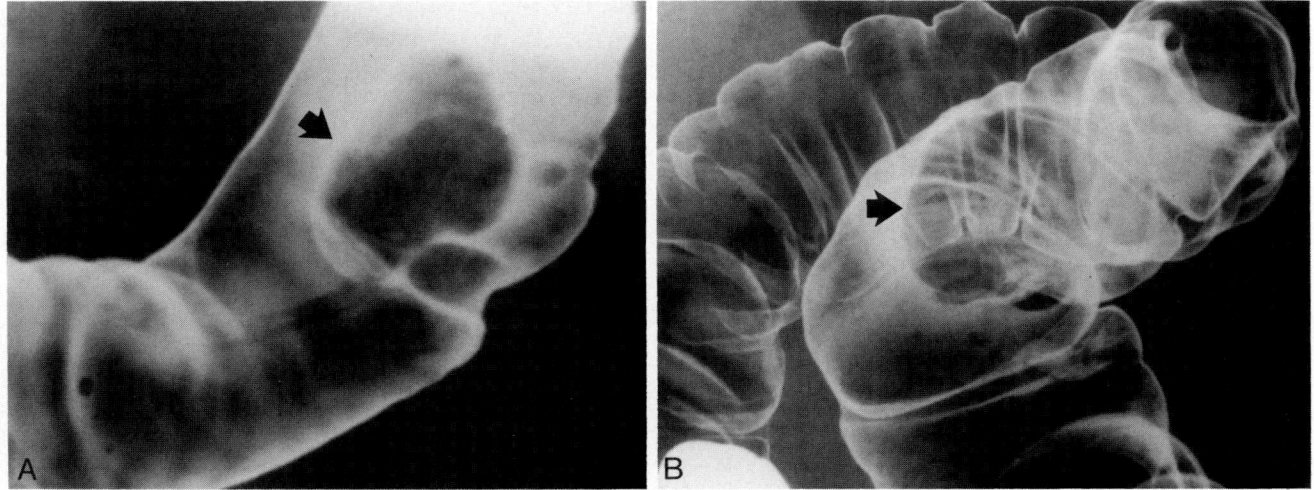

**Figure 66–15. Isolated juvenile polyps of childhood. A.** In a 4-year-old boy with rectal bleeding, a double contrast barium enema shows a large, pedunculated juvenile polyp *(arrow)* in the sigmoid colon. **B.** In a 10-year-old girl with rectal bleeding, a large, sessile, juvenile polyp *(arrow)* is seen in the proximal descending colon.

change.[200, 201] The lesions of juvenile polyposis are also considered to be hamartomas but are often characterized by histologic features that differ from isolated juvenile polyps. One such feature is the presence of foci of dysplasia.[201] These foci may be diffuse enough to justify the diagnosis of adenomas, because carcinoma can develop in such lesions.[200, 202–207]

## Isolated Juvenile Polyps of Childhood

The isolated juvenile polyp is the most common tumor of the colon in childhood; it occurs in approximately 1% of children between the ages of 4 and 14 years.[200, 205, 208, 209] They most often present with painless rectal bleeding and occasionally with a prolapsed rectal polyp.[210] The traditional concepts that isolated juvenile polyps are solitary and limited to the rectosigmoid colon have changed. On the basis of extensive colonoscopic studies, Mestre found that more than 50% of patients with juvenile polyps had more than one polyp and that 25% had four or more polyps. Furthermore, 60% of the polyps were located proximal to the rectum and sigmoid colon.[205, 211] Thus, in the present context, isolated juvenile polyps refer to the presence of one or more polyps, probably not more than five, evenly distributed throughout the rectum and colon.[200] The polyps are sessile or pedunculated, usually reddish, and often superficially ulcerated; they vary from 2 mm to more than 5 cm in diameter[205, 210] (Fig. 66–15). Most patients have no family history of polyposis, so that the lesions presumably result from environmental factors or genetic mutations.[212]

As previously indicated, the risk of malignant change in isolated juvenile polyps is low.[200] However, adenomas may coexist simultaneously with juvenile polyps, and there is a 3 to 5% chance that a particular polyp is an adenoma rather than a juvenile polyp.[203, 205, 210] Management strategies for these patients have changed, therefore. Colonoscopy or double contrast barium enemas should be performed for any child suspected of having a polyp. If a polyp is found, some authors advocate immediate removal by colonoscopy.[205] However, others favor observing otherwise healthy children with a single

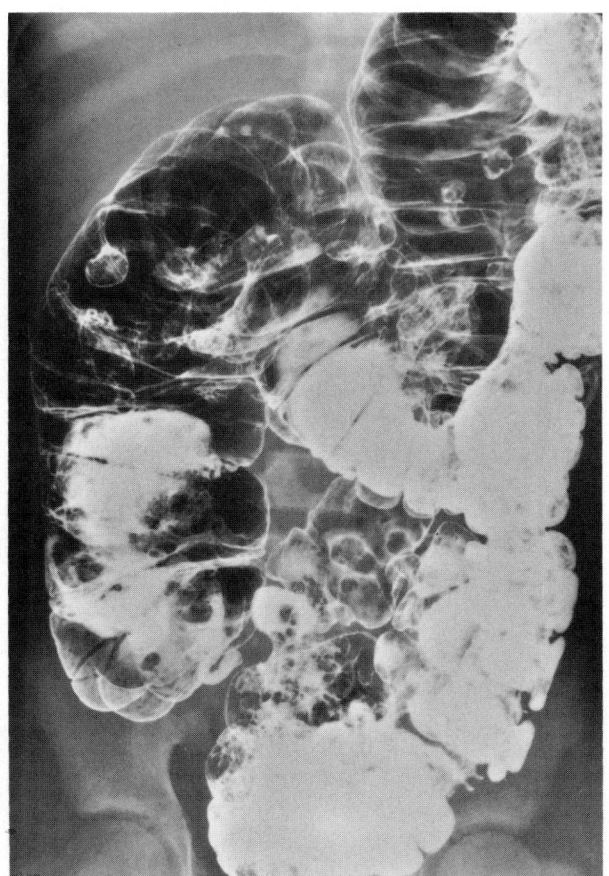

**Figure 66–16. Juvenile polyposis of the colon.** In a 15-year-old boy with rectal bleeding since 3 years of age, a double contrast barium enema shows multiple juvenile polyps throughout the colon.

polyp for up to 1 year, because many juvenile polyps characteristically undergo spontaneous autoamputation.[203] If at the end of 1 year the polyp remains, it should be removed. When multiple polyps are detected in the colon, however, they should be removed at the time of diagnosis.[203]

## Juvenile Polyposis of the Colon or Entire Gastrointestinal Tract

According to Jass and colleagues, the criteria for establishing the diagnosis of juvenile polyposis include 1) six or more juvenile polyps in the colon or rectum (Fig. 66–16), 2) juvenile polyps throughout the gastrointestinal tract (Fig. 66–17), and/or 3) any number of juvenile polyps in patients who have a family history of juvenile polyposis.[200] Juvenile polyposis is not as common as isolated juvenile polyps of childhood, but it is more common than juvenile polyposis of infancy. The age at onset is variable, but most cases present in the second decade.[200] Approximately 25% of cases are transmitted genetically as an autosomal dominant trait.[200, 204, 212–214] The nonfamilial cases may result from a new mutation, incomplete penetrance of the gene, or environmental factors.[204] The nonfamilial cases have a 25% incidence of associated congenital anomalies, including hydrocephalus and pulmonary arteriovenous malformations.[200, 204, 212, 215–217]

There is an increased risk for development of malignant neoplasms of the gastrointestinal tract in patients with juvenile polyposis and in their families. This risk usually applies only to patients with juvenile polyposis and not to patients with isolated juvenile polyps of childhood.[200] There are at least 26 reported cases of colorectal cancer occurring in patients with histologically confirmed juvenile polyposis.[200, 202, 207, 213, 218–221] The average age at which cancer developed was 32 years.[200, 207] Precancerous dysplasia within juvenile polyps in patients with juvenile polyposis has been well documented and provides strong evidence that carcinoma can arise in such polyps.[200–203, 205–207, 219, 221–227] Most malignant neoplasms of the colon occurring in juvenile polyposis have been poorly differentiated mucinous and signet ring carcinomas with a poor clinical prognosis.[200, 207, 219, 221] Carcinoma of the stomach, duodenum, and pancreas has also been reported in patients with juvenile polyposis of the entire gastrointestinal tract.[218, 228, 229] It is unclear whether the risk of colonic or other gastrointestinal malignant neoplasms is greater in familial cases of juvenile polyposis than in sporadic cases.[204, 207] Evidence now indicates that family members of patients with juvenile polyposis may also be at increased risk for developing malignant neoplasms of the colon and gastrointestinal tract.[204, 212, 218, 221]

Patients first diagnosed with juvenile polyposis of the colon should be further evaluated with double contrast radiographic studies or endoscopy for determining the presence of polyps elsewhere in the gastrointestinal

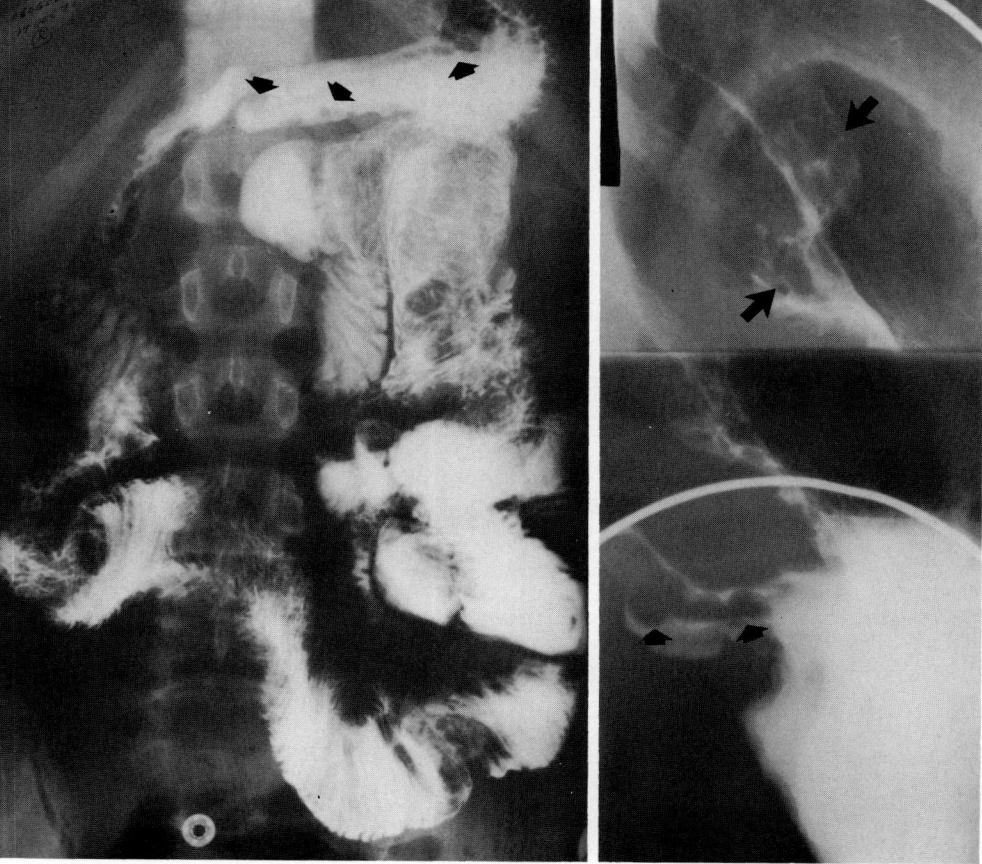

**Figure 66–17. Juvenile polyposis of the gastrointestinal tract in a 21-year-old man with diarrhea and rectal bleeding for 5 years. A.** An upper gastrointestinal study shows juvenile polyps in the stomach *(arrows)* and small bowel. **B.** Spot films of the stomach show large juvenile polyps in the fundus *(large arrows)* and smaller polyps in the antrum *(small arrows)*. Multiple juvenile polyps were also present in the colon.

A                                                                                                    B

tract. Because of the familial nature of the disease, management should be directed not only to the patient but also to the patient's family.[200]

## Juvenile Polyposis of Infancy

In 1974, Sachatello and associates described a rare, severe form of juvenile polyposis of the gastrointestinal tract in seven infants.[230] At least 14 cases are now documented in the literature.[215, 230–240] Most patients present with a severe, devastating diarrhea within the first 2 years of life.[239] The diarrhea may be either mucoid or bloody and leads to anemia, hypoproteinemia, and general failure to thrive. There is an increased susceptibility to bronchopulmonary infections. Recurrent episodes of rectal prolapse and small bowel intussusception are common.[230, 235, 237, 239, 240] Congenital anomalies such as clubbing of the fingers, brachydactyly, polydactyly, macrocephaly, and arachnoid cysts have been reported in a small number of cases, but the exact prevalence of these anomalies is unknown.[190, 233, 238] Ectodermal changes resembling Cronkhite-Canada syndrome have also been reported in a few cases.[190, 233, 238] In the majority of patients with juvenile polyposis of infancy, there is no family history.

The juvenile polyps are unevenly distributed throughout the gastrointestinal tract, with the small bowel and colon most severely involved.[230, 240] Polyps in the esophagus have not been described. The polyps vary from 2 to 3 mm in diameter, and the larger polyps are usually pedunculated.

The combination of repeated episodes of gastrointestinal bleeding, diarrhea, malnutrition, and intestinal obstruction results in death for the majority of patients before the age of 2 years.[235, 236, 239] Only four patients reported in the literature have survived beyond this age.[235, 236, 239]

## References

1. Gebert HF, Jagelman DG, McGannon E: Familial polyposis coli. Am Fam Physician 33:127–135, 1986.
2. Bussey JHR, Veale AMO, Morson BC: Genetics of gastrointestinal polyposis. Gastroenterology 74:1325–1330, 1978.
3. Pierce ER: Some genetic aspects of familial multiple polyposis of the colon in a kindred of 1,422 members. Dis Colon Rectum 11:321–327, 1968.
4. Leppert M, Dobbs M, Scambler P, et al: The gene for familial polyposis coli maps to the long arm of chromosome 5. Science 238:1411–1413, 1987.
5. Nakamura Y, Lathrop M, Lepert M, et al: Localization of the genetic defect in familial adenomatous polyposis within a small region of chromosome 5. Am J Hum Genet 43:638–644, 1988.
6. Leppert M, Burt R, Hughes JP, et al: Genetic analysis of an inherited predisposition to colon cancer in a family with a variable number of adenomatous polyps. N Engl J Med 322:904–908, 1990.
7. Bussey HJR: Familial Polyposis Coli. Baltimore: The Johns Hopkins University Press, 1975.
8. Lynch HT, Lynch PM, Follet K, et al: Familial polyposis coli: heterogenous polyp expression in 2 kindreds. J Med Genet 16:1–7, 1979.
9. Watne AL: The syndromes of intestinal polyposis. Curr Probl Surg 24:269–340, 1987.
10. Sarre RG, Jagelman DG, McGannon E, et al: Colectomy with ileorectal anastomosis for familial adenomatous polyposis: the risk of rectal cancer. Surgery 101:20–26, 1987.
11. Welling DR, Beart RW: Surgical alternatives in the treatment of polyposis coli. Semin Surg Oncol 3:99–104, 1987.
12. Bartram CI, Thornton A: Colonic polyp patterns in familial polyposis. AJR 142:305–308, 1984.
13. Hoffman DC, Goligher JC: Polyposis of the stomach and small intestine in association with familial polyposis coli. Br J Surg 58:126–128, 1971.
14. Bulow S, Lauritsen KB, Johansen A, et al: Gastroduodenal polyps in familial polyposis coli. Dis Colon Rectum 28:90–93, 1985.
15. Ushio K, Sasagawa M, Doi H, et al: Lesions associated with familial polyposis coli: studies of lesions of the stomach, duodenum, bones, and teeth. Gastrointest Radiol 1:67–80, 1976.
16. Utsunomiya J, Maki T, Iwama T, et al: Gastric lesion of familial polyposis coli. Cancer 34:745–754, 1974.
17. Burt RW, Berenson MM, Lee RG, et al: Upper gastrointestinal polyps in Gardner's syndrome. Gastroenterology 86:295–301, 1984.
18. Shemesh E, Bat L: A prospective evaluation of the upper gastrointestinal tract and periampullary region in patients with Gardner syndrome. Am J Gastroenterol 80:825–827, 1985.
19. Ranzi T, Castagnone D, Velio P, et al: Gastric and duodenal polyps in familial polyposis coli. Gut 11:363–367, 1981.
20. Tonelli F, Nardi E, Bechi P, et al: Extracolonic polyps in familial polyposis coli and Gardner's syndrome. Dis Colon Rectum 28:664–668, 1985.
21. Watanabe H, Enjoji M, Yao T, et al: Gastric lesions in familial adenomatosis coli. Hum Pathol 9:269–283, 1978.
22. Iida M, Yao T, Watanabe H, et al: Fundic gland polyposis in patients without familial adenomatosis coli: its incidence and clinical features. Gastroenterology 86:1437–1442, 1984.
23. Tatsuta M, Okuda S, Tamura H: Gastric hamartomatous polyps in the absence of familial polyposis coli. Cancer 45:818–823, 1980.
24. Nishiura M, Hirota T, Itabashi M, et al: A clinical and histopathological study of gastric polyps in familial polyposis coli. Am J Gastroenterol 79:98–103, 1984.
25. Sato T, Sakai Y, Ishiguro S, et al: Gastric hamartomatous polyp without polyposis coli: radiologic diagnosis. Gastrointest Radiol 13:19–23, 1988.
26. Iida M, Yao T, Itoh H, et al: Natural history of fundic gland polyposis in patients with familial adenomatous coli/Gardner's syndrome. Gastroenterology 89:1021–1025, 1985.
27. Itai Y, Kogure T, Okuyama Y, et al: Radiographic features of the gastric polyps in familial adenomatous coli. AJR 128:73–76, 1977.
28. Iida M, Yao T, Watanabe H, et al: Spontaneous disappearance of the fundic gland polyposis: report of three cases. Gastroenterology 79:725–728, 1980.
29. Denzler TB, Harned RK, Pergam CJ: Gastric polyps in familial polyposis coli. Radiology 130:63–66, 1979.
30. Yao T, Iida M, Ohsata K: Duodenal lesions in familial polyposis of the colon. Gastroenterology 73:1086–1092, 1977.
31. Qizilbash AH: Epithelial neoplasms of the duodenum and periampullary region. *In* Appelman HD (ed): Pathology of the Esophagus, Stomach and Duodenum. New York: Churchill Livingstone, 1984, p 145.
32. Schnur PL, David E, Brown PW, et al: Adenocarcinoma of the duodenum and the Gardner syndrome. JAMA 223:1229–1232, 1973.
33. Sugihara K, Muto T, Kamiya J, et al: Gardner's syndrome associated with periampullary carcinoma, duodenal and gastric adenomatosis: report of a case. Dis Colon Rectum 25:766–771, 1982.
34. Harned RK, Williams SM: Familial polyposis coli and periampullary malignancy. Dis Colon Rectum 25:227–229, 1982.
35. Bussey HJ: Extracolonic lesions associated with polyposis coli. Proc R Soc Med 65:294, 1972.
36. Ohsata K, Yao T, Watanabe H, et al: Small-intestinal involvement in familial polyposis diagnosed by operative intestinal fiberoscopy: report of four cases. Dis Colon Rectum 20:414–420, 1977.

37. Iida M, Yao T, Ohsata K, et al: Diagnostic value of intraoperative fiberoscopy for small-intestinal polyps in familial adenomatosis coli. Endoscopy 12:161–165, 1980.

38. Ross JE, Mara JE: Small bowel polyps and carcinoma in multiple intestinal polyposis. Arch Surg 108:736–738, 1974.

39. Phillips LG: Polyposis and carcinoma of the small bowel and familial colonic polyposis. Dis Colon Rectum 24:478–481, 1981.

40. Scully RE, Galdabini JJ, McNeely BU: Case 47–1978: presentation of case. Case records of the Massachusetts General Hospital. N Engl J Med 299:1237–1244, 1978.

41. Jarvinen HJ, Nyberg M, Peltokallio P: Biliary involvement in familial adenomatosis coli. Dis Colon Rectum 26:525–528, 1983.

42. Less CD, Hermann RE: Familial polyposis coli associated with bile duct cancer. Am J Surg 141:378–380, 1981.

43. Burney B, Assor D: Polyposis coli with adenocarcinoma associated with carcinoma in situ of the gallbladder. Am J Surg 132:100–102, 1976.

44. Willson SA, Princethal RA, Law B, et al: Gallbladder carcinoma in association with polyposis coli. Br J Radiol 60:771–773, 1987.

45. Gardner EJ, Richards RC: Multiple cutaneous and subcutaneous lesions occurring simultaneously with hereditary polyposis and osteomatosis. Am J Hum Genet 5:139–148, 1953.

46. Gardner EJ: Follow-up study of a family group exhibiting dominant inheritance for a syndrome including intestinal polyps, osteomas, fibromas and epidermal cysts. Am J Hum Genet 14:376–390, 1962.

47. Watne AL, Lai H, Carrier J, et al: The diagnosis of surgical treatment of patients with Gardner's syndrome. Surgery 82:327–333, 1977.

48. Lockhart-Mummery EH: Intestinal polyposis: the present position. Proc R Soc Med 60:381–388, 1967.

49. Cohen SB: Familial polyposis coli and its extracolonic manifestations. J Med Genet 19:193–203, 1982.

50. Jagelman DG: Extracolonic manifestations of familial polyposis coli. Cancer Genet Cytogenet 27:319–325, 1987.

51. Weary PE, Linthicum A, Cawley EP, et al: Gardner's syndrome. Arch Dermatol 90:20–30, 1964.

52. Gorlin RJ, Chaudhry AP: Multiple osteomatosis, fibromas, lipomas and fibrosarcomas of the skin and mesentery, epidermoid inclusion cysts of the skin, leiomyomas and multiple intestinal polyposis. N Engl J Med 263:1151–1158, 1960.

53. Chang CH, Piatt ED, Thomas KE, et al: Bone abnormalities in Gardner's syndrome. AJR 103:645–652, 1968.

54. Utsunomiya J, Nakamura T: The occult osteomatous changes in the mandible in patients with familial polyposis coli. Br J Surg 62:45–51, 1975.

55. Bülow S, Søndergaard JO, Witt I, et al: Mandibular osteomas in familial polyposis coli. Dis Colon Rectum 27:105–108, 1984.

56. Woods RJ, Sarre RG, Ctercteko GC, et al: Occult radiologic changes in the skull and jaw in familial adenomatous polyposis coli. Dis Colon Rectum 32:304–306, 1989.

57. Fader M, Kline SN, Spatz SS, et al: Gardner's syndrome (intestinal polyposis, osteomas, sebaceous cysts) and a new dental discovery. Oral Surg Oral Med Oral Pathol 15:153–172, 1962.

58. Søndergaard JO, Bulow S, Wolf J, et al: Dental anomalies in familial adenomatous polyposis coli. Acta Odontol Scand 45:61–63, 1987.

59. Hughes LE: Abdominal fibrodysplasia and polyposis coli. Dis Colon Rectum 13:121–123, 1970.

60. Jones IT, Fazio VW, Weakley FL, et al: Desmoid tumors in familial polyposis coli. Ann Surg 204:94–97, 1986.

61. Burke A, Sobin LH, Shekitka KM, et al: Intra-abdominal fibromatosis: a pathologic analysis of 130 tumors with comparison of clinical subgroups. Am J Surg Pathol 14:335–341, 1990.

62. Iwamma T, Mishima Y, Okamoto N, et al: Association of congenital hypertrophy of the retinal pigment epithelium with familial adenomatous polyposis. Br J Surg 77:273–276, 1990.

63. Traboulsi EI, Maumenee IH, Krush AJ, et al: Congenital hypertrophy of the retinal pigment epithelium predicts colorectal polyposis in Gardner's syndrome. Arch Ophthalmol 108:525–526, 1990.

64. Baker RH, Heinemann MH, Miller HH, et al: Hyperpigmented lesions of the retinal pigment epithelium in familial adenomatous polyposis. Am J Med Genet 31:427–435, 1988.

65. Romania A, Zakov ZN, McGannon E, et al: Congenital hypertrophy of the retinal pigment epithelium in familial adenomatous polyposis. Ophthalmology 96:879–884, 1989.

66. Baba S, Tsuchiya M, Watanabe I, et al: Importance of retinal pigmentation as a subclinical marker in familial adenomatous polyposis. Dis Colon Rectum 33:660–664, 1990.

67. Crail HW: Multiple primary malignancies arising in the rectum, brain and thyroid: report of a case. US Nav Med Bull 49:123–128, 1949.

68. Turcot J, Despres JP, Pierre F: Malignant tumors of the central nervous system associated with familial polyposis of the colon. Dis Colon Rectum 2:465–468, 1959.

69. Itoh H, Ohsato K, Yao T, et al: Turcot's syndrome and its mode of inheritance. Gut 20:414–419, 1979.

70. Jarvis L, Bathurst N, Mohan D, et al: Turcot's syndrome: a review. Dis Colon Rectum 31:907–914, 1988.

71. Costa O, Silva DM, Colnago FA, et al: Turcot syndrome: autosomal dominant or recessive transmission? Dis Colon Rectum 39:391–394, 1987.

72. Itoh H, Ohsato K: Turcot syndrome and its characteristic colonic manifestations. Dis Colon Rectum 28:399–402, 1985.

73. Chowdhary UM, Boehme DH, Al-Jishi M: Turcot syndrome (glioma polyposis): a case report. J Neurosurg 63:804–807, 1985.

74. Radin DR, Fortgang KC, Zee C, et al: Turcot syndrome: a case with spinal cord and colonic neoplasms. AJR 142:475–476, 1984.

75. Stevens MJ, Flanagan BT: Turcot's syndrome. Med J Aust 144:433–435, 1986.

76. Schroder S, Moehrs D, Von Weltzien J, et al: The Turcot syndrome. Dis Colon Rectum 26:533–538, 1983.

77. Plail RO, Bussey JH, Glazer G, et al: Adenomatous polyposis: an association with carcinoma of the thyroid. Br J Surg 74:377–380, 1987.

78. Delamarre J, Capron J, Armand A, et al: Thyroid carcinoma in two sisters with familial polyposis of the colon: case reports and review of the literature. J Clin Gastroenterol 10:659–662, 1988.

79. Schneider NR, Cubilla AL, Chaganti RS: Association of endocrine neoplasia with multiple polyposis of the colon. Cancer 51:1171–1175, 1983.

80. Perkins JT, Backstone MO, Riddell RH: Adenomatous polyposis coli and multiple endocrine neoplasia type 2b: a pathogenic relationship. Cancer 55:375–381, 1985.

81. Painter TA, Jagelman DG: Adrenal adenomas and adrenal carcinomas in association with hereditary adenomatosis of the colon and rectum. Cancer 55:2001–2004, 1985.

82. Bülow S: Familial adenomatous polyposis. Ann Med 21:299–307, 1989.

83. Schneider NR, Cubilla AL, Chaganti RS: Association of endocrine neoplasia with multiple polyposis of the colon. Cancer 51:1171–1175, 1983.

84. LeSher AR, Castronuovo JJ Jr, Filippone AL Jr: Hepatoblastoma in a patient with familial polyposis coli. Surgery 105:668–670, 1989.

85. Kingston JE, Herbert A, Draper GH, et al: Association between hepatoblastoma and polyposis coli. Arch Dis Child 58:959–962, 1983.

86. Jeghers H, McKusick VA, Katz KH: Generalized intestinal polyposis and melanin spots of the oral mucosa, lips, and digits. N Engl J Med 241:993–1005, 1031–1036, 1949.

87. Bartholomew LG, Moore CE, Dahlin DC, et al: Intestinal polyposis associated with mucocutaneous pigmentation. Surg Gynecol Obstet 115:1–11, 1962.

88. Linos DA, Dozols RR, Dahlin DC, et al: Does Peutz-Jeghers syndrome predispose to gastrointestinal malignancy? Arch Surg 116:1182–1184, 1981.

89. Jass JR, Sobin LH: Histological Typing of Intestinal Tumors (2nd ed). (WHO International Histological Classification of Tumors.) Berlin: Springer-Verlag, 1989, pp 22, 40.

90. Shepherd NA, Bussey HJR, Jass JR: Epithelial misplacement in Peutz-Jeghers syndrome. Am J Surg Pathol 11:743–749, 1987.

91. Foley TR, McGarrity TJ, Abt AB: Peutz-Jeghers syndrome: a clinicopathologic survey of the "Harrisburg family" with a 49-year follow-up. Gastroenterology 95:1535–1540, 1988.

92. Spiegelman AD, Murday V, Phillips RK: Cancer and the Peutz-Jeghers syndrome. Gut 30:1588–1590, 1989.

93. Dormandy TL: Gastrointestinal polyposis with mucocutaneous pigmentation (Peutz-Jeghers syndrome). N Engl J Med 256:1093–1103, 1141–1146, 1186–1187, 1957.

94. Godard JE, Dodds WJ, Phillips JC, et al: Peutz-Jeghers syndrome: clinical and roentgenographic features. AJR 113:316–324, 1971.

95. Erb RW: Inherited gastrointestinal polyposis syndrome. N Engl J Med 294:1101–1104, 1976.

96. Dozois RR, Judd ES, Dahlin DC, et al: The Peutz-Jeghers syndrome. Arch Surg 98:509–517, 1969.

97. McAllister AJ, Richard KF: Peutz-Jeghers syndrome. Experience with twenty patients in five generations. Am J Surg 134:717–720, 1977.

98. Dodds WJ: Clinical and roentgen features of the intestinal polyposis syndromes. Gastrointest Radiol 1:127–142, 1976.

99. Giardiello FM, Welsh SB, Hamilton SR, et al: Increased risk of cancer in the Peutz-Jeghers syndrome. N Engl J Med 315:1511–1514, 1987.

100. Narita T, Eto T, Ito T: Peutz-Jeghers syndrome with adenomas and adenocarcinomas in colonic polyps. Am J Surg Pathol 11:76–81, 1987.

101. Reid JD: Intestinal carcinoma in the Peutz-Jeghers syndrome. JAMA 229:833–834, 1974.

102. Utsunomiya J, Gocho H, Miyanaga T, et al: Peutz-Jeghers syndrome: its natural course and management. Johns Hopkins Med J 136:71–82, 1975.

103. Dodds WJ, Schulte WJ, Hensley GT, et al: Peutz-Jeghers syndrome and gastrointestinal malignancy. AJR 115:374–377, 1972.

104. Kyle J: Gastric carcinoma in Peutz-Jeghers syndrome. Scott Med J 29:187–191, 1984.

105. Shibata HR, Phillips MJ: Peutz-Jeghers syndrome with jejunal and colonic adenocarcinomas. Can Med Assoc J 103:285–287, 1970.

106. Matuchansky C, Babin P, Coutrot S, et al: Peutz-Jeghers syndrome with metastasizing carcinoma arising from a jejunal hamartoma. Gastroenterology 77:1311–1315, 1979.

107. Miller LJ, Bartholomew LG, Dozols RR, et al: Adenocarcinoma of the rectum arising in a hamartomatous polyp in a patient with Peutz-Jeghers syndrome. Dig Dis Sci 28:1047–1051, 1983.

108. Perzin KH, Bridge MF: Adenomatous and carcinomatous changes in hamartomatous polyps of the small intestine (Peutz-Jeghers syndrome). Cancer 49:971–983, 1982.

109. Bowlby LS: Pancreatic adenocarcinoma in an adolescent male with Peutz-Jeghers syndrome. Hum Pathol 17:97–99, 1986.

110. Konishi F, Wyse NE, Muto T, et al: Peutz-Jeghers polyposis associated with carcinoma of the digestive organs. Report of three cases and review of the literature. Dis Colon Rectum 30:790–799, 1987.

111. Thatcher BS, May ES, Taxier MS, et al: Pancreatic adenocarcinoma in a patient with Peutz-Jeghers syndrome: a case report and literature review. Am J Gastroenterol 81:594–597, 1986.

112. Scully RE: Sex cord tumor with annular tubules: a distinctive ovarian tumor of the Peutz-Jeghers syndrome. Cancer 25:1107–1121, 1970.

113. Young RH, Welch WR, Dickersin GR, et al: Ovarian sex cord tumor with annular tubules: review of 74 cases including 27 with Peutz-Jeghers syndrome and four with adenoma malignum of the cervix. Cancer 50:1384–1402, 1982.

114. Solh HM, Azoury RS, Najjar SS: Peutz-Jeghers syndrome associated with precocious puberty. J Pediatr 103:593–595, 1983.

115. Young RH, Dickersin GR, Scully RE: A distinctive ovarian sex cord-stromal tumor causing sexual precocity in the Peutz-Jeghers syndrome. Am J Surg Pathol 7:233–243, 1983.

116. Anderson NJ, Rivera ES, Flores DJ: Peutz-Jeghers syndrome with cervical adenocarcinoma and enteritis cystica profunda. West J Med 141:242–244, 1984.

117. Chen KTK: Female genital tract tumors in Peutz-Jeghers syndrome. Hum Pathol 17:858–861, 1986.

118. Kaku T, Hachisuga T, Toyoshima S, et al: Extremely well-differentiated adenocarcinoma ("adenoma malignum") of the cervix in a patient with Peutz-Jeghers syndrome. Int J Gynecol Obstet 4:266–273, 1985.

119. McGowan L, Young RH, Scully RE: Peutz-Jeghers syndrome with "adenoma malignum" of the cervix. Gynecol Oncol 10:125–133, 1980.

120. Young RH, Scully RE: Mucinous ovarian tumors associated with mucinous adenocarcinomas of the cervix. Int J Gynecol Pathol 7:99–111, 1988.

121. Cantu JM, Rivera H, Ocampo-Campos R, et al: Peutz-Jeghers syndrome with feminizing Sertoli cell tumor. Cancer 46:223–228, 1988.

122. Dubois RS, Hoffman WH, Krishnan THE, et al: Feminizing sex cord tumor with annular tubules in a boy with Peutz-Jeghers syndrome. J Pediatr 101:568–571, 1982.

123. Wilson DM, Pitts WC, Hintz RL, et al: Testicular tumors with Peutz-Jeghers syndrome. Cancer 57:2238–2240, 1986.

124. Riley E, Swift M: A family with Peutz-Jeghers syndrome and bilateral breast cancer. Cancer 46:815–817, 1980.

125. Lehur PA, Madarnas P, Devroede G, et al: Peutz-Jeghers syndrome: association of duodenal and bilateral breast cancers in the same patient. Dig Dis Sci 29:178–182, 1984.

126. Trau H, Schewach-Millet M, Fisher BK, et al: Peutz-Jeghers syndrome and bilateral breast cancer. Cancer 50:788–792, 1982.

127. Foster DR, Foster DBE: Gallbladder polyps in Peutz-Jeghers syndrome. Postgrad Med J 56:373–376, 1980.

128. Wada K, Tanaka M, Yamaguchi K: Carcinoma and polyps of the gallbladder associated with Peutz-Jeghers syndrome. Dig Dis Sci 32:943–946, 1987.

129. Jancu J: Peutz-Jeghers syndrome: involvement of the gastrointestinal and upper respiratory tracts. Am J Gastroenterol 56:545–549, 1971.

130. Keating MA, Young RH, Lillehei CW, et al: Hamartoma of the bladder in a 4 year old girl with hamartomatous polyps of the gastrointestinal tract. J Urol 138:366–369, 1987.

131. Sommerhaug RG, Mason T: Peutz-Jeghers syndrome and ureteral polyposis. JAMA 211:120–122, 1970.

132. Haggit RC, Reid BJ: Hereditary gastrointestinal polyposis syndromes. Am J Surg Pathol 10:871–887, 1986.

133. McKittrick JE, Lewis WM, Doane WA, et al: The Peutz-Jeghers syndrome. Arch Surg 103:57–62, 1971.

134. Starink TM, van Der Veen JW, De Waal LP, et al: The Cowden syndrome: a clinical and genetic study in 21 patients. Clin Genet 29:222–233, 1986.

135. Lloyd KM II, Dennis M: Cowden's disease. A possible new symptom complex with multiple system involvement. Ann Intern Med 58:136–142, 1963.

136. Salem OS, Steck WD: Cowden's disease (multiple hamartoma and neoplasia syndrome). A case report and review of the English literature. J Am Acad Dermatol 8:686–696, 1983.

137. Weary PE, Gorlin RJ, Gentry WC, et al: Multiple hamartoma syndrome (Cowden's disease). Arch Dermatol 106:682–690, 1972.

138. Gentry WC, Eskritt NR, Gorlin RJ: Multiple hamartoma syndrome. Arch Dermatol 109:521–525, 1974.

139. Siegel JM: Tuberous sclerosis (forme fruste) vs. Cowden syndrome. Arch Dermatol 110:476–477, 1974.

140. Burnett JW, Goldner R, Calton GH: Cowden disease: a report of two additional cases. Br J Dermatol 93:329–336, 1975.

141. Gentry WC, Reed WB, Siegel JM: Cowden disease. Birth Defects 11:137–141, 1975.

142. Siegel JM: Cowden disease: report of a case with malignant melanoma. Cutis 16:255–258, 1975.

143. Brownstein MH, Mehregan AH, Bikowski JB: Trichilemmomas in Cowden's disease. JAMA 238:26, 1977 (letter).

144. Mulivhill JJ, McKeen EA: Discussion: genetics of multiple primary tumors. A clinical etiologic approach illustrated by three patients. Cancer 40:1867–1871, 1977.

145. Brownstein MH, Wolf M, Bokowski JB: Cowden's disease. A cutaneous marker of breast cancer. Cancer 41:2393–2398, 1978.

146. Nuss DD, Aeling JL, Clemons DE, et al: Multiple hamartoma syndrome (Cowden's disease). Arch Dermatol 114:743–746, 1978.

147. Wade TP, Kopf AW: Cowden's disease: a case report and review of the literature. J Dermatol Surg Oncol 4:459–464, 1978.

148. Weinstock JV, Kawanishi H: Gastrointestinal polyposis with orocutaneous hamartomas (Cowden's disease). Gastroenterology 74:890–895, 1978.

149. Allen BS, Fitch MH, Smith JG Jr: Multiple hamartoma syndrome. A report of a new case with associated carcinoma of the

uterine cervix and angioid streaks of the eyes. J Am Acad Dermatol 2:303–308, 1980.

150. Emmerson RW: Epidermodysplasia verruciformis and punctate keratoderma. Br J Dermatol 103(suppl 18):50–52, 1980.

151. Gertzman GBR, Clark M, Gatson G: Multiple hamartoma and neoplasia syndrome (Cowden's syndrome). Oral Surg 49:314–316, 1980.

152. Gold BM, Bagla S, Zarrabi MH: Radiologic manifestations of Cowden disease. AJR 135:385–387, 1980.

153. Hauser H, Ody B, Piojoux O, et al: Radiological findings in multiple hamartoma syndrome (Cowden disease). A report of three cases. Radiology 137:317–323, 1980.

154. Ortonne JP, Lambert R, Daudet J, et al: Involvement of the digestive tract in Cowden's disease. Int J Dermatol 19:570–576, 1980.

155. Yuasa T, Hanano M, Ohshima F, et al: The association of myasthenia gravis with multiple hamartoma syndrome (Cowden disease). Ann Neurol 7:591–592, 1980.

156. Bart RS, Kopf AW: Cowden's disease (multiple hamartoma syndrome). J Dermatol Surg Oncol 7:378–380, 1981.

157. Elton R, Sroud J, Wagenberg H, et al: Cowden's syndrome. Int J Dermatol 20:617–618, 1981.

158. Thyresson HN, Doyle JA: Cowden's disease (multiple hamartoma syndrome). Mayo Clin Proc 56:179–184, 1981.

159. Ruschak PJ, Kauth YC, Luscombe HA: Cowden's disease associated with immunodeficiency. Arch Dermatol 117:573–575, 1981.

160. Russell JR, O'Brien M, Wells RS: Cowden's syndrome. Br J Dermatol 105(suppl 19):57–58, 1981.

161. Aylesworth R, Vance JC: Multiple hamartoma syndrome with endometrial carcinoma and the sign of Leser-Trélat. Arch Dermatol 118:136–138, 1982.

162. Aram H, Zidenbaum M: Multiple hamartoma syndrome (Cowden's disease). J Am Acad Dermatol 9:774–776, 1983.

163. Sogol PB, Sugawara M, Gordon HE, et al: Cowden's disease: familial goiter and skin hamartomas. A report of three cases. West J Med 139:324–328, 1983.

164. Camisa C, Bikowski JB, McDonald SG: Cowden's disease, association with squamous cell carcinoma of the tongue and perianal basal cell carcinoma. Arch Dermatol 120:677–678, 1984.

165. Carlson GJ, Nivatvongs S, Snover DC: Colorectal polyps in Cowden's disease (multiple hamartoma syndrome). Am J Surg Pathol 8:763–770, 1984.

166. Gorensek M, Matko I, Skralovnik A, et al: Disseminated hereditary gastrointestinal polyposis with orocutaneous hamartomatosis (Cowden's disease). Endoscopy 16:59–63, 1984.

167. Starink TM: Cowden's disease: analysis of fourteen new cases. J Am Acad Dermatol 11:1127–1141, 1984.

168. Gilbert HD, Plezia RA, Pietruk T: Cowden's disease (multiple hamartoma syndrome). J Oral Maxillofac Surg 43:457–460, 1985.

169. Halevy S, Sandbank M, Pick AI, et al: Cowden's disease in three siblings: electron-microscope and immunological studies. Acta Derm Venereol 65:126–131, 1985.

170. Swart JGN, Lekkas C, Alleard RHB: Oral manifestations in Cowden's syndrome. Oral Surg Oral Med Pathol 59:264–268, 1985.

171. Elston DM, James WD, Rodman OG, et al: Multiple hamartoma syndrome (Cowden's disease) associated with non-Hodgkins' lymphoma. Arch Dermatol 122:572–575, 1986.

172. Hover AR, Cawthern T, McDaniel W: Cowden's disease. J Clin Gastroenterol 8:576–579, 1986.

173. Walton BJ, Morain WD, Baughman RD, et al: Cowden's disease: a further indication for prophylactic mastectomy. Surgery 99:82–86, 1986.

174. Barax CN, Lebwohl M, Phelps RG: Multiple hamartomas syndrome. J Am Acad Dermatol 17:342–346, 1987.

175. Chen YM, Ott DJ, Wu WC, et al: Cowden's disease: a case report and literature review. Gastrointest Radiol 12:325–329, 1987.

176. Grattan CH, Hamburger J: Cowden's disease in two sisters, one showing partial expression. Clin Exp Dermatol 12:360–363, 1987.

177. Bardenstein DS, McLean IW, Nerney J, et al: Cowden's disease. Ophthalmology 95:1038–1041, 1988.

178. Taylor AJ, Dods WJ, Stewart ET: Alimentary tract lesions in Cowden's disease. Br J Radiol 62:890–892, 1989.

179. Wheeland RG, McGillis ST: Cowden's disease—treatment of cutaneous lesions using carbon dioxide laser vaporization: a comparison of conventional and superpulsed techniques. J Dermatol Surg Oncol 15:1055–1059, 1989.

180. Brownstein MH, Mehregan AH, Bikowski JB: The dermatopathology of Cowden's disease. Br J Dermatol 100:667–673, 1979.

181. Atarink TM, Meijer CM, Brownstein MH: The cutaneous pathology of Cowden's disease: new findings. J Cutan Pathol 12:83–93, 1985.

182. Greene SL, Thomas JR, Doyle JA: Cowden's disease with associated malignant melanoma. Int J Dermatol 23:466–467, 1984.

183. Shapiro SD, Lambert WC, Schwartz RA: Cowden's Disease, a marker for malignancy. Int J Dermatol 27:232–237, 1988.

184. Lashner BA, Riddell RH, Winans CS: Ganglioneuromatosis of the colon and extensive glycogenic acanthosis in Cowden's disease. Dig Dis Sci 31:212–216, 1986.

185. Jass JR, Sobin LH: Histological Typing of Intestinal Tumors (2nd ed). (WHO International Histological Classification of Tumors.) Berlin: Springer-Verlag, 1989, pp 22, 36, 126.

186. Snover DC: Cowden's disease. Surgery 101:119–120, 1987.

187. Cronkhite LW, Canada WJ: Generalized gastrointestinal polyposis: an unusual syndrome of polyposis, pigmentation, alopecia and onchytrophia. N Engl J Med 252:1011–1015, 1955.

188. Dachman AH, Buck JL, Burke AP, et al: Cronkhite-Canada syndrome: radiologic features. Gastrointest Radiol 14:285–290, 1989.

189. Daniel ES, Ludwig SL, Lewin KJ, et al: The Cronkhite-Canada syndrome: an analysis of clinical and pathologic features and therapy in 55 patients. Medicine (Baltimore) 61:293–309, 1982.

190. Scharf GM, Becker JHR, Laage NJ: Juvenile gastrointestinal polyposis or the infantile Cronkhite-Canada syndrome. J Pediatr Surg 21:953–954, 1981.

191. Burke AP, Sobin LH: The pathology of Cronkhite-Canada polyps. Am J Surg Pathol 13:940–946, 1989.

192. Parsa C: Cronkhite-Canada syndrome associated with systemic vasculitis: an autopsy study. Hum Pathol 13:758–760, 1982.

193. Russell D, Bhathal PS, St. John JB: Complete remission in Cronkhite-Canada syndrome. Gastroenterology 85:180–185, 1983.

194. Peart Jr AG, Sivak MV, Rankin GB, et al: Spontaneous improvement of Cronkhite-Canada syndrome in a postpartum female. Dig Dis Sci 29:470–474, 1984.

195. Ferney DM, Deschryver-Kecskemeti K, Clouse RE: Treatment of Cronkhite-Canada with home total parenteral nutrition. Ann Intern Med 104:588, 1986.

196. Kubo D, Hirose S, Aoki S, et al: Canada-Cronkhite syndrome associated with systemic lupus erythematosus. Arch Intern Med 146:995–997, 1986.

197. Kilcheski T, Kressel HY, Laufer I, et al: The radiographic appearance of the stomach in Cronkhite-Canada syndrome. Radiology 141:57–60, 1981.

198. Rappaport LB, Sperling HV, Stavrides A: Colon cancer in the Cronkhite-Canada syndrome. J Clin Gastroenterol 8:199–202, 1986.

199. Li CP: Cronkhite-Canada syndrome. Dig Dis Sci 32:109, 1987.

200. Jass JR, Williams CB, Bussey HR, et al: Juvenile polyposis: a precancerous condition. Histopathology 13:619–630, 1988.

201. Jass JR, Sobin LH: Histological Typing of Intestinal Tumors (2nd ed). (WHO International Histological Classification of Tumors.) Berlin: Springer-Verlag, 1989, pp 36, 40.

202. Goodman ZD, Yardley JH, Milligan FD: Pathogenesis of colonic polyps in multiple juvenile polyposis. Cancer 43:1906–1913, 1979.

203. Gryboski JD: All juvenile polyps are not benign. Am J Gastroenterol 82:397, 1986.

204. Haggit RC, Reid BJ: Hereditary gastrointestinal polyposis syndromes. Am J Surg Pathol 101:871–887, 1986.

205. Mestre JR: The changing pattern of juvenile polyps. Am J Gastroenterol 81:312–314, 1986.

206. Mills FE, Fechner RE: Unusual adenomatous polyps in juvenile polyposis coli. Am J Surg Pathol 6:177–183, 1982.

207. Longo WE, Touloukian RJ, West AB, et al: Malignant potential of juvenile polyposis coli: report of a case and review of the literature. Dis Colon Rectum 135:980–984, 1990.

208. Roth SI, Helwig EB: Juvenile polyps of the colon and rectum. Cancer 16:468–479, 1963.
209. Grosfeld JL, West KW: Generalized juvenile polyposis coli. Arch Surg 121:530–534, 1986.
210. Mazier WP, MacKeigan JM, Billingham RP, et al: Juvenile polyps of the colon and rectum. Surg Gynecol Obstet 154:829–832, 1982.
211. Douglas JR, Campbell CA, Salisbury DM, et al: Colonoscopic polypectomy in children. Br Med J 281:1386–1387, 1980.
212. Bussey HR, Veale AO, Morson BC: Genetics of gastrointestinal polyposis. Gastroenterology 74:1325–1330, 1978.
213. Smilow PC, Pryor CK, Swinton NW: Juvenile polyposis coli: a report of three patients in three generations of one family. Dis Colon Rectum 9:248–254, 1966.
214. Sachatello CR, Pickren JW, Grace JT: Generalized juvenile gastrointestinal polyposis: a hereditary syndrome. Gastroenterology 58:699–708, 1970.
215. Veale AM, Mecall I, Bussey HR, et al: Juvenile polyposis coli. J Med Genet 3:5–16, 1966.
216. Cox KL, Frates RC, Wong A: Hereditary generalized juvenile polyposis associated with pulmonary arteriovenous malformation. Gastroenterology 78:1566–1570, 1980.
217. Baert AL, Casteels-Van Daele M, Broeckx L, et al: Generalized juvenile polyposis with pulmonary arteriovenous malformations and hypertrophic osteoarthropathy. AJR 141:661–662, 1983.
218. Stemper TJ, Kent THE, Summers RW: Juvenile polyposis and gastrointestinal carcinoma: a study of a kindred. Ann Intern Med 83:639–646, 1975.
219. Grigioni WF, Alampi G, Martinelli G, et al: Atypical juvenile polyposis. Histopathology 5:361–376, 1981.
220. Rozen P, Baratz M: Familial juvenile polyposis with associated colon cancer. Cancer 49:1500–1503, 1982.
221. Jarvinen H, Franssila KO: Familial juvenile polyposis coli: increased risk of colorectal cancer. Gut 25:792–800, 1984.
222. Haggitt RC, Pitcock JA: Familial juvenile polyposis of the colon. Cancer 26:1232–1238, 1970.
223. Kaschula RC: Mixed juvenile adenomatous and intermediate polyposis coli. Dis Colon Rectum 14:368–374, 1971.
224. Velcek FT, Coopersmith IS, Chen CK, et al: Familial juvenile adenomatous polyposis. J Pediatr Surg 11:781–787, 1976.
225. Restrepo C, Moreno J, Dugue E, et al: Juvenile polyposis in Columbia. Dis Colon Rectum 21:600–612, 1978.
226. Lipper S, Kahn LB, Sandler RS, et al: Multiple juvenile polyposis; a study of the pathogenesis of juvenile polyps and their relationship to colonic adenomas. Hum Pathol 12:804–813, 1981.
227. Grotsky HW, Rickert RR, Smith WD, et al: Familial juvenile polyposis coli; a clinical and pathologic study of a large kindred. Gastroenterology 82:494–501, 1982.
228. Yoshida T, Haraguchi A, Tanaka A, et al: A case of generalized juvenile gastrointestinal polyposis associated with gastric carcinoma. Endoscopy 20:33–35, 1988.
229. Walpole IR, Cullity G: Juvenile polyposis: a case with early presentation and death attributable to adenocarcinoma of the pancreas. Am J Med Genet 32:1–8, 1989.
230. Sachatello CR, Song Hong II, Carrington CB: Juvenile gastrointestinal polyposis in a female infant: report of a case and review of the literature of a recently recognized syndrome. Surgery 75:107–113, 1974.
231. Ravitch MM: Polypoid adenomatosis of the entire gastrointestinal tract. Am Surg 128:283–298, 1948.
232. LeFevre HW, Jacques TF: Multiple polyposis in an infant of four months. Am Surg 77:90–91, 1951.
233. Ruymann FB: Juvenile polyp with cachexia: report of an infant and comparison with Cronkhite-Canada syndrome in adults. Gastroenterology 57:431–438, 1969.
234. Arbeter AM, Courtney RA, Gaynor MF: Diffuse gastrointestinal polyposis associated with chronic blood loss, hypoproteinemia, and anasarca in an infant. J Pediatr 70:609–611, 1970.
235. Berk RN, Rush JL, Elson EC: Multiple inflammatory polyps of the small intestine with cachexia and protein losing enteropathy. Radiology 95:611–612, 1970.
236. Ray JE, Heald RJ: Growing up with juvenile gastrointestinal polyposis: report of a case. Dis Colon Rectum 14:375–380, 1971.
237. Soper RT, Kent THE: Fatal juvenile polyposis in infancy. Surgery 169:692–698, 1971.
238. Koehler PR, Kyaw MM, Fenlon JW: Diffuse gastrointestinal polyposis with ectodermal changes: Cronkhite-Canada syndrome. Radiology 103:589–594, 1974.
239. Schwartz AM, McCauley RK: Juvenile gastrointestinal polyposis. Radiology 121:441–444, 1976.
240. LeLuyer B, LeBihan, Metayer P, et al: Generalized juvenile polyposis in an infant: report of a case and successful management by endoscopy. J Pediatr Gastroenterol Nutr 4:128–134, 1985.

# Large Bowel Obstruction

Richard M. Gore, M.D.
Ronald L. Eisenberg, M.D.

INTRODUCTION

PATHOPHYSIOLOGY

CLINICAL FINDINGS

RADIOLOGIC APPROACH TO SUSPECTED LARGE BOWEL OBSTRUCTION

MAJOR TYPES OF COLONIC OBSTRUCTION
Carcinoma of the Colon
Diverticulitis
Volvulus
Adult Intussusception
Adhesions

Hernias
Obturation Obstruction
Extrinsic Causes
Strictures

SUMMARY

## INTRODUCTION

Mechanical large bowel obstruction is four to five times less common than small bowel obstruction and differs significantly in terms of etiology (Table 67–1), pathophysiology (Table 67–2), therapy, and prognosis.[1–4] Prompt differentiation between these entities is important because large bowel obstruction is most often the result of a neoplasm (Table 67–3), whereas the majority of small bowel obstructions are due to adhesions.[5] This chapter discusses the major types of colonic obstruction as well as a generalized radiologic approach to the patient with suspected large bowel obstruction.

## PATHOPHYSIOLOGY

When colonic obstruction is caused by diverticulitis or cancer, symptoms are usually subacute or chronic. The swallowed air proximal to the obstruction causes dilatation, but the third spacing of fluid in the gut lumen characteristic of small bowel obstruction is not seen. Strangulation rarely occurs, except in occasional cases of volvulus.[1–4, 6]

Colonic response to the mechanical obstruction depends on the competency of the ileocecal valve (Fig. 67–1). The small bowel serves to decompress the colon when the valve is incompetent. A closed loop obstruction develops when the valve is competent because the

---

### TABLE 67–1. ETIOLOGY OF MECHANICAL LARGE BOWEL OBSTRUCTION

| INTRINSIC DEFECTS | EXTRINSIC DEFECTS |
|---|---|
| Neoplasms | Volvulus |
|   Benign |   Secondary |
|   Malignant |   Primary |
| Inflammatory | Hernias |
|   Diverticulitis |   Internal |
|   Ulcerative colitis |   External |
|   Crohn's disease | Adhesions |
|   Amebiasis | Mass Compression |
|   Tuberculosis |   Carcinomatosis |
| Intussusception |   Abscess |
| Obturation |   Pregnancy |
|   Gallstones |   Cysts |
|   Foreign bodies |   Pancreatitis |
|   Meconium |   Endometriosis |
|   Medications | |
|   Enteroliths | |
|   Bezoars | |
|   Worms | |
| Congenital | |
|   Atresia | |
|   Stenosis | |
|   Imperforate anus | |
|   Cysts and duplications | |
| Miscellaneous | |
|   Post-traumatic | |
|   Pneumatosis intestinalis | |

Adapted from Welch JP: General considerations and mortality. *In* Welch JP (ed): Bowel Obstruction. Philadelphia: WB Saunders, 1990, pp 59–95.

---

### TABLE 67–2. CLINICAL COMPARISON OF LARGE AND SMALL BOWEL OBSTRUCTION

| FEATURE | SMALL BOWEL OBSTRUCTION | LARGE BOWEL OBSTRUCTION |
|---|---|---|
| Onset | Acute | Gradual; complete obstruction may be abrupt |
| Distention | Moderate | Usually great |
| Vomiting | Common | Infrequent |
| Abdominal mass | Suggests strangulation | Suggests volvulus, cancer |
| Hematocrit | Hemoconcentration | Anemia common |
| Azotemia | Frequent | Infrequent |

Adapted from Welch JP: General considerations and mortality. *In* Welch JP (ed): Bowel Obstruction. Philadelphia: WB Saunders, 1990, pp 59–95.

### TABLE 67–3. ETIOLOGY OF COLONIC OBSTRUCTION: INCIDENCE BY CAUSE

| | |
|---|---|
| Carcinoma | 55% |
| Volvulus | 11% |
| Diverticulitis | 9% |
| Extrinsic cancer | 8% |
| Adhesions | 4% |
| Impaction | 3% |
| Hernia | 2% |
| Intrinsic | 4% |

Adapted from Welch JP: General considerations and mortality. *In* Welch JP (ed): Bowel Obstruction. Philadelphia: WB Saunders, 1990, pp 59–95.

colon cannot decompress. Because the cecum has the largest diameter of the colon, its walls develop the highest pressures owing to Laplace's law (tension on wall = intraluminal pressure × lumen caliber). Consequently, cecal "diastaltic" perforation can develop when intraluminal pressure increases to a range of 20 to 55 mm Hg. Ischemia, bacterial overgrowth, and mechanical mural tearing all combine to cause cecal perforation, which is most common when the cecum reaches a diameter of 9 to 12 cm. If colonic obstruction is due to a malignant neoplasm, the most common site is adjacent to the tumor, rather than the cecum.[7–9]

## CLINICAL FINDINGS

Most colonic obstructions are due to cancer. Consequently, most patients are elderly and have symptoms related to tumor location. Disease manifestation is often insidious with right colon lesions because the lumen is wide and the contents are semiliquid. Left-sided lesions cause progressive constipation and ultimately obstipation, abdominal distention, and abdominal pain. Lesions occurring at the ileocecal valve or ileocolic intussusception cause more acute symptoms of small bowel obstruction: abdominal pain, distention, vomiting, and obstipation.[10, 11] Patients with volvulus may develop pain and distention rapidly if a closed loop obstruction and bowel ischemia are present.[10–12] If the ileocecal valve is incompetent, retrograde decompression produces the

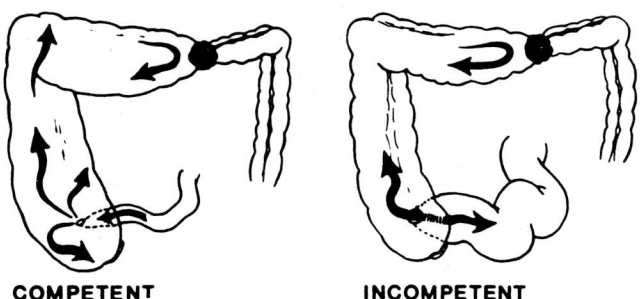

**COMPETENT**          **INCOMPETENT**

**Figure 67–1. The importance of the ileocecal valve in large bowel obstruction.** If the ileocecal valve is competent **(left)**, pronounced cecal dilatation can occur. An incompetent valve **(right)** allows retrograde decompression into the small bowel.

gradual onset of distention and eventually feculent vomiting.[10, 11]

On physical examination, an abdominal mass may be present (advanced right-sided colon cancer), and distention may be most marked in one region (the left upper quadrant in cecal volvulus). Bowel sounds are often hyperactive, particularly with superimposed small bowel obstruction. Marked tenderness or rebound suggests perforation or strangulation.[10, 11]

## RADIOLOGIC APPROACH TO SUSPECTED LARGE BOWEL OBSTRUCTION

Abdominal plain films obtained in the supine and erect or left lateral decubitus positions are the initial means of imaging patients with suspected obstruction.[12, 13] These radiographs serve to confirm the diagnosis, locate the site of obstruction, and in some cases identify the nature of the obstructing lesion.[14–18] The plain film findings in bowel obstruction are discussed in detail in Chapter 13.

Plain abdominal radiographs can correctly diagnose obstruction in 60 to 70% of cases. Up to 20% of patients, however, have no radiographic evidence of obstruction.[19, 20] In patients with suspected large bowel obstruction, or in patients in whom the level of obstruction is unknown, a contrast enema, preferably with water-soluble media, is the next step. Although barium is inherently a better contrast agent, it may interfere with future studies, such as computed tomography (CT) or colonoscopy.[21] If the patient proves to have pseudo-obstruction, rather than true obstruction, the barium may remain within the colon for days.[21] A water-soluble enema can also be therapeutic in patients with fecal impactions.[21]

There is a danger that oral barium can inspissate proximal to a partial or complete large bowel obstruction.[22, 23] Therefore, it is important to clear the colon of an obstructing lesion before the small bowel is examined with barium. After obstructive colonic lesions have been excluded, the next step has traditionally been the oral administration of barium, the conventional small bowel follow-through. This procedure is often prolonged and produces inconclusive results because in patients with long-standing obstruction, barium slowly percolates through the dilated, fluid-filled loops and may take many hours to reach the level of obstruction.[24–26] By this time the barium column is usually diluted, and dilated overlying loops may obscure the obstructing site.[24]

Enteroclysis, ultrasound, and CT have been advocated as more direct means of establishing the diagnosis of intestinal obstruction.[24, 26–34]

**Enteroclysis.** Enteroclysis has an accuracy of 85% in detecting small bowel obstruction and is a far shorter procedure than the conventional small bowel follow-through.[27, 28] It is favored in patients with subacute or intermittent small bowel obstruction.

**Computed Tomography.** In one study, CT proved useful as a primary imaging technique in patients with a history of abdominal malignancy (Fig. 67–2) and clinical symptoms suggestive of bowel obstruction. CT has a secondary role in postsurgical patients who most likely have adhesive obstruction.[24] In patients without a history of surgery, CT is most valuable when there are systemic signs suggesting infection, bowel infarction, or an associated palpable mass. CT can also reveal the cause of obstruction, such as diverticulitis and appendicitis.[24] CT identifies bowel obstruction as distended bowel loops seen proximal to collapsed loops. The transitional zone should be carefully evaluated for masses. When no masses are present, the obstruction is usually due to adhesions.[24]

**Ultrasound.** In patients with suspected large bowel obstruction, ultrasound can be useful in integrating abdominal plain film findings with clinical information, particularly in patients with obstruction who have gasless abdomens (Fig. 67–3), obstructions not evidenced on radiographs, extremely high obstruction, or clinically occult incarcerated femoral hernias. Ultrasound differentiates intestinal obstruction and ileus in postoperative patients.[30–35]

Bowel obstruction should be suspected sonographically when there are multiple fluid-filled loops of bowel, bowel dilatation greater than 3 cm, prominent valvulae conniventes in the fluid-filled jejunum, and vigorous peristalsis. In acute obstruction, peristalsis is often quite vigorous, but as the bowel decompensates, the degree of peristalsis diminishes. It may then become disordered and show nonpropulsive to-and-fro or swirling motion of intraluminal echoes. Intraluminal fluid can vary in echogenicity from anechoic to echogenic with internal debris. The cause of obstruction, such as a tumor or hernia, is occasionally visualized.[30–35]

# MAJOR TYPES OF COLONIC OBSTRUCTION

## Carcinoma of the Colon

Nearly 20% of colon cancers are complicated by some degree of obstruction; 5 to 10% are complicated by complete obstruction that requires emergent surgical intervention.[36] The hospital mortality rate is high, in the range of 15 to 30%, even with right-sided cancers, which is a reflection of advanced age of patients, malnutrition, sepsis, and surgical stress.[3] Mortality is even higher if there is concurrent perforation. Large bowel obstruction is caused by intrinsic colon carcinoma in approximately 55% of cases.[37, 38]

The sigmoid colon is the most common site of obstructive colon cancer because of its relatively narrow diameter and solid fecal contents. The incidence of obstructive site in one series was as follows: rectum, 13%; sigmoid colon, 35%; descending colon, 10%; splenic flexure, 12%; transverse colon, 11%; hepatic flexure, 3%; and right colon, 16%.[38] The ratio of obstructive carcinomas to total tumors is similar in both the right and left colons.[39] The risk of developing obstruction in tumors at a particular site has been estimated as follows: 50% for splenic flexure lesions; 25% for right- and left-sided ones; and 6% for rectal tumors.[39, 40] Perforation occurs in 2% of all patients with colonic obstruction but in 12 to 18% of those with malignant obstruction. Tumors of the transverse colon and splenic flexure are at particular risk for obstruction before clinical detection.[41]

The clinical presentation of obstructive colon cancer depends on its location, duration, and completeness of obstruction, as well as the competency of the ileocecal valve. Tumors located near the ileocecal valve can produce symptoms suggesting a distal small bowel obstruction. Some right colon tumors act as lead points for colocolic intussusceptions; others may perforate, causing abscess formation and obstruction by means of ileus and edema. Left-sided colon tumors tend to obstruct the lumen in an annular fashion or by a polypoid lesion that reaches a size sufficient to obstruct the lumen. Feces and intussusception can acutely obstruct the colonic lumen. The rectum is not a common source of obstruction because of its greater width and distensibility and the fact that rectal cancers often cause rectal bleeding early, prompting earlier medical attention. The rectosigmoid can also be obstructed by direct invasion by gynecologic and prostatic neoplasms, as well as drop metastases to the pouch of Douglas.[1–5, 36, 40, 42]

## Diverticulitis

Large bowel obstruction can be attributed to diverticular disease in about 12% of cases. Diverticulitis can

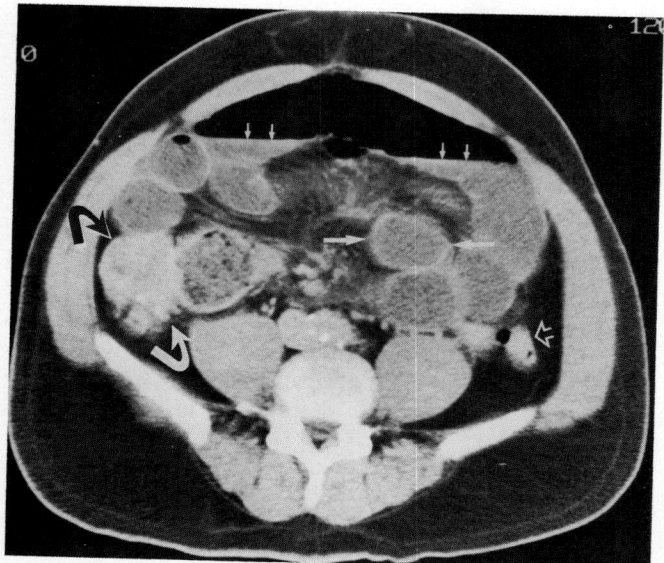

**Figure 67–2. The role of CT in bowel obstruction.** Plain films were normal for this patient who complained of distention, obstructive symptoms, and right lower quadrant pain. CT was the next examination obtained and showed a 3.5-cm mass *(curved arrows)* in the cecum. Dilated segments of fluid-filled small bowel *(large straight arrows)* are identified on this scan. One small bowel segment has a large air-fluid level *(small straight arrows)*. Note the normal-caliber descending colon *(open arrow)*.

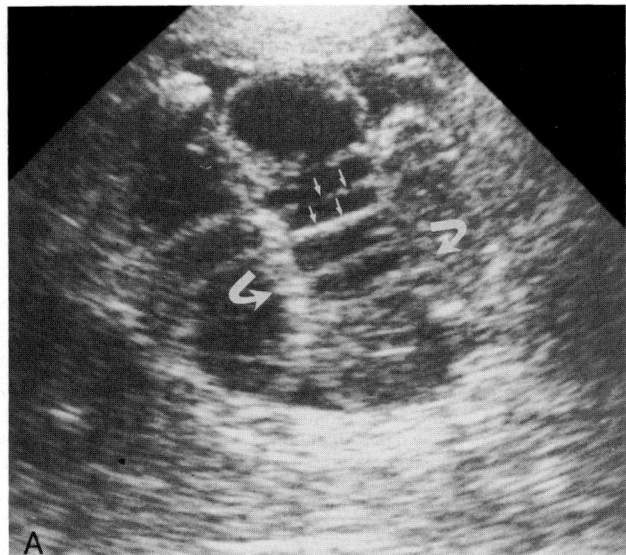

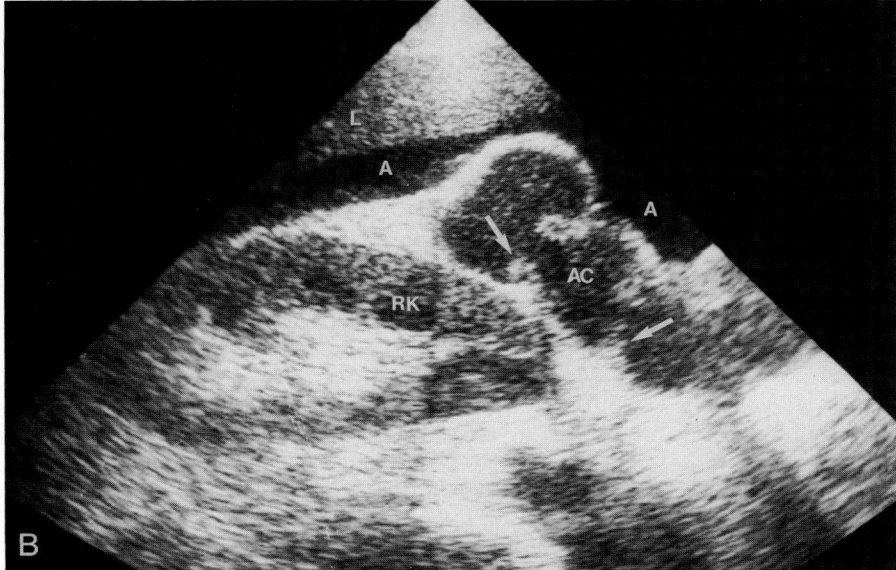

**Figure 67–3. The role of sonography in colonic obstruction.** This patient with carcinoma of the transverse colon presented with abdominal distention and a gasless abdomen on plain abdominal radiographs. **A.** Dilated, fluid-filled small bowel loops *(curved arrows)* are visualized on this periumbilical longitudinal sonogram. Individual valvulae conniventes *(straight arrows)* can be identified. **B.** Longitudinal sonogram demonstrates a dilated, fluid-filled ascending colon (AC). Individual haustra *(arrows)* are seen. A = ascites; L = liver; RK = right kidney.

cause both small and large bowel obstruction by mechanisms listed in Table 67–4. Partial colonic obstruction can complicate acute diverticulitis as a consequence of edema and pericolic inflammation or abscess formation. High-grade obstruction is uncommon; it is far more frequently caused by carcinoma of the colon. More commonly, obstruction follows recurrent attacks of diverticulitis with marked fibrosis of the colon wall leading to narrowing and eventually stricture formation. The site of obstruction is usually in the sigmoid colon, near the site of inflammation. Obstruction of the transverse or right colon attributable to diverticulitis is rare.[43, 44]

Clinically, patients with sigmoid diverticulitis complain of left lower quadrant pain, fever, and abnormal bowel habits. It is important for these symptoms to be differentiated from those of carcinoma of the colon, an often difficult task both clinically (Table 67–5) and radiologically (Table 67–6 and Fig. 67–4). Symptoms of rectal bleeding, constipation, and weight loss.[45–47]

Patients with suspected nonobstructing diverticulitis may benefit from CT examination as the initial study (Fig. 67–5). In the acutely obstructed patient, a water-soluble enema should be given to locate the site and cause of obstruction (see Chapter 61).[48, 49]

## Volvulus

Volvulus refers to torsion or twist of an organ on a pedicle to a degree sufficient to cause symptoms. Volvulus can affect the stomach, spleen, gallbladder, small bowel, right colon, transverse colon, splenic flexure, and sigmoid colon. Symptoms are caused by narrowing and obstruction of the gut or strangulation of the blood vessels, or both.[50]

## TABLE 67–4. FORMS OF INTESTINAL OBSTRUCTION COMPLICATING DIVERTICULAR DISEASE

Small bowel obstruction
  Localized ileus
  Adherence to inflammatory focus
  Twisting or kinking by adhesions
  Thickened or edematous bowel wall
Large bowel obstruction
  Angulated pelvic colon by adhesions
  Stricture after circumferential pericolic fibrosis
  Muscular contracture or spasm of redundant mucosa
  Volvulus of a giant sigmoid diverticulum
  Colonic pseudo-obstruction secondary to sepsis
  Compression by intramural or extramural abscesses
Combined small and large bowel obstruction

From Welch JP: Diverticular disease. *In* Welch JP (ed): Bowel Obstruction. Philadelphia: WB Saunders, 1990, pp 589–599.

## TABLE 67–6. SIGMOID DIVERTICULITIS VERSUS CARCINOMA: RADIOLOGIC DIFFERENTIATION

| DIVERTICULITIS | CARCINOMA |
| --- | --- |
| Spastic bowel | |
| Cone-shaped edges to narrowing | Normal adjacent bowel |
| Long segments | Sharp margins, shelf-like |
| Mucosa preserved | Short segments |
| Variable constriction between | Mucosa destroyed |
|   examinations | Progressive obstruction |
| Diverticular present | |
| Obstruction without tumor | Occasional diverticula |
| | Obstruction with tumor |

From Morton DL, Goldman L: Differential diagnosis of diverticulitis and carcinoma of the sigmoid colon. Am J Surg 103:55–61, 1962.

There are two major predisposing factors necessary for colonic volvulus: 1) a segment of redundant mobile colon and 2) relatively fixed point or points around which the volvulus may occur. Consequently, the sigmoid colon (50 to 75%), cecum (25 to 40%), and transverse colon (0 to 10%) are the most common sites of volvulus (Fig. 67–6). Other contributing factors include distention of the colon by feces or gas; increased muscular activity and changes in intraperitoneal relationships seen in pregnancy and parturition; previous abdominal surgery resulting in adhesions; congenital abnormalities, such as malrotation; and acquired obstructive lesions in the distal colon.[51–52] A more detailed discussion of colonic volvulus and its conventional radiographic features can be found in Chapter 13. On CT, a "whirl" sign has been described in volvulus (Fig. 67–7). The whirl is constituted by the afferent and efferent limbs leading into the volvulus. Tightly twisted mesentery and bowel compose the central portion of the whirl. The distal loop has a shape analogous to the "beak" sign seen on barium enema studies.[53, 54]

## Adult Intussusception

Intussusception is defined as the telescoping of one segment of the gastrointestinal tract into an adjacent

## TABLE 67–5. SIGMOID DIVERTICULITIS VERSUS CARCINOMA: CLINICAL DIFFERENTIATION

| FINDING | CARCINOMA | DIVERTICULITIS |
| --- | --- | --- |
| Previous attacks | Rare | Frequent |
| Illness onset | Gradual | Acute |
| Natural history of symptoms | Progressive | May subside |
| Lower abdominal pain | | |
|   Dull, constant | Rare | Common |
|   Cramping, intermittent | Common | Common |
| Rectal bleeding | Very frequent | Common, transient |
| Anemia | Common | Uncommon |
| Fever, leukocytosis | Uncommon | Common |

From Morton DL, Goldman L: Differential diagnosis of diverticulitis and carcinoma of the sigmoid colon. Am J Surg 103:55–61, 1962.

one (Fig. 67–8). It accounts for 80 to 90% of bowel obstruction in infants and children and ranks second only to appendicitis as the most common cause of an acute abdominal emergency in children. In children, the usual site of intussusception begins in the distal ileum; in 90% of cases, the cause is idiopathic.[1–4, 12] A complete discussion of childhood intussusception can be found in Chapter 78.

In contrast, intussusception in the adult is relatively

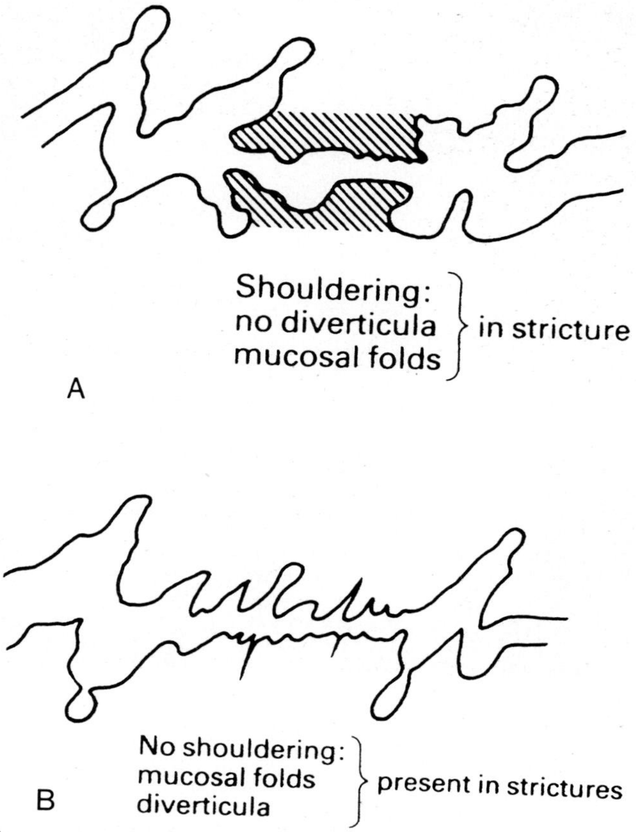

Shouldering:
no diverticula
mucosal folds } in stricture

A

No shouldering:
mucosal folds
diverticula } present in strictures

B

**Figure 67–4. Sigmoid diverticulitis versus carcinoma: barium enema findings. A.** Carcinoma in diverticular disease. **B.** Stricturing attributable to diverticular disease. (**A** and **B** from Bartram CT, Kumar P: Clinical Radiology in Gastroenterology. Oxford: Blackwell Scientific Publications, 1981, p 132.)

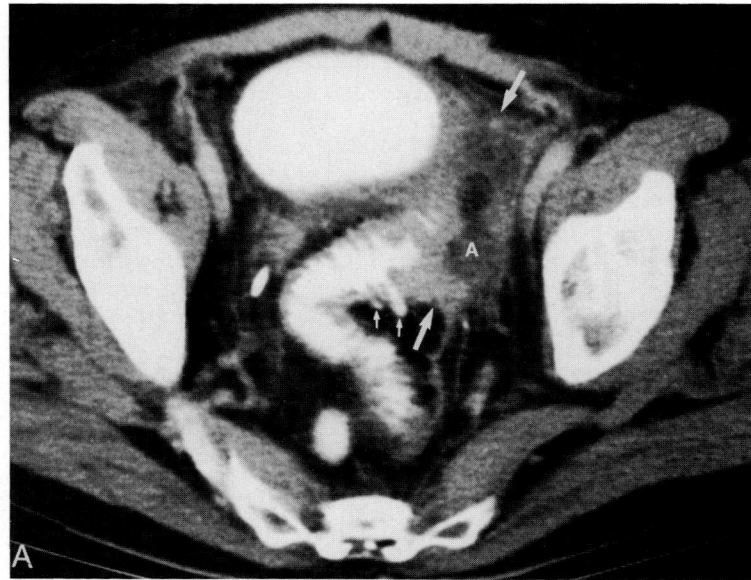

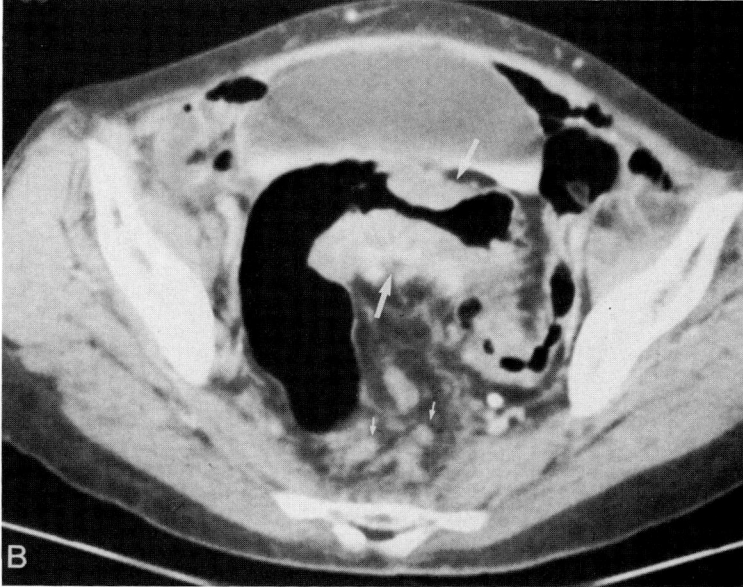

**Figure 67–5. Sigmoid diverticulitis versus carcinoma: CT findings. A**. Sigmoid diverticulitis. CT scan shows multiple diverticula *(small arrows)*, mural thickening, extensive inflammatory change *(large arrows)*, and an abscess (A) in the sigmoid mesocolon. **B**. Sigmoid cancer. The narrowing is over a more confined segment. An annular constricting mass *(large arrows)* and pelvic adenopathy *(small arrows)* are seen.

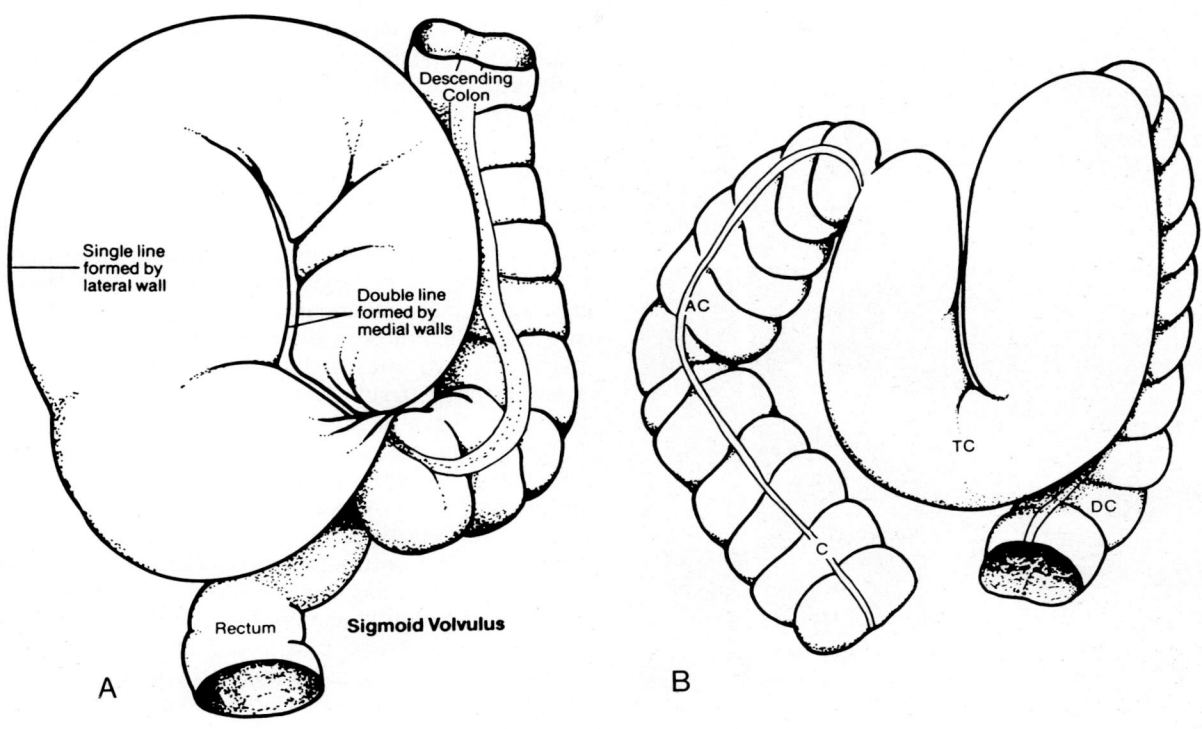

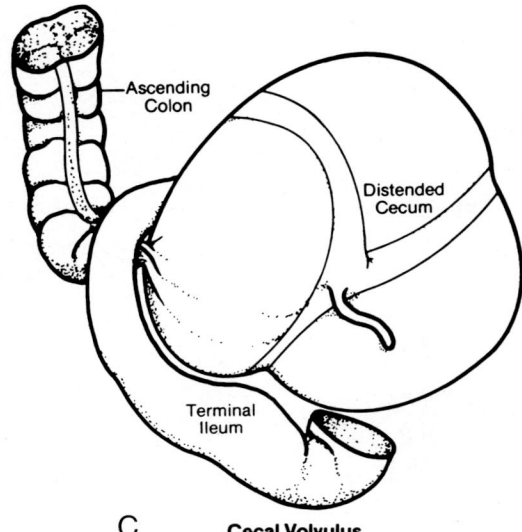

**Figure 67–6. The three major sites of colonic volvulus. A.** Sigmoid volvulus. Adjacent middle walls of the dilated sigmoid colon form a double line on plain films that converges on the point of twist in the sigmoid mesocolon. **B.** Transverse colonic volvulus. The caudal border of this ptotic colon is rounded, and the central double bowel wall does not extend to the sigmoid mesentery. AC = ascending colon; C = cecum; DC = descending colon; TC = transverse colon. **C.** Cecal volvulus. The dilated cecum twists clockwise, obstructing the ascending colon, while the terminal ileum swings around the dilated bowel. (**A**, **B**, and **C** from Rennell C, McCort JJ: Bowel gas and fluid. *In* McCort JJ [ed]: Abdominal Radiology. Baltimore: Williams & Wilkins, 1981, pp 97–180. © 1981, the Williams & Wilkins Co., Baltimore.)

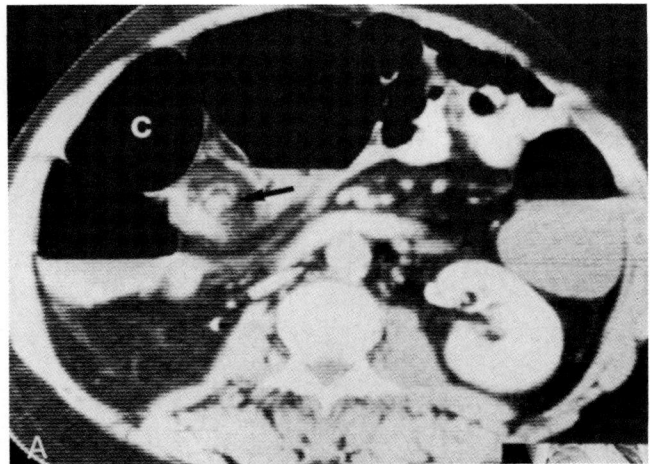

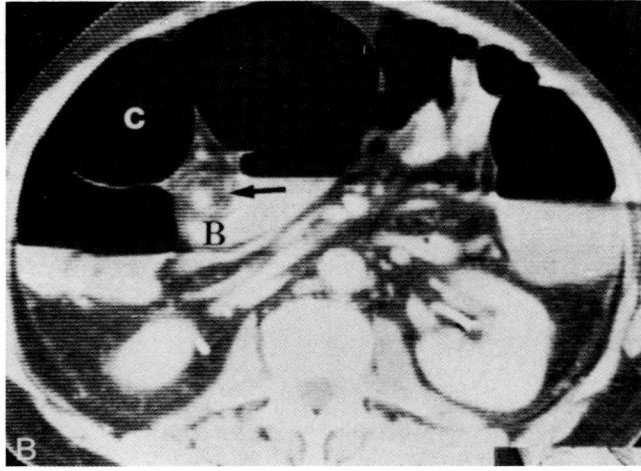

**Figure 67–7. CT of sigmoid volvulus. A** and **B**. Whirl sign of sigmoid volvulus. The central portion of the whirl is due to tightly twisted mesentery *(arrow)*. The distended proximal colon (C) demonstrates a beak sign (B) leading into the volvulus. (**A** and **B** from Shaff MI, Himmelfarb E, Sacks GA, et al: The whirl sign: a CT finding in volvulus of the large bowel. J Comput Assist Tomogr 9:410, 1985.)

rare; it accounts for only 5% of mechanical intestinal obstruction. A demonstrable cause is found in 80% of adult cases. Colonic intussusception is usually due to a primary colon cancer, whereas small bowel intussusception is usually related to a benign tumor and less often to a malignancy, most commonly a metastatic lesion.[55–65] Postoperative intussusceptions usually occur in the small bowel and are related to a number of factors: suture lines, ostomy closure, adhesions, long intestinal tubes, bypassed intestinal segments, submucosal edema, abnormal bowel motility, electrolyte imbalance, and chronic dilatation of the bowel.[65, 66]

Benign lesions that can serve as lead points in colonic intussusception include adenomatous polyp, lipoma, leiomyoma, appendiceal stump granulomas, and villous adenoma of the appendix.[65] The normal appendix may transiently intussuscept (see Chapter 69); clinically significant appendiceal intussusception usually occurs in the setting of appendiceal inflammation, infestation, neoplasm, or endometriosis deposition.[67] Intussuscep-

tion may develop in the postoperative adult patient owing to a suture line that serves as a lead point for the intussusception, adhesions, and the use of a long tube with balloon distention.[66]

General signs and symptoms of intestinal obstruction dominate the clinical picture of intussusception in the adult. The diagnosis is suggested by the presence of an abdominal mass and passage of blood per rectum. Because adult intussusception is often chronic and relapsing, the diagnosis is suggested by recurrent episodes of subacute obstruction and by variability of abdominal signs. During the height of an attack, a palpable mass may be present; this disappears completely when the patient is re-examined several hours later, by which time the symptoms have resolved.[3, 12]

If the intussusception is of the ileocolic or colocolic variety, the pathognomonic "crescent" sign (Fig. 67–9) may be seen. This sign is due to the fact that as the intussuscipiens invaginates into the intussusceptum, it stretches the outer wall; intraluminal gas trapped between the two intestinal surfaces can appear as a semilunar lucency, tracing haustral septa and valvulae conniventes. This lucent crescent is wider than normal bowel in diameter and is often superimposed on a round soft tissue density representing the mass created by the intussusception. A more central and less distinctive lucent arc may be seen as trapped gas situated in the lumen of the intussuscipiens. On supine views, the transverse colon gas shadow is often absent because this segment of colon is usually displaced distally.[13]

Whereas hydrostatic or pneumatic attempts at reducing intussusceptions in infants and young children should be attempted, the high incidence of organic, malignant lesions in adults precludes this approach.

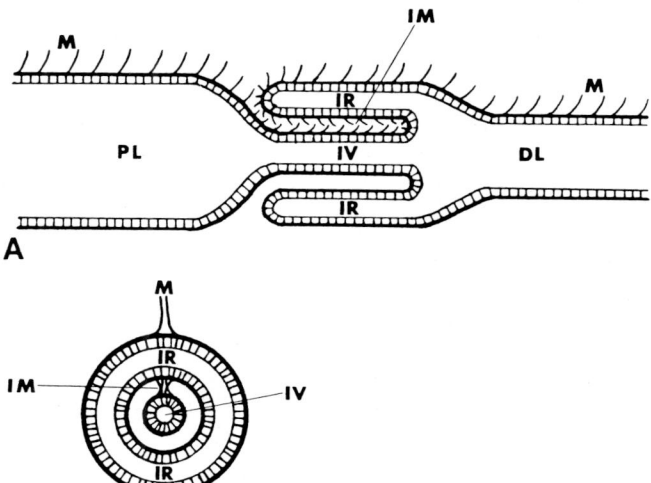

**Figure 67–8. Intussusception.** Longitudinal (**A**) and cross-sectional (**B**) diagrams of antegrade intussusception. IM = intussuscepted mesentery; IR = intussuscipiens; IV = intussusceptum; M = mesentery; PL and DL = proximal and distal intestinal loops. (**A** and **B** from BO Iko, JS Teal, SM Siram, et al, Computed tomography of adult colonic intussusception: clinical and experimental studies, AJR, 143, 4, 769–772, 1984, © by American Roentgen Ray Society.)

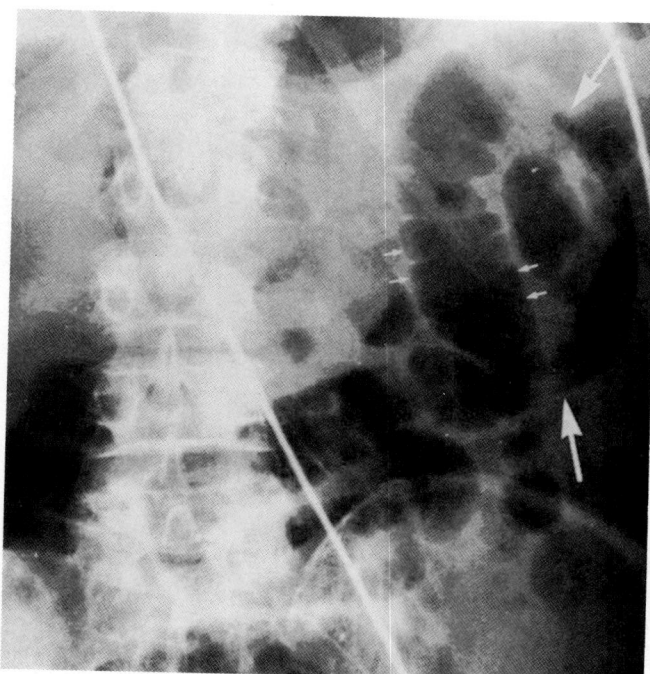

**Figure 67–9. Colonic intussusception: plain film findings**. Gas between the intussuscipiens and the stretched intussusceptum appears as a crescent *(large arrows)*. Within the arc of the crescent are nondescript collections of gas, which are present in the lumen of the intussuscipiens. The dilated small bowel loop *(small arrows)* indicates obstruction more distally. No gas is seen in the transverse colon because it is participating in the intussusception. (From Baker SR: The Abdominal Plain Film. East Norwalk, CT: Appleton & Lange, 1990, p 191.)

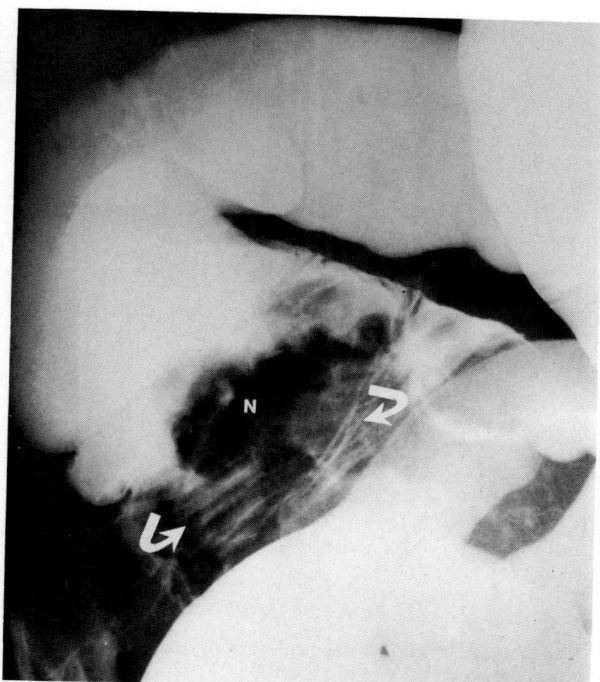

**Figure 67–10. Colonic intussusception: barium enema findings**. A cecal neoplasm (N) is intussuscepting into the ascending colon. Note the "coil spring" appearance *(arrows)*.

The classic appearance of intussusception on barium studies is the coil spring appearance as contrast is trapped between the intussusceptum and intussuscipiens (Fig. 67–10).

Ultrasound (Fig. 67–11) shows a target-like lesion, in which the hypoechoic halo is produced by the mesentery and the edematous wall of the intussuscipiens and the hyperechoic center is produced by multiple interfaces of compressed mucosal, submucosal, and serosal surfaces of the intussusceptum. Multiple concentric rings, best seen on transverse scans, are also characteristic. The corresponding appearance on longitudinal scans is that of multiple, thin, parallel, hypoechoic, and echogenic stripes.[68–71]

On CT scans (Fig. 67–12), intussusceptions appear as three different patterns, which reflect their severity and duration: 1) target sign; 2) sausage-shaped mass with alternating layers of low and high attenuation; and 3) reniform mass. Pathophysiologically, the target is the earliest stage of intussusception. As it progresses, a layering pattern, with alternating low-density (mesenteric fat) and high-attenuation areas (bowel wall), develops. If intussusception is untreated, edema and mural thickening develop. An intussusception with a reniform appearance is due to severe edema and vascular compromise, and this constitutes a surgical emergency. Intussusception is almost invariably associated with either acute intestinal obstruction or partial and recurrent

obstruction, air-fluid levels, and proximal bowel distention. The mesenteric arcade associated with the intussuscepted loop may show traction as it accompanies this eccentrically placed region of mesentery. If infarction occurs, this mass may be surrounded by intraperitoneal

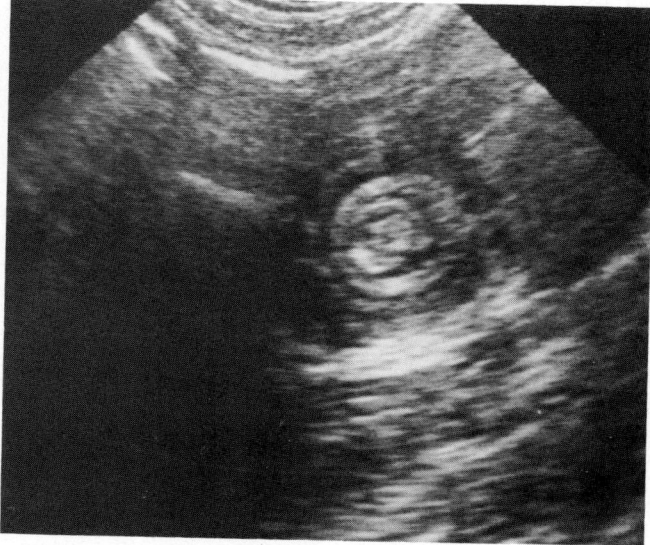

**Figure 67–11. Intussusception: sonographic findings**. On this axial image of the small bowel, the peripheral hypoechoic ring is due to the intussuscipiens, an intermediate hyperechoic area is caused by space between the intussuscipiens and intussusceptum, an internal hypoechoic ring is formed by the intussusceptum, and the central hypoechoic small area represents mucosa and the lumen of the intussusceptum. (Case courtesy of Stephanie A. Wilson, M.D., Toronto, Canada.)

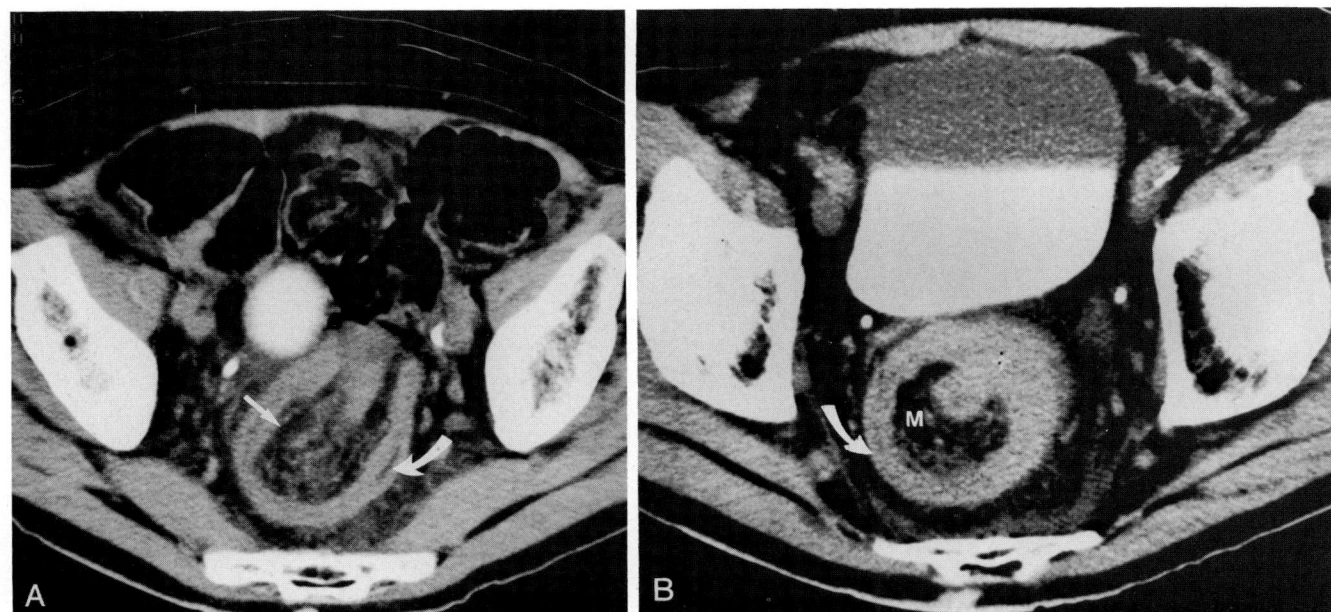

**Figure 67–12. Rectal intussusception: CT findings. This is the pathognomonic CT appearance of intussusception. A**. The curved arrow indicates the entering layer of intussusceptum, and the straight arrow demonstrates the mesentery. **B**. The arrow indicates the intussuscipiens. M = intussuscepted sigmoid mesocolon. (Case courtesy of Harvey M. Goldstein, M.D., San Antonio, Texas.)

fluid, edema and hemorrhage in the mesentery, and even perforation.[72–80]

## Adhesions

Adhesional large bowel obstruction is unusual because the colon is characteristically fixed and of large caliber; it is often thick walled and has protective appendices epiploicae. The small bowel, in contrast, has an inherently small caliber and a high degree of mobility; consequently, it is quite vulnerable to adhesional obstruction. As might be expected, the mobile, redundant portions of the colon are most likely to be involved by adhesive obstruction. Folding of the cecum on itself, the "cecal bascule," often occurs at the site of an adhesive band.[81–84]

The ascending colon can be obstructed by congenital bands or adhesions caused by inflammatory changes after colonoscopy and polypectomy.[85] Inflammation of the appendices epiploicae can rarely cause obstruction in the rectosigmoid, and ischemia and inflammation of the greater omentum can cause obstruction in the transverse colon.[86, 87]

## Hernias

Large bowel obstruction attributable to hernias (Fig. 67–13) is less common than small bowel obstruction because of the relatively fixed nature of the colon and its larger caliber.[88] Inguinal, femoral, umbilical, spigelian, incisional, and diaphragmatic hernias (congenital or post-traumatic) can all contain colon and cause bowel obstruction. Internal hernias, such as through the foramen of Winslow, can contain colon and cause obstruction as well.[89–95] A complete discussion of hernias can be found in Chapters 130 and 134.

## Obturation Obstruction

The terminal ileum is the narrowest portion of the gut and as a result is the most common site of obturation obstruction. In the large intestine, the sigmoid colon is the narrowest, measuring 2.5 cm in diameter (slightly wider than the distal ileum), followed by the hepatic and splenic flexures. These are the most likely points of colonic impaction of an intraluminal object.[96]

Some 3 to 5% of patients with gallstone ileus have colonic obstruction.[97] The gallstone most often bypasses the ileocecal valve through a cholecystocolic fistula and usually impacts in the sigmoid colon, which may be narrowed by prior diverticulitis.[96]

Bezoars, foods, and enteroliths usually do not affect the colon unless there is a stricture.[97–100] Patients with cystic fibrosis (see Chapter 118) tend to form large cecal masses of inspissated feces that can cause the meconium ileus equivalent syndrome.[101]

Sufficient amounts of various medications or diagnostic agents can cause colonic obturation obstruction. Antacid impactions containing nonabsorbable aluminum hydroxide antacid gels, given to prevent hyperphosphatemia, can develop in the right colons of patients having dialysis and renal transplantation. These impactions can be treated with orally or rectally administered hyperosmolar diatrizoate meglumine (Gastrografin).[96, 102]

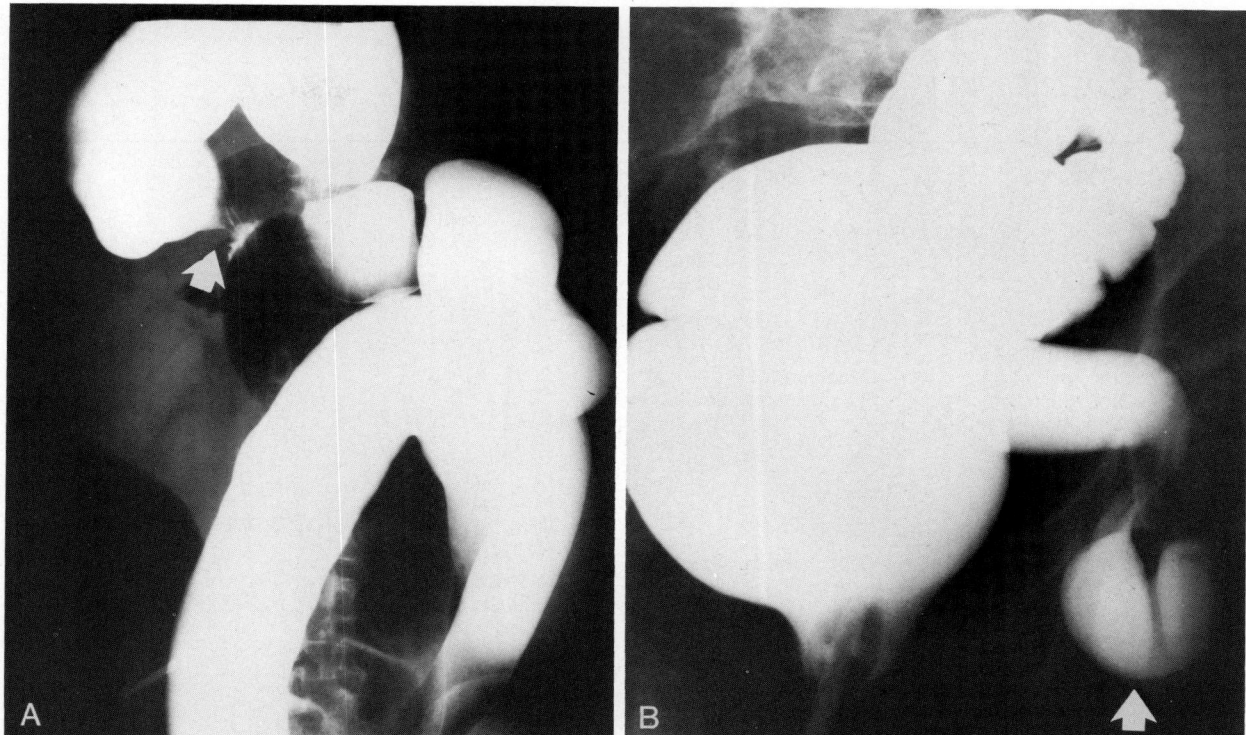

**Figure 67–13. Obstructive hernias. A.** The transverse colon is obstructed *(arrow)* by this diaphragmatic hernia. **B.** The sigmoid colon is obstructed in this older patient by an inguinal hernia *(arrow).*

Barium retained in the colon for several days is desiccated and can form impactions in any part of the colon, usually the proximal portion. These impactions can also be treated by hyperosmolar Gastrografin, which stimulates peristalsis and draws fluid into the bowel.[96, 103, 104] Foreign bodies entering via an oral or transanal route are becoming increasingly common and can cause obstruction or perforation.[105]

Elderly, inactive, debilitated, and mentally disturbed patients, drug addicts in methadone maintenance programs, transplantation and hemodialysis patients, and individuals with adult Hirschsprung's disease are at risk for developing fecal impaction. The most common sites are the rectum (70%) and sigmoid colon (20%). A fecaloma or stercoroma is a mass of fecal material that develops the characteristics of an intraluminal tumor. They are composed primarily of an accumulation of undigested food forming a nucleus around which fecal material accumulates. Obstruction, perforation, volvulus, stercoral ulceration, rectal prolapse, and rectal fissure are potential complications of fecalomas.[106, 107]

## Extrinsic Causes

The colon can be obstructed by diseases in adjacent organs. This most commonly occurs in the pelvis where the colon is fixed and confined by the bony pelvis. The transverse colon is another common location because of its omental and mesenteric attachments (see Chapter 65).

**Endometriosis.** The rectum and distal sigmoid colon are the most common sites of gastrointestinal involvement by endometriosis. These endometrial tissue implants can lead to obstruction by extrinsic compression or by inflammation and cicatrization. The obstruction is facilitated by tight adhesions to the uterus and edema and constriction of the bowel wall. Some 15 to 25% of women with rectosigmoid endometriosis have obstructive symptoms.[108] See Chapter 150 for a more detailed discussion of this disorder.

**Pancreatitis.** Approximately 1% of patients with acute pancreatitis have significant colonic problems (see Chapter 116). These complications usually occur 10 to 21 days after disease onset and may relate to compression caused by a pancreatic phlegmon or abscess and widespread fat necrosis or by mural thickening caused by edema and necrosis secondary to pancreatic enzymes dissecting down the transverse mesocolon or phrenicocolic ligament. Occasionally, a high-grade obstruction may occur that requires surgical intervention.[109–112]

**Metastases.** High-grade colonic obstruction is attributable much less often to metastatic than to primary tumors. Uterine, renal, and prostate neoplasms usually directly invade the colon. Gastric, ovarian, and pancreatic neoplasms can either directly invade the colon or narrow it by serosal metastases.[113]

Carcinoma of the prostate involves the rectum in 0.5 to 11% of cases and may simulate it clinically. Rectal obstruction occurs when there is direct extension through the thick, double-layered Denonvilliers' fascia

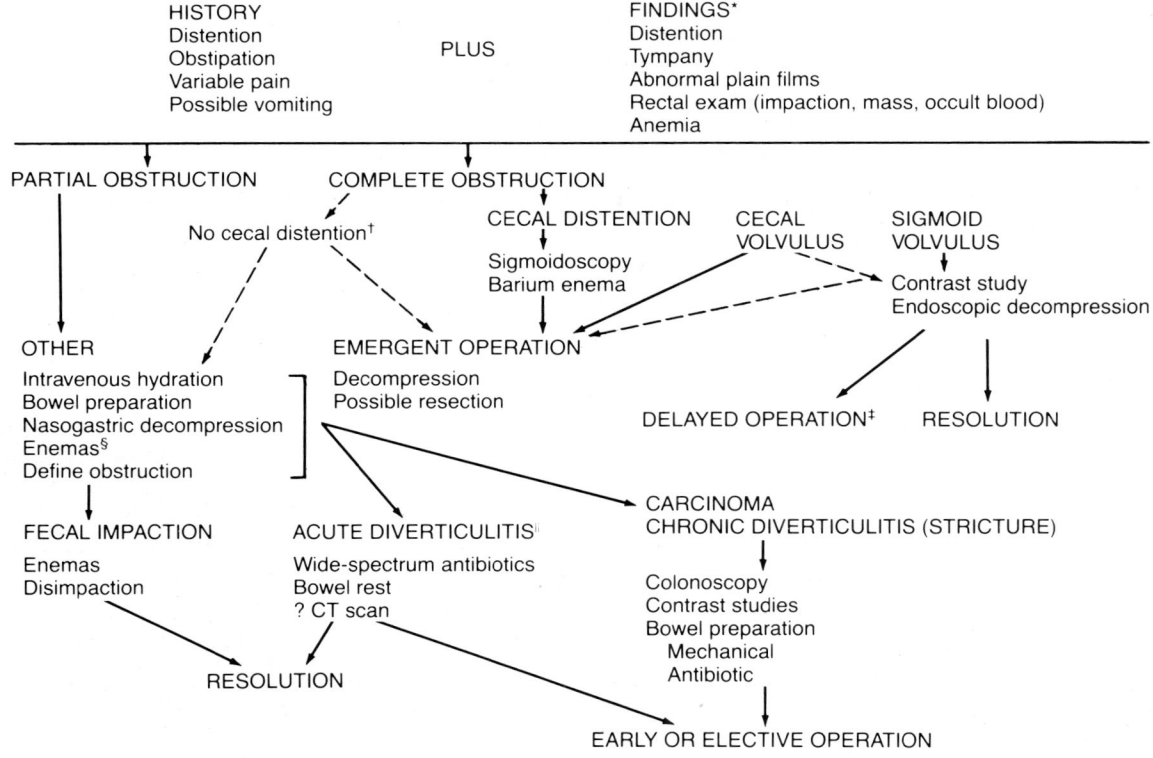

HISTORY
Distention
Obstipation                    PLUS
Variable pain
Possible vomiting

FINDINGS*
Distention
Tympany
Abnormal plain films
Rectal exam (impaction, mass, occult blood)
Anemia

PARTIAL OBSTRUCTION        COMPLETE OBSTRUCTION
                    No cecal distention†

CECAL DISTENTION    CECAL        SIGMOID
                    VOLVULUS     VOLVULUS

Sigmoidoscopy
Barium enema                     Contrast study
                                 Endoscopic decompression

OTHER                      EMERGENT OPERATION
Intravenous hydration      Decompression
Bowel preparation          Possible resection
Nasogastric decompression
Enemas§                                          DELAYED OPERATION‡    RESOLUTION
Define obstruction

FECAL IMPACTION        ACUTE DIVERTICULITIS‖

CARCINOMA
CHRONIC DIVERTICULITIS (STRICTURE)

Enemas                 Wide-spectrum antibiotics
Disimpaction           Bowel rest
                       ? CT scan            Colonoscopy
                                            Contrast studies
                                            Bowel preparation
                                              Mechanical
                                              Antibiotic
        RESOLUTION

                            EARLY OR ELECTIVE OPERATION

*If gangrene or perforation is suspected, emergent laparotomy is necessary.
†Seen with sigmoid volvulus, but rarely with obstructing cancer or diverticulitis.
‡Unless prohibitive operative risk.
§Avoid if perforation is suspected.
‖With or without abscess.

**Figure 67–14. An approach to mechanical large bowel obstruction.**

or by rectal compression caused by a massively enlarged prostate gland.[114, 115]

**Other Causes.** Pelvic lipomatosis, in which there is benign fatty tissue infiltration into the perirectal and perivesical spaces, usually causes straightening, narrowing, and rigidity of the rectum but occasionally can cause obstruction.[116] Pelvic masses such as large leiomyoma uteri, ovarian cyst and cancer, and pregnancy can also cause colonic obstruction. Mesenteric cysts, wandering spleen, retroperitoneal tumors, retractile mesenteritis, and retroperitoneal fibrosis are rarer causes of large bowel obstruction.[117–119]

## Strictures

Colonic strictures can result from a variety of disorders that are listed in Tables 70–4 to 70–6. These strictures often cause chronic obstructive symptoms and may cause acute obstruction owing to the presence of impacted feces or as a result of obturation in the stricture by some foreign object.

## SUMMARY

Bowel obstruction is a common and often difficult clinical problem. It requires the close cooperation of

internist, surgeon, and radiologist. One suggested approach to management of patients is given in Figure 67–14.

### Acknowledgment

Figures 67–1 and 67–14 are reproduced from Welch JP (ed): Bowel Obstruction. Philadelphia: WB Saunders, 1990.

## References

1. Welch JP: Mechanical obstruction of the small and large intestines. *In* Moody FG (ed): Surgical Treatment of Digestive Disease. Chicago: Year Book Medical Publishers, 1990, pp 624–654.
2. Cohn I: Intestinal obstruction. *In* Berk JE (ed): Bockus Gastroenterology (4th ed). Philadelphia: WB Saunders, 1985, pp 2056–2080.
3. Ellis H: Intestinal Obstruction. New York: Appleton-Century-Crofts, 1982.
4. Cohn I, Chappuis CW: Bowel obstruction. *In* Taylor MB (ed): Gastrointestinal Emergencies. Baltimore: Williams & Wilkins, 1992, pp 374–391.
5. Richards WO, Williams LF Jr: Obstruction of the large and small intestine. Surg Clin North Am 68:355–376, 1988.
6. Russell JC, Welch JP: Pathophysiology of bowel obstruction. *In* Welch JP (ed): Bowel Obstruction. Philadelphia: WB Saunders, 1990, pp 28–58.

7. Fielding LP: Implications of central and local hemodynamic changes during bowel obstruction. *In* Fielding LP, Welch JP (eds): Intestinal Obstruction. Edinburgh: Churchill Livingstone, 1987, pp 49–56.

8. Chappuis CW, Cohn J Jr: Pathophysiological effects on intraluminal contents. *In* Fielding LP, Welch JP (eds): Intestinal Obstruction. Edinburgh: Churchill Livingstone, 1987, pp 32–40.

9. Welch JP: General considerations and mortality. *In* Welch JP (ed): Bowel Obstruction. Philadelphia: WB Saunders, 1990, pp 59–95.

10. Nadrowski L: Clinical presentation and preoperative management of bowel obstruction. *In* Fielding LP, Welch JP (eds): Intestinal Obstruction. Edinburgh: Churchill Livingstone, 1987, pp 67–77.

11. Sugerman HJ: Systemic effects of intestinal obstruction. *In* Fielding LP, Welch JP (eds): Intestinal Obstruction. Edinburgh: Churchill Livingstone, 1987, pp 57–66.

12. Ellis H: Special forms of intestinal obstruction. *In* Schwartz SI, Ellis H (eds): Maingot's Abdominal Operations. East Norwalk, CT: Appleton & Lange, 1989, pp 905–932.

13. Baker SR: The Abdominal Plain Film. East Norwalk, CT: Appleton & Lange, 1990, pp 155–242.

14. Ziter FMH Jr: Radiologic diagnosis: small bowel. *In* Welch JP (ed): Bowel Obstruction. Philadelphia: WB Saunders, 1990, pp 96–107.

15. Markowitz KS: Radiologic diagnosis: colon. *In* Welch JP (ed): Bowel Obstruction. Philadelphia: WB Saunders, 1990, pp 108–122.

16. Gonzalez R, Siskind BN, Burrell MI: The role of radiology in the evaluation of intestinal obstruction. *In* Fielding LP, Welch JP (eds): Intestinal Obstruction. Edinburgh: Churchill Livingstone, 1987, pp 78–101.

17. Love L: Large bowel obstruction. Semin Roentgenol 8:299–321, 1973.

18. Levin B: Mechanical small bowel obstruction. Semin Roentgenol 8:281–297, 1983.

19. Lo AM, Evans WE, Carey LC: Review of small bowel obstruction at Milwaukee County General Hospital. Am J Surg 11:884–887, 1986.

20. Mucha P: Small intestinal obstruction. Surg Clin North Am 67:597–620, 1987.

21. Ott DJ, Gelfand DW: Gastrointestinal contrast agents. Indications, uses and risks. JAMA 249:2380–2384, 1983.

22. Grossman RI, Miller WT, Dann RW: Oral barium sulfate in partial large bowel obstruction. Radiology 136:327–331, 1980.

23. Frimann-Dahl JC: Administration of barium orally in acute obstructions: advantages and risks. Acta Radiol 42:285–288, 1954.

24. Megibow AJ, Balthazar EJ, Cho KC, et al: Bowel obstruction: evaluation with CT. Radiology 180:313–318, 1991.

25. Han SY, Laws HL, Aldrete JS: How and when to use barium for diagnosis of small bowel obstruction. South Med J 72:1519–1523, 1979.

26. Miller RE, Miller WJ: Small bowel obstruction: complete reflux small bowel examination. Am J Surg 10:572–577, 1985.

27. Caroline DF, Herlinger H, Laufer I, et al: Small bowel enema in the diagnosis of adhesive obstructions. AJR 142:1122–1139, 1984.

28. Maglinte DDT, Hall R, Miller RE, et al: Detection of surgical lesions of the small bowel by enteroclysis. Am J Surg 147:225–229, 1984.

29. Rubesin SE, Herlinger H: CT evaluation of bowel obstruction: a landmark article—implications for the future. Radiology 180:307–308, 1991.

30. Fukuya T, Hawes DR, Lo CC, et al: CT diagnosis of small-bowel obstruction: efficacy in 60 patients. AJR 158:765–769, 1992.

31. Meiser G, Meissner K: Ileus and intestinal obstruction: ultrasonographic findings as a guideline to therapy. Hepatogastroenterology 34:194–199, 1987.

32. Meiser G, Meissner K: Sonographic differential diagnosis of intestinal obstruction: result of a prospective study of 48 patients. Ultraschall Med 6:39–45, 1985.

33. Wilson SR: The gastrointestinal tract. *In* Rumack CM, Wilson SR, Charboneau JW (eds): Diagnostic Ultrasound. St. Louis: Mosby–Year Book, 1992, pp 181–207.

34. Carroll BR: US of the gastrointestinal tract. Radiology 172:605–608, 1989.

35. Seibert JJ, Williamson SL, Golladay ES, et al: The distended gasless abdomen: a fertile field for ultrasound. J Ultrasound Med 5:301–308, 1986.

36. Welch JP: Carcinoma of the colon. *In* Welch JP (ed): Bowel Obstruction. Philadelphia: WB Saunders, 1990, pp 546–574.

37. Phillips RKS, Hittinger R, Fry JS, et al: Malignant large bowel obstruction. Br J Surg 72:296–302, 1985.

38. Welch JP, Donaldson GA: Management of severe obstruction of the large bowel due to malignant disease. Am J Surg 127:492–499, 1974.

39. Vanek VW, Whitt CL, Abdu RA, et al: Comparison of right colon, left colon, and rectal carcinoma. Am Surg 52:504–509, 1986.

40. Turunen JM: Colorectal cancer obstruction: a challenge to improve diagnosis. Ann Chir Gynaecol 72:317–323, 1983.

41. Umpleby HC, Williamson RCN, Chir M: Survival in acute obstructing colorectal carcinoma. Dis Colon Rectum 27:299–304, 1984.

42. Irvin GL III, Horsely JS III, Caruana JA Jr: The morbidity and mortality of emergent operations for colorectal disease. Ann Surg 199:598–603, 1984.

43. Welch JP: Diverticular disease. *In* Welch JP (ed): Bowel Obstruction. Philadelphia: WB Saunders, 1990, pp 589–599.

44. Hughes LE: Complications of diverticular disease: inflammation, obstruction, and bleeding. Clin Gastroenterol 4:147–170, 1975.

45. Morton DL, Goldman L: Differential diagnosis of diverticulitis and carcinoma of the sigmoid colon. Am J Surg 103:55–61, 1962.

46. Schnyder P, Moss AA, Thoeni RF, et al: A double-blind study of radiologic accuracy in diverticulitis, diverticulosis, and carcinoma of the sigmoid colon. J Clin Gastroenterol 1:55–66, 1979.

47. Schatzki R: The roentgenologic differential diagnosis between cancer and diverticulitis of the colon. Radiology 34:651–662, 1940.

48. Balthazar EJ, Megibow A, Schinella RA, et al: Limitations in the CT diagnosis of acute diverticulitis: comparison of CT, contrast enema and pathologic findings in 16 patients. AJR 154:281–285, 1990.

49. Cho KC, Morehouse HT, Alterman DD, et al: Sigmoid diverticulitis: diagnostic role of CT—comparison with barium enema studies. Radiology 176:111–115, 1990.

50. Welch JP: Volvulus. *In* Welch JP (ed): Bowel Obstruction. Philadelphia: WB Saunders, 1990, pp 575–588.

51. Bubrick MP: Volvulus of the colon. *In* Gordon PH, Nivatvongs S (eds): Principles and Practice of Surgery for the Colon, Rectum, and Anus. St. Louis: Quality Medical Publishing, 1992, pp 799–816.

52. Kerry R, Ransom HK: Volvulus of the colon: etiology, diagnosis and treatment. Arch Surg 19:78–85, 1969.

53. Shaff MI, Himmelfarb E, Sacks GA, et al: The whirl sign: a CT finding in volvulus of the large bowel. J Comput Assist Tomogr 9:410, 1985.

54. Fisher JK: Computed tomographic diagnosis of volvulus in intestinal malrotation. Radiology 140:145–146, 1981.

55. Agha FP: Intussusception in adults. AJR 146:527–531, 1986.

56. Corang AG: Intussusception in adults. Am J Surg 177:735–738, 1969.

57. Dick A, Green CJ: Large bowel intussusception in adults. Br J Radiol 34:769–777, 1961.

58. Gupta S, Udupa KN, Gupta S: Intussusception in adults. Int Surg 61:231–233, 1976.

59. Briggs DF, Carpathios J, Zollinger RW: Intussusception in adults. Am J Surg 101:109–113, 1961.

60. Aston SJ, Machleder HI: Intussusception in the adult. Am Surg 41:576–580, 1975.

61. Lou CJ: Intussusception in adults: an analysis of 92 cases. Clin Med J 95:297–300, 1982.

62. Felix EL, Cohen MH, Bernstein AD, et al: Adult intussusception: case report and review of the literature. Am J Surg 131:758–761, 1976.

63. Stubenborg WT, Thorbjarnson B: Intussusception in adults. Ann Surg 172:306–310, 1970.

64. Burmeister RW: Intussusception in the adult: an elusive case of recurrent abdominal pain. Am J Dig Dis 7:360–374, 1962.

65. Orlando R III: Intussusception in adults. *In* Welch JP (ed): Bowel Obstruction. Philadelphia: WB Saunders, 1990, pp 229–240.

66. Sarr MG, Nagorney DM, McIlrath DC: Postoperative intussusception in the adult: a previous unrecognized entity? Arch Surg 116:144–148, 1981.

67. Levine MS, Trenkner SW, Herlinger H, et al: Coiled-spring sign of appendiceal intussusception. Radiology 155:41–44, 1985.

68. Verbanck JJ, Rutgeerts LJ, Douterlungne PH, et al: Sonographic and pathologic correlation intussusception of the bowel. J Clin Ultrasound 14:393–397, 1986.

69. Parienty RA, LePreux JF, Gruson B: Sonography and CT features of ileocolic intussusception. AJR 136:608–610, 1981.

70. Alessi V, Salerno G: The "hay-fork" sign in the ultrasonographic diagnosis of intussusception. Gastrointest Radiol 10:177–179, 1985.

71. Rao BK, Fleischer AC: Sonography of the gastrointestinal tract. Curr Opin Radiol 2:207–212, 1990.

72. Iko BO, Teal JS, Siram SM, et al: Computed tomography of adult colonic intussusception: clinical and experimental studies. AJR 143:769–772, 1984.

73. Lorigan JG, DuBrow RA: The computed tomographic appearances and clinical significance of intussusception in adults with malignant neoplasms. Br J Radiol 63:257–263, 1990.

74. Bar-Ziv J, Solomon A: Computed tomography in adult intussusception. Gastrointest Radiol 10:355–357, 1985.

75. Pottmeyer A, McDowell J, Lang EK: CT findings of a rectal intussusception. AJR 156:870, 1991.

76. Skaane P, Schindler G: Computed tomography of adult ileocolic intussusception. Gastrointest Radiol 10:355–357, 1985.

77. Yoshimitsuk F, Fukuya T, Onitsuka H, et al: Computed tomography of ileoileocolic intussusception caused by a lipoma. J Comput Assist Tomogr 13:704–706, 1989.

78. Styles RA, Larsen CR: CT appearance of adult intussusception. J Comput Assist Tomogr 7:331–333, 1983.

79. Balthazar EJ: CT of the gastrointestinal tract, principles and interpretation. AJR 156:23–32, 1991.

80. Hodgman CG, Lantz EJ, Maustr RJ, et al: Computed tomography of intussusception due to colon lipoma. J Comput Assist Tomogr 11:740–741, 1987.

81. Holt RW, Wagner RC: Adhesional obstruction of the colon. Dis Colon Rectum 27:314–315, 1984.

82. Twersky J, Himmelfarb E: Right colonic adhesions. Radiology 120:37–40, 1976.

83. Welch JP: Extrinsic causes. *In* Welch JP (ed): Bowel Obstruction. Philadelphia: WB Saunders, 1990, pp 640–653.

84. Brodey PA, Schuldt DR, Magnuson A, et al: Complete colonic obstruction secondary to adhesions. AJR 133:917–918, 1979.

85. Bonello JC, Kasten JM, Slezak FA: Large bowel obstruction following colonoscopic polypectomy. Contemp Surg 29:39–41, 1986.

86. Carmichael DH, Organ CH Jr: Epiploic disorders. Conditions of the epiploic appendages. Arch Surg 120:1167–1172, 1985.

87. Harte MS: Chronic partial intestinal obstruction due to intussusception of an appendix epiploica. Surgery 13:555–560, 1943.

88. Welch JP: Hernias causing bowel obstruction. *In* Welch JP (ed): Bowel Obstruction. Philadelphia: WB Saunders, 1990, pp 241–313.

89. Farrell B, Gerard PS, Bryk D: Paraesophageal hernia causing colonic obstruction. J Clin Gastroenterol 13:188–190, 1991.

90. Pritchard GA, Price-Thomas JM: Internal hernia of the transverse colon. Dis Colon Rectum 29:658–659, 1986.

91. Richardson JB, Anastopoulos HA: Hernia through the foramen of Winslow. MD State Med J 58:56–59, 1981.

92. Bryk D: Spigelian hernia containing sigmoid colon. AJR 99:71–73, 1962.

93. Javors BR, Bryk D: Colonic obstruction with inguinal hernia. J Can Assoc Radiol 32:162–163, 1981.

94. Blatt ES, Schneider H, Wiot JF, et al: Roentgen findings in obstructed diaphragmatic hernia. Radiology 79:649–657, 1962.

95. Gravier L, Freark RJ: Traumatic diaphragmatic hernia. Arch Surg 86:363–373, 1963.

96. Welch JP: Intrinsic causes. *In* Welch JP (ed): Bowel Obstruction. Philadelphia: WB Saunders, 1990, pp 654–671.

97. Holm-Nielsen P, Linnet-Jepsen P: Colon obstruction caused by gallstones. Acta Chir Scand 107:31–41, 1954.

98. Young WV Jr: Gallstone ileus of the colon. Report of an unusual type of colon obstruction. Arch Surg 82:333–336, 1961.

99. Price JE, Michel SL, Morgenstern L: Fruit pit obstruction. Arch Surg 111:773–775, 1976.

100. Cotner M: Fecal impaction due to bubblegum bezoar. South Med J 75:775–776, 1982.

101. Matseshe JW, Go VL, DiMagno EP: Meconium ileus equivalent complicating cystic fibrosis in post neonatal children and young adults. Gastroenterology 72:732–736, 1977.

102. Welch JP, Schweizer RT, Bartus SA: Management of antacid impactions in hemodialysis and renal transplant patients. Am J Surg 139:561–568, 1980.

103. Culp WC: Relief of severe rectal impactions with water-soluble contrast enemas. Radiology 115:9–12, 1975.

104. Zer M, Rubin M, Dintsman M: Dissolution of barium-impaction ileus by Gastrografin. Dis Colon Rectum 21:430–434, 1978.

105. Eftaiha M, Hambrick E, Abcarian H: Principles of management of colorectal foreign bodies. Arch Surg 112:691–695, 1977.

106. Segall H: Obstruction of large bowel due to fecaloma: successful medical treatment in two cases. Calif Med 108:54–56, 1968.

107. Welch JP: Constipation. *In* Welch JP (ed): Bowel Obstruction. Philadelphia: WB Saunders, 1990, pp 616–626.

108. Tate GT: Acute obstruction of the large bowel due to endometriosis. Br J Surg 50:771–773, 1963.

109. Aronson AR, Davis DA: Obstruction near hepatic flexure in pancreatitis. A rarely reported sign. JAMA 176:451–454, 1961.

110. Brearly S, Cambell DJ: Stenosis of the colon following acute pancreatitis. Postgrad Med J 58:293–296, 1982.

111. Thompson WM, Kelvin FM, Rice RP: Inflammation and necrosis of the transverse colon secondary to pancreatitis. AJR 128:943–948, 1977.

112. Mann NS: Colonic involvement in pancreatitis. Am J Gastroenterol 73:357–362, 1980.

113. Khilnani MT, Wolf BS: Late involvement of the alimentary tract by carcinoma of the kidney. Am J Dig Dis 5:529–540, 1960.

114. Fry DE, Amin M, Harbrecht PJ: Rectal obstruction secondary to carcinoma of the prostate. Ann Surg 189:488–492, 1979.

115. Ruggiero RP, Chang H: Rectal involvement by carcinoma of the prostate. Am J Gastroenterol 81:372–374, 1986.

116. Jones DJ, Dharmeratnam R, Langstaff RJ: Large bowel obstruction due to pelvic lipomatosis. Ann Surg 71:309–311, 1985.

117. Le Fall LD Jr, White JM, Mann M: Retroperitoneal fibrosis: two unusual cases. Arch Surg 89:1070–1076, 1964.

118. Williams RG, Nelson JA: Retractile mesenteritis: initial presentation as colonic obstruction. Radiology 126:35–37, 1978.

119. Sirinek KR, Livingston CD, Bova JG, et al: Bowel obstruction due to infarcted splenosis. South Med J 77:764–767, 1984.

# Rectum

Stephen E. Rubesin, M.D.
Mitchell D. Schnall, M.D., Ph.D.

## INTRODUCTION

The rectum is an organ of great social importance and interest. As an integral part of the colon, the rectum is prone to all diseases of the colon that have been discussed in Chapters 57 through 71. In addition, as a part of the gastrointestinal tract that communicates with the outside world, the rectum suffers traumatic and venereal diseases that do not involve the remainder of the colon. Disorders of defecation specific to the rectum are discussed in Chapter 58. Developmental disorders of the anus or rectum in Hirschsprung's disease are discussed in Chapter 78. Some conditions discussed in this chapter are more extensively discussed in chapters concerned with polyps, carcinoma, the polyposis syndromes, Crohn's disease, ulcerative colitis, other tumors of the colon, and inflammatory conditions of the colon.

Barium techniques for studying the rectum are extensively discussed in Chapter 57. Sonography and endoscopic ultrasonography are discussed in Chapters 7 and 10. High-resolution endorectal magnetic resonance (MR) imaging is an exciting new technique that allows the radiologist to see the anatomy within the rectal wall and may prove useful in evaluation of rectal carcinoma.[1, 2] Principles of MR imaging are discussed in Chapter 9.

## ANATOMY[3–6]

The rectum is 12 to 15 cm long, extending from the rectosigmoid junction to the anal canal. The rectum descends along the curve of the sacrum, from S-3 to slightly below the coccyx (Fig. 68–1). The location of the rectosigmoid junction is identified anatomically by the absence of the posterior peritoneum, appendices epiploicae, and haustral sacculations. The taeniae coli fuse at the rectosigmoid junction, approximately 6 cm from the anterior peritoneal reflection, to form a complete longitudinal muscle layer. Anterior and posterior thickenings of the longitudinal muscle layer cause rectal shortening resulting in three gross rectal flexures. The upper and lower rectal flexures are convex to the right; the middle flexure is convex to the left.

The upper third of the rectum is covered by peritoneum anteriorly and laterally, the middle third is covered by peritoneum only on its anterior surface, and the lower third is subperitoneal. In the female, the rectum is separated from the uterine cervix and the posterior fornix of the vagina by the rectouterine pouch (pouch of Douglas) (Fig. 68–2). The peritoneal reflection is lower in females than in males. In males, the rectovesical pouch separates the rectum from the seminal vesicles and the base of the urinary bladder. The peritoneal

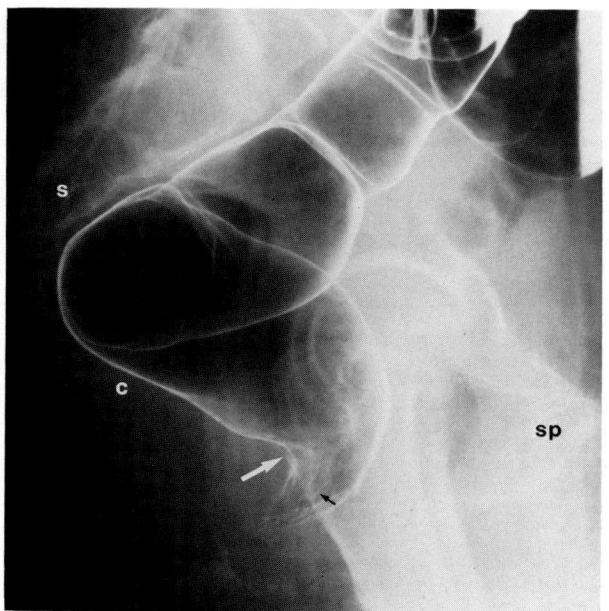

**Figure 68–1. Location of the rectum.** Prone, cross-table lateral view shows the rectum coursing anterior to the sacrum (s) and coccyx (c). The symphysis pubis (sp) is identified. The impression of the pubo-rectalis muscle (sling) is seen on the posterior wall of the rectum *(white arrow)*. Note that this patient with mild pelvic floor relaxation has a significant amount of air-distended rectum distal to the pubo-rectalis sling. The columns of Morgagni are seen faintly *(black arrow)*.

reflection is not fixed in position but extends cranially when the rectum is distended. The rectum can distend laterally into potential spaces—the pararectal fossae. The rectum has an inner circular muscle layer and a complete outer longitudinal muscle layer. In the distal rectum and anal canal, the inner circular muscle layer thickens to form a 2.5-cm-long involuntary internal anal sphincter.

The pelvic diaphragm is composed of a series of muscles that provide hammock-like support for the pelvic viscera (Figs. 68–3 to 68–5). The pelvic diaphragm is composed of two paired muscles: the levator ani and the coccygeus[3] (see Figs. 68–3 to 68–5). The paired levator ani muscles are composed of two main parts, the pubococcygeus and the iliococcygeus. The pubococcygeus is divided artificially into three parts. Its medial fibers attach to the prostate (the levator prostate) or vagina (pubovaginalis). The fibers of the midportion of the pubococcygeus form a U-shaped loop, the puborectalis, a sling-shaped muscle that supports the rectum and causes a 90-degree bend between the anteriorly coursing distal rectum and the posteriorly coursing anal canal. More laterally, the pubococcygeus proper inserts into the coccyx and anococcygeal ligament. The iliococcygeus is the most lateral and posterior part of the levator ani muscle. As the anal canal passes through the pelvic diaphragm, the levator ani muscle blends with the longitudinal muscle layer of the rectum. The fibers of the levator ani–internal longitudinal muscle layer of the colon then divide into tendinous insertions into both the internal and external anal sphincter (Fig. 68–6).

The external anal sphincter is a skeletal muscle surrounding the longitudinal layer of the anal canal (see Figs. 68–4 and 68–6). The external anal sphincter is divided into subcutaneous, superficial, and deep parts by various vascular structures (see Fig. 68–6).

Several arteries supply the rectum. The upper rectum is supplied by the superior rectal branch of the inferior mesenteric artery. The middle portion of the rectum is supplied by the middle rectal arteries from the internal iliac vessels. The lower rectum is supplied by the inferior rectal arteries from the internal pudendal vessels.

Above the pectinate line, venous drainage is into the internal rectal venous plexus in the submucosa (see Fig. 68–6). Drainage of the internal venous plexus is into the superior rectal vein, a tributary of the inferior mesenteric vein. Below the pectinate line, veins drain into the external venous plexus in the perianal space and hence into the internal pudendal vein and the inferior vena cava. The perimuscular plexus drains into the inconstant middle rectal veins.[3]

The lymphatic drainage of the rectum is important in understanding several inflammatory conditions involving the rectum, such as lymphogranuloma venereum and the pattern of metastasis of anorectal cancers. The lymphatic drainage of the upper rectum is along the course of the superior rectal vessels. Therefore, upper rectal cancers drain into the lymphatics coursing along the inferior mesenteric vessels. The lower portion of the rectum drains into three major lymph node sites. The lower rectum drains along the superior rectal vessels to

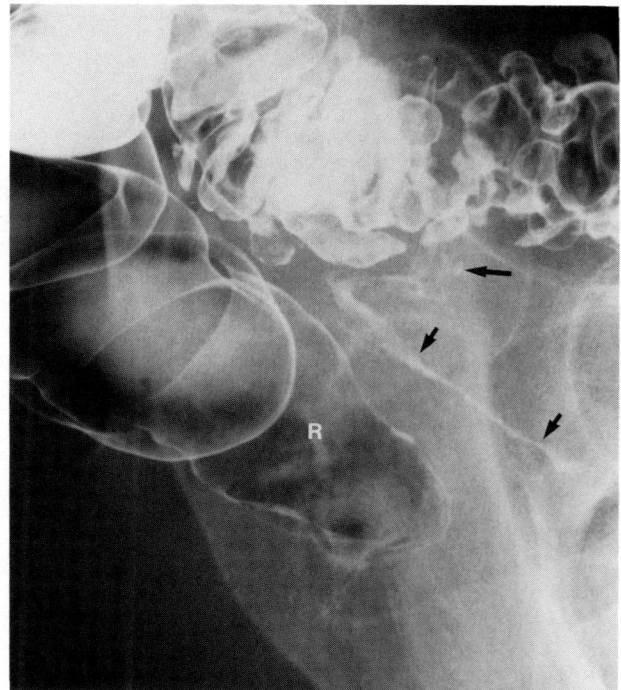

**Figure 68–2. Relationship of the rectum to the vagina.** Steep oblique view of the rectum shows the air-distended distal rectum (R) paralleling the course of the vagina *(short arrows)*. The vagina was filled with barium because a sigmoid-to-vaginal fistula *(long arrow)* was present, secondary to diverticulitis of the sigmoid colon.

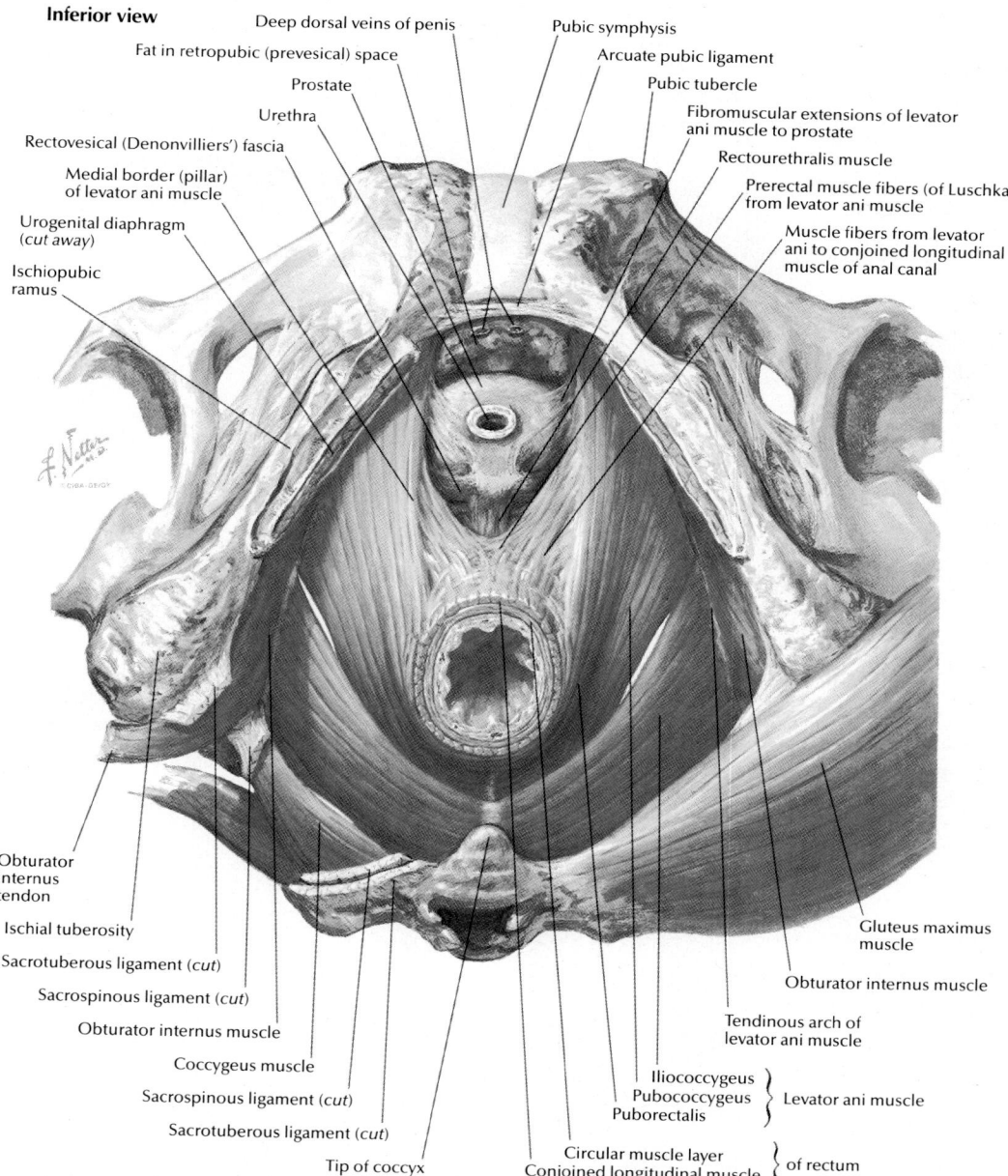

**Inferior view**

Deep dorsal veins of penis

Fat in retropubic (prevesical) space

Prostate

Urethra

Rectovesical (Denonvilliers') fascia

Medial border (pillar)
of levator ani muscle

Urogenital diaphragm
(cut away)

Ischiopubic
ramus

Pubic symphysis

Arcuate pubic ligament

Pubic tubercle

Fibromuscular extensions of levator
ani muscle to prostate

Rectourethralis muscle

Prerectal muscle fibers (of Luschka)
from levator ani muscle

Muscle fibers from levator
ani to conjoined longitudinal
muscle of anal canal

Obturator
internus
tendon

Ischial tuberosity

Sacrotuberous ligament (*cut*)

Sacrospinous ligament (*cut*)

Obturator internus muscle

Coccygeus muscle

Sacrospinous ligament (*cut*)

Sacrotuberous ligament (*cut*)

Tip of coccyx

Gluteus maximus
muscle

Obturator internus muscle

Tendinous arch of
levator ani muscle

Iliococcygeus
Pubococcygeus  } Levator ani muscle
Puborectalis

Circular muscle layer     } of rectum
Conjoined longitudinal muscle

**Figure 68–3. Inferior view of pelvic diaphragm.** The paired coccygeal and levator ani muscles form the pelvic diaphragm. Each levator ani is divided into two main parts: the iliococcygeus and the pubococcygeus. The pubococcygeus is artificially divided in three parts. Medial fibers of the pubococcygeus form a sling around the rectum—the puborectalis. This muscle directly supports the rectum. Other fibers of the pubococcygeus pass to the prostate in a male or vagina in a female. (© Copyright 1989 CIBA-GEIGY Corporation. Reproduced with permission from Atlas of Human Anatomy by Frank H. Netter, M.D. All rights reserved.)

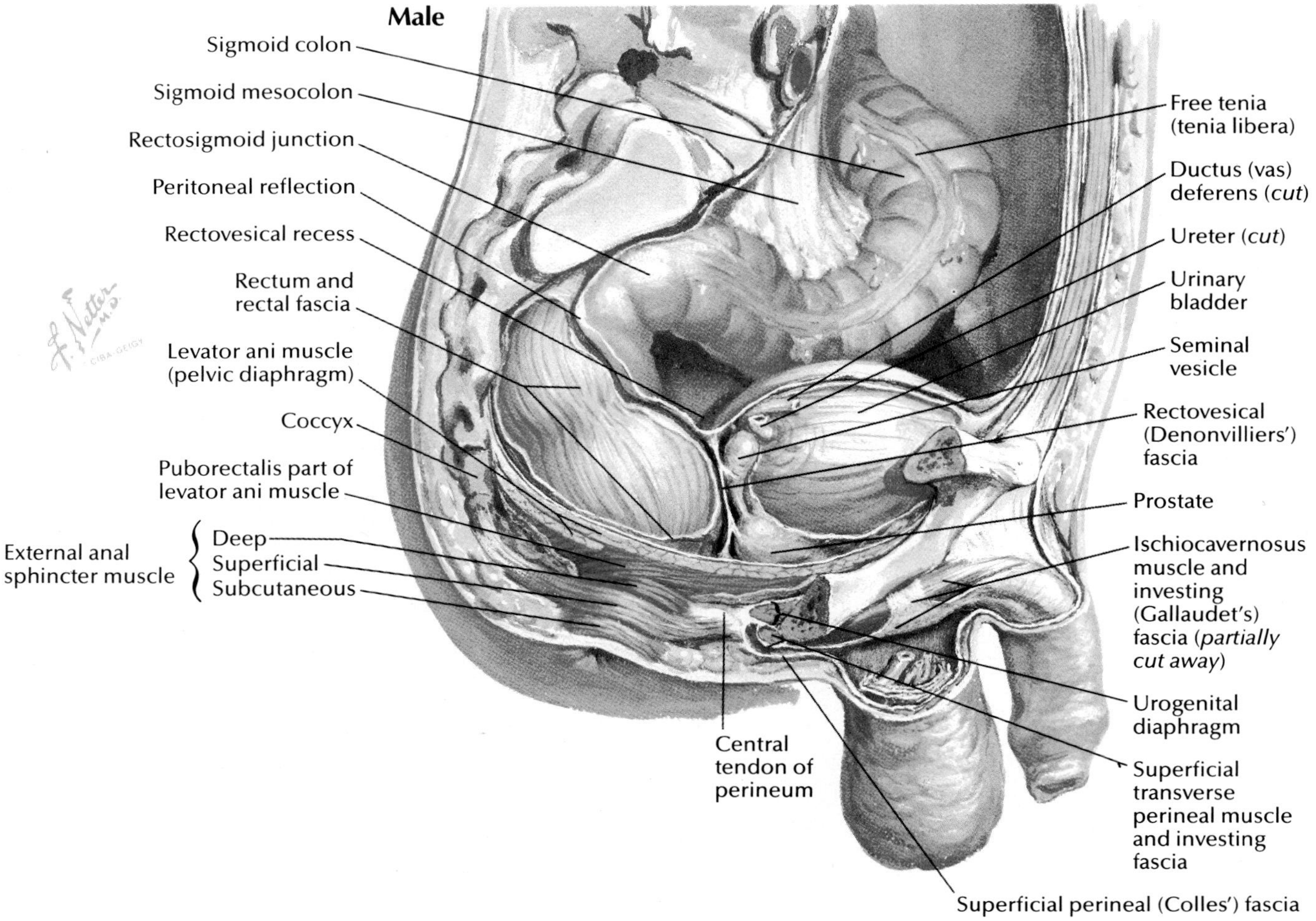

**Male**

Sigmoid colon

Sigmoid mesocolon

Rectosigmoid junction

Peritoneal reflection

Rectovesical recess

Rectum and rectal fascia

Levator ani muscle (pelvic diaphragm)

Coccyx

Puborectalis part of levator ani muscle

External anal sphincter muscle { Deep — Superficial — Subcutaneous —

Central tendon of perineum

Free tenia (tenia libera)

Ductus (vas) deferens (*cut*)

Ureter (*cut*)

Urinary bladder

Seminal vesicle

Rectovesical (Denonvilliers') fascia

Prostate

Ischiocavernosus muscle and investing (Gallaudet's) fascia (*partially cut away*)

Urogenital diaphragm

Superficial transverse perineal muscle and investing fascia

Superficial perineal (Colles') fascia

**Figure 68–4. Lateral view of the rectum.** Lateral view of the pelvis from the right side shows the rectum anterior to the sacrum and coccyx. The hammock-like sling of the levator ani muscle is demonstrated. (© Copyright 1989 CIBA-GEIGY Corporation. Reproduced with permission from Atlas of Human Anatomy by Frank H. Netter, M.D. All rights reserved.)

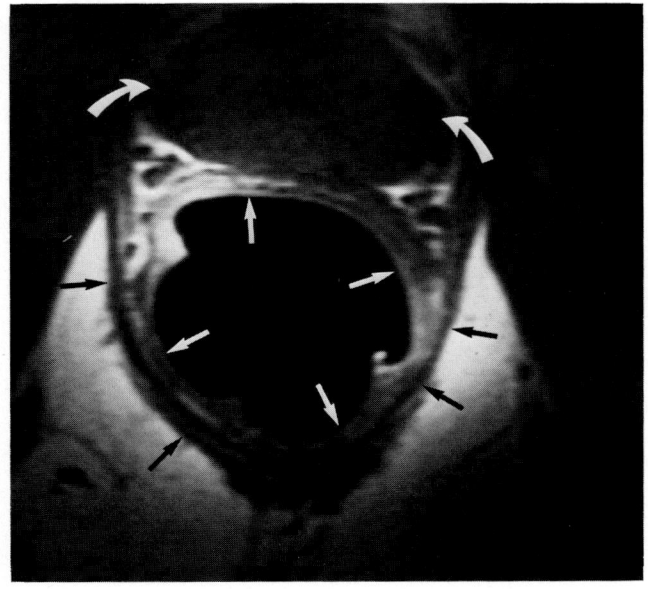

**Figure 68–5. The levator sling.** T1-weighted axial spin-echo image obtained with an endorectal surface coil shows the levator sling (*black arrows*) as a low signal curving around the rectal wall (*straight white arrows*). The prostate gland is identified (*curved white arrows*).

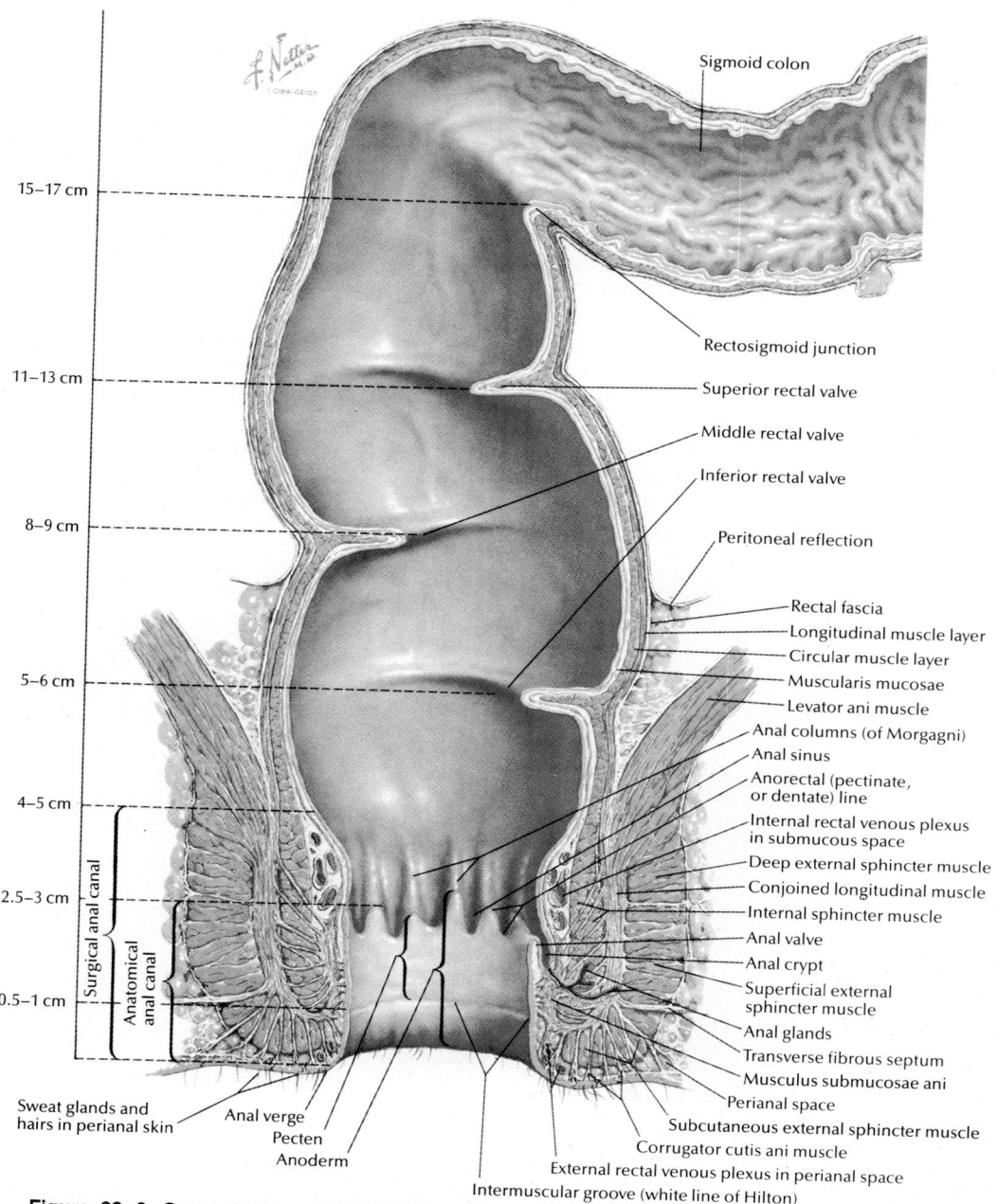

15–17 cm

11–13 cm

8–9 cm

5–6 cm

4–5 cm

2.5–3 cm

0.5–1 cm

Surgical anal canal

Anatomical anal canal

Sigmoid colon

Rectosigmoid junction

Superior rectal valve

Middle rectal valve

Inferior rectal valve

Peritoneal reflection

Rectal fascia

Longitudinal muscle layer

Circular muscle layer

Muscularis mucosae

Levator ani muscle

Anal columns (of Morgagni)

Anal sinus

Anorectal (pectinate, or dentate) line

Internal rectal venous plexus in submucous space

Deep external sphincter muscle

Conjoined longitudinal muscle

Internal sphincter muscle

Anal valve

Anal crypt

Superficial external sphincter muscle

Anal glands

Transverse fibrous septum

Musculus submucosae ani

Perianal space

Subcutaneous external sphincter muscle

Corrugator cutis ani muscle

External rectal venous plexus in perianal space

Intermuscular groove (white line of Hilton)

Sweat glands and hairs in perianal skin

Anal verge

Pecten

Anoderm

**Figure 68–6. Coronal view of the rectum.** The levator ani joins the longitudinal muscle of the rectum to form the conjoined longitudinal muscle of the rectum and anal canal. The external anal sphincter lies outside the conjoined muscle. The external sphincter is divided into deep, superficial, and subcutaneous parts. The internal anal sphincter is formed by a thickening of the circular muscle layer (smooth muscle) of the colon. The pectinate line lies at the approximate center of the internal anal sphincter. Also note the columns of Morgagni, anal crypts and sinuses, and the location of the internal and external rectal venous plexus. (© Copyright 1989 CIBA-GEIGY Corporation. Reproduced with permission from Atlas of Human Anatomy by Frank H. Netter, M.D. All rights reserved.)

some degree. However, the lower rectum also drains into lymphatics that course along the middle rectal vessels and hence to the internal iliac lymph nodes. In addition, lower rectal lymphatic drainage to the inguinal lymph nodes occurs via parasacral lymphatics. Thus, lower rectal disease can affect lymph nodes in the distribution of both the inferior mesenteric and internal iliac vessels and in the inguinal area.

Contrast radiology is most concerned with the mucosal structure of the anus and rectum. In the collapsed colon, at the rectosigmoid junction, the rugose mucosal membrane of the sigmoid colon merges with the smooth mucosal surface of the rectum. However, with distention during double contrast barium enema, the rugose mucosa of the sigmoid colon is stretched and it is difficult to tell the transition point between sigmoid colon and rectum.

The rectal mucosa is featureless except for three crescentic, transversely oriented folds that partially cross the rectum at sites corresponding to the rectal flexures (Fig. 68–7; see Fig. 68–6). These crescentic folds, known as the rectal valves of Houston, are composed of mucosa, submucosa, and smooth muscle from the circular muscle layer of the colon.

The anatomy of the anorectal region is confusing because the anorectal junction may be defined functionally by defecography, during double contrast barium enema, anatomically by the location of the intrinsic and extrinsic muscles, or histologically by the transition from rectal-type columnar mucosa of endodermal origin to anal squamous mucosa of ectodermal origin.

The transition between rectal-type columnar mucosa and squamous epithelium occurs at the pectinate (dentate) line (Fig. 68–8; see Fig. 68–6) in children. The pectinate line lies on a series of small, crescentic mucosal folds—the anal valves. These crescentic folds join the lower end of a series of 6 to 10 permanent, vertically oriented folds—the columns of Morgagni (Fig. 68–9; see Figs. 68–6 and 68–8). The anal glands empty into the anal sinuses, which are small recesses formed by the anal valves (Fig. 68–10; see Fig. 68–6). With advancing age, the transition between squamous and columnar epithelium extends cranially as the stratified squamous epithelium extends upward onto the columns of Morgagni.

Below the pectinate line lies the pecten, a simple squamous epithelium without appendages such as hair follicles or sweat glands[6] (see Figs. 68–6 and 68–8). The

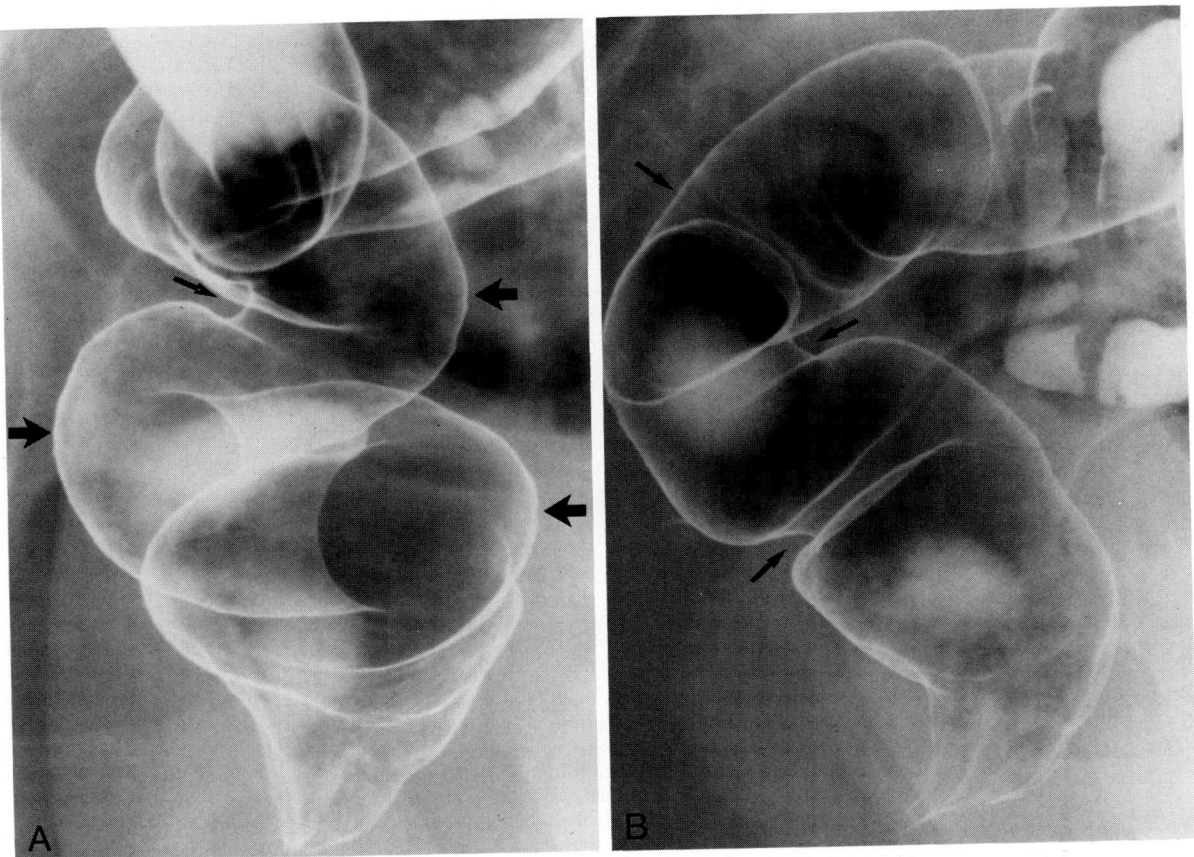

**Figure 68–7. Flexures of the rectum with corresponding rectal valves. A.** Supine view of the rectum shows three bends (flexures) *(large arrows)*. Only one rectal valve (of Houston) is seen faintly en face *(small arrow)* as parallel barium-etched lines. **B.** Lateral view of the same rectum shows the two lower rectal valves en face and the most superior valve at an angle. The rectal valves *(arrows)* correspond to the level of the three flexures of the rectum. Valves are composed of mucosa, submucosa, and a portion of the circular muscle layer.

lower limit of the anal canal, the anus, is marked by a change from the moist, hairless pecten to dry, hairy perianal skin. At the lower edge of the pecten, the squamous mucosa becomes keratinized.

Several definitions of *anorectal junction* lead to confusion. In some texts, the anorectal junction is defined as the sharp change in the direction of rectum to anus, which corresponds to the superior surface of the puborectalis portion of the levator ani muscle. This change in direction also corresponds to the proximal edge of the internal anal sphincter and the external anal sphincter. The transition from anteriorly coursing rectum and posteriorly coursing anal canal is well defined on double contrast barium enema examinations in the lateral view.

In other texts, however, the anorectal junction is defined as the transition from rectal-type columnar mucosa to nonkeratinized squamous mucosa at the pectinate line. The pectinate line corresponds to the midportion of the internal anal sphincter. The pectinate line is

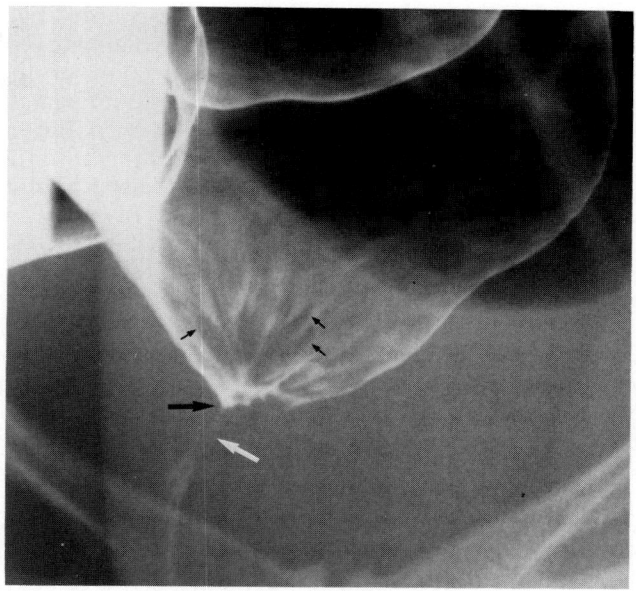

**Figure 68–9. Columns of Morgagni.** Right-side-down decubitus view of the rectum shows the anal canal *(white arrow)* closed by contraction of the internal and external anal sphincter. Radiolucent, tubular columns of Morgagni *(small black arrows)* extend cranially from the anorectal junction *(large black arrow).*

not seen on double contrast barium enema examination because this area is collapsed by active contraction of the sphincter muscles. However, on double contrast barium enema examination the upper portions of the columns of Morgagni are often seen. Thus, if radiologists accept the anorectal junction as the transition point in the angle between the rectum and anus, a portion of

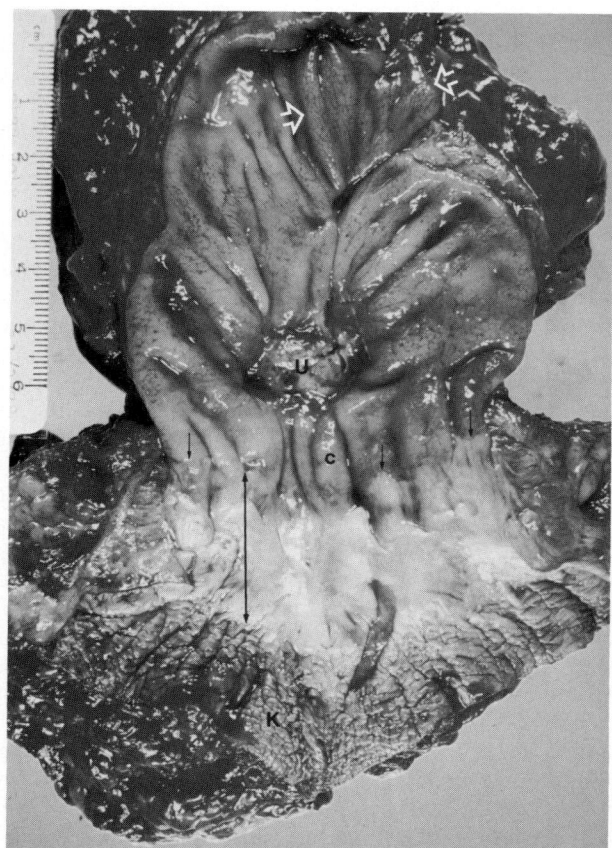

**Figure 68–8. Mucosa of the rectum and anal canal.** Specimen from an abdominal and perineal resection of the rectum and anus demonstrates the rectal mucosa en face. This region was resected because of an ulcerated adenocarcinoma of the rectum (U). The rectal mucosa glistens. In some areas, a fine reticular groove pattern is seen *(open arrows).* The columns of Morgagni (representative column labeled c) are covered by a columnar-rectal type of mucosa. The transition line between the columnar mucosa and nonkeratinized squamous epithelium is the serrated pectinate or dentate line *(small arrows).* The pecten *(double-headed arrow)* is nonkeratinized squamous epithelium. Keratinized and appendage-bearing squamous epithelium (skin) (K) lies inferiorly.

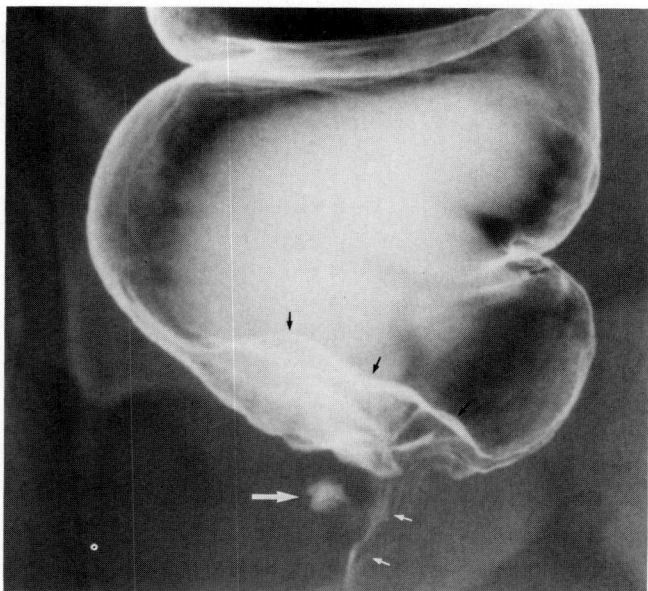

**Figure 68–10. Anal glands.** A small barium collection *(large white arrow)* arising from the anal canal *(small white arrows)* fills a small anal gland abscess. The anal glands mark the superior level of the pecten (the dentate line). Also note lobulated folds in the distal rectum *(black arrows)* representing internal hemorrhoids.

the anal canal is distended during double contrast barium enema and a portion is covered by columnar epithelium. If radiologists accept the definition of the anorectal junction as the dentate line, an extremely small portion of distal rectum is not imaged during double contrast barium enema examination because the sphincter mechanism contracts the most distal rectum and only the upper portions of the columns of Morgagni are visualized. In summary, the confusion about the definition of the anorectal junction lies in the transition between anus and rectum being defined either by the extrinsic muscles of the rectum or by the mucosa of the rectum. What the radiologist needs to know is that the columns of Morgagni are lined by rectal-type mucosa and that the most distal columns of Morgagni (and most distal columnar-type mucosa) are not visualized in the contracted anal canal during the barium enema examination. We prefer to define the anorectal junction functionally during barium enema study as the transition point between the collapsed, actively contracted anal canal and the distended distal rectum (Fig. 68–11).

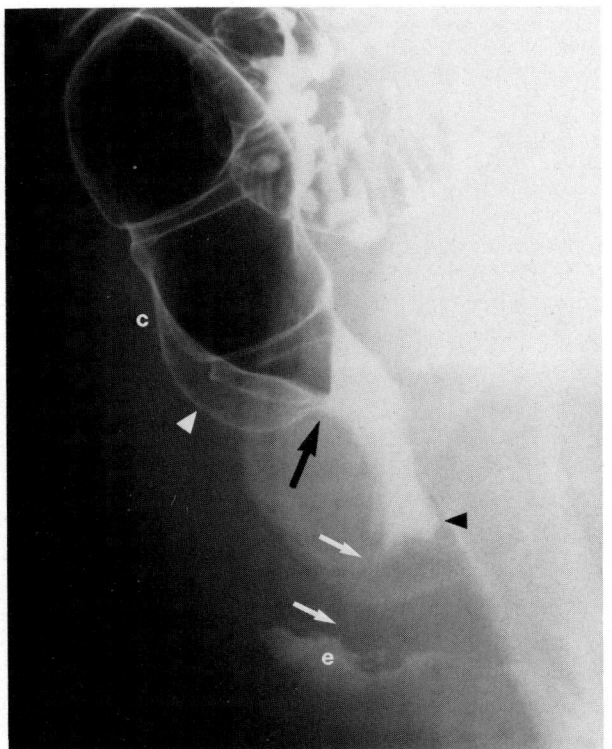

**Figure 68–11. Relationship of the puborectalis sling and the internal and external anal sphincters to the rectum.** Prone, cross-table lateral view of the rectum in a patient with moderate pelvic floor relaxation demonstrates small anterior *(black arrowhead)* and posterior *(white arrowhead)* rectoceles. The tip of the coccyx is identified (c). The puborectalis, a portion of the levator ani muscle, impresses the distal rectum *(black arrow)*. This muscular impression causes the rectum to change direction from an anteriorly to a posteriorly coursing structure. The anal canal *(white arrows)* is collapsed by the internal and external anal sphincters. Note that a small amount of barium has escaped (e) from the anal canal and marks the lower limit of the anal canal and sphincter mechanism. Note the separation, in this case, of the puborectalis and the internal and external anal sphincters, caused by the pelvic floor relaxation. Despite moderate pelvic floor relaxation, the internal and external anal sphincters functioned well enough that a double contrast barium enema examination was achieved.

High-resolution endorectal MR imaging demonstrates the layers of the rectal wall and the interface between the rectum and the perirectal fat (Fig. 68–12). T1-weighted images have high contrast between the rectal wall and the perirectal fat but provide little contrast between the various layers of the rectal wall itself. T2-weighted images demonstrate rectal wall anatomy. The mucus that covers the mucosa creates a high signal intensity layer. The mucosa causes a low signal intensity layer. The submucosa, which is composed predominantly of fat, causes a high signal intensity layer. The underlying muscularis propria is of intermediate signal intensity, and the perirectal fat is of high signal intensity.

## PHYSIOLOGY[4, 5]

In the conscious and mentally competent adult, defecation occurs at a socially acceptable time in a socially acceptable location. The normal number of bowel movements varies from two per day to two to three per week. Defecation is controlled at three primary levels, by intrinsic reflexes, extrinsic reflexes, and brain (voluntary) input.

The rectum is normally empty. A weak physiologic sphincter is present near the junction of the sigmoid colon and rectum. The smooth muscle internal sphincter of the anal canal is tonically contracted.

Defecation is initiated by a mass movement (peristaltic wave) of feces from the descending and sigmoid colon into the rectum. Rectal distention initiates a weak intrinsic reflex mediated through the myenteric plexus of the rectum and a strong extrinsic reflex mediated through pelvic parasympathetic nerves and the spinal cord. The weak intrinsic reflex is intensified by the extrinsic defecation reflex, which involves sacral segments of the spinal cord. When a peristaltic wave occurs, signals from the myenteric plexus cause weak contraction of the involuntary internal anal sphincter that prevents defecation temporarily. Parasympathetic signals from the spinal cord increase the peristaltic waves and relax the internal anal sphincter. Afferent signals from the pelvic nerves also go up the spinal cord to the brain. The conscious adult then either voluntarily relaxes the skeletal muscle–external anal sphincter to allow defecation or further contracts this muscle to prevent defecation. If the external anal sphincter is contracted voluntarily, the defecation reflex dissipates after a few minutes. Brain activity results not only in relaxation of the external anal sphincter but also in events that increase intra-abdominal pressure and pull the pelvic floor (the puborectalis sling–levator ani) downward to alter anorectal junction anatomy. Thus, defecation involves rectosigmoid mass movements; internal anal sphincter and external anal sphincter relaxation; puborectalis–levator ani contraction; and myenteric plexus, pelvic sympathetic nerves, conus medullaris, higher spinal cord, and brain function.

Destruction of the conus medullaris paralyzes defecation because the external anal sphincter cannot relax and the amplitude of peristaltic waves is relatively weak. Spinal cord damage between the conus medullaris and

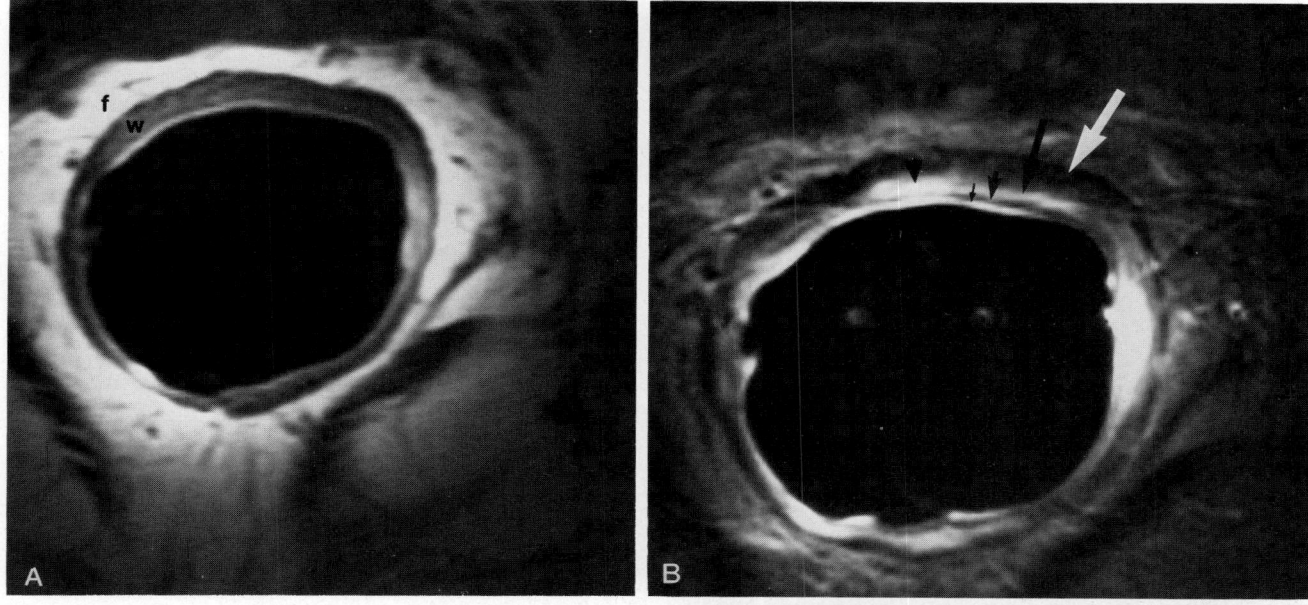

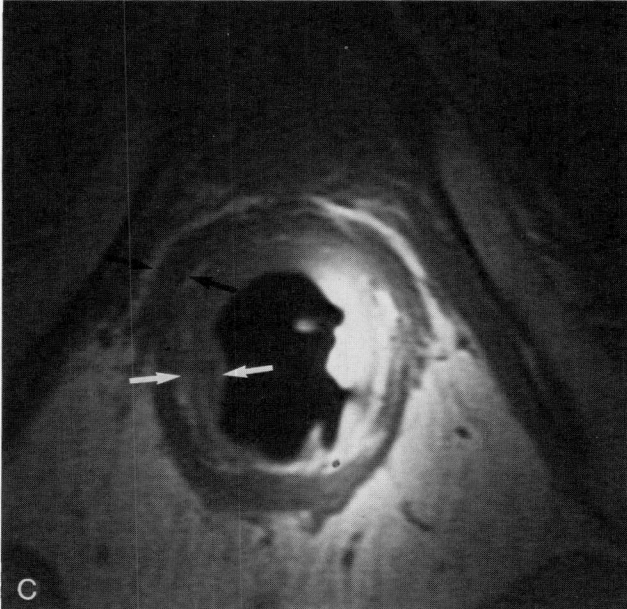

**Figure 68–12. MR imaging of rectal mucosa and anal sphincters. A.** T1-weighted endorectal surface coil spin-echo image of the rectal wall demonstrates excellent contrast between the rectal wall (w) and the perirectal fat (f). The intramural anatomy is not well visualized. **B.** T2-weighted endorectal surface coil fast spin-echo image demonstrates the intramural rectal anatomy: high signal intensity mucus *(small black arrow)*, low signal intensity mucosa *(medium-sized black arrow)*, high signal intensity submucosa *(large black arrow)*, and muscularis propria *(white arrow)*. An area of submucosal edema *(arrowhead)* is the result of a previous biopsy. **C.** T1-weighted axial spin-echo image obtained with an endorectal surface coil demonstrates the internal *(white arrows)* and external *(black arrows)* anal sphincters. The lumen of the anal canal is distended by the endorectal surface coil.

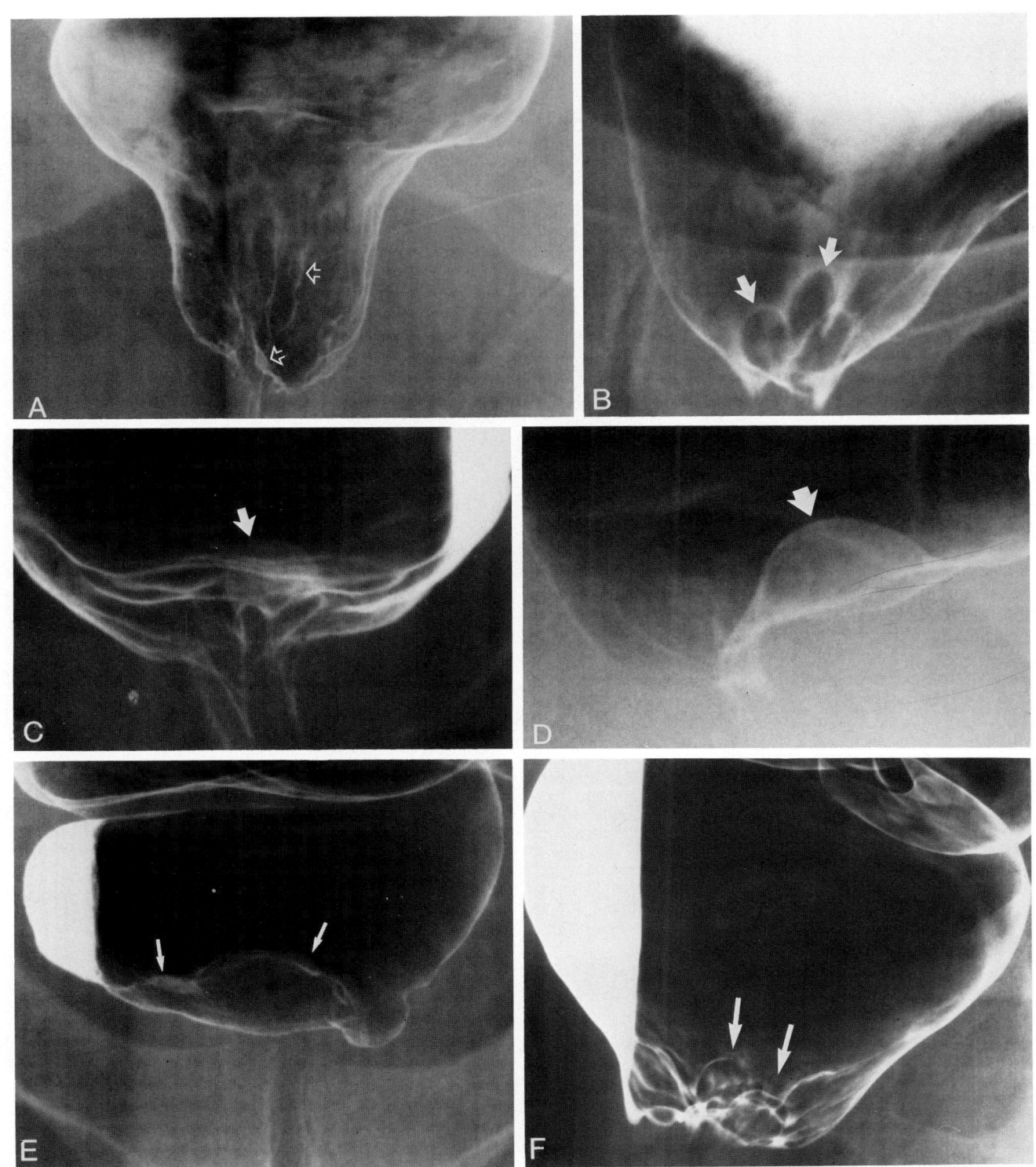

**Figure 68–13** *See legend on opposite page*

brain stem blocks the voluntary acts of defecation (external anal sphincter relaxation, pelvic floor descent, and elevated intra-abdominal pressure). Higher spinal cord or brain damage can be overcome by stimulation of the extrinsic sacral defecation reflex (i.e., through the use of enemas).

# VASCULAR LESIONS

## Internal Hemorrhoids[5-7]

Internal hemorrhoids are dilated vascular spaces of the internal hemorrhoidal plexus in the submucosal layer of the upper anal canal and lower rectum. Normally, the submucosa of the upper anal canal has three distinct vascular cushions—along the left lateral, right anterior, and right posterior wall.[6] It is postulated that these anal cushions aide in anal continence. The pathogenesis of hemorrhoids is multifactorial. With age, the connective tissue tethering the mucosa to the submucosa and muscular layer of the anal canal becomes lax. With excessive straining during defecation, prolapse of anal canal mucosa occurs, leading to congestion of vascular cushions and internal hemorrhoids. Pathologically, internal hemorrhoids appear as thick-walled submucosal veins with accompanying arteries and dilated capillaries. Abundant arteriovenous anastomoses are present.

Hemorrhoids (piles) are extremely common and usually result in brisk rectal bleeding, blood staining on toilet tissue, or painful swelling. With strangulation of hemorrhoids, mucosal infarction, necrosis, and superinfection may occur. Internal hemorrhoids may also be a complication of distal rectal carcinoma. Internal hemorrhoids are not varicose veins. Their incidence is not increased in patients with portal hypertension.

Hemorrhoids are frequently diagnosed by digital examination, anoscopy, and rigid or flexible sigmoidoscopy. Double contrast barium enema examination is a relatively accurate technique for diagnosing internal hemorrhoids, with a sensitivity and specificity of 83% and 88%, respectively.[8] However, the purpose of barium enema in patients with known or suspected internal hemorrhoids is to investigate the colon for a more serious cause of rectal bleeding or pain.

Internal hemorrhoids have a varying radiographic appearance.[9] When mild lobulation of anorectal folds (the columns of Morgagni) extends less than 3 cm from the radiographic anorectal junction, a radiographic diagnosis of internal hemorrhoids is confident (Fig. 68–13A). Another diagnostic appearance of internal hemorrhoids is a cluster of smooth-surfaced polyps less than 1 cm in size abutting the anorectal junction (Fig. 68–13B). Internal hemorrhoids may have nonspecific appearances as well, including a solitary polyp (Fig. 68–13C), a solitary submucosal mass (Fig. 68–13D), a mass (Fig. 68–13E), or large, infiltrative lobulated folds extending more than 3 cm from the anorectal junction (Fig. 68–13F). Internal hemorrhoids seen as solitary polyps cannot be distinguished from inflammatory, benign, or neoplastic rectal polyps. Internal hemorrhoids appearing as large, lobulated infiltrative folds extending more than 3 cm above the anorectal junction are indistinguishable from proctitis or infiltrating neoplasm.[9]

## Rectal Varices

Rectal varices are a rare cause of lower gastrointestinal bleeding and are usually seen in patients with portal hypertension. Rectal varices have been associated with adhesions.[10, 11] Radiologically, smooth serpiginous folds course along the rectal mucosa (Fig. 68–14). When seen in profile, rectal varices may appear as small, smooth-surfaced submucosal nodules. Like esophageal varices, rectal varices may change in size and shape with luminal distention.[12]

# NEOPLASMS

## Hyperplastic (Metaplastic) Polyps

The vast majority of hyperplastic polyps of the colon are seen in the rectum and sigmoid colon. Hyperplastic (metaplastic) polyps rarely cause symptoms. These tumors are usually detected during screening examinations or in patients with symptoms related to other colonic lesions. Hyperplastic polyps are usually small, sessile

**Figure 68–13. Radiographic appearances of internal hemorrhoids. A.** Lobulated folds. Mild lobulation of anorectal folds *(arrows)* that extend less than 3 cm above the anorectal junction is a typical radiographic finding for internal hemorrhoids. **B.** "Bunch of grapes." Three smooth-surfaced polyps *(arrows)* are clustered above the anorectal junction. This radiographic appearance is typical of internal hemorrhoids. **C.** Solitary polyp. A smooth-surfaced polyp *(arrow)* projects from mildly lobulated columns of Morgagni. This is a nonspecific radiographic appearance that requires endoscopy. **D.** Submucosal mass. A smooth-surfaced mass *(arrow)* with relatively abrupt angulation to the colonic contour is typical of a submucosal mass. Although this is a typical radiographic appearance of an internal hemorrhoid, other submucosal rectal masses include lymphoid polyps and solitary rectal ulcers. **E.** Mass-like internal hemorrhoid. A large mass *(arrows)* in the distal rectum has a focally irregular surface pattern. This huge internal hemorrhoid cannot be distinguished from other rectal masses such as carcinoma or cloacogenic carcinoma. Endoscopy and biopsy are necessary. **F.** Multiple polypoid folds. Large, polypoid folds *(arrows)* with a nodular surface pattern fill the distal rectum. Although these radiographic findings are typically seen with internal hemorrhoids, they may also be due to solitary rectal ulcer syndrome, various forms of proctitis, or an unusual infiltrating tumor.

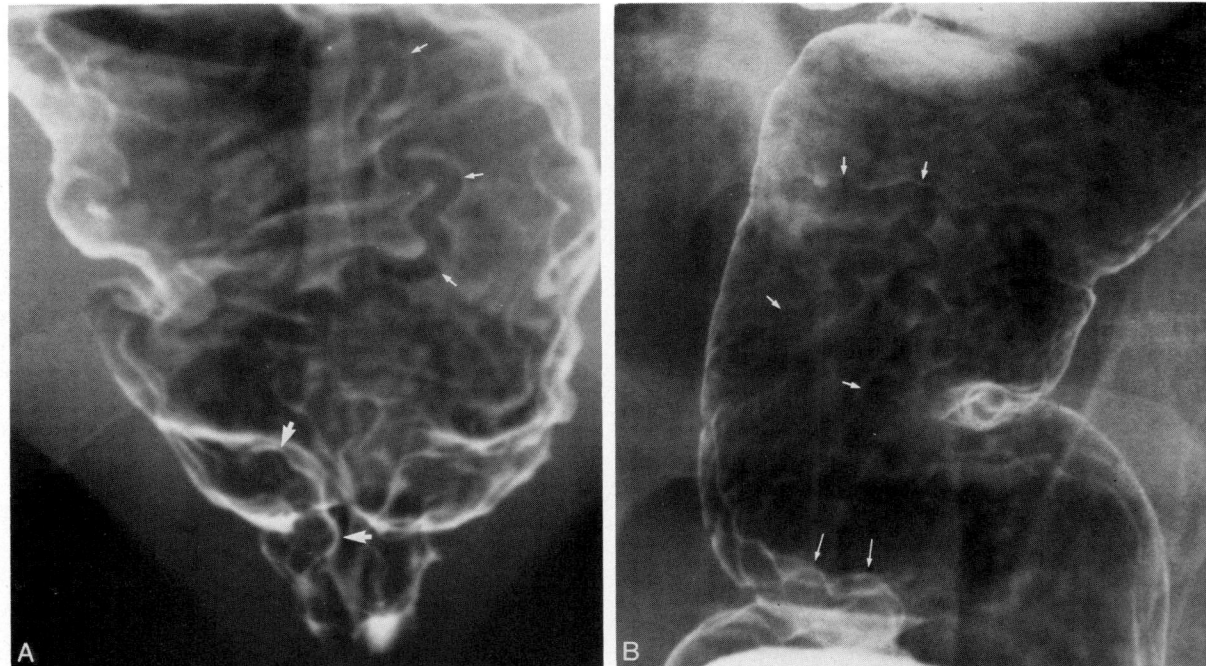

**Figure 68–14. Rectal varices. A.** Spot film of the distal rectum shows the en face appearance of rectal varices as serpentine folds etched in white *(small arrows)*. In profile, smooth, lobulated folds disrupt the contour of the bowel, extending from the anorectal junction proximally *(large arrows)*. **B.** In another patient, a spot film of the proximal rectum shows serpentine folds etched in white *(short arrows)*. In profile, a valve of Houston is expanded by a smooth, lobulated submucosal process compatible with a rectal varix *(long arrows)*. (**B** from Rubesin SE, Saul SH, Laufer I, et al: Carpet lesions of the colon. Radiographics 5:537–552, 1985.)

polyps less than 5 mm in size.[13–16] The polyps are smooth-surfaced elevations, the same color as rectal mucosa, typically lying on a mucosal crest.[13] Histologically, these tumors are composed of hyperplastic epithelial cells. The crypts are elongated and have prominent infoldings, producing a serrated or saw-toothed appearance.[5, 6] Hyperplastic polyps are not premalignant, although some polyps have both hyperplastic and adenomatous elements.

Radiologically, most hyperplastic polyps were thought to appear as smooth, sessile elevations less than 5 mm in size[17, 18] (Fig. 68–15). However, because subtle surface elevations less than 5 mm in size are difficult to detect during barium enema examination, only about one half of radiologically detected hyperplastic polyps fit the classic description. Fifty-two percent of hyperplastic polyps detected during barium enema study are greater than 5 mm in size, and 13% are greater than 1 cm.[19] The larger hyperplastic polyps often have a lobulated contour. A minority of hyperplastic polyps are pedunculated.[19]

A radiographic diagnosis of polyp is not histologically specific. The radiologist assumes the worst case, that a polyp is dysplastic and somewhere in the spectrum of adenomatous change. Pedunculation, a nodular mucosal surface, or indentation of the junction of the polyp and the colonic contour may be seen in hyperplastic as well as adenomatous polyps.

## Juvenile Polyps[5, 12, 13]

Juvenile polyps are non-neoplastic lesions often located in the rectum. These polyps are most frequently discovered in children but are occasionally found in adolescents and adults. The polyps are usually solitary, often pedunculated lesions, 1 to 3 cm in size. Patients usually complain of passage of bright red blood during defecation or rectal prolapse.

Pathologically, a single layer of flat to cuboidal to columnar mucus-secreting epithelial cells lines the polyp's surface. Tubules or cystically dilated tubules are embedded in the connective tissue stroma. The tubules are separated by a large amount of edematous or inflamed lamina propria. These polyps may be of inflammatory or hamartomatous etiology; they are not premalignant. If more than three to four juvenile polyps are found, one of the juvenile polyposis syndromes may be suspected (see Chapter 66).

## Lymphoid Polyps

Lymphoid polyps are uncommon, benign lesions occurring in the lower one third of the rectum. These tumors have been called "anal tonsils."[5] They are smooth, round, usually sessile polyps, varying from several millimeters up to 3 cm in size. The majority of

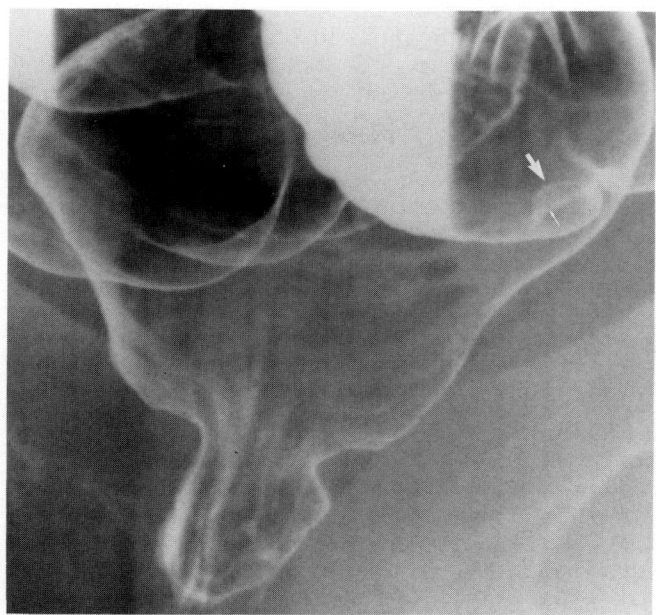

**Figure 68–15. Hyperplastic polyp.** Spot film of the distal rectum shows a "bowler hat" polyp. The dome of the bowler hat *(large arrow)* represents the surface of the polyp. The base of the polyp *(small arrow)* is shown by barium trapped between the polyp and the colon wall.

patients are asymptomatic. These solitary lesions are discovered incidentally during digital examination, endoscopy, or barium enema examination. They are submucosal tumors composed of benign lymphoid tissue with a prominent follicular pattern, covered by stretched, attenuated mucosa. Barium enema study is nonspecific and shows a smooth-surfaced, sessile or pedunculated rectal polyp (Fig. 68–16).

## Inflammatory Cloacogenic Polyps

Inflammatory cloacogenic polyps are benign protrusions occurring in the transition zone between the columnar and squamous mucosa of the anorectal junction.[20, 21] These polyps are usually sessile, although occasionally pedunculated, lesions 0.5 to 5 cm in size (Fig. 68–17). They are usually seen in adults in the fifth to seventh decades of life. Patients usually complain of intermittent rectal bleeding. These polyps are probably inflammatory or post-traumatic in nature and are associated with mucosal prolapse and/or solitary rectal ulcer syndrome. Pathologically, the surface epithelium is composed of a variable amount of stratified columnar, stratified cuboidal, or transitional epithelium.[20, 21] The mucosal surface is often inflamed or eroded. Crypt hyperplasia and a thickened muscularis mucosae are seen.

## Hemangiomas

Hemangiomas are discussed in Chapter 65.

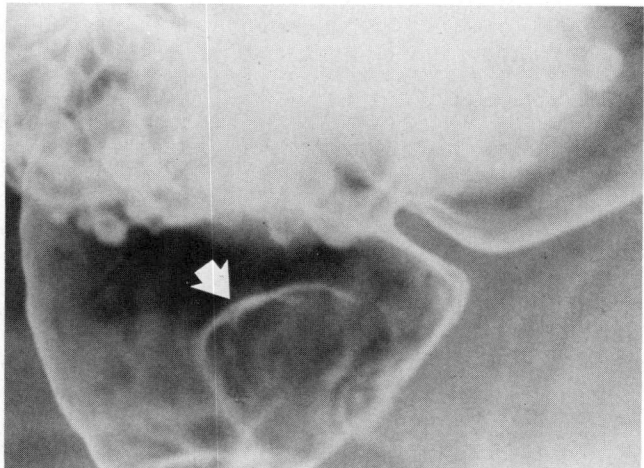

**Figure 68–16. Lymphoid polyp.** Spot film of the distal rectum shows a smooth-surfaced, finely lobulated polypoid mass *(arrow).*

## Carcinoid Tumors

The rectum is the most frequent site of carcinoid tumor occurring in the colon.[22–24] Rectal carcinoids are endocrine tumors of hindgut origin that manufacture, store, and secrete polypeptide hormones or biogenic amines. Rectal carcinoids do not secrete serotonin, and therefore carcinoid syndrome is rare in patients who have rectal carcinoid. Instead, rectal carcinoids manufacture polypeptide P, glucagon (glicentin), and somatostatin.[25] Most patients are asymptomatic, but some

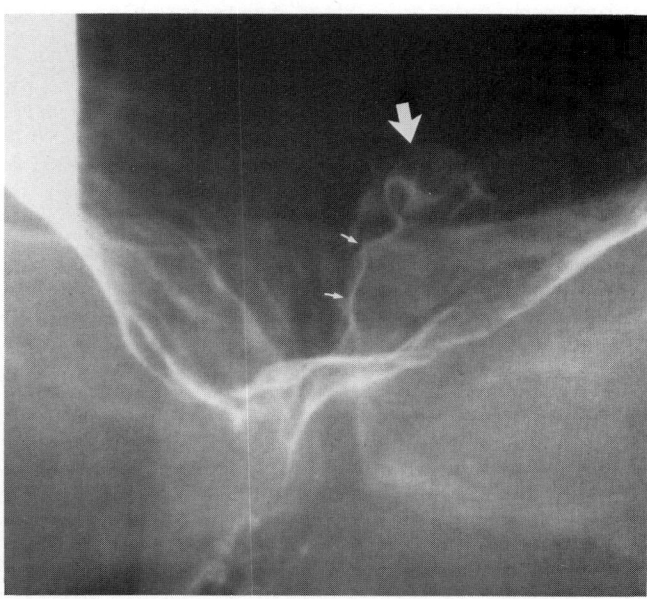

**Figure 68–17. Inflammatory cloacogenic polyp.** Right-side-down decubitus view of the rectum shows a relatively smooth-surfaced, finely lobulated polypoid lesion *(large arrow)* arising at the superior border of a column of Morgagni. Extension of the inflammatory reaction down the column of Morgagni is manifested as thickening of the column *(small arrows).*

may complain of rectal bleeding or discomfort.[26] These tumors are usually discovered incidentally during endoscopy or barium enema study and the histopathologic diagnosis is unexpected.[25]

Rectal carcinoids are manifest radiographically as solitary, small, smooth-surfaced polypoid lesions with a broad base (Fig. 68–18). The tumors are usually less than 2 cm in diameter and located in the lower two thirds of the rectum. More than one half of rectal carcinoids are less than 1 cm in diameter.[27] Larger lesions are manifest radiographically as bulky, infiltrative tumors or polypoid masses. Larger lesions have a significant malignant potential. Eighty-two percent of rectal carcinoids greater than 2 cm in size metastasize to lymph nodes or the liver.[22] Approximately 10% of lesions 1 to 2 cm and 2% of lesions less than 1 cm in size metastasize.

## Adenomas and Adenocarcinomas

The incidence of rectal carcinoma has been decreasing and the incidence of more proximal colonic adenomas and carcinomas increasing. The incidence of colonic carcinomas varies widely according to site, especially depending on geographic and ethnic variables.[13] Nevertheless, the rectum and the distal sigmoid colon are the most frequent sites of colonic adenomas and adenocarcinomas.

Most patients are older than 40 years of age. Colorectal carcinoma occurring before age 40 is more common in patients with inflammatory bowel disease, polyposis syndromes, and nonpolyposis family carcinoma syndromes.

Most rectal adenomas do not cause symptoms. Occasional rectal adenomas bleed if they are excoriated by

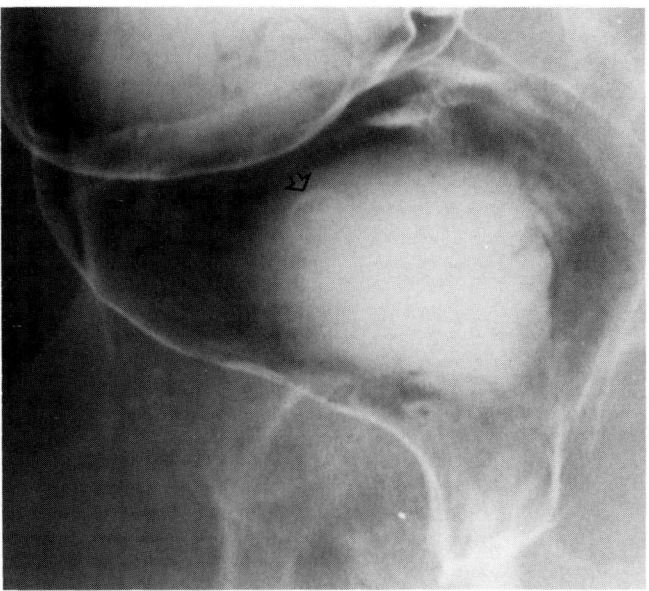

**Figure 68–18. Carcinoid tumor.** Oblique view of the distal rectum shows a polyp on the nondependent surface as a ring shadow etched in white *(arrow)*. The polyp is partly obscured by the barium pool on the dependent surface.

passage of hard stool. The severe fluid and electrolyte loss associated with villous adenoma is rare.

The majority of large bowel carcinomas arise in adenomas. Although the adenoma-to-carcinoma sequence is well accepted, it is more properly referred to as the dysplasia-to-carcinoma sequence.[28] In addition, tubular adenomas, tubulovillous adenomas, and villous adenomas are different macroscopic expressions of the same pathologic process. Although these tumors have gross structural differences, they have identical cytologic characteristics.[28] In tubular adenomas, multiple crypts are lined by adenomatous epithelium. In villous adenomas, papillary excrescences lined by adenomatous epithelium extend from the base of the mucosa toward the lumen. Tubular adenomas either have a flat surface or are divided into one to three lobules.[29] Tubulovillous adenomas can be divided into 3 to 10 lobules. Villous adenomas have innumerable lobules of smaller size, correlating with the frond-like excrescences.

The malignant potential of polyps increases with size, villous configuration, and degree of dysplasia. For the radiologist, polyp size is by far the most important criterion in assessing malignant potential. In one histologic study of 2487 adenomas, 1.3% of adenomas less than 1 cm in size were malignant, 9.5% of adenomas 1 to 2 cm were malignant, and 46% of adenomas greater than 2 cm were malignant.[30] In another series, approximately 4% of polypoid tumors had lymph node metastases, whereas 30% of sessile polyps had lymph node metastases.[31] In one series, if a polyp had a stalk greater than 3 mm in length, no metastases were seen. When a polyp is resected, the most significant prognostic factors for a carcinoma are depth of invasion, lymph node metastasis, and distant metastasis.

Radiographically, most tubular adenomas and tubulovillous adenomas in the rectum are small, spheric, pedunculated or sessile polyps (Fig. 68–19). A finely lobular surface is due to intercommunicating clefts. Basal indentation or lobulation of the polyp suggests malignancy only in polyps larger than 10 mm.[32] The radiologist assumes the worst case—that a rectal polyp is a possible adenoma with possible malignant potential. Clearly, polyps larger than 1 cm in size must be examined histologically.

Some adenomas grow as flat lesions spreading along the surface of the bowel. These sessile tumors, which show little protrusion into the bowel, are termed *carpet lesions*.[33, 34] Adenomas with carpet-like growth have a predilection for the rectum and ascending colon. En face, carpet lesions appear as a nodular or reticular surface disrupting the normally smooth colonic mucosa (Fig. 68–20). In profile, carpet lesions show slight irregularity of the mucosal contour (Fig. 68–21A). Disruption of the mucosal contour and asymmetric disruption of the tumor's surface pattern are signs that raise suspicion of malignancy arising in a carpet lesion. Despite their large size, many carpet lesions do not harbor malignancy[34] (Fig. 68–21B).

Rectal adenocarcinomas have the same morphology as adenocarcinomas in the rest of the colon. Adenocarcinomas may be polypoid masses (Fig. 68–22), bulky

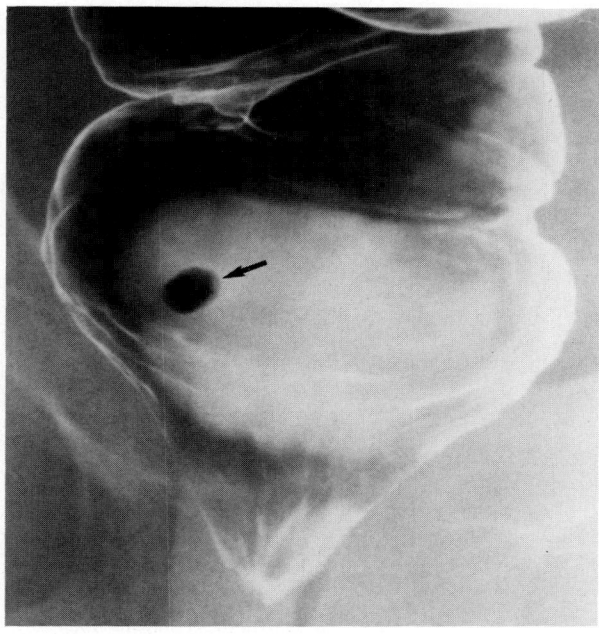

**Figure 68–19. Tubular adenoma.** A smooth-surfaced finely lobulated filling defect *(arrow)* is seen in the barium pool of the distal rectum.

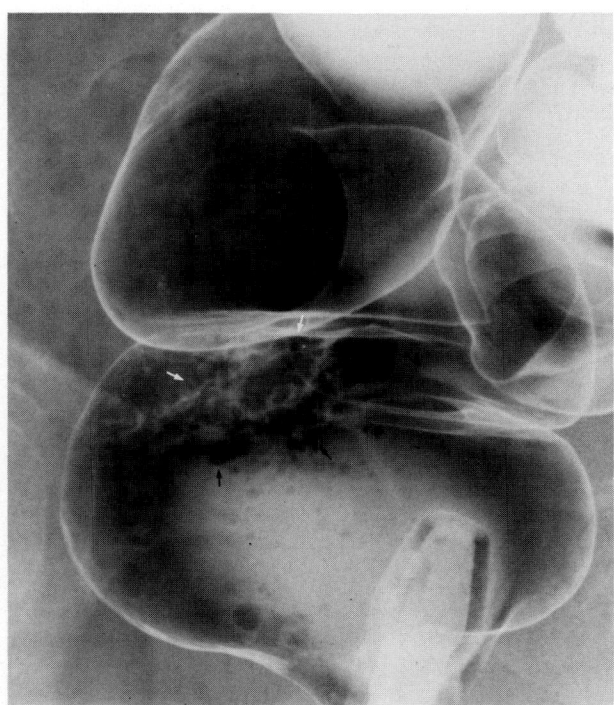

**Figure 68–20. Tubulovillous adenoma.** A flat, carpet-like lesion is seen in the distal rectum. In the barium pool, the tumor appears as fine, round, lobulated filling defects *(black arrows)*. When barium fills the interstices of the lesion, a nonuniform reticular pattern is seen *(white arrows)*. (From Rubesin SE, Saul SH, Laufer I, et al: Carpet lesions of the colon. Radiographics 5:537–552, 1985.)

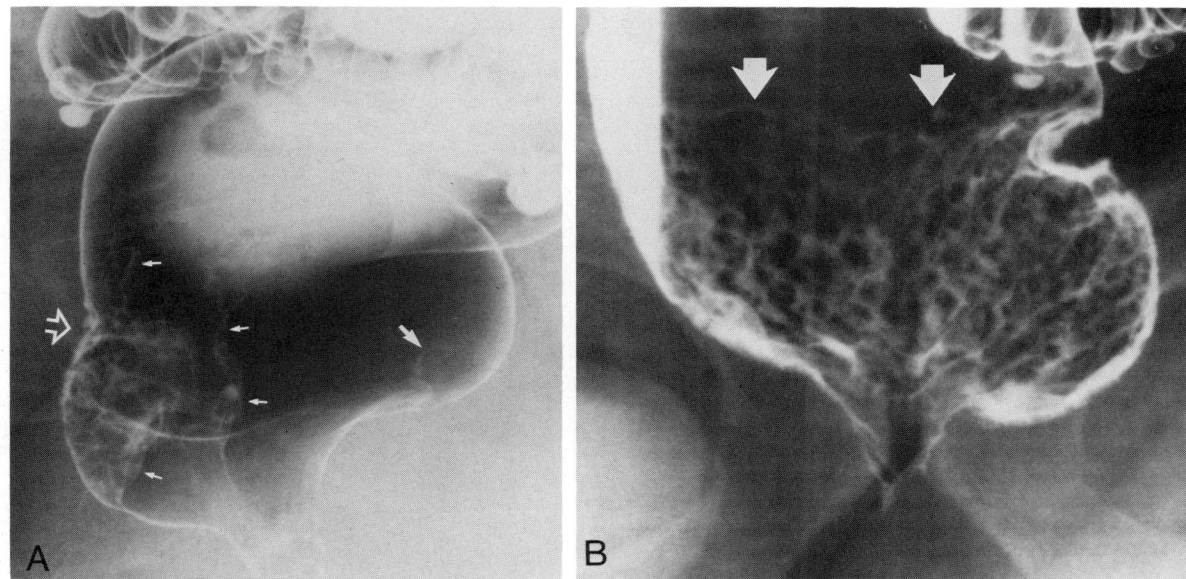

**Figure 68–21. Villous adenoma. A.** Barium filling the interstices between fronds of a villous adenoma shows a carpet lesion of the distal rectum manifested as a reticular pattern en face *(small arrows).* The colonic contour is only minimally disrupted by the tumor *(open arrow).* A small polyp (tubulovillous adenoma) is also noted *(large arrow).* **B.** A carpet lesion extends circumferentially around the distal rectum. En face the tumor is seen as a fine reticular and radiolucent nodular pattern *(arrows).* Note that the colonic contour is relatively intact. (**A** and **B** from Rubesin SE, Saul SH, Laufer I, et al: Carpet lesions of the colon. Radiographics 5:537–552, 1985.)

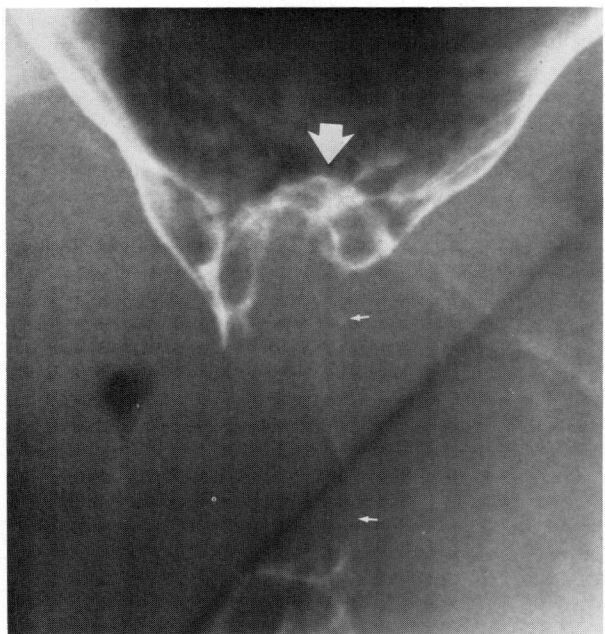

**Figure 68–22. Polypoid adenocarcinoma of the rectum.** A polypoid lesion *(large arrow)* of the anorectal junction is seen as a polypoid mass with a finely nodular surface pattern. Note infiltration of the anal canal seen as deviation of the barium-coated lumen *(small arrows).*

exophytic masses (Fig. 68–23), infiltrating plaque-like lesions (Fig. 68–24), or annular lesions (Fig. 68–25). The mucosal surface is irregular and nodular, with barium collecting in ulcerated surfaces or within tumor clefts.

Although technique is discussed more in Chapter 57, we would like to remind radiologists that the rectum is a difficult area to examine both endoscopically and radiologically. Endoscopic blind spots include the rectum just proximal to the anal verge and the regions behind the valves of Houston. Barium blind spots include the wall underneath the dense barium pool and the rectosigmoid junction obscured by overlapping bowel loops or involved by diverticulosis and circular muscle thickening. Any single contrast examination of the rectum in which palpation is not possible is not an optimal examination. Nevertheless, barium studies are as accurate as endoscopy in detection of rectal carcinoma.[35]

The ability of high-resolution endorectal surface coil MR imaging to demonstrate the anatomy of the rectal wall makes this a valuable tool in evaluation of rectal tumors. Early rectal cancer appears on endorectal MR images as an area of focal thickening of the mucosal layer.[2] Because the mucosa has low signal intensity on T2-weighted images, the epithelial component of the rectal carcinoma also has low signal intensity on T2-weighted images. As tumors grow, they often develop several different histologic components. In addition to low signal intensity epithelial components, high signal intensity mucin components of rectal tumors are often seen. Desmoplastic reaction to rectal tumors is seen as low signal intensity on T2-weighted images.

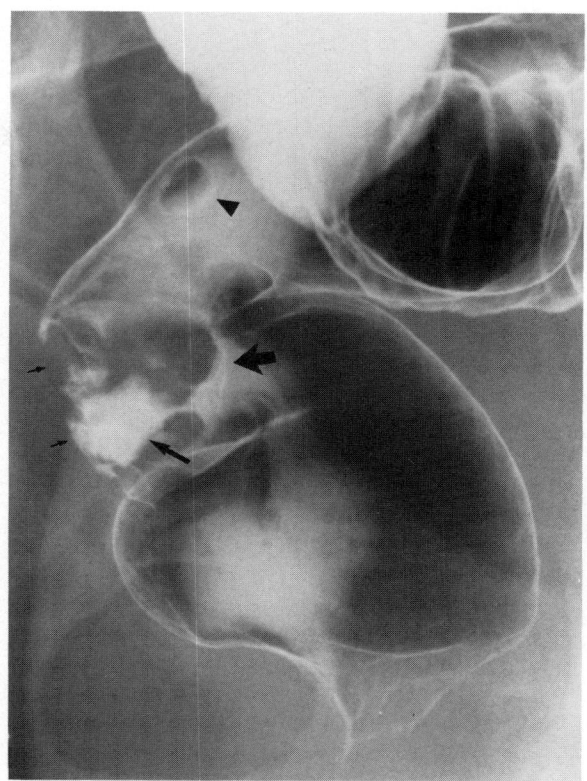

**Figure 68–23. Mass-like adenocarcinoma of the rectum.** Oblique spot film of the rectum shows a polypoid mass *(large arrow)* arising from the right posterolateral wall of the midrectum. Note central ulceration *(medium-sized arrow)* and disruption of the luminal contour *(small arrows)*. A "satellite" polyp is seen *(arrowhead)*.

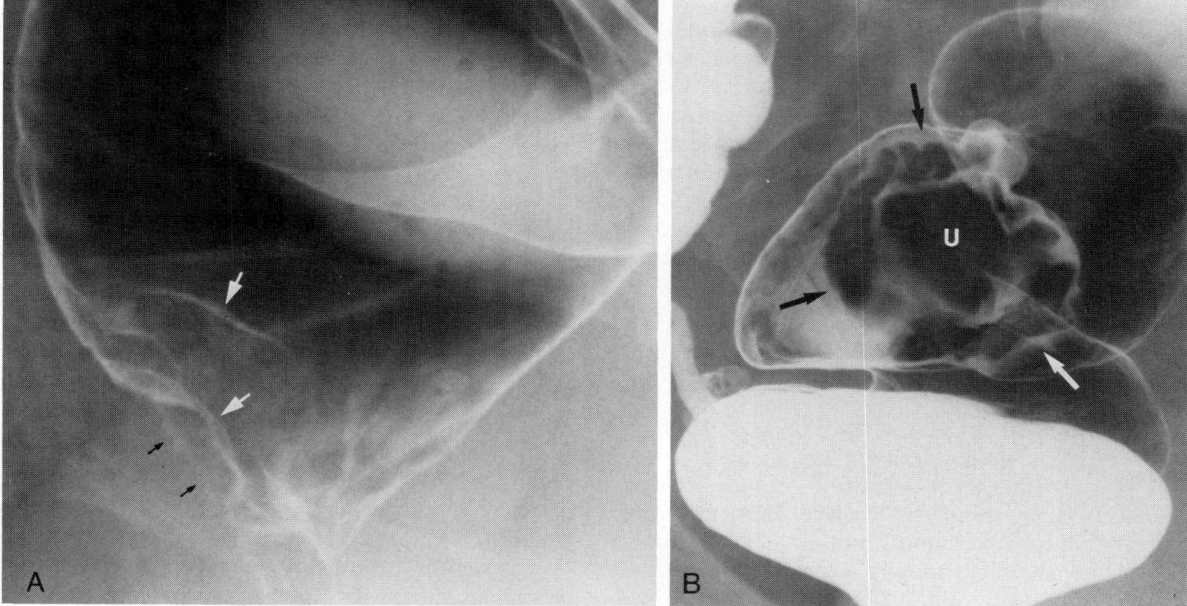

**Figure 68–24. Plaque-like adenocarcinomas of the rectum. A.** Spot film of the distal rectum shows barium-etched lines in an abnormal location *(white arrows)* and disruption of the luminal contour *(black arrows)*. **B.** A plaque-like tumor of the proximal rectum is seen. The plaque has a finely lobulated, rolled margin *(arrows)*. Centrally, a flat ulcer (U) is seen.

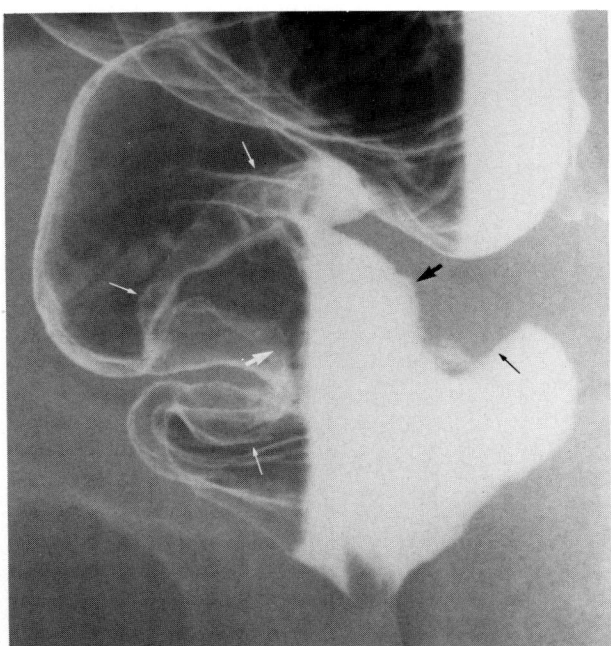

**Figure 68–25. Annular adenocarcinoma of the rectum.** Left-side-down decubitus view of the rectum shows an annular disruption of the luminal contour *(thick arrows)* and nodular shelf-like margins *(thin arrows).*

The transmural extent of rectal carcinoma is nicely demonstrated with high-resolution endorectal MR scanning (Fig. 68–26). The hallmark of a lesion confined to the mucosa and submucosa is visualization of a high signal intensity submucosal interface between the tumor and the muscularis propria. This confirms that the tumor has not yet invaded the muscularis propria. Tumor invasion of the muscularis propria is accompanied by obliteration of the high signal intensity submucosa on T2-weighted images and associated irregularity of the interface between the tumor and the muscularis propria. The invasion can be diagnosed only when tumor can be visualized completely obliterating the muscularis propria. Early results suggest that endorectal MR scanning is extremely accurate in demonstrating the transmural extent of rectal malignancies.[36] The precise clinical role of this technique has not yet been established.

## Stromal Tumors

Tumors composed of spindle or epithelioid cells have traditionally been termed leiomyomas or leiomyosarcomas.[37, 38] The current term is *gastrointestinal stromal tumor,* because only a minority of these tumors can be recognized as arising from smooth muscle cells by ultrastructural or histochemical means.[39, 40] Stromal tumors rarely arise in the colon. When they are present, however, the rectum is the most common site of colonic stromal lesions.[37]

Stromal tumors have two dominant forms: small polypoid lesions and large infiltrative masses.[41] Patients with small stromal tumors are usually asymptomatic. These lesions are usually sessile or pedunculated polyps discovered incidentally at endoscopy or during barium enema study. The lesions are histologically benign and do not recur after polypectomy. These tumors are probably true leiomyomas arising from the muscularis mucosae. Large stromal tumors usually cause perineal pain, tenesmus, bleeding per rectum, or a change in bowel habits. Macroscopically, the lesion appears as a submucosal mass (Fig. 68–27) with or without ulceration, a cavitary mass, or an annular lesion. These tumors are undifferentiated lesions arising in the circular muscle layer or internal anal sphincter. They have a poor prognosis, with a 5-year survival of approximately 25%.[41] These tumors frequently recur after local excision. Hematogenous metastases are frequent.

## Squamous Cell Carcinoma

Pure squamous cell carcinoma of the colon is rare. However, more than one half of colonic squamous cell carcinomas arise in the rectum.[42] Primary squamous cell carcinoma of the rectum must be distinguished from squamous cell carcinomas arising from 1) a hematogenous metastasis; 2) squamous cell carcinoma directly invading the rectum from the perineum, anal canal (Fig. 68–28), or a squamous mucosa–lined fistula; or 3) poorly differentiated adenocarcinoma showing extensive squamous differentiation.[6] Squamous cell carcinomas have been detected in patients with associated chronic ulcerative colitis, pelvic irradiation, and schistosomiasis. Thus, squamous cell carcinomas may arise in areas of chronic inflammation or of dysplastic glandular (adenomatous) epithelium.[5] These tumors are usually large, ulcerative tumors of the lower rectum, identical in appearance to adenocarcinomas. Hematogenous, lymphatic, and local metastases are frequent.

## Cloacogenic (Basaloid) Carcinoma

The transitional epithelium of the anal canal contains squamous, transitional, and stratified columnar epithelium, as well as scattered goblet cells. Various neoplasms of controversial origin arise in this transitional epithelium. The transitional zone has features of both urothelium and squamous epithelium consistent with a cloacogenic origin.[43] Hence, many tumors in this region were previously termed cloacogenic carcinomas. However, the transitional zone also has features suggesting that it is an area where metaplasia and reserve cell hyperplasia occur, similar to the transitional zone in the uterine cervix[44] or the transitional zone at the esophagogastric junction. Thus, it has also been postulated that tumors in this region are due to dysplasia and hence carcinoma arising in squamous metaplasia and reserve cell hyperplasia. For example, homosexual men have a high incidence of anal transitional cell carcinoma and squamous cell carcinoma. These tumors may be related to venereally transmissible agents such as oncogenic vi-

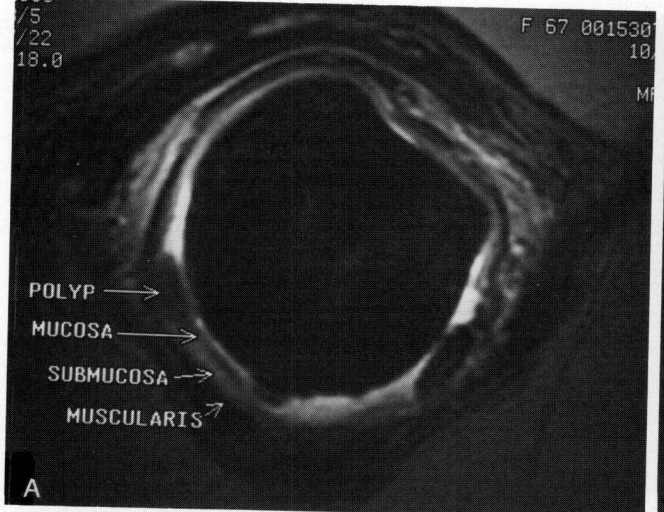

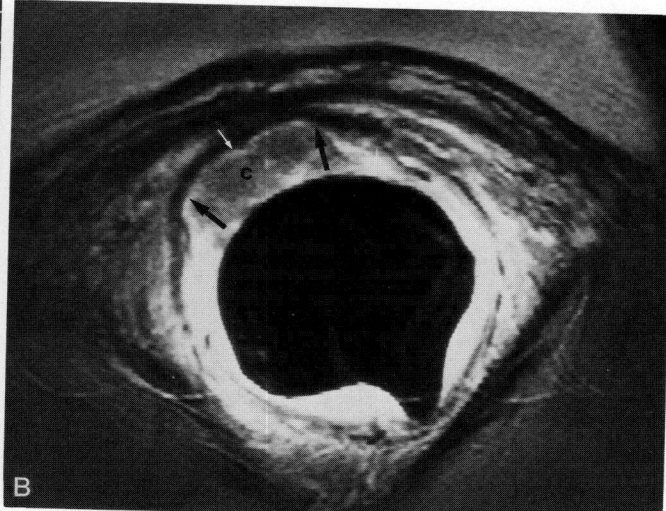

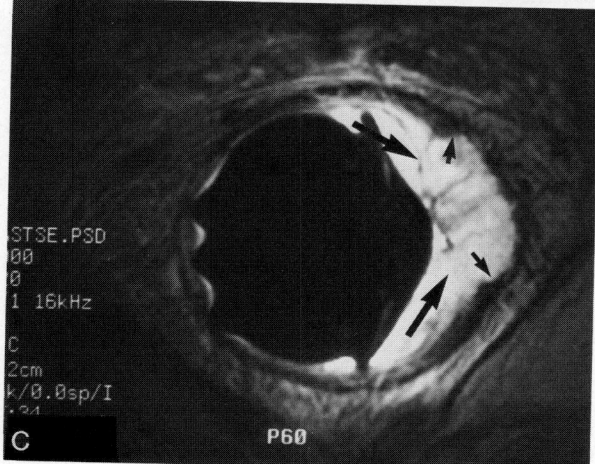

**Figure 68–26. MR imaging of rectal cancer. A.** T2-weighted endorectal surface coil fast spin-echo image demonstrates an area of focal thickening of the mucosa that was subsequently shown to represent an adenomatous polyp with focal carcinoma. **B.** Image obtained with the same technique demonstrates a villous carcinoma (c) invading the submucosa. The thin high signal intensity line *(arrows)* of submucosa between the lesion and the muscularis propria indicates absence of muscle invasion. **C.** Image obtained with the same technique demonstrates a high signal intensity rectal mass *(large arrows)* with invasion into the muscularis propria *(small arrows)*. The rectal cancer has high signal intensity because it produces a large amount of mucin; that is, it is a colloid carcinoma.

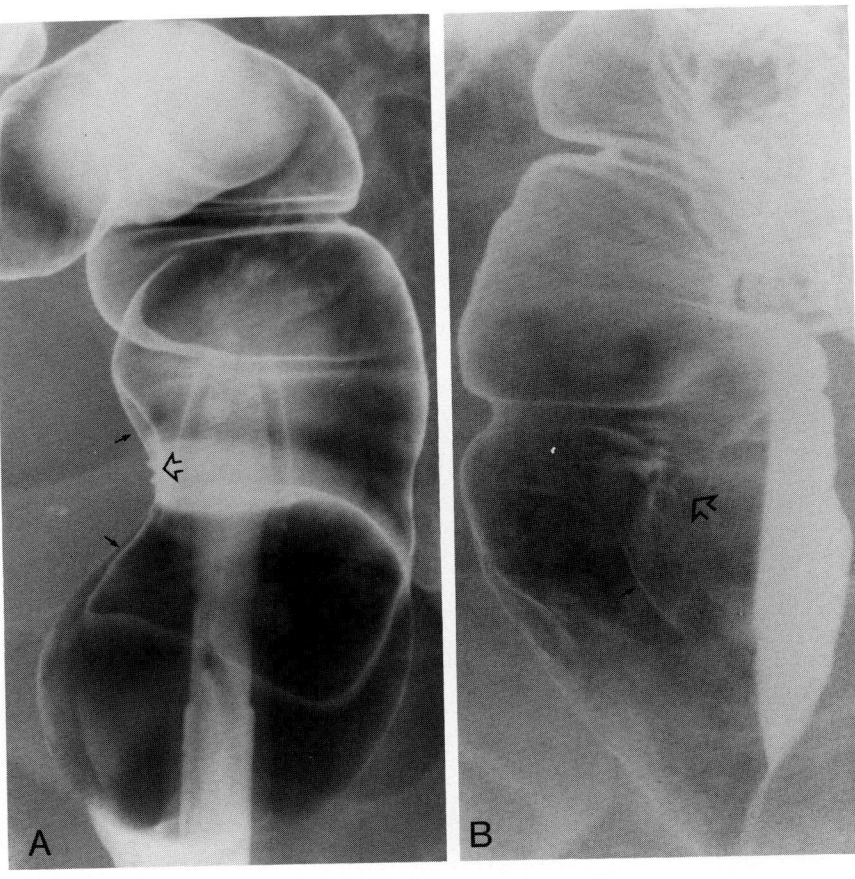

A

B

**Figure 68–27. Stromal tumor. A.** Oblique spot film of the rectum shows a broad-based mass *(solid arrows)* with central surface irregularity *(open arrow).* **B.** En face, small nodules are seen in the center of the surface of the lesion *(open arrow).* An abnormal line is also noted *(solid arrow).* With these radiographic findings it is difficult to distinguish a submucosal tumor infiltrating the mucosa from an extrinsic mass lesion invading the mucosa, such as prostatic carcinoma invading the rectum. At surgery, a submucosal tumor was seen. Histologically, a gastrointestinal stromal tumor with malignant features was diagnosed.

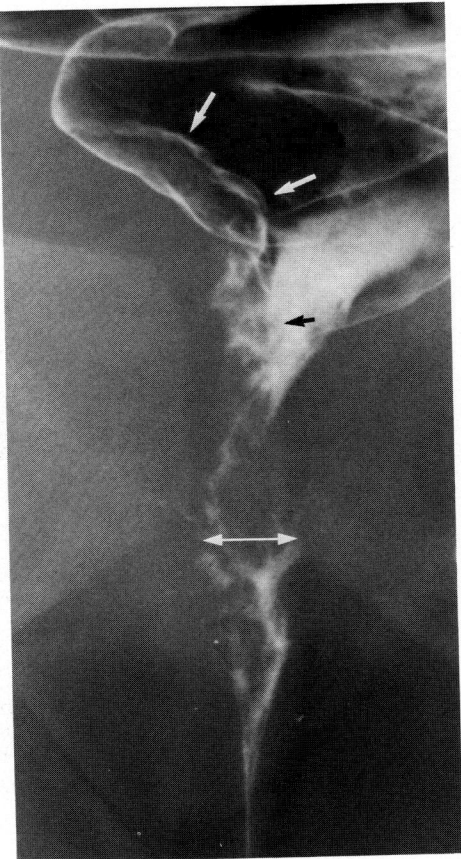

**Figure 68–28. Verrucous squamous cell carcinoma arising in a condyloma acuminatum.** This 24-year-old woman had been treated for 5 years for perianal, vaginal, cervical, and vulvar condylomata. A spot film of the distal rectum and anal canal shows a polypoid mass *(white arrows)* in the distal rectum and nodular mucosa extending to the anorectal junction *(black arrow)* and abnormal mucosa distending the anal canal *(double-headed white arrow).*

ruses, carcinogens in lubricants and cleansers, or mechanical irritation.[45-47] Tumors at the anorectal junction have been described by a wide variety of names, including squamous cell carcinoma, basaloid carcinoma, transitional cell carcinoma, mucoepidermoid carcinoma, adenoid cystic carcinoma, and verrucous carcinoma. Basaloid carcinoma and cloacogenic carcinoma are probably equivalent terms. Most tumors, however, have a mixture of growth patterns including basaloid areas, transitional cell carcinomas with squamous differentiation, adenoid cystic carcinoma, and mucoepidermoid carcinoma. The most common tumor of the anal canal is adenocarcinoma of the rectal mucosa invading the anal canal.

Cloacogenic (basaloid) carcinoma has no distinctive clinical, gross pathologic, or radiologic features. Patients usually complain of rectal bleeding, rectal pain, or a change in bowel habits. These tumors may be flat, infiltrative, annular, or ulcerative lesions with rolled borders. Radiographically, the tumor may appear as a submucosal mass with a smooth or ulcerated surface (Fig. 68–29), broad-based sessile polyps, or infiltrative lesions[48, 49] (Fig. 68–30).

Metastases occur in approximately 50% of patients to the sacral lymph nodes, internal and common iliac lymph nodes, and superficial inguinal lymph nodes. Venous drainage and hematogenous metastasis are both to the inferior vena cava and portal system. Five-year survival in patients with basaloid carcinoma is approximately 50%.[6]

## Metastases

Colonic metastases are discussed in Chapter 65. This section focuses on metastases to the rectum.

The rectum is involved by two primary forms of metastasis, direct invasion from a contiguous primary tumor or intraperitoneal seeding. Direct invasion of the rectum in males is primarily from tumors of the prostate, urinary bladder, and perineum and anus. In females, cervical and vaginal tumors may directly invade the rectum. Ovarian carcinoma may invade the rectum by intraperitoneal spread. Occasionally, perineal, uterine, or bladder cancers can directly invade the rectum. Rarely, primary neoplasms have lateral submucosal spread (Fig. 68–31).

### Prostatic Carcinoma

Prostatic carcinoma invades the rectum in 1 to 10% of all patients with prostatic carcinoma.[50, 51] Prostatic carcinoma invading the rectum causes symptoms identical to those of rectal carcinoma, including constipation and bleeding.[52] The diagnosis of prostatic carcinoma invading the rectum is often unknown at the time of initial barium enema examination or surgery.[53, 54]

Prostatic carcinoma usually spreads cranially into the seminal vesicles before it invades posteriorly. Therefore, most prostatic carcinomas invade the colon at the rectosigmoid junction, and the distal rectum is spared.[55] In some patients, however, prostatic cancer crosses Denon-

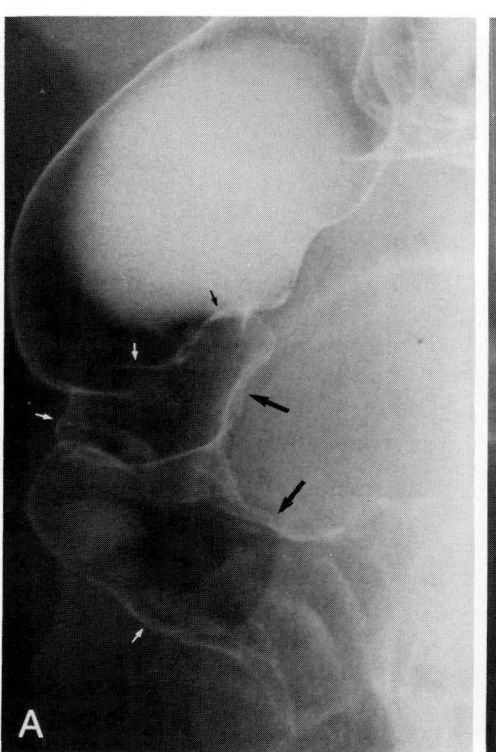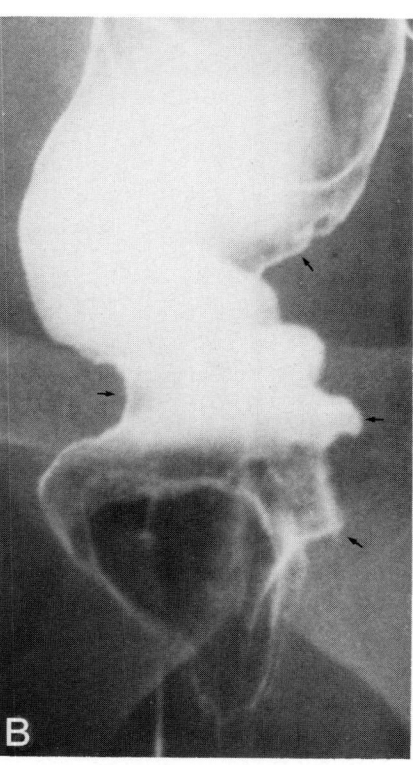

**Figure 68–29. Cloacogenic carcinoma. A.** Lateral spot view of the rectum shows a dominant, large submucosal mass *(large black arrows)* indenting the anterior wall of the midrectum. Diffuse infiltration of the remainder of the distal rectum is manifested by smooth narrowing of the distal rectum *(small arrows).* **B.** Supine view of the distal rectum shows diffuse narrowing of the rectal ampulla and a diffusely irregular contour *(arrows).*

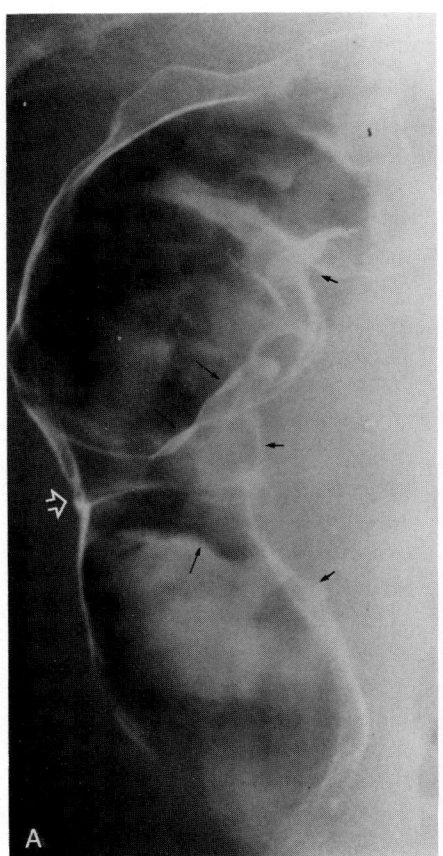 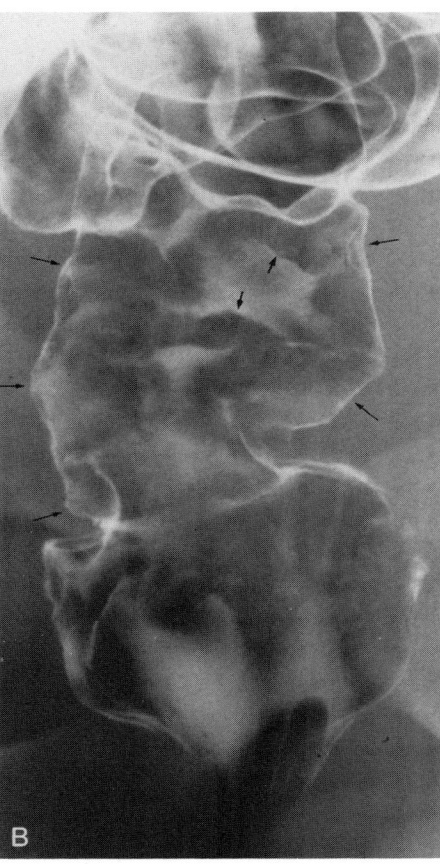

**Figure 68–30. Cloacogenic carcinoma. A.** Lateral view of the rectum demonstrates the infiltrative pattern of cloacogenic carcinoma. The anterior wall of the rectum is moderately flattened and lobulated *(short arrows)* and thick, nodular folds cross the rectum *(long arrows)*. The rectal mucosa is relatively smooth. Focal circumferential extension of tumor around the rectum is seen as flattening of the posterior rectal wall *(open arrow)*. **B.** Prone view of the rectum shows mild inbowing and irregularity of the contour of the lateral walls of the rectum *(long arrows)* and thick, nodular folds en face *(short arrows)*.

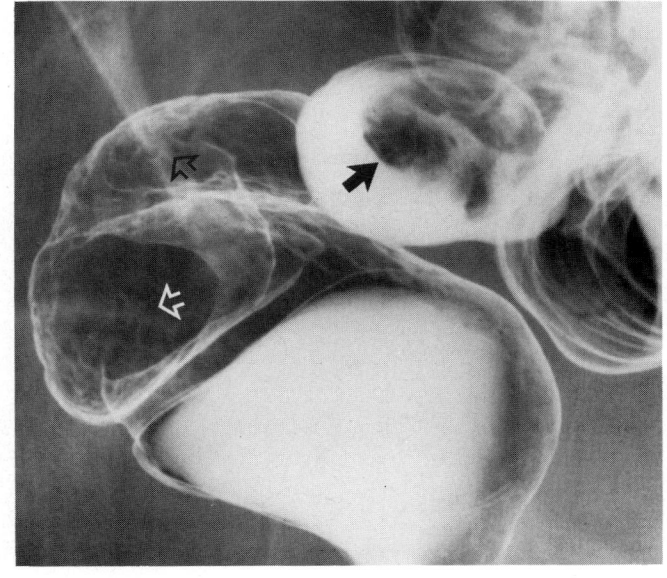

**Figure 68–31. Submucosal spread of tumor.** Diffuse nodularity of the proximal rectal mucosa *(open arrows)* is due to submucosal spread of tumor from an adjacent carcinoma in the sigmoid colon *(solid arrow)*. This radiographic appearance may mimic that of nonspecific proctitis or pseudomembranous colitis. (From Rubesin SE, Saul SH, Laufer I, et al: Carpet lesions of the colon. Radiographics 5:537–552, 1985.)

villiers' fascia to invade the lower rectum.[53, 55] Radiologically, prostatic carcinoma with seminal vesicle invasion may cause an extrinsic mass impression at the rectosigmoid junction. With direct invasion of the rectosigmoid junction serosa, pleating of the mucosa, spiculation of the luminal contour, and a mass effect are seen (Fig. 68–32). In advanced cases, the prostatic cancer extends circumferentially around the rectosigmoid junction, resulting in annular narrowing, spiculation of the contour, and a wide retrorectal (presacral) space (Fig. 68–33). Distal rectal invasion appears as a mild extrinsic mass effect along the anterior wall, spiculation of the luminal contour, and pleating of the mucosa[55] (Fig. 68–34). When barium enema examination has suggested the diagnosis, the work-up includes MR imaging, computed tomography (Fig. 68–35), transrectal sonography, and biopsy with stains for prostatic-specific antigen.

## Cervical Carcinoma

When cervical carcinoma invades the rectum, the rectosigmoid junction is usually involved. Barium enema findings are identical to those for prostatic carcinoma invading the rectum, including mass effect, spiculation of the luminal contour, and pleated colonic mucosa.

## Intraperitoneal Seeding

The rectovesical space in the male and the rectouterine space (pouch of Douglas) in the female are the most dependent portions of the peritoneal cavity when the

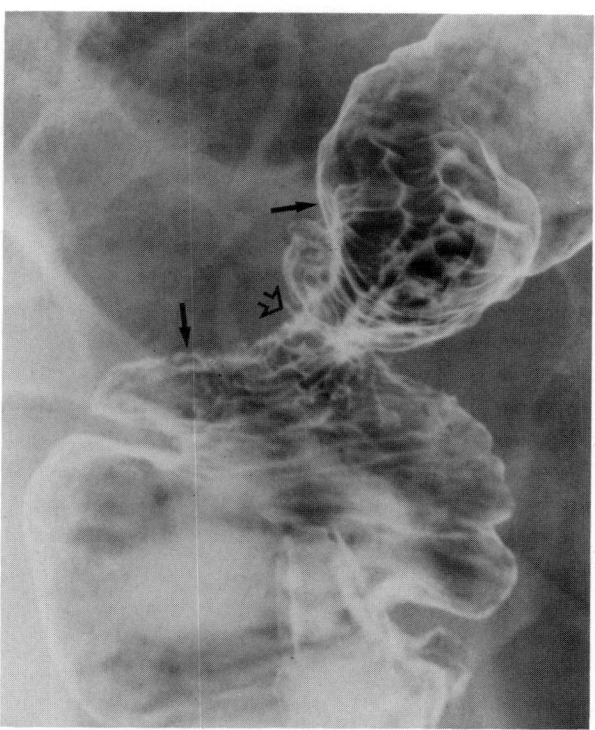

**Figure 68–32. Prostatic carcinoma invading the rectum.** An extrinsic mass impression at the rectosigmoid junction *(solid arrows)* is associated with pleating of smooth mucosal folds *(open arrow)*. (From SE Rubesin, MS Levin, M Bezzi, et al, Rectal involvement by prostatic carcinoma: barium enema findings, AJR, 152, 1, 53–57, 1989, © by American Roentgen Ray Society.)

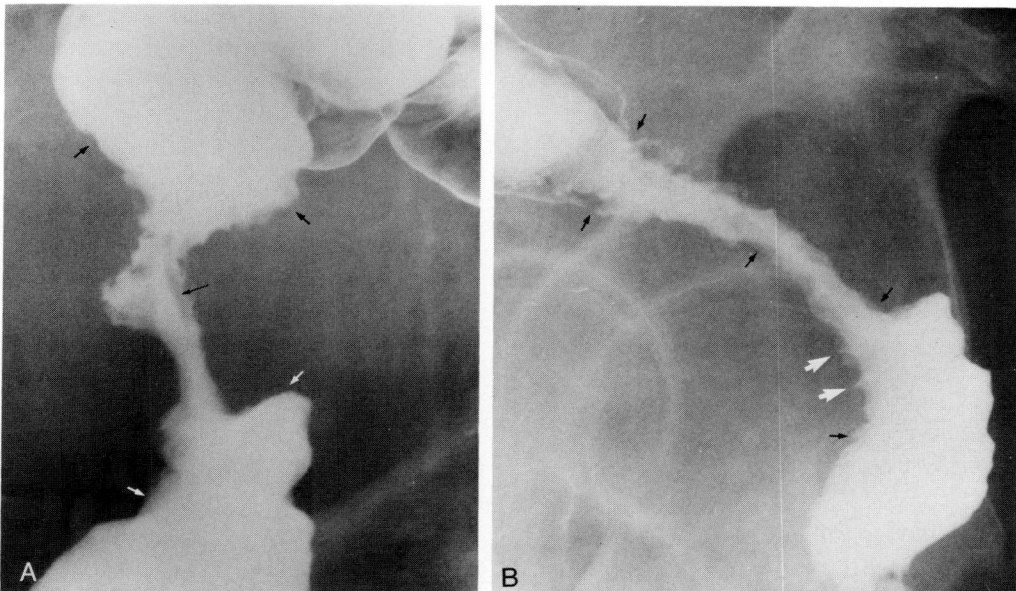

**Figure 68–33. Prostatic carcinoma invading the rectum. A.** Frontal view of the rectosigmoid junction shows a long, annular lesion *(short arrows)*. Mucosal folds are preserved in the center of the lesion *(long arrow).* **B.** Lateral view shows a long, circumferential lesion centered at the rectosigmoid junction *(small arrows)* with focal spiculation of the colonic contour *(large arrows).* In single contrast, this lesion is difficult to distinguish from a long, infiltrative scirrhous carcinoma of the colon or squamous carcinoma.

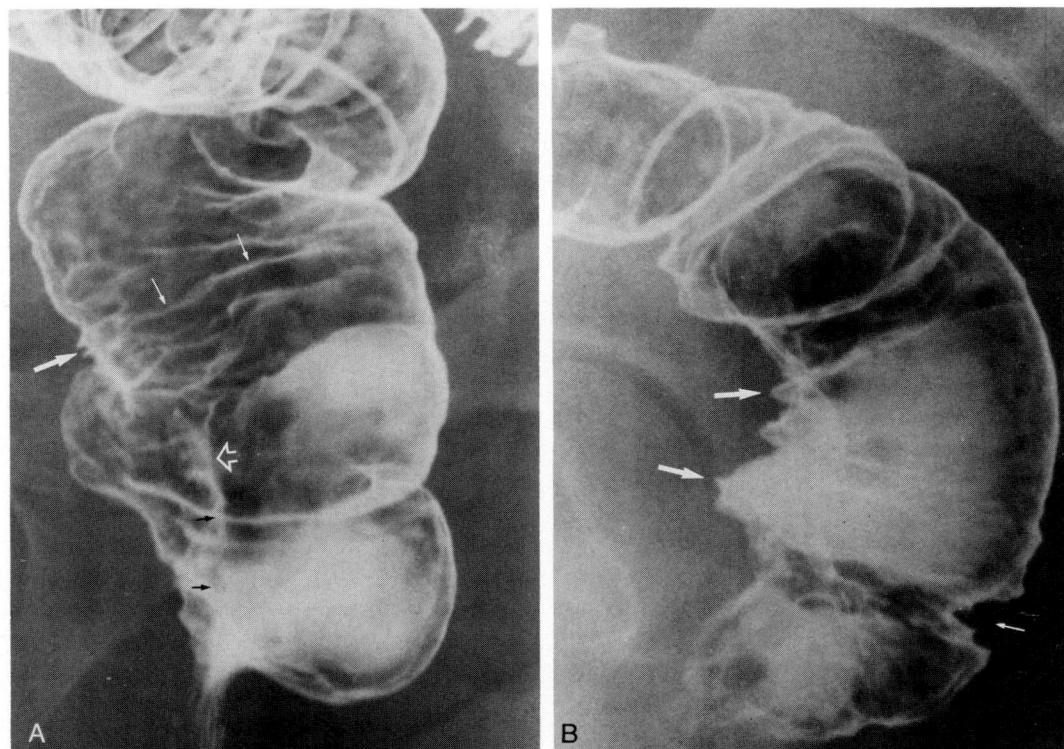

**Figure 68–34. Prostatic carcinoma invading the rectum. A.** Spot film of the rectum shows a mass effect along the right lateral wall of the rectum with obliteration of the rectal ampulla *(small black arrows)*, spiculation of the colonic contour *(large white arrow)*, and en face tethering of mucosal folds *(small white arrows)*. Focal nodularity of the rectal mucosa is seen *(open arrow)* at sites of muscularis propria and submucosal invasion by prostatic carcinoma. **B.** Lateral view of the rectum shows a mass effect along the distal anterior rectal wall and spiculation of the mucosal contour *(large arrows)*. Mild circumferential extension is seen distally *(small arrow)*. (**A** and **B** from SE Rubesin, MS Levine, M Bezzi, et al, Rectal involvement by prostatic carcinoma: barium enema findings, AJR, 152, 1, 53–57, 1989, © by American Roentgen Ray Society.)

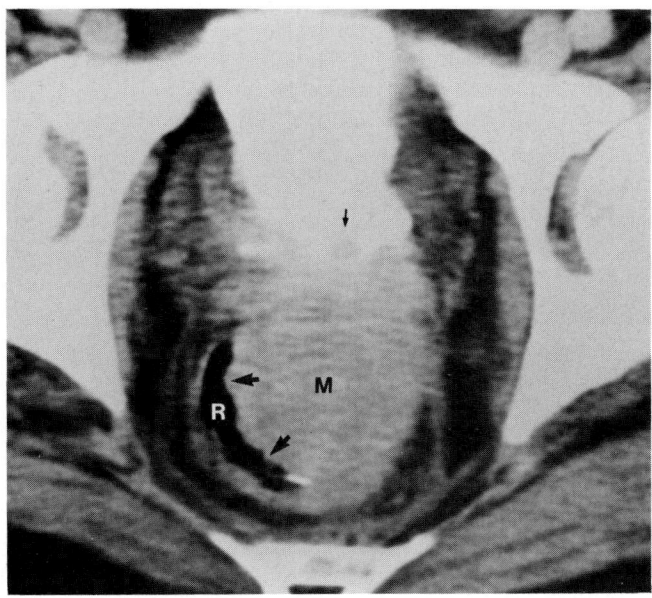

**Figure 68–35. Prostatic carcinoma invading the rectum.** Axial computed tomographic scan shows a large mass (M) arising in the prostate gland deviating the rectum (R) to the right. Infiltration of the rectal wall is shown by focal irregularity of the extrinsic mass impression *(large arrows)*. The prostatic mass also invades the urinary bladder *(small arrow)*.

patient is either erect or supine.[56] Both inflammatory and neoplastic processes extending to the intraperitoneal cavity may spread to the anterior wall of the rectosigmoid junction.[57] The neoplasm that most commonly spreads to the pouch of Douglas is ovarian carcinoma with peritoneal metastasis. Occasionally, uterine or bladder carcinomas spread peritoneally. The tumors in males that most commonly spread to the rectovesical space are gastrointestinal adenocarcinomas from the colon, stomach, and pancreas. With early intraperitoneal seeding, a smooth, extrinsic mass impression is seen radiographically on the anterior wall of the rectosigmoid junction. With direct invasion of the serosa, a desmoplastic reaction occurs, resulting in a radiographic appearance of spiculation of the colonic contour and pleating and angulation of smooth mucosal folds (Fig. 68–36). The radiographic findings are identical to those in endometriosis involving the colon, direct invasion by prostatic or cervical carcinoma, or a pelvic abscess resulting from tubo-ovarian abscess (Fig. 68–37), diverticulitis, appendicitis, or Crohn's disease secondarily affecting the colon. Circumferential extension of the desmoplastic process occurs most frequently with prostatic carcinoma, not intraperitoneal metastasis. The clinical history and age of the patient help to differentiate the causes of serosal desmoplastic disease involving the rectum.

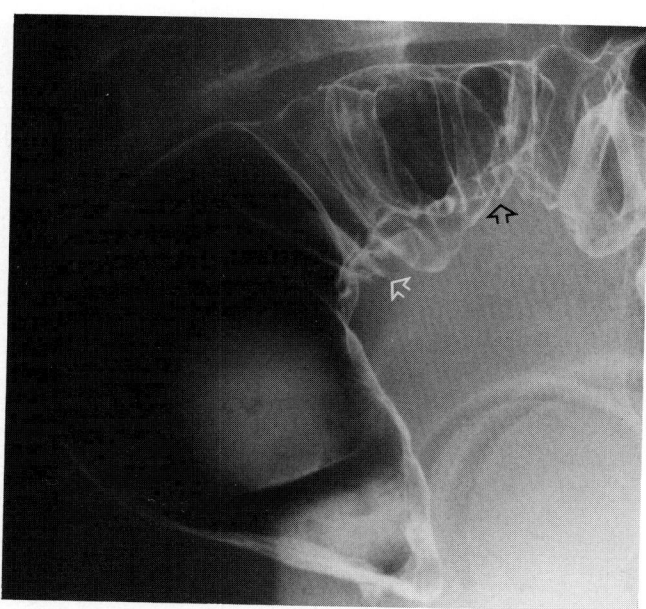

**Figure 68–37. Tubo-ovarian abscess with secondary inflammatory effects on the rectosigmoid junction.** Left lateral view of the rectum shows an extrinsic mass effect and spiculation of the colonic contour *(arrows)* in the pouch of Douglas. These radiographic findings are identical to those seen with peritoneal metastases involving the pouch of Douglas.

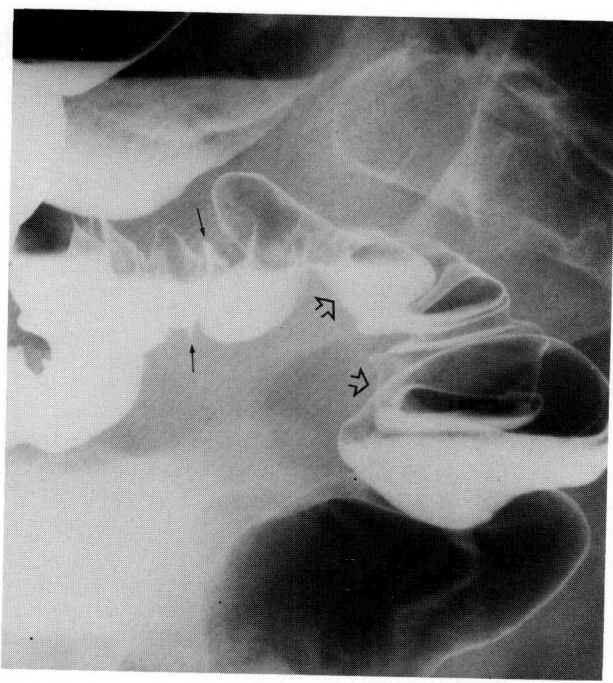

**Figure 68–36. Peritoneal metastasis to the pouch of Douglas by ovarian carcinoma.** Erect, right lateral spot film of the rectum shows a mass effect in the pouch of Douglas *(open arrows)*, spiculation of the colonic contour *(solid arrows)*, and mild, diffuse narrowing of the distal sigmoid colon. Note that the mucosa of the rectosigmoid colon is smooth.

## INFLAMMATORY DISORDERS

Many idiopathic, infectious, traumatic, and iatrogenic inflammatory disorders affect the rectum and colon. Most of these conditions are discussed in detail in Chapters 58, 61, 62, 63, and 70. This chapter highlights the main radiologic features of these disorders with respect to the rectum.

### Ulcerative Proctitis

Ulcerative proctitis is part of the spectrum of ulcerative colitis. Patients with ulcerative colitis confined to the rectum usually have mild diarrhea and mild rectal bleeding. Because the rectal mucosa is inflamed, bowel movements are usually frequent and of small volume. The rectum is almost always involved in all cases of ulcerative colitis, because the disease spreads retrogradely from the rectum to the more proximal colon. Inflammation begins at the anorectal junction and extends proximally, involving the entire circumference of bowel, and is without "skip" lesions.

Mild ulcerative colitis is manifest on double contrast barium enemas en face as finely granular mucosa—punctate dots of barium stippled on the colonic surface (Fig. 68–38). Granular mucosa is due to mucosal edema and hyperemia.[58, 59] In more chronic forms of ulcerative proctitis, the mucosa may become coarsely granular or finely nodular. With more severe inflammation, shallow

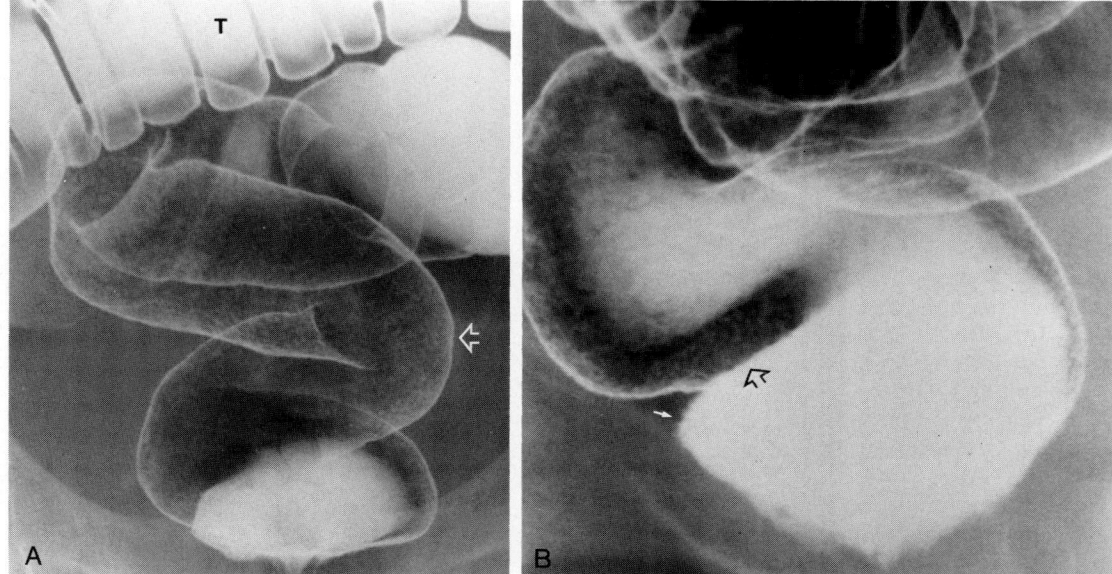

**Figure 68–38. Mucosal granularity in ulcerative proctosigmoiditis. A.** Punctate barium collections cover the entire circumference of the mucosa of the rectosigmoid colon (representative areas of granularity are identified by the arrow). The overlying transverse colon (T) has a smooth, normal mucosa. (From Rubesin SE, Laufer I, Dinsmore B: Radiologic investigation of inflammatory bowel disease. *In* MacDermott RP, Stenson WF [eds]: Inflammatory Bowel Disease. East Norwalk, CT: Appleton & Lange, 1992, pp 453–491.) **B.** In a different patient, punctate barium collections are seen only when the barium-coated mucosa is surrounded by air (representative area indicated by open arrow). En face, in the barium pool, shallow spiculation of the colonic contour is seen *(solid arrow).* The thick barium pool obscures the granular mucosa en face.

ulcers are seen as discrete punctate barium collections 1 to 3 mm in diameter on a background of granular mucosa.[60]

With advanced or chronic disease, changes in bowel configuration occur.[12] The rectum assumes a tubular configuration and the valves of Houston disappear (Fig. 68–39). With loss of colonic volume, perirectal fat proliferates, resulting in a widened presacral space. On lateral views, the posterior wall of the rectosigmoid junction appears more than 2 cm from the anterior wall of the sacrum.

Polypoid projections in ulcerative colitis may represent islands of residual mucosa between areas of ulceration (pseudopolyps) or inflammatory or hyperplastic tissue projecting into the lumen after the mucosal ulceration has healed (postinflammatory polyps) (Fig. 68–40). In patients with long-standing ulcerative colitis, some polypoid or plaque-like elevations may represent dysplastic epithelium (Fig. 68–41). Most dysplastic lesions in ulcerative colitis are flat and not demonstrated by barium enema examination.

Diagnosis of ulcerative colitis is based on clinical history, endoscopic and radiologic findings, and lack of positive culture results for enteric pathogens. Rectal infection by *Yersinia, Campylobacter, Shigella,* cytomegalovirus, and even amebae may mimic ulcerative proctitis endoscopically and radiologically.[61]

Ulcerative colitis has fewer complications if only the rectum is involved. Approximately one fourth of patients with ulcerative proctitis progress to left-sided colitis or pancolitis.[62] Although the lifetime risk of colorectal carcinoma in ulcerative colitis is 3 to 5%,[63–65] ulcerative proctitis probably does not predispose to colonic neoplasia.[12]

Because ulcerative proctitis may be extremely mild or a patient may have been treated with steroid enemas, the rectum may appear relatively normal. Mild ulcerative proctitis is the form of ulcerative colitis that may be missed on double contrast barium enema examinations.

## Crohn's Disease

Crohn's disease may be confined to the colon in up to 30% of patients.[66] The rectum is involved in approximately one half of patients with granulomatous colitis.[67, 68] Up to 40% of all other patients with Crohn's disease have both colonic and small bowel involvement,[66] but in these patients Crohn's disease typically involves the right side of the colon.

Patients with rectal Crohn's disease complain of low-volume diarrhea, tenesmus, and urgency. Although rectal bleeding is an infrequent complaint of all patients who have Crohn's disease, bleeding is not infrequent if Crohn's disease involves the rectum.

As in other intestinal sites, Crohn's disease involving the rectum has a patchy, asymmetric distribution. Aphthoid ulcers are separated by areas of normal or minimally erythematous mucosa.[69]

On double contrast barium enema examination, aphthoid ulcers are seen as punctate, round or oval

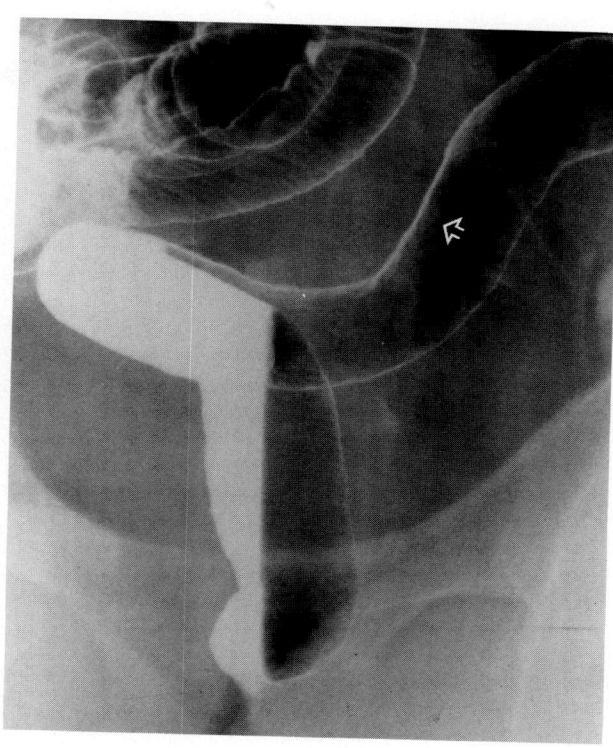

**Figure 68–39. Chronic ulcerative proctosigmoiditis.** Right-side-down decubitus view of the rectosigmoid colon shows diffuse, tubular narrowing, as well as loss of the valves of Houston and sigmoid folds. Coarse granularity of the sigmoid colon mucosa is present *(arrow)*.

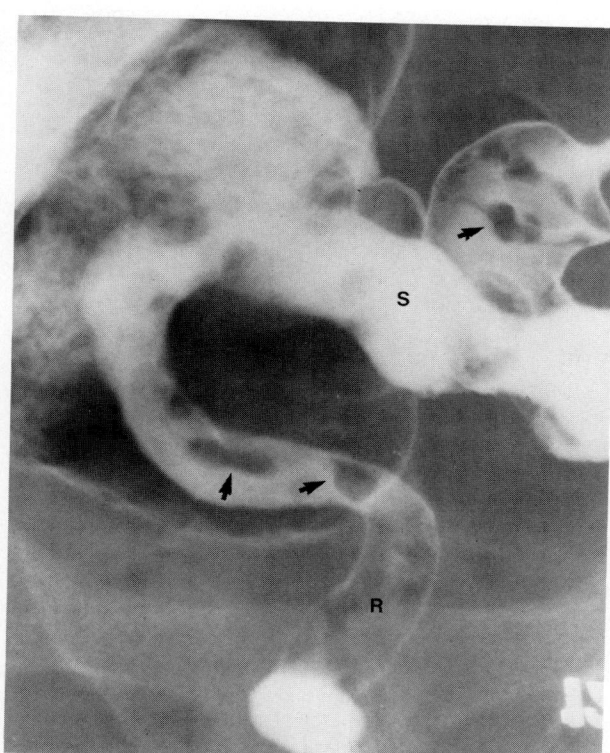

**Figure 68–40. Ulcerative colitis with postinflammatory polyps.** Diffuse narrowing of the rectum (R) and sigmoid colon (S) is seen in a patient with long ulcerative proctosigmoiditis. Ovoid and tubular radiolucent filling defects are seen in the barium pool *(arrows)*. Biopsy showed that these were postinflammatory polyps.

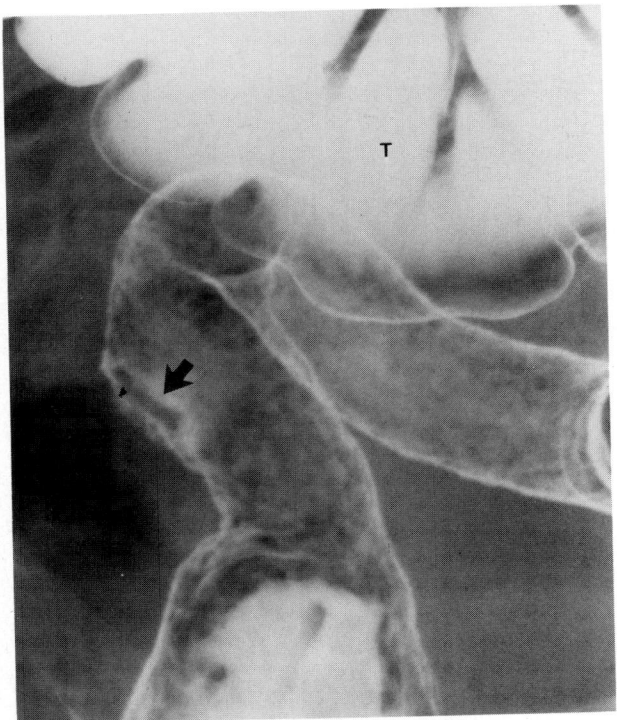

**Figure 68–41. Plaque-like dysplasia in ulcerative proctosigmoiditis.** Spot film of the rectosigmoid colon shows a slightly raised plaque *(arrow)* 1.5 cm in diameter. Also note diffuse, tubular narrowing of the rectosigmoid colon and coarsely granular mucosa. The transverse colon (T) is normal.

barium collections surrounded by radiolucent halos of edema[69, 70] (Fig. 68–42). With progression, deeper "collar button" ulcers may be seen (Fig. 68–43).

Strictures, perianal fissures (Fig. 68–44), and fistulas are serious and frequent complications of Crohn's disease, seen in 50 to 80% of patients with Crohn's colitis.[66, 71] Fistulas begin in deep rectal fissures or in the anorectal glands and extend through the rectal wall or external sphincter muscle. Perianal disease may be the initial clinical manifestation of Crohn's disease. Persistent perianal disease may result in strictures or fistulas such as rectovaginal fistulas (Fig. 68–45) or perianal abscess (Fig. 68–46). Destruction of the anal sphincter may result in fecal incontinence.[12] Pelvic abscesses caused by Crohn's disease may involve the rectum secondarily (Fig. 68–47).

Chronic enteric infections may mimic the clinical, endoscopic, and radiologic manifestations of rectal Crohn's disease. Enteric infections in which aphthoid-like ulcers occur include amebiasis (Fig. 68–48), *Yersinia* enterocolitis, cytomegalovirus colitis, and Behçet's disease. Infectious diseases typified by strictures or fistula formation include lymphogranuloma venereum, actinomycosis, and tuberculosis. Diagnosis of Crohn's disease relies on the clinical history, endoscopic and radiologic findings, and negative cultures and blood titers for various pathogens.

## Infectious Colitis

A wide variety of pathogens including *Shigella* species, *Campylobacter* species, and *Clostridium difficile* infect the rectum and colon.[72] These patients usually present with acute lower abdominal pain, tenesmus, and low-volume diarrhea with either bloody stools or passage of blood-stained mucus. The clinical considerations usually include an infectious colitis, acute ulcerative colitis, or rarely ischemic colitis. Diagnosis depends primarily on the clinical history, sigmoidoscopy, microscopic examination of stool for ova and parasites, stool cultures, and blood titers. Barium enemas are not usually performed for patients with acute watery or bloody diarrhea. If symptoms persist or intermittent, relapsing diarrhea occurs, barium enemas may be performed in patients with infectious colitis (Fig. 68–49).

## Shigella *Colitis*

Various species of *Shigella* may cause acute dysentery with passage of small, frequent bloody stools and bloody mucus discharge.[72, 73] Some patients develop a persistent, subacute form confused clinically, endoscopically, and radiologically with ulcerative colitis. Rectosigmoid involvement by ulceration and psuedomembrane formation is dominant, but disease may extend throughout

*Text continued on page 1293*

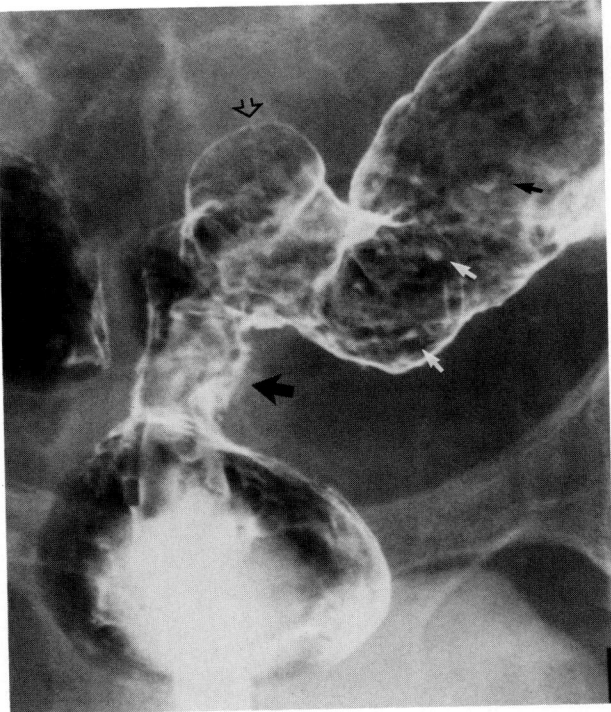

**Figure 68–42. Crohn's disease involving the rectosigmoid colon.** Numerous aphthoid ulcers *(small arrows)* are seen as punctate barium collections surrounded by radiolucent halos. Also note diffuse shortening of the rectosigmoid colon, focal stricture formation *(large arrow)*, and sacculation of relatively uninvolved colon wall *(open arrow)*.

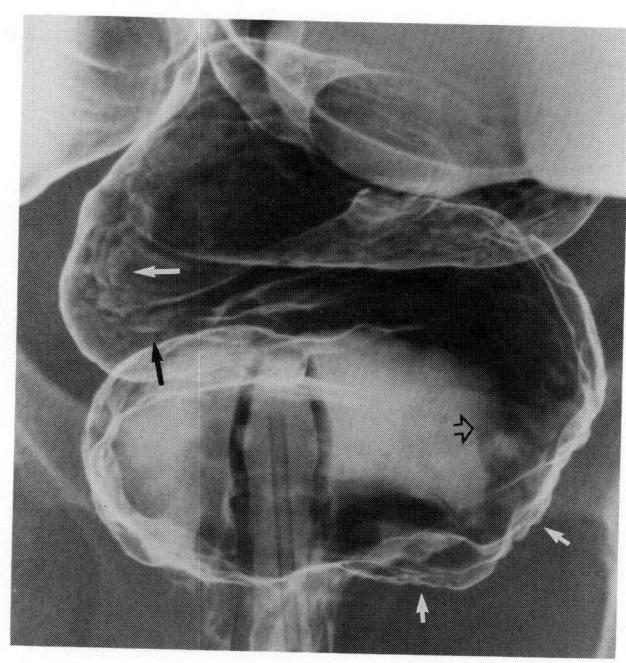

**Figure 68–43. Ulcers in Crohn's disease.** Spot film of the rectum shows relatively large ulcers *(large arrows)* seen as focal barium collections surrounded by radiolucent halos of edema. Note "boggy" rectal mucosa manifested as slight nodularity of the colonic contour *(small arrows)* and nonuniform barium coating *(open arrow)* of the rectal mucosa.

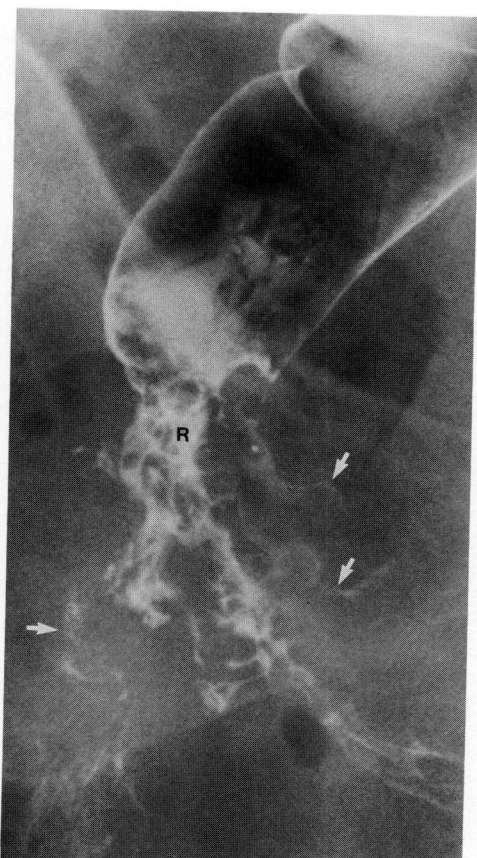

**Figure 68–44. Crohn's disease with perianal fissures.** Oblique spot film of the lower rectum shows numerous barium-filled tracks *(arrows)* extending from abnormal rectal mucosa into the perianal soft tissue. Note severe distal rectal narrowing and "cobblestone" appearance (R) of the mucosa.

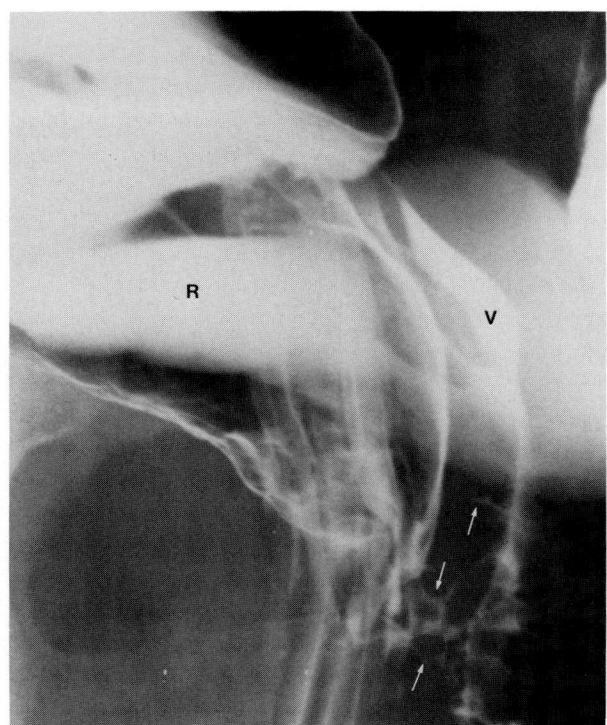

**Figure 68–45. Perianal Crohn's disease with distal rectovaginal fistula.**
Oblique spot film of the rectum (R) shows numerous barium-filled tracks
*(arrows)* extending from the distal rectum and anal canal into the lower
vagina. V = upper vagina.

**Figure 68–46. Crohn's disease with perianal fistula and abscess formation.** Spot film centered at the anorectal junction (A) shows fistulous tracks containing barium *(long arrow)* entering a tubular perianal abscess *(short arrows)*.

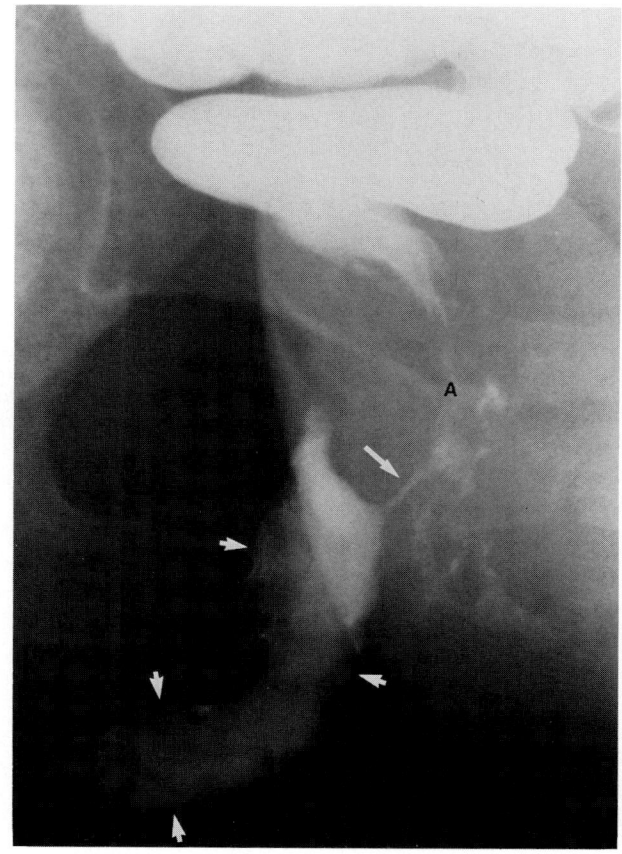

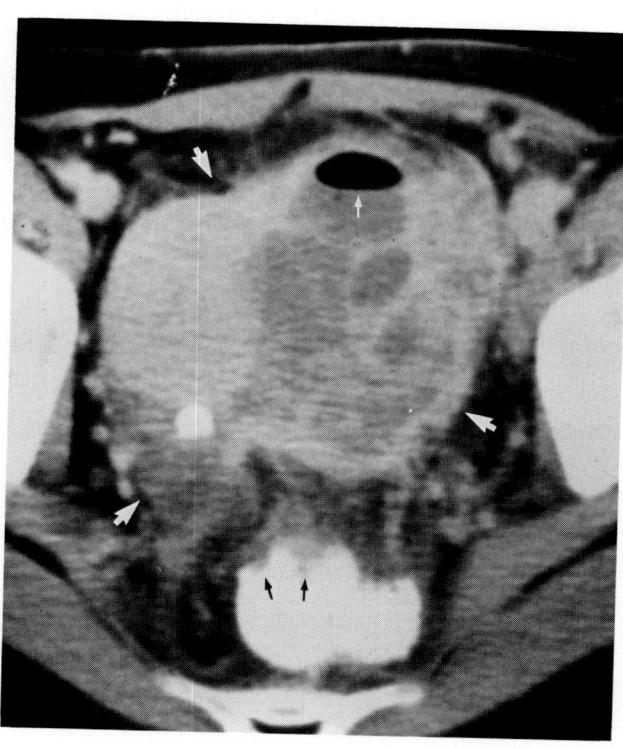

**Figure 68–47. Pelvic abscess in Crohn's disease secondarily involving the rectum.** A large soft tissue mass *(large white arrows)* with central fluid collections and air-fluid levels *(small white arrow)* is seen in the pelvis. The inflammatory reaction spreads from this abscess to involve the rectum *(black arrows)*.

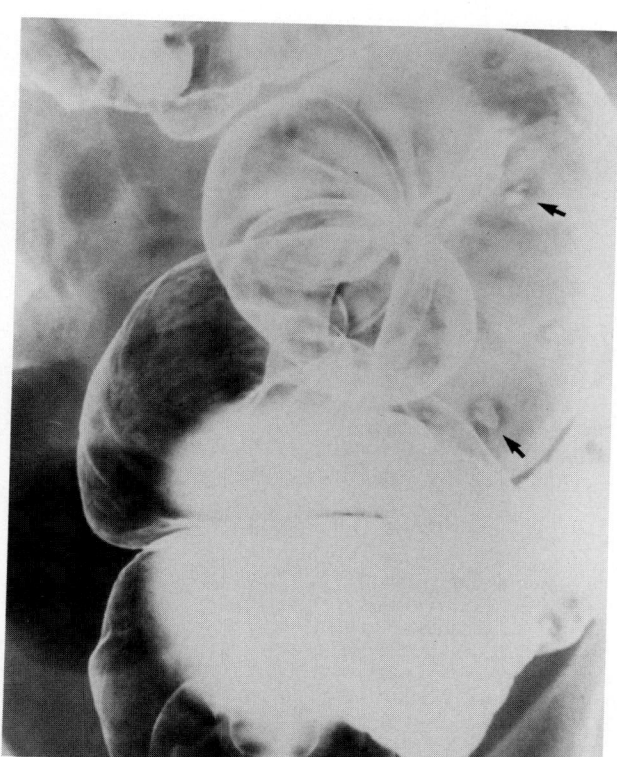

**Figure 68–48. Amebiasis involving the rectum.** Numerous small and large shallow ulcers are manifested as focal barium collections surrounded by radiolucent halos (of edema). (Representative ulcers are identified with arrows.) These ulcers mimic the aphthoid ulcers seen in Crohn's disease. (Courtesy of Harvey Goldstein, M.D., San Antonio, TX.)

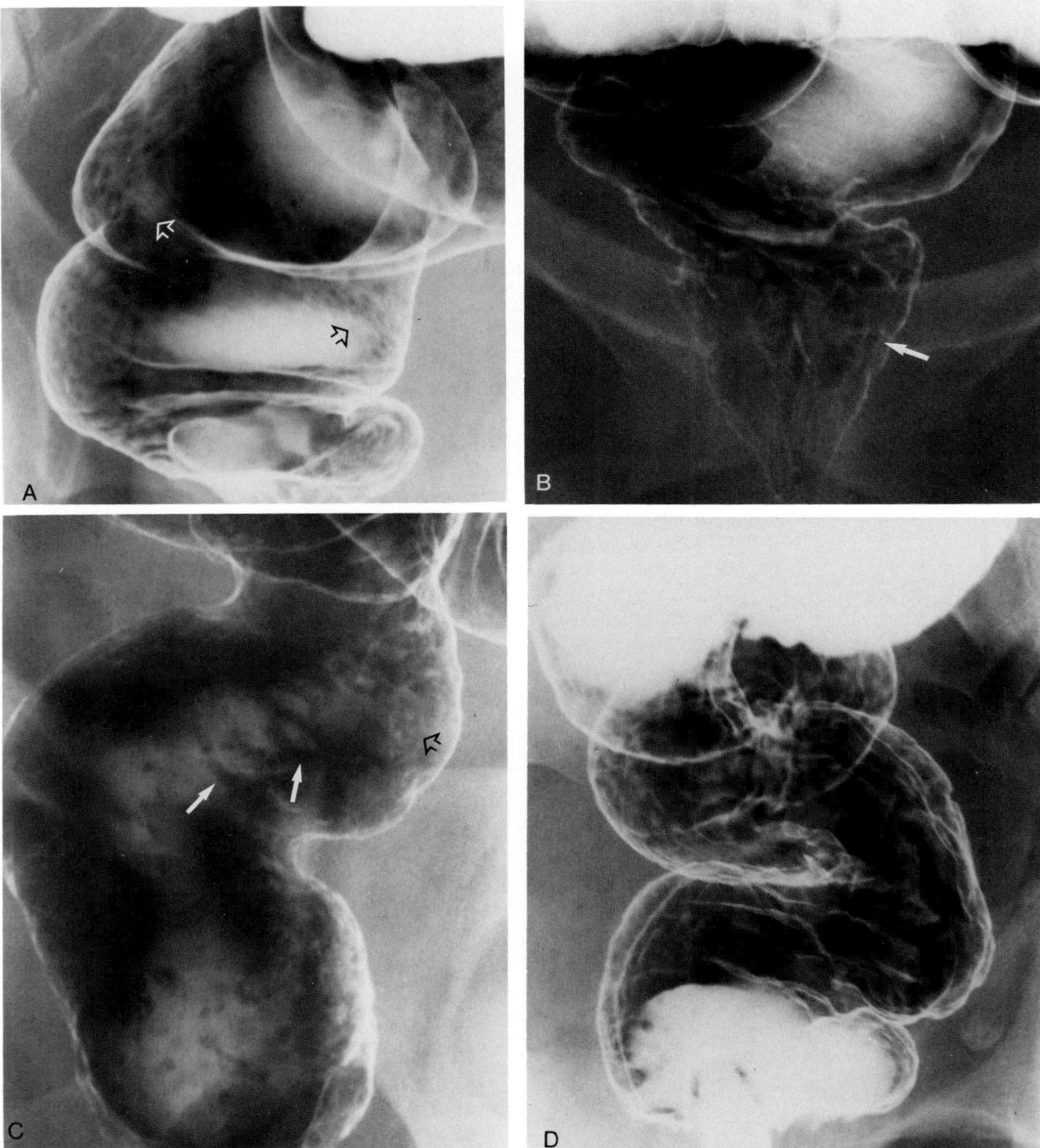

**Figure 68–49. Nonspecific proctitis. A.** Follicular proctitis. Numerous small, round, uniform radiolucent nodules *(arrows)* represent lymphoid follicles carpeting the distal rectum. This patient had chronic diarrhea. All culture results were negative. Lymphoid follicular hyperplasia was identified by biopsy. **B.** Nonspecific viral proctitis. The mucosa of the distal rectum shows raised, polygonal nodules (representative area identified by the arrow). A biopsy revealed viral inclusion bodies in the cytoplasm of epithelial cells. No cultures were performed. **C.** Nonspecific viral proctitis. Numerous small and large ulcers *(arrows)* are manifested as punctate barium collections surrounded by radiolucent halos of edema *(open arrow).* On biopsy specimens, viral inclusion bodies were identified in the cytoplasm of epithelial cells. **D.** Boggy mucosa in nonspecific proctitis. Coarse, nodular folds are present throughout the rectum. (**A** and **D** from Rubesin SE, Saul H, Laufer I, et al: Carpet lesion of the colon. Radiographics 5:537–552, 1985.)

the colon.[74] Barium enema examinations show spasm, mucosal edema, and ulceration.[75] *Shigella* colitis is discussed in detail in Chapter 63.

## Campylobacter *Colitis*

Colonic infection by *Campylobacter jejuni* results in a broad clinical spectrum from an asymptomatic carrier state to a fulminant colitis with toxic megacolon.[76] Barium enemas may be performed in patients with a chronic, relapsing course. Barium enema findings are those of a nonspecific colitis with granular mucosa, thickened interhaustral folds, and occasionally focal ulceration—findings confused with those of ulcerative colitis or Crohn's disease.[76–78] In patients with chronic diarrhea, diagnosis of *Campylobacter* colitis depends on positive culture results or immunofluorescent studies of rectal biopsies.[79]

## Clostridium difficile *Colitis*

Infection of the colon by *C. difficile,* a gram-positive bacillus, results in a broad spectrum of colitis, the most severe form being known as *pseudomembranous colitis.*[80] Although *C. difficile* is frequently found in neonates, the organism does not colonize the colon of older children and adults. However, *C. difficile* may colonize a colon whose endogenous microflora is altered by antibiotics, cancer chemotherapeutic agents, endogenous pathogens such as *Salmonella* or *Shigella,* or coexisting diseases such as ulcerative colitis or mild ischemia. Thus, *C. difficile* colitis is a common cause of antibiotic-induced colitis and a frequent primary nosocomial infection. *C. difficile* produces several endotoxins that cause both secretion of fluid into the colonic lumen and an inflammatory and necrotic response in the colonic epithelium. In a patient who is taking or has just completed a course of antibiotics, the most typical symptoms are watery, nonbloody diarrhea, crampy abdominal pain, fever, and leukocytosis. In this setting, the radiologist may review plain films of the abdomen. In patients with mild disease, the plain film of the abdomen is normal. In moderate to severe cases, the plain film shows diffuse dilatation of the colon, especially its most anterior portion, the transverse colon. Wide, transverse, slightly lobulated bands replace the normal interhaustral folds of the transverse colon.[81, 82] Thumbprinting may be seen.

If the clinical history of *C. difficile* colitis is suspected, the diagnosis relies on stool assay for cytotoxin and flexible sigmoidoscopy. At sigmoidoscopy, yellow-white, raised plaques, 2 to 5 mm in diameter, are scattered over the mucosal surface. These yellow plaques have given rise to the term pseudomembranous colitis. The plaques are composed of debris, fibrin, white blood cells, and mucus.[83] The underlying epithelium shows variable necrosis and acute inflammation.

However, there is a broad clinical, pathologic, endoscopic, and radiologic spectrum of *C. difficile* colitis. The radiologist is frequently the first physician to suggest the diagnosis in patients with an atypical clinical history

or nonspecific flexible sigmoidoscopy results. The radiologist most frequently encounters changes of pseudomembranous colitis in postoperative patients who have fever and leukocytosis, and a computed tomographic scan is performed to rule out an abdominal abscess. The scan shows a thick colonic wall with a scalloped, nodular luminal contour.[84–86]

Barium studies may be administered to patients with an atypical clinical history, such as bloody diarrhea or rectal bleeding without diarrhea. Barium studies may also be performed when sigmoidoscopic studies are normal or show mild, nonspecific colitis manifested solely by erythema and friability in the rectosigmoid colon. On barium enema examination, well-circumscribed, slightly raised, round to ovoid radiolucent plaques are seen both en face and in profile[87] (Fig. 68–50). Thick, mildly lobulated interhaustral folds corresponding to the folds seen on plain films may be present, especially in the transverse and ascending colon. The rectosigmoid colon is spared in 20 to 70% of patients with *C. difficile* colitis.[88–92] The rectosigmoid mucosa may be normal or show fine granularity in patients with rectosigmoid sparing.[93] However, the more proximal colon shows findings typical of pseudomembranous colitis.[93]

## Sexually Transmitted Proctitis

A wide variety of anorectal infections can result from homosexual or heterosexual anal intercourse.[94–98] The pathogens most frequently causing proctitis are *Neisseria gonorrhoeae, Treponema pallidum, Chlamydia trachomatis,* and herpes simplex virus. Multiple pathogens are found in many patients. The typical clinical history is that of anal discharge, bleeding, pain, tenesmus, and/or diarrhea. The clinician may have to elicit a clinical history of anal intercourse. Stools must be carefully cultured and special transport media are required for certain pathogens, especially *N. gonorrhoeae* and *C. trachomatis.*

### Gonorrheal Proctitis

Many patients who harbor *N. gonorrhoeae* in the rectum are asymptomatic or complain of mild systems such as anal itching. Other patients may complain of rectal bleeding, discharge, or constipation.[99–101] Flexible sigmoidoscopy may be normal or show mild nonspecific mucosal friability. The proctitis is usually confined to the anal canal, especially around anal crypts in the rectum. If untreated, disease may progress to perirectal abscess, stricture, or fistula formation.[102]

### Lymphogranuloma Venereum

*C. trachomatis,* an obligate intracellular organism, is the causative agent in lymphogranuloma venereum.[103] In males, infection is related to anal intercourse.[104] In women, proctitis is probably related to either anal intercourse or spread of infected vaginal discharge to the anal canal. A less likely mode of dissemination in

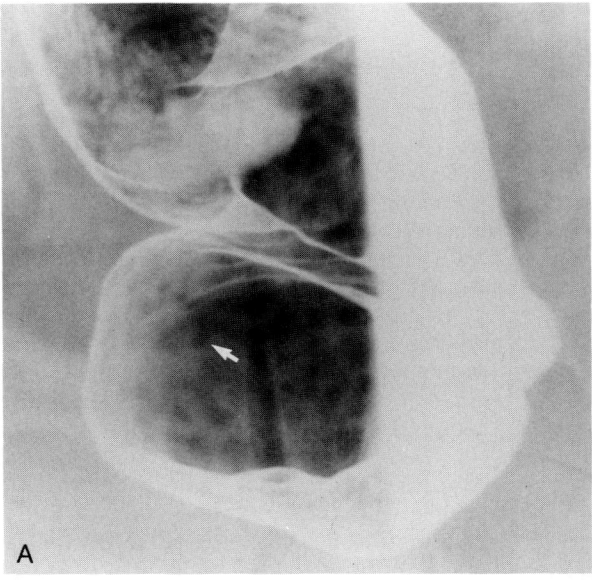

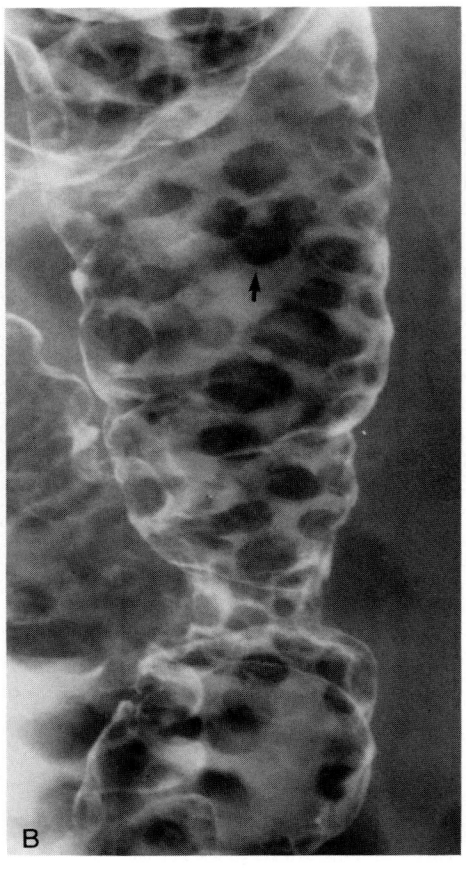

**Figure 68–50. Pseudomembranous colitis. A.** The pseudomembranous plaques in the rectum are manifested as numerous round, radiolucent filling defects *(arrow)* carpeting the rectal mucosa. These nodules are larger than those seen in lymphoid hyperplasia. **B.** Plaques in pseudomembranous colitis. A spot film of the splenic flexure shows numerous round, well-circumscribed, radiolucent filling defects in the shallow barium pool *(arrow)*.

females is spread of disease from inguinal lymphadenopathy.[12] The clinical spectrum ranges from an asymptomatic carrier state to bloody diarrhea with mucopurulent discharge, rectal pain, or tenesmus. If a chronic infection is present, the patient may complain of constipation. Clinical diagnosis requires a careful history, rectal culture using special transport media, immunofluorescent staining of biopsy material, and/or serologic diagnosis through public health laboratories. If the disease is untreated, chronic infection may lead to stricture formation.[105]

In the acute stage, sigmoidoscopy or barium enema examination shows a mild nonspecific proctitis with friable or granular mucosa, respectively. If it is untreated, deep ulceration, stricturing, and rectovaginal fistulas may occur.[106] Barium enema findings mimic those in Crohn's disease or nonspecific colitis, including granular mucosa, small ulcers (Fig. 68–51A), deep barium-filled clefts, diffuse narrowing of the rectosigmoid colon with loss of the valves of Houston (Fig. 68–51B), perianal fissures (Fig. 68–52), or a rectovaginal fistula.[106]

### Herpes Simplex Proctitis

Rectal infection with herpes simplex virus may be clinically manifest by abdominal pain, tenesmus, discharge, constipation, or inguinal lymphadenopathy.[107, 108] Many patients are asymptomatic. Flexible sigmoidoscopy may reveal small vesicles or focal ulceration. Bar-

ium enema examination shows marked spasm, edema, or mucosal ulcers resembling aphthoid ulcers[109] (Fig. 68–53). Diagnosis relies on virus isolation from swabs.

### Anorectal Syphilis

In most cases, anorectal syphilis is sexually transmitted.[110] Primary syphilis produces a chancre in the squamous epithelium of the anal canal or in the rectal mucosa. Patients complain of pain, discharge, and tenesmus.[111–113]

### Mucosal Prolapse Syndromes

Chronic prolapse of rectal mucosa may result in chronic inflammation, ulceration, and hyperplastic reparative response. During defecation, rectal mucosa passing inferiorly through a contracted puborectalis sling may experience trauma, especially along the anterior and anterolateral wall. Chronic intussusception may also result in mucosal damage. The mucosal response to chronic defecatory problems results in a spectrum of syndromes including solitary rectal ulcer syndrome, colitis cystica profunda, hypertrophied anal papilla, and inflammatory cloacogenic polyp.[114, 115] The latter two entities were described earlier. A similar histologic response may be seen with prolapsing internal hemorrhoids and prolapsing colostomies.[116]

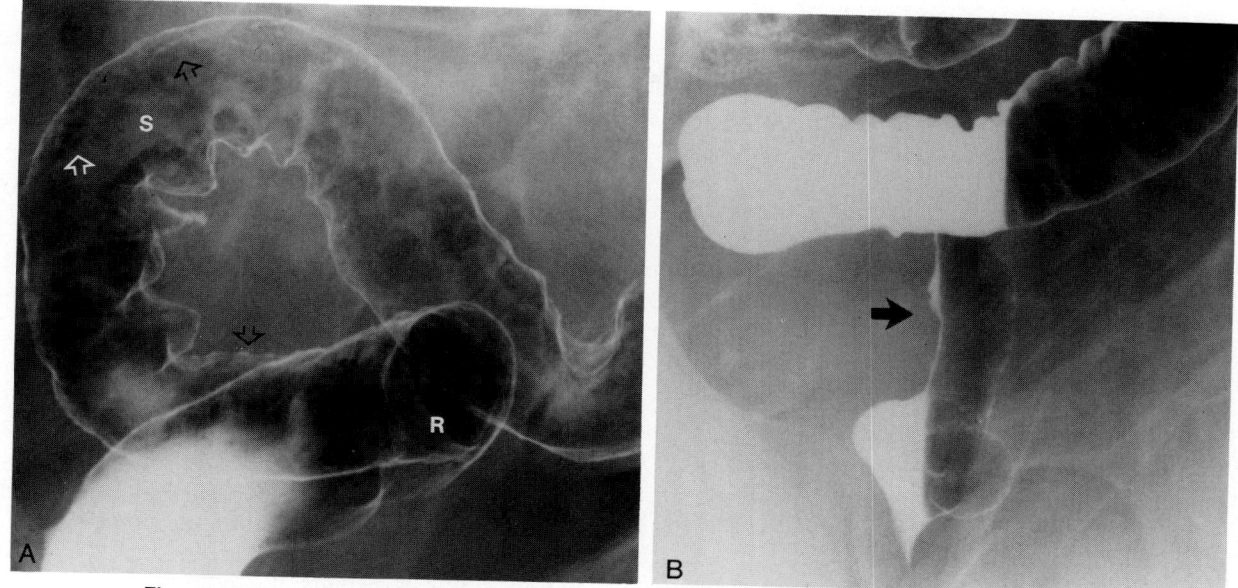

**Figure 68–51. Lymphogranuloma venereum. A.** Spot film of the distal sigmoid colon (S) and rectosigmoid junction (R) shows numerous, small punctate and linear barium collections *(arrows)* en face and in profile. This 49-year-old man had complained of diarrhea for 3 months. The initial clinical diagnosis was Crohn's disease. **B.** Three months later, the patient complained of passing narrow caliber stool. A barium enema was given, and a spot film of the rectosigmoid junction shows a smooth, tapered stricture *(arrow)*. A history of anal intercourse was elicited. Subsequent chlamydial titers were markedly elevated.

**Figure 68–52. Perianal fissures in lymphogranuloma venereum.** Supine **(A)** and oblique **(B)** views of the rectum show numerous barium-filled tracks *(arrows)* extending into the perirectal soft tissue. Diffuse rectal narrowing is present. This man had a long history of diarrhea and anal intercourse. Chlamydial titers were markedly elevated.

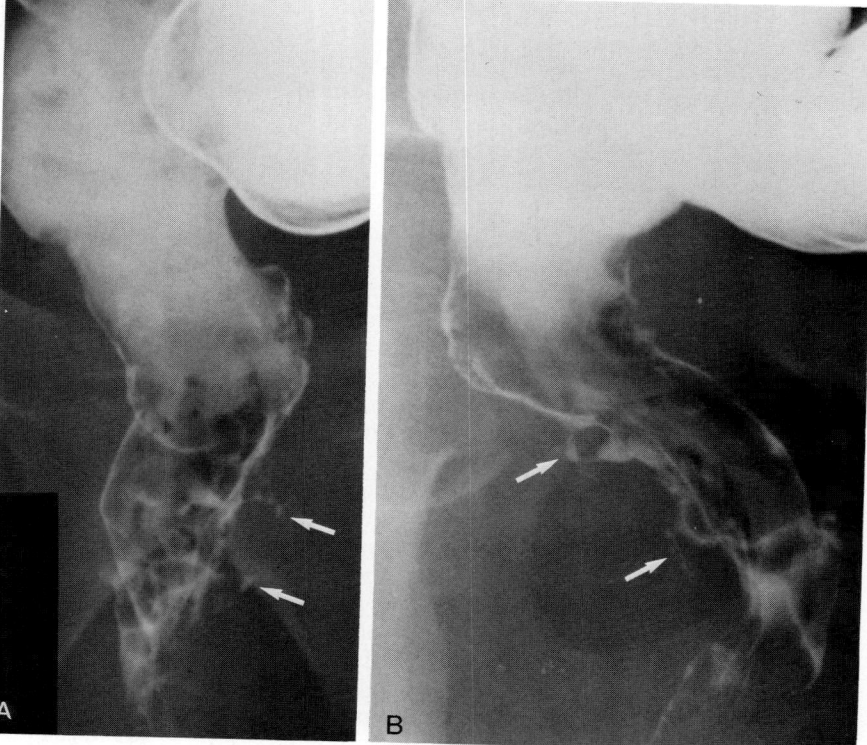

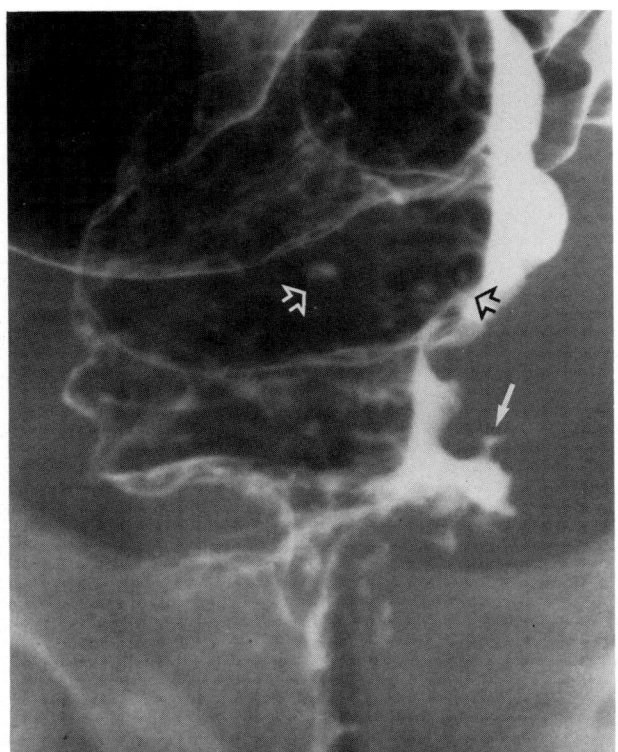

**Figure 68–53. Herpes simplex proctitis.** Numerous small, rectal ulcers *(open arrows)* are manifested as punctate barium collections surrounded by radiolucent halos. Also note deep extension of some ulcers into the rectal wall *(solid arrow)*. (Courtesy of Francis J. Scholz, M.D., Burlington, MA. From Shah SJ, Scholz FJ: Anorectal herpes: radiographic findings. Radiology 147:81–82, 1983.)

Solitary rectal ulcer syndrome and colitis cystica profunda are uncommon, chronic benign conditions. The name solitary ulcer syndrome is a misnomer because multiple small ulcers may be present, or the colon may not be grossly ulcerated at all. Although the syndrome is typically seen in young adults, it may occur at any age. Patients commonly complain of rectal bleeding, rectal pain, and passage of mucus.

At sigmoidoscopy, single or multiple well-demarcated, shallow ulcers may be found on the anterolateral or anterior wall of the distal half of the rectum.[117] An ulcer may not be visible; rather, the mucosa may appear diffusely erythematous, friable, or even polypoid.[118]

Pathologically, the mucosa is mildly inflamed. The glandular epithelium may be hyperplastic, occasionally showing villus formation, which may even be mistaken for villous adenoma.[119] The muscularis mucosae is disorganized, and there may be extension of the smooth muscle of the muscularis mucosae into the lamina propria. Mucin-filled glands may be trapped in the submucosa. When these glands become cystically dilated, a diagnosis of localized colitis cystica profunda may be made.[115] Solitary rectal ulcer syndrome and colitis cystica profunda have been confused with villous adenoma or infiltrating adenocarcinoma. However, the glandular ep-

ithelium is not dysplastic in solitary rectal ulcer syndrome and colitis cystica profunda.

The radiographic findings are variable.[120] The rectal mucosa may appear normal in up to 50% of cases.[121] Diffuse, finely nodular mucosa in the distal rectum may be seen, correlating with the friable, erythematous mucosa seen at proctoscopy (Fig. 68–54). A focal, small ulcer may be found on the anterior or anterolateral wall (Fig. 68–55). Redundant, prolapsing mucosa may appear as a polypoid mass. Localized colitis cystica profunda may have the appearance of a submucosal mass (Fig. 68–56). The valves of Houston may be markedly enlarged with a nodular contour[121, 122] (Fig. 68–57). Rarely, a stricture may be seen.[123]

## Radiation Proctosigmoiditis

Radiation proctosigmoiditis most frequently results from radiation therapy for cervical cancer. Radiation proctitis may also develop after radiotherapy for bladder, colon, uterine, or prostatic neoplasms. Acute radiation colitis is usually self-limited, occurring in the first week after radiotherapy because of a direct toxic effect of the radiation beam on the epithelial lining.[124] Patients complain of diarrhea, tenesmus, abdominal cramping, and occasionally bleeding. A barium enema examination during the episode of acute radiation damage may show spasm, edema, or granular mucosa, changes similar to those in ulcerative colitis.[124] Barium enemas, however, are rarely performed during this acute phase.

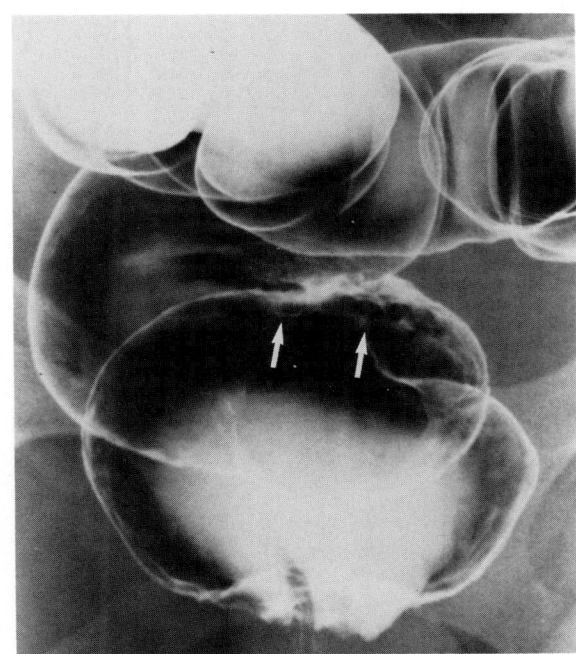

**Figure 68–54. Solitary rectal ulcer syndrome: mucosal nodularity.** Focal mucosal nodularity *(arrows)* is seen in the proximal rectum. (From Levine MS, Piccolello ML, Sollenberger LC, et al: Solitary rectal ulcer syndrome: a radiologic diagnosis? Gastrointest Radiol 11:187–193, 1986.)

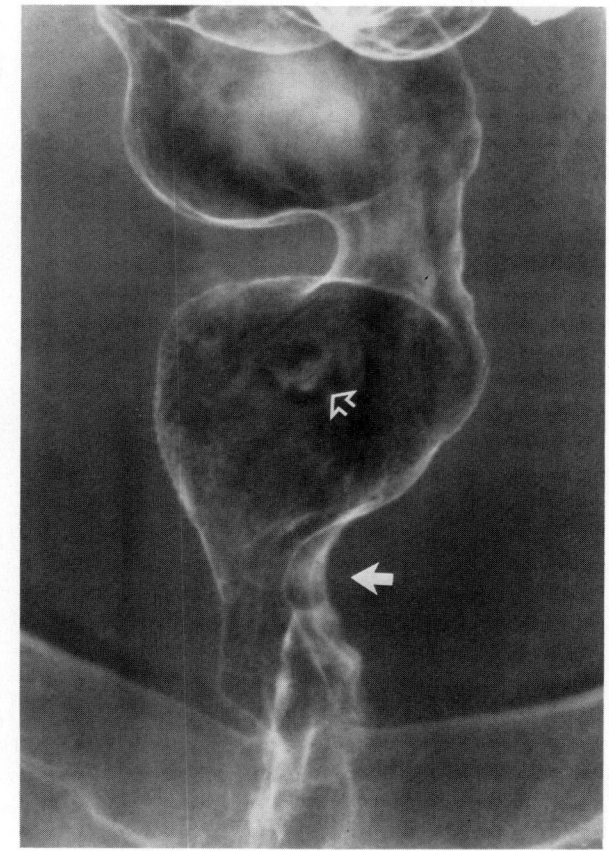

**Figure 68–55. Solitary rectal ulcer syndrome: solitary ulcer.** An irregular barium collection *(open arrow)* 1 cm in diameter is surrounded by a radiolucent halo (of edema). Also note mild granularity of distal rectal mucosa and focal submucosal mass effect *(solid arrow).*

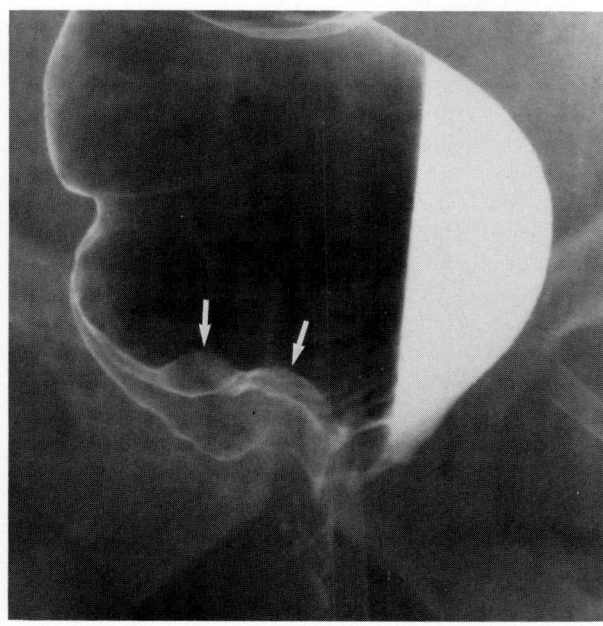

**Figure 68–56. Solitary rectal ulcer syndrome: submucosal masses.** Two smooth-surfaced, polypoid, submucosal-appearing masses *(arrows)* are seen in the distal rectum. These masses were due to mucus-filled, epithelium-lined cysts in the submucosa (colitis cystica profunda). (From Levine MS, Piccolello ML, Sollenberger LC, et al: Solitary rectal ulcer syndrome: a radiologic diagnosis? Gastrointest Radiol 11:187–193, 1986.)

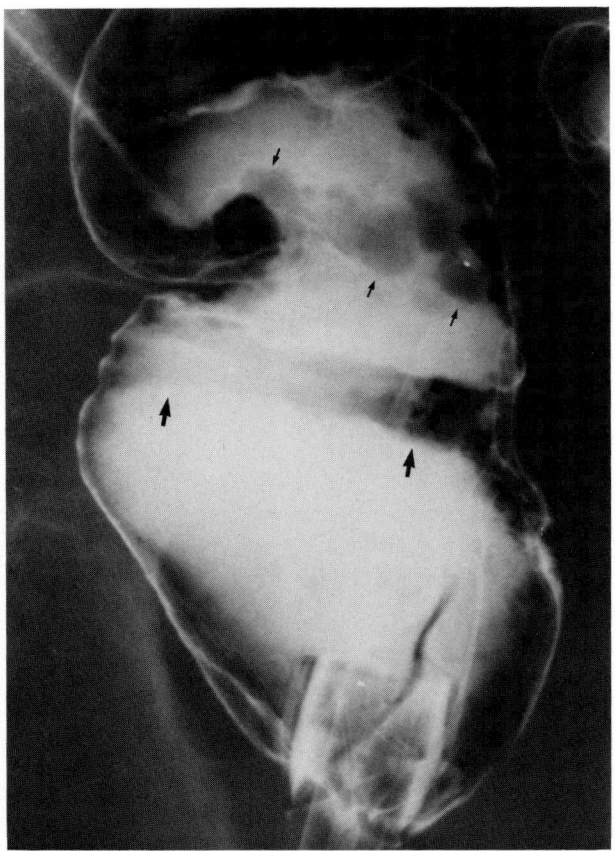

**Figure 68–57. Solitary rectal ulcer syndrome: enlarged valves of Houston.** The most distal valve of Houston *(large arrows)* is thickened and has a nodular contour. The middle valve of Houston is moderately thickened and shows mucosal nodularity en face *(small arrows).*

Chronic symptoms associated with progressive radiation damage are due to destruction of the colonic microvasculature. In the small arterioles of the submucosa, swelling of endothelial cells and intraluminal thrombosis are seen.[125] A progressive obliterative endarteritis develops, leading to ulceration and fissuring of the mucosa, fibrosis, and hypertrophy of the muscularis mucosae. Mucosal atrophy occurs with loss of goblet cells.

Chronic effects of radiotherapy are progressive and difficult to treat. Patients complain of lower abdominal pain, change in bowel habits, recurrent rectal bleeding, or recurrent bloody diarrhea, most frequently appearing 6 to 8 months after radiotherapy.[126] Radiation damage may be complicated by discrete ulceration, proctitis, rectovaginal fistula, stricture formation with obstructive symptoms, and colitis cystica profunda.[127, 128] In patients with chronic radiation enteritis, barium enema examinations are usually done to exclude other lesions as a cause of bloody diarrhea.

On barium enema examination, the rectosigmoid colon may have a smooth, featureless appearance. The haustra or valves of Houston are diminished in number or absent and the lumen is narrowed[129] (Fig. 68–58). The end result is a featureless, tubular rectosigmoid

colon (Fig. 68–59). The diffuse tubularity of the rectosigmoid colon mimics the appearance of the colon in pelvic lipomatosis (Fig. 68–60). Strictures may be long or short but have smooth, tapered margins.[130] Occasionally, the mucosa may appear granular, similar to the findings in ulcerative colitis (Fig. 68–61). Fistulas to the vagina or bladder may be apparent.

## Diversion Colitis

A nonspecific colitis may develop in a segment of colon that has been excluded from the fecal stream.[131, 132] This diversion colitis typically occurs in patients who have had operations for Crohn's disease, diverticulitis, or colonic carcinoma in whom an end-colostomy or end-ileostomy has been combined with a rectosigmoid pouch. The colitis may be confined to the distal rectum or involve the entire bypassed segment. The epithelial layer is abnormal, with distortion of the crypt architecture and crypt abscesses.[133] An acute and chronic inflammatory infiltrate is seen in the lamina propria.

Patients are usually asymptomatic but occasionally complain of bleeding.[134] Although the mechanism of colitis is unknown, symptoms and histologic abnormalities resolve after reanastomosis of the rectosigmoid pouch with either colon or small bowel.[135] It has been postulated that diversion of the fecal stream results in a

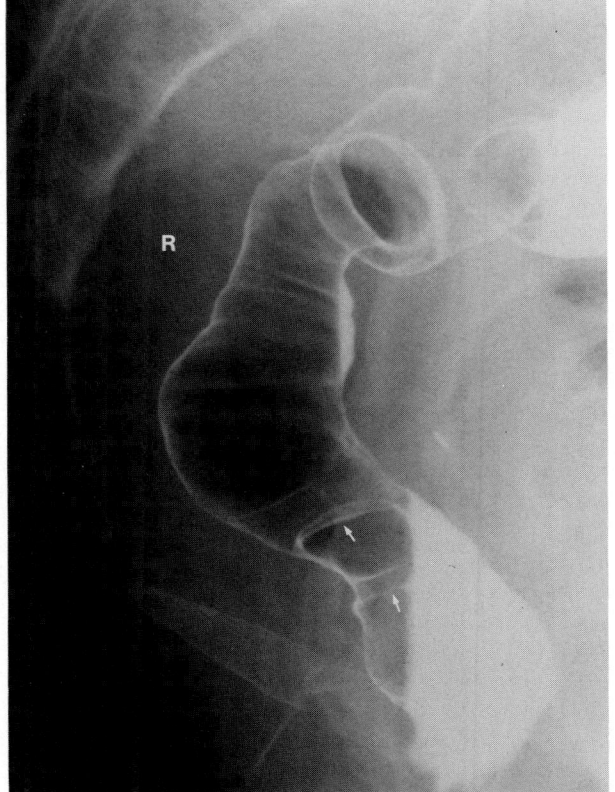

**Figure 68–58. Radiation proctitis.** Prone, cross-table lateral view of the rectum shows diffuse rectal narrowing. The valves of Houston are preserved *(arrows)*. The presacral space (R) is widened.

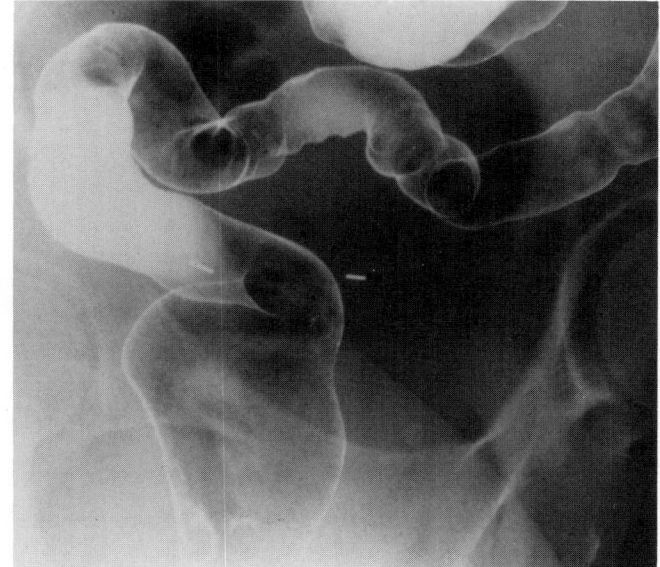

**Figure 68–59. Radiation proctosigmoiditis.** Diffuse narrowing of the rectum and sigmoid colon is seen. The valves of Houston are absent.

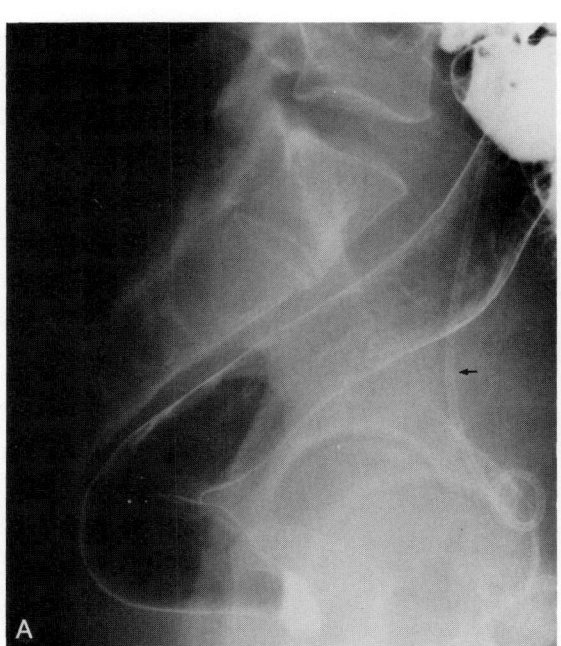

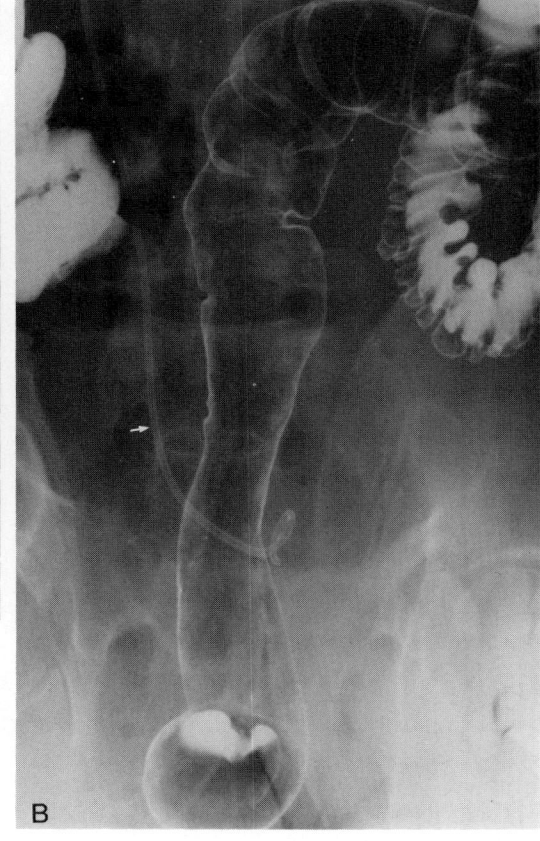

**Figure 68–60. Pelvic fibrolipomatosis.** A prone, cross-table lateral view **(A)** and a prone angle view **(B)** show diffuse, tubular narrowing of the rectosigmoid colon, loss of the valves of Houston, and distal sigmoid folds. A stent is seen in the distal right ureter *(arrows).*

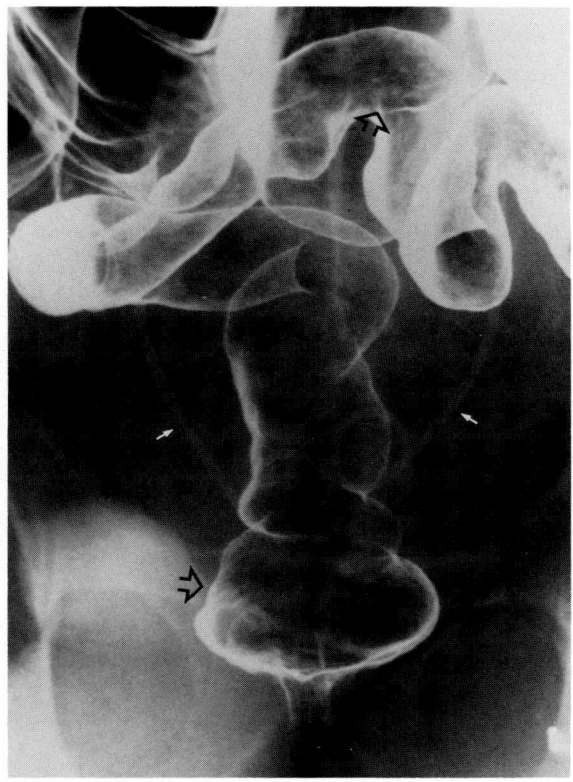

**Figure 68–61. Radiation proctosigmoiditis.** Diffuse mucosal granularity (representative areas identified with open arrows) is seen in the rectosigmoid colon. Also note diffuse tubular narrowing of the rectosigmoid colon, loss of the valves of Houston, and stents in the ureters *(solid arrows).*

nutritional deficiency of short chain fatty acids—the source of energy for colonic epithelial cells.[136] Instillation of short chain fatty acids into the rectosigmoid pouch leads to resolution of symptoms.[136]

If a barium enema is performed for symptoms or before reanastomosis of rectosigmoid colon to either colon or small bowel, the colonic mucosa will be abnormal. Barium enema may demonstrate fine or course nodularity of the mucosa, as well as a lymphoid follicular pattern[137] (Fig. 68–62).

## ENDOMETRIOSIS

Implants of endometrial tissue outside the uterus are common, occurring in up to 15% of menstruating women.[138] Of women with endometriosis, approximately 30% develop intestinal endometriosis. Most women with intestinal implants are asymptomatic; however, clinical complaints may occur, including infertility and crampy lower abdominal or pelvic pain. Bowel involvement is suggested by constipation, diarrhea, rectal bleeding, or tenesmus, sometimes of a cyclic nature.

The rectosigmoid junction abutting the pouch of Douglas is the most common site of bowel involvement because it is the most dependent portion of the peritoneal cavity in the erect and supine positions. Thus,

endometrial implants floating in the peritoneal cavity pool in the pouch of Douglas. Direct invasion of the inferior border of the sigmoid colon by left ovarian endometriosis may occur. Less frequently, peritoneal seeding affects other bowel sites, including the sigmoid colon, the cecum, the appendix, and the small intestine.

Other than direct inspection during laparoscopy, barium enema is the best examination for assessing bowel involvement by endometriosis. In the rectum, an extrinsic mass impression may be seen along the anterior wall of the rectosigmoid junction[139] (Fig. 68–63). With endometrial invasion of the subserosa and muscularis propria, inflammatory changes and hypertrophy of the muscularis propria occur. Endometrial invasion leads to distortion of the luminal contour and overlying mucosa that is radiographically manifest as spiculation of the colonic contour and pleating of overlying smooth mucosal folds[140] (Fig. 68–64). Severe hypertrophy of muscularis propria leads to the radiographic appearance of a submucosal or polypoid mass (Fig. 68–65). Polypoid endometriomas may occur in the sigmoid colon or cecum.[141] Occasionally, circumferential involvement may occur, but lack of mucosal nodularity or ulceration distinguishes circumferential endometrial involvement from a primary colonic carcinoma. However, the radiographic findings for serosal and subserosal involvement

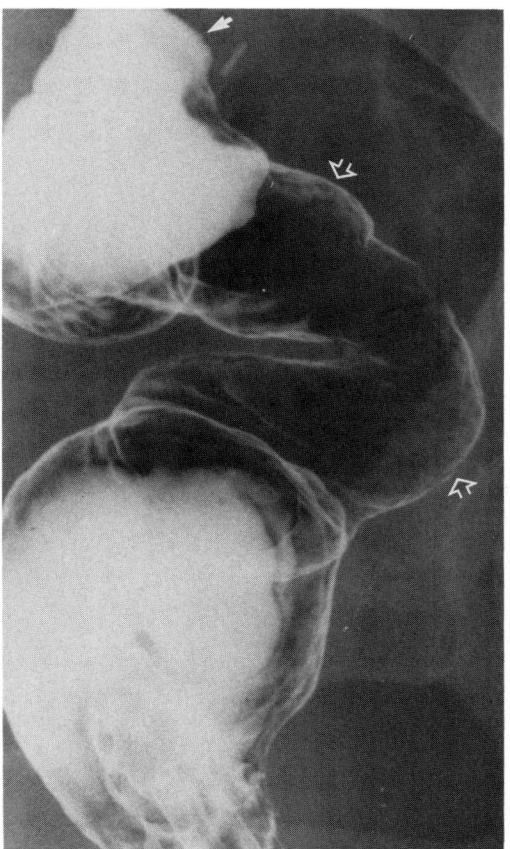

**Figure 68–62. Diversion colitis.** Oblique spot film of the rectum shows a lymphoid follicular pattern *(open arrows)* carpeting the rectal mucosa. Also note abrupt cutoff of the rectal pouch *(solid arrow).* (Courtesy of S. N. Glick, M.D., Philadelphia, PA.)

**Figure 68–63. Endometriosis involving the rectosigmoid junction.** Lateral view of the rectum shows a mass *(large solid arrow)* indenting the anterior wall of the rectosigmoid junction. Note abrupt angulation *(small solid arrow)* of the mass with the luminal contour, findings typical of an extrinsic or submucosal mass. Mild nodularity of the overlying rectal mucosal *(open arrow)* is seen in profile. Surgery showed endometriosis invading the rectal wall and causing muscular hypertrophy.

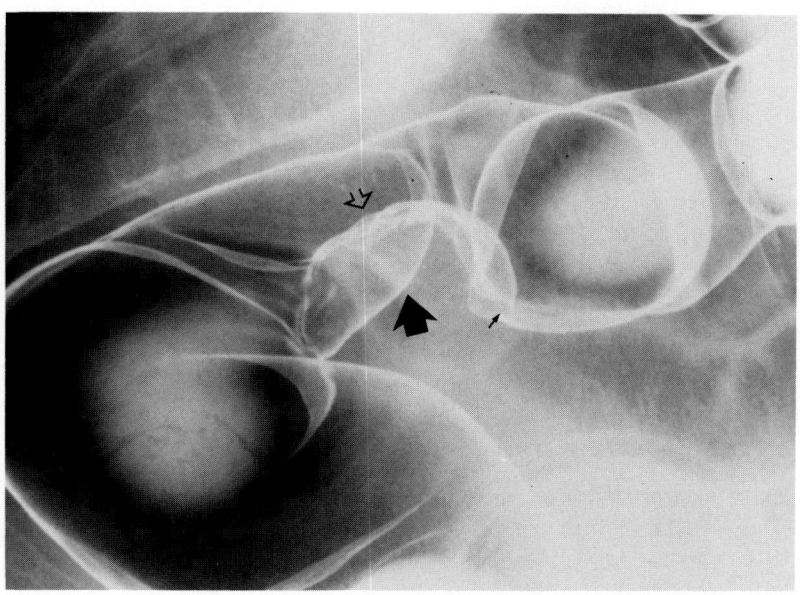

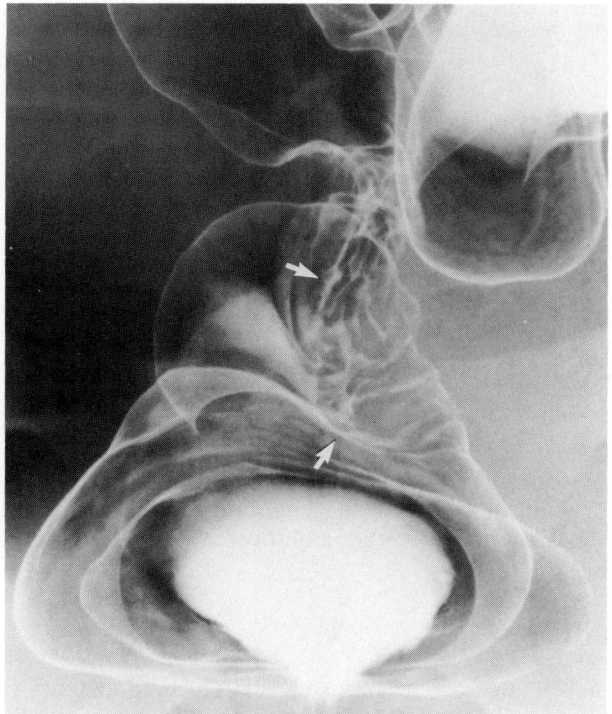

**Figure 68–64. Endometriosis.** Prone angle view of the rectosigmoid junction shows smooth, parallel, focally serpentine folds *(arrows),* a pattern termed mucosal pleating and seen in any extrinsic disease secondarily invading the colon. (From RL Gordon, K Evers, HY Kressel, et al, Double-contrast enema in pelvic endometriosis, AJR, 138, 3, 549–552, 1982, © by American Roentgen Ray Society.)

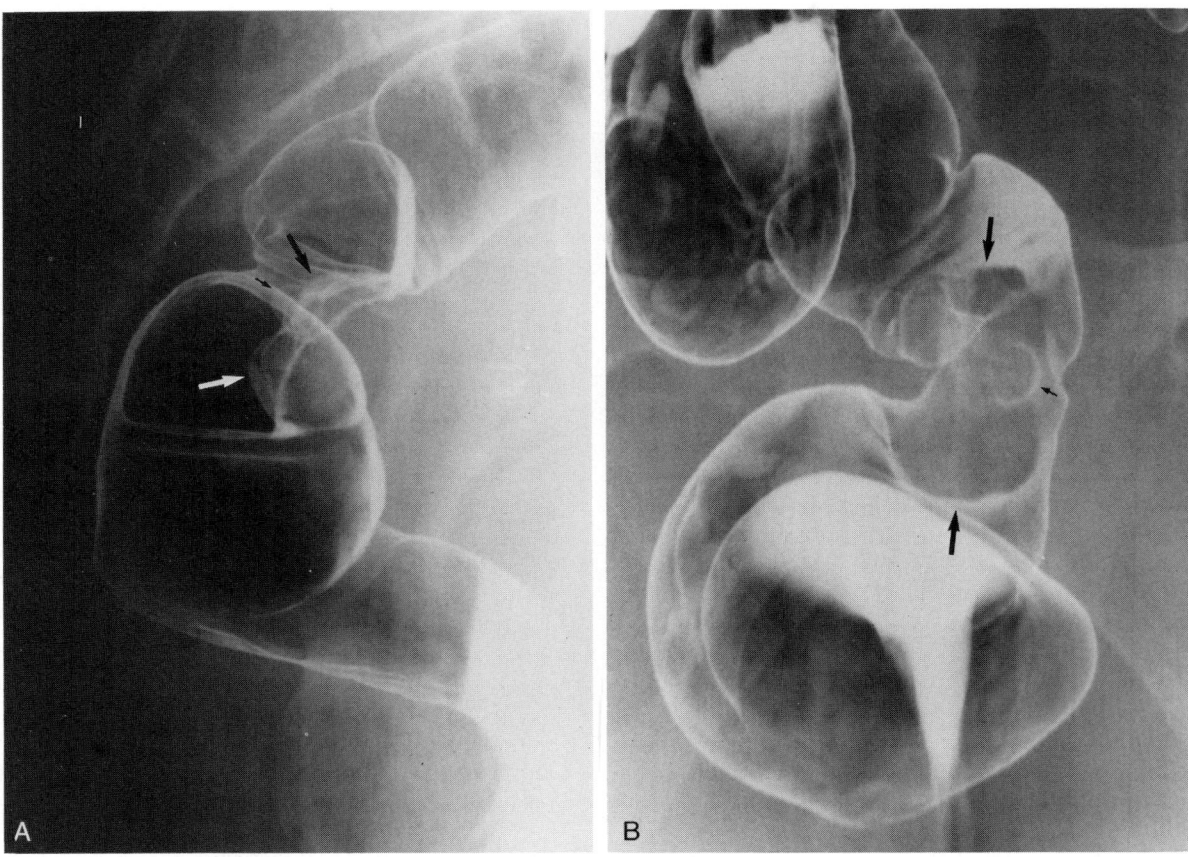

**Figure 68–65. Endometrioma, rectosigmoid junction.** A prone, cross-table lateral view **(A)** and a prone angle view **(B)** of the rectum show a well-circumscribed mass *(large arrows)* with focal lobulation *(small arrows).* Although the tumor has a bosselated contour, the mucosal surface is smooth.

by endometriosis are identical to those for peritoneal metastasis. The age of the patient and the clinical history help distinguish the two.

## FECAL IMPACTION

Lack of mobility and impaired anorectal sensation predispose to fecal impaction. Medications that depress bowel function are common, including tricyclic antidepressants, aluminum-containing antacids, narcotics, sucralfate, and antihypertensive agents with alpha-adrenergic, beta-adrenergic, and calcium channel–blocking properties.[142] Thus, fecal impaction typically occurs in the elderly who are bedridden or demented and in patients with psychiatric disorders or spinal cord injury or tumor.

Patients may complain of abdominal pain, tenderness, or diarrhea. They may have constipation or occasionally diarrhea caused by overflow incontinence. Both physical examination and barium enema examination are valuable in differentiating fecal impaction from an obstructive colonic neoplasm (Fig. 68–66).

## ANAL FISSURES AND ULCERATIONS, ANORECTAL FISTULAS, AND ANORECTAL ABSCESSES

An anal fissure is a linear ulcer in the anal canal. An anorectal fistula is an abnormal track between the anorectal mucosa and the perianal skin. Anorectal abscesses are collections of pus in the perianal area, usually arising from the epithelium of the anorectal canal. Various disorders, including trauma, infection, idiopathic inflammatory bowel disease, and immunocompromised states, may result in breaches of the lining of the anorectal canal with subsequent inflammation.[143]

### Anal Fissures

Anal fissures are usually small, linear tears extending below and perpendicular to the dentate line, usually along the posterior midline of the anal canal. These fissures are frequently seen in young adults or middle-

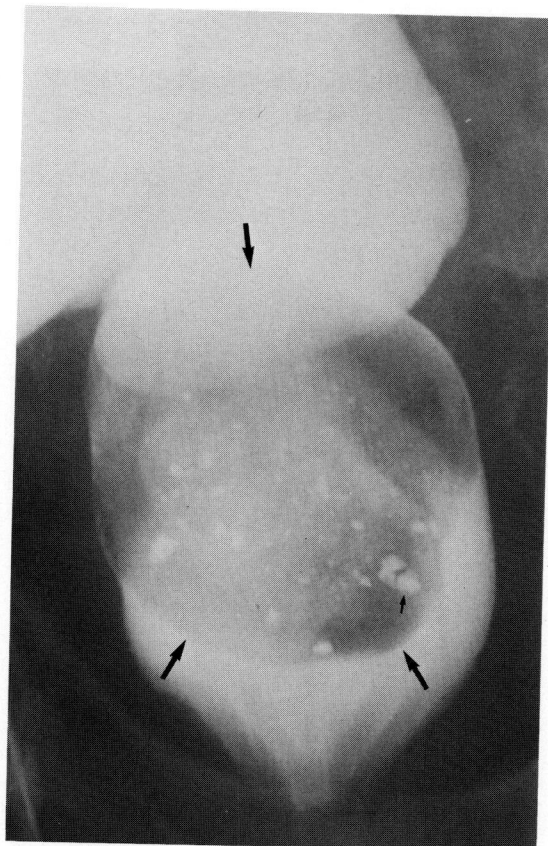

**Figure 68–66. Fecal impaction.** Spot film of the rectum from a single contrast barium enema examination shows a large fecolith as a radiolucent mass *(large arrows)*. Punctate collections of barium *(small arrow)* from a prior barium examination have been trapped within the fecolith.

aged adults who complain of severe rectal pain or bright red rectal bleeding. Anal fissures are frequently related to trauma resulting from constipation and passage of hard stool, the postpartum state, or hemorrhoidectomy.[144] However, a wide variety of infectious causes, idiopathic inflammatory bowel disease, or skin diseases may result in similar anal ulcerations. Specific infections include syphilis, gonorrhea, tuberculosis, *Chlamydia* infections (lymphogranuloma venereum), and granuloma inguinale (caused by a gram-negative bacillus, *Calymmatobacterium granulomatis*).[143] Crohn's disease and Behçets disease may result in anal ulcers or perianal fistulas. The neutropenia associated with various leukemic states may predispose to abscesses complicating anal fissures or fistulas.

If a barium enema is to be performed, the radiologist must gently insert the barium enema tip past the fissure or use a smaller and more compliant tube such as a Foley catheter. Barium enema examinations may demonstrate associated hypertrophied anal papillae or perirectal fistulas.

## Anorectal Fistulas and Abscesses

Traumatic causes of anorectal fistulas and abscesses include abnormal defecation, constipation with hard

stools, rectal stasis of feces, and diarrhea.[145] Other traumatic causes include anal intercourse and insertion of foreign bodies into the rectum. Infections complicating hemorrhoids, anal fissures, or the anal glands (Fig. 68–67) may progress to anorectal fistula and abscess formation.[143] Acute leukemia with neutropenia may predispose patients to anal gland infections. Specific inflammatory processes such as Crohn's disease, lymphogranuloma venereum, tuberculosis, and actinomycosis may involve the anal glands that arise at the level of the crypts of Morgagni.[144] Patients complain of perirectal pain, swelling, and prurulent discharge.

Anorectal fistulas are classified by their location in relation to the muscles of the pelvic floor. Intersphincteric fistulas are the most common type, arising below the level of the pectinate line and penetrating the internal sphincter, passing between the internal and external anal sphincters. Trans-sphincteric fistulas are less frequent, the internal opening above the pectinate line passing through both sphincters into the ischiorectal fossa.[144] Suprasphincteric fistulas pass upward in the intersphincteric plane over the puborectalis muscle into the ischiorectal fossa. Extrasphincteric fistulas (Fig. 68–68) arise in the distal rectum above the line of the levator ani muscle and extend into the ischiorectal fossa.

If multiple tracks are seen during barium enema examination, a diagnosis of Crohn's disease, hidradenitis suppurativa, or an infection complicating leukemia is suggested.[144]

## TRAUMATIC PROCTITIS

Various foreign bodies may be inserted into the rectum for medical diagnosis (Fig. 68–69) or treatment,

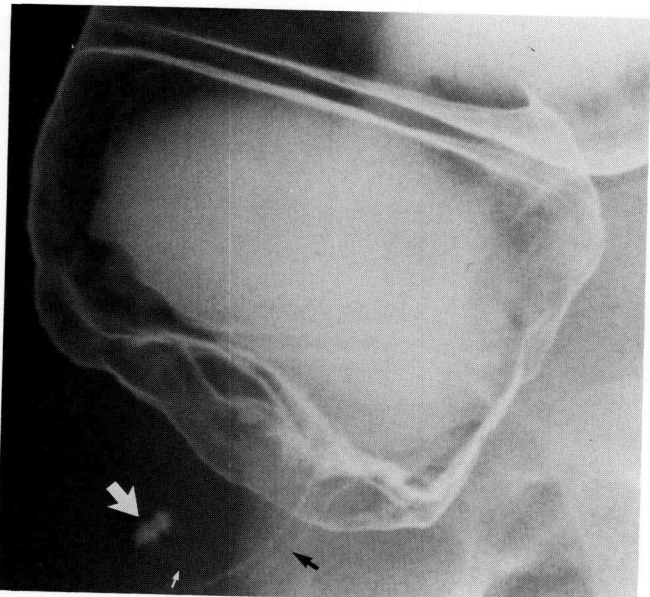

**Figure 68–67. Small anal gland abscess.** Oblique spot film of the distal rectum and anorectal junction *(black arrow)* shows a focal barium collection *(large white arrow)* arising in an anal gland. A faint track of barium extends to the anal canal *(small white arrow)*. The anal glands are at the level of the dentate line.

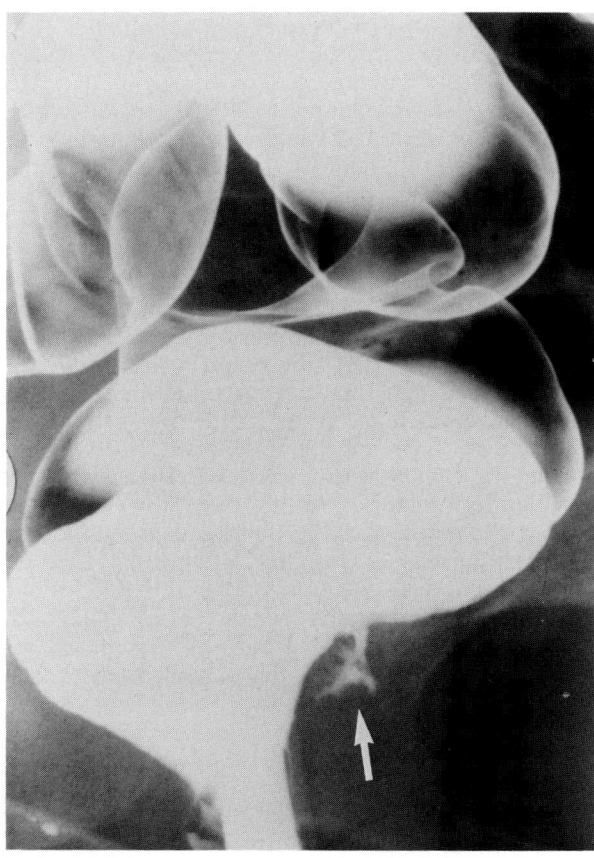

**Figure 68–68. Extrasphincteric fistula.** An irregular, barium-filled track *(arrow)* extends from the left lateral wall of the distal rectum into the perirectal soft tissue. (Courtesy of S. N. Glick, M.D., Philadelphia, PA).

**Figure 68–69. Traumatic proctitis from rectal biopsy.** The rectal biopsy site is identified by a barium-etched ring shadow *(solid arrow)*. A nodular surface pattern *(open arrow)* radiates from the central biopsy site. (Courtesy of Dr. H. DeGryse, Antwerp, Belgium. From Rubesin SE, Saul SH, Laufer I, et al: Carpet lesions of the colon. Radiographics 5:537–552, 1985.)

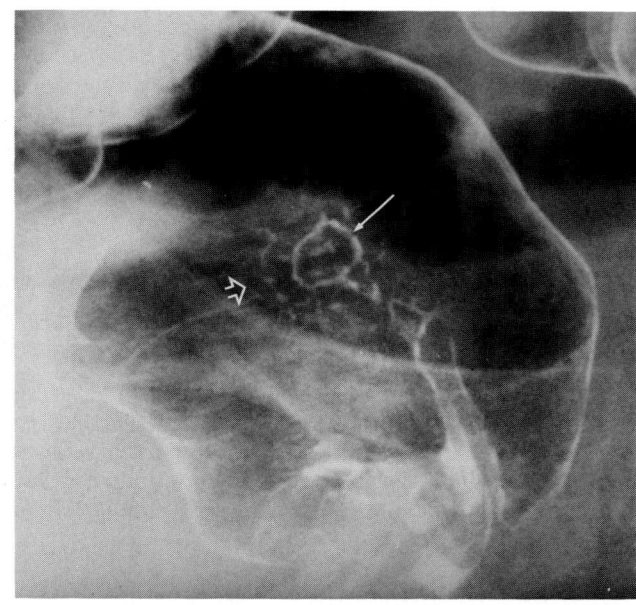

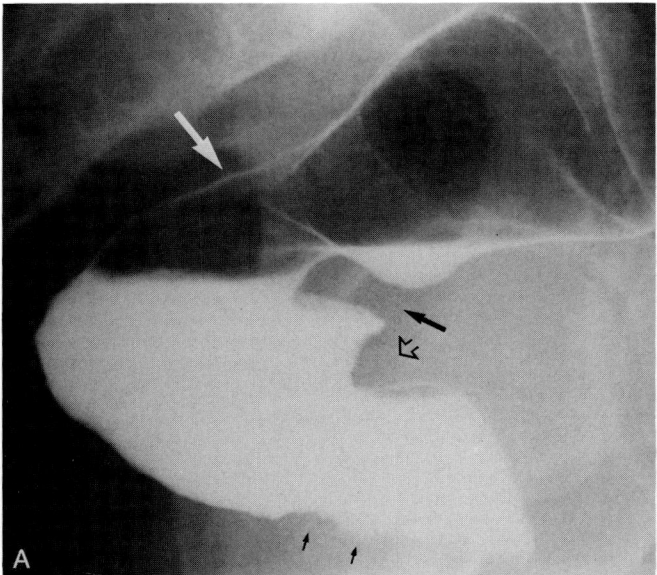

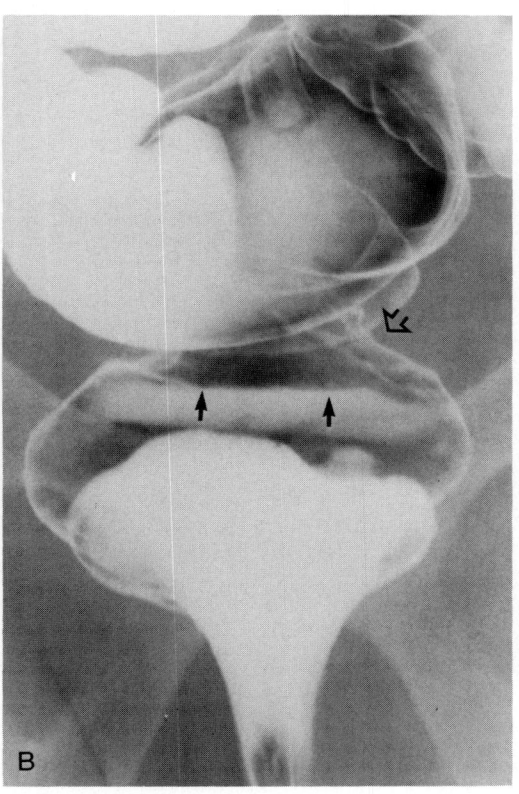

**Figure 68–70. Traumatic proctitis. A.** Erect lateral view of the rectum shows narrowing of the rectosigmoid colon *(white arrow)* and thickening of the middle *(large black arrow)* and lower *(open arrow)* valves of Houston. Mild mucosal nodularity is seen in profile *(small black arrows).* **B.** Prone view of the rectum shows a thick valve of Houston en face *(solid arrows)* and focal mucosal nodularity *(open arrow).* This young woman had been assaulted; a broomstick had been inserted into her rectum.

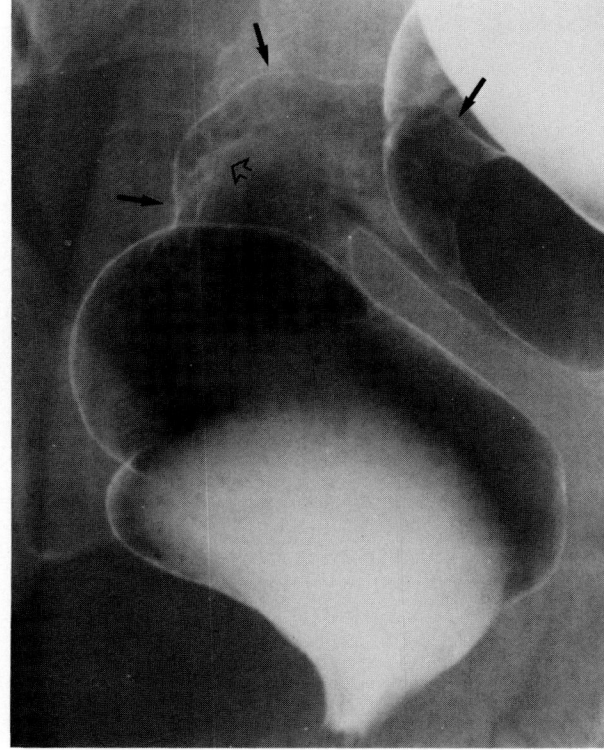

**Figure 68–71. Traumatic proctitis.** Focal, tubular narrowing of the rectosigmoid junction *(solid arrows)* is associated with fine mucosal nodularity (representative area identified by open arrow). A history of anal intercourse was elicited from this young woman. No organisms were identified by either culture or biopsy.

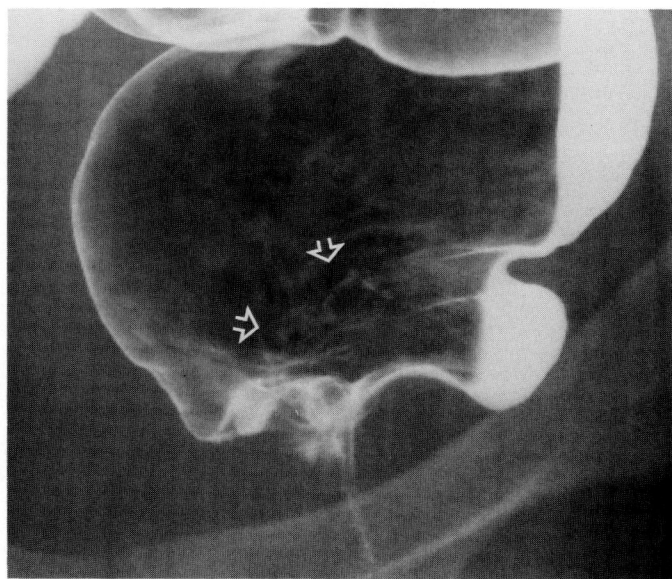

**Figure 68–72. Traumatic proctitis with focal scarring.** Left-side-down decubitus view of the rectum shows fine and coarse nodularity *(arrows)* of the distal rectal mucosa. This young woman had a history of anal intercourse. Biopsy showed chronic inflammation and fibrous scarring in the lamina propria.

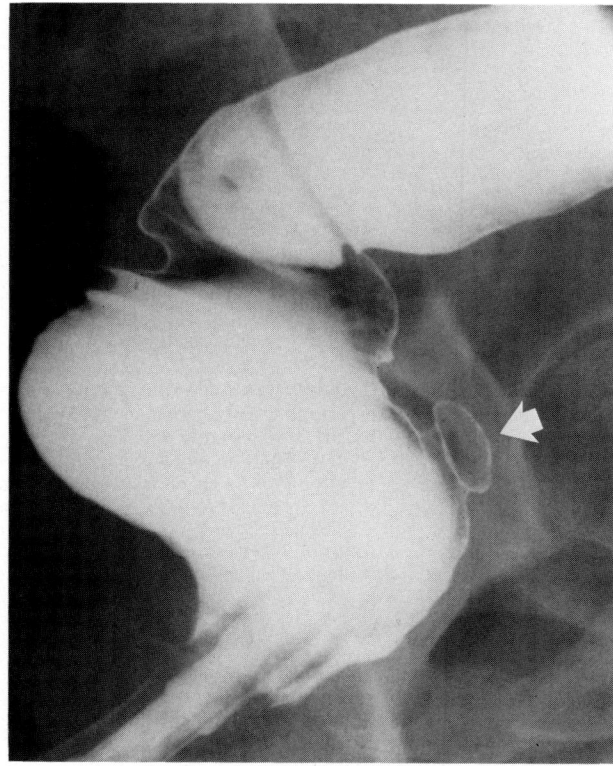

**Figure 68–73. Rectal diverticulum.** Steep oblique view of the rectum shows a diverticulum *(arrow)* 1.5 cm in diameter protruding from the anterior wall of the distal rectum.

concealment, assault, or sexual behavior. Patients may complain of bleeding or pain. Occasionally, a patient denies a history of insertion of a foreign body. Plain films may be valuable in detecting foreign bodies that are radiopaque. Barium enemas are rarely performed in patients with the history of suspected foreign body insertion.[146]

In traumatic proctitis, barium enema may show a focal or a diffuse proctitis. Mucosal nodularity (see Fig. 68–69) or coarse, lobulated folds (Fig. 68–70) may be seen, radiographic findings similar to those seen in solitary rectal ulcer syndrome. Rectal narrowing (Fig. 68–71) may represent spasm, edema, or stricture formation. Chronic, focal scarring may occur (Fig. 68–72).

## RECTAL DIVERTICULUM

Diverticula of the rectum are rare (Fig. 68–73), primarily because the longitudinal muscle of the colon envelops the rectum circumferentially. Thus, there are no areas of muscular weakness for mucosa to herniate through. Rectal diverticula probably represent duplications or post-traumatic outpouchings.

### Acknowledgment

Figure 68–18 is reproduced from Laufer I: Double Contrast Radiology with Endoscopic Correlation. Philadelphia: WB Saunders, 1979.

Figures 68–41 and 68–50B are reproduced from Laufer I, Levine MS (eds): Double Contrast Gastrointestinal Radiology (2nd ed). Philadelphia: WB Saunders, 1992.

## References

1. Bartolo DCC: Anorectal disease. Curr Opin Gastroenterol 9:66–74, 1993.
2. Imai Y, Kressel HY, Saul SH, et al: Colorectal tumors: an in vitro study of high-resolution MR imaging. Radiology 177:695–701, 1990.
3. Wyburn GM: The digestive system. *In* Romanes GJ (ed): Cunningham's Textbook of Anatomy (12th ed). London: Oxford University Press, 1972, pp 399–468.
4. Guyton AC: Textbook of Medical Physiology (8th ed). Philadelphia: WB Saunders, 1991, pp 706–707, 740.
5. Morson BC, Dawson IMP: Gastrointestinal Pathology. Oxford: Blackwell Scientific Publications, 1979, pp 485–735.
6. Heenan PF: Other tumors of the anal canal. *In* Whitehead R (ed): Gastrointestinal and Oesophageal Pathology. Edinburgh: Churchill Livingstone, 1989, pp 795–810.
7. James PP: The anal canal. *In* Whitehead R (ed): Gastrointestinal and Oesophageal Pathology. Edinburgh: Churchill Livingstone, 1989, pp 605–609.
8. Thoeni RF, Venbrux AC: The anal canal: distinction of internal hemorrhoids from small cancers by double-contrast barium enema examination. Radiology 145:17–19, 1982.
9. Levine MS, Kam LW, Rubesin SE, et al: Internal hemorrhoids: diagnosis with double contrast barium enema examinations. Radiology 177:141–144, 1990.
10. Manzi D, Samanta AK: Adhesion-related colonic varices. J Clin Gastroenterol 7:71–75, 1985.
11. McCormack TT, Bailey HR, Simms JM, et al: Rectal varices are not piles. Br J Surg 71:163, 1984.
12. Kelvin FM, Gardiner R: Clinical Imaging of the Colon and Rectum. New York: Raven Press, 1987, pp 422–460.
13. Fenoglio-Preiser CM, Pascal RR: Epithelial tumors. *In* Whitehead R (ed): Gastrointestinal and Oesophageal Pathology. Edinburgh: Churchill Livingstone, 1989, pp 747–767.
14. Williams GT, Arthur JF, Bussey HJR, et al: Metaplastic polyps and polyposis of the colorectum. Histopathology 4:155–170, 1980.
15. Estrada RG, Spjut HJ: Hyperplastic polyps of the large bowel. Am J Surg Pathol 4:127–133, 1980.
16. Tedesco FJ, Hendrix JC, Pickens CA, et al: Diminutive polyps: histopathology, spatial distribution, and clinical significance. Gastrointest Endosc 28:1–5, 1982.
17. Ott DJ, Gelfand DW: Colorectal tumors: pathology and detection. AJR 131:691–695, 1978.
18. Olmsted WW, Ros PR, Sobin LH, et al: The solitary colonic polyp: radiologic-histologic differentiation and significance. Radiology 160:9–16, 1986.
19. Levine MS, Barnes MJ, Bronner MP, et al: Atypical hyperplastic polyps on double-contrast barium enema. Radiology 175:691–694, 1990.
20. Saul SH: Inflammatory cloacogenic polyp: relationship to solitary rectal ulcer syndrome/mucosal prolapse and other bowel disorders. Hum Pathol 18:1120–1125, 1987.
21. Lobert PF, Appelman HD: Inflammatory cloacogenic polyp. A unique inflammatory lesion of the anal transitional zone. Am J Surg Pathol 8:761–766, 1981.
22. Bates HR II: Carcinoid tumors of the rectum—a statistical review. Dis Colon Rectum 9:90–94, 1966.
23. Godwin DJ: Carcinoid tumors. An analysis of 2837 cases. Cancer 36:560–569, 1975.
24. Balthazar EJ: Carcinoid tumors of the alimentary tract. Gastrointest Radiol 3:47–56, 1978.
25. Wilander E: Endocrine cell tumors. *In* Whitehead R (ed): Gastrointestinal and Oesophageal Pathology. Edinburgh: Churchill Livingstone, 1989, pp 629–641.
26. Martensson H, Nobin A, Sundler F: Carcinoid tumors in the gastrointestinal tract—an analysis of 156 cases. Acta Chir Scand 149:607–616, 1983.
27. Sato T, Sakai Y, Sonoyama A, et al: Radiologic spectrum of rectal carcinoid tumors. Gastrointest Radiol 9:23–26, 1984.
28. Morson BC, Konishi F: Contribution of the pathologist to the radiology and management of colorectal polyps. Gastrointest Radiol 7:275–281, 1982.
29. Thompson JJ, Enterline HT: The macroscopic appearance of colorectal polyps. Cancer 48:151–160, 1981.
30. Muto T, Bussey HJR, Morson BC: The evolution of cancer of the colon and rectum. Cancer 36:2251–2270, 1975.
31. Fenoglio CM, Pascal RR: Colorectal adenomas and cancer. Pathologic relationships. Cancer 50:2601–2608, 1982.
32. Ott DJ, Gelfand DW, Wu WC, et al: Colon polyp morphology on double-contrast barium enema: its pathologic predictive value. AJR 141:965–970, 1983.
33. Herman TE, Koehler RE, Lee JKT: Focal irregularity of the rectal mucosa. AJR 133:677–681, 1979.
34. Rubesin SE, Saul SH, Laufer I, et al: Carpet lesions of the colon. Radiographics 5:537–552, 1985.
35. Evers K, Laufer I, Gordon RL, et al: Double contrast examination for detection of rectal carcinoma. Radiology 140:635–639, 1981.
36. Chan TW, Kressel HY, Milestone B, et al: Rectal carcinoma: staging at MR imaging with endorectal coil. Work in progress. Radiology 181:461–467, 1991.
37. Rao BK, Kapur MM, Roy S: Leiomyosarcoma of the colon: a case report and review of literature. Dis Colon Rectum 23:184–190, 1980.
38. Akwari OE, Dozois RR, Weiland LH, et al: Leiomyosarcoma of the small and large bowel. Cancer 42:1375–1384, 1978.
39. Hendrickson MR, Kempson KL: Smooth muscle tumors. *In* Whitehead R (ed): Gastrointestinal and Oesophageal Pathology. Edinburgh: Churchill Livingstone, 1989, pp 619–628.
40. Saul SH, Rast ML, Brooks JJ: The immunohistochemistry of gastrointestinal stromal tumors. Evidence supporting an origin from smooth muscle. Am J Surg Pathol 11:464–473, 1987.
41. Walsh TH, Mann CV: Smooth muscle neoplasms of the rectum and anal canal. Br J Surg 71:597–599, 1984.
42. Williams GT, Blackshaw AJ, Morson BC: Squamous carcinoma of the colorectum and its genesis. J Pathol 129:139–147, 1979.

43. Gillespie JJ, MacKay B: Histogenesis of cloacogenic carcinoma. Fine structure of anal transitional epithelium and cloacogenic carcinoma. Hum Pathol 9:579–587, 1978.
44. Fenger C: The anal canal epithelium. A review. Scand J Gastroenterol 14(suppl):114–117, 1979.
45. Austin DF: Etiological clues from descriptive epidemiology: squamous carcinoma of the rectum or anus. Natl Cancer Inst Monogr 62:89–90, 1982.
46. Peters RK, Mack TM: Patterns of anal carcinoma by gender and marital status in Los Angeles County. Br J Cancer 48:629–636, 1983.
47. Daling JR, Weiss NS, Klopfenstein LL, et al: Correlates of homosexual behavior and the incidence of anal cancer. JAMA 247:1988–1990, 1982.
48. Kyaw MM, Gallagher T, Haines JO: Cloacogenic carcinoma of the anorectal junction: roentgenologic diagnosis. AJR 115:384–391, 1972.
49. Glickman MG, Margulis AR: Cloacogenic carcinoma. AJR 107:175–180, 1969.
50. Gengler L, Baer J, Finby N: Rectal and sigmoid involvement secondary to carcinoma of the prostate. AJR 125:910–917, 1975.
51. Winter CC: The problem of rectal involvement by prostatic cancer. Surg Gynecol Obstet 105:136–140, 1957.
52. Fry DE, Amin M, Harbrecht PJ: Rectal obstruction secondary to carcinoma of the prostate. Ann Surg 189:488–492, 1979.
53. Becker JA: Prostatic carcinoma involving the rectum and sigmoid colon. AJR 94:421–428, 1965.
54. Aigen AB, Schapira HE: Metastatic carcinoma of prostate and bladder causing intestinal obstruction. Urology 21:464–456, 1983.
55. Rubesin SE, Levine MS, Bezzi M, et al: Rectal involvement by prostatic carcinoma: radiographic findings. AJR 152:53–57, 1989.
56. Meyers MA: The spread and localization of acute intraperitoneal effusions. Radiology 95:547–554, 1970.
57. Meyers MA: Intraperitoneal spread of malignancies and its effect on the bowel. Clin Radiol 32:129–146, 1981.
58. Laufer I: The radiologic demonstration of early changes in ulcerative colitis by double contrast technique. J Can Assoc Radiol 26:116–121, 1975.
59. Welin S, Brahme F: The double contrast method in ulcerative colitis. Acta Radiol 55:257–271, 1961.
60. Bartram CI, Walmsley K: A radiological and pathological correlation of the mucosal changes in ulcerative colitis. Clin Radiol 29:323–328, 1978.
61. Tedesco FJ, Hardin RD, Harper RN, et al: Infectious colitis endoscopically simulating inflammatory bowel disease: a prospective evaluation. Gastrointest Endosc 27:195–197, 1983.
62. Powell-Tuck J, Ritchie JK, Lennard-Jones JE: The prognosis of idiopathic proctitis. Scand J Gastroenterol 12:727–732, 1977.
63. Prior P, Gyde SN, Macartney JC, et al: Cancer morbidity in ulcerative colitis. Gut 23:490–497, 1982.
64. Edwards FC, Truelove SC: The course and prognosis of ulcerative colitis: IV. Carcinoma of the colon. Gut 5:15–22, 1964.
65. Yardley JH, Ransohoff DF, Riddell RH, et al: Cancer in inflammatory bowel disease: how serious is the problem and what should be done about it? Gastroenterology 85:197–200, 1983 (editorial).
66. Farmer RG, Hawk WA, Turnbull RB: Clinical patterns in Crohn's disease: a statistical study of 615 cases. Gastroenterology 68:627–635, 1975.
67. Laufer I, Mullens JE, Hamilton J: Correlation of endoscopy and double-contrast radiography in the early stages of ulcerative and granulomatous colitis. Radiology 118:1–5, 1976.
68. Korelitz BI, Sommers SC: Differential diagnosis of ulcerative and granulomatous colitis by sigmoidoscopy, rectal biopsy and cell counts of rectal mucosa. Am J Gastroenterol 61:460–469, 1974.
69. Laufer I, Costopoulos L: Early lesions of Crohn's disease. AJR 130:307–311, 1978.
70. Rubesin SE, Bronner M: Radiologic-pathologic concepts in Crohn's disease. *In* Herlinger H, Megibow AJ (eds): Advances in Gastrointestinal Radiology, Volume 1. Chicago: Mosby–Year Book, 1991, pp 27–55.
71. DuBrow RA, Frank PH: Barium evaluation of anal canal in patients with inflammatory bowel disease. AJR 140:1151–1157, 1983.
72. Lamont JT: Bacterial infections of the colon. *In* Yamada T (ed): Textbook of Gastroenterology. Philadelphia: JB Lippincott, 1991, pp 1749–1768.
73. Mathan MM: Specific infections—Part 1, the large intestine. *In* Whitehead R (ed): Gastrointestinal Oesophageal Pathology. Edinburgh: Churchill Livingstone, 1989, pp 497–506.
74. Speelman P, Kabir I, Islam M: Distribution and spread of colonic lesions in shigellosis: a colonoscopic study. J Infect Dis 150:899–903, 1984.
75. Farman J, Rabinowitz JG, Meyers MA: Roentgenology of infectious colitis. AJR 119:375–381, 1973.
76. Kollitz JPM, Davis CB, Berk RN: *Campylobacter*: a common infectious form of acute colitis. Gastrointest Radiol 6:227–229, 1981.
77. Brodey PA, Fertig S, Aron JM: *Campylobacter* entercolitis: radiographic features. AJR 139:1199–1201, 1982.
78. Loss RW, Mangla JC, Pereira M: *Campylobacter* colitis presenting as inflammatory bowel disease with segmental colonic ulcerations. Gastroenterology 79:138–140, 1980.
79. Price AB, Dolby JM, Dunscombe PR, et al: Detection of *Campylobacter* by immunofluorescence in stools and rectal biopsies of patients with diarrhoea. J Clin Pathol 37:1107–1013, 1984.
80. Barlett JG, Moon N, Chang TW, et al: Role of *Clostridium difficile* in antibiotic-associated pseudomembranous colitis. Gastroenterology 75:778–782, 1978.
81. Stanley RJ, Tedesco FJ: Antibiotic-associated pseudomembranous colitis. Crit Rev Diagn Imaging 8:225–277, 1976.
82. Stanley RJ, Melson GL, Tedesco FJ, et al: Plain-film findings in severe pseudomembranous colitis. Radiology 118:7–11, 1976.
83. Price AB, Davies DR: Pseudomembranous colitis. J Clin Pathol 30:1–12, 1977.
84. Megibow AJ, Streiter ML, Balthazar EJ, et al: Pseudomembranous colitis: diagnosis by computed tomography. J Comput Assist Tomogr 8:281–283, 1984.
85. Brunner D, Feifarek C, McNeely D, et al: CT of pseudomembranous colitis. Gastrointest Radiol 9:73–75, 1984.
86. Letourneau JG, Day DL, Steely JW, et al: CT appearance of antibiotic-induced colitis. Gastrointest Radiol 12:257–261, 1987.
87. Strada M, Meregaglia D, Donzelli R: Double-contrast enema in antibiotic-related pseudomembranous colitis. Gastrointest Radiol 8:67–69, 1983.
88. Tedesco FJ: Antibiotic associated pseudomembranous colitis with negative proctosigmoidoscopy exam. Gastroenterology 77:295–297, 1979.
89. Tedesco FJ, Corless JK, Brownstein RE: Rectal sparing in antibiotic pseudomembranous colitis: a prospective study. Gastroenterology 83:1259–1260, 1982.
90. Burbige EJ, Radigan JJ: Antibiotic-associated colitis with normal appearing rectum. Dis Col Rectum 24:198–200, 1981.
91. Seppala K, Kjelt L, Sipponen P: Colonoscopy in the diagnosis of antibiotic-associated colitis. Scand J Gastroenterol 16:465–468, 1981.
92. Gerding DN, Olson MM, Peterson LR, et al: *Clostridium difficile*–associated diarrhea and colitis in adults: a prospective case-controlled epidemiologic study. Arch Intern Med 146:95–100, 1986.
93. Rubesin SE, Levine MS, Glick SN, et al: Pseudomembranous colitis with rectosigmoid sparing on barium studies. Radiology 170:811–813, 1989.
94. Quinn TC, Corey L, Chaffee RG, et al: The etiology of anorectal infections in homosexual men. Am J Med 71:395–406, 1981.
95. Phillips SC, Mildvan D, William DC, et al: Sexual transmission of enteric protozoa and helminths in a veneral-disease-clinic population. N Engl J Med 305:603–606, 1981.
96. Sohn N, Robilotti JG: The gay bowel syndrome. A review of colonic and rectal conditions in 200 male homosexuals. Am J Gastroenterol 67:478–484, 1977.
97. Weller IVD: The gay bowel. Gut 26:869–875, 1985.
98. Baker RW, Peppercorn MA: Gastrointestinal ailments of homosexual men. Medicine (Baltimore) 61:390–405, 1982.
99. Harkness AH: Anorectal gonorrhoea. Proc R Soc Med 41:476–478, 1948.
100. Lebedeff DA, Hochman EB: Rectal gonorrhea in men: diagnosis and treatment. Ann Intern Med 92:463–466, 1980.

101. Kilpatrick ZM: Gonorrheal proctitis. N Engl J Med 287:967–969, 1972.
102. Goodman KJ: Radiologic findings in anorectal gonorrhea. Gastrointest Radiol 3:223–224, 1978.
103. Quinn TC, Goodell SE, Mkrtichian E, et al: *Chlamydia trachomatis* proctitis. N Engl J Med 305:195–200, 1981.
104. Levine JS, Smith PD, Brugge WR: Chronic proctitis in male homosexuals due to lymphogranuloma venereum. Gastroenterology 79:563–565, 1980.
105. Levin I, Romano S, Steinberg M, et al: Lymphogranuloma venereum: rectal stricture and carcinoma. Dis Colon Rectum 7:129–134, 1964.
106. Annamunthodo H, Marryatt J: Barium studies in intestinal lymphogranuloma venereum. Br J Radiol 34:53–57, 1961.
107. Goldmeier D: Proctitis and herpes simplex virus in homosexual men. Br J Vener Dis 56:111–114, 1980.
108. Goodell SE, Quinn TC, Mkrtichian EE, et al: Herpes simplex virus proctitis in homosexual men: clinical, sigmoidoscopic, and histopathological features. N Engl J Med 308:868–871, 1983.
109. Shah SJ, Scholz FJ: Anorectal herpes: radiographic findings. Radiology 147:81–82, 1983.
110. Samenius B: Primary syphilis of anorectal region. Dis Colon Rectum 11:462–466, 1968.
111. Akdamar K, Martin RJ, Ichinose H: Syphilitic proctitis. Dig Dis 22:701–704, 1977.
112. Gluckman JB, Kleinman MS, May AG: Primary syphilis of rectum. N Y State J Med 74:2210–2211, 1974.
113. Cotton DWK, Kirkham N, Hicks DA: Rectal spirochaetosis. Br J Vener Dis 60:106–109, 1984.
114. Schweiger M, Alexander-Williams J: Solitary ulcer syndrome of the rectum. Its association with occult rectal prolapse. Lancet 1:170–171, 1977.
115. Rutter KR, Riddell RH: The solitary ulcer syndrome of the rectum. Clin Gastroenterol 4:505–530, 1975.
116. DuBoulay CEH, Fairbrother J, Isaacson PG: Mucosal prolapse syndrome—a unifying concept for solitary ulcer syndrome and related disorders. J Clin Pathol 36:1264–1268, 1983.
117. Madigan MR, Morson BC: Solitary ulcer of the rectum. Gut 10:871–881, 1969.
118. Feczko PJ, O'Connell DJ, Riddell RH, et al: Solitary rectal ulcer syndrome: radiologic manifestations. AJR 135:499–506, 1980.
119. DuBoulay CEH, James PD: Diverticular disease, solitary ulcer syndrome, anorectal prolapse and incontinence. *In* Whitehead R (ed): Gastrointestinal and Oesophageal Pathology. Edinburgh: Churchill Livingstone, 1989, pp 355–362.
120. Millward SF, Bayjoo P, Dixon MF, et al: The barium enema appearances in solitary rectal ulcer syndrome. Clin Radiol 36:185–189, 1985.
121. Levine MS, Piccolello ML, Sollenberger LC, et al: Solitary rectal ulcer syndrome: a radiologic diagnosis? Gastrointest Radiol 11:187–193, 1986.
122. Goldberg HI, Buchignani J, Rulon DB: Colitis cystica profunda. Radiology 96:447–452, 1970.
123. Chapa HJ, Smith HJ, Dickinson TA: Benign (solitary) ulcer of the rectum: another cause for rectal stricture. Gastrointest Radiol 6:85–88, 1981.
124. Gelfand MD, Tepper M, Katz LA, et al: Acute radiation proctitis in man. Gastroenterology 54:401–411, 1968.
125. Ackerman L: The pathology of radiation effect of normal and neoplastic tissue. AJR 114:447–459, 1972.
126. Kinsella TJ, Bloomer WD: Tolerance of the intestine to radiation therapy. Surg Gynecol Obstet 151:273–284, 1980.
127. Gardiner GW, McAuliffe N, Murray D: Colitis cystica profunda occurring in a radiation-induced colonic stricture. Hum Pathol 15:295–298, 1984.
128. Baratz M, Werbin N, Wiznitzer T, et al: Irradiation-induced colonic stricture and colitis cystica profunda. Report of case. Dis Colon Rectum 21:75–79, 1978.
129. Rogers LF, Goldstein HM: Roentgen manifestations of radiation injury to the gastrointestinal tract. Gastrointest Radiol 2:281–291, 1977.
130. Meyer JE: Radiography of the distal colon and rectum after irradiation of carcinoma of the cervix. AJR 136:691–699, 1981.
131. Glotzer DJ, Glick ME, Goldman H: Proctitis and colitis following diversion of the fecal stream. Gastroenterology 80:438–441, 1981.
132. Bosshardt RT, Abel ME: Proctitis following fecal diversion. Dis Colon Rectum 27:605–607, 1984.
133. Murray FE, O'Brien MJ, Birkett DH, et al: Diversion colitis—pathologic findings in a resected sigmoid colon and rectum. Gastroenterology 93:1404–1408, 1987.
134. Ona FV, Boger JN: Rectal bleeding due to diversion colitis. Am J Gastroenterol 80:40–41, 1985.
135. Korelitz BI, Cheskin LJ, Sohn N, et al: Proctitis after fecal diversion in Crohn's disease and its elimination with reanastomosis: implications for surgical management. Gastroenterology 87:710–713, 1984.
136. Harig JM, Soergel KH, Komorowski RA, et al: Treatment of diversion colitis with short-chain-fatty acid irrigation. N Engl J Med 320:23–28, 1989.
137. Scott RL, Pinstein ML: Diversion colitis demonstrated by double-contrast barium enema. AJR 143:767–768, 1984.
138. Croom RD, Donovan ML, Schwesinger WH: Intestinal endometriosis. Am J Surg 148:660–667, 1984.
139. Fagan CJ: Endometriosis: clinical and roentgenographic manifestations. Radiol Clin North Am 12:109–125, 1974.
140. Gordon RL, Evers K, Kressel HY, et al: Double-contrast enema in pelvic endometriosis. AJR 138:549–552, 1982.
141. Bashist B, Forde KA, McCaffrey RM: Polypoid endometrioma of the rectosigmoid. Gastrointest Radiol 8:85–88, 1983.
142. Wrenn K: Fecal impaction. N Engl J Med 321:658–662, 1989.
143. Lee FD: The anal region: specific and non-specific inflammatory lesions. *In* Whitehead R (ed): Gastrointestinal and Oesophageal Pathology. Edinburgh: Churchill Livingstone, 1989, pp 541–549.
144. Barnet JL, Raper SE: Anorectal diseases. *In* Yamada T (ed): Textbook of Gastroenterology. Philadelphia: JB Lippincott, 1991, pp 1813–1835.
145. Ramanujam PS, Prasad ML, Abcarian H, et al: Perianal abscesses and fistulas: a study of 1023 patients. Dis Colon Rectum 27:593–597, 1984.
146. Busch DB, Starling JR: Rectal foreign bodies: case reports and a comprehensive review of the world's literature. Surgery 100:512–519, 1986.

# Disorders of the Appendix

**Emil J. Balthazar, M.D.**

## INTRODUCTION

The vermiform appendix is the smallest and functionally most irrelevant segment of the gastrointestinal tract, yet diseases of the appendix are among the most common surgical emergencies in the Western world.[1-5] The appendix arises from the posteromedial aspect of the cecum at the junction of the three taeniae coli. It is a narrow, hollow organ that lacks a true mesentery and sacculations. It is supplied by the appendicular artery, which is a branch of the ileocolic artery. The worm-like appendix is contained in a peritoneal fold. The appendix has the same mural layers as the remainder of the gut but is distinguished by extremely rich lymphoid tissue in the mucosa and submucosa, which forms an entire layer of germinal follicles and lymphoid pulp in the young.[6] With age, this lymphoid tissue underlying the mucosal epithelium and glands undergoes progressive atrophy. The distal portion of the appendix sometimes undergoes fibrous obliteration in the elderly.[6]

## EMBRYOLOGY

During the sixth week of gestational life, the cecum begins to develop as a small bulge in the midgut at the level of the ileocolic junction. This diverticular structure continues to enlarge and assumes a conic shape. Its apex corresponds to the primitive appendix.[7-9] Because of differential growth rates, the development of the primitive appendix is slower than that of the rest of the cecum. It lengthens rapidly but fails to grow in thickness, soon assuming the configuration of a vermiform process. This gradual and continuous development occurs pari passu with cecal descent toward the right iliac fossa (Fig. 69–1). The fetal appendix (10 to 12 gestational weeks) is characterized by a distinctly funnel-shaped inferior cecal segment (Fig. 69–2). By birth the appendix has lengthened and shows a more abrupt transition zone at the junction with the cecum. At this time the appendix is still attached to the cecal apex. The fully developed adult appendix is uniformly narrow and arises from the left posterior wall of the cecum, rather than the cecal apex, about 2.5 to 3.5 cm below the ileocecal valve (Fig. 69–3). The process of migration of the root of the appendix from the cecal tip toward the left, on the same side as the ileocecal valve, is probably related to the upright posture of the child. The right and ventral walls of the cecum grow and distend at the expense of the left and posterior walls. The fixation at the ileocecal junction and the weight of the column of feces in the ascending colon explain this additional asymmetric development.

In adults, the root of the appendix can be located anywhere along the medioposterior wall of the cecum between the ileocecal valve and cecal tip. In addition, there is great variation in the position of the appendix in relation to the cecum and ascending colon[10, 11] (Fig. 69–4). A fully developed appendix varies in size and thickness, with an average length of 8 to 10 cm (range 4 to 25 cm). The location of the appendix in the peritoneal cavity depends on its length and relationship to cecum and the extreme variations in the mobility and location of the ascending colon and cecum.[12]

Examples of arrest in later phases of development of the appendix are common and can be recognized during barium enema examinations. An arrest in the fetal phase (see Fig. 69–2) of development is unusual. A conic configuration of the lower cecal segment signifies total absence or hypoplasia of the appendix. Agenesis of the appendix is rare; the reported incidence is about 1 in 100,000 individuals.[13]

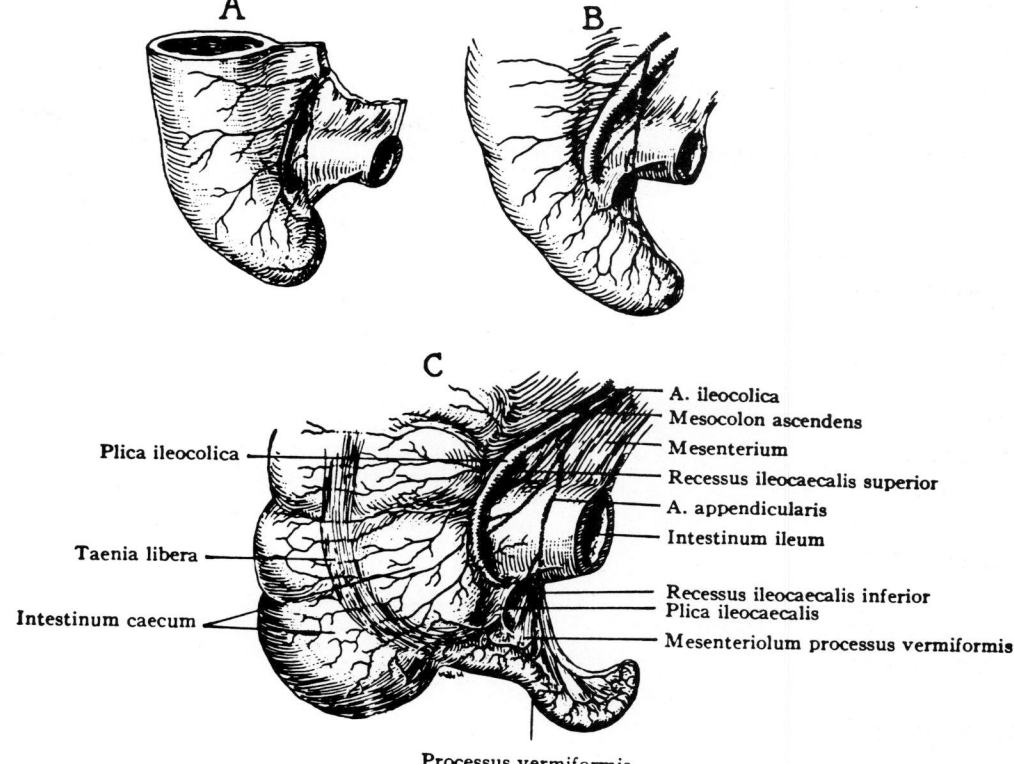

**Figure 69–1. Embryology of the appendix. A.** Growth of the inferior tip of the cecum lags during early intrauterine development. **B.** This produces the infantile appendix. **C.** Continued differential growth of the lateral cecal wall leads to the posteromedial position of the appendix in older children and adults.

Plica ileocolica

Taenia libera

Intestinum caecum

A. ileocolica
Mesocolon ascendens
Mesenterium
Recessus ileocaecalis superior
A. appendicularis
Intestinum ileum
Recessus ileocaecalis inferior
Plica ileocaecalis
Mesenteriolum processus vermiformis

Processus vermiformis

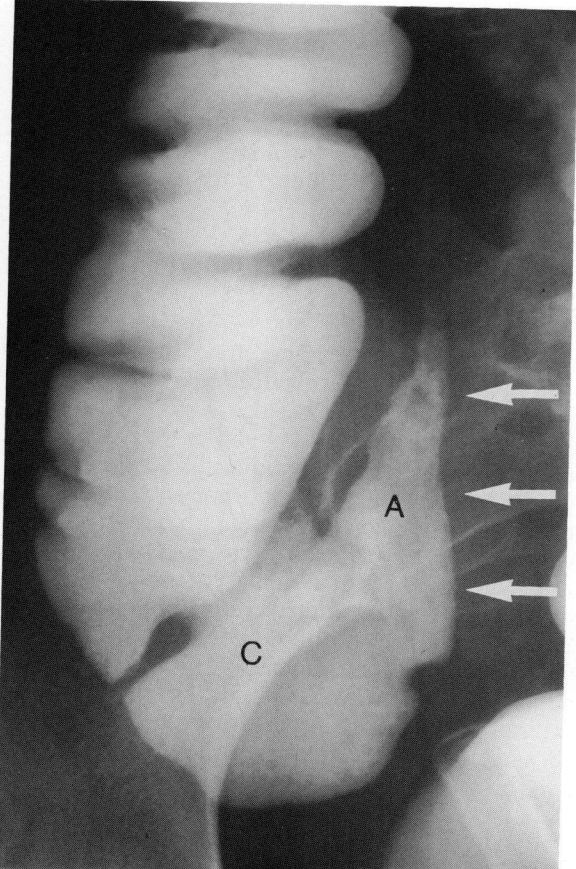

**Figure 69–2. Fetal appendix.** Barium enema examination in this 21-year-old woman shows arrest in the development of the appendix. The cecum (C) has a triangular, funnel-shaped inferior segment *(arrows)* with gradual transition into an incompletely developed appendix (A).

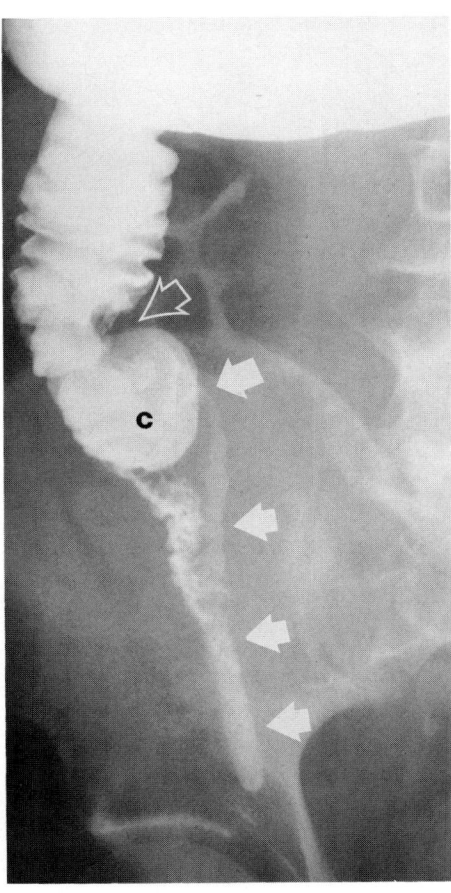

**Figure 69–3. Normal appendix: barium enema findings.** A long pelvic appendix is present, arising from the medial wall of the cecum (C) below the ileocecal valve *(open arrow)*. The appendix is uniformly narrow and completely filled with barium to the distal tip *(solid arrows)*. This finding rules out appendicitis.

## ACUTE APPENDICITIS

### Epidemiology

Appendicitis is the most common abdominal surgical emergency, affecting approximately 250,000 people annually in the United States. The incidence of acute appendicitis has been declining steadily during the past 50 years, and the current annual incidence is 10 per 100,000 population. The overall lifetime risk of developing appendicitis is approximately 7%. The comparable figures at the beginning of the century were 15 per 100,000 annual incidence and 15% lifetime risk.[1–5, 14]

Appendicitis is rare in infants but becomes increasingly common in childhood and reaches its peak incidence in the late teens and early 20s. There is a 3:2 male sex predilection in teen-agers and young adults that equalizes by the mid-30s.[1–5]

The mortality rate for acute appendicitis is less than 1 in 100,000 persons. The mortality risk of acute but not gangrenous appendicitis is less than 0.1% but rises to 0.6% in gangrenous appendicitis. Perforated appendicitis carries a 5% mortality risk, far better than the 50% mortality seen in the preantibiotic era.[1–5]

Complications occur in 1 to 5% of all patients with appendicitis, and wound infections account for nearly one third of all morbidity. Wound infection rates increase to 20 to 40% with perforated appendicitis; gangrene increases morbidity 5-fold and perforation 10-fold.[3] Clearly, delayed diagnosis and treatment account for much of the mortality and morbidity associated with this disorder.[15–19]

### Etiology

Like colonic diverticular disease, appendicitis appears to be a disease of prosperous Western nations. Low-fiber diets contribute to low-residue stool, which can become impacted within the appendiceal lumen. Improvements in hygiene greatly reduce the exposure of infants and children to enteric organisms, so these infections elicit an exaggerated lymphoid hyperplasia that may block the appendix or conceivably devitalize the appendiceal mucosa so that bacteria can invade.[20–23]

Obstruction of the appendiceal lumen followed by infection is the sine qua non of appendicitis (Fig. 69–5). The obstruction may be secondary to hyperplasia of the lymphoid follicles, fecalith, foreign body, stricture, Crohn's disease, tumor (carcinoid), kinks, and adhesions. At one time, prolonged retention of barium in the appendix was thought to be a risk factor for the development of appendicitis, but they have proved to be unrelated.[20–24]

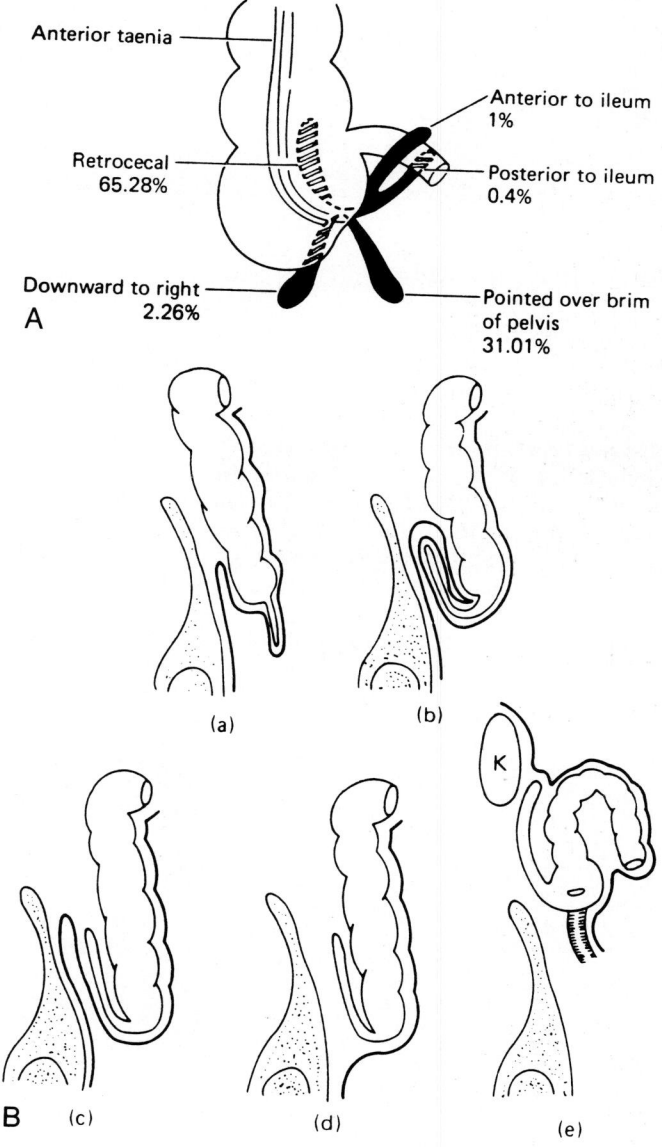

**Figure 69–4. Variations in position of the appendix. A.** Incidence of variations of positions of the appendix. (From Meyers MA: Dynamic Radiology of the Abdomen. New York: Springer-Verlag, 1988, p 403.) **B.** Normal variations in the position and peritoneal fixation of the appendix: (a) intraperitoneal, pointing over the brim of the pelvis; (b) intraperitoneal, ascending retrocecal; (c) extraperitoneal, ascending retrocecal, with a paracecal fossa present; (d) extraperitoneal, ascending retrocecal; (e) extraperitoneal, ascending retrocecal, lying anterior to the right kidney (K) deep to the liver, associated with an undescended subhepatic cecum. (The terminal ileum is also extraperitoneal and enters the cecum from behind.) (From Meyers MA, Oliphant M: Ascending retrocecal appendicitis. Radiology 110:295–299, 1974.)

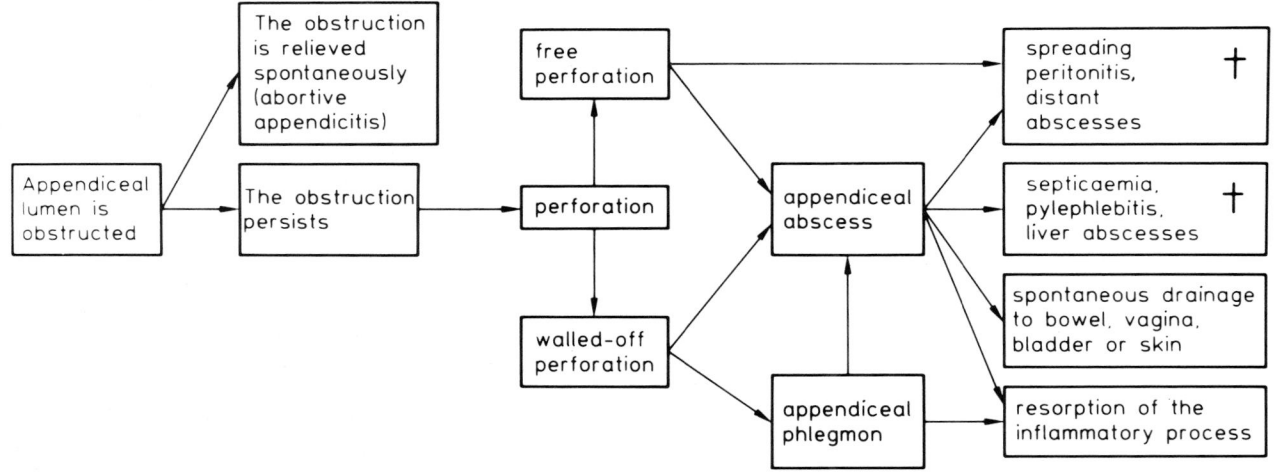

**Figure 69–5. Pathophysiologic pathways in untreated appendicitis.** (From Puylaert JBCM: Ultrasound of Appendicitis. Berlin: Springer-Verlag, 1990, p 5.)

## Pathophysiology

With obstruction, mucus accumulates within the appendiceal lumen and pressure within the organ increases. Bacteria that are normally present convert this accumulated mucus into pus, further increasing the pressure within the appendix because of the relative inelasticity of the serosa (Fig. 69–6A). This impedes lymphatic drainage of the appendix, leading to edema, mucosal ulceration, and diapedesis of bacteria. At this point, the patient perceives visceral epigastric or periumbilical pain, because the disease is still confined to the appendix.[1–5, 25]

With progressive secretion of mucus into the lumen, intraluminal pressure continues to rise, causing venous obstruction, increased edema, and appendiceal ischemia. Transmural spread of bacteria causes acute suppurative appendicitis. When the inflamed serosa of the appendix comes in contact with the parietal peritoneum, somatic pain is perceived with the classic shift of pain to the right lower quadrant.[1–5, 25]

Intramural venous and arterial thromboses ensue, resulting in gangrenous appendicitis. Infarcts permitting escape of pus into the peritoneal cavity then develop, resulting in perforating appendicitis (Fig. 69–6B and C). Perforation is the most serious complication and occurs in about 20% of patients, most often in the elderly and infant populations. Perforation can cause a localized or generalized peritonitis. Periappendiceal abscess or phlegmon occurs in 5% of all patients with appendicitis and is usually walled off by the adjacent greater omentum or small bowel loops. Inflammatory material can spread through the peritoneum to the paracolic gutters and subphrenic spaces, sigmoid colon, bladder, ovaries, or vagina. Infected thrombus may enter the portal vein, causing pylephlebitis, a rare occurrence in the antibiotic era.[1–5, 25]

## Clinical Findings

The diagnosis of appendicitis can usually be made on the basis of history and physical examination (Table 69–1). The pain is typically colicky and is initially located periumbilically or epigastrically. The pain subsequently shifts to the right lower quadrant, where it progressively becomes more severe. Nausea, vomiting, anorexia, and low-grade fever are common. Localized tenderness in the right lower quadrant is also common. An "appendiceal mass" implies abscess or phlegmon. Virtually all patients have leukocytosis.[26–29]

Despite the familiarity of the signs and symptoms of disease, some 20% of patients have an atypical presentation and there is a 20% surgical misdiagnosis rate. Clinical diagnosis is even more problematic in 1) the elderly, who may have minimal pain; 2) ovulating women 20 to 40 years of age, who have a misdiagnosis rate of 40% in some series because of diseases of the ovaries, fallopian tubes, uterus, or bladder; and 3) infants and young children, who cannot give an accurate

### TABLE 69–1. CLINICAL FEATURES OF ACUTE APPENDICITIS

| | |
|---|---|
| **History** | |
| Abdominal pain | 90–100% |
|     Beginning in epigastrium | 70% |
|     Migrating to right lower quadrant | 50% |
| Anorexia | 90% |
| Nausea | 80% |
| Vomiting | 60% |
| Fever | 20% |
| Diarrhea | 15% |
| **Physical findings** | |
| Right lower quadrant tenderness | 95–100% |
| Rectal tenderness | 45–60% |
| Abdominal guarding | 10–15% |
| Appendiceal mass | 10–15% |
| Positive psoas sign | 10–15% |
| **Laboratory findings** | |
| Leukocytosis: cell count > 10,000/mm³ | 80–90% |
| Bandemia | 90% |
| Leukocytosis or bandemia | 96% |
| Abnormal urinalysis | 25% |
| Abnormal abdominal x-ray film | 9.5% |

From Goldman LD: Acute appendicitis. *In* Taylor MB (ed): Gastrointestinal Emergencies. Baltimore: Williams & Wilkins, 1992, pp 426–436. © 1992, the Williams & Wilkins Co., Baltimore.

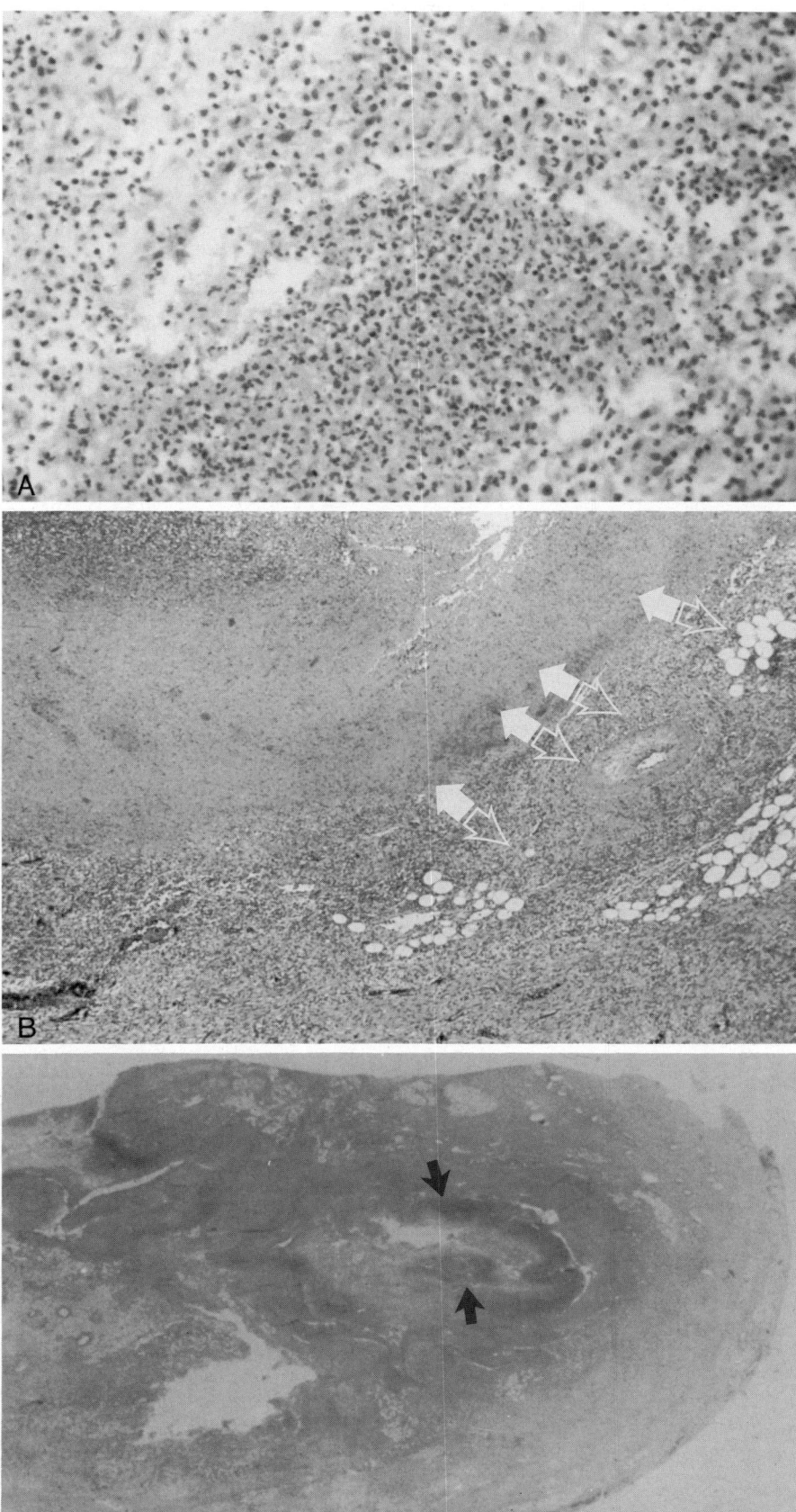

**Figure 69–6. Pathology of appendicitis.**
**A.** The lumen fills with purulent exudate.
Hematoxylin-eosin, × 150. **B.** Necrosis of
the muscularis propria *(solid arrows)* and
inflammation of the periappendiceal fat
*(open arrows)* are seen. Hematoxylin-eosin,
× 80. **C.** Transmural and periappendiceal
inflammation and fibrosis are present with
focal destruction *(arrows)* of the appendiceal
wall. Hematoxylin-eosin, × 6.

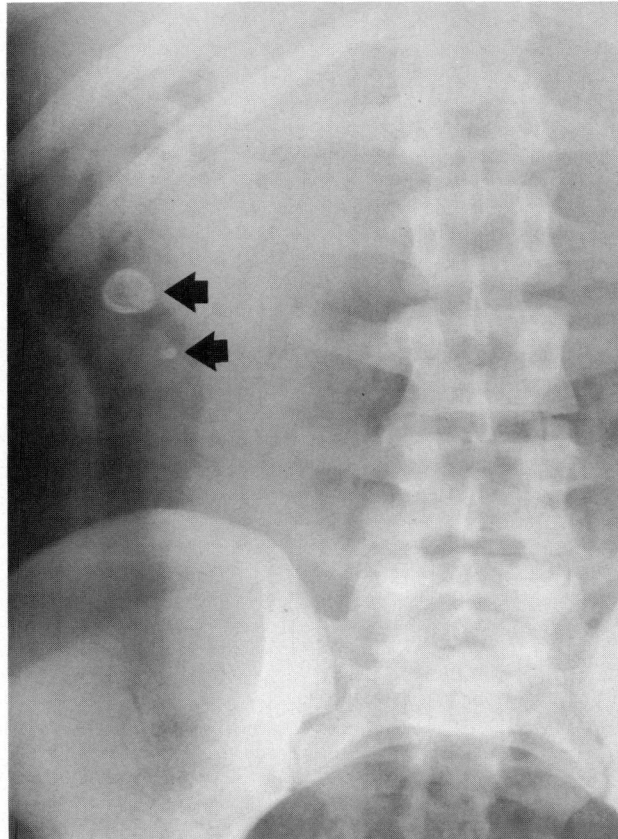

**Figure 69–7. Appendicoliths.** Two appendicoliths are present in the right upper quadrant *(arrows)*. The patient had a long retrocolic subhepatic appendix with acute appendicitis.

history.[30-35] The differential diagnosis of appendicitis is extensive (Table 69–2).

Radiology can reduce the number of misdiagnoses and negative laparotomies and can help in the management of appendiceal abscesses and postoperative complications.[36, 37]

### TABLE 69–2. CLINICAL DIFFERENTIAL DIAGNOSIS OF ACUTE APPENDICITIS

| | |
|---|---|
| Gynecologic disease | Acute cholecystitis |
| Pelvic inflammatory disease | Tuberculous ileitis |
| Torsion of an ovarian cyst | *Yersinia* ileitis |
| Rupture of an ovarian cyst | Infectious mononucleosis |
| | Ischemic colitis |
| Endometriosis | Adenocarcinoma of the appendix |
| Ectopic pregnancy | Adenocarcinoma of the cecum |
| Mesenteric adenitis | Small bowel obstruction |
| Regional ileitis | Urinary tract infection |
| Cecal diverticulitis | Pneumonia |
| Meckel's diverticulitis | Pancreatitis |
| Sigmoid diverticulitis | Helminthic infection |
| Ileal or cecal perforation | Perforated peptic ulcer |

From Goldman LD: Acute appendicitis. *In* Taylor MB (ed): Gastrointestinal Emergencies. Baltimore: Williams & Wilkins, 1992, pp 426–436. © 1992, the Williams & Wilkins Co., Baltimore.

### TABLE 69–3. APPENDICITIS: PLAIN FILM FINDINGS

Appendicolith
Cecal ileus
Right lower quadrant fluid levels
Paucity of right lower quadrant gas
Distortion of flank stripe
Loss of psoas margin
Loss of properitoneal flank stripe
Thickening of cecal wall
Scoliosis
Mottled gas collection in right lower quadrant
Pneumoperitoneum

## Radiologic Findings

In patients with the classic history and physical findings of acute appendicitis, it can be argued that imaging is not required. Imaging is advisable for the 20% of patients with atypical symptoms, infants and small children, the elderly, and young women.

### Plain Films

Plain films demonstrate some abnormality (Table 69–3) in up to 80% of patients with acute appendicitis. The

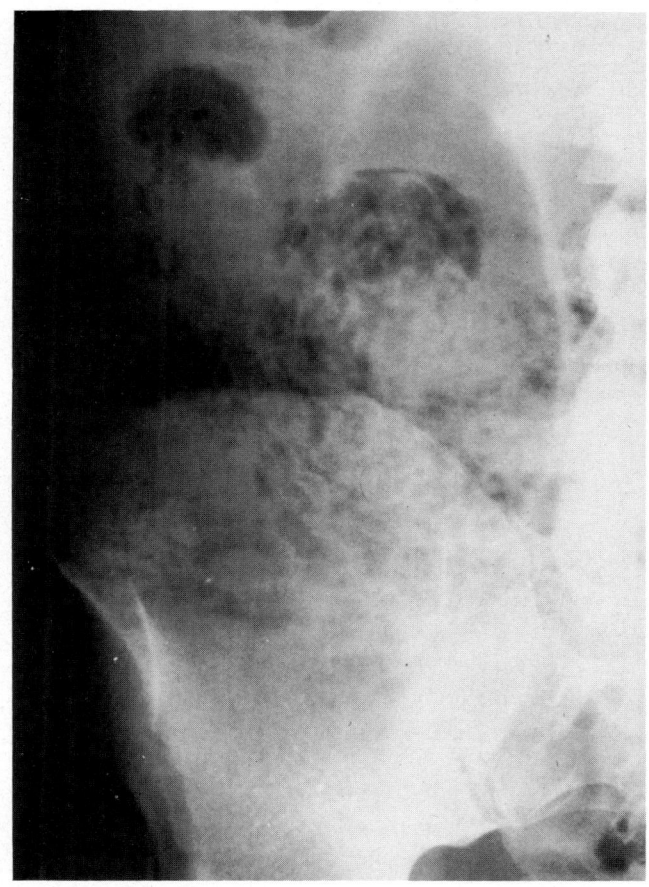

**Figure 69–8. Appendiceal abscess: plain film findings.** This abscess manifests as a bubbly collection of extraluminal gas in the right lower quadrant.

most specific plain film sign is the presence of an appendicolith (Fig. 69–7). They are found, however, in only 10% of patients with acute appendicitis and, when present, the incidence of perforation is nearly 50%. Appendicoliths are usually 0.5 to 2 cm in diameter and have a round or oval configuration and laminated rim. The calcified rim assists in differentiating them from bone islands, ureteral stones, and phleboliths. They may be obscured by the bone structures of the pelvis or may be ectopically located in the right upper abdomen in cases of retrocolic appendicitis. Appendicoliths are usually solitary, but two or three adjacent small calcifications are not unusual. Appendicoliths may be detected in asymptomatic individuals and, without associated clinical findings, are not indicative of appendicitis.[38–41]

Air in the appendix, particularly in the retrocecal location, is a normal finding. Extraluminal bubbles of air associated with an ill-defined soft tissue mass indicate an abscess (Fig. 69–8). Sometimes the inflammatory process in the right lower quadrant induces a severe localized ileus with dilatation and air-fluid levels in the ileal loops and cecum. When severe, this process can mimic the appearance of a mechanical distal small bowel obstruction (Fig. 69–9). Dilatation of the transverse colon in association with a gasless cecum and ascending colon may result from ileus of the transverse colon and spasm of the ascending colon. Free air in the peritoneal cavity is rare because the base of the appendix is usually occluded when perforation occurs.[38–52]

Other findings such as partial loss of the right psoas

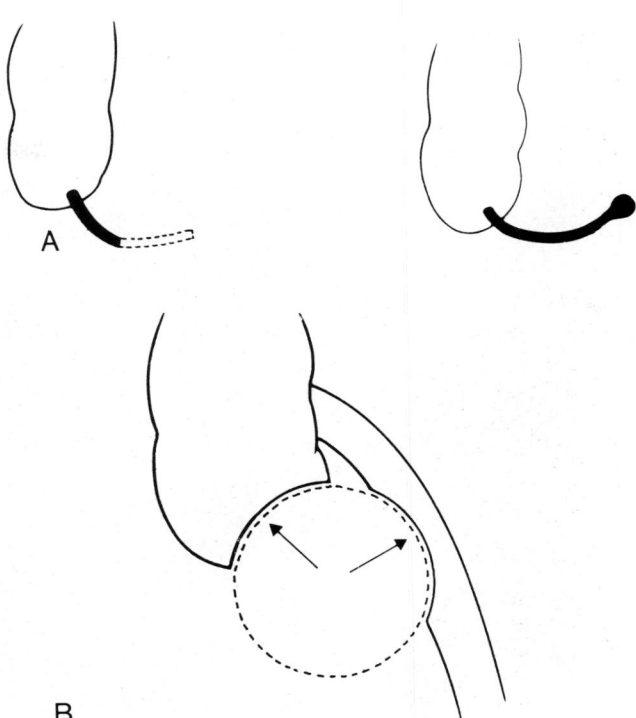

B

**Figure 69–10. Principles of barium enema diagnosis of acute appendicitis. A.** Only complete filling of the appendix to its bulbous tip excludes appendicitis. **B.** Ileocecal deformity caused by appendiceal abscess or phlegmon. (**A** and **B** from Bartram CI, Kumar P: Clinical Radiology in Gastroenterology. Oxford: Blackwell Scientific Publications, 1981, p 219.)

shadow and a lumbar scoliosis concave to the right are common, albeit nonspecific.[38–41]

## Barium Enema

Before the 1980s, the barium enema was the primary radiologic test used in the diagnosis of appendicitis. This examination can be performed quickly and safely with the single column technique. Appendicitis occurs in the setting of lumen obstruction, so complete filling of a normal appendix effectively excludes the diagnosis (Fig. 69–10A; see Fig. 69–3). Nonfilling or incomplete filling in the presence of a mass effect (Figs. 69–10B and 69–11) on the caput cecum and adjacent distal ileum do indicate inflammation, however[38–43, 50–60] (Table 69–4).

The barium enema study is also helpful in detecting other small bowel and colonic disease that can mimic the clinical presentation of acute appendicitis: neoplasm, Crohn's disease, ileal diverticulitis, and cecal diverticulitis.[38–43, 50–60]

Although the diagnostic accuracy of the barium enema study in patients with acute appendicitis is reportedly as high as 91.5%, this technique has several major drawbacks.[38–43, 50–60] Nonfilling of the appendix can be seen in 15 to 20% of normal patients, and it may be difficult to differentiate a partially filled from a completely filled appendix. Also, barium enema study provides only inferential information about extracolonic disease and cannot evaluate the nature of appendiceal phlegmons

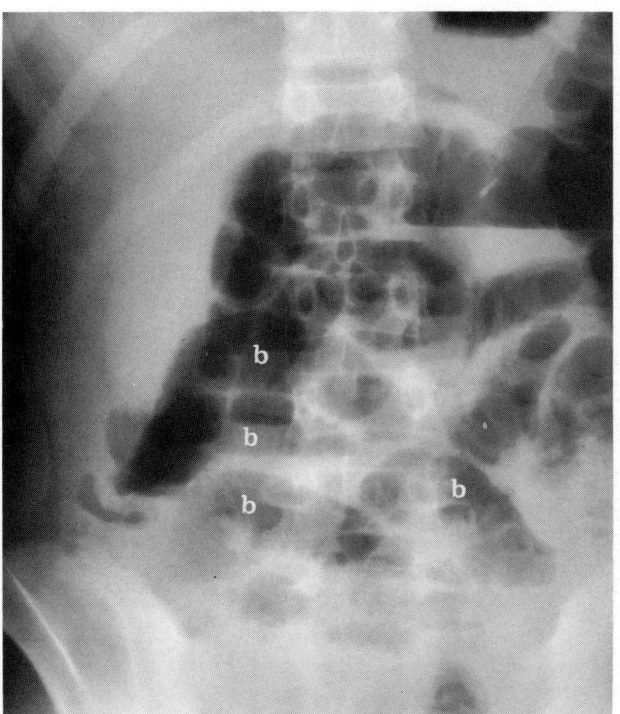

**Figure 69–9. Acute appendicitis mimicking partial small bowel obstruction.** Upright film shows dilatation and air-fluid levels in multiple lower abdominal small bowel loops (b). The patient presented with fever and leukocytosis, and gangrenous appendicitis was found at surgery.

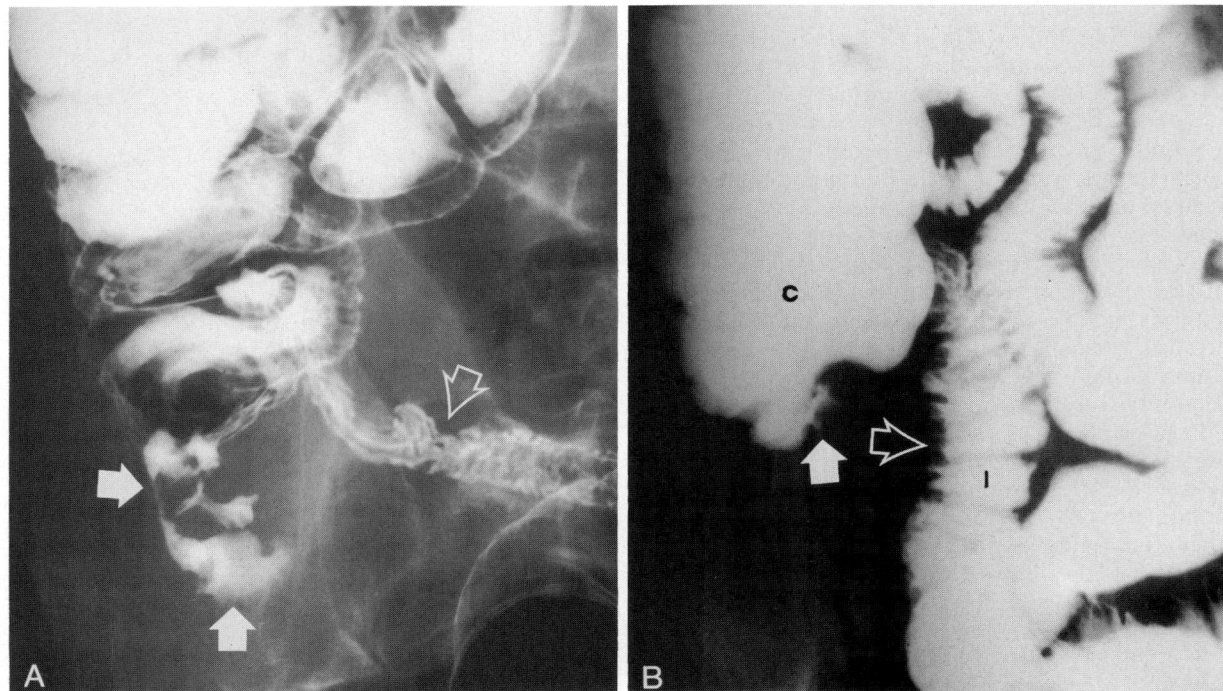

**Figure 69–11. Acute appendicitis: barium enema findings. A.** Extravasation of barium in a patient with sealed-off, perforative appendicitis *(solid arrows)*. The cecum and terminal ileum *(open arrow)* are unremarkable. **B.** Appendiceal abscess showing compression of the cecal caput, obstruction of the base of the appendix *(solid arrow)*, and a spiculated lateral contour *(open arrow)* of the terminal ileum. C = cecum; I = ileum.

and abscesses. The appendix can also intussuscept (Fig. 69–12) into the cecum, producing a cecal defect unrelated to appendicitis on barium enema studies (see later).[61–63]

In the past decade, ultrasound and computed tomography (CT) have gained acceptance as primary imaging techniques for acute appendicitis by virtue of their ability to image directly the appendix, adjacent fat, and gut.

## Computed Tomography

CT has the advantage of directly visualizing the appendix, as well as the periappendiceal and other intra-abdominal structures (Table 69–5). In so doing, CT not only images the abnormal appendix but also can evaluate the nature, severity, and extent of the associated inflammatory process. Furthermore, by detecting a normal appendix or other unsuspected abdominal pathology, CT is often able to allow an alternative diagnosis.[64–74]

### Technique

To maximize visualization of the appendix and diagnostic sensitivity of CT in acute appendicitis, a number of strategies are useful: 1) fast acquisition time (<2 seconds) CT scanners; 2) bolus intravenous contrast agent administration (I use 50 mL of 45% diatrizoate at 1.5 mL/s, followed by 140 mL at 0.8 mL/s); 3) filling of the terminal ileum and cecum with 800 to 1000 mL of dilute barium (1 to 2%) or diatrizoate meglumine (Gastrografin, 2%) given orally at least 1 hour before scanning; and 4) dynamic sequential scanning using 10 × 10 or 10 × 12 mm collimation in the upper abdomen and 5 × 8 mm over the cecum and upper pelvis.[69] If nonspecific abnormalities are seen and terminal ileal loops are not well filled, another examination of the pelvis 15 to 30 minutes later using 5 × 5 mm collimation over the region of interest is performed.

The use of intraluminal contrast medium may interfere with the visualization of an appendicolith. Recognition of the terminal ileal loops and cecum, however, is crucial for the detection of an abnormal appendix. In my experience, inadequate recognition of ileal loops is the most common cause of erroneous interpretation. By using different window settings, most appendicoliths can be visualized and differentiated from adjacent intestinal loops.

### Normal Appendix

Visualization of the appendix by CT depends on the quality of the examination, presence of mesenteric and retroperitoneal fat, and adequate visualization of terminal ileal loops and the cecum.[64, 68, 74] With high-resolution CT, utilizing 5 × 5 mm collimation, normal

---

#### TABLE 69–4. ACUTE APPENDICITIS: BARIUM ENEMA FINDINGS

Failure to fill appendix completely
Mass effect, caput cecum
Inflammatory changes: cecum, terminal ileum, and/or rectum

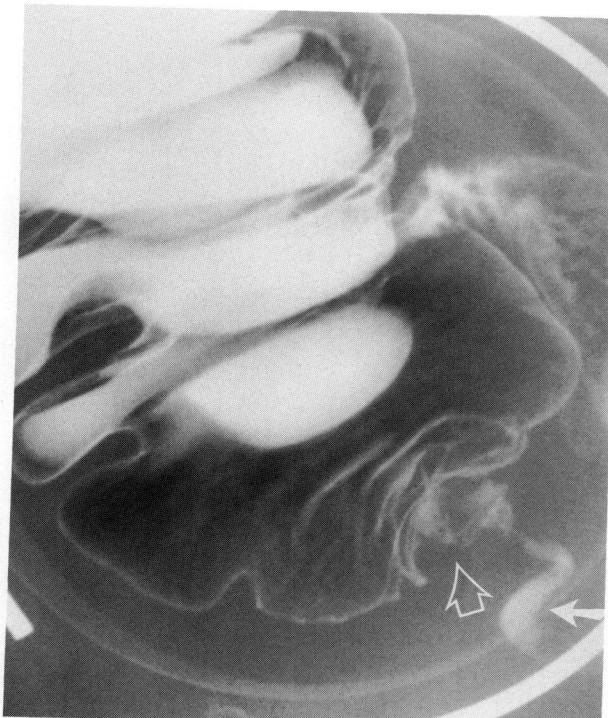

**Figure 69–12. Partial appendiceal intussusception.** The appendix is incompletely filled *(solid arrow)* and partially intussuscepting into the cecal caput *(open arrow).*

appendixes are seen in 50 to 60% of cases.[74] Because of the variable location of the cecum, the position of the appendix differs from individual to individual. Usually, it can be found in the right lower quadrant adjacent to the cecal caput, either caudal or posterior to it (Fig. 69–13). Depending on its orientation, the normal appendix appears as a small tubular or ring-shaped density. It may be collapsed or filled with fluid or air. It has an extremely thin wall and a sharp outer contour and is enveloped by the homogeneous fat density of the normal mesentery (see Fig. 69–13). Appendicoliths may be detected in asymptomatic individuals.[68] Without the associated inflammatory changes indicative of appendicitis, the presence of air, fecal matter, or calcifications in the appendix has no immediate clinical relevance.

## Computed Tomographic Diagnosis

The CT findings in acute appendicitis are variable, reflecting the type and severity of the pathologic proc-

### TABLE 69–5. ACUTE APPENDICITIS: COMPUTED TOMOGRAPHIC FINDINGS

Circumferential mural thickening of appendix
Mural contrast enhancement
Appendicolith
Hazy, streaky periappendiceal densities
Pericecal soft tissue mass (phlegmon)
Pericecal fluid collection (abscess)
Mural thickening, adjacent cecum and terminal ileum
Pneumoperitoneum

ess.[64, 68, 69] In milder forms, the appendix is only slightly distended and thickened, whereas in complicated appendicitis it is fragmented, destroyed, and replaced by a phlegmon or abscess. CT abnormalities can be divided into specific findings that provide a definite pathologic diagnosis and findings that are compatible and suggestive but not pathognomonic for appendicitis.

### SPECIFIC ABNORMALITIES

The diagnosis of acute appendicitis can be made with confidence when an abnormal appendix is identified or when an appendicolith associated with a phlegmon or abscess is detected in the right lower quadrant.

The abnormal appendix appears as a slightly distended, fluid-filled or collapsed tubular structure about 0.5 to 2 cm in diameter (Figs. 69–14 and 69–15). It does not exceed 3 to 4 cm, even when the appendix is severely distended (Fig. 69–16). The wall of the diseased appendix is circumferentially and asymmetrically thickened. It is homogeneously dense and is enhanced during the arterial phase of bolus administration because of inflammatory hyperemia (see Fig. 69–15). The inflamed wall is 1 to 3 mm thick and is demonstrated in almost all cases. Periappendiceal inflammation is the hallmark of appendicitis. The inflammatory response is variable: slightly increased hazy density of the mesenteric fat (Fig. 69–17), linear strands (see Fig. 69–16), fluid-containing abscesses (Fig. 69–18), or heterogeneous ill-defined soft tissue densities representing a phlegmon (Fig. 69–19). Secondary inflammatory and edematous changes can cause slight mural thickening of the small bowel or cecum (Fig. 69–20). These secondary findings often accompany acute appendicitis and should not be misinterpreted as primary ileocolic inflammatory disease. With high-resolution CT, an abnormal appendix can be identified in 75% of cases of acute appendicitis.[69]

Detection of an appendicolith in the right lower quadrant associated with a phlegmon or a pericecal abscess is indicative of complicated appendicitis (Fig. 69–21; see Fig. 69–18). The calcified appendicolith may be located in the appendiceal lumen, may be outside the appendix within an inflammatory mass, or may lie freely in a fluid-filled abscess cavity (see Fig. 69–21). In these cases, the appendix is fragmented and destroyed and cannot be specifically identified (Fig. 69–22; see Figs. 69–15 and 69–21). Detection of an appendicolith allows a specific etiologic diagnosis to be made. Appendicoliths are visualized in 28% (versus 10% for plain films) of adult patients with acute appendicitis by CT, reflecting the higher sensitivity of CT for detecting small intra-abdominal calcifications.[69] Detection of an intraluminal appendicolith is indicative of appendicitis only when there are associated inflammatory changes involving the appendix and/or periappendiceal fat (see Fig. 69–22).

### SUGGESTIVE ABNORMALITIES

Detection of right lower quadrant inflammation, phlegmon, and abscess adjacent to the cecum is highly suggestive but not pathognomonic for acute appendicitis (see Figs. 69–18 and 69–19). The differential diagnosis includes cecal diverticulitis (Fig. 69–23), perforated ce-

*Text continued on page 1324*

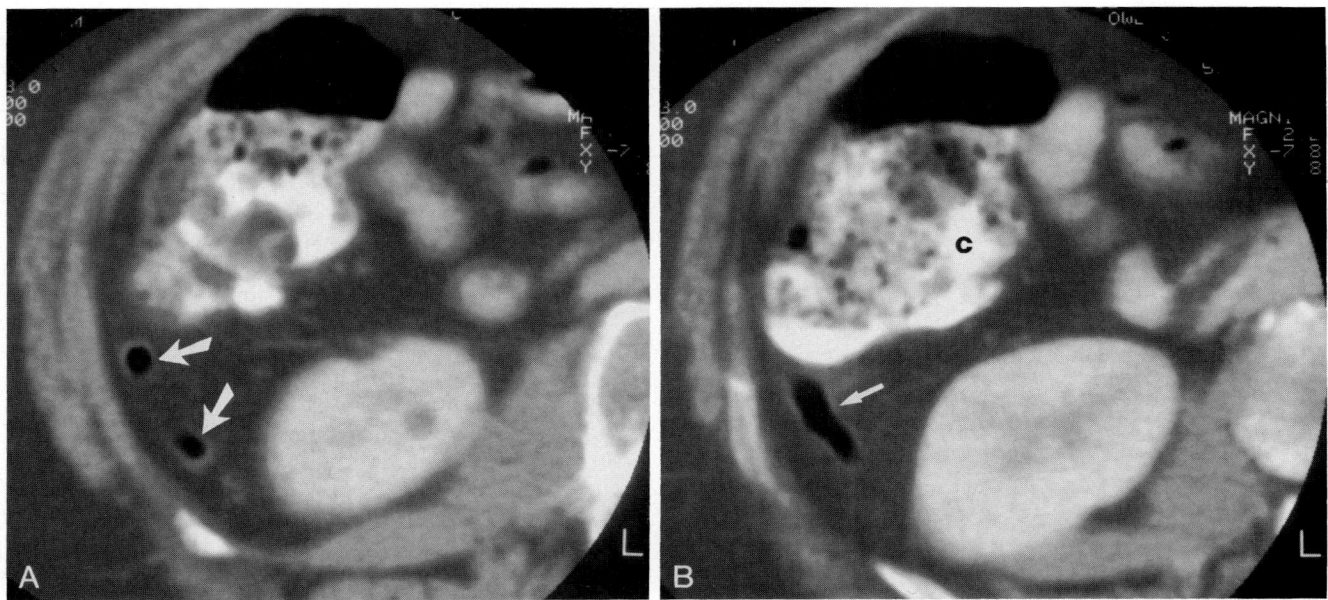

**Figure 69–13. Normal appendix: CT findings.** The air-filled appendix *(arrows)* is seen at two levels in the axial **(A)** and longitudinal **(B)** planes. The wall of the appendix is thin, and the periappendiceal mesenteric fat and retroperitoneal fat have a homogeneous, low density. C = cecum.

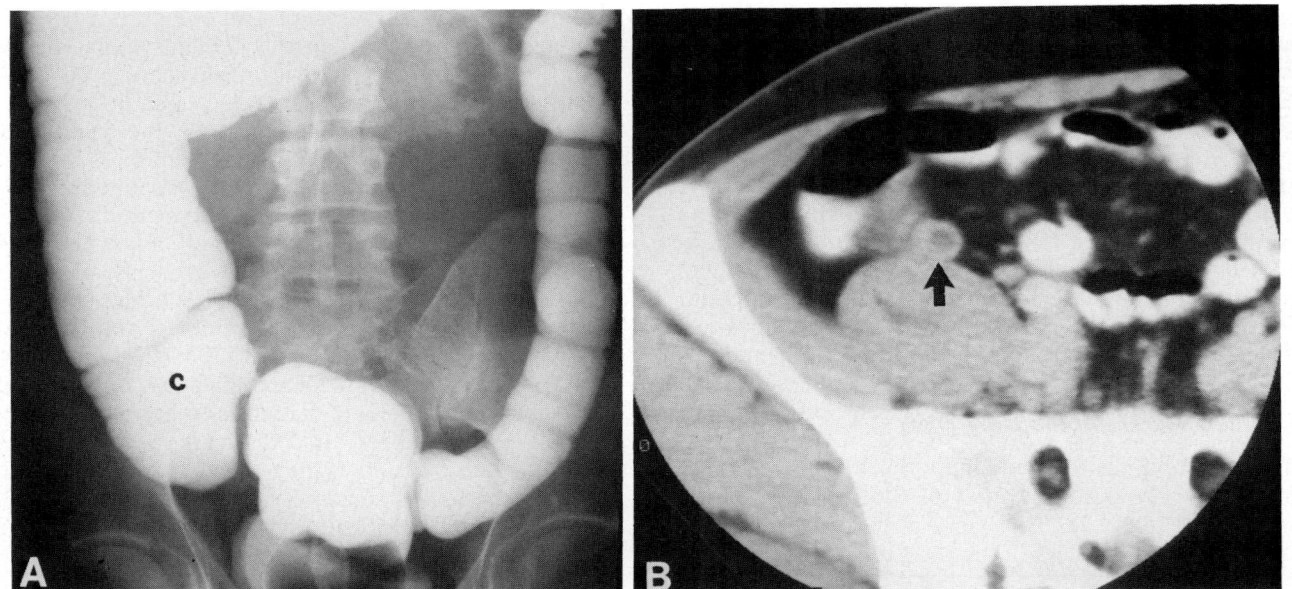

**Figure 69–14. Mild appendicitis. A.** Barium enema shows that the appendix is not visualized and there is a questionable mass effect in the caput cecum. **B.** CT scan shows a distended, fluid-filled appendix in cross section *(arrow)*. The appendix has a circumferentially thick wall that is enhanced homogeneously. There are no periappendiceal inflammatory changes.

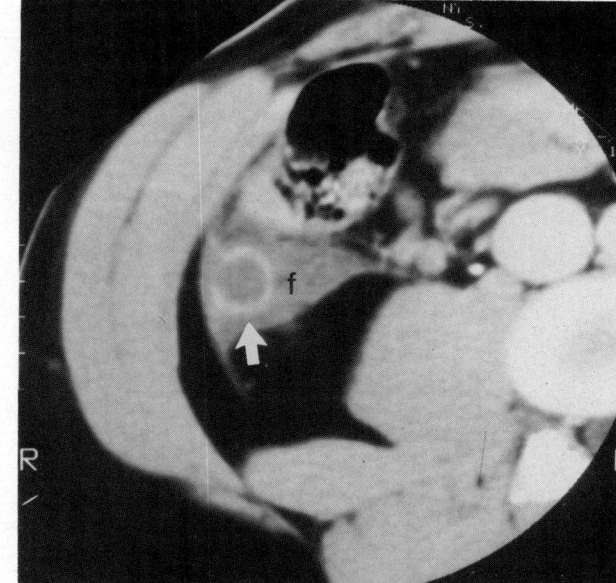

**Figure 69–15. CT scan in acute appendicitis.** The appendix is fluid filled and distended and shows an enhanced hyperemic wall *(arrow)*. A small amount of fluid is present around the appendix and in the mesoappendix (f).

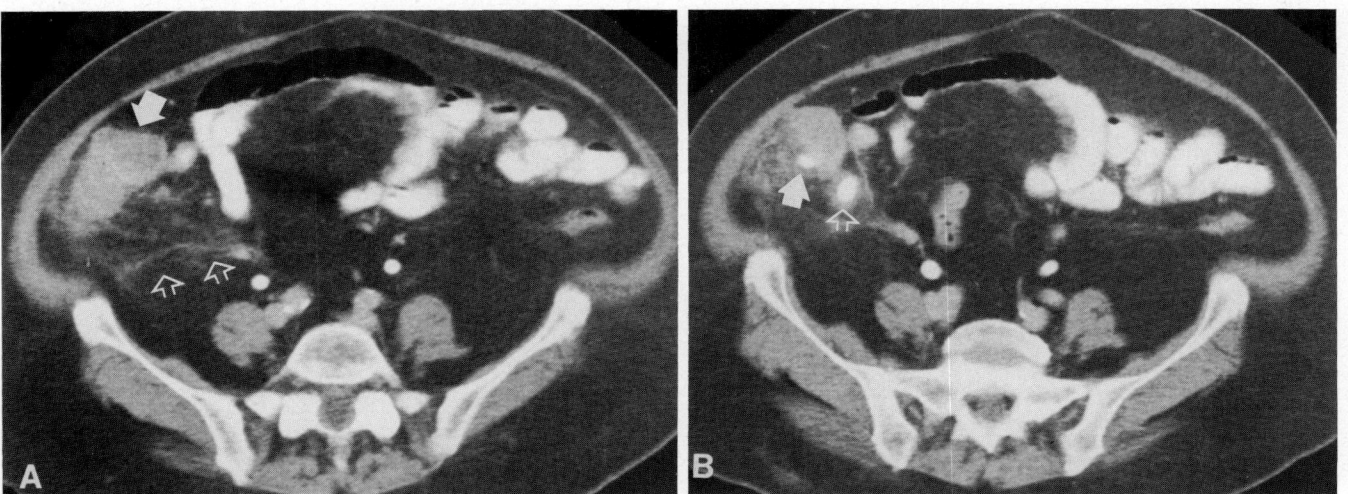

**Figure 69–16. CT scan in perforative appendicitis. A.** Appendix is fluid filled and markedly distended *(solid arrow)*. Linear strands and haziness are seen in the adjacent fat *(open arrows)*, indicating inflammation. **B.** At a more caudal level, the wall of the appendix is disrupted and one appendicolith is noted adjacent to the appendix *(solid arrow)*. A second calcified appendicolith is seen posteriorly *(open arrow)*.

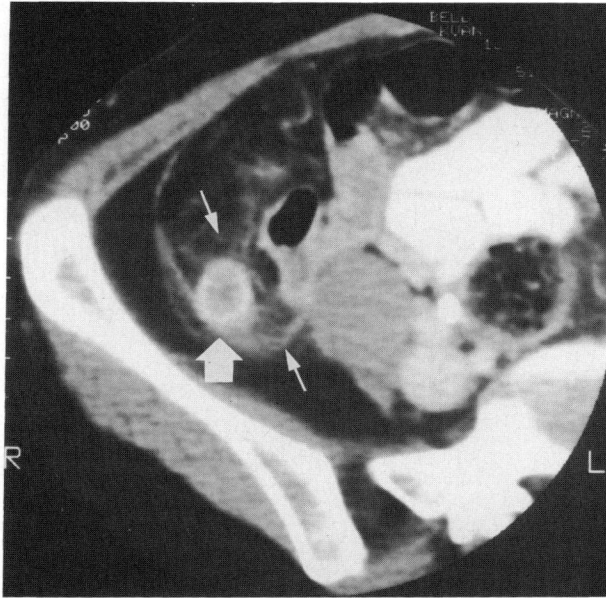

**Figure 69–17. CT scan in acute appendicitis.** The appendix is distended and fluid filled with a hyperemic, slightly thickened wall *(thick arrow)*. Periappendiceal fat has an increased hazy density containing a few linear strands *(thin arrows)*.

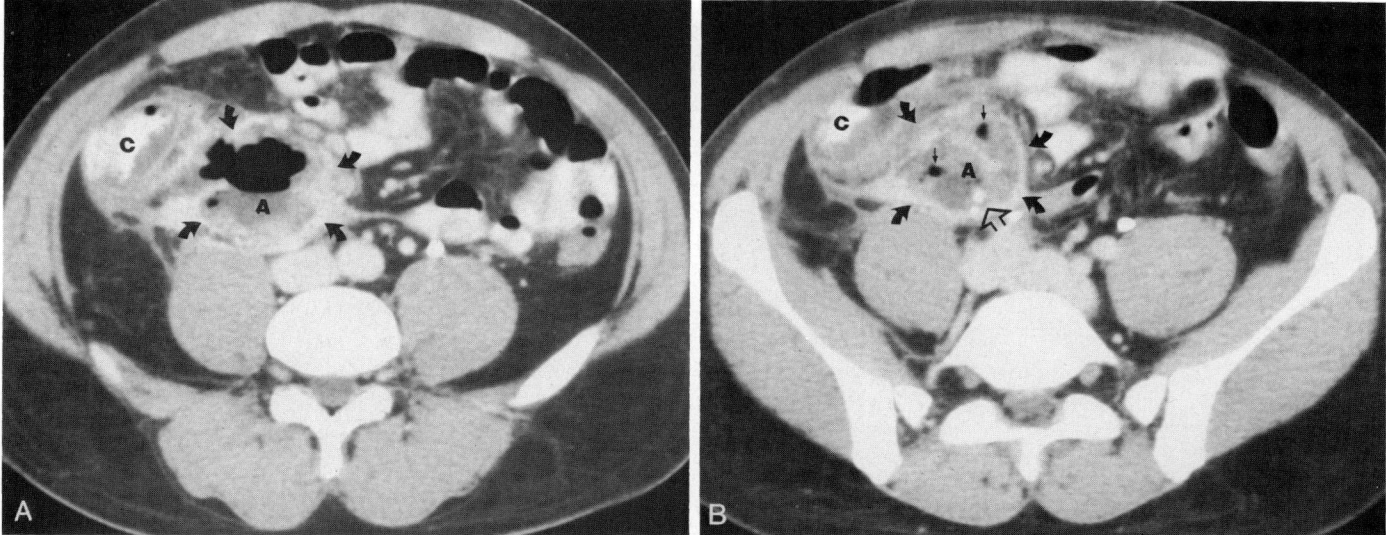

**Figure 69–18. Perforated appendicitis with appendiceal abscess.** The appendix is not visualized. **A.** Medial to cecum (C) and anterior to the psoas muscle, there is an air- and fluid-filled abscess (A). The abscess has a well-formed hyperemic (enhancing) capsule *(arrows)*. **B.** Abscess (A) containing a few bubbles of air *(straight black arrows)* is still seen at a more caudal level *(curved black arrows)*. Two small calcified appendicoliths are present in the abscess *(open arrow)*. C = cecum.

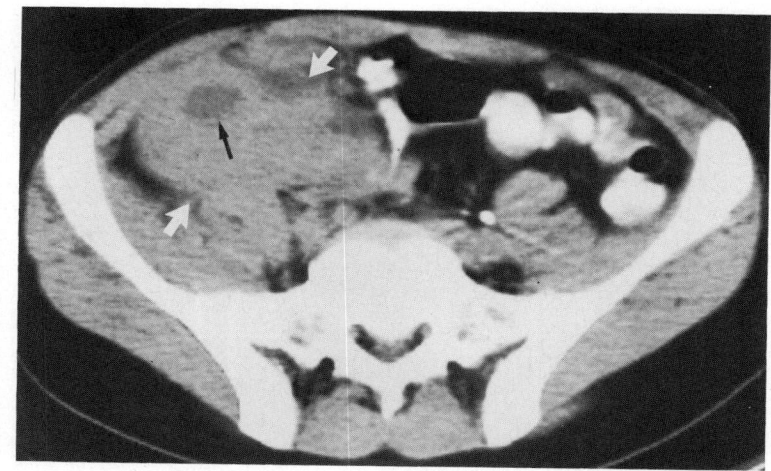

**Figure 69–19. Solid-appearing abscess in acute appendicitis.** A large ill-defined and lobulated soft tissue mass displaces adjacent small bowel loops *(white arrows)*. The phlegmon contains a low-density area of liquefaction representing fluid *(black arrow)*.

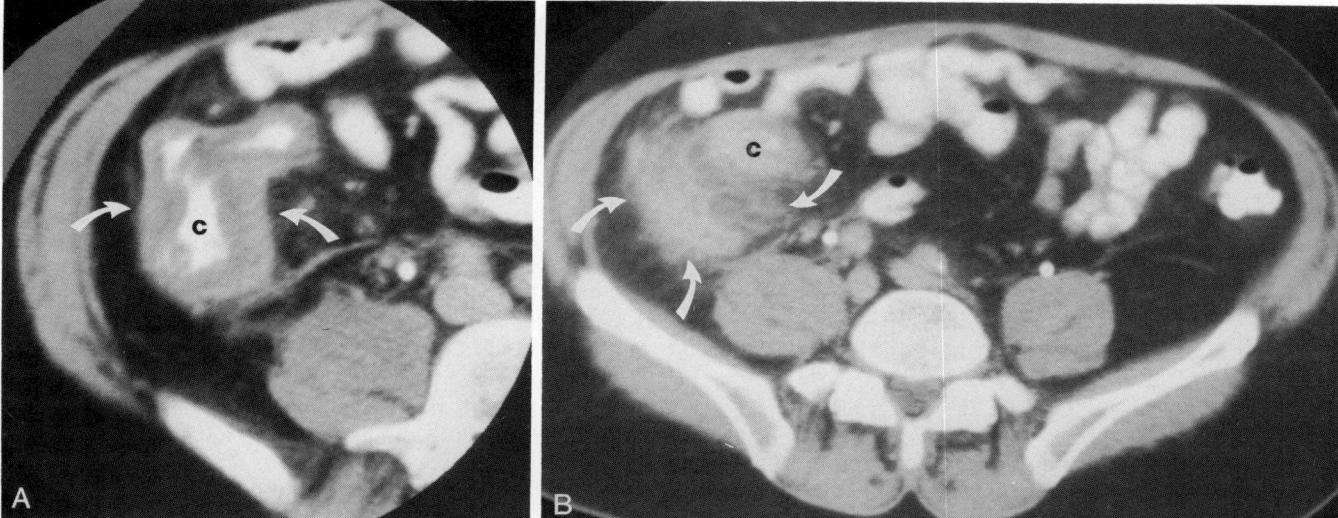

**Figure 69–20. Cecal edema in acute appendicitis. A.** The cecum (C) shows a circumferential thickened wall *(arrows)* having two concentric rings of low and high attenuation ("double halo" sign). Submucosal inflammation and edema were noted pathologically. **B.** At a slightly caudal level there is phlegmon *(arrows)* located posterior and lateral to cecal caput (C).

**Figure 69–21. Pericecal fluid and appendicolith characteristic of appendiceal abscess.** The appendix is not visualized. The abscess is poorly marginated *(open arrows)*, and the calcified appendicolith lies freely, posteriorly *(solid arrow)*.

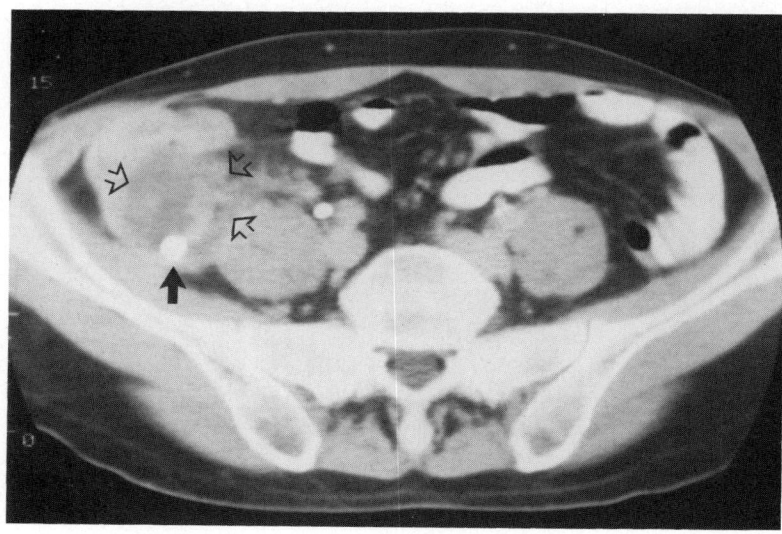

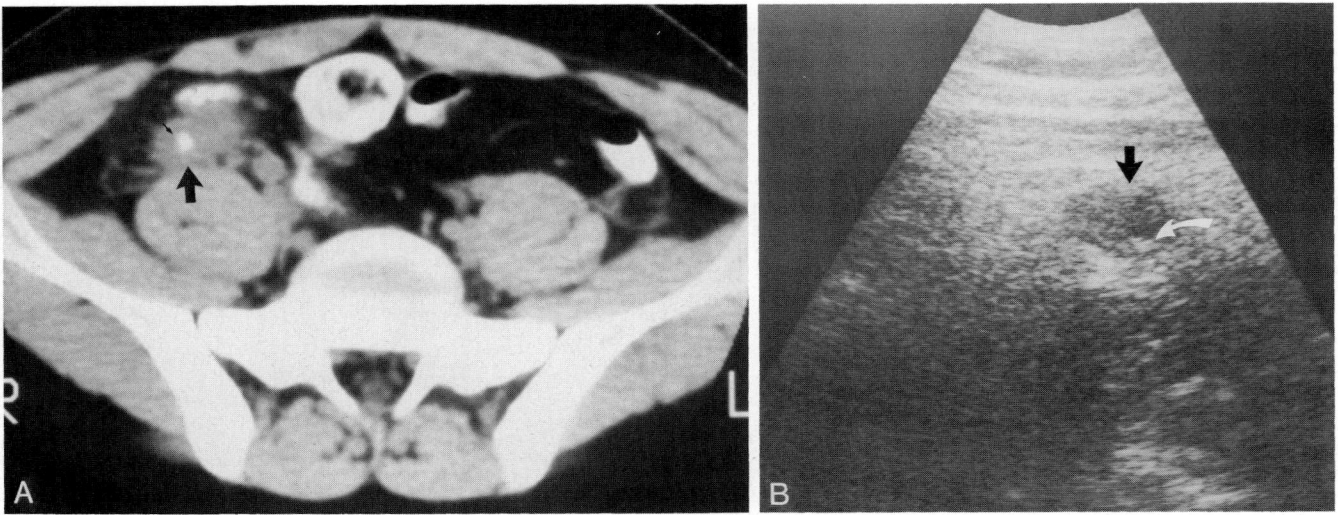

**Figure 69–22. Acute appendicitis with intraluminal appendicolith. A.** CT scan shows the thick-walled collapsed appendix *(large arrow)* with a calcified intraluminal appendicolith *(small arrow).* **B.** Sonography shows a thickened appendix 1 cm in diameter *(black arrow).* There is a questionable echogenic focus on its posterior wall *(white arrow).*

cal carcinoma, ileal diverticulitis, Crohn's disease, and, in young women, pelvic inflammatory disease. If an abnormal appendix or an appendicolith is not visualized, the etiology of the inflammatory process cannot be stated with certainty (see Fig. 69–23). These patients require a barium enema study to visualize a normal appendix (which rules out appendicitis) and evaluate the colon and terminal ileum for primary intestinal disease.

### Complicated Appendicitis

Perforation of the appendix can cause abnormalities ranging from a sealed-off abscess to widespread intraperitoneal contamination, which can be lethal if not promptly recognized. Perforation occurs in about 20% of cases of appendicitis.[15, 29] The inflammatory response is variable and depends on the size of the perforation,

virulence of the bacterial infection, and ability of the body to contain the infection.

Ill-defined heterogeneous soft tissue inflammatory masses seen on CT scans represent suppurative inflammations: phlegmons or solid abscesses (see Figs. 69–19 and 69–20). Liquefaction with recognizable fluid collections, either adjacent to or at a distance from the cecum, qualifies as an abscess (see Figs. 69–18 and 69–21). Abscesses are variable in size, have low attenuation numbers (10 to 30 Hounsfield units), and are poorly defined or partially encapsulated (see Figs. 69–18 and 69–21). The presence of an identifiable capsule signifies chronicity, indicating that the abscess is probably a few days to several weeks old (see Fig. 69–18). In 15% of cases, abscesses contain bubbles of air or air-fluid levels either from gas-forming bacteria or fistulization to bowel (see Fig. 69–18). High-density pus and necrotic tissue

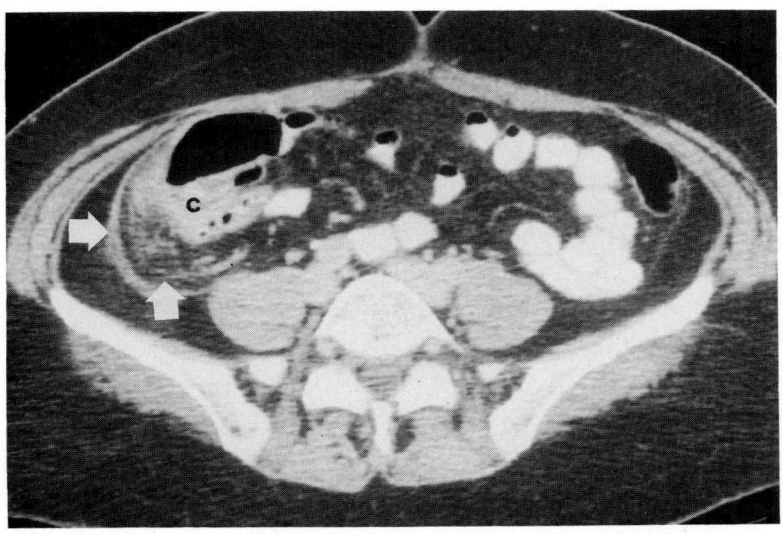

**Figure 69–23. Cecal diverticulitis.** CT scan shows thickening of the pericecal fascial plane and nonspecific retrocecal inflammatory changes *(arrows).* Sonography revealed no abnormalities. Surgery and pathologic study revealed cecal diverticulitis. C = cecum.

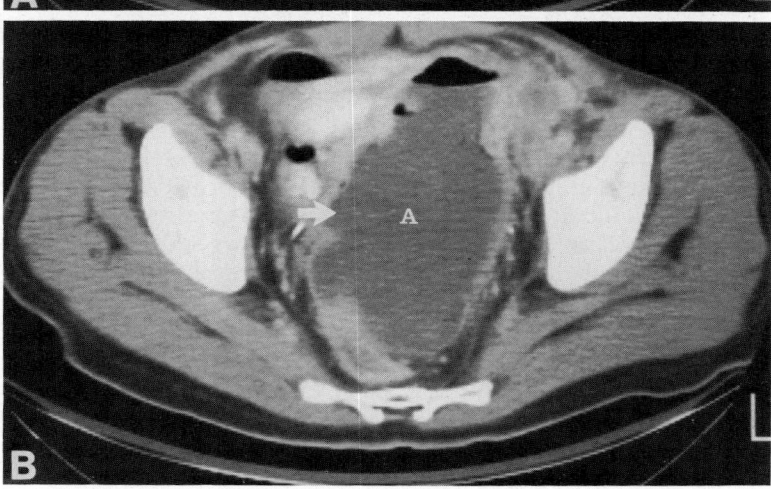

**Figure 69–24. Perforative appendicitis. A.** Several poorly defined interloop abscesses (A) are present in the upper pelvis *(arrows)*. **B.** There is a large abscess (A) with an air-fluid level *(arrow)* in the lower pelvis displacing adjacent loops of bowel. Neither the appendix nor an appendicolith is visualized. Surgery revealed perforation of the appendix and multiple abscesses.

may impart a solid appearance to the abscess (see Fig. 69–19).

Because of the length and position of the appendix and the patterns of fluid migration in the peritoneal cavity, abscesses may be found in locations distant from the cecum. Mesenteric interloop abscesses (Fig. 69–24) and pelvic or subhepatic fluid collections (Fig. 69–25) can develop in patients with perforative appendicitis. Most abscesses are located either inferior, medial, or posterior to the cecum or in the right paracolic gutter (see Figs. 69–18 to 69–21).

PERFORATIVE APPENDICITIS WITH EXTRALUMINAL AIR

Free intra-abdominal air is rarely seen in patients with perforative appendicitis. In most cases, obstruction of the appendix prevents free intraperitoneal leakage of colonic air. Even when air escapes, the perforation is usually sealed off or the amount of extraluminal air is minimal. CT can reveal minimal amounts of extraluminal air that are not recognized on conventional abdominal films. With free perforation, air can be seen under the right diaphragm (Fig. 69–26). When the tip of the inflamed appendix has a retroperitoneal location or is burrowed posteriorly, air is seen in the retroperitoneal fascial planes and may dissect into the abdominal

wall.[68] CT can reveal the extent and location of the air and also determine its origin in many instances (Fig. 69–27). An abnormal appendix or appendicolith or both are often demonstrated in these cases, allowing a specific diagnosis to be made (see Figs. 69–26 and 69–27).

ACCURACY OF COMPUTED TOMOGRAPHY

In a prospective evaluation of 100 consecutive patients with clinically suspected appendicitis, high-resolution CT had a sensitivity of 98%, specificity of 83%, and accuracy of 93%.[69] The positive and negative predictive values were greater than 90%.[69] In patients with pathologically proven appendicitis, the diagnosis was established by CT in 94% and right lower quadrant inflammatory changes were seen in 98%. Furthermore, in the group of patients who did not have appendicitis, high-resolution CT diagnosed other intra-abdominal conditions in 17 of 31.[69]

ADVANTAGES AND LIMITATIONS OF COMPUTED TOMOGRAPHY

The sensitivity and accuracy of high-resolution CT are superior to those of barium enema examination (see Fig. 69–14) and compare favorably with the reported data on graded compression sonography. Two additional

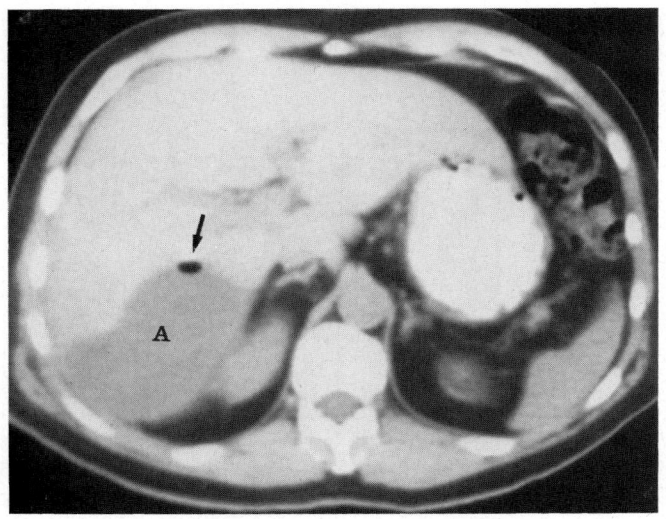

**Figure 69–25. Subhepatic abscess secondary to ruptured retrocecal appendicitis.** The fluid-filled abscess (A) contains a bubble of air *(arrow)* and is located between the upper pole of the right kidney and right lobe of the liver.

factors emphasize the value of CT imaging in patients with suspected acute appendicitis. First, CT can accurately differentiate mild inflammation from phlegmons and abscesses, as well as detect extension of disease distant from the appendiceal region. CT also provides a critical "road map" for surgical or percutaneous abscess drainage in cases of complicated appendicitis. Second, CT has a high sensitivity in the diagnosis of intra-abdominal disease unrelated to appendicitis that explains the patient's clinical symptoms (Fig. 69–28).

The limitations of CT are related to improper use of equipment, poor technique, radiation exposure, inadequate visualization of terminal ileal loops, and absence of retroperitoneal fat. Nonspecific inflammatory changes in the right lower quadrant are further relative limitations of CT because these changes are suggestive of but not specific for appendicitis.

## Ultrasound

Before 1986, sonography was used primarily to detect abscess and exclude cholecystitis and gynecologic and urologic diseases in patients with acute appendicitis. With the introduction of graded compression sonography (Fig. 69–29) by Puylaert, the role and utility of sonography in these cases have increased dramatically.[75–101]

### Sonographic Technique

A high-resolution, 5- or 7.5-MHz linear array transducer is used to perform the examination. The scan is obtained with the patient in the supine position over the area of maximal tenderness indicated by the patient. Pressure is applied slowly and gently to avoid pain or

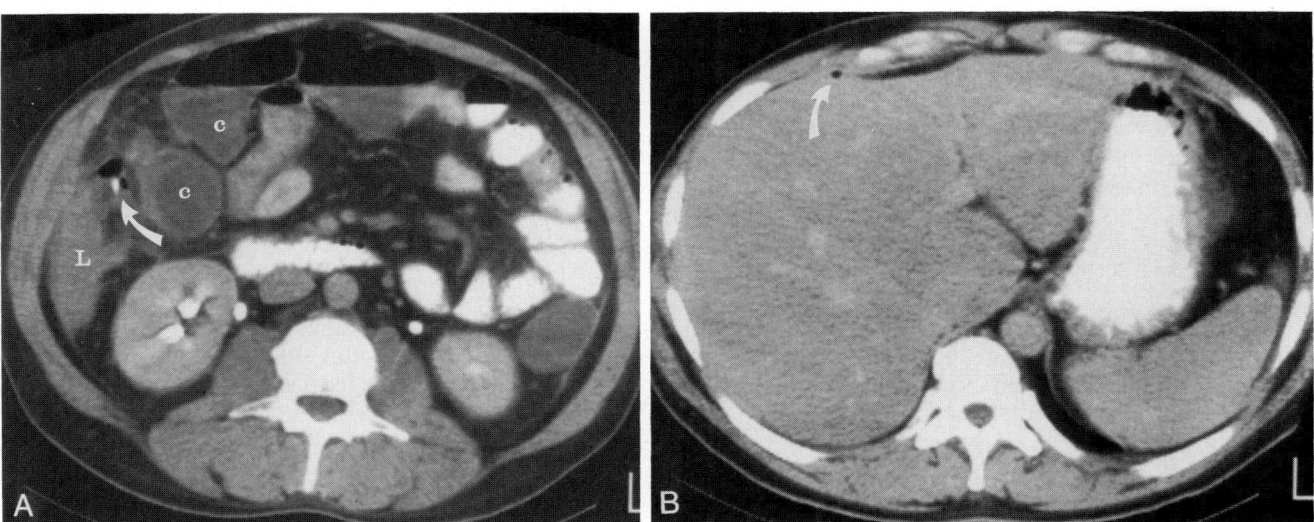

**Figure 69–26. Perforative appendicitis with free intraperitoneal air. A.** Perforation of a retrocolic appendix showing free air and an adjacent appendicolith *(arrow)*. Associated inflammatory changes are seen between the right lobe of the liver (L) and the hepatic flexure (c). **B.** A single bubble of free air is present under the diaphragm and above the liver *(arrow)*. The plain abdominal and chest films were normal.

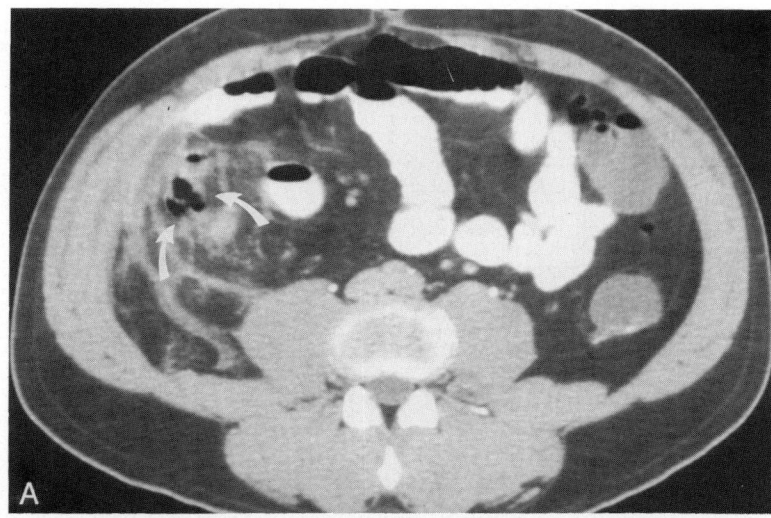

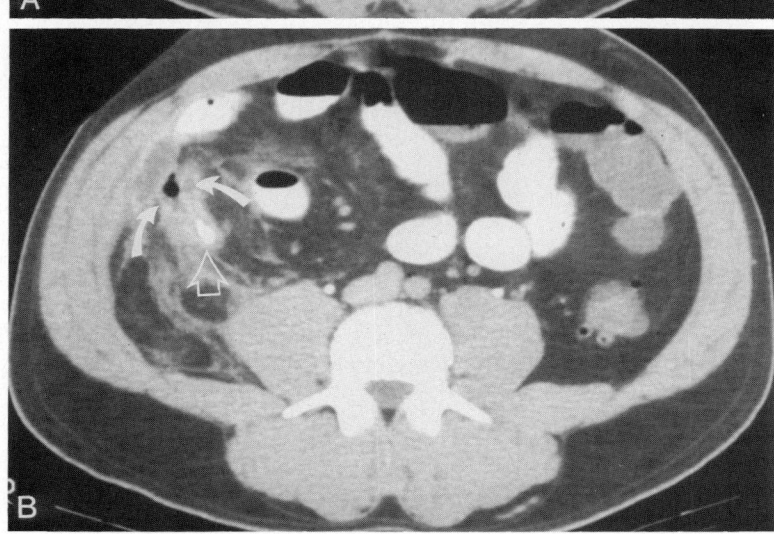

**Figure 69–27. Perforation of the appendix with extraluminal air. A.** Inflammatory changes and bubbles of air are present in the right lower abdomen *(arrows).* **B.** Adjacent section shows extraluminal air and inflammation *(solid arrows)* near a calcified appendicolith *(open arrow).*

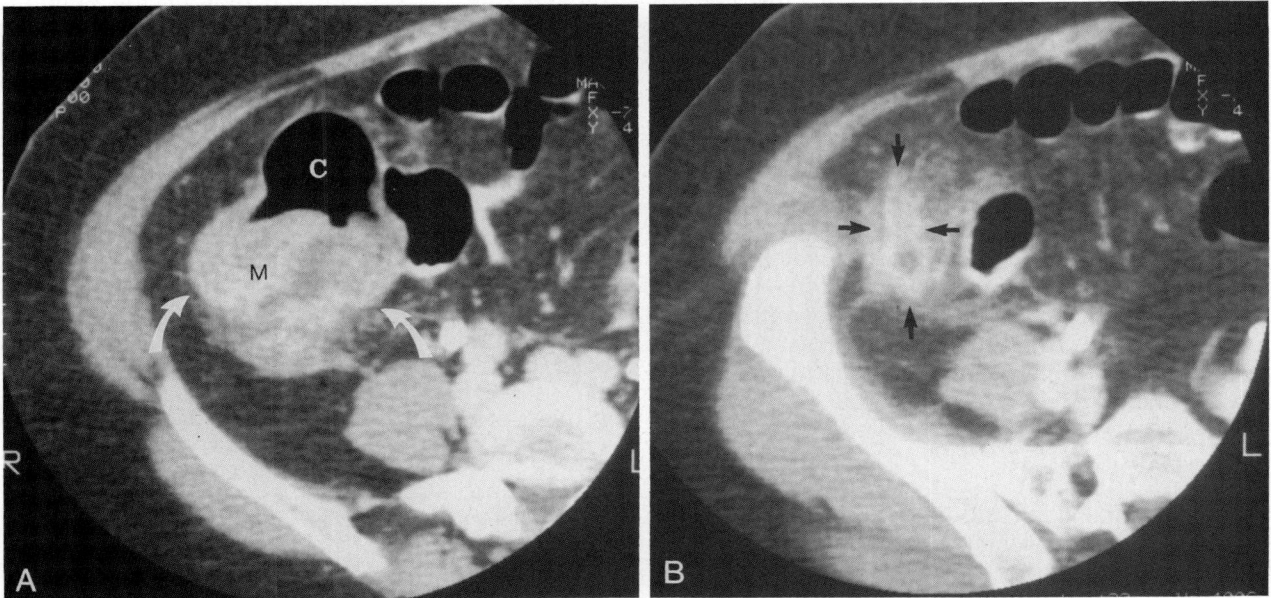

**Figure 69–28. Carcinoma of the cecum with associated acute appendicitis. A.** Soft tissue mass (M) on the inferior and posterior wall of the cecum (C) occludes the appendiceal orifice *(arrows).* **B.** Caudal section shows a thick-walled, hyperemic (enhancing) appendix with periappendiceal inflammation *(arrows).* Surgery showed cecal carcinoma with associated acute appendicitis.

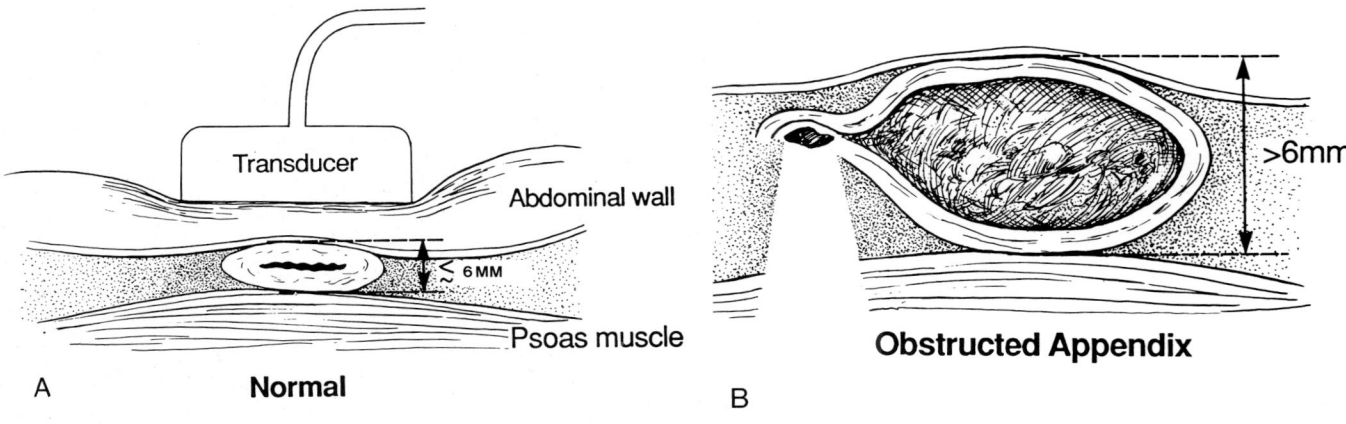

A          **Normal**                                          B          **Obstructed Appendix**

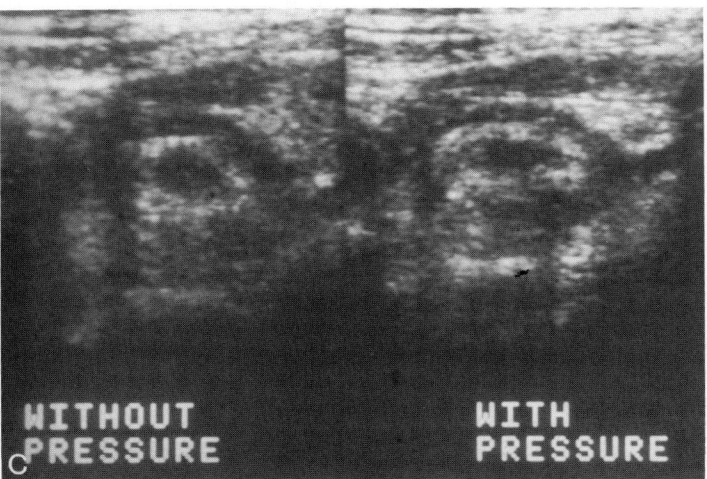

WITHOUT PRESSURE          WITH PRESSURE

**Figure 69–29. Principles of the sonographic diagnosis of appendicitis. A.** The normal appendix is usually not visualized on graded compression sonography. When visible, it should be compressible, with a diameter less than 6 mm. **B.** An incompressible appendix more than 6 mm in diameter is diagnostic of appendicitis. (**A** and **B** modified from Wilson SR: The gastrointestinal tract. *In* Rumack CM, Wilson SR, Charboneau JW [eds]: Diagnostic Ultrasound. St. Louis: Mosby–Year Book, 1991, p 186.) **C.** The diameter of the appendiceal lumen does not change with compression in this patient with acute appendicitis.

discomfort. Compression is used to reduce the distance from the transducer to the inflamed appendix; to displace bowel loops, fecal material, and gas that interfere with sound transmission; and to check the compressibility of the appendix and gut. Scans are obtained routinely in the transverse plane over the right lower quadrant; abnormal findings are confirmed in the longitudinal plane. A rapid survey of the liver, pancreas, gallbladder, and right kidney is also performed with the 3.5-MHz sector scanner. In female patients, the pelvic organs are examined and evaluated through the fluid-filled bladder. The normal appendix is visualized sonographically in less than 10 to 15% of normal individuals. It appears as a small, narrow (≤6 mm), blind-ended structure with a collapsed lumen and extremely thin wall.[75–101]

### Sonographic Diagnosis

The sonographic hallmark of acute appendicitis is the recognition of the abnormal appendix (Table 69–6). It is usually located inferior, medial, or posterior to the cecal caput and anterior to the psoas muscle and iliac vessels. The inflamed appendix is a noncompressible, tubular structure that shows no peristalsis in the longitudinal view[75–86] (Figs. 69–30 to 69–32; see Fig. 69–22). Its transverse diameter is in excess of 6 mm, and this

finding must be constant and reproducible. The abnormal appendix often has a "target" configuration in the transverse plane (see Fig. 69–27C). When the inflammation is mild and visualization is optimal, five distinct layers can be identified within the appendiceal wall similar to those in the other intestinal segments. In more advanced forms of suppurative appendicitis, the appendix is filled with fluid and is 1 to 2 cm in diameter. At this stage of the disease, the thickened appendiceal wall loses its stratification. An appendicolith is identified as an intraluminal echogenic focus with posterior shadowing (see Fig. 69–30). Appendicoliths are detected by ultrasound in approximately 30% of cases of acute

---

#### TABLE 69–6. ACUTE APPENDICITIS: SONOGRAPHIC FINDINGS

Noncompressible, blind-ending, aperistaltic tubular right lower quadrant structure (diseased appendix)
Target appearance of appendix
Appendiceal diameter greater than 6 mm
Lumen distended with anechoic, hyperechoic material
Appendicolith
Circumferential loss of submucosal layer of appendix
Loculated pericecal fluid
Prominent pericecal fat

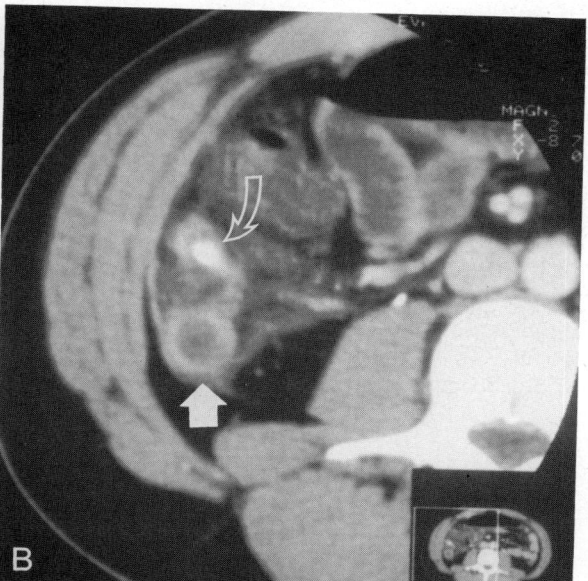

**Figure 69–30. Sonography of an inflamed appendix containing an appendicolith.** Longitudinal scan shows a thick-walled, fluid-filled appendix (A). The layers of the appendiceal wall are not well defined. Appendicolith *(thick arrow)* is identified as an echogenic focus with acoustic shadowing *(thin arrows)*.

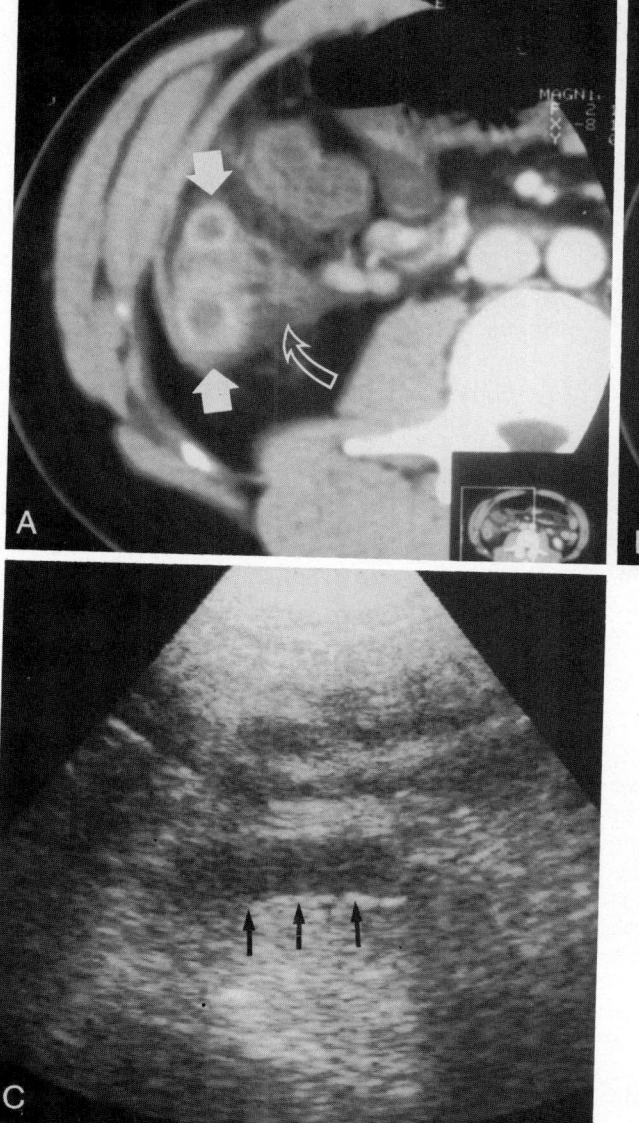

**Figure 69–31. Correlation of sonography and CT in acute appendicitis. A.** CT scan shows transverse sections in the two limbs of a fluid-filled distended appendix *(solid arrows)*. The appendix has a circumferentially thickened and hyperemic wall. Inflammation is present in the mesoappendix *(open arrow)*. **B.** Adjacent CT section shows similar findings *(solid arrow)* and a calcified intraluminal appendicolith *(open arrow)*. **C.** Longitudinal sonogram reveals a thick-walled, fluid-filled appendix *(arrows)*.

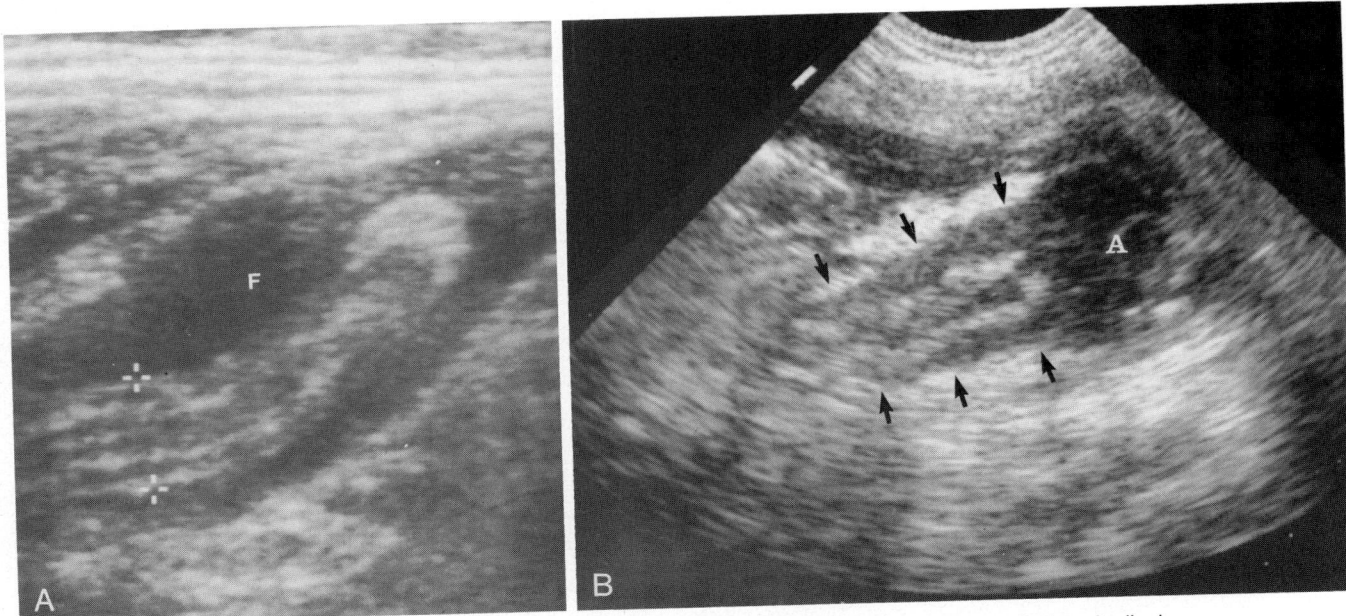

**Figure 69–32. Sonographic detection of periappendiceal fluid and abscess. A.** Longitudinal sonogram demonstrates a dilated appendix with a diameter of 10 mm *(cursors)*. Wall stratification is maintained and periappendiceal fluid (F) is visualized. **B.** A fluid-filled abscess (A) is visualized adjacent to the tip of the appendix *(arrows)*, in a different patient.

appendicitis.[85] They may be difficult to differentiate from gas, mucus, or debris in the appendiceal lumen.

High-resolution sonography can allow diagnosis of perforation and abscess formation, although less reliably than CT.[85, 86] Appendiceal abscess appears as a complex hypoechoic mass adjacent to the cecum or appendix (see Fig. 69–32). In these cases, the diseased appendix may not be recognized.

### Sonographic Accuracy

The reported sensitivity of high-resolution sonography in the diagnosis of acute appendicitis ranges from 80 to 89%; the specificity and accuracy are greater than 90%.[75–101] In an evaluation of 198 suspected cases, Abu-Yousef and Franken reported a sensitivity of 77%, specificity of 94%, and accuracy of 89%.[85]

### Advantages and Limitations of Sonography

In experienced hands, high-resolution sonography has proved valuable in detecting mild and severe suppurative appendicitis. Its advantages are related to the lack of radiation, particularly important in children and young women. The examination is also noninvasive and relatively fast and inexpensive. It produces pain or at least moderate discomfort but is accepted by most individuals.

The limitations of ultrasound are particularly obvious in obese patients or in patients with significant tenderness that prevents adequate compression. Fluid-filled bowel loops and fecal and gaseous distention of the colon interfere with adequate visualization of the appendiceal area. About 30% of cases missed sonographically

are due to a retrocecal appendix.[85, 86] In addition, sonography is less accurate than CT in evaluating the severity and extent of periappendiceal inflammation as well as identifying alternative abdominal and pelvic disease. Sonography is helpful in the diagnosis of various gynecologic diseases but is less accurate in identifying primary intestinal, mesenteric, or peritoneal disease.

### Computed Tomography Versus Ultrasound Versus Barium Enema

Sonography is recommended to establish the diagnosis of appendicitis in children, ovulating women, and pregnant women. Obese and elderly individuals and patients with more complicated forms of suppurative and perforative appendicitis (septic symptoms more than 2 to 3 days old) are better evaluated by CT. Contrast enema examination should be reserved for patients for whom CT and/or sonographic findings are nonspecific and the therapeutic approach is not clear.

### Alternative Diagnoses

Some 60 to 70% of patients referred for ultrasound and CT because of suspected acute appendicitis do not have this disease. Many have a viral gastroenteritis or other benign self-limited gastrointestinal disorder. In a small group of patients, however, cross-sectional imaging can suggest a specific alternative diagnosis.[87, 88, 95]

Marked mural thickening of the terminal ileum suggests Crohn's disease or infectious ileitis. Enlarged mesenteric lymph nodes suggest mesenteric adenitis or infectious ileitis (Fig. 69–33). Mural thickening of the cecum accompanied by visualization of an infected diverticulum indicates diverticulitis. Sonographically, the latter appears as a focus of high-amplitude echoes with acoustic shadowing. Adnexal cysts and masses and salpingitis are best appreciated by transvaginal ultrasound. The diagnosis of ureteral calculi and pyelonephritis can also be made by use of CT and ultrasound.[87, 88, 95]

### Nuclear Scintigraphy

[111]In-labeled leukocytes localize in abscesses and phlegmons in multiple sites for a variety of reasons. The optimal time for imaging is 17 to 24 hours after injection. In one study, tagged leukocyte scintigraphy performed 2 hours after injection had a sensitivity of 86%, specificity of 93%, and accuracy of 91% in detecting acute appendicitis.[102–104]

## Surgical Management

In patients with simple appendicitis, appendectomy is the treatment of choice, although some cases may resolve with simple antibiotics alone. A policy of nonoperative management, however, is risky because a delay in surgery can often lead to perforation.

Surgery is mandatory for perforative appendicitis with generalized or spreading peritonitis. These patients, however, are at high risk for postoperative abscess formation.

## Radiologic Management

There is ongoing controversy in the surgical literature about the management of patients with an appendiceal mass. This is related in part to inability in the past to assess the nature of the underlying inflammatory mass. CT, however, can differentiate areas of pus from a phlegmon and guide percutaneous drainage when appropriate.[105–111]

CT can be used to divide patients into three broad management categories: 1) patients with phlegmons or small abscesses, 2) patients with larger, well-defined abscesses confined to the right lower quadrant, and 3) patients with extensive, poorly defined multicompartmental abscesses. Patients in the first category do well with intravenous antibiotic therapy alone. After resolution of the inflammatory process, an interval appendectomy can be performed 4 to 6 weeks later through a clean operative field. This approach significantly reduces the number of postoperative complications such as abscess.[87, 88, 105–111]

Larger, well-defined abscesses can be drained percutaneously (Fig. 69–34), with a success rate of the order of 90%. Some 45% of these patients demonstrate communication between the abscess cavity and the caput cecum or appendix, but this does not pose a significant management problem. After defervescence with intravenous antibiotics, the patient can be discharged with the catheter in place and oral antibiotics. The fistula usually closes spontaneously, and when it does the catheter can be slowly withdrawn. At this point, interval appendectomy can be performed, again through a clean operative field.[87, 88]

Patients with a multicompartmental abscess are not appropriate candidates for percutaneous therapy and require early surgical drainage and débridement.

Postoperative complications occur in 5% of patients with nonperforative appendicitis and in 30 to 50% of patients with gangrenous or perforative appendicitis. The most common complications include wound infection, intra-abdominal abscess (20% in perforated or gangrenous appendicitis), fecal fistula, pylephlebitis, and intestinal obstruction. These grim statistics have prompted a growing number of surgeons to accept CT staging and therapy of periappendiceal inflammatory processes.[105]

## CROHN'S DISEASE

Approximately 20% of patients undergoing surgery for Crohn's ileocolitis demonstrate appendiceal involvement in the resected specimen. Primary Crohn's disease

**Figure 69–33. Sonographic differential diagnosis of appendicitis.** This diagram depicts the relative involvement of the terminal ileum, cecum, ascending colon, and mesenteric lymph nodes in bacterial ileocolitis caused by different organisms that can simulate appendicitis sonographically and clinically. (From Puylaert JBCM: Ultrasound of Appendicitis. Berlin: Springer-Verlag, 1990, p 66.)

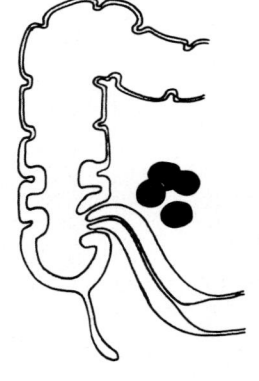

Yersinia enterocolitica
Yersinia pseudotuberculosis

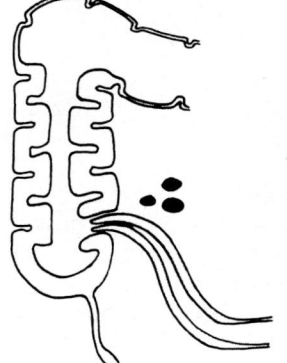

Campylobacter jejuni

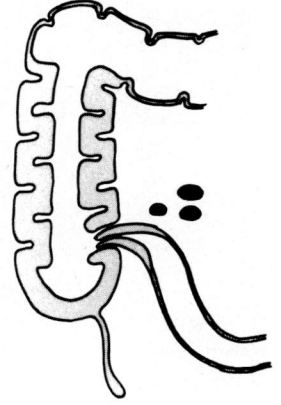

Salmonella enteritidis

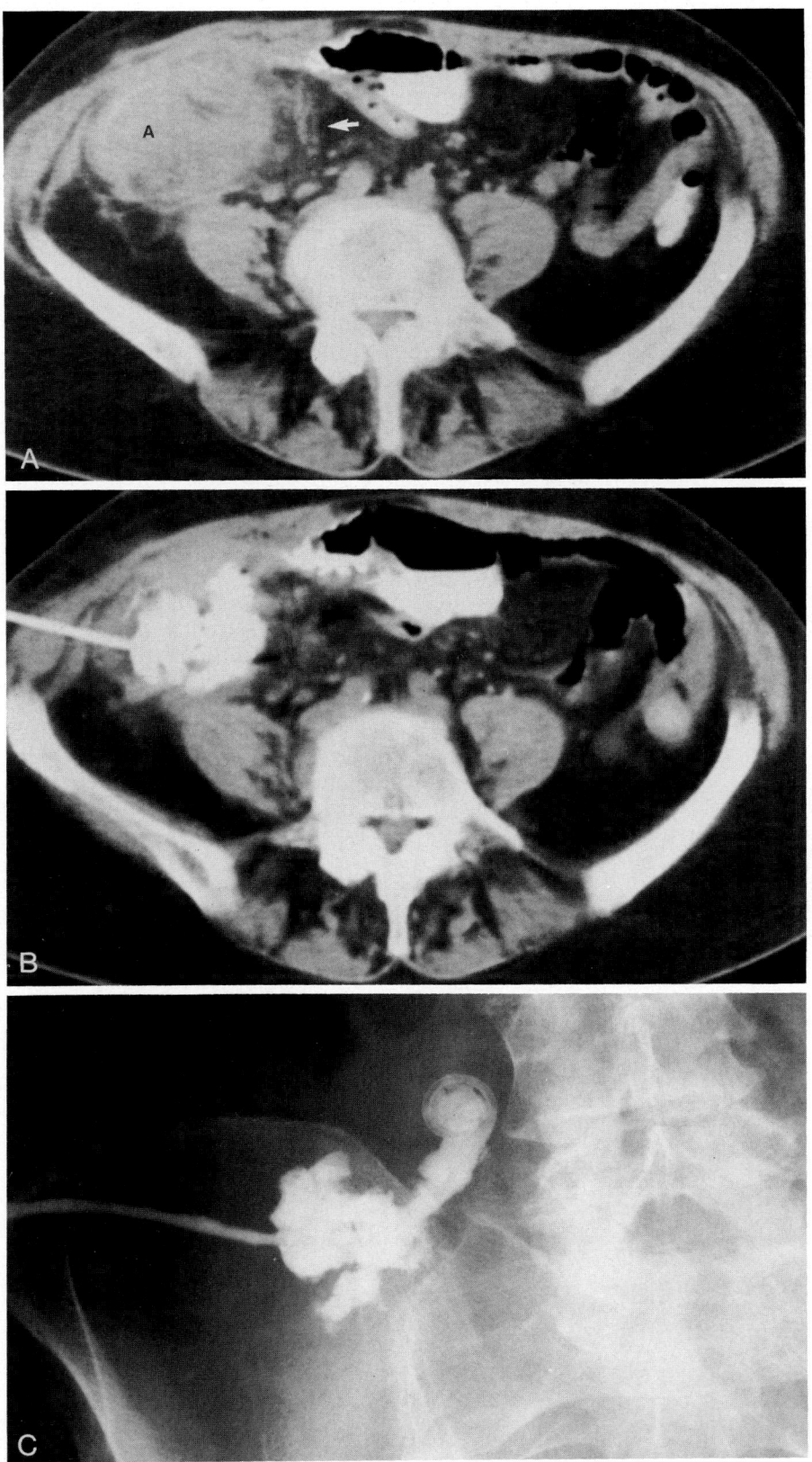

**Figure 69–34. CT-directed drainage of appendiceal abscess.** This patient presented with typical symptoms of appendicitis and an appendiceal mass in the right lower quadrant. **A.** A complex abscess (A) is visualized in the right iliac fossa. Note the inflammatory changes in the surrounding fat *(arrow)*. **B.** The abscess was percutaneously drained. Note communication with the gastrointestinal tract. **C.** Abscessogram 2 weeks later shows closing of this fistula. An interval appendectomy was performed 6 weeks after this study.

of the appendix is less common and clinically may mimic typical appendicitis.[112–116]

Some 20 to 25% of patients with Crohn's appendicitis have concurrent Crohn's disease elsewhere in the gastrointestinal tract, which can be helpful in the preoperative diagnosis. Crohn's disease develops elsewhere in the gut in about 10% of patients after resection of "isolated" Crohn's appendicitis.[112–115]

Radiographic findings in Crohn's appendicitis are usually identical to those in typical appendicitis. Occasionally, barium enema study may show a patent but irregularly narrowed appendiceal lumen (Fig. 69–35). If there are aphthae or other stigmata of Crohn's disease in the adjacent cecum or ileum, the diagnosis can be made preoperatively. Cross-sectional imaging may demonstrate a thickened incompressible appendix, inflamed right lower quadrant fat, and mural thickening of the ileum and colon.[112–115]

## MUCOCELE

### Epidemiology, Etiology, and Pathology

Mucocele of the appendix is a descriptive term used to indicate dilatation of the appendiceal lumen by mucinous secretions. The accumulation of mucin is slow, and if infection does not intervene the appendix becomes a large, thin-walled, mucin-filled cystic structure.[117–130] Mucoceles are uncommon, found in 0.3% of appendectomy specimens, with a 4:1 preponderance in females and a mean age of 55 years at presentation.[117]

Histologically, mucoceles are classified into three groups: 1) focal or diffuse hyperplasia, 2) mucinous cystadenoma, and 3) mucinous cystadenocarcinoma. A number of obstructing lesions can lead to mucocele formation: postappendicitis scarring (most common), fecalith, appendiceal carcinoma, appendiceal endometrioma, appendiceal carcinoid, carcinoma of the cecum or ascending colon, cecal bascule, appendiceal polyp, and appendiceal volvulus. It is unclear whether the cystadenoma or cystadenocarcinoma causes obstruction of the lumen as well or whether the mucosa of the obstructed appendix undergoes neoplastic change. Benign causes of obstruction outnumber malignant causes by a ratio of 4:1 to 10:1.[118–123]

Most mucoceles are between 3 and 6 cm in diameter. Calcifications may occur in the wall or lumen of the mucocele.[124–130]

Myxoglobulosis is a rare variant in which numerous small globules form in the appendix. They may calcify and produce numerous 1- to 10-mm round or oval mobile calcifications in the right lower quadrant. In myxoglobulosis, the appendiceal lumen has the consistency of tapioca or fish eggs.[38–40]

### Clinical Findings

The dominant complaint is chronic right lower quadrant pain in up to 64% of patients with mucoceles.

Nearly 23% of patients are asymptomatic. Abdominal swelling, anemia, or a mucous fistula may also be present. Physical examination discloses right lower quadrant tenderness in 38% and a palpable mass in 18 to 50% of patients.[117–123]

The major clinical significance of a mucocele lies in its complications: rupture or leakage leading to pseudomyxoma peritonei, torsion with gangrene and hemorrhage, and intussusception into the cecum causing various degrees of bowel obstruction. If pseudomyxoma peritonei results from rupture of a benign mucocele, only removal of the fluid is needed and the prognosis is good. When malignant, it behaves like an invasive neoplasm with adhesions and bowel obstruction and a 5-year survival of only 25%. Because cystadenoma and cystadenocarcinoma are usually indistinguishable radiologically, clinically, and on gross inspection, the surgeon must be warned of the presence of a mucocele preoperatively.[128, 129]

### Radiologic Findings

#### Plain Films

The plain abdominal film may be normal or show a well-defined right lower quadrant mass. Rim-like calcifications help establish the diagnosis but are uncommon. In myxoglobulosis, mobile calcifications may be present that must be differentiated from phleboliths, calcified mesenteric lymph nodes, and calcified metastases to the medial wall of the cecum.[38–40, 119–120a]

#### Barium Enema

The appendix fails to fill on barium enema examination and the cecum is indented on its medial aspect by a smooth-walled mass (Fig. 69–36). The cecum is distensible but inseparable from the mass. The terminal ileum is often displaced as well.[38–40, 119, 120–124]

#### Cross-sectional Imaging

Sonographically, mucoceles manifest as fluid-filled masses that may be completely anechoic or have septations and gravity-dependent echoes. These latter findings probably result from inspissated mucoid material that develops as the mucocele ages and matures. Increased through transmission is characteristic.[121, 122]

On CT scans, mucoceles appear as water density or, less often, soft tissue density masses. Calcification may be seen within the wall or lumen (Fig. 69–37; see Fig. 69–36).

When mucoceles contain predominantly fluid, they have long T1 and T2 relaxation times and low signal intensity on T1-weighted and high signal intensity on T2-weighted magnetic resonance images (Fig. 69–38). If their mucin content is high, mucoceles have a short T1 time and long T2 time, so they appear intense on both T1- and T2-weighted images.

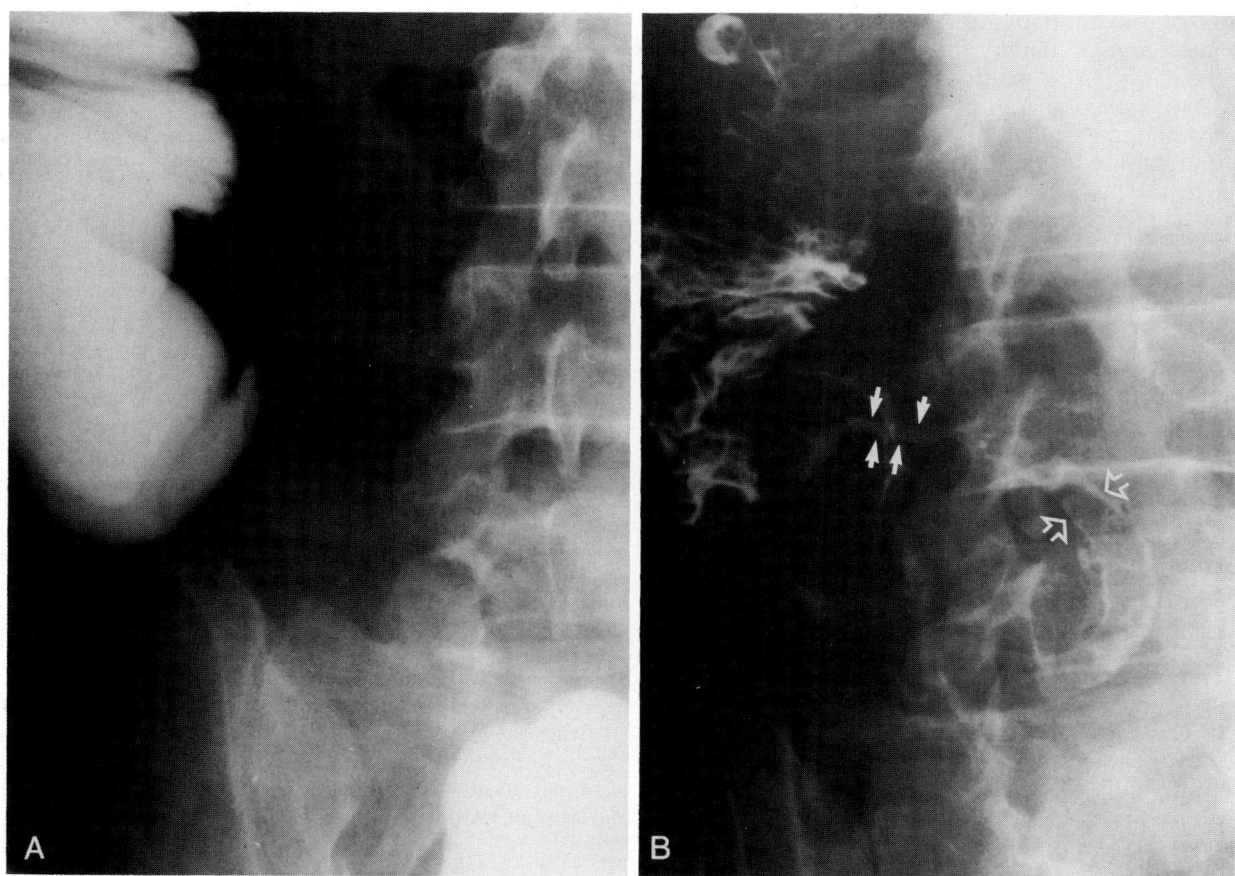

**Figure 69–35. Crohn's disease of the appendix.** Barium enema examination of a 27-year-old man with a 5-day history of right lower quadrant pain. **A.** During the initial part of the study the appendix did not reflux completely. **B.** On the postevacuation film, segmental narrowing *(solid arrows)* of the appendix is identified. Note the dilated appendix proximally *(open arrows)*. The patient's symptoms were unremitting and he underwent appendectomy. Pathologic examination demonstrated Crohn's appendicitis. The patient remains clinically and radiographically free of Crohn's disease elsewhere in the gut.

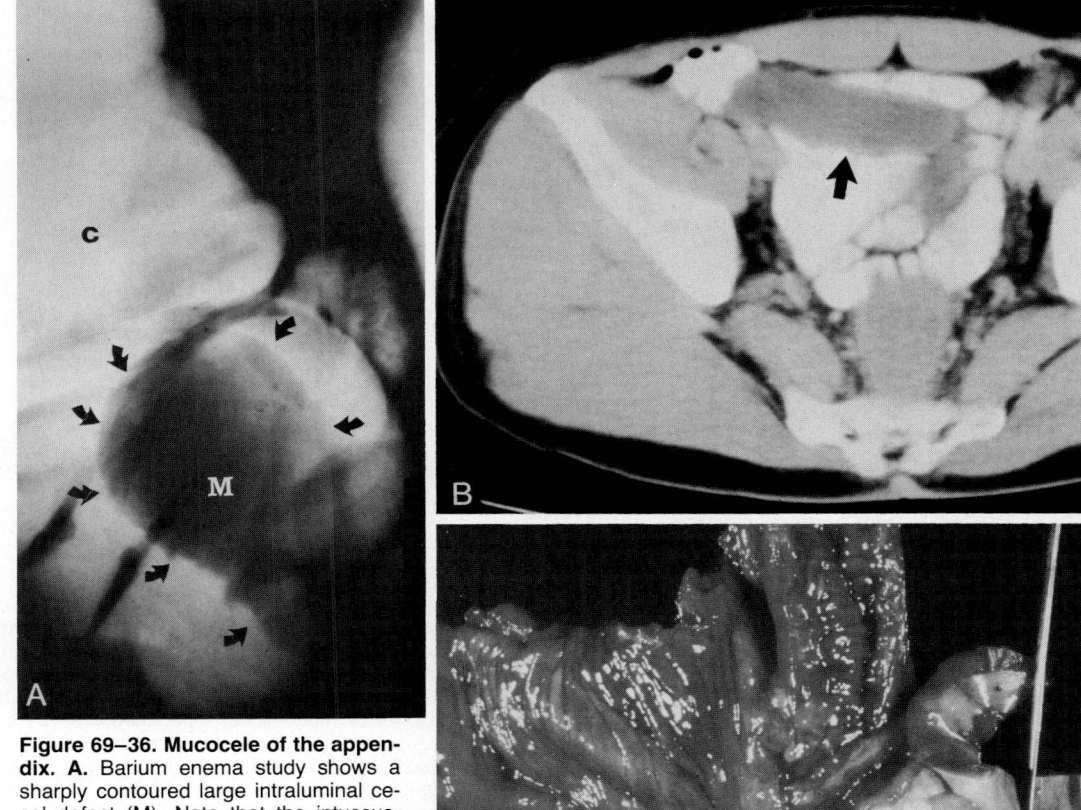

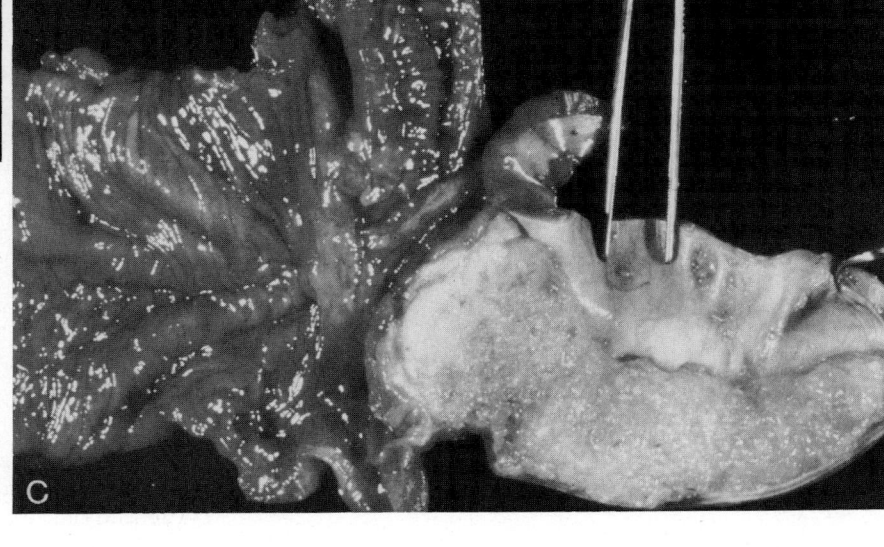

**Figure 69–36. Mucocele of the appendix. A.** Barium enema study shows a sharply contoured large intraluminal cecal defect (M). Note that the intussuscepting mucocele arises from the tip of the cecum (c) and the appendix is not filled *(arrows)*. **B.** CT scan shows the pericecal extension of the mucus-filled, distended appendix *(arrow)*. Note that there is no periappendiceal inflammation. **C.** Gross specimen reveals a markedly distended, mucus-filled appendix compressing the base of the cecum. Pathologic study showed benign mucocele.

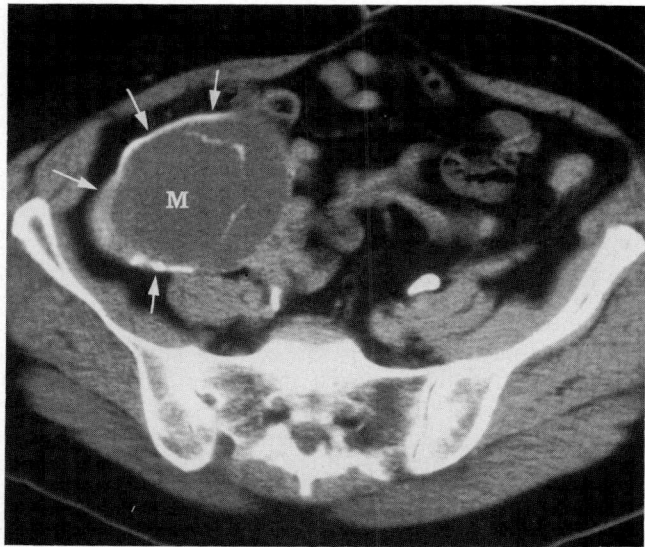

**Figure 69–37. Partially calcified mucocele of the appendix.** CT scan shows a round, fluid-filled cystic mass (M) with peripheral curvilinear calcifications in the right lower quadrant *(arrows)*. Pathologic study revealed a mucus-filled, benign cystadenoma of the appendix.

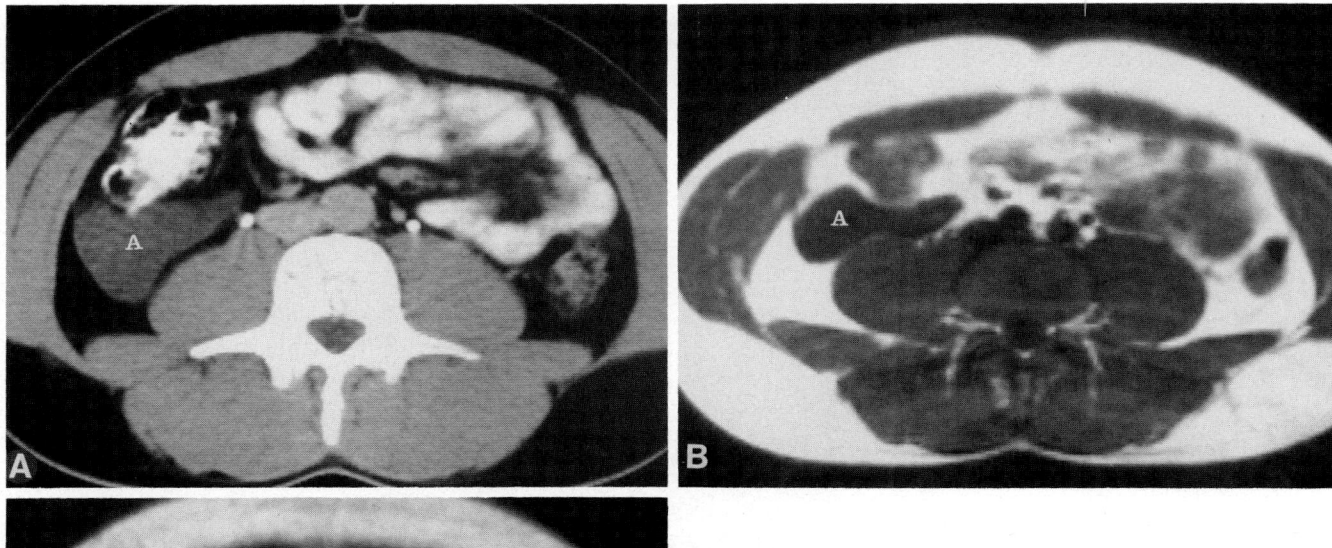

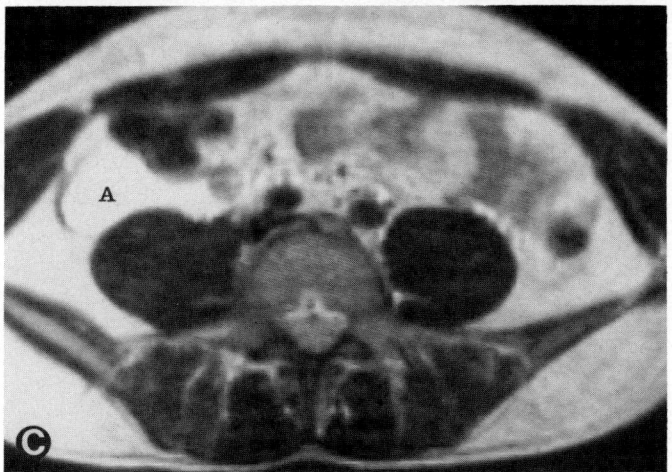

**Figure 69–38. Mucocele of appendix visualized by CT and magnetic resonance imaging. A.** CT scan shows a triangular, fluid-filled distended appendix (A). The appendix has a sharp outer contour, and there is no periappendiceal inflammation. **B.** T1-weighted magnetic resonance image (250/15) obtained at the same level reveals a low signal intensity, distended appendix (A). **C.** T2-weighted magnetic resonance image (2000/60) shows a bright, high signal intensity appendix (A) indicative of a fluid-filled structure. (Case courtesy of Charles A. Whelan, M.D., Montclair, NJ.)

When pseudomyxoma peritonei develops, malignant-appearing ascites and omental cakes are visualized[126, 130] (Fig. 69–39).

### Differential Diagnosis

The differential diagnosis of these imaging findings includes ovarian cysts and neoplasms, duplication cyst, mesenteric and omental cysts, mesenteric hematoma or tumor, and abdominal abscess.

## INTUSSUSCEPTION

Intussusception of the appendix can present clinically in five different ways: 1) acute appendicitis; 2) intussusception; 3) recurrent intermittent right lower quadrant pain; 4) intermittent painless rectal bleeding; or 5) asymptomatically, with incidental findings at laparotomy, barium enema, or colonoscopy.[131–134]

In the past, appendiceal intussusception was considered rare, found in only 0.01% of surgical cases. However, the fifth presentation is probably the most common. On double-contrast barium enema examination,

intussusception causes a characteristic "coil spring" appearance of the cecum with nonfilling of the appendix. These findings are best seen en face. In incidental cases, the intussusception usually disappears on delayed overhead or postevacuation films. The coil spring appearance can also be seen in appendicitis, but it is fixed in these cases and the patient is symptomatic in the right lower quadrant. There may be only partial intussusception of the appendix that produces an intraluminal filling defect on the medial wall of the cecum and nonfilling of the appendix. The defect may be mistaken for a polyp[131–134] (Fig. 69–40).

Most cases of significant appendiceal intussusception occur in children and are attributed to abnormal peristalsis caused by intraluminal or intramural irritants of the appendix. These include fecaliths, foreign bodies, endometriosis, lymphoid hyperplasia, carcinoid, adenocarcinoma, and mucoceles.[131–134]

Sonographically, the intussusception appears as multiple hypo- and hyperechoic rings, similar to intussusceptions elsewhere in the gut.[132, 133]

Hydrostatic reduction of appendiceal intussusceptions has been successful in children and adults. Asymptomatic transient intussusceptions probably does not require therapy or an extensive work-up, however.[131–134]

**Figure 69–39. Pseudomyxoma peritonei.** CT scan shows large amounts of intraperitoneal fluid (F) and thickening of the greater omentum *(solid arrows)* compatible with a malignant process. A fluid-filled cystic mass representing a malignant mucocele is seen in the right midabdomen *(open arrow)*. Surgery revealed mucocele and extensive mucinous ascites.

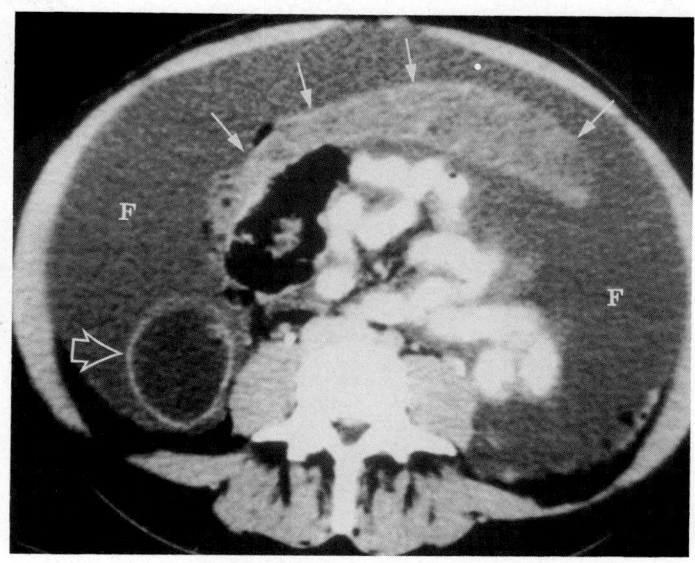

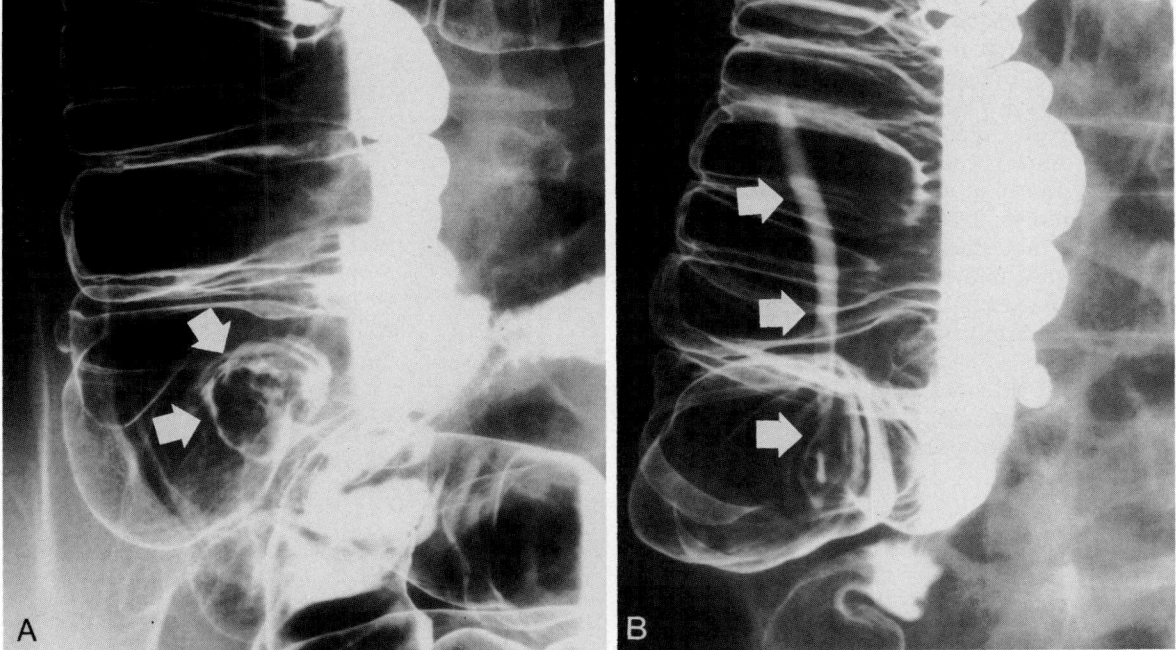

**Figure 69–40. Appendiceal intussusception. A.** The initial barium enema examination reveals a filling defect in the lower cecum that was interpreted as a polypoid mass *(arrows)*. Colonoscopy performed several days later revealed no abnormalities. **B.** A subsequent barium enema examination shows a normal rectrocecal appendix *(arrows)*.

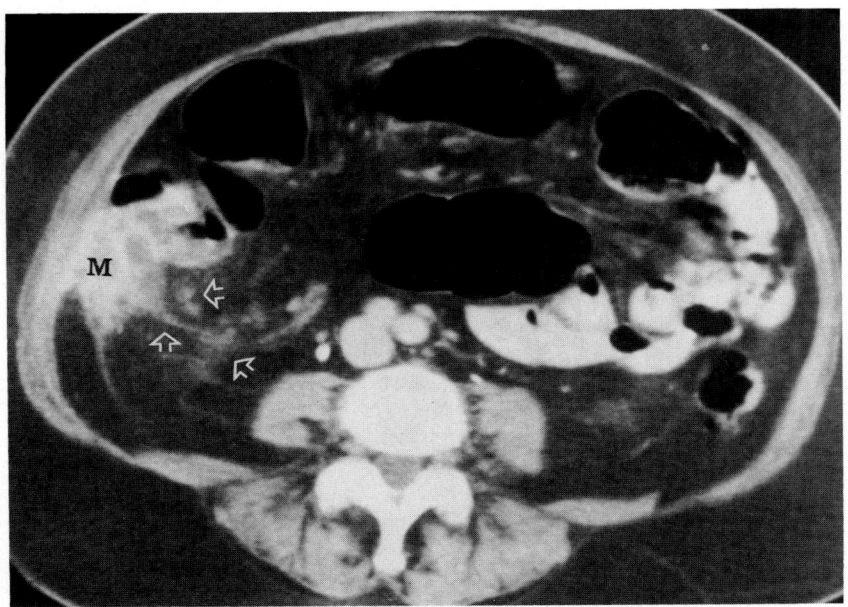

**Figure 69–41. CT scan of perforated carcinoma of the appendix.** A lobulated, heterogeneous complex mass (M) is seen posterior and caudal to the cecum. The mass has an irregular contour and periappendiceal inflammatory changes are present *(arrows)*.

## NEOPLASMS

Ninety per cent of all carcinoid tumors arise in the appendix and 90% of all appendiceal tumors are carcinoids.[25, 135–139] This tumor most frequently involves the distal tip of the appendix, where it produces a solid bulbous swelling 2 to 3 cm in diameter. Most are found incidentally at surgery for another procedure or for appendicitis. These tumors are histologically identical to other midgut carcinoids but appear sooner because they obstruct the narrow appendiceal lumen. Fortunately, because these tumors cause appendiceal obstruction, they are usually found at age 25 rather than age 55 (the norm for ileal tumors), interrupting their natural history. Not surprisingly, metastases are exceedingly rare, as is the carcinoid syndrome. A simple appendectomy is sufficient for localized tumors less than 2 cm in diameter. A right hemicolectomy may be needed for larger ones.[135–139]

Lymphoma and adenocarcinomas (Fig. 69–41) can also involve the appendix. As discussed previously, malignant mucoceles can lead to pseudomyxoma peritonei.[135–139]

## DIVERTICULOSIS

Appendiceal diverticula are found in 0.5 to 1.7% of patients. The majority are acquired because of either intrinsic mural weakness or abnormally raised intraluminal pressure secondary to increased muscular activity or closed loop obstruction.[140–142]

The presence of appendiceal diverticula may predispose to hemorrhage and diverticulitis. Accordingly, some surgeons recommend prophylactic appendectomy when diverticula are discovered during laparotomy for other disorders.[140, 142]

## Acknowledgment

Figure 69–1 is reproduced from McVay CB: Anson & McVay Surgical Anatomy (6th ed). Philadelphia: WB Saunders, 1984.

## References

1. Goldman LD: Acute appendicitis. *In* Taylor MB (ed): Gastrointestinal Emergencies. Baltimore: Williams & Wilkins, 1992, pp 426–436.
2. Telford GL, Condon RE: Appendix. *In* Zuidema GD (ed): Shackelford's Surgery of the Alimentary Tract (3rd ed). Philadelphia: WB Saunders, 1991, pp 133–141.
3. Condon RE: Appendicitis. *In* Moody FG (ed): Surgical Treatment of Digestive Disease (2nd ed). Chicago: Year Book Medical Publishers, 1990, pp 719–739.
4. Schrock TR: Acute appendicitis. *In* Sleisenger MH, Fordtran JS (eds): Gastrointestinal Disease: Pathophysiology, Diagnosis, Management (4th ed). Philadelphia: WB Saunders, 1989, pp 1382–1389.
5. Condon RE: Appendicitis. *In* Sabiston DC (ed): Textbook of Surgery (13th ed). Philadelphia: WB Saunders, 1986, pp 967–982.
6. Anson B, McVay CB: Surgical Anatomy (5th ed). Philadelphia: WB Saunders, 1971.
7. Arey LB: Developmental Anatomy: A Textbook of Laboratory Manual of Embryology (7th ed). Philadelphia: WB Saunders, 1974.
8. Voight AE: Embryology and anatomy of the appendix. Southwest Med 34:285–287, 1953.
9. Balthazar EJ, Gade M: The normal and abnormal development of the appendix. Radiology 121:599–604, 1976.
10. Wakeley CPG: The position of the vermiform appendix as ascertained by analysis of 10,000 cases. J Anat 67:277–283, 1933.
11. Maisel H: The position of the human vermiform appendix in fetal and adult age groups. Anat Rec 136:385–391, 1960.
12. Meyers MA: Dynamic Radiology of the Abdomen (3rd ed). New York: Springer-Verlag, 1988.
13. Collins DC: Agenesis of the vermiform appendix. Am J Surg 82:689–696, 1951.
14. Berry J Jr, Malt RA: Appendicitis near its centenary. Ann Surg 200:567–575, 1984.
15. Law D, Law R, Eiseman B: The continuing challenge of acute and perforated appendicitis. Am J Surg 131:533–535, 1976.

15a. Velanovich V, Satava R: Balancing the normal appendectomy rate with the perforated appendicitis rate—implications for quality assurance. Am Surg 58:264–269, 1992.

16. Lewis FR, Holcroft JH, Boey J, et al: Appendicitis: a critical review of diagnosis and treatment in 1,000 cases. Arch Surg 110:677–684, 1975.

17. Dueholm S, Bagi P, Bud M: Laboratory aid in the diagnosis of acute appendicitis. Dis Colon Rectum 32:855–859, 1989.

18. Gough IR: A study of diagnostic accuracy in acute appendicitis. Aust N Z J Surg 58:555–560, 1988.

19. Crabbe MM, Norwood SH, Robertson HD, et al: Recurrent and chronic appendicitis. Surg Gynecol Obstet 163:11–13, 1986.

20. Walker ARP, Segal I: What causes appendicitis? J Clin Gastroenterol 12:127–129, 1990 (editorial).

21. Larner AJ: The aetiology of appendicitis. Br J Hosp Med 38:540–542, 1988.

22. Wangensteen OH, Bowers WF: Significance of the obstructive factor in the genesis of acute appendicitis. Arch Surg 34:496–526, 1937.

23. Burkitt DP: The aetiology of appendicitis. Br J Surg 58:695–699, 1971.

24. Dunn EL, Moore EE, Elderling SC, et al: The unnecessary laparotomy for appendicitis: can it be decreased? Arch Surg 110:677–684, 1975.

25. Cotran RS, Kumar V, Robbins SL: Robbins Pathologic Basis of Disease. Philadelphia: WB Saunders, 1989, pp 902–904.

26. Pieper R, Kager L, Nasman P: Acute appendicitis: a clinical study of 1018 cases of emergency appendectomy. Acta Chir Scand 148:51–62, 1982.

27. Poole GV: Anatomic basis for delayed diagnosis of appendicitis. South Med J 83:771–773, 1990.

28. Kniskern JH, Eskin EM, Fletcher HS: Increasing accuracy in the diagnosis of acute appendicitis with modern diagnostic techniques. Arch Surg 52:222–225, 1986.

29. Andersen M, Lilja T, Lundell L, et al: Clinical and laboratory findings in patients subjected to laparotomy for suspected acute appendicitis. Acta Chir Scand 146:55–63, 1980.

30. Sumpio BE, Ballantyne GH, Zdon MJ, et al: Perforated appendicitis and obstructing colonic carcinoma in the elderly. Dis Colon Rectum 29:668–670, 1986.

31. Foss JF: Cecal carcinoma presenting as acute appendicitis. Postgrad Med 86:123–126, 1989.

32. Horowitz MD, Gomez GA, Santiesteban R, et al: Acute appendicitis during pregnancy. Arch Surg 120:1362–1367, 1985.

33. Marn CS, Bree RL: Advances in pelvic ultrasound: endovaginal scanning for ectopic gestation and graded compression sonography for appendicitis. Ann Emerg Med 18:1304–1309, 1989.

33a. Lim HK, Bae SH, Seo GS: Diagnosis of acute appendicitis in pregnant women: value of sonography. AJR 159:539–542, 1992.

34. Bongard F, Landers DV, Lewis F: Differential diagnosis of appendicitis and pelvic inflammatory disease. Am J Surg 150:90–96, 1985.

34a. Quillin SP, Siegel MJ: Appendicitis in children: color Doppler sonography. Radiology 184:745–747, 1992.

35. Cantrell JR, Stafford ES: The diminishing mortality from appendicitis. Ann Surg 141:749–758, 1955.

36. Soter CS: The contribution of the radiologist to the diagnosis of acute appendicitis. Semin Roentgenol 8:375–388, 1973.

37. Brown SJ: Acute appendicitis: the radiologist's role. Radiology 180:13–14, 1991.

38. Kelvin FM, Gardiner R: Clinical Imaging of the Colon and Rectum. New York: Raven Press, 1987, pp 460–491.

39. Marshak RH, Linder AH, Maklanky D: Radiology of the Colon. Philadelphia: WB Saunders, 1989, pp 491–515.

40. Long JA: The appendix. In Dreyfus JR, Janower ML (eds): Radiology of the Colon. Baltimore: Williams & Wilkins, 1980, pp 497–521.

41. Harding JA, Glick SN, Teplick SK, et al: Appendiceal filling by double-contrast barum enema. Gastrointest Radiol 11:105–107, 1986.

42. Sakover RP, Del Fava RL: Frequency of visualization of the normal appendix with the barium enema examination. Am J Roentgenol 121:312–317, 1974.

43. Cohen N, Modai D, Rosen A, et al: Barium appendicitis: fact or fancy? J Clin Gastroenterol 9:447–451, 1987.

44. Olutola PS: Plain film radiographic diagnosis of acute appendicitis: an evaluation of the signs. J Can Assoc Radiol 39:254–256, 1988.

45. Johnson JF, Coughlin WF: Plain film diagnosis of appendiceal perforation in children. Semin Ultrasound CT MR 10:306–313, 1989.

46. Mowji PJ, Jones MD, Cohen AJ: Localized ileus of the proximal jejunum: a new sign for acute appendicitis. Gastrointest Radiol 14:173–175, 1989.

47. Vaudagna JS, McCort JJ: Plain film diagnosis of retrocecal appendicitis. Radiology 117:533–536, 1975.

48. Fagenberg D: Fecoliths of the appendix: incidence and significance. Am J Roentgenol 89:752–759, 1963.

49. Beneventano TC, Schein CJ, Jacobson HG: The Roentgen aspects of some appendiceal abnormalities. Am J Roentgenol 96:344–360, 1966.

50. Shimkin PM: Radiology of acute appendicitis. AJR 130:1001–1004, 1978.

51. Harned RK: Retrocecal appendicitis presenting with air in the subhepatic space. Am J Roentgenol 126:416–418, 1976.

52. Meyers MA, Oliphant M: Ascending retrocecal appendicitis. Radiology 110:295–299, 1974.

53. Swischuk LE, Hayden CK: Appendicitis with perforation: the dilated transverse colon sign. AJR 135:687–689, 1980.

54. Smith DE, Kirchner NA, Stewart DR: Use of the barium enema in the diagnosis of acute appendicitis and its complications. Am J Surg 138:829–834, 1979.

55. Rajagopalan E, Mason JH, Kennedy M, et al: The value of the barium enema in the diagnosis of acute appendicitis. Arch Surg 112:531–533, 1977.

56. Garcia CJ, Rosenfield NS: The barium enema in the diagnosis of acute appendicitis. Semin Ultrasound CT MR 10:314–320, 1989.

57. Smith DE, Kirchmer NA, Stewart DR: Use of the barium enema in the diagnosis of acute appendicitis and its complications. AJR 138:829–834, 1979.

58. Rice RP, Thompson WM, Fedyshin PJ, et al: The barium enema in appendicitis: spectrum of appearances and pitfalls. Radiographics 4:393–409, 1984.

59. Fedyshin P, Kelvin FM, Rice RP: Nonspecificity of barium enema in acute appendicitis. AJR 143:99–102, 1984.

60. Totty WG, Koehler RE, Cheung LY: Significance of retained barium in the appendix. AJR 135:753–756, 1980.

61. Gorske K: Intussusception of the proximal appendix into the colon. Radiology 91:791, 1968.

62. Demos TC, Flisak ME: Coiled-spring sign of the cecum in acute appendicitis. AJR 146:45–48, 1986.

63. Halls JM, Meyers HI: Acute appendicitis with abscess simulating carcinoma of the sigmoid. AJR 129:1057–1059, 1977.

64. Balthazar EJ, Megibow AJ, Hulnick D, et al: CT of appendicitis. AJR 147:705–710, 1986.

65. Jones B, Fishman EK, Siegelman SS: Computed tomography and appendiceal abscess: special applicability in the elderly. J Comput Assist Tomogr 7:434–438, 1983.

66. Gale ME, Birnbaum S, Gerzof SG, et al: CT appearance of appendicitis and its local complications. J Comput Assist Tomogr 9:34–37, 1985.

67. Balthazar EJ, Megibow AJ, Gordon RB, et al: Computed tomography of the abnormal appendix. J Comput Assist Tomogr 12:595–601, 1988.

68. Balthazar EJ, Gordon RB: CT of appendicitis. Semin Ultrasound CT MR 10:326–340, 1989.

69. Balthazar EJ, Megibow AJ, Siegel SE, et al: High resolution CT in appendicitis. Prospective evaluation of 100 patients. Radiology 180:21–24, 1991.

70. Feldberg MAM, Hendriks MJ, Van Waes PFGM: Computed tomography in complicated acute appendicitis. Gastrointest Radiol 10:289–295, 1985.

71. Scatarige JC, Yousem DM, Fishman EK, et al: CT abnormalities in right lower quadrant inflammatory disease: review of findings in 26 patients. Gastrointest Radiol 12:156–162, 1987.

72. Barakos JA, Jeffrey RB, Federle MP, et al: CT in the management of periappendiceal abscess. AJR 146:1161–1164, 1986.

73. Clarke PD: Computed tomography of gangrenous appendicitis. J Comput Assist Tomogr 11:1081–1082, 1987.

74. Scatarige JC, DiSantis DJ, Allen HA III, et al: CT demonstration of the appendix in asymptomatic adults. Gastrointest Radiol 14:271–273, 1989.

75. Puylaert JBCM: Acute appendicitis: US evaluation using graded compression. Radiology 158:355–360, 1986.

75a. Spear R, Kimmey MB, Wang KY, et al: Appendiceal US scans: histologic correlation. Radiology 183:831–834, 1992.

76. Puylaert JBCM, Rutgers PH, Lalisang RI, et al: A prospective study of ultrasonography in the diagnosis of appendicitis. N Engl J Med 317:666–669, 1987.

77. Abu-Yousef MM, Phillips MR, Franken EA, et al: Sonography of acute appendicitis: a critical review. Crit Rev Diagn Imaging 29:381–408, 1989.

78. Abu-Yousef MM: Sonography of the right iliac fossa. Ultrasound Q 8:73–94, 1990.

79. Borushok KF, Jeffrey RB, Laing FC, et al: Sonographic diagnosis of perforation in patients with acute appendicitis. AJR 154:275–279, 1990.

79a. Hayden CK, Kuchelmeister J, Lipscomb TS: Sonography of acute appendicitis in childhood: perforation versus non-perforation. J Ultrasound Med 11:209–216, 1992.

80. Schwerk WB, Wichtrup B, Ruschoff J, et al: Acute and perforated appendicitis: Current experience with ultrasound aided diagnosis. World J Surg 14:271–276, 1990.

80a. Nghiem HV, Jeffrey RB: Acute appendicitis confined to the appendiceal tip: evaluation with graded compression sonography. J Ultrasound Med 11:205–207, 1992.

81. Finer RM, Merritt CRB: Ultrasonography of the appendix. Appl Radiol 20:29–32, 1991.

81a. Rioux M: Sonographic detection of the normal and abnormal appendix. AJR 158:773–778, 1992.

82. Adams DH, Fine C, Brooks DC: High resolution real-time ultrasonography: a new tool in the diagnosis of acute appendicitis. Am J Surg 155:93–97, 1988.

83. Jeffrey RB Jr, Laing FC, Lewis FC: Acute appendicitis: high-resolution real-time US findings. Radiology 163:11–14, 1987.

84. Abu-Yousef MM, Bleicher JJ, Maher JW, et al: High-resolution sonography of acute appendicitis. AJR 149:53–58, 1987.

85. Abu-Yousef MM, Franken EW: An overview of graded compression sonography in the diagnosis of acute appendicitis. Semin Ultrasound CT MR 10:352–363, 1989.

86. Jeffrey RB Jr, Laing FC, Townsend RR: Acute appendicitis: sonography criteria based on 250 cases. Radiology 167:327–329, 1988.

87. Jeffrey RB: CT and Sonography of the Acute Abdomen. New York: Raven Press, 1989, pp 234–246.

88. Jeffrey RB: Sonography and CT of acute right lower quadrant pain. In Gore RM (ed): Syllabus for Categorical Course on Gastrointestinal Radiology. Reston, VA: American College of Radiology, 1991, pp 133–138.

89. Schwerk WB, Wichtrup B, Rothmund M, et al: Ultrasonography in the diagnosis of acute appendicitis: a prospective study. Gastroenterology 97:630–639, 1989.

90. Larson JM, Peirce JC, Ellinger DM, et al: The validity and utility of sonography in the diagnosis of appendicitis in the community setting. AJR 153:687–691, 1989.

91. Siegel MJ, Carel C, Surrat S: Ultrasonography of acute abdominal pain in children. JAMA 266:1987–1989, 1991.

92. Kao S, Smith WL, Abu-Yousef MM, et al: Acute appendicitis in children: sonographic findings. AJR 153:375–379, 1989.

93. Vignault F, Filiatrault D, Brandt ML, et al: Acute appendicitis in children: evaluation with ultrasound. Radiology 176:501–504, 1990.

94. Bagi P, Dueholm S: Nonoperative management of the ultrasonically evaluated appendiceal mass. Surgery 101:602–605, 1987.

95. Gaensler EHL, Jeffrey RB, Laing FC, et al: Sonography in patients with suspected acute appendicitis: value in establishing alternative diagnoses. AJR 152:49–51, 1989.

96. Puylaert JBCM: Mesenteric adenitis and acute terminal ileitis: US evaluation using graded compression. Radiology 161:691–695, 1986.

97. Townsend RR, Jeffrey RB, Laing FC: Cecal diverticulitis differentiated from appendicitis using graded-compression sonography. AJR 152:1229–1230, 1989.

98. Blane CE, White SJ, Wesley JR, et al: Sonography of ruptured appendicitis. Gastrointest Radiol 11:357–360, 1986.

99. Baker DE, Silver TM, Coran AG, et al: Postappendectomy fluid collections in children: incidence, nature, and evolution evaluated using US. Radiology 161:341–344, 1986.

100. Machan L, Pon MS, Wood BJ, et al: The "coffee bean" sign in periappendiceal and peridiverticular abscess. J Ultrasound Med 6:373–375, 1987.

101. Poljak A, Jeffrey RB, Kernberg ME: The gas-containing appendix: potential sonographic pitfall in the diagnosis of acute appendicitis. J Ultrasound Med 10:625–628, 1991.

102. Navarro DA, Weber PM, Kang I, et al: Indium-111 leukocyte imaging in appendicitis. AJR 148:733–736, 1987.

103. Navarro DA, Weber PM: Indium 111 imaging in appendicitis. Semin Ultrasound CT MR 10:321–325, 1989.

104. DeLaney AR, Raviola CA, Weber PN, et al: Improving diagnosis of appendicitis. Arch Surg 124:1146–1152, 1989.

105. vanSonnenberg E, Wittich GR, Casola G, et al: Periappendiceal abscess: percutaneous drainage. Radiology 163:23–26, 1987.

106. Jeffrey RB, Tolentino CS, Federle MP, et al: Percutaneous drainage of periappendiceal abscess: review of 20 patients. AJR 149:59–62, 1987.

107. Nunez D, Huber JS, Yrizarry JM, et al: Nonsurgical drainage of appendiceal abscesses. AJR 146:587–589, 1986.

108. Pitkaranta P, Elonen E, Haapiainen R: Percutaneous drainage of periappendiceal abscess in a patients with acute leukemia. Acta Chir Scand 155:617–619, 1989.

109. Jeffrey RB: Management of the periappendiceal inflammatory mass. Semin Ultrasound CT MR 10:341–347, 1989.

110. Nunez D, Yrizarry JM, Casillas VJ, et al: Pericutaneous management of appendiceal abscesses. Semin Ultrasound CT MR 10:348–351, 1989.

111. Hoffman J, Lindhard A, Jensen HE: Appendix mass: conservative management without interval appendectomy. Am J Surg 148:379–382, 1986.

112. Threatt B, Appelman H: Crohn's disease of the appendix presenting as acute appendicitis. Radiology 110:313–317, 1974.

113. Rawlinson J, Hughes RG: Acute superative appendicitis. Dis Colon Rectum 28:608–609, 1985.

114. Simon M, Körner C, Mohr W: Granulomatöse Appendizitis: Differentialdiagnose zur "gemeinen" Appendizitis. Med Klin 85(suppl 1):137–140, 1990.

115. Agha FP, Ghahremani GG, Panella JS, et al: Appendicitis as the initial manifestation of Crohn's disease: radiologic features and prognosis. AJR 149:515–518, 1987.

116. Montgomery DP: A diagnostic approach to ileo-cecal abnormalities. In Simpkins KC (ed): A Textbook of Radiologic Diagnosis, Volume IV. London: HK Lewis, 1988, pp 559–578.

117. Wackym PA, Gray GF: Tumors of the appendix: I. Neoplastic and nonneoplastic mucoceles. South Med J 77:283–287, 1984.

118. Li YP, Morin ME, Tan A: Ultrasound findings in mucocele of the appendix. J Clin Ultrasound 9:406–408, 1981.

119. Fernandez Sanchez J, Bucklein W: Mukozele der Appendix. Radiologe 30:15–18, 1990.

120. Skaane P: Radiological features of mucocele of the appendix. ROFO 149:624–628, 1988.

120a. Isaacs KL, Warshauer DM: Mucocele of the appendix: computed tomographic, endoscopic, and pathologic correlation. Am J Gastroenterol 87:787–789, 1992.

121. Sandler MA, Pearlberg JL, Madrazo BL: Ultrasonic and computed tomographic features of mucocele of the appendix. J Ultrasound Med 3:97–100, 1984.

122. Kavakuc RJ: Unusual roentgenographic manifestations of mucocele of the appendix. Radiology 89:886–887, 1967.

123. Schmutzer KT, Bayar M, Zaki AE, et al: Tumors of the appendix. Dis Colon Rectum 18:324–331, 1975.

123a. Madwell D, Mindelzun R, Jeffrey RB: Mucocele of the appendix: imaging findings. AJR 159:69–72, 1992.

124. Hamilton DL, Stormont JM: The volcano sign of appendiceal mucocele. Gastrointest Endosc 35:453–456, 1989.

125. Higa E, Rosai J, Pizzimbono CA, et al: Mucosal hyperplasia, mucinous cystadenoma and mucinous cystadenocarcinoma of the appendix. A re-evaluation of appendiceal mucocele. Cancer 32:1525–1541, 1973.

126. Dachman AH, Lichtenstein JE, Friedman AC: Mucocele of the appendix and pseudomyxoma peritonei. AJR 144:923–929, 1985.

127. Novetsky GJ, Berlin L, Epstein AJ, et al: Pseudomyxoma peritonei. J Comput Assist Tomogr 6:398–399, 1982.

128. Mayes GB, Chuang VP, Fisher RG: CT of pseudomyxoma peritonei. AJR 136:807–808, 1981.

129. Miller DL, Udelsman R, Sugarbaker PH: Calcification of pseudomyxoma peritonei following intraperitoneal chemotherapy: CT demonstration. J Comput Assist Tomogr 9:1123–1124, 1985.

130. Balthazar EJ, Javors BR: Pseudomyxoma peritonei, clinical and radiographic features. Am J Gastroenterol 68:501–509, 1977.

131. Levine MS, Trenkner SW, Herlinger H, et al: Coiled-spring sign of appendiceal intussusception. Radiology 155:41–44, 1985.

132. Langsam LB, Raj PK, Galang CF: Intussusception of the appendix. Dis Colon Rectum 27:387–392, 1984.

133. Maglinte DDT, Fleischer AC, Chua GT, et al: Sonography of appendiceal intussusception. Gastrointest Radiol 12:163–165, 1987.

134. Kleinman PK: Intussusception of the appendix: hydrostatic reduction. AJR 134:1268–1270, 1980.

135. Andersson A, Bergdahl L, Boquist L: Primary carcinoma of the appendix. Ann Surg 183:53–60, 1976.

135a. Rutledge RH, Alexander JW: Primary appendiceal malignancies—rare but important. Surgery 11:244–250, 1992.

136. Collins DE: 71,000 human appendix specimens: a final report summarizing forty years study. Am J Proctol 4:365–381, 1963.

137. Mori M, Kusunoki T, Kikuchi M, et al: Primary lymphoma of the appendix. Jpn J Surg 15:230–233, 1985.

138. Stewart RJ, Mirakhur M: Primary malignant lymphoma of the appendix. Ulster Med J 55:187–189, 1986.

138a. Rao SK, Aydinalp N: Appendiceal lymphoma: a case report. J Clin Gastroenterol 13:588–590, 1992.

139. Carpenter BW: Lymphoma of the appendix. Gastrointest Radiol 16:256–258, 1991.

140. Sharp JF, Nicholson ML, Fossard DP: Diverticulosis of the appendix. Scott Med J 35:49–50, 1990.

141. Delikaris P, Teglbjaerg PS, Fisker-Sorensen P, et al: Diverticula of the veriform appendix. Dis Colon Rectum 26:374–376, 1983.

142. Buffo GC, Clair MR, Bonheim P: Diverticulosis of the vermiform appendix. Gastrointest Radiol 11:108–109, 1986.

# Postoperative Colon

**Francis J. Scholz, M.D.**

INTRODUCTION

SEGMENTAL RESECTION

SIDE-TO-SIDE ENTEROCOLIC
ANASTOMOSIS

COLOSTOMY
End Colostomy
Loop Colostomy

Double-barreled Colostomy
Divided Colostomy and Mucous
Fistula

CECOSTOMY

COLOANAL PULL-THROUGH
PROCEDURE

LOW ANTERIOR RESECTION

ABDOMINOPERINEAL RESECTION

HARTMANN'S PROCEDURE

MUCOUS FISTULA

APPENDECTOMY

ILEAL POUCH–ANAL
ANASTOMOSIS

## INTRODUCTION

Radiologists are often asked to evaluate the postoperative colon to exclude complications such as fistula, anastomotic dehiscence, stricture, and abscess formation. They are also called on to assess the colon in the asymptomatic patient for anastomotic healing or resolution of inflammatory disease before a colostomy is closed. The radiologist must be familiar with the details of the surgical procedure, terminology, and individual surgeon's modifications to render an intelligent consultation. This chapter discusses the major colonic surgical procedures. The minute intraoperative technical details are well described in classic surgical textbooks.[1–4]

## SEGMENTAL RESECTION

Segmental resection entails surgical removal of a diseased segment of the colon. Colonic continuity is usually restored with an end-to-end colocolic anastomosis (Fig. 70–1). An end-to-end enterocolic anastomosis (Fig. 70–2) is created for patients who undergo resection of the cecum or right colon. In some patients, the anastomotic line may be seen as a short segment ring-like indentation during contrast examination of the colon (Fig. 70–3), but in many patients the site of the anastomosis may not be discernible unless defined by surgical staples. Currently, surgeons have the option of hand sewing an anastomosis or using a stapling machine to re-establish bowel continuity. The stapling units usually create a uniform ring of staples, so disruption of the ring on a plain film of the abdomen may indicate disruption of the anastomosis.

## SIDE-TO-SIDE ENTEROCOLIC ANASTOMOSIS

A side-to-side enterocolic anastomosis (Fig. 70–4) may be created when a diseased segment of distal small bowel (in Crohn's disease or radiation enteritis) is bypassed or when the length of the functional small bowel is shortened for treatment of morbid obesity. This procedure is rarely performed now. Surgeons prefer to

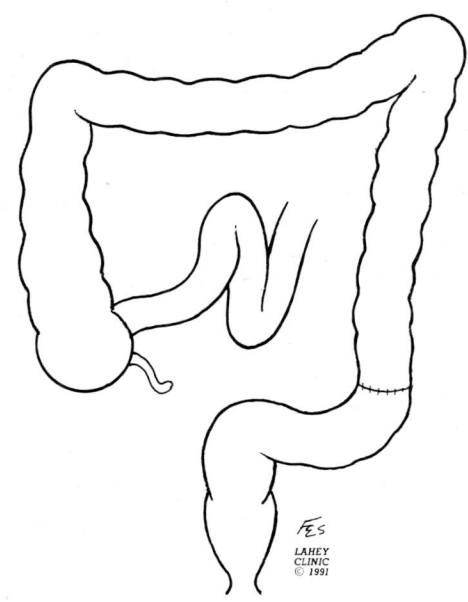

**Figure 70–1. Segmental sigmoid resection and end-to-end colocolic anastomosis.** Foreshortening of the sigmoid colon may or may not be radiographically apparent, depending on the length of colon resected. (Reprinted with the permission of the Lahey Clinic.)

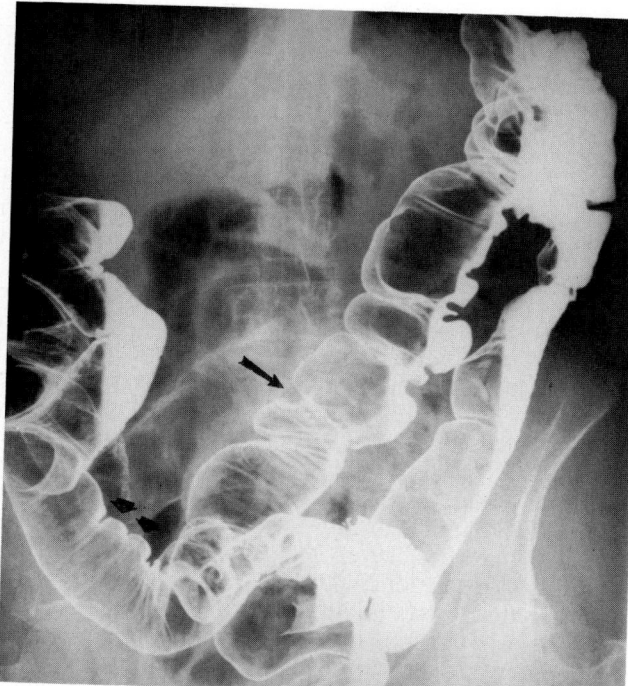

**Figure 70–2. Ileal–transverse colonic anastomosis.** The small bowel proximal to the anastomosis *(long arrow)* has an abnormal appearance with pseudohaustra *(short arrows)* and dilatation, an appearance termed colonization.

resect rather than bypass small bowel involved with Crohn's disease and gastric restrictive surgery is now preferred to a small bowel bypass procedure as therapy for morbid obesity.

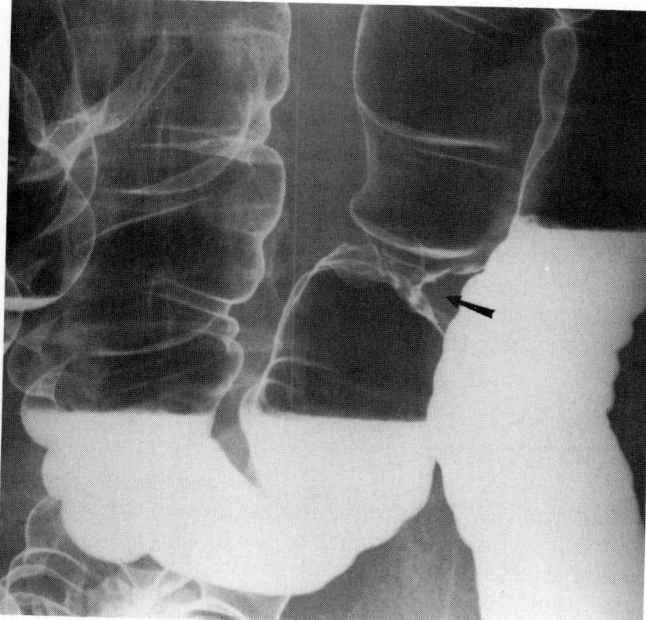

**Figure 70–3. Postoperative deformity after closure of prior diverting colostomy.** A prominent short segment annular constriction *(arrow)* is present in the transverse colon with intact mucosa. Serosal metastatic disease can have the same appearance.

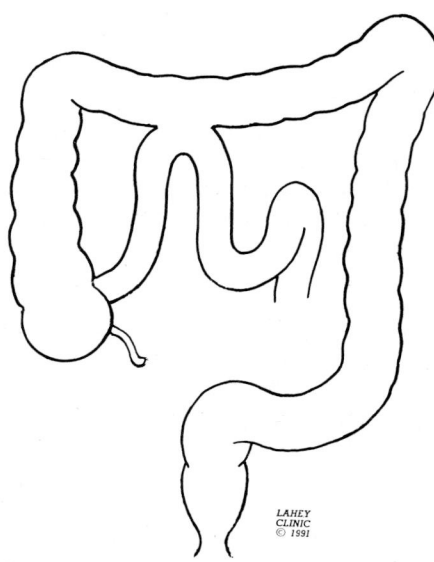

**Figure 70–4. Side-to-side enterocolic anastomosis.** Evaluation of the colon distal to the anastomosis may be technically difficult because of preferential filling of the small bowel rather than the right colon. (Reprinted with the permission of the Lahey Clinic.)

## COLOSTOMY

Colostomy is a colocutaneous anastomosis created to decompress a colonic obstruction or to divert the fecal stream away from the distal colon. Diverting colostomies (Fig. 70–5) are also created to protect a distal anastomosis that has just been created and requires time to heal or to direct the fecal stream away from a segment of distal colon that is too inflamed to be resected at the time of the initial operation. The surgeon may elect to

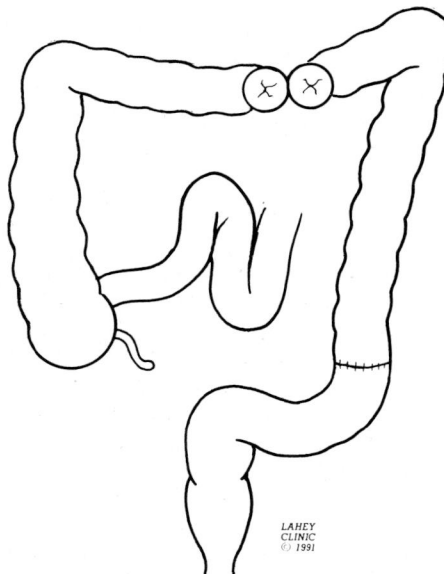

**Figure 70–5. Typical diverting transverse colostomy demonstrating fecal stoma, mucous fistula stoma, and end-to-end sigmoid anastomosis.** (Reprinted with the permission of the Lahey Clinic.)

resect the diseased segment, perform end-to-end anastomosis, and divert the fecal stream with a temporary colostomy. The colon proximal to the stoma is often evaluated radiologically to rule out additional colonic lesions; the distal colon is evaluated to assess the status of a distal anastomosis or a previously inflamed segment.

The choice of colostomy depends on whether it is to be permanent or temporary, the patient's body habitus and previous operations, and the surgeon's preference.

## End Colostomy

End colostomy may be performed as a permanent or long-term arrangement in patients with distal rectal carcinoma or as part of a two-stage procedure for diverticulitis. The stoma is usually in the left lower quadrant, and the descending colon is the portion forming the stomal opening. This procedure is performed in association with the Hartmann procedure to close off the rectal stump; therefore, only one stoma is present.

## Loop Colostomy

Loop colostomy is usually performed for the following indications: as a temporary procedure to relieve acute obstruction in the distal colon, to protect a new distal colonic anastomosis, and as a permanent procedure for unresectable advanced lesions. A loop of transverse or sigmoid colon is brought to the surface of the abdominal wall, sutured in place on the outside, and then opened up, creating afferent and efferent stomas. The mucosa connecting the two stoma openings is the posterior wall of the colon. Patients are usually aware of which stoma produces feces and are able to direct the radiologist to examine the correct portion of the colon.

## Double-barreled Colostomy

A double-barreled colostomy is created when the colon is divided completely and the two cut ends are sewn side by side to each other. This type of stoma is also seen with two openings, and the patient can usually tell which is the productive opening. This procedure is chosen because the stoma can be closed without reentering the abdomen. The apposed common walls are cut, and the stoma closes spontaneously or the margins of the two stomal openings can be pursed together with minimal suturing under local anesthesia.

## Divided Colostomy and Mucous Fistula

This operation creates two separate colostomies: one for the proximal colon, creating an efferent or productive stoma, and one for the distal colon, creating an afferent stoma. From the afferent stoma, the colon carries only mucus to the rectum, and this stoma has been termed a *mucous stoma* or *mucous fistula*. This procedure is not commonly performed but may be chosen to ensure that no fecal debris can pass into the distal colon.

After a few weeks or months, the colon is usually reexamined before closing the diverting colostomy to ensure that there is no leakage and that the regional inflammatory changes have subsided. When evaluating the colon to exclude fistula, a single contrast rather than double contrast barium enema study should be performed. It is safe to use barium in the asymptomatic patient because extravasation occurs in a well-sealed sinus tract and barium does not enter the peritoneal cavity. Also, barium has contrast characteristics superior to those of water-soluble contrast agents, which may not be sufficiently dense and can become diluted in a tract.

After diversion of the fecal stream with a colostomy, the distal colon may have an abnormal appearance when examined before closure. The unused segment of the colon may appear nondistensible and have an abnormal mucosal pattern with nodularity and lymphoid follicular hyperplasia.[5] This appearance is termed *diversion colitis*. The apparent lack of distensibility is probably the result of chronic lack of distention, and the mucosal irregularity may represent, in part, adherent mucus in a partly contracted and unprepared colon. Patients may be asymptomatic, and this entity may represent a radiographic phenomenon. With reconstitution of the fecal stream after closure of the colostomy, the morphologic features of the colon return to normal unless underlying colonic inflammatory disease is present.

Stoma creation is associated with a number of complications. Necrosis may occur if the blood supply is compromised by tension or compression during formation of the stoma. The stoma may become detached from the abdominal wall and migrate into the abdominal cavity. With stomal recession, the stoma may remain attached to the abdominal wall but retract into the abdomen, leading to inflammation of the surrounding skin. The bowel may prolapse or intussuscept through the stoma. Parastomal hernias may occur, with small or rarely large bowel passing through an enlarged fascial defect adjacent to the stoma. The hernia may remain in the subcutaneous tissues or may protrude completely externally beside the stoma. Stomal ulceration may occur because of mechanical irritation from the stomal appliance.

## CECOSTOMY

Cecostomy is an infrequently performed surgical procedure in which an opening of the cecum is created to relieve cecal distention produced by distal obstruction (e.g., tumor or cecal volvulus) or by profound paralytic ileus. Cecostomy is usually a temporizing measure in acutely ill patients and in those who would not tolerate definitive but more prolonged procedures, such as right hemicolectomy and ileal–ascending colonic (Fig. 70–6) or ileal–transverse colonic anastomosis or resection of a

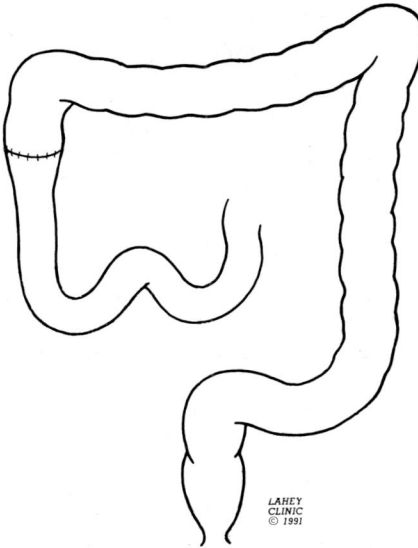

**Figure 70–6. Ileal–ascending colonic anastomosis.** This procedure is performed after resection of a right colonic tumor or ileocecal Crohn's disease. (Reprinted with the permission of the Lahey Clinic.)

distal colonic obstructive process. A tube is placed in the cecum and brought to the abdominal surface to relieve colonic distention. A definitive surgical procedure may be performed when the patient's condition permits. This procedure is rapidly being taken over by the interventional radiologist (see Chapter 60) and gastroenterologist.

## COLOANAL PULL-THROUGH PROCEDURE

The coloanal pull-through procedure (Fig. 70–7) consists of resection of an abnormal rectum with the distal colon pulled into the anal canal, where it is anastomosed to the dentate line of the anal canal. This procedure is performed when carcinoma of the midrectum is present or when a benign abnormality of the rectum is too low or too extensive for low anterior resection and colorectal anastomosis.[6] Examples of such benign diseases include extensive rectal villous edema, rectal radiation stricture or proctitis,[7] Hirschsprung's disease, and scarring from previous surgery. When the rectal disease does not involve the rectal muscles or nerves, a small cuff of rectum may be left with or without its mucosa. This latter technique may permit some sensation of rectal distention and nearly normal defecation.

## LOW ANTERIOR RESECTION

Low anterior resection is commonly performed for carcinoma of the proximal rectum and midrectum. It entails resection of the rectosigmoid and anastomosis of a cuff of the proximal colon to the distal rectum below the peritoneal reflection. This procedure involves an anastomosis deep within the pelvis and may be difficult

to perform. The surgeon must determine how low a resection to perform, and this depends on the patient's body habitus, the nature of the lesion to be resected, and the skill of the surgeon. Stapling devices greatly facilitate the technical performance of low anterior resection. A temporary, protective diverting transverse colostomy is occasionally used. Preoperatively, the surgeon usually wants to confirm the proctoscopic measurement of the distance from the anal canal to the lesion. Postoperatively, the status of the anastomosis may have to be evaluated with a water-soluble contrast enema before closure of the diverting colostomy. Leakage from a low anastomosis within the pelvis may produce a pelvic abscess, a perirectal abscess, or a colovaginal fistula (Fig. 70–8).

## ABDOMINOPERINEAL RESECTION

Lesions located below the levator ani muscles usually require an abdominoperineal resection. In this procedure, the rectum is removed and a permanent colostomy is created.

## HARTMANN'S PROCEDURE

With the Hartmann procedure, the tumor or segment of sigmoid diverticulitis is resected, a terminal end sigmoid colostomy is created, and the distal rectal stump is closed, leaving the distal rectum and anus intact. The resulting Hartmann pouch becomes a blind segment of colon from the anus to the sealed stump. Bowel continuity is re-established by a colorectal anastomosis. In some patients, however, the surgeon may elect not to re-establish continuity for medical or technical reasons.

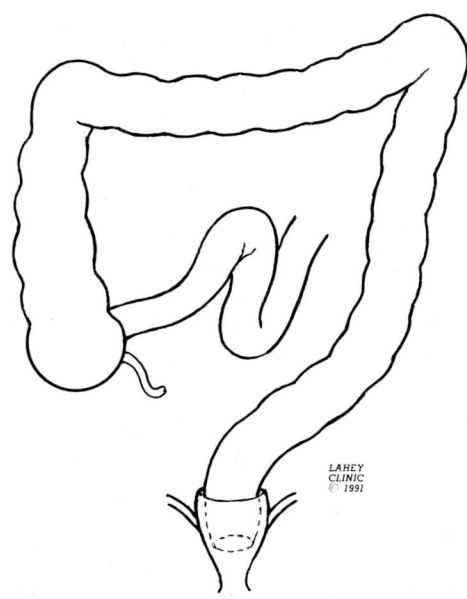

**Figure 70–7. Coloanal pull-through procedure with coloanal anastomosis.** (Reprinted with the permission of the Lahey Clinic.)

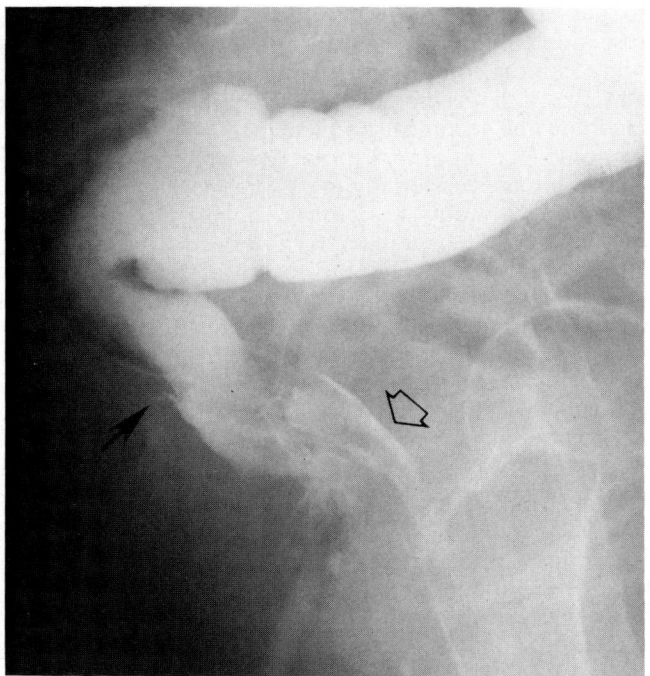

**Figure 70–8. Rectovaginal fistula.** Contrast material is identified in the vagina *(open arrow)*. Surgical clips *(solid arrow)* seen posteriorly define the level of the anastomosis and the level of the fistula.

The blind pouch may contain fecal debris, inspissated mucus, or enteroliths. Polyps or carcinoma can also develop in this segment.[8] Patients may be asymptomatic until the tumor has become far advanced. Although the classic Hartmann pouch involves only a portion of the rectum, in practice the pouch may be much longer and include part or all of the sigmoid colon. The Hartmann pouch may be created after total colectomy and creation of an ileostomy for familial polyposis or Crohn's disease (Fig. 70–9). The pouch can be closed by hand-sewn or stapled sutures. When stapling is used, the length of the pouch may be estimated on a film of the abdomen.

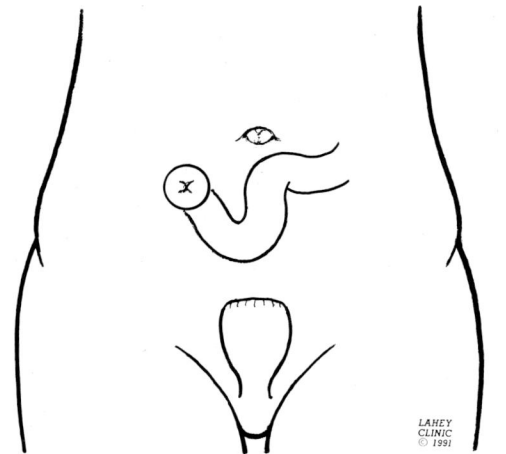

**Figure 70–9. Closed rectal pouch, Hartmann's pouch, with terminal ileostomy.** (Reprinted with the permission of the Lahey Clinic.)

## MUCOUS FISTULA

Rather than closing off the rectal stump, a rectosigmoid stoma or mucous fistula may be created. A mucous fistula is a stoma created by bringing out the proximal cut end of the distal sigmoid colon or rectum, which results in a stoma that produces only mucus. The distal colon extends from the stoma of the mucous fistula distally to the anus.

## APPENDECTOMY

Appendectomy is a simple procedure wherein the appendix is tied at its junction with the cecum and is resected. The stump is usually simply ligated and inverted. Occasionally, this operation may produce a sizable smooth polypoid defect in the base of the cecum (Fig. 70–10). The history of appendectomy and the location of the defect at the apex of the cecum prevent the mistaken diagnosis of cecal polyp. Nodularity, mucosal disruption, or a location away from the apex should arouse suspicion that this is a real polyp requiring colonoscopic evaluation.

When a diverting colostomy is closed to restore intestinal continuity, a deformity may be created at the site of the previous colostomy and may cause radiographic confusion when the history is not correlated with examination of the colon. The appearance is variable and may resemble that of a polypoid filling defect, a smooth or nodular annular lesion, or a submucosal or serosal process (see Fig. 70–3). Any colonic operative or endoscopic procedure may produce a persistent deformity that can mimic disease (Fig. 70–11). Careful review of the patient's history may prevent a misdiagnosis.

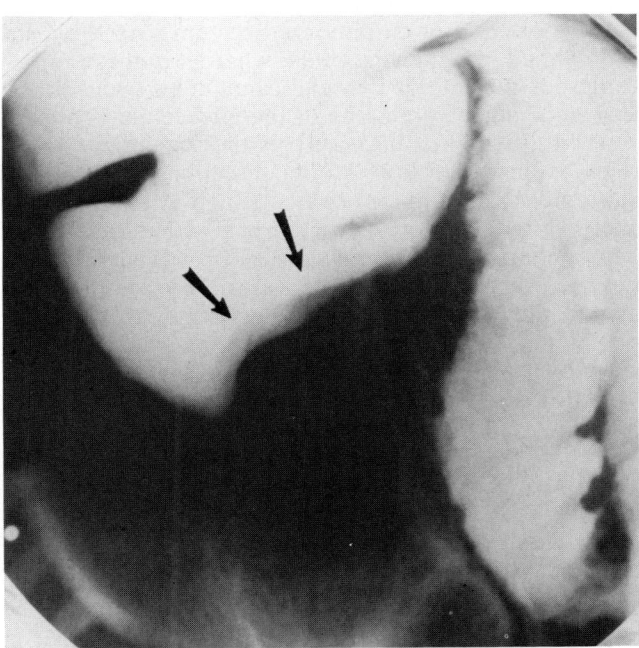

**Figure 70–10. Appendiceal stump deformity.** A broad-based defect *(arrows)* in the apex of the cecum is due to previous appendectomy. Most appendectomies produce minimal or no deformity of the cecum.

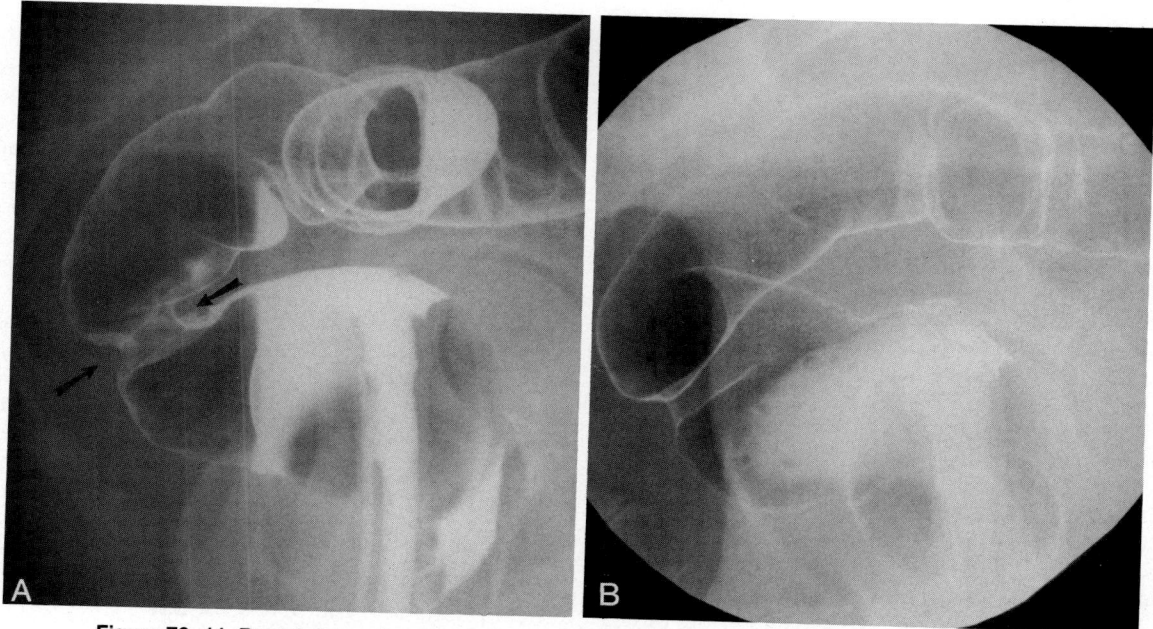

**Figure 70–11. Rectal deformity caused by prior abscess and drainage. A.** Examination performed because of a family history of colonic carcinoma demonstrates a short annular constriction *(arrows)* in the midrectum that was not present on an examination performed 6 years earlier. **B.** Endoscopy showed a normal mucosa in the contracted segment. Additional history was obtained before ordering further studies. It was found that an intervening appendectomy at another institution 4 years earlier required postoperative transrectal drainage of a perirectal abscess. This case represents residual deformity from that abscess and its treatment.

# ILEAL POUCH–ANAL ANASTOMOSIS

Ileal pouch–anal anastomosis is performed in patients who have ulcerative colitis (see Chapter 62) or familial polyposis (see Chapter 66).[9, 10] It is an alternative to proctocolectomy and offers the potential for nearly normal defecation through the intact anus. Careful radiographic and clinical evaluation of the patient to exclude Crohn's disease is essential. Patients with Crohn's disease may not tolerate extensive pelvic sur-

gery, and pelvic perineal fistulas and sinus tracts, inflammation of the pouch, and anastomotic stricture may develop. The procedure consists of colectomy, mucosal proctectomy, and creation of a small bowel reservoir. The colon and most of the rectum are removed, leaving the distal portion of the rectum in place. The mucosa is dissected from this rectal remnant, leaving a cuff of denuded rectum with intact muscularis propria. One of the several types of pouches, usually an S, J, or side-to-side (Fonkalsrud) pouch, may be created (Fig. 70–12).

The J pouch is formed when the distal ileum is closed and the ileum is doubled on itself, forming a J configuration. The apposed walls of the two limbs are stapled to each other, and the two segments are opened, creating a pouch having the volume of two limbs. The staples serve to delineate the length of the pouch. The pouch is placed into the rectal cuff, and a hole is created in the apex of the pouch for anastomosis to the anal mucosa.

The S pouch is created by apposing and suturing of three limbs of the distal ileum to each other. The common walls are opened, creating a pouch with the diameter of three segments of small bowel. This pouch and the Fonkalsrud pouch have an efferent limb that is brought into the rectal cuff, and its mucosa is sutured to the dentate line of the anal canal.

The Fonkalsrud pouch is created by resecting a segment of the distal ileum. That segment is placed next to the distal ileum, and a side-to-side anastomosis is created.

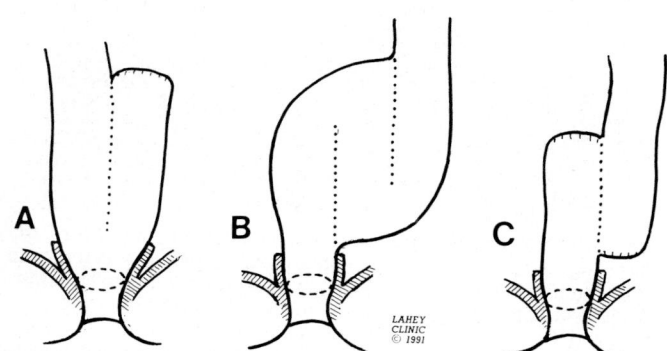

**Figure 70–12. Three major types of ileal pouch–anal anastomosis. A.** J pouch. **B.** S pouch. **C.** Side-to-side (Fonkalsrud) pouch. (Reprinted with the permission of the Lahey Clinic.)

All ileal pouch–anal anastomosis procedures leave a cuff of rectal wall in place with the theory that the intact sensory innervation of this segment permits the patient to sense bowel distention and the urge to defecate. Although bowel movements may be increased in frequency, patients may need to defecate no more often than they normally need to urinate. Although some patients have nocturnal soiling, the quality of life of patients who had ulcerative colitis is greatly enhanced and the risk of developing colon carcinoma is eliminated.

The ileal pouch–anal anastomosis procedure is usually performed in two stages, with initial colectomy, creation of the pouch and pouch-anal anastomosis, and creation of a protective ileostomy. At the second stage, the ileostomy is closed after 6 to 8 weeks to permit suture lines to mature. The radiologist may be called on before closure of the ileostomy to perform a contrast enema examination to be sure no leakage is occurring at any anastomosis or a computed tomographic examination to search for a pelvic abscess. Practice patterns and personal preference of the surgeon play an important role. Because some degree of narrowing is usual at the pouch-anal anastomosis, surgeons at the Lahey Clinic perform initial digital examination of the anus and adjacent pouch to dilate the anastomosis to the caliber of the index finger and to search for tender areas that may suggest small pelvic abscesses. A barium enema examination is performed. I use a 14 French Foley catheter that is inserted into the pouch but is not inflated. An inflated balloon may prevent barium from reaching the pouch-anal anastomosis. With care, the catheter rarely falls out. If it does, the balloon can be inflated under fluoroscopic observation and kept away from the pouch-anal anastomosis. The diameter of the inflated balloon should be less than the diameter of the pouch. The patient may have to be in the 45-degree upright position to place barium against the anteriorly positioned pouch-anal anastomosis and displace the air that is often present there (Fig. 70–13). Anteroposterior, oblique, and lateral views are obtained. These views must be low enough to include the pouch–anal canal junction. Leakage from the pouch or from the pouch-anal anastomosis requires that closure of the diverting ileostomy be postponed until healing has been confirmed. Small leakages and collections may be treated by endoscopic drainage, suturing, or antibiotic therapy if they do not resolve spontaneously.[11]

A three-stage procedure may be required when the patient is weakened by fulminant colitis and is receiving high-dose steroid therapy. The first stage consists of creation of a simple ileostomy, colectomy, and a Hartmann closure of the rectum. The second stage is performed a few months later, when healing and recovery of electrolyte and endocrine integrity after steroid withdrawal have occurred. The remainder of the rectum is resected, mucosal proctectomy is performed, and a pouch with pouch-anal anastomosis is created. The third stage is closure of the ileostomy, 6 to 8 weeks later.

Several complications may be encountered with this procedure that require radiographic evaluation.[8, 12] Any of the complications that attend all major abdominal operations may develop, including abscesses, ileus, or small bowel obstruction. The small bowel mesentery limits mobility of the ileum, and the small bowel may have to be manipulated extensively to create the pouch-anal anastomosis. This manipulation may play a role in the prolonged ileus seen in some patients. Small bowel obstruction can develop in the immediate postoperative period, in the period between creation of the pouch and closure of the ileostomy, or, as in all patients with abdominal surgery, at any time during the remainder of the patient's life. Mesenteric hematoma may occur if small mesenteric vessels rupture because of manipulation of or prolonged tension on the mesentery. The superior mesenteric artery syndrome can develop if tension placed on the mesentery in an attempt to position the pouch in the lowest portion of the pelvis pulls the superior mesenteric artery against the aorta.[12, 13] Prophylactic release of the small bowel mesentery at the ligament of Treitz, mesenteric lengthening incisions, and judicious suturing and resection of stretched branch mesenteric vessels facilitate mobilization of the terminal ileal pouch into the pelvis.[14]

Rarely, leakage may occur from the suture lines of the pouch (Fig. 70–14). More often, leakage is encountered at the pouch-anal anastomosis (Figs. 70–15 and

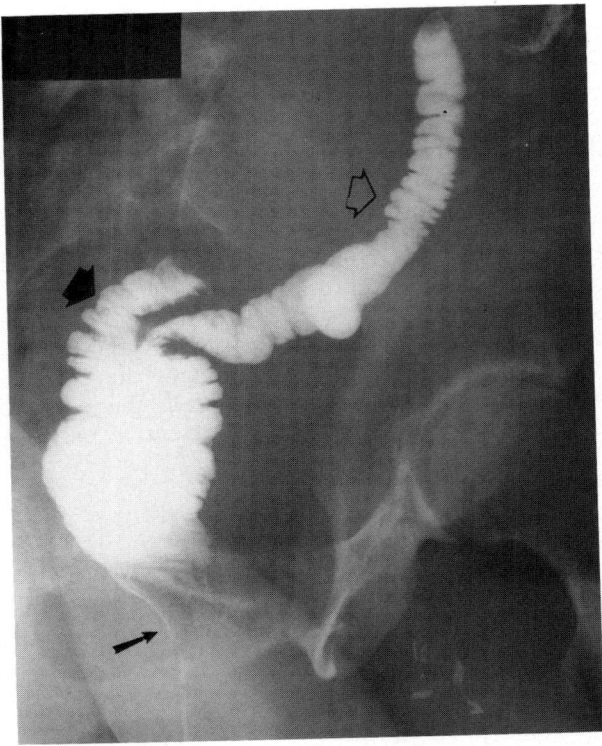

**Figure 70–13. Normal J pouch reservoir before closure of the diverting ileostomy.** Note the long J pouch appendage *(short solid arrow)* and the afferent limb *(open arrow)* leading from the ileostomy to the pouch. In this supine oblique view, air is present *(long solid arrow)* in the anterior portion of the pouch at the pouch-anal anastomotic region. Contrast material should be positioned at the pouch-anal anastomosis by placing the patient in the 45-degree erect position or turning the patient toward the prone position until air is displaced by contrast material.

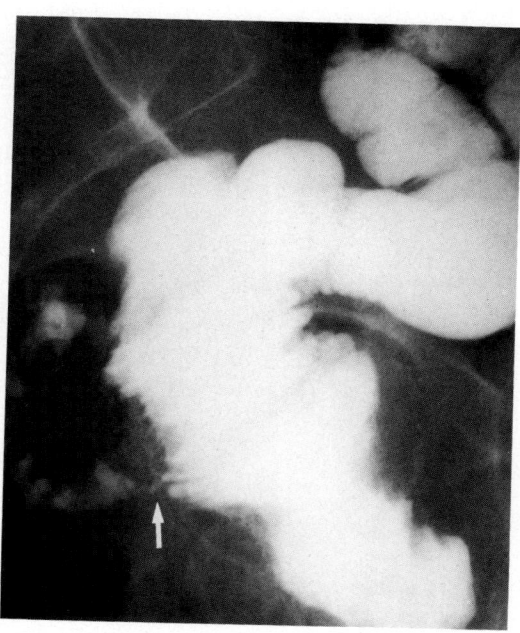

**Figure 70–14. Pouch leak.** Leakage *(arrow)* from a J pouch reservoir is seen. (From PW Kremers, FJ Scholz, DJ Schoetz Jr, et al, Radiology of the ileoanal reservoir, AJR, 145, 3, 559–567, 1985, © by American Roentgen Ray Society.)

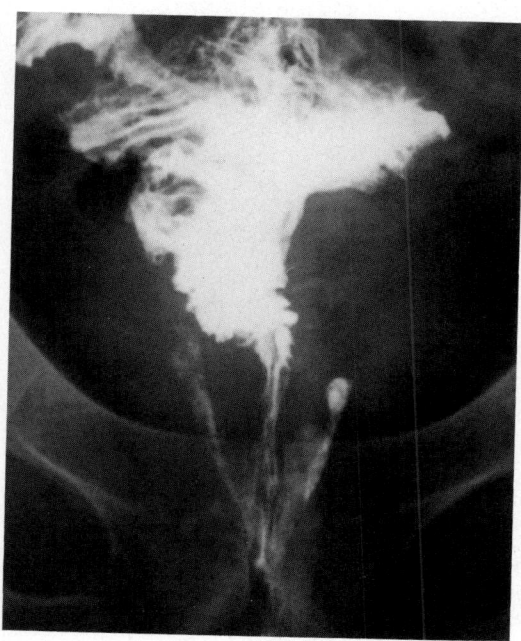

**Figure 70–15. Pouch leak.** Leakage from the pouch-anal anastomosis of a J pouch reservoir is seen. Leakage from any anal anastomosis has a typical chevron appearance resulting from tracking of the extravasated contrast material between the rectal cuff and the pouch or efferent limb inserted into the cuff. (From PW Kremers, FJ Scholz, DJ Schoetz Jr, et al, Radiology of the ileoanal reservoir, AJR, 145, 3, 559–567, 1985, © by American Roentgen Ray Society.)

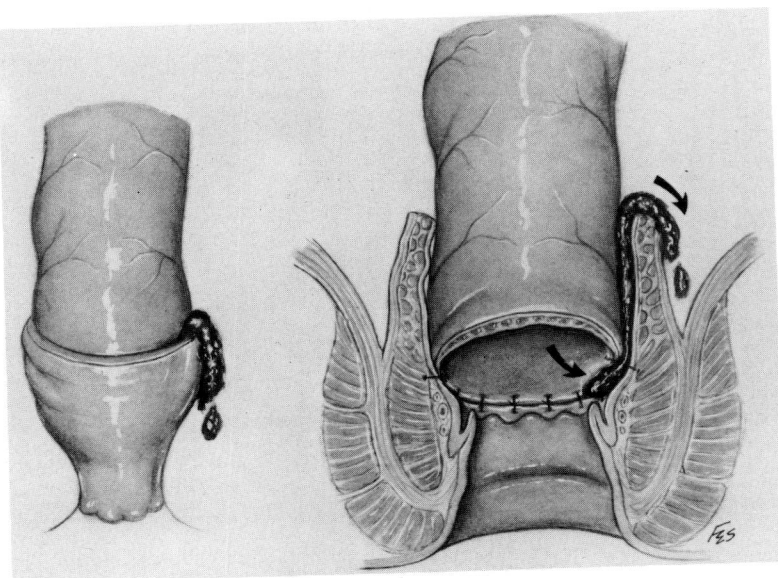

**Figure 70–16. Chevron configuration of ileoanal anastomotic leak.** Drawing illustrates the mechanism of extravasation from a pouch-anal anastomosis. Mucus (or contrast material) passes from the point of disruption *(lower curved arrow)* and courses between the pouch and the cuff of rectum, producing the chevron configuration seen in Figure 70–15. Purulent material will eventually dissect beyond the cuff and spill *(upper curved arrow)* into the perirectal soft tissues. (From PW Kremers, FJ Scholz, DJ Schoetz Jr, et al, Radiology of the ileoanal reservoir, AJR, 145, 3, 559–567, 1985, © by American Roentgen Ray Society.)

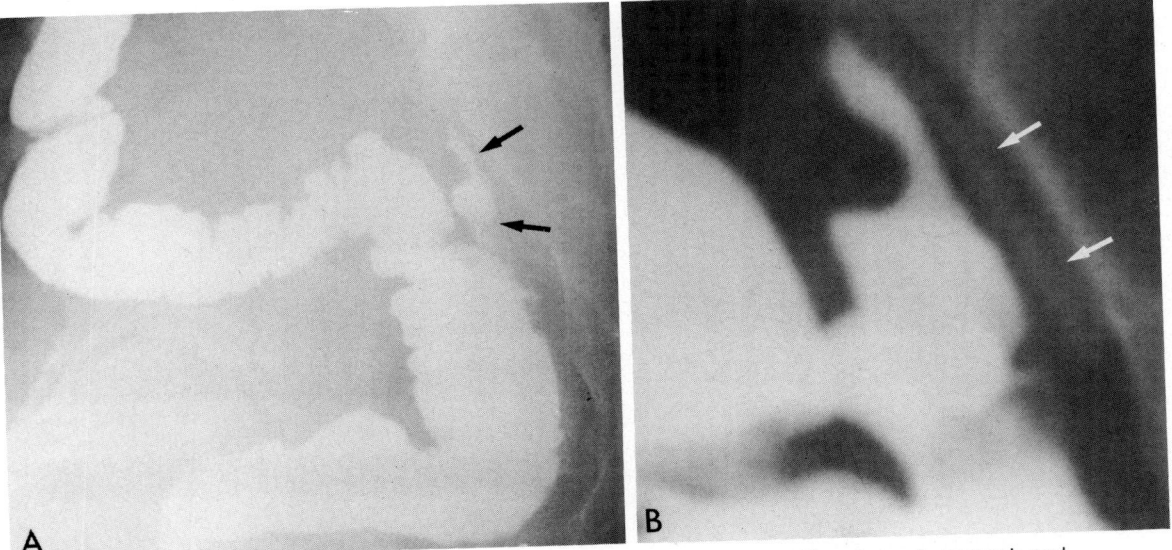

**Figure 70–17. Pseudoleakage.** This appearance is commonly seen with a J pouch reservoir and represents a potential radiographic pitfall. **A.** Initially, traces of contrast material *(arrows)* appear to extravasate from the proximal, posterior part of the J pouch reservoir. **B.** Detail from spot film after further distention shows contrast material surrounded by a faintly visible suture line *(arrows)* just anterior to the sacrum. The lateral view also demonstrates the anterior position of the lower portion of the pouch, which traps air in the supine position and makes visualization of the pouch-anal anastomosis difficult. (**A** and **B** from PW Kremers, FJ Scholz, DJ Schoetz Jr, et al, Radiology of the ileoanal reservoir, AJR, 145, 3, 559–567, 1985, © by American Roentgen Ray Society.)

70–16). A small length of closed reflected ileum is often not incorporated into the J pouch, and this is termed the *J pouch appendage* (Fig. 70–17; see Fig. 70–13). This appendage may leak, may be long enough to twist and necrose, or may simulate leakage[15] (see Fig. 70–17). The S pouch and the Fonkalsrud pouch have efferent limbs that pass between the pouch and the anus. These pouches, when distended with fecal contents, may press on the efferent limb and interfere with pouch emptying. Some patients may succeed in emptying their pouch in this condition by self-catheterization.

Patients who tolerate the complete procedure may return with "pouchitis," complaining of tenesmus and diarrhea, and rarely with bleeding, fever, arthralgias, and other systemic symptoms.[16, 17] Endoscopic examination of the pouch may reveal redness and ulceration.[18] Pouchitis is not associated with any consistent radiographic findings and its cause is unknown.

With time, an apparent accommodation of the small bowel to the pouch leads to an increase in capacity that leads to small bowel dilatation, which on a plain film simulates small bowel obstruction resulting from adhesions. When clinical and radiographic findings are confusing, enteroclysis or retrograde small bowel enema examination may be required to rule out mechanical obstruction.

# References

1. Corman ML: Colon and Rectal Surgery (2nd ed). Philadelphia: JB Lippincott, 1989.
2. Goligher J: Surgery of the Anus Rectum and Colon (5th ed). London: Bailliere Tindall, 1984.
3. Henry MM, Swash M (eds): Coloproctology and the Pelvic Floor (2nd ed). London: Butterworth-Heinemann, 1991.
4. Thomson JPS, Nicholls RJ, Williams CB: Colorectal Disease: An Introduction for Surgeons and Physicians. London: Heinemann, 1981.
5. Lechner GL, Frank W, Jantsch H: Lymphoid follicular hyperplasia in excluded colonic segments: a radiologic sign of diversion colitis. Radiology 176:135–136, 1990.
6. Haas PA, Fox TA: The fate of the forgotten rectal pouch after Hartmann's procedure without reconstruction. Am J Surg 159:106–111, 1990.
7. Gazet J-C: Parks' coloanal pull-through anastomosis for severe, complicated radiation proctitis. Dis Colon Rectum 28:110–114, 1985.
8. Hillard AE, Mann FA, Becker JM, et al: The ileoanal J pouch: radiographic evaluation. Radiology 155:591–594, 1985.
9. Schoetz DJ Jr, Coller JA, Veidenheimer MC: Proctocolectomy with ileoanal reservoir: an alternative to permanent ileostomy. Postgrad Med 75:123–138, 1984.
10. Schoetz DJ Jr, Coller JA, Veidenheimer MC: Ileoanal reservoir for ulcerative colitis and familial polyposis. Arch Surg 121:404–409, 1986.
11. Schoetz DJ Jr, Coller JA, Veidenheimer MC: Can the pouch be saved? Dis Colon Rectum 31:671–675, 1988.
12. Kremers PW, Scholz FJ, Schoetz DJ Jr, et al: Radiology of the ileoanal reservoir. AJR 145:559–567, 1985.
13. Ballantyne GH, Graham SM, Hammers L, et al: Superior mesenteric artery syndrome following ileal J-pouch anal anastomosis: an iatrogenic cause of early postoperative obstruction. Dis Colon Rectum 30:472–474, 1987.
14. Burnstein M, Schoetz DJ Jr, Coller JA, et al: Technique of mesenteric lengthening and ileal reservoir and anal anastomosis. Dis Colon Rectum 30:863–866, 1987.
15. Pezim ME, Taylor BA, Davis CJ, et al: Perforation of terminal ileal appendage of J-pelvic ileal reservoir. Dis Colon Rectum 30:161–163, 1987.
16. Franceschi D, Chen PF, Yuh J-N: Solitary J-pouch ulcer causing pouchitis-like syndrome. Dis Colon Rectum 29:515–517, 1986.
17. Knobler H, Ligumsky M, Okon E, et al: Pouch ileitis: recurrence of the inflammatory bowel disease in the ileal reservoir. Am J Gastroenterol 81:199–201, 1986.
18. Milsom JW: Surgery of colorectal cancer and inflammatory bowel disease. Curr Opin Gastroenterol 4:42–48, 1993.

# The Colon: Differential Diagnosis

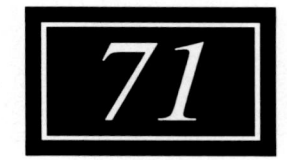

Richard M. Gore, M.D.

## TABLE 71–1. MULTIPLE COLONIC FILLING DEFECTS[1–4]

**ARTIFACTS**
Feces
Mucus strands
Oil droplets
Ingested foreign bodies
Air bubbles

**NEOPLASMS AND TUMORS**
Multiple adenomatous polyps
Hemangiomas
Familial polyposis
Gardner's syndrome
Cronkhite-Canada syndrome
Disseminated gastrointestinal polyposis
Juvenile polyposis coli
Turcot's syndrome
Neurocrest and colonic tumors
Ruvalcaba-Myhre-Smith syndrome
Lymphoma
Metastases
Multiple adenocarcinomas
Cowden's syndrome
Leukemic infiltration
Blue nevus syndrome
Neurofibromas, neurofibromatosis

**INFLAMMATORY DISORDERS**
Ulcerative colitis
Crohn's disease
Diversion colitis
Colitis cystica profunda
Malacoplakia
Behçet's syndrome

**INFECTIOUS DISORDERS**
Pseudomembranous colitis
Amebiasis
Schistosomiasis
Trichuriasis
*Strongyloides* infection
Cytomegalovirus infection
Ascariasis
Herpes zoster

**MISCELLANEOUS DISORDERS**
Lymphoid follicular pattern
Nodular lymphoid hyperplasia
Hemorrhoids
Diverticula
Pneumatosis intestinalis
Cystic fibrosis
Endometriosis
Colonic varices
Amyloidosis
Hemangiomas
Urticaria

## TABLE 71–2. SOLITARY COLONIC FILLING DEFECTS[1–4]

**BENIGN TUMORS**
Hyperplastic polyp
Adenomatous polyp
Villous adenoma
Villoglandular polyp
Hamartoma
Peutz-Jeghers polyp
Spindle cell tumor (lipoma, leiomyoma, fibroma, neurofibroma, cystic lymphangioma)
Traumatic neuroma
Carcinoid tumor

**MALIGNANT TUMORS**
Carcinoma
Lymphoma
Metastases
Kaposi's sarcoma

**INFECTIOUS DISORDERS**
Ameboma
Tuberculosis
Mucormycoma
Periappendiceal abscess
Diverticular abscess
Schistosomiasis (polypoid granuloma)
*Ascaris lumbricoides* (bolus of worms) infection
Intramural hematoma

**INFLAMMATORY DISORDERS**
Colitis cystica profunda
Solitary rectal ulcer syndrome
Foreign body perforation and abscess
Crohn's disease

**MISCELLANEOUS DISORDERS**
Endometrioma
Intussusception
Bezoar
Suture granuloma
Inverted appendiceal stump
Hypertrophied anal papilla
Stool, vegetable material
Amyloidosis
Varix, hemorrhoid

## TABLE 71–3. MOSAIC–SUBMUCOSAL EDEMA PATTERN[1–4]

| | |
|---|---|
| Colonic urticaria | Obstructive colon cancer |
| Herpes zoster | Cecal volvulus |
| *Yersinia* infection | Colonic ileus |
| Ischemia | |

## TABLE 71-4. SEGMENTAL COLONIC NARROWING[1-4]

**MALIGNANT DISORDERS**
Primary adenocarcinoma
Metastases
Kaposi's sarcoma
Lymphoma
Carcinoma
Carcinoid
Direct spread from renal, duodenal, pancreatic, ovarian tumor

**INFLAMMATORY DISORDERS**
Crohn's disease
Ulcerative colitis
Cathartic colon
Caustic colon
Retractile mesenteritis
Typhlitis
Solitary rectal ulcer syndrome

**INFECTIOUS DISORDERS**
Amebiasis
Schistosomiasis
*Strongyloides* infection
Tuberculosis
Gonorrheal proctitis
*Chlamydia* infection (lymphogranuloma venereum)
Herpes zoster
*Cytomegalovirus* infection
Bacillary dysentery
Actinomycosis
Giant anorectal condyloma acuminatum
Pericolic abscess

**VASCULAR DISORDERS**
Ischemic colitis
Radiation colitis
Intramural hematoma

**MISCELLANEOUS DISORDERS**
Pancreatitis
Pelvic lipomatosis
Endometriosis
Amyloidosis
Adhesive band
Postoperative deformity
Myochosis

## TABLE 71-5. ANNULAR "APPLE CORE" COLONIC LESION[1-4]

Carcinoma
Diverticulitis
Chronic Crohn's disease
Chronic ulcerative colitis
Ischemic colitis
*Chlamydia* infection (lymphogranuloma venereum)
Lymphoma
Tuberculosis
Villous adenoma
Helminthoma
Ameboma

## TABLE 71-6. CAUSES OF LARGE BOWEL OBSTRUCTION IN AN ADULT[1-4]

**INFLAMMATORY DISORDERS**
Diverticulitis
Inflammatory bowel disease
Retractile mesenteritis

**INFECTIOUS DISORDERS**
*Ascaris* bolus
Chagas' disease
Amebiasis
Schistosomiasis
Actinomycosis
Tuberculosis

**EXTRINSIC BOWEL LESIONS**
Adhesions
Hernias
Volvulus
Endometriosis
Neoplasms
Appendiceal abscess
Tubo-ovarian abscess
Distended bladder

**NEOPLASTIC LESIONS**
Adenocarcinoma of the colon
Lymphoma
Spindle cell tumor
Carcinoid
Metastases

**VASCULAR DISORDERS**
Intramural hematoma
Vascular occlusion, infarction

**OBTURATION OF LUMEN**
Bezoar
Fecal impaction
Foreign body
Intussusception

**MISCELLANEOUS DISORDERS**
Amyloidosis
Colonic pseudo-obstruction

## TABLE 71-7. INTESTINAL PSEUDO-OBSTRUCTION: OGILVIE'S SYNDROME[1-4]

**DRUG REACTION**
Phenothiazine
Antidepressants
Morphine
Antiparkinsonism

**PARALYTIC ILEUS**
Hypokalemia
Pancreatitis
Pneumonia
Myocardial infarction
Trauma

**ENDOCRINE DISEASE**
Myxedema
Diabetes
Hypoparathyroidism
Pheochromocytoma

**NEUROMUSCULAR DISORDERS**
Parkinson's disease
Chagas' disease
Myotonic dystrophy

**MISCELLANEOUS DISORDERS**
Amyloidosis
Sprue
Scleroderma
Retractile mesenteritis
Vitamin D deficiency

## TABLE 71–8. COLON DISTENTION WITHOUT OBSTRUCTION[1-4]

**PARALYTIC ILEUS**
After operation
Peritonitis
Appendicitis
Pancreatitis

**ELECTROLYTE IMBALANCE**
Hypokalemia
Hypochloremia
Calcium abnormality

**ENDOCRINE DISORDERS**
Diabetes
Adrenal insufficiency
Myxedema
Hypoparathyroidism

**NEUROMUSCULAR DISORDERS**
Hirschsprung's disease
Parkinson's disease
Multiple sclerosis
Riley-Day syndrome
Amyotonia congenita
Chagas' disease

**DRUG THERAPY**
Morphine, L-dopa, chlorpromazine, benztropine, atropine, propantheline bromide (Pro-Banthine)
Hexamethonium

**TRAUMA**
Spinal cord injury
Intramural hematoma
Lower rib injury
Retroperitoneal hemorrhage

**URINARY TRACT DISORDERS**
Ureteral colic
Renal failure, uremia
Urine retention

**COLLAGEN-VASCULAR DISEASE**
Scleroderma
Dermatomyositis
Polyarteritis nodosa
Kawasaki's syndrome

**ACUTE THORACIC DISEASE**
Myocardial infarction
Congestive heart failure

**MISCELLANEOUS DISORDERS**
Chronic constipation
Chronic laxative, cathartic abuse
Aerophagia
Mesenteric infarction
Shock
Septicemia
Toxic megacolon
Cystic fibrosis
Amyloidosis

## TABLE 71–9. LARGE BOWEL OBSTRUCTION IN A NEWBORN[1-4]

Congenital stenosis or atresia
Hernia, incarcerated, internal or external
Hirschsprung's disease
Imperforate anus
Rectal atresia
Intussusception
Midgut volvulus with malrotation
Small left colon syndrome
Megacystis-microcolon syndrome
Intraluminal web, diaphragm, or band
Duplication

## TABLE 71–10. INTESTINAL OBSTRUCTION IN A POSTNEONATAL CHILD[1-4]

| | |
|---|---|
| Hirschsprung's disease | Imperforate anus with fistula |
| Hernia | Cystic fibrosis |
| Appendicitis | Crohn's disease |
| Duplication | Fecal impaction |
| Intussusception | Foreign body, bezoar |
| Midgut volvulus | *Ascaris* bolus |
| Tuberculosis | Neoplasm |

## TABLE 71–11. TOXIC MEGACOLON[1-4]

| | |
|---|---|
| Ulcerative colitis | Cholera |
| Crohn's disease | Strongyloidiasis |
| Ischemic colitis | *Campylobacter* colitis |
| Amebic colitis | Pseudomembranous colitis |
| Bacillary dysentery | Behçet's disease |
| Typhoid fever | |

## TABLE 71–12. ENLARGED ILEOCECAL VALVE[1-4]

| | |
|---|---|
| Normal variant | Actinomycosis |
| Crohn's disease | Cathartic abuse |
| Amebiasis | Tuberculosis |
| Fatty infiltration, lipoma | Typhoid fever |
| Intussusception | Intramural hematoma |
| Villous adenoma | Anisakiasis |
| Adenocarcinoma | Ileocolic prolapse |
| Lymphoma | |

## TABLE 71-13. APPENDICEAL LESIONS[1-4]

| | |
|---|---|
| Abscess | Adenocarcinoma |
| Acute appendicitis | Spindle cell tumor |
| Calculus, fecalith | Carcinoid tumor |
| After operation (inverted stump, adhesions) | Diverticulosis |
| | Amebiasis |
| Crohn's disease | Ascariasis |
| Metastasis | Ulcerative colitis |
| Intussusception, invagination | Tuberculosis |
| Endometrial implantation | Lymphoma |
| Mucocele | Trichuriasis |
| Myxoglobulosis | Typhoid fever |

## TABLE 71-14. CONED CECUM[1-4]

| | |
|---|---|
| Crohn's disease | Tuberculosis |
| Amebiasis | Metastasis |
| Appendicitis | Anisakiasis |
| Carcinoma of the cecum | Typhoid fever |
| Ulcerative colitis | *Yersinia* enterocolitis |
| Diverticulitis | Cytomegalovirus infection |
| Cathartic abuse | Typhlitis |
| Actinomycosis | Radiation therapy |
| South American blastomycosis | |

## TABLE 71-15. CECAL FILLING DEFECTS[1-4]

Appendiceal lesions
Metastases
General causes of colonic filling defects
Intussusception of appendix, Meckel's diverticulum, lymphoma, distal ileum
Diverticulitis
Endometriosis
Solitary benign ulcer
Adherent fecalith (cystic fibrosis)
Burkitt's lymphoma
Ameboma
Lipomatous ileocecal valve

## TABLE 71-16. GAS IN THE COLON WALL[1-4]

| | |
|---|---|
| Ischemic colitis | Toxic megacolon |
| Necrotizing enterocolitis | Large bowel obstruction |
| Pseudomembranous colitis | |

## TABLE 71-17. PNEUMATOSIS CYSTOIDES COLI (NON-NECROTIZING)[1-4]

Colonoscopy
Colonic irrigation or enema
Pneumomediastinum with abdominal extension
Emphysema, asthma
Scleroderma
Dermatomyositis
Juvenile rheumatoid arthritis
Pyloric obstruction
Imperforate anus
Hirschsprung's disease
After operation (intestinal bypass)
Blunt abdominal trauma
Cystic fibrosis
Peptic ulcer with intramural perforation
Hydrogen peroxide enema

## TABLE 71-18. FISTULA INVOLVING THE COLON[1-4]

**INFLAMMATORY DISORDERS**
Crohn's disease
Diverticulitis
Biliary fistula
Peptic ulcer, marginal ulcer
Pancreatitis

**INFECTIOUS DISORDERS**
Actinomycosis
Pelvic inflammatory disease
Tuberculosis
Amebiasis
*Chlamydia* infection (lymphogranuloma venereum)
Appendiceal abscess
Renal abscess

**MALIGNANT DISORDERS**
Adenocarcinoma of the colon
Lymphoma
Metastasis

**MISCELLANEOUS DISORDERS**
After operation
Ischemic colitis
Infarction
Foreign body (pin, bone, toothpick)
Abdominal trauma
Iatrogenic trauma

## TABLE 71–19. RECTOVAGINAL FISTULA[1–4]

**INFLAMMATORY DISORDERS**
Crohn's disease
Diverticulitis

**NEOPLASTIC DISORDERS**
Carcinoma of the rectum
Carcinoma of the cervix
Carcinoma of the vagina

**INFECTIOUS DISORDERS**
*Chlamydia* infection (lymphogranuloma venereum)
Appendiceal abscess
Tubo-ovarian abscess
Actinomycosis
Schistosomiasis
Tuberculosis

**TRAUMA**
External
Sexual
Puerperal
Iatrogenic

**MISCELLANEOUS DISORDERS**
Endometriosis
Radiation therapy
Foreign body
Imperforate anus or other cloacal anomaly

## TABLE 71–20. DOUBLE TRACKING IN THE SIGMOID COLON[1–4]

Diverticulitis
Crohn's disease
Carcinoma of the colon

## TABLE 71–21. COLONIC THUMBPRINTING[1–4]

**VASCULAR DISORDERS**
Occlusive vascular disease
Intramural hemorrhage (anticoagulants, bleeding diathesis)
Traumatic intramural hematoma
Hemolytic-uremic syndrome
Hereditary angioneurotic edema

**INFLAMMATORY DISORDERS**
Ulcerative colitis
Crohn's disease
Retractile mesenteritis

**INFECTIOUS DISORDERS**
Amebiasis
Schistosomiasis
Cytomegalovirus infection
Strongyloidiasis
Pseudomembranous colitis
Typhlitis
*Staphylococcus* colitis

**NEOPLASTIC DISORDERS**
Lymphoma
Metastases

**MISCELLANEOUS DISORDERS**
Amyloidosis
Endometriosis
Diverticulosis or diverticulitis
Mesenteric or peritoneal lesions
Pneumatosis cystoides coli

## TABLE 71–22. LARGE LYMPHOID FOLICLES[1–4]

**INFLAMMATORY DISORDERS**
Crohn's disease
Behçet's syndrome
Nodular lymphoid hyperplasia

**INFECTIOUS DISORDERS**
*Campylobacter* colitis
*Yersinia* colitis
Amebic colitis
Herpes colitis
*Salmonella* colitis
*Shigella* colitis
Tuberculosis

**NEOPLASTIC DISORDERS**
Lymphoma
Adenocarcinoma
Adenoma
Leukemia

**IMMUNOLOGIC DISORDERS**
Acquired immunodeficiency syndrome
Immunoglobulin E deficiency

### TABLE 71–23. APHTHOID ULCERATIONS

| | |
|---|---|
| Crohn's disease | Lymphoma |
| *Yersinia* enterocolitis | *Salmonella* colitis |
| Amebic colitis | *Shigella* colitis |
| Behçet's disease | Herpes colitis |
| Ischemic colitis | Cytomegalovirus colitis |

### TABLE 71–24. ULCERATIVE COLONIC LESIONS[1-4]

**INFLAMMATORY DISORDERS**
Ulcerative disorders
Crohn's disease
Caustic colitis
Behçet's syndrome
Diversion colitis
Solitary rectal ulcer syndrome
Diverticulitis
Pancreatitis
Stercoral colitis

**INFECTIOUS DISORDERS**
Pseudomembranous colitis
Amebiasis
*Campylobacter* colitis
Schistosomiasis
Shigellosis
Tuberculosis
Gonorrhea
Staphylococcal colitis
*Yersinia* colitis
*Chlamydia* infection (lymphogranuloma venereum)
Herpes zoster
Herpes simplex
Rotavirus infection
Cytomegalovirus infection
Strongyloidiasis
Histoplasmosis
Candidiasis
Actinomycosis
Mucormycosis

**VASCULAR DISORDERS**
Ischemic colitis
Uremic colitis
Hemolytic-uremic syndrome

**MALIGNANT DISORDERS**
Carcinoma
Lymphoma
Leukemic infiltration

**MISCELLANEOUS DISORDERS**
Drug-induced colitis (steroids, antibiotics, chemotherapy)
Inorganic mercury poisoning
Chemical (paraldehyde) proctitis
Amyloidosis

### TABLE 71–25. SMOOTH COLON

| | |
|---|---|
| Ulcerative colitis | Amyloidosis |
| Crohn's disease | Radiation colitis (late) |
| Cathartic or enema abuse | Schistosomiasis |
| Ischemic colitis (late) | |

### TABLE 71–26. PERICOLIC ABSCESS[1-4]

| | |
|---|---|
| Diverticulitis | Amebiasis |
| Appendicitis | Schistosomiasis |
| Crohn's disease | Helminthoma |
| Peforated primary or | *Chlamydia* infection |
| metastatic neoplasm | (lymphogranuloma |
| Tubo-ovarian abscess | venereum) |
| Pancreatitis | Actinomycosis |
| Trauma | Tuberculosis |
| Foreign body perforation | Renal infection |
| Ischemic colitis | |

### TABLE 71–27. WIDENED PRESACRAL SPACE[1-4]

**NORMAL VARIANT**

**INFLAMMATORY DISORDERS**
Ulcerative colitis
Crohn's disease
Retroperitoneal fibrosis
Pelvic lipomatosis
Colitis cystica profunda
Chemical (paraldehyde) proctitis

**INFECTIOUS DISORDERS**
Presacral abscess
Diverticulitis
Appendicitis
Tuberculosis
Amebiasis
*Chlamydia* infection (lymphogranuloma venereum)
Pelvic abscess (diverticular, appendiceal)
Gonorrheal proctitis

**TUMORS**
Primary rectal tumors (adenocarcinoma, lymphoma, sarcoma, cloacogenic carcinoma)
Invasion by adjacent tumors (bladder, prostate, ovary, cervix, myeloma)
Sacral or coccygeal neoplasm (osteogenic sarcoma, chondrosarcoma, giant cell tumor) or teratoma
Neurogenic tumors (chordoma, neurofibroma, schwannoma)
Multiple myeloma
Sacral metastases
Ovarian cyst or neoplasm

**VASCULAR DISORDERS**
Hematoma
Radiation fibrosis
Inferior vena cava obstruction (pelvic edema)
Hemorrhoidal injection

**MISCELLANEOUS DISORDERS**
Urinoma
Lymphocele
Inguinal hernia with rectal traction
Amyloidosis

## TABLE 71–28. ANTERIOR INDENTATION ON THE RECTOSIGMOID JUNCTION

| | |
|---|---|
| Peritoneal metastases (stomach, colon, pancreas, ovary, Blumer's shelf) | Iliac artery aneurysm |
| | Pelvic lipomatosis, |
| Extrinsic invasion from prostate, uterus, bladder, vagina, neoplasms | retroperitoneal fibrosis |
| | Lymphadenopathy |
| Abscess | Surgical sling repair |
| Hematoma | Lymphocele |
| Ascites | Hematocolpos |

## TABLE 71–29. CONGENITAL SYNDROMES ASSOCIATED WITH COLONIC MALROTATION[1-4]

| | |
|---|---|
| Marfan's syndrome | Thoracoabdominal wall defect |
| Mobile cecum | Eagle-Barrett syndrome |
| Prune-belly syndrome | Cornelia de Lange's syndrome |
| Asplenia or polysplenia | Abdominal heterotaxy |
| Trisomy 21 | |

## TABLE 71–30. MURAL THICKENING OF THE COLON ON COMPUTED TOMOGRAPHY, ULTRASOUND, MAGNETIC RESONANCE IMAGING

**NEOPLASMS**
Carcinoma
Lymphoma
Polyposis syndromes
Metastases
Leiomyoma, leiomyosarcoma

**INFLAMMATORY DISORDERS**
Ulcerative colitis
Crohn's disease
Behçet's disease
Diverticulosis, diverticulitis
Typhlitis

**INFECTIOUS DISORDERS**
Pseudomembranous colitis
Amebic colitis

**MISCELLANEOUS DISORDERS**
Intussusception
Hematoma
Low-protein states

## References

1. Chapman S, Nakielny R: Aids to Radiological Differential Diagnosis (2nd ed). London: Bailliere Tindall, 1990.
2. Eisenberg RL: Gastrointestinal Radiology. A Pattern Approach. Philadelphia: JB Lippincott, 1990.
3. Reeder MM: Reeder and Felson's Gamuts in Radiology (3rd ed). New York: Springer-Verlag, 1993.
4. Dähnert W: Radiology Review Manual. Baltimore: Williams & Wilkins, 1991.

# Pediatric Diseases

*Section Editor*

Sandra K. Fernbach, M.D.

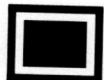

# Applied Embryology of the Gastrointestinal Tract

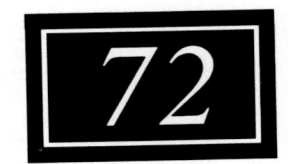

Bruce R. Javors, M.D.
James H. Sloves, M.D.

# INTRODUCTION

The complex anatomy of the gastrointestinal tract and the peritoneal cavity arises from much simpler origins. The transition from the primitive straight tubular alimentary canal to the elongated and tortuous gut (and its accessory organs) suspended by mesenteries and encased by peritoneal reflections can readily be explained by a well-defined series of events. These include cell differentiation and maturation, sometimes rapid and asymmetric rates of growth, turning about multiple axes of rotation, and the partial resorption of tissues.

Although these processes are summarized individually in the following pages, it should be kept in mind that some of these multiple events are occurring simultaneously and with complex interactions. All illustrations have been drawn to correspond to the usual computed tomographic orientation of being viewed from below; this is the reverse of what is usually depicted in anatomy and embryology texts.

# EARLY DEVELOPMENT

After fertilization, the zygote rapidly undergoes repeated mitotic divisions that result in an increased number of cells. This occurs without a corresponding increase in the cell mass.

Approximately 3 days after fertilization, a solid ball of cells (the morula) develops. The following day, central cavities appear, which separate the cells into the trophoblast (from which part of the placenta develops) and the embryoblast. Two days later, endometrial implantation begins.

During the second week of development, the spheric mass of cells flattens into a bilaminar disk. A primitive yolk sac also develops. During the third week, the embryonic disk rapidly develops into the embryo (gastrulation). The cells differentiate into the three classic germ cell layers (endoderm, mesoderm, and ectoderm).

The endoderm gives rise to the lining epithelium of the respiratory and gastrointestinal tracts as well as the glandular elements of the liver and pancreas. From the mesoderm arise the smooth muscle of the gastrointestinal tract, the connective tissues, and their associated blood vessels. Blood cells and their progenitors as well as striated muscles, bone, cartilage, and the reproductive and genitourinary tract are also mesodermal in origin. The ectoderm is the source of the epidermis and the nervous system.

Clefts appear within the lateral aspects of the developing intermediate mesodermal layer, forming the intraembryonic coelom. These open laterally into the yolk sac. They lie between and separate the more dorsal somatic mesoderm from the ventral splanchnic mesoderm.[1] The somatic mesoderm, in association with the ectodermal layer, forms the embryonic body wall (somatopleure); the splanchnic mesoderm, along with the endoderm, forms the embryonic gut (splanchnopleure) (Fig. 72–1).

As the lateral margins of the embryonic disk move

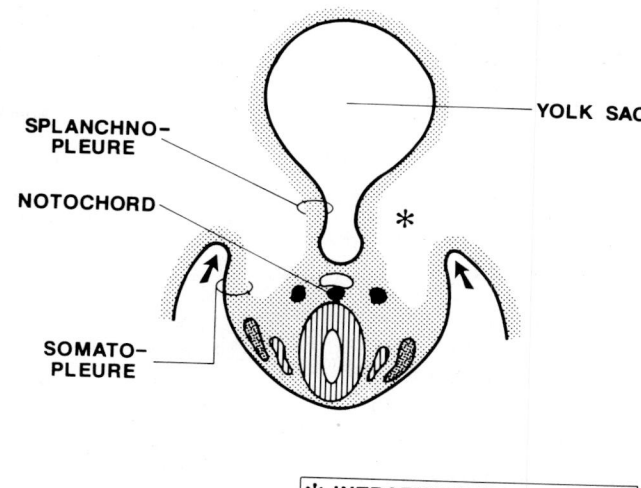

**Figure 72–1. Embryologic development: early fourth week.** Cross section through the midportion of an embryo early in the fourth week shows infolding of the somatopleure as it begins to encase the intraembryonic coelom. This will eventually encompass the body cavity. The splanchnopleure's contribution to the formation of the midgut is evident as well.

ventrally and medially, they begin to pinch off the yolk sac and the more laterally placed intraembryonic coelom. Continued growth by the somatopleure and its eventual midline fusion complete the encompassment of the intraembryonic coelom with formation of a cylindric body cavity. The more centrally placed splanchnopleure also starts to close ventrally, partially separating the primary yolk sac into the gut and the secondary yolk sac (separated by the yolk stalk) (Fig. 72–2).

Thus, a primitive alimentary tube is formed within the larger surrounding body cavity. The dorsal mesentery and its visceral peritoneum are derived from the splanchnopleure. The ventral mesentery is also derived from this structure except about the yolk stalk, where the fusion of the lateral margins of the splanchnopleure is still incomplete. Most of the ventral mesentery (except in the caudal foregut) degenerates with time, leaving a large embryonic body (coelomic) cavity.[2]

# DIVISION OF THE INTRAEMBRYONIC COELOM AND FORMATION OF THE DIAPHRAGM

During the fourth to sixth weeks, the large common intraembryonic coelomic cavity is partitioned into the pleural, pericardial, and peritoneal spaces. By the fourth week, a large pericardial cavity is connected to the peritoneal cavity by two smaller pericardioperitoneal canals. The pressure of the developing head fold (convex curvature and growth of the cranial end of the embryo) causes the heart and pericardial cavity to be displaced caudally and ventrally. The pericardioperitoneal canals exit from the pericardium along its dorsal aspect to enter the peritoneum.

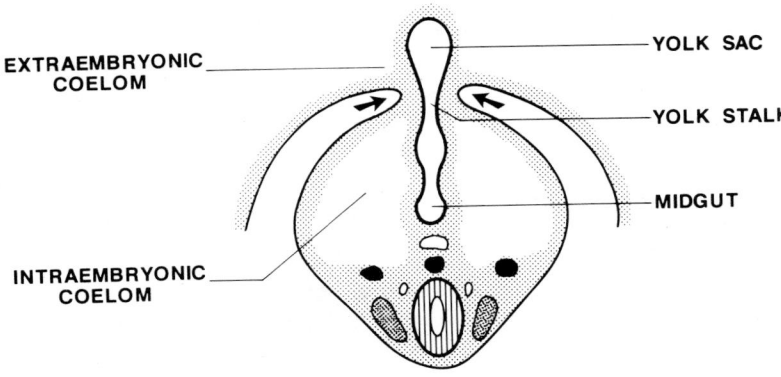

EXTRAEMBRYONIC
COELOM

YOLK SAC

YOLK STALK

MIDGUT

INTRAEMBRYONIC
COELOM

**Figure 72–2. Embryologic development: late fourth week.** Similar cross section as in Figure 72–1 but at the end of the fourth week of development. The envelopment of the intraembryonic coelom is almost complete. The yolk sac has now separated into a more definitive yolk stalk and midgut as well.

As the lung buds develop, they grow into the paired pericardioperitoneal canals. This produces two pairs of ridges. The cranial pair gives rise to the pleuropericardial membrane that eventually separates the primitive pericardial cavity into the definitive pericardial and pleural spaces.

The more caudal pair gives rise to the pleuroperitoneal membrane. This plays an important role in the development of the diaphragm. As the lung buds grow superiorly and the liver and peritoneal space expand inferiorly, these membranes become more prominent. They attach themselves to the abdominal wall along their dorsal and lateral margins. Their free edges project into the pericardioperitoneal canals.

During the sixth week, these free edges of the dorsolateral pleuroperitoneal membrane fuse with the midline dorsal mesentery of the esophagus (now forming part of the primitive mediastinum). The anterior half of the primitive diaphragm is formed by the septum transversum. This structure first arises in the third week as a condensation of mesoderm. By the fourth week, it has thickened to form an incomplete division anteriorly between the pericardium and the peritoneal cavity (Fig. 72–3).

From the 6th to the 12th weeks, many changes take place in the relative contributions of these structures to the diaphragm that exists at birth. The large dorsolateral component formed by the pleuroperitoneal membranes decreases in size. Myoblasts from the abdominal wall migrate into the peripheral aspects of the membranes, which contributes to the growth of the diaphragm. These muscular elements eventually give rise to the costophrenic sulci. Myoblasts also grow into the primitive dorsal esophageal mesentery, forming the diaphragmatic crura. Thus, four separate elements (septum transversum, pleuroperitoneal membranes, dorsal mesentery of the esophagus, and the body wall) all contribute to the final formation of the diaphragm.

In addition to its complex formation, the diaphragm markedly shifts in position. Initially (in the fourth week), the septum transversum is at the level of the third to fifth cervical somites. The myoblasts and associated nerve innervation arise from these levels as well. From the fourth to the sixth weeks, the dorsal part of the embryo grows rapidly, which causes an apparent descent or inferior migration of the diaphragm. The mesenchyme of the septum transversum contributes its own myoblasts to the diaphragm, continuing its original C-3 to C-5 innervation. Thus, in its definitive state, the diaphragm lies at the level of the thoracolumbar junction while maintaining its phrenic nerve innervation from the midcervical level.

## ANOMALIES OF DIAPHRAGMATIC DEVELOPMENT

### Diaphragmatic Hernia

If the pleuroperitoneal membrane fails to close entirely, a patent canal may persist between the pleural and peritoneal cavities. If this dorsal and laterally placed canal is still present at the time of the reduction of the physiologic herniation of the midgut (week 10; see later), the returning bowel may herniate through this patent foramen of Bochdalek into the chest. This occurs most frequently on the left side.[2]

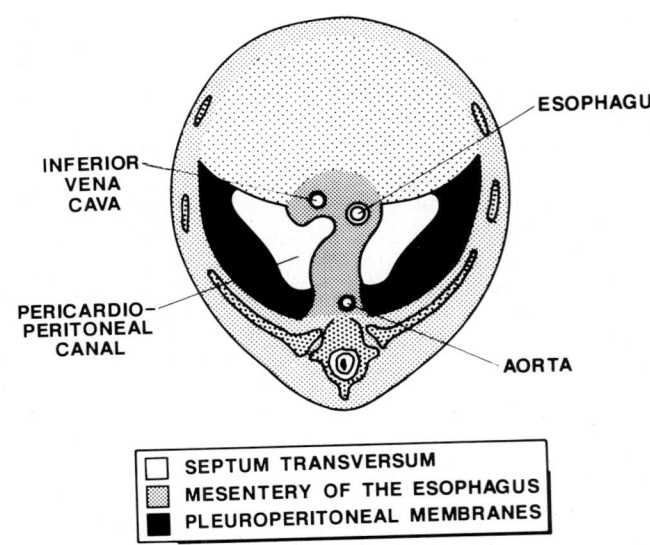

ESOPHAGUS

INFERIOR
VENA
CAVA

PERICARDIO-
PERITONEAL
CANAL

AORTA

☐ SEPTUM TRANSVERSUM
▨ MESENTERY OF THE ESOPHAGUS
■ PLEUROPERITONEAL MEMBRANES

**Figure 72–3. Embryologic development: fifth week.** Diagram of a 5-week embryo as seen from below. The relative contributions of the septum transversum, esophageal mesentery, and pleuroperitoneal membranes will change with further development.

## Foramen of Morgagni Hernia

A natural weakness in the anteromedial portion of the diaphragm (retrosternal) is caused by the passage of the superior epigastric vessels. Herniation of omentum or intestines may occur at this site. This occurs most frequently on the right side.[3]

## Eventration

Defective muscular development of the dome of the diaphragm may lead to structural weakness and subsequent ballooning. Only a thin aponeurotic sheet of tissue then separates the pleural cavity from the peritoneal space. With the increased intra-abdominal pressure, abdominal contents bulge into the thoracic cavity. This does not represent a true herniation, but it may be difficult to differentiate from that entity.

## NORMAL LIVER DEVELOPMENT

During the fourth week of development, the caudal portion of the foregut develops a ventral bud of endoderm called the liver bud (primordial hepatic diverticulum). The liver bud enlarges and grows into and between the two layers of the ventral mesentery. More superiorly, it grows in contact with and into the mass of mesenchyme, the septum transversum, which also contributes to the formation of the diaphragm (see earlier). The ventral liver bud divides into cranial and caudal portions within the mesentery. The cranial portion gives rise to the liver and intrahepatic bile ducts; the caudal portion forms the gallbladder and cystic duct.[4]

The cranial liver bud further divides into right and left lobes, which are initially of equal size. The right lobe eventually becomes much larger than the left. The distal branches of the right and left lobe cords undergo canalization to become the definitive main right and left hepatic ducts. The intrahepatic biliary tree is thought to arise from the hepatic parenchyme. These cords of tissue extend along the randomly created pattern of portal vein tributaries (see later). Consequently, the pattern of intrahepatic bile ducts is quite variable.

In the embryo, the liver is a major site of hematopoiesis, which begins in the sixth week. By the fourth to fifth month, bile is formed and passes into the duodenum. This gives meconium its characteristic color.

The mature liver has two ligaments that represent remnants of embryologic vascular channels. These are the ligamentum teres (round ligament) within the falciform ligament and the ligamentum venosum. These develop from the vitelline and umbilical veins, respectively. The paired vitelline veins drain the yolk sac, pass through the developing liver and septum transversum, and empty into the right side of the primitive heart (sinus venosus). The vitelline veins within the liver create a mesh-like network of vascular channels that become the hepatic sinusoids. Some of the lining cells of the sinusoids later differentiate into macrophages (Kupffer cells), the reticuloendothelial component of the liver.[5] The segments of the vitelline veins proximal and distal to the sinusoids become, respectively, the hepatic veins and hepatic portion of the portal vein.[6]

The paired umbilical veins drain the placenta and chorion. They pass through the septum transversum, contributing minimally to hepatic sinusoidal development, and then empty into the sinus venosus. The entire right umbilical vein and a segment of the left proximal (cephalad) to the liver atrophy. A large venous channel, the ductus venosus, arises from the hepatic sinusoidal network and carries blood from the distal (caudal) left umbilical vein into the sinus venosus, bypassing the liver. Eventually the lumen of the ductus venosus is obliterated, and the structure becomes the ligamentum venosum. The distal portion of the left umbilical vein migrates medially to the liver edge, and its lumen closes. It then becomes the round ligament (ligamentum teres). This ligament, which connects the ligamentum venosum to the umbilicus, is encased within the most anterior portion of the ventral mesentery, the falciform ligament[7] (Fig. 72–4).

The mesenchymal septum transversum contributes to the ventral mesentery that surrounds the liver and gallbladder. The fibrous tissue of the liver including Glisson's capsule, embryonal hepatic hematopoietic tissues, and the Kupffer cells lining the sinusoids are also derived from the septum transversum.[7]

The membranous ventral mesentery is a double layered structure that encloses the liver and gallbladder to become their visceral peritoneum. The cephalic portion of the liver directly contacts the septum transversum (part of the future diaphragm) and therefore is not enveloped by the ventral mesentery. This region is devoid of a peritoneal covering and is known as the bare area of the liver (see Fig. 72–4). The visceral peritoneum reflects off the liver onto the undersurface of the diaphragm as the coronary ligaments outlining this region.

## ABNORMAL LIVER DEVELOPMENT

### Atypical Segmentation

Although congenital malformations of the liver are rare, variations of lobulation are not infrequent. A bipartite liver results from an exaggerated separation of the lobes, which may actually represent congenital absence of the medial segment of the left lobe.[8]

An absent right lobe of the liver may be secondary to maldevelopment of the portal vein or the primordial hepatic diverticulum proper.[9, 10] A portal venous abnormality may account for an absent left lobe. Multilobar livers (as many as 16) may also be seen.[7] Hepatic anomalies are further discussed in Chapter 104.

### Atypical Location

Hepatic lobes can develop in the thorax, and when they have a separate mesentery, they may undergo

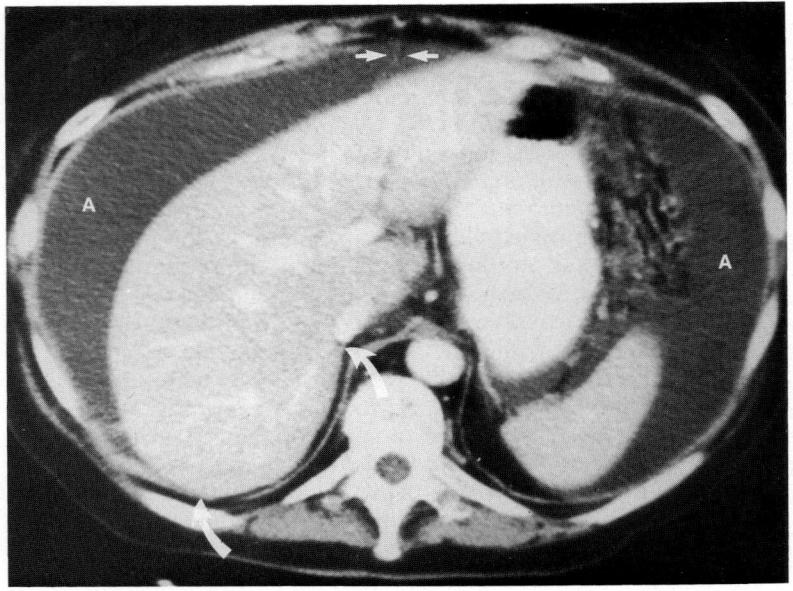

**Figure 72–4. Falciform ligament and bare area of liver.** Computed tomographic scan of the upper abdomen shows a large amount of ascites (A) outlining the falciform ligament _(arrows)_. Along the posterior aspect of the right lobe, there is a region not surrounded by the fluid, the bare area _(curved arrows)_. This represents that portion of the liver that developed in contact with the septum transversum and thus is not covered by the peritoneum.

torsion.[11] Heterotopic liver tissue can also be found within structures that share a common site of embryologic development: gallbladder, pancreas, umbilical cord, and gastrohepatic ligament.[12]

## NORMAL GALLBLADDER AND BILE DUCT DEVELOPMENT

As noted, the fourth week of embryogenesis is marked by the appearance of the hepatic diverticulum. This is then divided into both cranial and caudal buds. The caudal bud forms the gallbladder, the cystic duct, and the extrahepatic bile ducts. The development of these structures precedes that of the intrahepatic ducts by several weeks.

The common bile duct develops as a cord connecting the cystic duct and main hepatic ducts to the descending duodenum (second portion). The hollow gallbladder and common bile duct primordia become occluded with proliferating endoderm during the fifth week. They recanalize by vacuolization and cell degeneration by the end of that week. The recanalization of the common bile duct precedes that of the gallbladder and duodenum. As the duodenum rotates 90 degrees to the right, the common bile duct rotates an additional 180 degrees along with the ventral pancreatic anlage. Thus, the common duct is carried from its original ventral position to the right, then posteriorly, and finally to the medial aspect of the duodenal sweep.

The gallbladder and intrahepatic ducts also communicate via the cystohepatic ducts of Luschka during fetal life. These ducts usually atrophy in the adult but may remain patent in some patients. When they persist and are not recognized during cholecystectomy, a significant bile leak may result.[13]

Vacuoles in the wall of the duodenum coalesce to form two separate channels and then one single lumen

for the adjacent common bile and main pancreatic ducts. Within the wall of the duodenum are primitive ampullary tissues that enlarge and displace the junction of the two ducts away from the duodenal lumen. However, this displacement is impeded and actually reversed by the growth of the smooth muscle layer of the duodenal wall. These factors account for the considerable variability seen in the junction of these two structures.[14, 15]

## ABNORMAL GALLBLADDER AND BILE DUCT DEVELOPMENT

### Phrygian Cap

This abnormal shape of the gallbladder actually represents a folding of the fundus on itself and is not truly pathologic.

### Gallbladder Diverticulum

This true diverticulum (containing all normal wall elements) probably is the remnant of the cystohepatic duct. It can be a site of bile stasis and stone formation (see Chapter 89).[16]

### Positional Anomalies

The most common anomaly of gallbladder position is that of a "wandering" or "floating" gallbladder. These represent elongation of the mesenteric attachment of the gallbladder to the undersurface of the liver with subsequent excessive mobility. The gallbladder may be left sided, herniate into the lesser sac, undergo torsion, or be located in the transverse mesocolon, in the falciform ligament, in the perihepatic spaces, or intrahepatically (see Chapter 89).[7, 16–19]

## Bifid Gallbladder/Duplication

A bifid gallbladder has two cavities but only one cystic duct. Duplicated or even triplicated gallbladders each have their own cystic duct. These entities may be secondary to a persistent outpouching of the extrahepatic duct or incomplete recanalization of the gallbladder.[5, 7, 16, 18] Incomplete recanalization may also give rise to a septated gallbladder (see Chapter 87).[7, 20]

## Agenesis

This rare entity is secondary to lack of development of the caudal portion of the liver bud or improper recanalization of the gallbladder.[6, 7, 18, 21] It may be associated with a host of other anomalies affecting many other organ systems (see Chapter 89).

## Tracheobiliary Fistula

In this entity, the biliary tree (usually the left main hepatic duct) is connected to the carinal region. The combination of bile-stained sputum and pneumobilia is characteristic.[7, 18, 22]

## Biliary Atresia

In this disorder, the number of intrahepatic bile ducts is decreased. This may develop primarily or secondary to alpha$_1$-antitrypsin deficiency, cystic fibrosis, and viral hepatitis (see Chapter 137).[23]

## Alagille's Syndrome

This autosomal dominant syndrome of arteriohepatic dysplasia is characterized by paucity of bile ducts, peripheral pulmonic stenosis, vertebral anomalies, and mental and physical retardation (see Chapter 137).[24]

## Cystic Disease

There is an entire spectrum of diseases ranging from intrahepatic cysts or fibrosis to renal disease. Various patterns of inheritance are also present. Within the liver, cysts attributable to defective development of the intrahepatic ducts may be present. In other forms, bile duct hyperplasia and portal fibrosis may predominate (see Chapters 89 and 137).

## Caroli's Disease

This nonfamilial entity is characterized by segmental cystic dilatation of the intrahepatic bile ducts. It may represent an intermediate form of disease between congenital hepatic fibrosis and choledochal cysts.[18] A possible cause is perinatal hepatic artery occlusion.[25] Multiple episodes of cholangitis may occur secondary to bile stasis (see Chapter 89).

## Choledochal Cysts

Multiple theories have been proposed to explain the etiology of choledochal cysts.[26–28] These include distal biliary ductal obstruction with subsequent weakening and ballooning of the wall, an anomalous course of the bile duct through the duodenal wall, and a deficient development of the bile duct wall. Additional theories include a high junction of the bile and pancreatic ducts, which allows reflux of pancreatic enzymes up the common bile duct with resultant cholangitis and dilatation. Yet another theory suggests an excess quantity of epithelial cells in the primitive choledochus followed by recanalization leading to cyst formation. Viral infection leading to infantile obstructive cholangiopathy is a widely favored theory.

Whatever the theory, choledochal cysts are found more often in Asians and in females. Five classic radiographic types have been identified.[29] The most common type is aneurysmal dilatation of the common duct, often seen extending into the cystic duct and the main hepatic ducts as well. The second and rarest form is that of a diverticulum that projects off the distal common duct. The third form is that of a choledochocele, which represents a dilatation of the distal common bile duct that protrudes into the duodenum. This last form may also be explained by its being a congenital duplication cyst of the duodenum through which the common duct courses (see Chapter 89).[30]

Two other types may be included in the classification of choledochal cysts. One is multifocal segmental dilatation involving both the intra- and extrahepatic ducts. The other is Caroli's disease (see earlier).

# NORMAL DEVELOPMENT OF THE ESOPHAGUS

During the latter half of the fourth week of embryonic development, the respiratory system develops as a ventral bud of the foregut. The laryngotracheal groove forms along the caudal end of the primitive pharynx. This groove deepens and evaginates to form the laryngotracheal diverticulum. Longitudinal (tracheoesophageal) folds eventually separate the primordial ventral respiratory apparatus from the dorsal gastrointestinal tract (esophagus).

When initially formed, the esophagus is relatively short. Changes in body growth in general and in the heart and lungs in particular contribute to the elongation of the esophagus.

The endodermal elements of the esophagus (epithelium and epithelial glands) proliferate, which leads to obliteration of the hollow lumen. This cellular plug is successfully resorbed by the end of the fetal period (eighth week).

# ABNORMAL DEVELOPMENT OF THE ESOPHAGUS

## Tracheoesophageal Fistula

Partial fusion of the tracheoesophageal folds leads to incomplete separation of the respiratory and gastrointestinal tracts (tracheoesophageal fistula). This is usually accompanied by some narrowing of the associated lumens (esophageal atresia). This common anomaly is further discussed in Chapter 74.

## Duplication

During the period of recanalization, there may be incomplete resorption of the endothelial plug.[31] This may result in a duplication of the esophagus (see Chapters 75 and 79). The usual noncommunicating duplication cyst resembles any other submucosal mass on routine esophagrams. Computed tomography or endoscopic sonography can document its cystic nature. The lumen of the cyst will rarely open into the normal esophagus (communicating duplication).

## Stenosis

Either web-like narrowing or long segmental strictures may occur in the distal esophagus from incomplete recanalization (see Chapter 75).[32]

## Esophageal Bronchus

The development of an esophageal bronchus is further evidence of the common origin of the respiratory and gastrointestinal tracts. In this entity, a branching bronchus arises from the esophagus. This is usually in association with a pulmonary sequestration.[33]

## Congenital Short Esophagus

If the esophagus does not proportionally elongate as the body grows, a congenital short esophagus occurs.[32] This is seen at birth in association with a hiatal hernia. This markedly differs in pathogenesis from the acquired form of hiatal hernia found in the adult.

# NORMAL DEVELOPMENT OF THE STOMACH, DUODENUM, AND LESSER OMENTUM

At the midpoint of the fetal period (end of the fourth week), the primitive stomach is still a straight, hollow tube in the midsagittal plane. During the next 2 weeks, the site of the future stomach starts to dilate. This dilatation starts in a fusiform manner but then accelerates with preferential growth of its dorsal wall. This

causes the formation of a marked dorsal bulge (the origin of the greater curvature).

During the sixth to eighth weeks of development, the stomach rotates along two different axes simultaneously. The first and major rotation is about the longitudinal axis, which causes the dorsal bulge to now form the lateral border of the stomach. The former ventral aspect now forms the medial wall (lesser curvature) of the stomach.[32] This rotation accounts for the fact that the left vagus nerve in the adult innervates the anterior wall of the stomach, whereas the right innervates the posterior wall (Fig. 72–5).

The second rotation is about the anteroposterior axis. The pressure from the enlarging liver in the abdomen contributes to this rotation. In this stage, the stomach shifts from a purely longitudinal orientation to one more transverse. This results in the greater curvature convexity's being directed inferiorly and laterally; the lesser curvature is concave superiorly and medially. There is great variability in the final configuration of the stomach, ranging from a transverse position just underneath the diaphragm to a longitudinal one, with the greater curvature reaching and even descending below the level of the iliac crest.

The ventral mesentery persists in the distal foregut into adulthood. The role of this structure in the forma-

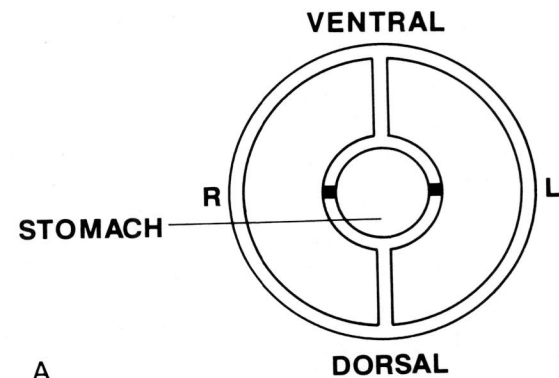

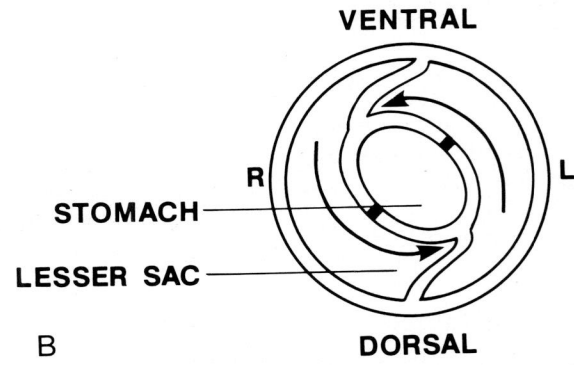

**Figure 72–5. Gastric rotation and formation of lesser sac. A** and **B.** Schematic cross-sectional diagrams depicting the rotation of the stomach about the body's longitudinal axis. The left vagus nerve is carried to the anterior wall of the stomach. The extension of the right peritoneal space posterior to the stomach starts the formation of the lesser sac.

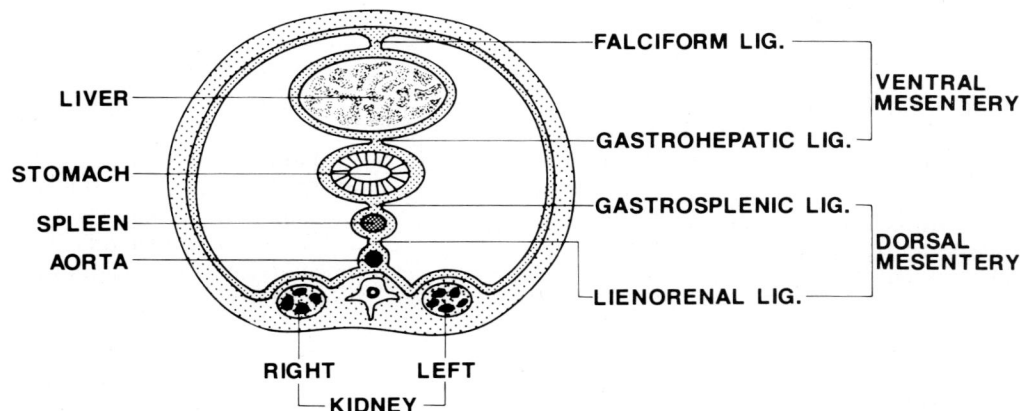

**Figure 72–6. Embryologic origins of mesenteries and supporting ligaments.** A cross section through a 5-week embryo at the level of the liver shows the paired superior peritoneum (right and left) separated by both the ventral and dorsal mesenteries. Even at this stage of development, the origins of many of the suspensory ligaments of the adult are clearly demonstrated.

tion of the liver and the falciform ligament is discussed in the preceding. However, the ventral mesentery also continues to connect the lesser curvature of the stomach (former ventral wall) to the undersurface of the liver at the junction of the caudate lobe and the lateral segment of the left lobe as the gastrohepatic ligament[34] (Fig. 72–6). Within this structure lie the left gastric artery, coronary veins, and multiple lymph nodes. In the duodenum, the more caudal portion of the lesser omentum forms the hepatoduodenal ligament. Within the free edge of the lesser omentum lie the hepatic artery, portal vein, common hepatic and bile ducts, and lymph nodes.[35] This free edge forms one of the borders of the foramen of Winslow, which separates the lesser peritoneal sac from the greater peritoneal cavity.

The dorsal mesentery likewise persists into adulthood and has a major role in the formation of the greater omentum and lesser sac (see later). The major blood supply of the foregut (celiac axis) arises from the dorsal aorta and passes through the dorsal mesentery.

As the stomach forms as a dorsal bulge in the fourth and fifth weeks, the duodenum forms as a ventral bulge. The proximal portion of the duodenum (from the pylorus to just past the papilla) is derived from the foregut. Therefore, it maintains its blood supply from the celiac axis (the major foregut artery). The remainder of the duodenum is derived from the midgut. Consequently, it is supplied by the superior mesenteric artery (major artery of the midgut).

With gastric rotation, the duodenum also changes in position. The concave border formerly directed dorsally now is open to the left (the classic C loop) as the convexity points to the right. The dorsal mesentery is subsequently resorbed, leaving a covering of visceral peritoneum along its anterior surface. This loss of mesenteric attachment accounts for the final "retroperitoneal" location of the duodenum distal to the bulb.

## ABNORMAL DEVELOPMENT OF THE STOMACH AND DUODENUM

### Antral Web

This thin, concentric narrowing of the antrum is composed of mucosa and submucosa (Fig. 72–7). It may be congenital in origin (recanalization error) or be associated with peptic ulcer disease.[36]

### Gastric Diverticula

These usually occur high on the posterior wall of the fundus. Some are true diverticula, and others are pseudodiverticula with an absence of a muscular wall.[36] The constancy of position suggests an underlying, perhaps congenital basis.

### Duplications

Usually found along the greater curvature, these noncommunicating cystic masses may vary greatly in size (see Chapter 79).[36, 37]

### Duodenal Stenosis

Duodenal stenosis manifests as a narrowing of variable length, usually in the third and fourth portions. It may result from faulty recanalization (see Chapter 76).[32]

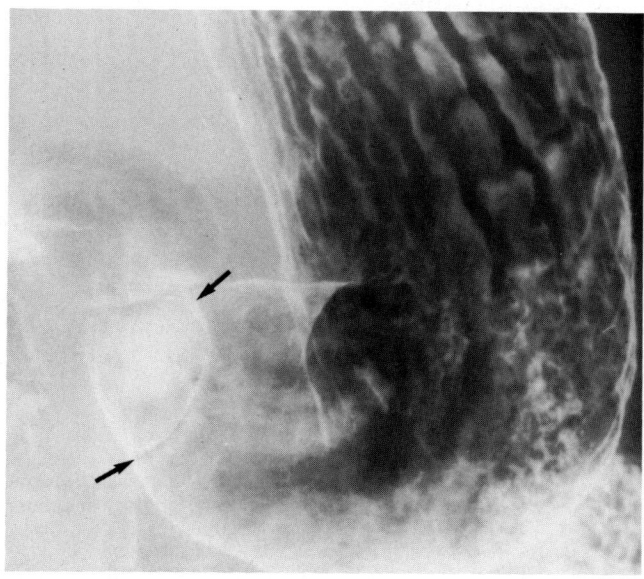

**Figure 72–7. Antral web.** There is a thin, linear, nonobstructive defect *(arrows)* in the gastric antrum.

## Duodenal Web and Inverted Diverticulum

As in the antrum, a thin, narrow band of tissue may partially block the duodenum. With the continued pressure of peristalsis propelling intestinal contents, this web may stretch and balloon into a sac-like structure within the normal duodenal lumen. This has been called an inverted diverticulum or "wind sock" deformity (see Chapter 76).[38]

## NORMAL DEVELOPMENT OF THE PANCREAS

The endoderm of the caudal foregut also produces both dorsal and ventral pancreatic buds during the fourth week of development. The dorsal bud appears first and lies cephalad to the ventral anlage. The dorsal bud rapidly grows into the dorsal mesentery (mesoduodenum). It gives rise to the body and tail of the pancreas. The more caudal ventral pancreatic bud develops from the hepatic diverticulum. This bud is originally bifid, but the left side atrophies while the right side persists to form the uncinate process and the head of the pancreas.[39, 40]

As the duodenum rotates 90 degrees to the right, the dorsal pancreatic bud and its mesentery are carried along in the concavity of the primitive duodenal sweep (see earlier). They are ultimately situated along the left (medial) margin of the descending duodenum. The common bile duct and the right side of the ventral pancreatic anlage also complete this 90-degree rotation while undergoing an additional 180-degree rotation of their own. Therefore, they too come to lie along the

concavity of the duodenal sweep after rotating through a total of 270 degrees (Fig. 72–8A and B).

Eventually, the dorsal mesentery of the duodenum (mesoduodenum) fuses with the posterior peritoneal wall. This results in the retroperitoneal location of the pancreas. However, a small portion of the tail of the pancreas lies in a portion of the mesogastrium (dorsal mesentery of the stomach) that sometimes is not fully resorbed and therefore maintains its intraperitoneal location near the hilum of the spleen.[39]

During the sixth week of embryogenesis, the parenchyma of the ventral and dorsal buds as well as their ducts unite. The main pancreatic duct (Wirsung), which empties through the main papilla, is therefore derived from the ventral anlage in the head of the pancreas and the dorsal anlage in the body and tail (Fig. 72–8C). The accessory duct (Santorini's) is derived from the distal aspect of the dorsal anlage and in 10% of patients empties via the minor papilla.[39] In the remaining cases, the main pancreatic duct is the predominant excretory pathway as the two ductal systems communicate.

The exocrine pancreatic tissue is derived from both pancreatic buds that produce tubules. Vesicles form at the ends of these tubules, which give rise to acini. The endocrine islets of Langerhans also derive from the endoderm.[39] The splanchnic mesenchyme adjacent to the pancreas provides the connective tissue stroma of the pancreas.[32]

## ABNORMAL DEVELOPMENT OF THE PANCREAS

### Annular Pancreas

In this unusual anomaly, the descending duodenum is surrounded by a band of pancreatic tissue[39, 40] (Fig. 72–

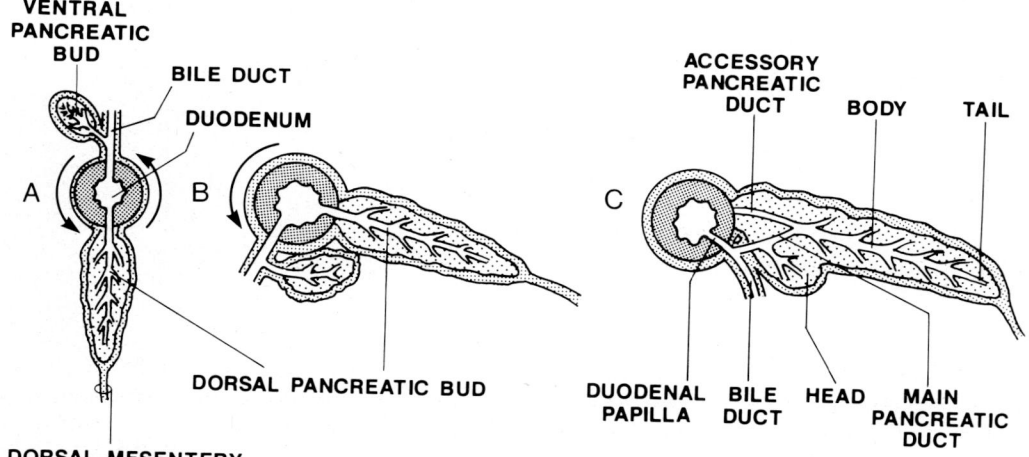

**Figure 72–8. Stages of pancreatic development: superior perspective. A.** Starting in the fourth week, the ventral pancreatic anlage rotates 180 degrees (first to the right and then posteriorly) as the duodenum rotates 90 degrees as well. This results in a total rotation of 270 degrees, with the original ventral anlage coming to the left of the duodenum. This rotation also carries the distal common bile duct posterior to the duodenum. **B.** The dorsal anlage is carried along by the duodenal rotation so that it too lies to the left of the duodenum. **C.** By the seventh to eighth week, the ducts of the two pancreatic buds fuse with the ventral pancreas, contributing the distal portion of the main pancreatic duct. Most of the proximal main duct arises from the dorsal anlage.

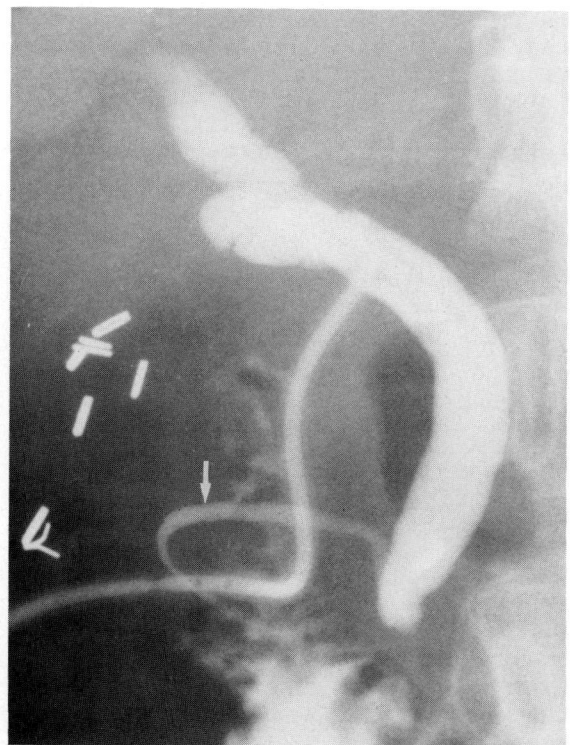

**Figure 72–9. Annular pancreas.** T tube cholangiogram shows reflux into a circumduodenal pancreatic duct *(arrow)*, confirming the presence of an annular pancreas.

9). In approximately 15% of cases, other levels of the duodenum may be involved. Annular pancreas is most often found in males and may be associated with other congenital anomalies in up to 75% of cases (see Chapter 115).

The originally bifid ventral pancreatic bud is thought to be the cause of this abnormality. In one theory, the left bud persists and helps contribute to the ring of tissue around the duodenum.[41] Another theory proposes that the tip of the right bud abnormally adheres to the duodenum as both it and the anlage rotate, thereby stretching and wrapping the pancreatic tissue around the duodenum.[39, 40]

## Pancreas Divisum

This entity is caused by failure of the dorsal and ventral pancreatic buds to unite. This allows the uncinate process and a portion of the head to be drained by a short and narrow caliber main pancreatic duct (Wirsung's) via the major papilla. The tail, the body, and a small portion of the head are drained by the accessory pancreatic duct (Santorini's) via the minor papilla that lies cephalad and ventral to the major papilla. Although pancreas divisum may be an incidental finding, the narrow opening of the minor papilla may predispose these patients to pancreatitis (see Chapter 115).[42]

## Ectopic Pancreatic Tissue

Small islands of pancreatic tissue may grow along the greater curvature of the antrum or medial aspect of the duodenal sweep with formation of submucosal nodules.[36, 38] Other sites of involvement, including the omentum, have also been reported (see Chapter 115). Fully developed ducts are extremely rare.

## NORMAL DEVELOPMENT OF THE LESSER SAC AND GREATER OMENTUM

With the resorption of the ventral mesentery along the midgut and its persistence along the distal foregut, the abdomen is divided into paired (left and right) cephalic peritoneal spaces and a larger, common one more caudally.

As the primitive stomach develops and its dorsal bulge occurs (see earlier), the dorsal mesentery (mesogastrium) with its accompanying vascular supply starts to elongate markedly. The dorsal bulge of the stomach along with its elongated mesogastrium is carried along during the gastric rotation described before. This causes the right half of the paired cephalic peritoneal space to extend posterior to the stomach into the left upper quadrant, forming the lesser sac (see Fig. 72–5).

The most dorsal aspect of this elongated mesogastrium (containing the spleen) eventually fuses partially with the posterior abdominal wall, which accounts for the retroperitoneal course of the splenic artery[35] (Fig. 72–10). The more ventral portion of the elongated and now

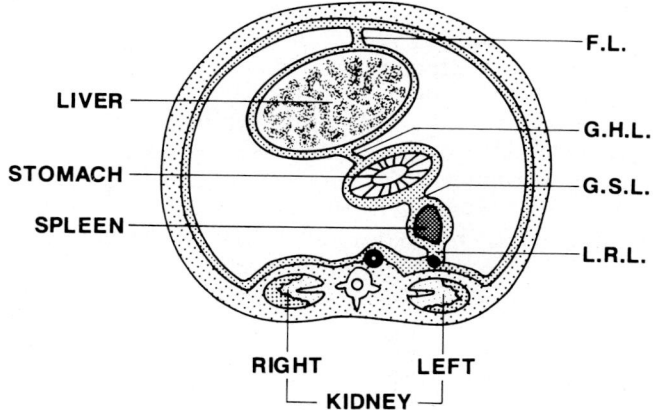

**Figure 72–10. Rotation of the mesogastrium.** Schematic cross-sectional diagram through the upper abdomen reveals continued rotation of the elongated mesogastrium containing the splenic bud. This rotation brings the dorsal mesentery to lie along the posterior abdominal wall. Eventual involution and fusion of the mesentery leaves the lienorenal ligament (L.R.L.) as its remnant. The gastrosplenic ligament (G.S.L.) forms one of the lateral borders of the lesser sac. The gastrohepatic ligament (G.H.L.) persists as the lesser omentum. The falciform ligament (F.L.) continues to separate the right side of the peritoneum from the left, anteriorly and superiorly in the subphrenic space.

redundant mesogastrium projects anteriorly and inferiorly. It hangs from the greater curvature (former dorsal wall) of the stomach and overlies the transverse colon and mesenteric small bowel. It then loops back on itself to rejoin its already fused dorsal component at the posterior abdominal wall (Fig. 72–11A).

With the fusion of the two leaves of this redundant apron of mesentery, the space between the two layers (inferior recess of the lesser sac) is eventually obliterated. Thus, a single thick structure, the greater omentum (composed of four layers of peritoneum), hangs like an apron over much of the peritoneal cavity. As it passes over the transverse colon and its dorsal mesentery (mesocolon), the greater omentum partially fuses with these two structures[32, 35] (Fig. 72–11B). Ventrally, this gives rise to the gastrocolic ligament as the greater omentum adheres to the superior aspect of the transverse colon. Dorsally, the mesogastrium and mesocolon fuse to form the definitive transverse mesocolon.[32, 35] This delineates the inferior border of the lesser sac. The transverse mesocolon takes rise over the pancreas and may act as a pathway for the spread of disease from the retroperitoneal pancreas to the intraperitoneal colon.[43]

The entry point from the greater peritoneum into the lesser sac is the foramen of Winslow. This is bordered by the free edge of the hepatoduodenal ligament (lesser omentum) ventrally, the caudate lobe of the liver superiorly, the inferior vena cava posteriorly, and a reflection of peritoneum from the pyloroduodenal region inferiorly.[44]

The spleen also develops within the elongated mesogastrium. The spleen divides the stomach's dorsal mesentery into two components. These both contribute to the lateral borders of the lesser sac. The lienorenal ligament represents the fusion of the dorsal portion of the spleen containing mesogastrium to the retroperitoneum. The gastrosplenic ligament represents the more ventral remnant of the spleen's mesenteric origin between the stomach and posterior abdominal wall[44] (see Fig. 72–10).

The course of the left gastric artery and the raised peritoneal ridge overlying it divide the lesser sac into two compartments. The smaller, medial compartment contains the submerged (subdiaphragmatic) portion of the esophagus. Therefore, inflammatory exudate in the medial lesser peritoneal sac may extend transdiaphragmatically through the esophageal hiatus into the mediastinum.

## ABNORMAL DEVELOPMENT OF THE LESSER SAC AND GREATER OMENTUM

### Infracardiac Bursa

Rarely, a persistent communication exists at the level of the diaphragm, with the medial lesser peritoneal sac extending into the mediastinum. This forms an infracardiac cystic space medial to the right lung.[32]

### Omental Cyst

A mesenchyme-lined omental cyst can develop within the leaves of the greater omentum. It most likely represents incomplete obliteration of the inferior recess of the greater omentum during the fusion of its redundant layers. Histologic differentiation of mesenteric, omental, duplication, and neurenteric cysts is based on their respective cell linings as well as their wall constituents.[45, 46]

## NORMAL DEVELOPMENT OF THE SPLEEN

The spleen develops from the mesenchyme within the dorsal mesentery of the stomach (mesogastrium) during the fifth week of development. Initially, several distinct clusters of mesenchyme are formed. These masses coalesce and fuse to form the spleen, which develops its characteristic shape by the third month. The fusion of the mesenchymal clusters leads to a lobulated contour of the spleen. Before birth, the splenic contour smoothes; only a few notches are left along its anterosuperior border. The mesenchyme forms the reticular framework, trabeculae, and capsule of the spleen. The T and B lymphocytes migrate to the spleen after arising

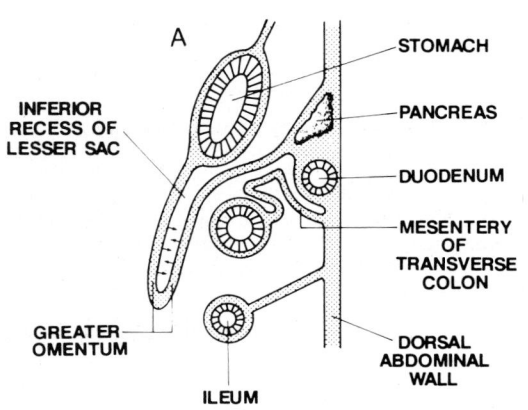

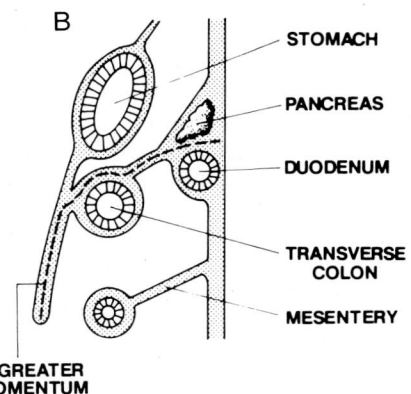

**Figure 72–11. Formation of the greater omentum. A.** Longitudinal schematic drawing showing the fusion of the two leaves of the greater omentum with obliteration of the inferior recess of the lesser sac. **B.** Fusion of the greater omentum with the transverse colon and its dorsal mesentery gives rise to the definitive gastrocolic ligament and transverse mesocolon.

in the bone marrow. By the fourth month, the spleen is producing megakaryocytes and other blood cell precursors as part of its hematopoietic activity. The level of this production decreases during the eighth month, but this capacity is retained in the adult mature spleen. The formation of the ligamentous attachments of the spleen is discussed earlier.

## ABNORMAL DEVELOPMENT OF THE SPLEEN

### Accessory Spleen

Accessory spleen refers to congenitally derived ectopic splenic tissue (see Chapter 124). This is separate and distinct from splenosis, which is ectopic splenic tissue secondary to trauma and subsequent implantation and growth of splenic fragments. Accessory spleens may result from failure of the splenic mesenchymal clusters to fuse within the dorsal mesentery (mesogastrium).[47] Alternatively, exaggerated lobulation of the spleen may cause tissue to be pinched off and separated from the main spleen.[48] Some 10 to 30% of the population has accessory splenic tissue.[32, 47] It is most commonly found in the splenic hilum. Other common sites include the splenic ligaments, pancreas, and elsewhere in the retroperitoneum.[49] Usually only one accessory spleen is present. In some patients, there is an association between an accessory spleen and hematologic disorder.[50]

### Wandering Spleen

This rare anomaly occurs in less than 0.2% of all patients.[47] It is most commonly found in multiparous women.[51, 52] In this entity, the spleen has an unusual degree of mobility within the abdominal cavity and often has an atypical location (see Chapter 124). Wandering spleen has been associated with incomplete fusion or even absence of the gastrosplenic and lienorenal ligaments (remnants of the primitive mesogastrium).[53, 54] However, its association with splenomegaly and its increased frequency in postpartum women suggests an acquired cause.[55] The exaggerated mobility of the spleen may predispose to torsion and subsequent infarction.

### Asplenia

When isolated absence of the spleen is encountered without accompanying abnormalities, it is usually of an acquired nature.[56, 57] However, it occurs more frequently in males with a complex constellation of congenital abnormalities involving the cardiovascular, gastrointestinal, pulmonary, and urogenital systems (see Chapter 124).[58] Although the etiology is unclear, one theory suggests a link with maldevelopment of the body curvature in the embryo.[59] This accounts for the frequent

observation of situs abnormalities (especially dextroisomerism) in conjunction with asplenia.[47]

### Polysplenia

This rare syndrome is also defined by a host of accompanying abnormalities (see Chapter 124). Unlike asplenia, polysplenia is most often found in females and is associated with levoisomerism.[47, 60] The similarities between the two entities are great, with multiple organ system anomalies probably being related to abnormal development of the embryo's body curvature.[59]

### Splenic-Gonadal Fusion

In this rare entity, there is ectopic splenic and gonadal tissue or an anomalous connection between the spleen and the gonad. It is almost exclusively seen in males and involves the left side.[61, 62] Both continuous and discontinuous forms are seen with equal frequency. The continuous form involves a band of fibrous and splenic tissue connecting the left gonad to the spleen proper.[61] Approximately 25% of these patients have cryptorchidism. In the discontinuous form, ectopic splenic tissue is located in the gonad.

The origin of this unusual entity is clearly congenital. The developing gonad arises during the sixth week of embryogenesis from the mesonephros, which is adjacent to the splenic precursor in the dorsal mesentery.[63] The gonadal tissue normally descends during the eighth week of development. Failure of these two anlages to separate completely may account for this anomaly.

## NORMAL MIDGUT ROTATION AND FIXATION

The final position of both the small and large bowel depends on many interrelated factors. Only anthropoid apes and humans have partial obliteration of the primitive dorsal mesentery. This is most likely due to their upright posture.[64]

During the third and fourth weeks of development, the embryo starts to grow much more rapidly than the yolk sac. By the fifth week, the intra- and extraembryonic coelomic cavities connect via a narrow stalk (omphalomesenteric or vitellointestinal duct; yolk stalk) (see Fig. 72–2).

Within the intraembryonic coelom, the midgut starts to change from a straight tube with parallel walls to a more complex shape. As this tube elongates, it loops ventrally into the yolk sac. This midgut loop can be divided into two segments, originally of roughly equal length. The axis of this loop is the superior mesenteric artery (SMA), and its apex is marked by the omphalomesenteric duct. The prearterial segment starts at the foregut-midgut junction and ends at the apex of the loop. This gives rise to the duodenum distal to the papilla, the jejunum, and most of the ileum. The post-

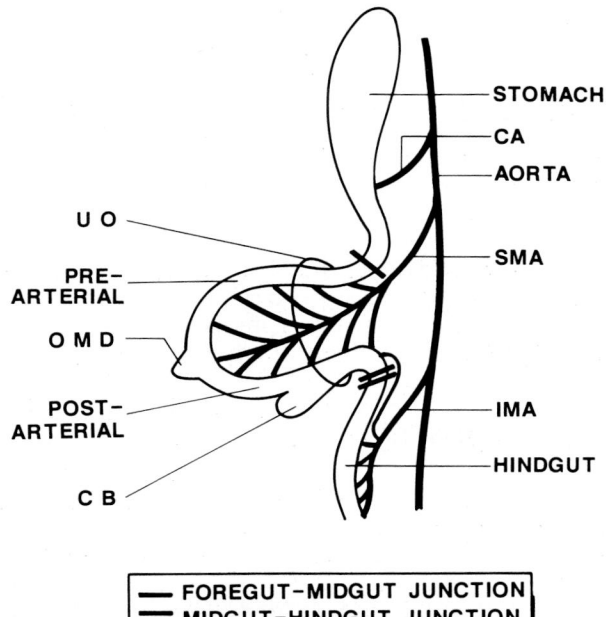

**Figure 72–12. Intestinal tract development at 6 weeks.** Longitudinal view of the intestinal tract at 6 weeks of development. The superior mesenteric artery (SMA) acts as the axis for midgut rotation. The omphalomesenteric duct (OMD) divides the midgut into pre- and postarterial limbs. Also seen is the physiologic herniation of the midgut through the umbilical orifice (UO). Heavy lines mark the foregut-midgut ( / ) and the midgut-hindgut ( // ) junctions. The celiac axis (CA) is the major artery of the foregut; the inferior mesenteric artery (IMA) supplies the hindgut. CB = cecal bud.

arterial limb extends from the apex of the loop to the midgut-hindgut junction. From this segment arise the very distal and terminal ileum, cecum and appendix, ascending colon, and most of the transverse colon. The transition to the hindgut is usually in the distal third of the transverse colon, where the changeover from SMA (middle colic) to inferior mesenteric artery (left colic) distribution occurs (Fig. 72–12).

By the fifth week, a small swelling may be noted in the proximal postarterial segment just distal to the apex of the umbilical loop. This cecal bud marks the beginning of the differentiation between the small and large bowel.

The entire midgut was originally thought to elongate, herniate, rotate, and return to the abdomen as a single unit. The pioneering work of Snyder and Chaffin in the early 1950s prompted a major revision of this theory.[65, 66]

The herniation of the midgut takes place in the sixth week of development. It is limited by dense condensations of the dorsal mesentery that bind the more proximal prearterial and more distal postarterial segments to the posterior peritoneum.[67] Within this hernia, the midgut now undergoes a dramatic increase in length. The growth is asymmetric, however, and predominantly involves the prearterial segment. Pressure from the enlarging right lobe of the liver along with the rapid elongation forces the prearterial segment down and to the right.[32, 67] The increase in length is accommodated

by the coiling of the prearterial midgut into a series of convolutions and small loops. The postarterial segment now occupies the left side of the umbilical hernia. Viewed from the front, this represents a 90-degree counterclockwise rotation.

By the 10th week, the relative changes created by further growth in the peritoneal cavity and less rapid increase in the liver size allow sufficient room for the physiologic herniation of the midgut to reduce itself.

First to return is the elongated, convoluted prearterial limb.[32, 65–67] These right-sided (originally cranial-located) loops enter the abdomen on the right side of the SMA but then pass behind that artery to occupy the left side of the abdomen. The cecal bud (now more a diverticulum) may impede the return of the postarterial (originally caudal), now left-sided midgut until the prearterial return is complete[32] (Fig. 72–13).

During the 11th week, the more slowly growing postarterial segment returns. As the herniation is reduced, the colon continues to rotate, first in front of and then to the right of the SMA (Fig. 72–14). By the 12th week, the colon completes a 270-degree counterclockwise rotation. These 270 degrees comprise 90 degrees occurring during the umbilical herniation and an additional 180 degrees during its reduction. Because of the flexion of the embryo, the cecum "descends" to the level of the iliac crest. Its final position in the right lower quadrant is a result of the continued growth of the ascending colon and not further midgut rotation.[32]

The development of the appendix is a separate and distinct process.[68] Differential rates of growth between the base of the primitive cecum and its apex result in

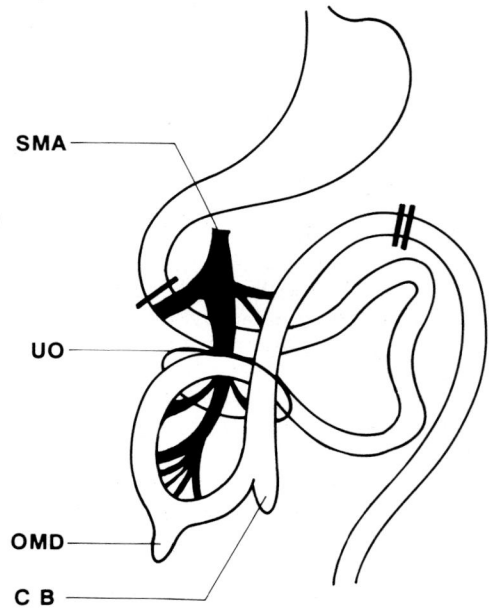

**Figure 72–13. Intestinal tract development at 10 weeks.** Frontal view of a 10-week fetus. The elongated redundant prearterial limb has re-entered the abdomen and crossed to the left of and behind the SMA. This displaces the hindgut to the left. Heavy lines mark the foregut-midgut ( / ) and the midgut-hindgut ( // ) junctions. CB = cecal bud; OMD = omphalomesenteric duct; UO = umbilical orifice.

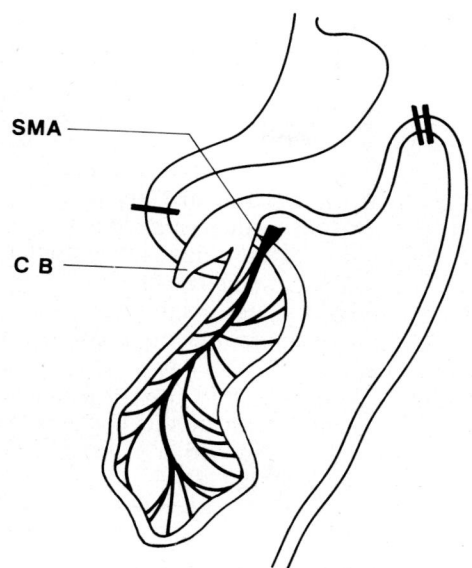

**Figure 72–14. Intestinal tract development at 11 weeks.** One week later, the reduction of the physiologic herniation is complete. The postarterial limb has partially completed its 180-degree rotation. The cecum now lies in the upper abdomen on its way to the right side. CB = cecal bud.

the rapid but thin development of a vermiform appendage (the appendix). Additional asymmetric growth of the lateral wall of the cecum after birth causes the appendix to migrate from the midline to the same side of the cecum as the ileocecal valve. The growth of the medial wall may be hindered by the presence of the ileum and its vascular pedicle.[68]

From the 11th week to the end of the fifth month, a gradual, partial resorption of the dorsal mesentery occurs. The postarterial segments attaching the ascending and descending colon agglutinate with the parietal peritoneum of the posterior abdominal wall, which leads to their final so-called retroperitoneal location. In reality, they are usually covered by peritoneum on their anterior, medial, and lateral borders; only their posterior walls are truly retroperitoneal.

The transverse colon mesentery (mesocolon) persists into adulthood. It partially fuses with the greater omentum, forming the gastrocolic ligament. The distal end of the transverse mesocolon serves as an anchor that fixes the splenic flexure in the left upper quadrant. This portion is called the phrenicocolic ligament. It also serves to seal the left paracolic gutter, preventing the spread of disease into the left upper quadrant from below.[35, 69]

In the small bowel, the thick proximal attachment of the prearterial segment lies to the left of the second lumbar vertebra, marking the duodenal-jejunal junction. This dorsal mesenteric remnant of the duodenum is also resorbed into the posterior abdominal wall, which results in a similar "retroperitonealization" of the duodenum. The distal end of the small bowel dorsal mesentery is carried into the right lower quadrant, ending at the level of the fourth or fifth lumbar vertebra. Thus, the mesenteric small bowel is suspended from a short

posterior attachment along the posterior abdominal wall.

The sigmoid colon maintains its dorsal mesenteric attachment as the sigmoid mesocolon. Its short length in comparison to the variable length of attached colon may be a contributing factor in the development of sigmoid volvulus.

## ABNORMAL MIDGUT ROTATION AND FIXATION

### Duplication

Because of errors in recanalization, a second intestinal lumen may form parallel to the primary one.[32, 46, 70] The duplication usually does not communicate with the primary lumen but does share a common muscular wall and, more important, a common blood supply. They are more often found in the ileum (see Chapters 77 and 79).[32, 45]

### Ileal Atresia

Atresias of all levels of the small bowel from duodenum to ileum have usually been attributed to in utero ischemic processes (see Chapters 74, 77, and 79).[71, 72] However, some authors implicate intrauterine inflammatory disease in cases of multiple intestinal atresias.[73]

### Mesenteric Cyst

Cysts within the mesentery are of various origins, including lymphangiomas, duplications, enteric or mesothelial cysts, and pancreatic pseudocysts. Their differentiation depends on the histologic elements of their wall constituents as well as their lining cells.[45, 46]

### Nonrotation

Although commonly called malrotation, this entity represents an abnormal arrest of the midgut rotation after the first 90 degrees of rotation.[32, 46, 74] At this point, the prearterial midgut lies to the right of the SMA and the postarterial limb to the left. The postarterial limb is then first to return to the abdomen. Consequently, it lies in the left hemiabdomen. The returning prearterial segment is forced to remain on the right (Fig. 72–15). Both segments continue to share a common dorsal mesentery, which lies in the midline. This allows considerable mobility of both the small and large bowel and predisposes to midgut volvulus.

### Reversed Rotation

In this rare entity, the order of the midgut return is reversed, with the postarterial limb preceding the

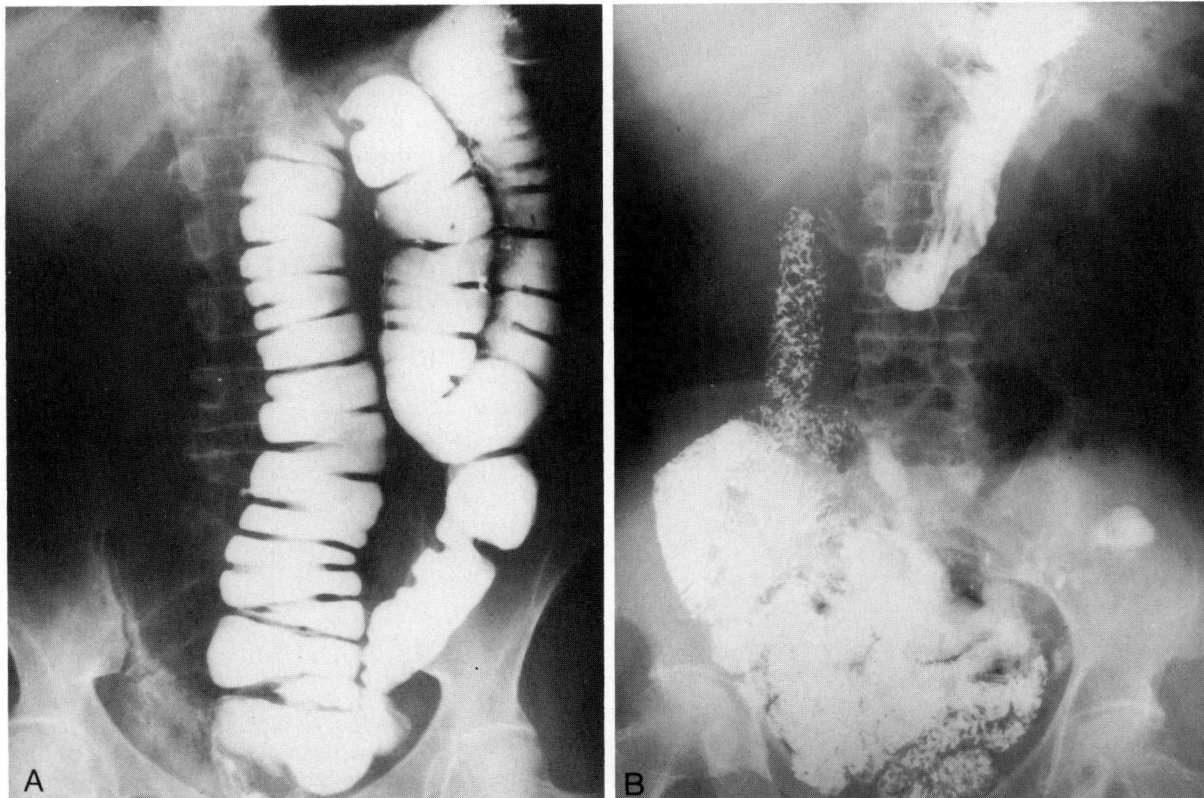

**Figure 72–15. Nonrotation of the gut. A.** A single contrast barium enema shows the entire colon to lie in the left hemiabdomen. This reflects the premature return of the postarterial limb of the midgut after the first 90 degrees of rotation. **B.** An upper gastrointestinal series in the same patient demonstrates incomplete formation of the duodenal sweep. The jejunum and most of the small bowel lie in the right hemiabdomen. The prearterial limb of midgut must remain on the right after the postarterial limb occupies the left.

prearterial.[32, 46] This causes the colon to lie posterior to the SMA; the duodenum and small bowel cross anteriorly. Abnormal mesenteric bands may cause obstruction.

## Incomplete Rotation and Malfixation

Although rotation and fixation are two separate and distinct stages of development, abnormalities of rotation are frequently associated with malfixation.[32, 46, 64, 74] Most often the colon fails to complete its final 180-degree rotation, ending in the right upper quadrant. In addition, there may be incomplete resorption of the dorsal mesentery that allows formation of elongated and mobile segments of colon (Fig. 72–16). Many different variations and combinations of abnormal rotation and fixation may be encountered. It should be noted that the presence of an abnormally rotated proximal limb does not necessarily imply an abnormally rotated lower tract, yet the presence of an abnormal lower tract almost always is associated with abnormal proximal rotation.

Multiple congenital anomalies of both the gastrointestinal tract and other organ systems have been reported with abnormal intestinal rotation and fixation.[74]

## Hyper-rotation

In this abnormality, an elongated colon continues to rotate past its usual 270-degree stopping point.[32, 46] The cecum may cross the midline, sometimes reaching the left upper quadrant. Because the prearterial segment is normal in length and rotation, it lies in its normal position and is not affected in this entity.

## Internal Herniations

Abnormalities in formation and resorption of the dorsal mesentery may allow fossae to develop into which loops of bowel may herniate (see Chapter 134). The most common of these fossae are those near the duodenum.[32, 46]

Left paraduodenal hernias are much more common than those on the right. The fossa of Landzert is formed by incomplete fusion of the descending colon mesentery.[46] Bowel loops may herniate under the colon and in front of the inferior mesenteric vein. A similar defect in the small bowel mesentery (fossa of Waldeyer, mesentericoparietal fossa) allows loops to herniate from the

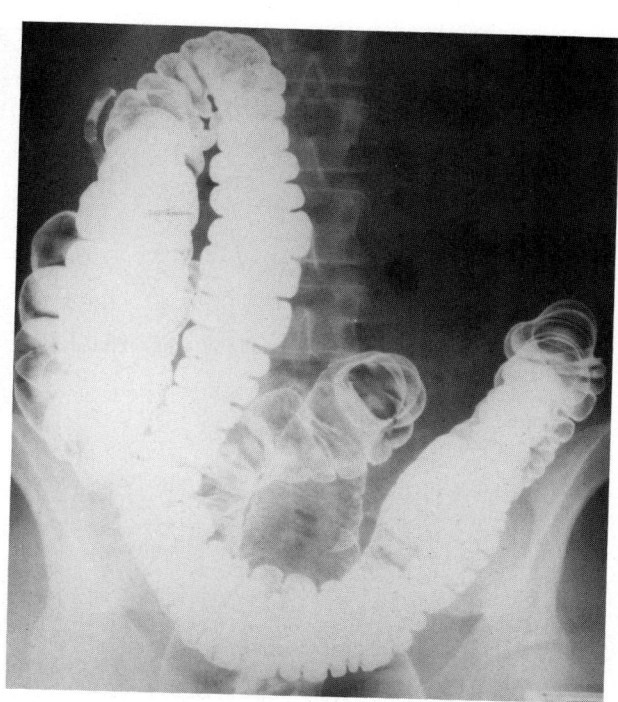

**Figure 72–16. Incomplete rotation and malfixation.** A double contrast barium enema reveals a short descending colon with a long, redundant transverse colon. This represents incomplete fusion of the descending colon mesentery, with its remnant allowing excessive mobility. In addition, the cecum is pointed superiorly in the right upper quadrant, which represents premature arrest of the postarterial midgut rotation.

left upper quadrant beneath the SMA to the right.[46] This is a right paraduodenal hernia.

Similar but less common defects may exist in the pericecal region, within the sigmoid mesocolon, and even in the transverse colon mesentery, which allows many different types and positions of internal herniations.

## Meckel's Diverticulum

If the omphalomesenteric duct fails to be completely obliterated, a persistent outpouching of the bowel may persist. Its location at the apex of the physiologic herniation accounts for the location of Meckel's diverticula in the distal ileum (see Chapter 77).

There is a wide spectrum of variation within the overall entity of Meckel's diverticulum.[46] There may be cystic remnants between the small bowel and umbilicus or fibrous bands. Communication with the bowel is the most common (Fig. 72–17), but draining umbilical sinuses have been reported. The fibrous cord may act as an axis of rotation, allowing volvulus to develop.

These diverticula can contain ectopic gastric or pancreatic tissue. The presence of ectopic gastric tissue may lead to peptic ulceration and bleeding. Rare neoplasms

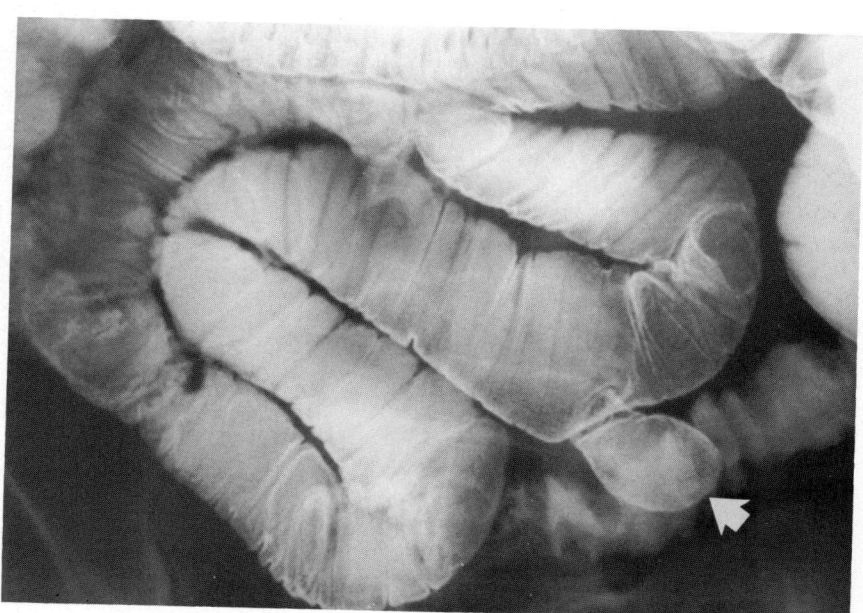

**Figure 72–17. Meckel's diverticulum.** Coned down view from an enteroclysis shows a Meckel diverticulum *(arrow)* arising from the antimesenteric border of an ileal loop. This represents the remnant of the omphalomesenteric duct.

have been reported within the mucosal lining. In addition, stasis of intestinal contents within the diverticulum may give rise to enterolith formation. Rarely, the diverticulum may invert and act as the leading edge of an intussusception. In Littre's hernia, the diverticulum enters a hernia sac.[46]

# References

1. Moore KL: The Developing Human (4th ed). Philadelphia: WB Saunders, 1988, pp 50–59.
2. Moore KL: The Developing Human (4th ed). Philadelphia: WB Saunders, 1988, pp 159–169.
3. Monie IW: Embryology. *In* Margulis AR, Burhenne HJ (eds): Alimentary Tract Roentgenology (3rd ed). St. Louis: CV Mosby, 1983, pp 275–291.
4. DuBois AM: The embryonic liver. *In* Roviller CH (ed): The Liver: Morphology, Biochemistry and Physiology. New York: Academic Press, 1963, pp 1–32.
5. Kelly DE, Wood RL, Enders AC: Bailey's Textbook of Microscopic Anatomy. Baltimore: Williams & Wilkins, 1984, pp 590–593.
6. Netter FH: Digestive System. Part III: Liver, Biliary Tract and Pancreas. The Ciba Collection of Medical Illustrations, Volume 3. Summit, NJ: Ciba Pharmaceutical Products, 1957, pp 2–3.
7. Giovannelli AS, Friedman A: Liver: embryology, anatomy, histology and variations. *In* Friedman AC (ed): Radiology of the Liver, Biliary Tract, Pancreas and Spleen. Baltimore: Williams & Wilkins, 1987, pp 3–36.
8. Li YP, Morin ME, Tan A: Bipartite liver as a cause of 99m Tc liver scan defect. Appl Radiol 1:97–98, 1982.
9. Radin DR, Colletti PM, Ralls PW, et al: Agenesis of the right lobe of the liver. Radiology 164:639–642, 1987.
10. Champetier J, Yuer R, Letoublon C, et al: A general review of anomalies of hepatic morphology and their clinical implications. Anat Clin 7:285–299, 1985.
11. Pujari BD, Deodhare SG: Symptomatic accessory lobe of the liver with review of the literature. Postgrad Med J 52:234–236, 1976.
12. Rappaport AM: Physioanatomic considerations. *In* Schiff L, Schiff ER (eds): Diseases of the Liver. Philadelphia: JB Lippincott, 1987, pp 1–46.
13. Hayes NA, Goldenberg IS, Bishop CC: The developmental basis for bile duct anomalies. Surg Gynecol Obstet 107:447–456, 1958.
14. Snell RS: Clinical Anatomy for Medical Students (2nd ed). Boston: Little, Brown, 1981, pp 202–205.
15. Schwegler RA Jr, Boyden EA: Development of pars intestinalis of common bile duct in human fetus with special reference to origin of ampulla of Vater and sphincter of Oddi. Anat Rec 67:441–467, 1937.
16. Pontes JF, Pinotti WH: Anomalies of the gallbladder and biliary system. *In* Bockus HL, Berk JE, Haubrich WS, et al (eds): Gastroenterology (3rd ed). Philadelphia: WB Saunders, 1976, pp 651–665.
17. Berk RM: Oral cholecystography. *In* Berk RN, Ferrucci JT Jr, Leopold GR (eds): Radiology of the Gallbladder and Bile Ducts, Diagnosis and Intervention. Philadelphia: WB Saunders, 1983, pp 121–142.
18. Singleton E: Pediatric diseases of the gallbladder and bile ducts. *In* Berk RN, Ferrucci JT Jr, Leopold GR (eds): Radiology of the Gallbladder and Bile Ducts, Diagnosis and Intervention. Philadelphia: WB Saunders, 1983, pp 513–546.
19. Youndwith JD, Peters JC, Perry MC: The suprahepatic gallbladder. Radiology 149:57–58, 1983.
20. Croce ES: The multiseptate gallbladder. Arch Surg 107:104–108, 1973.
21. Hatfield PM, Wise RE: Anatomic variation in the gallbladder and bile ducts. Semin Roentgenol 11:157–164, 1976.
22. Neuhauser EBD, Elkin M, Landing BH: Congenital direct communication between biliary system and respiratory tract. Am J Dis Child 83:654–658, 1952.
23. Witzleben CL: Bile duct paucity ("intrahepatic atresia"). Perspect Pediatr Pathol 7:185–200, 1982.
24. Alagille D: Intrahepatiac biliary atresia (hepatic ductal hypoplasia). *In* Berenberg SR (ed): Liver Disease in Childhood. Baltimore: Williams & Wilkins, 1976, p 129.
25. Doppman JL, Dunnick NR, Girton M, et al: Bile duct cysts secondary to liver infarcts: report of a case and experimental production by small vessel hepatic artery occlusion. Radiology 130:1–5, 1979.
26. Berger PE, Kuhn JP: Computed tomography of the hepatobiliary system in infancy and childhood. Radiol Clin North Am 19:431–441, 1981.
27. Babbitt DP, Starshak RJ, Clemett A: Choledochal cyst: a concept of etiology. AJR 119:57–62, 1973.
28. Ghahremani GG, Lu CT, Woodlief RM, et al: Choledochal cyst in adults. A clinical and radiologic study in ten cases. Gastrointest Radiol 1:305–313, 1977.
29. Todani T, Watanabe Y, Narusue M, et al: Congenital bile duct cysts. Am J Surg 134:263–268, 1977.
30. Sherlock S: Diseases of the Liver and Biliary System (6th ed). Oxford: Black Scientific, 1981, pp 406–412.
31. Dodds WJ: Radiology (esophagus and esophagogastric region). *In* Margulis AR, Burhenne HJ (eds): Alimentary Tract Roentgenology (3rd ed). St. Louis: CV Mosby, 1983, pp 529–603.
32. Moore KL: The Developing Human (4th ed). Philadelphia: WB Saunders, 1988, pp 217–245.
33. Franken EA Jr, Smith WL: Pediatric esophagus. *In* Levine MS: Radiology of the Esophagus. Philadelphia: WB Saunders, 1989, pp 337–362.
34. Balfe DM, Mauro MA, Koehler RE, et al: Gastrohepatic ligament: normal and pathologic CT anatomy. Radiology 150:485–490, 1984.
35. Balfe DM, Peterson RR, van Dyke JA: Normal abdominal and pelvic anatomy. *In* Lee JKT, Sagel SS, Stanley RJ (eds): Computed Body Tomography with MRI Correlation (2nd ed). New York: Raven Press, 1989, pp 415–475.
36. Seaman WB: Nonneoplastic lesions (stomach and duodenum). *In* Margulis AR, Burhenne HJ (eds): Alimentary Tract Roentgenology (3rd ed). St. Louis: CV Mosby, 1983, pp 529–603.
37. Koehler RE, Balfe DM, Stanley RJ: Gastrointestinal tract. *In* Lee JKT, Sagel SS, Stanley RJ (eds): Computed Body Tomography with MRI Correlation (2nd ed). New York: Raven Press, 1989, pp 477–520.
38. Op den Orth JO: Duodenum. *In* Margulis AR, Burhenne HJ (eds): Alimentary Tract Roentgenology (3rd ed). St. Louis: CV Mosby, 1983, pp 800–831.
39. Friedman AC, Birns MT: Embryology, anatomy, histology and physiology (pancreas). *In* Friedman AC (ed): Radiology of the Liver, Biliary Tract, Pancreas and Spleen. Baltimore: Williams & Wilkins, 1987, pp 619–642.
40. Ravitch MM: The pancreas in infants and children. Surg Clin North Am 55:377–385, 1975.
41. Glazer GM, Margulis AR: Annular pancreas: etiology and diagnosis using ERCP. Radiology 133:303–306, 1979.
42. Richter JM, Schapiro RM, Mulley AG, et al: Association of pancreas divisum and pancreatitis and its treatment by sphincteroplasty of the accessory ampulla. Gastroenterology 81:1104–1110, 1981.
43. Stanley RJ, Koslin B, Lee JKT: Pancreas. *In* Lee JKT, Sagel SS, Stanley RJ (eds): Computed Body Tomography with MRI Correlation (2nd ed). New York: Raven Press, 1989, pp 543–592.
44. Dodds WJ, Foley WD, Lawson TL, et al: Anatomy and imaging of the lesser peritoneal sac. AJR 144:567–575, 1985.
45. Ros PR, Olmsted WJ, Moser RP Jr, et al: Mesenteric and omental cysts: histologic classification with imaging correlation. Radiology 164:327–332, 1987.
46. Maglinte DDT, Herlinger H: Congenital and developmental anomalies in adolescents and adults. *In* Herlinger H, Maglinte D (eds): Clinical Radiology of the Small Intestine. Philadelphia: WB Saunders, 1989, pp 249–273.
47. Dachman AH: Anomalies and congenital disorders (spleen). *In* Friedman AC (ed): Radiology of the Liver, Biliary Tract, Pancreas and Spleen. Baltimore: Williams & Wilkins, 1987, pp 913–930.
48. Blaustein A: The Spleen. New York: McGraw-Hill, 1963, p 45.

49. Halpert B, Gyorkey F: Lesions observed in accessory spleens of 311 patients. Am J Clin Pathol 32:165–168, 1959.
50. Olsen WR, Beaudoin DE: Increased incidence of accessory spleens in hematologic disease. Arch Surg 98:762–763, 1969.
51. Malins E: Rotation of the spleen; removal; recovery. Lancet 2:607, 1894.
52. McClain GH, Lebherz TB: Radiographic evidence of splenic torsion: report of a case. Obstet Gynecol 29:475–478, 1967.
53. Gordon DH, Burrell MI, Levin DC, et al: Wandering spleen: the radiological and clinical spectrum. Radiology 125:39–46, 1977.
54. Vermylen C, Lebecque P, Claus D, et al: The wandering spleen. Eur J Pediatr 140:112–115, 1983.
55. Kelly KJ, Chusid MJ, Camitta BM: Splenic torsion in an infant associated with secondary disseminated Hemophilus influenzae infection. Clin Pediatr 21:365–366, 1982.
56. Monie IW: The asplenia syndrome: an explanation for absence of the spleen. Teratology 25:212–219, 1982.
57. Honigman R, Lanzkowsky P: Isolated congenital asplenia: an occult case of overwhelming sepsis. Am J Dis Child 133:552–553, 1979.
58. Ivemark BI: Implications of agenesis of the spleen on the pathogenesis of cono-truncus anomalies in childhood. An analysis of the heart malformations in the splenic agenesis syndrome with fourteen new cases. Acta Paediatr 44(suppl 104):1–110, 1955.
59. Hutchins GM, Morre GW, Lipford EH, et al: Asplenia and polysplenia malformation complexes explained by abnormal embryonic body curvature. Pathol Res Pract 177:60–76, 1983.
60. Rose V, Izukawa T, Moes CAF: Syndromes of asplenia and polysplenia: a review of cardiac and non-cardiac malformations in 60 cases with special reference to diagnosis and prognosis. Br Heart J 37:840–852, 1975.
61. Bearss RW: Splenic-gonadal fusion. Urology 16:277–279, 1980.
62. Ceccacci L, Tosi S: Splenic-gonadal fusion: case report and review of the literature. J Urol 126:387–389, 1981.
63. Putschar WGJ, Manion WC: Congenital absence of the spleen and associated anomalies. Am J Clin Pathol 26:429–445, 1956.
64. Balthazar EJ: Congenital positional anomalies of the colon: radiographic diagnosis and clinical implications. II. Abnormalities of fixation. Gastrointest Radiol 2:49–56, 1977.
65. Snyder WH Jr, Chaffin L: Intermediate stage in return of the intestines from the umbilical cord. Anat Rec 113:451–457, 1952.
66. Snyder WH Jr, Chaffin L: Embryology and pathology of intestinal tract: presentation of 40 cases of malrotation. Ann Surg 140:368–379, 1954.
67. Maglinte DDT, Herlinger H: Embryology of the small intestine. In Herlinger H, Maglinte D (eds): Clinical Radiology of the Small Intestine. Philadelphia: WB Saunders, 1989, pp 3–6.
68. Balthazar EJ, Gade M: The normal and abnormal development of the appendix. Radiology 121:599–604, 1976.
69. Heiken JP: Abdominal wall and peritoneal cavity. In Lee JKT, Sagel SS, Stanley RJ (eds): Computed Body Tomography with MRI Correlation (2nd ed). New York: Raven Press, 1989, pp 661–705.
70. Kottra JJ, Dodds WJ: Duplication of the large bowel. AJR 113:310–315, 1971.
71. Earlam RJ: A study of the aetiology of congenital stenosis of the gut. Ann R Coll Surg Engl 51:126–130, 1972.
72. de Sa DJ: Congenital stenosis and atresia of the jejunum and ileum. J Clin Pathol 25:1063–1070, 1972.
73. Puri P, Fujimoto T: New observations on the pathogenesis of multiple atresias. J Pediatr Surg 23:221–225, 1988.
74. Balthazar EJ: Congenital positional anomalies of the colon: radiographic diagnosis and clinical implications. I. Abnormalities of rotation. Gastrointest Radiol 2:49–56, 1977.

# Pediatric Gastrointestinal Radiology: An Approach to the Child

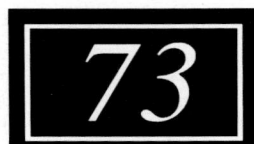

Sandra K. Fernbach, M.D.

Kate A. Feinstein, M.D.

Rita Littlewood Teele, M.D.

Jane Chrestman Share, M.D.

## CONTRAST EXAMINATION OF THE PEDIATRIC GASTROINTESTINAL TRACT

The radiologist performing gastrointestinal studies in children must be familiar with the appearance of the common congenital abnormalities both before and after surgery as well as acquired lesions of the pediatric age group. Because gastrointestinal malignant neoplasms are rare in children, gastrointestinal studies are directed more toward solving the specific presenting problem, with less concern about missing an incidental cancer. In this chapter, methods of immobilization, positioning techniques, choices of contrast material, and preparation regimens are presented.

## Immobilization of the Patient

Immobilization is key to successful radiography in infants and young children. It optimizes positioning of the patient, decreases voluntary and involuntary motion, and shortens the study, thereby decreasing the radiation dose. Whereas some institutions achieve immobilization by swaddling the baby in sheets, we use the commercially available Octostop board, which is a flat board affixed to the midportion of two eight-sided rings (Fig. 73–1A). After the board is covered with sheets, the child is placed on the board and then wrapped with the sheets. The wrapped child is held in place on the board with broad Velcro straps about the arms, chest, and legs. The head is also stabilized with padding placed on the forehead and Velcro straps placed over the padding to secure the head. The Octostop board can be rotated into various positions (Fig. 73–1B). Older infants requiring less restraint can be positioned by the technologist and radiologist working together (Fig. 73–2).

Swaddling works less well after infancy, but toddlers can be immobilized on the Octostop board. Remote control fluoroscopy is impractical for studying infants or young children because they require assistance in eating and positioning.

Older children are usually cooperative when the study is explained to them in simply understood terms. Educational material is useful in this regard. The child is told about changing into hospital clothing; the size, position, and noises of the camera; and how the barium or other contrast medium is to be administered. The information sheets should also reinforce the appropriate preparation for the study (fasting, enemas, laxatives).

Larger cradle devices are useful in examining older handicapped children who are difficult to move and position.

For prevention of hypothermia, infants must be kept warm during fluoroscopy, and radiant heating devices should be directed at the infant when fluoroscopy is not being performed.

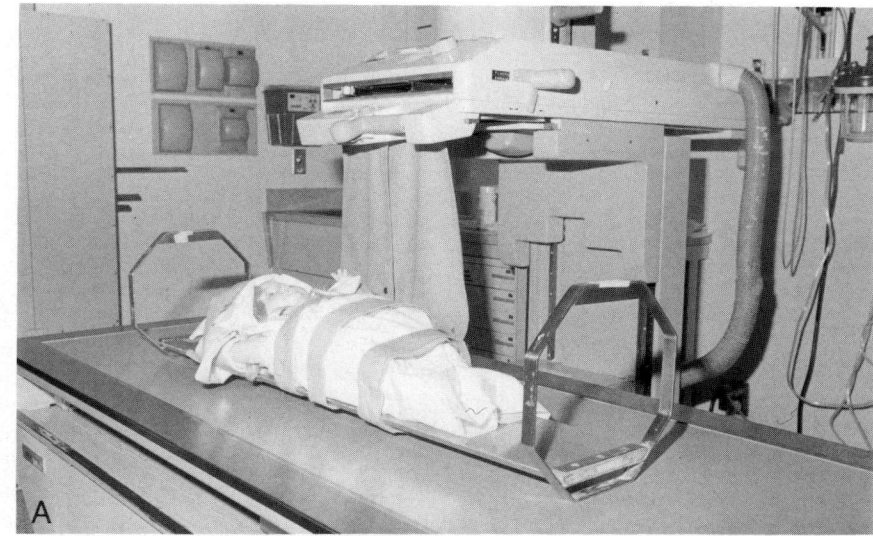

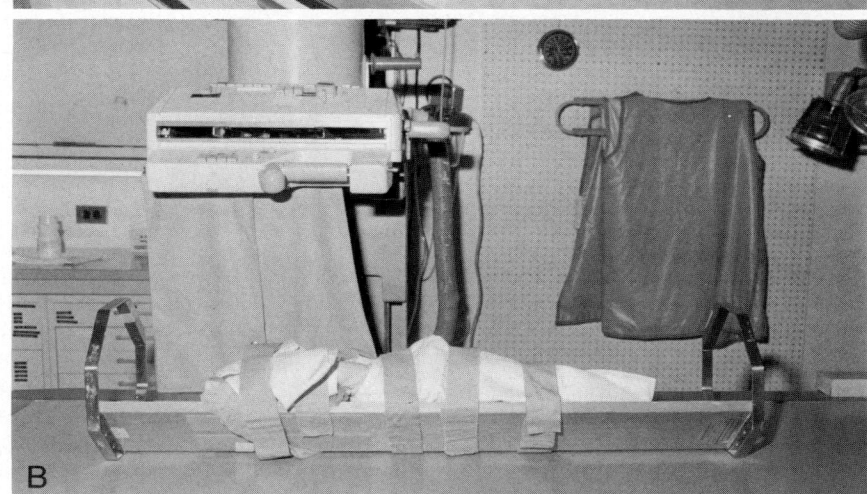

**Figure 73–1. Octostop immobilization board.**
**A.** The infant is placed supine on the board, swaddled, and held in place with Velcro straps. **B.** Once secured on the board, the child can be rotated into oblique, lateral, and prone positions.

## Noncontrast Radiography

When a child presents with acute onset of abdominal signs and symptoms, both supine and upright or decubitus views are mandatory. Because it may be difficult to distinguish thoracic from abdominal processes on physical examination alone, especially in the neonate, chest films may be useful.

A plain abdominal radiograph is routinely obtained before contrast studies to search for the presence of skeletal abnormalities, calcification, and evidence of a mass and to assess the abdominal gas pattern. If an abnormality is detected, additional views should be performed before the administration of contrast medium.[1, 2]

## Contrast Radiography

### Oral Barium Administration

There are several ways to feed barium to an infant. The most widely used method is to place the barium in a bottle and let the infant suck through the nipple, which has been slightly enlarged to facilitate flow (see Fig. 73–2). Lead shielding is placed under the infant's head to protect the technologist who is feeding and holding the child. Because the lead may interfere with visualization of the swallowing mechanism, it should be used only when no swallowing problems are suspected or after swallowing problems have been excluded.

Another successful method is the feeding device created by Poznanski and later modified by others.[3, 4] An 8 French feeding tube is placed through a standard or premature nipple, depending on the size of the child to be fed. The end of the feeding tube is snipped off, which creates a single end hole. The nipple is inserted in the baby's mouth and taped in place. The other end of the feeding tube is attached to barium-filled syringes, which can be used to actively deliver the barium. When the child has a strong suck, the barium is easily drawn from the syringe. Older children can drink barium directly from a cup or through a straw. When an older child is unable to use a cup or straw, barium can be given orally through a catheter-tipped syringe. To avoid aspiration, care must be taken not to exceed the rate at which the

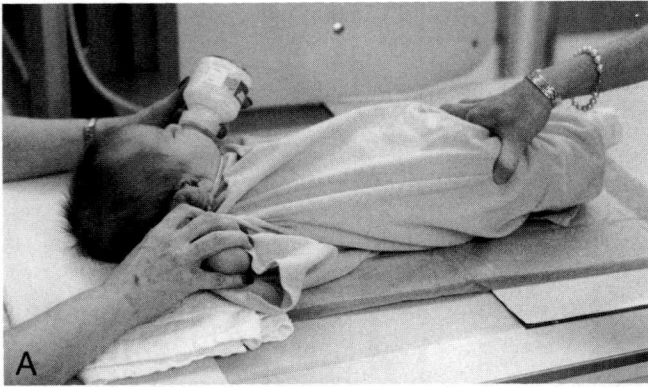

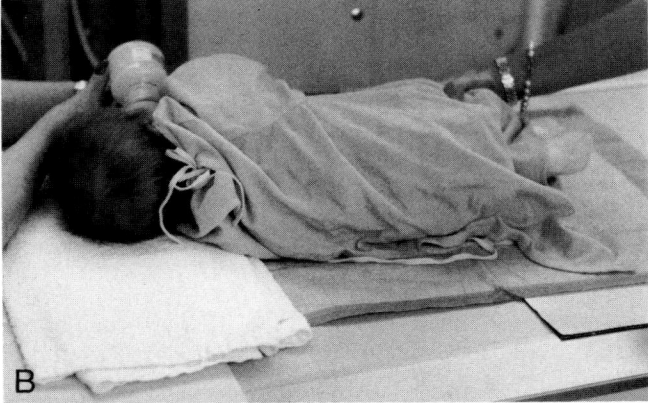

**Figure 73–2. Nonswaddled infant: fluoroscopic positioning and feeding. A.** The infant is immobilized by the technologist and radiologist. Barium is administered through a standard bottle and a nipple with slightly enlarged holes. **B.** Working together, the technologist and radiologist are able to position the infant as necessary for the study.

child can safely handle the fluid. If a large amount of barium must be given to exclude gastroesophageal reflux or to perform a small bowel study, it may be preferable to give barium through a nasogastric tube.

Several techniques are available to create double contrast studies of the upper gastrointestinal tract. In the very young, air can be injected through a nasogastric tube placed in the stomach. In the toddler or slightly older child, a small hole cut into the side of the straw will increase the amount of air ingested with the barium. Children older than 6 years of age will usually take gas-producing granules.

### Rectal Barium Administration

A variety of barium enema tips are available; the choice for any particular study depends on the size of the child, the lesion suspected, and the child's ability to retain the barium (Fig. 73–3). In general, we prefer to use the smallest tip that will allow the study to be properly performed. Small tips are more comfortable and are less likely to produce artifacts, which can obscure a small polyp or dilate an aganglionic rectum.

The thick barium used for double contrast studies requires a large bore for easy flow. A large bore catheter

is also necessary to transmit hydrostatic pressure. Accordingly, when an intussusception is suspected, we place a noninflated Foley catheter of 20 French or greater in the rectum before vigorously taping the tube in place and the buttocks in close apposition. This permits us to inflate the balloon of the catheter, if necessary, for help in keeping the colon sealed, without having to stop, change catheters, and retape the buttocks.

### Choice of Oral Contrast Material

In most settings, commercially available flavored barium sulfate preparations are used.[5] These can be purchased as a powder and resuspended in fluid as desired, or they can be purchased in unit dose, ready-to-use containers. We do not favor the suspension of large amounts of barium at one time because the typical "barium kitchen" has been shown to be an easily contaminated environment. Neonates and infants receive sterilized fluids at home and in the hospital, and the same should be true within the radiology department. Although barium is generally well tolerated, there have been reports of an allergic-type reaction to both oral and rectal barium in adults.[6, 7] We have observed a few minor skin reactions in children undergoing oral barium study at sites where the contrast agent came into direct contact with the skin.

The first generation of oral nonbarium, water-soluble contrast agents was developed to allow radiologic examination of children with possible gastrointestinal tract discontinuity. When extravasated, these agents (diatrizoate meglumine or diatrizoate sodium [Gastrografin, Renografin]) are readily absorbed from the adjacent tissues. Extravasated barium remains at the site of perforation or in spaces continuous with the perforation (extrapleural space, peritoneal cavity) unless it is mechanically removed. Unfortunately, these early water-soluble agents are hyperosmolar and produce electrolyte disturbances when they are systemically absorbed and

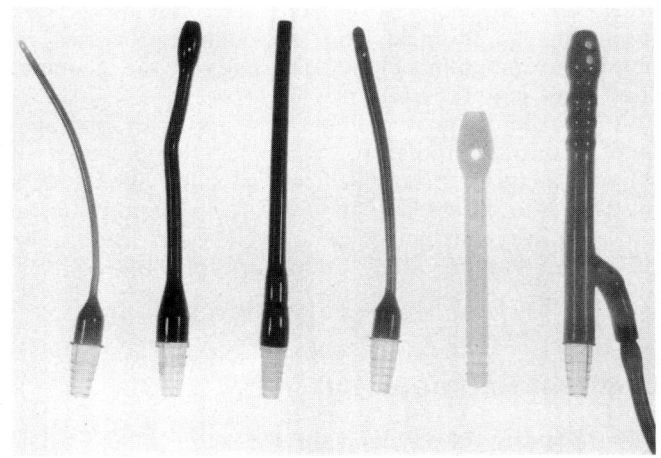

**Figure 73–3. Catheters available for rectal administration of contrast material.**

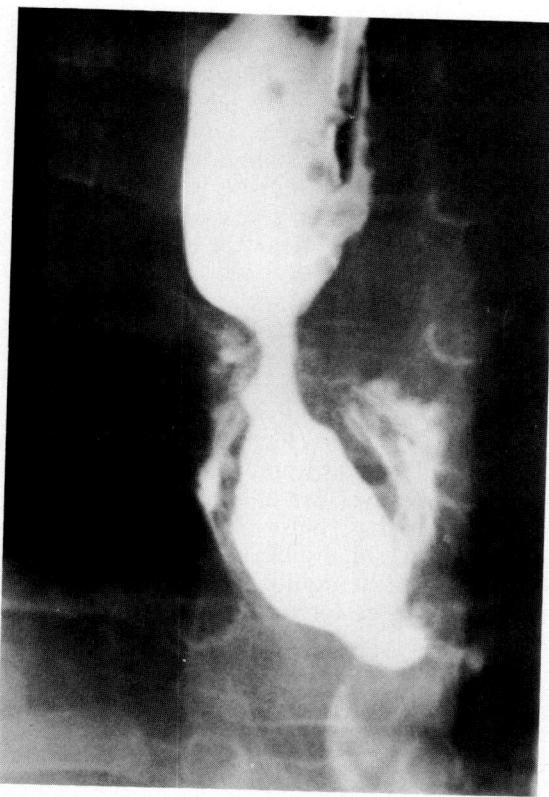

**Figure 73–4. Nonionic contrast esophagram: distal perforation.** This child with severe esophagitis from gastroesophageal reflux had undergone a Nissen fundoplication. Dilation of the tight gastric wrap was necessary but complicated by perforation of the distal esophagus.

dehydration when they cause third spacing of fluid in the gut.[8, 9]

Nonionic water-soluble contrast agents can be safely ingested and are recommended for excluding a tracheo-esophageal fistula; an anastomotic leak; or an esophageal perforation from foreign body and esophageal dilation or other manipulation[10] (Fig. 73–4). Small bowel studies in cases of suspected necrotizing enterocolitis can be safely performed with nonionic agents.[11–14] Unfortunately, both high- and low-osmolality nonionic contrast agents cause diarrhea in almost 50% of the patients.[14] In addition, these agents are expensive and provide inherently inferior gut mucosal contrast, compared with barium. We presently limit the gastrointestinal use of nonionic contrast agents to the situations described earlier.

Barium paste is used as an adjunct to regular barium when the swallowing mechanism is evaluated and when demonstration of esophageal varices is attempted.

## Choice of Rectal Contrast Agent

Barium is the contrast agent of choice for most pediatric colonic studies. It can be purchased as a powder and mixed with water in the department or as a ready-to-use liquid. In most studies of the colon, a routine preparation of barium is employed. For children with known or suspected Hirschsprung's disease, the

powdered barium is mixed with normal saline rather than tap water to prevent overhydration in the event that the fluid is retained above the aganglionic segment. For neonates or infants, the powdered barium is mixed with warm tap water for prevention of hypothermia. High-density barium preparations are used for performing double contrast studies.

Ionic and nonionic water-soluble contrast agents are indicated in several clinical situations. Ionic contrast media are employed in the diagnosis and treatment of neonates with meconium ileus. Enema with these agents is not entirely without hazard; mucosal changes and necrotizing enterocolitis have been reported subsequent to ionic enema.[15–17] The contrast medium is therapeutic because it will draw fluid into the lumen and aid in the passage of retained meconium and feces.[18] Ionic agents should also be used to image the colon in the teen-ager with meconium ileus equivalent.

Water-soluble agents should be used for studying the distal limb of the colon in a child with imperforate anus for excluding fistula to the urinary tract before corrective surgery.

The more expensive nonionic agents are indicated in the following situations: possible colonic leak or perforation; neonates recovering from necrotizing enterocolitis; and those children with recent surgery for imperforate anus or Hirschsprung's disease in whom a complication is suspected (Fig. 73–5).

Large studies have shown that rectal insufflation of air is a safe and effective way of diagnosing and treating children with ileocolic or colocolic intussusception.[19, 20] This technique is discussed in Chapter 78.

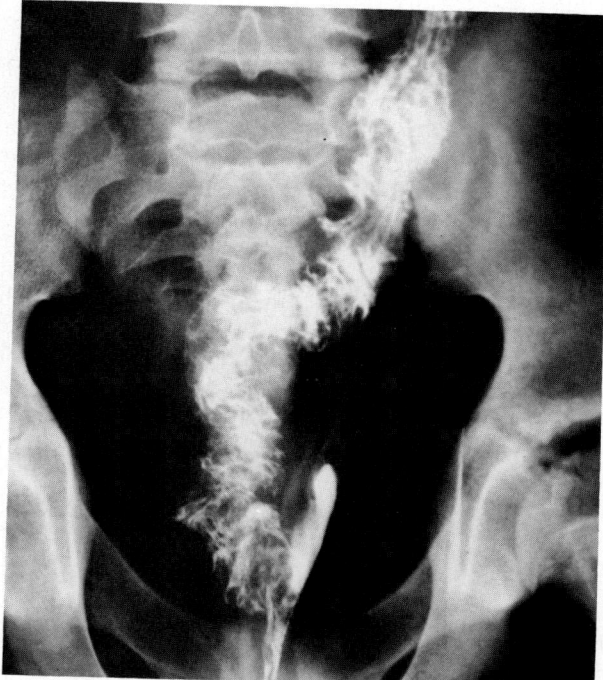

**Figure 73–5. Nonionic contrast enema: perforation.** Nonionic contrast is filling the nonused segment of colon recently pulled through to create a neoanus. Contrast material extravasates into the pelvis.

## Catheter Injection

When the position of a gastrostomy tube is in doubt, the initial injections should be done with a water-soluble, preferably nonionic, medium or air. This will prevent peritoneal spillage of barium if the tube is improperly placed or has become dislodged. Anteroposterior and lateral views of the tube relative to the stomach should also be obtained. Failure of the injected air or contrast medium to fill the stomach indicates that 1) the tube is extragastric; 2) the tube is plugged or cracked; or 3) the tube is past the pylorus or, rarely, within the esophagus. If the tube is in good position and there is no leakage of the air or water-soluble contrast medium, barium can be used for the remainder of the study.

## Preparation of the Patient

### Esophagram, Upper Gastrointestinal Series, Small Bowel Study

Infants will not swallow barium if they are not hungry. They should not, however, be fasted longer than their typical interval between feedings. This is usually 3 to 4 hours in the first 3 months of life. Premature infants, who are quite fragile, should not be fasted longer than 2 to 3 hours unless they are receiving parenteral nutrition. Children older than age 2 years should be fasted at least 6 hours. They should not chew gum in this period because this encourages salivary and gastric secretion, which interferes with mucosal coating.

The amount of contrast agent given varies with the age of the patient and the length of gut to be examined. In studying infants or children for gastroesophageal reflux, the child should receive the same volume as a normal feeding. If less is given, the lower gastroesophageal sphincter is not adequately challenged, and the study may be falsely negative. In performing a small bowel follow-through, greater amounts of barium are given to distend the small bowel and to encourage peristalsis.

Enteroclysis has not been popular in pediatric radiology departments because of the need to premedicate the children, the implicit difficulty of intubating the duodenum, the radiation exposure, the necessity for keeping special barium products at hand, and the relative rarity of small bowel disease in children. This technique has been successful in detecting small bowel obstruction or inflammatory bowel disease in children.[21–23] The diagnostic yield of a routine small bowel follow-through study depends on the frequency of fluoroscopic palpation and the sequence and number of overhead films.[24–26]

### Barium Enema

The preparation for the barium enema examination in children depends on the clinical urgency of the study and the clinical problem to be resolved. In the child with suspected intussusception, contrast enema is performed without any preparation of the colon. Similarly, no preparation is recommended before study of the child with possible Hirschsprung's disease. When a child presents with a history of rectal bleeding, the colon should be cleansed before the double contrast barium enema. A thorough preparation is necessary to minimize residual feces that might mimic a juvenile polyp.

In children younger than 2 years of age with a history of active or recent bleeding, the preparation may be minimal because bowel evacuation is frequent in this age group and is enhanced with active bleeding.

Older children with a history of prior rectal bleeding and suspected polyp should receive a more vigorous bowel cleansing regimen. GoLYTELY or other volume lavage agents can be used to cleanse the colon. They should be given at least 16 hours before the study to allow the colonic mucus to reconstitute. Dietary manipulation and purgatives are another means of preparing the colon. Four days before the enema, the child is begun on a low-residue diet. In the 24 hours preceding the study, only clear liquids are ingested. On the day before the study, castor oil is given (in proportion to the weight of the patient) in the late afternoon. Commercially available enemas are to be given the night before and the morning of the examination.

When the child is actively bleeding per rectum, no laxatives or cleansing enemas are given lest the bleeding worsen. Because blood in the bowel acts to increase peristalsis, the need for preparation of the colon is decreased. Whereas the diagnosis of inflammatory bowel disease is less accurate in the unprepared colon, active disease can frequently be seen. If there is no evidence of inflammatory disease, the child can be restudied after a more complete bowel preparation.[27]

## CROSS-SECTIONAL IMAGING OF THE PEDIATRIC GASTROINTESTINAL TRACT

### Ultrasound

The advantages of sonography in imaging the pediatric patient are many: portability, lack of ionizing radiation, and the infrequent need for preparation or sedation of the patient. These virtues, combined with the diagnostic range of this technique, have placed sonography at the forefront of pediatric abdominal imaging. Sonography has been used to study the alimentary tract from the posterior pharyngeal spaces to the anus.[28–38] It can detect and characterize congenital (meconium cysts, duplications) and acquired (hematoma, appendicitis, intussusception) lesions of the gastrointestinal tract.[39, 40]

In certain clinical situations, supplemental techniques may be needed to enhance the diagnostic yield of ultrasound. For example, in searching for the thickened muscle of pyloric stenosis, it may be necessary to drain the stomach or to feed the child so that passage of fluid from the stomach can be visualized. In studying the pelvis, filling the bladder, vagina, or rectum with water may help define the anatomy. Graded compression is needed to establish the diagnosis of appendicitis.[39]

With the advent of real-time scanning and high-frequency transducers, ultrasound can demonstrate dynamic processes: gastroesophageal reflux, gastric and bowel peristalsis, and portal venous gas bubbling through the liver. Differentiation of bowel wall layers and detection of mucosal ulceration is also possible. Normal values have been established for stomach and bowel wall thickness, bowel contour and size, appearance of the appendix, and thickness of the omentum.[34, 41] Small amounts of free fluid can be detected, and meconium peritonitis can be differentiated from ascites.

Duplex and color flow Doppler sonography can detect varices in children with portal hypertension and aid in the diagnosis of bowel ischemia. Vascular ultrasound can also be useful in the diagnosis of malrotation.[42, 43] Doppler evaluation of the kidneys in children with hemolytic-uremic syndrome may provide the first concrete evidence of returning renal function.[44]

## Nuclear Medicine

Most scintigraphic studies of the gut are performed with technetium Tc 99m pertechnetate alone or coupled with an agent that determines how it is handled within the gastrointestinal tract. Studies devised to evaluate esophageal function, gastroesophageal reflux, and gastric emptying require that the isotope be ingested mixed with water, juice, or other fluid. Gastroesophageal reflux and gastric emptying can be sensitively quantified with significantly less radiation than with standard fluoroscopic techniques.[45, 46]

Ectopic gastric mucosa in a duplication, Meckel's diverticulum, or other site will take up free pertechnetate.[47, 48] Active gastrointestinal bleeding can be similarly demonstrated by labeled red blood cell studies or sulfur colloid scans.[49, 50]

Indium 111 scans can highlight segments of gut with active inflammatory bowel disease, but this technique has not been widely used.[51] Appendicitis can be diagnosed with technetium-labeled leukocytes.[52] Gallium citrate Ga 67 is sometimes used to stage a tumor or to detect a source of infection in a child with persistent fever of unknown origin. However, the radiation dose of a gallium scan is not trivial, so this examination is usually limited to children with known or suspected malignant neoplasms.

## Computed Tomography

Oral, rectal, and intravenous contrast media may be necessary to optimize visualization of intra-abdominal processes with computed tomography.[53, 54] Sedation is given to infants and young children so that motion of the patient, which would degrade the image, is decreased. Medication to diminish intestinal peristalsis may also be given.[55]

Computed tomography has been of value in demon-strating complications of inflammatory bowel disease, appendicitis, and prior surgery. It has been used to evaluate children with congenital lesions (alimentary duplication, imperforate anus) and neoplasms. Special technical concerns and a more extended discussion of the uses of computed tomography in the pediatric population are presented in Chapter 136.

## Magnetic Resonance Imaging

The pediatric applications of magnetic resonance have evoked considerable interest because this technique uses no ionizing radiation. Solid organs and retroperitoneal structures are more successfully imaged than are the bowel or mesentery.[56, 57] Visualization of the gut is limited by peristalsis, which degrades the magnetic resonance image, and the lack of a satisfactory agent to opacify the bowel.[58]

Magnetic resonance has been used to evaluate the pelvic musculature and spinal canal in children with imperforate anus and the great vessels in children with suspected vascular rings.[59–63]

## References

1. Lorenzo RL, Harolds JA: The use of prone films for suspected bowel obstruction in infants and children. AJR 129:617–622, 1977.
2. Seibert JJ, Parvey LS: The telltale triangle: use of the supine cross table lateral radiograph of the abdomen in early detection of pneumoperitoneum. Pediatr Radiol 5:209–210, 1977.
3. Poznanski A: Technical note: a simple device for administering barium to infants. Radiology 93:1106, 1969.
4. Becker MH, Genieser NB: A new device for feeding infants during fluoroscopy. J Pediatr 80:291, 1972.
5. Cohen MD: Choosing contrast media for the evaluation of the gastrointestinal tract of neonates and infants. Radiology 162:447–456, 1987.
6. Janower ML: Hypersensitivity reactions after barium studies of the upper and lower gastrointestinal tract. Radiology 161:139–140, 1986.
7. Feczko PJ: Increased frequency of reactions to contrast materials during gastrointestinal studies. Radiology 174:367–368, 1990.
8. Poole CA, Rowe MI: Clinical evidence of intestinal absorption of Gastrografin. Radiology 118:151–153, 1976.
9. Harris PD, Neuhauser EBD, Gerth R: The osmotic effect of water soluble contrast media on circulating plasma volume. AJR 91:694–698, 1964.
10. Brick SH, Caroline DF, Lev-Toaff AS, et al: Esophageal disruption: evaluation with Iohexol esophagography. Radiology 169:141–143, 1988.
11. Cohen M, Smith WL, Smith JA, et al: Use of metrizamide (Amipaque) to visualise the gastrointestinal tract in children: a preliminary report. Clin Radiol 31:635–641, 1980.
12. Cohen MD, Weber T: Metrizamide in neonatal and childhood small bowel obstruction. AJR 139:689–692, 1982.
13. Cohen MD, Weber TR, Grosfeld JL: Bowel perforation in the newborn: diagnosis with metrizamide. Radiology 150:65–69, 1984.
14. Cohen MD, Towbin R, Baker S, et al: Comparison of Iohexol with barium in gastrointestinal studies of infants and children. AJR 156:345–350, 1991.
15. Wood BP, Katzberg RW, Ryan DH, et al: Diatrizoate enemas: facts and fallacies of colonic toxicity. Radiology 126:441–444, 1978.
16. Wood BP, Katzberg RW: Tween 80/diatrizoate enemas in bowel obstruction. AJR 130:747–750, 1978.
17. Leonidas JC, Burry VF, Fellows RA, et al: Possible adverse effect

of methylglucamine diatrizoate compounds on the bowel of new-born infants with meconium ileus. Radiology 121:693–696, 1976.

18. Hanly JG, Fitzgerald MX: Meconium ileus equivalent in older patients with cystic fibrosis. BMJ 286:1411–1413, 1983.

19. Katz M, Phelan E, Carlin JB, et al: Gas enema for the reduction of intussusception: relationship between clinical signs and symptoms and outcome. AJR 160:363–366, 1993.

20. Phelan E, de Campo JF, Malecky G: Comparison of oxygen and barium reduction of ileocolic intussusception. AJR 150:1349–1352, 1988.

21. Baath L, Ekberg O, Borulf S, et al: Small bowel barium examination in children. Diagnostic accuracy and clinical value as evaluated from 331 enteroclysis and follow-through examinations. Acta Radiol 30:621–626, 1989.

22. Ratcliffe JF: The small bowel enema in children: a description of technique. Clin Radiol 34:287–289, 1983.

23. Eklöf O, Erasmie U: The small bowel enema. An improved method of examination and its indications in children. Ann Radiol 21:143–148, 1978.

24. Gyepes MT, Smith LE, Ament ME: Fiberoptic endoscopy and upper gastrointestinal series: comparative analysis in infants and children. AJR 128:53–56, 1977.

25. Winthrop JD, Balfe DM, Shackelford GD, et al: Ulcerative and granulomatous colitis in children. Comparison of double- and single-contrast studies. Radiology 154:657–660, 1985.

26. Stringer DA, Sherman P, Liu P, et al: Value of the peroral pneumocolon in children. AJR 146:763–766, 1986.

27. Stringer DA, Sherman PM, Jakowenko N: Correlation of double-contrast high-density barium enema, colonoscopy, and histology in children with special attention to disparities. Pediatr Radiol 16:298–301, 1986.

28. Miller JH, Kemberling CR: Ultrasound scanning of the gastrointestinal tract in children: subject review. Radiology 152:671–677, 1984.

29. Carroll BA: US of the gastrointestinal tract. Radiology 172:605–608, 1989.

30. Teele RL, Smith EH: Ultrasound diagnosis of idiopathic hypertrophic pyloric stenosis. N Engl J Med 296:1149–1150, 1977.

31. Blumhagen JD, Maclin L, Krauter D, et al: Sonographic diagnosis of hypertrophic pyloric stenosis. AJR 150:1367–1370, 1988.

32. Breaux CW, Georgeson KE, Royal SA, et al: Changing patterns in the diagnosis of hypertrophic pyloric stenosis. Pediatrics 81:213–217, 1988.

33. Hayden CK Jr, Swischuk LE, Rytting JE. Gastric ulcer disease in infants: US findings. Radiology 164:131–134, 1987.

34. Fleischer AC, Muhletaler CA, James AE: Sonographic assessment of the bowel wall. AJR 136:887–891, 1981.

35. Merritt CRB, Goldsmith JP, Sharp MJ: Sonographic detection of portal venous gas in infants with necrotizing enterocolitis. AJR 143:1059–1062, 1984.

36. Alexander JE, Williamson SL, Seibert JJ: The ultrasonographic diagnosis of typhlitis (neutropenic colitis). Pediatr Radiol 18:200–204, 1988.

37. Shanon A, Martin DJ, Feldman W: Ultrasonographic studies in the management of recurrent abdominal pain. Pediatrics 86:35–38, 1990.

38. Cohen HL, Haller JO, Mestel AL, et al: Neonatal duodenum: fluid aided US examination. Radiology 164:805–809, 1987.

39. Puylaert JBCM: Appendicitis: US evaluation using graded compression sonography. Radiology 158:355–360, 1986.

40. Swischuk LE, Hayden CK, Boulden T: Intussusception: indications for ultrasonography and an explanation of the doughnut and pseudokidney sign. Pediatr Radiol 15:338–391, 1985.

41. Patriquin H, Tessier G, Grignon A, et al: Lesser omental thickness in normal children: baseline for detection of portal hypertension. AJR 145:693–696, 1985.

42. Loyer E, Eggli KD: Sonographic evaluation of superior mesenteric vascular relationship in malrotation. Pediatr Radiol 19:173–175, 1989.

43. Leonidas JC, Magid N, Soberman N, et al: Midgut volvulus in infants: diagnosis with US. Work in progress. Radiology 179:491–493, 1991.

44. Patriquin HB, O'Regan S, Robitaille P, et al: Hemolytic-uremic syndrome: intrarenal arterial Doppler patterns as a useful guide to therapy. Radiology 172:625–628, 1989.

45. Miller JH: Upper gastrointestinal tract evaluation with radionuclides in infants. Radiology 178:326–327, 1991.

46. Gelfand MJ, Wagner GG: Gastric emptying in infants and children: limited utility of 1-hour measurement. Radiology 178:379–381, 1991.

47. Sfakianakis GN, Haase GM: Abdominal scintigraphy for ectopic gastric mucosa: a retrospective analysis of 143 studies. AJR 138:7–12, 1982.

48. Ohba S, Fukuda A, Kohno S, et al: Ileal duplication and multiple intraluminal diverticula: scintigraphy and barium meal. AJR 136:992–994, 1981.

49. Som P, Oster ZH, Atkins HL, et al: Detection of gastrointestinal blood loss with 99mTc-labelled, heat-treated red blood cells. Radiology 138:207–209, 1981.

50. Alavi A, Ring EJ: Localization of gastrointestinal bleeding of 99mTc sulfur colloid compared with angiography. AJR 137:741–748, 1981.

51. Dawson DJ, Khan AN, Miller V, et al: Detection of inflammatory bowel disease in adults and children: evaluation of a new isotopic technique. BMJ 291:1227–1230, 1985.

52. Henneman PL, Marcus CS, Inkelis SH, et al: Evaluation of children with possible appendicitis using technetium 99-m leukocyte scan. Pediatrics 85:838–843, 1990.

53. Siegel MJ, Evans SJ, Balfe DM: Small bowel disease in children: diagnosis with CT. Radiology 169:127–130, 1988.

54. Yousem DM, Fishman EK, Jones B: Crohn disease: perirectal and perianal findings at CT. Radiology 167:331–334, 1988.

55. Thoeni RF, Filson RG: Abdominal and pelvic CT: use of oral metoclopramide to enhance bowel opacification. Radiology 169:391–393, 1988.

56. Stark DD, Fahlvik AK, Klaveness J: Abdominal imaging. JMRI 3:285–295, 1993.

57. Gerscovich EO, McGahan JP, Buonocore MH, et al: The rediscovery of infant feeding formula with magnetic resonance imaging. Pediatr Radiol 20:147–151, 1990.

58. Harris TM, Cohen MD: Abdominal magnetic resonance imaging. Pediatr Radiol 20:10–19, 1989.

59. Sheldon C, Cormier M, Crone K, et al: Occult neurovesical dysfunction in children with imperforate anus and its variants. J Pediatr Surg 26:49–54, 1991.

60. Sachs TM, Applebaum H, Touran T, et al: Use of MRI in evaluation of anorectal anomalies. J Pediatr Surg 25:817–821, 1990.

61. Fletcher BD, Cohn RC: Tracheal compression and the innominate artery: MR evaluation in infants. Radiology 170:103–107, 1989.

62. Bisset GS, Strife JL, Kirks DR, et al: Vascular rings: MR imaging. AJR 149:251–256, 1987.

63. Vogl T, Wilimzig C, Hofmann U, et al: MRI in tracheal stenosis by innominate artery in children. Pediatr Radiol 21:89–93, 1991.

# Neonatal Gastrointestinal Radiology

Sandra K. Fernbach, M.D.

## INTRODUCTION

In this chapter, the broad spectrum of gastrointestinal malformations that present during the neonatal period is discussed. Some malformations are grossly apparent at birth (gastroschisis, omphalocele, diaphragmatic hernia); others generally present within the first hours or days of life (jejunal, ileal, or colonic atresia; meconium ileus; meconium plug; Hirschsprung's disease); and still others cause symptoms shortly after birth (esophageal atresia). Many of these diagnoses can be suggested by prenatal ultrasound.

## ROTATIONAL ANOMALIES

### Embryology

During the sixth gestational week, rapid elongation of the mid- and hindgut results in herniation of these portions of the gut into a sac in the midline of the anterior abdominal wall.[1] During the ninth week of fetal life, the bowel begins to return to the peritoneal cavity. Before it does so, the midgut revolves 90 degrees around the superior mesenteric artery. After the bowel returns to the abdominal cavity, it rotates an additional 180 degrees, which positions the duodenojejunal junction to the left of the spine at the level of the stomach, the jejunum in the left upper quadrant, and the ileum in the right hypochondrium or right lower quadrant.[1–3] The colon undergoes a separate counterclockwise rotation of 270 degrees, which brings the cecum into the right lower quadrant. When normal rotation occurs, the mesentery is attached with a broad base that extends from the left upper quadrant to the right lower quadrant. In addition to the mesenteric base, there are normal attachments that are vital for keeping the normally rotated bowel fixed in position: the ligament of Treitz at the duodenojejunal junction and an attachment at the cecal base.

Deviation from normal rotation and fixation occurs universally in children with omphalocele, gastroschisis, and diaphragmatic hernia.[1–3] Variations of rotation may also be present in asplenia and polysplenia syndromes, duodenal stenosis or atresia, and Hirschsprung's disease. However, the process of rotation may founder even when the remainder of the embryologic development proceeds normally.

The spectrum of rotational abnormalities is broad[4–14] (Figs. 74–1 to 74–3). In some children, the process of rotation may take place, but fixation fails to occur. In others, there are only minor variations from the normal position. Complete nonrotation is said to be present when the jejunum is to the right of the spine and the ileum is in the pelvis or to the left of the spine (see Fig. 74–1). Most clinical problems arise in children with the greatest deviation from the normal rotational pattern. In children with classic malrotation, the cecum lies in the midabdomen or left of the midline (see Fig. 74–2) and may be fixed in place by broad bands that emanate from the undersurface of the liver. These so-called Ladd's bands cross the duodenum and may cause extrin-

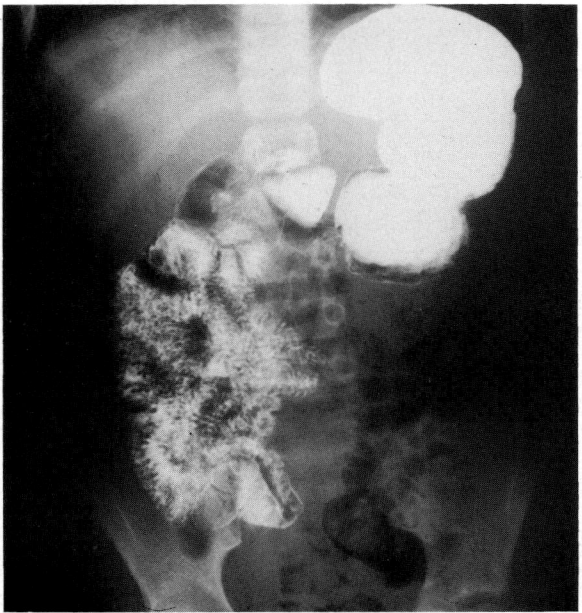

**Figure 74–1. Rotational variation.** The duodenal bulb overlies the spine, and multiple jejunal loops are seen throughout the right side of the abdomen.

sic compression and obstruction of the gut at this level (see Fig. 74–3).

## Clinical Findings

The majority of children with malrotation present in the first few months of life either with chronic vomiting and failure to thrive because of obstructing Ladd's bands (see Fig. 74–3) or with acute volvulus if there has been twisting of the bowel on its shortened mesentery. Midgut volvulus may produce vascular compromise, which can lead to gangrene of the entire small bowel if it is not promptly diagnosed and treated[7–12, 15, 16] (Fig. 74–4).

In some children, the malrotation abnormality is not detected until later, when studies are done for other purposes.[5, 17–19] Even more rarely, malrotation can be associated with chronic volvulus that interferes with lymphatic and venous drainage, which produces malabsorption or failure to thrive.[20–22] The older child and adult with rotational anomalies can rarely experience acute volvulus with infarction of bowel with the same consequences as in the younger patient.[5, 18] Motility abnormalities may persist after corrective surgery.[22a]

There is a high incidence of other duodenal abnormalities in children with malrotation: duodenal atresia, annular pancreas, and preduodenal portal vein.

## Radiologic Findings

Plain films are of little value in the child with an uncomplicated rotational abnormality because the ligament of Treitz and the position of the cecum are usually not well seen. Occasionally, there is abnormal configuration of the gas in the right hypochondrium, "the duodenal triangle," which may suggest the diagnosis of malrotation.[23] Normal radiographs also do not exclude the diagnosis of malrotation with volvulus.[6–9]

In the neonate or child with abdominal pain or vomiting, plain films may suggest a high obstruction if there is gaseous distention of the stomach and duodenal bulb. This appearance, referred to as the "double bubble," can also be seen in duodenal atresia and annular pancreas. A contrast study may be necessary for differentiation between the relatively benign complication of Ladd's bands (see Fig. 74–3) and the surgical emergency of volvulus (see Fig. 74–4).

In the child with midgut volvulus, the abdominal gas pattern may be normal or show high or low obstruction, or the abdomen may be gasless.[7–12] Because of the variable appearance of the plain films and the grim consequences of delayed diagnosis, contrast studies should be performed emergently when volvulus is suspected clinically or radiographically.

An upper gastrointestinal and small bowel series should be performed first to detect the malrotation and its complications: Ladd's bands and volvulus. The barium enema can show a malpositioned or malfixed cecum (see Fig. 74–2), but a normal study does not always exclude malrotation. For this reason, it

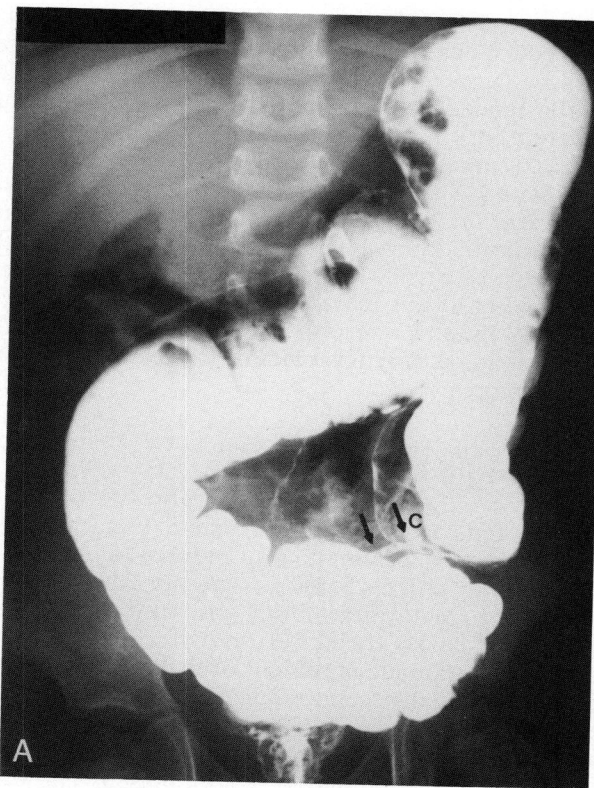

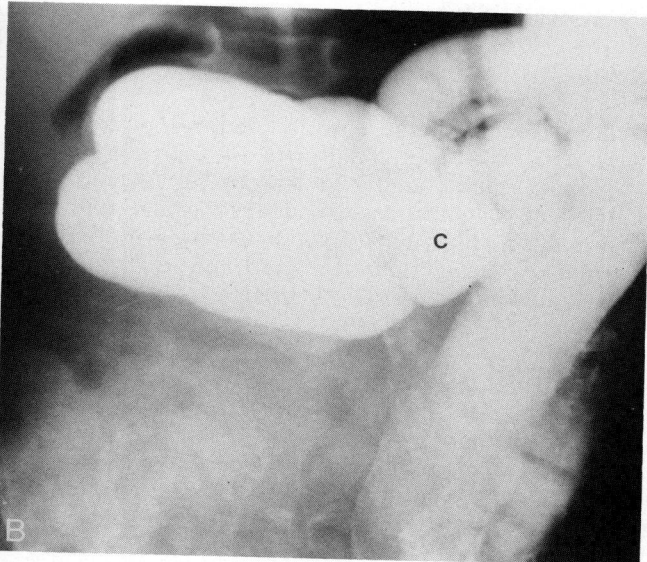

**Figure 74–2. Malrotation demonstrated on barium enema. A.** The cecum (C) lies in the left lower quadrant. Note contrast medium in the appendix *(arrows)*. **B.** In a different child, the cecum (C) is in the left upper quadrant.

may be necessary for an upper gastrointestinal series to be performed after the enema if a low obstructive lesion is not found and malrotation is still considered.

The diagnosis of malrotation can be made sonographically, although it is usually an incidental finding on studies performed for other reasons.[24–27] The failure of the bowel to rotate normally produces an abnormal relationship between the superior mesenteric artery and vein.[28] Computed tomography (CT) can also show these vascular changes as well as malpositioned and twisted bowel.[29, 29a, 30]

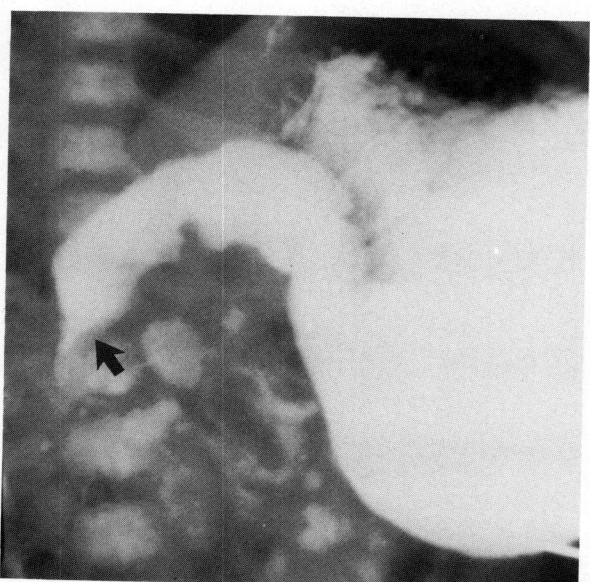

**Figure 74–3. Malrotation with Ladd's bands.** This upper gastrointestinal series shows a partially obstructing, extrinsic defect *(arrow)* in the duodenum.

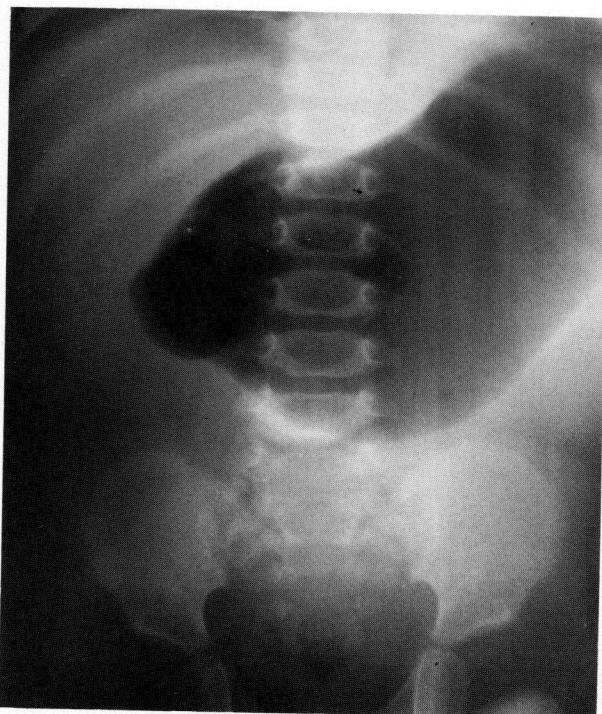

**Figure 74–4. Midgut volvulus.** Plain film demonstrates air only in the stomach and duodenum in this acutely ill infant with midgut volvulus.

# GASTROSCHISIS

## General Considerations

The development of the anterior abdominal wall is complex, with the orderly ingrowth of four separate folds (cranial, caudal, and two lateral) necessary for normal closure.[31-33] Gastroschisis defines a parasagittal defect, usually to the right of the normally positioned and normal-appearing umbilical cord, through which bowel herniates into the amniotic fluid.[34, 35]

## Clinical Findings

In contrast to the omphalocele, the gastroschisis defect has no covering membrane or sac and is associated with a rise in the maternal serum alpha-fetoprotein. Gastroschisis occurs seven times more often in infants of mothers younger than 20 years than of those older than 25 years of age.[36] Occurring in about 1 of 6000 live births, the abnormality can be diagnosed prenatally with sonography.[2, 37-41] At birth, the defect and the herniated bowel are apparent and not easily confused with other abdominal wall defects.

Malrotation or nonrotation of the bowel is the rule in gastroschisis, but this rarely leads to complications. Bowel atresia is present in up to 20% of cases, but gastroschisis is usually seen as an isolated finding.[32, 41-50]

## Treatment

Although only a small amount of bowel is usually herniated through a usually small defect, surgical repair is associated with a postoperative mortality between 7 and 25%, with major complications of sepsis and electrolyte problems.[42-50] Antenatal exposure to amniotic fluid produces bowel wall edema and inflammatory thickening of the serosa, which interferes with peristaltic function, even after repair. In utero, the exposed bowel and mesentery may become shortened and coiled, which also affects postnatal function. Short gut syndrome may decrease intestinal absorption and cause diminished constitutional growth.[51] Children with short gut or hypoperistalsis can be supported with parenteral hyperalimentation, but this, too, can create management problems: venous thrombosis, liver disease, and cholelithiasis.[52] It appears that cesarean delivery of affected infants several weeks before term impedes the development of a "peel" on the bowel and helps to minimize mesenteric changes.[49] The postoperative period in this group of infants also has fewer complications.

The type of surgical correction depends on the size of the defect and the presence of other complications such as atresia and short gut.[32, 42-51] Primary closure is performed if it will not produce high intra-abdominal pressure that causes respiratory distress and vascular compromise of the gut.[53] Alternatively, a protective Silastic silo can be placed over the bowel loops, and the abdominal wall defect can be closed at a later time. With either approach, postoperative ventilatory assistance is usually needed. When there is associated intestinal atresia, it may be necessary to create a stoma for decompression of the dilated proximal bowel as well as to provide a covering for the herniated bowel.

After surgery, motility changes are universal in children with gastroschisis.[54-56] Initially, there is postoperative paralytic ileus; later, marked prolongation of intestinal transit is common. These children also have a high incidence of significant gastroesophageal reflux. Necrotizing enterocolitis (NEC) occurs in up to 23% of cases at 1 to 4 months after repair despite the fact that these children are usually term infants and have fairly normal Apgar scores.[55]

## Radiologic Findings

The prenatal sonographic diagnosis of gastroschisis is based on the observation of normal umbilical cord insertion in a fetus with an anterior abdominal wall defect through which bowel has herniated.[2, 37-41] No membrane covers the bowel, so that if fetal ascites or a covering membrane is present or if the liver is detected in the herniated viscera, omphalocele is the more likely diagnosis.[38, 39] Thickening of the exteriorized bowel loops is strongly suggestive of gastroschisis and indicates that later bowel function may be compromised. The volume of amniotic fluid is usually normal.

Postnatal plain films show the normally positioned umbilical clamp separated from herniated bowel loops, which are outlined by air (Fig. 74–5). Plain abdominal films should be carefully scrutinized throughout the

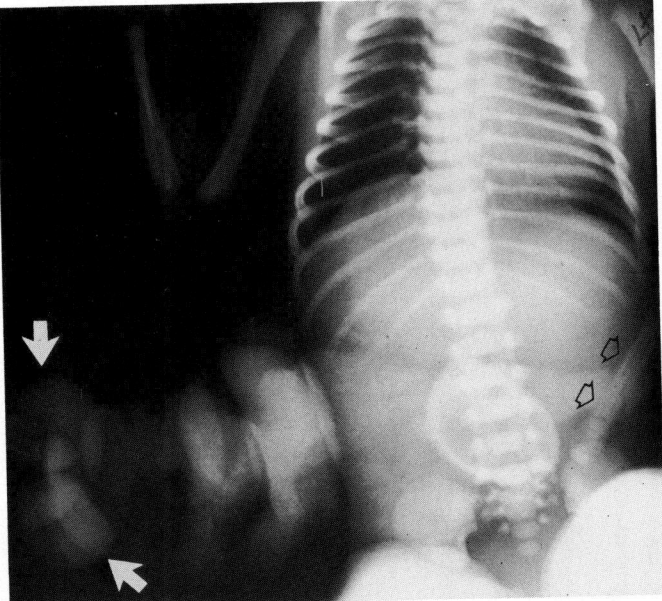

**Figure 74–5. Gastroschisis.** Exteriorized bowel loops (white arrows) extend lateral to the abdominal wall in this neonate with gastroschisis. Because the loops lack a covering membrane, each is clearly outlined by air. The normally inserted umbilical cord is in the midline, defined by the umbilical clamp to the left of midline (open arrows).

postoperative course as well. Although the radiographic pattern of late-developing NEC is typical (ileus, dilated bowel loops, intramural air), the clinical pattern is not; only 36% of the children have blood-streaked stools.[55]

Barium studies after birth are used to document gastroesophageal reflux, the degree of bowel loop dilatation, the presence of obstructive adhesions, the amount of bowel present, and abnormalities of position or transit time.

## OMPHALOCELE

### Clinical Findings

Omphalocele is present in about 1 of 5000 live births. It is a midline defect of variable size through which bowel, liver, spleen, pancreas, and even uterus may protrude. A membrane or sac usually covers the herniated organs, but the sac may be ruptured at birth. The umbilical cord inserts into the apex of the sac. The bowel is malrotated, and 8 to 20% of these children have Meckel's diverticulum. Abnormal development of both lateral folds is necessary for an isolated omphalocele; if the cephalic fold also develops abnormally, there will be ectopia cordis.

The diagnosis of omphalocele can be made with prenatal ultrasound.[2, 38–40, 57–60] Maternal alpha-fetoprotein levels may be elevated, but because of the covering sac, the levels are generally not as elevated as those found with gastroschisis defects.

Associated anomalies are seen in about 50 to 80% of infants with omphalocele, including tetralogy of Fallot and the secundum type of atrial septal defect, as well as other cardiac, central nervous system, and gastrointestinal anomalies.[47, 48, 50, 58–61] Detection of certain anomalies may influence the management or outcome of the pregnancy.[58]

Children with small anterior abdominal defects (gastroschisis, small omphalocele) tend to have a normally developed thorax. With giant omphaloceles that contain liver and bowel, the thorax is small; there is an increased incidence of pulmonary hypoplasia and an extended period of respiratory insufficiency requiring ventilatory support after surgery.[53, 62, 63]

Surgical management may take many forms.[42, 47, 49, 50, 64] In children with other life-threatening anomalies, the sac is painted with Mercurochrome to toughen it and prevent rupture. In most children, an attempt is made to correct the defect by primary skin closure or closure with Silastic halo. The surgical method chosen is based on the size of the defect; larger defects may even require a staged reduction.

Children with Beckwith-Wiedemann syndrome account for nearly 12% of the population with omphalocele.[58, 64] These children are large at birth and have a large tongue that may interfere with breathing or eating and require partial glossectomy. A specific pancreatic abnormality, nesidioblastosis, predisposes the children to hypoglycemia. An increased number of children with trisomy 13 and trisomy 18 also occur in the population with omphalocele.[42, 47, 48, 50, 58, 64]

## Radiologic Findings

Prenatal sonographic diagnosis of omphalocele is based on visualization of the umbilical cord inserting into the membrane covering structures anterior to the abdominal wall of the fetus.[2, 38–40, 58–60] Fetal ascites, abnormal amounts of amniotic fluid, and associated congenital defects are supportive ancillary findings.[65–67] When the exteriorized bowel loops are thickened or if no membrane or sac is detected, the fetus is likely to have gastroschisis.

Postnatal plain films of the abdomen (Fig. 74–6) demonstrate the omphalocele as a soft tissue density whose margins are well defined by the adjacent air. In contrast to gastroschisis, in which separate bowel loops are outlined by air (see Fig. 74–5), the bowel loops are not individually seen unless there has been rupture of the omphalocele.

## DIAPHRAGMATIC HERNIA: FORAMEN OF BOCHDALEK HERNIA

### Embryology

In early fetal life, the peritoneal cavity and the pleural space are in continuity. At week 8, just before the return of the bowel to the abdominal cavity, the communication between these two spaces is closed by the development of the diaphragm.[68] If the bowel returns to the abdomen prematurely or if the diaphragm develops late or incompletely, a diaphragmatic hernia (DH) develops. Affected children have malrotation of the bowel because there is interruption of the normal rotation that occurs as the bowel returns to the abdomen. A membrane covering the herniated gut is found in only 10% of Bochdalek hernias.

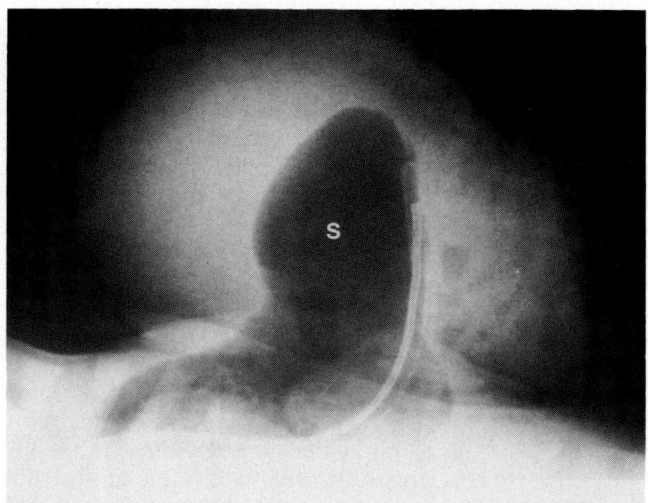

**Figure 74–6. Omphalocele.** Lateral plain film of the abdomen reveals a membrane-covered omphalocele. The walls of the membrane are outlined by air and clearly seen, but individual bowel loops cannot be identified because they are not exposed to air, in contrast to the situation in gastroschisis. The air-filled stomach (S) protrudes into the omphalocele.

## Clinical Findings

The posterolateral or Bochdalek hernia occurs in approximately 1 per 3000 live births. Reports based on CT scans of adult patients suggest a much greater prevalence of 6%.[68-71] This larger number may be due to the fact that CT readily detects asymptomatic, small hernias that are not recognized on standard radiographs. In addition, some of the hernias may be acquired secondary to trauma or infection.[72, 73] In the neonatal period, noncongenital DH can develop on the right in association with group B streptococcal infection.[74] No etiologic agent or risk factor has been linked to congenital DH.

Congenital DH occurs six to nine times more often on the left, presumably owing to the fact that the pleuroperitoneal canal closes earlier on the right; about 3% of children have bilateral DH.[69] Left-sided hernias usually contain portions of the gastrointestinal tract. The liver may extend into the thorax with right-sided hernias, which accounts for much of the morbidity and mortality associated with DH.

DH should be suspected clinically when a neonate with severe respiratory distress has a scaphoid abdomen. Because bowel contents are in the thorax, the abdomen lacks its normal protuberant appearance. Most children with DH are rapidly intubated and resuscitated; when stable, they undergo surgical repair.[68, 75, 76] All children are carefully inspected for the exclusion of associated anomalies including midline defects (cleft lip and palate, spina bifida, and omphalocele) and cardiac lesions (ventricular septal defects and tetralogy of Fallot).[69, 71, 75-77]

Regardless of the side on which the hernia occurs, both the ipsilateral lung and the contralateral lung are compressed, and the most critical factor in determining the infant's outcome is the degree of pulmonary hypoplasia.[78, 78a, 79]

Despite ventilatory support and pharmacologic manipulations to decrease the common additional complication of persistent fetal circulation, early postnatal mortality rates range between 20 and 80%.[77-79] To improve survival, a new postnatal treatment called extracorporeal membrane oxygenation (ECMO) is used in infants who, after surgery, experience significant respiratory insufficiency because of pulmonary hypoplasia. This lung bypass system entails placing large vascular cannulas into the right atrium and aortic arch via the right common carotid artery. Heparinization is routine, as it is with other cardiopulmonary bypass procedures. The bypass removes carbon dioxide and oxygenates the blood; the lungs are minimally ventilated and given the chance to mature and grow. ECMO therapy can extend up to 10 days. The technique has increased postsurgical survival to over 80%.[80] It is, however, not without complications: bleeding at the neck wounds, intracerebral hemorrhage, and difficulty with later central line placement.[80-87]

## Radiologic Findings

The prenatal sonographic diagnosis of DH is made when the heart and other mediastinal contents are shifted from the midline and a "mass" that consists of liver or unaerated gut is present in the thorax. Fetal ascites, fetal pleural effusion, and polyhydramnios have also been reported in association with DH.[88-90]

Diagnosis with ultrasound has contributed to the development of still experimental prenatal surgery for correction of the hernia.[91] In utero surgery has been performed to remove the pressure on the lung. Because pulmonary hypoplasia is the key cause of neonatal mortality in those with DH, it is hoped that early intervention enhances pulmonary maturation and growth.[91]

When not diagnosed prenatally, the affected infant will be detected shortly after birth because of respiratory distress. Chest and abdominal films are obtained to determine the amount of bowel present in the abdomen and to exclude causes of neonatal respiratory distress such as pulmonary hypoplasia, congenital cystic adenomatoid malformation, and neonatal pneumonia. On early films, the herniated bowel loops may appear as a soft tissue mass. With time and air swallowing, the chest radiographs will have a more typical appearance (Fig. 74-7). Right-sided hernias that contain liver appear more solid and may be accompanied by a pleural collection.[92]

The first set of radiographs should be evaluated for alternative diagnoses, complications of resuscitation, and other congenital abnormalities that might affect management. Pneumothorax is common and requires prompt treatment. Abnormal position of the endotracheal tube or vascular catheters needs to be corrected before surgery. The detection of bony or somatic changes of certain syndromes might prompt less aggressive treatment.

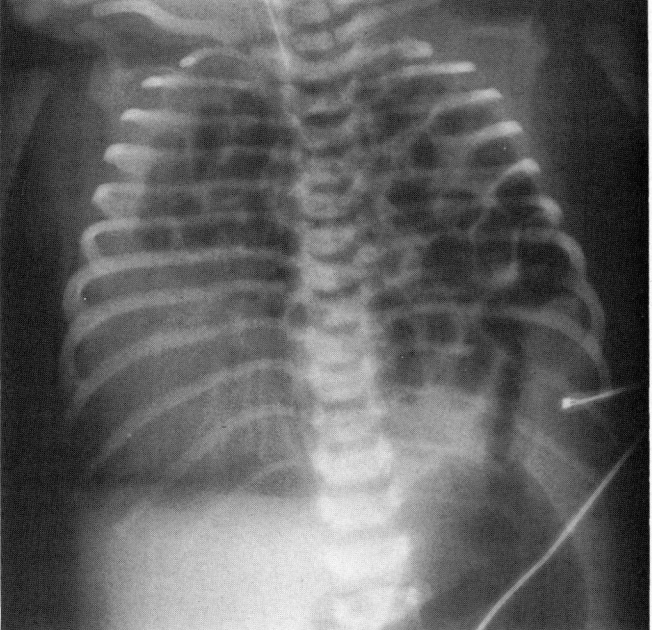

**Figure 74–7. Left Bochdalek hernia.** Left foramen of Bochdalek hernia manifests as multiple air-filled bowel loops that fill the left thorax and right apex. The mediastinum is shifted to the right, and the soft tissue densities of the heart and the hypoplastic right lung merge.

If there is question about the nature of the thoracic contents, a nasogastric tube should be inserted to define the stomach and to distend the bowel with air. Contrast studies are occasionally needed to visualize the upper or lower gastrointestinal tract before surgery (Fig. 74–8). Abdominal ultrasound should be performed to determine the location of the spleen, kidneys, and liver.

The mediastinum remains shifted to the side opposite the hernia on postoperative chest radiographs. Attempts to bring the mediastinum to the midline may result in overexpansion of the hypoplastic contralateral lung and cause pneumothorax. The ipsilateral lung appears as a soft tissue density outlined with air, close to the mediastinum. Pneumothorax on the side of the hernia repair is expected, and because of the long-standing mediastinal shift, it may simulate tension pneumothorax. During the first few postoperative days, as the ipsilateral lung grows and expands, fluid may occupy a portion of the pleural space and produce unilateral haziness in the thorax.

Before a child is placed on ECMO, cardiac, cranial, and abdominal ultrasound studies are performed to select those children who can safely receive this treatment. Children with prior intracranial hemorrhage or with a lethal deformity are excluded.

Once ECMO is begun, the infants receive a daily chest radiograph. Careful evaluation of line placement is necessary because kinking and dislodgment may occur and compromise treatment. Chest radiographs commonly show mediastinal air or fluid mass in the midline, which is the esophagus dilated from gastroesophageal reflux and increased pulmonary density.[93, 94, 94a]

The most striking finding on the radiographs of many long-term survivors is the degree to which the hypoplastic lungs can develop. In many children, a chest film at age 2 or 3 years has a near-normal appearance.[95]

## DIAPHRAGMATIC HERNIA: FORAMEN OF MORGAGNI HERNIA

Herniation of colon, omentum, or other structures into the retrosternal space is rare and occurs when there is faulty development of the anteromedial aspect of the

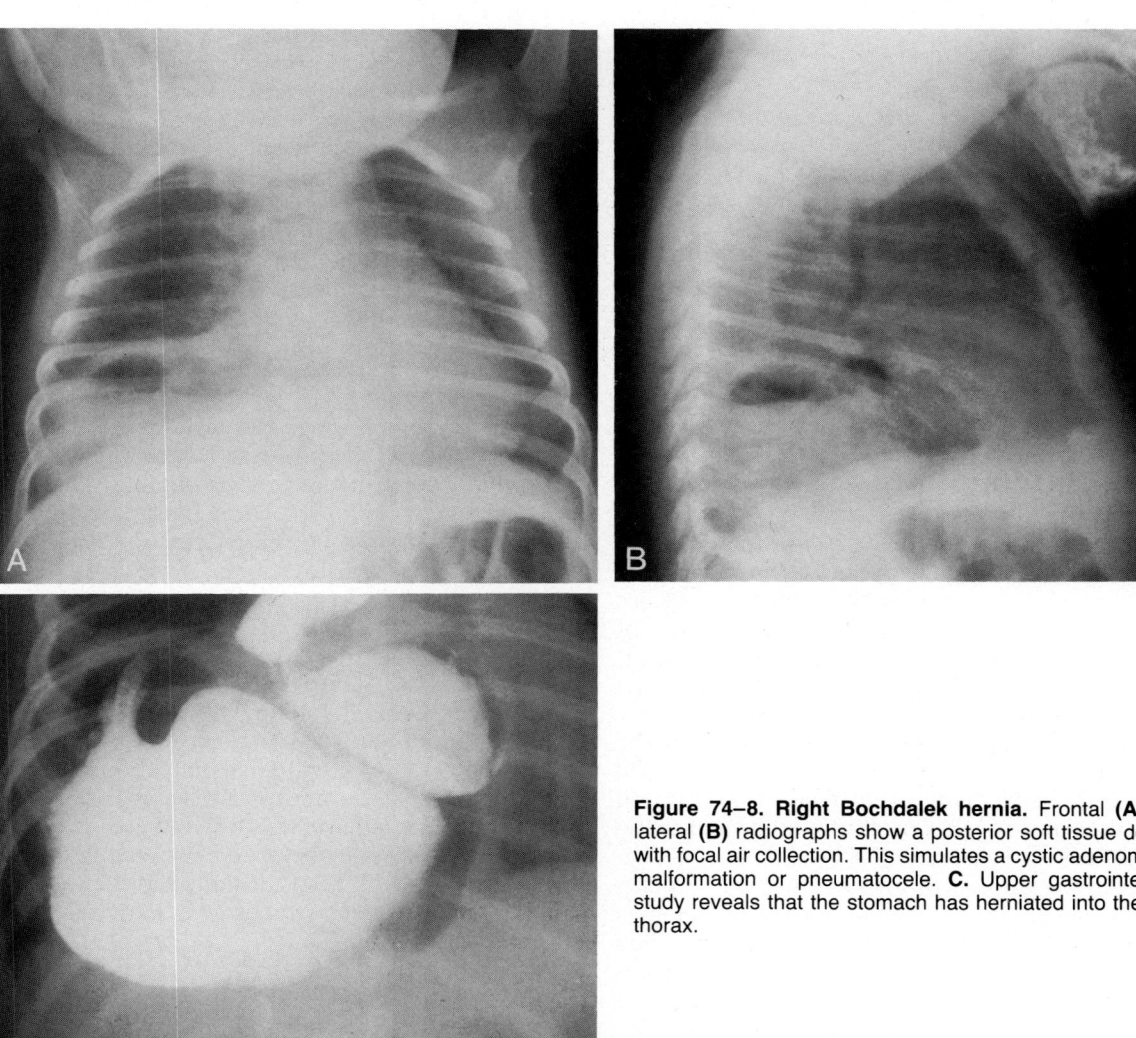

**Figure 74–8. Right Bochdalek hernia.** Frontal **(A)** and lateral **(B)** radiographs show a posterior soft tissue density with focal air collection. This simulates a cystic adenomatoid malformation or pneumatocele. **C.** Upper gastrointestinal study reveals that the stomach has herniated into the right thorax.

diaphragm.[68, 69, 71, 96] The so-called foramen of Morgagni hernia accounts for about 2 to 4% of all DH.[68, 69, 71]

Respiratory and gastrointestinal complaints are common but not necessarily related to the hernia.[96–99] The child may be asymptomatic, and the abnormality may be detected on a chest film done for a nonrelated purpose. Indeed, only 50% are detected by age 5 years.[96–101]

Although the amount of bowel herniated into the chest in Morgagni hernias is usually much less than in Bochdalek hernias, malrotation or malfixation is common. In contrast to Bochdalek hernias, Morgagni hernias usually are right sided and have a covering or sac.[97–101]

The differential diagnosis of air-containing Morgagni hernias includes pneumonia, atelectasis, pneumatocele, abscess, and cystic adenomatoid malformation. If the liver is herniated, the solid appearance may simulate a tumor of the diaphragm, a pericardial mass, or an anterior mediastinal mass.

Morgagni hernias are corrected even in asymptomatic children because there is always the potential for incarceration and strangulation.

## Radiologic Findings

Anteroposterior chest films may show a soft tissue or air density along the heart border (Fig. 74–9). On the lateral projection, the anterior location of the hernia and visualization of bowel markings establish the diagnosis. In some cases, additional imaging with sonography, barium studies, CT, and magnetic resonance (MR) may be needed to identify the nature and extent of the hernia.[101–103]

## NORMAL AND ABNORMAL NEONATAL BOWEL GAS

With the first breath, the neonate begins to aerate the previously fluid-filled respiratory and gastrointestinal tracts.[104] Unless there is obstruction, these processes tend to parallel each other.[104] However, the degree of lung expansion and the amount of gastrointestinal air are not equal, especially in the first minute post partum.[104]

Several problems delay the passage of air into the gastrointestinal tract. The most obvious is a mechanical obstruction in the oral cavity or esophagus, most often esophageal atresia. Drugs given during labor and delivery complications can depress the swallowing mechanism, diminish the amount of air swallowed, and delay passage of air distally into the small bowel and colon.[105]

Abdominal films that are initially normal but then become gasless raise the possibility that the child has become toxic, has developed electrolyte imbalance, is receiving gastric suction, or is being paralyzed with curariform agents while being ventilated.[105–108] These processes decrease the amount of air swallowed and/or decrease the amount available for passage into distal bowel.

The bowel gas pattern should be carefully scrutinized in any neonate with respiratory or gastrointestinal symptoms. Gas should be symmetrically distributed throughout the abdomen. Paucity or malposition of the abdominal gas may suggest a DH in the proper clinical setting. An abdominal mass may also displace bowel loops and, through pressure on the diaphragm, cause respiratory distress. When there is high intestinal obstruction, few loops of bowel are distended with air and fluid in the upper abdomen (Fig. 74–10). With distal obstruction, many loops of dilated bowel fill the abdomen (Fig. 74–11).

In the very young child, it may be difficult to differentiate small from large bowel because haustral markings are poorly developed in neonates. Whereas some authors report that location will also allow differentiation of small from large bowel, very distended small bowel may fill the space usually occupied by the colon.[109, 110]

It is important to determine the most distal extent of gastrointestinal air because the differential diagnosis varies with the level of the obstruction. Additional views may be necessary for detecting air within the colon. Oblique views of the abdomen should be obtained before distention causes small bowel to displace the airless colon or obliterates the haustral markings.[110] Prone lateral rectal views may be useful if an extremely distal lesion is suspected. In many cases, a contrast study of the colon may be performed to determine whether there is an obstruction or to identify the level and nature of the obstruction.[111]

## ABDOMINAL MASSES

The differential diagnosis of abdominal mass in the newborn is extensive: ovarian cyst or tumor; alimentary tract duplication; mesenteric or omental lymphangioma; cyst or tumor of the spleen or liver; lymphoma; choledochal cyst; cystic meconium peritonitis; hydrometrocolpos; and retroperitoneal masses.[112–117] In the neonatal period, the majority of abdominal masses originate in the genitourinary tract; ureteropelvic junction obstruction and multicystic dysplastic kidneys are the most common causes. Gastrointestinal lesions account for 8 to 15% of neonatal abdominal masses.[118–121]

The abdominal mass may be detected by prenatal sonography or by abdominal palpation after birth. In some neonates, the mass is sufficiently large to distend or distort the abdominal wall and cause respiratory distress. Ascites may be present or simulated.[122–124] Pain or obstruction will result if the mass is producing pressure on an adjacent structure or if there is torsion of the mass.

A bruit over the liver in an infant with congestive heart failure suggests a hepatic hemangioma. If a mass is present over the buttocks, the abdominal mass may represent internal extension of a sacrococcygeal teratoma.[125]

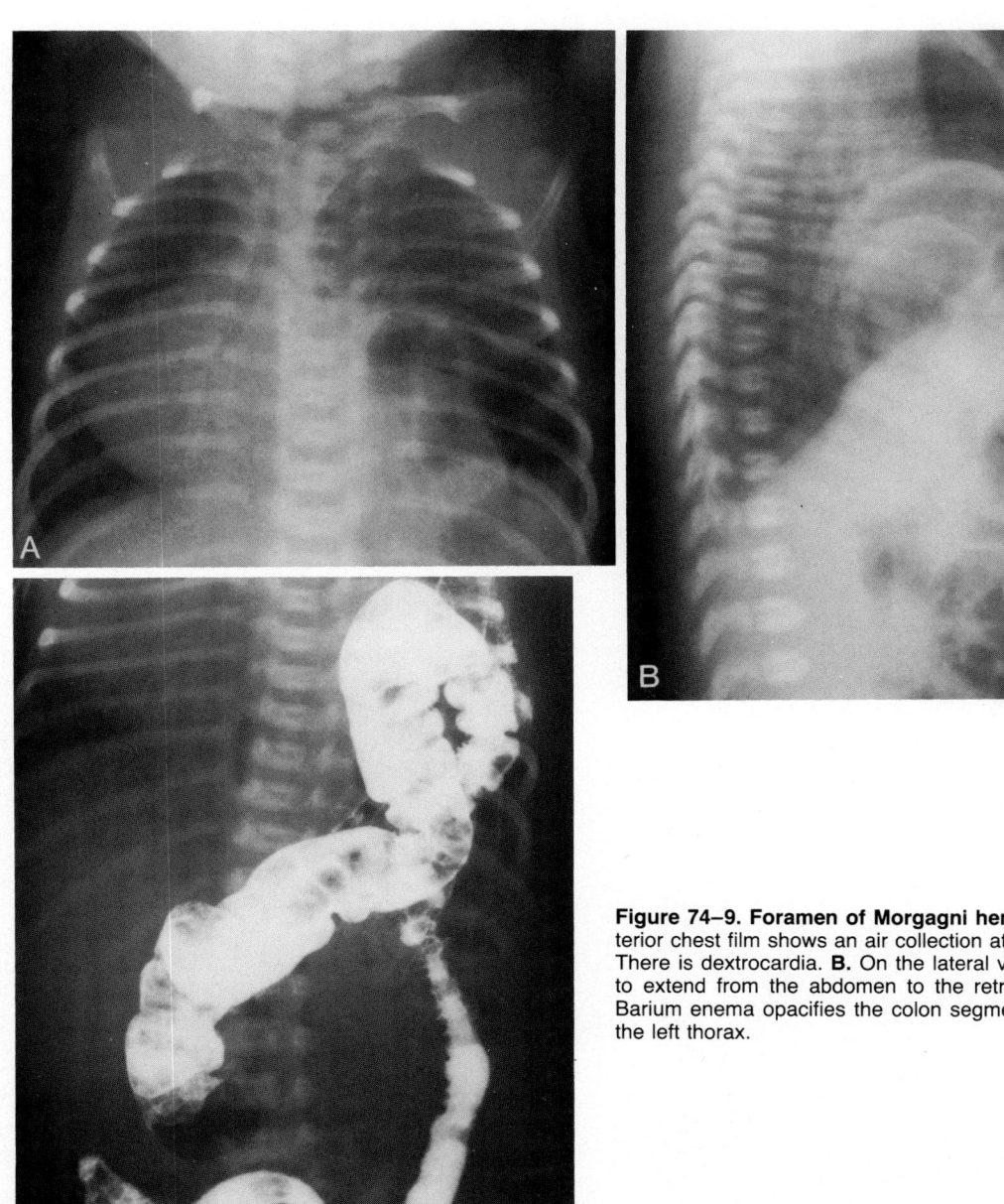

**Figure 74–9. Foramen of Morgagni hernia. A.** Anteroposterior chest film shows an air collection at the left lung base. There is dextrocardia. **B.** On the lateral view, bowel is seen to extend from the abdomen to the retrosternal space. **C.** Barium enema opacifies the colon segments, which occupy the left thorax.

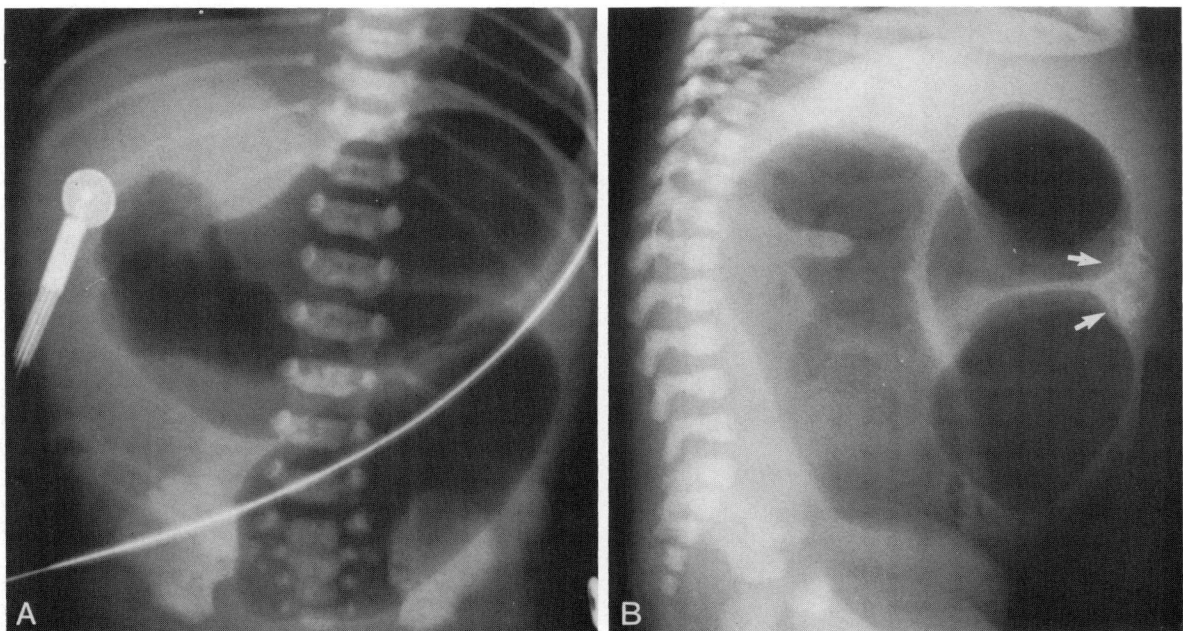

**Figure 74–10. High obstruction.** Anteroposterior **(A)** and lateral **(B)** abdominal radiographs in this child with jejunal atresia show several markedly distended bowel loops that fill the abdomen. The calcification along the anterior abdominal wall *(arrows)* indicates prior bowel perforation and meconium peritonitis.

## Radiologic Findings

Plain films may show bowel obstruction or bowel displacement, although these findings are relatively nonspecific. Calcifications suggest meconium peritonitis, teratoma, and hepatoblastoma; congenital bone abnormal-

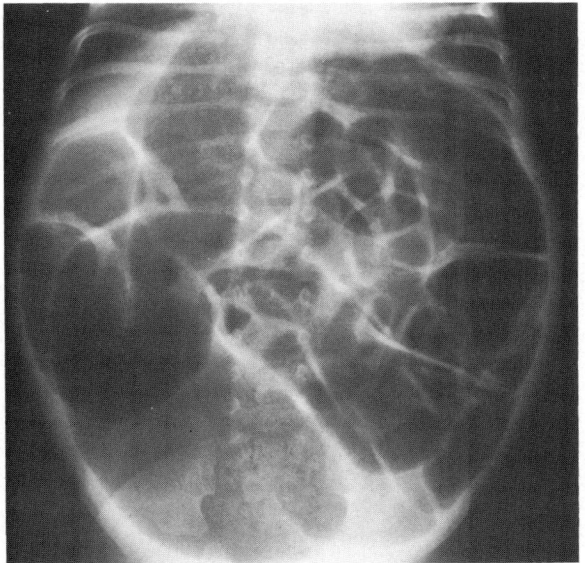

**Figure 74–11. Low obstruction.** Colonic obstruction from Hirschsprung's disease has produced dilatation of multiple bowel loops throughout the abdomen. Discrete haustral markings cannot be identified, so it is difficult to appreciate that the colon is dilated in addition to the entire small bowel.

ities suggest anterior sacral meningocele, obstructed cloacal deformity, or sacrococcygeal teratoma with an internal component.[125]

Ultrasound is the premier imaging technique for abdominal and pelvic masses in neonates. The following issues should be addressed. From what compartment or organ does the mass originate? Is the mass solid, cystic, or septated? Is there a wall, membrane, or capsule around it? Do the structures surrounding the mass look normal? Is there ascites? Are there any sites of spread or extension within the abdomen or retroperitoneum? On the basis of the information obtained, the child may proceed to surgery, undergo further radiologic evaluation, or be clinically observed and restudied after a period of observation.[126–129]

## NECROTIZING ENTEROCOLITIS

### Clinical Findings

NEC is a life-threatening process that primarily affects the gastrointestinal tracts of premature infants. The following signs and symptoms usually develop in the first 2 weeks of life: rising gastric residual volume, abdominal distention, bloody stools, lethargy, and even changing respiratory status.[130–134]

The exact etiology is unknown, but the pathologic changes in the bowel wall are believed to be due to intestinal ischemia. Shunting of blood from the mesenteric system may be a reflex event or result from other aberrations of physiology such as low left ventricular output and patent ductus arteriosus.[134–139] Ischemic bowel perforation has also been reported in neonates exposed to cocaine in utero.[139a] The epidemic nature of some cases suggests that a bacterial or viral agent may predispose the bowel to ischemic change. Dietary agents and gut hormones have also been implicated, and about 90% of neonates with NEC have been receiving enteral feeding; larger volumes are associated with a greater incidence of NEC.[140] The amount of carbohydrate fermentation that occurs within the neonatal colon influences intraluminal pH and the pattern of bacterial colonization, important links in the development of NEC.[130–134]

On pathologic examination, there is ulceration that begins in the mucosa and then extends to the submucosa; inflammatory cells may be present in multiple bowel layers.[141] Pneumatosis intestinalis is seen in the subserosa. In 50% of cases, there are normal areas of bowel between diseased segments. Inflammatory pseudomembranes are uncommon and are seen in less than 10%. Many specimens concurrently show acute changes and reparative changes in the same bowel segment, which suggests that subclinical disease precedes the clinically apparent acute process.

Complications of NEC include perforation with peritonitis or enterocyst formation and stricture.[130–134, 142–145] Erythema of the abdominal wall, positive results of paracentesis, or palpation of an abdominal mass suggests bowel perforation and mandates surgical treatment. Specific plain film changes are also considered to be indications for surgery: pneumoperitoneum, fixed bowel loop on sequential studies, and portal venous gas.

Strictures are late findings; 80% occur in the colon, and 15% are multiple. The terminal ileum is involved in 15% of affected infants.[145]

Strictures develop in 6 to 33% of children with NEC. They can present after a delay of up to 20 months. Children whose NEC-induced bowel perforations are treated with bowel diversion or percutaneous peritoneal drainage have a higher rate of stricture formation than do those who received only medical management.[142, 145–148] For this reason, children with diversions should undergo a contrast study of the bypassed bowel for excluding a stricture before bowel continuity is re-established.[148, 149]

Medical management of infants with suspected NEC includes parenteral nutrition and antibiotic therapy.[130–134] Even infants who undergo surgery require parenteral nutrition, which predisposes to fungal sepsis and gallbladder disease.[150, 151]

The survival rate for children with NEC has risen dramatically for those treated both medically and surgically. The majority of children with NEC now survive. Late complications include short gut syndrome, abdominal abscess, recurrent NEC, and stricture formation.[151a]

## Radiologic Findings

Plain film findings include gastric dilatation, a persistently dilated bowel loop, or an unchanging bowel gas pattern.[130–134, 152–163] Pneumatosis intestinalis (Figs. 74–12

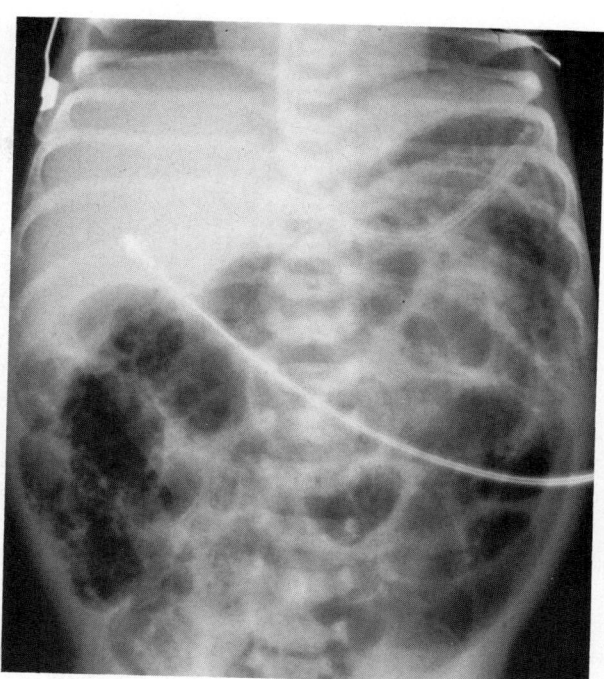

**Figure 74–12. NEC with pneumatosis intestinalis.** The bubbly appearance of the abdomen is due to the air within the bowel wall. In some segments, the intramural air clearly parallels the lumen; in other segments, it is seen as a circular pattern surrounding the lumen.

and 74–13) presents later, and large collections of intramural gas create a linear streaky pattern that parallels the bowel wall. When these collections are seen en face, their circular appearance confirms their mural rather than intraluminal location. Although the bubbly appearance of the bowel may suggest feces, the premature infant rarely has stool seen in the colon in the first 2 weeks of life.[164]

Gas can enter the mesenteric veins and be carried to the intrahepatic branches of the portal vein. The air produces streaky lucencies radiating over the liver (see Fig. 74–13). This is an evanescent sign in most children, but some physicians advocate surgery when intrahepatic portal gas is identified.[133]

Perforation is the most serious complication of NEC and is manifested by free air. When the amount of air is large, a diffuse lucency appears over the liver or midabdomen, the "football" sign. Air outlining the falciform ligament (Fig. 74–14) represents the laces of the football. Both the inner and outer bowel walls may be clearly seen. In a few children, the umbilical vessels are visible because of the surrounding air, which produces an inverted V sign in the pelvis. Air in Morison's pouch produces a triangular lucency.[155]

In searching for free air, cross-table lateral films are more easily obtained on these ill neonates than are upright films. Free air is visible over the liver and stomach or as small triangular lucencies projecting downward from the abdominal wall between the bowel loops.[162]

Although ultrasound is not the primary imaging technique for NEC, it can show mural thickening of affected

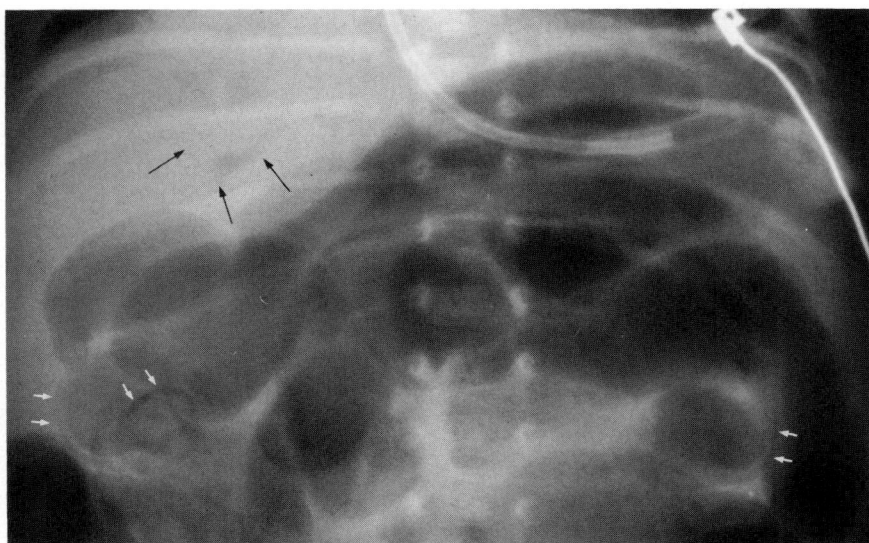

**Figure 74–13. NEC with portal venous air.** Branching lucencies throughout the liver represent gas within the portal venous system *(black arrows)*. Intramural air is also present *(white arrows)*.

loops and portal venous gas before their detection on plain films.[165–167] Intrahepatic portal venous gas is seen as bright reflectors bubbling through the liver. The hepatic parenchyma develops unusually bright echoes in a patchy distribution. The sonographic detection of portal gas is thought to be less significant than its detection on abdominal radiographs.

Early diagnosis of NEC prompts therapy that in most cases aborts the process. When NEC is suspected, but none of the radiographic signs is present, the child should be treated for presumed NEC, or studies should be obtained to confirm the diagnosis. In this setting, gastrointestinal imaging should be performed with oral, water-soluble, nonionic contrast agents.[168] Because of the success in treating children with suspected NEC, the classically described radiographic signs are seen with decreasing frequency.

The strictures that occur later in the natural history of NEC can cause clinical and radiographic signs of bowel obstruction. Contrast enema (Fig. 74–15) should

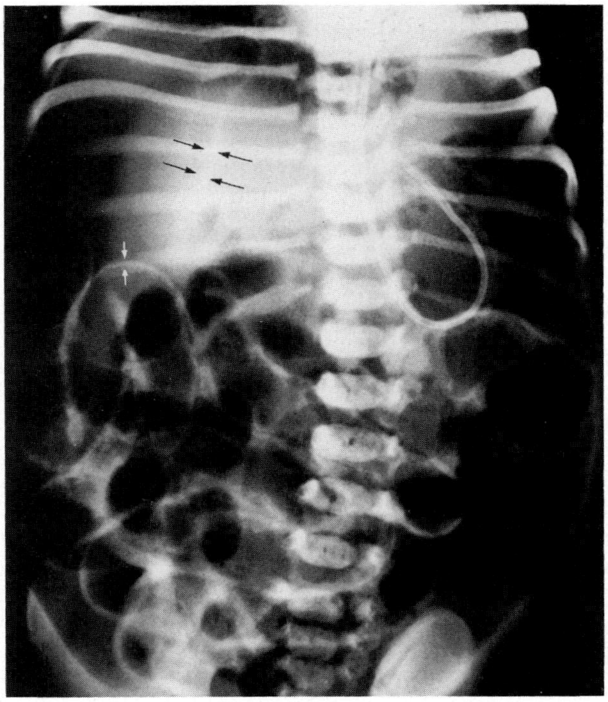

**Figure 74–14. NEC with perforation—the football sign.** A large amount of free peritoneal air clearly outlines the falciform ligament *(black arrows)*. The air has also given the entire right upper quadrant an unusual lucent appearance. Both the inner and the outer walls *(white arrows)* of multiple bowel loops are visible, another sign of free peritoneal air.

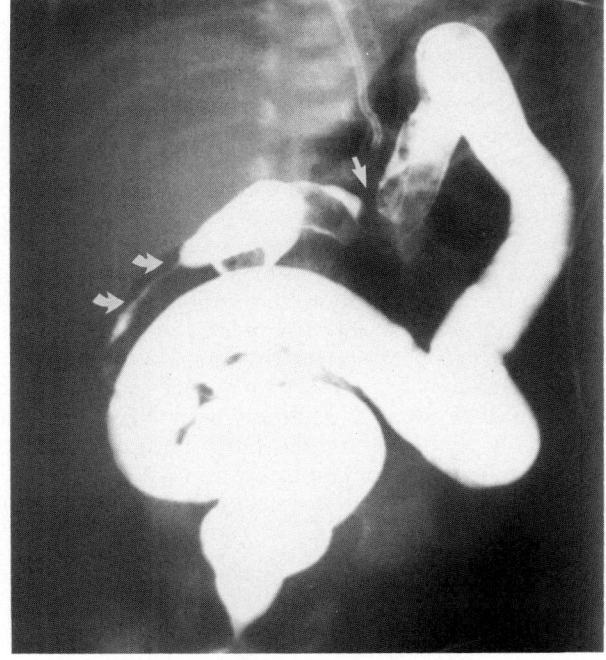

**Figure 74–15. Colonic stricture from NEC.** Water-soluble enema depicts an area of minor narrowing in the midtransverse colon *(straight arrow)* and a more severely narrowed segment at the hepatic flexure *(curved arrows)*.

be used to evaluate the entire colon and terminal ileum, where more than 90% of strictures occur. Although some of the strictures may spontaneously regress, most are either resected surgically or dilated with balloon catheters.[148, 168, 169]

## ESOPHAGEAL ATRESIA

Esophageal atresia (EA) occurs in about 1 in 5000 live births; males and females are equally affected. Most commonly there is an associated tracheoesophageal fistula (TEF), but in about 10% of children, the atresia is complete (Fig. 74–16).

EA is in the differential diagnosis of polyhydramnios.[170] At birth, the infant has difficulty handling secretions and may have severe respiratory distress with the first feeding. Attempts to pass a nasogastric tube are usually unsuccessful, although rarely the tube may pass from the trachea to the distal esophagus through the fistula and then into the stomach. Prompt diagnosis of EA is necessary to protect the lungs. A small drainage tube should be placed into the upper segment; oral feeding, of course, should be withheld.

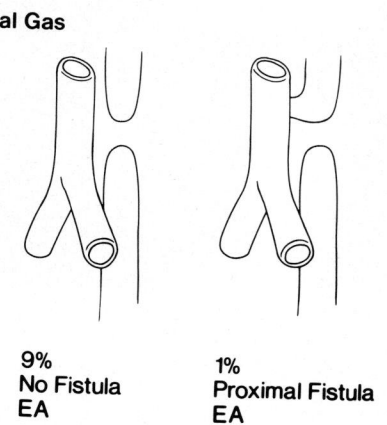

**Distal Gas**

82%
Distal Fistula
EA

6%
H-Type Fistula

2%
Proximal Fistula
Distal Fistula
EA

**No Distal Gas**

9%
No Fistula
EA

1%
Proximal Fistula
EA

**Figure 74–16.** Diagram depicting the common forms of esophageal atresia (EA).

The neonate with EA or EA and TEF must be evaluated for exclusion of other disorders including trisomy 21 and the VATER anomaly.[171–178] The acronym VATER or VACTERL association emphasizes the fact that vertebral, anorectal, cardiac, tracheoesophageal, renal, and limb anomalies may present together. There is a higher incidence of additional anomalies in those children whose EA is complete. Physical examination, radiographic studies, and ultrasound are performed before surgery to find other anomalies that need emergency correction (duodenal atresia) or that influence the standard surgical correction of TEF (right aortic arch).[179, 180]

The presence of a distal fistula can be diagnosed clinically (see Fig. 74–16) because neonates with TEF have a rounded abdomen and bowel sounds. The infant with EA without a fistula has a scaphoid abdomen and absent bowel sounds.

In the absence of prematurity or aspiration, surgical correction of EA with TEF is done in the first few days of life. Because the proximal and distal segments are usually close enough for apposition without tension, a simple anastomosis may be all that is necessary. Parenteral nutrition is then provided for a few days until postoperative studies confirm that the anastomosis is intact and oral feedings can be given safely. Gastrostomy is generally not necessary.[181, 182]

Primary correction in the neonatal period is not attempted in the child with EA and no TEF because there is too large a gap between the proximal and distal segments of the esophagus.[181–184] The infant undergoes gastrostomy placement for long-term nutritional support, and the proximal esophageal segment is brought to the skin as a "spit fistula" (cervical esophagostomy) so that secretions will be diverted and not aspirated.

When there is a small gap between the segments, the distal pouch can be dilated by bougienage or balloon catheters passed through the gastrostomy. If the gap between the proximal and distal segments is too great for simple anastomosis, the distance is bridged by interposing a segment of bowel brought into the chest on its vascular pedicle. Definitive correction is often delayed until the child is 1 year of age.

Postoperative complications are numerous regardless of the timing and type of repair performed. An anastomotic leak is seen in up to 27% of children who undergo primary repair in the neonatal period[185–188] (Fig. 74–17). Narrowing or stricture formation (Figs. 74–18 and 74–19) at the anastomosis occurs in over one third of cases. The strictures result from anastomotic leaks attributable to vascular change at the anastomosis or gastroesophageal reflux. Bougienage and, more recently, balloon dilatation are used to treat the strictures.[181, 185–190]

Development of a fistula at the surgical site (Fig. 74–20) or a proximal pouch fistula (Fig. 74–21), present in 3 to 5% of children with EA, may cause continued feeding difficulty simulating aspiration.[181, 191–194] The proximal fistula may be sought before surgery with carefully performed injections of a water-soluble contrast agent or air into the proximal pouch. Many institutions do not attempt to demonstrate the proximal

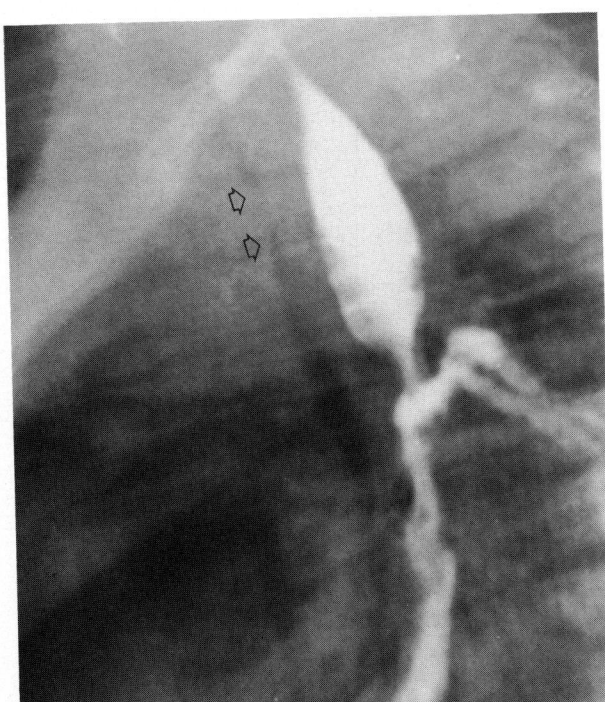

**Figure 74–17. Anastomotic leak after TEF repair.** As contrast medium reaches the anastomosis, it passes into the distal esophagus and into the posteriorly directed leak. Note the narrowing of the proximal trachea *(arrows)*.

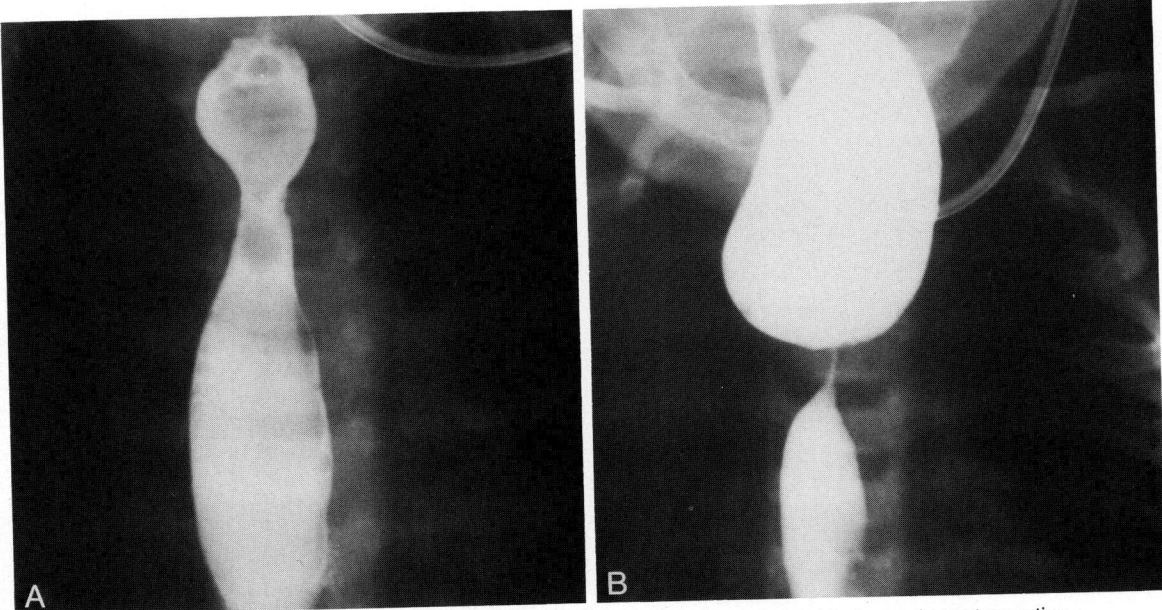

**Figure 74–18. Stricture formation after TEF repair. A.** A study performed in the early postoperative period demonstrates mild narrowing at the anastomotic site. This can be normal. **B.** Several months later, a study shows a severe stricture causing dilatation of the proximal esophagus.

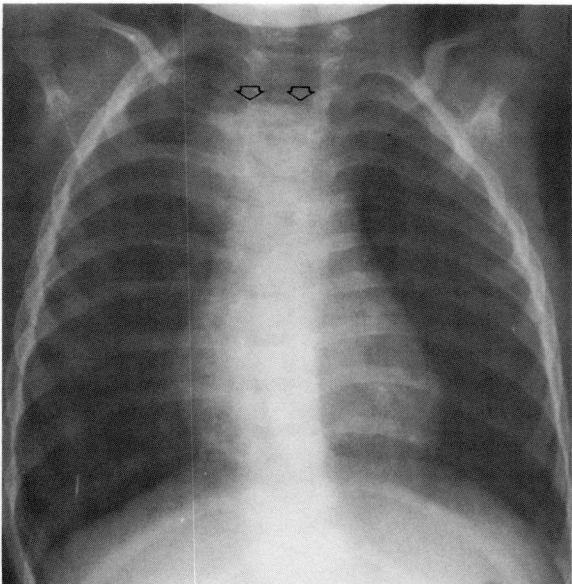

**Figure 74–19. Anastomotic stricture after TEF repair.** A soft tissue density with air-fluid level *(arrows)* deviates the trachea to the left. This is the dilated upper pouch above a narrowed anastomosis. The child is acutely symptomatic as food is impacted at the anastomosis.

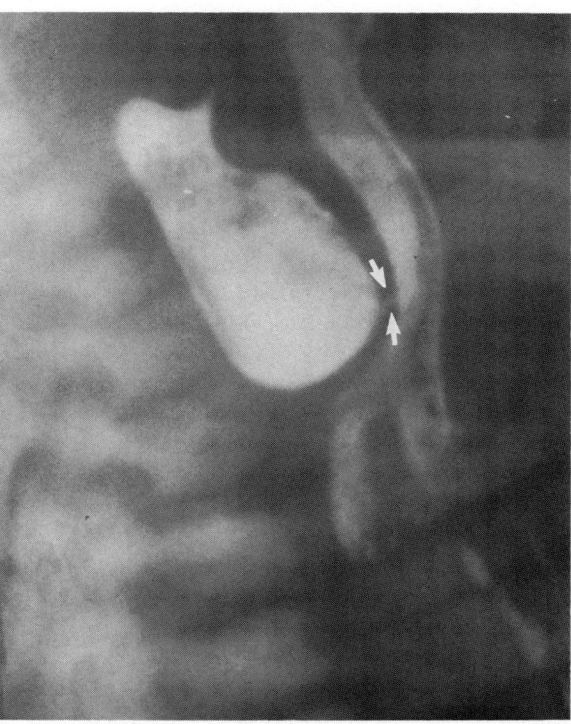

**Figure 74–21. Upper pouch fistula.** The upper pouch is filled with a small amount of contrast medium. The trachea is being filled through a tiny fistula *(arrows)*.

fistula because of its rarity, the possible complications of the pouch study, or the fact that the fistula may not be seen even when present because its muscular wall may be contracted and prevent contrast material from passing through it.

Children with an H-type fistula (Fig. 74–22) may have only intermittent feeding problems; the anomaly can remain undetected for years, until a barium swallow is performed to evaluate the cause of multiple pneumonias. The muscular wall of the fistula may contract or

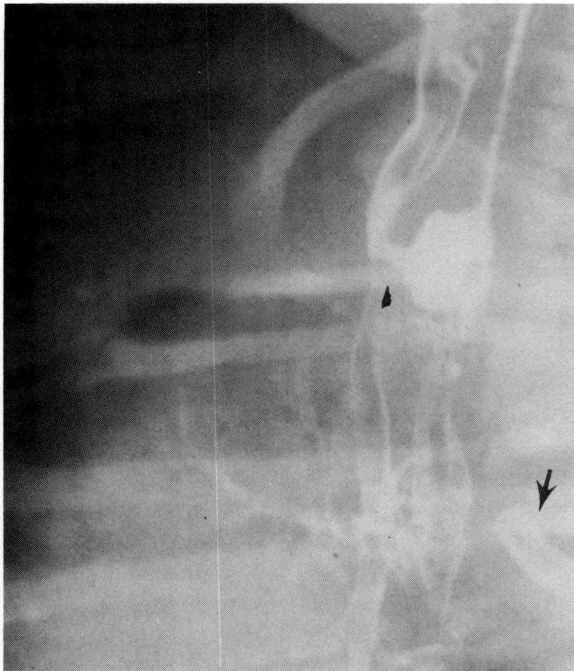

**Figure 74–20. Postsurgical TEF.** This fistula is demonstrated several days after surgery. Contrast medium instilled into the upper esophagus passes through a fistula *(arrowhead)* into the trachea. Arrow = pleural drain.

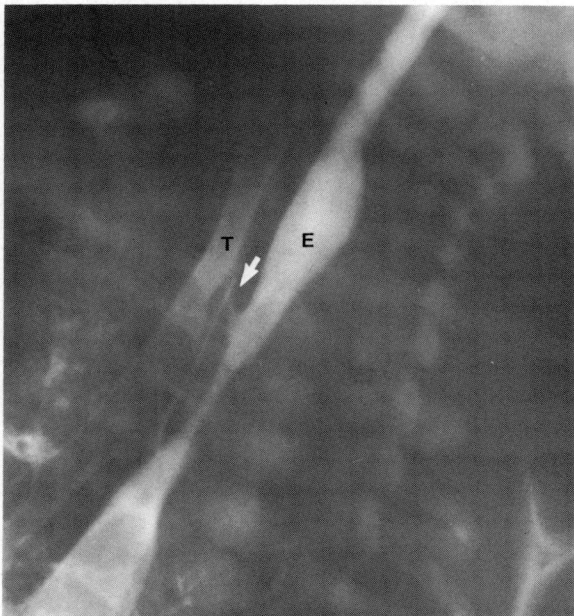

**Figure 74–22. H-type TEF.** Contrast agent injected into the upper esophagus fills the esophagus (E), the fistula *(arrow)*, and the trachea (T).

the fistula may become impacted with mucus or food, which allows the child intermittently to eat without difficulty.

Gastroesophageal reflux with dysphagia, retrosternal pain, and pulmonary disease are common throughout the lives of children with EA and TEF. Reflux may derive from a primary abnormality of the distal esophagus or may be caused by postsurgical changes in the anatomy of the gastroesophageal junction.[181, 188, 195] Reflux of gastric acid may contribute to the tendency to stricture formation at the anastomotic site or distal esophagus (Fig. 74–23). The gastroesophageal reflux is complicated by poor antegrade peristalsis. If a fundoplication is performed to treat the reflux, care must be taken so that the poorly emptying esophagus will not become obstructed by the newly competent gastroesophageal junction.[181, 195]

CT studies done years after repair have documented structural and functional abnormalities of the trachea and puddling of fluid in the dilated upper esophagus.[196] The tracheal abnormalities may be due to congenital underdevelopment of the foregut as well as the surgical changes.[196a, 197] The resultant laryngomalacia can cause stridor.

## Radiologic Findings

The prenatal diagnosis of EA with TEF is suggested by the presence of polyhydramnios with absence of fluid in the stomach. At times, the fluid-filled upper pouch may be detected. When duodenal atresia is associated

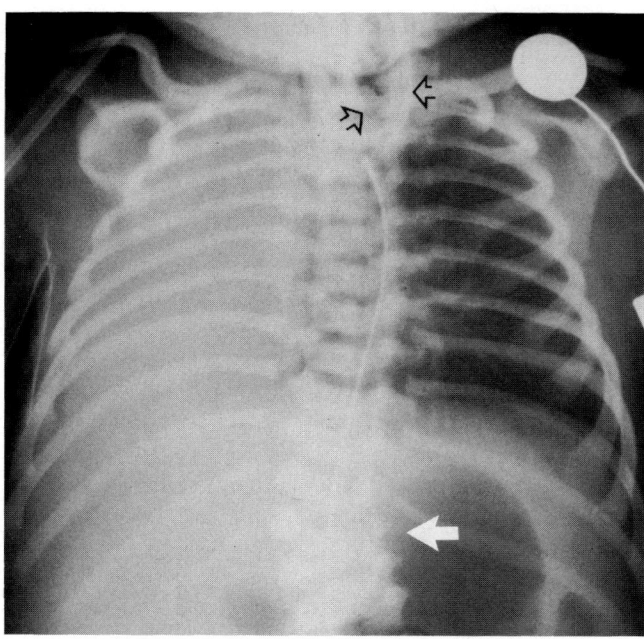

**Figure 74–24. The VATER association.** A feeding tube is coiled in the upper esophageal pouch *(open black arrows)*. Eleven ribs are present on the left and 12 on the right. Segmentation anomalies including a hemivertebra are noted at the thoracolumbar level *(solid white arrow)*. The right hemithorax is opacified, and the mediastinal contents are shifted to the right because the right lung is agenetic. This child also had unilateral renal agenesis.

with the TEF, fluid may be seen in both stomach and duodenum but not in distal loops of bowel.

### Plain Films

Chest and abdominal radiographs should be scrutinized for vertebral segmentation and limb anomalies as part of the VATER association (Fig. 74–24); tetralogy of Fallot and right-sided aortic arch, for avoidance of injury during the thoracotomy, which is usually performed on the right; and bowel gas, to search for other gut atresias and to detect the presence of TEF.[171–179, 198]

### Contrast Studies

In the child with EA and no TEF, barium studies are done through the gastrostomy tube to define the length of the lower esophageal segment before surgery. This tends to extend above the diaphragm for only a small distance (Fig. 74–25). For identifying any proximal fistulas, cross-table films of the upper esophagus are obtained during manual injection of a few milliliters of nonionic water-soluble contrast agent through a feeding tube placed in the upper pouch. The examination can also be performed with the child supported in a semi-upright position. When a fistula is identified, no additional contrast medium is injected (see Fig. 74–21). When there is no fistula, the contrast material is removed via a feeding tube (Fig. 74–26). Air may also be injected into the upper pouch to detect the proximal fistula.

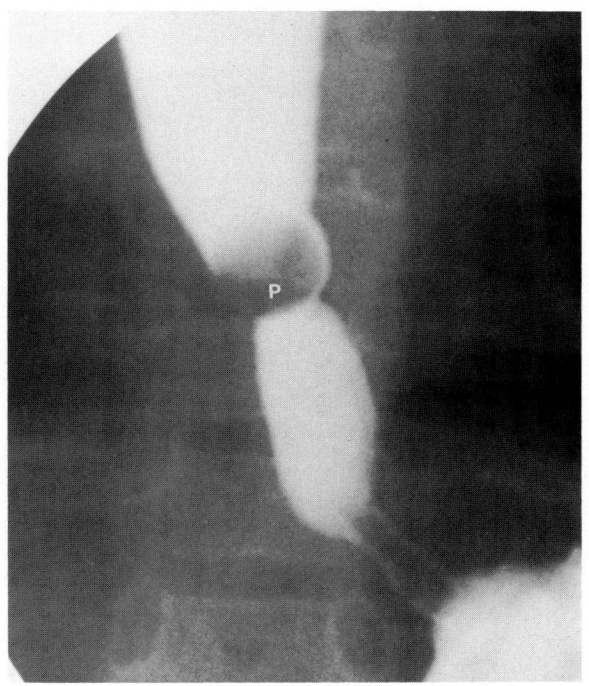

**Figure 74–23. Gastroesophageal reflux after TEF repair.** The reflux has produced such severe narrowing of the distal esophagus that a pea (P), swallowed whole, could not pass into the stomach.

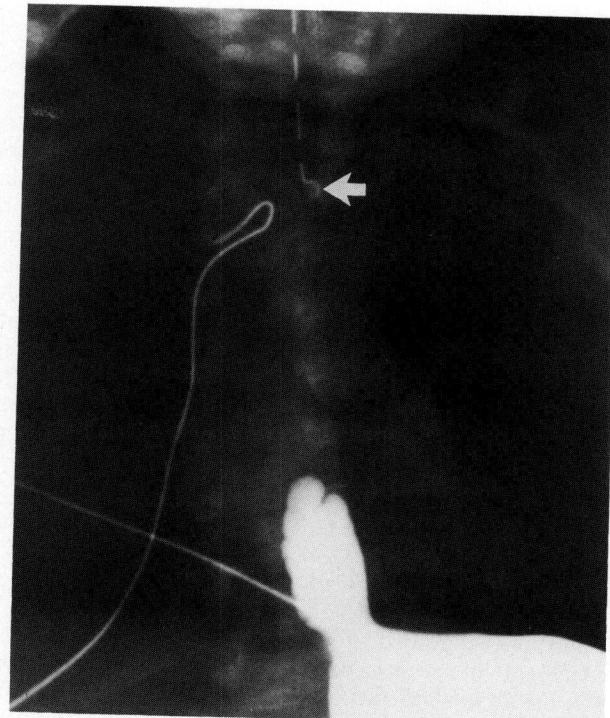

**Figure 74–25. Esophageal atresia without TEF.** Gastrostomy injection of an esophageal atresia without fistula. A feeding tube is in the upper esophageal pouch *(arrow)*. Contrast medium injected into the stomach through a gastrostomy has refluxed into the short distal esophageal segment. The distance between the distal aspect of the upper pouch and the proximal aspect of distal esophagus is approximately the height of five vertebral bodies.

It may be difficult to demonstrate an H-type TEF because the anomalous channel is not always patent. The esophagus must be distended, and in some children, a second or third barium esophagram may be necessary before the fistula is seen. When a repeated examination is performed, it is advisable to place a feeding tube in the upper esophagus and to give a bolus injection of contrast medium manually. As the fistula passes anteriorly, it passes superiorly as well, which gives the appearance of an N rather than an H to the fistula (see Fig. 74–22).

## Ultrasound Studies

Sonography is performed to search for genitourinary malformations including the VATER association.[173, 199]

## Postoperative Studies

In evaluating the anastomosis (see Fig. 74–17) for leakage, nonionic water-soluble contrast agent should be used for the first few observed swallows, and the remainder of the study can be performed with barium if the esophagus is intact.

Because there is a tendency toward narrowing or stricture formation at the anastomotic site, a barium esophagram should be performed whenever there is a change in the child's eating pattern. A refusal of solid food may be the first indication of significant narrowing. At the time of examination, the child must take swallows adequate to distend the esophagus. Small amounts of liquid may pass through a narrowed segment with relative ease, causing this abnormal segment to be overlooked. A child who presents with drooling or complete refusal to eat may have a foreign body or food impacted above the anastomosis or distal esophagus (see Figs. 74–19 and 74–23). Studies done with water-soluble contrast agent are usually performed after endoscopic retrieval of food or a foreign body or dilatation of an esophageal stricture.

## LARYNGOTRACHEAL CLEFT

Laryngotracheal cleft is a more severe failure of foregut division that has a slight male predominance. The cleft is of variable length and is frequently associated with EA and TEF.[200–208] The EA and TEF may mask the laryngotracheal cleft because the symptoms are similar: coughing, inability to handle secretions, and recurrent pneumonias.[201, 203–205] This anomaly, which causes a toneless cry, is also associated with anal anomalies, malrotation and malfixation of the bowel, meconium ileus, hypospadias, renal agenesis, lung hypoplasia, tracheomalacia, ventricular septal defect, coarctation of the aorta, and transposition of the great vessels.[204, 205]

The diagnosis of laryngotracheal cleft is confirmed with endoscopy. Radiologic studies should be performed with small amounts of contrast agent given slowly so that the cleft can be differentiated from the usual types of aspiration.[202, 203]

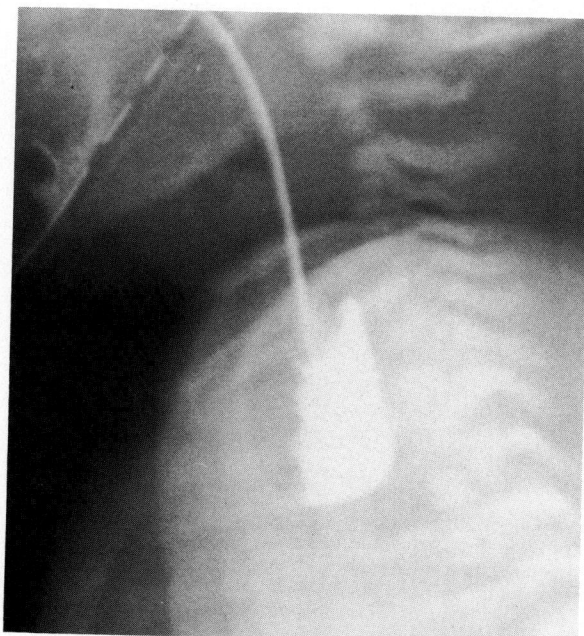

**Figure 74–26. Esophageal atresia, no TEF.** The upper pouch is filled with a small amount of contrast medium. No fistula is identified.

Surgery is necessary to divide the trachea from the esophagus. Unfortunately, the extent of the cleft and associated tracheomalacia make reconstruction difficult in many children. The mortality rate is also high because of the associated lesions in other organ systems.

## JEJUNAL AND ILEAL STENOSIS AND ATRESIA

Small bowel atresia occurs in about 1 of 5000 births. The diagnosis can be suggested by prenatal ultrasound, which shows polyhydramnios in 50% of cases, or the condition may be diagnosed after birth when vomiting and abdominal distention develop.[170, 209, 210]

Jejunal and ileal atresia are thought to be secondary to a vascular insult to the bowel by focal pressure (as in gastroschisis); by compromise of the mesenteric root (as in volvulus); by intravascular thrombosis (as in fetal demise in twin pregnancy); or by failure of complete recanalization of the bowel.[210–218] Multiple levels of atresia are seen in 5 to 22% of affected neonates.[216, 217, 219] Most cases occur sporadically, although hereditary syndromes of multiple gastrointestinal atresias have been described.[220–223]

Bowel atresias are classified by differences in the bowel lesions and differences of the mesentery[211, 217] (Fig. 74–27). Atresia is about six times more frequent than congenital stenosis.[216, 217]

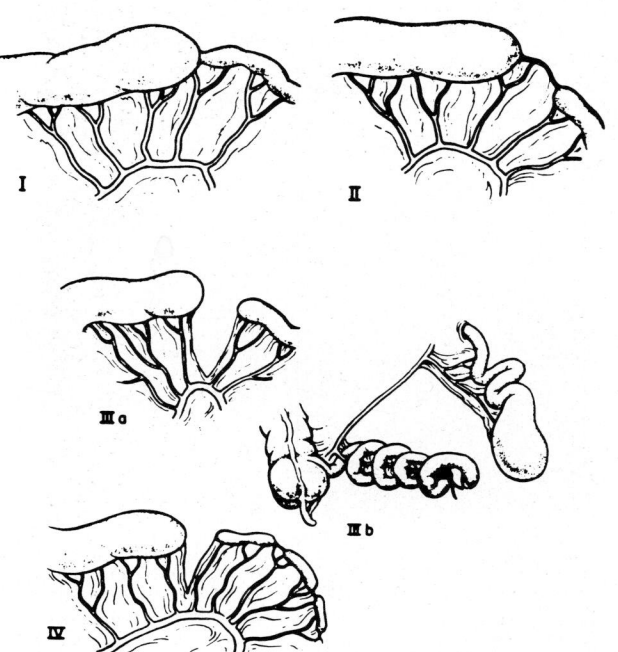

**Figure 74–27. Classification of bowel atresia.** Type I: there is a web or diaphragm between adjacent bowel loops. Type II: there is a discontinuity of bowel, usually with dilatation of the proximal segment. The mesentery is intact. Type IIIa: there is a gap in the mesentery and a discontinuity between the bowel loops. Type IIIb: there is a long segment of atretic small bowel. The remaining small bowel has a corkscrew or "apple peel" appearance. Type IV: there are multiple areas of intestinal atresia. (From Grosfeld JL, Ballantine TVN, Shoemaker R: Operative management of intestinal atresia and stenosis based on pathologic findings. J Pediatr Surg 3:368–375, 1979.)

## Treatment

Improvements in operative technique and postoperative care have significantly enhanced the outcome of patients with small bowel atresia.[224, 225] The choice of operation depends on the site and extent of atresia, the type of atresia, and the extent of proximal bowel dilatation.[211, 216, 217, 224–226] Short gut, defined as a bowel with less than half of its normal length of 200 cm, has been a consistent cause of morbidity and mortality.[51] When short gut is present, total parenteral nutrition is routine because it allows the bowel to rest in the immediate postoperative period and also allows the bowel, if shortened, to grow before being called on to meet all of the child's metabolic needs. Surgical treatment of the atretic bowel may be compromised by associated anomalies as well as by prematurity or meconium peritonitis.

## Radiologic Findings

Plain films demonstrate dilated, air-filled bowel loops proximal to the atretic or stenotic segment. The proximal loop nearest to the obstruction may be dilated out of proportion to the other segments and have a rounded edge: "the bulbous bowel segment" sign[227] (see Fig. 74–10). No distal bowel gas is noted in atresia, whereas a paucity of distal air is found in neonates with stenosis. Peritoneal calcifications are supportive evidence that the atresia is complicated by meconium peritonitis (Fig. 74–28; see also Fig. 74–10). However, meconium peritonitis can be present even when no calcifications are noted radiographically or at surgery (Fig. 74–29). Intramural calcifications have been reported in children with intestinal atresia.[228, 229] Intraluminal calcification suggests but is not diagnostic of atresia.[220, 223, 229, 230]

Air usually provides adequate contrast for determining the level of obstruction. With jejunal atresia, few loops are filled with air or with air-fluid levels (see Fig. 74–10). When multiple dilated loops are present, the obstruction is more likely to be in the ileum (see Fig. 74–28). When there is an extremely low ileal obstruction, the dilated loops may fill the entire abdomen and make differentiation from colonic obstruction impossible. Occasionally, a dilated bowel loop may simulate the stomach both in location and in contour.[231] In this setting, or to exclude a second distal obstruction in the child with suspected jejunal atresia, a contrast enema may be performed. Because of the inherent risk of perforation, the author prefers to use nonionic water-soluble contrast agents for these studies.[232]

A normal caliber colon is present when the obstruction is high because the secretions of the bowel distal to the obstruction are passed into the colon, which preserves its reservoir function. A small caliber colon implies that the obstruction is in the distal small bowel and that little small bowel contents has entered the colon (see Fig. 74–28). However, microcolon can develop in children with complete luminal patency when meconium is prevented from passing into distal bowel because of extrinsic compression.[233]

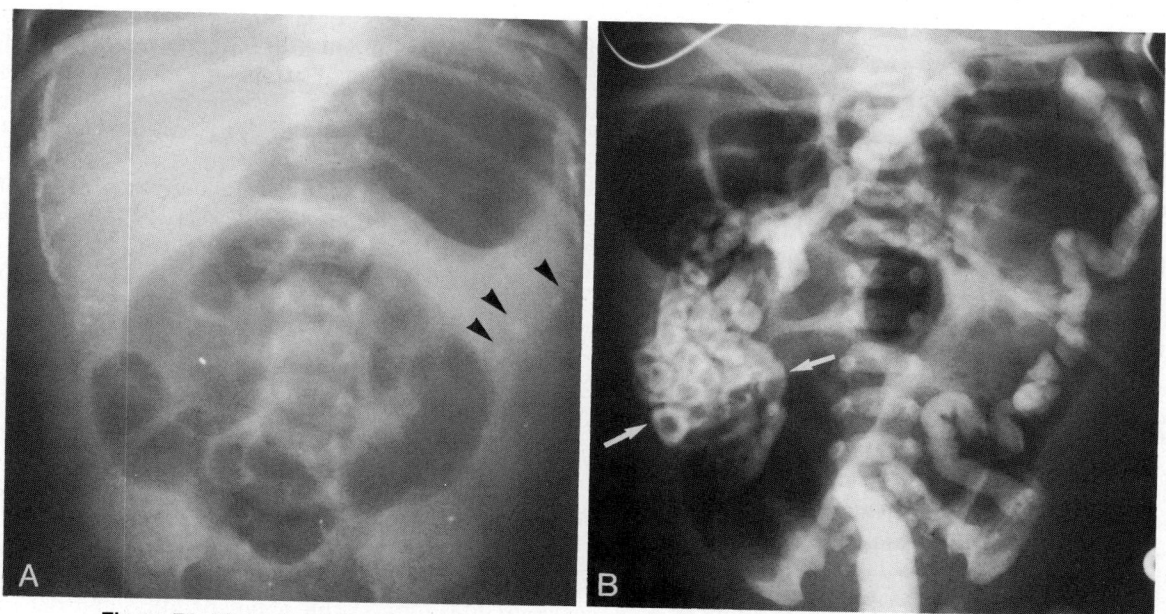

**Figure 74–28. Ileal atresia. A.** Dense calcifications *(arrowheads)* rim the lateral aspect of the upper abdomen. Note the dilated bowel loops proximal to a surgically proven high ileal atresia. **B.** Contrast enema in a different patient with ileal atresia shows a small caliber colon and reflux of contrast into a meconium-filled terminal ileum *(arrows)*.

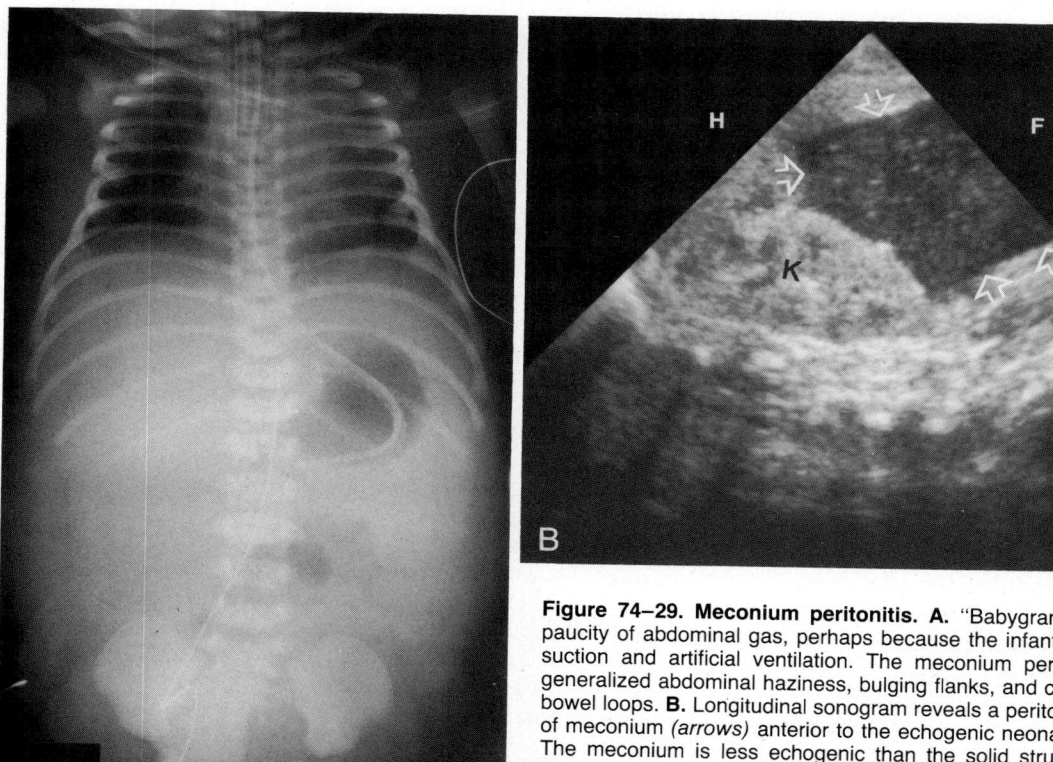

**Figure 74–29. Meconium peritonitis. A.** "Babygram." There is a paucity of abdominal gas, perhaps because the infant is undergoing suction and artificial ventilation. The meconium peritonitis causes generalized abdominal haziness, bulging flanks, and centralization of bowel loops. **B.** Longitudinal sonogram reveals a peritoneal collection of meconium *(arrows)* anterior to the echogenic neonatal kidney (K). The meconium is less echogenic than the solid structures are but contains more echoes than a simple transudative ascites. H = superior; F = inferior.

Ultrasound may be useful if meconium peritonitis or other intraperitoneal process is suspected. Free fluid, free meconium, or enterocysts may be detected (see Fig. 74–29). Meconium is echogenic because it is a complex substance composed of secretions, desquamated cells, and lanugo hairs.

If a large amount of bowel is atretic or resected, postoperative barium studies of the small bowel may show many changes that represent the bowel's attempting to compensate for its loss of length.[51, 234] The small bowel becomes dilated, the folds become thicker than usual, and transit time may be increased. Bacterial overgrowth may develop and interfere with absorptive function.[233, 234]

## MECONIUM PERITONITIS

When bowel perforation occurs in utero, sterile meconium leaks into the peritoneal cavity and creates a chemical peritonitis, meconium peritonitis (MP). The perforation is due to ischemia that is secondary to volvulus, internal hernia, intussusception, or meconium ileus with or without cystic fibrosis.[118, 235–242] The peritonitis is associated with atresia, adhesions, intra-abdominal cystic masses, ascites, scrotal masses, and, in many cases, calcifications.[118, 235–242] MP occurs in 1 of 35,000 live births.

On the basis of early surgical descriptions, MP has been categorized into several distinct forms: fibroadhesive, cystic, and generalized. Fibroadhesive MP is defined by dense bands and membranes that form around and across bowel loops in response to the peritoneal process. Cystic MP develops when the perforation of bowel is contained by inflammatory tissue and adjacent loops of bowel that are matted together.[118, 236–238] After birth, the "cyst" may be filled with fluid if the perforation has sealed or with air and bowel contents if the cavity remains in continuity with the bowel lumen. In the generalized form of MP, loosely adherent or free-floating plaques of calcium are scattered throughout the peritoneal cavity. The calcifications may not be seen on plain films but noted only at surgery.

### Clinical Findings

Seventy percent of children with MP present within the first 24 hours of life with abdominal distention and bilious vomiting resulting from adhesive bands, discontinuity of bowel, or meconium ascites[242–250] (see Fig. 74–29). Asymptomatic children may not be diagnosed until later when abdominal radiographs done for other reasons demonstrate calcification.[240]

MP and cystic fibrosis may occur independently, and calcification of meconium often occurs in the absence of cystic fibrosis.[240, 242] Children with cystic fibrosis and MP often do not have abdominal calcifications because fewer pancreatic enzymes are available to propagate the inflammatory process, and the abnormally thick meconium is less likely to pass from the bowel lumen and initiate the inflammation.

The differential diagnosis of abdominal calcifications in the neonatal period is limited: tumors such as neuroblastoma, hepatoblastoma, teratoma; calcification in the walls or lumen of a distended bowel loop; and retroperitoneal calcifications from prenatal adrenal hemorrhage or renal vein thrombosis. Whereas all children with MP should undergo a sweat chloride test to exclude cystic fibrosis, less than 10% will have the disease.[245] Despite advances in neonatal surgery and postoperative support, the prognosis for children with MP is still guarded.

### Radiologic Findings

The sonographic criteria for MP include fetal ascites that may have echogenic debris, echogenicity along the peritoneal surfaces, abnormal cystic abdominal masses, and bowel thickening dilatation.[242–250]

Plain radiography may show classic peritoneal calcifications (see Figs. 74–10 and 74–28), intestinal obstruction, and less commonly pneumoperitoneum.

Sonography should be used if there is ascites or a palpable mass in the pelvis or abdomen because it can define the size of the mass and exclude other masses or obstructive lesions: gastrointestinal duplication, hydrocolpos, neonatal intussusception, and volvulus. Sonography can also show meconium in the peritoneal cavity and differentiate it from the more usual ascites (see Fig. 74–29).

Plain films of the skeleton may show focal bands of density in the metaphysis, growth arrest lines that develop at the time of the perforation.[251]

## COLONIC ATRESIA

The incidence of colonic atresia is lower than in other portions of the gut; it occurs in about 1 of 40,000 live births.[252] The transverse colon is more frequently involved than other sites, and there is a slight female predominance.[253–255] In contrast to the increased rate of prematurity found with other intestinal atresias, children with colonic atresia are more likely to be born at term.

The neonate with colonic atresia presents with vomiting and abdominal distention.[252–257] The meconium may have passed normally. The less common colonic stenosis may produce all of these findings and can cause rectal prolapse.[258, 259]

The differential diagnosis of colonic atresia includes other causes of low obstruction: Hirschsprung's disease, duplication, meconium plug, small left colon syndrome, intussusception, and even distal ileal processes. A contrast enema should be performed to limit the diagnostic possibilities and to direct additional testing and therapy.

### Radiologic Findings

Plain films show changes of a low obstruction, and the dilated bowel loops may have air-fluid levels or a bubbly appearance because of intraluminal meconium.[252]

The plain film diagnosis of colonic atresia is difficult, particularly in the first few hours of life because air may not yet have reached the most distal bowel segment.

Sonography is useful for excluding the presence of ascites or mass lesion. Sonographic diagnosis of colonic atresia has been reported, but the contrast enema is the diagnostic study of choice.[257]

A water-soluble agent, preferably nonionic, is recommended because of an increased incidence of colonic rupture in patients with atresia. The contrast column will end abruptly and may taper or have a rounded, "cobra head" or club deformity if a membrane is present.[252, 256, 260] The colon may be normal or small in caliber, depending on the time when luminal occlusion occurred.

## IMPERFORATE ANUS

### Clinical Findings

This complex anomaly occurs in about 1 of 5000 live births with a slight predominance of males.[261–263] The distal extent of the rectum must be delineated soon after birth; this will determine whether the child needs immediate colostomy and the probability that other malformations are present.[264, 265] The position of the distal rectal pouch in relation to the levator muscle is used to categorize grossly the different type of imperforate anus (IA). When the rectum ends above the levator ani muscles, the child has a "high" or supralevator IA. When the rectum ends below these muscles, the child has a "low" or infralevator IA. Radiologic and clinical data are used to differentiate high from low lesions.

The spectrum of anorectal malformations is great and varies with the patient's sex (Fig. 74–30). Numerous attempts at categorizing the multiple variants of IA have been made; the most recent is called the Wingspread classification.[261, 262] Male infants are more apt to have enterourinary fistulas than are female infants because they lack interposed genital structures (see Fig. 74–30). Female infants have a high incidence of enterovaginal fistulas, and radiologic evaluation is recommended especially to define the internal anatomy, which may be inaccurately determined on the basis of external appearance alone.[263]

When there is any uncertainty about the level of the distal colon, imaging studies should be performed. Plain films, ultrasound, CT, and MR may be used, depending on the clinical setting.

A low lesion is suggested when there is a fistula, perineal pearls, a corrugated appearance of the extrinsic sphincter, or normal-appearing female urethra and vagina.[264] Children with low lesions undergo anoplasty or temporary enlargement of the fistula.[265–267] High lesions should be suspected when there is no fistula, when there is a smooth perineum, or when a female child has a single opening for both vagina and urethra (cloacal anomaly). Children with high lesions need a colostomy. Corrective surgery, a pull-through procedure, is performed at about 1 year of age.[265–267]

Genitourinary abnormalities are common in infants with IA.[263, 268–273] Renal anomalies (absence, agenesis, ectopia, horseshoe kidney) are more frequent and more severe in children with high IA.[272] A fistula to the vagina may be quite large and provide adequate decompression of the colon. A fistulous connection to the urinary tract, usually the urethra or the bladder, is present in about 23% of children with supralevator IA. The fistula may be diagnosed at birth when there is meconium in the urine or when there is air in the bladder on early postnatal plain films of the abdomen. Otherwise the fistula is sought with contrast studies before colostomy closure. In children with the VATER association, there is an increased incidence of congenital urethral lesions: duplications, stricture, and megalourethra.[199]

The incidence of cardiovascular malformations, especially tetralogy of Fallot and ventricular septal defect, is increased in children with otherwise isolated IA.[269, 274] The cardiac anomalies contribute significantly to the mortality rate of children with IA.

### Treatment

The definitive corrective procedure depends on the anatomy of the congenital lesion and surgical preference.[265–267] The posterior sagittal anorectoplasty, abdominoperineal procedure, and sacroperineal procedure are the most common. The goal of all surgical procedures is to preserve and, if necessary, enhance the mechanisms of continence.[265–267, 275] Urinary abnormalities are usually repaired at the time of corrective rectal surgery.

Children with low IA tend to have better development of the levator sling, a more intact neural arc, and, hence, more normal evacuation patterns after surgery than do children with high IA. The incidence of spinal deformity and intraspinal lesions is also lower in children with low IA.[276–286]

After the corrective surgery, girls have greater success at achieving continence than do boys. This is probably due to the fact that more than 90% of boys but only 69% of affected girls have supralevator IA.[286]

### Radiologic Findings

#### Prenatal Diagnosis: Ultrasound

Prenatal ultrasound may suggest bowel obstruction in patients with IA; however, dilated bowel is seen only in the later stages of gestation.[170, 287] Because infants with jejunal and ileal atresia have few extragastrointestinal abnormalities, detection of any of the stigmata of the VATER association in a fetus with multiple dilated bowel loops is suggestive of IA.

#### Plain Radiographs

A number of associated anomalies of IA can be visualized on plain films of the chest and abdomen: spinal deformity with absent, additional, or fused segments; scimitar sacrum; tetralogy of Fallot; ventricular septal defect.[269, 274, 276–280] The bowel gas pattern may show little except changes of distal obstruction. Intra-

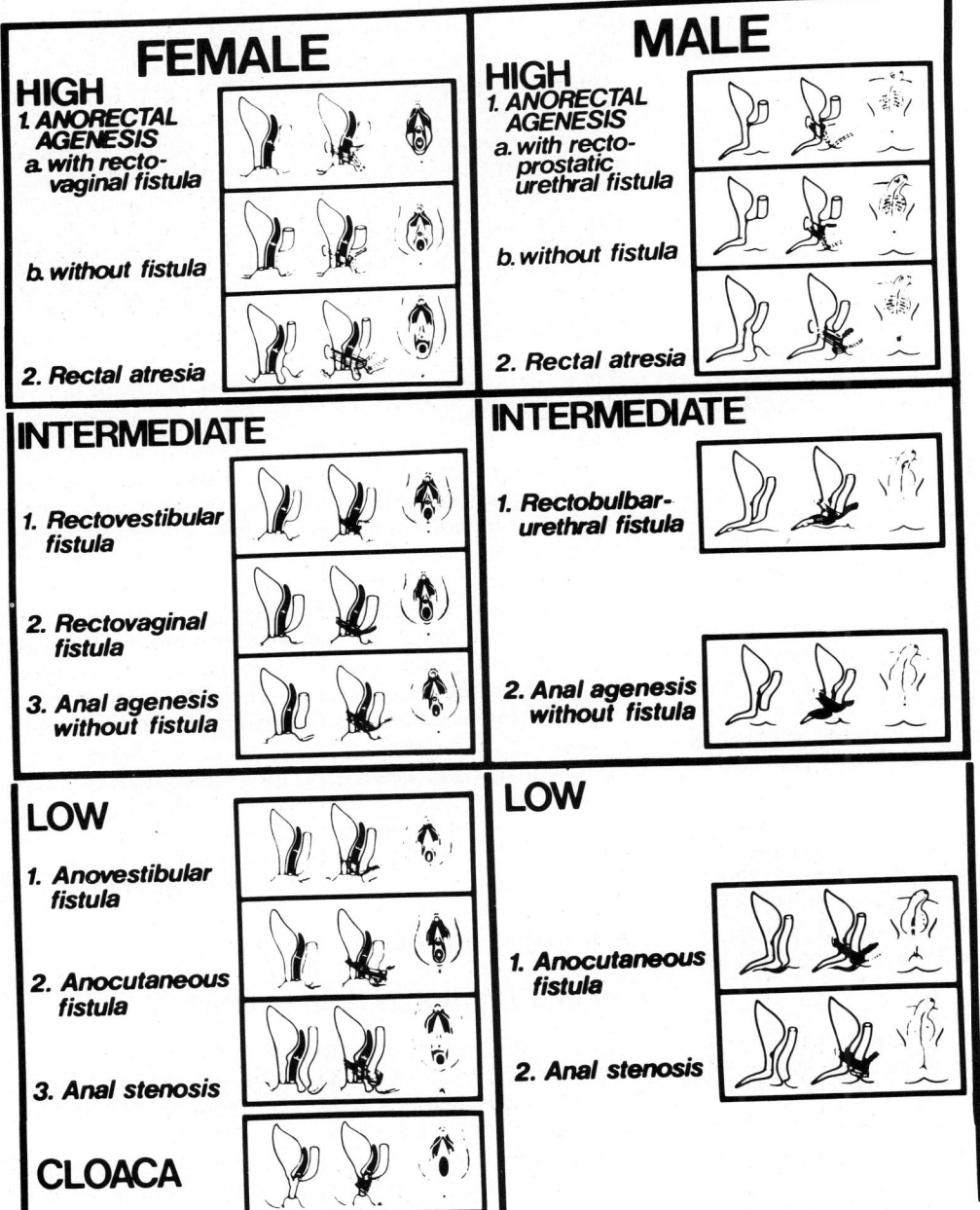

**Figure 74–30. Classification of imperforate anus (IA).** This diagram shows many of the possible relationships of the IA to the internal organs in children of both sexes. (Modified from Grosfeld JL, Ballantine TVN, Shoemaker R: Operative management of intestinal atresia and stenosis based on pathologic findings. J Pediatr Surg 3:368–375, 1979.)

luminal calcification has been reported in a small number of infants with IA. This may be due to prenatal mixture of urine and colon contents, although intraluminal calcification can occur in the absence of obstruction or fistulous communication between the gut and the genitourinary tract[288–291] (Fig. 74–31).

When the physical examination does not provide enough information about the level of the distal pouch, it must be defined radiographically. A lateral film of the rectum obtained with the child inverted, the "invertogram," was the standard way of assessing rectal position.[292] The level of the levator sling was determined to be the same as the pubococcygeal line: a line drawn from the junction of the superior third of the pubis with the middle third to the inferior aspect of the fifth sacral vertebra. If the rectal air stopped proximal to this line, the lesion was considered to be high; if below, low. Falsely high lesions were misdiagnosed when the colonic air had not yet passed to the rectal pouch or when the air escaped through a fistula. Falsely low lesions were misdiagnosed when the child was crying or otherwise straining and depressing the levator muscles. These problems as well as difficulty with positioning of the patient and the inexact construction of the pubococcygeal line when there is sacral deformity have led to dissatisfaction with the standard invertogram.

One variant of the invertogram that is less difficult to perform and less physiologically stressful for the infant is the cross-table lateral rectal film with the infant prone[293] (Fig. 74–32). The child can comfortably stay in this modified Trendelenburg position for a long period. This position encourages colonic gas to pass to the rectum and, at the same time, tends to prevent distal air from escaping through a fistula. The landmarks used are the same as on the standard invertogram.

The CT invertogram (actually done with the patient prone or in the knee-chest position) provides better

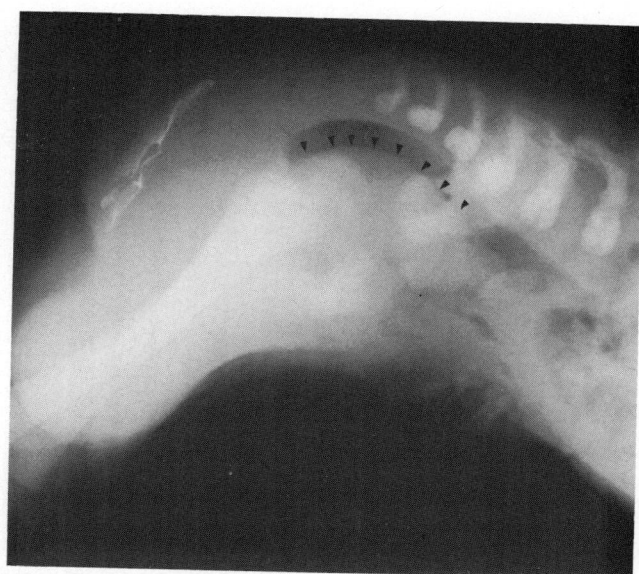

**Figure 74–32. Trendelenburg position invertogram demonstrating an IA.** The child is positioned prone with the hips elevated on a cloth roll. Barium paste marks the anus. Meconium *(arrowheads)* in the rectal pouch is outlined by air.

delineation of the anatomy than do plain film studies.[294] On direct sagittal imaging, the distal colon can be seen in relation to the midline bony structures even if it has not yet been filled with air.

When plain films fail to reveal the level of the distal pouch, some advocate blindly passing a needle cephalad from the region of the anus.[295] Small amounts of contrast medium are injected as the needle is advanced, filling the distal pouch once it is reached. At some centers, this technique has become routine; at others, it is never used because certain surgeons prefer the tissue in the region of later pull-through to remain untouched.

## Ultrasound Studies

Ultrasound can be used to identify the distal rectal pouch because the pouch contains echogenic meconium (Fig. 74–33). If this pouch is greater than 15 mm above the skin surface, the patient has a high IA, and diverting colostomy is created. If the pouch is seen within 10 mm of the skin, the child has a low IA that can be treated with a simple perineal anoplasty. If the pouch ends in between these two points, it is considered indeterminate. Most of these children are subsequently found to have high IA.[296–298]

Ultrasound of the kidneys should be routine in all children with IA, although the yield will be greater in those with high IA. Spinal ultrasound may show intraspinal lesions, if present, but spinal ultrasound is usually reserved for children with bone deformity of the spine or high IA.

## Gastrointestinal and Genitourinary Contrast Studies

Voiding cystourethrography is routinely performed to exclude vesicoureteral reflux, which occurs in close to

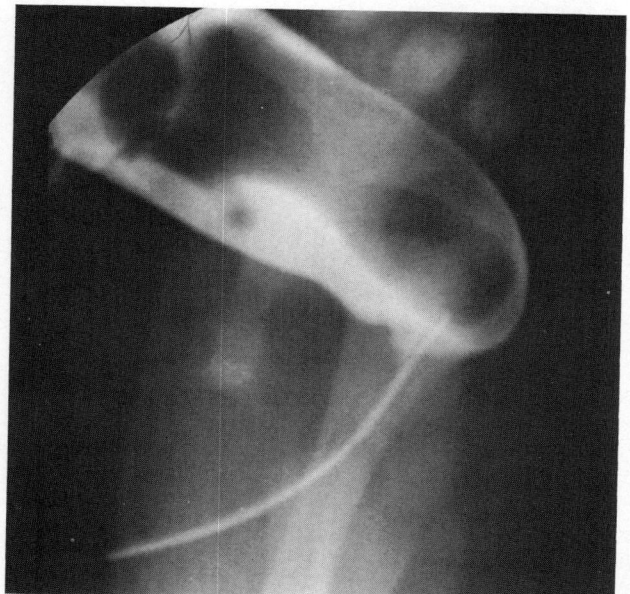

**Figure 74–31. Rectourethral fistula.** A catheter placed in the urethra for a voiding cystourethrogram passed into the rectourethral fistula. Contrast medium outlines the distal rectal segment.

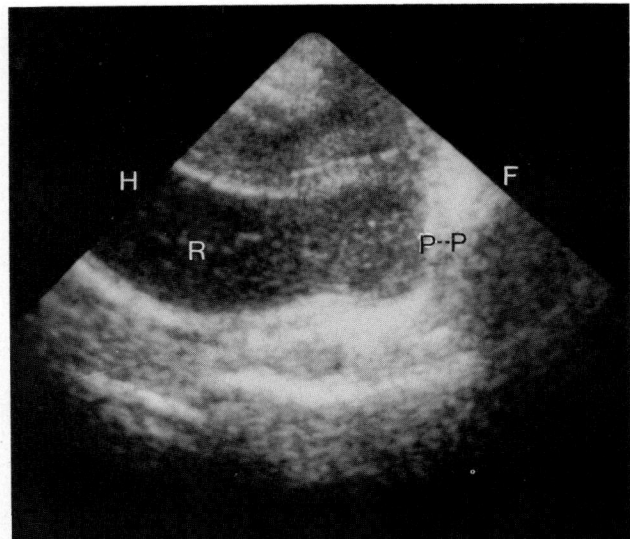

**Figure 74–33. Imperforate anus.** Longitudinal sonogram of the rectal pouch in an infant with IA. The echogenic meconium distends and defines the distal rectal (R) pouch. The pouch to perineum distance (P—P) is only a few millimeters. H = superior; F = inferior.

50% of children with high IA and in 35% of children with low IA.[272] In male infants, voiding cystourethrography is also necessary for excluding rectourinary fistula, which requires ligation at the time of pull-through surgery. Even if no fistula is seen in the neonatal period, the study should be repeated just before corrective surgery, usually at age 1 year, because the fistula may not always fill on the initial examination.

At this later time, a contrast study of the distal colon is also performed because the fistula sometimes is demonstrated only with the antegrade flow of contrast medium.[272a] Water-soluble contrast agents should be used to fill this unused segment so that no barium is introduced into the urinary tract if there is a fistula and so that retained barium will not impact in the unused colon. The fistula is best seen when the distal colon segment is distended and the child is in the lateral position (Fig. 74–34).

## Computed Tomography and Magnetic Resonance

Preoperative evaluation of the levator sling can be performed with CT or MR.[276, 278, 281–283, 285] In the neonate, MR displays the sphincteric muscle complex (SMC) better than CT, which is limited by the small amount of fat present in the very young. Because of its inherent multiplanar capabilities, MR can better demonstrate those muscles best imaged in the coronal or sagittal planes. When there is insufficient intrinsic muscle to produce continence, surgical results may be disappointing unless special procedures to buttress the muscles are also performed. MR studies are therefore valuable in determining what additional surgery may be necessary at the time of pull-through. As the children grow and

develop, it is easier to visualize the pelvic muscles with both CT and MR.

When there is spinal deformity, MR may be useful in evaluating the spinal cord because there is an increased incidence of lesions that tether the spinal cord in patients with IA.[278] In the neonatal period, MR also displays the distal portion of the colon well; the impacted meconium produces an intense signal.

## Postoperative Studies

After surgery, studies are done when there is concern that there may be an anastomotic leak. Later contrast studies are performed if there is fecal soiling or severe constipation. In some instances, CT and MR are better for defining postsurgical problems[284, 299, 300] (Figs. 74–35 and 74–36). Both can show the position of the colon pull-through in relation to the SMC. For the muscles to work properly, the rectum should be centrally positioned within the SMC. In children with a well-developed SMC, incontinence has been associated with surgical malposition of the rectum. Poor centralization of the neorectum is more common in children with poorly developed SMC than in those with normally developed muscles (see Fig. 74–35). Some children evacuate well initially but later develop incontinence caused by a lesion that puts traction on the spinal cord as the child grows.

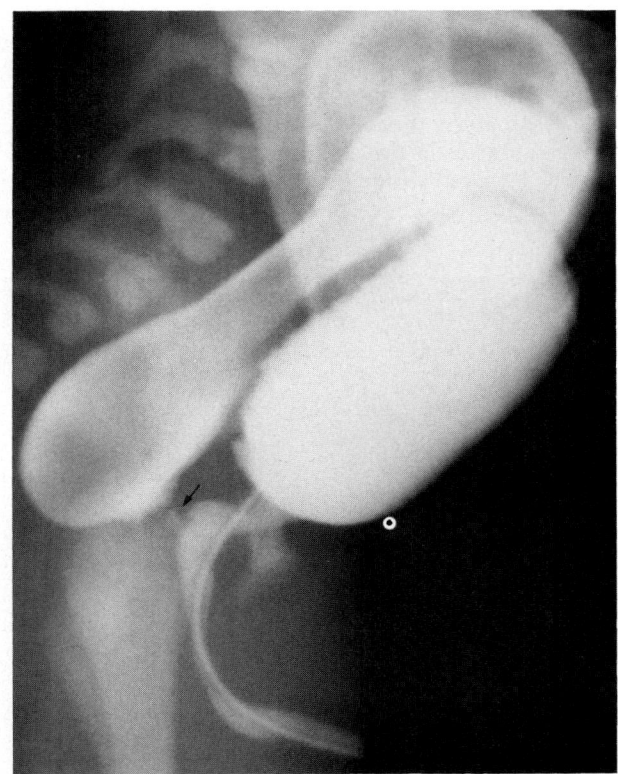

**Figure 74–34. IA with rectourethral fistula.** A rectourethral fistula is demonstrated on this voiding cystourethrogram. As the child voids and fills the urethra, contrast medium passes through the fistula (*arrow*) into the blind-ending rectum. The fistula is demonstrated best on lateral films.

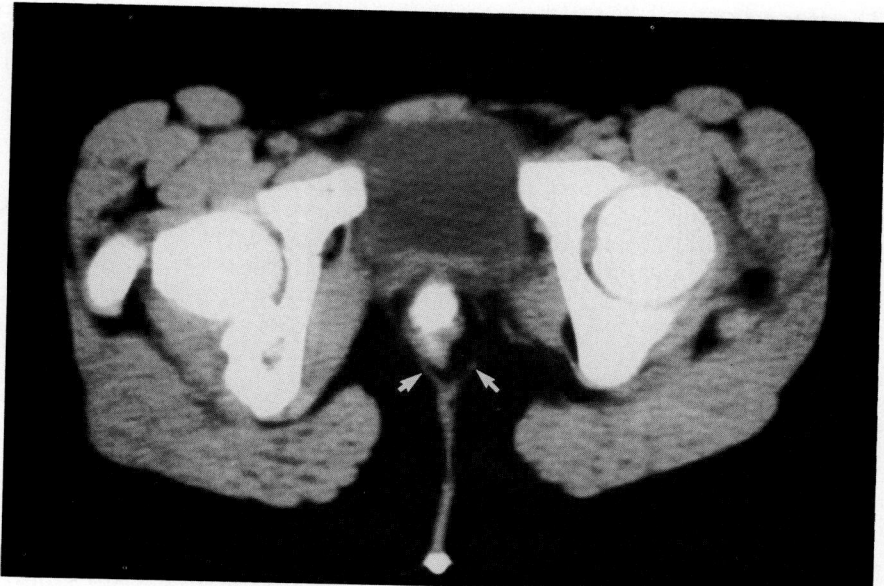

**Figure 74–35. IA: postsurgical CT.** Postoperative evaluation of the sphincter muscle in an infant with IA. Pelvic CT scan shows that the sphincter muscles *(arrows)* are extremely thin and underdeveloped.

# IMPERFORATE ANUS VARIANTS

## Cloacal Malformation

In female infants, there is a less common variant of IA associated with more profound renal, vaginal, and uterine abnormalities, the cloacal malformation.[301–308] It occurs in 1 of every 40,000 to 50,000 births. This anomaly can be diagnosed at birth when a "bland" or "featureless" perineum with only one opening is detected. This opening is usually beneath an enlarged clitoris, which has a phallus-like appearance. The external anatomy indicates that there is a confluence, at some levels, of the bladder/urethra, vagina, and rectum into a common distal channel of variable length. The numerous possible configurations depend on which distal channel is dominant.[301–307]

In one third of neonates with cloaca, the vaginal opening of the confluent channel is stenotic, which causes hydrocolpos with resultant abdominal mass.[301–307] If the bladder cannot drain freely or if there is associated reflux, the child may develop urinary sepsis. Management in the neonatal period requires that these urinary tract abnormalities be corrected and that the fecal stream be diverted. The colostomy is usually placed in the transverse colon, well away from the site of later corrective surgery, and has two distinct stomas so that the fecal stream will have no contact with the distal loop.

Genitourinary tract anomalies such as solitary kidney, renal ectopia, ureteral obstruction, vesicoureteral reflux, bladder diverticula, duplication of the vagina, a vaginal septum, and uterine duplication are common.[301–308] Cardiac, skeletal, and other gastrointestinal anomalies are also seen with increased frequency.[306, 307]

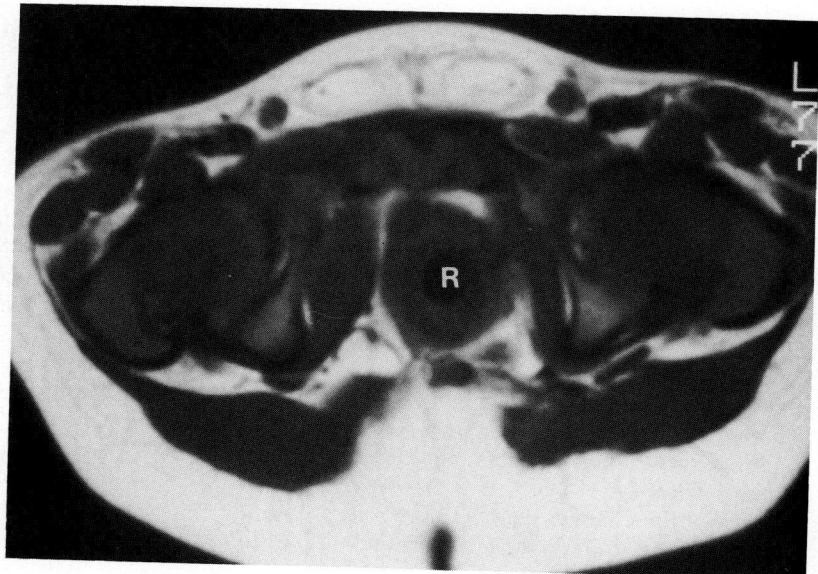

**Figure 74–36. IA: MR of pull-through.** Axial MR shows the anal pull-through in good position. The rectum (R) is centrally placed within a well-developed sphincteric muscle complex.

## Treatment

Corrective surgery is delayed until after 1 year of age.[301, 303] In some children, the anatomy lends itself to a one-stage correction. Other girls, especially those with a long common channel, will need a staged repair for creation of a urethra, a separate vagina, and a functioning anus. As with repair of IA, the goal of surgery is to achieve fecal and urinary continence as well as normal sexual function. A posterior sagittal approach is most commonly used to correct the anorectal malformation.[301]

## Radiologic Findings

It is vital to delineate the internal anatomy accurately in the neonatal period so that urinary tract injury is minimized.

A plain abdominal radiograph provides much information. It is important to document presence or absence of a pelvic mass (dilated vagina), a vertebral deformity, or abdominal calcifications.

Water-soluble contrast studies are needed to visualize the length of the common channel and the relationship of each of the systems above the channel. These studies are performed with catheters introduced through the perineal opening with devices that occlude the opening while the contrast agent is being injected; the catheter is introduced from above if colostomy, vesicostomy, or vaginostomy has been created.[306] Any secondary or accessory openings should also be injected with contrast medium.

Ultrasound is useful for detecting renal, uterine, or vaginal abnormalities. The common channel is difficult to visualize with ultrasound or CT, however.[306]

MR is helpful in evaluating the spinal cord; tethering of the cord is common, as in children with IA, and this will affect later bowel and bladder function.

## CAUDAL REGRESSION

This rare association of severe malformations of the lower spine, lower limbs, genitourinary tract, and anorectum occurs in about 1% of the offspring of diabetic mothers.[309–312] No other predisposing factor or agent has been identified. There is a spectrum of the anomalies in each system. When there is fusion of the lower limbs into a single structure, the child is said to have a specific form of caudal regression, sirenomelia, or mermaid deformity; this is a lethal variant often associated with complete renal agenesis.[309, 313]

Other children with milder changes of caudal regression present with many of the classic stigmata of the VATER association. The lower limbs may be atrophied, malrotated, or contracted. The genitourinary anomalies are the same as those seen in IA, and the degree of bladder dysfunction reflects but does not parallel the spinal deformity.

Many of the changes can be diagnosed prenatally.[287, 312] The spinal and limb changes are usually apparent earlier than the anorectal anomaly. It is easier to appreciate bowel dilatation on sonograms done later in pregnancy; in one study of 12 fetuses with anorectal anomalies, no lesion was detected in those younger than 27 menstrual weeks.[287]

## CURRARINO TRIAD

Another variant of anorectal malformations is the Currarino triad, which additionally includes a sacral deformity and presacral mass.[314–316] The anorectal lesion has been described as being anal stenosis, anal ectopia, IA, or Hirschsprung's disease. Sacral lesions are not uncommon in children with anorectal malformations, but presacral masses (anterior meningocele, duplication, teratoma) are. In some children, the presacral mass is detected years after the anal lesion has been repaired (Fig. 74–37).

To some, this combination of abnormalities represents a form of the split notochord syndrome that is more frequently seen in the thorax. However, thoracic manifestations of the split notochord syndrome are not usually associated with malformations of the esophagus or trachea other than the enteric duplication.[316]

## OTHER LOW OBSTRUCTIVE LESIONS

There is a long list of disorders, which are often interrelated, that produce signs and symptoms of low bowel obstruction. Many of the "obstructive" lesions are functional rather than mechanical.[317] When a contrast enema is performed in a child with signs of Hirschsprung's disease, the diseases described in the following sections should be considered. In addition, many other processes, including generalized sepsis, can produce ileus and obstruction and should be excluded clinically.[318–323]

### Meconium Ileus

#### Clinical Findings

Eighty percent of cases of meconium ileus develop in patients with cystic fibrosis. The lumen of the bowel, especially the ileum, is obstructed with abnormally thickened meconium or meconium pellets. The neonate does not pass meconium or stool.[324, 325] Survival of infants with meconium ileus has dramatically improved in the last 20 years as first-year mortality rates have declined from 50 to 10%.[326] A more complete discussion of the gastrointestinal manifestations of cystic fibrosis can be found in Chapters 79 and 118.

#### Therapy

At one time, meconium ileus was treated by laparotomy with manual removal of the meconium through an

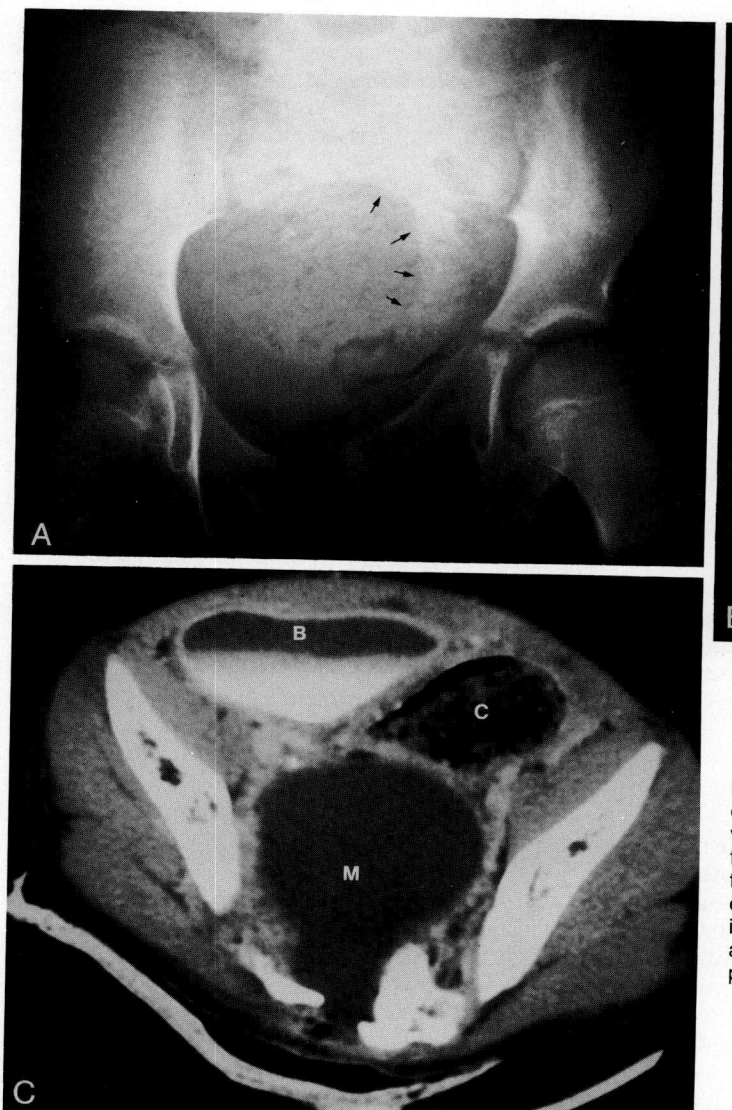

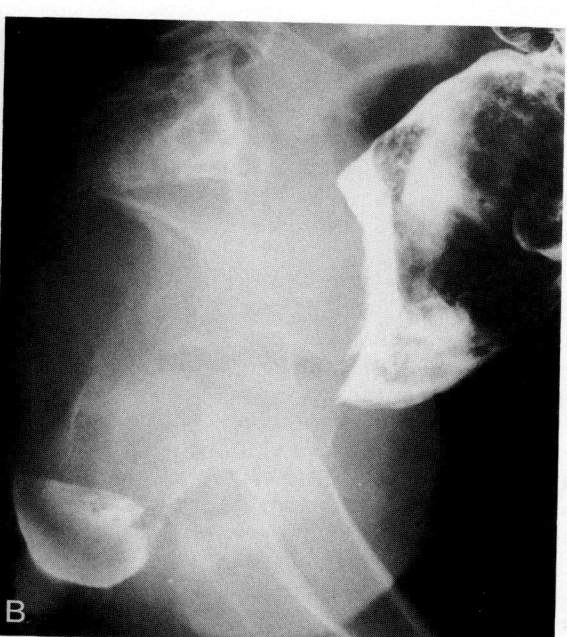

**Figure 74–37. Currarino triad. A.** An anteroposterior film of the pelvis shows a large amount of feces obscuring visualization of the sacrum. The sacrum is abnormally formed and is scimitar shaped *(arrows).* **B.** Lateral film from a barium enema shows that the rectal channel is effaced by a posterior extrinsic mass. The proximal colon is dilated. **C.** Axial CT scan demonstrates a water density anterior sacral meningocele (M) compressing and displacing both the bladder (B) and the colon (C).

enterotomy. Cleansing enemas of hypertonic water-soluble contrast media are now used both to diagnose and to treat this disorder.[327–329] The method is not without hazard because the contrast medium can irritate the mucosa and produce fluid shifts from the intravascular compartment to the colon, which can dehydrate the infant.[330–333] The necessity of refluxing contrast medium into the obstructed terminal ileum has been associated with bowel perforation.[334] However, most children with perforation do well, despite the need for immediate surgery.[334]

### Radiologic Findings

Plain films show multiple dilated small bowel loops consistent with the diagnosis of low obstruction[324] (Fig. 74–38). A granular appearance of the right lower quadrant and the absence of air-fluid levels in this region are due to the thickened intraluminal meconium, which does not change position with gravity.[335]

Contrast enema demonstrates a colon with a small caliber that is malrotated in 33 to 50% of patients. Contrast medium refluxed into the terminal ileum outlines the impacted meconium (see Fig. 74–38). To avoid perforation, the author does not attempt to fill the entire obstructed segment with the first contrast enema. When some of the terminal ileum is filled, the study is concluded. The child is returned to the nursery and followed clinically. If symptoms clear, no additional enemas are performed. If there is continued obstruction, additional enemas are given generally 1 day apart. Each time, it is necessary to observe that the retrograde flow reaches the impacted meconium.

Sonography, although not generally used for diagnosis, can show the inspissated meconium or meconium in the dilated proximal bowel loops (Fig. 74–39).

## Meconium Plug Syndrome

Delayed passage of meconium and abdominal distention are the presenting findings in neonates with meconium plug syndrome. This syndrome is seen in about 1 in 500 to 1000 neonates, of which 25% have cystic fibrosis and another 5 to 10% have Hirschsprung's disease.[336–340] Other factors associated with meconium plug include prematurity or maternal treatment with magnesium sulfate.[341–343] In many children, meconium plug is an isolated process without specific cause.

The majority of children are promptly and completely relieved by contrast enema, which stimulates passage of the plug. If the obstruction does not clear after passage of the meconium plug, a rectal biopsy for excluding Hirschsprung's disease should be performed. The differential diagnosis of meconium plug includes other causes of low obstruction: ileal atresia, duplication, meconium ileus, Hirschsprung's disease, and small left colon syndrome.

If obstructive symptoms develop after an uneventful perinatal period, a contrast enema done to exclude Hirschsprung's disease may show filling defects in the terminal ileum. In this setting, milk curd syndrome should be considered. This is treated with diatrizoate meglumine (Gastrografin) or other "cleansing" enema.[318, 319] For unknown reasons, boys are affected with milk curd syndrome about five times more frequently than are girls.

### Radiologic Findings

In the meconium plug syndrome, plain films demonstrate multiple dilated bowel loops (Fig. 74–40A). Contrast enema, performed with a water-soluble agent, outlines the adherent plug, which fills the lumen (Fig. 74–40B). The colon may be normal in caliber or have a diminished caliber up to the splenic flexure, as seen in neonates with small left colon syndrome.[340]

## Small Left Colon Syndrome

The small left colon syndrome is an uncommon functional obstruction seen primarily in infants of diabetic mothers.[344–347] This temporary obstruction usually passes within a few days without surgery, although in rare cases perforation may occur. Microscopic examination of the colon reveals an increased number of small cells and a decreased number of larger multipolar cells in the intermyenteric plexus. This pathologic change is typical of an immature colon and can be normally observed in premature infants. Within a few days to weeks, this immaturity is outgrown, and normal colon function develops. Small left colon syndrome has also been reported in cystic fibrosis and neonates with a history of maternal substance abuse.[348, 349]

A meconium plug is occasionally present in children with small left colon, which makes differentiation from the meconium plug syndrome difficult.[347] Most children with meconium plug syndrome are not infants of a diabetic mother, and most children with small left colon syndrome do not get immediate relief of symptoms after passage of a meconium plug.

### Clinical Findings

The infant with small left colon syndrome presents with delayed passage of meconium, abdominal distention, and vomiting. The differential diagnosis includes aganglionosis, the meconium plug syndrome, ileal or colonic atresia, and other low obstructive lesions including microcolon of prematurity.

### Radiologic Findings

The plain film of the abdomen shows nonspecific changes of a distal bowel obstruction. The thickness of the soft tissues over the lower thorax may be increased, a sign that the child is an infant of a diabetic mother.[350] If the obstruction has caused perforation, free air may be present.[347]

Contrast enema demonstrates a distal colon with a small caliber that becomes more normal at the level of

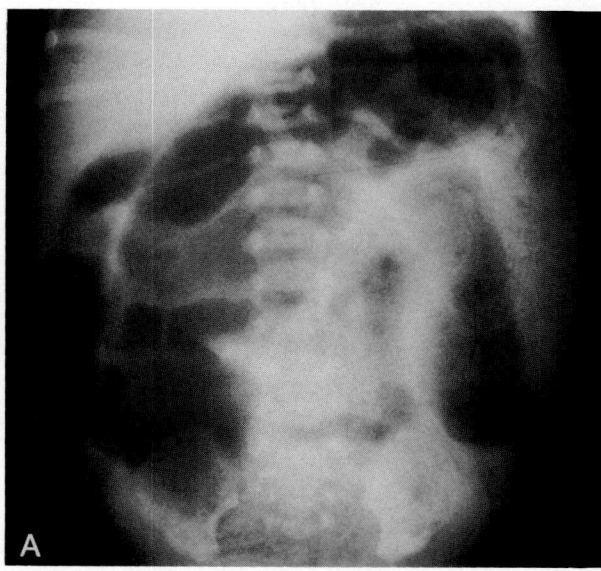

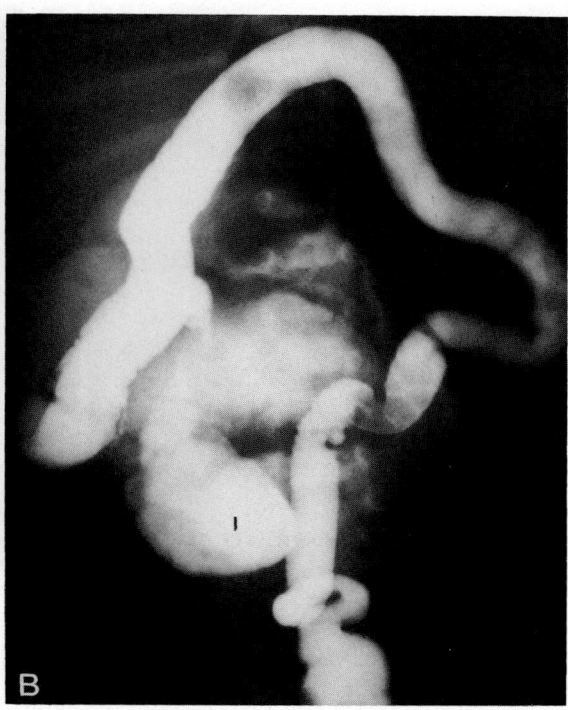

**Figure 74–38. Meconium ileus. A.** Air-filled, dilated bowel loops are present throughout the abdomen. Multiple loops of meconium-filled gut are seen above the distal meconium impaction. **B.** The caliber of the colon is slightly diminished on contrast enema. As contrast medium refluxes into the dilated and obstructed terminal ileum (I), it is diluted by the intraluminal meconium.

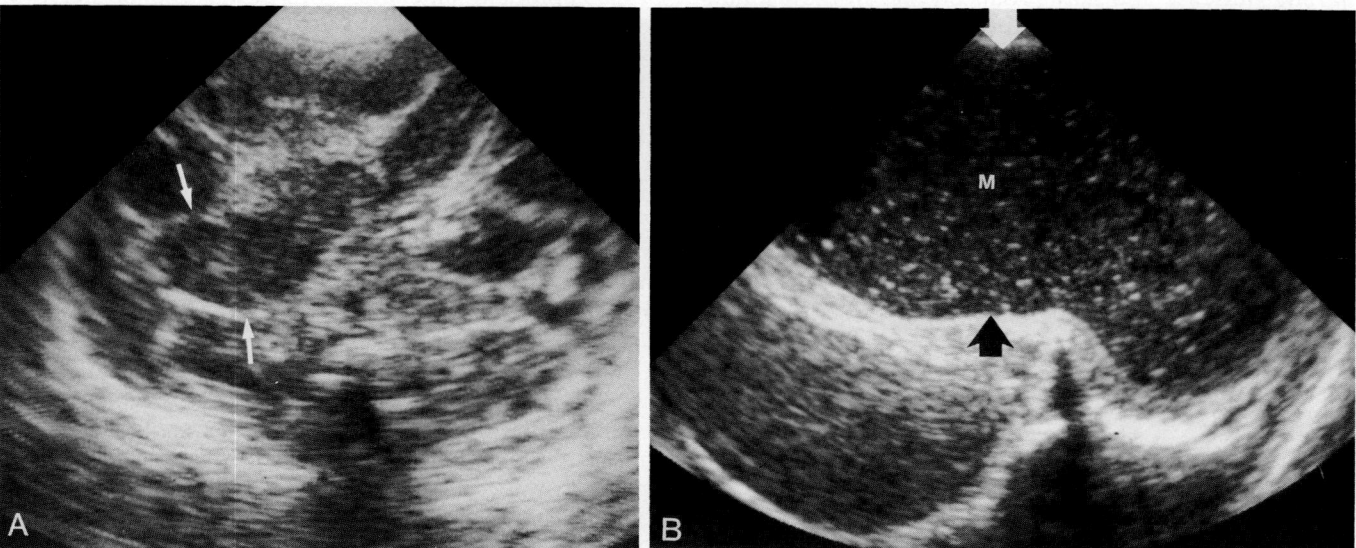

**Figure 74–39. Ultrasound appearance of meconium ileus. A.** Rounded loops of bowel *(arrows)* full of echogenic meconium are visualized on this transverse scan. **B.** Echogenic meconium (M) fills this very dilated bowel loop *(arrow)*.

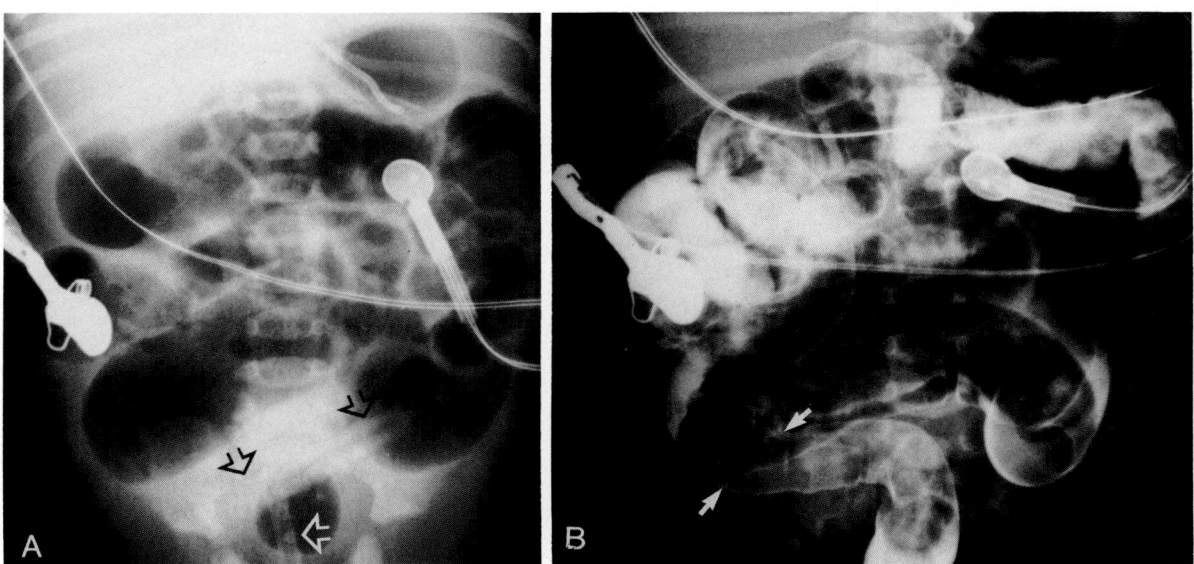

**Figure 74–40. Meconium plug in Hirschsprung's disease. A.** Multiple dilated bowel loops fill the abdomen. None can be specifically identified as the colon. The umbilical clamp projects *(open black arrows)* over the lower abdomen. A rectal enema tip is in place *(open white arrow).* **B.** An intraluminal tubular defect *(arrows)* extends from the descending colon to the rectum. There is a subtle change in the caliber of the colon, with the sigmoid colon being larger than the rectum.

the splenic flexure (Fig. 74–41). A meconium plug is present in about 5% of the neonates and can be cleared by performing an ionic contrast enema with an emulsifying agent. Not only does this expedite the passage of the meconium, but it should be used when the diagnosis is uncertain. Water-soluble enemas will not interfere with diagnosis of small left colon syndrome or Hirschsprung's disease and may produce relief in the neonate who has meconium plug syndrome as well.

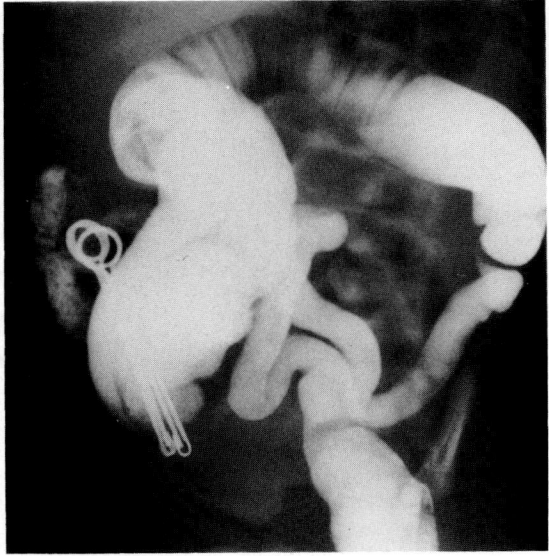

**Figure 74–41. Small left colon syndrome.** The rectum is large, but the descending colon and sigmoid colon are much smaller than normal. There is an abrupt change in caliber at the level of the splenic flexure, a classic finding.

The rectosigmoid colon and descending colon are nondistensible, but the mucosa is normal, and there is no spasm or difficulty filling the left colon. A transition in lumen caliber is invariably found at the splenic flexure, although the reason for this consistently reproducible location is unclear. Interestingly, the same morphologic changes in the colon are present in up to 50% of asymptomatic neonates born to diabetic mothers.[345]

Although the narrow caliber of the descending colon simulates the changes seen in Hirschsprung's disease, the splenic flexure transition zone makes this diagnosis unlikely. Also, children with small left colon syndrome do not develop colitis, whereas those with Hirschsprung's disease do. Rectal biopsy is recommended when the diagnosis is in question.[347]

## Megacystis-Microcolon—Intestinal Hypoperistalsis Syndrome

The pathophysiology of megacystis-microcolon–intestinal hypoperistalsis syndrome (MMIH) is not understood. Although there may be abnormalities of autonomic inhibitory input to the smooth muscle cells of the small intestine and imbalance of gut peptides, there are normal numbers of normal-appearing ganglion cells present.[351, 352]

### Clinical Findings

This rare condition is seen almost exclusively in female infants.[351–355] Most cases are sporadic, but in some there has been a pattern of autosomal recessive inheritance.[353–358]

The affected infant presents shortly after birth with abdominal distention and vomiting. The lax, wrinkled appearance of the abdomen, similar to that of the prune-belly syndrome, may be first appreciated after the huge bladder is catheterized and drained.

Virtually all children with MMIH die in infancy. Chemical stimulation of the gastrointestinal tract fails to improve function, and ileostomy or colostomy does not enhance drainage. Hyperalimentation improves nutritional status, but this is only a temporizing measure because bowel function does not improve with age. The small bowel does tend to increase in size over time.

The main alternative diagnosis to MMIH is Hirschsprung's disease, which is not usually associated with microcolon or dilated bladder. In some children, biopsy of the colon may be necessary to exclude the diagnosis.

## Radiologic Findings

The MMIH syndrome can be suggested in utero by finding a markedly dilated bladder and upper urinary tract in a female infant.[359–361] Unlike other syndromes in which bladder distention and upper urinary tract changes are associated with oligohydramnios, the amount of amniotic fluid is usually normal in MMIH. Male infants with a distended bladder and upper tract abnormalities are more likely to have posterior urethral valves or prune-belly syndrome.

Postnatal radiologic studies may show the dilated upper urinary tract but fail to disclose any site of mechanical obstruction in either the gastrointestinal or the genitourinary tract. Contrast agent used for contrast enema fills the microcolon, which also has a tendency to be abnormally rotated or fixed.

Contrast studies of the genitourinary tract are routinely performed to exclude obstruction. Sonography can show the dilated bladder and upper tracts and exclude other causes of abdominal mass.

## Hirschsprung's Disease

Hirschsprung's disease typically presents in the neonatal period. This disorder is discussed in Chapter 78.

## References

1. Snyder WH, Chaffin L: Embryology and pathology of the intestinal tract: presentation of 40 cases of malrotation. Ann Surg 140:368–379, 1954.
2. Cyr DR, Mack LA, Schoenecker SA, et al: Bowel migration in the normal fetus: US detection. Radiology 161:119–121, 1986.
3. Parulekar SG: Sonography of normal fetal bowel. J Ultrasound Med 10:211–220, 1991.
4. Ablow RC, Hoffer FA, Seashore JH, et al: Z-shaped duodenojejunal loop: sign of mesenteric fixation anomaly and congenital bands. AJR 141:461–464, 1983.
5. Balthazar EJ: Intestinal malrotation in adults. Roentgenographic assessment with emphasis on isolated complete and partial nonrotations. AJR 126:358–367, 1976.
6. Katz ME, Siegel MJ, Shackelford GD, et al: The position and mobility of the duodenum in children. AJR 148:947–951, 1987.
7. Houston CS, Wittenborg MH: Roentgen evaluation of anomalies of rotation and fixation of the bowel in children. Radiology 84:1–18, 1965.
8. Simpson AJ, Leonidas JC, Krasna IH, et al: Roentgen diagnosis of midgut malrotation: value of upper gastrointestinal radiographic study. J Pediatr Surg 7:243–252, 1972.
9. Berdon WE, Baker DH, Bull S, et al: Midgut malrotation and volvulus. Which films are most helpful? Radiology 96:375–383, 1970.
10. Filston HC, Kirks DR: Malrotation: the ubiquitous anomaly. J Pediatr Surg 16:614–620, 1981.
11. Stewart DR, Colodny AL, Daggett WC: Malrotation of the bowel in infants and children: a 15 year review. Surgery 79:716–720, 1976.
12. Allen RP, Akers DR, Shopfner CE: Midgut volvulus. Radiology 74:784–789, 1960.
13. Firor HV, Harris VJ: Rotational abnormalities of the gut. Reemphasis of a neglected facet, isolated incomplete rotation of the duodenum. AJR 120:315–321, 1974.
14. DePrima SJ, Hardy DC, Brant WE: Reversed intestinal rotation. Radiology 157:603–604, 1985.
15. Frye TR, Mah CL, Schiller M: Roentgenographic evidence of gangrenous bowel in midgut volvulus with observations in experimental volvulus. AJR 114:394–401, 1972.
16. Janik JS, Ein SH: Normal intestinal rotation with non-fixation: a cause of chronic abdominal pain. J Pediatr Surg 14:670–674, 1979.
17. Spigland N, Brandt ML, Yazbeck S: Malrotation presenting beyond the neonatal period. J Pediatr Surg 25:1139–1142, 1990.
18. Firor HV, Steiger E: Morbidity of rotational abnormalities of the gut beyond infancy. Cleve Clin Q 50:303–309, 1983.
19. Kassner EG, Kottmeier PK: Absence and retention of small bowel gas in infants with midgut volvulus: mechanisms and significance. Pediatr Radiol 4:28–30, 1975.
20. Mori H, Hayashi K, Futagawa S, et al: Vascular compromise in chronic volvulus with midgut malrotation. Pediatr Radiol 17:277–281, 1987.
21. Verma TR, Bankole MA: Lymphovenous obstruction in anomalous midgut rotation. Arch Dis Child 48:154–156, 1973.
22. Symbas PN, Puayu FA, Scott HW: Malabsorption syndrome secondary to jejunal stenosis and incomplete rotation of the colon. Ann Surg 159:574–580, 1964.
22a. Coombs RC, Buick RG, Gornall PG, et al: Intestinal malrotation: The role of small intestinal dysmotility in the cause of persistent symptoms. J Pediatr Surg 26:553–556, 1991.
23. Potts SR, Thomas PS, Garstin WIH, et al: The duodenal triangle: a plain film sign of midgut malrotation and volvulus in the neonate. Clin Radiol 36:47–49, 1985.
24. Cloutier MG, Fried AM, Selke AC: Antenatal observation of midgut volvulus by ultrasound. JCU 11:286–288, 1983.
25. Loyer E, Eggli KD: Sonographic evaluation of superior mesenteric vascular relationship in malrotation. Pediatr Radiol 19:173–175, 1989.
26. Gaines PA, Saunders AJS, Drake D: Midgut malrotation diagnosed by ultrasound. Clin Radiol 38:51–55, 1987.
27. Leonidas JC, Magid N, Soberman N, et al: Midgut volvulus in infants: diagnosis with US. Radiology 179:491–493, 1991.
28. Griska LB, Popky GL: Angiography in mid-gut malrotation with volvulus. AJR 135:1055–1056, 1980.
29. Nichols DM, Li DK: Superior mesenteric vein rotation: a CT sign of midgut malrotation. AJR 141:707–708, 1983.
29a. Zerin JM, Di Pietro MA: Mesenteric vascular anatomy at CT: normal and abnormal appearances. Radiology 179:739–742, 1991.
30. Jaramillo D, Raval B: CT diagnosis of primary small-bowel volvulus. AJR 147:941–942, 1986.
31. Franken EA: Anomalies of the anterior abdominal wall: classification and roentgenology. AJR 112:58–67, 1971.
32. Tibboel D, Raine P, McNee M, et al: Developmental aspects of gastroschisis. J Pediatr Surg 21:865–869, 1986.
33. Duhamel B: Embryology of exomphalos and allied malformation. Arch Dis Child 38:142–147, 1963.
34. Hoyme HE, Jones MC, Jones KL: Gastroschisis: abdominal wall disruption secondary to early gestational interruption of the omphalomesenteric artery. Semin Perinatol 7:294–298, 1983.

35. Glick PL, Harrison MR, Adzick NS, et al: The missing link in the pathogenesis of gastroschisis. J Pediatr Surg 20:406–409, 1985.

36. Torfs C, Curry C, Roeper P: Gastroschisis. J Pediatr 116:1–6, 1990.

37. Giulian BB, Alvear DT: Prenatal ultrasonographic diagnosis of fetal gastroschisis. Radiology 129:473–475, 1978.

38. Bair JH, Russ PD, Pretorius DH, et al: Fetal omphalocele and gastroschisis: a review of 24 cases. AJR 147:1047–1051, 1986.

39. Lindfors KK, McGahan JP, Walter JP: Fetal omphalocele and gastroschisis: pitfalls in the sonographic diagnosis. AJR 147:797–800, 1986.

40. Mann L, Ferguson-Smith MA, Desai M, et al: Prenatal assessment of anterior abdominal wall defects and their prognosis. Prenat Diagn 4:427–435, 1984.

41. Grossman M, Fischermann EA, German J: Sonographic findings in gastroschisis. JCU 6:175–176, 1978.

42. Mayer T, Black R, Matlak ME, et al: Gastroschisis and omphalocele. An eight-year review. Ann Surg 192:783–787, 1980.

43. Muraji T, Tsugawa C, Nishijima E, et al: Gastroschisis: a 17 year experience. J Pediatr Surg 24:343–345, 1990.

44. Gornall P: Management of intestinal atresia complicating gastroschisis. J Pediatr Surg 24:522–524, 1989.

45. Caniano DA, Brokaw B, Ginn-Pease ME: An individualized approach to the management of gastroschisis. J Pediatr Surg 25:297–300, 1990.

46. Luck SR, Sherman JO, Raffensperger JG, et al: Gastroschisis in 106 consecutive newborn infants. Surgery 98:677–683, 1985.

47. Meller JL, Reyes HM, Loeff DS: Gastroschisis and omphalocele. Clin Perinatol 16:113–122, 1989.

48. Kohn MR, Shi ECP: Gastroschisis and exomphalos: recent trends and factors influencing survival. Aust N Z J Surg 60:199–202, 1990.

49. Fitzsimmons J, Nyberg DA, Cyr DR, et al: Perinatal management of gastroschisis. Obstet Gynecol 71:910–912, 1988.

50. Kirk EP, Wah RM: Obstetric management of the fetus with omphalocele or gastroschisis: a review of one hundred twelve cases. Am J Obstet Gynecol 146:512–518, 1983.

51. Pokorny WJ, Harberg FJ, McGill CW: Gastroschisis complicated by intestinal atresia. J Pediatr Surg 16:261–263, 1981.

52. Stewart BA, Karrer FM, Hall RJ, et al: The blind loop syndrome in children. J Pediatr Surg 25:905–908, 1990.

53. Schuck RJ, Sturm B, Deeg KH, et al: Intra-abdominal pressure monitoring in newborns with gastroschisis, omphalocele, and diaphragmatic hernia. Pediatr Surg Int 4:245–248, 1989.

54. Oh KS, Dorst JP, Dominguez R, et al: Abnormal intestinal motility in gastroschisis. Radiology 127:457–460, 1978.

55. Blane CE, Wesley JR, DiPietro MA, et al: Gastrointestinal complications of gastroschisis. AJR 144:589–591, 1985.

56. Touloukian RJ, Spackman TJ: Gastrointestinal function and radiographic appearance following gastroschisis repair. J Pediatr Surg 6:427–434, 1971.

57. Oldham KT, Coran AG, Drongowski RA, et al: The development of necrotizing enterocolitis following repair of gastroschisis: a surprisingly high incidence. J Pediatr Surg 23:945–949, 1988.

58. Hughes MD, Nyberg DA, Mack LA, et al: Fetal omphalocele: prenatal US detection of concurrent anomalies and other predictors of outcome. Radiology 173:371–376, 1989.

59. Curtis JA, Watson L: Sonographic diagnosis of omphalocele in the first trimester of fetal gestation. J Ultrasound Med 7:97–100, 1988.

60. Weinstein L, Anderson C: In utero diagnosis of Beckwith-Wiedemann syndrome by ultrasound. Radiology 134:474, 1980.

61. Greenwood RD, Rosenthal A, Nadas AS: Cardiovascular malformations associated with omphalocele. J Pediatr 85:818–821, 1974.

62. Argyle JC: Pulmonary hypoplasia in infants with giant abdominal wall defects. Pediatr Pathol 9:43–55, 1989.

63. Hershenson MB, Brouillette RT, Klemka L, et al: Respiratory insufficiency in newborns with abdominal wall defects. J Pediatr Surg 20:348–353, 1985.

64. Knight PJ, Sommer A, Clatsworthy HW: Omphalocele: a prognostic classification. J Pediatr Surg 16:599–604, 1981.

65. Salzman L, Kuligowska E, Semine A: Pseudoomphalocele: pitfall in fetal sonography. AJR 146:1283–1285, 1986.

66. Oh KS, Strife JL, Fischer KC, et al: Pyloroduodenal deformity due to liver malformation associated with omphalocele. AJR 128:957–960, 1977.

67. Pickney LE, Moskowitz PS, Lebowitz RL, et al: Renal malposition associated with omphalocele. Radiology 129:677–682, 1978.

68. Cullen MC, Klein MD, Philippart AI: Congenital diaphragmatic hernia. Surg Clin North Am 65:1115–1138, 1985.

69. David TJ, Illingworth CA: Diaphragmatic hernia in the southwest of England. J Med Genet 13:253–262, 1976.

70. Gale ME: Bochdalek hernia: prevalence and CT characteristics. Radiology 156:449–452, 1985.

71. Leck I, Record RG, McKeown T, et al: The incidence of malformations in Birmingham, England, 1950–1959. Teratology 1:263–280, 1959.

72. Gaisie G, Young LW, Oh KS: Late-onset Bochdalek's hernia with obstruction: radiologic spectrum of presentation. Clin Radiol 34:267–270, 1983.

73. Berman L, Stringer D, Ein SH, et al: The late-presenting diaphragmatic hernia: a 20 year review. J Pediatr Surg 23:735–739, 1988.

74. McCarten KM, Rosenberg HK, Borden S, et al: Delayed appearance of right diaphragmatic hernia associated with Group B Streptococcal infection in newborns. Radiology 139:385–389, 1981.

75. Reynolds M, Luck SR, Lappen R: The "critical" neonate with diaphragmatic hernia: a 21 year perspective. J Pediatr Surg 19:364–369, 1984.

76. Benjamin DR, Juul S, Siebert JR: Congenital posterolateral diaphragmatic hernia: associated malformations. J Pediatr Surg 23:899–903, 1988.

77. Wiener ES: Congenital posterolateral diaphragmatic hernia: new dimensions in management. Surgery 92:670–679, 1982.

78. Touloukian RJ, Markowitz RI: A preoperative X-ray scoring system for risk assessment of newborns with congenital diaphragmatic hernia. J Pediatr Surg 19:252–257, 1984.

78a. Cloutier R, Fournier L, Major D: Index of pulmonary expansion: A new method to estimate lung hypoplasia in congenital diaphragmatic hernia. J Pediatr Surg 27:456–458, 1992.

79. Vacanti JP, Crone RK, Murphy JD, et al: The pulmonary hemodynamic response to perioperative anesthesia in the treatment of high-risk infants with congenital diaphragmatic hernia. J Pediatr Surg 19:672–679, 1984.

80. Taylor GA, Glass P, Fitz CR, et al: Neurologic status in infants treated with extracorporeal membrane oxygenation: correlation of imaging with developmental outcome. Radiology 165:679–682, 1987.

81. Adolph V, Ekelund C, Smith C, et al: Developmental outcome of neonates treated with extracorporeal membrane oxygenation. J Pediatr Surg 25:43–46, 1990.

82. Taylor GA, Fitz CR, Miller MK, et al: Intracranial abnormalities in infants with extracorporeal membrane oxygenation: imaging with US and CT. Radiology 165:675–678, 1987.

83. Taylor GA, Walker LK: Intracranial venous system in newborns treated with extracorporeal membrane oxygenation: Doppler US evaluation after ligation of the right jugular vein. Radiology 183:453–456, 1992.

84. Lewin JS, Masaryk TJ, Modic MT, et al: Extracorporeal membrane oxygenation in infants: angiographic and parenchymal evaluation of the brain with MR imaging. Radiology 173:361–365, 1989.

85. Ford E, Kitagawa H, Atkinson JB: Vascular access in the neonate following extracorporeal membrane oxygenation. J Pediatr Surg 25:594–595, 1990.

86. Boedy RF, Goldberg AK, Howell CG, et al: Incidence of hypertension in infants on extracorporeal membrane oxygenation. J Pediatr Surg 25:258–261, 1990.

87. Connors RH, Tracy T Jr, Bailey PV, et al: Congenital diaphragmatic hernia repair on ECMO. J Pediatr Surg 25:1043–1047, 1990.

88. Chinn DH, Filly RA, Callen PW, et al: Congenital diaphragmatic hernia diagnosed prenatally by ultrasound. Radiology 148:119–123, 1983.

88a. Natch EI, Kendall J, Blumhagen J: Stomach position as an in utero predictor of neonatal outcome in left-sided diaphragmatic hernia. J Pediatr Surg 27:778–779, 1992.

89. Benacerraf BR, Greene MF: Congenital diaphragmatic hernia:

US diagnosis prior to 22 weeks gestation. Radiology 15:809–810, 1986.

90. Benacerraf BR, Adzick NS: Fetal diaphragmatic hernia: ultrasound diagnosis and clinical outcome in 19 cases. Am J Obstet Gynecol 156:573–576, 1987.

91. Harrison MR, Langer JC, Adzick NS, et al: Correction of diaphragmatic hernia in utero. V. Initial clinical experience. J Pediatr Surg 25:47–57, 1990.

92. Gilsanz V, Emons D, Hansmann M, et al: Hydrothorax, ascites, and right diaphragmatic hernia. Radiology 158:243–246, 1986.

93. Stoler CJH, Berdon WE, Dillon PW, et al: Esophageal dilatation and reflux in neonates supported by ECMO after diaphragmatic hernia repair. AJR 151:135–137, 1988.

94. Taylor GA, Short BL, Kriesmer P: Extracorporeal membrane oxygenation: radiographic appearance of the neonatal chest. AJR 146:1257–1260, 1986.

94a. Kelly RE Jr, Phillips JD, Foglia RP, et al: Pulmonary edema and fluid mobilization as determinants of duration of ECMO support. J Pediatr Surg 26:1016–1022, 1991.

95. Taylor GA, Lotze A, Kapur S, et al: Diffuse pulmonary opacification in infants undergoing extracorporeal membrane oxygenation: clinical and pathologic correlation. Radiology 161:347–350, 1986.

96. Thomas GG, Clitherow NR: Herniation through the foramen of Morgagni in children. Br J Surg 64:215–217, 1977.

97. Baran EB, Houston HE, Lynne HB, et al: Foramen of Morgagni hernias in children. Surgery 62:1076–1081, 1967.

98. Mandell GA, Finkelstein MS, Hallowell M: Delayed presentation of a symptomatic Morgagni hernia. South Med J 82:1299–1302, 1989.

99. Pokorny WJ, McGill CW, Harberg FJ: Morgagni hernias during infancy: presentation and associated anomalies. J Pediatr Surg 19:394–397, 1984.

100. Groff DB: Diagnosis of a Morgagni hernia complicated by a previous normal chest x-ray. J Pediatr Surg 25:556–557, 1990.

101. Merten DF, Bowie JD, Kirks DR, et al: Anteromedial diaphragmatic defects in infancy: current approaches to diagnostic imaging. Radiology 142:361–365, 1982.

102. Yeager BA, Guglielmi GE, Schiebler ML, et al: Magnetic resonance imaging of Morgagni hernia. Gastrointest Radiol 12:296–298, 1989.

103. Newman B, Davis PL: Sonographic and magnetic resonance imaging of an anterior diaphragmatic hernia. Pediatr Radiol 20:110–112, 1989.

104. Boreadis AG, Gershon-Cohen J: Aeration of the respiratory and gastrointestinal tracts during the first minute of neonatal life. Radiology 67:407–409, 1956.

105. Burko H: Toxic depression of the newborn causing deficient intestinal gas pattern. AJR 88:575–578, 1962.

106. Eklöf O, Lette E: Scanty intestinal gas in infants and children. Acta Radiol Diagn 19:259–267, 1978.

107. Coradello H, Ponhold W, Lubec G, et al: Disappearance of bowel gas in newborn infants on mechanical ventilation. Pediatr Radiol 12:11–14, 1982.

108. Siegle RL: Neonatal gasless abdomen: another cause. AJR 133:522–523, 1979.

109. Davis WS, Allen RP: Conditioning value of the plain film examination in the diagnosis of neonatal Hirschsprung's disease. Radiology 93:129–133, 1969.

110. Kleinman PK, Winchester P, Meyers MA, et al: The neonatal colon: an anatomic approach to plain films. AJR 128:61–64, 1977.

111. Cohen MD, Jansen R, Lemons J, et al: Evaluation of the gasless abdomen in the newborn and young infant with metrizamide. AJR 142:393–396, 1984.

112. Wedge JJ, Grosfeld JL, Smith JP: Abdominal masses in the newborn: 63 cases. J Urol 106:770–774, 1971.

113. Griscom NT: Roentgenology of neonatal abdominal masses. AJR 93:447–463, 1965.

114. Kirks DR, Rosenberg ER, Johnson DG, et al: Integrated imaging of neonatal renal masses. Pediatr Radiol 15:147–156, 1985.

115. Effmann EL, Griscom NT, Colodny AH, et al: Neonatal gastrointestinal masses arising late in gestation. AJR 135:681–686, 1980.

116. Nussbaum AR, Sanders RD, Benator R, et al: Spontaneous resolution of neonatal ovarian cysts. AJR 148:175–176, 1987.

116a. Croitoru DP, Aaron LE, Laberge JM: Management of complex ovarian cysts presenting in the first year of life. J Pediatr Surg 26:1366–1368, 1991.

117. Brandt ML, Luks FI, Filiatrault D, et al: Surgical indications in antenatally diagnosed ovarian cysts. J Pediatr Surg 26:276–282, 1991.

118. Effmann EL, Griscom NT, Colodny AH, et al: Neonatal gastrointestinal masses arising late in gestation. AJR 135:681–686, 1980.

119. Ratcliffe J, Tait J, Lisle D, et al: Segmental dilatation of the small bowel: report of three cases and a literature review. Radiology 171:827–830, 1989.

120. Mahaffey SM, Ryckman FC, Martin LW: Clinical aspects of abdominal masses in children. Semin Roentgenol 23:161–174, 1988.

121. Teele RL, Share JC: The abdominal mass in the neonate. Semin Roentgenol 23:175–184, 1988.

122. Griscom NT, Colodny AH, Rosenberg HK, et al: Diagnostic aspects of neonatal ascites: report of 27 cases. AJR 128:961–970, 1977.

123. Daneman A, Stringer D, Reilly BJ: Neonatal ascites due to lysosomal storage disease. Radiology 149:463–467, 1983.

124. Gyeves-Ray K, Hernandez RJ, Hillemeir AC: Pseudoascites: unusual presentation of omental cyst. Pediatr Radiol 20:560–561, 1990.

125. Sheth S, Nussbaum A, Sanders RC, et al: Prenatal diagnosis of sacrococcygeal teratoma: sonographic-pathologic correlation. Radiology 169:131–136, 1988.

126. Feldman M, Byrne P, Johnson MA, et al: Neonatal sacrococcygeal teratoma: multiimaging modality assessment. J Pediatr Surg 25:675–678, 1990.

127. Ros PR, Olmsted WW, Moser RP, et al: Mesenteric and omental cysts: histologic classification with imaging correlation. Radiology 164:327–332, 1987.

128. Dietrich RB, Kangarloo H: Pelvic abnormalities in children: assessment with MR imaging. Radiology 163:367–372, 1987.

129. Wu A, Siegel MJ: Sonography of pelvic masses in children: diagnostic predictability. AJR 148:1199–1202, 1987.

130. Bell RS, Graham CB, Stevenson JK: Roentgenologic and clinical manifestations of neonatal necrotizing enterocolitis. AJR 112:123–134, 1971.

131. Rabinowitz JG, Siegle RL: Changing clinical and roentgenographic patterns of necrotizing enterocolitis. AJR 126:560–566, 1976.

132. Kliegman RM, Fanaroff AA: Necrotizing enterocolitis. N Engl J Med 310:1093–1103, 1984.

133. Kosloske AM, Musemeche CA: Necrotizing enterocolitis of the neonate. Clin Perinatol 16:97–111, 1989.

134. Andrews DA, Sawin RS, Ledbetter DJ, et al: Necrotizing enterocolitis in term neonates. Am J Surg 159:507–509, 1990.

135. Van Bel F, Van Zwieten PHT, Guit G, et al: Superior mesenteric artery blood flow velocity and estimated volume flow: duplex Doppler US study of preterm and term neonates. Radiology 174:165–169, 1990.

136. Palder SB, Schwartz MZ, Tyson KR, et al: Association of closure of patent ductus arteriosus and development of necrotizing enterocolitis. J Pediatr Surg 23:422–423, 1988.

137. Cassady G, Crouse DT, Kirklin JW, et al: A randomized, controlled trial of very early prophylactic ligation of the ductus arteriosus in babies who weighed 1000 g or less at birth. N Engl J Med 320:1511–1516, 1989.

138. Kleinman PK, Winchester P, Brill P: Necrotizing enterocolitis after open heart surgery employing hypothermia and cardiopulmonary bypass. AJR 127:757–760, 1976.

139. Allen HA, Haney PJ: Left ventricular outflow obstruction and necrotizing enterocolitis. Radiology 150:401–402, 1984.

139a. Hall TH, Zaninova A, Lewin D, et al: Neonatal intestinal ischemia with bowel perforation: an in utero complication of maternal cocaine abuse. AJR 158:1303–1304, 1992.

140. Ansley-Green A, Lucas A, Lawson GR, et al: Gut hormones and regulatory peptides in relation to enteral feeding, gastroenteritis, and necrotizing enterocolitis in infancy. J Pediatr 117:S24–S32, 1990.

141. Ballance WA, Dahms BA, Shenker N, et al: Pathology of neonatal necrotizing enterocolitis: a ten year experience. J Pediatr 117:S6–S13, 1990.

142. Costin BS, Singleton EB: Bowel stenosis as a late complication of acute necrotizing enterocolitis. Radiology 128:435–438, 1978.

143. Frey EE, Smith W, Franken EA, et al: Analysis of bowel perforation in necrotizing enterocolitis. Pediatr Radiol 17:380–382, 1987.

144. Ball TI, Wyly JB: Enterocyst formation: a late complication of neonatal necrotizing enterocolitis. AJR 147:806–808, 1986.

145. Janik JS, Ein SH, Mancer K: Intestinal stricture after necrotizing enterocolitis. J Pediatr Surg 16:438–443, 1981.

146. Janik JS, Ein SH: Peritoneal drainage under local anesthesia for necrotizing enterocolitis (NEC) perforation: a second look. J Pediatr Surg 15:565–568, 1980.

147. Ein SH, Shandling B, Wesson D, et al: A 13-year experience with peritoneal drainage under local anesthesia for necrotizing enterocolitis perforation. J Pediatr Surg 25:1034–1037, 1990.

148. Hartman GE, Grugas GT, Shocat SJ: Post-necrotizing enterocolitis strictures presenting with sepsis of perforation: risk of clinical observation. J Pediatr Surg 23:562–566, 1988.

149. Tonkin ILD, Bjelland JC, Hunter TB, et al: Spontaneous resolution of colonic strictures caused by necrotizing enterocolitis: therapeutic implications. AJR 130:1077–1081, 1978.

150. Smith SD, Tagge EP, Miller J, et al: The hidden mortality in surgically treated necrotizing enterocolitis: fungal sepsis. J Pediatr Surg 25:1030–1033, 1990.

151. Matos C, Avni EF, Van Gansbeke D, et al: Total parenteral nutrition and gallbladder disease in neonates. J Ultrasound Med 6:243–248, 1987.

151a. Georgeson KE, Breaux CW Jr: Outcome and intestinal adaptation in neonatal short-bowel syndrome. J Pediatr Surg 27:344–350, 1992.

152. Robinson AE, Grossman H, Brumley GW: Pneumatosis intestinalis in the neonate. AJR 120:333–341, 1974.

153. Gupta A: Pneumatosis intestinalis in children. Br J Radiol 51:589–595, 1978.

154. Wexler HA: The persistent loop sign in neonatal necrotizing enterocolitis: a new indication for surgical intervention? Radiology 126:201–204, 1978.

155. Brill PW, Olson SR, Winchester P: Neonatal necrotizing enterocolitis: air in Morison pouch. Radiology 174:469–471, 1990.

156. Johnson JF: Pneumatosis in the descending colon: preliminary observations on the value of prone positioning. Pediatr Radiol 19:25–27, 1988.

157. Kogutt MS: Necrotizing enterocolitis of infancy. Early roentgen patterns as a guide to prompt diagnosis. Radiology 130:367–370, 1979.

158. Daneman A, Woodward S, deSilva M: The radiology of neonatal necrotizing enterocolitis. A review of 47 cases and the literature. Pediatr Radiol 7:70–77, 1978.

159. Weinstein MM: The persistent loop sign in neonatal necrotizing enterocolitis: a new cause. Pediatr Radiol 16:71–72, 1986.

160. Leonard T, Johnson JF, Pettett PG: Critical evaluation of the persistent loop sign in necrotizing enterocolitis. Radiology 142:385–386, 1982.

161. Odita JC, Omene JA, Okolo AA: Gastric distention in neonatal necrotizing enterocolitis. Pediatr Radiol 17:202–205, 1987.

162. Seibert JJ, Parvey LS: The telltale triangle: use of the supine cross table lateral radiograph of the abdomen in early detection of pneumoperitoneum. Pediatr Radiol 5:209–210, 1977.

163. Gross GW, Ehrlich SM, Wang Y: Diagnostic quality of portable abdominal radiographs in neonates with necrotizing enterocolitis: digitized vs nondigitized images. AJR 154:779–783, 1990.

164. Patriquin HB, Fisch CH, Bureau M, et al: Radiologically visible fecal gas patterns in "normal" newborn and young infants. Pediatr Radiol 14:87–90, 1984.

165. Merritt CRB, Goldsmith JP, Sharp MJ: Sonographic detection of portal venous gas in infants with necrotizing enterocolitis. AJR 143:1059–1062, 1984.

166. Kodroff MB, Hartenberg MA, Goldschmidt RA: Ultrasonographic diagnosis of gangrenous bowel in neonatal necrotizing enterocolitis. Pediatr Radiol 14:168–170, 1984.

167. Patel U, Leonidas JC, Furie D: Sonographic detection of necrotizing enterocolitis in infancy. J Ultrasound Med 9:673–675, 1990.

168. Cohen MD, Smith JA, Slabaugh RD, et al: Neonatal necrotizing enterocolitis shown by oral metrizamide (Amipaque). AJR 138:1019–1023, 1982.

169. Ball WS, Seigel RS, Goldthorn JF, et al: Colonic strictures in infants following intestinal ischemia. Treatment by balloon catheter dilatation. Radiology 149:469–472, 1983.

170. Langer JC, Adzick NS, Filly RA, et al: Gastrointestinal tract obstruction in the fetus. Arch Surg 124:1183–1187, 1989.

171. Quan L, Smith DW: The VATER association, Vertebral defects, Anal atresia, T-E fistula with esophageal atresia, Radial and renal dysplasia: a spectrum of associated defects. J Pediatr 82:104–107, 1973.

172. Barnes JC, Smith WL: The VATER association. Radiology 126:445–449, 1978.

173. Berkhoff WBC, Scholtmeyer RJ, Tibboel D, et al: Urogenital tract abnormalities associated with esophageal atresia and tracheoesophageal fistula. J Urol 141:362–363, 1989.

174. Benson JE, Olsen MM, Fletcher BD: A spectrum of bronchopulmonary anomalies associated with tracheoesophageal malformations. Pediatr Radiol 15:377–380, 1985.

175. Landing BH: Syndromes of congenital heart disease with tracheobronchial anomalies. Edward B.D. Neuhauser lecture, 1974. AJR 123:679–686, 1975.

176. Kirks DR, Filston HC: The association of esophageal duplication cyst with esophageal atresia. Pediatr Radiol 11:214–216, 1981.

177. Chittmittrapap S, Spitz L, Kiely EM, et al: Oesophageal atresia and associated anomalies. Arch Dis Child 64:364–368, 1989.

178. Chetcuti P, Dickens DRV, Phelan PD: Spinal deformity in patients with oesophageal atresia and tracheo-oesophageal fistula. Arch Dis Child 64:1427–1430, 1989.

179. Day DL: Aortic arch in neonates with esophageal atresia: preoperative assessment using CT. Radiology 155:99–100, 1985.

180. Stringel G, Coln D, Guertin L: Esophageal atresia and right aortic arch. Right or left thoracotomy? Pediatr Surg Int 5:103–105, 1990.

181. Beasley SW, Auldist AW, Myers NA: Current surgical management of oesophageal atresia and/or tracheo-esophageal fistula. Aust N Z J Surg 59:707–712, 1989.

182. Randolph JG, Newman KD, Anderson KD: Current results in repair of esophageal atresia with tracheoesophageal fistula using physiologic status as a guide to therapy. Ann Surg 209:526–531, 1989.

183. Mehrabi V, Nezakatgoo N, Ansari MJ: Further look at colon-patch esophagoplasty in benign strictures of the esophagus in children. Z Kinderchir 44:221–227, 1989.

184. Mitchell IM, Goh DW, Roberts KD, et al: Colon interposition in children. Br J Surg 76:681–686, 1989.

185. Stringer DA, Ein S: Recurrent tracheo-esophageal fistula: a protocol for investigation. Radiology 151:637–641, 1984.

186. Chittmittrapap S, Spitz L, Kiely EM, et al: Anastomotic stricture following repair of esophageal atresia. J Pediatr Surg 25:508–511, 1990.

187. Gilsanz V, Boechat IM, Birnberg FA, et al: Scoliosis after thoracotomy for esophageal atresia. AJR 141:457–460, 1983.

188. Poenaru D, Laberge JM, Neilson IR, et al: A more than 25 year experience with end-to-end versus end-to-side repair for esophageal atresia. J Pediatr Surg 26:472–477, 1991.

189. Kleinman PK, Waite RJ, Cohen IT, et al: Atretic esophagus: transgastric balloon-assisted hydrostatic dilatation. Radiology 171:831–833, 1989.

190. Sato Y, Frey EE, Smith WL, et al: Balloon dilatation of esophageal stenosis in children. AJR 150:639–642, 1988.

191. Kirks DR, Briley CA, Currarino G: Selective catheterization of tracheoesophageal fistula. AJR 133:763–764, 1979.

192. Berdon WE, Baker DH: Radiographic findings in esophageal atresia with proximal pouch fistula (type B). Pediatr Radiol 3:70–74, 1975.

193. Morgan CL, Grossman H, Leonidas J: Roentgenographic findings in a spectrum of uncommon tracheo-oesophageal anomalies. Clin Radiol 30:353–358, 1979.

194. van der Zee DC, van der Staak FHJ, Severijnen RSVM, et al: Proximal fistula in esophageal atresia: pitfall in routine procedure. Pediatr Surg Int 3:23–26, 1988.

195. Curci MR, Dibbins AW: Problems associated with a Nissen fundoplication following tracheoesophageal fistula and esophageal atresia repair. Arch Surg 123:618–620, 1988.

196. Griscom NT, Martin TR: The trachea and esophagus after repair of esophageal atresia and distal fistula: computed tomographic observations. Pediatr Radiol 20:447–450, 1990.

196a. Rideout DT, Hayashi AH, Gillis DA, et al: The absence of clinically significant tracheomalacia in patients having esophageal atresia without tracheoesophageal fistula. J Pediatr Surg 26:1303–1305, 1991.

197. Kluth D, Steding G, Seidl W: The embryology of foregut malformations. J Pediatr Surg 22:389–393, 1987.

198. Fernbach SK, Glass RBJ: The expanded spectrum of limb anomalies in the VATER association. Pediatr Radiol 18:215–220, 1988.

199. Fernbach SK: Urethral anomalies in male neonates with VATER association. AJR 156:137–140, 1991.

200. Ogawa T, Yamataka A, Miyano T, et al: Treatment of laryngotracheal cleft. J Pediatr Surg 24:341–342, 1989.

201. Ure BM, Holschneider AM, Holski J, et al: Congenital laryngo-tracheo-esophageal cleft. Z Kinderchir 44:237–242, 1989.

202. Frates RE: Roentgen signs in laryngotracheoesophageal cleft. Radiology 88:484–486, 1967.

203. Griscom NT: Persistent esophagotrachea. The most severe degree of laryngotracheal-esophageal cleft. AJR 97:211–215, 1966.

204. Dubois JJ, Pokorny WJ, Harberg FJ, et al: Current management of laryngeal and laryngotracheoesophageal clefts. J Pediatr Surg 25:855–860, 1990.

205. Donahoe PK, Hendren WH: The surgical management of laryngotracheal cleft with tracheoesophageal fistula and esophageal atresia. Surgery 71:363–368, 1972.

206. Pettersson G: Laryngotracheoesophageal cleft. Z Kinderchir 7:43–49, 1969.

207. Verloes A, LeMerrer M, Briard ML: BBBG syndrome or Opitz syndrome: new family. Am J Clin Genet 34:313–316, 1989.

208. Wilson GN, Oliver WJ: Further delineation of the G syndrome: a manageable genetic cause of infantile dysphagia. J Med Genet 25:157–163, 1988.

209. Fletman D, McQuown D, Kanchanapoom, et al: "Apple peel" atresia of the small bowel: prenatal diagnosis of the obstruction by ultrasound. Pediatr Radiol 9:118–119, 1980.

210. Patten RM, Mack LA, Nyberg DA, et al: Twin embolization syndrome: prenatal sonographic detection and significance. Radiology 173:685–689, 1990.

211. Louw JH: Jejunoileal atresia and stenosis. J Pediatr Surg 1:8–23, 1966.

212. Heij HA, Moorman-Voestermans CGM, Vos A: Atresia of jejunum and ileum: is it the same disease? J Pediatr Surg 25:635–637, 1990.

213. Moorman-Voestermans CGM, Heij HA, Vos A: Jejunal atresia in twins. J Pediatr Surg 25:638–639, 1990.

214. Gibson MF: Familial multiple jejunal atresia with malrotation. J Pediatr Surg 22:1013–1014, 1987.

215. Dickson JAS: Apple peel small bowel: an uncommon variant of duodenal and jejunal atresia. J Pediatr Surg 5:595–600, 1970.

216. Nixon HH, Tawes R: Etiology and treatment of small intestinal atresia: analysis of a series of 127 jejunoileal atresias and comparison with 62 duodenal atresias. Surgery 69:41–51, 1971.

217. Grosfeld JL, Ballantine TVN, Shoemaker R: Operative management of intestinal atresia and stenosis based on pathologic findings. J Pediatr Surg 14:368–375, 1979.

218. Adejuyigbe O, Odesaami WO: Intrauterine intussusception causing intestinal atresia. J Pediatr Surg 25:562–563, 1990.

219. Weiss RG, Ryan DP, Ildstad ST, et al: A complex case of jejunoileocolic atresia. J Pediatr Surg 25:560–561, 1990.

220. Martin CE, Leonidas JC, Amoury RA: Multiple gastrointestinal atresia, with intraluminal calcifications and cystic dilatation of bile ducts: a newly recognized entity resembling "a string of pearls." Pediatrics 576:268–271, 1976.

221. Puri P, Guiney EJ, Carroll R: Multiple gastrointestinal atresias in three consecutive siblings: observations on pathogenesis. J Pediatr Surg 20:22–24, 1985.

222. Shen-Schwarz S, Fitko R: Multiple gastrointestinal atresias with imperforate anus: pathology and pathogenesis. Am J Med Genet 36:451–455, 1990.

223. Daneman A, Martin DJ: A syndrome of multiple gastrointestinal atresias with intraluminal calcification. A report of a case and a review of the literature. Pediatr Radiol 8:227–231, 1979.

224. Smith GHH, Glasson M: Intestinal atresia: factors affecting survival. Aust N Z J Surg 59:151–156, 1989.

225. Patrapinyokul S, Brereton RJ, Spitz L, et al: Small bowel atresia and stenosis. Pediatr Surg Int 4:390–395, 1989.

226. Manning C, Strauss A, Gyepes MT: Jejunal atresia with "apple peel" deformity. A report of eight survivors. J Perinatol 9:281–286, 1989.

227. Gaisie G, Odagiri K, Oh KS, et al: The bulbous bowel segment: a sign of congenital small bowel obstruction. Radiology 135:331–334, 1980.

228. Aharon M, Kleinhaus U, Lichtig C: Neonatal intramural intestinal calcifications associated with bowel atresia. AJR 130:999–1000, 1978.

229. Winchester P, Heheghan M, Brill PW, et al: Neonatal intramural bowel calcification without atresia. AJR 136:826–827, 1981.

230. Cook PL: Calcified meconium in the newborn. Clin Radiol 29:541–546, 1978.

231. Lee FA: Small bowel dilatation mimicking gastric dilatation. Pediatr Radiol 12:109–110, 1982.

232. Wolfson JJ, Williams H: A hazard of barium enema studies in infants with small bowel atresia. Radiology 95:341–343, 1970.

233. Leonidas JC: Microcolon in the absence of small bowel obstruction in the newborn. J Pediatr Surg 24:180–182, 1989.

234. Kalifa G, Devred PH, Riccour C, et al: Radiological aspects of the small bowel after extensive resection in children. Pediatr Radiol 8:70–75, 1979.

235. Tibboel D, Molenaar JC: Meconium peritonitis: a retrospective prognostic analysis of 69 patients. Z Kinderchir 39:25–28, 1984.

236. Berdon WE, Baker DH, Becker J, et al: Scrotal masses in healed meconium peritonitis. N Engl J Med 277:585–587, 1967.

237. Fujioka M, Bowen A: Cystic meconium peritonitis. Radiology 140:380, 1981.

238. Kolawole TM, Bamkole MA, Olurin EO, et al: Meconium peritonitis presenting as giant cysts in neonates. Br J Radiol 46:964–967, 1973.

239. Olsen MM, Luck SM, Lloyd-Still J, et al: The spectrum of meconium disease in infancy. J Pediatr Surg 17:479–481, 1982.

240. Pan EY, Chen LY, Zang JZ, et al: Radiographic diagnosis of meconium peritonitis. Pediatr Radiol 13:199–205, 1983.

241. Finkel LI, Slovis TL: Meconium peritonitis, intraperitoneal calcifications and cystic fibrosis. Pediatr Radiol 12:92–93, 1982.

242. Ya-Xiong S, Lia-Chen S: Meconium peritonitis: observation in 115 cases and antenatal diagnosis. Z Kinderchir 37:2–5, 1982.

243. Garb M, Riseborough J: Meconium peritonitis presenting as fetal ascites on ultrasound. Br J Radiol 53:602–604, 1979.

244. Schwimer SR, Vanley GT, Reinke RT: Prenatal diagnosis of meconium peritonitis. JCU 12:37–39, 1984.

245. Foster MA, Nyberg DA, Mahony BS, et al: Meconium peritonitis: prenatal sonographic findings and their clinical significance. Radiology 165:661–665, 1987.

246. Blumenthal DG, Rushovich AM, Williams RK, et al: Prenatal sonographic findings of meconium peritonitis with pathologic correlation. JCU 10:350–352, 1982.

247. Nancarrow PA, Mattrey RF, Edwards DK, et al: Fibroadhesive meconium peritonitis: in utero sonographic diagnosis. J Ultrasound Med 4:213–215, 1985.

248. Foster MA, Nyberg DA, Mahony BS, et al: Meconium peritonitis: prenatal sonographic findings and their clinical significance. Radiology 165:661–665, 1987.

249. Dillard JP, Edwards DK, Leopold GR: Meconium peritonitis masquerading as fetal hydrops. J Ultrasound Med 6:49–51, 1987.

250. Lawrence PW, Chrispin A: Sonographic appearances in two neonates with generalised meconium peritonitis: the snowstorm sign. Br J Radiol 57:340–342, 1984.

251. Wolfson JJ, Engel RR: Anticipating meconium peritonitis from metaphyseal bands. Radiology 92:1055–1060, 1969.

252. Bley WR, Franken EA: Roentgenology of colon atresia. Pediatr Radiol 1:105–108, 1973.

253. Sturim HS, Ternberg JL: Congenital atresia of the colon. Surgery 59:458–464, 1966.

254. Pohlson EC, Hatch EI Jr, Glick PL, et al: Individualized management of colonic atresia. Am J Surg 155:690–692, 1988.

255. Davenport M, Bianchi A, Doig CM, et al: Colonic atresia: current results of treatment. J R Coll Surg Edinb 35:25–28, 1990.

256. Blank E, Afshani E, Girdany BR, et al: "Windsock sign" of congenital membranous atresia of the colon. AJR 120:330–332, 1974.

257. Pasto ME, Deiling JM, O'Hara AE, et al: Neonatal colonic atresia: ultrasound findings. Pediatr Radiol 14:346–348, 1984.

258. Pai GK, Pai P: A case of congenital colonic stenosis presenting as rectal prolapse. J Pediatr Surg 25:699–700, 1990.

259. Erskine JM: Colonic stenosis in the newborn: the possible thromboembolic etiology of intestinal stenosis and atresia. J Pediatr Surg 5:321–333, 1970.

260. Selke AC Jr, Jona JZ: The hook sign in type 3 congenital colonic atresia. AJR 131:350–351, 1978.

261. Santulli TV, Kiesewetter WB, Bill AH: Anorectal anomalies: a suggested international classification. J Pediatr Surg 5:281–287, 1970.

262. Stephens FD: Wingspread anomalies, rarities, and super rarities of the anorectum and cloaca. Birth Defects 24:581–585, 1988.

263. Fleming SE, Hall R, Gysler M, et al: Imperforate anus in females: frequency of genital tract involvement, incidence of associated anomalies, and functional outcome. J Pediatr Surg 21:146–150, 1986.

264. Siebert JJ, Golladay ES: Clinical evaluation of imperforate anus: clue to type of anal-rectal anomaly. AJR 133:289–292, 1979.

265. Kiesewetter WB, Nixon HH: Imperforate anus. I. Its surgical anatomy. J Pediatr Surg 2:60–68, 1967.

266. Kiesewetter WB, Bill AH, Nixon HH, et al: Imperforate anus. Arch Surg 111:518–525, 1976.

267. Hedlund H, Peña A: Does the distal rectal muscle in anorectal malformations have the functional properties of a sphincter? J Pediatr Surg 25:985–989, 1990.

268. Thompson W, Grossman H: The association of spinal and genitourinary abnormalities with low anorectal anomalies (imperforate anus) in female infants. Radiology 113:693–698, 1974.

269. Smith ED, Saeki M: Associated anomalies. Birth Defects 24:501–509, 1988.

270. Smith ED: Urinary anomalies and complications in imperforate anus and rectum. J Pediatr Surg 3:337–348, 1968.

271. Hoekstra WJ, Scholtmeijer RJ, Molenaar JC, et al: Urogenital tract abnormalities associated with congenital anorectal anomalies. J Urol 130:962–963, 1983.

272. Belman AB, King LR: Urinary tract abnormalities associated with imperforate anus. J Urol 108:823–824, 1972.

272a. Gross GW, Wolfson PJ, Pena A: Augmented-pressure colostogram in imperforate anus with fistula. Pediatr Radiol 21:560–562, 1991.

273. Uehling DT, Gilbert E, Chesney R: Urologic implications of the VATER association. J Urol 129:352–354, 1983.

274. Greenwood RD, Rosenthal A, Nadas AS: Cardiovascular malformations associated with imperforate anus. J Pediatr 86:576–579, 1975.

275. Rintala R, Lindahl H, Sariola H, et al: The rectourogenital connection in anorectal malformations is an ectopic anal canal. J Pediatr Surg 25:665–668, 1990.

276. Sheldon C, Cormier M, Crone K, et al: Occult neurovesical dysfunction in children with imperforate anus and its variants. J Pediatr Surg 26:49–54, 1991.

277. Carson JA, Barnes PD, Tunell WP, et al: Imperforate anus: the neurologic implication of sacral abnormalities. J Pediatr Surg 19:838–842, 1984.

278. Karrer FM, Flannery AM, Nelson MD, et al: Anorectal malformations: evaluation of associated spinal dysraphic syndromes. J Pediatr Surg 23:45–48, 1988.

279. Berdon WE, Hochberg B, Baker DH, et al: The association of lumbosacral spine and genitourinary anomalies with imperforate anus. AJR 98:181–191, 1966.

280. Denton JR: The association of congenital spinal anomalies with imperforate anus. Clin Orthop 162:90–98, 1982.

281. Kohda E, Fujioka M, Ikawa H, et al: Congenital anorectal anomaly: CT evaluation. Radiology 157:349–352, 1985.

282. Sato Y, Pringle KC, Bergman RA, et al: Congenital anorectal anomalies: MR imaging. Radiology 168:157–162, 1988.

283. Mezzacappa PM, Price AP, Haller JO, et al: MR and CT demonstration of levator sling in congenital anorectal anomalies. J Comput Assist Tomogr 11:273–275, 1987.

284. Taccone A, Martucciello G, Fondelli P, et al: CT of anorectal malformation: a postoperative evaluation. Pediatr Radiol 19:375–378, 1989.

285. Sachs TM, Applebaum H, Touran T, et al: Use of MRI in evaluation of anorectal anomalies. J Pediatr Surg 25:817–821, 1990.

286. Ong NT, Beasley SW: Comparison of clinical methods for the assessment of continence after repair of high anorectal anomalies. Pediatr Surg Int 5:234–237, 1990.

287. Harris RD, Nyberg DA, Mack LA, et al: Anorectal atresia: prenatal sonographic diagnosis. AJR 149:395–400, 1987.

288. Yousefzadeh DK, Jackson JH Jr, Smith WL, et al: Intraluminal meconium calcification without distal obstruction. Pediatr Radiol 14:23–27, 1984.

289. Berdon WE, Baker DH, Wigger HJ, et al: Calcified intraluminal meconium in newborn males with imperforate anus. Enterolithiasis in the newborn. AJR 125:449–455, 1975.

290. Grant T, Newman M, Gould R, et al: Intraluminal colonic calcifications associated with anorectal atresia. J Ultrasound Med 9:411–413, 1990.

291. Wagensteen OH, Rice CO: Imperforate anus: method of determining surgical approach. Arch Surg 92:77–91, 1930.

292. Berdon WE, Baker DH: The inherent errors in measurements of inverted films in patients with imperforate anus. Ann Radiol 10:235–240, 1967.

293. Narasimharao KL, Prasad GR, Katariya S, et al: Prone cross-table lateral view: an alternative to the invertogram in imperforate anus. AJR 140:227–229, 1983.

294. Leighton DM, deCampo M: CT invertograms. Pediatr Radiol 19:176–178, 1989.

295. Wagner ML, Harberg FJ, Kumar APM, et al: The evaluation of imperforate anus utilizing percutaneous injection of water-soluble iodide contrast material. Pediatr Radiol 1:34–40, 1973.

296. Schuster SR, Teele RL: An analysis of ultrasound scanning as a guide in determining "high" or "low" imperforate anus. J Pediatr Surg 14:798–800, 1979.

297. Oppenheimer DA, Carroll BA, Shochat SJ: Sonography of imperforate anus. Radiology 148:127–128, 1983.

298. Donaldson JS, Black CT, Reynolds M, et al: Ultrasound of the distal pouch in infants with imperforate anus. J Pediatr Surg 24:465–468, 1989.

299. Vade A, Reyes H, Wilbur A, et al: The anorectal sphincter after rectal pull-through surgery for anorectal anomalies: MRI evaluation. Pediatr Radiol 19:179–183, 1989.

300. Ong NT, de Campo M, Fowler R Jr: Computerised tomography in the management of imperforate anus patients following rectoplasty. Pediatr Surg Int 5:241–245, 1990.

301. Peña A: The surgical management of persistent cloaca: results in 54 patients treated with a posterior sagittal approach. J Pediatr Surg 24:590–598, 1989.

302. Thomas DFM: Cloacal malformations: embryology, anatomy and principles of management. Prog Pediatr Surg 23:135–143, 1989.

303. Hendren WH: Urological aspects of cloacal malformations. J Urol 140:1207–1213, 1988.

304. Stephens FD: Embryology of the cloaca and embryogenesis of anorectal malformations. Birth Defects 24:177–209, 1988.

305. Raffensperger JG: The cloaca in the newborn. Birth Defects 24:111–123, 1988.

306. Jaramillo D, Lebowitz RL, Hendren WH: Cloacal malformations: radiologic findings. Radiology 177:441–448, 1990.

307. Kay R, Tank ES: Principles of management of the persistent cloaca in the female newborn. J Urol 117:102–104, 1977.

308. Wood BP: Cloacal malformations and exstrophy syndromes. Radiology 177:326–327, 1990.

309. Duhamel B: From the mermaid to anal imperforation: the syndrome of caudal regression. Arch Dis Child 36:152–155, 1961.

310. Assemany SR, Muzzo S, Gardner LI: Syndrome of phocomelic diabetic embryopathy (caudal dysplasia). Am J Dis Child 123:489–491, 1972.

311. Cousins L: Congenital anomalies among infants of diabetic mothers. Am J Obstet Gynecol 147:333–338, 1983.

312. Loewy JA, Richards DG, Toi A: In utero diagnosis of the caudal regression syndrome: report of three cases. JCU 15:469–474, 1987.

313. Sitori M, Chidini A, Romero R, et al: Prenatal diagnosis of sirenomelia. J Ultrasound Med 8:83–88, 1989.

314. Kennedy RLJ: An unusual rectal polyp: anterior sacral meningocele. Surg Gynecol Obstet 43:803–804, 1926.

315. Currarino G, Coln D, Votteler T: Triad of anorectal, sacral, and presacral anomalies. AJR 137:395–398, 1981.

316. Kirks DR, Merten DF, Filston HC, et al: The Currarino triad: complex of anorectal malformation, sacral bony deformity and presacral mass. Pediatr Radiol 14:220–225, 1984.

317. Le Quesne GW, Reilly BJ: Functional immaturity of the large bowel in the newborn infant. Radiol Clin North Am 13:331–342, 1975.

318. Cremin BJ, Smythe PM, Cywes S: The radiological appearance of the "inspissated milk syndrome": a cause of intestinal obstruction in infants. Br J Radiol 43:856–858, 1970.

319. Konvolinka CW, Frederick J: Milk curd syndrome in neonates. J Pediatr Surg 24:497–498, 1990.

320. Ueda T, Okamoto E, Seki Y: Nonmechanical intestinal obstruction simulating surgical emergency in the newborn infant. J Pediatr Surg 3:676–681, 1968.

321. Merten DF, Grossman H: Intestinal obstruction associated with cholestyramine therapy. AJR 134:827–828, 1980.

322. McIlhenny J, Sutphen JL, Block CA: Food allergy presenting as obstruction in an infant. AJR 150:373–375, 1988.

323. Abrahamson J, Shandling B: Intestinal hemangiomata in childhood and a syndrome for diagnosis: a collective review. J Pediatr Surg 8:487–495, 1973.

324. Leonidas JC, Berdon WE, Baker DH, et al: Meconium ileus and its complications. A reappraisal of plain film roentgen diagnosis. AJR 108:598–608, 1970.

325. Siegel MJ, Shackelford GD, McAlister WH: Neonatal meconium blockage in the ileum and proximal colon. Radiology 132:79–82, 1979.

326. Rescorla FJ, Grosfeld JL, West KJ, et al: Changing patterns of treatment and survival in neonates with meconium ileus. Arch Surg 124:837–840, 1989.

327. Noblett HR: Treatment of uncomplicated meconium ileus by Gastrografin enema: a preliminary report. J Pediatr Surg 4:190–197, 1969.

328. Wagget J, Bishop HC, Koop CE: Experience with Gastrografin enema in the treatment of meconium ileus. J Pediatr Surg 5:649–654, 1970.

329. Bowring AC, Jones RFC, Kern IB: The use of solvents in the intestinal manifestations of mucoviscidosis. J Pediatr Surg 5:338–343, 1970.

330. Leonidas JC, Burry VF, Fellows RA, et al: Possible adverse effect of methylglucamine diatrizoate compounds on the bowel of newborn infants with meconium ileus. Radiology 121:693–696, 1976.

331. Wood BP, Katzberg RW, Ryan DH, et al: Diatrizoate enemas: facts and fallacies of colonic toxicity. Radiology 126:441–444, 1978.

332. Grantmyre EB, Butler GJ, Gillis DA: Necrotizing enterocolitis after Renografin-76 treatment of meconium ileus. AJR 136:990–991, 1981.

333. Harris PD, Neuhauser EBD, Gerth R: The osmotic effect of water soluble contrast media on circulation plasma volume. AJR 91:694–698, 1964.

334. Ein SH, Shandling B, Reilly BJ, et al: Bowel perforation with nonoperative treatment of meconium ileus. J Pediatr Surg 22:146–147, 1987.

335. White H: Meconium ileus: a new roentgen sign. Radiology 66:567–571, 1956.

336. Clatworthy HW Jr, Howard HR, Lloyd J: The meconium plug syndrome. Surgery 39:131–142, 1956.

337. Ellis DG, Clatworthy HW Jr: The meconium plug syndrome revisited. J Pediatr Surg 1:54–61, 1966.

338. Hen J, Dolan TF, Touloukian RJ: Meconium plug syndrome associated with cystic fibrosis and Hirschsprung's disease. Pediatrics 66:466, 1980.

339. Rosenstein BJ: Cystic fibrosis presenting with the meconium plug syndrome. Am J Dis Child 132:167–169, 1978.

340. Berdon WE, Slovis TL, Campbell JB, et al: Neonatal left colon syndrome: its relationship to aganglionosis and meconium plug syndrome. Radiology 125:457–462, 1977.

341. Cremin BJ: Functional intestinal obstruction in premature infants. Pediatr Radiol 1:109–112, 1973.

342. Amodio J, Berdon W, Abramson S, et al: Microcolon of prematurity: a form of functional obstruction. AJR 146:239–244, 1986.

343. Sokal MM, Koenigsberger MR, Rose JS, et al: Neonatal hypermagnesemia and the meconium plug syndrome. N Engl J Med 286:823–825, 1972.

344. Davis WS, Allen RP, Favara BE, et al: Neonatal small left colon syndrome. AJR 120:322–329, 1974.

345. Davis WS, Campbell JB: Neonatal small left colon syndrome. Occurrence in asymptomatic infants of diabetic mothers. Am J Dis Child 129:1024–1027, 1975.

346. Philipart AI, Reed JO, Georgeson KE: Neonatal small left colon syndrome: intramural not intraluminal obstruction. J Pediatr Surg 10:733–740, 1975.

347. Nixon GW, Condon VR, Stewart DR: Intestinal perforation as a complication of the neonatal small left colon syndrome. Radiology 125:75–80, 1975.

348. Falterman CG, Richardson CJ: Small left colon syndrome associated with maternal ingestion of psychotropic drugs. J Pediatr 97:308–310, 1980.

349. Ellerbroek C, Smith WL: Neonatal small left colon in an infant with cystic fibrosis. Pediatr Radiol 16:162–163, 1986.

350. Kuhns LR, Berger PE, Poznanski AK, et al: Fat thickness in the neonatal small left colon syndrome. AJR 126:538–541, 1976.

351. Kubota M, Ikeda K, Shono T, et al: Autonomic innervation of the intestine from a baby with megacystis microcolon intestinal hypoperistalsis syndrome. I. Immunohistochemical study. J Pediatr Surg 24:1264–1266, 1989.

352. Kubota M, Ikeda K, Ito Y: Autonomic innervation of the intestine from a baby with megacystis microcolon intestinal hypoperistalsis syndrome. II. Electrophysiological study. J Pediatr Surg 24:1267–1270, 1989.

353. Wiswell TE, Rawlings JS, Wilson JL, et al: Megacystis-microcolon–intestinal hypoperistalsis syndrome. Pediatrics 63:805–808, 1979.

354. Patel R, Carty H: Megacystis-microcolon–intestinal hypoperistalsis syndrome: a rare cause of intestinal obstruction in the newborn. Br J Radiol 53:249–252, 1980.

355. Young LW, Yunis EJ, Girdany BR, et al: Megacystis-microcolon–intestinal hypoperistalsis syndrome: additional clinical, radiological, surgical, and histopathologic aspects. AJR 137:749–755, 1981.

356. Penman DG, Lilford RJ: The megacystis-microcolon–intestinal hypoperistalsis syndrome: a fatal autosomal recessive condition. J Med Genet 26:66–67, 1989.

357. Berdon WE, Baker DH, Blanc WA, et al: Megacystis-microcolon–intestinal hypoperistalsis syndrome: a new cause of intestinal obstruction in the newborn. Report of radiologic findings in five newborn girls. AJR 126:957–964, 1976.

358. Amoury RA, Fellows RA, Goodwin CD, et al: Megacystis-microcolon–intestinal hypoperistalsis syndrome: a cause of intestinal obstruction in the newborn period. J Pediatr 12:1063–1065, 1977.

359. Vezina WC, Morin FR, Winsberg F: Megacystis-microcolon–intestinal hypoperistalsis syndrome: antenatal ultrasound appearance. AJR 133:749–750, 1979.

360. Farrell SA: Intrauterine death in megacystis-microcolon–intestinal hypoplasia syndrome. J Med Genet 25:350–351, 1988.

361. Manco LG, Osterdahl P: The antenatal diagnosis of megacystis-microcolon–intestinal hypoperistalsis syndrome. JCU 12:595–598, 1984.

# Congenital and Acquired Lesions of the Esophagus

**Sandra K. Fernbach, M.D.**

**CONGENITAL ANOMALIES OF THE ESOPHAGUS**
Swallowing Disorders
Vascular Rings

**ACQUIRED ABNORMALITIES OF THE ESOPHAGUS**
Gastroesophageal Reflux
Achalasia

Esophageal Varices
Foreign Body and Caustic Ingestion
Other Esophageal Injuries

## CONGENITAL ANOMALIES OF THE ESOPHAGUS

Many congenital lesions affect esophageal morphology and function. Duplications may be asymptomatic or may manifest with respiratory or swallowing problems. Esophageal atresia is a complex anomaly that is frequently accompanied by abnormalities of other organ systems. These disorders are described in Chapters 74 and 79.

Some malformations of the primitive foregut, such as agenesis of the trachea or esophageal bronchus, are rare[1-3] (Figs. 75-1 and 75-2). Webs and diverticula may occur in early childhood with mucosal inflammation and dysphagia[4-7] (Fig. 75-3). Esophageal diverticulum has been reported both as an isolated finding and as a manifestation of Ehlers-Danlos syndrome.[8] In neonates, a posteriorly positioned diverticulum should be differentiated from a cavity acquired from a traumatically introduced endotracheal or nasogastric tube.[9]

Ectopic gastric or respiratory epithelium and tracheal cartilage in the esophagus are other congenital causes of dysphagia.[10-13] Clinically, such cases are uncommon, but the incidence of ectopic gastric mucosa in the upper esophagus approaches 21% in pediatric autopsy series.[10] Intramural leiomyomas in children may be familial, syndromic or isolated, and idiopathic.[14-16] Leiomyoblastomas may arise in the esophageal wall in association with other pathologic anomalies, such as pulmonary chondromas.[17]

### Swallowing Disorders

Many congenital and acquired abnormalities are associated with the derangement of the voluntary or reflex segments of swallowing.[18-23] Structural lesions associated with abnormal swallowing include absence of the tongue, macroglossia, palatal clefts, and micrognathia. Neurologic disorders causing abnormal swallowing include cranial nerve lesions, cerebral palsy, and meningomyelocele.

In studying a child with a suspected swallowing disorder, all stages of the swallowing process should be observed.[24-26] In older children, age-appropriate foods should be given to assess completeness of mastication and the ability to centralize the food within the oral cavity. Some children handle liquids and puréed foods well but have difficulty swallowing solids. Variation in the quantity of food and serving utensils may affect the ability to swallow in some children.[27] Although routine esophagrams are done with the child horizontal, the swallowing mechanism is studied with the child in a supported semiupright position, because it simulates the way the child usually eats (Fig. 75-4). For children with neuromuscular disorders, the support of a special chair decreases intrinsic spasticity and enhances the ability to swallow. Maneuvers to augment swallowing (e.g., stroking the cheek, additional chin and head support) are more easily performed in this position as well.

The neonate makes several sucking motions for each swallow, a pattern that normally disappears by the age of 2 to 3 months. It persists in children with neuromuscular disorders who continue to need a pumping motion before bolus formation. Neuromuscular disorders can affect the tongue, causing poor bolus formation; the palate, with resultant nasopharyngeal aspiration (Fig. 75-5A); the epiglottis, with secondary tracheal aspiration; pharyngeal emptying, causing laryngeal "spill" despite relatively normal epiglottic function; and cricopharyngeal muscle relaxation, interfering with the passage of the bolus. Failure of cricopharyngeal muscle relaxation is called *cricopharyngeal spasm* or *cricopharyngeal bar* and occurs transiently in some normal children[20] (Fig. 75-5B). Persistent failure of relaxation of the cricopharyngeal muscle can be treated with calcium channel blockers but may require myotomy.

Swallowing studies should be performed in conjunction with the speech or occupational therapist.[24] The therapist can observe the optimal food volume, feeding implements, and any compensatory maneuvers that as-

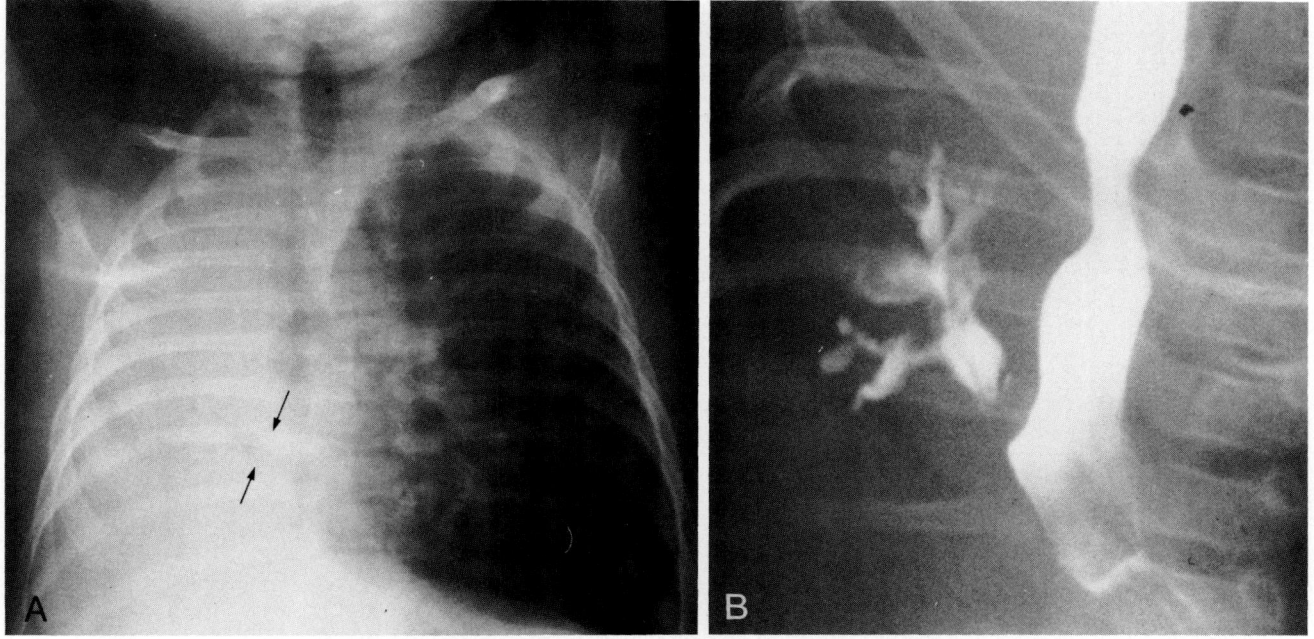

**Figure 75–1. Esophageal origin of right main stem bronchus. A.** The mediastinum is shifted to the opacified right hemithorax. An air collection is seen in the midline over the lower third of the thorax *(arrows).* **B.** The bronchus to the right lung fills with contrast from the esophagus.

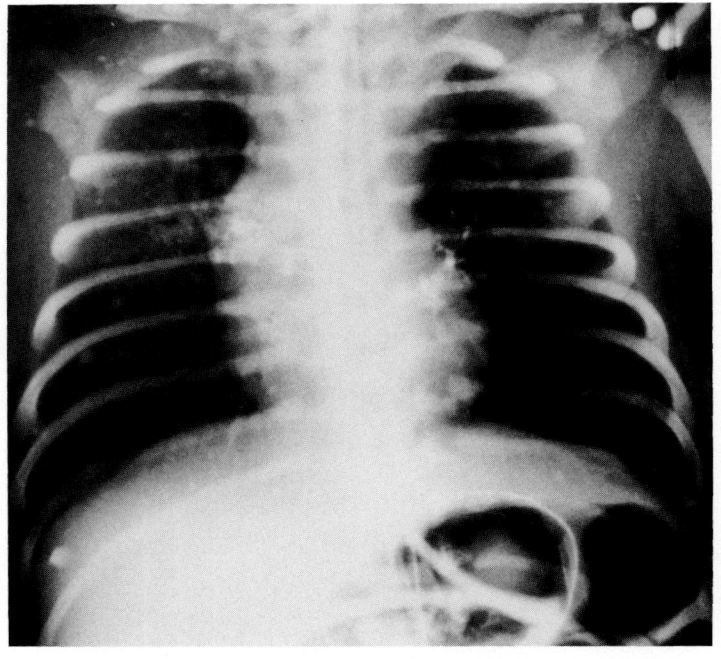

**Figure 75–2. Tracheal agenesis.** Despite apparent aeration and development of both lungs, the child had marked respiratory distress. Endoscopy performed after several unsuccessful attempts at intubation revealed tracheal agenesis. The intraoperative study shows that both main bronchi contain barium because they are arising from the esophagus.

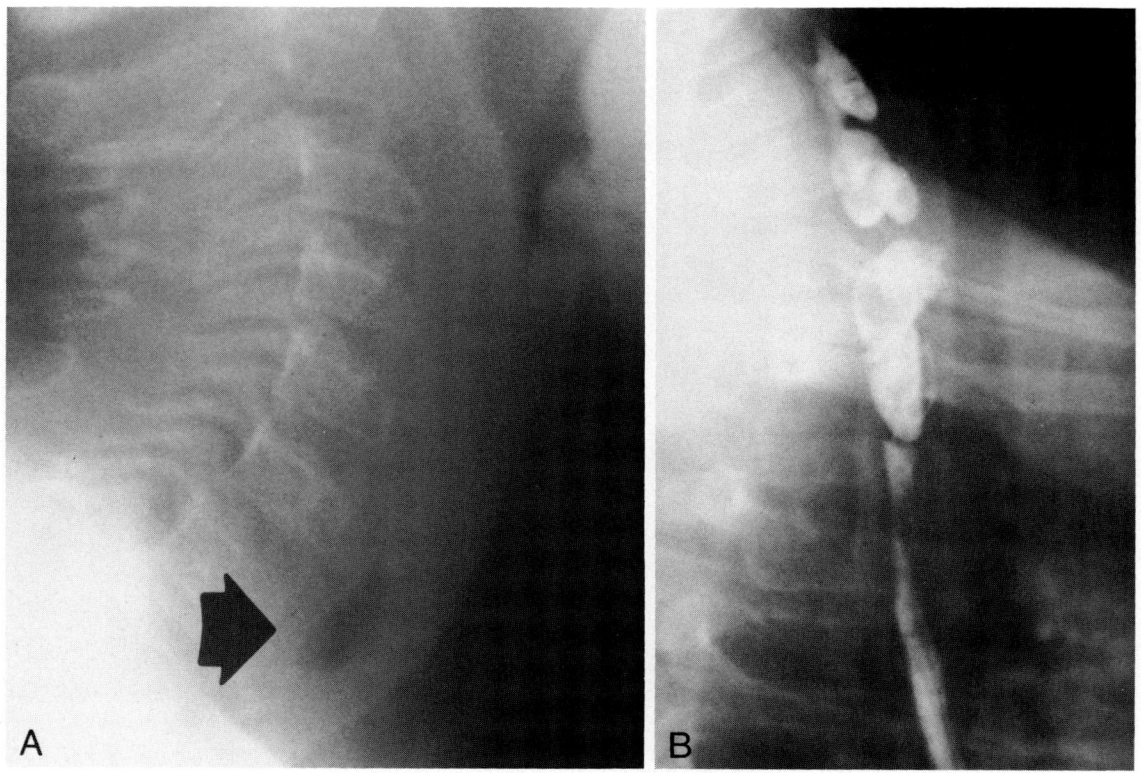

**Figure 75–3. Esophageal webs. A.** On the lateral projection, a small air collection is seen in the retrotracheal space *(arrow)*. **B.** Barium fills discrete segments as multiple webs obstruct and deform the upper esophagus.

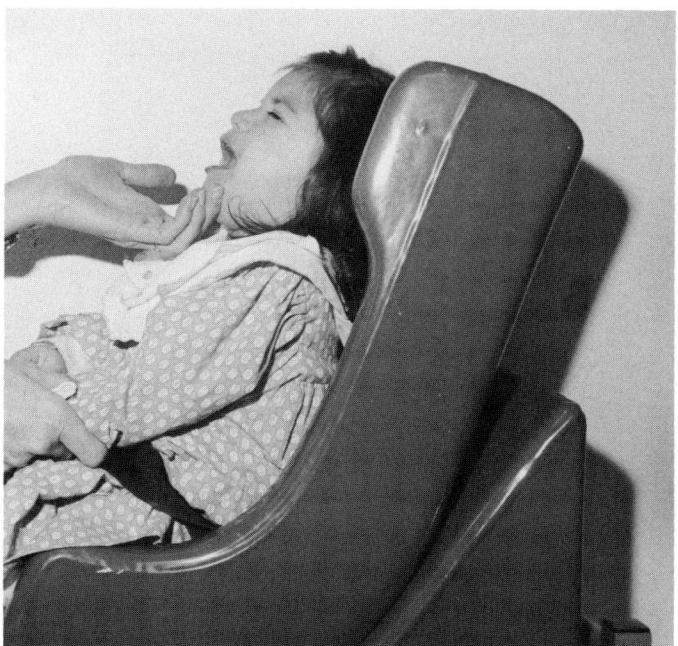

**Figure 75–4. Custom chair for esophageal studies.** A contoured chair supports the child and facilitates feeding and fluoroscopic observation. The chin can be supported, and swallowing can be enhanced with facial, oral, or neck stimulation.

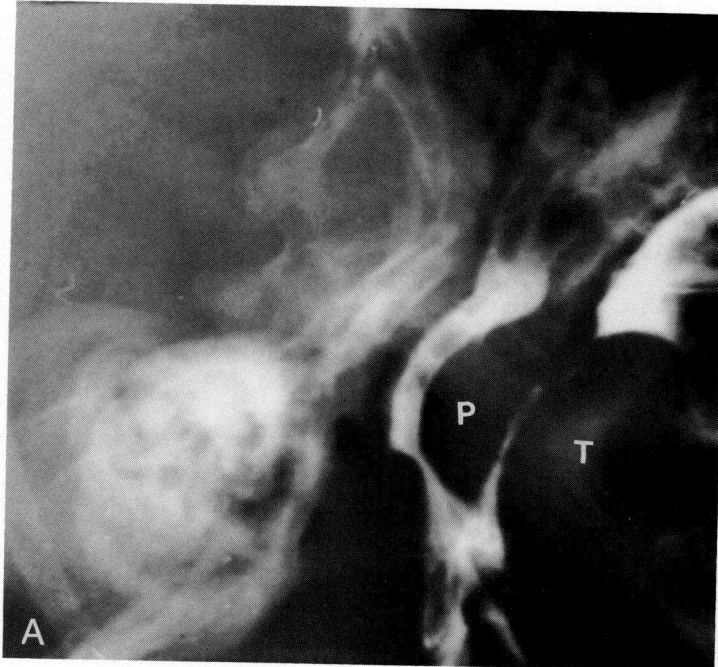
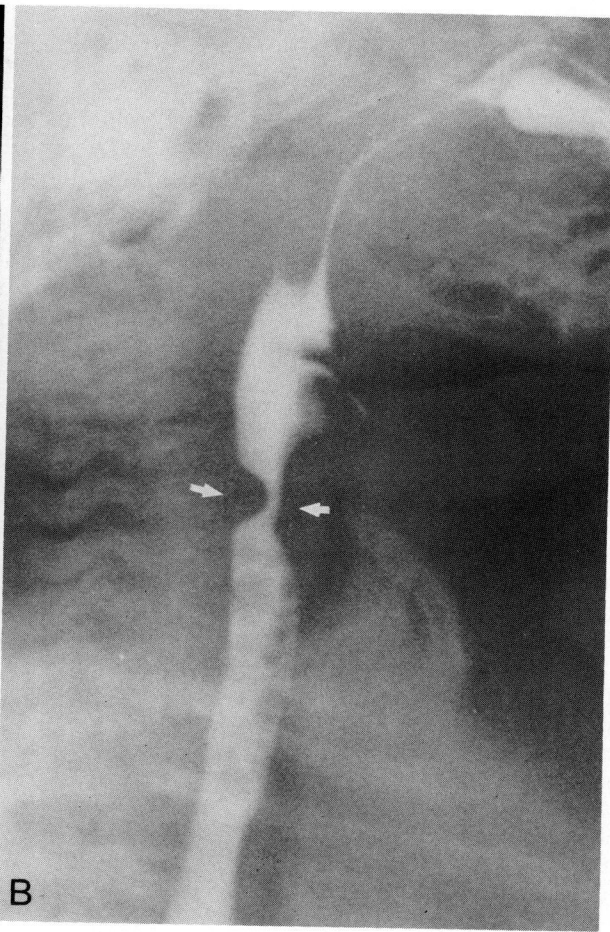

**Figure 75–5. Abnormal swallowing. A.** Nasopharyngeal aspiration. As barium passes over the tongue (T), the palate (P) does not close off the nasopharynx, which is filling with barium. **B.** Cricopharyngeal spasm. There is narrowing of the esophagus at the C-5 level, at the upper esophageal sphincter, which is the cricopharyngeal muscle *(arrows)*.

sist swallowing. The examination should be videotaped to allow immediate and repeated review, sparing the child repeated swallows and radiation exposure. Structural abnormalities, such as webs and cricopharyngeal bars, and aspiration should be recorded on radiographs.

## Vascular Rings

Vascular rings occur when the esophagus and trachea are encircled, displaced, or compressed by the aorta, its branches, or remnants of the fetal circulation.[28–39] Some of these rings are incomplete, but others, like the double aortic arch, completely surround and frequently compress the esophagus and trachea.

Many asymptomatic rings are incidentally discovered on chest films. Others cause symptoms, with stridor a common presenting complaint. Respiratory distress may develop during feeding as the esophagus dilates with passage of the food bolus, causing additional tracheal compression. Reflex apnea is a third presentation of vascular rings and may prompt urgent surgery. Approximately 12 to 25% of these children also have congenital heart disease.[29]

The double aortic arch is the most common vascular ring. It is formed by the larger and more cephalad right aortic arch and the smaller and more caudal left aortic

arch. The second most common ring occurs if the right subclavian artery arises as the last branch of a left aortic arch rather than the first. To reach its normal position, this vessel must pass from left to right in an oblique, cephalad direction, indenting the posterior aspect of the esophagus. A similar ring develops if the left subclavian artery arises as the last branch of a right aortic arch. This ring causes more tracheal and esophageal impingement, because the subclavian originates from the usually small but space-occupying diverticulum of Kommerell, and the normal left-sided ligamentum arteriosum persists.

The right innominate artery, even if it is the first vessel to arise from the aorta, originates completely or partially to the left of midline in almost all children.[37] As it crosses from left to right, it passes anteriorly and may compress and indent the trachea. Because many children with this deviation are asymptomatic and many symptomatic children outgrow the symptoms, the aberrant right innominate artery is thought by some physicians to be a normal variant.[37] However, some children are severely symptomatic and respond dramatically to innominopexy, a surgical procedure that elevates and fixes the artery from the trachea.[30, 33, 36, 38]

A vascular sling is an anomaly of the pulmonary artery in which the main pulmonary artery gives rise to the right pulmonary artery, which gives rise to the left pulmonary artery.[28, 33, 35, 39] The left pulmonary artery courses from the right side to the left in the space between the trachea and esophagus. There is an increased incidence of intracardiac and bronchial anomalies in children with pulmonary sling, including variations in the normal branching pattern and ventricular septal defects.

### Radiologic Findings

Plain films can often suggest the diagnosis. On the frontal view of the airway or chest, the position of the aortic arch and trachea should be carefully evaluated (Fig. 75–6). The presence of a right aortic arch in a child with respiratory symptoms suggests that there may be a double aortic arch or right aortic arch with an aberrant left subclavian artery. In this setting, lateral views of the airway should be scrutinized to determine if there is anterior indentation of the airway. If the frontal chest radiograph is normal, lateral airway views showing anterior displacement of the trachea suggest a pulmonary sling, although enlarged lymph nodes or bronchogenic cyst can produce similar findings.

The barium esophagram frequently is the next examination obtained in children with suspected vascular rings. Lateral views of the barium-filled esophagus are most useful. Each type of ring has a characteristic appearance (Fig. 75–7). Because these vascular anomalies are related to the upper esophagus, this region should be meticulously examined. The frontal view of the esophagus shows specific changes in a child with a double aortic arch or aberrant subclavian artery.

Angiography was once considered mandatory before corrective surgery.[29] Computed tomographic scans of the upper thorax obtained during the intravenous bolus

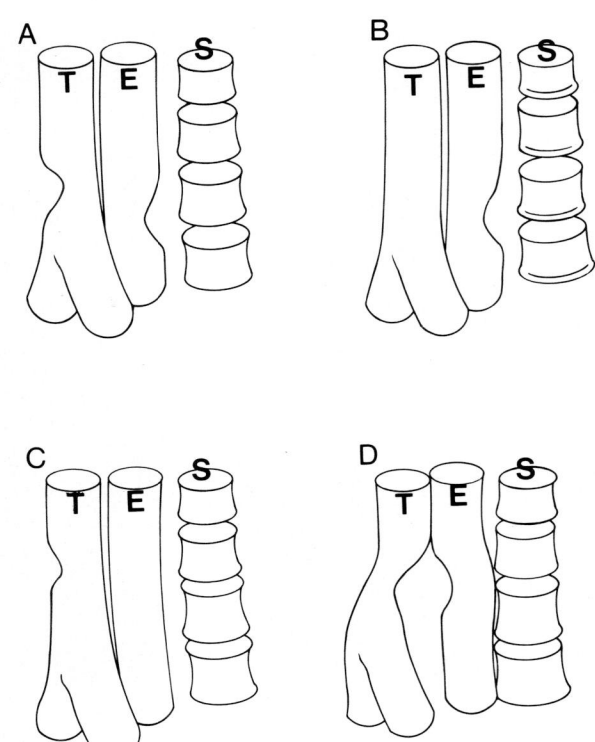

**Figure 75–7. Tracheoesophageal anomalies: lateral view. A.** Double aortic arch. The trachea is indented by the anterior portion of the arch and the esophagus by the posterior. **B.** Aberrant subclavian artery. The trachea has a normal appearance. The esophagus is indented posteriorly by the anomalous vessel. **C.** Anomalous innominate artery. The trachea is flattened anteriorly by the innominate artery. The esophagus has a normal appearance. **D.** Vascular sling. The trachea is displaced anteriorly and the esophagus posteriorly by the left pulmonary artery, which is passing between them. E = esophagus; S = spine; T = trachea. (**A** to **D** modified from Berdon WE, Baker DH: Vascular anomalies and the infant lung: rings, slings, and other things. Semin Roentgenol 7:39–64, 1972.)

injection of contrast medium (Fig. 75–8) and digital subtraction angiography have supplanted routine angiography.[32] Although both show the anomalous vascular structures, computed tomography has an advantage by virtue of its ability to demonstrate compression of the airway.

Despite the need for patient sedation and the longer scanning time, magnetic resonance may soon replace computed tomography in the study of children with suspected vascular rings. Magnetic resonance provides excellent multiplane images of the great vessels and does not require intravenous contrast[30, 35, 36] (Figs. 75–9 and 75–10). The coronal and sagittal depictions of the anomalies greatly enhance preoperative planning.

## ACQUIRED ABNORMALITIES OF THE ESOPHAGUS

### Gastroesophageal Reflux

#### Clinical Findings

Gastroesophageal reflux (GER) is a common, almost physiologic process that occurs in infants and children.[40]

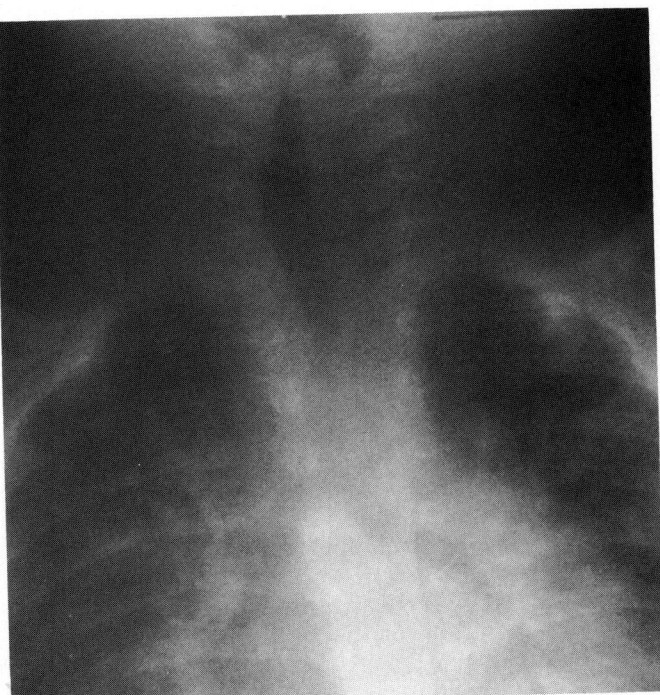

**Figure 75–6. Double aortic arch.** The larger and higher right arch is indenting and displacing the trachea toward the left.

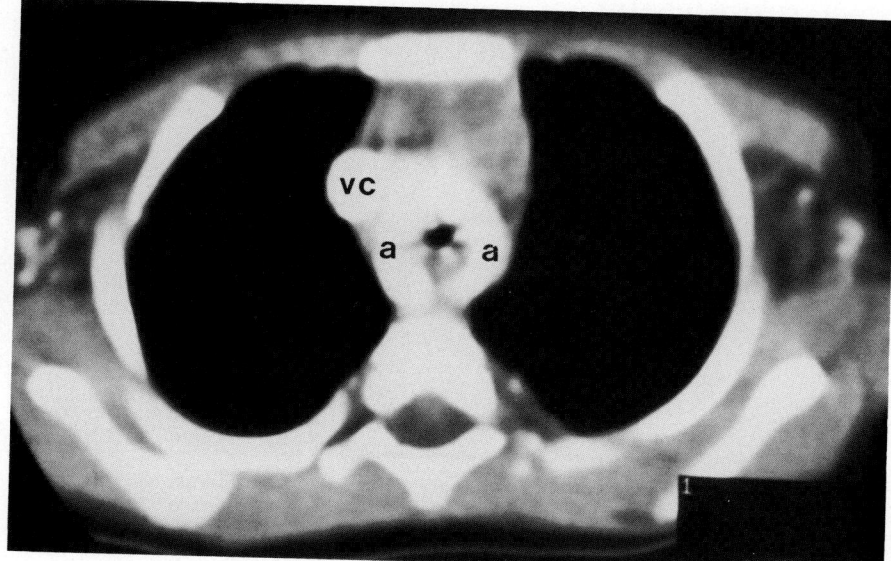

**Figure 75–8. Double aortic arch.** During the bolus injection of contrast medium, computed tomographic scan demonstrates both segments of the double aortic arch (a), which encircle the trachea and esophagus. The superior vena cava is opacified (vc).

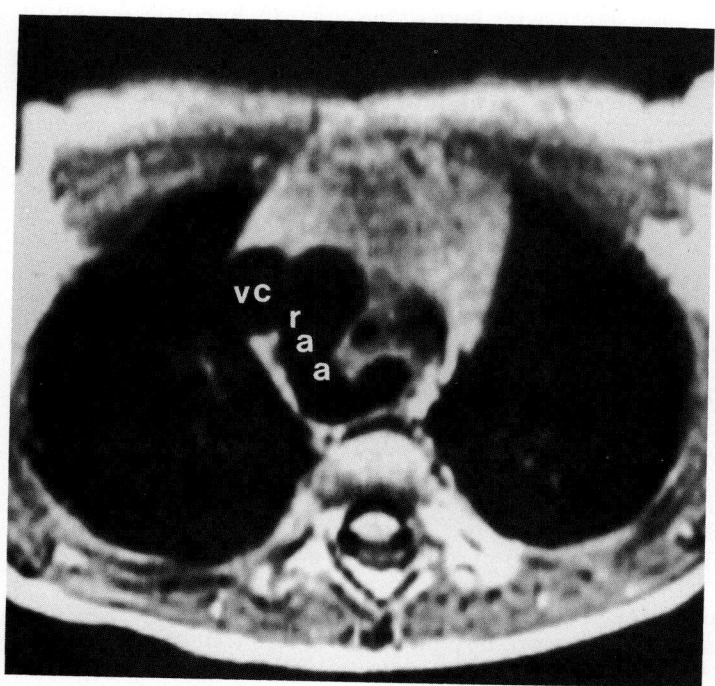

**Figure 75–9. Right aortic arch and aberrant left subclavian artery.** The right aortic arch (raa) is medial to the superior vena cava (vc) on this axial magnetic resonance scan. The anomalous subclavian artery courses posteriorly and to the left, close to the spine.

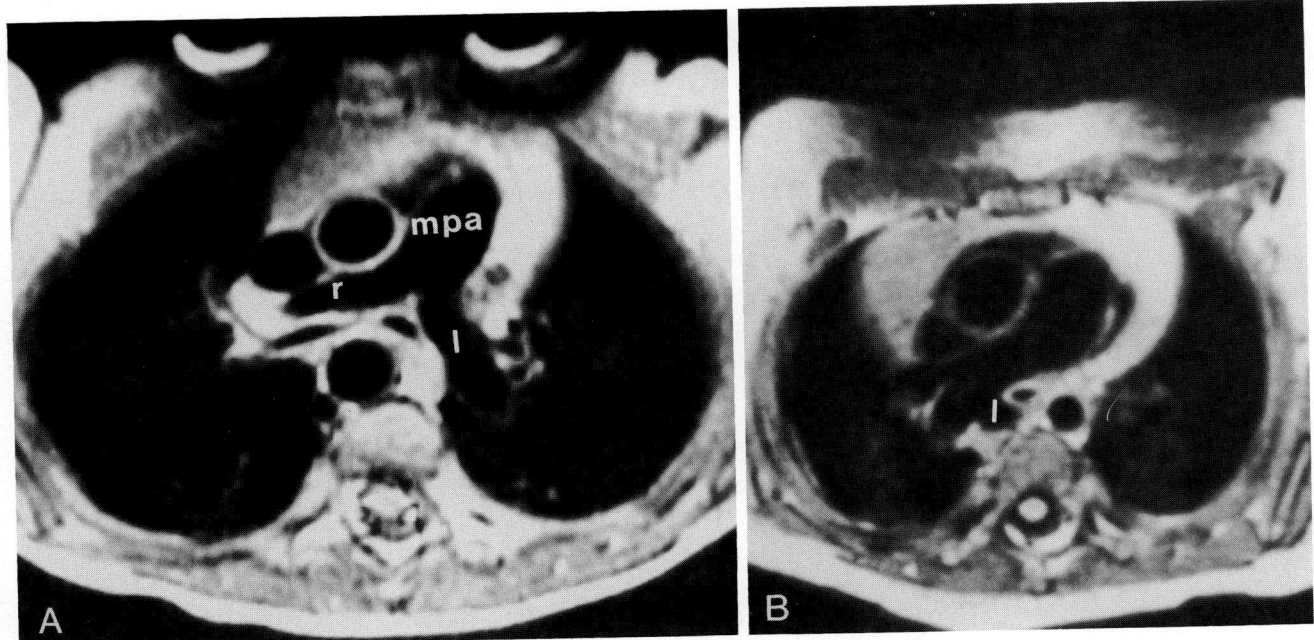

**Figure 75–10. Pulmonary sling: magnetic resonance findings. A.** Normal anatomy: the main pulmonary artery (mpa) divides into the right (r) and left (l) pulmonary arteries. **B.** The anomalous left (l) pulmonary artery arises from the right.

It is the result of the failure of the lower esophageal sphincter to maintain an adequate resting pressure. GER is pathologic when it is associated with hematemesis, failure to thrive, apnea, bradycardia, or stricture formation.[41–45] GER has been implicated in some cases of sudden infant death syndrome, asthma, and recurrent upper respiratory tract infections.[46–49] GER is also responsible for the development of Barrett's mucosa in the esophagus.

Gastroesophageal reflux can be an isolated problem, but it occurs with increased frequency in children with neuromuscular disorders, repair of tracheoesophageal fistula, cystic fibrosis, and collagen-vascular diseases. In one large series, 35% of the children with GER had additional disorders of esophageal motility.[50] Some medications reduce lower esophageal sphincter pressure, which facilitates GER. For example, theophylline, given to decrease bronchial spasm and enhance aeration in children with bronchopulmonary dysplasia and asthma, may cause or worsen GER and exacerbate respiratory symptoms.[51] Secondary GER occurs in infants and children with gastric outlet obstruction and may disappear after the obstruction is corrected.[52–58] Primary GER and delayed gastric emptying coexist in as many as 50% of children.[59]

Although the diagnosis of GER can be made on clinical grounds (i.e., infant who vomits after every feeding), most pediatricians prefer to document and quantify the reflux before beginning therapy.[43–45] The barium esophagram is the most commonly used test. It is inexpensive, readily available, and familiar to most clinicians. Radionuclide scintigraphy, manometry, and pH probe monitoring of the esophagus provide additional information about the frequency and duration of reflux.[44, 53, 60–63] Endoscopy can document the presence and severity of esophagitis.

Most children with isolated GER outgrow the process, but those with underlying abnormalities are less likely to do so.[40] Symptomatic GER can be treated by thickening the infant's formula, giving smaller amounts at each meal, and positioning the infant appropriately after eating. Discontinuing potentially provocative medications or correcting an upper gastrointestinal obstruction may also eliminate GER.

Some children require surgical augmentation of the lower esophageal sphincter with a gastric wrap around the lower esophagus, called a *fundoplication.*[64–66] In children with poor motility (Fig. 75–11), a relatively loose wrap is formed that does not obstruct antegrade peristalsis.[64–66] Corrective surgery produces less morbidity and is more successful in children with isolated GER than in those with a complex medical or surgical history.[50, 64, 66, 67] Before performing fundoplication, it is important to exclude a lesion that interferes with gastric emptying. If one is found, the antireflux surgery should be complemented by pyloroplasty. Children may lose the ability to perform some normal physiologic maneuvers, such as burping or vomiting, after fundoplication.[67a] Although these losses are usually well tolerated, small bowel distention may result if excessive air is swallowed, as commonly occurs in children with cerebral palsy or other neuromuscular disorders.

In some children, GER is associated with torticollis and abnormal movements of the trunk, head, and neck, producing a neurologic abnormality called Sandifer's syndrome.[68] The abnormal movements and posturing cease after the GER is corrected, and they may be the result of the pain caused by the GER or represent attempts to minimize reflux.

A rare association is the Herbst triad.[69] Children with this diagnosis have digital clubbing and hypoproteinemia associated with their GER. After the GER is corrected, the other abnormalities disappear.

## Radiographic Findings

### Barium Studies

If the child refuses to drink the desired amount of barium, the necessary volume can be instilled into the stomach through a nasogastric tube, which is then removed. If the child has ingested almost as much barium as necessary and then refuses to drink more, formula or juice may be given to supplement the volume. The slight dilution of barium does not affect the quality of the reflux study. If there is a gastrostomy tube, barium should be injected at a rate and volume that reproduce the child's usual feeding.[70, 71]

For children with neurologic impairment of swallowing, it is desirable to document GER before placing a gastrostomy tube. In this setting, I include a limited study of the swallowing mechanism. Some children, who on clinical grounds are thought to aspirate, may be found to swallow normally and thus may not require a gastrostomy.[24] To achieve sufficient gastric volume safely in the child who does aspirate, the stomach may be directly filled through a nasogastric tube, which is removed before the fluoroscopic evaluation of GER.

Fluoroscopy is used to define the cephalad extent of the GER (Fig. 75–12) and document aspiration. Aspiration only rarely occurs as a result of GER but may be demonstrated during the swallowing portion of the barium esophagram. The rate at which the barium clears from the esophagus should be evaluated. Children whose reflux clears rapidly are less likely to aspirate or develop esophagitis. GER esophagitis is rarely seen on standard single contrast studies.[70, 71]

To optimize the barium study, the gastroesophageal junction should be challenged by an adequate amount of liquid in the stomach, observation should be continued for several minutes, and the child should be calm during the period of observation. The increased intra-abdominal pressure associated with crying does not appear to increase the frequency of GER.[72]

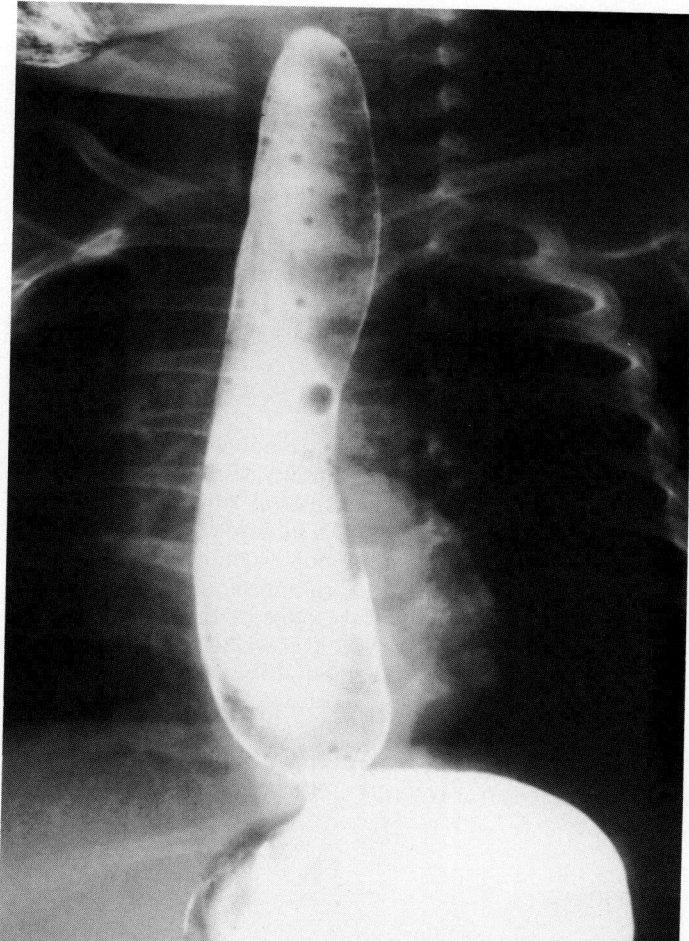

**Figure 75–11. Abnormal esophageal motility.** During antegrade study, the esophagus is large and lacks clearly defined stripping waves in a child who had massive GER.

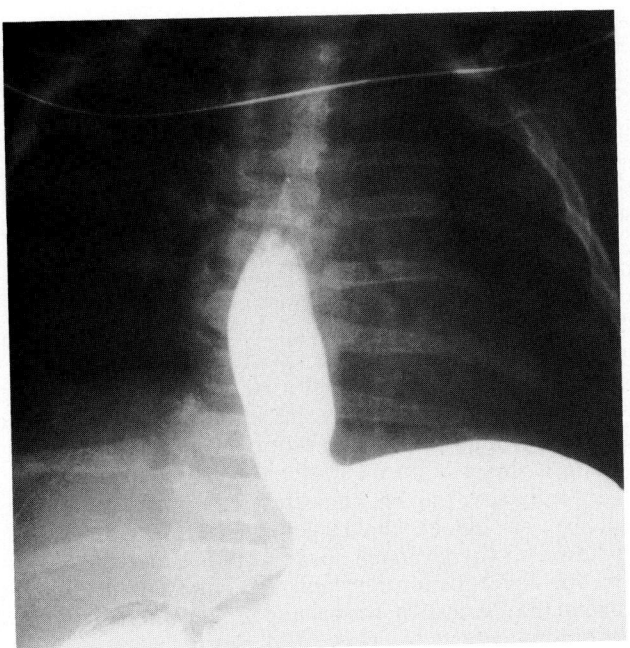

**Figure 75–12. GER.** A large volume of contrast material refluxes to the level of the carina. The gastroesophageal junction is patulous.

Provocative maneuvers (e.g., gastric compression, water siphonage) are usually not performed in children because the clinical significance of reflux induced by these nonphysiologic techniques is minimal.[73] An indwelling nasogastric tube compromises the function of the lower esophageal sphincter, and the tube should be removed before the child is observed for reflux.

After the question of reflux has been addressed, the stomach and duodenum should be observed to exclude gastric outlet obstruction, duodenal obstruction, or malrotation. All studies should include a film of the ligament of Treitz.

### Nuclear Scintigraphy

The radionuclide scan is extremely sensitive in the diagnosis of GER.[53, 60–63] The child is given formula or juice containing technetium Tc 99m sulfur colloid and is continuously scanned. This is a major advantage over fluoroscopy, which must be intermittent to minimize exposure of the patient to radiation. This technique documents the number of episodes of reflux in a given period with greater accuracy. Rarely, aspiration can be seen when the lungs are imaged at the conclusion of the study.[74] Gastric emptying can also be calculated with this technique.[52–58, 61] There is little evidence that delayed gastric emptying causes the GER, but this information is important for correcting both conditions during surgery.[62]

### Ultrasound

Ultrasound can accurately demonstrate episodes of GER and correlates well with the results of barium studies and esophageal pH monitoring.[75, 76] The gastroesophageal junction is visualized through adjacent solid organs. After feeding, GER is seen as retrograde passage of highly echogenic material toward the esophagus. Unfortunately, sonography cannot document the cephalad extent of the GER. Although sonography is unlikely to replace other tests in the primary diagnosis of GER, it can be used to assess the efficacy of therapy. Ultrasound can also be used to identify GER in infants whose sonogram for hypertrophic pyloric stenosis is negative.

### Postsurgical Studies

The indications for postsurgical studies include dysphagia, which may indicate that the fundoplication is too tight, and continued reflux symptoms, which suggest that gastric wrap is too loose or has become undone.[77–79] Radiographically, the intact wrap produces a mass effect at the gastroesophageal junction (Fig. 75–13). Breakdown of the wrap may be associated with paraesophageal hernia or GER (Fig. 75–14).

## Achalasia

Children account for only 3% of patients with achalasia.[80–83] Achalasia has been associated with Down's syndrome, familial dysautonomia, the triple A syndrome (i.e., achalasia, alacrima, corticotropin [ACTH] insensitivity), and a microcephaly syndrome.[84–85]

These children typically present with vomiting or regurgitation of undigested food or difficulty in swallowing.[80–83] Recurrent pneumonia may be the result of aspiration of esophageal contents at night by the recumbent, sleeping child whose airway protective mechanisms are not fully activated. Other airway symptoms may result from compression of the trachea by the enlarged esophagus.[86, 87] Weight loss or failure to thrive may bring the child to clinical attention.

Although pneumatic dilation of the esophagus has been successful in some patients, it is more commonly used in affected adults than children.[88] Surgical treatment with the modified Heller myotomy usually provides complete relief.[89] Approximately 25% of patients may need a fundoplication performed at the time of myotomy or later to control GER.[89, 90]

### Radiologic Findings

The radiologic findings of achalasia in children are similar to those of adults (see Chapter 23). Chest radiographs may show a dilated, fluid-filled esophagus, evidence of chronic aspiration, no gastric air bubble, and tracheal compression or displacement. Barium studies reveal a dilated, fluid-filled, atonic or poorly contractile esophagus that ends in a tapered, narrowed segment (i.e., "beaking").

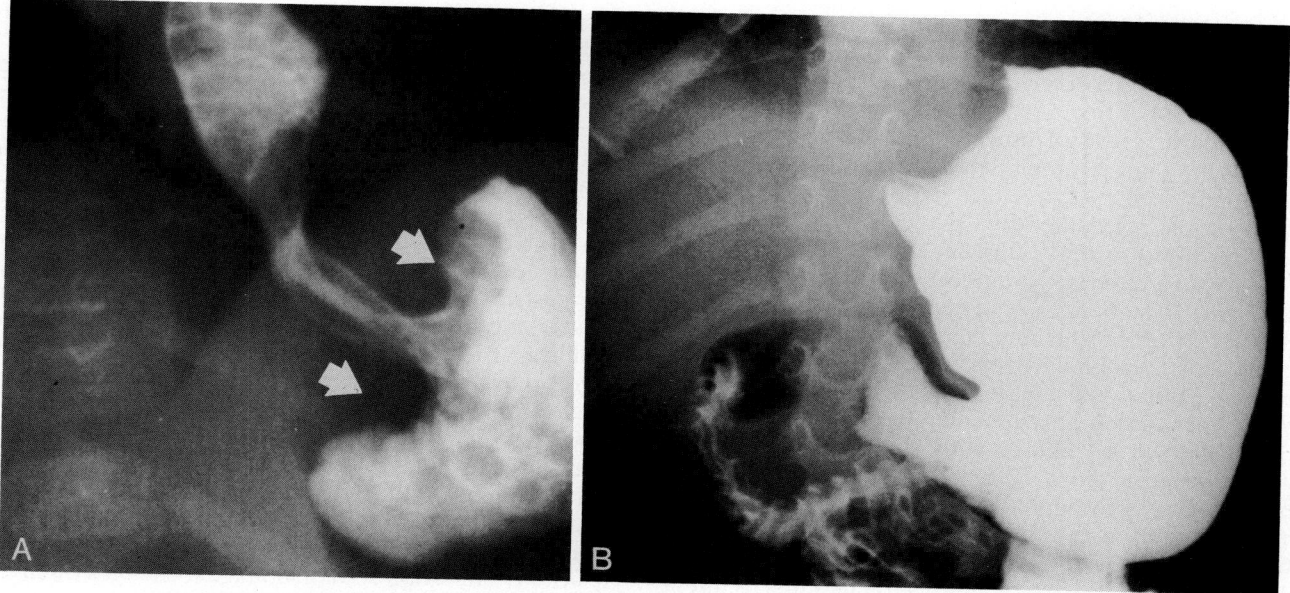

**Figure 75–13. Barium esophagram after fundoplication. A.** The gastric wrap has produced narrowing of the distal esophagus and mass effect on the gastric fundus *(arrows).* **B.** The concavity of the fundus is at the site of fundoplication.

## Esophageal Varices

In children, esophageal varices are usually a consequence of extrahepatic obstruction of the portal vein rather than parenchymal liver disease.[91] Although the cause of the portal venous thrombosis is unknown in most children, there are several predisposing risk factors: dehydration, intra-abdominal infection, and umbilical venous catheterization.[91] Intrahepatic portal venous obstruction is due to congenital or acquired diseases that produce hepatic fibrosis: biliary atresia, alpha$_1$-antitrypsin deficiency, polycystic kidney disease, and cystic fibrosis.[91, 92]

Clinical diagnosis is often problematic. Splenomegaly may or may not exist. Liver function tests and liver biopsy may be normal if the portal hypertension is due to extrahepatic obstruction. Children with intrahepatic causes of portal hypertension usually present earlier and

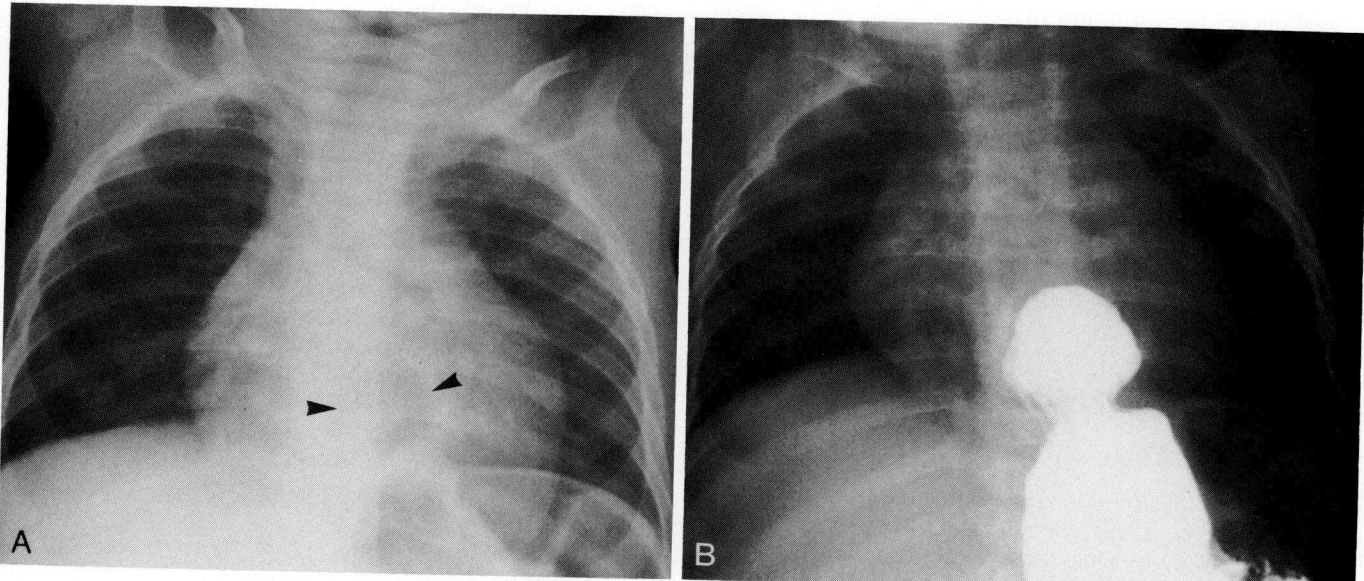

**Figure 75–14. Failed Nissen fundoplications. A.** A rounded retrocardiac air collection *(arrowheads)* on the chest film represents the herniated stomach. **B.** The abnormally located gastric fundus is filled with barium. The indentation indicates the remnants of the gastric wrap.

appear sicker, with jaundice, ascites, and other signs of liver disease.[91] The diagnosis of varices is based on visualization at endoscopy, barium studies, angiography, or cross-sectional imaging.[93] Because esophageal varices are the major cause of upper gastrointestinal bleeding in children, their prompt detection and treatment are vital.[94]

Endoscopic sclerotherapy, pioneered in adults, has been successful in the treatment of bleeding varices in children.[95-97] Transient complications, such as hiccups, dysphagia, dysmotility, or focal ulceration, generally pass quickly. More serious complications are rare and include sepsis, esophageal stricture, and esophageal perforation. Endoscopic ligation of varices has been successfully performed and has side effects similar to those of sclerotherapy.[98] Children with repeated severe bleeding may require more extreme surgery: esophagogastrectomy or gastroesophageal devascularization. If the varices are due to intrahepatic fibrosis, liver transplantation may be curative. The small size of the inferior vena cava makes mesocaval shunt surgery a less frequent option for children.[91]

## Radiologic Findings

Plain films of the abdomen may be normal or show splenomegaly. Varices can be demonstrated indirectly with barium studies or directly through contrast enhancement.[93, 94] On the barium esophagram, varices appear as tortuous, linear filling defects extending cephalad into the esophagus from the gastric fundus (Fig. 75-15A). The varices may be directly filled via splenoportography (Fig. 75-15B). Delayed films of an injection of the celiac axis show the collateral veins, especially if subtraction techniques are used. Enlarged collateral veins are also demonstrable on computed tomographic scans (Fig. 75-15C).

Sonographic evaluation of the thickness of the lesser omentum is recommended for detecting children with portal hypertension.[99] The ratio of the lesser omental thickness to the aortic diameter is increased in children with esophageal varices. Measurement of the portal vein diameter and its relationship to the body surface appear to have a predictive value.[100] These measurements are being supplanted by color flow and duplex Doppler ultrasound, which can reveal varices directly and assess the direction and rate of flow in the splanchnic circulation and in surgically created portosystemic shunts.[101]

## Foreign Body and Caustic Ingestion

### Clinical Findings

Young children instinctively place objects in their mouths, and it is not surprising that most caustic and foreign body ingestions occur in children younger than 5 years of age. Few ingestions occur in children younger than 6 or 7 months of age, because these children lack the ability to place grasped objects in their mouths. If they occur in a young infant, child abuse should be suspected.[102] In older children, caustic and foreign body ingestions may be suicide attempts.

With caustic ingestion, the type and location of mucosal injury depend on the pH of the agent.[103-105] Caustic agents such as lye and laundry detergents have a high pH and cause most damage in the mouth and upper esophagus (Fig. 75-16). Most children recover without sequelae; perforation or stricture formation occurs in about 3% of patients.[105a] Acids and other low pH corrosive agents (e.g., toilet bowl cleaners) primarily injure the gastric antrum. Contact between the acid and upper airway can produce life-threatening epiglottitis in some children. Bleaches have a neutral pH of 7 and generally cause only transient irritation of the esophagus without long-term complications.[103] In one series, however, deep circular lesions were found endoscopically in four children after documented bleach ingestion.[106]

In patients with suspected perforation or stricture, endoscopy is used to determine the depth and extent of injury. Approximately one third of children with a history of ingestion have esophageal changes discovered by endoscopy. In one series, clinical findings, such as oral burns, stridor, drooling, and vomiting, did not correlate with the extent of injury found endoscopically. A later series, however, correlated the number of clinical findings and the degree of mucosal damage.[107, 108]

Children with esophageal damage have routinely been treated with antibiotics and steroids, but certain studies indicate that this may not be necessary.[106] In one series, 11 children with documented moderate to severe mucosal injury were treated only with a modified nasogastric tube to function as an intraluminal stent. One child developed a mild and easily dilatable stricture.[106]

Foreign bodies are easy to detect if they contain radiodense metal. Coins are the most frequently seen foreign bodies on chest radiographs.[109-111] Aluminum foreign bodies, especially the ring from pop-top soda cans, may be difficult to see, as are some foreign coins made from metals that are only slightly radiodense.[112] Visualization of glass depends on the size of the piece ingested and on the presence of overlying structures.

Most swallowed objects (e.g., food and small plastic toys) are not opaque and can be detected only with contrast radiography or endoscopy.[103, 112] These tests should be performed after a witnessed ingestion or for a child with acute onset of dysphagia, drooling, or wheezing that is not responsive to the usual bronchodilators.

Button batteries for hearing aids, cameras, and watches are easy to swallow and can produce a traumatic tracheoesophageal fistula or a lethal fistula to the aorta (Fig. 75-17). Acid leaking from an impacted battery can cause severe tissue damage within a few hours. Battery impaction can be also associated with low-voltage electrical tissue damage and pressure necrosis at the site of impaction.[113-115]

Several physiologic sites of narrowing can trap ingested foreign bodies: the thoracic inlet, the level of the aortic knob, and the gastroesophageal junction. Foreign body impaction at any other level should raise the suspicion of intrinsic stricture or vascular ring.

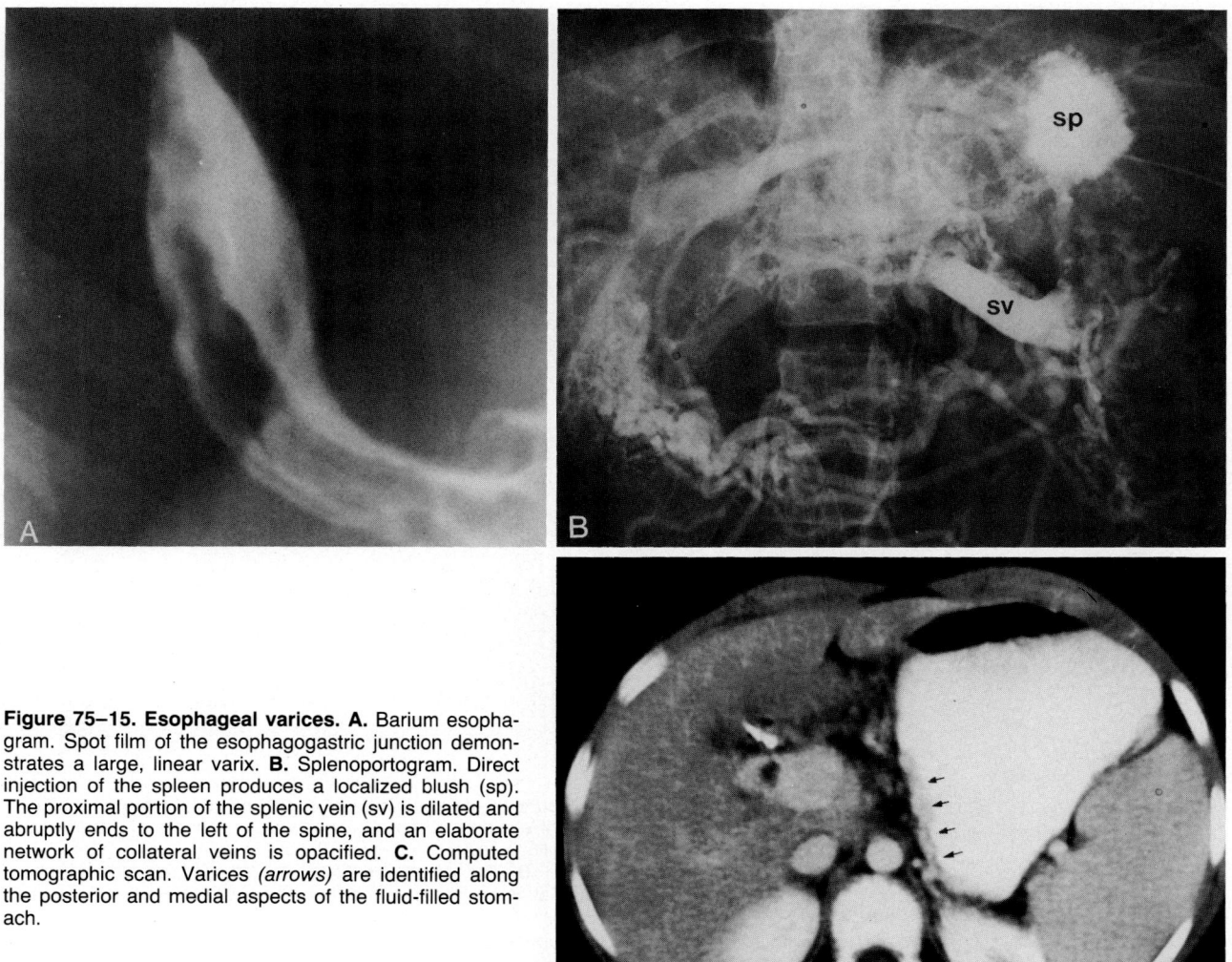

**Figure 75–15. Esophageal varices. A.** Barium esophagram. Spot film of the esophagogastric junction demonstrates a large, linear varix. **B.** Splenoportogram. Direct injection of the spleen produces a localized blush (sp). The proximal portion of the splenic vein (sv) is dilated and abruptly ends to the left of the spine, and an elaborate network of collateral veins is opacified. **C.** Computed tomographic scan. Varices *(arrows)* are identified along the posterior and medial aspects of the fluid-filled stomach.

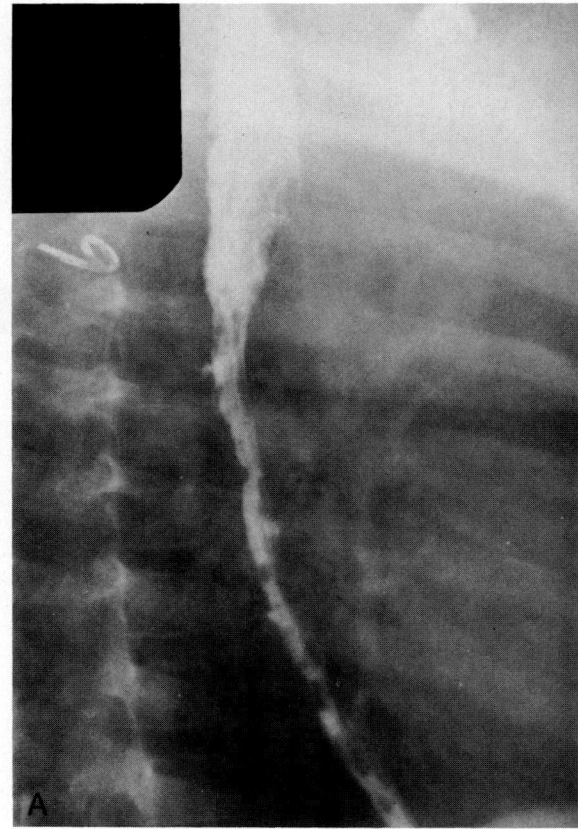

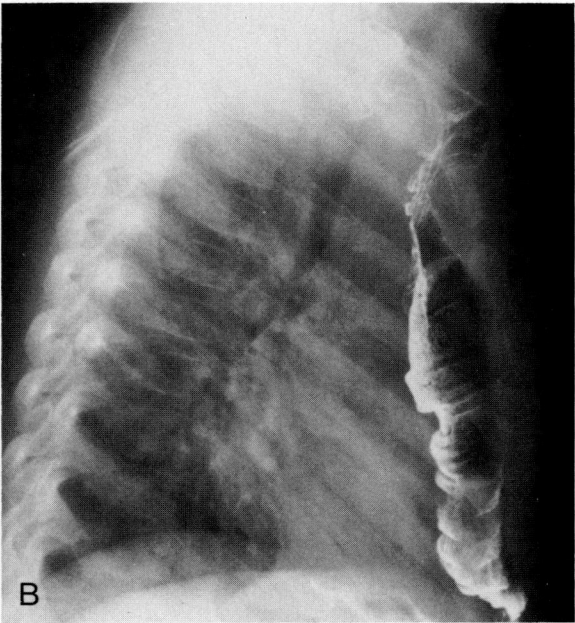

**Figure 75–16. Lye ingestion and surgical correction.**
**A.** Irregularity of the distal esophagus and lack of distensibility indicate the degree of damage done by the ingestion. **B.** The interposed colon, coated with contrast material, is positioned in the retrosternal space.

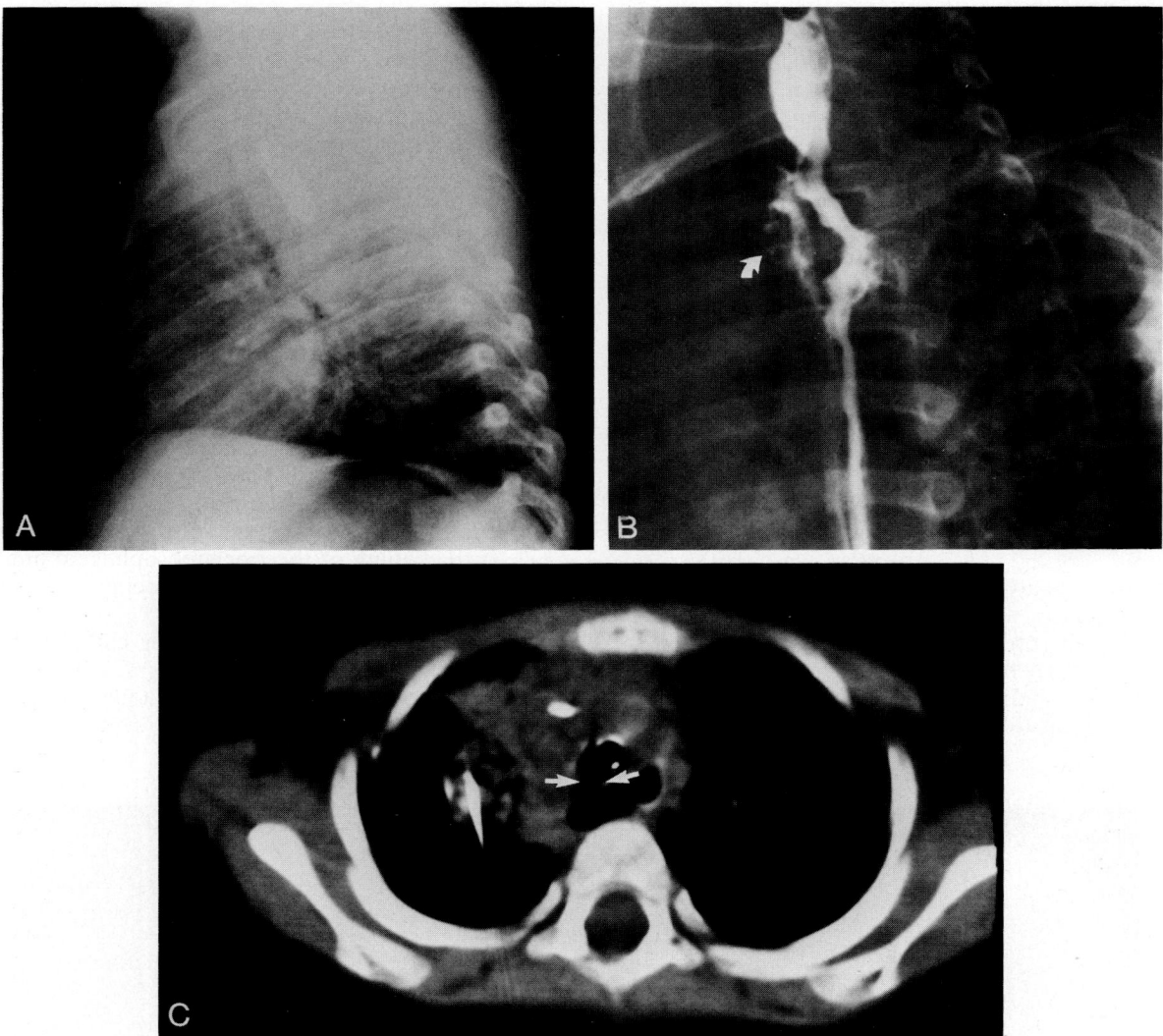

**Figure 75–17. Battery-induced tracheoesophageal fistula. A.** Lateral chest radiograph. The lodged radiopaque battery is associated with thickening of the soft tissue between the trachea and esophagus and anterior bowing of the trachea. **B.** Esophagram. Water-soluble contrast material passes from the normal cervical esophagus into the irregular-appearing region where the battery was previously seen. The anterior collection *(arrow)* of contrast indicates that perforation occurred. **C.** Computed tomographic scan. After several days of antibiotics and feeding through a gastrostomy tube, the child developed a fever. A fistula *(arrows)* was identified between the trachea and traumatically widened esophagus.

Radiologic diagnosis can be coupled with treatment if the radiologist is skillful in removing foreign bodies with a combined balloon catheter and fluoroscopic technique.[116-118] Button batteries can be removed with fluoroscopic guidance after being coupled to a magnetic-tipped catheter.[115] Magnetic retrieval of metallic foreign bodies from the stomach can be performed with a magnetic orogastric tube.[119] Physicians performing this procedure must be skilled at intubation in case the foreign body obstructs the airway. Endoscopy has again become popular for foreign body extraction. It may be less traumatic and safer, despite the need for general anesthesia, and it can provide information about the esophagus at the site of impaction.[120]

In asymptomatic children, the swallowed coin may be allowed to pass without intervention. Coin removal is necessary if symptoms develop or serial radiographs show that the position of the coin has not changed.

## Radiologic Findings

After caustic ingestion, airway and chest films should be obtained. Any swelling of the epiglottis or edema of the airway should be viewed with alarm, and measures to ensure airway patency should be implemented. Lung damage, although rare, may occur. Mediastinal air, indicating perforation of the esophagus, may not develop acutely but should be sought on both early and later films.

Barium studies are not useful in diagnosis or management immediately after caustic ingestion. Endoscopic evaluation of the esophagus is more precise during this period. In the early recuperative period, contrast studies may show abnormalities of predictive value. Retention of contrast within the wall of the esophagus and persis-tent gaseous dilatation of the esophagus usually signify severe injury and may precede perforation. Caustic-induced dysmotility may be associated with the appearance of transverse folds in the esophagus, and strictures can develop at these sites.[104, 121, 122] Barium studies are of value in detecting late changes of the esophagus, such as stricture, or abnormalities in sites not visualized during endoscopy.[123] If the stricture is long and does not respond to dilatation, colon interposition may be necessary to allow adequate oral intake (see Fig. 75-16).

Postingestion changes in esophageal function have been analyzed scintigraphically. Orally administered [81m]Kr and uncoupled [99m]Tc can demonstrate motility disturbances, which correlate well with the degree of mucosal damage.[124] Late clinical symptoms such as dysphagia often do not correlate with the degree of stenosis or delay in esophageal transit.

Plain films of the airway or chest may be entirely normal despite the presence of an esophageal foreign body. The mediastinum should be carefully analyzed on the lateral projection, with particular attention to the soft tissue thickness between the esophagus and the trachea. Thickening of the soft tissues in this region may be a sign of esophageal edema, which decreases the likelihood of successful retrieval of the foreign body via catheter. Thickening or anterior bowing of the esophagus may be due to mediastinitis, which develops after esophageal perforation[125, 126] (Fig. 75-18; see Fig. 75-17). If thickening of the tracheoesophageal line is present, endoscopic removal of the foreign body is recommended.

If an otherwise healthy appearing child presents with recent onset of drooling or dysphagia, a barium study is recommended to exclude a nonopaque foreign body, a congenital lesion that has become symptomatic, or ac-

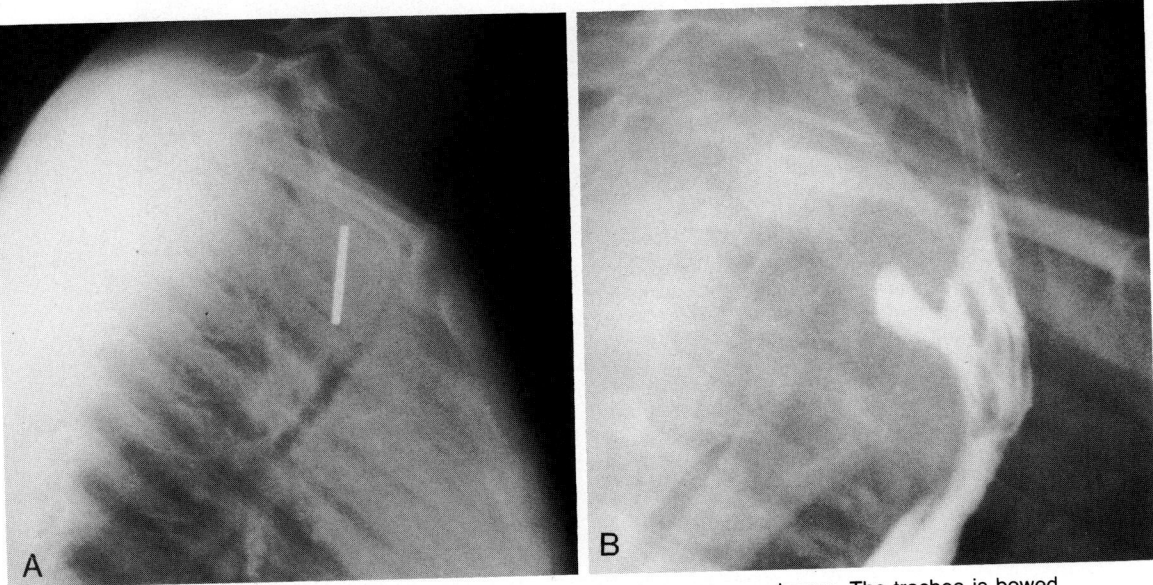

**Figure 75-18. Coin ingestion. A.** The coin is seen in the upper esophagus. The trachea is bowed anteriorly and is narrowed. **B.** After removal of the coin, the contrast study demonstrates that the coin had perforated the esophagus posteriorly and that the esophagus was pushed anteriorly by the inflammatory process surrounding the site of perforation.

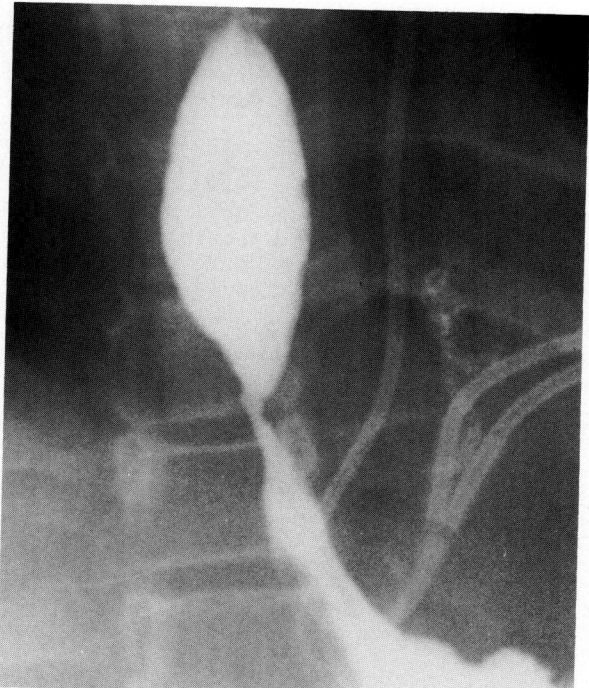

**Figure 75–19. Radiation- and chemotherapy-associated esophagitis.** This teen-age girl received chemotherapy and radiotherapy for a lower thoracic primitive neuroectodermal tumor. The esophagram performed because of dysphagia demonstrates a long, narrowed segment.

quired inflammatory lesions. The swallowing mechanism and common locations of physiologic narrowing should be scrutinized as previously described, because these sites are where foreign bodies are most likely to lodge (see Fig. 75–18).

After the foreign body has been removed, a contrast study should be performed to exclude intrinsic esophageal disease and to detect any secondary changes caused by the foreign body.

## Other Esophageal Injuries

Radiation therapy, particularly if combined with certain chemotherapeutic agents, can produce esophagitis, stricture, and fistula formation[127-128] (Fig. 75–19). Motility and mucosal abnormalities are also seen acutely in children receiving chemotherapy alone. Because of immunosuppression, esophageal infections by opportunistic organisms such as herpesvirus, *Candida,* and cytomegalovirus are common.[129]

Many oral medications can produce focal esophageal injury, presumably caused by direct mucosal contact with the tablet.[130]

Esophageal narrowing requiring dilatation has been described as part of the Stevens-Johnson syndrome.[131] Esophageal involvement in epidermolysis bullosa usually takes the form of short or long, multiple or single strictures. Webs, pseudodiverticula, and overall esophageal shortening may occur in this cutaneous disorder.[132-140]

## References

1. Leithiser RE, Capitanio MA, MacPherson RI, et al: "Communicating" bronchopulmonary foregut malformations. AJR 146:227–231, 1986.
2. Lacasse JE, Reilly BJ, Mancer K: Segmental esophageal trachea: a potentially fatal type of tracheal stenosis. AJR 134:829–831, 1980.
3. Reilly BJ, McDonald P, Cumming WA, et al: Three cases of bronchopulmonary foregut malformation. Ann Radiol 16:281–285, 1973.
4. Maclean AD, Houghton-Allen BW: Upper oesophageal web in childhood. Pediatr Radiol 3:240–241, 1975.
5. Theander G: Congenital posterior midline pharyngo-esophageal diverticula. Pediatr Radiol 1:153–155, 1973.
6. Braun P, Nussle D, Roy CC, et al: Intramural diverticulosis of the esophagus in an eight-year-old boy. Pediatr Radiol 6:235–237, 1978.
7. Nosher JL, Campbell WL, Seaman WB: The clinical significance of cervical esophageal and hypopharyngeal webs. Radiology 117:45–47, 1975.
8. Toyohara T, Kaneko T, Araki H, et al: Giant epiphrenic diverticulum in a boy with Ehlers-Danlos syndrome. Pediatr Radiol 19:437, 1989.
9. Lucaya J, Herrera M, Salcedo S: Traumatic pharyngeal pseudodiverticulum in neonates and infants. Two case reports and review of the literature. Pediatr Radiol 8:65–69, 1979.
10. Variend S, Howat AJ: Upper oesophageal heterotopia: a prospective necropsy study in children. J Clin Pathol 4:742–745, 1988.
11. Anderson LS, Shackelford GD, Mancilla-Jimenez R, et al: Cartilaginous esophageal ring: a cause of esophageal stenosis in infants and children. Radiology 108:665–666, 1973.
12. Wolf Y, Katz S, Lax E, et al: Dysphagia in a child with aggressive fibromatosis of the esophagus. J Pediatr Surg 24:1137–1139, 1989.
13. Powell RW, Luck SR: Cervical esophageal obstruction by ectopic gastric mucosa. J Pediatr Surg 23:632–634, 1988.
14. Cochat P, Guibaud P, Garcia-Torres R, et al: Diffuse leiomyomatosis in Alport syndrome. J Pediatr 113:339–343, 1988.
15. Rabushka LS, Fishman EK, Kuhlman JE, et al: Diffuse esophageal leiomyomatosis in a patient with Alport syndrome: CT demonstration. Radiology 179:176–178, 1991.
16. Bourque MD, Spigland N, Bensoussan AL, et al: Esophageal leiomyoma in children: two case reports and review of the literature. J Pediatr Surg 24:1103–1107, 1989.
17. Mazas-Artasona L, Romeo M, Felices R, et al: Gastro-oesophageal leiomyoblastomas and multiple pulmonary chondromas: an incomplete variant of Carney's triad. Br J Radiol 61:1181–1184, 1988.
18. Fisher SE, Painter M, Milmoe G: Swallowing disorders in infancy. Pediatr Clin North Am 28:845–853, 1981.
19. Williams DJ, Mitchell DP: Pharyngoesophageal dysphagia in infancy. Int J Pediatr Otorhinolaryngol 2:231–242, 1980.
20. Ekberg O, Nylander G: Dysfunction of the cricopharyngeal muscle. Radiology 143:481–486, 1982.
21. Grunebaum M, Nutman J, Nitzan M: The pharyngo-laryngeal deficit in the acute form of infantile spinal muscular atrophy (Werdnig-Hoffmann disease). Pediatr Radiol 11:67–70, 1981.
22. Fernbach SK, McLone DG: Derangement of swallowing in children with myelomeningocele. Pediatr Radiol 15:311–314, 1985.
23. Bowie JD, Clair MR: Fetal swallowing and regurgitation: observation of normal and abnormal activity. Radiology 144:877–878, 1982.
24. Zerilli KS, Stefans VA, DiPietro MA: Protocol for the use of videofluoroscopy in pediatric swallowing dysfunction. Am J Occup Ther 44:441–446, 1990.
25. Dodds WJ, Logemann JA, Stewart ET: Radiologic assessment of abnormal oral and pharyngeal phases of swallowing. AJR 154:965–974, 1990.
26. Dodds WJ, Stewart ET, Logemann JA: Physiology and radiology of the normal oral and pharyngeal phases of swallowing. AJR 154:953–963, 1990.
27. Dodds WJ, Man KM, Cook IJ, et al: Influence of bolus volume

on swallow-induced hyoid movement in normal subjects. AJR 150:1307–1309, 1988.

28. Berdon WE, Baker DH: Vascular anomalies and the infant lung: rings, slings, and other things. Semin Roentgenol 7:39–64, 1972.

29. Tonkin IL, Elliot LP, Bargeron LM: Concomitant axial cineangiography and barium esophagography in the evaluation of vascular rings. Radiology 135:69–76, 1980.

30. Vogl T, Wilimzig C, Hofmann U, et al: MRI in tracheal stenosis by innominate artery in children. Pediatr Radiol 21:89–93, 1991.

31. Gross RE: Arterial malformations which cause compression of the trachea and esophagus. Circulation 11:124–134, 1966.

32. Tonkin ILD, Gold RE, Moser D, et al: Evaluation of vascular rings with digital subtraction angiography. AJR 142:1287–1291, 1984.

33. Backer CL, Ilbawi MN, Idriss FS, et al: Vascular anomalies causing tracheoesophageal compression. Review of experience in children. J Thorac Cardiovasc Surg 97:725–731, 1989.

33a. Lowe GM, Donaldson JS, Backer CL: Vascular rings: 10-year review of imaging. Radiographics 11:637–646, 1991.

34. Rivilla F, Utrilla JG, Alvarez F; Surgical management and follow-up of vascular rings. Z Kinderchir 44:199–202, 1989.

35. Bisset GS, Strife JL, Kirks D, et al: Vascular rings: MR imaging. AJR 149:251–356, 1987.

36. Fletcher BD, Cohn RC: Tracheal compression and the innominate artery: MR evaluation in infants. Radiology 170:103–107, 1989.

37. Strife JL, Baumel AS, Dunbar JS: Tracheal compression by the innominate artery in infancy and childhood. Radiology 139:73–75, 1981.

38. Berdon WE, Baker DH, Bordiuk J, et al: Innominate artery compression of the trachea in infants with stridor and apnea. Radiology 92:272–278, 1969.

39. Capitanio MA, Ramos R, Kirkpatrick JA: Pulmonary sling. Roentgen observations. AJR 112:28–34, 1971.

40. Boix-Ochoa J, Canals J: Maturation of the lower esophagus. J Pediatr Surg 11:749–756, 1976.

41. Walsh JK, Farrell MK, Keenan WJ, et al: Gastroesophageal reflux in infants: relation to apnea. J Pediatr 99:197–201, 1981.

42. Darling DB, McCauley RGK, Leape LL, et al: The child with peptic esophagitis: a correlation of radiologic signs with esophageal pathology. Radiology 145:673–676, 1982.

43. Bowen AD: The vomiting infant: recent advances and unsettled issues in imaging. Radiol Clin North Am 26:377–391, 1988.

44. Sondheimer JM: Gastroesophageal reflux: update on pathogenesis and diagnosis. Pediatr Clin North Am 35:103–116, 1988.

44a. Gomes H, Lallemano PH: Infant apnea and gastroesophageal reflux. Pediatr Radiol 22:8–11, 1992.

45. Itani Y, Fujioka M, Nishimura G, et al: Upper GI examinations in older premature infants with persistent apnea: correlation with simultaneous cardiorespiratory monitoring. Pediatr Radiol 18:464–467, 1988.

46. Darling DB, McCauley RGK, Leonidas JC, et al: Gastroesophageal reflux in infants and children: correlation of radiological severity and pulmonary pathology. Radiology 127:735–740, 1978.

47. Nielson DW, Heldt GP, Tooley WH: Stridor and gastroesophageal reflux in infants. Pediatrics 85:1034–1039, 1990.

48. Jolley SG, Halpern CT, Sterling CE, et al: The relationship of respiratory complications from gastroesophageal reflux to prematurity in infants. J Pediatr Surg 25:755–757, 1990.

49. Malfroot A, Vandenplas Y, Verlinden M, et al: Gastroesophageal reflux and unexplained chronic respiratory disease in infants and children. Pediatr Pulmonol 3:208–213, 1987.

50. Caniano DA, Ginn-Pease MA, King DR: The failed antireflux procedure: analysis of risk factors and morbidity. J Pediatr Surg 25:1022–1026, 1990.

51. Berquist WE, Rachelefsky GS, Kadden M, et al: Effect of theophylline on gastroesophageal reflux in normal adults. J Allergy Clin Immunol 67:407–411, 1981.

52. Di Lorenzo C, Piepsz A, Ham H, et al: Gastric emptying with gastro-oesophageal reflux. Arch Dis Child 62:449–452, 1987.

53. Blumhagen JD, Rudd TG, Christie DL: Gastroesophageal reflux in children: radionuclide gastroesophagography. AJR 135:1001–1004, 1980.

54. Gelfand MJ, Wagner GG: Gastric emptying in infants and children: limited utility of 1-hour measurement. Radiology 178:379–381, 1991.

55. Moore JG, Christian PE, Taylor AT, et al: Gastric emptying measurements: delayed emptying patterns without appropriate correction. J Nucl Med 26:1206–1210, 1985.

56. Seibert JJ, Byrne WJ, Euler AR: Gastric emptying in children: unusual patterns detected by scintigraphy. AJR 141:49–51, 1983.

57. Cucchiara S, Bortolotti M, Minella R, et al: Fasting and postprandial mechanisms of gastroesophageal reflux in children with gastroesophageal reflux disease. Dig Dis Sci 38:86–92, 1993.

58. Papaila JG, Wilmot D, Grosfeld JL, et al: Increased incidence of delayed gastric emptying in children with gastroesophageal reflux. Arch Surg 124:933–936, 1989.

59. Swischuk LE, Hayden CK, Fawcett HD, et al: Gastroesophageal reflux: how much imaging is required? Radiographics 8:1137–1145, 1988.

60. Heyman S: Esophageal scintigraphy (milk scans) in infants and children with gastroesophageal reflux. Radiology 144:891–893, 1982.

61. Rudd TG, Christie DL: Demonstration of gastroesophageal reflux in children by radionuclide gastroesophagography. Radiology 131:483–486, 1979.

62. Miller JH: Upper gastrointestinal tract evaluation with radionuclides in infants. Radiology 178:326–327, 1991.

63. Seibert JJ, Byrne WJ, Euler AR, et al: Gastroesophageal reflux—the acid test: scintigraphy or the pH probe? AJR 140:1087–1090, 1983.

64. Fonkalsrud EW, Foglia RP, Ament ME, et al: Operative treatment for the gastroesophageal reflux syndrome in children. J Pediatr Surg 24:525–529, 1989.

65. Stringel G: Gastrostomy with antireflux properties. J Pediatr Surg 25:1019–1021, 1990.

66. Curci MR, Dibbins AW: Problems associated with a Nissen fundoplication following tracheoesophageal fistula and esophageal atresia repair. Arch Surg 123:618–620, 1988.

67. Pearl RH, Robie DK, Ein SH, et al: Complications of gastroesophageal antireflux surgery in neurologically impaired versus neurologically normal children. J Pediatr Surg 25:1169–1173, 1990.

67a. Martinez DA, Ginn-Pease ME, Caniano DA: Sequelae of antireflux surgery in profoundly disabled children. J Pediatr Surg 27:267–273, 1992.

68. Sutcliffe J: Torsion spasms and abnormal postures in children with hiatal hernia: Sandifer's syndrome. Prog Pediatr Radiol 2:190–197, 1969.

69. Sacher P, Stauffer UG: The Herbst triad: report of two cases. J Pediatr Surg 25:1238–1239, 1990.

70. Cleveland RH, Kushner DC, Schwartz AN: Gastroesophageal reflux in children: results of a standardized fluoroscopic approach. AJR 141:53–56, 1983.

71. Darling DB: Hiatal hernia and gastroesophageal reflux in infancy and childhood. Analysis of the radiologic findings. AJR 123:724–736, 1975.

72. McCauley RGK, Darling DB, Leonidas JC, et al: Gastroesophageal reflux in infants and children: a useful classification and reliable physiologic technique for its demonstration. AJR 130:47–50, 1978.

73. Blumhagen JD, Christie DL: Gastroesophageal reflux in children: evaluation of the water siphon test. Radiology 131:345–349, 1979.

74. Fawcett HD, Hayden CK, Adams JC, et al: How useful is gastroesophageal reflux in suspected childhood aspiration? Pediatr Radiol 18:311–313, 1988.

75. Westra SJ, Wolf BHM, Staalman CR: Ultrasound diagnosis of gastroesophageal reflux and hiatal hernia in infants and young children. JCU 18:477–485, 1990.

76. Naik DR, Bolia A, Moore DJ: Comparison of barium swallow and ultrasound in diagnosis of gastro-oesophageal reflux in children. Br Med J 290:1943–1945, 1985.

77. Blane CE, Turnage RH, Oldham KT, et al: Long-term radiographic follow-up of the Nissen fundoplication in children. Pediatr Radiol 19:523–526, 1989.

78. Thoeni RF, Moss AA: The radiographic appearance of complications following Nissen fundoplication. Radiology 131:17–21, 1979.

79. Hatfield M, Shapir J: The radiologic manifestations of failed antireflux operations. AJR 144:1209–1214, 1985.

80. Magilner AD, Isard HJ: Achalasia of the esophagus in infancy. Radiology 98:81–82, 1971.

81. Willich E: Achalasia of the cardia in children. Manometric, cinematographic and pharmacoradiologic studies. Pediatr Radiol 1:229–236, 1973.

82. Starinsky R, Berlovitz I, Mares AJ, et al: Infantile achalasia. Pediatr Radiol 14:113–115, 1984.

83. Taylor RG, Myers NA: Achalasia of the cardia in children. A retrospective review of 20 cases. Pediatr Surg Int 4:386–389, 1989.

84. Nihoul-Fekete C, Bawab F, Lortat-Jacob S, et al: Achalasia of the esophagus in childhood: surgical treatment in 35 cases with special reference to familial cases and glucocorticoid deficiency association. J Pediatr Surg 24:1060–1063, 1989.

85. Khalifa MM: Familial achalasia, microcephaly, and mental retardation. Case report and review of the literature. Clin Pediatr 27:509–512, 1988.

86. Akhter J, Newcomb RW: Tracheal obstruction secondary to esophageal achalasia. J Pediatr Gastroenterol Nutr 7:769–772, 1988.

87. Dodds WJ, Stewart ET, Kishk SM: Radiologic amyl nitrite test for distinguishing pseudoachalasia from idiopathic achalasia. AJR 146:21–23, 1986.

88. Agha FP, Lee HH: The esophagus after endoscopic pneumatic balloon dilatation for achalasia. AJR 146:25–29, 1986.

89. Vane DW, Cosby K, West K, et al: Late results following esophagomyotomy in children with achalasia. J Pediatr Surg 23:515–519, 1988.

90. Stewart ET, Miller WN, Hogan WJ, et al: Desirability of roentgen esophageal examination immediately after pneumatic dilatation for achalasia. Radiology 130:589–591, 1979.

91. Fonkalsrud EW: Treatment of variceal hemorrhage in children. Surg Clin North Am 70:475–487, 1990.

92. Berk RN, Lee FA: The late gastrointestinal manifestations of cystic fibrosis of the pancreas. Radiology 106:377–381, 1973.

93. Cockerill EM, Miller RE, Chernish SM, et al: Optimal visualization of esophageal varices. AJR 126:512–523, 1976.

94. Buonocore E, Collmann IR, Kerley HE, et al: Massive upper gastrointestinal hemorrhage in children. AJR 115:289–296, 1972.

95. Hassall E, Berquist WE, Ament ME, et al: Sclerotherapy for extrahepatic portal hypertension in childhood. J Pediatr 115:69–74, 1989.

96. Sarin SK, Misra SP, Singal AK, et al: Endoscopic sclerotherapy for varices in children. J Pediatr Gastroenterol Nutr 7:662–666, 1988.

97. Stringer MD, Howard ER, Mowat AP: Endoscopic sclerotherapy in the management of esophageal varices in 61 children with biliary atresia. J Pediatr Surg 24:438–442, 1989.

98. Hall RJ, Lilly JR, Stiegmann GV: Endoscopic esophageal varix ligation: technique and preliminary results in children. J Pediatr Surg 23:1222–1223, 1988.

99. Patriquin H, Tessier G, Grignon A, et al: Lesser omental thickness in normal children: baseline for detection of portal hypertension. AJR 145:693–696, 1985.

100. DeGiacomo C, Tomasi G, Gatti C, et al: Ultrasonographic prediction of the presence and severity of esophageal varices in children. J Pediatr Gastroenterol Nutr 9:431–435, 1989.

101. Patriquin H, Lafortune M, Weber A, et al: Surgical portosystemic shunts in children: assessment with duplex Doppler US. Radiology 165:25–28, 1987.

102. Ablin DS, Reinhart MA: Esophageal perforation with mediastinal abscess in child abuse. Pediatr Radiol 20:524–525, 1990.

103. Friedman EM: Caustic ingestions and foreign bodies in the aerodigestive tract of children. Pediatr Clin North Am 36:1403–1410, 1989.

104. Martel W: Radiologic features of esophagogastritis secondary to extremely caustic agents. Radiology 103:31–36, 1972.

105. Franken EA: Caustic damage of the gastrointestinal tract: roentgen features. AJR 118:77–85, 1973.

105a. Gündoğdu HZ, Tanyel FC, Bükyükpamkçu N, et al: Conservative treatment of caustic esophageal strictures in children. J Pediatr Surg 27:767–170, 1992.

106. Wijburg FA, Heymans HSA, Urbanus NAM: Caustic esophageal lesions in childhood: prevention of stricture formation. J Pediatr Surg 24:171–173, 1989.

107. Gaudreault P, Parent M, McGuigan MA, et al: Predictability of esophageal injury from signs and symptoms: a study of caustic ingestion in 378 children. Pediatrics 71:767–770, 1983.

108. Crain EF, Gershel JC, Mezey AP: Caustic ingestions. Symptoms as predictors of esophageal injury. Am J Dis Child 138:863–865, 1984.

109. Caravati EM, Bennett DL, McElwee NE: Pediatric coin ingestion. A prospective study on the utility of routine roentgenograms. Am J Dis Child 143:549–551, 1989.

110. Schunk JE, Corneli H, Bolte R: Pediatric coin ingestions. A prospective study of coin location and symptoms. Am J Dis Child 143:546–548, 1989.

111. Banerjee A, Rao KS, Khanna SK, et al: Laryngo-tracheo-bronchial foreign bodies in children. J Laryngol Otol 10:1029–1032, 1988.

112. Eggli KD, Potter BM, Garcia V, et al: Delayed diagnosis of esophageal perforation by aluminum foreign bodies. Pediatr Radiol 16:511–516, 1986.

113. Vaishnav A, Spitz L: Alkaline battery-induced tracheo-oesophageal fistula. Br J Surg 76:1045, 1989.

114. Sigalet D, Lees G: Tracheoesophageal injury secondary to disc battery ingestion. J Pediatr Surg 23:996–998, 1988.

115. Volle E, Beyer P, Kaufmann HJ: Therapeutic approach to ingested button-type batteries. Magnetic removal of ingested button-type batteries. Pediatr Radiol 19:114–119, 1989.

116. Campbell JB, Davis WS: Catheter technique for extraction of blunt esophageal foreign bodies. Radiology 108:438–440, 1973.

117. Campbell JB, Condon VR: Catheter removal of blunt foreign bodies in children. Survey of the Society for Pediatric Radiology. Pediatr Radiol 19:361–365, 1989.

118. Shackelford GD, McAlister WH, Robertson CL: The use of a Foley catheter for removal of blunt esophageal foreign bodies from children. Radiology 105:455–456, 1972.

119. Paulson EK, Jaffe RB: Metallic foreign bodies in the stomach: fluoroscopic removal with a magnetic orogastric tube. Radiology 174:191–194, 1990.

120. Myer CM III: Potential hazards of esophageal foreign body extraction. Pediatr Radiol 20:97–98, 1991.

121. Cadranel S, Di Lorenzo C, Rodesch P, et al: Caustic ingestion and esophageal function. J Pediatr Gastroenterol Nutr 10:164–168, 1990.

122. Reeder JD, Kramer SS, Dudgeon DL: Transverse esophageal folds: association with corrosive injury. Radiology 155:303–304, 1985.

123. Subbarao KS, Kakar AK, Chandrasekhar V, et al: Cicatricial gastric stenosis caused by corrosive ingestion. Aust N Z J Surg 58:143–146, 1988.

124. Mughal MM, Marples M, Bancewicz J: Scintigraphic assessment of esophageal motility: what does it show and how reliable is it? Gut 27:946–953, 1986.

125. Towbin R, Lederman HM, Dunbar JS, et al: Esophageal edema as a predictor of unsuccessful balloon extraction of esophageal foreign body. Pediatr Radiol 19:359–360, 1989.

126. van der Zee DC, Festen C, Severijnen RS, et al: Management of pediatric esophageal perforation. J Thorac Cardiovasc Surg 95:692–695, 1988.

127. Boal DKB, Newburger PE, Teele RL: Esophagitis induced by combined radiation and Adriamycin. AJR 132:567–570, 1979.

128. Lepke RA, Libshitz HI: Radiation-induced injury of the esophagus. Radiology 148:375–378, 1983.

129. Levine MS, Laufer I, Kressel HY, et al: Herpes esophagitis. AJR 136:863–866, 1981.

130. Fiedorek SC, Casteel HB: Pediatric medication-induced focal esophagitis. Case report and review. Clin Pediatr 27:455–456, 1988.

131. Howell CG, Mansberger HA, Parrish RA: Esophageal stricture secondary to Stevens-Johnson syndrome. J Pediatr Surg 22:994–995, 1987.

132. Kern IB, Eisenberg M, Willis S: Management of oesophageal stenosis in epidermolysis bullosa dystrophica. Arch Dis Child 64:551–556, 1989.

133. Becker MH, Swinyard CA: Epidermolysis bullosa dystrophica in children. Radiology 90:124–128, 1968.

134. Agha FP, Francis IR, Ellis CN: Esophageal involvement in epidermolysis bullosa dystrophica: clinical and roentgenographic manifestations. Gastrointest Radiol 8:111–117, 1983.

135. El Shafie M, Stidham GL, Klippel CH, et al: Pyloric atresia and epidermolysis bullosa letalis: a lethal combination in two premature newborn siblings. J Pediatr Surg 14:446–449, 1979.

136. Korber JS, Glasson MJ: Pyloric atresia associated with epidermolysis bullosa. J Pediatr 14:600–601, 1977.

137. Orense M, García Hernández JB, Celorio C, et al: Pyloric atresia associated with epidermolysis bullosa. Pediatr Radiol 17:435, 1987.

138. Mauro MA, Parker LA, Hartley WS, et al: Epidermolysis bullosa: radiographic findings in 16 cases. AJR 149:925–927, 1987.

139. Tishler JM, Han SY, Helman CA: Esophageal involvement in epidermolysis bullosa dystrophica. AJR 141:1283–1286, 1983.

140. Orlando RC, Bozymski EM, Briggaman, et al: Epidermolysis bullosa: gastrointestinal manifestations. Ann Intern Med 81:203–206, 1974.

# Diseases of the Stomach and Duodenum

Rita Littlewood Teele, M.D.

Jane Chrestman Share, M.D.

## CONGENITAL ANOMALIES

Most anomalies affecting the stomach and duodenum are evident on abdominal plain film studies: complete atresia of the pylorus results in a single bubble of air, atresia of the duodenum manifests as the well-known radiographic "double bubble," and duplication cysts can displace or obstruct bowel. Microgastria is associated with cardiovascular and splenic anomalies, and duodenal stenosis occurs with greater frequency among children with trisomy 21. Whenever an anomaly of stomach or duodenum is encountered, careful clinical and radiologic searches for other anomalies are mandatory.

## Pyloric and Antral Atresias

Pyloric and antral atresias are rare anomalies in which the neonate is unable to feed without vomiting. The abdomen is gasless except for a single bubble of air (Fig. 76-1). Sonograms performed on infants with pyloric atresia do not show a normal canal or muscle.[1] This contrasts with neonates with pyloric stenosis, in whom the obstruction is incomplete and sonography can reveal a lumen and thick musculature. A complete prepyloric membrane is another cause of congenital gastric outlet obstruction, but a pyloric channel should be seen sonographically.[2] Differentiation between atresia and membrane usually rests with the surgeon because plain films, showing complete obstruction in the first day of life, mandate an operation.

There is an association between pyloric atresia and epidermolysis bullosa, although the exact relationship is unclear.[3, 4] In affected patients, minimal trauma to the skin results in blisters and erosions, and this may happen in utero. Similarly, pyloric atresia in these patients can be congenital or acquired if it presents after the newborn period.

## Antral Mucosal Diaphragm

Complete mucosal diaphragm of the antrum is an uncommon anomaly that is usually discovered in infancy or old age.[5] In infants, the antral diaphragm or web may cause vomiting or failure to thrive. On upper gastrointestinal studies, the thin membrane presents as filling defect across the antrum (Fig. 76-2) and is best seen on the right anterior oblique view when surrounded by the barium pool. Air-contrast views are not as helpful. Strands of tenaciously adherent mucus can occasionally simulate an antral web.[6] Strands of mucus, however, do not cause obstruction and do not impart a double-chambered appearance to the antrum.

Adult patients become symptomatic from their web only if the central aperture of the diaphragm is less than 1 cm.[5] In symptomatic infants, the aperture is often less than or equal to 5 mm.[7] The size of the aperture cannot accurately be judged on fluoroscopic examination. Theoretically, gastric ultrasonography could directly assess aperture size when the stomach is distended with water. Endoscopic confirmation and transection of a web have been reported in an adolescent patient.[5] Asymptomatic, incidentally discovered webs probably do not require intervention according to some authors.[8] Others support a more aggressive approach.[7]

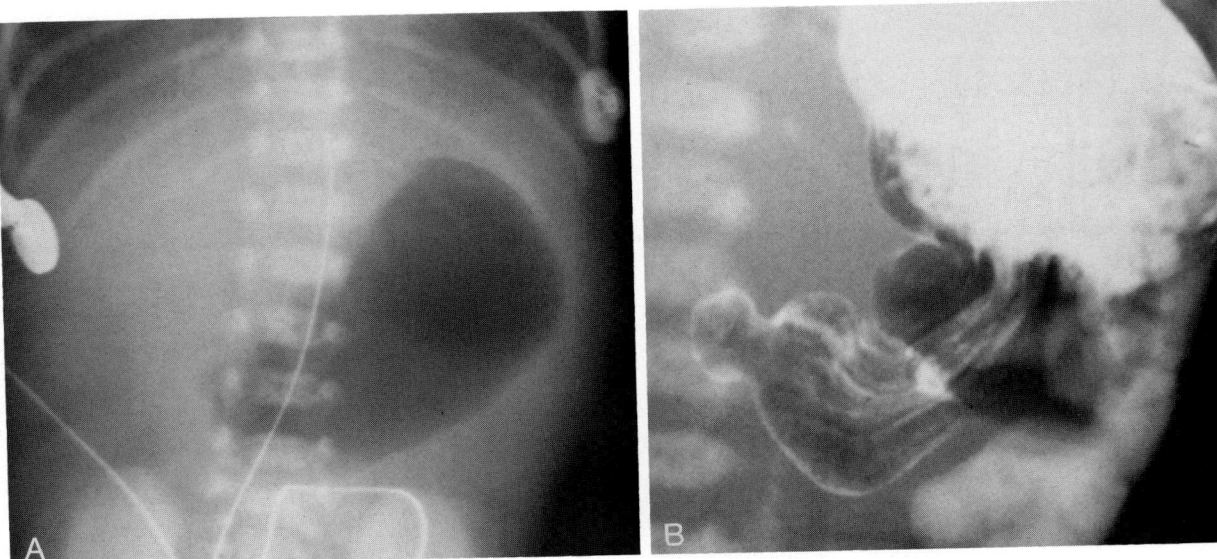

**Figure 76–1. Pyloric atresia. A.** An abdominal radiograph obtained 48 hours after birth shows gas in the stomach and no air distally. **B.** Contrast medium given orally demonstrates complete obstruction at the pylorus. The intraluminal contrast area to the left of the stomach is in the colon, which was opacified during a previous barium enema. Maternal polyhydramnios developed prenatally. (Case courtesy of Michael DiPietro, M.D., Ann Arbor, MI.)

## Microgastria

Microgastria is an anomaly that is often associated with absence of the spleen and mesenteric abnormalities.[9] These patients present with vomiting and failure to thrive. Radiographically, there is no gastric air bubble, and the esophagus is often dilated (Fig. 76–3) as it functions as an accessory stomach through reflux.[10] The miniature stomach empties into a normal caliber duodenum that may be in an abnormal position. Treatment

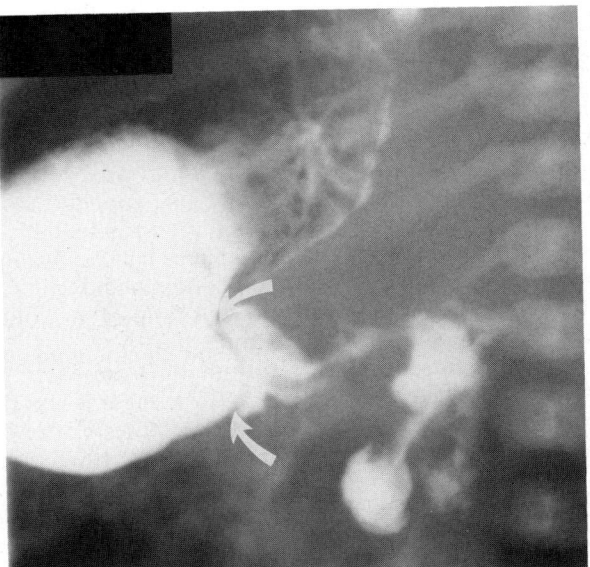

**Figure 76–2. Antral web.** Single contrast view of the stomach in the prone, right anterior oblique position demonstrates a thin, linear filling defect across the barium-filled antrum *(arrows)*. The infant presented a few hours after birth with postprandial projectile vomiting.

is directed toward increasing gastric capacity by creating and attaching a jejunal pouch.[11]

## Duodenal Atresia, Stenosis, and Annular Pancreas

Atresia and stenosis are related anomalies of the proximal duodenum. They develop if there is failure of normal canalization of this portion of the gut during the 8th to 10th weeks in utero. Approximately one third of infants with atresia or stenosis have trisomy 21.[12] If the obstruction is complete, the diagnosis is usually apparent on the first or second day of life. The newborn typically has bilious vomiting, because the atresia is located distal to the ampulla of Vater in 75% of patients.[12] The abdominal plain film usually shows the classic double bubble, with gas filling a distended stomach and proximal duodenum (Fig. 76–4). The film may be nondiagnostic if severe vomiting empties the stomach and proximal duodenum or a decompressing nasogastric tube is inserted immediately after birth. Immediate nasogastric decompression is becoming more common, because obstruction of the fetal gastrointestinal tract is being diagnosed in utero with greater frequency sonographically.[13, 14] To confirm the diagnosis of duodenal atresia, air or barium can be injected through the nasogastric tube.

Associated anomalies are common in patients with duodenal atresia and stenosis, and some physicians advocate a contrast enema to identify possible colonic atresia or abnormalities in the position of the cecum, because malrotation is more common in this population. It has been postulated that a large, ectatic proximal duodenum impedes normal gut rotation in utero.

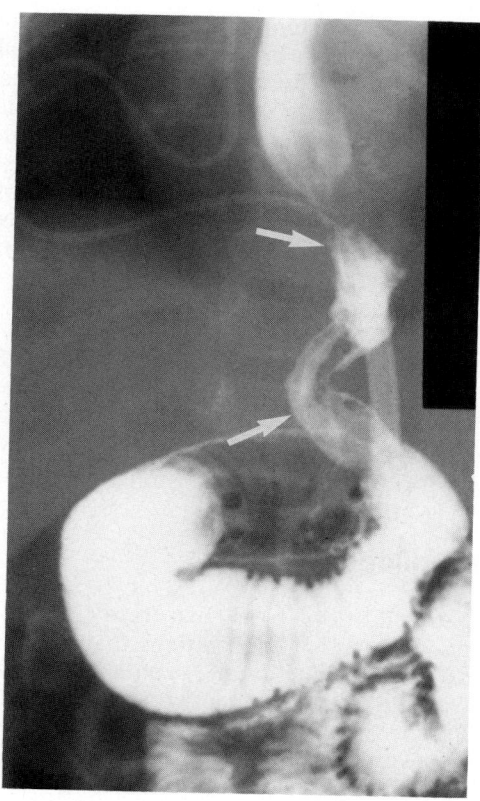

**Figure 76–3. Microgastria.** Supine frontal view shows a miniature stomach *(arrows).* The moderately dilated duodenum is in the normal position. The infant had marked gastroesophageal reflux during the examination. This upper gastrointestinal series was done as part of an evaluation of the failure to thrive of an 8-month-old infant. The overlying catheter is a central venous line.

Partial duodenal obstruction often develops in patients with duodenal stenosis, duodenal diaphragm, and annular pancreas. A double bubble may be apparent on plain films, but distal gas is also present. These disorders may not become clinically evident until later in life. The small lumen may become obstructed with food after the infant graduates from a liquid to a solid diet. Children with trisomy 21 and significant mental retardation are notorious for ingesting foreign bodies, and their duodenal narrowing may become apparent only after the duodenum becomes completely obstructed by fruit pits, coins, or other items.[15]

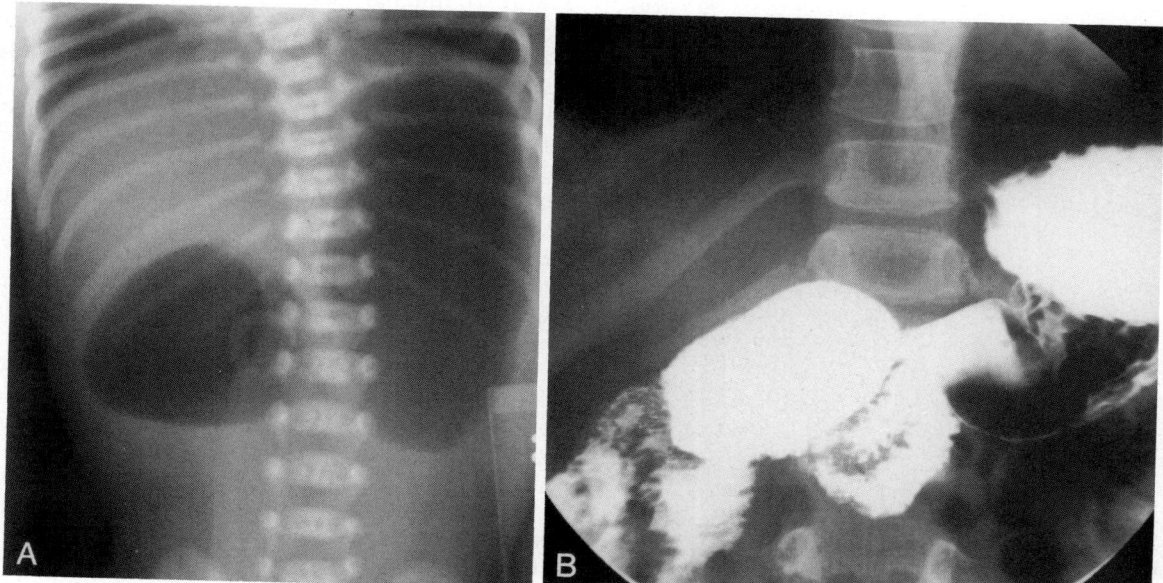

**Figure 76–4. Duodenal atresia. A.** Upright abdominal radiograph of this 2-day-old neonate shows the classic double bubble of duodenal atresia. **B.** Duodenal jejunostomy was performed to bypass the atresia. A postoperative study shows barium in the stomach and proximal bowel. Note that the duodenum remains dilated after surgery.

Duodenal diaphragm, or "windsock duodenum," also carries the confusing label of intraluminal diverticulum. It presents on fluoroscopy as a fine linear filling defect within the lumen of the barium-filled duodenum[16] (Fig. 76–5). The diagnosis has also been made with ultrasonography.[17] The partial obstruction caused by its small aperture results in variable dilatation of the proximal duodenum and forward ballooning of the diaphragm so that it resembles a windsock. Situs inversus and malrotation are associated anomalies.[17]

Annular pancreas usually occurs in the setting of intrinsic duodenal stenosis. This association should be remembered whenever duodenal stenosis is encountered (Fig. 76–6). Because the surgical approach to duodenal stenosis does not differ significantly if annular pancreas is present, an extensive preoperative evaluation is unnecessary.

## Duplication Cyst

Duplication cysts are rare in the stomach and duodenum.[18, 19] Duplications that arise from the gastroesophageal junction may contain respiratory and enteric tissue, and they probably represent a bronchopulmonary foregut malformation.[18] Therefore, if a cystic mass is discovered at the gastroesophageal junction, chest radiographs should be scrutinized for a mediastinal or pulmonary component to the cyst. Duplication cysts of the distal stomach and duodenum are enteric or neurenteric in origin.[18a]

In early intrauterine life, a neurenteric canal connects ectoderm to endoderm and passes through dorsal neural folds. Persistence of this or an accessory canal (i.e., split

notochord syndrome) gives rise to a series of anomalies, including diastematomyelia, hemivertebrae, and enteric cysts.[20] Therefore the vertebrae must be carefully assessed in patients with suspected enteric or neurenteric cysts.

Most gastric and distal cysts were thought to arise as a result of failure of normal canalization of the intestinal tract at 8 weeks in utero.[21] This theory, however, does not explain a case report in which respiratory tract mucosa was found in a huge duodenal duplication.[22] No existing theory can easily explain concomitant cysts of the esophagus, stomach, and duodenum that have been reported in one child.[23]

The common clinical features of gastric or duodenal duplication cysts include obstruction, palpable upper abdominal mass, gastrointestinal bleeding, and respiratory distress. Most are diagnosed during the first year of life, and the combination of findings observed on sonography and upper gastrointestinal series (Figs. 76–7 and 76–8) is diagnostic.[24, 25] At fluoroscopy, a "beak" appearance results at the gastric outlet when contrast medium surrounds the proximal portion of an obstructive duodenal duplication cyst.[28] A complete discussion of gastrointestinal duplications can be found in Chapter 79.

## Malrotation

The developing gastrointestinal tract normally has two zones that have the ability to actively pull adjacent bowel along with them. These zones correspond to the duodenojejunal segment and the cecocolic segment. Before the 10th week of intrauterine life, the duodenojejunal segment returns to the peritoneal cavity from the omphalos, having coursed counterclockwise, to the left of the midline, under the superior mesenteric artery. The cecocolic segment undergoes a counterclockwise rotation to lie finally in the right lower quadrant. The cecum may be in a normal position despite an incompletely rotated duodenum.[27, 28] There is a spectrum of rotational anomalies, ranging from nonrotation, in which the small bowel lies to the right of the mesenteric vessels and the colon to the left, to minor degrees of cecal elevation. Malrotation is an incomplete rotation resulting in formation of abnormal mesenteric attachments (i.e., Ladd's bands) and shortening of the mesenteric base that normally lies obliquely across the retroperitoneum.

The ligament of Treitz is a suspensory ligament of connective tissue and smooth muscle that runs from the root of superior mesenteric artery to the third and fourth portions of the duodenum.[29] Its presence is manifested by a normal position of duodenojejunal junction in relation to the stomach, proximal duodenum, and spine. Normal duodenal position is characterized by a pylorus located to the right of midline, the duodenojejunal flexure situated left of the medial margin of the left-sided vertebral pedicles, and a primarily left-sided jejunum. Cephalocaudal position of the duodenojejunal flexure is considered normal if it is superior to the L-2

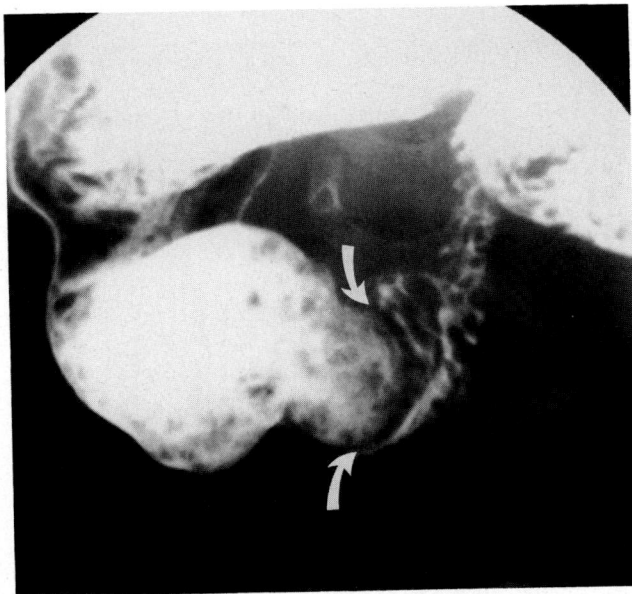

**Figure 76–5. Windsock duodenum.** Corn kernels, which had been ingested the evening before the contrast study, filled the duodenum proximal to an obstructive duodenal web in this 18-month-old boy. Intermittent vomiting was the only symptom. An oblique view of the transverse duodenum demonstrates the thin duodenal web *(arrows)*.

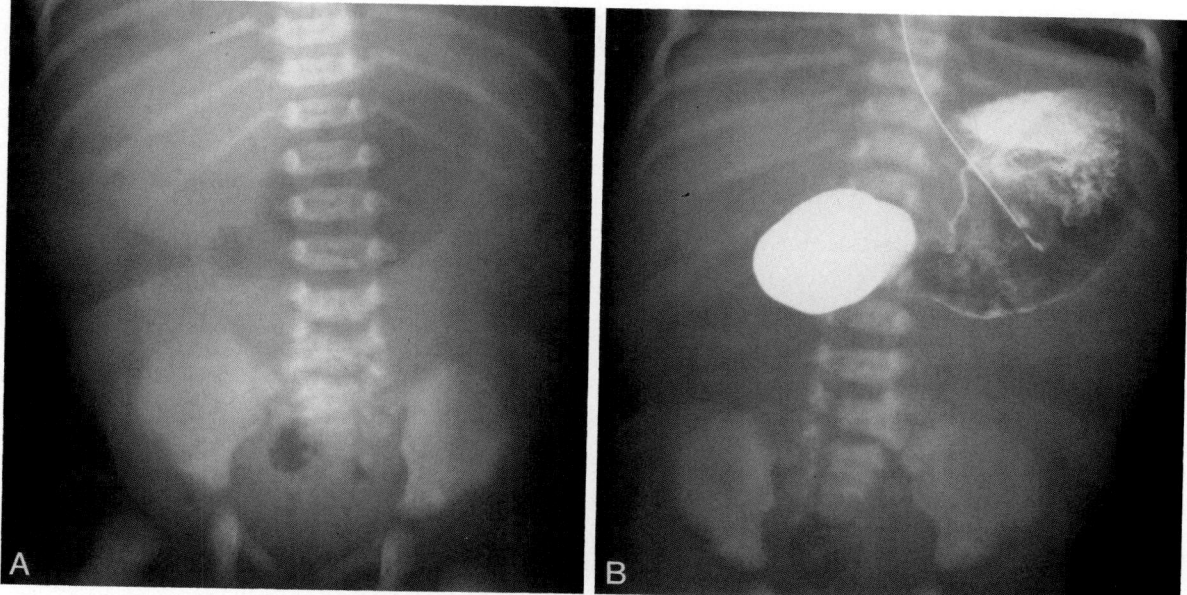

**Figure 76–6. Intrinsic duodenal stenosis with annular pancreas. A.** Abdominal radiograph of this 3-day-old infant shows gas in the stomach, with a paucity of distal gas. The dilated duodenal bulb is filled with fluid. **B.** Contrast medium administered via an esophagogastric catheter demonstrates high-grade obstruction of the postbulbar duodenum. The infant had been vomiting since birth. Although annular pancreas cannot be diagnosed from this study, the association between duodenal stenosis and annular pancreas should always be considered.

superior end plate and at the level (with minor variation) of the apex of the duodenal bulb.[30] The duodenojejunal flexure is mobile in children younger than 4 years of age. This explains the common plain film finding of nasogastric tubes causing marked distortion of duodenal anatomy in infants with no intestinal anomaly.[30] The duodenojejunal junction can also be inferiorly displaced by a distended intestine in children with distal obstruction of the intestinal tract.[31]

Malrotation alone does not cause the symptoms, but obstruction may result from Ladd's bands across the duodenum or from midgut volvulus around the narrow superior mesenteric vascular pedicle. Volvulus is a life-threatening emergency.[32] Bilious vomiting in an otherwise healthy infant is the classic presentation. Occasionally, a child may tolerate obstruction from intermittent volvulus and come to medical attention with episodic pain or symptoms of malabsorption.[33, 34] Because the lymphatics course with the blood vessels, chronic intermittent volvulus is a cause of secondary lymphangiectasia and chylous ascites.

There is considerable debate in the literature concerning the best diagnostic approach to midgut volvulus: barium studies or ultrasound.[35–38] We advocate a carefully controlled upper gastrointestinal series, because the diagnosis of a subtle abnormality of duodenal position is difficult even with contrast medium. In these cases, sonography, which assesses the relative location of the superior mesenteric artery and vein, may be falsely negative and delay diagnosis. It is worthwhile, however, to identify the superior mesenteric vasculature in children undergoing ultrasonography as part of an

evaluation for nonspecific abdominal pain. In malrotation, the superior mesenteric vein lies on the left and more ventrally than normal[39] (Fig. 76–9). The sensitivity of this finding in malrotation has not been established. Preduodenal portal vein can be diagnosed sonographically and serve as a clue to malrotation and duodenal stenosis, anomalies with which it is commonly associated.[40]

Plain films of patients with malrotation may be normal or show an unusual position of the air-filled stomach or intestinal loops, paucity of distal bowel gas, dilatation of duodenal cap, or grossly distended air-filled loops with mural thickening if there is ischemia from volvulus. If midgut volvulus is suspected, we place a nasogastric tube in the stomach, inject some air, which may be diagnostic, and then inject barium if it is not. Contrast medium should be aspirated if an obstruction is identified. Ladd's bands typically cause a Z-type configuration of duodenum and proximal jejunum.[41] Midgut volvulus causes a corkscrew appearance of the duodenum and jejunum, with proximal dilatation of the duodenum from the obstructing twist (Fig. 76–10).

## Paraduodenal Hernia

Paraduodenal hernia is an internal hernia of loops of small bowel. A congenital defect in development of the peritoneum is thought to encourage the entrapment of intestine in a sac adjacent to the duodenum. The duodenum may be distorted by the hernia, which is typically in a left-sided location.[42] The diagnosis is usually made

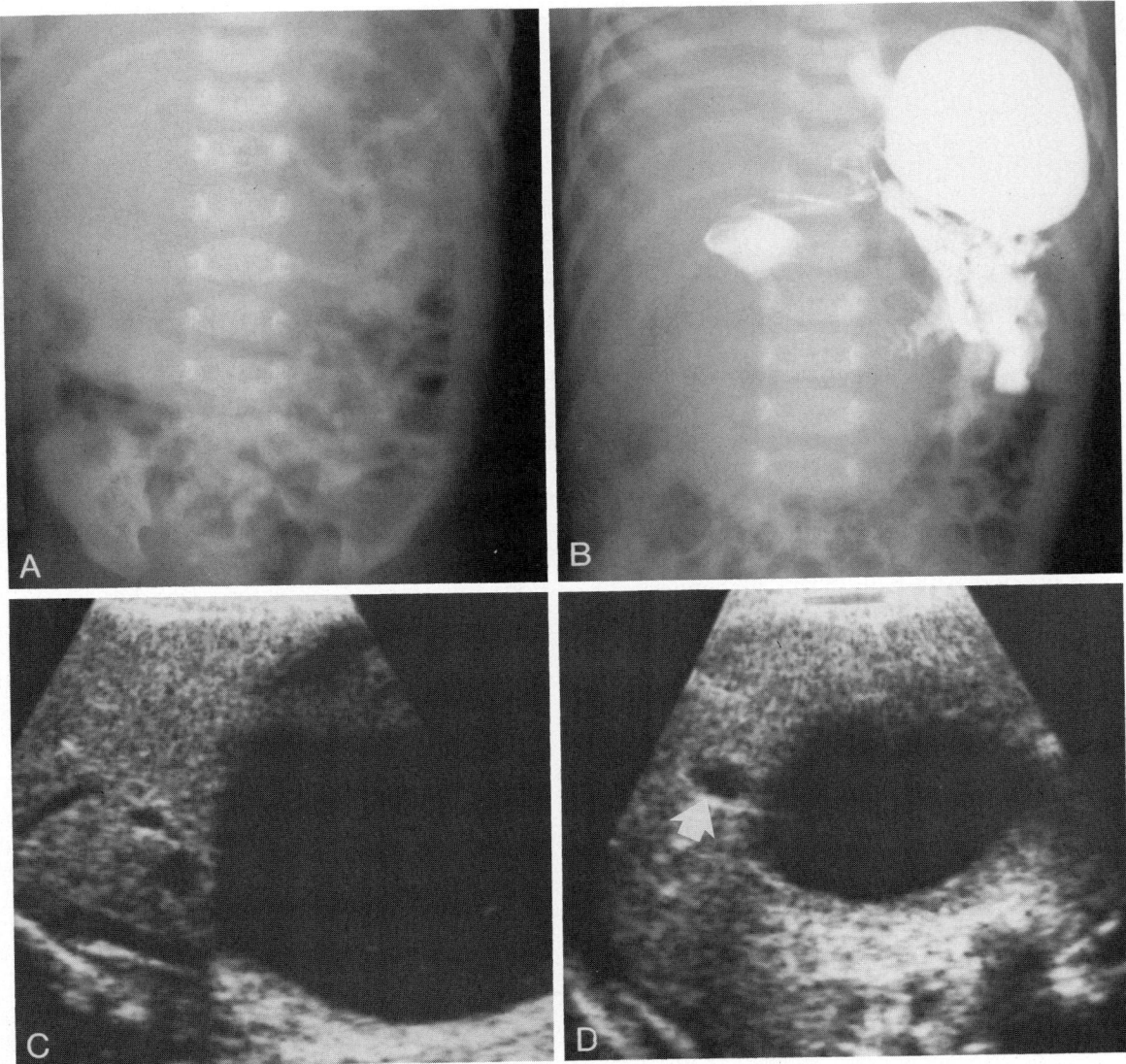

**Figure 76–7. Gastric duplication. A.** Abdominal radiograph of this 5-week-old infant with postprandial vomiting since birth shows an opacity in the right side of the abdomen displacing bowel loops inferiorly and to the left. **B.** Duodenal and jejunal loops are draped around this mass on the upper gastrointestinal series. The antrum is also compressed by the mass. Longitudinal **(C)** and transverse **(D)** sonograms of the right upper quadrant show a cystic mass, separate from the gallbladder *(arrow)* and bile duct.

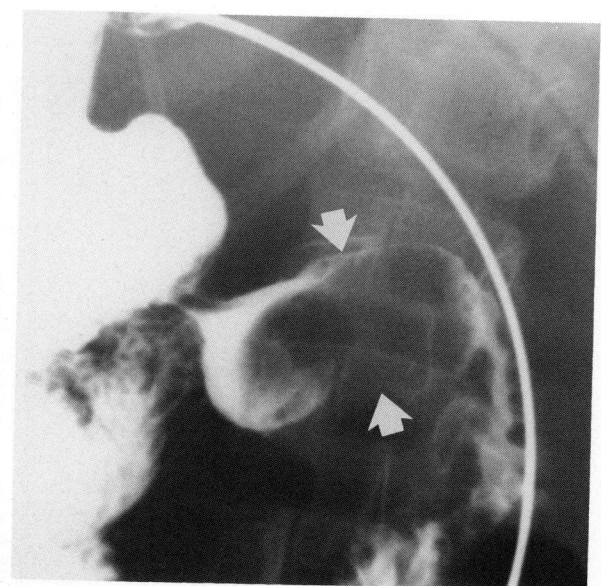

**Figure 76–8. Antral duplication cyst.** Compression view of the antrum shows a submucosal mass *(arrows)*. This 17-year-old boy presented with a 3-month history of intermittent nausea and vomiting.

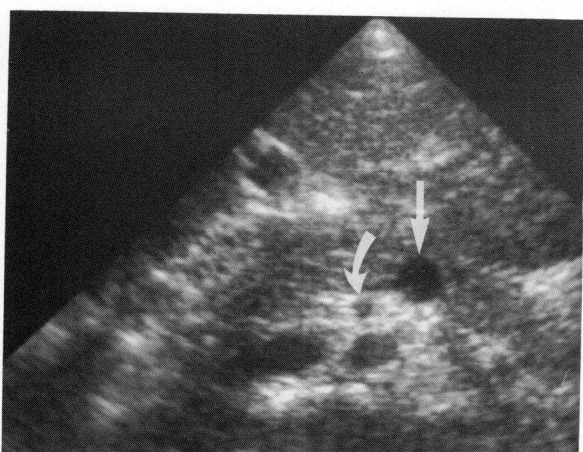

**Figure 76–9. Malrotation with reversal of the position of the superior mesenteric vein and artery.** Transverse sonogram demonstrates the superior mesenteric vein *(straight arrow)* at the 1 o'clock position relative to the superior mesenteric artery *(curved arrow)*, a reversal of the normal relationship.

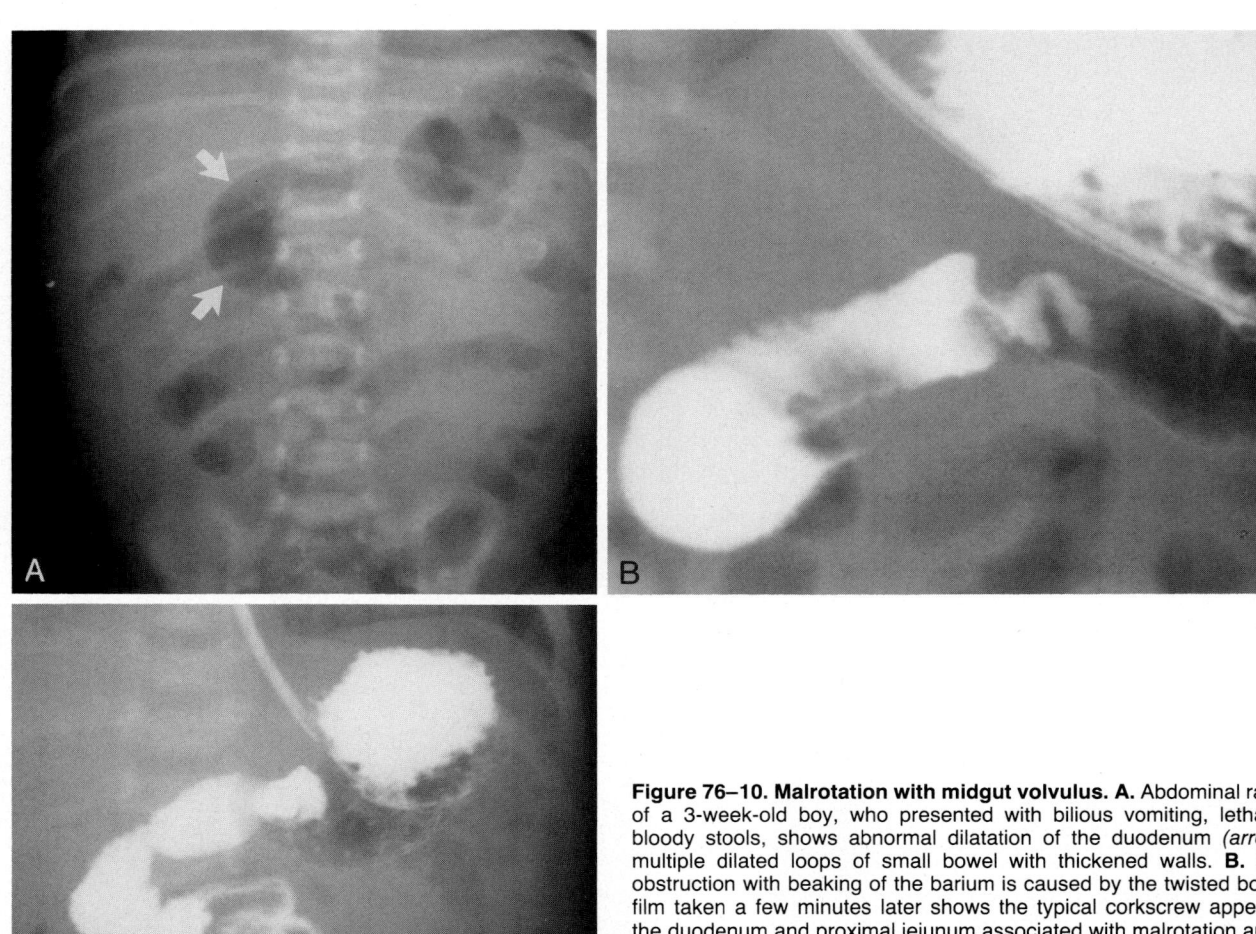

**Figure 76–10. Malrotation with midgut volvulus. A.** Abdominal radiograph of a 3-week-old boy, who presented with bilious vomiting, lethargy, and bloody stools, shows abnormal dilatation of the duodenum *(arrows)* and multiple dilated loops of small bowel with thickened walls. **B.** Duodenal obstruction with beaking of the barium is caused by the twisted bowel. **C.** A film taken a few minutes later shows the typical corkscrew appearance of the duodenum and proximal jejunum associated with malrotation and midgut volvulus.

in adolescence or adulthood; we have seen only one child for whom an upper gastrointestinal series was diagnostic.

## "Apple Peel" or "Christmas Tree" Bowel

When the superior mesenteric artery fails to develop or becomes occluded in utero, a rotational anomaly of the duodenum may develop that is associated with deficiency of the mesentery, luminal stenoses, a short gut, and a tenuous vascular supply to the gut via the left branch of the ileocolic artery. The affected newborn presents with duodenal or jejunal obstruction. Contrast enema demonstrates a microcolon (Fig. 76–11) that usually is in an abnormal position.[43] Surgery is complicated by the short gut and the need to relieve areas of obstruction in the face of limited blood supply.

## ACQUIRED DISEASES

### Gastric Perforation

The incidence of acute gastric rupture is declining.[44] There are several predisposing factors: acute distention of the stomach; ischemic necrosis associated with perinatal asphyxia; and distal obstruction, such as annular pancreas or duodenal stenosis.[44–47] Plain radiographs of infants who have had gastric perforation show pneumoperitoneum and absence of a gastric air-fluid level on upright views.[48] Neonatal duodenal perforation is rare.[49]

Gastric perforation in older children occurs in the following clinical settings: perforated peptic ulcer, dermatomyositis (although duodenal perforation is more common), migration of tubes and catheters through the gastric wall, and prior ingestion of corrosive substances.[50–54] A life-threatening complication of the Nissen and other fundoplications is gastric rupture or infarction in patients with a distal small bowel obstruction.[55] Blunt trauma to the upper abdomen when the stomach is distended occasionally results in gastric rupture.

## Pyloric Stenosis

Hypertrophic pyloric stenosis is the most common indication for surgery in infants. This disorder has a 5:1 male predominance and randomly occurs in 3 of 1000 infants. A parental history increases the offspring's chance to 6.9%.[56, 57] Projectile, bile-free emesis in a previously healthy 6-week-old infant is the classic presentation of pyloric stenosis.

There has been increasing reliance on barium radiography and ultrasonography in children with suspected pyloric stenosis.[57–59] With new generations of residents less vigorously trained in the art of clinical examination, there is little likelihood of reversing this trend. Ideally, imaging should be reserved for the 20% of infants with pyloric stenosis in whom an experienced examiner cannot palpate the classic "olive," which represents the hypertrophied pyloric muscle.

Ultrasound and barium studies are well established and accurate for the diagnosis of pyloric stenosis. The mode of examination depends on equipment, expertise,

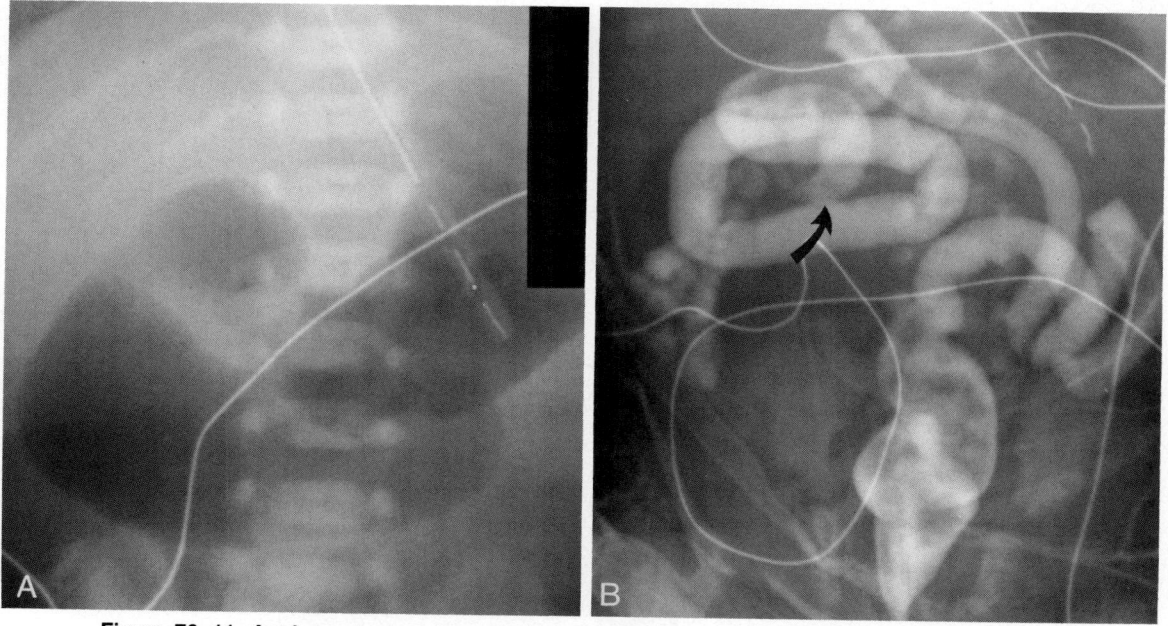

**Figure 76–11. Apple peel mesentery. A.** Abdominal radiograph in this 1-day-old neonate shows gas in the stomach and a dilated duodenum. A prenatal diagnosis of intestinal obstruction prompted evaluation of the infant's gastrointestinal tract shortly after birth. **B.** Contrast enema in the same patient shows a microcolon and abnormal location of the cecum *(arrow).* At surgery, jejunal atresia and an apple peel mesentery were found.

and examiner comfort level. If equipment and expertise are available, ultrasonography is the fastest and least invasive method.

The classic barium meal features of pyloric stenosis include partial or complete gastric outlet obstruction; hyperperistalsis of the stomach or, if there is a prolonged history, gastric atony; elongation of the pyloric channel; single ("string" sign) or double ("train track" sign) streaks of barium within the compressed lumen of the channel; the shoulder sign of a pyloric mass indenting the barium-filled stomach with peristalsis abutting the mass; and indentation of the base of the duodenal bulb from a pyloric mass (Fig. 76–12). The sonographic criteria for diagnosis vary slightly among institutions.[36, 56, 60–63] Some authorities rely primarily on measurements of muscle thickness;[60] others depend on channel length.[62] We use a composite score, which includes muscle thickness greater than 3.5 mm, channel length 17 mm or

greater, little or no passage of gastric contents, and gastric peristalsis that stops abruptly at the pyloric muscle (Fig. 76–13). To allow adequate distention of the antrum with fluid, we turn the infant to right posterior oblique position and give glucose water through a nipple if the stomach has been emptied by vomiting (Fig. 76–14). Questionable cases can be rescanned in 24 to 36 hours or investigated with an upper gastrointestinal series.

## Gastric and Duodenal Hematomas

Trauma to the upper abdomen may injure the stomach but more commonly results in a duodenal hematoma. The typical history is that of a child falling onto the handlebars of a bicycle or being struck in the abdomen during play or an athletic event.[64, 65] Child abuse should

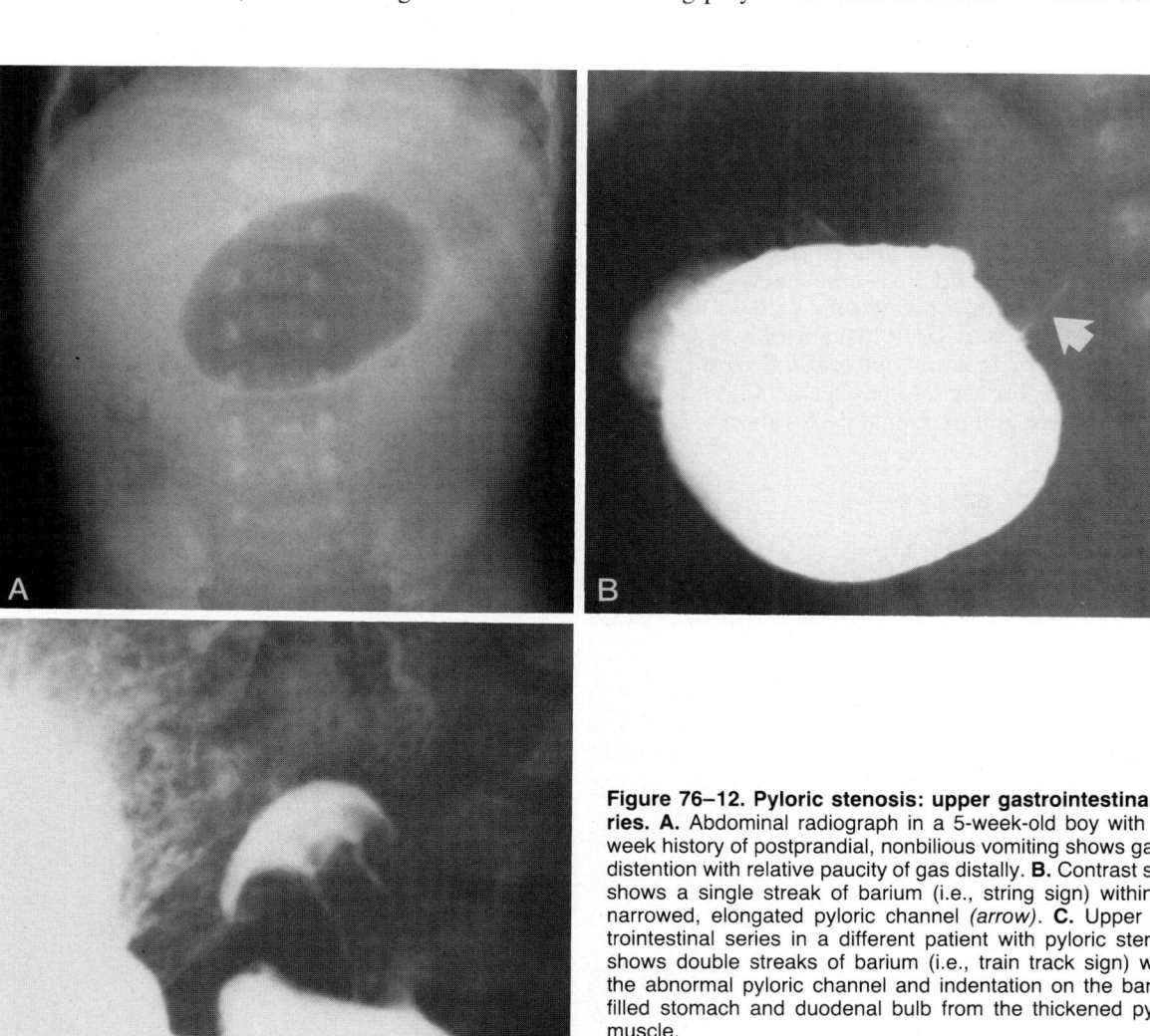

**Figure 76–12. Pyloric stenosis: upper gastrointestinal series. A.** Abdominal radiograph in a 5-week-old boy with a 1-week history of postprandial, nonbilious vomiting shows gastric distention with relative paucity of gas distally. **B.** Contrast study shows a single streak of barium (i.e., string sign) within the narrowed, elongated pyloric channel *(arrow).* **C.** Upper gastrointestinal series in a different patient with pyloric stenosis shows double streaks of barium (i.e., train track sign) within the abnormal pyloric channel and indentation on the barium-filled stomach and duodenal bulb from the thickened pyloric muscle.

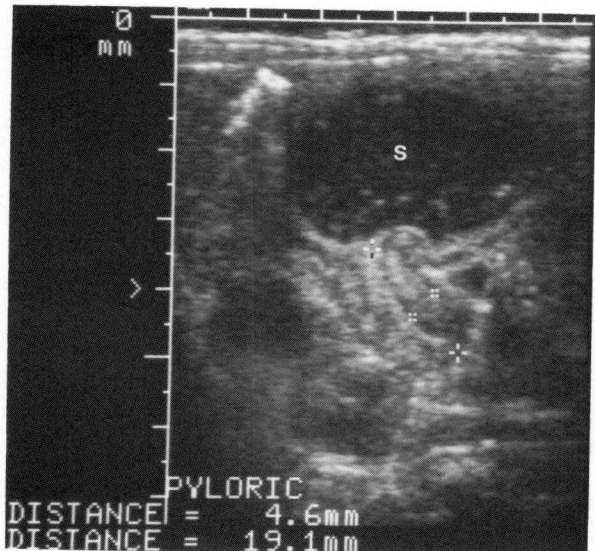

**Figure 76–13. Pyloric stenosis: ultrasound.** Sonography of the pylorus showed no peristalsis during the examination. Echogenic material in the stomach (S) represents retained gastric contents in this 3-week-old boy with a 48-hour history of projectile vomiting. The thickness of one wall of the pyloric muscle is 4.6 mm; the length of the channel is 19.1 mm.

be considered for any child who has a suspicious history of accidental trauma.[66] Other risk factors include Henoch-Schönlein purpura, bleeding associated with leukemia, coagulopathies, idiopathic thrombocytopenia purpura, endoscopic biopsy, and anticoagulant therapy.[67]

The diagnosis of gastric and duodenal hematoma can be suggested by plain films if gastric distention, a soft tissue mass in the right hemiabdomen, and sparse distal gas are all present. Coexisting duodenal perforation must be excluded, because operation is reserved only for children with perforation.[64] Occasionally, retroperitoneal air can be seen on the plain films or computed tomographic scan as a sign of transmural leakage.[68]

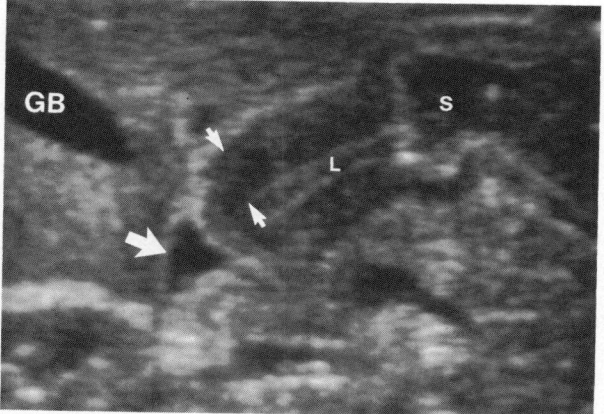

**Figure 76–14. Pyloric stenosis: ultrasound.** This infant was given glucose water before the scans. Enough fluid passed through the pylorus to outline the duodenal bulb *(large arrow)*. The thickened pyloric wall *(small arrows)* is also visible. GB = gallbladder; L = pyloric lumen; S = stomach.

Barium studies show the intramural mass effect of the hematoma (Fig. 76–15A) but may not demonstrate the perforation if the hematoma is plugging the rent. As the hematoma and its tamponade effect resolve, perforation and duodenal diastasis may become apparent. Therefore, every child with a duodenal hematoma must be carefully watched during the first 7 to 10 days after trauma.[68a]

Ultrasonography can demonstrate and follow to resolution the hematoma and adjacent pancreatic injury that are commonly present (Fig. 76–15B), but it cannot reliably demonstrate perforation.[69] Computed tomography is preferred if there has been severe upper abdominal trauma, especially crush injury, because it can image all organs well. However, computed tomography can miss subtle duodenal rupture.[70]

## Gastric and Duodenal Masses

Bezoars and ingested foreign bodies account for many gastric masses. The most common bezoar in childhood is a trichobezoar, or hairball. The parents of young children, when questioned, are usually aware of the ingestion of hair and can occasionally produce a bald infant sister or brother as proof. Some physicians consider trichobezoar an indicator of an underlying psychologic problem. The trichobezoar is usually confined to the stomach (Fig. 76–16), but a tail may extend into the duodenum and rarely throughout the small bowel.[71] Lactobezoars have been described in premature infants, and they probably form as a result of immature mechanisms of gastric emptying.[72] Phytobezoars are uncommon because children generally do not have the predisposing gastric conditions, nor are they great consumers of vegetables. The symptoms of bezoars are those of insidious obstruction, although some are discovered incidentally by plain films, ultrasonography, or physical examination. Complications include bleeding, perforation, obstructive jaundice, intussusception, and appendicitis.[71]

Foreign body ingestion is common in children between the ages of 6 months and 3 years and in older children with psychologic problems. Most foreign bodies probably pass through the intestinal tract without the parents' being aware of their ingestion. Most foreign bodies that cause symptoms become lodged in the esophagus. Of foreign bodies that reach the stomach, 90 to 95% pass spontaneously if the stomach and duodenum are normal.[73] Prior gastric surgery, antral web, and duodenal stenosis are predisposing abnormalities that prevent passage of objects. Open safety pins, bobby pins, and objects larger than 6 cm long should be endoscopically removed if located in the stomach.[74] Because most objects pass without problem, even in small children, a conservative approach is taken by surgeons and pediatricians. If the object is retained in the stomach or duodenum for more than 1 week, further evaluation and intervention (Fig. 76–17) are required. Although button batteries are small, they have the potential for causing injury because of their contents. Five percent of children

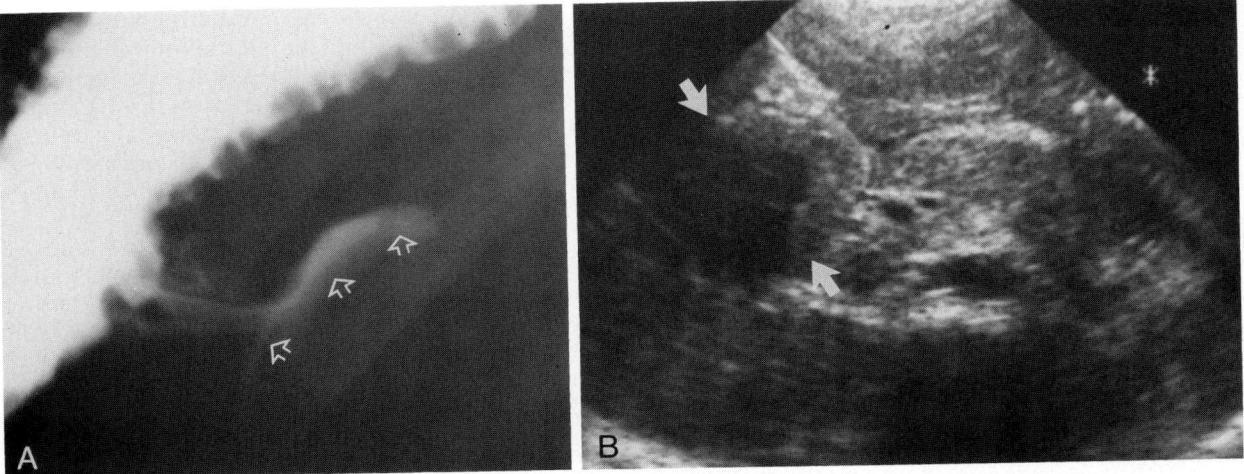

**Figure 76–15. Duodenal hematoma. A.** Prone oblique view from an upper gastrointestinal series shows duodenal obstruction with barium *(arrows)* outlining a duodenal "mass." **B.** Transverse sonogram of the upper abdomen demonstrates the mass to be a duodenal hematoma *(arrows)* in this 10-year-old child who sustained a bicycle handlebar injury to the upper abdomen. The complete sonographic study also demonstrated pancreatic swelling and peripancreatic fluid from injury (not shown).

who have swallowed button batteries have swallowed more than one.[75] Therefore, in this and all cases of foreign body ingestion, the gut from the mouth to the anus must be radiographed.

## Neoplasms

Gastric and duodenal neoplasms are rare in childhood (Fig. 76–18). Gastric teratoma is a tumor of infants. Virtually all of these patients present with upper abdominal masses during the first year of life.[76] Plain radio-

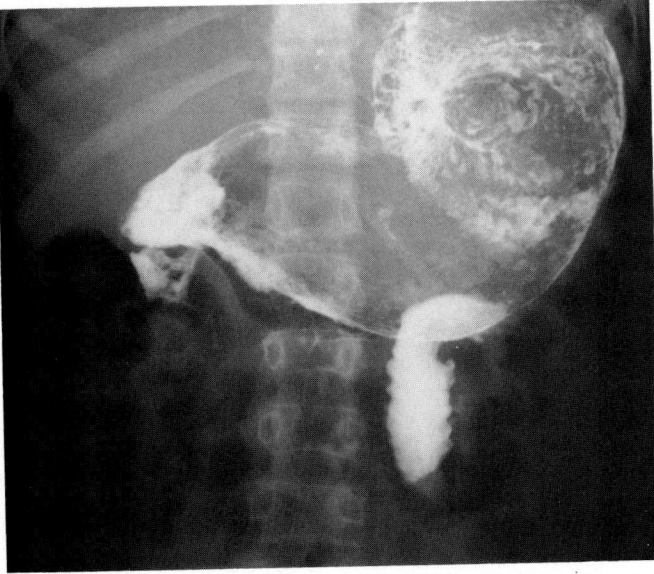

**Figure 76–16. Trichobezoar.** There is a large filling defect within the barium-filled stomach of this 12-year-old girl with a 2-year history of trichophagia, which left bald patches on her head. At surgery, a 500-g mass of matted, brunette hair was removed from the stomach.

graphs typically show calcification within a mass that displaces the gastric air bubble.[77] Without cross-sectional imaging, differentiation from retroperitoneal neuroblastoma may be difficult in some patients. Only 2 of 59 patients reported in the world's literature have been girls.[78]

Leiomyomas and leiomyosarcomas look similar on gross inspection and produce a similar appearance on barium studies: lobulated or polypoid filling defects arising from the gastric wall.[78a] They can be differentiated only by histologic examination.[79] Leiomyoblastoma is a rare tumor of the gastric wall that tends to grow in an intraluminal fashion, causing ulceration of the overlying mucosa. Its biologic behavior is generally benign, but metastases have been reported, with the liver being the most frequent site.[80] Lymphoma of the stomach may be a primary lesion or, rarely, part of generalized involvement with Burkitt's lymphoma.[81] In either case, the appearance is similar: diffuse infiltration of the gastric wall, mucosal thickening, ulcerations, and a discrete gastric mass. Lymphoma, leiomyosarcoma, and gastric adenocarcinoma have a similar appearance on studies done with contrast material.[82] Gastric carcinomas are extremely rare in children and have been associated with ataxia-telangiectasia and immunodeficiency.[83] Gastric sarcoma may be a late complication of radiation therapy.[84]

Gastric inflammatory pseudotumor can simulate a malignant tumor on radiographic studies. This disorder should be considered if a mass encompasses an ulcer or confined perforation, if the child has another unusual associated problem such as retroperitoneal fibrosis or sclerosing cholangitis, or if the child has Castleman's syndrome.[85] Large pancreatic pseudocysts or hepatic masses indent the stomach on conventional radiographic studies or cross-sectional imaging.

Familial polyps of the stomach and duodenum are most commonly hamartomatous and part of the Peutz-

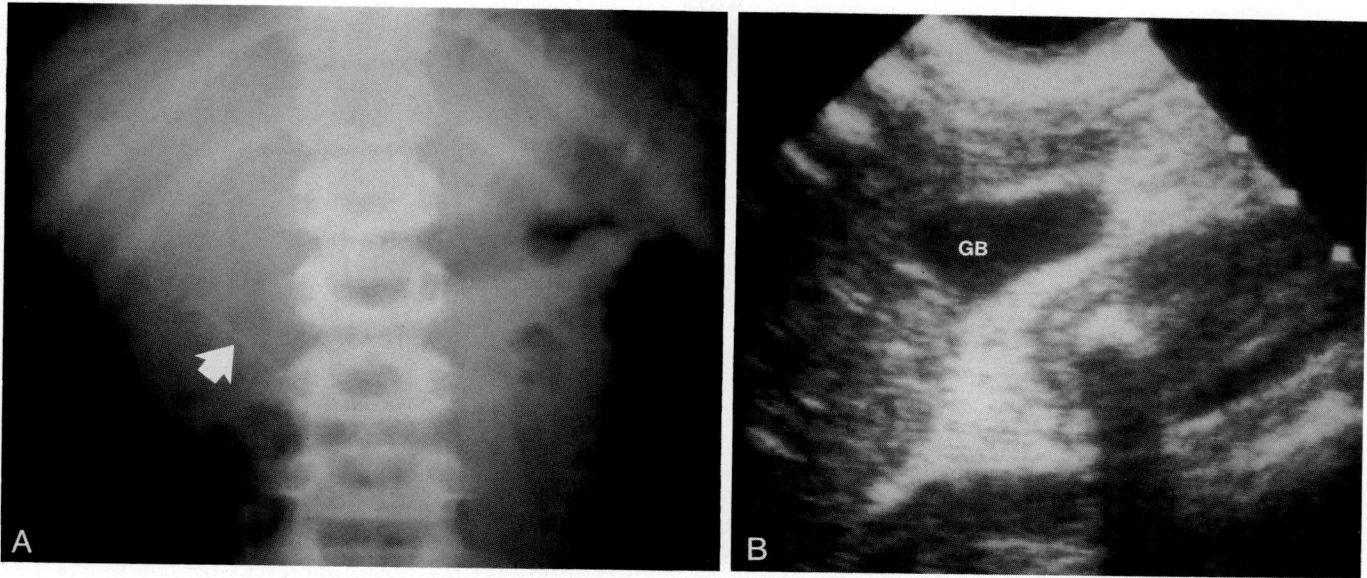

**Figure 76–17. Duodenal foreign body.** This child was chewing on a pencil, which she accidentally swallowed. Months later, she presented with upper abdominal discomfort and early satiety. **A.** Plain film shows the pencil as a faint, linear density in the right upper quadrant *(arrow).* **B.** Oblique sonogram of the right upper quadrant demonstrates the echogenic, shadowing pencil and the surrounding inflammatory mass. The imbedded pencil was removed endoscopically without complication. GB = gallbladder. (Case courtesy of Susan Craw, M.D., Dunedin, New Zealand.)

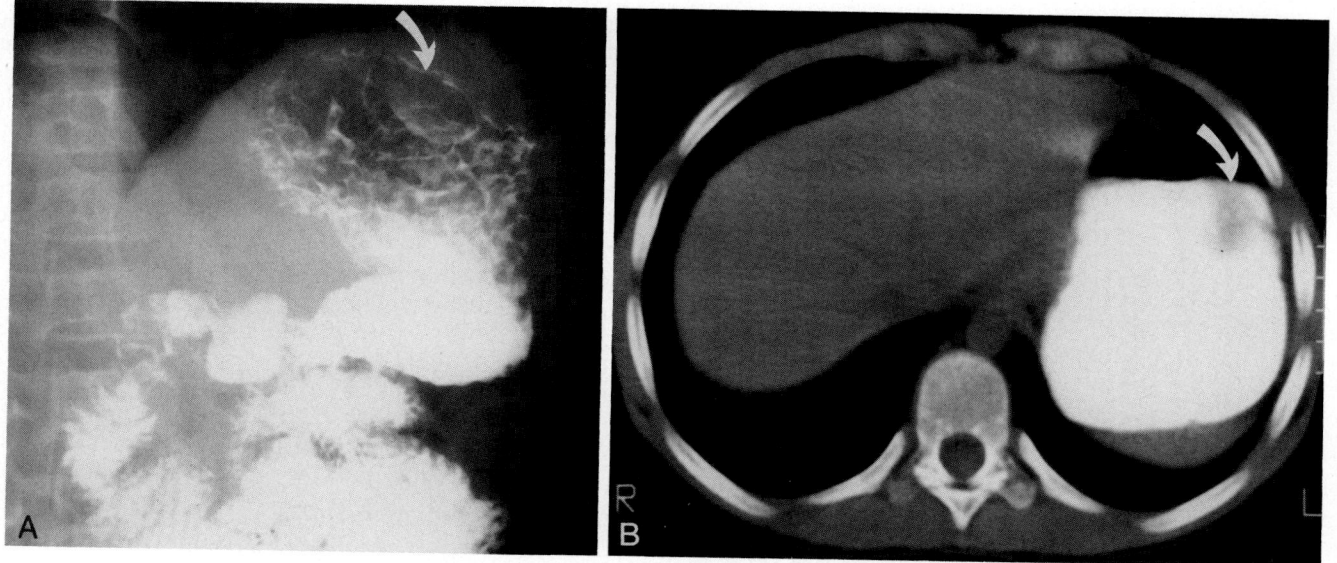

**Figure 76–18. Spindle cell tumor of stomach.** This 10-year-old boy presented with melena and anemia. **A.** Upper gastrointestinal series demonstrates a submucosal mass in the gastric fundus *(arrow).* **B.** It is confirmed by a CT scan *(arrow).* At surgery, a benign spindle cell tumor was resected in toto.

Jeghers syndrome (Fig. 76–19). Fundic gland polyposis has been described in children and adults who have familial adenomatosis coli and Gardner's syndrome.[86] A complete discussion of the gastroduodenal manifestations of the polyposis is presented in Chapter 66. Other gastric polyps in children include inflammatory fibroid polyp, solitary hyperplastic polyp, and polypoid focal foveolar hyperplasia.[87–90]

Neurofibromas can develop in the gastric or duodenal wall. Although these lesions are generally benign, they may cause vomiting, jaundice, and hematemesis.[91] Neurofibromas usually occur with other stigmata of von Recklinghausen's disease.

Varices result in compressible filling defects of the gastric and duodenal walls. They are most obvious in children who have had idiopathic obstruction of portal venous flow (e.g., cavernous transformation of portal vein) but can occur in cirrhosis. Downhill varices occur when the superior vena cava is obstructed close to the right atrium and flow is redirected down the azygos-hemiazygos system. Other compressible masses of the gastric and duodenal walls include lymphangiomas and hemangiomas.[92]

Pancreatic rests, manifesting as masses along the greater curvature of the stomach or inner margin of the duodenum, are congenital abnormalities that are rarely diagnosed in infancy.[93] They are described in detail in Chapter 115. Choledochocele may manifest as a smooth, well-defined mass at the ampulla of Vater. This abnormality is discussed in Chapter 89.

Intussusception of the duodenum or stomach can occur when a large hamartomatous polyp, gastrostomy tube, or Foley catheter acts as a lead point.[94]

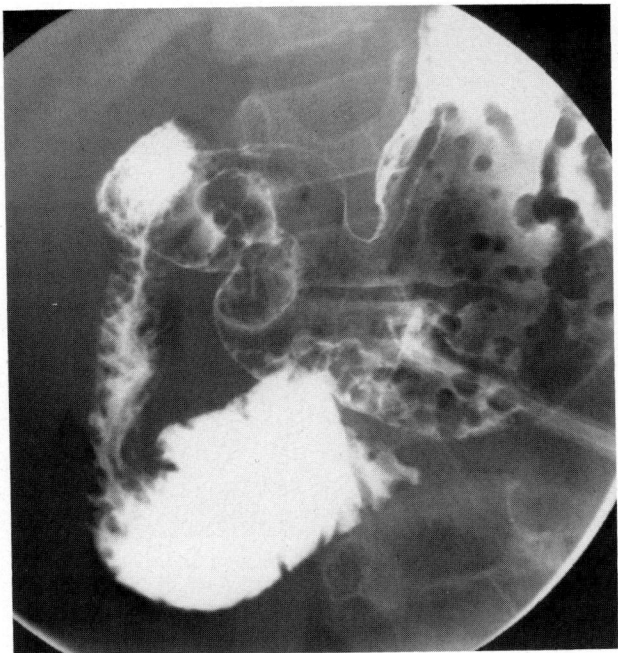

**Figure 76–19. Peutz-Jeghers syndrome.** Barium and air administered through a gastrostomy tube in this patient with known Peutz-Jeghers syndrome outline multiple filling defects representing hamartomatous polyps.

## Peptic Ulcer Disease

Peptic ulcer disease is rare in childhood, and there is often a positive family history.[95] Stress ulcers account for at least 80% of peptic disease encountered in infancy and early childhood.[96] Shock, respiratory failure, sepsis, hypoglycemia, severe burns (i.e., Curling's ulcer), intracranial lesions (i.e., Cushing's ulcer), and chronic systemic disease have been implicated in addition to aspirin, other nonsteroidal anti-inflammatory drugs, corticosteroids, and tolazoline.[50]

Hayden and associates reported that thickening of antral mucosa to greater than 4 mm (mean, 5.5 ± 1.41) was a common correlate of ulcer disease.[97]

A retrospective review of endoscopy procedures in children revealed a poor correlation with barium studies if an ulcer was present.[73] Although double contrast techniques would be expected to be more sensitive, there are no prospective comparative studies in children. Good double contrast examination is difficult in young children who have severe underlying illness or who are bleeding from their ulcers. Pediatric patients are often poorly compliant, coating of gastric and duodenal mucosa is hindered by secretions, and adequate manipulation during fluoroscopy is limited by the child's generally poor condition. In adolescents, who are more likely to have primary ulcer disease and present with abdominal pain, an adequate radiologic examination is far easier to accomplish. Its accuracy in detecting ulcers depends on the skill and experience of the fluoroscopist and the size of the ulcer. We concur with the practice of immediate endoscopy for a child presenting with acute upper gastrointestinal hemorrhage.

Angiographic intervention is rarely necessary, because most children can be stabilized with intensive medical management. For a few patients with brisk bleeding, diagnostic arteriography followed by therapeutic vasopressin (Pitressin) or absorbable gelatin sponge (Gelfoam) embolization is required.

Zollinger-Ellison syndrome is rare in children, and the registry tabulating this disease recorded only 28 children in 21 years.[50] Peptic ulceration, gastric acid hypersecretion, and hypergastrinemia have occasionally occurred in children with antral G cell hyperplasia.[50]

The association of a gram-negative, motile bacteria called *Helicobacter pylori* with gastritis and peptic ulcer has renewed interest in peptic disease. Children with primary gastritis appear to have a high probability of antral colonization with *H. pylori*.[98] In the future, children with upper abdominal pain may be serologically, rather than fluoroscopically, screened for peptic ulcer disease.[98a]

## Inflammatory Disorders Other Than Peptic Disease

Menetrier's disease is an inflammatory disorder characterized by enlarged gastric folds, predominantly in the body and fundus, and proliferation of gastric glands.[99] Clinically, this disease is acute and self-limited. Affected children present with upper abdominal pain, nausea, and vomiting that is occasionally complicated by hematemesis, anemia, and marked hypoproteinemia. The association between Menetrier's disease and cytomegalovirus has been documented, but it is uncertain whether the virus is etiologic or opportunistic.[99–101] Ultrasonography has shown thickened rugal folds in a 2-year-old boy with Menetrier's disease who had increased cytomegalovirus titers during his illness.[102]

Children with allergic gastroenteritis often present with asthma, failure to thrive, and peripheral eosinophilia. The gastric antrum and small bowel are primarily involved. Radiographic findings include a lacy antral mucosa pattern and a variably abnormal small bowel pattern. Remission induced by steroids results in a return of mucosal pattern to normal.[103]

Chronic granulomatous disease is a hematologic disorder in which polymorphonuclear leukocytes are unable to destroy some types of bacteria. In this disease, which usually affects boys, there is a defect in the mechanism for producing superoxide, resulting in ineffective lysis of certain bacteria. Macrophages and other granulomatous responses are then mobilized. This granulomatous response classically occurs in the gastric antrum, and narrowing of the gastric outlet is evident sonographically and on barium studies[104, 105] (Fig. 76–20).

Upper gastrointestinal tract Crohn's disease is unusual in children and is generally found in patients with well-established small bowel and colonic disease.[106–108] Mucosal nodularity and ulceration, fistula and sinus tracts, and irregular narrowing and pseudodiverticula forma-

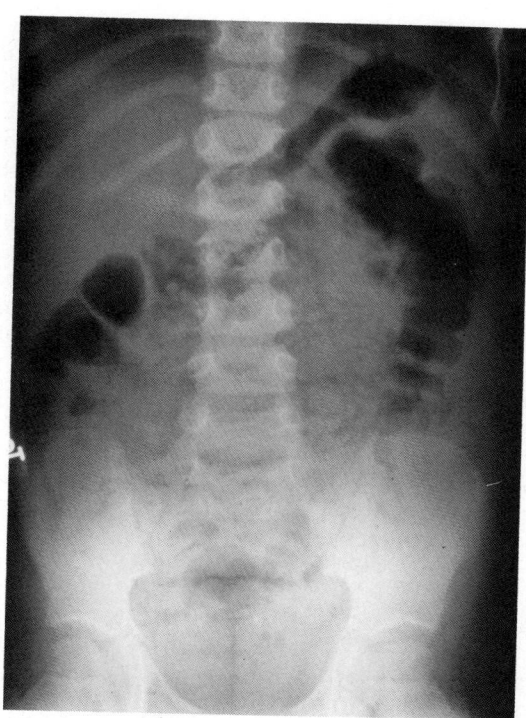

**Figure 76–21. Ascariasis.** This 5-year-old girl from Puerto Rico had a 2-month history of abdominal pain. Diarrhea was accompanied by vomiting, and the vomitus contained worms. Note the unusual gas pattern in the midduodenum and jejunum.

tion are the major radiographic findings in gastroduodenal Crohn's disease[106] (see Chapters 79 and 159). Pyloroduodenal tuberculosis can cause irregular stenosis, ulceration, and mass effects on the stomach and duodenum that resemble Crohn's disease. Enlarged nodes surrounding the outlet of the stomach and the duodenum are responsible for many of these radiographic findings.[109]

Twenty-five percent of the world's population harbor *Ascaris lumbricoides*, and most infected people are children.[110] This is the only parasite that ingests barium, and worms in the stomach or duodenum manifest as filling defects streaked with barium.[110] When the worm burden is sufficiently large, obstruction can result, and radiologists working in endemic areas become skilled at differentiating clumps of intraluminal worms from stool and other masses (Fig. 76–21). More than 75% of children with obstruction from ascaris have abnormal radiographs.[110]

Gastric mucosal penetration by the larvae of *Anisakis*, ingested with a meal of infected raw fish, causes acute, severe abdominal pain. Double contrast barium studies can be diagnostic: thread-like filling defects associated with a mound of mucosal edema at the site of larval penetrations of gastric wall.[111] Endoscopic removal of the larvae results in resolution of abdominal pain.

Although giardiasis classically occurs in the setting of dysgammaglobulinemia, immunocompetent children can be infected if the water source is contaminated. Duodenal spasm, thickening of the mucosa, and increased intraluminal fluid are characteristic, albeit nonspecific,

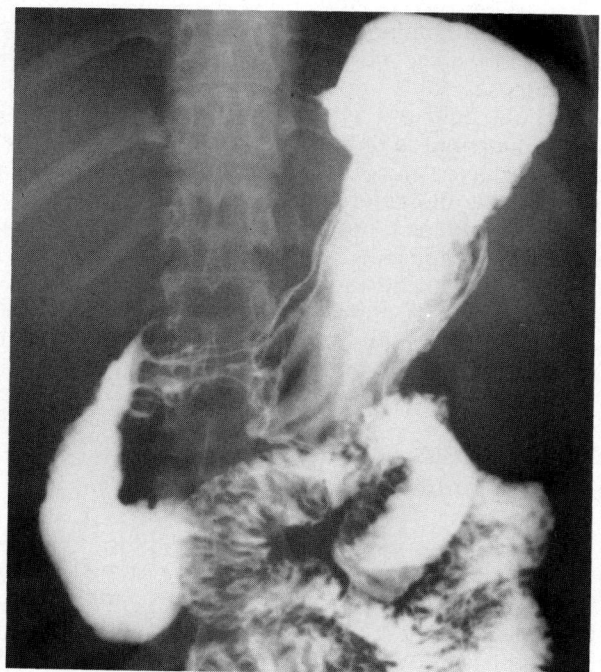

**Figure 76–20. Chronic granulomatous disease.** Thickened gastric folds with marked antral narrowing are seen in this patient with a long-standing history of chronic granulomatous disease. This study was prompted by symptoms of epigastric discomfort and vomiting.

radiologic features of infection.[112] *Strongyloides* also affects duodenal mucosa and provokes an inflammatory response. Chronic disease results in a fixed, narrowed, and featureless duodenum.[113]

Liquefaction necrosis of the esophagus and to a lesser degree the stomach occurs with lye ingestion, but the coagulation necrosis induced by acids primarily involves the stomach (see Chapter 75). After corrosive ingestion, esophageal folds may be thickened or ulcerated, and peristalsis in the esophagus and stomach may be absent.[114] Inflammation of the mucosal surface of the stomach develops acutely, and variable degrees of gastric outlet obstruction develop later (Fig. 76–22). Involvement of duodenal mucosa with edema and ulceration has also been described.[115] Radiology is more useful in the follow-up of prior corrosive injury. Scarring takes weeks to months to occur. Stenosis and contraction of stomach and rigidity of duodenal loop are characteristic of prior caustic ingestion.

## Gastric or Duodenal Distention

Gaseous distention of the stomach is seen in several disorders peculiar to the pediatric population. Many children swallow air when crying or nervous. There is overt aerophagia in some groups of mentally retarded youngsters, which may predispose these patients to gastric volvulus.[116, 117] Volvulus is also associated with deficient mesenteric and ligamentous attachments and diaphragmatic defects.[116, 117] Mesenteroaxial volvulus is a twist along an axis joining the lesser and greater curvature of the stomach. It has a characteristic appearance on plain radiographs[116] (Fig. 76–23). Organoaxial volvulus is a twist along the gastric axis.[118] Intrathoracic

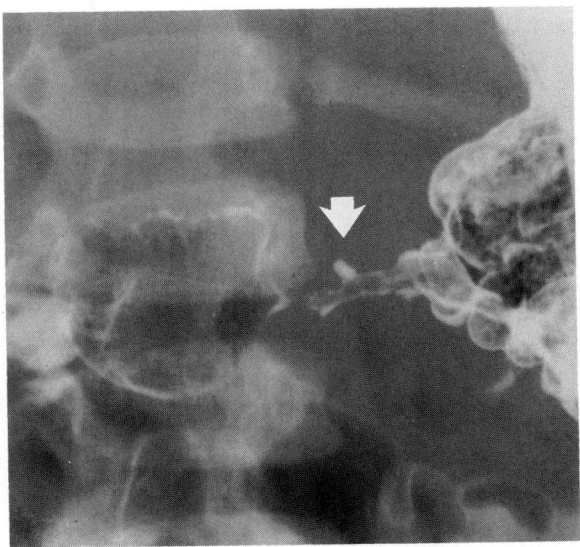

**Figure 76–22. Corrosive gastritis.** Marked antral narrowing and irregularity *(arrow)* are seen in this 7-year-old boy who accidentally swallowed sulfuric acid. This was the only case we could find in our files during the last 10 years, a testimony to the fact that child-proof containers and consumer education have resulted in corrosive gastritis' becoming a rarity.

gastric volvulus may accompany a large congenital hiatal hernia.[119, 120]

Gastric distention with air occurs with tracheoesophageal fistula, with or without esophageal atresia, or after an endotracheal tube is inadvertently placed in the esophagus. Diabetes mellitus and prior starvation are causes of gastric dilatation that are probably due to atony.

Superior mesenteric artery syndrome is obstructive compression of the third and fourth parts of the duodenum by the superior mesenteric artery and the root of the mesentery.[121–124] It may follow surgery and casting for correction of scoliosis (cast syndrome) or occur after severe weight loss. Plain radiographs and upper gastrointestinal series show distention of the stomach and proximal duodenum and a sharp cutoff in the midtransverse portion of the duodenum. In our experience, operative treatment is rarely necessary. Feeding in the prone position or hyperalimentation alleviates the symptoms in most patients. However, in one series of 13 affected pediatric patients, surgical repair was required in 9.[118–124]

Idiopathic megaduodenum is part of the spectrum of chronic intestinal pseudo-obstruction and may occur sporadically or in families.[125, 126] The condition is due to disease of the smooth muscle, abnormal extrinsic or intrinsic nerves, or alteration of their neuroendocrine environment (see Chapter 158). Dilatation of sections of the gastrointestinal tract without anatomic obstruction is characteristic. Bacterial overgrowth and diarrhea are common problems. Secondary megaduodenum from diabetes, scleroderma, and amyloidosis are always mentioned in differential diagnoses, but they are virtually never encountered in pediatric patients.

Radiographically demonstrable abnormalities of the duodenum are common in cystic fibrosis and are most prevalent in the second portion of duodenum.[127] Thickened mucosal folds, nodular mucosa, and increased intraluminal fluid are typical features. These findings have been attributed to hyperplasia of Brunner's glands, tenacious mucus, mucosal edema, or inappropriate contraction of the muscularis mucosae.[128] Because an ulcer is difficult to detect on this background of abnormal mucosa radiographically, endoscopy is recommended in patients with cystic fibrosis who have symptoms of peptic ulcer disease.[128] A more complete discussion of the gastrointestinal manifestations of cystic fibrosis can be found in Chapters 79 and 118.

## Postoperative Appearances of Stomach and Duodenum

The postoperative appearance of the Nissen and other types of fundoplications in children is similar to that seen in adults. This is also true for pyloroplasty, the Billroth I and II procedures (rarely performed in children), gastrostomy, and gastric reductions. However, pyloromyotomy for pyloric stenosis is surgery peculiar to children. The radiographic appearance in the immediate postoperative period looks similar to that of preoperative studies (Fig. 76–24). By 6 weeks, however,

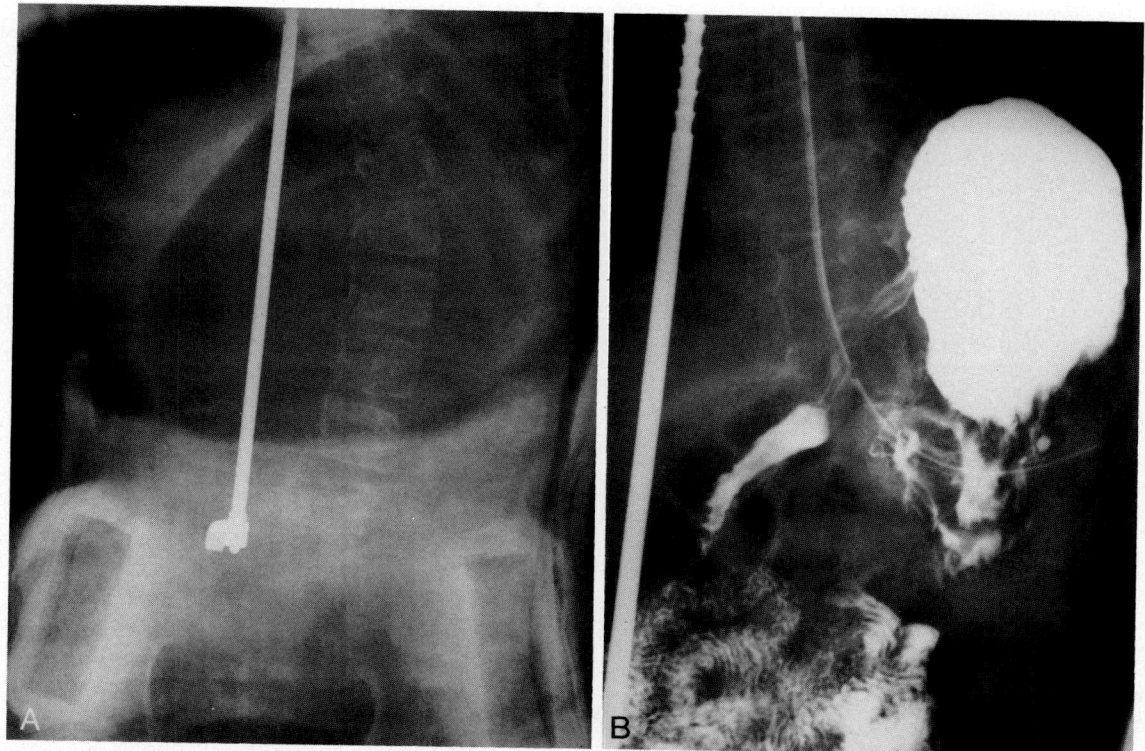

**Figure 76–23. Gastric volvulus. A.** Abdominal radiograph, taken 11 days after posterior spinal fusion in a patient who complained of nausea, shows marked gastric distention. The patient is in a body cast. **B.** Mesenteroaxial volvulus is the cause of this patient's symptoms. The gastric outlet is cephalad to the esophagogastric junction, as identified by the nasogastric tube. The underlying malrotation probably predisposed him to gastric volvulus. Note the abnormal position of the duodenum.

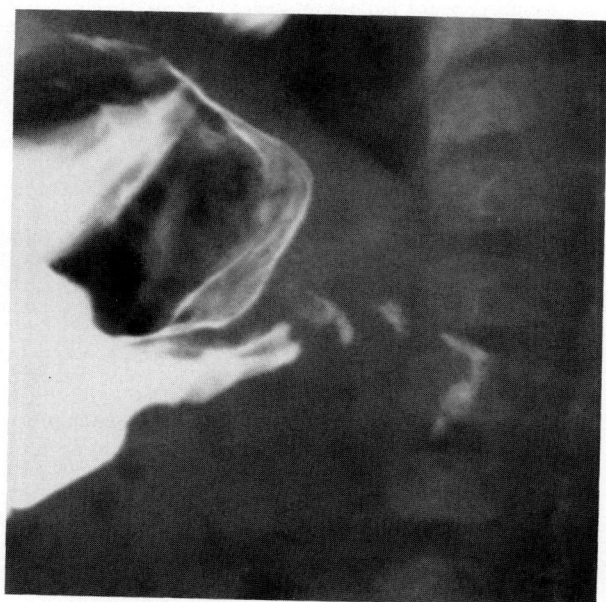

**Figure 76–24. Postoperative pyloromyotomy.** There is residual deformity of the pylorus but normal gastric emptying after surgery for pyloric stenosis. The follow-up examination was done for persistent "spitting" postoperatively. The patient responded to conservative medical therapy.

the sonographic and radiographic appearance should be normal for most patients. Until then, there is asymmetry of the channel as the mucosa eventrates through the defect of the "cracked" muscle. Incomplete pyloromyotomy results in persistence of an elongated, narrowed channel with poor gastric emptying.[129] Patients who have had a past history of successful pyloromyotomy may be left with some antropyloric dysfunction. Swallowed foreign bodies, such as coins, may have prolonged retention in the stomachs of these patients.[130]

# References

1. Grunebaum M, Kornreich L, Ziv N, et al: The imaging diagnosis of pyloric atresia. Z Kinderchir 40:308–311, 1985.
2. Gerber BC, Aberdeen SD: Prepyloric diaphragm: an unusual abnormality. Arch Surg 90:472–480, 1965.
3. Korber JS, Glasson MJ: Pyloric atresia associated with epidermolysis bullosa. J Pediatr 90:600–601, 1977.
4. Orense M, Garcia Hernandez JB, Celorio C, et al: Pyloric atresia associated with epidermolysis bullosa. Pediatr Radiol 17:435, 1987.
5. Berr F, Rienmueller R, Sauerbruch T: Successful endoscopic transection of a partially obstructing antral diaphragm. Gastroenterology 89:1147–1151, 1985.
6. Fujioka M, Fisher S, Young LW: Pseudoweb of the gastric antrum in infants. Pediatr Radiol 9:73–75, 1980.
7. Blazek FD, Boeckman CR: Prepyloric antral diaphragm: delays in treatment. J Pediatr Surg 22:948–949, 1987.
8. Tunnell WP, Smith EI: Antral web in infancy. J Pediatr Surg 15:152–155, 1980.
9. Mandell GA, Heyman S, Alavi A, et al: A case of microgastria in association with splenic-gonadal fusion. Pediatr Radiol 13:95–98, 1983.
10. Gorman B, Shaw DG: Congenital microgastria. Br J Radiol 57:260–262, 1984.
11. Dorney SF, Middleton AW, Kozlowski K, et al: Congenital agastria. J Pediatr Gastroenterol Nutr 6:307–310, 1987.
12. Fonkalsrud EW, deLorimier AA, Hays DM: Congenital atresia and stenosis of the duodenum: A review compiled from the members of the Surgical Section of the American Academy of Pediatrics. Pediatrics 43:79–83, 1969.
13. Hancock BJ, Wiseman NE: Congenital duodenal obstruction: the impact of an antenatal diagnosis. J Pediatr Surg 24:1027–1031, 1989.
14. Miro J, Bard H: Congenital atresia and stenosis of the duodenum: The impact of a prenatal diagnosis. Am J Obstet Gynecol 158:555–559, 1988.
15. Smith GV, Teele RL: Delayed diagnosis of duodenal obstruction in Down syndrome. AJR 120:315–321, 1980.
16. Karoll MP, Ghahremani GG, Port RB, et al: Diagnosis and management of intraluminal duodenal diverticulum. Dig Dis Sci 28:411–416, 1983.
17. Cremin BJ, Solomon DJ: Ultrasonic diagnosis of duodenal diaphragm. Pediatr Radiol 17:489–490, 1987.
18. Heithoff KB, Sane SM, Williams JH, et al: Bronchopulmonary foregut malformations: a unifying etiological concept. AJR 126:46–55, 1976.
18a. Murty TVM, Bhargava RK, Rakas FS: Gastroduodenal duplication. J Pediatr Surg 27:515–517, 1992.
19. Bower RJ, Sieber WK, Kiesewetter WB: Alimentary tract duplications in children. Ann Surg 188:669–674, 1978.
20. Neuhauser EBD, Harris GBC, Berret A: Roentgenographic features of neurenteric cysts. AJR 79:235–240, 1958.
21. Inouye WY, Farrell C, Fitts WT Jr, et al: Duodenal duplication: case report and literature review. Ann Surg 162:910–916, 1965.
22. Sommerschild H, Maurseth K, Skarstein A, et al: Duodenal duplication—a case with special features. Z Kinderchir 41:52–55, 1986.
23. Egelhoff JC, Bisset GS III, Strife JL: Multiple enteric duplications in an infant. Pediatr Radiol 16:160–161, 1986.
24. Teele RL, Henschke CI, Tapper D: The radiographic and ultrasonographic evaluation of enteric duplication cysts. Pediatr Radiol 10:9–14, 1980.
25. Lamont AC, Starinsky R, Cremin BJ: Ultrasonic diagnosis of duplication cysts in children. Br J Radiol 57:463–467, 1984.
26. Blake NS: Beak sign in duodenal duplication cyst. Pediatr Radiol 14:232–233, 1984.
27. Firor HV, Harris VJ: Rotational anomalies of the gut. Reemphasis of a neglected facet, isolated incomplete rotation of the duodenum. AJR 120:315–321, 1974.
28. Berdon WE, Baker DH, Bull S, et al: Midgut malrotation and volvulus. Which films are most helpful? Radiology 96:375–383, 1970.
29. Jit I: The development and the structure of the suspensory muscle of the duodenum. Anat Rec 113:395–407, 1952.
30. Katz ME, Siegel MJ, Shackelford GD, et al: The position and mobility of the duodenum in children. AJR 148:947–951, 1987.
31. Taylor GA, Teele RL: Chronic intestinal obstruction mimicking malrotation in children. Pediatr Radiol 15:392–394, 1985.
32. Rescoria FJ, Shedd FJ, Grosfeld JL, et al: Anomalies of intestinal rotation in childhood: analysis of 447 cases. Surgery 108:710–715, 1990.
33. Kullendorff CM, Mikaelsson C, Ivancev K: Malrotation in children with symptoms of gastrointestinal allergy and psychosomatic abdominal pain. Acta Paediatr Scand 74:296–299, 1985.
34. Brandt ML, Pokorny WJ, McGill CW, et al: Late presentations of midgut malrotation in children. Am J Surg 150:767–771, 1985.
35. Blumhagen JD: The role of ultrasonography in the evaluation of vomiting in infants. Pediatr Radiol 16:324–327, 1986.
36. Bowen AD: The vomiting infant: recent advances and unsettled issues in imaging. Radiol Clin North Am 26:377–392, 1988.
37. Cohen HL, Haller JO, Mestel AL, et al: Neonatal duodenum: fluid-aided US examination. Radiology 164:805–809, 1987.
38. Hayden CK Jr, Boulden TF, Swischuk LE, et al: Sonographic demonstration of duodenal obstruction with midgut volvulus. AJR 143:9–10, 1984.
39. Gaines PA, Saunders AJS, Drake D: Midgut malrotation diagnosed by ultrasound. Clin Radiol 38:51–53, 1987.
40. McCarten KM, Teele RL: Preduodenal portal vein: venography, ultrasonography, and review of the literature. Ann Radiol 21:155–160, 1978.
41. Ablow RC, Hoffer FA, Seashore JH, et al: Z-shaped duodenojejunal loop: sign of mesenteric fixation anomaly and congenital bands. AJR 141:461–464, 1983.
42. Brigham RA, Fallon WF, Saunders JR, et al: Paraduodenal hernia: diagnosis and surgical management. Surgery 96:498–502, 1984.
43. Schiavetti E, Sassotti G, Torricelli M, et al: "Apple peel" syndrome. A radiological study. Pediatr Radiol 14:380–383, 1984.
44. Shaw A, Blanc WA, Santulli TV, et al: Spontaneous rupture of the stomach in the newborn: a clinical and experimental study. Surgery 58:561–571, 1965.
45. Lloyd JR: The etiology of gastrointestinal perforation in the newborn. J Pediatr Surg 4:77–84, 1969.
46. Odita JC, Omene JA, Okolo AA: Gastric distension in neonatal necrotising enterocolitis. Pediatr Radiol 17:202–205, 1987.
47. Ibach JR, Inouye WY: Neonatal gastric perforation secondary to annular pancreas. Am J Surg 110:985–987, 1965.
48. Pochaczevsky R, Bryk DK: New roentgenographic signs of neonatal gastric perforation. Radiology 102:145–147, 1972.
49. Miller BM, Kumar A: Neonatal duodenal perforation. J Pediatr Gastroenterol Nutr 11:407–410, 1990.
50. Nord KS: Peptic ulcer disease in the pediatric population. Pediatr Clin North Am 35:117–140, 1988.
51. Magill HL, Hixson SD, Whitington G, et al: Duodenal perforation in childhood dermatomyositis. Pediatr Radiol 14:28–30, 1984.
52. Schullinger JN, Jacobs JC, Berdon WE: Diagnosis and management of gastrointestinal perforations in childhood dermatomyositis with particular reference to perforations of the duodenum. J Pediatr Surg 20:521–524, 1985.

53. Oi SZ, Shose Y, Asano N, et al: Intragastric migration of a ventriculoperitoneal shunt catheter. Neurosurgery 21:255–257, 1987.

54. Estrera A, Taylor W, Mills LF, et al: Corrosive burns of the esophagus and stomach: a recommendation for an aggressive surgical approach. Ann Thorac Surg 41:276–283, 1986.

55. Glick PL, Harrison MR, Adzick NS, et al: Gastric infarction secondary to small bowel obstruction: a preventable complication after Nissen fundoplication. J Pediatr Surg 22:941–943, 1987.

56. Haller JO, Cohen HL: Hypertrophic pyloric stenosis: diagnosis using ultrasound. Radiology 161:335–339, 1986.

57. Davies RP, Linke RJ, Robinson RG, et al: Sonographic diagnosis of infantile hypertrophic pyloric stenosis. J Ultrasound Med 11:603–605, 1992.

58. Breaux CH Jr, Georgeson KE, Royal SA, et al: Changing patterns in the diagnosis of hypertrophic pyloric stenosis. Pediatrics 81:213–217, 1988.

59. Forman HP, Leonidas JC, Kronfeld GD: A rational approach to the diagnosis of hypertrophic pyloric stenosis: do the results match the claims? J Pediatr Surg 25:262–266, 1990.

60. Blumhagen JD, Maclin L, Krauter D, et al: Sonographic diagnosis of hypertrophic pyloric stenosis. AJR 150:1367–1370, 1988.

61. Carver RA, Okorie M, Steiner GM, et al: Infantile hypertrophic pyloric stenosis—diagnosis from the pyloric muscle index. Clin Radiol 38:625–627, 1987.

62. Stunden RJ, LeQuesne GW, Little KET: The improved ultrasound diagnosis of hypertrophic pyloric stenosis. Pediatr Radiol 16:200–205, 1986.

63. Finkelstein MS, Mandell GA, Tarbell KV: Hypertrophic pyloric stenosis: volumetric measurement of nasogastric aspirate to determine the imaging modality. Radiology 177:759–761, 1990.

64. Jewett TC Jr, Caldarola V, Karp MP, et al: Intramural hematoma of the duodenum. Arch Surg 123:54–58, 1988.

65. Hernanz-Schulman M, Genieser NB, Ambrosino M: Sonographic diagnosis of intramural duodenal hematoma. J Ultrasound Med 8:273–276, 1989.

66. Kleinman PK, Brill PW, Winchester P: Resolving duodenal-jejunal hematoma in abused children. Radiology 160:747–750, 1986.

67. Ben-Baruch D, Powsner E, Cohen M, et al: Intramural hematoma of duodenum following endoscopic intestinal biopsy. J Pediatr Surg 22:1009–1010, 1987.

68. Tu RK, Starshak RJ, Brown B: CT diagnosis of gastric rupture following blunt abdominal trauma in a child. Pediatr Radiol 22:146–147, 1992.

68a. Touloukian RJ: Protocol for the nonoperative treatment of obstructing intramural duodenal hematoma during childhood. Am J Surg 145:330–334, 1983.

69. Foley C, Teele RL: Duodenal and pancreatic injuries following blunt trauma: evaluation by ultrasound. AJR 132:593–598, 1979.

70. Cook DE, Walsh JW, Vick CW, et al: Upper abdominal trauma: pitfalls in CT diagnosis. Radiology 159:65–69, 1986.

71. Wolfson PJ, Fabius RJ, Leibowitz AN: The Rapunzel syndrome: an unusual trichobezoar. Am J Gastroenterol 82:365–367, 1987.

72. Yoss BS: Human milk lactobezoars. J Pediatr 105:819–822, 1984.

73. Ament ME, Berquist WE, Vargas J, et al: Fiberoptic upper intestinal endoscopy in infants and children. Pediatr Clin North Am 35:141–155, 1988.

74. Welch KJ, Randolph JG, Ravitch MM, et al (eds): Pediatric Surgery (4th ed). Chicago: Year Book Medical Publishers, 1986, pp 907–908.

75. David TJ, Ferguson AP: Management of children who have swallowed button batteries. Arch Dis Child 61:321–322, 1986.

76. Niedzwiecki G, Wood BP: Radiological cases of the month. Gastric teratoma. Am J Dis Child 144:1147–1148, 1990.

77. Atwell JD, Claireaux AE, Nixon HH: Teratoma of the stomach in the newborn. J Pediatr Surg 2:197–204, 1967.

78. Earnshaw JJ: Gastric teratoma in infancy. J R Coll Surg Edinb 30:199–200, 1985.

78a. Ablin DS, Brant WE: Cystic leiomyosarcoma of the stomach in a child. J Clin Ultrasound 20:72–76, 1992.

79. Wurlitzer FP, Mares AJ, Isaacs H Jr, et al: Smooth muscle tumors of the stomach in childhood and adolescence. J Pediatr Surg 8:421–427, 1973.

80. Van Steenbergen W, Kojima T, Geboes K, et al: Gastric leiomyoblastoma with metastases to the liver. A 36-year follow-up study. Gastroenterology 89:875–881, 1985.

81. Krudy AG, Long JL, Magrath IT, et al: Gastric manifestations of North American Burkitt's lymphoma. Br J Radiol 56:697–702, 1983.

82. Mahour GH, Isaacs H Jr, Chang L: Primary malignant tumors of the stomach in children. J Pediatr Surg 15:603–608, 1980.

83. Haerer AF, Jackson JF, Evers CG: Ataxia-telangiectasia with gastric adenocarcinoma. JAMA 210:1884–1887, 1969.

84. Schneider K, Dickerhoff R, Bertele RM: Malignant gastric sarcoma—diagnosis by ultrasound and endoscopy. Pediatr Radiol 16:69–70, 1986.

85. Maves CK, Johnson JF, Bove D, et al: Gastric inflammatory pseudotumor in children. Radiology 173:381–383, 1989.

86. Iida M, Yao T, Itoh H, et al: Natural history of fundic gland polyposis in patients with familial adenomatosis coli/Gardner's syndrome. Gastroenterology 89:1021–1025, 1985.

87. Schroeder BA, Wells RG, Sty JR: Inflammatory fibroid polyp of the stomach in a child. Pediatr Radiol 17:71–72, 1987.

88. Buts J-P, Gosseye S, Claus D, et al: Solitary hyperplastic polyp of the stomach. Am J Dis Child 135:846–847, 1981.

89. Katz ME, Blocker SH, McAlister WH: Focal foveolar hyperplasia presenting as an antral-pyloric mass in a young infant. Pediatr Radiol 15:136–137, 1985.

90. McAlister WH, Katz ME, Perlman JM, et al: Sonography of focal foveolar hyperplasia causing gastric obstruction in an infant. Pediatr Radiol 18:79–81, 1988.

91. Tishler JM, Han SY, Colcher H, et al: Neurogenic tumors of the duodenum in patients with neurofibromatosis. Radiology 149:51–53, 1983.

92. Plavsic B, Jereb-Provic B: Radiologic and endoscopic diagnosis of duodenal angioma. Acta Radiol 28:735–738, 1987.

93. Kilman WJ, Berk RN: The spectrum of radiographic features of aberrant pancreatic rests involving the stomach. Radiology 123:291–296, 1977.

94. Lamont AC, Rode H: Retrograde jejuno-duodeno-gastric intussusception. Br J Radiol 58:559–561, 1985.

95. Drumm B, Rhoads JM, Stringer DA, et al: Peptic ulcer disease in children: etiology, clinical findings and clinical course. Pediatrics 82(part 2):410–414, 1988.

96. Rosioru C, Glassman MS, Berezin SH, et al: Treatment of *Helicobacter pylori*–associated gastroduodenal disease in children. Dig Dis Sci 38:123–128, 1993.

97. Hayden CK Jr, Swischuk LE, Rytting JE: Gastric ulcer disease in infants: US findings. Radiology 164:131–134, 1987.

98. Ordera G, Vaira D, Holton J, et al: *Helicobacter pylori* in children with peptic ulcer and their families. Dig Dis Sci 36:572–576, 1991.

98a. Mitchell JD, Mitchell HM, Tobias V: Acute *Helicobacter pylori* in recurrent, functional abdominal pain in children. Am J Gastroenterol 87:347–349, 1992.

99. Marks MP, Lanza MV, Kahlstrom EJ, et al: Pediatric hypertrophic gastropathy. AJR 147:1031–1034, 1986.

100. Coad NA, Shah KJ: Menetrier's disease in childhood associated with cytomegalovirus infection: a case report and review of the literature. Br J Radiol 59:615–620, 1986.

101. Day DL, Allan BT, Young LW: Radiological case of the month. Menetrier's disease. Am J Dis Child 142:91–92, 1988.

102. Gassner I, Strasser K, Bart G, et al: Sonographic appearance of Menetrier's disease in a child. J Ultrasound Med 9:537–539, 1990.

103. Teele RL, Katz AJ, Goldman H, et al: The radiographic features of eosinophilic gastroenteritis (allergic gastroenteropathy) of childhood. AJR 132:575–580, 1979.

104. Griscom NTG, Kirkpatrick JA Jr, Girdany BR, et al: Gastric antral narrowing in chronic granulomatous disease of childhood. Pediatrics 54:456–460, 1974.

105. Kopen PA, McAlister WH: Upper gastrointestinal and ultrasound examinations of gastric antral involvement in chronic granulomatous disease. Pediatr Radiol 14:91–93, 1984.

106. Ross TM, Fazio VW, Farmer RG: Long-term results of surgical treatment for Crohn's disease of the duodenum. Ann Surg 197:399–406, 1993.

107. Kirschner BS: Inflammatory bowel disease in children. Pediatr Clin North Am 35:189–208, 1988.

108. Manson DE, Stringer DA, Durie PR, et al: The radiologic and endoscopic investigation and etiologic classification of gastritis in children. Can Assoc Radiol J 41:201–206, 1990.

109. Bateson EM: Pyloro-duodenal gland tuberculosis in an aboriginal child. Australas Radiol 29:26–28, 1985.

110. Palmer PES: Diagnostic imaging in parasitic infections. Pediatr Clin North Am 32:1019–1040, 1985.

111. Sugimachi K, Inokuchi K, Ooiwa T, et al: Acute gastric anisakiasis. Analysis of 178 cases. JAMA 253:1012–1013, 1985.

112. Marshak RH, Ruoff M, Lindner AE: Roentgen manifestations of giardiasis. AJR 104:557–560, 1968.

113. Berkmen YM, Rabinowitz J: Gastrointestinal manifestations of the strongyloidiasis. AJR 115:306–311, 1972.

114. Martel WM: Radiologic features of esophagogastritis secondary to extremely caustic agents. Radiology 103:31–36, 1972.

115. Goldman LP, Weigert JM: Corrosive substance ingestion: a review. Am J Gastroenterol 79:85–90, 1984.

116. Ziprkowski MN, Teele RL: Gastric volvulus in childhood. AJR 132:921–925, 1979.

117. Cameron AEP, Howard ER: Gastric volvulus in childhood. J Pediatr Surg 22:944–947, 1987.

118. Senocak ME, Buyukpamukcu N, Hicsonmez A: Chronic gastric volvulus in children—a ten-year experience. Z Kinderchir 45:159–163, 1990.

119. Bonadio WA, Wood BP: Radiological case of the month. Intrathoracic stomach with volvulus. Am J Dis Child 143:503–504, 1989.

120. Reddy ER, Onyett H, Fitzgerald GW: Gastric torsion. Can Assoc Radiol J 40:47–48, 1989.

121. Moskovich R, Cheong-Leen P: Vascular compression of the duodenum. J R Soc Med 79:465–467, 1986.

122. McClenahan JH, Wood BP: Radiological case of the month. Hyperthyroidism as a cause of superior mesenteric artery syndrome. Am J Dis Child 142:685–686, 1988.

123. Ortiz C, Cleveland RH, Blickman JG, et al: Familial superior mesenteric artery syndrome. Pediatr Radiol 20:588–589, 1990.

124. Marchant EA, Alvear DT, Fagelman KM: True clinical entity of vascular compression of the duodenum in adolescence. Surg Gynecol Obstet 168:381–386, 1989.

125. Eaves ER, Schmidt GT: Chronic idiopathic megaduodenum in a family. Aust N Z J Med 15:1–6, 1985.

126. Milla PJ: Gastrointestinal motility disorders in children. Pediatr Clin North Am 35:311–330, 1988.

127. Phelan MS, Fine DR, Zentler-Munro PL, et al: Radiographic abnormalities of the duodenum in cystic fibrosis. Clin Radiol 34:573–577, 1983.

128. Fiedorek SC, Schulman RJ, Klish WJ: Endoscopic detection of peptic ulcer disease in cystic fibrosis. Clin Pediatr 25:243–246, 1986.

129. Jamroz GA, Blocker SH, McAlister WH: Radiographic findings after incomplete pyloromyotomy. Gastrointest Radiol 11:139–141, 1986.

130. Cass DT: Gastric retention of a swallowed coin after surgical treatment of pyloric stenosis. Aust Paediatr J 25:299–301, 1989.

# Pediatric Small Bowel Pathology

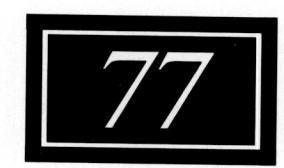

### Sandra K. Fernbach, M.D.

| MECKEL'S DIVERTICULUM | INTESTINAL LYMPHANGIECTASIA | HENOCH-SCHÖNLEIN PURPURA |
|---|---|---|
| Clinical Findings | Clinical Findings | Clinical Findings |
| Radiologic Findings | Radiologic Findings | Radiologic Findings |

## MECKEL'S DIVERTICULUM

In early fetal life, the primitive midgut communicates with the yolk sac through the omphalomesenteric or vitelline duct. Usually this duct involutes, but failure of complete regression can produce abnormalities anywhere along the course of the duct (Fig. 77–1). The most common anomaly is Meckel's diverticulum (MD), with omphalomesenteric or mesodiverticular bands, vitelline fistula, omphalomesenteric cyst, and umbilical polyps occurring less frequently.[1–6]

MD is a true diverticulum, comprising all bowel layers. Unlike alimentary duplications and most diverticula, MD is on the antimesenteric border of the bowel and has a separate blood supply. Ectopic gastric mucosa is found in 20 to 55% of patients with MD.[1]

## Clinical Findings

Almost half of the children with MD are seen before the age of 2 years because of intussusception or rectal bleeding.[1–7] Indeed, the diverticulum is the most common "lead point" found in children who come to surgery for an irreducible intussusception.[7] There is a 2:1 to 3:1 male predominance in this anomaly.

Painless lower gastrointestinal bleeding is a major complication of MD containing gastric mucosa; the production of gastric acid in a site where there is little secretion of buffering material leads to adjacent small bowel ulceration and hemorrhage. Approximately 90% of Meckel's diverticula that bleed contain gastric mucosa. At times the nourishing blood vessels in the diverticulum wall are the source of the bleeding.

Giant MD can serve as a lead point for volvulus and may present in the left upper quadrant.[8, 9] These enormous diverticula lead to stasis with bacterial overgrowth resulting in malabsorption.[9] Persistence of the omphalomesenteric duct as the omphalomesenteric cord or mesodiverticular band produces obstruction in a number of ways.[5, 6] Volvulus can occur around the cord or band, bowel can herniate beneath it, or the band may cause obstruction directly by extrinsically applied pressure. As in MD, there is a male predominance of these anomalies.

## Radiologic Findings

### Standard Radiography

Plain abdominal films are usually normal in MD but may show obstruction if there is an intussusception. MD is rarely filled on routine barium studies, but the higher pressures of enteroclysis may opacify the diverticulum or provide other suggestive evidence. A mucosal triangular plateau or a triradiate fold pattern in the right lower quadrant has been described in patients with MD and persistent omphalomesenteric band.[4] Air-filled giant diverticula (Fig. 77–2) may fill with contrast medium on delayed studies. Whenever MD is suspected clinically, barium studies should be postponed until after the pertechnetate scan because residual barium would absorb the emitted gamma rays and cause a false-negative study.

Children with symptomatic mesodiverticular bands often show findings of small bowel obstruction[1, 4, 5] (Fig. 77–3). Barium studies of the colon may be normal. Small bowel studies can show the level of obstruction, but few such studies are done because the clinical presentation and plain film findings are generally sufficient to prompt surgery, even when the exact diagnosis is uncertain.

### Nuclear Medicine

Technetium Tc 99m pertechnetate scintigraphy is the most widely used method for diagnosing MD and has a sensitivity of 85%.[10–13] The isotope localizes in the right lower quadrant or hypochondrium (Fig. 77–4) on positive scans. Pentagastrin should be used to stimulate MD gastric mucosal uptake if the result of a prior study has been negative or equivocal and MD is still strongly suspected.[14]

False-negative studies occur when there is residual barium in the region of the diverticulum, when there is profound ulceration with destruction of the offending gastric mucosa, or when the isotope is incorrectly considered to be within the genitourinary tract. Lateral scans of the abdomen should be performed routinely to minimize this last error.

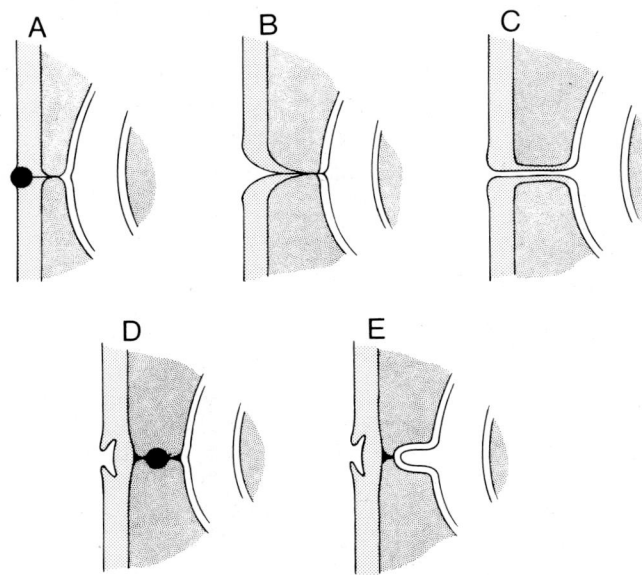

**Figure 77–1. Abnormalities of regression of the omphalomesenteric duct. A.** Umbilical polyp. **B.** Mesodiverticular or omphalomesenteric band. **C.** Patent omphalomesenteric duct or vitelline fistula. **D.** Vitelline cyst. **E.** Meckel's diverticulum.

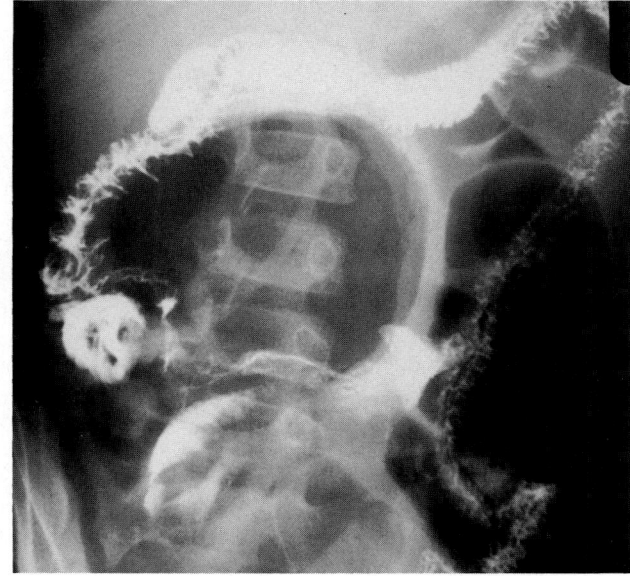

**Figure 77–2. Giant MD.** A film obtained after barium enema demonstrates residual contrast within colon and several small bowel loops. The large, rounded gas collection in the midabdomen, causing proximal small bowel obstruction, is a giant MD.

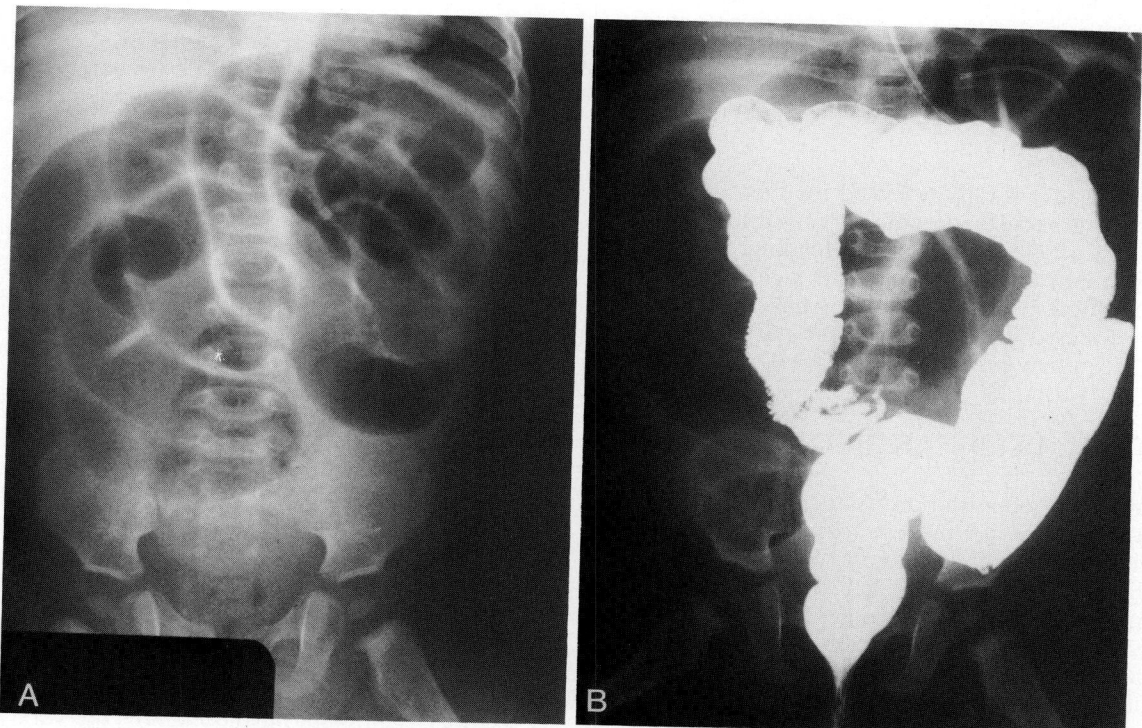

**Figure 77–3. Omphalomesenteric band. A**. Multiple dilated small bowel loops suggest a low obstruction on the plain abdominal film of an infant. **B**. The colon was normal except that the right colon was displaced from the lateral abdominal wall and it was impossible to distend the cecum. At surgery, small bowel that had herniated beneath the omphalomesenteric duct was found to be entrapped.

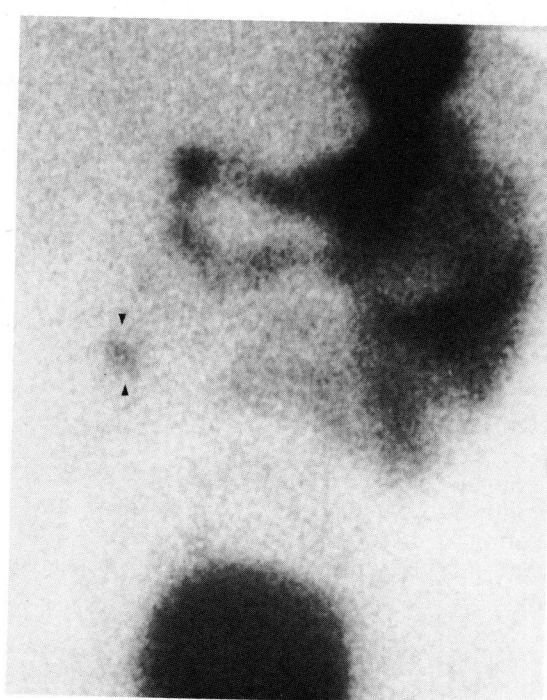

**Figure 77–4. Nuclear scintiscan—MD.** Technetium pertechnetate has passed from stomach into the proximal small bowel. A small region of activity in the right lower quadrant *(arrowheads)* is isotope localizing within the MD.

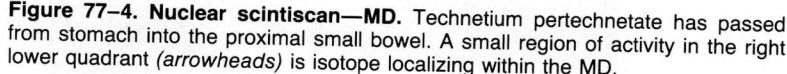

False-positive studies can also occur but are easier to recognize. Ectopic gastric mucosa in gastrointestinal cysts is responsible for most of the false-positive studies. Inflammatory processes may rarely localize the tracer as well, despite the absence of gastric mucosa.

### Angiography

Angiograms are usually reserved for the rare cases in which bleeding persists after negative barium or radionuclide studies.[15, 16] With active bleeding, a blush of contrast medium may be seen in the right lower quadrant. When there is no active hemorrhage, angiography should be directed to detection of the persistence of an abnormal primitive vascularity to the MD.

## INTESTINAL LYMPHANGIECTASIA

Congenital and acquired disorders of the small bowel lymphatics can produce protein loss, diarrhea, and decreased immunoglobulin levels.[17-21] Small bowel biopsy reveals dilated lymphatics in all bowel layers that may be accompanied by villous changes and infiltration of the mucosa by inflammatory cells. The process can involve large amounts of bowel or be focal.[22] Segmental enlargement of the lymphatic channels of the bowel and mesentery (lymphangioma) is a different entity that tends to present as a mass rather than with diarrhea or malabsorption.

### Clinical Findings

Because of the protein loss through the small bowel, the child may fail to thrive. Lymph cells may also be lost into the bowel lumen with resulting lymphopenia. Complaints of nausea and abdominal pain are common. Lymphatic abnormalities are also found in other organs.[17-21, 23] Swelling of the limbs may be due to abnormally developed lymphatics or hypoalbuminemia-induced edema and is more frequently seen in children with congenital intestinal lymphangiectasia than in adults who acquire the disease. The secondary form of lymphangiectasia develops in the setting of constrictive pericarditis, pancreatitis, retroperitoneal fibrosis, and inflammatory bowel disease.[24, 25]

### Radiologic Findings

Small bowel series show thickening of the valvulae conniventes, nodularity of the mucosa, and excess secretions if there is malabsorption. The caliber of the gut is normal. Barium enema examination may show thickening of the affected colonic folds.

The abnormal, dilated lymphatics have been observed sonographically.[26] Sonography can also demonstrate ascites and the thickened bowel walls and mesentery. The latter changes may be primary or secondary to the hypoproteinemia caused by this protein-losing enteropathy.

Findings on lymphangiography include hypoplasia or atresia of normal lymphatics in the extremities and abnormal lymphatics and lymph nodes in the abdomen, with occasional leakage of contrast medium into the peritoneal cavity. These tests, however, are rarely performed to diagnose intestinal lymphangiectasia.[27]

## HENOCH-SCHÖNLEIN PURPURA

### Clinical Findings

Vasculitis underlies the symptoms and complications of Henoch-Schönlein purpura. Skin, bowel, gut, and kidney are commonly involved.[27, 28] Brain involvement may take many forms: seizures, blindness, or headache.[29] Arthralgias typically occur in a few large joints and can precede the skin lesions and obscure the diagnosis. The associated rash may evolve from an urticarial to a maculopapular rash to become the classically described palpable purpuric lesions. The skin lesions are most prominent over the buttocks and lower extremities. Biopsy of the skin lesions shows granulocytes around arterioles and venules.[28] Renal disease manifests as hematuria, but a significant decline in renal function is uncommon. Renal biopsy may document glomerulonephritis or changes of immunoglobulin A nephritis.[30]

Henoch-Schönlein purpura spares the very young and is most common in children between 3 and 10 years of age, with a slight male predominance. As many as 30% of affected patients may be older than 20 years.[28] It occurs more often in the winter than in other seasons.

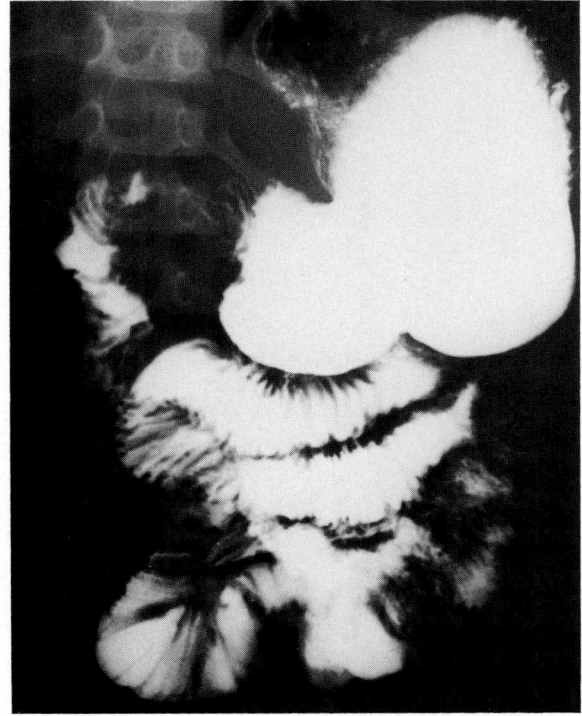

**Figure 77–5. Upper gastrointestinal series—Henoch-Schönlein purpura.** The valvulae are thickened in the jejunum. Contrast medium is being diluted as it passes into more distal, fluid-filled loops.

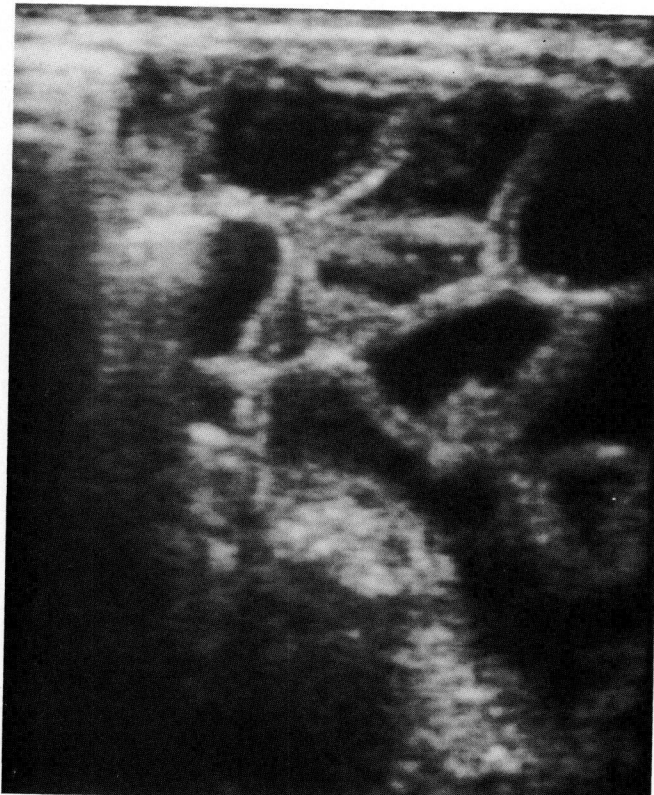

**Figure 77–6. Longitudinal ultrasound—Henoch-Schönlein purpura.** The bowel loops are distended with fluid and the walls are thickened.

The abdominal pain may be intense, simulating that of a surgical abdomen. Unfortunately, 3 to 5% of children with Henoch-Schönlein purpura develop bowel perforation or irreducible intussusception.[28] These intussusceptions are as likely to be ileoileal as the more usual ileocolic. Gastrointestinal bleeding is present in about half of the pediatric patients but is self-contained and unlikely to require transfusion. Such bleeding is less common in older patients. Relapse may follow initial clearing of symptoms. Most children recover completely without residua of the acute process.

## Radiologic Findings

Plain films of the abdomen are usually normal unless there has been perforation, intussusception with small bowel obstruction, or sufficient bowel wall thickening to produce thumbprinting of segments distended with air.[27] Studies of the upper gastrointestinal tract done with contrast material show mucosal thickening and submucosal edema (Fig. 77–5) that tend to be localized. Obstruction or ileal intussusception may be detected.[31–34] Sonography demonstrates mural thickening of affected bowel (Fig. 77–6). These loops are often distended with fluid.[33] Sonography is also useful in excluding other abdominal processes such as intussusception.

## References

1. Rutherford RB, Akers DR: Meckel's diverticulum: a review of 148 pediatric patients with special reference to the pattern of bleeding and to mesodiverticular bands. Surgery 59:618–626, 1966.
2. Berne AS: Meckel's diverticulum. X-ray diagnosis. N Engl J Med 260:690–696, 1959.
3. Dalinka MK, Wunder JF: Meckel's diverticulum and its complications with emphasis on roentgenologic demonstration. Radiology 106:295–298, 1973.
4. Maglinte DDT, Elmore MF, Isenberg M, et al: Meckel diverticulum: radiologic demonstration by enteroclysis. AJR 134:925–932, 1980.
5. Johnson GF, Verhagen AD: Mesodiverticular band. Radiology 123:409–412, 1977.
6. Gaisie G, Curnes JT, Scatliff JH, et al: Neonatal intestinal obstruction from omphalomesenteric duct remnants. AJR 144:109–112, 1985.
7. Mok PM, Humphry A: Ileo-ileocolic intussusception: radiologic features and reducibility. Pediatr Radiol 12:127–131, 1982.
8. Galifer RB, Noblet D, Ferran JL: "Giant Meckel's diverticulum": report of an unusual case in a child with preoperative x-ray diagnosis. Pediatr Radiol 11:217–218, 1981.
9. Orenstein SR, Magill HL, Whitington PF: Ileal dysgenesis presenting with anemia and growth failure. Pediatr Radiol 14:59–61, 1984.
10. Conway JJ: Radionuclide diagnosis of Meckel's diverticulum. Gastrointest Radiol 5:209–213, 1980.
11. Rosenthall L, Henry JH, Murphy DA, et al: Radiopertechnetate imaging of the Meckel's diverticulum. Radiology 105:371–373, 1972.
12. Fries M, Mortensson W, Robertson B: Technetium pertechnetate scintigraphy to detect ectopic gastric mucosa in Meckel's diverticulum. Acta Radiol Diagn 25:417–422, 1984.
13. Sfakianakis GN, Haase GM: Abdominal scintigraphy for ectopic gastric mucosa: a retrospective analysis of 143 studies. AJR 138:7–12, 1982.
14. Treves S, Grand RJ, Eraklis AJ: Pentagastrin stimulation of technetium-99m uptake by ectopic gastric mucosa in a Meckel's diverticulum. Radiology 128:711–712, 1978.
15. Bree RL, Reuter SR: Angiographic demonstration of a bleeding Meckel's diverticulum. Radiology 108:287–288, 1973.
16. Routh WD, Lawdahl RB, Lund E, et al: Meckel's diverticula: angiographic diagnosis in patients with non-acute hemorrhage and negative scintigraphy. Pediatr Radiol 20:152–156, 1990.
17. Waldmann TA, Steinfeld JL, Dutcher TF, et al: The role of the gastrointestinal system in "idiopathic hypoproteinemia." Gastroenterology 41:197–207, 1961.
18. Gorske K, Winchester P, Grossman H: Unusual protein-losing enteropathies in children. Radiology 92:739–744, 1969.
19. Olmsted WW, Madewell JE: Lymphangiectasia of the small intestine: description and pathophysiology of roentgenographic signs. Gastrointest Radiol 1:241–243, 1976.
20. Marshak RH, Lindner AE, Maklansky D: Lymphoreticular disorders of the gastrointestinal tract: roentgenographic features. Gastrointest Radiol 4:103–120, 1979.
21. Kingham JG, Moriarty KJ, Furness M, et al: Lymphangiectasia of the colon and small intestine. Br J Radiol 55:774–77, 1982.
22. Simpson AJ, Amer H: Segmental lymphangiectasia of the small bowel. Am J Gastroenterol 72:95–100, 1979.
23. Lanning P, Simila S, Sioramo I, et al: Lymphatic abnormalities in Noonan's syndrome. Pediatr Radiol 7:106–109, 1978.
24. Wilkinson P, Pinto B, Senior JR: Reversible protein-losing enteropathy with intestinal lymphangiectasia secondary to chronic constrictive pericarditis. N Engl J Med 273:1178–1181, 1965.
25. Abramowsky C, Hupertz V, Kilbridge P, et al: Intestinal lymphangiectasia in children: a study of upper gastrointestinal endoscopic biopsies. Pediatr Pathol 9:289–297, 1989.
26. Dorne HL, Jequier S: Sonography of intestinal lymphangiectasia. J Ultrasound Med 5:13–16, 1986.
27. Glasier CM, Siegel MJ, McAlister WH, et al: Henoch-Schönlein syndrome in children: gastrointestinal manifestations. AJR 136:1081–1085, 1981.

28. Mills JA, Michel BA, Bloch DA, et al: The American College of Rheumatology 1990 criteria for the classification of Henoch-Schönlein purpura. Arthritis Rheum 33:1114–1121, 1990.

29. Elinson P, Foster KW, Kaufman DB: Magnetic resonance imaging of central nervous system vasculitis. A case report of Henoch-Schönlein purpura. Acta Paediatr Scand 79:710–713, 1990.

30. Waldo FB: Is Henoch-Schönlein purpura the systemic form of IgA nephropathy? Am J Kidney Dis 12:373–377, 1988.

31. Mir E: Surgical complications in Henoch-Schönlein purpura in childhood. Z Kinderchir 43:391–393, 1988.

32. Cull DL, Rosario V, Lally KP, et al: Surgical implications of Henoch-Schönlein purpura. J Pediatr Surg 25:741–742, 1990.

33. Miyamoto Y, Fukuda Y, Urushibara K, et al: Ultrasonographic findings in duodenum caused by Schönlein-Henoch purpura. JCU 17:299–303, 1989.

34. Katz S, Borst M, Seekri I, et al: Surgical evaluation of Henoch-Schönlein purpura. Arch Surg 126:849–854, 1991.

# Radiology of the Pediatric Colon

Sandra K. Fernbach, M.D.

## LYMPHOID FOLLICULAR PATTERN AND LYMPHOID HYPERPLASIA

Lymphoid follicles are a normal feature of the gastrointestinal tract and are much more prominent in children than adults. The lymphoid follicular pattern is best appreciated on double contrast barium enema studies and may be seen in 50 to 70% of such examinations in children[1–5] (Fig. 78–1). Normal follicles are 2 mm in diameter, are uniform in size, and often have central umbilications. They can simulate familial polyposis in the way they carpet the colon. Follicles larger than 2 to 3 mm are associated with nodular lymphoid hyperplasia, which occurs in response to a number of immunologic, infectious, inflammatory, or allergic stimuli.[6–9]

## ANTERIOR ANUS

In the late 1970s, the anterior anus was recognized as another organic cause of constipation. Children with this anomaly were previously said to have psychogenic constipation or suspected of having Hirschsprung's disease (HD).[10, 11] The anterior anus is considered by some to be a mild variant of imperforate anus with perineal fistula.[10–12] As with other forms of imperforate anus, an anomaly of the distal sphincter seen at surgery seems to explain the radiologic changes.[13]

Although physical examination would seem to be the preferred method of diagnosis, the amount of displacement may be minimal and hard to appreciate even when sought. The external changes may be harder to discern in boys than in girls. Measurements can be made of fixed sites on the perineum to determine whether anal position is normal, but these are not widely used because position alone does not determine alteration in function.[14] Some girls with an anus displaced so far anteriorly that it abuts the vagina have normal evacuation; in others, a small amount of displacement is associated with severe constipation.

Affected children may have an abnormal evacuation history that begins at birth or may evacuate normally for several months. A long interval between bowel movements, straining with defecation, and fecal soiling are also common complaints.[10, 11]

Treatment is surgical. The anorectal canal and internal anal sphincter are mobilized and a neoanus is created at the more normal location, usually determined by visualizing a pigmented region in the midline of the perineum. Reports document a low complication rate and development of near-normal evacuation patterns.[10–12]

The differential diagnosis of anterior anus is as follows: Hirschsprung's disease, neurologic constipation, and psychogenic constipation. These other disorders can usually be excluded on the basis of physical examination, spine films, rectal manometry, and rectal biopsy.

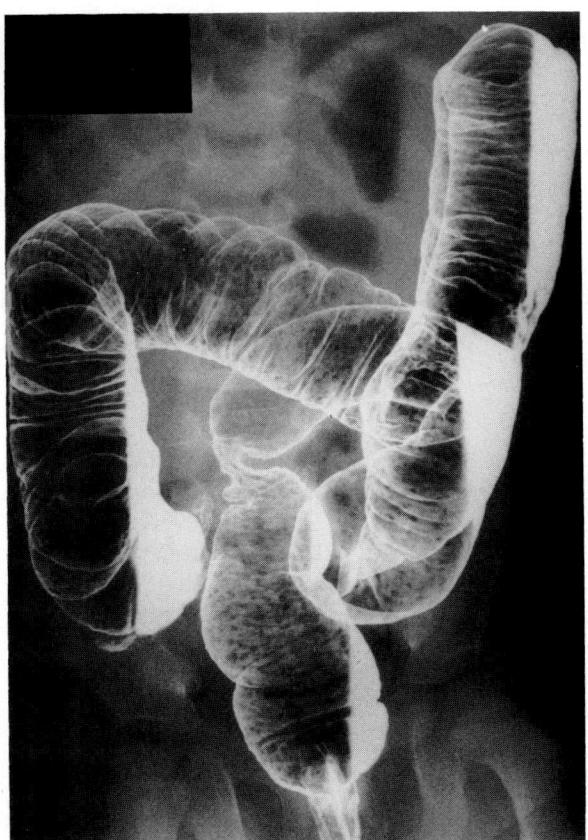

**Figure 78–1. Lymphoid follicular pattern.** Fine nodules of similar size are seen throughout the colon on this double contrast barium enema study.

## Radiologic Findings

Plain films should be obtained to evaluate the amount of stool present and to detect spinal anomalies. If a large amount of stool obscures the sacrum, a lateral spine film may be necessary to exclude deformities that may be associated with neurogenic rectal dysfunction.

When a barium enema examination is performed, it is helpful to mark the location of the anus with barium paste. The lateral rectal view is, as in children with HD, key in diagnosis. In children with anterior anus, there is a deep posterior recess or shelf behind the rectal catheter (Fig. 78–2). The rectum descends below the last turn of the colon as it passes anteriorly to become the anus.[13] Postevacuation films, with the rectal tube removed, show that the anus is more anterior than usual and lies at an angle to the posterior rectal shelf, which is in a normal position a few millimeters anterior to the sacrum.[14]

## HIRSCHSPRUNG'S DISEASE

## Pathologic Findings

HD is characterized by absence of ganglion cells in Auerbach's and Meissner's plexus in the affected

bowel.[15] The process is believed to be due to arrest of the usual craniocaudal migration of primitive neuroblasts, which in some children is associated with other abnormalities of the neural crest.[16–18] The involved segment is of variable length and is always distal. Approximately 85% of cases are limited to the descending colon and distal segments; 55% of all cases involve the rectosigmoid colon and distal segments.[15, 19] Total colonic aganglionosis, with or without small bowel involvement, is seen in 8% of affected children.[15–19] Zonal aganglionosis is reported but is rare.[20–22] It may be an acquired lesion or have a different embryologic basis. Extensive aganglionosis is a rare, usually lethal variant in which the entire small bowel and even the stomach lack normal ganglion cells.[23, 24] Two thirds to three quarters of affected patients are male.

## Clinical Findings

HD is the most common cause of neonatal obstruction of the colon and more than 70% of cases are diagnosed in this period.[24] Neonates present with delayed passage of meconium, abdominal distention, and/or vomiting. Delay in diagnosis can lead to bowel perforation or potentially fatal enterocolitis. In one series, 4.7% of children with HD died of enterocolitis, usually within the first 3 months of life, and in another, 10% of children with HD developed enterocolitis before surgery.[25] Pseudomembranous colitis may also develop in these children even without recent exposure to antibiotics and can lead

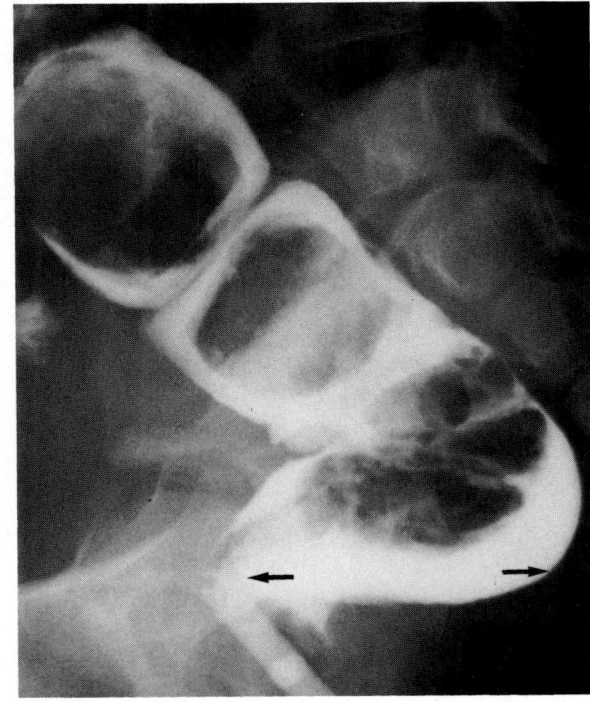

**Figure 78–2. Anterior anus.** Barium enema study shows that the rectum is capacious and contains much fecal debris. A deep posterior segment of the rectum *(arrows)* far behind the anus is identified by the catheter tip.

to perforation of the appendix and proximal colon in 4.4% of cases. Because pseudomembranous colitis is treatable, some authors recommend that stool cultures be obtained in children with HD and "typical" colitis.[25]

Older children with undiagnosed HD usually have an abnormal neonatal stooling history and unremitting constipation. Occasionally the diagnosis is delayed until the second and third decades of life, leading to chronic constipation, chronic laxative abuse, and colonic distention, which predispose the colon to volvulus.

Clinical history and physical examination are generally quite specific. In contrast to children with psychogenic constipation, whose symptoms begin at the time of toilet training, children with HD have an abnormal stooling history from birth and rarely have fecal soiling of their undergarments. On physical examination the rectal ampulla is full in children with psychogenic constipation and empty in those with HD.[15]

Rectal manometry is performed to differentiate between these two groups of children if the diagnosis remains uncertain. Distention of the rectum fails to produce normal reflex relaxation of the internal sphincter in children with HD.[26–32] Rectal manometry is a relatively noninvasive way to screen children with suspected HD but may give equivocal or incorrect results in approximately 16% of those tested.[31]

Biopsy of the rectum establishes the diagnosis definitively. Rarely, this procedure can lead to a stricture.[30]

Ultrashort segment HD is a controversial variant in which the clinical, radiologic, and pathologic criteria of classical HD are lacking.[33–36] The symptoms are milder and the children tend to be older at presentation. There may be a full rectal ampulla, fecal soiling, and ganglion cells present on rectal biopsy specimens. Manometric studies, however, are abnormal, showing failure of the internal sphincter to relax in response to rectal stimulation as in classic HD.[35] These children do not require the more complicated surgical procedures performed in children with classic HD but instead do well with a simple anal myomectomy.[36]

In most children, HD is an isolated finding, but there is an increased incidence of this disorder in children with trisomy 21, Waardenburg's syndrome, Smith-Lemli-Opitz syndrome, and several other syndromes. In some families, HD appears to be genetically transmitted.[37–39]

There is an increased incidence of malrotation in children with HD.[40, 41] In utero, this malrotation may lead to volvulus and ischemia and contribute to the increased incidence of intestinal atresia in children with HD.[42, 43] The association of HD with intestinal atresia also suggests that the ischemic event that produced the atresia may have interfered with the craniocaudal migration of neuroblasts.

## Therapy

Initial treatment of HD is directed toward decompressing the colon to prevent enterocolitis. Although this can be achieved with saline enemas, colostomy above the aganglionic segment, with intraoperative pathologic guidance to define the true transition zone, is the more common treatment.

Definitive or corrective surgery is usually delayed until the child is 1 year of age. All operations (e.g., the Swenson, the Soave, and the Duhamel procedures) attempt to restore normal function by removing or bypassing the aganglionic segment.[15, 19]

When diagnosis is made in an older child, a colostomy is performed before corrective surgery to enable the enlarged colon to normalize in caliber. This makes later surgery easier. Postoperative complications include leakage at the anastomosis, continued obstruction, or, rarely, development of aganglionosis in a previously normal segment.[22, 23, 44]

Children with total colonic aganglionosis undergo ileostomy, again under histologic intraoperative guidance so that the ileostomy is placed in a segment that contains ganglion cells. Later these children undergo total colectomy and ileoanal, endorectal pull-through.

## Radiologic Findings

The early diagnosis of HD can be lifesaving. Unfortunately, radiologic diagnosis is more difficult in the neonatal period than in later life. Plain films show changes of distal bowel obstruction.[45–49] Rarely, calcifications may be present in bowel lumen.[50]

Contrast enema examination is necessary to visualize the colon and to exclude other causes of distal obstruction such as meconium plug, small left colon syndrome, and colonic atresia. When HD is suspected, powdered barium should be reconstituted with normal saline because retention and absorption of tap water above an aganglionic segment can cause overhydration and serious electrolyte disturbances. A small caliber enema tip should be used so as not to dilate the rectum.[32, 42]

The enema is begun with the infant or child in the left lateral decubitus position to improve visualization of the segments most likely to be abnormal: the rectum and the rectosigmoid (Fig. 78–3). In infants, a funnel- or cone-shaped appearance suggests HD (Fig. 78–4). I discourage filling the colon above such an abnormal configuration, despite reports that delayed abdominal films demonstrating retained barium are valuable in confirming the diagnosis, for fear of possible barium impaction. A lateral film of the rectum obtained after the enema tip has been removed may be key to appreciating the abnormally small rectal vault and demonstrating the abnormal rectosigmoid index.[51–53]

In the neonate with total colonic aganglionosis, the colon may fill easily with rapid reflux into the small bowel, a transition zone between normal and dilated bowel in the ileum, and loss of the normal colonic redundancy.[45–47] These neonates may present with a meconium plug or the colon may have a normal appearance.[48]

Barium enemas in neonates with active colitis demonstrate a spastic colon that is difficult to distend (Fig. 78–5). When the mucosa has a spiculated or saw-toothed

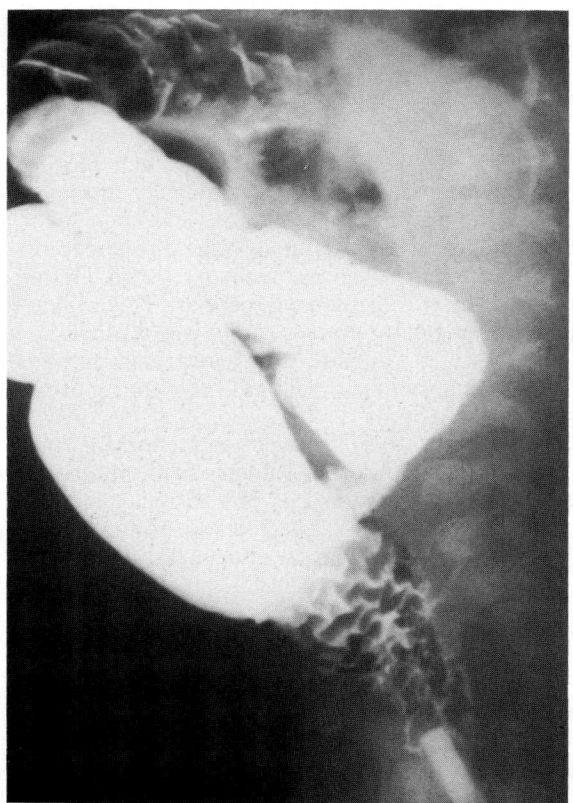

**Figure 78–3. Hirschsprung's disease.** On this lateral view from a barium enema study the rectum is smaller than the sigmoid colon. The corrugated àppearance of the rectum has also been described in HD.

pattern, the diagnosis of HD with colitis should be considered.[44] When there is active colitis, barium is rapidly expelled, which accounts for false-negative post-evacuation films in children with HD.

In the older child with a history of constipation, I prefer to study the unprepared colon. Decompression of the dilated colon and enema-produced dilation of the rectum may decrease the abrupt changes that produce the classic transition zone. *Transition zone* is the term applied to the region in which there is a marked change in caliber, with the dilated normal colon above and the narrowed aganglionic colon below.[54] There may be aganglionic bowel in the dilated segment; the massively enlarged colon pushes its contents distally and dilates the abnormal segment. Therefore, surgical and pathologic confirmation of the true transition zone is always obtained before palliative or corrective surgery is performed.

When barium enema examination shows a dilated rectum and sigmoid colon, classic HD has been excluded and there is little value in filling the more proximal colon. Ultrashort HD must be diagnosed with an alternative method. Limited filling of the colon in the severely constipated child also minimizes the need for vigorous colon cleansing to prevent barium impaction. When the child undergoes a bypass procedure as the initial part of surgical therapy, the distal segment is usually studied before re-establishing gastrointestinal continuity. On barium enema study this segment is poorly distensible and rigid with mucosal thickening, nodularity, and polypoid lymphoid hyperplasia. Redundancy is often seen as a result of prior inflammation and dilatation of the ganglionic portion of this segment.[55, 56]

After definitive corrective surgery, there is no routine time or indication for radiologic study. If the child is septic, a gentle injection of water-soluble contrast medium into the rectum through a tiny catheter is useful to exclude leakage. In the absence of symptoms, studies done with contrast material may be delayed until the child has had several months to heal.

## INFLAMMATORY BOWEL DISEASE

The pathology, epidemiology, and radiographic findings in ulcerative colitis are discussed extensively in Chapter 62 and Crohn's colitis is covered in Chapters 62 and 159. This discussion focuses on special aspects of ulcerative colitis in the child. Pediatric Crohn's disease is presented in Chapter 79.

Ulcerative colitis is rare during the first and uncommon in the second decade of life. The symptoms of diarrhea with blood and/or mucus, abdominal pain, and fever suggest a juvenile polyp, Meckel's diverticulum, or infectious or allergic colitis. Anemia and weight loss may also develop.[57–59]

The radiographic findings in children with ulcerative colitis are identical to those in adults. Toxic megacolon, however, occurs much less commonly in children.[57–59]

## OTHER COLITIDES AND CAUSES OF DIARRHEA

Persistent bloody or watery diarrhea is unusual in children and a cause for concern because it can cause electrolyte abnormalities, protein and weight loss, and irritation of the buttocks. Viral, bacterial, or parasitic processes are frequently the source of the problem.[60–63] Celiac disease, which is usually considered to be a small bowel disorder, may be the most common noninfectious form of diarrhea. Diagnosis is based on response to a gluten-free diet and small bowel biopsy.

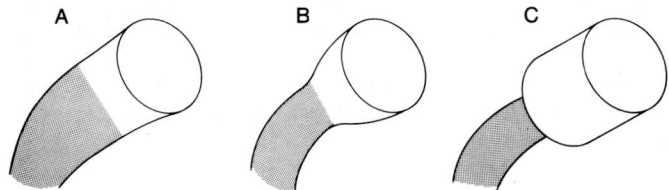

**Figure 78–4. Hirschsprung's disease.** Diagram depicting the varied appearance of the transition zone in the rectum in HD, lateral view. **A.** In the very young, the transition zone may have a cone shape with the caliber imperceptibly decreasing as it goes from sigmoid colon to rectum. **B** and **C.** A discrete change in caliber is more typical, with the radiologic transition zone more clearly defined in **C.**

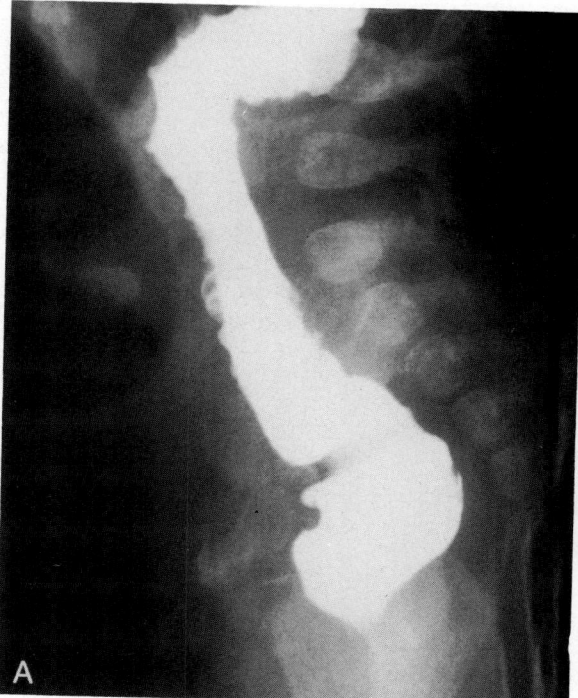
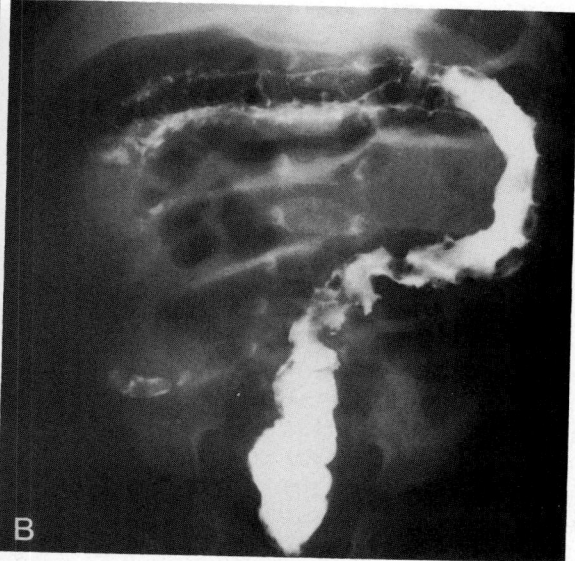

**Figure 78–5. Total colonic Hirschsprung's disease.** Frontal **(A)** and lateral **(B)** views from a barium enema study show that the rectum is larger than the more proximal colon. Intense spasm from colitis prevents colonic distention. Spiculation and mucosal ulcerations are present throughout except in the rectum.

Milk allergy and lactose intolerance are two other causes of diarrhea in children. Inability to digest lactose can cause diarrhea in the first year of life. Removal of the offending disaccharide results in remission of symptoms. The proteins in cow's milk and soy-based milk can damage the gastrointestinal mucosa in some children with allergy to these foods. Rectal biopsy shows diagnostic histologic changes.[64, 65] Barium enema examination may show nonspecific changes of colitis: narrowing, thumbprinting, and spasm.[64] Although these changes usually involve the entire colon, segmental changes have been described.[65] The wall of the small bowel may also be affected, producing thickening of the valvulae conniventes or narrowing of involved segments.

An even more unusual cause of diarrhea in children is collagenous colitis, an entity described in adults before it was reported in children.[66–68] This form of colitis is associated with watery diarrhea and colicky pain. Microscopic analysis of biopsy specimens of mucosa is necessary for diagnosis. Widening of the collagen band of the basement membrane, few inflammatory cells, and edema of the lamina propria are observed. Symptoms usually respond to corticosteroids or sulfasalazine but may recur after the medications have been withdrawn.

Watery diarrhea may also be a sign of tumor. A small fraction of ganglioneuroblastomas and ganglioneuromas secrete vasoactive intestinal polypeptide, which, as its name suggests, produces increased intestinal motility.[69] This disorder is often unsuspected but the diagnosis is made when the plain film preceding barium enema reveals paravertebral calcifications. About two thirds of tumors that secrete the polypeptide in children are in the paravertebral region and about 50% have visible calcification. Plasma levels of vasoactive intestinal poly-

peptide can be measured to confirm the diagnosis and computed tomography (CT) or sonography may be useful in better delineating tumor size and tissue of origin. Removal of the tumor is followed by cessation of the diarrhea.

Cleansing enemas may cause colitis if performed with inappropriate agents. Alkaline detergents can cause severe mucosal damage and rectal bleeding acutely. Submucosal damage manifests later as lack of distensibility or narrowing of the colon.[70]

Kawasaki's disease may cause a variety of physical and physiologic changes: abdominal pain, serum abnormalities indicative of liver disease, frank organ necrosis, and atypical colitis simulating ischemic colitis disease.[71]

In up to 28% of children, the etiology of the diarrhea may elude diagnosis despite a battery of diagnostic tests.[60]

# HEMOLYTIC-UREMIC SYNDROME

## Clinical Findings

Hemolytic-uremic syndrome is a pathologic entity of unknown etiology characterized by an acute microangiopathic hemolytic anemia, oliguric renal failure, and thrombocytopenia.[72–77] It usually occurs in infants and children who present with an influenza-like illness, gastroenteritis, and bloody diarrhea that precede the more striking renal and hematologic manifestations by several days or weeks.[75] The gastrointestinal manifestations of the prodromal period are protean, requiring differentiation from ulcerative colitis, pseudomembranous colitis, granulomatous colitis, shigellosis, salmonellosis, cecal polyp, and intussusception.[76] Diagnosis is often delayed until anemia, thrombocytopenia, or renal failure appears.[72–80] Urinalysis provides vital information because the majority of patients have proteinuria, hemoglobinuria, or hematuria (microscopic or gross) early in the course of the disease. The peripheral blood smear is also suggestive when schistocytes and burr cells are present.

Infants younger than 6 months of age appear to be spared. Few with hemolytic-uremic syndrome are younger than 2 years or older than 10 years at presentation.

The vigorous fluid therapy given to children with active peritoneal signs typical of hemolytic-uremic syndrome results in overhydration and causes peripheral and pulmonary edema when acute renal failure develops. Prompt recognition of the clinical and radiologic appearance of the syndrome may avert an unwarranted laparotomy and contribute to the proper management of fluid needs. Dialysis is necessary until renal function resumes.

Most patients recover without sequelae. Death, more frequent in children with anuria, is attributable not to the anuria but to the manner in which the thrombotic process affects other organs.

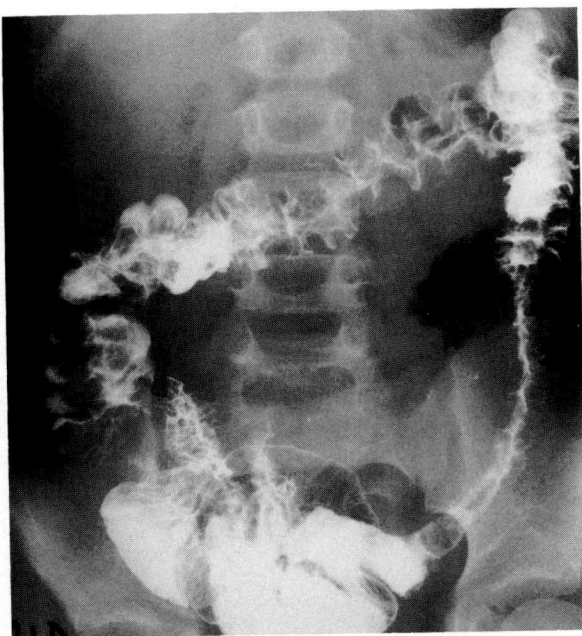

**Figure 78–6. Hemolytic-uremic syndrome.** Spasm and ulceration are present in the descending colon and mild thumbprinting deforms the transverse colon on this barium enema study.

## Radiologic Findings

Plain film findings are often abnormal but nondiagnostic.[77–79] A disordered bowel gas pattern and thickening or thumbprinting of affected bowel loops may be noted.

The colon may demonstrate spasm, thumbprinting, ulceration, straightening, and narrowing of edematous segments (Fig. 78–6) on barium enema examination.[76, 77, 79] Later, strictures may form.

Ultrasound is useful in excluding causes of a surgical abdomen and in showing changes that suggest the diagnosis: peritoneal fluid, bowel wall thickening, and increased echogenicity of the renal parenchyma. During periods of oliguria or anuria, there are profound abnormalities of systolic and diastolic blood flow on Doppler studies. A return of normal blood flow heralds impending diuresis, useful information in children undergoing dialysis.[80]

## APPENDICITIS

### Clinical Findings

The most common indication for emergency laparotomy in children is an inflamed or ruptured appendix. The diagnosis is based on symptoms (abdominal pain, vomiting, low-grade fever), signs (pain on palpation of the right lower quadrant, rebound tenderness), and laboratory data (low-grade leukocytosis, absence of urinary tract infection). When the presentation is classic, surgery is usually performed without radiologic studies.

A large number of children present atypically with a history of fever of unknown origin, change in bowel habits, or hepatomegaly.[81] In these cases, the diagnosis of appendicitis is made only after imaging studies are performed. Misdiagnosis occurs in about 10% of patients and other significant abdominal disease clinically simulating appendicitis is present in another 5%.[82, 83] These diagnostic difficulties occur more often in teen-age girls, in whom ovarian cysts and teratomas, pelvic inflammatory disease, and ectopic pregnancies may produce localized pain and gastrointestinal symptoms.[83a] Pancreatitis, bowel perforation, mesenteric lymphadenopathy, and inflammatory bowel disease may produce diagnostic error in children of both sexes.[83]

Rupture or perforation occurs in about 25% of cases of appendicitis and is more common in the pediatric population.[84, 85] In children, a normal appendix may become inflamed and rupture within 3 hours. After rupture, the abdominal symptoms sometimes diminish temporarily, which obscures the diagnosis.

If rupture has occurred, the inflammation of the local soft tissues (bowel, omentum) is termed a *phlegmon*. Phlegmon or periappendiceal abscess is reported in as many as 7% of children with acute appendicitis. An appendiceal mass may be palpated in both.[86–88] A complete discussion of the diagnosis, treatment, and prognosis of appendiceal abscess is presented in Chapter 69.

## Radiologic Findings

The radiographic findings in children with appendicitis are identical to those in adults and are presented in detail in Chapter 69. Certain features of pediatric appendicitis should be noted. First, appendicoliths are more common in children than adults with appendicitis and, when present, are more likely to be associated with appendiceal rupture (Figs. 78–7 to 78–9). When cross-sectional imaging is indicated, ultrasound (Fig. 78–10) is superior to CT in most cases because children have a relative paucity of fat.[86–91] If an abscess is suspected and possible drainage is contemplated, CT is useful. Ultrasound and CT are helpful in differentiating *Yersinia* enterocolitis from appendicitis (Fig. 78–11). Scintigraphy using white blood cells tagged with technetium has also been reported as a sensitive test for diagnosing appendicitis.[92]

## TYPHLITIS

Typhlitis is acute inflammation of the cecum that occurs in immunosuppressed patients.[93–95] It occurs more commonly in children than in adults regardless of the degree of immunosuppression, usually in the setting of acute myelogenous leukemia. Acute lymphogenous leukemia, renal transplantation, and acquired immunodeficiency syndrome are other significant risk factors.[96]

### Clinical Findings

Children with typhlitis present with right lower quadrant pain, leukopenia, fever, peritoneal signs, and occasionally an inflammatory mass and lower gastrointestinal hemorrhage. Prompt diagnosis is vital because delay may lead to sepsis and death. Perforation of the cecum may occur but is not necessarily lethal. Surgical resection of affected bowel, granulocyte transfusions, and antibiotics are useful for stopping the progress of the inflammation.[97]

The differential diagnosis of typhlitis includes appendicitis clinically and pneumatosis intestinalis radiologically. Sonography is useful in excluding appendicitis. Pneumatosis intestinalis may develop in immunocompromised patients but may have a benign clinical presentation and course.[98]

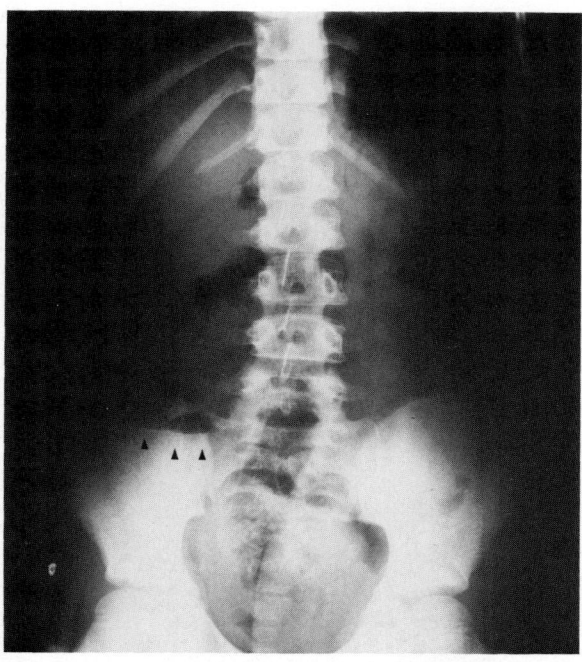

**Figure 78–8. Appendicitis.** Mild left lumbar scoliosis may be due to right psoas spasm. A few air-fluid levels are present in right lower quadrant loops *(arrowheads)*, a sign of focal ileus.

### Radiologic Findings

Plain films in typhlitis may show an abnormal amount of bowel gas or a soft tissue mass in the right lower quadrant, ascites, and/or pneumatosis. Free intraperitoneal air is a more ominous sign and indicates the need

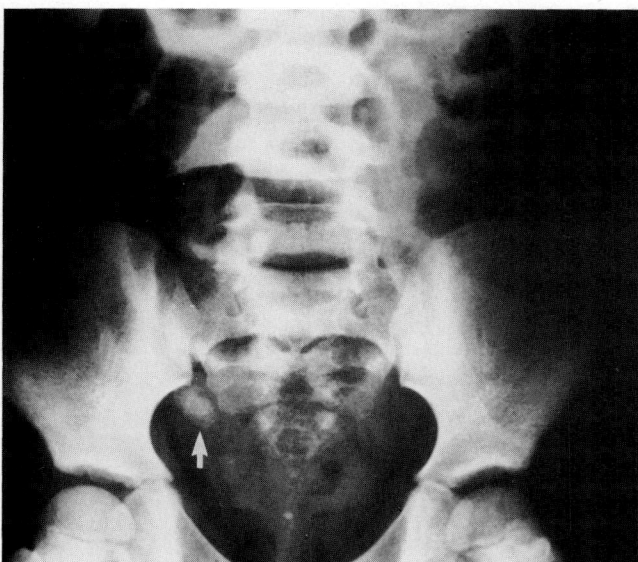

**Figure 78–7. Fecalith.** A large calcified fecalith is seen below the right sacroiliac joint *(arrow)*.

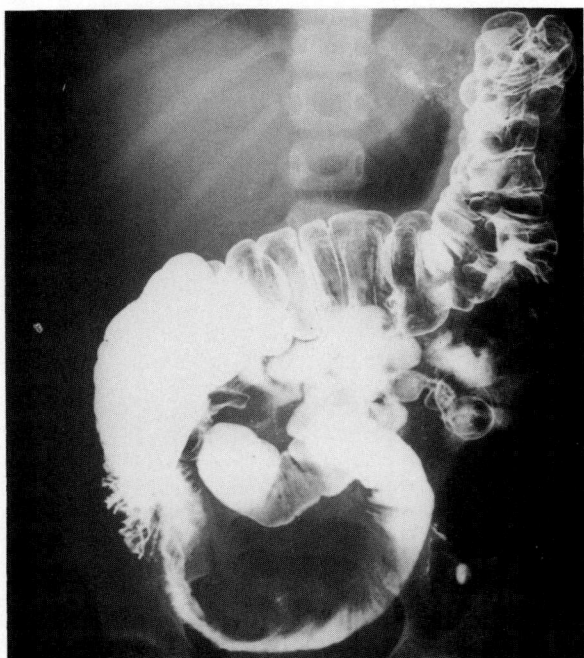

**Figure 78–9. Appendiceal abscess.** The terminal ileum is extrinsically compressed by and displaced around an appendiceal abscess in this small bowel series.

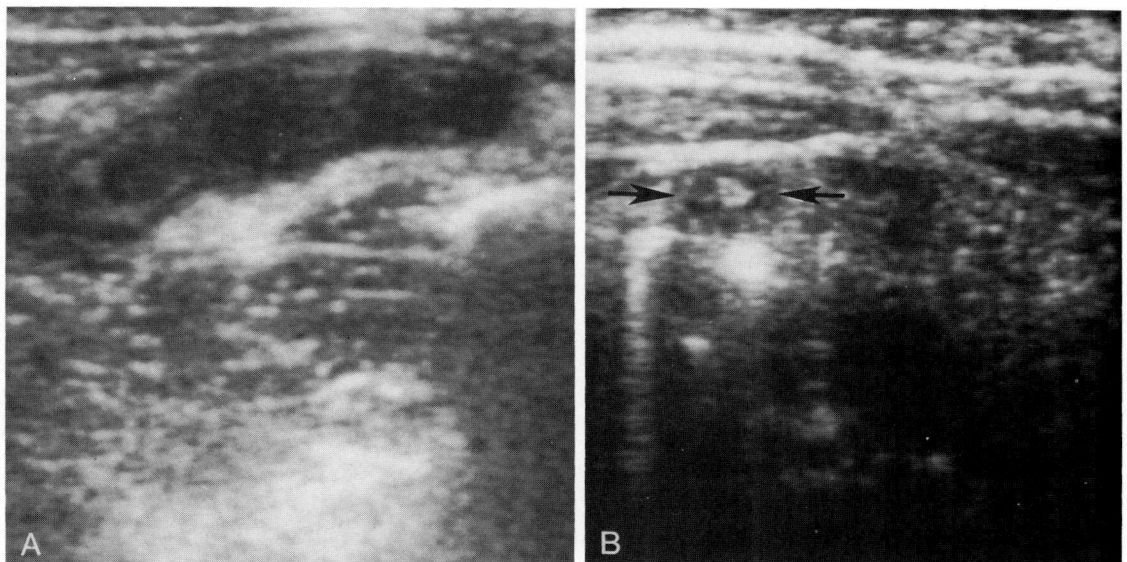

**Figure 78–10. Appendicitis. A.** A dilated, incompressible appendix lies beneath the abdominal musculature on this longitudinal scan. **B.** Transverse scan of the right lower quadrant in a different child shows a widened appendix suggesting appendicitis. The echogenic focus in the center causing distal shadowing is a fecalith.

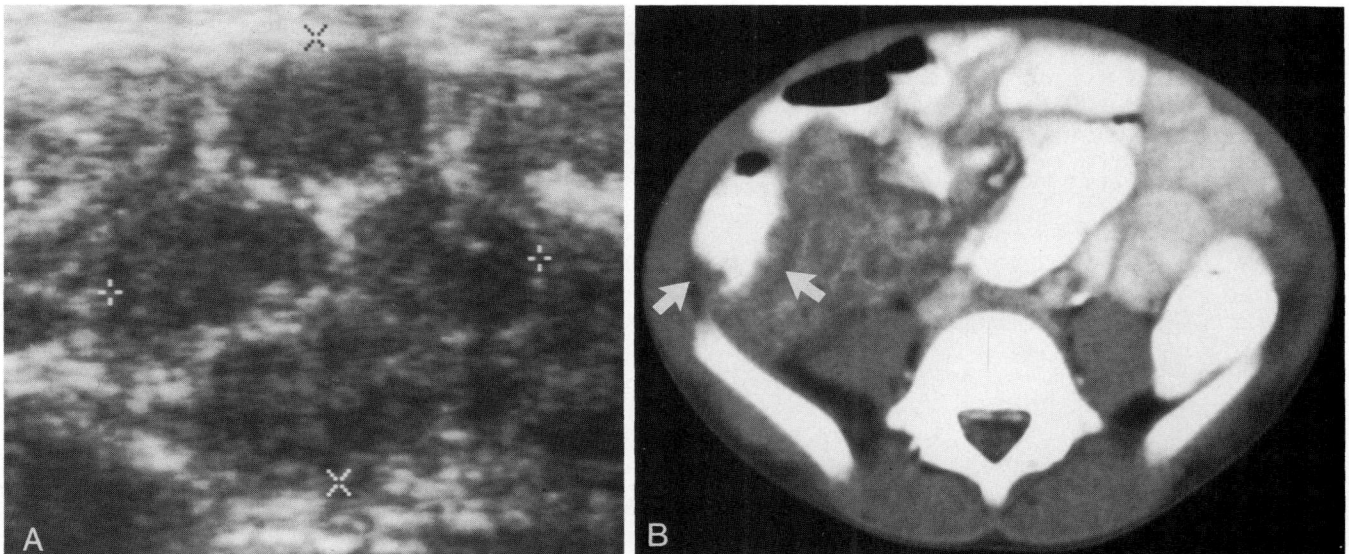

**Figure 78–11. *Yersinia* enterocolitis. A.** Several enlarged lymph nodes *(cursors)* are seen on this sagittal sonogram of a child whose appendix appeared normal. **B.** The enlarged lymph nodes produce an inhomogeneous mass in the right iliac fossa. The wall of the cecum *(arrows)* is thickened on this CT scan.

for surgery unless another source (e.g., mediastinal leak) of the air is apparent.

On barium enema examination, the cecum may be difficult to fill because of spasm and show mural thickening accompanied by mucosal thumbprinting. These secondary changes are helpful in differentiating typhlitis from appendicitis.[93, 95–99]

Angiography demonstrates hyperemic changes of the mucosa, staining at sites of ulceration, and arteriovenous shunting. Although angiography is no longer needed for diagnosis, embolotherapy may be useful if bleeding is massive.

Sonography shows mural thickening of the cecum, ascending colon, and ileum in patients with typhlitis.[100–103] It is also useful in identifying abscesses and in excluding appendiceal inflammation.

CT can identify similar changes but has been used less as a screening technique because it cannot be performed at the bedside and is more expensive than ultrasound.[104]

# INTUSSUSCEPTION

Intussusception occurs when a proximal segment of bowel passes into the lumen of a more distal segment and, through peristalsis, is propelled distally. The proximal segment is referred to as the intussusceptum and the distal segment, the intussuscipiens. Intussusceptions are named by the segments involved. The most common form (70 to 90%) is ileocolic, in which the ileum is prolapsed into the colon for a variable distance. Other less common types of intussusceptions are ileoileocolic, ileoileal, and jejunoileal.

Despite a seasonal variation in the incidence, which suggests that there may be a predisposing viral agent, the majority of children with intussusception have no prodrome or discernible cause. Only 3 to 10% of children have an intrinsic bowel abnormality that serves as the "lead point" for the intussusception: duplication, hemangioma, polyp, Meckel's diverticulum, or lymphoma.[105–109]

Most intussusceptions occur in children between 3 months and 3 years of age with a 2:1 male predominance. Nearly one third of children who develop an intussusception outside this age range have a pathologic lead point.[106–109] Nevertheless, radiologic reduction of the intussusception should be attempted in these children because the majority do not have a lead point.

## Clinical Findings

Children with intussusceptions present with colicky abdominal pain that waxes and wanes. The stools may test positive for occult blood or have the classic, but infrequent, "currant jelly" appearance. Vomiting, diarrhea, and other gastrointestinal symptoms occur in more than 90% of cases. An abdominal mass may be palpated in slightly more than half of the affected children. A few children are lethargic and/or dehydrated. In neo-

nates, vomiting is usually the most striking clinical finding. Rectal bleeding is also more frequent in the neonate with intussusception than in the older child and may suggest necrotizing enterocolitis rather than the correct diagnosis.

## Therapeutic Considerations

The barium enema has traditionally been used to diagnose and to treat ileocolic intussusception. The hydrostatic pressure of the barium column is used to drive the infolded segment of bowel in a retrograde direction to its normal position. Surgery is required to reduce intussusceptions that do not respond to hydrostatic pressure and to treat children whose clinical status precludes radiologic intervention. Children with fever, elevated white blood cell count, peritoneal signs, or marked systemic toxicity should have immediate surgery because these findings suggest perforated bowel or gangrenous gut. Spontaneous reduction may occur, often as a result of general anesthesia, and about 14% of children with documented intussusception may have none present at surgery.[110, 111] Relative contraindications to attempted radiologic reduction include extremes of a patient's age, evidence of a small bowel obstruction, or presence of symptoms for more than 24 hours. In these settings, the success rate for reduction is decreased.[112–117] Whereas the success rate may be greater than 60% in children seen acutely, it is reported to be as high as 31% in those who have symptoms for more than 48 hours. No single factor, such as the patient's age, duration of symptoms, or radiographic signs of small bowel obstruction, is associated with a significant decrease in reducibility. The presence of two or more of these factors, however, decreases the success rate.[115, 116] Because the only alternative to hydrostatic or pneumatic reduction is surgery, with its increased morbidity and cost, I attempt reduction in all children who do not have the medical problems described previously.

Recurrent intussusception develops in 7 to 10% of the children who have been successfully reduced.[106, 113] Second and even third episodes of intussusception do not necessarily indicate that there is a lead point. In large series, only 10 to 20% of children with recurrence had lead points found at surgery.[106, 108, 109, 113] For this reason, hydrostatic or air reduction should be attempted despite recurrence.

Children with Henoch-Schönlein purpura, recent abdominal surgery, and cystic fibrosis have an increased incidence of intussusception.[118, 119] Standard reduction methods may work in these populations as well but are usually less successful in children with Henoch-Schönlein purpura.[119]

## Radiologic Findings

The diagnosis of intussusception can often be made on abdominal plain films.[120–123] In many children with intussusception, the amount of intestinal gas is subnormal and there is displacement of bowel loops from the right hypochondrium. The appendix, if air filled, may be in an abnormal location and the intussusceptum can be identified as a soft tissue mass.[122, 122a] When there is a strong suspicion of intussusception, a contrast enema with barium, air, or water-soluble agents is performed for both diagnosis and treatment.

Barium enema examination is performed only in the medically stable child. Surgical consultation should be obtained before the study in case reduction is unsuccessful or a complication occurs. The lethargic or dehydrated child should be stabilized before beginning the examination. A large bore catheter (with or without inflatable balloon) is placed securely in the rectum and the buttocks are firmly taped shut. The bag of contrast medium is suspended 36 to 39 inches above the fluoroscopy table.

Flow of contrast medium is continued until the colon is filled and there is free reflux into the small bowel or until the intussusceptum is encountered (Fig. 78–12). The barium bag remains open to the patient throughout the study to maintain a constant pressure in an attempt to push the gut to its original position. Manual pressure on the abdomen should be avoided because it is associated with an increased risk of perforation. The barium

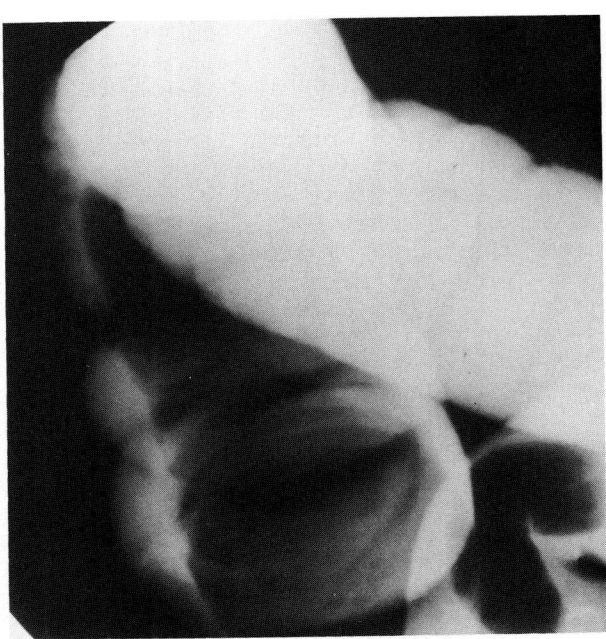

**Figure 78–13. Dissection sign of intussusception on barium enema study.** Contrast medium is seen along the sides of the intussusception, which has a "coil spring" appearance. When this sign is observed, the likelihood of successful reduction is diminished although reduction is still possible.

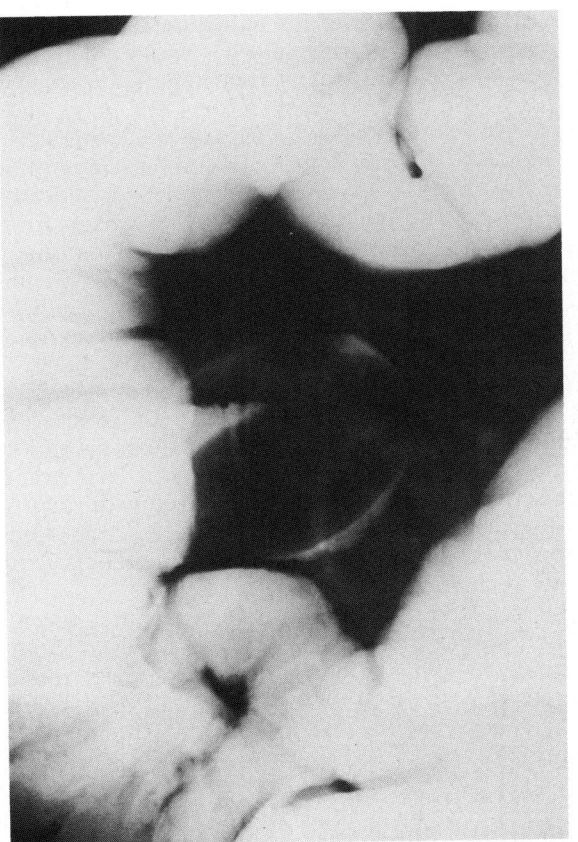

**Figure 78–12. Intussusception.** A persistent filling defect is seen on barium enema examination in the ileum in this child who had a normal-appearing colon. Because the sonogram that preceded this study showed the intussusception, it was necessary to reflux into more ileal loops than usual to confirm and treat the problem.

flow continues as long as there is retrograde motion of the intussusceptum. When there is a standstill, the barium bag should remain open to the patient another 3 to 5 minutes. If there is no movement during this period, the barium is drained from the colon and the child is allowed to rest for a few minutes. Enema reduction is attempted again and this sequence is followed up to three times. If incomplete or no reduction has occurred, surgery is indicated. Successful reduction with this technique occurs in 60 to 90% of children.

Analgesia or sedation may be given if the first reduction attempt is unsuccessful.[105, 110, 111] This tends to make the child more comfortable and may prompt spontaneous reduction. I use meperidine hydrochloride, 2 mg/kg given intravenously over a 2- to 3-minute period, and wait 10 minutes before additional attempts. I do not routinely sedate children with suspected intussusception before beginning a contrast enema because the medication may obscure the nature of the abdominal process in children who do not have an intussusception. Glucagon, an effective smooth muscle relaxant during the adult barium enema, has not proved helpful in intussusception reduction in children.[124]

Barium dissecting between the intussusceptum and the intussuscipiens has been reported as a sign of nonreduction[125] (Fig. 78–13). There is an increased incidence of necrotic bowel in children with this sign. However, reduction is possible in as many as 40% of these children and a nonvigorous attempt, perhaps with water-soluble contrast medium, may avoid surgery.

Reduction is considered to be present only when there is free reflux of barium into small bowel loops. These should be carefully evaluated at fluoroscopy and on overhead filled and postevacuation films in an attempt to find a lead point (see Fig. 78–13).

After reduction, a residual mass effect in the region of the cecum may simulate a focal lesion.[126] The ileocecal valve is often quite prominent because of edema, and it may simulate a persistent intussusception or lead point. In older children, a delayed abdominal film is helpful in identifying a residual cecal mass that may represent lymphoma or other lead point.

Perforation can occur during the reduction procedure at the site of the intussusception, the distal colon, or the rectum if the balloon is overinflated.[114, 115, 127–129] Perforation is rare, occurring in less than 1% of studies.

Water-soluble contrast medium should be used if there is concern about the viability of the underlying bowel, if symptoms have been present for more than 48 hours, and in neonates and infants. Water-soluble contrast medium exerts less hydrostatic pressure than barium, so the enema bag can be raised higher than the standard 3 ft.[130]

Intussusception reduction by air enema with room air or oxygen is becoming increasingly popular.[131–135] This technique has an impressive success rate, few complications, and many advantages: no foreign agent is introduced if there is perforation into the peritoneal cavity, reduction attempts are less messy, and radiation exposure is reduced because fluoroscopy time is often shorter and lower fluoroscopic techniques can be used. This technique has a learning curve, and the novice, particularly with limited pediatric experience, may have difficulty in defining normal anatomy, diagnosing an intussusception, and feeling confident that reduction has occurred. Indeed, air may pass into and distend the small bowel before complete reduction has occurred.[136–138]

Air reduction has many of the same requirements as hydrostatic reduction: placement of a rectal tube, a good

seal of the rectum, and fluoroscopy. Air can be delivered by intermittent manual insufflation or through a continuous delivery system. Rather than controlling the height of the barium bag, it is imperative to measure the pressure at which the air is introduced. Manometry must be incorporated into the system so that the desired pressures are reached but not exceeded. Low pressure (60 mm Hg) and a low flow rate (1 L/min) may aid visualization of the intussusception at the beginning of the study, but pressures between 80 and 120 mm Hg are used routinely during most of the study.[131–135]

Several reports have described the sonographic findings of intussusception.[136–142] The mass of infolded bowel and the layering of the bowel walls produce a "target" or "doughnut" appearance on transverse scans (Fig. 78–14A) and a pseudokidney or "sandwich" sign on longitudinal scans (Fig. 78–14B). Sonography is only a diagnostic technique and the patient still requires a reduction procedure.

Ultrasound is most useful when clinical suspicion of intussusception is low and there is reluctance to perform a barium enema examination or when the child is extremely ill and surgery is contemplated. Pitfalls of sonographic diagnosis include false-positives produced when the bowel is thickened for other reasons, such as lymphoma or Crohn's disease, and false-negatives when the amount of bowel gas present precludes a complete abdominal examination. Detection of false lead points has also been reported.[142]

The CT appearance of intussusception has been described in a few adults (see Chapters 44, 59, and 67).[143] CT should not be used as a screening technique because it is expensive and cannot be used to treat the intussusception when found. CT or sonography may be of use in the child with no visible intussusceptum but a competent ileocecal valve. In this setting, it is important to

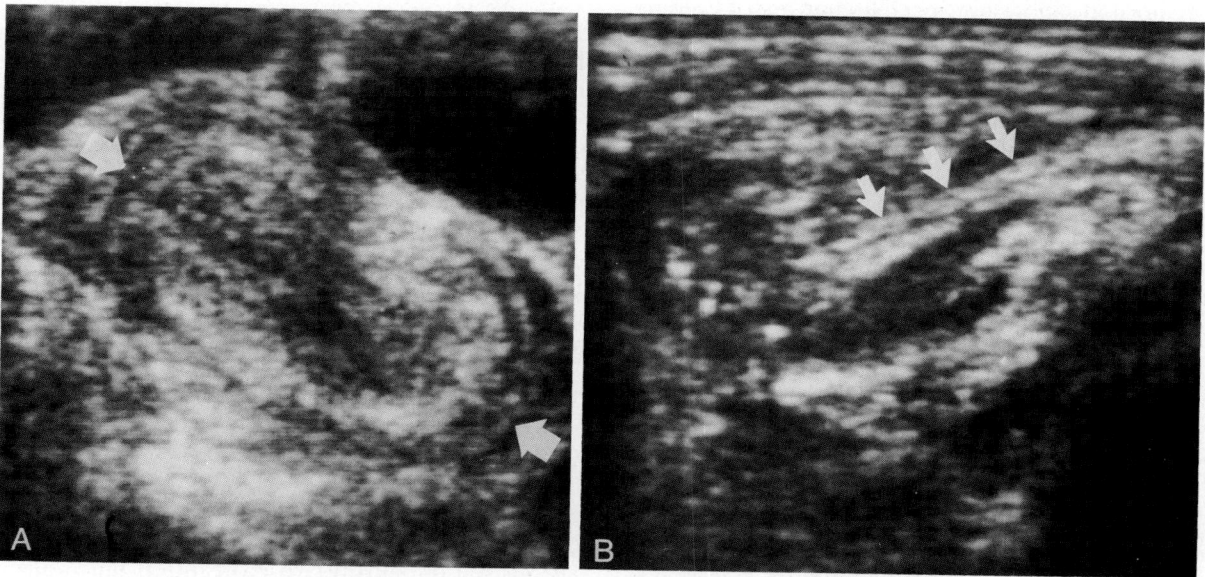

**Figure 78–14. Intussusception. A.** The pseudokidney *(arrows)* sign of intussusception is demonstrated on this longitudinal sonogram. The sonolucent structures anteriorly are dilated bowel loops. **B.** Transverse scan of a different patient shows parallel echogenic mucosa *(arrows)* of the intussuscipiens and intussusceptum.

differentiate the child with no intussusception from the child with ileoileal or other intussusception variant.

## VOLVULUS OF THE COLON

### Clinical Findings

Volvulus of the colon is rare in children and occurs most commonly in the setting of malrotation and other anomalies of mesenteric attachment; constipation associated with mental retardation, HD, or cystic fibrosis; or aerophagia.[144–152] Cecal volvulus includes twisting of the adjacent small bowel.[151]

The very young are spared and the mean age of childhood volvulus is approximately 7 years.[147] Both colonic volvulus generally and sigmoid volvulus specifically occur two to three times more frequently in boys than in girls. At presentation, the child has abdominal pain and, less frequently, vomiting accompanying the physical findings of abdominal distention and tenderness. This presentation may simulate that of an intussusception, although the latter diagnosis would be unlikely in an older child.

Treatment consists of a diagnostic enema and proctoscopy or colonoscopy with or without insertion of a large bore catheter for decompression. Operative treatment is needed if decompression is not achieved or if the volvulus recurs, which it does in one third of cases. If there are signs of peritonitis, surgery is indicated because gangrenous bowel can result from vascular compromise of the involved gut.

### Radiologic Findings

In patients with volvulus, plain films may be interpreted as normal, show nonspecific changes of colonic or small bowel obstruction, or, less commonly, demonstrate the bean-shaped abnormally twisted loop. Cecal volvulus may present as an air-filled structure in the left midabdomen or left upper quadrant.[144] Plain films are most useful for excluding other causes of abdominal pain and free air.

Contrast enema study characteristically demonstrates the narrowing, twisting, or "bird-beak" deformity of the volvulus (Fig. 78–15). The pressure of the enema may untwist the affected segment. A more detailed discussion of volvulus can be found in Chapter 67.

## JUVENILE POLYPS

### Clinical Findings

Juvenile polyps are benign "inflammatory" polyps that occur slightly more commonly in males but are not hereditary or associated with inflammatory bowel disease. In about 80% of cases, the polyp is a solitary lesion that is usually pedunculated.[153–158] These polyps are rare in the neonate and present in the second and third years of life with blood in the stools. The bleeding

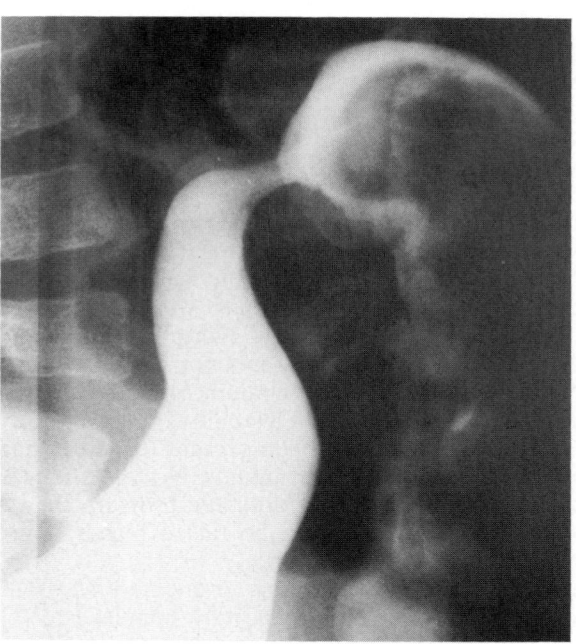

**Figure 78–15. Sigmoid volvulus.** The twisting of the colon produces narrowing just above the rectum. The segment above the volvulus is dilated and full of feces.

is not accompanied by diarrhea or extragastrointestinal symptoms to suggest infectious or inflammatory bowel disease. Inspection of the anus can exclude fissure or tear as a cause of blood. Occasionally, the polyp may manifest as a prolapsing rectal mass.

Although most polyps can be removed easily by endoscopic polypectomy, many children are treated expectantly because the polyp often sloughs spontaneously with resolution of symptoms.[159, 160]

### Radiologic Findings

Juvenile polyps are best demonstrated on double contrast barium enema studies.[160, 161] Most juvenile polyps are left sided and the majority are smooth and pedunculated (Fig. 78–16). The radiologic criteria for differentiating benign and malignant polyps in adults are of little value in children because virtually all these polyps are benign regardless of their appearance. Demonstration of one polyp should not detract from the search for an additional one because approximately 20% of children have more than one juvenile polyp.

## COLON CARCINOMA

Primary colon cancer is exceedingly rare in children.[162–171] In contrast to adult carcinomas, pediatric lesions pathologically are more often mucinous or colloid variants. Most of these tumors occur in the rectum and sigmoid colon. These cancers may arise spontaneously or be secondary to ulcerative colitis or familial polyposis.

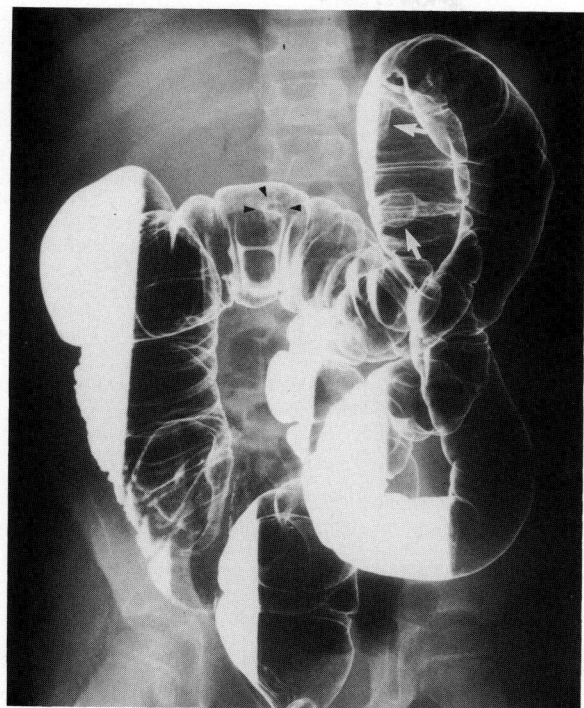

**Figure 78–16. Juvenile polyps.** Double contrast barium enema examination demonstrates three polyps: two on stalks in the region of the splenic flexure *(arrows)* and the third en face *(arrowheads)* in the transverse colon.

## Clinical Findings

A mass is palpable in about 10% of patients. The symptoms of colon cancer (vomiting, pain, constipation, bleeding) would seem to warrant early and complete evaluation. However, the rarity of this neoplasm in children tends to delay a thorough diagnostic work-up. Consequently, the disease is often advanced at the time of diagnosis. Patients tend to do poorly despite surgery and adjuvant chemotherapy.

The differential diagnosis of colon cancer is limited. Non-neoplastic lesions such as intussusception, appendicitis, gastroenteritis, and even parasitic infestations should be considered and excluded with appropriate tests. Obstruction, mass, and rectal bleeding can also be the presenting signs of a number of other neoplasms: hemangioma, lymphoma, leiomyomas, and other spindle cell tumors.

## Radiologic Findings

The single and double contrast barium enema characteristics of colon cancer are identical to those found in adults (see Chapter 64). Mucosal irregularity or narrowing of the caliber of the colon with a typical "apple core" deformity may be present. As in adults, sonography or CT is useful in looking for local, metastatic, or recurrent disease.

## References

1. Capitanio MA, Kirkpatrick JA: Lymphoid hyperplasia of the colon in children. Roentgen observations. Radiology 94:323–327, 1970.
2. Theander G, Tragardh B: Lymphoid hyperplasia of the colon in childhood. Acta Radiol Diagn 17:631–640, 1976.
3. Franken EA Jr: Lymphoid hyperplasia of the colon. Radiology 94:329–334, 1970.
4. Jona JZ, Belin RP, Burke JA: Lymphoid hyperplasia of the bowel and its surgical significance in children. J Pediatr Surg 11:997–1006, 1976.
5. Laufer I, de Sa D: Lymphoid follicular pattern: a normal feature of the pediatric colon. AJR 130:51–55, 1978.
6. Kenney PJ, Koehler RE, Shackelford GD: The clinical significance of large lymphoid follicles of the colon. Radiology 142:41–46, 1982.
7. Lechner GL, Frank W, Jantsch H, et al: Lymphoid follicular hyperplasia in excluded colonic segments: a radiologic sign of diversion colitis. Radiology 176:135–136, 1990.
8. Glick S, Teplick SK, Ross WM: Colonic lymphoid follicles associated with colonic neoplasms. Radiology 168:603–607, 1988.
9. Crooks DJM, Brown WR: The distribution of intestinal nodular lymphoid hyperplasia in immunoglobulin deficiency. Clin Radiol 31:701–706, 1980.
10. Hendren WH: Constipation caused by anterior location of the anus and its surgical correction. J Pediatr Surg 13:505–512, 1978.
11. Leape LL, Ramenofsky ML: Anterior ectopic anus: a common cause of constipation in children. J Pediatr Surg 13:627–630, 1978.
12. Tuggle DW, Perkins TA, Tunnell WP, et al: Operative treatment of anterior ectopic anus: the efficacy and influence of age on results. J Pediatr Surg 25:996–998, 1990.
13. Upadhyaya P: Mid–anal sphincteric malformation, cause of constipation in anterior perineal anus. J Pediatr Surg 19:183–186, 1984.
14. Reisner SH, Sivan Y, Nitzan M, et al: Determination of anterior displacement of the anus in newborn infants and children. Pediatrics 73:216–217, 1984.
15. Swenson O, Sherman JO, Fisher JH: Diagnosis of congenital megacolon: an analysis of 501 patients. J Pediatr Surg 8:587–594, 1983.
16. Gaisie G, Oh KS, Young LW: Coexistent neuroblastoma and Hirschsprung's disease—another manifestation of neurocristopathy? Pediatr Radiol 8:161–163, 1979.
17. Roshow JE, Haller JO, Berdon WE, et al: Hirschsprung's disease, Ondine's curse, and neuroblastoma—manifestations of neurocristopathy. Pediatr Radiol 19:45–49, 1988.
18. Michna BA, McWilliams NB, Krummel TM, et al: Multifocal ganglioneuroblastoma coexistent with total colonic aganglionosis. J Pediatr Surg 23:57–59, 1988.
19. Foster P, Cowan G, Wrenn EL Jr: Twenty-five years' experience with Hirschsprung's disease. J Pediatr Surg 25:531–534, 1990.
20. de Chadarevian JP, Slim M, Akel S: Double zonal aganglionosis in long segment Hirschsprung's disease with a "skip area" in transverse colon. J Pediatr Surg 17:195–197, 1982.
21. Haney PJ, Hill JL, Sun CCJ: Zonal colonic aganglionosis. Pediatr Radiol 12:258–261, 1982.
22. Cogbill TH, Lilly JR: Acquired aganglionosis after Soave's procedure for Hirschsprung's disease. Arch Surg 117:1346–1347, 1982.
23. West KW, Grosfeld JL, Rescorla FJ, et al: Acquired aganglionosis: a rare occurrence following pull-through procedures for Hirschsprung's disease. J Pediatr Surg 25:104–108, 1990.
24. Senyuz OF, Buyukunal C, Danismend N, et al: Extensive intestinal aganglionosis. J Pediatr Surg 24:453–456, 1989.
25. Kleinhaus S, Boley SC, Sheran M, et al: Hirschsprung's disease: a survey of the members of the surgical section of the American Academy of Pediatrics. J Pediatr Surg 14:588–597, 1979.
26. Brearly S, Armstrong GR, Nairn R, et al: Pseudomembranous colitis: a lethal complication of Hirschsprung's disease unrelated to antibiotic usage. J Pediatr Surg 22:257–259, 1987.
27. Newman B, Nussbaum A, Kirkpatrick JA Jr: Bowel perforation in Hirschsprung's disease. AJR 148:1195–1197, 1987.

28. Arliss J, Holgerson LO: Neonatal perforation and Hirschsprung's disease. J Pediatr Surg 25:694–695, 1990.

29. Wheatley MJ, Wesley JR, Coran AG, et al: Hirschsprung's disease in adolescents and adults. Dis Colon Rectum 33:622–629, 1990.

30. Lefebvre MP, Leape LL, Pohl DA, et al: Total colonic aganglionosis diagnosed in an adolescent. Gastroenterology 87:1364–1366, 1984.

31. Penninckx F, Lestar B, Kerremans R: Pitfalls and limitations of testing the rectoanal inhibitory reflex in screening for Hirschsprung's disease. Pediatr Surg Int 5:260–265, 1990.

32. Aaronson I, Nixon HH: A clinical evaluation of anorectal pressure studies in the diagnosis of Hirschsprung's disease. Gut 13:138–146, 1972.

33. Neilson IR, Yazbeck S: Ultrashort Hirschsprung's disease: myth or reality. J Pediatr Surg 25:1135–1138, 1990.

34. Wilder WM, Melhem RE: Balloon dilatation of post-surgical ano-rectal strictures in two infants. Pediatr Radiol 19:527–529, 1989.

35. Mahboubi S, Schnaufer L: The barium-enema examination and rectal manometry in Hirschsprung disease. Radiology 130:643–647, 1979.

36. Scobey WG, Mackinlay GA: Anorectal myectomy in treatment of ultrashort segment Hirschsprung's disease. Arch Dis Child 52:713–715, 1977.

37. Lipson AH, Harvey J: Three-generation transmission of Hirschsprung's disease. Clin Genet 32:175–178, 1987.

38. Schiller M, Levy P, Shawa RA, et al: Familial Hirschsprung's disease—a report of 22 affected siblings in four families. J Pediatr Surg 25:322–325, 1990.

39. Shaw KS, Rubin SZ: Anatomically identical short-segment Hirschsprung's disease in three male siblings. Pediatr Surg Int 5:359–360, 1990.

40. Filston HC, Kirks DR: The association of malrotation and Hirschsprung's disease. Pediatr Radiol 12:6–10, 1982.

41. Stannard VA, Fowler C, Robinson L, et al: Familial Hirschsprung's disease: report of autosomal dominant and probable X-linked kindreds. J Pediatr Surg 26:591–594, 1991.

42. Johnson JF, Dean BL: Hirschsprung's disease coexisting with colonic atresia. Pediatr Radiol 11:97–98, 1981.

43. Moore SW, Rode H, Millar AJW, et al: Intestinal atresia and Hirschsprung's disease. Pediatr Surg Int 5:182–184, 1990.

44. James AE, Greenfield JB, Pfister RC, et al: The roentgenologic appearance of postoperative congenital megacolon (Hirschsprung's disease). AJR 109:351–366, 1970.

45. Chandler NW, Zwiren GT: Complete reflux of the small bowel in total colon Hirschsprung's disease. Radiology 94:335–339, 1970.

46. DeCampo JF, Mayne V, Boldt DW, et al: Radiological findings in total aganglionosis coli. Pediatr Radiol 14:205–209, 1984.

47. Berdon WE, Koontz P, Baker DH: The diagnosis of colonic and terminal ileal aganglionosis. AJR 91:680–689, 1984.

48. Cremin BJ: The early diagnosis of Hirschsprung's disease. Pediatr Radiol 2:23–28, 1974.

49. Berdon WE, Baker DH: The roentgenographic diagnosis of Hirschsprung's disease in infancy. AJR 93:432–446, 1965.

50. Fletcher BD, Yulish BS: Intraluminal calcifications in the small bowel of newborn infants with total colonic aganglionosis. Radiology 126:451–455, 1978.

51. Rosenfield NS, Ablow RC, Markowitz RI, et al: Hirschsprung disease: accuracy of the barium enema examination. Radiology 139:393–400, 1984.

52. Pochaczevsky R, Leonidas JC: The "recto-sigmoid index." A measurement for the early diagnosis of Hirschsprung's disease. AJR 123:770–777, 1975.

53. Siegel MJ, Shackelford GD, McAlister WH: The rectosigmoid index. Radiology 139:497–499, 1981.

54. Johnson JF, Cronk RL: The pseudotransition zone in long segment Hirschsprung's disease. Pediatr Radiol 10:87–89, 1980.

55. Leonidas JC, Krasna IH, Strauss L, et al: Roentgen appearance of the excluded colon after colostomy for infantile Hirschsprung's disease. AJR 112:116–122, 1971.

56. Oestrich AE: Ultrasound diagnosis of Hirschsprung disease in the infant with distended abdomen. Radiologe 30:19–20, 1990.

57. Kirschner BS: Medical management of inflammatory bowel disease in children. _In_ Kirsner JB, Shorter RG (eds): Inflammatory Bowel Disease (3rd ed). Philadelphia: Lea & Febiger, 1988, pp 503–512.

58. Grand RJ, Motil KJ: Inflammatory bowel disease in childhood and adolescence. _In_ Korelitz BI, Sohn N (eds): Inflammatory Bowel Disease: Experience and Controversy. Orlando, FL: Grune & Stratton, 1985, pp 9–30.

59. Stenson WF, MacDermott RP: Inflammatory bowel disease. _In_ Yamada T (ed): Textbook of Gastroenterology. Philadelphia: JB Lippincott, 1991, pp 1588–1644.

60. Larcher VF, Shepherd R, Francis DEM, et al: Protracted diarrhoea in infancy. Arch Dis Child 52:597–605, 1977.

61. Hamilton JR: Viral enteritis. Pediatr Clin North Am 35:89–101, 1988.

62. Bishop WP, Ulshen MH: Bacterial gastroenteritis. Pediatr Clin North Am 35:69–87, 1988.

63. Berger LA, Wilkinson D: The investigation of colitis in infancy. Pediatr Radiol 2:145–154, 1974.

64. Richards DG, Somers S, Issenman RM, et al: Cow's milk protein/soy protein allergy: gastrointestinal imaging. Radiology 167:721–723, 1988.

65. Swischuk LE, Hayden CK Jr: Barium enema findings (?segmental colitis) in four neonates with bloody diarrhea—possible cow's milk allergy. Pediatr Radiol 15:34–37, 1985.

66. Perisic VN, Kokai G: Diarrhoea caused by collagenous colitis. Arch Dis Child 64:867–869, 1989.

67. Busuttil A: Collagenous colitis in a child. Am J Dis Child 143:998–1000, 1989.

68. Palmer KR, Berr H, Wheeler PJ, et al: Collagenous colitis: a relapsing and remitting disease. Gut 27:578–580, 1986.

69. Davies RP, Slavotinek JP, Dorney SFA: VIP secreting tumours in infancy. Pediatr Radiol 20:504–508, 1990.

70. Kirschner SG, Buckspan GS, O'Neill JA, et al: Detergent enema: a cause of caustic colitis. Pediatr Radiol 6:141–146, 1977.

71. Fan ST, Lau WY, Wong KK: Ischemic colitis in Kawasaki disease. J Pediatr Surg 21:964–965, 1986.

72. Smith CD, Schuster SR, Gruppe WE, et al: Hemolytic-uremic syndrome: a diagnostic and therapeutic dilemma for the surgeon. J Pediatr Surg 13:597–604, 1978.

73. Whitington PF, Friedman AL, Chesney RW: Gastrointestinal disease in the hemolytic-uremic syndrome. Gastroenterology 76:728–733, 1979.

74. Seror D, Szold A, Udassin R, et al: Surgical complications in hemolytic-uremic syndrome: gangrenous appendicitis. Pediatr Surg Int 5:214–215, 1990.

75. Drummond KN: Hemolytic uremic syndrome—then and now. N Engl J Med 312:116–118, 1985.

76. Siegler RL: Management of hemolytic-uremic syndrome. J Pediatr 112:1014–1020, 1988.

77. Kirks DR: The radiology of the enteritis due to the hemolytic-uremic syndrome. Pediatr Radiol 12:179–183, 1982.

78. Brandt ML, O'Reagan S, Rousseau E, et al: Surgical complications of the hemolytic-uremic syndrome. J Pediatr Surg 25:1109–1112, 1990.

79. Peterson RB, Meseroll WP, Shrago GG, et al: Radiographic features of colitis associated with the hemolytic-uremic syndrome. Radiology 118:667–671, 1976.

80. Patriquin HB, O'Reagan S, Robitalle P, et al: Hemolytic-uremic syndrome: intrarenal arterial Doppler patterns as a useful guide to therapy. Radiology 172:625–628, 1989.

81. Picus D, Shackelford GD: Perforated appendix presenting as severe diarrhea. Findings on barium-enema examination. Radiology 149:141–143, 1983.

82. Rubin SZ, Martin DJ: Ultrasonography in the management of possible appendicitis in childhood. J Pediatr Surg 25:737–740, 1990.

83. Neilson IR, Laberge JM, Nguyen LT, et al: Appendicitis in children: current therapeutic recommendations. J Pediatr Surg 25:1113–1116, 1990.

83a. Gilchrist BF, Lobe TE, Schropp KP, et al: Is there a role for laparascopic appendectomy in pediatric surgery? J Pediatr Surg

84. Rappaport WD, Peterson M, Stanton C: Factors responsible for the high perforation rate seen in early childhood appendicitis. Am Surg 55:602–605, 1989.

85. Ceres L, Alonso I, Lopez P, et al: Ultrasound study of acute

appendicitis in children with emphasis upon the diagnosis of retrocecal appendicitis. Pediatr Radiol 20:258–261, 1990.

86. Vignault F, Filiatrault D, Brandt ML, et al: Acute appendicitis in children: evaluation with US. Radiology 176:501–504, 1990.

87. Puri P, O'Donnell B: Management of appendiceal mass in children. Pediatr Surg Int 4:306–308, 1989.

88. Riddlesberger MM Jr, Afshani E, Kuhn JP, et al: Unusual presentation of appendiceal abscess on barium contrast studies. Pediatr Radiol 7:15–18, 1978.

89. Kao SCS, Smith WL, Abu-Yousef MM, et al: Acute appendicitis in children: sonographic findings. AJR 153:375–379, 1989.

89a. Quillen SP, Siegel MJ, Coffin CM: Acute appendicitis in children: value of sonography in detecting perforation. AJR 159:1265–1268, 1992.

89b. Quillen SP, Siegel MJ: Appendicitis in children: color Doppler sonography. Radiology 184:745–747, 1992.

89c. Sivit CJ, Newman KD, Boenning DA, et al: Appendicitis: usefulness of US in diagnosis in a pediatric population. Radiology 185:549–552, 1992.

90. Baker DE, Silver TM, Coran AG, et al: Postappendectomy fluid collections in children: incidence, nature, and evolution evaluated using US. Radiology 161:341–344, 1986.

91. Slovis TL, Haller JO, Cohen HL, et al: Complicated appendiceal inflammatory disease in children: pylephlebitis and liver abscess. Radiology 171:823–825, 1989.

92. Henneman PL, Marcus CS, Inkelis SH, et al: Evaluation of children with possible appendicitis using technetium 99m leukocyte scan. Pediatrics 85:838–843, 1990.

93. Abramson SJ, Berdon WE, Baker DH: Childhood typhlitis: its increasing association with acute myelogenous leukemia. Radiology 146:61–64, 1983.

94. Meyerovitz MF, Fellows KE: Typhlitis: a cause of gastrointestinal hemorrhage in children. AJR 143:833–835, 1984.

95. McNamara MJ, Chalmers AG, Morgan M, et al: Typhlitis in acute childhood leukemia: radiological features. Clin Radiol 37:83–87, 1986.

96. Merine DS, Fishman EK, Jones B, et al: Right lower quadrant pain in the immunocompromised patient: CT findings in 10 cases. AJR 149:1177–1179, 1987.

97. Koea JB, Shaw JH: Surgical management of neutropenic enterocolitis. Br J Surg 76:821–824, 1989.

98. Keats TE, Smith TH: Benign pneumatosis intestinalis in childhood leukemia. AJR 122:150–152, 1974.

99. Archibald RB, Nelson JA: Necrotizing enterocolitis in acute leukemia: radiographic findings. Gastrointest Radiol 3:63–65, 1978.

100. Gootenberg JE, Abbondanzo SL: Rapid diagnosis of neutropenic enterocolitis (typhlitis) by ultrasonography. Am J Pediatr Hematol Oncol 9:222–227, 1987.

101. Glass-Royal MC, Choyke PL, Gootenberg JE, et al: Sonography in the diagnosis of neutropenic colitis. J Ultrasound Med 6:671–673, 1987.

102. Teefey SA, Montana MA, Goldfogel GA, et al: Sonographic diagnosis of neutropenic typhlitis. AJR 149:731–733, 1987.

103. Alexander JE, Williamson SL, Seibert JJ, et al: The ultrasonographic diagnosis of typhlitis (neutropenic colitis). Pediatr Radiol 18:200–204, 1988.

104. Bankoff MS, Sarno RC, Bonica AJ, et al: CT detection of necrotising enterocolitis. Br J Radiol 58:495–497, 1985.

105. Schuh S, Wesson DE: Intussusception in children 2 years of age or older. Can Med Assoc J 136:269–272, 1987.

106. Patriquin HB, Afshani E, Effman E, et al: Neonatal intussusception. Report of 12 cases. Radiology 125:463–466, 1977.

107. Newman J, Schuh S: Intussusception in babies under 4 months of age. Can Med Assoc J 136:266–269, 1987.

108. Ong NT, Beasley SW: The leadpoint in intussusception. J Pediatr Surg 25:640–643, 1990.

109. Eklöf OA, Johanson L, Lohr G: Childhood intussusception: hydrostatic reducibility and incidence of leading points in different age groups. Pediatr Radiol 10:83–86, 1980.

110. Touloukian RJ, O'Connell JB, Markowitz RI, et al: Analgesic premedication in the management of ileocolic intussusception. Pediatrics 79:432–434, 1987.

111. Collins DL, Pickney LE, Miller KE, et al: Hydrostatic reduction

of ileocolic intussusception: a second attempt in the operating room with general anesthesia. J Pediatr 115:204–207, 1989.

112. Jennings C, Kelleher J: Intussusception: influence of age on reducibility. Pediatr Radiol 14:292–294, 1984.

113. Ein SH: Recurrent intussusception in children: J Pediatr Surg 10:751–755, 1975.

114. Mok PM, Humphry A: Ileo-ileocolic intussusception: radiological features and reducibility. Pediatr Radiol 12:127–131, 1982.

115. Stephenson CA, Seibert JJ, Strain JD, et al: Intussusception: clinical and radiographic factors influencing reducibility. Pediatr Radiol 20:57–60, 1989.

116. Leonidas JC: Treatment of intussusception with small bowel obstruction: application of decision analysis. AJR 145:665–669, 1985.

117. Barr LL, Stansberry SD, Swischuk LE: Significance of age, duration, obstruction and the dissection sign in intussusception. Pediatr Radiol 20:454–456, 1990.

118. Holsclaw DS, Rocmans C, Shwachman H: Intussusception in patients with cystic fibrosis. Pediatrics 48:51–58, 1971.

119. Glasier CM, Siegel MJ, McAlister WH, et al: Henoch-Schönlein syndrome in children: gastrointestinal manifestation. AJR 136:1081–1085, 1981.

120. White SJ, Blane CE: Intussusception: additional observations on the plain radiograph. AJR 139:511–513, 1982.

121. Gilsanz V: Displacement of the appendix in intussusception. AJR 142:407–408, 1984.

122. Eklöf O, Hartelius H: Reliability of the abdominal plain film diagnosis in pediatric patients with suspected intussusception. Pediatr Radiol 9:199–206, 1980.

122a. Ratcliffe JF, Fong S, Cheong I, et al: Plain film diagnosis of intussusception: prevalence of the target sign. AJR 158:619–621, 1992.

123. Johnson JF, Woisard KK: Ileocolic intussusception: new sign on the cross-table radiograph. Radiology 170:483–486, 1989.

124. Franken EA, Smith WL, Chernish SM, et al: The use of glucagon in hydrostatic reduction of intussusception: a double blind study of 30 patients. Radiology 146:687–689, 1983.

125. Fishman MC, Borden S, Cooper A: The dissection sign of nonreducible ileocolic intussusception. AJR 143:5–8, 1984.

126. Devred PH, Faure F, Padovani J: Pseudotumoral cecum after hydrostatic reduction of intussusception. Pediatr Radiol 14:295–298, 1984.

127. Humphry A, Ein SH, Mok PM: Perforation of the intussuscepted colon. AJR 137:1135–1138, 1981.

127a. Bramson RT, Blickman JG: Perforation during hydrostatic reduction of intussusception: proposed mechanism and review of the literature. J Pediatr Surg 27:589–591, 1992.

128. Campbell JB: Contrast media in intussusception. Pediatr Radiol 19:293–296, 1989.

129. Armstrong EA, Dunbar JS, Graviss ER, et al: Intussusception complicated by distal perforation of the colon. Radiology 136:77–81, 1980.

130. Kuta AJ, Benator RM: Intussusception: hydrostatic pressure equivalents for barium and meglumine sodium diatrizoate. Radiology 175:125–126, 1990.

131. Palder SB, Ein SH, Stringer DA, et al: Intussusception: barium or air? J Pediatr Surg 26:271–275, 1991.

132. Gu L, Alton DJ, Daneman A, et al: Intussusception reduction in children by rectal insufflation of air. AJR 150:1345–1348, 1988.

133. Katz M, Phelan E, Carlin JB, et al: Gas enema reduction of intussusception: relationship between clinical signs and symptoms. AJR 160:363–366, 1993.

133a. Beasley SW, Glover J: Intussusception: prediction of outcome of gas enema. J Pediatr Surg 27:474–475, 1992.

134. Hedlund GL, Johnson JF, Strife JL: Ileocolic intussusception: extensive reflux of air preceding pneumatic reduction. Radiology 174:187–189, 1990.

135. Guo J, Ma X, Zhou Q: Results of air pressure enema reduction of intussusception: 6,396 cases in 13 years. J Pediatr Surg 21:1201–1203, 1986.

136. Bolia AA: Case report: diagnosis and hydrostatic reduction of an intussusception under ultrasound guidance. Clin Radiol 36:655–657, 1985.

136a. Woo SK, Kim JS, Sun SJ, et al: Childhood intussusception: US-guided hydrostatic reduction. Radiology 182:77–80, 1992.

137. Morin ME, Blumenthal DH, Tan A, et al: The ultrasonic appearance of ileocolic intussusception. J Clin Ultrasound 9:516–518, 1981.

138. Bowerman RA, Silver TM, Jaffe MH: Real-time ultrasound diagnosis of intussusception in children. Radiology 143:527–529, 1982.

139. Swischuk LE, Hayden CK, Boulden T: Intussusception: indications for ultrasonography and an explanation of the doughnut and pseudokidney signs. Pediatr Radiol 15:388–391, 1985.

139a. Verschelden P, Filiatrault D, Garel L, et al: Intussusception in children: reliability of US in diagnosis—a prospective study. Radiology 184:741–744, 1992.

140. Alessi V, Salerno G: The "hay-fork" sign in the ultrasonographic diagnosis of intussusception. Pediatr Radiol 10:177–179, 1985.

140a. Bhisitkud DM, Listernick R, Shkolnik A, et al: Clinical application of ultrasonography in the diagnosis of intussusception. J Pediatr 121:182–186, 1992.

141. Pracros JP, Tran-minh VA, Morin de Finfe CH, et al: Acute intestinal intussusception in children. Contribution of ultrasonography (145 cases). Ann Radiol 30:525–530, 1987.

142. Kenney IJ: Ultrasound in intussusception: a false cystic lead point. Pediatr Radiol 20:348, 1990.

143. Parienty RA, Lepreux JF, Gruson B: Sonographic and CT features of ileocolic intussusception. AJR 136:608–610, 1981.

144. Allen RP, Nordstrom JE: Volvulus of the sigmoid in children. AJR 91:690–693, 1964.

145. Trillis F, Gauderer MWL, Ponsky JL, et al: Transverse colon volvulus in a child with pathologic aerophagia. J Pediatr Surg 21:966–968, 1986.

146. Berger RB, Hillemeir AC, Stahl RS, et al: Volvulus of the ascending colon: an unusual complication of non-rotation of the midgut. Pediatr Radiol 12:298–300, 1982.

147. Smith SD, Golladay ES, Wagner C, et al: Sigmoid volvulus in childhood. South Med J 83:778–781, 1990.

148. Andersen JF, Eklöf O, Thomasson B: Large bowel volvulus in children. Pediatr Radiol 11:129–138, 1981.

149. Leeba JM, Boas RN: Simultaneous intussusception and sigmoid volvulus in a child. Pediatr Radiol 16:248–249, 1986.

150. Schwab FJ, Glick SN, Teplick SK: Reduction of cecal volvulus by multiple barium enemas. Gastrointest Radiol 10:185–187, 1985.

151. Kirks DR, Swischuk LE, Merten DF, et al: Cecal volvulus in children. AJR 136:419–422, 1981.

152. Neilson IR, Youssef S: Delayed presentation of Hirschsprung's disease: acute obstruction secondary to megacolon with transverse colonic volvulus. J Pediatr Surg 25:1177–1179, 1990.

153. Shermeta DW, Morgan WW, Eggleston J, et al: Juvenile retention polyps. J Pediatr Surg 4:211–215, 1969.

154. Holgerson M, Miller RE, Zintel HA: Juvenile polyps of the colon. Surgery 69:288–293, 1971.

155. Cynamon HA, Milov DE, Andres JM: Diagnosis and management of colonic polyps in children. J Pediatr 114:593–596, 1989.

155a. Jalihal A, Misra SP, Arvind AS, et al: Colonoscopic polypectomy in children. J Pediatr Surg 27:1220–1222, 1992.

156. Toccalino H, Guastavino E, DePinni F, et al: Juvenile polyps of the rectum and colon. Acta Pediatr Scand 62:337–340, 1973.

157. Cremin BJ, Louw JH: Polyps in the large bowel in children. Clin Radiol 21:195–200, 1970.

158. Harris JW: Polyps of the colon and rectum in children. Dis Colon Rectum 10:267–272, 1967.

159. Euler AR, Seibert JJ: The role of sigmoidoscopy, radiographs, and colonoscopy in the diagnostic evaluation of pediatric age patients with suspected juvenile polyps. J Pediatr Surg 16:500–502, 1981.

160. Daum F, Zucker P, Boley SJ, et al: Colonoscopic polypectomy in children. Am J Dis Child 131:566–567, 1977.

161. Feczko PJ, Halpert RD: Limiting overhead views in double-contrast colon examinations does not affect diagnostic accuracy. Gastrointest Radiol 12:175–177, 1987.

162. Steinberg JB, Tuggle DW, Postier RG: Adenocarcinoma of the colon in adolescents. Am J Surg 156:460–462, 1988.

163. Andersson A, Bergdahl L: Carcinoma of the colon in children: a report of six new cases and a review of the literature. J Pediatr Surg 11:967–971, 1976.

164. Enker WE, Paloyan E, Kirsner JB: Carcinoma of the colon in the adolescent—a report of survival and an analysis of the literature. Am J Surg 133:737–741, 1977.

165. Hoerner MT: Carcinoma of the colon and rectum in persons under twenty years of age. Am J Surg 96:47–53, 1958.

166. Alaghemand A: Carcinoma of the colon and rectum in children. Am Surg 28:784–789, 1962.

167. Buchman JA, Calhoun JD: Colloid carcinoma of the colon in children. Am Surg 25:280–286, 1958.

168. Cremin BJ, Brown RA: Carcinoma of the colon: diagnosis by ultrasound and enema. Pediatr Radiol 17:319–320, 1987.

169. Lewis CTP, Riley E, Georgeson K, et al: Carcinoma of the colon and rectum in patients less than 20 years of age. South Med J 83:383–385, 1990.

170. Middelkamp JN, Haffner H: Carcinoma of the colon in children. Pediatrics 32:558–571, 1963.

171. Lamego CMB, Torloni H: Colorectal adenocarcinoma in childhood and adolescence. Report of 11 cases and review of the literature. Pediatr Radiol 19:504–508, 1989.

# Lesions Involving Multiple Areas of the Gastrointestinal Tract

Sandra K. Fernbach, M.D.

## GASTROINTESTINAL DUPLICATIONS

Duplications can occur in any portion of the gastrointestinal tract, from tongue to anus, but are most common in the region of the terminal ileum. Failure of recanalization, intrauterine vascular insults, and incomplete twinning have been proposed as possible embryologic defects that produce duplication. Multiple theories have developed because no one theory can explain the protean clinical and pathologic findings.

Duplications are located in continuity with or in close apposition to the gut. The duplication may contain the mucosa of any segment of the gastrointestinal tract and even pancreas, regardless of its location. It can also contain more than one type of mucosa. Heterotopic gastric mucosa is found in 20 to 50% of duplications even though gastric duplications per se account for less than 10% of all duplications.[1-3]

A communicating duplication shares a wall or lumen with the adjacent gastrointestinal tract. The communication may be proximal, be distal, or run the entire length of the duplication. A noncommunicating duplication is adjacent to a segment of the gastrointestinal tract but does not share a lumen. Noncommunicating duplications are four times more common than communicating ones.[1] Noncommunicating duplications tend to be rounded and cystic but may also have a dumbbell configuration. Elongated tubular duplications are more likely to communicate with adjacent bowel than are cystic duplications. In the abdomen, duplications are located on the mesenteric side of the bowel.[4-6]

### Clinical Findings

Duplications are manifested in a variety of ways, and most are diagnosed by age 2 years. Some duplications are detected by prenatal sonography; others present in the neonatal period, causing bowel obstruction, intussusception, mass, or bleeding[7, 8] (Fig. 79–1). In later childhood, duplications often manifest as a mass or with hemorrhage. Oral or esophageal duplications may cause airway narrowing and respiratory symptoms or may be an incidental finding on a chest radiograph.[9, 10] Esophageal duplications cannot be differentiated clinically or radiographically from bronchogenic cysts.[11-13] These are both malformations of the primitive foregut that share a similar cause, presentation, and location. Microscopic examination of the mucosal lining is necessary to determine whether the lesion arose from the respiratory or gastrointestinal tract. Approximately 15% of esophageal duplications straddle the esophageal hiatus.[11]

Pyloric duplications are rare and clinically simulate hypertrophic pyloric stenosis.[14, 15] Intrapancreatic or duodenal duplications can obstruct pancreatic drainage and cause pancreatitis or perforation of adjacent bowel from pressure and vascular compromise.[16-19]

Colonic duplication is a more complex lesion[20-23] (Fig. 79–2). The typical segmental duplication as described in the preceding is the most common type. The entire colon including appendix may be duplicated, however, with the distal portions fusing or one portion developing into a form of imperforate anus (Fig. 79–3). Some rare forms of colonic duplication are associated with duplications of the bladder, genitalia, and sacrum. Colonic and rectal duplications may present as an anal fistula or with bleeding, focal infection, or rectal prolapse.[20-25]

Most affected children have only one duplication, although multiple duplications may be present in up to 15%.[1-5] Children with multiple duplications are more likely to have additional congenital malformations than are those with solitary ones.[3]

Neurenteric cysts are a rare form of duplication in which a gastrointestinal abnormality is associated with a

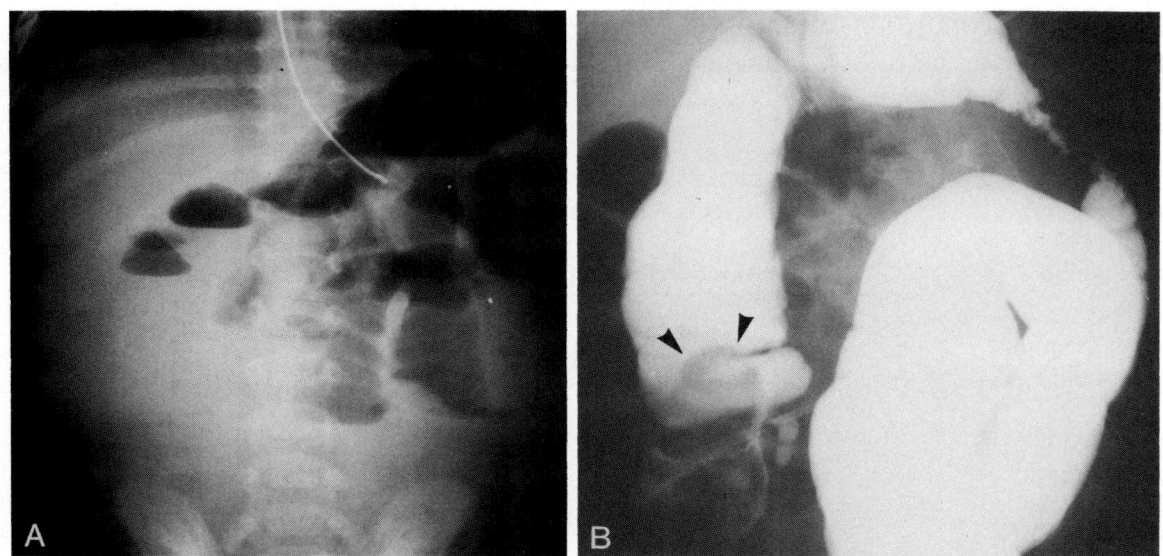

**Figure 79–1. Ileal duplication causing intussusception in a neonate. A.** Dilated bowel loops with air-fluid levels are seen proximal to the intussusception on this plain film. **B.** Barium enema could not reduce the intussuscepted mass in the cecum *(arrowheads)* and at surgery a duplication was found as the lead point.

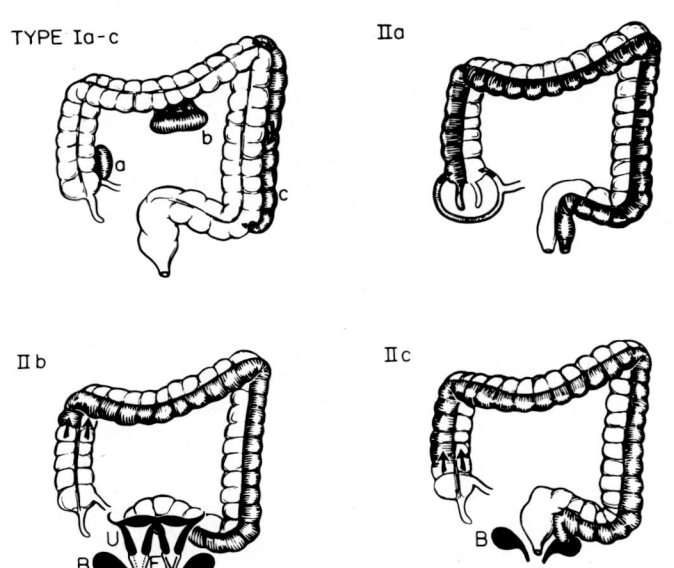

**Figure 79–2. Types of colonic duplication.** Type I, segmental colonic duplication without other caudal duplication: a, noncommunicating spheric duplication; b, noncommunicating tubular duplication; c, communicating tubular duplication. Type II, complete or segmental colonic duplication with genitourinary duplication: a, duplication with two perineal openings; b, duplication with one or both segments ending as a fistula to the vagina, bladder, or perineum; c, duplication with one or both segments imperforate and no fistula. B = bladder; F = fistula; U = uterus; V = vagina. (Reprinted from, by permission of the publisher, Carr SL, Shaffer HA, de Lange EE: Duplication of the colon: varied presentations of a rare congenital anomaly. Can Assoc Radiol J, Vol 39, pp 29–32, March 1988.)

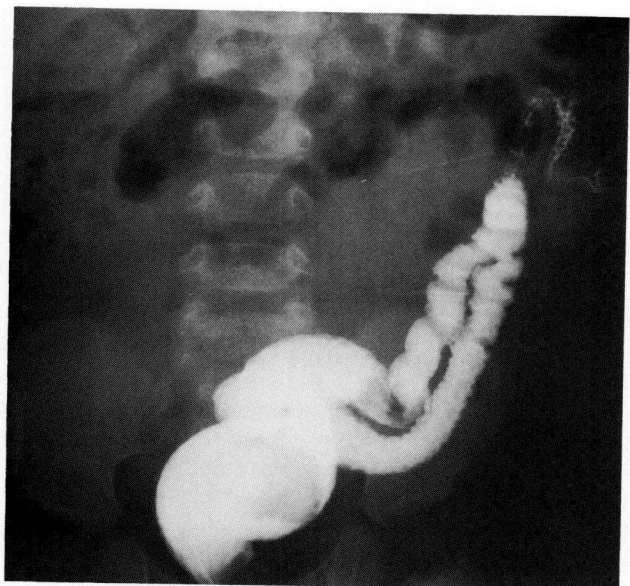

**Figure 79–3. Colonic duplication.** Contrast medium instilled through a stoma in the left upper quadrant fills both limbs of a distal duplication. This child with imperforate anus had both segments ending blindly in the pelvis. The nonfused rectum was surgically created by excising the wall between the segments.

vertebral anomaly, usually some form of spinal dysraphism (Fig. 79–4A). The cysts develop owing to an abnormal persistence of the primitive connection of ectoderm with the endoderm. An adhesion occurs in

the midline of the back, which divides the spinal canal and gives rise to the term *split notochord syndrome.* An intraspinal component may also be present (Fig. 79–4B). The duplicated esophageal segment usually projects from the thoracic spine into the posterior mediastinum, although these cysts can occur in the abdominal cavity. The duplication usually lies caudal to the vertebral changes because of differential growth of the two structures. Vertebral anomalies are seen more frequently in children with thoracic than abdominal duplications even in the absence of neurenteric cyst formation.[26–28]

Physical examination is often unremarkable. If the duplication causes tracheal or bronchial compression, abnormal air exchange or wheezing may be detected. In the abdomen, the fluid-filled duplication can be mobile and elude palpation.

## Treatment

The management of duplication is based on a number of factors: location and size, presenting symptoms, and the presence of communication with adjacent structures.[1–3] Most duplications are treated with simple excision. In some children, a staged repair is necessary. The shared blood supply of abdominal duplications must be recognized, and the vascular supply of the normal bowel must not be compromised. A seldom used approach is percutaneous aspiration of the fluid within the duplication.[29] Internal drainage of duplications containing gastric mucosa is potentially dangerous because acidic gas-

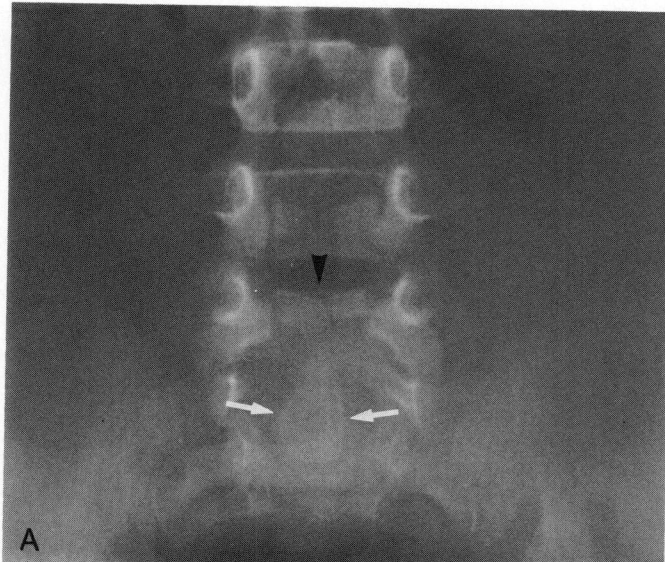

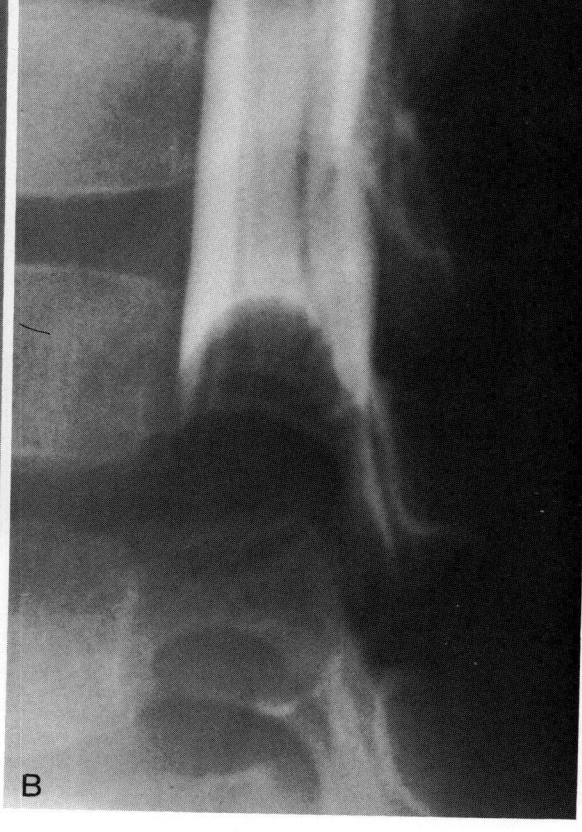

**Figure 79–4. Neurenteric cyst. A.** There is a midline bony fusion mass at the lumbosacral junction *(white arrows)* in addition to the spina bifida in the lower lumbar spine *(black arrowhead).* **B.** Myelography demonstrates the intradural component of the intra-abdominal duplication.

tric secretions can ulcerate the mucosa of adjacent bowel.

## Differential Diagnosis

The differential diagnosis of alimentary duplication depends on the patient's age and sex. A choledochal cyst can be excluded by a hepatobiliary scan. An obstructed renal duplication can be identified by careful sonography. Ovarian cysts may be quite large in the fetus and neonate and present in any quadrant of the abdomen. Serial sonography may be useful because many ovarian cysts decrease in size in the first few months of postnatal life. Mesenteric cysts and omental cysts are less common and are often multilocular or septate.

## Radiologic Findings

When prenatal ultrasound reveals a fluid-filled structure in the abdominal cavity, postnatal scanning should be performed to assess change in its size and echogenicity and to detect any secondary characteristics that can assist in diagnosis.[6, 30, 31] Many duplications have an echogenic muscular rim that is not present in other cystic lesions[31] (Fig. 79–5). The fluid within the duplication cyst may become echogenic if there is hemorrhage or communication with adjacent bowel.

Esophageal duplications manifest as soft tissue masses (Figs. 79–6 and 79–7) on chest radiographs, simulating adenopathy or posterior mediastinal tumors, although some appear to arise from the middle mediastinum. They occur five times more often on the right than on the left and are only rarely calcified.

When chest films demonstrate a mediastinal mass,

chest computed tomography (CT) should be the next examination obtained. On CT, the density of the fluid within the duplication depends on protein content and the presence of hemorrhage and communication with the gut. CT or magnetic resonance shows the full extent of the duplication, excludes noncystic masses, and diagnoses additional foregut abnormalities that occur with increased frequency in children with esophageal duplication. A barium esophagram may need to be obtained to better assess communication between the lumen and the duplication.[3, 13, 29, 32]

Plain films of the abdomen are of little value in the diagnosis of duplication because calcification and mass effect are rarely present.[33] Plain film calcification is most often associated with genitourinary or adrenal diseases. Duplications may be unexpected findings on barium studies performed for the presenting or unrelated symptoms (Fig. 79–8; see also Figs. 79–1 and 79–6). Sonography should then be performed and the work-up can stop if the classic muscular rim of duplication is identified.[31] CT may be required if the patient has atypical symptoms or if the diagnosis remains uncertain after ultrasound (Fig. 79–9).

Duplications that present with gastrointestinal bleeding usually contain gastric mucosa. In this setting, technetium Tc 99m pertechnetate scintigraphy should be performed because it will identify gastric mucosa even in aberrant locations.[4, 34]

Imaging of the spinal canal and cord is recommended when there are spinal changes associated with a suspected duplication. CT depicts the structural bone abnormalities to best advantage, whereas magnetic resonance is superior in demonstrating associated spinal cord disease.[27, 28] The detection of anomalies of the central nervous system is desirable so that excision of the duplication will not produce trauma or infection of the spinal cord.

## CYSTIC FIBROSIS

Cystic fibrosis (CF) is the most common lethal genetic abnormality in the white population. The recessive gene is carried by about 5% of this group, and CF is seen in 1 per 2000 live births. Mucoviscidosis, the older name for cystic fibrosis, gives a clue to the underlying pathologic process. All mucus-producing glands manifest an abnormality of exocrine function by making unusually thick secretions. The disease affects multiple organs, but the degree of involvement is not parallel in all organs. Many children with severe lung disease have little gastrointestinal disease, and some children with minimal lung disease are diagnosed because of gastrointestinal disease or hepatic fibrosis. A more detailed discussion of the etiology and pathogenesis of this disorder is presented in Chapter 118.[35–42]

## Clinical Findings

The first postnatal intestinal manifestations of CF relate to abnormal meconium: meconium peritonitis,

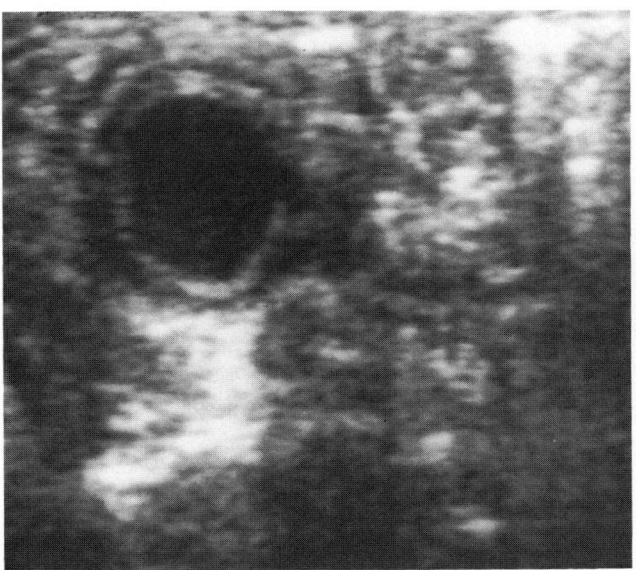

**Figure 79–5. Small bowel duplication.** This transverse sonogram shows a rounded, fluid-filled mass that has a well-defined echogenic edge, which represents the classic muscular rim of alimentary duplications.

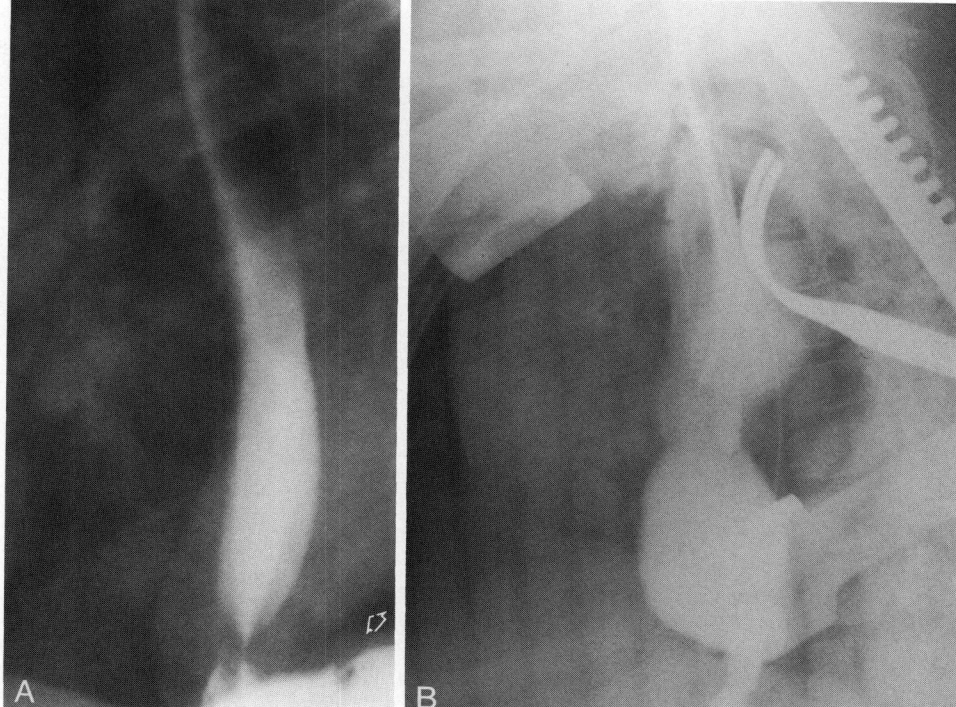

**Figure 79–6. Noncommunicating esophageal duplication. A**. The barium-filled esophagus is normal in caliber. On this lateral projection, an oblique soft tissue structure is extending from above to the diaphragm *(arrow)*. **B**. Intraoperative injection of the tubular duplication demonstrates that it extends the length of the thorax.

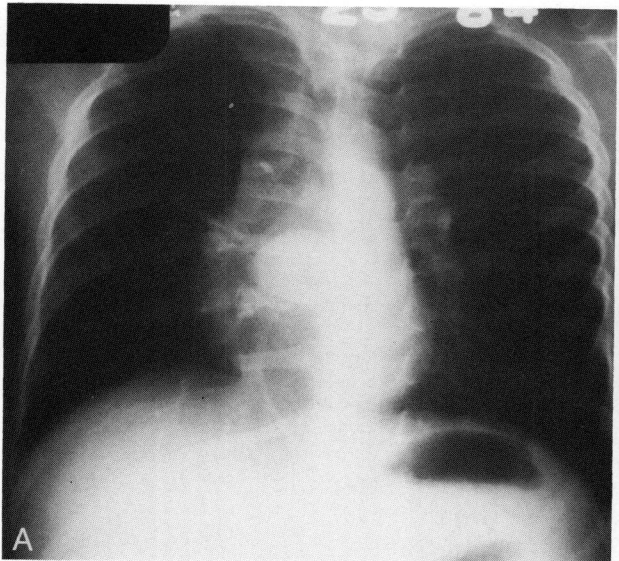

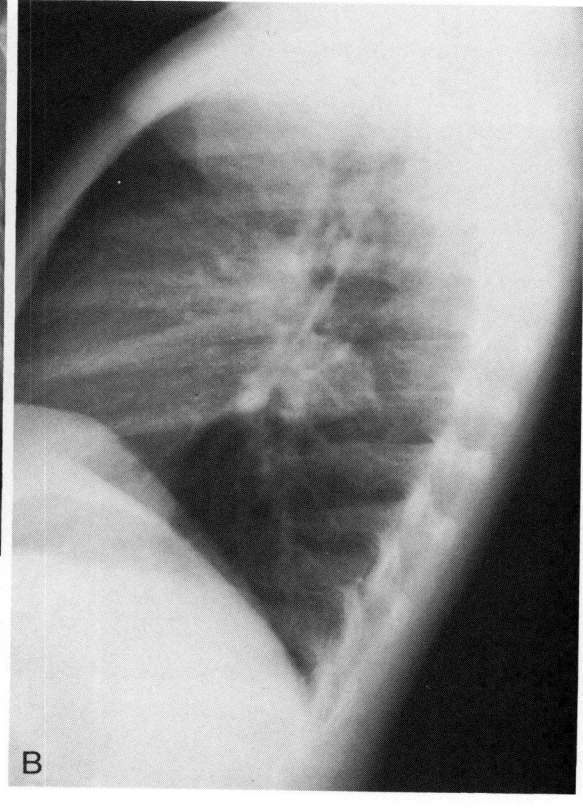

**Figure 79–7. Esophageal duplication.** Posteroanterior **(A)** and lateral **(B)** chest films reveal a well-circumscribed, rounded soft tissue mass that projects posteriorly and to the right.

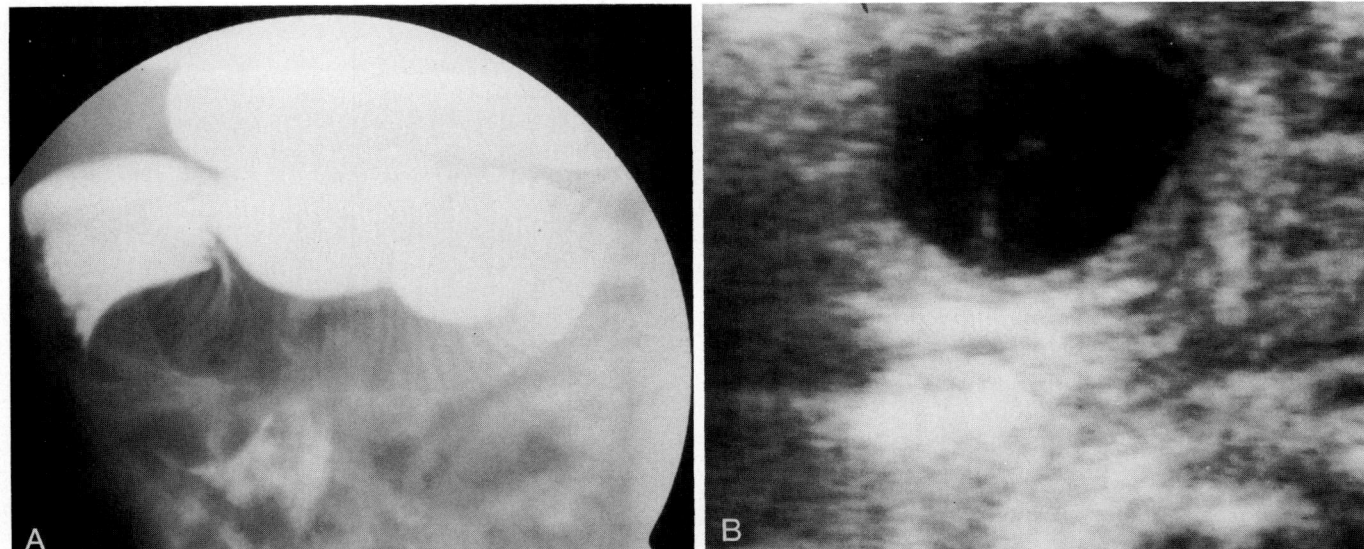

**Figure 79–8. Jejunal duplication. A**. An upper gastrointestinal series performed on a neonate who presented with vomiting shows a filling defect in the jejunum that was only intermittently observed. For this reason, sonography was performed. **B**. A longitudinal scan of the upper abdomen demonstrates a fluid-filled structure with a muscular rim that could only be identified in the deepest portion of the duplication.

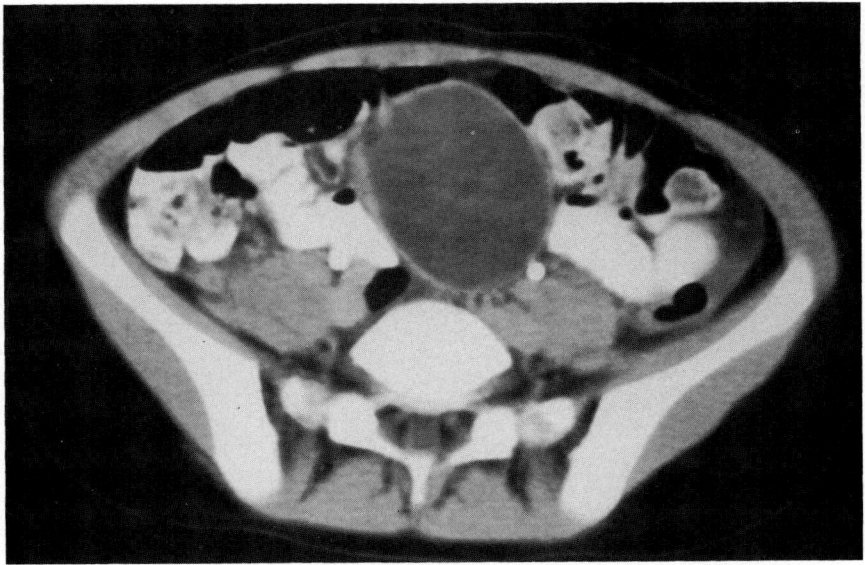

**Figure 79–9. Ileal duplication.** CT scan shows a spherical cystic mass with a perceptible wall that enhances to the same degree as adjacent muscular structures.

meconium ileus, and meconium plug (see Chapter 74). Meconium ileus, which occurs in 10 to 15% of CF children, is due to impaction of thick meconium or pellets of meconium in the distal ileum (Fig. 79–10). At one time, meconium ileus was associated with a 50% mortality, but the survival rate has increased to greater than 90% in the past two decades.[37–41] A meconium ileus–like syndrome has been described in 16 children, none of whom had CF.[41a] Improved survival can be attributed to nonsurgical management of the meconium ileus itself and better pulmonary and nutritional therapy.[42] There is a higher incidence of hepatic fibrosis in CF children who present with meconium ileus than in those who do not.[42]

A meconium plug is the first manifestation of CF in 25% of CF neonates (see Chapter 74).[43] In the majority of neonates, meconium plug is a self-limited condition, but it may also herald Hirschsprung's disease. CF and Hirschsprung's disease can coexist, and in some infants, the small left colon syndrome may be the first sign of CF.[43, 44]

Changes in thoracic configuration resulting from the underlying lung disease predispose CF children to gastroesophageal reflux.[45–48] Reflux and aspiration, in turn, aggravate the underlying pulmonary disease. Retrosternal pain caused by the reflux may secondarily limit caloric intake by the infant, which compounds nutritional problems.

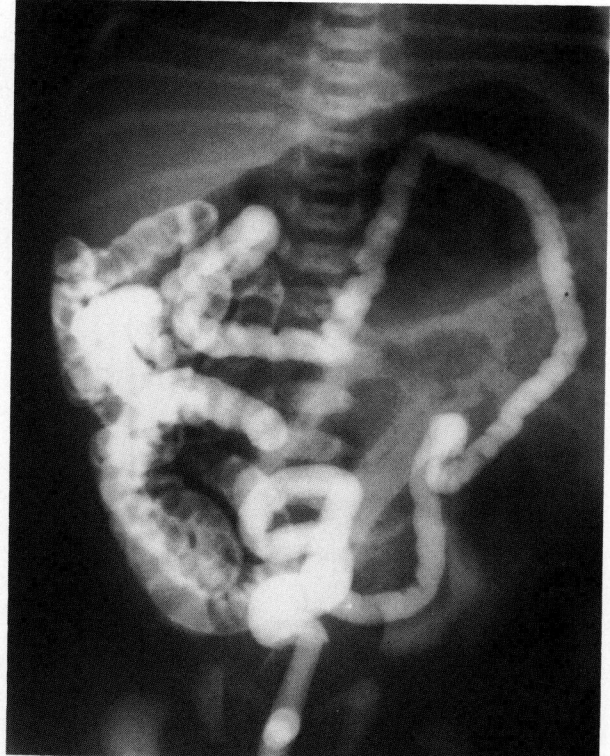

**Figure 79–10. Meconium ileus demonstrated on water-soluble enema.** The colon is small in caliber, similar in diameter to the small bowel, which is impacted with multiple small, rounded pellets of meconium.

Malabsorption and steatorrhea resulting from pancreatic insufficiency can be minimized with oral pancreatic enzyme replacement. Persistent symptoms of abdominal pain, bloating, diarrhea, or malabsorption in a child whose enzyme replacement is at proper levels suggest that there may be an additional gastrointestinal problem such as inflammatory bowel disease, giardiasis, or lactose intolerance.[48–50]

Children with CF can present with abdominal pain resulting from several different processes. Intussusception may develop in older children and teen-agers with cystic fibrosis.[51] Appendiceal disease may take the usual form of appendicitis or a more unusual but symptomatic mucous distention of the appendix.[52] Hypersecretion of gastric acid may cause ulceration or other mucosal changes in the duodenum and proximal small bowel.[53] Meconium ileus equivalent occurs in about 1 to 15% of the CF population and is discussed in Chapter 118. Rectal prolapse may be an initial indication of CF or develop while children are being treated.[54, 55] In one series, 11% of children with rectal prolapse were found to have CF.[55] Children with rectal prolapse without underlying abnormality (constipation, diarrhea, meningomyelocele) should undergo sweat chloride analysis for exclusion of CF.

## Radiologic Findings

The prenatal diagnosis of CF is based on a number of nonspecific ultrasonographic findings: polyhydramnios, meconium peritonitis, intra-abdominal cyst, ascites, or dilated bowel.[56] These findings take on particular significance when there is a sibling with CF. Meconium peritonitis and meconium ileus are described and illustrated in Chapter 74.[57, 58]

Barium esophagrams should be performed to identify varices in children with signs of portal hypertension or children with hemoptysis. When these studies are being performed, it is also important to look for gastroesophageal reflux and its complications, such as esophagitis and stricture. Portal venous flow should also be documented by Doppler sonography when portal hypertension is suspected.[59]

Pulmonary inflammation may be a source of active bleeding that can be confused with variceal bleeding. Pulmonary bleeders are identified via bronchial arteriography and are treated with intravascular embolization techniques or segmental lung resection.

Plain films of the abdomen in CF children may reveal peritoneal or, in older patients, pancreatic calcifications. In patients with hepatic fibrosis, the spleen is often enlarged. Large amounts of bubbly stool or small bowel obstruction can be seen in children with meconium ileus equivalent[40] (Fig. 79–11). Intussusception may be difficult to differentiate from meconium ileus equivalent syndrome. Benign pneumatosis intestinalis may be present in older patients who have other abnormal air collections in the thorax or abdomen.[60, 61] This benign pneumatosis is not associated with underlying bowel necrosis or ulceration.

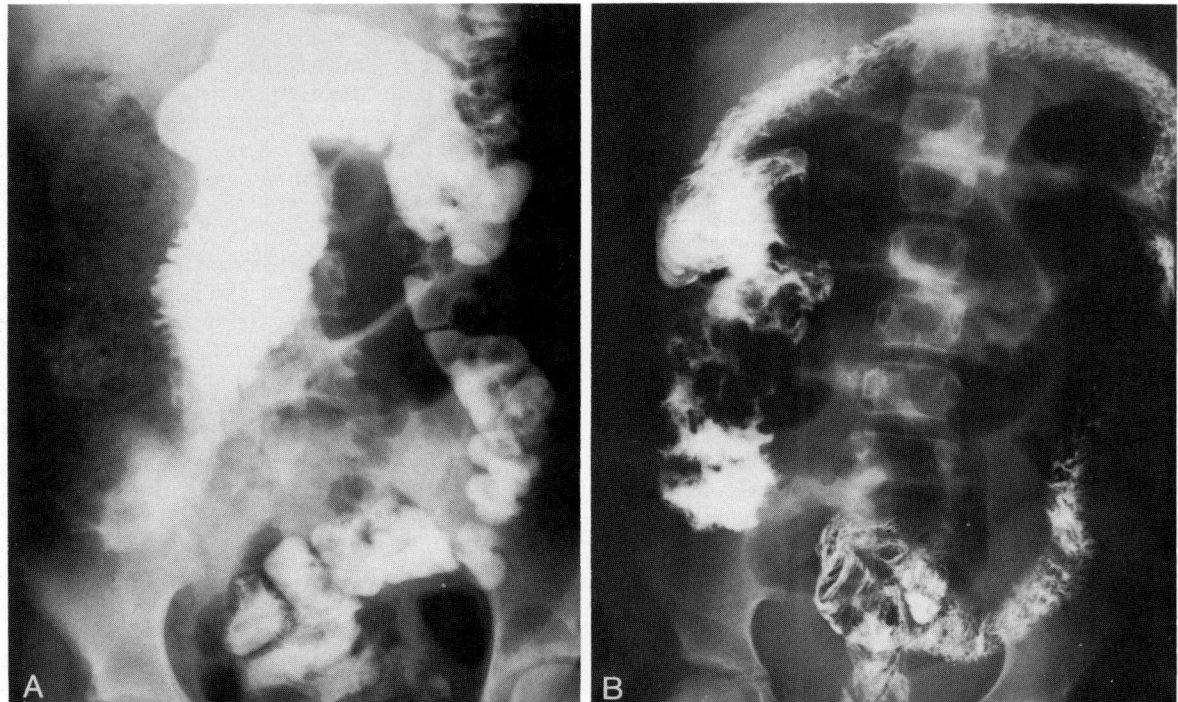

**Figure 79–11. Meconium ileus equivalent syndrome. A**. Meconium ileus equivalent syndrome diagnosed and treated with a diatrizoate meglumine (Cystografin) enema. **B**. In a different child, the postevacuation film demonstrates residual fecal material in the dilated ascending colon. The colonic mucosa has an abnormal spiculated appearance.

Studies of the duodenum (see Chapter 76) and small bowel performed with contrast medium often demonstrate dilatation, prolonged transit time, and prominent valvulae conniventes. Poor coating of the duodenum is due to abnormal quantity and quality of mucus. Filling defects can also result from enlarged Brunner's glands or paraduodenal varices. Thickened mucus becomes impacted in the mucosal crypts, causing them to enlarge. If these ectatic crypts fill with barium, the mucosal coating of the small bowel becomes irregular and spiculated. Duodenal mucosal injury is aggravated by gastric hypersecretion that is insufficiently buffered by the subnormal pancreatic secretions.

## SMALL BOWEL AND COLONIC INFECTIONS

Bacterial, viral, and parasitic gastroenteritis is a major cause of pediatric morbidity and mortality worldwide. The fever, diarrhea, and abdominal pain that accompany the intestinal infection result from enterotoxin release, mucosal invasion, and damage to enterocytes.[62–66] Most children are successfully treated with oral rehydration. Medications to decrease gut motility or antibiotics to control specific infections are used in specific settings.[62, 67, 68]

Infections with *Helicobacter pylori* have been implicated in the development of peptic ulcer disease. The same organism is seen in association with a diarrheal illness in both adults and children and may produce lactose intolerance.

*Yersinia* enterocolitis may produce symptoms that simulate appendicitis or Crohn's disease.[67, 69] Barium studies show changes in the terminal ileum reminiscent of Crohn's disease. Ultrasound is useful in this setting because it can identify the enlarged lymph nodes that often accompany *Yersinia* infection.

Most children with the clinical picture of gastroenteritis do not need imaging.[70] Studies are required when the child presents with an acute abdomen or when symptoms persist and laboratory tests fail to provide a specific diagnosis.

## GASTROINTESTINAL PERFORATION

### Clinical Findings

Perforation of the gastrointestinal tract is associated with serious morbidity and significant mortality. Perforation may be due to ischemia (intussusception, volvulus, vasculitis, necrotizing enterocolitis), inflammation (infections, peptic ulceration, appendicitis, regional enteritis) or trauma (blunt, sharp, iatrogenic).[71–88]

In neonates, perforation most commonly occurs in the small bowel and colon and usually is due to necrotizing enterocolitis. Prematurity, birth asphyxia, low birth weight, Hirschsprung's disease, and meconium ileus are all associated with high rates of neonatal perforation. Idiopathic gastric perforation is believed to be caused by the splanchnic ischemia that attends the redirection of blood from mesenteric blood supply, the so-called diving reflex. The relative incidence of gastric perforation is declining in relationship to small bowel perforation as more very premature infants survive the perinatal period to subsequently develop necrotizing enterocolitis.

Pharyngeal and esophageal perforations are usually due to instrumentation at delivery. The infant may present with fever, blood-tinged mucus or emesis, or difficulty eating. With acute presentation, plain films may show air in the soft tissues of the neck. A study with water-soluble contrast medium should be performed when perforation is suspected. A perforation appears as a cavity of variable size with irregular walls, whereas a congenital diverticulum has smooth walls (Fig. 79–12). The symptoms and the radiologic findings allow the traumatically induced cavity to be differentiated from a congenital diverticulum. Occasionally, neonates and children will reflux or vomit so forcefully that they will produce an esophageal tear, Boerhaave's syndrome.[89–93]

In older children, pharyngeal perforation is usually due to falling with a ruler, pencil, or other stiff object in the mouth. In a few children, pharyngeal perforation is a sign of child abuse.

Gastrointestinal perforations present in a variety of ways in children. In the neonatal period, respiratory distress often accompanies necrotizing enterocolitis and may dominate the clinical picture. Fever, malaise, and other nonspecific symptoms often make early diagnosis of perforation difficult. Prompt diagnosis is critical, especially for iatrogenic perforations, which have a mortality approaching 50% in some series.[71]

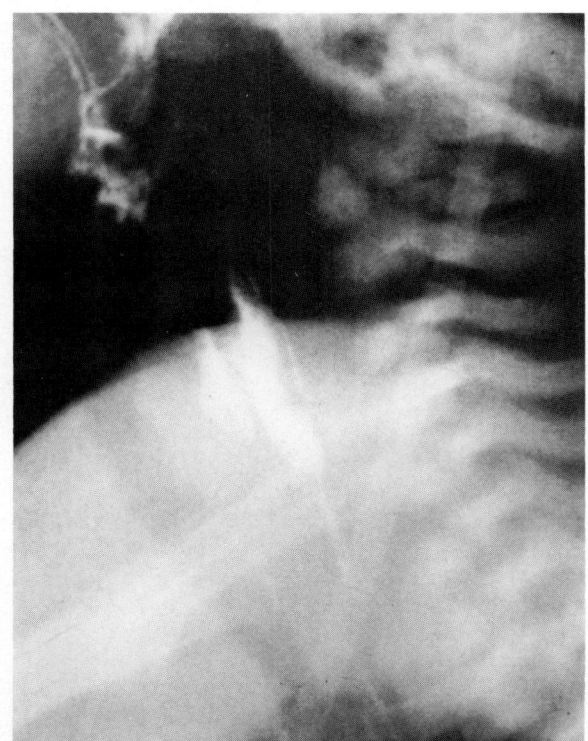

**Figure 79–12. Esophageal perforation demonstrated on a water-soluble esophagram.** At the thoracic inlet, there is an extraluminal collection of contrast medium anterior to the esophagus. The collection is irregular and is associated with soft tissue swelling that is bowing the trachea anteriorly.

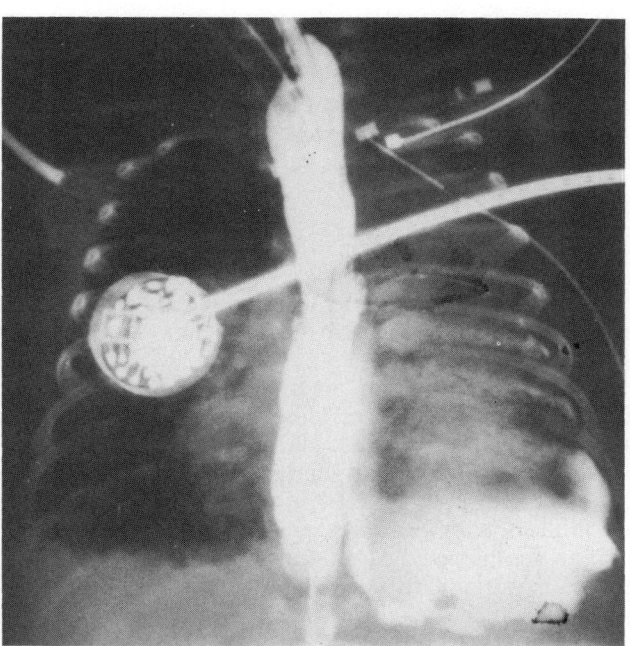

**Figure 79–13. Esophageal perforation.** The side holes of the nasogastric tube permitted water-soluble contrast medium to flow into the esophagus. Because of the perforation, contrast medium spills into the mediastinum and pleural space.

## Radiologic Findings

Esophageal perforation is associated with streaky air collections in the mediastinum that can extend into the neck or abdomen.[94] Acute rupture of the esophagus can cause pneumothorax.[89–92] Free intraperitoneal air can outline the falciform ligament and remnants of the umbilical vessels, define both sides of the bowel wall, or collect centrally with creation of the "football" sign.

Abnormal position or configuration of a nasogastric or nasoduodenal feeding tube suggests that there has been perforation, although duodenal feeding tubes often take a "nonanatomic" course even in the absence of perforation.[83–85] Plain films, including cross-table lateral views, may be useful in determining the position of the catheter. If the catheter tip location is uncertain, it can be determined by injecting a small amount of water-soluble contrast medium through the tube.

Changes of inflammation caused by leakage of gastrointestinal contents into adjacent tissues will appear next. Mediastinal widening and increased soft tissue density may follow esophageal rupture. Pleural effusion and hydropneumothorax may be noted on chest radiographs. Peritoneal fluid, seen with horizontal beam radiography or ultrasound, occurs when intraperitoneal portions of the gut perforate. Lack of visible air-fluid levels does not exclude perforation. If only a small amount of fluid has passed into the peritoneal cavity, air-fluid levels may be absent.[72]

When perforation is suspected, gastrointestinal studies should be performed only with water-soluble contrast agents (Fig. 79–13; see Fig. 79–12). Initially, small amounts of nonionic contrast medium should be given with close fluoroscopic monitoring so that the site and size of the perforation can be identified before it is obscured by peritoneal spill.[95]

Gastrointestinal injuries may be demonstrated by CT performed to exclude trauma to the aorta, liver, or spleen.[96–98] CT is rarely indicated as the first test when isolated perforation of the gut is suspected, however.

## CROHN'S DISEASE

Approximately 12% of cases of Crohn's disease occur in children under the age of 15 years, whereas 28% develop between the ages of 15 and 20 years.[99–110] The radiology, epidemiology, and pathology of pediatric and adult Crohn's disease are identical and are discussed in detail in Chapters 26, 36, 62, and 159. This discussion focuses on the special clinical features of pediatric Crohn's disease.

Children with regional enteritis may present in a fashion similar to that of adults, with diarrhea, abdominal pain, perianal fistulas, and fever, or with age-related symptoms such as failure to thrive and growth retardation.[111–116] Growth retardation may precede the development of gastrointestinal symptoms, and it occurs in up to 30% of children with disease onset before puberty.[110, 111] Anorexia can accompany the disease; in the teen-aged girl, it may be incorrectly attributed to psychologic illness. Children with anorexia nervosa show no evidence of declining growth, however, in contrast to the growth failure in children with inflammatory bowel disease. Anemia is seen in about 25% at the time of presentation.

Arthritis, erythema nodosum, and pyoderma gangrenosum are uncommon initial complaints.[100, 112, 113] Transient arthritis of the larger joints may appear later.

Crohn's disease can affect any portion of the alimentary canal, and in contrast to adults, in whom oral and esophageal involvement is rare, lesions of the upper gastrointestinal tract are seen in about one third of children on radiologic or endoscopic studies.[99–110, 114, 115] Dysphagia or nausea and vomiting are the initial complaints of upper gastrointestinal tract disease. Delay in diagnosis is common because these symptoms are nonspecific. Involvement of the upper gastrointestinal tract is more frequent in children with ileocolitis. Crohn's disease isolated to the upper gastrointestinal tract is rare in children, as is isolated granulomatous colitis. In the very young, the pattern of small bowel disease differs from that of adolescents and adults; there may be jejunal and ileal disease with sparing of the terminal ileum.[110, 115]

Children with upper gastrointestinal tract disease seem to require longer steroid treatment and are more likely to require exogenous nutrition (intravenous or nasogastric). Surgical resection of limited disease may give symptomatic relief.[104, 108] Bone age delay is present in about 30% of affected children, and these individuals also reach an adult height below the expected mean. There is no significant difference in the height of children who have received surgical therapy, compared with medical treatment.[108, 111] Steroid treatment can produce bone changes leading to vertebral body collapse and avascular necrosis of the femoral head.

## LYMPHOMA

Although rare, lymphoma occurs throughout childhood at a rate of about 14 cases per million per year.[117] In this population, there is a slight preponderance of non-Hodgkin's lymphoma over Hodgkin's disease, and there is a 3:1 male to female predilection. In addition, there is an increased incidence of lymphoma in children with Wiskott-Aldrich syndrome, ataxia-telangiectasia, acquired immunodeficiency syndrome, renal transplant, hypogammaglobulinemia, and other immunocompromised states.[117–119]

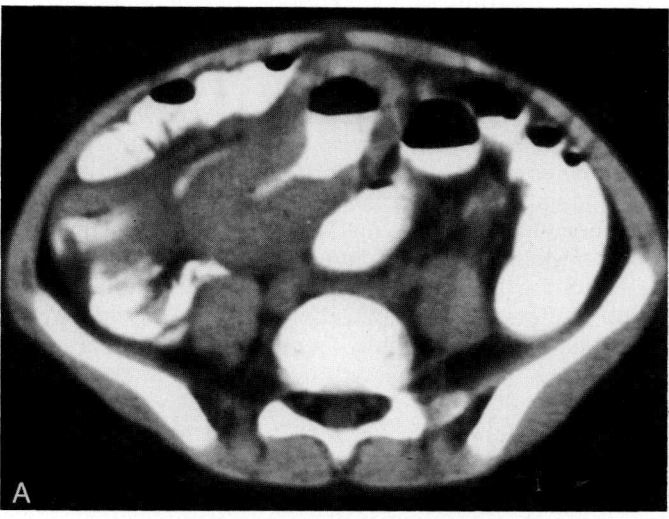 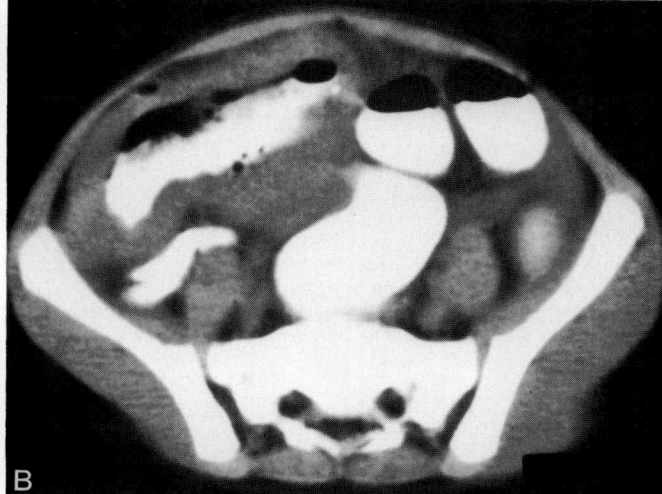

**Figure 79–14. Abdominal lymphoma. A**. Infiltration of the bowel wall causes mural thickening and lumen narrowing on this CT scan. **B**. This more caudal scan shows a thickened wall as well as aneurysmal dilatation.

Approximately 50% of children with lymphoma will either present with abdominal disease or develop it during the course of their illness.[120] Abdominal lymphoma may present clinically with abdominal fullness or functional change, such as bowel obstruction. Occasionally, the lymphoma will act as a lead point for ileocolic intussusception or present as a rectal polyp.[121, 122] The abdominal disease may also produce no symptoms and be discovered only because of radiologic studies done for extra-abdominal lymphoma .

## Radiologic Findings

Plain films of the abdomen yield little information about the extent of disease. Hepatosplenomegaly may be noted. A haziness to the abdomen suggests the presence of ascites. Barium studies show the following abnormalities in lymphoma: nodularity, focal mass, polyp formation, narrowing, obstruction, or focal aneurysmal dilatation of a bowel loop (see Chapter 151).

CT and ultrasound have replaced barium studies and excretory urography for staging. On ultrasound scans, lymphomatous masses within bowel can be complex or relatively sonolucent.[123–127] Lymphomatous involvement of bowel may cause focal or diffuse thickening of the wall. If the lumen is compressed by the lymphoma, the intraluminal contents may be intensely echogenic.

Lymphomatous lymph nodes are generally sonolucent as well. Lymphangiography has shown that not all enlarged lymph nodes contain lymphoma and that some normal-appearing lymph nodes may be infiltrated with tumor. Therefore, both negative and positive results should be interpreted with caution and with attention to other pertinent findings.

CT has the advantage of staging the chest, abdomen (Fig. 79–14), and pelvis at one examination and is also superb in revealing complications of treatment such as fatty replacement of the liver or fungal microabscesses of the solid organs.[128–132]

## References

1. Holcomb GW III, Gheissari A, O'Neill JA Jr, et al: Surgical management of alimentary tract duplications. Ann Surg 209:167–174, 1989.
2. Ildstad ST, Tollerud DJ, Weiss RG, et al: Duplication of the alimentary tract. Clinical characteristics, preferred treatment, and associated malformations. Ann Surg 208:184–189, 1988.
3. Bower RJ, Sieber WK, Kiesewetter WB: Alimentary tract duplications in children. Ann Surg 188:669–674, 1978.
4. Gilchrist AM, Sloan JM, Logan CJH, et al: Case report: gastrointestinal bleeding due to multiple ileal duplications diagnosed by scintigraphy and barium studies. Clin Radiol 41:134–136, 1990.
5. Egelhoff JC, Bisset GS III, Strife JL: Multiple enteric duplications in an infant. Pediatr Radiol 16:160–161, 1986.
6. Bidwell JK, Nelson A: Prenatal diagnosis of congenital duplication of the stomach. J Ultrasound Med 5:589–591, 1986.
7. Patriquin HB, Afshani E, Effman E, et al: Neonatal intussusception. Report of 12 cases. Radiology 125:463–466, 1977.
8. Sonada N, Matsuzaki S, Ono A, et al: Duplication of the caecum in a neonate simulating intussusception. Pediatr Radiol 15:427–428, 1985.
9. Winslow RE, Dykstra G, Scholten DJ, et al: Duplication of the cervical esophagus. An unrecognized cause of respiratory distress in infants. Am Surg 50:506–508, 1984.
10. Lister J, Zachary RB: Cystic duplications in the tongue. J Pediatr Surg 3:491–493, 1968.
11. Hall CM: Transdiaphragmatic jejunal duplication: a report of five cases. Radiology 131:663–667, 1979.
12. Fitch SJ, Tonkin ILD, Tonkin AK: Imaging of foregut duplication cysts. Radiographics 6:189–201, 1986.
13. Hernandez RJ: Role of CT in evaluation of children with foregut cyst. Pediatr Radiol 17:265–268, 1987.
14. Mogilner JG, Vinograd I, Presman A, et al: Pyloric duplication in children. Pediatr Surg Int 5:61–63, 1990.
15. Bommen M, Singh MP: Pyloric duplication in a preterm infant. J Pediatr Surg 19:158–159, 1984.
16. Lavine JE, Harrison M, Heyman MD: Gastrointestinal duplications causing relapsing pancreatitis in children. Gastroenterol 97:1556–1558, 1989.
17. Case records of the Massachusetts General Hospital (case 48–1982). N Engl J Med 307:1438–1443, 1982.
17a. Archer D, Somers S: Duodenal duplication cysts—case report and review of the current literature. J Can Assoc Radiol 43:49–51, 1992.
18. Royle SG, Doig CM: Perforation of the jejunum secondary to a duplication cyst lined with ectopic gastric mucosa. J Pediatr Surg 23:1025–1026, 1988.
18a. Murty TVM, Bhargava RK, Rakas FS: Gastroduodenal duplication. J Pediatr Surg 27:515–517, 1992.
19. Kremer RM, Lepoff RB, Izant RJ: Duplication of the stomach. J Pediatr Surg 5:360–364, 1970.
20. Kottra JJ, Dodds WJ: Duplication of the large bowel. AJR 113:310–315, 1971.
21. Carr SL, Shaffer HA Jr, de Lange EE: Duplication of the colon: varied presentations of a rare anomaly. Can Assoc Radiol J 39:29–32, 1988.
22. Yousefzadeh DH, Bickers GH, Jackson JH Jr, et al: Tubular colonic duplication—review of 1876–1981 literature. Pediatr Radiol 13:65–71, 1983.
23. Yucesan S, Zorludemir U, Olcay I: Complete duplication of the colon. J Pediatr Surg 21:962–963, 1986.
24. LaQuaglia MP, Feins N, Eraklis A, et al: Rectal duplications. J Pediatr Surg 25:980–984, 1990.
25. Boothroyd AE, Christine MH: Rectal duplications in children: a presentation of four cases. Eur J Radiol 10:38–41, 1990.
26. Bentley JFR, Smith JR: Developmental posterior enteric remnants and spinal malformations. The split notochord syndrome. Arch Dis Child 35:76–78, 1960.
27. Alrabeeah A, Gillis DA, Giacomantonio M, et al: Neurenteric cysts—a spectrum. J Pediatr Surg 23:752–754, 1988.
28. Gilchrist BF, Harrison MW, Campbell JR: Neurenteric cyst: current management. J Pediatr Surg 25:1231–1233, 1990.
29. Kuhlman JE, Fishman EK, Wang KP, et al: Esophageal duplication cyst: CT and transesophageal needle aspiration. AJR 145:531–532, 1985.
30. Lamont AC, Starinsky R, Cremin BJ: Ultrasonic diagnosis of duplication cysts in children. Br J Radiol 57:463–467, 1984.
31. Barr LL, Hayden CK, Stansberry SD, et al: Enteric duplication cysts in children: are their ultrasonographic wall characteristics diagnostic? Pediatr Radiol 20:326–328, 1990.
32. Rhee RS, Ray CG III, Kravetz MH, et al: Cervical esophageal duplication cyst: MR imaging. J Comput Assist Tomogr 12:693–695, 1988.
33. Alford BA, Armstrong P, Franken EA, et al: Calcification associated with duodenal duplications in children. Radiology 134:647–648, 1980.
34. Chaudhuri TK, Polak JJ: Autoradiographic studies of distribution in the stomach of 99m Tc-pertechnetate. Radiology 123:223–224, 1977.
35. Rosenstein BJ: Cystic fibrosis presenting with the meconium plug syndrome. Am J Dis Child 132:167–169, 1978.
36. Park RW, Grand RJ: Gastrointestinal manifestations of cystic fibrosis: a review. Gastroenterology 81:1143–1161, 1981.
37. Rescorla FJ, Grosfeld JL, West KJ, et al: Changing patterns of treatment and survival in neonates with meconium ileus. Arch Surg 124:837–840, 1989.

38. Djurhuus MJ, Lykkegaard E, Pock-Steen OC: Gastrointestinal radiological findings in cystic fibrosis. Pediatr Radiol 1:113–117, 1973.

39. Olson MM, Luck SR, Lloyd-Still J, et al: The spectrum of meconium disease in infancy. J Pediatr Surg 17:479–481, 1982.

40. Maurage C, Lenaerts C, Weber A, et al: Meconium ileus and its equivalent as a risk factor for the development of cirrhosis: an autopsy study in cystic fibrosis. J Pediatr Gastroenterol Nutr 9:17–20, 1989.

41. Kerem E, Corey M, Kerem B, et al: Clinical and genetic comparisons of patients with cystic fibrosis, with or without meconium ileus. J Pediatr 114:767–773, 1989.

41a. Chang PY, Huang FY, Yeh ML, et al: Meconium ileus–like condition in Chinese neonates. J Pediatr Surg 27:1217–1219, 1992.

42. Wheeler WB, Colten HR: Cystic fibrosis: current approach to diagnosis and management. Pediatr Rev 9:241–248, 1988.

43. Hen J, Dolan TF, Touloukian RJ: Meconium plug syndrome associated with cystic fibrosis and Hirschsprung's disease. Pediatrics 66:466–471, 1980.

44. Ellerbroek C, Smith WL: Neonatal small left colon in an infant with cystic fibrosis. Pediatr Radiol 16:162–163, 1986.

45. Bendig DW, Seilheimer DK, Wagner ML, et al: Complications of gastroesophageal reflux in patients with cystic fibrosis. J Pediatr 100:536–540, 1982.

46. Scott BR, O'Loughlin EV, Gall DG: Gastroesophageal reflux in patients with cystic fibrosis. J Pediatr 106:223–227, 1984.

47. Stringer DA, Sprigg A, Juodis E, et al: The association of cystic fibrosis, gastroesophageal reflux and reduced pulmonary function. Can Assoc Radiol J 39:100–102, 1988.

48. Baxter PS, Dickson JA, Variend S, et al: Intestinal disease in cystic fibrosis. Arch Dis Child 63:1496–1497, 1988.

49. Behrens R, Segerer H, Bowing B, et al: Crohn's disease in cystic fibrosis. J Pediatr Gastroenterol Nutr 9:528–531, 1989.

50. Hill SM, Phillips AD, Mearns M, et al: Cows' milk sensitive enteropathy in cystic fibrosis. Arch Dis Child 64:1251–1255, 1989.

51. Holsclaw DS, Rocmans C, Shwachman H: Intussusception in patients with cystic fibrosis. Pediatrics 48:51–58, 1971.

52. Coughlin JP, Gauderer MLW, Stern RC, et al: The spectrum of appendiceal disease in cystic fibrosis. J Pediatr Surg 25:835–839, 1990.

53. Cox KL, Isenberg JN, Ament ME: Gastric acid hypersecretion in cystic fibrosis. J Pediatr Gastroenterol Nutr 1:559–565, 1982.

54. Stern RC, Izant RJ, Boat TF, et al: Treatment and prognosis of rectal prolapse in cystic fibrosis. Gastroenterology 82:707–710, 1982.

55. Zempsky WT, Rosenstein BJ: The cause of rectal prolapse in children. Am J Dis Child 142:338–339, 1988.

56. Nyberg DA, Hastrup W, Watts H, et al: Dilated fetal bowel. A sonographic sign of cystic fibrosis. J Ultrasound Med 6:257–260, 1987.

57. Finkel LI, Slovis TL: Meconium peritonitis, intraperitoneal calcifications and cystic fibrosis. Pediatr Radiol 12:92–93, 1982.

58. Pan EY, Chen LY, Yang JZ, et al: Radiographic diagnosis of meconium peritonitis. A report of 200 cases including six fetal cases. Pediatr Radiol 13:199–205, 1983.

59. Vergesslich KA, Gotz M, Mostbeck G, et al: Portal venous blood flow in cystic fibrosis: assessment by duplex Doppler sonography. Pediatr Radiol 19:371–374, 1989.

60. Hernanz-Schulman M, Kirkpatrick J, Shwachman H, et al: Pneumatosis intestinalis in cystic fibrosis. Radiology 160:497–499, 1986.

61. Olmsted WW, Madewell JE: Pneumatosis cystoides intestinalis: a pathophysiologic explanation of the roentgenographic signs. Gastrointest Radiol 1:177–181, 1976.

62. Radetsky M: Laboratory evaluation of acute diarrhea. Pediatr Infect Dis 5:230–238, 1986.

63. Bishop WP, Ulshen MH: Bacterial gastroenteritis. Pediatr Clin North Am 35:69–87, 1988.

63a. Gracey M: Gastrointestinal infections in children. Curr Opin Gastroenterol 9:107–111, 1993.

64. Hamilton JR: Viral enteritis. Pediatr Clin North Am 35:89–101, 1988.

65. Ho MS, Glass RI, Pinsky PF, et al: Rotavirus as a cause of diarrheal morbidity and mortality in the United States. J Infect Dis 158:1112–1116, 1988.

66. Pizarro D, Posada G, Mahalanabis D, et al: Comparison of efficacy of a glucose/glycerine/glycylglycine electrolyte solution versus the standard WHO/ORS in diarrheic dehydrated children. J Pediatr Gastroenterol Nutr 7:882–888, 1988.

67. Atkinson GO Jr, Gay BB Jr, Ball TI Jr, et al: *Yersinia enterocolitica* colitis in infants: radiographic changes. Radiology 148:113–116, 1983.

68. McShane A, Gillespie SH, Corkery CWB: Neonatal campylobacterenteritis with secondary lactose intolerance. Acta Paediatr Scand 77:603, 1988.

69. Matsumoto T, Iida M, Sakai T, et al: *Yersinia* terminal ileitis: sonographic findings in eight patients. AJR 156:965–967, 1991.

70. Ho MS, Glass RI, Pinsky PF, et al: Diarrheal deaths in American children. Are they preventable? JAMA 260:3281–3285, 1988.

71. Borzotta AP, Groff DB: Gastrointestinal perforation in infants. Am J Surg 155:447–452, 1988.

72. Kaufman RA, Kuhns LR, Poznanski AK, et al: Gastrointestinal perforation without intraperitoneal air-fluid level in neonatal pneumoperitoneum. AJR 127:915–921, 1976.

73. Gugliantini P, Caione P, Rivosecchi M, et al: Intestinal perforation in newborn following intrauterine meconium peritonitis. Pediatr Radiol 8:113–115, 1979.

74. Lloyd JR: The etiology of gastrointestinal perforations in the newborn. J Pediatr Surg 4:77–84, 1969.

75. Tucker AS, Soine L, Izant RJ Jr: Gastrointestinal perforations in infancy. Anatomic and etiologic gamuts. AJR 123:755–763, 1975.

76. Tan CEL, Kiely EM, Agrawal M, et al: Neonatal gastrointestinal perforation. J Pediatr Surg 24:888–892, 1989.

77. Wardhan H, Gangopadhayay AN, Singhal GD: Intestinal perforation in children. Aust Paediatr 25:99–100, 1989.

78. Puglisi BS, Kauffman HM, Stewart ET, et al: Colonic perforations in renal transplant patients. AJR 145:555–558, 1985.

79. Taylor GA, Eichelberger MR: Abdominal CT in children with neurologic impairment following blunt trauma. Abdominal CT in comatose children. Ann Surg 210:229–233, 1989.

80. Bulas DI, Taylor GA, Eichelberger MR: The value of CT in detecting bowel perforation in children after blunt abdominal trauma. AJR 153:561–564, 1989.

81. Grosfeld JL, Rescorla FJ, West KW, et al: Gastrointestinal injuries in childhood: analysis of 53 patients. J Pediatr Surg 24:580–583, 1989.

82. Leonidas J, Berdon WE, Baker DH, et al: Perforation of the gastrointestinal tract and pneumoperitoneum in newborns treated with continuous lung distending pressures. Pediatr Radiol 1:241–246, 1974.

83. Siegle RL, Rabinowitz JG, Sarasohn C: Intestinal perforation secondary to nasojejunal feeding tubes. AJR 126:1229–1232, 1976.

84. McAlister WH, Siegel MJ, Shackelford GD, et al: Intestinal perforations by tube feedings in small infants: clinical and experimental studies. AJR 146:687–691, 1985.

85. Merten DF, Mumford L, Filston HC, et al: Radiologic observations during transpyloric tube feeding in infants of low birth weight. Perforation of the duodenum and variations in normal duodenal anatomy. Radiology 136:67–75, 1980.

86. Zahran M, Eklöf O, Thomasson B: Blunt abdominal trauma and hollow viscus injury in children: the diagnostic value of plain radiography. Pediatr Radiol 14:304–309, 1984.

87. Mandell GA, Finkelstein M: Gastric pneumatosis secondary to an intramural feeding catheter. Pediatr Radiol 18:418–420, 1988.

88. Azimi F, Dinn WM, Naumann RA: Intestinal perforation. An infrequent complication of ventriculo-peritoneal shunts. Radiology 121:701–702, 1976.

89. Kimura K, Kubo M, Okasora T, et al: Esophageal perforation in a neonate associated with gastroesophageal reflux. J Pediatr Surg 19:191–193, 1984.

90. Jawad J, Al-Muzrachi AM, Al-Samarrai AI: Spontaneous esophageal perforation in a newborn. Z Kinderchir 44:370–372, 1989.

91. Dubos JP, Bouchez MC, Kacet N, et al: Spontaneous rupture of the esophagus in the newborn. Pediatr Radiol 16:317–319, 1986.

92. Harell GS, Friedland GW, Daily WJ, et al: Neonatal Boerhaave's syndrome. Radiology 95:665–668, 1970.

93. Aaronson LA, Cywes S, Louw JH: Spontaneous esophageal rupture in the newborn. J Pediatr Surg 10:459–466, 1975.

94. Amodio JB, Berdon WE, Abramson SJ, et al: Retrocardiac pneumomediastinum in association with tracheal and esophageal perforations. Pediatr Radiol 16:380–383, 1986.

95. Cohen MD, Weber TR, Grosfeld JL: Bowel perforation in the newborn: diagnosis with metrizamide. Radiology 150:65–69, 1984.

96. Taylor GA, Fallat ME, Eichelberger MR: Hypovolemic shock in children: abdominal CT manifestations. Radiology 164:479–481, 1987.

97. Bulas DI, Taylor GA, Eichelberger MR: The value of CT in detecting bowel perforation in children after blunt abdominal trauma. AJR 153:561–564, 1989.

98. Rizzo MJ, Federle MP, Griffiths BG: Bowel and mesenteric injury following blunt abdominal trauma: evaluation with CT. Radiology 173:143–148, 1989.

99. Moseley JE, Marshak RH, Wolf BS: Regional enteritis in children. AJR 84:532–539, 1960.

100. Kelts DG, Grand RJ: Inflammatory bowel disease in children and adolescents. Curr Probl Pediatr 10:1–40, 1980.

101. O'Donoghue DP, Dawson AM: Crohn's disease in childhood. Arch Dis Child 52:627–632, 1977.

102. Dubois RS, Rothchild J, Silverman A, et al: The varied manifestations of Crohn's disease in children and adolescents. Am J Gastroenterol 69:203–211, 1978.

103. Sherman NJ, Swanson V, Fleisher D, et al: Regional enteritis in childhood. J Pediatr Surg 7:585–589, 1972.

104. Guttman FM: Granulomatous enterocolitis in childhood and adolescence. J Pediatr Surg 9:115–121, 1974.

105. Gryboski JD, Spiro HM: Prognosis in children with Crohn's disease. Gastroenterology 74:807–817, 1978.

106. Kirschner BS: Inflammatory bowel disease in children. Pediatr Clin North Am 35:189–208, 1988.

107. Lenaerts C, Roy CC, Vaillancourt M, et al: High incidence of upper gastrointestinal tract involvement in children with Crohn disease. Pediatrics 83:777–781, 1989.

108. Castile RG, Telander RL, Cooney DR, et al: Crohn's disease in children: assessment of the progression of disease, growth, and prognosis. J Pediatr Surg 15:462–469, 1980.

109. Manson DE, Stringer DA, Durie PR, et al: The radiologic and endoscopic investigation and etiologic classification of gastritis in children. Can Assoc Radiol J 41:201–206, 1990.

110. Kirks DR, Currarino G: Regional enteritis in children: small bowel disease in children with normal terminal ileum. Pediatr Radiol 7:10–14, 1978.

111. Chong SKF, Grossman A, Walker-Smith JA, et al: Endocrine dysfunction in children with Crohn's disease. J Pediatr Gastroenterol Nutr 3:529–534, 1984.

112. Lindsley CB, Schaller JG: Arthritis associated with inflammatory bowel disease in children. J Pediatr 84:16–20, 1974.

113. Israel DM, Olson AD, Ilowite NT, et al: Arthritis as the initial manifestation of inflammatory bowel disease. J Pediatr Gastroenterol Nutr 9:123–125, 1989.

114. Treem WR, Ragsdale BD: Crohn's disease of the esophagus: a case report and review of the literature. J Pediatr Gastroenterol Nutr 7:451–455, 1988.

115. Stringer DA: Imaging inflammatory bowel disease in the pediatric patient. Radiol Clin North Am 25:93–113, 1987.

116. Lipson A, Bartram CI, Williams CB, et al: Barium studies and ileoscopy compared in children with suspected Crohn's disease. Clin Radiol 41:5–8, 1990.

117. Young J, Miller R: Incidence of malignant tumors in U.S. children. J Pediatr 86:254–258, 1975.

118. Muller-Weihrich ST, Henze G, Schwarze EW, et al: Childhood non-Hodgkin's lymphoma: strategies for diagnosis and therapy. Monogr Paediatr 18:169–186, 1986.

119. Ritter J, Schellong G, Wannamacher M: Treatment of Hodgkin's disease in children. Monogr Paediatr 18:187–205, 1986.

120. Dragosics B, Bauer P, Radaszkiewicz T: Primary gastrointestinal non-Hodgkin's lymphomas: a retrospective clinicopathologic study of 150 cases. Cancer 55:1060–1073, 1985.

121. Hirakata K, Nakata H, Nakayama T, et al: Primary malignant lymphoma of the rectum. Pediatr Radiol 19:474–476, 1989.

122. Pais RC, Hammami A, Kim H, et al: Non-Hodgkin's lymphoma presenting as a rectal polyp in a child. J Pediatr Surg 25:1280–1282, 1990.

123. Miller JH, Hindman BW, Lam AHK: Ultrasound in the evaluation of small bowel lymphoma in children. Radiology 135:409–415, 1980.

124. Cohen MD, Siddiqui A, Weetman R, et al: Hodgkin disease and non-Hodgkin lymphomas in children: utilization of radiologic modalities. Radiology 158:499–505, 1986.

125. Mueller PR, Ferrucci JT, Harbin WP, et al: Appearance of lymphomatous involvement of the mesentery by ultrasonography and body computed tomography: the "sandwich sign." Radiology 134:467–473, 1980.

126. Carroll BA, Ta HN: The ultrasonic appearance of extranodal abdominal lymphoma. Radiology 136:419–425, 1980.

127. Goerg C, Schwerk WB, Goerg K: Gastrointestinal lymphoma: sonographic findings in 54 patients. AJR 155:795–798, 1990.

128. Lee JKT, Stanley RJ, Sagel SS, et al: Accuracy of computed tomography in detecting intra-abdominal and pelvic adenopathy in lymphoma. AJR 131:311–315, 1978.

129. Redman HC, Glatstein E, Castellino RA, et al: Computed tomography as adjunct in the staging of Hodgkin's disease and non-Hodgkin's lymphomas. Radiology 124:381–385, 1977.

130. Breiman RS, Castellino RA, Harell GS, et al: CT-pathologic correlations in Hodgkin's disease and non-Hodgkin's lymphoma. Radiology 126:159–166, 1978.

131. Pastakia B, Shawker TH, Thaler M, et al: Hepatosplenic candidiasis: wheels within wheels. Radiology 166:417–421, 1988.

132. Yoshikawa J, Matsui O, Takashima T, et al: Focal fatty change of the liver adjacent to the falciform ligament: CT and sonographic findings in five surgically confirmed cases. AJR 149:491–494, 1987.

# Index

Note: Page numbers in *italics* refer to illustrations;
page numbers followed by t refer to tables.